西医经典名著集成

菲兹帕里克皮肤病学

FITZPATRICK'S DERMATOLOGY

9TH EDITION

VOLUME 3

Sewon Kang
Masayuki Amagai
Anna L. Bruckner
Alexander H. Enk
David J. Margolis
Amy J. McMichael
Jeffrey S. Orringer

第9版（双语版）

编译委员会主任委员　陈翔　粟娟

下 册

 湖南科学技术出版社

CONTENTS

目 录

Volume 1
上　册

PART 1 FOUNDATIONS OF CLINICAL DERMATOLOGY
第一篇　临床皮肤病学基础

1. Fundamentals of Clinical Dermatology: Morphology and Special Clinical Considerations 1
   Erin H. Amerson, Susan Burgin, & Kanade Shinkai
   第一章　临床皮肤病学基本原理：形态学和特殊的临床考虑

2. Pathology of Skin Lesions 19
   Rosalie Elenitsas & Emily Y. Chu
   第二章　皮疹的病理学

3. Epidemiology and Public Health in Dermatology 42
   Junko Takeshita & David J. Margolis
   第三章　皮肤病流行病学和公共卫生学

PART 2 STRUCTURE AND FUNCTION OF SKIN
第二篇　皮肤的结构和功能

4. Developmental Biology of the Skin 53
   Luis Garza
   第四章　皮肤发育生物学

5. Growth and Differentiation of the Epidermis 67
   Terry Lechler
   第五章　表皮生长和分化

6. Skin Glands: Sebaceous, Eccrine, and Apocrine Glands 76
   Christos C. Zouboulis
   第六章　皮肤腺体：皮脂腺、小汗腺和顶泌汗腺

7. Biology of Hair Follicles 96
   George Cotsarelis & Vladimir Botchkarev
   第七章　毛囊生物学

8. Nail 114
   Krzysztof Kobielak
   第八章　甲

9. Cutaneous Vasculature 124
   Peter Petzelbauer, Robert Loewe, & Jordan S. Pober
   第九章　皮肤血管系统

10. The Immunological Structure of the Skin 139
    Georg Stingl & Marie-Charlotte Brüggen
    第十章　皮肤免疫系统

11. Cellular Components of the Cutaneous Immune System 153
    Johann E. Gudjonsson & Robert L. Modlin
    第十一章　皮肤免疫系统的细胞成分

12. Soluble Mediators of the Cutaneous Immune System 170
    Allen W. Ho & Thomas S. Kupper
    第十二章　皮肤免疫系统的可溶性介质

13. Basic Principles of Immunologic Diseases in Skin (Pathophysiology of Immunologic/Inflammatory Skin Diseases) 204
    Keisuke Nagao & Mark C. Udey
    第十三章　皮肤免疫性疾病发生的基本原理（免疫性/炎症性皮肤病的病理生理学）

14. Skin Barrier 219
    Akiharu Kubo & Masayuki Amagai
    第十四章　皮肤屏障

15. Epidermal and Dermal Adhesion 246
    Leena Bruckner-Tuderman & Aimee S. Payne
    第十五章　表皮和真皮的黏附

16. Microbiome of the Skin 268
    Heidi H. Kong
    第十六章　皮肤微生物组学

17 Cutaneous Photobiology · · · · · · · · · · 280
Thomas M. Rünger
第十七章　皮肤光生物学

18 Genetics in Relation to the Skin · · · · · · · 305
Etienne C. E. Wang, John A. McGrath,
& Angela M. Christiano
第十八章　皮肤遗传学

19 Carcinogenesis and Skin · · · · · · · · · · · · 328
Kenneth Y. Tsai & Andrzej A. Dlugosz
第十九章　癌变与皮肤

20 Pigmentation and Melanocyte Biology · · · · · · · 347
Stephen M. Ostrowski & David E. Fisher
第二十章　色素沉着和黑素细胞生物学

21 Neurobiology of the Skin · · · · · · · · · · · 371
Sonja Ständer, Manuel P. Pereira,
& Thomas A. Luger
第二十一章　皮肤神经生物学

PART 3 DERMATITIS

第三篇　皮炎

22 Atopic Dermatitis · · · · · · · · · · · · · · · 383
Eric L. Simpson, Donald Y. M. Leung,
Lawrence F. Eichenfield, & Mark Boguniewicz
第二十二章　特应性皮炎

23 Nummular Eczema, Lichen Simplex Chronicus, and Prurigo Nodularis · · · · · · · 406
Jonathan I. Silverberg
第二十三章　钱币状湿疹、慢性单纯性苔藓和结节性痒疹

24 Allergic Contact Dermatitis · · · · · · · · · · 416
Jake E. Turrentine, Michael P. Sheehan,
& Ponciano D. Cruz, Jr.
第二十四章　变应性接触性皮炎

25 Irritant Dermatitis · · · · · · · · · · · · · · 436
Susan T. Nedorost
第二十五章　刺激性皮炎

26 Seborrheic Dermatitis · · · · · · · · · · · · 451
Dae Hun Suh
第二十六章　脂溢性皮炎

27 Occupational Skin Diseases · · · · · · · · · · 462
Andy Chern, Casey M. Chern, & Boris D. Lushniak
第二十七章　职业性皮肤疾病

PART 4 PSORIASIFORM DISORDERS

第四篇　银屑病样皮肤疾病

28 Psoriasis · · · · · · · · · · · · · · · · · · · 483
Johann E. Gudjonsson & James T. Elder
第二十八章　银屑病

29 Pityriasis Rubra Pilaris · · · · · · · · · · · 525
Knut Schäkel
第二十九章　毛发红糠疹

30 Parapsoriasis and Pityriasis Lichenoides · · · · · 533
Stefan M. Schieke & Gary S. Wood
第三十章　副银屑病和苔藓样糠疹

31 Pityriasis Rosea · · · · · · · · · · · · · · · 547
Matthew Clark & Johann E. Gudjonsson
第三十一章　玫瑰糠疹

PART 5 LICHENOID AND GRANULOMATOUS DISORDERS

第五篇　苔藓样皮炎和肉芽肿性皮炎

32 Lichen Planus · · · · · · · · · · · · · · · · 557
Aaron R. Mangold & Mark R. Pittelkow
第三十二章　扁平苔藓

33 Lichen Nitidus and Lichen Striatus · · · · · · · 585
Aaron R. Mangold & Mark R. Pittelkow
第三十三章　光泽苔藓和线状苔藓

34 Granuloma Annulare · · · · · · · · · · · · · 595
Julie S. Prendiville
第三十四章　环状肉芽肿

35 Sarcoidosis · · · · · · · · · · · · · · · · · 603
Richard Marchell
第三十五章　结节病

PART 6 NEUTROPHILIC, EOSINOPHILIC, AND MAST CELL DISORDERS

第六篇　中性粒细胞、嗜酸性粒细胞、肥大细胞相关性疾病

36 Sweet Syndrome · · · · · · · · · · · · · · · 619
Philip R. Cohen & Razelle Kurzrock
第三十六章　Sweet综合征

37 Pyoderma Gangrenosum · · · · · · · · · · · · · · · · · · · 638
   Natanel Jourabchi & Gerald S. Lazarus
   第三十七章　坏疽性脓皮病

38 Subcorneal Pustular Dermatosis
   (Sneddon-Wilkinson Disease) · · · · · · · · · · · · · · · 651
   Franz Trautinger & Herbert Hönigsmann
   第三十八章　角层下脓疱病

39 Autoinflammatory Disorders · · · · · · · · · · · · · · · · 656
   Takashi K. Satoh & Lars E. French
   第三十九章　自身炎症性疾病

40 Eosinophilic Diseases · 685
   Hideyuki Ujiie & Hiroshi Shimizu
   第四十章　嗜酸性粒细胞疾病

41 Urticaria and Angioedema · · · · · · · · · · · · · · · · · · 721
   *Michihiro Hide, Shunsuke Takahagi,
   & Takaaki Hiragun*
   第四十一章　荨麻疹和血管性水肿

42 Mastocytosis · 748
   Michael D. Tharp
   第四十二章　肥大细胞增生症

PART 7　REACTIVE ERYTHEMAS
第七篇　反应性红斑

43 Erythema Multiforme · 763
   Jean-Claude Roujeau & Maja Mockenhaupt
   第四十三章　多形红斑

44 Epidermal Necrolysis (Stevens-Johnson
   Syndrome and Toxic Epidermal Necrolysis) · · · · 774
   Maja Mockenhaupt & Jean-Claude Roujeau
   第四十四章　表皮坏死松解症（Stevens-
   　　　　　　Johnson综合征和中毒性表皮
   　　　　　　坏死松解症）

45 Cutaneous Reactions to Drugs · · · · · · · · · · · · · · 791
   Kara Heelan, Cathryn Sibbald, & Neil H. Shear
   第四十五章　药物所致皮肤反应

46 Erythema Annulare Centrifugum and Other
   Figurate Erythemas · 808
   Christine S. Ahn & William W. Huang
   第四十六章　离心性环状红斑和其他形态
   　　　　　　红斑

PART 8　DSORDERS OF CORNIFICATION
第八篇　角化异常性疾病

47 The Ichthyoses · 819
   Keith A. Choate & Leonard M. Milstone
   第四十七章　鱼鳞病

48 Inherited Palmoplantar Keratodermas · · · · · · · · 861
   Liat Samuelov & Eli Sprecher
   第四十八章　遗传性掌跖角化病

49 Keratosis Pilaris and Other Follicular
   Keratotic Disorders · 913
   Anna L. Bruckner
   第四十九章　毛周角化病和其他毛囊性
   　　　　　　角化疾病

50 Acantholytic Disorders of the Skin · · · · · · · · · · · 924
   Alain Hovnanian
   第五十章　棘层松解性皮肤病

51 Porokeratosis · 949
   *Cathal O'Connor, Grainne M. O'Regan,
   & Alan D. Irvine*
   第五十一章　汗孔角化症

PART 9　VESICULOBULLOUS DISORDERS
第九篇　水疱大疱性疾病

52 Pemphigus · 957
   Aimee S. Payne & John R. Stanley
   第五十二章　天疱疮

53 Paraneoplastic Pemphigus · · · · · · · · · · · · · · · · · · 983
   Grant J. Anhalt & Daniel Mimouni
   第五十三章　副肿瘤性天疱疮

54 Bullous Pemphigoid · 994
   Donna A. Culton, Zhi Liu, & Luis A. Diaz
   第五十四章　大疱性类天疱疮

55 Mucous Membrane Pemphigoid · · · · · · · · · · · · 1011
   Kim B. Yancey
   第五十五章　黏膜类天疱疮

56 Epidermolysis Bullosa Acquisita · · · · · · · · · · · · 1023
   David T. Woodley & Mei Chen
   第五十六章　获得性大疱性表皮松解症

57 Intercellular Immunoglobulin (Ig)
   A Dermatosis (IgA Pemphigus) · · · · · · · · · · · · · 1034
   Takashi Hashimoto
   第五十七章　细胞间IgA皮病（IgA天疱
   　　　　　　疮）

58 Linear Immunoglobulin A Dermatosis and
   Chronic Bullous Disease of Childhood · · · · · · · 1046
   *Matilda W. Nicholas, Caroline L. Rao,
   & Russell P. Hall III*
   第五十八章　线状IgA皮病和儿童慢性大
   　　　　　　疱性皮病

59 Dermatitis Herpetiformis · · · · · · · · · · · · · · · · · · 1057
Stephen I. Katz

第五十九章　疱疹样皮炎

60 Inherited Epidermolysis Bullosa · · · · · · · · 1067
M. Peter Marinkovich

第六十章　遗传性大疱性表皮松解症

PART 10 AUTOIMMUNE CONNECTIVE TISSUE AND RHEUMATOLOGIC DISORDERS

第十篇　自身免疫结缔组织病和风湿病

61 Lupus Erythematosus · 1093
Clayton J. Sontheimer, Melissa I. Costner, & Richard D. Sontheimer

第六十一章　红斑狼疮

62 Dermatomyositis · 1118
Matthew Lewis & David Fiorentino

第六十二章　皮肌炎

63 Systemic Sclerosis · 1144
Pia Moinzadeh, Christopher P. Denton, Carol M. Black, & Thomas Krieg

第六十三章　系统性硬皮病

64 Morphea and Lichen Sclerosus · · · · · · · · · · 1165
Nika Cyrus & Heidi T. Jacobe

第六十四章　硬斑病和硬化性萎缩性苔藓

65 Psoriatic Arthritis and Reactive Arthritis · · · · · 1187
Ana-Maria Orbai & John A. Flynn

第六十五章　银屑病性关节炎和反应性关节炎

66 Rheumatoid Arthritis, Juvenile Idiopathic Arthritis, Adult-Onset Still Disease, and Rheumatic Fever · 1207
Warren W. Piette

第六十六章　类风湿性关节炎、幼年特发性关节炎、成人Still病和风湿热

67 Scleredema and Scleromyxedema · · · · · · · · · · 1225
Roger H. Weenig & Mark R. Pittelkow

第六十七章　硬肿症和硬化性黏液水肿

68 Sjögren Syndrome · 1232
Akiko Tanikawa

第六十八章　干燥综合征

69 Relapsing Polychondritis · · · · · · · · · · · · · · · · · 1249
Camille Francès

第六十九章　复发性多软骨炎

PART 11 DERMAL CONNECTIVE TISSUE DISORDERS

第十一篇　真皮结缔组织异常

70 Anetoderma and Other Atrophic Disorders of the Skin · 1255
Catherine Maari & Julie Powell

第七十章　斑状萎缩和其他萎缩性皮病

71 Acquired Perforating Disorders · · · · · · · · · · · 1265
Garrett T. Desman & Raymond L. Barnhill

第七十一章　获得性穿通性皮病

72 Genetic Disorders Affecting Dermal Connective Tissue · 1275
Jonathan A. Dyer

第七十二章　影响真皮结缔组织的遗传性疾病

PART 12 SUBCUTANEOUS TISSUE DISORDERS

第十二篇　皮下脂肪疾病

73 Panniculitis · 1315
Eden Pappo Lake, Sophie M. Worobec, & Iris K. Aronson

第七十三章　脂膜炎

74 Lipodystrophy · 1360
Abhimanyu Garg

第七十四章　脂肪营养不良

Volume 2
中　册

PART 13 MELANOCYTIC DISORDERS

第十三篇　色素细胞性疾病

75 Albinism and Other Genetic Disorders of Pigmentation · 1375
Masahiro Hayashi & Tamio Suzuki

第七十五章　白化病和其他遗传性色素性疾病

76 Vitiligo · 1397
Khaled Ezzedine & John E. Harris

第七十六章　白癜风

77 Hypermelanoses · 1419
Michelle Rodrigues & Amit G. Pandya

第七十七章　色素沉着过度性疾病

PART 14 ACNEIFORM DISORDERS
第十四篇 痤疮样皮肤病

78 Acne Vulgaris · 1461
Carolyn Goh, Carol Cheng, George Agak, Andrea L. Zaenglein, Emmy M. Graber, Diane M. Thiboutot, & Jenny Kim
第七十八章 寻常痤疮

79 Rosacea · 1490
Martin Steinhoff & Jörg Buddenkotte
第七十九章 玫瑰痤疮

80 Acne Variants and Acneiform Eruptions · · · · · 1520
Andrea L. Zaenglein, Emmy M. Graber, & Diane M. Thiboutot
第八十章 痤疮异型和痤疮样疹

PART 15 DISORDERS OF ECCRINE AND APOCRINE SWEAT GLANDS
第十五篇 汗腺疾病

81 Hyperhidrosis and Anhidrosis · · · · · · · · · · 1531
Anastasia O. Kurta & Dee Anna Glaser
第八十一章 多汗症和无汗症

82 Bromhidrosis and Chromhidrosis · · · · · · · · · 1543
Christos C. Zouboulis
第八十二章 腋臭和色汗

83 Fox-Fordyce Disease · · · · · · · · · · · · · · · · · 1551
Powell Perng & Inbal Sander
第八十三章 Fox-Fordyce病

84 Hidradenitis Suppurativa · · · · · · · · · · · · · · 1557
Ginette A. Okoye
第八十四章 化脓性汗腺炎

PART 16 DISORDERS OF THE HAIR AND NAILS
第十六篇 毛发和甲疾病

85 Androgenetic Alopecia · · · · · · · · · · · · · · · · 1575
Ulrike Blume-Peytavi & Varvara Kanti
第八十五章 雄激素性脱发

86 Telogen Effluvium · · · · · · · · · · · · · · · · · · · 1588
Manabu Ohyama
第八十六章 休止期脱发

87 Alopecia Areata · 1599
Nina Otberg & Jerry Shapiro
第八十七章 斑秃

88 Cicatricial Alopecias · · · · · · · · · · · · · · · · · 1607
Nina Otberg & Jerry Shapiro
第八十八章 瘢痕性脱发

89 Hair Shaft Disorders · · · · · · · · · · · · · · · · · · 1621
Leslie Castelo-Soccio & Deepa Patel
第八十九章 毛干疾病

90 Hirsutism and Hypertrichosis · · · · · · · · · · · 1640
Thusanth Thuraisingam & Amy J. McMichael
第九十章 多毛和多毛症

91 Nail Disorders · 1655
Eckart Haneke
第九十一章 甲疾病

PART 17 DISORDERS DUE TO THE ENVIRONMENT
第十七篇 环境引起的皮肤病

92 Polymorphic Light Eruption · · · · · · · · · · · · 1699
Alexandra Gruber-Wackernagel & Peter Wolf
第九十二章 多形性日光疹

93 Actinic Prurigo · 1716
Travis Vandergriff
第九十三章 光化性痒疹

94 Hydroa Vacciniforme · · · · · · · · · · · · · · · · · 1723
Travis Vandergriff
第九十四章 种痘样水疱病

95 Actinic Dermatitis · 1728
Robert S. Dawe
第九十五章 光化性皮炎

96 Solar Urticaria · 1740
Marcus Maurer, Joachim W. Fluhr, & Karsten Weller
第九十六章 日光性荨麻疹

97 Phototoxicity and Photoallergy · · · · · · · · · · 1747
Henry W. Lim
第九十七章 光毒性与光过敏

98 Cold Injuries · 1756
Ashley N. Millard, Clayton B. Green, & Erik J. Stratman
第九十八章 冻伤

99 Burns · 1769
Benjamin Levi & Stewart Wang
第九十九章 烧伤

PART 18 PSYCHOSOCIAL SKIN DISEASE
第十八篇 心理社会性皮肤病

100 Delusional, Obsessive-Compulsive, and Factitious Skin Diseases 1783
Mio Nakamura, Josie Howard, & John Y. M. Koo
第一百章 妄想、强迫症和人为皮肤病

101 Drug Abuse 1796
Nicholas Frank, Cara Hennings, & Jami L. Miller
第一百零一章 药物滥用

102 Physical Abuse 1809
Kelly M. MacArthur & Annie Grossberg
第一百零二章 身体虐待

PART 19 SKIN CHANGES ACROSS THE SPAN OF LIFE
第十九篇 皮肤在人一生中的变化

103 Neonatal Dermatology 1819
Raegan Hunt, Mary Wu Chang, & Kara N. Shah
第一百零三章 新生儿皮肤病学

104 Pediatric and Adolescent Dermatology 1844
Mary Wu Chang
第一百零四章 儿科和青少年皮肤病学

105 Skin Changes and Diseases in Pregnancy 1861
Lauren E. Wiznia & Miriam Keltz Pomeranz
第一百零五章 妊娠期的皮肤变化和疾病

106 Skin Aging 1877
Michelle L. Kerns, Anna L. Chien, & Sewon Kang
第一百零六章 皮肤老化

107 Caring for LGBT Persons in Dermatology 1892
Howa Yeung, Matthew D. Mansh, Suephy C. Chen, & Kenneth A. Katz
第一百零七章 关于LGBT人群的皮肤病学

PART 20 NEOPLASIA
第二十篇 皮肤肿瘤

108 Benign Epithelial Tumors, Hamartomas, and Hyperplasias 1901
Jonathan D. Cuda, Sophia Rangwala, & Janis M. Taube
第一百零八章 良性上皮肿瘤、错构瘤和增生性病变

109 Appendage Tumors of the Skin 1923
Ruth K. Foreman & Lyn McDivitt Duncan
第一百零九章 皮肤附属器肿瘤

110 Epithelial Precancerous Lesions 1961
Markus V. Heppt, Gabriel Schlager, & Carola Berking
第一百一十章 上皮癌前病变

111 Basal Cell Carcinoma and Basal Cell Nevus Syndrome 1989
Jean Y. Tang, Ervin H. Epstein, Jr., & Anthony E. Oro
第一百一十一章 基底细胞癌和基底细胞痣综合征

112 Squamous Cell Carcinoma and Keratoacanthoma 2006
Anke S. Lonsdorf & Eva N. Hadaschik
第一百一十二章 鳞状细胞癌和角化棘皮瘤

113 Merkel Cell Carcinoma 2026
Aubriana McEvoy & Paul Nghiem
第一百一十三章 梅克尔细胞癌

114 Paget's Disease 2041
Conroy Chow, Isaac M. Neuhaus, & Roy C. Grekin
第一百一十四章 佩吉特病

115 Melanocytic Nevi 2052
Jonathan D. Cuda, Robert F. Moore, & Klaus J. Busam
第一百一十五章 黑素细胞痣

116 Melanoma 2090
Jessica C. Hassel & Alexander H. Enk
第一百一十六章 黑色素瘤

117 Histiocytosis 2127
Astrid Schmieder, Sergij Goerdt, & Jochen Utikal
第一百一十七章 组织细胞增生症

118 Vascular Tumors 2152
Kelly M. MacArthur & Katherine Püttgen
第一百一十八章 血管性肿瘤

119 Cutaneous Lymphoma 2182
Martine Bagot & Rudolf Stadler
第一百一十九章 皮肤淋巴瘤

120 Cutaneous Pseudolymphoma 2219
Werner Kempf, Rudolf Stadler, & Martine Bagot
第一百二十章 皮肤假性淋巴瘤

121 Neoplasias and Hyperplasias of Muscular and Neural Origin 2242
Hansgeorg Müller & Heinz Kutzner
第一百二十一章 肌肉和神经源性肿瘤与增生

122 Lipogenic Neoplasms · 2285
Thomas Mentzel & Thomas Brenn

第一百二十二章　脂肪源性肿瘤

PART 21 METABOLIC, GENETIC, AND SYSTEMIC DISEASES

第二十一篇　代谢性、遗传性和全身性疾病

123 Cutaneous Changes in Nutritional Disease · 2313
Albert C. Yan

第一百二十三章　营养性疾病的皮肤改变

124 The Porphyrias · 2349
Eric W. Gou & Karl E. Anderson

第一百二十四章　卟啉病

125 Amyloidosis · 2374
Peter D. Gorevic & Robert G. Phelps

第一百二十五章　淀粉样变性

126 Xanthomas and Lipoprotein Disorders · · · · · · · 2390
Vasanth Sathiyakumar, Steven R. Jones, & Seth S. Martin

第一百二十六章　黄色瘤和脂蛋白紊乱

127 Fabry Disease · 2410
Atul B. Mehta & Catherine H. Orteu

第一百二十七章　Fabry病

128 Calcium and Other Mineral Deposition Disorders · 2426
Janet A. Fairley & Adam B. Aronson

第一百二十八章　钙和其他矿物沉积紊乱

129 Graft-Versus-Host Disease · · · · · · · · · · · · · · · · 2440
Kathryn J. Martires & Edward W. Cowen

第一百二十九章　移植物抗宿主病

130 Hereditary Disorders of Genome Instability and DNA Repair · 2463
John J. DiGiovanna, Thomas M. Rünger, & Kenneth H. Kraemer

第一百三十章　基因组不稳定性和DNA修复障碍的遗传性疾病

131 Ectodermal Dysplasias · · · · · · · · · · · · · · · · · · 2494
Elizabeth L. Nieman & Dorothy Katherine Grange

第一百三十一章　外胚层发育不良

132 Genetic Immunodeficiency Diseases · · · · · · · · 2517
Ramsay L. Fuleihan & Amy S. Paller

第一百三十二章　遗传性免疫缺陷病

133 Skin Manifestations of Internal Organ Disorders · 2549
Amy K. Forrestel & Robert G. Micheletti

第一百三十三章　内脏疾病的皮肤表现

134 Cutaneous Paraneoplastic Syndromes · · · · · · · 2566
Manasmon Chairatchaneeboon & Ellen J. Kim

第一百三十四章　皮肤副肿瘤综合征

135 The Neurofibromatoses · · · · · · · · · · · · · · · · · · 2590
Robert Listernick & Joel Charrow

第一百三十五章　神经纤维瘤病

136 Tuberous Sclerosis Complex · · · · · · · · · · · · · · 2606
Thomas N. Darling

第一百三十六章　结节性硬化症

137 Diabetes and Other Endocrine Diseases · · · · · · 2620
April Schachtel & Andrea Kalus

第一百三十七章　糖尿病和其他内分泌疾病

Volume 3
下　册

PART 22 VASCULAR DISEASES

第二十二篇　血管性疾病

138 Cutaneous Necrotizing Venulitis · · · · · · · · · · · · 2655
Nicholas A. Soter

第一百三十八章　皮肤坏死性静脉炎

139 Systemic Necrotizing Arteritis · · · · · · · · · · · · · 2669
Peter A. Merkel & Paul A. Monach

第一百三十九章　系统性坏死性动脉炎

140 Erythema Elevatum Diutinum · · · · · · · · · · · · · 2694
Theodore J. Alkousakis & Whitney A. High

第一百四十章　持久性隆起性红斑

141 Adamantiades–Behçet Disease · · · · · · · · · · · · 2701
Christos C. Zouboulis

第一百四十一章　白塞病

142 Kawasaki Disease · 2716
Anne H. Rowley

第一百四十二章　川崎病

143 Pigmented Purpuric Dermatoses · · · · · · · · · · · 2728
Alexandra Haden & David H. Peng

第一百四十三章　色素性紫癜性皮病

144 Cryoglobulinemia and
Cryofibrinogenemia 2739
Julio C. Sartori-Valinotti & Mark D. P. Davis

第一百四十四章　冷球蛋白血症和冷
纤维蛋白原血症

145 Raynaud Phenomenon 2755
Drew Kurtzman & Ruth Ann Vleugels

第一百四十五章　雷诺现象

146 Malignant Atrophic Papulosis
(Degos Disease) 2774
Dan Lipsker

第一百四十六章　恶性萎缩性丘疹病

147 Vascular Malformations 2782
*Laurence M. Boon, Fanny Ballieux,
& Miikka Vikkula*

第一百四十七章　血管畸形

148 Cutaneous Changes in Arterial, Venous, and
Lymphatic Dysfunction 2817
Sabrina A. Newman

第一百四十八章　动脉、静脉和淋巴管功
能障碍的皮肤表现

149 Wound Healing 2850
Afsaneh Alavi & Robert S. Kirsner

第一百四十九章　伤口愈合

PART 23　BACTERIAL DISEASES

第二十三篇　细菌性疾病

150 Superficial Cutaneous Infections and
Pyodermas 2871
Lloyd S. Miller

第一百五十章　浅部皮肤感染和脓皮病

151 Cellulitis and Erysipelas 2899
David R. Pearson & David J. Margolis

第一百五十一章　蜂窝织炎和丹毒

152 Gram-Positive Infections Associated with
Toxin Production 2911
Jeffrey B. Travers

第一百五十二章　产毒素革兰氏阳性细菌
感染

153 Necrotizing Fasciitis, Necrotizing Cellulitis,
and Myonecrosis 2924
Avery LaChance & Daniela Kroshinsky

第一百五十三章　坏死性筋膜炎、坏死性
蜂窝组织炎和肌坏死

154 Gram-Negative Coccal and
Bacillary Infections 2937
Breanne Mordorski & Adam J. Friedman

第一百五十四章　革兰氏阴性球菌和细菌
感染

155 The Skin in Infective Endocarditis, Sepsis,
Septic Shock, and Disseminated
Intravascular Coagulation 2971
Joseph C. English III & Misha Rosenbach

第一百五十五章　感染性心内膜炎、脓毒
血症、脓毒性休克和弥
散性血管内凝血中的皮
肤表现

156 Miscellaneous Bacterial Infections with
Cutaneous Manifestations 2983
Scott A. Norton & Michael A. Cardis

第一百五十六章　混杂细菌感染引起的皮
肤表现

157 Tuberculosis and Infections with Atypical
Mycobacteria 3015
Aisha Sethi

第一百五十七章　结核和非典型分枝杆菌
感染

158 Actinomycosis, Nocardiosis, and
Actinomycetoma 3034
*Francisco G. Bravo, Roberto Arenas,
& Daniel Asz Sigall*

第一百五十八章　放线菌病、诺卡氏菌病
和放线菌瘤

159 Leprosy 3051
*Claudio Guedes Salgado, Arival Cardoso de Brito,
Ubirajara Imbiriba Salgado, & John Stewart Spencer*

第一百五十九章　麻风病

PART 24　FUNGAL DISEASES

第二十四篇　真菌性疾病

160 Superficial Fungal Infection 3085
Lauren N. Craddock & Stefan M. Schieke

第一百六十章　浅部真菌感染

161 Yeast Infections 3113
Iris Ahronowitz & Kieron Leslie

第一百六十一章　酵母菌感染

162 Deep Fungal Infections 3127
Roderick J. Hay

第一百六十二章　深部真菌感染

PART 25　VIRAL DISEASES

第二十五篇　病毒性疾病

163 Exanthematous Viral Diseases 3151

Vikash S. Oza & Erin F. D. Mathes

第一百六十三章　病毒疹性疾病

164 Herpes Simplex ··················3184
Jeffrey I. Cohen

第一百六十四章　单纯疱疹

165 Varicella and Herpes Zoster ···········3199
Myron J. Levin, Kenneth E. Schmader,
& Michael N. Oxman

第一百六十五章　水痘–带状疱疹

166 Poxvirus Infections ················3230
Ellen S. Haddock & Sheila Fallon Friedlander

第一百六十六章　痘病毒感染

167 Human Papillomavirus Infections ········3261
Jane C. Sterling

第一百六十七章　人乳头瘤病毒感染

168 Cutaneous Manifestations of HIV
and Human T-Lymphotropic Virus ········3274
Adam D. Lipworth, Esther E. Freeman,
& Arturo P. Saavedra

第一百六十八章　HIV和人类嗜T细胞病毒感染的皮肤表现

169 Mosquito-Borne Viral Diseases ·········3303
Edwin J. Asturias & J. David Beckham

第一百六十九章　蚊媒病毒性疾病

PART 26 SEXUALLY TRANSMITTED DISEASES

第二十六篇　性传播疾病

170 Syphilis ·······················3315
Susan A. Tuddenham & Jonathan M. Zenilman

第一百七十章　梅毒

171 Endemic (Nonvenereal) Treponematoses ····3345
Francisco G. Bravo, Carolina Talhari,
& Khaled Ezzedine

第一百七十一章　地方性（非性病性）密螺旋体病

172 Chancroid ·····················3360
Stephan Lautenschlager & Norbert H. Brockmeyer

第一百七十二章　软下疳

173 Lymphogranuloma Venereum ··········3369
Norbert H. Brockmeyer & Stephan Lautenschlager

第一百七十三章　性病性淋巴肉芽肿

174 Granuloma Inguinale ···············3380
Melissa B. Hoffman & Rita O. Pichardo

第一百七十四章　腹股沟肉芽肿

175 Gonorrhea, Mycoplasma, and Vaginosis·····3387
Lindsay C. Strowd, Sean McGregor, & Rita O. Pichardo

第一百七十五章　淋病、支原体感染和细菌性阴道病

PART 27 INFESTATIONS, BITES, AND STINGS

第二十七篇　虫媒叮咬和感染性疾病

176 Leishmaniasis and Other Protozoan
Infections ·····················3405
Esther von Stebut

第一百七十六章　利什曼病和其他原虫感染

177 Helminthic Infections ···············3434
Kathryn N. Suh & Jay S. Keystone

第一百七十七章　蠕虫感染

178 Scabies, Other Mites, and Pediculosis ········3458
Chikoti M. Wheat, Craig N. Burkhart,
Craig G. Burkhart, & Bernard A. Cohen

第一百七十八章　疥疮、其他螨类和虱病

179 Lyme Borreliosis··················3472
Roger Clark & Linden Hu

第一百七十九章　莱姆病

180 The Rickettsioses, Ehrlichioses, and
Anaplasmoses ··················3492
Maryam Liaqat, Analisa V. Halpern, Justin J. Green,
& Warren R. Heymann

第一百八十章　立克次体病、埃氏立克次体病和无浆体病

181 Arthropod Bites and Stings ···········3511
Robert A. Schwartz & Christopher J. Steen

第一百八十一章　节肢动物咬伤和蜇伤

182 Bites and Stings of Terrestrial and
Aquatic Life ····················3526
Camila K. Janniger, Robert A. Schwartz,
Jennifer S. Daly, & Mark Jordan Scharf

第一百八十二章　陆生和水生生物的叮咬和蜇伤

PART 28 TOPICAL AND SYSTEMIC TREATMENTS

第二十八篇　外用和系统药物治疗

183 Principles of Topical Therapy ···········3553
Mohammed D. Saleem,
Howard I. Maibach, & Steven R. Feldman

第一百八十三章　外用药物的治疗原则

184 Glucocorticoids······3573
Avrom Caplan, Nicole Fett, & Victoria Werth
第一百八十四章　糖皮质激素

185 Retinoids······3587
Anna L. Chien, Anders Vahlquist,
Jean-Hilaire Saurat, John J. Voorhees, & Sewon Kang
第一百八十五章　维甲酸类药物

186 Systemic and Topical Antibiotics······3600
Sean C. Condon, Carlos M. Isada,
& Kenneth J. Tomecki
第一百八十六章　系统使用和外用抗生素

187 Dapsone······3617
Chee Leok Goh & Jiun Yit Pan
第一百八十七章　氨苯砜

188 Antifungals······3631
Mahmoud Ghannoum, Iman Salem,
& Luisa Christensen
第一百八十八章　抗真菌药

189 Antihistamines······3647
Michael D. Tharp
第一百八十九章　抗组胺药

190 Cytotoxic and Antimetabolic Agents······3659
Jeremy S. Honaker & Neil J. Korman
第一百九十章　细胞毒性和抗代谢药

191 Antiviral Drugs······3690
Zeena Y. Nawas, Quynh-Giao Nguyen,
Khaled S. Sanber, & Stephen K. Tyring
第一百九十一章　抗病毒药

192 Immunosuppressive and
Immunomodulatory Drugs······3715
Drew Kurtzman, Ruth Ann Vleugels, & Jeffrey Callen
第一百九十二章　免疫抑制药和免疫调节药

193 Immunobiologics: Targeted Therapy Against
Cytokines, Cytokine Receptors, and Growth
Factors in Dermatology······3730
Andrew Johnston, Yoshikazu Takada, & Sam T. Hwang
第一百九十三章　免疫生物制剂：皮肤病学中针对细胞因子、细胞因子受体和生长因子的靶向治疗

194 Molecular Targeted Therapies······3758
David Michael Miller, Bobby Y. Reddy, & Hensin Tsao
第一百九十四章　分子靶向治疗

195 Antiangiogenic Agents······3790
Adilson da Costa, Michael Y. Bonner,
& Jack L. Arbiser
第一百九十五章　抗血管生成抑制药

196 Other Topical Medications······3810
Shawn G. Kwatra & Manisha Loss
第一百九十六章　其他外用药

197 Photoprotection······3824
Jin Ho Chung
第一百九十七章　光保护剂

PART 29 PHYSICAL TREATMENTS
第二十九篇　物理治疗

198 Phototherapy······3837
Tarannum Jaleel, Brian P. Pollack, & Craig A. Elmets
第一百九十八章　光疗

199 Photochemotherapy and Photodynamic
Therapy······3867
Herbert Hönigsmann, Rolf-Markus Szeimies,
& Robert Knobler
第一百九十九章　光化学疗法和光动力疗法

200 Radiotherapy······3891
Roy H. Decker & Lynn D. Wilson
第二百章　放疗

PART 30 DERMATOLOGIC SURGERY
第三十篇　皮肤外科

201 Cutaneous Surgical Anatomy······3903
Arif Aslam & Sumaira Z. Aasi
第二百零一章　皮肤外科解剖学

202 Perioperative Considerations in
Dermatologic Surgery······3913
Noah Smith, Kelly B. Cha, & Christopher Bichakjian
第二百零二章　皮肤科手术的围手术期注意事项

203 Excisional Surgery and Repair,
Flaps, and Grafts······3934
Adele Haimovic, Jessica M. Sheehan,
& Thomas E. Rohrer
第二百零三章　肿物切除术和修复、皮瓣和皮片移植

204 Mohs Micrographic Surgery······3970
Sean R. Christensen & David J. Leffell
第二百零四章　莫氏显微外科

205 Nail Surgery······3984
Robert Baran & Olivier Cogrel
第二百零五章　甲部手术

206 Cryosurgery and Electrosurgery······4002

Justin J. Vujevich & Leonard H. Goldberg
　　第二百零六章　冷冻疗法和电疗法

PART 31 COSMETIC DERMATOLOGY
第三十一篇　美容皮肤学

207 Cosmeceuticals and Skin Care in Dermatology ······················ 4015
Leslie Baumann
　　第二百零七章　化妆品和皮肤护理

208 Fundamentals of Laser and Light-Based Treatments ················ 4033
Omer Ibrahim & Jeffrey S. Dover
　　第二百零八章　激光原理和光学治疗

209 Laser Skin Resurfacing: Cosmetic and Medical Applications ············ 4048
Bridget E. McIlwee & Tina S. Alster
　　第二百零九章　激光皮肤表皮重建：美容和医疗应用

210 Nonablative Laser and Light-Based Therapy: Cosmetic and Medical Indications ············ 4061
Jeffrey S. Orringer
　　第二百一十章　非剥脱激光和以光为基础的治疗：美容和医学适应证

211 Noninvasive Body Contouring ············ 4073
Murad Alam
　　第二百一十一章　无创塑形

212 Treatment of Varicose Veins and Telangiectatic Lower-Extremity Vessels ······ 4088
Daniel P. Friedmann, Vineet Mishra, & Jeffrey T. S. Hsu
　　第二百一十二章　下肢静脉曲张和毛细血管扩张的治疗

213 Chemical Peels and Dermabrasion ·········· 4113
Gary Monheit & Bailey Tayebi
　　第二百一十三章　化学剥脱术和磨削术

214 Liposuction Using Tumescent Local Anesthesia ····················· 4125
C. William Hanke, Cheryl J. Gustafson, William G. Stebbins, & Aimee L. Leonard
　　第二百一十四章　局部麻醉下的肿胀吸脂术

215 Soft-Tissue Augmentation ················ 4130
Lisa M. Donofrio & Dana L. Ellis
　　第二百一十五章　软组织填充术

216 Botulinum Toxin ······················ 4142
Richard G. Glogau
　　第二百一十六章　肉毒杆菌毒素

217 Hair Transplantation ··················· 4153
Robin H. Unger & Walter P. Unger
　　第二百一十七章　毛发移植

Vascular Diseases PART 22

第二十二篇 血管性疾病

Chapter 138 :: Cutaneous Necrotizing Venulitis :: Nicholas A. Soter

第一百三十八章 皮肤坏死性静脉炎

中文导读

皮肤坏死性静脉炎/血管炎（CNV）是累及皮肤小静脉的坏死性血管炎，CNV可能局限于皮肤，也可能与潜在的慢性病相关，可能由感染或药物诱发，或可能为特发性（表138-1）。本章节从历史视角、流行病学、临床特征、病因和发病机制、诊断、鉴别诊断和治疗对该病进行了详细阐述。

1. 历史视角 坏死性血管炎最初被描述是在19世纪，但最初对于静脉或动脉受累，小血管或大血管受累命名较混乱，直到20世纪70年代才明确CNV为皮肤小静脉受累的血管炎。

2. 流行病学 CNV每年的总体发病率约为4.5/100000。最常见的亚型是皮肤小血管血管炎和IgA血管炎，分别占45%和30%，IgA血管炎是儿童CNV最常见的表现形式。最常见的病因为特发性，伴系统受累约占4%，有一定的复发率。

3. 临床特征 CNV的皮损多形，可触及的紫癜是其特征性损害（图138-1A），其他表现包括斑疹、丘疹、荨麻疹/血管性水肿、水泡、脓疱、血性大疱（图138-1B）、坏死和溃疡（图138-1C）以及网状青斑。最常累及下肢或受压部位，如背部和臀部。患者自觉症状包括瘙痒或灼烧感，疼痛感不常见，在疾病活动期可伴有发热、不适、关节痛或肌痛。接下来，作者对CNV相关的系统性疾病，CNV的常见诱因（感染和药物）进行了详细阐述。

特发型CNV的疾病种类主要包括IgA血管炎（原Henoch-Schonlein紫癜）、婴儿急性出血性水肿、荨麻疹静脉炎（荨麻疹血管炎）、持久性隆起性红斑、结节性血管炎（硬红斑）、青斑样血管病（青斑样血管炎、青斑血管炎、节段透明性血管炎、白色萎缩）、Sneddon综合征和嗜酸性粒细胞性血管炎。作者将上述疾病的流行病学及临床特征总结列在表138-2。

4．病因和发病机制　主要从免疫复合物的参与、淋巴细胞的激活和炎症因子的级联释放所致的组织损伤对CNV的发病机制进行了详细阐述。此外，作者提及ANCAs和小血管坏死性血管炎之间也存在密切关联，另有少数针对HLA的研究表明遗传因素可能在CNV的发生中起作用。

5．诊断

（1）实验室检查：作者列出了与CNV相关的实验室检查（表138-3），并建议根据患者病史和临床表现以及所合并的系统性疾病选择性完善。红细胞沉降率往往普遍升高，白细胞增多、贫血、血小板增多、尿沉渣异常、循环免疫复合物、类风湿因子和抗核抗体在特发性CNV中也偶尔出现。

（2）组织学病理学：临床上可触及性紫癜和荨麻疹性血管炎的皮肤活检标本中，诊断CNV的组织病理学标准包括血管壁的坏死和纤维蛋白样物质沉积、真皮内伴核尘的中性粒细胞和单核细胞浸润及红细胞外溢（图138-6A）。小动脉往往不受累。提及CNV皮损中浸润的炎症细胞有两种不同的类型：一种富含中性粒细胞，另一种富含淋巴细胞。中性粒细胞的浸润会随着单核细胞浸润的持续而消退，提示了疾病发展过程中炎症细胞的演变。

通过直接免疫荧光技术，常可见到小静脉壁中纤维蛋白沉积，而免疫球蛋白和补体蛋白的沉积情况则各不相同。作者提及IgA沉积与自身免疫和炎症性疾病的消失有关，IgM沉积与自身免疫和炎症性疾病的出现有关，而IgG沉积与ANCA阳性有关。C3是CNV中最常出现的补体蛋白。

6．鉴别诊断　表138-4概述了CNV的鉴别诊断，主要包括血小板减少引起的瘀点或紫癜；老年人血管脆性增加、皮肤光老化、长期服用阿司匹林和内源性或医源性皮质功能亢进的皮肤创伤；坏血病；弥散性血管内凝血（fulminans紫癜）；脓毒性栓子；动脉粥样硬化栓塞；皮肤钙质沉着。

7．治疗　坏死性血管炎的治疗包括减少免疫复合物的沉积、抑制炎症反应、调节潜在的免疫病理机制和局部治疗。若有明确的诱发因素，去除诱因如停止用药或治疗感染可使皮肤病变消退。如果同时存在慢性疾病，治疗潜在疾病可能会改善皮肤血管病变。总的来说，CNV是一种自限性疾病，且目前缺乏循证级别高的药物。表138-5列出了被报道用于CNV治疗的药物，建议疾病治疗需对皮损情况（疾病类型）以及药物的毒副作用进行综合考量后按阶梯进行。

〔黄莹雪〕

AT-A-GLANCE

- The signature lesions of cutaneous necrotizing venulitis (CNV) are palpable purpura, erythematous to violaceous papules that do not blanch when the skin is pressed.
- Palpable purpura persist for 1 to 4 weeks and resolve at times with transient hyperpigmentation and/or atrophic scars.
- CNV may be associated with episodes of recurrent and chronic urticaria and angioedema.
- Lesions may occur anywhere on the skin but are most common on the lower extremities or over dependent areas such as the back and gluteal regions.
- CNV may be associated with connective tissue diseases, malignant conditions, cryoglobulinemia, antineutrophil cytoplasmic or antiphospholipid antibody syndromes.
- CNV has many precipitating causes, but infections and drugs are most common.
- The most widely recognized subgroup of idiopathic cutaneous necrotizing vasculitis in children is immunoglobulin A vasculitis.
- Histopathologic criteria include necrosis of the blood vessels with the deposition of fibrinoid material and dermal cellular infiltrates that consist of neutrophils with nuclear debris, mononuclear cells, and extravasated erythrocytes.
- Therapeutic approaches are divisible into removal of antigen, treatment of any underlying disorder, and treatment of CNV.

Necrotizing angiitis or vasculitis comprises a diverse group of disorders that combine inflammation with necrosis of the blood vessels. The vascular damage may result from immunologic and/or inflammatory mechanisms. Clinical syndromes are based on criteria that include the gross appearance and the histopathologic alterations of the vascular lesions, the caliber of the affected blood vessels, the frequency of involvement of specific organs, and laboratory abnormalities. Necrotizing vasculitis may be a primary disease, may develop as a feature of a systemic disorder, or may be idiopathic. Although there is no standard classification of the vasculitides, the American College of Rheumatology classification and the International Chapel Hill Consensus criteria are widely used.[1,2]

Necrotizing vasculitis in the skin predominantly involves venules and is known as cutaneous necrotizing venulitis/vasculitis (CNV), cutaneous small-vessel vasculitis, and leukocytoclastic vasculitis. The occurrence of CNV in association with systemic involvement of the small blood vessels has been termed *hypersensitivity angiitis/vasculitis*, *systemic polyangiitis*, and *microscopic polyangiitis* (see Chap. 139). CNV may be restricted to the skin, may occur in association with an underlying chronic disease, may be precipitated by infections or drugs, or may develop for unknown reasons (Table 138-1). Systemic forms of necrotizing vasculitis that affect larger blood vessels are considered in Chap. 139, "Systemic Necrotizing Arteritis."

HISTORICAL PERSPECTIVE

Various syndromes of necrotizing vasculitis were described in the 19th century, including necrotizing vasculitis of small blood vessels, described by Schönlein in 1837 and by Henoch in 1847. In 1952, Zeek differentiated systemic hypersensitivity angiitis that involved small blood vessels from polyarteritis nodosa. In various countries, different diagnostic terms were used to describe necrotizing vasculitis of the small blood vessels in the skin, which were perceived to be arterioles in the 1960s but were shown to be venules in the 1970s by multiple investigators.

EPIDEMIOLOGY

In a population-based study in Minnesota, the overall incidence of CNV was 4.5 per 100,000 person-years. The most common subtypes were cutaneous small-vessel vasculitis in 45% and immunoglobulin (Ig) A vasculitis in 30% of persons with CNV. The most common etiology was idiopathic. CNV was accompanied by systemic involvement in 4%.[3] In a study in France, the 5-year survival rate was 75.6%. Age older than 65 years at the outset of vasculitis was the only factor that was significantly associated with a shorter survival.[4] In this

TABLE 138-1
Cutaneous Necrotizing Venulitis: Associated Disorders and Events

Associated Chronic Disorders
- Rheumatoid arthritis
- Sjögren syndrome
- Systemic lupus erythematosus
- Hypergammaglobulinemic purpura
- Paraneoplastic vasculitis
- Cryoglobulinemia
- Ulcerative colitis
- Cystic fibrosis
- Antineutrophil cytoplasmic or antiphospholipid antibody syndromes

Precipitating Events
- Bacterial, viral, mycobacterial, and rickettsial infections
- Therapeutic and diagnostic agents

Idiopathic Disorders
- Immunoglobulin A vasculitis (Henoch-Schönlein purpura)
- Acute hemorrhagic edema of infancy
- Urticarial venulitis
- Erythema elevatum diutinum
- Nodular vasculitis
- Livedoid vasculopathy
- Genetic complement deficiencies
- Eosinophilic vasculitis
- Idiopathic

study, 18% of patients experienced relapses, especially when vascular thrombosis was identified in the skin biopsy specimen, when an antineutrophil cytoplasmic antibody (ANCA) was present, when hepatic liver enzymes were elevated, and when peripheral neuropathy was present. When the skin was the single organ involved, there were no relapses. IgA vasculitis is the most common form of CNV in children. Geographic variations in vasculitis may reflect an environmental influence, and seasonal variations in the incidence of vasculitis may suggest an infectious etiology.

CLINICAL FEATURES

The skin lesions of CNV are polymorphous. Erythematous to violaceous papules that do not blanch when the skin is pressed, known as *palpable purpura*, are the signature lesions (Fig. 138-1A). Macules, papules, urticaria/angioedema, pustules, vesicles, hemorrhagic blisters (Fig. 138-1B), necrosis and ulcers (Fig. 138-1C), and livedo reticularis may be present. Occasionally, there is subcutaneous edema below the area of the dermal lesions.

The eruption most often appears on the lower extremities or over dependent areas, such as the back and gluteal regions. The lesions may occur anywhere on the skin but are uncommon on the face, palms, soles, and mucous membranes. The clinical lesions are episodic and may recur over weeks to years. Palpable purpura persist for 1 to 4 weeks and resolve at times with transient hyperpigmentation and/or atrophic scars. Lesional symptoms include pruritus or burning and, less commonly, pain.

Fever, malaise, arthralgias, or myalgias may accompany an episode of cutaneous vascular lesions, irrespective of a defined underlying cause or associated disease. Systemic involvement of the small blood vessels most commonly occurs in the synovia, GI tract, voluntary muscles, peripheral nerves, and kidneys.

ASSOCIATED CHRONIC DISORDERS

CNV is associated with connective tissue diseases, notably rheumatoid arthritis, Sjögren syndrome, systemic lupus erythematosus (SLE), and hypergammaglobulinemic purpura. It rarely occurs in mixed connective tissue disease, relapsing polychondritis, polymyositis/dermatomyositis, ankylosing spondylitis,[5] and scleroderma. In patients with rheumatoid arthritis and CNV, the development of vascular lesions is related to the severity of the disease, which is generally, but not always, seropositive. Patients with rheumatoid arthritis often have involvement of larger vessels with associated peripheral neuropathy, nailfold infarcts, and digital gangrene.

In patients with SLE, CNV is associated with exacerbations of the underlying disease. Patients with anti-Ro antibody have a greater risk for the development of CNV. Vasculitis, however, is rare in patients with subacute cutaneous lupus erythematosus. Some women with necrotizing vasculitis without connective tissue disease have anti-Ro antibodies, and their infants may be born with neonatal lupus erythematosus.

In patients with Sjögren syndrome, the vascular lesions are located predominantly on the lower extremities and appear after exercise. Both hyperpigmentation and cutaneous ulcers are common features. Patients with Sjögren syndrome and CNV have a higher prevalence of articular involvement, peripheral neuropathy, Raynaud phenomenon, and

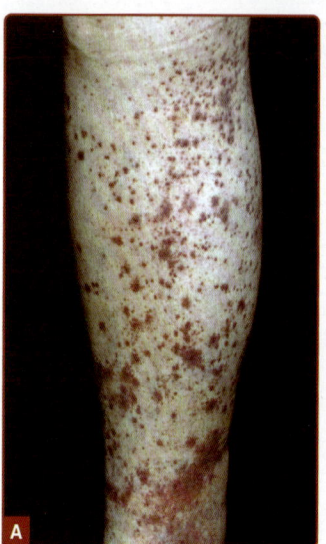
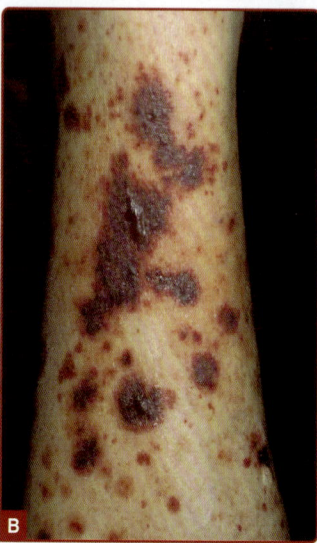
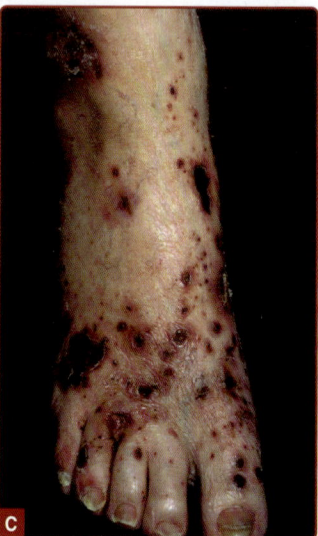

Figure 138-1 **A,** Palpable purpura on the lower leg in a patient with Henoch-Schönlein purpura. **B,** Palpable purpura with more-severe tissue damage with hemorrhagic vesicles and bullae. **C,** With even more tissue damage, multiple necrosis, and ulcers.

renal involvement, as well as the presence of anti-Ro antibody. Hypergammaglobulinemic purpura occurs in older women and may be associated with Sjögren syndrome, SLE, or a lymphoproliferative disorder. Dermatomyositis in children, but not in adults, may be associated with vasculitis of the GI tract.

Paraneoplastic vasculitis[6] describes CNV with associated malignant conditions. Hematologic disorders constitute the most common group of malignant disorders, especially chronic myelomonocytic leukemia, non-Hodgkin lymphoma, Hodgkin disease, chronic lymphocytic leukemia, myelodysplastic syndrome, and acute myelogenous leukemia. Less commonly, CNV is related to solid tumors, especially renal, lung, colon, breast, and prostate. However, the association between CNV and neoplasia is rare. It is not necessary to evaluate all patients with CNV for associated malignant conditions.

Cryoglobulins (see Chap. 144), especially mixed Types II and III, may be found in patients with idiopathic CNV and in patients with CNV that is associated with connective tissue diseases, lymphoproliferative disorders, propylthiouracil administration, and hepatitides A, B, and C virus infections. Hepatitis C virus is the most common infection, especially when it is associated with cryoglobulinemia. CNV occurs in patients with cystic fibrosis, inflammatory bowel diseases of the colon, and Behçet disease.

ANCAs are associated with various forms of necrotizing vasculitis. ANCAs are present in patients with microscopic polyangiitis and cutaneous vasculitis with hepatitis C virus infection (see Chap. 139). The most common cutaneous feature in patients with ANCAs is palpable purpura. Microscopic polyangiitis is associated with small-vessel systemic vasculitis that involves the cutaneous venules and arterioles, the kidneys with necrotizing and crescentic glomerulonephritis, the lungs with pulmonary hemorrhage or interstitial pneumonia, and perinuclear ANCAs (pANCAs). Erythematous macules, purpura, and livedo reticularis are cutaneous manifestations in microscopic polyangiitis. IgA ANCAs are present in acute IgA vasculitis in children.

Various subtypes of antiphospholipid antibodies occur in patients with necrotizing vasculitis. IgA anticardiolipin antibodies were detected in some patients with idiopathic CNV. IgA anticardiolipin, IgA and IgM anti–phosphatidyl serine–prothrombin complex, and IgA antibody-β_2 glycoprotein antibodies were detected in adults with IgA vasculitis. IgM anti–phosphatidyl serine–prothrombin complex antibodies were detected in adults with CNV. IgG and IgM anticardiolipin antibodies were detected in some individuals with livedoid vasculitis.

PRECIPITATING INFECTIONS AND DRUGS

Infections[7] and drugs[8-10] may precipitate episodes of CNV. The most commonly recognized infectious agents are β-hemolytic *Streptococcus*, *Staphylococcus aureus*, *Mycobacterium leprae*, and hepatitides B and C viruses. Transient episodes of urticaria may occur early in the course of hepatitis B virus infection and represent immune complex–induced vasculitis. Cutaneous vasculitis has been recognized in a limited number of individuals with HIV infection; the skin lesions consisted of palpable purpura, which at times had a follicular localization, and cutaneous ulcers.

Erythema nodosum leprosum, which appears as cutaneous nodules in lepromatous leprosy, is a form of necrotizing vasculitis that involves capillaries, venules, arterioles, small-to-medium-size arteries, and veins. The vascular lesions occur spontaneously or are precipitated by the administration of chemotherapeutic agents. They may be accompanied by fever, malaise, arthralgias, lymphadenopathy, and polyneuritis.

Necrotizing vasculitis that is caused by the direct invasion of the blood vessel wall occurs in septicemia caused by *Neisseria meningitidis*, *Neisseria gonorrhoeae*, *Pseudomonas*, *Haemophilus influenzae*, *Rickettsia*, *Candida*, and infectious endocarditis; in Rocky Mountain spotted fever; and in infections localized at the site of a catheter.

Palpable purpura is one of the less-common forms of drug reactions. The most commonly incriminated therapeutic agents were antibiotics, especially β-lactam agents, penicillin, and cephalosporins; nonsteroidal antiinflammatory agents; acetaminophen (paracetamol); allopurinol; anticonvulsants; propylthiouracil; hydralazine; granulocyte colony-stimulating factor/granulocyte-macrophage colony-stimulating factor; penicillamine; phenytoin; isotretinoin; methotrexate; and levamisole in cocaine.[11] Propylthiouracil[12] and hydralazine may cause vasculitis in association with ANCAs. Cutaneous vasculitis also has occurred after the administration of streptokinase, radiocontrast media, and staphylococcal protein A column immunoadsorption therapy. CNV is one of the most frequent autoimmune disorders triggered by anti–tumor necrosis factor biologic agents.[13]

IDIOPATHIC DISORDERS

Table 138-2 summarizes idiopathic small vessel vasculitides.

IMMUNOGLOBULIN A VASCULITIS

The most widely recognized subgroup of idiopathic CNV is IgA vasculitis,[14-18] which formerly was known as anaphylactoid purpura and Henoch-Schönlein purpura. It comprises 75% of CNV in children and 25% of CNV in adults. Most cases occur in the autumn and winter, and often are preceded by a history of a recent upper respiratory tract infection, especially in children. Sites of involvement include the skin, synovia, GI tract, and kidneys. Symptoms may include abdominal pain, melena, arthralgia, and hematuria.

TABLE 138-2
A Summary of Idiopathic Small Vessel Vasculitides

	EPIDEMIOLOGY	MANIFESTATIONS
IgA vasculitis (formerly Henoch-Schönlein purpura)	75% of CNV in children; 25% of CNV in adults	History of recent upper respiratory tract infection; involvement of skin, synovia, GI tract, kidneys; associated with abdominal pain, melena, arthralgia and hematuria; risk for progressive renal disease
Acute hemorrhagic edema of infancy	Infants and children <2 years of age	Painful, edematous petechiae and ecchymoses on head and distal extremities; may have associated facial edema; lesions may appear targetoid with bullae and necrosis; resolves within 1 to 3 weeks without sequelae
Urticarial venulitis (*urticarial vasculitis*)	Women most often affected; may be associated with serum sickness, connective tissue disorders, hematologic and malignant conditions, infections, or may be idiopathic	Erythematous, indurated wheals with a foci of purpura; may be associated with macular erythema, angioedema, livedo reticularis, nodules and bullae; persists for as long as 5 days; episodes may be chronic and recurrent
Erythema elevatum diutinum	Rare; most common in 4th to 6th decades	Symmetric, persistent, red-purple or red-brown plaques over joints or extensors and over gluteal area
Nodular vasculitis (*erythema induratum*)	More common in women between 30 and 40 years of age; may be associated with *Mycobacterium tuberculosis* infection (Erythema induratum) and hepatitis C virus infection	Tender, red, subcutaneous nodules over calves without systemic manifestations; may be recurrent
Livedoid vasculopathy (livedoid vasculitis, livedo vasculitis, segmental hyalinizing vasculitis, atrophie blanche)	More common in women; may occur in association with connective tissue disorders, malignancies, hypercoagulable states, thrombophilia	Chronic recurrent episodic exacerbations; arteriosclerosis or stasis of the lower extremities
Sneddon syndrome	May be associated with SLE	Livedo racemosa and livedoid vasculopathy are associated with ischemic cerebrovascular lesions, hypotension, and extracerebral arterial and venous thromboses
Eosinophilic vasculitis	Idiopathic	Recurrent, pruritic, purpuric papular skin lesions, urticarial plaques, and angioedema

CNV, cutaneous necrotizing venulitis; IgA, immunoglobulin A; SLE, systemic lupus erythematosus.

Long-term morbidity from progressive renal disease depends on the degree of initial renal damage. The distribution of skin lesions on the upper and lower extremities is a predictive factor for long-term renal involvement. Adults with onset after 60 years of age have a worse prognosis, owing to an increased risk of renal disease. Approximately 23% of IgA vasculitis patients experience a relapse. Longer duration of the initial episode, abdominal pain, joint manifestations, and the lack of an infectious cause were associated with relapses. Complete recovery occurred in 82.7% of those with relapses.

ACUTE HEMORRHAGIC EDEMA OF INFANCY

This uncommon disorder affects infants and children younger than 2 years of age, with a slight predominance in boys.[19] It has been classified by some as a variant of IgA vasculitis, while others consider it is a distinct clinical entity. The lesions appear as painful, edematous petechiae and ecchymoses that affect the head and distal portions of the extremities. Facial edema may be the initial sign. The skin lesions may be associated with a target-like appearance and may develop bullae and necrosis. Infections, drugs, or immunizations may be triggering factors. Acute hemorrhagic edema of infancy is distinguished from IgA vasculitis by its age distribution, lack of systemic features, and resolution within 1 to 3 weeks without sequelae.

URTICARIAL VENULITIS

Episodes of recurrent and chronic urticaria and angioedema may be a clinical manifestation of CNV.[20] Known as *urticarial vasculitis/venulitis*, this edematous form of necrotizing venulitis occurs in patients with serum sickness, connective tissue disorders, hematologic and other malignant conditions, an IgM_κ M component, infections, and, rarely, physical urticarias; after the administration of a variety of therapeutic agents; and as an idiopathic disorder.[21] The term *hypocomplementemic urticarial vasculitis syndrome* (HUVS) has been used to describe patients with more severe systemic manifestations, hypocomplementemia with low Clq levels, and an autoantibody to the collagen-like region of Clq.[22]

The skin lesions appear as erythematous, occasionally indurated, wheals that may contain foci of purpura (Fig. 138-2). Other skin manifestations include angioedema, macular erythema, livedo reticularis, nodules, and bullae. Although the individual urticarial lesions may last for fewer than 24 hours, they often persist for up to 3 to 5 days. The lesions are pruritic or possess a burning or painful quality; they usually resolve without residua although some individuals may develop contusions or hyperpigmentation. The episodes of urticaria are chronic, range in duration from months to years, and vary in frequency. Approximately 70% of affected individuals are women. The prevalence of this disorder remains unknown. General features include fever, malaise, and myalgia; the lymph nodes, liver, and spleen may be enlarged. Extracutaneous features involve the synovium, kidneys, GI tract, lungs, eyes, heart, CNS, peripheral nerves, and blood vessels. These extracutaneous features are more extensive in patients with HUVS.

The natural history of urticarial vasculitis is unknown, although individuals have been described with historic episodes of cutaneous lesions for up to 25 years. In one series of patients followed for 1 year, 40% experienced complete resolution of skin lesions; in another series of individuals followed for as long as 14 years, resolution occurred in only 1 patient. Sjögren syndrome and SLE have developed. Deaths have been reported from pulmonary disease, sepsis, and myocardial infarction.

The prevalence of urticarial vasculitis in individuals with chronic idiopathic urticaria is unknown, although series have reported rates that range from 1% to 50%. Most of these data have been reported from histopathologic studies in tertiary referral centers. The prevalence of urticarial vasculitis in a prospective clinical study in a university hospital in India was 11.4%.

Schnitzler syndrome[23,24] consists of episodes of urticarial vasculitis that is characterized by an infiltrate of neutrophils in the dermis and, less commonly, CNV that occur in association with a monoclonal IgM_K M component. Associated features include fever, lymphadenopathy, hepatosplenomegaly, bone pain, a sensorimotor neuropathy, and renal failure. It is a recurrent disorder with periods of spontaneous remission. Evolution into hematologic malignant conditions has been reported in 15% of Schnitzler syndrome patients.

ERYTHEMA ELEVATUM DIUTINUM

Erythema elevatum diutinum occurs as symmetric, persistent, red-purple or red-brown plaques that are predominantly distributed over the joints of extensor surfaces and over the gluteal area (see Chap. 140).

NODULAR VASCULITIS

Nodular vasculitis appears as tender, red, subcutaneous nodules over the lower extremities, especially the calves, without systemic manifestations (Fig. 138-3). At times, lesions develop on the thighs, buttocks, trunk, and arms, and ulcerated nodules may be present. Recurrent episodes are common. It is more common in women and has a peak incidence in individuals between 30 and 40 years of age. Erythema induratum is a form of nodular vasculitis, which has been associated with *Mycobacterium tuberculosis* infection, as demonstrated by polymerase chain reaction amplification

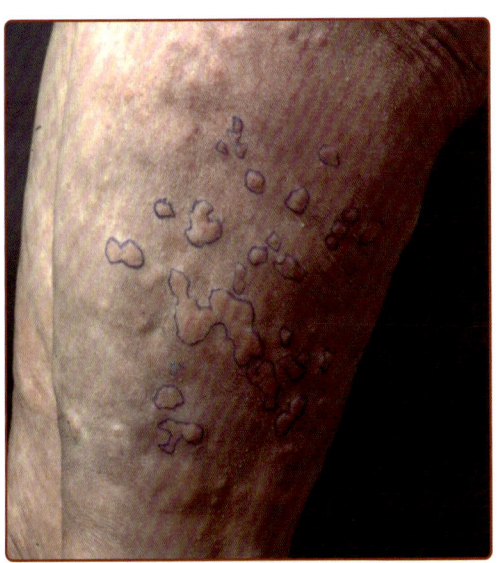

Figure 138-2 Urticarial venulitis. Some of the wheals have been marked 24 hours previously to demonstrate persistent character of the urticaria.

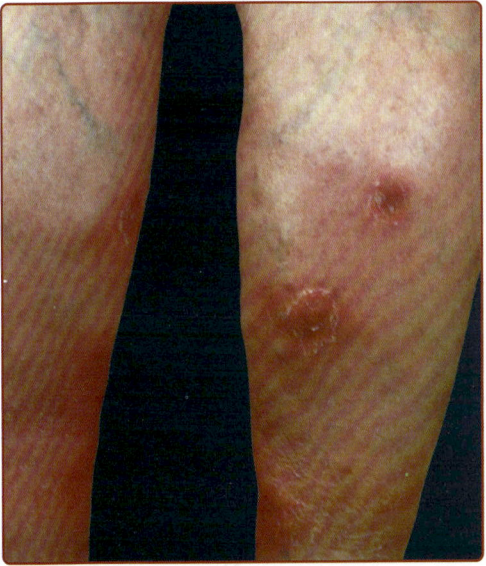

Figure 138-3 Nodular vasculitis with ulcers on lower legs.

for *M. tuberculosis* DNA in skin biopsy specimens. Various sizes of blood vessels, including venules, are affected. Erythema induratum also is associated with hepatitis C virus infection.

LIVEDOID VASCULOPATHY AND SNEDDON SYNDROME

Livedoid vasculopathy (Fig. 138-4), also known as livedoid vasculitis, livedo vasculitis, segmental hyalinizing vasculitis, and atrophie blanche, occurs as recurrent, painful ulcers of the lower extremities in association with persistent livedo reticularis (livedo racemosa) that often is deep purple in color. Healing results in sclerotic pale areas that are surrounded by telangiectasias termed *atrophie blanche* (Fig. 138-5). The clinical course is chronic with recurrent episodic exacerbations. Systemic involvement is not a feature of idiopathic livedoid vasculopathy. Many patients have arteriosclerosis or stasis of the lower extremities. Livedoid vasculopathy is more common in women and may occur in patients with connective tissue disorders, in malignant conditions, hypercoagulable states, in thrombophilia, and as an idiopathic disorder.[25] Protein C and protein S deficiencies, factor V Leiden gene mutation, activated protein C resistance, prothrombin gene mutation, hyperhomocysteinemia, and antithrombin deficiency have been reported. Atrophie blanche, however, probably represents the end stage of a variety of forms of vascular damage in the skin. Elevated levels of fibrinopeptide A, homocysteine, and plasminogen activator inhibitor may occur. Pathogenesis has focused on a hypercoagulable state with fibrin thrombi in the lumina of the superficial blood vessels. Some consider this condition to be a thrombogenic vasculopathy rather than a small-vessel vasculitis. Antiphospholipid antibodies have been detected in a few individuals.

Sneddon syndrome is a condition in which livedo racemosa and livedoid vasculopathy are associated with ischemic cerebrovascular lesions, hypotension, and extracerebral arterial and venous thromboses.[26,27] This condition may be associated with SLE. Antiendothelial cell antibodies, antiphospholipid antibodies, anti–β_2-glycoprotein antibodies, and antiprothrombin antibodies were detected in some patients.

GENETIC COMPLEMENT DEFICIENCIES

Genetic C2 deficiency has been recognized in association with CNV in 3 children and in 2 siblings with human leukocyte antigen (HLA)-A25, HLA-B18, and HLA-DR2 (w15) haplotype. C4 deficiency was present in 1 child with CNV and in 1 adult with CNV, and augmented C4 messenger RNA expression.[28] Deficiencies of C4A and C4B isotypes were found in some children and adults with IgA vasculitis. A partial C4B deficiency with C4A1, C4A3, and C4B1, and a null allele B*QO was reported in a 51-year-old woman with CNV.[29] A complete deficiency of complement factor 1 with a homozygous missense mutation in exon 2 of the *CF1* gene was reported in a 25-year-old woman with CNV.[29]

EOSINOPHILIC VASCULITIS

Eosinophilic vasculitis has been described as an idiopathic syndrome in individuals with recurrent, pruritic, and purpuric papular skin lesions, urticarial plaques, and angioedema. Skin biopsy specimens showed an infiltrate that is composed of eosinophils that express CD40 and vascular cell adhesion molecule (VCAM)-1 on endothelial cells of involved vessels. Eosinophilic vasculitis also has been described in some individuals with the hypereosinophilic syndrome (see

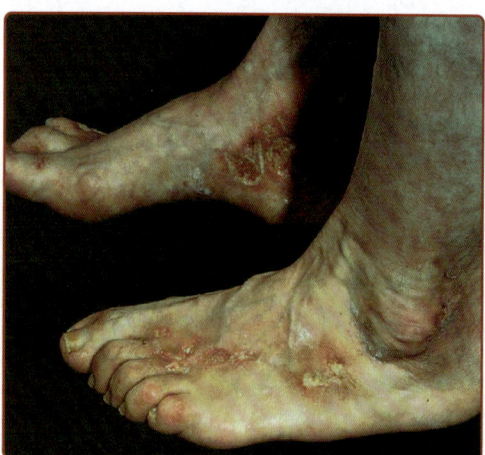

Figure 138-4 Livedoid vasculitis with recurrent, painful ulcers and livedo reticularis.

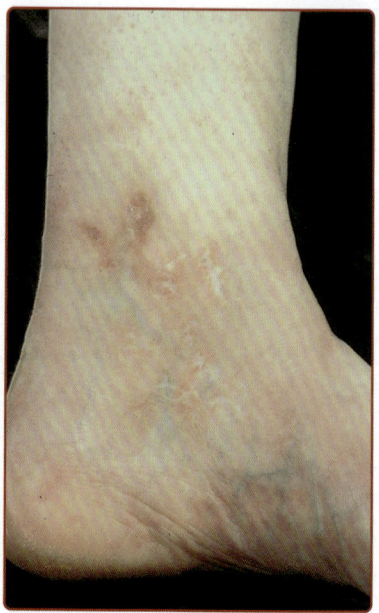

Figure 138-5 Atrophie blanche over the medial malleolus with porcelain-white atrophy, telangiectases, and ulcers.

Chap. 40) and in others with connective tissue disorders. There may be depressed complement levels, peripheral eosinophilia, elevated major basic protein levels, and a prolonged eosinophil survival time.

IDIOPATHIC

CNV that does not meet the criteria for a recognized syndrome is classified as idiopathic. Most cases are idiopathic.

ETIOLOGY AND PATHOGENESIS

Experimental studies in animal models and observations in humans implicate immune complexes as a major pathobiologic mechanism in the production of CNV. Data obtained in animal models suggest that the localization of immune complexes in venules is related to vasoactive amines and subsequent vasopermeability alterations. Additional factors that are operative in the localization of immune complexes include endothelial cell surface receptors and the defective clearance of immune complexes by the reticuloendothelial system.

The most frequently postulated mechanisms in the production of CNV are the local deposition of circulating immune complexes that are formed during antigen excess or the formation of immune complexes in situ in the skin. Immune complexes may activate the complement system and lead to the generation of C5a anaphylatoxin that degranulates mast cells and attracts neutrophils, which release lysosomal enzymes that damage tissue. The neutrophil superoxide-generating system may produce reactive oxygen products, which also cause tissue injury. The generation of the chemoattractant leukotriene B_4 from infiltrating neutrophils enhances the influx of neutrophils. The initial neutrophilic infiltrate contains few CD3, CD4, CD1a, and CD36 cells as these cells are prominent in the later phase, with the adhesion receptors intercellular adhesion molecule-1 (ICAM-1) and lymphocyte function-associated antigen-1. In IgA vasculitis, the fragmentation of neutrophils was attributed to apoptosis on the basis of the detection of inducible nitric oxide synthase and nitrotyrosine in the infiltrates and the detection of interleukin (IL)-8 on vascular endothelial cells. Long penetration PTX3, which inhibits phagocytosis of apoptotic neutrophils by macrophages, was detected in skin biopsy specimens of idiopathic CNV and of IgA vasculitis about blood vessels and at sites of infiltrates with leukocytoclasia.

In CNV, circulating immune complexes have been demonstrated in serum as mixed-type cryoglobulins and indirectly by assays that detect C1q precipitins, materials that bind to complement receptors on human lymphocytoid (Raji) cells, materials that bind to monoclonal rheumatoid factor, and substances that function in the antibody-dependent cellular cytotoxicity inhibition assay. The presence of immune complexes is inferred from the occurrence of serum hypocomplementemia with activation of the classic activating pathway and by the detection of increased plasma levels of C4a and C3a anaphylatoxins.

In CNV, immune complexes have been detected in lesional tissues by their ultrastructural observation as electron-dense subendothelial deposits; the membrane-attack complex, C5b-9, of the complement system has been detected on the surface of endothelial cells and infiltrating neutrophils. Decay-accelerating factor, which is a regulatory complement protein that prevents the assembly of the membrane-attack complex, was not present on the surface of endothelial cells of the superficial dermal microvasculature. Tissue immune complexes also have been detected by direct immunofluorescence techniques as deposited immunoglobulins and complement proteins. In time–course studies of the evolution of cutaneous vascular lesions, immune reactants have been identified in lesions that are less than 24 hours old. Antigens have been identified only in a few instances as bacterial, viral, mycobacterial, or rickettsial proteins by direct immunofluorescence techniques or by the polymerase chain reaction.

A role for lymphocytes in the production of CNV is suggested by a perivenular infiltrate in skin lesions that is rich in lymphocytes with large and hyperchromatic nuclei. The lymphocytes express CD3, CD4, CD1a, CD36, ICAM-1, and lymphocyte function-associated antigen-1. Lymphocytes may be activated by immune complexes, by cellular immune mechanisms, and by primary activation in autoimmune disease to produce lymphokines. In CNV, there were increased numbers of factor XIIIa+–derived dendrocytes, which are involved in antigen presentation to T cells. Endothelial cells also can present antigens to and activate T lymphocytes. Activated macrophages secrete chemokines and lysosomal enzymes. γ/δ T cells have been detected in CNV with a neutrophil-rich pattern and with an infectious etiology. In these specimens, a 72-kDa heat shock protein was expressed by endothelial cells and antigen-presenting cells.

The participation of mast cells in CNV is suggested by hypogranulated mast cells with shed extracellular granules and by the development of vascular lesions after the intracutaneous injection of histamine in patients with active episodes of CNV. Mast cells can be activated directly by immune complexes through FcγRIII or by C5a. Through the production of histamine, prostaglandin D_2, and cysteinyl leukotrienes, the mast cell could alter venular permeability; interendothelial cell gaps have been noted in venules in patients with CNV. Eosinophils and neutrophils may be recruited by mast cell–derived chemotactic factors. The neutral proteases and acid hydrolases of mast cells may facilitate tissue damage, and the release of tumor necrosis factor-α (TNF-α) may increase expression of E-selectin on endothelial cells and facilitate neutrophil recruitment.

Evidence for the role of the mast cell also is provided by time–course analyses of the sequential histopathologic changes in individuals with physical urticaria. In a patient with circulating immune complexes and hypocomplementemia, in whom cold and trauma elicited CNV, initial mast cell degranulation was followed by the infiltration of neutrophils, the deposition of fibrin, and venular endothelial cell necrosis. A postulated sequence of events would be the activation of the mast cell by physical stimuli, the release of vasoactive mediators, the deposition of circulating immune complexes with activation of the complement system, the influx of neutrophils, and the development of CNV. Another example of the time–course analysis of CNV in human skin was provided by an individual with exercise-induced vasculitis. At 3 hours, the number of mast cells decreased, and the eosinophil was the first cell to appear around the venules with the deposition of eosinophil peroxidase. TNF-α levels were elevated, E-selectin was expressed on endothelial cells, and an influx of neutrophils appeared with the deposition of neutrophil elastase and the development of CNV.

In a study of 10 adult patients with CNV,[30] skin biopsy specimens were obtained from early petechial lesions and the later lesions of palpable purpura. The number of mast cells that contained tryptase and chymase were decreased in the early lesions, which suggested degranulation. The levels of chymase as well as $α_1$-antichymotrypsin continued to decrease with the progression of vasculitis, which suggested inhibition by antichymotrypsin. IgG, IgM, IgA, and fibrin increased in palpable purpura.

Early in the course of necrotizing venulitis, endothelial cells show increased expression of ICAM-1 and E-selectin without the expression of VCAM-1 in response to TNF-α. Because E-selectin is an adhesion molecule for neutrophils and for skin-homing, memory T lymphocytes, the increase in E-selectin is associated with an infiltrate of neutrophils that express CD11b within the first 24 hours.

In the acute phase of IgA vasculitis, endothelin-1, serum insulin-like growth factor-1,[31] insulin-like growth factor–binding protein-3, plasma matrix metalloproteinase-9, ICAM-1, VCAM-1, TNF-α, tumor necrosis factor-like inducer of apoptosis weak,[32] IL-1β, IL-2 receptor, IL-6, IL-8, IL-33,[33] transforming growth factor-β, vascular endothelial cell growth factor, high-mobility group box-1,[34] visfatin,[35] CCL5, CXCL1b, CX_3CL,[36] and urine leukotriene E_4 levels were elevated. However, the pathogenic roles of these mediators remain undefined. IgA antiendothelial cell antibodies bind to endothelial cells and enhance endothelial cell production of IL-8 via the mitogen-activated protein kinase/extracellular signal-regulated kinase pathways.

In skin biopsy specimens from patients with idiopathic CNV, hypersensitivity vasculitis, urticarial vasculitis, and IgA vasculitis, E-selectin was detected on endothelial cells of lesions that were less than 48 hours old and was associated with an infiltrate of neutrophils that expressed CD11b. The endothelial cells expressed HLA-DR and very-late-activating antigen-1 but not P-selectin, and the perivascular cells expressed VCAM-1 and HLA-DR. Diminished cutaneous fibrinolytic activity with reduced release of plasminogen activator from venular endothelial cells occurs in patients with CNV; the subsequent reduction in fibrinolytic activity leads to fibrin deposition. Increased levels of plasma thrombomodulin, tissue-type plasminogen activator, and plasminogen activator inhibitor-1 were detected in patients with IgA vasculitis.

Cutaneous nerve fibers can release neuropeptides that cause vasodilation, such as substance P, neurokinin A, and calcitonin gene-related peptide. Substance P activates mast cells and macrophages and increases fibrinolytic activity that is mediated by plasminogen activator. Calcitonin gene-related peptide induces expression of E-selectin on endothelial cells and is chemotactic for T lymphocytes.

Eosinophils are minor infiltrating cells in CNV except in eosinophilic vasculitis and drug-induced CNV. Eosinophils produce leukotriene C_4 and platelet-activating factor, which increase vascular permeability. Eosinophil granule proteins are toxic to endothelial cells and cause the release of mediators from mast cells.

Associations have been recognized between small-vessel necrotizing vasculitis and ANCAs, which have specificity for proteins of the cytoplasmic granules of neutrophils and the lysosomes of monocytes. Two forms are recognized: cytoplasmic (cANCAs) that are directed against proteinase 3 and perinuclear (pANCAs) that are directed against myeloperoxidase. TNF-α facilitates neutrophil activation and cell-surface expression of proteinase 3 and myeloperoxidase, which bind to ANCAs and increase the adherence of neutrophils to endothelial cells resulting in endothelial cell injury. Antiendothelial cell antibodies have been detected in the sera of patients with systemic vasculitis, rheumatoid arthritis with vasculitis, microscopic polyangiitis, and Sneddon syndrome.

An increased prevalence of the HLA haplotype HLA-A11, Bw35 in patients with CNV and associated connective tissue disorders suggests that genetic factors may be operative. HLA-DRB1 genotype associations were detected in patients with CNV and IgA vasculitis in Spain.

DIAGNOSIS

LABORATORY TESTING

The laboratory evaluation of patients with CNV depends on information obtained from the history and physical examination (Table 138-3). An elevated erythrocyte sedimentation rate is the most consistent abnormal laboratory finding. The platelet count usually is normal. Other abnormalities reflect either a coexistent chronic disorder or the involvement of additional organ systems. Occasionally, leukocytosis, anemia, thrombocytosis, abnormal urine sediment, circulating immune complexes, rheumatoid factor, and antinuclear antibodies have been reported in idiopathic disease.

Serum complement levels are usually normal. Hypocomplementemia may develop in patients with concomitant connective tissue diseases or cryoglobu-

TABLE 138-3
Laboratory Evaluation of Cutaneous Necrotizing Venulitis

- Erythrocyte sedimentation rate
- Complete blood count with differential analysis
- Platelet count
- Urinalysis
- 24-Hour urine protein and creatinine clearance
- Blood chemistry profile
- Serum protein electrophoresis
- Immunoelectrophoresis
- Hepatitis B antigen and hepatitis A and C antibodies
- Cryoglobulins
- CH_{50} (50% hemolytic complement)
- Antinuclear antibody
- Rheumatoid factor
- Antineutrophil cytoplasmic antibodies
- Antiphospholipid antibodies
- Circulating immune complexes
- Stool guaiac test
- Skin biopsy

linemia and reflects the associated disease or the composition of the cryoglobulin. Hypocomplementemia also occurs in some individuals with idiopathic CNV and in 40% of individuals with urticarial venulitis.

In patients with the HUVS, a low-molecular-weight 7s C1q precipitin, which has been identified as an IgG autoantibody against the collagen-like region of C1q, was detected. Autoantibodies to vascular endothelial cells were detected in patients with HUVS, in patients with SLE and urticarial vasculitis, and in patients with urticarial vasculitis alone. In IgA purpura, serum IgA_1 levels are elevated, IgA ANCAs may be present, and urinary endothelin-1 levels may be elevated. In patients with CNV, various types of circulating immune complexes and IgA ANCAs have been described. IgG autoantibodies to IgE and to FcεRIα also have been identified in some patients with urticarial venulitis.

HISTOPATHOLOGY

In skin biopsy specimens of palpable purpura and urticarial vasculitis stained with hematoxylin and eosin, the histopathologic criteria requisite for the diagnosis of CNV include necrosis of the blood vessels with deposition of fibrinoid material and dermal cellular infiltrates that consist of neutrophils with nuclear debris, mononuclear cells, and extravasated erythrocytes (Fig. 138-6A). The dermal inflammatory infiltrates vary in intensity and are usually perivenular in location, but may be dispersed widely. In patients with CNV associated with bacterial infections, the biopsy specimens showed a greater number of neutrophils.[37] Some patients with connective tissue disorders and cutaneous vasculitis have an infiltrate of inflammatory cells composed of eosinophils with deposited major basic protein and decreased numbers of mast cells. Eosinophils may be present in increased numbers in drug-induced CNV. The fibrinoid material consists of fibrin, necrotic endothelial cells, immunoreactants, and antigens.

Studies with 1-µm–thick sections[38] show 2 distinct cellular patterns in CNV: one rich in neutrophils and the other in lymphocytes. The infiltrate of neutrophils regresses with the persistence of an infiltrate of mononuclear cells; repeat biopsy specimens in some patients consistently demonstrated an infiltrate of mononuclear cells. In a time–course study over 6 days of the evolution of experimentally induced CNV in a patient with physical urticaria, the number of infiltrating neutrophils decreased without a concomitant increase in lymphocytes although the number of monocytes/macrophages was increased at 48 hours and 72 hours. Other features in both cell patterns of

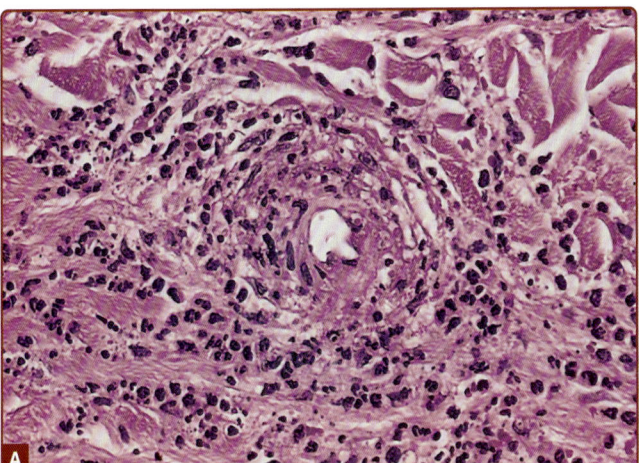
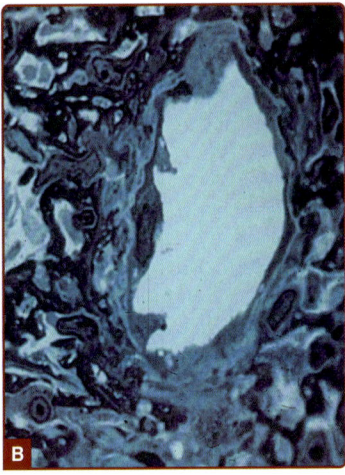

Figure 138-6 **A,** Perivenular infiltrate of neutrophils with fibrin deposition (hematoxylin and eosin stain, ×50 in the original magnification). **B,** Endothelial cell necrosis of a venule with perivenular fibrin and neutrophils (1-µm section, Giemsa stain, ×1000 in the original magnification).

CNV include hypogranulated mast cells, macrophages containing debris, and the perivenular and interstitial deposition of fibrin. Venular alterations in both cell patterns consist of endothelial-cell swelling, activation of nuclei, wrinkling of nuclear membranes, necrosis (see Fig. 138-6B), and basement membrane reduplication and thickening. The arterioles are not affected.

By direct immunofluorescence techniques, fibrin deposition in venules is routinely identified in biopsy specimens, whereas the deposition of immunoglobulins and complement proteins varies widely.[39,40] IgG, IgM, and IgA have been detected. In one study,[41] IgA deposits were related to absence of autoimmune and inflammatory disorders, IgM deposits to the presence of autoimmune and inflammatory disorders, and IgG deposits to a positive ANCA. IgA is deposited about blood vessels in the skin, intestines, and kidneys in IgA vasculitis and has become an immunopathologic marker of this condition (Fig. 138-7). In the skin in IgA vasculitis, IgA_1 is the dominant subclass that is deposited. C3 is the most frequently detected immunoreactant, but it is the only complement protein that has been sought with frequency in CNV.

DIFFERENTIAL DIAGNOSIS

Table 138-4 outlines the differential diagnosis of CNV.

MANAGEMENT

Therapeutic approaches may be divided into removal of the antigen, treatment of an underlying disorder, and treatment of CNV. Therapeutic approaches in the treatment of necrotizing vasculitis consist of prevention of the deposition of immune complexes, suppression of the inflammatory response, modulation of underlying immunopathologic mechanisms, and local therapy. When the eruption is associated with a precipitating event, withdrawal of the medication or treatment of the infection results in resolution of the cutaneous lesions. If a coexistent chronic disease is present, treatment of the underlying disease may be associated with improvement in the cutaneous vascular lesions. In many cases, CNV is a self-limited condition, and double-blind, placebo-controlled, prospective trials of therapeutic agents are usually lacking.

The treatment of CNV (Table 138-5) depends on an analysis of the cutaneous disability as well as on the toxicity and side effects of the therapeutic agents. H_1 antihistamines are used in patients with palpable purpura to alleviate lesional symptoms and perhaps to reduce tissue deposition of circulating immune complexes. Nonsteroidal antiinflammatory agents are combined with the H_1 antihistamine. Depending on

TABLE 138-4
Differential Diagnosis of Cutaneous Necrotizing Venulitis

DISORDER	CLINICAL CONSIDERATIONS
Petechiae or purpura caused by thrombocytopenia	The lesions are flat
Trauma to skin of elderly individuals with vascular fragility, dermatoheliosis, chronic aspirin ingestion, and endogenous or iatrogenic hypercorticism	The lesions are flat
Scurvy	Hemorrhagic follicular papules with corkscrew hairs over the lower extremities
Disseminated intravascular coagulation (purpura fulminans)	Extensive areas of purpura with a slate-gray color
Septic emboli	Finite numbers of hemorrhagic papules, pustules, and vesicles that are distributed over the acral areas
Atheromatous embolism	Purpura, livedo reticularis, nodules, and ulcers distributed over acral areas with blue or discolored toes
Calcinosis cutis	Indurated purpura, livedo reticularis, nodules and ulcers

TABLE 138-5
Agents Used in the Treatment of Cutaneous Necrotizing Venulitis

- H_1 antihistamines
- Nonsteroidal antiinflammatory agents
- Colchicine
- Hydroxychloroquine sulfate
- Systemic glucocorticoids
- Methotrexate
- Cyclosporine
- Mycophenolate mofetil
- Intravenous gammaglobulin
- Plasmapheresis
- Infliximab
- Etanercept
- Adalimumab
- Rituximab

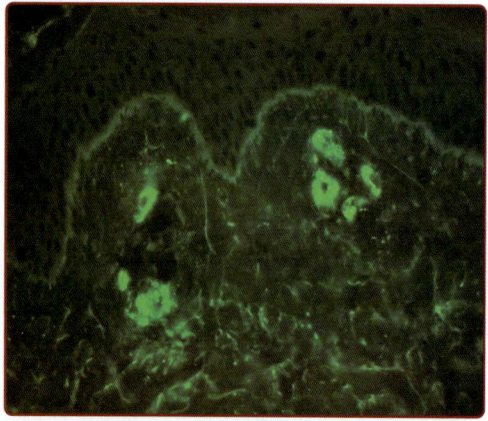

Figure 138-7 Immunofluorescence study of the skin showing deposition of IgA in the venules of the superficial dermis. (Image courtesy of Dr. James E. Fitzpatrick and used with permission.)

the therapeutic response, colchicine can be added to or substituted for these agents. However, colchicine was shown to have no significant therapeutic effect in a prospective, randomized, controlled trial. If there is no benefit, dapsone or hydroxychloroquine sulfate can be used. If there still is no therapeutic response, a major decision must be made because systemic glucocorticoids, azathioprine, methotrexate, cyclosporine, mycophenolate mofetil, cyclophosphamide, plasmapheresis, intravenous immunoglobulin, infliximab, adalimumab, etanercept, and rituximab are associated with serious side effects. Although all of these agents are reported to benefit some patients, controlled clinical trials are not available. The administration of interferon-α is associated with clearing of cutaneous vasculitis in patients with hepatitis C virus infection.

The treatment of patients with urticarial vasculitis is similar to those with palpable purpura. Additional case reports exist on the treatment of patients with intramuscular gold therapy, cyclophosphamide-dexamethasone pulse therapy, mycophenolate mofetil, thalidomide, anakinra, cinnarizine, and psoralen plus ultraviolet A photochemotherapy. In an open-label pilot study in 10 patients with urticarial venulitis, improvement was noted after a single, subcutaneous dose of canakinumab.[42] In patients with Schnitzler syndrome, IL-1 inhibition is the only completely efficient treatment with the use of anakinra, canakinumab, or rilonacept.

In the treatment of livedoid vasculitis, support stockings are useful. Empiric trials of aspirin and dipyridamole, colchicine, dapsone, danazol, low-dose heparin, systemic glucocorticoids, nicotinic acid, low-molecular-weight dextran, phenformin, ethylestrenol, nifedipine, pentoxifylline, and rivaroxaban[43] have been used. Infusions of prostacyclin, prostaglandin E_1, intravenous immunoglobulin, rituximab, tissue plasminogen activator, hyperbaric oxygen therapy, and psoralen plus ultraviolet A photochemotherapy have been used successfully in a few patients.

REFERENCES

1. Calabrese LH, Michel BA, Bloch DA, et al. The American College of Rheumatology 1990 criteria for the classification of hypersensitivity vasculitis. *Arthritis Rheum*. 1990;33(8):1108-1113.
2. Jennette JC, Falk RJ, Bacon PA, et al. 2012 Revised International Chapel Hill Consensus Conference nomenclature of vasculitides. *Arthritis Rheum*. 2013;65(1):1-11.
3. Arora D, Wetter DA, Gonzalez-Santiago TM, et al. Incidence of leukocytoclastic vasculitis, 1996-2010: a population-based study in Olmsted County, Minnesota. *Mayo Clin Proc*. 2014;89(11):1515-1524.
4. Bouiller K, Audia S, Devilliers H, et al. Etiologies and prognostic factors of leukocytoclastic vasculitis with skin involvement: a retrospective study in 112 patients. *Medicine (Baltimore)*. 2016;95(28):e4238.
5. Kobak S, Yilmaz H, Karaarsian A, et al. Leukocytoclastic vasculitis in a patient with ankylosing spondylitis. *Case Rep Rheumatol*. 2014;2014:653837.
6. Loricera J, Calvo-Rio V, Ortiz-Sanjuán F, et al. The spectrum of paraneoplastic cutaneous vasculitis in a defined population: incidence and clinical features. *Medicine (Baltimore)*. 2013;92(6):331-343.
7. Loricera J, Blanco R, Hernandez JL, et al. Cutaneous vasculitis associated with severe bacterial infections: a study of 27 patients from a series of 766 cutaneous vasculitis. *Clin Exp Rheumatol*. 2015;33(2)(suppl 89):536-543.
8. Ortiz-Sanjuán F, Blanco R, Hernandez JL, et al. Drug-associated cutaneous vasculitis: study of 239 patients from a single referral center. *J Rheumatol*. 2014;41(11):2201-2207.
9. Loricera J, Blanco R, Oritz-Sanjuán F, et al. Single-organ cutaneous small-vessel vasculitis according to the 2012 revised International Chapel Hill Consensus Conference nomenclature of vasculitides: a study of 60 patients from a series of 766 cutaneous vasculitis cases. *Rheumatology (Oxford)*. 2015;54(1):77-82.
10. Khetan P, Sethuraman G, Khaitan BK, et al. An aetiological & clinicopathological study on cutaneous vasculitis. *Indian J Med Res*. 2012;135(1):107-113.
11. Patnaik S, Balderia P, Vanchhawng L, et al. Is levamisole-induced vasculitis a relegated diagnostic possibility? A case report and review of literature. *Am J Case Rep*. 2015;16:658-662.
12. Zivanovic D, Dobrosavljevic D, Nikolic M, et al. Cryoglobulins and multispecific antineutrophil cytoplasmic antibodies in propylthiouracil-induced necrotizing cutaneous vasculitis-a new association. *Eur J Dermatol*. 2012;22(5):707-709.
13. Ramos-Casals M, Roberto-Perez-Alvarez, Diaz-Lagares C, et al; BIOGEAS Study Group. Autoimmune diseases induced by biological agents: a double-edged sword? *Autoimmun Rev*. 2010;9(3):188-193.
14. Park SJ, Suh J-S, Lee JH, et al. Advances in our understanding of the pathogenesis of Henoch-Schönlein purpura and the implications for improving its diagnosis. *Expert Rev Clin Immunol*. 2013;9(12):1223-1238.
15. Calvo-Rio V, Hernández JL, Ortiz-Sanjuán F, et al. Relapses in patients with Henoch-Schönlein purpura: analysis of 417 patients from a single center. *Medicine (Baltimore)*. 2016;95(28):e4217.
16. Linskey KR, Kroshinsky D, Mihm MC Jr, et al. Immunoglobulin-A-associated small-vessel vasculitis: a 10-year experience at the Massachusetts General Hospital. *J Am Acad Dermatol*. 2012;66(5):813-822.
17. Hong S, Ahn S, Lim D, et al. Late-onset IgA vasculitis in adult patients exhibits distinct clinical characteristics and outcomes. *Clin Exp Rheumatol*. 2016;34(3)(suppl 97):S77-S83.
18. Calvo-Rio V, Loricera J, Mata C, et al. Henoch-Schönlein purpura in Northern Spain: clinical spectrum of the disease in 417 patients from a single center. *Medicine (Baltimore)*. 2014;93(2):106-113.
19. Ting TV. Diagnosis and management of cutaneous vasculitis in children. *Pediatr Clin North Am*. 2014;61(2):321-346.
20. Moreno-Suárez F, Pulpillo-Ruiz A, Zulucta Dorado T, et al. Urticaria vasculitis: estudio retrospectivo de 15 casos. *Actas Dermosifiliogr*. 2013;104(7):579-585.
21. Loricera J, Calvio-Rio V, Mata, et al. Urticarial vasculitis in Northern Spain: clinical study of 21 cases. *Medicine (Baltimore)*. 2014;93(1):53-60.
22. Jachiet M, Flaguel B, Deroux A, et al. The clinical spectrum and therapeutic management of hypocomplementemic urticarial vasculitis: data from a French nationwide

22. study of fifty-seven patients. *Arthritis Rheum*. 2015; 67(2):527-534.
23. Simon A, Asli B, Braun-Falco M, et al. Schnitzler's syndrome: diagnosis, treatment, and follow-up. *Allergy*. 2013;68(5):562-568.
24. Gameiro A. Gouveia M, Pereira M, et al. Clinical characterization and long-term follow-up of Schnitzler syndrome. *Clin Exp Immunol*. 2016;41(5):461-467.
25. Vasudevan B, Neema S, Verma R. Livedoid vasculopathy: a review of pathogenesis and principles of management. *Indian J Dermatol Venereol Leprol*. 2016; 82(5):478-488.
26. Wu S, Xu Z, Liang H. Sneddon's syndrome: a comprehensive review of the literature. *Orphanet J Rare Dis*. 2014;9:215.
27. Bersano A, Morbin M, Ciceri E, et al. The diagnostic challenge of Divry van Bogaert and Sneddon syndrome: report of three cases and literature review. *J Neurol Sci*. 2016;364:77-83.
28. Kosada S, Osada S, Kaneko T, et al. Cutaneous vasculitis and glomerulonephritis associated with C4 deficiency. *Clin Exp Dermatol*. 2013;38(5):492-495.
29. Bay JT, Katzenstein TL, Kofoed K, et al. Novel CF1 mutation in a patient with leukocytoclastic vasculitis may redefine the clinical spectrum of Complement factor 1 deficiency. *Clin Immunol*. 2015;160(2):315-318.
30. Lipitsa T, Naukkarinen A, Harvima IT. Mast cell tryptase and chymase in the progress of cutaneous vasculitis. *Arch Dermatol Res*. 2015;307(10):917-924.
31. Chen T, Guo ZP, Zhang Y-H, et al. Elevated serum heme oxygenase-1 and insulin-like growth factor-1 levels in patients with Henoch-Schönlein purpura. *Rheumatol Int*. 2011;31(3):321-326.
32. Chen T, Guo Z-p, Li L, et al. TWEAK enhances E-selection and ICAM-1 expression, and may contribute to the development of cutaneous vasculitis. *PLoS One*. 2013;8(2):e56830.
33. Chen T, Jia R-z, Guo Z-p, et al. Elevated serum interleukin-33 levels in patients with Henoch-Schönlein purpura. *Arch Dermatol Res*. 2013;305(2):173-177.
34. Chen T, Guo Z-p, Wang W-j, et al. Increased serum HMGB1 levels in patients with Henoch-Schönlein purpura. *Exp Dermatol*. 2014;23(6):419-423.
35. Cao N, Chen T, Guo Z-P, et al. Elevated levels of visfatin in patients with Henoch-Schönlein purpura. *Ann Dermatol*. 2014;26(3):303-307.
36. Chen T, Guo Z-p, Jiao X-y, et al. CCL5, CXCL16, and CX3CL1 are associated with Henoch-Schönlein purpura. *Arch Dermatol Res*. 2011;303(10):715-725.
37. Loricera J, González-Vela C, Blanco R, et al. Histopathologic differences between cutaneous vasculitis associated with severe bacterial infection and cutaneous vasculitis secondary to other causes: study of 52 patients. *Clin Exp Rheumatol*. 2016;34(3)(suppl 97): 93-97.
38. Soter NA, Mihm MC Jr, Gigli I, et al. Two distinct cellular patterns in cutaneous necrotizing angiitis. *J Invest Dermatol*. 1976;66(6):344-350.
39. Nandeesh B. Tirumalae R. Direct immunofluorescence in cutaneous vasculitis: experience from a referral hospital in India. *Indian J Dermatol*. 2013;58(1):22-25.
40. Alalwani M, Billings SD, Gota CE. Clinical significance of immunoglobulin deposition in leukocytoclastic vasculitis: a 5-year retrospective study of 88 patients at Cleveland Clinic. *Am J Dermatopathol*. 2014;36(9): 723-729.
41. Takatu CM, Heringer APR, Aoki V, et al. Clinicopathologic correlation of 282 leukocytoclastic vasculitis cases in a tertiary hospital: a focus on immunofluorescence findings at the blood vessel wall. *Immunol Res*. 2017;65(1):395-401.
42. Krause K, Mahamed A, Weller K, et al. Efficacy and safety of canakinumab in urticarial vasculitis: an open-label study. *J Allergy Clin Immunol*. 2013;132(3):751-754.
43. Lee JM, Kim IH. Case series of recalcitrant livedoid vasculopathy treated with rivaroxaban. *Clin Exp Dermatol*. 2016;41(5):559-561.

Chapter 139 :: Systemic Necrotizing Arteritis
Peter A. Merkel & Paul A. Monach

第一百三十九章

系统性坏死性动脉炎

中文导读

本章首先对血管炎和系统性血管炎进行了定义,并指出皮肤血管炎可能是系统性疾病的表现。本章重点介绍系统性血管炎中的皮肤病变,主要从血管炎的分类、流行病学、临床表现、病因和发病机制、诊断、常见病种、临床过程和预后及治疗八个方面进行了详细阐述。

1. 血管炎的分类　作者对血管炎的分类标准现状进行了介绍,提出最普遍接受的方法是按血管的管径大小进行分类(中等、小型、中型或大型),再视情况细分或分组(图139-1)。

2. 流行病学　在美国,各种形式的特发性血管炎属于罕见疾病(患病人数少于200,000),在欧洲和其他地方也存在类似情况。作者就部分疾病的好发人群进行了举例,并提出某些地域差异与HLA的遗传易感性有关。

3. 临床表现

(1) 皮肤表现:血管炎的皮肤表现与受累血管的大小和深度、炎症和红细胞外渗的严重程度、受损血管的密度和导致的组织破坏有关。皮肤中小血管血管炎的典型表现是可触及的紫癜,也可出现不可触及的紫癜、丘疹、荨麻疹病变、大小和深度不同的结节、大疱性病变和溃疡(图139-3、139-4、139-6至139-12)。结节和溃疡常伴有疼痛感。

(2) 非皮肤表现:病史和体格检查往往能发现多器官系统受累的线索。表139-1列出了各种形式血管炎的重要体征和症状。

4. 病因和发病机制　除了与感染有关的血管炎和药物引起的血管炎外,大多数类型的血管炎的病因尚不清楚,作者总结其发病机制主要涉及以下两种途径:免疫复合物沉积或与ANCA相关的非免疫复合物介导的病理过程。

5. 诊断流程　发现患者可能与血管炎有关的皮肤病变时,作者建议按图139-2流程来识别血管炎诊断,并判断血管炎的类型及严重程度。

6. 系统回顾　全面系统回顾是对怀疑血管炎患者早期评估的重要组成部分。表139-1列出了各种形式的血管炎的重要体征和症状。建议详细询问血管炎患者的病史,包括同时存在的其他疾病和感染、用药史、职业接触或其他接触非药物性毒物的情况。

7. 体格检查　除了对皮肤进行仔细和全面的评估外,多系统体格检查有助于确定血管炎的诊断并发现之前所忽视的损害。作者对于血管炎的体格检查的重点进行了阐述和建议。

8. 皮肤活检　皮肤活检对于血管炎的诊断至关重要,皮肤活检的深度通常取决于所涉血管的大小,建议选择48小时以内的病变进行活检，最大程度发现急性中性粒细胞性血管炎的典型特征。

9. 其他组织活检　血管炎可通过对肾脏、肺、肌肉或周围神经，甚至从手术标本中进行活检明确诊断（图139-5），肾脏或肺活检对某些疾病的诊断比皮肤活检更重要，但仍建议行皮肤活检，以免不必要的侵入性活检。

10. 实验室检查　主要包括肾功能、肝功能、血细胞计数、急性期指标、自身免疫血清学、ANCA、抗核抗体、类风湿因子、副球蛋白、补体、感染性疾病的相关检查及药物滥用，作者对于上述检查需重点关注的情况进行了详细阐述。

11. 影像　主要包括胸部影像、鼻窦影像学和血管造影，建议对于任何怀疑血管炎的患者，都应筛查胸部X光片，并视情况进行计算机断层扫描（CT）检查。

12. 其他诊断试验　主要包括神经传导检查与肌电图和听力测试。

13. 血管炎总结　本章在这一部分将血管炎疾病分病种进行了疾病特点和临床表现的详细介绍，包括显微镜下多脉管炎、肉芽肿性多血管炎、嗜酸性肉芽肿型多脉管炎、冷球蛋白血症性血管炎、IgA血管炎、自身免疫性疾病相关的血管炎、恶性疾病相关的血管炎、皮肤白细胞碎裂性血管炎、药物诱发血管炎、白塞病、结节性多动脉炎、川崎病、中枢神经系统的原发性血管炎、巨细胞性多动脉炎和大动脉炎。

14. 临床过程和预后　作者对于不同血管炎疾病的预后、复发及并发症情况进行了介绍。

15. 治疗　系统性血管炎的治疗概况、具体流程如图139-14所示，对于预期病程较长和/或病情严重的血管炎，治疗通常是分两个阶段进行：诱导缓解和维持缓解。诱导缓解通常需使用大剂量糖皮质激素逐步减量并结合短疗程（3~6个月）的快速强效免疫抑制药，如环磷酰胺、利妥昔单抗和甲氨蝶呤。维持缓解通常涉及长期使用非环磷酰胺的治疗方案，以使糖皮质激素完全停药或维持低剂量（例如每天≤10mg泼尼松）。对于其他非重症血管炎则单独使用糖皮质激素就足以控制病情。此外对于血管炎治疗的时机及治疗过程中的注意事项也进行了强调，并指出对这类患者进行随访的重要性。本章分别介绍了糖皮质激素、免疫抑制药、生物制剂及其他治疗药物在系统性血管炎中的应用及进展。系统性血管炎的诊治误区主要指出三大问题：误诊；系统性血管炎患者免疫抑制治疗不足或不及时；中高剂量糖皮质激素的适应症把握不当。系统性血管炎通常会损害器官或威胁生命或迅速进展为医疗紧急情况。表139-2概述了几种最常见的需要紧急处理的情况。

〔黄莹雪〕

AT-A-GLANCE

- Cutaneous vasculitis can be a presenting feature of a systemic disease affecting other organ systems. Thus, all patients with cutaneous vasculitis need to be evaluated for possible systemic vasculitis including all forms of small- and medium-vessel vasculitis.
- Additional testing for vasculitis is guided by findings from medical history and physical examination, but should usually include routine laboratory testing of renal function, evaluating for hepatitis B and C viral infections, serologic testing for ANA and ANCA, selected radiographic imaging, and other tests as indicated by presentation.
- Skin biopsy is nearly always essential to establish a diagnosis of vasculitis and biopsies can help determine the type of vasculitis.
- Mimics of idiopathic vasculitis need to be considered, especially including infection, malignancy, thrombosis, or embolic disease.
- Drug-induced vasculitis frequently presents with skin lesions. However, all patients with suspected drug-induced disease should still be evaluated for other possible causes or types of vasculitis.
- Treatment of vasculitis that involves the skin is guided by the disease and the organ systems involved. For the systemic necrotizing vasculitides, glucocorticoids are always used, initially at high doses for severe disease. Additional immunosuppressive medications depend on the type of vasculitis, extent of disease, and comorbidities of the patient.
- Treatment of suspected drug-induced vasculitis may include discontinuing the suspected etiologic agent and careful observation but could also involve treatment with glucocorticoids or other drugs.
- Use of immunosuppressive medications should be overseen by physicians experienced with the use of this class of drugs.
- Comprehensive clinical followup of all patients with vasculitis is an essential aspect of management.

INTRODUCTION

The term *vasculitis* can be defined broadly to mean inflammation of blood vessels. Although vasculitis sometimes affects a single organ, particularly the skin, to most clinicians *vasculitis* connotes a group of diseases in which inflammation of the blood vessels is the major, but not the only, pathologic process. The systemic vasculitides are a wide-ranging set of diseases that are mostly idiopathic, rare, and multisystemic. These diseases involve such variety of clinical presentations and pathologies that all clinicians in every medical and surgical specialty will encounter such patients.

Vasculitis of the skin is fairly common, and skin disease is a frequent manifestation in many forms of vasculitis, especially small- and medium-vessel arteritis where skin lesions may be the presenting symptom of a systemic illness.

This chapter focuses on skin disease in the systemic vasculitides. Isolated forms of skin vasculitis and some of the systemic vasculitides are covered in Chap. 138. In addition to outlining the skin manifestations of vasculitis in general and for specific types of vasculitis, this chapter will provide an approach to patients with skin disease in which vasculitis is a diagnostic consideration.

Multiple systems for classifying vasculitis exist, a situation that reflects a lack of clear understanding of the underlying pathophysiology and the overlap of clinical features among many types of vasculitis.[1-6] The most commonly accepted approach is to sort them by the size(s) of the predominant vessel involved (small, medium, or large) and then subdivide or group diseases, as appropriate (Fig. 139-1).

Classification criteria and definitions have been developed for many, but not all, specific types of vasculitis. These systems were designed for use in clinical research to create fairly homogenous study cohorts and were not meant to be used as "diagnostic" criteria.[2] Nonetheless, clinicians will find these criteria helpful in their approach to the field. The most widely used criteria for vasculitis are from the classification criteria of the American College of Rheumatology[4,5] and the disease definitions of the Chapel Hill Consensus Conference.[6] Furthermore, some classes are no longer advised for use (eg, *hypersensitivity vasculitis* is a term that has lost specific meaning). It should be emphasized that the term *leukocytoclastic vasculitis* does not refer to a specific disease but is a pathologic description that often, but not always, applies to vasculitis in the skin or other organs. There are also some separate sets of criteria for pediatric patients.[7]

An important extension of the Chapel Hill Consensus Conference process is the recently completed Addendum that provides a comprehensive set of definitions for vasculitis of the skin.[8]

A new international initiative is under way to reconsider the classification of the vasculitides and take into consideration data regarding the clinical and pathophysiologic aspects of vasculitis not available when the prior systems were created; such new elements include testing for antineutrophil cytoplasmic autoantibodies (ANCA) and greater availability of advanced imaging techniques for large arterial disease.[2]

EPIDEMIOLOGY

With the probable exception of drug/toxin-induced vasculitis, all forms of idiopathic vasculitis are considered rare, "orphan" diseases in the United States (prevalences of less than 200,000 people); similar designations exist in Europe and elsewhere.

Vasculitis occurs in people of both sexes, all ages,

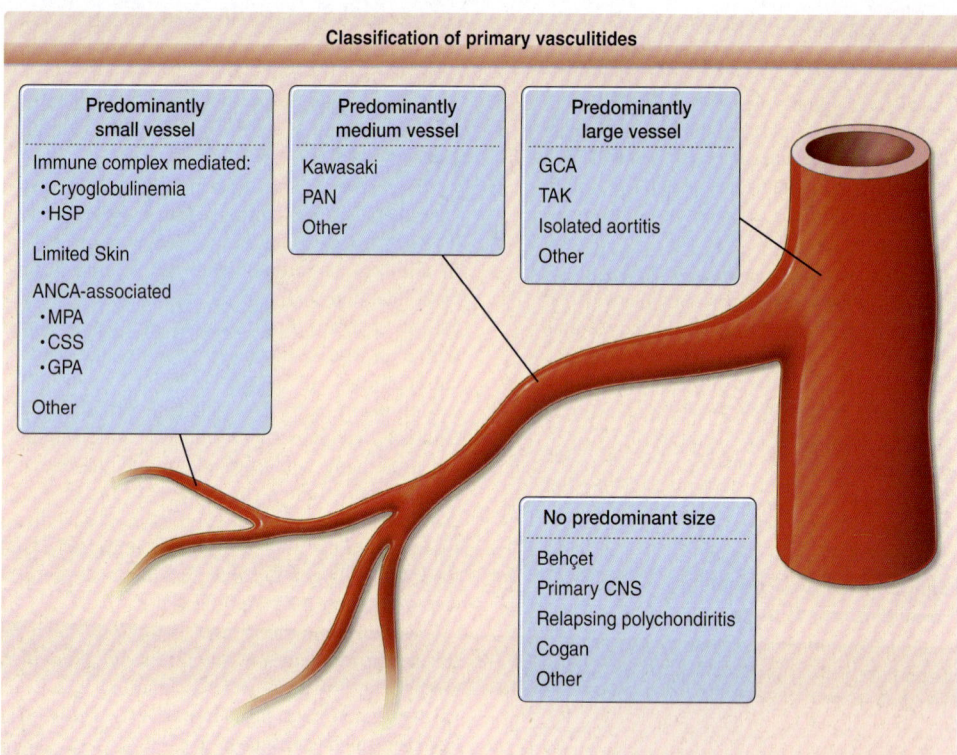

Figure 139-1 Classification of the primary vasculitides. ANCA, antineutrophil cytoplasmic antibodies; CSS, Churg–Strauss syndrome; GCA, giant cell arteritis; GPA, granulomatosis with polyangiitis (Wegener); HSP, Henoch–Schönlein purpura; MPA, microscopic polyangiitis; PAN, polyarteritis nodosa; TAK, Takayasu arteritis. (Redrawn from Watts RA et al: Systemic vasculitis—Is it time to reclassify? Rheumatology (Oxford). 2011;50(4):643-645.)

and all major racial/ethnic groups. However, some forms are more common in certain groups. For example, Takayasu arteritis is substantially more common in women than men, Kawasaki disease is almost exclusively a disease of young children, and giant cell arteritis is limited to older adults. Granulomatosis with polyangiitis (Wegener) mostly occurs in whites and Behçet disease is markedly more common in countries in the Eastern Mediterranean as well as Japan and Korea. The demographic differences among the vasculitides are of scientific interest as clues to etiology and can be helpful in developing a differential diagnosis.[9] Not surprisingly, vasculitides in which there is strong regional variation have genetic risk factors in the HLA region.[10-13] However, the epidemiologic tendencies, including genetics, are not so strong as to fully exclude the diagnosis of a specific form of vasculitis in any one person, and exceptions to the typical epidemiology occur regularly.

CLINICAL FEATURES

CUTANEOUS FINDINGS

The appearance of cutaneous vasculitis reflects the size and depth of the involved vessels, the severity of inflammation and red blood cell extravasation, and the density of damaged vessels and resulting tissue destruction. For example, vasculitis caused by immune complexes in the dermal microvasculature often first appears as a tiny, bright red circle due to red blood cell extravasation, which becomes palpable once it reaches about 2 mm in diameter. A high density of such lesions, however, may produce areas of confluent purpura and/or central necrosis or ulceration. Vasculitis of small arteries (also referred to confusingly as "medium-vessel"), which lie deeper in the skin and subcutaneous tissues, produces nodules that are often erythematous but not as bright red as purpura, or livedo racemosa if the involved vessels are predominantly parallel to the surface. Ulceration and digit ischemia are more readily produced in medium-vessel than in small-vessel vasculitis.

The classic presentation of small-vessel vasculitis in the skin is palpable purpura, but other presentations are common. These include nonpalpable purpura that can be either round or have angular borders (retiform purpura), papules, urticarial lesions, nodules of different sizes and at different depths, bullous lesions, and ulcers (Figs. 139-3, 139-4, 139-6 to 139-12). Edema in and near visibly affected areas is common.

Symptoms attributable to cutaneous vasculitis vary widely. Purpura or livedo may be asymptomatic or produce pain that is often described as stinging or burning but sometimes as itching. Nodules and ulcers are usually painful. Severe pain in a region not affected by nodules, ulcers, or confluent purpura should raise suspicion for neuropathy or inflammatory arthritis.

NONCUTANEOUS FINDINGS

It is the presence or absence of particular features in the history and physical examination that give the first clue whether a patient has a disease involving multiple organ systems. A list of important signs and symptoms in different forms of vasculitis is shown in Table 139-1.

ETIOLOGY AND PATHOGENESIS

With the exception of infection-related vasculitis (eg, hepatitis B virus in many cases of polyarteritis nodosa and hepatitis C virus in most cases of cryoglobulinemic vasculitis) and drug-induced vasculitis, the etiology of most types of vasculitis is unknown. Similarly, the pathogenesis of the vasculitides remains an area of active investigation. This section summarizes the current thinking on causes and mechanisms of vasculitis with the caveat that although much of the evidence outlined in this section is strong, the pathogenesis of these diseases is almost certainly even more complex.

Broadly speaking, the small-vessel vasculitides follow one of 2 pathways: (1) immune complex deposition or (2) non–immune complex mediated pathology that likely involves ANCA. Immune complexes consist of immunoglobulins, the antigens they are bound to, and complement components, and can form in a wide range of immune responses to microbes, autoantigens, or drugs. In a small percentage of antibody responses, the concentrations and properties of antibody and antigen favor deposition in the microvasculature, which may lead to activation of neutrophils and necrotizing vasculitis with destruction of endothelial cells. ANCA are directed against the neutrophil proteins myeloperoxidase (MPO) or proteinase-3 (PR3), which are primarily contained in intracellular granules but are also translocated to the cell surface or released via degranulation or excretion of neutrophil extracellular traps (NETs), allowing access to ANCA, activation of neutrophils, involvement of complement components, and necrotizing vasculitis. Genetics appear to contribute modestly to ANCA-associated vasculitis, with the genes identified so far being associated with the specificity of the antibody to PR3 or MPO.[10,11] Although the humoral immune system plays key roles in the pathogenesis of small-vessel vasculitis, there is evidence for the additional importance of cellular immune responses in these diseases.

Large-vessel vasculitides, in contrast, are thought to be mediated by T cells activating macrophages in the walls of large arteries. In giant cell arteritis (GCA), both IL-17-secreting (Th17) and interferon-γ–secreting (Th1) cells are prominent. T cells enter the artery wall by the vasa vasorum, so the endothelium remains intact. Multiple studies implicating different infectious agents in GCA have not been reproducible, so it continues to be regarded as an autoimmune disease, as is Takayasu arteritis. Although these diseases have similar microscopic pathology, they have quite different epidemiology, moderately different vessel distributions, and different genetics. Genetics contributes modestly to both diseases via the HLA locus, but that is in the class II region in GCA and class I in Takayasu arteritis, with little overlap otherwise.[12,13]

The etiology and pathogenesis of polyarteritis nodosa (PAN) that is not associated with hepatitis B virus infection are unclear, including uncertainty about whether it is mediated by antibodies and whether it is a syndrome with many rare causes or has 1 or a few major causes. No genetic studies have been published; an HLA association would support the existence of a predominant target antigen but would not identify the target as an autoantigen or a microbe. Individual lesions may clearly show neutrophils with necrosis and destruction of the endothelium or may show a more mixed infiltrate with an intact endothelium, but it is uncertain whether the latter finding represents a different disease process or healing from a recent necrotizing lesion. This uncertainty is reflected in application of new nomenclature such as "macular arteritis" for the latter situation when it is limited to the skin, leading to the counterproposal that it be considered a subtype of "cutaneous PAN."

DIAGNOSIS

DIAGNOSTIC ALGORITHM

When a patient presents with skin lesions that are concerning for possible vasculitis, answers to 3 questions should be sought quickly:

1. *Is the lesion due to vasculitis?*
2. *Are other organ systems involved in the illness?*
3. *Are there additional findings on medical interview, physical examination, laboratory testing, or radiographic imaging that can help establish a specific diagnosis?*

If a diagnosis of vasculitis is obtained, then it is imperative to ask 2 more questions:

4. *Is it possible to make a diagnosis of a specific type of vasculitis for the patient?*
5. *Does the patient need immediate treatment and/or hospitalization?*

A suggested approach to a patients with skin lesions suspected of being due to vasculitis is shown in Fig. 139-2. The answer to the first question is often obtained by skin biopsy, a procedure indicated in many cases of palpable purpura or other lesions when a diagnosis of vasculitis is not otherwise easily established. The second question is addressed by a thorough review of systems and physical examination and routine laboratory testing that can usually be completed rapidly. The third question is addressed by more specialized laboratory tests for which results typically take several days to return. It is important to

TABLE 139-1
Major Signs, Symptoms, and Disease Processes of the Primary Vasculitides[a]

ORGAN SYSTEM	SIGNS AND SYMPTOMS	DISEASE PROCESS	TYPE OF VASCULITIS
General			
	Fever	Systemic inflammation	Many of the systemic vasculitides
	Fatigue/malaise	Systemic inflammation	Most of the systemic vasculitides
	Weight loss	Systemic inflammation	Most of the systemic vasculitides
Eye			
	Red eye	Episcleritis, scleritis, uveitis, conjunctivitis	GPA, MPA, RPC, BD, others
	Acute visual loss or amaurosis fugax	Arterial insufficiency	GCA, TAK
	Proptosis	Orbital granuloma ("pseudotumor")	GPA
	Tearing	Dacryocystitis with lacrimal duct occlusion	GPA, EGPA
Ear			
	Hearing loss	Sensorineural hearing loss	GPA, MPA, EGPA, GCA
		Conductive hearing loss	GPA, EGPA, RPC
	Ear pain and fullness	Mastoiditis and/or other inflammation of upper airway, auditory tube, middle ear	GPA, EGPA
	External ear redness, tenderness, swelling	Chondritis	RPC, GPA, EGPA
Nose and Sinuses			
	Epistaxis, nasal crusting and discharge	Nasal mucosal inflammation	GPA, EGPA
	Nasal bridge collapse (saddle nose deformity)	Nasal cartilage inflammation	GPA, RPC
	Nasal polyps	Eosinophilic nasal inflammation	EGPA
	Facial pain/tooth pain	Sinusitis	GPA, EGPA
	Anosmia	Olfactory epithelium/cells damage	GPA, EGPA
Oral Cavity			
	Painful oral ulcers	Aphthous ulcers	BD, GPA
	Gingival pain and swelling	Gingival inflammation	GPA
	Jaw claudication	Arterial insufficiency to muscles of mastication	GCA
Pulmonary			
	Hemoptysis	Alveolar hemorrhage	GPA, MPA
		Pulmonary artery rupture	BD
		Pulmonary embolus	GPA, MPA, EGPA, BD
		Pulmonary nodules	GPA, EGPA
	Dyspnea/cough	(See causes of hemoptysis above)	GPA, MPA, EGPA
		Pulmonary infiltrates	GPA, RPC
		Bronchitis/large airway collapse	GPA, EGPA
		Pleuritis	
	Stridor/dyspnea	Subglottic stenosis	GPA, RPC
	Wheezing	Asthma	EGPA
		Large airway collapse	GPA, RPC
Cardiovascular			
	Angina	Coronary arteritis	TAK
		Aortic root/valvular disease	TAK, GCA, BD, RPC
	Congestive heart failure	Myocarditis	EGPA, GPA
		Aortic valve insufficiency	TAK, GCA
	Limb claudication	Large artery stenosis	TAK, GCA
GI			
	Abdominal ischemic pain	Arterial insufficiency	PAN, IGAV, GCA, TAK
	Lower GI bleeding	Mucosal ulcers or infarction	IGAV, EGPA, GPA, MPA, PAN

(Continued)

TABLE 139-1
Major Signs, Symptoms, and Disease Processes of the Primary Vasculitides[a] (Continued)

ORGAN SYSTEM	SIGNS AND SYMPTOMS	DISEASE PROCESS	TYPE OF VASCULITIS
Renal			
	Gross hematuria	Renal infarction	PAN
		Glomerulonephritis (rare cause of gross hematuria)	GPA, MPA, EGPA, IGAV, Cryo
CNS			
	Headache, scalp tenderness	Cranial arteritis	GCA, TAK
	Lightheadedness/syncope	Arterial insufficiency to brain	GCA, TAK
	Cranial neuropathy	Inflammation of nerves; rarely mass lesion	GCA, GPA, MPA
Peripheral Nervous System			
	Sensory/motor dysfunction	Inflammation of nerves; rarely mass lesion	EGPA, GPA, MPA, PAN, Cryo
Musculoskeletal			
	Polyarthralgia	Polyarthritis	GPA, GCA, TAK, Cryo, IGAV, BD
	Shoulder and hip girdle pain	Polymyalgia rheumatica	GCA
	Muscle weakness	Myositis	EGPA
Skin			
	Purpura	Small-vessel vasculitis	GPA, MPA, EGPA, PAN, IGAV, Cryo
	Painful nodules, deep ulcers	Medium-vessel vasculitis	PAN, GPA, MPA, Cryo
	Digital ischemia/gangrene	Medium-large artery stenosis	GCA, TAK, PAN, GPA, MPA, Cryo
	Superficial nodules	Granulomas	GPA, EGPA
	Papules, acnelike lesions	Papulopustular lesions	BD
	Painful, red nodules	Erythema nodosum	BD, TAK
	Peripheral edema	Deep vein thrombosis	GPA, MPA, EGPA, BD

[a]This list is not inclusive of all manifestations for all diseases.

BD, Behçet disease; Cryo, cryoglobulinemic vasculitis; EGPA, eosinophilic granulomatosis with polyangiitis; GCA, giant cell arteritis; GPA, granulomatosis with polyangiitis; IgAV, IgA vasculitis (Henoch–Schönlein); MPA, microscopic polyangiitis; PAN, polyarteritis nodosa; RPC, relapsing polychondritis; TAK, Takayasu arteritis. RPC, an autoimmune disease defined by destruction of cartilage, is included in this table because several of its features overlap with those of GPA. As with BD, about 30% of patients with RPC also have vasculitis, with a wide range of vessel sizes involved.

quickly identify organ system involvement and how "sick" the patient is (or might soon be), because some causes of cutaneous vasculitis require no treatment but others require immediate hospitalization for initiation of immune-suppressive and supportive therapy.

Given the broad range of entities that fall under the category "vasculitis," and the even larger number of diseases that are also reasonably considered when evaluating a patient suspected of having vasculitis, a vast number and range of diagnostic tests are often considered in such cases. However, obtaining a thorough medical history and conducting a detailed physical examination should enable the clinician to limit the types of vasculitis under consideration and prioritize the ordering of diagnostic tests. Not all tests need to be ordered for all patients suspected of having vasculitis. This approach must of course be balanced by a desire to be open-minded to atypical presentations of vasculitis as well as a range of infections, malignancies, and other diseases in the differential diagnosis of such patients. Evaluation for possible vasculitis usually occurs in parallel to evaluation for other processes.

REVIEW OF SYSTEMS

A full review of systems with assessment of the overall severity of illness is the single most important component of the early evaluation of a patient suspected of having vasculitis. Together, the diseases that cause cutaneous vasculitis can affect all organ systems, and in most cases that involvement will cause symptoms, renal disease being a prominent exception. Although some symptoms are clearly more concerning than others (hemoptysis vs dry cough, painful red eye vs mild arthralgias), even relatively mild symptoms can be a clue that disease is not limited to the skin. A list of important signs and symptoms in different forms of vasculitis is shown in Table 139-1.

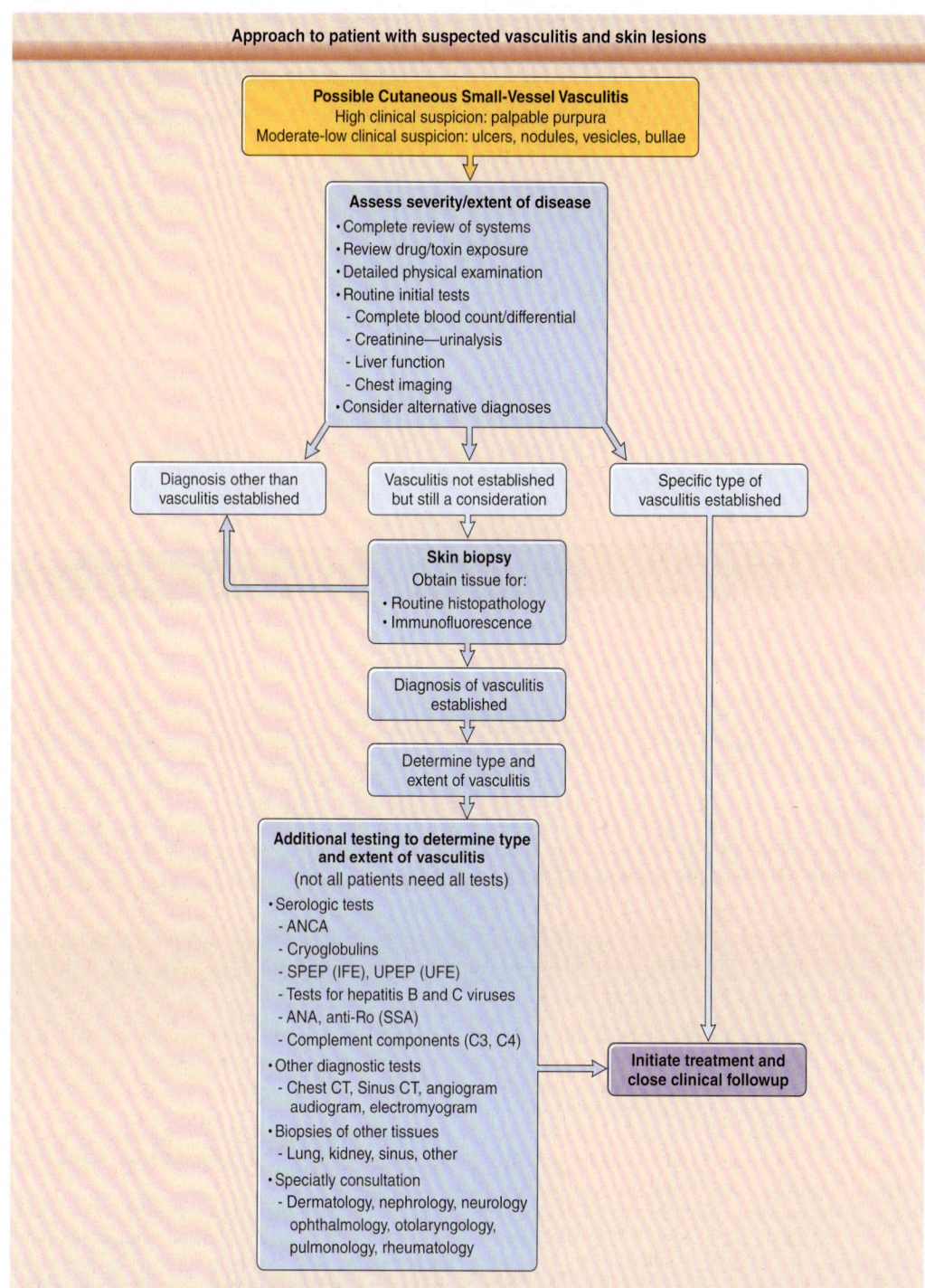

Figure 139-2 Approach to the patient with suspected vasculitis and skin lesions. ANCA, antineutrophil cytoplasmic antibodies; ANA, antinuclear antibodies; CT, computed tomography; IFE, immunofixation electrophoresis; SPEP, serum protein electrophoresis; UPEP, urine protein electrophoresis.

MEDICAL HISTORY, MEDICATION USE, AND EXPOSURES TO TOXINS OR INFECTIOUS DISEASES

It is critical to know the full medical history of any patient suspected of having vasculitis. Other diseases may either have vasculitis as a component of the illness (eg, lupus) or may cause skin lesions that mimic vasculitis. Drug-induced vasculitis is common, and skin lesions, usually but not always purpura, are the most common manifestation of drug-induced vasculitis.[14] The list of drugs reported to cause vasculitis is enormous, with almost every class of medication implicated in possible cases of drug-induced vasculitis. It is useful to ask about prescription, nonprescription, and "alternative" or herbal mediation use in the prior 6 to 12 months since the effect of some mediations may persist after usage ends. Patients should also be asked about use of illegal or recreational drugs because several such agents, including methamphetamines, cocaine, and others have been implicated in cases of vasculitis. Occupational or other exposure to nondrug toxins should be asked about.

The patient should be asked about not only usual signs and symptoms of infection but also recent travel, sick contacts, and risks for sexually transmitted diseases.

PHYSICAL EXAMINATION

Beyond a careful and full assessment of the skin, a multisystem examination is useful to determine whether symptoms are associated with objective abnormalities, or whether there are findings that a patient has not noticed. Vital signs are essential, but a patient with normal blood pressure can still have severe glomerulonephritis. The eyes should be inspected for redness and proptosis. The anterior nasal cavity can be easily visualized with an otoscope. Evidence of lymphadenopathy should be sought. Cardiac, lung, and abdominal examinations can give clues to underlying disease, but normal examinations do not rule out pathology. Similarly, absent pulses, asymmetric blood pressure readings, and bruits are helpful but imperfect measures to screen for large-vessel vasculitis. A complete joint examination is important and any findings suggestive of synovitis (joint swelling, warmth, redness) must be further investigated; however, many patients with vasculitis will have arthralgias without joint effusions. A full neurologic examination is one of the most valuable components of the evaluation and triage of a patient suspected of having vasculitis; subtle sensory and even motor abnormalities are often missed on initial evaluation.

The more detailed and expert examinations that can be performed by ophthalmologists and otolaryngologists are often extremely helpful in evaluating patients suspected of having vasculitis. Urgent referral is often indicated in patients with concerning symptoms such as new visual impairment, painful or red eyes, hoarseness or stridor, or hearing loss.

SUPPORTIVE STUDIES

SKIN BIOPSY

The method for diagnosing vasculitis depends on the type of vasculitis suspected, which is often based on size of vessel involved. Vasculitides affecting the skin usually involve small and medium-sized vessels, and these vessels are amenable to biopsy (Fig. 139-3). Given the ease and low risk of skin biopsies, they play an important role in diagnosing vasculitis, and an equally important role in establishing a diagnosis other than vasculitis. A standard punch biopsy is sufficient to diagnose small-vessel vasculitis, but a deeper and wider excision may be necessary to capture information on medium-sized vessels.[15,16] Lesions that should be approached with a deeper biopsy include subcutaneous nodules, livedo racemosa, or deep ulcers (Fig. 139-4). Many types of small-vessel vasculitis may also involve medium-sized skin vessels. It is important to realize that the difference between "small" and "medium" vessels is somewhat subjective, and skin pathologists often make such distinctions more than other pathologists who see larger biopsy specimens.

Sometimes the presence of a typical clinical syndrome makes biopsy unnecessary. For example, IgA vasculitis (Henoch-Schönlein) in children is often diagnosed on clinical grounds alone and some cases of ANCA-associated or cryoglobulinemic vasculitis can be diagnosed confidently by combining clinical features with specific serologic tests. Behçet disease and Kawasaki disease are diagnosed based on the clinical syndromes; biopsy is usually not performed on the skin lesions that are common in these diseases, and such biopsies are often nondiagnostic.

It is generally recommended to biopsy a skin lesion that has been clinically apparent for less than 48 hours, if possible, to maximize the chance of finding the typical features of acute neutrophilic vasculitis, including fibrinoid necrosis, extravasation of erythrocytes, extravasation of neutrophils with release of nuclear debris (leukocytoclasia), and the presence of immune deposits.[15,16] Processing of tissue is different for conventional histopathology or immunofluorescence testing; if immunofluorescence is desired, then either 2 biopsies need to be performed or a single biopsy needs to be divided before processing. The latter approach may damage the tissue.[15]

As discussed throughout this chapter, the histologic finding of leukocytoclastic vasculitis is helpful in confirming the diagnosis of vasculitis but does nothing to establish an etiology from among the broad number of possibilities. Microscopy sometimes reveals features that are suggestive but not diagnostic of vasculitis,

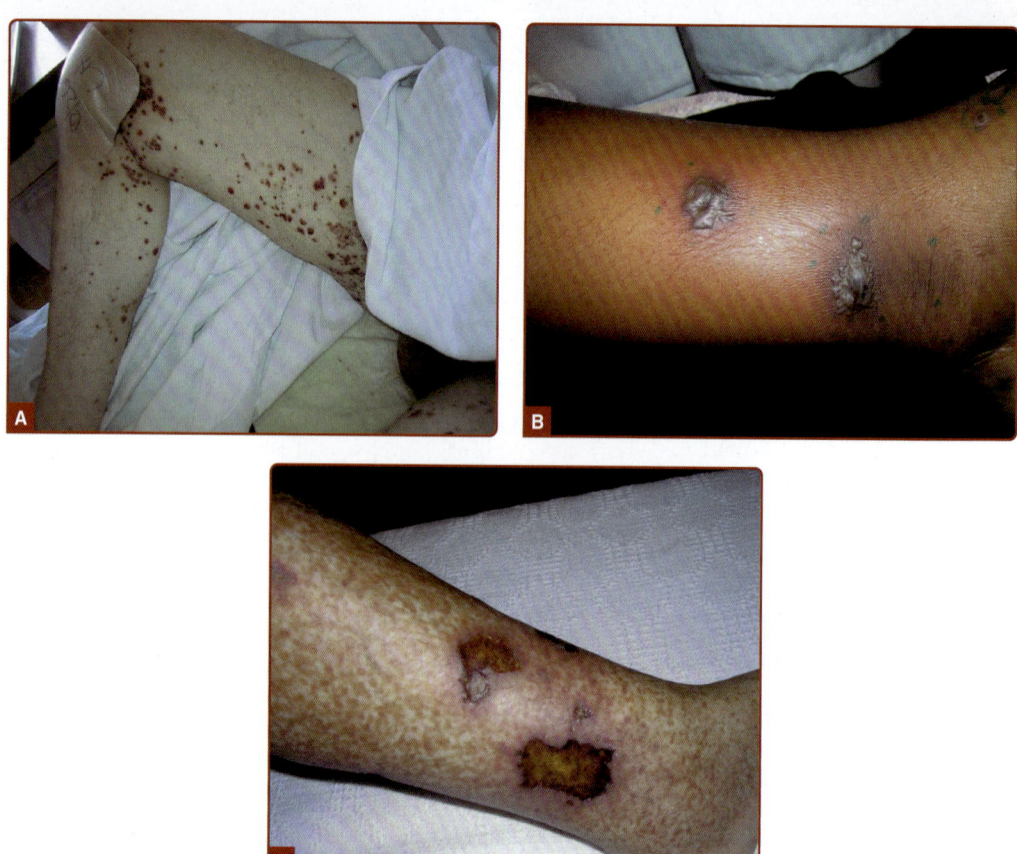

Figure 139-3 Different skin manifestations of systemic vasculitis. **A,** Purpura. **B,** Bullae. **C,** Ulcer.

such as leukocytoclasia without fibrinoid necrosis. The finding of a perivascular infiltrate, particularly if it consists predominantly of mononuclear cells but even if it is neutrophilic, is also nonspecific. Certain features, when seen in addition to leukocytoclastic vasculitis, are strongly suggestive of particular diseases, such as extravascular granulomas with geographic necrosis (granulomatosis with polyangiitis), or eosinophil-rich extravascular granulomas (eosinophilic granulomatosis with polyangiitis),[17] but these features are seen in a minority of biopsies in these diseases.

A predominance of IgA over IgG/IgM by immunofluorescence is suggestive but not diagnostic of IgA vasculitis (Henoch–Schönlein). The presence of

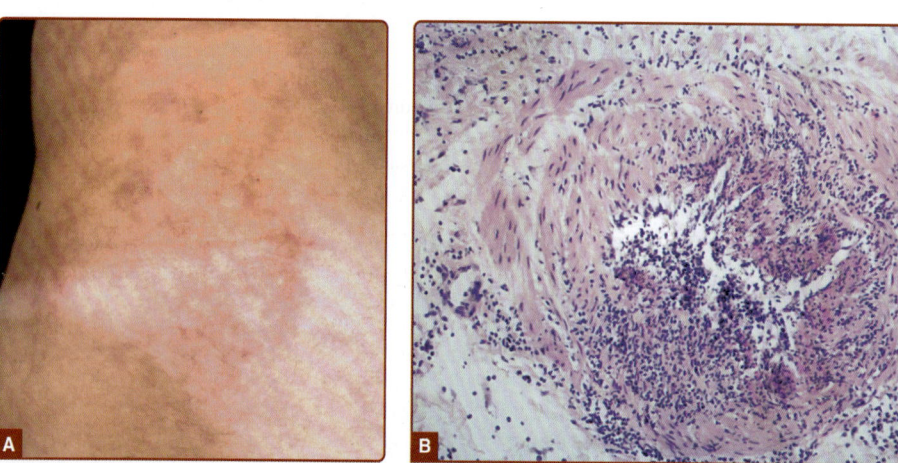

Figure 139-4 **A,** A patient with polyarteritis nodosa with "starburst" livedo made up of a cluster of nodular lesions. **B,** Histopathology of skin lesions in polyarteritis nodosa showing segmental necrotizing arteritis.

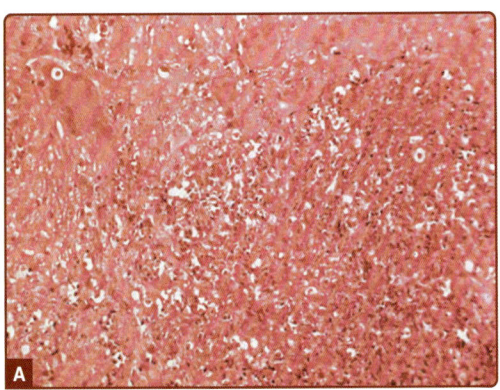 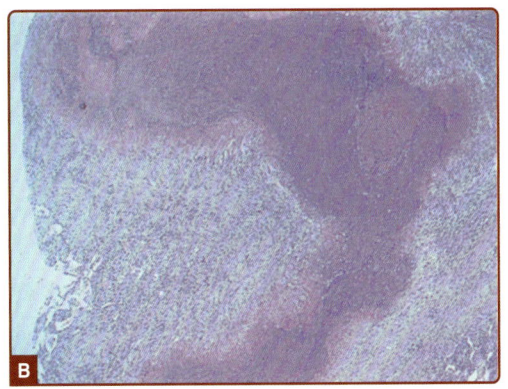

Figure 139-5 **A,** Lung histopathology from a patient with granulomatosis with polyangiitis (Wegener) demonstrating necrosis, giant cells, and mixed cellular inflammation. **B,** "Geographic necrosis" in a low-power view of an open lung biopsy specimen from a patient with granulomatosis with polyangiitis (Wegener).

deposits of IgG, IgM, and/or complement is suggestive of one of several immune complex–mediated etiologies, including drug hypersensitivity, postinfectious vasculitis, cryoglobulinemia, and vasculitis secondary to systemic lupus erythematosus, Sjögren syndrome, or rheumatoid arthritis.[17]

OTHER BIOPSIES

Vasculitis is often diagnosed by biopsy of other organs, such as kidney, lung, muscle, or peripheral nerve or even from surgical specimens (Fig. 139-5). Kidney or lung biopsies are more likely than skin biopsies to show pathology diagnostic of a particular disease. Nonetheless, a skin biopsy establishing the diagnosis of vasculitis may preclude the need for more invasive biopsies.

LABORATORY TESTING

Although individual laboratory tests on their own are almost never diagnostic for vasculitis, such tests are essential in the evaluation of a patient in whom cutaneous vasculitis is being considered. Laboratory testing may identify organ systems involved in the disease process, especially renal disease. Furthermore, in the proper setting, selected serologic tests may establish an etiology for vasculitis. However, serologic tests usually complement rather than substitute for biopsy, particularly in a patient with skin lesions that can be readily biopsied.

TESTS OF RENAL FUNCTION

Tests for renal disease are the most important to order in evaluating a patient suspected of having vasculitis because renal disease is common in many vasculitides and is rarely accompanied by signs or symptoms until end-stage renal failure occurs. Urinalysis, including both dipstick and microscopic examinations, should be performed on all patients in whom vasculitis is suspected and repeated in patients in whom vasculitis of small or medium-sized vessels is established in another organ system. The presence of any blood on the routine dipstick tests needs to be followed by an examination for red blood cell casts by someone specifically trained to look for casts (many nephrologists, some rheumatologists, but few laboratory technicians in North America). Measurement of serum creatinine is critical to estimate the glomerular filtration rate (GFR). Small changes in creatinine, even within the normal range, may be early evidence of decline in GFR. Although small-vessel vasculitis affecting the glomeruli is expected to produce hematuria, usually accompanied by red blood cell casts and proteinuria, vasculitis affecting only medium-sized vessels (eg, polyarteritis nodosa) typically produces either isolated hematuria or a normal urinalysis. Urinalysis and serum creatinine are equally important tests and are complementary; neither alone is sufficient to exclude renal disease in vasculitis.

TESTS OF LIVER FUNCTION

Vasculitis, particularly polyarteritis nodosa, can involve the liver, but significant hepatic dysfunction is rare. Liver function tests are thus of limited value in diagnosing vasculitis, but they do provide a baseline against which future values can be compared if, as is often the case, potentially hepatotoxic drugs are to be used for treatment. Liver function tests can also provide an early hint at infection with hepatitis B or C viruses, both of which are associated with vasculitis, but do not substitute for serologic testing for these infections. Normal liver function tests do not rule out infectious hepatitis.

COMPLETE BLOOD COUNT

A complete blood count should be ordered on all patients suspected of having vasculitis. Many patients with active vasculitis have anemia and/or thrombocytosis, but the same is true of a wide range of inflammatory diseases. Severe anemia can be a clue to serious GI involvement from various forms of vasculitis. The white blood cell count and differential also can be clues to the presence of infection or hematologic malignancy. However, leukocytosis is usually nonspecific and is also commonly caused by use of glucocorticoids. An elevated absolute eosinophil is found in most untreated patients with eosinophilic granulomatosis with polyangiitis (Churg–Strauss), and a count greater than 1000 cells/µL helps differentiate this disease from asthma and atopy.

ACUTE PHASE REACTANTS

The erythrocyte sedimentation rate (ESR) and levels of C reactive protein (CRP) are elevated in many patients with vasculitis, but the diagnostic sensitivity and specificity of these tests are not particularly high. Thus, these tests are not particularly helpful in either establishing or excluding a diagnosis of vasculitis. Furthermore, the levels of ESR and CRP do not correlate well with stage or severity of disease. ESR and CRP are often elevated in conditions that mimic vasculitis in the skin, as well as in many serious systemic diseases, including infections and malignancies. Patients with active vasculitis can have normal ESR and CRP values, and patients may remain in clinical remission despite persistent elevation of these markers after treatment.

AUTOIMMUNE SEROLOGIES

Testing for autoantibodies is often a critical component of establishing the type of vasculitis present, but it is important to recognize that serologic testing on its own is never diagnostic and should never substitute for clinical judgment.

Testing for ANCA and anti–glomerular basement membrane (GBM) antibodies, as well as antinuclear antibodies (ANA) to address the alternative possibility of systemic lupus erythematosus, is advised for any patient presenting with pulmonary hemorrhage and/or acute renal insufficiency with an active urinary sediment. ANCA-associated vasculitis (AAV) and lupus can present with vasculitis of the skin, but anti-GBM disease does not, so the latter topic will not be discussed further.

ANTINEUTROPHIL CYTOPLASMIC ANTIBODIES (ANCA)

Approximately 90% of patients with microscopic polyangiitis, 75% of patients with granulomatosis with polyangiitis, and 40% of patients with eosinophilic granulomatosis with polyangiitis will test positive for ANCA.[18-21] Modern ANCA testing includes both immunofluorescence staining of neutrophils for the cytoplasmic (c-ANCA) or perinuclear (p-ANCA) patterns and enzyme-linked immunosorbent assays (ELISAs) for specific autoantigens (PR3 and MPO).[21-23] Specificity of positive testing for anti-PR3 and anti-MPO antibodies for AAV is quite high,[22-24] but specificity of p-ANCA staining in the absence of anti-MPO antibodies is low. Thus, positive tests for ANCA by ELISA are essential to consider ANCA testing positive for purposes of diagnosing vasculitis.

The predictive value of positive ANCA testing depends on the setting. In cases of biopsy-proven vasculitis or clinical "surrogates" of a biopsy of vasculitis, such as diffuse alveolar hemorrhage or acute renal failure with an "active" urinary sediment, positive testing for anti-PR3/MPO ANCA is highly specific. In the setting of nonspecific constitutional and musculoskeletal symptoms, the positive predictive value of ANCA testing is lower.

ANTINUCLEAR ANTIBODIES (ANA)

Testing for ANA and related autoantibodies is useful when there is suspicion of systemic lupus or Sjögren syndrome. ANA testing is extremely sensitive (>95%) but not specific for the diagnosis of lupus. With the exception of anti-Ro (SSA) antibodies, additional tests for specific nuclear antigens, including double-stranded DNA, Smith, RNP, and La (SSB), should only be ordered if the ANA is positive and lupus is still under consideration. Only 80% of patients with Sjögren syndrome test positive for either rheumatoid factor, anti-Ro (SSA), or anti-La (SSB) antibodies, so negative tests do not rule out this diagnosis.

RHEUMATOID FACTOR (RF)

Testing for rheumatoid factor is rarely useful in establishing either the diagnosis or specific type of vasculitis. The sensitivity and specificity of rheumatoid factor for Sjögren syndrome or cryoglobulinemic vasculitis are low. Although at least 70% of patients with rheumatoid arthritis test positive for rheumatoid factor, the test is positive in more than 95% of patients with rheumatoid vasculitis.[25] However, because rheumatoid vasculitis typically occurs in patients with longstanding, severe rheumatoid arthritis, such testing has little additive value.

PARAPROTEINS (ABNORMAL IMMUNOGLOBULINS, INCLUDING CRYOGLOBULINS)

Cryoglobulins are immune complexes (immunoglobulins and their target antigens) that precipitate in the cold and are associated with clinical syndromes in which vasculitis is a prominent component (see Chap. 144). Cryoglobulinemia most commonly results from chronic infection with hepatitis C virus, but rheumatoid arthritis, systemic lupus erythematosus, Sjögren syndrome, and hematologic malignancies are also all associated with cryoglobulinemia. Testing for cryoglobulins requires careful attention to specimen handling and processing since incorrect practice at any one of several steps results in a high false-negative rate. Similarly, standard serum protein electrophoresis testing may not pick up some immunoglobulin clones, and immunofixation electrophoresis is a more comprehensive screen for clonal immunoglobulins.

Vasculitis also has been associated with monoclonal gammopathies (myeloma, plasmacytoma, or lymphoma) in the absence of cryoglobulinemia.[26]

COMPLEMENT

Total hemolytic complement is measured using the CH50, but since this assay is cumbersome and suffers from variability between laboratories, measurement in serum of the complement proteins C3 and C4 is usually sufficient, and is useful for assessing patients with cutaneous vasculitis in several settings. In patients with cryoglobulinemic vasculitis, C4 levels are usually severely depleted whereas C3 levels are less depleted or even normal.[27,28] One or both of these components are low in 70% of patients with rheumatoid vasculitis,[25] which is useful because rheumatoid arthritis is generally not associated with low circulating complement. In contrast, because systemic lupus erythematosus is commonly associated with low complement in a variety of settings, low complement helps to raise the suspicion for lupus but is not specific for vasculitis in SLE. A subset of patients whose cutaneous vasculitis presents as urticaria (hence the term *urticarial vasculitis*), but who cannot be diagnosed with lupus or another underlying disease, have depletion of complement (Chap. 138).

SELECTED TESTING FOR INFECTIOUS DISEASES

Many infections can cause skin lesions that either include vasculitis or mimic vasculitis. Chronic infection with hepatitis C virus is strongly associated with cryoglobulinemic vasculitis, and it also can be associated with polyarteritis nodosa in the absence of cryoglobulins.[29] Chronic hepatitis B virus infection was the cause of many cases of polyarteritis nodosa before the widespread adoption of vaccination programs.[30] Thus, patients with known or suspected vasculitis affecting small or medium-sized arteries should be screened for hepatitis B and C infections.

Endocarditis can cause both true vasculitis, presumably through deposition of immune complexes, and lesions that mimic vasculitis, through septic emboli. Blood cultures are appropriate for some patients suspected of small-vessel vasculitis. Interestingly, bacteremia can be a cause of a positive test for ANCA that is not associated with vasculitis.[31]

Numerous and diverse infections have been implicated in causing secondary vasculitis, usually of small vessels and limited to the skin. Testing for specific organisms should therefore be based on a history of exposure or a suspicious clinical syndrome (eg, sore throat or acute diarrhea).

Several uncommon infections directly infect and damage vascular endothelial cells and thus produce lesions that can either be regarded as vasculitis or as mimics of vasculitis; numerous organisms have been implicated, mostly in the form of case reports.

SCREENING FOR DRUGS OF ABUSE

Toxicology screens for commonly used drugs of abuse may be appropriate for some clinical situations where vasculitis is suspected. In particular, both cocaine and methamphetamines have been associated with cutaneous vasculitis and/or arterial vasospasm, and nasal inhalation of cocaine can produce destructive nasal disease as severe as that seen in ANCA-associated vasculitis, although certain clinical features may help distinguish the 2 causes.[32,33] There is a now well-recognized form of destructive vasculopathy/vasculitis associated with exposure to levamisole, an antihelminthic and immunomodulatory agent that is an adulterant of illegal cocaine, especially in North America. Levamisole can lead to characteristic gangrenous lesions as well as positive tests for both anti-MPO and anti-PR3 ANCA.[34] Levamisole use can be confirmed by testing in urine.

IMAGING

CHEST IMAGING

A chest radiograph is an appropriate screening test for any patient suspected of having vasculitis. For a patient with pulmonary symptoms, computed tomography (CT) is usually indicated, because plain radiographs will frequently not detect small nodules or subtle but significant infiltrates. In patients diagnosed with granulomatosis with polyangiitis, microscopic polyangiitis, or eosinophilic granulomatosis with polyangiitis (Churg–Strauss), a screening CT is indicated for staging purposes and to establish a baseline, even in asymptomatic patients.

If subglottic stenosis is suspected, CT of the neck/trachea can be a helpful adjunct to direct laryngoscopy.

SINUS IMAGING

Sinus involvement is extremely common in granulomatosis with polyangiitis and eosinophilic granulomatosis with polyangiitis, and the ability to evaluate the sinuses on physical examination is limited even for an otolaryngologist. CT of the sinuses can help assess the possibility of granulomatosis with polyangiitis or eosinophilic granulomatosis with polyangiitis and is useful in staging and restaging disease once one of those diagnoses is made and treatment is initiated. However, the CT appearance of sinus inflammation in these diseases does not allow discrimination from other causes of sinusitis, and patients with prior damage from vasculitis often have persistent abnormalities. Nasal inflammation is better assessed by physical examination than by CT.

ANGIOGRAPHY

Angiography has a central role in the diagnosis and management of large- and medium-vessel vasculitis. Conventional catheter-based dye angiography has the highest resolution but is an invasive procedure and still does not allow visualization of most small vessels. Angiography based on CT and magnetic resonance (MR) are increasingly replacing the use of catheter-based angiography.[35]

The role of angiography in the diagnosis of vasculitis of the skin is limited to either establishing the underlying type of vasculitis (eg, abdominal angiography demonstrating multiple aneurysms and stenoses in polyarteritis nodosa) or evaluating the arterial supply in patients with gangrene.

OTHER DIAGNOSTIC STUDIES

NERVE CONDUCTION STUDIES AND ELECTROMYOGRAPHY

Nerve conduction studies should never replace a full neurologic examination, and most patients with neurologic manifestations of vasculitis do not need such testing. Thus, nerve conduction testing is not recommended for screening asymptomatic patients, but can be useful for providing objective evidence of neuropathy and for distinguishing between compressive (ie, mechanical) and non-compressive neuropathy, with the latter type including neuropathy due to vasculitis and many other medical causes. Electromyography (EMG) can establish the presence of myopathy, but not the cause. Nerve conduction studies are painful and require expertise not always readily available.

AUDIOLOGY TESTING

An audiogram is critical in diagnosing and distinguishing between conductive and/or sensorineural hearing loss. Hearing loss is a commonly missed manifestation of small-vessel vasculitis, including among elderly patients.[36] Sensorineural hearing loss is a cranial neuropathy and may rapidly lead to irreversible hearing loss. Although an audiogram is not generally indicated for screening an asymptomatic patient, a baseline audiogram is advised for all patients with an established diagnosis of ANCA-associated vasculitis (granulomatosis with polyangiitis, microscopic polyangiitis, or eosinophilic granulomatosis with polyangiitis).

SUMMARIES OF THE VASCULITIDES

MICROSCOPIC POLYANGIITIS

Microscopic polyangiitis (MPA) is a multisystem vasculitis of small and also sometimes medium-sized vessels.[37,38] Pauci-immune glomerulonephritis develops in the majority of patients, and pulmonary hemorrhage, peripheral and cranial neuropathy, musculoskeletal, and constitutional symptoms are also common; cardiac and GI involvement are less common. Most patients with microscopic polyangiitis are positive for ANCA, usually with specificity for antibodies to myeloperoxidase (MPO).[39] Although rapidly progressive glomerulonephritis and/or diffuse alveolar hemorrhage commonly lead to diagnosis, microscopic polyangiitis often features a prolonged prodrome limited to musculoskeletal and constitutional symptoms.[40]

The skin is frequently involved in microscopic polyangiitis.[20] The most common cutaneous lesion is palpable purpura and the pathology is indistinguishable from other types of leukocytoclastic vasculitis[17,41] (Fig. 139-6). Vasculitis of medium-sized vessels, leading to digital ischemia, subcutaneous nodules, livedo reticularis, and deep ulcers, can rarely occur in microscopic polyangiitis.

GRANULOMATOSIS WITH POLYANGIITIS

Granulomatosis with polyangiitis encompasses all the features of microscopic polyangiitis but also many additional manifestations caused by necrotizing granulomatous inflammation, and the 2 syndromes are currently considered distinct entities. Chronic inflammation of the upper airway (nasal cavity, sinuses, auditory tube, and middle ear) is present in about

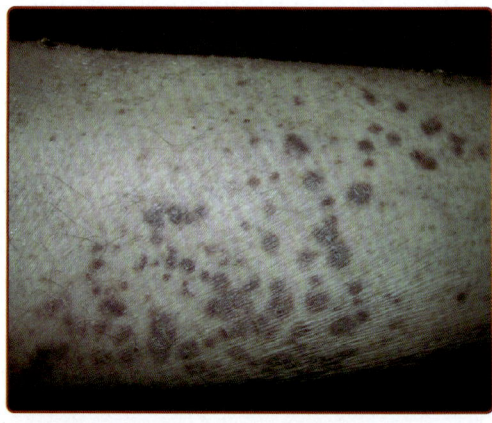

Figure 139-6 Purpura in a patient with microscopic polyangiitis.

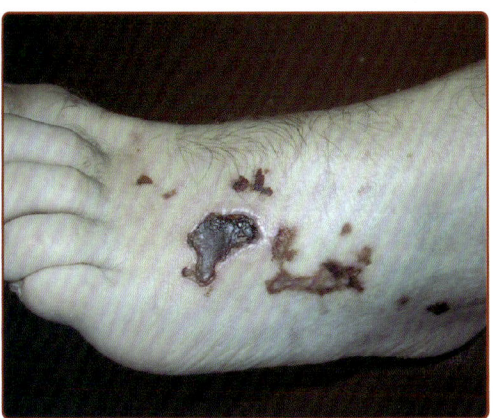

Figure 139-7 Skin ulcer in a patient with granulomatosis with polyangiitis (Wegener).

90% of patients, often but not always as the initial manifestation.[18,42,43] Cavitary pulmonary nodules, orbital pseudotumor, and subglottic stenosis are also common and important features. Vasculitis of the eye (scleritis and episcleritis) is also much more common in granulomatosis with polyangiitis than in microscopic polyangiitis.[18,37,42-44] Most patients with granulomatosis with polyangiitis who have involvement of multiple organ systems will test positive for ANCA.[44,45] The majority ANCA type in this disease is C-ANCA/anti-PR3; however, P-ANCA/anti-MPO is also not uncommon. Patients with disease seemingly restricted to the upper airway are only ANCA-positive in about 70% of cases, which can make diagnosis more challenging.[21,44]

In addition to palpable purpura and other presentations typical of small-vessel vasculitis, additional skin lesions occur in granulomatosis with polyangiitis and reflect a combination of vasculitis and necrotizing granulomatous disease, including neutrophilic and granulomatous dermatitis with papules (particularly on the extensor surfaces of the elbows), subcutaneous nodules, and ulcers[17,46-49] (Figs. 139-7 and 139-8). Vasculitis and extravascular granulomatous disease are sometimes seen in the same biopsy, facilitating diagnosis. As with MPA, manifestations attributable to involvement of medium-sized vessels also can be seen (Fig. 139-9).

EOSINOPHILIC GRANULOMATOSIS WITH POLYANGIITIS

Eosinophilic granulomatosis with polyangiitis is often included among the ANCA-associated vasculitides since approximately 40% of patients test positive for ANCA,[50] and there is considerable overlap in features of eosinophilic granulomatosis with polyangiitis with both granulomatosis with polyangiitis and microscopic polyangiitis. However, eosinophilic granulomatosis with polyangiitis has unique features, the most prominent being a history of asthma (often severe or poorly controlled), and blood eosinophilia. Nasal polyps, constitutional symptoms, and rashes, all typical of atopy, are also common. The presence of pulmonary infiltrates on chest imaging (eosinophilic pneumonia) provides an important distinction from asthma. The most common presentation of severe vasculitis in eosinophilic granulomatosis with polyangiitis is acute peripheral neuropathy with involvement of the heart, GI tract, brain, and eyes less commonly. Glomerulonephritis and pulmonary hemorrhage occur in about 10% and less than 5%, respectively, of patients with eosinophilic granulomatosis with polyangiitis.[19,51,52]

Cutaneous disease is more common in eosinophilic granulomatosis with polyangiitis than in systemic granulomatous vasculitis or microscopic polyangiitis.[19,51,52] Palpable and nonpalpable purpura, reflecting vasculitis histologically, comprise about 50% of cutaneous lesions.[17] Eosinophilic dermatitis and granulomatous dermatitis rich in both neutrophils and eosinophils are also common and produce erythematous macules, papules, and nodules. As with granulomatosis with polyangiitis, small-vessel vasculitis and extravascular eosinophilic and/or granulomatous

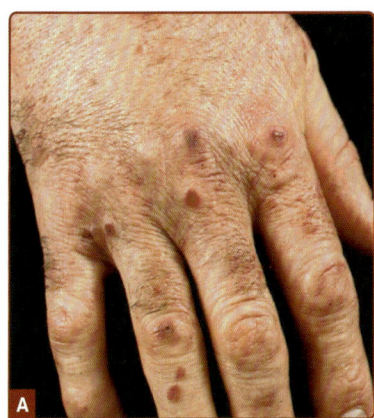
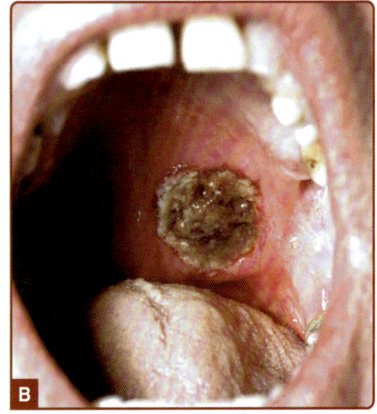

Figure 139-8 Granulomatosis with polyangiitis (Wegener). **A,** Palpable purpura **B,** Deep ulcer on the soft palate.

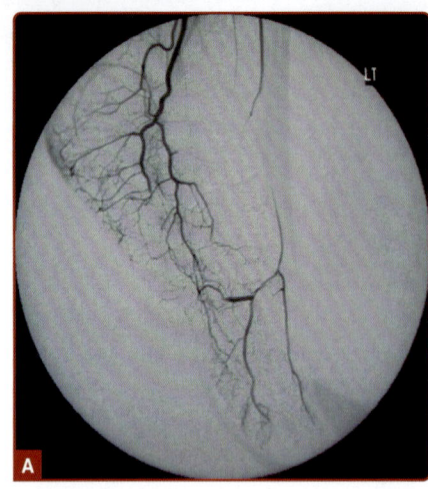 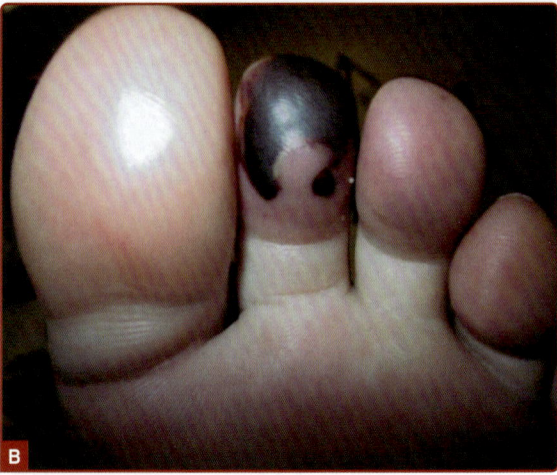

Figure 139-9 Granulomatosis with polyangiitis (Wegener). **A,** Vasculitis and occlusion of the dorsal pedal artery. **B,** Gangrenous toe secondary to the occlusion in panel A.

disease are sometimes seen in the same biopsy. While the skin lesions of eosinophilic granulomatosis with polyangiitis often contain eosinophils, with or without vasculitis, eosinophil-rich skin biopsies are not unique to this disease and can be seen in other types of vasculitis.

CRYOGLOBULINEMIC VASCULITIS

See Chap. 144 "Cryoglobulinemia and Cryofibrinogenemia."

IGA VASCULITIS (HENOCH–SCHÖNLEIN)

See Chap. 138 "Cutaneous Necrotizing Venulitis."

VASCULITIS ASSOCIATED WITH OTHER AUTOIMMUNE DISEASES

Vasculitis is seen relatively commonly in patients with systemic lupus (10% to 36%)[53,54] and Sjögren syndrome (10%)[55] but is now extremely uncommon in rheumatoid arthritis.[56,57] Vasculitis in these diseases affects mostly small vessels, with some medium-vessel disease. The vasculitis may cause peripheral neuropathy, GI ischemia, and CNS disease, with other visceral involvement being rare. Inflammatory bowel disease and relapsing polychondritis[58] also have been associated with vasculitis involving small, medium, or large vessels.

MALIGNANCY-ASSOCIATED VASCULITIS

Vasculitis temporally associated with a solid malignancy has been described in many case reports and a few larger series.[59] Diverse malignancies have been implicated. Small-vessel vasculitis of the skin appears to be most common, and reports of remission of vasculitis after surgical resection of the tumor (and no other therapy) are suggestive of a causal relationship. Hematologic malignancies with or without associated paraproteinemias can result in vasculitis.[26] On the other hand, the comprehensive medical testing and imaging associated with evaluating a patient with possible vasculitis can lead to discovery of a malignancy in a patient with vasculitis, and the 2 diagnoses may be unrelated.

CUTANEOUS LEUKOCYTOCLASTIC ANGIITIS

All of the diseases and syndromes described to this point are defined by a combination of clinical and laboratory parameters. Cutaneous leukocytoclastic angiitis, in contrast, is a histologic term defined by the absence of evidence of systemic disease. The term undoubtedly encompasses many etiologies, and appears in this list only to serve as a reminder that cutaneous vasculitis is not always a marker of systemic disease. If, and only if, a patient has biopsy-proven vasculitis, has no evidence of involvement of other organ systems by vasculitis, and has no clinical of laboratory evidence to support a specific form of vasculitis or a coexisting autoimmune inflammatory disease, should the diagnosis of cutaneous leukocytoclastic angiitis be tentatively made. This term appears in the nomenclature of the Chapel Hill Consensus Conference of 1994 to acknowledge that vasculitis limited to the skin is relatively common.[7] It has been estimated that about 20% of such cases follow a wide range of infections, and another 20% are associated with drug exposure.[17] However, it is quite problematic to label skin-only vasculitis as a separate disease entity, and all such patients should be followed carefully for the possible evolution to a more systemic form of vasculitis.

DRUG-INDUCED VASCULITIS

Reactions to drugs have been implicated in about 20% of cases of cutaneous small-vessel vasculitis,[15] but the exact frequency of drug-induced disease is hard to establish due to incomplete reporting of cases and difficulty in firmly establishing causality of any one agent. Most categories of drugs have been implicated as causing vasculitis, but the number of reports for a given drug may represent reporting bias rather than relative risk.[14,60] Cutaneous small-vessel disease is the norm, but medium-vessel vasculitis and visceral involvement have been reported. The literature is undoubtedly biased toward severe cases, but there are numerous reports of serious or fatal internal organ involvement (particularly renal, pulmonary, and hepatic). There is also a now well-accepted subset of drug-induced ANCA-associated vasculitis (antibodies usually directed against myeloperoxidase), especially involving propylthiouracil and related agents, hydralazine, but also other drugs.[61,62]

The cutaneous presentation of drug-induced vasculitis is indistinguishable from other causes of small-vessel vasculitis (ie, usually purpura but sometimes with other lesions) (Fig. 139-10).

It is essential that a comprehensive review of all prescription, nonprescription, illegal, and "alternative" drugs and supplements be undertaken for all patients suspected of having vasculitis.

Establishing a diagnosis of drug-induced vasculitis may lead to avoidance of treatment with glucocorticoids and immunosuppressive drugs in favor of clinical followup after drug discontinuation. However, 2 important caveats must be kept in mind in such cases: (1) drug discontinuation alone may not resolve the disease and severe disease may be present necessitating treatment, and (2) the diagnosis of drug-induced vasculitis may be wrong and the patient really has another form of vasculitis; thus, careful and prolonged followup of all patients is required.

BEHÇET DISEASE

See Chap. 141 "Adamantiades-Behçet Disease."

POLYARTERITIS NODOSA

Idiopathic vasculitis of medium-sized vessels (ie, small or medium-sized muscular arteries) can present in one or multiple organ systems. "Classic" polyarteritis nodosa involves multiple organ systems and presents with some combination of skin disease, myalgia, hypertension (from renal artery involvement), abdominal pain, neuropathy, and/or testicular pain. However, many patients do not present with the full set of manifestations, and disease limited to muscle and nerve, single internal organs, or to the skin are well-described variants. When the disease is limited to the skin, it is sometimes referred to as cutaneous polyarteritis nodosa; however, some of these patients will later manifest disease in other organs.

Interpreting the literature on polyarteritis nodosa is problematic since the term was formerly used to describe several forms of vasculitis now considered to be distinct diseases (particularly microscopic polyangiitis).[63,64] Historically, many cases of polyarteritis nodosa were associated with chronic infection with hepatitis B, but that association has declined markedly in countries in which vaccination against hepatitis B has become routine.[64] Whether the remaining, rare entity still known as polyarteritis nodosa represents one, a few, or many etiologies, or even whether there is a unified fundamental pathophysiology (eg, immune complex disease), is unclear.

The most common cutaneous features of polyarteritis nodosa are livedo reticularis/racemosa (a lacy pattern of cutaneous blood vessels on the legs, and not always easy to distinguish from a benign consequence of vasoconstriction of more superficial vessels) (Fig. 139-11), painful cutaneous nodules or ulcers (Fig. 139-12), and digital ischemia.[65,66] These manifestations reflect vasculitis of "medium-sized" arteries in the subcutis, which are frequently too deep to be sampled in a routine punch biopsy.[15]

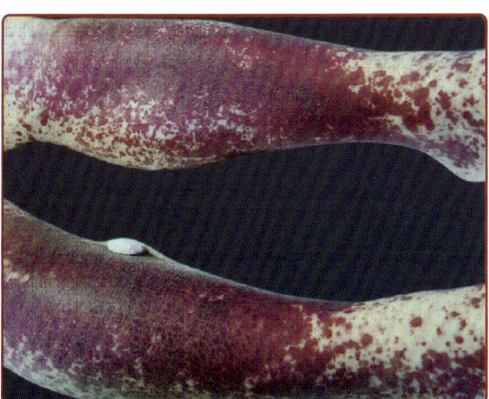

Figure 139-10 Leukocytoclastic vasculitis after administration of granulocyte macrophage colony-stimulating factor for aplastic anemia.

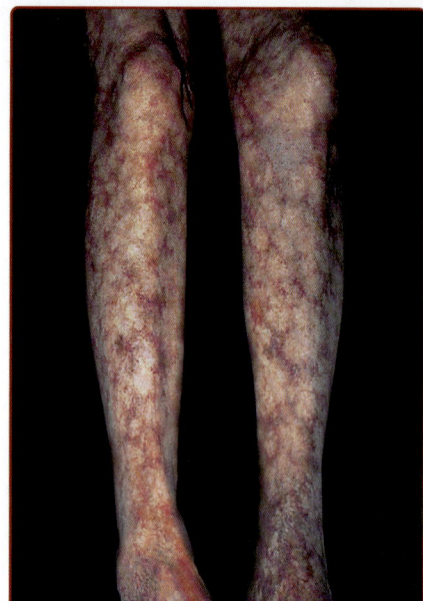

Figure 139-11 Livedo reticularis.

KAWASAKI DISEASE

See Chap. 142 "Kawasaki Disease."

PRIMARY VASCULITIS OF THE CNS

This rare disease is limited to the CNS (hence, no cutaneous findings) and presents with symptoms of encephalopathy, multiple small strokes, and often headache.[67,68]

GIANT CELL ARTERITIS

Giant cell arteritis (temporal arteritis) is currently considered strictly a disease of adults older than 50 years that is markedly more common with advancing age. It is mostly a disease of people of Northern European ancestry. Cranial arteritis is a common feature with this term indicating stenosis or occlusion of 1 or more branches of the carotid artery to produce headache (70% to 80%), jaw claudication (50%), and monocular (and rarely binocular) blindness (15%). Polymyalgia rheumatica, which includes pain and stiffness of the shoulder and hip girdles, is seen in at least 30% to 40% of patients and may occur without cranial disease. Constitutional symptoms are common, including fever, malaise, and weight loss. Involvement of the aorta and its major branches produces symptoms similar to Takayasu arteritis and is present in 15% to 20% of patients. Diagnosis of GCA is usually confirmed by temporal artery biopsy (Fig. 139-13).

Palpable nodularity of the temporal artery is present in 30% to 40% of cases and is the only cutaneous manifestation of GCA apparent on examination. Scalp necrosis and digital ischemia are rare complications.[69,70]

TAKAYASU ARTERITIS

Takayasu is a rare form of vasculitis (prevalence <1:100,000) involving the aorta and its major branches.[71-76] Many patients are diagnosed as young adults, and 90% are female. The typical presentation of Takayasu is limb claudication. Dizziness, constitutional symptoms, and severe hypertension (from renal artery stenosis) are also common. Cerebral infarction can occur. Coronary occlusions with angina or infarction and bowel ischemia are less common but life-threatening complications. Absent pulse(s), abnormal blood pressure readings, and arterial bruits are common but not universal findings. Diagnosis is made by angiography.

Lesions resembling erythema nodosum or pyoderma gangrenosum[77] have been described repeatedly in Takayasu, with pathology of nodular lesions often, but not always, showing vasculitis and thereby differing from typical erythema nodosum.[78,79] Although complete occlusion of subclavian arteries is common, digital ischemia is rare.

CLINICAL COURSE AND PROGNOSIS

The severity of vasculitis varies widely, but all of the named diseases have the potential to cause permanent damage to vital organs. All forms of vasculitis

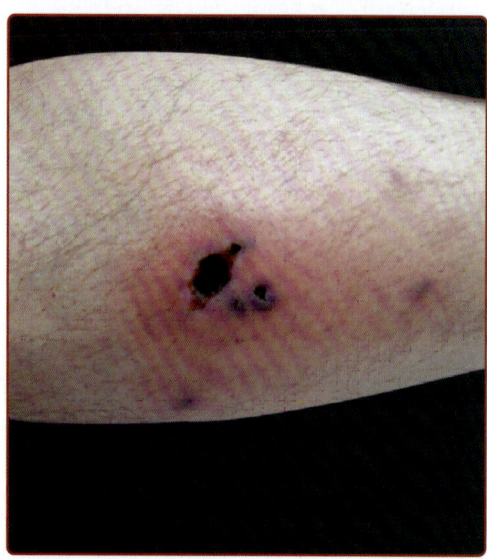

Figure 139-12 Leg ulcer in a patient with polyarteritis nodosa.

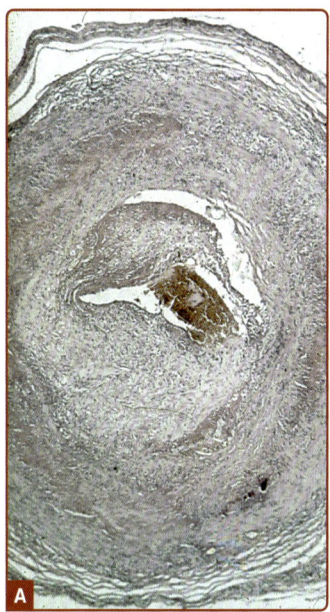
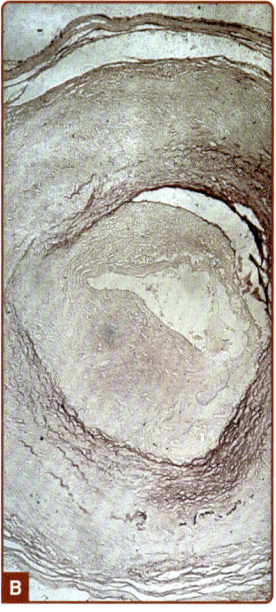

Figure 139-13 **A,** Histopathology of the temporal artery from a patient with giant cell arteritis shows necrosis of the media, inflammatory infiltrates consisting of lymphocytes, and giant cells. There is also subintimal proliferation of fibroblasts and fibrosis. **B,** Elastic tissue stain reveals destruction of the lamina interna and externa.

are treatable, and the goal is to make the diagnosis and start treatment before damage has occurred. After successful treatment with immune-suppressive drugs, some forms of vasculitis are more likely to recur than others. Granulomatosis with polyangiitis with anti-PR3 antibodies recurs in well over 50% of cases in the absence of long-term treatment, whereas microscopic polyangiitis with anti-MPO antibodies recurs in fewer than 50%. Polyarteritis nodosa and eosinophilic granulomatosis with polyangiitis also recur in fewer than 50% of patients, although in eosinophilic granulomatosis with polyangiitis, chronic asthma and/or sinonasal disease recur in most patients and require long-term treatment. IgA vasculitis is usually monophasic or resolves after a few episodes in children but is more likely to be chronic in adults. Cryoglobulinemic vasculitis secondary to hepatitis C virus is usually, but not always, cured by eradication of the virus, whereas it usually recurs in the absence of eradication. Vasculitis associated with connective tissue diseases can be monophasic, episodic, or chronic and varies widely in severity.

Treatment is also a source of morbidity. Glucocorticoids are used in almost all forms of severe vasculitis and carry numerous risks at high doses or with long-term use even at moderate or low doses. Almost all other medications used to treat vasculitis increase risk of infection but are considered preferable to glucocorticoids on those grounds and others.

Mortality in the first 3 to 6 months of severe vasculitis affecting vital organs is around 10%, because of either complications of vasculitis (eg, pulmonary hemorrhage, bowel perforation, or cardiomyopathy) or to infection. After that, as treatment is reduced and vasculitis usually remains in control, mortality is reduced dramatically but appears to remain somewhat higher than expected.[80] Other than advanced age, the predictors of higher risk of mortality reflect prior organ damage: kidney damage in the case of granulomatosis with polyangiitis and microscopic polyangiitis,[81] and cardiac damage in the case of eosinophilic granulomatosis with polyangiitis.[82]

MANAGEMENT

GENERAL APPROACH TO TREATMENT OF SYSTEMIC VASCULITIS

When establishing a treatment regimen for a patient with vasculitis, consideration must be given to both the severity of the current presentation and the likelihood of disease progression and recurrence. An overview is presented in Fig. 139-14. For an increasing number of vasculitides, treatment is guided by results of relatively large randomized controlled trials. However, for many situations, clinicians still rely upon either extrapolation from trials in other diseases or empiric treatment based on small case series or personal experience.

For vasculitides expected to have extended courses and/or to include severe manifestations, the general approach is to plan for 2 phases of treatment: remission induction and remission maintenance.[83,84] Remission induction usually involves use of high-dose glucocorticoids with steady dose taper combined with a short course (3-6 months) of a fairly rapid-acting and potent immunosuppressive agent. For example,

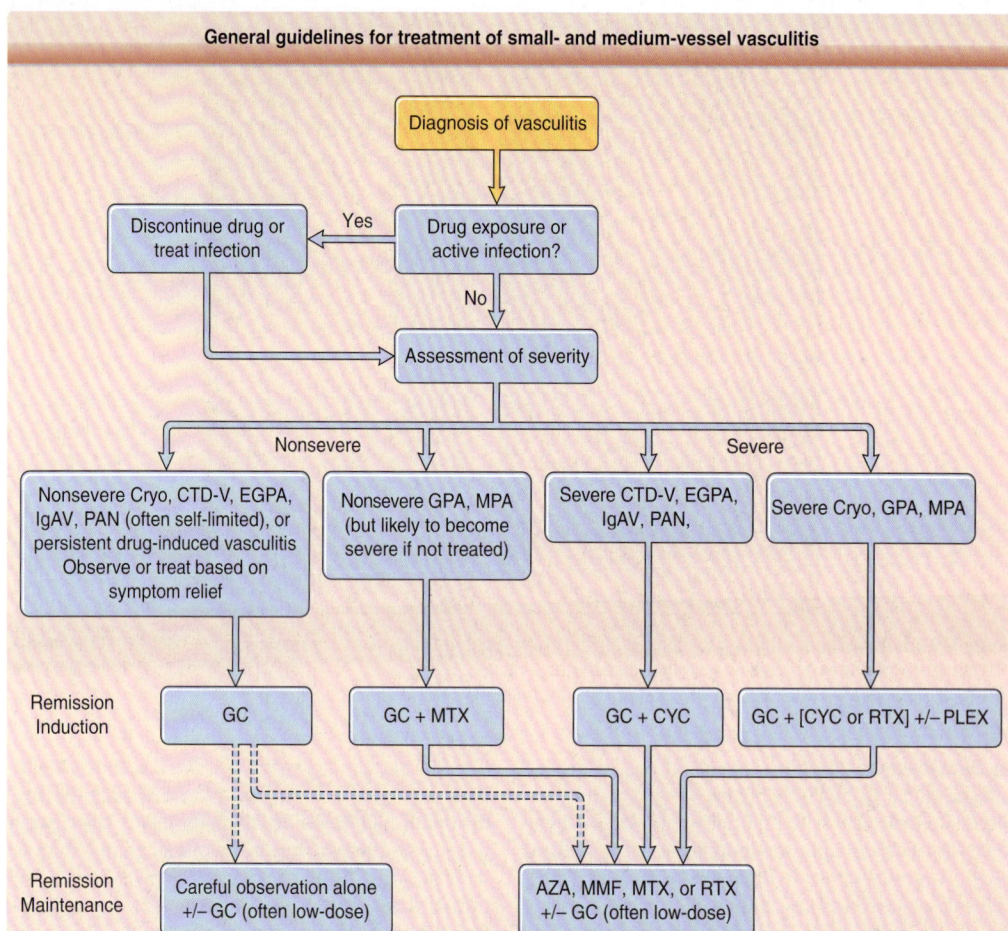

Figure 139-14 General guidelines for treatment of small- and medium-vessel vasculitis. It is important to recognize that approaches will vary substantially based on severity and comorbidity, and high-quality data are not available to guide treatment of many forms of vasculitis. Once the diagnosis is established and treatable causes are identified or excluded, severity is assessed by the organ systems involved and the severity of disease in that organ system. For example: CNS and cardiac involvement are always considered severe; GI, renal, and peripheral nerve disease usually severe; skin manifestations usually not severe; musculoskeletal not severe. Dashed lines indicate where multiple options exist. CTD-V, vasculitis associated with a systemic connective tissue disease (eg, systemic lupus erythematosus, Sjögren syndrome, rheumatoid arthritis); Cryo, cryoglobulinemic vasculitis; EGPA, eosinophilic granulomatosis with polyangiitis (Churg–Strauss); GPA, granulomatosis with polyangiitis (Wegener); IgAV, IgA vasculitis (Henoch–Schönlein); MPA, microscopic polyangiitis; PAN, polyarteritis nodosa; GC, glucocorticoids; AZA, azathioprine; CYC, cyclophosphamide; MMF, mycophenolate; MTX, methotrexate; PLEX, plasma exchange; RTX, rituximab. Treatment of giant cell arteritis and Takayasu arteritis includes GC, but the options for glucocorticoid-sparing drugs differ from the algorithm shown here. The approach to treatment for Behçet disease is complex and does not fit readily into algorithms with other vasculitides.

cyclophosphamide, rituximab, and methotrexate all have roles in remission induction for ANCA-associated vasculitis. Remission maintenance usually involves prolonged use of a non–cyclophosphamide-based regimen to allow for glucocorticoids to be either fully discontinued or maintained at a low dose (eg, ≤10 mg prednisone daily). However, although the above approach is usual for the ANCA-associated vasculitides, polyarteritis nodosa, and some other forms of severe systemic disease for which there are data from clinical trials to guide treatment, it is less commonly used for other vasculitides in which glucocorticoids alone may suffice as therapy.

Clinicians must always remain alert to the possibilities of (1) a different diagnosis (either a different form of vasculitis or an entirely different disease); (2) development of additional manifestations of vasculitis; and (3) treatment-related side effects, some of which can mimic vasculitis (infections, skin reactions, etc).

An important aspect of caring for patients with vasculitis is determining who and when *not* to treat. "Watchful waiting" may be a reasonable management approach when (1) a diagnosis is not clear and no major organ system appears threatened; (2) there is an obvious cause or etiology for the vasculitis that is either reversible (toxin/drug) or self-limited (some infections); (3) uncertainty exists as to whether the patient's symptoms are due to a flare of disease or the result of either chronic damage or another process.

A critical component to the care of patients with vasculitis is close, regular clinical followup. Vasculitis often progresses rapidly, and most forms of vasculitis have high rates of relapse. Depending on the form of vasculitis, regular office visits should be accompanied by laboratory and radiographic monitoring. Close followup should occur not only at the start of the disease process, but also for years following diagnosis.

TREATMENTS FOR SYSTEMIC VASCULITIS

A comprehensive list of drugs used in the treatment of the various systemic vasculitides and details of treatment regimens is beyond the scope of this chapter (additional information about specific agents is available in Chaps. 184, "Glucocorticoids," 190, "Cytotoxic and Antimetabolic Agents," 192, "Immunosuppressive and Immunomodulatory Drugs," and 193, "Immunobiologicals: Targeted Therapy Against Cytokines, Cytokine Receptors, and Growth Factors in Dermatology").

GLUCOCORTICOIDS

Glucocorticoids remain the mainstay of therapy for vasculitis given the rapidity of action, reliability of response, and physicians' familiarity with dosing and side effects. Glucocorticoids are usually the initial drug used to treat vasculitis and may be the only agent used for some forms of the disease. However, additional agents are often prescribed because either the dose of glucocorticoids needed to maintain disease control is unacceptably high or disease control is not attained by glucocorticoids alone. The acute and chronic toxicities are often underappreciated and the potential cumulative damage from chronic or recurrent use of glucocorticoids may be substantial.

OTHER IMMUNOSUPPRESSIVE AGENTS

A wide variety of additional immunosuppressive agents are used for treatment of the vasculitides. The proven effectiveness of the alkylating agent cyclophosphamide for the ANCA-associated vasculitides and, to a lesser extent, other forms of vasculitis, have helped establish this drug as the standard of care for initial treatment of severe forms of vasculitis.[42,85-87] Other alkylating agents are now rarely prescribed for vasculitis. Although effective in many, but certainly not all, cases, cyclophosphamide is also associated with serious toxicities, many of which are related to total cumulative dose (eg, female and male infertility, bladder cancer). Therefore, the past 3 decades have seen the emergence of "cyclophosphamide-sparing" regimens that usually have patients transition from an initial course of treatment with cyclophosphamide to a more prolonged course of a less toxic immunosuppressive agent, especially either methotrexate[88,89] or azathioprine.[86,90] Mycophenolate, cyclosporine A, and other agents also have been used for maintenance therapy.

Apremilast has now been demonstrated to have efficacy in the treatment of mucocutaneous manifestations of Behçet disease.[91,92]

BIOLOGIC AGENTS

More recently, "biologic" agents, drugs created using recombinant DNA techniques to target specific components of the immune system, have been studied for use in treating vasculitis, often with a goal of being either cyclophosphamide-sparing or glucocorticoid-sparing. The recent demonstration that rituximab, a B cell–depleting therapy, is as effective as cyclophosphamide for induction of remission in AAV is considered a major advance for the field.[93-95] Mepolizumab, a monoclonal antibody to anti-interleukin 5, has been demonstrated to have efficacy in the treatment of eosinophilic granulomatosis with polyangiitis.[96] Two trials have demonstrated the efficacy of tocilizumab, a monoclonal antibody to interleukin 6, for the treatment of giant cell arteritis.[97,98] Promising data on the use of abatacept, a CTLA-4 immunoglobin, to treat giant cell arteritis also has been published.[99] However, studies examining the efficacy of anti-TNF agents for either granulomatosis with polyangiitis or giant cell arteritis have been highly disappointing.[100,101] There are many new biologic agents under consideration for use in the treatment of vasculitis, and clinical trials are needed to properly evaluate these new treatments.

OTHER TREATMENTS

Although a variety of other drug classes, including colchicine, antibiotics (dapsone and others), and "alternative" therapies have been promoted for treatment of various forms of vasculitis, good evidence is generally lacking for the efficacy of these agents.

The role of plasma exchange in the treatment of vasculitis remains controversial. There is some evidence for efficacy of plasma exchange in patients with AAV and severe renal disease[102] and possibly forms of cryoglobulinemic vasculitis. A large international multicenter, but randomized, trial of plasma exchange for AAV is nearing completion.

COMMON ERRORS IN THE DIAGNOSIS AND TREATMENT OF SYSTEMIC VASCULITIS

Given the huge spectrum of disease manifestations in vasculitis, the potential toxicities of treatments for vasculitis, and the serious ramifications of missing alternative diagnoses, especially infections, diagnostic misclassification is a major concern. Establishing a firm diagnosis of vasculitis based on physical examination and laboratory findings alone is a common problem. This is especially true for skin disease since not all purpura is due to vasculitis and not all skin disease in vasculitis is purpuric. Clinicians are cautioned against making a diagnosis of vasculitis in the skin without a biopsy; the exception to this guideline is if the patient has a clearly established diagnosis of vasculitis based on other evidence, but even then, it may be necessary to know what is causing a skin lesion. Many types of skin lesions improve with treatment with glucocorticoids so response to empiric use of this treatment is not diagnostically useful.

Undertreatment or delayed initiation of immunosuppressive therapy is a common problem for patients with systemic vasculitis. Undertreatment may take the form of failure to recognize multiorgan system disease, delay or reluctance to initiate immunosuppressive medications other than glucocorticoids for those forms of vasculitis for which such therapy has been shown to be useful, or underdosing of immunosuppressive agents.

Another common mistake is extending the course of treatment with medium-high doses of glucocorticoids beyond what is necessary to control an acute flare of vasculitis or the more serious manifestations.

MEDICAL EMERGENCIES RELATED TO THE PRIMARY VASCULITIDES

The systemic vasculitides vary greatly in their rate of progression and level of medical severity. However, it is imperative that all clinicians caring for patients with vasculitis understand that these diseases are often organ- and life-threatening and that progression to emergency situations may be rapid. Furthermore, vasculitis can accelerate rapidly even after a long period of slowly changing or even indolent disease. Table 139-2 outlines several of the most common situations in which patients require emergency care but this list is incomplete and clinicians must be vigilant about considering these and other potentially rapidly progressive problems.

TABLE 139-2
Medical Emergencies Related to the Primary Vasculitides

EMERGENCY MANIFESTATIONS OF VASCULITIS	TYPE OF VASCULITIS
Ophthalmologic	
Threatened vision; monocular blindness	GCA, TAK
▪ Scleritis	GPA, MPA, RPC
▪ Uveitis	BD
Pulmonary	
Subglottic stenosis	GPA, RPC
▪ Alveolar hemorrhage	GPA, MPA, EGPA
▪ Diffuse inflammatory infiltrates	GPA, MPA, EGPA
▪ Pulmonary embolus	GPA, MPA, EGPA, BD
Cardiovascular	
Malignant hypertension—Renal arterial stenoses	TAK, GCA, PAN
▪ Rapid-onset cardiomyopathy/heart failure	EGPA
▪ Angina/myocardial infarction	TAK, GCA
▪ Gangrene—digital ischemia	GCA, TAK, PAN, GPA, MPA
▪ Aneurysm dissection (aorta or branches)	PAN, BD, GCA, TAK
GI	
Mesenteric ischemia	PAN, IgAV, GCA, TAK
Renal	
Glomerulonephritis/rising creatinine/renal failure	GPA, MPA, EGPA, IgAV, PAN, Cryo
Neurologic	
Headache	GCA
▪ Syncope	GCA, TAK
▪ Stroke	GPA, MPA, EGPA, BD, GCA, TAK
▪ Sensorineural hearing loss or other cranial neuropathies	GPA, MPA
▪ Mononeuritis multiplex	EGPA, PAN, GPA, MPA
Other Organ-Threatening Disease	Any systemic vasculitis

BD, Behçet disease; Cryo, cryoglobulinemic vasculitis; EGPA, eosinophilic granulomatosis with polyangiitis; GCA, giant cell arteritis; GPA, granulomatosis with polyangiitis; IgAV, IgA vasculitis (Henoch–Schönlein); MPA, microscopic polyangiitis; PAN, polyarteritis nodosa; RPC, relapsing polychondritis; TAK, Takayasu arteritis.

REFERENCES

1. Basu N, Watts R, Bajema I, et al. EULAR points to consider in the development of classification and diagnostic criteria in systemic vasculitis. *Ann Rheum Dis.* 2010;69(10):1744-1750.
2. Watts RA, Suppiah R, Merkel PA, et al. Systemic vasculitis—is it time to reclassify? *Rheumatology (Oxford).* 2011;50(4):643-645.
3. Lie JT. Nomenclature and classification of vasculitis: plus ca change, plus c'est la meme chose. *Arthritis Rheum.* 1994;37(2):181-186.
4. Hunder GG, Arend WP, Bloch DA, et al. The American College of Rheumatology 1990 criteria for the

4. classification of vasculitis. Introduction. *Arthritis Rheum*. 1990;33(8):1065-1067.
5. Fries JF, Hunder GG, Bloch DA, et al. The American College of Rheumatology 1990 criteria for the classification of vasculitis. Summary. *Arthritis Rheum*. 1990;33(8):1135-1136.
6. Jennette JC, Falk RJ, Bacon PA, et al. 2012 revised International Chapel Hill Consensus Conference Nomenclature of Vasculitides. *Arthritis Rheum*. 2013;65(1):1-11.
7. Ozen S, Ruperto N, Dillon MJ, et al. EULAR/PReS endorsed consensus criteria for the classification of childhood vasculitides. *Ann Rheum Dis*. 2006; 65(7):936-941.
8. Sunderkötter CH, Zelger B, Chen KR, et al. Nomenclature of Cutaneous Vasculitis: Dermatologic Addendum to the 2012 Revised International Chapel Hill Consensus Conference Nomenclature of Vasculitides. *Arthritis Rheumatol*. 2018;70(2):171-184.
9. Mahr AD, Neogi T, Merkel PA. Epidemiology of Wegener's granulomatosis: Lessons from descriptive studies and analyses of genetic and environmental risk determinants. *Clin Exp Rheumatol*. 2006;24(2) (suppl 41):S82-S91.
10. Lyons PA, Rayner TF, Trivedi S, et al. Genetically distinct subsets within ANCA-associated vasculitis. *N Engl J Med*. 2012;367(3):214-223.
11. Merkel PA, Xie G, Monach PA, et al. Identification of functional and expression polymorphisms associated with risk for antineutrophil cytoplasmic autoantibody-associated vasculitis. *Arthritis Rheumatol*. 2017;69(5):1054-1066.
12. Carmona FD, Vaglio A, Mackie SL, et al. A Genome-wide Association Study Identifies Risk Alleles in Plasminogen and P4HA2 Associated with Giant Cell Arteritis. *Am J Hum Genet*. 2017;100(1):64-74.
13. Carmona FD, Coit P, Saruhan-Direskeneli G, et al. Analysis of the common genetic component of large-vessel vasculitides through a meta-Immunochip strategy. *Sci Rep*. 2017;7:43953.
14. Merkel PA. Drug-induced vasculitis. *Rheum Dis Clin North Am*. 2001;27(4):849-862.
15. Carlson JA, Ng BT, Chen KR. Cutaneous vasculitis update: diagnostic criteria, classification, epidemiology, etiology, pathogenesis, evaluation and prognosis. *Am J Dermatopathol*. 2005;27(6):504-528.
16. Carlson JA. The histological assessment of cutaneous vasculitis. *Histopathology*. 2010;56(1):3-23.
17. Carlson JA, Chen KR. Cutaneous vasculitis update: small vessel neutrophilic vasculitis syndromes. *Am J Dermatopathol*. 2006;28(6):486-506.
18. WGET Research Group. Limited versus severe Wegener's granulomatosis: baseline data on patients in the Wegener's granulomatosis etanercept trial. *Arthritis Rheum*. 2003;48(8):2299-2309.
19. Guillevin L, Cohen P, Gayraud M, et al. Churg-Strauss syndrome. Clinical study and long-term follow-up of 96 patients. *Medicine (Baltimore)*. 1999;78(1):26-37.
20. Guillevin L, Durand-Gasselin B, Cevallos R, et al. Microscopic polyangiitis: clinical and laboratory findings in eighty-five patients. *Arthritis Rheum*. 1999; 42(3):421-430.
21. Hoffman GS, Specks U. Antineutrophil cytoplasmic antibodies. *Arthritis Rheum*. 1998;41(9):1521-1537.
22. Merkel PA, Polisson RP, Chang Y, et al. Prevalence of antineutrophil cytoplasmic antibodies in a large inception cohort of patients with connective tissue disease. *Ann Intern Med*. 1997;126(11):866-873.
23. Savige J, Gillis D, Benson E, et al. International consensus statement on testing and reporting of Antineutrophil Cytoplasmic Antibodies (ANCA). *Am J Clin Pathol*. 1999;111(4):507-513.
24. Choi HK, Liu S, Merkel PA, et al. Diagnostic performance of antineutrophil cytoplasmic antibody tests for idiopathic vasculitides: metaanalysis with a focus on antimyeloperoxidase antibodies. *J Rheumatol*. 2001;28(7):1584-1590.
25. Voskuyl AE, Hazes JM, Zwinderman AH, et al. Diagnostic strategy for the assessment of rheumatoid vasculitis. *Ann Rheum Dis*. 2003;62(5):407-413.
26. Wooten MD, Jasin HE. Vasculitis and lymphoproliferative diseases. *Semin Arthritis Rheum*. 1996;26(2):564-574.
27. Sene D, Ghillani-Dalbin P, Thibault V, et al. Long-term course of mixed cryoglobulinemia in patients infected with hepatitis C virus. *J Rheumatol*. 2004; 31(11):2199-2206.
28. Rieu V, Cohen P, Andre MH, et al. Characteristics and outcome of 49 patients with symptomatic cryoglobulinaemia. *Rheumatology (Oxford)*. 2002;41(3):290-300.
29. Ramos-Casals M, Munoz S, Medina F, et al. Systemic autoimmune diseases in patients with hepatitis C virus infection: characterization of 1020 cases (The HISPAMEC Registry). *J Rheumatol*. 2009;36(7):1442-1448.
30. Guillevin L, Lhote F, Gayraud M, et al. Prognostic factors in polyarteritis nodosa and Churg-Strauss syndrome. A prospective study in 342 patients. *Medicine (Baltimore)*. 1996;75(1):17-28.
31. Mahr A, Batteux F, Tubiana S, et al. Brief report: prevalence of antineutrophil cytoplasmic antibodies in infective endocarditis. *Arthritis Rheumatol*. 2014;66(6):1672-1677.
32. Trimarchi M, Gregorini G, Facchetti F, et al. Cocaine-induced midline destructive lesions: clinical, radiographic, histopathologic, and serologic features and their differentiation from Wegener granulomatosis. *Medicine (Baltimore)*. 2001;80(6):391-404.
33. Trimarchi M, Nicolai P, Lombardi D, et al. Sinonasal osteocartilaginous necrosis in cocaine abusers: experience in 25 patients. *Am J Rhinol*. 2003;17(1):33-43.
34. Pearson T, Bremmer M, Cohen J, et al. Vasculopathy related to cocaine adulterated with levamisole: a review of the literature. *Dermatol Online J*. 2012;18(7):1.
35. Kissin EY, Merkel PA. Diagnostic imaging in Takayasu arteritis. *Curr Opin Rheumatol*. 2004;16(1):31-37.
36. Bakthavachalam S, Driver MS, Cox C, et al. Hearing loss in Wegener's granulomatosis. *Otol Neurotol*. 2004;25(5):833-837.
37. Villiger PM, Guillevin L. Microscopic polyangiitis: clinical presentation. *Autoimmun Rev*. 2010;9(12):812-819.
38. Savage CO, Winearls CG, Evans DJ, et al. Microscopic polyarteritis: presentation, pathology and prognosis. *Q J Med*. 1985;56(220):467-483.
39. Niles JL, Bottinger EP, Saurina GR, et al. The syndrome of lung hemorrhage and nephritis is usually an ANCA-associated condition. *Arch Intern Med*. 1996 26;156(4):440-445.
40. Agard C, Mouthon L, Mahr A, et al. Microscopic polyangiitis and polyarteritis nodosa: how and when do they start? *Arthritis Rheum*. 2003;49(5):709-715.
41. Niiyama S, Amoh Y, Tomita M, et al. Dermatological manifestations associated with microscopic polyangiitis. *Rheumatol Int*. 2008;28(6):593-595.
42. Hoffman GS, Kerr GS, Leavitt RY, et al. Wegener granulomatosis: an analysis of 158 patients. *Ann Intern Med*. 1992;116(6):488-498.

43. Reinhold-Keller E, Beuge N, Latza U, et al. An interdisciplinary approach to the care of patients with Wegener's granulomatosis: long-term outcome in 155 patients. *Arthritis Rheum*. 2000;43(5):1021-1032.
44. Stone JH. Limited versus severe Wegener's granulomatosis: baseline data on patients in the Wegener's granulomatosis etanercept trial. *Arthritis Rheum*. 2003;48(8):2299-2309.
45. Finkielman JD, Lee AS, Hummel AM, et al. ANCA are detectable in nearly all patients with active severe Wegener's granulomatosis. *Am J Med*. 2007;120(7):643.e9-643.e14.
46. Frances C, Du LT, Piette JC, et al. Wegener's granulomatosis. Dermatological manifestations in 75 cases with clinicopathologic correlation. *Arch Dermatol*. 1994;130(7):861-867.
47. Daoud MS, Gibson LE, DeRemee RA, et al. Cutaneous Wegener's granulomatosis: clinical, histopathologic, and immunopathologic features of thirty patients. *J Am Acad Dermatol*. 1994;31(4):605-612.
48. Barksdale SK, Hallahan CW, Kerr GS, et al. Cutaneous pathology in Wegener's granulomatosis. A clinicopathologic study of 75 biopsies in 46 patients. *Am J Surg Pathol*. 1995;19(2):161-172.
49. Hu CH, O'Loughlin S, Winkelmann RK. Cutaneous manifestations of Wegener granulomatosis. *Arch Dermatol*. 1977;113(2):175-182.
50. Sable-Fourtassou R, Cohen P, Mahr A, et al. Antineutrophil cytoplasmic antibodies and the Churg-Strauss syndrome. *Ann Intern Med*. 2005;143(9):632-638.
51. Solans R, Bosch JA, Perez-Bocanegra C, et al. Churg-Strauss syndrome: outcome and long-term follow-up of 32 patients. *Rheumatology (Oxford)*. 2001;40(7):763-771.
52. Lanham JG, Elkon KB, Pusey CD, et al. Systemic vasculitis with asthma and eosinophilia: a clinical approach to the Churg-Strauss syndrome. *Medicine (Baltimore)*. 1984;63(2):65-81.
53. Calamia KT, Balabanova M. Vasculitis in systemic lupus erythematosus. *Clin Dermatol*. 2004;22(2):148-156.
54. Drenkard C, Villa AR, Reyes E, et al. Vasculitis in systemic lupus erythematosus. *Lupus*. 1997;6(3):235-242.
55. Ramos-Casals M, Anaya JM, Garcia-Carrasco M, et al. Cutaneous vasculitis in primary Sjogren syndrome: classification and clinical significance of 52 patients. *Medicine (Baltimore)*. 2004;83(2):96-106.
56. Watts RA, Mooney J, Lane SE, et al. Rheumatoid vasculitis: becoming extinct? *Rheumatology (Oxford)*. 2004;43(7):920-923.
57. Bartels C, Bell C, Rosenthal A, et al. Decline in rheumatoid vasculitis prevalence among US veterans: a retrospective cross-sectional study. *Arthritis Rheum*. 2009;60(9):2553-2557.
58. Frances C, el Rassi R, Laporte JL, et al. Dermatologic manifestations of relapsing polychondritis. A study of 200 cases at a single center. *Medicine (Baltimore)*. 2001;80(3):173-179.
59. Solans-Laque R, Bosch-Gil JA, Perez-Bocanegra C, et al. Paraneoplastic vasculitis in patients with solid tumors: report of 15 cases. *J Rheumatol*. 2008;35(2):294-304.
60. ten Holder SM, Joy MS, Falk RJ. Cutaneous and systemic manifestations of drug-induced vasculitis. *Ann Pharmacother*. 2002;36(1):130-147.
61. Choi HK, Merkel PA, Walker AM, et al. Drug-associated antineutrophil cytoplasmic antibody-positive vasculitis: prevalence among patients with high titers of antimyeloperoxidase antibodies. *Arthritis Rheum*. 2000;43(2):405-413.
62. Choi HK, Merkel PA, Niles JL. ANCA-positive vasculitis associated with allopurinol therapy. *Clin Exp Rheumatol*. 1998;16(6):743-744.
63. Adu D, Howie AJ, Scott DG, et al. Polyarteritis and the kidney. *Q J Med*. 1987;62(239):221-237.
64. Guillevin L, Mahr A, Callard P, et al. Hepatitis B virus-associated polyarteritis nodosa: clinical characteristics, outcome, and impact of treatment in 115 patients. *Medicine (Baltimore)*. 2005;84(5):313-322.
65. Daoud MS, Hutton KP, Gibson LE. Cutaneous periarteritis nodosa: a clinicopathological study of 79 cases. *Br J Dermatol*. 1997;136(5):706-713.
66. Chen KR. Cutaneous polyarteritis nodosa: a clinical and histopathological study of 20 cases. *J Dermatol*. 1989;16(6):429-442.
67. Moore PM, Cupps TR. Neurological complications of vasculitis. *Ann Neurol*. 1983;14(2):155-167.
68. Calabrese LH, Duna GF, Lie JT. Vasculitis in the central nervous system. *Arthritis Rheum*. 1997;40(7):1189-1201.
69. Tsianakas A, Ehrchen JM, Presser D, et al. Scalp necrosis in giant cell arteritis: case report and review of the relevance of this cutaneous sign of large-vessel vasculitis. *J Am Acad Dermatol*. 2009;61(4):701-706.
70. Baum EW, Sams WM Jr, Payne RR. Giant cell arteritis: a systemic disease with rare cutaneous manifestations. *J Am Acad Dermatol*. 1982;6(6):1081-1088.
71. Kerr GS, Hallahan CW, Giordano J, et al. Takayasu arteritis. *Ann Intern Med*. 1994;120(11):919-929.
72. Vanoli M, Daina E, Salvarani C, et al. Takayasu's arteritis: A study of 104 Italian patients. *Arthritis Rheum*. 2005;53(1):100-107.
73. Jain S, Kumari S, Ganguly NK, et al. Current status of Takayasu arteritis in India. *Int J Cardiol*. 1996;54(suppl):S111-S116.
74. Ishikawa K, Maetani S. Long-term outcome for 120 Japanese patients with Takayasu's disease. Clinical and statistical analyses of related prognostic factors. *Circulation*. 1994;90(4):1855-1860.
75. Lupi-Herrera E, Sanchez-Torres G, Marcushamer J, et al. Takayasu's arteritis. Clinical study of 107 cases. *Am Heart J*. 1977;93(1):94-103.
76. Maksimowicz-McKinnon K, Clark TM, Hoffman GS. Limitations of therapy and a guarded prognosis in an American cohort of Takayasu arteritis patients. *Arthritis Rheum*. 2007;56(3):1000-1009.
77. Ujiie H, Sawamura D, Yokota K, et al. Pyoderma gangrenosum associated with Takayasu's arteritis. *Clin Exp Dermatol*. 2004;29(4):357-359.
78. Perniciaro CV, Winkelmann RK, Hunder GG. Cutaneous manifestations of Takayasu's arteritis. A clinicopathologic correlation. *J Am Acad Dermatol*. 1987;17(6):998-1005.
79. Pascual-Lopez M, Hernandez-Nunez A, Aragues-Montanes M, et al. Takayasu's disease with cutaneous involvement. *Dermatology*. 2004;208(1):10-15.
80. Flossman O, Berden A, de Groot K, et al. Long-term patient survival in ANCA-associated vasculitis. *Ann Rheum Dis*. 2011;70(3):488-494.
81. Westman K, Flossmann O, Gregorini G. The long-term outcomes of systemic vasculitis. *Nephrol Dial Transplant*. 2015;30(suppl 1):i60-i66.
82. Comarmond C, Pagnoux C, Khellaf M, et al. Eosinophilic granulomatosis with polyangiitis (Churg-Strauss): clinical characteristics and long-term followup

of the 383 patients enrolled in the French Vasculitis Study Group cohort. *Arthritis Rheum*. 2013;65:270-281.
83. Yates M, Watts RA, Bajema IM, et al. EULAR/ERA-EDTA recommendations for the management of ANCA-associated vasculitis. *Ann Rheum Dis*. 2016;75(9):1583-1594.
84. Mukhtyar C, Guillevin L, Cid MC, et al. EULAR recommendations for the management of large vessel vasculitis. *Ann Rheum Dis*. 2009;68(3):318-323.
85. Fauci AS, Katz P, Haynes BF, et al. Cyclophosphamide therapy of severe systemic necrotizing vasculitis. *N Engl J Med*. 1979;301(5):235-238.
86. Jayne D, Rasmussen N, Andrassy K, et al. A randomized trial of maintenance therapy for vasculitis associated with antineutrophil cytoplasmic autoantibodies. *N Engl J Med*. 2003;349(1):36-44.
87. Gayraud M, Guillevin L, Cohen P, et al. Treatment of good-prognosis polyarteritis nodosa and Churg-Strauss syndrome: comparison of steroids and oral or pulse cyclophosphamide in 25 patients. French Cooperative Study Group for Vasculitides. *Br J Rheumatol*. 1997;36(12):1290-1297.
88. De Groot K, Rasmussen N, Bacon PA, et al. Randomized trial of cyclophosphamide versus methotrexate for induction of remission in early systemic antineutrophil cytoplasmic antibody-associated vasculitis. *Arthritis Rheum*. 2005;52(8):2461-2469.
89. Sneller MC, Hoffman GS, Talar-Williams C, et al. An analysis of forty-two Wegener's granulomatosis patients treated with methotrexate and prednisone. *Arthritis Rheum*. 1995;38(5):608-613.
90. Pagnoux C, Mahr A, Hamidou MA, et al. Azathioprine or methotrexate maintenance for ANCA-associated vasculitis. *N Engl J Med*. 2008;359(26):2790-2803.
91. Hatemi G, Melikoglu M, Tunc R, et al. Apremilast for Behçet's syndrome—a phase 2, placebo-controlled study. *N Engl J Med*. 2015;372(16):1510-1518.
92. A phase 3 randomized, double-blind study to evaluate the efficacy and safety of Apremilast (CC-10004) in subjects with active Behcet's disease. ClinicalTrials.gov Identifier: NCT02307513.
93. Jones RB, Tervaert JW, Hauser T, et al. Rituximab versus cyclophosphamide in ANCA-associated renal vasculitis. *N Engl J Med*. 2010;363(3):211-220.
94. Stone JH, Merkel PA, Spiera R, et al. Rituximab versus cyclophosphamide for ANCA-associated vasculitis. *N Engl J Med*. 2010;363(3):221-232.
95. Guillevin L, Pagnoux C, Karras A, et al. Rituximab versus azathioprine for maintenance in ANCA-associated vasculitis. *N Engl J Med*. 2014;371(19):1771-1780.
96. Wechsler ME, Akuthota P, Jayne D, et al. Mepolizumab or placebo for eosinophilic granulomatosis with polyangiitis. *N Engl J Med*. 2017;376(20):1921-1932.
97. Villiger PM, Adler S, Kuchen S, et al. Tocilizumab for induction and maintenance of remission in giant cell arteritis: a phase 2, randomised, double-blind, placebo-controlled trial. *Lancet*. 2016;387(10031):1921-1927.
98. Stone JH, Tuckwell K, Dimonaco S, et al. Trial of tocilizumab in giant-cell arteritis. *N Engl J Med*. 2017;377(4):317-328.
99. Langford CA, Cuthbertson D, Ytterberg SR, et al. A randomized, double-blind trial of abatacept (CTLA-4Ig) for the treatment of giant cell arteritis. *Arthritis Rheumatol*. 2017;69(4):837-845.
100. WGET Research Group. Etanercept plus standard therapy for Wegener's granulomatosis. *N Engl J Med*. 2005;352(4):351-361.
101. Hoffman GS, Cid MC, Rendt-Zagar KE, et al. Infliximab for maintenance of glucocorticosteroid-induced remission of giant cell arteritis: a randomized trial. *Ann Intern Med*. 2007;146(9):621-630.
102. Jayne DR, Gaskin G, Rasmussen N, et al. Randomized trial of plasma exchange or high-dosage methylprednisolone as adjunctive therapy for severe renal vasculitis. *J Am Soc Nephrol*. 2007;18(7):2180-2188.

Chapter 140 :: Erythema Elevatum Diutinum
:: Theodore J. Alkousakis & Whitney A. High

第一百四十章
持久性隆起性红斑

中文导读

持久性隆起性红斑（EED）是一种罕见的慢性白细胞碎裂性血管炎（LCV），主要表现为对称的丘疹和斑块分布在关节伸侧，呈粉红色、红斑、棕色、紫色或黄色。本章首先对该病的命名由来和演变进行了介绍，并对该病的流行病学、临床特征、发病机制、相关疾病、诊断、鉴别诊断和治疗进行了详细阐述。

1. 流行病学　EED罕见，文献中仅报道了250例，最常见于40～60岁，尚不能确定明确的性别倾向或种族偏好。

2. 临床特征　EED通常首先表现为水肿性红色到紫色丘疹、结节或斑块，相对对称地分布在手指、脚趾和手关节处（图140-1）或肘部（图140-2）、腕部、膝盖（图140-3）、脚踝、腿部及跟腱伸侧表面的皮肤。EED的单个病变为圆形至椭圆形，通常光滑无鳞屑（图140-4），不能推动。EED病变可能无症状，也可能出现瘙痒、疼痛、烧灼感、刺痛、感觉异常或神经病。若在皮疹发展期，可能会伴有系统症状如关节痛和发热。EED的早期病变通常较软且可能很软，但陈旧性病变可能坚实也可能柔软。EED的病灶可能在晚上会变得更加坚硬、隆起或更红。

随着疾病的发展，皮损会变成深褐色或紫红色，并可能会发生纤维化，也可能会观察到黄色，类似于黄瘤表现。HIV感染患者的慢性EED表现更为多样，可模拟卡波济肉瘤或杆菌性血管瘤。

EED的自然病程不尽相同，疾病发生5到10年后可自发消退，有时也会持续数十年。症状可能会反复出现，或者在数周或数月内突然爆发。链球菌感染可诱发疾病发作，寒冷的天气会加剧症状或引起新的病变。

3. 发病机制　EED的发病机制不明，有假说认为是由于抗原-抗体复合物的形成导致免疫复合物在血管壁中的沉积引起白细胞碎裂血管炎，而血管炎的反复发作导致纤维化和其他疾病晚期的后遗症。本章罗列了这些假说的依据。

4. 相关疾病　EED与多种疾病有关：感染（链球菌、乙型肝炎、梅毒、结核、HIV）、单克隆和多克隆丙种球蛋白血症、炎症性肠病和乳糜泻、结缔组织病（类风湿关节炎、强直性脊柱炎、红斑狼疮、皮肌炎、复发性多软骨炎、肉芽肿性多血管炎）以及淋巴增殖和骨髓增生异常（骨髓增生异常、淋巴瘤、白血病、骨髓瘤）（请参见表140-1）。提及IgA副蛋白血症是EED最常合并的疾病。

5. 诊断　诊断主要依靠皮肤活检，组织学表现取决于疾病过程。白细胞碎裂性血管炎是整个疾病过程的主要特征。早期的EED常表现为真皮浅中层血管周围嗜中性粒细胞浸润，伴核尘及纤维蛋白（图140-5），可能伴有淋巴细胞、组织细胞甚至少数嗜酸性粒细胞。晚期EED会逐渐出现纤维化，甚至硬化。在某些晚期病例中，可能难以找到血管炎。此外，在晚期疾病中可能偶尔会看到组织细胞内脂质沉积和罕见的胆固醇裂隙。直接免疫荧光可见IgG、IgM、IgA、C3和纤维蛋白在血管周围非特异性沉积。由于与EED相关的疾病范围很广，因此作者建议完善以下实验室检查：全血细胞计数，全面的代谢检查，HIV筛查，免疫固定电泳，链酶检测，乙肝和丙肝病毒筛查，抗核抗体（ANA），抗中性粒细胞胞浆抗体，抗磷脂抗体和尿液分析（表140-2）。提倡免疫固定电泳，而不是血清蛋白电泳，并完善胸片。

6．鉴别诊断　表140-3中列出了需要鉴别的诊断，及临床和组织学特征的鉴别点。

特别提及EED在组织学上最应该与面部肉芽肿（GF）相鉴别。二者组织学上的共同点包括白细胞碎裂性血管炎及晚期病变中血管周围同心圆性纤维化。一些皮肤病理学家主张使用术语"局部慢性纤维化性血管炎"来代表GF和EED的晚期共同终点。

7．治疗　治疗目标包括症状缓解，清除病灶和合理治疗相关疾病。虽然早期EED治疗反应好，提倡持续治疗以防止复发。基于砜的疗法（包括氨苯砜和磺胺吡啶）是一线治疗药物，通常可在48小时内或数周或数月内使所有病变完全消失。但是，症状通常会因停药而迅速复发。其他报道有效的药物包括烟酰胺和四环素、秋水仙碱、非甾体类药物抗炎药（双氯芬酸）、羟氯喹、二甲双胍、氯法齐明、环磷酰胺，它们可作为单一药物或与血浆置换联合使用。

系统使用皮质类固醇可用于顽固性病例或出现氨苯砜相关的贫血时，但是需考虑潜在的基础疾病。皮损内使用皮质类固醇或强效皮质类固醇外用制剂可以有效治疗局限性皮损。作者建议同时治疗潜在的相关疾病或感染，可以加快皮疹消退。还指出EED有一定的复发率，也有部分患者对治疗反应差。此外，慢性纤维化病变缺乏有效治疗手段。

〔黄莹雪〕

AT-A-GLANCE

- Rare disorder, with around 250 case reports in literature.
- A chronic leukocytoclastic vasculitis typified by a distinctive clinical pattern of symmetric, erythematous, violaceous, or yellow–brown papules, nodules, or plaques.
- Sites of involvement often include the skin overlying the joints of the hands and fingers, or extensor surfaces like the elbows, knees, legs, and Achilles tendon. The trunk is usually spared.
- Coexisting diseases include monoclonal paraproteinemia, lymphoproliferative disorders, chronic infections, autoimmune conditions, and connective tissue disease.
- Histopathology reveals a leukocytoclastic vasculitis in early-stage disease, and mixed inflammation and fibrosis in late-stage disease.

Erythema elevatum diutinum (EED) is a rare, chronic leukocytoclastic vasculitis (LCV) that presents as largely symmetric papules and plaques, chiefly over joints and upon extensor surfaces, with a pink, erythematous, brown, violaceous, or yellow hue. Cases now recognized as EED were first reported by Hutchinson[1,2] in 1878, and Bury[3] in 1889. The current nosology, EED, was proposed by Radcliffe-Crocker and Williams in 1894,[4] with the last part of the name, *diutinum*, meaning "long-lasting."

Radcliffe-Crocker and Williams proposed a division of cases into "Bury-type" (more often seen in young women with a personal and/or family history rheumatism), and "Hutchinson-type" (more often seen in older men with gout). In 1932, so-called extracellular cholesterosis of Urbach[5] was proposed as a third form. In 1929, Weidman and Besancon classified EED as a vasculitis,[6] and this conclusion is now widely held. EED is no longer subdivided, and all forms are considered a spectrum of the disorder.

EPIDEMIOLOGY

The incidence of EED is unknown, with only about 250 cases reported in the literature.[7] A case series, culled from a tertiary care center, and spanning 60 years, contained only 13 cases.[8] EED may present at any age but is most common in the fourth through sixth decades of life. One of the original cases reported occurred in a 6-year-old.[2] Men were thought to be affected more often, but with so few cases reported, it is difficult to ascertain any definitive sexual or ethnic predilection.

CLINICAL FEATURES

EED typically first presents as edematous, erythematous to violaceous papules, nodules, and plaques, distributed relatively symmetrically upon the skin overlying the joints of the fingers, toes, and hands (Fig. 140-1), or upon the extensor surfaces, such as the elbows (Fig. 140-2), wrists, knees (Fig. 140-3), ankles, legs, and Achilles tendon. Purpura, petechiae, vegetative lesions,[9] ulcerations, and bullous appearance may occur in association with EED.[10]

Individual lesions of EED are round to oval, usually smooth and without scale (Fig. 140-4). The lesions are not fixed to the underlying structures. EED is uncommon on the face, ears, buttocks, and genitals. The torso and mucosal membranes are also typically spared. Involvement of the retroauricular area or the palmoplantar skin is uncommon.[11-13]

Lesions of EED may be asymptomatic, or the condition may be associated with pruritus, pain, burning, stinging, paresthesia, or neuropathy.[14] Systemic symptoms, such as arthralgia and fever, may be experienced with the eruption. Over time, EED can coalesce into irregular patterns. Although early lesions of EED are often soft and possibly tender, older lesions may be firm or doughy. Lesions of EED may become more firm, raised, and erythematous in the evening hours.[8,15,16]

Over time, lesions of EED can become darker brown or violaceous in color. Fibrosis may ensue. Yellow hues may be observed, with the latter resembling xanthomata. The varied appearance of chronic EED may be even more pronounced in HIV-infected persons, and the condition can resemble Kaposi sarcoma or bacillary angiomatosis.

The natural course of EED varies. Spontaneous resolution can transpire, usually after 5 to 10 years of

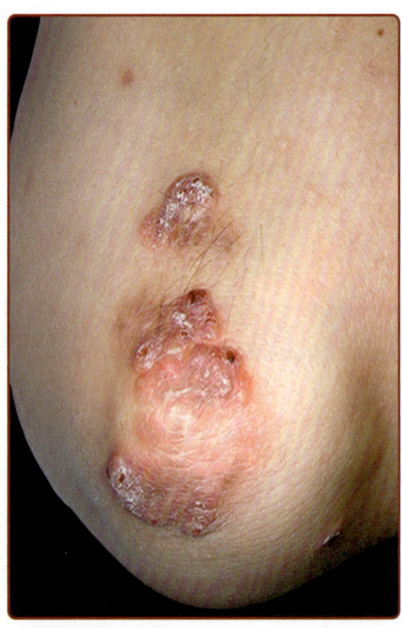

Figure 140-2 Multiple erythematous scaly papules coalescing into plaques on extensor elbow.

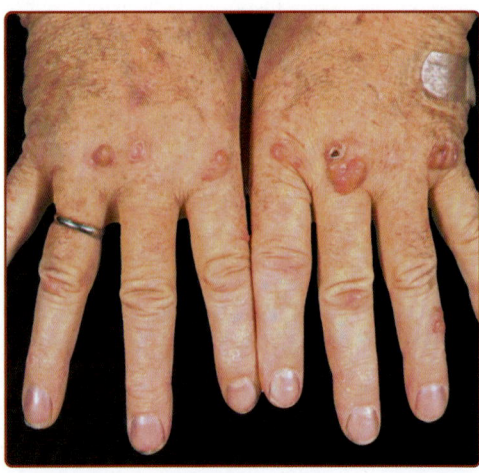

Figure 140-1 Erythema elevatum diutinum. Nodular lesions on dorsal hand present for several years.

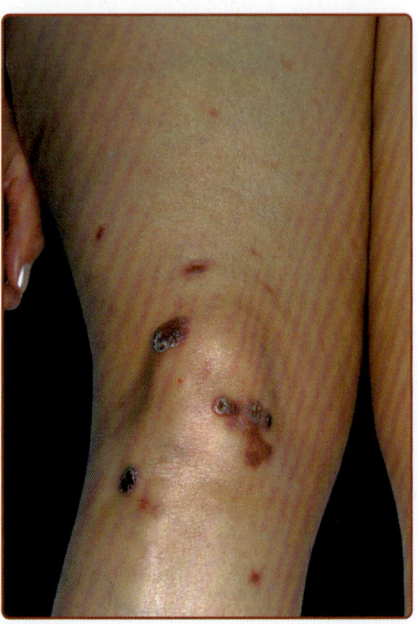

Figure 140-3 Crusted brown and violaceous papules over knee and anterior thigh.

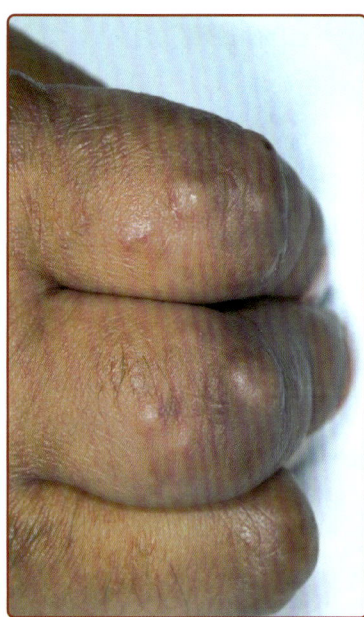

Figure 140-4 Smooth, flesh-colored to slightly erythematous papules on extensor fingers over proximal interphalangeal joints.

disease activity, while in other cases, fixed lesions last decades.[17,18] The condition may wax and wane slowly, or flares or crops of disease can erupt rapidly, over weeks or months. Streptococcal infections can precipitate outbreaks. Cold weather can exacerbate symptoms or cause new lesions.

PATHOGENESIS

The pathogenesis of EED is not fully understood. A hypothesis is the formation of antigen-antibody complexes leads to deposition of immune complexes in blood vessel walls.[19] This leads to complement activation, with chemotaxis of neutrophils, the latter perhaps due to overexpression of IL-8.[20] A leukocytoclastic vasculitis ensues, and repeated episodes of this vasculitis lead to fibrosis and other sequelae of late disease.

Evidence in support of this proposed mechanism includes (1) the inducing of lesions with injection of streptokinase, leading to streptokinase-streptodornase complexes[21]; (2) deposition of IgG, IgM, IgA, and fibrin in vascular and perivascular locations on direct immunofluorescence examination[19]; and (3) increased C1q-binding activity and enhanced IL-8 responses in the sera of affected patients.[20,22]

ASSOCIATED CONDITIONS

EED has been associated with a variety of medical conditions: infections (streptococcal, hepatitis B, syphilis, tuberculosis, HIV), monoclonal and polyclonal gammopathies, inflammatory bowel disease and celiac disease, connective tissue disease (rheumatoid arthritis, ankylosing spondylitis, lupus erythematosus, dermatomyositis, relapsing polychondritis, granulomatous polyangiitis), and lymphoproliferative and myelodysplastic conditions (myelodysplasias, lymphoma, leukemia, myeloma) (see Table 140-1). In some series, the most frequent association with EED was an IgA paraproteinemia,[8] although the severity of EED did not appear dependent on total paraprotein levels.

TABLE 140-1

Entities Associated with Erythema Elevatum Diutinum

DISEASE CATEGORY	SPECIFIC CONDITIONS
Autoimmune/Connective Tissue Disorders	Rheumatoid arthritis
	Ankylosing spondylitis
	Relapsing polychondritis
	Cutaneous or systemic lupus erythematosus
	Granulomatosis with polyangiitis
	Myasthenia gravis
	Celiac disease
	Dermatitis herpetiformis
	Sjogren syndrome
	Autoimmune keratolysis of the eye
Infectious diseases	Chronic bacterial infections
	HIV-1, HIV-2
	Streptococcal infection/rheumatic fever
	Measles virus
	Human herpesvirus 6
	Syphilis
	Tuberculosis
	Hepatitis B
Inflammatory disorders	Crohn disease
	Ulcerative colitis
	Mixed cryoglobulinemia
	Pyoderma gangrenosum
Malignancy	IgA/IgG paraproteinemia (monoclonal gammopathy/monoclonal gammopathy of undetermined significance/myeloma)
	Myelodysplasia
	Polycythemia vera
	Hairy-cell leukemia
	Chronic lymphocytic leukemia
	B-cell lymphoma/non-Hodgkin lymphoma
	Lymphadenopathy-associated virus/human T-cell lymphotrophic virus Type 3
	Lung cancer
	Prostate cancer
Medications	Rifampin
	Pyrazinamide
	Isoniazid
	Streptomycin
Miscellaneous	Pulmonary infiltrates/pleural effusions
	Hypothyroidism
	Mosquito bites
	Insulin-dependent diabetes mellitus
	Hyper-IgD D syndrome
	Hypereosinophilic syndrome
	Acro-osteolysis
	Hemophilia
	Peripheral ulcerative keratitis

DIAGNOSIS

The diagnosis of EED is suspected when appropriate clinical findings are present, but it is established via skin biopsy. A biopsy to establish EED should contain the full thickness of the dermis and extend into the upper subcutis. Most often, a deep punch technique is utilized.

The histologic findings by light microscopy depend on the temporal course. Leukocytoclastic vasculitis is a central feature of disease process. Early EED often demonstrates neutrophilic infiltrates and neutrophilic pyknotic debris, as well as fibrin, surrounding the upper and middermal vascular plexii (Fig. 140-5). Lymphocytes, histiocytes, and even a few eosinophils, may accompany this neutrophilic infiltrate. Late EED becomes progressively more fibrotic, and perhaps even sclerotic, on occasion.[23] In some late-stage cases, it can be difficult to appreciate a vasculitis. In addition, intracellular lipid deposition and rare cholesterol clefts may be seen, especially in admixed histiocytes, may be seen in late-stage disease.[24]

Direct immunofluorescence studies of EED often reveal the non-specific deposition of IgG, IgM, IgA, C3, and fibrin in perivascular locations.[25]

There are no laboratory studies to confirm a diagnosis of EED. Because of the range of conditions associated with EED, it is common to consider the following lab tests: complete blood count, comprehensive metabolic panel, HIV screening, immunofixation electrophoresis, streptozyme test, hepatitis B and C screening, antinuclear antibody (ANA), antineutrophil cytoplasmic antibodies, antiphospholipid antibodies, and urinalysis (Table 140-2). Immunofixation electrophoresis has been advocated, over serum protein electrophoresis.[8] A chest radiograph should also be considered.

DIFFERENTIAL DIAGNOSIS

The clinical differential diagnosis of EED depends on the chronicity and symptomatology of the lesions. The main conditions to consider and their differentiating clinical and histologic features are reviewed in Table 140-3.

In the setting of HIV-positive persons, the clinical appearance EED can mimic various stages of Kaposi sarcoma (patch, plaque, or nodular disease) and bacillary angiomatosis.

Of special mention in the histologic differential diagnosis of EED is granuloma faciale (GF). GF is a rare disorder, characterized by red-brown to violaceous papules and plaques, often with a *peau d'orange* appearance. The face is the most common location for GF. Histologic similarities between GF and EED include a leukocytoclastic vasculitis with concentric perivascular fibrosis in later lesions. GF is more likely to demonstrate admixed plasma cells and eosinophils, whereas EED is more likely to demonstrate histiocytes and granulomatous areas. Indeed, some dermatopathologists have advocated for the term "localized chronic fibrosing vasculitis" to represent a late-stage common endpoint of GF and EED.[26,27]

MANAGEMENT

Treatment of early EED can facilitate a dramatic response, and continued therapy is advocated to prevent recrudescence. The goals of therapy include symptomatic relief, clearing of lesions, and appropriate management of associated conditions.

Sulfone-based therapies, including dapsone and sulfapyridine, represent first-line agents.[10,15,19,21] Rapid improvement may transpire in the first 48 hours, with complete resolution of all lesions over weeks or months. However, lesions often recur rapidly with discontinuation. Although not completely elucidated, it is thought the mechanism of action involves the inhibition of chemotaxis and function of neutrophils.

Additional anecdotal therapies, culled from case reports and with varied success and reproducibility, include niacinamide and tetracyclines,[28] colchicine,[29]

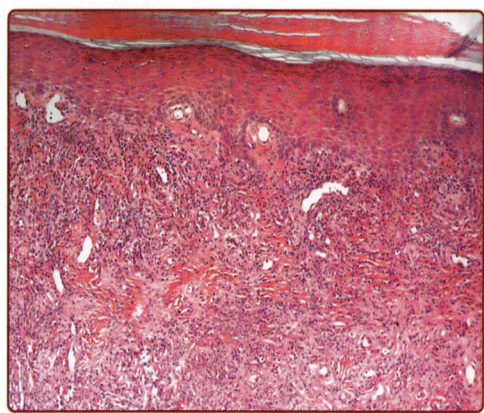

Figure 140-5 Early-stage lesion of erythema elevatum diutinum: Focal leukocytoclastic vasculitis with a fairly dense perivascular and interstitial infiltrate composed of neutrophils, lymphocytes, histiocytes, and leukocytoclastic debris. Mild capillary proliferation is also evident.

TABLE 140-2
Laboratory Tests to Consider for a Patient with Erythema Elevatum Diutinum

Complete blood count
Comprehensive metabolic panel
HIV screening
Immunofixation electrophoresis
Streptozyme test
Hepatitis B and C panel
Antinuclear antibodies (ANA)
Antineutrophil cytoplasmic antibodies
Antiphospholipid antibodies
Urinalysis
Chest radiograph

TABLE 140-3
The Differential Diagnosis of Erythema Elevatum Diutinum

DISEASE STAGE	DIAGNOSIS	DIFFERENTIATING CLINICAL FEATURES	DIFFERENTIATING HISTOLOGIC FEATURES
Early	Granuloma Annulare	Expanding, annular lesions overlying joints. Disseminated GA more often associated with diabetes.	Palisaded and/or interstitial granulomatous infiltrate without vasculitis.
	Acute febrile neutrophilic dermatosis (Sweet syndrome)	Reactive condition characterized by tender, erythematous, edematous papules and plaques on the head/neck, upper trunk, and extremities.	Papillary dermal edema with sheets of neutrophils, but without a frank vasculitis.
	Rheumatoid neutrophilic dermatitis	Associated with rheumatoid arthritis. Presents with asymptomatic papules, plaques, or nodules, on the hands, forearms, neck and trunk.	Dense dermal neutrophilic infiltrate without vasculitis.
	Palisaded and granulomatous neutrophilic dermatosis	Rare. Associated with rheumatoid arthritis, connective tissue disease, and lymphoproliferative disorders. Presents as erythematous papules on the extensor surfaces of the upper extremities.	Sparse mixed perivascular infiltrate, to interstitial and/or palisaded granulomas with fibrosis, but without vasculitis.
	Neutrophilic dermatosis of the hands	A localized variant of acute febrile neutrophilic dermatosis and/or pyoderma gangrenosum. Papules, pustules, and ulcerations, typically of the dorsal hands.	Sheets of neutrophils. Although vessels may be affected, not considered a primary vasculitis.
Chronic	Dermatofibroma	Limited lesions, typically on lower extremities. Sudden eruptive dermatofibromata may be associated with lupus erythematosus.	Fibrohistiocytic cells intercalated between and among collagen bundles with overlying epidermal induction.
	Xanthoma (particularly tuberous xanthomas)	Occur on extensor surfaces and overlying tendons (like the Achilles tendon).	Foamy, lipid laden histiocytes with minimal fibrosis.
	Rheumatoid nodules	Associated with rheumatoid arthritis. Found in the deeper soft tissue over the elbow	Deeply situated palisaded granulomas with fibrinoid degeneration, but without frank vasculitis.
	Multicentric reticulohistiocytoma	Associated with destructive arthropathy and telescoping digits.	Histiocytic cells with characteristic "muddy rose" or "ground glass" cytoplasm.

addition of nonsteroidal antiinflammatory drugs (diclofenac),[30] chloroquine,[31] phenformin,[32] clofazimine,[15] and cyclophosphamide[33] as a single agent or combined with plasma exchange.[34]

Systemic corticosteroids are of variable efficacy. The addition of prednisone may be helpful in recalcitrant cases or when faced with dapsone-associated anemia.[35] However, in the setting of certain underlying associated illnesses, systemic steroids might be best avoided. Intralesional corticosteroids or high-potency topical corticosteroids can be effective in limited disease.

When EED is associated with an underlying condition or infection, appropriate management of that illness can hasten resolution. For example, in HIV-positive patients, antiretroviral therapy should be added to sulfone-based therapy. The treatment of underlying paraproteinemias also improves the symptoms of EED.[15]

Lastly, even with appropriate treatment, EED may remain nonresponsive or it may recur at various points across a lifetime. Moreover, chronic, fibrotic lesions are unlikely to respond to any therapy.[8]

REFERENCES

1. Hutchinson J. *Illustrations of Clinical Surgery*. Vol. 1. London: J and A Churchill Ltd; 1878:42.
2. Hutchinson J. On two remarkable cases of symmetrical purple congestion of the skin in patches, with induration. *Br J Dermatol*. 1888;1:10.
3. Bury JS. A case of erythema with remarkable nodular thickening and induration of the skin associated with intermittent albuminuria. *Illus Med News*. 1889;3:145.
4. Radcliffe-Crocker H, Williams C. Erythema elevatum diutinum. *Br J Dermatol*. 1894;6:1-9, 33-38.
5. Urbach E, Epstein E, Lorenz K. Extazelluläre cholesterinose. *Arch Dermat Syph (Berlin)*. 1932;166:243-272.
6. Weidman FD, Besancon JH. Erythema elevatum diutinum. *Arch Derm Syphilol*. 1929;20:593-620.
7. Patnala GP, Sunandini AP, Yandapalli PS. Erythema elevatum diutinum in association with IgA monoclonal gammopathy: a rare case report. *Indian Dermatol Online J*. 2016;7:300-303.
8. Yiannias JA, El-Azhary RA, Gibson LE. Erythema elevatum diutinum: a clinical and histopathologic study of 13 patients. *J Am Acad Dermatol*. 1992;26:38-44.
9. Stevanovich DV. Erythema elevatum diutinum (a vegetating and ulcerative variant). *Dermatol Monatchr*. 1971;157:345-355.
10. Vollum Dl. Erythema elevatum diutinum—vesicular lesions and sulphone response. *Br J Dermatol*. 1968;80: 178-183.
11. Gibson LE, El-Azhary R. Erythema elevatum diutinum. *Clin Dermatol*. 2000;18:295.
12. Dowd PM, Munro DD. Erythema elevatum diutinum. *J R Soc Med*. 1983;76:310.
13. Chowdhury MM, Inaloz HS, Motley RJ, et al. Erythema elevatum diutinum and IgA paraproteinaemia: "a pre-

clinical iceberg." *Int J Dermatol.* 2002;41:368.
14. Nguyen GH, Guo EL, Norris D. A rare case of erythema elevatum diutinum presenting as diffuse neuropathy. *JAAD Case Rep.* 2016;3(1):1-3.
15. Farella V, Lotti T, Difonzo EM, et al. Erythema elevatum diutinum. *Int J Dermatol.* 1994;33(9):638-640.
16. Katz SI, Gallin JI, Hertz KC, et al. Erythema elevatum diutinum: skin and systemic manifestations, immunologic studies, and successful treatment with dapsone. *Medicine (Baltimore).* 1977;56(5):443-455.
17. High WA, Hoang MP, Stevens K, et al. Late-stage nodular erythema elevatum diutinum. *J Am Acad Dermatol.* 2003;49:764-767.
18. Wilkinson SM, English JC, Smith NP, et al. Erythema elevatum diutinum: a clinicopathological study. *Clin Exp Dermatol.* 1992;17:87-93.
19. Gibson LE, Su WP. Cutaneous vasculitis. *Rheum Dis Clin North Am.* 1990;16(2):309-324.
20. Grabbe J, Haas N, Moller A, et al. Erythema elevatum diutinum—evidence for disease-dependent leucocyte alterations and response to dapsone. *Br J Dermatol.* 2000;143(2):415-420.
21. Wolff H, Shever R, Maciejewski W, et al. Erythema elevatum diutinum: immunoelectromicroscopical study of leukocytoclastic vasculitis within the intracutaneous test reaction induced by streptococcal antigen [in German]. *Arch Dermatol Res.* 1978;261(11):17-26.
22. Katz SI, Gallin JI, Hertz KC, et al. Erythema elevatum diutinum: skin and systemic manifestations, immunologic studies, and successful treatment with dapsone. *Medicine.* 1977;56:443-455.
23. High WA, Stewart D, Essary LR, et al. Sclerotic fibroma-like change in various neoplastic and inflammatory skin lesions: is sclerotic fibroma a distinct entity? *J Cutan Pathol.* 2004;31:373-378.
24. Kanitakis J, Cozzani E, Lyonnet S, et al. Ultrastructural study of chronic lesions of erythema elevatum diutinum: "extracellular cholesterosis" is a misnomer. *J Am Acad Dermatol.* 1993;29:363-367.
25. Shimizu S, Nakamura Y, Togawa Y, et al. Erythema elevatum diutinum with primary Sjögren syndrome associated with IgA antineutrophil cytoplasmic antibody. *Br J Dermatol.* 2008;159:733-735.
26. Carlson JA, LeBoit PE. Localized chronic fibrosing vasculitis of the skin: an inflammatory reaction that occurs in settings other than erythema elevatum diutinum and granuloma faciale. *Am J Surg Pathol.* 1997;21:698-705.
27. Navarro R, de Argila D, Fraga J, et al. Erythema elevatum diutinum or extrafacial granuloma faciale? *Actas Dermosifiliogr.* 2010;101:814-815.
28. Kohler IK, Lorincz AL. Erythema elevatum diutinum treated with niacinamide and tetracycline. *Arch Dermatol.* 1980;116(6):693-695.
29. Henriksson R, Hofer PA, Hornqvist R. Erythema elevatum diutinum—a case successfully treated with colchicine. *Clin Exp Dermatol.* 1989;14(6):451-453.
30. Yıldız F, Karakaş T. Erythema elevatum diutinum coexisting with ankylosing spondylitis. *Eur J Rheumatol.* 2015;2(2):73-75.
31. Kint A, de Cuyper C. Erythema elevatum diutinum. *Hautarzt.* 1980;31(8):447-449.
32. Schumacher H, Carroll E, Taylor F, et al. Erythema elevatum diutinum: Cutaneous vasculitis, impaired clot lysis and response to phenformin. *J Rheumatol.* 1977;4(1):103-112.
33. Krrok G, Waldenström JG. Relapsing annular erythema and myeloma successfully treated with cyclophosphamide. *Acta Med Scand.* 1978;203(4):289-292.
34. Chow RK, Benny WB. Erythema elevatum diutinum associated with IgA paraproteinemia successfully controlled with intermittent plasma exchange. *Arch Dermatol.* 1996;132(11):1360-1364.
35. Delgado J, Gómez-Cerezo J, Sigüenza M, et al. Relapsing polychondritis and erythema elevatum diutinum: an unusual association refractory to dapsone. *J Rheumatol.* 2001;28(3):634-635.

Chapter 141 :: Adamantiades–Behçet Disease
:: Christos C. Zouboulis

第一百四十一章
白塞病

中文导读

白塞病（Adamantiades-Behçet）是一种病因不明的累及所有血管类型的系统性血管炎。本章节从历史视角、流行病学、病因和发病机制、临床特征、诊断、鉴别诊断、临床过程和预后、治疗及预防对该病进行了详细阐述。

1. 历史视角　该病以希腊眼科医师BenediktosAdamantiades和土耳其皮肤科医生HulûsiBehçet的名字命名，作者对该病的由来进行了介绍。

2. 流行病学　该病在全世界范围内的患病率不同，在东亚、中亚以及东地中海国家（沿所谓的丝绸之路）流行，作者详细介绍了该病在不同地区的患病情况。该病最常累及20多岁和30多岁患者，男女患病率的差异因不同地区存在区别，不同种族群体的青少年中发生率在2%至21%之间。

3. 病因和发病机制　该病的病因不明，与遗传因素、感染、环境污染、免疫学机制以及血管内皮和凝血因子有关，目前比较公认的观点是遗传因素和环境的触发下导致疾病的发生。

白塞病没有特定的孟德尔遗传模式。家族性发病具有地区差异，与患病父母相比，子女患病的时间更早，青少年的家族性发病率比成人高。

接下来作者对人类白细胞抗原-B51（HLA-B51）与该病之间的关联性以及新近关于GWAS研究和基因多态性研究的结果进行了综述，并提出相关基因的多态性可能会与疾病的易感性和/或疾病的严重性有关。

白塞病不具有传染性，但病毒和细菌感染与机体启动该病的免疫病理学途径有关，触发疾病的症状。

（1）病毒：主要介绍了单纯疱疹病毒1型（HSV-1）与该病的相关研究。

（2）细菌：该病的活动与细菌感染有关，作者主要介绍了链球菌感染与该病的相关性证据，并提及发酵支原体可能参与该病的发生。细菌感染在该病中的作用可能与Toll样受体2激活单核细胞有关。

（3）免疫机制：该疾病目前已归类于自身炎症性疾病中，主要与固有免疫系统的原发性功能障碍有关。

（4）自身免疫：在大多数疾病活动部位的主要微观变化是免疫介导的闭塞性血管炎。该疾病被认为是典型的Th1介导的炎症性疾病。新近的研究表明，Th17细胞和IL17/IL23途径可能在该病的发病机制中也起了重要作用。除了T细胞免疫缺陷外，B细胞激活也受到影响。

（5）热休克蛋白：介绍了热休克蛋白（HSP）与该病的研究进展。

（6）细胞因子：白塞病患者的血清中存

在各种促炎细胞因子，作者特别提出IL-8在该病中起着重要的作用，并且可作为疾病活动的敏感标志。

（7）血管内皮细胞：血管内皮是该病的主要靶器官，作者详细介绍了该病相关的血管内皮细胞研究进展。

（8）表观遗传学：对该病存在的甲基化异常、组蛋白修饰及miRNA的调控进行了简要描述。

4．临床特征　复发性口腔溃疡、复发性生殖器溃疡、皮肤表现、眼部病变以及关节炎是最常见的临床表现。对该病的少见表现也进行了介绍（图141-1），并指出该病可呈急性发作过程也可长期慢性存在，符合国际诊断标准即可确定诊断。

（1）皮肤黏膜损害：最常见的黏膜表现是复发性口腔溃疡和生殖器溃疡，作者对于这两种表现的发生率、具体特征、持续时间及预后进行了详细介绍。对该病具有诊断价值的皮肤表现主要包括脓疱性血管性病变（含针刺改变图141-4A）、结节性红斑样病变（图141-4B）、Sweet样病变、坏疽性脓皮病样病变和坏死性静脉炎的可触及紫癜性病变（图141-5）。提及目前存在用于标准化评估皮肤黏膜严重程度的皮肤黏膜活动指数，但尚未推广。

（2）系统损害：眼部受累是引起该病并发症的主要原因，最具诊断价值的病变是后葡萄膜炎（也称为视网膜血管炎），严重时可能导致失明（图141-6A）。对其他眼部表现及并发症进行了详细介绍。

特征性关节炎是非侵蚀性、不对称的无菌性血清阴性的单关节炎。作者建议必须排除HLA-B27阳性的侵蚀性关节炎。

系统性血管受累是该病的重要表现，包括静脉阻塞和静脉曲张、动脉阻塞和动脉瘤。其中大静脉血栓形成（下腔静脉、颅静脉窦）或大动脉瘤的情况可能致命。作者在该部分对该病的血管、心脏及肾脏受累情况进行了介绍。

接下来对胃肠道、神经系统及其他少见的系统受累表现及结局进行了详细介绍。

5．诊断　白塞病的诊断基于临床特征，按照国际标准进行诊断（表141-1）。

（1）组织病理学：白塞病的典型组织病理学特征是中性粒细胞血管炎和血栓形成（图141-5）。对该病的早期和晚期病理特点进行了介绍。

（2）特殊检查：针刺试验。介绍了针刺试验的操作方法和判读，及其他可解释为高反应性的广义的针刺试验阳性现象，但也指出针刺试验对于本病的诊断并不特异。

（3）影像学表现：在这一部分介绍了一些支持该病的特征性影像学表现。

6．鉴别诊断　请参阅表141-2。

7．临床过程和预后　白塞病的临床过程可轻可重。作者对该病的并发症及提示严重并发症的危险因素进行了介绍，并指出中枢神经系统、肺及大血管受累以及肠穿孔是威胁生命的主要并发症，免疫抑制治疗所致的并发症也可能导致死亡。

8．治疗　根据该病的临床表现部位和严重程度，提供了不同的治疗建议并介绍了治疗进展，对局部治疗抵抗的皮肤黏膜损害、系统受累以及预后不良的患者可考虑系统治疗，根据不同循证级别证据（表141-4和表141-5），可选择的药物包括系统使用糖皮质激素、免疫抑制药、秋水仙碱、氨苯砜、柳氮磺吡啶或干扰素-α单独或联合使用。

9．预防　作者建议患有严重或进行性复发性阿弗他口腔溃疡的患者应随访多年，怀疑患有白塞病的患者应及早转诊以获得专科医生意见。

〔黄莹雪〕

AT-A-GLANCE

- Rare disease with worldwide distribution but strongly varying prevalence; certain ethnic groups are mainly affected.
- A genetically determined disorder with a probable environmental triggering factor.
- Multisystem occurrence, with oral aphthous ulcers, genital ulcers, papulopustules, erythema nodosum–like lesions, uveitis, and arthropathy as the most common signs.
- Inflammatory disease representing a neutrophilic vascular reaction or vasculitis.
- Chronic, relapsing, and progressive course with a potentially poor prognosis (especially in males with systemic presenting signs; mortality, 0%-6%).

Adamantiades–Behçet disease is a multisystem inflammatory disease of unknown etiology. It is classified as a systemic vasculitis involving all types and sizes of blood vessels and characterized clinically by recurrent oral aphthous and genital ulcers, skin lesions, iridocyclitis/posterior uveitis, and arthritis. These findings are occasionally accompanied by vascular, GI, neurologic, or other manifestations.[1,2]

HISTORICAL ASPECTS

Hippocrates of Kos (460-377 BC) used the designation "στοματα αφθωδεα, ελκωδεα" (oral aphthous ulcers) in a probable first description of a patient with the disease (*Epidemion Book III*, Case 7). The disease is named after Benediktos Adamantiades, a Greek ophthalmologist and Hulûsi Behçet, a Turkish dermatologist, who, in 1931 and 1937, respectively, described patients with the characteristic clinical complex.[3] The first international multidisciplinary conference was organized by 2 dermatologists, Drs M. Monacelli and P. Nazarro, in 1964 in Rome, Italy.

EPIDEMIOLOGY

Adamantiades–Behçet disease occurs worldwide with varying prevalence, being endemic in the Eastern and Central Asian and the Eastern Mediterranean countries (along the so-called Silk Road) and rare in Northern European countries, Central and Southern Africa, the Americas, and Australia.[4] A prevalence of 80 to 420 patients per 100,000 inhabitants has been reported in Turkey,[5] 7 to 30 patients per 100,000 inhabitants in the rest of the Asian continent (Japan, 14-31:100,000; Korea, 35:100,000; Northern China, 14:100,000; Saudi Arabia, 20:100,000; Iran, 17:100,000), and 1.5 to 7.5 per 100,000 in Southern Europe.[4] In Northern Europe (0.27-1.18:100,000) and the United States (0.75:100,000), the disease is rare.[6,7] The increasing prevalence of the disease is due to its chronic nature.

Its annual incidence is low; 0.75 to 1.0 new cases per 100,000 inhabitants were assessed in Japan (1990) and Germany (2005).[6] Adamantiades–Behçet disease most often affects patients in their 20s and 30s; however, early and late onsets (first year of life to 72 years) have been reported. Juvenile disease rates are 2% to 21% in different ethnic groups. Its prevalence was estimated to be 0.17:100,000 in France.[8,9] In contrast to old Japanese and Turkish reports of male predominance, the male-to-female ratio drastically decreased in the last 20 years.[10] Currently, both genders are equally affected overall; however, male predominance is still observed in Arab populations, and female predominance is evident in Korea, China, some Northern European countries, and the United States.

ETIOLOGY AND PATHOGENESIS

The etiology of the disease remains unknown, although genetic factors, infectious agents, environmental pollution, immunologic mechanisms, and endothelial and clotting factors have been implicated and studied intensively.[1,2,11] The endemic occurrence along the historical Silk Road, the major involvement of certain ethnic groups (mostly of Turkmenic and Mongol descent), and associated immunogenetic data support the hypothesis that the disease followed the migration of these old nomadic tribes.[2,11] On the other hand, the wide variation of the disease prevalence in the same ethnic group in association with different geographic areas of residence indicates an additional environmental triggering factor. Therefore, transfer of genetic material and/or of an unknown exogenous agent may have been responsible for the expansion of the disease.[2,11]

GENETICS AND IMMUNOGENETICS

There is no specific mode of Mendelian transmission in Adamantiades–Behçet disease.[2,11-15] Familial occurrence with regional differences has been reported, being more frequent in Korea (15%) than in Japan or China (2%-3%), and in Arab countries, Israel, and Turkey (2%-18%) than in Europe (0%-5%).[4,13,14] An earlier disease onset in children compared with their parents, and a higher frequency of familial cases in juveniles than in adults, has been observed.[8,13,14]

A significant association exists between the disease and human leukocyte antigen-B_{51} (HLA-B_{51}) in Japan, the Middle East, and the Mediterranean countries; however, this relationship is not as strong in Western countries.[12,15,16] The allele also seems to be associated with a more severe prognosis and ocular involvement.[4,13,17] Its exact role in the disease mechanism is still unknown; however, it may be involved in the disease development through specific antigen presentation, molecular mimicry with microbial antigens, or participation in linkage disequilibrium with a presently unknown susceptibility gene.[14]

In an effort to explain the disease process, it has been suggested that Adamantiades–Behçet disease constitutes one of a newly termed group of diseases, the "MHC-I-opathies."[18] Recent work analyzing the peptidome of HLA-B_{51} suggests that altered peptide presentation by HLA-B_{51} is vital to the disease process. It is likely that (1) natural killer or other cell interactions, perhaps mediated by leucocyte immunoglobulin-like receptor or killer immunoglobulin-like receptor, are culpable in pathogenesis, or (2) HLA misfolding may lead directly to inflammation.

Among the 24 currently described alleles, HLA-B_{5101} and -B_{5108} have most frequently been associated with Adamantiades–Behçet disease.[19] Shared amino acid residues (defining the Bw4 epitope) are crucial for antigen binding and natural killer cell interactions,[20] and Bw_4 was also reported to contribute to the severity of the disease.[21] Genes possibly associated with the disease have been localized on chromosome 6 in the region between the *tumor necrosis factor* gene and *HLA-B* or *HLA-C* genes, including the *major histocompatibility complex class I chain A* gene (A6 allele) and genes for heat shock proteins.[14-17,19,22] In addition, a susceptibility locus mapped to 6p22-23 was detected.[19] Lately, associations on chromosomes 1p31.3 [interleukin (IL) 23R-IL12RB2] and 1q32.1 (IL10) were found by genomewide association studies.[20,23] A haplotype association of *IL-8* gene with Adamantiades–Behçet disease was also detected.[24] Polymorphisms in genes encoding for host effector molecules may contribute to the disease susceptibility and/or severity of the disease, such as in IL-23R reported in a Chinese Han population.[25] New gene associations with *ERAP-1*, *CCR1-CCR3*, *KLRC4*, and *STAT4* genes have been reported.[26]

INFECTIOUS PRECIPITANTS

Adamantiades–Behçet disease is not considered contagious as no horizontal transmission has ever been reported. However, viral and bacterial infections have been implicated in initiating immunopathologic pathways, leading to the onset of the disease.[2,11,27]

VIRAL AGENTS

Early theories of the pathogenesis of Adamantiades–Behçet disease proposed a viral or other infectious etiology.[11] Partial transcription of herpes simplex virus Type 1 (HSV-1) DNA in patients' peripheral blood lymphocytes was reported. HSV-1 DNA was detected in patients' saliva and oral and genital ulcers, and HSV-1 antibodies were found in patients' serum.

BACTERIAL AGENTS

The disease activity has been known to correlate with bacterial infection, particularly *Streptococci*.[11,27] *Streptococcus sanguinis* dominates the flora of the oral mucosa in patients with the disease and appears to be the most relevant *Streptococcus* strain as a provoking factor for initiation of the disease.[27] *Streptococcus* antigens and antistreptococcal antibodies are frequently found in the oral mucosa and serum of patients. The involvement of immunoglobulin A protease-producing *S. sanguinis* is proposed as an explanation for chronic infection leading to initiation of Adamantiades–Behçet disease. High titers of the immunogenic *S. sanguinis* antigen KTH-1 have been detected in patients. In addition, exposure of the patients to *Streptococcus* antigens may be a major provoking factor for disease activity. The lipoprotein of *Mycoplasma fermentans* MALP-404 was found in the serum of patients with Adamantiades–Behçet disease but not in healthy controls.[28] Interestingly, MALP-404 contains a peptide motif, which can be presented by HLA-B_{51}. A possible role for bacterial stimulation of monocytes via Toll-like receptor-2 producing neutrophil-stimulating proinflammatory factors in Adamantiades–Behçet disease was detected.[29]

IMMUNOLOGIC MECHANISMS

Immunologic mechanisms are considered to play a major role in the pathogenesis of Adamantiades–Behçet disease.[2,11,27] The disease has currently been classified among the autoinflammatory disorders,[30] which are caused by primary dysfunction of the innate immune system.

AUTOIMMUNE MECHANISMS

The major microscopic finding at most sites of active disease is an immune-mediated occlusive vasculitis. The pathergy reaction (see section "Clinical Findings") is induced by the rapid accumulation of neutrophils (hyperchemotaxis) and later by T lymphocytes and monocytes/macrophages at needle prick sites. The disease has been considered to be a typical Th1-mediated inflammatory disease, characterized by elevated levels of Th1 cytokines such as IFN-γ, IL-2, and TNF-α. Recently, some studies reported that Th17-associated cytokines were increased; thus, Th17 cells and the IL17/IL23 pathway may play important roles in the pathogenesis of Adamantiades–Behçet disease.[31] T cells in the peripheral blood and in the involved tissues are increased, and a predominant T helper 1 immune response induced by IL-12 has been demonstrated.[32] Patients' lymphocytes also express CD29 molecules and bind to endothelial cells in active disease. In addition to defective T-cell immunity, B-cell activation is impaired. Circulating immune complexes, together with enhanced neutrophil migration, may be involved; diversity of T cells indicates that specific T-cell responses to several antigens may lead to the variety of symptoms.[33] Tropomyosins and the 160-kDa polypeptide kinectin have been detected as autoantigens in Adamantiades–Behçet disease.[34,35]

HEAT SHOCK PROTEINS

Increased levels of heat shock protein (HSP)–specific antibodies in serum have been found in Adamantiades–Behçet disease.[36,37] T cells respond to 60-kDa HSP, and 4 different peptide determinants within 60-kDa HSP identified by T-cell epitope mapping have been suggested to be involved in the pathogenesis of the disease.

CYTOKINE MEDIATORS

Various proinflammatory cytokines, such as IL-1, -8, -12, -17, -23, and tumor necrosis factor-α, are elevated in the sera of patients with Adamantiades–Behçet disease.[38-42] In particular, IL-8 seems to play an important role, can also be released by endothelial cells, has a potent effect on the inflammatory response, and is a sensitive marker of disease activity.[38-40] Cytokine release may be dependent on the involved organ.[38,39,41]

ENDOTHELIAL CELLS

The endothelium seems to be the primary target; however, it may just be subject to the bizarre behavior of the immune system.[43] An immunoglobulin M-type, 47-kDa cell surface HSP against endothelial α-enolase was identified in the serum of patients with Adamantiades–Behçet disease.[44] Plasma endothelin-1 concentrations were found significantly increased, perhaps indicating vasoconstriction and being the direct result of elevated synthesis by injured vascular endothelial cells. Thrombomodulin, a cell surface glycoprotein of vascular endothelium, which is also increased in the plasma of patients with active disease, potentially damages the endothelial cells.

EPIGENETICS

Epigenetic studies on Adamantiades–Behçet disease have shown the role of alterations in the methylation level of interspersed repetitive sequence elements, histone modifications such as H3K4me27 and H3K4me3, upregulation of miR-182 and miR-3591-3p as well as downregulation of miR-155, miR-638, and miR-4488 in the pathogenesis of the disease.[45]

CLINICAL FINDINGS

Adamantiades–Behçet disease is a chronic, recurrent, multisystem, and, occasionally, life-threatening disorder.[1,2,4] Recurrent oral aphthous ulcers, recurrent genital ulcers, skin manifestations, ocular lesions, and arthritis/arthropathy are the most frequent clinical manifestations.[1,6] Vascular, GI, neurologic, psychiatric, pulmonary, renal, and cardiac manifestations; epididymitis; and other findings can also occur (Fig. 141-1). The clinical picture usually develops within a few months after the presenting sign; both an acute multisystem presentation and long-term development of the disease over the years are possible. The fulfillment of the International Diagnostic Criteria[46] supports the diagnosis.

MUCOCUTANEOUS LESIONS

Recurrent oral aphthous and genital ulcers are the most frequently observed mucosal manifestations. Oral aphthous ulcers are the presenting sign in more than 80% of the cases.[1,4,6] Although recurrent aphthous stomatitis is a common disorder, only a few patients progress to Adamantiades–Behçet disease, and it is not possible to determine in whom or when the transition may occur. Typically, lesions are multiple, painful, 1 to 3 cm in diameter, and sharply margined with a fibrin-coated base and surrounding erythema (Fig. 141-2). Oral aphthous ulcers usually heal without scarring (92%). Genital ulcers may not recur as often and usually heal with a characteristic scar (64%-88%; Fig. 141-3). Spontaneous healing of aphthae occurs within 4 days to 1 month; genital ulcers may persist longer. Large oral ulcerations can also be associated with problems such as pharyngeal involvement, dysphagia, and dyspnea or fistulae involving the pharynx, larynx, trachea, or esophagus. Genital ulcers can occur on the penis, scrotum, vagina, labia, and urethra, and also in the anal, perineal, and inguinal regions.

Skin lesions that should be accepted as diagnostically relevant in Adamantiades–Behçet disease should be confined to pustular vasculitic lesions (including pathergy lesions, see Fig. 141-4A), erythema nodosum–like lesions (Fig. 141-4B), Sweet-like lesions, pyoderma gangrenosum–like lesions, and palpable purpuric lesions of necrotizing venulitis (Fig. 141-5).[47-49] All of these lesions are characterized in their early stages by a neutrophilic vascular reaction.[48] Single acneiform lesions or follicle-based pustules should not be considered relevant.[50]

To standardize the evaluation of mucocutaneous severity, a Mucocutaneous Activity Index has currently been established.[51] This is a specific score that

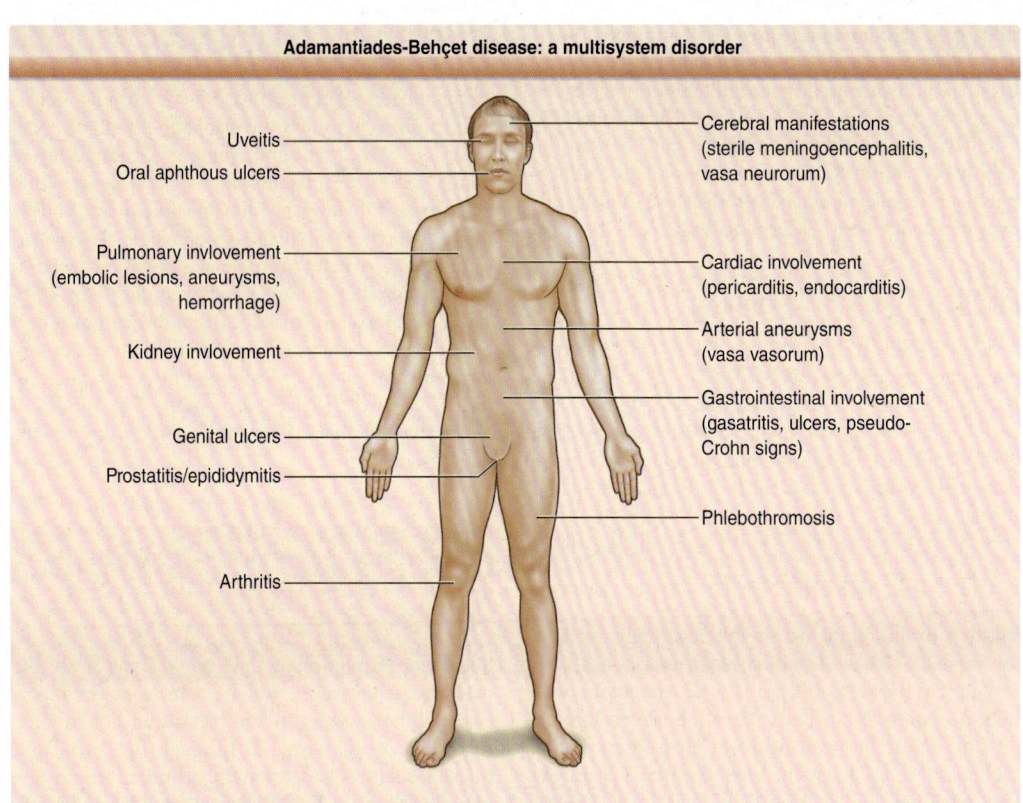

Figure 141-1 Adamantiades–Behçet disease: a multisystem disorder.

can help with therapeutic decisions and reduce morbidity; however, it still lacks validation.

SYSTEMIC LESIONS

Ocular involvement is the major cause of morbidity in patients with Adamantiades–Behçet disease. The most diagnostically relevant lesion is posterior uveitis (also called *retinal vasculitis*), which can lead to blindness (Fig. 141-6A). Other ocular lesions include anterior uveitis, hypopyon (pus in the anterior chamber of the eye, which is now—due to early treatment—uncommon; see Fig. 141-6B), and secondary complications such as cataract, glaucoma, and neovascular lesions.[52] Retinal inflammation can lead to vascular occlusion and, ultimately, tractional retinal detachment. Severe vitreous involvement, chronic cystoid macular edema, and

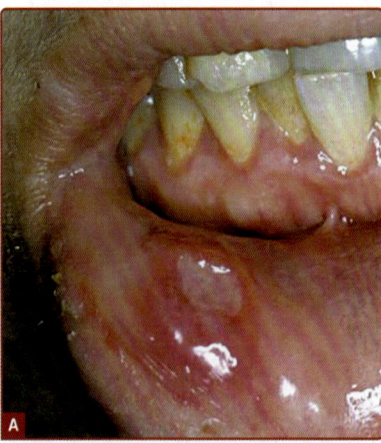
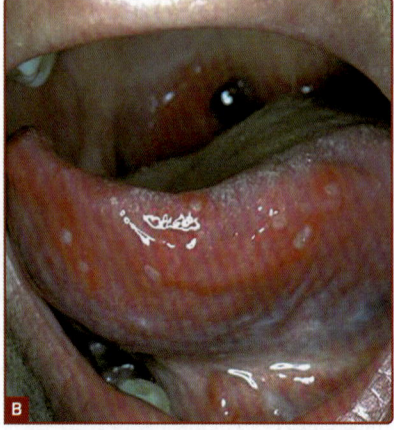

Figure 141-2 (**A**) Single and (**B**) multiple oral aphthous ulcers. (**A** from Altenburg A et al. Epidemiology and clinical manifestations of Adamantiades-Behçet disease in Germany—current pathogenetic concepts and therapeutic possibilities. *J Dtsch Dermatol Ges*. 2006;4:49, with permission. Copyright © 2006 John Wiley & Sons.)

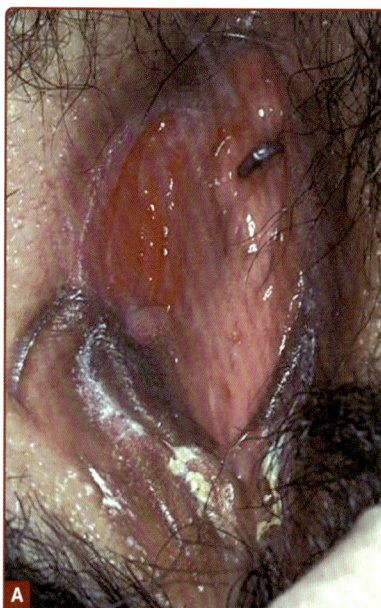

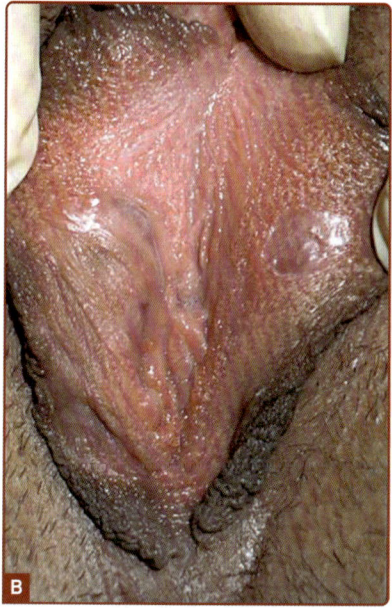

Figure 141-3 (**A**) Genital ulcer healing with (**B**) a demarcated flat scar.

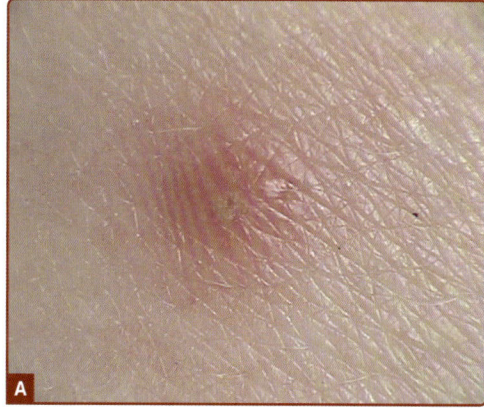

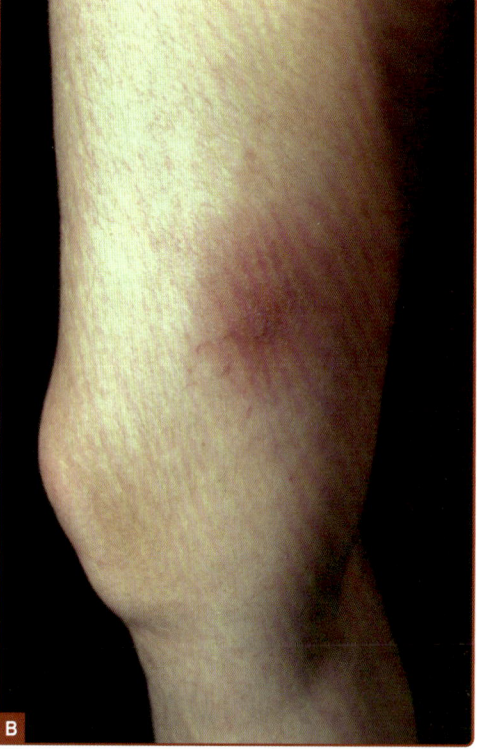

Figure 141-4 (**A**) Positive pathergy test and (**B**) erythema nodosum–like lesion in Adamantiades–Behçet disease.

possible—presumably also vasculitic—involvement of the optic nerve can result in vision loss.[53] Recurrent vasculitic changes can ultimately lead to ischemic optic nerve atrophy.

The characteristic arthritis is a nonerosive, asymmetric, sterile, seronegative oligoarthritis; however, symmetric polyarticular involvement is common. Joint manifestations frequently occur first in one knee or ankle and then the other as migratory monoarthritis, then in both joints simultaneously, and finally affecting nearly all joints.[1] An HLA-B27-positive, erosive sacroiliitis has to be excluded.

Systemic vascular involvement can be significant and includes venous occlusions and varices, arterial occlusions, and aneurysms, often being migratory. Cases of large-vein thrombosis (inferior vena cava, cranial venous sinuses) or large-artery aneurysms are potentially fatal.[1,2,4,6] Arterial involvement is rather rare and usually presents in the form of thromboses and, less often, of aneurysms, resulting from multicentric arteritis. Aneurysms may develop in large arteries as a result of vasculitis of the vasa vasorum with penetration of the lamina elastica. Pulmonary artery aneurysms are the principal feature of pulmonary involvement in Adamantiades–Behçet disease, occasionally resulting in coughing and hemoptysis. Cardiac involvement can

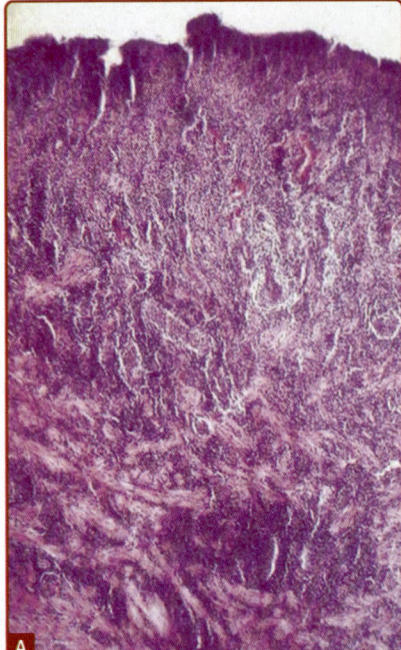

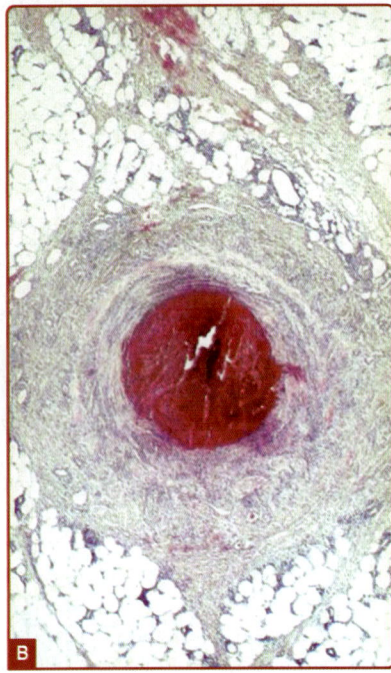

Figure 141-5 A, Abundant mixed inflammatory infiltrate dominated by neutrophils in an oral ulcer of Adamantiades–Behçet disease. **B,** Vessel thrombosis in an erythema nodosum–like lesion.

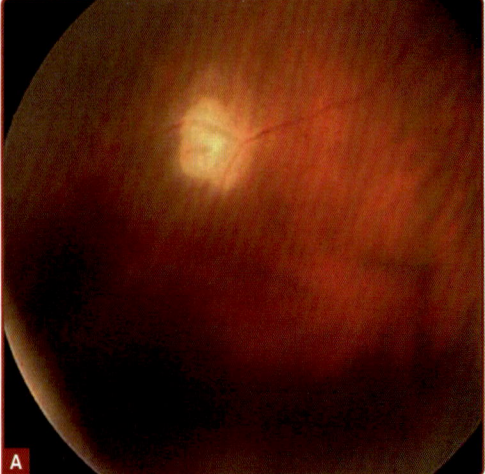

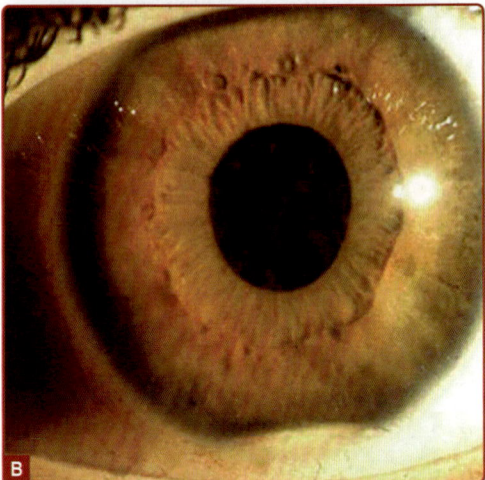

Figure 141-6 A, Posterior uveitis. **B,** Hypopyon iritis. (From Altenburg A et al. Epidemiology and clinical manifestations of Adamantiades-Behçet disease in Germany—current pathogenetic concepts and therapeutic possibilities. *J Dtsch Dermatol Ges*. 2006;4:49, with permission. Copyright © 2006 John Wiley & Sons.)

include myocarditis, coronary arteritis, endocarditis, and valvular disease. A wide spectrum of renal manifestations can occur, varying from minimal-change disease to proliferative glomerulonephritis and rapidly progressive crescentic glomerulonephritis. Immune complex deposition is thought to be responsible for the underlying pathogenesis of glomerulonephritis in some cases. Carotid plaques, pulse-wave velocity, and flow-mediated dilation represent clinical biomarkers of prognosis.[54]

GI complaints can be a symptom for aphthae throughout the GI tract and can rarely result in perforation and peritonitis (0.5%). On the other hand, GI involvement has an acute exacerbating course with ulcers, most commonly in the ileocolonic area.[55] These ulcers can be large and deep, causing perforation and massive bleeding. Inflammatory bowel disease has to be excluded.

Sterile prostatitis and epididymitis can be present in male patients without genital ulcers.[56] Significant neurologic manifestations occur in approximately 10% of patients and may be delayed in onset.[2,4,6] Meningoencephalitis, cerebral venous sinus thrombosis, benign intracranial hypertension, cranial nerve palsies, brainstem lesions, and pyramidal or extrapyramidal lesions have been described. Poor prognosis is associated with a progressive course, relapses after treatment, repeated attacks, and cerebellar symptoms or parenchymal disease. Neurologic manifestations usually present with severe headache. Further symptoms include gait disturbance, dysarthria, vertigo, and diplopia as well as hyperreflexia, epileptic seizures, hemiplegia, ataxia, or a positive Babinski reflex. Psychiatric symptoms, such as depression, insomnia, or memory impairment, are also signs of neurologic involvement.

DIAGNOSIS

The diagnosis of Adamantiades–Behçet disease is based on clinical signs, as pathognomonic laboratory tests or histologic characteristics are absent. There are several sets of diagnostic criteria with the current International Criteria[46] being the most accurate among them (Table 141-1).

HISTOPATHOLOGY

Characteristic histopathologic features of Adamantiades–Behçet disease are vasculitis and thrombosis (Fig. 141-5). Biopsies from early mucocutaneous lesions show a neutrophilic vascular reaction with endothelial swelling, extravasation of erythrocytes, and leukocytoclasia or a fully developed leukocytoclastic vasculitis with fibrinoid necrosis of blood vessel walls.[1,6] Although there are reports of lesions that consist primarily of a lymphocytic perivasculitis, most of these lesions are likely older. The neutrophilic vascular reaction should be considered the predominant histopathologic finding.[7,49,57]

TABLE 141-1
International Criteria for Behçet Disease[46]

SYMPTOM	POINTS
Ocular lesions (recurrent)	2
Oral aphthosis (recurrent)	2
Genital aphthosis (recurrent)	2
Skin lesions (recurrent)	1
CNS	1
Vascular manifestations	1
Positive pathergy test[b]	1

[a]BCD scoring: score ≥4 indicates Adamantiades–Behçet disease.
[b]Though the main scoring system does not require the pathergy test, if it *is* conducted, a positive result may be included for 1 extra point.

SPECIAL TESTS

PATHERGY TEST

A positive pathergy test (hyperreactivity reaction) manifests within 48 hours as an erythematous papule (>2 mm) or pustule at the site of a skin needle prick or after intracutaneous injection of 0.1-mL isotonic saline using a 20-gauge needle without prior disinfection of the injection site (Fig. 141-4A). The skin prick is generally placed at an angle of 45°, 3 to 5 mm intracutaneously on the volar forearm. Erythema without infiltration is considered a negative finding. Provoked oral aphthae and genital ulcers after injection or injury (such as chorioretinitis in the corneal region of the eye after photocoagulation of the ocular fundus region) can also be considered as positive pathergy phenomenon. Broader pathergy phenomena also include the occurrence of aneurysms around vascular anastomoses as well as local recurrence of ulcers after resection of affected bowel segments. Although a positive pathergy reaction is a sign of Adamantiades–Behçet disease, it is not pathognomic, as it can also occur in patients with pyoderma gangrenosum, rheumatoid arthritis, Crohn disease, and genital herpes infection.

RADIOLOGIC FINDINGS

Scintigraphic evidence of arthritis is found in 50% of the patients.[6] Cranial MRI allows documentation of hypodense or atrophic changes in the brain. Electroencephalographic detection of diffuse α-waves is considered a positive finding. Vascular lesions can be detected by angiography. Because of the rarity of disease, documentation of characteristic imaging can be supportive for the diagnosis.[58]

DIFFERENTIAL DIAGNOSIS

Refer to Table 141-2.[6,59]

CLINICAL COURSE AND PROGNOSIS

The clinical course of Adamantiades–Behçet disease is variable. There can be a delay of up to several years before the diagnosis is made, and this may influence the prognosis. Mucocutaneous and joint manifestations usually occur first. Recurrent erythema nodosum and $HLAB_{51}$ positivity are risk factors for the development of superficial thrombophlebitis and vision loss,[4,13,53] and superficial thrombophlebitis, ocular lesions, and male gender are risk factors for the development of systemic vessel involvement.[4,13,56,60] A severe course, including blindness, meningoencephalitis, hemoptysis, intestinal perforation, and severe

TABLE 141-2
Differential Diagnosis of Adamantiades–Behçet Disease[6,50]

- Oculocutaneous/mucocutaneous syndromes
  - Erythema multiforme exudativum and variants, including Stevens–Johnson syndrome
  - Vogt–Koyanagi–Harada syndrome
  - Reiter disease
  - Bullous autoimmune diseases: Pemphigus vulgaris, cicatricial mucous membrane pemphigoid, epidermolysis bullosa acquisita
  - Viral infections (herpes, coxsackie, echo)
  - Syphilis
- Articulomucocutaneous syndromes
  - Systemic lupus erythematosus
  - MAGIC syndrome (mouth and genital ulcers with inflamed cartilage)
  - Yersiniosis
  - Arthropathic psoriasis
- GI/mucocutaneous syndromes
  - Ulcerative colitis, Crohn disease
  - Tuberculosis
  - Bowel-associated dermatitis-arthritis syndrome
- Aphthae
  - Recurrent aphthous stomatitis (RAS)
  - Cyclic neutropenia
  - Herpes simplex infection
- Genital ulcers
  - Ulcus vulvae acutum (Lipschütz ulcer)
  - Herpes simplex infection
  - Sexually transmitted infections
- Uveitis
  - Other forms of uveitis
- Arthritis
  - Ankylosing spondylitis
  - Juvenile rheumatoid arthritis
- CNS manifestation
  - Multiple sclerosis
  - Neuro-Sweet disease
- Lung manifestation
  - Sarcoidosis

arthritis, occurs in approximately 10% of patients. Blindness often can be prevented with early aggressive therapy of posterior uveitis. Lethal outcome has been seen in 0 to 6% of affected patients in different ethnic groups. CNS and pulmonary and large vessel involvement, as well as bowel perforation, are the major life-threatening complications; death may also result as a complication of immunosuppressive therapy. Markers of severe prognosis include HLA-B_{51} positivity, male gender, and early development of systemic signs.[4] Indeed, there is an association of male gender with ocular involvement, vascular involvement, superficial and deep venous thrombosis, cardiac involvement, folliculitis, and papulopustular lesions, whereas females present more often genital ulcers, erythema nodosum, and joint involvement.[56] Onset in childhood does not necessarily predict a poor prognosis.[8] Spontaneous remissions of certain or all manifestations of the disease have been observed. Ophthalmic and neurologic sequelae are leading causes of morbidity, followed by severe vascular and GI manifestations, and their effects on morbidity may be cumulative.

TREATMENT

The choice of treatment for patients with Adamantiades–Behçet disease depends on the site and severity of the clinical manifestations of the disease. Recurrent aphthae are most often treated with palliative agents, such as mild diet, avoidance of irritating agents, and potent topical glucocorticoids and local anesthetics[61-63]; recently, topical hyaluronic acid 0.2% gel 2 times a day over 30 days was found effective[64] (Table 141-3). For the topical treatment of genital ulcers and skin lesions, corticosteroid and antiseptic creams can be applied for up to 7 days. Painful genital ulcerations can be managed by topical anesthetics in cream. Corticosteroid injections (triamcinolone acetonide, 0.1-0.5 mL/lesion) can be helpful in recalcitrant ulcerations. They can also be beneficial on panuveitis and cystoid macular edema as a single intravitreal injection (triamcinolone acetonide 4 mg).[65,66]

Patients with mucocutaneous lesions resistant to topical treatment, those with systemic involvement, and patients with markers of poor prognosis are

TABLE 141-3
Topical Treatment of Oral Aphthous Ulcers[63]

- Mild diet
- Avoidance of hard, spicy, or salty nutrients and irritating chemicals, such as toasted bread, nuts, oranges, lemons, tomatoes, spices (pepper, paprika, curry), alcohol- or CO_2-containing drinks, mouthwashes, toothpastes containing sodium lauryl sulfate[a]
- Topical treatment of the aphthous oral ulcers includes:
  - Caustic solutions (silver nitrate, 1%-2%; tinctura myrrha, 5%-10% weight/volume; H_2O_2, 0.5%; methyl violet, 0.5%) 1-2 times a day
  - Antiseptic and anti-inflammatory preparations (amlexanox, 5% in oral paste[a]; triclosan, 0.1% mouthwash solution and in toothpastes[a]; amyloglucosidase- and glucoseoxidase-containing toothpastes[a]; hexetidine, 1%, chlorhexidine, 1%-2% mouthwash solutions; benzydamine; camomile extracts); 3% diclofenac in 2.5% hyaluronic acid[a]; hyaluronic acid 0.2% gel; tetracycline mouthwash (as glycerine solution 250 mg/5 mL glycerine) 2 min 4-6 times a day[a] (caveat: pregnancy); doxycycline in isobutylcyanoacrylate[a]
  - Corticosteroids (triamcinolone mucosal ointment, dexamethasone mucosal paste, betamethasone pastilles) 4 times a day or during the night (ointment/paste) or intrafocal infiltrations with triamcinolone suspension 0.1-0.5 mL per lesion
  - Anesthetics (lidocaine, 2%-5%; mepivacaine, 1.5%; tetracaine, 0.5%-1% gels or mucosal ointments) 2-3 times a day (caveat: allergy)
  - 5-Aminosalicylic acid (5% cream) 3 times a day (reduces the duration of lesions and the pain intensity)
  - Cyclosporine A, 500 mg solution for mouthwash 3 times a day (effective as topical immunosuppressive drug)
  - Sucralfate suspension, 5 mL × 4 times a day[a] (for oral aphthous and genital ulcers)
  - A close association of smoking with a decrease of recurrences of oral aphthous ulcers has been described.

[a]Small, randomized, double-blind, placebo-controlled trial against placebo.

candidates for systemic treatment.[61-63,67-69] Several compounds have been found effective in randomized, double-blind, placebo-controlled trials[70-90] (Table 141-4). Additional treatments have been successful in studies with a lower grade of evidence (Table 141-5).[2,16,48,71-83] Oral and intravenous prednisolone can be combined with other immunosuppressants, colchicine, dapsone, sulfasalazine, or interferon-α. A synergistic effect with cyclosporine A has been described in patients with ocular involvement. Prednisolone is one of the few medications that can be used during pregnancy. Colchicine can be combined with immunosuppressants and interferon-α. A rapid relapse often occurs after discontinuing cyclosporine A, interferon-α, dapsone, or infliximab.[73,76,78]

PREVENTION

- Patients with severe or progressive recurrent aphthous stomatitis should be followed up for years as potential candidates for Adamantiades–Behçet disease, particularly those patients with familial occurrence of the disease.
- Patients with suspected Adamantiades–Behçet disease should be referred early for specialist advice.
- Male patients with systemic involvement as a presenting sign and/or an early age of onset should be treated systemically because of the poor prognosis.

TABLE 141-4
Studied Systemic Treatments of Adamantiades–Behçet Disease[a]

DRUG	DOSE	INDICATION	REF.
Methylprednisolone	40 mg every 3 wk IM	Erythema nodosum (but not orogenital ulcers)	70
Rebamipide	300 mg/d orally (caveat: pregnancy, lactation)	Oral ulcers	71
Colchicine	1-2 mg/d orally (caveat: pregnancy, lactation—induces oligozoospermia)	Oral aphthous ulcers, genital ulcers, folliculitis, erythema nodosum	72
	1.5 mg/d	Erythema nodosum, arthritis, genital ulcers, (oral ulcers in females)	73
		Ineffective	74
Dapsone	100 mg/d orally (caveat: pregnancy, lactation—methemoglobin increase: ascorbic acid, 500 mg/d)	Oral ulcers, genital ulcers, skin lesions, pathergy test	75
Azathioprine	2.5 mg/kg/d (caveat: pregnancy, lactation, severe liver disease, bone marrow depression, severe infection, children)	Recent-onset ocular disease	76
Interferon-α 2a	6×10^6 IU 3 times a week SC (caveat: pregnancy, lactation—induces psychotic signs, psoriasis, myopathy)	Oral ulcers, genital ulcers, papulopustular lesions	77
Interferon-α	1000 and 2000 IU/d orally	Ineffective	78
Thalidomide	100 or 300 mg/d (caveat: pregnancy, lactation—induces polyneuropathy: minimized at 25 mg/d)	Oral ulcers, genital ulcers, papulopustular lesions	79
Cyclosporine A	10 mg/kg/d orally (against colchicine, 1 mg/d orally) (caveat: lactation, renal insufficiency—induces pathologic CNS findings)	Ocular manifestations, oral ulcers, skin lesions, genital ulcers	80
	5 mg/kg/d orally (against cyclophosphamide pulses)	Visual acuity	81
	5 mg/d orally (against conventional treatment)	Ocular attacks	82
Adalimumab	80 mg SC (initial dose), 40 mg SC every other week starting 1 wk after the initial dose	Intermediate uveitis, posterior uveitis and panuveitis	83,84
Daclizumab	1 mg/kg BW IV every 2 wk	Ineffective	85
Etanercept	25 mg 2 times a week orally (caveat: pregnancy, lactation)	Oral ulcers, nodular lesions, papulopustular lesions (not pathergy test)	86
Secukinumab	300 mg SC every 2 wk	Ineffective	87
Apremilast	30 mg 2 times a day orally over 12 wk	Oral ulcers	88
Aciclovir	5×800 mg for 1 wk + 2×400 mg/d for 11 wk	Ineffective	89
Azapropazone	900 mg/d over 3 wk orally	Arthritis, ineffective	90

[a]Evidence grade A—randomized, double-blind, placebo-controlled trials except otherwise mentioned.

TABLE 141-5
Other Systemic Treatments of Adamantiades-Behçet Disease[a]

DRUG	DOSE	INDICATION
Corticosteroids	5-60 mg/d prednisolone equivalent orally 100-1000 mg/d IV over 1-3 d (alone or in combination) (caveat: diabetes —induce psychosis)	Active disease Acute exacerbation (particularly uveitis, neurologic manifestations)
Indomethacin	100 mg/d PO	mucocutaneous lesions, arthritis
Pentoxifylline Oxpentifylline	300 mg × 1-3/d PO 400 mg × 3/d PO	oral ulcers (particularly in children)
Irsoglandine	2-4 mg/d PO	Recurrent oral ulcers
Cyclosporin A	3-6 mg/kg/d PO (serum levels: 100-150 ng/mL) (caveat: lactation, renal insufficiency—induces pathologic CNS findings)	Uveitis, mucocutaneous signs, thrombophlebitis, acute hearing loss
Tacrolimus	0.05-0.2 mg/kg/d PO (serum levels: 15-25 ng/mL)	Refractory uveitis
Interferon-α	9×10^6 IU 3 times a week / $3-9 \times 10^6$ IU 5 times a week SC (3×10^6 IU 3 times a week maintenance dose) (caveat: pregnancy, lactation—induces psychotic signs, psoriasis, myopathy) $1.5-3 \times 10^6$ IU 3 times a week according to body weight	Ocular lesions, long-term visual prognosis, arthritis, vascular lesions Corticodependent uveitis in children
Cyclophosphamide	1 g/mo IV bolus (caveat: hemorrhagic cystitis: mesna 200 mg)	Uveitis, neurologic manifestations
Chlorambucil	0.1 mg/d orally (2 mg/d maintenance dose) (caveat: cumulative toxicity)	Neurologic manifestations, uveitis, thrombosis, mucocutaneous lesions
Methotrexate	7.5-20 mg once a week orally (caveat: pregnancy, lactation, severe bone marrow depression, liver dysfunction, acute infections, GI ulcers, kidney insufficiency)	Severe mucocutaneous lesions, arthritis, progressive psychosis or dementia
Infliximab	5 mg/kg IV days 1, 7, 14, 28 or days 1, 14 / 1, 30 / 1, 45 (caveat: pregnancy, lactation)	Acute uveitis, refractory posterior uveitis, neurologic manifestations, intestinal involvement, vascular involvement
Adalimumab		Refractory ocular lesions, GI lesions
Anakinra	100 mg/d SC; escalation to 200 mg/d after 1 mo and 300 mg/d after 6 mo in partial responders (caveat: mild infections)	Oral ulcers, ocular lesions
Canakinumab		Ocular lesions
Gevokizumab	30 or 60 mg once in 4 wk IV or SC (on top of a stable immunosuppressive regimen).	Ocular lesions
Ustekinumab	90 mg SC at weeks 0, 4, and every 12 wk (caveat: headache)	oral ulcers
Alemtuzumab	12 mg/d IV (caveat: infusion reactions, onset of symptomatic thyroid disease)	Ocular lesions
Allicin	20 mg 3 times a day orally over 12 wk (caveat: unpleasant smell, nausea, vomiting, abdominal pain, allergic reaction)	Oral ulcers, skin lesions
Sulfasalazine	1.5-3 g/d orally	GI ulcers
Thalidomide	2 mg/kg/d orally; increased to 3 mg/kg/d if necessary or decreased to 1-0.5 mg/kg/d according to the response (caveat: neurotoxicity)	Intestinal involvement (in children)

[a]Evidence grade B—well-conducted open clinical trial.

REFERENCES

1. Davatchi F, Chams-Davatchi C, Shams H, et al. Behçet's disease: epidemiology, clinical manifestations, and diagnosis. *Expert Rev Clin Immunol.* 2017;13(1):57-65.
2. Alpsoy E. Behçet's disease: a comprehensive review with a focus on epidemiology, etiology and clinical features, and management of mucocutaneous lesions. *J Dermatol.* 2016;43(6):620-632.
3. Zouboulis CC, Keitel W. A Historical review of early descriptions of Adamantiades-Behçet's disease. *J Invest Dermatol.* 2002;119(1):201-205.
4. Zouboulis CC. Epidemiology of Adamantiades-Behçet's disease. In: Zierhut M, Ohno S, eds. *Immunology of Behçet's Disease.* Lisse, PA: Swets & Zeitlinger; 2003:1.
5. Azizlerli G, Koese AK, Sarica R, et al. Prevalence of Behçet's disease in Istanbul, Turkey. *Int J Dermatol.* 2003;42(10):803-806.
6. Altenburg A, Mahr A, Maldini C, et al. Epidemiology and clinical aspects of Adamantiades-Behçet disease in Germany [in German]. Current data. *Ophthalmologe.* 2012;109(6):531-541.
7. Wessman LL, Andersen LK, Davis MDP. Incidence of diseases primarily affecting the skin by age group:

7. population-based epidemiologic study in Olmsted County, Minnesota, and comparison with age-specific incidence rates worldwide [published online ahead of print January 29, 2018]. *Int J Dermatol.* doi:10.1111/ijd.13904.
8. Vaiopoulos AG, Kanakis MA, Kapsimali V, et al. Juvenile Adamantiades-Behçet disease. *Dermatology.* 2016;232(2):129-136.
9. Koné-Paut I. Behçet's disease in children, an overview. *Pediatr Rheumatol Online J.* 2016;14(1):10.
10. Kim DY, Choi MJ, Cho S, et al. Changing clinical expression of Behçet disease in Korea during three decades (1983–2012): chronological analysis of 3674 hospital-based patients. *Br J Dermatol.* 2014;170(2):458-461.
11. Zouboulis CC, May T. Pathogenesis of Adamantiades-Behçet's disease. *Adv Exp Med Biol.* 2003;528:161-171.
12. Durrani K, Papaliodis GN. The genetics of Adamantiades-Behcet's disease. *Semin Ophthalmol.* 2008;23(1):73-79.
13. Zouboulis CC, Turnbull JR, Martus P. Univariate and multivariate analyses comparing demographic, genetic, clinical, and serological risk factors for severe Adamantiades-Behçet's disease. *Adv Exp Med Biol.* 2003;528:123-126.
14. Morton LT, Situnayake D, Wallace GR. Genetics of Behçet's disease. *Curr Opin Rheumatol.* 2016;28(1):39-44.
15. Fietta P. Behçet's disease: familial clustering and immunogenetics. *Clin Exp Rheumatol.* 2005;23(suppl 38):S96.
16. de Menthon M, Lavalley MP, Maldini C, et al. HLA-B51/B5 and the risk of Behçet's disease: a systematic review and meta-analysis of case-control genetic association studies. *Arthritis Rheum.* 2009;61(10):1287-1296.
17. Horie Y, Meguro A, Ohta T, et al. HLA-B51 carriers are susceptible to ocular symptoms of Behçet disease and the association between the two becomes stronger towards the east along the Silk Road: a literature survey. *Ocul Immunol Inflamm.* 2017;25(1):37-40.
18. Giza M, Koftori D, Chen L, et al. Is Behçet's disease a "class 1-opathy"? The role of HLA-B*51 in the pathogenesis of Behçet's disease. *Clin Exp Immunol.* 2018;191(1):11-18.
19. Zierhut M, Mizuki N, Ohno S, et al. Immunology and functional genomics of Behçet's disease. *Cell Mol Life Sci.* 2003;60(9):1903-1922.
20. Remmers EF, Cosan F, Kirino Y, et al. Genome-wide association study identifies variants in the MHC class I, IL10, and IL23R-IL12RB2 regions associated with Behçet's disease. *Nat Genet.* 2010;42(8):698-702.
21. Papoutsis N, Bonitsis N, Altenburg A, et al. HLA-antigens and their importance as prognostic-marker in Adamantiades-Behçet's disease (ABD)—Is HLA-Bw4 a new prognostic marker? Abstracts of the 14th International Conference on Behçet's disease, London, UK, 2010:163.
22. Escudier M, Bagan J, Scully C. Behçet's disease (Adamantiades syndrome). *Oral Dis.* 2006;12(2):78-84.
23. Mizuki N, Meguro A, Ota M, et al. Genome-wide association studies identify IL23R-IL12RB2 and IL10 as Behçet's disease susceptibility loci. *Nat Genet.* 2010;42(8):703-706.
24. Lee EB, Kim JY, Zhao J, et al. Haplotype association of IL-8 gene with Behcet's disease. *Tissue Antigens.* 2007;69(2):128-132.
25. Jiang Z, Yang P, Hou S, et al. IL-23R gene confers susceptibility to Behcet's disease in a Chinese Han population. *Ann Rheum Dis.* 2010;69(7):1325-1328.
26. Hatemi G, Seyahi E, Fresko I, et al. Behçet's syndrome: a critical digest of the 2012–2013 literature. *Clin Exp Rheumatol.* 2013;31(3)(suppl 77):108-117.
27. Kaneko F, Tojo M, Sato M, et al. The role of infectious agents in the pathogenesis of Behçet's disease. *Adv Exp Med Biol.* 2003;528:181-183.
28. Zouboulis CC, Turnbull JR, Mühlradt PF. High seroprevalence of anti-Mycoplasma fermentans antibodies in patients with malignant aphthosis. *J Invest Dermatol.* 2003;121(1):211-212.
29. Neves FS, Carrasco S, Goldenstein-Schainberg C, et al. Neutrophil hyperchemotaxis in Behçet's disease: a possible role for monocytes orchestrating bacterial-induced innate immune responses. *Clin Rheumatol.* 2009;28(12):1403-1410.
30. Gül A. Behçet's disease as an autoinflammatory disorder. *Curr Drug Targets Inflamm Allergy.* 2005;4(1):81-83.
31. Nanke Y, Yago T, Kotake S. The role of Th17 cells in the pathogenesis of Behçet's disease. *J Clin Med.* 2017;6(7):E74.
32. Yanagihori H, Oyama N, Nakamura K, et al. Role of IL-12B promoter polymorphism in Adamantiades-Behçet's disease susceptibility: an involvement of Th1 immunoreactivity against *Streptococcus sanguinis* antigen. *J Invest Dermatol.* 2006;126(7):1534-1540.
33. Freysdottir J, Hussain L, Farmer I, et al. Diversity of γδ T cells in patients with Behçet's disease is indicative of polyclonal activation. *Oral Dis.* 2006;12(3):271-277.
34. Mahesh SP, Li Z, Buggage R, et al. Alpha tropomyosin as a self-antigen in patients with Behçet's disease. *Clin Exp Immunol.* 2005;140(2):368-375.
35. Lu Y, Ye P, Chen SL, et al. Identification of kinectin as a novel Behçet's disease autoantigen. *Arthritis Res Ther.* 2005;7(5):R1133-R1139.
36. Direskeneli H, Saruhan-Direskeneli G. The role of heat shock proteins in Behçet's disease. *Clin Exp Rheumatol.* 2003;21(4)(suppl 30):S44-S48.
37. Birtas-Atesoglu E, Inanc N, Yavuz S, et al. Serum levels of free heat shock protein 70 and anti-HSP70 are elevated in Behçet's disease. *Clin Exp Rheumatol.* 2008;26(suppl 50):S96-S98.
38. Katsantonis J, Adler Y, Orfanos CE, et al. Adamantiades-Behçet's disease: serum IL-8 is a more reliable marker for disease activity than C-reactive protein and erythrocyte sedimentation rate. *Dermatology.* 2000;201(1):37-39.
39. Durmazlar SP, Ulkar GB, Eskioglu F, et al. Significance of serum interleukin-8 levels in patients with Behcet's disease: high levels may indicate vascular involvement. *Int J Dermatol.* 2009;48(3):259-264.
40. Polat M, Vahaboglu G, Onde U, et al. Classifying patients with Behçet's disease for disease severity, using a discriminating analysis method. *Clin Exp Dermatol.* 2009;34(2):151-155.
41. Chi W, Zhu X, Yang P, et al. Upregulated IL-23 and IL-17 in Behcet patients with active uveitis. *Invest Ophthalmol Vis Sci.* 2008;49(7):3058-3064.
42. Habibagahi Z, Habibagahi M, Heidari M. Raised concentration of soluble form of vascular endothelial cadherin and IL-23 in sera of patients with Behçet's disease. *Mod Rheumatol.* 2010;20(2):154-159.
43. Kalayciyan A, Zouboulis CC. An update on Behçet's disease. *J Eur Acad Dermatol Venereol.* 2007;21(1):1-10.
44. Lee KH, Chung HS, Kim HS, et al. Human alpha-enolase from endothelial cells as a target antigen of anti-endothelial cell antibody in Behçet's disease. *Arthritis Rheum.* 2003;48(7):2025-2035.

45. Alipour S, Nouri M, Sakhinia E, et al. Epigenetic alterations in chronic disease focusing on Behçet's disease: review. *Biomed Pharmacother.* 2017;91:526-533.
46. International Team for the Revision of the International Criteria for Behçet's Disease (ITR-ICBD). The International Criteria for Behçet's Disease (ICBD): a collaborative study of 27 countries on the sensitivity and specificity of the new criteria. *J Eur Acad Dermatol Venereol.* 2014;28(3):338-347.
47. Kienbaum S, Zouboulis CC, Waibel M, et al. Papulopustular skin lesions in Adamantiades-Behçet's disease show a similar histopathological pattern as the classical mucocutaneous manifestations. In: Wechsler B, Godeau P, eds. *Behçet's disease, International Congress Series 1037.* Amsterdam: Excerpta Medica; 1993:331.
48. Oh SH, Han EC, Lee JH, et al. Comparison of the clinical features of recurrent aphthous stomatitis and Behçet's disease. *Clin Exp Dermatol.* 2009;34(6):e208-e212.
49. Jorizzo JL, Abernethy JL, White WL, et al. Mucocutaneous criteria for the diagnosis of Behçet's disease: an analysis of clinicopathologic data from multiple international centers. *J Am Acad Dermatol.* 1995;32(6):968-976.
50. Rogers RS 3rd. Pseudo-Behçet's disease. *Dermatol Clin.* 2003;21(1):49-69.
51. Scherrer MAR, Rocha VB, Garcia LC. Behçet's disease: review with emphasis on dermatological aspects. *An Bras Dermatol.* 2017;92(4):452-464.
52. Krause L, Köhler AK, Altenburg A, et al. Ocular involvement in Adamantiades-Behçet's disease in Berlin, Germany. *Graefes Arch Clin Exp Ophthalmol.* 2009;247(5):661-666.
53. Sakamoto M, Akazawa K, Nishioka Y, et al. Prognostic factors of vision in patients with Behçet disease. *Ophthalmology.* 1995;102(2):317-321.
54. Protogerou AD, Nasothimiou EG, Sfikakis PP, et al. Non-invasive vascular biomarkers in patients with Behçet's disease: review of the data and future perspectives. *Clin Exp Rheumatol.* 2017;35(suppl 108):100-107.
55. Hatemi I, Hatemi G, Çelik AF. Gastrointestinal involvement in Behçet disease. *Rheum Dis Clin North Am.* 2018;44(1):45-64.
56. Bonitsis NG, Luong Nguyen LB, LaValley MP, et al. Gender-specific differences in Adamantiades-Behçet's disease manifestations: an analysis of the German registry and meta-analysis of data from the literature. *Rheumatology (Oxford).* 2015;54(1):121-133.
57. Kienbaum S. Chemotactic neutrophilic vasculitis: a new histopathological pattern of vasculitis found in mucocutaneous lesions of patients with Adamantiades-Behçet's disease. In: Wechsler B, Godeau P, eds. *Behçet's disease, International Congress Series 1037.* Amsterdam: Excerpta Medica; 1993:337.
58. Mehdipoor G, Davatchi F, Ghoreishian H, et al. Imaging manifestations of Behçet's disease: key considerations and major features. *Eur J Radiol.* 2018;98:214-225.
59. Kaneko F, Togashi A, Nomura E, Nakamura K. Behçet's disease and diseases for its differential diagnosis in dermatology. An annual report of the Behçet's Disease Research Committee of Japan, 1999;128.
60. Coskun B, Öztürk P, Saral Y. Are erythema nodosum-like lesions and superficial thrombophlebitis prodromal in terms of visceral involvement in Behçet's disease? *Int J Clin Pract.* 2005;59(1):69-71.
61. Zouboulis CC. Adamantiades-Behçet's disease. In: Katsambas AD, Lotti TM, Dessinioti C, et al, eds. *European Handbook of Dermatological Treatments.* 3rd ed. New York: Springer; 2015:33.
62. Bonitsis NG, Altenburg A, Krause L, et al. Current concepts in the treatment of Adamantiades-Behçet's disease. *Drugs Future.* 2009;34:749.
63. Altenburg A, El-Haj N, Micheli C, et al. The treatment of chronically recurring aphthous mouth ulcers. *Dtsch Arztebl Int.* 2014;111:665-673.
64. Lee JH, Jung JY, Bang D. The efficacy of topical 0.2% hyaluronic acid gel on recurrent oral ulcers: comparison between recurrent aphthous ulcers and the oral ulcers of Behçet's disease. *J Eur Acad Dermatol Venereol.* 2008;22(5):590-595.
65. Atmaca LS, Yalçindağ FN, Ozdemir O. Intravitreal triamcinolone acetonide in the management of cystoid macular edema in Behçet's disease. *Graefes Arch Clin Exp Ophthalmol.* 2007;245(3):451-456.
66. Tuncer S, Yilmaz S, Urgancioglu M, et al. Results of intravitreal triamcinolone acetonide (IVTA) injection for the treatment of panuveitis attacks in patients with Behçet disease. *J Ocul Pharmacol Ther.* 2007;23(4):395-401.
67. Pipitone N, Olivieri I, Cantini F, et al. New approaches in the treatment of Adamantiades-Behçet's disease. *Curr Opin Rheumatol.* 2006;18(1):3-9.
68. Hatemi G, Silman A, Bang D, et al. Management of Behçet disease: a systematic literature review for the European League Against Rheumatism evidence-based recommendations for the management of Behçet disease. *Ann Rheum Dis.* 2009;68(10):1528-1534.
69. Sota J, Rigante D, Lopalco G, et al. Biological therapies for the treatment of Behçet's disease-related uveitis beyond TNF-alpha blockade: a narrative review. *Rheumatol Int.* 2018;38(1):25-35.
70. Mat C, Yurdakul S, Uysal S, et al. A double-blind trial of depot corticosteroids in Behçet's syndrome. *Rheumatology (Oxford).* 2006;45(3):348-352.
71. Matsuda T, Ohno S, Hirohata S, et al. Efficacy of rebamipide as adjunctive therapy in the treatment of recurrent oral aphthous ulcers in patients with Behçet's disease: a randomised, double-blind, placebo-controlled study. *Drugs R D.* 2003;4(1):19-28.
72. Davatchi F, Sadeghi Abdollahi B, Tehrani Banihashemi A, et al. Colchicine versus placebo in Behçet's disease: randomized, double-blind, controlled crossover trial. *Mod Rheumatol.* 2009;19(5):542-549.
73. Yurdakul S, Mat C, Tüzün Y, et al. A double-blind trial of colchicine in Behçet's syndrome. *Arthritis Rheum.* 2001;44(11):2686-2892.
74. Aktulga E, Altaç M, Müftüoglu A, et al. A double blind study of colchicine in Behcet's disease. *Haematologica.* 1980;65(3):399-402.
75. Sharquie KE, Najim RA, Abu-Raghif AR. Dapsone in Behçet's disease: a double-blind, placebo-controlled, cross-over study. *J Dermatol.* 2002;29(5):267-279.
76. Yazici H, Pazarli H, Barnes CG, et al. A controlled trial of azathioprine in Behçet's disease. *N Engl J Med.* 1990;322(5):281-285.
77. Alpsoy E, Durusoy C, Yilmaz E, et al. Interferon alfa-2a in the treatment of Behçet's disease: a randomized placebo-controlled and double-blind study. *Arch Dermatol.* 2002;138(4):467-471.
78. Kiliç H, Zeytin HE, Korkmaz C, et al. Low-dose natural human interferon-alpha lozenges in the treatment

of Behçet's syndrome. *Rheumatology (Oxford)*. 2009;48(11):1388-1391.
79. Hamuryudan V, Mat C, Saip S, et al. Thalidomide in the treatment of the mucocutaneous lesions of the Behçet syndrome. A randomized, double-blind, placebo-controlled trial. *Ann Intern Med*. 1998;128(6):443-450.
80. Masuda K, Nakajima A, Urayama A, et al. Double-masked trial of cyclosporin versus colchicine and long-term open study of cyclosporin in Behçet's disease. *Lancet*. 1989;1(8647):1093-1096.
81. Ozyazgan Y, Yurdakul S, Yazici H, et al. Low dose cyclosporin A versus pulsed cyclophosphamide in Behçet's syndrome: a single masked trial. *Br J Ophthalmol*. 1992;76:241-243.
82. BenEzra D, Cohen E, Chajek T, et al. Evaluation of conventional therapy versus cyclosporine A in Behçet's syndrome. *Transplant Proc*. 1988;20(suppl 4):136-143.
83. Jaffe GJ, Dick AD, Brézin AP, et al. Adalimumab in patients with active noninfectious uveitis. *N Engl J Med*. 2016;375(10):932-943.
84. Nguyen QD, Merrill PT, Jaffe GJ, et al. Adalimumab for prevention of uveitic flare in patients with inactive non-infectious uveitis controlled by corticosteroids (VISUAL II): a multicentre, double-masked, randomised, placebo-controlled phase 3 trial. *Lancet*. 2016;388(10050):1183-1192.
85. Buggage RR, Levy-Clarke G, Sen HN, et al. A double-masked, randomized study to investigate the safety and efficacy of daclizumab to treat the ocular complications related to Behçet's disease. *Ocul Immunol Inflamm*. 2007;15(2):63-70.
86. Melikoglu M, Fresko I, Mat C, et al. Short-term trial of etanercept in Behçet's disease: a double blind, placebo controlled study. *J Rheumatol*. 2005;32(1):98-105.
87. Dick AD, Tugal-Tutkun I, Foster S, et al. Secukinumab in the treatment of noninfectious uveitis: results of three randomized, controlled clinical trials. *Ophthalmology*. 2013;120(4):777-787.
88. Hatemi G, Melikoglu M, Tunc R, et al. Apremilast for Behçet's syndrome—a phase 2, placebo-controlled study. *N Engl J Med*. 2015;372(16):1510-1518.
89. Davies UM, Palmer RG, Denman AM. Treatment with acyclovir does not affect orogenital ulcers in Behçet's syndrome: a randomized double-blind trial. *Br J Rheumatol*. 1988;27(4):300-302.
90. Moral F, Hamuryudan V, Yurdakul S, Yazici H. Inefficacy of azapropazone in the acute arthritis of Behçet's syndrome: a randomized, double blind, placebo controlled study. *Clin Exp Rheumatol*. 1995;13:493-495.

Chapter 142 :: Kawasaki Disease
:: Anne H. Rowley

第一百四十二章

川崎病

中文导读

川崎病（KD）是一种多系统炎症性疾病，主要累及血管，尤其是冠状动脉，是发达国家儿童获得性心脏病的主要原因。本章节从历史视角、流行病学、临床特征、病因和发病机制、诊断、临床过程和预后及治疗对该病进行了详细阐述。

1. 历史视角　KD是以日本儿科医生Tomisaku Kawasaki博士的名字来命名的，作者详细介绍了该病的认识过程及如何确定为一种新的独立疾病。

2. 流行病学　KD主要是幼儿疾病，其中80%的病例发生在6个月至5岁的儿童中。男孩与女孩受累比例通常为3∶2。日本人中KD的发病率比白人儿童高约10倍。KD具有一定的遗传易感性，其流行病学特征支持感染为可能的病因。

3. 临床特征

（1）皮肤表现：全身性发疹常见，在躯干和四肢最明显，通常表现为以下3种形式中的一种：麻疹样（图142-1A）、靶样（图142-1B）或猩红热样（弥散性红斑，图142-1C）。在疾病的急性发热期，通常会观察到腹股沟的红斑和脱屑（图142-2），并且可能被误诊为念珠菌性尿布皮炎甚至葡萄球菌烫伤的皮肤综合征。典型的手指和足趾的甲周脱屑通常在发热后的第二到第三周才开始出现，并且会逐渐累及整个手部和足部（图142-3）。在患病后的第三至第六周，通常会出现横跨指甲的横线（Beau线）。

（2）非皮肤表现：该病具有5种典型临床特征：结膜充血、口腔黏膜变化、手和足部改变、皮疹和颈淋巴结病。作者详细介绍了这几个主要表现的特点，并提出了一些提示该病的线索。该病通常分为三个阶段：急性发热期、亚急性期和恢复期。由于KD是一个多系统炎症过程，因此许多器官和组织都参与了炎症过程，文中详细列出了各种相关的临床特征（表142-1）。

（3）并发症：如上所述，大约25%的未治疗儿童发展为冠状动脉异常，包括扩张和动脉瘤（图142-7），这可能导致心肌梗塞、动脉瘤破裂和猝死。超过50%的KD患者在急性发热期间患有心肌炎，临床表现为与发烧不成比例的心动过速。在疾病的急性期，也可能会出现可自发缓解的心包积液。

4. 病因和发病机制　KD的病因不明。最符合临床、免疫学和流行病学特征的假说是KD是具有遗传易感性的个体感染普通病原体所致。首先对KD的遗传易感基因进行了简单介绍，并指出KD血管病变是三个密切相关的病理过程：嗜中性坏死性动脉炎、亚急性/慢性血管炎以及与亚急性/慢性血管炎密切相关的管腔肌纤维母细胞增生。接下来对KD的免疫学机制进行了阐述，并提出导致KD的病原体可能为病毒。

5. 诊断　急性KD的实验室检查结果无特异性，但具有一定的特征性。对血细胞计数、尿液分析、肝功能、急性期反应物［例如C反应蛋白（CRP）和ESR］等可能出现的异常结果及时进行了总结。

（1）病理：皮肤和淋巴结活检无特异性。

（2）影像：建议所有怀疑患有KD的儿童均应在诊断时、发热后2～3周以及发热后6～8周进行超声心动图检查，对于发生冠状动脉扩张的患者，在急性期和随访期间需要更频繁的超声心动图检查，警惕冠状动脉血栓形成的风险。

（3）诊断流程：介绍了典型KD的诊断标准为持续发烧5天或以上的情况下，出现以下5个临床特征中的4个，且无法用其他疾病来解释：①非化脓性球结膜充血；②嘴唇发红、肿胀和干燥，可能会开裂和流血；③手足发红和肿胀；④皮疹；⑤直径大于或等于1.5厘米的颈部淋巴结肿大（表142-2）。由于KD患者（尤其是婴儿）在疾病的高热期并不总是符合经典的诊断标准，但可能出现冠状动脉异常。美国心脏协会委员会发布了不完全型KD的诊断流程，强调诊断时应结合临床特征、实验室检查和超声心动图检查（表142-3）。对几种应完善超声心动图的发热患儿提出了建议。

（4）鉴别诊断：建议对于具有某些KD临床特征或临床不够典型患者，必须仔细考虑其他诊断（表142-4）。将麻疹、A组链球菌感染（猩红热）、单纯腺病毒及其他病毒感染、药物超敏反应、葡萄球菌烫伤性皮肤综合征、中毒性休克综合征、类风湿关节炎与KD的鉴别要点进行了总结。

6. 临床过程和预后　在患病的前10天内接受IVIG和阿司匹林治疗的KD儿童中，约有85%对发烧和其他临床症状有快速缓解的反应，还有大约15%的KD儿童有出现冠脉异常的风险。建议根据冠状动脉异常的严重程度应定期进行心血管风险评估。

7. 治疗

（1）药物：急性KD患儿应在诊断后尽快给予2g/kg IVIG和阿司匹林（80～100 mg/kg/d，每6小时口服一次）（表142-5），建议在发热的前10天使用。对不同情况下IVIG和阿司匹林的疗程、减量方法进行了详细介绍。对初次治疗反应较差的"难治性" KD患者，再次使用IVIG、大剂量激素或英夫利昔单抗是可替代的选择。

（2）会诊：建议伴冠状动脉受累的患者接受儿科心脏病专家的随访和建议。

（3）治疗流程：表142-5概述了治疗KD的方法。

〔黄莹雪〕

AT-A-GLANCE

- Kawasaki disease (KD) is a multisystem inflammatory process of unknown but suspected infectious etiology.
- Highest incidence is in Asian children; 1 in 80 Japanese children develops KD by age 5 years.
- KD is the most common cause of acquired heart disease in children in developed nations.
- KD affects all blood vessels in the body, but primarily damages medium-sized muscular arteries such as the coronary arteries.
- Major symptoms are prolonged high fever, conjunctival injection, oral mucosal changes such as red lips and pharynx and strawberry tongue, redness and swelling of the hands and feet, erythematous polymorphic rash, and cervical lymphadenopathy.
- Inflammation in the coronary arteries can lead to aneurysms with subsequent myocardial infarction, aneurysm rupture, and sudden death.
- Treatment with intravenous immunoglobulin (IVIG) and aspirin, when given in the first 10 days of fever, reduces the prevalence of coronary artery abnormalities from 25% in those treated with aspirin alone, to 5% in those who receive IVIG with aspirin.
- Long-term complications are confined to the heart and vascular tree, primarily thrombosis and stenosis of the major coronary arteries with myocardial ischemia.

Kawasaki disease (KD), the leading cause of acquired heart disease in children in developed nations, is a multisystem inflammatory illness that particularly affects blood vessels, especially the coronary arteries. Approximately 25% of untreated children develop coronary artery abnormalities, including dilation and aneurysms that can lead to myocardial infarction and sudden death.[1,2] The etiology is unknown, but clinical and epidemiologic data support an infectious cause. In KD, an intense inflammatory cell response develops in a wide array of organs and tissues[3]; in medium-sized arteries such as the coronary arteries, this response can damage collagen and elastin fibers in the vessel walls and lead to loss of their normal structural integrity with resultant ballooning or aneurysm formation. Despite a limited understanding of KD pathogenesis, a very effective therapy exists in the form of intravenous immunoglobulin (IVIG) with aspirin; when given in the first 10 days of fever, this therapy reduces the prevalence of coronary artery abnormalities from 25% in untreated patients to 5% in those who receive the therapy.[4] Because the etiology is unknown, no diagnostic test exists, and the diagnosis is made clinically. Classic KD is diagnosed in a patient with prolonged fever and 4 of 5 other clinical features. However, incomplete forms of illness, in which a child manifests prolonged fever with fewer than 4 other clinical features of the illness and subsequently develops coronary artery abnormalities, are well-recognized. The existence of these incomplete forms of illness results in a major diagnostic dilemma for physicians in establishing the diagnosis accurately in children with prolonged fever of uncertain cause.

HISTORICAL PERSPECTIVE

KD is named for Dr. Tomisaku Kawasaki, a Japanese pediatrician who first recognized the clinical features of the illness. He described 50 cases of a new illness in 1967 in the Japanese-language literature that he termed *mucocutaneous lymph node syndrome*.[5] It was not until later that some of the children with this newly described illness experienced sudden death; autopsy revealed myocardial infarction from thrombosis of coronary artery aneurysms. Prior to Dr. Kawasaki's description of the clinical features, KD was recognized only by pathologists at autopsy, who called the disease *infantile periarteritis nodosa*.[6] Dr. Kawasaki described the illness in the English-language literature in 1974; this report was closely followed by a description of the same illness, observed independently in the early 1970s in Hawaii by Dr. Marian Melish and colleagues.[7,8] Since that time, it has become clear that although the attack rate of KD is highest in Asian, particularly Japanese, Korean, and Chinese children, all racial and ethnic groups around the world are affected by the illness.

EPIDEMIOLOGY

KD is predominantly an illness of young children, with 80% of cases occurring in children ages 6 months to 5 years.[9,10] However, infants younger than 6 months of age can be affected, often manifest incomplete forms of the illness, and can have particularly severe KD.[11,12] Similarly, KD can occur in older children and teenagers, in whom the diagnosis is often delayed, and who may also have more-severe KD with a higher prevalence of coronary artery abnormalities.[11-13] Therefore, the diagnosis must be considered in all pediatric age groups.

Boys are more commonly affected than girls at a ratio of 3:2. The incidence of KD is approximately 10-fold higher in Japanese than in white children.[9,10] Approximately 1 in 80 Japanese children develop KD by the age of 5 years; the peak age of illness is 9 to 11 months of age in both Japan and the United States.[9,10] The higher attack rate in Japanese children persists in those who adopt a Western diet and lifestyle, and is likely related to a genetic predisposition to KD among Asian children.[14] The risk of KD in siblings is 10-fold higher than in the general population, and the incidence of KD in children born to parents who had KD is twice as high as in the general population.[15,16] Recurrence is rare, occurring in approximately 3% of cases in Japan.[10]

Many epidemiologic features of KD suggest an infectious agent is the cause. Among these are the well-described epidemics of illness[14,17-19] and the geographic wave-like spread of illness during an epidemic, compatible with spread of an infectious agent.[19] Cases in the United States are more common in the winter and spring.[9]

CLINICAL FEATURES

CUTANEOUS FINDINGS

A generalized exanthem is commonly observed in KD, is most pronounced on the trunk and extremities, and generally takes 1 of 3 forms: morbilliform (Fig. 142-1A), targetoid (Fig. 142-1B), or scarlatiniform (diffuse erythema, Fig. 142-1C). Bullae, vesicles, and ulcerative lesions are not observed, but a fine micropustular rash, especially on the extensor surfaces, occasionally occurs. The rash may be pruritic. In the acute febrile phase of illness, groin erythema and desquamation are commonly observed (Fig. 142-2), and can be mistaken for candidal diaper dermatitis or even a staphylococcal scalded skin syndrome. The skin changes in the groin can be seen both in children in diapers and toilet-trained children. Classic periungual desquamation of the fingers and toes does not begin until the second to third week after fever begins, and can progress to involve the entire hand and foot (Fig. 142-3); treatment should be administered well before its appearance. In the third to sixth week after illness, transverse lines across the fingernails (Beau lines) are often apparent. These grow out with the nail.

In countries where bacille Calmette-Guérin vaccine is routinely administered, such as in Japan, a common finding in children with KD is erythema and swelling at the site of bacille Calmette-Guérin vaccine administration; the mechanism is unknown but the process resolves with treatment of KD. Although KD results in a vasculitis affecting all arteries and veins in the body, blood vessels in the skin are not prominently affected, and skin biopsy is not useful for diagnosis because pathologic findings are nonspecific.

NONCUTANEOUS FINDINGS

KD should be considered in the differential diagnosis of any child with prolonged fever without other explanation. In KD, all clinical features may not be present simultaneously. Therefore, it is important to query parents and physicians who saw the patient during the course of a prolonged febrile illness as to the presence of the other 5 clinical features of the illness: conjunctival injection, oral mucosal changes, changes of the hands and feet, rash, and cervical adenopathy. Children with KD often have significant enough swelling and discomfort of the hands and feet that they will refuse to pick up objects or to walk (Fig. 142-4). This is not commonly observed in children with most other illnesses in the differential diagnosis of KD, and can provide an important clue to the diagnosis. Similarly, extreme irritability is common in KD, and not as common in

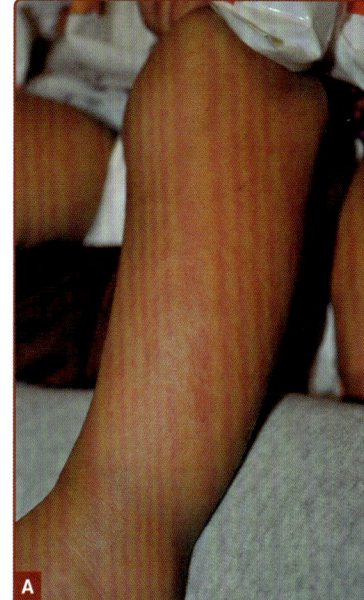

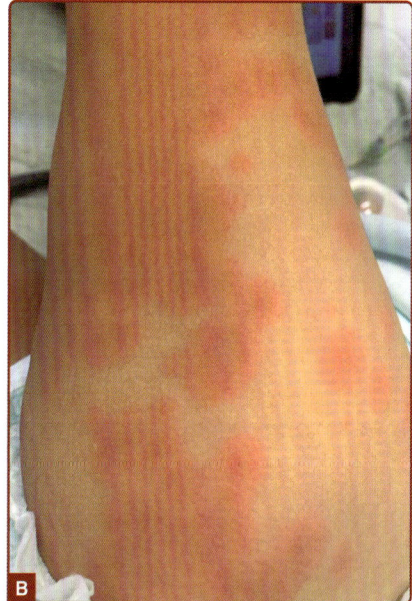

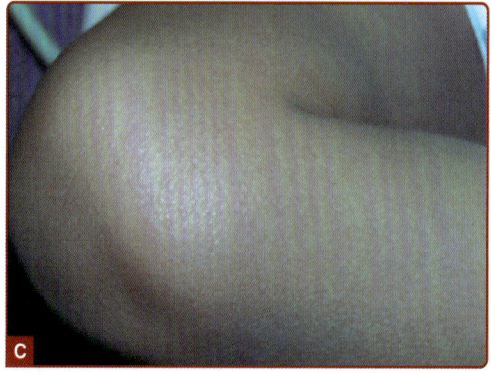

Figure 142-1 The exanthems observed acute in Kawasaki disease. **A,** Erythematous morbilliform exanthem; **B,** targetoid or urticarial changes; **C,** diffuse erythema.

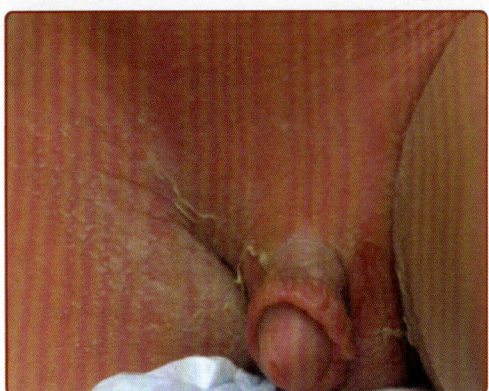

Figure 142-2 Erythematous desquamating groin rash of acute Kawasaki disease.

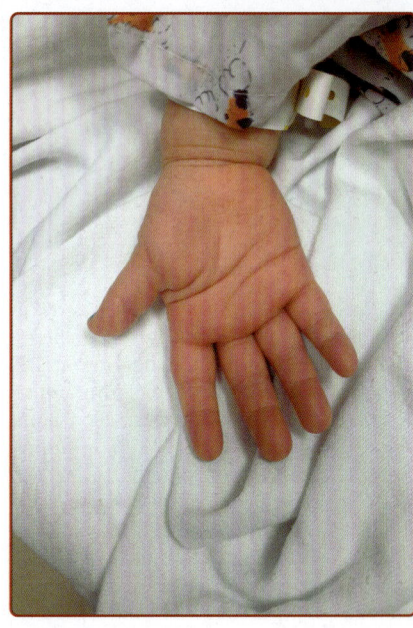

Figure 142-4 Erythema and edema of the hands in Kawasaki disease.

most other illnesses in the differential diagnosis. Without specific therapy, fever in KD is daily, high spiking, intermittent, and lasts for 1 to 2 weeks. The illness is often divided into 3 stages: the acute febrile phase, the subacute phase (that begins when fever resolves and continues until all clinical features have normalized), and the convalescent phase (that follows the subacute phase and continues until the erythrocyte sedimentation rate [ESR] normalizes, usually at 6 to 8 weeks after the onset of fever).

Conjunctival injection in KD is bilateral and nonexudative. There may be limbal sparing (Fig. 142-5). Photophobia is a common accompanying feature. Oral findings include red, swollen, dry, cracked lips that may bleed (Fig. 142-6), a "strawberry" tongue, and erythema of the mouth and throat. Oral ulcers are not a feature of KD. Palmar and plantar erythema is a common feature, and there can be an abrupt transition from marked erythema to normal skin at the wrists and ankles. The hands and feet can be edematous and painful. Cervical adenopathy is the least commonly observed clinical feature, occurring in approximately 75% of children with classic KD, but can be the most prominent feature in a subset of patients who are often treated with multiple different courses of antibiotic therapy without improvement before the correct diagnosis is made.[20] Cervical adenopathy is usually unilateral, may or may not be associated with superficial erythema and/or tenderness to palpation, and is nonfluctuant. Because KD is a multisystem inflammatory process, many organs and tissues are involved in the inflammatory process, leading to a variety of associated clinical features (Table 142-1). In particular, arthritis can occur during the acute febrile phase, involving the small interphalangeal joints and larger joints, or may occur during the subacute phase of illness, usually involving the larger joints such as the knees and ankles. Aseptic meningitis is a common finding in patients who undergo lumbar puncture.

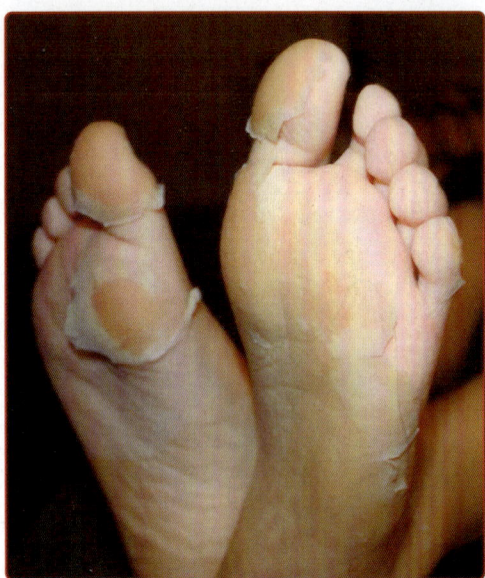

Figure 142-3 Desquamation of the feet in the subacute phase of Kawasaki disease; this process began periungually and progressed to involve the entire soles.

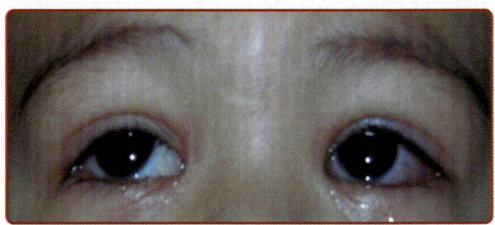

Figure 142-5 Conjunctival injection with limbal sparing in acute Kawasaki disease.

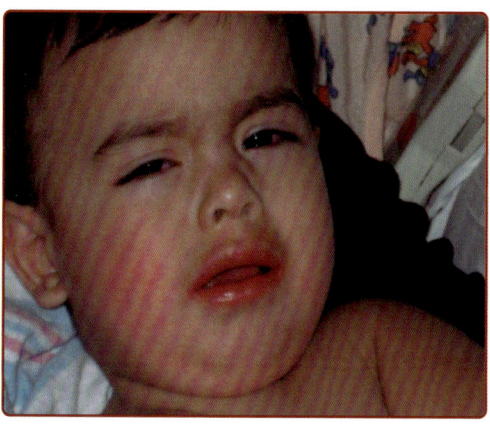

Figure 142-6 Typical facial features of acute Kawasaki disease showing conjunctival injection and red dry lips.

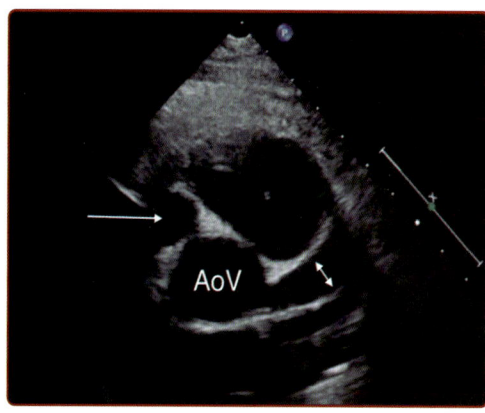

Figure 142-7 Coronary artery aneurysms in Kawasaki disease demonstrated by echocardiography. *AoV*, aortic valve; *double arrow*, aneurysm of proximal left anterior descending coronary artery; *single arrow*, large aneurysm of proximal right coronary artery.

COMPLICATIONS

As noted above, approximately 25% of untreated children develop coronary artery abnormalities, including dilation and aneurysms (Fig. 142-7), which can result in myocardial infarction, aneurysm rupture, and sudden death. Myocardial infarction can occur from thrombosis of an aneurysm, which is most common in the first few months after the onset, or from coronary artery stenosis, which occurs months to years following the illness. Aneurysm rupture is less common and usually occurs within the first month after the onset. More than 50% of KD patients have myocarditis during the acute febrile phase, manifested clinically as tachycardia disproportionate to fever, which generally improves rapidly with IVIG therapy. In the acute phase of illness, a pericardial effusion can be present; this resolves spontaneously. In patients with the most-severe coronary artery aneurysms, aneurysms of other medium-sized arteries can also be observed, most commonly in the iliac, femoral, and axillary arteries. Valvulitis significant enough to require valve replacement is rarely reported. Although KD is a systemic inflammatory disease affecting multiple organs and tissues, there are no known long-term consequences of the disease outside of the heart and blood vessels.

TABLE 142-1
Associated Clinical Features of Kawasaki Disease

Cardiovascular
- Coronary artery aneurysms
- Myocarditis
- Pericardial effusion
- Aneurysms of other medium-sized arteries (uncommon)
- Valvular disease (rare)
- Peripheral gangrene (rare)

Respiratory
- Pneumonitis: interstitial or peribronchial infiltrates on chest X-ray, usually without respiratory distress
- Pulmonary nodules (rare)

Gastrointestinal
- Hepatitis
- Obstructive jaundice
- Gallbladder hydrops
- Diarrhea

Musculoskeletal
- Arthritis

Genitourinary
- Urethritis
- Hydrocele

Neurologic
- Marked irritability
- Aseptic meningitis
- Facial palsy (uncommon)
- Sensorineural hearing loss (uncommon)

Other
- Anterior uveitis
- Erythema and induration at the site of a bacille Calmette-Guérin (BCG) vaccine

ETIOLOGY AND PATHOGENESIS

The etiology of KD remains unknown. The hypothesis that best fits the available clinical, immunologic, and epidemiologic data is that KD results from infection with a ubiquitous etiologic agent that usually results in asymptomatic infection, but causes KD in a small subset of genetically predisposed individuals. Genetic predisposition is a common theme in susceptibility and host response to infectious diseases. It is likely that KD is polygenic. Intensive investigation of genetic factors influencing susceptibility to KD is ongoing by several international collaborative groups. A functional polymorphism in the *ITPKC* gene, which is a negative regulator of T-cell activation, is associated with KD susceptibility and risk of developing coronary artery abnormalities[21]; other immune genes, such as *CASP3*,

BLK, CD40, FCGR2A, and ORAI1, also appear to be associated with KD susceptibility.[22-24]

Three linked pathologic processes are characteristic of KD vasculopathy, which most significantly affects the coronary arteries: neutrophilic necrotizing arteritis, which occurs in the first 2 weeks after fever onset; subacute/chronic vasculitis, which begins in the first 2 weeks but can persist for months to years and is comprised of lymphocytes (predominately CD8 T lymphocytes[25]), plasma cells (particularly immunoglobulin [Ig] A plasma cells[26,27]), eosinophils, and macrophages; and luminal myofibroblastic proliferation, which is closely associated with subacute/chronic vasculitis and can result in progressive arterial stenosis.[28] These 3 processes explain the potential adverse outcomes of KD. Necrotizing arteritis can result in necrosis and sloughing of the intima and media; in its most severe form only a thin layer of adventitia may remain, resulting in giant aneurysms that occasionally rupture, but more commonly accumulate layers of thrombi, which can become occlusive and cause myocardial infarction. Subacute/chronic arteritis is associated with luminal myofibroblastic proliferation and progressive arterial stenosis, which with or without overlying thrombi can lead to myocardial infarction.[28] Adaptive immune responses in KD have been demonstrated to be antigen-driven.[29-31] The presence of IgA plasma cells and CD8 T cells as primary components of the inflammatory infiltrate in acute KD suggests an immune response to an intracellular pathogen with a respiratory portal of entry. Synthetic versions of these oligoclonal IgA antibodies identify antigen in acute KD tissues, which appears to reside in intracytoplasmic inclusion bodies containing protein and RNA, and are highly suggestive of a viral etiology, although the specific agent has so far eluded identification, perhaps because of a lack of homology to known viral families.[32-35] The immune transcriptional profile of KD arteritis has features of an antiviral immune response, such as activated cytotoxic T-lymphocyte and Type I interferon-induced gene upregulation;[36] this information should help guide the development of new immunomodulatory therapies for KD arteritis.

RISK FACTORS

Asian children, particularly Japanese, Chinese, and Korean children, have the highest attack rates of KD.[10,14] Infants and older children have the highest prevalence of coronary artery abnormalities following KD.[11-13] Risk-scoring systems have been developed in Japan that are useful in determining those KD children who are at highest risk of developing coronary artery disease and allowing for selective intensification of primary KD therapy.[37] However, these scoring systems do not accurately predict risk of coronary artery disease in non-Japanese, multiethnic populations.[38]

DIAGNOSIS

In the absence of knowledge of the etiology of KD, a diagnostic test is not available. Laboratory findings in acute KD are nonspecific but quite characteristic. A complete blood count reveals either a normal or elevated white blood cell count with a neutrophil predominance. A low white blood cell count with lymphocyte predominance would be distinctly unusual in KD. A normochromic, normocytic anemia can be present, and resolves spontaneously with resolution of KD. The platelet count is normal in the first week of illness, although thrombocytopenia has been reported to be associated with a more severe outcome. Thrombocytosis, with platelet counts sometimes exceeding 1,000,000/mm^3, is characteristic of the subacute phase of KD, peaking in the second to third week after the onset of fever. This feature, like periungual desquamation, is not useful in making a diagnosis of KD in the first week of fever. Patients with anemia and low albumin levels may be at higher risk of developing coronary artery disease. A mild elevation of the liver transaminases is commonly observed in acute KD. Occasionally, obstructive jaundice occurs. Gallbladder hydrops, with accompanying right upper quadrant abdominal pain, resolves spontaneously and does not require surgical intervention. Sterile pyuria is also commonly observed. Acute-phase reactants such as the C-reactive protein (CRP) and the ESR are characteristically elevated in patients with acute KD, and the CRP is sometimes used to follow clinical response in patients refractory to IVIG therapy. Once IVIG is given, the ESR cannot be used to follow clinical response, because IVIG itself transiently increases the ESR. A complete blood count and CRP or ESR should be performed at baseline, and the CRP repeated at 2 to 3 weeks and 6 to 8 weeks after onset to monitor for resolution of inflammation.

PATHOLOGY

Skin and lymph node biopsies reveal nonspecific findings in KD and are not useful in establishing the diagnosis.

IMAGING

Echocardiography should be performed in all children with suspected KD, and should be performed at diagnosis, at 2 to 3 weeks after fever onset, and at 6 to 8 weeks after fever onset.[39] The peak time to detect coronary artery dilation is 2 to 3 weeks after onset of fever, during the subacute phase of illness. Patients who do not manifest coronary artery abnormalities on any of these 3 echocardiograms may not require additional studies, although some centers perform 1 additional echocardiogram at 1 year after the onset. In patients who develop coronary artery dilation, more frequent echocardiograms will be needed during the acute phase and in followup; these should be scheduled in consultation with a pediatric cardiologist. In particular, frequent echocardiograms are advisable in the first few weeks in patients in whom coronary artery luminal diameters are continuing to expand; these patients are at particularly high risk of developing coronary artery thrombosis. Electrocardiogram in the acute febrile phase of illness most often shows a prolonged PR interval and/or nonspecific ST- and T-wave changes. CT angiography or magnetic resonance angiography can be useful in evaluating the coronary arteries of teenagers in whom adequate images of the coronary arteries may be difficult to obtain by echocardiography, and of children with particularly severe coronary artery disease.[40,41]

DIAGNOSTIC ALGORITHM

A diagnosis of classic KD is made in the presence of prolonged fever lasting 5 or more days, with 4 of the following 5 clinical features in the absence of another explanation for the illness: (a) nonpurulent bulbar conjunctival injection; (b) red, swollen, dry lips, which may crack and bleed; (c) redness and swelling of the hands and feet; (d) rash; and (e) cervical lymphadenopathy, 1.5 cm or larger in diameter (Table 142-2). Experienced physicians can make a diagnosis of KD before the fifth day of fever in children with classic features. A patient with prolonged fever and fewer than 4 of the other features of the illness can be diagnosed with KD if coronary artery abnormalities develop.

Incomplete (or atypical) KD refers to children with prolonged fever and fewer than 4 of the other features of illness who have a laboratory profile compatible with KD. Such patients should undergo echocardiography and be considered for treatment with IVIG because KD patients, particularly infants, do not always manifest classic diagnostic criteria during the acute febrile phase of illness, yet can develop coronary artery abnormalities. The American Heart Association Committee on Rheumatic Fever, Endocarditis, and Kawasaki Disease has published an algorithm to assist the clinician in diagnosing incomplete KD.[39] This algorithm emphasizes the importance of combining clinical features, laboratory findings, and echocardiographic findings in making a diagnosis (Table 142-3). In difficult cases, consultation with a KD expert should be considered. If the patient is not treated for KD but develops typical periungual desquamation after fever has resolved, and an alternative diagnosis that could explain this clinical finding has not been established (such as scarlet fever), an echocardiogram should be repeated. Infants 6 months of age or younger can have mild or subtle clinical findings with KD, but have a

TABLE 142-2
Diagnostic Criteria for Classic Kawasaki Disease

Fever ≥5 days,[a] high spiking and intermittent, with at least 4 of the 5 clinical features[b]:
1. Bilateral, nonexudative conjunctival injection.
2. Oral mucosal changes, including red, dry, cracked lips, pharyngeal erythema, and/or strawberry tongue.
3. Changes of the hands and feet: erythema of palms and soles and/or swelling of the hands and feet during the acute phase, and/or periungual desquamation of the fingers and toes during the subacute phase.
4. Rash: erythematous morbilliform, scarlatiniform, or targetoid.
5. Cervical lymphadenopathy ≥1.5 cm in diameter.

[a]The diagnosis can be made before the fifth day of fever by experienced physicians if the patient has the other clinical features of the illness.
[b]In the absence of another explanation for the illness.

TABLE 142-3
Criteria for Diagnosis of Incomplete Kawasaki Disease

Fever for ≥5 days with 2 or 3 compatible clinical features of KD and
- ESR ≥40 mm/h and/or CRP ≥3.0 mg/dL
  - If patient has at least 3 compatible laboratory features,[a] perform echocardiogram and begin treatment.
  - If patient has fewer than 3 compatible laboratory features,[a] but has dilated coronary arteries by echocardiogram (Z score of LAD or RCA ≥2.5), begin treatment.
  - If patient has fewer than 3 compatible laboratory features[a] and LAD and RCA Z scores <2.5, but has at least 3 supportive echocardiographic features,[a] begin treatment.
  - If patient has fewer than 3 compatible laboratory features,[a] LAD and RCA Z scores <2.5, and fewer than 3 supportive echocardiographic features,[b] then follow patient and consider other diagnoses. If fevers persist and no other diagnosis is established, consider repeating laboratory tests and echocardiogram and consider consulting a KD expert. If fever resolves, KD is unlikely.
- ESR <40 mm/h and/or CRP <3.0 mg/dL
  - Follow patient. If fever continues, reevaluate clinically and consider repeating ESR and CRP. If fever resolves but patient develops typical periungual desquamation, perform echocardiogram.

[a]Compatible laboratory features:
1. Albumin ≤3.0 g/dL
2. Anemia for age
3. Elevated alanine aminotransferase
4. Platelet count ≥450,000/mm³ after the 7th day of illness
5. White blood cell (WBC) ≥15,000/mm³
6. Urinalysis with ≥10 WBC/high-power field

[b]Supportive echocardiographic features:
1. Lack of tapering
2. Decreased left ventricular function
3. Mitral regurgitation
4. Pericardial effusion
5. Z scores of LAD or RCA of 2.0 to 2.5

CRP, C-reactive protein; *ESR*, erythrocyte sedimentation rate; *LAD*, left anterior descending coronary artery; *RCA*, right coronary artery.

Data from Newburger JW, Takahashi M, Gerber MA, et al. Diagnosis, treatment, and long-term management of Kawasaki disease: a statement for health professionals from the Committee on Rheumatic Fever, Endocarditis and Kawasaki Disease, Council on Cardiovascular Disease in the Young, American Heart Association. *Circulation*. 2004;110(17):2747-2771.

high risk of developing coronary artery abnormalities. Therefore, infants with fever for 1 week or longer without other explanation should have laboratory testing performed. If evidence of an inflammatory process is present, an echocardiogram should be ordered and KD considered, even in the absence of other clinical features of the illness.

DIFFERENTIAL DIAGNOSIS

The KD child with prolonged high fever, marked conjunctival injection, red, swollen hands and feet, erythematous rash, and red, cracked, bleeding lips who has a markedly elevated ESR and/or CRP and an elevated peripheral white blood cell count with a neutrophil predominance has a very distinctive illness and usually does not pose any difficulties in diagnosis. In other patients who have only some of the clinical features of KD, or in whom clinical findings are not as dramatic, other diagnoses must be carefully considered (Table 142-4).

In areas where measles is still prevalent, differentiating the 2 disorders can be difficult. Classically, patients with measles have rash that begins on the face behind the ears and Koplik spots in the mouth; neither of these features is observed in KD. Later in the course of measles infection, the rash becomes diffuse and Koplik spots are no longer visible. Conjunctival injection and edema of the hands and feet can be observed in both disorders. In uncomplicated measles, the peripheral white blood cell count and the ESR are generally low. The measles IgM antibody is virtually always positive by the appearance of the measles rash, and is the best single test to differentiate the two conditions.

Group A streptococcal infection should be considered in the differential diagnosis of a KD patient with a scarlatiniform rash, and can be excluded by a negative throat culture. Diagnostic uncertainty could arise in a KD patient who is a group A streptococcal carrier. Administration of antibiotic therapy followed by reevaluation in 24 to 48 hours generally clarifies the diagnosis; children with group A streptococcal pharyngitis have a rapid response to therapy, while antibiotics are ineffective in KD. Adenovirus infection can mimic KD. The presence of exudative conjunctivitis and exudative pharyngitis suggests adenovirus as the most likely diagnosis. Other viruses can occasionally cause prolonged fever, such as enterovirus; in differentiating KD patients from those with uncomplicated viral infection, laboratory tests such as the ESR, CRP, and urinalysis can be helpful, as pyuria and markedly elevated acute-phase reactants are more typical of KD.

Drug hypersensitivity reactions can mimic KD. Oral and mucosal ulcers observed in Stevens–Johnson syndrome are absent in KD. Edema of the face, particularly around the eyes, is much more suggestive of drug reaction than KD. In general, the ESR and CRP are either normal or only mildly elevated in drug hypersensitivity reactions.

Staphylococcal scalded skin syndrome is easily distinguished by the classic finding of painful skin in staphylococcal scalded skin syndrome, which is not observed in KD, and by flaccid blisters, desquamation, and a positive Nikolsky sign, which is present in staphylococcal scalded skin syndrome and absent in KD.

Although hypotension is unusual in KD, a KD shock syndrome occurs rarely,[42,43] and toxic shock syndrome is in the differential diagnosis of such patients. Renal involvement and elevated creatinine phosphokinase are more likely to be observed in toxic shock syndrome than in KD. IVIG administered for a possible diagnosis of KD may serve as adjunctive therapy for toxic shock syndrome.

Juvenile rheumatoid arthritis is a diagnosis of exclusion, and an occasional patient with this disorder might initially be diagnosed with and treated for incomplete KD. The correct diagnosis may become apparent when fever recurs following reduction of high-dose aspirin therapy, implying an original clinical response to aspirin rather than to IVIG.

CLINICAL COURSE AND PROGNOSIS

Approximately 85% of KD children treated with IVIG and aspirin within the first 10 days of illness respond with rapid resolution of fever and other clinical signs. The vast majority of KD patients who are promptly diagnosed and treated do well, without developing cardiac complications. However, approximately 15% of KD children treated within the first 10 days of illness continue to have fever following a single infusion of IVIG with aspirin and require additional therapy; these patients have a higher risk of developing coronary artery abnormalities.[44] A study assessing KD patients treated within the first 10 days of illness indicated that 18% had a coronary artery Z score higher than 2 at week 5 after the onset.[45] The larger the aneurysm, the less likely that the luminal diameter will return to normal over time. Very large or "giant" coronary artery aneurysms are associated with the most-severe

---

TABLE 142-4
Differential Diagnosis of Kawasaki Disease

- Measles
- Adenovirus infection
- Enterovirus infection
- Scarlet fever
- Staphylococcal scalded skin syndrome
- Toxic shock syndrome
- Drug hypersensitivity reaction
- Juvenile rheumatoid arthritis

If patient has epidemiologic risk factor:
- Rocky Mountain spotted fever
- Leptospirosis

outcomes.[46] A decrease in luminal diameter of an aneurysm can result from thrombosis or luminal myofibroblastic proliferation, which can lead to coronary artery stenosis and myocardial infarction.[28] In young infants and children, myocardial infarction usually presents as shock, emesis, and/or abdominal pain.[47] Patients with significant coronary artery disease may require catheter intervention procedures,[48] coronary artery bypass surgery,[49] or, rarely, heart transplantation.[50] Cardiovascular risk assessment should be performed at intervals dependent upon the severity of coronary artery abnormalities.[39]

MANAGEMENT

INTERVENTIONS

MEDICATIONS

A single infusion of IVIG 2 g/kg with aspirin (80-100 mg/kg/day given every 6 hours orally) should be administered to children with acute KD as soon as possible after diagnosis (Table 142-5) as demonstrated in a study by Newburger and colleagues.[51] This regimen, when administered to children with KD within the first 10 days of fever, was shown to reduce the prevalence of coronary artery abnormalities from 25% in untreated patients to 5% in those who receive the therapy. However, this study was performed prior to use of coronary artery Z scores to identify coronary artery dilation, and more recent studies suggest a higher prevalence of coronary artery dilation in KD patients overall than was previously appreciated.[45,52] Most children experience rapid resolution of fever and other clinical signs following treatment, as well as improvement in acute-phase reactants. The mechanism of action of IVIG in KD is unknown.

Aspirin is given in high doses during acute KD for antiinflammatory effect. It is generally continued at 80 to 100 mg/kg/day until the 14th illness day, or until the patient has been afebrile for at least 2 days. Aspirin is then reduced to 3 to 5 mg/kg/day given in a single daily dose, for its antithrombotic effect. Aspirin is discontinued at 6 to 8 weeks after onset if all echocardiograms have been normal and acute-phase reactants have normalized. If coronary artery abnormalities develop, low-dose aspirin is continued. Depending upon the severity of coronary artery disease, other therapies, such as clopidogrel and warfarin, may be indicated[39]; such decisions should be made in consultation with a pediatric cardiologist.

IVIG and aspirin is also given to KD patients who present after the 10th day of illness if fever and/or clinical and laboratory signs of ongoing inflammation are present, although the efficacy of the therapy in this clinical situation is uncertain. In Japan, risk-scoring systems have been developed that can predict which Japanese children are at highest risk of developing coronary artery abnormalities with good accuracy, and the "RAISE" study showed that primary therapy with IVIG and a tapering course of prednisolone over 2 to 3 weeks improved outcomes in high-risk patients.[37] Unfortunately, risk-scoring systems have thus far performed poorly in multiethnic populations such as in North America, making the selection of patients in non-Japanese populations for intensified primary therapy more problematic.[38]

Approximately 15% of acute KD patients do not respond to initial therapy; optimal therapy for these patients with "refractory" KD is unknown. Most of these patients will respond to a second 2 g/kg IVIG infusion.[44] In patients who do not respond to initial therapy and are already in a high-risk category because of the presence of coronary artery dilation, a second dose of IVIG given with prednisolone in a tapering regimen over 2 to 3 weeks should be considered.[53] Other options for IVIG nonresponders include high-dose intravenous methylprednisolone once daily for 3 days or infliximab.[54,55] More specific therapy awaits the identification of the cause of KD.

COUNSELING

Patients who do not develop coronary artery abnormalities are not known to develop any long-term sequelae. Patients who have coronary artery abnormalities with normalization of the luminal diameter over time should be followed by a pediatric cardiologist; these patients may be at risk of developing arterial stenoses in the future. Patients with significant persisting coronary artery abnormalities should be followed by a pediatric cardiologist who can make recommendations about long-term therapy and activity restrictions based upon guidelines established by the American Heart Association.[39]

TREATMENT ALGORITHM

Table 142-5 outlines the approach to treatment of KD.

TABLE 142-5
Treatment of Acute Kawasaki Disease

- Intravenous gammaglobulin (IVIG) 2 g/kg infused over 10 to 12 hours; monitor vital signs carefully during infusion, with aspirin 80 to 100 mg/kg/day divided every 6 hours orally until the 14th illness day or until patient is afebrile for at least 2 days, then reduce dose to 3 to 5 mg/kg/day as a single daily dose.
- Aspirin is discontinued if echocardiograms at 2 to 3 weeks and 6 to 8 weeks are normal and when acute-phase reactants have normalized.

REFERENCES

1. Amano S, Hazama F, Hamashima Y. Pathology of Kawasaki disease: II. Distribution and incidence of the vascular lesions. *Jpn Circ J*. 1979;43(8):741-748.
2. Amano S, Hazama F, Hamashima Y. Pathology of Kawasaki disease: I. Pathology and morphogenesis of the vascular changes. *Jpn Circ J*. 1979;43(7):633-643.
3. Amano S, Hazama F, Kubagawa H, et al. General pathology of Kawasaki disease. On the morphological alterations corresponding to the clinical manifestations. *Acta Pathol Jpn*. 1980;30(5):681-694.
4. Newburger JW, Takahashi M, Burns JC, et al. The treatment of Kawasaki syndrome with intravenous gamma globulin. *N Engl J Med*. 1986;315(6):341-347.
5. Kawasaki T. Acute febrile mucocutaneous syndrome with lymphoid involvement with specific desquamation of the fingers and toes in children [in Japanese]. *Arerugi*. 1967;16(3):178-222.
6. Landing BH, Larson EJ. Are infantile periarteritis nodosa with coronary artery involvement and fatal mucocutaneous lymph node syndrome the same? Comparison of 20 patients from North America with patients from Hawaii and Japan. *Pediatrics*. 1977;59(5):651-662.
7. Kawasaki T, Kosaki F, Okawa S, et al. A new infantile acute febrile mucocutaneous lymph node syndrome (MLNS) prevailing in Japan. *Pediatrics*. 1974;54(3):271-276.
8. Melish ME, Hicks RM, Larson EJ. Mucocutaneous lymph node syndrome in the United States. *Am J Dis Child*. 1976;130(6):599-607.
9. Holman RC, Belay ED, Christensen KY, et al. Hospitalizations for Kawasaki syndrome among children in the United States, 1997-2007. *Pediatr Infect Dis J*. 2010;29(6):483-488.
10. Makino N, Nakamura Y, Yashiro M, et al. Descriptive epidemiology of Kawasaki disease in Japan, 2011-2012: from the results of the 22nd nationwide survey. *J Epidemiol*. 2015;25(3):239-245.
11. Burns JC, Wiggins JW Jr, Toews WH, et al. Clinical spectrum of Kawasaki disease in infants younger than 6 months of age. *J Pediatr*. 1986;109(5):759-763.
12. Momenah T, Sanatani S, Potts J, et al. Kawasaki disease in the older child. *Pediatrics*. 1998;102(1):e7.
13. Rosenfeld EA, Corydon KE, Shulman ST. Kawasaki disease in infants less than one year of age. *J Pediatr*. 1995;126(4):524-529.
14. Dean AG, Melish ME, Hicks R, et al. An epidemic of Kawasaki syndrome in Hawaii. *J Pediatr*. 1982;100(4):552-557.
15. Fujita Y, Nakamura Y, Sakata K, et al. Kawasaki disease in families. *Pediatrics*. 1989;84(4):666-669.
16. Uehara R, Yashiro M, Nakamura Y, et al. Kawasaki disease in parents and children. *Acta Paediatr*. 2003;92(6):694-697.
17. Bell DM, Brink EW, Nitzkin JL, et al. Kawasaki syndrome: description of two outbreaks in the United States. *N Engl J Med*. 1981;304(26):1568-1575.
18. Salo E, Pelkonen P, Pettay O. Outbreak of Kawasaki syndrome in Finland. *Acta Paediatr Scand*. 1986;75(1):75-80.
19. Yanagawa H, Nakamura Y, Kawasaki T, et al. Nationwide epidemic of Kawasaki disease in Japan during winter of 1985-86. *Lancet*. 1986;2(8516):1138-1139.
20. Stamos JK, Corydon K, Donaldson J, et al. Lymphadenitis as the dominant manifestation of Kawasaki disease. *Pediatrics*. 1994;93(3):525-528.
21. Onouchi Y, Gunji T, Burns JC, et al. ITPKC functional polymorphism associated with Kawasaki disease susceptibility and formation of coronary artery aneurysms. *Nat Genet*. 2008;40(1):35-42.
22. Onouchi Y, Ozaki K, Buns JC, et al. Common variants in CASP3 confer susceptibility to Kawasaki disease. *Hum Mol Genet*. 2010;19(14):2898-2906.
23. Onouchi Y, Ozaki K, Burns JC, et al. A genome-wide association study identifies three new risk loci for Kawasaki disease. *Nat Genet*. 2012;44(5):517-521.
24. Onouchi Y, Fukazawa R, Yamamura K, et al. Variations in ORAI1 gene associated with Kawasaki disease. *PLoS One*. 2016;11(1):e0145486.
25. Brown TJ, Crawford SE, Cornwall ML, et al. CD8 T lymphocytes and macrophages infiltrate coronary artery aneurysms in acute Kawasaki disease. *J Infect Dis*. 2001;184(7):940-943.
26. Rowley AH, Eckerley CA, Jack HM, et al. IgA plasma cells in vascular tissue of patients with Kawasaki syndrome. *J Immunol*. 1997;159(12):5946-5955.
27. Rowley AH, Shulman ST, Mask CA, et al. IgA plasma cell infiltration of proximal respiratory tract, pancreas, kidney, and coronary artery in acute Kawasaki disease. *J Infect Dis*. 2000;182(4):1183-1191.
28. Orenstein JM, Shulman ST, Fox LM, et al. Three linked vasculopathic processes characterize Kawasaki disease: a light and transmission electron microscopic study. *PLoS One*. 2012;7(6):e38998.
29. Choi IH, Chwae YJ, Shim WS, et al. Clonal expansion of CD8+ T cells in Kawasaki disease. *J Immunol*. 1997;159(1):481-486.
30. Lee HH, Shin JS, Kim DS. Immunoglobulin V(H) chain gene analysis of peripheral blood IgM-producing B cells in patients with Kawasaki disease. *Yonsei Med J*. 2009;50(4):493-504.
31. Rowley AH, Shulman ST, Spike BT, et al. Oligoclonal IgA response in the vascular wall in acute Kawasaki disease. *J Immunol*. 2001;166(2):1334-1343.
32. Rowley AH, Baker SC, Shulman ST, et al. Cytoplasmic inclusion bodies are detected by synthetic antibody in ciliated bronchial epithelium during acute Kawasaki disease. *J Infect Dis*. 2005;192(10):1757-1766.
33. Rowley AH, Baker SC, Shulman ST, et al. RNA-containing cytoplasmic inclusion bodies in ciliated bronchial epithelium months to years after acute Kawasaki disease. *PLoS One*. 2008;3(2):e1582.
34. Rowley AH, Baker SC, Shulman ST, et al. Detection of antigen in bronchial epithelium and macrophages in acute Kawasaki disease by use of synthetic antibody. *J Infect Dis*. 2004;190(4):856-865.
35. Rowley AH, Baker SC, Shulman ST, et al. Ultrastructural, immunofluorescence, and RNA evidence support the hypothesis of a "new" virus associated with Kawasaki disease. *J Infect Dis*. 2011;203(7):1021-1030.
36. Rowley AH, Wylie KM, Kim KY, et al. The transcriptional profile of coronary arteritis in Kawasaki disease. *BMC Genomics*. 2015;16(1):1076.
37. Kobayashi T, Saji T, Otani T, et al. Efficacy of immunoglobulin plus prednisolone for prevention of coronary artery abnormalities in severe Kawasaki disease (RAISE study): a randomised, open-label, blinded-endpoints trial. *Lancet*. 2012;379(9826):1613-1620.
38. Son MB, Newburger JW. Management of Kawasaki disease: corticosteroids revisited. *Lancet*. 2012;379(9826):1571-1572.
39. McCrindle BW, Rowley AH, Newburger JW, et al. Diagnosis, Treatment, and Long-Term Management of Kawasaki Disease: A Scientific Statement for Health

Professionals From the American Heart Association. *Circulation*. 2017;135(17):e927-e999.
40. Tacke CE, Romeih S, Kuipers IM, et al. Evaluation of cardiac function by magnetic resonance imaging during the follow-up of patients with Kawasaki disease. *Circ Cardiovasc Imaging*. 2013;6(1):67-73.
41. Kanamaru H, Sato Y, Takayama T, et al. Assessment of coronary artery abnormalities by multislice spiral computed tomography in adolescents and young adults with Kawasaki disease. *Am J Cardiol*. 2005;95(4):522-525.
42. Dominguez SR, Friedman K, Seewald R, et al. Kawasaki disease in a pediatric intensive care unit: a case-control study. *Pediatrics*. 2008;122(4):e786-e790.
43. Kanegaye JT, Wilder MS, Molkara D, et al. Recognition of a Kawasaki disease shock syndrome. *Pediatrics*. 2009;123(5):e783-e789.
44. Wallace CA, French JW, Kahn SJ, et al. Initial intravenous gammaglobulin treatment failure in Kawasaki disease. *Pediatrics*. 2000;105(6):E78.
45. Printz BF, Sleeper LA, Newburger JW, et al. Noncoronary cardiac abnormalities are associated with coronary artery dilation and with laboratory inflammatory markers in acute Kawasaki disease. *J Am Coll Cardiol*. 2011;57(1):86-92.
46. Suda K, Iemura M, Nishiono H, et al. Long-term prognosis of patients with Kawasaki disease complicated by giant coronary aneurysms: a single-institution experience. *Circulation*. 2011;123(17):1836-1842.
47. Nakano H, Saito A, Ueda K, et al. Clinical characteristics of myocardial infarction following Kawasaki disease: report of 11 cases. *J Pediatr*. 1986;108(2):198-203.
48. Ishii M, Ueno T, Akagi T, et al. Guidelines for catheter intervention in coronary artery lesion in Kawasaki disease. *Pediatr Int*. 2001;43(5):558-562.
49. Kitamura S, Tsuda E, Kobayashi J, et al. Twenty-five-year outcome of pediatric coronary artery bypass surgery for Kawasaki disease. *Circulation*. 2009;120(1):60-68.
50. Checchia PA, Pahl E, Shaddy RE, et al. Cardiac transplantation for Kawasaki disease. *Pediatrics*. 1997;100(4):695-699.
51. Newburger JW, Takahashi M, Beiser AS, et al. A single intravenous infusion of gamma globulin as compared with four infusions in the treatment of acute Kawasaki syndrome. *N Engl J Med*. 1991;324(23):1633-1639.
52. Dominguez SR, Anderson MS, El-Adawy M, et al. Preventing coronary artery abnormalities: a need for earlier diagnosis and treatment of Kawasaki disease. *Pediatr Infect Dis J*. 2012;31(12):1217-1220.
53. Kobayashi T, Morikawa A, Ikeda K, et al. Efficacy of intravenous immunoglobulin combined with prednisolone following resistance to initial intravenous immunoglobulin treatment of acute Kawasaki disease. *J Pediatr*. 2013;163(2):521-526.
54. Burns JC, Best BM, Mejias A, et al. Infliximab treatment of intravenous immunoglobulin-resistant Kawasaki disease. *J Pediatr*. 2008;153(6):833-838.
55. Wright DA, Newburger JW, Baker A, et al. Treatment of immune globulin-resistant Kawasaki disease with pulsed doses of corticosteroids. *J Pediatr*. 1996;128(1):146-149.

Chapter 143 :: Pigmented Purpuric Dermatoses
Alexandra Haden & David H. Peng

第一百四十三章

色素性紫癜性皮病

中文导读

色素性紫癜性皮疹（也称为色素性紫癜性皮病[PPD]）是一组以瘀斑和色素沉着为特征的皮肤病，最常见于下肢也可能累及躯干和上肢。这组疾病可分为几个临床亚类，包括进行性色素性皮肤病（Schamberg病）、毛细血管扩张性环状紫癜（Majocchipurpura）、Gougerot和Blum的色素性紫癜性苔藓样皮病、Doucas和Kapetanakis的类湿疹样紫癜以及金黄色苔藓（表143-1）。本章节从流行病学、临床特征、病因和发病机制、诊断、鉴别诊断、临床过程和预后及治疗对该组疾病进行了详细阐述。

1. 流行病学　PPD相对不常见，最常见于中年（见表143-1），无明显种族倾向，一般而言，PPD在男性中的发病率更高。

2. 临床特征

（1）进行性色素性皮肤病（Schamberg病）：该病由Schamberg首先描述，具体表现为下肢不规则形状的红褐色斑块伴有"针头大小的红色出血点，非常类似于辣椒粉"，是儿童色素性紫癜性皮病中最常见类型，慢性病程，常以发作期和缓解期交替持续存在。

（2）毛细血管扩张性环状紫癜（Majocchipurpura）：Majocchi于1896年首先描述，这种PPD的亚型以其独特的环状分布为特征（图143-3）。每个病变都是从点状毛细血管扩张开始，逐渐向外周扩散，中央出现色素减退或轻度萎缩。病变可为单发或多发，下肢是最常见的受累部位。与PPD的其他亚型不同，Majocchipurpura最常见于成年女性。

（3）Gougerot和Blum的色素性紫癜性苔藓样皮病：1925年由Gougerot和Blum首先报道，在临床上以红褐色的圆形或多边形苔藓样丘疹或斑块为特征，并伴有紫癜或毛细血管扩张的背景（图143-4）。该病最常见于下肢，呈慢性病程。

（4）Doucas和Kapetanakis的类湿疹样紫癜：1953年由Doucas和Kapetanakis首先描述，临床上伴有瘙痒性红色斑片或斑块，上方覆盖轻薄的鳞屑。在组织病理学上，除了典型的PPD组织病理学特征外，还存在海绵水肿。该亚型往往在15～30天的时间内迅速扩散，即使不进行治疗也可在几个月至几年后逐渐消失，但有复发的可能性。

（5）金黄色苔藓：该亚型以局限性和持续性金色、铁锈或橙色的斑片或丘疹为表现（图143-5）。组织学上可见致密的带状炎细胞呈苔藓样浸润。病变通常无症状，常发生于一侧下肢，多见于成年男性，在20~40岁发病率最高，往往呈稳定或缓慢进展的慢性病程。

（6）瘙痒性紫癜（弥漫性瘙痒性血管皮炎）：表现为急性泛发的伴有严重瘙痒的橙棕色至紫癜性损害。病变首先出现在足背或下肢，沿腰线、腋窝、肘前窝和腘窝的区域更为明显，呈慢性病程，有自发缓解趋势。

（7）单侧线状毛细血管炎（节段性色素性紫癜）：该亚型在临床上通过其线性或节段分布来定义，倾向于良好的预后，与其他PPD亚型相比，其自发缓解可能性更高。

（8）肉芽肿性色素性紫癜：PPD的肉芽肿变异型首次由Saito和Matsuoka于1996年提出，中年人好发。在临床上，最常表现为下肢和足背的紫癜性和褐色斑，在组织病理学上除了PPD的经典组织病理学特征外，还存在肉芽肿浸润。作者特别指出这类患者必须排除系统性肉芽肿性疾病和感染（分枝杆菌和深部真菌）。此外，肉芽肿性色素性紫癜与高脂血症存在相关性。

（9）色素性紫癜性皮病/蕈样肉芽肿重叠：提及有一些证据认为PPD的苔藓样变体可能是MF的早期表现，文献中报道了二者3种不同的关系：MF在临床上模拟色素性紫癜，色素性紫癜演变成MF，以及色素性紫癜在组织学上模拟MF。接下来作者对于二者在组织学上和免疫标记上的相似性进行了详细描述，并提出PPD皮损出现大面积融合、网状排列、叠加紫罗兰色调或伴瘙痒且持续存在或复发数年需怀疑MF的可能，建议长期随访监测。

3. 病因和发病机制 关于PPD的发病机制有3种不同的观点。首先是皮肤血管被破坏导致毛细血管脆性和红细胞外渗。第二种理论是PPD从体液免疫反应发展而来。第三个理论是PPD是细胞免疫反应的结果。本章对支持这三种理论的证据进行了详细阐述。PPD还可被多种药物诱发（表143-2），作者对药物诱发的PPD的特点进行了总结。此外，遗传性因素以及重力和静脉压升高也被认为与PPD相关，但总体而言大多数PPD为特发性。

4. 诊断 通常通过临床诊断，组织病理学检查可支持诊断，应该询问患者的病史、药物和可能的接触过敏原。

（1）实验室检查：实验室检查通常用于排除其他疾病。

（2）病理：所有PPD均具有相似的组织病理学特征，真皮乳头中存在淋巴细胞性围血管浸润，并伴有内皮肿胀和红细胞外渗，以及巨噬细胞内铁血黄素沉积（图143-6）。对于不同亚型的特异性改变作者也进行了介绍。

（3）鉴别诊断：表143-4概述了PPD的鉴别诊断。

5. 临床过程和预后 PPD是良性无症状的慢性疾病，单侧线状毛细血管炎和药物引起的PPD总体预后更好。

6. 治疗

（1）药物：常见的一线治疗包括局部类固醇和抗组胺药，以及使用压缩袜治疗相关的静脉功能不全。除局部类固醇外，也可外用吡美莫司。作者对已报道的系统用于治疗PPD的药物进行了综述，不建议对该病进行过于激进的治疗，除非全身泛发或伴有严重的症状。

（2）光疗和激光治疗：补骨脂素和紫外线A光化学疗法（PUVA）和窄波紫外线B（nbUVB）均被报道可用于清除皮损。595nm染料脉冲激光治疗Schamberg病也有个案报道。

（3）建议：应告知患者疾病的良性性质和慢性复发性过程，建议持续随访来监测疾病的进展。

〔黄莹雪〕

AT-A-GLANCE

- A group of dermatoses characterized by petechiae, pigmentation, and occasionally, telangiectasia.
- Found most commonly on the lower extremities; however, lesions may involve the upper body but rarely become generalized.
- Benign, generally asymptomatic eruptions that tend to be chronic with flares and remissions.
- Common histopathologic features include a superficial lymphocytic infiltrate, erythrocyte extravasation, and hemosiderin deposition.
- Clinical variation between eruptions led to their subclassification into eponymic groups; however, frequent overlap may make differentiation difficult.

Pigmented purpuric eruptions (also called *pigmented purpuric dermatoses* [PPDs]) are a group of dermatoses that are characterized by petechiae, pigmentation, and, occasionally, telangiectasia. They are most commonly located on the lower extremities; however, lesions may involve the trunk and upper extremities, or, rarely, become generalized. They are subdivided into clinical subcategories, which include progressive pigmentary dermatosis (Schamberg disease), purpura annularis telangiectodes (Majocchi purpura), pigmented purpuric lichenoid dermatosis of Gougerot and Blum, eczematid-like purpura of Doucas and Kapetanakis, and lichen aureus (Table 143-1). These dermatoses are benign and generally asymptomatic, but tend to run a chronic course with flares and remissions. Despite differing clinical presentations, the subtypes of PPDs share common histopathologic features, including a superficial lymphocytic infiltrate, erythrocyte extravasation and hemosiderin deposition.

EPIDEMIOLOGY

PPDs are relatively uncommon. They may present at any age, including in children, and are most common in middle age (see Table 143-1). There is no ethnic predisposition, although the granulomatous variant has been reported more commonly in patients of Asian descent.[1] In general, PPDs occur more frequently in males, except for the Majocchi subtype, which is seen more frequently in females.[2]

CLINICAL FEATURES

PROGRESSIVE PIGMENTARY DERMATOSIS (SCHAMBERG DISEASE)

Schamberg first described an eruption of irregularly shaped reddish-brown patches with "pin head sized reddish puncta, closely resembling grains of cayenne pepper" over the legs of a 15-year-old boy in 1901.[3] Schamberg disease is the most common of the PPDs to occur in children. It is, however, more common overall in adults with a peak incidence in the fifth decade.[4] The lesions are insidious in their development and are usually asymptomatic. The lower extremities are the most common site of involvement. Lesions can involve the trunk or the upper extremities (Figs. 143-1 and 143-2). Schamberg disease is chronic and persistent with flares and remissions occurring indefinitely.

PURPURA ANNULARIS TELANGIECTODES (MAJOCCHI PURPURA)

Majocchi described the first case of purpura annularis telangiectodes in 1896 in a 21-year-old male who presented with annular patches of follicular and punctate reddish-brown macules with telangiectasias and purpura on the lower extremities.[5] This subtype of PPD is characterized by its distinctive annular pattern (Fig. 143-3). Individual lesions begin as punctate telangiectatic macules that extend peripherally with central hypopigmentation or slight atrophy.[1] Lesions may be solitary or multiple in number. The lower extremities are the most common site of involvement and lesions can extend to involve the upper extremities and trunk. Majocchi purpura are generally asymptomatic and last several months with flares and remissions. As opposed to other subtypes of PPDs, Majocchi purpura presents most commonly in young adult females.[2,6]

PIGMENTED PURPURIC LICHENOID DERMATOSIS OF GOUGEROT AND BLUM

In 1925, Gougerot and Blum reported a pigmented eruption on the lower extremity of a 41-year-old man.[7] This subtype is clinically distinguished by the presence of reddish-brown round or polygonal lichenoid papules and plaques, with a background of purpura or telangiectasias (Fig. 143-4). The term *lichenoid* describes this clinical appearance of lichenoid papules and plaques rather than the underlying histology. Its clinical appearance can be mistaken for Kaposi sarcoma. Similar to other subtypes of PPDs, pigmented purpuric lichenoid dermatosis of Gougerot and Blum is most commonly found on the lower extremities, occasionally involves the trunk and upper extremities, and runs a chronic course.

TABLE 143-1
Subtypes of Pigmented Purpuric Dermatoses

	SCHAMBERG	MAJOCCHI	GOUGEROT AND BLUM	DOUCAS AND KAPETANAKIS	ITCHING PURPURA	LICHEN AUREUS
Average age of presentation	40s	30s	40s	40s	50s	20s-30s
Sex	M > F	F > M	M > F	M > F	M > F	M > F
Onset	Insidious	Abrupt	Insidious	Abrupt	Abrupt	Abrupt
Primary lesion	Red-brown macule with pinpoint petechiae ("cayenne pepper")	Annular plaques with border of telangiectasia and purpura	Lichenoid papule	Red-brown macule + scale	Red-brown macule	Orange-brown papule or plaque

F, female; M, male.

ECZEMATID-LIKE PURPURA OF DOUCAS AND KAPETANAKIS

Eczematid-like purpura was first described by Doucas and Kapetanakis in 1953 in a group of patients with an asymptomatic seasonal eruption occurring in the spring and summer.[8] It is distinguished clinically by mild scaling overlying pinpoint erythematous macules and patches with associated pruritus. Lichenification can occur from repeated scratching. Histopathologically, spongiosis is present, in addition to the classic histopathologic features of PPD. This subtype spreads rapidly over a period of 15 to 30 days and will subsequently fade without treatment over several months to years, although recurrence is possible.

LICHEN AUREUS

In 1958, Martin first reported this subtype of PPD under the term *lichen purpuricus*, which was later named *lichen aureus* in 1960 by Calnan to emphasize its vivid yellow-orange color.[9,10] As opposed to

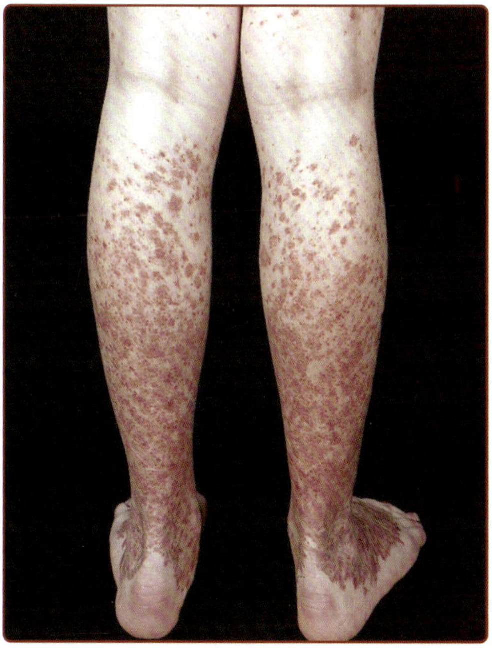

Figure 143-1 Pigmented purpuric dermatosis: Schamberg disease. Multiple, discrete, and confluent nonpalpable, nonblanching purpuric lesions of many months' duration on the legs. Acute microhemorrhages resolve with deposition of hemosiderin, creating a disfiguring dark-brown peppered stain.

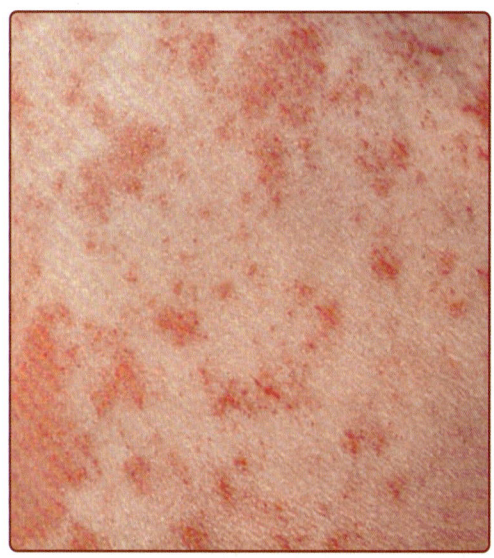

Figure 143-2 "Cayenne pepper" appearance of Schamberg disease. (From Wolff K, Johnson R, Saavedra AP, et al. *Fitzpatrick's Color Atlas and Synopsis of Clinical Dermatology*, 8th ed. New York, NY: McGraw-Hill; 2017, with permission.)

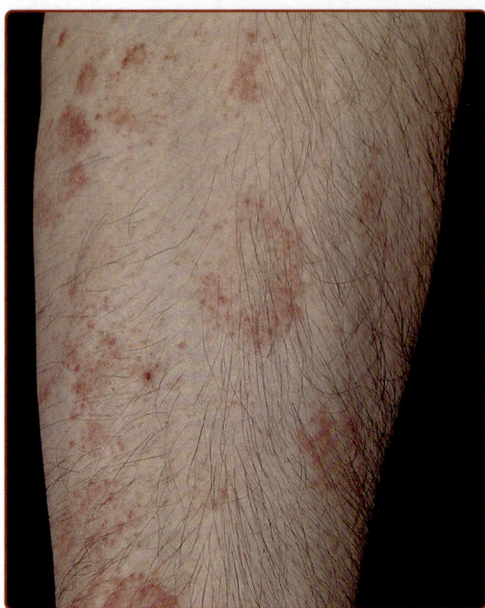

Figure 143-3 Pigmented purpuric dermatosis: Majocchi disease. Multiple nonpalpable, nonblanching purpuric lesions arranged in annular configurations and associated with tiny telangiectasias. Note brownish discoloration of older lesions.

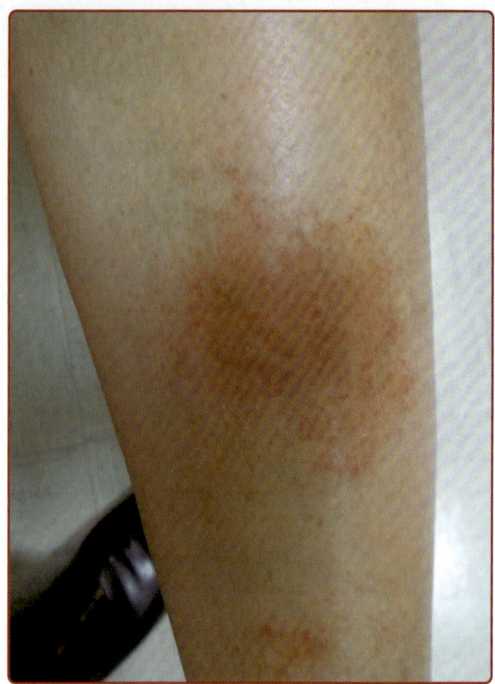

Figure 143-5 Lichen aureus. (Used with permission from Dr. Ashley Crew.)

pigmented purpuric lichenoid dermatosis of Gougerot and Blum, where lichenoid refers to the clinical morphology of the lesions, in lichen aureus, *lichen* refers to both its clinical and histopathologic features. This subtype presents with more localized and persistent lesions with circumscribed macules or papules that are a distinctive gold, rust, or orange color (Fig. 143-5). Histologically a dense, band-like lichenoid infiltrate of inflammatory cells is seen. The lesions are generally asymptomatic but at times are intensely pruritic. They are most commonly localized to one lower extremity, but other body sites can be involved, and a segmental distribution has been reported.[11,12] This disorder has a predilection for young adult males, with a peak incidence in the second and third decades. It runs a chronic course, with stable or slowly progressing lesions.

ITCHING PURPURA (DISSEMINATED PRURIGINOUS ANGIODERMATITIS)

Itching purpura, also known as disseminated pruriginous angiodermatitis, presents acutely with widely disseminated orange-brown to purpuric lesions associated with severe pruritus.[13,14] The lesions first appear on the dorsal feet or lower extremities and then spread upward, sometimes with involvement of the trunk. Purpuric lesions are more apparent along the waistline, axilla, antecubital and popliteal fossae. Although this subtype of PPD has a chronic course, spontaneous remissions are possible.

UNILATERAL LINEAR CAPILLARITIS (SEGMENTAL PIGMENTED PURPURA)

In 1990, a transient PPD in a segmental distribution on the lower trunk of a middle-aged woman was reported. Later, Riordan and colleagues reported PPDs in 4 young men with linear and pseudodermatomal

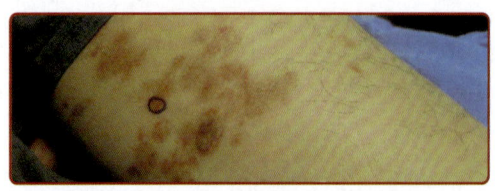

Figure 143-4 Lichenoid dermatosis of Gougerot and Blum. (Used with permission from Dr. April Armstrong.)

patterns, which they termed *unilateral linear capillaritis*.[15] Both "segmental pigmented purpura" and "quadrantic capillaropathy" are considered subtypes of unilateral linear capillaritis.[16,17] This PPD is clinically distinguished by its linear or segmental distribution. It tends to have a favorable prognosis, with spontaneous resolution occurring more commonly than in the other subtypes of PPDs.

GRANULOMATOUS PIGMENTED PURPURA

The first report of the granulomatous variant of PPDs was in 1996 by Saito and Matsuoka and since then more than 17 cases have been reported.[18-20] It is most common in middle age and has been reported more commonly in patients of Asian descent.[1,20] Clinically, the lesions appear similar to other PPDs with purpuric and brown macules developing most commonly on the lower extremities and dorsal feet. This subtype is distinguished by its histopathologic findings. In addition to the classic histopathologic features of a PPD, a granulomatous infiltrate is present. The granulomatous infiltrate is most commonly located in the papillary dermis, but may be in the mid to deep dermis separate from a more superficially located lichenoid infiltrate. Systemic granulomatous disorders and infectious processes (mycobacterial and deep fungal) must be ruled out in these patients. Hyperlipidemia is a relatively common association with granulomatous pigmented purpura with 9 of 17 reported cases showing elevated cholesterol levels in a review from 2014.[19]

PIGMENTED PURPURIC DERMATOSIS/MYCOSIS FUNGOIDES OVERLAP

In 1988, Barnhill and Braverman reported the first cases of pigmented purpura-like eruptions progressing to mycosis fungoides.[21] Furthermore, the first patient diagnosed with lichen aureus in the United States was later diagnosed with mycosis fungoides (MF; see Chap. 119). Some evidence supports the idea that lichenoid variants of PPD may be precursors of MF, with similar histologic findings and clonal populations of lymphocytes.[22-29] Although there is no clear connection between these 2 diseases, and the occurrence of MF in the setting of a PPD is rare, 3 different relationships have been reported: MF mimicking pigmented purpura clinically, pigmented purpura evolving into MF, and pigmented purpura that simulates MF histologically.

In a study of T-cell clonality and markers, T-cell monoclonality of PPD was most likely to predict progression to MF, whereas the absence of certain T-cell markers was a less reliable predictor.[30] It is important to note that both MF and PPD can display clonality. Histologic clues of MF are subtle and include greater lymphoid atypia in the intraepidermal lymphocytes compared to dermal lymphocytes, large intraepidermal groups of lymphocytes anywhere in the epidermis, or many lymphocytes in the spinous layer.[30,31] Santucci and colleagues suggested that to distinguish early MF from its inflammatory mimickers the most important feature is lymphocytes with extremely convoluted, medium to large nuclei, that are single or clustered in the epidermis and in small sheets in the dermis.[32] Ackerman compared the histologic features of lichenoid purpuric eruptions with plaque stage MF and noted many similarities, concluding that it may be impossible to differentiate these two on a histologic basis alone.[33]

The differentiation between PPD and MF can be difficult and requires the integration of clinical, histologic and immunophenotypic information.[30,33] PPDs with large areas of confluence, reticular arrangements, a superimposed violaceous hue, or pruritus that has been present or relapsing for several years are suspicious for MF. There is a predominance in adult males.[21,34] For selected patients, long-term followup is needed to monitor for evolution into MF, even though the overall incidence of MF occurring in association with PPD is rare.

ETIOLOGY AND PATHOGENESIS

There are 3 different views on the pathogenesis of PPDs. The first is that there is a disturbance or weakness of cutaneous blood vessels, leading to capillary fragility and erythrocyte extravasation. This proposed mechanism, however, does not account for the inflammatory infiltrate that is also seen in these eruptions. The second theory is that PPDs develop from a humoral immune response. This theory is supported by direct immunofluorescence studies showing vascular deposition of C3, C1q, immunoglobulin M, or immunoglobulin A.[35,36] The final theory is that PPDs develop as a result of a cellular immune response.[37,38] This theory suggests that the inflammatory infiltrate, consisting of lymphocytes, macrophages, and Langerhans cells, leads to vascular fragility and subsequent extravasation of erythrocytes. Aiba and Tagami used immunohistologic studies in 8 cases of Schamberg disease to demonstrate that the dermal infiltrate was predominantly composed of helper-inducer T-cells and OKT6-reactive cells, whereas the epidermis showed intercellular staining with human leukocyte antigen-DR antibody and OKT6 antibody.[39] Based on this study, they concluded that a cellular immune reaction, specifically with Langerhans cell, likely plays an important role in the pathogenesis. Additionally, Ghersetich and colleagues showed that cell-mediated mechanisms may be important in the development of Schamberg disease as CD4+ T cells and CD1a dendritic cells predominate in early lesions and this infiltrate clears with potent topical steroid therapy.[38]

PPD may be induced by multiple drugs (Table 143-2).[1,40-53] These drug-induced eruptions are more likely to be generalized, but still present with lower-extremity involvement. They are often transient, with a mean duration of 3 to 4 months, with many cases resolving within a few weeks.[53] A temporal relationship may be difficult to establish as patients can be taking the culprit medication for months to years prior to the onset of the eruption. Rechallenge has been used to confirm diagnosis.

In addition to medications, other causes also have been implicated (Table 143-3).[54-61] A handful of cases show familial involvement, with one report of an autosomal dominant inheritance pattern.[62] Gravity and increased venous pressure may account for the lesions localizing to the lower extremities. Overall, the majority of cases of PPDs are idiopathic.

TABLE 143-2
Drugs Implicated in Pigmented Purpuric Dermatoses

- Acetaminophen
- Aminoglutethimide
- Ampicillin
- Aspirin
- Bezafibrate
- Bufexamac
- Carbamazepine
- Carbromal
- Carbutamide
- Chlordiazepoxide
- Diltiazem
- Dipyridamole
- Topical fluorouracil
- Furosemide
- Glipizide
- Glybuzole
- Hydralazine
- Infliximab
- Interferon-α
- Isotretinoin
- Medroxyprogesterone acetate
- Meprobamate
- Minocycline
- Nitroglycerin
- Nonsteroidal antiinflammatory drugs
- Phenobarbital
- Pseudoephedrine
- Raloxifene
- Reserpine
- Sildenafil
- Tartrazine (food additive)
- Thiamine
- Trichlormethiazide
- Zomepirac sodium

TABLE 143-3
Other Implicated Causes of Pigmented Purpuric Dermatoses

- Contact dermatitis
    - Disperse dyes
    - Paraphenylenediamine
    - Black rubber
    - Cobalt
    - Benzoyl peroxide
    - Epoxy resin
    - Methylmethacrylate
    - Eutectic mixture of local anesthetics
- Venous stasis/acroangiodermatitis
- Step aerobics
- Strenuous exercise
- Rheumatoid arthritis
- Systemic lupus erythematosus
- Diabetes mellitus
- Thyroid dysfunction
- Hyperlipidemia
- Benign hyperglobulinemic purpura (of Waldenstrom)/dysproteinemic purpura)
- Hodgkin disease
- Hepatitides B and C
- Odontogenic infection
- Polycythemia
- Hereditary spherocytosis
- Porphyrias
- Purpuric mycosis fungoides

DIAGNOSIS

Diagnosis is generally made clinically and may be supported by histopathologic examination. The clinical measurement of capillary fragility by application of a sphygmomanometer (Hess test) does not appear to be reliable, as increased capillary fragility is not consistently seen in PPD. The patient's medical history, medications, and potential contact allergens should be reviewed. MF should be considered if the lesions are chronic and unremitting.

SUPPORTIVE STUDIES

LABORATORY TESTING

Laboratory testing is not required for diagnosis. In selected cases, laboratory testing may include a complete blood cell count with peripheral smear (to rule out thrombocytopenia or other hematologic disorders), coagulation studies (to rule out other causes of purpura), as well as an antinuclear antibody, rheumatoid factor, and hepatitis serologies.[1]

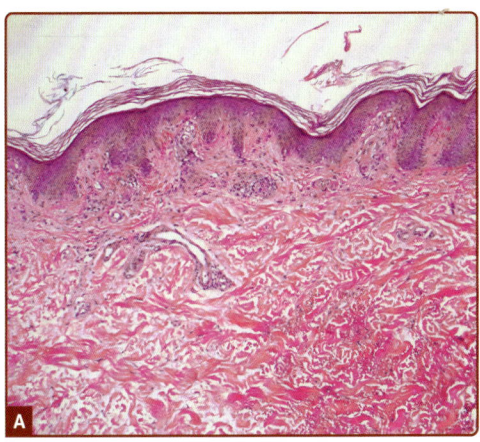
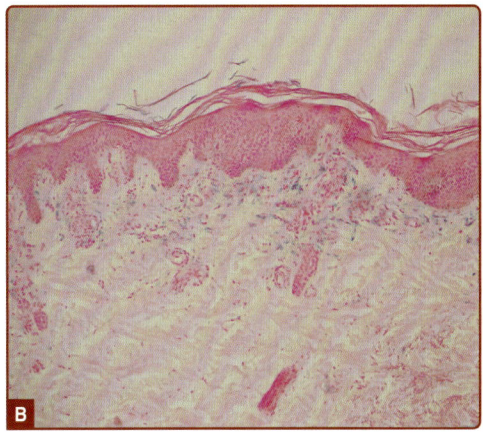

Figure 143-6 **A,** Pigmented purpuric dermatosis showing superficial perivascular lymphocytes and extravasated erythrocytes. **B,** Hemosiderin deposition highlighted by Prussian Blue staining. (Used with permission from Gene H. Kim, MD.)

PATHOLOGY

All PPDs share similar histopathology. A lymphocytic perivascular infiltrate is present in the papillary dermis with endothelial swelling and extravasated erythrocytes and hemosiderin deposition within macrophages (Fig. 143-6). In older lesions, there is less inflammation, and extravasated red cells may no longer be present. Although there is no consensus on whether a capillaritis is present, Ackerman asserts that there is no true capillaritis because of the lack of fibrin in the luminal walls and absence of thrombi.[1] The epidermis may show spongiosis and parakeratosis, particularly in pigmented purpuric lichenoid dermatitis of Gougerot and Blum and eczematid-like purpura of Doucas and Kapetanakis. In lichen aureus, there is a band-like mononuclear infiltrate in the upper dermis separated from the epidermis by a thin rim of uninvolved collagen. In granulomatous pigmented purpura, a granulomatous infiltrate is present either in the papillary dermis, or in the mid to deep dermis, which separated from a more superficially located lichenoid infiltrate.

DIFFERENTIAL DIAGNOSIS

Table 143-4 outlines the differential diagnosis of PPD.

CLINICAL COURSE AND PROGNOSIS

PPDs are benign and commonly asymptomatic. In general, PPDs are chronic with flares and remissions. Exceptions to this chronic course include unilateral linear capillaritis and drug-induced PPDs, which tend to have shorter clinical courses and more favorable overall prognoses.

MANAGEMENT

Management of PPD is challenging, as treatments are often ineffective. The patient's medical history, medications, and potential contact allergens should be reviewed. If the eruption is induced by a drug or contact allergen, discontinuation of the causative agent can lead to complete resolution. However, residual pigmentation may persist for years.

INTERVENTIONS

MEDICATIONS

Common initial therapies include topical steroids and antihistamines, which are particularly helpful in treating associated pruritus, as well as the use of compression stockings to treat associated venous insufficiency. In addition to topical steroids, topical pimecrolimus has been used. Treatment with topical pimecrolimus twice daily for 10 weeks cleared lichen aureus lesions in a 10-year-old boy. The patient had a minor flare after discontinuation that responded to 2 weeks of repeat treatment.[63] Intralesional corticosteroids have

TABLE 143-4

Differential Diagnosis of Pigmented Purpuric Dermatoses

- Contact dermatitis
- Leukocytoclastic vasculitis
- Stasis dermatitis and purpura
- Angioma serpiginosum
- Kaposi sarcoma (Gougerot-Blum)
- Mycosis fungoides
- Sarcoidosis
- Scurvy
- Hypergammaglobinemic purpura

also led to improvement, although tissue atrophy may develop and the development of new lesions is not prevented.[6]

Oral bioflavonoid (rutoside, 50 mg twice daily) and ascorbic acid (500 mg twice daily) given to 3 patients with chronic PPD in an open trial led to clearance in all 3 patients within 4 weeks with maintenance of remission 3 months after treatment.[64] In a pilot study, calcium dobesilate, 500 mg twice daily, was given to 9 patients for 3 months.[65] Seven patients had mild-to-moderate improvement that was sustained at 1 year after cessation of therapy. Griseofulvin, 500 mg to 750 mg daily, improved existing lesions within a week and stopped new lesions within a mean of 33 days in an open trial of 6 patients.[66] Colchicine, 0.5 mg twice daily, cleared a 28-year-old woman with recalcitrant Schamberg disease.[67] Minocycline also has been reported to be beneficial.

Pentoxifylline, which inhibits T-cell adherence to endothelial cells and keratinocytes, may be helpful. A randomized, investigator-blinded trial compared pentoxifylline, 400 mg 3 times daily, with topical betamethasone dipropionate cream, 0.05% twice daily, for 2 months. Patients treated with pentoxifylline had significantly greater improvement than those treated with the topical steroid. However, the response was not sustained after discontinuation of the medication.[68]

Immunosuppressants, such as systemic corticosteroids, cyclosporine, and methotrexate are often effective but are rarely indicated because of the benign nature of the disorder as well as recurrence upon discontinuation of these medications.[6,69] Methotrexate was reported to clear a patient with Majocchi purpura with just 15 mg weekly dosing for 4 weeks, although she had reoccurrence when the medication was discontinued. Again, aggressive therapy is not often warranted for this benign condition unless a generalized eruption or severe symptoms occur.

PHOTOTHERAPY AND LASER THERAPY

Psoralen and ultraviolet A light (PUVA) and narrowband ultraviolet B (nbUVB) have both been reported to clear lesions.[70-79] The phototherapy-induced immunosuppression of the cell-mediated response is the proposed mechanism.[6]

Gudi and White were the first to report the effectiveness of nbUVB in treating a patient with Schamberg disease.[70] In a report by Lasocki and Kelly, nbUVB was used to maintain disease suppression while tapering oral prednisolone. The patient remained clear on a once-every-2-week dosing, but had recurrence when UVB was completely stopped.[71] Additional cases have reported effectiveness of nbUVB in the treatment of PPD.[72-75]

PUVA inhibits T-cell interleukin-2 production and leads to resolution of the perivascular lymphocytic infiltrate.[76] Krisa and colleagues treated 7 patients with PUVA with clearance after 7 to 20 treatments.[77] Five of these patients remained in remission and 2 patients relapsed, but responded to a second course of PUVA. In another report, a cohort of 11 patients with PPDs responded to PUVA.[78]

Photodynamic therapy has been reported as beneficial as it affects both immunomodulation and vascular destruction.[80] In addition, successful clearance of Schamberg disease with the use of a 595-nm pulsed-dye laser after 5 monthly treatments has been reported.[81]

COUNSELING

Patients should be counseled about the benign but chronic and relapsing nature of these eruptions. Ongoing follow up may be warranted to monitor disease progression. Setting the expectation of treating symptoms, rather than aiming to cure the condition, may lead to improved patient satisfaction, as treatments to clear the eruption are often ineffective.

ACKNOWLEDGMENTS

The authors acknowledge the contributions of Theresa Schroeder Devere and Anisha B. Patel, the former authors of this chapter.

REFERENCES

1. Sardana K, Sarkar R, Sehgal VN. Pigmented purpuric dermatoses: an overview. *Int J Dermatol*. 2004;43(7): 482-488.
2. Kim DH, Seo SH, Ahn HH, et al. Characteristics and clinical manifestations of pigmented purpuric dermatosis. *Ann Dermatol*. 2015;27(4):404-410.
3. Schamberg JF. A peculiar progressive pigmentary disease of the skin. *Br J Dermatol*. 1901;13:1.
4. Torrela A, Requena C, Mediero IG, et al. Schamberg's purpura in children: a review of 13 cases. *J Am Acad Dermatol*. 2003;48(1):31-33.
5. Majocchi D. Sopra una dermatosi telangiectode non ancora descritta: purpura annularis. *G Ital Mal Venl*. 1896;31:263.
6. Hoesly FJ, Hueter CJ, Shehan JM. Purpura annularis telangiectodes of Majocchi: case report and review of the literature. *Int J Dermatol*. 2009;48(10):1129-1133.
7. Gougerot H, Blum P. Purpura angioscleux prurigeneux avec elements lichenoides. *Bull Soc Fr Dermatol Syphiligr*. 1925;32:161.
8. Doucas C, Kapetenakis J. Eczematid-like purpura. *Dermatologica*. 1953;106(2):86-95.
9. Marten RH. Case for diagnosis. *Trans St Johns Hosp Dermatol Soc*. 1958;30:98.
10. Calnan CD. Lichen aureus. *Br J Dermatol*. 1960;72: 373-374.
11. Mishra D, Maheshwari V. Segmental lichen aureus in child. *Int J Dermatol*. 1991;30(9):654-655.
12. Ruiz-Esmenjaud J, Dahl MV. Segmental lichen aureus: onset associated with trauma and puberty. *Arch Dermatol*. 1988;124(10):1572-1574.
13. Mosto SJ, Casala AM. Disseminated pruriginous angiodermatitis (itching purpura). *Arch Dermatol*. 1965; 91(4):351-356.

14. Pravda DJ, Moynihan GD. Itching purpura. *Cutis*. 1980; 25:147.
15. Riordan CA, Darley C, Markey AC, et al. Unilateral linear capillaritis. *Clin Exp Dermatol*. 1992;17(3):182-185.
16. Higgins EM, Cox NH. A case of quadrantic capillaropathy. *Dermatologica*. 1990;180(2):93-95.
17. Pock L, Capkova S. Segmental pigmented purpura. *Pediatr Dermatol*. 2002;19(6):517-519.
18. Saito R, Matsuoka Y. Granulomatous pigmented purpuric dermatosis. *J Dermatol*. 1996;23(8):551-555.
19. Battle LR, Shalin SC, Gao L. Granulomatous pigmented purpuric dermatosis. *Clin Exp Dermatol*. 2015; 40(4):387-390.
20. MacKenzie AI, Biswas A. Granulomatous pigmented purpuric dermatosis: report of a case with atypical clinical presentation including dermoscopic findings. *Am J Dermatopathol*. 2015;37(4):311-314.
21. Barnhill RL, Braverman IM. Progression of pigmented purpura-like eruptions to mycosis fungoides: report of three cases. *J Am Acad Dermatol*. 1998;19(1, pt 1): 25-31.
22. Martinez W, del Pozo J, Vázquez J, et al. Cutaneous T-cell lymphoma presenting as disseminated, pigmented, purpura-like eruption. *Int J Dermatol*. 2001;40(2):140-144.
23. Ugajin T, Satoh T, Yokozeki H, et al. Mycosis fungoides presenting as pigmented purpuric eruption. *Eur J Dermatol*. 2005;15(6):489-491.
24. Kazakov DV, Burg G, Kempf W. Clinicopathological spectrum of mycosis fungoides. *J Eur Acad Dermatol Venereol*. 2004;18(4):397-415.
25. Georgala S, Katoulis AC, Symeonidou S, et al. Persistent pigmented purpuric eruption associated with mycosis fungoides: a case report and review of the literature. *J Eur Acad Dermatol Venereol*. 2001;15(1): 62-64.
26. Puddu P, Ferranti G, Frezzolini A, et al. Pigmented purpura-like eruption as cutaneous sign of mycosis fungoides with autoimmune purpura. *J Am Acad Dermatol*. 1999;40(2, pt 2):298-299.
27. Cather JC, Farmer A, Jackow C, et al. Unusual presentation of mycosis fungoides as pigmented purpura with malignant thymoma. *J Am Acad Dermatol*. 1998;39 (5, pt 2):858-863.
28. Toro JR, Sander CA, LeBoit PE. Persistent pigmented purpuric dermatitis and mycosis fungoides: stimulant, precursor, or both: a study by light microscopy and molecular methods. *Am J Dermatopathol*. 1997; 19(2):108-118.
29. Lor P, Krueger U, Kempf W, et al. Monoclonal rearrangement of the T cell receptor gamma-chain in lichenoid pigmented purpuric dermatitis of Gougerot-Blum responding to topical corticosteroid therapy. *Dermatology*. 2002;205(2):191-193.
30. Magro CM, Schaefer JT, Crowson AN, et al. Pigmented purpuric dermatosis: classification by phenotypic and molecular profiles. *Am J Clin Pathol*. 2007;128(2): 218-229.
31. Hanna S, Walsh N, D'Intino Y, et al. Mycosis fungoides presenting as pigmented purpuric dermatitis. *Pediatr Dermatol*. 2006;23(4):350-354.
32. Santucci M, Biggeri A, Feller AC, et al. Efficacy of histologic criteria for diagnosing early mycosis fungoides: an EORTC Cutaneous Lymphoma Study Group investigation. *Am J Clin Pathol*. 2000;24(1):40-50.
33. Ameen M, Darvay A, Black MM, et al. CD8-positive mycosis fungoides presenting as capillaritis. *Br J Dermatol*. 2000;142(3):564-567.
34. Lipsker D, Cribier B, Heid E, et al. Cutaneous lymphoma manifesting as pigmented, purpuric capillaries [in French]. *Ann Dermatol Venereol*. 1999;126(4):321-326.
35. Ratnam KV, Su WP, Peters MS. Purpura simplex (inflammatory purpura without vasculitis): a clinicopathologic study of 174 cases. *J Am Acad Dermatol*. 1991;25(4): 642-647.
36. Iwatsuki K, Aoshima T, Tagami H, et al. Immunofluorescence study in purpura pigmentosa chronica. *Acta Derm Venereol*. 1980;60(4):341-345.
37. von den Driesch P, Simon M Jr. Cellular adhesion antigen modulation in purpura pigmentosa chronica. *J Am Acad Dermatol*. 1994;30(2, pt 1):193-200.
38. Ghersetich I, Lotti T, Bacci S, et al. Cell infiltrate in progressive pigmented purpura (Schamberg's disease): immunophenotype adhesion receptors, and intercellular relationships. *Int J Dermatol*. 1995;34(12):846-850.
39. Aiba S, Tagami H. Immunohistologic studies in Schamberg's disease: evidence for cellular immune reaction in lesional skin. *Arch Dermatol*. 1988;124(7):1058-1062.
40. Nishioka K, Katayama I, Masuzawa M, et al. Drug-induced chronic pigmented purpura. *J Dermatol*. 1989;16(3): 220-222.
41. Kwon SJ, Lee CW. Figurate purpuric eruptions on the trunk: acetaminophen-induced rashes. *J Dermatol*. 1998;25(11):756-758.
42. Stratakis CA, Chrousos GP. Capillaritis (purpura simplex) associated with use of aminoglutethimide in Cushing's syndrome. *Am J Hosp Pharm*. 1994;51(20):2589-2591.
43. Voelter WW. Pigmented purpuric dermatosis-like reaction to topical fluorouracil. *Arch Dermatol*. 1983; 119(11):875-876.
44. Gupta G, Holmes SC, Spence E, et al. Capillaritis associated with interferon-alfa treatment of chronic hepatitis C infection. *J Am Acad Dermatol*. 2000;43(5, pt 2): 937-938.
45. Yung A, Gouldern V. Pigmented purpuric dermatosis (capillaritis) induced by bezafibrate. *J Am Acad Dermatol*. 2005;53(1):168-169.
46. Adams BB, Gadenne AS. Glipizide-induced pigmented purpuric dermatosis. *J Am Acad Dermatol*. 1999;41 (5, pt 2):827-829.
47. Tsao H, Lerner LH. Pigmented purpuric eruption associated with injection medroxyprogesterone acetate. *J Am Acad Dermatol*. 2000;43(2, pt 1):308-310.
48. Erbagci Z, Tuncel A, Erkilic S, et al. Progressive pigmentary purpura related to raloxifene. *Saudi Med J*. 2005;26(2):314-316.
49. Kalinke DU, Wuthrich B. Purpura pigmentosa progressive in type III cryoglobulinemia and tartrazine intolerance. A follow-up over 20 years [in German]. *Hautarzt*. 1999;50(1):47-51.
50. Inui S, Itami S, Yoshikawa K. A case of lichenoid purpura possibly caused by diltiazem hydrochloride. *J Dermatol*. 2001;28(2):100-102.
51. Waltermann K, Marsch WCh, Kreft B. Bufexamac-induced pigmented purpuric eruption [in German]. *Hautarzt*. 2009;60(5):424-427.
52. Díaz-Jara M, Tornero P, Barrio MD, et al. Pigmented purpuric dermatosis due to pseudoephedrine. *Contact Dermatitis*. 2002;46(5):300-301.
53. Kaplan R, Meehan SA, Leger M. A case of isotretinoin-induced purpura annularis telangiectodes of Majocchi and review of substance-induced pigmented purpuric dermatosis. *JAMA Dermatol*. 2014;150(2):182-184.
54. Komericki P, Aberer W, Arbab E, et al. Pigmented purpuric contact dermatitis from Disperse Blue 106 and 124 dyes. *J Am Acad Dermatol*. 2001;45(3):456-458.

55. Foti C, Elia G, Filotico R, et al. Purpuric clothing dermatitis due to Disperse Yellow 27. *Contact Dermatitis*. 1998;39(5):273.
56. Koch P, Baum HP, John S. Purpuric patch test reaction and venulitis due to methyl methacrylate in a dental prosthesis. *Contact Dermatitis*. 1996;34(3):213-215.
57. De Waard-van der Spek FB, Oranje AP. Purpura caused by EMLA is of toxic origin. *Contact Dermatitis*. 1997;36(1):11-13.
58. van Joost T, van Ulsen J, Vuzevski VD, et al. Purpuric contact dermatitis to benzoyl peroxide. *Contact Dermatitis*. 1990;22(2, pt 2):359-361.
59. Wahba-Yahav AV. Schamberg's purpura: association with persistent hepatitis B surface antigenemia and treatment with pentoxifylline. *Cutis*. 1994;54(3):205-206.
60. Dessoukey MW, Abdel-Dayem H, Omar MF, et al. Pigmented purpuric dermatosis and hepatitis profile: a report on 10 patients. *Int J Dematol*. 2005;44(6):486-488.
61. Satoh T, Yokozeki H, Nishioka K. Chronic pigmented purpura associated with odontogenic infection. *J Am Acad Dermatol*. 2002;46(6):942-944.
62. Sethuraman G, Sugandhan S, Bansal A, et al. Familial pigmented purpuric dermatoses. *J Dermatol*. 2006;33(9):639-641.
63. Böhm M, Bonsmann G, Luger TA. Resolution of lichen aureus in a 10-year-old child after topical pimecrolimus. *Br J Dermatol*. 2004;151(2):519-520.
64. Reinhold U, Seiter S, Ugurel S, et al. Treatment of progressive pigmented purpura with oral bioflavonoids and ascorbic acid: an open pilot study in 3 patients. *J Am Acad Dermatol*. 1999;41(2, pt 1):207-208.
65. Agrawal SK, Gandhi V, Bhattacharya SN. Calcium dobesilate (Cd) in pigmented purpuric dermatosis (PPD): a pilot evaluation. *J Dermatol*. 2004;31(2):98-103.
66. Tamaki K, Yasaka N, Osada A, et al. Successful treatment of pigmented purpuric dermatosis with griseofulvin. *Br J Dermatol*. 1995;132(1):159-160.
67. Geller M. Benefit of colchicine in the treatment of Schamberg's disease. *Ann Allergy Asthma Immunol*. 2000;85(3):246.
68. Panda S, Malakar S, Lahiri K. Oral pentoxifylline vs topical betamethasone in Schamberg disease: a comparative randomized investigator-blinded parallel-group trial. *Arch Dermatol*. 2004;140(4):491-493.
69. Okada K, Ishikawa O, Miyachi Y. Purpura pigmentosa chronica successfully treated with oral cyclosporin A. *Br J Dermatol*. 1996;134(1):180-181.
70. Fathy H, Abdelgaber S. Treatment of pigmented purpuric dermatoses with narrow-band UVB: a report of six cases. *J Eur Acad Dermatol Venereol*. 2011;25(5):603-606.
71. Lasocki AL, Kelly RI. Narrowband UVB therapy as an effective treatment for Schamberg's disease. *Australas J Dermatol*. 2008;49(1):16-18.
72. Kocaturk E, Kavala M, Zindanci I, et al. Narrowband UVB treatment of pigmented purpuric lichenoid dermatitis (Gougerot-Blum). *Photodermatol Photoimmunol Photomed*. 2009;25(1):55-56.
73. Karadag AS, Bilgili SG, Onder S, et al. Two cases of eczematid-like purpura of Doucas and Kapetanakis responsive to narrow band ultraviolet B treatment. *Photodermatol Photoimmunol Photomed*. 2013;29(2):97-99.
74. Gudi VS, White MI. Progressive pigmented purpura (Schamberg's disease) responding to TL01 ultraviolet B therapy. *Clin Exp Dermatol*. 2004;29(6):683-684.
75. Dhali TK, Chahar M, Haroon MA. Phototherapy as an effective treatment for Majocchi's disease—case report. *An Bras Dermatol*. 2015;90(1):96-99.
76. Ling TC, Gouldern V, Goodfield MJ. PUVA therapy in lichen aureus. *J Am Acad Dermatol*. 2001;45(1):145-146.
77. Krisa J, Hunyadi J, Dobozy A. PUVA treatment of pigmented purpuric lichenoid dermatitis (Gougerot-Blum). *J Am Acad Dermatol*. 1992;27(5, pt 1):778-780.
78. Seckin D, Yazici Z, Senol A, et al. A case of Schamberg's disease responding dramatically to PUVA treatment. *Photodermatol Photoimmunol Photomed*. 2008;24(2):95-96.
79. Wong WK, Ratnam KV. A report of two cases of pigmented purpuric dermatosis treated with PUVA therapy. *Acta Derm Venereol*. 1991;71(1):68-70.
80. Kim SK, Kim EH, Kim YC. Treatment of pigmented purpuric dermatosis with topical photodynamic therapy. *Dermatology*. 2009;219(2):184-186.
81. D'Ambrosia RA, Rajpara VS, Glogau RG. The successful treatment of Schamberg's disease with the 595nm vascular laser. *Dermatol Surg*. 2011;37(1):100-101.

Chapter 144 :: Cryoglobulinemia and Cryofibrinogenemia
:: Julio C. Sartori-Valinotti & Mark D. P. Davis

第一百四十四章
冷球蛋白血症和冷纤维蛋白原血症

中文导读

本章重点介绍导致微血管闭塞（Ⅰ型冷球蛋白血症和冷纤维蛋白原血症）或中小血管炎（Ⅱ型和Ⅲ型冷球蛋白血症）的疾病，按照冷球蛋白血症和冷纤维蛋白原血症分别描述。

一、冷球蛋白血症

1. 概况　首先对冷球蛋白血症的定义及发现过程进行了介绍，并指出冷球蛋白血症可以是无症状的，或者可以引起闭塞性血管病，或引起以血管炎为特征的冷球蛋白血症性综合征。

表144-1列出了冷球蛋白血症的Brouet分类方案，并对Ⅰ、Ⅱ和Ⅲ型冷球蛋白血症的分子特性进行了详细介绍。其中Ⅱ型和Ⅲ型冷球蛋白是免疫复合物，通常被称为"混合性冷球蛋白血症"。

2. 流行病学　冷球蛋白血症的估计患病率为（1~7）/100,000。据报道75%的患者与感染相关，24%与自身免疫性疾病有关，7%与血液系统疾病有关。

3. 临床特征

（1）皮肤表现：皮肤病变是最常见的表现，多达90%的患者会发生。

Ⅰ型冷球蛋白血症通常无症状，其皮肤症状与诱发缺血性血管病有关，可表现为雷诺现象、肢端缺血（图144-2）并可能发展为坏疽（图144-3）、网状青斑、肢端紫绀（图144-4）或网状紫癜，这些病变通常由冷诱发的。

Ⅱ、Ⅲ型冷球蛋白性血管炎最常见的表现为间歇性体位性可触及的紫癜，主要累及下肢（图144-5），临床症状可从零星孤立的瘀点或红斑到严重的带有溃疡的血管病变。白细胞碎裂性血管炎是混合性冷球蛋白血症的标志性病理特征。

（2）非皮肤表现：混合性冷球蛋白性血管炎患者最常见的皮外表现为乏力和关节痛或关节炎。此外，也可发生严重的内脏器官受累，详细介绍了肾、神经系统、骨骼肌肉及肺部等内脏受累的表现。

4. 病因和发病机制　Ⅰ型冷球蛋白血症与血液病有关。在许多感染性或系统性疾病中，通常可检测到循环混合（Ⅱ型和Ⅲ型）冷球蛋白（参见表144-1），其中以HCV感染和冷球蛋白血症的关系最为密切。

5. 诊断　四肢末端的紫癜、四肢发绀和坏死常提示诊断冷球蛋白血症或冷球蛋白血症性综合征的可能性。建议从靶器官受累或鉴别诊断的方向有针对性地进行系统检查。实验室检查应该包括与冷球蛋白血症和重要的鉴别诊断有关的指标。表144-2列出了针对可疑患者的诊断流程。

6．鉴别诊断　有关冷球蛋白血症（和冷纤维蛋白原血症）的鉴别诊断，请参见表144-3。

7．临床过程和预后　预后主要由冷球蛋白血症性综合征（系统受累）的严重程度及引起冷球蛋白血症的基础疾病所决定。对不同类型冷球蛋白血症的早晚期并发症及预后进行了介绍。

8．治疗　包括三种水平的治疗：①病因治疗；②病理生理学治疗；③对症治疗。建议治疗应以症状的严重性为依据，无症状的冷球蛋白血症通常不必治疗。

（1）Ⅰ型冷球蛋白血症：主要是治疗潜在的血液系统疾病，在潜在疾病的治疗显效之前可通过血浆置换或冷冻过滤作为过渡疗法。

（2）HCV相关的轻中度Ⅱ型和Ⅲ型冷球蛋白血症：主要的治疗方法取决于疾病的严重程度，最好的方法是使用抗病毒药物治疗。作者详细介绍了抗病毒的治疗方法及优缺点。

（3）HCV相关的重度Ⅱ型和Ⅲ型冷球蛋白血症：如果出现了器官衰竭，需要通过免疫抑制或生物制剂显著降低冷球蛋白水平。作者详细比较了生物制剂和抗病毒治疗的有效率及优缺点。

（4）与HCV无关的Ⅱ型和Ⅲ型冷球蛋白血性血管炎：对于轻度至中度的疾病，采取保守措施。对于更严重的病例，作者建议采用以利妥昔单抗为基础的治疗方案。

二、冷纤维蛋白原血症

1．流行病学　本章对冷纤维蛋白原血症的患病率进行了综述，在住院患者中的患病率从3.4%～22.2%不等，患者往往在40~70岁被诊断，女性可能更高发。

2．临床特征　部分患者无症状，而另一部分则具有血栓形成的临床特征，如果不及时治疗可能会危及生命。

（1）皮肤表现：通常位于寒冷暴露区域，可触及的紫癜伴潜在的白细胞碎裂性血管炎是最常见的临床表现。

（2）非皮肤表现：发热和不适常见，还可出现包括血管（血栓事件）、肾脏、肌肉骨骼和/或神经元受累的临床表现。

3．病因和发病机制　冷纤维蛋白原血症可分为原发性或继发性。继发性冷纤维蛋白原血症最常见的原因包括恶性肿瘤、感染、结缔组织和自身免疫性疾病（请参阅表144-4）。对冷纤维蛋白原的组成及病理学进行了阐述，并提及免疫学机制可能在该病的病理生理中起重要作用。

4．诊断

（1）实验室检查：对实验室检查冷纤维蛋白的方法及注意事项进行了详细描述，并特别指出应平行地对冷球蛋白进行检测。

（2）组织学特征：冷纤维蛋白血症可出现血管腔内闭塞性血栓形成。肾沉积物检查显示肾小球毛细血管腔和肾小管内独特形态的纤维性物质。

5．鉴别诊断　表144-3列出了冷球蛋白血症和冷纤维蛋白原血症的鉴别诊断。

6．临床过程和预后　关于冷纤维蛋白原血症的预后的资料很有限。

7．并发症　由血栓形成事件引起的经典并发症包括坏疽（5%）、败血病（5%）和小腿截肢（3.3%），在某些情况下，原发性冷纤维蛋白原血症可能继发淋巴瘤。

8．治疗　戒烟、避免冷暴露和停用血管收缩药是非药物干预措施。在继发性冷纤维蛋白原血症中，对基础疾病的特异性治疗可改善相关症状。对于原发性冷纤维蛋白原血症，主要介绍了纤维蛋白溶解药物和免疫抑制药的使用。

〔黄莹雪〕

Cryoglobulins are circulating immunoglobulins found in both serum and plasma that reversibly precipitate or gel upon cold exposure. Cryofibrinogens result from precipitation of fibrinogens on cold exposure and are detectable only in plasma samples, not serum. This chapter focuses on conditions that lead to either microvascular occlusion (Type I cryoglobulinemia and cryofibrinogenemia) or small- and medium-sized vessel vasculitis (Type II and III cryoglobulinemia) with emphasis on lesion morphology and cutaneous manifestations.

CRYOGLOBULINEMIA

AT-A-GLANCE

- Cryoglobulins are circulating immunoglobulin complexes found in plasma or serum that reversibly precipitate in cold temperatures.
- Cryoglobulinemia may be asymptomatic or cause a clinical syndrome involving the skin: purpura at distal sites is the hallmark. Livedo reticularis, acrocyanosis, ulceration, or gangrene also may be seen.
- Cryoglobulins are classified based on molecular properties into Types I, II, III (Brouet classification).
- Type I cryoglobulins consist of a single monoclonal immunoglobulin (typically IgG) or light chain. They occur with hematologic malignancies such as multiple myeloma. If symptomatic, they present with a noninflammatory occlusive vasculopathy.
- Type II cryoglobulins consist of a monoclonal immunoglobulin (typically IgM) complexed with a polyclonal immunoglobulin (typically IgG).
- Type III cryoglobulins consist of purely polyclonal immunoglobulin complexes; Type II-III refers to an intermediate state with oligoclonal immunoglobulin.
- Types II and III are also referred to as mixed cryoglobulinemias. They are caused by chronic hepatitis C virus (HCV) infection in >90% of cases, whereas in a minority of cases no etiology can be identified, designating them as "essential mixed" cryoglobulinemias. They present as the cryoglobulinemic vasculitis syndrome, an immune complex vasculitis involving the skin, neural, and renal tissues.
- Therapy primarily consists of controlling the underlying disease. In addition, immunosuppressants, plasma exchange, or targeting of cryoglobulin-producing B-cell clones may alleviate the cryoglobulin burden.

INTRODUCTION

DEFINITIONS AND HISTORICAL PERSPECTIVES

In 1933, Wintrobe and Buell first noted the in vitro phenomenon of cryoprecipitation, the cold-induced precipitation of plasma or serum proteins that is reversible upon rewarming at 37°C (98.6°F).[1] In 1947, Lerner and Watson described immunoglobulins and mixtures of immunoglobulins with other proteins that precipitate in the cold and called them cryoglobulins.[2] In 1974, Brouet introduced the classification of cryoglobulins based on molecular properties that is widely used.[2] Cryoglobulinemia describes the presence of cryoglobulins in a patient's serum (Fig. 144-1). It can be asymptomatic, meaning that its presence usually goes clinically undetected, or it can cause occlusive vasculopathy or the so-called cryoglobulinemic syndrome, which is characterized by immune-complex deposition causing vasculitis that involves the skin and other tissues.

The classification scheme of Brouet, estimated frequency, and composition of cryoglobulins is depicted in Table 144-1. Type I cryoglobulins consist of a single monoclonal immunoglobulin (Ig), typically IgM, less commonly IgG, IgA, or free Ig light chains (Bence Jones proteins). Complement components are not routinely found in Type I cryoprecipitates. Type I cryoglobulins are often present in substantial amounts, ranging from 1 to 30 mg/mL. The large molecular size of monoclonal IgM and other molecular characteristics, such as absence of sialic acid moieties, deficient carbohydrate side chains, and weak noncovalent factors may predispose these immunoglobulins to precipitation.[3]

Type II and Type III cryoglobulins are immune complexes composed of polyclonal IgGs and mono- or polyclonal IgMs classically referred to as "mixed cryoglobulinemias." Type II and Type III cryoglobulins are typically present in relatively small amounts and generally result from chronic inflammatory states. Type II and Type III cryoglobulins may fix complement.

Type II cryoglobulins represent a mixture of 2 Ig components: polyclonal immunoglobulins are associated with a monoclonal Ig that exhibits rheumatoid factor (RF) activity. Typically, a monoclonal IgM RF is complexed with a polyclonal IgG. HCV infection is the classical underlying disease.

A mixture of polyclonal immunoglobulins or polyclonal Ig-nonimmunoglobulin cryoprecipitates results in detection of Type III cryoglobulins. Polyclonal IgM–IgG cryoglobulins with complement as an integral component are the most frequent scenario in Type III cryoglobulinemia that is commonly associated with HCV infection or connective tissue diseases.

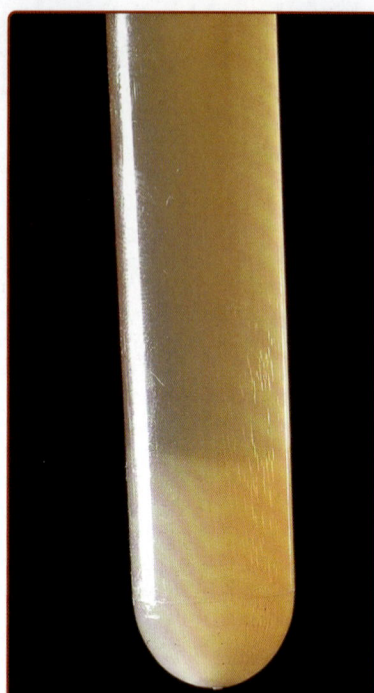

Figure 144-1 Whitish cryoprecipitates after keeping tube at 4°C (39.2°F) for 48 hours and centrifugation.

A new type of cryoglobulins, not included in the original Brouet classification, called Type II-III cryoglobulin, containing polyclonal IgG associated with a mixture of polyclonal and monoclonal (oligoclonal) IgM, has been described.[4] This type of cryoprecipitate describes an intermediate, developing state between Types III and II, suggesting a continuous transition from a purely polyclonal to a partially monoclonal composition by a process of successive clonal selection.

EPIDEMIOLOGY

Because of the heterogeneity of clinical presentations, including nonclinically apparent disease, the overall prevalence of this syndrome is probably underreported but has been estimated at 1 to 7 in 100,000.[5] Geographic differences in the distribution of hepatitis C infection are responsible for the predominance of mixed cryoglobulinemia in Southern Europe as compared to Northern Europe or the United States.[6] "Essential mixed cryoglobulinemia," or mixed cryoglobulinemia without an identifiable cause, is more common in females than males with a 3:1 ratio. The average age at onset is 54 years. Many cases formerly known as "essential" have been found to be associated with HCV and other infectious etiologies.[7]

An association with infectious diseases has been reported in 75% of patients, autoimmune disease in 24%, and hematologic diseases in 7%.[8] The vast majority (>90%) of mixed cryoglobulinemias occurs in association with chronic HCV infection. On average, 30% of chronically HCV-infected subjects develop cryoglobulinemia, and this proportion can go up to 90% when patients with very longstanding disease are examined.[9-11] On average, symptomatic cryoglobulinemic vasculitis syndrome is present in only 2% to 5% of chronically HCV-infected patients,[12] though figures as high as 15% have been proposed.[13,14] More recently, non–HCV-related infectious cryoglobulinemic vasculitis has been reported in association with hepatitis B virus (HBV), cytomegalovirus, Epstein–Barr virus, parvovirus B19, HIV, and bacterial, fungal, and mycobacterial infections.[15]

CLINICAL FEATURES

CUTANEOUS FINDINGS

Cutaneous lesions are the most frequent manifestation, occurring in up to 90% of patients.

Type I cryoglobulinemia per se is often asymptomatic and cutaneous signs are related to hyperviscosity and/or thrombosis that induce ischemic vasculopathy presenting as Raynaud phenomenon, digital ischemia (Fig. 144-2) that may progress to gangrene (Fig. 144-3), livedo reticularis, acrocyanosis (Fig. 144-4) or retiform purpura. These vascular occlusive lesions are typically cold induced. Infarction, hemorrhagic crusts, ulcers, and lesions on the head and oral or nasal mucosa are relatively more common in Type I than in mixed cryoglobulinemia.[16]

Type II and III cryoglobulinemic vasculitis is mediated by deposition of antigen–antibody complexes in small and medium-sized arteries, leading to inflammation of, preferentially, small blood vessel walls (capillaries, venules, or arterioles). Intermittent orthostatic palpable purpura, frequently observed late in the afternoon when highest cryoglobulin concentrations are present, is the most common presentation and particularly affects the lower extremities (Fig. 144-5). The face and the trunk, with the exception of the lower abdomen, are usually spared.[2] The clinical signs can vary from sporadic isolated petechiae or erythematous macules to severe vasculitic lesions with ulcerations. Leukocytoclastic vasculitis is the histopathologic hallmark of mixed cryoglobulinemia and is easily detectable by skin biopsy. Approximately 15% of individuals with circulating cryoglobulins have symptomatology consistent with cryoglobulinemic vasculitis. Erythematous papules, ecchymosis, and dermal nodules also can be seen.[14] Postinflammatory hyperpigmentation is also common (40% of patients).[7] Nail-fold capillary abnormalities are common and include dilation, altered orientation, capillary shortening, and neoangiogenesis.[17]

TABLE 144-1
Types of Cryoglobulins, Composition of Cryoprecipitates, and Disease Associations

TYPE OF CRYOGLOBULINEMIA (ESTIMATED FREQUENCY)	COMPOSITION OF CRYOPRECIPITATES	DISEASE ASSOCIATIONS
Type I (25%)	Monoclonal IgM (sometimes IgG, IgA), immunoglobulin light chain, complexed to other proteins	Hematologic disorders - Multiple myeloma - Waldenström macroglobulinemia - Plasma cell dyscrasias, monoclonal gammopathy of undetermined significance (MGUS) - Other lymphoproliferative diseases with M components
Type II (25%)	Combination of monoclonal (usually IgM with rheumatoid factor activity) and polyclonal (usually IgG) immunoglobulins	Chronic infection - Viral (HCV) Autoimmune diseases - Sjögren syndrome - Cold agglutinin disease Hematologic disorders - Waldenström macroglobulinemia - Chronic lymphocytic leukemia - B-cell non-Hodgkin lymphoma
Type III (50%)	Polyclonal immunoglobulins	Chronic infection - Viral (HCV, HIV, HBV) - Bacterial (subacute bacterial endocarditis, leprosy, spirochetal) - Fungal, parasitic Autoimmune diseases - Systemic lupus erythematosus - Rheumatoid arthritis - Dermatomyositis/polymyositis - Inflammatory bowel diseases - Biliary cirrhosis
Type II and III (frequency unknown)	Oligoclonal IgM, intermediate state between the entirely polyclonal Type III and the monoclonal, polyclonal Type II	Chronic infection (HCV) Autoimmune diseases Lymphoproliferative diseases Chronic liver disease Proliferative glomerulonephritis

Data from Crowson AN et al. Cutaneous vasculitis: A review. *J Cutan Pathol*. 2003;30:161-173; and Kallemuchikkal U, Gorevic PD. Evaluation of cryoglobulins. *Arch Pathol Lab Med*. 1999;123:119-25.

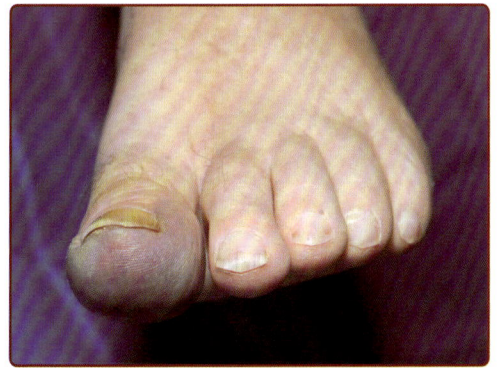

Figure 144-2 Blue discoloration of the distal aspect of the left first toe as the earliest finding of impending digital ischemia in a patient with cryoglobulinemia.

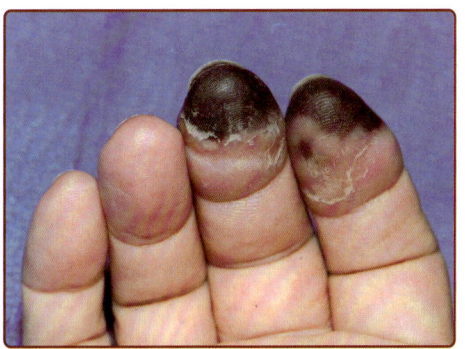

Figure 144-3 Digital gangrene of the distal right second and third fingers in a patient with cryoglobulinemia Type I. Note the well-demarcated color changes and absence of inflammation (erythema).

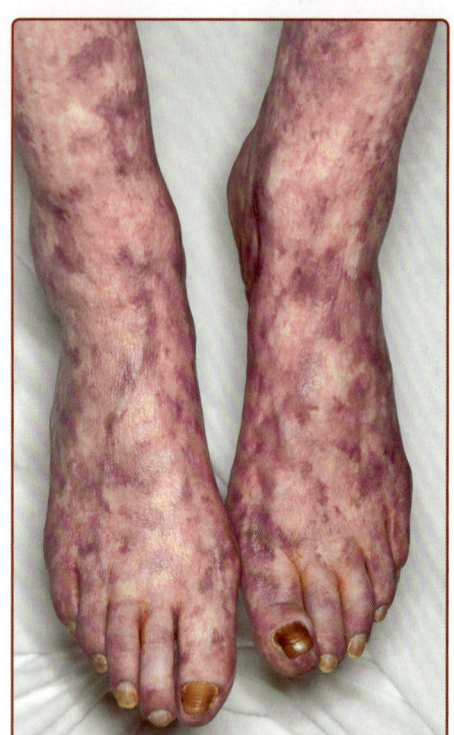

Figure 144-4 Acrocyanosis and livedo reticularis in a patient with cryoglobulinemia in the setting of multiple myeloma.

NONCUTANEOUS FINDINGS

The most common extracutaneous manifestations in patients with mixed cryoglobulinemic vasculitis are weakness and arthralgias or arthritis[14] but serious internal organ involvement also occur. The association of purpura, arthralgias, and weakness, known as

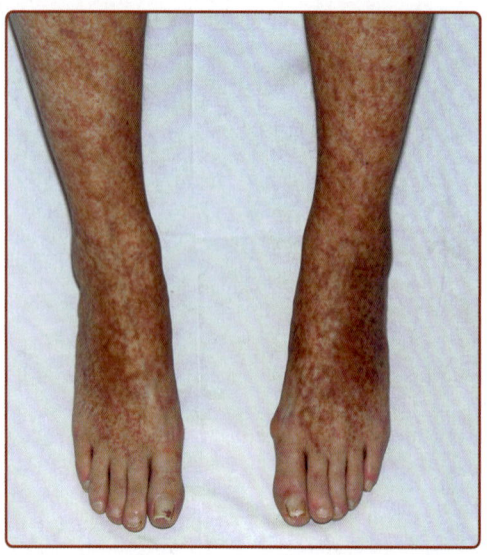

Figure 144-5 Leukocytoclastic vasculitis in a patient with mixed cryoglobulinemia manifested as palpable purpura.

the "Meltzer triad," is seen in about 25% to 30% of patients.[18,19]

Renal involvement is a serious complication, typically manifests early in the course of the disease and can present as a broad range of clinical findings, including hematuria with or without renal insufficiency (41%), isolated proteinuria, nephrotic syndrome (21%) or acute nephritic syndrome.[20] Chronic renal insufficiency without significant renal abnormalities and acute renal failure are less common. The incidence of renal disease in cryoglobulinemia varies from 5% to 60% and is typically immune complex mediated (Type II and III), but may also occur secondary to thrombosis (Type I). Membranoproliferative glomerulonephritis (MPGN) is more common in mixed cryoglobulinemia.

Neurologic manifestations, typically affecting the sensory peripheral nervous system secondary to epineural vasculitis, frequently complicate the clinical course of patients with mixed cryoglobulinemia. Patients typically describe paresthesias with burning symptoms in the lower limbs, often with nocturnal exacerbation, leading to severely compromised quality of life. Electromyographic and nerve conduction studies demonstrated peripheral neuropathy in up to 80% of patients with mixed cryoglobulinemia,[21,22] but many symptom-based demographic studies report prevalence of only 5% to 45%. Isolated polyneuropathy is more common with Type II than Type III cryoglobulinemia, but multifocal neuropathy and polyneuropathy are the most common form in Type III cryoglobulinemia.[23] Restless leg syndrome may be the major manifestation of peripheral neuropathy in middle-aged women with mixed cryoglobulinemia.[24] Peripheral neurologic disease manifests as a progressive, chronic distal mild sensory neuritis and only rarely as acute mononeuritis. Clinically apparent CNS dysfunction is rare. Hyperviscosity due to high levels of monoclonal cryoglobulins in Type I cryoglobulinemia, typically seen in Waldenström macroglobulinemia and less frequently in multiple myeloma, can induce microcirculation impairment and neurologic symptoms: blurring or loss of vision, headache, vertigo, nystagmus, dizziness, sudden deafness, diplopia, ataxia, confusion, dementia, disturbances of consciousness, stroke, seizures, somnolence, or coma. A characteristic retinal venous engorgement ("sausaging") on funduscopic inspection can serve as a diagnostic clue.

Musculoskeletal complaints, typically arthralgias and myalgias, are described in more than 70% of persons with cryoglobulinemia, predominantly in Type II and III disease. Arthralgias classically affect the proximal interphalangeal and metacarpophalangeal joints of the hands, the knees, and ankles. Clear clinical signs of myositis or arthritis are rare.[25]

Pulmonary involvement. Approximately 40% of patients are symptomatic with dyspnea, cough, or pleuritic pain. Pulmonary function tests often reveal evidence of small airways disease and chest radiographs sometimes show interstitial infiltrates or signs of subclinical alveolitis.[26,27] Severe pulmonary disease, for example, bronchiolitis obliterans organizing pneumonia (BOOP), or pulmonary vasculitis are very uncommon.[28] Pulmonary-renal syndrome also has been described.[29]

Other. Thyroid disorders and diabetes mellitus seem to be associated with cryoglobulinemia.[30] Nonspecific abdominal pain can affect 2% to 22%. Intestinal vasculitis of the small mesenteric vessels leading to acute abdomen has been reported.

ETIOLOGY AND PATHOGENESIS

Type I cryoglobulinemia is associated with hematologic disorders, such as Waldenström macroglobulinemia, multiple myeloma, or lymphoproliferative diseases. Non-Hodgkin B-cell lymphoma is the most frequently encountered hematologic malignancy.

Circulating mixed (Types II and III) cryoglobulins are commonly detected in a great number of infectious or systemic disorders (see Table 144-1). The term *essential* is reserved for instances of mixed cryoglobulinemia in the absence of a well-defined underlying disease and accounts for only a minority of cryoglobulinemic patients.

Prevalence of serum anti-HCV antibodies and/or HCV RNA in cryoglobulinemic patients ranges from 70% to 100%. Type II cryoglobulinemia is more strongly associated with HCV than Type III (90% vs 70%, respectively). Presence of cryoglobulins increases with duration of HCV infection: cryoglobulins are found in 55% to 90% of patients with longstanding infection. However, overt cryoglobulinemic syndrome develops in only 2% to 5% of these cases.[12] The precise role of viral or host factors contributing to this discrepancy remains largely unknown. Specific HCV genotypes or distinct HLA subtypes, like HLA-DR11 or HLA-DR6 may predispose to extrahepatic systemic manifestations of cryoglobulinemia.[31,32] Pathogenesis of mixed cryoglobulinemia is probably a multifactorial and multistep process. Viral HCV antigens exert a chronic stimulus on the host immune system, resulting in specific immune dysregulatory mechanisms with B-cell proliferation and autoantibody production. HCV-related B-cell lymphoproliferative disorders comprise a spectrum of disease, ranging from asymptomatic clonal B-cell expansions to pathogenic cryoglobulinemia and lymphoma. From that perspective, HCV-associated mixed cryoglobulinemia is a benign lymphoproliferative B-cell disease with a potential for subsequent development of B-cell lymphoma.[19,33] Development of HCV-associated cryoglobulinemic vasculitis syndrome is associated with longstanding infection, old age, Type II cryoglobulins, higher cryoglobulin levels, and clonal B-cell expansion.[34] The mechanism for B-cell activation and proliferation may be explained in part due to the presence of a t(14;18) translocation involving a rearrangement of *bcl-2* and inhibition of apoptosis.[6]

In cases of HCV-associated mixed cryoglobulinemia, there is complex interaction between several inflammatory cytokines that amplifies and perpetuates the autoimmune process. Elevated serum levels of interleukin (IL)-1beta, IL-6, and tumor necrosis factor (TNF)-alpha have been found in these patients[35] in addition to T-helper 1 chemokines, CXCL11 and CXCL10.[36] High levels of CXCL10 are found in patients with clinically active vasculitis and autoimmune thyroiditis.[37]

Using environmental scanning electron microscopy and energy dispersive X-ray spectroscopy microanalysis, higher concentration of microparticles and nanoparticles were found in HCV-associated mixed cryoglobulinemia than in controls, further supporting a role for environmental factors in the pathogenesis of this condition.[38]

The group of non-HCV-induced mixed cryoglobulinemias is small. An association of cryoglobulinemia with other infectious viral agents, for example, hepatitis B virus,[39] and HIV, with or without HCV coinfection, has been demonstrated.[40] HIV infection does seem to play a role in the generation of circulating cryoglobulins.[41] Parvovirus B19 has been implicated in a mild form of cryoglobulinemic syndrome.[42] Another important and well-known association is the one with Sjögren syndrome. According to one study, 16% of patients with primary Sjögren syndrome had cryoglobulins, and of those, 56% had cryoglobulinemic syndrome.[43,44] Importantly, Sjögren syndrome patients who meet diagnostic criteria for cryoglobulinemic vasculitis at the time of diagnosis have increased mortality.[45] A study by the same group found cryoglobulinemia in 25% of patients with systemic lupus erythematosus.[46] A rare association between antiphospholipid syndrome and cryoglobulinemia has recently been reported.[47]

DIAGNOSIS

In almost all cases, the possibility of a diagnosis of cryoglobulinemia or cryoglobulinemic syndrome is primarily suggested by the presence of purpura of the distal extremities or by acral cyanosis and necrosis, depending on the potential presence of Type I or Types II and III cryoglobulinemia. Alternatively, the potential diagnosis may be suggested by the presence of a candidate underlying disease. A targeted review of systems and subsequent clinical examination will guide the physician toward the entire picture of organ involvement or differential diagnoses. The laboratory panel must include parameters relevant to both cryoglobulinemia and important differential diagnoses. Table 144-2 presents an algorithm for the diagnostic approach to the patient, including laboratory testing.

LABORATORY TESTING

In clinical practice, cryoglobulin testing is underutilized, most probably due to the expenditure of time and stringent temperature requirements. They can be

TABLE 144-2
Algorithm for Patients with Suspected Cryoglobulinemia

History and Examination (Including Optional Technical Methods)

Ask for
- Cold sensitivity
- Weakness, musculoskeletal complaints, arthralgia
- Alcohol consumption, hereditary liver disease, history of hepatitis
- Known infections (HCV, HBV, HIV)
- Urine abnormalities (hematuria, foamy urine, edema)
- Paresthesias
- Difficulties in concentrating (suggesting CNS involvement)

Look for
- Acrocyanosis, Raynaud phenomenon (suggesting Type I cryoglobulinemia)
- Purpura of distal extremities (suggesting Type II and III cryoglobulinemia)
- Peripheral neuropathy (consider electromyographic testing)
- Joint swelling (suggestive for rheumatoid arthritis, SLE)
- Lymph node enlargement (suggesting lymphoma)

Technical examination (optional)
- Ultrasonography: Liver abnormalities, splenomegaly (suggesting lymphoma)
- Electrocardiography, echocardiography (suggesting SLE)
- Ophthalmology: Eye involvement, chorioretinitis (suggesting Behçet disease or sarcoidosis)

Mandatory Laboratory Testing in Cryoglobulinemia
- Cryoglobulins (establishing the diagnosis when positive; stringent laboratory workup at 37°C is needed)
- Complete blood count, including differential
- Creatinine, BUN
- Complement levels
- IgA level (suggestive for liver disease or Henoch–Schönlein Purpura)
- ANA, SS-B, SS-A (positive in SLE- and Sjögren syndrome–associated cryoglobulinemia)
- ANCA (possibly positive, or suggesting granulomatosis with polyangiitis [Wegener] or microscopic polyangiitis)
- Rheumatoid factor RF (positive in Type II cryoglobulinemia with a very high titer)
- Urinalysis. If positive, add microscopic examination of urinary sediment
- Hepatitis A, B, C serology
- Look for other viruses, such as parvovirus B19, HIV, if appropriate
- Further workup for hepatic failure if appropriate

Histology
- Consider skin biopsy
  - To confirm leukocytoclastic vasculitis (stain for complement and immune complexes)
  - To rule out other forms of vasculitis
- Consider renal biopsy (discern between MPGN I and other forms)
- Consider hepatic biopsy

---

falsely negative and should be obtained during active flares and repeated several weeks apart. By current standard laboratory techniques, most healthy individuals will have undetectable circulating cryoglobulins.

Serum must be obtained in warm tubes at 37°C in the absence of anticoagulants. Temperature should be kept at 37°C up until laboratory processing. After clotting and centrifugation at 37°C, the separated serum is stored at 4°C and inspected daily for a precipitate. Type I cryoglobulins tend to precipitate within the first 24 hours (at concentrations >5 mg/mL), whereas Type III cryoglobulins may require 7 days (Fig. 144-1). For calculation of cryocrit (volume of packed cryoglobulins as percentage of original serum volume), the cryoprecipitate has to be spun in a graded (Wintrobe) tube. A cryocrit ≥2% is considered to be positive. Cryocrit levels usually do not correlate with severity and prognosis of disease.

Some authors recommend proof of reversibility of the cryoprecipitate by rewarming an aliquot at 37°C for 24 hours.[7] For phenotyping and identification of cryoglobulin components, specific immunologic assays are performed at 37°C.

Clinical diagnosis of hyperviscosity can be established by measuring serum viscosity with an Oswald-type viscometer. Reference serum viscosity, measured as flow time through the viscometer of the patient's serum divided by that of water or saline, is between 1.4 and 1.8, whereas most symptomatic patients have values between 5 and 8. Again, clinical manifestations are often not proportional to serum viscosity.

As hypocomplementemia (with the typical pattern of low or undetectable C4 and normal or relatively normal C3 levels) occurs in up to 90% of patients with mixed cryoglobulinemia, C3 and C4 levels, usually measured in nephelometric immunoassays, should be routinely determined. A sudden increase in complement C4, raised to abnormally high levels, can be observed in some patients developing a B-cell lymphoma.[48]

RF is often positive in Type II and III cryoglobulinemia. Testing for antinuclear antibodies (ANAs, SS-A, SS-B) and other autoantibodies is indicated when there is a clinical suspicion of underlying systemic connective tissue disease, such as SLE or Sjögren syndrome. Although the immunofluorescence ANA assay is the current diagnostic gold standard, titer and specificity of ANAs may vary considerably.

Serological studies for hepatitis C and HIV should be conducted. Confirmation of other viral (hepatitis B, Epstein–Barr virus, and cytomegalovirus) or bacterial agents should be considered and may be warranted in the appropriate clinical scenario.

DIFFERENTIAL DIAGNOSIS

See Table 144-3 for an overview on differential diagnosis of cryoglobulinemia (and cryofibrinogenemia).

CLINICAL COURSE AND PROGNOSIS

Prognosis is defined by the severity of the cryoglobulinemic syndrome and by the treatability of the underlying disease causing cryoglobulinemia.

In Type I cryoglobulinemia, this will depend on the nature and stage of the hematologic disease.

TABLE 144-3
Differential Diagnosis of Cryoglobulinemia and Cryofibrinogenemia

CONDITION	DIFFERENTIAL DIAGNOSIS	COMMENTS
Type I cryoglobulinemia Cryofibrinogenemia	Thromboembolic conditions: ■ Inheritable or acquired hypercoagulable states (protein C or S deficiency, antiphospholipid syndrome, lupus anticoagulant) ■ Thrombocytopenic disorders (thrombotic thrombocytopenic purpura, idiopathic thrombocytopenic purpura) ■ Paroxysmal nocturnal hemoglobinuria ■ Disseminated intravascular coagulation ■ Atherosclerotic peripheral vascular disease ■ Thromboangiitis obliterans ■ Livedoid vasculopathy ■ Drug-induced (ie, heparin, warfarin) ■ Atheroemboli, cholesterol emboli, septic emboli, atrial myxoma Hyperviscosity due to: ■ Thrombocytosis (essential or secondary) ■ Polyclonal or monoclonal gammapathies that are not cryoglobulins (ie, multiple myeloma, Waldenstrom macroglobulinemia) Primary cutaneous disorders: ■ Urticaria ■ Livedo or livedoid vasculitis ■ Neutrophilic dermatoses ■ Lipodermatosclerosis ■ Panniculitis ■ Idiopathic perniosis (chilblains) Oxalosis Calciphylaxis Hemoglobinopathies Infections (malaria, babesiosis)	Conditions that present with Raynaud phenomenon, noninflammatory retiform purpura, digital ischemia, gangrene and/or acrocyanosis due to vascular occlusion
Types II and III cryoglobulinemia	Small- and medium-vessel vasculitis: ■ IgA vasculitis ■ ANCA-associated (granulomatosis with polyangiitis, eosinophilic granulomatosis with polyangiitis, microscopic polyangiitis, polyarteritis nodosa) ■ Rheumatic vasculitides (lupus erythematosus, rheumatoid arthritis, dermatomyositis, Sjögren syndrome) ■ Drug-induced ■ Infection-related (bacterial endocarditis, Rickettsia rickettsia, Neisseria meningitidis)	Conditions that primarily present with palpable purpura due to small- and medium-vessel vasculitis

A favorable prognosis in a patient with Type I cryoglobulinemia can only be expected when control of the underlying disease can be achieved. In contrast, patients with cryoglobulinemic vasculitis (Type II or III), have increased associated morbidity and mortality. Consequently, 10-year-survival rates are significantly lower than in the normal population because of renal involvement, intestinal vasculitis and widespread vasculitis, liver and cardiac disease, cardiovascular complications, and myeloproliferative disorders.[49-51] These data integrate a heterogeneous population that included hepatitis C–associated cases that were treated by differing approaches ranging from symptomatic steroid therapy to antiviral treatment.

Recent studies better elucidate the differences in prognosis and long-term complications in patients with mixed cryoglobulinemia based on HCV status. It seems that patients with non-HCV mixed cryoglobulinemia have lower gammaglobulin levels, increased frequency of renal involvement, 4-fold increased risk of developing B-cell lymphoma, and overall higher mortality rate than their HCV-positive counterparts.[33] These observations may be explained in part by the fact that HCV-associated cryoglobulinemic vasculitis can be treated with antivirals. Indeed, in this group of patients, response to antiviral therapy significantly reduces the mortality rate and changes the spectrum of complications. Infection is the most common cause of death in HCV patients with mixed cryoglobulinemia, followed by complications related to liver and cardiac involvement.[52]

COMPLICATIONS

Acute severe complications directly caused by cryoglobulins are rare with any type of cryoglobulinemia. The organs most vulnerable to complications are the nervous system and the kidneys. In Type I cryoglobulinemia, they are mostly related to an acute vaso-occlusive crisis caused by increased serum viscosity leading to acute acral ischemia or to cerebral and renal ischemia, causing stroke or acute renal failure, respectively. In addition, the underlying hematologic disease of Type I cryoglobulinemia can directly cause renal failure (myeloma kidney). At advanced stages, complications are defined by the underlying hematologic disease itself: immunosuppression leading to infection and sepsis, coagulation disorders with severe bleeding, and side effects of hematologic disease–specific treatments.

Renal involvement remains a poor prognostic sign in patients with cryoglobulinemic vasculitis, with 15% progressing to end-stage renal disease (ESRD).[49] MPGN I from any cause including noncryoglobulinemic ones has a poor prognosis: 50% progress to ESRD within 10 years. Small studies report successful treatment of MPGN I by antiviral strategies.[53,54] The prognosis of cryoglobulinemia with no identified underlying disease (essential mixed cryoglobulinemia) is not predictable, and, again, renal involvement is associated with poor prognosis (renal failure in 10% of patients).[55] In cases of noninfectious mixed cryoglobulinemic glomerulonephritis, severe infectious and new-onset lymphoma severely impacted long-term outcome.[56]

Mixed cryoglobulinemic vasculitis may involve the peripheral nerves, leading to life-threatening situations or cause acute-on-chronic renal failure. Advanced stages of the underlying disease (mostly hepatitis C or other types of liver disease) can result in acute liver failure or problems associated with hepatic insufficiency, such as coagulation disorders, malnutrition, ascites, and the hepatorenal syndrome. Skin necrosis and vasculitic lesions can be entry sites for infection. Catastrophic individual patient courses have been described.[57]

MANAGEMENT

Three levels of treatment can be considered when treating cryoglobulinemia: (1) etiologic treatment, which is aimed at the cure or safe containment of the underlying disease; (2) pathophysiologic treatment, which is aimed at reducing the production of cryoglobulins although the underlying etiology remains untreated; and (3) symptomatic treatment that is aimed at reducing the cryoglobulin burden by removal from plasma or at mitigating the tissue's vasculitic reaction. Sometimes a combination of these approaches is used. The decision for initiation of a therapy should be informed by the severity of the symptoms, with benefits outweighing risks. Cryoglobulinemia without symptoms does not justify treatment, unless there is an underlying condition that merits therapy.

TYPE I CRYOGLOBULINEMIA

Etiologic treatment is the treatment of choice. The underlying hematologic disease, typically multiple myeloma, Waldenström macroglobulinemia, or lymphoma must be treated with chemotherapy directed by a hematologist according to current standards of care. In addition to this, severely symptomatic hyperviscosity syndrome of Type I cryoglobulinemia can be reduced by repeated plasma exchange or by cryofiltration. This may be necessary as a bridging therapy until therapy of the underlying disease shows an effect. In plasma exchange, the patient's plasma is removed by an apheresis membrane and substituted using approximately 3.5 L of donor plasma per session. Cryofiltration operates by passing the patient's cooled plasma through a specialized membrane unit designed to remove cryoprecipitates without necessitating plasma substitution.[58] However, this latter approach may be hampered by rapid clogging of the membrane in the setting of high cryoglobulin concentrations. In severe cases of Type I cryoglobulinemia, it may be necessary that these removal procedures be performed daily over a period of 2 weeks or more.

HCV-ASSOCIATED TYPE II AND III CRYOGLOBULINEMIA IN PATIENTS WITH MILD TO MODERATE DISEASE

The primary therapeutic approach depends on disease severity. Patients with mild to moderate cryoglobulinemic vasculitis without major organ failure are best treated using antiviral agents. Although the effects of the treatment exhibit some delay, the approach has the advantage of offering a potentially complete and sustained remission of the vasculitic syndrome. This has been shown by a series of pioneering studies employing regimens of interferon alone or in combination with ribavirin in patients with HCV and cryoglobulinemia.[59-62] Among those therapeutic regimens, the highest response rates were found using the current gold standard of therapy, PEGylated interferon α-2b and ribavirin.[59,63] Recovery rates for symptoms are as follows: purpura 87.5%, arthralgia 82%, peripheral neuropathy 74%, and nephropathy 50%. The rate of sustained viral response was similar to large study populations without cryoglobulinemia: 62.5%. The regimen is detailed in the current statements on the management of hepatitis C of the American Gastroenterological Association.[64] There are several limitations of antiviral combination therapy. Applicability in renal insufficiency is reduced because of drug accumulation. Recommendations for dosage adjustment have been published in the current Kidney Disease: Improving Global Outcomes (KDIGO) guidelines.[65] Although ribavirin is contraindicated at an estimated GFR <50 mL/min, it is a desirable drug rendering interferon therapy markedly more powerful.[63,66] Therefore, a dosage regimen guided by plasma levels has been proposed that could allow for off-label administration in settings of a GFR <50 mL/min.[67] Of note, ribavirin can cause hemolytic anemia requiring pausing or dosage adjustments. Interdisciplinary collaboration with expert hepatologists and nephrologists is recommended.

HCV-ASSOCIATED TYPE II AND III CRYOGLOBULINEMIA IN PATIENTS WITH SEVERE DISEASE

In the case of organ failure, such as overt renal failure, possibly accompanied by the nephrotic syndrome or neuropathy, initial pathophysiologic and symptomatic therapy are required to achieve a reasonably rapid response. Traditionally, an immunosuppressive combination therapy using steroids possibly followed by cyclophosphamide, azathioprine, or chlorambucil has been used.[68] The use of the chimeric anti-CD20 antibody, rituximab, has recently emerged as a powerful alternative to classic immunosuppression.[69] The antibody targets B-lymphocytes, leading to a depletion of 95% of the B-lymphocytic population. Thereby, the cryoglobulin-producing B lymphocytic clone is markedly reduced, leading to marked cryoglobulin level reduction and consecutive remission. Taken together, this represents a pathophysiologic approach to treatment. One recent clinical trial compared the efficacy and safety profile of a combination of pegylated interferon-α (Peg-IFN-α) and ribavirin, with or without rituximab. More patients in the rituximab group had complete response and greater than 80% had sustained clearance of HCV RNA for up to 3 years compared to only 40% of patients in the Peg-IFN-α and ribavirin only group.[70] Another similar study found that patients in the Peg-IFN-α/ribavirin/rituximab arm had a shorter time to clinical remission, better renal response rates, and higher rates of cryoglobulin clearance.[71] In light of these findings, some authors recommend rituximab combined with Peg-IFN-α/ribavirin as the preferred therapeutic regimen in patients with severe or refractory/relapsing disease, renal involvement, and in those in whom rapid clinical response is needed.[72,73] Though reported to be generally well tolerated in patients with cryoglobulinemic syndrome, rituximab has several limitations. It should not be used in patients with overt skin ulceration because of interference with wound healing. A recent report has pointed to a severe complication with worsening of cryoglobulinemic vasculitis syndrome in patients with high baseline levels of mixed cryoglobulins receiving rituximab.[74]

TYPE II AND III CRYOGLOBULINEMIC VASCULITIS NOT ASSOCIATED WITH HCV

In Type II and III cryoglobulinemic vasculitis not associated with HCV, therapeutic regimens have not been extensively studied. In mild to moderate disease, conservative measures including the avoidance of cold temperatures, resting, and the use of nonsteroidal antiinflammatory drugs such as colchicine may be sufficient. For more severe cases, a combination of rituximab and oral prednisone showed greater efficacy at achieving complete clinical, renal, and immunologic responses compared to the combination of alkylating agents and prednisone at the expense of more severe infections in the rituximab group. Mortality rates, however, were similar in both groups.[75] Therefore, rituximab-based regimens are more effective but should be used judiciously because of the high prevalence of infections.

CRYOFIBRINOGENEMIA

AT-A-GLANCE

- Cryofibrinogenemia results from cryoprecipitation of patients' native fibrinogen or fibrin by-products in plasma but not serum.
- Cryofibrinogenemia is classified as essential or secondary (associated with malignancies, collagen vascular diseases, and thrombotic disorders).
- Cryofibrinogenemia is rare, but probably underestimated in clinical practice.
- Typical clinical features result from thrombosis (thrombotic phenomena of skin and viscera) and are often life-threatening.

EPIDEMIOLOGY

Cryofibrinogenemia is often clinically asymptomatic. Of note, 2% to 9% of healthy persons may have demonstrable amounts of cryofibrinogen, usually in concentrations less than 50 mg/L. In the past, cryofibrinogenemia was considered rare, but recent single-center studies indicate that this disorder is possibly underrecognized because of the infrequency with which it causes symptoms, and inconsistencies in laboratory investigations producing falsely negative results. Patients are usually diagnosed between the fifth and seventh decades of life. Initial studies noted the prevalence of cryofibrinogenemia among hospitalized patients between 3.4% and 13%, with a female predilection (female–male ratio 4:1) without age or racial differences. In a study by Saadoun and coworkers, 2312 hospitalized patients were tested for cryofibrinogenemia between 1996 and 2006.[76] A total of 515 (22.2%) patients had positive test results, of whom 88% had secondary and 12% had essential cryofibrinogenemia. Another retrospective, single-hospital, 10-year report identified 61 patients having cryofibrinogenemia, which was essential in 18 (29.5%) and secondary in 43 (70.5%) patients.[77]

CLINICAL FEATURES

Some people with cryofibrinogenemia are asymptomatic, whereas others have clinical features resulting from thrombosis that can be life-threatening when untreated.

CUTANEOUS FINDINGS

Patients with cryofibrinogenemia typically report a temporal association between cold exposure and onset of symptoms. Clinical signs in cryofibrinogenemia are mostly cutaneous and are typically located on cold-exposed areas (hands, feet, buttocks, ear, nose). These cold-sensitive lesions often reflect cold-induced thromboses, increased viscosity, and/or vascular reactivity. Palpable purpura with underlying leucocytoclastic vasculitis is the most frequent clinical presentation. Other cutaneous features can include painful ulcerations, livedo racemosa, Raynaud phenomenon, segmental swelling, lower extremity nodules, painful or pruritic erythema (perniosis) of the extremities, and cold urticaria. Cryofibrinogenemia may clinically simulate calciphylaxis, which is usually seen in patients with ESRD.

NONCUTANEOUS FINDINGS

Nonspecific constitutional complaints of fever and malaise are common. Cryofibrinogenemia has a broad spectrum of clinical manifestations including vessel, kidney, musculoskeletal, and/or neuronal involvement. Various thrombotic events, nephritic or nephrotic syndrome, arthralgia, myalgia, multineuritis, and fever have been reported.[78] In a recent study, the main clinical manifestations included purpura (46.6%), skin necrosis (36.6%), and arthralgia (31.6%), with cold sensitivity in 40% and overall thrombotic events occurring in up to 40% of cases. A high cryofibrinogen plasma concentration was a significant predisposing factor for thrombotic events.[76] Thrombotic events include cerebrovascular accidents (stroke, ocular thrombi, including retinal arterial and/or venous occlusions), myocardial infarction, limb and bowel ischemia or infarction, and pulmonary emboli, although a causal relationship has not been proven for all described cases.

ETIOLOGY AND PATHOGENESIS

Precipitation of patients' native fibrinogen or fibrin byproducts in plasma, but not serum, was first described by Korst and Kratochvil in 1955.[79] Cryofibrinogenemia can be classified as primary (also named essential or idiopathic) or secondary. Diagnosis of primary cryofibrinogenemia requires the presence of cryofibrinogens in plasma, absence of cryoglobulins, and one or more compatible clinical features, such as cold-induced thromboses, increases in blood viscosity and/or vascular reactivity, in an otherwise healthy individual. Some authors hypothesize that essential cryofibrinogenemia might be a prerequisite for a secondary disease.

Secondary cryofibrinogenemia is diagnosed when an associated disease or drug is present. The most frequently associated disorders include malignancy, infections, and connective tissue and autoimmune diseases (see Table 144-4).

Cryofibrinogen is characteristically composed of fibrinogen, fibrin, fibronectin, and/or fibrin degradation products. Other components include albumin, cold-insoluble globulin, factor VIII, and plasma proteins, as well as the plasmin activity inhibitors α1-antitrypsin and α2-macroglobulin. Pathology in cryofibrinogenemia is attributed to "in situ" thrombosis, leading to thrombotic occlusion of small and medium-sized dermal vessels and resultant ischemia. Defects in the fibrinolysis process might lead to further clotting in small and medium arteries. Additional immunologic mechanisms may play a significant role in the pathophysiology of cryofibrinogenemia.

Secondary forms of cryofibrinogenemia are significantly more frequent in patients with combined cryofibrinogenemia and cryoglobulinemia than in those with isolated cryofibrinogenemia (79 vs 47%).[80] Among HCV-infected patients, cryofibrinogenemia is common, and closely correlated with cryoglobulinemia. In a study of 143 patients with HCV infection, 53 (37%) had cryofibrinogen levels >50 mg/L. Forty-seven of these cryofibrinogen-positive patients (89%) had positive tests for cryoglobulins.[81]

TABLE 144-4
Conditions Associated with Cryofibrinogenemia

Endocrine Disorders
Diabetes mellitus
Hypothyroidism (Hashimoto disease)
Graves disease

Infections
Viral (VZV, EBV, HC)
Bacterial (*Klebsiella pneumoniae, Mycoplasma pneumoniae*)
Severe sepsis

Malignancy
Adenocarcinoma (gastric, lung)
Hepatocarcinoma
Ovarian cancer
Prostate cancer

Hematologic Disorders
Multiple myeloma
Waldenstrom macroglobulinemia
Lymphoma (follicular, B cell, T cell)
Chronic myelomonocytic leukemia

Autoimmune Diseases
Mixed connective tissue disease
Sjögren syndrome
Dermatomyositis
Polymyositis
Rheumatoid arthritis
Systemic lupus erythematosus
Systemic sclerosis

Vasculitis
ANCA-associated vasculitis
Giant cell arteritis
Behçet disease
Polyarteritis nodosa
Henoch–Schönlein purpura

Cutaneous Disorders
Psoriasis
Pyoderma gangrenosum

Drugs
Oral contraceptive agents

Miscellaneous
Sarcoidosis
Spondyloarthropathy
Inflammatory bowel disease.

EBV, Epstein–Barr virus; HCV, hepatitis C virus; VZV, varicella-zoster virus.

DIAGNOSIS

LABORATORY TESTING

Laboratory workup is critical for the accuracy of cryofibrinogen detection and ideally includes separation in a temperature-controlled centrifuge.

The warm blood specimen should be anticoagulated with citrate, EDTA, or oxalate, but not heparin, which nonspecifically precipitates fibrinogen and may result in a false positive result. The formation of a cryoprecipitate may also lead to a false negative result if the sample was not collected at 37°C. The sample should be processed within an hour. After centrifugation at 37°C, the plasma is placed in a Wintrobe tube, refrigerated at 4°C, and observed for the formation of a precipitate for 72 hours. The cryocrit is quantitated by centrifuging the specimen while it remains cooled to 4°C. Each millimeter of visible precipitate in the Wintrobe tube represents 1% of cryocrit.

In parallel, a cryoglobulin test is simultaneously performed in a sample without anticoagulants, to ensure that the plasma precipitate is cryofibrinogen and not cryoglobulin.

Affinity-chromatography, immunodiffusion, and/or electrophoresis are used for quantitation and/or identification of the individual cryofibrinogen components using antifibrinogen, anti–heavy-chain and anti–light-chain antibodies.[80,82]

HISTOLOGIC FEATURES

Irrespective of the anatomic site, cryofibrinogenemia shows an occlusive thrombotic diathesis comprising eosinophilic refractile deposits within vessel lumina with extension into the vessel intima, with or without an accompanying characteristic granulomatous vasculitis.[77,83] Cryofibrinogen precipitates have a cylindrical configuration in ultrastructural analysis, which is often displayed within the vessel lumina. Examination of renal deposits showed fibrillary material within glomerular capillary lumina and tubules with unique morphologic features not previously described.[78]

DIFFERENTIAL DIAGNOSIS

Table 144-3 provides a comprehensive list of differential diagnosis of cryoglobulinemia and cryofibrinogenemia.

CLINICAL COURSE AND PROGNOSIS

Clinical data regarding prognosis in cryofibrinogenemia are limited. In one study, 3 of 60 patients with essential cryofibrinogenemia died after a mean followup of 85 months.

COMPLICATIONS

Typical complications due to thrombotic events include gangrene (5%), septicemia (5%), and leg amputation (3.3%).[76] In some cases, essential cryofibrinogenemia might suggest a secondary disease, particularly lymphomas.[84] In a 2008 report, 27% of patients with primary cryofibrinogenemia developed lymphoma after a 5-year followup period.[77]

MANAGEMENT

Smoking cessation, avoidance of cold exposure, and eliminating the use of vasoconstricting drugs are nonpharmacologic interventions that are recommended but are only partially effective. In secondary cryofibrinogenemia, specific treatment of the underlying disease can lead to improvement in related symptoms.

For essential cryofibrinogenemia, various pharmacologic agents including fibrinolytic approaches and immunosuppressive agents have been proposed. Oral stanozolol (2-4 mg twice daily), a synthetic derivative of testosterone with substantial fibrinolytic properties, has been effective after several days of treatment.[85] Streptokinase (sometimes in combination with streptodornase), given intravenously (25,000-200,000 U/d) has a more rapid onset of action than stanozolol. The use of colchicine (0.6 mg twice daily) in combination with high-dose pentoxifylline (800 mg 3 times daily) has been described.[86]

Combinations of glucocorticoids (prednisone 10-60 mg/d) with low-dose aspirin, for nonsevere cases, or other immunosuppressive agents, for severe disease (azathioprine 150 mg/d or chlorambucil 10 mg/d) also have been used in small studies with some benefit, including successful treatment of acute attacks.[87,88]

Plasmapheresis might be considered when high levels of cryofibrinogens are present and are associated with monoclonal proteins (as seen in myeloma, Waldenström macroglobulinemia), hyperviscosity, or clinically significant thrombosis. Long-term repeated plasmaphereses and antiimmunoglobulin adsorption improved the symptoms in one patient with secondary cryofibrinogenemia.[89]

Regular followups are mandatory because of the high risk of symptom recurrence and development of lymphoma years after the initial diagnosis.[77,90]

ACKNOWLEDGMENTS

The authors acknowledge the significant contributions of Holger Schmid and Gerald S. Braun, the former authors of this chapter.

REFERENCES

1. Wintrobe MM, Buell MV. Hyperproteinemia associated with multiple myeloma. With report of a case in which an extraordinary hyperproteinemia was associated with thrombosis of the retinal veins and symptoms suggesting Raynaud's disease. *Bull Johns Hopkins Hosp.* 1933;52:156-165.
2. Brouet JC, Clauvel JP, Danon F, et al. Biologic and clinical significance of cryoglobulins. A report of 86 cases. *Am J Med.* 1974;57(5):775-788.
3. Zinneman HH. Cryoglobulins and pyroglobulins. *Pathobiol Annu.* 1980;10:83-104.
4. Tissot JD, Schifferli JA, Hochstrasser DF, et al. Two-dimensional polyacrylamide gel electrophoresis analysis of cryoglobulins and identification of an IgM-associated peptide. *J Immunol Methods.* 1994;173(1):63-75.
5. Roccatello D, Fornasieri A, Giachino O, et al. Multicenter study on hepatitis C virus-related cryoglobulinemic glomerulonephritis. *Am J Kidney Dis.* 2007;49(1):69-82.
6. Ferri C, Mascia MT. Cryoglobulinemic vasculitis. *Curr Opin Rheumatol.* 2006;18(1):54-63.
7. Ferri C. Mixed cryoglobulinemia. *Orphanet J Rare Dis.* 2008;3:25.
8. Trejo O, Ramos-Casals M, García-Carrasco M, et al. Cryoglobulinemia: study of etiologic factors and clinical and immunologic features in 443 patients from a single center. *Medicine (Baltimore).* 2001;80(4):252-262.
9. Lunel F, Musset L, Cacoub P, et al. Cryoglobulinemia in chronic liver diseases: role of hepatitis C virus and liver damage. *Gastroenterology.* 1994;106(5):1291-1300.
10. Pawlotsky JM, Ben Yahia M, Andre C, et al. Immunological disorders in C virus chronic active hepatitis: a prospective case-control study. *Hepatology.* 1994;19(4):841-848.
11. Santagostino E, et al. High prevalence of serum cryoglobulins in multitransfused hemophilic patients with chronic hepatitis C. *Blood.* 1998;92(2):516-519.
12. Cacoub P, Poynard T, Ghillani P, et al. Extrahepatic manifestations of chronic hepatitis C. MULTIVIRC Group. Multidepartment Virus C. *Arthritis Rheum.* 1999;42(10):2204-2212.
13. Cacoub P, Costedoat-Chalumeau N, Lidove O, et al. Cryoglobulinemia vasculitis. *Curr Opin Rheumatol.* 2002;14(1):29-35.
14. Fiorentino DF. Cutaneous vasculitis. *J Am Acad Dermatol.* 2003;48(3):311-340.
15. Terrier B, Marie I, Lacraz A, et al. Non HCV-related infectious cryoglobulinemia vasculitis: results from the French nationwide CryoVas survey and systematic review of the literature. *J Autoimmun.* 2015;65:74-81.
16. Cohen SJ, Pittelkow MR, Su WP. Cutaneous manifestations of cryoglobulinemia: clinical and histopathologic study of seventy-two patients. *J Am Acad Dermatol.* 1991;25(1, pt 1):21-27.
17. Rossi D, Mansouri M, Baldovino S, et al. Nail fold videocapillaroscopy in mixed cryoglobulinaemia. *Nephrol Dial Transplant.* 2004;19(9):2245-2249.
18. Meltzer M, Franklin EC. Cryoglobulinemia—a study of twenty-nine patients. I. IgG and IgM cryoglobulins and factors affecting cryoprecipitability. *Am J Med.* 1966;40(6):828-836.
19. Monti G, Galli M, Invernizzi F, et al. Cryoglobulinaemias: a multi-centre study of the early clinical and laboratory manifestations of primary and secondary disease. GISC. Italian Group for the Study of Cryoglobulinaemias. *Q J Med.* 1995;88(2):115-126.
20. Perico N, Cattaneo D, Bikbov B, et al. Hepatitis C infection and chronic renal diseases. *Clin J Am Soc Nephrol.* 2009;4(1):207-220.
21. Ferri C, La Civita L, Cirafisi C, et al. Peripheral neuropathy in mixed cryoglobulinemia: clinical and electrophysiologic investigations. *J Rheumatol.* 1992;19(6):889-895.
22. Manganelli P, Pavesi G, Fiocchi A, et al. Peripheral neuropathy with mixed cryoglobulinemia [in Italian]. *Recenti Prog Med.* 1990;81(11):681-685.
23. Gemignani F, Pavesi G, Fiocchi A, et al. Peripheral neuropathy in essential mixed cryoglobulinaemia. *J Neurol Neurosurg Psychiatry.* 1992;55(2):116-120.
24. Gemignani F, Marbini A, Di Giovanni G, et al. Cryoglobulinaemic neuropathy manifesting with restless legs syndrome. *J Neurol Sci.* 1997;152(2):218-223.
25. Weinberger A, Berliner S, Pinkhas J. Articular manifestations of essential cryoglobulinemia. *Semin Arthritis Rheum.* 1981;10(3):224-229.
26. Viegi G, Fornai E, Ferri C, et al. Lung function in essential mixed cryoglobulinemia: a short-term follow-up. *Clin Rheumatol.* 1989;8(3):331-338.
27. Bertorelli G, et al. Subclinical pulmonary involvement in essential mixed cryoglobulinemia assessed by bronchoalveolar lavage. *Chest.* 1991;100(5):1478-1479.
28. Zackrison LH, Katz P. Bronchiolitis obliterans organizing pneumonia associated with essential mixed cryoglobulinemia. *Arthritis Rheum.* 1993;36(11):1627-1630.
29. Abdulkarim T, Saklayen M, Yap J. Cryoglobulinemia due to hepatitis C with pulmonary renal syndrome. *Case Rep Nephrol.* 2013;2013:278975.
30. Antonelli A, Ferri C, Fallahi P, et al. Type 2 diabetes in hepatitis C-related mixed cryoglobulinaemia patients. *Rheumatology (Oxford).* 2004;43(2):238-240.
31. Cacoub P, Renou C, Kerr G, et al. Influence of HLA-DR phenotype on the risk of hepatitis C virus-associated mixed cryoglobulinemia. *Arthritis Rheum.* 2001;44(9):2118-2124.
32. Sebastiani GD, Bellisai F, Caudai C, et al. Association of extrahepatic manifestations with HLA class II alleles and with virus genotype in HCV infected patients. *J Biol Regul Homeost Agents.* 2005;19(1-2):17-22.
33. Saadoun D, Sellam J, Ghillani-Dalbin P, et al. Increased risks of lymphoma and death among patients with non-hepatitis C virus-related mixed cryoglobulinemia. *Arch Intern Med.* 2006;166(19):2101-2108.
34. Sene D, Ghillani-Dalbin P, Thibault V, et al. Long-term course of mixed cryoglobulinemia in patients infected with hepatitis C virus. *J Rheumatol.* 2004;31(11):2199-2206.
35. Antonelli A, Ferri C, Ferrari SM, et al. Serum levels of proinflammatory cytokines interleukin-1beta, interleukin-6, and tumor necrosis factor alpha in mixed cryoglobulinemia. *Arthritis Rheum.* 2009;60(12):3841-3847.
36. Antonelli A, Fallahi P, Ferrari SM, et al. Parallel increase of circulating CXCL11 and CXCL10 in mixed cryoglobulinemia, while the proinflammatory cytokine IL-6 is associated with high serum Th2 chemokine CCL2. *Clin Rheumatol.* 2013;32(8):1147-1154.
37. Mazzi V, Ferrari SM, Giuggioli D, et al. Role of CXCL10 in cryoglobulinemia. *Clin Exp Rheumatol.* 2015;33(3):433-436.
38. Artoni E, Sighinolfi GL, Gatti AM, et al. Micro and nanoparticles as possible pathogenetic co-factors in mixed cryoglobulinemia. *Occup Med (Lond).* 2017;67(1):64-67.
39. Levo Y, Gorevic PD, Kassab HJ, et al. Association between hepatitis B virus and essential mixed cryoglobulinemia. *N Engl J Med.* 1977;296(26):1501-1504.

40. Dimitrakopoulos AN, Kordossis T, Hatzakis A, et al. Mixed cryoglobulinemia in HIV-1 infection: the role of HIV-1. *Ann Intern Med*. 1999;130(3):226-230.
41. Fabris P, Tositti G, Giordani MT, et al. Prevalence and clinical significance of circulating cryoglobulins in HIV-positive patients with and without co-infection with hepatitis C virus. *J Med Virol*. 2003;69(3):339-343.
42. Chiche L, Grados A, Harlé JR, et al. Mixed cryoglobulinemia: a role for parvovirus b19 infection. *Clin Infect Dis*. 2010;50(7):1074-1075.
43. Ramos-Casals M, Anaya JM, García-Carrasco M, et al. Cutaneous vasculitis in primary Sjogren syndrome: classification and clinical significance of 52 patients. *Medicine (Baltimore)*. 2004;83(2):96-106.
44. Ramos-Casals M, Cervera R, Yagüe J, et al. Cryoglobulinemia in primary Sjogren's syndrome: prevalence and clinical characteristics in a series of 115 patients. *Semin Arthritis Rheum*. 1998;28(3):200-205.
45. Retamozo S, Gheitasi H, Quartuccio L, et al. Cryoglobulinaemic vasculitis at diagnosis predicts mortality in primary Sjogren syndrome: analysis of 515 patients. *Rheumatology (Oxford)*. 2016;55(8):1443-1451.
46. Garcia-Carrasco M, Ramos-Casals M, Cervera R, et al. Cryoglobulinemia in systemic lupus erythematosus: prevalence and clinical characteristics in a series of 122 patients. *Semin Arthritis Rheum*. 2001;30(5):366-373.
47. Shachaf S, Yair M. The correlation between antiphospholipid syndrome and cryoglobulinemia: case series of 4 patients and review of the literature. *Rev Bras Reumatol Engl Ed*. 2016;56(1):2-7.
48. Vitali C, Ferri C, Nasti P, et al. Hypercomplementaemia as a marker of the evolution from benign to malignant B cell proliferation in patients with type II mixed cryoglobulinaemia. *Br J Rheumatol*. 1994;33(8):791-792.
49. Ferri C, Sebastiani M, Giuggioli D, et al. Mixed cryoglobulinemia: demographic, clinical, and serologic features and survival in 231 patients. *Semin Arthritis Rheum*. 2004;33(6):355-374.
50. Della Rossa A, Marchi F, Catarsi E, et al. Mixed cryoglobulinemia and mortality: a review of the literature. *Clin Exp Rheumatol*. 2008;26(5)(suppl 51):S105-S108.
51. Saccardo E, Novati P, Sironi D, et al. Causes of death in symptomatic cryoglobulinemia: 30 years of observation in a Department of Internal Medicine. *Dig Liver Dis*. 2007;39(suppl 1):S52-S54.
52. Landau DA, Scerra S, Sene D, et al. Causes and predictive factors of mortality in a cohort of patients with hepatitis C virus-related cryoglobulinemic vasculitis treated with antiviral therapy. *J Rheumatol*. 2010;37(3):615-621.
53. Bruchfeld A, Lindahl K, Ståhle L, et al. Interferon and ribavirin treatment in patients with hepatitis C-associated renal disease and renal insufficiency. *Nephrol Dial Transplant*. 2003;18(8):1573-1580.
54. Sabry AA, Sobh MA, Sheaashaa HA, et al. Effect of combination therapy (ribavirin and interferon) in HCV-related glomerulopathy. *Nephrol Dial Transplant*. 2002;17(11):1924-1930.
55. Gorevic PD, Kassab HJ, Levo Y, et al. Mixed cryoglobulinemia: clinical aspects and long-term follow-up of 40 patients. *Am J Med*. 1980;69(2):287-308.
56. Zaidan M, Terrier B, Pozdzik A, et al; CryoVas study group. Spectrum and prognosis of noninfectious renal mixed cryoglobulinemic GN. *J Am Soc Nephrol*. 2016;27(4):1213-1224.
57. Monti G, Saccardo F. Emergency in cryoglobulinemic syndrome: what to do? *Dig Liver Dis*. 2007;39(suppl 1):S112-S115.
58. Siami GA, Siami FS, Ferguson P, et al. Cryofiltration apheresis for treatment of cryoglobulinemia associated with hepatitis C. *ASAIO J*. 1995;41(3):M315-M318.
59. Cacoub P, Saadoun D, Limal N, et al. PEGylated interferon alfa-2b and ribavirin treatment in patients with hepatitis C virus-related systemic vasculitis. *Arthritis Rheum*. 2005;52(3):911-915.
60. Casato M, Agnello V, Pucillo LP, et al. Predictors of long-term response to high-dose interferon therapy in type II cryoglobulinemia associated with hepatitis C virus infection. *Blood*. 1997;90(10):3865-3873.
61. Mazzaro C, Zorat F, Caizzi M, et al. Treatment with peginterferon alfa-2b and ribavirin of hepatitis C virus-associated mixed cryoglobulinemia: a pilot study. *J Hepatol*. 2005;42(5):632-638.
62. Naarendorp M, Kallemuchikkal U, Nuovo GJ, et al. Longterm efficacy of interferon-alpha for extrahepatic disease associated with hepatitis C virus infection. *J Rheumatol*. 2001;28(11):2466-2473.
63. Saadoun D, Resche-Rigon M, Thibault V, et al. Antiviral therapy for hepatitis C virus--associated mixed cryoglobulinemia vasculitis: a long-term followup study. *Arthritis Rheum*. 2006;54(11):3696-3706.
64. Ghany MG, Strader DB, Thomas DL, et al. Diagnosis, management, and treatment of hepatitis C: an update. *Hepatology*. 2009;49(4):1335-1374.
65. Kidney Disease: Improving Global Outcomes (KDIGO). KDIGO clinical practice guidelines for the prevention, diagnosis, evaluation, and treatment of hepatitis C in chronic kidney disease. *Kidney Int Suppl*. 2008;(109):S1-S99.
66. Dienstag JL, McHutchison JG. American Gastroenterological Association technical review on the management of hepatitis C. *Gastroenterology*. 2006;130(1):231-264; quiz 214-217.
67. Bruchfeld A, Lindahl K, Schvarcz R, et al. Dosage of ribavirin in patients with hepatitis C should be based on renal function: a population pharmacokinetic analysis. *Ther Drug Monit*. 2002;24(6):701-708.
68. Saadoun D, Delluc A, Piette JC, et al. Treatment of hepatitis C-associated mixed cryoglobulinemia vasculitis. *Curr Opin Rheumatol*. 2008;20(1):23-28.
69. Cacoub P, Delluc A, Saadoun D, et al. Anti-CD20 monoclonal antibody (rituximab) treatment for cryoglobulinemic vasculitis: where do we stand? *Ann Rheum Dis*. 2008;67(3):283-287.
70. Dammacco F, Tucci FA, Lauletta G, et al. Pegylated interferon-alpha, ribavirin, and rituximab combined therapy of hepatitis C virus-related mixed cryoglobulinemia: a long-term study. *Blood*. 2010;116(3):343-353.
71. Saadoun D, Resche Rigon M, Sene D, et al. Rituximab plus Peg-interferon-alpha/ribavirin compared with Peg-interferon-alpha/ribavirin in hepatitis C-related mixed cryoglobulinemia. *Blood*. 2010;116(3):326-334; quiz 504-505.
72. Terrier B, Cacoub P. Cryoglobulinemia vasculitis: an update. *Curr Opin Rheumatol*. 2013;25(1):10-18.
73. Saadoun D, Resche-Rigon M, Sene D, et al. Rituximab combined with Peg-interferon-ribavirin in refractory hepatitis C virus-associated cryoglobulinaemia vasculitis. *Ann Rheum Dis*. 2008;67(10):1431-1436.
74. Sene D, Ghillani-Dalbin P, Amoura Z, et al. Rituximab may form a complex with IgMkappa mixed cryoglobulin and induce severe systemic reactions in patients with hepatitis C virus-induced vasculitis. *Arthritis Rheum*. 2009;60(12):3848-3855.
75. Terrier B, Krastinova E, Marie I, et al. Management of noninfectious mixed cryoglobulinemia vasculitis: data

76. Saadoun D, Elalamy I, Ghillani-Dalbin P, et al. Cryofibrinogenemia: new insights into clinical and pathogenic features. *Am J Med.* 2009;122(12):1128-1135.
77. Belizna CC, Tron F, Joly P, et al. Outcome of essential cryofibrinogenaemia in a series of 61 patients. *Rheumatology (Oxford).* 2008;47(2):205-207.
78. Singh A, Gaber LW. Nephrotic syndrome and chronic renal insufficiency associated with essential cryofibrinogenemia. *Nephrol Dial Transplant.* 2007;22(6):1772-1775.
79. Korst DR, Kratochvil CH. Cryofibrinogen in a case of lung neoplasm associated with thrombophlebitis migrans. *Blood.* 1955;10(9):945-953.
80. Blain H, Cacoub P, Musset L, et al. Cryofibrinogenaemia: a study of 49 patients. *Clin Exp Immunol.* 2000;120(2):253-260.
81. Delluc A, Saadoun D, Ghillani-Dalbin P, et al. Cryofibrinogen in patients with hepatitis C virus infection. *Am J Med.* 2008;121(7):624-631.
82. Musset L, Diemert MC, Taibi F, et al. Characterization of cryoglobulins by immunoblotting. *Clin Chem.* 1992;38(6):798-802.
83. Nash JW, Ross P Jr, Neil Crowson A, et al. The histopathologic spectrum of cryofibrinogenemia in four anatomic sites. Skin, lung, muscle, and kidney. *Am J Clin Pathol.* 2003;119(1):114-122.
84. Lee J, Apisarnthanarax N, Jordon RE, et al. Cryofibrinogenemia in a patient with B-cell lymphoma. *Clin Lymphoma.* 2000;1(3):234-237; discussion 238-239.
85. Kirsner RS, Eaglstein WH, Katz MH, et al. Stanozolol causes rapid pain relief and healing of cutaneous ulcers caused by cryofibrinogenemia. *J Am Acad Dermatol.* 1993;28(1):71-74.
86. Chartier M, Falanga V. Healing of ulcers due to cryofibrinogenemia with colchicine and high-dose pentoxifylline. *Am J Clin Dermatol.* 2009;10(1):39-42.
87. Amdo TD, Welker JA. An approach to the diagnosis and treatment of cryofibrinogenemia. *Am J Med.* 2004;116(5):332-337.
88. Michaud M, Pourrat J. Cryofibrinogenemia. *J Clin Rheumatol.* 2013;19(3):142-148.
89. Euler HH, Zeuner RA, Béress R, et al. Monoclonal cryo-antifibrinogenemia. *Arthritis Rheum.* 1996;39(6):1066-1069.
90. Belizna C, Loufrani L, Subra JF, et al. A 5-year prospective follow-up study in essential cryofibrinogenemia patients. *Autoimmun Rev.* 2011;10(9):559-562.

Chapter 145 :: Raynaud Phenomenon
:: Drew Kurtzman & Ruth Ann Vleugels

第一百四十五章

雷诺现象

中文导读

雷诺现象（RP）是一种常见的反复发作的因动脉血管收缩导致肢端组织灌注不足的疾病。经典的RP表现为手和/或足的肢端颜色按一定的顺序发生一连串变化：界限清楚的苍白（对应于血管收缩和局部缺血），然后发绀（静脉淤滞），最后是红斑（代偿性再灌注）。根据潜在疾病的存在与否，可分为原发性和继发性。本章节从流行病学、临床特征、相关疾病、病因和发病机制、诊断、临床过程和预后及治疗对该病进行了详细阐述。

1. 流行病学　缺乏有关RP的准确流行病学数据，原发性RP的病例约占90%。RP的症状通常在生命的第二个十年中出现，女性与男性的患病率估计为4：1，某些病例存在家族聚集性。

2. 临床特征　RP患者常抱怨冷暴露和情绪刺激后引起的肢端白色或蓝色发作性变化。从患者的角度对RP发作的持续时间、特点和好发部位进行了详细描述。

（1）皮肤表现：详细介绍了RP可能出现的皮肤改变，最主要的皮肤表现是从肢端延伸到手指或足趾近端部分的边界清楚的苍白或紫绀（图145-1）。其他皮肤改变包括萎缩、营养不良性甲变化、肢端背侧的毛发脱落和肢端硬化，可出现溃疡（图145-2），严重时可能发生坏疽或远端截断。

（2）其他表现：除了进行仔细的皮肤检查外，建议还应评估外周血管搏动、两臂的血压，并进行Allen测试以评估手的动脉和毛细血管功能。详细的神经系统检查评估可以帮助识别潜在的神经系统疾病。

3. 相关情况　作者提出原发性RP患者的长期结局有进展为继发性疾病的可能，其中最常见的是结缔组织病。继发性RP则可在各种疾病、职业因素和/或药物和毒物暴露的情况下发生（表145-1和145-2），文中对此分别进行了详细讲述。

4. 病因和发病机制　RP的发病机理尚未完全阐明，目前的观点认为血管系统、神经系统和细胞因子之间的复杂相互作用是其发展的原因。

5. 诊断　该部分提出了原发性RP的诊断标准（表145-3），并介绍了基于三步法诊断原发性RP的专家共识。指出对于继发性RP需识别潜在病因，并介绍了可提示继发性RP的临床线索。

（1）实验室检查：建议所有RP患者均应进行全血细胞计数、红细胞沉降率、尿液分析和抗核抗体检测。根据病史和体格检查的结果，对可选择完善的检查进行了举例。

（2）特殊检查：甲皱襞毛细血管镜检查对于预测RP进展SSc的可能性有辅助价值。作者对原发性RP和继发性RP的甲皱襞毛细血管形态变化进行了详细的介绍。热成像是一种较新的诊断技术，可通过测量肢端表面温度来区分原发性RP和SSc相关的RP。作者对于该技术的价值及局限性进行了介绍。

6. 鉴别诊断　需与RP鉴别的主要血管性疾病见表145-4，对这些疾病的鉴别诊断要点进行了详细阐述。

7. 临床过程和预后　原发性RP预后较好，继发性RP的预后较差且易出现肢端溃疡等并发症。还介绍了一种可靠的评估RP活动性量表，即Raynaud条件评分（RCS）。对该量表的详细内容、意义及适用情况进行了详细介绍。

8. 治疗　RP的治疗目标在于减轻或减少发作的频率、严重性和持续时间以及治疗与缺血相关的并发症上。当确定存在继发性RP的原因时，应祛除病因。表145-5概述了有效的行为改变，详细介绍了这些行为。表145-6概述了雷诺现象的药物治疗。

（1）血管扩张剂：钙通道阻滞剂（CCBs）是RP的首选一线治疗药物。对该类药物的疗效、不良反应及代表性药物进行了介绍。此外，还介绍了一些新型血管扩张剂在RP中的应用进展。

（2）血管收缩抑制药：在该部分对血管收缩抑制药包括血管紧张素转化酶抑制药和血管紧张素Ⅱ受体拮抗药、选择性5-羟色胺再摄取抑制药（SSRIs）、内皮素受体拮抗药、α-肾上腺素能阻滞药、Rho激酶抑制药治疗RP的现状进行了综述。

（3）其他药物：对阿司匹林和其他抗血小板疗法、己酮可可碱等改变血液黏度和血液动力学的药物、抗凝剂和溶栓剂及抗氧化剂治疗RP的进展和适用情况进行了介绍。

（4）手术干预：①对肉毒杆菌毒素治疗RP的疗效、作用机制及治疗方法进行了综述。②交感神经切除术。分别介绍了一种传统的和新型的手术方法，并对疗效和不良反应进行了阐述。③手术清创与截肢。对于慢性不愈合的溃疡或出现失活的坏死组织，可能需要手术清创术。如果出现坏疽或继发骨髓炎，则可能需要截肢。④血管重建。适用于近端动脉闭塞的情况。

（5）特殊建议：①溃疡护理。着重强调了疼痛控制、伤口处理、改善循环及控制感染的护理原则。②严重缺血。主要指雷诺危象时的严重缺血，详细介绍了对于严重缺血的正确识别和治疗建议。③治疗流程。图145-4概述了RP患者的治疗流程。

〔黄莹雪〕

AT-A-GLANCE

- Raynaud phenomenon is a vascular disorder characterized by recurrent episodic attacks of digital ischemia provoked by exposure to cold or emotional stress.
- Affects up to 10% of the population, 4:1 female-to-male ratio.
- Classified as primary (idiopathic) and secondary (underlying disease or cause present) forms; severity ranges from mild/benign to severe with loss of tissue and risk of amputation.
- Connective tissue diseases, particularly systemic sclerosis, are among the most common underlying causes of secondary Raynaud phenomenon.
- Behavioral modification, pharmacologic therapies, and surgical interventions are effective at reducing the frequency and severity of attacks.

Raynaud phenomenon (RP) is a common disorder characterized by recurrent attacks of arterial vasoconstriction resulting in hypoperfusion of the digits and acral tissues. Episodes of RP are triggered by exposure to cold or, less commonly, emotional stress. Classically,

RP exhibits a triphasic sequence of color changes of the digits of the hands and/or feet: well-demarcated pallor (corresponding to vasoconstriction and ischemia), followed by cyanosis (venous stasis), and, finally, erythema (compensatory reperfusion) upon rewarming.[1] However, not all patients demonstrate this classic triad of color changes.

Depending on the presence or absence of an underlying disorder, 2 forms of RP are recognized and usually display divergent disease courses. Primary (idiopathic) RP represents an exaggerated physiologic response to cold or emotional stimuli caused by functional changes in blood vessels and their innervation.[2] By definition, primary RP does not result in tissue injury. Secondary RP, which occurs as a result of a systemic disorder or drug exposure, is distinguished by a more aggressive course that can lead to profound tissue ischemia and eventuate in cutaneous ulceration, scarring, or digital gangrene. Management of RP centers on behavioral changes to avoid attacks and on pharmacologic and nonpharmacologic therapies to allay symptoms and reduce morbidity. When present, treatment of the underlying cause remains a critical component of managing secondary disease.

EPIDEMIOLOGY

Precise epidemiologic data on RP are lacking. True estimates are biased by underreporting because many patients with RP never seek medical attention and by the greater attention that has been given to secondary forms of the disease. RP likely affects up to 10% of the general population and 90% of patients with systemic sclerosis (SSc).[3-5] Despite study biases, cases of primary RP far outnumber those of secondary disease and comprise up to 90% of all cases.[6,7] Symptoms of RP often develop during the second decade of life, and there is a strong female predominance, with an estimated 4:1 female-to-male prevalence ratio. Increases in the frequency and severity of attacks during menstrual cycles suggest that female hormones play a role in the pathogenesis of RP.[8] Differences in seasonal skin temperatures, alcohol use, age, smoking status, and marital status between women and men also explain the sex differences observed.[9,10] Familial aggregation has been noted in some series, substantiating a role for genetic predisposition.[11] Other associations reported in epidemiologic studies include living in a cold climate, certain occupations, cardiovascular disease, low body mass index, and use of vibratory tools.

CLINICAL FEATURES

HISTORY

A clear description of vasospastic attacks is fundamental to the diagnosis of RP. Patients with RP report episodic attacks of white or blue digits induced by cold exposure and, less commonly, by emotional stimuli. Often, only a portion of the digit is affected, and the thumbs are typically spared. Patients rarely volunteer the classic tri-sequence color change, and most only recognize the pallor phase. During attacks, affected digits are numb and, upon rewarming, become bright red and may be accompanied by throbbing pain. If pain is prominent during the ischemic (pallor) phase, a secondary cause is more likely. Other features suggestive of secondary disease are cutaneous ulceration or thumb involvement, as these are rarely seen in primary RP.[2] Episodes of RP usually last for 30 minutes, but can persist for hours. Although the fingers and toes are classically affected, attacks may involve the nose, earlobes, or nipples.

A careful review of systems is needed to screen for symptoms that point to an underlying disorder as a cause for secondary RP. Arthralgias, dysphagia, muscle weakness, photosensitivity, gastroesophageal reflux, shortness of breath, or sicca symptoms suggest a connective tissue disorder. Claudication indicates atherosclerotic arterial disease. A careful review of medications allows for identification of a potential drug cause. Use of vibratory tools or perpetual hand trauma helps to establish an occupational exposure or hobby as the cause for RP.

CUTANEOUS FINDINGS

Well-demarcated pallor or cyanosis extending from the tip to the more proximal segments of the digits of the fingers or toes typifies the skin changes seen in RP (Fig. 145-1). The skin distal to the line of ischemia is cold and pale, while the proximal skin is often pink and warm. As digits rewarm, blanched skin becomes cyanotic, secondary to low blood flow and deoxygenation, and then transitions to bright red, due to reactive hyperemia. Persistent ischemic discoloration in spite of rewarming suggests secondary disease.

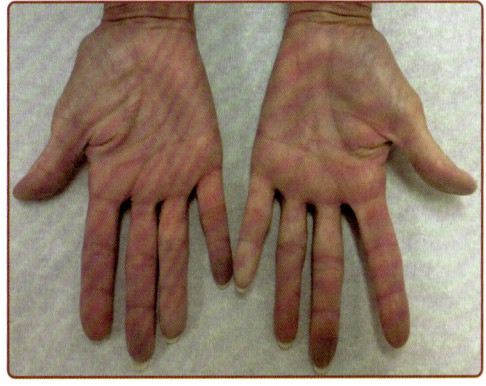

Figure 145-1 Triphasic color changes on the fingers of a patient with primary Raynaud phenomenon.

Trophic changes of the digits are signs of prolonged attacks of RP and also point to secondary disease. Other skin changes may include atrophy, dystrophic nail changes, and alopecia on the dorsal surfaces of the digits. If present, true sclerodactyly warrants a high degree of suspicion for SSc. In the setting of longstanding RP with repeated bouts of ischemia, digital tapering may occur, which can be challenging to distinguish from sclerodactyly for many clinicians. Ulcerations, which can be extremely painful and punctuated at night, favor the pulp of the finger and the nail unit. Ulcers heal slowly, leaving characteristic small, pitted scars (Fig. 145-2). Ulcers may become infected and can even result in digital osteomyelitis. Although rare, gangrene and autoamputation of distal portions of the digits can occur.

Careful inspection of the proximal nailfold, giving attention to the capillaries with the aid of microscopy (or handheld dermoscopy), is a critical part of evaluating the patient with RP. In a large, single institution study prospectively following 586 patients with RP, the presence of an abnormal nailfold capillary pattern (capillary enlargement and/or capillary loss) at baseline predicted the development of SSc in 151 (25.8%) of patients during a 15-year followup period.[12] When accompanied by an SSc-specific autoantibody, abnormal capillaries portended a 60-fold increased risk for progression to SSc among subjects in their cohort. The authors concluded that microvascular damage, which can be assessed by evaluating the proximal nailfold capillaries, is an independent predictor for progression to SSc, highlighting the importance of this examination finding.

The presence of hand edema (puffy hands), sclerodactyly, mat telangiectasias, or calcinosis in a patient with RP points to a potential diagnosis of SSc. Other cutaneous findings may imply a specific secondary disorder, for example, purpura, indicating a blood dyscrasia, or jaundice, suggesting viral hepatitis.

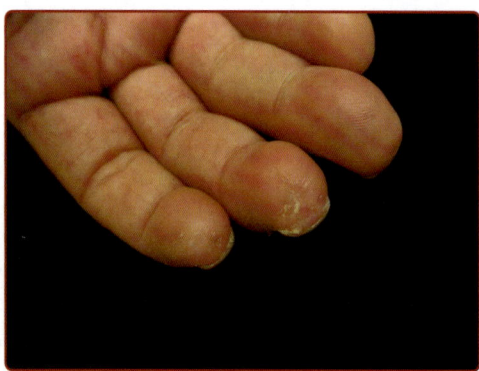

Figure 145-2 Pitted scarring involving fourth and fifth fingertips in a patient with Raynaud phenomenon in the setting of systemic sclerosis.

OTHER FINDINGS

In addition to a careful skin examination, peripheral pulses should be evaluated and blood pressure obtained in both arms. An Allen test also should be performed to assess arterial and capillary function of the hands. In this test, the examiner simultaneously compresses the radial and ulnar arteries, while the patient opens and closes the fist to induce blanching of the palm. Selective arterial filling is judged by the rate of color return as pressure is sequentially released from the radial and ulnar arteries. Abnormal filling implies structural disease of the microcirculation, raising the suspicion for a secondary form of RP or the presence of a thrombus. A positive Allen test should be confirmed with a more definitive diagnostic evaluation such as a Doppler study or angiogram. Vascular obstruction from the thoracic outlet syndrome can be assessed by the Adson maneuver, which tests for diminution of the radial pulse with exaggerated movement of the neck and shoulder. A careful neurologic examination looking for signs of sympathetic nervous system hyperactivity, abnormal reflexes, or muscular weakness or atrophy can help identify an underlying neurologic disorder.

ASSOCIATIONS

By definition, primary RP develops without an identifiable systemic or drug cause. Several studies have examined the long-term outcome of patients with primary RP.[6,12-14] Progression to a secondary form, most commonly a connective tissue disease such as SSc or systemic lupus erythematosus, is as high as 15% during the first decade of onset. Features predictive of progression include nailfold capillary abnormalities, hand edema (puffy hands), positive Allen's test, and antinuclear antibodies.[12,14]

Secondary RP develops in the context of various disorders and/or drug and toxin exposures (Tables 145-1 and 145-2).

CONNECTIVE TISSUE DISEASES

The connective tissue diseases are the most common cause of secondary RP. Among patients with SSc, 80% to 90% manifest symptoms of RP. It is the presenting sign in approximately one-third of patients with SSc and may be the only manifestation of the disease for years. Among patients with systemic lupus erythematosus, autoimmune myositis, and systemic vasculitis, RP develops in up to a third. Interestingly, although patients with rheumatoid arthritis often complain of mottled skin changes accompanying cold hands, the incidence of RP appears to be equal to that of the general population.[15] Arteriograms of patients with

TABLE 145-1
Causes of Secondary Raynaud Phenomenon

Connective Tissue Disease
- Systemic sclerosis (SSc)
- Systemic lupus erythematosus
- Dermatomyositis and polymyositis
- Mixed connective tissue disease
- Systemic vasculitis
- Sjögren syndrome

Obstructive Arterial Disease
- Atherosclerosis
- Thromboangiitis obliterans (Buerger disease)
- Thromboembolism
- Thoracic outlet syndrome

Neurologic Disorders
- Carpal tunnel syndrome
- Reflex sympathetic dystrophy
- Hemiplegia
- Poliomyelitis
- Multiple sclerosis
- Syringomyelia

Occupation/Environmental Exposure
- Vibration injury (lumberjacks, pneumatic hammer operators)
- Posttraumatic injury (hypothenar hammer syndrome, crutch pressure)
- Vinyl chloride exposure
- Cold injury

Hyperviscosity Disorders
- Cryoproteins (cryoglobulins, cryofibrinogens)
- Cold agglutinins
- Macroglobulins
- Polycythemia
- Thrombocytosis

Miscellaneous
- Hypothyroidism
- Infections (bacterial endocarditis, Lyme disease, viral hepatitis)
- Malignancy
- Primary pulmonary hypertension
- Arteriovenous fistula

TABLE 145-2
Drugs Associated with Raynaud Phenomenon

- β-Adrenergic blockers
- Ergotamines
- Oral contraceptives
- Methysergide
- Bleomycin
- Vinblastine
- Clonidine
- Bromocriptine
- Cyclosporine
- Amphetamines
- Interferon-α and interferon-β
- Imatinib

connective tissue diseases often show digital and sometimes ulnar or radial artery obstructions.

NEUROLOGIC DISORDERS

Any neurologic condition that results in impaired use of a limb may be associated with sympathetic nervous system disturbances and RP. Although distinct from RP, thermoregulatory changes may be a prominent feature of reflex sympathetic dystrophy and can simulate RP.[16] Nerve root compression may also cause RP. RP infrequently complicates carpal tunnel syndrome, but if it does develop, the pattern of involvement conforms to the innervation of the median nerve, affecting the first, index, and middle fingers.[17,18] RP may also develop from neurovascular compression at the thoracic outlet by cervical ribs, scalene muscles, bony defects of the cervical vertebrae or clavicle, or shoulder compression syndromes.[19,20]

OCCUPATIONAL FACTORS

RP is common among individuals with certain occupations. Specifically, individuals who work with vibratory tools, such as air hammers, chainsaws, and rivet guns, and those who experience prolonged exposure to cold temperatures, such as butchers, ice cream workers, and fish packers, are at risk for RP. The prevalence of RP appears to correlate with the vibration level of the tool used, duration of use, and the duration of exposure to cold temperatures.[21] Vinyl chloride manufacturing in the polymer industry also confers a risk for developing RP.[22]

MEDICATIONS AND TOXINS

A variety of medications can cause or exacerbate RP (see Table 145-2). Mechanistically, drugs may cause peripheral vasoconstriction, endothelial injury, neurotoxicity, or local enhancement of blood viscosity.[23] β-Adrenergic blockers, a widely prescribed class of antihypertensives, are the most common cause of iatrogenic RP.[24,25] Unopposed peripheral vasoconstriction likely accounts for the development of RP, and specific drugs within the class, for example, propranolol, exhibit a higher propensity to cause disease than do other drugs.[25] Other drugs capable of causing RP by vasoconstrictive mechanisms include clonidine, ergot alkaloids (for migraine headaches), dopaminergic agonists, centrally acting stimulants such as methylphenidate and dextroamphetamine, cyclosporine, sympathomimetics (pseudoephedrine, phenylephrine), and cocaine.[26-35]

Chemotherapies, in particular bleomycin, cisplatin, and vinblastine, are also well-known causes of RP, likely precipitating symptoms by toxin-mediated endothelial dysfunction.[36-39] Although the risk of developing RP appears to be commensurate with the cumulative dose of chemotherapy, there are reports of RP after a single injection of bleomycin for the treatment of common warts, supporting the concept that idiosyncratic reactions may also account for some cases.[40]

RP is a known side effect of treatment with interferon.[23,41] Administration of both isotypes of interferon (α and β) can cause severe RP, and some interferon-induced cases have even required surgical amputation because of the ischemic injury sustained.[42] The pathophysiology of interferon-induced RP is potentially related to several mechanisms, including a direct vasospastic effect, an increase in blood viscosity, a deposition of immune complexes, and arterial occlusion by thrombi.[43-45]

Sulfasalazine, propofol, amphotericin B, and, more recently, the tyrosine kinase inhibitors, also have been reported to cause RP.[23]

In cases of drug-induced RP, discontinuation of the offending medication usually reverses symptoms, but in some instances, the vascular changes are permanent and may require disease-specific interventions. Notably, in patients with preexisting RP, many of these medications can exacerbate disease symptoms. Careful attention to a patient's medication regimen allows for appropriate substitutions to be made to mitigate disease activity.

MISCELLANEOUS DISORDERS

Patients with hyperviscosity from cryoglobulins, cryofibrinogens, macroglobulins, cold agglutinins, and polycythemia can develop RP. Endocrine disorders, infections, and a variety of malignancies, may also manifest with symptoms of RP.

ETIOLOGY AND PATHOGENESIS

Although the pathogenesis of RP is incompletely understood, it appears that complex interactions between the vasculature, nervous system, and circulating cytokines are responsible for its development.[2,46]

VASCULAR ABNORMALITIES

Several studies have demonstrated that endothelial-dependent vasodilation is reduced in both primary and SSc-related RP.[47-50] Inadequate production of vasodilatory mediators, including nitric oxide and prostacyclin, appears to be critical for this impaired vasodilation.[51]

In addition, excessive vasoconstriction, partly caused by high circulating levels of endothelin-1 and angiotensin II, contributes to acral hypoperfusion.[52,53] Inhibition of the endothelin-1 receptor with bosentan attenuates symptoms of SSc-associated RP, substantiating the pathogenic role of this vasoconstrictor in RP.[54,55] These functional blood vessel abnormalities (impaired vasodilation and enhanced vasoconstriction) are present in both forms of RP. Structural derangements of the microvasculature and digital arteries also occur in secondary RP and augment impaired digital perfusion.[2,56] Microangiopathy and intimal wall hyperplasia characterize these structural changes and promote ongoing vascular injury, likely accounting for the progressive nature of some cases of secondary RP.

NEURAL ABNORMALITIES

Aberrant signals from the autonomic nervous system, afferent sensory nerves, and the CNS are implicated in the pathogenesis of RP.[2] Blood vessels receive innervation from 3 primary sources including sympathetic, parasympathetic, and sensory neurons.[46] An imbalance favoring the activation of neurally mediated vasoconstrictive pathways has been demonstrated in RP. Calcitonin gene-related peptide–immunoreactive sensory neurons are reduced in the skin of fingers in patients with SSc-associated RP and primary RP compared to healthy controls, and by altering the neurovascular axis, this deficiency contributes to defective vasodilation.[57] Moreover, hyperresponsive $α_2$-adrenoceptors that govern vasoconstriction in response to cold stimuli have been detected in the digital arteries of individuals with RP.[58,59] Central mechanisms may also contribute to RP, as attacks can be elicited by emotional stress. The inability to habituate to episode-provoking stimuli has been cited as a cause for CNS-mediated RP.[60,61]

INTRAVASCULAR ABNORMALITIES

Platelet activation, increased thrombin generation, defective fibrinolysis, reduced red cell deformability, aberrant white blood cell activation, and increased viscosity collectively constitute the intravascular alterations seen in RP.[2] Secondary forms of the disease display a higher likelihood of several of these abnormalities being present simultaneously.[62] Oxidative stress imposed on endothelial cells through peroxidation of cell membranes and hypoxia-reperfusion injury, as a result of recurrent ischemic and hyperemic insults, also contribute to SSc-associated RP and, to a lesser extent, to primary RP.[2]

OTHER MECHANISMS

A variety of other factors likely play a role in the genesis of RP, but are poorly defined. Among those described, hormonal influences from estrogen and genetic predisposition have the strongest data supporting an etiologic association.[62] Polymorphisms in genes encoding portions of the neuromuscular acetylcholine receptor and serotonin 1B and serotonin 1E receptors may confer genetic susceptibility to developing primary RP.[63]

DIAGNOSIS

Primary RP is common, and although a large subset of patients never seek medical attention, many with primary RP do so out of concern for the possibility of an underlying connective tissue disorder.[2] Criteria for the diagnosis of primary RP have been developed and validated (Table 145-3).[64-66] An expert consensus definition of primary RP has been proposed based on a 3-step algorithm.[67] To satisfy a diagnosis of primary RP, patients must have evidence of their fingers having unusual cold sensitivity, experience at least biphasic color changes during vasospastic episodes (white and blue), and have a minimum of 3 of the following features present: attacks triggered by stimuli other than cold (eg, emotional stress); involvement of both hands, even if asymmetric; attacks accompanied by numbness or paresthesias; color changes characterized by a well-demarcated border between affected and unaffected skin; photographs that strongly support a diagnosis of RP; episodes occurring at other body sites (eg, nose, ears, feet, and nipples); and triphasic color changes (white, blue, red).

In addition to classic symptoms, the diagnosis of secondary RP requires the simultaneous identification of a systemic disorder, medication, or toxin exposure known to cause the disease. Secondary RP is more likely in the following settings: an age at onset of 30 years or older; episodes that are intense, painful, asymmetric, or associated with ischemic skin lesions; clinical signs suggestive of a connective tissue disease, such as arthritis or abnormal lung function; specific autoantibodies; and evidence of microvascular disease seen on nailfold microscopy, particularly capillary dropout and giant capillary loops.[68-70]

LABORATORY STUDIES

In all patients with RP, a complete blood count, erythrocyte sedimentation rate, urinalysis, and antinuclear antibody testing should be obtained.[68] In patients with abnormal antinuclear antibody titers, testing for antibodies to specific nuclear antigens, for example, centromere or topoisomerase, are helpful to identify specific connective tissue diseases such as SSc. Notably, a positive antinuclear antibody without antigen specificity carries a lower risk of a concomitant connective tissue disorder, as compared to antigen-specific autoantibodies.[13,71,72]

Additional laboratory studies may be warranted based on findings from the history and physical examination and include a comprehensive chemistry panel; thyroid function tests; measurement of C3 and C4 complement levels; serum protein electrophoresis and immunofixation electrophoresis; testing for rheumatoid factor; and evaluation for cryoglobulins. A chest radiograph may detect a cervical rib in patients with symptoms of thoracic outlet obstruction. If proximal large vessel disease is suspected, for example in the case of unilateral RP or when peripheral pulses are difficult to palpate, arterial Doppler investigations are necessary.[2] Abnormal Doppler studies require further evaluation with appropriate imaging and/or referral to a vascular specialist.

SPECIAL TESTING

Nailfold capillaroscopy is a helpful adjunctive tool to predict progression to SSc. Whereas normal nailfolds consisting of uniformly sized capillaries with regular spacing are reassuring and are present in the majority of cases of primary RP, capillary dilation (giant capillaries) with focal hemorrhage and areas of avascularity (capillary dropout) are highly specific for and can predict transition to SSc (Fig. 145-3).[2,70,73] In SSc-associated RP, serial nailfold capillary microscopy examinations show progressive decreases in the total number of nailfold capillary loops, and end-stage changes, which include haphazardly arranged vessels (telangiectasia) and near total loss of capillaries, correlate with advanced sclerodactyly.[74] These dynamic nailfold changes are not observed in primary RP.

Thermal imaging (thermography) is a newer diagnostic technique that measures digital and acral surface temperatures and may be able to distinguish between patients with primary RP and those with SSc.[75] By determining the temperature differences between

---

TABLE 145-3
Criteria for Primary Raynaud Phenomenon

- Vasospastic attacks precipitated by exposure to cold or emotional stimuli
- Bilateral involvement of extremities
- Normal vascular examination with symmetric peripheral pulses and normal nailfold capillary microscopy
- Absence of gangrene or, if present, limited to the skin of the fingertips
- No evidence of an underlying disease, drug, or occupational exposure that could be responsible for vasospastic attacks
- Negative antinuclear antibody test
- Normal erythrocyte sedimentation rate
- History of symptoms for at least 2 years

Combined criteria of Allen and Brown[64] and Le Roy and Medsger.[65]

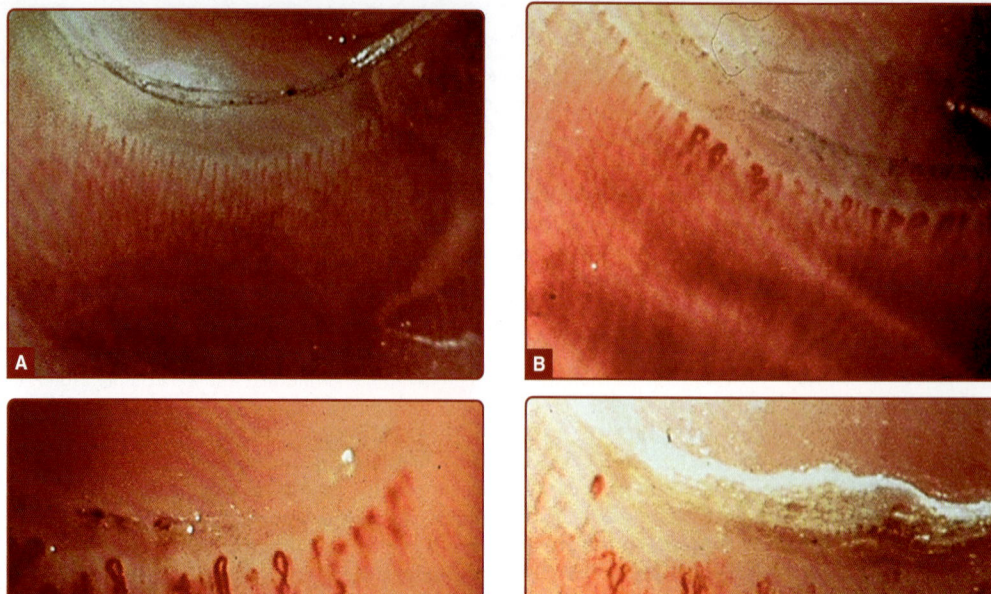

Figure 145-3 Nailfold capillary microscopy in a normal patient (**A**) compared to 3 patients with systemic sclerosis showing dilated capillaries (**B**), capillary tortuosity with dropout (**C**), and a telangiectatic pattern (**D**).

distal fingertips and the dorsal hand ("distal–dorsal difference"), parameters derived from thermography appear to reliably predict whether a structural vascular defect (eg, related to SSc) is present. Thermography awaits further validation, and its usefulness is limited by its cost and availability.

Other techniques that have been used to diagnose RP include laser Doppler imaging, plethysmography, and finger systolic pressure measurements.[76-78] As of this writing, such tests are not routinely used in clinical practice, but may ultimately provide practical, noninvasive methods to assist in the diagnosis of RP.

DIFFERENTIAL DIAGNOSIS

The major forms of vascular disease that must be distinguished from RP are physiologic cold fingers, acrocyanosis, pernio, erythromelalgia, livedo reticularis, and reflex sympathetic dystrophy (Table 145-4).

Many patients experience cold, sometimes painful digits without a color change in response to cold temperature exposure. This condition is physiologic and, although pronounced in some individuals, represents normal sympathetic nervous system activity. This type of response to cold exposure is not synonymous with RP.

Acrocyanosis is a functional vascular condition characterized by blue-violet discoloration of acral skin as a result of diminished oxyhemoglobin.[79,80] Defects in central oxygenation, as seen in cardiac and pulmonary diseases, or local hypoxia are responsible for the manifestations of the disorder. Acrocyanosis is much less common than RP, and by definition, the color changes seen in acrocyanosis are persistent, irrespective of exposure to cold temperature or other stimuli. Triphasic color changes are not seen in acrocyanosis.

Pernio is an acral, inflammatory dermatosis that develops in response to exposure to cold, wet conditions. Lesions of pernio appear as erythematous to violaceous macules, papules, or plaques that symmetrically involve the toes and/or fingers. Rarely, the heels, thighs, nose, and ears may be affected. Hemorrhagic lesions, bullae, loss of the nails, and ulcerations may complicate severe cases. If ulcerations develop, secondary infections may supervene. Pain, pruritus, and a burning sensation may accompany lesions of pernio. The disorder is typically benign and self-limiting, and lesions last approximately 1 to 3 weeks. Uncomplicated cases of pernio do not require treatment, but

TABLE 145-4
Differential Diagnosis of Raynaud Phenomenon

- Physiologic response to cold temperature
- Acrocyanosis
- Pernio
- Erythromelalgia
- Livedo reticularis
- Reflex sympathetic dystrophy

when present in patients with concomitant connective tissue disease, it may be more challenging to manage and necessitate disease-specific therapy.

Erythromelalgia is a rare, functional vascular disease characterized by pain, burning, edema, and erythema, most often of the extremities. Unlike RP, affected limbs are characteristically warm. Exercise, standing, walking, limb dependency, and warm exposure trigger episodes of erythromelalgia. Attacks of erythromelalgia tend to occur in the evening and at night, and can disrupt sleep. The feet are affected in 90% of patients, whereas the hands are involved in only 25%.[81] Rarely, the face and the ears may be involved. Because of the extreme warmth and burning pain experienced, patients seek various ways to cool the affected area, and often find relief with limb elevation or immersion in ice water. Immersion in ice water causes reactive vasoconstriction that may lead to skin breakdown and cold water tissue injury, eventuating in infection and, rarely, autoamputation. Erythromelalgia may be primary, or may occur as a result of a systemic disorder. Although the etiology and pathogenesis of erythromelalgia are poorly understood, it is thought to relate to abnormalities of platelet function, changes in vascular dynamics, and dysfunction of voltage-gated sodium channels.[82,83] Cases of coexisting erythromelalgia and RP have been described, and some investigators view the 2 disorders as existing on a spectrum, with RP representing the excessive vasoconstrictive form and erythromelalgia representing the exaggerated vasodilatory form.[82]

Livedo reticularis is a very common skin change resulting from a localized physiologic response to cold exposure and appears as a mottled, well-formed reticulated (net-like) vascular pattern that blanches with pressure. Although any body site may be affected, lesions preferentially occur on the limbs, particularly the lower extremities. Livedo reticularis develops from alterations in blood flow through the cutaneous microvasculature.[84] It may be a primary physiologic response or, less commonly, associated with an underlying condition, especially disorders that alter blood viscosity or cause intraluminal vascular obstruction.

Reflex sympathetic dystrophy is a rare, painful disorder accompanied by vasomotor instability that results from autonomic nervous system dysfunction.[85] Most cases arise after injury to a limb. Consequently, changes seen in reflex sympathetic dystrophy favor the upper and lower extremities, as well as the hands. Complex alterations in nociceptive nerve terminals amplify pain signals from the CNS and are thought to cause the disorder. Reflex sympathetic dystrophy characteristically progresses through various stages that ultimately result in soft-tissue destruction.[85] The second stage of disease, which is characterized by pain and vasomotor instability, develops months after nerve injury has occurred and may resemble RP. Distinguishing features include disproportionate levels of pain, hypotrichosis or hypertrichosis, nail changes, hyperhidrosis or anhidrosis, and, in advanced stages, soft-tissue atrophy.

CLINICAL COURSE AND PROGNOSIS

The clinical course of RP is largely dictated by whether the disorder is primary or secondary. The vast majority of cases of primary RP exhibit an indolent course. Simple behavioral modifications alone usually suffice to control the disease. Complications such as digital ulceration, soft-tissue atrophy, and bone loss rarely occur in primary RP.

In contrast, secondary RP has a more guarded prognosis. In secondary disease, repeated bouts of prolonged digital ischemia result in skin breakdown, soft-tissue injury, ulceration, and, occasionally, autoamputation. These complications are more frequent in inadequately treated patients. Digital pulp cellulitis (felon) and osteomyelitis may also complicate secondary RP, especially after the development of cutaneous ulceration.

Raynaud crisis is a rapidly progressive form of RP that is characterized by acute, potentially catastrophic tissue ischemia and is considered a medical emergency. Without intervention, Raynaud crisis results in digital infarction and may lead to digit loss. Patients with secondary RP should be alerted to the possibility of developing this rare complication, which is heralded by extreme pain and persistent white-blue color changes in a digit that will not rewarm. Susceptibility to Raynaud crisis is highest among patients with SSc with coexisting macrovascular disease and positive anti-centromere antibodies.[86]

RP can have a profound impact on a patient's quality of life. When controlling for severe pulmonary and GI disease in a study examining RP activity in SSc patients, patient-reported health assessment questionnaire pain and disability scores, as well as visual analog scale severity scores were greater for RP and digital ulcers compared to breathing and intestinal complaints, indicating a more substantial impact on quality of life.[87] High levels of depressed mood and feelings of anxiety related to attacks of RP were also found in the study's cohort.

The development of digital ulcers is a poor prognostic sign. Apart from morbidity directly related to digital ulcers, higher incidences of disability, pain, and limited hand function accompany this complication.[87]

A validated, reliable measure of RP activity, the Raynaud Condition Score (RCS), has been developed.[87] The score represents a global composite of objective metrics (number of attacks per day, length of each attack) and a subjective, patient-reported severity score. The severity score component is administered on either a visual analog scale (0 to 100) or an 11-point Likert scale, averaged over a 1- or 2-week period. While primarily used to assess response to therapy in clinical trials, implementation of the RCS as a practice tool has gained popularity, allowing clinicians to assign a severity score to patients in order to gauge suitability for an intervention and to objectively follow their outcome. The RCS and other RP measures, including the health assessment questionnaire's pain and disability scale and mood scales, are highly sensitive to changes in RP activity and can discriminate between subjects with and without digital ulcers.[87] Recently, the minimally important difference, representing the smallest improvement in a score that patients perceive as beneficial, and the Patient Acceptable Symptom State, defined as the absolute value beyond which patients consider themselves well, have been established for the RCS.[88] These estimates, a 14- to 15-point improvement (0 to 100, visual analog scale) and a score of 34 points or less for the minimally important difference and Patient Acceptable Symptom State, respectively, will assist with objectively evaluating the success of treatments for RP using meaningful end points in future clinical trials.

MANAGEMENT

The management of RP centers on attenuating the frequency, severity, and duration of attacks as well as treating ischemia-related complications. These goals can be achieved through the implementation of behavioral modification, pharmacologic therapies, and procedural interventions. In some cases, a combination approach is necessary. When causes of secondary RP are identified, treatment of the underlying disorder may result in improvement of RP. When a drug or occupational exposure is suspected, cessation of the culprit medication or removing the patient from the causal environment is necessary.

BEHAVIORAL MODIFICATION

Table 145-5 outlines effective behavior modifications. Mild RP is generally amenable to lifestyle changes that minimize exposure to the cold. Dressing warmly with layered clothing and maintaining a higher-than-normal thermostat setting while indoors are easy habits for patients to implement. Limiting time spent outdoors during the winter, wearing insulated mittens or gloves and thick socks, and using hand or foot warmers, are also helpful. Patients should be taught to recognize and terminate attacks of RP promptly by returning to a warmer environment and applying heat to affected digits if symptoms persist after acclimating. In addition, counseling to maintain a warm core temperature (including wearing hats and additional layers centrally) should be reinforced at each patient encounter. This measure prevents the reflexive, peripheral vasoconstriction that accompanies a drop in core temperature, as blood shunts centrally to rewarm the body. Smoking cessation in smokers with RP and counseling to avoid secondhand smoke in nonsmokers should be emphasized because nicotine induces cutaneous vasoconstriction and can provoke attacks of RP. Caffeine has mixed vasoactive properties, but one of its major downstream effects is to enhance vasoconstriction by blocking adenosine receptors. Consequently, limiting caffeine consumption should also be considered in caffeine-sensitive patients. Stress modification is important to minimize vasoconstriction in those with hyperactivity of the sympathetic nervous system. Counseling, training in relaxation, biofeedback techniques, and, in anxiety-provoked cases, anxiolytics may be beneficial.

PHARMACOLOGIC INTERVENTIONS

Table 145-6 outlines pharmacologic therapies for Raynaud phenomenon.

VASODILATORS

Calcium channel blockers (CCBs) are the preferred first-line therapy for both primary and SSc-associated RP in patients who do not respond to behavioral modification alone.[89-91] The dihydropyridine class of CCBs (nifedipine, amlodipine, nicardipine, and felodipine) are the least cardioselective and appear to be the most efficacious in terms of reducing the frequency and severity of attacks of RP.[46] Their beneficial effect has been confirmed in several randomized, blinded, placebo-controlled trials. Diltiazem, a nondihydropyridine CCB, also reduces vasospastic episodes in both primary and secondary RP.[92] A metaanalysis of 18 trials evaluating CCBs as a primary intervention for RP demonstrated an average decrease of 2.8 to 5 attacks and a 33% reduction of symptom severity during a 1-week period.[89] Adverse side effects from CCBs occur in up to 15% of users and include headache, flushing, hypotension, and lower-extremity edema.[93] Side effects can be dose-dependent or idiosyncratic. In SSc patients with esophageal dysmotility, CCBs can also exacerbate gastroesophageal reflux symptoms.[46,94] Commencing treatment with a low dose followed by a gradual escalation until the desired response is achieved is the most effective approach. Furthermore, selection of a once-daily, sustained-release preparation is preferable to shorter-acting formulations and encourages patient compliance. In addition, when the sustained-release dose is given nightly, CCBs are better tolerated, even in patients with low baseline blood pressures.

Studies implicating the pathogenic deficiency of

TABLE 145-5
Behavioral Modification

1. Dress warmly and layer clothing
2. Maintain higher-than-normal thermostat settings indoors
3. Limit time spent outdoors during winter
4. Use hand or foot warmers
5. Recognize and terminate attacks early
6. Smoking cessation and/or avoidance of secondhand smoke
7. Limit caffeine consumption

TABLE 145-6
Pharmacologic Therapies for Raynaud Phenomenon

CLASS	DRUGS	DOSE & ADMINISTRATION
Vasodilators	Nifedipine	30 to 89 mg by mouth each evening
	Amlodipine	5 to 20 mg by mouth every day
	Diltiazem	30 to 120 mg by mouth thrice daily
	Tadalafil	20 mg by mouth every day
	Sildenafil	20 mg by mouth thrice daily
	L-Arginine	2 to 8 g by mouth every day
Inhibitors of vasoconstriction	Losartan	25 to 100 mg by mouth every day
	Enalapril	5 to 20 mg by mouth twice daily
	Quinapril	20 to 80 mg by mouth every day
	Fluoxetine	20 to 40 mg by mouth every day
	Bosentan	62.5 mg by mouth twice daily × 2 weeks, then increase to 125 mg by mouth twice daily
	Prazosin	1 to 5 mg by mouth twice daily
Other medications	Aspirin	150 to 325 mg by mouth every day
	Pentoxifylline	400 to 800 mg by mouth thrice daily
Infusions[a]	Sodium nitroprusside	0.3 to 10 mcg/kg/min
	Iloprost	0.5 to 2 ng/kg/min
	Alprostadil	6 to 10 ng/kg/min

[a]Typically reserved for Raynaud crisis.

More recently, the phosphodiesterase (PDE) inhibitors have emerged as a promising class of medications for managing patients with CCB-refractory RP. These vasodilators exert their biologic effects by enhancing nitric oxide signaling via inhibition of cyclic guanosine monophosphate degradation, resulting in improved tissue perfusion. In a double-blind, randomized, placebo-controlled trial examining the effect of the PDE inhibitor tadalafil in individuals with CCB-refractory RP, those receiving tadalafil had significant improvements in multiple outcome measures including frequency and duration of RP attacks, RCS, digital ulcer healing time, prevention of digital ulcers, physician and patient global assessments, health assessment questionnaire disability and pain scales, and several quality-of-life domains at the end of a 6-week period.[97] Similar results have been published for sildenafil, a shorter-acting PDE inhibitor, with a comparable safety and tolerability profile.[98] PDE inhibitors are usually well tolerated, but occasional side effects include headache, dyspepsia, dizziness, and, rarely, visual disturbances. Interestingly, not every placebo-controlled trial evaluating the utility of PDE inhibitors for secondary RP has demonstrated benefit.[99,100] The issue of reproducibility among these null trials has been ascribed to insufficient powering, as many trials used small sample sizes and each showed trends favoring PDE inhibitor over placebo. A recent metaanalysis examining the data across all studies has substantiated the efficacy of PDE inhibitors for treating secondary RP.[101] In the authors' experience, the addition of sildenafil to a CCB-based therapeutic regimen has typically resulted in disease improvement, including the amelioration of digital ulcers.

Prostaglandins and their analogs possess potent vasodilatory properties and have been used successfully to treat both primary and SSc-associated RP. As of this writing, iloprost, a chemically stable synthetic prostacyclin analog that dilates the peripheral vasculature and inhibits platelet adhesion and aggregation, has been the most rigorously studied. Intravenous administration of iloprost attenuates the severity and number of attacks of RP and leads to more rapid digital ulcer healing time in patients with SSc-associated RP.[102,103] In some trials, the effects of iloprost were sustained and led to a decreased requirement for ongoing therapies. In fact, in a 12-month prospective, parallel-group trial assessing the outcomes of subjects with SSc-associated RP assigned to receive either iloprost infusions at 6-week intervals or conventional vasodilator therapy, individuals in the iloprost intervention arm had significant reductions in RP severity scores and required fewer ancillary therapies.[104] Additional end points of significance favoring the iloprost treatment group, while controlling for immunomodulatory therapy, included improvement in modified Rodnan skin scores and diffusion capacity for carbon monoxide, reflecting reduced cutaneous sclerosis and enhanced pulmonary function, respectively. As a result of their findings, the authors concluded that iloprost might act as a disease-modifying agent in SSc-associated RP. Owing to the expense and occasional hypersensitivity associated with intravenous administration, an oral formulation

nitric oxide in RP have led to an interest in strategies that increase tissue levels of nitric oxide as a therapeutic approach. Nitric oxide stimulates smooth muscle relaxation by increasing intracellular concentrations of cyclic guanosine monophosphate, and results in vasodilation and increased digital perfusion. Initial studies exploiting this pathway showed promise, as topical nitrates attenuated symptom severity and improved digital ulcer healing times in patients with connective tissue disease–associated RP in a randomized, placebo-controlled trial.[95] Subsequent studies have validated the efficacy of other nitric oxide substitutes such as L-arginine and sodium nitroprusside.[96] Although promising, difficulty associated with their administration (eg, sodium nitroprusside requires intravenous infusion) and the limited availability of some these agents has hindered their routine use in clinical practice.

of iloprost has been developed. A single randomized, placebo-controlled trial confirmed the efficacy of oral iloprost for RP,[105] but this finding was not replicated in a larger, multicenter study.[106] Consequently, intravenous, but not oral, iloprost is recommended for the management of refractory RP in the setting of SSc.[107]

INHIBITORS OF VASOCONSTRICTION

Angiotensin-converting enzyme inhibitors and angiotensin II receptor antagonists have been investigated for treating RP. Both act on the renin–angiotensin system and impede vasoconstriction by reducing the downstream activity of angiotensin. Despite mixed results with enalapril[108,109] and quinapril,[110] a greater treatment response using once-daily losartan was observed when compared to nifedipine in a parallel-group trial over a 12-week period in participants with both primary and secondary RP.[111] This data supports the use of direct angiotensin receptor inhibitors over indirect inhibitors (angiotensin-converting enzyme inhibitors) for managing RP, although both are effective. In select circumstances, for example, scleroderma renal crisis, angiotensin-converting enzyme inhibitors may be the preferred option.

Several studies have implicated serotonin as an important mediator in the development of RP.[112,113] An in vivo human experiment infusing serotonin into the brachial artery reproduced the characteristic color changes seen in RP, confirming that serotonin is a potent vasoconstrictor in the peripheral circulation under physiologic circumstances.[114] In the periphery, selective serotonin reuptake inhibitors (SSRIs) block serotonin uptake by platelets, which decreases arterial vasoconstriction. Centrally, serotonin acts as a vasodilator, and by increasing the availability of serotonin in the CNS, SSRIs facilitate centrally mediated peripheral vasodilation. The results of 1 randomized, controlled trial demonstrated that the SSRI fluoxetine was more efficacious than nifedipine in terminating attacks and decreasing the severity of RP over a 6-week period.[115] SSRIs may, therefore, represent a rational choice in patients who have not adequately responded to CCBs. Given their anxiolytic properties, SSRIs may be especially desirable in patients with anxiety and RP triggered by emotional stimuli.

As previously mentioned, endothelin-1 contributes to the pathogenesis of RP by inducing vasoconstriction. Bosentan, an oral endothelin receptor antagonist, has demonstrated efficacy for treating SSc-associated RP.[55] Apart from improving symptoms of RP, bosentan decreased ulcer healing time and prevented the formation of new ulcers in 2 similar cohorts of patients with SSc-associated digital ulcers.[116,117] Dose-dependent elevation of hepatic transaminases is seen during treatment with bosentan in up to 10% of individuals, and rare occurrences of cirrhosis and fulminant liver failure have been reported with its use. Although prescribers should exercise caution prior to choosing this agent, in carefully selected circumstances, bosentan may prove to be an indispensable option, particularly in the setting of refractory digital ulcers.

α-Adrenergic blockers, in particular the α_1-adrenoceptor inhibitor prazosin, can also effectively treat RP. In a Cochrane database review, investigators found high-quality evidence from 2 randomized, controlled trials that demonstrated a beneficial effect of prazosin over placebo in patients with SSc-associated RP.[118] Side effects, including postural hypotension, drowsiness, and fatigue, were common among treatment participants, but were mild overall and could be avoided by nighttime administration.[119] A recent Phase II, randomized, placebo-controlled trial investigating the effect of a novel, high-potency α_2-adrenoceptor antagonist in subjects with SSc-associated RP showed no benefit over placebo in terms of recovery from a cold challenge test.[120] For unclear reasons, it appears that selective blockade of α_1-adrenergic but not α_2-adrenergic receptors is an effective treatment strategy for RP.

Recent advancements in our understanding of cold-induced vasoconstriction have identified the Rho family of kinases as putative targets for RP. Cold exposure initiates a cascade of events involving the activation of the sympathetic nervous system and release of norepinephrine, ultimately resulting in cutaneous vasoconstriction. Norepinephrine stimulates vascular smooth muscle cells to contract, and this latter process is controlled in part by activation of the Rho kinase pathway.[121] Rho kinases play a central role in regulating actin-dependent and myosin-dependent vasoconstriction,[122] which created interest in exploiting this pathway as a mechanism-based approach to treating RP. Unfortunately, results from a randomized, placebo-controlled trial using the Rho kinase inhibitor fasudil failed to show benefit in terms of skin temperature recovery time and digital blood flow following a cold challenge in individuals with SSc-associated RP.[123] The trial's investigators attributed the study design and selection of participants with advanced disease as possible explanations for its failure. Future studies will seek to address whether Rho kinase inhibition is relevant for treating RP.

OTHER MEDICATIONS

Aspirin and other antiplatelet therapies are routinely used in RP, despite a paucity of data to support their use. These agents likely exert benefit by reducing local thrombosis and platelet-mediated vasoconstriction, the latter of which results from the release of vasoactive mediators by platelets. Occasionally, aspirin therapy can worsen RP. This phenomenon may be explained by its effect on reducing the production of vasodilatory prostaglandins.[46]

Agents that alter blood viscosity and the hemorrheologic dynamics of red cells, such as pentoxifylline, also have been used to treat RP.[124,125] These are preferable in select settings, such as in cases of cryoprecipitable disorders or Waldenström macroglobulinemia in which vascular sludging contributes to the development of RP, or in individuals with a baseline low blood pressure who are intolerant of CCBs. Pentoxifylline also can be added to an existing drug regimen to enhance therapeutic efficacy.

Anticoagulants and thrombolytic agents are most useful when treating RP secondary to an embolus or vasoocclusive event. In Raynaud crisis, heparin may be indicated during the acute phase of ischemia to prevent irreversible tissue injury. A pilot study showed benefit from adding low-molecular-weight heparin to a conventional RP treatment protocol in a cohort of patients with primary and secondary RP, the effect of which was maximal by 20 weeks of daily use.[126] When considering heparin for RP, the risk of serious bleeding must be balanced against any potential benefit it may confer. Anticoagulation with warfarin is not routinely recommended to treat RP. Notable exceptions include cases in which a thrombotic diathesis exists, or in cases of SSc in which warfarin is specifically selected to treat associated calcinosis cutis.[127]

As oxidative stress likely contributes to RP, there is ongoing interest in using antioxidants to placate the symptoms and sequelae of the disorder. Intravenous N-acetylcysteine significantly reduced the frequency and severity of RP attacks as well as the number of digital ulcers in a cohort of 20 patients with SSc.[128] The therapy was well tolerated, and no substantial side effects were observed. Other studies have also supported the role of antioxidant therapy for RP.[129] The benefits of antioxidants are potentially greatest when used early in the course of disease.[46]

Several complementary and alternative medicines have been used for RP with no demonstrable benefit as of this writing.[130]

PROCEDURAL INTERVENTIONS

BOTULINUM NEUROTOXIN

Interest in botulinum neurotoxin (BoNT) as a treatment of RP emerged after a series of ex vivo experiments demonstrated a blunting effect on arterial contraction following incubation with modest concentrations of BoNT.[131] A seminal clinical report followed, in which 2 patients with severe, multidrug-resistant RP were given local injections of BoNT and subsequently experienced substantial improvements in both patient-reported disease activity and digital perfusion, as measured by laser Doppler interferometry.[132] A larger, prospective study comprised of 11 patients with pharmacologically refractory RP secondary to connective tissue disease supported these findings.[133] According to the study results, after digital injections with BoNT, each subject achieved clinically meaningful improvement in RP-associated pain, 9 of the 11 reported decreased severity and frequency of vasospastic episodes, and previously nonhealing ulcers spontaneously healed following therapy in 9 subjects. Benefit was observed as early as 24 hours after injection, and all subjects experienced pain relief within 48 hours. Numerous subsequent studies, including 1 placebo-controlled trial, have further validated BoNT as an effective option for RP, particularly in the setting of multiple medication failures.[134,135] Complications related to BoNT injections include dysesthesia and transient hand weakness, but the rate is acceptably low. The effect of BoNT usually lasts for months, but some reports have indicated ongoing benefit for up to a year.

Mechanistically, BoNT decreases muscle tone by preventing the presynaptic release of acetylcholine at the neuromuscular endplate. This results in paralysis of both striated and smooth muscle, including the musculature encasing blood vessels.[136] Chemodenervation with BoNT therefore enhances digital perfusion via toxin-mediated vasodilation. In addition to its direct effect on muscle, BoNT blocks the recruitment of α_2-adrenoceptors and decreases C-fiber nociceptor density, which raises the threshold of smooth muscle reactivity to cold stimuli and attenuates pain, respectively.[131,137]

A standardized technique for injecting BoNT has been reported and is easy to perform because it uses reliable anatomic landmarks.[138] At the metacarpophalangeal flexion crease, 5 to 10 units of onabotulinumtoxinA (BoNT type A) are injected while aiming proximally toward the neurovascular plexus. Approximately 40 to 100 units of onabotulinumtoxinA are used per hand, and in most instances, injection of the thumb is unnecessary. In some highly responsive individuals, pain relief is felt almost instantaneously. Use of a topical anesthetic under occlusion prior to injections makes the procedure more tolerable.

In the authors' experience, use of BoNT as an adjunctive therapy for RP has resulted in notable improvements in patient and physician global assessments, particularly among those who have failed multiple medical interventions.

SYMPATHECTOMY

In rare instances, aggressive medical therapies are insufficient to adequately control RP. In such scenarios, surgical intervention may be warranted. The most commonly performed surgery is a sympathectomy, which serves to permanently sever vasoconstrictive signals from the sympathetic nervous system innervating the hands. As of this writing, 2 techniques, either a thoracocervical or a digital approach, are used and appear to be comparable in terms of benefit.

Thoracocervical sympathectomy is the traditional approach for RP and can be performed in either an open fashion or using an endoscopic technique. The goal of the procedure is to transect postganglionic fibers that exit via the thoracic sympathetic chain and fuse with the cervical stellate ganglion to innervate the hand. Outcomes data are mixed. Although early reports documented poor long-term outcomes with high rates of symptom recurrence and postoperative complications,[139] advances in surgical techniques have yielded better results. A review collating the most recent outcomes data indicated that short-term improvement after thoracic sympathectomy was achieved in 92% and 89% of patients with primary and secondary RP, respectively.[140] Healing of refractory digital ulcers following the procedure was also high, with 98% of patients deriving benefit, the majority of which had complete resolution. Data from the same review showed that long-term improvement (on the order of years) was higher among patients with secondary RP (89%) compared to those with primary RP (58%). While promising, complications related to thoracic sympathectomy are not uncommon and can include the development of hyperhidrosis, Horner syndrome, and persistent neuropathic pain.[139] If the procedure proves unsuccessful, the recurrence of symptoms generally occurs after 6 months.

Localized digital sympathectomy is an alternative procedure that appears to have comparable efficacy to the thoracocervical approach. The operation involves careful stripping of the adventitia containing the autonomic nerve plexus from the palmar arterial arch, common digital arteries, and/or proper digital arteries.[141,142] As a result of the meticulous nature of the procedure, its availability is limited to specialized centers. Serious complications are very infrequent. Postoperative pain and scar formation constitute the major cause for procedure-related morbidity. A novel 2-step incision technique for performing digital artery sympathectomy for RP has been published, with similar results in terms of symptom improvement and lower rates of scar formation, faster postoperative recovery time, and better aesthetic outcomes.[143]

SURGICAL DEBRIDEMENT AND AMPUTATION

Surgical debridement may be needed for chronic, nonhealing ulcers and if devitalized necrotic tissue develops. If gangrene supervenes, amputation may be required. Osteomyelitis developing in the context of a digital ulcer may also mandate partial digit amputation.

VASCULAR RECONSTRUCTION

Surgical reconstruction of the digital arteries is rarely indicated for RP. It may provide relief of symptoms and improve digital perfusion if proximal artery occlusion develops, which is most often seen in the setting of severe SSc, advanced atherosclerosis, or chronic thromboembolic disease.[144]

SPECIAL CONSIDERATIONS

ULCER CARE

Digital ulcers from RP can be extremely painful and often take weeks or months to heal. Pain control is important because pain may lead to vasospasm and provoke additional bouts of ischemia. In some instances, opioids are needed to control symptoms.

Digits with ulcers should be soaked in a tepid antiseptic solution twice daily to soften or loosen crusts or eschars. After drying, plain petrolatum is applied to the ulcer, and the digit is covered with an occlusive dressing. Maximum tolerated pharmacologic therapies should be employed throughout treatment of an ulcer to promote wound healing by improving blood flow to the area. Importantly, local wound care alone without pharmacologic intervention to improve digital blood flow is unlikely to result in ulcer resolution.

Infection is a common complication of digital ulcers and typically manifests with increasing pain, erythema, swelling, or purulent drainage. Cultures usually demonstrate *Staphylococcus* species, and treatment with cephalosporins, or in the case of methicillin-resistant *Staphylococcus aureus*, trimethoprim-sulfamethoxazole, clindamycin, or a tetracycline, are usually effective. Antimicrobial therapy should be directed by the local antibiogram when available.

CRITICAL ISCHEMIA

Raynaud crisis is typified by critical ischemia and always requires urgent intervention. The guiding principle for managing Raynaud crisis is early diagnosis and intervention to preempt irreversible tissue injury. Patients with critical ischemia require hospitalization and intravenous prostaglandin therapy.[2,145] Iloprost dosed 0.5 to 2 ng/kg by continuous infusion should be given over several hours on 3 consecutive days. Intraarterial phentolamine also has been successfully used in cases of Raynaud crisis, but its administration requires monitoring in an acute care setting given the risk for hemodynamic instability. Analgesics and antibiotics are often coadministered when digital ulcers are present. Skilled nursing and podiatry care (for toe involvement) is an important element of ulcer care, and wound assessments should be performed at routine intervals. It is essential to exclude competing diagnoses when evaluating the patient with critical ischemia. Medium-vessel vasculitis, thromboembolism, and severe atherosclerotic disease may mimic Raynaud crisis, but their management differs substantially. Anticoagulation therapy with heparin may be considered if signs of tissue ischemia continue despite aggressive medical therapy. A digital block with lidocaine or bupivacaine can provide pain relief and serves as a chemical sympathectomy to reverse vasoconstriction. Surgical interventions may be considered as a salvage effort in unresponsive patients.

TREATMENT ALGORITHM

Figure 145-4 outlines a treatment algorithm for managing the patient with RP.

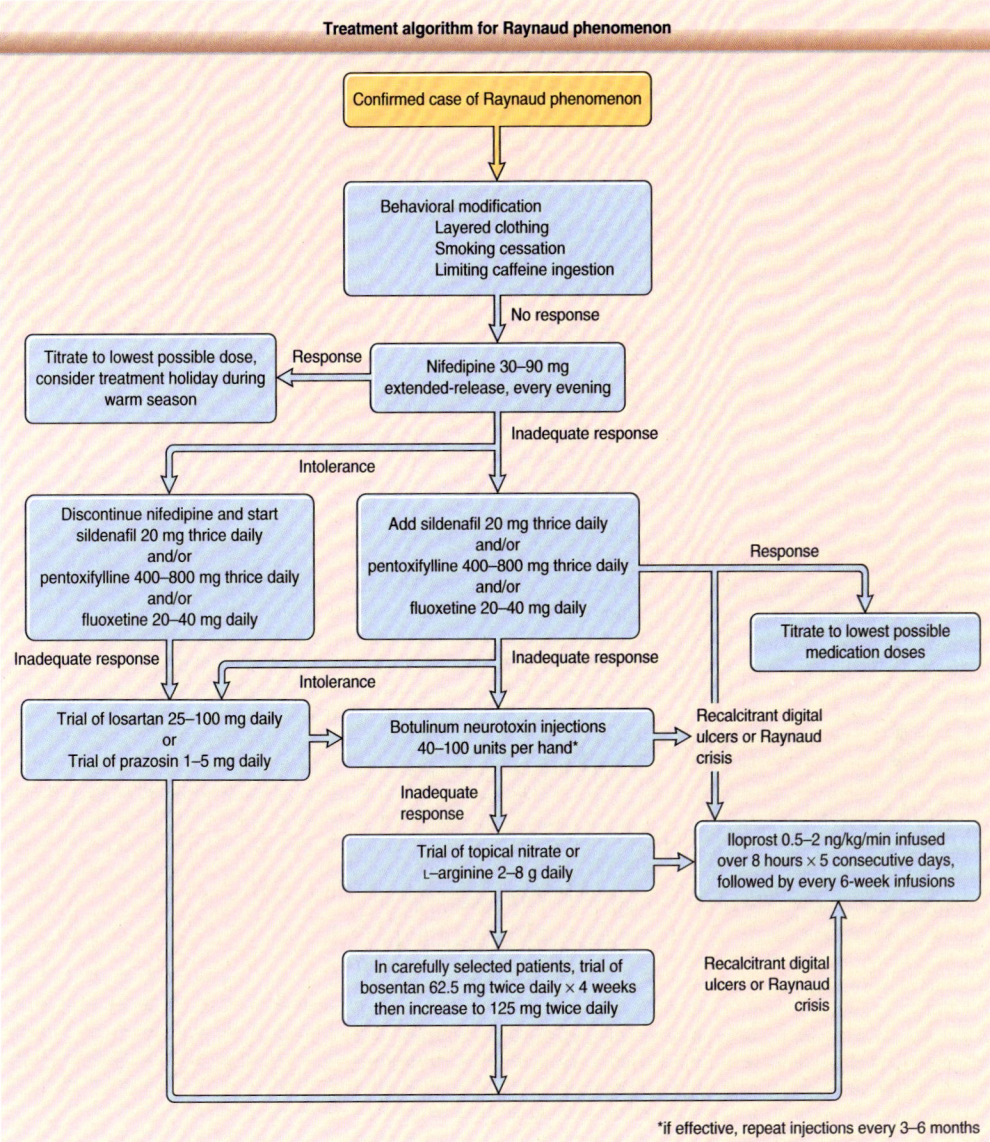

Figure 145-4 Treatment algorithm for Raynaud phenomenon.

REFERENCES

1. Block JA, Sequeira W. Raynaud's phenomenon. *Lancet.* 2001;357(9273):2042-2048.
2. Herrick AL. The pathogenesis, diagnosis and treatment of Raynaud phenomenon. *Nat Rev Rheumatol.* 2012;8(8):469-479.
3. Brand FN, Larson MG, Kannel WB, et al. The occurrence of Raynaud's phenomenon in a general population: the Framingham Study. *Vasc Med.* 1997;2(4):296-301.
4. Gelber AC, Wigley FM, Stallings RY, et al. Symptoms of Raynaud's phenomenon in an inner-city African-American community: prevalence and self-reported cardiovascular comorbidity. *J Clin Epidemiol.* 1999;52(5):441-446.
5. Medsger TA Jr. Natural history of systemic sclerosis and the assessment of disease activity, severity, functional status, and psychologic well-being. *Rheum Dis Clin North Am.* 2003;29(2):255-273, vi.
6. Hirschl M, Kundi M. Initial prevalence and incidence of secondary Raynaud's phenomenon in patients with Raynaud's symptomatology. *J Rheumatol.* 1996;23(2):302-309.
7. Riera G, Vilardell M, Vaque J, et al. Prevalence of Raynaud's phenomenon in a healthy Spanish population. *J Rheumatol.* 1993;20(1):66-69.
8. Greenstein D, Jeffcote N, Ilsley D, et al. The menstrual cycle and Raynaud's phenomenon. *Angiology.* 1996;47(5):427-436.
9. Gardner-Medwin JM, Macdonald IA, Taylor JY, et al. Seasonal differences in finger skin temperature and microvascular blood flow in healthy men and women

are exaggerated in women with primary Raynaud's phenomenon. *Br J Clin Pharmacol.* 2001;52(1):17-23.
10. Fraenkel L, Zhang Y, Chaisson CE, et al. Different factors influencing the expression of Raynaud's phenomenon in men and women. *Arthritis Rheum.* 1999;42(2):306-310.
11. Freedman RR, Mayes MD. Familial aggregation of primary Raynaud's disease. *Arthritis Rheum.* 1996; 39(7):1189-1191.
12. Koenig M, Joyal F, Fritzler MJ, et al. Autoantibodies and microvascular damage are independent predictive factors for the progression of Raynaud's phenomenon to systemic sclerosis: a twenty-year prospective study of 586 patients, with validation of proposed criteria for early systemic sclerosis. *Arthritis Rheum.* 2008;58(12):3902-3912.
13. Spencer-Green G. Outcomes in primary Raynaud phenomenon: a meta-analysis of the frequency, rates, and predictors of transition to secondary diseases. *Arch Intern Med.* 1998;158(6):595-600.
14. Hirschl M, Hirschl K, Lenz M, et al. Transition from primary Raynaud's phenomenon to secondary Raynaud's phenomenon identified by diagnosis of an associated disease: results of ten years of prospective surveillance. *Arthritis Rheum.* 2006;54(6):1974-1981.
15. Hartmann P, Mohokum M, Schlattmann P. The association of Raynaud's syndrome with rheumatoid arthritis—a meta-analysis. *Clin Rheumatol.* 2011; 30(8):1013-1019.
16. Herrick A, el-Hadidy K, Marsh D, et al. Abnormal thermoregulatory responses in patients with reflex sympathetic dystrophy syndrome. *J Rheumatol.* 1994; 21(7):1319-1324.
17. Chung MS, Gong HS, Baek GH. Prevalence of Raynaud's phenomenon in patients with idiopathic carpal tunnel syndrome. *J Bone Joint Surg Br.* 1999;81(6): 1017-1019.
18. Hartmann P, Mohokum M, Schlattmann P. The association of Raynaud's syndrome with carpal tunnel syndrome: a meta-analysis. *Rheumatol Int.* 2012;32(3):569-574.
19. Grassi W, De Angelis R, Lapadula G, et al. Clinical diagnosis found in patients with Raynaud's phenomenon: a multicentre study. *Rheumatol Int.* 1998;18(1):17-20.
20. Pistorius MA, Planchon B. Incidence of thoracic outlet syndrome on the epidemiology and clinical presentation of apparently primary Raynaud's phenomenon. A prospective study in 570 patients. *Int Angiol.* 1995;14(1):60-64.
21. Palmer KT, Griffin MJ, Syddall H, et al. Prevalence of Raynaud's phenomenon in Great Britain and its relation to hand transmitted vibration: a national postal survey. *Occup Environ Med.* 2000;57(7):448-452.
22. Laplanche A, Clavel F, Contassot JC, et al. Exposure to vinyl chloride monomer: report on a cohort study. *Br J Ind Med.* 1987;44(10):711-715.
23. Khouri C, Blaise S, Carpentier P, et al. Drug-induced Raynaud's phenomenon: beyond beta-blockers. *Br J Clin Pharmacol.* 2016;82(1):6-16.
24. Mohokum M, Hartmann P, Schlattmann P. The association of Raynaud syndrome with beta-blockers: a meta-analysis. *Angiology.* 2012;63(7):535-540.
25. Khouri C, Jouve T, Blaise S, et al. Peripheral vasoconstriction induced by beta-blockers: a systematic review and a network meta-analysis. *Br J Clin Pharmacol.* 2016;82(2):549-560.
26. Flavahan NA. A vascular mechanistic approach to understanding Raynaud phenomenon. *Nat Rev Rheumatol.* 2015;11(3):146-158.
27. Robb LG. Severe vasospasm following ergot administration. *West J Med.* 1975;123(3):231-235.
28. Duvoisin RC. Digital vasospasm with bromocriptine. *Lancet.* 1976;2(7978):204.
29. Rudnick A, Modai I, Zelikovski A. Fluoxetine-induced Raynaud's phenomenon. *Biol Psychiatry.* 1997;41(12): 1218-1221.
30. Bell C, Coupland N, Creamer P. Digital infarction in a patient with Raynaud's phenomenon associated with treatment with a specific serotonin reuptake inhibitor. A case report. *Angiology.* 1996;47(9):901-903.
31. Peiro AM, Margarit C, Torra M. Citalopram-induced Raynaud's phenomenon. *Rheumatol Int.* 2007;27(6): 599-601.
32. Goldman W, Seltzer R, Reuman P. Association between treatment with central nervous system stimulants and Raynaud's syndrome in children: a retrospective case-control study of rheumatology patients. *Arthritis Rheum.* 2008;58(2):563-566.
33. Deray G, Le Hoang P, Achour L, et al. Cyclosporin and Raynaud phenomenon. *Lancet.* 1986;2(8515): 1092-1093.
34. Arinsoy T, Derici U, Yuksel A, et al. Cyclosporine—a treatment and a rare complication: Raynaud's phenomenon. *Int J Clin Pract.* 2005;59(7):863-864.
35. Balbir-Gurman A, Braun-Moscovici Y, Nahir AM. Cocaine-Induced Raynaud's phenomenon and ischaemic finger necrosis. *Clin Rheumatol.* 2001;20(5): 376-378.
36. Berger CC, Bokemeyer C, Schneider M, et al. Secondary Raynaud's phenomenon and other late vascular complications following chemotherapy for testicular cancer. *Eur J Cancer.* 1995;31A(13-14): 2229-2238.
37. Glendenning JL, Barbachano Y, Norman AR, et al. Long-term neurologic and peripheral vascular toxicity after chemotherapy treatment of testicular cancer. *Cancer.* 2010;116(10):2322-2331.
38. Fossa SD, Lehne G, Heimdal K, et al. Clinical and biochemical long-term toxicity after postoperative cisplatin-based chemotherapy in patients with low-stage testicular cancer. *Oncology.* 1995;52(4):300-305.
39. Brydoy M, Oldenburg J, Klepp O, et al. Observational study of prevalence of long-term Raynaud-like phenomena and neurological side effects in testicular cancer survivors. *J Natl Cancer Inst.* 2009;101(24): 1682-1695.
40. Epstein E. Intralesional bleomycin and Raynaud's phenomenon. *J Am Acad Dermatol.* 1991;24(5, pt 1): 785-786.
41. Mohokum M, Hartmann P, Schlattmann P. Association of Raynaud's syndrome with interferons. A meta-analysis. *Int Angiol.* 2012;31(5):408-413.
42. Schapira D, Nahir AM, Hadad N. Interferon-induced Raynaud's syndrome. *Semin Arthritis Rheum.* 2002; 32(3):157-162.
43. Zeidman A, Dicker D, Mittelman M. Interferon-induced vasospasm in chronic myeloid leukaemia. *Acta Haematol.* 1998;100(2):94-96.
44. Roy V, Newland AC. Raynaud's phenomenon and cryoglobulinaemia associated with the use of recombinant human alpha-interferon. *Lancet.* 1988; 1(8591):944-945.
45. Rot U, Ledinek AH. Interferons beta have vasoconstrictive and procoagulant effects: a woman who developed livedo reticularis and Raynaud phenomenon in association with interferon beta

treatment for multiple sclerosis. *Clin Neurol Neurosurg.* 2013;115(suppl 1):S79-S81.
46. Bakst R, Merola JF, Franks AG Jr, et al. Raynaud's phenomenon: pathogenesis and management. *J Am Acad Dermatol.* 2008;59(4):633-653.
47. Bedarida G, Kim D, Blaschke TF, et al. Venodilation in Raynaud's disease. *Lancet.* 1993;342(8885):1451-1454.
48. Herrick AL. Pathogenesis of Raynaud's phenomenon. *Rheumatology (Oxford).* 2005;44(5):587-596.
49. Anderson ME, Moore TL, Hollis S, et al. Endothelial-dependent vasodilation is impaired in patients with systemic sclerosis, as assessed by low dose iontophoresis. *Clin Exp Rheumatol.* 2003;21(3):403.
50. Gunawardena H, Harris ND, Carmichael C, et al. Maximum blood flow and microvascular regulatory responses in systemic sclerosis. *Rheumatology (Oxford).* 2007;46(7):1079-1082.
51. Rajagopalan S, Pfenninger D, Kehrer C, et al. Increased asymmetric dimethylarginine and endothelin 1 levels in secondary Raynaud's phenomenon: implications for vascular dysfunction and progression of disease. *Arthritis Rheum.* 2003;48(7):1992-2000.
52. Zamora MR, O'Brien RF, Rutherford RB, et al. Serum endothelin-1 concentrations and cold provocation in primary Raynaud's phenomenon. *Lancet.* 1990;336(8724):1144-1147.
53. Duprez DA. Role of the renin-angiotensin-aldosterone system in vascular remodeling and inflammation: a clinical review. *J Hypertens.* 2006;24(6):983-991.
54. Vancheeswaran R, Azam A, Black C, et al. Localization of endothelin-1 and its binding sites in scleroderma skin. *J Rheumatol.* 1994;21(7):1268-1276.
55. Ramos-Casals M, Brito-Zeron P, Nardi N, et al. Successful treatment of severe Raynaud's phenomenon with bosentan in four patients with systemic sclerosis. *Rheumatology (Oxford).* 2004;43(11):1454-1456.
56. Bukhari M, Herrick AL, Moore T, et al. Increased nail-fold capillary dimensions in primary Raynaud's phenomenon and systemic sclerosis. *Br J Rheumatol.* 1996;35(11):1127-1131.
57. Bunker CB, Terenghi G, Springall DR, et al. Deficiency of calcitonin gene-related peptide in Raynaud's phenomenon. *Lancet.* 1990;336(8730):1530-1533.
58. Coffman JD, Cohen RA. Role of alpha-adrenoceptor subtypes mediating sympathetic vasoconstriction in human digits. *Eur J Clin Invest.* 1988;18(3):309-313.
59. Flavahan NA, Cooke JP, Shepherd JT, et al. Human postjunctional alpha-1 and alpha-2 adrenoceptors: differential distribution in arteries of the limbs. *J Pharmacol Exp Ther.* 1987;241(2):361-365.
60. Edwards CM, Marshall JM, Pugh M. Lack of habituation of the pattern of cardiovascular response evoked by sound in subjects with primary Raynaud's disease. *Clin Sci (Lond).* 1998;95(3):249-260.
61. Edwards CM, Marshall JM, Pugh M. The cutaneous vasoconstrictor response to venous stasis is normal in subjects with primary Raynaud's disease. *Clin Auton Res.* 1999;9(5):255-262.
62. Pamuk GE, Turgut B, Pamuk ON, et al. Increased circulating platelet-leucocyte complexes in patients with primary Raynaud's phenomenon and Raynaud's phenomenon secondary to systemic sclerosis: a comparative study. *Blood Coagul Fibrinolysis.* 2007; 18(4):297-302.
63. Susol E, MacGregor AJ, Barrett JH, et al. A two-stage, genome-wide screen for susceptibility loci in primary Raynaud's phenomenon. *Arthritis Rheum.* 2000;43(7):1641-1646.
64. Allen EV, Brown GE. Raynaud's disease: a clinical study of one hundred and forty-seven cases. *JAMA.* 1932;99(18):1472-1478.
65. LeRoy EC, Medsger TA Jr. Raynaud's phenomenon: a proposal for classification. *Clin Exp Rheumatol.* 1992;10(5):485-488.
66. Brennan P, Silman A, Black C, et al. Validity and reliability of three methods used in the diagnosis of Raynaud's phenomenon. The UK Scleroderma Study Group. *Br J Rheumatol.* 1993;32(5):357-361.
67. Maverakis E, Patel F, Kronenberg DG, et al. International consensus criteria for the diagnosis of Raynaud's phenomenon. *J Autoimmun.* 2014;48-49:60-65.
68. Wigley FM. Clinical practice. Raynaud's phenomenon. *N Engl J Med.* 2002;347(13):1001-1008.
69. Pavlov-Dolijanovic S, Damjanov NS, Vujasinovic Stupar NZ, et al. Late appearance and exacerbation of primary Raynaud's phenomenon attacks can predict future development of connective tissue disease: a retrospective chart review of 3,035 patients. *Rheumatol Int.* 2013;33(4):921-926.
70. Ingegnoli F, Boracchi P, Gualtierotti R, et al. Improving outcome prediction of systemic sclerosis from isolated Raynaud's phenomenon: role of autoantibodies and nail-fold capillaroscopy. *Rheumatology (Oxford).* 2010;49(4):797-805.
71. Kallenberg CG, Wouda AA, Hoet MH, et al. Development of connective tissue disease in patients presenting with Raynaud's phenomenon: a six year follow up with emphasis on the predictive value of antinuclear antibodies as detected by immunoblotting. *Ann Rheum Dis.* 1988;47(8):634-641.
72. Wollersheim H, Thien T, Hoet MH, et al. The diagnostic value of several immunological tests for antinuclear antibody in predicting the development of connective tissue disease in patients presenting with Raynaud's phenomenon. *Eur J Clin Invest.* 1989;19(6):535-541.
73. Maricq HR, LeRoy EC. Patterns of finger capillary abnormalities in connective tissue disease by "wide-field" microscopy. *Arthritis Rheum.* 1973;16(5):619-628.
74. ter Borg EJ, Piersma-Wichers G, Smit AJ, et al. Serial nailfold capillary microscopy in primary Raynaud's phenomenon and scleroderma. *Semin Arthritis Rheum.* 1994;24(1):40-47.
75. Anderson ME, Moore TL, Lunt M, et al. The "distal-dorsal difference": a thermographic parameter by which to differentiate between primary and secondary Raynaud's phenomenon. *Rheumatology (Oxford).* 2007;46(3):533-538.
76. Murray AK, Moore TL, Manning JB, et al. Noninvasive imaging techniques in the assessment of scleroderma spectrum disorders. *Arthritis Rheum.* 2009;61(8):1103-1111.
77. Rosato E, Borghese F, Pisarri S, et al. Laser Doppler perfusion imaging is useful in the study of Raynaud's phenomenon and improves the capillaroscopic diagnosis. *J Rheumatol.* 2009;36(10):2257-2263.
78. Herrick AL, Clark S. Quantifying digital vascular disease in patients with primary Raynaud's phenomenon and systemic sclerosis. *Ann Rheum Dis.* 1998;57(2):70-78.
79. Das S, Maiti A. Acrocyanosis: an overview. *Indian J Dermatol.* 2013;58(6):417-420.
80. Heidrich H. Functional vascular diseases: Raynaud's syndrome, acrocyanosis and erythromelalgia. *Vasa.* 2010;39(1):33-41.

81. Kelly R, Baker C. Other vascular disorders. In: Bolognia JL, Jorizzo JL, Schaffer JV, editors. *Dermatology*. 3rd ed. Philadelphia, PA: Elsevier Saunders; 2012:1747-1756.
82. Berlin AL, Pehr K. Coexistence of erythromelalgia and Raynaud's phenomenon. *J Am Acad Dermatol*. 2004;50(3):456-460.
83. Yang Y, Wang Y, Li S, et al. Mutations in SCN9A, encoding a sodium channel alpha subunit, in patients with primary erythermalgia. *J Med Genet*. 2004;41(3):171-174.
84. Gibbs MB, English JC 3rd, Zirwas MJ. Livedo reticularis: an update. *J Am Acad Dermatol*. 2005;52(6):1009-1019.
85. Phelps GR, Wilentz S. Reflex sympathetic dystrophy. *Int J Dermatol*. 2000;39(7):481-486.
86. Youssef P, Englert H, Bertouch J. Large vessel occlusive disease associated with CREST syndrome and scleroderma. *Ann Rheum Dis*. 1993;52(6):464-466.
87. Merkel PA, Herlyn K, Martin RW, et al. Measuring disease activity and functional status in patients with scleroderma and Raynaud's phenomenon. *Arthritis Rheum*. 2002;46(9):2410-2420.
88. Khanna PP, Maranian P, Gregory J, et al. The minimally important difference and patient acceptable symptom state for the Raynaud's condition score in patients with Raynaud's phenomenon in a large randomised controlled clinical trial. *Ann Rheum Dis*. 2010;69(3):588-591.
89. Thompson AE, Pope JE. Calcium channel blockers for primary Raynaud's phenomenon: a meta-analysis. *Rheumatology (Oxford)*. 2005;44(2):145-150.
90. Thompson AE, Shea B, Welch V, et al. Calcium-channel blockers for Raynaud's phenomenon in systemic sclerosis. *Arthritis Rheum*. 2001;44(8):1841-1847.
91. Ennis H, Hughes M, Anderson ME, et al. Calcium channel blockers for primary Raynaud's phenomenon. *Cochrane Database Syst Rev*. 2016;2:CD002069.
92. Rhedda A, McCans J, Willan AR, et al. A double blind placebo controlled crossover randomized trial of diltiazem in Raynaud's phenomenon. *J Rheumatol*. 1985;12(4):724-727.
93. Comparison of sustained-release nifedipine and temperature biofeedback for treatment of primary Raynaud phenomenon. Results from a randomized clinical trial with 1-year follow-up. *Arch Intern Med*. 2000;160(8):1101-1108.
94. Kahan A, Bour B, Couturier D, et al. Nifedipine and esophageal dysfunction in progressive systemic sclerosis. A controlled manometric study. *Arthritis Rheum*. 1985;28(5):490-495.
95. Franks AG Jr. Topical glyceryl trinitrate as adjunctive treatment in Raynaud's disease. *Lancet*. 1982;1(8263):76-77.
96. Freedman RR, Girgis R, Mayes MD. Acute effect of nitric oxide on Raynaud's phenomenon in scleroderma. *Lancet*. 1999;354(9180):739.
97. Shenoy PD, Kumar S, Jha LK, et al. Efficacy of tadalafil in secondary Raynaud's phenomenon resistant to vasodilator therapy: a double-blind randomized cross-over trial. *Rheumatology (Oxford)*. 2010;49(12):2420-2428.
98. Fries R, Shariat K, von Wilmowsky H, et al. Sildenafil in the treatment of Raynaud's phenomenon resistant to vasodilatory therapy. *Circulation*. 2005;112(19):2980-2985.
99. Herrick AL, van den Hoogen F, Gabrielli A, et al. Modified-release sildenafil reduces Raynaud's phenomenon attack frequency in limited cutaneous systemic sclerosis. *Arthritis Rheum*. 2011;63(3):775-782.
100. Schiopu E, Hsu VM, Impens AJ, et al. Randomized placebo-controlled crossover trial of tadalafil in Raynaud's phenomenon secondary to systemic sclerosis. *J Rheumatol*. 2009;36(10):2264-2268.
101. Roustit M, Blaise S, Allanore Y, et al. Phosphodiesterase-5 inhibitors for the treatment of secondary Raynaud's phenomenon: systematic review and meta-analysis of randomised trials. *Ann Rheum Dis*. 2013;72(10):1696-1699.
102. Wigley FM, Seibold JR, Wise RA, et al. Intravenous iloprost treatment of Raynaud's phenomenon and ischemic ulcers secondary to systemic sclerosis. *J Rheumatol*. 1992;19(9):1407-1414.
103. Wigley FM, Wise RA, Seibold JR, et al. Intravenous iloprost infusion in patients with Raynaud phenomenon secondary to systemic sclerosis. A multicenter, placebo-controlled, double-blind study. *Ann Intern Med*. 1994;120(3):199-206.
104. Scorza R, Caronni M, Mascagni B, et al. Effects of long-term cyclic iloprost therapy in systemic sclerosis with Raynaud's phenomenon. A randomized, controlled study. *Clin Exp Rheumatol*. 2001;19(5):503-508.
105. Black CM, Halkier-Sorensen L, Belch JJ, et al. Oral iloprost in Raynaud's phenomenon secondary to systemic sclerosis: a multicentre, placebo-controlled, dose-comparison study. *Br J Rheumatol*. 1998;37(9):952-960.
106. Wigley FM, Korn JH, Csuka ME, et al. Oral iloprost treatment in patients with Raynaud's phenomenon secondary to systemic sclerosis: a multicenter, placebo-controlled, double-blind study. *Arthritis Rheum*. 1998;41(4):670-677.
107. Pope J, Fenlon D, Thompson A, et al. Iloprost and cisaprost for Raynaud's phenomenon in progressive systemic sclerosis. *Cochrane Database Syst Rev*. 2000(2):CD000953.
108. Challenor VF, Waller DG, Hayward RA, et al. Subjective and objective assessment of enalapril in primary Raynaud's phenomenon. *Br J Clin Pharmacol*. 1991;31(4):477-480.
109. Janini SD, Scott DG, Coppock JS, et al. Enalapril in Raynaud's phenomenon. *J Clin Pharm Ther*. 1988;13(2):145-150.
110. Gliddon AE, Dore CJ, Black CM, et al. Prevention of vascular damage in scleroderma and autoimmune Raynaud's phenomenon: a multicenter, randomized, double-blind, placebo-controlled trial of the angiotensin-converting enzyme inhibitor quinapril. *Arthritis Rheum*. 2007;56(11):3837-3846.
111. Dziadzio M, Denton CP, Smith R, et al. Losartan therapy for Raynaud's phenomenon and scleroderma: clinical and biochemical findings in a fifteen-week, randomized, parallel-group, controlled trial. *Arthritis Rheum*. 1999;42(12):2646-2655.
112. Seibold JR. Serotonin and Raynaud's phenomenon. *J Cardiovasc Pharmacol*. 1985;7(suppl 7):S95-S98.
113. Dees C, Akhmetshina A, Zerr P, et al. Platelet-derived serotonin links vascular disease and tissue fibrosis. *J Exp Med*. 2011;208(5):961-972.
114. Halpern A, Kuhn PH, Shaftel HE, et al. Raynaud's disease, Raynaud's phenomenon, and serotonin. *Angiology*. 1960;11:151-167.
115. Coleiro B, Marshall SE, Denton CP, et al. Treatment of Raynaud's phenomenon with the selective serotonin reuptake inhibitor fluoxetine. *Rheumatology (Oxford)*. 2001;40(9):1038-1043.
116. Humbert M, Cabane J. Successful treatment of systemic sclerosis digital ulcers and pulmonary arterial hypertension with endothelin receptor antag-

117. Korn JH, Mayes M, Matucci Cerinic M, et al. Digital ulcers in systemic sclerosis: prevention by treatment with bosentan, an oral endothelin receptor antagonist. *Arthritis Rheum.* 2004;50(12):3985-3993.
118. Pope J, Fenlon D, Thompson A, et al. Prazosin for Raynaud's phenomenon in progressive systemic sclerosis. *Cochrane Database Syst Rev.* 2000(2):CD000956.
119. Surwit RS, Gilgor RS, Allen LM, et al. A double-blind study of prazosin in the treatment of Raynaud's phenomenon in scleroderma. *Arch Dermatol.* 1984;120(3):329-331.
120. Herrick AL, Murray AK, Ruck A, et al. A double-blind, randomized, placebo-controlled crossover trial of the alpha2C-adrenoceptor antagonist ORM-12741 for prevention of cold-induced vasospasm in patients with systemic sclerosis. *Rheumatology (Oxford).* 2014;53(5):948-952.
121. Bailey SR, Eid AH, Mitra S, et al. Rho kinase mediates cold-induced constriction of cutaneous arteries: role of alpha2C-adrenoceptor translocation. *Circ Res.* 2004;94(10):1367-1374.
122. Flavahan NA. Regulation of vascular reactivity in scleroderma: new insights into Raynaud's phenomenon. *Rheum Dis Clin North Am.* 2008;34(1):81-87; vii.
123. Fava A, Wung PK, Wigley FM, et al. Efficacy of Rho kinase inhibitor fasudil in secondary Raynaud's phenomenon. *Arthritis Care Res (Hoboken).* 2012;64(6):925-929.
124. Neirotti M, Longo F, Molaschi M, et al. Functional vascular disorders: treatment with pentoxifylline. *Angiology.* 1987;38(8):575-580.
125. Goldberg J, Dlesk A. Successful treatment of Raynaud's phenomenon with pentoxifylline. *Arthritis Rheum.* 1986;29(8):1055-1056.
126. Denton CP, Howell K, Stratton RJ, et al. Long-term low molecular weight heparin therapy for severe Raynaud's phenomenon: a pilot study. *Clin Exp Rheumatol.* 2000;18(4):499-502.
127. Cukierman T, Elinav E, Korem M, et al. Low dose warfarin treatment for calcinosis in patients with systemic sclerosis. *Ann Rheum Dis.* 2004;63(10):1341-1343.
128. Sambo P, Amico D, Giacomelli R, et al. Intravenous N-acetylcysteine for treatment of Raynaud's phenomenon secondary to systemic sclerosis: a pilot study. *J Rheumatol.* 2001;28(10):2257-2262.
129. Denton CP, Bunce TD, Dorado MB, et al. Probucol improves symptoms and reduces lipoprotein oxidation susceptibility in patients with Raynaud's phenomenon. *Rheumatology (Oxford).* 1999;38(4):309-315.
130. Malenfant D, Catton M, Pope JE. The efficacy of complementary and alternative medicine in the treatment of Raynaud's phenomenon: a literature review and meta-analysis. *Rheumatology (Oxford).* 2009;48(7):791-795.
131. Morris JL, Jobling P, Gibbins IL. Differential inhibition by botulinum neurotoxin A of cotransmitters released from autonomic vasodilator neurons. *Am J Physiol Heart Circ Physiol.* 2001;281(5):H2124-H2132.
132. Sycha T, Graninger M, Auff E, et al. Botulinum toxin in the treatment of Raynaud's phenomenon: a pilot study. *Eur J Clin Invest.* 2004;34(4):312-313.
133. Van Beek AL, Lim PK, Gear AJ, et al. Management of vasospastic disorders with botulinum toxin A. *Plast Reconstr Surg.* 2007;119(1):217-226.
134. Iorio ML, Masden DL, Higgins JP. Botulinum toxin A treatment of Raynaud's phenomenon: a review. *Semin Arthritis Rheum.* 2012;41(4):599-603.
135. Jenkins SN, Neyman KM, Veledar E, et al. A pilot study evaluating the efficacy of botulinum toxin A in the treatment of Raynaud phenomenon. *J Am Acad Dermatol.* 2013;69(5):834-835.
136. Clemens MW, Higgins JP, Wilgis EF. Prevention of anastomotic thrombosis by botulinum toxin a in an animal model. *Plast Reconstr Surg.* 2009;123(1):64-70.
137. Matic DB, Lee TY, Wells RG, et al. The effects of botulinum toxin type A on muscle blood perfusion and metabolism. *Plast Reconstr Surg.* 2007;120(7):1823-1833.
138. Neumeister MW. Botulinum toxin type A in the treatment of Raynaud's phenomenon. *J Hand Surg Am.* 2010;35(12):2085-2092.
139. Gordon A, Zechmeister K, Collin J. The role of sympathectomy in current surgical practice. *Eur J Vasc Surg.* 1994;8(2):129-137.
140. Coveliers HM, Hoexum F, Nederhoed JH, et al. Thoracic sympathectomy for digital ischemia: a summary of evidence. *J Vasc Surg.* 2011;54(1):273-277.
141. el-Gammal TA, Blair WF. Digital periarterial sympathectomy for ischaemic digital pain and ulcers. *J Hand Surg Am.* 1991;16(4):382-385.
142. Balogh B, Mayer W, Vesely M, et al. Adventitial stripping of the radial and ulnar arteries in Raynaud's disease. *J Hand Surg Am.* 2002;27(6):1073-1080.
143. Jeon SB, Ahn HC, Ahn YS, et al. Two-step incision for periarterial sympathectomy of the hand. *Arch Plast Surg.* 2015;42(6):761-768.
144. Taylor MH, McFadden JA, Bolster MB, et al. Ulnar artery involvement in systemic sclerosis (scleroderma). *J Rheumatol.* 2002;29(1):102-106.
145. Hummers LK, Wigley FM. Management of Raynaud's phenomenon and digital ischemic lesions in scleroderma. *Rheum Dis Clin North Am.* 2003;29(2):293-313.

Chapter 146 :: Malignant Atrophic Papulosis (Degos Disease)
:: Dan Lipsker

第一百四十六章
恶性萎缩性丘疹病

中文导读

本章首先介绍了恶性萎缩性丘疹病的识别过程，并指出Degos病既可作为一种特发性疾病，包括经典的Degos病或其良性变异型，又可作为临床线索提示某些结缔组织病如抗磷脂综合征、红斑狼疮、皮肌炎和系统性硬化症等。本章节从流行病学、病因和发病机制、临床表现、实验室检查、诊断、鉴别诊断、预后和治疗对该病进行了详细阐述。

1. 流行病学　经典的Degos病很少见，文献报道约有250例，几乎都发生在白人身上，最常见于30~40岁之间，但可以发生在任何年龄。男性比女性更容易受累（比例为3∶1）。大多数病例为散发性的，但也有家族性病例报道，其中大多数呈常染色体显性遗传。

2. 病因和发病机制　Degos病的病因不明。组织病理学表现提示原发性血管闭塞过程，血管内凝血病和/或内皮细胞损伤被视为主要的致病机制。对Degos病的发病机制进行了综述，并指出促血栓形成因子的联合作用可能在触发疾病中起作用。

3. 临床表现

（1）皮肤和眼部皮损：皮肤病变最初约2~10毫米大小玫瑰色斑片，大部分无症状或轻度瘙痒，迅速发展为圆形、光滑的坚固丘疹，通常呈圆顶状（图146-2）。部分病变表现出中央的脐凹和/或坏死（图146-3）。这些病变会在几天或几周内演变成瓷白色的萎缩性丘疹，边缘呈玫瑰色红斑和/或毛细血管扩张（图146-4）。成熟病变与白色萎缩非常相似。Degos病的病变通常是孤立的，但可能会融合成多环状萎缩或溃疡。病变最常发生于躯干和四肢，局限于肢端往往提示结缔组织疾病。眼部可受累，最常见的表现是结膜上的无血管性斑块。

（2）经典的Degos病：在经典的Degos疾病中，皮肤病变的数量从几个到100多个不等。皮肤发现通常先于系统表现。胃肠道表现包括肠穿孔和腹膜炎，中枢神经系统表现包括出血性或缺血性中风。尸检研究表明，小血管血栓形成可累及多个器官。部分典型Degos病患者具有抗磷脂抗体，提示与原发性抗磷脂综合征可能存在相关性。

（3）良性Degos病：Degos疾病的良性型现已广泛被认同。这种类型仅有皮肤受累，大多数家族发病均为良性型。目前尚无可预测患者是否会出现皮外受累的方法。

（4）Degos病样皮损或继发性Degos病：Degos病样皮损可能发生在红斑狼疮患者尤其是抗磷脂抗体阳性的患者、皮肌炎、系统性硬化症、肉芽肿性多血管炎（韦格纳肉芽肿病）、克罗恩病、阿片类药物引起的血栓性微血管病以及细小病毒B19所致的病毒血症期间。

4. 实验室检查

(1) 组织病理学：成熟的Degos病灶表现为从真皮乳头延伸至真皮网状深层轻至重度的少细胞性楔形坏死区，伴有真皮水肿和大量黏蛋白沉积（图146-5）。在病变的底部可以发现闭塞性血管，偶有血栓形成，血管壁增厚伴内膜纤维化，内皮细胞增生，以及稀疏的血管周淋巴细胞浸润（图146-6）。表皮可出现大量继发性改变：角化过度、界面皮炎、散在的坏死角质形成细胞和萎缩。

(2) 其他实验室检查和特殊检查：应对每位患者进行抗核抗体、狼疮抗凝物、抗心磷脂抗体及冷球蛋白的筛查。如果存在结缔组织病或抗磷脂综合征的迹象，可考虑继发性Degos病。进行凝血功能的全面检查有时会发现异常。若疾病发作突然，应排查细小病毒B19感染的可能。若临床评估发现肠或脑受累的迹象（疼痛、腹泻、偏瘫、视力模糊及感觉异常），则必须进行影像学评估，包括脑MRI和/或内窥镜评估/腹腔镜检查。

5. 诊断　由于皮肤病变极具特征性，通常临床即可诊断，但仍应完善活检明确诊断。

6. 鉴别诊断　表146-1概述了严重萎缩性丘疹病（Degos病）的鉴别诊断。

7. 预后和临床过程　在诊断后的2或3年内，约30%的患者会出现皮外表现。如果在诊断后7年内未发生皮外表现，则单纯皮肤受累良性型的可能性大于90%。如果存在皮外受累，致死率大于50%，主要死因是严重的肠管受累。家族性Degos病预后较好。

8. 治疗　由于Degos病的罕见性，尚无对照的临床试验。对经典Degos病的患者应进行心血管危险因素的干预，如停止吸烟，筛查和控制其血脂水平。一线治疗应包括抗血小板集聚药物（阿斯匹林、氯吡格雷、双嘧达莫，表146-2）。特别指出对结缔组织病患者继发性Degos疾病的治疗应在结缔组织病标准治疗的基础上加用抗血小板药。其他被报道有效的药物包括抗生素、羟氯喹、免疫抑制药、苯基丁氮酮和纤溶剂。文中提到全身性类固醇会加重病情，不宜使用。低分子量肝素和新型抗凝药仅用于对抗血小板药无反应的急性疾病患者。对其他药物无反应或病情严重的患者应考虑静脉注射免疫球蛋白。由于补体攻击复合体C5b-9可能参与了Degos病的发病过程，靶向C5的依库丽单抗可考虑用于急性血栓形成阶段。此外，前列环素类似物曲前列环素在个案报道中有效。

〔黄莹雪〕

AT-A-GLANCE

- Malignant atrophic papulosis (Degos disease) is a rare, primary vasoocclusive disorder, affecting mainly the skin, the GI tract, and the CNS.
- Diagnosis relies on clinical and pathologic evaluation and correlation.
- Characterized by numerous, typical, porcelain-white, atrophic papules, with a rim of rosy erythema and/or telangiectasia.
- Pathology shows a wedge-shaped area of dermal necrosis with edema and mucin deposition.
- Benign forms without extracutaneous involvement are possible.

Köhlmeier first described malignant atrophic papulosis in the early 1940s, and Degos, Delort, and Tricot recognized it as a specific entity a year later.[1-3] We now know that the clinically distinctive lesion of so-called Degos disease is a marker of cutaneous thrombobliterative vasculopathy rather than of a specific disease per se. Such lesions can be found in at least 2 distinctive clinical settings: (a) as an apparent idiopathic disease, either classic Degos disease or its benign variant, or (b) as a surrogate clinical finding in some connective tissue diseases such as the antiphospholipid syndrome, lupus erythematosus, dermatomyositis, and systemic sclerosis.

EPIDEMIOLOGY

Classic Degos disease is rare, with approximately 250 reported cases in the literature. It almost always occurs in whites, but cases have been observed in African American patients and in Japan. The disease most commonly presents between the third and fourth decades but can occur at any age. Men are more often affected than women (ratio: 3:1). The majority of cases are sporadic, but familial cases have been described, and most of these cases are consistent with an autosomal dominant pattern of inheritance.[4]

ETIOLOGY AND PATHOGENESIS

The etiology of Degos disease is poorly understood. The histopathologic findings suggest a primary vasoocclusive process, and vascular coagulopathy and/or endothelial cell damage should be considered as the major pathogenic mechanism. Several disease processes may converge to produce the clinical and histologic findings. A combination of prothrombotic factors possibly plays a role in triggering the full-blown disease. Extensive studies of prothrombotic factors have been performed in patients with Degos disease, and no single abnormality has been repeatedly identified. Assier and colleagues did not find antiphospholipid or antiendothelial cell antibodies in their series of 15 patients.[5] Inhibition of fibrinolysis and platelet abnormalities, including increased platelet adhesiveness and spontaneous aggregation, have been reported in some patients.[5-8] Strong stromal cell–derived factor-1/CXCL12 expression of the inflammatory cells was reported in 2 Japanese patients. This could contribute to platelet aggregation via the CXCR4 receptor.[9] Magro and colleagues suggested that Degos disease could be an interferon-α–mediated endotheliopathy syndrome,[10] and that the membranolytic complement attack complex C5b-9 could contribute to the thrombogenic microangiopathy.[10,11] However, complement-mediated injury is probably a late event, explaining why targeted treatment with an anti-C5 antibody, eculizumab, can effectively rescue the acutely ill, but has no effect on occlusive fibrointimal arteriopathy.[11]

CLINICAL FINDINGS

Figure 146-1 outlines an approach to the patient with suspected Degos disease.

HISTORY

Patients present with small cutaneous lesions that are usually neither pruritic nor painful. In some, history and/or review of systems will reveal signs indicative of extracutaneous involvement: abdominal pain, diarrhea, melena, nausea, blurred vision, hemiparesis, paresthesia, or any other sign indicative of an ischemic event. History can also give a clue to previous thromboembolic or obstetrical events suggestive of

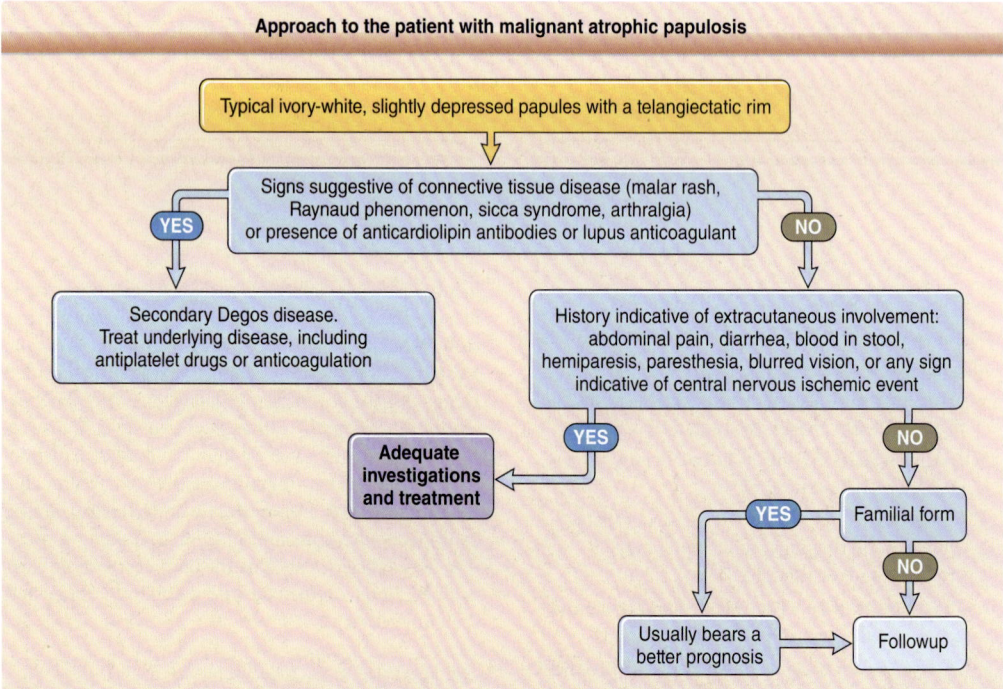

Figure 146-1 Approach to the patient with malignant atrophic papulosis (Degos disease).

the antiphospholipid antibody syndrome. A preceding infection is sometimes reported.[12]

CUTANEOUS AND OCULAR LESIONS

Cutaneous lesions start as crops of 2 to 10 mm, largely asymptomatic or mildly pruritic, rose-colored macules that progress quickly to round, smooth, often dome-shaped, firm papules (Fig. 146-2). Some lesions display central umbilication and/or necrosis (Fig. 146-3). These lesions evolve over days or weeks to porcelain-white, atrophic papules with a rim of rosy erythema and/or telangiectasias (Fig. 146-4). A fully developed lesion closely resembles the changes of atrophie blanche. In time, the reddish border disappears, and only a varicelliform white scar remains. The lesions of Degos disease are typically discreet, but they may coalesce, leading to polycyclic atrophic areas or ulcerations.

The lesions are most often located on the trunk and limbs. Palms, soles, face, scalp, and genitalia are usually spared, although exceptions occur. Exclusive acral localization is suggestive of connective tissue disease rather than Degos disease. A linear distribution has been reported.[13] Eye involvement is possible. The most common manifestation is an avascular patch on the conjunctivae, but sclerae, episclera, retina, choroids, and optic nerves may be affected.

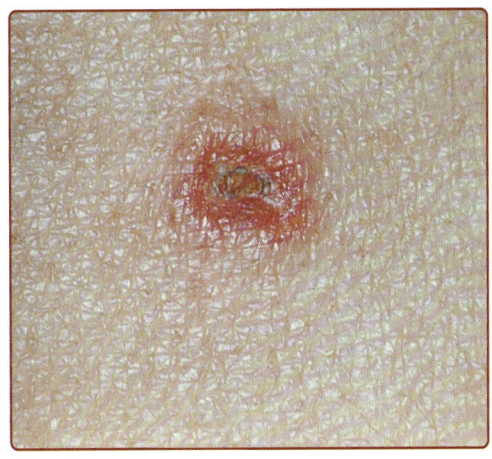

Figure 146-3 Papule with central ulceration in a patient with malignant atrophic papulosis (Degos disease).

CLASSIC DEGOS DISEASE

In classic Degos disease, the number of cutaneous lesions varies from a few to more than 100. Cutaneous findings usually precede the systemic manifestations. GI findings include bowel perforation and peritonitis, and the CNS findings include hemorrhagic or ischemic stroke. Cutaneous lesions rarely occur simultaneously or after GI or CNS involvement. Postmortem studies have revealed small-vessel thrombotic involvement of many organs, including kidney, bladder, prostate, liver, pleura, pericardium, lung, and eyes.[14] Some patients with classic Degos disease have antiphospholipid antibodies, which raises the possibility of a relationship with a primary antiphospholipid syndrome.

BENIGN DEGOS DISEASE

A benign form of Degos disease is now widely recognized. In this form, only skin involvement is found,

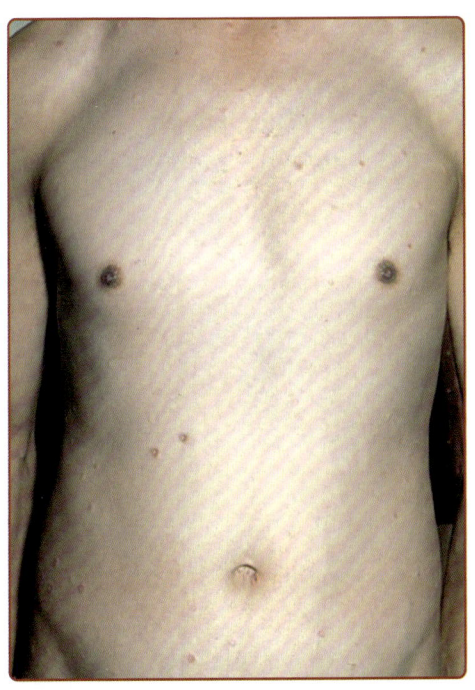

Figure 146-2 Numerous typical papules of malignant atrophic papulosis (Degos disease) in a young man.

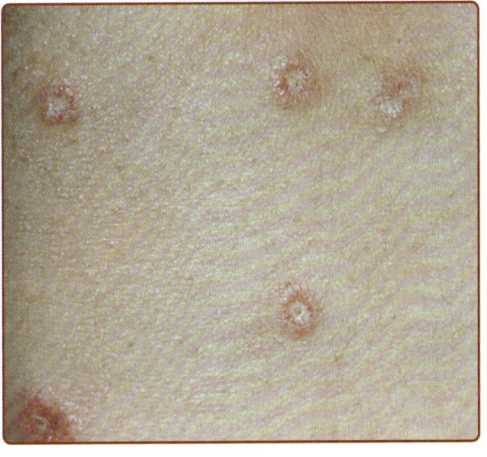

Figure 146-4 Typical pathognomonic papules of malignant atrophic papulosis (Degos disease) with a porcelain-white center and an erythematous raised border.

and most of the familial cases are benign.[4] Development during pregnancy has been reported in a patient with antiphospholipid antibodies,[15] as well as a case occurring in a patient with AIDS.[16] Skin changes consistent with Degos disease have been described at the sites of injection of interferon, a drug known to induce atrophie blanche–like lesions.[17-19] There is no clearcut distinction between the classic and the benign form of Degos disease, and there is no way to predict which patients will develop extracutaneous involvement.

DEGOS DISEASE–LIKE LESIONS OR SECONDARY DEGOS DISEASE

Degos disease–like lesions can occur in patients with lupus erythematosus, especially those with antiphospholipid antibodies, dermatomyositis, systemic sclerosis, granulomatosis with polyangiitis (Wegener granulomatosis), Crohn disease, opioid-induced thrombotic microangiopathy, and during parvovirus B19 viremia, a virus with a known affinity for endothelial cells.[20-25]

LABORATORY TESTS

HISTOPATHOLOGY

Fully developed lesions of Degos disease demonstrate a cell-poor, wedge-shaped area of mild-to-severe dermal necrosis with dermal edema and copious mucin deposition, extending from the papillary dermis to the deep reticular dermis (Fig. 146-5). At the base of the lesion, occluded vessels with occasional thrombosis, thickened vessel walls with intimal fibrosis, proliferating endothelial cells, and a sparse perivascular lymphocytic infiltrate can be found (Fig. 146-6). A full-blown leukocytoclastic, neutrophilic vasculitis is never found in patients with malignant atrophic papulosis, signifying this entity should not be classified as vasculitis. Numerous secondary, epidermal changes can be found: hyperkeratosis, interface dermatitis, scattered necrotic keratinocytes, and atrophy. An associated sclerosing panniculitis was reported in one patient.[26] Results of direct immunofluorescence studies have been inconsistent. Electron microscopy occasionally reveals tubuloreticular aggregates within endothelial cells of uncertain significance.

Because some of the histopathologic findings, such as mucinous infiltration of the dermis, interface dermatitis, and a perivascular lymphocytic dermal infiltrate, are shared by lupus erythematosus and dermatomyositis, Degos disease is considered by some as a possible variant of lupus erythematosus.[22]

OTHER LABORATORY TESTS AND SPECIAL TESTS

There is no diagnostic or prognostic marker of the disease. A search for antinuclear antibodies, lupus anticoagulant, and anticardiolipin antibodies should be performed in each patient. All patients should be screened for the presence of antiphospholipid antibodies/lupus anticoagulant and cryoglobulins. An extensive exploration of hemostasis will sometimes reveal abnormalities. When the disease starts with sudden onset, parvovirus B19 infection should be suspected and circulating viral DNA should be searched for by polymerase chain reaction.[23]

Clinical evaluation can confirm secondary Degos disease if signs suggestive of connective tissue disease or antiphospholipid syndrome are present. If the clinical evaluation reveals signs of intestinal or cerebral involvement (pain, diarrhea, hemiparesis, blurred vision, paresthesia), imaging studies, including cerebral MRI and/or endoscopic evaluation/laparoscopy, are mandatory.

DIAGNOSIS

The diagnosis is usually established clinically, because of the distinctive skin lesions. A confirmatory biopsy should always be performed.

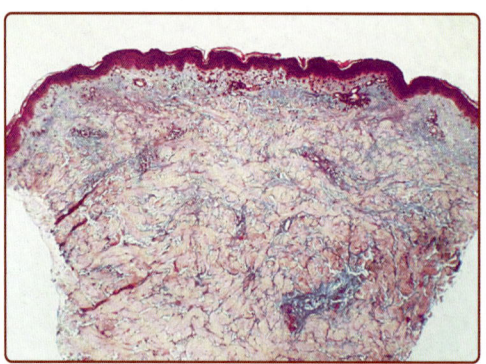

Figure 146-5 A wedge-shaped, cell-poor area of dermal necrosis, with copious mucin deposition, extending from the papillar dermis to the deep part of the reticular dermis (hematoxylin-eosin-saffron-Astra blue stain, ×40 magnification).

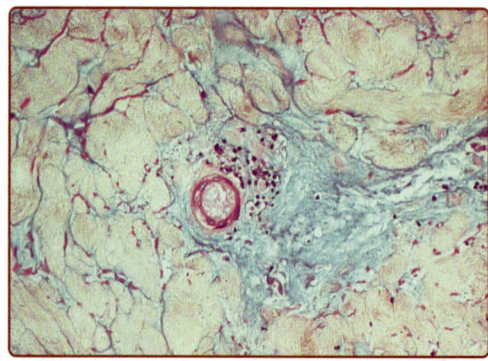

Figure 146-6 In the deeper reticular dermis, prominent mucin deposition and a sparse lymphocytic infiltrate is seen around a blood vessel (hematoxylin-eosin-saffron-Astra blue, ×200 magnification).

DIFFERENTIAL DIAGNOSIS

Table 146-1 outlines the differential diagnosis of malignant atrophic papulosis (Degos disease).

COMPLICATIONS

GI hemorrhage, perforation, and peritonitis are the most frequent complications of the disease and are the major ominous events, occurring in up to 73% of the 30% of patients with the systemic form of the disease.[27] Neurologic complications, including hemiparesis, aphasia, multiple cranial nerve involvement, monoplegia, sensory disturbances, and seizures, are less common. Rarely, progressive neurologic involvement can lead to death, especially in children. Exceptionally, death can result from respiratory failure or myocardial infarction. Thus, death related to an ischemic cerebral or GI event is the major complication of Degos disease, conferring a 5-year survival rate in patients with systemic disease of approximately 54%.[27]

PROGNOSIS AND CLINICAL COURSE

Extracutaneous manifestations will occur in approximately 30% of patients within 2 or 3 years after diagnosis.[27] Although absence of visceral involvement 2 years after diagnosis portends a better prognosis, systemic involvement can occur many years after the initial presentation of cutaneous lesions, making it impossible to predict the outcome. Nevertheless, if no extracutaneous manifestations have occurred 7 years after diagnosis, the probability of a benign monosymptomatic cutaneous course is greater than 90%.[27] Lethality is greater than 50% if patients present with extracutaneous involvement, and most of these patients die within 2 to 3 years, mainly because of severe intestinal involvement. Familial Degos disease bears a better prognosis.[4]

TREATMENT

As a consequence of the rarity of Degos disease, there are no controlled clinical trials of therapy, but only anecdotal reports. As some aspects of Degos disease resemble livedoid vasculopathy, some treatments reported to be effective in patients with livedoid vasculopathy are worth trying (see table below). The treatment of secondary Degos disease occurring in patients with known connective tissue disease should involve the introduction of antiplatelet agents in addition to the standard treatments otherwise required by those patients.

Patients with classic Degos disease should be screened for all known preventable cardiovascular risk factors. Patients should cease smoking, and their lipid levels should be screened and lowered, if necessary, using statins.

First-line treatment of patients with Degos disease should include platelet aggregation inhibitors (aspirin, clopidogrel, dipyridamole; Table 146-2). A substantial number of patients responded to aspirin and dipyridamole.[6,7,16] A number of anecdotal treatments, including antibiotics, chloroquine, immunosuppressive agents, phenylbutazone, and fibrinolytics, have been reported and have had variable success. Systemic steroids have been reported to exacerbate the disease and should not be prescribed.[28] The tumor necrosis factor inhibitor infliximab was not effective in one report.[29] Heparin and other anticoagulation strategies, such as vitamin K inhibitors (warfarin, fluindione) have variable success rates. Yet, borrowing from livedoid vasculopathy, low-molecular-weight heparin and the newer anticoagulants might warrant a trial in the acutely ill patient who is not responding to antiplatelet agents.[30] Intravenous immunoglobulins should be considered in patients who are not responding to

TABLE 146-1
Differential Diagnosis of Malignant Atrophic Papulosis (Degos Disease)

Conditions with White and/or Necrotic Papules
Common
- Atrophie blanche

Less Common
- Cutaneous lichen sclerosus
- Pityriasis lichenoides
- Lymphomatoid papulosis
- Syphilids, tuberculids
- Cutaneous Kikuchi disease (histiocytic necrotizing lymphadenitis)
- Clear-cell papulosis
- Calcinosis cutis
- Fibroelastolytic papulosis of the neck
- White lentiginosis
- Scar, artifactual disease

Always Rule Out
- Connective tissue disease with Degos disease–like lesions
- Crohn disease
- Granulomatosis with polyangiitis (Wegener granulomatosis)
- Opioid-induced thrombotic microangiopathy
- Parvovirus B19 infection

TABLE 146-2
Treatment of Malignant Atrophic Papulosis (Degos Disease)

First-line treatment	Aspirin (100-325 mg) and dipyridamole (3 × 400 mg)
Second-line treatment	Heparin and other anticoagulation strategies
Unresponsive or acutely ill patients	Intravenous immunoglobulins (1 g/kg/day for 2 days or 0.4 g/kg/day for 5 days) Eculizumab, treprostinil
Adjunctive measures	Control of cardiovascular risk factors

other treatments or are the acutely ill.[23,31] As the membranolytic complement attack complex C5b-9 seems involved in the pathogenesis of Degos disease, there is a rationale for using the monoclonal antibody eculizumab.[10-12] Eculizumab targets C5 and inhibits its cleavage to C5a and C5b by the C5 convertase, preventing the generation of the terminal complement complex C5b-9. A few patients treated with eculizumab had a substantial response, especially in the acute thrombotic phase,[11] but others did not respond or progress under treatment.[32-34] Treprostinil, a prostacyclin analog, was found to be effective in 1 patient with systemic sclerosis/lupus erythematosus overlap and Degos disease–like skin lesions and in a 17-year-old patient with severe Degos disease progressing on eculizumab.[34]

REFERENCES

1. Köhlmeier W. Multiple Hautnekrosen bei thrombangiitis obliterans. *Arch Dermatol Syph*. 1941;181:783.
2. Degos R, Delort J, Tricot R. Dermatite papulosquameuse atrophiante. *Bull Soc Fr Dermatol Syphiligr*. 1942;49:148.
3. Degos R, Delort J, Tricot R. Papulose atrophiante maligne (syndrome cutaneo-intestinal mortel). *Bull Mem Soc Med Hop Paris*. 1948;64:803.
4. Pinault AL, Barbaud A, Weber-Muller F, et al. Forme familiale bénigne de maladie de Degos. *Ann Dermatol Venereol*. 2004;131:989.
5. Assier H, Chosidow O, Piette JC, et al. Absence of antiphospholipid antibodies and anti-endothelial cell antibodies in malignant atrophic papulosis: a study of 15 cases. *J Am Acad Dermatol*. 1995;33:831.
6. Caux F, Aractingi S, Scrobohaci ML, et al. Anomalies de la fibrinolyse dans la maladie de Degos. *Ann Dermatol Venereol*. 1994;121:537.
7. Drucker CR. Malignant atrophic papulosis: response to antiplatelet therapy. *Dermatologica*. 1990;180:90.
8. Torrelo A, Sevilla J, Mediero IG, et al. Malignant atrophic papulosis in an infant. *Br J Dermatol*. 2002;146:916.
9. Meephansan J, Komine M, Hosoda S, et al. Possible involvement of SDF-1/CXCL12 in the pathogenesis of Degos disease. *J Am Acad Dermatol*. 2013;68(1):138-143.
10. Magro CM, Poe JC, Kim C, et al. Degos disease: a C5b-9/interferon-α-mediated endotheliopathy syndrome. *Am J Clin Pathol*. 2011;135(4):599.
11. Magro CM, Wang X, Garrett-Bakelman F, et al. The effects of eculizumab on the pathology of malignant atrophic papulosis. *Orphanet J Rare Dis*. 2013;8:185.
12. Pati S, Muley SA, Grill MF, et al. Post-streptococcal vasculopathy with evolution to Degos' disease. *J Neurol Sci*. 2011;300(1-2):157.
13. Kirkup ME, Hunt SJ, Pawade J, et al. Inflammatory linear vasculopathy mimicking Degos' disease. *Br J Dermatol*. 2004;150:1212.
14. Howsden SM, Hodge SJ, Herndon JH, et al. Malignant atrophic papulosis of Degos. *Arch Dermatol*. 1976;112:1582.
15. Bogenrieder T, Kuske M, Landthaler M, et al. Benign Degos' disease developing during pregnancy and followed for 10 years. *Acta Derm Venereol*. 2002;82:284.
16. Requena L, Farina C, Barat A. Degos disease in a patient with acquired immunodeficiency syndrome. *J Am Acad Dermatol*. 1998;38:852.
17. Bugatti L, Filosa G, Nicolini M, et al. Atrophie blanche associated with interferon-alfa adjuvant therapy for melanoma: a cutaneous side effect related to the procoagulant activity of interferon? *Dermatology*. 2002;204:154.
18. Zuber J, Martinez F, Droz D, et al. Alpha-interferon-associated thrombotic microangiopathy: a clinicopathologic study of 8 patients and review of the literature. *Medicine (Baltimore)*. 2002;81:321.
19. Zaharia D, Truchot F, Ronger-Savle S, et al. Benign form of atrophic papulosis developed at injection sites of pegylated-alpha-interferon: is there a pathophysiological link? *Br J Dermatol*. 2014;170(4):992.
20. Stephansson EA, Niemi KM, Jouhikainen T, et al. Lupus anticoagulant and the skin. A longterm follow-up study of SLE patients with special reference to histopathological findings. *Acta Derm Venereol*. 1991;71:416.
21. High WA, Aranda J, Patel SB, et al. Is Degos' disease a clinical and histological end point rather than a specific disease? *J Am Acad Dermatol*. 2004;50:895.
22. Ball E, Newburger A, Ackerman AB. Degos' disease: a distinctive pattern of disease, chiefly of lupus erythematosus, and not a specific disease per se. *Am J Dermatopathol*. 2003;25(4):308-320.
23. Dyrsen ME, Iwenofu OH, Nuovo G, et al. Parvovirus B19-associated catastrophic endothelialitis with a Degos-like presentation. *J Cutan Pathol*. 2008;35:20-25.
24. Guhl G, Diaz-Ley B, Delgado Y, et al. Wegener's granulomatosis: a new entity in the growing differential diagnosis of Degos' disease. *Clin Exp Dermatol*. 2009;34:e(1).
25. Magro CM, Toledo-Garcia A, Pala O, et al. Opioid associated intravenous and cutaneous microvascular drug abuse (skin-popping) masquerading as Degos disease (malignant atrophic papulosis) with multiorgan involvement. *Dermatol Online J*. 2015;21(9).
26. Grilli R, Soriano ML, Izquierdo MJ, et al. Panniculitis mimicking lupus erythematosus profundus: a new histopathologic finding in malignant atrophic papulosis (Degos disease). *Am J Dermatopathol*. 1999;21:365.
27. Theodoridis A, Konstantinidou A, Makrantonaki E, et al. Malignant and benign forms of atrophic papulosis (Köhlmeier-Degos disease): systemic involvement determines the prognosis. *Br J Dermatol*. 2014;170:110-115.
28. Burg G, Vieluf D, Stolz W, et al. Malignant atrophic papulosis (Köhlmeier-Degos disease [in German]). *Hautarzt*. 1989;40:480-485.
29. De Breucker S, Vandergheynst F, Decaux G. Inefficacy of intravenous immunoglobulins and infliximab in Degos' disease. *Acta Clin Belg*. 2008;63(2):99.
30. Hairston BR, Davis MD, Gibson LE, et al. Treatment of livedoid vasculopathy with low-molecular-weight heparin: report of 2 cases. *Arch Dermatol*. 2003;139:987.
31. Zhu KJ, Zhou Q, Lin AH, et al. The use of intravenous immunoglobulin in cutaneous and recurrent perforating intestinal Degos disease (malignant atrophic papulosis). *Br J Dermatol*. 2007;157(1):206.
32. Scheinfeld N. Commentary on "Degos disease: a C5b-9/interferon-α-mediated endotheliopathy syndrome" by Magro et al: a reconsideration of Degos disease as hematologic or endothelial genetic disease. *Dermatol Online J*. 2011;17(8):6.

33. Theodoridis A, Makrantonaki E, Zouboulis CC. Malignant atrophic papulosis (Köhlmeier-Degos disease)—a review. *Orphanet J Rare Dis*. 2013;8:10.

34. Shapiro LS, Toledo-Garcia AE, Farrell JF. Effective treatment of malignant atrophic papulosis (Köhlmeier-Degos disease) with treprostinil-early experience. *Orphanet J Rare Dis*. 2013;8:52.

Chapter 147 :: Vascular Malformations
:: Laurence M. Boon, Fanny Ballieux, & Miikka Vikkula

第一百四十七章

血管畸形

中文导读

血管畸形是在胚胎发育的第4~第10周内发生的血管发育异常，常根据受累的血管类型来命名。本章节首先对血管畸形进行了总体描述，接下来分别阐述了毛细血管畸形、静脉畸形、淋巴管畸形及动静脉畸形，从流行病学、临床特征、病因和发病机制、诊断、鉴别诊断、临床过程和预后及治疗对这些类型的血管畸形进行了详细介绍。

1. 血管畸形 血管畸形累及约0.3%的人口，其中大多数为毛细血管畸形（CM）。在流变学上，血管畸形分为慢流和快流（表147-2），通常只影响美观，少数情况下可导致功能受损甚至威胁生命。目前已确定遗传性血管畸形的相关基因突变（表147-3）。诊断常基于临床表现。组织学上，血管畸形由扩大的迂曲血管组成。多普勒超声检查可为区分血管畸形的类型提供线索。磁共振成像（MRI）可用于确定病变的范围和精确定位。血管畸形的治疗取决于受累血管类型、病变位置、患者年龄和症状，广泛或复杂的病变需多学科合作。

2. 毛细血管畸形 毛细血管畸形主要是散发病例，与遗传相关时，它们通常是毛细血管畸形-动静脉畸形（CM-AVM）的一部分。CM患病率为0.3%，可能是综合征的一部分，作者在该小节对出现CM表现的综合征概况进行了介绍。

接下来作者对CM的皮肤表现、非皮肤表现及并发症进行了详细阐述。

面部CM被认为是源自神经嵴的异常细胞的克隆增生，对于该病相关的遗传学机制也进行了详细介绍。组织学上，CM表现为乳头和真皮网状上层的毛细血管扩张及部分区域正常形态的毛细血管数目增加（图147-8）。建议对于多灶性病变（CM-AVM1和2）的患者应行基因检测。对于需与CM相鉴别的疾病，列于表147-4。CM通常在出生时就存在，随着时间的推移会逐渐变厚和变暗、或凸起形成结节（见图147-7），可出现化脓性肉芽肿以及软组织或骨肥大。

治疗目的是监测并预防并发症，并最大程度地降低CM对生活质量的影响。遮盖疗法是有效的治疗方式（图147-9），同时提出了骨科干预、激光治疗及多学科治疗建议。

3. 静脉畸形（VM） VM是由皮肤黏膜的静脉血管构成的先天性病变。首先介绍了该病的流行病学特点及可出现静脉异常的综合征。临床特征包括皮肤表现、非皮肤表现和并发症表现，作者将这些特征总结在表147-5中。在发病机制上，作者主要介绍了VM不同临床亚型及综合征的遗传学机制，对多灶性病变患者可进行基因检测。在实验室检查上，建议对于单纯VM或伴有综合征的任何患者，均应进行血小板计数、纤维蛋白原和D-二聚体水平的凝血分析，警惕LIC及DIC等严重并发症，并对VM的组织学特征进行了详细描述。对于需与VM相鉴别的疾病，列于表147-6。VM常随患者长大而成比例地增长，主要并发症是危及生命的胃肠道出血和气道压迫。治疗常需多学科合作，治疗指征是疼痛和功能障碍。治疗措施主要包括压力服装、药物、手术及多学科会诊。

4．淋巴管异常 该部分介绍了淋巴管畸形（LM）和原发性淋巴水肿两种淋巴管异常。LM是指淋巴管的局部形态异常，大多数LM在婴儿期或2岁之前出现。原发性淋巴水肿是指淋巴液积聚在组织间隙，下肢最常受累。这两种淋巴管异常都可以是一种独立的疾病，也可以是综合征的一部分。从流行病学、疾病症候群、皮肤表现、非皮肤表现、并发症、所涉及的遗传学机制、病理改变、鉴别诊断及预后对这两种淋巴管异常进行了详细介绍。治疗上，雷帕霉素治疗LM有效，淋巴水肿最好用弹性长袜、按摩和气压装置治疗，同时也提出了手术和会诊建议。

5．动静脉畸形 快速流动的血管畸形即AVM和AVF，是最严重和最具破坏性的血管畸形。在该部分从流行病学、疾病症候群、皮肤表现、非皮肤表现、并发症、所涉及的遗传学机制、病理改变、影像学检查价值、鉴别诊断及预后对动静脉畸形进行了详细介绍。治疗AVM的目标是闭塞（通过血管栓塞术）和完全清除病灶。治疗手段主要包括弹力袜、药物、手术，同时提供了对某些综合征的治疗建议。

〔黄莹雪〕

VASCULAR MALFORMATIONS

AT-A-GLANCE

- The worldwide prevalence is roughly 0.3%, mostly accounted for by capillary malformations.
- Congenital, localized (although sometimes extensive or multifocal), and well-demarcated lesions of malformed vessels of various types: capillary, venous, lymphatic, arteriovenous, and combined
- Histologically consist of enlarged, tortuous vessels of various types.
- Caused by inherited or somatic mutations in various gene
- Can be isolated, combined, or part of a syndrome
- Management: multidisciplinary approach

INTRODUCTION

DEFINITION

Vascular malformations are believed to arise because of errors in the development of vessels that occur during the 4th to 10th weeks of intrauterine life. Most vascular malformations are sporadic, although several families with inherited forms have been identified. They are very heterogeneous.[1]

CLASSIFICATION

For many years, vascular anomalies were grouped under the term *angioma*, hampering precise classification and leading to incorrect diagnosis and improper management. For example, the term *hemangioma* has been used both for vascular malformations, often venous (cavernous hemangioma), as well as for vascular tumors (strawberry hemangioma). This nomenclature changed in 1982 with the development of a biologic classification by Mulliken and Glowacki.[2,3] This classification system organized vascular anomalies based on clinical, hemodynamic, radiologic, and histologic features. It divided vascular anomalies into two major categories: (1) vascular tumors (with cellular proliferation, hemangioma being the most common; see Chap. 118), and (2) vascular malformations (structural anomalies of blood vessels) that are subsequently subdivided, depending on the affected vessel type, into arterial, capillary, lymphatic, or venous malformations (VMs). In 1996, this classification was adopted and further developed by the International Society for the Study of Vascular Anomalies (ISSVA; Table 147-1).[4]

Vascular malformations mostly affect a single vessel type (Fig. 147-1), yet combined malformations also exist. They are named according to the affected vessel types, capillary-venous or venolymphatic malformation, for instance. In addition to isolated forms, vascular malformations occur in syndromes such as Klippel-Trenaunay syndrome (KTS, capillary-lymphatic-VM with limb hypertrophy), Maffucci syndrome (multiple enchondromas associated with multiple venous anomalies and high incidence of malignancy), CLOVES (congenital lipomatous overgrowth with vascular malformations, epidermal nevi, and spinal or skeletal anomalies or scoliosis) syndrome, or Parkes Weber syndrome (high-flow vascular malformation of the extremity with soft tissue hypertrophy).[4]

TABLE 147-1
Classification of Vascular Anomalies

VASCULAR TUMORS	VASCULAR MALFORMATIONS
Hemangiomas	**Capillary**
Infantile hemangioma	Capillary malformation (CM, also called port-wine stain)
Congenital hemangioma	Telangiectasia (hereditary benign telangiectasia, essential telangiectasia)
Rapidly-involuting congenital hemangioma (RICH)	Hereditary hemorrhagic telangiectasia (HHT)
Noninvoluting congenital hemangioma (NICH)	Capillary malformation–arteriovenous malformation (CM-AVM)
	Sturge-Weber syndrome
Hemangioendotheliomas	**Venous**
Kaposiform hemangioendothelioma	Venous malformation (VM)
Tufted angioma	Familial form: cutaneo-mucosal venous malformation (VMCM)
	Glomuvenous malformation (GVM)
	Blue rubber bleb nevus or Bean syndrome (BRBN)
Angiosarcoma	**Lymphatic**
	Lymphatic malformation (LM)
	Primary Lymphedemas
	Arterial
	Arteriovenous malformation (AVM)
	Capillary malformation–arteriovenous malformation (CM-AVM)
	Arteriovenous fistula (AVF)
	Syndromic Malformations
	Slow flow
	Klippel-Trenaunay syndrome (capillary–lymphatic–venous malformation with limb hypertrophy)
	Maffucci syndrome
	CLOVES (congenital lipomatous overgrowth with vascular malformations, epidermal nevi, and spinal or skeletal anomalies or scoliosis) syndrome
	Fast flow
	Parkes Weber syndrome

EPIDEMIOLOGY

Vascular malformations affect about 0.3% of the population with most of these being capillary malformations (CMs). Vascular malformations are mostly congenital, even though they may be diagnosed later in life.[5]

CLINICAL FEATURES

Vascular malformations grow proportionately with the patient. Usually they do not regress. Most frequently, they are well-demarcated and localized. They can affect any part of the body, including the viscera. In rare instances, they can be the stigmata of deep lesions or the first sign of a syndrome. Vascular malformations are rheologically divided into *slow flow* (capillary, lymphatic, venous, and combined) and *fast flow* (arterial, arteriovenous, and combined) (Table 147-2).[4] They can lead to esthetic or functional impairment or even threaten life in rare instances.[6]

ETIOLOGY AND PATHOGENESIS

Several genes have been identified to be mutated in the inherited forms of vascular malformations (Table 147-3). Somatic genetic mutations have also been unraveled as the cause of many common sporadic lesions.[7-15]

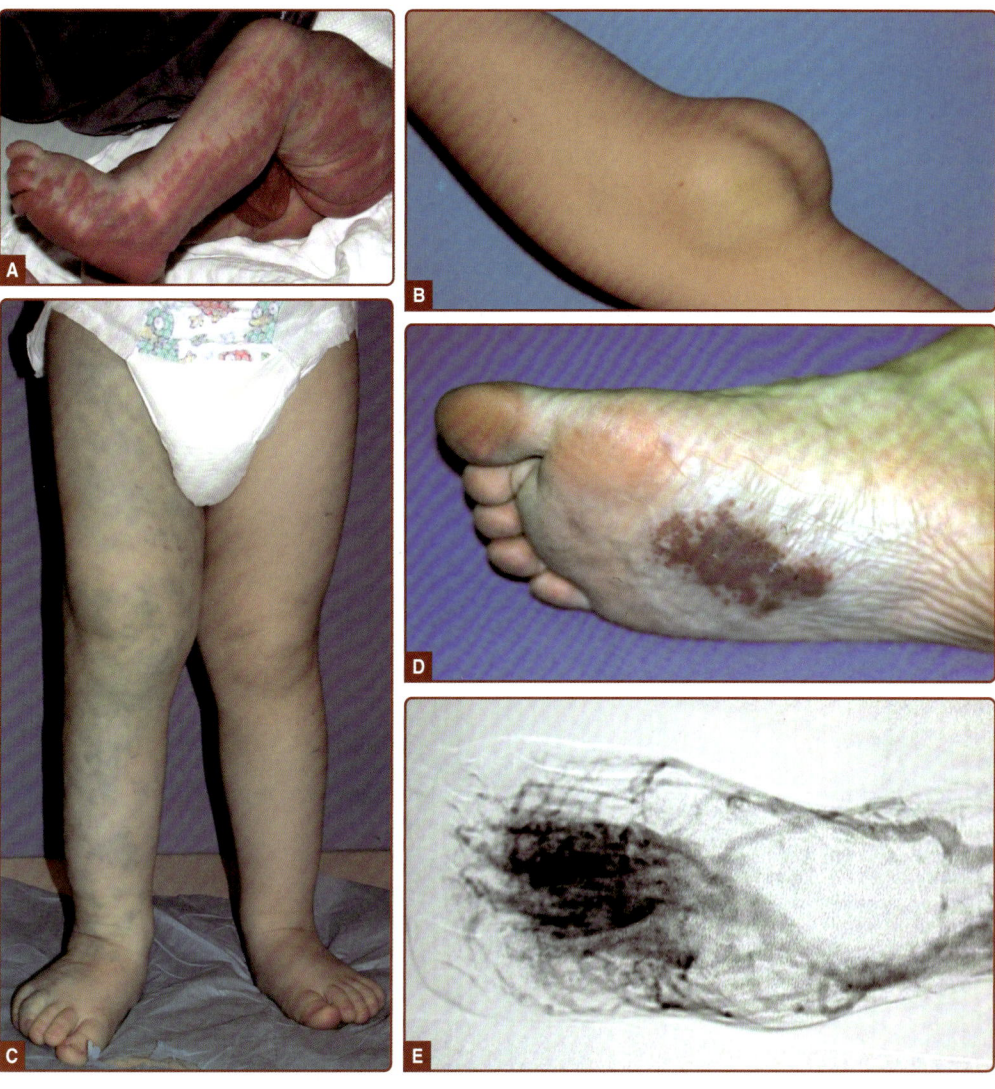

Figure 147-1 Vascular malformations of various vessel types. **A,** Capillary malformation of left lower extremity and genitalia. **B,** Subcutaneous lymphatic malformation invading the cubital nerve. **C,** Extensive venous malformation of right lower extremity, causing pain, swelling, and coagulopathy. **D,** Arteriovenous malformation of the sole. **E,** Nidus of the lesion on arteriography.

TABLE 147-2
Clinical Characteristics of Vascular Malformations

	CAPILLARY	VENOUS	LYMPHATIC	ARTERIOVENOUS
Skin color	Red	Normal-bluish-purple	Normal to yellowish-purple	Normal to red
Aspect	Flat	Flat to raised	Raised to vesicular	Flat to raised
Temperature	Normal	Normal	Normal	Warm
Palpation	Normal	Compressible	Firm, noncompressible	Thrill, bruit
Associations	—	Phleboliths, deformation	—	Ulceration, deformation
Radiology	No flow	Slow flow	Slow flow, cyst	Fast flow
Histology	Dilated capillaries D2-40 negative	Thin-walled venous channels D2-40 negative	Cystic lymphatic channels D2-40 positive	Arterialized veins D2-40 negative
Etiology	See Table 147-3			
Treatment	Pulsed-dye laser	Sclerotherapy, surgery, sirolimus medication	Surgery, sclerotherapy, sirolimus medication	Embolization followed by surgical resection of nidus

TABLE 147-3
The Genetic Causes of Vascular Anomalies

SPORADIC MALFORMATIONS		INHERITED MALFORMATIONS	
DIAGNOSIS	MUTATED GENE	DIAGNOSIS	MUTATED GENE
Capillary Malformations (CMs)			
CM	*GNAQ*	CM-AVM1	*RASA1*
Sturge-Weber syndrome		CM-AVM2	*EPHB4*
Phakomatosis pigmentovascularis (PPV)	*GNAQ* or *GNA11*		
Macrocephaly–capillary malformation (M-CM)	*AKT3, PIK3CA, PIK3R2*		
Venous Malformations (VMs)			
VM	*TIE2* (60%) *PIK3CA* (20%)	Mucocutaneous venous malformations (VMCM)	*TIE2*
Blue rubber bleb nevus (BRBN)	*TIE2*	Glomuvenous malformation (GVM)	*GLOMULIN*
Multifocal venous malformation (MVM)			
Verrucous venous malformation (VVM)	*MAP3K3*		
Maffucci syndrome	*IDH1, IDH2*		
Lymphatic Malformations (LMs)			
LM	*PIK3CA*	Nonne-Milroy lymphedema	*VEGFR3*
CLOVES (congenital lipomatous overgrowth with vascular malformations, epidermal nevi, and spinal or skeletal anomalies or scoliosis)		Nonne-Milroy–like lymphedema	*VEGF-C*
Klippel-Trenaunay syndrome (KTS)		Lymphedema distichiasis	*FOXC2*
		Microcephaly, chorioretinopathy, lymph-edema, mental retardation	*KIF11*
		Hypotrichosis–lymphedema–telangiectasia	*SOX18*
		Hennekam lymphedema–lymphangiectasia 1	*CCBE1*
		Hennekam lymphedema–lymphangiectasia 2	*FAT4*
		Hennekam lymphedema–lymphangiectasia 3	*ADAMTS3*
		Emberger syndrome	*GATA2*
		Fetal chylothorax	*ITGA9*
		Lymphedema–choanal atresia	*PTPN14*
		Four-limb lymphedema	*GJC2 (CX47)*
Arteriovenous Malformations (AVMs)			
Extracranial AVM	*MAP2K1*	Hereditary hemorrhagic telangiectasia (HHT)1	*ENG*
Brain AVM	*KRAS*	HHT2	*ACVRL1 (ALK1)*
		HHT3	*SMAD4, GDF2*
		Phosphatase and tensin (PTEN) homolog (protein encoded by PTEN gene)	*PTEN*

DIAGNOSIS

The diagnosis is usually based on clinical features in 90% of superficial malformations.

SUPPORTIVE STUDIES

Pathology: Histologically, vascular malformations consist of enlarged, tortuous vessels with quiescent endothelium. In contrast to hemangioma, there is neither a parenchymal mass nor overt cellular proliferation.

Imaging: Radiologic investigation is needed to delineate the extent of a malformation but rarely for diagnosis unless the malformation is deeply located. Doppler ultrasonography is a very useful noninvasive radiologic examination that provides clues for differentiating the various types. Magnetic resonance imaging (MRI) details the extension and precise location of the lesion.[16]

Genetic Testing: Because a germline or somatic genetic cause is known for a large number of vascular anomalies, genetic testing can be used to confirm or help make the precise diagnosis. For somatic mutations, a biopsy of the affected tissue is needed. For inherited mutations, a blood test is sufficient to make the diagnosis.

MANAGEMENT

Treatment of vascular malformations depends on the affected vessel type, the location of the lesion, the age of the patient, and the symptoms. Because many lesions are extensive, patients should be aware that a complete cure is often not possible and that recurrence occurs. Treatment can be difficult and with severe complications. Extensive or complex lesions should always be managed by a multidisciplinary team.

CAPILLARY MALFORMATIONS

AT-A-GLANCE

- Worldwide occurrence. Prevalence is roughly 0.3%.
- Congenital, slow-flow malformations of the capillary bed
- Pinkish-red to purple in color; tend to darken and thicken with time
- Can be part of a sporadic syndrome, such as Sturge-Weber syndrome or KTS
- Can be part of the inherited capillary malformation-arteriovenous malformation phenotype
- Pathology: capillaries that are increased in size and number with abnormal innervation.

Capillary malformations mainly occur sporadically, although there are well-documented pedigrees showing autosomal dominant inheritance.[17] When inherited, they are usually multiple and part of the capillary malformation–arteriovenous malformation (CM-AVM) phenotype, which associates atypical CMs with arteriovenous malformation (AVM, see Arteriovenous Malformations later).[18-23]

EPIDEMIOLOGY

CMs, commonly called *port-wine stain*, is a slow-flow vascular malformation with a prevalence of 0.3%.[5] There is no sex preponderance.

Although most often an isolated finding, in rare instances, CM can be the cutaneous hallmark of occult spinal dysraphism, especially if located in the lumbosacral area.[24] Other blanchable, pink patches, known as *stork bite, angel's kiss, salmon patch, nevus simplex,* or *nevus flammeus neonatorum*, are often confused with CM. They are located on the nape of the neck (81%), the eyelids (45%), or the glabella (33%).[25] When located on the occiput, the moniker *Unna nevus* may be used (Fig. 147-2). These patches have a much higher incidence (42%) in white infants than in black infants (31%).[26] They are also present in various syndromes, such as Beckwith-Wiedemann and Rubinstein-Taybi syndromes. These lesions (with the exception of the Unna nevus) disappear spontaneously around the age of 1 to 4 years. In contrast, true CMs persist lifelong.

SYNDROMIC DISORDERS

CMs can be part of a syndrome, such as phakomatosis pigmentovascularis (PPV), Sturge-Weber

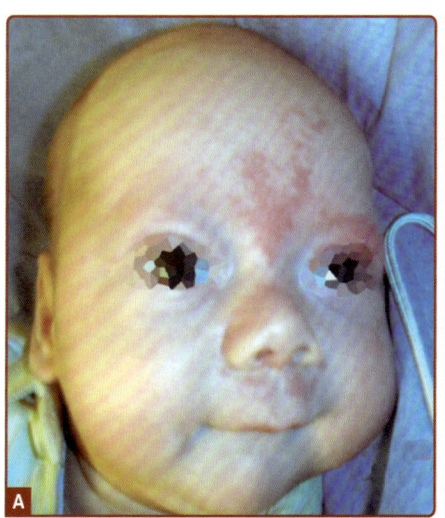 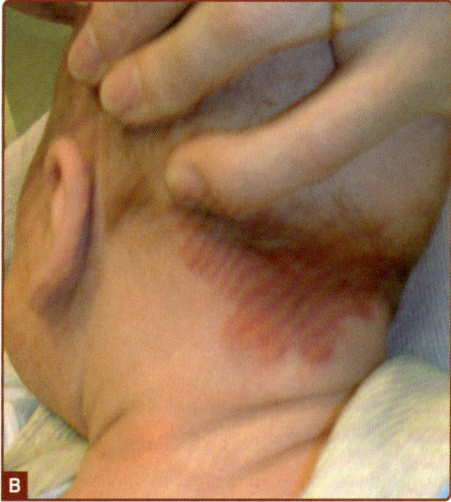

Figure 147-2 Nevus flammeus neonatorum (also called nevus simplex) on the glabella, upper eyelids, and upper lip (**A**) of a 6-week-old neonate who also has an Unna nevus on the occiput (**B**).

syndrome (SWS), KTS, Parkes Weber syndrome, CLOVES syndrome, PTEN (phosphatase and tensin homolog) Hamartoma tumor syndrome, diffuse capillary malformation with overgrowth (DCMO), and macrocephaly–capillary malformation (M-CM, also called megalencephaly–capillary malformation–polymicrogyria syndrome). None of these syndromes is inherited.

PHAKOMATOSIS PIGMENTOVASCULARIS

PPV is thought to be an embryogenic anomaly affecting the vasomotor nerves and the melanocytes, both derived from neural crest. It manifests as a large, metameric CMs, usually located on the trunk or the extremities, in association with pigmented cutaneous lesions, such as a pigmented nevus, a nevus spilus, a café-au-lait patch, or an atypical Mongolian spot (see Chap. 77) that is not located on the sacrum (Fig. 147-3).[27] Nevus anemicus can also be seen in the vicinity as a twin spot.[28]

STURGE-WEBER SYNDROME

When located in the frontopalpebral area, CM can be part of SWS (Fig. 147-4A). This neuro-oculo-cutaneous syndrome associates a cutaneous CM of the ophthalmic branch of the trigeminal nerve (V1) with a homolateral leptomeningeal capillary-venous malformation (CVM) and a choroid CVM. Glaucoma is often present (Fig. 147-4B). SWS is associated with a high risk of epilepsy and mental retardation because of anomalies of the venous drainage of the encephalon, as well as with glaucoma, buphthalmos, and sometimes retinal detachment.[29]

DIFFUSE CAPILLARY MALFORMATION WITH OVERGROWTH

Patients with DCMO have hemihypertrophy, which can be total, regional, or contralateral. CM can be diffuse over the entire body. This entity is characterized by a reticulated, ill-defined CM.[30] The lesions do not follow the lines of Blaschko (Fig. 147-5A).

MACROCEPHALY–CAPILLARY MALFORMATION

A well-delineated, dark CM of the vermillion border, the tip of the nose, or both associated with macrocephaly is often pathognomonic of M-CM. These patients have megalencephaly and are at risk of mental retardation.[31] There are two reports of M-CM associated with Wilms tumor in the literature.[32]

CLINICAL FEATURES

CUTANEOUS FINDINGS

CM is a red, homogenous, congenital lesion that is often unilateral, sometimes bilateral, but usually not median. CMs involve skin and subcutis and sometimes mucosa (see Fig. 147-5). Their color varies from pinkish-red to deep purple with a geographic contour or a dermatomal distribution. Lesions are flat and painless, do not bleed spontaneously, and are never warm on palpation in contrast to AVM (see later). Acquired CM can be seen after trauma.[33]

Fifty percent of CMs are located on the face, where they follow the distribution of the trigeminal nerve: ophthalmic branch V1 (front and upper eyelid), maxillary branch V2 (lower eyelid, cheek, and upper lip) (see Figs. 147-4A and 147-5B), or mandibular V3 (lower lip, chin, and mandible). CM can be diffuse over the entire body, often with associated hemihypertrophy (see Fig. 147-5A). This entity is called *diffuse capillary malformation with overgrowth* (see earlier discussion).

When inherited, CMs are usually small and multifocal, such as in CM-AVM1 and 2. These small CMs vary in size from a couple mm to several centimeters in size. They are often round-to-oval, pink, red, or brown in color and are often surrounded with a pale halo (Fig. 147-6).[18,34] The lesions are well-circumscribed and blanch on pressure with a diascopy. Some of them are

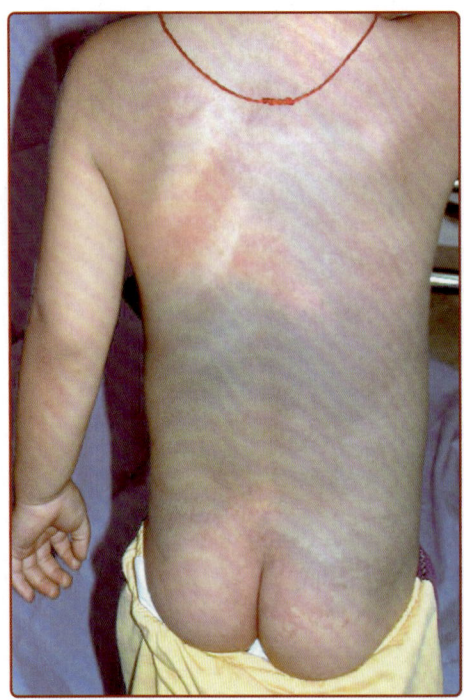

Figure 147-3 Clinical characteristics of phakomatosis pigmentovascularis. A large metameric capillary malformation with atypical extensive dermal melanocytosis located on the back.

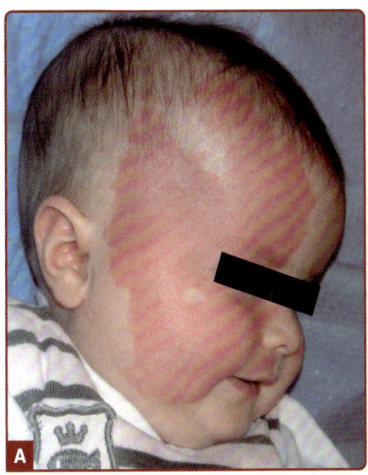
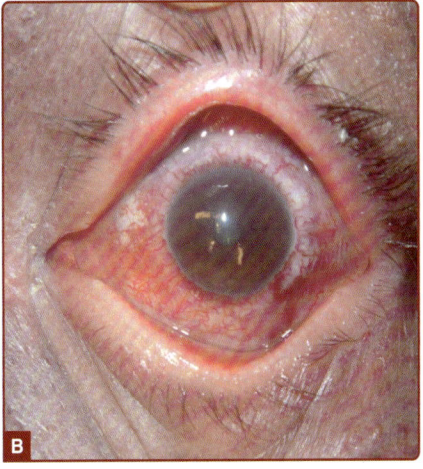

Figure 147-4 Extensive right facial capillary malformation. **A,** Involving the ophthalmic and maxillary branches of the trigeminal nerve in a 6-month-old girl with Sturge-Weber syndrome. **B,** Choroid capillary–venous malformation causing vision loss in a 50-year-old man with Sturge-Weber syndrome.

present at birth, but others appear later. They grow with the child and are asymptomatic. Bier spots, white cutaneous spots surrounded by a pale halo of redness, are seen in both entities. In contract to CM-AVM1, CMs in CM-AVM2 can be more telangiectatic in appearance, especially periorally and on the upper thorax.[23] CM-AVM1 is characterized by the presence of CMs in 97%, AVMs or arteriovenous fistulas (AVFs) in 24% (10% intra–central nervous system [CNS], 13% extra-CNS), and Parkes Weber phenotype in 8% of patients.[21,35] In CM-AVM2, the risk of a fast-flow lesion seems to be less frequent because the respective penetrances are 93% (CM), 19% (AVM), and 7% (Parkes Weber).

NONCUTANEOUS FINDINGS

In rare instances, CM can be the stigmata of an underlying anomaly such as lumbar dysraphism underneath a sacral CM. Cutaneous lesions of PPV can be associated with systemic, visceral (hypoplasia of the larynx, intestinal polyposis), muscular (scoliosis), or neurologic (mental retardation, epilepsy, intracranial) signs and symptoms in 60% of cases.[36]

SWS is associated with a high risk of epilepsy and mental retardation because of anomalies of the venous drainage of the encephalon, as well as with glaucoma, buphthalmos, and sometimes retinal detachment.[29] Patients with DCMO have hemihypertrophy, which can be total, regional, or contralateral. They have also associated toe anomalies (in 30%) and prominent veins.[30] In CM-AVM1 or 2, there is a 20% to 30% risk of an associated AVM located on the skin, the brain, or the spine.[21,35] A well-delineated dark CM of the vermillion border or the tip of the nose associated with macrocephaly is often pathognomonic of M-CM, and these patients have megalencephaly and are at risk of mental retardation.[31]

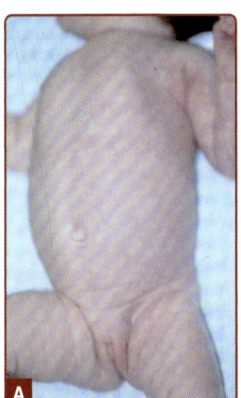
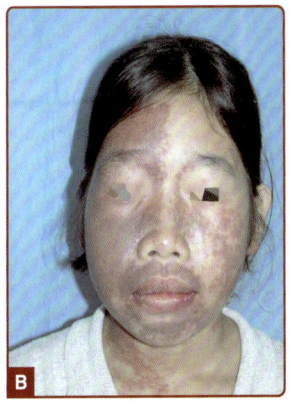
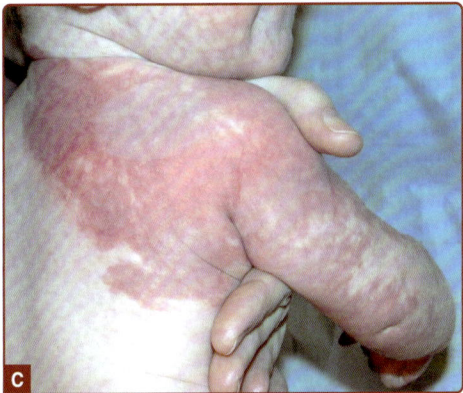

Figure 147-5 Several aspects of capillary malformations. **A,** Light red lesions involving half of the body. **B,** Dark red lesions on the face with mucosal involvement and soft tissue hypertrophy. **C,** More localized on the shoulder and arm.

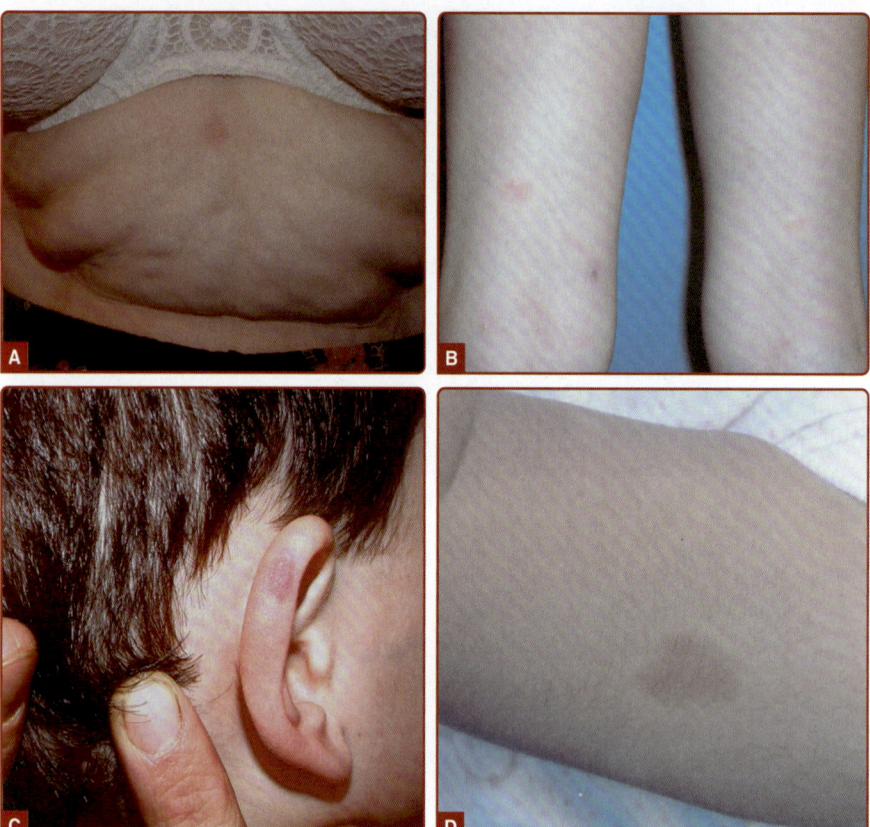

Figure 147-6 A–D, Examples of small atypical capillary malformations which belong to CM-AVM (capillary malformation-arteriovenous malformation). **D,** Note the pale halo surrounding the lesion.

COMPLICATIONS

The major concern for a patient with a CM is cosmetic because of the visible discoloration. *Hypertrophy* of soft (often lips and gums) and underlying hard tissues can occur with time, especially when the CM affects the V2 and V3 dermatomes or the extremities (Fig. 147-7D and 147-7). *Overgrowth* of the maxilla or mandible leads to skeletal asymmetry, occlusal tilt, and open-bite deformity. When the child has atopic dermatitis, psoriasis, or acne, lesions are worse in the area of CM, a finding known as the Meyerson phenomenon.[37] Evenly thickened skin, purple nodules, and pyogenic granulomas can develop by adolescence (Fig. 147-7B and 147-7C).[38,39]

ETIOLOGY AND PATHOGENESIS

Facial CM is thought to be caused by clonal expansion of abnormal cells originating from the neural crest.[40] Somatic activating mutations in *GNAQ* have been identified as the cause of facial CM with hypertrophy as well as of SWS.[13] GNAG is a q class of G-protein α subunits that mediates signals between G protein–coupled receptors and their downstream effectors. Mutations in *GNAQ* and *GNA11* have also been identified in pigmented lesions such as blue nevi, nevus of Ota, uveal melanoma, and PPV.[41,42]

The inherited CM-AVM1 is caused by inactivating mutations in *RASA1*.[21] This gene encodes a GTPase-activating protein, which negatively regulates Ras activity. CM-AVM2 is caused by inactivating mutations in *EPHB4*.[23] EPHB4 is usually expressed in venous endothelial cells and its ligand EPHINB2 on arterial endothelial cells. They regulate arteriovenous identity. EPHB4 interacts with RASA1 to regulate RAS-MAPK signaling, and loss of EPHB4 or RASA1 in CM-AVM likely activates this signaling pathway. M-CM is caused by activating mutations in *AKT3*, *PIK3CA*, and *PIK3R2*.[43]

DIAGNOSIS

SUPPORTIVE STUDIES

Pathology: Histologically, CM is characterized by dilated capillaries of the papillary and upper reticular dermis combined with areas of increased number of

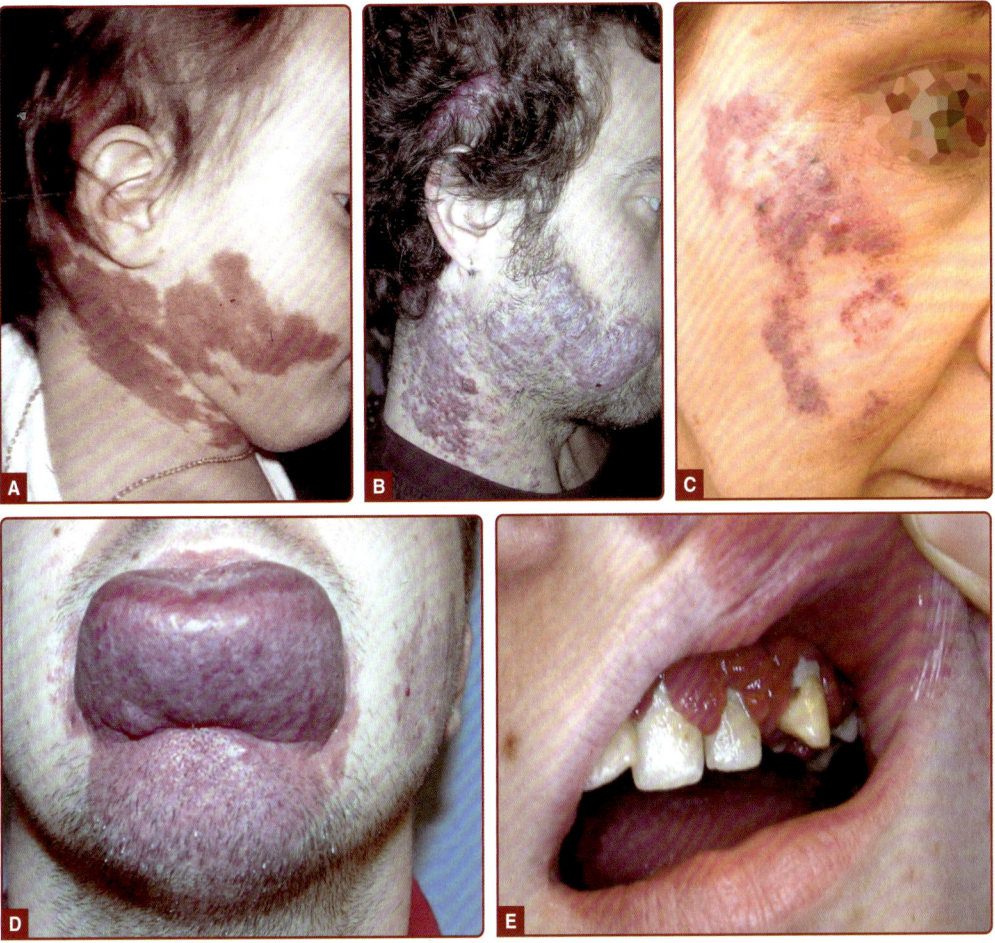

Figure 147-7 Clinical evolution of capillary malformation: darkening and thickening with time. **A,** At age 6 months. **B,** At age 33 years. **C,** Development of pyogenic granuloma. **D,** Soft tissue hypertrophy. **E,** Mucosal hypertrophy.

normal-looking capillaries (Fig. 147-8).[44] Endothelial cells are flat. Factor VIII, fibronectin, and basement membrane protein are normal, but S100 staining shows abnormal innervation.[45,46]

Imaging: No imaging studies are mandatory for a CM except in rare situations. If a so-called "CM" is painful, warm, or spontaneously bleeds, Doppler ultrasound is indicated to exclude the diagnosis of a fast-flow malformation, such as an AVM, Parkes Weber syndrome, or a proliferating hemangioma.

CM located in the frontopalpebral area, especially if the inner part of the upper eyelid is involved, can be part of SWS. Therefore, for these CMs, an ophthalmologic and neurologic examination is mandatory. They need to be done during the first months of life and repeated once a year until puberty, even if normal at younger age.[47] A brain MRI should also be done to evaluate the occurrence of associated leptomeningeal CVM. In patients with PPV, ophthalmologic, neurologic, and orthopedic follow-up is mandatory because of the common association of CM with systemic lesions. In patients with extensive CMs of the lower extremity, such as in DCMO, a scaniometry study (leg length films) is needed to evaluate possible progressive growth discrepancy around the age of 4 to 6 years and needs to be repeated until the end of growth to allow the orthopedist to correct the discrepancy at the adequate time. Serial renal ultrasound examinations are also indicated to rule out the appearance of a Wilms tumor. MRI of the spinal cord is indicated in the presence of a lumbosacral CM. Brain and spinal MRI should be considered in patients with CM-AVM.

Genetic Testing: Genetic testing is indicated, especially in patients with multifocal lesions (CM-AVM1 and 2) because of increased risk for intracerebral fast-flow lesions. These patients should be screened for *RASA1* and *EPHB4*. Pale, uncharacteristic, and inconspicuous CMs can be sign of PHTS, especially if these vascular lesions are associated with macrocephaly (see AVM later). Because of increased cancer risk, such patients should be screened for *PTEN* mutations.

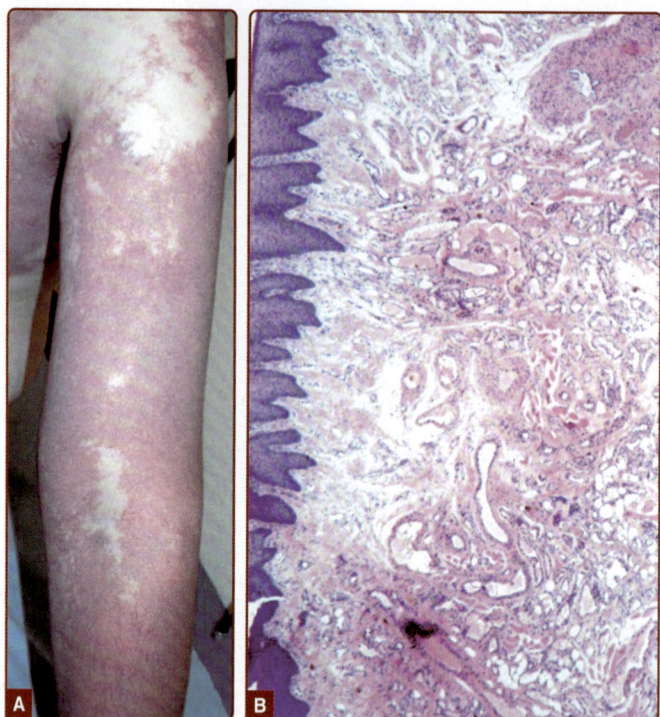

Figure 147-8 **A,** Extensive capillary malformation of upper extremity. **B,** Histologically, capillary malformation is characterized by dilated capillaries of normal number in the papillary and upper reticular dermis in combination with areas of increased number of normal-looking capillaries (hematoxylin and eosin staining).

Identification of a germline mutation would enable precise counseling and surveillance.

DIFFERENTIAL DIAGNOSIS

See Table 147-4.

CLINICAL COURSE AND PROGNOSIS

CM is present at birth and never regresses spontaneously. During the first weeks of life, they can slightly fade, as the hemoglobin level of the newborn decreases. Subsequently, the red hue stabilizes, and the lesion grows in proportion to the rest of the body. Around puberty, as well as later in life, CM slowly thickens and darkens with time. It often becomes raised and nodular (see Fig. 147-7).[38] Pyogenic granuloma can occur with time, as well as soft tissue or bony hypertrophy.[39]

MANAGEMENT

The goal of management is to monitor for associated complications and minimize the impact of the CM on self-esteem and quality of life. Camouflage using a foundation such as Covermark is still an effectively approach (Fig. 147-9)

INTERVENTIONS

Orthopedic Considerations: In the presence of leg-length discrepancy, an early-adapted shoe lift is needed if leg-length discrepancy is over 1.5 cm to prevent compensatory tilting of the pelvis. Epiphysiodesis is sometimes necessary when the child is approximately 11 to 13 years old.

Procedures: Laser treatment is the gold standard therapy for most CM. Pulsed-dye laser with its specific wavelength (585 or 595 nm) and a short pulse duration (400–1500 ms) currently gives the best results in infants and children by lightening the red color of the CM. There are few complications. Multiple sessions (6–12) are

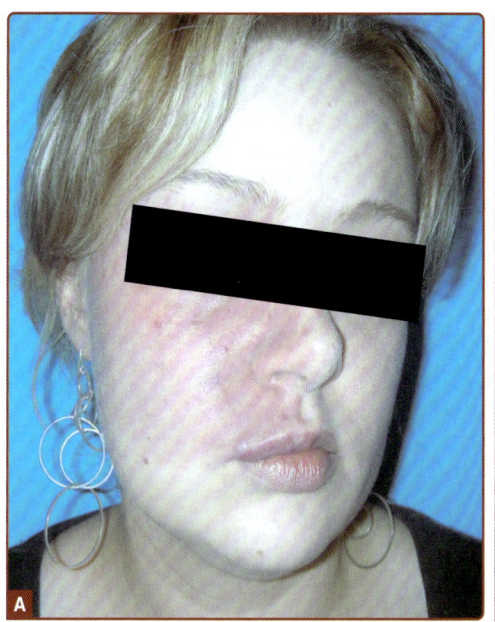 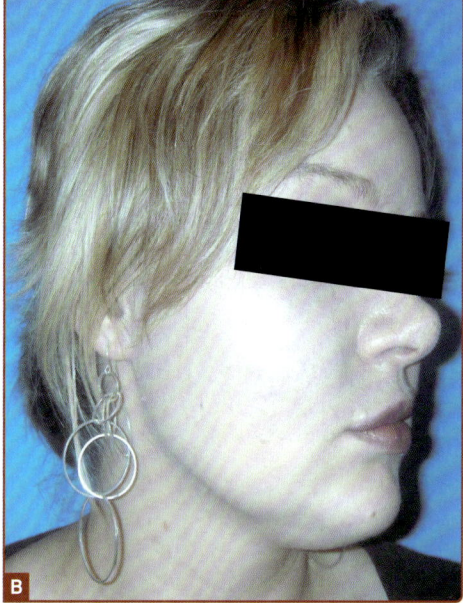

Figure 147-9 Efficient noninvasive management of facial capillary malformation using cosmetic makeup.

needed, and general anesthesia may be necessary as the procedure is painful. Laser treatment is more efficient on the cervicofacial and trunk area than on the extremities. Early treatment during childhood does not reduce the number of laser sessions.[48] The use of a dynamic cooling system to avoid heating the epidermis allows higher laser fluencies, resulting in optimal lightening of the lesion. Recurrence can occur after cessation of therapy.[49] Laser has no impact on associated hypertrophy.[6,50]

Contour resection is considered to treat complications such as pyogenic granuloma or lip hypertrophy.[6]

Counseling: Genetic and psychological counseling for the patients and their families are part of multidisciplinary management. Patient organizations dedicated to vascular anomalies also have an important role in supporting patients and their families.

PREVENTION

In patients with SWS, ophthalmologic follow-up, started immediately after birth is essential because reducing visual impairment will depend on the promptness of treatment. Prophylactic antiepileptic medication to prevent neural cell death has also been advocated, although randomized prospective studies to support efficacy are lacking at this time.[51,52]

VENOUS ANOMALIES

AT-A-GLANCE

- Most common referral to specialized centers for vascular anomalies; incidence unknown but is substantially lower than for CM and estimated at 1 in 10,000
- Congenital slow-flow malformation of the venous bed
- Bluish in color, localized or extensive, solitary or multifocal
- Compressible on palpation; presence of phleboliths
- Associated with consumptive coagulation abnormalities in about 40% of cases
- Histologically consists of ectatic venous-like channels with anomalies in mural cells
- Mainly sporadic but can be inherited as an autosomal dominant trait
- Inherited venous anomalies: cutaneomucosal venous malformation (1%), glomuvenous malformation (>5%)
- Syndromic venous malformation: KTS, blue rubber bleb nevus, Maffucci syndrome.

TABLE 147-4
Differential Diagnosis of Capillary Malformation

Based on Morphology
Most Likely
Faint pink median patch
- Unna nevus
- Nevus flammeus neonatorum (nevus simplex)

Multiple, inherited
- CM of CM-AVM

Telangiectatic patch
- CMTC
- HHT
- CM-AVM2
- Essential telangiectasia
- Unilateral nevoid telangiectasia

Warm on palpation
- Proliferating hemangioma
- AVM
- AVF

Ulcerated or painful
- AVM
- AVF

Rule Out
Small, multiple
- Mastocytosis
- CM of CM-AVM

Based on Location
Most Likely
Occiput
- Unna nevus

Glabella, upper eyelid, nape of neck
- Stork bite, angel's kiss, salmon patch

Consider
Extremity
- CMTC
- Klippel-Trenaunay syndrome
- Parkes Weber syndrome

Faint on trunk
- M-CM

Rule Out
Scalp
- Adams-Oliver syndrome
- Multiple telangiectasia near canthus
- Ataxia telangiectasia

AVF, arteriovenous fistula; AVM, arteriovenous malformation; CM, capillary malformation; CM-AVM, capillary malformation-arteriovenous malformation; CMTC, cutis marmorata telangiectatica congenita; HHT, hereditary hemorrhagic telangiectasia; M-CM, macrocephaly capillary malformation.

INTRODUCTION

A VM is a congenital lesion made up of venous-type vessels of the skin or mucosa but can involve any structure (subcutis, muscles, bones, and nerves) and any organ (CNS, gastrointestinal [GI] tract). Fifty percent of VMs are located in the cervicofacial area, and 37% are on the extremities. VMs are mainly isolated but can be part of complex vascular disorders, such as the KTS, Maffucci, and blue rubber bleb nevus (BRBN) syndromes.[53,54]

EPIDEMIOLOGY

Venous anomalies are the most common VMs referred to specialized center with an overall incidence of 1 in 10,000 in the population.[54] They mainly occur sporadically, although 1% are inherited mucocutaneous venous malformations (VMCMs) and 5% are inherited glomuvenous malformations (GVMs). No sex preponderance is reported.[55] Both VMCM and GVM have an age-dependant variation in penetrance, which reaches its maximum by 20 years of age (87% for VMCM and 92.7% for GVM).[56] Large VMCMs and GVMs are present at birth. However, 17% of affected individuals develop new small lesions over time.[55] BRBN syndrome is rare and occurs sporadically with about 200 cases reported in the literature.

SYNDROMIC DISORDERS

Syndromes with a venous anomaly include BRBN syndrome, KTS (see Lymphatic Malformations later), and Maffucci syndrome.

BLUE RUBBER BLEB NEVUS SYNDROME

BRBN is characterized by numerous malformations of the venous system that involve the skin and visceral organs. It is commonly characterized by one large "dominant" VM lesion associated with multiple small, dark blue, nipple-like lesions, the latter being typically located on the palm and soles (Fig. 147-10).[15] These cutaneous lesions are associated with

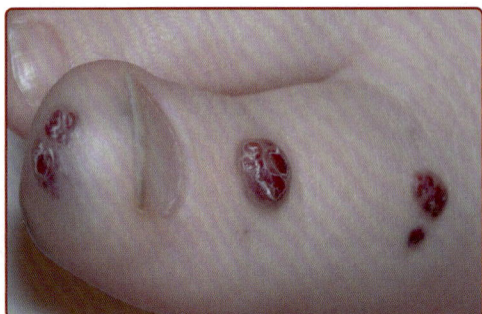

Figure 147-10 Blue rubber bleb nevus syndrome. Pathognomonic multiple small, dark blue, nipple-like lesions on the toe.

TABLE 147-5
Characteristics of Venous Anomalies

	VENOUS MALFORMATION	VENOUS MALFORMATION CUTANEOMUCOSAL	GLOMUVENOUS MALFORMATION	BLUE RUBBER BLEB NEVUS SYNDROME
Location	50% head and neck	Extremities, mucosa	70% extremities	Especially palms and soles
Skin color	Normal to bluish-purple	Bluish	Bluish-red-purple	Bluish-dark-blue
Aspect	Flat to raised	Raised, dome shaped	Raised, cobblestone Plaquelike, hyperkeratotic	Dome shaped, nipple-like
	Single, large	Multiple, small	Multiple	Multiple, small, often + 1 large lesion
Palpation	Phleboliths	Compressible	Noncompressible, painful	Firm, rubbery, spongy
Associated	Coagulopathy	—	—	Visceral venous malformation, coagulopathy
Radiologic	Phleboliths	Venous channels	No phlebolith	Venous channels
Tissue involved	Often deep location	Cutis, subcutis	Cutis, subcutis	Often deep component
Histology	Thin-walled venous channels	Thin-walled venous channels	Glomus cells	Thin-walled venous channels
Inheritance	Sporadic	Autosomal dominant	Autosomal dominant	Sporadic

multiple small GI VMs, often responsible for chronic anemia.[15,57]

MAFFUCCI SYNDROME

Maffucci syndrome is a rare disorder characterized by multiple enchondromas associated with subcutaneous VMs of the distal extremities (Fig. 147-11). The disease starts during childhood with the development of enchondromas of the bones of hands and feet, as well as of the long bones. Deformities and shortening of extremities often occur. Subcutaneous vascular nodules appear later, around puberty, on the fingers and the toes. Phleboliths may become present.[58]

CLINICAL FEATURES

The features of venous anomalies are summarized in Table 147-5.

CUTANEOUS FINDINGS

VMs are usually solitary but can be multifocal, the latter suggesting an inheritable disorder in most instances.[54] They may be relatively localized or extensive within an anatomic region. The most common location is the head and neck area (Fig. 147-12A and 147-12D–F). VMs can affect any tissue or organ (Figs. 147-12 to 147-14).

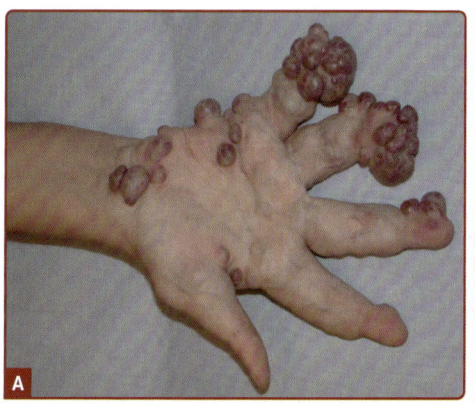 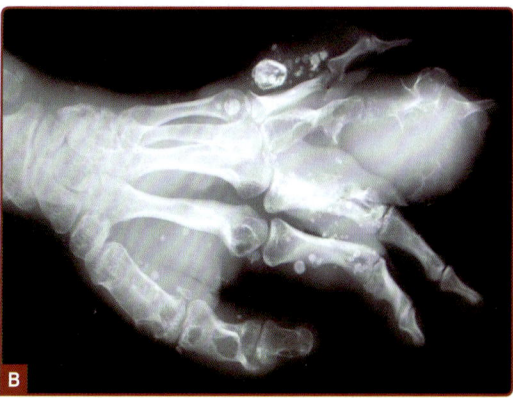

Figure 147-11 Clinical (**A**) and radiologic (**B**) aspects of Maffucci syndrome. Multiple venous malformations and enchondromas deforming the hand and fingers.

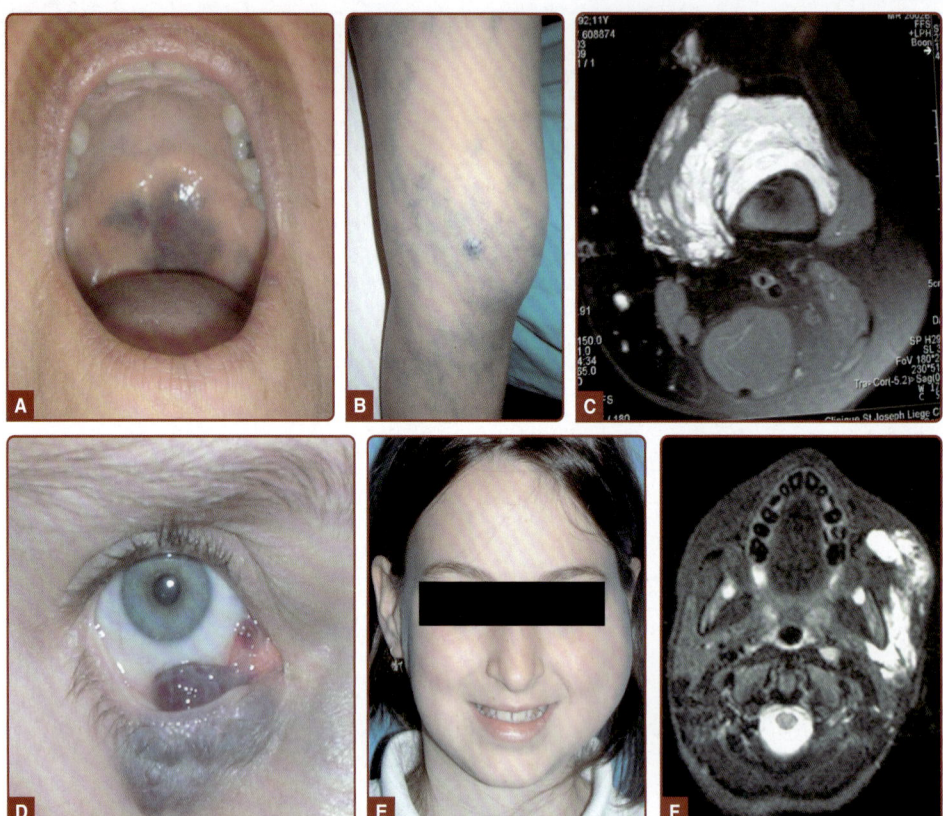

Figure 147-12 Various venous malformations. **A.** Of the soft palate, causing sleeping apnea. **B** and **C,** Of the knee, causing hemarthroses; confirmed by T2-weighted images. **D.** Of the mucosal eyelid. **E** and **F,** Of the cheek, causing facial asymmetry and pain.

VMs are congenital, light to dark bluish lesions. Deep VM has a normal overlying skin color and is often diagnosed only at puberty or later in life with the onset of pain. Size varies from small spongy blebs to large lesions of several centimeters in diameter. Skin temperature is normal. There is no thrill or bruit. VMs are larger when in a dependent position and can easily be emptied by compression or facilitating venous drainage. Palpation is not painful unless thrombosis occurs.[54,59]

VM lesions in VMCM are small and multifocal. They are more reminiscent of small sporadically occurring VMs than BRBNs. They can enlarge with time and are often asymptomatic. The VMs are generally small (<5 cm), and more than 80% of patients have more than two lesions. Some are present at birth; most lesions appear by puberty. Mucosal lesions involve the lips, tongue, and buccal mucosa.[60,61]

In rare instances, VM can be sporadic yet multiple. These multifocal venous malformations (MVMs) are very similar to the VMCM lesions, yet there is no family history of the same findings.[15]

GVM is a bluish to purple, raised venous anomaly characterized by multifocality, hyperkeratosis, and nodularity with a cobblestone surface (see Fig. 147-13C). In rare cases (especially in newborns), the lesions may be flat and purple in color, mimicking CM[62]; this plaque-like GVM usually darkens with time. GVMs are usually present at birth and slowly expand during childhood. New small lesions appear with time. In contrast to VM, GVM is often painful on palpation and cannot be completely emptied by compression. GVMs are usually multifocal and located on the extremities, involving the skin and subcutis. They are rarely encountered in mucosae, and intestinal hemorrhage is not present. Patients with GVMs have normal mental and physical development. Diagnosis of GVM is based on clinical and histologic evaluation of the cutaneous lesions. Genetic testing can differentiate small multifocal GVMs from VMCMs.[55]

Verrucous Venous Malformation:

Verrucous venous malformation (VVM), previously known as verrucous hemangioma, is a rare congenital vascular anomaly. Although VVM expresses an immunohistochemical profile similar to vascular neoplasms (Wilms tumor 1 and GLUT-1 positive), it is distinct from infantile hemangioma because it is usually noted at birth and never spontaneously involutes. Mainly located on the legs, VVM can also be found on the head and the trunk. It initially appears as a bluish macule that later becomes erythematous-violaceous in color and after trauma and secondary infections often evolves into a verrucous nodule (see Fig. 147-14). It never involves muscles or deep tissues.[63]

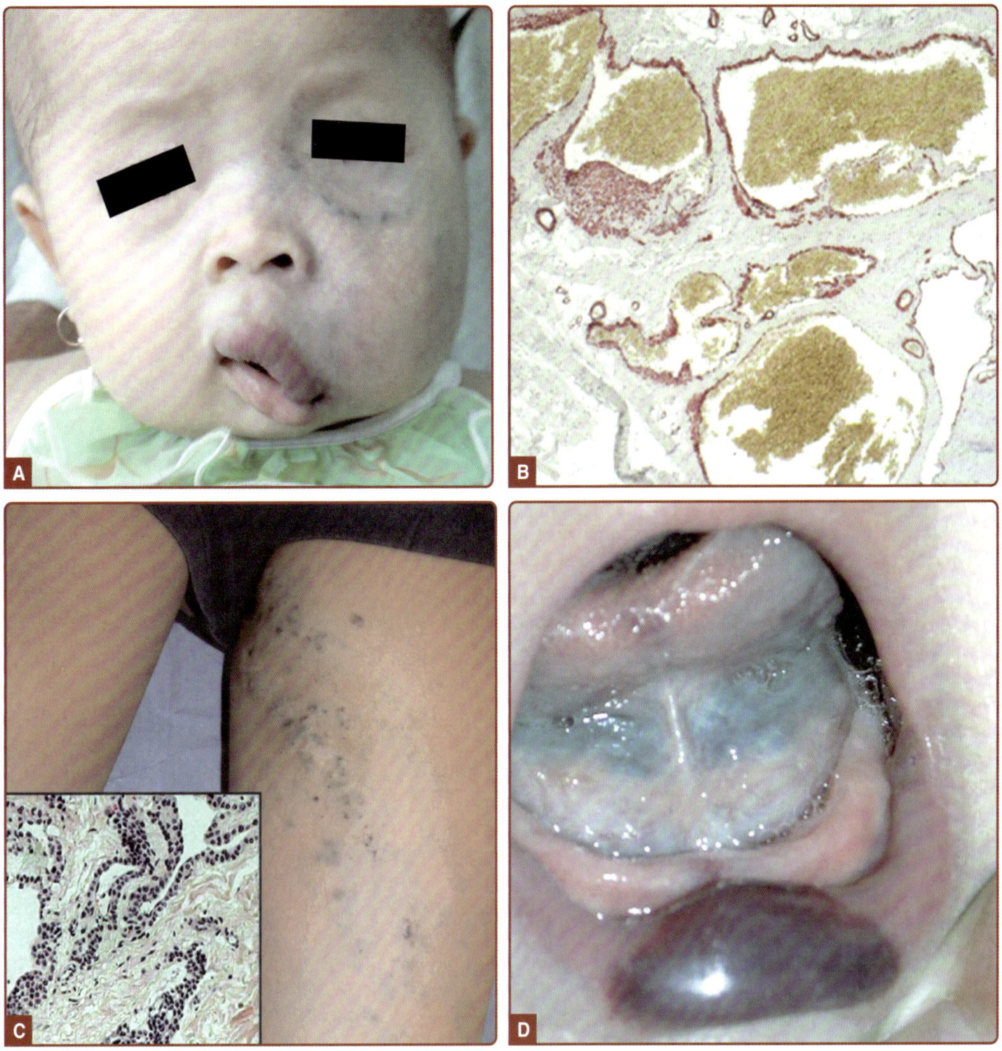

Figure 147-13 Venous malformations (VMs). **A,** Extensive hemifacial VM causing soft tissue hypertrophy and lip deformation in a 6-month-old boy. **B,** Histologically, VM consists of ectatic venous-like channels with anomalies in mural cells (hematoxylin and eosin). **C,** Superficial glomuvenous malformation of the inner thigh. Note the presence of mural glomus cells on histology (hematoxylin and eosin). **D,** Mucosal VM involving the lower lip and floor of the mouth.

NONCUTANEOUS FINDINGS

Patients with VMCM, like those with sporadically occurring MVM, seldom have VMs located in internal organs, such as the lungs, kidneys, brain, or GI tract.[15] Extracutaneous manifestations of BRBN include GI tract involvement. The small bowel is the predominant region; however, VMs can occur in any site from the oral cavity to the anal mucosa. In rare instances, VMs can also be seen in brain, lungs, and kidneys, as well as other organs.[57]

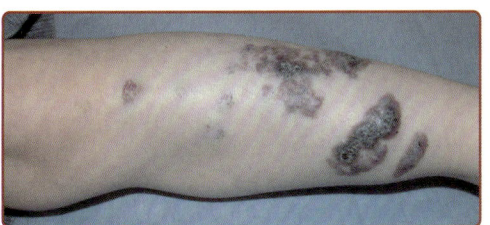

Figure 147-14 Verrucous venous malformation (previously known as verrucous hemangioma) on the lower extremity, causing oozing. It is purple-red in color and slightly raised, with hyperkeratosis.

COMPLICATIONS

VM is usually unilateral, causing asymmetry and progressive, slowly worsening distortion (see Figs. 147-12 and 147-13). Depending on their size and location, VMs can cause pain, particularly in the morning on awakening, and anatomic distortion and can even threaten life because of bleeding, expansion, or obstruction of vital structures. Migraine is a common feature when VM is located in the temporal muscle. Whereas oropharyngeal

VM can impair speech and cause difficulties in swallowing, pharyngeal or laryngeal lesions can compromise the airway and cause snoring and sleeping apnea.[54]

On the extremities, VMs often involve muscles and joints. They cause *muscle weakness, hypotrophy*, and sometimes hypertrophy, resulting in leg-length discrepancy, which is less severe than in KTS. Intraarticular bleeding, if the malformation is located in the knee joint, leads to early-onset arthrosis.[64] Genital VM often occurs with limb VM and can cause dyspareunia. GI VM may lead to chronic anemia.

Local thrombosis is usually responsible for acute pain that lasts for several days and resolves as phleboliths, which can be identified by palpation or by radiography. VM rarely causes pulmonary embolism, although this complication can occur when large draining veins exist.[65,66]

Chronic localized intravascular coagulopathy (LIC) is associated with solitary or syndromic spongy VMs. It is characterized by elevated D-dimer level (>500 ng/mL) in 40% of patients. Severe LIC with low fibrinogen levels is common in large VMs of the extremities and rare in the cervicofacial area. A number of events, such as surgery, sclerotherapy, and hormonal influences, can trigger the conversion of LIC to disseminated intravascular coagulopathy (DIC).[67]

In contrast to skin lesions, GI lesions, as seen in patients with BRBN, have a tendency to bleed. They may spontaneously rupture, causing acute hemorrhage and even death. However, most of the bleeding tends to progress slowly, resulting in chronic and occult blood loss that can lead to iron-deficiency anemia. Other complications include intussusception, volvulus, and bowel infarction, which are to be considered in patients with BRBN and abdominal pain. Morbidity depends on the extent of GI involvement.[57] VVM often ulcerates.[63]

ETIOLOGY AND PATHOGENESIS

VMCM is inherited as an autosomal dominant disorder caused by germline mutations in the *TEK* gene, which encodes the angiopoietin receptor, TIE2.[68,69] The inherited mutations cause hyperphosphorylation of the receptor even in the absence of a ligand. Somatic second hits have been found in VMCM tissues of two patients: one caused loss of membranous expression of the second, wild-type, allele; two others occurred on the allele with the inherited mutation, causing an increase in hyperphosphorylation.[15,70] These mutations activate the PI3K/AKT signaling pathway in endothelial cells.[71,72]

GVM is caused by dominant, loss-of-function mutations in the *glomulin* gene.[73] In addition, a somatic second hit is required for lesions to form, leading to complete loss of function of glomulin. The most common second hit is acquired uniparental isodisomy, which leads to homozygosity of the inherited mutation.[73,74] This explains the variable expressivity regarding penetrance, the extent of the lesions, and the number of lesions within family members.[75] So far, a mutation in *glomulin* has been found in almost all GVM families tested, demonstrating locus homogeneity.[75-77] Glomulin seems to be expressed in vascular smooth muscle cells, but its exact function remains unknown.

Sporadic VMs are also caused by genetic mutations. Sixty percent are caused by activating somatic mutations in *TIE2*.[70] The mutations differ from the inherited ones seen in VMCM. The most common mutation in VMs (L914F) has not been identified in VMCM, and the most common inherited mutation in VMCM (R849W) has not been identified in single somatic VM. This suggests that whereas the recurrent somatic mutations have effects too detrimental to be supported in the germline and probably cause lethality, the inherited ones have weaker effects that require additional changes (somatic second hits).[70-72]

Another 20% of sporadically occurring VMs are caused by somatic mutations in the *PIK3CA* gene.[10] The same mutations are seen in cancers. They activate the PI3K/AKT signaling pathway, as do the mutations in *TIE2*, underscoring perturbations in this signaling activity to underlie pathogenesis of VMs.[10,11]

MVM is also caused by *TIE2* mutations. Similar to VMCM, these patients often have two *TIE2* mutations. Most frequently, a R915C mutation is present as a mosaic change, and a somatic Y897C mutation occurs on top of the R915C change on the same allele. This explains the lack of family history (the first mutation has appeared de novo in a mosaic fashion in the patient), multifocality (the mosaic mutation is a predisposing change, like the inherited mutations are in VMCM), and the clinical similarity with VMCM lesions (both have similar, albeit not the same, double cis mutations).[15] VVM is caused by somatic *MAP3K3* mutations.[78] BRBN syndrome, like VMCM, MVM, and 60% of VMs, is also caused by mutations in *TIE2*. BRBN mutations are not detectable in the blood; they are somatic.[15] Yet in distinct, distally located lesions of the same patient with BRBN, the same double mutations can be identified with equal allele frequencies. The most common is a T1105N–T1106P double mutation. This suggests that the separate and even newly appearing lesions are formed by endothelial cells that originate form a single common site, such as the dominant lesion or bone marrow. The BRBN-causing *TIE2* mutations cause strong hyperphosphorylation of the receptor, and the endothelial cells acquire increased colony-forming capacity, survival, and faster migration.[15]

Maffucci syndrome is caused by somatic mutations in *IDH1 and 2*.[79-81]

DIAGNOSIS

SUPPORTIVE STUDIES

Laboratory Testing: A coagulation profile with platelet count, fibrinogen, and D-dimer level should be done in any patients with a pure VM or complex malformation with a venous component because the D-dimer level is elevated in about 40% of VMs. This blood test, done at the first consultation, should be repeated around puberty and whenever the malformation becomes painful. This is never the case in a patient with GVM or other simple vascular anomalies. Associated low fibrinogen is pathognomonic of severe LIC. Severe LIC can easily decompensate to DIC with severe bleeding during interventional or surgical procedures.[67,82-84]

Pathology: VMs are histologically composed of ectatic vascular channels of venous type with flat endothelium. The vascular walls are thin and lined by a discontinuous layer of mural smooth muscle cells positive for smooth muscle-α-actin.[85] Basement membranes are also thin. In contrast, GVM is histologically characterized by distended venous channels surrounded by mural "glomus cells," which are aberrantly differentiated smooth muscle cells. Glomus cells are round or polygonal, instead of being elongated, like the normal vascular smooth muscle cells.[86] By immunohistochemistry, glomus cells stain positively for smooth muscle-α-actin and vimentin, but they are negative for desmin, von Willebrand factor, and S100.[87] By in situ hybridization, they are also negative for glomulin.[76]

VVM is characterized by hyperkeratotic epidermis on top of small blood vessels with a multilaminated membrane located in the dermis and the subcutis. Focal positive staining for GLUT-1 is seen.[63] Histopathologic examination of patients with Maffucci syndrome shows features of spindle cell hemangioendothelioma.

Imaging: Plain radiography can identify the calcification of phleboliths, which are pathognomonic of LIC in a VM. It can also show the presence of multiple enchondromas in patients with Maffucci syndrome (see Fig. 147-11). Doppler ultrasonography is noninvasive and can confirm the slow-flow nature of the lesion. In contrast to lymphatic malformations (LMs), the venous channels are compressible with the probe.[88] MRI imaging with spin-echo T1- and T2-weighted and fat-saturation sequences depicts the exact anatomic location of the lesion (see Fig. 147-12).[89] This will highlight the more cellular component, as well as the more superficial location of GVM compared with VM. Atypical MRI findings require a biopsy to rule out a sarcoma or neurofibroma.

In the presence of palmar-plantar multifocal lesions typical of BRBN (see Fig. 147-10), an endoscopy, colonoscopy, or wireless capsule endoscopy should be performed to detect GI lesions.

These radiologic examinations are mandatory for pretherapeutic evaluation of any venous anomaly.

Genetic Testing: Consider genetic testing for *TIE2* and *glomulin* mutations in patients with multifocal lesions. This differentiates the conditions and enables genetic counseling.

DIFFERENTIAL DIAGNOSIS

See Table 147-6.

An unusual pathway of cerebral drainage, a cerebral developmental venous anomaly that consists of dilated intramedullary veins converging into a larger draining vein, can be seen in 0.5% of the population. In contrast, it is present in 20% of patients with extensive head and neck VMs. Although usually asymptomatic, this anomaly can cause headache.

TABLE 147-6
Differential Diagnosis of Venous Malformation

Based on Morphology

Most Likely

Bluish subcutaneous mass, noncompressible
- Infantile hemangioma (deep)
- Lymphatic malformation

With multiple enchondromas
- Maffucci syndrome

Consider

Hyperkeratotic
- GVM, if on extremity
- Cutaneous lesions of CCM
- VVM

Rule Out

Superficial, collateral normal veins
- Deep venous insufficiency, iatrogenic stenosis, or congenital agenesis

Bluish nonvascular lesion

Based on Location

Consider

Base of the nose
- Normal prominent veins

Scalp or forehead
- Sinus pericranii
- Underlying Galen malformation

Subungual
- Solitary glomus tumor

Cheek
- Blue nevus

Brain
- Developmental venous anomaly
- CCM

Rule Out

Neck; deep mass
- Thyroglossal duct
- Bronchogenic cyst

CCM, cerebral cavernous malformation; GVM, glomuvenous malformation; VVM, verrucous venous malformation

CLINICAL COURSE AND PROGNOSIS

VMs grow proportionately with the patient. They never regress spontaneously. Initially, asymptomatic lesions often become painful in response to trauma or in altered hormonal states (puberty or pregnancy). They may also expand following thrombosis. No oncogenic transformation of this condition has been described. The major complications are life-threatening GI hemorrhage and airway compression. Patients with inherited venous anomalies, as well as BRBN and MVM, tend to develop additional small lesions with time.[15] Patients with Maffucci syndrome have a high incidence of malignancies (40%), mainly chondrosarcoma but also glioma, fibrosarcoma, and angiosarcoma.[58]

MANAGEMENT

Treatment of venous anomalies is warranted when lesions are symptomatic or for cosmetic purposes. The most common indications for treatment are pain and functional impairment.[54] Their management is often multidisciplinary, involving hematologists, surgeons, and interventional radiologists.

INTERVENTIONS

Medical Management: Compression garments can be helpful to decrease swelling and pain in VMs of the extremity by decreasing venous pressure. In contrast, compression increases pain in GVM patients and is not indicated in this situation.

Low-molecular-weight heparin (LMWH; LMWH, 100 IU anti-Xa/kg/day) is usually given to patients with signs of LIC 24 hours before and for another 5 days after surgical procedures to minimize hemorrhagic risk. The same treatment is given to patients with painful episodes of local thrombosis. In this circumstance, the duration of treatment is usually 2 weeks.[54,67,84]

Bleeding from GI BRBN lesions can be managed conservatively with iron supplementation and blood transfusions.

With the understanding of the underlying pathophysiologic mechanisms (activation of the PI3K-AKT signaling), targeted molecular therapies are becoming possible. *Rapamycin* (sirolimus) was promising in a preclinical VM-mouse model trial.[90] A phase II clinical trial for difficult-to-treat extensive VMs or complex slow-flow vascular anomalies not amenable to conventional management also gave encouraging results.[90,91] Patients experienced almost complete relief of pain and symptoms, reduced coagulopathy when present, improved function, and increased self-perceived quality of life. Bleeding in sporadic VM as well as in BRBN stopped within 24 hours. Side effects were minor and included mucositis, mild headache, fatigue, and diarrhea. Moreover, a statistically significant reduction in volume was observed with MRIs in most patients that reached 1-year follow-up. A multicentric European Study (VASE; NCT 02638389) is ongoing to determine which subtypes of VMs are best suited for rapamycin treatment and for how long the treatment should be continued. Rapamycin should not be considered as treatment for small, localized, and asymptomatic slow-flow vascular malformations that respond to standard of care.[92]

Procedures: Percutaneous intralesional sclerotherapy is the primary treatment for VM, in contrast to GVM. Absolute ethanol is the most efficient sclerosing agent.[93] Local compression or intralesional coils are used to prevent dissemination of ethanol into the systemic circulation. Local complications include inflammation, edema, blistering, necrosis, chronic drainage, and temporary or permanent nerve deficit. Systemic complications, such as renal or pulmonary toxicity, myocardial depression, and cardiac arrest, have been reported. Multiple sclerotherapy sessions are often needed because VMs have a propensity to recanalize and recur. Alternatives to ethanol sclerotherapy are sodium tetradecyl-sulphate foam or lauromacrogol that are effective for small VMs and cause fewer local adverse effects. Positive response was seen in 49.5% (for pain) and 52.7% (for mass reduction), within the 86 patients (91 VMs) involved in one study.[94] Detergent sclerosants have been used as microfoams, using air bubbles or carbon dioxide to increase volume and surface contact with endothelium. However, neurologic complications have been described in 2% of cases. A modified radiopaque ethanol sclerosing agent was therefore developed. It traps ethanol within a mesh of ethylcellulose to increase viscosity.[95,96]

Surgical resection is often performed after sclerotherapy.[53] In patients with BRBN, endoscopic coagulation with Nd:YAG (neodymium-doped yttrium aluminum garnet)laser, bipolar or argon plasma coagulation, and band-ligation are useful. An open surgery allowing surgical resection of all GI lesions can eradicate the need for blood transfusion as well as the common intermittent abdominal pain caused by intussusception.[97,98] In patients with GVM, skin graft is often needed if excision is undertaken. VVM is also best treated with surgical resection. Closure often necessitates a skin graft.

Counseling: In patients with VMCM or GVM, genetic counseling should be provided for affected families, informing patients of a 50% risk of inheriting the disease-causing mutation and of the variability in clinical expression. Psychosocial counseling and patient organizations dedicated to vascular anomalies are also an important asset for patients and their families.

LYMPHATIC ANOMALIES

AT-A-GLANCE

- Worldwide occurrence of LM is unknown, but it is less frequent than that of VM.
- Congenital, sporadic, slow-flow malformations of lymphatic vessels
- LMs consist of micro- or macrocysts filled with lymphatic fluid.
- Histologically consist of dilated lymphatic channels with flat endothelium that expresses D2-40.
- Primary lymphedema can be inherited as an autosomal trait.
- Infection is the most common complication that can lead to septicemia.

INTRODUCTION

LMs are localized morphogenic errors of the lymphatic vessels. They consist of small vesicles or large cysts filled with lymphatic fluid. Macrocystic LM can be diagnosed in utero as early as the first trimester of pregnancy.[99] However, most LMs are diagnosed during infancy, before the age of 2 years. Some can manifest only at puberty or during adulthood. They can be isolated, combined with other vascular anomalies, or be part of a syndrome.

Primary lymphedema is not a localized lesion but a more generalized condition, in which the lymph fluid accumulates in the interstitial tissue. Lower extremities are most commonly affected. It can be uni- or bilateral. Primary lymphedema can be an isolated condition or part of a syndrome, and it can occur sporadically or as an inherited disorder.

EPIDEMIOLOGY

LM is a congenital disorder of unknown incidence. It occurs sporadically in contrast to primary lymphedema, which can be inherited, usually as an autosomal dominant trait, in up to 20% of cases. Primary lymphedema is divided into congenital (Milroy disease, Online Mendelian Inheritance in Man [OMIM] #153100) and late onset (presenting at puberty, Meige disease, OMIM #153200). It can be isolated or part of a syndrome, such as in Turner and Noonan syndromes.[100]

SYNDROMIC DISORDERS

KLIPPEL-TRENAUNAY SYNDROME

Klippel-Trenaunay syndrome is a combined capillary–lymphatic–venous malformation associated with hypertrophy of the affected limb. Lower limbs are affected in 70% of cases. It is characterized by a geographic, widespread CM associated with lymphatic vesicles. The persistence of a persistent embryonic vein located on the lateral side of the thigh is pathognomonic.[101,102]

CLOVES SYNDROME

CLOVES syndrome is an eponym for congenital lipomatous overgrowth with vascular malformations, epidermal nevi, and skeletal anomalies.[103] This nonhereditary disorder is characterized by progressive asymmetric hypertrophy, multiple truncal lipomatous masses with paraspinal fast-flow or slow-flow vascular anomalies (or both), epidermal nevus or nevi, acral lesions, and skeletal or spinal anomalies (Fig. 147-15). The most important differential diagnoses are other

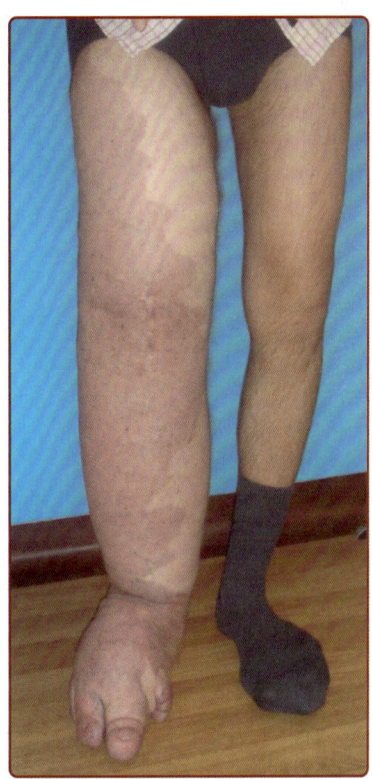

Figure 147-15 Capillary–lymphatic–venous malformation of right lower extremity with soft tissue hypertrophy (CLOVES syndrome).

overgrowth syndromes, such as the Proteus syndrome and Proteus-like syndrome.[104]

GENERALIZED LYMPHATIC ANOMALY

Generalized lymphatic anomaly (GLA) is a rare condition in which LMs can invade several organs such as the mediastinum, lungs, pleura, GI tract, bones, and soft tissue.[105]

GORHAM-STOUT SYNDROME

Gorham-Stout syndrome, or "vanishing bone disease," is an aggressive rare lymphatic disorder characterized by progressive demineralization and destruction of bones, which are replaced by lymphatic vessels and capillaries.[106]

CLINICAL FEATURES

CUTANEOUS FINDINGS

LMs are composed of microcysts (Figs. 147-16 and 147-17), previously termed *lymphangioma circumscriptum*) or macrocysts (>1 cm in diameter, previously known as *cystic hygroma*) that grow proportionally with the child (see Figs. 147-1B, 147-16, and 147-17). They are filled with clear or serosanguineous fluid (see Fig. 147-17B). Whereas macrocystic LM manifests as a soft, multilobulated, well-defined mass, microcystic LMs are ill-defined and often invade adjacent structures. Dermal LMs can manifest as small, millimeter-sized vesicles, clear (see Figs. 147-16D and 147-17A) or dark red in color (when there is intracystic bleeding), that can bleed and become purple and nodular.

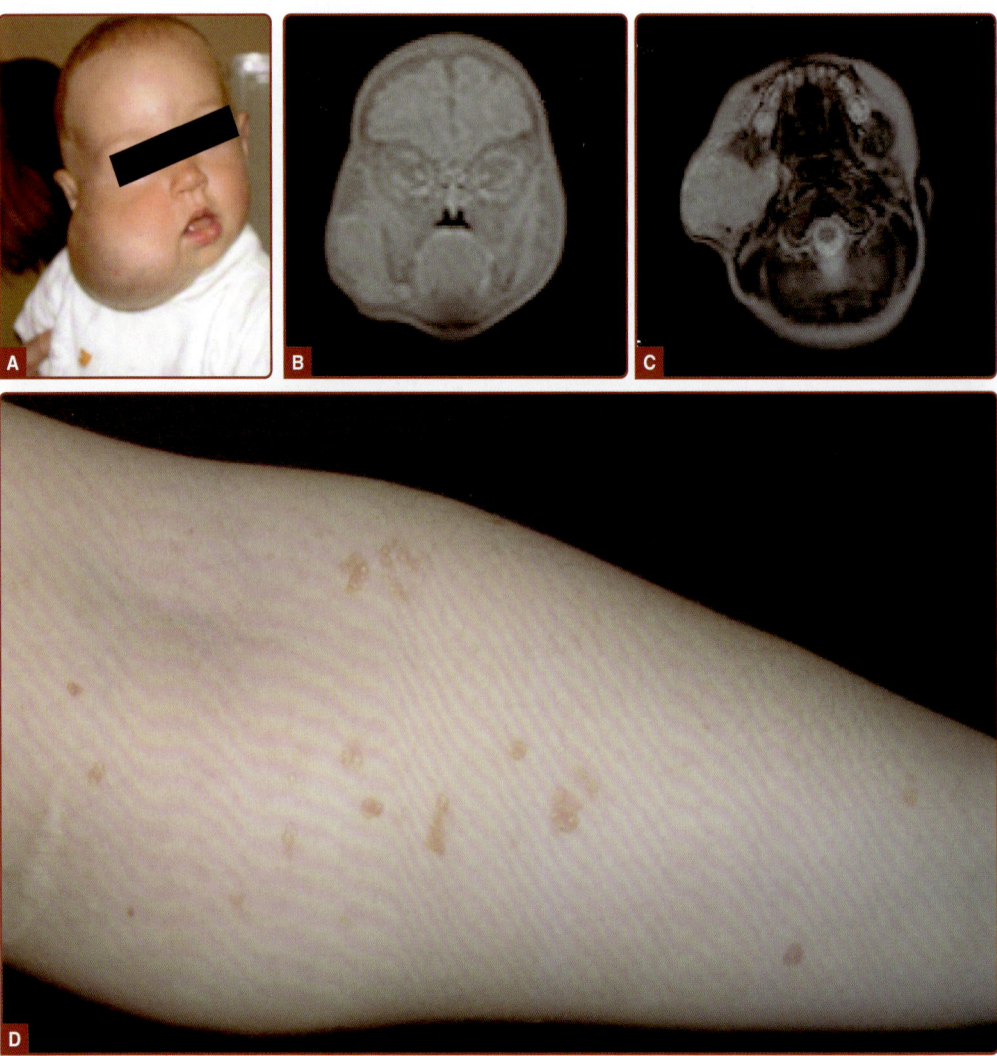

Figure 147-16 Various aspects of lymphatic malformation (LM). Bluish discoloration (**A**) of extensive LM of cheek, as seen on computed tomography scan (**B** and **C**). Small clear vesicles of dermal LM (**D**).

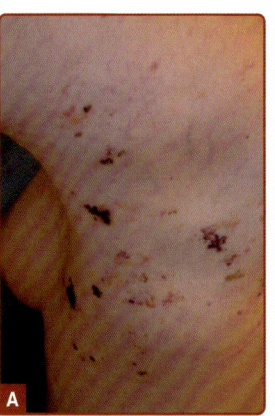 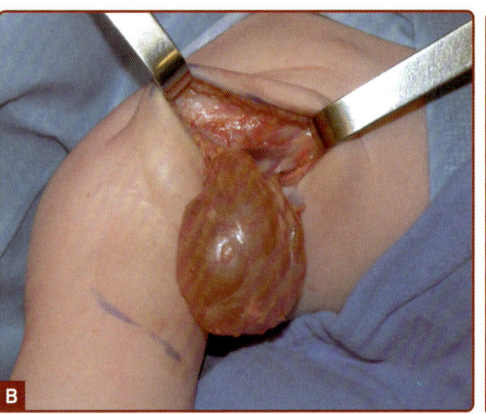 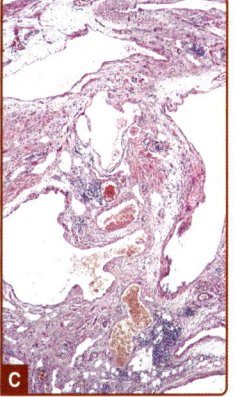

Figure 147-17 **A,** Microcystic, dermal lymphatic malformation (LM) consisting of clear and dark-red vesicles. **B,** Intraoperative view of a macrocystic LM of axilla showing a well-delineated cyst filled with clear lymph fluid. **C,** Histologically, LM consists of dilated lymphatic channels with flat endothelium (hematoxylin and eosin).

Angiokeratoma Circumscriptum: Angiokeratoma circumscriptum, or capillary-lymphatic malformation (CLM), is a combined, well-demarcated lesion often located on an extremity. The lesion is pink to bluish-red in color, slightly raised, and usually hyperkeratotic. Clinically, angiokeratoma circumscriptum, angiokeratoma of Mibelli (circumscribed, dark-red, hyperkeratotic plaques on distal extremities), and angiokeratoma of Fordyce (very common hyperkeratotic, blue-black papules on the scrotum of elderly men) are recognized. They are to be differentiated from angiokeratomas of Fabry disease (see Chap. 127) and from VVM (previously known as verrucous hemangioma; see earlier VM section).

Lymphedema: Lymphedema is characterized by swelling of the affected body part, usually a lower extremity, and caused by accumulation of lymphatic fluid into the extracellular space caused by intrinsic lymphatic dysfunction (Fig. 147-18). Various phenotypes exist depending on the age of onset, location, and associated anomalies.[107,108]

Congenital Lymphedema: Milroy disease is suspected in the presence of swelling of the dorsum of the feet with a family history of lymphedema. Lymphedema is present at birth, often bilateral, and affects the lower limbs below the knees.[109] Other features can be associated with congenital lymphedema, such as hydrocele (37% of males), prominent veins (23%), upslanting toenails (14%), papillomatosis (10%), or urethral abnormalities in males (4%).

NONCUTANEOUS FINDINGS

Pulmonary embolism can occur in patients with KTS or CLOVES syndrome.[110] Depending on the affected organ, symptoms such as pleural effusion, ascites, and malabsorption can occur in patients with GLA.[105] Painful pathological fractures are common in patients with Gorham-Stout syndrome.[106]

COMPLICATIONS

LM can suddenly enlarge in response to cough, inflammation, fever, viral or bacterial infection, or intralesional bleeding (Fig. 147-19). Recurrent cellulitis is the major complication, especially in patients with KTS, and it can evolve into septicemia if not promptly treated. Local redness and warmth appear, and the lesion becomes painful.

Facial asymmetry, especially of the mandible, is commonly associated with microcystic LM (see Fig. 147-16). Intraorbital LM is responsible for ocular dystopia and exophthalmia, as well as orbital enlargement. LM on the tongue impairs speech and produces oozing and halitosis. Airway obstruction is common when the base of the tongue or the cervicofacial area is affected.[111] Extensive limb LM can cause elephantiasis. Extension into the pleura can occur and cause chylothorax. Visceral LM can cause protein-losing enteropathy and hypoalbuminemia. Patients with KTS as well as patients with CLOVES are at high risk of pulmonary embolism because of the persistent embryonic vein and the presence of ectatic thoracic veins, respectively.[110]

Lymphedema is complicated by cellulitis in 20% of cases. More rarely, pleural effusion, even in utero; hydrops fetalis; and chylous ascites can be observed.[108,112,113]

ETIOLOGY AND PATHOGENESIS

LMs, as well as KTS and CLOVES syndrome, are caused by mosaic or somatic mutations in *PIK3CA* that activate the PI3K/AKT/mTor signaling pathway.[11,12,114,115]

More than 20 genes have been identified to be mutated in various forms primary lymphedema.[108] Milroy disease is caused by inherited loss-of-function mutations in vascular endothelial growth factor receptor 3 (*VEGFR3*).[116-118] Mutations in the same gene

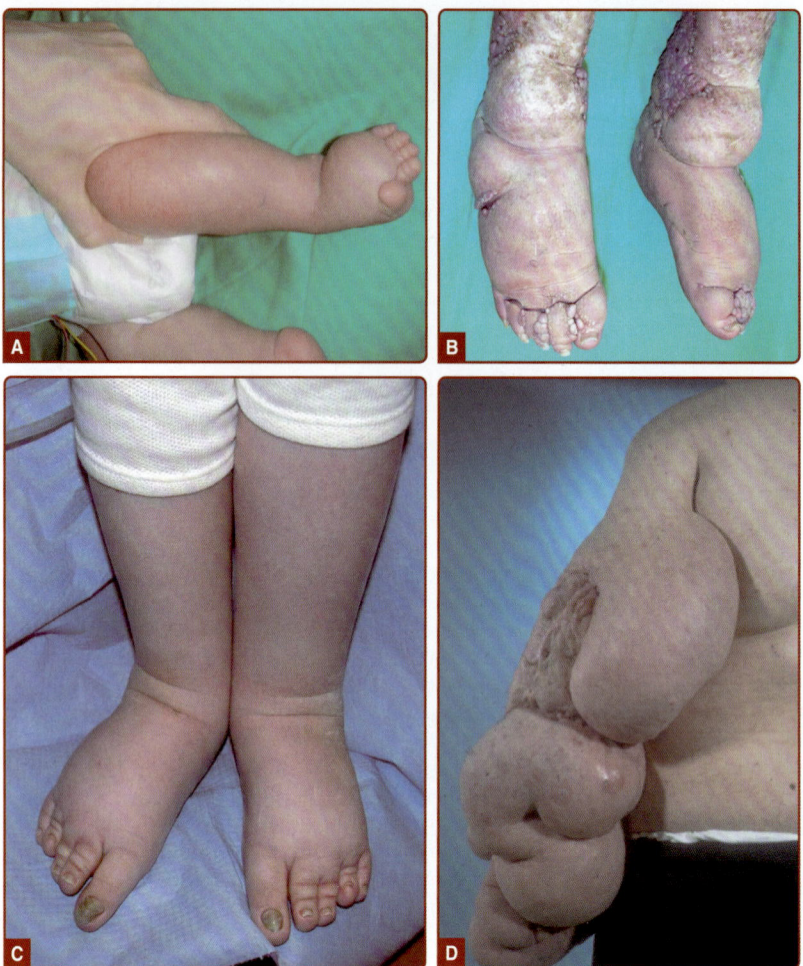

Figure 147-18 Various types of congenital primary lymphedema characterized by lymphedema of lower limb, below the knees (**A**); with papillomatosis (**B**); with upslanting toenails (**C**); that can evolve into elephantiasis (**D**).

are also responsible for sporadic hydrops fetalis and generalized subcutaneous edema.[119] Lymphedema-distichiasis is caused by loss-of-function mutations in the FOXC2 transcription factor.[120] Lymphedema associated with microcephaly, with or without chorioretinopathy or developmental delay, is caused

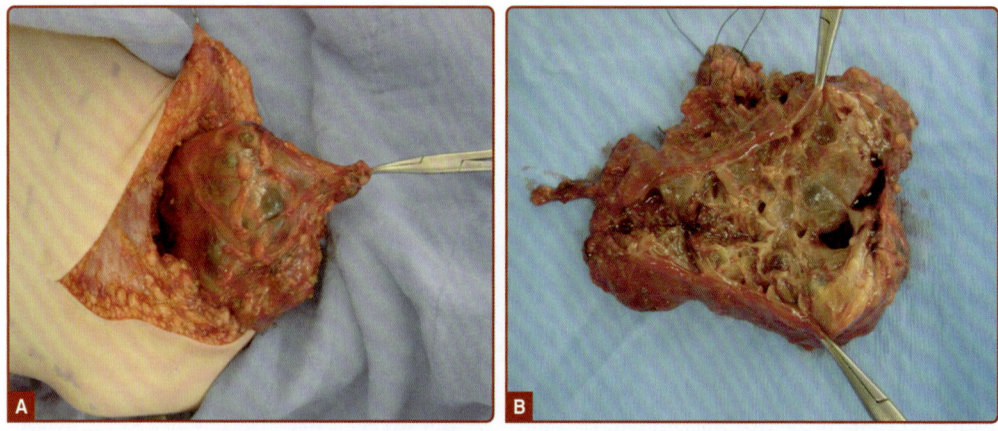

Figure 147-19 Intraoperative view of an axillary lymphatic malformation that had suddenly increased in size because of intracystic bleeding.

by dominantly inherited mutations in *KIF11*.[121,122] Hypotrichosis–lymphedema–telangiectasia, which has an autosomal-dominant or -recessive pattern of inheritance, is caused by mutations in *SOX18*.[118] Hennekam syndrome (OMIM #235510) is an autosomal recessive generalized lymphatic dysplasia characterized by intestinal lymphangiectasia with severe and progressive lymphedema of the limbs, genitalia, and face, as well as severe mental retardation.[123] Mutations have been identified in *CCBE1* (collagen and calcium-binding EGF domains 1).[107,124] Lymphedema is associated with hematologic malignancies in Emberger syndrome caused by *GATA2* mutations.[125] In about 35% to 40% of patients with familial primary lymphedema, a germline mutation can be identified.[108,126]

TABLE 147-7

Differential Diagnosis of Lymphatic Malformation

Most Likely
- Infantile hemangioma

Consider
- Venous malformation
- Teratoma
- Fibrosarcoma or rhabdomyosarcoma

Rule Out
Vulvar
- Acquired lymphangiectasia caused by radiotherapy
- Acquired lymphangiectasia caused by Crohn disease

DIAGNOSIS

SUPPORTIVE STUDIES

Pathology: LMs are characterized by dilated, flat-endothelium-lined channels of variable wall thickness (see Fig. 147-8C). No blood cells are seen in these spaces, except after intracystic bleeding or in the presence of a combined lymphatic-venous malformation. Macrocystic LM consists of a single or multiple lymphatic cysts surrounded by a thick fibrous membrane. The cysts do not communicate with each other. Endothelial cells express specific lymphatic markers, such as podoplanin, D2-40, and VEGFR-3.[44,127] Lymphedema is characterized by abnormalities in the primary peripheral lymphatic capillaries, collecting lymphatic vessels, or lymphatic valves and lymphovenous valves. This is pronounced in the affected limb but is sometimes also seen on the contralateral side. Extensive dermal fibrosis is often present.[44]

Imaging: Doppler ultrasound shows microcysts, macrocysts, or both separated by thin septa. In contrast to VMs, they are not compressible by the probe. MRI also demonstrates the cystic nature of the lesion, with often discernable fluid-fluid levels.[128,129] Computed tomography (CT) is the best study to show bony involvement.

Doppler ultrasonography of the deep venous system of the affected lower limb and the pelvic area is needed in patients with KTS and CLOVES. Moreover, because CLOVES syndrome is characterized by progressive overgrowth during infancy, careful follow-up every 6 months is recommended until the end of puberty. Follow-up consists of clinical examination, scaniometry (leg length films), and abdominal ultrasonography because of the increased risk of cryptorchidism, hydrocele, renal atrophy, and Wilms tumor.[130] Additional investigations should be done according to symptoms.

Genetic Testing: Genetic panel–based testing is available in accredited diagnostic laboratories. Such screens help identify germline mutations and can aid management. For example, identification of a germline *GATA2* mutation indicates specific cancer surveillance programs, and a *KIF11* mutation implies a need for detailed ophthalmologic and developmental examination.

DIFFERENTIAL DIAGNOSIS

See Table 147-7.

CLINICAL COURSE AND PROGNOSIS

LM usually grows with the child. It can cause asymmetry with bony overgrowth. Increases in size can be seen during infection or intralesional bleeding. Episodic reports of spontaneous involution exist. Because regression is commonly seen after local infection, it may be caused by postinflammatory autosclerosis. Patients with Gorham-Stout syndrome have a poor prognosis; it is lethal in 16% of cases.

MANAGEMENT

INTERVENTIONS

Medical Management: Systemic antibiotics should be used to treat intralesional bacterial infection as well as early cellulitis in both isolated and syndromic LM. Antiinflammatory drugs may be required to alleviate pain. Patients with CLOVES or KTS syndrome need to receive LMWH at prophylactic dosages of 100 anti-Xa/kg/day before any surgical procedure; this should be continued for another 10 to 20 days postoperatively to avoid perioperative decompensation of their coagulation abnormalities, and more importantly, to reduce the risk of life-threatening postoperative pulmonary embolism.[110] Rapamycin has been effectively

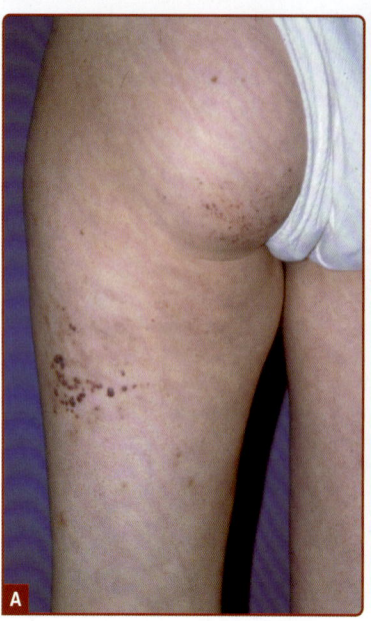 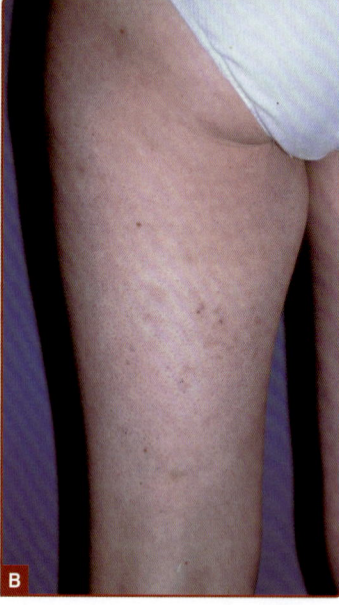

Figure 147-20 Dermal lymphatic malformation (**A**) efficiently treated with carbon dioxide laser (**B**).

used for extensive LMs resistant to standard treatment, as well as for patients with KTS and GLA. Although none had complete resolution, several patients experienced cessation of lymphatic leakage and infection and reduction of volume of the malformation. Side effects were minor.[131,132]

Lymphedema is best treated with elastic stockings, massage, and pneumatic compression devices. Sildenafil was suggested as effective in the treatment of LM,[133] but further studies have not confirmed its efficacy and highlighted potential side effects, such as infections and bleeding.[134,135]

Procedures: Nd:YAG laser or carbon dioxide laser photocoagulation has been used to treat dermal LM vesicles that cause oozing (Fig. 147-20). Macrocystic LM is treated with fluid aspiration followed by percutaneous, intralesional injection of sclerosing agents performed by an interventional radiologist. Sclerosing agents include sodium tetradecyl sulfate, pure ethanol, OK432 (extract from a killed strain of group A *Streptococcus pyogenes*: picibanil), doxycycline, and bleomycin. Side effects vary from fever and erythema to edema.[136,137]

Surgical resection is another alternative for LM, CLOVES, and KTS syndrome.[138,139] Results depend on the anatomical site and extension of the lesion. Recurrence is frequent because it is difficult to differentiate microcystic LM from adjacent normal tissue. This leads to either incomplete resection or unnecessary sacrifice of normal structures.

Counseling: Family and patient education regarding the cause and treatment is necessary for primary lymphedema because it can be inherited and associated with other important medical problems, necessitating inclusion in special surveillance programs. Psychosocial counseling and patient organizations dedicated to vascular anomalies are also an important help for patients and their families.

ARTERIOVENOUS MALFORMATIONS

AT-A-GLANCE

- Worldwide occurrence; rare but exact frequency unknown
- Congenital, fast-flow malformations that can be occult until puberty
- Histologically consist of direct communications between arteries and veins
- Usually sporadic but can have a genetic predisposition as in CM-AVM, hereditary hemorrhagic telangiectasia, or PHTS
- Most difficult vascular malformation to treat; need a multidisciplinary approach

INTRODUCTION

Fast-flow vascular malformations, namely AVM and AVF, are the most severe and devastating malformations. AVF is usually the result of trauma. AVM is characterized by the presence of a "nidus," the epicenter of the lesion that is composed of direct communications between multiple feeding arteries and draining veins without an intervening normal capillary bed. AVMs are present at birth, although they are not always visible. They can be localized or extensive and evolve with age.

EPIDEMIOLOGY

The incidence of AVM is unknown. No sex preponderance has been identified. It is a rare, usually sporadic, fast-flow vascular malformation. Hereditary hemorrhagic telangiectasia (HHT) is an autosomal inherited disorder with a prevalence of 1 in 5000 individuals.[140] CM-AVM is another familial form with autosomal dominant inheritance and a similar prevalence estimate.[19-23]

SYNDROMIC DISORDERS

BONNET-DECHAUME-BLANC OR WYBURN-MASON SYNDROME

Bonnet-Dechaume-Blanc or Wyburn-Mason syndrome is a sporadic, syndromic AVM located in the centrofacial or hemifacial area (or both), with oculo-orbital and cerebral involvement.[141] It rarely follows a trigeminal distribution like SWS. Intracerebral AVMs are common in Bonnet-Dechaume syndrome and can cause epistaxis, exophthalmos, and hemianopia. Mental retardation can also occur.

COBB SYNDROME

Cobb syndrome is another sporadic, syndromic AVM that associates cutaneous and spinal cord AVMs of the same metamere.[142] The cutaneous lesion masquerades as a CM, although it is warm on palpation. Cobb syndrome manifests in childhood with a sudden onset of back or lower extremity pain associated with sensory disturbance. Other neurologic complications (pain, sensory and motor disturbances, and neurogenic bladder) can occur depending on the location and extension of the AVM.

HEREDITARY HEMORRHAGIC TELANGIECTASIA

Individuals with HHT demonstrate combinations of the following triad: multiple cutaneous and mucosal telangiectasias, often located on the mucosal lip; epistaxis; and a positive family history.[143] The diagnosis is clinical, in accordance with the Curaçao criteria. The estimated frequencies of manifestations in HHT patients are spontaneous, recurrent epistaxis, 90%; skin telangiectasia, 75%; hepatic or pulmonary AVMs, 30%; and GI bleeding, 15%.[144] In 30% of patients with HHT, a hepatic, pulmonary, or cerebral AVM (or a combination of any of these AVMs) can be seen.[144] In contrast, in 23% of patients with CM-AVM1 and 13% of patients with CM-AVM2, an intracerebral or intraspinal AVM is present.[18,19,22,23,35]], but there is no risk for visceral AVM as in HHT. Vein of Galen aneurysmal malformation is also part of the phenotype. Recurrent epistaxis is typically the initial manifestation of HHT. The nosebleeds can be severe enough to require blood transfusions. Pulmonary AVMs affect approximately 30% of patients with HHT and are particularly common in HHT1. These patients are at higher risk of stroke and brain abscess than in the healthy population because the normal filtering function of the lung is lost. Migraine headaches occur in 13% to 50% of cases. Recurrent painless GI bleeding occurs in 10% to 40% of patients. Symptoms may include abdominal pain, jaundice, symptoms of high-output cardiac failure, and bleeding from esophageal varices.[145]

PARKES WEBER SYNDROME

Parkes Weber syndrome is characterized by a large, congenital, cutaneous, red vascular stain on an extremity in association with soft tissue and skeletal hypertrophy of the affected limb and underlying multiple arteriolar-venular microfistulas.[146] The affected extremity, often the lower one, is longer and larger than the contralateral one. Although often sporadic, it can be part of CM-AVM. In these cases, there are small, multifocal CMs located on other parts of the body. The signs and symptoms worsen with age. Affected patients can develop congestive heart failure.

PHOSPHATASE AND TENSIN HOMOLOG HAMARTOMA TUMOR SYNDROME

PHTS is an autosomal-dominant disorder that includes patients with Bannayan-Riley-Ruvalcaba syndrome and Cowden syndrome because 60% and 81% of them, respectively, have a mutation in *PTEN*.[147] These patients typically have macrocephaly, penile freckling, multiple developmental venous anomalies in the brain, fast-flow VMs (54%), and an increased risk of malignancy. The VMs are often multifocal (57%) and musculoskeletal and associated with ectopic fat deposition and disruption of the normal tissue architecture.[147,148]

CLINICAL FEATURES

CUTANEOUS FINDINGS

AVMs usually manifest as cutaneous, faint, red to purple, ill-defined masses with a thrill, a bruit, or a pulsation of increased amplitude (Figs. 147-21 to 147-23; see also Figs. 147-1D and 147-1E). About one third of AVMs are present at birth, another -third appear during childhood or at puberty, and the rest

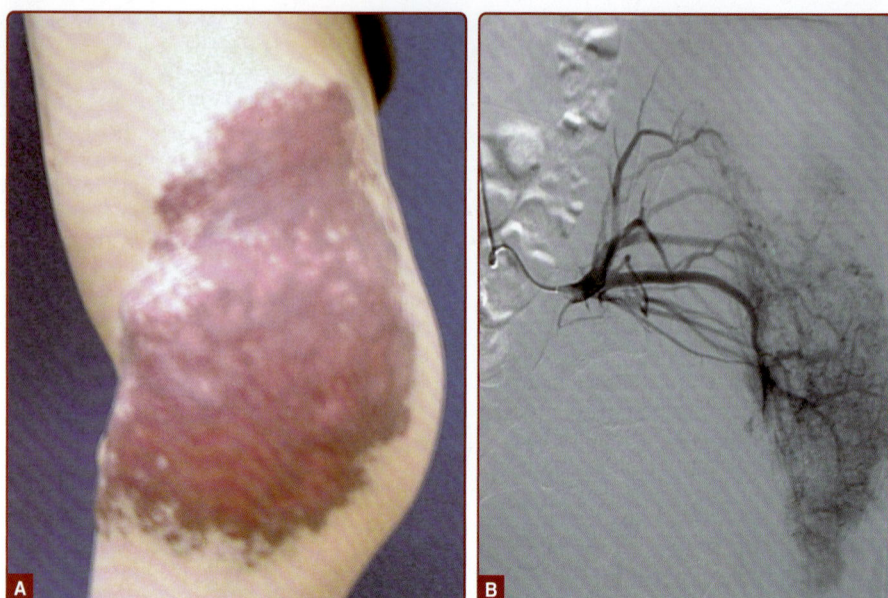

Figure 147-21 Stage 2 arteriovenous malformation of the left thigh mimicking an infantile hemangioma that did not disappear at 8 years of age (**A**). Arteriography showing the nidus confirmed the diagnosis (**B**).

manifest in adulthood because hormonal changes and trauma usually trigger the growth of an AVM. AVMs can affect any tissue and organ. Seventy percent of AVMs are located on the head and neck. They never regress spontaneously and get worse with time.[149] In 1985, Schobinger staged AVMs according to their severity. Schobinger stage I is a red stain with bruit and pulses of increased amplitude. With age, puberty, or trauma, AVM can worsen, and veins become prominent and tortuous (Schobinger stage II; Fig. 147-22) and subsequently darker and painful, and they ulcerate and bleed (Schobinger stage III; see Fig. 147-23). The final stage of a large AVM is cardiac failure (Schobinger stage IV; see Fig. 147-23).[150] The patient often reports hearing his or her cardiac pulse.

CM-AVM (see earlier discussion of CM-AVM) manifests as multiple atypical CMs that are randomly distributed (see Fig. 147-6) and associated with fast-flow lesions—AVM, AVF, or Parkes Weber syndrome—in 30% (CM-AVM1) or 20% (CM-AVM2) of patients. The expressivity is highly variable within families, from small, asymptomatic CMs to life-threatening AVMs. The fast-flow lesions (AVM or AVF) are either cutaneous or subcutaneous, with or without intramuscular and intraosseous involvement. About 10% to 15% of patients with CM-AVM have a Parkes Weber phenotype affecting the lower (two thirds of such cases) or the upper extremity. The AVMs can be asymptomatic, but complications occur depending on the location and size.[19-21]

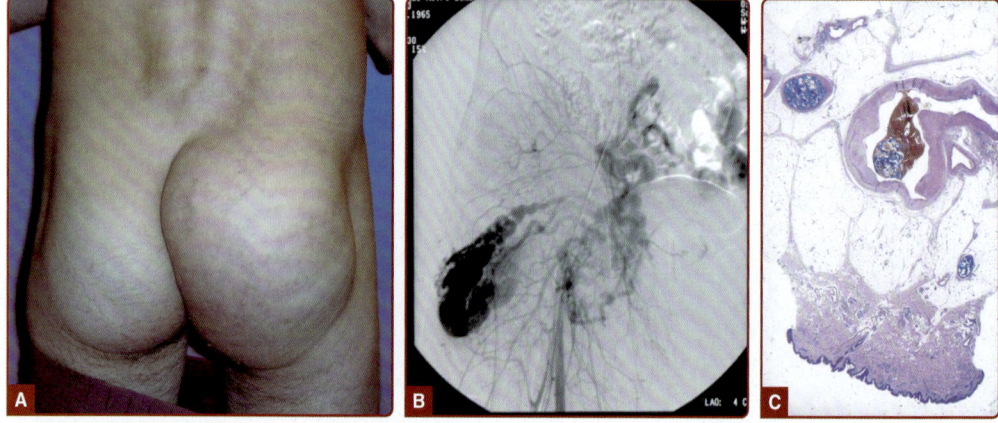

Figure 147-22 **A,** Extensive arteriovenous malformation deforming the right buttock. **B,** Arteriography showing nidus of the malformation. **C,** Histology shows direct connection between artery and vein, with thrombotic material secondary to embolization procedure.

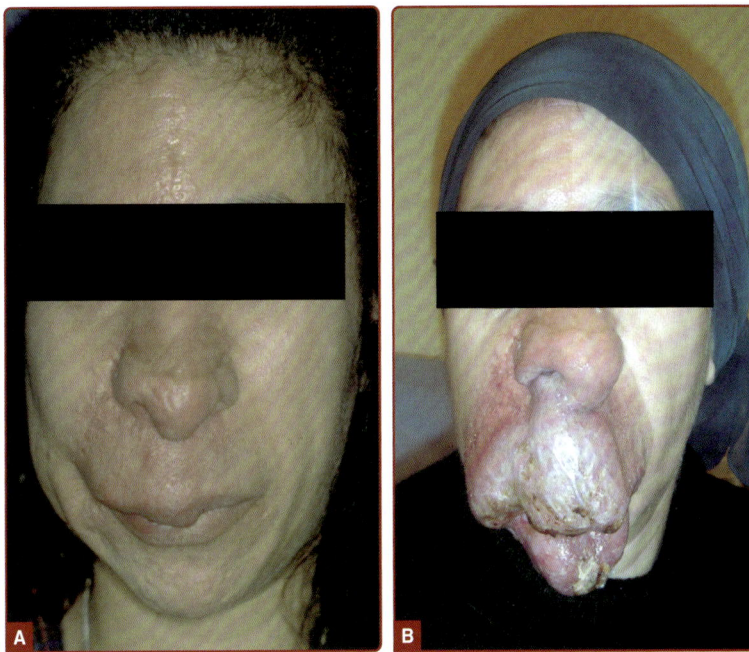

Figure 147-23 Stage 2 arteriovenous malformation (AVM; **A**) evolving into stage 4 AVM (**B**).

NONCUTANEOUS FINDINGS

In 30% of patients with HHT, a hepatic, pulmonary, or cerebral AVM (or a combination of any of these AVMs).[144] In 23% of patients CM-AVM1 and 13% of patients with CM-AVM2, an intracerebral or intraspinal AVM (or both) is present.[18,19,22,23,35]

COMPLICATIONS

AVMs involving the face can as well destroy the bone structure underneath and can cause gingival bleeding or epistaxis as well as hypertrophic asymmetry. Bony hypertrophy is a common feature of facial AVM, which causes asymmetry. AVM of an extremity often causes peripheral ischemia due to blood flow steel phenomenon. Cardiac failure is rare (Schobinger stage IV), especially during childhood. Puberty and trauma as well as hormonal influence can trigger appearance of AVMs. Intracerebral AVM such as in Bonnet-Dechaume syndrome, can cause epistaxis, exophthalmos, and hemianopia. Mental retardation can also occur.

Cobb syndrome manifests in childhood with a sudden onset of back or lower extremity pain associated with sensory disturbance. Other neurologic complications (pain, sensory and motor disturbances, and neurogenic bladder) can occur depending on the location and extension of the AVM.

Recurrent epistaxis is typically the initial manifestation of HHT. The nosebleeds can be severe enough to require blood transfusions. The prevalence of brain AVM is 1000-fold higher in patients with HHT1 than in the general population (1 in 10,000) and 100-fold higher in patients with HHT2. A similar increased risk is seen in CM-AVM1 and 2. Patients with HHT with pulmonary AVMs and telangiectasia of the GI tract are at risk for life-threatening hemorrhage. Other sites of bleeding may include sites in the kidney, spleen, bladder, liver, meninges, and brain. Strokes may be either hemorrhagic or ischemic.

These patients are at higher risk of stroke and brain abscess than in the healthy population because the normal filtering function of the lung is lost. Migraine headaches occur in 13% to 50% of the cases. Recurrent painless GI bleeding occurs in 10% to 40% of patients. Symptoms may include abdominal pain, jaundice, symptoms of high-output cardiac failure, and bleeding from esophageal varices.[145]

Patients with CM-AVM can exhibit intrauterine life-threatening intracerebral bleeding caused by vein of Galen aneurysmal malformation.[22,151] The brain and medullary AVMs can also bleed postnatally.[22,35,151]

ETIOLOGY AND PATHOGENESIS

Underlying genetic defects have been identified for the fast-flow vascular malformations of CM-AVM (OMIM #608354), HHT (OMIM #187300), and PHTS (OMIM #153480 and 158350). These disorders are inherited as an autosomal-dominant pattern with a penetrance of about 95% for the cutaneous CMs or telangiectasias.[18,19,22,151]

HHT is caused by alterations in the transforming growth factor-β signaling pathway. The genes implicated in HHT are *ENG*, encoding endoglin (HHT type 1), and *ACVRL1* (formerly called *ALK1*, HHT type 2); *SMAD4*, and *GDF2* are less frequently involved.[152-155]

Endoglin and ACVL1 are type III and type I transforming growth factor-β receptors, and both are well-expressed on vascular endothelial cells. Loss-of-function of this signaling concomitantly increases PI3K-AKT signaling.[156]

CM-AVM1 is caused by loss-of-function mutations in *RASA1*.[18,20] RASA1 encodes P120RASGAP, a GTPase regulating RAS activity. It converts the active GTP-bound RAS into its inactive GDP-bound form.[61,62,157] The high intrafamilial phenotypic variability is explained by the necessity of a somatic second-hit mutation to occur.[21,158] In 30% of patients with CM-AVM1, the mutation is de novo. CM-AVM2 is caused by loss-of-function mutation in *EPHB4*, which encodes an endothelial cell receptor in venous vessels. The ligand EPHRINB2, in contrast to EPHB4, is expressed in arterial endothelial cells. This bidirectional ligand–receptor system is important for arteriovenous identity and separation. EPHB4 signals using p120RASGAP, and the loss of function of either gene causes increased RAS-MAPK signaling.[18,159-162]

AVM can also be caused by loss-of-function mutation in *PTEN*, a tumor suppressor gene, as seen in patients with PHTS.[163] PTEN regulates PI3K-AKT activity, and this seems to be regulated at least in part by the HHT receptor complex (see earlier). Loss of function of one of the partners of this complex or of PTEN itself leads to activation of PI3K.

Sporadic extracranial AVMs are caused by somatic activating *MAP2K1 (MEK)* mutations.[14] Brain AVM are caused by another activating mutation in *KRAS*, which is also involved in the RAS-MAPK signaling pathway.[164]

DIAGNOSIS

SUPPORTIVE STUDIES

Pathology: Histologically, AVMs are poorly demarcated and consist of distorted arteries and veins with thickened muscle walls caused by arteriovenous shunting and fibrosis (see Fig. 147-22C).

Imaging: Ultrasonography and color Doppler show no mass but an aggregation of high-velocity arterial and pulsatile venous flow with low resistance. Vessels are tortuous. On the extremities, noninvasive follow-up is performed by comparing the arterial outflow of the affected limb with the unaffected one. MRI is preferred over CT to delineate the extent of an AVM and differentiate AVM from hemangiomas and other VMs. Flow voids, corresponding to fast-flow vessels, are pathognomonic of AVM. Arteriography is needed before any treatment to determine feeding arteries and the nidus (see Figs. 147-1E and 147-22B).

Genetic Testing: Genetic testing is indicated in patients with an AVM that is associated with multifocal cutaneous CMs (CM-AVM) or telangiectasias (HHT). Molecular diagnosis helps genetic counseling and guide further imaging for eventual undetected malformations. Patients with AVM with associated macrocephaly should be screened for *PTEN* mutations. Identification of a germline mutation would enable precise counseling and inclusion in cancer surveillance programs.

DIFFERENTIAL DIAGNOSIS

See Table 147-8.

During childhood, AVM is often mistaken for a CM or hemangioma because of its presentation as a faint, ill-defined, macular red stain. However, disproportionate warmth on palpation is a clue to its fast-flow component. A pulse, thrill, and bruit are other signs supporting AVM. Doppler ultrasonography can help differentiate a slow-flow CM from a fast-flow AVM or hemangioma. Hemangiomas have equatorial feeding arteries, peripheral veins, variable echogenicity, and fast flow but no true arteriovenous shunting.

Other dermatologic lesions can mimic AVM. Epithelioid hemangioendothelioma occurs in the extremity as a purple and locally aggressive lesion. Tumid lupus erythematosus, sarcoidosis of the face, and Melkersson-Rosenthal syndrome of the lip can mimic AVM. Dabska tumor can simulate an AVM on a child when it is located in the ear.

CLINICAL COURSE AND PROGNOSIS

AVMs tend to worsen with time, causing local destruction or life-threatening bleeding. Puberty and trauma trigger growth of the lesion. Improper management, often because of misdiagnosis, such as ligation of feeding arteries, or partial resection of the nidus, can have

---

TABLE 147-8

Differential Diagnosis of Arteriovenous Malformation

Most Likely

At birth
- Congenital hemangioma
- Infantile fibrosarcoma
- Other sarcoma

Rapid growth after birth
- Infantile hemangioma

Rule Out

Ear, nose
- Lupus erythematosus tumidus
- Sarcoidosis
- Dabska tumor

Lip
- Melkersson-Rosenthal syndrome

dramatic consequences and expansion of the AVM (see Fig. 147-23). The CMs in CM-AVM are harmless and usually of only cosmetic importance, although flow characteristics are commonly abnormal.

MANAGEMENT

This fast-flow VM is the most complex and difficult vascular anomaly to treat. Its management is multidisciplinary. AVMs should be followed by periodic evaluation. The goal of cure of an AVM is based on obliteration (by embolization) and complete removal of the nidus. Partial resection and proximal ligation of the feeding arteries lead to severe complications, recurrence, and reexpansion over time. Furthermore, ligature of the proximal arteries prevents access to the nidus for embolization, stimulates recruitment of new feeding arteries, and therefore expands the malformation. Mismanagement of AVM can lead to amputation.[19]

INTERVENTIONS

Medications: In a limb AVM or multiple AVFs, elastic stockings can stabilize the lesion and protect the skin, especially in the early stage. Because AVM is difficult to eradicate, the focus of management is often to control the evolution of the malformation rather than to cure the patient.[40,45] A pharmacologic approach with Marimastat, a synthetic matrix metalloproteinase inhibitor, has been used to treat extensive AVMs with good results. It reduced extension of the malformation and decreased pain and bruit.[46] Unfortunately, the drug is no longer available. Thalidomide was successfully used to reduce the frequency and duration of nosebleeds in patients with HHT.[165] It has also been used in unresectable stage 3 AVMs for which standard treatment had not been successful. For some patients, it was used in combination with embolization to improve efficacy.

Procedures: *Superselective embolization*: In contrast to AVF, superselective arterial embolization alone is only palliative and is done only in unresectable, complicated AVM. The embolized particles need to reach the epicenter of the lesion to avoid refilling of the nidus through new collaterals.[166] Direct puncture of the nidus is another possibility in patients with previous arterial ligation or embolization.[167] The most common materials are liquids (ethanol, isobutylcyanoacrylate), particles (Ivalon), foam, and implantable devices (coils, microspheres). Embolization is rarely curative unless performed for an arteriovenous fistula. Embolization can be used alone (palliative approach) or followed by complete surgical excision (curative approach). The site of injection must be as close as possible to the nidus to permit a superselective approach. Proximal occlusion is responsible of secondary refilling of the nidus through collateral arteries.[24]

Radical excision: Surgical resection is usually done only after embolization to minimize perioperative bleeding.[168] Excision should be complete and radical with carcinologic margins when possible. It is preceded with superselective embolization to occlude the nidus and reduce intraoperative bleeding.[19,26] The overlying skin can be saved if normal; otherwise, it is widely excised. Coverage options include tissue expansion or a local or free flap.[29] Cutaneous expansion can be done before embolization or surgery but may act as a trigger to stimulate growth of the malformation. Early intervention for "quiescent AVM" (Schobinger stage I) is debatable and should be considered only if complete resection is possible.[169] Follow-up for at least 5 years with annual Doppler ultrasonography or MRI (or both) is mandatory after any treatment.

For patients with Parkes Weber syndrome, treatment should be as conservative as possible. Epiphysiodesis may be necessary to control leg-length discrepancy. This procedure can sometimes aggravate the AVM.[146] For patients with HHT, multiple treatments have been tried to reduce bleeding, including topical application of antiinflammatory drugs, laser, or surgery. Because of the extensiveness of the lesions, they all give limited symptom-free intervals.

Counseling: Genetic counseling is mandatory in CM-AVM, HHT, and PHTS.

REFERENCES

1. Boon LM, Ballieux F, Vikkula M. Pathogenesis of vascular anomalies. *Clin Plast Surg*. 2011;38(1):7-19.
2. Mulliken JB, Glowacki J. Hemangiomas and vascular malformations in infants and children: a classification based on endothelial characteristics. *Plast Reconstr Surg*. 1982;69(3):412-422.
3. Mulliken JB. *Mulliken and Young's Vascular Anomalies: Hemangiomas and Malformations*. 2nd ed. New York: Oxford University Press; 2013.
4. Wassef M, Blei F, Adams D, et al. Vascular anomalies classification: recommendations from the International Society for the Study of Vascular Anomalies. *Pediatrics*. 2015;136(1):e203-e214.
5. Jacobs AH, Walton RG. The incidence of birthmarks in the neonate. *Pediatrics*. 1976;58(2):218-222.
6. Elajmi A, Clapuyt P, Hammer F, et al. Management of vascular anomalies in children. *Ann Chir Plast Esthet*. 2016;61(5):480-497.
7. Brouillard P, Vikkula M. Genetic causes of vascular malformations. *Hum Mol Genet*. 2007;16(Spec No. 2):R140-R149.
8. Limaye N, Boon LM, Vikkula M. From germline towards somatic mutations in the pathophysiology of vascular anomalies. *Hum Mol Genet*. 2009;18(R1):R65-R74.
9. Nguyen HL, Boon LM, Vikkula M. Genetics of vascular malformations. *Semin Pediatr Surg*. 2014;23(4):221-226.
10. Limaye N, Kangas J, Mendola A, et al. Somatic activating PIK3CA mutations cause venous malformation. *Am J Hum Genet*. 2015;97(6):914-921.
11. Boscolo E, Coma S, Luks VL, et al. AKT hyperphosphorylation associated with PI3K mutations in lymphatic endothelial cells from a patient with lymphatic malformation. *Angiogenesis*. 2015;18(2):151-162.

12. Luks VL, Kamitaki N, Vivero MP, et al. Lymphatic and other vascular malformative/overgrowth disorders are caused by somatic mutations in PIK3CA. *J Pediatr*. 2015;166(4):1048-54 e1-e5.
13. Shirley MD, Tang H, Gallione CJ, et al. Sturge-Weber syndrome and port-wine stains caused by somatic mutation in GNAQ. *N Engl J Med*. 2013;368(21):1971-1979.
14. Couto JA, Huang AY, Konczyk DJ, et al. Somatic MAP2K1 mutations are associated with extracranial arteriovenous malformation. *Am J Hum Genet*. 2017;100(3):546-554.
15. Soblet J, Kangas J, Natynki M, et al. Blue rubber bleb nevus (BRBN) syndrome is caused by somatic TEK (TIE2) mutations. *J Invest Dermatol*. 2017;137(1):207-216.
16. Burrows PE, Laor T, Paltiel H, et al. Diagnostic imaging in the evaluation of vascular birthmarks. *Dermatol Clin*. 1998;16(3):455-488.
17. Eerola I, Boon LM, Watanabe S, et al. Locus for susceptibility for familial capillary malformation ("port-wine stain") maps to 5q. *Eur J Hum Genet*. 2002;10(6):375-380.
18. Eerola I, Boon LM, Mulliken JB, et al. Capillary malformation-arteriovenous malformation, a new clinical and genetic disorder caused by RASA1 mutations. *Am J Hum Genet*. 2003;73(6):1240-1249.
19. Boon LM, Mulliken JB, Vikkula M. RASA1: variable phenotype with capillary and arteriovenous malformations. *Curr Opin Genet Dev*. 2005;15(3):265-269.
20. Revencu N, Boon LM, Mulliken JB, et al. Parkes Weber syndrome, vein of Galen aneurysmal malformation, and other fast-flow vascular anomalies are caused by RASA1 mutations. *Hum Mutat*. 2008;29(7):959-965.
21. Revencu N, Boon LM, Mendola A, et al. RASA1 mutations and associated phenotypes in 68 families with capillary malformation-arteriovenous malformation. *Hum Mutat*. 2013;34(12):1632-1641.
22. Revencu N, Boon LM, Mulliken JB, et al. RASA1 and capillary malformation-arteriovenous malformation. In: Erickson RP, Wynshaw-Boris A, eds. *Inborn Errors of Development: The Molecular Basis of Clinical Disorders of Morphogenesis*. New York: Oxford University Press; 2016:1423-1428.
23. Amyere M, Revencu N, Helaers R, et al. Germline loss-of-function mutations in EPHB4 cause a second form of capillary malformation–arteriovenous malformation (CM-AVM2) deregulating RAS-MAPK signaling. *Circulation*. 2017;136(11):1037-1048.
24. Enjolras O, Boukobza M, Jdid R. Cervical occult spinal dysraphism: MRI findings and the value of a vascular birthmark. *Pediatr Dermatol*. 1995;12(3):256-259.
25. Leung AK, Telmesani AM. Salmon patches in Caucasian children. *Pediatr Dermatol*. 1989;6(3):185-187.
26. Pratt AG. Birthmarks in infants. *AMA Arch Derm Syphilol*. 1953;67(3):302-305.
27. Ruiz-Maldonado R, Tamayo L, Laterza AM, et al. Phacomatosis pigmentovascularis: a new syndrome? Report of four cases. *Pediatr Dermatol*. 1987;4(3):189-196.
28. Happle R. Phacomatosis pigmentovascularis revisited and reclassified. *Arch Dermatol*. 2005;141(3):385-388.
29. Boukobza M, Enjolras O, Cambra M, et al. Sturge-Weber syndrome. The current neuroradiologic data. *J Radiol*. 2000;81(7):765-771.
30. Lee MS, Liang MG, Mulliken JB. Diffuse capillary malformation with overgrowth: a clinical subtype of vascular anomalies with hypertrophy. *J Am Acad Dermatol*. 2013;69(4):589-594.
31. Toriello HV, Mulliken JB. Accurately renaming macrocephaly-cutis marmorata telangiectatica congenita (M-CMTC) as macrocephaly-capillary malformation (M-CM). *Am J Med Genet A*. 2007;143A(24):3009.
32. Peterman CM, Vadeboncoeur S, Mulliken JB, et al. Wilms tumor screening in diffuse capillary malformation with overgrowth and macrocephaly-capillary malformation: a retrospective study. *J Am Acad Dermatol*. 2017;77(5):874-878.
33. Adams BB, Lucky AW. Acquired port-wine stains and antecedent trauma: case report and review of the literature. *Arch Dermatol*. 2000;136(7):897-899.
34. Larralde M, Abad ME, Luna PC, et al. Capillary malformation-arteriovenous malformation: a clinical review of 45 patients. *Int J Dermatol*. 2014;53(4):458-461.
35. Thiex R, Mulliken JB, Revencu N, et al. A novel association between RASA1 mutations and spinal arteriovenous anomalies. *Am J Neuroradiol*. 2010;31(4):775-779.
36. Segatto MM, Schmitt EU, Hagemann LN, et al. Phacomatosis pigmentovascularis type IIa—case report. *Ann Bras Dermatol*. 2013;88(6 suppl 1):85-88.
37. Hofer T. Meyerson phenomenon within a nevus flammeus. The different eczematous reactions within port-wine stains. *Dermatology*. 2002;205(2):180-183.
38. Klapman MH, Yao JF. Thickening and nodules in port-wine stains. *J Am Acad Dermatol*. 2001;44(2):300-302.
39. Valeyrie L, Lebrun-Vignes B, Descamps V, et al. Pyogenic granuloma within port-wine stains: an alarming clinical presentation. *Eur J Dermatol*. 2002;12(4):373-375.
40. Etchevers HC, Vincent C, Le Douarin NM, et al. The cephalic neural crest provides pericytes and smooth muscle cells to all blood vessels of the face and forebrain. *Development*. 2001;128(7):1059-1068.
41. Van Raamsdonk CD, Bezrookove V, Green G, et al. Frequent somatic mutations of GNAQ in uveal melanoma and blue naevi. *Nature*. 2009;457(7229):599-602.
42. Thomas AC, Zeng Z, Riviere JB, et al. Mosaic activating mutations in GNA11 and GNAQ are associated with phakomatosis pigmentovascularis and extensive dermal melanocytosis. *J Invest Dermatol*. 2016;136(4):770-778.
43. Riviere JB, Mirzaa GM, O'Roak BJ, et al. De novo germline and postzygotic mutations in AKT3, PIK3R2 and PIK3CA cause a spectrum of related megalencephaly syndromes. *Nat Genet*. 2012;44(8):934-940.
44. Wassef M, Vanwijck R, Clapuyt P, et al. Vascular tumours and malformations, classification, pathology and imaging. *Ann Chir Plast Esthet*. 2006;51(4-5):263-281.
45. Finley JL, Clark RA, Colvin RB, et al. Immunofluorescent staining with antibodies to factor VIII, fibronectin, and collagenous basement membrane protein in normal human skin and port wine stains. *Arch Dermatol*. 1982;118(12):971-975.
46. Breugem CC, Hennekam RC, van Gemert MJ, et al. Are capillary malformations neurovenular or purely neural? *Plast Reconstr Surg*. 2005;115(2):578-587.
47. Enjolras O, Riche MC, Merland JJ. Facial port-wine stains and Sturge-Weber syndrome. *Pediatrics*. 1985;76(1):48-51.
48. van der Horst CM, Koster PH, de Borgie CA, et al. Effect of the timing of treatment of port-wine stains with the flash-lamp-pumped pulsed-dye laser. *N Engl J Med*. 1998;338(15):1028-1033.

49. Michel S, Landthaler M, Hohenleutner U. Recurrence of port-wine stains after treatment with the flashlamp-pumped pulsed dye laser. *Br J Dermatol*. 2000;143(6):1230-1234.
50. Passeron T, Salhi A, Mazer JM, et al. Prognosis and response to laser treatment of early-onset hypertrophic port-wine stains (PWS). *J Am Acad Dermatol*. 2016;75(1):64-68.
51. Ville D, Enjolras O, Chiron C, et al. Prophylactic antiepileptic treatment in Sturge-Weber disease. *Seizure*. 2002;11(3):145-150.
52. Arzimanoglou AA, Andermann F, Aicardi J, et al. Sturge-Weber syndrome: indications and results of surgery in 20 patients. *Neurology*. 2000;55(10):1472-1479.
53. Boon LM, Vanwijck R. Medical and surgical treatment of venous malformations. *Ann Chir Plast Esthet*. 2006;51(4-5):403-411.
54. Dompmartin A, Vikkula M, Boon LM. Venous malformation: update on aetiopathogenesis, diagnosis and management. *Phlebology*. 2010;25:224-235.
55. Boon LM, Mulliken JB, Enjolras O, et al. Glomuvenous malformation (glomangioma) and venous malformation: distinct clinicopathologic and genetic entities. *Arch Dermatol*. 2004;140(8):971-976.
56. Brouillard P, Boon LM, Mulliken JB, et al. Mutations in a novel factor, glomulin, are responsible for glomuvenous malformations ("glomangiomas"). *Am J Hum Genet*. 2002;70(4):866-874.
57. Ballieux F, Boon LM, Vikkula M. Blue bleb rubber nevus syndrome. *Handb Clin Neurol*. 2015;132:223-230.
58. Kaplan RP, Wang JT, Amron DM, et al. Maffucci's syndrome: two case reports with a literature review. *J Am Acad Dermatol*. 1993;29(5 Pt 2):894-899.
59. Boon L, Mulliken J, Enjolras O, et al. Glomuvenous malformation ("glomangioma") is a distinct clinicopathologic and genetic entity. *Eur J Hum Genet*. 2002;10:123.
60. Boon LM, Vikkula M. Multiple cutaneous and mucosal venous malformations. In: Pagon RA, Bird TD, Dolan CR, Stephens K, eds. *GeneReviews*. Seattle; 1993.
61. Vikkula M, Boon LM, Carraway KL 3rd, et al. Vascular dysmorphogenesis caused by an activating mutation in the receptor tyrosine kinase TIE2. *Cell*. 1996;87(7):1181-1190.
62. Mallory SB, Enjolras O, Boon LM, et al. Congenital plaque-type glomuvenous malformations presenting in childhood. *Arch Dermatol*. 2006;142(7):892-896.
63. Tennant LB, Mulliken JB, Perez-Atayde AR, et al. Verrucous hemangioma revisited. *Pediatr Dermatol*. 2006;23(3):208-215.
64. Hein KD, Mulliken JB, Kozakewich HP, et al. Venous malformations of skeletal muscle. *Plast Reconstr Surg*. 2002;110(7):1625-1635.
65. Berenguer B, Burrows PE, Zurakowski D, et al. Sclerotherapy of craniofacial venous malformations: complications and results. *Plast Reconstr Surg*. 1999;104(1):1-11; discussion 12-15.
66. Rodriguez-Manero M, Aguado L, Redondo P. Pulmonary arterial hypertension in patients with slow-flow vascular malformations. *Arch Dermatol*. 2010;146(12):1347-1352.
67. Dompmartin A, Acher A, Thibon P, et al. Association of localized intravascular coagulopathy with venous malformations. *Arch Dermatol*. 2008;144(7):873-877.
68. Wouters V, Limaye N, Uebelhoer M, et al. Hereditary cutaneomucosal venous malformations are caused by TIE2 mutations with widely variable hyper-phosphorylating effects. *Eur J Hum Genet*. 2010;18(4):414-420.
69. Wouters V, Boon LM, Mulliken JB, et al. TIE2 and cutaneomucosal venous malformation. In: Epstein C, Erickson RP, Wynshaw-Boris A, eds. *Inborn Errors of Development: The Molecular Basis of Clinical Disorders of Morphogenesis*. 2nd ed. New York: Oxford University Press; 2008:491-494.
70. Limaye N, Wouters V, Uebelhoer M, et al. Somatic mutations in angiopoietin receptor gene TEK cause solitary and multiple sporadic venous malformations. *Nat Genet*. 2009;41(1):118-124.
71. Uebelhoer M, Natynki M, Kangas J, et al. Venous malformation-causative TIE2 mutations mediate an AKT-dependent decrease in PDGFB. *Hum Mol Genet*. 2013;22(17):3438-3448.
72. Nätynki M, Kangas J, Miinalainen I, et al. Common and specific effects of TIE2 mutations causing venous malformations. *Hum Mol Genet*. 2015;24(22):6374-6389.
73. Brouillard P, Ghassibé M, Boon L, et al. Identification of novel glomulin gene mutations responsible for inherited glomuvenous malformations (glomangiomas). *Am J Hum Genet*. 2002;71(4):521.
74. Amyere M, Aerts V, Brouillard P, et al. Somatic uniparental isodisomy explains multifocality of glomuvenous malformations. *Am J Hum Genet*. 2013;92(2):188-196.
75. Brouillard P, Ghassibe M, Penington A, et al. Four common glomulin mutations cause two thirds of glomuvenous malformations ("familial glomangiomas"): evidence for a founder effect. *J Med Genet*. 2005;42(2):e13.
76. Brouillard P, Enjolras O, Boon LM, et al. Glomulin and glomuvenous malformation. In: Epstein CJ, Erickson RP, Wynshaw-Boris A, eds. *Inborn Errors of Development: The Molecular Basis of Clinical Disorders of Morphogenesis*. 2nd ed. New York: Oxford University Press; 2008:1561-1565.
77. Brouillard P, Boon LM, Revencu N, et al. Genotypes and phenotypes of 162 families with a glomulin mutation. *Mol Syndromol*. 2013;4(4):157-164.
78. Couto JA, Vivero MP, Kozakewich HP, et al. A somatic MAP3K3 mutation is associated with verrucous venous malformation. *Am J Hum Genet*. 2015;96(3):480-486.
79. Couvineau A, Wouters V, Bertrand G, et al. PTHR1 mutations associated with Ollier disease result in receptor loss of function. *Hum Mol Genet*. 2008;17(18):2766-2775.
80. Pansuriya TC, van Eijk R, d'Adamo P, et al. Somatic mosaic IDH1 and IDH2 mutations are associated with enchondroma and spindle cell hemangioma in Ollier disease and Maffucci syndrome. *Nat Genet*. 2011;43(12):1256-1261.
81. Amyere M, Dompmartin A, Wouters V, et al. Common somatic alterations identified in Maffucci syndrome by molecular karyotyping. *Mol Syndromol*. 2014;5(6):259-267.
82. Mazoyer E, Enjolras O, Laurian C, et al. Coagulation abnormalities associated with extensive venous malformations of the limbs: differentiation from Kasabach-Merritt syndrome. *Clin Lab Haematol*. 2002;24(4):243-51.
83. Hermans C, Dessomme B, Lambert C, et al. Venous malformations and coagulopathy. *Ann Chir Plast Esthet*. 2006;51(4-5):388-393.
84. Dompmartin A, Ballieux F, Thibon P, et al. Elevated D-dimer level in the differential diagnosis of venous malformations. *Arch Dermatol*. 2009;145(11):1239-1244.

85. Wassef M, Enjolras O. Superficial vascular malformations: classification and histopathology. *Ann Pathol*. 1999;19(3):253-264.
86. Kato N, Kumakiri M, Ohkawara A. Localized form of multiple glomus tumors: report of the first case showing partial involution. *J Dermatol*. 1990;17(7):423-428.
87. Goodman TF, Abele DC. Multiple glomus tumors. A clinical and electron microscopic study. *Arch Dermatol*. 1971;103(1):11-23.
88. Paltiel HJ, Burrows PE, Kozakewich HP, et al. Soft-tissue vascular anomalies: utility of US for diagnosis. *Radiology*. 2000;214(3):747-754.
89. Konez O, Burrows PE. Magnetic resonance of vascular anomalies. *Magn Reson Imaging Clin North Am*. 2002;10(2):363-388, vii.
90. Boscolo E, Limaye N, Huang L, et al. Rapamycin improves TIE2-mutated venous malformation in murine model and human subjects. *J Clin Invest*. 2015;125(9):3491-3504.
91. Boon LM, Hammer J, Seront E, et al. Rapamycin as novel treatment for refractory-to-standard-care slow-flow vascular malformations. *Plast Reconstr Surg*. 2015;136(4 suppl):38.
92. Yuksekkaya H, Ozbek O, Keser M, et al. Blue rubber bleb nevus syndrome: successful treatment with sirolimus. *Pediatrics*. 2012;129(4):e1080-e1084.
93. Hammer FD, Boon LM, Mathurin P, et al. Ethanol sclerotherapy of venous malformations: evaluation of systemic ethanol contamination. *J Vasc Interv Radiol*. 2001;12(5):595-600.
94. Park HS, Do YS, Park KB, et al. Clinical outcome and predictors of treatment response in foam sodium tetradecyl sulfate sclerotherapy of venous malformations. *Eur Radiol*. 2016;26(5):1301-1310.
95. Sannier K, Dompmartin A, Théron J, et al. A new sclerosing agent in the treatment of venous malformations. *Study on 23 cases Intervent Radiol*. 2004;10:113-127.
96. Dompmartin A, Blaizot X, Théron J, et al. Radio-opaque ethylcellulose-ethanol is a safe and efficient sclerosing agent for venous malformations. *Eur Radiol*. 2011;21(12):2647-2656.
97. Fishman SJ, Fox VL. Visceral vascular anomalies. *Gastrointest Endosc Clin North Am*. 2001;11(4):813-834, viii.
98. Fishman SJ, Smithers CJ, Folkman J, et al. Blue rubber bleb nevus syndrome: surgical eradication of gastrointestinal bleeding. *Ann Surg*. 2005;241(3):523-528.
99. Marler JJ, Fishman SJ, Upton J, et al. Prenatal diagnosis of vascular anomalies. *J Pediatr Surg*. 2002;37(3):318-326.
100. Sybert VP, McCauley E. Turner's syndrome. *N Engl J Med*. 2004;351(12):1227-1238.
101. Cohen MM Jr. Klippel-Trenaunay syndrome. *Am J Med Genet*. 2000;93(3):171-175.
102. Oduber CE, van der Horst CM, Hennekam RC. Klippel-Trenaunay syndrome: diagnostic criteria and hypothesis on etiology. *Ann Plast Surg*. 2008;60(2):217-223.
103. Alomari AI, Thiex R, Mulliken JB. Hermann Friedberg's case report: an early description of CLOVES syndrome. *Clin Genet*. 2010;78(4):342-347.
104. Biesecker LG, Happle R, Mulliken JB, et al. Proteus syndrome: diagnostic criteria, differential diagnosis, and patient evaluation. *Am J Med Genet*. 1999;84(5):389-395.
105. Lala S, Mulliken JB, Alomari AI, et al. Gorham-Stout disease and generalized lymphatic anomaly—clinical, radiologic, and histologic differentiation. *Skeletal Radiol*. 2013;42(7):917-924.
106. Moller G, Priemel M, Amling M, et al. The Gorham-Stout syndrome (Gorham's massive osteolysis). A report of six cases with histopathological findings. *J Bone Joint Surg Br*. 1999;81(3):501-506.
107. Connell F, Kalidas K, Ostergaard P, et al. Linkage and sequence analysis indicate that CCBE1 is mutated in recessively inherited generalised lymphatic dysplasia. *Hum Genet*. 2010;127(2):231-241.
108. Brouillard P, Boon L, Vikkula M. Genetics of lymphatic anomalies. *J Clin Invest*. 2014;124(3):898-904.
109. Brice G, Child AH, Evans A, et al. Milroy disease and the VEGFR-3 mutation phenotype. *J Med Genet*. 2005;42(2):98-102.
110. Alomari AI, Burrows PE, Lee EY, et al. CLOVES syndrome with thoracic and central phlebectasia: increased risk of pulmonary embolism. *J Thorac Cardiovasc Surg*. 2010;140(2):459-463.
111. Edwards PD, Rahbar R, Ferraro NF, et al. Lymphatic malformation of the lingual base and oral floor. *Plast Reconstr Surg*. 2005;115(7):1906-1915.
112. Ghalamkarpour A, Morlot S, Raas-Rothschild A, et al. Hereditary lymphedema type I associated with VEGFR3 mutation: the first de novo case and atypical presentations. *Clin Genet*. 2006;70(4):330-335.
113. Daniel-Spiegel E, Ghalamkarpour A, Spiegel R, et al. Hydrops fetalis: an unusual prenatal presentation of hereditary congenital lymphedema. *Prenat Diagn*. 2005;25(11):1015-1018.
114. Osborn AJ, Dickie P, Neilson DE, et al. Activating PIK3CA alleles and lymphangiogenic phenotype of lymphatic endothelial cells isolated from lymphatic malformations. *Hum Mol Genet*. 2015;24(4):926-938.
115. Kurek KC, Luks VL, Ayturk UM, et al. Somatic mosaic activating mutations in PIK3CA cause CLOVES syndrome. *Am J Hum Genet*. 2012;90(6):1108-1115.
116. Irrthum A, Karkkainen MJ, Devriendt K, et al. Congenital hereditary lymphedema caused by a mutation that inactivates VEGFR3 tyrosine kinase. *Am J Hum Genet*. 2000;67(2):295-301.
117. Evans AL, Bell R, Brice G, et al. Identification of eight novel VEGFR-3 mutations in families with primary congenital lymphoedema. *J Med Genet*. 2003;40(9):697-703.
118. Irrthum A, Devriendt K, Chitayat D, et al. Mutations in the transcription factor gene SOX18 underlie recessive and dominant forms of hypotrichosis-lymphedema-telangiectasia. *Am J Hum Genet*. 2003;72(6):1470-1478.
119. Ghalamkarpour A, Holnthoner W, Saharinen P, et al. Recessive primary congenital lymphoedema caused by a VEGFR3 mutation. *J Med Genet*. 2009;46(6):399-404.
120. Mansour S, Brice GW, Jeffery S, et al. Lymphedema-distichiasis syndrome. In: Pagon RA, Adam MP, Ardinger HH, et al, eds. *GeneReviews*. Seattle; 1993.
121. Ostergaard P, Simpson MA, Mendola A, et al. Mutations in KIF11 cause autosomal-dominant microcephaly variably associated with congenital lymphedema and chorioretinopathy. *Am J Hum Genet*. 2012;90(2):356-362.
122. Schlogel MJ, Mendola A, Fastre E, et al. No evidence of locus heterogeneity in familial microcephaly with or without chorioretinopathy, lymphedema, or mental retardation syndrome. *Orphanet J Rare Dis*. 2015;10:52.
123. Hennekam RC, Geerdink RA, Hamel BC, et al. Autosomal recessive intestinal lymphangiectasia and lymphedema, with facial anomalies and mental retardation. *J Med Genet Am J Med Genet*. 1989;34(4):593-600.

124. Alders M, Hogan BM, Gjini E, et al. Mutations in CCBE1 cause generalized lymph vessel dysplasia in humans. *Nat Genet*. 2009;41(12):1272-1274.
125. Ostergaard P, Simpson MA, Connell FC, et al. Mutations in GATA2 cause primary lymphedema associated with a predisposition to acute myeloid leukemia (Emberger syndrome). *Nat Genet*. 2011;43(10):929-931.
126. Mendola A, Schlogel MJ, Ghalamkarpour A, et al. Mutations in the VEGFR3 signaling pathway explain 36% of familial lymphedema. *Mol Syndromol*. 2013;4(6):257-266.
127. Galambos C, Nodit L. Identification of lymphatic endothelium in pediatric vascular tumors and malformations. *Pediatr Dev Pathol*. 2005;8(2):181-189.
128. Dubois J, Garel L, Abela A, et al. Lymphangiomas in children: percutaneous sclerotherapy with an alcoholic solution of zein. *Radiology*. 1997;204(3):651-654.
129. Dubois J, Garel L, Grignon A, et al. Imaging of hemangiomas and vascular malformations in children. *Acad Radiol*. 1998;5(5):390-400.
130. Peterman CM, Fevurly RD, Alomari AI, et al. Sonographic screening for Wilms tumor in children with CLOVES syndrome. *Pediatr Blood Cancer*. 2017;64(12).
131. Hammill AM, Wentzel M, Gupta A, et al. Sirolimus for the treatment of complicated vascular anomalies in children. *Pediatr Blood Cancer*. 2011;57(6):1018-1024.
132. Adams DM, Trenor CC 3rd, Hammill AM, et al. Efficacy and safety of sirolimus in the treatment of complicated vascular anomalies. *Pediatrics*. 2016;137(2):1-10.
133. Swetman GL, Berk DR, Vasanawala SS, et al. Sildenafil for severe lymphatic malformations. *N Engl J Med*. 2012;366(4):384-386.
134. Rankin H, Zwicker K, Trenor CC 3rd. Caution is recommended prior to sildenafil use in vascular anomalies. *Pediatr Blood Cancer*. 2015;62(11):2015-2017.
135. Koshy JC, Eisemann BS, Agrawal N, et al. Sildenafil for microcystic lymphatic malformations of the head and neck: a prospective study. *Int J Pediatr Otorhinolaryngol*. 2015;79(7):980-982.
136. Mathur NN, Rana I, Bothra R, et al. Bleomycin sclerotherapy in congenital lymphatic and vascular malformations of head and neck. *Int J Pediatr Otorhinolaryngol*. 2005;69(1):75-80.
137. Claesson G, Kuylenstierna R. OK-432 therapy for lymphatic malformation in 32 patients (28 children). *Int J Pediatr Otorhinolaryngol*. 2002;65(1):1-6.
138. Harsha WJ, Perkins JA, Lewis CW, et al. Pediatric admissions and procedures for lymphatic malformations in the United States: 1997 and 2000. *Lymphat Res Biol*. 2005;3(2):58-65.
139. Ballieux F, Modarressi A, Hammer F, et al. Reconstructive surgery in the management of a patient with CLOVES syndrome. *J Plast Reconstr Aesthet Surg*. 2013;66(12):1813-1815.
140. Hosman AE, Devlin HL, Silva BM, et al. Specific cancer rates may differ in patients with hereditary haemorrhagic telangiectasia compared to controls. *Orphanet J Rare Dis*. 2013;8:195.
141. Lester J, Ruano-Calderon LA, Gonzalez-Olhovich I. Wyburn-Mason syndrome. *J Neuroimaging*. 2005;15(3):284-285.
142. Rodesch G, Hurth M, Alvarez H, et al. Classification of spinal cord arteriovenous shunts: proposal for a reappraisal—the Bicetre experience with 155 consecutive patients treated between 1981 and 1999. *Neurosurgery*. 2002;51(2):374-379; discussion 379-380.
143. Letteboer TG, Mager HJ, Snijder RJ, et al. Genotype-phenotype relationship for localization and age distribution of telangiectases in hereditary hemorrhagic telangiectasia. *J Med GenetAm J Med Genet A*. 2008;146A(21):2733-2739.
144. Morgan T, McDonald J, Anderson C, et al. Intracranial hemorrhage in infants and children with hereditary hemorrhagic telangiectasia (Osler-Weber-Rendu syndrome). *Pediatrics*. 2002;109(1):E12.
145. Govani FS, Shovlin CL. Hereditary haemorrhagic telangiectasia: a clinical and scientific review. *Eur J Hum Genet*. 2009;17(7):860-871.
146. Enjolras O, Chapot R, Merland JJ. Vascular anomalies and the growth of limbs: a review. *J Pediatr Orthop B*. 2004;13(6):349-357.
147. Tan WH, Baris HN, Burrows PE, et al. The spectrum of vascular anomalies in patients with PTEN mutations: implications for diagnosis and management. *J Med Genet*. 2007;44(9):594-602.
148. Cohen MM Jr. Vasculogenesis, angiogenesis, hemangiomas, and vascular malformations. *J Med GenetAm J Med Genet*. 2002;108(4):265-274.
149. Enjolras O, Logeart I, Gelbert F, et al. Arteriovenous malformations: a study of 200 cases. *Ann Dermatol Venereol*. 2000;127(1):17-22.
150. Kohout MP, Hansen M, Pribaz JJ, et al. Arteriovenous malformations of the head and neck: natural history and management. *Plast Reconstr Surg*. 1998;102(3):643-654.
151. Revencu N, Boon LM, Mulliken JB, et al. RASA1 and capillary malformation-arteriovenous malformation. In: Epstein C, Erickson R, Wynshaw-Boris A, eds. *Inborn Errors of Development: The Molecular Basis of Clinical Disorders of Morphogenesis*. 2nd ed. Oxford, UK: Oxford University Press; 2008:647-650.
152. Johnson DW, Berg JN, Baldwin MA, et al. Mutations in the activin receptor-like kinase 1 gene in hereditary haemorrhagic telangiectasia type 2. *Nat Genet*. 1996;13(2):189-195.
153. McAllister KA, Grogg KM, Johnson DW, et al. Endoglin, a TGF-beta binding protein of endothelial cells, is the gene for hereditary haemorrhagic telangiectasia type 1. *Nat Genet*. 1994;8(4):345-351.
154. Gallione CJ, Repetto GM, Legius E, et al. A combined syndrome of juvenile polyposis and hereditary haemorrhagic telangiectasia associated with mutations in MADH4 (SMAD4). *Lancet*. 2004;363(9412):852-859.
155. Wooderchak-Donahue WL, McDonald J, O'Fallon B, et al. BMP9 mutations cause a vascular-anomaly syndrome with phenotypic overlap with hereditary hemorrhagic telangiectasia. *Am J Hum Genet*. 2013;93(3):530-537.
156. Ola R, Dubrac A, Han J, et al. PI3 kinase inhibition improves vascular malformations in mouse models of hereditary haemorrhagic telangiectasia. *Nat Commun*. 2016;7:13650.
157. Blume-Peytavi U, Adler YD, Geilen CC, et al. Multiple familial cutaneous glomangioma: a pedigree of 4 generations and critical analysis of histologic and genetic differences of glomus tumors. *J Am Acad Dermatol*. 2000;42(4):633-639.
158. Macmurdo CF, Wooderchak-Donahue W, Bayrak-Toydemir P, et al. RASA1 somatic mutation and variable expressivity in capillary malformation/arteriovenous malformation (CM/AVM) syndrome. *J Med GenetAm J Med Genet A*. 2016;170(6):1450-1454.

159. van der Geer P, Henkemeyer M, Jacks T, et al. Aberrant Ras regulation and reduced p190 tyrosine phosphorylation in cells lacking p120-Gap. *Mol Cell Biol*. 1997;17(4):1840-1847.
160. Henkemeyer M, Rossi DJ, Holmyard DP, et al. Vascular system defects and neuronal apoptosis in mice lacking ras GTPase-activating protein. *Nature*. 1995;377(6551):695-701.
161. Kawasaki J, Aegerter S, Fevurly RD, et al. RASA1 functions in EPHB4 signaling pathway to suppress endothelial mTORC1 activity. *J Clin Invest*. 2014;124(6):2774-2784.
162. Xiao Z, Carrasco R, Kinneer K, et al. EphB4 promotes or suppresses Ras/MEK/ERK pathway in a context-dependent manner: implications for EphB4 as a cancer target. *Cancer Biol Ther*. 2012;13(8):630-637.
163. Zhou XP, Marsh DJ, Hampel H, et al. Germline and germline mosaic PTEN mutations associated with a Proteus-like syndrome of hemihypertrophy, lower limb asymmetry, arteriovenous malformations and lipomatosis. *Hum Mol Genet*. 2000;9(5):765-768.
164. Nikolaev SI, Vetiska S, Bonilla X, et al. Somatic activating KRAS mutations in arteriovenous malformations of the brain. *N Engl J Med*. 2018;378(3):250-261.
165. Lebrin F, Srun S, Raymond K, et al. Thalidomide stimulates vessel maturation and reduces epistaxis in individuals with hereditary hemorrhagic telangiectasia. *Nat Med*. 2010;16(4):420-428.
166. Burrows PE, Fellows KE. Techniques for management of pediatric vascular anomalies. In: Cope C, ed. *Current Techniques in Interventional Radiology*. Philadelphia: Current Medicine; 1995:12-27.
167. Yakes WF, Rossi P, Odink H. How I do it. Arteriovenous malformation management. *Cardiovasc Intervent Radiol*. 1996;19(2):65-71.
168. Wu JK, Bisdorff A, Gelbert F, et al. arteriovenous malformation: evaluation, management, and outcome. *Plast Reconstr Surg*. 2005;115(4):985-995.
169. Liu AS, Mulliken JB, Zurakowski D, et al. Extracranial arteriovenous malformations: natural progression and recurrence after treatment. *Plast Reconstr Surg*. 2010;125(4):1185-1194.

Chapter 148 :: Cutaneous Changes in Arterial, Venous, and Lymphatic Dysfunction
:: Sabrina A. Newman

第一百四十八章
动脉、静脉和淋巴管功能障碍的皮肤表现

中文导读

本章共分为7节：①阻塞性外周动脉疾病；②动脉粥样性栓塞；③闭塞性血栓脉管炎（Buerger病）；④网状青斑和葡萄状青斑；⑤红斑肢痛症；⑥慢性静脉疾病；⑦淋巴水肿。

1. 阻塞性外周动脉疾病　外周动脉疾病（PAD）主要是由于动脉粥样硬化导致远端主动脉以及下腹、骨盆和腿部大动脉狭窄或闭塞所致。其患病率在65岁以上的人群中高达20%。男性更高发，女性绝经后的发病率上升。

（1）临床特征：继发于血管血栓或栓塞的急性肢体缺血表现为：①剧烈疼痛，通常在休息时持续存在；②苍白；③无搏动；④感觉异常；⑤瘫痪（"5Ps"）。异形体温（四肢冰凉）也可加到这一组临床表现中（表148-1）。神经系统症状的存在往往提示缺血严重，需要紧急评估。接下来对于PAD患者的皮肤症状、非皮肤表现以及并发症进行了详细介绍。

（2）病因和发病机制：动脉粥样硬化的危险因素包括糖尿病、高血压、高脂血症、吸烟、血管疾病家族史和肥胖症。详细介绍了动脉粥样硬化的不同时期的病理表现及形成机制。

（3）诊断：图148-3为诊断PAD的流程。

（4）鉴别诊断：PAD的鉴别诊断包括局部因素和全身性疾病（表148-3）。

（5）临床过程和预后：PAD最严重的后果是肢体缺血导致截肢。此外，PAD患者心血管疾病和死亡的风险较高。

（6）治疗：医疗管理的目标包括阻止疾病进展和减轻症状。对该病的非药物一般治疗措施、药物治疗和手术治疗方法和适应症进行了介绍。

2．动脉粥样性栓塞

（1）流行病学：动脉粥样硬化栓塞的发生率在0.15%～4%之间。男性比女性更为常见，平均发病年龄为66～72岁。

（2）病因和发病机制：动脉粥样硬化栓塞的发病机制是近端动脉粥样硬化斑块上脱落的动脉粥样碎片（所谓的胆固醇晶体）阻塞小动脉（直径为50～900μm）并继发异物炎症反应，这种炎症过程导致血栓形成。接下来对动脉粥样硬化栓塞的危险因素进行了描述。

（3）临床特征：动脉粥样硬化栓塞可自发生，但侵入性操作常常是诱因。临床表现与栓塞的位置以及下游血流的模式和分布有关。对该病的皮肤表现、相关体格检查及并发症进行了详细介绍。

（4）特异性检查：对诊断本病具有确诊

价值的检查作了详细介绍，并总结了其鉴别诊断（表148-8）。

（5）临床过程和预后：胆固醇栓塞的预后通常较差，1年死亡率高达20%～30%，其临床结局还取决于受累的器官系统。

（6）治疗和预防：治疗的主要手段包括预防进一步的缺血性损伤、支持性护理和去除动脉粥样硬化来源。作者对目前可能有帮助的药物进行了详细介绍，并提出了针对动脉粥样硬化栓塞的建议。

3．闭塞性血栓脉管炎（Buerger病） 闭塞性血栓脉管炎（TAO），也称为Buerger病，是一种罕见的进行性炎症性血栓性疾病，主要累及四肢的中小动脉。对该病的流行病学、临床特征、病因和发病机制、诊断和鉴别诊断、治疗进行了详细阐述。

4．网状青斑和葡萄状青斑 网状青斑是一种良性的累及年轻至中年女性的原发性疾病，表现为对称的可逆的且均匀的颜色改变。葡萄状青斑是一种继发性的病理性和永久性的病变，这种颜色改变是不对称的不可逆的且"不完整的"，是抗磷脂综合征患者最常见的皮肤表现。在该部分对这两种类型的青斑改变的皮肤损害、病因和发病机制、诊断要点、预后及治疗方法进行了详细介绍，提及临床医生区分网状青斑和葡萄状青斑至关重要，并建议所有表现为葡萄状青斑的患者都应该完善抗磷脂抗体相关检查。

5．红斑肢痛症 肢端发红、灼热、剧烈疼痛和灼痛是红斑肢痛症的特征，最常累及下肢，通常由增加体温的活动（例如运动、环境温度或晚上使用厚毛毯）引起。红斑肢痛症的病因和发病机制尚不清楚，可能与动静脉分流和小纤维神经病变有关。继发性红斑肢痛症可发生在红细胞增多症、血小板增多症和自身免疫性疾病患者中。在该部分对红斑肢痛症的病因和发病机制、诊断和鉴别诊断、预后及治疗方法进行了详细介绍，并指出治疗的重点是预防发作和控制症状。对于继发性红斑肢痛患者，阿司匹林通常有效。

6．慢性静脉疾病 外周静脉的慢性疾病包括从毛细血管扩张到网状静脉和静脉曲张的一系列变化，其临床表现可以从早期的水肿、压痛到晚期的静脉溃疡（Table148-14）。在该部分对慢性静脉疾病的流行病学、皮肤损害、并发症、病因和发病机制、诊断和鉴别诊断要点、预后及治疗方法进行了详细介绍，提出压迫疗法应作为治疗慢性静脉功能不全的任何治疗方案的一部分，并指出湿性疗法对于静脉溃疡的重要性。

7．淋巴水肿 淋巴水肿是指因淋巴管畸形或功能障碍导致淋巴转运能力受损所致的身体某一部分肿胀，可分为原发性和继发性。在这一部分对于存在原发性淋巴水肿的综合征从临床特征、病因及发病机制的角度进行了介绍。对于继发性淋巴水肿，指出丝虫病是最常见的原因，并从流行病学、临床特征、诊断和鉴别诊断、预后及治疗方法进行了详细介绍。

最后，对局限在面部、外阴和阴茎的局限性淋巴水肿的病因及治疗原则进行了简单介绍。

〔黄莹雪〕

OBSTRUCTIVE PERIPHERAL ARTERIAL DISEASE

AT-A-GLANCE

- Most commonly caused by atherosclerosis of the vessels supplying the lower extremity.
- Affects 15% of the U.S. adult population older than age 65 years.
- Stenosis or obstruction of the large arteries to the lower extremities leading to supply–demand mismatch, initially with exertion, but may progress to occur at rest.
- Intermittent claudication with exertional muscle pain or fatigue, critical limb ischemia with rest pain or tissue compromise, and acute limb ischemia.
- Cutaneous findings from hypoperfusion range from dry skin, hair loss, and malformed toenails to ulceration and gangrene.

Peripheral arterial disease (PAD) occurs when atherosclerosis causes stenosis or occlusion in the distal aorta and large arteries of the lower abdomen, pelvis, and legs. Patients may be asymptomatic, experience exertional ischemic leg symptoms (intermittent claudication), or develop critical limb ischemia. The most classic symptom of PAD is intermittent claudication, which is usually described as pain, fatigue, or tiredness in a defined muscle group distal to the diseased vascular segment upon walking that is relieved by rest. The location of the pain differs depending on the anatomical location of the arterial lesions. Because the disease is most common in the distal superficial femoral artery, patients most commonly present with claudication in the calf muscle area (the muscle group just distal to the arterial disease). When the disease affects the more proximal aortoiliac vessels, thigh and buttock muscle claudication predominates. The discomfort tends to be highly reproducible within the same muscle groups and is precipitated by the same level of exertion. It is crucial to determine the amount of walking distance, a standard measure that quantifies severity and response to treatment, before the onset of symptoms. Resolution within several minutes of rest is an expected finding. Patients with inadequate collateral circulation may complain of cold extremities, hyperesthesia, rest pain, discolored toes, or skin breakdown. Ischemic rest pain typically affects the foot and may interfere with sleep or necessitate sleeping with the leg in a dependent position. Peripheral edema may then occur.

EPIDEMIOLOGY

Although atherosclerotic obstructive PAD has a prevalence of only 3% in patients 40 to 59 years of age, this rises to up to 20% in the older than age 65 years group. This translates into approximately 8.5 million cases in the United States, and this number is expected to increase along with aging demographics.[1-3] PAD is often unrecognized clinically, and more than one-half of all patients are asymptomatic. Gender predisposition shows preponderance in males, although the incidence in females rises rapidly after menopause. Anatomically, superficial femoral artery disease predominates, with development of symptoms typically in the seventh decade. Interestingly, symptoms from aortoiliac disease usually present a decade earlier.

CLINICAL FEATURES

Acute limb ischemia secondary to vessel thrombosis or embolism presents more dramatically with (a) severe pain, usually persistent at rest, (b) pallor, (c) pulselessness, (d) paresthesias, and (e) paralysis (the "5 Ps"). Poikilothermia (a cold extremity) may be added to this pentad of clinical findings (Table 148-1). The presence of neurologic symptoms indicates severe ischemia and need for emergent evaluation.

Because atherosclerosis is a systemic disease process, patients who present with claudication attributable to PAD can be expected to have atherosclerosis elsewhere. Hence, it is common for patients to present with symptoms related to disease affecting the other vascular territories.

CUTANEOUS FINDINGS

The cutaneous findings in PAD will vary depending on the severity of arterial obstruction and tissue ischemia (Table 148-2). Limbs in patients with intermittent claudication may appear normal, although associated clinical findings may include hair loss, coldness, cyanosis,

---

TABLE 148-1
Acute Limb Ischemia: 6 Ps

1. Pain
2. Pallor
3. Pulselessness
4. Paresthesia
5. Paralysis
6. Poikilothermia

TABLE 148-2
Cutaneous Findings in Peripheral Arterial Disease

- Pallor
- Coolness of the extremities
- Dependent rubor
- Subcutaneous atrophy
- Hair loss
- Brittle toenails
- Absence of sweating
- Ulceration
- Gangrene
- Tenderness
- Regional edema

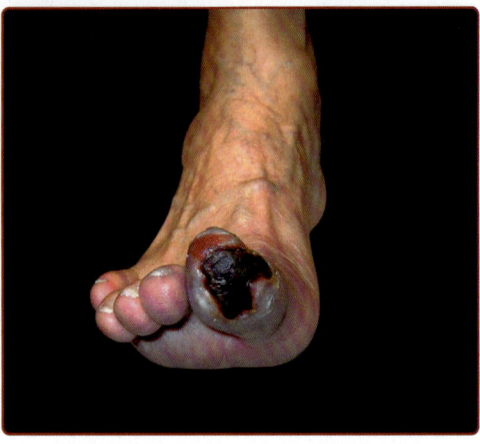

Figure 148-2 Necrotic toe in a patient with peripheral arterial obstructive disease. There is marked dependent rubor of the toes and distal aspect of the foot.

and/or thickened and malformed toenails. In patients with severe ischemia, the skin is apt to be atrophic, dry, and shiny. In patients with rest pain, the foot is usually bright red and cold in dependency. Ulcerations most often start at the tips of the toes or on the heel of the foot and are extremely painful, except when diabetic neuropathy is also present (Fig. 148-1). Ulcers also occasionally start on the lower calves or lateral aspect of the heel. They frequently demonstrate irregular borders and a pale base. The heels may show cracks in the skin with numerous fissures. When gangrene occurs, usually 1 or more toes become black, dry, and mummified (Fig. 148-2). Superimposed infection is a major concern. Important associated signs of infection include purulent discharge or decay (wet gangrene), and (often) surrounding tissue erythema and swelling.

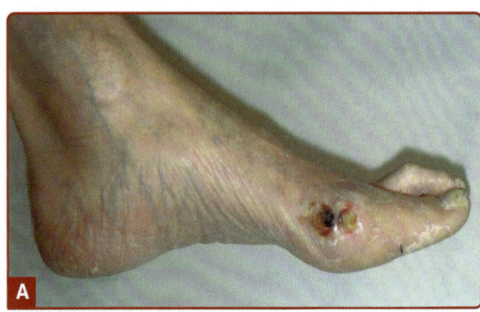

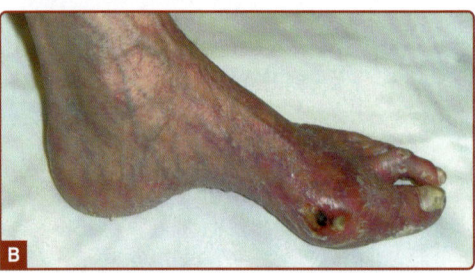

Figure 148-1 Obstructive peripheral arterial disease. An ulcer is seen on the medial aspect of the foot at the base of the great toe. **A,** Foot pallor with elevation of limb suggests severe ischemia. **B,** Foot erythema with the leg in a dependent position, termed *dependent rubor*, also suggests severe ischemia.

NONCUTANEOUS FINDINGS

Decreased or absent pulses distal to the stenotic arterial segment are the hallmark noncutaneous finding in PAD. Bruits on auscultation over the diseased segment of vessel as a result of turbulent flow also may be present. It is also possible to find normal palpable pulses in a patient who presents with symptoms suggestive of intermittent claudication. In such a case, the clinician can have the patient walk around the office (or perform toe raises) until the symptoms are reproduced and then palpate for pulses. Exercise may "unmask" the stenosis, causing the atherosclerotic lesion to become significant, and should diminish the strength of the pulses distal to the lesion. The collateral circulation to limbs affected by PAD can be evaluated by simple bedside examination. With the patient supine, elevation of the limb at a 45-degree angle for 2 minutes should not produce pallor. Collateral circulation is deemed inadequate if the toes and feet become pale. The patient then assumes a sitting position with the legs dependent, and the time for filling of the foot veins and flushing of the feet is measured. The veins should fill within 20 seconds and the feet flush immediately in a warm environment. When these times exceed 30 seconds, the collateral circulation is deemed inadequate, and the patient must be observed frequently for the development of rest pain, ulcers, or gangrene. Venous filling times are of limited value when varicose veins coexist.

COMPLICATIONS

The major direct complications of PAD relate to limb loss from progressive severe ischemia or superimposed infection. In patients with rest pain or tissue loss, the risk of infection is high and wound healing slow or absent. Under these circumstances, the need for revascularization is more urgent to avoid the need for amputation. Superimposed infection needs to be aggressively treated with antibiotics, wound debridement, and local foot care; if the infection is rapidly progressive, it presents a medical emergency.

ETIOLOGY AND PATHOGENESIS

Atherosclerotic risk factors are similar to those identified for coronary artery disease and include diabetes mellitus, hypertension, hyperlipidemia, smoking, family history of vascular disease, and obesity. Among these, diabetes mellitus and smoking are the most significant and are associated with a doubling of relative risk. Patients with diabetes mellitus develop the disease at an earlier age than nondiabetic patients, and have more-severe and progressive disease. The anatomic distribution of obstruction differs from nondiabetic patients with less aortoiliac involvement and more extensive disease of the run-off vessels below the knees. However, superficial femoral artery disease is similar in both populations. Approximately 50% of patients have hyperlipidemia. PAD is also more commonly encountered in patients with hypertension.

The pathologic findings in atherosclerosis occur in large- and medium-sized arteries, and are morphologically diverse, with focal accumulation of lipids and lipoproteins, mucopolysaccharides and collagen, smooth muscle cells and macrophages, and calcium deposits in variable quantities. Localized areas of intimal thickening secondary to smooth muscle cell proliferation and lipid-laden macrophages are seen in early stages with disruption of the internal elastic lamina. The media is often atrophic with thin strands of smooth muscle, lipid pools, collagen tissue, and calcium deposits. Enlarging plaques encroach on the lumen despite dilation of the artery, and the plaques may ulcerate. Hemorrhages occur in the arterial wall. Thrombi may also form and occlude the narrowed arterial lumen.

The etiology of atherosclerosis is complex and multifactorial, but progressive buildup of plaque narrows the vessel lumen, and complete occlusion may develop acutely secondary to thrombosis. Because disease progression is usually over an extended time period, collateral blood vessels have time to develop and are usually robust. Tissue perfusion to the affected limb is often adequate at rest, but the blood pressure distal to the occlusions is decreased secondary to high resistance and limited flow through collateral vessels. Under resting conditions, normal blood flow to extremity muscle groups averages 300 to 400 mL/min. Once exercise begins, blood flow increases up to 10-fold owing to the increase in cardiac output and compensatory vasodilation at the tissue level. When exercise ceases, the blood flow returns to normal within minutes. In patients with PAD, resting blood flow may be similar to that of a healthy person. However, during exercise, blood flow cannot maximally increase in muscle tissue because of fixed proximal arterial stenoses. When the metabolic demands of the muscle exceed blood flow, claudication symptoms ensue. At the same time, a longer recovery period is required for blood flow to return to baseline once exercise is terminated. Dermatologic changes imply severe compromise of tissue perfusion, often secondary to tandem high-grade stenoses or occlusions present at multiple levels in the arterial tree.

DIAGNOSIS

Figure 148-3 outlines an approach to diagnosing PAD. An ankle-brachial index (ABI) is the recommended diagnostic test to assess for PAD. It is the ratio of the blood pressure at the ankle to the blood pressure in the upper arm (brachium). The ankle systolic pressure in the supine, resting position should be equal to, or greater than, the brachial artery systolic pressure. Thus, a normal ABI range is 1.00 to 1.40. A value less than or equal to 0.90 is considered abnormal, and values of 0.91 to 0.99 are defined as "borderline." Of note, patients with heavily calcified or "noncompressible" vessels, most commonly persons with diabetes or of advanced age, may have falsely elevated ABIs (greater than 1.4) despite the presence of significant PAD. Under these circumstances, a toe-brachial index should be used to establish the diagnosis of PAD, as smaller vessels are rarely affected. When the ABI is borderline or normal despite symptoms suggestive of claudication, an exercise ABI is recommended.[4,5]

ABI values are of prognostic use for determination of wound healing or the need for revascularization. Other vascular diagnostic methods include segmental pressures, Doppler waveform analysis, pulse volume recordings, or ABI with duplex ultrasonography to document the presence and location of PAD in the lower extremity.

Magnetic resonance angiography and computed tomographic angiography are competitive technologies used to demonstrate precise anatomic location and extent of disease in the arteries, but supply limited hemodynamic information. Magnetic resonance angiography is often preferred because of lack of ionizing radiation or need for iodine-based contrast dye, but may not be tolerated by claustrophobic individuals. Conventional catheter-based arteriography is usually reserved for definitive evaluation in patients about to undergo vascular surgery, or as a necessary component of percutaneous angioplasty or stenting procedures (Fig. 148-4).

DIFFERENTIAL DIAGNOSIS

The diagnosis of PAD can usually be made by the typical history of intermittent claudication and palpation

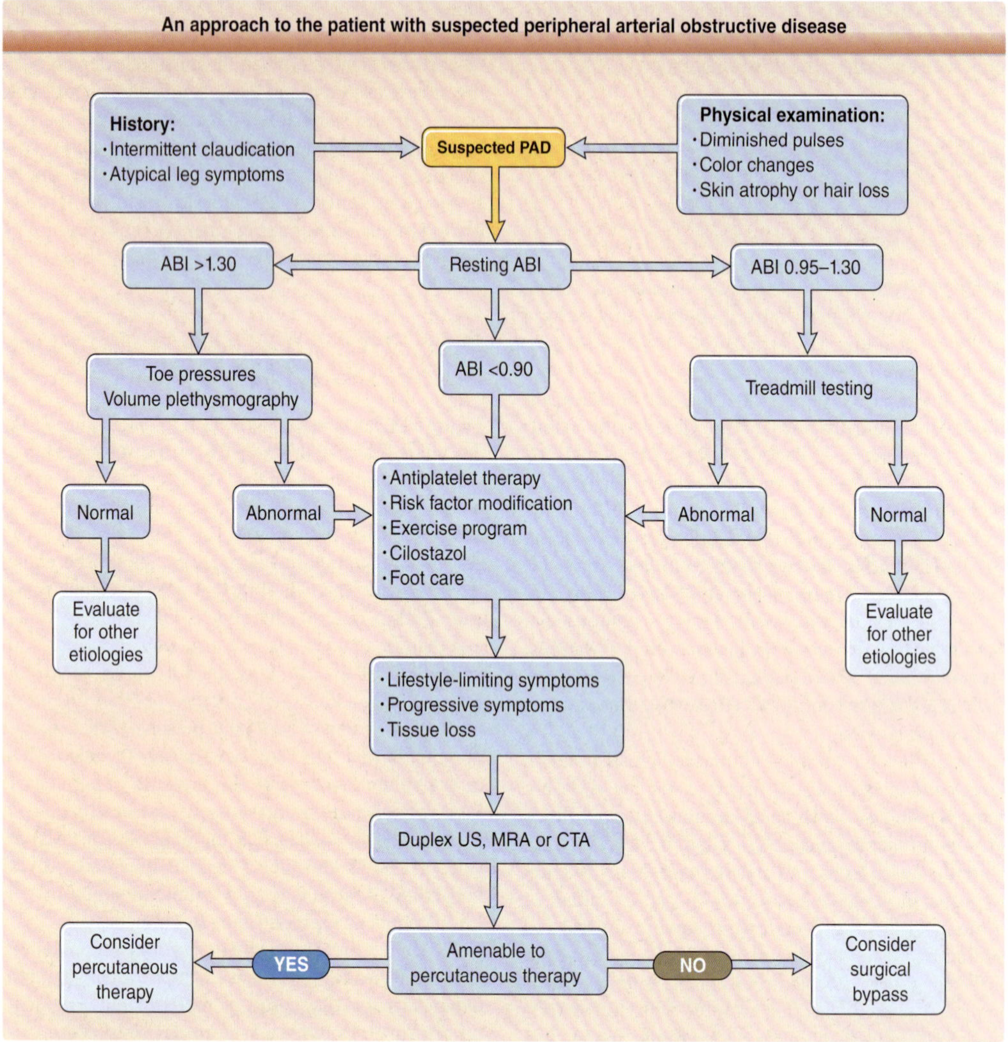

An approach to the patient with suspected peripheral arterial obstructive disease

```
History:                    Suspected PAD          Physical examination:
• Intermittent claudication                        • Diminished pulses
• Atypical leg symptoms                            • Color changes
                                                   • Skin atrophy or hair loss
                                   ↓
                             Resting ABI
         ↙                         ↓                         ↘
   ABI >1.30                   ABI <0.90               ABI 0.95–1.30
       ↓                           ↓                         ↓
Toe pressures                                          Treadmill testing
Volume plethysmography
    ↙       ↘                                            ↙      ↘
Normal   Abnormal  →  • Antiplatelet therapy  ←  Abnormal   Normal
   ↓                  • Risk factor modification                ↓
Evaluate              • Exercise program                    Evaluate
for other             • Cilostazol                          for other
etiologies            • Foot care                           etiologies
                             ↓
                      • Lifestyle-limiting symptoms
                      • Progressive symptoms
                      • Tissue loss
                             ↓
                      Duplex US, MRA or CTA
                             ↓
Consider           Amenable to            Consider
percutaneous  ← YES  percutaneous  NO →   surgical
therapy            therapy                bypass
```

Figure 148-3 An approach to the patient with suspected peripheral arterial obstructive disease. ABI, ankle-brachial index; CTA, computed tomographic angiography; duplex US, duplex ultrasonography; MRA, magnetic resonance angiography; PAD, peripheral arterial disease.

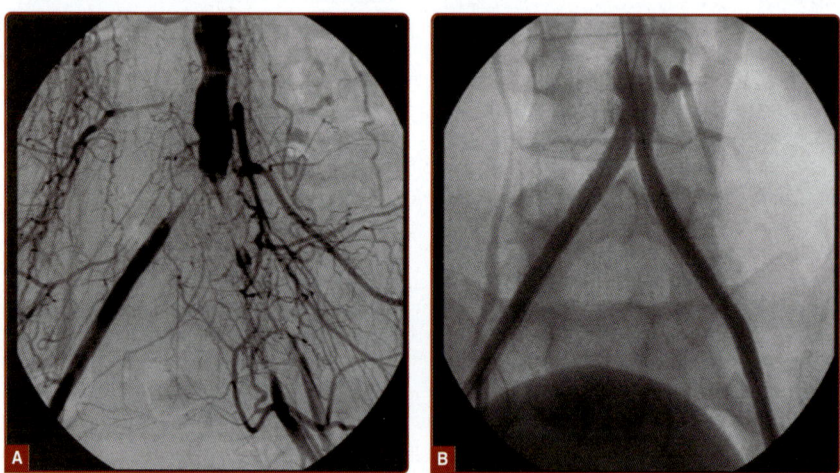

Figure 148-4 **A,** Contrast angiography demonstrating extensive peripheral artery occlusive disease involving the bilateral iliac arteries with stenoses and occlusions. **B,** Recanalization of the iliac arteries after placement of bilateral iliac artery stents.

TABLE 148-3
Differential Diagnosis of Obstructive Peripheral Arterial Disease

Local Factors
- Trauma (including iatrogenic)
- Arterial dissection
- Cystic adventitial disease
- Thrombosed popliteal artery aneurysm
- Arterial entrapment syndromes
- Extrinsic compression

Systemic Disease
- Primary thrombotic disorder (thrombophilia)
- Embolic
- Thromboangiitis obliterans
- Vasculitic disorders (particularly giant cell arteritis or Takayasu arteritis)

TABLE 148-4
Differential Diagnosis of Foot Ulcers

- Obstructive peripheral arterial disease
- Microvascular disease
- Chronic venous insufficiency
- Neuropathic (particularly diabetic neuropathy)
- Infection (diabetes or fungal)
- Trauma

---

for diminished or absent pulses in the limbs. The ABI is usually diminished, although occasional patients may have normal values at rest. When the diagnosis remains in doubt, a helpful provocative maneuver to increase blood flow is to exercise the patient. Postexercise blood flow may be limited by the arterial obstructive disease, and repeat ABI will then be diminished.

The differential diagnosis of PAD includes both local factors and systemic disorders (Table 148-3). Arterial obstructive disease is just one of several potential etiologies for the development of a foot ulcer (Table 148-4). However, ulcer location and associated symptoms can be helpful in differentiating some of the causes (Table 148-5). In particular, diabetic neuropathic foot ulcers, or other diseases resulting in neuropathy, may develop on the heel, toes, or shin in the presence of normal pulses. These painless (neurotrophic) ulcers are caused by repetitive trauma not noticed by the patient because of the peripheral neuropathy. With regard to the foot, ulcers often occur over pressure points with a surrounding callus. Arterial limb ulcers differ; they are exquisitely tender, do not have a preference for pressure points on the foot, and lack a surrounding callus.

Thromboangiitis obliterans also causes intermittent claudication, ulcers, and gangrene. It occurs in young smokers (onset of symptoms before the age of 45 years) and is often associated with superficial thrombophlebitis and vasospasm. In contrast to PAD, it affects medium-sized and smaller arteries, most commonly in the upper extremities.

Occlusive vascular disease confined to focal anatomic locations in young patients with minimal traditional risk factors for atherosclerosis should raise suspicion for alternative etiologies. For example, popliteal artery occlusion may occur secondary to entrapment by calf muscles or cystic adventitial disease. In popliteal artery occlusion, an abnormal anatomical insertion of the medial gastrocnemius muscle head causes compression of the popliteal artery, with the tibial pulses disappearing on plantar (or dorsi) flexion of the foot and full extension of the knee. Pain is aggravated with walking but less so with running because knee extension is not as severe with running as it is with walking. In cystic adventitial disease, adventitial cysts of unclear etiology compress the vessel lumen, most commonly in the popliteal artery (85%) or, rarely, in the external iliac or femoral arteries, presenting as intermittent claudication. Surgical excision of the cysts usually alleviates symptoms although, in the event of complete vessel occlusion, an interposition graft may be necessary.

Neurogenic claudication (pseudoclaudication) is often a difficult diagnosis to distinguish and is caused by compression or intermittent ischemia of the lower spinal cord or cauda equina with exercise. Etiologic factors are prolapsed intervertebral discs, congenital stenosis, or hypertrophic bony ridging of the spinal canal. In contrast to PAD, leg pain may occur in the erect position without exercise and be affected

TABLE 148-5
Comparison of Different Leg Ulcer Types

	ARTERIAL	VENOUS	NEUROPATHIC
Common sites	Tips of toes, lateral heel, lower calves	Below the knee; commonly the medial malleolar area	Heels, toes, shins, pressure points
Characteristic appearance	Very tender ulcer, with irregular borders and a pale base; gangrene and a superimposed infection may be present	Tender, shallow ulcer with an irregular red base	Painless ulcer with a surrounding callus
Appearance of nearby skin	Atrophic, dry, and shiny	Hyperpigmented; may have accompanying stasis dermatitis or edema, visible varicosities	Smooth; may have accompanying anhidrosis and sensory deficiency

by changes in posture, neurologic signs may be present before or after exercise, and peripheral pulses are normal. The pain is frequently relieved by leaning forward against a solid surface or by sitting. Dilemmas in diagnosis and management can occur when both conditions coexist. MRI or CT scan of the spine is used to confirm the diagnosis.

CLINICAL COURSE AND PROGNOSIS

The most feared consequence of PAD is severe limb-threatening ischemia leading to amputation. Fortunately, the peripheral vascular outcomes in patients with intermittent claudication as a consequence of PAD tend to be relatively benign, with studies showing that 60% to 90% of such patients remained stable over a period of 5 to 9 years.[6] In a large prospective study of 1440 patients with intermittent claudication, only 176 patients (12.2%) were reported to require amputation during a followup period of 10 years. Occasional patients show spontaneous improvement in symptoms, most likely secondary to enhanced collateral blood flow, although plaque regression is possible. However, patients with diabetes mellitus tend to have progressive disease, and their amputation rate is fourfold greater than for patients without diabetes. In patients with diabetic neuropathy, trauma to the limbs must be avoided, and special shoes may be required. Ongoing smokers also have greater amputation and vascular graft occlusion rates than nonsmokers.

In contrast with the limb-related outcomes, the risk of associated cardiovascular morbidity and mortality is high in patients with PAD because they often have advanced atherosclerosis present in multiple vascular beds.[1,5] The 5-year mortality in patients with intermittent claudication is 30%, with death largely attributed to cardiovascular causes. In addition, another 20% of patients will incur a nonfatal myocardial infarction or stroke. The association between PAD and cardiovascular morbidity and mortality is independent of prior history of cardiovascular disease and independent of known cardiovascular risk factors. Studies also show that more-severe PAD, as indicated by a lower ABI value, is associated with greater risk of cardiovascular mortality than mild PAD, as evidenced by a higher ABI value. It should be emphasized that PAD of any severity (as documented by an abnormal ABI) may be used to identify the individuals with an increased risk of cardiovascular events and mortality.[7]

MANAGEMENT

The goal of medical management should include measures to halt the progression of the disease as well as to alleviate the symptoms. The measures to halt the progression of disease include cessation of smoking and optimization of risk factors, such as diabetes mellitus, hypertension, and hyperlipidemia. For patients with symptoms of intermittent claudication, an exercise program is often the treatment of choice (Table 148-6). Patients are instructed to exercise to the threshold of tolerable pain, briefly rest, and then exercise again for a total duration of 30 to 60 minutes a day in excess of their normal activity, 3 or more times a week.[1,8] The exercise period must be performed in 1 session, with walking being the preferred modality. Drawing on data from several studies, approximately 80% of patients may be expected to show significant improvements in exercise tolerance through these techniques. Even though the exact mechanism for improvement in walking distance with exercise remains unknown, regular exercise is thought to condition the muscles to work more efficiently (more extraction of blood) and increase collateral vessel formation. The magnitude of benefit associated with exercise programs for claudication appears to be greater than that reported for clinical trials of pharmacologic therapy. Patients should be further instructed to keep their feet warm, clean, and dry; and extremes of temperature should be avoided because ischemic tissue is more susceptible to burning and to frostbite than normal tissue. Cuts or severe bruises of the limbs or feet should be treated immediately. Conventional vasodilators appear to have no value in treatment.

Two agents have been approved for the indication of intermittent claudication in the United States. Cilostazol, a phosphodiesterase inhibitor with antiplatelet and vasodilatory properties, is an effective treatment to improve symptoms and increase walking distance.[1] Cilostazol improves maximal walking distance by 40% to 60% after 12 to 24 weeks of therapy.[1,9] Side effects include GI symptoms and headaches. It is contraindicated in patients with congestive heart failure.

TABLE 148-6
Treatment of Obstructive Peripheral Arterial Disease

	SYMPTOM RELIEF	RISK REDUCTION
First-line therapy	Exercise program Cilostazol (Pletal) Pentoxifylline (Trental)	Smoking cessation Statin therapy (target low-density lipoprotein <100 mg/dL) Aspirin Glycemic control Antihypertensive therapy Other lipid therapy
Second-line therapy	Percutaneous revascularization (angioplasty, stent, atherectomy, cryotherapy) Surgical revascularization (endarterectomy or bypass)	Clopidogrel (Plavix)

Pentoxifylline affects red cell deformability and blood viscosity and can be considered as second-line alternative therapy to cilostazol. Although it improves pain-free and maximal walking distance, the degree of improvement varies among studies.[10] Other agents, such as propionyl-L-carnitine, L-arginine, and ginkgo biloba are not well established.

Endovascular intervention with angioplasty or stenting is highly effective for aortoiliac disease and is often indicated for moderate, or lifestyle-limiting claudication. Angioplasty, or stenting, of the superficial femoral artery is technically feasible but limited in applicability by high restenosis rates, particularly in the setting of long occlusions, a common scenario in this location. Despite this limitation, it is a valid therapeutic option for patients with focal disease, severe claudication, or tissue loss. Endovascular management of infrapopliteal (below the knee) disease is associated with extremely high restenosis rates, and is usually a temporizing measure to allow increased blood flow for wound healing. Surgical bypass techniques are effective but are generally high-risk procedures in a population with frequent comorbidities, and are usually reserved for patients with severe intermittent claudication or rest pain, or to allow healing of ulcers and gangrene. Sympathectomy is not of value for intermittent claudication, but has been used in the past to allow small ulcers or areas of gangrene to heal. In patients with rest pain, ulcers, or gangrene who are technically unrevascularizable or a very high risk for surgery, treatment options are limited. A period of rest with legs dependent may improve some patients, but amputation is a frequent outcome. Parenterally administered prostacyclin or prostaglandin E_1, despite some favorable reports of success, has not yet been thoroughly evaluated and is an expensive mode of therapy.

Dry gangrene of the digits or lower limbs should be allowed to spontaneously demarcate. Soaking or ointments are unnecessary. The edges of the gangrenous areas should be kept open if possible and observed frequently for infection. Pain medication is usually necessary for 2 to 3 months with digital gangrene. A conservative approach and patience will save many digits and extremities. Infected (wet) gangrenous areas must be actively debrided and appropriate antibiotics administered. Amputations may be necessary.

PREVENTION

The grim statistics regarding cardiovascular outcomes in these patients emphasize the need for aggressive secondary prevention by modifying appropriate cardiovascular risk factors when possible. Tobacco smoking is absolutely contraindicated. Continued smoking has been identified as the most consistent adverse risk factor associated with the progression of the disease. Smoking even 1 or 2 cigarettes a day can interfere with PAD treatments. Smokers also have significantly higher rates of amputation compared with nonsmokers. The rate of in-hospital amputation was 23% in smokers and 10% in nonsmokers. On the other hand, quitting smoking slows the progress of PAD and also reduces the rates of amputation required. Hypertension and diabetes mellitus should be controlled, and hyperlipidemias should be treated with a target low-density lipoprotein of less than 100 mg/dL (or <70 mg/dL with uncontrolled or multiple risk factors) as per recent guidelines for secondary prevention. All patients with PAD should be on a statin with the goal of preventing progression of PAD, in addition to prevention of myocardial infarction and stroke. Antiplatelet therapy is also indicated to reduce the risk of myocardial infarction, stroke, or vascular death in individuals with atherosclerotic lower extremity PAD.[11]

The use of thienopyridines, such as clopidogrel, may be of additional benefit, but may be associated with higher bleeding rates (particularly with combined therapy) and expense. Use of antiplatelet therapy is a must for those with PAD but should be individualized.

ATHEROMATOUS EMBOLISM

AT-A-GLANCE

- Atheromatous embolism is the embolization of small pieces of atheromatous debris from the more proximal arteries to the smaller distal arteries.
- Synonyms include *cholesterol embolism*, *atheroembolism*, *blue toe syndrome*, and *pseudovasculitis syndrome*.
- More common with advanced age and after invasive procedures.
- Manifestations include blue or discolored toes, livedo racemosa, gangrene, necrosis, ulceration, and fissure.
- Renal failure and stroke from systemic involvement.
- Diagnosis confirmed by cholesterol clefts in skin, kidney, or skeletal muscle biopsies.
- Treatment focuses on prevention during invasive procedures and elimination of the embolic source. Medical therapy may include antiplatelet therapy and statin agents; the use of anticoagulation is controversial and often avoided.

EPIDEMIOLOGY

The epidemiology of atheromatous embolism is poorly defined as a consequence of underreporting and difficulties establishing a clinical diagnosis.[12] Routine autopsy series of the adult population suggest an incidence of atheromatous embolism of between 0.15% and approximately 4%.[13] The incidence increases dramatically in the presence of severe atherosclerotic disease. Atheromatous embolism has been found in more than 20% of deaths following cardiac surgery or angiography. However, it should be emphasized that the rate of clinically detected atheromatous embolism appears to be reasonably low (less than 1%). The atheromatous embolism appears to be more common in males than in females, with a reported male-to-female ratio of approximately 3.4:1.[12,13] It is strongly associated with older age, with the mean age reported to range from 66 to 72 years.[13]

ETIOLOGY AND PATHOGENESIS

The pathogenesis of atheromatous embolism involves the occlusion of small arteries and arterioles (50 to 900 μm in diameter) by atheromatous debris (so-called cholesterol crystals) that is dislodged from a proximal atherosclerotic plaque, followed by a foreign-body inflammatory cascade. This inflammatory process leads to further occlusion with thrombus formation, endothelial cell proliferation, and intimal fibrosis, which may result in ischemia, infarction, and necrosis. The clinical picture is characterized by impaired perfusion of the skin and muscle as a result of small vessel occlusion, although nearly any organ of the body may be involved.

The major risk factor for the development of atheromatous embolism is atherosclerotic disease of the thoracic or abdominal aorta. The risk is higher with more extensive atheroma burden (defined by thickness above 4 mm) or unfavorable plaque features, such as protruding mobile plaque.[14] Coexistent vascular disease, including coronary artery disease, PAD, and even an abdominal aortic aneurysm are risk factors. The more traditional atherosclerotic risk factors also increase the risk of atheromatous embolism, with older age (older than 60 years) being prominent.

Atheromatous embolism often occurs after an invasive procedure.[13,15] Angiography, endovascular procedures, and both cardiac and vascular surgical procedures may create mechanical trauma to the vessel and destabilize an atherosclerotic plaque. Anticoagulation, primarily with warfarin, and thrombolytic therapy are potential risk factors. It has been postulated that anticoagulation may delay the healing of irregular or ulcerated plaques. Embolic events may occur spontaneously, although minor stressors, such as coughing or straining, may be provocative factors.

CLINICAL FINDINGS

HISTORY

The clinical presentation of atheromatous embolism, although it can occur spontaneously, usually follows an invasive procedure such as an invasive angiographic or vascular surgical procedure. The clinical manifestations may be immediate, or delayed by several days to weeks after the inciting event. The precise clinical syndrome depends on the location of the source of embolism and the pattern and distribution of flow downstream. This may range from subtle clinical findings to catastrophic systemic embolic complications. Nearly any organ of the body may be involved. Involvement of the ascending aorta may result in systemic complications, including transient ischemic attacks, strokes, or retinal manifestations, and involvement of the descending or abdominal aorta may lead to lower-extremity ischemia, renal failure, mesenteric ischemia, or hemorrhagic pancreatitis. As the more common sites for severe atheromatous disease are in the abdominal aorta and iliac arteries, the signs and symptoms more often result from embolism to the lower half of the body. Lower-extremity involvement typically presents with manifestations of discolored or ulcerated painful toes and tender calf muscles.

In addition, constitutional symptoms, including fever and weight loss, may be seen as a result of hypermetabolism associated with the inflammatory process.

CUTANEOUS LESIONS

The dermatologic manifestations are often the presenting complaint (Table 148-7). The most common of these findings are related to tissue or digital ischemia and include cyanosis, necrosis, gangrene, ulcerations, and fissures. The finding of tender, cool, blue, or purple toes with normal pulses, found in the "blue toe syndrome," is common (Fig. 148-5A). Approximately 50% of patients will have livedo racemosa, which typically involves the foot and leg, but may extend onto the trunk or buttocks. Erythematous lesions are often seen on the lateral aspect of the foot and calcaneal region. Although advanced ischemic manifestations, such as ulcers or gangrene, may be present (Fig. 148-5B), the surrounding areas are normally perfused tissue. There may be other cutaneous manifestations, often hemorrhagic in nature, including petechiae, ecchymosis, purpura, and splinter hemorrhages. Raised, painful, inflammatory nodules may occur.

TABLE 148-7
Cutaneous Findings in Atheromatous Embolism

- Blue or purple toes
- Livedo racemosa
- Gangrenous digits
- Ulcers
- Fissures
- Nodules
- Petechiae
- Purpura
- Splinter hemorrhages

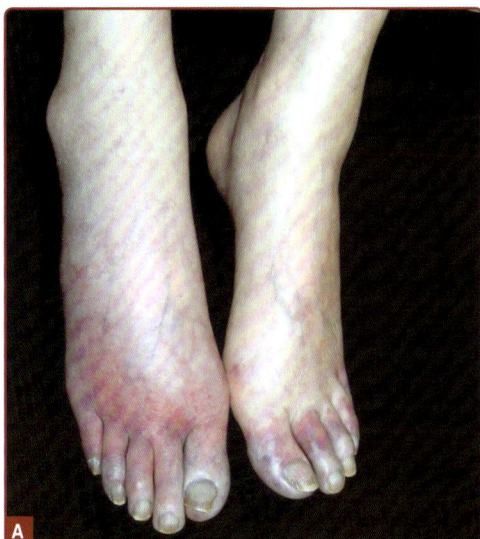

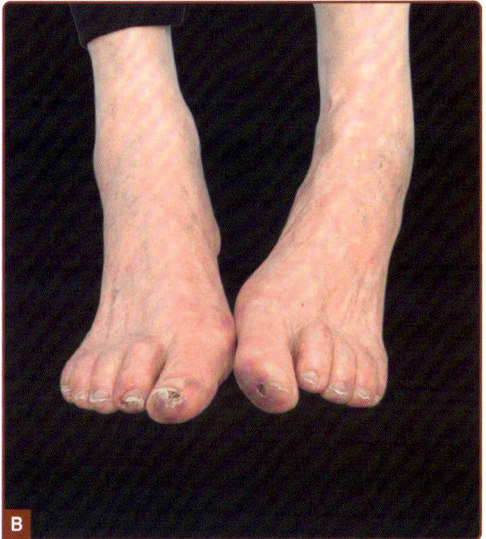

Figure 148-5 **A,** Typical appearance of blue toes caused by multiple atheromatous emboli to the lower limbs in a patient with extensive atheromatous disease of the aorta. **B,** Development of ulceration of the tip of the toes caused by atheromatous embolism with a faint reticular pattern on the forefoot typical of livedo racemosa.

from a source distal to the aortic arch. Fever may be present.

COMPLICATIONS

There are numerous ischemic complications depending upon the organ involved. These include the kidneys, mesenteric circulation, and CNS. Renal atheroembolic disease is a consequence of showering of emboli to the renal parenchymal branch vessels. An intense inflammatory process may ensue, producing glomerular sclerosis, tubular atrophy, and interstitial fibrosis. Although there is variable timing of onset and progression of disease, there typically is a several-week delay after the inciting event before the development of renal dysfunction. New onset of hypertension or overt renal failure may ensue. It is rare to develop gross hematuria or frank renal infarction. The development of renal failure is one of the more ominous complications with a high mortality in affected individuals.

The CNS is another feared site of involvement with atheromatous embolism. There is concern for ischemic manifestations such as transient ischemic attacks, stroke, and paralysis. However, other less-readily appreciated manifestations may ensue, such as encephalopathy or a progressive neurologic decline.

The GI tract is perhaps the third most common organ system involved with atheromatous embolism. The manifestations may be nonspecific abdominal complaints such as abdominal pain, nausea, vomiting, or diarrhea. More-severe ischemic manifestations may be seen with GI bleeding or bowel infarction. The colon is the most common site in the GI tract to be affected. Establishing a diagnosis may be difficult as endoscopy findings are often nonspecific, and biopsy may miss the classic findings. Splenic infarction, cholecystitis, gangrene of the gall bladder, pancreatitis, and pancreatic necrosis also have been reported.

RELATED PHYSICAL FINDINGS

Examination of the vascular system often reveals normal pedal and proximal pulses, because the small arteries are occluded with cholesterol emboli, rather than the larger superficial arteries. However, systolic bruits may be heard on auscultation over the aorta or common femoral arteries. Tenderness of skeletal muscles, particularly in the calf, may be detected. Funduscopic examination, revealing cholesterol embolus within branching points of the retinal arteries (Hollenhorst plaques), is a specific but insensitive finding because most atheromatous emboli arise

DIAGNOSIS

LABORATORY TESTS

The laboratory tests are typically nonspecific and depend upon the organ involved and the severity of disease. An elevated erythrocyte sedimentation rate, thrombocytopenia, hypocomplementemia, leukocytosis, and anemia may all be seen as a consequence of the systemic inflammatory response. Azotemia, proteinuria, microscopic hematuria, eosinophilia, and even eosinophiluria may be seen with renal involvement. Transient eosinophilia has been reported in up to 80% of those with renal involvement. Involvement of the GI tract may lead to anemia and blood in the stool. Injury to the liver, gallbladder, or pancreas may lead to abnormal liver function tests and elevated pancreatic enzymes.

SPECIAL TESTS

Contrast angiography may reveal diffuse atherosclerotic involvement of the vessels proximal to the lesions, but is typically avoided due to the risk of precipitating further embolic events. Noninvasive imaging techniques such as computed tomographic angiography or magnetic resonance angiography are useful to evaluate for atherosclerotic disease within the aorta or other large vessels. Although stenotic atherosclerotic disease is the most common finding, aneurysmal disease also may be present. Transthoracic echocardiography is often helpful to evaluate for a cardiac source, but the more definitive transesophageal echocardiography can also assess the thoracic aorta for plaque.

Definitive diagnosis of cholesterol embolization requires demonstration of cholesterol crystals, which are birefringent under polarized light. However, as a result of the solubility of cholesterol with typical solvents used in processing of tissue for histopathology, cholesterol crystals appear as empty clefts. Skin, muscle, or renal biopsies may reveal these characteristic elongated, needle-shaped clefts in small arterial vessels. There also may be inflammatory infiltrates, intimal thickening, and perivascular fibrosis, as well as giant cells. The sensitivity of the biopsy depends upon the site. Muscle biopsy seems to be the most sensitive test, reportedly being positive in more than 95% of cases, but is technically difficult, painful, and risky to obtain. The sensitivity of skin biopsy has varied from 40% to 90%. Skin biopsies offer maximum yield when obtained directly from areas of suspected emboli, such as those with livedo racemosa, but should be cautiously obtained or avoided in areas of more overt ischemic injury.

DIFFERENTIAL DIAGNOSIS

Because of its clinical similarity to other systemic diseases, atheromatous embolism is often misdiagnosed. Blue or ulcerated painful digits, livedo racemosa, petechiae, and tender calf muscles in the presence of normal pulses suggest the diagnosis of atheromatous emboli. However, it is difficult to establish the diagnosis, when the clinical features are subtle and nonspecific. Thus, a high index of suspicion is needed, especially in the setting of a history of preexisting atherosclerotic disease and a specific precipitating event. Definitive diagnosis can be made by skin, muscle, or even renal biopsies. Several other entities must be considered in

TABLE 148-8
Differential Diagnosis of Atheromatous Embolism

- Antiphospholipid antibodies
- Atrial myxoma
- Calciphylaxis
- Chilblains (or pernio)
- Cryoglobulinemia
- Heparin-induced thrombocytopenia
- Malignancies
- Multiple myeloma
- Nonbacterial thrombotic endocarditis
- Polyarteritis nodosa
- Subacute bacterial endocarditis
- Thrombocytopenia, polycythemia
- Thrombotic embolism
- Vasculitis
- Warfarin-induced skin necrosis

the differential diagnosis of atheromatous embolism (Table 148-8).

Moreover, among patients who develop acute renal failure, it is important to distinguish from contrast nephropathy, which is typically reversible. Renal failure caused by atheromatous emboli usually develops over 1 to 4 weeks after an angiographic procedure and shows partial recovery, whereas contrast-induced renal failure typically appears soon after testing and begins to recover within 3 to 5 days.

CLINICAL COURSE AND PROGNOSIS

The prognosis of cholesterol embolism is generally poor, in part because of the severe underlying atherosclerosis. The outcome also depends upon the organ system affected with the emboli. Estimates of mortality range from 20% to 30% for 1-year mortality. The poorest outcomes have been reported in those with emboli arising from a suprarenal location.

The syndrome usually subsides, and lesions heal following successful surgical or medical treatment, although spontaneous resolution may occur. Recurrent embolism may result in limb loss in the absence of surgical or interventional management options. In the "malignant multisystem" disease, most patients die within 1 year if treatment is unsuccessful. The prognosis is extremely poor in the presence of systemic complications, particularly renal failure or stroke. The development of end-stage renal disease due to atheromatous embolism is a strong predictor of death.

MANAGEMENT

Early recognition is essential to minimize end-organ damage and improve the clinical outcomes.[13] Preventing further ischemic insult, supportive care, and removal of the atheromatous source are the mainstays of therapy.[14] Elimination of the source of the emboli can often be accomplished by surgical bypasses or endarterectomy although many of these patients have contraindications to major surgery. Endovascular procedures with covered stents also may be considered; however, this approach may carry significant risk with the potential to exacerbate further embolization.

Medical therapies have not been well studied, and recommendations are based on the results from small series or anecdotal reports. Antiplatelet agents, such as aspirin, dipyridamole, or clopidogrel, are most often tried, and if successful, should be continued long-term. Antithrombotic therapy such as subcutaneous heparin or low-molecular-weight heparin may be beneficial with some patients, suggesting that these agents may reduce the secondary small-vessel thrombosis. Warfarin is usually avoided because of potential for exacerbating the process, but this concern has a limited basis. There is even a proposed beneficial effect of long-term anticoagulation to prevent embolic events in those with extensive mobile aortic atheroma. The use of statins may aid in plaque stabilization and has clear established benefits in prevention of cardiovascular ischemic events in those with vascular disease. Other agents, such as iloprost and cilostazol, have limited evidence to suggest benefit, but have been tried in those with renal dysfunction (iloprost) and cutaneous lesions (cilostazol). Systemic corticosteroids are not recommended. As most of these patients have severe underlying atherosclerosis, they should be aggressively treated for secondary prevention of cardiovascular disease with optimization of the risk factors.

PREVENTION

Because of the rarity of the disease and the difficulties in establishing the diagnosis, increased awareness of the problem is important. Primary prevention in high-risk patients, targeted to avoid the development of atherosclerotic plaque, should be performed. Once atherosclerosis develops, avoiding unnecessary invasive procedures is advised. When angiography is necessary, more cautious techniques with the use of soft-tipped guidewires and more flexible catheters help to reduce the risk. In addition, protective devices, such as filters, baskets, and balloon occlusion, have been used. In patients with atheromatous disease of the abdominal aorta and iliac arteries, use of a brachial artery approach is often considered. Surgical techniques also have been refined with less aortic manipulation and circulation arrest, which may help to minimize the chance of developing this disorder.

THROMBOANGIITIS OBLITERANS (BUERGER DISEASE)

AT-A-GLANCE

- Rare inflammatory occlusive disease affecting medium and small arteries and veins, most commonly in the extremities.
- Predominantly affects males, at age 20 to 40 years.
- Extremely strong association with smoking; often abates with smoking cessation.
- Clinical manifestations include ischemia, cold sensitivity, or claudication of the foot, leg, or hand, which progress to ischemic ulcers, peripheral cyanosis, gangrene, or superficial thrombophlebitis.

Thromboangiitis obliterans (TAO), also known as Buerger disease, is a rare, progressive, inflammatory and thrombotic disease that predominately affects small- and medium-sized arteries of the extremities. It is strongly associated with the use of tobacco products, and seen mostly in men between the ages of 20 and 40 years.

EPIDEMIOLOGY

The prevalence of this disease is greatest in Mediterranean countries, the Middle East, and Asia, and it is relatively less common in people of northern European descent.[16] Males are afflicted with a higher prevalence than females (with a male-to-female ratio of 3:1), although an increased incidence in females has occurred in recent years, likely reflecting the pattern of tobacco use.[17] Patients are usually between the ages of 20 and 40 years. Since 1990 there has been a marked decline in the reported prevalence of TAO in the United States, possibly reflecting the impact of adoption of strict diagnostic criteria for this disease entity, although declining smoking prevalence may also play a role. In 1947, the prevalence of the disease in the United States was estimated at 104 cases per 100,000 population; however, the prevalence has been estimated at 12 to 20 cases per 100,000 population more recently.[16]

CLINICAL FEATURES

CUTANEOUS FINDINGS

The most common initial complaints are claudication of the foot or lower calf, digital cyanosis or gangrene, or rest pain. Involvement of multiple limbs is typical. Patients may present with ulcers of the toes or fingers. Although the lower extremities are affected most often, more than one-third of patients have upper-extremity involvement. Ulcerations or gangrenous areas are characteristically extremely painful. Superficial thrombophlebitis, often migratory, may occur in up to 40% of patients.[16] Cold sensitivity or even classical Raynaud phenomenon may be observed.

The cutaneous findings of TAO are similar to that of PAD. Common findings include ulceration or gangrene of digits (feet worse than hands; Fig. 148-6), peripheral cyanosis or Raynaud phenomenon, and superficial thrombophlebitis, often migratory, with indurated red nodules.

The hands and feet of patients with the disease are usually cold and mildly edematous. They may develop cyanotic, ulcerated, or gangrenous and very painful digits. Typically, the distal pulses (dorsalis pedis, posterior tibial, and ulnar pulses) are absent, while the more proximal pulses are preserved. During episodes of thrombophlebitis, small-indurated red, tender nodules will be found, which follow the course of superficial veins and are common on the thigh or calf. Typical changes of Raynaud phenomenon, with well-demarcated pallor or cyanosis of the digits, may be seen on exposure to cold; one or more extremities may be involved. Sensory abnormalities reflecting ischemic neuropathy have been observed in advanced cases. Nailfold examination with capillaroscopy may reveal multiple dilated capillary loops.

ETIOLOGY AND PATHOGENESIS

The etiology of TAO remains unknown. The disease occurs almost exclusively in smokers and often abates with the cessation of tobacco smoking. Increased cellular sensitivity to types I and III collagen has been reported in comparison to a group of normal individuals and patients with atherosclerotic disease. An increased prevalence of human leukocyte antigen (HLA)-A9, HLA-A54, and HLA-B5 has been observed in these patients, suggesting a genetic component to the disease.[18] Tissue ischemia is produced by an inflammatory reaction involving medium- and small-sized arteries of the extremities and superimposed obstruction by thrombi. Despite the inflammatory process, TAO is considered serologically silent, and even during active disease, inflammatory markers, such as erythrocyte sedimentation rate and C-reactive protein levels, are usually normal. In one report, serum anti-endothelial cell antibody titers were found to be high, and impaired endothelial-dependent vasodilation to acetylcholine has been demonstrated to occur even in nonobstructed limbs. Veins also may be involved. Occasionally, cardiac, intestinal, and cerebral vessels are involved.

DIAGNOSIS

Even though a variety of diagnostic criteria have been published, a uniform criterion does not exist. Figure 148-7 presents an approach to TAO. Diagnosis of TAO typically relies on the clinical presentation and arteriography findings. Arteriography findings, in particular findings of corkscrew-shaped collaterals, are typical, but not pathognomonic for the condition. Because TAO is not limited to a single limb, abnormal arteriography findings are often bilateral. Exclusion of arteriosclerosis, or risk factors of other occlusive vasculopathies is crucial to establishing the diagnosis of TAO.

Histopathologic findings of arteries and veins on biopsy demonstrate inflammatory thrombus infiltrated with polymorphonuclear leukocytes and multinucleated giant cells.[19] A biopsy is not required to make the diagnosis, but can be used in atypical presentations.

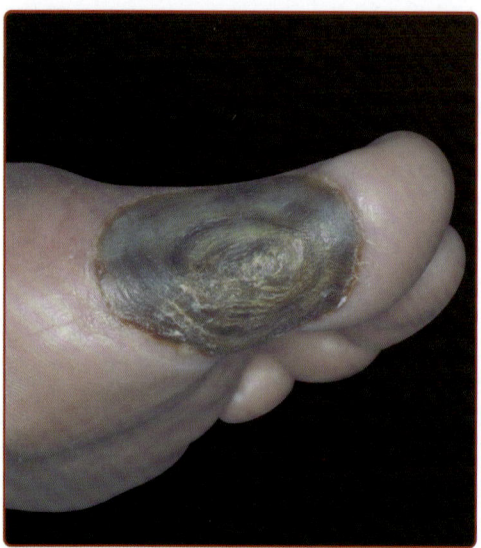

Figure 148-6 Necrotic toe in a patient with thromboangiitis obliterans; this appearance may be seen with other arterial occlusive processes.

DIFFERENTIAL DIAGNOSIS

Table 148-9 outlines the differential diagnosis for TAO.

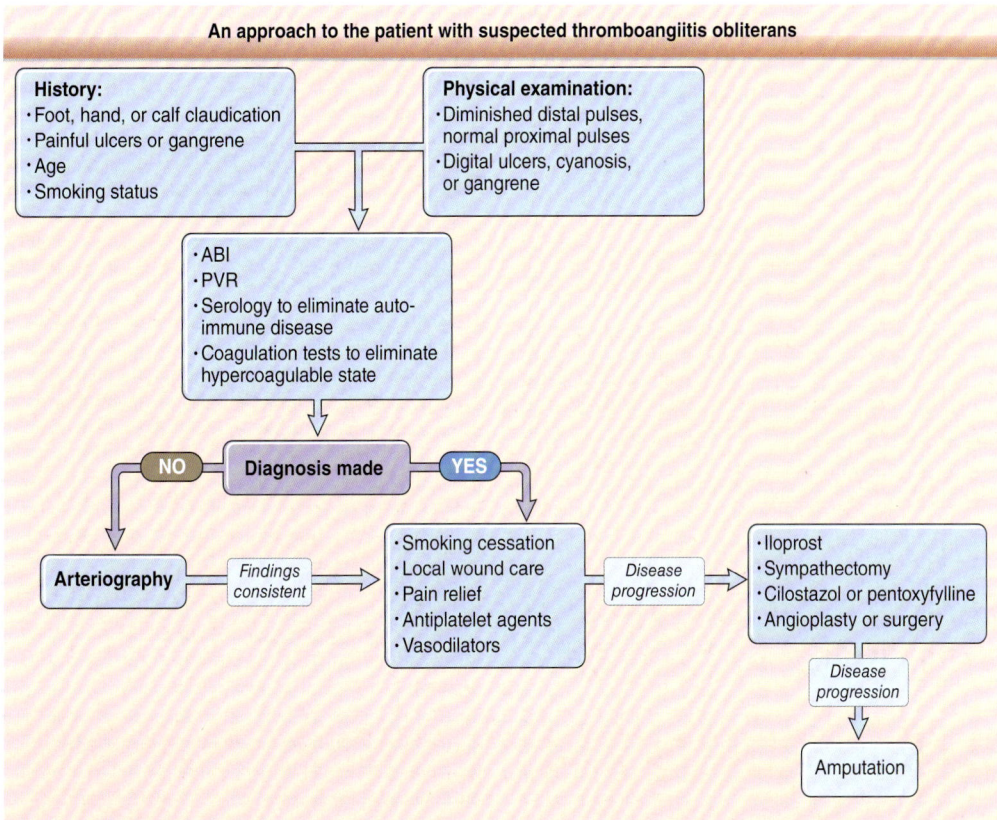

Figure 148-7 An approach to the patient with suspected thromboangiitis obliterans. ABI, ankle-brachial index; PVR, pulse-volume recording.

MANAGEMENT

Table 148-10 presents management options for TAO. Smoking cessation results in dramatic improvement. Avoidance of smokeless (chewing) tobacco and nicotine-containing patches is also necessary for disease abatement. A *Cochrane Database Review* revealed that, compared to aspirin, the IV prostacyclin analog, iloprost, improves ulcer healing and eliminates rest pain.[15] In addition to pharmacologic agents, local wound care and adequate analgesic therapy is imperative. Cilostazol, clopidogrel, pentoxifylline, or oral prostanoid is often initiated in the treatment of TAO, despite the absence of data from large randomized trials. Bypass surgery and angioplasty have been reported, but are suboptimal therapeutic options because of the small size and distal location of the vessels affected. Sympathectomy may help patients with a prominent vasospastic component. Vascular endothelial growth

TABLE 148-9
Differential Diagnosis of Thromboangiitis Obliterans

- Warfarin necrosis
- Livedoid vasculopathy
- Disseminated intravascular coagulation
- Purpura fulminans
- Cryoglobulinemia type 1
- Cryofibrinogenemia
- Cholesterol emboli
- Antiphospholipid syndrome
- Thrombotic thrombocytopenic purpura
- Levamisole-adulterated cocaine thrombotic vasculopathy

TABLE 148-10
Treatment of Thromboangiitis Obliterans

	IMPROVE BLOOD FLOW	SYMPTOM RELIEF
First-line therapy	Smoking cessation IV iloprost	Local wound care Analgesics
Second-line therapy	Antiplatelet agents Oral vasodilators Cilostazol (Pletal) Pentoxifylline (Trental)	
Third-line therapy	Angioplasty Surgical endarterectomy or bypass	Sympathectomy Amputation

factor gene therapy may prove of value, but has not yet been well studied. In those with refractory disease with nonhealing ulcers, gangrene, or intractable pain, surgical amputation of the affected distal limbs is often unavoidable.

PREVENTION

Absolute discontinuation of tobacco use is the only strategy proven to prevent the progression of TAO. Smoking as few as 1 or 2 cigarettes daily, using chewing tobacco, or even using nicotine replacements may keep the disease active.[20] The following strategies are important in prevention of complications from the disease: use of well-fitting protective footwear to prevent foot trauma and thermal or chemical injury, avoidance of cold environments, and avoidance of drugs that lead to vasoconstriction.

LIVEDO RETICULARIS AND LIVEDO RACEMOSA

AT-A-GLANCE

- Livedo is an ischemic dermopathy characterized by a violaceous reticular or "net-like" mottling of the skin.
- Livedo reticularis is a primary disorder affecting young to middle-aged females that is benign. The livid conical discoloration is symmetric, reversible, and uniform.
- Livedo racemosa is a secondary disorder that is pathologic and permanent. The livid conical discoloration is asymmetric, irreversible, and "broken."
- Differentiating benign livedo reticularis from pathologic livedo racemosa is imperative.
- Antiphospholipid antibody testing should be obtained on all patients presenting with livedo racemosa.

EPIDEMIOLOGY

Livedo reticularis is typically a primary disorder that affects young to middle-aged females (20 to 50 years of age) who are otherwise healthy.[21] Amantadine-induced livedo reticularis is also more common in females. The epidemiologic factors of livedo racemosa are dependent on the underlying condition. It is the most frequent dermatologic manifestation in patients with antiphospholipid syndrome, present in 25% of patients with primary antiphospholipid syndrome, and in up to 70% of patients with systemic lupus erythematosus–associated antiphospholipid syndrome.[22] The distinction between livedo racemosa and livedo reticularis is an evolving concept that is neither universally quoted nor referred to in most of the older literature.

CLINICAL FEATURES

With the exception of a subjective feeling of coldness, the majority of patients with livedo reticularis are asymptomatic (Table 148-11). Patients often present with concerns regarding their skin discoloration. A minority describe mild pain and numbness. The symptoms are worse during winter months. Livedo racemosa-associated symptoms are related to the causative secondary disorder.

CUTANEOUS LESIONS

In livedo reticularis, a symmetric, fishnet-like red or purple mottling surrounds a pallorous conical core (Fig. 148-8). This discoloration is aggravated by cold exposure and may completely dissipate with warming. The livid rings are most pronounced on the lower extremities yet the abdomen and upper extremities can be affected.

In contradistinction to the symmetric and uniform reticular pattern of livedo reticularis, the discoloration of livedo racemosa is asymmetric, irregular, and "broken" (Fig. 148-9; see Table 148-11). Although it may improve with warming, it does not resolve completely. Attendant skin manifestations of livedo racemosa may include purpura, nodules, macules, ulcerations,

TABLE 148-11
Comparison of Livedo Reticularis and Livedo Racemosa

	LIVEDO RETICULARIS	LIVEDO RACEMOSA
Condition	Benign	Pathologic
Associated conditions	Occasionally drug-related (amantadine)	See Table 148-12
Symptoms	Asymptomatic; mild pain or numbness	Symptoms related to associated causative disorder
Characteristic appearance	Symmetric, fishnet-like red or purple mottling with a pale conical core over lower extremities, abdomen or upper extremities (see Fig. 148-8)	Asymmetric, irregular, and "broken" (see Fig. 148-9)
Surrounding skin	Unaffected	Purpura, nodules, macules, ulcerations, atrophie blanche–type scarring
Aggravating/relieving factors	Aggravated by cold, relieved by warming	May improve with warming but no complete resolution

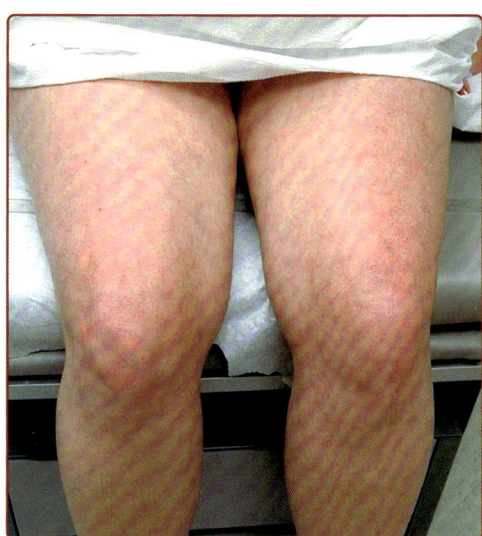

Figure 148-8 Symmetric and relatively uniform, conical rings of primary, reversible livedo reticularis (cutis marmorata).

and/or atrophie blanche-type scarring. When associated with livedoid vasculitis, painful ulcerations of the ankles and forefeet may occur.

In both livedo reticularis and racemosa, the skin is palpably cool.

NONCUTANEOUS FINDINGS

Livedo reticularis and livedo racemosa are often associated with vasospastic digits or acrocyanosis. With exception of the characteristic skin changes, the examination in livedo reticularis is otherwise unremarkable. Patients with livedo racemosa may have concurrent abnormal physical findings related to their underlying disease (eg, aphasia and lateralizing neurologic signs associated with Sneddon syndrome).

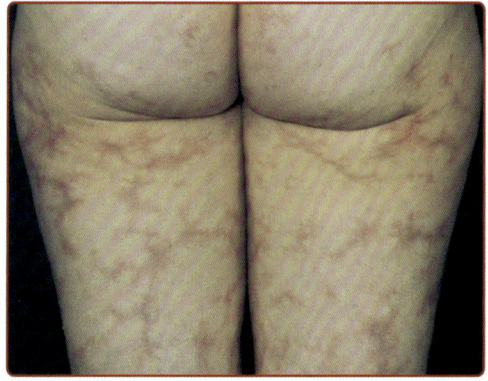

Figure 148-9 Permanent and "broken" rings of secondary livedo racemosa on the buttocks and thighs in a woman who had cerebrovascular thrombosis. This is an example of Sneddon syndrome.

ETIOLOGY AND PATHOGENESIS

In both disorders, the characteristic ring-like mottling results from (patho)physiologic changes within the cutaneous microvascular system. Anatomically, the dermis is perfused via perpendicularly oriented ascending arterioles. Individual arterioles arborize into a capillary bed at the skin surface. Ultimately, the capillary beds empty into a conical-appearing, peripherally located subpapillary venous plexus.

Pathophysiologically, livedo arises from either deoxygenation or venodilation within the venous plexus.[23] Decreased arteriolar perfusion is the predominant cause of deoxygenation within the venous plexus. Diminished arteriolar flow can result from vasospasm, hyperviscosity, and/or thrombosis. Physiologic arteriolar vasospasm produces the reversible cutaneous discoloration of livedo reticularis. The livedo reticularis can occur as a physiologic reaction to cold exposure, when it is known as cutis marmorata, or the skin color changes may be unrelated to ambient temperature. Protracted arteriolar vasospasm, thrombosis, and/or hyperviscosity underlie the pathologic skin changes of livedo racemosa. Venodilation of the venous plexus may be provoked by hypoxia or autonomic dysfunction.

A possible role for endothelial cells also has been suggested in the subset of patients with antiphospholipid syndrome with livedo racemosa. The interaction of antiphospholipid antibodies with endothelial cells could induce livedo racemosa and also lead to increased production of procoagulant substances such as tissue factor, plasminogen activator inhibitor-1, and endothelin. Increased tissue factor expression on endothelial cells induced by antiphospholipid antibodies could be responsible, in part, for hypercoagulability and might explain the thrombosis in both arterial and venous circulation that characterizes these patients.[22]

Amantadine-induced livedo reticularis has traditionally been ascribed to catecholamine provoked arteriolar vasospasm; however, an interaction between amantadine and N-methyl-D-aspartic acid receptors in the skin may be responsible in some unexplained fashion.[24]

Livedoid vasculopathy is a rare ulcerative subtype of livedo racemosa caused by fibrinolytic abnormalities and microcirculatory thrombosis.

DIAGNOSIS

LABORATORY TESTING

In livedo reticularis, laboratory testing is typically negative and consequently is unwarranted. An antiphospholipid antibody panel should be obtained on all patients presenting with livedo racemosa. A complete thrombophilia panel is warranted in the rare patient with livedoid vasculopathy (see Chap. 138). The need for additional laboratory analysis in a patient with livedo racemosa should be directed by the clinical assessment.

A skin biopsy is not required in livedo reticularis as the findings are nonspecific. A large punch or wedge biopsy of the deep reticular dermis and subcutaneous fat is sometimes helpful in identifying the secondary cause of livedo racemosa. Selection of the correct biopsy site (seemingly uninvolved skin in the center of the lesion) is essential for detection of relevant vascular pathology. The biopsy findings are highly variable and reflect the associated livedo racemosa etiology. For instance, cholesterol clefts suggest atheroembolic disease, calcification of the vessels and interstitium indicate calciphylaxis, noninflammatory arteriolar obstruction occurs with Sneddon syndrome, livedoid vasculopathy is associated with extensive fibrin deposition and microthrombi (see Chap. 138), whereas fibrinoid necrosis is present in polyarteritis nodosa (see Chap. 139).

DIFFERENTIAL DIAGNOSIS

Identifying the characteristic mottled skin discoloration easily makes the diagnosis of livedo. It is paramount that the clinicians distinguish between livedo reticularis and livedo racemosa. Once a diagnosis of livedo racemosa is established, the secondary cause (Table 148-12) should be sought by appropriate clinical laboratory tests. Diagnostic difficulties may occur when no other pathologic signs except livedo racemosa are found. This clinical condition, known as *idiopathic livedo racemosa*, may represent a very early stage of Sneddon syndrome.

TABLE 148-12
Conditions Associated with Livedo Racemosa

- Antiphospholipid antibody syndrome
- Atheroembolic disease
- Atrial myxoma
- Calciphylaxis
- Chronic pancreatitis
- Collagen vascular disease
- Cryoglobulinemia/cryofibrinogenemia/cold agglutinin disease
- Erythema ab igne
- Hyperoxaluria
- Infections
- Livedoid vasculopathy
- Myeloproliferative syndromes (polycythemia vera, essential thrombocytosis)
- Paraproteinemias
- Sneddon syndrome
- Vasculitis (especially polyarteritis nodosa)

CLINICAL COURSE AND PROGNOSIS

The prognosis for livedo reticularis is excellent as this is primarily a cosmetic condition. Livedo racemosa–associated prognosis is less favorable and parallels the associated disease. Of interest, livedo racemosa has been identified as a marker for predicting multisystem thrombosis in the antiphospholipid antibody syndrome. Additionally, up to 40% of patients manifest livedo racemosa as the initial sign of the antiphospholipid antibody syndrome.[25] In addition, an increased rate of pregnancy loss has been recognized in patients with widespread livedo racemosa who were seronegative for antiphospholipid antibodies, suggesting that livedo racemosa may be an independent risk factor for pregnancy loss in the absence of antiphospholipid syndrome. Livedoid vasculopathy tends to be a relapsing condition marked by recurrent painful ulcerations and subsequent atrophie blanche-type scars.

MANAGEMENT

Other than cold avoidance, medical treatment for primary livedo reticularis is typically unwarranted. As a last resort, vasodilator therapy may be tried in the patient who is socially inhibited by the cosmetic appearance of the disorder. The symptoms may improve spontaneously with age.

Therapy of livedo racemosa should be directed toward the underlying disorder. Patients with livedo racemosa and the antiphospholipid antibody syndrome with thrombosis require anticoagulation. Treatment of livedoid vasculopathy is often unsatisfactory, but potentially beneficial medications include anticoagulants, antiplatelet agents, immunosuppressants, pentoxifylline, danazol, and tissue plasminogen activator. Alternatively, hyperbaric oxygen and psoralen plus ultraviolet A light therapy also have been successfully used to treat livedoid vasculopathy.

ERYTHROMELALGIA (ERYTHERMALGIA)

AT-A-GLANCE

- Intense, burning pain with marked erythema, typically of the lower extremity.
- Typically intermittent. May be precipitated by exercise.
- Primary disorder or secondary to a myeloproliferative disorder.

(Continued)

AT-A-GLANCE (Continued)

- Cutaneous manifestations are often a result of attempts to alleviate the symptoms with immersion and thermal injury.
- Aspirin may be effective for secondary erythromelalgia.

Red, hot, painful extremities with characteristic intense, burning pain characterize erythromelalgia. It most commonly affects the lower extremities but may affect the upper extremities as well as other body parts, such as the face and ears. Involvement is usually symmetric, although it can be unilateral in secondary cases. The symptoms are typically intermittent in nature, but may become constant. Onset can be gradual or abrupt, and usually is precipitated by activities that increase the body temperature, such as exercise, ambient temperature, or the use of heavy blankets at night. The episodes also can be triggered by dependency of the limb, wearing socks, or tight shoes, and sometimes with the ingestion of alcohol or spicy foods. There are also reports of episodes triggered by ingestion of some drugs, such as pergolide, bromocriptine, and calcium channel blockers (nifedipine, felodipine, and nicardipine). In contrast, cold exposure (eg, standing on a cold floor) or immersion in ice water often relieves the flares.

Patients with both erythromelalgia and Raynaud phenomenon also have been described. During the hyperemic phase of Raynaud phenomenon, patients often complain of erythromelalgic-like symptoms. It is postulated that both syndromes have a common basis in a dysfunction of the regulation of vasomotor tone.[24]

EPIDEMIOLOGY

This is a rare disorder with limited epidemiologic data available. In Norway, the incidence is estimated to be 0.25 per 100,000 population with a prevalence of 2 per 100,000 population.[26] In the United States, extrapolation from a series of erythromelalgia patients at the Mayo Clinic suggests an incidence of 1.3 case per 100,000 patients.[27] Primary erythromelalgia may occur at any age with an uncertain gender predilection, although recent studies seem to suggest a female predominance.[27] In contrast, secondary erythromelalgia has an equal sex distribution and occurs mostly after the third decade.[28]

CLINICAL FEATURES

CUTANEOUS LESIONS

Examination during attacks reveals warm, red, extremely sensitive extremities with normal pulses (Fig. 148-10). Between flares, the extremities may

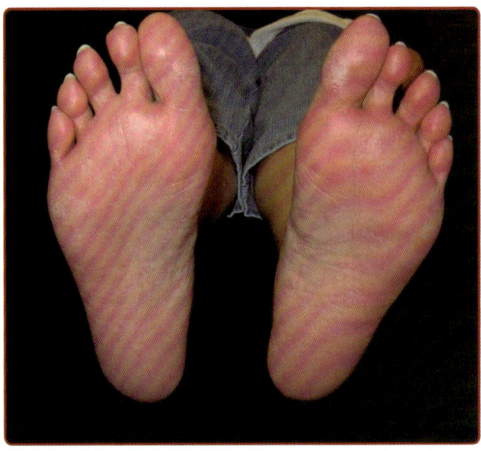

Figure 148-10 Intense erythema of the feet with associated burning pain typical of erythromelalgia.

appear normal. The constant use of ice water leads to maceration of the skin, secondary infection, ulcers, and necrosis.

NONCUTANEOUS FINDINGS

Physical examination is usually unremarkable in primary erythromelalgia; however, it may reveal signs of an underlying disorder in the secondary erythromelalgia. The peripheral pulses are usually normal or bounding.

ETIOLOGY AND PATHOGENESIS

The etiology and pathogenesis of the erythromelalgia are unknown. Several mechanisms have been postulated for primary erythromelalgia, including arteriovenous shunting and a small fiber neuropathy. It has been speculated that precapillary sphincters may be constricted while arteriovenous shunts are open, leading to an increased total perfusion but a deficient nutritive blood flow.[29] Substances produced by local hypoxia lead to increased local blood flow, warmth, redness, and pain. In contrast, the genetics of erythromelalgia appears to be supporting a neuropathic basis. A mutation in *SCN9A*, the gene encoding voltage-gated sodium channels of sensory nerves, has been reported in inherited erythromelalgia.[30]

Secondary erythromelalgia occurs in polycythemia, thrombocythemia, and autoimmune disorders, and is hypothesized to be caused by platelet breakdown products based on the response to aspirin therapy.

DIAGNOSIS

Erythromelalgia is diagnosed based on evaluation of the characteristic symptoms and signs of the disease.

TABLE 148-13
Differential Diagnosis of Erythromelalgia

- Complex regional pain syndrome
- Peripheral neuropathy
- Raynaud phenomenon (hyperemic phase)
- Systemic lupus erythematosus

There is often a delay in diagnosis given the intermittent nature of the condition. Photos taken by the patient during a flare can be beneficial. Alternatively, provoking a flare with use of exercise or immersion of the affected area in hot water for at least 10 minutes may be required to assist with definitive diagnosis. Family history is necessary to assess for inherited primary erythromelalgia.

Secondary erythromelalgia, caused by polycythemia vera or essential thrombocythemia, should be ruled out by first obtaining a laboratory test for a complete blood count. If abnormalities are present, additional specialized testing may be required.

DIFFERENTIAL DIAGNOSIS

Table 148-13 outlines the differential diagnosis for erythromelalgia.

CLINICAL COURSE AND PROGNOSIS

The natural history of erythromelalgia is extremely variable.[31] Symptoms may be mild for several years or totally disabling within weeks. It has been reported that with long-term followup, symptoms were worse in 32%, unchanged in 27%, improved in 31%, and resolved in 10% of patients. Many patients become disabled, being unable to work or carry on daily activities. As a result of the profound impact upon their life with intractable symptoms, patients have even been known to commit suicide. There is a decrease in survival compared with age- and gender-matched controls.

MANAGEMENT

Limited data is available to guide therapy, primarily based upon case reports or small series. Treatment is focused on prevention of flares and symptom control. Behavioral modifications should include efforts to keep the limbs cool and avoid the use of ice water or prolonged soaking. Cool air, such as from air conditioners or fans, can provide symptom relief, although prolonged exposure is not recommended. Topical therapies, such as a lidocaine patch, can be of tremendous help. Topical formulations that contain a combination of amitriptyline, ketamine, and gabapentin may also provide relief.

Pharmacologic therapy has varied, but often has focused on vasoactive drugs and drugs that affect the nervous system. Most vasoactive drugs, including calcium-channel blockers and β blockers, have been minimally effective in treating this disorder. Drugs used to treat neuropathy, such as serotonin reuptake inhibitors, tricyclic antidepressants, and gabapentin, have been used and may provide some relief. Combinations of these medications are often required, and starting with a low dose is advised to avoid side effects. Numerous other agents, including misoprostol, antihistamines, IV iloprost, lorazepam, cycloheptadine, piroxicam, and pizotifen, have been tried in selected cases. The prostaglandin E_1 analog misoprostol was evaluated in a double-blind crossover trial and found to be superior to placebo.

Surgical or medical sympathectomies also have been tried but have had mixed results. As a result of the chronic pain that can be associated with erythromelalgia, pain rehabilitation with the use of biofeedback, and even hypnosis, may be beneficial.

In secondary erythromelalgia, aspirin is often of great benefit.

PREVENTION

There are no established measures to prevent the development of erythromelalgia. The focus has been to prevent flares once the disorder occurs. The key to prevention is to avoid exacerbating factors and to prophylactically cool the involved extremity. The other preventive measures are to prevent the development of secondary complications often as a result of prolonged cold exposure, either from ice water or excessive cold blowing air.

CHRONIC VENOUS DISEASE

AT-A-GLANCE

- One percent to 3% of U.S. health care expenses are for peripheral venous diseases and their complications.
- Venous ulcers are the most common.
- Risk factors include genetics, obesity, female gender, pregnancy, and occupations requiring prolonged standing, surgery, trauma, and malignancies.
- Peripheral venous disease should be considered part of a spectrum including the following:
  - Early signs: tenderness, edema, hyperpigmentation, and varicose veins.
  - Late signs: atrophie blanche, lipodermatosclerosis, and venous ulcers.

(Continued)

AT-A-GLANCE (Continued)

- Venous ulcers are located exclusively below the knee after venous pump failure, most often secondary to prior thrombosis.
- Treatment for all stages includes leg elevation, compression, treatment of infection and dermatitis.
- Deep venous disease is associated with thromboembolism.

Chronic venous disease of the peripheral veins includes a spectrum of findings ranging from telangiectasias to reticular veins and varicose veins. Chronic venous insufficiency is a result of persistent ambulatory venous hypertension of the lower-extremity venous system, which results in a spectrum of clinical findings from edema and tenderness to venous ulceration (Table 148-14).

EPIDEMIOLOGY

Chronic venous disease is extremely common and has a prevalence in the adult population of up to 30%.[32] Although estimated cost and time lost from work have not been objectively assessed in more than 2 decades, estimates state that 25 million adults in the United States have varicose veins and 6 million have evidence of advanced disease.[33] Venous ulcers, as a result of chronic venous insufficiency, cause significant disability and are estimated to be 1% of the adult population. The care of venous ulcers is estimated to cost $3 billion annually.[34]

Risk factors for chronic venous disease include heredity, age, female sex, obesity, pregnancy, prolonged standing, phlebitis, previous leg injury, and greater height.[34]

TABLE 148-14
Common Signs and Symptoms of Peripheral Venous Disease

Symptoms
- Leg fullness
- Aching discomfort
- Heaviness
- Nocturnal leg cramps
- Bursting pain on standing

Signs
Very Early
- Tenderness to palpation

Early
- Edema
- Hyperpigmentation
- Stasis dermatitis
- Varicose veins

Late
- Venous ulcers
- Atrophie blanche
- Lipodermatosclerosis
- Acroangiodermatitis of Mali
- Postphlebitic syndrome

CLINICAL FINDINGS

CUTANEOUS LESIONS

There is a spectrum of clinical manifestations of chronic venous disease starting with telangiectasias and reticular veins on one end of the spectrum, and advanced chronic venous insufficiency, including skin ulcerations and fibrosis, at the other end. Once there is chronic venous insufficiency, findings include dilated veins (varicose veins), edema, leg pain, and cutaneous changes. The earliest finding is perimalleolar edema that ascends up the leg, followed by soft tissue tenderness, even of normal appearing skin. Tenderness if often elicited when palpating for the presence of edema.

Varicose veins, especially noticeable when the patient is standing, and smaller varicosities appear about the dorsum of the foot and ankle (see Chap. 212). Although they are usually asymptomatic, patients may complain of aching, cramping, itching, fatigue, and swelling that are worse with prolonged standing. Superficial thrombophlebitis can develop along the course of the varicose vein and present with an area of induration, erythema, warmth, and tenderness.

Stasis dermatitis, characterized by erythema, scaling, pruritus, erosions, crusting, and occasional vesicles and serous drainage may occur during any stage of chronic venous insufficiency (Fig. 148-11). It typically occurs in the medial supramalleolar region where microangiopathy is most intense. Over time, lesions may lichenify. It is important to evaluate for coexisting allergic contact dermatitis, as up to 80% of patients

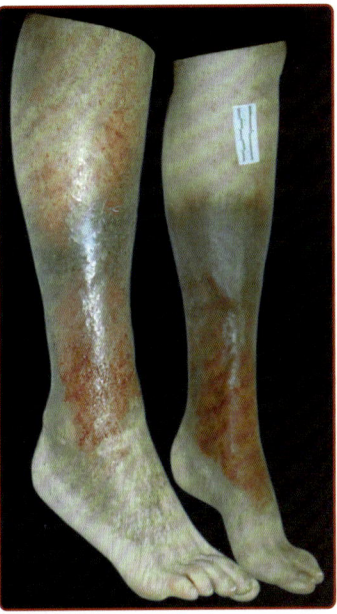

Figure 148-11 Bilateral venous disease with dermatitis and extensive hemosiderosis.

with venous leg ulcers develop contact sensitization to topical therapies.

In lipodermatosclerosis (sclerosing panniculitis, hypodermatitis sclerodermiformis), pliable subcutaneous fat is gradually replaced by fibrosis, and the skin begins to feel firm and indurated. This is a fibrosing panniculitis characterized by a bound down plaque that begins at the medial ankle and extends circumferentially around the entire distal lower leg.[35] As the fibrosis increases, it may constrict and strangle the lower leg further, impeding venous and lymphatic flow and leading to brawny edema above and below the fibrosis. These late changes resemble an inverted champagne bottle (see Fig. 148-11).

Occasionally, lipodermatosclerosis can present acutely with bright red erythema and tenderness and mimics cellulitis, except systemic signs and symptoms are lacking. Lack of response to oral antibiotics and a relapsing nature eventually lead to the diagnosis. This is a result of acute inflammation of the subcutaneous fat, and a septal panniculitis can be seen histopathologically in this setting (see Chap. 73).

Atrophie blanche refers to skin overlying areas of fibrosis that often appears porcelain white and atrophic. Fully established lesions of atrophie blanche consist of irregular, smooth, atrophic stellate plaques with surrounding hyperpigmentation and telangiectasias (Fig. 148-12). Although mostly related to venous stasis, atrophie blanche also may be associated with an underlying disorder of hypercoagulation (eg, antiphospholipid syndrome, inherited coagulopathies), livedoid vasculitis (see Chap. 138), or autoimmune disease (eg, scleroderma, lupus erythematosus).[36] Acroangiodermatitis (pseudo-Kaposi sarcoma, congenital dysplastic angiopathy, arteriovenous malformation with angiodermatitis) has purple macules, nodules, or verrucous plaques on the dorsal feet and toes of patients with longstanding venous insufficiency and mimics Kaposi sarcoma clinically and histologically. Identical lesions have been described in arteriovenous malformations of the legs, arteriovenous shunts for hemodialysis, paralyzed limbs, and amputation stumps.

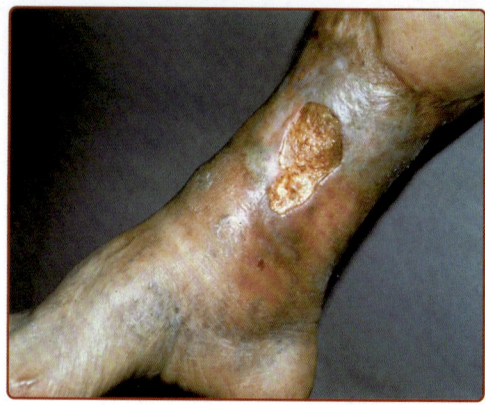

Figure 148-13 Venous ulceration in an area of lipodermatosclerosis, hemosiderosis, inflammation, and varicosities on the foot. Note lipodermatosclerosis constricts lower leg below the calf ("inverted champagne bottle").

The soft-tissue injury that precedes ulceration begins in the subcutis, and visible changes may not appear for some time. Frequently one notes the appearance of petechial lesions, which have the appearance of cayenne pepper sprinkled about the gaiter area. As the hemoglobin in the petechial lesions breaks down, the iron remains in the skin as hemosiderin, which may lead to impressive discoloration (see Fig. 148-11).

Although ulceration is classically located in the gaiter area (Fig. 148-13), *venous ulcers* have been described as ulcers occurring anywhere below the knee. Venous ulcers are typically tender, shallow, irregular, and have a red-base (Figs. 148-13 and 148-14). They are usually located on the medial ankle or along the line of the long or short saphenous veins. Clinical distinction should be made with other common ulcers of the lower extremity (see Table 148-5) as shown in Table 148-15.

COMPLICATIONS

Recurrent ulceration is frequent. Any open wound provides a portal of entry for bacteria, and cellulitis, although infrequent, may develop at any time. Stasis dermatitis is itchy and the skin is easily excoriated and may become infected. In addition, these patients are easily sensitized to the topical agents they apply, and contact dermatitis is common, especially that caused by topical antibiotics. The dermatitis of venous disease may become generalized as an id reaction and may rarely produce an exfoliative erythroderma. Many of these individuals are predisposed to thrombi,

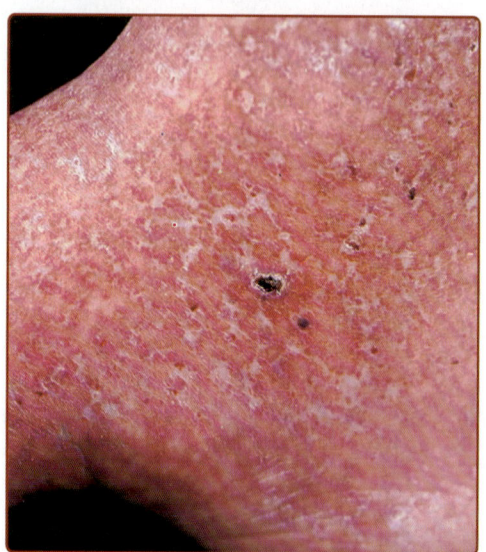

Figure 148-12 Atrophie blanche with irregular porcelain-white atrophic scars, small ulcerations, and crusting.

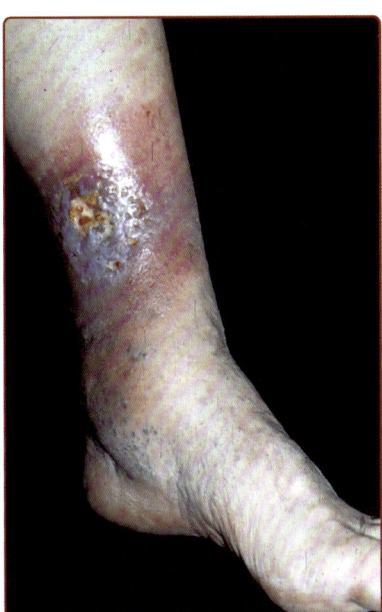

Figure 148-14 Venous ulceration with stasis dermatitis, edema, and varicosities.

TABLE 148-15
Differential Diagnosis of Leg Ulcers

Vascular Diseases
- Arterial (hypertensive atherosclerotic, vasospastic)
- Venous (venous stasis ulcer)

Metabolic Disorders
- Diabetes mellitus
- Gout
- Necrobiosis lipoidica diabeticorum
- Pancreatic (pancreatitis, carcinoma)
- Porphyria cutanea tarda

Infections
- Bacterial (especially *Staphylococcus aureus*, *Streptococcus*)
- Fungal (deep fungal, mycetoma)
- Opportunistic in immunocompromised
- Spirochetal (syphilis)
- Viral

Vasculitis
- Granulomatosis with polyangiitis (Wegener granulomatosis)
- Hypersensitivity vasculitis
- Lymphomatoid granulomatosis
- Polyarteritis
- Rheumatoid vasculitis
- Systemic lupus erythematosus

Lymphedema
- Congenital
- Postinfectious
- Postirradiation
- Postsurgical

Drugs
- Anticoagulant necrosis (Coumadin, heparin)
- Drug-induced vasculitis
- Ergotism
- Halogens (bromide, iodide)
- Hydroxyurea

Hematologic Abnormalities
- Dysproteinemia (cryoglobulinemia, macroglobulinemia)
- Hypercoagulable states (protein C, protein S, antithrombin III deficiency, activated protein C resistance, prothrombin gene polymorphism)
- Leukemia
- Lupus anticoagulant syndrome
- Paroxysmal nocturnal hemoglobinuria
- Polycythemia vera
- Sickle cell anemia
- Thalassemia

Tumors
- Cutaneous (basal cell cancer, squamous cell cancer, sarcoma, malignant melanoma, Merkel cell)
- Kaposi sarcoma
- Secondary (metastatic carcinoma, lymphoma)

Miscellaneous
- Bullous diseases (epidermolysis bullosa)
- Burns
- Idiopathic
- Insect bites (brown recluse spider)
- Pressure ulcers, neuropathic ulcers
- Pyoderma gangrenosum
- Sweet syndrome
- Trauma (including factitial)
- Ulcerative lichen planus

and recurrent episodes of venous thrombosis are not uncommon.

All patients with advanced venous disease have some degree of lymphatic impairment, though lymphatic impairment may also result from inherited defects in lymphatic development or destruction of lymphatics after cellulitis, lymphangitis, surgical interruption, or radiation. Loss of lymphatic drainage from the lower leg may lead to verrucous changes and cutaneous hypertrophy, called elephantiasis nostras (see section "Secondary Lymphedema").

ETIOLOGY AND PATHOGENESIS

A venous ulcer occurs after failure of the calf muscle pump. The heart pumps blood down to the foot; the calf muscle pump (when upright) returns venous blood to the heart. Venous blood from the skin and subcutis collects in the superficial venous system, including the greater and lesser saphenous veins and its tributaries, moves through the fascia in a series of "perforating" or "communicating" veins, and fills the muscle-enveloped deep venous system. With muscle contraction, the deep veins are compressed; one-way valves in the deep system allow the now high-pressure flow to move against gravity, and one-way valves in the perforators close to prevent–pressure injury in the skin (Fig. 148-15). In all patients with venous disease there is failure of these one-way valves, and this can result in varicose veins (Fig. 148-16). The severity of venous disease is influenced by the number and

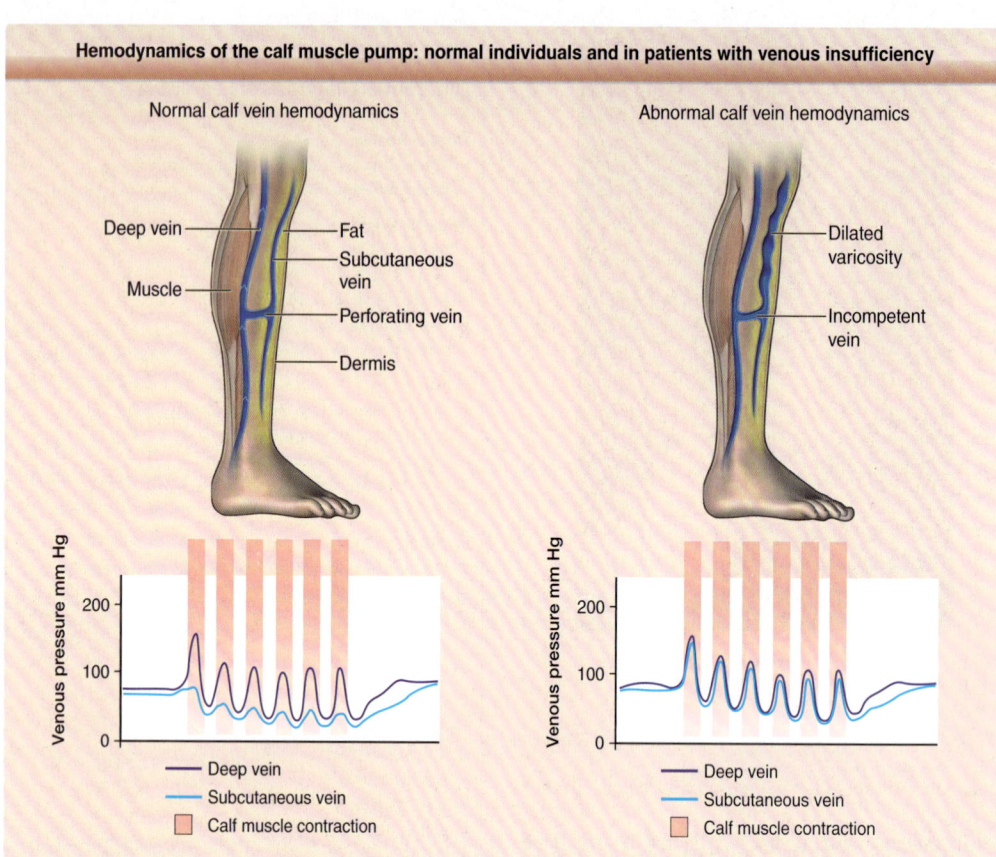

Figure 148-15 Anatomy and hemodynamics of the calf muscle pump in normal individuals and in patients with venous insufficiency. Venous insufficiency is characterized by high-pressure reflux from deep veins into the superficial veins and small vessels of the skin.

distribution of incompetent valves and is worsened by any impairment of leg muscle function or ankle joint range of motion—all critical components of the calf muscle pump. Any obstruction to venous return (eg, thrombosis, radiation fibrosis) or elevation of right atrial pressure (eg, pulmonary hypertension, heart failure) further compromises venous return. Chap. 212 provides a more detailed description of the anatomy and hemodynamics of the venous system of the lower extremities.

The most common cause of venous valvular failure is thrombosis. The nidus for venous thrombosis is typically the valve cusp, and when the thrombus is lysed by plasmin, valve function is often lost as well. Calf muscle pump failure after deep venous thrombosis is often referred to as the *postphlebitic syndrome*.[33]

Once valves fail, especially those in the perforators, high-pressure blood in the deep system refluxes into the unsupported veins of the skin. There is then vascular leakage of fibrinogen producing "fibrin cuffs" that may interfere with tissue nourishment. In addition, white blood cell trapping leads to soft-tissue injury, inflammation, and, eventually, fibrosis, as the subcutaneous fat is replaced by scar, resulting in lipodermatosclerosis.

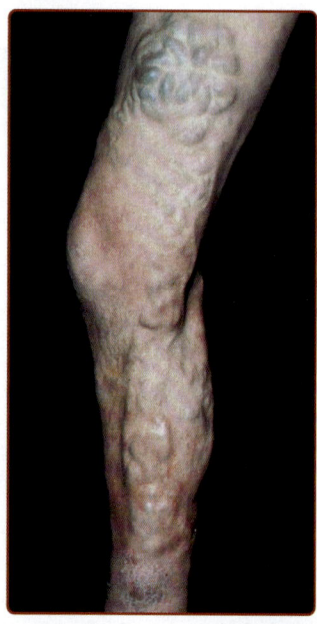

Figure 148-16 Extensive varicose veins on the calf and thigh.

DIAGNOSIS

LABORATORY TESTS AND IMAGING STUDIES

It is crucial to exclude arterial disease as a cause of ulceration. A useful bedside screening test for PAD is to calculate the ratio of the systolic blood pressure in the ankle (as measured by Doppler) to the systolic pressure in the brachial artery (also measured by Doppler). This ankle-brachial index is greater than or equal to 1 in normal individuals. Anything less than 1 is an indication of PAD. The lower the ratio, the more severe the arterial obstruction. An ankle-brachial index is reliable except in the presence of calcified vessels, which are noncompressible and therefore a true systolic pressure cannot be measured.

Having excluded arterial disease as a cause of ulceration, a clinical diagnosis of venous disease is sufficient for the initiation of empiric therapy in most cases (Fig. 148-17). When the diagnosis is in doubt, skin biopsy may be useful. Tissue should be sent for both histology and tissue culture. Functional testing of calf muscle pump function and venous valvular function using plethysmography is occasionally useful. Duplex Doppler ultrasonography can be useful to document valvular incompetence and to evaluate patients for possible sclerotherapy or surgery (see Chap. 212).

Histologic signs of venous hypertension include hemosiderin deposition, lobular superficial and/or deep dermal neovascularization, and fibrosis of the dermis and subcutaneous tissue in later stages. These histologic findings are found in all clinical manifestations of chronic venous disease.

DIFFERENTIAL DIAGNOSIS

Together Tables 148-5 ("Comparison of Different Leg Ulcer Types") and 148-15 ("Differential Diagnosis of Leg Ulcers") outline the differential diagnosis of chronic venous disease.

CLINICAL COURSE AND PROGNOSIS

The prognosis for healing areas of ulceration and inflammation is excellent in the absence of comorbid illness that interferes with healing. The vast majority of patients with uncomplicated chronic venous disease respond well to ambulatory outpatient therapy as outlined in "Management" below. Permanent changes include hemosiderosis and fibrosis that develop before the initiation of therapy. Loss of valvular function is irreversible. In the absence of continual lifelong cutaneous support in the form of inelastic wraps or elastic stockings, skin and soft-tissue injury continues.

MANAGEMENT

Table 148-16 outlines the treatment of chronic venous insufficiency. Treatment for all clinical manifestations of chronic venous insufficiency includes therapies that lower venous pressure and improve venous and lymphatic flow by mechanical means, dressings, drugs, and surgery.

Given the limitations of bed rest as an effective therapy, the focus is now on an ambulatory outpatient approach to the management of venous ulceration. Most experts agree on the essential role of compression in treating chronic venous insufficiency.[37] Hence, unless there are contraindications (arterial occlusive disease or abnormal ankle, brachial indexes), compression therapy should remain part of any treatment regimen for chronic venous disease.

Toward the end of the 19th century, Paul Gerson Unna recognized that by providing a compression bandage to the distal extremity he could heal venous ulcers in an ambulatory patient population using a zinc-impregnated gauze wrap, the "Unna boot." Although the literature over the years continued to document the success of this approach, it proved difficult to achieve

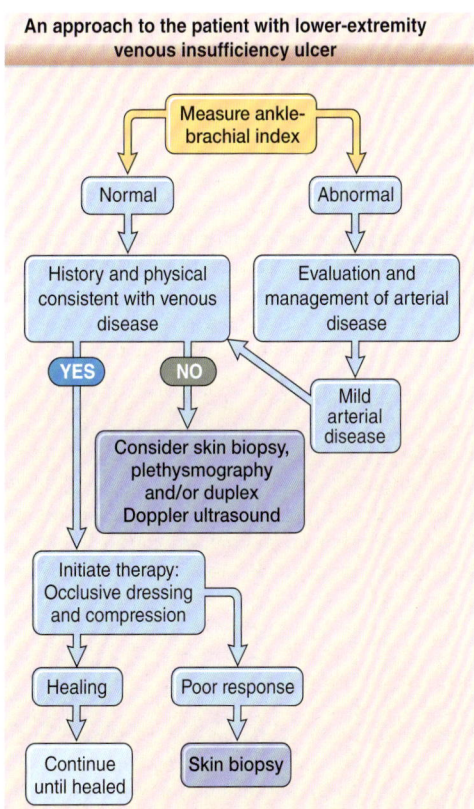

Figure 148-17 An approach to the patient with lower-extremity venous insufficiency ulcer.

TABLE 148-16
Treatment of Chronic Venous Insufficiency

Mechanical
- Compression bandages
- Compression stockings
- Intermittent pneumatic compression pumps
- Leg elevation

Drug Therapy
- Aspirin
- Horse chestnut seed extract
- Pentoxifylline
- Topical steroids (for stasis dermatitis)

Dressings
- Occlusive hydrocolloid or gel dressings
- Wet and dry nonadherent dressings
- Zinc paste-impregnated bandages (Unna boot)

Surgery
- Calf varicosity avulsions
- Endovenous laser therapy
- Long saphenous vein stripping
- Radiofrequency ablation
- Saphenofemoral/saphenopopliteal junction disconnection
- Sclerotherapy
- Subfascial endoscopic perforator vein ligation

---

graduated compression with this wrap, and compliance was poor. Eventually, the addition of a self-adherent second layer (Coban, for example) over a zinc wrap was introduced as the "Duke boot" (Fig. 148-18). This has proven to be easy to apply with reproducible, graduated, inelastic compression to counter the outflow from perforator incompetence, and is the cornerstone of venous ulcer management.[38]

In 1962, George Winter reported the use of an occlusive layer enhanced healing in a pig model of acute wounds. His data suggested a roughly 100% improvement in the rate of wound healing simply by providing a moist environment. The impact on wound care has been dramatic. There are now thousands of such dressings on the market and although they differ in composition, absorption, gas exchange, and cost, all provide a moist environment. Underneath such dressings, fibrinopurulent and necrotic debris, aided by host and bacterial enzymes, dissolves painlessly. One can take advantage of these dressings to provide the best local environment for the wound, followed by a compression wrap to address the underlying hemodynamic disturbance (see Chap. 149).

Mechanical therapy is the mainstay of treatment for all clinical manifestations of chronic venous insufficiency. Daily use of elastic compression stockings reduces swelling in some patients with post-thrombotic syndrome, and may prevent worsening of established postthrombotic syndrome and reduce recurrence of healed venous ulcers.[38] Each pharmaceutical therapy targets a specific clinical aspect of chronic venous insufficiency. Diuretics may be used in the short-term for treating severe edema. Aspirin (300 to 325 mg/day)[39,40] and pentoxifylline[41,42] may improve healing of chronic venous ulcers, although data is insufficient to recommend in all cases. Finally, topical steroids and emollients aid resolution of stasis dermatitis.

Although all wounds harbor potential pathogens, there is no evidence that routine use of antibiotics is helpful in patients with venous ulcer. If cellulitis is suspected, empiric therapy with coverage for *Staphylococcus aureus* and streptococci is warranted. Topical antibiotics, especially mupirocin, are useful for folliculitis due to *S. aureus* and streptococci. With the increasing incidence of community acquired methicillin-resistant *S. aureus* in this population, culture and sensitivity are suggested for suspected skin and soft tissue infections. Horse chestnut seed extract (*Aesculus hippocastanum* L.), often standardized to 50 mg escin twice daily, is an herbal remedy that appears to be safe and effective as a short-term treatment for leg pain and swelling.[43]

Venous disease is progressive and irreversible. Patients must be educated about the need for continual hemodynamic support after the wound has healed. Graduated stockings that provide a minimum of 30 to 40 mm Hg at the ankle should be carefully fitted to all patients and worn for their lifetime. It is a mistake to place elastic stockings on edematous limbs, especially those limbs that are tender. Compression bandaging should be used until all edema, inflammation, and tenderness have resolved before fitting the patient with stockings.

In carefully selected cases, sclerotherapy or surgical techniques, especially endovenous ablation, may close incompetent perforators and correct the hemodynamic abnormalities that lead to venous ulcer (see Chap. 212).[44,45]

PREVENTION

Prevention of venous thrombosis prevents venous insufficiency. Because many thrombotic traits are genetic, it is likely those patients at extra risk for thrombosis may be identified and treated for this risk before an event, and efforts to prevent thrombosis during elective surgery and hospitalization should reduce the

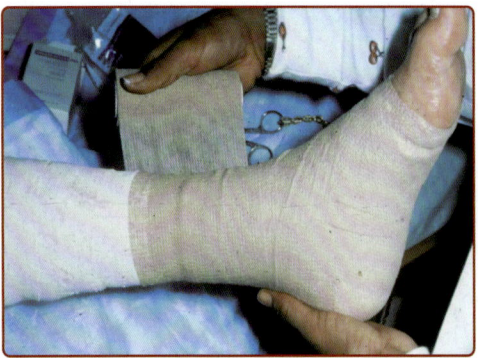

Figure 148-18 Compression bandage using a zinc paste primary layer (Unna boot) followed by Coban at full stretch.

numbers of postphlebitic limbs. Once a patient develops venous thrombosis, elastic compression stockings are the only proven method to reduce the risk of postthrombotic syndrome.[38]

Valvular failure may develop during pregnancy. Therefore, the use of supportive stockings throughout maternity, although not proven, can be recommended. If one's occupation or lifestyle involves long periods of immobility (long-distance flights appear to be especially risky), stockings are advisable.

LYMPHEDEMA

AT-A-GLANCE

- Lymphatics are essential for the clearing of extravascular fluids and debris and as conduits for transport of immunocompetent cells during the initiation of an immune response.
- Genetic defects causing lymphedema in childhood or early adult life are often caused by defects in the genes *VEGFR3* (encoding vascular growth factor receptor) and *FOXC2*, a transcription factor.
- Lymphedema acquired in adult life is often related to chronic venous disease, after mastectomy with radiation and node removal, and, in certain geographic locations, filariasis.
- Cellulitis may complicate all forms of lymphedema and should be aggressively treated.

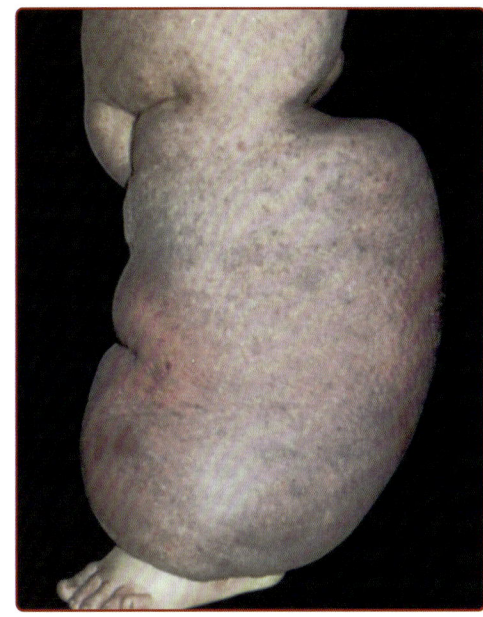

Figure 148-19 Lymphedema of the left leg in a 47-year-old firefighter. The extreme swelling began at birth and was painless. Note the lack of stasis pigmentation or ulceration. The patient functioned normally at work and wanted no treatment.

The lymphatic vasculature plays a crucial role in the return of interstitial fluid to the bloodstream, absorption of dietary lipids, and trafficking of immune cells. Valves in collecting lymphatic vessels allow lymph to be efficiently returned to the bloodstream, and their formation is a key event during maturation of the lymphatic vasculature. Defects in lymphatic valve formation contribute to aberrant lymphatic function in lymphedema syndromes.[46]

Edema is an excess of fluid in the body tissues. Although most of this fluid is in the interstitial spaces, there is usually excess fluid both in the vascular bed and within cells. When this becomes chronic, inflammatory cells and their cytokines lead to an irreversible state. This chronic accumulation of protein-rich fluid may occur as a consequence of conditions that predispose to chronic edema, such as venous stasis; or it may occur because of lymphatic failure secondary to trauma, malignancy, disease, or genetic mutations that give rise to nonfunctional lymphatics.

Lymphedema refers specifically to swelling of a part of the body due to impaired lymph transport capacity as a consequence of a malformation or malfunction of the lymphatics.

Primary lymphedema is a congenitally determined intrinsic or constitutional fault in lymphatic drainage. This is most commonly due to mutations in specific genes that are critical to lymphatic development or function, but may arise as a result of a developmental abnormality due to unknown causes *in utero*. Depending on the cause, primary lymphedema may present at any age (Fig. 148-19).

Secondary lymphedema occurs when previously normal lymphatics suffer an external insult such as disease, infection (eg, repeated episodes of erysipelas), trauma, or surgery, and subsequently lose their functional capability, giving rise to lymphedema. The most common cause worldwide is parasitic infection. In industrialized countries, secondary lymphedema occurs following trauma, infection, surgery, malignancy, or radiation therapy.[47]

In all the clinical disorders discussed, lymphedema may be transient and pitting with pressure, but with time becomes fixed, and is accompanied by adipose tissue hypertrophy, fibrosis, and epidermal hyperplasia (Fig. 148-20) that eventually makes pitting less evident.[48]

Patients with lymphedema are susceptible to recurrent erysipelas, physical impairment, and psychosocial stigmatization, and may be at increased risk of malignancy such as lymphangiosarcoma.

PRIMARY LYMPHEDEMA

EPIDEMIOLOGY

Primary lymphedema is thought to occur in approximately 1 to 3 of every 10,000 live births.[49] It also can be

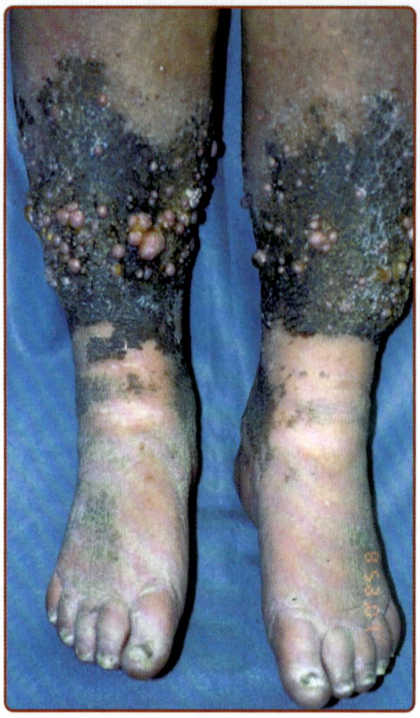

Figure 148-20 Verrucous skin changes in chronic lymphedema.

a feature of certain inherited chromosomal conditions, such as Aagenaes syndrome (cholestasis and lymphedema), Noonan syndrome, Klinefelter syndrome, Turner syndrome, and Prader-Willi syndrome.[50]

EMBERGER SYNDROME

Emberger syndrome (OMIM [Online Mendelian Inheritance in Man]: 614038) is the cooccurrence of primary lymphedema and myelodysplasia/acute myeloid leukemia.

Clinical Features: In addition to unilateral or bilateral lymphedema of the lower extremities, patients with Emberger syndrome also have a low CD4:CD8 ratio, immune dysfunction (widespread cutaneous warts), sensorineural deafness, and genital lymphedema.[51] These patients require monitoring because of their predisposition to acute myeloid leukemia. Lymphedema precedes the hematologic abnormalities.

Etiology and Pathogenesis: Emberger syndrome is an autosomal dominant primary lymphedema syndrome caused by mutations in *GATA2*, which regulates the transcription of genes that are important for both development and maintenance of lymphovenous and lymphatic vessel valves.[52] Transcription factor GATA2 is also crucial for hematopoietic stem cell development during both embryogenesis and adulthood. It is known now that deficiency in this transcription factor encompasses a broad phenotype that includes immunodeficiency, bone marrow failure, pulmonary disease, and vascular/lymphatic dysfunction.[53]

MILROY SYNDROME

Milroy syndrome (OMIM: 153100) is a congenital primary lymphedema that leads to disability and disfiguring swelling of the lower extremities. It is also known as hereditary lymphedema IA and Nonne-Milroy lymphedema. Onset is usually at birth or in early childhood, and the severity can vary but often progresses with time.[54,55] It is a relatively rare condition with an estimated frequency of approximately 1 in 6000 live births, and there is a 2.3:1 female predominance in pedigrees.[55] This sex ratio may be the result of more-severe disease in males that leads to hydrops fetalis and fetal death.[56]

Clinical Features: Bilateral lower-limb asymmetric swelling is most common with deep creases noted over the toes. Large superficial veins can be visible during infancy. Nail and skin changes all occur, such as toenail upslanting ("ski jump") dysplasia or skin papillomatosis (greatest over second toe). Skin infections and hydroceles are also common. Hypoproteinemia from intestinal loss of albumin via intestinal lymphangiectasias, chylous ascites, and scrotal edema are known complications.[54] Thickening of the skin overlying the digits leads to a positive Kaposi-Stemmer sign (inability to pinch up a fold of skin between the second and third toe on the dorsum of the foot).

Etiology and Pathogenesis: Milroy syndrome is an autosomal dominant disease caused by a mutation in *VEGFR3* (also called the *FLT4* gene).[55] This causes impaired tyrosine kinase activity of the VEGFR3 receptor, which disrupts lymphangiogenesis. Prenatal ultrasonography can show edematous legs in the fetus. Skin biopsy from swollen feet of patients who possess the *VEGFR3* mutation reveals abundant skin lymphatics that are confirmed to be nonfunctional by fluorescence microlymphangiography.[57] Interestingly, lymphangiography also demonstrates dysplastic lymphatics in both clinically affected and clinically normal extremities, emphasizing the complexity of the pathophysiology that ultimately leads to disease.

The mechanism by which Milroy lymphedema develops appear to be the result of functional failure of the lymphatics as opposed to absence of initial lymphatics.[57] Penetrance is relatively high (80%), but not complete, suggesting a role of additional genetic or environmental factors resulting in variation of clinical expression.

LYMPHEDEMA-DISTICHIASIS

Clinical Features: Lymphedema typically develops during puberty, but may be delayed until early adulthood, especially in females. The lymphedema will commonly worsen in severity over time, and may be complicated by recurrent infection and eventual papillomatosis. A double row of eyelashes (*distichiasis*) are aberrant eyelashes arising along the posterior border of the eyelid margin, which frequently leads to eyelash irritation of the cornea and photophobia. Other associated findings of this syndrome include cardiac defects, varicose veins, cleft palate, spinal extradural cysts, and other ophthalmologic complications. Given the complexity of this disorder and the possibility of systemic involvement, treatment of this disorder frequently requires a multidisciplinary approach, including dermatologists, pediatricians, and geneticists.[58]

Etiology and Pathogenesis: Autosomal dominant nonsense and frameshift mutations in the forkhead transcription factor FoxC2 cause abnormalities in morphogenesis of the lymphatic valves in this disease.[59] Radiographic studies of patients with lymphedema-distichiasis show lymph and venous reflux of the lower limbs, illustrating the primary valve failure. Distichiasis, a double row of eyelashes, develops as a result of failure of proper differentiation of eyelid follicles into meibomian glands.[58] Although the *FOXC2* mutation is specific for lymphedema-distichiasis,[59] further investigation has illustrated that lymphedema with ptosis may actually be one of the variable manifestations of *FOXC2* mutations, rather than a distinct disorder.[60]

SECONDARY LYMPHEDEMA

EPIDEMIOLOGY

The prevalence of chronic edema in a community sample in London was 1.33 per 1000 people and 5.4 per 1000 persons older than the age of 65 years.[61] Twenty-five percent of chronic edema was related to malignancy; 29% of patients had at least 1 episode of cellulitis during the year before the survey; and 70% to 80% of patients were female.[61]

Worldwide, lymphedema caused by filariasis is estimated to affect 100 million individuals and is considered to be the second leading cause of permanent disability in the world.[62,63] For the epidemiology, clinical manifestations, and treatment of filariasis, see Chap. 177.

Other infectious diseases with lymphedema are much less common and include lymphogranuloma venereum, granuloma inguinale (see Chaps. 173 and 174), and tuberculosis (see Chap. 157).

In regions of tropical Africa, Central America, and the Indian subcontinent where filariasis is uncommon, there is a condition of chronic lymphedema called *podoconiosis* or *nonfilarial elephantiasis*. This condition causes edematous feet and legs, and is usually bilateral. Podoconiosis is not infectious in origin. It is caused by chronic inoculation of microparticles of silica through the soles of barefoot walkers.[64]

CLINICAL FEATURES

Typically, patients will present with a persistently edematous extremity without concurrent pain or inflammation (Table 148-17). The foot is often involved first, and initially lesions pit with pressure. Patients presenting later in the disease course may present with nonpitting edema. Feet may illustrate swollen toes with upturned nails. Thickening of the skin over the digits may be present, as may the Kaposi-Stemmer sign. If the condition has been longstanding, the skin overlying the affected extremity may show generalized thickening, papillomatosis, or verrucous tissue overgrowth (see Fig. 148-20). Fungal and bacterial infections, or viral warts also may be present.

Unilateral lymphedema suggests localized obstructing factors, but bilateral lymphedema does not rule out anatomic obstruction, as the obstruction may be in the pelvis or abdomen.

Inflammation as manifested by redness, pain, and swelling is not lymphedema, but can be pyogenic infection, most commonly with *S. aureus* or *Streptococcus pyogenes*. Systemic antibiotics should be started before waiting for red lymphangitic streaking. A common complication is contact dermatitis from the use of topical antibiotics or multiple emollients and antiinflammatory creams. However, itch is often the dominant symptom in this case.

Prolonged lymphedema leads to fibrosis and epidermal hyperplasia with verrucous hyperkeratosis. Ulceration rarely occurs, although the edema and hyperkeratotic changes may be profound. Lymphangiosarcoma, called Stewart-Treves syndrome when associated with postmastectomy lymphedema, is a potential complication in chronically lymphedematous locations (see Chap. 118).

DIAGNOSIS

If there is doubt regarding the clinical diagnosis of lymphedema, especially when trying to differentiate from edema, there are various studies that may be employed for diagnostic confirmation. Isotopic lymphoscintigraphy is recommended, but radiocontrast

TABLE 148-17
Signs and Symptoms of Lymphedema

Symptoms
- Edematous extremity
- Heaviness
- Indentations from socks on standing
- Indentations improve overnight
- Painless

Signs
Early
- Erysipelas
- Pitting edema

Late
- Nonpitting edema
- Papillomatosis
- Secondary infections (bacterial, fungal, viral warts)
- "Ski-jump" upturned toe nails
- Thickened, woody skin
- Verrucous tissue overgrowth

lymphangiography also can be used.[65,66] CT and MRI are other radiographic options, although not ideal. MRI is preferred over CT because of its ability to detect water. These modalities should reveal the characteristic "honeycomb" pattern of the subcutaneous tissue present in chronic lymphedema.[65] This pattern is not present in other types of edema. Venous duplex ultrasonography may be required to rule out concomitant deep venous thrombosis and to assess for chronic venous insufficiency as a cause for swelling.

Special Tests: Diagnosis of filariasis (see Chap. 177) includes assays to detect filarial antigens, and ultrasonography to visualize living adult worms, even in the absence of microfilaremia.[67]

DIFFERENTIAL DIAGNOSIS

Chronic venous insufficiency can present with very similar features of early lymphedema. In this clinical context, both conditions will have pitting edema, and the characteristic skin changes of late-stage lymphedema have not yet developed. However, chronic venous insufficiency is typically bilateral, rather than unilateral as in lymphedema. It is imperative to exclude medical causes of lower-extremity swelling (Table 148-18). An uncommon clinical mimic to lymphedema is lipedema of the leg. This syndrome is caused by bilateral adipose deposition, usually in the buttocks and lower extremities. This leads to enlargement that stops abruptly at the level of the malleoli, characteristically sparing the feet. This distinctive clinical presentation is referred to as "armchair legs."[47] This condition predominates among overweight women who spend the majority of their time with their legs in a dependent position. Chronic immobility leads to decreased lymphatic drainage and subsequent lymphedema.

CLINICAL COURSE AND PROGNOSIS

Lymphedema is chronic and can be disabling. Pain, heaviness, and discomfort in the affected limb are common symptoms as lymphedema progresses. Extremities affected by lymphedema are at increased risk of skin breakdown, lymph fluid leakage, and infections. Cellulitis, erysipelas, tinea pedis, and lymphangitis are common complications of longstanding lymphedema and can subsequently worsen lymphedema.

MANAGEMENT

There is no cure for lymphedema; thus the goal is to improve mobility of the limb and minimize secondary complications. A combination of elevation, exercise, compression garments/devices, skin care aimed at preventing infection, and manual lymphatic drainage, usually via massage, are the mainstays of management (Table 148-19).[47,68] In patients with primary and secondary lymphedema, in the absence of venous or arterial disease, manual lymphatic drainage and sequential pneumatic pumps, in addition to compression wraps and garments, may be useful.

Exercise under compression is beneficial for lymphedema by enhancing lymph flow and potentially improving protein resorption. Lymph moves faster during limb activity and exercise. A combination of flexibility training, aerobic training, and strengthening exercises—while wearing compression garments or devices—significantly improve lymphedema.[68]

Drug therapy for lymphedema, in general, has been inadequate. Diuretics are frequently prescribed, and not only do they not alleviate the symptoms, they may actually worsen the condition and should not be used as a primary treatment for lymphedema. There is some evidence to suggest the efficacy of coumarin therapy. Coumarin apparently reduces capillary filtration as well as reduces fibrotic tissue deposition.[47]

Recurrent cellulitis, erysipelas, and lymphangitis are a significant problem in lymphedematous sites, and there is both a rationale and results that encourage long-term antibiotic use (eg, 2.4 million units of benzathine-penicillin G IM every 2 weeks, or cephalexin).[69] Interdigital maceration and tinea pedis create a portal of entry for bacteria. Thus prompt antifungal management and avoidance of web space moisture is necessary.

Lymphatic microsurgery to bypass obstructed nodes can be considered if nonsurgical treatments are unsuccessful. This procedure is not commonly performed in the United States, but the literature from studies of this procedure performed in Europe is considerable. The surgery consists of the formation of multiple end-to-end lymphatic–venous anastomoses.[68,70] Congenital

---

TABLE 148-18
Differential Diagnosis of Secondary Lymphedema

- Chronic venous insufficiency
- Filariasis
- Medical disease
  - Congestive Heart Failure
  - Drug-induced edema
  - Hypoalbuminemia
  - Lipedema "armchair sign"
  - Obesity
  - Pregnancy
  - Protein-losing nephropathy
  - Renal Failure
- Podoconiosis
- Postphlebitic syndrome
- Recurrent infection

TABLE 148-19
Therapeutic Options

- Compression by multilayered wrappings or compression garments
- Elevation
- Exercise (under compression)
- Manual lymphatic drainage
- Skin care
- Surgery

lymphatic disorders have been treated with this intervention in the early childhood years with dramatic results.[68,70]

Low-level laser therapy, either in combination with pneumatic compression or as a solo intervention, has been studied in patients with postoperative lymphedema, primarily in postmastectomy lymphedema. Results are encouraging, and patients have had improvements in the total volume of affected limbs at followup analysis of up to 1 year.[71]

Excisional or suction-assisted lipectomy (liposuction) may be an option in selected patients who are not eligible for other treatment options, or in whom other therapeutic modalities have failed.

Prevention: Any patient with lymphedema, whatever the cause, should keep their feet dry, nails trimmed, and prevent and aggressively treat pyogenic infection. Use of topical antifungal therapy is encouraged.

LOCALIZED AREAS OF LYMPHEDEMA

Lymphedema is common in some locations, especially on the face, vulva, and penis, and can lead to superficial lesions termed *lymphangiectasia*. These focal areas of lymphedema occur from obstruction of previously normal lymphatics, progressing to lymphatic valve incompetence, lymph reflux, and retrograde lymph flow to the skin. This leads to blister-like lesions full of lymphatic fluid called *lymphangiectasias*. These most commonly occur after trauma, treatment for malignancy, or infection. These lesions are highly symptomatic and distressing. They are frequently painful, pruritic, and exudative. Carbon dioxide laser ablation is a currently favored treatment modality for superficial lesions.[72] Because the underlying obstructed lymph vessels are not corrected by laser ablation, recurrences are common.[73] Other options for treatment include surgical excision, superficial radiotherapy, and sclerotherapy.[73-75]

ACKNOWLEDGMENTS

The author acknowledges the contributions of Veerendra Chadachan, Steven M. Dean, Robert T. Eberhardt, Craig N. Burkhart, Chris Adigun, and Claude S. Burton, the former authors of this chapter.

REFERENCES

1. Rooke TW, Hirsch AT, Misra S, et al. 2011 ACCF/AHA focused update of the guideline for the management of patients with peripheral artery disease (updating the 2005 guidelines): a report of the American College of Cardiology Foundation/American Heart Association Task Force on Practice Guidelines. *J Am Coll Cardiol*. 2011;58(19):2020-2045.
2. Hirsch AT, Haskal ZJ, Hertzer NR, et al. ACC/AHA 2005 guidelines for the management of patients with peripheral arterial disease (lower extremity, renal, mesenteric, and abdominal aortic): executive summary a collaborative report from the American Association for Vascular Surgery/Society for Vascular Surgery, Society for Cardiovascular Angiography and Interventions, Society for Vascular Medicine and Biology, Society of Interventional Radiology, and the ACC/AHA Task Force on Practice Guidelines (Writing Committee to Develop Guidelines for the Management of Patients With Peripheral Arterial Disease) endorsed by the American Association of Cardiovascular and Pulmonary Rehabilitation; National Heart, Lung, and Blood Institute; Society for Vascular Nursing; TransAtlantic Inter-Society Consensus; and Vascular Disease Foundation. *J Am Coll Cardiol*. 2006;47(6):1239-1312.
3. Fowkes FG, Rudan D, Rudan I, et al. Comparison of global estimates of prevalence and risk factors for peripheral artery disease in 2000 and 2010. *Lancet*. 2013;382(9901);1329-1340.
4. Skelly CL, Cifu AS. Screening, evaluation and treatment of peripheral arterial disease. *JAMA*. 2016;316(14): 1486-1487.
5. Conte MS, Pomposelli FB, Clair DG, et al. Society for Vascular Surgery practice guidelines for atherosclerotic occlusive disease of the lower extremity. *J Vasc Surg*. 2015;61(suppl 3);2S-41S.
6. Imparato AM, Kim GE, Davidson T, et al. Intermittent claudication: its natural course. *Surgery*. 1975;78(6): 795.
7. O'Hare AM, Katz R, Shlipak MG, et al. Mortality and cardiovascular risk across the ankle-arm index spectrum: results from the Cardiovascular Health Study. *Circulation*. 2006;113(3):388-393.
8. Malgor RD, Alahdab F, Elraiyah TA, et al. A systemic review for the screening for peripheral arterial disease in asymptomatic patients. *J Vasc Surg*. 2015;61(suppl 3): 42S-53S.
9. Dawson DL, Cutler BS, Meissner MH, et al. Cilostazol has beneficial effects in treatment of intermittent claudication: results from a multicenter, randomized, prospective, double-blind trial. *Circulation*. 1998; 98(7):678-686.
10. Salhiyyah K, Senanayake E, Abdel-Hadi M, et al. Pentoxifylline for intermittent claudication. *Cochrane Database Syst Rev*. 2012;1:CD005262.
11. Mozaffarian D, Benjamin EJ, Go AS, et al. Executive summary: heart disease and stroke statistics—2016 update: a report from the American Heart Association. *Circulation*. 2016;133(4):447-454.
12. Liew YP, Bartholomew JR. Atheromatous embolization. *Vasc Med*. 2005;10(4):309-326.
13. Fukumoto Y, Tsutsui H, Tsuchihashi M, et al. The incidence and risk factors of cholesterol embolization syndrome, a complication of cardiac catheterization: a prospective study. *J Am Coll Cardiol*. 2003;42(2):211-216.
14. Ismail I, Agarwal A, Aggarwal S, et al. Aortic atherosclerosis: a common source of cerebral emboli, often overlooked! *Am J Ther*. 2016;23(1):e268-e272.
15. Saric M, Kronzon I. Cholesterol embolization syndrome. *Curr Opin Cardiol*. 2011;26(6):472-479.
16. Rivera-Chavarría IJ, Brenes-Gutierrez JD. Thromboangiitis obliterans (Buerger's disease). *Ann Med Surg (Lond)*. 2016;29(7):79-82.
17. Gallagher K, Tracci M, Scovell S. Vascular arteritides in women. *J Vasc Surg*. 2013;57(4)(suppl):27S-36S.

18. McLoughlin GA, Helsby CR, Evans CC, et al. Association of HLA-A9 and HLA-B5 with Buerger's disease. *Br Med J*. 1976;13(2):1165-1166.
19. Del Conde I, Peña C. Buerger disease (thromboangiitis obliterans). *Tech Vasc Interv Radiol*. 2014;17(4):234-240.
20. Olin JW, Shih A. Thromboangiitis obliterans (Buerger's disease). *Curr Opin Rheumatol*. 2006;18(1):18-24.
21. Gibbs MB, English JC, Zirwas, MJ. Livedo reticularis: an update. *J Am Acad Dermatol*. 2005;52(6):1009-1019.
22. Uthman IW, Khamastha MA. Livedo racemosa: a striking dermatological sign for the antiphospholipid syndrome. *J Rheumatol*. 2006;33(12):2379-2382.
23. Vollum DI, Parkes JD, Doyle D. Livedo reticularis during amantadine treatment. *Br Med J*. 1971;12(2):627-628.
24. Berlin AL, Pehr K. Coexistence of erythromelalgia and Raynaud's phenomenon. *J Am Acad Dermatol*. 2004;50(3):456.
25. Toubi E, Krause I, Fraser A, et al. Livedo reticularis is a marker for predicting multi-system thrombosis in antiphospholipid syndrome. *Clin Exp Rheumatol*. 2005;23(4):499-504.
26. Cohen JS. Erythromelalgia: new theories and new therapies. *J Am Acad Dermatol*. 2000;43(5, pt 1):841-847.
27. Andersen LK, Davis MD. Sex differences in the incidence of skin and skin-related diseases in Olmsted County, Minnesota, United States, and a comparison with other rates published worldwide. *Int J Dermatol*. 2016;55(9):939-955.
28. Reed KB, Davis MD. Incidence of erythromelalgia: a population-based study in Olmsted County, Minnesota. *J Eur Acad Dermatol Venereol*. 2009;23(1):13-15.
29. Cook-Norris RH, Tollefson MM, Cruz-Inigo BA, et al. Pediatric erythromelalgia: a retrospective review of 32 cases evaluated at Mayo Clinic over a 37-year period. *J Am Acad Dermatol*. 2012;66(3):416-423.
30. McDonnell A, Schulman B, Ali Z, et al. Inherited erythromelalgia due to mutations in SCN9A: natural history, clinical phenotype and somatosensory profile. *Brain*. 2016;139(pt 4):1052-1065.
31. Tang Z, Chen Z, Tang B, et al. Primary erythromelalgia: a review. *Orphanet J Rare Dis*. 2015;30(10):127.
32. Beebe-Dimmer JL, Pfeifer JR, Engle JS, et al. The epidemiology of chronic venous insufficiency and varicose veins. *Ann Epidemiol*. 2005;15(3):175-184.
33. Bergan JJ, Schmid-Schönbein GW, Smith PD, et al. Chronic venous disease. *N Engl J Med*. 2006; 355(5):488-498.
34. Fowkes FG, Evans CJ, Lee AJ. Prevalence and risk factors for chronic venous insufficiency. *Angiology*. 2001;52(suppl 1):S5-S15.
35. Barron GS, Jacob SE, Kirsner RS. Dermatologic complications of chronic venous disease: medical management and beyond. *Ann Vasc Surg*. 2007;21(5):652-662.
36. Gibson GE, Su WP, Pittelkow MR. Antiphospholipid syndrome and the skin. *J Am Acad Dermatol*. 1997;36(6, pt 1):970-982.
37. Gloviczki P, Comerota AJ, Dalsing MC, et al. The care of patients with varicose veins and associated chronic venous diseases: clinical practice guidelines of the Society for Vascular Surgery and the American Venous Forum. *J Vasc Surg*. 2011;53(5 suppl):2S-48S.
38. Subbiah R, Aggarwal V, Zhao H, et al. Effect of compression stockings on post thrombotic syndrome in patients with deep vein thrombosis: a meta-analysis of randomised controlled trials. *Lancet Haematol*. 2016;3(6):e293-e300.
39. de Oliveira Carvalho PE, Magolbo NG, De Aquino RF, et al. Oral aspirin for treating venous leg ulcers. *Cochrane Database Syst Rev*. 2016;2:CD009432.
40. Ibbotson SH, Layton AM, Davies JA, et al. The effect of aspirin on haemostatic activity in the treatment of chronic venous leg ulceration. *Br J Dermatol*. 1995;132(3):422-426.
41. Jull A, Waters J, Arroll B. Pentoxifylline for treatment of venous leg ulcers: a systematic review. *Lancet*. 2002;359(9317):1550.
42. Jull AB, Arroll B, Parag V, et al. Pentoxifylline for treating venous leg ulcers. *Cochrane Database Syst Rev*. 2012;12:CD001733.
43. Pittler MH, Ernst E. Horse chestnut seed extract for chronic venous insufficiency. *Cochrane Database Syst Rev*. 2012;11:CD003230.
44. Tenbrook JA Jr, Iafrati MD, O'donnell TF Jr, et al. Systematic review of outcomes after surgical management of venous disease incorporating subfascial endoscopic perforator surgery. *J Vasc Surg*. 2004;39(3):583-589.
45. Chaby G, Viseux V, Ramelet AA, et al. Refractory venous leg ulcers: a study of risk factors. *Dermatol Surg*. 2006;32(4):512-519.
46. Petrova TV, Karpanen T, Norrmén C, et al. Defective valves and abnormal mural cell recruitment underlie lymphatic vascular failure in lymphedema distichiasis. *Nat Med*. 2004;10(9):974-981.
47. Kerchner K, Fleischer A, Yosipovitch G. Lower extremity lymphedema update: pathophysiology, diagnosis, and treatment guidelines. *J Am Acad Dermatol*. 2008;59(2):324-331.
48. Murdaca G, Cagnati P, Gulli R, et al. Current views on diagnostic approach and treatment of lymphedema. *Am J Med*. 2012;125(2):134-140.
49. Kurland LT, Molgaard CA. The patient record in epidemiology. *Sci Am*. 1981;245(4):54-63.
50. Saito Y, Nakagami H, Kaneda Y, et al. Lymphedema and therapeutic lymphangiogenesis. *Biomed Res Int*. 2013;2013:804675.
51. Ostergaard P, Simpson MA, Connell FC, et al. Mutations in GATA2 cause primary lymphedema associated with a predisposition to acute myeloid leukemia (Emberger syndrome). *Nat Genet*. 2011;43(10):929-931.
52. Kazenwadel J, Betterman KL, Chong C, et al. GATA2 is required for lymphatic vessel valve development and maintenance. *J Clin Invest*. 2015;125(8):2979-2994.
53. Spinner MA, Sanchez LA, Hsu AP, et al. GATA2 deficiency: a protean disorder of hematopoiesis, lymphatics and immunity. *Blood*. 2014;123(6):809-821.
54. Gordon K, Schulte D, Brice G, et al. Mutation in vascular endothelial growth factor-C, a ligand for vascular endothelial growth factor receptor-3, is associated with autosomal dominant Milroy-like primary lymphedema. *Circ Res*. 2013;112(6):956-960.
55. Balboa-Beltran E, Fernandez-Seara MJ, Perez-Munuzuri A, et al. A novel stop mutation in the vascular endothelial growth factor-C gene (VEGFC) results in Milroy-like disease. *J Med Genet*. 2014;51(7):475-478.
56. Ghalamkampour A, Morlot S, Raas-Rothschild A, et al. Hereditary lymphedema type I associated with VEGFR 3 mutation: the first de novo case and atypical presentations. *Clin Genet*. 2006;70(4):330-335.
57. Connell F, Brice G, Mortimer P. Phenotypic characterization of primary lymphedema. *Ann N Y Acad Sci*. 2008;1131:140-146.
58. Brice G, Mansour S, Bell R, et al. Analysis of the phenotypic abnormalities in lymphoedema-distichiasis

58. ...syndrome in 74 patients with FOXC2 mutations or linkage to 16q24. *J Med Genet.* 2002;39(7):478-483.
59. Mellor RH, Brice G, Stanton AW, et al. Mutations in FOXC2 are strongly associated with primary valve failure in veins of the lower limb. *Circulation.* 2007;115(14):1912-1920.
60. Rezaie T, Ghoroghchian R, Bell R, et al. Primary non-syndromic lymphedema (Meige disease) is not caused by mutations in FOXC2. *Eur J Hum Genet.* 2008;16(3):300-304.
61. Moffatt CJ, Franks PJ, Doherty DC, et al. Lymphoedema: an underestimated health problem. *Q J Med.* 2003;96(10):731-738.
62. Shenoy RK, Bockarie MJ. Lymphatic filariasis in children: clinical features, infection burdens and future prospects for elimination. *Parasitology.* 2011;138(12):1559-1568.
63. Rizzo JA, Belo C, Lins R, et al. Children and adolescents infected with *Wuchereria bancrofti* in Greater Recife, Brazil: a randomized, year-long clinical trial of single treatments with diethylcarbamazine or diethylcarbamazine-albendazole. *Ann Trop Med Parasitol.* 2007;101(5):423-433.
64. Bekele K, Deribe K, Amberbir T, et al. Burden assessment of podoconiosis in Wayu Tuka Woreda, East Wollega zone, western Ethiopia: a community-based cross-sectional study. *BMJ Open.* 2016;6:e012308.
65. Dimakakos E, Koureas A, Koutoulidis V, et al. Interstitial magnetic resonance lymphography: the clinical effectiveness of a new method. *Lymphology.* 2008;41(3):116-125.
66. Liu N, Zhang Y. Magnetic resonance lymphangiography for the study of lymphatic system in lymphedema. *J Reconstr Microsurg.* 2016;32(1):66-71.
67. Thomsen EK, Sanuku N, Baea M, et al. Efficacy, safety, and pharmacokinetics of coadministered diethylcarbamazine, albendazole, and ivermectin for treatment of bancroftian filariasis. *Clin Infect Dis.* 2016;62(3):334-341.
68. Ogawa Y. Recent advances in medical treatment for lymphedema. *Ann Vasc Dis.* 2012;5(2):139-144.
69. Vignes S, Dupuy A. Recurrence of lymphedema associated cellulitis (erysipelas) under prophylactic antibiotherapy: a retrospective cohort study. *J Eur Acad Dermatol Venereol.* 2006;20(7):818-822.
70. Baumeister RG, Mayo W, Notohamiprodjo M, et al. Microsurgical lymphatic vessel transplantation. *J Reconstr Microsurg.* 2016;32(1):34-41.
71. Smoot B, Chiavola-Larson L, Lee J, et al. Effect of low-level laser therapy on pain and swelling in women with breast cancer-related lymphedema: a systematic review and meta-analysis. *J Cancer Surviv.* 2015;9(2):287-304.
72. Savas JA, Ledon J, Franca K, et al. Carbon dioxide laser for the treatment of microcystic lymphatic malformations (lymphangioma circumscriptum): a systematic review. *Dermatol Surg.* 2013;39:1147-1157.
73. Niti K, Manish P. Microcystic lymphatic malformation (lymphangioma circumscriptum) treated using a minimally invasive technique of radiofrequency ablation and sclerotherapy. *Dermatol Surg.* 2010;36:1711-1717.
74. Yoon G, Kim HS, Lee YY, et al. Clinical outcomes of primary surgical treatment for acquired vulvar lymphangioma circumscriptum. *Arch Gynecol Obstet.* 2016;293:157-162.
75. Wiegand S, Eivazi B, Zimmermann AP, et al. Sclerotherapy of lymphangiomas of the head and neck. *Head Neck.* 2011;33:1649-1655.

Chapter 149 :: Wound Healing
:: Afsaneh Alavi & Robert S. Kirsner

第一百四十九章

伤口愈合

中文导读

伤口愈合涉及一系列旨在恢复屏障的复杂又相互重叠的序列事件，从凝血到炎症、增殖和重塑。伤口可以根据创伤的深度来分类，这有助于预测疤痕发生的可能性，图149-1展示了不同深度的伤口差别。

1. 不同类型的伤口愈合 一期愈合，是指伤口形成后不久的闭合，如外科伤口和清洁伤口的愈合过程。

延迟的一期愈合，是伤口的轻微延迟闭合，一般是几天后。例如污染伤口通常会先使用抗菌药物杀灭细菌，结果往往导致愈合延迟。

在二期愈合中，开放性伤口愈合需经过肉芽组织形成和上皮化过程。通常见于软组织大面积缺失，如严重创伤或严重烧伤。二期愈合可导致伤口挛缩，甚至造成功能受限。

三期愈合是指最初一期愈合的伤口裂开后形成二期愈合。

作者提及伤口完全愈合的时间与许多因素有关，如伤口的深度、伤口的位置、血供、是否存在感染和伤口形状。

2. 伤口愈合的机制

（1）伤口愈合阶段：将伤口愈合总结成四个阶段，分别为凝血、炎症、增殖（和迁移）和重塑，并在这一部分对各阶段进行了详细阐述。图149-2以图表形式阐述了这几个阶段，图149-3展示了在各个阶段发生的特定事件。指出血小板、嗜中性粒细胞、巨噬细胞、成纤维细胞、内皮细胞和上皮细胞是参与伤口愈合的主要细胞，并受多种细胞因子和生长因子的影响。此外，直接或间接发挥作用的淋巴细胞也越来越被重视。

（2）胎儿伤口愈合：在早期胚胎发生过程中，受伤胎儿组织愈合过程中无纤维化发生，而纤维调节蛋白是在影响瘢痕形成的众多因素中介导胎儿皮肤无瘢痕愈合的一种小分子糖蛋白。

（3）生长因子和细胞因子：伤口愈合受伤口处释放的多种生长因子和细胞因子的调节。表149-1列出了与愈合相关的主要生长因子和细胞因子及其各自的作用。详细介绍了EGF、TGF-β、FGF、PDGF、VEGF、GM-CSF、促炎因子和趋化因子在伤口愈合中所起的作用，并提出虽然从治疗角度来看这些生长因子在伤口愈合过程中很重要，但临床上只有PDGF-BB、bFGF和粒细胞-巨噬细胞集落刺激因子（GM-CSF）用于伤口治疗，只有PDGF被美国食品和药物管理局（FDA）批准用于伤口愈合。

3. 伤口愈合的临床问题

（1）创面床准备：尽管大多数伤口均能正常愈合，但有一定比例的伤口并没有遵循愈合的序列过程。愈合不良的伤口需要创面床准备以促进愈合。将创面床准备的概念用"TIME"进行总结：T-组织清创，I-感染/炎症，M-水分平衡，E-上皮边缘组织。组织清创术是指去除坏死组织和致病细菌的过程，表149-3列出了用于组织清创术的技术。尽管炎症是伤口愈合的生理过程，但是不适当的炎症会导致延迟愈合。治疗感染和炎症是指评估局部使用抗菌剂和/或全身性抗生素的指征来控制感染及继发的炎症。提及由于抗生素耐药的风险，不建议将抗生素局部用于慢性伤口，而是通过各种现代含抗菌剂的敷料来减少敷料以及伤口表面的微生物数量，表149-4列出了这些抗菌敷料。水分不平衡是指对伤口渗出液的评估和处理。表149-5列出了敷料的主要类型，在确定某一伤口最合适的敷料时，必须考虑对渗出液的吸收需求，对额外水分的需求以及伤口及其边缘上皮是否可以耐受去除粘性敷料所致的微小的创伤。边缘评估主要指识别无进展的伤口边缘，并适当使用治疗手段如清创术来推进伤口边缘的愈合。

（2）皮肤移植：皮肤移植物按移植的组织量进行分类，介绍了不同厚度移植皮片的特点，并指出皮肤移植物愈合的显著特征是移植物依赖受体的创面床进行血运重建，其余过程则与正常伤口愈合大致相同。接下来对皮肤移植后期存活所涉及的细胞及分子机制进行了简要阐述。

（3）皮肤替代物：皮肤替代物可分为两大类：细胞类产品和脱细胞基质类产品（表149-6）。对于各种皮肤替代物的代表产品、获批适应症及治疗进展进行了介绍。

（4）干细胞治疗：干细胞在伤口处理中的应用旨在用新的细胞替代伤口残留细胞，这些细胞有可能对伤口愈合过程的信号作出反应。目前大多数干细胞治疗人类伤口的研究使用的都是骨髓间充质干细胞，对干细胞应用伤口愈合的进展进行了介绍。

（5）慢性伤口和愈合不良：慢性伤口愈合不良可能与缺血、压迫、感染或多种因素共同作用有关。作者提及静脉性溃疡是真正的伤口愈合不良，并对其原因和可能的机制进行了阐述。

（6）创面愈合的年龄相关改变：提及对于急性和慢性伤口，延迟愈合都与衰老有关，并对其原因进行了分析。

（7）伤口护理的基本标准：治疗在一定程度上依赖于伤口原因。详细的病史和体查，以及辅助诊断试验，如伤口活检、血管研究、影像学、组织培养和实验室检查可能有助于病因诊断。

（8）预测伤口闭合的方法：用于预测伤口闭合的方法包括简单的测量伤口大小（宽度和长度）和伤口面积变化，到计算机平面分析和评估伤口边缘移动。提及在治疗的前4周预测伤口是否能及时闭合非常重要，临床医生可基于预测结果来确定当前的治疗是否应该继续或需要调整。

4．结论 伤口愈合是一个复杂又具有一定重叠性的炎症、增殖和重塑的过程。作者对于伤口愈合未来的治疗方向如智能生物敷料、组织工程皮肤和干细胞治疗等方面进行了展望。

〔黄莹雪〕

AT-A-GLANCE

- While acute and chronic wounds are different, all chronic wounds start as an acute wound.
- In acute wounds, there is an orderly progression from injury to coagulation, inflammation, cell and matrix proliferation, cell migration, and tissue remodeling.
- In the initial phases, a wide range of growth factors, including platelet-derived growth factor and transforming growth factor-β_1, play an important role. In the proliferation/migration and modeling phases, tissue matrix metalloproteinases (MMPs), integrins, basic fibroblast growth factor, and epidermal growth factor are critical. MMP-1, MMP-9, and MMP-10 are essential for remodeling.
- For acute wounds, moist wounds heal faster, and a variety of wound dressings are available, including hydrogels, polyurethane films, hydrocolloids, foams, alginates, superabsorbent dressings, and collagen-based products.
- In chronic wounds, the linear progression between the sequential phases of acute wound healing is lost. Chronic wounds are often the result of ischemia, pressure, and infection; healing, in part, is dependent on addressing these factors.
- Healing after skin grafting is also different, as it depends on revascularization, either neovascularization or inosculation.

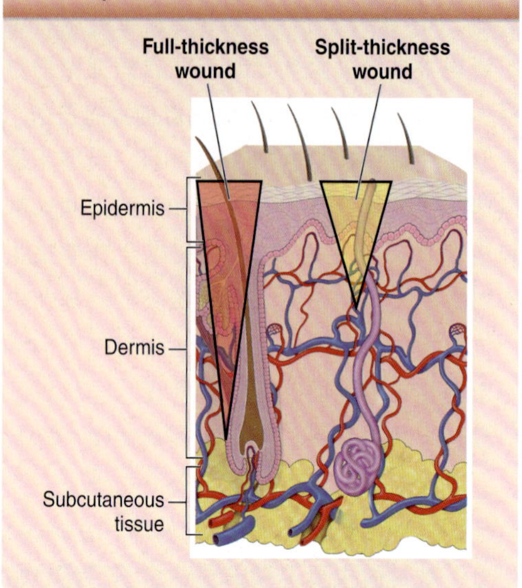

Figure 149-1 Diagrammatic representation of the skin, with 2 inverted triangles representing either a split-thickness or full-thickness wound. Extending the injury below the reservoir of keratinocytes present in skin appendages (full-thickness wound) removes the capability of the keratinocytes to populate the defect from within the wound bed, which means healing has to occur from the wound edges and more scarring takes place.

Wound healing involves a complex but overlapping sequential series of events aimed at barrier restoration, from hemostasis to inflammation, proliferation, and remodeling. Many mediators, such as platelets, neutrophils, macrophages, cytokines, growth factors, matrix metalloproteinases, and their inhibitors regulate these events.[1] Some wounds fail to move through these stages in an orderly and timely fashion and become chronic wounds. All these components play a role in healing, and alteration in one or more of these components may impair healing and/or lead to abnormal scar formation, such as a hypertrophic scar or keloid.[2] Wounds can be categorized by the depth of the wound, which helps predict the amount of scarring that will occur. Greater scarring occurs in full-thickness versus partial or spilt-thickness wounds. Figure 149-1 outlines these differences.

DIFFERENT TYPES OF WOUND HEALING

Primary healing, also called healing by primary or first intention, is the closure of the wound soon after wound creation, as seen in surgical wounds and clean lacerations. Wound closure is aided by approximation of the wound edges using sutures, glues, tapes, or mechanical devices, and in side-to-side closure and with grafts and flaps.

Delayed primary healing is the slightly delayed closure of a wound, typically by a few days. As an example, a contaminated wound may first be treated with antimicrobials to assure eradication of bacteria that might delay healing.

In healing by *secondary intention*, the open wound heals through a process that includes granulation tissue formation and epithelialization. Commonly employed after an excessive loss of soft tissue, such as major trauma or severe burns, the large defect requires ingrowth of granulation tissue and extracellular matrix (ECM) formation. Myofibroblasts plays a major role in this type of healing,[1] appearing 3 days after the injury and reaching a maximum level 10 to 21 days postinjury. Secondary intention healing may result in wound contracture and can cause functional restriction.

Tertiary intention occurs when a wound originally closed by primary intention dehisces and then heals by secondary intention.

The time to complete healing depends on many factors such as the depth of the wound, location of the wound (eg, facial wounds heal faster than acral wounds), vascular supply, presence of infection, and wound shape (smaller diameter wounds heal faster than larger diameter wounds of the same size/area.)[3]

MECHANISMS OF WOUND HEALING

PHASES OF WOUND HEALING

Tissue injury triggers a cascade of sequential, overlapping events that have been categorized into several phases, including: (a) coagulation, (b) the inflammatory phase, (c) the proliferative (and migratory) phase, and (d) the remodeling phase. Figure 149-2 illustrates these phases in diagrammatic form, and Fig. 149-3 shows specific events that take place during the various phases. The cell types primarily involved in wound healing are platelets, neutrophils, and macrophages, fibroblasts, endothelial cells, and epithelial cells. More recently, increasing importance is accumulating for the role, either directly or indirectly, of lymphocytes.[4,5]

COAGULATION

Immediately after injury, disruption of blood vessels leads to local release of blood cells and bloodborne elements, resulting in clot formation and activation of the intrinsic and extrinsic coagulation cascade.[3] While the blood clot within the vessel lumen provides hemostasis, the clot within the injury site acts as a provisional matrix for cell migration, leads to further formation of ECM,[6] and provides a reservoir for cytokines and growth factors.[7,8] Platelets degranulate and release α granules which secret growth factors including platelet-derived growth factors, insulin-like growth factors, epidermal growth factors, transforming growth factor-β, and platelet factor 4. Platelets also release a number of chemotactic factors that attract other platelets, leukocytes, and fibroblasts to the site of injury.[8,9] The clot also contains fibrin, fibronectin, vitronectin, von Willebrand factor, and thrombospondin, which provide a matrix for cell migration. Vasoactive amines released from platelets, such as serotonin, facilitate cell migration by increased microvascular permeability. Hageman factor XII is a specific enzyme released following platelet aggregation to initiate the intrinsic coagulation cascade. Prothrombin transforms into thrombin, converting soluble fibrinogen to insoluble fibrin. Additionally, injured tissue releases a tissue factor that activates the extrinsic coagulation pathway.[9]

INFLAMMATION

Inflammation begins with activation of classic and alternative complement cascades and subsequent neutrophil infiltration to the wound site within 24 to 48 hours of injury. White cells have multiple functions, including phagocytosis of necrotic material and bacteria, as well as the production of certain critical cytokines.[10,11] Leukocytes adhere to the adjacent blood vessels (margination) and actively move through the vessel wall via diapedesis. Leukocytes release enzymes and oxygen-derived free radicals. After the first few days, the constituency of white cells changes as neutrophils are replaced by macrophages.[12]

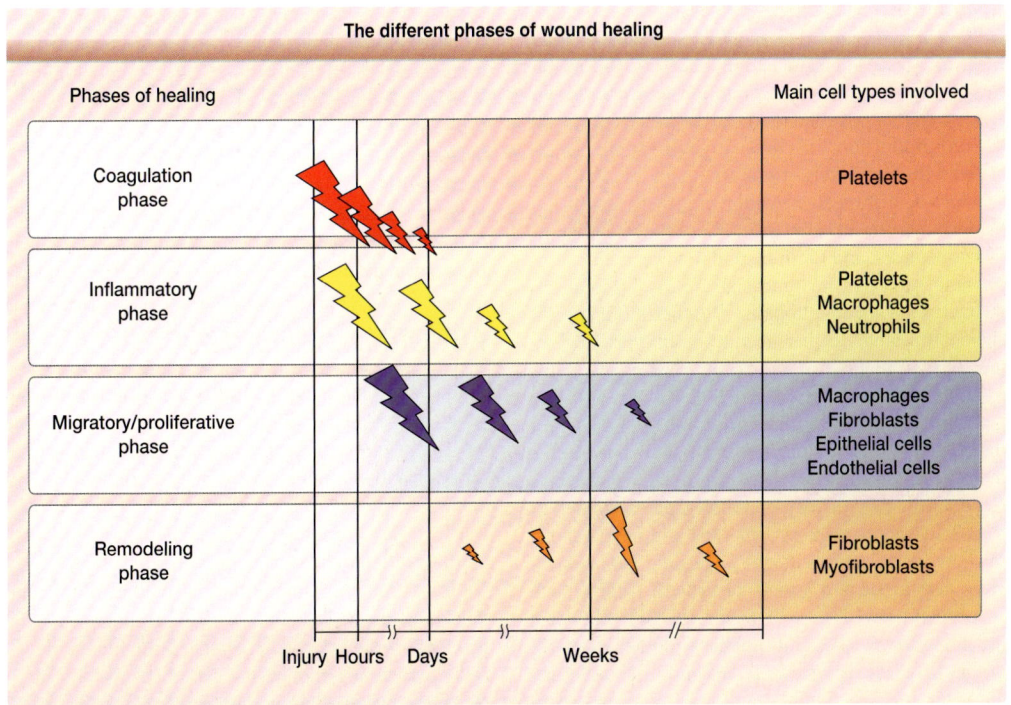

Figure 149-2 Schematic, different of the different phases of wound healing.

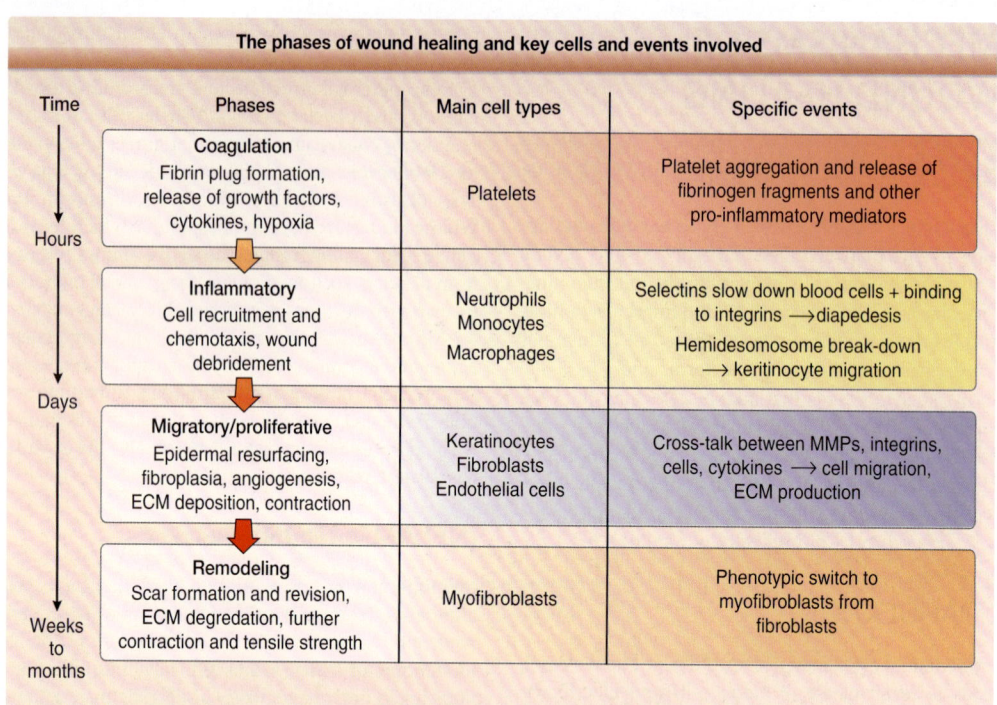

Figure 149-3 The phases of wound healing, and key cells and events involved. (Reprinted from Falanga V. Wound healing and its impairment in the diabetic foot. *The Lancet*. 2005;366:1736-1743; with permission. Copyright © Elsevier.)

Macrophages, often considered the most important regulatory cells in the wound healing inflammatory process, typically appear in the wound site 72 hours after the injury. Macrophages, key regulator cells for repair, are the main phagocytic cells and release proteolytic enzymes such as a variety of collagenases. Macrophages also produce growth factors responsible for the smooth muscle proliferation and endothelial cell and fibroblast proliferation, all of which contribute to ECM production. This hypoxic environment is associated with high levels of proteases and low pH, both of which contribute to activation of growth factors.[11]

Monocytes are attracted to the injury site by kallikrein, fibrinopeptides, and fibrin-degradation products; some of these same chemoattractants are also responsible for recruitment of neutrophils.[13,14] Other more specific chemoattractants further recruit monocytes, including collagen fragments, fibronectin, elastin, and transforming growth factor (TGF)-β_1. Monocytes undergo a phenotypic change to tissue macrophages critical for the progression of healing.[15,16] Macrophages release chemotactic factors to attract fibroblasts to the wound area. Importantly, they display impressive plasticity, and at least 2 subsets of macrophages exist and have distinct phenotypes in various stages of healing (see below). They also produce a variety of growth factors, such as platelet-derived growth factor (PDGF), fibroblast growth factors (FGFs), and vascular endothelial growth factors (VEGFs), as well as TGF-β and TGF-α. Alterations in tissue macrophages or circulating monocytes lead to poor intrinsic debridement, delay proliferation of fibroblasts, and allow for inadequate angiogenesis and overall poor healing.[17]

Macrophages are divided into M1 (or classically activated) and M2 (or alternatively activated) macrophages. M1 phenotype macrophages are activated by interferon-γ and tumor necrosis factor (TNF)-α following wound formation. They release interleukin (IL)-12 and promote a proinflammatory T-helper (Th)-1 immune response early on. Subsequently, M2 macrophages, activated by IL-4 and IL-13, work to downregulate inflammation by releasing antiinflammatory cytokines such as IL-10. These M2 macrophages present later in healing during granulation tissue formation.[17-19]

ABNORMAL INFLAMMATORY PHASE

Immediately after injury, local vasodilation, extravasation of blood and fluid, and lymphatic drainage blockage (in some cases) can lead to cardinal symptoms of inflammation such as heat, redness, pain, and swelling. The acute inflammatory response may last 2 weeks; however, prolongation of inflammation (chronic inflammation) may delay healing.[20]

With chronic inflammation, the wound often contains necrotic tissue and pathogenic organisms. In this case, granulocytes disappear and mononuclear cells, particularly monocytes, lymphocytes, and macrophages, become the predominant cells at the site of inflammation.

From the clinical standpoint, certain wounds, such as pyoderma gangrenosum, have excessive inflammation and treatment, with corticosteroids for example, leads to downregulation of inflammation and healing. Fine-tuning the inflammatory response may represent a therapeutic target for other wounds as well.[21]

PROLIFERATION

The proliferative phase, characterized by fibroblast migration, deposition of ECM, and formation of granulation tissue, normally starts at about day 3 after wounding and lasts for 2 to 4 weeks. Figure 149-4 illustrates events that occur in the proliferative/migratory and remodeling phases. An important event in this phase is reepithelialization. This critical event also involves migration of keratinocytes and the interdependence between keratinocyte movement over the provisional fibrin matrix, recruitment of fibroblasts and endothelial cells, and ECM formation.[22]

Growth factors, such as PDGF and TGF-β, attract fibroblasts to the wound. Fibroblasts subsequently proliferate and produce a matrix consisting of fibronectin and hyaluronan initially, and collagen and proteoglycans later. These components are essential for new ECM formation and tissue repair. ECM serves both as turgor of soft tissue and as a scaffold and regulator of cell adhesion and growth. It is made of an interstitial matrix of adhesive proteins embedded in proteoglycan and glycosaminoglycan gel as well as the fibrinous structural proteins collagen and elastin.[23]

Fibroblasts make collagen, the most abundant protein in the body, and noncollagenous proteins. During the proliferative phase, collagen synthesis is induced by PDGF, basic FGF (bFGF), TGF-β, IL-1, and TNF. There are 18 different types of collagen. Fibrillar collagens, such as I, III, and V, form the connective tissue in the healing wound, and nonfibrillar forms, such as collagen IV, form the basement membrane.

Collagen gene expression is regulated by multiple factors such as TGF-β and FGF. TGF-β stimulates production of collagen I and collagen III. The overexpression of matrix metalloproteinases (MMPs) and/or impaired counteraction of tissue inhibitor of metalloproteinases (TIMPs) contributes to delayed healing and fibrosis. Interaction between these cytokines is extremely important. The fibroblasts in patients with longstanding diabetic foot ulcers show a decreased response to TGF-$β_1$ and decreased expression of TGF-β receptors. Although overexpression may be problematic, tissue matrix MMPs and other enzymes, such as plasminogen activator inhibitor, are critical to the movement of cells through provisional structural matrix components.

Adhesive proteins, including fibronectin (FN), laminin, thrombospondin, and integrins, help guide cellular migration.[24] FN is a large heterodimer linked to cell surfaces, basal membranes, and the ECM. FN can attach to ECM components such as collagen, fibrin, and proteoglycan, or to integrins and directly mediate the cell migration. FN also activates intracellular signaling pathways to increase the sensitivity of certain cells, such as endothelial cells, to growth factors.[25]

Integrins are important in cell–cell and cell–matrix adhesion, serving to regulate interaction between ECM and the cytoskeleton. The integrins, consisting of at least 24 αβ heterodimers (18 α and 8 β subunits), are transmembrane cell surface receptors that bind the ECM to cytoskeletal structures.[25] The integrin profile is very dynamic during the repair process. For example, dermal fibroblasts undergo a switch from $α_2$ to $α_3$ and $α_5$ integrin subunits. As another example, endothelial cells cannot respond to angiogenic stimuli without the expression of $αvβ_5$ integrin. Certain polypeptide

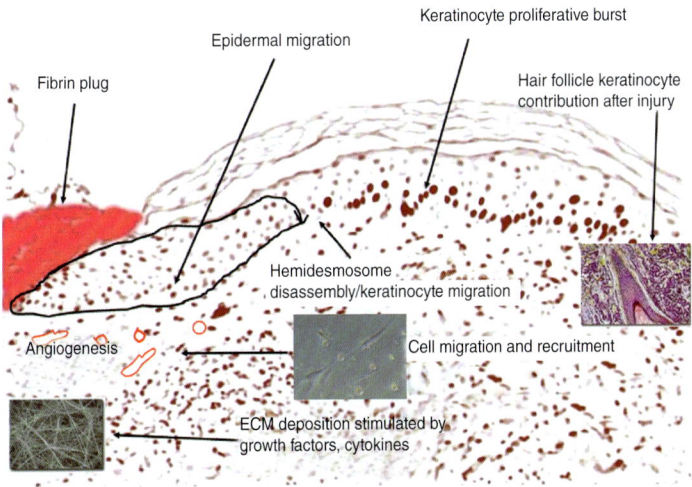

Figure 149-4 Schematic, using a modified photomicrograph section, of the events taking place shortly after injury, including formation of a fibrin plug, epidermal migration, and extracellular matrix deposition.

growth factors are essential to angiogenesis, including bFGF and VEGF.[25,26] Table 149-1 highlights the main cytokines and growth factors shown to play a role in the repair process.

Another constituent of ECM are noncollagenous proteins such as proteoglycans, which are glycosaminoglycans (dermatan sulfate, heparin sulfate) linked to a protein backbone that modulate cell growth and differentiation. Additionally, glycosaminoglycans without a protein core (hyaluronan) are also important components of the ECM.

Histopathology of a granulating wound bed shows proliferation of fibroblasts and capillaries in a loose ECM. Neovascularization, or formation of new blood vessels, is characteristic of this stage. Several factors induce angiogenesis as a part of granulation tissue development; new capillaries sprout, invading the fibrin and FN-rich clot. The density of blood vessels is reduced over time with scar formation and as the wound moves toward the remodeling phase.[26] Fibroblast replication and longevity are enhanced in hypoxia, and low oxygen tension stimulates clonal expansion of dermal fibroblasts seeded as single cells.[27] Moreover, the synthesis of a number of growth factors is enhanced in hypoxic cells.

After a provisional matrix has formed, keratinocytes migrate to epithelize the wound. MMP function is critical for allowing keratinocytes at the edge of the wound to detach from their hemidesmosomal and desmosomal attachments and migrate across the provisional matrix. Other proteins play important roles, including plasminogen activator inhibitor, a serine protein inhibitor that functions as the main inhibitor of tissue plasminogen activator, and urokinase plasminogen activator.[28]

Upregulation of tissue plasminogen activator and urokinase plasminogen activator are important for keratinocyte migration, which may depend on crosstalk and interactions between $\alpha_3\beta_1$, keratinocytes, and collagen. These events lead to the induction of MMP-1 (collagenase-1 or interstitial collagenase), which is important for keratinocyte migration and epithelialization.[6] MMP-9 plays a fundamental role in "cutting" Type IV and Type VII collagen, which are essential

TABLE 149-1
The Major Growth Factors Involved in Wound Healing and Their Functions[39]

GROWTH FACTOR	MAJOR SOURCES	FUNCTION
Epidermal growth factor (EGF)	Platelets, macrophages, fibroblasts	Epithelialization Fibroblast proliferation Keratinocyte proliferation Angiogenesis
Transforming growth factor (TGF)-α	Keratinocytes, macrophages, fibroblasts, lymphocytes	Keratinocyte migration
TGF-β	Macrophages, fibroblasts, keratinocytes, platelets	Inflammation, angiogenesis, reepithelialization, connective tissue regeneration, remodeling TGF-β_1, TGF-β_2: promote fibrosis and scar formation TGF-β_3: antiscar properties
Activins	Fibroblasts, keratinocytes	Epithelialization
Fibroblast growth factor (FGF)	Keratinocytes, fibroblasts, smooth muscle cells, chondrocytes, endothelial cells, mast cells	FGF-2: granulation tissue formation, reepithelialization, tissue remodeling, fibroblast migration, collagen formation FGF-7, FGF-10: increase transcription factors, detoxification of reactive oxygen species FGF-7: neovascularization
Platelet-derived growth factor	Platelets, macrophages, vascular endothelium, fibroblasts	Fibroblast proliferation Angiogenesis Matrix formation
Vascular endothelial growth factor (A-E)	Keratinocytes, endothelial cells, fibroblasts, smooth muscle cells, platelets, neutrophils, macrophages	Angiogenesis
Granulocyte-macrophage colony-stimulating factor	Macrophages Fibroblasts Endothelial cells Natural killer cells Mast cells	Keratinocyte proliferation Epithelialization Cell migration Chemotaxis Angiogenesis
Interleukin (IL)-1	Monocytes Macrophages Keratinocytes	Keratinocyte proliferation Fibroblast proliferation Angiogenesis Neutrophil chemotaxis
IL-6	Neutrophils Monocytes	Keratinocytes proliferation Neutrophil chemotaxis

components of the basement membrane and anchoring fibrils, and promotes inflammation and neutrophil migration. For keratinocyte migration to occur, a necessity exists to break down these complex structures anchoring the basal keratinocytes to the basement membrane and neighboring keratinocytes. This process is as complex as the structure itself, and involves interactions between MMPs, integrins, growth factors, and structural proteins. In the normal resting state, laminin-332 is bound to $\alpha_6\beta_4$-integrin, the latter linking the intracellular keratin filaments of keratinocytes to the basement membrane. As a result of the interaction of integrins (including their phosphorylation status) with the ECM and their receptor clustering on the surface of keratinocytes, important morphologic changes, such as lamellipodia formation, occur for keratinocyte locomotion.[29-31] Migration of keratinocytes is essential for resurfacing of the wound.[26,32]

Keratinocytes begin to migrate from the wound edge and from skin appendages within the first 24 hours. The hair bulge, the germinative portion of the hair, is an important reservoir for keratinocytes in partial thickness wounds. A series of events in migration involves elongation of keratinocytes, development of pseudopod-like projection of lamellipodia, loss of cell-to-cell adhesion, retraction of intracellular tonofilaments, and formation of actin filaments at the edge of the cytoplasm, all of which occur while the proliferative ability of keratinocytes is inhibited.

To facilitate migration, there is a marked increase in mitotic activity within the basal epithelial cells of the wound edge from 12 hours, extending lamellipodia along the wound edges. Subsequently keratinocytes lose their attachment to the underlying dermis to migrate in a leapfrog fashion. Eventually a new basement membrane forms and further growth and differentiation of epithelial cells establishes the stratified epithelium. The process of epithelialization is facilitated in a moist environment, serving as the biologic basis for modern occlusive dressings.

REMODELING

The final phase, remodeling, is typically the longest phase, involving the continuous synthesis and breakdown of collagen as the ECM evolves. Starting early in the healing process, wound remodeling may continue for months. The interaction of ECM and fibroblasts causes wound contraction and is influenced by multiple cytokines, including TGF-β, PDGF and bFGF.

The remodeling of the ECM, as well as the movement of cells, is highly dependent on MMPs and serine proteases.[33] An important component of this dependence on MMPs is MMP-driven degradation of ECM and the resulting exposure of selective bioactive ECM segments that influence cell behavior, including migration and proliferation.[6,33]

Metalloproteinases produced by fibroblasts, neutrophils, keratinocytes, and macrophages, include interstitial collagenase (degrades collagen Types I, II, and III), gelatinases (degrades denatured collagen and FN) and stromelysins (degrades proteoglycans, laminin, FN, and amorphous collagen). MMP-10 (stromelysin) breaks down other noncollagenous ECM components and facilitates migration.[6,11,34] Other mediators, such as thymosin-β, upregulate MMPs during wound repair.[35] The activity of MMPs are tightly regulated because they may degrade essential collagens and impair healing. They are activated by certain proteins (plasmin) and inhibited by specific tissue inhibitors of metalloproteinases. Table 149-2 summarizes certain MMPs and their prominent effect in wound healing.

During the remodeling process, a phenotypic switch occurs in certain cell subpopulations from fibroblasts to myofibroblasts.[36] Although the early process of healing relies largely on matrix accumulation, which, in turn, facilitates cell migration, later healing requires a dampening of ECM formation to a level that at least approximates the preinjury state. However, the remodeling phase is more than a breakdown of excess macromolecules formed during the proliferative phase of wound healing. During this phase, cells within the wound are returned to a stable phenotype, ECM material is altered (ie, collagen Type III to collagen Type I), and granulation tissue disappears.[11,26] Granulation tissue evolves to a scar composed of less-active fibroblasts, dense collagen, and fragments of elastic tissue along with the rest of ECM. Scar matures and the tensile strength increases to a maximum of 80% strength of noninjured skin. In full-thickness wounds, contraction is responsible for 40% of the decrease in wound size.

FETAL HEALING

During early embryogenesis, wounded fetal tissue heals without fibrosis. Regeneration, as opposed to repair, occurs. Later in embryogenesis (last trimester) and after childbirth, repair (as opposed to regeneration) occurs, with resulting fibrosis. Among factors that affect scarring, fibromodulin is a small glycoprotein that mediates scarless healing in fetal skin.[37]

GROWTH FACTORS AND CYTOKINES

Wound healing is regulated by multiple growth factors and cytokines released at the wound site. Growth factors are biologically active polypeptides that can alter the growth, differentiation and metabolism of a target cell. They are important elements in the healing of wounds. Table 149-1 lists the major growth factors and cytokines involved in healing and their respective roles.[38-40] Although potentially important in healing

TABLE 149-2
Matrix Metalloproteinases Proteinases with Well-Established, Functional Effects on Wound Healing

EFFECT	COMMON NAMES	CORRESPONDING MMP DESIGNATION	SOME SPECIFIC EFFECTS
Keratinocyte proliferation and migration	Collagenase 1 Gelatinase A Stromelysin 2 Matrilysin-1 Epilysin	MMP-1 MMP-2 MMP-10 MMP-7 MMP-28	Increased migration
Endothelial cell (EC) migration	Collagenase 3 Gelatinase A MT1-MMP	MMP-13 MMP-2 MMP-14	Increases EC migration Needed for angiogenesis Needed for angiogenesis
Cell migration	Stromelysin 1 Stromelysin 2 Matrilysin-2	MMP-3 MMP-10 MMP-26	Required for excisional wounds
Inflammation	Collagenase 2 Gelatinase A Gelatinase B Matrilysin-1	MMP-8 MMP-2 MMP-9 MMP-7	Antiinflammatory Antiinflammatory Promotes inflammation
Neutrophil migration	Gelatinase B MT6-MMP	MMP-9 MMP-25	Increases neutrophil migration
Apoptosis	Collagenase 2 MT1-MMP MT2-MMP MT6-MMP	MMP-8 MMP-14 MMP-15 MMP-25	Prevents apoptosis Antiapoptotic

MMP, matrix metalloprotease; MT, membrane type.

from a therapeutic standpoint, only PDGF-BB, bFGF, and granulocyte-macrophage colony-stimulating factor (GM-CSF) are used clinically in the management of wounds, and only PDGF is approved for wound healing by the U.S. Food and Drug Administration (FDA).

EPIDERMAL GROWTH FACTOR FAMILY

Epidermal growth factor (EGF) family members bind to a tyrosine kinase transmembrane protein or EGF receptor.[41] EGFR normally localizes throughout the epidermis with its membranous presence being more prominent in the basal layer. EGFR plays an important role in reepithelialization by increasing keratinocyte proliferation and cell migration.[42,43]

EGF is secreted in a paracrine fashion by platelets, macrophages and fibroblasts and acts on keratinocytes. Faulty location of the EGF receptor may be problematic in some nonhealing wounds. An in vitro study demonstrated the presence of EGFR in the cytoplasm, rather than the extracellular membrane, of cells in non-healing wounds, suggesting receptor downregulation within chronic wounds.[42-44] TGF-α is another member of the EGF family that is secreted by keratinocytes, macrophages, fibroblasts, and lymphocytes, and works in an autocrine fashion.[45,46] TGF-α induces expression of keratin 6 and keratin 16 (present in proliferating keratinocytes) and increases keratinocyte migration.[47]

TRANSFORMING GROWTH FACTOR-β FAMILY

TGF-β family members include TGF-β_1 to TGF-β_3, bone morphogenic proteins, and activins. TGF-β_1, TGF-β_2, and TGF-β_3 promote the migration of fibroblasts and endothelial cells and deposition of extracellular matrices by fibroblasts during granulation tissue formation. TGF-β_1 predominates in wound healing.[48] Interestingly, TGF-β_1 and TGF-β_2 promote fibrosis and scar formation, whereas TGF-β_3 has antifibrotic properties.[49] TGF-β, produced by macrophages, fibroblasts, keratinocytes, and platelets, is important in the wound healing processes of inflammation, angiogenesis, reepithelialization, and connective tissue regeneration.[48,50] TGF-β_1 facilitates recruitment of inflammatory cells, and promotes macrophage mediated debridement and granulation tissue formation. During reepithelialization, TGF-β_1 shifts keratinocyte integrin expression toward a more migratory subtype.[51] In the remodeling phase, TGF-β_1 plays a major role in collagen production and inhibits collagen breakdown by inhibiting MMP-1, MMP-3, and MMP-9, and promoting TIMP-1.[52,53]

TGF-β₁ plays an important role in the formation of hypertrophic scars and keloids by overexpression of connective tissue growth factor.[54] In fetal wounds, deceases in TGF-β₁ transcription help explain the scarless healing that is seen.[55]

Activins are members of the TGF-β family produced by fibroblasts and keratinocytes and play role in reepithelization. Activin inhibits keratinocyte proliferation and induces terminal differentiation of keratinocytes. bone morphogenic proteins are another member of the family involved in keratinocyte differentiation. Overexpression of bone morphogenic protein-6 is associated with delayed healing.[39,56]

FIBROBLAST GROWTH FACTOR FAMILY

The 3 main members of the FGF family involved in wound healing are FGF-2, FGF-7, and FGF-10. FGFs are produced by keratinocytes, fibroblasts, smooth muscle cells, chondrocytes, endothelial cells, and mast cells.[57] FGF receptors 1 to 4 are tyrosine kinase transmembrane proteins that work like EGFR.[45]

bFGF or FGF-2 plays a role in granulation tissue formation, reepithelialization, and tissue remodeling.[58] FGF-2 regulates the synthesis of ECM components, and facilitates keratinocyte and fibroblast migration and collagenase formation. bFGF is decreased in chronic wounds.[59]

FGF-7 or keratinocyte growth factor-1 and FGF 10 or keratinocyte growth factor-2. FGF-7 and FGF-10 are secreted in a paracrine fashion, found only on keratinocytes, and have a role in reepithelialization. FGF-7 and FGF-10 increase transcription factors involved in detoxification of reactive oxygen species. FGF-7 is a strong mitogen of vascular endothelial cells and is important during neovascularization.[60]

PLATELET-DERIVED GROWTH FACTOR FAMILY

PDGFs, produced by platelets, macrophages, vascular endothelium, fibroblasts, and keratinocytes, bind to 2 different transmembrane tyrosine kinase receptors (α and β).[61] Upon injury PDGF is released from degranulating platelets. PDGF, chemotactic for monocytes, macrophages, and neutrophils, is a mitogen for fibroblasts and smooth muscle cells in vitro. PDGF also stimulates macrophages to produce growth factors such as TGF-β.[62] PDGF plays an important role in blood vessel maturation and works synergistically with hypoxia to stimulate VEGF formation in vitro. However, PDGF angiogenic activity is less than FGF and VEGF.[63] While not directly affecting keratinocyte migration, PDGF plays role in reepithelialization by in vitro production of insulin-like growth factor-1 and thrombospondin-1. PDGF also enhances the proliferation of fibroblasts and, in turn, the production of ECM. Recombinant human PDGF-BB (becaplermin) is the only FDA-approved drug for nonhealing neuropathic diabetic foot ulcers.[64,65]

VASCULAR ENDOTHELIAL GROWTH FACTOR FAMILY

Members of the VEGF family include VEGF-A to VEGF-E and placental growth factor.[66] VEGF-A, which is secreted by keratinocytes, endothelial cells, fibroblast smooth muscle cells, platelets, neutrophils, and macrophages, binds to a tyrosine kinase surface receptor that is located on the endothelial surface of blood vessels, early in wound healing angiogenesis.[67] Platelets release VEGF-A upon injury. Macrophages release VEGF-A directly but also release TNF-α, which induces VEGF-A expression on keratinocytes and fibroblasts. Hypoxia is a major stimulus for release of VEGF-A, and the VEGF-A gradient parallels the hypoxia gradient. VEGF-A is also involved mainly in the inflammatory stage of wound healing. Placental growth factor is expressed by keratinocytes and endothelial cells as a proangiogenic molecule. Placental growth factor stimulates cultured fibroblast migration and stimulates granulation tissue formation.[68]

GRANULOCYTE-MONOCYTE COLONY-STIMULATING FACTOR

GM-CSF has particular importance in the inflammatory stage of wound healing by increasing keratinocyte proliferation and enhancing reepithelialization. GM-CSF promotes proliferation and differentiation of neutrophils and hence increases host defenses.[69] GM-CSF indirectly upregulates IL-6. In 2 studies on diabetic foot ulcers, in total 67 patients with infected diabetic foot ulcers were treated either with placebo or topical GM-CSF. Although GM-CSF improved neutrophil function and increased absolute neutrophil numbers, the addition of topical GM-CSF to standard care had no additional beneficial clinical effect.[69]

PROINFLAMMATORY CYTOKINES

Proinflammatory cytokines, including IL-1, IL-6, and TNF-α, are upregulated in the inflammatory phase of wound healing. IL-1 is produced by monocytes, macrophages, monocytes, and keratinocytes, with both paracrine and autocrine functions. IL-1 induces expression of keratin 6 and keratin 16 in migrating keratinocytes, and activates fibroblasts to secrete FGF-7.[70] IL-6 is produced by neutrophils and monocytes with mitogenic and proliferative effect on keratinocytes and chemoattractive effects on neutrophils. TNF-α and IL-1β are increased in chronic wounds. The effect of exogenous TNF is dependent on the concentration and duration of exposure.[70,71] TNF-α at low levels promotes healing by stimulating inflammation and increasing macrophage-produced growth factors, whereas at higher levels TNF-α impairs wound healing by suppressing production of ECM and TIMP and increasing MMPs. Chronic inflammation stimulates production of TNF-α and IL-1β that synergistically increases production of MMPs and suppress production of TIMPs.[72]

CHEMOKINES

Chemokines are a family of small cytokines or signaling proteins that attract neutrophils to the site. Macrophage chemoattractant protein-1 (or CCL2) is induced by keratinocytes and is chemoattractant for monocyte/macrophages, T cells, and mast cells.[73]

Interferon-inducible protein 10 (or CXCL10) is another cytokine that negatively impacts wound healing. Interferon-inducible protein 10 inhibits migration of fibroblasts. IL-8 increases keratinocyte migration and proliferation, and is a chemoattractant of neutrophils.[74]

CLINICAL ISSUES IN WOUND HEALING

WOUND BED PREPARATION

Although the majority of wounds heal in a timely manner, a proportion of wounds stall and do not follow the stages of healing. A nonhealing wound needs wound bed preparation to promote healing. The concept of wound bed preparation has been summarized using the pneumonic *TIME*: *T*issue debridement, *I*nfection/inflammation, *M*oisture balance, *E*pithelia edge tissue.[21,32,75]

Tissue debridement plays a key role in tissue preparation by removing nonviable tissue and pathogenic bacteria. Multiple techniques to debride exist, including surgical, enzymatic, biologic, mechanical, and autolytic techniques. Newer tools, such as low-frequency ultrasound and hydrosurgery devices, have been developed.[76] Table 149-3 lists techniques used for tissue debridement.

Treating infection and inflammation implies assessment of the need for topical antiseptic and/or systemic antibiotic use to control infection and subsequent inflammation. Although inflammation is a physiologic process in wound healing, inappropriate inflammation can cause delayed healing. Infection may be classically seen as a host response, as in cellulitis. Bacteria may also delay healing through formation of biofilm, seen in 60% of chronic wounds. Biofilms are colonies of microorganisms that protect themselves through community living, in part by a surrounding glycocalyx (Fig. 149-5). Disruption of biofilms with debridement, with or without antimicrobial agents, helps alleviate persistent inflammation.[77]

The term *antimicrobial* includes disinfectants, antiseptics, and antibiotics. Antiseptics are broad spectrum with less risk of bacterial resistance. The difference between antibiotics and antiseptics is that antiseptics are nonspecific, while antibiotics work specifically on

TABLE 149-3
Debridement Techniques

DEBRIDEMENT TECHNIQUES	ADVANTAGES	DISADVANTAGES
Surgical, sharp (with scissors and/or scalpel)	High speed Selectivity	Painful procedure, expensive Needs skilled professionals Contraindicated in ischemic tissue and bleeding disorders
Enzymatic (collagenase)	Low pain	Medium cost and low selectivity Some patients are allergic to the enzyme preparation
Biologic (larval therapy)	High speed and high selectivity Medium pain	High cost Contraindicated in bleeding diathesis and deep, tunneling wounds
Mechanical (wet to dry dressings, hydrotherapy, ultrasonography)	Medium speed	Painful Nonselective
Autolytic (endogenous enzymes with moisture-retentive dressings)	Low pain	Low speed Low selectivity Relatively high cost Contraindicated in infected wounds Risk of exposed bone/tendon and friable skin

bacteria functions or processes such as disputing cell wall function but also can allow bacteria opportunity to mutate and develop resistance. As a result, topical antibiotics are not recommended for chronic wounds because of the risk of antibiotic resistance. A variety of modern antiseptic-impregnated dressings have been used to reduce microorganism numbers in the dressings and, in theory, on the wound surface. Their effect on biofilm organisms is less-well defined. Table 149-4 lists these antiseptics.

Moisture imbalance involves the assessment and management of wound exudate. While acute wound fluid promotes cell growth and is rich in cytokines and growth factors, chronic wound fluid inhibits cell growth and contains high levels of proteases and pro-inflammatory cytokines. Thus, acute wounds benefit from contact with wound fluid, whereas chronic wounds do not. Moisture can hinder wound healing in other ways as well: extra moisture can damage periwound skin, and lack of moisture can hinder keratinocyte migration.

The major dressing types (Table 149-5) include hydrogels, transparent polyurethane films, hydrocolloids, gelling fibers, alginates, foams, superabsorbents, and collagen products. In determining the most appropriate dressing for a particular wound,

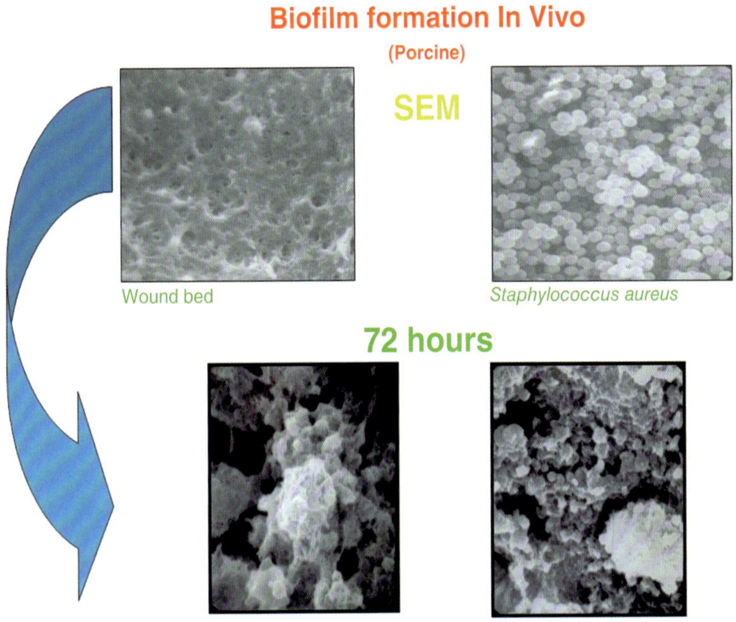

Figure 149-5 Biofilm formation. Colonies of microorganisms with a surrounding glycocalyx. SEM, scanning electron micrograph.

one must consider the need for absorption of exudate (foams and alginates), the need for additional moisture (hydrogels), and whether the wound and its epithelial edges can tolerate the often subtle (but important) trauma that comes from removal of adhesive dressings such as films. Thin contact layers, consisting of different polymeric materials, some with perforations, allow wound fluid to escape and are useful in preventing tissue injury upon dressing changes.

Edge assessment involves the assessment of nonadvancing wound edges and proper use of therapies to advance the wound edge.[21] Keratinocytes from the edge of chronic wounds often abnormally express *c-myc* and treatments, such as debridement, which remove or reverse this cellular biomarker, can promote keratinocyte migration.[78-80]

SKIN GRAFTS

Skin grafts are categorized by the amount of tissue being grafting. For example, split-thickness grafts include a portion of dermis and full-thickness grafts contain the entire dermis. The likelihood of the survival

TABLE 149-4
Common Antiseptics Used in Wound Healing[109,110,125,126]

ANTISEPTICS	MAIN ADVANTAGES	MAIN DISADVANTAGES
Iodine Based:		
▪ Povidine-iodine 10% ▪ Cadexomer iodine ▪ Inadine	▪ Broad spectrum ▪ Good penetration to biofilm ▪ Proinflammatory	▪ Toxic to granulation tissue in high concentration ▪ Risk of thyroid dysfunction ▪ Risk of contact dermatitis
Chlorhexidine Based:		
▪ PHMB (polyhexamethylene biguanide)—foam, gauze	▪ Broad spectrum ▪ 0.02% concentration use for wound irrigation	▪ May damage cartilage/ear toxicity
Silver-Based:		
▪ Microcrystalline silver ▪ Silver sulfadiazine cream ▪ Silver nitrate sticks	Antiinflammatory, antibacterial, antifungal, antiviral	Silver toxicity, argyria with silver sulfasalazine; silver sulfadiazine + silver nitrate sticks may produce pseudoeschar/delay healing
Honey-Based:		
▪ Honey alginate ▪ Honey gel	Antiinflammatory, best for hard adherent eschar	Risk of botulism; may promote bacterial growth

TABLE 149-5
Main Categories of Dressings[109,110,125,126]

DRESSING CATEGORY	INGREDIENTS	FUNCTION	COMMENTS
Hydrogels	- Polymers with high water content	- Provide moisture - Nonpainful	- Needs secondary dressings - Contraindicated in infected wounds - Needs frequent dressing change
Films	- Semipermeable adhesive sheets of elastic polyurethane - Impermeable to water and bacteria	- Transparent	- Adherent (trauma when removed) - Nonabsorbent
Hydrocolloids	- Hydrophilic colloid particles bound to polyurethane film - Some composed of gelatin, pectin, and carboxy methylcellulose	- Long wear time - Autolytic debridement	- Nonabsorptive - Trauma with removal - Allergy to adhesives - Smell
Calcium alginates	- Sheets (wick laterally) - Ropes (wick upward) - From seaweed-kelp	- Hemostatic - Absorptive - Autolytic debridement	- Need secondary dressing
Gelling fibers	- Sheets or ribbons	- Absorptive - Autolytic debridement	- Needs secondary dressing
Foams	- Polyurethane foam fluid exchange with partial fluid retention if variable pore size	- Absorbent	- Bulky and may macerate surrounding skin
Superabsorbent dressings	- Fiber technology/conducts moisture	- Absorbent - Diaper technology	- Bulky
Collagen-based dressings	- Bovine-derived collagen dressings	- Promote healing - Reduce matrix metalloproteinases	- Cost

and whether wound contracture is reduced depends on the amount of dermis in the graft. Split-thickness skin grafts can survive in areas with less vascularity but also are less likely to prevent wound contracture, whereas full-thickness skin grafts require better vascularity for survival and but can better prevent contracture.

While skin grafting is centuries old, modern grafting is thought to have begun with the first skin autotransplant done in 1869 by Reverdin and then in 1929 by Brown and colleagues who introduced the technique of the split-thickness skin graft.[81] The healing of a skin graft, however, is different from the description provided earlier of the events after acute injury. One distinguishing feature of skin graft "take" or healing is the dependence of the graft on the recipient wound bed for revascularization, which requires several unique physiologic events.

Much of the remainder of skin graft healing involves events in common with the normal wound healing process. Infiltration by fibroblasts in the graft occurs 3 to 5 days after grafting, followed by a progressive increase in both graft and recipient fibroblasts within the graft.[82,83] Although graft "take" allows for donor tissue to replace missing tissue in the recipient wound, skin grafts may also stimulate wound healing of the recipient site, and this ability can be augmented. For example "prewounding" of the donor site skin prior to grafting enhances the graft's ability to stimulate healing.[83,84] Ki67 antibody and β_1-integrin expression after grafting has been noted, as has production of stimulatory growth factors and cytokines, implying that healing stimuli were provided by the grafts.[85]

SKIN SUBSTITUTES

Skin substitutes are divided into 2 main groups of cellular and acellular matrix products (Table 149-6).[86]

CELLULAR PRODUCTS

The cellular skin substitute products with best available evidence are the bilayered living cellular construct (BLCC), Apligraf (Organogenesis, Canton, MA) and cellular dermal matrix, Dermagraft (Organogenesis, Canton, MA). BLCC is a tissue-engineered cellular matrix composed of bovine Type I collage with neonatal foreskin fibroblasts for dermal component and human neonatal keratinocytes for epidermis.[87] BLCC has FDA approval for venous leg ulcers (VLUs) greater than 4 weeks' duration and for full-thickness diabetic foot ulcers present for longer than 3 weeks. The evidence supports the safety and efficacy of up to 5 applications of BLCC. An example of its efficacy is 47% of chronic, hard-to-heal VLUs present longer than 1 year treated with BLCC healed after 24 weeks compared to 19% in the group with compression alone.[88]

Cellular dermal matrix is composed of human neonatal foreskin fibroblasts cultured onto a bioabsorbable glycolic acid scaffold. The fibroblasts secrete collagen, matrix proteins, growth factors, and cytokines. It has FDA approval for diabetic foot ulcers of longer than 6 weeks' duration.

Human placental products also are used to speed healing of chronic wounds. The 2 supported by

TABLE 149-6
Cellular and Acellular Matrices[86]

NAMES	ADVANTAGE	FDA APPROVAL
Cellular Matrices:		
Bilayered living cellular construct (Apligraf, Organogenesis, Canton, MA)	Dermal part: Bovine Type I collagen with human neonatal foreskin fibroblasts Epidermal part: keratinocytes	Noninfected partial- and full-thickness venous leg ulcers, >1 month duration Full-thickness diabetic foot ulcers, >3 weeks' duration
Cellular dermal matrix (Dermagraft, Organogenesis, Canton, MA)	Human neonatal foreskin fibroblasts cultured onto a bioresorbable glycolic acid scaffold (polyglactin 910)	Full-thickness diabetic foot ulcers >6 weeks' duration that do not involve tendon, muscle, joint capsule, or bones
Dehydrated human amnion/chorion membrane (DHACM) (Epifix, MiMedx Group Inc., Marietta, GA)	DHACM is composed of a single layer of epithelial cells, a basement membrane, and an avascular connective tissue matrix	DHACM is composed of a single layer of epithelial cells, a basement membrane, and an avascular connective tissue matrix
Cryopreserved placental membrane (Grafix, Osiris Therapeutics, Inc., Columbia, MD)	Human viable wound matrix provides the wound with mesenchymal stem cells, neonatal fibroblasts, epithelial cells, growth factors, and angiogenic factors	Human viable wound matrix provides the wound with mesenchymal stem cells, neonatal fibroblasts, epithelial cells, growth factors, and angiogenic factors
Acellular Matrices:		
Dermal regeneration matrix (Integra Dermal Regeneration Template, Integra, Life Sciences, Plainsboro, NJ)	Composed of a crosslinked bovine tendon collagen and glycosaminoglycan dermal equivalent, and a semipermeable polysiloxane (silicone) epidermal equivalent	FDA-approved device (510[k] for diabetic foot ulcers)
Porcine small intestinal submucosa (Cook Biotech, West Lafayette, Indiana)	Derived from small intestinal submucosa of porcine; 3-dimensional extracellular matrix that acts as a scaffold to allow for cellular migration, formation of granulation tissue, and vascularization of the wound	FDA-approved 510(k)-cleared medical device
Cadaveric allograft (AlloDerm Regenerative Tissue Matrix [RTM], LifeCell, Branchburg, NJ)	Cadaveric human skin that has been processed to remove the epidermis and cells that lead to tissue rejection and graft failure	Regulated by the FDA as human tissue for transplantation
Poly-N-acetyl glucosamine–derived membrane (Talymed, Marine Polymer Technologies Inc., Danvers, MA)	Composed of poly-N-acetyl glucosamine shortened fibers that are derived from microalgae	FDA approved—510(k)

evidence (albeit less robust) include dehydrated human amnion/chorion membrane (Epifix, MiMedx, Marietta, GA) and cryopreserved placental membrane (Grafix, Osiris Therapeutics Inc.). Epifix is composed of a single layer of epithelial cells, a basement membrane, and a connective tissue matrix. Grafix is composed of placental membrane, a source of mesenchymal stem cells, neonatal fibroblasts, epithelial cells, growth factors, and angiogenic cells.[89-92]

ACELLULAR PRODUCTS

Acellular products function as a scaffold for cellular migration, proliferation, and matrix formation. Examples of acellular products include dermal regeneration matrix, porcine small intestinal submucosa, cadaveric allograft, and poly-N-acetyl glucosamine.[86]

INTEGRA Dermal Regeneration Template (Integra LifeSciences Corp.) is a bilayered acellular matrix composed of crosslinked bovine tendon collagen, a glycosaminoglycan dermal equivalent, and a semipermeable polysiloxane epidermal equivalent. It is approved for burns and diabetic foot ulcers. In a recent study on diabetic foot ulcer patients, 51% of patients on Dermal Regeneration Template achieved complete healing, compared to 32% of controls.[93,94] Porcine small intestine submucosa (Oasis, Smith, & Nephew) is a scaffold for cellular migration, granulation tissue formation and neovascularization. The evidence supports the successful use of small intestine submucosa in patients with diabetic foot ulcers and VLUs.[95] Cadaveric allograft is made of cadaveric human skin. It is indicated for tissue repair in abdominal wall and breast reconstruction.[96] Poly-N-acetyl glucosamine (Talymed) is derived from microalgae and has FDA approval for a variety of wounds. Poly-N-acetyl glucosamine has also antibacterial properties.[97]

STEM CELL THERAPY

The use of stem cells in the management of wounds aims to replace the wound resident cells with new cells with the potential to respond to wound healing process signals. Numerous animal studies and a small number of pilot studies in human have shown that bone marrow mesenchymal cells can promote wound healing.[98,99] In 2003, freshly applied autologous bone marrow aspirate and cultured bone marrow cells helped 3 wounds heal.[100,101] In animal models, the use of stem cells is associated with healing and increase in tensile strength. In addition to bone marrow–derived cells, other sources of stem cells, such as fat and hair follicles, may be beneficial.[98]

However, most studies of adult stem cell therapy for human wounds have used cultured bone marrow–derived mesenchymal stem cells.[102] The improvement of wounds with adult stem cells may be a result of either integration of the stem cells or their paracrine effects.[103] Topically applied autologous mesenchymal stem cells accelerate the healing of human and murine wounds.[104] The first randomized, controlled trial reported the use of bone marrow mesenchymal stem cell application via IM and subcutaneous injection to chronic nonhealing wounds with success compared to standard care.[105]

CHRONIC WOUNDS AND IMPAIRED HEALING

Acute wounds, such as those created by surgery or by trauma, have a predictable time-frame for healing and generally heal quite readily when not interrupted. Impaired healing in chronic wounds may be a consequence of many factors.

Some chronic wounds are the result of ischemia, pressure, and infection or a combination, thereof.[26] There is still considerable controversy whether hyperglycemia itself plays a pathophysiologic role in the development of ulcers in patients with diabetes mellitus, although neutrophil function is impaired in this setting, and the propensity to infection is enhanced in the diabetic state.[26] Importantly, the notion of "small vessel disease" in diabetes mellitus has not been shown to be an obstructive phenomenon. Revascularization of the diabetic foot is now viewed as standard care in the presence of large vessel disease and good run-off circulation.

Perhaps the best example of truly impaired healing, not related to undue pressure and poor arterial supply, is venous ulceration. The underlying abnormality in the development of venous ulcers is the presence of sustained ambulatory venous pressure, also known as *venous hypertension*, which refers to the inability of venous pressure in the leg and feet to decrease in response to exercise.[106] It should also be recognized that the tissue surrounding chronic wounds is not normal and has been altered by the primary pathogenic mechanisms or inability to heal readily. Clinically, the best example of this is the intense fibrosis surrounding venous ulcers, as seen in lipodermatosclerosis.[107,108] Lipodermatosclerosis is a risk factor for ulceration, and venous ulcers surrounded by lipodermatosclerosis are more difficult to heal.[109,110]

Evidence suggests an alteration of the cellular makeup of wounds that do not heal. Fibroblasts derived from venous ulcers are unresponsive to certain selected cytokines and growth factors.[111] For example, venous ulcer fibroblasts are unresponsive to the action of TGF-β_1 and PDGF.[111,112] The lack of response to stimuli such as TGF-β_1 may be because of decreased expression of Type II TGF-β receptors. This receptor abnormality also leads to decreased phosphorylation of key TGF-β signaling proteins, including Smad2, Smad3, and mitogen-activated protein kinases.[113] Cells in diabetic ulcers are altered, such that chronic wounds are said to be "stuck" in a certain phases of the repair process.[114] An association has been reported between some of these cellular alterations and the inability to heal.[115,116]

AGE-RELATED CHANGES IN WOUND HEALING

The population is aging, and older adults are more prone to develop all type of wounds, including VLUs, arterial ulcers, and pressure ulcers. For both acute and chronic wounds, aging is associated with delayed healing. The healing response by ECM changes throughout life.[117] Overexpression of MMPs has been shown in elderly skin.[117] The vasoregulation in aged skin includes fewer progenitor cells, impaired perfusion and changes in temperature regulation. Age-associated aberrations in macrophage function delay vascularization, collagen formation, and remodeling. Mitochondrial dysfunction and lower levels of antioxidants also are associated with aging. Comorbidities and polypharmacy may also factor into delayed healing in the elderly population.[118-120]

BASIC STANDARDS OF WOUND CARE

Reversing or treating the underlying cause of impaired healing is the focus of wound care treatment. Treatment relies in part on wound etiology. A thorough history and examination, along with adjunctive diagnostic tests, such as wound biopsy, vascular studies, imaging, tissue culture, and laboratory analysis may help with diagnosis.[121,122] The most common lower extremity ulcers are venous, diabetic, and arterial ulcers. Chronic wounds are common. VLUs have a 2% prevalence in developed countries, and diabetic foot ulcers occur in 1 in 4 patients with diabetes mellitus over their lifetime.[17,123,124]

Using VLUs as an example, the fundamental of treatment is compression therapy with adjunctive medical and surgical therapies.[109,110,125,126] With regard to medical therapy, pentoxifylline has been tested in several large randomized trials for its ability to accelerate the healing of venous ulcers. The results have varied, and it may be that a high dose of pentoxifylline, 800 mg 3 times a day, is more effective than 400 mg 3 times a day.[127] Whether the use of pentoxifylline should be considered standard therapy for venous ulcers is unclear at the moment. The anabolic steroid stanozolol has been effective in diminishing the induration of lipodermatosclerosis, and in the acute and painful phase of lipodermatosclerosis, when compression bandages and stockings are too painful to use.[128] Danazol may be a useful substitute for stanozolol if it is not available. Recent studies show an effect of statins in the healing of VLUs (and possibly diabetic foot ulcers).[129,130] The only known medical approach for decreasing recurrence of venous ulcers seems to be graded elastic stockings, with a pressure at the ankle in the range of 40 mm Hg along. Surgical therapy is an adjunct, if indicated. Stockings should be considered a lifelong therapy to help prevent ulcer recurrence and the other manifestations of venous disease.

PREDICTING WOUND CLOSURE

Several recent studies now allow the prediction of whether a wound will heal in a timely fashion from simple observation in the first 3 to 4 weeks of therapy. The methods used to predict wound closure range from simple measurements of wound size (width and length) and change in wound area, to computerized planimetric analysis and assessment of migration of the wound edge.[131] In a study of 56,488 wounds, it was shown that a percent change of approximately 30% at 4 weeks could predict wound closure with a sensitivity of 0.67, a specificity of 0.69, and had a positive and negative predictive value of 0.80 and 0.52, respectively.[132] In practical terms, the appearance of the wound edge is important. Steep edges imply no progress of the wound, while the edges of healing wounds become less steep and begin to migrate toward the center. The implications of the ability to predict closure are very important. By 4 weeks, the clinician should be able to determine whether the current therapy should be continued or whether a change is required, including a complete reassessment of the clinical situation. The prognostic value of the healing rate by 4 weeks of therapy has been confirmed.[132,133]

CONCLUSIONS

Wound healing is a complex process of overlapping phases of inflammation, proliferation and remodeling. The burden of wounds on millions of people is globally underappreciated. There are still challenges, in terms of improving the fundamentals of care in limited-resource countries, as well as research gaps in smart biologic dressings, bioengineered skin, and stem cell therapy. We need continued and increased understanding of the science involved. It is also possible that lessons learned from failure to heal, as in chronic wounds, will provide valuable lessons for the general principles of surgical and acute wound healing.

REFERENCES

1. Enoch S, Leaper DJ. Basic science of wound healing. *Surgery (Oxford)*. 2008;26:31-37.
2. Li J, Chen J, Kirsner R. Pathophysiology of acute wound healing. *Clin Dermatol*. 2007;25:9-18.
3. Kirsner RS, Eaglstein WH. The wound healing process. *Dermatol Clin*. 1993;11:629-640.
4. Nosbaum A, Prevel N, Truong HA, et al. Cutting edge: regulatory T cells facilitate cutaneous wound healing. *J Immunol*. 2016;196(5):2010-2014.
5. Vatankhah N, Jahangiri Y, Landry GJ, et al. Predictive value of neutrophil-to-lymphocyte ratio in diabetic wound healing. *J Vasc Surg*. 2017;65(2):478-483.
6. Xue M, Le NT, Jackson CJ. Targeting matrix metalloproteases to improve cutaneous wound healing. *Expert Opin Ther Targets*. 2006;10:143-155.
7. Werner S, Grose R. Regulation of wound healing by growth factors and cytokines. *Physiol Rev*. 2003;83:835-870.
8. Patel S, Maheshwari A, Chandra A. Biomarkers for wound healing and their evaluation. *J Wound Care*. 2016;25:46-55.
9. Golebiewska EM, Poole AW. Platelet secretion: From haemostasis to wound healing and beyond. *Blood Rev*. 2015;29:153-162.
10. Leaper D. Perfusion, oxygenation and warming. *Int Wound J*. 2007;4(suppl 3):4-8.
11. Ramasastry SS. Acute wounds. *Clin Plast Surg*. 2005;32:195-208.
12. Rothwell SW, Sawyer E, Dorsey J, et al. Wound healing and the immune response in swine treated with a hemostatic bandage composed of salmon thrombin and fibrinogen. *J Mater Sci Mater Med*. 2009;20:2155-2166.
13. Frechette JP, Martineau I, Gagnon G. Platelet-rich plasmas: growth factor content and roles in wound healing. *J Dent Res*. 2005;84:434-439.
14. Martin P, Leibovich SJ. Inflammatory cells during wound repair: the good, the bad and the ugly. *Trends Cell Biol*. 2005;15:599-607.
15. Baum CL, Arpey CJ. Normal cutaneous wound healing: clinical correlation with cellular and molecular events. *Dermatol Surg*. 2005;31:674-686; discussion 686.
16. Pull SL, Doherty JM, Mills JC, et al. Activated macrophages are an adaptive element of the colonic epithelial progenitor niche necessary for regenerative responses to injury. *Proc Natl Acad Sci U S A*. 2005;102:99-104.
17. Snyder RJ, Lantis J, Kirsner RS, et al. Macrophages: a review of their role in wound healing and their therapeutic use. *Wound Repair Regen*. 2016;24:613-629.
18. Pradhan L, Cai X, Wu S, et al. Gene expression of pro-inflammatory cytokines and neuropeptides in diabetic wound healing. *J Surg Res*. 2011;167:336-342.
19. Pradhan L, Nabzdyk C, Andersen ND, et al. Inflammation and neuropeptides: the connection in diabetic wound healing. *Expert Rev Mol Med*. 2009;11:e2.
20. Katz MH, Alvarez AF, Kirsner RS, et al. Human wound fluid from acute wounds stimulates fibroblast

and endothelial cell growth. *J Am Acad Dermatol.* 1991;25:1054-1058.
21. Panuncialman J, Falanga V. The science of wound bed preparation. *Surg Clin North Am.* 2009;89:611-626.
22. Laplante AF, Germain L, Auger FA, Moulin V. Mechanisms of wound reepithelialization: hints from a tissue-engineered reconstructed skin to long-standing questions. *FASEB J.* 2001;15:2377-2389.
23. Chandler LA, Gu DL, Ma C, et al. Matrix-enabled gene transfer for cutaneous wound repair. *Wound Repair Regen.* 2000;8:473-479.
24. Becchetti A, Arcangeli A. Integrins and ion channels in cell migration: implications for neuronal development, wound healing and metastatic spread. *Adv Exp Med Biol.* 2010;674:107-123.
25. Zhou HM, Wang J, Elliott C, et al. Spatiotemporal expression of periostin during skin development and incisional wound healing: lessons for human fibrotic scar formation. *J Cell Commun Signal.* 2010;4:99-107.
26. Falanga V. Wound healing and its impairment in the diabetic foot. *Lancet.* 2005;366:1736-1743.
27. Lokmic Z, Musyoka J, Hewitson TD, et al. Hypoxia and hypoxia signaling in tissue repair and fibrosis. *Int Rev Cell Mol Biol.* 2012;296:139-185.
28. Ghosh AK, Vaughan DE. PAI-1 in tissue fibrosis. *J Cell Physiol.* 2012;227:493-507.
29. Choma DP, Milano V, Pumiglia KM, et al. Integrin alpha3beta1-dependent activation of FAK/Src regulates Rac1-mediated keratinocyte polarization on laminin-5. *J Invest Dermatol.* 2007;127:31-40.
30. Choma DP, Pumiglia K, DiPersio CM. Integrin alpha-3beta1 directs the stabilization of a polarized lamellipodium in epithelial cells through activation of Rac1. *J Cell Sci.* 2004;117:3947-3959.
31. Yan C, Grimm WA, Garner WL, et al. Epithelial to mesenchymal transition in human skin wound healing is induced by tumor necrosis factor-alpha through bone morphogenic protein-2. *Am J Pathol.* 2010;176:2247-2258.
32. Falanga V. Wound bed preparation: future approaches. *Ostomy Wound Manage.* 2003;49:30-33.
33. Schultz GS, Wysocki A. Interactions between extracellular matrix and growth factors in wound healing. *Wound Repair Regen.* 2009;17:153-162.
34. Toy LW. Matrix metalloproteinases: their function in tissue repair. *J Wound Care.* 2005;14:20-22.
35. Philp D, Scheremeta B, Sibliss K, et al. Thymosin beta4 promotes matrix metalloproteinase expression during wound repair. *J Cell Physiol.* 2006;208:195-200.
36. Shephard P, Martin G, Smola-Hess S, et al. Myofibroblast differentiation is induced in keratinocyte-fibroblast co-cultures and is antagonistically regulated by endogenous transforming growth factor-beta and interleukin-1. *Am J Pathol.* 2004;164:2055-2066.
37. Leavitt T, Hu MS, Marshall CD, et al. Scarless wound healing: finding the right cells and signals. *Cell Tissue Res.* 2016;365:483-493.
38. Bao P, Kodra A, Tomic-Canic M, et al. The role of vascular endothelial growth factor in wound healing. *J Surg Res.* 2009;153:347-358.
39. Barrientos S, Stojadinovic O, Golinko MS, et al. Growth factors and cytokines in wound healing. *Wound Repair Regen.* 2008;16:585-601.
40. Tomic-Canic M, Ayello EA, Stojadinovic O, et al. Using gene transcription patterns (bar coding scans) to guide wound debridement and healing. *Adv Skin Wound Care.* 2008;21:487-492; quiz 493-494.
41. Oda K, Matsuoka Y, Funahashi A, et al. A comprehensive pathway map of epidermal growth factor receptor signaling. *Mol Syst Biol.* 2005;1:2005.0010.
42. Yahata Y, Shirakata Y, Tokumaru S, et al. A novel function of angiotensin II in skin wound healing. Induction of fibroblast and keratinocyte migration by angiotensin II via heparin-binding epidermal growth factor (EGF)-like growth factor-mediated EGF receptor transactivation. *J Biol Chem.* 2006;281:13209-13216.
43. Tokumaru S, Sayama K, Shirakata Y, et al. Induction of keratinocyte migration via transactivation of the epidermal growth factor receptor by the antimicrobial peptide LL-37. *J Immunol.* 2005;175:4662-4668.
44. Pullar CE, Baier BS, Kariya Y, et al. Beta4 integrin and epidermal growth factor coordinately regulate electric field-mediated directional migration via Rac1. *Mol Biol Cell.* 2006;17:4925-4935.
45. Bennett SP, Griffiths GD, Schor AM, et al. Growth factors in the treatment of diabetic foot ulcers. *Br J Surg.* 2003;90:133-146.
46. Hashimoto K. Regulation of keratinocyte function by growth factors. *J Dermatol Sci.* 2000;24(suppl 1):S46-S50.
47. White LA, Mitchell TI, Brinckerhoff CE. Transforming growth factor beta inhibitory element in the rabbit matrix metalloproteinase-1 (collagenase-1) gene functions as a repressor of constitutive transcription. *Biochim Biophys Acta.* 2000;1490:259-268.
48. Rolfe KJ, Irvine LM, Grobbelaar AO, et al. Differential gene expression in response to transforming growth factor-beta1 by fetal and postnatal dermal fibroblasts. *Wound Repair Regen.* 2007;15:897-906.
49. Tyrone JW, Marcus JR, Bonomo SR, et al. Transforming growth factor beta3 promotes fascial wound healing in a new animal model. *Arch Surg.* 2000;135:1154-1159.
50. Eppley BL, Woodell JE, Higgins J. Platelet quantification and growth factor analysis from platelet-rich plasma: implications for wound healing. *Plast Reconstr Surg.* 2004;114:1502-1508.
51. Mitra R, Khar A. Suppression of macrophage function in AK-5 tumor transplanted animals: role of TGF-beta1. *Immunol Lett.* 2004;91:189-195.
52. Papakonstantinou E, Aletras AJ, Roth M, et al. Hypoxia modulates the effects of transforming growth factor-beta isoforms on matrix-formation by primary human lung fibroblasts. *Cytokine.* 2003;24:25-35.
53. Zeng G, McCue HM, Mastrangelo L, et al. Endogenous TGF-beta activity is modified during cellular aging: effects on metalloproteinase and TIMP-1 expression. *Exp Cell Res.* 1996;228:271-276.
54. Colwell AS, Phan TT, Kong W, et al. Hypertrophic scar fibroblasts have increased connective tissue growth factor expression after transforming growth factor-beta stimulation. *Plast Reconstr Surg.* 2005;116:1387-1390; discussion 1391-1392.
55. Lin RY, Sullivan KM, Argenta PA, et al. Exogenous transforming growth factor-beta amplifies its own expression and induces scar formation in a model of human fetal skin repair. *Ann Surg.* 1995;222:146-154.
56. Shimizu A, Kato M, Nakao A, et al. Identification of receptors and Smad proteins involved in activin signalling in a human epidermal keratinocyte cell line. *Genes Cells.* 1998;3:125-134.
57. Ceccarelli S, Cardinali G, Aspite N, et al. Cortactin involvement in the keratinocyte growth factor and fibroblast growth factor 10 promotion of migration

58. Sogabe Y, Abe M, Yokoyama Y, et al. Basic fibroblast growth factor stimulates human keratinocyte motility by Rac activation. *Wound Repair Regen.* 2006;14:457-462.
59. Powers CJ, McLeskey SW, Wellstein A. Fibroblast growth factors, their receptors and signaling. *Endocr Relat Cancer.* 2000;7:165-197.
60. Ornitz DM, Xu J, Colvin JS, et al. Receptor specificity of the fibroblast growth factor family. *J Biol Chem.* 1996;271:15292-15297.
61. Niessen FB, Andriessen MP, Schalkwijk J, et al. Keratinocyte-derived growth factors play a role in the formation of hypertrophic scars. *J Pathol.* 2001;194:207-216.
62. Uutela M, Wirzenius M, Paavonen K, et al. PDGF-D induces macrophage recruitment, increased interstitial pressure, and blood vessel maturation during angiogenesis. *Blood.* 2004;104:3198-3204.
63. Edelberg JM, Aird WC, Wu W, et al. PDGF mediates cardiac microvascular communication. *J Clin Invest.* 1998;102:837-843.
64. Margolis DJ, Crombleholme T, Herlyn M, et al. Clinical protocol. Phase I trial to evaluate the safety of H5.020CMV.PDGF-b and limb compression bandage for the treatment of venous leg ulcer: trial A. *Hum Gene Ther.* 2004;15:1003-1019.
65. Margolis DJ, Crombleholme T, Herlyn M. Clinical protocol: phase I trial to evaluate the safety of H5.020CMV.PDGF-B for the treatment of a diabetic insensate foot ulcer. *Wound Repair Regen.* 2000;8:480-493.
66. Saaristo A, Tammela T, Farkkilä A, et al. Vascular endothelial growth factor-C accelerates diabetic wound healing. *Am J Pathol.* 2006;169:1080-1087.
67. Jazwa A, Loboda A, Golda S, et al. Effect of heme and heme oxygenase-1 on vascular endothelial growth factor synthesis and angiogenic potency of human keratinocytes. *Free Radic Biol Med.* 2006;40:1250-1263.
68. Cianfarani F, Zambruno G, Brogelli L, et al. Placenta growth factor in diabetic wound healing: altered expression and therapeutic potential. *Am J Pathol.* 2006;169:1167-1182.
69. Kastenbauer T, Hornlein B, Sokol G, et al. Evaluation of granulocyte-colony stimulating factor (filgrastim) in infected diabetic foot ulcers. *Diabetologia.* 2003;46:27-30.
70. Komine M, Rao LS, Kaneko T, et al. Inflammatory versus proliferative processes in epidermis. Tumor necrosis factor alpha induces K6b keratin synthesis through a transcriptional complex containing NFkappa B and C/EBPbeta. *J Biol Chem.* 2000;275:32077-32088.
71. Finnerty CC, Herndon DN, Przkora R, et al. Cytokine expression profile over time in severely burned pediatric patients. *Shock.* 2006;26:13-19.
72. Wallace HJ, Stacey MC. Levels of tumor necrosis factor-alpha (TNF-alpha) and soluble TNF receptors in chronic venous leg ulcers—correlations to healing status. *J Invest Dermatol.* 1998;110:292-296.
73. Wetzler C, Kampfer H, Stallmeyer B, et al. Large and sustained induction of chemokines during impaired wound healing in the genetically diabetic mouse: prolonged persistence of neutrophils and macrophages during the late phase of repair. *J Invest Dermatol.* 2000;115:245-253.
74. Dipietro LA, Reintjes MG, Low QE, et al. Modulation of macrophage recruitment into wounds by monocyte chemoattractant protein-1. *Wound Repair Regen.* 2001;9:28-33.
75. Schultz GS, Sibbald RG, Falanga V, et al. Wound bed preparation: a systematic approach to wound management. *Wound Repair Regen.* 2003;11(suppl 1):S1-S28.
76. Gethin G, Cowman S, Kolbach DN. Debridement for venous leg ulcers. *Cochrane Database Syst Rev.* 2015;CD008599.
77. Wolcott RD, Rumbaugh KP, James G, et al. Biofilm maturity studies indicate sharp debridement opens a time-dependent therapeutic window. *J Wound Care.* 2010;19:320-328.
78. Woo K, Ayello EA, Sibbald RG. The edge effect: current therapeutic options to advance the wound edge. *Adv Skin Wound Care.* 2007;20:99-117; quiz 118-119.
79. Kirsner RS, Warriner R, Michela M, et al. Advanced biological therapies for diabetic foot ulcers. *Arch Dermatol.* 2010;146:857-862.
80. Veves A, Falanga V, Armstrong DG, et al. Graftskin, a human skin equivalent, is effective in the management of noninfected neuropathic diabetic foot ulcers: a prospective randomized multicenter clinical trial. *Diabetes Care.* 2001;24(2):290-295.
81. Alrubaiy L, Al-Rubaiy KK. Skin substitutes: a brief review of types and clinical applications. *Oman Med J.* 2009;24:4-6.
82. Shimizu R, Kishi K. Skin graft. *Plast Surg Int.* 2012;2012:563493.
83. Kirsner RS, Falanga V, Eaglstein WH. The biology of skin grafts. Skin grafts as pharmacologic agents. *Arch Dermatol.* 1993;129:481-483.
84. Zell D, Hu S, Kirsner RS. A paradigm shift in the mechanisms of graft rejection. *J Invest Dermatol.* 2008;128:1874.
85. Kirsner RS, Falanga V, Kerdel FA, et al. Skin grafts as pharmacological agents: pre-wounding of the donor site. *Br J Dermatol.* 1996;135:292-296.
86. Hughes OB, Rakosi A, Macquhae F, et al. A review of cellular and acellular matrix products: indications, techniques, and outcomes. *Plast Reconstr Surg.* 2016;138:138S-147S.
87. Hu S, Kirsner RS, Falanga V, et al. Evaluation of Apligraf persistence and basement membrane restoration in donor site wounds: a pilot study. *Wound Repair Regen.* 2006;14:427-433.
88. Falanga V, Sabolinski M. A bilayered living skin construct (APLIGRAF) accelerates complete closure of hard-to-heal venous ulcers. *Wound Repair Regen.* 1999;7:201-207.
89. Serena TE, Carter MJ, Le LT, et al. A multicenter, randomized, controlled clinical trial evaluating the use of dehydrated human amnion/chorion membrane allografts and multilayer compression therapy vs. multilayer compression therapy alone in the treatment of venous leg ulcers. *Wound Repair Regen.* 2014;22:688-693.
90. Zelen CM, Gould L, Serena TE, et al. A prospective, randomised, controlled, multi-centre comparative effectiveness study of healing using dehydrated human amnion/chorion membrane allograft, bioengineered skin substitute or standard of care for treatment of chronic lower extremity diabetic ulcers. *Int Wound J.* 2015;12:724-732.
91. Zelen CM, Serena TE, Snyder RJ. A prospective, randomised comparative study of weekly versus biweekly application of dehydrated human amnion/

chorion membrane allograft in the management of diabetic foot ulcers. *Int Wound J.* 2014;11:122-128.
92. Lavery LA, Fulmer J, Shebetka KA, et al. The efficacy and safety of Grafix(®) for the treatment of chronic diabetic foot ulcers: results of a multi-centre, controlled, randomised, blinded, clinical trial. *Int Wound J.* 2014;11:554-560.
93. Yao M, Attalla K, Ren Y, et al. Ease of use, safety, and efficacy of integra bilayer wound matrix in the treatment of diabetic foot ulcers in an outpatient clinical setting: a prospective pilot study. *J Am Podiatr Med Assoc.* 2013;103:274-280.
94. Driver VR, Lavery LA, Reyzelman AM, et al. A clinical trial of Integra Template for diabetic foot ulcer treatment. *Wound Repair Regen.* 2015;23:891-900.
95. Mostow EN, Haraway GD, Dalsing M, et al. Effectiveness of an extracellular matrix graft (OASIS Wound Matrix) in the treatment of chronic leg ulcers: a randomized clinical trial. *J Vasc Surg.* 2005;41: 837-843.
96. Brigido SA. The use of an acellular dermal regenerative tissue matrix in the treatment of lower extremity wounds: a prospective 16-week pilot study. *Int Wound J.* 2006;3:181-187.
97. Kelechi TJ, Mueller M, Hankin CS, et al. A randomized, investigator-blinded, controlled pilot study to evaluate the safety and efficacy of a poly-N-acetyl glucosamine-derived membrane material in patients with venous leg ulcers. *J Am Acad Dermatol.* 2012; 66:e209-e215.
98. Dabiri G, Heiner D, Falanga V. The emerging use of bone marrow-derived mesenchymal stem cells in the treatment of human chronic wounds. *Expert Opin Emerg Drugs.* 2013;18:405-419.
99. Derakhshani A, Raoof M, Dabiri S, et al. Isolation and evaluation of dental pulp stem cells from teeth with advanced periodontal disease. *Arch Iran Med.* 2015;18:211-217.
100. Quesenberry P, Colvin G, Lambert JF, et al. Marrow stem cell potential within a continuum. *Ann N Y Acad Sci.* 2003;996:209-221.
101. Quesenberry PJ, Colvin GA, Abedi M, et al. The marrow stem cell: the continuum. *Bone Marrow Transplant.* 2003;32(suppl 1):S19-S22.
102. Fu X, Sun X. Can hematopoietic stem cells be an alternative source for skin regeneration? *Ageing Res Rev.* 2009;8:244-249.
103. Templin C, Grote K, Schledzewski K, et al. Ex vivo expanded haematopoietic progenitor cells improve dermal wound healing by paracrine mechanisms. *Exp Dermatol.* 2009;18:445-453.
104. Falanga V, Iwamoto S, Chartier M, et al. Autologous bone marrow-derived cultured mesenchymal stem cells delivered in a fibrin spray accelerate healing in murine and human cutaneous wounds. *Tissue Eng.* 2007;13:1299-1312.
105. Dash A, Maiti R, Akantappa Bandakkanavar TK, et al. Intramuscular drotaverine and diclofenac in acute renal colic: a comparative study of analgesic efficacy and safety. *Pain Med.* 2012;13:466-471.
106. Falanga V, Eaglstein WH. The "trap" hypothesis of venous ulceration. *Lancet.* 1993;341:1006-1008.
107. Kirsner RS, Pardes JB, Eaglstein WH, et al. The clinical spectrum of lipodermatosclerosis. *J Am Acad Dermatol.* 1993;28:623-627.
108. Miteva M, Romanelli P, Kirsner RS. Lipodermatosclerosis. *Dermatol Ther.* 2010;23:375-388.
109. Alavi A, Sibbald RG, Phillips TJ, et al. What's new: management of venous leg ulcers: treating venous leg ulcers. *J Am Acad Dermatol.* 2016;74:643-664; quiz 665-666.
110. Alavi A, Sibbald RG, Phillips TJ, et al. What's new: management of venous leg ulcers: approach to venous leg ulcers. *J Am Acad Dermatol.* 2016;74:627-640; quiz 641-642.
111. Kim BC, Kim HT, Park SH, et al. Fibroblasts from chronic wounds show altered TGF-beta-signaling and decreased TGF-beta Type II receptor expression. *J Cell Physiol.* 2003;195:331-336.
112. Agren MS. Matrix metalloproteinases (MMPs) are required for re-epithelialization of cutaneous wounds. *Arch Dermatol Res.* 1999;291:583-590.
113. Pastar I, Stojadinovic O, Krzyzanowska A, et al. Attenuation of the transforming growth factor beta-signaling pathway in chronic venous ulcers. *Mol Med.* 2010;16:92-101.
114. Loots MA, Lamme EN, Zeegelaar J, et al. Differences in cellular infiltrate and extracellular matrix of chronic diabetic and venous ulcers versus acute wounds. *J Invest Dermatol.* 1998;111:850-857.
115. Mendez MV, Stanley A, Park HY, et al. Fibroblasts cultured from venous ulcers display cellular characteristics of senescence. *J Vasc Surg.* 1998;28:876-883.
116. Mendez MV, Stanley A, Phillips T, et al. Fibroblasts cultured from distal lower extremities in patients with venous reflux display cellular characteristics of senescence. *J Vasc Surg.* 1998;28:1040-1050.
117. Gould L, Abadir P, Brem H, et al. Chronic wound repair and healing in older adults: current status and future research. *J Am Geriatr Soc.* 2015;63:427-438.
118. Gurtner GC, Werner S, Barrandon Y, et al. Wound repair and regeneration. *Nature.* 2008;453:314-321.
119. Ashcroft GS, Horan MA, Herrick SE, et al. Age-related differences in the temporal and spatial regulation of matrix metalloproteinases (MMPs) in normal skin and acute cutaneous wounds of healthy humans. *Cell Tissue Res.* 1997;290:581-591.
120. Ashcroft GS, Kielty CM, Horan MA, et al. Age-related changes in the temporal and spatial distributions of fibrillin and elastin mRNAs and proteins in acute cutaneous wounds of healthy humans. *J Pathol.* 1997; 183:80-89.
121. Morton LM, Phillips TJ. Wound healing and treating wounds: differential diagnosis and evaluation of chronic wounds. *J Am Acad Dermatol.* 2016;74: 589-605; quiz 605-606.
122. Powers JG, Higham C, Broussard K, et al. Wound healing and treating wounds: Chronic wound care and management. *J Am Acad Dermatol.* 2016:74:607-625; quiz 625-626.
123. Grey JE, Harding KG, Enoch S. Venous and arterial leg ulcers. *BMJ.* 2006;332:347-350.
124. VanGilder C, Amlung S, Harrison P, et al. Results of the 2008-2009 International Pressure Ulcer Prevalence Survey and a 3-year, acute care, unit-specific analysis. *Ostomy Wound Manage.* 2009;55:39-45.
125. Alavi A, Sibbald RG, Mayer D, et al. Diabetic foot ulcers: part II. Management. *J Am Acad Dermatol.* 2014; 70:21.e21-21.e24; quiz 45-46.
126. Alavi A, Sibbald RG, Mayer D, et al. Diabetic foot ulcers: part I. Pathophysiology and prevention. *J Am Acad Dermatol.* 2014;70:1.e1-1.e18; quiz 19-20.
127. Falanga V, Fujitani RM, Diaz C, et al. Systemic treatment of venous leg ulcers with high doses of pentoxifylline: efficacy in a randomized, placebo-controlled trial. *Wound Repair Regen.*

128. Helfman T, Falanga V. Stanozolol as a novel therapeutic agent in dermatology. *J Am Acad Dermatol.* 1995;33:254-258.
129. Fox JD, Baquerizo-Nole KL, Macquhae F, et al. Comment on Yang et al. Association of statin use and reduced risk of lower-extremity amputation among patients with diabetes: a nationwide population-based cohort observation. *Diabetes Care* 2016;39:e54-e55. Diabetes Care. 2016;39:e159-e160.
130. Yang TL, Lin LY, Huang CC, et al. Association of statin use and reduced risk of lower-extremity amputation among patients with diabetes: a nationwide population-based cohort observation. *Diabetes Care.* 2016;39:e54-55.
131. Tallman P, Muscare E, Carson P, et al. Initial rate of healing predicts complete healing of venous ulcers. *Arch Dermatol.* 1997;133:1231-1234.
132. Gelfand JM, Hoffstad O, Margolis DJ. Surrogate endpoints for the treatment of venous leg ulcers. *J Invest Dermatol.* 2002;119:1420-1425.
133. Cardinal M, Eisenbud DE, Phillips T, et al. Early healing rates and wound area measurements are reliable predictors of later complete wound closure. *Wound Repair Regen.* 2008;16:19-22.

Bacterial Diseases PART 23

第二十三篇 细菌性疾病

Chapter 150 :: Superficial Cutaneous Infections and Pyodermas :: Lloyd S. Miller

第一百五十章

浅部皮肤感染和脓皮病

中文导读

正常人的皮肤在出生后不久就被细菌定植，大量细菌生存于表皮和皮肤附属器（即皮肤微生物组），在一定条件下，这些寄生菌会出现致病性，或一些特殊的细菌可以引起皮肤感染，本章主要讨论浅表皮肤感染和脓皮病。本章共分5节：①葡萄球菌皮肤感染；②链球菌皮肤感染；③窝状角质松解症；④皮肤红癣；⑤毛霉菌病。全面讨论了各种类型细菌感染的皮肤问题，分别就这几大类皮肤感染的流行病学、临床特征、危险因素、病因和发病机制、诊断、鉴别诊断、临床病程和预后、临床管理进行了全面的阐释和讨论。

〔汪 犇〕

Normal human skin is colonized soon after birth by a large number of bacteria that live as commensals on the epidermis and in epidermal appendages (ie, the skin microbiome). For example, coagulase-negative *Staphylococci* (*Staphylococcus epidermidis*) are inoculated during vaginal passage and coryneform bacteria take up residence on neonatal skin shortly after birth. Within weeks after birth, neonatal skin is colonized with many different species of bacteria, fungi and viruses that comprise the human skin microbiome (see Chap. 16).

This chapter discusses superficial cutaneous infections and pyodermas. Pyodermas are infections of the skin that are pyogenic (ie, filled with pus). The majority of the cutaneous pyodermas are caused by *Staphylococcus aureus* or group A *Streptococcus* (GAS) (also known as *Streptococcus pyogenes*). These Gram-positive bacteria cause a broad clinical spectrum of infections ranging from superficial pyodermas to more invasive skin and soft-tissue infections (SSTIs; see Chaps. 151 to 153) depending on the organism, the anatomic location of infections, and on host factors. In addition, this chapter also discusses other common superficial bacterial skin infections, including pitted keratolysis, which is thought to be caused by *Kytococcus sedentarius*, *Dermatophilus congolensis* or other *Corynebacterium* spp., erythrasma, which is caused by *Corynebacterium minutissimum*, and trichobacteriosis, which is caused by *Corynebacterium* spp.

STAPHYLOCOCCAL SKIN INFECTIONS

AT-A-GLANCE

- *Staphylococcus aureus* is the most common cause of superficial purulent skin infections (pyodermas).
- Thirty percent of individuals are continuously colonized with *S. aureus*, and occasional carriage is found in up to 60% of healthy people. This represents a common source and risk factor for infection.
- Contributing factors include immunosuppressive disorders, diabetes mellitus, atopic dermatitis, and preexisting tissue injury.
- Local manifestations include impetigo, ecthyma, folliculitis, and furunculosis.
- Systemic reactions include staphylococcal scalded-skin syndrome, staphylococcal scarlet fever, and staphylococcal toxic shock syndrome.
- Pathology: dense neutrophilic infiltration.
- Treatment: topical, oral, or parenteral antibiotics; change predisposing conditions, if possible. When planning therapy, consider antimicrobial resistance patterns.

Staphylococci are classified into 2 major groups: (a) coagulase-negative *Staphylococci* (*S. epidermidis*) and (b) coagulase-positive *Staphylococci* (*S. aureus*). Whereas *S. epidermidis* is primarily a harmless commensal bacterium found on the surface of human skin, *S. aureus* can be found as both a harmless commensal bacterium as well as an aggressive and deadly pathogen. In 1928, Alexander Fleming found that golden-colored *S. aureus* colonies were seen growing throughout a petri dish, except in one area contaminated by the mold *Penicillium chrysogenum* (also known as *Penicillium notatum*). This led to Fleming's important discovery of penicillin and started the golden age of antibiotics. However, as antibiotic use became widespread so did the development of antibiotic resistance, which has complicated treatment of bacterial infections. These antibiotic-resistant bacteria include the widespread emergence of hospital-acquired and community-acquired methicillin-resistant *S. aureus* (MRSA) strains, as well as antibiotic resistance developing in commensal bacteria such as *S. epidermidis*. As a result, this chapter provides current recommended treatments to cover for antibiotic resistance.

EPIDEMIOLOGY

S. epidermidis is a major commensal bacterium found on the surface of human skin. Individuals carry many transient and resident colonizing strains of *S. epidermidis*, the most common coagulase-negative strain. *S. epidermidis* is a common colonizer of the skin but is capable of causing superficial and invasive infections, particularly on implanted foreign materials such as surgical implants and catheters or in cases of immunosuppression.

Using traditional microbiologic techniques, *S. aureus* is found permanently colonized in the anterior nares in approximately 30% of the population.[1] Carriage is transient in other individuals. Approximately 60% of healthy individuals are intermittent carriers of *S. aureus* at some site in the skin or mucosa.[1] Common sites of colonization typically include moist areas of the skin, such as the inguinal region, axillae, and perirectal skin, as well as the nasal, pharynx, or rectal mucosa.[2] Conditions predisposing to *S. aureus* colonization include atopic dermatitis, diabetes mellitus, renal insufficiency patients on dialysis, intravenous drug use, liver dysfunction, and certain genetic or acquired immunosuppressive disorders, including HIV infection.[3] Colonization by *S. aureus* is found at some body site in up to 37% of patients presenting with purulent community-acquired methicillin-resistant *S. aureus* (CA-MRSA) infections.[2]

S. aureus is the most common cause of primary pyodermas and SSTIs, as well as of secondary infections (superinfections) on disease-altered skin (Table 150-1). In the United States, SSTIs cause approximately 14.2 million outpatient and emergency department visits and nearly 870,000 hospital admissions per year.[4,5] In addition, CA-MRSA is the most frequent cause of SSTIs that present to emergency departments in the United States.[6,7] *S. aureus* pyodermas and SSTIs can invade the bloodstream, producing bacteremia and metastatic infection such as osteomyelitis, acute infective endocarditis, and abscesses in many organs and tissues. Antibiotic resistance has become an emerging problem, especially with MRSA, which causes between 80,000 and 111,000 invasive infections per year in the United States.[8,9] Some strains of *S. aureus* also produce exotoxins, which can cause constellations of cutaneous and systemic symptoms, such as staphylococcal scalded-skin syndrome, staphylococcal scarlet fever, and staphylococcal toxic shock syndrome (see Chap. 152).

Transfer of *S. aureus* bacteria to patients occurs predominantly via contact with skin of other persons or fomites rather than through the air.[10] Any individuals with open staphylococcal infections are high-risk potential carriers and transmitters of infection. Nasal

TABLE 150-1
Infections and Toxin Syndromes Involving the Skin and Soft Tissues Caused By *Staphylococcus aureus*

Sites of Colonization (Carrier State)
- Anterior nares
- Throat
- Axillae, perineum
- Hands
- Involved skin in individuals with atopic dermatitis

Sites of Colonization in Neonates (and Sites of Infection)
- Skin
- Umbilicus
- Circumcision site
- Conjunctivae

Superficial Pyodermas
- Primary pyodermas
  - Skin
    - Impetigo
    - Bullous impetigo
    - Ecthyma
    - Botryomycosis
  - Hair follicles
    - Superficial folliculitis (follicular or Bockhart impetigo)
    - Folliculitis (sycosis barbae)
    - Furuncle (boil)
    - Carbuncle
  - Intertriginous sites
    - Intertrigo
    - Perianal dermatitis
  - Digital infections
    - Paronychia
    - Whitlow or felon
    - Blistering distal dactylitis
  - After skin disruption
    - Trauma (physical, thermal)
    - Foreign body (intravascular catheter, prosthetic device)
- Secondary pyodermas
  - Impetiginization of dermatoses such as atopic dermatitis, herpes simplex (superinfection)
  - Certain primary immunodeficiency disorders (eg, Job's syndrome, chronic granulomatous disease)

Invasive Infections
- Acute lymphangitis, lymphadenitis
- Erysipelas
- Cellulitis
- Abscesses (dermal and subcutaneous)
- Necrotizing fasciitis
- Pyomyositis
- Bacteremia, septicemia

Metastatic Skin Infections Associated With Bacteremia (Often *S. aureus* Acute Infectious Endocarditis)
- Abscesses (superficial and deep)
- Septic vasculitis (pustular purpura)

Purpura Fulminans
- Disseminated intravascular coagulation associated with staphylococcal bacteremia
- Meningococcemia-like syndrome

Staphylococcal Toxin-Associated Syndromes
- Staphylococcal scalded-skin syndrome
- Staphylococcal scarlet fever
- Staphylococcal toxic shock syndrome

---

carriage of *S. aureus* appears to be a major risk factor for postoperative surgical wound infections.[11] Nasal colonization among neonates is associated with *S. aureus* infections in newborns in nurseries and neonatal and pediatric intensive care units.[12] The rate of *S. aureus* bacteremia is also higher in nasal carriers of *S. aureus*.[12] There are particular concerns with increasing rates with antibiotic-resistant *S. aureus* strains such as hospital-acquired MRSA, which has been endemic in hospitals worldwide beginning in the 1960s. Careful handling of patients, strict hand-washing procedures, and isolation of patients with open draining staphylococcal infections are important in the reduction of transmission of *Staphylococci*. In addition, since the late 1990s there has been an epidemic of CA-MRSA strains, such as US300 in the United States, which are causing SSTIs in healthy individuals outside hospital settings and without known risk factors for infection.[13-15]

CLINICAL FEATURES

CUTANEOUS FINDINGS

Impetigo: Two clinical patterns of impetigo are recognized: nonbullous and bullous. Nonbullous accounts for 70% of impetigo cases and can be caused by *S. aureus* (most commonly), or GAS, or both in combination. It is more often seen in children, but can be seen in adults of all ages. Typically, nonbullous impetigo arises on the face (especially around the nares) or extremities after trauma. It starts as erythematous papules that become vesicles and pustules that rupture and lead to honey-colored crusted papules on an erythematous base (Fig. 150-1). In nares carriers of *S. aureus*, nonbullous impetigo often presents with a transient papule or pustule in or around the nares with associated pruritus or soreness (Fig. 150-2), which evolves into the typical honey-colored crusted papules and plaques.

Bullous impetigo is caused by *S. aureus* strains that express certain exfoliative toxins (see section "Etiology and Pathogenesis") that cleave desmoglein 1 in the epidermis, resulting in clusters of thin-roofed bullae, vesicles, and/or pustules. Bullae usually arise on areas of grossly normal skin and can easily rupture, creating crusted and erythematous erosions that may have a residual collarette of scale that represent remnants of the bullae and vesicles. Bullous impetigo occurs most commonly in newborns and older infants, and is characterized by the rapid progression of vesicles to flaccid bullae (Fig. 150-3). Decades ago, extensive bullous impetigo (archaic terms: pemphigus neonatorum or Ritter disease) occurred in epidemics within neonatal nurseries. Bullae usually arise on areas of grossly normal skin. The Nikolsky sign (sheet-like removal of epidermis by shearing pressure) is not present. Bullae initially contain clear yellow fluid that subsequently becomes dark yellow and turbid (Fig. 150-3A), and their margins are sharply demarcated without an erythematous halo. The bullae are superficial and within

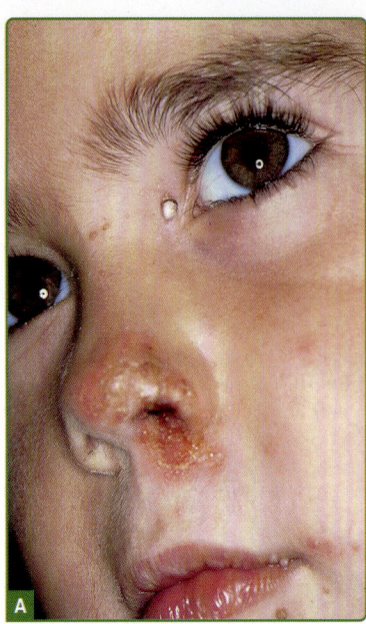
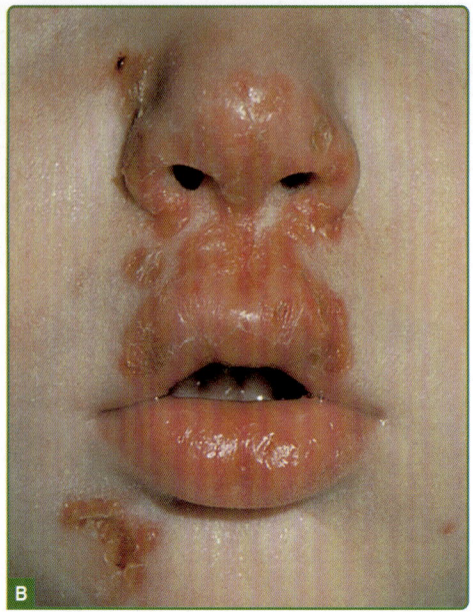

Figure 150-1 *Staphylococcus aureus:* impetigo. Erythema and honey-colored crusting on the nose and upper lip area (**A**), which can spread to involve the entire centrofacial region (**B**).

a day or two they rupture and collapse, forming thin, light-brown to golden-yellow crusts (Fig. 150-3B). So-called *bullous varicella* represents superinfection of varicella lesions by *S. aureus* strains that express exfoliative toxins (bullous impetiginization).

Intact skin is usually resistant to "impetiginization." However, conditions with disrupted epidermal barrier or integrity are predisposed to *S. aureus* impetiginization such as atopic dermatitis, insect bites, epidermal dermatophytoses, herpes simplex, varicella, abrasions, lacerations, and thermal burns. Constitutional symptoms are absent. Regional lymphadenopathy may be present in up to 90% of patients with prolonged, untreated infections. If untreated, the lesions may slowly enlarge and involve new sites over several weeks. In some individuals, lesions resolve spontaneously; in others, the lesions extend into the dermis, forming an ulcer (see "Ecthyma" below).

Ecthyma: Ecthyma can be caused by *S. aureus* and/or GAS and classically evolves from untreated impetigo occluded by footwear and clothing and extends more deeply, penetrating the epidermis and producing "punched-out" ulcers in which dirty grayish-yellow crust and purulent material can be debrided (Fig. 150-4). The margin of the ulcers are indurated, raised, and violaceous, and the granulating base extends deeply into the dermis. There is typically surrounding edema. Untreated ecthymatous lesions enlarge over weeks to months to a diameter of 2 to 3 cm or more, and unlike impetigo, often heal with scarring. Ecthyma occurs most commonly on the lower extremities of children, neglected elderly patients, and individuals with diabetes. Poor hygiene and neglect are key elements in pathogenesis. Ecthymatous lesions can also evolve from a primary pyoderma or within a preexisting dermatosis or site of trauma. Ecthyma should be distinguished from ecthyma gangrenosum, which is a cutaneous ulcer caused by *Pseudomonas aeruginosa* and resembles staphylococcal or streptococcal ecthyma (see Chap. 154).

Folliculitis: Folliculitis is a pyoderma that begins within the hair follicle, and is classified according to the depth of invasion (superficial and deep), and microbial etiology (Table 150-2). Superficial folliculitis also has been termed *follicular* or *Bockhart impetigo*. A small, fragile, dome-shaped pustule occurs at the infundibulum (ostium or opening) of a hair follicle, often on the scalps of children and in the beard area (Fig. 150-5), axillae, extremities, and buttocks of adults. Isolated staphylococcal folliculitis is particularly common on

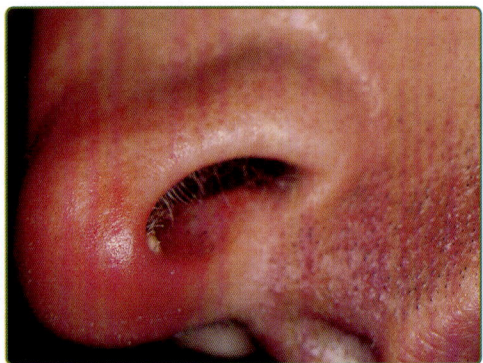

Figure 150-2 *Staphylococcus aureus*: nasal carriage with impetigo. Erythema with a small pustule on the tip of the nose and nares in an individual whose nares are colonized by *S. aureus*.

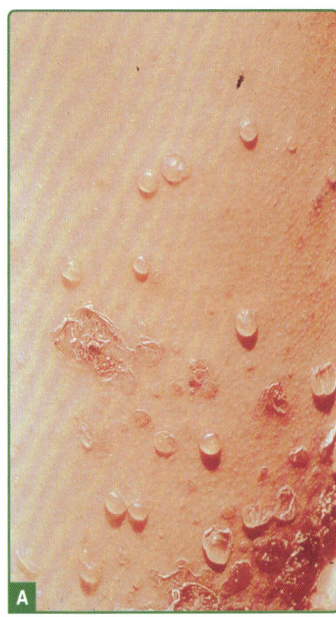
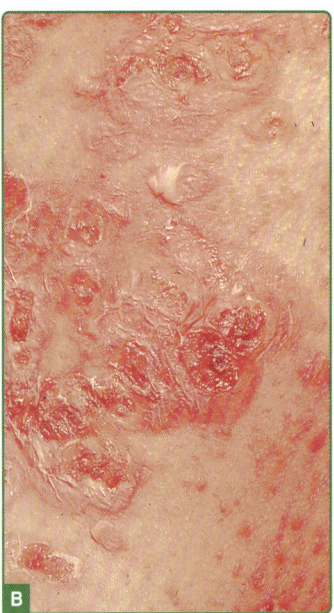

Figure 150-3 *Staphylococcus aureus*: bullous impetigo. Multiple vesicles with clear and turbid contents (**A**) that rapidly coalesce to form flaccid bullae (**B**).

the buttocks of adults. *Periporitis staphylogenes* refers to secondary infection of miliaria of neonates by *S. aureus*. Staphylococcal blepharitis is a *S. aureus* infection of the eyelids, presenting with scaling or crusting of the eyelid margins, often with associated conjunctivitis; the differential diagnosis includes seborrheic dermatitis and rosacea of the eyelid. Sycosis barbae is a deep folliculitis with perifollicular inflammation occurring in the bearded areas of the face and upper lip (Fig. 150-6). If untreated, the lesions may become more deeply seated and chronic. Lupoid sycosis is a deep, chronic form of sycosis barbae associated with scarring, usually occurring as a circinate lesion. A central cicatrix surrounded by pustules and papules gives the appearance of lupus vulgaris (see Chap. 157).

S. aureus folliculitis must be differentiated from other folliculocentric infections. These include 3 noninfectious and inflammatory follicular disorders that are more common in black men: (a) pseudofolliculitis barbae, which occurs on the lower beard area (Fig. 150-7); (b) folliculitis keloidalis or acne keloidalis nuchae, on the nape of the neck; and (c) perifolliculitis capitis, on the scalp. *S. aureus* can cause secondary infection in these inflammatory disorders. Exposure to mineral oils, tar products, and cutting oils can cause an irritant folliculitis. Acne vulgaris, drug-induced

Figure 150-4 *Staphylococcus aureus*: ecthyma. Multiple thickly crusted ulcers on the leg of a patient with diabetes and renal failure. Ecthymatous lesions were also present on the other leg, the arms, and the hands.

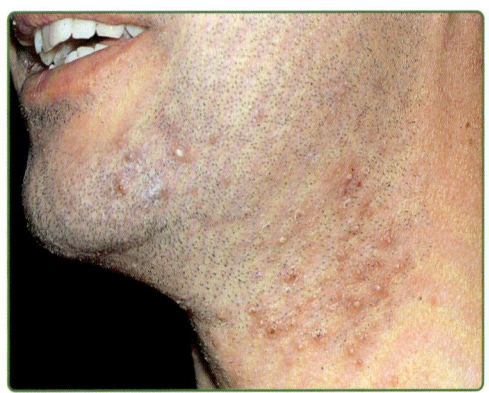

Figure 150-5 *Staphylococcus aureus*: superficial folliculitis. Multiple pustules confined to the beard area.

TABLE 150-2
Classification of Infectious Folliculitis

Bacterial Folliculitis
- *Staphylococcus aureus* folliculitis
  - Periporitis staphylogenes
  - Superficial (follicular or Bockhart impetigo)
  - Deep (eg, sycosis barbae) (may progress to furuncle [boil], carbuncle, or abscess)
- *Pseudomonas aeruginosa* folliculitis ("hot tub" folliculitis)
- Gram-negative folliculitis (often occurring in acne vulgaris patients on the face or back while on antibioitc therapy)
- Syphilitic folliculitis (secondary; acneiform)

Fungal Folliculitis
- Dermatophytic folliculitis
  - Tinea capitis
  - Tinea barbae
  - Majocchi granuloma
- *Malassezia* folliculitis (formerly *Pityrosporum* folliculitis)
- *Candida* folliculitis

Viral Folliculitis
- Herpes simplex virus folliculitis
- Follicular molluscum contagiosum

Infestation
- Follicular molluscum contagiosum
- Demodicidosis

acneiform eruptions, rosacea, hidradenitis suppurativa, acne necrotica of the scalp, and eosinophilic folliculitis of HIV disease must be distinguished from infectious folliculitis as well. Also, "hot tub" folliculitis may be caused by *P. aeruginosa* (see Chap. 154). Dermatophytic folliculitis must be differentiated from *S. aureus* folliculitis. In fungal infections, hairs are usually broken or loosened, and there are suppurative or granulomatous nodules rather than pustules. Also, in dermatophytic folliculitis, plucking of hairs is usually painless (see Chap. 160).

Furuncles: A furuncle or boil is a deep-seated inflammatory nodule that develops around a hair follicle, usually from a preceding, more superficial folliculitis and often evolves into an abscess. A furuncle starts as a hard, tender, red folliculocentric nodule in hair-bearing skin that enlarges and becomes painful and fluctuant after several days (ie, undergoes abscess formation; Fig. 150-8A). Rupture occurs with discharge of pus, and often a core of necrotic material. The pain surrounding the lesion then subsides, and the redness and edema diminish over several days to several weeks. Furuncles may occur as solitary lesions or as multiple lesions in sites such as the buttocks (Fig. 150-8B). Furuncles typically arise in hair-bearing sites, particularly in regions subject to friction, occlusion, and perspiration, such as the neck, face, axillae, and buttocks. They may complicate preexisting lesions such as atopic dermatitis, excoriations, abrasions, scabies, or pediculosis, but occur more often in the absence of any local predisposing causes. In addition, a variety of systemic host factors are associated with furunculosis, including obesity, blood dyscrasias, defects in neutrophil function, and immunosuppression caused by systemic glucocorticoids, chemotherapy, or immunoglobulin deficiency states. The process is often more extensive in patients with diabetes. However, the majority of patients with problems of furunculosis appear to be otherwise healthy.

Carbuncles: A carbuncle is a more extensive, deeper, communicating, infiltrated, and serious inflammatory lesion that develops when suppuration occurs in thick inelastic skin when multiple, closely set furuncles coalesce. A carbuncle characteristically presents as an extremely painful lesion at the nape of the neck, the back, or thighs (Fig. 150-9). Fever and malaise are often present, and the patient may appear quite ill. The involved area is red and indurated, and multiple

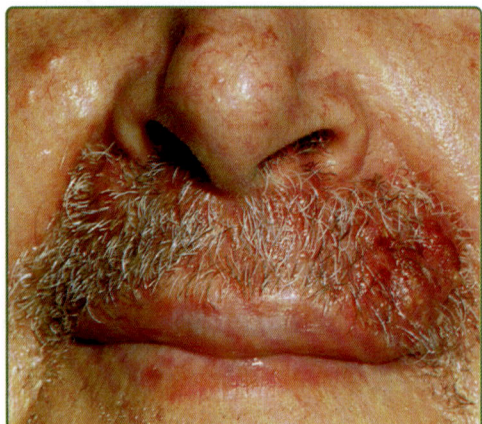

Figure 150-6 Sycosis barbae. Deep staphylococcal folliculitis of the mustache region.

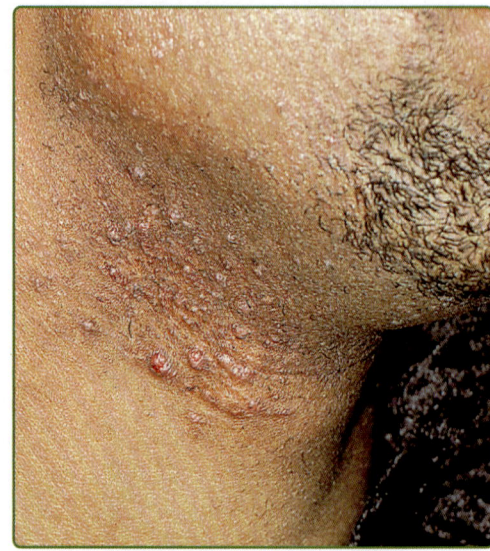

Figure 150-7 Pseudofolliculitis barbae. Multiple papules in the lower beard area caused by ingrowing of the curved hair shaft in a black man who shaves. If pustules are present, secondary *Staphylococcus aureus* infection must be ruled out.

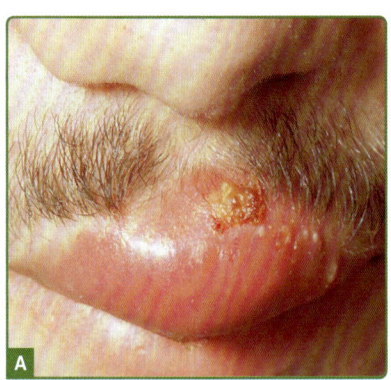

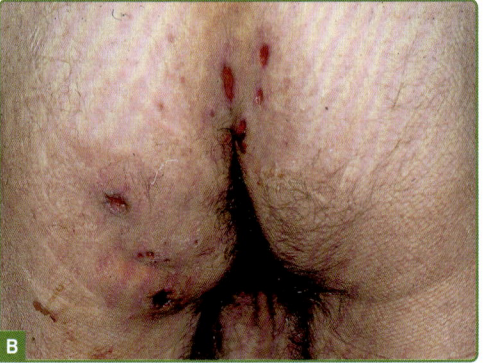

Figure 150-8 **A,** Furuncle of the upper lip. The lesion is nodular, and the central necrotic plug is covered by purulent crust. Several small pustules are seen lateral to the center of the lesion. **B,** Multiple furuncles. Multiple abscesses on the buttocks of long standing in a young man with inflammatory bowel disease. The lesions healed with scarring after a prolonged course of systemic antibiotics.

pustules soon appear on the surface, draining externally around multiple hair follicles. The lesion soon develops a yellow-gray irregular crater at the center, which may then heal slowly by granulating, although the area may remain deeply violaceous for a prolonged period. The resulting permanent scar is often dense and readily evident.

Abscesses: *S. aureus* dermal and subcutaneous abscesses commonly occur in folliculocentric infections—that is, folliculitis, furuncles, and carbuncles as described earlier. Abscesses can also occur at sites of trauma, foreign bodies, burns, or sites of insertion of intravenous catheters. The initial lesion is an erythematous nodule. If untreated, the lesion often enlarges, with the formation of a pus-filled cavity (Fig. 150-10). CA-MRSA should be suspected in all patients with a skin abscess as this is a common presentation for these virulent *S. aureus* strains.[15,16]

Botryomycosis: Botryomycosis is a rare pyogenic disease that presents as a purulent, chronic, subcutaneous infection. Predisposing factors include trauma, immunosuppression (HIV disease, hyperimmunoglobulin E syndrome), chronic alcoholism, and diabetes mellitus. Lesions (usually solitary) can occur in skin, bone, and liver. Cutaneous botryomycosis usually presents as a solitary lesion or a few lesions, often occurring in the genital area. The lesion has the gross appearance of a ruptured epidermal inclusion cyst (an erythematous circumscribed tender nodule), or prurigo nodularis (Fig. 150-11). In the majority of reported cases, a foreign body has played a role in initiating or perpetuating the lesion.

Staphylococcal Paronychia: Individuals exposed to hand trauma or chronic moisture are predisposed to staphylococcal paronychia, as well as to other causes of paronychia (eg, *Candida, Pseudomonas, Streptococcus,* dermatophytes). *S. aureus* is the major infectious cause of acute paronychia, usually around the fingernails, often originating from a break in the skin, such as a hangnail. Clinically, skin and soft tissue of the proximal and lateral nailfold are red, hot, and tender, and can progress to abscess formation if not treated (Fig. 150-12). In contrast, chronic or recurrent paronychia caused by *Candida albicans* is an infection of the space created by separation of the proximal dorsal nail plate

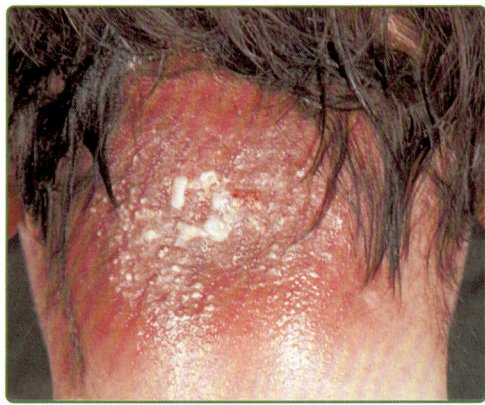

Figure 150-9 Carbuncle. This lesion represents multiple confluent furuncles draining pus from multiple openings.

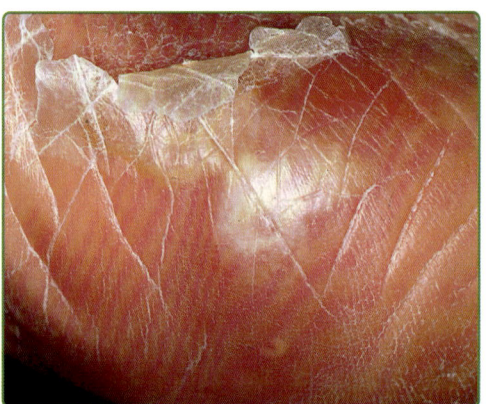

Figure 150-10 *Staphylococcus aureus* abscess. A large painful abscess on the heel of a patient with diabetes improved clinically; however, the severe pain persisted. Radiographs of the heel revealed a broken-off sewing needle. The patient had sensory neuropathy and was unaware of stepping on this foreign body.

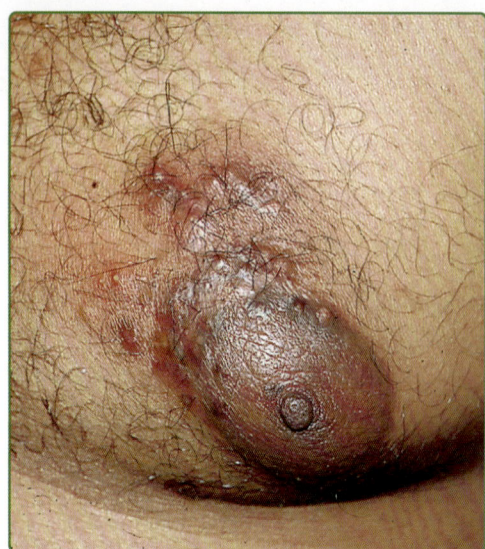

Figure 150-11 *Staphylococcus aureus* botryomycosis. A plaque on the chest had been present for several months in this HIV-infected individual. The diagnosis was confirmed on lesional biopsy findings and culture.

and the undersurface of the proximal nailfold. Candidal paronychia is most common in individuals who have their hands in water for a great deal of time (see Chap. 161).

Staphylococcal Whitlow: A whitlow (or felon) is a purulent infection or abscess involving the bulbous distal end of a finger. The most common causes are *S. aureus* and herpes simplex virus. The portal of entry of *S. aureus* is a traumatic injury or possible extension of an acute paronychia. This infection is usually very painful. An obvious portal of entry is often apparent. The finger bulb is red, hot, tender, and edematous, with possible abscess formation (Fig. 150-13). In contrast, individuals with herpetic whitlows usually have a history of lesions occurring in the same site and present with grouped hemorrhagic vesicles, which may become confluent and form a single bulla (see Chap. 164).

NONCUTANEOUS FINDINGS

In response to more-severe *S. aureus* SSTIs, which typically occur with deep furunculosis and abscesses, there might be signs of a systemic infection (eg, fever, chills, rigors, myalgias, mental status changes, hemodynamic instability) or systemic inflammatory response syndrome, which includes temperature higher than 38°C (100.4°F) or lower than 36°C (96.8°F), tachypnea exceeding 24 breaths per minute, tachycardia exceeding 90 beats per minute, or white blood cell count higher than 12,000 or less than 400 cells/μL.[6,17] These cases require immediate systemic antibiotic therapy (see section "Management").

COMPLICATIONS

If untreated, invasive infection can complicate all of these *S. aureus* skin infections and result in cellulitis, lymphangitis, and bacteremia, which can lead to life-threating *S. aureus* infections in many organs and tissues, including osteomyelitis, septic arthritis, abscesses

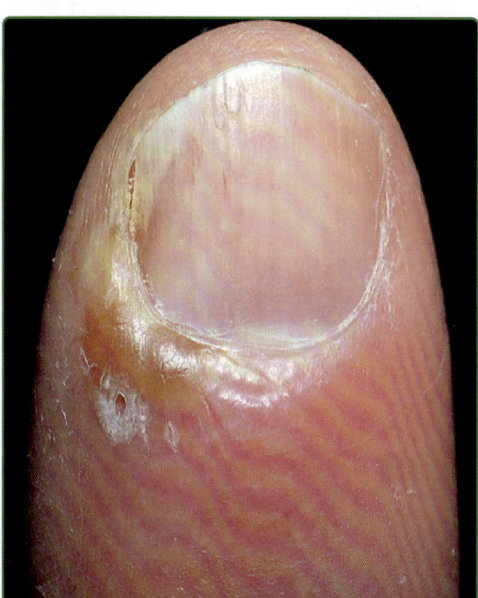

Figure 150-12 *Staphylococcus aureus* paronychia. An abscess is seen in the dorsum of the finger, beginning in a small break in the cuticle. In contrast, *Candida* paronychia is a space infection, occurring in the space created by the separation of the proximal dorsal nail plate and the overlying proximal nailfold.

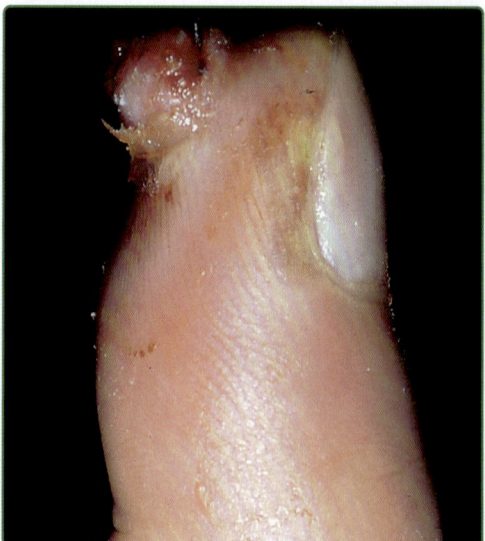

Figure 150-13 *Staphylococcus aureus* whitlow (felon). A pyogenic granuloma arose 1 week after trauma to the bulb of the thumb. A week later, the bulb became swollen, erythematous, and very tender. Abscess formation is seen with loculation of pus. Radiographs showed early osteomyelitis complicating the whitlow.

of various organs (brain, liver, etc), endocarditis, pneumonia, and sepsis. Lesions about the lips and nose raise the specter of spread via the facial and angular emissary veins to the cavernous sinus. Fortunately, these complications are uncommon. However, the risk for invasive infection is higher with deeper infections, such as furuncles, carbuncles, and abscesses, in an unpredictable fashion, and manipulation of such lesions is particularly dangerous and may facilitate spread of the infection via the bloodstream. *S. aureus* exotoxins can result in staphylococcal scalded-skin syndrome, staphylococcal scarlatiniform eruption, toxic shock syndrome, recalcitrant erythematous, desquamating disorders, and recurrent toxin-mediated perineal erythema (see Chap. 152). Staphylococcal scalded-skin syndrome is more likely to occur in infants and in adults who are immunocompromised or have impaired renal function.

ETIOLOGY AND PATHOGENESIS

Risk factors for *S. aureus* SSTIs, include colonization by *S. aureus* in mucosal sites (especially the nares) and on the skin, which may be transient or represent a prolonged carrier state. In addition, patients with preexisting tissue injury or inflammation (surgical wounds, burns, trauma, atopic dermatitis, retained foreign body) all are at higher risk of *S. aureus* SSTIs.[18] Patients with immunodeficiency disorders, such as HIV and AIDS, or who are on systemic corticosteroids are also predisposed to *S. aureus* SSTI. Any condition that results in defective neutrophil number or function, including genetic (eg, chronic granulomatous disease) or acquired (eg, persons with diabetes, cancer patients on chemotherapy) disorders are highly susceptible to *S. aureus* SSTIs as well as to *S. aureus* invasive and systemic infections.[18] Finally, rare patients with genetic or acquired deficiency of interleukin (IL)-17 responses (eg, Job's syndrome) are also susceptible to *S. aureus* SSTIs.[19]

The pathogenesis of *S. aureus* SSTIs involves many different virulence factors that promote colonization and infection and evade host immune detection and function.[1,20-22] For example, *S. aureus* secretes pore-forming toxins that lyse host cells such as neutrophils and macrophages, thereby preventing the host defense function of these cells.[20] There are 2 main families of *S. aureus* pore-forming toxins: (a) single-component α-hemolysin (also known as α-toxin) and (b) biocomponent leukotoxins, including Panton–Valentine leukocidin (PVL or LukSF–PV), γ-hemolysin AB and γ-hemolysin CB (HlgAB and HlgCB), leukocidin ED (LukED) and leukocidin AB (LukAB; also known as LukGH).[20] These toxins have specific host cell targets. For example, α-toxin targets ADAM10, PVL targets C5a receptors, LukAB targets CD11b and LukED targets CCR5, CXCR1, and CXCR2.[20] In particular, α-toxin and PVL are associated with the virulence of *S. aureus*, including CA-MRSA.[1] High serum antibody titers against α-toxin correlate with protection against recurrent *S. aureus* SSTIs.[23] In addition, *S. aureus* secretes phenol-soluble modulins (PSMs), including PSMα$_1$-PSMα$_4$, PSMβ$_1$, PSMβ$_2$, and PSMδ (δ-toxin), which lyse human leukocytes and erythrocytes.[24] PSMα is associated with the enhanced virulence of CA-MRSA.[24]

Certain *S. aureus* strains produce and secrete exfoliative toxins. Bullous impetigo is caused certain types of exfoliative toxins (including types ETA, ETB, and ETD [ETC has no activity in humans]). These exfoliative toxins are serine proteases that target desmoglein 1,[25] the desmosomal cadherin that is also the target of autoantibodies in pemphigus foliaceus (see Chap. 52).[26] ETA and ETB are the most common and are located in *S. aureus* bacteriophages (ie, phage group II) whereas ETD is located in the bacterial chromosome.[25] These exfoliative toxins result in intraepithelial bullae formation in bullous impetigo when the toxin is secreted locally in the skin, and in staphylococcal scalded-skin syndrome when the toxin is present systemically (see Chap. 152).[25]

There are at least 24 different superantigens produced by *S. aureus* that are enterotoxins (also called pyrogenic toxin superantigens), including toxic shock syndrome toxin-1 (TSST-1), enterotoxins (serotypes A, B$_n$, C$_n$, D, E, and G [n refers to multiple variants]), SE-like (SE-1) superantigens (serotypes H, I, J, and K).[21] Superantigens have the ability to nonspecifically activate T cells by interacting with the human leukocyte antigen–DR molecules (major histocompatibility complex II) on antigen-presenting cells and the variable region of the β subunit of the T-cell receptor without antigen present, resulting in nonspecific activation of CD4+ T cells. TSST-1 is the toxin largely responsible for *S. aureus* toxic shock syndrome, which is characterized by high fever, hypotension, scarlet fever–like rash, desquamation of skin, and multiorgan dysfunction. With relevance to *S. aureus* SSTIs, *S. aureus* superantigens (especially SEB) can increase the severity of atopic dermatitis by driving cutaneous inflammation, promoting T-helper type 2 (Th2) responses, and inducing production of immunoglobulin (Ig) E antibodies (some of the IgE is directed against the superantigens themselves).[21]

S. aureus has many different mechanisms to inhibit neutrophil function, therapy increasing virulence and pathogenicity, and these are described in detail elsewhere.[22] However, some examples include *S. aureus* inhibition of neutrophil chemotaxis through production of chemotaxis inhibitory protein of *S. aureus* (CHIPS) or staphopain A (ScpA), which block complement and formyl peptide receptors or CXCR2 neutrophil-attracting chemokines, respectively. *S. aureus* also inhibits neutrophil extravasation from blood vessels via its production of staphylococcal superantigen-like 5 and 11 (SSL5, SSL11) and extracellular adherence protein (Eap), which block P-selectin and intercellular adhesion molecule (ICAM)-1, respectively, to inhibit neutrophil rolling and adhesion to endothelium.[22] *S. aureus* also produces several virulence factors that inhibit neutrophil function, including catalase, alkyl hydroperoxide reductase and staphyloxanthin (the yellow carotenoid pigment responsible for the golden color of *S. aureus* colonies), which all inhibit reactive oxygen-mediated killing. *S. aureus* also produces adenosine synthase A (AdsA) and staphylococcal nuclease (Nuc), which degrade neutrophil extracellular traps (NETs) to prevent NETosis-mediated killing of *S. aureus*.[22] Finally, *S. aureus* expresses protein A on its surface, which binds antibody in the incorrect orientation, which effectively blocks antibody-mediated phagocytosis by neutrophils and macrophages.[22]

IMMUNITY

The skin has innate immune mechanisms that protect against *S. aureus* colonization and infection. These include the constitutive and inducible production of antimicrobial peptides (by keratinocytes and other resident stromal and immune cells in the skin), which have bacteriostatic or bactericidal activity against *S. aureus* (eg, human β-defensins 2 and 3, cathelicidin, and RNase7).[18] In addition, resident and recruited skin and immune cells express pattern recognition receptors that recognize components of *S. aureus* during an infection to initiate inflammatory immune responses, especially neutrophil recruitment and abscess formation, which are required for control of the infection and bacterial clearance.[27] These include Toll-like receptor 2 (TLR2), which recognizes *S. aureus* lipoproteins, lipoteichoic acid and peptidoglycan, and nucleotide-binding oligomerization domain-containing protein 2 (NOD2), which recognizes muramyl dipeptide (a breakdown product of *S. aureus* peptidoglycan). In addition, *S. aureus* activates the inflammasome via its pore-forming toxins and phagosomal rupture, resulting in caspase-1 activation and proteolytic processing of IL-1β into its active and secreted form.[18] IL-1β is a critical cytokine for inducing neutrophil recruitment and abscess formation to a site of *S. aureus* infection in the skin.[18] In addition, IL-17 likely produced by Th17 cells (which is in part induced by IL-1β) also plays a key role in promoting neutrophil recruitment during a *S. aureus* skin infection.[18] Recurrent *S. aureus* skin infections are common, suggesting that the adaptive immune responses, such as antibody responses and T-cell responses, are not entirely capable of preventing all *S. aureus* skin reinfections. This is highlighted by the failure of antibody-based vaccination strategies in clinical trials that target *S. aureus* surface components to facilitate antibody-mediated phagocytosis.[18] However, it is thought that generation of Th17 cells and Th1 cells likely provide some degree of protection against recurrent *S. aureus* skin infections.[18]

DIAGNOSIS

LABORATORY TESTING

For impetigo and ecthyma, the diagnosis is typically made on clinical appearance. However, Gram stain and culture of pus or exudates are generally recommended to diagnose the cause of the infection as *S. aureus* (including MRSA) and/or GAS.[17] For typical and uncomplicated cases of impetigo or ecthyma, empiric therapy can be started without performing these tests. For large furuncles, carbuncles, and abscesses, the diagnosis is also made clinically. However, and culture of pus following incision and drainage or from open draining lesions is strongly recommended.[17] Gram stain will typically reveal Gram-positive cocci in clusters (*S. aureus*) or chains (GAS) or a combination of cocci in clusters and chains when both organisms are involved. Bacterial culture and sensitivity testing will provide important information to direct appropriate antibiotic coverage and to help monitor for potential complications of *S. aureus* (see section "Complications") or GAS infections (see section "Streptococcal Skin Infections - Complications"). In patients with extensive furuncles, carbuncles, or abscesses, body temperature, respiratory rate, and blood counts should be obtained to evaluate for systemic infection or systemic inflammatory response syndrome (see "Noncutaneous Findings" section) as these patients require more aggressive parenteral antibiotic therapy.[17] These extensive infections are most commonly caused by CA-MRSA strains, which often are multidrug resistant strains and the antibiotic susceptibility testing is exceedingly important to determine adequate antibiotic coverage. Blood cultures can also be obtained if there is a suspicion for bacteremia or invasive infection.

PATHOLOGY

In general, skin biopsies are not typically performed in uncomplicated cases of impetigo, ecthyma, folliculitis/furunculosis, carbuncles, or abscesses. However, biopsy or aspiration of extensive furuncles, carbuncles, or abscesses are recommended in immunocompromised patients and in patients with fever and neutropenia for histologic evaluation (including microorganism staining), and microbiology cultures and antibiotic sensitivities to help with the diagnosis and to determine antibiotic susceptibility.[17] Histologic examination of a furuncle shows a dense polymorphonuclear inflammatory process in the dermis and subcutaneous fat. In carbuncles, multiple abscesses that separated by connective-tissue trabeculae are present in the dermis (especially along the edges of the hair follicles) and reach the surface of the skin through openings in the undermined epidermis.

IMAGING

Imaging is not typically indicated except in cases of febrile neutropenic patients with extensive furuncles, carbuncles, or abscesses. Ultrasonography can be used to direct needle aspiration of a furuncle, carbuncle, or abscess for culture and antibiotic susceptibility testing. In addition, radiographic imaging (X-ray, CT, or MRI) can be performed to determine the depth and extent of an infection. This is particularly important if there is a concern for underlying osteomyelitis (eg, in cases of *S. aureus*-infected foot ulcers in diabetic patients) or if there is a suspected indolent pulmonary site of *S. aureus* infection, which can spread to the overlying skin and soft tissues.[17]

DIAGNOSTIC ALGORITHM

Figure 150-14 shows a diagnostic and management algorithm for *S. aureus* and GAS SSTIs.

DIFFERENTIAL DIAGNOSIS

Table 150-3 outlines the differential diagnoses of impetigo, ecthyma, and furunculosis.

CLINICAL COURSE AND PROGNOSIS

Most *S. aureus* superficial skin infections and pyodermas can successfully be treated with appropriate management (see "Management" below). However, there is a high rate of recurrent *S. aureus* skin infections that can continue for many years. This is especially the case with furunculosis and skin abscesses caused by CA-MRSA, which are reported to recur in 30% to 50% of patients.[28-31] If untreated, there is a potential for invasive spread of the infection, resulting in cellulitis, lymphangitis, and bacteremia. From the bloodstream, *S. aureus* can disseminate and cause infections of many organs and tissues such as osteomyelitis, septic arthritis, abscesses of various organs, endocarditis, pneumonia and sepsis.

MANAGEMENT

A major problem in treating staphylococcal infections has been the emergence of antibiotic-resistant strains.[13-15] Hospital-acquired MRSA and CA-MRSA strains are resistance to methicillin, which indicates that these strains are resistant to all β-lactam antibiotics (ie, penicillins and cephalosporins). Many of these strains are also multidrug resistant and have variable resistance to macrolides, fluoroquinolones, tetracyclines, clindamycin, and trimethoprim-sulfamethoxazole (TMP-SMX).[13-15] There is an increasing number of reports of vancomycin intermediate-resistant *S. aureus* strains, which have impacted the effectiveness of vancomycin therapy. However, true vancomycin-resistant *S. aureus* strains are exceeding rare with only several cases reported.

TABLE 150-3
Differential Diagnosis of *Staphylococcus aureus* Pyodermas

Nonbullous Impetigo (*Staphylococcus aureus* or Group A *Streptococcus*)[a]
- Herpes simplex (*always rule out*)
- Herpes zoster/Varicella (*always rule out*)
- Scabies (*always rule out*)
- Seborrheic dermatitis
- Atopic dermatitis
- Allergic contact dermatitis
- Epidermal dermatophyte infections
- Tinea capitis
- Insect bite reaction
- Burns
- Erythema multiforme
- Pemphigus foliaceous
- Cellulitis
- Pediculosis capitis

Bullous Impetigo (*Staphylococcus aureus*)[a]
- Herpes simplex (*always rule out*)
- Herpes zoster/Varicella (*always rule out*)
- Bullous tinea (*always rule out*)
- Bullous fixed-drug eruption (*always rule out*)
- Bullous drug eruption
- Contact dermatitis
- Bullous insect bites
- Staphylococcal scalded skin syndrome
- Thermal burns
- Pemphigus vulgaris
- Bullous pemphigoid
- Erythema multiforme
- Dermatitis herpetiformis

Ecthyma (*Staphylococcus aureus* or Group A *Streptococcus*)
- Ecthyma gangrenosum
- Sporotrichosis
- Nontuberculosis mycobacterial skin infection (eg, *Mycobacterium marinum*)
- Papulonecrotic tuberculids
- Insect bites
- Pyoderma gangrenosum
- Leishmaniasis
- Anthrax
- Orf
- Other causes of ulcers (eg, vasculitis)

Furunculosis (*Staphylococcus aureus*)
- Cystic acne
- Kerion
- Hidradenitis suppurativa
- Ruptured epidermal inclusion cysts
- Furuncular myiasis
- Apical dental abscess
- Osteomyelitis

[a]Any of these disorders may occur primarily and become secondarily impetiginized with *S. aureus* or group A *Streptococcus*.

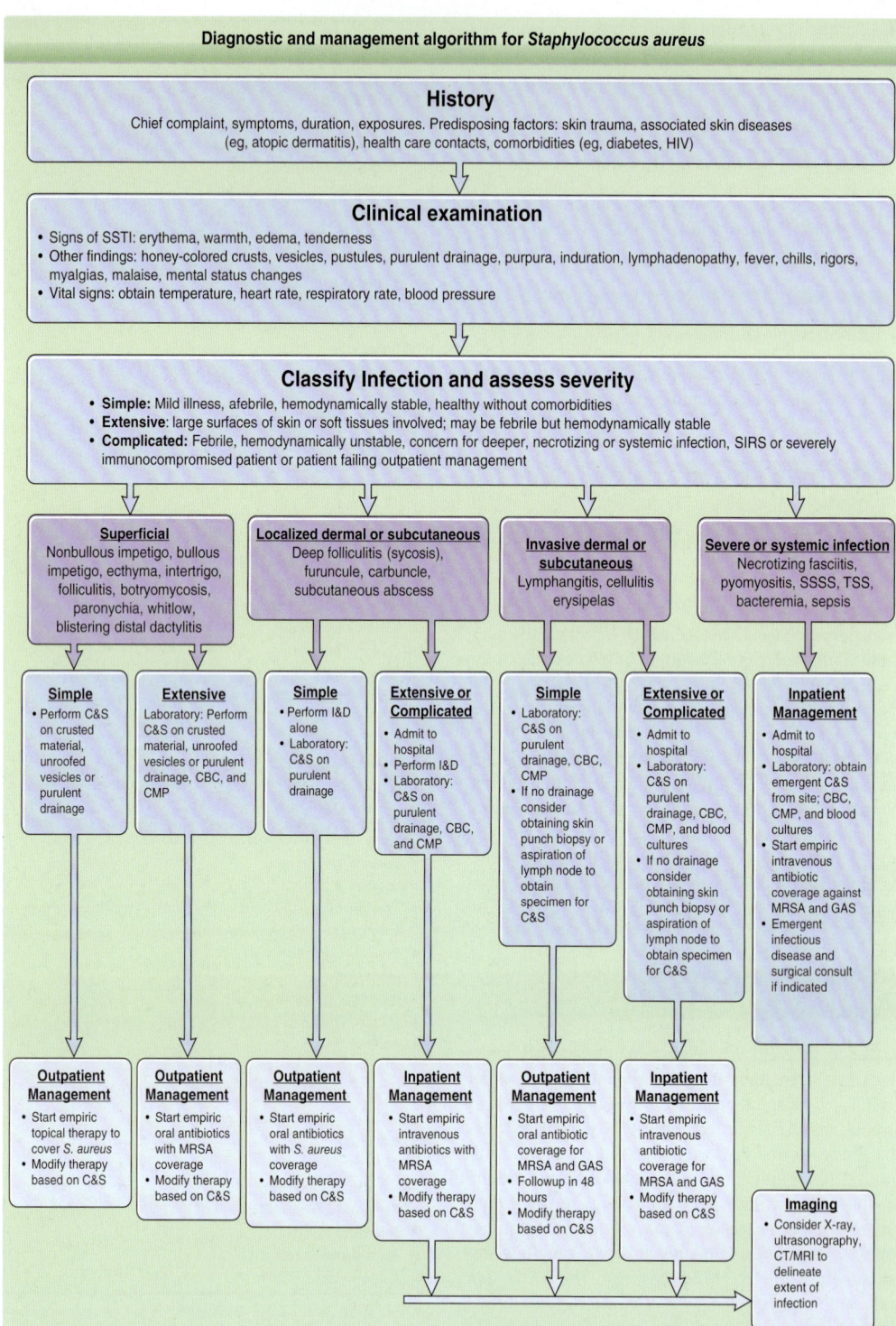

Figure 150-14 Diagnostic and management algorithm for *Staphylococcus aureus* and group A *Streptococcus* (GAS) skin and soft tissue infections (SSTIs). *Abbreviations:* C&S, culture and sensitivity; CBC, complete blood count; CMP, comprehensive metabolic panel; I&D, incision and drainage; MRSA, methicillin-resistant *S. aureus*; SIRS, severe inflammatory response syndrome; SSSS, staphylococcal scalded-skin syndrome; TSS, toxic shock syndrome.

INTERVENTIONS, MEDICATIONS, AND PROCEDURES

Impetigo, Ecthyma, and Folliculitis: Impetigo (nonbullous and bullous) can be treated with oral or topical antimicrobials (Table 150-4). Local topical treatments include mupirocin 2% topical ointment or retapamulin 1% ointment twice daily for 5 to 7 days, along with gentle physical removal of the superficial crusts by cleansing with soap and water.[17] Fusidic acid is an equally effective topical agent for localized impetigo and has few adverse side effects, but it is currently unavailable in the United States. Oral therapy can be used for impetigo and is recommended for ecthyma and uncomplicated folliculitis.[17] Because *S. aureus* isolates from impetigo, ecthyma and folliculitis are more frequently caused by methicillin-sensitive *S. aureus*, dicloxacillin (or similar penicillinase-resistant semisynthetic penicillin) (adults: 250 to 500 mg orally 4 times a day; not typically used in children) or cephalexin (adults: 500 mg orally 4 times a day; children 50 to 100 mg/kg/day divided 3 to 4 times per day) is recommended.[17] In general, oral antibiotic treatment should be continued 7 days (10 days if streptococci are isolated; see below). For patients allergic to penicillin or β-lactams, erythromycin could serve as a substitute (adults: 250 to 500 mg orally 4 times a day; children: 40 mg/kg/day divided 3 to 4 times per day).[17] However, erythromycin-resistant *S. aureus* is common among isolates that cause impetigo in children.[17] Other oral treatment options for *S. aureus* impetigo in children include amoxicillin plus clavulanic acid (25 mg/kg/day given 3 times a day) or clindamycin (15 mg/kg/day 3 or 4 times a day). If CA-MRSA is suspected as the causative organism, doxycycline (adults: 100 mg twice daily; children: not recommended for children younger than age 8 years), clindamycin (adults: 300 to 450 mg 3 to 4 times a day; children: 20 to 40 mg/kg/day in divided doses) or TMP-SMX (1 double-strength tablet twice daily; children: 8 to 12 mg/kg/day [trimethoprim component] divided 2 times per day) are recommended for initial empiric therapy, but the choice of antibiotic might need to be changed based on the clinical response and antibiotic sensitivity results.[17] Of note, tetracyclines (including doxycycline) should not be used in children younger than 8 years old, and a recent study found that clindamycin and TMP-SMX were equally and highly effective for uncomplicated SSTIs in pediatric patients.[30]

Furuncles, Carbuncles, and Abscesses: For simple furuncles, carbuncles, and abscesses, incision and drainage (I&D) alone is often performed and is likely to be adequate but additional antibiotic coverage has a better cure rate (see Table 150-4).[17] Local application of moist heat, which helps promote drainage, can also be helpful. Although I&D can be effective alone without antibiotic therapy, adjunctive antibiotic therapy should be added as described above for impetigo/ecthyma/folliculitis if the patients failed prior treatment with I&D alone, if there is severe or extensive disease with multiple sites of infection, surrounding cellulitis or signs of systemic infection or inflammation (see section "Noncutaneozus Findings") and in patients predisposed to SSTIs such as immunosuppressed patients (eg, HIV/AIDS, diabetic patients, cancer chemotherapy patients, and patients on systemic immunosuppressive agents, and if the patients are very young or very old), and in areas in which I&D is difficult (eg, face, hands, and genitalia).[6,17] The addition of systemic antibiotics does appear to have an added benefit as patients with skin abscesses treated with I&D plus TMP-SMX had a better cure rate than I&D plus placebo.[32] For severe infections or infections in a dangerous area, maximal antibiotic dosage should be employed by the parenteral route. CA-MRSA should be suspected in all serious purulent infections.[6] Vancomycin or other systemic parenteral agents (eg, daptomycin, linezolid, or ceftaroline), which all have anti–CA-MRSA activity, are indicated for these patients.[6] Linezolid is also available as an oral agent and has excellent (100%) bioavailability when given orally or intravenously.[6] Other parenteral agents with activity against MRSA, such as telavancin and quinupristin-dalfopristin, are reserved only for salvage therapy for treatment failures and complicated cases.[6] Of note, with vancomycin intermediate-resistant *S. aureus* strains in which the vancomycin minimal inhibitory concentration is equal to or greater than 2 μg/mL, an alternative to vancomycin should be used such as linezolid or daptomycin.[6] Antibiotic treatment should be continued for at least 7 to 14 days and, in general, antimicrobial therapy should be continued until all evidence of inflammation has regressed. The choice of antibiotic might have to be changed when culture sensitivity results become available. Draining lesions should be covered with dry bandages to prevent auto-inoculation and diligent hand-washing performed.

For recurrent furuncles, carbuncles, and abscesses at the same site of prior infection, a source for other etiologies should be considered, such as hidradenitis suppurativa, a pilonidal cyst, or a foreign body.[17] Children or adults with recurrent abscesses that began in childhood should be evaluated for neutrophil disorders or other primary immunodeficiency syndromes.[17] Treatment of recurrences should be based on antibiotic susceptibility results, typically with a 5- to 10-day course of an oral antibiotic against the causative pathogen, although the duration of the course should be individualized and based on the clinical response.[6,17] Decolonization regimens should be considered in patients who suffer recurrent infections (see "Prevention/Screening" below).

Botryomycosis, Paronychia, and Whitlow: For botryomycosis, local treatment with warm saline compresses to promote drainage and local antibiotics (eg, mupirocin or clindamycin) may be sufficient to control infection. More extensive cases require systemic antibiotic therapy as described above (see Table 150-4). Management of paronychia caused by *S. aureus* includes oral and topical antibiotics, and I&D

TABLE 150-4
Management of *Staphylococcus aureus* Skin Infections

INFECTION	TREATMENT	ADULT DOSING	PEDIATRIC DOSING	DURATION
Impetigo (localized and simple)	Mupirocin 2% ointment	Twice daily	Twice daily	5- to 7-day course
	Retapamulin 1% ointment	Twice daily	Twice daily	
	Fusidic acid 1% cream (not available in U.S.)	2-4 times daily	2-4 times daily	
Impetigo, ecthyma, folliculitis (methicillin-sensitive *S. aureus* [MSSA])	Dicloxacillin	250-500 mg po 4 times daily	Not typically used in children	7-day course recommended, depending on clinical response
	Cephalexin	500 mg po 4 times daily	50-100 mg/kg/day (3-4 divided doses)	
	Erythromycin	200-500 mg po 4 times daily	30-50 mg/kg/day (3-4 divided doses)	
	Amoxicillin/clavulanic acid	875/125 mg po twice daily	25 mg/kg/day (3 divided doses)	
	Clindamycin	300-450 mg po 3-4 times daily	20-30 mg/kg/day (3-4 divided doses)	
Impetigo, ecthyma, folliculitis (methicillin-resistant *S. aureus* [MRSA])	Clindamycin	300-450 mg po 3-4 times daily	20-40 mg/kg/day (3-4 divided doses)	7-day course recommended, depending on clinical response
	Trimethoprim-sulfamethoxazole (TMP-SMX)	1 double-strength (DS) tab twice daily	8-12 mg/kg/day (TMP dose) (divided twice daily)	
	Doxycycline	100 mg po twice daily	Not for children <8 years old	
	Minocycline	200 × 1 + 100 mg po twice daily	Not for children <8 years old	
Furuncles, carbuncles, abscesses (simple)	Incision and drainage (consider oral antibiotics in below row)	Not applicable	Not applicable	
Furuncles, carbuncles, abscesses that are not drainable and are associated with cellulitis	Incision and drainage	Not applicable	Not applicable	7- to 14-day course recommended, depending on clinical response
	Clindamycin	300-450 mg po 3-4 times daily	20-40 mg/kg/day (3-4 divided doses)	
	TMP-SMX	1 double-strength (DS) tab po twice daily	8-12 mg/kg/day (TMP dose) (divided twice daily)	
	Doxycycline	100 mg po twice daily	Not for children <8 years old	
	Minocycline	200 × 1 + 100 mg po twice daily	Not for children <8 years old	
	Linezolid	600 mg po twice daily	10 mg/kg/dose po thrice daily (maximum: 600 mg/dose)	
Complicated MRSA skin and soft-tissue infection (SSTI)	Vancomycin	15-20 mg/kg IV q8-12h	40 mg/kg/day IV (4 divided doses q6h)	7- to 14-day course recommended, depending on clinical response
	Linezolid	600 mg po or IV twice daily	10 mg/kg/dose po or IV thrice daily (maximum: 600 mg/dose)	
	Daptomycin	4 mg/kg IV daily	Not determined	
	Ceftaroline	600 mg IV q12h	8-12 mg/kg/dose IV q8h	
	Clindamycin	600 mg po or IV thrice daily	10-13 mg/kg/dose po or IV q6-8h (maximum: 40 mg/kg/day)	
	Telavancin	10 mg/kg IV daily	Not determined	
	Quinupristin-dalfopristin	7.5 mg/kg IV q8-12h	Not determined	
Nares and skin decolonization	Mupirocin 2% ointment	Twice daily × 5 to 10 days		Can be repeated monthly × 3 months
	Chlorhexidine soap	Daily × 5 to 14 days		
	Bleach baths	Twice weekly × 3 months		
	Rifampin (included *only in combination* with an oral antibiotic regimen above)	300 mg twice daily + other oral antibiotic × 7-14 days		

Information derived from the clinical practice guidelines for the treatment of skin and soft-tissue infections (available at http://www.idsociety.org/uploadedFiles/IDSA/Guidelines-Patient_Care/PDF_Library/Skin%20and%20Soft%20Tissue.pdf) and MRSA infections (available at http://www.idsociety.org/uploadedFiles/IDSA/Guidelines-Patient_Care/PDF_Library/MRSA.pdf) from the Infectious Diseases Society of America (IDSA).[18,19]

O, orally; IV, intravenous; q, every; h, hours.

of abscesses. Management of a staphylococcal whitlow requires I&D of loculated abscess(es) within the tissue and intravenous antibiotic therapy. X-ray (or MRI) imaging of the involved finger is indicated to determine the presence of osteomyelitis. CA-MRSA should be suspected in all cases.

TREATMENT ALGORITHM

Table 150-4 outlines the management of *S. aureus* skin infections.

PREVENTION/SCREENING

All patients with *S. aureus* SSTIs should be educated about preventive measures to prevent autoinoculation and spread of *S. aureus* infections to other close contacts and individuals.[6,17] Draining wounds should be kept clean and covered with clean and dry bandages. Frequent cleansing of hands with soap and water and/or alcohol-based hand gels is especially important after contacting infected skin. Patients should avoid using or sharing personal hygiene items that have come in contact with infected skin, such as disposable razors, linens, and towels. Because fomites in the environment can serve as a reinfection source, surfaces that are frequently touched by bare skin, including door knobs, countertops, bath tubs, and toilet seats, should be routinely and repeatedly cleaned with antimicrobial commercial cleansers and detergents.[6]

In cases of recurrent *S. aureus* SSTIs despite appropriate treatment and the aforementioned personal and environmental hygienic measures, decolonization of the patients can be attempted.[6] Nasal decolonization of *S. aureus* can be achieved with mupirocin ointment administered to the nares twice daily for 5 to 10 days along with body decolonization with either daily chlorhexidine cleansing solution for 5 to 14 days or bleach baths. The nares and body decolonization procedures can be repeated on a monthly basis for 3 months. A typical regimen for bleach baths is 1 teaspoon of bleach per 1 gallon of water or one-quarter cup of bleach per one-quarter bathtub of water (approximately 13 gallons of water) and can be performed for 15 minutes twice weekly for 3 months. If these decolonization measures are ineffective, oral antibiotic treatment according to the treatment regimens above could be used in conjunction with rifampin (typically 300 mg twice daily). Importantly, rifampin can only be used in combination with other systemic antibiotics because rapid antibiotic resistance develops if rifampin is used as a single agent.

In cases in which there is evidence for household or interpersonal transmission, in addition to the personal and environmental hygiene measures described above, symptomatic contacts should be treated and decolonization of asymptomatic household contacts can also be performed according to the above procedures for nasal and body decolonization. Surveillance cultures of nares or body sites following decolonization regimens are typically not necessary in the absence of recurrent infections.

STREPTOCOCCAL SKIN INFECTIONS

AT-A-GLANCE

- Group A *Streptococcus* (ie, *Streptococcus pyogenes*) is a common cause of superficial purulent skin infections (pyodermas). Skin infections are less commonly caused by non-Group A *Streptococcal* spp.
- Group A *Streptococcus* is the leading cause of bacterial pharyngitis and approximately 20% to 30% of individuals recovering from an infection are asymptomatic carriers and can serve as sources of transmission and recurrent infection.
- Local manifestations include impetigo, ecthyma, intertrigo, and blistering distal dactylitis.
- Invasive skin infections, such as erysipelas, cellulitis, and necrotizing fasciitis, can occur.
- Pathology: abundant neutrophilic infiltration.
- Treatment: topical, oral, or parenteral antibiotics; change predisposing conditions. Cover empirically for *S. aureus* (as antibiotic resistance is more common) until etiology is known.

GAS is a Gram-positive extracellular bacterial pathogen that is a common cause of pyogenic skin infections, consistent with its scientific name *Streptococcus pyogenes* from the Latin for "pus-generating." Superficial skin infections caused by GAS include impetigo, ecthyma, intertrigo, and blistering distal dactylitis, and is the most common cause of bacterial pharyngitis (ie, "strep throat") (Table 150-5).[33] Scarlet fever is most commonly associated with GAS pharyngitis and includes a morbilliform rash, strawberry tongue, and desquamation of skin that is caused by streptococcal pyrogenic exotoxins (see Chap. 152).[33] GAS also causes more-invasive SSTIs, such as erysipelas, which is an infection of the superficial layers of the skin and lymphatics, and cellulitis, which is an infection that spreads through deep dermal and subcutaneous tissues (see Chap. 151).[33] GAS can also cause necrotizing fasciitis, which is a deep soft-tissue infection resulting in necrosis of subcutaneous fat and fascia, often leading to sepsis, shock, multiorgan failure, and death (see Chap. 153). Other severe infections caused by GAS include lymphangitis, bacteremia, septic arthritis, osteomyelitis, pneumonia, meningitis, and streptococcal toxic shock syndrome.[33] After a GAS infection, immunologic-mediated diseases such as guttate psoriasis, acute

TABLE 150-5
Infections and Toxin Syndromes Involving the Skin and Soft Tissues Caused By Group A *Streptococcus*

Sites of Colonization (Carrier State)
- Nasopharyngeal mucosa
- Upper airways
- Skin

Superficial Pyodermas
- Nonintertriginous skin
  - Impetigo (nonbullous)
  - Ecthyma
  - Blistering distal dactylitis
- Intertriginous skin
  - Perianal streptococcal cellulitis
  - Streptococcal vulvovaginitis
  - Streptococcal intertrigo

Invasive Infections
- Acute lymphangitis, lymphadenitis
- Erysipelas
- Cellulitis
- Necrotizing fasciitis
- Bacteremia, septicemia

Streptococcal Toxin-Associated Syndromes
- Scarlet fever
- Streptococcal toxic shock syndrome
- Streptococcal gangrene

Nonsuppurative Complications
- Poststreptococcal glomerulonephritis
- Rheumatic fever
- Rheumatic heart disease
- Guttate psoriasis

Other Associated Cutaneous Reactions
- Erythema nodosum
- Erythema multiforme
- Vasculitis

---

rheumatic fever, rheumatic heart disease, and glomerulonephritis may ensue.[33]

Lancefield grouping uses antigenic differences in cell wall carbohydrates and has identified 20 different species of coagulase-negative, β-hemolytic streptococcal species. GAS is classified as group A whereas *Streptococcus agalactiae* and *Enterococcus faecalis* are classified as group B and group D, respectively. GAS isolates can be further classified using serotyping against the M protein, a key virulence factor of GAS infection.[34] With advances in molecular biology, GAS strains are currently classified using sequences of the 5′ variable region of the *emm* gene that codes for the M protein and more than 200 *emm* types have been identified. Although there is substantial temporal and geographic variability of *emm* types, certain *emm* types are associated with various different disease manifestations. For example, impetigo is associated with *emm* types 33, 41, 42, 52, 53, and 70, and necrotizing fasciitis is associated with *emm* types 1, 3, and 28.[34]

EPIDEMIOLOGY

Globally, the World Health Organization estimates that each year there are more than 100 million superficial skin infections caused by GAS and more than 600 million cases of pharyngitis.[33] The major source of GAS transmission is from respiratory droplets from patients with infections or colonization in the upper respiratory tract.[35,36] It is estimated that 15% of school-age children and 4% to 10% of adults in industrialized countries suffer from GAS pharyngitis, which could be more than 5 times higher in developing countries.[35,36] After recovery from GAS pharyngitis, GAS may persist in approximately 20% to 30% of individuals and these asymptomatic carriers can serve as sources for GAS transmission.[35,36] Another source of GAS infection is from patients with GAS skin infections such as impetigo and infected wounds. The major factor in the spread from a carrier or an infected person is the proximity to the individual disseminating the bacteria. Thus, family members or close contacts are at a greater risk of infection than the general population during outbreaks. GAS impetigo predominantly in preschool-age children and is more common in warmer, more humid climates than in temperate zones. Its peak seasonal incidence is in the late summer and early fall. Non–group A streptococci (eg, groups B, C, and G) are less-common causes of impetigo, such as group B streptococci, which can cause impetigo in newborns.

CLINICAL FEATURES

CUTANEOUS FINDINGS

Impetigo: GAS is a common cause of nonbullous impetigo that presents as a crusted superficial infection of the skin with the same clinical appearance as *S. aureus* impetigo (see "Impetigo" above) (see Fig. 150-1). The inflammatory process of impetigo is superficial and begins with a unilocular vesicopustule located between the stratum corneum above and the stratum granulosum below and is usually situated near the opening of a hair follicle. Organisms, as well as leukocytes and cell debris, then fill the vesicopustules, which rapidly evolve into honey-colored crusted papules. Pruritus and burning may occur, but the lesions are usually painless. Preexisting lesions, such as scabies, varicella, or eczema, predispose to superinfection with GAS impetigo. Crowding, poor hygiene, and neglected minor skin trauma contribute to the spread of streptococcal impetigo in families. Minor outbreaks have also occurred among athletes involved in contact sports. Although the majority of cases occur in children of preschool age, older children and adults of all ages can be affected.

Streptococcal Ecthyma: GAS is also a cause of ecthyma that is indistinguishable from *S. aureus* ecthyma (see "Ecthyma" above).

Intertriginous Streptococcal Infections: GAS pyodermas can occur in occluded sites, such as the perineum/perianal region, vulva/vagina, axillae (Fig. 150-15), inframammary region, groin, preputial sac, and web spaces of the feet. Perianal (group A) streptococcal "cellulitis" occurs principally in children, presenting with intense perianal erythema (Fig. 150-16), pain on defecation, blood-streaked stools associated with anal fissures, and chronicity if untreated.[37] It is often confused with psoriasis, candidiasis, seborrheic dermatitis, inflammatory bowel disease, pinworm infection, or a behavioral problem. The infection can also involve the penis and vulva.

Blistering Distal Dactylitis: GAS and *S. aureus* are responsible for the majority of cases of blistering distal dactylitis, also called *bulla repens*, usually occurring in children and adolescents. However, group B *Streptococcus* has reported to rarely cause this infection. A large, tense blister develops, filled with seropurulent fluid, over the volar skin pad of distal fingers or toes (Fig. 150-17). The blisters are often surrounded by an erythematous base. The lesion may be more proximally located on the finger or extend to involve the nailfolds.

Acute Lymphangitis: Acute lymphangitis is an inflammatory process involving the subcutaneous lymphatic channels. It is usually caused by GAS, but occasionally may be caused by *S. aureus* or other organisms, such as *Pasteurella multocida* (eg, from an animal bite) or herpes simplex virus. The portal of entry of the infectious organism is commonly a wound on an extremity, an infected blister, or paronychia. Clinically, acute lymphangitis presents as the rapid onset of red linear streaks, which may be a few millimeters to several centimeters in width, extending from the local portal of entry toward the regional lymph nodes, which

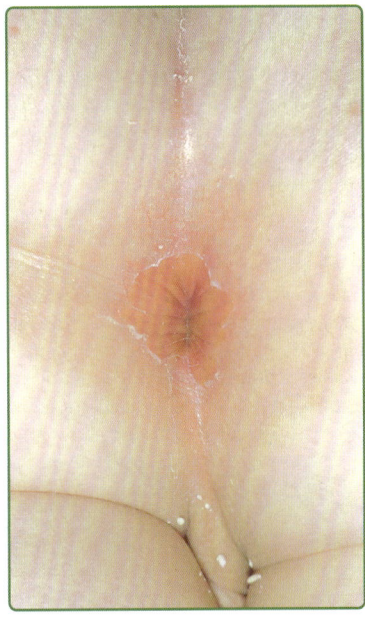

Figure 150-16 Group A streptococcal intertrigo: perianal streptococcal cellulitis. Well-demarcated erosive erythema in the perianal region and perineum in an 8-year-old boy who complained of soreness.

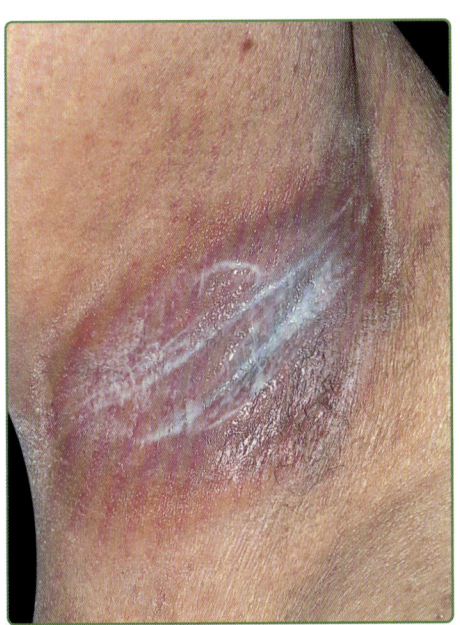

Figure 150-15 Group A streptococcal intertrigo. A sharply marginated erythematous and oozing plaque in the axilla, which was also present in the other axilla, inframammary area, and inguinal folds, was painful in this HIV-infected woman.

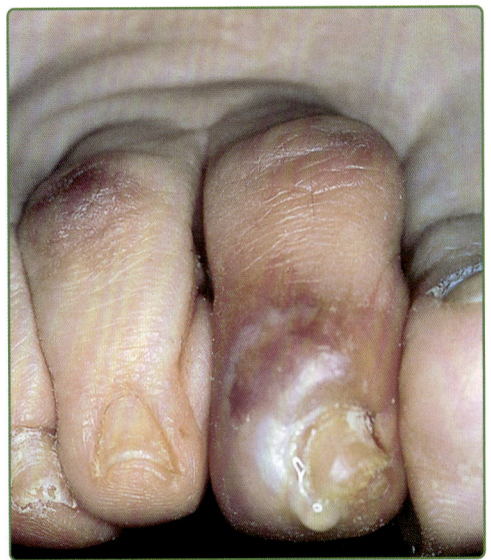

Figure 150-17 Group A streptococcal blistering dactylitis. A blister is seen on a toe adjacent to the nailfold; the patient also had group A streptococcal intertrigo of an abdominal skin fold.

are usually enlarged and tender (Fig. 150-18). Systemic manifestations of infection may occur either before any evidence of infection that is present at the site of inoculation or after the initial lesion has subsided. The patient may notice pain over an area of redness proximal to the original break in the skin. Systemic symptoms are often more prominent than expected from the degree of local pain and erythema. In the upper extremities, acute lymphangitis usually can be differentiated from subacute or chronic sporotrichoid syndrome caused by organisms such as *Sporothrix schenckii*. In the lower extremities, superficial thrombophlebitis may produce somewhat similar linear areas of tender erythema. The absence of a portal of entry and of tender regional adenopathy is helpful in distinguishing superficial thrombophlebitis from acute lymphangitis.

An unusual spread of GAS or *S. aureus* lymphangitis infection of the thumb (paronychia) or of the interdigital webs between the thumb and index finger may occur occasionally. Lymphatic drainage from this area can bypass the lymph nodes at the elbow and drain into the axillary nodes, which, in turn, communicate with the subpectoral nodes and the pleural lymphatics. As a consequence, subpectoral abscesses and pleural effusion can develop. The subpectoral infection may dissect downward and appear over the lower chest and upper abdomen as an area of cellulitis. This is a very serious illness. The clinical clues to the development of this sequence of events are provided by the location of the original infection on the thumb or medial surface of the index finger and the early occurrence of axillary pain.

NONCUTANEOUS FINDINGS

In response to more severe GAS pyodermas, there might be signs and symptoms of systemic infection or inflammation and these are the same as the noncutaneous findings of *S. aureus* pyodermas (see "Clinical Features" above).

COMPLICATIONS

GAS superficial skin infections can become more invasive and result in GAS erysipelas and cellulitis (see Chap. 151) or severe infections such as streptococcal gangrene and necrotizing fasciitis (see Chap. 153). Other associated cutaneous sequelae, include erythema nodosum (see Chap. 73), erythema multiforme–like lesions (which may occur during GAS or *S. aureus* bacteremia in infants and young children) (see Chap. 43), and erythema marginatum (ie, cutaneous lesions of acute rheumatic fever) (see Chap. 152). Scarlet fever and toxic streptococcal syndromes caused by GAS toxins can also occur during and following GAS pharyngitis or skin infections (see Chap. 152). Rarely, during or following GAS pharyngitis or skin infections, patients (especially children and adolescents) can develop acute guttate psoriasis (see Chap. 28).

After GAS pharyngitis or skin infection, endemic and epidemic acute poststreptococcal glomerulonephritis can occur as well as acute rheumatic fever and rheumatic heart disease.[38] Poststreptococcal glomerulonephritis typically occurs 1 to 3 weeks following GAS pharyngitis and 3 to 6 weeks following GAS impetigo.[38] The disease is rare in developed countries (occurring in 0.3 per 100,000 individuals) and is more common in developing countries (occurring in 9.5 to 28.5 per 100,000 individuals). However, the frequency of occurrence of acute poststreptococcal glomerulonephritis from a known GAS nephritogenic strains is 10% to 15% overall and is higher following a GAS skin infection (25%) than following GAS pharyngitis (approximately 5%). Poststreptococcal glomerulonephritis is the most common cause of acute nephritis in children (typically 3 to 12 years old), but can also occur in adults. Clinically, it typically presents with edema, hematuria, and hypertension. Even though this entity usually resolves without specific treatment, renal failure can occur in some cases.[38]

Acute rheumatic fever occurs in less than 1% of patients with a GAS infection, and typically occurs 2 weeks following a GAS pharyngitis infection. In rare instances or certain geographic locations, rheumatic fever has been reported to occur after a GAS skin infection. Diagnosis is made according to Jones criteria, consisting of major manifestations in organs and tissues (joints [arthritis], heart [endocarditis], brain [chorea], skin [erythema marginatum], and subcutaneous tissue [nodules]) as well as minor criteria.[38] Although carditis can occur in up to 60% of cases of acute rheumatic fever (with mitral and aortic valves typically involved), the progression to rheumatic heart disease is poorly understood, but does seem to correlate with the severity of the course of the acute rheumatic

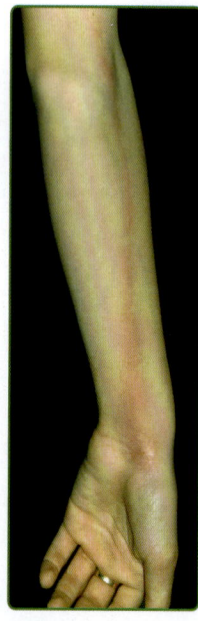

Figure 150-18 Acute lymphangitis of forearm due to *Staphylococcus aureus*. There is a tender linear streak extending proximally from a small area of cellulitis on the volar wrist.

fever and the frequency of recurrences.[38] Rheumatic heart disease has a variable clinical course from asymptomatic valvular disease to heart failure, and has long-term complications of acute infectious endocarditis, thromboembolic disease, atrial fibrillation, and progressive valvular stenosis or incompetence, requiring lifelong medical and surgical management. Sydenham chorea (involuntary, rapid, and purposeless movements of the face or limbs associated with emotional lability) can appear with acute rheumatic fever and up to 6 months after the preceding GAS infection. Finally, it should be mentioned that pediatric autoimmune neuropsychiatric disorders with streptococcal infection (PANDAS) with symptoms of choreoathetosis, obsessive-compulsive disorder, or tic disorder (eg, Tourette syndrome) has been hypothesized to be associated with an antecedent GAS infection.[38]

ETIOLOGY AND PATHOGENESIS

The primary invasive streptococcal pyodermas are almost exclusively a result of GAS, which is usually considerably more invasive than of other streptococci. Nonsuppurative postinfectious complications are limited mostly to those produced by GAS. Risk factors for GAS skin infections include colonization by GAS in the nasopharynx and skin, as well as crowding, poor hygiene, and poverty.[33] Like *S. aureus*, individuals with preexisting tissue injury or inflammation (surgical wounds, burns, trauma, atopic dermatitis, scabies, dermatophyte infection, retained foreign body) all are at higher risk for GAS skin infections.[33] Blunt trauma into muscle is a risk factor for GAS necrotizing fasciitis.[33]

Lancefield classification uses cell wall carbohydrates to distinguish 20 different species of coagulase-negative, β-hemolytic streptococcal species (A to H and K to V).[34] The presence of streptococci of groups other than A in skin lesions may represent either surface colonization or actual secondary infection in preexisting dermatoses. Group C streptococci and group G streptococci occasionally have been implicated in impetiginous lesions, secondarily infected dermatitis, and wound infections with lymphangitis, and even in erysipelas and cellulitis (see Chap. 151). Streptococci of groups B (eg, *S. agalactiae*) and D (eg, *E. faecalis*) have been isolated from infections of skin lesions secondary to ischemia or venous stasis, and have particularly involved the perineal area and operative wound sites. As with most secondary infections, those caused by group B and group D streptococci are frequently mixed infections with enteric bacteria or *S. aureus*. Group B streptococci may cause cellulitis and otitis in neonates and, sometimes, in adults. Group L streptococci (*Streptococcus dysgalactiae*) (often carried by pigs, cattle, and poultry) have been responsible for impetigo, secondarily infected wounds, and paronychias in meat handlers.

As mentioned above, there are more than 200 subtypes of GAS that can be classified by sequencing the 5′ region of the *emm* gene, which codes for the M protein, a fibrillate structure extending from the bacterial cell surface.[34] In addition, chromosomal arrangements of the *emm* gene can also be classified into patterns A to E.[34] Patterns A, B, and C are associated with pharyngitis; pattern D is associated with skin infections; and pattern E is associated with both pharyngitis and skin infections.[34] The M protein is an important virulence factor of GAS and it is a multifunctional protein that can inhibit different host immune defenses.[34] For example, the M protein can bind to regulators of the complement system (including factor H and factor H–like protein 1 and C4-binding protein), which results in decreased activation of the classic and alternative complement pathways, as well as in inhibition of complement (C3b)-mediated phagocytosis.[34] The M protein also interacts with Fc region of IgG, which results in inhibition of antibody-mediated phagocytosis.[34] The M protein can induce inflammation by interacting with TLR2 on human monocytes leading to production of proinflammatory cytokines (eg, IL-6, IL-1β, and tumor necrosis factor–α).[34] Finally, the M protein can facilitate invasion of host cells by binding to components of the extracellular matrix, such as fibronectin, and these complexes can be recognized by integrins expressed on host cells, resulting in host-cell invasion and pathogenicity.[34] Another mechanism by which M protein can facilitate invasion into host cells is through its binding of CD46 on human keratinocytes, which results in invasion of these cells.[34]

Similar to *S. aureus*, GAS also produces pore-forming toxins. Two of the key pore-forming toxins are streptolysin O and streptolysin S.[34] Streptolysin O and streptolysin S contribute to GAS-mediated β-hemolysis on blood agar medium.[34] Streptolysin O produces large pores in host-cell membranes, leading to apoptosis of neutrophils, macrophages, and epithelial cells.[34] Streptolysin S has cytolytic activity against many different host-cell types, including neutrophils, lymphocytes, erythrocytes, and platelets, which leads to defective immune function and increased inflammation that contribute to vascular injury and tissue necrosis.[34]

GAS produces up to 11 known superantigens (also called streptococcal pyrogenic exotoxins). These include streptococcal pyrogenic exotoxin serotypes A, C, and G to M, as well as the streptococcal mitogenic exotoxin SMEZ$_n$.[21] These GAS superantigens nonspecifically activate T cells and contribute to the pathogenesis these infections. In addition, GAS superantigens are also responsible for both streptococcal toxic shock syndrome and manifestations of scarlet fever, and they are thought to contribute to the pathogenesis of erysipelas and more-invasive GAS infections.[21]

Neutrophils are an important cell type in host defense against GAS and *S. aureus* infections. Like *S. aureus*, GAS has several mechanisms to evade neutrophil immune function. For example, GAS produces glutathione peroxidase, superoxide dismutase, alkylhydroperoxidase and alkylhydroperoxidase reductase, which all inhibit reactive oxygen-mediated killing. Furthermore, both the cell wall–anchored nuclease A (SpnA) and the bacteriophage-encoded DNase Sda1 degrade NETs to prevent NETosis-mediated killing of GAS.[33]

IMMUNITY

The innate immune response against GAS, involves antimicrobial peptides and is similar to *S. aureus* (see "Immunity" in section "Etiology and Pathogenesis" of Staphylococcal skin infections). Of note, GAS is susceptible to killing by human β-defensins 1 to 3 and cathelicidin.[33,39] However, in addition to recognition of GAS components by TLR2, NOD2, and the inflammasome, TLR9 appears to play a key role in host defense against GAS skin infections.[33,39] TLR9 is found in endosomal membranes of host cells and recognizes hypomethylated DNA from bacteria, as well as GAS DNA, to elicit a Type I interferon (IFNα/β)-mediated immune response. In addition, TLR9 promotes oxidative burst and clearance of GAS infections.[33,39] Neutrophil recruitment to the site of infection is an important immune response to control GAS (and *S. aureus*) SSTIs, which is in part mediated by the pattern recognition receptors TLR2, NOD2, and TLR9.[33,39] Regarding adaptive immunity against GAS, both antibody and T-cell responses likely contribute to host defense.[33] In particular, antibodies and T-cell responses directed against the M protein of GAS protect against colonization and protection.[40,41] This antibody response is effective against a particular strain expressing the same M protein. However, because there are more than 200 different *emm* types identified among clinical isolates, immunity against a single M protein type does not necessarily confer protection to M proteins comprised of a different amino acid sequence.[40,41] Similarly, an effective human vaccine against M protein and other components or toxins of GAS has been challenging because of the substantial genetic diversity among clinical isolates.[40,41]

DIAGNOSIS

LABORATORY TESTING

As with *S. aureus*, for impetigo and ecthyma caused by GAS, the diagnosis is typically made on clinical appearance. However, Gram stain and bacterial culture and sensitivity of pus or exudates are generally recommended to diagnose the cause of the infection.[17] This is important because GAS requires a longer treatment course and is associated with immunologic-mediated sequelae that need to be monitored. Gram stain will typically reveal Gram-positive cocci in chains (GAS), or clusters (*S. aureus*), or a combination of both in infections involving both pathogens.[17] In patients with extensive infection, concerns for systemic infection, or in cases of acute lymphangitis, body temperature, respiratory rate, and peripheral blood counts should be obtained to evaluate for systemic infection or inflammation (systemic inflammatory response syndrome), as these patients would require more aggressive systemic antibiotic therapy.[17] In cases of acute lymphangitis, cultures from the skin are often negative (because the infection is restricted to lymphatic channels), but a culture from aspirated fluid or from a biopsy of the portal of entry or a suppurative lymph node might reveal the etiologic agent. Blood cultures can also be obtained in all cases of lymphangitis or if there is a suspicion for bacteremia or invasive infection. In patients developing poststreptococcal glomerulonephritis, rheumatic fever, rheumatic heart disease or guttate psoriasis, antistreptolysin O and anti-deoxyribonuclease B antibody titers are helpful to determine whether or not there was an antecedent GAS infection.[42] Of note, high antistreptolysin O titers are more common after GAS pharyngitis, whereas high antideoxyribonuclease B titers are more common following GAS skin infections and at least 1 of the antibodies is typically positive in 95% of cases.[42]

PATHOLOGY

In general, skin biopsies are not typically performed in uncomplicated cases of impetigo, ecthyma, intertriginous infections, blistering distal dactylitis or acute lymphangitis. However, biopsies are recommended in immunocompromised patients or in patients with fever and neutropenia for histologic evaluation (including microorganism staining) and microbiology cultures and antibiotic sensitivities to diagnose the pathogenic organism and to help direct appropriate antibiotic therapy.[17]

IMAGING

Imaging is not typically indicated except in cases of acute lymphangitis in which there is evidence of spread into the axillary nodes, which would raise suspicion of a subpectoral abscesses and pleural effusion, especially if cellulitis is observed over the lower chest and upper abdomen. In these cases, radiographic imaging (ie, chest X-ray or CT imaging) is indicated to determine the extent of chest infection.

DIAGNOSTIC ALGORITHM

Figure 150-14 shows a diagnostic and management algorithm for *S. aureus* and GAS SSTIs.

DIFFERENTIAL DIAGNOSIS

Table 150-3 outlines the differential diagnoses for impetigo and ecthyma. Table 150-6 outlines the differential diagnoses of intertrigo, blistering distal dactylitis, and acute lymphangitis.

TABLE 150-6
Differential Diagnosis of Group A *Streptococcus* Pyodermas

Intertrigo (Group A *Streptococcus* or *Staphylococcus aureus*)
- *Candida* intertrigo
- Contact dermatitis
- Seborrheic dermatitis
- Atopic dermatitis
- Erythrasma
- Inverse psoriasis
- Scabies
- Tinea cruris or tinea corporis
- Familial benign pemphigus (Hailey-Hailey disease)
- Keratosis follicularis (Darier disease)
- Pemphigus vegetans
- Extramammary Paget disease
- Mycosis fungoides
- Acrodermatitis enteropathica
- Langerhans cell histiocytosis

Blistering Distal Dactylitis (Group A *Streptococcus* or *Staphylococcus aureus*)
- Bullous impetigo
- Herpes simplex
- Traumatic/friction blister
- Burn
- Bullous drug eruption
- Bullous cellulitis
- Bullous pemphigoid (localized)
- Insect bite reaction
- Epidermolysis bullosa
- Porphyria cutanea tarda
- Pseudoporphyria

Acute Lymphangitis (Group A *Streptococcus* or *Staphylococcus aureus*)
- Contact dermatitis
- Cellulitis
- Superficial thrombophlebitis
- Sporotrichosis
- *Mycobacterium marinum* infection
- Filariasis
- Leishmaniasis
- *Nocardia* infection
- Myositis

CLINICAL COURSE AND PROGNOSIS

If untreated, GAS impetigo may persist and new lesions may develop over the course of several weeks. Thereafter, the infection tends to resolve spontaneously unless there is some underlying cutaneous disorder such as atopic dermatitis. If untreated, some lesions become chronic and deeper, such as ecthyma. Complicating erysipelas, cellulitis, or bacteremia are unusual. GAS ecthyma, intertrigo, and blistering distal dactylitis usually can be successfully treated with appropriate management (see "Management"). However, GAS may persist in approximately 20% to 30% of individuals and these asymptomatic carriers can serve as common sources for GAS transmission and potential recurrent infection.[35,36] If infections are untreated or neglected, there is a potential for invasive spread of the infection, resulting in erysipelas, cellulitis, lymphangitis, bacteremia, and necrotizing fasciitis. Acute lymphangitis is a serious invasive infection that requires prompt treatment because it can frequently lead to bacteremia with metastatic infection of various organs. Other potential complications of GAS skin infections are discussed above (see "Clinical Features").

MANAGEMENT

INTERVENTIONS, MEDICATIONS, AND PROCEDURES

Topical therapy for GAS impetigo is the same as for *S. aureus* (mupirocin 2% topical ointment or retapamulin 1% ointment twice daily for 5 days with removal of the superficial crusts by cleansing with soap and water).[17] By clinical findings alone, the cause of nonbullous impetigo cannot be accurately distinguished between GAS and *S. aureus*. As most cases of nonbullous impetigo are caused by *S. aureus*, and if the etiology is unknown and systemic therapy is desired, it is reasonable to empirically cover for *S. aureus* using dicloxacillin or cephalexin (described above).[17] However, in contrast to *S. aureus*, the systemic antibiotic treatment of superficial pyodermas (eg, impetigo, ecthyma, and intertrigo) known to be caused by GAS is penicillin and treatment should be continued for 10 days to ensure eradication of the infection (Table 150-7). A 10-day course of oral penicillin V potassium (penicillin VK) can be given to adults (250 to 500 mg 4 times a day) or children (250 to 500 mg 2 to 3 times daily [25 to 45 mg/kg/day divided 2 to 3 times/day]).[17] In young children, a 10-day course amoxicillin-clavulanic acid (250 to 500 mg twice daily [25 to 45 mg/kg/day of the amoxicillin component twice daily]) can be used in place of oral penicillin V. As an alternative, a single dose of long-acting benzathine penicillin G can be given intramuscularly (1,200,000 units for adults or 600,000 units for children). In patients with penicillin or β-lactam hypersensitivity/allergy, a 10-day course of erythromycin can be administered for adults (250 to 500 mg orally 4 times/day) or children (30 to 50 mg/kg/day by mouth in divided doses 4 times/day), which is acceptable given that erythromycin resistance among GAS isolates in most areas of the United States is less than 7%.[33] However, it should be noted that 20% or more of GAS strains are resistant to erythromycin in certain geographic areas (eg, Poland [42%], Hong Kong [28%], Italy [25%], Portugal [24%], and Spain [21%])[33] and other alternatives should be used, such as clindamycin orally for 10 days in adults (300 to 450 mg 3 times a day) or children (20 to 30 mg/kg/day divided 3 to 4 times a day). Blistering distal dactylitis can be treated the same way as GAS pyodermas but I&D is often required to release subungual pus.

For acute GAS lymphangitis, children older than age 3 years or adults without comorbidities that appear nontoxic can be treated with the above antibiotics in an outpatient setting. However, if patients have signs

TABLE 150-7
Management of Skin Infections Caused by Group A *Streptococcus*

INFECTION	TREATMENT	ADULT DOSING	PEDIATRIC DOSING	DURATION
Impetigo (localized and simple)	Mupirocin 2% ointment	Twice daily	Twice daily	5- to 7-day course
	Retapamulin 1% ointment	Twice daily	Twice daily	
	Fusidic acid 1% cream (not available in U.S.)	2-4 times daily	2-4 times daily	
Impetigo, ecthyma (group A *Streptococcus* [GAS])	Penicillin VK	250-500 mg po 4 times daily	25-45 mg/kg/day (2-3 divided doses)	10-day course recommended, depending on clinical response
	Amoxicillin-clavulanic acid	875/125 mg po twice daily	25-45 mg/kg/day (amoxicillin dose) twice daily	
	Benzathine penicillin G	1.2 million units IM × 1 dose	600,000 units IM × 1 dose	
	Cephalexin	500 mg po 4 times daily	50-100 mg/kg/day (3-4 divided doses)	
	Erythromycin	200-500 mg po 4 times daily	30-50 mg/kg/day (3-4 divided doses)	
	Clindamycin	300-450 mg po thrice daily	20-30 mg/kg/day (3-4 divided doses)	
Lymphangitis (GAS)	Penicillin	2-4 million units IV q4-6h	60,000-100,000 units/kg/dose IV q6h	10- to 14-day course recommended, depending on clinical response
	Clindamycin	600-900 mg IV q8h	10-13 mg/kg/dose IV q8h	
	Nafcillin	1-2 g IV q4-6h	50 mg/kg/dose IV q6h	
	Cefazolin	1 g IV q8h	33 mg/kg/dose IV q8h	
	Vancomycin	15-20 mg/kg IV q8-12h	40 mg/kg/day IV (4 divided doses q6h)	
	Linezolid	600 mg po or IV twice daily	10 mg/kg/dose po or IV thrice daily (maximum: 600 mg/dose)	
	Daptomycin	4 mg/kg IV daily	Not determined	
	Telavancin	10 mg/kg IV daily	Not determined	
Recurrent GAS infections	Clindamycin	350-450 mg po thrice daily	20-30 mg/kg/day (3-4 divided doses)	10-day course recommended depending on clinical response
	Amoxicillin-clavulanic acid	875/125 mg po twice daily	25-45 mg/kg/day (amoxicillin dose) twice daily	

Information derived from the "Clinical Practice Guidelines for the Treatment of Skin and Soft-Tissue Infections"[17] (available at http://www.idsociety.org/uploadedFiles/IDSA/Guidelines-Patient_Care/PDF_Library/Skin%20and%20Soft%20Tissue.pdf) and Clinical Practice Guideline for the Diagnosis and Management of Group A Streptococcal Pharyngitis: 2012 Update (available at https://www.idsociety.org/uploadedFiles/IDSA/Guidelines-Patient_Care/PDF_Library/2012%20Strep%20Guideline.pdf) from the Infectious Diseases Society of America (IDSA).[43]

O, orally; IV, intravenous; q, every; h, hours.

of systemic infection (eg, fever, chills, rigors, myalgias, mental status changes, hemodynamic instability) or inflammation (systemic inflammatory response syndrome), they should admitted to the hospital and treated aggressively with intravenous antibiotics as required for complicated erysipelas or cellulitis (see Chap. 151).

TREATMENT ALGORITHM

Table 150-7 outlines the management of skin infections caused by GAS.

PREVENTION/SCREENING

In general, patients hospitalized with GAS infections should be isolated until the organisms have been eradicated by antibiotic treatment. Although the initial treatment antibiotic courses can clear the lesions of GAS pyodermas and prevent recurrence for a short time, GAS can persist on or newly colonize unaffected skin in spite of this therapy. Individuals with a single reoccurrence can be treated with same oral antibiotic therapy as an initial GAS pyoderma (see Table 150-7). However, patients with recurrent episodes of GAS infections can also be treated with a 10-day course of clindamycin (adults: 300 to 450 mg twice daily; children: 20 to 30 mg/kg/day in 3 equally divided doses) or amoxicillin-clavulanic acid (adults: 875/125 mg twice daily; children: 40 mg/kg/day in 3 equally divided doses). Clindamycin or amoxicillin-clavulanic acid also have been used effectively as secondary prophylaxis against recurrent GAS pharyngitis.[43] In addition, prophylactic penicillin (or other appropriate GAS antibiotics) is indicated for close family contacts (particularly children) of patients with recurrent GAS skin or pharyngitis.

There is no evidence to suggest that treatment of GAS pyoderma can prevent subsequent poststreptococcal glomerulonephritis in any individual. However, systemic antibiotics should be used for all GAS infections during outbreaks of poststreptococcal glomerulonephritis to help eliminate nephritogenic strains of GAS from the community.[17]

PITTED KERATOLYSIS

AT-A-GLANCE

- Pitted keratolysis involves the formation of small crateriform pits that coalesce to form a large, discrete defect with serpiginous borders on the plantar surface of the foot.
- More commonly found in young men and is associated with warm moist skin and occlusive shoes.
- The etiologic agent is not entirely clear but many include *Kytococcus sedentarius* (formerly *Micrococcus sedentarius*), *Dermatophilus congolensis*, and *Corynebacterium* spp.
- Treatment typically includes measures and agents to keep the feet dry and decrease hyperhidrosis in combination with topical antibiotics (eg, clindamycin or erythromycin) and keratolytics.

Pitted keratolysis involves the stratum corneum of the web spaces and plantar surface of the feet. Originally named *keratoma plantare sulcatum* by Castellani in 1910, this disease has become more commonly called by its current name after Taplin and Zaias coined it in 1967. The disease was first seen in those who went barefooted during the rainy season.

EPIDEMIOLOGY

Pitted keratolysis occurs in adults and children of both sexes, but adult males with sweaty feet are most susceptible (approximately 90% of cases) with a male-to-female ratio of approximately 8:1.[44] Pitted keratolysis is much more common in tropical climates than in temperate ones.

CLINICAL FEATURES

Pitted keratolysis presents as a superficial erosion of the stratum corneum, composed of numerous small crateriform pits coalescing to form a large discrete defect with serpiginous borders on the plantar surface of the foot. The pits are usually larger than 0.7 mm in diameter, but at times are smaller than 0.5 mm in diameter. The pits have elongated configurations along the plantar furrows and are located predominantly on the pressure-bearing hyperkeratotic areas of the feet, such as the ventral aspect of the toe, ball of the foot, and the heel, but they also are seen on non–pressure-bearing areas.[44] The web spaces between the toes also are commonly involved sites, and may be the only manifestation (Fig. 150-19). The diagnosis is made clinically. Sliminess of the skin, often manifests by the foot sticking to the socks, is also a common complaint (70% of cases). The feet are typically very malodorous (two-thirds of patients) and one-third of patients complain of pain, burning, or irritation.

ETIOLOGY AND PATHOGENESIS

The specific bacterial species that causes pitted keratolysis is not entirely clear. However, *K. sedentarius* (formerly *Micrococcus sedentarius*), *D. congolensis* and *Corynebacterium* spp. have been implicated as the etiologic agents of this disease. It is thought that warm, moist skin as a consequence of protective or occlusive shoes in warmer climates leads to softening of the stratum corneum and a more neutral pH of the surface of this skin, which enhances proteolytic activity of these bacteria to allow them to invade the stratum corneum and produce the characteristic clinical lesions. By electron microscopy, the bacterial organisms can be found inside keratinocytes in the stratum corneum and stratum granulosum.

DIAGNOSIS

The diagnosis is made clinically. However, Gram staining of scrapings may detect the microorganism more readily than potassium hydroxide examination. Bacterial cultures are often not helpful as multiple species of bacteria grow out. A biopsy is usually unnecessary but if one is performed, Gram, periodic acid–Schiff, and methenamine silver stains reveal the bacterial organisms in the walls and bases of the crateriform defects in the upper layer of the stratum corneum. The organisms appear as coccoid forms located more superficially and

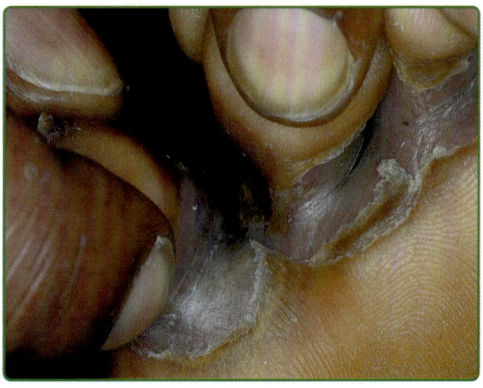

Figure 150-19 Pitted keratolysis. The web spaces between the toes are sharply eroded. Interdigital tinea pedis and erythrasma may occur concurrently.

filamentous forms with branches and septa are seen in deeper locations.[44]

DIFFERENTIAL DIAGNOSIS

Interdigital tinea pedis can present with erosive lesions in the web spaces as is often misdiagnosed in cases of pitted keratolysis. Erythrasma in the web spaces is usually hyperkeratotic but can be erosive.

MANAGEMENT

Prophylactic measures are aimed at keeping the feet as dry as possible and wearing well-fitted and nonocclusive shoes as much as possible.[44] Inert antiseptic foot powders often help. Socks and shoes should also be changed often and socks should be washed at least at 60°C (140°F) to help kill the bacteria.[44] Aluminum chloride 20% solution to decrease hyperhidrosis is often helpful. Similarly, botulinum toxin has been used to decrease hyperhidrosis to help treat pitted keratolysis. A benzoyl peroxide cleanser or 5% gel/cream are effective therapies in most cases as well. Other commonly used topical adjunctive agents include clindamycin and erythromycin solutions, as well as imidazole derivatives (eg, miconazole) and fusidic acid.[44] These topical agents can be combined with keratolytics to decrease the hyperkeratosis and enhance the topical drug penetration into the skin.[44] Systemic use of clindamycin and erythromycin can be attempted in severe cases.[44]

ERYTHRASMA

AT-A-GLANCE

- Erythrasma is a superficial bacterial infection of the skin characterized by well-defined but irregular reddish-brown patches, occurring in the intertriginous areas, or by fissuring and white maceration in the toe clefts.
- It is more common in tropical climates and in patients with obesity, diabetes, or immunosuppression (eg, HIV disease).
- The etiologic agent is *Corynebacterium minutissimum*, which produces coproporphyrin III and a coral red fluorescence that can be seen on Wood's lamp evaluation.
- Treatment typically includes topical clindamycin or erythromycin, and oral antibiotics, such as a 2-week course of oral erythromycin or a single dose of clarithromycin, can be used for widespread involvement or cases not responding to topical therapy.

Erythrasma is a common superficial bacterial infection of the skin characterized by well-defined but irregular reddish-brown patches, occurring in the intertriginous areas, or by fissuring and white maceration in the toe clefts. In the groin, it is commonly misdiagnosed as tinea cruris for many months before proper diagnosis is made.

EPIDEMIOLOGY

C. minutissimum, the etiologic agent of erythrasma, is a short, Gram-positive rod with subterminal granules. The infection is more common in tropical than in temperate climates and in obese and diabetic patients. Generalized erythrasma is much more common in the tropics. Erythrasma is more common in males and may occur in an asymptomatic form in the genitocrural area. In cases involving immunocompromised patients, such as patients with HIV disease, *C. minutissimum* may progress to bacteremia, cellulitis, costochondral abscess, and pyelonephritis.[44]

CLINICAL FEATURES

The most common site of involvement are the web spaces of the feet, where erythrasma presents as a hyperkeratotic white macerated plaque (Fig. 150-20), especially between the fourth and fifth toes. In the genitocrural, axillary, and inframammary regions, the lesions present as well-demarcated, reddish-brown, superficial, finely scaled, and finely wrinkled patches appearing as thin as cigarette paper (Fig. 150-21). In these sites, the patches have a relatively uniform appearance as compared with tinea corporis or cruris, which often have central clearing.

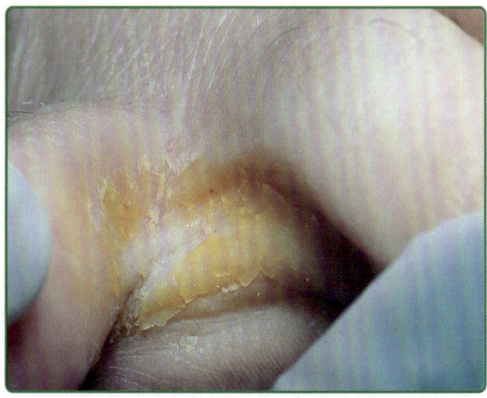

Figure 150-20 Erythrasma. Hyperkeratosis with a yellowish hue in the web space of the foot. The 3 lateral web spaces of both feet were involved. The potassium hydroxide preparation was negative; Wood's lamp examination showed a bright coral red fluorescence.

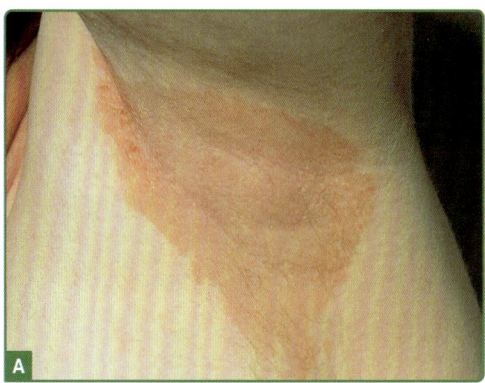

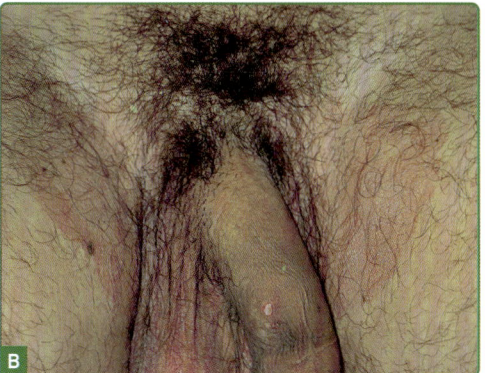

Figure 150-21 Erythrasma. Well-demarcated reddish-brown patches in the axilla (**A**) and groin (**B**). The potassium hydroxide preparations were negative; Wood's lamp examination showed a bright coral red fluorescence.

Concomitant infection can occur with *Candida* or dermatophytes. Wood's lamp examination of erythrasma reveals a coral-red fluorescence caused by coproporphyrin III production by the bacteria. The fluorescence may persist after eradication of the *Corynebacterium* as the pigment remains within a thick stratum corneum. Symptoms vary from a completely asymptomatic form, through a genitocrural form with considerable pruritus, to a generalized form with scaly lamellated plaques on the trunk, inguinal area, and web spaces of the feet. When pruritic, irritation of lesions may cause secondary changes of excoriations and lichenification.

ETIOLOGY AND PATHOGENESIS

Warm and moist skin in areas of skin folds create an environment in which erythrasma can develop.

DIAGNOSIS

Culture of the specific *Corynebacterium* in abundance from the lesion corroborates the diagnosis. Gram-stained imprints of the stratum corneum show rod-like, Gram-positive organisms in large numbers. The bacteria in the stratum corneum can also be seen on skin biopsies stained with periodic acid–Schiff, methenamine silver, or Gram stain. The diagnosis is strongly suggested by the location and superficial character of the process, but can be confirmed by demonstration of the characteristic coral-red fluorescence with Wood's lamp illumination.

DIFFERENTIAL DIAGNOSIS

Tinea versicolor is distinguished from erythrasma by the lesions on the trunk being most numerous at non-intertriginous sites. Tinea cruris tends to have an active scaling border with central clearing. Inverse psoriasis usually presents as sharply demarcated plaques with a shiny red color in the intergluteal cleft, inguinal folds, and axillae.

CLINICAL COURSE AND PROGNOSIS

The disease may remain asymptomatic for years or may undergo periodic exacerbations. Relapses occasionally occur even after successful antibiotic treatment.

MANAGEMENT

For localized erythrasma, especially of the web spaces of the feet, benzoyl peroxide cleanser and 5% gel are effective in most cases.[44,45] Clindamycin or erythromycin (2% solution) or azole creams are several of the many effective topical agents. Fusidic acid has been used outside the United States. For widespread involvement, oral erythromycin 250 mg 4 times a day for 14 days is effective. Alternatives, including clarithromycin 1 g given as a single oral dose, as well as oral tetracycline or chloramphenicol, have been used successfully.[44,45] For secondary prophylaxis, an antibacterial benzoyl peroxide cleanser when showering is effective.

TRICHOBACTERIOSIS

AT-A-GLANCE

- Trichobacteriosis is a bacterial infection of the hair shaft.
- Clinically, it typically affects the axillary or pubic hair and consists of tan, reddish, yellow, or black concretions on the surface of the hair shaft, which represent biofilms of *Corynebacterium* spp.
- Trichobacteriosis is asymptomatic other than its appearance.
- Treatment involves removing the hair by shaving, decreasing hyperhidrosis, and topical benzoyl peroxide, antibiotics, and antiperspirants.

CLINICAL FEATURES

Trichobacteriosis (formerly called *trichomycosis*) is a bacterial infection of the hair shaft (not fungal as its previous name had implied) characterized by what appears to be nodular thickenings on the hair shaft that are composed of colonies of aerobic *Corynebacterium* spp. Trichobacteriosis more commonly occurs in the axillae, but can also occur in the pubic area. The bacteria produce various pigments, giving the nodules a range of colors. The concretions on the hair shaft are usually a tan color but may be reddish, yellow, or black (Fig. 150-22). Lesions are most dense and may be present only in the central portion of the axillary hair. Trichobacteriosis is asymptomatic except for the patient's concern regarding their appearance and because they are malodorous.

ETIOLOGY AND PATHOGENESIS

Although the exact etiology is unclear, disturbances in sweat production and bacterial proliferation are likely needed for trichobacteriosis development. In addition, a warm moist environment and poor hygiene are predisposing factors. The nodules themselves are caused by encapsulated biofilms of corynebacteria adherent to the hair shaft without penetration.

DIAGNOSIS

The diagnosis is usually made on the basis of the clinical findings. The concretions can be visualized using a potassium hydroxide preparation. Wood's lamp can often reveal a pale yellowish fluorescence. Ultraviolet light enhanced visualization represents a newer diagnostic modality and highlights in white the presence of the corynebacteria biofilms on the hair shaft. Pediculosis pubis infestation with multiple eggs on the hair shaft should be considered in the differential diagnosis and ruled out.

MANAGEMENT

The involved hair can be removed by shaving. Benzoyl peroxide cleansers and gels/creams are effective as treatment and prevention against recurrence of trichobacteriosis. Topical clindamycin or erythromycin solutions (and imidazole derivatives) can be used as well. Improved hygiene and cleansing practices and regular use of antiperspirants such as aluminum chloride might reduce recurrences.

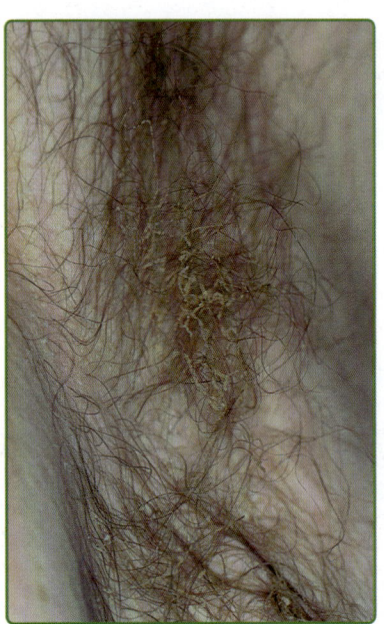

Figure 150-22 Trichobacteriosis. Tan-yellow concretions on the hair shafts of the axilla.

REFERENCES

1. Tong SY, Chen LF, Fowler VG Jr. Colonization, pathogenicity, host susceptibility, and therapeutics for *Staphylococcus aureus*: what is the clinical relevance? *Semin Immunopathol*. 2012;34(2):185-200.
2. Yang ES, Tan J, Eells S, et al. Body site colonization in patients with community-associated methicillin-resistant *Staphylococcus aureus* and other types of *S. aureus* skin infections. *Clin Microbiol Infect*. 2010;16(5): 425-431.
3. Montgomery CP, David MZ, Daum RS. Host factors that contribute to recurrent staphylococcal skin infection.

Curr Opin Infect Dis. 2015;28(3):253-258.
4. Edelsberg J, Taneja C, Zervos M, et al. Trends in US hospital admissions for skin and soft tissue infections. *Emerg Infect Dis*. 2009;15(9):1516-1518.
5. Hersh AL, Chambers HF, Maselli JH, et al. National trends in ambulatory visits and antibiotic prescribing for skin and soft-tissue infections. *Arch Intern Med*. 2008;168(14):1585-1591.
6. Liu C, Bayer A, Cosgrove SE, et al. Clinical practice guidelines by the infectious diseases society of america for the treatment of methicillin-resistant *Staphylococcus aureus* infections in adults and children. *Clin Infect Dis*. 2011;52(3):e18-e55.
7. Moran GJ, Krishnadasan A, Gorwitz RJ, et al. Methicillin-resistant *S. aureus* infections among patients in the emergency department. *N Engl J Med*. 2006;355(7):666-674.
8. Dantes R, Mu Y, Belflower R, et al. National burden of invasive methicillin-resistant Staphylococcus aureus infections, United States, 2011. *JAMA Intern Med*. 2013;173(21):1970-1978.
9. Klevens RM, Morrison MA, Nadle J, et al. Invasive methicillin-resistant *Staphylococcus aureus* infections in the United States. *JAMA*. 2007;298(15):1763-1771.
10. Miller LG, Diep BA. Clinical practice: colonization, fomites, and virulence: rethinking the pathogenesis of community-associated methicillin-resistant *Staphylococcus aureus* infection. *Clin Infect Dis*. 2008;46(5):752-760.
11. Bode LG, Kluytmans JA, Wertheim HF, et al. Preventing surgical-site infections in nasal carriers of *Staphylococcus aureus*. *N Engl J Med*. 2010;362(1):9-17.
12. Zacharioudakis IM, Zervou FN, Ziakas PD, et al. Meta-analysis of methicillin-resistant *Staphylococcus aureus* colonization and risk of infection in dialysis patients. *J Am Soc Nephrol*. 2014;25(9):2131-2141.
13. David MZ, Daum RS. Community-associated methicillin-resistant *Staphylococcus aureus*: epidemiology and clinical consequences of an emerging epidemic. *Clin Microbiol Rev*. 2010;23(3):616-687.
14. DeLeo FR, Otto M, Kreiswirth BN, et al. Community-associated meticillin-resistant *Staphylococcus aureus*. *Lancet*. 2010;375(9725):1557-1568.
15. Elston DM. Community-acquired methicillin-resistant *Staphylococcus aureus*. *J Am Acad Dermatol*. 2007;56(1):1-16; quiz 17-20.
16. Daum RS. Clinical practice. Skin and soft-tissue infections caused by methicillin-resistant *Staphylococcus aureus*. *N Engl J Med*. 2007;357(4):380-390.
17. Stevens DL, Bisno AL, Chambers HF, et al. Practice guidelines for the diagnosis and management of skin and soft tissue infections: 2014 update by the Infectious Diseases Society of America. *Clin Infect Dis*. 2014;59(2):e10-e52.
18. Miller LS, Cho JS. Immunity against *Staphylococcus aureus* cutaneous infections. *Nat Rev Immunol*. 2011;11(8):505-518.
19. Patel DD, Kuchroo VK. Th17 cell pathway in human immunity: lessons from genetics and therapeutic interventions. *Immunity*. 2015;43(6):1040-1051.
20. Alonzo F 3rd, Torres VJ. The bicomponent pore-forming leucocidins of *Staphylococcus aureus*. *Microbiol Mol Biol Rev*. 2014;78(2):199-230.
21. Spaulding AR, Salgado-Pabon W, Kohler PL, et al. Staphylococcal and streptococcal superantigen exotoxins. *Clin Microbiol Rev*. 2013;26(3):422-447.
22. Thammavongsa V, Kim HK, Missiakas D, et al. Staphylococcal manipulation of host immune responses. *Nat Rev Microbiol*. 2015;13(9):529-543.
23. Fritz SA, Tiemann KM, Hogan PG, et al. A serologic correlate of protective immunity against community-onset *Staphylococcus aureus* infection. *Clin Infect Dis*. 2013;56(11):1554-1561.
24. Peschel A, Otto M. Phenol-soluble modulins and staphylococcal infection. *Nat Rev Microbiol*. 2013;11(10):667-673.
25. Bukowski M, Wladyka B, Dubin G. Exfoliative toxins of *Staphylococcus aureus*. *Toxins (Basel)*. 2010;2(5):1148-1165.
26. Amagai M, Matsuyoshi N, Wang ZH, et al. Toxin in bullous impetigo and staphylococcal scalded-skin syndrome targets desmoglein 1. *Nat Med*. 2000;6(11):1275-1277.
27. van Kessel KP, Bestebroer J, van Strijp JA. Neutrophil-mediated phagocytosis of *Staphylococcus aureus*. *Front Immunol*. 2014;5:467.
28. Fritz SA, Camins BC, Eisenstein KA, et al. Effectiveness of measures to eradicate *Staphylococcus* aureus carriage in patients with community-associated skin and soft-tissue infections: a randomized trial. *Infect Control Hosp Epidemiol*. 2011;32(9):872-880.
29. Fritz SA, Hogan PG, Hayek G, et al. Household versus individual approaches to eradication of community-associated *Staphylococcus aureus* in children: a randomized trial. *Clin Infect Dis*. 2012;54(6):743-751.
30. Miller LG, Daum RS, Creech CB, et al. Clindamycin versus trimethoprim-sulfamethoxazole for uncomplicated skin infections. *N Engl J Med*. 2015;372(12):1093-1103.
31. Miller LG, Quan C, Shay A, et al. A prospective investigation of outcomes after hospital discharge for endemic, community-acquired methicillin-resistant and -susceptible *Staphylococcus aureus* skin infection. *Clin Infect Dis*. 2007;44(4):483-492.
32. Talan DA, Mower WR, Krishnadasan A, et al. Trimethoprim-sulfamethoxazole versus placebo for uncomplicated skin abscess. *N Engl J Med*. 2016;374(9):823-832.
33. Walker MJ, Barnett TC, McArthur JD, et al. Disease manifestations and pathogenic mechanisms of group A streptococcus. *Clin Microbiol Rev*. 2014;27(2):264-301.
34. Metzgar D, Zampolli A. The M protein of group A streptococcus is a key virulence factor and a clinically relevant strain identification marker. *Virulence*. 2011;2(5):402-412.
35. Carapetis JR, Steer AC, Mulholland EK, et al. The global burden of group A streptococcal diseases. *Lancet Infect Dis*. 2005;5(11):685-694.
36. Ralph AP, Carapetis JR. Group A streptococcal diseases and their global burden. *Curr Top Microbiol Immunol*. 2013;368:1-27.
37. Clegg HW, Giftos PM, Anderson WE, et al. Clinical perineal streptococcal infection in children: epidemiologic features, low symptomatic recurrence rate after treatment, and risk factors for recurrence. *J Pediatr*. 2015;167(3):687-693.e1-e2.
38. Martin WJ, Steer AC, Smeesters PR, et al. Post-infectious group A streptococcal autoimmune syndromes and the heart. *Autoimmun Rev*. 2015;14(8):710-725.
39. Fieber C, Kovarik P. Responses of innate immune cells to group A Streptococcus. *Front Cell Infect Microbiol*. 2014;4:140.

40. Dale JB, Fischetti VA, Carapetis JR, et al. Group A streptococcal vaccines: paving a path for accelerated development. *Vaccine*. 2013;31(suppl 2):B216-B222.
41. Henningham A, Gillen CM, Walker MJ. Group A streptococcal vaccine candidates: potential for the development of a human vaccine. *Curr Top Microbiol Immunol*. 2013;368:207-242.
42. Sen ES, Ramanan AV. How to use antistreptolysin O titre. *Arch Dis Child Educ Pract Ed*. 2014;99(6):231-238.
43. Bisno AL, Gerber MA, Gwaltney JM Jr, et al. Practice guidelines for the diagnosis and management of group A streptococcal pharyngitis. Infectious Diseases Society of America. *Clin Infect Dis*. 2002;35(2):113-125.
44. Blaise G, Nikkels AF, Hermanns-Lê T, et al. Corynebacterium-associated skin infections. *Int J Dermatol*. 2008;47(9):884-890.
45. Holdiness MR. Management of cutaneous erythrasma. *Drugs*. 2002;62(8):1131-1141.

Chapter 151 :: Cellulitis and Erysipelas
:: David R. Pearson & David J. Margolis

第一百五十一章

蜂窝织炎和丹毒

中文导读

蜂窝织炎是真皮深层和皮下组织的常见感染，通常是由细菌引起的，表现出典型的炎症迹象。丹毒是蜂窝织炎的一种变体，主要影响浅表淋巴管和周围组织。丹毒不同于典型的蜂窝织炎的特征不清的斑块，丹毒表现出边缘明显的水肿斑块。诊断可能具有挑战性，并且主要取决于临床发现。本章就蜂窝织炎和丹毒的定义、流行病学、病因与发病机制、临床特征、微生物学特征、诊断、鉴别诊断、临床病程和预后、临床管理进行了全面的阐释和讨论。

〔汪 犇〕

AT-A-GLANCE

- Common infection of the deep dermis and subcutaneous tissue most often caused by streptococcal and staphylococcal species, resulting in erythema, swelling, warmth, and pain of the affected site.
- Unilateral lower-extremity involvement is typical and systemic symptoms are usually absent.
- Important local risk factors include compromise of the skin barrier or underlying lymphovascular system.
- Diagnosis is most often made clinically because of frequently equivocal or negative workups.
- Treatment consists of antibiotics, but multiple recurrences may be observed.
- Common variants:
  - *Erysipelas:* sharply demarcated, bright red, edematous plaques resulting from superficial lymphatic infiltration.
  - *Purulent cellulitis:* localized pustules or abscesses associated with cellulitis.

Cellulitis is a common infection of the deep dermis and subcutaneous tissue, most often caused by bacteria, that presents with the classic signs of inflammation as described by the Roman scholar Celsus in the first century CE: redness (*rubor*), swelling (*tumor*), heat (*calor*), and pain (*dolor*). *Erysipelas* is a variant of cellulitis that predominantly affects the superficial lymphatic vessels and surrounding tissue. Unlike the ill-defined plaques characterizing classic cellulitis, erysipelas demonstrates sharply marginated edematous plaques and is strikingly red in color. Diagnosis may be challenging and relies predominantly on clinical findings as laboratory, serologic, microbiologic, histopathologic, and imaging studies are often equivocal or negative. For these reasons, despite the high prevalence of these infections, misdiagnosis is common and may lead to both treatment-related morbidity and significant health care costs.

DEFINITIONS

Most modern studies group classic cellulitis and erysipelas together under the simple term *cellulitis* when evaluating pathogenesis, risk factors, diagnosis, and treatment; this chapter follows that convention. Other cutaneous bacterial infections, including pyodermas (Chap. 150), toxin-mediated infections (Chap. 152), and necrotizing soft-tissue infections (Chap. 153) are considered separately.

HISTORICAL PERSPECTIVE

Skin and soft-tissue infections have been described for thousands of years.[1] In the preantibiotic era, cellulitis had a mortality rate of approximately 11% and only two-thirds of patients treated were cured with treatment.[2] Early therapies in the antibiotic era, including ultraviolet light, penicillin, and sulfonamide, significantly reduced mortality, although study designs were comparatively simpler than modern clinical trials.[2] In recent years, the emergence of community-acquired methicillin-resistant *Staphylococcus aureus* (MRSA), an increasingly common cause of cellulitis, has affected the epidemiology and treatment of this infection.

EPIDEMIOLOGY

Cellulitis is common and has increased in prevalence: in 1997 there were 4.6 million ambulatory visits for cellulitis or abscess in the United States, and this increased to 9.6 million in 2005.[3] The incidence rate increased from 17.3 to 32.5 per 1000 population during this time period, which parallels the rise of community-acquired MRSA.[3,4] In the United States, rates appear to have stabilized, although they continue to rise in other economically developed nations.[5,6] More than 10% of hospitalizations for infectious diseases in the Unites States are because of cellulitis, and hospitalizations for cellulitis in the United States have increased from approximately 300,000 in 1999 to more than 530,000 in 2013, with an estimated cost of $3.7 billion.[7,8]

Recurrent cellulitis represents 22% to 49% of patients, but its specific epidemiology is not well characterized.[9,10] Each reoccurrence increases the risk of subsequent episodes, because of local and systemic risk factors (see section "Risk Factors").[11,12] Most patients with recurrent cellulitis can be managed in the ambulatory setting and only a minority require hospitalization.[10]

CLINICAL FEATURES

CUTANEOUS FINDINGS

Classic cellulitis presents acutely with spreading, ill-defined erythema and edema, and is often warm and painful. The lower extremity is the most common site in adults, but the upper extremities, trunk, and head and neck may be involved (Fig. 151-1). Children are more likely than adults to have facial involvement. It is unilateral in the vast majority of cases, and bilateral involvement should prompt consideration of an alternative diagnosis, except in rare circumstances.[13] Linear streaking, lymphangiitis, and tender regional

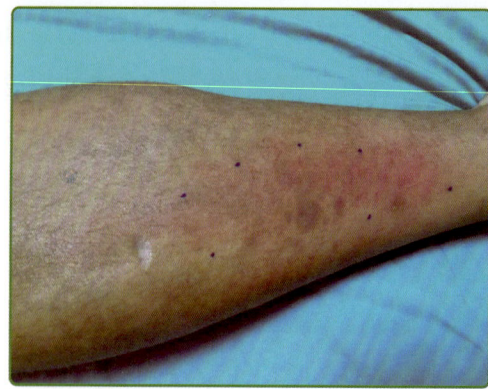

Figure 151-1 Cellulitis with ill-defined erythema on the lower leg. Note the subtle, streaky lymphangiitis extending proximally.

lymphadenopathy may be observed, as well as small areas of spared intervening skin, so-called "skip areas." When there is significant involvement of the lymphatics or superficial edema, the skin may acquire a peau d'orange appearance. Bulla formation and superficial necrosis can result in epidermal sloughing or erosions (Fig. 151-2). Hemorrhage may be observed as the result of disruption of superficial vessels by inflammation and edema. The presence of crepitus, anesthesia, or pain disproportionate to clinical findings should

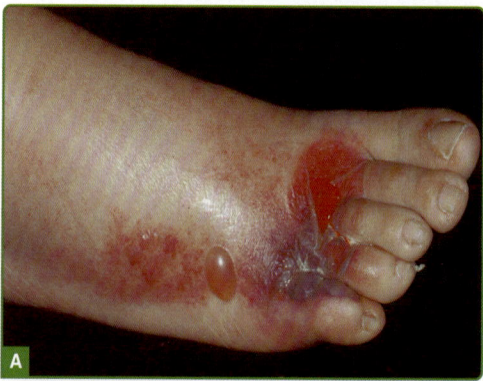

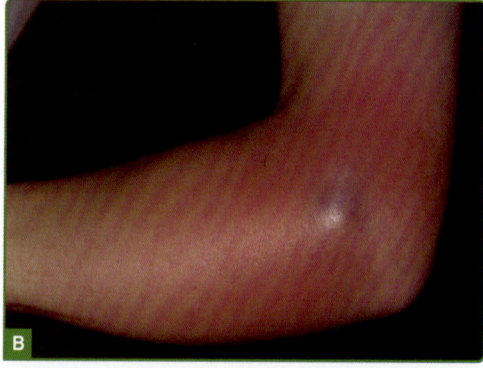

Figure 151-2 Cellulitis with swelling, erythema, and tenderness. **A,** Note blister formation on the lower extremity. **B,** Cellulitis emanating from an upper-extremity abscess.

raise concern for a necrotizing soft-tissue infection (see Chap. 153).

NONCUTANEOUS FINDINGS

Fever is an inconsistent complication of cellulitis and may be present in 12% to 71% of hospitalized patients; it may be even less common in patients who require only outpatient management.[13,14] Tachycardia may be observed.[13] Hemodynamic instability should prompt assessment for complicating sepsis, toxin-mediated systemic illness, or other serious infection.

COMPLICATIONS

Lymphatic damage leading to lymphedema is a frequent complication of cellulitis that increases the risk of recurrence (Fig. 151-3).[9,11,12] Superficial thrombophlebitis may be seen in the acute setting, but the risk of deep venous thrombosis is low.[15] More serious complications in treated patients are uncommon, but may include bacteremia, which occurs in approximately 5% of patients, and its sequelae, including sepsis, bacterial endocarditis, postinfectious glomerulonephritis, and toxin-mediated systemic syndromes (see Chaps. 152 and 155).[16,17] Spread of infection to deeper tissues is rare in the absence of other risk factors or chronic systemic disease.

CLINICAL VARIANTS

Erysipelas shares many clinical features with classic cellulitis, but the area of involvement is sharply demarcated and bright red in color. The most common site of involvement is the leg in 76% to 90% of cases, followed by the face and upper extremity (Figs. 151-4 and 151-5).[18,19] Fever is more common than in classic cellulitis.[18] Recurrence may be observed but systemic complications are uncommon.

Purulent cellulitis is defined by the presence of pustules or abscess development, which may precede or follow cellulitis (Fig. 151-6A). There should be a higher suspicion for *Staphylococcus aureus* as the causative organism.[20] If purulent collections are identified by physical examination or ultrasonography, there should be strong consideration for incision and drainage in addition to culture-directed and sensitivity-directed antibiotics (see also Chap. 150).

Surgical site infections localize to the site of surgery and are often accompanied by purulence (see Fig. 151-6B). *S. aureus* is commonly cultured, but other organisms may predominate depending upon the anatomic location and type of surgery.

Bite wounds may give rise to cellulitis at the site of inoculation in 20% to 30% of cases (see Chap. 182).[21] Dog bites are usually associated with crush injuries, whereas cat bites, because of the sharper teeth of cats, inject organisms into deeper tissue spaces, including joint spaces, tendon sheaths, and bone. Human bites are often polymicrobial and can result from direct biting or indirectly from contact of a fist to another person's teeth ("fight bite").

Periorbital or *preseptal cellulitis* is an infection anterior to the orbital septum, and demonstrates erythema, swelling, warmth, and pain in a periorbital distribution. Like classic cellulitis, there may be a clear portal of entry for infection. Patients may or may not have systemic symptoms, and neurologic sequelae are absent.[22]

Orbital cellulitis, in contrast, is infection posterior to the septum with involvement of the orbit proper. It usually results from direct extension of sinusitis, and may manifest with similar cutaneous findings to

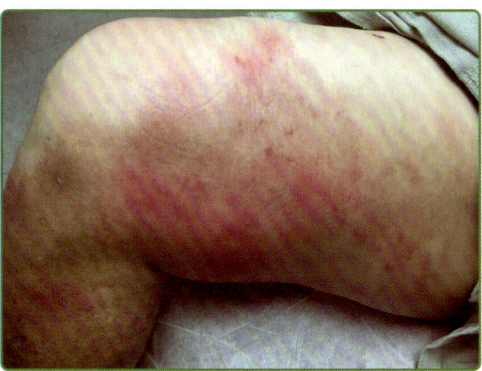

Figure 151-3 Recurrent cellulitis. Note the patchy, ill-defined erythema with "skip areas" on the medial thigh and lower leg. This pattern may be observed more frequently in recurrent cellulitis as a result of underlying lymphatic damage.

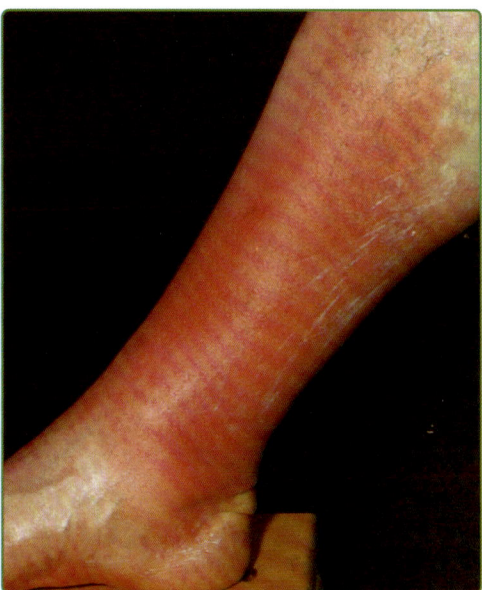

Figure 151-4 Erysipelas. There is painful, warm erythema of the lower extremity with well-defined borders.

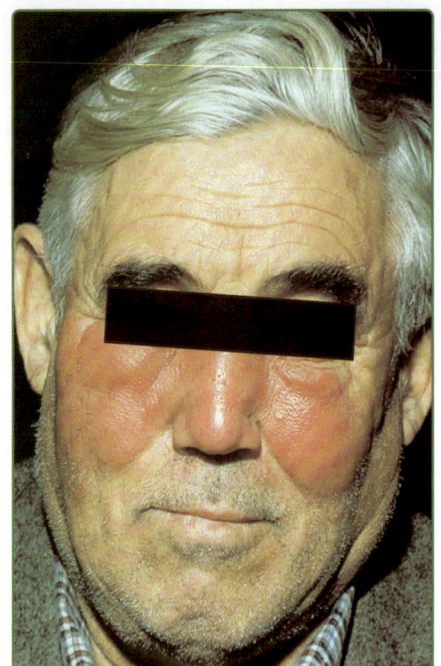

Figure 151-5 Erysipelas. Painful, edematous erythema with sharp margination on both cheeks and the nose. There is tenderness, and the patient has fever and chills.

periorbital cellulitis.[22] Proptosis, bulbar conjunctival edema, ophthalmoplegia, and decreased visual acuity are important clues to diagnosis, and necessitate rapid evaluation and treatment.[22] Orbital cellulitis may be complicated by permanent vision loss or posterior spread of infection into the brain.

Bilateral cellulitis, where infection occurs simultaneously on both extremities, is rare in the absence of predisposing factors such as penetrating trauma. Most of these patients are misdiagnosed (see section "Differential Diagnosis"); however, patients with deficient cellular immunity, such as solid organ transplantation recipients or individuals with HIV, may be at greater risk of true bilateral infection. In this patient population atypical causes of cellulitis should be considered, including disseminated cryptococcosis.[23,24]

ETIOLOGY AND PATHOGENESIS

Microbial pathogens gain access to the deep dermal and subcutaneous tissues through breaks in the skin, where they can spread into lymphatics, blood vessels, and interstitial spaces. A portal of entry can be identified in up to 62% of patients, with toe web infections as the most common etiology.[19] Disseminated infection with secondary seeding of the skin is a rare cause of cellulitis that may occur in immunocompromised patients.

Given the difficulty in culturing or identifying causative pathogens, cellulitis may be relatively paucimicrobial, with a significant portion of the clinical symptoms and signs due to host inflammatory responses to killed bacteria and bacterial exotoxins.

MICROBIOLOGY

Group A β-hemolytic streptococci (*Streptococcus pyogenes*) and staphylococci (particularly *S. aureus*) are the most commonly identified pathogens, but the specific incidence is difficult to characterize as identification of the causative organism occurs in less than one-third of cases.[16,19,25,26] Historically, erysipelas was attributed solely to streptococci, but recent studies have found a microbial profile that is similar to the microbial

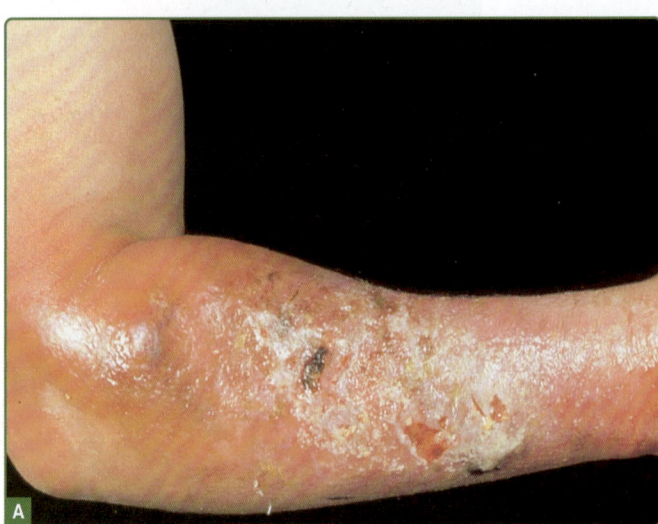
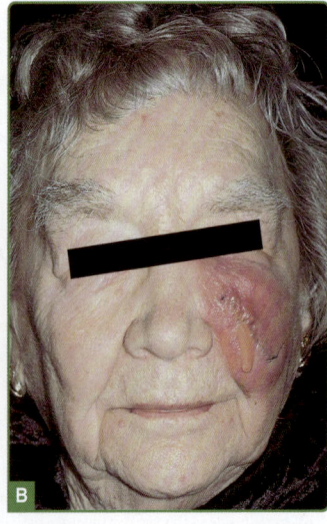

Figure 151-6 **A,** Cellulitis after puncture trauma. The forearm is swollen, erythematous, and tender; there is abscess formation. **B,** Cellulitis, caused by *Staphylococcus aureus* infection, arising at the site of a surgical excision. Note discharge of pus.

TABLE 151-1
Microbiology of Cellulitis

TYPE OF INFECTION	MOST COMMON CAUSE (S)	SELECT UNCOMMON CAUSES
Cellulitis and erysipelas (including periorbital/orbital cellulitis)	Group A streptococci (*Streptococcus pyogenes*); *Staphylococcus aureus*	Groups B, C, or G streptococci; coagulase-negative staphylococci; *Streptococcus iniae*; *Streptococcus pneumoniae*; *Haemophilus influenzae* (children); *Escherichia coli*, *Proteus* spp., other Enterobacteriaceae, and other Gram-negative anaerobes; *Neisseria* spp.; *Moraxella* spp.; *Campylobacter jejuni*; *Cryptococcus* spp. and other disseminated fungal organisms (immunocompromised); *Legionella pneumophila*, *Legionella micdadei*; *Pseudomonas aeruginosa* (secondary to bacteremia)
Cellulitis from animal and human bites (see Chap. 182)	*Pasteurella* spp.; streptococci, staphylococci	*Bacteroides* spp.; *Bartonella henselae* (cat); *Capnocytophaga canimorsus* (dog); *Eikenella* spp. (human); *Fusobacterium* spp.; *Moraxella* spp.
Cellulitis from aquatic trauma (exposure-specific)	*Aeromonas* spp.; *Erysipelothrix rhusiopathiae*; *Mycobacterium marinum* and other atypical mycobacteria; *Vibrio vulnificus*	

profile of classic cellulitis.[16] Other streptococcal species (groups B, C, and G) and coagulase-negative staphylococci are less-often encountered, but may be of increasing importance in hospitalized patients. Prior to widespread vaccination, which began in the late 1980s, *Haemophilus influenzae* Type B was observed in up to 6% of children with any systemic infection.[27] Surgical site infections, pressure or diabetic ulcers, and those with cellular immunodeficiency may be at greater risk for polymicrobial or atypical infections, including enterococci, *Pseudomonas* spp., Gram-negative anaerobes, mycobacteria, and disseminated fungal infections such as cryptococcosis. Cellulitis resulting from bite wounds may be polymicrobial and include Gram-negative anaerobes such as *Pasteurella* spp., *Eikenella* spp., and *Capnocytophaga canimorsus* (see Chap. 182). Aquatic trauma may lead to cellulitis from atypical organisms including *Aeromonas* spp., *Erysipelothrix rhusiopathiae*, *Mycobacterium marinum* or other atypical mycobacteria, and *Vibrio vulnificus*.[28]

Table 151-1 lists common and uncommon causes of cellulitis and variants.

RISK FACTORS

Cellulitis is more common in men than women, and its incidence rises during summer months and markedly with increasing patient age.[6,8] Other systemic or epidemiologic risk factors include obesity, renal or hepatic disease, connective tissue disease, and malignancy, but immunodeficiency (including iatrogenic or from systemic conditions such as HIV or diabetes) as a predisposing factor for routine cellulitis is controversial.[6,29-31] Compromise of the skin barrier or underlying lymphovascular system are important local risk factors, and may result from lymphedema, toe web infection, inflammatory dermatoses, peripheral vascular disease, or iatrogenic causes, including IV line placement, surgical site intervention (which may disrupt both the skin barrier and underlying lymphovascular system), and postradiation changes.[6,29,31] Of these, lymphedema confers the highest risk at more than 70-fold, followed by disruption of the skin barrier at nearly 24-fold.[31]

Recurrent cellulitis has similar risk factors to primary infection. Lymphedema, age, obesity, and prior surgical site intervention are among the most important.[32] Like primary cellulitis, recurrent infection is frequently misdiagnosed (see section "Diagnosis" and "Differential Diagnosis").

Table 151-2 summarizes both systemic and local risk factors for primary and recurrent cellulitis.

DIAGNOSIS

The diagnosis of cellulitis is most often made by clinical history and physical examination as there are no reliably accurate diagnostic studies. The cardinal symptoms and signs of erythema, swelling, warmth, and pain, even when accompanied by fever, leukocytosis, or elevated inflammatory markers, may be observed in clinical mimics of cellulitis known collectively as *pseudocellulitis* (see section "Differential Diagnosis").[29]

TABLE 151-2
Systemic and Local Risk Factors for Primary and Recurrent Cellulitis

Systemic/Environmental	Local
▪ Age ▪ Obesity ▪ Systemic disease: renal, hepatic, or autoimmune connective tissue diseases, malignancy; immunosuppression[a] (including diabetes, HIV, and iatrogenic) ▪ Summer season	▪ Disrupted skin barrier (toe web infections such as tinea pedis, inflammatory dermatoses, penetrating trauma, including iatrogenic causes) ▪ Compromised lymphovascular system (edema/lymphedema, venous insufficiency, peripheral arterial disease)

[a]Controversial as a risk factor for routine cellulitis. Immunosuppression should prompt consideration of unusual presentations or atypical pathogens and may require more aggressive treatment.

Misdiagnosis rates of greater than 30% have been observed in acute care settings (emergency department or hospital) and lead to hundreds of millions of dollars in avoidable health care spending.[33-36] Consultation of a dermatologist improves diagnostic accuracy, shortens duration of unnecessary antibiotic use, and improves short-term clinical outcomes.[35,37] Despite its high prevalence, there is clear need for improved diagnostic testing for cellulitis.

SUPPORTIVE STUDIES

LABORATORY TESTING

Leukocytosis (≥10,000 cells/µL) is present in 34% to 50% of patients, and inflammatory markers such as the erythrocyte sedimentation rate and C-reactive protein are elevated in more than 75% of patients, but these laboratory findings are nonspecific and also may be seen in pseudocellulitis.[13,19,38] Procalcitonin has been reliably used in serious systemic bacterial infections, but its usefulness as a surrogate biomarker in localized cellulitis has not been consistent, and additional prospective studies are necessary.[39-41]

Serologic tests for cellulitis are controversial, as they may not reliably distinguish acute infection from prior exposure. Antistreptolysin O responses are more limited in cutaneous than upper respiratory tract infections, typically appear after 1 week, peak at 3 to 6 weeks, and decline at less-well-defined rates, thereby complicating the diagnosis of both primary and recurrent cellulitis.[42] The anti-DNase B test peaks at 6 to 8 weeks, later than is useful for clinical decision making in the acute setting.[42]

MICROBIAL CULTURE

Skin swabs and surface wound cultures are often unhelpful, as they are commonly polymicrobial and determination of colonization versus true pathogenicity is challenging.[14,29] Positive polymerase chain reaction swabs for MRSA carriage have correlated with an increased overall risk of cellulitis, but their usefulness in acute infection is debated.[43] Needle aspiration followed by aspirate culture has shown widely disparate diagnostic usefulness, ranging from less than 5% to 40%, but may be more useful in patients with underlying systemic risk factors.[14,44] Blood cultures are not routinely performed in uncomplicated cellulitis as they are positive in only approximately 5% of cases.[16,17] However, in certain high-risk populations, such as the elderly, the immunocompromised, the systemically ill, and those with penetrating trauma, or if there is concern for atypical or severe systemic infection, blood cultures should be drawn. The 2014 update to the Infectious Diseases Society of America (IDSA) guidelines on the diagnosis and management of skin and soft-tissue infections does not recommend routinely culturing blood or cutaneous aspirates or swabs.[26] In contrast, pustules, abscesses, or other fluid collections associated with purulent cellulitis should be drained and cultured early during diagnostic workup.[26,29]

PATHOLOGY

Because the histopathologic findings of cellulitis are nonspecific, biopsy is not routinely performed. A sparse to moderately dense superficial and deep perivascular lymphocytic infiltrate with variable amounts of neutrophils may be seen, sometimes with background dermal edema, but Gram stains are frequently negative. Skin biopsy can be useful in evaluating for pseudocellulitis, depending upon the underlying etiology. Submission of skin biopsies for tissue culture is not routinely recommended, as the biopsies are positive in only 20% to 30% of cases.[26] If there is concern for an atypical causative organism, including mycobacteria, fungi, or viruses, or in immunocompromised or other high-risk patient populations, a biopsy for histopathologic evaluation and tissue culture should be performed.

Molecular techniques for microbe detection, including polymerase chain reaction of skin biopsies, do not reliably differentiate clinically involved from uninvolved skin and are often negative.[26,39] Routine use has not been widely adopted.

IMAGING

For uncomplicated cellulitis, imaging studies are not diagnostic. Ultrasonography or MRI can be helpful in identifying localized fluid collections in purulent cellulitis for guidance of incision and drainage. MRI also may be used to identify involvement of deeper tissues, such as pyomyositis or osteomyelitis, rare complications of severe or longstanding cellulitis. CT or MRI can be useful in differentiating cellulitis from necrotizing soft-tissue infections.

EMERGING DIAGNOSTIC MODALITIES

Given the high rate of misdiagnosis and lack of accurate and reliable studies, there is interest in finding better diagnostic methods for cellulitis. The ALT-70 (Table 151-3), a risk prediction model generated to

TABLE 151-3
ALT-70 Risk Prediction for Cellulitis

Asymmetry (unilateral)	3 points[a]
Leukocytosis ≥10,000 cells/µL	1 point
Tachycardia ≥90 beats/min	1 point
70 years of age or older	2 points

[a]A score of 0 to 2 = ≥83.3% likelihood of pseudocellulitis; a score of ≥5 points = ≥82.2% likelihood of true cellulitis.

predict the likelihood of lower-extremity cellulitis among admitted patients, is based on asymmetry (unilaterality) of infection, leukocytosis equal to or greater than 10,000 cells/µL, tachycardia equal to or greater than 90 beats/min, and patient age equal to or greater than 70 years.[13] A score of 0 to 2 points indicates a negative predictive value greater than 83.3%, and 5 points or higher indicates a positive predictive value greater than 82.2% for cellulitis.[13] A skin surface temperature gradient greater than 0.47°C (0.85°F) between a patient's involved and uninvolved skin, as determined by thermal imaging, has also shown promise, with a sensitivity of 96.6% for the diagnosis of cellulitis, but additional confirmatory studies are needed.[45] Genetic testing may prove useful; a recent pilot study found that HLA-DQA1 expression was 34-fold higher among cases with cellulitis than controls.[39]

DIFFERENTIAL DIAGNOSIS

The differential diagnosis for cellulitis is broad, and includes causes of pseudocellulitis as well as causes of other infectious etiologies (Table 151-4). In difficult cases, skin biopsy or other laboratory markers may be useful for diagnosis when placed into the clinical context of the patient.

The most common cause of pseudocellulitis is stasis dermatitis.[29,30,46,47] Stasis dermatitis is commonly bilateral, which may aid in differentiating it from cellulitis; however, it is often asymmetric and may be unilateral (Fig. 151-7A). The chronicity, association of scaling and pruritus, absence of fever or leukocytosis, and response to compression, elevation, and topical corticosteroids can assist in diagnosis. Other lymphovascular diseases and sequelae, including deep venous thrombosis, hematoma, lipodermatosclerosis, and chronic edema or lymphedema, are commonly encountered and may mimic cellulitis. Eczematous dermatitides, such as allergic or irritant contact and asteatotic dermatitis, are usually discriminated by the presence of scaling and pruritus and absence of fever or leukocytosis. Bilateral involvement or geometric borders may be observed and aid diagnosis. Gout or pseudogout may mimic localized, early cellulitis, and can be accompanied by fever and leukocytosis, but typically overlies a joint. Erythema nodosum and small-vessel vasculitides tend to present as multifocal eruptions, but fever and leukocytosis are variably present (Fig. 151-7B).

Erythema migrans is an important infectious mimic of cellulitis in endemic areas, may not present in the classic annular configuration, and can be accompanied by fever or systemic symptoms. The patient may not

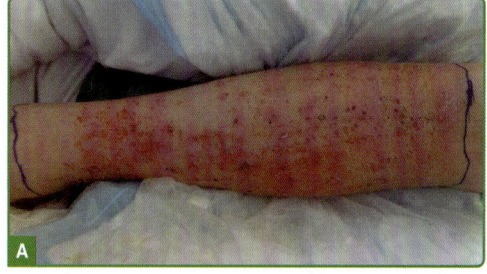

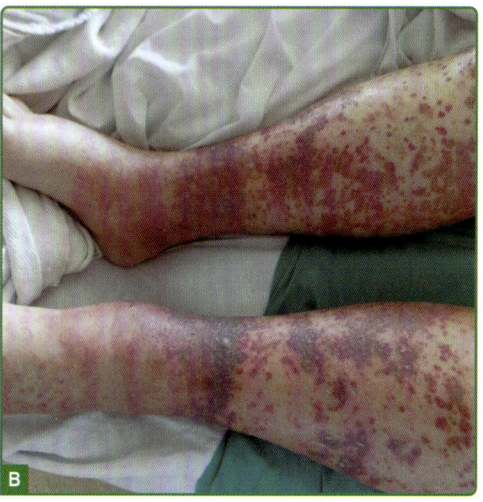

Figure 151-7 **A,** Stasis dermatitis with linear excoriations. The eruption is eczematous with evidence of scratching (because of pruritus), which would be atypical in cellulitis. Note the "marker sign," commonly observed in hospitalized patients seen by dermatology consultants, which is testament to the difficulty of diagnosis. **B,** Cutaneous small-vessel vasculitis attributed to naproxen use. The purpuric eruption is bilateral and located in areas of dependency, consisting of coalescing papules and plaques with secondary blister formation. This patient has low-grade elevated temperatures.

TABLE 151-4
Differential Diagnosis of Cellulitis[a]

Inflammatory	Infectious
- **Stasis dermatitis** - **Irritant/allergic contact dermatitis and other eczematous dermatitides** - Drug eruption - Vasculitides - Panniculitides (eg, lipodermatosclerosis, erythema nodosum) - Neutrophilic dermatoses (eg, pyoderma gangrenosum, Sweet syndrome) - Follicular occlusion (eg, hidradenitis suppurativa) - Sarcoidosis - Autoimmune connective tissue diseases - Radiation dermatitis	- **Dermatophytoses** - Cutaneous candidiasis - Erythema migrans - Necrotizing soft-tissue infections - Acute/chronic paronychia - Cutaneous mycobacterial infections
Vascular	**Neoplastic/Paraneoplastic**
- **Edema/lymphedema** - Deep venous thrombosis - Superficial thrombophlebitis - Hematoma	- Cutaneous lymphoma - Paget disease - Carcinoma erysipeloides - Erythromelalgia
	Miscellaneous
	- **Arthropod bite** - Gout/pseudogout - Calciphylaxis - Wells syndrome (eosinophilic cellulitis) - Hereditary periodic fever syndromes (eg, familial Mediterranean fever)

[a]Commonly misdiagnosed pseudocellulitides are highlighted in bold.

recall a history of tick bite. Other arthropod bites are usually multifocal without systemic symptoms. It is important to exclude necrotizing soft-tissue infections when evaluating cellulitis, as they require emergent surgical evaluation and debridement.

CLINICAL COURSE AND PROGNOSIS

The natural history of acute cellulitis is rarely observed in the modern era, however prior to use of antibiotics, therapeutic cure was achieved in approximately two-thirds of patients with an 11% mortality rate.[2] Cure rates are difficult to estimate in clinical trials because of the lack of definitive biomarkers for infection, but average approximately 80% to 85%, and are interestingly higher in complicated cellulitis than uncomplicated cases.[48] These relatively low cure rates may be related to inadvertent inclusion of pseudocellulitis into antimicrobial trials, or prolonged time to complete recovery beyond the usual clinical assessment period.[48,49] Without treatment, infection can spread into the bloodstream and become life-threatening.

Prognosis for treated cellulitis is good and modern mortality rates are negligible in uncomplicated cases treated with antibiotics. The recovery period is usually several weeks, although by 30 days as many as 20% of patients have not yet returned to normal activities.[49] Recurrence occurs in more than 10% of patients.[11] This risk increases with number of previous reoccurrences, which is suggestive of predisposing systemic or local risk factors for infection.

The common practice of outlining the involved area of cellulitis may be useful to monitor response to treatment, although indistinct margins, presence of "skip areas," and occasional transient progression of erythema despite other evidence of clinical improvement may make interpretation difficult in some patients.[50] Serial high-quality photographs can provide an alternative, reliable method to monitor treatment response, particularly in the inpatient setting where the primary provider may change during a patient's hospitalization.[50]

MANAGEMENT

Empiric antibiotic therapy directed against streptococcal and staphylococcal species is recommended for the treatment of cellulitis, but the evidence of superiority for one regimen over another has not been definitively established.[51] Treatment recommendations vary based upon the presence of purulence, systemic symptoms, and overall clinical assessment, the patient's underlying risk factors, and community rates of drug-resistant pathogens. Outpatient therapy with oral antibiotics is appropriate in hemodynamically stable patients without evidence of systemic infection, but hospitalization may be required in the seriously ill, immunocompromised patients, or with failure of outpatient therapy.

Table 151-5 outlines the treatments for bacterial cellulitis.

ANTIBIOTICS

NONPURULENT CELLULITIS

Nonpurulent cellulitis without systemic evidence of infection should be treated with oral antistreptococcal antibiotics such as cephalexin, dicloxacillin, or penicillin V. In cases of true Type I hypersensitivity reactions to penicillins or cephalosporins, clindamycin or macrolides should be considered.[26,29] No difference in failure rate between β-lactams and non–β-lactams has been demonstrated, although some studies have shown higher rates of treatment-related adverse events (predominantly GI symptoms) among patients treated with non–β-lactams.[52,53] Addition of clindamycin or trimethoprim-sulfamethoxazole, both agents with activity against MRSA, to β-lactam antibiotics have not demonstrated significant benefits over β-lactam coverage alone for uncomplicated nonpurulent cellulitis.[49,54]

Patients with evidence of systemic infection, including 2 or more systemic inflammatory response syndrome criteria (temperature >38°C [100.4°F] or <36°C [96.8°F]; pulse >90 beats/min; respiratory rate >20 breaths/min; or leukocyte count >12,000 cells/μL or <4000 cells/μL), or those who fail outpatient treatment should receive parenteral antibiotics such as cefazolin, ceftriaxone, or penicillin G.[26] Clindamycin should be used in patients with true Type I hypersensitivity reactions to penicillins or cephalosporins. If there is associated penetrating trauma, including injection drug use, or known MRSA colonization or infection elsewhere, empiric coverage with vancomycin may be indicated. Severe infections with rapid progression, hypotension, end-organ dysfunction, or in immunocompromised patients or in those suspected of having atypical or resistant organisms should be treated with broad-spectrum parenteral antibiotics and narrowed according to culture and sensitivity results.[26,29]

PURULENT CELLULITIS

Patients with purulent cellulitis should be cultured and fluid collections incised and drained. In mild disease, empiric therapy with oral anti-staphylococcal antibiotics should be initiated while awaiting culture and sensitivity results. The decision to treat for methicillin-sensitive *S. aureus* (MSSA) versus MRSA should depend upon clinical suspicion based on host or environmental factors, including history of known MRSA colonization, patient risk factors, and local rates of MRSA infections. Cephalexin and dicloxacillin are first-line agents of choice in MSSA, whereas clindamycin, tetracyclines, and trimethoprim-sulfamethoxazole are used in MRSA. In these cases, concomitant

TABLE 151-5
Treatments for Bacterial Cellulitis

DISEASE	SEVERITY	FIRST-LINE ANTIBIOTICS	ALTERNATIVE ANTIBIOTICS
Nonpurulent cellulitis	Mild (no evidence of systemic disease); outpatient setting with oral therapy	• Cephalexin • Dicloxacillin • Penicillin V	• Clindamycin • Macrolides (azithromycin, erythromycin)
	Moderate (≥2 SIRS criteria or failure of outpatient therapy); acute care setting with IV therapy	• Cefazolin • Ceftriaxone • Penicillin G	• Clindamycin • Consider vancomycin if associated IVDU or known MRSA colonization/infection
	Severe (≥2 SIRS criteria with rapid progression, hypotension, or evidence of end-organ damage) or immunocompromised; hospitalization with IV therapy • Consider surgical evaluation for necrotizing soft-tissue infection • Cultures and sensitivities	• Broad-spectrum with vancomycin and piperacillin-tazobactam • Narrow as appropriate per cultures and sensitivities	
Purulent cellulitis	Mild (no evidence of systemic disease); outpatient setting with oral therapy • Incise and drain; consider cultures and sensitivities	MSSA suspected: • Cephalexin • Dicloxacillin MRSA suspected: • Clindamycin • Tetracyclines (doxycycline, minocycline, tetracycline) • Trimethoprim-sulfamethoxazole	• Clindamycin
	Moderate (≥2 SIRS criteria or failure of outpatient therapy); acute care setting with IV therapy • Incise and drain; cultures and sensitivities	MSSA suspected: • Oxacillin • Nafcillin • Cefazolin MRSA suspected: • Vancomycin • Clindamycin	• Clindamycin • Linezolid (MRSA)
	Severe (≥2 SIRS criteria with rapid progression, hypotension, or evidence of end-organ damage) or immunocompromised; hospitalization with IV therapy • Consider surgical evaluation for necrotizing soft-tissue infection • Incise and drain; cultures and sensitivities	• Broad-spectrum with vancomycin and piperacillin-tazobactam • Narrow as appropriate per cultures and sensitivities	• Clindamycin • Daptomycin • Ceftaroline • Telavancin • Tigecycline

IVDU, IV drug use; MRSA, methicillin-resistant *Staphylococcus aureus*; MSSA, methicillin-sensitive *Staphylococcus aureus*; SIRS, systemic inflammatory response syndrome (temperature >38°C [100.4°F] or <36°C [96.8°F]; pulse >90 beats/min; respiratory rate >20 breaths/min; or leukocyte count >12,000 cells/μL or <4000 cells/μL).

coverage for streptococcal species may be required.[26,29] If penicillin or cephalosporin allergy exists, clindamycin is an alternative. Note some geographic regions demonstrate high rates of inducible clindamycin resistance in *S. aureus* isolates.

Patients with systemic infection or failure of outpatient treatment require parenteral antibiotics (Table 151-6). Oxacillin, nafcillin, and cefazolin, or clindamycin in penicillin-allergic or cephalosporin-allergic patients, are appropriate for MSSA.[26,29] Vancomycin, clindamycin, or linezolid are preferred

TABLE 151-6
Indications for Parenteral Administration of Antibiotics

At least 2 or more of the following
- Temperature >38°C (100.4°F) or <36°C (96.8°F)
- Pulse >90 beats/min
- Respiratory rate >20 breaths/min
- Leukocyte count >12,000 cells/μL or <4000 cells/μL

or

Failed outpatient treatment

in MRSA.[26,29] Severe infections or infections in special patient populations require broad-spectrum parenteral antibiotic coverage, including against MRSA, while awaiting culture and sensitivity results.

DURATION

The optimal duration of antibiotic therapy has not been identified in clinical trials. The IDSA guidelines recommend 5 days for uncomplicated patients, with extension of therapy if signs of infection persist.[26] In general, 5 to 10 days are recommended for uncomplicated patients with slightly longer courses (7 to 14 days) for immunocompromised patients.[29] Reassessment at 24 to 72 hours is important to assess response to therapy.

RECURRENT CELLULITIS AND PROPHYLAXIS

Recurrent episodes of cellulitis may require longer treatment courses or hospitalization, although the majority can be managed in the ambulatory setting. Risk factors for recurrence should be addressed (see section "Prevention"). Although controversial, prophylactic antibiotics, such as low-dose penicillin or erythromycin, should be considered if there are 3 to 4 recurrences per year despite these efforts.[26] Prophylaxis may reduce both the incidence of first reoccurrence after primary cellulitis and subsequent recurrences, but these effects diminish after discontinuation of therapy.[55-58] Optimal type, dosing, and duration of antibiotics require further investigation. Prophylaxis has demonstrated cost-effectiveness, but long-term tolerability data is lacking and its effects on antibacterial resistance patterns are unknown.[59]

ADJUNCTIVE TREATMENTS

Combination therapy with antibiotics and adjunctive antiinflammatories, including nonsteroidal antiinflammatory drugs (NSAIDs) and systemic corticosteroids, may be beneficial in some patients. NSAIDs may reduce time to regression of inflammation.[60,61] However, there are concerns over their effects on neutrophil chemotaxis as NSAID use has been correlated with an increased risk of skin infection in children with varicella.[62,63]

Despite concerns over immunosuppressive effects, the addition of prednisolone to antibiotics has demonstrated shortened time to healing in uncomplicated erysipelas with a trend toward decreased relapse, and oral corticosteroids in combination with parenteral antibiotics reduced resolution time and ocular complications in orbital cellulitis.[64-66] The IDSA guidelines recommend consideration of systemic corticosteroids in nondiabetic adult patients with cellulitis.[26]

PREVENTION

Treatment of predisposing factors, including lymphedema, toe web infections, and local skin barrier defects, and underlying medical conditions is recommended to prevent primary and recurrent episodes of cellulitis. Decolonization strategies for MRSA carriage are controversial and their effectiveness in reducing the risk of cellulitis requires further study.[67]

ACKNOWLEDGMENTS

The author acknowledges the contributions of Adam D. Lipworth, Arturo P. Saavedra, Arnold N. Weinberg, and Richard Allen Johnson, the former authors of this chapter.

REFERENCES

1. Stevens D. Antimicrobial agents for complicated skin and skin-structure infections: noninferiority margins, placebo-controlled trials, and the complexity of clinical trials. *Clin Infect Dis.* 2009;49:392-394.
2. Spellberg B, Talbot GH, Boucher HW, et al. Antimicrobial agents for complicated skin and skin-structure infections: justification of noninferiority margins in the absence of placebo-controlled trials. *Clin Infect Dis.* 2009;49:383-391.
3. Hersh AL, Chambers HF, Maselli JH, et al. National trends in ambulatory visits and antibiotic prescribing for skin and soft-tissue infections. *Arch Intern Med.* 2008;168:1585-1591.
4. Como-Sabetti K, Harriman KH, Buck JM, et al. Community-associated methicillin-resistant *Staphylococcus aureus*: trends in case and isolate characteristics from six years of prospective surveillance. *Public Health Rep.* 2009;124(3):427-435.
5. Marcelin JR, Challener DW, Tan EM, et al. Incidence and effects of seasonality on nonpurulent lower extremity cellulitis after the emergence of community-acquired methicillin-resistant *Staphylococcus aureus*. *Mayo Clin Proc.* 2017;92(8):1227-1233.
6. Cannon J, Rajakaruna G, Dyer J, et al. Severe lower limb cellulitis: defining the epidemiology and risk factors for primary episodes in a population-based case-control study. *Clin Microbiol Infect.* 2018. [Epub ahead of print]
7. Yorita KL, Holman RC, Sejvar JJ, et al. Infectious disease hospitalizations among infants in the United States. *Pediatrics.* 2008;121(2):244-252.
8. Peterson R, Polgreen L, Cavanaugh J, et al. Increasing incidence, cost, and seasonality in patients hospitalized for cellulitis. *Open Forum Infect Dis.* 2017;4(1):ofx008.
9. Jorup-Ronstrom C, Britton S. Recurrent erysipelas: predisposing factors and costs of prophylaxis. *Infection.* 1987;15(2):105-106.
10. St John J, Strazzula L, Vedak P, et al. Estimating the health care costs associated with recurrent cellulitis managed in the outpatient setting. *J Am Acad Dermatol.* 2018;78(4):749-753.

11. Cannon J, Dyer J, Carapetis J, et al. The epidemiology and risk factors for recurrent severe lower limb cellulitis: a longitudinal cohort study. *Clin Microbiol Infect.* 2018. [Epub ahead of print]
12. Cox NH. Oedema as a risk factor for multiple episodes of cellulitis/erysipelas of the lower leg: a series with community. *Br J Dermatol.* 2006;155(5):947-950.
13. Raff AB, Weng QY, Cohen JM, et al. A predictive model for diagnosis of lower extremity cellulitis: a cross-sectional study. *J Am Acad Dermatol.* 2017;76(4):618-625.e2.
14. Hirschmann JV, Raugi GJ. Lower limb cellulitis and its mimics: part I. Lower limb cellulitis. *J Am Acad Dermatol.* 2012;67(2):163.e1-e12.
15. Gunderson CG, Chang JJ. Risk of deep vein thrombosis in patients with cellulitis and erysipelas: a systematic review and meta-analysis. *Thromb Res.* 2013;132(3):336-340.
16. Gunderson CG, Martinello RA. A systematic review of bacteremias in cellulitis and erysipelas. *J Infect.* 2012;64(2):148-155.
17. Perl B, Gottehrer NP, Raveh D, et al. Cost-effectiveness of blood cultures for adult patients with cellulitis. *Clin Infect Dis.* 1999;29(6):1483-1488.
18. Bonnetblanc JM, Bédane C. Erysipelas: recognition and management. *Am J Clin Dermatol.* 2003;4(3):157-163.
19. Krasagakis K, Valachis A, Maniatakis P, et al. Analysis of epidemiology, clinical features and management of erysipelas. *Int J Dermatol.* 2010;49(9):1012-1017.
20. Moran GJ, Krishnadasan A, Gorwitz RJ, et al. Methicillin-resistant S. aureus infections among patients in the emergency department. *N Engl J Med.* 2006;355(7):666-674.
21. Rothe K, Tsokos M, Handrick W. Animal and human bite wounds. *Dtsch Arztebl Int.* 2015;112(25):433-443.
22. Givner LB. Periorbital versus orbital cellulitis. *Pediatr Infect Dis J.* 2002;21(12):1157-1158.
23. Chakradeo K, Paul Chia Y, Liu C, et al. Disseminated cryptococcosis presenting initially as lower limb cellulitis in a renal transplant recipient-a case report. *BMC Nephrol.* 2018;19:18.
24. Nishioka H, Takegawa H, Kamei H. Disseminated crytococcosis in a patient taking tocilizumab for Castleman's disease. *J Infect Chemother.* 2018;24:138-141.
25. Chira S, Miller LG. Staphylococcus aureus is the most common identified cause of cellulitis: a systematic review. *Epidemiol Infect.* 2010;138(3):313-317.
26. Stevens DL, Bisno AL, Chambers HF, et al. Practice guidelines for the diagnosis and management of skin and soft tissue infections: 2014 update by the Infectious Diseases Society of America. *Clin Infect Dis.* 2014;59(2):e10-e52.
27. Inamadar AC, Palit A. Blue cellulitis: a rare entity in the era of Hib conjugate vaccine. *Pediatr Dermatol.* 2004;21(1):90-91.
28. Diaz JH, Lopez FA. Skin, soft tissue and systemic bacterial infections following aquatic injuries and exposures. *Am J Med Sci.* 2015;349(3):269-275.
29. Raff AB, Kroshinsky D. Cellulitis: a review. *JAMA.* 2016;316(3):325-337.
30. Bailey E, Kroshinsky D. Cellulitis: diagnosis and management. *Dermatol Ther.* 2011;24(2):229-239.
31. Dupuy A, Benchikhi H, Roujeau JC, et al. Risk factors for erysipelas of the leg (cellulitis): case-control study. *BMJ.* 1999;318(7198):1591-1594.
32. Karppelin M, Siljander T, Vuopio-Varkila J, et al. Factors predisposing to acute and recurrent bacterial non-necrotizing cellulitis in hospitalized patients: a prospective case-control study. *Clin Microbiol Infect.* 2010;16(6):729-734.
33. Weng QY, Raff AB, Cohen JM, et al. Costs and consequences associated with misdiagnosed lower extremity cellulitis. *JAMA Dermatol.* 2017;153(2):141-146.
34. Levell NJ, Wingfield CG, Garioch JJ. Severe lower limb cellulitis is best diagnosed by dermatologists and managed with shared care between primary and secondary care. *Br J Dermatol.* 2011;164(6):1326-1328.
35. Ko L, Garza-Mayers A, St John J, et al. Effect of dermatology consultation on outcomes for patients with presumed cellulitis: a randomized clinical trial. *JAMA Dermatol.* 2018;154(5):529-536.
36. Li D, Xia F, Khosravi H, et al. Outcomes of early dermatology consultation for inpatients diagnosed with cellulitis. *JAMA Dermatol.* 2018;154(5):537-543.
37. Arakaki RY, Strazzula L, Woo E, et al. The impact of dermatology consultation on diagnostic accuracy and antibiotic use among patients with suspected cellulitis seen at outpatient internal medicine offices: a randomized clinical trial. *JAMA Dermatol.* 2014;150(10):1056-1061.
38. Lazzarini L, Conti E, Tositti G, et al. Erysipelas and cellulitis: clinical and microbiological spectrum in an Italian tertiary care hospital. *J Infect.* 2005;51(5):383-389.
39. Pallin DJ, Bry L, Dwyer RC, et al. Toward an objective diagnostic test for bacterial cellulitis. *PLoS One.* 2016;11(9):e0162947.
40. Rast AC, Knobel D, Faessler L, et al. Use of procalcitonin, C-reactive protein and white blood cell count to distinguish between lower limb erysipelas and deep vein thrombosis in the emergency department: a prospective observational study. *J Dermatol.* 2015;42(8):778-785.
41. Noh SH, Park SD, Kim EJ. Serum procalcitonin level reflects the severity of cellulitis. *Ann Dermatol.* 2016;28(6):704-710.
42. Shet A, Kaplan EL. Clinical use and interpretation of group A streptococcal antibody tests: a practical approach for the pediatrician or primary care physician. *Pediatr Infect Dis J.* 2002;21(5):420-426.
43. Chen CJ, Wang SC, Chang HY, et al. Longitudinal analysis of methicillin-resistant and methicillin-susceptible Staphylococcus aureus carriage in healthy adolescents. *J Clin Microbiol.* 2013;51(8):2508-2514.
44. Sachs MK. The optimum use of needle aspiration in the bacteriologic diagnosis of cellulitis in adults. *Arch Intern Med.* 1990;150(9):1907-1912.
45. Ko LN, Raff AB, Garza-Mayers AC, et al. Skin surface temperatures measured by thermal imaging aid in the diagnosis of cellulitis. *J Invest Dermatol.* 2018;138(3):520-526.
46. Hirschmann JV, Raugi GJ. Lower limb cellulitis and its mimics: part II. Conditions that simulate lower limb cellulitis. *J Am Acad Dermatol.* 2012;67(2):177.e1-177.e9.
47. Strazzula L, Cotliar J, Fox LP, et al. Inpatient dermatology consultation aids diagnosis of cellulitis among hospitalized patients: a multi-institutional analysis. *J Am Acad Dermatol.* 2015;73(1):70-75.
48. Obaitan I, Dwyer R, Lipworth AD, et al. Failure of antibiotics in cellulitis trials: a systematic review and meta-analysis. *Am J Emerg Med.* 2016;34(8):1645-1652.
49. Brindle R, Williams OM, Davies P, et al. Adjunctive clindamycin for cellulitis: a clinical trial comparing flucloxacillin with or without clindamycin for the treat-

ment of limb cellulitis. *BMJ Open*. 2017;7(3):e013260.
50. Kak V, Miller L, Lessing JN, et al. Therapy for cellulitis. *JAMA*. 2016;316(19):2045-2046.
51. Kilburn SA, Featherstone P, Higgins B, et al. Interventions for cellulitis and erysipelas. *Cochrane Database Syst Rev*. 2010;(6):CD004299.
52. Madaras-Kelly KJ, Remington RE, Oliphant CM, et al. Efficacy of oral β-Lactam versus non-β-lactam treatment of uncomplicated cellulitis. *Am J Med*. 2008;121(5):419-425.
53. Ferreira A, Bolland M, Thomas M. Meta analysis of randomised trials comparing a penicillin or cephalosporin with a macrolide or lincosamide in the treatment of cellulitis or erysipelas. *Infection*. 2016;44:607-615.
54. Moran GJ, Krishnadasan A, Mower WR, et al. Effect of cephalexin plus trimethoprim-sulfamethoxazole vs cephalexin alone on clinical cure of uncomplicated cellulitis: a randomized clinical trial. *JAMA*. 2017;317(20):2088-2096.
55. Thomas KS, Crook AM, Nunn AJ, et al. Penicillin to prevent recurrent leg cellulitis. *N Engl J Med*. 2013;368(18):1695-1703.
56. UK Dermatology Clinical Trials Network's PATCH Trial Team, Thomas K, Crook A, et al. Prophylactic antibiotics for the prevention of cellulitis (erysipelas) of the leg: results of the UK Dermatology Clinical Trials Network's PATCH II trial. *Br J Dermatol*. 2012;166:169-178.
57. Dalal A, Eskin-Schwartz M, Mimouni D, et al. Interventions for the prevention of recurrent erysipelas and cellulitis. *Cochrane Database Syst Rev*. 2017;6:CD009758.
58. Oh CC, Ko HC, Lee HY, et al. Antibiotic prophylaxis for preventing recurrent cellulitis: a systematic review and meta-analysis. *J Infect*. 2014;69(1):26-34.
59. Mason JM, Thomas KS, Crook AM, et al. Prophylactic antibiotics to prevent cellulitis of the leg: economic analysis of the PATCH I & II trials. *PLoS One*. 2014;9(2):e82694.
60. Dall L, Peterson S, Simmons T, et al. Rapid resolution of cellulitis in patients managed with combination antibiotic and anti-inflammatory therapy. *Cutis*. 2005;75(3):177-180.
61. Davis JS, Mackrow C, Binks P, et al. A double-blind randomised controlled trial of ibuprofen compared with placebo for uncomplicated cellulitis of the upper or lower limb. *Clin Microbiol Infect*. 2017;23(4):242-246.
62. Chosidow O, Saiag P, Pinquier L, et al. Nonsteroidal anti-inflammatory drugs in cellulitis: a cautionary note. *Arch Dermatol*. 1991;127:1845-1846.
63. Mikaeloff Y, Kezouh A, Suissa S. Nonsteroidal anti-inflammatory drug use and the risk of severe skin and soft tissue complications in patients with varicella or zoster disease. *Br J Clin Pharmacol*. 2008;65(2):203-209.
64. Bergkvist PI, Sjöbeck K. Antibiotic and prednisolone therapy of erysipelas: a randomized, double blind, placebo-controlled study. *Scand J Infect Dis*. 1997;29(4):377-382.
65. Bergkvist PI, Sjöbeck K. Relapse of erysipelas following treatment with prednisolone or placebo in addition to antibiotics: a 1-year follow-up. *Scand J Infect Dis*. 1998;30(2):206-207.
66. Pushker N, Tejwani LK, Bajaj MS, et al. Role of oral corticosteroids in orbital cellulitis. *Am J Ophthalmol*. 2013;156(1):178-183.e1.
67. Loeb M, Main C, Walker-Dilks C, et al. Antimicrobial drugs for treating methicillin-resistant Staphylococcus aureus colonization. *Cochrane Database Syst Rev*. 2003;(4):CD003340.

Chapter 152 :: Gram-Positive Infections Associated with Toxin Production
:: Jeffrey B. Travers

第一百五十二章

产毒素革兰氏阳性细菌感染

中文导读

革兰氏阳性细菌、金黄色葡萄球菌和A组链球菌（化脓性链球菌）引起的皮肤感染是发病率和死亡率的重要来源。这些细菌通过表达毒素的能力发挥许多作用，这些毒素可以诱导特征性综合征，包括葡萄球菌烫伤皮肤综合征和中毒性休克综合征。该章节重点介绍了全身性葡萄球菌烫伤皮肤综合征（SSSS）的临床表现、治疗和预后等内容。同时，还就超抗原毒素引起的疾病进行了阐述，分别就中毒性休克综合征、顽固性红斑剥脱病、猩红热、毒素介导的红斑等少见类型进行了简单的介绍和分析。

〔汪 犇〕

AT-A-GLANCE

- Gram-positive infections are caused by *Staphylococcus aureus* and/or Group A *Streptococcus* toxin-producing bacteria.
- Characteristic syndromes (all with skin manifestations): can be divided into 3 categories depending the predominant clinical presentation:
  - Predominantly cutaneous
    - Local: bullous impetigo
    - Generalized: *Staphylococcus* scalded-skin syndrome
  - Cutaneous and systemic
    - Local: recurrent toxin mediated erythema (recurrent perineal erythema)
    - Generalized: recalcitrant erythematous desquamating disorder
    - Other abortive hybrids of predominantly systemic manifestations
- Predominately systemic
  - Generalized: toxic shock syndrome *Staphylococcus* (predominantly) or *Streptococcus*
  - Scarlet fever: *Streptococcus* (predominantly) or *Staphylococcus*

Skin infections with the Gram-positive bacteria *Staphylococcus aureus* and group A *Streptococcus* (*Streptococcus pyogenes*) are an important source of morbidity and mortality. These bacteria exert many of their effects via their ability to express toxins which can induce characteristic syndromes including staphylococcal scalded-skin syndrome and toxic shock syndrome. Moreover, the production of these toxins is thought to be behind the ability of infection with these bacteria to initiate and/or propagate inflammatory and neoplastic skin diseases. As is outlined in this chapter, the clinician needs to be aware that there are not only classical syndromes, but, also partial ones in which Gram-positive toxins are likely inducing effects.

EPIDEMIOLOGY

FACTORS IN TOXIN-MEDIATED DISEASE

Staphylococcal and streptococcal pathogenicity are caused by production of a repertoire of immunomodulatory proteins, including toxins, exoenzymes, and adhesins (reviewed in Dinges and colleagues[1]). Among the best characterized of these are the toxins, which are outlined in Table 152-1.

Many risk factors play a role in the ability of a toxin-forming *Staphylococcus* or *Streptococcus* to produce disease. The development of disease is related to the resistance of the host to infection and to the virulence of the organism. The host's resistance depends, among other factors, on intact skin and mucous membranes serving as barriers to invasion and the host's ability to mount an immune response (eg, neutralizing antibodies) against such toxins. Colonization by virulent *Staphylococcus* or *Streptococcus* toxin-producing organisms exposed to optimal, focal conditions for growth and toxin production (eg, menstruation plus tampon use or abscess) allows these bacteria to initiate and/or propagate infection.

Thus, minor defects in these barriers, such as those produced by superficial excoriations, toe web fungal infections, or, alternatively, major defects produced by surgery, trauma, burns, or foreign substances (packing, sutures, intravascular catheters, shunts), increase the risk of infection. In addition to these factors, the host response is important. For example, if a patient has an underlying immunodeficiency and cannot produce adequate neutralizing antibodies or as in chronic granulomatous disease where neutrophils lack the oxidative burst to destroy catalase-positive bacteria (eg, *S. aureus*), the patient would be at increased risk for colonization/infection by toxin-producing bacteria. Finally, the types of immune cells activated play an important role in the subsequent host response, especially as it relates to toxins that act as superantigens. As is detailed in this chapter, the ability of a superantigen to activate numerous T cells is based upon the variable region of the T-cell receptor. This could result in various types of responses, depending on the specificity of the individual T-cell that is activated.

DISEASES CAUSED BY EXFOLIATIVE TOXINS

S. aureus–mediated production of exfoliative toxin results in a spectrum of blistering skin disorders ranging from localized bullous impetigo to a severe generalized form, staphylococcal scalded-skin syndrome (SSSS). SSSS is a generalized exanthematous disease consisting of cutaneous tenderness and widespread superficial blistering and denudation.

ETIOLOGY AND PATHOGENESIS

Exfoliative toxins (ETs) are made by certain strains of *S. aureus* (usually phage group 2). Exfoliatin A and B (ETA and ETB) are 2 serologically distinct proteins produced by *S. aureus*.[2] ETs are serine proteases that bind to the cell-adhesion molecule desmoglein-1 and cleave it resulting in a loss of cell–cell adhesion.[3] Consistent with the pattern of desmoglein-1 protein expression, which is found in the upper part of the epidermis, the epidermolysis takes place usually between the stratum spinosum and granulosum. This results in a very-thin-walled, flaccid blister that is easily disrupted, exhibiting a positive Nikolsky sign. The pathophysiology of ET resembles that of the autoimmune blistering disease pemphigus foliaceus, with both diseases targeting desmoglein-1. Presumably, staphylococcal bacteria have evolved this toxin to allow the bacteria to proliferate and spread beneath the stratum corneum barrier of the skin. There are 2 forms of ET-mediated disease: localized bullous impetigo and systemic SSSS. Studies suggest that the majority of localized bullous impetigo are caused by ETA and systemic forms, such as

TABLE 152-1
Toxins and Diseases Caused by *Staphylococcus aureus* and Group A *Streptococcus*

BACTERIA	TOXIN	TOXIN TYPE	CLINICAL DISEASE
Staphylococcus aureus	Exfoliatin type A (ETA)	Epidermolytic	Bullous impetigo Staphylococcal scalded skin syndrome (SSSS)
	Exfoliatin type B (ETB)	Epidermolytic	SSSS Bullous impetigo
	Toxic shock syndrome toxin 1 (TSST-1)	Superantigen	Toxic shock syndrome (TSS) (menstrual >> nonmenstrual), food poisoning
	Staphylococcal enterotoxins A to C (SEA, SEB, SEC)	Superantigen	TSS (nonmenstrual > menstrual), food poisoning
Streptococcus pyogenes	Streptococcal pyrogenic exotoxins A and C (SPEA, SPEC)	Superantigen	TSS (nonmenstrual), scarlet fever

SSSS, are caused by ETB, possibly because of a lower titer of anti–ETB-neutralizing antibodies in the general population.[4] Although some reports suggest that ETs can also act as superantigens (see below) in addition to their epidermolytic activities,[5] this has been questioned.[6]

CLINICAL FEATURES

LOCALIZED FORM (BULLOUS IMPETIGO)

Figures 152-1 and 152-2 show the blisters of bullous impetigo in a child.

Infection of the upper part of the skin (epidermis) by *S. aureus* or *S. pyogenes* results in impetigo contagiosum. Impetigo, which may account for up to 10% of all pediatric skin problems, consists of honey-colored crusts on an erythematous base. Approximately 25% of cases of impetigo are bullous as a result of local ET-expressing *Staphylococcus* without hematogenous dissemination. As is the case with SSSS, bullous impetigo tends to be a disease of children, although adult cases can also occur. The early lesions of bullous impetigo are cloudy vesicles or bullae surrounded by an erythematous rim. These blisters often rupture leaving superficial erosions. Lesions at various stages can often be seen. The lesions tend to be found around exposed parts of body and around orifices. Diagnosis is usually based upon clinical appearance. In contrast to SSSS, confirmation of diagnosis can be easily obtained by aspiration of blister fluid for Gram stain and cultures will reveal *S. aureus*.

GENERALIZED FORM (STAPHYLOCOCCAL SCALDED-SKIN SYNDROME)

Figures 152-3 and 152-4 depict clinical findings of SSSS in children.

The clinical features of SSSS were first described in 1878 by the German physician Baron Gotfried Ritter von Rittershain, who reported almost 300 cases of "dermatitis exfoliativa neonatorum" among young children.[7] The term *Ritter disease* is still used to denote generalized SSSS in neonates. Outbreaks of SSSS tend to occur in clusters as a consequence of cross-infection. Typically, neonatal or maternity hospital staff colonized or infected with ET-producing staphylococci is the source of these outbreaks. Although more commonly seen in infants and children, SSSS also can be seen in adults. The risk factors for adults include a compromised immune response allowing for growth of the *S. aureus* and possibly impaired amounts of toxin-neutralizing antibodies or renal insufficiency decreasing the clearance of the toxin. Affected individuals initially exhibit a faint, orange-red macular exanthem sparing mucosal surfaces in association with a purulent conjunctivitis, otitis media, nasopharyngeal infection or occasionally pyogenic skin infection such as from an umbilical stump or boil (carbuncle). Periorificial and flexural accentuation of the exanthema is often noted. Although the early rash is not distinctive in appearance, the concomitant cutaneous tenderness is usually present at this early stage. Tenderness can be often so severe that an infant will refuse to lie down or allow anyone to hold them. Within 1 to 2 days the rash progresses from an exanthematous scarlatiniform to a blistering eruption. Characteristic, very superficial, tissue-paper-like wrinkling of the epidermis progresses to large flaccid bullae in flexural and periorificial surfaces. A positive Nikolsky sign can be elicited by stroking the skin, resulting in a superficial blister. Large sheets of epidermal surface are typically shed, revealing a moist underlying erythematous base.

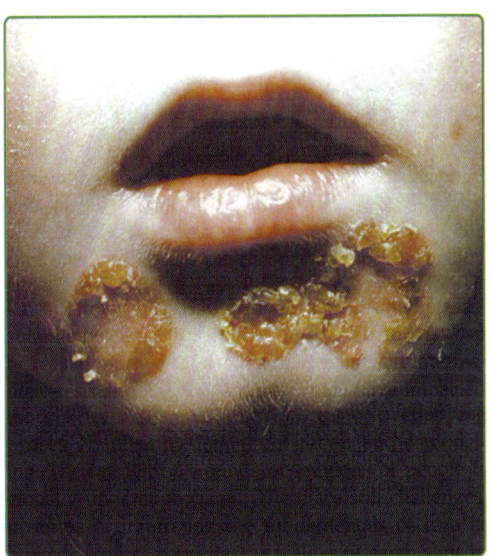

Figure 152-1 Bullous impetigo in a child. Blisters are initially filled with cloudy fluid and later rupture, resulting in erosions and crusting.

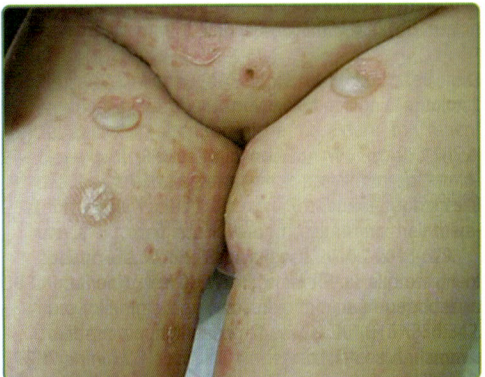

Figure 152-2 Bullous impetigo in a child. Note blisters filled with cloudy fluid and lesions that have ruptured, leading to erosions and crusting.

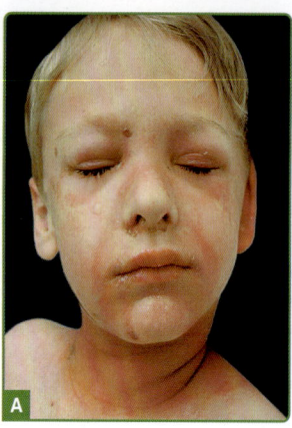
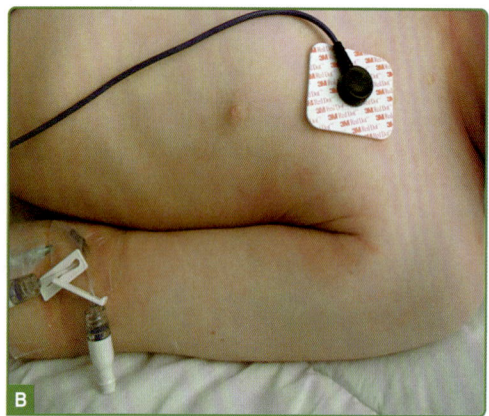
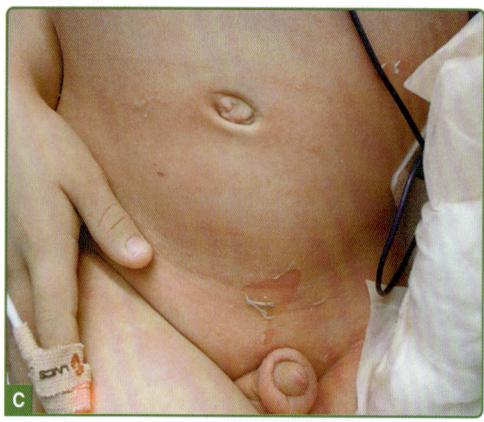

Figure 152-3 Staphylococcal scalded-skin syndrome (SSSS). Pictures of early SSSS demonstrating the development of indistinct erythema with positive Nikolsky sign and superficial erosions.

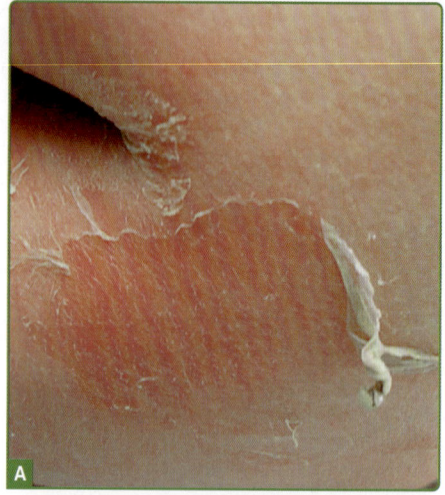
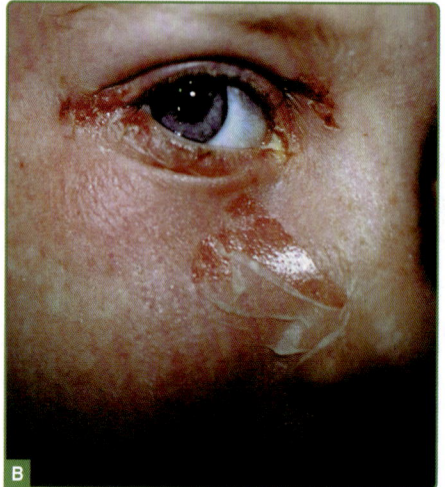
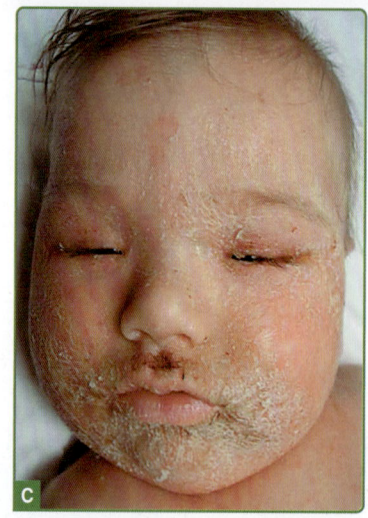

Figure 152-4 Staphylococcal scalded-skin syndrome (SSSS). Pictures of later SSSS. **A,** The same patient as in Figure 156-3A, 24 hours later, with erythema and more superficial blisters with desquamation of large sheets. **B,** Superficial erosions with underlying denuded skin. **C,** Characteristic crusting with superficial erosions noted on face of this 10-month-old with SSSS.

At this stage, the disease looks very worrisome, as if a generalized scalding burn had occurred. Although fevers are often present, the infants and children do not usually appear toxic. The cutaneous process usually resolves by use of antibiotics, with superficial desquamation and healing complete within 5 to 7 days. Cultures obtained from an intact blister are usually sterile, consistent with the pathogenesis of a hematogenously disseminated toxin originating from a distant focus of infection inducing the disease.

INTERMEDIATE (ABORTIVE) FORMS

In addition to localized bullous impetigo and generalized SSSS, intermediate forms of staphylococcal-mediated eruptions in which blistering can be apparent can be encountered. One scenario is that localized bullous impetigo evolves to produce regionally limited bullae and denuded areas that may or may not actually harbor *S. aureus*. A possibly abortive form of SSSS known as the scarlatiniform variant with features of the early erythrodermic and final desquamative stages yet very little blister formation also has been described (see section "Staphylococcal Scarlet Fever").[8] Again, because *S. aureus* bacteria strains can produce both exfoliative and other superantigenic toxins, and ETs could potentially have superantigenic activity,[5] it is not surprising that rarely overlapping syndromes with features of toxic shock and scalded skin can be observed (see sections "Toxic Shock Syndrome" and "Staphylococcal Scarlet Fever").

DIAGNOSIS AND DIFFERENTIAL DIAGNOSIS

All forms of SSSS are characterized by intraepidermal cleavage with splitting beneath and within the stratum granulosum (see histology in Fig. 152-5). The cleavage space may contain either partially or totally unattached acantholytic cells. However, the remainder of the epidermis is usually unremarkable and the dermis contains few inflammatory cells. In localized bullous impetigo, more inflammatory cells including neutrophils can be often visualized.

The principal diagnostic problem is distinguishing generalized SSSS from toxic epidermal necrolysis (TEN) (see Chap. 44). It should be noted that the cases that represented Lyell's first description of TEN actually included some that were probably SSSS.[9] The age distributions of SSSS (neonates, children) and TEN tend to be different, yet much overlap occurs. Use of frozen sections that can rapidly differentiate the superficial subgranular epidermolysis in SSSS versus the characteristic full-thickness epidermal necrosis and dermal–epidermal separation seen in TEN can be very helpful.

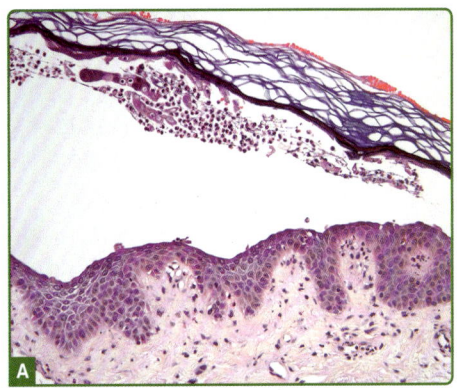
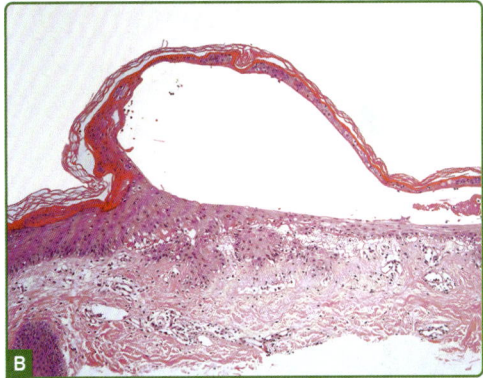

Figure 152-5 Histology of (**A**) bullous impetigo (×200 magnification) versus (**B**) staphylococcal scalded-skin syndrome (SSSS) (×100 magnification). In both conditions, the intraepidermal cleavage induced by the epidermolytic toxin occurs within or just below the stratum granulosum. Note paucity of cells in generalized disease (SSSS) in comparison to the large numbers of leucocytes found in the localized form (bullous impetigo).

TREATMENT AND PROGNOSIS

Therapy for bullous impetigo may constitute topical mupirocin ointment therapy alone and/or oral antibiotics. Prognosis for recovery is excellent. Therapy for SSSS should be directed toward eradication of *S. aureus*, which generally requires hospitalization and intravenous antistaphylococcal antibiotics. For uncomplicated cases, oral antibiotics can usually be substituted after several days. The use of suitable antibiotics combined with supportive skin care and management of potential fluid and electrolyte abnormalities resulting from the widespread disruption of barrier function will usually be sufficient to ensure rapid recovery. Neonates benefit from incubators to maintain body temperature and humidity. Nonadherent dressings, including petrolatum-impregnated gauze, placed over the widespread areas of superficial blistering are helpful. Antibiotic mupirocin ointment applied several times each day to clearly impetiginized areas, including the original source, is often a helpful adjunct to the systemic antibiotics.

Major complications of SSSS are serious fluid and electrolyte disturbances. The mortality in uncomplicated pediatric SSSS is very low (2%) and is not usually associated with sepsis. Adult mortality is higher (approximately 10%) as a result of the concomitant morbidity factors and increased likelihood of sepsis.

DISEASES CAUSED BY SUPERANTIGENIC TOXINS

ETIOLOGY AND PATHOGENESIS

Superantigens are a group of microbial and viral proteins that differ in several important respects from conventional peptide antigens (Fig. 152-6) (reviewed in McCormick and colleagues[10] and Brosnahan and Schlievert[11]). First, unlike conventional protein antigens, which are taken up and processed by antigen-presenting cells, superantigens exert their effects as globular extracellular intact proteins. Similar to peptide antigens, class II major histocompatibility complex (MHC) molecules are involved; however, they do not interact with the MHC peptide β-antigen-binding groove, but instead bind to conserved amino acid residues that are on the outer walls of the peptide antigen-binding groove. Thus, whereas recognition of conventional peptide antigens by the T-cell receptor is restricted by MHC alleles, recognition of superantigens is generally not MHC restricted. Second, superantigens primarily recognize and bind to the variable region of the T-cell receptor β chain (Vβ). This is in contrast to nominal peptide antigens, which require recognition by all 5 variable elements (ie, Vβ, Dβ, Jβ, Vα, and Jα) of the T-cell receptor. Therefore, the responding frequency of a superantigen for resting T cells is several orders of magnitude greater (up to 30%) than a conventional peptide antigen (0.01% to 0.1%) The unique ability of a superantigen to bind directly to (and signal through) MHC class II molecules, and crosslink (and thus activate) a large percentage of T cells expressing relevant T-cell receptor Vβ chains, provides an explanation for the potent immune stimulation seen with these molecules. Of note, in comparison to nominal antigens, activation of superantigen-mediated T cells tends to generate increased numbers of T cells expressing the skin homing receptor cutaneous lymphocyte antigen (CLA).[12] Given that CLA-positive T cells are the T-cell type that traffics readily to the skin, the increased numbers of CLA-positive T cells generated by these agents is thought to be responsible for the high propensity of cutaneous manifestations in these conditions. Superantigens lead to a massive release of cytokines, including tumor necrosis factor α, interleukin-1, and interleukin-6. This cytokine "storm" is in great part responsible for a capillary leak syndrome and accounts for the majority of the clinical manifestations seen in superantigen-mediated diseases. The prototypical disease caused by superantigens is toxic shock syndrome (TSS) caused by staphylococcal or streptococcal toxins (see next). Although specific syndromes, such as TSS and scarlet fever, have characteristic findings, overlap syndromes have been described. Given that the individual clinical findings are the summation of amount(s) and type(s) of toxins and the types of cells responding to activation, it should not be surprising that heterogeneity in clinical presentations could occur.

Unlike syndromes associated with ETs, which usually do not exhibit significant systemic symptoms, those resulting from superantigens are characterized by systemic manifestations. Superantigen-mediated toxin syndromes can be divided into *intermediate cutaneous and systemic* or *predominantly systemic* based on the relative amounts of systemic toxicity. Disorders that have predominantly systemic manifestations are scarlet fever and the most ominous toxin-mediated disease, TSS The *intermediate cutaneous and systemic* category would include syndromes such as recalcitrant erythematous desquamating disorder (REDD) and toxin-mediated erythema, which are less systemic versions of TSS and scarlet fever, respectively. All of these superantigen-mediated disorders are diagnosed based on clinical findings, and can be

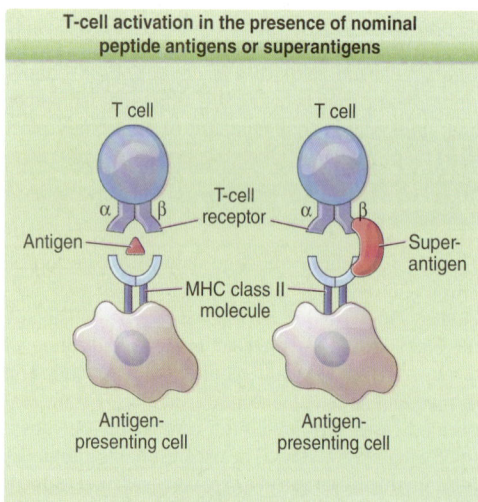

Figure 152-6 T-cell activation in the presence of nominal peptide antigens (*left*) or superantigens (*right*). The peptide antigen binds in the groove of the major histocompatibility complex (MHC) class II molecule and activates only antigen-specific T cells through the T-cell receptor. In contrast, a superantigen is a large globular protein that binds to the MHC class II molecule outside the antigen-binding groove and directly crosslinks the MHC class II molecule and the Vβ chain of the T-cell receptor, leading to polyclonal T-cell activation.

caused by toxins produced by either *S. aureus* or group A *Streptococcus*.

TOXIC SHOCK SYNDROME

Figure 152-7 illustrates TSS caused by *S. aureus*.

TSS is an inflammatory response characterized by fever, rash, hypotension, and multiorgan involvement representing the severe end of the spectrum of superantigen-mediated diseases. Although first described in 1978 in a series of children with *S. aureus* infection,[13] TSS became recognized with reports of epidemics associated with use of highly absorbent tampons in menstruating women in the early 1980s.[14] Presumably the tampon served as a nidus for infection, the blood adding protein and neutralizing the normally bactericidal acidic vaginal pH. Since the first descriptions, TSS has been shown to be associated with many types of staphylococcal and streptococcal infections.

CLINICAL FINDINGS

Staphylococcal Toxic Shock Syndrome: The most common staphylococcal toxin associated with TSS is TSS toxin-1 (TSST-1), and is the predominant toxin associated with menstrual-associated cases. TSST-1 appears unique among superantigens in its ability to cross mucosal surfaces. With the removal of highly absorbent tampons from the market and patient education, the numbers of menstruation-associated TSS have decreased steadily, and at present the incidence of nonmenstrual TSS exceeds that of menstrual-associated cases. Nonmenstrual TSS is associated with postsurgical wounds, sinusitis, osteomyelitis, influenza, intravenous drug use, burn wounds, and gynecologic infection (especially in the postpartum period). Other staphylococcal toxins, including staphylococcal enterotoxin B (SEB) and enterotoxin C (SEC), also can be found. SEB and SEC superantigenic toxins comprise approximately 50% of nonmenstrual TSS. The host response is an important factor in the development of TSS as studies have shown an increased susceptibility in patients who do not have neutralizing antibodies against TSST-1.[15]

The symptoms of TSS begin with acute onset of fever, sore throat, and myalgia. Diarrhea is common, and vomiting may also occur. The rash is most often a macular erythema but a scarlatiniform type can sometimes be seen. The eruption usually begins on the trunk and spreads to the extremities, and can involve palms and soles. Especially if the patient is hypotensive, the eruption tends to be more prominent on the trunk than extremities. Symptoms of hypotension include orthostatic dizziness, fainting, and overt shock. Nonpurulent conjunctival hyperemia, pharyngeal inflammation and strawberry tongue (see section "Scarlet Fever") are invariably present. Signs of decreased mentation can also occur. The rash will desquamate within 1 to 2 weeks after beginning. Table 152-2 lists the Centers for Disease Control and Prevention (CDC) criteria for TSS. Cases of lesser severity that do not meet the full definition probably do occur frequently, especially with earlier recognition and treatment. In nonmenstruation cases, especially those associated with postoperative infections, the classic signs of a localized infection, such as erythema, pain, and purulence, can be absent (often in contrast to streptococcal TSS).

Streptococcal Toxic Shock Syndrome: Streptococcal TSS was described in the late 1980s as a disease similar to staphylococcal TSS, but caused by invasive group A *Streptococcus*. Streptococcal TSS is more commonly encountered than the staphylococcal form (2 to 4 cases vs 0.3 to 0.5 cases per 100,000 population, respectively).[16] The majority of cases of streptococcal TSS are caused by streptococcal pyrogenic exotoxin A (SPEA), yet other superantigenic toxins including streptococcal pyrogenic exotoxin B (SPEB), streptococcal pyrogenic exotoxin C (SPEC), and involvement of other non–group A *Streptococcus* also have been reported. Although not associated with tampon use, streptococcal TSS can result from nearly any type of group A streptococcal infection. The most common types of infections appear to be wounds, and streptococcal TSS has been well-described as a complication of varicella and influenza A. However, in many cases the route of infection cannot be determined. The initial presentation is skin pain often localized to an extremity. The localized pain often progresses over several days to localized erythema and edema to cellulitis associated with necrotizing fasciitis and myositis with concomitant streptococcal invasion of the bloodstream. It should be noted that blood cultures are positive in more than half of patients with streptococcal TSS, in contrast to only 10% of patients with staphylococcal TSS. Thus, a patient with signs of TSS and a localized cellulitis should suggest streptococcal TSS, as soft-tissue infections are not usually seen with staphylococcal TSS. Although very young, elderly, diabetic or

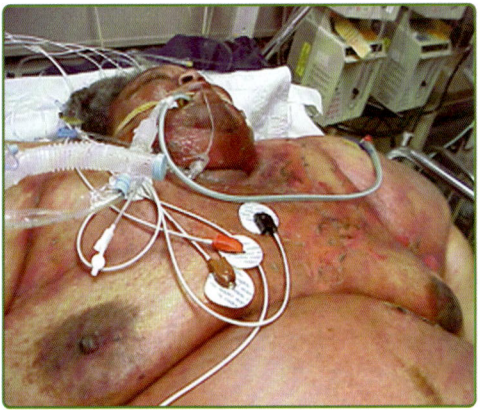

Figure 152-7 Toxic shock syndrome (TSS). Patient in intensive care unit with TSS caused by *Staphylococcus aureus*. Note patient's eruption is nonspecific erythema around intertriginous areas and face. The eruption associated with staphylococcal TSS varies and could be morbilliform, scarlatiniform, or even pustular.

TABLE 152-2
Centers for Disease Control and Prevention 2011 Case Definition of Staphylococcal Toxic Shock Syndrome

MAJOR CRITERIA (ALL 4 MUST BE MET)	MULTISYSTEM INVOLVEMENT (3 OR MORE MUST BE MET)	NORMAL TEST RESULTS (IF PERFORMED)
Fever: temperature >38.9°C (102°F) **Rash:** diffuse macular erythroderma **Desquamation:** 1 to 2 weeks after onset of illness, particularly on palms/soles **Hypotension:** systolic blood pressure <95 mm Hg for adults, or less than 5th percentile by age for children <16 years of age, or orthostatic syncope	**GI:** vomiting or diarrhea at onset of illness **Muscular:** severe myalgia or creatine kinase level twice upper limit of normal **Mucous membrane:** oropharyngeal, conjunctival or vaginal hyperemia **Renal:** blood urea nitrogen or creatinine level twice upper limit of normal, or >5 white blood cells per high-power field in urine in absence of urinary tract infection **Hepatic:** total bilirubin, aspartate aminotransferase, or alanine aminotransferase level at least twice upper limit of normal **Hematologic:** platelets <100,000/mm³ **CNS:** disorientation or alterations in consciousness without focal neurologic signs when fever and hypotension are absent	Blood, throat, or cerebrospinal fluid cultures (blood cultures may be positive for *Staphylococcus aureus*) Rise in titer in antibody tests for Rocky Mountain spotted fever, leptospirosis, or measles

Probable TSS: A case that meets the laboratory criteria and in which 4 of the 5 clinical criteria described above are present.
Confirmed TSS: A case that meets the laboratory criteria and in which all 5 clinical criteria described above are present, including desquamation (unless the patient dies before desquamation takes place).

immunocompromised patients would be more susceptible to streptococcal TSS, the majority of cases have occurred in otherwise healthy adults.

DIFFERENTIAL DIAGNOSIS

Table 152-3 outlines the differential diagnoses of TSS. The differential diagnosis of staphylococcal TSS includes exclusion of septic shock, staphylococcal exfoliative syndromes, Rocky Mountain spotted fever, viral hemorrhagic shock, measles, leptospirosis, and Stevens-Johnson syndrome. Although Kawasaki syndrome has many similar clinical findings, including swelling of extremities and desquamation of palms and soles during convalescence, Kawasaki syndrome differs in that the course of fever is prolonged and diarrhea and hypotension are absent. Streptococcal-mediated syndromes, including scarlet fever and, especially, streptococcal TSS, can mimic staphylococcal TSS.

TABLE 152-3
Differential Diagnoses of Toxic Shock Syndrome

Septic shock
Staphylococcal exfoliative syndromes
Rocky Mountain spotted fever
Viral hemorrhagic shock
Measles
Leptospirosis
Stevens-Johnson syndrome
Kawasaki syndrome

In a patient with fever, rash, and hypotension, a thorough search for possible sites of staphylococcal and streptococcal infection is critical. Surgical wounds should be carefully examined even if no clinical signs of infection are apparent. Vaginal examination and removal of tampon or other foreign body should be done, and vaginal irrigation with saline or povidone-iodine has been recommended.

TREATMENT AND PROGNOSIS

The treatment of TSS is supportive (and usually in the intensive care setting) as well as to eradicate the offending *S. aureus*. Large doses of a beta-lactamase–resistant, antistaphylococcal antibiotic (eg, nafcillin) have been historically used. Because these agents have been known to increase TSST-1 in vitro (probably as a result of cell lysis), concomitant clindamycin or linezolid (both of which will inhibit bacterial protein toxin production) treatment is often used. Given the increasing amounts of methicillin-resistant staphylococci in the community, vancomycin is often recommended. Beta-lactamase–resistant penicillins are of lesser value, not only because of emerging resistance, but also because they have less effect on high levels of bacteria (in contrast to clindamycin or vancomycin). Todd has recommended a combination of vancomycin and clindamycin for suspected serious staphylococcal infections pending culture and sensitivity.[17] Intravenous immunoglobulin (IVIG; which presumably acts in part by neutralizing antibodies against toxins) has been used and appears to have significant promise.[18] As of this writing, IVIG is used in severe or recalcitrant cases. Contraindications to IVIG include previous hypersensitivity to it or immunoglobulin A deficiency. Systemic corticosteroids are controversial, and probably are of lesser impact, possibly because of the report that superantigen-mediated immune cell activation is associated with corticosteroid resistance.[19]

Although clearly a life-threatening disease, the mortality rate of staphylococcal TSS is only approximately 5%, probably because the majority of cases are in otherwise healthy young individuals, as well as because increased recognition of this entity has resulted in earlier intervention. Unfortunately, recurrences can be seen in up to 20% TSS patients. Women who have had TSS should avoid using tampons during menstruation as it will increase the likelihood of reinfection. Diaphragms and contraceptive sponges should also be avoided in this population.

The treatment of streptococcal TSS is similar to staphylococcal TSS. For cases associated with necrotizing fasciitis/myositis, rapid recognition and conservative surgical debridement of devitalized tissue are imperative. IVIG is becoming more recognized as an important part of treatment of streptococcal TSS, especially as the mortality rate in this disease can be greater than 30%.[18] One study has confirmed that IVIG treatment in streptococcal TSS results in statistically significant decreased mortality.[18]

RECALCITRANT ERYTHEMATOUS DESQUAMATING DISORDER

A new presentation of a toxin-mediated disorder, termed *recalcitrant erythematous, desquamating disorder* (REDD), was first described in 1992.[20] The clinical findings include fever and hypotension. The rash of REDD consists of diffuse macular erythema with delayed desquamation. Other findings in common with TSS include ocular and oral mucosal injection and strawberry tongue. Staphylococci producing TSST-1, SEA or SEB have been isolated from various places, including nasal sinuses, soft tissues, and blood. Although the majority of cases described as of this writing had AIDS, some REDD patients without AIDS have been reported. In contrast to TSS, this is a prolonged disease (measured in weeks to several months) in which only several of the TSS criteria are met. Again, the diagnosis is often established by careful examination for occult colonization/infection in a susceptible individual.

SCARLET FEVER

Figure 152-8 illustrates the enanthem and exanthem of Streptococcal scarlet fever.

Scarlet fever is a syndrome characterized by exudative pharyngitis, fever, and scarlatiniform rash. It is most commonly caused by pyrogenic exotoxin-producing group A *Streptococcus*, although staphylococcal infections can produce a similar-appearing disease. The exact mechanism by which toxins produce the symptomology is unclear. Compelling studies by Schlievert that the scarlatiniform eruption could only be induced in mice that were previously sensitized against toxins, suggests that a combination of a conventional delayed type and superantigen-mediated processes are occurring.[21] It should be noted that streptococcal toxins, especially SPEA has areas of significant homology with collagen, which could provide a mechanism for rare autoimmune sequelae of streptococcal scarlet fever, including renal failure and rheumatic fever.[22,23] It should be noted that scarlet fever is no longer the major public health threat it was in the past; not only because of antibiotic treatment but that most streptococcal isolates causing scarlet fever express the less virulent SPEB and SPEC rather than SPEA.

STREPTOCOCCAL SCARLET FEVER

Streptococcal scarlet fever is a childhood disease, and is most common in winter and early spring. It is estimated that up to 10% of childhood group A streptococcal pharyngitis patients develop scarlet fever. Approximately 12 hours to 5 days after exposure, an abrupt prodrome consisting of pharyngitis, headache, vomiting, abdominal pain, and fever develops. The rash appears 1 to 2 days after onset of the illness, first on the neck and then extending to the trunk and extremities, although sparing the palms and soles. The exanthem texture is usually coarse like fine-grade sandpaper, and the erythema blanches with pressure. The skin can be mildly pruritic, but usually is not painful. A few days following generalization of the exanthem, it becomes more intense around skinfolds and lines of confluent petechiae resulting from increased capillary fragility (the Pastia sign) can be seen. The generalized exanthem begins to fade 3 to 4 days after onset and a desquamative phase begins, usually starting with the face. Peeling from the palms and fingers and sometimes soles occurs approximately a week later and can last for as long as 1 month.

Oral findings of streptococcal scarlet fever include edematous, erythematous tonsils sometimes covered with a yellow, gray, or white exudate and tender anterior cervical lymphadenopathy is common. Petechiae and punctuate red macules are seen on the soft palate and uvula (Forchheimer spots). A flushed face with circumoral pallor is also commonly noted. The tongue in scarlet fever has characteristic changes. During the first 2 days of the disease, the tongue has a white coat through which the red and edematous papillae project (white strawberry tongue). After 2 days, the tongue desquamates resulting in a red tongue with prominent papillae (red strawberry tongue).

The diagnosis of scarlet fever is made by the characteristic clinical signs and confirmed by rapid streptococcal test or throat culture. Scarlet fever usually follows a benign course and any undue morbidity/mortality is likely to be from suppurative complications, including peritonsillar abscess, sinusitis,

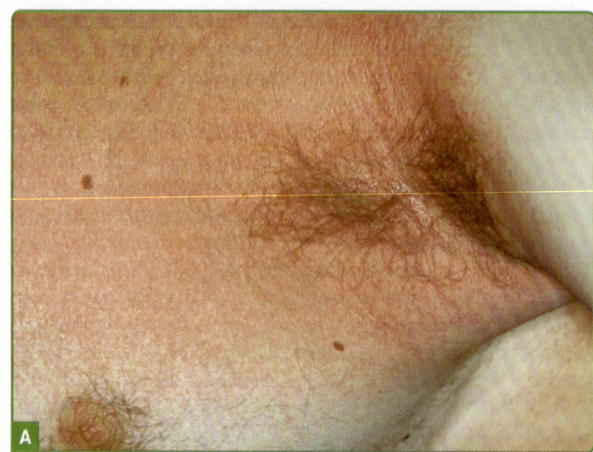
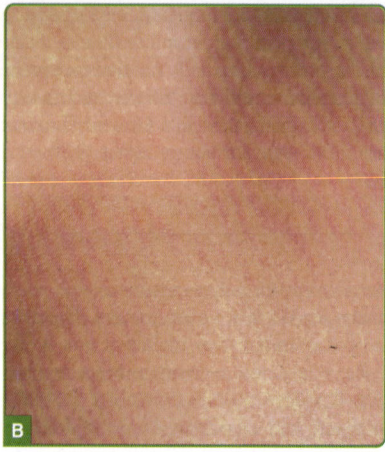
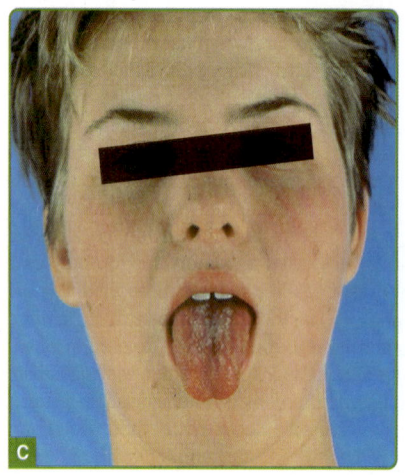
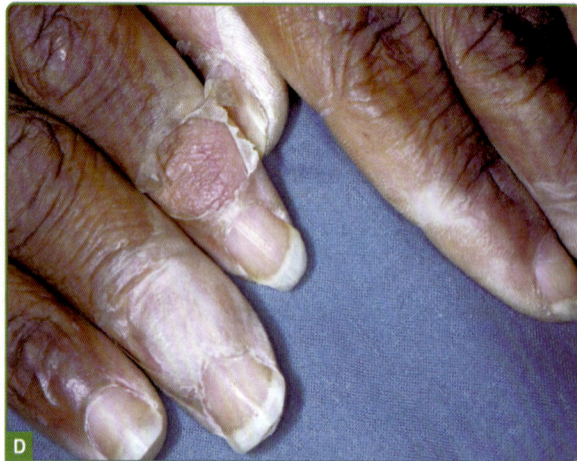

Figure 152-8 Scarlet fever: exanthem and enanthem. **A** and **B,** Significant erythema with a sandpaper texture is noted on trunk. **C,** Beefy "strawberry" red tongue. **D,** Poststreptococcal desquamation.

pneumonia, and meningitis, or from nonsuppurative complications associated with immune-related rheumatic fever or glomerulonephritis. The risk of acute rheumatic fever following an untreated group A streptococcal infection is estimated to be approximately 3% in epidemics, and 0.3% in endemic scenarios. The risk of glomerulonephritis can be up to 15% after infection with nephritogenic group A streptococcal strain. In addition to pharyngitis, group A *Streptococcus* can cause scarlet fever–like eruptions from skin (often surgical wounds) or uterine infections.

Treatment of scarlet fever is by antibiotics (penicillin or erythromycin for a 10-day course) and supportive care. Fever usually abates within 12 to 24 hours after initiation of antibiotic therapy. Recurrences are common.

STAPHYLOCOCCAL SCARLET FEVER

Staphylococcal scarlet fever, also known as scarlatiniform erythroderma/rash, was first described in 1927 and until recently was considered to be a milder or abortive form of SSSS.[21] Patients usually develop a generalized erythroderma with a roughened, sandpaper-like texture. The exanthem of staphylococcal scarlet fever tends to be more tender than corresponding streptococcal scarlet fever. Systemic signs, including malaise and fever, are invariably present. Within a few days of initiation of rash, thick flakes develop and the entire skin desquamates over the next week. Unlike generalized SSSS, the scarlatiniform eruption is not associated with the formation of bullae or superficial exfoliation and can be very difficult to differentiate from other infectious erythrodermal causes, such as TSS and streptococcal scarlet fever. Scarlet fever induced by staphylococci differs from streptococcal-mediated disease by the lack of pharyngitis. A study by Wang and colleagues examined the clinical characteristics and toxin(s) detected from 20 children with staphylococcal scarlet fever.[23] They found that all of the patient's staphylococcal infections arose from the skin; 16 of 20 cases from furuncles/carbuncles; 2 each from abscesses or wound infections. All of the *S. aureus* strains expressed SEB. Of note, SEB shows significant protein sequence homology with SPEA, a known exotoxin associated with streptococcal scarlet fever. Yet other studies have implicated other staphylococcal enterotoxins.[24] One explanation for this heterogeneity of toxins associated with this disorder is that the diagnosis is made upon clinical grounds. It is possible that staphylococcal scarlet fever represents an incomplete form of TSS, in which toxins spread from the skin and thus activating the skin-associated lymphoid tissue rather than mucosal-associated lymphoid tissue. Because most cases of streptococcal scarlet fever arise from a pharyngitis, the lack of pharyngitis in a patient with characteristic rash and other clinical signs of scarlet fever should alert the clinician to look for a localized nidus of infection (eg, furuncle) that could be cultured to establish the diagnosis.

DIFFERENTIAL DIAGNOSIS

The diagnosis of scarlet fever is made upon clinical grounds with supporting positive bacterial cultures. The differential diagnosis of scarlet fever would include other toxin-mediated disorders, including SSSS. Although Kawasaki syndrome has many similar clinical findings, including mucosal involvement (eg, strawberry tongue), and swelling of extremities and desquamation of palms and soles during convalescence, Kawasaki syndrome differs in that the course of fever is prolonged and cultures would be expected to be negative. Atypical drug hypersensitivity reactions can have some cutaneous but less likely mucosal features and there is usually a history of an offending drug and peripheral eosinophilia. Scarlet fever from group A *Streptococcus* can usually be differentiated from that induced by *S. aureus* as the usual nidus of infection in streptococcal scarlet fever is from a pharyngitis whereas the staphylococcal variant usually has its infectious nidus in the skin.

TREATMENT AND PROGNOSIS

The treatment of scarlet fever includes antibiotics to eradicate the offending bacteria. If the localized nidus of infection is an abscess or furuncle/carbuncle, then this should be drained. Acute rheumatic fever or glomerulonephritis are not associated with staphylococcal scarlet fever. For situations in which more systemic signs resembling TSS are becoming apparent, then the treatment could resemble TSS (see above).

TOXIN-MEDIATED ERYTHEMA (RECURRENT TOXIN-MEDIATED PERINEAL ERYTHEMA)

In 1996, Manders and colleagues recognized a previously unreported toxin-mediated disorder, which they termed *recurrent toxin-mediated perineal erythema*.[25] Recurrent toxin-mediated perineal erythema is characterized by a striking diffuse macular perineal erythema that occurs within 24 to 48 hours after a pharyngitis with a toxin-producing group A *Streptococcus* or *S. aureus*. Clinical findings seen in scarlet fever, including a strawberry tongue, as well as erythema, edema, and, later, palmoplantar desquamation, are commonly found in recurrent perineal erythema. Fever, hypotension, and other systemic signs of scarlet fever or TSS are characteristically absent, although diarrhea is a common feature. Recurrences are more frequently found in this localized form. It has been proposed by Manders that that the term *toxin-mediated erythema* be used to describe the following clinical settings in which a toxin-producing *Staphylococcus* or *Streptococcus* can be found: recurrent erythroderma associated with a preceding bacterial pharyngitis; isolated episodes of toxin-mediated erythema without recurrences; and patients with episodic mild hypotension, fever, and typical mucocutaneous findings in the absence of full criteria for TSS.[26]

OTHER DISEASES INITIATED AND/OR EXACERBATED BY SUPERANTIGENS

In addition to the ability of superantigens to induce characteristic diseases including TSS, scarlet fevers, and gastroenteritis, recent evidence is accumulating indicating that these potent immunomodulatory agents can initiate and/or exacerbate other skin disorders.

PSORIASIS

Psoriasis (see Chap. 28) is an autoimmune T-cell–driven keratinocyte hyperproliferative disease involving skin and, rarely, joints. Superantigens have been implicated in psoriasis in at least 2 settings, the guttate (acute eruptive) form and where psoriasis flares in response to becoming secondarily infected.[27,28]

The acute guttate form of psoriasis is characterized by the rapid onset of small erythematous psoriasiform papules which can be generalized. This form can develop during or most commonly right after a group A streptococcal infection (usually pharyngitis). More commonly found in children and young adults, guttate psoriasis has been estimated to be the initiation of psoriasis in up to 20% of patients. Studies examining a series of guttate psoriasis patients have demonstrated the association of an SPEC-expressing group A *Streptococcus* along with expansion of the appropriate T-cell receptor β Vβ pattern in the skin lesions and in perilesional skin.[27] These and other supporting studies do suggest that the superantigen-mediated systemic activation of T cells and MHC II–expressing accessory cells, resulting in the uncovering of the specific oligoclonal activation seen in chronic lesions, is a plausible explanation for how infection could initiate this form of psoriasis.

In addition to the ability of systemic activation by a superantigen to initiate psoriasis, accumulating evidence has emerged that a localized infection with a superantigen-secreting microbe could be the trigger for worsening of psoriasis. For example, patients with psoriasis have an increased cutaneous reactivity to the topical application of small (nanogram) amounts of superantigens, which is caused by the increased levels of keratinocyte MHC II expression seen in patients with activated psoriasis.[28] Thus, guttate psoriasis and flaring of existing psoriasis should prompt a careful examination and treatment of microbial infections. In women, a history of possible menstrual-associated flares of psoriasis (especially with tampon use) should prompt appropriate investigations and treatment.

AUTOECZEMATIZATION (ID) RESPONSE

The autoeczematization (id) response is an acute, generalized skin reaction to a variety of stimuli. This stimulus may be a preexisting or new dermatitis (most often on the lower leg), or skin infection with fungi, bacteria, viruses, or parasites. The erythematous and papular pruritic rash often develops at distant sites and tends to be symmetric. No concomitant systemic toxicities are usually seen. One common clinical scenario is a patient with known stasis dermatitis who develops an allergic skin reaction to topical agent (neomycin-containing antibiotic) used on the leg. Given the ability of superantigens to stimulate significantly high numbers of T cells expressing CLA and thus use these homing receptors to traffic to skin, localized bacterial infection with a superantigen-producing *S. aureus* or group A *Streptococcus* could result in an autoeczematization response. Thus, careful examination of a patient with autoeczematization response for a microbial trigger is warranted.

ATOPIC DERMATITIS

Secondary infection with *S. aureus* or group A *Streptococcus* is a well-known trigger for atopic dermatitis (see Chap. 22). It is estimated that *S. aureus* can be cultured from essentially all subjects with atopic dermatitis (reviewed in Ong and Leung[29]). Studies demonstrate that skin from subjects with active atopic dermatitis have decreased levels of antimicrobial proteins.[30] This lack of antimicrobial proteins may provide one explanation for the almost universal bacterial infection associated with flaring atopic dermatitis. The mechanism(s) by which bacterial infection can worsen atopic dermatitis is an active area of study and, not surprisingly, superantigens have been implicated. In addition to the "usual" mechanism of crosslinking T-cell receptor and MHC-II molecules, it has been shown that many atopic dermatitis patients have immunoglobulin E antibodies that recognize these globular proteins.[31] Thus, in addition to being a superantigen, these toxins can act as allergens in this population. Other gram-positive bacterial products have been associated with the worsening of atopic dermatitis. This includes the lytic toxin staphylococcal delta-toxin, which has been shown to trigger mast cell degranulation.[32] High levels (mcg/cm^2) of the bacterial cell wall constituent lipoteichoic acid are found on clinically impetiginized atopic skin,[33] which could have clinical significance as lipoteichoic acid acts on both toll-like receptor 2 as well as the platelet-activating factor receptor.[34]

CUTANEOUS T-CELL LYMPHOMA

Although potential infectious causes for cutaneous T-cell lymphoma (CTCL; see Chap. 119) have been extensively investigated, the etiology for this rare T-cell dyscrasia remains as yet unknown (reviewed in Mirvish and colleagues[35]). However, several observations suggest that staphylococcal toxins could be playing a role in the clinical progression of CTCL. First, CTCL patients exhibit high levels of *S. aureus* colonization, and this bacteria is a major source of both local and systemic infections in this population. Second, *S. aureus* infection is reported to correlate with CTCL disease severity. Consistent with this notion, antibiotic treatment of *S. aureus* is reported to improve CTCL disease activity in this population of infected patients.

Multiple studies have taken advantage of the fact that superantigens activate specific β patterns to examine CTCL T-cell β patterns as supporting evidence for a role for toxin involvement. In particular, the Duvic group reported that in erythrodermic CTCL patients, those culture-positive for a TSST-1–expressing *S. aureus* exhibited overrepresentation of the β pattern associated with TSST-1 (T-cell receptor β 2.1).[36] The most likely interpretation of these studies is that superantigens are not causing CTCL, but, can worsen disease activity. Thus, patients with CTCL need to be closely monitored and treated appropriately for secondary infection.

REFERENCES

1. Dinges MM, Orwin PM, Schlievert PM. Exotoxins of *Staphylococcus aureus*. *Clin Microbiol Rev.* 2000;13:16.
2. Ladhani S, Joannou CL, Lochrie DP, et al. Clinical, microbial, and biochemical aspects of the exfoliative toxins causing staphylococcal scalded-skin syndrome. *Clin Microbiol Rev.* 1999;12:224.
3. Amagai M, Matsuyoshi N, Wang ZH, et al. Toxin in bullous impetigo and staphylococcal scalded-skin syndrome targets desmoglein I. *Nat Med.* 2000;6:1275.
4. Yamasaki O, Yamaguchi T, Sugai M, et al. Clinical manifestations of staphylococcal scalded skin syndrome depend on serotypes of exfoliative toxins. *J Clin Microbiol.* 2005;43:1890.
5. Rago JV, Vath GM, Bohach GA, et al. Mutational analysis of the superantigen staphylococcal exfoliative toxin A (ETA) *J Immunol.* 2000;164:2207.

6. Plano LR, Gutman DM, Woischnik M, et al. Recombinant *Staphylococcus aureus* exfoliative toxins are not bacterial superantigens. *Infect Immun.* 2000;68:3048.
7. Ritter von Rittershain G. Die exfoliative Dermatitis jüngerer Sauglinge. *Zentralzeitung fur Kinderheilkunde.* 1878;2:3.
8. Melish ME, Glasgow A. The staphylococcal scalded skin syndrome: development of an experimental mouse model. *N Engl J Med.* 1970;282:1114.
9. Lyell A. Toxic epidermal necrolysis: An eruption resembling scalding of the skin. *Br J Dermatol.* 1956;68:355.
10. McCormick JK, Yarwood JM, Schlievert PM. Toxic shock syndrome and bacterial superantigens: an update. *Annu Rev Microbiol.* 2001;55:77.
11. Brosnahan AJ, Schlievert PM. Gram-positive bacterial superantigen outside-in signaling causes toxic shock syndrome. *FEBS J* 2011;278:4649.
12. Leung DY, Gately M, Trumble A, et al. Bacterial superantigens induce T cell expression of the skin-selective homing receptor, the cutaneous lymphocyte-associated antigen, via stimulation of interleukin 12 production. *J Exp Med.* 1995;181(2):747.
13. Todd JK, Kapral FA, Fishaut M, et al. Toxic shock syndrome associated with phage group I staphylococci. *Lancet.* 1978;2:1116.
14. Shands KN, Schmid GP, Dan BB, et al. Toxic shock syndrome in menstruating women: association with tampon use and *Staphylococcus aureus* and clinical features in 52 cases. *N Engl J Med.* 1980;303:1436.
15. Rosten PM, Bartlett KH, Chow AW. Serologic responses to toxic shock syndrome (TSS) toxin-1 in menstrual and nonmenstrual TSS. *Clin Invest Med.* 1988; 11(3):187.
16. Lappin E, Ferguson AJ. Gram-positive toxic shock syndromes. *Lancet Infect Dis.* 2009;9(5):281.
17. Todd JK. Staphylococcal infections. *Pediatr Rev.* 2005;26:444.
18. Linner A, Darenberg J, Sjolin J, et al. Clinical efficacy of polyspecific intravenous immunoglobulin therapy in patients with streptococcal toxic shock syndrome: a comparative observational study. *Clin Infect Dis.* 2014;59:851.
19. Li LB, Goleva E, Hall CF, et al. Superantigen-induced corticosteroid resistance of human T cells occurs through activation of the mitogen-activated protein kinase kinase/extracellular signal-regulated kinase (MEK-ERK) pathway. *J Allergy Clin Immunol.* 2004;114:1059.
20. Cone LA, Woodard DR, Byrd RG, et al. A recalcitrant, erythematous, desquamating disorder associated with toxin-producing staphylococci in patients with AIDS. *J Infect Dis.* 1992;165(4):638.
21. Schlievert PM. Staphylococcal scarlet fever: role of pyrogenic exotoxins. *Infect Immun.* 1981;31(2):732.
22. Reid SD, Hoe NP, Smoot LM, et al. Group A streptococcus: allelic variation, population genetics, and host-pathogen interactions. *J Clin Invest.* 2001;107: 393.
23. Wang CC, Lo WT, Hsu CF, et al. Enterotoxin B is the predominant toxin involved in staphylococcal scarlet fever in Taiwan. *Clin Infect Dis.* 2004;38(10):1498.
24. Jarraud S, Cozon G, Vandenesch F, et al. Involvement of enterotoxins G and I in staphylococcal toxic shock syndrome and staphylococcal scarlet fever. *J Clin Microbiol.* 1999;37:2446.
25. Manders SM, Heymann WR, Atillasoy E, et al. Recurrent toxin-mediated perineal erythema. *Arch Dermatol.* 1996;132(1):57.
26. Manders SM. Toxin-mediated streptococcal and staphylococcal disease. *J Am Acad Dermatol.* 1998;39:383.
27. Leung DY, Travers JB, Giorno R, et al. Evidence for a streptococcal superantigen-driven process in acute guttate psoriasis. *J Clin Invest.* 1995;96:2106.
28. Travers JB, Hamid QA, Norris DA, et al. Epidermal HLA-DR and the enhancement of cutaneous reactivity to superantigenic toxins in psoriasis. *J Clin Invest.* 1999;104(9):1181.
29. Ong PY, Leung DY. Bacterial and viral infections in atopic dermatitis: a comprehensive review. *Clin Rev Allergy Immunol.* 2016;51(3):329-337.
30. Ong PY, Ohtake T, Brandt C, et al. Endogenous antimicrobial peptides and skin infections in atopic dermatitis. *N Engl J Med.* 2002;347(15):1151.
31. Leung DY, Harbeck R, Bina P, et al. Presence of IgE antibodies to staphylococcal exotoxins on the skin of patients with atopic dermatitis. Evidence for a new group of allergens. *J Clin Invest.* 1993;92(3):1374.
32. Nakamura Y, Oscherwitz J, Cease KB, et al. Staphylococcus δ-toxin promotes allergic skin disease by inducing mast cell degranulation. *Nature.* 2013;503(7476):397.
33. Travers JB, Kozman A, Mousdicas N, et al. Infected atopic dermatitis lesions contain pharmacologic amounts of lipoteichoic acid. *J Allergy Clin Immunol.* 2010; 125:146.
34. Zhang Q, Mousdicas N, Yi Q, et al. Staphylococcal lipoteichoic acid inhibits delayed-type hypersensitivity reactions via the platelet-activating factor receptor. *J Clin Invest.* 2005;115:2855.
35. Mirvish JJ, Pomerantz RG, Falo LD Jr, et al. Role of infectious agents in cutaneous T-cell lymphoma: facts and controversies. *Clin Dermatol.* 2013;31:423.
36. Jackow CM, Cather JC, Hearne V, et al. Association of erythrodermic cutaneous T-cell lymphoma, superantigen-positive Staphylococcus aureus, and oligoclonal T-cell receptor V beta gene expansion. *Blood.* 1997;89:32.

Chapter 153 :: Necrotizing Fasciitis, Necrotizing Cellulitis, and Myonecrosis
:: Avery LaChance & Daniela Kroshinksy

第一百五十三章
坏死性筋膜炎、坏死性蜂窝组织炎和肌坏死

中文导读

本章节介绍的三种细菌感染性疾病，均属于比较严重的类型。坏死性筋膜炎是一种罕见的皮肤和皮下软组织的快速进展性感染，其沿筋膜平面追踪并迅速扩散。该病的特征是进行性坏死和高死亡率。坏死性或坏疽性蜂窝组织炎是坏死性感染，有或无气体形成局限于皮肤和皮下组织，但延伸的深度不足以累及基础筋膜或肌肉。肌坏死包括的2种主要感染是化脓性肌炎和梭菌性气体坏疽，这两个疾病的特征都是来自皮下肌肉内部和周围的坏死感染。本章节全面讨论了它们的流行病学、临床特征、病因和发病机制、诊断、鉴别诊断、临床病程和预后、临床管理等内容。

〔汪 犇〕

AT-A-GLANCE

This chapter discusses necrotizing, gangrenous, and purulent bacterial infections of the skin, soft tissue, fascia, and muscle. Broadly speaking, the different entities can be characterized by anatomic depth of infection with necrosis extending to the skin (gangrenous cellulitis), fascia (necrotizing fasciitis), and muscle (pyomyositis). However, it should be noted that there is significant overlap between these entities in terms of presentation, clinical course, and treatment. Given this, some current literature groups these infections (as well as necrotizing fungal infections) into 1 larger, overarching subgroup of *necrotizing soft-tissue infections*.[1] Trends in how the medical community chooses to approach and classify these disease entities may change with time and this broader, all-encompassing nomenclature may become the favored terminology in the future. Given the clinical and management nuances for each of these categories, as well as the fact that the term *necrotizing soft-tissue infections* has not been broadly accepted, this chapter describes the clinical features intrinsic to each separately here. The reader is encouraged to follow how classification for this group of infections may evolve in the literature in the years to come.

NECROTIZING FASCIITIS
HISTORICAL PERSPECTIVES

Necrotizing fasciitis is a rare, rapidly progressive infection of the skin and subcutaneous soft tissue that tracks down to and spreads rapidly along the fascial plane. The disease is characterized by progressive necrosis and high mortality rates in the absence of prompt diagnosis and management.

Initial signs and symptoms of necrotizing fasciitis were described by Hippocrates in the fifth century BC.[2] In 1871, this group of infections was named "hospital gangrene" by Joseph Jones, a surgeon who served in the Confederate Army and subsequently went on to become the Secretary of the Southern Historical Society where he spent time chronicling disease states he encountered in the war.[1,3] In 1918, Pfanner diagnosed a patient with a necrotizing beta-hemolytic streptococcal infection and coined the term *necrotizing erysipelas*.[4] In 1924, a case series of necrotizing infection of the skin and subcutaneous tissue described as "streptococcal gangrene" was reported by Melany.[4] The term *necrotizing fasciitis* was finally introduced by Wilson in 1951 to 1952 to encompass both gas-forming and non–gas-forming necrotizing soft-tissue infections encompassing and spreading along the fascial plane.[2,3] Only recently was necrotizing fasciitis thought to represent part of a larger group of necrotizing and gangrenous soft-tissue infections. More recent literature includes necrotizing fasciitis as one of several necrotizing soft-tissue infections, that are grouped together given similarities in behavior, diagnosis, management, and poor prognosis without prompt intervention.[1,3]

EPIDEMIOLOGY

Data surrounding current necrotizing fasciitis epidemiology is limited. A 2013 study by Psoinos and colleagues utilized the Nationwide Inpatient Sample Database to examine necrotizing soft-tissue infection epidemiology as a group within the United States.[5] This study found 56,527 admissions for necrotizing soft-tissue infections during the period 1998 to 2010, which is an average of 3800 to 5800 admissions for necrotizing soft-tissue infections annually in the United States.[5] Over this time, the incidence peaked in 2004 and demonstrated a downtrend from 2004 to 2010.[5] Conversely, a 2015 study by Oud and Watkins that evaluated data for all inpatient admissions for necrotizing fasciitis in Texas demonstrated, a rise in hospitalization for necrotizing fasciitis over time from 59 cases of necrotizing fasciitis per 1 million patient-years in 2001 to 2002 to 76 cases of necrotizing fasciitis per 1 million patient-years in 2009 to 2010.[6] Studies of the pediatric population are limited. One small study showed the worldwide prevalence of pediatric necrotizing fasciitis between 2010 and 2015 to be 0.8 per 1 million patient-years.[7]

From 2003 to 2013, a total of 9871 deaths from necrotizing fasciitis were reported in the United States, or approximately 4.8 deaths per 1 million patient-years.[8] Arif and colleagues, in a study of these deaths, determined that deaths were higher in black, Hispanic, and Native American individuals than in whites.[8] Death was also found to be lower among Asian American individuals.[8]

ETIOLOGY, MICROBIOLOGY, PATHOGENESIS

The majority of necrotizing fasciitis and other necrotizing soft-tissue infections are community acquired via bacterial introduction through a break in the skin.[9] Although prior surgical sites can be portals of entry, pathogens are often introduced into the skin and subcutaneous tissue through cuts, scrapes, or sites of minor prior trauma, such as bug bites, animal bites, or injection sites in intravenous drug users.[9] In more tropical climates, numerous cases of necrotizing fasciitis have been described following snake bites with a particularly high incidence from the *Naja atra* snake.[10] In a minority of patients, the site of bacterial introduction is never identified, and, in some cases, infection is attributed to prior nonpenetrating trauma (ie, bruise).[9]

Once the bacterial pathogen enters the skin, infection quickly tracks down to and spreads along the fascia. This tracking process is assisted by bacterial release of enzymes that cause tissue breakdown and assist with rapid progression of disease. Although necrotizing fasciitis can involve underlying muscle, often infection tracks along the superficial fascia overlying the muscle without significant muscle involvement.

Although some cases of necrotizing fasciitis occur in otherwise healthy patients, a majority of cases are found in patients with predisposing comorbidities which are thought to place patients at increased risk for developing necrotizing fasciitis.[11] Comorbidities found at increased rates in patients with necrotizing fasciitis include diabetes, cardiovascular disease, IV drug abuse, peripheral vascular disease, venous stasis, vascular insufficiency, obesity, smoking, alcohol abuse, cirrhosis, malignancy, corticosteroid use, and chronic kidney disease.[2,3,9,11] In particular, cardiovascular disease and diabetes are thought to portend the highest risk of necrotizing fasciitis.[2,3] Additionally, patients who are either postpartum or postabortion can develop necrotizing fasciitis along the uterus or at sites of prior episiotomies.[9]

Necrotizing fasciitis in the adult population is often polymicrobial with up to 5 pathogens identified in many cases.[11] Polymicrobial infections are particularly high in 4 specific clinical scenarios: (a) bowel-associated infections (perianal abscesses, penetrating abdominal traumas, or bowel surgery associated); (b) decubitus ulcers; (c) IV drug users; and (d) spread from genital sites.[9] Alternatively, pediatric populations have a higher incidence of monomicrobial infections when compared with infections in adults.[7]

Table 153-1 lists the numerous pathogens identified as causative of or contributors to necrotizing soft-tissue infections/necrotizing fasciitis. Among these, the most common isolate found in community-acquired necrotizing soft-tissue infections is *Streptococcus pyogenes*,

TABLE 153-1
Bacterial Subspecies Isolated in Patients Presenting with Necrotizing Fasciitis

Gram Positive
- Bacillus spp.[2]
- Coagulase-negative Staphylococcus[41]
- Enterococcus spp.[2]
- Group B Streptococcus[41]
- Group D Streptococcus[41]
- Non-A, non-B, non-D Streptococcus[41]
- Staphylococcus aureus[11]
- Streptococcus milleri group
- Streptococcus pneumoniae[2]
- Streptococcus pyogenes[11]
- Viridans streptococci[41]

Gram Negative
- Acinetobacter spp.[2]
- Aeromonas spp.[9]
- Eikenella corrodens
- Enterobacter cloacae[2]
- Escherichia coli[2,11]
- Haemophilus influenzae
- Klebsiella spp.[2]
- Morganella spp.[25]
- Proteus spp.[2]
- Pseudomonas spp.[11]
- Salmonella group B factors 4 and 5[41]
- Serratia Marcescens[2]
- Stenotrophomonas maltophilia[2]
- Vibrio spp.[41]

Anaerobic Bacteria
- Anaerobic gram-negative rods[2]
- Bacteroides spp.[25]
- Citrobacter freundii[2]
- Clostridium spp.[2]
- Fusobacterium necrophorum[16]
- Lactobacillus spp.[16]
- Peptostreptococcus spp.[41]
- Prevotella spp.[16]
- Propionibacterium acnes[16]

and in hospital-acquired infections, the most common isolates are *Staphylococcus aureus*, followed by *Escherichia coli* and *Pseudomonas* spp.[11,12] For patients with diabetes, necrotizing infection caused by *Klebsiella pneumoniae* is described with increased frequency.[13]

CLINICAL FEATURES

CUTANEOUS FEATURES

Early cutaneous changes of necrotizing fasciitis can be quite subtle, and, in the early stages, defining features of erythema, pain, and surrounding edema often mimic classic cellulitis.[2,9] As disease progresses, cutaneous findings can become much more pronounced with more dramatic changes in color (deep erythema or violaceous changes), bullae, and eventually gangrenous or necrotic changes of the skin and subcutaneous tissues.[2,9] Additionally, as lesions worsen, edema can become much more pronounced, occasionally with subcutaneous emphysema and/or firm, woody induration of the surrounding skin and subcutaneous tissue.[2,9] Severe focal pain can precede any identifiable cutaneous changes with pain often spreading outward as disease progresses. During more advanced stages of infection, early sites of involvement can lose this initial sensation of pain and develop progressive anesthesia over involved areas.[2,9] Approximately 66% of cases are reported to begin in the lower extremities with proximal spread following inoculation.[9]

NONCUTANEOUS FEATURES

Although symptoms often start locally at the site of infection, as the disease progresses severe systemic symptoms commonly arise. Often, patients develop systemic illness shortly after the development of cutaneous findings with early complaints of malaise, fever, nausea, and vomiting.[2] Eventually, tachycardia, disorientation, and lethargy often develop as patients progress to take on a septic physiology.[2,9] Given this, many patients progress to require intensive care unit level of care.

SUBTYPES OF NECROTIZING FASCIITIS

MICROBIOLOGIC SUBTYPING OF NECROTIZING FASCIITIS INFECTIONS

Subtyping of necrotizing fasciitis, particularly that based on microbiology, is a source of debate in the literature with no general consensus surrounding classification guidelines. Furthermore, much of the literature does not use any standardized classification system for these infections with a majority of current publications dividing necrotizing fasciitis into simply "monomicrobial" or "polymicrobial" without labeling infections with a standard specific subclassification title. We favor this broader "monomicrobial" versus "polymicrobial" subgrouping; however, given that several subtypes based on microbiology are described in the literature, these subtypes are outlined here to familiarize the reader with these proposed classification systems.

Some authors propose subtyping necrotizing fasciitis infections into 4 major groups based on the microbial pathogens identified within the infection (Table 153-2).[2] Of note, when this classification system is used, the frequency of these subtypes varies regionally. For example, Type III infections, caused by *Vibrio* spp., have increased in frequency in Asian and Australian populations where there is increased exposure to tropical waters.[2] However, using this classification system for populations with less marine-based activity results in a majority of cases being caused by Type I or Type II necrotizing fasciitis. In these non–aquatic-based populations, Type I necrotizing fasciitis predominates

TABLE 153-2
Proposed Cutaneous Variants of Necrotizing Fasciitis

CUTANEOUS VARIANT	DEFINING FEATURES
Type I necrotizing fasciitis	▪ 1 or more anaerobic species ▪ 1 or more facultative anaerobic streptococci (streptococci other than *Streptococcus pyogenes*) ▪ Members of the aerobic Gram-negative rod grouping Enterobacteriaceae[2]

Type II necrotizing fasciitis	▪ Often monomicrobial
	▪ Hemolytic *Streptococcus*
	  ▪ Group A *Streptococcus* (*S. pyogenes*)
	  ▪ Rarely hemolytic *Streptococcus* group C or group G
	▪ ± Coinfection (or monoculture) with *Staphylococcus aureus*[2]

Type III necrotizing fasciitis	▪ *Vibrio* subspecies ▪ Result of puncture wound caused by fish or marine insect[2]
Type IV necrotizing fasciitis	▪ Fungal cases caused by candidal necrotizing fasciitis ▪ Very rare[2]

with approximately 60% of necrotizing fasciitis being caused by pathogens in this grouping, and the remaining approximately 40% being caused by subspecies in Type II necrotizing fasciitis.[2]

More frequently, groups simplify the classification scheme into grouping all polymicrobial infections into *Type I necrotizing fasciitis* and all monomicrobial infections into *Type II necrotizing fasciitis*.[2,3] From this subgroup, some of the older literature describes an entity called *synergistic necrotizing cellulitis*, which is defined by a Type I necrotizing fasciitis with necrosis extending down to and involving the muscle.[14] However, this term has not been used in newer literature; instead, the term *necrotizing soft-tissue infections* has been adopted. *Meleney gangrene* was used to describe polymicrobial cases of necrotizing fasciitis resulting from the synergistic relationship of multiple bacterial species and is also no longer used.[15]

ANATOMIC SUBTYPING OF NECROTIZING FASCIITIS INFECTIONS

Cervical and Craniofacial Necrotizing Fasciitis: *Cervical and craniofacial necrotizing fasciitis* describes a very rare subtype of disease that has an anatomic predilection for the head and neck region.[4] Although trauma is the most common source of infection in these patients, odontogenic, pharyngeal, or tonsillar infections as well as nasal malignancy have been described as additional sources.[4] A few studies have proposed a clinical staging system specifically for cervical necrotizing fasciitis with Stage 1 characterized by tenderness, erythema, swelling, and heat; Stage 2 characterized by blistering and bullae; and Stage 3 characterized by crepitus, anesthesia, and skin necrosis.[16] This staging system has not been adopted more broadly for necrotizing fasciitis at other anatomic locations.

Fournier Gangrene: *Fournier gangrene* refers to necrotizing fasciitis localized to the genitalia, perineum, anus, and, occasionally, skin of the lower abdomen.[3,17] Age at presentation is generally 50 to 60 years, and a majority of these adult patients with Fournier gangrene have significant underlying comorbidities, particularly diabetes mellitus or underlying immunocompromised status.[9,17] Rarely, Fournier gangrene also is noted in the pediatric population, particularly before the age of 3 years, which is thought possibly to be secondary to introduction of infection through underlying diaper dermatitis.[7] Generally, infection stems from underlying retroperitoneal or perianal infection, untreated perirectal abscess, severe urinary tract infection, or trauma to the genital area; given the mechanism of bacterial spread, cases are nearly always polymicrobial (with mixed aerobic and anaerobic pathogens) in nature.[9,17] Additionally, it is important to note that, although the focus of this chapter is on necrotizing bacterial infection of the skin, cases of fungal-mediated Fournier gangrene have been reported in the literature.[18]

Depending on the clinical scenario, infection can begin slowly or progress rapidly and the constellation of symptoms at onset includes erythema, edema, and pain involving the genitalia and surrounding skin.[9] As with cases of necrotizing fasciitis at other sites, clinical findings at onset can be subtle and characterized solely by focal swelling in the genital area with little to no cutaneous changes.[17] Systemic symptoms can include septic shock (like in other forms of necrotizing fasciitis) as well as urinary retention. A CT scan can be obtained fairly rapidly to help delineate anatomic areas of involvement prior to surgical treatment in this sensitive area.[17] Akin to other forms of necrotizing fasciitis, surgical intervention is the first line of therapy and, importantly for patients with extensive rectal involvement, diverting colostomy can be considered to help minimize fecal contamination of surgical wounds and to assist with wound healing following surgical debridement.[17]

DIAGNOSIS

Given the surgical urgency for treating necrotizing fasciitis, surgical consultation and exploration of the concerning site remain the gold standard for diagnosis.[9,19] Firm diagnosis hinges on the unveiling of fascial involvement during surgical exploration and a defining feature of necrotizing fasciitis is notable easy dissection along the superficial fascial planes in attempts made to probe along the edge of an open wound.[2,9] Deep debridement will demonstrate a gray, dusky, edematous fascial plane.[9] Additionally, dissection should reveal underlying necrosis often with a thin, stringy-brown exudate from sites of dissection.[9] Scoring systems and other alternative diagnostic tests as of this writing have been more useful in ruling out necrotizing soft-tissue infection than aiding with confirming diagnosis.[9]

A thorough cutaneous examination can play a key role in helping to determine which patients warrant prompt surgical evaluation for diagnosis and/or debridement. If diagnosis is unclear during clinical examination, a small exploratory incision can be made into the center of the site in question to look for underlying diagnostic features as listed in "Clinical Features" section.[9] If not already performed while awaiting surgical consultation, tissue culture should be obtained during the first surgical debridement to help guide antimicrobial therapy.[3] Deep tissue cultures are preferred to superficial swabs given the increased sensitivity of deep tissue cultures in identifying the culprit organism(s).[9]

In situations in which surgical evaluation is delayed, biopsy can be performed to determine the architecture of involved tissue and for tissue culture. Given the emergent nature of this process, any biopsies taken for standard processing should be sent for frozen sectioning and rush histopathologic reading.[9] In general, it is thought that if the index of suspicion is high enough to warrant biopsy for necrotizing fasciitis, the patient is better served by proceeding straight to gross surgical examination by dissection, if this option is available in the practice setting.[9]

In 2004 a laboratory scoring system, the Laboratory Risk Indicator for Necrotizing Fasciitis (LRINEC), was proposed to help detect early cases of necrotizing fasciitis and allow for expedient surgical intervention.[20] This score combines values for C-reactive protein, white blood cell count, hemoglobin, sodium, creatinine, and glucose as predictive markers for early-onset necrotizing fasciitis, as outlined in Table 153-3.[20] Early clinical suspicion for necrotizing fasciitis with a score of 6 points or more with this LRINEC system had a positive predictive value of 92% and negative predictive value of 96% in initial studies evaluating the diagnostic accuracy of this scoring system.[20] Despite this, the scoring system has not been adequately studied in larger patient populations, limiting its generalizability and widespread acceptance as a first-line diagnostic tool. These initial rates for sensitivity and specificity were shown to be lower in a followup study investigating these parameters, but the study was limited by the retrospective nature of the study design.[2]

It is prudent to draw blood cultures in patients with necrotizing fasciitis as part of the initial workup even though bacteremia is present only in a minority of these patients.[11] As discussed above, superficial wound cultures have a low sensitivity and specificity for determining culprit pathogens causing infection, but needle aspirate of fluid from involved sites of skin and subcutaneous tissue can be used in cases where surgical intervention is delayed to help identify the causative pathogen.[9]

Certain key features, such as thickening and inflammation of fascial planes, can be seen on MRI and CT and help support a diagnosis of necrotizing fasciitis.[9] However, the sensitivity and specificity of these tests have not been determined. Additionally, if clinical suspicion is high, these studies are thought to just delay time to surgical diagnosis.[9] Radiology may be a useful investigative tool as part of a full workup in cases where clinical suspicion for necrotizing fasciitis is low to help avoid unnecessary surgical intervention for patients without necrotizing fasciitis.

DIFFERENTIAL DIAGNOSIS

Table 153-4 outlines the differential diagnosis of necrotizing fasciitis.

CLINICAL COURSE AND PROGNOSIS

Although some progress has been made in recent years in management of necrotizing fasciitis, mostly

TABLE 153-3
Laboratory Risk Indicator for Necrotizing Fasciitis (LRINEC) Score

LABORATORY TEST	VALUE	SCORE
C-reactive protein (mg/L)	<150	0
	≥150	4
Leukocyte count (10⁹/L)	<15	0
	15-25	1
	>25	2
Hemoglobin (mmol/L)	>8.4	0
	6.8-8.4	1
Sodium (mmol/L)	≥135	0
	<135	2
Creatinine (μmol/L)	≤141	0
	>141	2
Glucose (mmol/L)	≤10	0
	>10	1
Total		13

Score of 6 points or greater thought to be consistent with necrotizing fasciitis.[20]

TABLE 153-4
Differential Diagnoses for Necrotizing Fasciitis

Infectious Differential Diagnosis
- Abscess[2]
- Cellulitis[2]
- Erysipelas[16]
- Invasive/deep fungal infection[21]

Noninfectious Differential Diagnosis
- Necrotizing Sweet syndrome[23,24]
- Pyoderma gangrenosum[22]

in increased awareness of the need for prompt surgical intervention, adult mortality rates remain high at 20% to 30%.[2,3,5,11,19,25] Pediatric mortality is generally reported to be lower with recent literature demonstrating mortality rates of approximately 10% to 15%.[7] Most deaths in necrotizing fasciitis are secondary to underlying bacteremia, septic shock, and/or multiorgan failure.[13,25] Given the high risks of morbidity and mortality, patients with confirmed or suspected necrotizing fasciitis should be managed as an inpatient and management attempts should not be made to care for these patients in the outpatient setting.[9]

Table 153-5 identifies the patient factors, clinical parameters, and disease characteristics that are associated with an increased risk of mortality for patients with necrotizing fasciitis. On a systems level, delayed surgical intervention and interhospital transfer are associated with an increased risk of mortality; given this, efforts should be made to have patients undergo at least initial surgical debridement at their presenting hospital.[19,26] In general, anatomic location of disease has not been found to be a risk factor for mortality.

Of note, for patients who survive, morbidity remains high given aggressive surgical interventions and prolonged hospital course. Amputation is common for patients with limb disease and patients with underlying diabetes mellitus have an increased risk of requiring surgical amputation as treatment of limb necrotizing fasciitis.[13] Additionally, following discharge, the recovery process for patients who survive necrotizing fasciitis is often long and laborious.

MANAGEMENT

Even though prompt initiation of appropriate antibiotics is crucial, rapid surgical intervention remains the mainstay of therapy for patients with necrotizing fasciitis.[11] Surgical intervention less than 24 hours following onset is associated with improved clinical outcomes.[20] Despite this, in reality, delays in surgical management are persistent, with a significant subset of patients receiving delayed (longer than 24 hours) surgical intervention demonstrating need for continued education on diagnosis, workup, and treatment of this surgical emergency.[2]

Surgical interventions include radical debridement of necrotic tissue at baseline with possible amputation for severe limb disease.[2] Ultimately, full surgical debridement of all necrotic areas involved in the underlying infection is essential to achieving therapeutic success.[9] Generally, this is not achieved in one debridement, but rather by staged, daily debridings until no further areas of involvement are found on surgical exploration.[9] Following surgical debridement, wound closure is often achieved through vacuum-assisted closure devices and skin grafting.[2] There is insufficient data to support hyperbaric oxygen therapy in these patients at this point in time; however, research toward this end is ongoing.[9,16]

Although not the first-line treatment of necrotizing fasciitis, antibiotics are a crucial adjunctive therapy. In 2014, the Infectious Diseases Society of America (IDSA) published updated guidelines surrounding antimicro-

TABLE 153-5
Factors Found in Literature to Be Associated with a High Mortality Risk in Patients with Necrotizing Fasciitis

PATIENT CHARACTERISTICS	CLINICAL PRESENTATION	DISEASE CHARACTERISTICS
Older age[11,19,41-43]	Acute renal failure[42,44]	Hospital-acquired necrotizing fasciitis[11]
Female gender[43]	Severe sepsis or septic shock[11,42]	Sacral involvement[25]
Low body mass index[3]	Less pain at presentation[25]	Multifocal infection[11,25,45]
Race[8]	Lower frequency of fever at presentation[25]	Air in the involved soft tissue or surrounding infection[41]
Increased comorbidities or immunosuppression at baseline[3,8,11,19,41,43,46,47]: • Coronary artery disease • Malignancy • Peripheral vascular disease • Hemodialysis-dependent chronic kidney disease • Cirrhosis • Congestive heart failure • History of gout • Obesity • Diabetes mellitus	Laboratory abnormalities at presentation[25,41,45,46]: • Lower hemoglobin • Lower platelet count • Higher creatinine • Greater LRINEC score • Greater SOFA score • Increased band polymorphonuclear neutrophils • Activated partial thromboplastin time >60 s • Serum albumin <2.5 mg/dL • Serum protein <6 g/dL	Specific microbiology characteristics: • Monobacterial Gram-negative infections[25] • Polybacterial infections • Pseudomonal infections[25] • *Proteus* infections[25] • *Aeromonas* infection[41]
	Bacteremia	Traumatic injuries leading to infection[25,45]
	Hypotension on admission[43,46]	Skin necrosis on presentation[43,44,48]
	Pulse >130 beats/min[43]	Hemorrhagic bullae at presentation[48]

LRINEC, Laboratory Risk Indicator for Necrotizing Fasciitis; SOFA, Sequential Organ Failure Assessment.

bial selection for patients with necrotizing infections of the skin, fascia, and muscle (Table 153-6).[9] These guidelines are applicable to all infections covered in this chapter. As with most aggressive infections, broad-spectrum antibiotics are recommended initially, with narrowing based on data from tissue culture obtained from biopsy or during surgical debridement. The IDSA recommends initial broad-spectrum antimicrobial therapy with either vancomycin, linezolid, or daptomycin used in conjunction with either piperacilling-tazobactam, carbapenem, ceftriaxone plus metronidazole, or fluoroquinolone plus metronidazole while awaiting culture data.[9] Antibiotics should be continued until final surgical debridement has been completed, patient is afebrile for 48 to 72 hours, and patient has clinically stabilized.[9]

Lesions of necrotizing fasciitis release a significant amount of drainage. As such, fluid resuscitation and close monitoring of vitals and underlying electrolyte balance is crucial.[9] Early studies suggest some benefit to the use of IV immunoglobulin in patients with necrotizing fasciitis; however, data is limited and there is no strong evidence to support its routine use in patients with necrotizing fasciitis.[9]

TABLE 153-6
Infectious Diseases Society of America 2014 Guidelines for Antimicrobial Management for Patients with Necrotizing Soft-Tissue Infections[9]

TYPE OF INFECTION	FIRST-LINE ANTIMICROBIAL AGENT	ADULT DOSAGE	PEDIATRIC DOSAGE BEYOND NEONATAL PERIOD	AGENTS FOR PATIENTS WITH SEVERE PENICILLIN ALLERGY
Mixed infections	Piperacillin-tazobactam plus vancomycin	3.37 g q6-8h IV; 30 mg/kg/day in 2 divided doses	60 to 75 mg/kg/dose of the piperacillin component q6h IV; 10 to 13 mg/kg/dose q8h IV	Clindamycin or metronidazole with an aminoglycoside or fluoroquinolone
	Imipenem-cilastatin	1 g q6-8h IV	Not available (n/a)	n/a
	Meropenem	1 g q8h IV	20 mg/kg/dose q8h IV	n/a
	Ertapenem	1 g daily IV	15 mg/kg/dose q12h IV for children 3 months to 12 years of age	n/a
	Cefotaxime plus metronidazole or clindamycin	2 g q6h IV; 500 mg q6h IV; 600 to 900 mg q8h IV	50 mg/kg/dose q6h IV; 7.5 mg/kg/dose q6h IV; 10 to 13 mg/kg/dose q8h IV	n/a
Streptococcus	Penicillin plus clindamycin	2 to 4 million units q4-6h IV (adult); 600 to 900 mg q8h IV	60,000 to 100,000 units/kg/dose q6h IV; 10 to 13 mg/kg/dose q8h IV	Vancomycin, linezolid, quinupristin/dalfopristin, daptomycin
Staphylococcus aureus	Nafcillin	1 to 2 g q4h IV	50 mg/kg/dose q6h IV	Vancomycin, linezolid, quinupristin/dalfopristin, daptomycin
	Oxacillin	1 to 2 g q4h IV	50 mg/kg/dose q6h IV	
	Cefazolin	1 g q8h IV	33 mg/kg/dose q8h IV	
	Vancomycin (for resistant strains)	30 mg/kg/day in 2 divided doses IV	15 mg/kg/dose q6h IV	
	Clindamycin	600 to 900 mg q8h IV	10 to 13 mg/kg/dose q8h IV	Bacteriostatic; potential cross-resistance and emergence of resistance in erythromycin-resistant strains; inducible resistance in methicillin-resistant *S. aureus*
Clostridium spp.	Clindamycin plus penicillin	600 to 900 mg q8h IV; 2 to 4 million units q4-6h IV (adult)	10 to 13 mg/kg/dose q8h IV; 60,000 to 100,000 units/kg/dose q6h IV	n/a
Aeromonas hydrophila	Doxycycline plus ciprofloxacin or ceftriaxone	100 mg q12h IV; 500 mg q12h IV; 1 to 2 g q24h IV	Not recommended for children but may need to use in life-threatening situations	n/a
Vibrio vulnificus	Doxycycline plus ceftriaxone or cefotaxime	100 mg q12h IV; 1 g 4 times daily IV; 2 g thrice daily IV	Not recommended for children but may need to use in life-threatening situations	n/a

Adapted from Stevens DL, Bisno AL, Chambers HF, et al. Practice guidelines for the diagnosis and management of skin and soft tissue infections: 2014 update by the Infectious Diseases Society of America. *Clin Infect Dis.* 2014;59(2):e10-e52. By permission of Oxford University Press on behalf of the Infectious Diseases Society of America.

GANGRENOUS OR NECROTIZING CELLULITIS

Necrotizing or gangrenous cellulitis accounts for necrotizing infections with or without gas formation localized to the skin and subcutaneous tissue but not extending deep enough to involve the underlying fascia or muscles. In recent literature, these more superficial infections are also grouped into the larger umbrella term *necrotizing soft-tissue infections*, and broadly speaking, the same bacterial subspecies responsible for necrotizing fasciitis and pyomyositis can cause a similar necrotizing, rapidly progressive infection of the skin and subcutaneous tissue. Given this, there is relatively sparse current literature focusing on "gangrenous or necrotizing cellulitis" exclusively rather than grouping these diseases into larger groups of necrotizing soft-tissue infections.

Some prior literature grouped gangrenous or necrotizing cellulitis infections into either clostridial or nonclostridial crepitant or gangrenous cellulitis.[27] The *Clostridium* spp. are known more widely for causing severe crepitant myonecrosis or "gas gangrene" as discussed in "Clostridial Gas Gangrene" section.[27] The term *clostridial crepitant cellulitis* arose to describe cases of limited, superficial, and focal infections of the skin, often without severe systemic symptoms and caused by this same bacterial subgroup.[27] These clostridial crepitant cellulitis infections, as opposed to traditional cellulitis, were characterized by extensive subcutaneous emphysema with often minimal overlying skin changes.[27] Tissue necrosis in these cases was limited to superficial skin and subcutaneous tissue.[27]

Nonclostridial necrotizing cellulitis can be either gas forming or non gas forming. Aside from the *Clostridium* spp., gas can also be produced by other anaerobic or facultative bacterial species. These include *Peptostreptococcus* spp., *Bacteroides* spp., *Enterobacteriaceae*, and *Klebsiella* spp.[27] The defining feature for infections caused by each of these gas-forming bacteria is subcutaneous emphysema and each of these bacterial species can cause infection confined to the skin or extending more deeply into the muscle or fascia.

Gram-negative bacilli are common pathogens identified in patients with non–gas-forming necrotizing cellulitis, many of which are acquired by exposure to marine animals or aquatic environments.[28] Marine-associated necrotizing skin infections are most commonly caused by *Vibrio* spp. or *Aeromonas* spp.,[28] but a number of other less-common aquatic pathogens can cause similar presentations (Table 153-7). *Vibrio vulnificus* is the most virulent of this group of curved Gram-negative bacilli found in coastal waters.[28] Again, infection is often the result of inoculation through prior wound or site of trauma.[28] Clinically, bullae are a common defining feature found in patients with infection secondary to *Vibrio* spp. Not uncommonly, patients with *Vibrio* spp. infection can develop fulminant sepsis/shock. Patients with underlying renal disease, liver dysfunction, or immunosuppression at baseline are at increased risk for more-severe infection and fulminant sepsis associated with *Vibrio* spp. infection, also termed *vibriosis*.[28]

For each of these entities, the same management guidelines as those used in necrotizing fasciitis as outlined above can be followed. Surgical debridement, albeit more limited than for necrotizing fasciitis, in conjunction with antimicrobial therapy as outlined by the IDSA guidelines, remains the cornerstone of therapy.[27] Overall, it is clear that there is significant overlap in clinical presentation, microbiology, management, and treatment between necrotizing fasciitis and gangrenous or necrotizing cellulitis, suggesting that these forms of necrotizing or gangrenous cellulitis are thought to represent one point on a spectrum of severity within the larger group of necrotizing soft-tissue infections.

MYONECROSIS

The 2 major infections included within the group of myonecrosis are pyomyositis and clostridial gas gangrene. Both entities are characterized by necrotic infections stemming from within and around the subcutaneous muscle. Although these infections can involve the more superficial structures—fascia, skin, and subcutaneous soft tissue—the focus of the infection and associated necrosis is located within the confines of the muscle itself. Each is described separately below.

PYOMYOSITIS

HISTORICAL PERSPECTIVES

Pyomyositis is an infection characterized by bacterial infection leading to collections of purulent material within the body of 1 or more muscles in affected patients.[9] Early reports of symptoms and surgical findings reflecting the disease we now refer to as pyomyositis were found in reports of Julius Scriba, a German surgeon, dating back to 1885 while working abroad in Japan.[29] However, pyomyositis was first classified as a disease entity in the 19th century by Virchow, who called the disease "spontaneous acute myositis."[29] Literature for this disease was then increased by a Japanese surgeon Miyake Hayari who published a case

TABLE 153-7
Causes of Marine-Based Necrotizing Cellulitis[28]

- *Aeromonas* spp.
- *Edwardsiella tarda*
- *Erysipelothrix rhusiopathiae*
- *Plesiomonas shigelloides*
- *Streptococcus iniae*
- *Vibrio* spp.

Data from Vinh DC, Embil JM. Severe skin and soft tissue infections and associated critical illness. *Curr Infect Dis Rep*. 2007;9(5):415-21.

series of 33 patients with this disease.[29] In the early 20th century, additional cases were recognized in populations from warmer, more tropical climates, giving the disease the label tropical pyomyositis, which is still used commonly today.[29]

EPIDEMIOLOGY

Pyomyositis is described more frequently in tropical climates with the majority of cases reported in Asia, Africa, the Caribbean, and Oceania; additionally, even in these warmer climates, the infection has been described to occur with increased frequency during warmer, more humid months.[29] More recently, infections have been described with increased frequency in more temperate climates, which is thought to be possibly linked to increased frequency of community-acquired cases of methicillin-resistant *Staphylococcus aureus* in these climates.[29,30] One recent study estimated that the prevalence of pyomyositis in the developed world ranges from 1 per 1145 to 1 per 4000 emergency department hospital admissions.[30] A Brazilian study found that pyomyositis accounted for approximately 1% of all hospital admissions.[31]

As opposed to most other entities discussed in this chapter, pyomyositis in tropical climates occurs more frequently in children than adults.[30,31] In temperate climates, however, pyomyositis is more common in adult populations with multiple medical comorbidities.[31]

ETIOLOGY, MICROBIOLOGY, PATHOGENESIS

In addition to patients who live in warmer/tropical climates, pyomyositis occurs with increased frequency in patients who are immunosuppressed (eg, HIV) or have diabetes mellitus.[9] Additionally, bacteremia or other local skin and soft-tissue infections preceding cases of pyomyositis are thought to increase risk for subsequent development of this type of infection.[30] Pyomyositis infections demonstrate a predilection for the lower extremities and pelvic girdle, and occur more commonly following localized trauma or muscle overuse.[9]

A majority of pyomyositis infections (90%) are caused by *S. aureus*.[9] It has been postulated that Panton-Valentine leukocidin, which is a cytotoxin secreted by some staphylococcal strains, plays a role in pyomyositis development and the ability for *Staphylococcus* organisms to create intramuscular abscesses in this disease.[29] Nonstaphylococcal infections can be caused by *S. pneumoniae* or Gram-negative enteric bacteria.[9] Table 153-8 lists the bacterial causes of pyomyositis. Less commonly, pyomyositis can be caused by viral, parasitic, or fungal pathogens.[29]

CLINICAL FEATURES

Cutaneous Features: Given the depth of infection, there may be very few cutaneous changes seen in early pyomyositis.[32] Because of this, diagnosis is often delayed.[32] As lesions progress, patients often develop more focal pain that can be reproduced by palpation to this area.[32] Eventually, patients may develop a firm, woody induration over areas of involvement, demonstrate fluctuance, or develop areas of overlying cutaneous erythema and inflammation.[9,32]

TABLE 153-8
Microbiology of Pyomyositis

- *Escherichia coli*[29]
- *Klebsiella pneumoniae*[51]
- *Mycobacterium tuberculosis*[50]
- *Salmonella*[49]
- *Staphylococcus aureus*
- *Streptococcus pneumoniae*

Noncutaneous Features: Presenting symptoms for patients with infectious myositis are often vague or nonspecific and can include focal limb pain, muscle tenderness, and fever.[9] Focal pain can manifest itself as limp or restricted limb movement, particularly for those infections found in the pelvic girdle region.[30] As the disease progresses, however, patients with a delay in diagnosis can become progressively sicker, eventually developing sepsis and disseminated systemic infection.[32]

A clinical staging system for this disease has been suggested to describe the progression of symptoms found in patients with pyomyositis. Stage I involves inflammation and pain surrounding the infected muscle with associated leukocytosis. At this point there may be mild induration of the subcutaneous tissue structures; however, cutaneous changes are typically absent.[29] Stage II is characterized by suppuration with abscess formation within the muscle belly; this stage is associated with severe focal pain, fever, and swelling overlying the affected muscle.[29] This stage generally lasts 1 to 3 weeks. Stage III is characterized by progression to systemic disease with septic physiology, shock, and multifocal abscess formation.[29]

DIAGNOSIS

As opposed to some of the more superficial necrotizing processes, given the depth of this infection, MRI remains the gold standard for pyomyositis diagnosis.[9] Patients with pyomyositis will demonstrate muscle inflammation and intramuscular abscess formation on MRI. CT scan and ultrasonography are other helpful imaging modalities that can be used for this entity when MRI is not available or not practical to use to establish a diagnosis.[9,32] However, CT scan is limited by lack of definition of soft-tissue structures and ultrasonography is helpful only to characterize superficial abscesses.[9] Plain X-ray can give clues to suggest soft-tissue swelling, but lacks the capability to define underlying soft-tissue structures.[9] Interventional radiology-guided drainage of purulent material can help confirm the diagnosis and identify causative pathogens with culture, after which appropriate narrowing of antimicrobial therapy can occur. For persistently febrile patients despite ongoing antimicrobial therapy, repeat, serial imaging studies can be used to assess for remaining collections of purulence.[9]

Blood cultures in pyomyositis are crucial, but positivity rates are low, ranging from 5% to 30% of cases.[9] Leukocytosis, elevated erythrocyte sedimentation rate, and elevated C-reactive protein can also be seen in patients with pyomyositis; these tests can help to suggest a diagnosis for patients presenting with vague early symptoms.[32]

DIFFERENTIAL DIAGNOSIS

Table 153-9 outlines the differential diagnosis of pyomyositis.

CLINICAL COURSE AND PROGNOSIS

Mortality rates are reportedly lower (0.89% to 10%) in pyomyositis than some of the other disease entities covered in this chapter.[31,37,38] Factors shown to increase risk of mortality for patients with pyomyositis include septic physiology, hypotension, tachycardia, lower Glasgow coma score, higher Sequential Organ Failure Assessment (SOFA) score, elevated laboratory markers, including blood urea nitrogen, creatinine, bilirubin, and serum glutamic pyruvate transaminase.[37]

MANAGEMENT

Management options for pyomyositis involve both antimicrobials as well as surgical interventions. However, as opposed to many of the other entities in this chapter which are considered surgical emergencies, surgical intervention is not always required for pyomyositis; some patients are able to be managed conservatively with antibiotics alone or antibiotics with percutaneous abscess drainage.[30] The need for surgical intervention depends on extent and severity of disease.[30] When surgical intervention is required, orthopedic surgical specialists are often called upon for operative wash out and abscess decompression at sites of infection.[32]

Antimicrobial treatment of pyomyositis should also start broadly with vancomycin. Piperacillin-tazobactam, ampicillin-tazobactam, or carbapenem should be added to vancomycin empirically for patients who have multiple comorbidities, are immunocompromised, or developed infection as the result of a penetrating wound.[9] Again, once causative pathogens are identified, narrowing of antimicrobials to oral agents can be achieved with a goal of a 2- to 3-week course of treatment.[9] Based on the severity of infection and the clinical response to antibiotics, antibiotic regimens often can be changed from IV to oral.[30] Patients with pyomyositis whose cultures are positive for methicillin-sensitive *S. aureus* should be narrowed to either cefazolin or an antistaphylococcal penicillin (eg, nafcillin or oxacillin).[9]

CLOSTRIDIAL GAS GANGRENE

HISTORICAL PERSPECTIVES

Clostridium subspecies are a group of anaerobic or aerotolerant, Gram-positive, toxin-producing bacterial rods commonly found in soil and human and animal feces.[28] As opposed to the more superficial infection of "clostridial crepitant cellulitis," clostridial gas gangrene is a much deeper infection characterized by severe necrosis of skeletal muscle caused by the *Clostridium* subspecies.[28] The disease is rapidly progressive, often accompanied by severe systemic symptoms with risk for progression to multiorgan system shock. The disease became infamous in World War II when soldiers were found to develop soft-tissue infections at sites of contaminated prior battle wounds that were characterized by crepitus or gas release upon surgical intervention.[28]

ETIOLOGY, MICROBIOLOGY, PATHOGENESIS

Similar to what was discovered in World War II, today clostridial myonecrosis is most often found at sites of localized trauma or prior surgical intervention.[28] Infections can also occur in the postpartum period or following medical or spontaneous abortion.[28] Spontaneous (nontraumatic) cases of clostridial gas gangrene occur most frequently in patients with underlying gastric malignancy or underlying neutropenic gastritis.[9,28] GI cancers, such as colon cancer, can allow for bowel perforation and hematogenous spread of *Clostridium* organisms to previously healthy, nontraumatized sites of seeding.[9]

TABLE 153-9
Differential Diagnosis of Pyomyositis

Infectious Differential Diagnosis
- Bacterial meningitis[35]
- Cellulitis
- Osteomyelitis[33]
- Septic arthritis[34]

Noninfectious Differential Diagnosis
- Deep vein thrombosis[36]
- Hematoma
- Malignancy[33]
- Transient synovitis[33]

The most common causative organisms of clostridial myonecrosis are *Clostridium perfringens*, *Clostridium novyi*, *Clostridium histolyticum*, and *Clostridium septicum*.[9] *Clostridium sordellii* myonecrosis can be found in myonecrotic infections of the uterus and perineum in the postpartum and postabortive periods.[28] Cases related to trauma are most commonly caused by *C. perfringens* and spontaneous non–trauma-related cases are most commonly caused by *C. septicum*.[9,28] Clostridial myonecrosis in IV drug users is most commonly caused by *C. sordellii* and *C. novyi* subspecies.[28]

CLINICAL FEATURES

Patients with spontaneous, nontraumatic forms of clostridial myonecrosis can develop acute abdominal pain followed by pain localized to a limb where the infection has seeded.[28] Once infection has seeded, lesions of clostridial myonecrosis progress rapidly over the course of 24 hours to develop pronounced color changes to overlying skin. The lesions begin with pallor and progress on to other color changes, including a deep bronze followed by purple-red mottling.[9,28] The rapid doubling time of *Clostridium* species (as little as 10 minutes) is thought to contribute to the rapid progression of these diseases, with time from inoculation to fulminant disease ranging from a few hours to 3 days.[28] Disease progression and muscle necrosis can move at a rate of a few inches per hours.[28] Overlying skin can become edematous, tense, and firm with overlying bullae filled with a red-blue fluid.[9] Pain is often severe and is a prominent feature of clostridial myonecrosis.[28] Gas collection in tissue manifests as overlying crepitus and is the cardinal feature of clostridial myonecrosis as it is in clostridial crepitant cellulitis.[9] A brownish discharge with a foul smell, described as "dishwater exudate," can be noted.[28] Given depth of infection and structures involved, postpartum and post abortive patients often do not have associated skin findings.[28]

Overall, given the speed of progression of infection, patients with clostridial myonecrosis or gas gangrene become sick rapidly. They can develop an influenza-like prodrome and then develop tachycardia, fever, diaphoresis, tachypnea, hypotension, and a feeling of impending doom shortly after the start of these infection.[9,28] Also, as swelling spreads up the extremity, patients can develop intense edema localized to the extremity involved and risk for compartment syndrome is high.[28] Progressive myonecrosis can lead to myoglobinuria and subsequent renal failure.[28] Ultimately, systemic symptoms often progress to shock and multiorgan system failure.[9]

DIAGNOSIS

The triad of soft-tissue crepitus, severe pain, and tachycardia disproportionate to the fever is thought to be diagnostic of clostridial myonecrosis.[28] In reality, however, the diagnosis is often suggested clinically when gas collections are noted overlying the cutaneous findings described above and then confirmed with surgical exploration.[9,28] Surgical exploration reveals myonecrosis on gross surgical examination.[28] Tissue or exudate retrieved during surgical exploration and sent for microbiologic studies will reveal large Gram-positive or Gram-variable "blunt-end" rods from sites of infection.[9,28]

Laboratory studies are not required for the diagnosis of this infection. However, cases of clostridial myonecrosis are often associated with leukocytosis (leukemoid reaction), hemoconcentration, and laboratory evidence of end-organ damage.[28] With shock, patients can develop associated disseminated intravascular coagulopathy.[28] Similar to necrotizing fasciitis, imaging studies for clostridial myonecrosis are discouraged out of concern that the studies may only serve to delay treatment. However, if imaging studies are pursued, MRI or CT scan may demonstrate gas pockets or collections in the soft tissue surrounding infection.[9]

CLINICAL COURSE AND PROGNOSIS

Given rapid progression and associated systemic toxicity, cases of clostridial myonecrosis are associated with a high rate of morbidity and mortality. As with necrotizing fasciitis, morbidity is aggravated by delay in surgical intervention.[39] When occurring in limbs, the amputation rate is high; early amputation has been shown to decrease morbidity overall.[39] For patients who avoid amputation, limb function for affected limbs is rarely preserved.[39] Mortality rates for clostridial myonecrosis are reported to be as high as 100% and are highest among patients who initially present in shock.[39]

MANAGEMENT

Similar to necrotizing fasciitis, surgical debridement is the mainstay of therapy for patients with clostridial myonecrosis.[9] Additionally, these patients also often require multiple surgical debridements, and amputations of involved limbs may be necessary.[28] Given the clinically tenuous nature of these patients, intensive care unit–level care is often needed to closely monitor and replete fluids and electrolytes as necessary.[9] Broad-spectrum antibiotics should be started based on the IDSA guidelines, as outlined in Table 153-6, pending confirmation of clostridial pathogens.[9] Once diagnosis is confirmed to be secondary to a *Clostridium* subspecies, antibiotics of choice are clindamycin plus high-dose penicillin.[9,28] Combined therapy has been recommended given that approximately 5% of *Clostridium* subspecies will demonstrate resistance to clindamycin monotherapy.[9] Patients with penicillin allergy can be treated with clindamycin monotherapy or with metronidazole.[9] However, penicillin and metronidazole are thought to have opposing factors and their concomitant use is not recommended.[28]

As with necrotizing fasciitis, there is insufficient evidence to support hyperbaric oxygen therapy for patients with clostridial myonecrosis and it is thought that these procedures, which often require transporting patients to another facility or building, only delay or interrupt surgery and antibiotics, which are the cornerstones of therapy for these patients. Given this, the IDSA discouraged use of hyperbaric oxygen therapy in these patients in their 2014 guidelines for managements of skin and soft-tissue infections.[9] This notion received further support in the 2015 Cochrane review of treatment options for clostridial gas gangrene, which, again, demonstrated no overall benefit for patients receiving adjunctive hyperbaric oxygen therapy as a part of their overall care.[40]

REFERENCES

1. Hussein QA, Anaya DA. Necrotizing soft tissue infections. *Crit Care Clin*. 2013;29(4):795-806.
2. van Stigt SF, de Vries J, Bijker JB, et al. Review of 58 patients with necrotizing fasciitis in the Netherlands. *World J Emerg Surg*. 2016;11:21.
3. Park SJ, Kim DH, Choi CI, et al. Necrotizing soft tissue infection: analysis of the factors related to mortality in 30 cases of a single institution for 5 years. *Ann Surg Treat Res*. 2016;91(1):45-50.
4. Adekanye AG, Umana AN, Offiong ME, et al. Cervical necrotizing fasciitis: management challenges in poor resource environment. *Eur Arch Otorhinolaryngol*. 2016;273(9):2779-2784.
5. Psoinos CM, Flahive JM, Shaw JJ, et al. Contemporary trends in necrotizing soft-tissue infections in the United States. *Surgery*. 2013;153(6):819-827.
6. Oud L, Watkins P. Contemporary trends of the epidemiology, clinical characteristics, and resource utilization of necrotizing fasciitis in Texas: a population-based cohort study. *Crit Care Res Pract*. 2015;2015:618067.
7. Zundel S, Lemarechal A, Kaiser P, et al. Diagnosis and treatment of pediatric necrotizing fasciitis: a systematic review of the literature. *Eur J Pediatr Surg*. 2017;27(2):127-137.
8. Arif N, Yousfi S, Vinnard C. Deaths from necrotizing fasciitis in the United States, 2003-2013. *Epidemiol Infect*. 2016;144(6):1338-1344.
9. Stevens DL, Bisno AL, Chambers HF, et al. Practice guidelines for the diagnosis and management of skin and soft tissue infections: 2014 update by the Infectious Diseases Society of America. *Clin Infect Dis*. 2014;59(2):e10-e52.
10. Mao YC, Liu PY, Hung DZ, et al. Bacteriology of *Naja atra* snakebite wound and its implications for antibiotic therapy. *Am J Trop Med Hyg*. 2016;94(5):1129-1135.
11. Hua C, Sbidian E, Hemery F, et al. Prognostic factors in necrotizing soft-tissue infections (NSTI): A cohort study. *J Am Acad Dermatol*. 2015;73(6):1006-1012.e8.
12. Zarb P, Coignard B, Griskeviciene J, et al. The European Centre for Disease Prevention and Control (ECDC) pilot point prevalence survey of healthcare-associated infections and antimicrobial use. *Euro Surveill*. 2012;17(46).
13. Cheng NC, Tai HC, Chang SC, et al. Necrotizing fasciitis in patients with diabetes mellitus: clinical characteristics and risk factors for mortality. *BMC Infect Dis*. 2015;15:417.
14. Sada A, Misago N, Okawa T, et al. Necrotizing fasciitis and myonecrosis "synergistic necrotizing cellulitis" caused by *Bacillus cereus*. *J Dermatol*. 2009;36(7):423-426.
15. Meleney FL. Bacterial synergism in disease processes: with a confirmation of the synergistic bacterial etiology of a certain type of progressive gangrene of the abdominal wall. *Ann Surg*. 1931;94(6):961-81.
16. Elander J, Nekludov M, Larsson A, et al. Cervical necrotizing fasciitis: descriptive, retrospective analysis of 59 cases treated at a single center. *Eur Arch Otorhinolaryngol*. 2016;273(12):4461-4467.
17. Lohsiriwat V. Anorectal emergencies. *World J Gastroenterol*. 2016;22(26):5867-5878.
18. Crowell W, Roberts R, Tarry S. Fungal Fournier's gangrene in an immunocompromised patient. *Urol Case Rep*. 2016;4:1-3.
19. Holena DN, Mills AM, Carr BG, et al. Transfer status: a risk factor for mortality in patients with necrotizing fasciitis. *Surgery*. 2011;150(3):363-370.
20. Wong CH, Khin LW, Heng KS, et al. The LRINEC (Laboratory Risk Indicator for Necrotizing Fasciitis) score: a tool for distinguishing necrotizing fasciitis from other soft tissue infections. *Crit Care Med*. 2004;32(7):1535-1541.
21. Aytekin S, Guder H, Goktay F, et al. Pyoderma gangrenosum and necrotizing fasciitis-like opportunistic invasive cutaneous fungal infection. *Int J Dermatol*. 2016;55(10):e563-e565.
22. de Souza EF, da Silva GA, Dos Santos GR, et al. Pyoderma gangrenosum simulating necrotizing fasciitis. *Case Rep Med*. 2015;2015:504970.
23. Kroshinsky D, Alloo A, Rothschild B, et al. Necrotizing Sweet syndrome: a new variant of neutrophilic dermatosis mimicking necrotizing fasciitis. *J Am Acad Dermatol*. 2012;67(5):945-954.
24. de Moya MA, Wong JT, Kroshinsky D, et al. Case records of the Massachusetts General Hospital. Case 28-2012. A 30-year-old woman with shock and abdominal-wall necrosis after cesarean section. *N Engl J Med*. 2012;367(11):1046-1057.
25. Jabbour G, El-Menyar A, Peralta R, et al. Pattern and predictors of mortality in necrotizing fasciitis patients in a single tertiary hospital. *World J Emerg Surg*. 2016;11:40.
26. Hadeed GJ, Smith J, O'Keeffe T, et al. Early surgical intervention and its impact on patients presenting with necrotizing soft tissue infections: a single academic center experience. *J Emerg Trauma Shock*. 2016;9(1):22-27.
27. Bryant P, Carapetis J, Matussek J, et al. Recurrent crepitant cellulitis caused by *Clostridium perfringens*. *Pediatr Infect Dis J*. 2002;21(12):1173-1174.
28. Vinh DC, Embil JM. Severe skin and soft tissue infections and associated critical illness. *Curr Infect Dis Rep*. 2007;9(5):415-421.
29. Verma S. Pyomyositis in children. *Curr Infect Dis Rep*. 2016;18(4):12.
30. Moriarty P, Leung C, Walsh M, et al. Increasing pyomyositis presentations among children in Queensland, Australia. *Pediatr Infect Dis J*. 2015;34(1):1-4.
31. Borges AH, Faragher B, Lalloo DG. Pyomyositis in the upper Negro river basin, Brazilian Amazonia. *Trans R Soc Trop Med Hyg*. 2012;106(9):532-537.
32. Kumar MP, Seif D, Perera P, et al. Point-of-care ultrasound in diagnosing pyomyositis: a report of three cases. *J Emerg Med*. 2014;47(4):420-426.
33. Chong X, Ashik M, Arjandas M. Obturator internus pyomyositis in a child: a case report. *Malays Orthop J*. 2014;8(1):69-70.
34. Ghazala CG, Fatone E, Bentley R, et al. Primary bacterial gluteal pyomyositis: a rare disease in temperate

climates presenting as suspected septic arthritis of the hip. *J Emerg Med*. 2016;51(3):319-321.
35. Itaya S, Kobayashi Z, Tomimitsu H, et al. Pneumococcal pyomyositis of the neck muscles. *Intern Med*. 2016;55(15):2069-2071.
36. Narayanan M, Mookherjee S, Spector TB, et al. MSSA brain abscess and pyomyositis presenting as brain tumour and DVT. *BMJ Case Rep*. 2013;2013.
37. Sharma A, Kumar S, Wanchu A, et al. Clinical characteristics and predictors of mortality in 67 patients with primary pyomyositis: a study from North India. *Clin Rheumatol*. 2010;29(1):45-51.
38. Drosos G. Pyomyositis. A literature review. *Acta Orthop Belg*. 2005;71(1):9-16.
39. Aggelidakis J, Lasithiotakis K, Topalidou A, et al. Limb salvage after gas gangrene: a case report and review of the literature. *World J Emerg Surg*. 2011;6:28.
40. Yang Z, Hu J, Qu Y, et al. Interventions for treating gas gangrene. *Cochrane Database Syst Rev*. 2015(12):CD010577.
41. Huang KF, Hung MH, Lin YS, et al. Independent predictors of mortality for necrotizing fasciitis: a retrospective analysis in a single institution. *J Trauma*. 2011;71(2):467-473.
42. Kao LS, Lew DF, Arab SN, et al. Local variations in the epidemiology, microbiology, and outcome of necrotizing soft-tissue infections: a multicenter study. *Am J Surg*. 2011;202(2):139-145.
43. Khamnuan P, Chongruksut W, Jearwattanakanok K, et al. Necrotizing fasciitis: risk factors of mortality. *Risk Manag Healthc Policy*. 2015;8:1-7.
44. Krieg A, Dizdar L, Verde PE, et al. Predictors of mortality for necrotizing soft-tissue infections: a retrospective analysis of 64 cases. *Langenbecks Arch Surg*. 2014;399(3):333-341.
45. Lee YC, Hor LI, Chiu HY, et al. Prognostic factor of mortality and its clinical implications in patients with necrotizing fasciitis caused by *Vibrio vulnificus*. *Eur J Clin Microbiol Infect Dis*. 2014;33(6):1011-1018.
46. Yeung YK, Ho ST, Yen CH, et al. Factors affecting mortality in Hong Kong patients with upper limb necrotising fasciitis. *Hong Kong Med J*. 2011;17(2):96-104.
47. Nisbet M, Ansell G, Lang S, et al. Necrotizing fasciitis: review of 82 cases in South Auckland. *Intern Med J*. 2011;41(7):543-548.
48. Khamnuan P, Chongruksut W, Jearwattanakanok K, et al. Clinical predictors for severe sepsis in patients with necrotizing fasciitis: an observational cohort study in northern Thailand. *Infect Drug Resist*. 2015;8:207-216.
49. Gandhi A, Phadke P. *Salmonella* pyomyositis with concurrent osteomyelitis presenting as piriformis syndrome. *J Assoc Physicians India*. 2016;64(1):55.
50. Osorio J, Barreto J, Benavides J, et al. Tuberculous pyomyositis in an immunosuppressed patient. *Biomedica*. 2016;36(0):23-28.
51. Liao WH, Lai CC, Huang SH, et al. Rectus femoris pyomyositis caused by *Klebsiella pneumoniae*. *Surg Infect (Larchmt)*. 2014;15(4):464-465.

Chapter 154 :: Gram-Negative Coccal and Bacillary Infections
:: Breanne Mordorski & Adam J. Friedman

第一百五十四章
革兰氏阴性球菌和细菌感染

中文导读

革兰氏阴性细菌可按其形态和代谢能力进行分类。在临床分离物中发现的革兰氏阴性球菌通常代表奈瑟氏球菌，取决于麦芽糖发酵活性，可鉴定为脑膜炎奈瑟氏球菌或淋病奈瑟氏球菌。另一方面，革兰氏阴性杆菌可根据形态进行细分，包括球菌、逗号形杆菌、梭形杆菌和棒状杆菌。这一章节，重点介绍其他章节未涵盖的感染的皮肤表现，共分为6节：①脑膜炎奈瑟菌引起的感染；②铜绿假单胞菌引起的感染；③巴氏杆菌属物种引起的感染；④沙门氏菌引起的肠炎；⑤克雷伯氏菌引起的鼻窦炎；⑥流感嗜血杆菌引起的蜂窝织炎。分别介绍了这些特殊感染的流行病学、临床特征、危险因素、病因和发病机制、诊断、鉴别诊断、临床病程和预后、临床管理。

〔汪 犇〕

The Gram stain, developed in the late 1800s by Hans Christian Gram, is used to distinguish 2 major categories of bacteria. Gram-positive bacteria retain the purple hue of the initial crystal violet stain, whereas Gram-negative bacteria are decolorized and subsequently stain red by safranin or carbol fuchsin. While Gram-positive bacteria have thick walls of peptidoglycan and secondary polymers that are relatively impermeable and resist decolorization, Gram-negative bacteria have a thin peptidoglycan layer with an outer lipid membrane bilayer that is readily disrupted by this process.[1]

Gram-negative bacteria may be further categorized by their morphology and metabolic capabilities. Gram-negative cocci found in clinical isolates typically represent *Neisseria* spp., which may be identified as *Neisseria meningitidis* or *Neisseria gonorrhoeae* depending on maltose fermenting activity. On the other hand, Gram-negative bacilli may be subdivided based on morphology, including coccobacilli, comma-shaped bacilli, fusiform bacilli, and rods. Gram-negative rods, for example, can be further subdivided by lactose fermenting activity, oxidase positivity, and so on.[2] This chapter focuses on cutaneous manifestations of Gram-negative infections not already covered in other chapters. Many manifestations occur from direct invasion of the skin or subcutaneous tissues, and may be accompanied by signs such as fever or hypotension attributable to the patient's immune response.

INFECTIONS CAUSED BY *NEISSERIA MENINGITIDIS*

AT-A-GLANCE

- Worldwide, *Neisseria meningitidis* is responsible for 1.2 million cases of infection and 135,000 deaths annually.
- Disseminated meningococcal infection may present as (a) meningitis alone, (b) acute meningococcemia with or without meningitis, or (c) chronic meningococcemia.
- In acute meningococcemia, a classic petechial rash is present in approximately 60% of patients, most commonly on the extremities. In severe cases, necrosis of the skin and underlying tissue may necessitate amputation.
- The rash of chronic meningococcemia more commonly consists of rose-colored macules and papules, although petechiae, nodules, vesicles, and pustules may be present. The rash may wax and wane with periodic fevers.
- Mortality rates for meningococcal infection in the United States are 10% to 15% with 11% to 19% of survivors suffering from long-term sequelae.
- The gold standard for diagnosis is culture isolation of *N. meningitidis* from blood, cerebrospinal fluid, other bodily fluids, or skin biopsy tissues. Polymerase chain reaction is useful when cultures are negative.
- The single most important factor in the treatment of acute meningococcal infection is early initiation of antibiotics.
- In the United States, vaccination with a capsular polysaccharide conjugate vaccine against serogroups A, C, W135, and Y is recommended for all patients at 11 or 12 years of age with a booster at age 16 years.

INTRODUCTION AND BACTERIOLOGY

N. meningitidis is a maltose-fermenting aerobic Gram-negative diplococcus. It is a fastidious organism, meaning it has complex nutritional requirements and will die within hours on nonliving surfaces. It grows on blood agar, trypticase soy agar, chocolate agar, and modified Thayer-Martin agar, which consists of a chocolate agar base with growth factors and antibiotics that select for pathogenic *Neisseria* spp. On blood agar, colonies are light gray, nonhemolytic, round, and glistening, and have a clearly defined edge.[3,4]

While some strains do not have a capsule, pathogenic *N. meningitidis* is almost always encapsulated, allowing differentiation into serogroups based on capsular polysaccharides. At least 13 serogroups have been identified; however, only 6 (A, B, C, W-135, X, and Y) cause life-threatening disease. The capsule is vital for *N. meningitidis* survival in the blood as it inhibits antibody-mediated and complement-mediated killing, as well as phagocytosis. Capsules decrease the visibility of *N. meningitidis* to the host immune system via molecular mimicry, a phenomenon perhaps best illustrated by serogroup B, whose capsular polysaccharides closely resemble those found on human neuronal cells. Vaccination against *N. meningitidis* serogroup B has proven especially challenging, as the capsular antigen is poorly immunogenic, necessitating the use of alternate antigens in the creation of vaccines.[5]

As with other Gram-negative bacteria, *N. meningitidis* has a subcapsular envelope comprised of an outer membrane bilayer, a peptidoglycan layer and a cytoplasmic membrane bilayer. The outer membrane bilayer contains pili, opacity proteins (Opa, Opc), factor H binding protein, and lipooligosaccharide (LOS). Pili and opacity proteins enable *N. meningitidis* adherence to host cells and tissues, and both undergo phase and antigenic variation. Pili may also undergo posttranscriptional glycosylation, promoting secretion of soluble pilin units that compete with antipilin antibodies. Type IV pili drive initial *N. meningitidis* adherence to nasopharyngeal epithelium and aggregation into microcolonies. Later in the bloodstream, Type IV pili enable adherence to endothelial cells, mediate vascular damage, and facilitate the breach of the blood–brain barrier.[4,6,7] Factor H binding protein binds factor H, a downregulator of the alternative complement pathway, to the surface of *N. meningitidis*, where it serves to degrade complement component C3.[8] In the setting of infection, LOS binds a variety of receptors on dendritic and monocytic cells, including lipopolysaccharide binding protein, CD14, and myeloid differentiation protein 2, part of the toll-like receptor (TLR)-4 complex. Together, LOS and other outer membrane components trigger downstream production of proinflammatory cytokines and chemokines, activation of complement, and simultaneous activation and inhibition of coagulation pathways.[9] Studies show a direct correlation between serum levels of LOS and severity of meningococcal infection, and high serum LOS is correlated with poor prognosis.

EPIDEMIOLOGY

There are approximately 1.2 million cases of *N. meningitidis* infection each year, leading to 135,000 deaths worldwide. Infections continue to occur in both developed and developing countries. Of note, the "meningitis belt" in sub-Saharan Africa encompasses 18 countries from Ethiopia to Senegal and is characterized by large epidemics of primarily meningococcal meningitis, which have occurred approximately every 8 to 10 years since 1905. The cause of these epidemics is poorly understood, although it is thought that humidity and dust play a role. Interestingly, peak *N. meningitidis* infection in developed countries typically corresponds with viral respiratory illnesses during winter months, whereas N. meningitidis infection in Africa occurs during the dry season.[4,10]

Humans are the exclusive natural host for N. meningitidis, and approximately 6% of the population develops nasopharyngeal carriage each year. Nasopharyngeal carriage persists for weeks to months and distribution varies with age: 0.5 to 1% carriage in infants and young children, 5% in adolescents, and 20% to 40% in young adults. The containment of infection to the nasopharynx is mediated by undetermined host and environmental factors, as well as host immunity. Sporadic N. meningitidis infection occurs most frequently in young children as a consequence of waning levels of protective maternal antibodies. However, in epidemics, older children, especially those living in crowded living quarters such as college dormitories, have higher infection rates. Overall, males have a higher risk of infection, whereas females have higher mortality.[4,10,11]

N. meningitidis infection is primarily caused by serogroups A, B, C, W-135, X, and Y. Serogroup A has been responsible for the largest and most devastating outbreaks in sub-Saharan Africa, whereas serogroups B and C most frequently cause disease in developed countries. Serogroup B accounts for 30% to 40% of cases in the United States and up to 80% in Europe, whereas serogroup C is responsible for approximately 30% of cases in both the United States and Europe. W-135 has caused infections with high mortality in sub-Saharan Africa, and since the 1990s it has been known to affect travelers to Saudi Arabia during the Hajj pilgrimage. Serogroup Y has emerged in the United States, accounting for approximately 25% of disease, particularly meningococcal pneumonia in older adults, as well as meningitis and meningococcemia in infants younger than 6 months old. Serogroup X is the most recent serogroup to emerge as a cause of disease in sub-Saharan Africa.[4,11]

CLINICAL FEATURES

N. meningitidis carriage is often asymptomatic, although upper respiratory tract infection–like symptoms may occur.[12] If N. meningitidis breaches the nasopharyngeal epithelium, patients may develop acute meningococcemia with or without meningitis, or meningitis alone. Acute meningococcemia is characterized by fever and a petechial rash, which may progress to fulminant septicemia within a matter of hours. More rarely, patients may develop chronic meningococcemia, which presents over weeks to months with recurrent fevers, migratory arthralgias, and a rash of varied morphology.[13,14]

CUTANEOUS FINDINGS

Acute meningococcemia is known to produce a petechial rash; however, this hallmark is not always present. In a study of 752 patients in the Netherlands, 601 had cutaneous exam data, of which 363 (60%) had petechiae on presentation. Petechiae were more common in children ages 1 to 18 (74%) than infants (48%) or adults (45%).[15] When present, petechiae are small and irregular with a "smudged" appearance, and may occur all over the body, including palms, soles, mucous membranes, and conjunctiva, although the extremities are the most common location (Fig. 154-1).[11] Extensive petechiae with central necrosis or bullae may also develop. Although the presence of petechiae do not predict the risk of mortality, a rapid increase in their number and size correlates with fulminant dis-

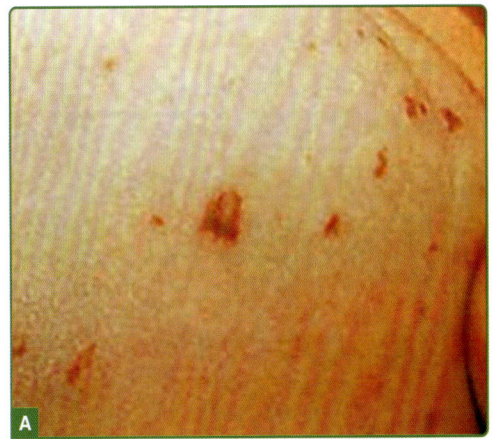

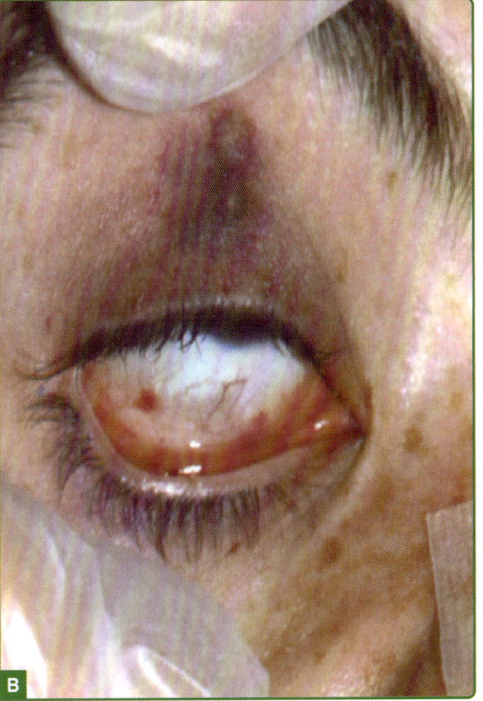

Figure 154-1 Acute meningococcemia may be accompanied by petechial lesions of the skin (**A**), mucous membranes and conjunctiva (**B**). (Reproduced with permission from Baselga E, Drolet BA, Esterly NB. Purpura in infants and children. *J Am Acad Dermatol*. 1997;37[5]:673-705. Copyright © American Academy of Dermatology.)

ease progression.[15] Purpura fulminans may occur with severe disseminated intravascular coagulation (DIC) caused by sepsis, characterized by retiform purpura and necrosis of the skin, which may extend to subcutaneous tissues and, occasionally, muscle and bone (Fig. 154-2). Patients affected by DIC and purpura fulminans tend to have low levels of protein C.[13,16] In some cases of acute meningococcemia, patients may display transient macular or papular eruptions, similar to those seen in viral exanthems.[17]

Cutaneous manifestations of chronic meningococcemia are polymorphous, and may fade and recur with intermittent fevers. Skin findings often occur around painful joints or pressure points, and, from most common to least common, include (a) rose-colored macules and papules, (b) slightly indurated and tender erythema nodosum-like nodules, (c) petechiae, (d) petechiae with vesicular or pustular centers, (e) minute hemorrhages with an areola of paler erythema, and (f) grossly hemorrhagic areas with pale blue-gray centers.[18]

NONCUTANEOUS FINDINGS

Patients with acute meningococcemia may present with lethargy, anorexia, headache, nausea/vomiting, myalgias, arthralgias, cold or discolored extremities, hypotension, altered mental status, renal failure, acute respiratory distress syndrome, and DIC.[9,13] With severe DIC, the patient is at risk for Waterhouse-Friderichsen syndrome, a life-threatening condition characterized by adrenal hemorrhage and ensuing adrenal crisis, often accompanied by purpura fulminans.[13,16] With breach of the blood–brain barrier, patients may develop meningococcal meningitis, which is marked by meningism (nuchal rigidity, headache, photophobia), fever, nausea/vomiting, and altered mental status. Kernig and Brudzinski signs may become positive.[9] Rarely, meningococcemia may lead to septic foci in other locations, including septic arthritis, purulent pericarditis, and bacterial endocarditis. More commonly, a delayed immune complex-mediated syndrome can occur while patients are in recovery, which may include a range of symptoms due to sterile arthritis, vasculitis, pleuritis, pericarditis, or episcleritis.[19,20]

COMPLICATIONS

Severe cases of meningococcemia may require amputation of digits or extremities, as well as extensive skin grafting.[9] Purpura fulminans, in particular, frequently leads amputation and scarring, and may even cause abnormal bone growth in children.[13] Survivors of severe meningococcemia may require weeks of mechanical ventilation or dialysis.[9] With meningitis, the most common sequela is sensorineural hearing loss or deafness, although seizures, motor problems, hydrocephalus, mental retardation, and cognitive and behavioral problems may also occur.[9,13]

In some cases, chronic meningococcemia can evolve into acute meningococcemia, meningitis or carditis.[14,21] In one case report, a patient thought to have Sweet syndrome was treated with corticosteroids and subsequently developed meningococcal meningitis. Retrospective, nonroutine polymerase chain reaction (PCR) and silver staining of skin biopsy specimens revealed chronic meningococcemia.[14]

ETIOLOGY AND PATHOGENESIS

N. meningitidis is known to reside in the nasopharynx of healthy individuals, and can be transferred from person to person via respiratory droplets or by direct contact, such as kissing. When invasive

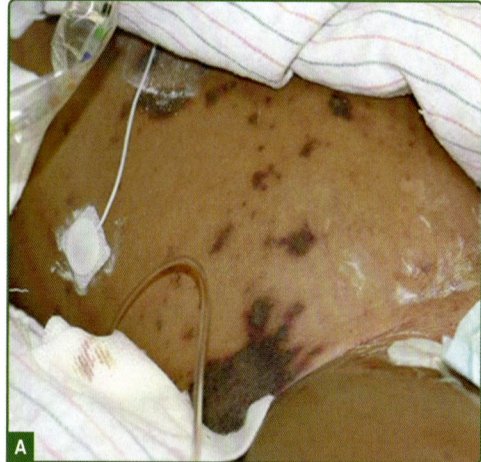
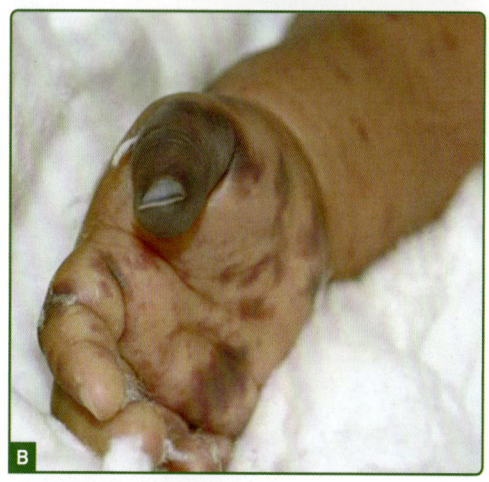

Figure 154-2 Acute meningococcemia with disseminated intravascular coagulation may produce purpura fulminans, characterized by retiform purpura and necrosis of the skin (**A**), which may progress to gangrene of the digits and distal extremities (**B**). (Reproduced with permission from Mishkin DR, Rosh AJ. Female infant with fever and rash. *Ann Emerg Med.* 2009;54[2]:155-180. Copyright © Elsevier; and David R. Mishkin, MD.)

disease occurs, it typically arises within 2 weeks of acquisition.[11]

Meningococci adherent to the nasopharyngeal epithelium undergo phase variation of Type IV pili and opacity proteins. In the development of invasive disease, N. meningitidis traverses epithelial cells via parasite directed endocytosis, entering capillaries and small veins in the underlying submucosal tissue.[4] Once in the bloodstream, N. meningitidis preferentially adheres to microvessel endothelium where it proliferates rapidly, forming microcolonies. Type IV pili facilitate both adherence and crosstalk with endothelial cells, ultimately leading to reshaping of endothelial cell membranes with formation of filopodia-like protrusions.[7] N. meningitidis adherence and presence of LOS triggers the production of proinflammatory cytokines of the innate immune system, including interleukin (IL)-6, IL-8, and tumor necrosis factor-α, which also contribute to endothelial damage.[22] Vascular damage alters endothelial antithrombotic properties, leading to widespread thrombosis. This is associated with blood flow alterations, red blood cell congestion, vessel engorgement, and leakage. Edema, infarction of overlying skin, and red blood cell extravasation are responsible for the cutaneous findings associated with acute meningococcemia. Of note, even though N. meningitidis is tightly adherent to endothelial cells, it may not always be present in the bloodstream to a great extent. Thus, some patients may show negative blood cultures despite large quantities of bacteria adherent to the microvessels.[22]

In some patients, N. meningitidis develops a remarkably tight interaction with endothelial cells of the brain microvasculature, characterized by the assembly of "cortical plaques," comprised of actin and other proteins, beneath the adherent bacteria. This interaction, also mediated by Type IV pili, facilitates compromise of the blood–brain barrier, enabling infection of the subarachnoid space.[6,9] N. meningitidis continues to proliferate in the cerebrospinal fluid (CSF) to levels 10^3 to 10^5 times those seen in the blood, leading to production of proinflammatory cytokines and meningism.[9] While other causes of bacterial meningitis, such as Streptococcus pneumoniae, may seed the brain, leading to focal neurologic signs, this typically does not happen with N. meningitidis.

In chronic meningococcemia, bacteria adhere to microvasculature endothelium, and although nonpurpuric lesions do not reveal disruption of microvasculature under light microscopy, both purpuric and nonpurpuric lesions reveal N. meningitidis in the extravascular space. Studies indicate a role for N. meningitidis–driven remodeling of interendothelial junctions, leading to meningococcal perivascular invasion via the paracellular route in chronic meningococcemia.[23]

RISK FACTORS

The single greatest risk factor for disseminated meningococcal disease is a lack of bactericidal antibodies.[9] Patients with anatomic or functional asplenia, HIV infection, or defects in the terminal (C5 to C9) or alternative complement pathways are at increased risk, as well. Specifically, a deficiency in properdin, a positive regulator of the alternative complement pathway confers increased susceptibility.[6] Other at-risk groups include adolescents and young adults living in crowded conditions, such as military barracks or college dormitories, infants and young children in daycare centers, and those exposed to tobacco smoke.[4,11]

DIAGNOSIS

Initial diagnosis of N. meningitidis infection is typically clinical, as systemic infection constitutes a medical emergency, and treatment should not be delayed waiting for test results. Blood cultures should be swiftly collected and empiric antimicrobial therapy administered immediately. Lumbar puncture is also warranted, in addition to fluid collection from other bodily sites of suspected dissemination; however, such tests should never delay therapy.[13]

LABORATORY TESTING

The gold standard for diagnosis is culture isolation of N. meningitidis from blood, CSF, synovial fluid, pleural fluid, pericardial fluid, or skin biopsy tissues. This enables etiologic confirmation as well as determination of antibiotic susceptibility.[11] In acute meningococcemia, blood cultures may be positive in 40% to 80% of patients, and sensitivity declines quickly following initiation of antibiotics.[24] Cultures from CSF and other organ sites may also have a low sensitivity, especially once antibiotics are started. In one study of 9 children with positive CSF cultures, 1 child had sterile CSF within 15 minutes of antibiotic administration, 3 had sterile CSF within 1 hour, and all were sterile within 2 hours. By comparison, CSF sterilization in pneumococcal or group B streptococcal infection typically takes several hours.[25] In the setting of meningococcal meningitis, CSF leukocytes typically exceed $100 \times 10^6/L$ with elevated protein and decreased glucose; however, 1 or more of these classic findings may be absent.[9]

The skin may provide another site for bacterial isolation, either via needle aspiration of cutaneous lesions or punch biopsy. One study isolated N. meningitidis from 86% of meningococcemia patients via needle aspiration,[26] and another study found 72% sensitivity among patients evaluated with either needle aspiration or biopsy.[21] In contrast to blood and CSF, meningococci have been cultured from skin lesions up to 13 hours following antibiotic administration.[9] In a prospective study of 31 patients and 12 controls, the sensitivities of blood, CSF, and skin biopsy cultures were 56%, 50%, and 36%, respectively. When culture and Gram staining were combined, the sensitivities were 56% (blood), 64% (CSF), and 56% (skin biopsy). In 3 patients, the diagnosis was made on positive skin biopsy results alone.[27]

Given suboptimal sensitivities of cultures and Gram staining, patients with a high suspicion for infection despite negative workup may benefit from PCR. Although PCR cannot determine antibiotic sensitivities, it can quickly type *N. meningitidis* strains. PCR is highly sensitive (96%) and specific (100%), and because live bacteria are not required, sensitivity is not diminished by initiation of antibiotics. Additionally, PCR takes less than 4 hours, and in-house test results are typically available the same day as collection.[28] Despite these advantages, cultures have not been replaced by PCR given that it cannot determine sensitivities and does not have widespread availability. For these reasons, PCR for blood and CSF is indicated when cultures are uninformative and is not typically employed in initial diagnostic workup.[21]

PCR is also being investigated in skin biopsy specimens, which may offer even higher sensitivity compared to PCR of blood or CSF samples.[11] This testing modality may be especially useful in chronic meningococcemia as skin lesions are nonspecific, and positive cultures may be more difficult to come by because of waxing and waning bacterial levels. At least 4 cases of chronic meningococcemia have been reported with negative blood cultures, and diagnosis was established based on PCR of skin biopsies alone.[14,21,23] Silver staining and immunohistochemical staining of skin lesions also may be useful in both acute and chronic cases of meningococcal disease.[14,29]

Additional tests used in meningococcal meningitis include a latex agglutination assay and rapid dipstick test. Agglutination kits use latex beads with antibodies to capsular antigens, capable of detecting serogroups A, C, W135, and Y, with significantly lower sensitivity for serogroup B. This is problematic given the high proportion of serogroup B infections in the United States and Europe, and for this reason, latex agglutination tests are not routinely performed.[30] The rapid dipstick test, developed to detect serogroups A, C, W135, and Y in CSF, was found to detect 90% of meningitis cases caused by A and W135 in Niger when compared to PCR. Given the favorable sensitivity and ability to be administered by nonspecialized staff members, this test is especially valuable in developing countries.[31]

PATHOLOGY

Routine pathology of skin biopsy specimens may reveal findings consistent with necrotizing vasculitis,[32] including perivascular infiltrates comprised of neutrophils and monocytes with microvascular thrombosis and perivascular hemorrhage.[13,22] Gram stain may reveal Gram-negative cocci.[32] In the setting of chronic meningococcemia, perivascular infiltrates are comprised of lymphocytes and neutrophils, and leukocytoclastic vasculitis may be appreciated in petechial lesions.[12]

DIFFERENTIAL DIAGNOSIS

Table 154-1 outlines the differential diagnosis for acute and chronic meningococcemia.

CLINICAL COURSE AND PROGNOSIS

If untreated, acute meningococcal infection usually ends fatally and is capable of killing previously heathy children and adults in as few as 12 hours.[4] *N. meningitidis* proliferates rapidly, leading to shock and multiple organ failure, which is the direct cause of death in 9 of 10 patients who die from acute meningococcal infection in developed countries. Far fewer patients die from meningitis leading to brain edema and herniation.[9] With chronic meningococcemia, some patients may spontaneously recover, although without treatment the infection is more likely to worsen, potentially progressing to affect vital functions and lead to death. For treated chronic meningococcemia, prognosis is excellent.[21]

As of 2012, mortality rates for meningococcal infection were 10 to 15% in the United States, and among survivors, 11% to 19% suffered from long-term sequelae such as limb loss, hearing loss, cognitive dysfunction, visual impairment, educational difficulties, motor nerve deficits, seizure disorders, and behavioral problems.[4,33] In a study of 752 patients in the Netherlands presenting with meningococcal disease over a 28-month period, case fatality rate was 6.7% overall, but reached 16% in adults older than age 50 years. Approximately half of all fatalities died within 12 hours of arriving at the hospital, with two-thirds passing away within 24 hours.[15]

MANAGEMENT

The single most important factor in the treatment of acute meningococcal infection is early initiation of antibiotics. Ideally, no more than 30 minutes should pass between a presumptive diagnosis and administration of intravenous therapy. Diagnostic testing should never be a reason for delayed treatment.[34] Although less emergent, chronic meningococcemia is treated with similar antibiotic regimens and all patients should be offered a comprehensive immunologic workup including complement pathway deficiencies after the infection has been effectively treated.[14]

TABLE 154-1
Differential Diagnosis for Acute and Chronic Meningococcemia

CONDITIONS	CONSIDERATIONS
Acute Meningococcemia	
Enteroviral infection	Patients may present with fever, aseptic meningitis, and petechial rash.
Sepsis caused by another bacterial organism	Although classically associated with *Neisseria meningitidis*, purpura fulminans may occur with *Streptococcus pneumoniae*, *Haemophilus influenzae*, *Staphylococcus aureus*, and groups A and B β-hemolytic streptococci.
Acute bacterial endocarditis	Mucous membrane and conjunctival lesions, as well as subungual splinter hemorrhages, may be present. Petechial eruptions may be seen in acute *S. aureus* endocarditis.
Toxic shock syndrome	Presents with fever, rash (macular erythema), and hypotension.
Rocky Mountain spotted fever	Patients present with fever, myalgias, and headache. A rash may follow 3 to 5 days later; petechiae are seen in 50% of cases.
Leptospirosis	Patients have fevers and myalgias, may develop meningitis and/or petechial rash.
Chronic Meningococcemia	
Disseminated gonococcemia	Triad of "dermatitis", migratory polyarthritis, and tenosynovitis may be present.
Sweet syndrome	Fever, neutrophilia, arthralgias, and painful erythematous plaques, which may be recurrent.
Subacute bacterial endocarditis	May include a polymorphous petechial rash and/or joint symptoms in the setting of prolonged fever.
Cutaneous small vessel vasculitis	Occurs in Henoch-Schönlein purpura, or may be secondary to connective tissue disease (rheumatoid arthritis, Sjögren syndrome, systemic lupus erythematosus), infections, or drugs. Characterized by palpable purpura, although eruption may be polymorphous and episodic, occurring with fever and arthralgias. Henoch-Schönlein purpura may include abdominal pain, melena, and hematuria.
Rat-bite fever	Paroxysmal fever, migratory polyarthritis in 50% of cases, and rash 2 to 4 days following fever onset; classically, red-purple macules and papules.
Rheumatic fever	Fever, migratory polyarthritis, and cutaneous findings (erythema marginatum may occur in recurrent crops).

MEDICATIONS

Prior to obtaining antibiotic sensitivity results, patients should be treated with a third-generation cephalosporin such as ceftriaxone or cefotaxime. If testing reveals a penicillin minimum inhibitory concentration less than 0.1 µg/mL, penicillin G or ampicillin may be used.[30] For patients who are allergic to penicillin and cephalosporin, chloramphenicol is an alternative.[34] During outbreaks in sub-Saharan Africa a single dose of intramuscular long-acting chloramphenicol or ceftriaxone may be used.[35] As a result of significant antibiotic resistance, ciprofloxacin and sulfonamides are no longer recommended.[4] Standard antibiotic duration is 7 days.[11,30]

For cases complicated by septic shock, patients may require large volumes of fluids, as well as vasoactive drugs.[9] Although not widely available, patients with purpura fulminans may benefit from protein C concentrate, which has improved survival and limited amputations in small studies.[36] Although useful in pneumococcal meningitis, dexamethasone has not shown any benefit in meningococcal meningitis and should not be given in these patients.[37]

PROCEDURES

Patients with extensive necrosis and limb ischemia may require surgical debridement, skin grafting, muscular flap coverage for limb salvage, and/or amputation of digits or limbs.[13]

PREVENTION

Meningococcal disease can be prevented through population-wide vaccination and antibiotic chemoprophylaxis in close contacts of infected patients. Droplet precautions should be maintained from presumptive diagnosis until at least 24 hours after initiation of an effective antibiotic regimen.[11,30]

Chemoprophylaxis: Close contacts are defined as those who have had prolonged contact (>8 hours) within close proximity (<3 feet) of an infected patient, or those who have had direct exposure to the patient's oral secretions from 7 days before the onset of symptoms until 24 hours following initiation of effective antibiotics.[11] This may include family, friends, romantic partners, roommates, colleagues, contacts at school or daycare centers, contacts in college dormitories or military training centers, or travelers seated directly next to the patient on a long flight. As chemoprophylaxis is not warranted in those with brief contact, most health care workers do not require treatment, unless they have had direct exposure to respiratory secretions via suctioning or intubation.[33]

In ideal situations, chemoprophylaxis in those meeting criteria should be initiated within 24 hours of identification of an index patient. Otherwise, treatment should be initiated as soon as possible. Chemoprophylaxis administered more than 14 days after exposure is not recommended.[33] Antibiotics recommended for chemoprophylaxis include rifampin (children and adults; 4 doses given over 2 days), ciprofloxacin (adults; single dose), and ceftriaxone (children, adults, and pregnant women; single intramuscular dose). Rifampin and ciprofloxacin are not recommended in pregnancy.[11,33,34]

Vaccination: In the United States, there are several meningococcal vaccines available (Table 154-2). The Advisory Committee on Immunization Practices recommends immunization with a conjugate quadrivalent vaccine, Menactra or Menveo, for all patients 11 to 18 years old. Ideally, patients should be vaccinated at 11 or 12 years old with a booster at age 16 years. If the first dose is given at age 16 years or older, a booster is not needed.[33,38] In adolescents receiving Menactra, the effectiveness of inducing immunity is estimated to be approximately 80% to 85%.[39] Serogroup B meningococcal vaccines, Bexsero and Trumenba (licensed by the FDA in 2015 and 2014, respectively), are also recommended in the United States for certain high-risk patients age 10 years and older. For patients who are not high-risk, routine vaccination has not been recommended. However, clinical discretion may be used for elective administration in patients 16 to 23 years old, with preferred ages for vaccination between 16 years and 18 years.[38,40] The Advisory Committee on Immunization Practices outlines special vaccination guidelines for high-risk individuals, including those with asplenia, complement deficiencies (C3, C5 to C9, properdin, factor D, factor H), HIV, microbiologists routinely working with *N. meningitidis*, military recruits, college freshmen living in dormitories, and those traveling or residing in areas where meningococcal disease is epidemic or hyperendemic (eg, countries in the meningitis belt of sub-Saharan Africa during dry season or Mecca, Saudi Arabia, during the annual Hajj).[33,38]

INFECTIONS CAUSED BY *PSEUDOMONAS AERUGINOSA*

AT-A-GLANCE

- *Pseudomonas aeruginosa* is a ubiquitous Gram-negative rod, with a predilection for aqueous environments. It may be recognized by its sweet, grape-like odor and blue-green color conferred by pyocyanin pigment.
- *P. aeruginosa* is an important cause of nosocomial and ventilator-acquired pneumonia, cystic fibrosis lung infections, urinary tract infections in catheterized patients, and secondary cutaneous infection of burns, diabetic foot ulcers, surgical incision sites, and puncture wounds.
- Primary cutaneous infections, such as green nail syndrome, toe web infection, folliculitis, hot-foot syndrome, external otitis, and perichondritis typically necessitate a breach in skin integrity.
- Pseudomonal folliculitis and hot-foot syndrome are self-limited. The majority of other localized *P. aeruginosa* infections improve rapidly with topical or oral therapy, except for malignant otitis externa, which is invasive with a mortality rate of approximately 20%.
- Bacteremia and ecthyma gangrenosum typically affect hospitalized immunocompromised hosts, especially those with neutropenia.
- *P. aeruginosa* bacteremia is associated with higher mortality than bacteremia caused by other Gram-negative organisms. Mortality for patients with ecthyma gangrenosum ranges from 30% to 70%.
- Patients with serious *P. aeruginosa* infection require prompt initiation of systemic antibiotics with antipseudomonal activity. Drug resistance, including multidrug-resistant *P. aeruginosa* is a major challenge for therapy.

TABLE 154-2
Meningococcal Vaccines Available in the United States

VACCINE	SEROGROUPS	TYPE OF VACCINE
Menactra (MenACWY-DT)	A, C, W-135, Y	Polysaccharide conjugate with diphtheria toxoid
Menveo (MenACWY-CRM)	A, C, W-135, Y	Polysaccharide conjugate with mutant diphtheria toxin (CRM197)
Menomune (MPSV4)	A, C, W-135, Y	Polysaccharide, unconjugated
MenHibrix (HibMenCY)	C, Y, *Haemophilus influenzae* **type b**	Polysaccharide conjugate with tetanus toxoid
Bexsero (MenB-4C)	B	Includes 3 recombinant proteins—neisserial adhesion A (NadA), factor H binding protein (FHbp), and neisserial heparin binding antigen (NHBA)—as well as outer membrane vesicles (OMV) from a New Zealand epidemic strain (NZ98/254)
Trumenba (MenB-FHbp)	B	Includes 2 recombinant FHbp antigens

INTRODUCTION AND BACTERIOLOGY

Pseudomonas aeruginosa is an oxidase-positive, non-lactose fermenting, obligately aerobic Gram-negative rod with motility conferred by a single flagellum. It has a characteristic blue-green color and grape-like odor and can grow at temperatures up to 42°C (107.6°F). *P. aeruginosa* produces pyoverdin, a green-yellow pigment that fluoresces under a Wood lamp and is common to all fluorescent *Pseudomonas* species. It also produces pyocyanin, a blue-green nonfluorescent pigment specific to *P. aeruginosa*. It grows on blood, tryptic soy, and cetrimide agar, as well as MacConkey agar, where colonies appear white because of an absence of lactose fermentation.[41,42]

P. aeruginosa cutaneous infections typically necessitate a breach in skin integrity, as caused by maceration, dermatophyte infection, indwelling catheters, trauma or burns. Invasion of the skin and subcutaneous tissues is attributed to alkaline protease, protease IV, and elastases, which degrade cutaneous structures, and components of the host immune system. When *P. aeruginosa* makes contact with host cells, a Type III secretion may be activated by which exoenzymes (ExoS, ExoT, ExoU, and ExoY) are directly translocated into the host cell. ExoS interacts with TLRs to induce tumor necrosis factor-α production, ExoT binds adenosine diphosphate–ribosyltransferase, ExoU damages cell membranes, and ExoY binds adenylate cyclase.[43,44] *P. aeruginosa* also secretes exotoxin A, which inhibits eukaryotic elongation factor 2 via adenosine diphosphate–ribosylation, similar to diphtheria toxin, thereby inhibiting elongation of polypeptides during protein synthesis, leading to cell death.[43] Patients with higher serum levels of anti–exotoxin A antibodies experience milder *P. aeruginosa* septicemia.[44] Additional *P. aeruginosa* virulence factors include lipopolysaccharide, a TLR4 agonist and septic shock mediator common to other Gram-negative bacteria[45]; pyocyanin, which exerts proinflammatory and oxidative effects[46]; pyoverdin and pyochelin iron scavengers; and quorum sensing, which involves intercellular signaling to coordinate gene transcription and mediation of other virulence factors, such as biofilm formation.[44]

During prolonged colonization, *P. aeruginosa* may convert to a mucoid phenotype via overproduction of alginate, which scavenges macrophage free radicals, impairs phagocytosis, inhibits neutrophil chemotaxis and complement activation, and enables biofilm formation. Biofilms are particularly important in the setting of wound infections and osteomyelitis, vascular and urinary catheter-associated infections, lung infections in cystic fibrosis, and endocarditis in intravenous drug users where they confer resistance to antibiotics, as well as host immunity. Other mechanisms of antibiotic resistance include multidrug efflux pumps, beta-lactamases and downregulation of porins in the outer membrane bilayer.[43]

EPIDEMIOLOGY

P. aeruginosa is a ubiquitous bacterium, with a predilection for aqueous environments. It can be recovered from virtually any environmental water source, and its hardiness enables survival even under the nutritionally stringent conditions of distilled water where it uses dissolved gases and residual ions for growth. *P. aeruginosa* has been identified in the conjunctival microflora and feces of healthy patients, and has been isolated from practically every source within hospitals, from water reservoir systems to the hands of health care workers.[42,43]

While *P. aeruginosa* can cause minor infections in otherwise healthy patients with a compromised skin barrier, *P. aeruginosa* is an important cause of major, life-threatening infections in immunocompromised patients, such as those with uncontrolled diabetes, neutropenia, hematologic disorders, cancer, or transplanted organs, or those receiving prolonged treatment with steroids or antibiotics.[44] *P. aeruginosa* accounts for 4% to 6% of all hospital-acquired bloodstream infections, although rates may be as high as 20% in intensive care units.[43] It is the number one pathogen responsible for lung injury among ventilator-dependent patients and those with cystic fibrosis, the second most common cause of nosocomial pneumonia, and the third most common cause of urinary tract infection, especially in catheterized patients. *P. aeruginosa* is frequently isolated from burn wounds, diabetic foot ulcers, surgical incision sites, and puncture wounds.[43,44,47] The growing presence of *P. aeruginosa*, especially in hospital settings, has been attributed to antibiotic use. Among 200 hospitals in the United States, *P. aeruginosa* multidrug resistance was 22% in the setting of pneumonia and 15% among bloodstream infections.[48]

CLINICAL FEATURES

P. aeruginosa cutaneous infection may occur from direct inoculation, typically in the setting of skin-barrier compromise, or secondary to *P. aeruginosa* bacteremia. Local conditions associated with direct inoculation include green nail syndrome, toe web infection, folliculitis, hot-foot syndrome, external otitis, and perichondritis, whereas ecthyma gangrenosum and nonspecific cutaneous findings, most commonly subcutaneous nodules, are associated with bacteremia (Table 154-3).

CUTANEOUS FINDINGS

Green Nail Syndrome and Toe Web Infection: Green nail syndrome, or chloronychia, is characterized by nail dyspigmentation that may be greenish-yellow, greenish-blue, greenish-brown, or greenish-black. Dyspigmentation results from the accumulation of debris and pyocyanin, which adheres to the underside of the nail plate. It may affect the entire or partial nail and is typically limited to one or two dig-

TABLE 154-3
Summary Table for *Pseudomonas aeruginosa* Infection

	CLINICAL FEATURES	RISK FACTORS	LABORATORY TESTS	COURSE AND PROGNOSIS	MANAGEMENT
Green nail syndrome	Greenish-yellow, greenish-blue, greenish-brown, or greenish-black dyspigmentation of the nail (chloronychia)	Prolonged submersion in fresh water	Nail specimens for culture Wood lamp: white and green fluorescence	Responsive to treatment	Detachment of nail plate and topical antimicrobial for 1 to 4 months; acetic acid soaks Preventive measures
Pseudomonas toe web infection	Thickened, macerated skin with moth eaten appearance and yellow-green purulence; web space and sole of foot may be affected	Persistently wet feet in heat and humidity			Usually, both antifungal and antibacterial therapy are required; topical antibacterials (gentamicin) or oral antibacterials; Castellani paint, gentian violet, acetic acid soaks
Pseudomonas folliculitis	Discrete, follicular papules and pustules of sudden onset (24 hours following exposure); upper trunk, axillary folds, hips and buttocks typically affected	Recreational use of hot tubs, whirlpools, swimming pools	Unroofing pustule and bacterial culture Punch biopsy of nodules (for hot-foot syndrome) Water sample of suspected sources	Self-limited	Avoidance of predisposing factors; symptomatic care Oral antibiotics (ciprofloxacin) for protracted cases or significant discomfort
Hot-foot syndrome	Acute painful, erythematous, warm plantar nodules				
External otitis and perichondritis	Acute-onset edema, erythema, and discoloration of the external auditory canal; tenderness with tragal pressure; severe pain disproportionate to examination findings may indicate malignant otitis externa	Swimmers with prolonged excess moisture in the ear canal, use of ear-occluding devices; dermatologic conditions affecting skin integrity of the auditory canal	Otoscopy (to rule out otitis media) Cultures of ear discharge Blood cultures (if constitutional symptoms present)	Malignant otitis externa is invasive with 20% mortality	Antimicrobial ear drops, wick placement for severe disease; oral antibacterials (ciprofloxacin) for severe cases or immunocompromised patients; perichondritis: drainage and extended antibacterial therapy (6 to 8 weeks); malignant otitis externa warrants referral to a surgical otolaryngology service
Bacteremia and ecthyma gangrenosum	Subcutaneous nodules, cellulitis, pustules, absent	Neutropenia, hematologic malignancy, CD4+ lymphocyte count <50 cells/mm^3	Biopsies reveal necrotizing or hemorrhagic vasculitis, epidermal and dermal necrosis	Bacteremia: 30-day mortality rate of 39%; ecthyma gangrenosum: 30% to 70% mortality rate	Prompt intravenous empiric therapy with an antipseudomonal β-lactam

its. Many patients present with a triad of dyspigmentation, onycholysis, and paronychia (Fig. 154-3).[41,42,49]

P. aeruginosa toe web infection presents with thickened, macerated skin with a characteristic moth-eaten appearance and yellow-green purulence.[12,41] Vesicles, pustules, and erosions may be present with a hyperkeratotic rim. The infection can affect toe web spaces, as well as the sole of the foot, and patients sometimes complain of burning and pain.[42]

Folliculitis and Hot-Foot Syndrome:

P. aeruginosa folliculitis, commonly "hot tub folliculitis," presents with discrete, follicular papules and pustules that heal with fine desquamation and hyperpigmented macules. Urticarial lesions may occur in some patients. Onset is sudden, approximately 24 hours following exposure to contaminated hot tubs or whirlpools and may be associated with pruritus or pain. Commonly affected areas include the upper trunk, axillary folds, hips, and buttocks, typically including areas covered by the patient's bathing suit (Fig. 154-4A). The Montgomery (areolar) glands may be affected in both sexes.[41,42] Of note, acne patients treated with long courses of tetracycline antibiotics occasionally may develop folliculitis caused by Gram-negative bacteria, including *P. aeruginosa*.

A related entity, hot-foot syndrome, has been described following emersion in contaminated wading pools and hot tubs, usually in children. It presents with acute painful, erythematous, warm plantar nodules. One report described an outbreak of hot-foot syndrome among 40 children within approximately 40 hours of spending time in a wading pool with a rough, abrasive floor.[50] Another report described similar findings on both the soles and palms of 33 children following use of a contaminated hot tub (see Fig. 154-4B, C).[51]

External Otitis and Perichondritis:

Otitis externa, or "swimmer's ear," is characterized by acute onset of edema and erythema or discoloration of the external auditory canal, sometimes with maceration, discharge and/or regional lymphadenopathy. There is often tenderness with tragal pressure or movement of the pinna, and patients may complain of pruritus.[41,52] Although the condition is most common among children 5 to 14 years of age, it can occur in all age groups following submersion of the head in water.[53]

In elderly patients, especially those with diabetes, external otitis may progress to life-threatening malignant otitis externa, an invasive condition leading to skull-base osteomyelitis. Malignant otitis externa is characterized by an insidious onset with edema, erythema, and persistent discharge from the ear canal with severe pain that appears disproportionate to examination findings. Early cases usually lack fever or constitutional symptoms. The presence of granulation tissue in the floor of the external auditory canal at the bony–cartilaginous junction is a classic finding, and frank necrosis of the canal also may be present. Tympanic membrane visualization is often blocked by discharge and granulation tissue.[41,42]

Perichondritis of the ear helix or tragus may be caused by *P. aeruginosa* following commercial piercings as a result of contaminated cleansing agents, as well as following trauma or acupuncture.[42] The ear is typically swollen, erythematous, and tender, and prompt treatment is essential because of rapid progression to cartilage necrosis.

Bacteremia and Ecthyma Gangrenosum:

P. aeruginosa bacteremia is associated with cutaneous manifestations in approximately one-third of cases, the most recognized of which include subcutaneous nodules, ecthyma gangrenosum, and gangrenous cellulitis, although pustules, abscesses, vesicles, bullae, petechiae, and maculopapular eruptions also have been reported. Subcutaneous nodules are typically warm, erythematous, indurated, usually nonfluctuant, and they may be painful or painless. They have been reported on the face, neck, chest, abdomen, back, and extremities.[41,42]

Ecthyma gangrenosum is responsible for necrotic cutaneous lesions associated with *P. aeruginosa* bacteremia, especially in neutropenic patients, although, rarely, bacteremia may be absent. It begins with a painless, infarcted gunmetal gray macule or papule with surrounding erythema. As the ecthyma develops, the lesion becomes more indurated and pustules or hemorrhagic bullae may develop. Over a rapid course of 12 to 18 hours the patient is left with a necrotic, ulcerative eschar with a halo of tender erythema (Fig. 154-5). Ecthyma gangrenosum may be solitary or numerous, with lesions

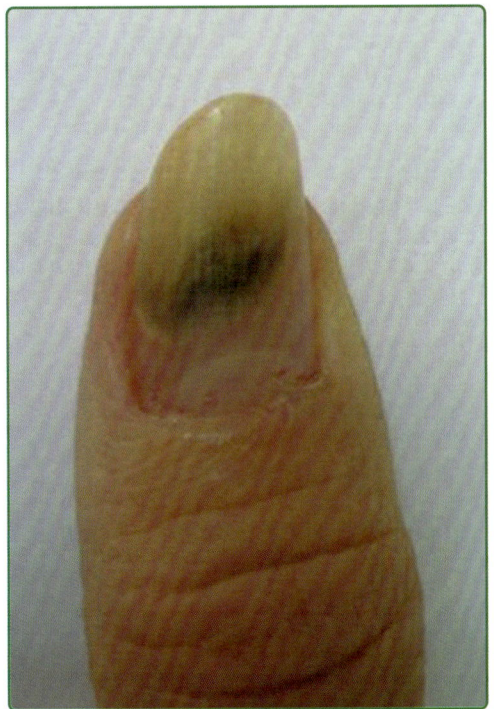

Figure 154-3 *Pseudomonas* green nail syndrome often occurs in those with preexisting onycholysis, especially when frequently submerged in fresh water. (Reproduced with permission from Shemer A, Daniel CR. Common nail disorders. *Clin Dermatol*. 2013;31(5):578-586. Copyright © Elsevier.)

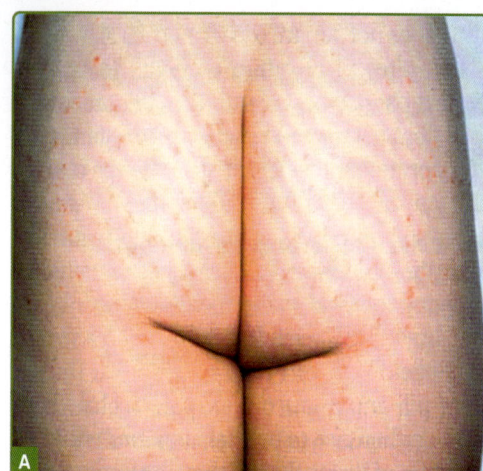
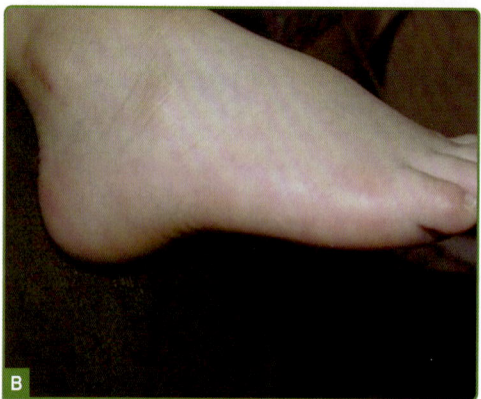
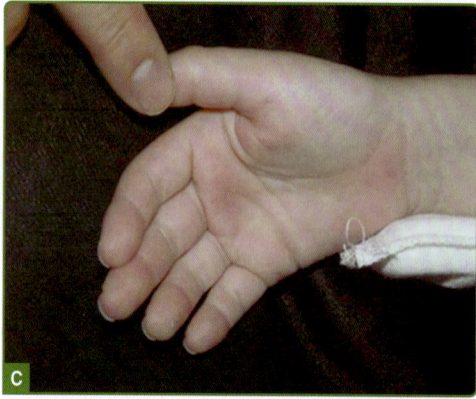

Figure 154-4 Exposure to contaminated hot tubs, whirlpools, or wading pools may lead to pseudomonal folliculitis, typically affecting areas covered by the patient's bathing suit (**A**). Children may present with hot-foot syndrome, characterized by painful, erythematous plantar nodules (**B**), which may also affect the palms (**C**). (Image **A**, Used with permission from Kenneth E. Greer, MD. Previously published in Wortman PD. Bacterial infections of the skin. *Curr Probl Dermatol.* 1993;5[6]:197-224; and Images **B** and **C**, from Yu Y, Cheng AS, Wang L, et al. Hot tub folliculitis or hot hand–foot syndrome caused by *Pseudomonas aeruginosa*. *J Am Acad Dermatol.* 2007;57[4]:596-600.)

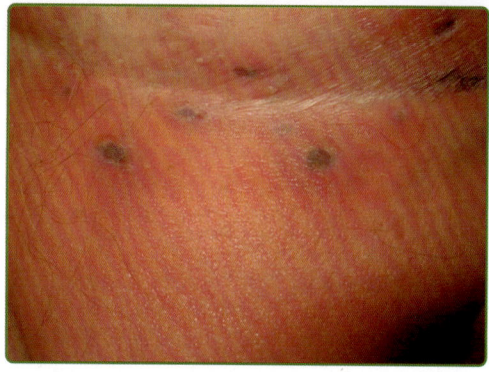

Figure 154-5 This patient with ecthyma gangrenosum has multifocal gunmetal gray, necrotic ulcers scattered across the suprapubic area with halos of erythema. (Reproduced with permission from Cresce N, Marchetti MA, Russell M. A sea sickness? Ecthyma gangrenosum. *Am J Med.* 2014; 127[7]:592-594. Copyright © Elsevier.)

most commonly affecting the anogenital region (57%), extremities (30%), trunk (6%), and face (6%).[42,54,55]

NONCUTANEOUS FINDINGS

Even in the absence of bacteremia, mild *P. aeruginosa* infections, such as folliculitis or otitis externa, may present with fever and malaise. As bacteremic patients progress to sepsis, they may present with fever, tachycardia, tachypnea, altered mental status, and hypotension. Most patients with ecthyma gangrenosum present with fever and other constitutional signs, although sometimes these may be absent.

Both otitis externa and malignant otitis externa may lead to severe swelling of the external auditory canal, producing conductive hearing loss. As necrosis and osteomyelitis associated with malignant otitis externa progresses, patients may experience cranial nerve palsies, most commonly affecting the facial nerve, as well as trismus, or lockjaw, when the temporomandibular joint is affected.[42]

ETIOLOGY AND PATHOGENESIS

GREEN NAIL SYNDROME AND TOE WEB INFECTION

Green nail syndrome typically occurs in patients whose digits are subjected to prolonged submersion in fresh water, especially with soap or detergents. Patients whose nailbeds are more easily accessible to pathogens due to onycholysis, chronic paronychia or other nail disorders, such as psoriasis, are particularly at risk.[49]

Pseudomonas toe web infection is found in patients with persistently wet feet as a consequence of closed-toe, tight-fitting shoes, occupational or recreational exertion, and/or warm, humid weather. Infection may also occur secondarily in the setting of tinea pedis.[41]

FOLLICULITIS AND HOT-FOOT SYNDROME

Pseudomonal folliculitis and hot-foot syndrome occur following recreational use of hot tubs, whirlpools, and, less commonly, swimming pools that lack adequate halogenation. Folliculitis outbreaks most commonly occur following submersion in water heated above 38 °C, as *P. aeruginosa* is heat tolerant, and infection risk increases with duration of bathing. The most frequent *P. aeruginosa* serotype isolated from pseudomonal folliculitis is O-11, although serotypes O-4, O-6, and O-9 also have been implicated.[41,42]

EXTERNAL OTITIS

Pathogenesis of external otitis is best understood through examination of basic anatomy and physiology of the external auditory canal. The outer cartilaginous portion is lined with skin containing cerumen glands, sebaceous glands, and hair follicles. The inner bony portion contains thin skin devoid of adnexal structures and a dermis that is in direct contact with underlying periosteum. Cerumen provides a sticky, hydrophobic protective layer that repels water and traps fine debris, as well as an antimicrobial lysozyme and pH of 6.9, which discourage microbial growth. The canal is self-cleaning by lateral epithelial migration, a process that slows with age.

Those at risk for external otitis include swimmers with prolonged excess moisture in their ear canal, those who scratch or aggressively clean their ears, use ear-occluding devices such as earphones or hearing aids, or suffer from dermatologic conditions such as psoriasis, atopic dermatitis or seborrheic dermatitis. Any of these factors may contribute to breakdown of the skin-cerumen barrier in the external auditory canal. This breakdown then triggers inflammation, pruritus (with further scratching), edema and obstruction, ultimately leading to changes in the quantity and quality of cerumen production, impaired epithelial migration and increased pH of the canal, creating an environment hospitable to microorganisms. *P. aeruginosa* is involved in approximately 50% of external otitis cases, and is by far the most common etiologic agent. The next most common cause is *Staphylococcus aureus*, followed by a variety of other aerobic bacteria, anaerobes, and fungi.[56,57]

In malignant otitis externa, *P. aeruginosa* invades the soft tissues at the bony–cartilaginous junction of the external canal, which may lead to infection and necrosis of the cartilage, mastoid process, temporal bone, and, eventually, the base of the skull. The predominance of malignant otitis externa in elderly diabetic patients may be the result of microangiopathy of the ear canal, as well as an increased pH of diabetic cerumen. Although elderly diabetics are the most commonly affected group, malignant otitis externa has also been reported in younger, nondiabetic patients with HIV, as well as in nondiabetic elderly people following aural surgery or water irrigation. Overall, more than 95% of cases are caused by *P. aeruginosa*, although malignant otitis externa in HIV patients also may be caused by *Aspergillus* spp.[58]

BACTEREMIA AND ECTHYMA GANGRENOSUM

P. aeruginosa bacteremia is usually seen in hospitalized patients, especially those with neutropenia, hematologic malignancy, CD4+ lymphocyte count less than 50 cells/mm^3, or other immunocompromised states. Those with recent courses of antimicrobial therapy, chemotherapy, invasive devices, or surgical procedures are also at higher risk.[43,59] Bacteremia may occur as a result of direct bloodstream inoculation, such as through an intravenous catheter, or secondary to invasive infection. Primary infection sites commonly leading to bacteremia include the lungs, urinary and GI tracts, and skin and soft tissues, especially wound infections.[60] Pseudomonal skin infections that typically remain localized in immunocompetent patients may become a source of bacteremia in immunocompromised patients. For example, pseudomonal toe web infection may progress to cellulitis, osteomyelitis and sepsis, especially in overweight persons with diabetes.[61]

Approximately 1.3% to 3% of patients with *P. aeruginosa* bacteremia develop ecthyma gangrenosum from perivascular bacterial invasion of the media and adventitia of small veins and arteries. Rarely, ecthyma gangrenosum caused by *P. aeruginosa* has been reported in the absence of bacteremia.[55,62] Although *P. aeruginosa* is the most well-known cause of ecthyma gangrenosum, cases also have been reported as being caused by a variety of Gram-negative (*Aeromonas hydrophila, Escherichia coli, Burkholderia cepacia*) and Gram-positive (group A streptococci, *S. aureus*) bacteria, as well as fungi (*Candida, Aspergillus, Mucor, Fusarium* spp.).[12,55]

DIAGNOSIS

LABORATORY TESTING

Green Nail Syndrome and Toe Web Infection: In patients with green nail syndrome, nail specimens collected for cultures frequently reveal *P. aeruginosa*, as well as fungi associated with onycholysis. *P. aeruginosa* also can be cultured from toe web infections, and illumination under a Wood lamp may reveal that the infection fluoresces white and green. Toe web infections that are scraped and subjected to a potassium hydroxide preparation may reveal dermatophytes associated with tinea pedis.[41]

Folliculitis and Hot-Foot Syndrome: Pseudomonal folliculitis may be diagnosed via unroofing and culture of pustules, and bacterial subtyping frequently reveals serotype O-11.[42] When the diagnosis of hot-foot syndrome is uncertain, a punch biopsy of a nodule may be performed for pathology and culture.[50] Water samples from suspected sources, such as hot-tubs and wading pools, also may be tested for *P. aeruginosa* contamination.

External Otitis and Perichondritis: The diagnosis of uncomplicated external otitis is typically clinical and should include otoscopy to distinguish from otitis media. Cultures should be collected when external otitis is severe, chronic, recurrent, nonresponsive to treatment, or occurring after aural surgery or in immunocompromised patients.[63] Perichondritis should be cultured following incision and drainage.[64]

Suspicion for malignant otitis externa warrants prompt referral to a surgical otolaryngology service. Ear discharge should be sent for cultures, and blood cultures should be collected, especially when constitutional symptoms or fevers are present. Routine laboratory test results are often normal, except for erythrocyte sedimentation rate and C-reactive protein, which are usually elevated and may be used to monitor disease activity.[41,65]

Bacteremia and Ecthyma Gangrenosum: Blood cultures should be collected from any patient with suspected *P. aeruginosa* bacteremia and/or ecthyma gangrenosum. Cutaneous findings associated with bacteremia should be cultured whenever possible, and subcutaneous nodules in bacteremic patients are frequently biopsied. Suspected ecthyma gangrenosum warrants a culture of any lesion exudates, as well as a biopsy for pathology and culture.[41,42]

PATHOLOGY

Hot-Foot Syndrome: If biopsied, hot-foot syndrome may reveal perivascular, interstitial, and periadnexal infiltration of neutrophils that extend to the lobules of subcutaneous fat, and may include deep dermal or subcutaneous abscesses. Specimens may also show focal areas of vasculitis with thrombi.[50]

Bacteremia and Ecthyma Gangrenosum: Subcutaneous nodules associated with *P. aeruginosa* bacteremia reveal an acute vasculitis and suppurative panniculitis with visible Gram-negative rods.[42] Ecthyma gangrenosum is characterized by a necrotizing hemorrhagic vasculitis, a necrosed epidermis and upper dermis, and variable inflammatory infiltrates depending on the hematologic status of the patient. Gram-negative bacteria may be visualized between the collagen bundles, as well as in the media and adventitia of small vessels, classically with intimal sparing.[32,41,42]

IMAGING

Malignant Otitis Externa: CT or MRI may be used in malignant otitis externa patients to visualize disease extension into the bony structures. If the infectious nature of the disease is uncertain following examination and laboratory testing, patients may require a biopsy, as imaging cannot differentiate squamous cell carcinoma of the external auditory canal from malignant otitis externa.[65]

DIFFERENTIAL DIAGNOSIS

Table 154-4 outlines the differential diagnosis for *Pseudomonas aeruginosa* infections.

CLINICAL COURSE AND PROGNOSIS

Pseudomonal folliculitis and hot-foot syndrome are benign and self-limited, and the majority of other localized *P. aeruginosa* infections improve rapidly with topical or oral therapy. Malignant otitis externa is invasive and carries a mortality rate of approximately 20%.[66]

P. aeruginosa bacteremia is associated with higher mortality than bacteremia caused by other Gram-negative organisms. In one study, the 30-day mortality rate was 39%.[67] In another study, a comparison between *P. aeruginosa* bacteremia patients who received timely, appropriate therapy and those who experienced a 1- to 2-day delay in treatment had cure rates of 74% and 46%, respectively.[68] For patients with ecthyma gangrenosum, the mortality rate ranges from 30% to 70%, with multiple lesions, prolonged neutropenia, and delayed therapy correlating with a poor prognosis.[41]

MANAGEMENT

When required, systemic treatment of *P. aeruginosa* infection is limited to select antibiotics with antipseudomonal activity, including certain penicillins (ticarcillin-clavulanic acid, piperacillin-tazobactam), cephalosporins (cefepime, ceftazidime, cefoperazone), monobactams (aztreonam), carbapenems (meropenem, doripenem, imipenem/cilastatin), fluoroquinolones (ciprofloxacin, levofloxacin), aminoglycosides (gentamicin, tobramycin, amikacin), and polymyxins (colistin). However, *P. aeruginosa* may develop resistance to any of these agents, typically as a consequence of previous exposure. Resistance development is especially rapid against

TABLE 154-4
Differential Diagnosis for *Pseudomonas aeruginosa* Infections

P. AERUGINOSA INFECTION	DIFFERENTIAL DIAGNOSIS
Green nail syndrome	Subungual hematoma Melanocytic nevus Melanoma Onychomycosis caused by *Aspergillus*, *Candida*, or dermatophytes Infection with other Gram-negative or Gram-positive bacteria
Pseudomonal toe web infection	Toe web infection caused by dermatophytes, *Aspergillus*, *Candida*, or other Gram-negative or Gram-positive bacteria Erythrasma Pitted keratolysis Atopic dermatitis Psoriasis
Pseudomonal folliculitis	Other bacterial folliculitis Eosinophilic folliculitis Papular urticaria Acne vulgaris Steroid acne Insect bites Miliaria rubra
Hot-foot syndrome	Plantar urticaria Palmoplantar eccrine hidradenitis Chilblains Erythema multiforme Erythema nodosum
External otitis	Chronic suppurative otitis media External otitis caused by other aerobic bacteria, anaerobic bacteria, or fungi Contact, atopic, or seborrheic dermatitis Psoriasis Squamous cell carcinoma
Malignant external otitis	Malignant otitis externa caused by *Aspergillus* spp. (especially in HIV patients) Squamous cell carcinoma with temporal bone involvement
Ecthyma gangrenosum	Ecthyma gangrenosum caused by other Gram-negative or Gram-positive bacteria or fungi Pyoderma gangrenosum Calciphylaxis Septic emboli Cutaneous anthrax Cutaneous aspergillosis Acute meningococcemia

imipenem/cilastatin because of downregulation of a carbapenem-specific porin in the outer membrane bilayer, as well as ciprofloxacin as a consequence of drug efflux and mutation of drug targets (DNA gyrase, topoisomerase IV).[43]

GREEN NAIL SYNDROME AND TOE WEB INFECTION

Green nail syndrome should be treated via removal of detached nail plate, followed by application of a topical antimicrobial for 1 to 4 months. Topical antimicrobials may include 2% sodium hypochlorite, aminoglycosides (eg, tobramycin, gentamicin), fluoroquinolones (eg, ciprofloxacin, nadifloxacin), polymyxin B, or bacitracin. Acetic acid soaks also have been used. When patients do not respond to topical treatment or topical therapy is not preferred, oral ciprofloxacin may be used for 2 to 3 weeks. Any topical or oral intervention should be accompanied by avoidance of chronic moisture or submersion in water.[12,41,42,49]

Pseudomonal toe web infections typically require both antibacterial and antifungal therapy, in addition to debridement of any necrotic tissue. Topical antibacterial treatment, such as with gentamicin cream, may be sufficient in mild cases, whereas more fulminant cases require oral antibacterials (eg, ciprofloxacin) and severe cases, especially in persons with diabetes, warrant intravenous therapy. Application of Castellani (carbol-fuchsin) paint, gentian violet, or acetic acid soaks also may be employed.[42,69]

FOLLICULITIS AND HOT-FOOT SYNDROME

Given the self-limited nature of pseudomonal folliculitis and hot-foot syndrome, most patients are treated with exposure removal and symptomatic care. Oral ciprofloxacin can be used in protracted cases or those associated with significant discomfort. Use of topical gentamicin or tobramycin cream with diluted acetic acid baths also have been reported.[42]

EXTERNAL OTITIS AND PERICHONDRITIS

External otitis treatment should include gentle removal of canal debris, followed by administration of antimicrobial ear drops, which may be selected from a variety of antibiotic, antiseptic, or combination antibiotic/glucocorticoid solutions. Meta-analyses have not revealed significant differences between topical interventions, except that acetic acid antiseptic was less effective than combination antibiotic–glucocorticoid solution among patients with unresolved symptoms after 1 week.[52,70] Wick placement should be pursued for patients with severe disease or a completely occluded canal. Oral ciprofloxacin should be given for 7 to 10 days for coverage of *P. aeruginosa* and *S. aureus* in immunocompromised patients or those with extended infection beyond the external canal (eg, periaural cellulitis).[63]

Patients with perichondritis require prompt culture and drainage with through-and-through incisions, initiation of oral ciprofloxacin, and follow up of sensitivity data to ensure adequate treatment. Extended therapy may be required as cartilaginous ear structures have poor blood supply. Timely, appropriate therapy is essential because of the risk of cartilage necrosis and permanent ear deformity.[71]

Malignant otitis externa warrants prompt referral to a surgical otolaryngology service. Treatment includes debridement of necrotic tissue and a prolonged course of systemic antibiotics, as required for osteomyelitis. Ciprofloxacin may be used for 6 to 8 weeks against sensitive strains. Fluoroquinolone-resistant strains require 6 to 10 weeks of an antipseudomonal β-lactam, such as piperacillin-tazobactam, ceftazidime, or cefepime. Mastoidectomy or other surgical intervention may be required in extensive cases.[41,42,72]

BACTEREMIA AND ECTHYMA GANGRENOSUM

In patients with suspected *P. aeruginosa* bacteremia, the primary site of infection should always be addressed, if known, and any infected catheters should be removed. Patients require prompt intravenous empiric therapy, typically with an antipseudomonal β-lactam. When empiric combination therapy is desired, especially in those with neutropenia, burn wounds, ecthyma gangrenosum or signs of sepsis, an aminoglycoside is commonly added. In patients with renal insufficiency, a fluoroquinolone may be added instead. Once susceptibility results are available, patients may be switched to an appropriate monotherapy, as combination regimens have not been shown to improve mortality or prevent emergence of antibiotic resistant *P. aeruginosa*. Aminoglycosides should never be used as monotherapy when other options are available. Alternative antibiotics for multidrug-resistant infections include ceftazidime-avibactam, ceftolozane-tazobactam, and colistin. Because colistin is the only option against some multidrug-resistant strains, it is increasingly used despite very high rates of nephrotoxicity.[41-43,73-75]

PREVENTION

Green nail syndrome can be prevented by wearing gloves while dishwashing and discarding or sterilizing contaminated sponges. Toe web infection may be avoided by keeping feet dry and treating underlying fungal infections. To prevent recurrence of pseudomonal folliculitis, hot tubs should be drained and superchlorinated or scrubbed with quaternary ammonium compounds.[42,49] Patients prone to external otitis should be advised not to clean the ear with fingers, cotton swabs, or other foreign objects. Following submersion of the head in water, ears can be dried noninvasively by tilting the head or using a blow dryer (1 foot away from the ear, on low setting). Homemade ear drops comprised of 1:1 5% acetic acid (white vinegar) and isopropyl alcohol (rubbing alcohol) have been employed after water exposure as a preventive measure.[41]

Given the prevalence of *P. aeruginosa* in inpatient settings, hospital-acquired infections may be minimized via handwashing, sterile technique, cleaning shared equipment, and strict contact isolation of patients with multidrug resistant infection. Burn patients should receive wound care that reduces colonizing bacteria, including wound cleaning, debridement, dressings, and application of silver sulfadiazine.[43]

INFECTIONS CAUSED BY *BARTONELLA* SPECIES

AT-A-GLANCE

- *Bartonella* are facultative intracellular Gram-negative bacilli, that parasitize erythrocytes.
- *Bartonella henselae* is responsible for cat scratch disease, bacillary angiomatosis, and endocarditis. The vector is the cat flea (*Ctenocephalides felis*), cats are reservoir hosts, and infection in humans is incidental.
- *Bartonella quintana* causes trench fever, bacillary angiomatosis, and endocarditis. Humans serve as reservoir hosts, and the human body louse (*Pediculus humanus*) is the vector.
- *Bartonella bacilliformis* is the etiologic agent of Carrion disease, a biphasic infection with an acute phase known as *Oroya fever*, followed by a chronic phase, verruga peruana. Humans are the only known reservoir hosts, and the vector is the sand fly (*Lutzomyia verrucarum*).
- *Bartonella* species cause prolonged intraerythrocytic bacteremia in natural reservoir hosts, but not incidental hosts, thereby positioning themselves to be spread from reservoir to reservoir via blood-sucking arthropods.
- *Bartonella* may generate angiomatous lesions in bacillary angiomatosis and verruga peruana by stimulating angiogenesis and inhibiting endothelial cell apoptosis in the setting of an immunocompromised host.
- Cat scratch disease typically occurs in immunocompetent hosts. Rather than generating angiomatous lesions, *B. henselae* may instigate granuloma formation by inhibiting phagocytic uptake and delaying bacterial death within macrophages.
- Culture isolation of *Bartonella* is difficult in clinical practice, and specimens may require weeks of incubation. An indirect fluorescent antibody assay is frequently used.

INTRODUCTION AND BACTERIOLOGY

Bartonella is a genus of fastidious, facultative intracellular Gram-negative bacilli, which frequently parasitize erythrocytes because of their inability to synthesize heme or protoporphyrin X. They are best cultured on 5% rabbit or sheep blood agar at 35°C to 37°C (95°F to 98.6°F) with 5% to 10% carbon dioxide and 40% humidity. Even under ideal conditions, primary isolates require several days or weeks for visible growth, which in practice makes diagnosis challenging.[76,77]

Bartonella belong to the α_2 subgroup of the class *Proteobacteria*, which includes other intracellular parasites, such as *Brucella*, *Rickettsia*, and *Ehrlichia*. The *Bartonella* genus includes more than 30 species, many of which reside in animals, and only some cause human disease. *Bartonella* infection is often arthropod borne (flea, louse, sand fly), but it also can be transmitted via animal scratches or bites.[76]

The 3 most clinically relevant *Bartonella* species are *Bartonella henselae*, *Bartonella quintana*, and *Bartonella bacilliformis* (Table 154-5). *B. henselae* is responsible for cat scratch disease (CSD), as well as some cases of bacillary angiomatosis (BA) and endocarditis. The vector is the cat flea (*Ctenocephalides felis*), and cats are reservoir hosts, and infection in humans is incidental. *B. quintana* causes trench fever, BA, and endocarditis. Humans serve as reservoir hosts, and the human body louse (*Pediculus humanus*) is the vector. *B. bacilliformis* is the etiologic agent of Carrion disease, a biphasic infection with an acute phase known as Oroya fever, followed by a chronic phase, verruga peruana. Humans are the only known reservoir hosts of *B. bacilliformis*, and the vector is the sand fly (*Lutzomyia verrucarum*).[76,77]

EPIDEMIOLOGY

CAT SCRATCH DISEASE

CSD is the most common *Bartonella* infection. Although the disease has a worldwide distribution, there is an increased prevalence in warm, humid climates where cat fleas (*C. felis*) are most abundant, and peak occurrence is in fall and winter. CSD typically affects immunocompetent patients, especially children and young adults, with a median age of 15 years. There is typically a history of cat contact, scratches, or bites, although this is not always found. Although cats are the main reservoir for the causative agent, *B. henselae*, rare cases have been associated with dogs.

In the United States, more than 40,000 cases of CSD and more than 2000 associated hospitalizations are reported each year. The findings of 2 California studies indicate a substantial rate of cat infection. One study isolated *B. henselae* from the blood in 25 (41%) of 61 healthy impounded or pet cats, while the other study found *B. henselae* antibodies in 166 (81%) of 205 cats.[76,78,79]

TRENCH FEVER

Trench fever was perhaps the most widespread *Bartonella* infection of the past. It is best known for affecting soldiers throughout World War I, during which an estimated 1 million people were infected. Infections rose again, but to a lesser extent, during World War II, after which the incidence of trench fever became rare. Currently, trench fever is considered a reemerging disease among homeless people in urban areas, sometimes termed *urban trench fever*. The classic patient is a homeless, alcoholic man with poor hygiene, and patients are often immunocompetent.

The etiologic agent, *B. quintana*, is passed from person to person via the human body louse (*P. humanus*) vector. As with *B. henselae* in cats, *B. quintana* may cause a chronic, asymptomatic bacteremia in human reservoirs. In a 1997 study in Marseilles, France, *B. quintana* bacteremia was identified in 10 (14%) of 71 homeless people evaluated in an emergency department, who lacked any clinical signs or symptoms of infection.[76,78,80]

BACILLARY ANGIOMATOSIS

BA was first described as a new condition in HIV-infected patients in 1983, especially those with CD4+ lymphocyte counts less than 100 cells/mm³. It is occasionally reported in other immunocompromised patients, including patients after cardiac or renal transplantation and those receiving chemotherapy for hematologic malignancies. It is rarely reported in immunocompetent patients. Currently, BA is uncommon given the widespread use of antiretroviral

TABLE 154-5
Bartonella Species Infections

SPECIES	DISEASE	VECTOR	RESERVOIR
Bartonella bacilliformis	Carrion disease (Oroya fever and verruga peruana)	*Lutzomyia verrucarum* (sand fly)	Human
Bartonella henselae	Cat scratch disease, bacillary angiomatosis, endocarditis	*Ctenocephalides felis* (cat flea)	Cat
Bartonella quintana	Trench fever, bacillary angiomatosis, endocarditis	*Pediculus humanus* (human body louse)	Human

therapy. In a study in Germany, the incidence was estimated to be 1.2 cases per 1000 HIV-infected patients.[81]

BA may be caused by either *B. henselae* or *B. quintana*, and each accounts for roughly half of all cases in the United States. By contrast, *B. quintana* has been the main etiologic agent in Europe; *B. henselae* has only recently been documented as an etiologic agent of BA in Europe.[78]

BA lesions have been identified in the skin, as well as in visceral organs, bone, and lymph nodes. Epidemiologic studies indicate that the skin is the most common site of disease, ranging from 55% to 90% of total cases. *B. henselae* and *B. quintana* have an approximately equal tendency to cause cutaneous lesions, while *B. henselae* is the primary cause of liver, splenic, and lymph node lesions, and *B. quintana* is the primary cause of lesions in the subcutis and bone.[76,77]

CARRION DISEASE

Carrion disease, which includes Oroya fever and verruga peruana, is typically found in the Andean valleys of Peru, Colombia, and Ecuador. This corresponds with the ecologic distribution of the sand fly vector (*L. verrucarum*) for *B. bacilliformis*. Recently, however, the disease was identified outside of these river valleys, presenting public health problems across various areas of Peru, Columbia, and Ecuador, which have been attributed to climate change. Cases also have been reported in Bolivia, Chile, and Guatemala.[76,78,82]

Humans are the only known reservoirs of *B. bacilliformis*, and those native to endemic regions may serve as carriers, with prolonged asymptomatic bacteremia. Compared to travelers who often develop severe infection, natives with Carrion disease are more likely to experience a mild course, and may frequently present with only the chronic phase of disease, verruga peruana, without a history of Oroya fever. One study in a Peruvian valley community found a 0.5% baseline prevalence of asymptomatic *B. bacilliformis* bacteremia, and Carrion disease occurred in the community at a rate of 12.7 per 100 person-years over a 2-year period. Children younger than age 5 years had the highest incidence of disease, which declined linearly with age and was attributed to acquired immunity. In the community, the disease followed a cluster pattern with 70% of cases arising in 18% of households. This pattern is seen in other endemic diseases, such as malaria and leishmaniasis, and is consistent with the "20/80 rule," which states that approximately 80% of the disease burden will be found in 20% of households.[78,83]

CLINICAL FEATURES

Table 154-6 summarizes the diseases caused by *Bartonella* species.

CUTANEOUS FINDINGS

Cat Scratch Disease: Three to 10 days following inoculation via cat exposure, CSD begins with an erythematous papule at the inoculation site. The papule typically persists for 1 to 3 weeks, during which time it may become vesicular, followed by a crusted papule of 2 to 6 mm in diameter. Less commonly, the lesion may be pustular or nodular. Three to 50 days following inoculation, patients develop regional lymphadenomegaly, most commonly affecting the axillary, cervical, inguinal, epitrochlear or preauricular nodes. At first, lymph nodes are soft but become firm and tender, often with erythema of the overlying skin. Suppuration occurs in 10% to 15% of patients. Lymphadenitis is typically the presenting sign, although the inoculation site lesion may still be appreciable at presentation (Fig. 154-6). Examination should include thorough inspection of interdigital spaces, skin creases, and scalp. In 5% to 10% of cases the inoculation site may include the eye (nonsuppurative conjunctivitis, ocular granuloma) or mucous membranes (oral ulceration). Specifically, the Parinaud oculoglandular syndrome can arise when the inoculation site occurs near the eye, characterized by unilateral granulomatous conjunctivitis with ipsilateral preauricular and submandibular lymphadenopathy. Other, less common, cutaneous findings associated with CSD include morbilliform eruptions, urticaria, erythema nodosum, erythema multiforme, and erythema marginatum.[76,78,84]

Trench Fever: Five to 20 days following exposure to human body louse (*P. humanus*), patients may develop trench fever, also known as 5-day fever, quintan fever, shinbone fever, shank fever, and His-Werner disease. It is characterized by cyclic fevers of approximately 5 days' duration, and as many as 90% of patients may develop crops of erythematous macules or papules, which may be found across the abdomen, chest, and back.[76,78,85]

Bacillary Angiomatosis: The characteristic BA lesion is a reddish-purple, angiomatous papule approximately 1 cm in diameter. The lesion also may be nodular or pedunculated. The surface is smooth or verrucous and may ulcerate and occasionally bleed (Fig. 154-7). Less-common BA variants include subcutaneous nodules and hyperkeratotic plaques. When present, subcutaneous nodules are deep-seated and tender with overlying erythematous or normal-colored skin, sometimes with ulceration. Lesions may be solitary or multiple, occurring in a localized area or, rarely, disseminated across the body. BA may also affect the mucosa, and oral lesions have been reported with and without the presence of cutaneous findings, specifically affecting the gingiva, buccal mucosa, oral labial mucosa, hard palate, and posterior pharynx.[78,86,87]

Carrion Disease: Following sand fly (*L. verrucarum*) exposure in an endemic area of South America, there is

TABLE 154-6
Summary Table of Diseases Caused by *Bartonella* Species

DISEASE	CUTANEOUS FINDINGS & DISEASE COURSE	NONCUTANEOUS FINDINGS	LABORATORY TESTS	COURSE & PROGNOSIS	TREATMENT
Cat scratch disease (CSD)	Erythematous papule at inoculation site (3 to 10 days after inoculation) Papule becomes vesicular and crusts (1 to 3 weeks) Regional lymphadenopathy (3 to 50 days postinoculation), with suppuration in 10% to 15% Parinaud oculoglandular syndrome (inoculation near eye)	Fever, chills, malaise, headache, weight loss, nausea, vomiting or splenomegaly Liver and spleen may develop granulomatous inflammation CSD neuroretinitis may develop	Serology: indirect fluorescent antibody assay Lymph node biopsy: Warthin-Starry staining and polymerase chain reaction (PCR) may identify organisms Skin cultures usually negative	Lymphadenopathy resolves in a median of 7 weeks; CSD lymphadenitis is benign and self-limited, disseminated manifestations may be life threatening	Mild to moderate cases: no treatment recommended Large, bulky lymphadenopathy: azithromycin, doxycycline, erythromycin; needle aspiration of suppurative lymph nodes Liver or spleen involvement: rifampicin alone or in combination with gentamicin or trimethoprim-sulfamethoxazole Ocular CSD: doxycycline, or doxycycline + rifampicin
Trench fever	Fever (of approximately 5 days duration) occurs 5 to 20 days after exposure and recurs cyclically Cutaneous features include erythematous macules or papules over abdomen, chest, and back	Accompanying chills, malaise, anorexia, or diaphoresis, as well as retroorbital pain, headache, muscle aches, joint or shin pain; conjunctival injection and splenomegaly may occur	Blood culture is confirmatory, but often difficult Indirect fluorescent antibody assay; PCR blood tests	Course is often mild	Oral doxycycline × 28 days + IV gentamicin × 14 days or oral doxycycline or erythromycin or azithromycin × 4 to 6 weeks
Bacillary angiomatosis	Nodular or pedunculated papule that may ulcerate or bleed; lesions may be solitary or multiple; mucosa also affected	Liver (peliosis hepatis), spleen (splenic peliosis), bone (most commonly radius and tibia) and lymph nodes may be affected Respiratory tract, GI tract, and brain may be involved	Skin biopsy often diagnostic; additional staining for Warthin-Starry; PCR Indirect fluorescent antibody assay	Responsive to antibiotic therapy within 1 week, with clearance within 1 month Relapses may occur when antibiotics are given for <3 months	Uncomplicated BA, peliosis and osteomyelitis: oral doxycycline or erythromycin × 3 to 4 months Severe cases: oral doxycycline or erythromycin, + rifampicin HL? *Bartonella* endocarditis: doxycycline + gentamicin × 2 weeks
Carrions disease	After ~60 days of incubation, symptoms of Oroya fever develop: acute bacteremic syndrome, hemolytic anemia; verruga peruana develops 2 months later, with eruptive angiomatous lesions resembling bacillary angiomatosis	Nonspecific prodrome (fever, chills, malaise, headache, anorexia, myalgias, arthralgias) Severe hemolytic anemia with jaundice, dyspnea and confusion may occur, with hepatosplenomegaly and generalized lymphadenopathy	Blood smear with Giemsa staining for presence of blue-colored intraerythrocytic or extraerythrocytic bacilli	Oroya fever lasts 1 to 4 weeks	Uncomplicated Oroya fever: ciprofloxacin alone or chloramphenicol + β-lactam × 14 days Severe disease: ciprofloxacin + ceftriaxone HL? Transfusions (red blood cells) should be considered Verruga peruana: rifampicin × 14 to 21 days or streptomycin IM

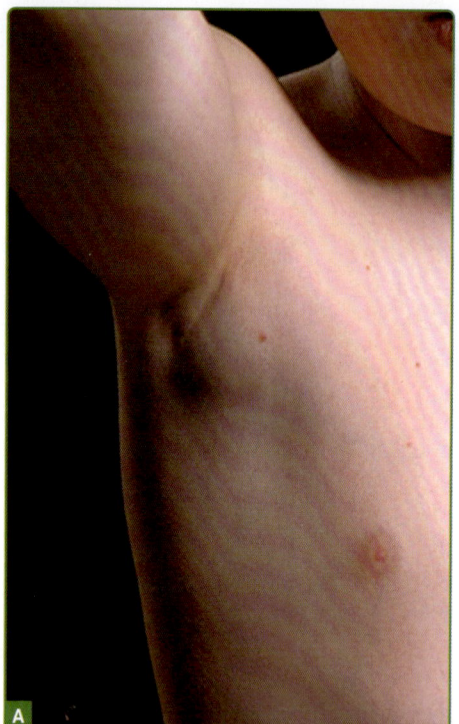
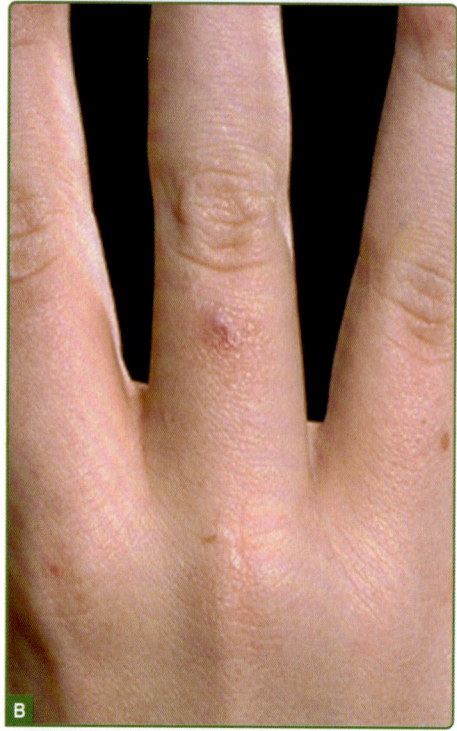

Figure 154-6 Regional lymphadenitis is frequently the presenting sign of cat scratch disease (**A**). An inoculation site papule (**B**) persists for 1 to 3 weeks and may be present at the time of initial presentation. (Reproduced with permission from Stutchfield CJ, Tyrrell J. Evaluation of lymphadenopathy in children. *Paediatr Child Health*. 2012;22[3]:98-102. Copyright © Elsevier.)

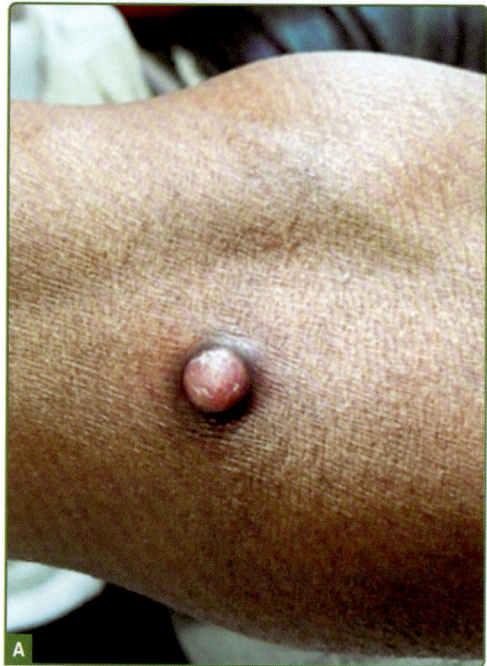
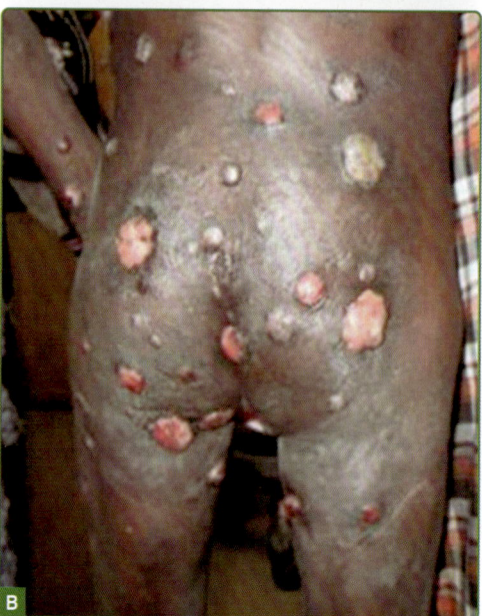

Figure 154-7 Bacillary angiomatosis may be solitary or multifocal, and feature angiomatous papules and nodules with smooth (**A**) or verrucous (**B**) surfaces that may ulcerate and occasionally bleed. (Image **A,** Reproduced from Claasens S, Schwartz IS, Jordaan HF, et al. Bacillary angiomatosis presenting with polymorphic skin lesions. *IDCases*. 2016;6:77-78; Image **B,** Rodriguez O, Campbell LR, Bacha JM, et al. Successful treatment of bacillary angiomatosis with oral doxycycline in an HIV-infected child with skin lesions mimicking Kaposi sarcoma. *JAAD Case Rep*. 2016;2[1]:77-79. Copyright © Elsevier.)

an incubation period of approximately 60 days (range: 1 to 30 weeks) before patients may exhibit symptoms of Oroya fever, an acute bacteremic syndrome and hemolytic anemia, with an associated increase in development of opportunistic infections. Approximately 2 months (range: 2 weeks to several years) following Oroya fever, patients may develop verruga peruana, an eruptive angiomatous cutaneous condition that resembles BA.

Verruga peruana, or Peruvian wart, is characterized by eruptive crops of angiomatous nodular and/or verrucous lesions, primarily on the head and distal extremities. Mucous membranes of the mouth, conjunctiva and nose may be affected, as well. Lesions range from red to purple and vary in size from papules of only a few millimeters in diameter to pedunculated or sessile plaques, several centimeters in size. In many patients, the lesions bleed, ulcerate, or become complicated with secondary infection (Fig. 154-8).[76,78,88,89]

NONCUTANEOUS FINDINGS

Cat Scratch Disease: Some patients with CSD may have fever, chills, malaise, headache, weight loss, nausea, vomiting, or splenomegaly. A variety of uncommon, extranodal manifestations of CSD may also occur, which often lack characteristic lymphadenitis and an inoculation site papule, making diagnosis especially challenging. Atypical manifestations include granulomatous hepatitis or splenitis, neuroretinitis, encephalitis, myelitis, peripheral neuropathy, facial nerve palsy, arthritis, osteomyelitis, mediastinal masses, and atypical pneumonia.

CSD may affect the liver, spleen or both with granulomatous inflammation. Symptoms may include fever, abdominal pain, and weight loss. On examination, the liver and/or spleen may be enlarged and tender, and liver function tests may be mildly abnormal. The erythrocyte sedimentation rate and C-reactive protein levels are frequently elevated. Hepatosplenic CSD should not be confused with BA-associated peliosis hepatis or splenic peliosis, which usually affects HIV-infected or other immunocompromised patients. CSD neuroretinitis is characterized by acute unilateral blurred vision resulting from optic nerve edema, often with an afferent pupillary defect. Funduscopic examination may reveal hemorrhages, cotton wool spots, and a stellate macular exudate or "macular star."[76,90-92]

Trench Fever: Trench fever is characterized by sudden-onset febrile episodes of approximately 5 days' duration, associated with chills, malaise, anorexia, or diaphoresis, as well as retroorbital pain, headache, muscle aches, joint pain, or shin pain. In addition to a truncal rash, patients may exhibit conjunctival injection and splenomegaly. Fevers may occur over a course of 4 to 6 weeks during which patients may experience up to 8 episodes of fever, lasting approximately 5 days each. Although the names "5-day fever" and "quintan fever" denote this cyclic pattern, which is most commonly seen, patients also may have only a single febrile episode lasting 4 to 5 days or a persistent fever lasting 2 to 6 weeks.[76,78,85]

Bacillary Angiomatosis: BA may cause extracutaneous angiomatous proliferation, with or without concurrent angiomatous skin lesions. Typical sites include the liver (peliosis hepatis), spleen (splenic peliosis), bone and lymph nodes. Rarely affected sites include the respiratory tract, GI tract, and brain. Regardless of the site of disease, BA patients may have fever, chills, malaise, headache, or anorexia.

Peliosis hepatis is characterized by abdominal pain, hepatomegaly, and splenomegaly. Patients often have elevated alkaline phosphatase and normal or slightly elevated bilirubin and aminotransferases. With splenic peliosis, thrombocytopenia and pancytopenia have been reported.[76,93,94] Bony involvement is characterized by painful, isolated, lytic lesions. The radius or tibia are most commonly affected, and may be accompanied by overlying cellulitis.[76,86,95]

Carrion Disease: Patients with Oroya fever present with a nonspecific prodrome of fever, chills, malaise, headache, anorexia, myalgias, and arthralgias. This is followed by a rapid deterioration with pallor, jaundice, dyspnea, and/or confusion, associated with a severe hemolytic anemia caused by a parasitic erythrocyte infection. Patients may also exhibit hepatosplenomegaly and generalized lymphadenopathy. Severe cases may include heart failure, convulsions, coma,

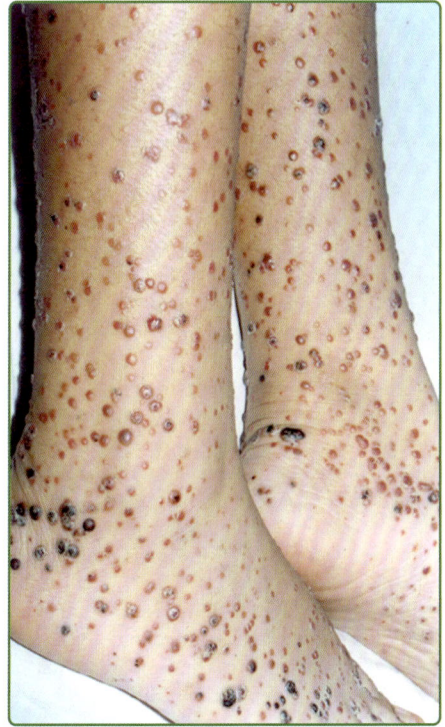

Figure 154-8 Verruga peruana features eruptive crops of angiomatous nodular and/or verrucous lesions, which may be pedunculated or sessile, ranging from red to purple and varying from a few millimeters to several centimeters in size. (Reproduced with permission from Maguiña C, Guerra H, Ventosilla P. Bartonellosis. *Clin Dermatol.* 2009;27[3]:271-280. Copyright © Elsevier.)

anasarca, and multiorgan failure. With verruga peruana, the eruption of cutaneous lesions may be accompanied by nonspecific constitutional symptoms.[76,78]

COMPLICATIONS

Infection with *B. henselae* or *B. quintana* may be complicated by endocarditis, often termed *culture-negative endocarditis*, as repeat cultures are frequently negative. *Bartonella* endocarditis usually occurs in those with underlying heart valve abnormalities. Patients have a chronic clinical course characterized by fever, and vegetations are visible in 90% of patients undergoing echocardiography.[93]

During the hemolytic phase of Oroya fever, patients are predisposed to infection by a number of opportunistic pathogens. Infections may include *Salmonella* spp. (typhoidal and nontyphoidal strains), *Shigella dysenteriae*, *S. aureus*, *Enterobacter* spp., toxoplasmosis reactivation, disseminated histoplasmosis, *Pneumocystis jiroveci* pneumonia, and malaria, to name a few.[89] One study of 68 patients with Oroya fever in Peru found that 36 (53%) had cardiovascular complications. Among the patients with complications, rates of heart failure, pericardial effusion, pulmonary edema, cardiogenic shock, cardiac tamponade and myocarditis were 91%, 44%, 36%, 17%, 11%, and 11%, respectively.[96]

ETIOLOGY AND PATHOGENESIS

A common theme among *Bartonella* species is their propensity to cause prolonged intraerythrocytic bacteremia in natural reservoir hosts, but not incidental hosts, thereby positioning themselves to be spread from reservoir to reservoir via bloodsucking arthropods. Rather than spreading through the bites of arthropods, *Bartonella* is transmitted via arthropod feces, coupled with superficial scratching of the skin. As an example, cat fleas harboring *B. henselae* feed on cats, during which time they excrete feces containing *Bartonella*. As the cat scratches its skin in an area infested with fleas, a cat may inoculate itself intradermally with *B. henselae* and, simultaneously contaminate its claws with feces. Cats may also contaminate their saliva by eating fleas. Subsequently, humans become incidental hosts of *B. henselae* after being scratched, bitten, or licked by a cat whose claws and/or saliva have been contaminated with flea feces. Humans serve as reservoir hosts for both *B. quintana* and *B. bacilliformis*. Similarly, bacteria are transmitted from person to person via human body lice and sandflies, respectively, specifically when bacteria in the arthropod feces is inoculated through the skin via scratching.[76,77]

Once reservoir hosts have been inoculated with *Bartonella*, a prolonged, subclinical intraerythrocytic bacteremia may occur. This has been documented in cats with *B. henselae*,[79] homeless people with *B. quintana*,[80] and members of a Peruvian valley community with *B. bacilliformis*.[83] One 2-year study that followed a naturally infected cat showed that the animal had persistent *B. henselae* bacteremia for the first 5 months postinoculation. Following a 2-month abacteremic period, the bacteremia reoccurred. For the remainder of the study, the cat became cyclically bacteremic for 2-month intervals with interspersed abacteremic periods of approximately 2 months each.[97]

The tendency to produce prolonged, subclinical bacteremic infections indicate that *Bartonella* have adapted to circumvent the immune systems of their reservoir hosts. The mechanisms by which they achieve this feat have been investigated in detail.[77] Briefly, *Bartonella* express lipopolysaccharide that is only weakly recognized by TLR4, a receptor known to activate the innate immune system and mediate septic shock following recognition of lipopolysaccharide borne by Gram-negative bacteria. In fact, *B. quintana* lipopolysaccharide does not stimulate the production of proinflammatory cytokines in human monocytes and may actually act as a TLR4 antagonist.[98] Furthermore, some *Bartonella* species, including *B. bacilliformis*, express flagella that have undergone amino acid changes, while preserving motility. Thus, their flagella are not recognized by TLR5, a receptor of the innate immune system responsible for recognizing an evolutionarily conserved portion of bacterial flagellin.[99]

In addition to evading hosts' innate immune systems, *Bartonella* may subvert adaptive immunity via antigenic variation. This has been demonstrated by several *Bartonella* antigens, including cell-adhesion molecules, Vomps and BadA, as well as Trw-T4SS, a Type 4 secretion system involved in erythrocyte adhesion. Vomp-specific antibodies are the most frequently detected human immunoglobulins against *B. quintana*, and the Vomp locus has been shown to undergo extensive genetic rearrangements in vivo.[100] Additionally, cat models have demonstrated the development of genetically distinct *B. henselae* clones at different peaks of relapsing bacteremia.[101] Sometimes, the cats demonstrated bacteremia even in the presence of high specific titers, and at one point in the experiment no increase in specific immunoglobulin G was observed during a subsequent bacteremic episode. Finally, *Bartonella* elude both humoral and cellular immunity by naturally parasitizing host erythrocytes. As a consequence of a lack of major histocompatibility complexes, erythrocytes cannot present antigens on their surfaces, thereby offering a protective environment, at least for the life span of the erythrocyte.[77]

Besides interacting closely with erythrocytes, *Bartonella* are known to have an affinity for endothelial cells. This affinity plays an important role, not only in promoting vascular proliferation in the setting of disease, but also in maintaining the carrier state in natural reservoir hosts. Multiple observations point to the existence of a primary niche within reservoir hosts where *Bartonella* persist and can be periodically seeded into the circulation. Although a few theories exist as to the primary niche of *Bartonella*, the endothelial cell hypothesis is the most widely accepted.[77,102] *B. henselae*,

B. quintana, and *B. bacilliformis* have all been shown to adhere to and invade endothelial cells.[77]

To demonstrate the role of *Bartonella* in the generation of angiomatous lesions, one study showed that *B. henselae* increased cell migration and secretion of vascular endothelial growth factor in human, but not feline, endothelial cells.[103] Further investigations have indicated that *Bartonella*-mediated vascular endothelial growth factor upregulation occurs via activation of hypoxia-inducible factor-1, a transcription factor and mediator of vascular endothelial growth factor expression, via cellular hypoxia induced by intracellular bacterial replication.[77] *Bartonella* also have been hypothesized to secrete their own angiogenic factor; stimulate endothelial growth factors, IL-1b, IL-8, and angiopoietin 2 from macrophages and endothelial cells; and downregulate endothelial apoptosis via decreased IL-12 and interferon-γ. Inoculation of endothelial cells with *B. henselae* or *B. quintana* is known to increase their life span, and inhibit in vitro actinomycin D–induced apoptosis.[76,77,93]

In addition to these mechanisms by which *Bartonella* promotes vascular proliferation, the formation of angiomatous lesions such as BA and verruga peruana appears to necessitate a host immunocompromised state. For example, *B. henselae* and *B. quintana* infection lead to BA in those with diminished CD4+ lymphocyte counts and phagocytic dysfunction.[78] This could be compared with the immunologic dysfunction caused by Oroya fever, which is known to put hosts at risk for opportunistic infection.[78] During *B. bacilliformis* infection, erythrocytes have demonstrated a significant increase in IL-10 production, which downregulates cytokines, CD4+ cells, macrophages, and dendritic cells.[104] This is accompanied by decreased CD4+ lymphocytes and increased CD8+ lymphocytes in the peripheral blood with an inversion of the CD4+-to-CD8+ ratio and impaired cellular immunity.[78]

Given these observations, it is thought that host immune responses to *Bartonella*, as well as differing virulence across bacterial strains, influence the pathologic processes and clinical manifestations that occur in different patients infected with the same *Bartonella* species.[78] For example, *B. henselae* in patients with a low CD4+ lymphocyte count leads to BA, whereas *B. henselae* in immunocompetent patients leads to CSD, characterized by granulomatous lymphadenitis, as well as granulomatous inflammation in visceral organs. Studies of *B. henselae*–macrophage interaction indicate that BadA adhesion molecules inhibit phagocytic uptake. When successfully phagocytized, *B. henselae* enter macrophages via a specialized vacuolar compartment, termed a *Bartonella*-containing vacuole, which lacks early endocytic marker proteins. In later stages of infection, *Bartonella*-containing vacuoles fuse with lysosomes, eventually leading to bacterial destruction.[77]

DIAGNOSIS

LABORATORY TESTING

Table 154-6 summarizes the laboratory tests for diseases caused by *Bartonella* species.

Cat Scratch Disease: CSD is typically diagnosed via serology, specifically an indirect fluorescent antibody (IFA) assay. Although not routinely required in patients with a classic presentation, a lymph node biopsy may be sent for histology, Warthin-Starry staining, and PCR. PCR also may be performed on lymph node aspirates. Although tissue samples may be sent for culture, they are frequently negative. Skin testing for CSD is no longer performed. Biopsies of liver and spleen have also fallen out of favor when involvement is suspected, as imaging findings in the setting of a positive IFA are often adequate.[76,105]

Trench Fever: Trench fever may be confirmed by isolating *B. quintana* from the blood. However, given the difficulty associated with *Bartonella* culture isolation, IFA assay is often used. In some settings, PCR blood tests are also available. Biopsy does not play a role in the diagnosis of trench fever.[76,80]

Bacillary Angiomatosis: BA is often diagnosed via skin biopsy, which should be sent for histology, Warthin-Starry staining, and PCR. IFA may be used. BA lesions associated with peliosis hepatis and splenic peliosis may be biopsied, as well.[76,78]

Carrion Disease: In the diagnosis of Carrion disease, *B. bacilliformis* identification is often attempted by inspecting a Giemsa-stained blood smear for blue-colored intraerythrocytic or extraerythrocytic bacilli. Blood cultures are often collected during the acute phase (Oroya fever), when as many as 71% of patients may yield positive results within 2 to 4 weeks. The successful isolation of *B. bacilliformis* drops dramatically during the chronic phase (verruga peruana).[89] Skin biopsy of verruga peruana lesions may be sent for histology, and Warthin-Starry or Giemsa stains to enhance *B. bacilliformis* visualization. IFA assay and PCR are available, although these may not be feasible in resource-poor settings.[76]

PATHOLOGY

Cat Scratch Disease: The inoculation-site papule of CSD features areas of stellate necrosis surrounded by rims of histiocytes, neutrophils, and occasional giant cells. Epidermal changes may include acanthosis or ulceration.[32] Warthin-Starry silver stain may show bacilli within the area of necrosis, although the bacteria are diminished as the lesion resolves. Similar findings are also seen on lymph node biopsy, with lymphoid hyperplasia and arteriolar proliferation (Fig. 154-9).[76,106]

Bacillary Angiomatosis: BA is characterized by a lobular accumulation of rounded blood vessels featuring plump endothelial cells with cell necrosis, atypia, and mitoses. There is a mixed inflammatory infiltrate with a neutrophil predominance and intermittent leukocytoclasia. Bacilli maybe seen in intracellular or extracellular clumps with Warthin-Starry silver stain (Fig. 154-10).[76,78]

Liver biopsy in peliosis hepatis may reveal cystic, blood-filled spaces within the hepatic parenchyma. There may be an excess of misshapen endothelial cells forming capillary-like sprouts and a mixed inflammatory infiltrate of histiocytes and neutrophils. Warthin-Starry silver stain may identify bacilli.[77,94]

Carrion Disease: Verruga peruana features an intense angioblastic proliferation with sheets of endothelial cells and neutrophils comprising most of the cellular infiltrate. Interspersed macrophages, lymphocytes and plasma cells may be seen. Warthin-Starry or Giemsa stain are used to visualize *Bartonella* organisms, which may be found as intracellular inclusions, as well as free organisms in the extracellular matrix.[76]

IMAGING

Cat Scratch Disease: An abdominal CT of patients with hepatic or splenic CSD will show scattered, multiple hypodense areas, which are hypoechoic on ultrasonography.[107]

Bacillary Angiomatosis: An abdominal CT of patients with peliosis hepatis and/or splenic peliosis shows organomegaly and scattered hypodense lesions.[94] In patients with bony involvement, radiographs reveal lytic lesions with cortical destruction and periosteal reaction. Technetium scans demonstrate increased uptake.[86,95]

DIFFERENTIAL DIAGNOSIS

Table 154-7 outlines the differential diagnosis for *Bartonella* infections.

CLINICAL COURSE AND PROGNOSIS

Table 154-6 summarizes the clinical courses and prognoses for diseases caused by *Bartonella* species.

CAT SCRATCH DISEASE

Inoculation-site lesions persist for 1 to 3 weeks and lymphadenopathy resolves in a median of 7 weeks, although 6 to 24 months of prolonged lymphadenopathy occur in 20% of cases. Cutaneous manifestations heal without scarring. CSD lymphadenitis is benign and self-limited, while disseminated manifestations may be life threatening.[76]

TRENCH FEVER

Trench fever typically follows a mild course, although some cases may be fairly debilitating. Death is rare.[76]

BACILLARY ANGIOMATOSIS

BA responds well to antibiotic therapy, with lesions improving within 1 week and full clearance often occurring within 1 month. However, BA may become life-threatening in the absence of treatment. Relapses

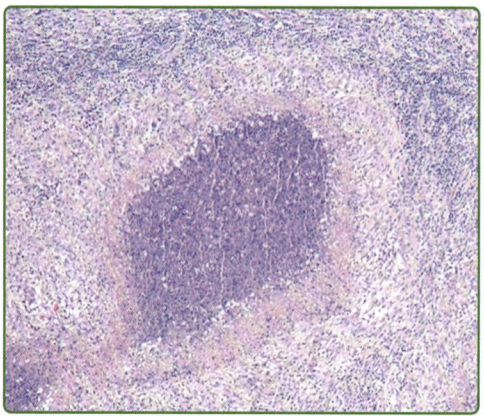

Figure 154-9 Lymph nodes affected by cat scratch disease reveal inflammatory, granulomatous changes featuring central microabscesses surrounded by rings of histiocytes and occasional giant cells, as seen here at ×100 magnification. (Reproduced with permission from Angelakis E, Raoult D. Pathogenicity and treatment of *Bartonella* infections. *Int J Antimicrob Agents*. 2014;44[1]:16-25. Copyright © Elsevier.)

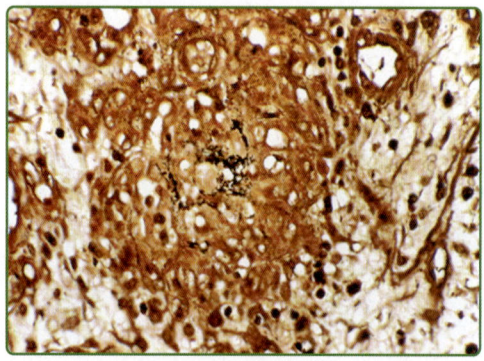

Figure 154-10 Bacillary angiomatosis is characterized by lobular proliferations of endothelial cells with mixed, neutrophil-predominant infiltrates and bacilli seen in intracellular or extracellular clumps on Warthin-Starry silver stain, as shown here at ×1000 magnification. (Reproduced with permission from Angelakis E, Raoult D. Pathogenicity and treatment of *Bartonella* infections. *Int J Antimicrob Agents*. 2014;44[1]:16-25. Copyright © Elsevier.)

TABLE 154-7
Differential Diagnosis for *Bartonella* Infections

BARTONELLA INFECTION	DIFFERENTIAL DIAGNOSIS
Cat scratch disease	Sporotrichosis, paracoccidioidomycosis, histoplasmosis
	Tuberculosis, atypical mycobacteria
	Sarcoidosis
	Nocardiosis
	Foreign-body granuloma
	HIV infection
	Syphilis
	Lymphogranuloma venereum
	Epstein-Barr virus
	Lymphoma
	Kikuchi-Fujimoto disease
Trench fever	Enteric fever
	Brucellosis
	Leptospirosis
	Dengue
	Relapsing fever
	Typhus
	Malaria
	Viral exanthem
Bacillary angiomatosis	Kaposi sarcoma
	Epithelioid hemangioma
	Pyogenic granuloma
	Angiokeratoma
	Cherry angioma
	Dermatofibroma
	Tuberculosis, atypical mycobacteria, or dimorphic fungi
	Verruga peruana
Carrion disease	Oroya fever
	Malaria
	Brucellosis
	Viral hepatitis
	Leptospirosis
	Hematologic malignancy
	Aplastic or hemolytic anemia
	Verruga peruana
	Pyogenic granuloma
	Hemangioma
	Warts
	Bacillary angiomatosis
	Kaposi sarcoma
	Yaws
	Lymphomatoid papulosis
	Malignant lymphoma
	Angiolymphoid hyperplasia with eosinophilia

suspected.[93] Severe cases are more likely to occur in travelers versus patients native to endemic regions. When deaths occur, they are usually associated with opportunistic infection[76,89]

In addition to a milder disease course, patients native to endemic regions frequently present with verruga peruana in the absence of any history of Oroya fever. Lesions of verruga peruana usually erupt over a course of 3 to 6 months, although they may continue to appear for years if left untreated. In the absence of complications, lesions heal without scarring.[76]

MANAGEMENT

Table 154-6 summarizes the management of diseases caused by *Bartonella* species.

CAT SCRATCH DISEASE

Classic CSD is benign, self-limited, and responds poorly to antimicrobial therapy. Consequently, no treatment is recommended for mild to moderate disease. In patients with large, bulky lymphadenopathy, azithromycin, doxycycline, and erythromycin have been used. When lymph nodes suppurate, needle aspiration is likely to be beneficial, and surgical removal may be considered in those with large, painful nodes unresponsive to an extended course of treatment. For those with liver and/or spleen involvement, rifampicin alone or in combination with gentamicin or trimethoprim-sulfamethoxazole should be used. Ocular CSD is typically treated with doxycycline because of superior ocular penetration; a combination of doxycycline and rifampicin also has been employed.[76,93,108,109]

TRENCH FEVER

A randomized trial supports the use of 28 days of oral doxycycline plus 14 days of IV gentamicin for the treatment of trench fever. Treatment of uncomplicated disease also may be attempted with a 4- to 6-week course of oral doxycycline, erythromycin, or azithromycin. Because of unreliable activity, trimethoprim-sulfamethoxazole, fluoroquinolones, penicillins, and first-generation cephalosporins should not be used.[76,110,111]

BACILLARY ANGIOMATOSIS

Erythromycin or doxycycline for 3 or more months may be used to treat uncomplicated BA, peliosis, and osteomyelitis. Azithromycin and clarithromycin are alternative therapies. In severe cases, combination therapy should be employed with erythromycin or doxycycline plus a rifamycin, and intravenous therapy may initially be required. *Bartonella* endocarditis should be treated with doxycycline with the addition of gentamicin for 2 weeks; a rifamycin can be substituted for gentamicin in the setting of renal insufficiency.[112] Rifampicin, a potent cytochrome P450

are not uncommon, especially when antibiotic treatment is given for less than 3 months.[76]

CARRION DISEASE

Oroya fever lasts 1 to 4 weeks. Clinical severity ranges from mild to severe with 44% to 88% mortality among untreated patients. When treated with antibiotics, mortality is less than 10%, although if symptoms fail to resolve within 72 hours, complications should be inducer, requires dose adjustments in patients who are also receiving antiretroviral therapy. Because of unreliable activity, trimethoprim-sulfamethoxazole, fluoroquinolones, penicillins, and first-generation cephalosporins should not be used.[76]

CARRION DISEASE

First-line treatment of uncomplicated Oroya fever includes ciprofloxacin or combination therapy with chloramphenicol and a β-lactam. Fourteen days is a common duration of treatment. Success also has been reported with trimethoprim-sulfamethoxazole, macrolides, and norfloxacin. For severe disease, ciprofloxacin plus ceftriaxone may be used, and red blood cells should be transfused if the hematocrit falls below 20%. Patients with complications, such as coma, convulsions, and edema, are often given short courses of dexamethasone.[76,89,93,113]

Verruga peruana may be treated with rifampicin for 14 to 21 days. Intramuscular streptomycin is an alternative.[93,108] Other antibiotics that have demonstrated successful treatment include azithromycin, ciprofloxacin, and erythromycin. Chloramphenicol and penicillins are not effective against verruga peruana.[76]

ENTERIC FEVER CAUSED BY *SALMONELLA*

AT-A-GLANCE

- Worldwide, approximately 13.5 million cases of enteric fever occur each year.
- Disease is spread by chronic carriers and contracted following ingestion of contaminated water or food.
- Regions with the greatest density of enteric fever include south-central and southeastern Asia and areas of southern Africa.
- Rose spots are the classic cutaneous manifestation, occurring in 30% of cases. They are most commonly seen when antibiotic treatment has been delayed.
- Symptoms include fever, abdominal pain, and constipation or diarrhea.
- The most common complications are intestinal bleeding, ileal perforation, and encephalopathy.
- With antibiotics, death from enteric fever occurs in less than 1% of cases.

INTRODUCTION AND BACTERIOLOGY

Salmonella is a genus of Gram-negative, oxidase-negative, flagellate rods that do not ferment lactose and grow best on MacConkey or *Salmonella-Shigella* agar. Currently, there are only 2 identified species of *Salmonella*, *Salmonella enterica* and *Salmonella bongori*. Although previous classification systems have included more *Salmonella* species, genetic analysis has since indicated that they are more appropriately classified as subspecies and serovars. Thus, *S. enterica* has been divided into 6 subspecies, one of which is *S. enterica* subsp. *enterica*. Within subspecies *enterica* there are more than 1000 serovars, differentiated by O (somatic) and H (flagellar) antigens.[114]

Salmonella is responsible for 2 major clinical syndromes: enteric fever and gastroenteritis; enteric fever is the focus of this chapter. The classic cause of enteric fever is *S. enterica* subsp. *enterica* serovar Typhi (*Salmonella typhi*), although *Salmonella paratyphi* A, *S. paratyphi* B, *S. paratyphi* C, and *Salmonella choleraesuis* also have been implicated. Thus, the term *enteric fever* encompasses both typhoid and paratyphoid fever.

EPIDEMIOLOGY

Worldwide, approximately 13.5 million cases of enteric fever occur each year,[115] with the greatest prevalence among children and young adults. Approximately 350 cases occur annually in the United States, most of which are associated with travel to endemic regions; only approximately 18% are domestically acquired. Infections attained in endemic areas are more likely to be drug-resistant. Enteric fever is endemic in many developing countries, especially resource-poor areas with overcrowding and inadequate sanitation. Regions with the greatest density of disease include south-central and southeastern Asia and areas of southern Africa.

Humans are the only hosts of *S. typhi*, while other serovars are widespread in nature and can be carried by mammals, poultry, and reptiles. Although worldwide studies indicate that *S. typhi* is the most frequent cause of enteric fever, *S. paratyphi* A appears to be responsible for a growing portion of disease in multiple Asian countries. In some studies, *S. paratyphi* A has accounted for 50% of *Salmonella* bloodstream isolates among enteric fever patients. This finding is concerning, as current available vaccines have either limited or no protection against paratyphoid fever.[115-118]

CLINICAL FEATURES

Traditionally, it has been thought that typhoid fever has a more robust presentation that is associated with greater severity and rates of complications compared to paratyphoid fever. However, this hypothesis has not held true in recent investigations, which show that it is not possible to predict the etiologic organism of enteric fever based on clinical presentation.[119-122]

CUTANEOUS FINDINGS

Rose spots are the classic cutaneous manifestation of enteric fever, presenting several days following the onset of symptoms. They are estimated to occur in approximately 30% of cases, and are more likely to be observed in patients where antibiotic treatment has been delayed. Rose spots are described as asymptomatic, blanching, erythematous to pale-pink papules, usually on the abdomen, chest, or back. They occur in crops that fade over 3 to 5 days and can easily be missed on darkly pigmented skin. Other cutaneous manifestations of enteric fever may include erythema multiforme, Sweet syndrome, hemorrhagic bullae, pustular dermatitis, or erythema typhosum, a generalized erythematous eruption.[12,123,124] In rare cases, ulcerative lesions of the vulva or scrotum have been the presenting symptom of enteric fever.[125,126]

Of note, rose spots may be seen to a lesser extent in psittacosis, leptospirosis, brucellosis, rat-bite fever, and shigellosis, although in these contexts they are not well-described.[124]

NONCUTANEOUS FINDINGS

Following an incubation period of 1 to 2 weeks, patients present with fever and nonspecific flu-like symptoms (malaise, anorexia, nausea, myalgias, headache). Fever is initially low and rises in a stepwise fashion, often reaching 39°C to 40°C (102.2°F to 104°F), and may be accompanied by relative bradycardia. Over time, patients develop abdominal pain, and diarrhea or constipation. Diarrhea is common in children and HIV patients, while constipation is more likely to occur in adults. On examination, patients may have abdominal tenderness or hepatosplenomegaly. Patients can also experience intermittent confusion or apathy, and convulsions have been described in young children.

White cell counts, hemoglobin, and platelets may all be reduced, although children are prone to leukocytosis. Liver enzymes are frequently 2 to 3 times the upper limit of normal. In one study of 60 patients with enteric fever, rose spots, relative bradycardia, splenomegaly, thrombocytopenia, and elevated aspartate aminotransferase were found to have the strongest predictive value for enteric fever.[116,127]

COMPLICATIONS

Complications arise in 10% to 15% of patients and may include GI bleeding, intestinal perforation, and encephalopathy. GI bleeding occurs most frequently, and although most patients do not require a blood transfusion, this complication may be fatal in some cases. The most serious complication is intestinal perforation, which occurs in 1% to 3% of hospitalized patients and usually affects the ileum. It may present overtly as an acute abdomen, or in a more surreptitious fashion with simple worsening of abdominal pain, a rising heart rate, and falling blood pressure.

In 1% to 4% of cases, infection persists as a chronic carrier state, defined by excretion of *Salmonella* in the stool for more than 12 months after infection. Less commonly, patients may exhibit chronic urinary carriage, especially in those with urinary tract abnormalities or concurrent *Schistosoma haematobium* bladder infection. Chronic carriage most frequently occurs in women, elderly patients, and patients with cholelithiasis. In some patients, infection may proceed directly to a chronic carrier state, as up to 25% of long-term carriers have no history of enteric fever. Carriers pose a major infection risk to others, especially when they are involved in food preparation, and carriage confers an increased risk of gallbladder carcinoma, as well as other cancers. Eradication should be attempted in these patients with antimicrobial therapy to decrease the infection risk to others; however, it is unclear how eradication may impact the risk of carcinogenesis.[116,128]

ETIOLOGY AND PATHOGENESIS

Typhoidal *Salmonella* is acquired by ingesting contaminated water or food, usually while traveling or residing in developing countries. Following ingestion, bacteria survive passage through gastric acid and arrive in the small bowel, where they are able to breach the epithelium via 1 of 2 pathways. Bacteria may enter the mucosa via M cells, an antigen-presenting cell associated with lymphoid tissue throughout the gut, or via uptake by epithelial cells, as mediated by the cystic fibrosis transmembrane conductance regulator (CFTR) protein that is mutated in cystic fibrosis. Thus, variation in the *CFTR* gene is correlated with a degree of protection against enteric fever.

Following penetration of the epithelium, bacteria replicate in the submucosa and cause hypertrophy of Peyer patches. Hypertrophy and necrosis of the small intestine may cause abdominal pain and microscopic or macroscopic compromise of the mucosal barrier, potentially leading to secondary bacteremia, intestinal bleeding, or ileal perforation.[129] From the small intestine, *Salmonella* disseminate via the blood and lymphatic system, leading to systemic infection.[130,131] Ultimately, bacteria infiltrate tissue macrophages of the liver, spleen, and bone marrow, which may serve as sources for infection relapse or facilitate rare manifestations such as pericarditis, visceral abscesses, or osteomyelitis. The bone marrow is a potential source for diagnostic cultures, even after the initiation of antimicrobial therapy.[132]

DIAGNOSIS

LABORATORY TESTING

Blood cultures are the standard mode of diagnosis, and are positive in 40% to 80% of cases, depending on prior antimicrobial therapy. Cultures of bone marrow are more sensitive, yielding positive results in 80% to 95% of cases even after several days of antibiotics; however, this is invasive and should be reserved for complicated cases where the diagnosis remains uncertain. Other potential culture sources include rose spots, stool, urine, and intestinal secretions (via duodenal string capsule). One study of enteric fever patients demonstrated positive culture rates from rose spots, stool, and urine of 63%, 37%, and 7%, respectively.[116,133] Serologic tests are of limited utility, except in the diagnosis of chronic carriers, who may be identified by measuring serum antibodies against the Vi polysaccharide antigen.[128]

PATHOLOGY

Biopsy of rose spots may reveal dilated capillaries with edema and perivascular infiltrates of histiocytes and few neutrophils.[124,134]

DIFFERENTIAL DIAGNOSIS

The differential diagnosis for enteric fever comprises a variety of infectious and some noninfectious diseases. Such conditions include malaria, amebiasis, dengue fever, visceral leishmaniasis, brucellosis, typhus, miliary tuberculosis, influenza, slow-onset appendicitis, and lymphoproliferative disease.

CLINICAL COURSE AND PROGNOSIS

With antibiotics, fever resolves in 3 to 5 days with full recovery occurring over weeks to months. Enteric fever may relapse in 5% to 10% of patients, even with adequate therapy, usually 2 to 3 weeks following the resolution of fever. Death occurs in less than 1% of cases, although mortality may be significantly higher in resource-poor regions. The mortality rate associated with ileal perforation ranges from 10% to 32%.[116]

MANAGEMENT

MEDICATIONS

Enteric fever should be treated with systemic antimicrobial therapy. Commonly used treatments include ciprofloxacin, ofloxacin, azithromycin, and ceftriaxone. However, ciprofloxacin is no longer recommended as a first-line empiric treatment for patients returning from South Asia because of rising resistance in this region. In cases of suspected ciprofloxacin resistance, ofloxacin or azithromycin may be used. Ceftriaxone is especially useful in the treatment of severe or complicated enteric fever. Typhoidal organisms demonstrate significant resistance to ampicillin, trimethoprim-sulfamethoxazole, and chloramphenicol, and thus these agents are no longer routinely employed.[135]

PREVENTION

Two vaccines available for enteric fever include Ty21a, a live attenuated oral vaccine, as well as a parenteral Vi polysaccharide vaccine. Because *S. paratyphi* serovars do not display the Vi antigen, it is assumed that the Vi polysaccharide vaccine does not offer protection against paratyphoid fever. There is some evidence that the Ty21a vaccine offers limited protection against *S. paratyphi* A and *S. paratyphi* B.[118]

RHINOSCLEROMA CAUSED BY *KLEBSIELLA RHINOSCLEROMATIS*

Klebsiella rhinoscleromatis is a subspecies of *Klebsiella pneumoniae* (*K. pneumoniae* subsp. *rhinoscleromatis*), a lactose-fermenting Gram-negative rod. It is known to cause rhinoscleroma, a rare chronic granulomatous disease affecting the nose and upper respiratory tract. Endemic areas include Africa, the Middle East, Central and South America, Central and Eastern Europe, China, India, and Indonesia. *K. rhinoscleromatis* are contracted by inhaling contaminated respiratory droplets, and infection begins in the nasal mucosa, although it may spread to affect the nasopharynx, pharynx, oral cavity, paranasal sinuses, orbit, larynx, trachea, and even bronchi. Iron deficiency and defective cellular immunity are predisposing factors, with defective cellular immunity explaining the presence of Mikulicz cells that have phagocytosed and retained *K. rhinoscleromatis* bacilli.[136-138]

Rhinoscleroma progresses through 3 phases of disease. First, the atrophic phase, which lasts several months, is characterized by symptoms of the common cold. Patients may experience nasal blockage accompanied by a purulent, foul-smelling discharge. Next, the proliferative phase lasts months to years and is marked by the development of granulomatous nodules, nasal deformity, hyposmia, dysphagia, dysphonia, stridor, and difficulty breathing. In the final cicatricial stage, areas of involvement undergo extensive sclerosis (Fig. 154-11).[138]

Rhinoscleroma may be diagnosed via culture isolation of *K. rhinoscleromatis* from nasal swabs, blood, or biopsy specimens. Biopsied tissue reveals plasma cells, lymphocytes, Russell bodies, and pathognomonic Mikulicz cells, which are large vacuolated histiocytes containing *K. rhinoscleromatis*. Mikulicz cells can be visualized with CD68 immunostaining, and Warthin-Starry silver stain may show *K. rhinoscleromatis* residing in Mikulicz cells. Periodic acid–Schiff staining can be used to enhance Russell bodies. A CT scan may show nonenhancing homogeneous soft-tissue crypt-like irregular masses with nodular deformity and distinct edge definition. Lesions of the larynx and trachea appear as concentric irregular airway narrowing. Rhinoscleroma must be differentiated from tuberculosis, leprosy, sarcoidosis, mucocutaneous leishmaniasis, dimorphic fungal infection, granulomatosis with polyangiitis, lymphoma, and basal or squamous cell carcinoma. The condition is treated with antimicrobial therapy and surgical correction of airway obstructions. In the absence of established guidelines, commonly used antibiotics include tetracycline, rifampicin, ciprofloxacin, and trimethoprim-sulfamethoxazole. Antibiotic therapy should continue for 3 to 6 months until repeat histology and cultures are negative. Despite prolonged therapy, rhinoscleroma has a high incidence of relapse.[138-140]

CELLULITIS CAUSED BY *HAEMOPHILUS INFLUENZAE*

Haemophilus influenzae is a fastidious, Gram-negative coccobacillus that grows on chocolate agar and requires hemin (factor X) and nicotinamide adenine dinucleotide (factor V) for growth. The bacteria may be rough or encapsulated, and encapsulated strains are divided into 6 types based on capsular polysaccharide antigens (a through f). Rough strains are primarily responsible for acute otitis media, pneumonia and chronic bronchitis exacerbations. Prior to the widespread use of *H. influenzae* type b (Hib) vaccines, this organism was a well-known cause of meningitis, epiglottitis, and cellulitis, especially facial cellulitis in children.[141] Although Hib-associated infections have fallen dramatically since the implementation of vaccines, they may still be seen in developing countries or other areas with low rates of vaccination.

Typical Hib facial cellulitis presents in children between 3 and 24 months of age, usually following a

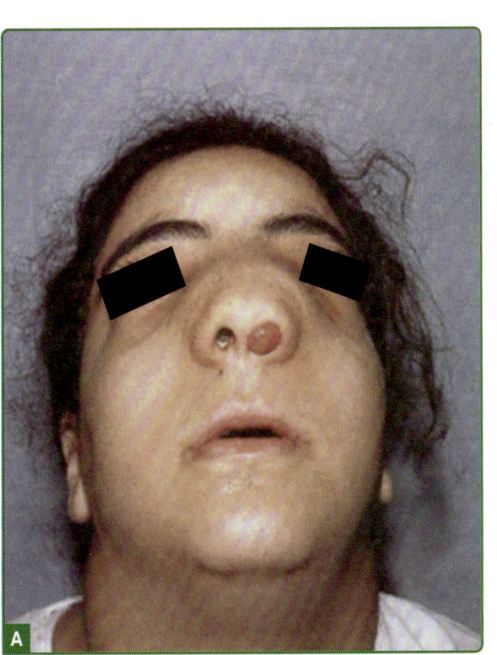
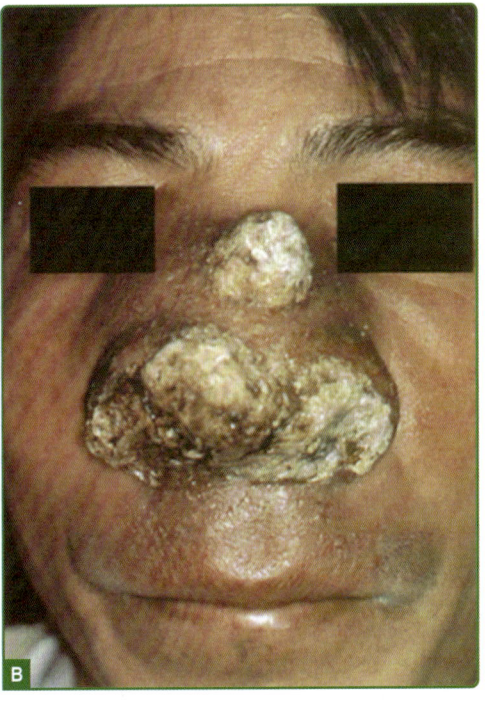

Figure 154-11 Rhinoscleroma in an Egyptian woman (**A**) with pronounced deformity of the nose and cheeks, as well as in a Guatemalan man (**B**) presenting 17 years following initial onset. (Reproduced with permission from Friedmann I. Ulcerative/necrotizing diseases of the nose and paranasal sinuses. *Curr Diagn Pathol*. 1995;2[4]:236-255; and Sedano HO, Koutlas IG. Respiratory scleroma: a clinicopathologic and ultrastructural study. *Oral Surg Oral Med Oral Pathol Oral Radiol Endod*. 1996;81[6]:665-671. Copyright © Elsevier.)

mild upper respiratory tract infection. Patients rapidly develop high fever, irritability and unilateral facial swelling, especially in the buccal or periorbital region. The affected area is usually warm, edematous and erythematous, classically with a violaceous hue. In contrast to other causes of cellulitis, Hib cellulitis was frequently associated with bacteremia, with positive blood cultures in approximately 75% of patients. This was especially significant because of the propensity of this organism to cause secondary infection, particularly meningitis. For this reason, lumbar puncture was once a routine measure in the evaluation of facial cellulitis in children; however, this measure has since been discontinued.[142] Recent reports have indicated a decline in *H. influenzae*–associated facial cellulitis. When identified, nontypeable strains have been implicated, which have not been associated with bacteremia.[143,144] *H. influenzae*–associated facial cellulitis is diagnosed by culture of the affected area to rule out other common organisms, including streptococci and staphylococci. Third-generation cephalosporins, such as ceftriaxone or cefotaxime, are the drugs of choice.

REFERENCES

1. Beveridge TJ. Use of the Gram stain in microbiology. *Biotech Histochem.* 2001;76(3):111-118.
2. Jorgensen JH, Pfaller MA, Carroll KC. *Manual of Clinical Microbiology.* Washington, DC: ASM Press; 2015.
3. Mahon CR, Lehman DC, Manuselis G. *Textbook of Diagnostic Microbiology.* 5th ed. Philadelphia, PA: Elsevier Saunders; 2014.
4. Rouphael NG, Stephens DS. *Neisseria meningitidis*: biology, microbiology, and epidemiology. *Methods Mol Biol.* 2012;799:1-20.
5. Green LR, Eiden J, Hao L, et al. Approach to the discovery, development, and evaluation of a novel *Neisseria meningitidis* serogroup B vaccine. *Methods Mol Biol.* 2016;1403:445-469.
6. Kolappan S, Coureuil M, Yu X, et al. Structure of the *Neisseria meningitidis* type IV pilus. *Nat Commun.* 2016;7:13015.
7. Imhaus AF, Duménil G. The number of *Neisseria meningitidis* type IV pili determines host cell interaction. *EMBO J.* 2014;33(16):1767-1783.
8. Madico G, Welsch JA, Lewis LA, et al. The meningococcal vaccine candidate GNA1870 binds the complement regulatory protein factor H and enhances serum resistance. *J Immunol.* 2006;177(1):501-510.
9. Brandtzaeg P, van Deuren M. Classification and pathogenesis of meningococcal infections. *Methods Mol Biol.* 2012;799:21-35.
10. Scheld MW, Marra CM, Whitley RJ. *Infections of the Central Nervous System.* 4th ed. Philadelphia, PA: Lippincott Williams & Wilkins; 2014.
11. Takada S, Fujiwara S, Inoue T, et al. Meningococcemia in adults: a review of the literature. *Intern Med.* 2016;55(6):567-572.
12. Bolognia JL, Jorizzo JI, Schaffer JV, eds. *Dermatology.* 3rd ed. Philadelphia, PA: Elsevier Saunders; 2012.
13. Sabatini C, Bosis S, Semino M, et al. Clinical presentation of meningococcal disease in childhood. *J Prev Med Hyg.* 2012;53(2):116-119.
14. Wenzel M, Jakob L, Wieser A, et al. Corticosteroid-induced meningococcal meningitis in a patient with chronic meningococcemia. *JAMA Dermatol.* 2014;150(7):752-755.
15. De Greeff S, de Melker H, Schouls L, et al. Pre-admission clinical course of meningococcal disease and opportunities for the earlier start of appropriate intervention: a prospective epidemiological study on 752 patients in the Netherlands, 2003-2005. *Eur J Clin Microbiol Infect Dis.* 2008;27(10):985-992.
16. Hale AJ, LaSalvia M, Kirby JE, et al. Fatal purpura fulminans and Waterhouse-Friderichsen syndrome from fulminant *Streptococcus pneumoniae* sepsis in an asplenic young adult. *IDCases.* 2016;6:1-4.
17. Feldman H. Meningococcal infections. *Adv Intern Med.* 1972;18:117.
18. Cohen MS, Rutala W, Weber D. Gram-negative coccal and bacillary infections. In: Goldsmith LA, Katz SI, Gilchrest BA, et al, eds. *Fitzpatrick's Dermatology in General Medicine.* 8th ed. New York, NY: McGraw-Hill; 2012:2183-2186.
19. Van Deuren M, Brandtzaeg P, van der Meer JW. Update on meningococcal disease with emphasis on pathogenesis and clinical management. *Clin Microbiol Rev.* 2000;13(1):144-166.
20. Goedvolk C, Von Rosenstiel I, Bos A. Immune complex associated complications in the subacute phase of meningococcal disease: incidence and literature review. *Arch Dis Child.* 2003;88(10):927-930.
21. Parmentier L, Garzoni C, Antille C, et al. Value of a novel *Neisseria meningitidis*–specific polymerase chain reaction assay in skin biopsy specimens as a diagnostic tool in chronic meningococcemia. *Arch Dermatol.* 2008;144(6):770-773.
22. Melican K, Veloso PM, Martin T, et al. Adhesion of *Neisseria meningitidis* to dermal vessels leads to local vascular damage and purpura in a humanized mouse model. *PLoS Pathog.* 2013;9(1):e1003139.
23. Dupin N, Lecuyer H, Carlotti A, et al. Chronic meningococcemia cutaneous lesions involve meningococcal perivascular invasion through the remodeling of endothelial barriers. *Clin Infect Dis.* 2012;54(8):1162-1165.
24. Strelow VL, Vidal JE. Invasive meningococcal disease. *Arq Neuropsiquiatr.* 2013;71(9B):653-658.
25. Kanegaye JT, Soliemanzadeh P, Bradley JS. Lumbar puncture in pediatric bacterial meningitis: defining the time interval for recovery of cerebrospinal fluid pathogens after parenteral antibiotic pretreatment. *Pediatrics.* 2001;108(5):1169-1174.
26. Van Deuren M, Van Dijke BJ, Koopman R, et al. Rapid diagnosis of acute meningococcal infections by needle aspiration or biopsy of skin lesions. *BMJ.* 1993;306(6887):1229-1232.
27. Arend S, Lavrijsen A, Kuijken I, et al. Prospective controlled study of the diagnostic value of skin biopsy in patients with presumed meningococcal disease. *Eur J Clin Microbiol Infect Dis.* 2006;25(10):643-649.
28. Bryant PA, Li HY, Zaia A, et al. Prospective study of a real-time PCR that is highly sensitive, specific, and clinically useful for diagnosis of meningococcal disease in children. *J Clin Microbiol.* 2004;42(7):2919-2925.
29. Guarner J, Greer PW, Whitney A, et al. Pathogenesis and diagnosis of human meningococcal disease using immunohistochemical and PCR assays. *Am J Clin Pathol.* 2004;122(5):754-764.

30. Tunkel AR, Hartman BJ, Kaplan SL, et al. Practice guidelines for the management of bacterial meningitis. *Clin Infect Dis.* 2004;39(9):1267-1284.
31. Collard J-M, Wang X, Mahamane AE, et al. A five-year field assessment of rapid diagnostic tests for meningococcal meningitis in Niger by using the combination of conventional and real-time PCR assays as a gold standard. *Trans R Soc Trop Med Hyg.* 2014;108(1):6-12.
32. Busam K. *Dermatopathology*. 2nd ed. Philadelphia, PA: Elsevier Saunders; 2015.
33. Cohn AC, MacNeil JR, Clark TA, et al. Prevention and control of meningococcal disease: recommendations of the Advisory Committee on Immunization Practices (ACIP). *MMWR Recomm Rep.* 2013;62(RR-2):1-28.
34. Mandell GL, Bennett JE, Dolin R. *Mandell, Douglas, and Bennett's Principles and Practice of Infectious Diseases*. 7th ed. Philadelphia, PA: Churchill Livingstone; 2010.
35. Nathan N, Borel T, Djibo A, et al. Ceftriaxone as effective as long-acting chloramphenicol in short-course treatment of meningococcal meningitis during epidemics: a randomised non-inferiority study. *Lancet.* 2005;366(9482):308-313.
36. White B, Livingstone W, Murphy C, et al. An open-label study of the role of adjuvant hemostatic support with protein C replacement therapy in purpura fulminans–associated meningococcemia. *Blood.* 2000;96(12):3719-3724.
37. Brouwer MC, McIntyre P, Prasad K, et al. Corticosteroids for acute bacterial meningitis. *Cochrane Database Syst Rev.* 2015;(9):CD004405.
38. Robinson CL. Advisory Committee on Immunization Practices recommended immunization schedules for persons aged 0 through 18 years—United States, 2016. *Am J Transplant.* 2016;16(6):1928-1929.
39. MacNeil JR, Cohn AC, Zell ER, et al. Early estimate of the effectiveness of quadrivalent meningococcal conjugate vaccine. *Pediatr Infect Dis J.* 2011;30(6):451-455.
40. Folaranmi T, Rubin L, Martin SW, et al. Use of serogroup B meningococcal vaccines in persons aged ≥10 years at increased risk for serogroup B meningococcal disease: Recommendations of the Advisory Committee on Immunization Practices, 2015. *MMWR Morb Mortal Wkly Rep.* 2015;64(22):608-612.
41. Agger WA, Mardan A. *Pseudomonas aeruginosa* infections of intact skin. *Clin Infect Dis.* 1995;20(2):302-308.
42. Wu DC, Chan WW, Metelitsa AI, et al. *Pseudomonas* skin infection. *Am J Clin Dermatol.* 2011;12(3):157-169.
43. Driscoll JA, Brody SL, Kollef MH. The epidemiology, pathogenesis and treatment of Pseudomonas aeruginosa infections. *Drugs.* 2007;67(3):351-368.
44. Andonova M, Urumova V. Immune surveillance mechanisms of the skin against the stealth infection strategy of *Pseudomonas aeruginosa*—review. *Comp Immunol Microbiol Infect Dis.* 2013;36(5):433-448.
45. Lavoie EG, Wangdi T, Kazmierczak BI. Innate immune responses to *Pseudomonas aeruginosa* infection. *Microbes Infect.* 2011;13(14):1133-1145.
46. Hall S, McDermott C, Anoopkumar-Dukie S, et al. Cellular effects of pyocyanin, a secreted virulence factor of *Pseudomonas aeruginosa*. *Toxins (Basel).* 2016;8(8):236.
47. Solomon S, Horan T, Andrus M, et al. National Nosocomial Infections Surveillance (NNIS) system report, data summary from January 1992 through June 2003, issued August 2003. *Am J Infect Control.* 2003;31(8):481-498.
48. Zilberberg MD, Shorr AF. Prevalence of multidrug-resistant *Pseudomonas aeruginosa* and carbapenem-resistant *Enterobacteriaceae* among specimens from hospitalized patients with pneumonia and bloodstream infections in the United States from 2000 to 2009. *J Hosp Med.* 2013;8(10):559-563.
49. Chiriac A, Brzezinski P, Foia L, et al. Chloronychia: green nail syndrome caused by *Pseudomonas aeruginosa* in elderly persons. *Clin Interv Aging.* 2015;10:265.
50. Fiorillo L, Zucker M, Sawyer D, et al. The *Pseudomonas* hot-foot syndrome. *N Engl J Med.* 2001;345(5):335-338.
51. Yu Y, Cheng AS, Wang L, et al. Hot tub folliculitis or hot hand–foot syndrome caused by *Pseudomonas aeruginosa*. *J Am Acad Dermatol.* 2007;57(4):596-600.
52. Rosenfeld RM, Schwartz SR, Cannon CR, et al. Clinical practice guideline acute otitis externa. *Otolaryngol Head Neck Surg.* 2014;150(1)(suppl):S1-S24.
53. Centers for Disease Control and Prevention. Estimated burden of acute otitis externa--United States, 2003-2007. *MMWR Morb Mortal Wkly Rep.* 2011;60(19):605.
54. Ishikawa T, Sakurai Y, Tanaka M, et al. Ecthyma gangrenosum-like lesions in a healthy child after infection treated with antibiotics. *Pediatr Dermatol.* 2005;22(5):453-456.
55. Sarkar S, Patra AK, Mondal M. Ecthyma gangrenosum in the periorbital region in a previously healthy immunocompetent woman without bacteremia. *Indian Dermatol Online J.* 2016;7(1):36.
56. Osguthorpe JD, Nielsen DR. Otitis externa: review and clinical update. *Am Fam Physician.* 2006;74(9):1510-1516.
57. Lee H, Kim J, Nguyen V. Ear infections: otitis externa and otitis media. *Prim Care.* 2013;40(3):671-686.
58. Driscoll P, Ramachandrula A, Drezner D, et al. Characteristics of cerumen in diabetic patients: a key to understanding malignant external otitis? *Otolaryngol Head Neck Surg.* 1993;109(4):676.
59. Schechner V, Nobre V, Kaye KS, et al. Gram-negative bacteremia upon hospital admission: when should *Pseudomonas aeruginosa* be suspected? *Clin Infect Dis.* 2009;48(5):580-586.
60. Sifuentes-Osornio J, González R, Ponce-de-Leon A, et al. Epidemiology and prognosis of *Pseudomonas aeruginosa* bacteremia in a tertiary care center. *Rev Invest Clin.* 1997;50(5):383-388.
61. Atzori L, Zucca M, Lai M, et al. Gram-negative bacterial toe web intertrigo. *Eur Med J Dermatol.* 2014;2:106-111.
62. El Baze P, Thyss A, Caldani C, et al. *Pseudomonas aeruginosa* O-11 folliculitis: development into ecthyma gangrenosum in immunosuppressed patients. *Arch Dermatol.* 1985;121(7):873-876.
63. Llor C, McNulty CA, Butler CC. Ordering and interpreting ear swabs in otitis externa. *BMJ.* 2014;349:g5259.
64. Rowshan HH, Keith K, Baur D, et al. *Pseudomonas aeruginosa* infection of the auricular cartilage caused by "high ear piercing": a case report and review of the literature. *J Oral Maxillofac Surg.* 2008;66(3):543-546.
65. Rubin J, Victor LY. Malignant external otitis: insights into pathogenesis, clinical manifestations, diagnosis, and therapy. *Am J Med.* 1988;85(3):391-398.
66. Loh S, Loh WS. Malignant otitis externa an Asian perspective on treatment outcomes and prognostic factors. *Otolaryngol Head Neck Surg.* 2013;148(6):991-996.

67. Kang C-I, Kim S-H, Kim H-B, et al. *Pseudomonas aeruginosa* bacteremia: risk factors for mortality and influence of delayed receipt of effective antimicrobial therapy on clinical outcome. *Clin Infect Dis*. 2003;37(6):745-751.
68. Bodey GP, Jadeja L, Elting L. *Pseudomonas* bacteremia: retrospective analysis of 410 episodes. *Arch Intern Med*. 1985;145(9):1621-1629.
69. Aste N, Atzori L, Zucca M, et al. Gram-negative bacterial toe web infection: a survey of 123 cases from the district of Cagliari, Italy. *J Am Acad Dermatol*. 2001;45(4):537-541.
70. Kaushik V, Malik T, Saeed SR. Interventions for acute otitis externa. *Cochrane Database Syst Rev*. 2010;(1):CD004740.
71. Noel SB, Scallan P, Meadors MC, et al. Treatment of *Pseudomonas aeruginosa* auricular perichondritis with oral ciprofloxacin. *J Dermatol Surg Oncol*. 1989;15(6):633-637.
72. Mion M, Bovo R, Marchese-Ragona R, et al. Outcome predictors of treatment effectiveness for fungal malignant external otitis: a systematic review. *Acta Otorhinolaryngol Ital*. 2015;35(5):307.
73. Vardakas KZ, Tansarli GS, Bliziotis IA, et al. β-Lactam plus aminoglycoside or fluoroquinolone combination versus β-lactam monotherapy for *Pseudomonas aeruginosa* infections: a meta-analysis. *Int J Antimicrob Agents*. 2013;41(4):301-310.
74. van Duin D, Bonomo RA. Ceftazidime/avibactam and ceftolozane/tazobactam: second-generation β-lactam/β-lactamase combinations. *Clin Infect Dis*. 2016;63(2):234-241.
75. Sabuda DM, Laupland K, Pitout J, et al. Utilization of colistin for treatment of multidrug-resistant *Pseudomonas aeruginosa*. *Can J Infect Dis Med Microbiol*. 2008;19(6):413-418.
76. Maguiña C, Guerra H, Ventosilla P. Bartonellosis. *Clin Dermatol*. 2009;27(3):271-280.
77. Pulliainen AT, Dehio C. Persistence of *Bartonella* spp. stealth pathogens: from subclinical infections to vasoproliferative tumor formation. *FEMS Microbiol Rev*. 2012;36(3):563-599.
78. Chian CA, Arrese JE, Piérard GE. Skin manifestations of *Bartonella* infections. *Int J Dermatol*. 2002;41(8):461-466.
79. Chomel BB, Kasten RW, Floyd-Hawkins K, et al. Experimental transmission of Bartonella henselae by the cat flea. *J Clin Microbiol*. 1996;34(8):1952-1956.
80. Brouqui P, Lascola B, Roux V, et al. Chronic *Bartonella quintana* bacteremia in homeless patients. *N Engl J Med*. 1999;340(3):184-189.
81. Plettenberg A, Lorenzen T, Burtsche B, et al. Bacillary angiomatosis in HIV-infected patients—an epidemiological and clinical study. *Dermatology*. 2000;201(4):326-331.
82. Clemente NS, Ugarte-Gil CA, Solórzano N, et al. *Bartonella bacilliformis*: a systematic review of the literature to guide the research agenda for elimination. *PLoS Negl Trop Dis*. 2012;6(10):e1819.
83. Chamberlin J, Laughlin LW, Romero S, et al. Epidemiology of endemic *Bartonella bacilliformis*: a prospective cohort study in a Peruvian mountain valley community. *J Infect Dis*. 2002;186(7):983-990.
84. Lappin MR, Davis WL, Hawley JR, et al. A flea and tick collar containing 10% imidacloprid and 4.5% flumethrin prevents flea transmission of *Bartonella henselae* in cats. *Parasit Vectors*. 2013;6(1):26.
85. Varela G, Vinson J, Molina-Pasquel C. Trench fever. III. Induction of clinical disease in volunteers inoculated with Rickettsia quintana propagated on blood agar. *Am J Trop Med Hyg*. 1969;18(5):713-722.
86. Koehler JE, Tappero JW. Bacillary angiomatosis and bacillary peliosis in patients infected with human immunodeficiency virus. *Clin Infect Dis*. 1993;17(4):612-624.
87. Monteil R, Michiels J-F, Hofman P, et al. Histological and ultrastructural study of one case of oral bacillary angiomatosis in HIV disease and review of the literature. *Eur J Cancer B Oral Oncol*. 1994;30(1):65-71.
88. Maguiña C, Ugarte-Gil C, Breña P, et al. Actualización de la Enfermedad de Carrión. Update of Carrion's disease. *Rev Medica Hered*. 2008;19(1):036-041.
89. Maguiña C, García PJ, Gotuzzo E, et al. Bartonellosis (Carrion's disease) in the modern era. *Clin Infect Dis*. 2001;33(6):772-779.
90. Fretzayas A, Papadopoulos NG, Moustaki M, et al. Unsuspected extralymphocutaneous dissemination in febrile cat scratch disease. *Scand J Infect Dis*. 2001;33(8):599-603.
91. Reed JB, Scales DK, Wong MT, et al. *Bartonella henselae* neuroretinitis in cat scratch disease: diagnosis, management, and sequelae. *Ophthalmology*. 1998;105(3):459-466.
92. Arisoy ES, Correa AG, Wagner ML, et al. Hepatosplenic cat-scratch disease in children: selected clinical features and treatment. *Clin Infect Dis*. 1999;28(4):778-784.
93. Angelakis E, Raoult D. Pathogenicity and treatment of *Bartonella* infections. *Int J Antimicrob Agents*. 2014;44(1):16-25.
94. Perkocha LA, Geaghan SM, Yen TB, et al. Clinical and pathological features of bacillary peliosis hepatis in association with human immunodeficiency virus infection. *N Engl J Med*. 1990;323(23):1581-1586.
95. Baron A, Steinbach L, LeBoit P, et al. Osteolytic lesions and bacillary angiomatosis in HIV infection: radiologic differentiation from AIDS-related Kaposi sarcoma. *Radiology*. 1990;177(1):77-81.
96. Maguiña Vargas C, Ordaya Espinoza E, Ugarte-Gil C, et al. Compromiso cardiovascular en la fase aguda de la enfermedad de Carrión o bartonelosis humana: 20 años de experiencia en Hospital Nacional Cayetano Heredia. *Acta Médica Peruana*. 2008;25(1):30-38.
97. Abbott RC, Chomel BB, Kasten RW, et al. Experimental and natural infection with Bartonella henselae in domestic cats. *Comp Immunol Microbiol Infect Dis*. 1997;20(1):41-51.
98. Popa C, Abdollahi-Roodsaz S, Joosten LA, et al. *Bartonella quintana* lipopolysaccharide is a natural antagonist of Toll-like receptor 4. *Infect Immun*. 2007;75(10):4831-4837.
99. Andersen-Nissen E, Smith KD, Strobe KL, et al. Evasion of toll-like receptor 5 by flagellated bacteria. *Proc Natl Acad Sci U S A*. 2005;102(26):9247-9252.
100. Boonjakuakul JK, Gerns HL, Chen Y-T, et al. Proteomic and immunoblot analyses of *Bartonella quintana* total membrane proteins identify antigens recognized by sera from infected patients. *Infect Immun*. 2007;75(5):2548-2561.
101. Kabeya H, Maruyama S, Irei M, et al. Genomic variations among *Bartonella henselae* isolates derived from naturally infected cats. *Vet Microbiol*. 2002;89(2):211-221.
102. Dehio C. *Bartonella*–host-cell interactions and vascular tumour formation. *Nat Rev Microbiol*.

103. Berrich M, Kieda C, Grillon C, et al. Differential effects of *Bartonella henselae* on human and feline macro- and micro-vascular endothelial cells. *PLoS One*. 2011;6(5):e20204.
104. Harms A, Dehio C. Intruders below the radar: molecular pathogenesis of *Bartonella* spp. *Clin Microbiol Rev*. 2012;25(1):42-78.
105. Vermeulen MJ, Diederen BM, Verbakel H, et al. Low sensitivity of *Bartonella henselae* PCR in serum samples of patients with cat-scratch disease lymphadenitis. *J Med Microbiol*. 2008;57(8):1049-1050.
106. Piérard-Franchimont C, Quatresooz P, Piérard GE. Skin diseases associated with Bartonella infection: facts and controversies. *Clin Dermatol*. 2010;28(5):483-488.
107. van Ierland-van Leeuwen M, Peringa J, Blaauwgeers H, et al. Cat scratch disease, a rare cause of hypodense liver lesions, lymphadenopathy and a protruding duodenal lesion, caused by *Bartonella henselae*. *BMJ Case Rep*. 2014;2014.
108. Prutsky G, Domecq JP, Mori L, et al. Treatment outcomes of human bartonellosis: a systematic review and meta-analysis. *Int J Infect Dis*. 2013;17(10):e811-e819.
109. King KY, Hicks MJ, Mazziotti MV, et al. Persistent cat scratch disease requiring surgical excision in a patient with MPGN. *Pediatrics*. 2015;135(6):e1514-e1517.
110. Foucault C, Raoult D, Brouqui P. Randomized open trial of gentamicin and doxycycline for eradication of *Bartonella quintana* from blood in patients with chronic bacteremia. *Antimicrob Agents Chemother*. 2003;47(7):2204-2207.
111. Ohl ME, Spach DH. *Bartonella quintana* and urban trench fever. *Clin Infect Dis*. 2000;31(1):131-135.
112. Panel on Antiretroviral Guidelines for Adults and Adolescents. Guidelines for the use of antiretroviral agents in HIV-1-infected adults and adolescents. Department of Health and Human Services. May 30, 2018. Available at http://aidsinfo.nih.gov/contentfiles/lvguidelines/AdultandAdolescentGL.pdf
113. Rolain J, Brouqui P, Koehler J, et al. Recommendations for treatment of human infections caused by *Bartonella* species. *Antimicrob Agents Chemother*. 2004;48(6):1921-1933.
114. Grimont PA, Weill F-X. *Antigenic Formulae of the Salmonella Serovars*. 9th ed. Paris, France: WHO Collaborating Centre for Reference and Research on Salmonella; 2007. Available at http://docplayer.net/1605957-Antigenic-formulae-of-the-salmonella-serovars.html
115. Imanishi M, Newton A, Vieira A, et al. Typhoid fever acquired in the United States, 1999-2010: epidemiology, microbiology, and use of a space–time scan statistic for outbreak detection. *Epidemiol Infect*. 2015;143(11):2343-2354.
116. Parry CM, Hien TT, Dougan G, et al. Typhoid fever. *N Engl J Med*. 2002;347:1770-1782.
117. Crump JA, Luby SP, Mintz ED. The global burden of typhoid fever. *Bull World Health Organ*. 2004;82(5):346-353.
118. Crump JA, Mintz ED. Global trends in typhoid and paratyphoid fever. *Clin Infect Dis*. 2010;50(2):241-246.
119. Maskey AP, Day JN, Tuan PQ, et al. *Salmonella enterica* serovar *Paratyphi* A and *S. enterica* serovar *Typhi* cause indistinguishable clinical syndromes in Kathmandu, Nepal. *Clin Infect Dis*. 2006;42(9):1247-1253.
120. Vollaard AM, Ali S, Widjaja S, et al. Identification of typhoid fever and paratyphoid fever cases at presentation in outpatient clinics in Jakarta, Indonesia. *Trans R Soc Trop Med Hyg*. 2005;99(6):440-450.
121. Meltzer E, Schwartz E. Enteric fever: a travel medicine oriented view. *Curr Opin Infect Dis*. 2010;23(5):432-437.
122. Patel TA, Armstrong M, Morris-Jones SD, et al. Imported enteric fever: case series from the hospital for tropical diseases, London, United Kingdom. *Am J Trop Med Hyg*. 2010;82(6):1121-1126.
123. Burns T, Breathnach S. *Rook's Textbook of Dermatology*, Vol. 4. London, UK: Blackwell Scientific; 1992.
124. Litwack KD, Hoke AW, Borchardt KA. Rose spots in typhoid fever. *Arch Dermatol*. 1972;105(2):252-255.
125. Cohen JI, Bartlett JA, Corey GR. Extra-intestinal manifestations of salmonella infections. *Medicine (Baltimore)*. 1987;66(5):349-388.
126. Raveendran KM, Viswanathan S. Typhoid fever, below the belt. *J Clin Diagn Res*. 2016;10(1):OD12-OD13.
127. Kuvandik C, Karaoglan I, Namiduru M, et al. Predictive value of clinical and laboratory findings in the diagnosis of enteric fever. *New Microbiol*. 2009;32(1):25.
128. Shukla VK, Singh H, Pandey M, et al. Carcinoma of the gallbladder—is it a sequel of typhoid? *Dig Dis Sci*. 2000;45(5):900-903.
129. Toapanta FR, Bernal PJ, Fresnay S, et al. Oral wild-type *Salmonella typhi* challenge induces activation of circulating monocytes and dendritic cells in individuals who develop typhoid disease. *PLoS Negl Trop Dis*. 2015;9(6):e0003837.
130. Kohbata S, Yokoyama H, Yabuuchi E. Cytopathogenic effect of *Salmonella typhi* GIFU 10007 on M cells of murine ileal Peyer's patches in ligated ileal loops: an ultrastructural study. *Microbiol Immunol*. 1986;30(12):1225-1237.
131. van de Vosse E, de Visser AW, Al-Attar S, et al. Distribution of CFTR variations in an Indonesian enteric fever cohort. *Clin Infect Dis*. 2010;50(9):1231-1237.
132. Gasem M, Dolmans W, Isbandrio B, et al. Culture of *Salmonella typhi* and *Salmonella paratyphi* from blood and bone marrow in suspected typhoid fever. *Trop Geogr Med*. 1994;47(4):164-167.
133. Gilman R, Terminel M, Levine M, et al. Relative efficacy of blood, urine, rectal swab, bone-marrow, and rose-spot cultures for recovery of *Salmonella typhi* in typhoid fever. *Lancet*. 1975;305(7918):1211-1213.
134. Hornick RB, Greisman S, Woodward T, et al. Typhoid fever: pathogenesis and immunologic control. *N Engl J Med*. 1970;283(14):739-746.
135. Dave J, Sefton A. Enteric fever and its impact on returning travellers. *Int Health*. 2015;7(3):163-168.
136. Fernández Vozmediano J, Armario Hita J, Cabrerizo AG. Rhinoscleroma in three siblings. *Pediatr Dermatol*. 2004;21(2):134-138.
137. Hart C, Rao S. Rhinoscleroma. *J Med Microbiol*. 2000;49(5):395-396.
138. Mukara B, Munyarugamba P, Dazert S, et al. Rhinoscleroma: a case series report and review of the literature. *Eur Arch Otorhinolaryngol*. 2014;271(7):1851-1856.
139. Bailhache A, Dehesdin D, François A, et al. Rhinoscleroma of the sinuses. *Rhinology*. 2008;46(4):338-341.
140. Talwar A, Patel N, Chen L, et al. Rhinoscleroma of the tracheobronchial tree: bronchoscopic, PET, and CT correlation. *Indian J Chest Dis Allied Sci*. 2008;50(2):225.

141. Leibovitz E, Jacobs MR, Dagan R. *Haemophilus influenzae*: a significant pathogen in acute otitis media. *Pediatr Infect Dis J.* 2004;23(12):1142-1152.
142. Fisher RG, Benjamin DK Jr. Facial cellulitis in childhood: a changing spectrum. *South Med J.* 2002;95(7):672-675.
143. Rimon A, Hoffer V, Prais D, et al. Periorbital cellulitis in the era of *Haemophilus influenzae* type B vaccine: predisposing factors and etiologic agents in hospitalized children. *J AAPOS.* 2008;45(5):300-304.
144. Sharma A, Liu ES, Le TD, et al. Pediatric orbital cellulitis in the *Haemophilus influenzae* vaccine era. *J AAPOS.* 2015;19(3):206-210.

Chapter 155 :: The Skin in Infective Endocarditis, Sepsis, Septic Shock, and Disseminated Intravascular Coagulation
:: Joseph C. English III & Misha Rosenbach

第一百五十五章

感染性心内膜炎、脓毒血症、脓毒性休克和弥散性血管内凝血中的皮肤表现

中文导读

本章节主要围绕三类全身性细菌感染的疾病进行阐述，分为3节：①感染性心内膜炎；②脓毒血症和脓毒性休克；③弥散性血管内凝血。感染性心内膜炎（IE）定义为由细菌或真菌感染引起的心脏心内膜和植入材料的炎症。严重的可以发展为脓毒血症，即因宿主对感染的反应失调而导致的危及生命的器官功能障碍，脓毒性休克属于脓毒血症的一个子集。弥散性血管内凝血是脓毒血症最常见的结果，是凝血级联反应的系统性激活产生的结果。本章节全面讨论了它们的流行病学、病因和发病机制、诊断、鉴别诊断、临床病程和预后、临床管理等内容。

〔汪 犇〕

AT-A-GLANCE

- *Infective endocarditis:* staphylococcal, streptococcal, and enterococcal bacteria cause 80% of cases; intravenous drug use is the most common cause of right-sided infective endocarditis.
- *Sepsis:* Gram-positive and Gram-negative bacteria, fungi, and viruses may cause sepsis; 10th leading cause of death in the United States for all races and sexes at age 45 years and older.
- *Disseminated intravascular coagulation:* most commonly a consequence of sepsis; results from systemic activation of the coagulation cascade.
- *Cutaneous manifestations of these entities include:* splinter hemorrhages, Janeway lesions, Osler nodules, erythroderma, cellulitis, purpura, hemorrhage, purpura fulminans, and skin necrosis.

INFECTIVE ENDOCARDITIS

DEFINITION AND HISTORICAL PERSPECTIVE

Infective endocarditis (IE) is defined as inflammation of the endocardial lining of the heart (naïve or prosthetic heart valves, mural endocardium) and implanted material caused by infection from bacteria or fungus.[1,2] The historical definitions of IE as acute, subacute, and chronic IE have been discarded for a more appropriate description based on infectious agent and the infected endocardial structure.[3,4]

EPIDEMIOLOGY

The incidence of IE is 3 to 10 cases per 100,000 people.[4,5] The male-to-female ratio is 2:1 and the incidence peaks at 194 cases per million in men 75 to 79 years of age.[5] Pediatric cases are rare. Rheumatic heart disease in the setting oral cavity procedures is the most-common cause in low-income countries; however, IE is now more commonly seen in health care–associated cases in the setting of valvular heart disease, prosthetic valves, implantable pacemakers and defibrillators, hemodialysis, IV lines, and invasive procedures in higher-income countries.[5] In addition, risk factors include a history of IE, diabetes, cancer, congenital heart disease, dental procedures, HIV disease, IV drug abuse.[1,4-6]

CLINICAL FEATURES

The most common clinical presentations of IE include fever and a new cardiac murmur; consequently, IE should be considered in the differential diagnosis of all fevers, embolic events of unknown origin, and patients with persistently positive blood cultures.[5] The modified Duke criteria (Table 155-1),[7] help make the diagnosis of IE. Newer reviews of the Duke criteria for diagnosing IE note its continual importance in identifying IE.[2]

TABLE 155-1
Modified Duke Criteria for Infective Endocarditis

- A clinically definite case is defined as fulfilling 2 major, 1 major plus 3 minor, or 5 minor criteria.
- A clinically suspicious case is defined as fulfilling 1 major and 1 minor, or 3 minor criteria

Major Criteria
1. **Microbiologic**
   a. Two separate blood cultures positive for typical microorganism
   or
   b. Persistently positive blood culture for typical microorganism
   or
   c. Single positive blood culture for *Coxiella burnetii* or a Phase I immunoglobulin G antibody titer to *C. burnetii* ratio greater than 1:800
2. **Evidence of endocardial involvement**
   a. New valvular regurgitation
   or
   b. Positive echocardiogram showing oscillating echogenic intracardiac mass at the site of endocardial injury, a periannular abscess, or new dehiscence of a prosthetic valve

Minor Criteria
1. Predisposition to infective endocarditis
2. Fever
3. Vascular phenomena such as Osler nodes or Roth spots
4. Immunologic factors such as a positive rheumatoid factor or glomerulonephritis
5. Serologic evidence of active infection not meeting microbiologic major criteria

CUTANEOUS

Cutaneous signs of IE (splinter hemorrhages, petechiae/purpura, Janeway lesions, Osler nodes) are nonspecific but may help the dermatologist in assisting the primary medical team in diagnosing IE during the inpatient consultation.[8-10] Cutaneous findings are caused either by embolic events, thrombosis, or focal vasculitis, and are more commonly found in left-sided IE.[6] IE patients with skin manifestations had higher rates of cerebral emboli without increased mortality, whereas Janeway lesions were more frequently associated with extracerebral emboli, and if purpura was present, larger valvular vegetations occurred.[10]

Splinter hemorrhages (Fig. 155-1) are 1- to 2-mm red-brown or black longitudinal streaks under the nail plate. They are seen in approximately 15% of patients with IE and are considered to be of greater diagnostic value if proximally located. Splinter hemorrhages associated with IE are the result of small capillary vasculitis, or from microemboli. In the absence of other signs or symptoms of IE, the mere presence of splinter hemorrhage is not specific enough evidence to warrant a workup. Crops of petechiae are commonly seen in the buccal membrane, conjunctival mucosa, soft palate and extremities.

Janeway lesions are painless, irregular, nonblanchable, erythematous maculopapules that appear on the palms and soles and last days to weeks (Fig. 155-2). Histologically, thrombi are found in small vessels in the absence of vasculitis. Neutrophilic microabscesses can be seen in the dermis with occasional Gram-positive organisms. Osler nodes present as painful red papulonodules with a pale center on the fingertips lasting days to weeks. Osler nodes are painful, perhaps because of involvement of the glomus bodies located in the fingertips. Histologically, neutrophilic microabscesses are present in the dermis, and arteriolar microemboli may contain Gram-positive cocci.

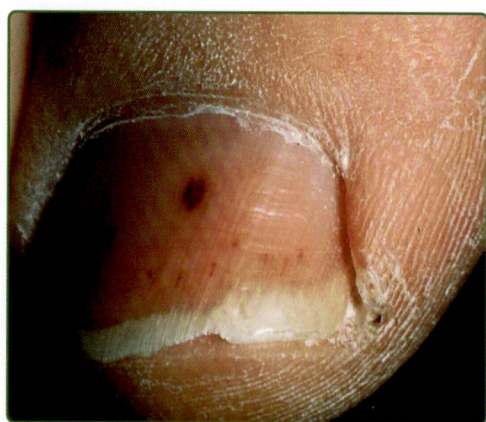

Figure 155-1 Globular proximal splinter hemorrhage and several distal linear splinter hemorrhages in a patient with infective endocarditis. (Image used with permission from William James, MD, and James Fitzpatrick, MD.)

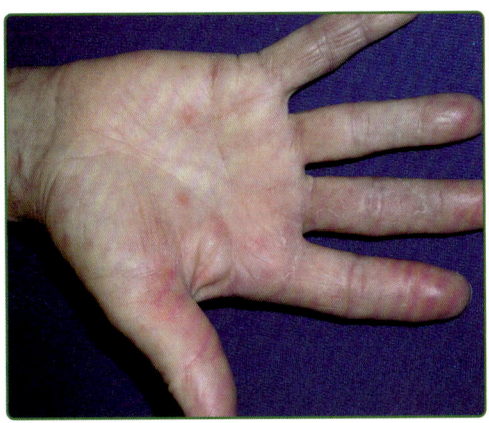

Figure 155-2 Janeway lesions of infectious endocarditis.

Septic emboli of valvular vegetation fragments can cause ischemia of distal extremities. Toes are most commonly involved, followed by fingers, and this condition presents as reticulated purpura or purple digit similar to that seen in cholesterol emboli syndrome (see Chap. 148). Although this condition generally resolves without sequelae, tissue necrosis or gangrene can result. In addition patients may have nonspecific acrocyanosis from hypoxemia and livedo reticularis from sepsis and embolization.[11,12]

NONCUTANEOUS FINDINGS

In addition to fever and new cardiac murmur, patients may have anorexia, weight loss, and malaise. More commonly, signs of stroke, meningitis, congestive heart failure, myocardial infarction, renal failure, pneumonitis, acute abdomen, peripheral emboli, and metastatic infections are present.[5,6] Splenomegaly and ocular findings (conjunctival hemorrhage or Roth spots) are less often present.

COMPLICATIONS

Most concerning and severe complications of IE are neurologic in nature.[4] Up to 50% of nervous system complications are ischemic lesions.[13] In addition hemorrhagic strokes, transient ischemic attack, brain abscess, and meningitis may occur.

ETIOLOGY AND PATHOGENESIS

IE is classified based on valve (native valve vs prosthetic valve), and source of infection (community or health care acquired). The causative organisms in 80% of IE cases are staphylococci, streptococci (coagulase negative and viridans group) or enterococci.[5] The most common cause of IE in high-income countries is *Staphylococcus aureus* for both naïve and prosthetic valves.[5] Rare causes may be from HACEK (*Haemophilus, Aggregatibacter, Cardiobacterium, Eikenella, Kingella*) organisms, as well as *Bartonella, Brucella,* and *Coxiella* species, and fungi (ie, *Candida*). Culture-negative IE (5% to 10%) occurs in the setting of patients receiving antibiotics before cultures obtained or infection with fastidious bacterium.[4]

Endothelial damage can occur in setting of electrodes or catheter trauma, from particles in IV drugs or chronic inflammation.[4] After injury, the release of inflammatory mediators and tissue factor leads to a platelet-fibrin thrombus that easily allows bacterial adherence.[5] Bacterial adhesion proteins help induce the formation of bacterial biofilms on the valves that potentiate antibiotic resistance, resulting in the development of valvular vegetations that can cause local tissue destruction and embolic events.[5]

Native valve endocarditis occurs most commonly in the setting of valvular disease or in people who use IV drugs.[6] IV drug users are particularly susceptible to IE even though most have no preexisting structural heart disease.[6] More than half of the cases of IE in injection drug users are right-sided, involving the tricuspid valve. Prosthetic valve endocarditis can be classified as early (in the first 2 months following valve replacement) or late (2 months or later). Early prosthetic valve endocarditis is most commonly caused by coagulase-negative streptococci or by *S. aureus* and late prosthetic valve endocarditis can be caused by any of the infectious organism that can cause IE.[6]

DIAGNOSIS

SUPPORTIVE STUDIES

Laboratory Testing: Bacterial cultures (3 sets prior to antibiotics) detect bacteremia and guide appropriate antibiotic therapy. If unable to culture and surgery is performed, removed valves also can be cultured and, along with broad-ranged polymerase chain reaction sequencing and immunostaining techniques, can help identify the organism.[4] Erythrocyte sedimentation rate, C-reactive protein, antineutrophilic cytoplasmic antibody (ANCA), and rheumatoid factor elevation, as well as anemia and red cell casts/pyuria on urinalysis, are laboratory findings.[5]

Pathology: Histologic findings of the cutaneous manifestations of IE are nonspecific.

Clinical pathologic correlation of systemic symptoms and skin lesions with findings of extravasated red blood cells, fibrinoid degeneration of vasculature, karyorrhexis, and Gram-positive/negative organisms in microemboli on pathology are suggestive of IE.

Imaging: An EKG baseline is necessary to monitor for changes in conduction that may indicate worsening disease.[5] Echocardiography allows the visualization of the valves and can provide information as to the level of myocardial involvement. Transthoracic echocardiography is less invasive and less expensive than transesophageal echocardiography. When these imaging modalities are used in combination valvular vegetations can be detected in the majority of cases.[4] Other potential imaging studies include high-resolution cardiac CT and ^{18}F-fluorodeoxyglucose positron emission tomography CT.[1,5] Vegetations larger than 10 mm are associated with a greater embolic risk.[5] Emboli to the CNS leads to stroke; brain abscess and meningitis and can be identified with MRI.[1]

DIFFERENTIAL DIAGNOSIS

The differential diagnosis of IE includes noninfectious endocarditis from neoplastic or immunologic sources.[1] Examples include atrial myxomas, other cardiac tumors and nonbacterial thrombotic endocarditis, such as Libman-Sacks endocarditis from systemic lupus erythematosus, and hypercoagulable states (eg, cancer, antiphospholipid antibody syndrome).[6] Table 155-2 outlines the differential diagnosis of splinter hemorrhages. Janeway lesions and Osler nodes can be similar in appearance to septic emboli and neutrophilic eccrine hidradenitis. Cases of culture-negative, ANCA-positive bacterial endocarditis, particularly in the presence of cutaneous manifestations such as purpura, may mimic ANCA-associated vasculitis.[14]

CLINICAL COURSE AND PROGNOSIS

The prognosis and clinical course of IE varies per patient based on the variable infecting organisms and associated clinical comorbidities (presence of emboli and the extent of cardiac damage).[4] Poor prognostic indicators are left-sided IE, vegetation size (>10 mm), prosthetic valves, older age, diabetes, immunosuppression, heart failure, renal failure, septic shock, brain hemorrhage, and infections from methicillin-resistant *S. aureus*,
fungi, or polymicrobial infections.[4,6] The 5-year mortality rate of IE is approximately 40%.[4,6] Right-sided IE (tricuspid valve) has a better prognosis.[5,6] Right-sided IV drug user IE has a 5% to 9% mortality rate and recurring IE is seen most often in IV drug users. A person with a prosthetic (mechanical and biologic heart valve has a 3% to 4% chance of developing IE, and if the person develops IE, the person has up to a 50% 1-year mortality.[5] Multidisciplinary management, early diagnosis, and treatment improve outcomes.[15] Neurologic failure is a major determinant of short-term prognosis.[13] Cerebral embolic disease and congestive heart failure are the most common causes of death.[16]

MANAGEMENT

INTERVENTIONS

The goal of IE treatment should focus on eliminating infection with the appropriate antibiotic, early surgical intervention, and the treatment of complications.

Medications: Appropriate antibiotic therapy should be initiated in suspected cases of IE after blood cultures have been drawn and sensitivities have been identified. Long-term (4 to 6 weeks) parenteral antibiotics, usually with a penicillin derivative (eg, penicillin G, ceftriaxone, gentamycin, vancomycin) are used to treat both streptococcal and staphylococcal IE. Enterococcal IE requires ampicillin or penicillin with gentamycin or streptomycin and others based on antibiotic resistance.[3,17] Duration, frequency, and antibiotics also vary based on Native or prosthetic valve IE. Antibiotic treatment reduces the risk of subsequent embolism and decreases sepsis, organ damage, and death. Treatment of IE caused by other organisms is reviewed elsewhere.[3]

Procedures: Recent data suggest surgical intervention within 48 hours of diagnosing IE and when vegetations are larger than 10 mm decreases the risk of death in IE.[16,18] Failure of parenteral antibiotic therapy, perivulvar abscess, valvular destruction/dysfunction with heart failure, persistent fever, and ischemic neurologic complications are settings that require surgery.[1,4,5] Surgery should be avoided for 3 weeks if IE is complicated by hemorrhagic strokes or if cerebral damage is severe.[13]

PREVENTION/SCREENING

Good oral, dental, and skin hygiene are important for patients at risk for IE.[4] Currently, prophylactic antibiotics for skin surgery are not indicated for procedures performed on noninfected surgically scrubbed skin regardless of cardiac history. Guidelines issued by the American Heart Association in May 2007 shifted from recommending antibiotic prophylaxis for patients at increased risk for IE, to recommending IE prophylaxis

TABLE 155-2
Differential Diagnosis of Splinter Hemorrhages

- Atopic dermatitis
- Cryoglobulinemia
- Drug-induced
  - Vascular endothelial growth factor receptor inhibitors
  - Tetracyclines
- Endocarditis
- Idiopathic
- Internal malignancy
- Psoriasis
- Scurvy
- Thyrotoxicosis
- Trauma
- Trichinosis
- Vasculitis

for patients who have a high risk of an adverse outcome associated with IE and who are to have a procedure that involves a contaminated or infected wound, or surgery on oral or nasal mucosa.[19] For dermatologists, this would include patients with a prosthetic heart valve, a personal history of IE, valvulopathy in a cardiac transplant patient, or an unrepaired cyanotic heart defect.

SEPSIS AND SEPTIC SHOCK

DEFINITION AND HISTORICAL PERSPECTIVE

The Third International Consensus Definitions for Sepsis and Septic Shock, which was published in *JAMA* in 2016 after a literature review and expert deliberation, has redefined sepsis and eliminated the historical terms *sepsis syndrome*, *septicemia*, and *severe sepsis*. Sepsis is defined as life-threatening organ dysfunction that results from a dysregulated host response to infection.[20] Septic shock is a subset of sepsis in which vasopressor therapy is required to maintain a mean arterial pressure of 65 mm Hg or greater, and having a serum lactate level greater than 2 mmol/L persisting after fluid resuscitation.[21]

EPIDEMIOLOGY

Sepsis is a leading cause of critical illness, morbidity, and mortality.[22] A review of U.S. hospitalizations from 2004 to 2009 revealed the annual incidence of sepsis varied from 300 to 1031 per 100,000 population with an annual average increase of 13%.[23] In 2011, the 1.1 million cases of sepsis was the most expensive condition treated in the United States by all payers, accounting for roughly $20 billion of hospital costs.[24] In 2020, sepsis cases are estimated to reach 2 million.[25] The increased incidence is associated with the aging populations, an increase in syndrome recognition, and specific use of billing codes that can easily be tabulated. Over the next several years, with the newer consensus definition, a more uniform and consistent methodology may be instituted to enable an assessment of the true incidence of this syndrome of physiologic, pathologic, and biochemical reactions to infection.[22,23,26]

CLINICAL FEATURES

CUTANEOUS

The causative organism in sepsis is not always identifiable by routine culture. The use of real-time polymerase chain reaction, fluorescence in situ hybridization, and matrix-assisted laser desorption ionization time of flight mass spectrometry will enhance quicker identification; however, differentiating the cause of organ dysfunction is often clinically difficult.[25,26] In some cases, the cutaneous examination and histologic evaluation of diseased skin can provide clues to the identity of the responsible pathogen, providing a valuable clinical tool in the management of the septic patient and the critical role for skin evaluation by the dermatologist in the intensive care unit.

Erythroderma in the septic patient suggests staphylococcal or streptococcal toxic shock syndrome (TSS).[27] Patients with TSS are usually young and otherwise healthy. Patients with staphylococcal TSS are much more likely to be erythrodermic but much less likely to have positive blood culture than are patients with streptococcal TSS. Streptococcal TSS is commonly associated with a necrotizing soft-tissue infection.

The finding of pustules on the skin of a septic patient, particularly in the neonate or immunocompromised individual, may be suggestive of fungal infection, particularly with *Candida* species. Congenital candidiasis, most often seen in infants born to mothers with vaginal candidiasis, is generally a skin-limited disease. However, in the septic infant with pustules, candidemia should be considered.

The vasculitis[28] and coagulopathy[29] that can occur in the septic patient may cause purpura, sometimes prominent in the nailfold small capillaries (Fig. 155-3). Purpura is particularly prominent in those patients with thrombocytopenia. Such infections are seen most commonly in oncology patients undergoing bone marrow transplantation. In the immunocompromised host, opportunistic fungal infection, such as with *Aspergillus* spp., *Fusarium* spp., and *Candida* spp., often presents as erythematous papules, petechiae or pustules that progress to purpuric lesions (Fig. 155-4).[30]

Pustules resulting from disseminated gonococcemia are acrally located, typically tender and a characteristic gun-metal gray color, hemorrhagic or black, and are most commonly seen in the otherwise healthy adolescent or young adult. Gram staining of the pustule will reveal intracellular Gram-negative diplococci. In its

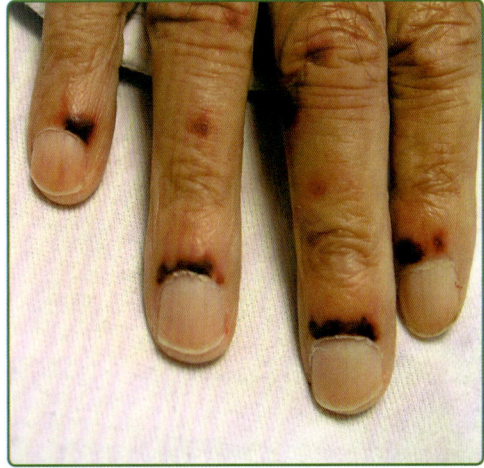

Figure 155-3 Proximal nailfold purpura from leukocytoclastic vasculitis caused by *Clostridium difficile* sepsis.

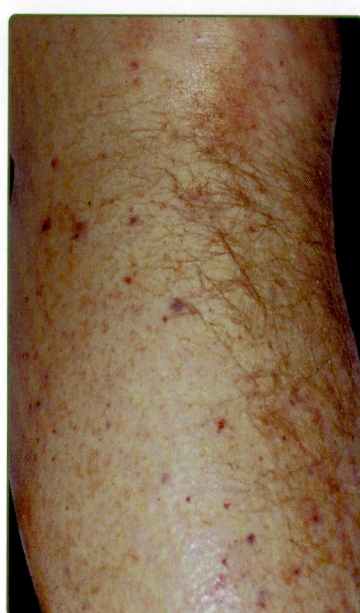

Figure 155-4 Petechiae from *Fusarium* sepsis in an immunosuppressed patient.

most extreme form, meningococcemia can cause stellate purpura (Fig. 155-5) and retiform to purpura fulminans (Fig. 155-6). Pustules also may be secondary to a local inoculation site, as in the case of staphylococcal sepsis.

Cellulitis is characterized by intense local inflammation in the presence of relatively few infectious organisms, and blood cultures are rarely positive (see Chap. 153).[31] Most commonly occurring on the legs, the affected extremity is typically erythematous, hyperemic, and edematous. The most common causes of cellulitis are *S. aureus* and group A *Streptococcus*. Rarely, anaerobic organisms, including clostridial species and other anaerobic bacteria species such as *Bacteroides*, *Peptostreptococcus*, and *Peptococcus*, are the causative organism. In immunosuppressed patients, *Cryptococcus neoformans* can also cause cellulitis, particularly in the setting of AIDS, although rates are increasing in the organ transplant population. Patients with liver compromise can develop hemorrhagic bullous cellulitis from *Vibrio vulnificus*, a Gram-negative bacterium that lives in warm marine environments and becomes concentrated in filter-feeding shellfish. Infection occurs either via consumption of contaminated organisms, such as raw oysters, or through contact with infected water. Mortality rates exceed 40% in those with *V. vulnificus* sepsis.[32]

A more aggressive local soft-tissue infection, necrotizing fasciitis or necrotizing soft-tissue infection, can be associated with positive blood cultures later in the course of the disease because of hematogenous seeding by the organisms.[33] Clinically, necrotizing fasciitis is rapidly progressive, initially painful, and accompanied by fever and leukocytosis (see Chap. 153). Necrotic soft-tissue infections have a higher mortality rate when associated with hospital-acquired infections, patients older than age 75 years, severe peripheral vascular disease, and coexistent sepsis/septic shock.[34]

Ecthyma gangrenosum (see Chap. 154) begins as an erythematous papule that expands and eventually becomes a necrotic bulla. Lesions are most commonly seen between the umbilicus and the knees. Classic ecthyma gangrenosum represents cutaneous seeding of bacteria, usually *Pseudomonas aeruginosa*, from a hematogenous source and is seen almost exclusively in neutropenic patients, often in association with an underlying malignancy. Nonclassical cases have been reported with *Aeromonas hydrophila*, *Escherichia coli*, *Citrobacter freundii*, and *Corynebacterium diphtheriae*, fungal infection including *Candida*, *Aspergillus*, *Fusarium*, and mucormycosis-causing species, and even herpes simplex virus.[35]

NONCUTANEOUS

The septic patient presents with fever, prostration, oliguria, tachycardia, and tachypnea. Signs of pneumonia,

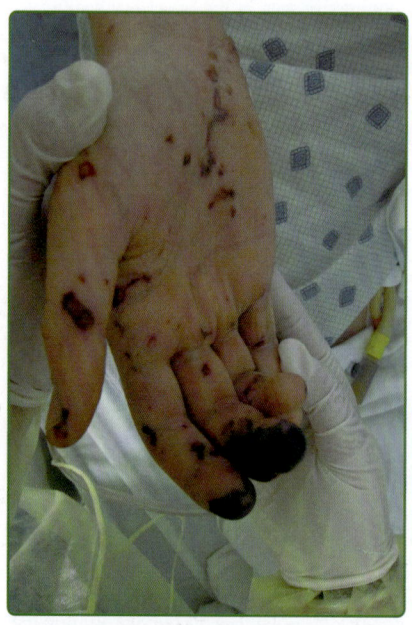

Figure 155-5 Stellate purpura from meningococcemia.

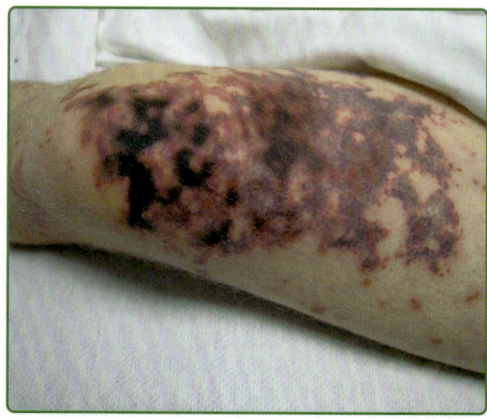

Figure 155-6 Retiform or purpura fulminans from meningococcemia.

meningitis, or peritonitis may occur.[36] The qSOFA (quick Sequential [sepsis-related] Organ Failure Assessment) score criteria (consisting of a respiratory rate greater than 22 breaths/min, altered mental status, and systolic blood pressure less than 100 mm Hg) is a new bedside index to identify patients outside of critical care units to help determine if the patient is transitioning from infection to sepsis.[22,26] The differentiation of sepsis from infection is the presence of organ dysfunction. New-onset organ dysfunction should raise the possibility of underlying infection. The organ systems commonly affected in sepsis include the renal, hepatic, central nervous, pulmonary, GI, and cardiovascular systems. The presentation of sepsis can be highly variable (the depth of which cannot be reviewed adequately in this format) and is shaped by type of pathogen, sex, age, race, genomics, preexisting acute illness overlapping with long-term comorbidities, immunosuppression, drug use, environment, medications, and interventions.[22]

COMPLICATIONS

Complications of sepsis and septic shock include death, loss of limbs from hypoperfusion, and permanent organ dysfunction. Septic patients may also develop acute respiratory distress syndrome and often fall into coma.[25] Sepsis and septic shock can lead to complications of disseminated intravascular coagulation (DIC), which is a devastating coagulopathy that adds to the already significant mortality of sepsis and septic shock.[25]

ETIOLOGY AND PATHOGENESIS

Sepsis and septic shock are initiated by a complex interaction through the infectious agent (Gram-negative and Gram-positive bacteria, fungi, viruses), cytokines (interleukin [IL]-1 IL-18) and Toll-like receptors on immune and nonimmune cells. Activation of stress-responsive transcription factors (eg, nuclear factor κB, activator protein-1) causes nuclear activation of inflammatory genes (sepsis response signatures), which causes a "genomic storm" from increased production of multiple mediators (eg, tumor necrosis factor-α, IL-6, IL-8, cyclooxygenase-2, nitric oxide, interferon-B). Subsequent microvascular dysfunction, injury, and apoptosis leads to organ dysfunction.[25,26,37] Hypotension in septic shock is most likely produced by overproduction of cyclooxygenase-2 and nitric oxide.[25]

DIAGNOSIS

SUPPORTIVE STUDIES

Recently, the Third International Consensus Definitions for Sepsis and Septic Shock, on assessment of clinical criteria for sepsis, recommended the use of the SOFA score in the critical care setting for its greater predictive value.[20] This criteria includes scores from 0 to 4 for the patient's partial pressure arterial oxygen/fraction of inspired oxygen, mean arterial pressure, platelet count, bilirubin, Glasgow coma scale score, urine output, and creatinine. SOFA scores greater than 2 are suggestive of a 10% mortality risk in the general hospitalized patient with suspected infections.[20,22] A patient with septic shock requires vasopressors to maintain a mean arterial pressure of 65 mm Hg and have a serum lactate level of greater than 2 mmol/L.[21]

Laboratory Testing: Blood cultures can be helpful in guiding treatment of septic patients; however, only 30% to 50% of septic patients will have positive blood cultures. Decreasing thrombocytopenia (below $150 \times 10^9/L$) is a strong and independent predictor of adverse outcomes in this clinical setting.[38] Hyperbilirubinemia (>1.2 mg/dL), renal insufficiency (creatinine >1.2 mg/dL) and urine output (<500 mL) are concerning for a worse prognosis.[22] Serum lactate is not part of the SOFA criteria but can be a clinical outcome predictor of mortality in septic shock.[39] The septic patient will generally have a white blood cell count greater than $12 \times 10^9/L$ or less than $4 \times 10^9/L$, or a bandemia of greater than 10%, and elevated C-reactive protein and procalcitonin levels.

Pathology: Histologic analysis of the cutaneous findings in the setting of sepsis and septic shock is very important. It can help determine the infectious agent, signs of vasculopathy or vasculitis that can be pertinent in patient care.

Imaging: The use of chest radiography, ultrasonography, CT, and MRI, is used by critical care physicians to help locate potential infection sources, as well as to monitor organ dysfunction. Brain MRI in septic shock may identify leukoencephalopathy and ischemic stroke[40] and contrast-enhanced CT scan has been used in to evaluate renal volume and attenuation can increase or decrease as the severity of the sepsis increases or decreases.[41] Noninvasive optical monitoring and transcutaneous oximetry are used in sepsis patients to monitor for microcirculatory collapse and subsequent sepsis shock.[42]

DIFFERENTIAL DIAGNOSIS

Table 155-3 outlines the differential diagnosis of skin findings in the septic patient.

CLINICAL COURSE AND PROGNOSIS

Sepsis precedes septic shock in up to 50% of affected patients.[43] Sepsis enters the top 10 leading causes of death for all races and sexes at age 45 years and older in 2013 data.[44] In-hospital mortality has ranged from 15% to 30% in different studies.[23] Septic shock is

TABLE 155-3
Differential Diagnosis of Skin Findings in the Septic Patient

- Erythroderma
  - Staphylococcal or streptococcal toxic shock syndrome
  - Severe cutaneous adverse reactions (drug reactions)
  - Cutaneous T-cell lymphoma
  - Psoriasis
- Papules and pustules
  - Candidemia
  - Disseminated gonococcemia
  - Folliculitis
  - Miliaria
  - Acute generalized exanthematous pustulosis
- Purpura
  - Invasive fungal infection, especially in thrombocytopenic patient
  - Disseminated intravascular coagulation
  - Vasculitis (infectious, neoplastic, drug-induced, or autoimmune)
  - Trauma induced
  - Heparin or Coumadin necrosis
  - Thrombotic thrombocytopenic purpura
  - Cryoglobulinemia
  - Calciphylaxis
- Cellulitis
  - Infectious cellulitis
  - Necrotizing fasciitis
  - Stasis dermatitis
- Ecthyma gangrenosum
  - Pseudomonal ecthyma gangrenosum
  - Nonpseudomonal bacterial or fungal ecthyma gangrenosum
  - Herpes simplex infection in immunosuppressed patient
  - Necrotizing vasculitis
  - Cryoglobulinemia

associated with a higher risk of mortality (up to 50%) then sepsis alone.[21]

MANAGEMENT

INTERVENTIONS

A recent metaanalysis showed that early goal-directed therapy (the *Surviving Sepsis Campaign*) reduces the risk of mortality among patients with sepsis and septic shock.[45,46] Early goal-directed therapy focuses on improving blood volume, cellular hypoxia, and tissue and organ perfusion within the first 6 hours. This includes early recognition of the diagnosis, timely hemodynamic support focusing on fluid resuscitation, vasopressors and inotropic medication, blood transfusion, and adequate antibiotic administration.[45,46] Although initial therapy may occur in the emergency department or hospital wards, patients need to go to an intensive care unit for extensive hemodynamic monitoring (ie, central line) and individualized care. Even though the use of anticoagulant therapy has not shown benefits in sepsis or sepsis-induced coagulopathy, decreased mortality was found in the sepsis-induced DIC population.[47] Recombinant human soluble thrombomodulin improves organ dysfunction in the setting of sepsis-induced DIC.[48,49] The development of biomarkers that can identify a specific inflammatory source of sepsis may in the future direct therapy in sepsis and septic shock as it has in the field of oncology.[26]

PREVENTION

The prevention of sepsis in a hospital setting is achieved by the implementation of basic infection-control measures, including routine hand washing and the minimization and regular replacement of indwelling catheters. In patients who are immunocompromised, particularly in the setting of organ transplantation or AIDS, the use of prophylactic antibiotics can help to reduce the incidence of sepsis. The use of vaccinations (eg, *Streptococcus pneumoniae*, *Haemophilus influenzae*, *Neisseria meningitidis*) also has been shown to decrease hospitalizations and sepsis.[25]

DISSEMINATED INTRAVASCULAR COAGULATION

DEFINITION AND HISTORICAL PERSPECTIVE

Since the late 1990s DIC has been defined as an acquired reactive syndrome of consumptive hypercoagulation, insufficient anticoagulation, hemorrhage, systemic vascular inflammation, and endothelial dysfunction.[50,51] The physiologic abnormalities of simultaneous bleeding and thrombosis may lead to organ dysfunction and eventual death. DIC is caused most commonly caused by infection and sepsis but has multiple other etiologies, several of which can overlap within a given patient's disease course (Table 155-4).[52] The onset of

TABLE 155-4
Settings in Which Disseminated Intravascular Coagulation Can Occur

- Hepatic failure
- Immunologic reaction to drugs or toxins
- Malignancy
- Obstetrical complication (amniotic fluid embolism, placental abruption)
- Protein C or protein S deficiency
- Sepsis
- Transfusion reactions
- Transplant reaction
- Trauma
- Vascular abnormalities (aortic aneurysm, cardiac arrest)

DIC in the neonatal period is suggestive of protein C or protein S deficiency.

EPIDEMIOLOGY

The true incidence is DIC is unknown. However, a recent population-based retrospective study from 2004 to 2010 performed in the United States, noted that the incidence of DIC had decreased during this time frame.[53] The incidence increased with age in men and women, with men having a greater incidence then women. The overall incidence rate, however, declined from 26.2 to 18.6 per 100,000 population, which was significant for men but not for women.[53] The mortality rate remained the same. Approximately 30% to 50% of septic patients, 7% of cancer patients with solid malignancy, and 15% to 20% of patients who present with acute lymphoblastic leukemia develop DIC.[52,54]

CLINICAL FEATURES

CUTANEOUS

The most characteristic cutaneous finding in DIC is diffuse noninflammatory retiform purpura from extensive microvascular occlusion, which is referred to as purpura fulminans.[29] Skin lesions may develop bullae, active hemorrhage, and necrosis (Fig. 155-7). Patients with purpura fulminans may present with ischemic digits or extremities (Fig. 155-8) that if left untreated can progress to gangrene.

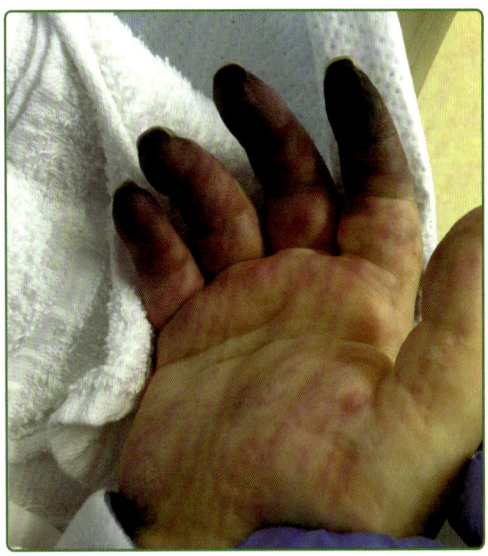

Figure 155-8 Acral ischemic changes from sepsis-associated disseminated intravascular coagulation. (Image used with permission from Kaitlin V. Peters, MD.)

NONCUTANEOUS FINDINGS

DIC can affect all organ systems. It commonly can cause chest pains, shortness of breath, headache, speech changes, paralysis, pain, and swelling of extremities as a consequence of clotting. The bleeding diathesis of DIC will cause hematuria and hematochezia.

COMPLICATIONS

Complications of DIC include tissue necrosis and infection, often requiring amputation of limbs or digits, multiorgan failure, and death. In its most extreme form, patients with DIC can develop the Waterhouse-Friderichsen syndrome, most commonly seen in meningococcal sepsis (see Chap. 154). This is a syndrome of multiorgan failure characterized by a petechiae or purpura, coagulopathy, cardiovascular collapse, and bilateral adrenal hemorrhage.[55] DIC also can be associated with obstetric complications, including preeclampsia, abruption, and amniotic fluid embolism. In these cases, the placenta appears to play a central role in the hemostatic pathway.[56]

ETIOLOGY AND PATHOGENESIS

DIC represents systemic activation of the coagulation cascade. This leads to fibrin deposition in the vasculature which can cause organ ischemia and death. In addition, the consumption of platelets and coagulation factors can lead to bleeding. In DIC, coagulation activation is a tissue factor dependent. Inflammatory cytokines such as tumor necrosis factor-α promote damage

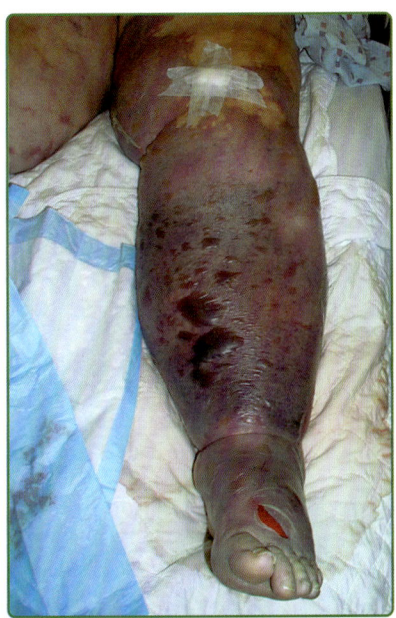

Figure 155-7 Purpura fulminans with bullae from *Escherichia coli* sepsis-induced disseminated intravascular coagulation.

to endothelial cells and activation of mononuclear cells. These cells then produce tissue factor, which binds to factor VIIa and activates downstream coagulation cascades. Thrombin generation is amplified by defective anticoagulant mechanisms and results in increased fibrin deposition. The fibrin that is generated fails to be degraded by the fibrinolytic system. In the healthy state, antithrombin regulates thrombin activity. In DIC, antithrombin levels are low as a result of continuous consumption, degradation by neutrophil elastase, and impaired synthesis caused by liver failure in some settings. Fibrinolysis is inhibited by plasminogen activator inhibitor Type I (PAI-1). Studies show that individuals with high plasma levels of PAI-1 are at higher risk of mortality in DIC.[52] This correlates with a mutation in PAI-1 that is associated with higher PAI-1 plasma concentrations. Thus, some individuals may be genetically predisposed (4G4G genotype of PAI-1 promoter polymorphism) to fatal outcomes from DIC because of a point mutation in PAI-1.[57]

DIAGNOSIS

SUPPORTIVE STUDIES

Several diagnostic scoring algorithms exist that assign numerical values to particular laboratory findings. These allow the calculation of a single numerical score that is helpful in predicting the presence of and mortality from DIC, but uniformity in clinical practice varies and is reviewed elsewhere.[58]

Laboratory Testing: Routine laboratory testing in DIC is characterized by decreased platelet count (<100 × 10^9/L), prolonged prothrombin and activated partial thromboplastin time, elevated fibrin degradation products (eg, D-dimer), and decreased protease inhibitors (protein C, protein S, antithrombin) and fibrinogen.[52] Other laboratory testing used may include decreased ADAMTS13 (a disintegrin and metalloprotease with a thrombospondin Type 1 motif member 13) activity, and elevated PAI-1, van Willebrand factor, thrombomodulin, thrombin–antithrombin complex, and plasmin–plasmin inhibitor complex.[59,60] Unfortunately, no one laboratory test can diagnosis DIC.

Pathology: Histologic evaluation of purpura fulminans reveals occlusive microthrombi, extravasated red blood cells, and varying degrees of epidermal death and necrosis.

Imaging: As with laboratory testing, no one study can diagnosis DIC. However, the use of ultrasonography, CT, and MRI can be used as needed by intensivists in determining underlying etiologies that can initiate DIC.

DIFFERENTIAL DIAGNOSIS

The differential diagnosis of DIC includes massive blood loss, thrombocytopenic thrombotic purpura, the hemolytic uremic syndrome, the HELLP (hemolysis, elevated liver enzymes, low platelets) syndrome seen in obstetric patients, heparin-induced thrombocytopenia, vitamin K deficiency, and liver insufficiency.[52] The differential of purpura fulminans includes catastrophic antiphospholipid antibody syndrome, calciphylaxis, and monoclonal cryoglobulinemia.[29]

CLINICAL COURSE AND PROGNOSIS

The abnormalities in hemostasis in DIC vary by the underlying cause and several clinical expressions may occur, such as bleeding or hyperfibrinolysis type (leukemia, obstetric disease, aortic aneurysms); organ failure or hypercoagulation type (sepsis); massive bleeding or consumptive with hypercoagulation and hyperfibrinolysis type (bleeding after major surgery, trauma, or obstetric disease); and nonsymptomatic type.[59] Shifts may occur between types of DIC within a given patient's illness.

DIC is an independent predictor for organ failure and mortality. Patients with thrombocytopenia (<50 × 10^9/L) and DIC have a greater risk of bleeding.[52] The mortality risk is doubled in patients with DIC who are septic or have experienced trauma.

MANAGEMENT

INTERVENTIONS

Medications: A review of published management of DIC demonstrates a limited and heterogeneous approach for both diagnosis and management among clinicians.[58,61] Although there is no treatment consensus, the basic tenets of treatment include treatment of the underlying disease and treatment of hemostatic abnormalities. Platelets, plasma transfusion, anticoagulation (low-molecular-weight heparin, recombinant human soluble thrombomodulin), or fibrinolytics based on the type of DIC can be initiated by intensivists.[52,62]

There is very little published experience regarding the treatment of the cutaneous necrosis seen in DIC. Skin necrosis secondary to DIC is similar to that seen in full-thickness cutaneous burns. Possible excision of necrotic tissue and coverage with autografts, and/or amputation of extremities are treatment options.

PREVENTION

Most interventions in DIC are aimed at minimizing organ damage and bleeding. Prevention of DIC itself can be achieved by the prompt diagnosis and treatment of its causes, particularly sepsis.

REFERENCES

1. Thuny F, Grisoli D, Cautela J, et al. Infective endocarditis: prevention, diagnosis and management. *Can J Cardiol.* 2014;30:1046-1057.
2. Topan A, Carstina D, Slavcovich A, et al. Assessment of the Duke criteria for the diagnosis of infective endocarditis after 20 years. *Clujul Med.* 2015;88:321-326.
3. Chopra T, Kaatz GW. Treatment strategies for infective endocarditis. *Expert Opin Pharmacother.* 2010;11: 345-360.
4. Hoen B, Duval X. Infective endocarditis. *N Engl J Med.* 2013;368:1425-1433.
5. Cahill TJ, Prendergast BD. Infective endocarditis. *Lancet.* 2016;387(10021):882-893.
6. Colville T, Sharma V, Albouaini K. Infective endocarditis in intravenous drug users: a review article. *Postgrad Med J.* 2016;92:105-111.
7. Li JS, Sexton DJ, Mick N, et al. Proposed modifications to Duke criteria for the diagnosis of infective endocarditis. *Clin Infect Dis.* 2000;30:633-638.
8. Hirai T, Koster M. Osler's nodes, Janeway lesions and splinter hemorrhages. *BMJ Case Rep.* 2013;2013.
9. Seth K, Buckley J, deWolff J. Splinter hemorrhages, Osler's nodes, Janeway lesions and Roth spots: the peripheral stigmata of endocarditis. *Br J Hosp Med (Lond).* 2013;74:C139-C142.
10. Servy A, Valeyrie-Allanore L, Alla F, et al. Prognostic value of skin manifestations of infective endocarditis. *JAMA Dermatol.* 2014;150:494-500.
11. Brown PJ, Zirwas MJ, English JC 3rd. The purple digit: an algorithmic approach to diagnosis. *Am J Clin Dermatol.* 2010;11:103-116.
12. Gibbs MB, English JC 3rd, Zirwas MJ. Livedo reticularis: an update. *J Am Acad Dermatol.* 2005;52: 1009-1019.
13. Novy E, Sonneville R, Mazighi M, et al. Neurologic complications of infective endocarditis: new breakthrough in diagnosis and management. *Med Mal Infect.* 2013; 43:443-450.
14. Ying CM, Yao DT, Ding HH, et al. Infective endocarditis with antineutrophil cytoplasmic antibody: report of 13 cases and literature review. *PLoS One.* 2014;9: e89777.
15. Chirillo F, Scotton P, Rocco R, et al. Impact of a multidisciplinary management strategy on the outcome of patients with native valve infective endocarditis. *Am J Cardiol.* 2013;112:1171-1176.
16. Kang DH, Kim YJ, Kim SH, et al. Early surgery versus conventional treatment for infective endocarditis. *N Engl J Med.* 2012;366:2466-2473.
17. Sabe MA, Shrestha NK, Menon V. Contemporary drug treatment of infective endocarditis. *Am J Cardiovasc Drugs.* 2013;13:251-258.
18. Okonta KE, Adamu YB. What size of vegetation is an indication for surgery in endocarditis. *Interact Cardiovasc Thorac Surg.* 2012;15:1052.
19. Wilson W, Taubert KA, Gewitz M, et al. Prevention of infective endocarditis: guidelines from the American Heart Association: a guideline from the American Heart Association Rheumatic Fever, Endocarditis, and Kawasaki Disease Committee, Council on Cardiovascular Disease in the Young, and the council on Clinical Cardiology, Council on Cardiovascular Surgery and Anesthesia, and the Quality of Care and Outcomes Research Interdisciplinary Working Group. *Circulation.* 2007;116:1736-1754.
20. Seymour CW, Liu VX, Iwashyna TJ, et al. Assessment of clinical criteria for sepsis for the third international consensus definitions for sepsis and septic shock. *JAMA.* 2016;315:762-774.
21. Shankar-Hari M, Phillips GS, Levy ML, et al. Developing a new definition and assessing new clinical criteria for septic shock for the third international consensus definitions for sepsis and septic shock. *JAMA.* 2016;315:775-787.
22. Singer M, Deutschman CS, Seymour CW, et al. The third international consensus definitions for sepsis and septic shock. *JAMA.* 2016;315:801-810.
23. Gaieski DF, Edwards JM, Kallan MJ, et al. Benchmarking the incidence and mortality of severe sepsis in the United States. *Crit Care Med.* 2013;41:1167-1174.
24. Torio CM, Andrews RM. *National Inpatient Hospitals Costs: the Most Expensive Conditions by Payer, 2011.* Healthcare Cost and Utilization Project, Statistical Brief #160. Rockville, MD: Agency for Health Care Policy and Research; 2013. Available at: http://www.ncbi.nlm.nih.gov/books/NBK169005.
25. Hawiger J, Veach A, Zienkiewicz J. New paradigms in sepsis: from prevention to protection of failing microcirculation. *J Thromb Haemost.* 2015;13: 1743-1756.
26. Abraham E. New definitions for sepsis and septic shock continuing evolution but with much still to be done. *JAMA.* 2016;315:757-759.
27. Lappin E, Ferguson AJ. Gram-positive toxic shock syndromes. *Lancet.* 2009;9:281-290.
28. Forentino DF. Cutaneous vasculitis. *J Am Acad Dermatol.* 2003;48:311-340.
29. Thornsberry LA, Losicco KI, English JC 3rd. The skin and hypercoagulable states. *J Am Acad Dermatol.* 2013;69:450-462.
30. Gaona-Flores VA, Campos-Navarro LA, Cervantes-Tovar RM, et al. The epidemiology of fungemia in an infectious disease hospital in Mexico City. *Med Mycol.* 2016;54(6):600-604.
31. Hirschman JV, Raugi GJ. Lower limb cellulitis and its mimics. Part I. Lower limb cellulitis. *J Am Acad Dermatol.* 2012;67:e1-e12.
32. Horseman MA, Surani S. A comprehensive review of vibrio vulnificus: an important cause of sever sepsis and skin and soft-tissue infections. *Int J Infect Dis.* 2011;15:e157-e166.
33. Hakkarainen TW, Kopari NM, Pham TN, et al. Necrotizing soft tissue infections: review and current concepts in treatment, systems of care and outcomes. *Curr Probl Surg.* 2014;51:344-362.
34. Hua C, Sbidian E, Hemery F, et al. Prognostic factors in necrotizing soft-tissue infections (NTSI): a cohort study. *J Am Acad Dermatol.* 2015;73:1006-1012.
35. Reich HL, Fadeyi DW, Naik NS, et al., Nonpseudomonal ecthyma gangrenosum. *J Am Acad Dermatol.* 2004;50:S114-S117.
36. Vincent JL, Mira JP, Antonelli M. Sepsis: older and newer concepts. *Lancet.* 2016;4:237-240.
37. Davenport EE, Burnham KL, Radhakrishnan J, et al. Genomic landscape of the individual host response and outcomes in sepsis: a prospective cohort study. *Lancet.* 2016;4(4):259-271.
38. Levi M. Platelets in critical illness. *Semin Thromb Hemost.* 2016;42(3):252-257.
39. Chertoff J, Chisum M, Garcia B, et al. Lactate kinetics in sepsis and septic shock: a review of the literature and rationale for further research. *J Intensive Care.* 2015; 3:39.

40. Polito A, Eischwald F, Maho AL, et al. Pattern of brain injury in the acute setting of human septic shock. *Crit Care*. 2013;17:R204.
41. Sasaguri K, Yamaguchi K, Nakazono T, et al. Sepsis patients' renal manifestations on contrast-enhanced CT. *Clin Radiol*. 2016:71:617.e1-e7.
42. Lima A. Current status of tissue monitoring in the management of shock. *Curr Opin Crit Care*. 2016;22: 274-278.
43. Rocha LL, Pessoa CMS, Correa TD, et al. Current concepts on hemodynamic support and the therapy in septic shock. *Rev Bras Anestesiol*. 2015;65:395-402.
44. Heron M. Deaths: leading cause for 2013. *Natl Vital Stat Rep*. 2016;65:1-95.
45. Lu J, Wang X, Chen Q, et al. The effect of early goal-directed therapy on mortality in patients with severe sepsis and septic shock: a meta-analysis. *J Surg Res*. 2016;202(2):389-397.
46. Dellinger RP, Levy MM, Rhodes A, et al. Surviving sepsis campaign: international guidelines for management of severe sepsis and septic shock: 2012. *Crit Care Med*. 2013;41:580-637.
47. Umemura Y, Yamakawa K, Ogura H, et al. Efficacy and safety of anticoagulant therapy in three specific populations with sepsis: a meta-analysis of randomized controlled trials. *J Thromb Haemost*. 2016;14(3): 518-530.
48. Yamakawa K, Fujimi S, Mohri T, et al. Treatment effects of recombinant human soluble thrombomodulin in patients with severe sepsis: a historical control study. *Crit Care*. 2011;25:R123.
49. Ogawa Y, Yamakawa K, Ogura H, et al. Recombinant human soluble thrombomodulin improves mortality and respiratory dysfunction in patients with severe sepsis. *J Trauma Acute Care Surg*. 2012;72: 1150-1157.
50. Gando S, Meziani F, Levi M. What's new in the diagnostic criteria of disseminated intravascular coagulation? *Intensive Care Med*. 2016;42:1062-1064.
51. Levi M, Ten Chate H. Disseminated intravascular coagulation. *N Engl J Med*. 1999;341:586-592.
52. Levi M, van der Poll T. Disseminated intravascular coagulation: a review for the internist. *Intern Emerg Med*. 2013;8:23-32.
53. Singh B, Hanson AC, Alhurani R, et al. Trends in the incidence and outcomes of disseminated intravascular coagulation in critically ill patients (2004-2010): a population based study. *Chest*. 2013;143: 1235-1242.
54. Marcel L. Management of cancer-associated disseminated intravascular coagulation. *Thromb Res*. 2016; 140(suppl 1):566-570.
55. Sonavane A, Baradkar V, Salunkhe P, et al. Waterhouse-Friderichsen syndrome in an adult patient with meningococcal meningitis. *Indian J Dermatol*. 2011;56: 326-328.
56. Cunningham FG, Nelson DB. Disseminated intravascular coagulation syndromes in obstetrics. *Obstet Gynecol*. 2015;126:999-1011.
57. Binder A, Endler G, Muller M, et al. 4G4G genotype of the plasminogen activator inhibitor-1 promoter polymorphism associated with disseminated intravascular coagulation in children with systemic meningococcemia. *J Thromb Haemost*. 2007;10:2049-2054.
58. Di Nisio M, Thachil J, Squizzato A. Management of disseminated intravascular coagulation: A survey of the international society on thrombosis and haemostasis. *Thromb Res*. 2015:136:239-242.
59. Wada H, Matsumoto T, Yamashita Y. Diagnosis and treatment of disseminated intravascular coagulation (DIC) according to four DIC guidelines. *J Intensive Care*. 2014;2:15-22.
60. Iba T, Ito T, Maruyama I, et al. Potential diagnostic markers for disseminated intravascular coagulation of sepsis. *Blood Rev*. 2016;30(2):149-155.
61. Squizzato A, Hunt BJ, Kinasewitz GT, et al. Supportive management strategies for disseminated intravascular coagulation. An international consensus. *Thromb Haemost*. 2016;115(5):896-904.
62. Itoh S, Shirabe K, Kohnoe S, et al. Impact of recombinant human soluble thrombomodulin for disseminated intravascular coagulation. *Anticancer Res*. 2016:36:2493-2496.

Chapter 156 :: Miscellaneous Bacterial Infections with Cutaneous Manifestations
Scott A. Norton & Michael A. Cardis

第一百五十六章
混杂细菌感染引起的皮肤表现

中文导读

除了上述章节中普通常见的细菌感染以外，还有很多其他少见细菌引起的疾病，这些细菌感染疾病也可以引起皮肤的改变。本章共分为11节：①炭疽热；②兔热病（土拉弗朗西斯菌感染）；③鼠疫；④布鲁氏菌病；⑤鼻疽病；⑥出血败血性巴斯德氏菌感染；⑦鼠咬热；⑧海豹指；⑨李氏杆菌病（李斯特菌单核细胞增生性感染）；⑩创伤弧菌感染；⑪其他少见感染，如嗜水气单胞菌感染、类鼻疽病、类丹毒、猪链球菌感染、青紫色素杆菌感染等。

〔汪 犇〕

ANTHRAX

AT-A-GLANCE

- A large Gram-positive rod, *Bacillus anthracis*, changes into dormant spores under environmentally harsh conditions. Spores are infectious particles that revert to active bacillary form in host tissues.
- Natural pathogen of livestock, especially sheep, goats, and cattle. Most human diseases are occupationally related to exposure to live animals or animal products.
- Cutaneous anthrax is the most common form and is associated with the lowest morbidity. Inhalational and GI anthrax are more virulent and frequently lethal.
- Cutaneous lesions arise from percutaneous spore inoculation, usually unnoticed. They present as painless edematous papules or plaques that develop jet-black central eschars.
- The organism is a Centers for Disease Control and Prevention Category A bioweapon in aerosolizable micropowder form. There is no potential for human-to-human transmission of inhalational anthrax.

ETIOLOGY AND EPIDEMIOLOGY

Anthrax (Fig. 156-1) is a zoonotic infectious disease caused by *Bacillus anthracis*, a large aerobic, spore-forming Gram-positive rod.[1] Anthrax occurs naturally in ruminant mammals, such as sheep, cattle, and goats. Human disease is seen most often in agrarian, livestock-dependent regions. Consequently, human anthrax usually follows agricultural or industrial exposure, either through direct handling of infected

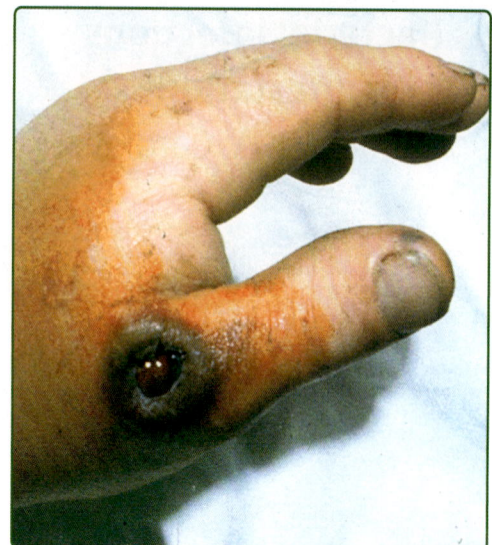

Figure 156-1 Anthrax. The classic cutaneous lesion of a primary infection in anthrax is a painless papule that evolves into a hemorrhagic bulla with surrounding brawny non-pitting edema. Note the typical localization on the hand. The name *anthrax* comes from the Greek word ανθραξ *(anthrax)*, meaning coal, which refers to the coal-black hue of the lesions of cutaneous anthrax.

animals or contaminated soil or through the processing of hides, wool, hair, or meat.[2] Anthrax has potential as a class A bioweapon (Table 156-1) because it is easily aerosolized and often lethal.

The clinical presentation of human anthrax depends on the route of inoculation. Each of anthrax's forms has distinctive clinical, epidemiologic, and prognostic features.[3]

In 95% of human cases, the disease is acquired through percutaneous inoculation of anthrax spores. Human anthrax also can be acquired as inhalational and GI disease. Recent cases in the United States of both forms were associated with recreational use of drums made of unprocessed animal hides imported from West Africa.[4,5]

In 2009, a novel mode of anthrax transmission known as "*injectional anthrax*," which resulted from exposure to contaminated heroin, emerged in Europe. Injectional anthrax has a distinct clinical course that is more insidious than cutaneous anthrax because it presents without an eschar. It is more virulent, too, with a much higher mortality rate than cutaneous disease.[6-8]

Outbreaks still occur in endemic areas.[9-14] During the late 20th century, thousands of people in the African nations of Zambia and Zimbabwe developed anthrax.[15] More than 90% of cases were cutaneous and the remainder represented an equal mix of inhalational and GI disease. Dying animals typically release vegetative bacilli into the environment, which then convert into the dormant, yet infectious, spores. There are ongoing outbreaks of animal anthrax among free-ranging wood bison (Athabaskan buffalo) in Northern Canada,[16] several species of antelope in Zambia,[17] hippopotami in Uganda, and domesticated grazing animals in North Dakota.[18]

The major virulence factors of the bacterium are its poly-γ-D-glutamic acid capsule, and the tripartite anthrax toxin that contains 3 proteins: protective antigen, lethal factor, and edema factor.[19] The protective antigen is the best target for vaccines or immunotherapy.

CLINICAL FINDINGS

HISTORY

After an incubation period of 1 to 7 days, patients may experience low-grade fever and malaise, and develop a painless papule at the exposed site. As the lesion enlarges, the surrounding skin becomes increasingly edematous. Pain, if present, is usually the result of edema-associated pressure or secondary infection.

CUTANEOUS LESIONS

Cutaneous anthrax develops when spores enter minor breaks in the skin, especially on exposed parts of the hands, legs, and face (see Fig. 156-1). In the hospitable environment of human skin, spores revert to their rod forms and produce their toxins. A dermal papule, often resembling an arthropod bite reaction, develops over several days, and then progresses through vesicular, pustular, and escharotic phases. Lesions are surrounded by varying degrees of edema. Depending on the manner of inoculation, 1 to several lesions may appear, and there may be regional lymphadenitis, malaise, and fever. Individual lesions may appear pustular, leading to the name "malignant pustule," but they do not suppurate. In anthrax, true pustules are rare; a primary pustular lesion is unlikely to be cutaneous anthrax.

The lesion enlarges into a glistening pseudobulla that becomes hemorrhagic with central necrosis and may be umbilicated (see Fig. 156-1). The necrotic ulcer is usually painless, which is an important feature for differentiating it from a brown recluse spider bite. There may be small satellite papules and vesicles that may extend along lymphatics in a sporotrichoid manner. An area of brawny, nonpitting edema ("malignant edema") often surrounds the main lesion. Lesional progression is caused by toxins and is unaffected by antibiotic therapy. Fatigue, fever, chills, and tender regional adenopathy may cause an ulceroglandular syndrome. The eschar dries and separates in 1 to 2 weeks.[20-24]

RELATED PHYSICAL FINDINGS

Cutaneous anthrax may cause fever, tachycardia, and hypotension.

HISTOPATHOLOGY

The prominent features are hemorrhagic edema, dilated lymphatics, and epidermal necrosis. Bacilli

TABLE 156-1
Overview of Bacterial Infections

INFECTION	EXPECTED DEMOGRAPHIC DISTRIBUTION	TYPICAL PRESENTATION (SKIN)[a]	TYPICAL EXPOSURE	BIOWEAPON POTENTIAL[b]	TREATMENT
Anthrax	Worldwide, especially developing agrarian areas	Painless edematous plaque with central black ulcer or eschar	Goats, sheep, cattle, or products made from them	A	Penicillin, doxycycline, ciprofloxacin
Tularemia	North America, Europe	Ulceroglandular: painful papule that ulcerates and forms eschar	Tick bites, rabbits, rodents	A	Aminoglycoside, fluoroquinolone, doxycycline
Plague	Worldwide, especially southwestern United States and India	Buboes (tender regional lymphadenopathy) followed by purpura and gangrene	Flea bites, spread from infected rodents	A	Aminoglycoside, doxycycline, cotrimoxazole
Brucellosis	Worldwide, especially developing agrarian areas	Variable; skin manifestations present in <5% of patients	Cattle, sheep, goats, or untreated milk	B	Doxycycline plus aminoglycoside or rifampin
Glanders	Rare and focal in Asia, Middle East	Nodule with cellulitis that ulcerates; later, deep abscesses and sinuses	Donkeys, mules, horses	B	Sulfadiazine, gentamycin, doxycycline
Pasteurella infection	Worldwide	Rapid onset of cellulitis at bite site followed by necrosis	Dog or cat bite	NR	Amoxicillin plus clavulanic acid
Rat-bite fever (streptobacillary)	Worldwide, especially Asia	Morbilliform eruption with fever followed by arthritis	Rats or their excreta	NR	Amoxicillin plus clavulanic acid
Seal finger	Cool coastal regions worldwide	Extremely painful nodule on finger	Seals or sea lions	NR	Tetracycline, ceftriaxone
Listeriosis	Worldwide	In neonates, generalized petechiae, papules, and pustules	In neonates, infected mother with transfer in utero or shortly after birth	NR	Ampicillin or penicillin IV
Vibrio vulnificus infection	Worldwide	Necrotizing fasciitis, hemorrhagic bullae often beginning as a wound infection	Warm saltwater or brackish water or undercooked seafood	NR	Doxycycline and ceftazidime IV, debridement of lesions
Aeromonas hydrophila infection	Worldwide	Cellulitis evolving to abscess formation; often beginning as a wound infection	Fresh or brackish water, contaminated fish	NR	Third-generation cephalosporins, fluoroquinolones; debridement
Melioidosis	Wet tropical areas, especially Southeast Asia and northern Australia	Indolent abscesses; suppurative parotitis (in children)	Wet soil (classically rice paddies), flooded regions	B	Ceftazidime plus a carbapenem IV, then prolonged oral amoxicillin clavulanic acid or TMP-SMX
Erysipeloid	Worldwide	Tender violaceous plaque on hand at site of injury	Contaminated fish, shellfish, poultry, meat, and animal products	NR	Penicillin, ampicillin, ceftriaxone, fluoroquinolone
Streptococcus iniae infection	Worldwide, especially freshwater fish farms	Rapid onset of hand cellulitis following a puncture wound	Contaminated farm-raised fish	NR	Penicillin, cephalosporin
Leptospirosis	Worldwide, especially the tropics	Papules, petechiae, jaundice	Contaminated freshwater, moist soil, or animal urine	NR	Doxycycline, penicillin
Diphtheria	Worldwide where immunization is not practiced	Pustule or superinfected abrasion, evolving to an ulcer with gray membrane at base	Asymptomatic human carriers	NR	Penicillin IV or erythromycin plus antitoxin

[a]For many entities, multiple presentations are possible depending on the route of inoculation (percutaneous entry, oral ingestion, or inhalation). See text.
[b]If aerosolized, per criteria of the Centers for Disease Control and Prevention.
A, highest (systemic disease, often fatal); B, substantial (severe systemic disease, sometimes fatal); NR, not rated; TMP-SMX, trimethoprim-sulfamethoxazole.

may be found in the eschar. Anthrax is toxin-mediated and induces scant inflammatory infiltrate. Immunohistochemical stains are quite useful.[25]

TREATMENT

Naturally occurring anthrax is treated with penicillin or doxycycline. Weaponized anthrax, on the other hand, may be resistant to these antibiotics; consequently, a fluoroquinolone is recommended for the initial treatment of confirmed or suspected bioterrorism-associated anthrax, even in pregnant women and children. Once drug sensitivities have been established, the patient may be switched to another antibiotic as clinically indicated. Antibiotics will kill activated *B. anthracis* bacilli but will not alter tissue damage already caused by toxins.[26,27] To neutralize the anthrax toxins, the Centers for Disease Control and Prevention (CDC) now possesses human antianthrax immunoglobulin and monoclonal antibodies directed against the toxins are in development. The U.S. Food and Drug Administration (FDA) has licensed a humanized monoclonal antibody, raxibacumab, that has specificity for the bacterial protective antigen, to be used in cases of inhalational anthrax.

Although cutaneous anthrax is usually an uncomplicated and readily treatable infection, public health concerns warrant hospitalization. Standard universal precautions are appropriate but specific measures against secondary respiratory transmission are unnecessary because anthrax is not transmitted from person-to-person.

Parenteral crystalline penicillin G (2 million units every 6 hours) was the treatment of choice prior to the 2001 bioterrorism outbreak. In one study, smears and cultures from vesicles or from the necrotic tissue beneath the eschar became negative within 6 hours of initiation of penicillin therapy. Treatment of primary cutaneous anthrax is continued with parenteral therapy until the local edema disappears or the lesion dries up over 1 to 2 weeks. When the edema resolves, the patient may complete the 60-day treatment with oral therapy.

Other than to obtain material for culture or histopathology, incision and debridement of the cutaneous lesion is unnecessary. First, the lesions contain no purulent material needing evacuation and, second, without effective antibiotics, these procedures increase the risk of bacteremic spread of the disease.

PROGNOSIS AND CLINICAL COURSE

Untreated cutaneous anthrax, particularly if nonedematous, is a largely self-resolving disease. In contrast, some lesions, especially ones with massive edema, pose the risk of bacteremia with subsequent septicemia. Thus, the mortality rate of untreated cutaneous anthrax is roughly 5% to 20%. With prompt and appropriate antibiotics, there is rapid defervescence and clinical improvement. Massive facial edema associated with cutaneous lesions of the head or neck may lead to respiratory compromise, requiring intubation or tracheostomy and systemic corticosteroids. Palpebral lesions may scar the eyelids and edema-associated seventh-nerve palsy may occur.[28] Because of high mortality rates, patients with injectional, inhalational, or GI anthrax should be placed in intensive care units.

PREVENTION

In nonendemic areas, any case of anthrax requires immediate reporting to public health authorities and a prompt public health response because of the threat of intentional criminal or terrorist release. Although anthrax is a dangerous disease, it is not transmitted from person-to-person. Instead, the spore is the infectious propagule. Therefore patients with anthrax—of whatever clinical presentation—do not require isolation.

An anthrax vaccine has been in use since 1954 for people with occupational exposure to natural anthrax (eg, veterinarians, wildlife biologists). The CDC recently released new guidelines on its use in the post-9/11 era for routine occupational use and for preoutbreak and postoutbreak exposure use.[29]

Although cutaneous anthrax is usually an uncomplicated and readily treatable infection, public health concerns warrant hospitalization. Standard universal precautions are appropriate but specific measures against secondary respiratory transmission are unnecessary because anthrax is not transmitted from person-to-person.

TULAREMIA (*FRANCISELLA TULARENSIS* INFECTIONS)

AT-A-GLANCE

- Caused by *Francisella tularensis*, a Gram-negative coccobacillus found in rabbits, rodents, other mammals, and their immediate environments in temperate and cold regions of North America.
- Has diverse clinical presentations related to route of transmission. Ulceroglandular disease after tick bites is most common.
- Bacteria are easily aerosolized and highly infectious in small inocula; consequently, tularemia poses risks of laboratory accidents or use as a bioweapon.

ETIOLOGY AND EPIDEMIOLOGY

Tularemia is a zoonotic infectious disease caused by *Francisella tularensis*, a pleomorphic Gram-negative coccobacillus found in nearly 200 species of mammals and their immediate environments. The most important groups known to carry the bacterium are lagomorphs (rabbits and hares) and rodents. The bacteria are highly virulent and require a low inoculum for infection. They can be transmitted in multiple ways, and cause 6 major clinical presentations, which are defined by their route of transmission and are known as glandular, ulceroglandular, oculoglandular, oropharyngeal, typhoidal, and pneumonic forms of tularemia.[30]

Tularemia, also known as deerfly fever, rabbit plague, and rabbit fever, was first described in the United States in the early 20th century. It occurs solely in temperate and cold regions of the Northern Hemisphere. The most common form in the United States is ulceroglandular disease in which organisms are inoculated directly into the skin by minor trauma or by bites of infected arthropods that maintain the enzootic cycle. Before 1950, most U.S. infections occurred in hunters who handled infected rabbits and hares. Two incidence peaks each year corresponded with summer and winter hunting seasons. Currently, 100 to 150 U.S. cases occur each year, mostly in Arkansas, Missouri, and Oklahoma, with transmission of the organism largely via tick bites. The most common tick vectors are *Dermacentor variabilis*, *Amblyomma americanum*, and, in Europe, *Ixodes* sp.[31-35]

Of several subspecies, the most virulent (*F. tularensis* subspecies *tularensis*) lives only in the North America. A more benign one (*F. tularensis* subspecies *holarctica*) is the only subspecies in Eurasia. Although these bacteria do not produce spores, they can survive environmentally—and maintain infectivity—for months.[33,34]

Tularemia is transmitted in other ways, too. Other arthropod vectors include the deerfly (*Chrysops discalis*) in the Western United States, and mosquitoes in Scandinavia and the Baltic region.[36] An outbreak of pulmonary tularemia on Martha's Vineyard, Massachusetts, was associated with springtime mowing of tall grass.[37] The precise environmental source was not clear, perhaps aerosolization of animal excreta in the grass. Domestic cats may spread the organism via direct contact, bite, or aerosol. In parts of Europe, aquatic rodents (muskrats and beavers), household rodents, and drinking water contaminated by these animals are the major sources of infection. *F. tularensis holarctica* can maintain a long-term aquatic lifecycle, leading to waterborne disease, and in some European countries, mosquitos may serve as mechanical vectors of the disease.[38]

Rarely, direct inoculation into conjunctivae or ingestion of poorly cooked, contaminated meat causes infection. There is no human-to-human transmission. A second species, *Francisella philomiragia*, can infect patients with inherited defects in phagocytosis such as chronic granulomatous disease.

CLINICAL FINDINGS

HISTORY

Duration of incubation varies with size of inoculum, ranging from 2 to 10 days. All forms of tularemia present as a sudden flu-like illness characterized by fever, headache, malaise, and myalgia.

CUTANEOUS LESIONS

In ulceroglandular tularemia, a painful red papule appears at the inoculation site (Fig. 156-2). It enlarges rapidly and evolves into a necrotic chancriform ulcer often covered by a black eschar. Regional lymph nodes are large and tender.[37] Bacteremia may cause sepsis and virulent pneumonia. In 2 recent Scandinavian outbreaks with the less-virulent *F. tularensis holarctica* type of tularemia, primarily caused by mosquitoborne ulceroglandular disease, approximately one-third of nearly 300 patients developed nonspecific secondary cutaneous manifestations, such as erythema nodosum, erythema multiforme, or an asymptomatic id-like papular eruption on the extremities.[36,39]

Tularemia is a chancre-like ulcer with raised margins on the dorsum of the fourth digit with accompanying axillary lymphadenopathy. The rash on the chest is unrelated and is pityriasis versicolor.

RELATED PHYSICAL FINDINGS

In oculoglandular tularemia, organisms are introduced directly into the conjunctivae, for example, after handling an infected tick or rabbit. This causes purulent conjunctivitis with pain, edema, and local adenopathy. In a recent outbreak in Bulgaria, more than 90% of cases were oropharyngeal, reflecting transmission via contaminated well water. Swallowing the organism may cause ulcerative pharyngotonsillitis with cervical adenopathy or may cause "typhoidal" tularemia.[40] Pulmonary tularemia may be primary (ie, caused by

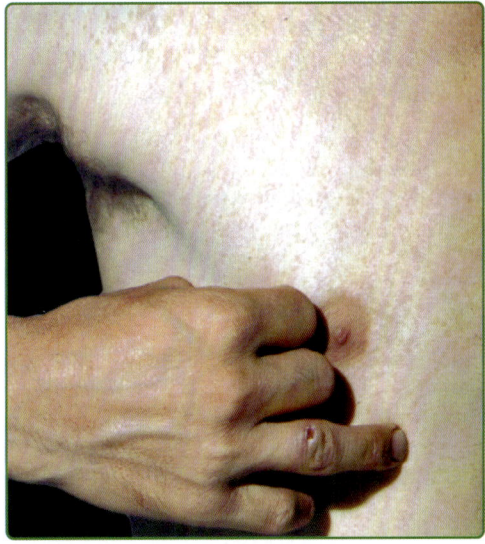

Figure 156-2 Tularemia. A chancre-like ulcer with raised margins on the dorsum of the fourth digit with accompanying axillary lymphadenopathy. The rash on the chest is unrelated and is pityriasis versicolor.

inhalation of organisms) but is more often because of bacteremic spread from another focus.

LABORATORY FINDINGS

Laboratories should be notified of suspected tularemia so that cultures can be set under biohazard conditions to avoid aerosolization. *F. tularensis* grows best on cysteine-supplemented blood agar, producing nonmotile, nonsporulating, pleomorphic, Gram-negative coccobacilli. Some reference laboratories also use animal inoculation techniques.

HISTOPATHOLOGY

The pathogen survives intracellularly in phagocytes, and small granulomas develop in lymph nodes, liver, and spleen. Some lesions may caseate and progress to frank abscess formation. Hepatic granulomas may resemble tuberculosis or brucellosis.

DIFFERENTIAL DIAGNOSIS

The primary lesion of tick-transmitted tularemia resembles a pyogenic infection (such as a furuncle, paronychia, or common ecthyma), the initial lesion of anthrax, *Pasteurella multocida* infection, or sporotrichosis. Prominent regional adenopathy may suggest cat-scratch disease, plague, or melioidosis. Fever after a tick bite might suggest Rocky Mountain spotted fever, but that usually has an exanthem rather than a chancriform lesion. Other tickborne febrile diseases include other rickettsioses, ehrlichiosis, babesiosis, and viral tick fevers. Because *F. tularensis* is difficult to grow, the diagnosis is usually made by serologic tests showing a rise in titers. Although the subspecies of *F. tularensis* are clinically and epidemiologically distinct, they are serologically indistinguishable.[33]

TREATMENT

A presumptive diagnosis of tularemia on clinical and epidemiologic grounds is sufficient to initiate treatment while awaiting serologic confirmation (see Table 156-1). Treatment consists of an aminoglycoside antibiotic, such as gentamicin (or streptomycin, if available), or a fluoroquinolone; these should be given for at least 10 days. A tetracycline antibiotic, such as doxycycline, given for at least 15 days is an acceptable alternative. Patients improve within 24 to 48 hours, but treatment should continue for at least 7 to 10 afebrile days to reduce the risk of relapse.

COURSE, PROGNOSIS, AND COMPLICATIONS

Untreated pulmonary and typhoidal tularemia have mortality rates of approximately 30%. Without antibiotics, ulceroglandular disease lasts many weeks and has a mortality rate of 5%. Brief courses of antibiotics may permit relapse but, with proper treatment, uncomplicated recovery is expected.

PREVENTION

Hunters and animal handlers should wear impervious gloves when handling game, especially rabbits. Game meat should be cooked thoroughly, even if stored frozen for long periods. A live-attenuated (but rarely used) vaccine was developed in Russia; the U.S. government is currently funding vaccine research. The disease is reportable in the United States and any cluster of pulmonary tularemia cases should raise concerns of bioterrorism.[34,41] Antibiotic prophylaxis with ciprofloxacin is useful in patients with proven exposure.[38]

PLAGUE

AT-A-GLANCE

- Focal enzootic sites worldwide, including the southwestern United States. Human disease is caused by bites from infected fleas or direct contact with rodent reservoirs.
- The bubonic form is the most common, producing large tender lymph nodes (buboes) proximal to the site of fleabite. All forms can lead to sepsis, distal gangrene (origin of the term *black death*), and death.
- Pneumonic plague because of respiratory spread of aerosolized *Yersinia pestis* has a high mortality and is a possible weapon of bioterrorism.

ETIOLOGY AND EPIDEMIOLOGY

Plague is a severe, acute, febrile zoonosis caused by the aerobic Gram-negative bacillus *Yersinia pestis*. Plague is found on every continent except Antarctica, and exists in an enzootic cycle, infecting humans through contact with rodent reservoirs or flea vectors. Human plague has 3 clinical forms: (a) bubonic; (b) bubonic-septicemic, a more virulent form resulting from secondary bacteremia and sepsis; and (c) pneumonic (fulminant disease resulting from respiratory spread). Distal purpura and gangrene associated with septicemic plague likely gave rise to the term *black death*. The plague bacillus likely evolved from the fecal–oral pathogen, *Yersinia pseudotuberculosis*, by acquiring several virulence plasmids.[42]

Endemic or sylvatic plague occurs in wild rodents in the western United States, parts of South America, much of sub-Saharan Africa, and across Southern Asia.

In most places, plague is sporadic but Madagascar currently has epidemic plague.[43,44] There are several thousand cases of plague worldwide each year and the disease prevalence is increasing across Africa; Madagascar alone accounts for nearly half the number of human cases each year.[42,45]

In the United States, human disease is almost always transmitted by fleas. Direct handling of infected rodents, rabbits, or their carcasses can also transmit plague. Some cases are transmitted by direct contact with pet dogs or cats that become ill after contact with infected wild animals. Between 1990 and 2005, 107 plague cases, more than 80% bubonic, were reported in the United States, averaging 7 per year, mostly in summertime. In western states, winter cases are often linked with handling of animal carcasses while hunting. In recent years, epizootics have occurred among prairie dogs, and sporadic human cases were seen on several Indian reservations, associated with ground squirrels.[46] Rarely, bacteremic bubonic disease may evolve into pneumonic plague and further initiate respiratory spread to others.[47,48]

The flea associated with epidemic plague in the Old World is *Xenopsylla cheopis*, but fleas in other genera (eg, *Anomiopsyllus*, *Aetheca*, *Pulex*) are also vectors in the United States.

Plague is an historically important disease, causing more than 100 million deaths during several pandemics over the past 15 centuries. Because *Y. pestis* can be aerosolized, it is devastatingly lethal, and can spread from person-to-person; it is considered a Category A biologic weapon (see Table 156-1). *Y. pestis* produces an intracellular toxin and virulence factors.

CLINICAL FINDINGS

HISTORY

Bubonic plague incubates for roughly 2 to 6 days, followed by the sudden onset of high fever, prostration, malaise, myalgia, backache, and tachycardia. Primary pneumonic plague has a shorter incubation time.

CUTANEOUS LESIONS

In bubonic plague, the initial skin lesion is related to the fleabite and may appear as papular urticaria. However, the hallmark of bubonic plague is prominent, exquisitely tender regional lymphadenopathy with extensive subcutaneous edema. Inguinal buboes are most common in adults; cervical and axillary buboes are more common in children.[42]

Any form of plague can lead to overwhelming endotoxic septicemia accompanied by disseminated intravascular coagulopathy (see Chap. 155). Subsequent purpura and gangrene are most severe on distal extremities.[49]

RELATED PHYSICAL FINDINGS

Primary septicemic plague lacks buboes and presents with typical Gram-negative sepsis. Many patients also have severe abdominal pain, nausea, vomiting, and bloody diarrhea. Pneumonic plague has an abrupt onset with high fever, tachycardia, tachypnea, chest pain, and dyspnea. Within 24 hours of onset, the patient is critically ill and producing bloody sputum laden with *Y. pestis*. Meningitis may complicate all forms of plague.

LABORATORY FINDINGS

In bubonic plague, organisms can be cultured from lymph node aspirates and blood; in pneumonic plague, sputum or tracheal washes. Lymph node aspirates are obtained by using a sterile syringe to inject 1 mL of saline into the center of a bubo and withdrawing purulent material until the pus is tinged with blood. Special transport medium (eg, Cary-Blair medium) is helpful but the culture may be performed in standard brain–heart nutrient broth. The organisms appear as Gram-negative coccobacilli with a Gram stain but their bipolar bacillary appearance is more distinctive with Wright-Giemsa or Wayson stain.[42,50] Bacilli can sometimes be seen on stained buffy coat smears. Leukocytosis occurs in all forms of the disease. Renal failure and disseminated intravascular coagulopathy may occur in severe cases. Bacteria can be cultured on standard blood agar media. Direct fluorescent antibody assays, enzyme-linked immunosorbent assay, and polymerase chain reaction testing are useful when available, but serologic tests are less reliable.[49,51] Histopathologically, acute inflammatory changes are seen in the involved nodes. Immunohistochemical stains of tissue biopsy specimens may show organisms.[52]

DIFFERENTIAL DIAGNOSIS

Most patients with bubonic plague present with the rapid onset of a toxic febrile illness, painful buboes, and evidence of an arthropod bite without surrounding cellulitis. Bubonic plague should be distinguished from tularemia, lymphogranuloma venereum, cat-scratch disease, chancroid, Kikuchi disease, and suppurative lymphadenitis caused by staphylococcal or streptococcal infection. Pneumonic plague must be differentiated from other acute bacterial pneumonias. Epidemiologic considerations and the tempo of the illness are major points in the differential diagnosis. The diagnosis is made by examining Gram-stained (or specific fluorescent antibody–stained) smears of infected material or by culturing organism from blood, sputum, or aspirated buboes. Serologic methods help retrospectively by demonstrating a fourfold or greater rise in titers. A convalescent passive hemagglutination titer of greater than 1:16 suggests the diagnosis.

TREATMENT

Because the original drug of choice, streptomycin, is not widely available, another aminoglycoside antibiotic, gentamicin, is the preferred treatment (although the FDA has not approved it for this indication; see Table 156-1). Doxycycline is also effective and may be the treatment of choice when oral therapy is required or to use as postexposure prophylaxis. Cotrimoxazole is useful when combination therapy is desired.[50] Patients with pneumonic plague must be placed in respiratory isolation to prevent further transmission. The course of treatment, irrespective of medication, is 10 days. Ordinarily, buboes should not be drained until they are well-localized and antibiotic therapy has been started.[53]

PROGNOSIS AND CLINICAL COURSE

Pneumonic and septicemic plague, if untreated, are nearly always fatal. Untreated bubonic plague has a mortality rate of approximately 50% but early antibiotic therapy has reduced this to 5% to 10%. Because primary septicemic plague lacks telltale buboes, the clinical suspicion of plague is often delayed, hence antibiotics are started late and mortality is high.

PREVENTION

Most cases in the United States are acquired peridomestically so it is important in endemic areas to control rodents around homes. Children should be taught to avoid rodent nests, burrows, and dead animals. Pets should be given regular flea treatments, examined properly when ill, and trained not to hunt small mammals or eat sick or dead mammals. Rabbit hunters should wear gloves when handling carcasses. With pneumonic cases, respiratory isolation is mandatory and close contacts should receive antibiotic prophylaxis with doxycycline or cotrimoxazole. Plague vaccine is no longer available. Because the disease is a zoonosis, it is considered ineradicable, so prevention through rodent control is the most important way to prevent plague.[42,45]

BRUCELLOSIS

> ### AT-A-GLANCE
> - Zoonosis transmitted by contact with infected animals or consumption of contaminated dairy products.
> - May be transmitted via aerosolized bacteria, hence the concern regarding the use of *Brucella* in bioterrorism.
>
> *(Continued)*

> ### AT-A-GLANCE (Continued)
> - Usually presents with undulant fever and can involve all organ systems, especially the joints, reproductive organs, liver, and CNS. Endocarditis can be fatal.
> - Cutaneous lesions are seen in fewer than 5% of patients, usually children. Variable morphologies include vasculitis, erythema nodosum, panniculitis, abscesses, and polymorphous papules, pustules, and papulosquamous lesions. Children with acute brucellosis may have a violaceous papulonodular eruption primarily on the trunk and lower extremities.

ETIOLOGY AND EPIDEMIOLOGY

Brucellosis is caused by any of 4 species of *Brucella*, which ordinarily infect livestock, especially cattle, sheep, and goats. It is transmitted to humans by contact with infected animals or animal products, ingestion of unpasteurized or contaminated dairy products, and, rarely, by inhalation of aerosolized bacteria. There are approximately 500,000 human cases per year worldwide, making it one of the most common zoonoses worldwide. The highest incidence is in underdeveloped agrarian areas where there are poor health controls for herds, where people consume raw dairy products, and the populations are nomadic with less access to medical care. These regions include East Africa, grazing areas of upland South and Central America, and the belt of nations extending from Spain and Portugal across the Mediterranean basin, through Asia from Turkey and the Middle East, and across the former Soviet republics to Mongolia. Domesticated animals are reservoirs for *Brucella*, and the 2 species that most commonly infect humans are *Brucella melitensis* ("from Malta," where the disease was first described) and *Brucella abortus*. *Brucella suis*, and *Brucella canis* are less common pathogens.[54-58]

In the United States, brucellosis has largely been eliminated by proper animal husbandry practices. Still, there are 100 to 200 cases annually, mostly in travelers who ate raw dairy products in endemic areas or in people who consume illegally imported unpasteurized Mexican dairy products. Those at high risk include herders, farmers, veterinarians, and abattoir workers. Hunters who handle carcasses of large game, such as deer, elk, and wild pigs, are also at risk.

People can become infected by ingestion or inhalation of the pathogens or via contact through conjunctiva or open skin. The bacteria then invade reticuloendothelial tissues and typically evade host defenses as intracellular pathogens.[58]

Contaminated unpasteurized milk or cheese is the most common source for human infection. Also, direct contact with infected animals, their placentae, or excreta may allow organisms to enter through abraded skin. Droplet inhalation can occur in abattoir workers. *Brucella* multiply intracellularly in many tissues and may persist for prolonged periods, leading to acute and chronic disease. Although *Brucella* is an intracellular pathogen, AIDS patients do not have more frequent or severe disease.

In the past, most U.S. infections were caused by *B. abortus* after contact with infected cattle and dairy products. This species may cause bovine abortions and stillbirths, so handling infected fetuses or placentae is risky. Dog owners are at increased risk of infections with *B. canis*.[56]

CLINICAL FINDINGS

HISTORY

The incubation period varies and is usually 1 to 3 weeks, but may be 2 months or longer. The disease presents either as an acute febrile, flu-like bacteremic syndrome or as a chronic disease with nonspecific signs and symptoms such as weakness, anorexia, headache, and low-grade fever. Relapses occur in approximately 15% of patients, often after an ineffective antibiotic regimen.

CUTANEOUS LESIONS

Skin manifestations occur in fewer than 5% of patients and are more common in children than in adults. Furthermore, skin lesions, when present, vary widely, appearing as vasculitis, erythema nodosum, panniculitis, abscesses, and polymorphous papules, pustules, and papulosquamous lesions. This is because cutaneous brucellosis can be related to direct inoculation, hematogenous spread, deposition of antigen–antibody complexes, or hypersensitivity reactions. Children with acute cutaneous brucellosis typically have a violaceous papulonodular eruption primarily on the trunk and lower extremities. Rarely, *Brucella*-related osteomyelitis or suppurative lymph nodes may create cutaneous abscesses or sinuses.[59-64]

A rare but distinctive dermatosis is seen in veterinarians or farmers who handle infected animals or tissues[65] and develop a severe contact hypersensitivity reaction to *Brucella* antigens. This presents with discrete, elevated, red papules on the hands or arms that may ulcerate. Needle-stick injuries while handling the live-attenuated *Brucella* vaccine also causes local reactions.[51]

RELATED PHYSICAL FINDINGS

Brucellosis can involve every organ system, although there are no pathognomic clinical findings. The disease can be debilitating but it is rarely fatal. Joints, reproductive organs, liver, and the CNS are, in order, the most frequently involved. Nearly all patients have a characteristic undulant fever (alternating pattern of several febrile days followed by several afebrile days). Arthritis can be axial (eg, sacroiliitis) or peripheral. The disease shows a predilection for reproductive organs, which leads to miscarriages, stillbirths, mastitis, prostatitis, orchitis, and epididymitis. Spinal osteomyelitis is well described, and endocarditis can be fatal. Persistent neuropsychiatric findings occur in 5% of patients.[58]

LABORATORY FINDINGS

Patients often have leukopenia, anemia, and elevated liver enzymes. Blood cultures may be positive during the acute illness. Because organisms are easily aerosolized and highly infectious, culture must be under Biosafety Level III conditions. *Brucella* are nonmotile, coccobacillary, Gram-negative rods that grow best in enriched media and hypercapnic conditions with 8% to 10% CO_2. Serodiagnosis is challenging.[58]

HISTOPATHOLOGY

The papulonodular eruption shows focal perivascular and periadnexal lymphohistiocytic granulomatous inflammation. Macular lesions have a nonspecific, mild, lymph perivascular infiltrate. The panniculitis usually shows septolobular inflammation with abundant plasma cells. Hepatic and splenic lesions contain small, noncaseating granulomas. Caseation necrosis and calcification may occur in *B. suis* infections.[55,56]

DIFFERENTIAL DIAGNOSIS

The clinical diagnosis of brucellosis is challenging and the epidemiologic suspicion is often delayed. Confirmation by culture or by serological techniques is necessary but the laboratory techniques are difficult.[58] The diagnosis is usually made on the basis of epidemiologic information, coupled with isolation of the organism, finding high or rising agglutination titers, or detecting organisms from a clinical specimen by direct fluorescent antibody technique. For cultures, bone marrow specimens have the highest yield. An agglutination titer of greater than 1:160 is sufficient to begin treatment. Confirmatory titers should be obtained 7 to 14 days later. In chronic disease, immunoglobulin G antibodies indicate continuing or recrudescent infection. Cross-reactions with *F. tularensis*, the cause of tularemia, are known, and recent cholera vaccination may stimulate a false-positive *Brucella* agglutination.

The differential diagnosis includes other acute bacterial infections, such as salmonellosis, listeriosis, tuberculosis, and endocarditis. Hodgkin disease may mimic many findings of brucellosis. Vertebral osteomyelitis is sometimes the sole manifestation of brucellosis.

TREATMENT

Brucellosis requires prolonged multidrug therapy with antimicrobials that penetrate into cells. Optimal therapy consists of doxycycline combined with either streptomycin, which is difficult to obtain, or gentamicin. The World Health Organization recommends an oral–oral regimen of doxycycline and rifampin (see Table 156-1). Treatment should last at least 6 weeks; shorter courses carry a risk for relapse.[58]

PROGNOSIS AND CLINICAL COURSE

Perhaps 5% of brucellosis patients die, mostly because of *B. melitensis* endocarditis. Early treatment results in rapid improvement but relapses occur in approximately 10% to 15% of patients with suboptimal treatment. Chronic brucellosis can cause disabling fevers, arthritis, fatigue, and nonspecific neuropsychiatric changes.[57]

PREVENTION

In Western nations, brucellosis is largely preventable through occupational precautions such as wearing gloves when handling game or products of conception from livestock. People should avoid unpasteurized dairy products and be especially vigilant when traveling in endemic countries. Vaccines exist for animals but not humans. Brucellosis is a reportable disease and any occurrence should initiate a search for—and possible destruction of—the animal or food source. The CDC categorizes *Brucella* as a Category B bioweapon, so a criminal source also must be considered.[56,58]

GLANDERS

AT-A-GLANCE

- Rare zoonosis caused by the Gram-negative bacillus *Burkholderia mallei* (formerly *Pseudomonas mallei*), found focally in Asia and the Middle East.
- Animal glanders occurs in horses, mules, and donkeys. Humans are infected through direct occupational exposure to animal reservoirs.
- Most human cases are acquired by direct inoculation into skin or contact of open skin with an infected animal or its secretions. Inhalational transmission is rare.
- A cutaneous ulcer develops after a 1- to 5-day incubation period, followed by several presentations: ulceroglandular syndrome, localized abscesses (acute or chronic), or bacteremic dissemination (often fatal).

ETIOLOGY AND EPIDEMIOLOGY

Glanders is a rare zoonosis caused by the Gram-negative bacillus *Burkholderia mallei* (formerly *Pseudomonas mallei*). Glanders occurs mostly in horses, mules, donkeys, and related species, and exists focally in Asia and the Middle East.[66] The disease is usually fatal in donkeys and mules, but may cause a chronic suppurative condition, called *farcy*, in horses. Human cases are usually the result of direct exposures to animal reservoirs. In endemic areas, animal handlers, veterinarians, and abattoir workers have the greatest risks of exposure.[67-69]

CLINICAL FINDINGS

HISTORY

Human glanders may present in several ways, depending whether the disease is transmitted via cutaneous inoculation or respiratory inhalation: acute localized infection, chronic cutaneous infection, acute pulmonary disease, and septicemia.[70,71] Most cases are acquired transcutaneously, and a local ulcer develops within 1 to 5 days. Regional lymph nodes may then enlarge, producing a ulceroglandular syndrome.

CUTANEOUS LESIONS

The 2 types of cutaneous glanders are (a) an acute, febrile, disseminated, infectious process that may resolve in a few weeks and (b) an indolent, relapsing, chronic infection, with multiple cutaneous or subcutaneous abscesses and draining sinuses. Abscesses may develop in muscle, liver, or spleen.

In acute glanders, a nodule surrounded by cellulitis appears at the site of inoculation (see Table 156-1). Local swelling and suppuration occur, the lesion ulcerates, and regional lymphadenopathy develops. The ulcer is painful and has irregular edges with a gray-yellow base. Nodules rapidly develop along lymphatics that drain the initial lesion. These become necrotic and ulcerated, forming sinuses. Widespread dissemination quickly follows, with multiple nodular necrotic abscesses in subcutaneous tissues and muscle. Lesions frequently coalesce into gangrenous areas.

During bacteremic spread, patients have fevers, rigors, and night sweats. The characteristic eruption is composed of crops of papules, bullae, and pustules. These may be generalized or localized to the face and neck, in which case involvement of the nasal mucosa, either initially or by secondary spread, is prominent. Mucopurulent, bloody nasal discharge is common. Infection may spread to the paranasal sinuses, pharynx, and lungs.

In chronic glanders, cutaneous and subcutaneous nodules appear on the extremities and occasionally on the face. The lesions ulcerate, and draining sinuses develop. Ulceration of the hard palate and perforation of the nasal septum can occur. If the organisms are inhaled, pulmonary disease may produce pneumonia, pulmonary abscesses, or pleural effusions. Septicemic glanders is usually fatal.

LABORATORY FINDINGS

Histopathologic examination of the skin and other involved organs shows a suppurative, necrotic process containing numerous intracellular and extracellular bacteria. Chronic glanders causes granulomatous changes.

DIFFERENTIAL DIAGNOSIS

The diagnosis is made on an epidemiologic basis, examination of Gram-stained smears of pus, and isolation of the organism from abscesses. Furthermore, in the pulmonary and septicemic forms, organisms may be recovered from blood, sputum, or urine. Acute glanders may resemble miliary tuberculosis. The multiple subcutaneous abscesses suggest staphylococcal or deep fungal infections or melioidosis. Lymphonodular disease resembles sporotrichosis, nocardiosis, tularemia, New World leishmaniasis, and *Mycobacterium marinum* infection.

TREATMENT

The CDC recommends treatment with sulfadiazine, although in vitro data indicate that *B. mallei* is susceptible to ceftazidime, gentamicin, doxycycline, imipenem, and ciprofloxacin. Patients with subcutaneous or visceral abscesses may require treatment for up to 1 year.[70-72] Because the disease has largely disappeared, few evidence-based recommendations are available.

PROGNOSIS, CLINICAL COURSE, AND COMPLICATIONS

Untreated septicemic glanders causes widespread abscesses in lungs, liver, spleen, muscles, and is nearly always fatal.

PREVENTION

The usual way to control zoonotic or epizootic glanders has been to destroy infected animals. Such measures have nearly eradicated this once common equine infection and eliminated transmission to humans in industrialized countries. In the United States, glanders is a reportable disease. There are no vaccines against *B. mallei* infection for humans or animals. However, vaccines might be developed because of the bioweapon potential of this pathogen.[69]

PASTEURELLA MULTOCIDA INFECTIONS

AT-A-GLANCE

- Normal flora in oropharynx of many domestic animals. Most human infections are from dog or cat bites.
- Local pain and swelling appear rapidly, usually less than 2 days after exposure.
- Gram-negative organism; nevertheless, infection is treated with penicillin or presumptively with amoxicillin/clavulanic acid.

ETIOLOGY AND EPIDEMIOLOGY

Pasteurella multocida is a small, ovoid, Gram-negative rod that can cause local skin infection with regional adenitis after a superficial animal bite, scratch, or lick,[73] or septic arthritis and osteomyelitis after a deeper animal bite. Respiratory tract infections unassociated with trauma occur in rare cases, and bacteremia may accompany meningitis or osteomyelitis.

P. multocida commonly colonizes the oropharynx and nasopharynx of healthy cats, dogs, rats, mice, pigs, and other livestock, and poultry. Nearly all patients with *P. multocida* infection have had animal exposure, most commonly a dog or cat bite. Cat teeth are often longer and sharper than those of dogs and therefore may penetrate more deeply to cause septic arthritis or osteomyelitis. Compromising conditions such as cirrhosis, malignancy, and chronic obstructive pulmonary disease coexist in most severe cases.[74-79]

Neonatal pasteurellosis can be acquired by exposure to animals, usually pet dogs and cats in the household, even without known or recognized traumatic contact, possibly via respiratory droplets from the animal, or via vertical transmission from an asymptomatic mother.[80]

CLINICAL FINDINGS

HISTORY

Local pain and swelling occur within a few days of an animal bite or contact exposure. Fever is uncommon.

CUTANEOUS LESIONS

Redness, swelling, ulceration, and seropurulent drainage develop at the bite site. Cellulitis may progress rapidly and extensively, producing lymphangitis or local necrosis. Purpura fulminans and necrotizing fasciitis with septic shock have been reported.[74,81]

RELATED PHYSICAL FINDINGS

Regional adenopathy may be present. Deep bites may introduce organisms into a joint or beneath periosteum and cause septic arthritis or osteomyelitis.

LABORATORY FINDINGS

Mild leukocytosis is present. After several weeks, a radiograph of underlying bone may show osteomyelitis. The organism is Gram-negative, and Wright-Giemsa stain reveals a bipolar appearance. Histopathologically, an acute pyogenic response is seen.[75]

DIFFERENTIAL DIAGNOSIS

The diagnosis is suspected when a painful infection develops rapidly (<2 days) at the site of an animal bite. Approximately 75% of infected cat bites are caused by *P. multocida*. Local ulceration and proximal lymphadenitis mimic ulceroglandular tularemia, but *P. multocida* characteristically produces a necrotizing cellulitis and not chancriform syndrome. The diagnosis is confirmed by isolation of the organism, although treatment is often initiated according to an animal bite protocol or based on the history of a rapidly appearing painful cellulitis after a dog or cat bite.[81,82]

TREATMENT

Because most animal bite wounds show polymicrobial contamination, an amoxicillin-clavulanic acid preparation should be started after a dog or cat bite. Although *P. multocida* is a Gram-negative organism, most strains are susceptible to penicillin, which is the drug of choice if only *Pasteurella* is cultured. If one suspects that the bite reached periosteum, oral penicillin should be given until the local lesion is well healed. *P. multocida* is also susceptible to doxycycline, later-generation cephalosporins, and trimethoprim-sulfamethoxazole (see Table 156-1).

PROGNOSIS AND CLINICAL COURSE

Infection usually responds promptly to antibiotic therapy. Osteomyelitis, abscesses, and remnant foreign bodies should be treated surgically as well as medically. *P. multocida* infections may be more severe or lead to sepsis in immunocompromised or AIDS patients.

PREVENTION

A great many animal bites are unprovoked by family pets onto a child's hand, therefore judicious selection of pets and instruction to children are useful, but not guaranteed, ways to reduce domestic animal bites.[83]

RAT-BITE FEVER

AT-A-GLANCE

- Rat-bite fever refers to 2 clinically similar zoonoses caused by *Streptobacillus moniliformis* and *Spirillum minus*.
- Infection is usually acquired through rat bite or ingestion of rat-contaminated food or drink.
- The disease is characterized by the classic triad of fever, polyarthralgias, and rash.

ETIOLOGY AND EPIDEMIOLOGY

The term *rat-bite fever* applies to 2 clinically similar zoonoses that are both attributable to contact with rats or their excreta. The more common form is caused by *Streptobacillus moniliformis*, a pleomorphic Gram-negative rod found in the nasopharyngeal flora of most wild and laboratory rats, which are asymptomatic carriers, and is excreted in their urine.[84] Carnivores that prey on wild rodents may also transmit infection. Infections with *S. moniliformis* arise in 1 of 2 ways: (a) direct contact with infected animals, usually through a bite, or (b) ingestion of food or drink contaminated by rat urine, feces, or other secretions.[85] In both forms, patients have an acute flu-like infection characterized by a clinical triad of fever, polyarthralgias or arthritis, and rash. In 1926, an outbreak in Haverhill, Massachusetts, caused by consumption of milk tainted by rat excreta led to the designation *Haverhill fever* or *erythema arthriticum epidemicum*.

The other pathogen implicated in rat-bite fever is *Spirillum minus*, a Gram-negative spirochete. Spirillary rat-bite fever differs in its geographic distribution, incubation period, and milder arthritis. It occurs almost exclusively in East Asia. Its Japanese name is *sodoku*.[83]

Both diseases are most common where people live in crowded, unsanitary conditions ideal for rats. Although streptobacillary fever occurs worldwide, it is most common in Asia. Most U.S. cases occur in children with a new pet rat. Person-to-person transmission is unknown. Rat-bite fever is nonreportable so its exact incidence is not known.[86]

CLINICAL FINDINGS

HISTORY

Streptobacillary disease has an asymptomatic incubation period of 1 to 7 days, and, in rare cases, as long as 3 weeks. Often, the rat bite has healed by the time a flu-like illness begins with fever, chills, headache, stiff neck, nausea and vomiting, and myalgia. A rash begins to appear several days later. Spirillary rat-bite fever has an incubation period of longer than 14 days.

CUTANEOUS LESIONS

Approximately 75% of patients with streptobacillary fever develop a morbilliform eruption, usually 2 to 3 days after the fever. Individual lesions can be macular, morbilliform, or petechial. Lesions are most prominent on the palms, soles, and around joints but may become generalized, resembling measles.[86-88] There can be hemorrhagic acral vesicles, resembling lesions of leukocytoclastic vasculitis or gonococcemia.[89] Notably, when the rash appears, the rat bite has usually healed and only rarely shows evidence of infection, inflammation, or regional adenopathy. A week or so after resolution of the disease, the palms and soles have a characteristic desquamation that may resemble Kawasaki disease.

In contrast, the bite producing spirillary fever is usually tender, red, indurated, or ulcerated when the rash appears.[90] Cutaneous lesions are larger and are prominent on the abdomen, thus resembling the rose spots of typhoid. There can be tender regional lymphadenopathy and lymphangitis.[91]

RELATED PHYSICAL FINDINGS

Within a week of the febrile symptoms, arthritis usually develops, predominantly involving large joints. The arthritis may be an asymmetric polyarthritis resembling rheumatoid arthritis but is rarely suppurative. Regional lymphadenopathy may be present. Infection may involve the liver, kidneys, meninges, and heart valves.[84] Arthritis is uncommon in *S. minus* infection.[89]

LABORATORY FINDINGS

Gram stains of *S. moniliformis* shows Gram-negative filamentous branching chains, interspersed with bead-like swellings, hence the name *moniliformis,* meaning "necklace-shaped." The organisms, however, are pleomorphic in shape and staining qualities, possibly resembling Gram-positive rods.[84] If cultured properly, the organism can be recovered from blood, joint fluid, or palmar pustules. It is fastidious in culture; growth is inhibited by the sodium polyanethol sulfonate found in most aerobic blood-culture bottles. It grows best on trypticase-soy broth or supplemented thioglycolate broth in which characteristic "puffball" colonies are seen. Anaerobic culture media, which lack the sulfonates, permits slow growth and should be held for several additional days. Histopathologic examination of purpuric lesions shows a lymphocytic vasculitis with focal intravascular thrombi.[88] In fulminant cases, filamentous organisms have been seen in silver-stained tissues.[86] Approximately one-third of patients have false-positive Venereal Disease Research Laboratory tests, but no specific serologic tests are currently available.

S. minus cannot be cultured in vitro. Darkfield microscopy may reveal characteristic spirochetes.

DIFFERENTIAL DIAGNOSIS

The diagnosis should be suspected in any person with unexplained fevers and recent rat exposure.[86] The triad of fever, arthritis, and acral rash, accompanied by a history of a recent rat bite, should raise suspicion. The differential diagnosis should also include other causes of fever, rash, and arthralgia, such as meningococcemia, disseminated gonococcemia, acute rheumatic fever, rheumatoid arthritis, endocarditis, Lyme disease, viral exanthems (eg, from coxsackievirus), ehrlichiosis and rickettsioses, leptospirosis, secondary syphilis, typhoid, and *P. multocida* infection.

Blood cultures are the best way to confirm the diagnosis of streptobacillary rat-bite fever. Several features help differentiate the 2 types of rat-bite fever. In *S. moniliformis* infection the incubation period is shorter (usually <10 days vs >14 days),[91] the bite site usually heals before systemic symptoms begin, the rash is more peripheral, and arthritis is more common (60% vs 20%).

TREATMENT

The treatment of choice for someone who becomes ill after a rat bite is amoxicillin-clavulanic acid. In patients allergic to penicillins, doxycycline is acceptable. Once *S. moniliformis* is identified, penicillin is the drug of choice. In general, rat bites should be cleansed promptly and thoroughly. Tetanus immunization status should be checked. Although there are no established guidelines, one might consider a prompt prophylactic course of penicillin or doxycycline after any rat bite.[85]

PROGNOSIS, CLINICAL COURSE, AND COMPLICATIONS

Untreated disease may last for a few days to several weeks and 10% to 20% are fatal, usually from endocarditis. If diagnosed early, appropriate antibiotics produce a prompt clinical response although migratory arthritis may persist after bacteriologic cure.

PREVENTION

To prevent rat-bite fever, dwellings should be rat proofed and open water supplies should be protected from contamination by rat excreta. Persons who handle rats should wear gloves, wash their hands frequently, and avoid hand-to-mouth contact when around rats. Children with pet rats should be taught these simple precautions.[87]

SEAL FINGER

AT-A-GLANCE

- Occupational zoonosis after contact with seals or sea lions. Occurs worldwide in marine environments.
- Usually presents as an exquisitely painful nodule on the distal phalanx of the finger that may progress to tenosynovitis or joint destruction.
- The pathogen is likely to be a marine *Mycoplasma* found in the seal's normal oropharyngeal flora. The infection responds quickly to tetracyclines.

ETIOLOGY AND EPIDEMIOLOGY

Seal finger is an occupational zoonosis that occurs only after direct contact with seals, sea lions, and similar marine mammals (order Pinnipedia), transmitted via bites or through open skin after handling seals or their carcasses. Seal finger is characterized by intensely painful red nodules, usually on the distal phalanx. Untreated, it can evolve into tenosynovitis, osteitis, and joint destruction.[92,93] Although this has not been fully confirmed, seal finger appears to be caused by a group of *Mycoplasma* that is part of the normal oropharyngeal flora of pinnipeds.[94]

CLINICAL FINDINGS

People at risk include hunters, zookeepers, and marine biologists. Seal finger is common in cold water coastal areas around Scandinavia, Greenland, Newfoundland, and similar environments in the Southern Hemisphere. Most cases occur during the spring sealing season. Incubation is usually approximately 4 days, rarely as long as 3 weeks. A furuncle-like lesion appears at the inoculation site, followed by severe pain, marked swelling, and stiffness.[92,93]

DIFFERENTIAL DIAGNOSIS

The differential diagnosis includes other pathogens transmitted in a cold marine environment. Erysipeloid is less painful, has a more violaceous hue, and usually extends beyond the original entry site. *M. marinum* infection is usually painless and indolent. Seal pox is an orthopoxvirus infection transmitted through contact with mouths of seals and other pinnipeds. Staphylococcal or streptococcal pyodermas may have a similar picture. Herpetic whitlow can also cause a painful distal phalanx. Culture should be attempted on special *Mycoplasma* media.

TREATMENT

Seal finger does not respond to the β-lactam antibiotics frequently prescribed presumptively for cellulitis caused by *Staphylococcus*, *Streptococcus*, or *Erysipelothrix*. The lack of response to β-lactams further suggests seal finger. Tetracyclines are the treatment of choice and must be continued for 4 to 6 weeks (see Table 156-1). Older accounts describe occasional sealers who amputated their own fingers to rid themselves of the excruciatingly painful digit.[95]

LISTERIOSIS (*LISTERIA MONOCYTOGENES* INFECTIONS)

AT-A-GLANCE

- Caused by anaerobic Gram-positive bacillus transmitted in fecal–oral manner through consumption of contaminated dairy products.
- Human listeriosis is most common in pregnant women, neonates, and patients with AIDS, and in foodborne outbreaks. May cause miscarriages, stillbirths, and virulent neonatal infections.
- Generalized petechiae, papules, or pustules may be seen in neonatal listeriosis, especially in meconium-stained newborns.

ETIOLOGY AND EPIDEMIOLOGY

Listeria monocytogenes is an anaerobic Gram-positive bacillus found widely in soil, water, vegetation, and the gut flora of humans and other animals. Exposure to this organism occurs through fecal–oral contamination, but the disease has an opportunistic nature, appearing in very young, very old, pregnant, and immunocompromised individuals. *L. monocytogenes* is found in the feces of many domestic and wild animals and birds, and is widespread in the environment.[96] Typically, livestock become infected by eating manure-contaminated silage; this can cause abortions, septicemia, and a peculiar form of encephalitis called *circling disease*.[97]

Human listeriosis is uncommon but occurs in 3 typical settings: (a) sporadic disease in pregnant women and neonates; (b) sporadic disease in AIDS patients; and (c) foodborne outbreaks.[98] Humans usually become infected by eating contaminated, unpasteurized, or improperly pasteurized dairy products. In adults, the disease can present as septicemia, meningitis, vaginal infection, pneumonitis, or oculoglandular syndrome, and can cause miscarriages and stillbirths.[70] Infantile listeriosis presents acutely with septicemia, meningitis and meningoencephalitis, and septic granulomatosis (granulomatosis infantiseptica).

Primary cutaneous listeriosis is rare and usually follows occupational exposure where there has been direct cutaneous inoculation from animal products of conception.[99] Typically, skin infections manifest as nonpainful, nonpruritic, self-limited, localized, papulopustular, or vesiculopustular eruptions in healthy persons. Less commonly, skin lesions may arise from hematogenous dissemination in compromised hosts with invasive disease.[100]

Approximately 5% of humans are fecal carriers of *Listeria*. Higher rates of carriage have been observed in family contacts of patients with listeriosis. Several outbreaks have implicated unpasteurized soft cheeses imported from Mexico or vegetables from farms that fertilize crops with manure.[101]

The highest incidence of human listeriosis is seen among infants in the perinatal period, which suggests that the transmission occurs in utero or at birth. One-fourth of adult cases occur in pregnant women. Many other adult cases occur in patients with altered cellular immunity, such as those with Hodgkin disease, leukemia, or AIDS, and in those who have undergone organ transplantation. Hepatic disorders, such as cirrhosis and iron overload, also predispose to infection. Recent reports suggest that biologic therapies that interfere with tumor necrosis factor activity, such as treating psoriatic arthritis with infliximab, may increase the risk for listeriosis.[102]

CLINICAL FINDINGS

HISTORY

Early-onset neonatal listeriosis develops in infants infected in utero by untreated bacteremic mothers shortly before labor begins. Findings are evident at birth or become apparent within the first few days. These neonates are acutely ill and have generalized pustular, papular, or petechial skin lesions. Late-onset neonatal listeriosis occurs several weeks after a healthy birth, is presumably acquired postpartum, and usually presents as meningitis.[101,103,104]

Listeriosis from foodborne organisms usually causes outbreaks of acute gastroenteritis in families or communities. Patients have fever, vomiting, and nonbloody diarrhea, but this form lacks skin lesions.

CUTANEOUS LESIONS

In septic infants, cutaneous lesions appear as generalized petechiae, papules, or pustules. Veterinarians or farmers who handle infected bovine fetuses may develop an acute febrile illness with headache, malaise, and regional adenopathy. Tender red papules develop on exposed surfaces and may evolve into pustules over 2 to 3 days. These contain the characteristic Gram-positive rods.

RELATED PHYSICAL FINDINGS

Neonates with early-onset listeriosis are often meconium-stained at birth, lethargic, and have an enlarged liver and spleen. CNS listeriosis has a spectrum of neurologic manifestations, ranging from typical acute bacterial meningitis, abscesses, encephalitis, and infarcts.[104]

LABORATORY FINDINGS

L. monocytogenes is a small pleomorphic bacillus that often appears coccoid in infected tissues and body fluids. Pustules, meconium, cerebrospinal fluid, or blood cultures reveal the characteristic Gram-positive rods. The organism is β-hemolytic when cultured on sheep blood agar and exhibits a characteristic tumbling motility when grown in broth. In adults with meningitis, the cerebrospinal fluid contains neutrophils, but about one-third of meningitic infants have a mononuclear response.

HISTOPATHOLOGY

Skin lesions show focal necrosis, neutrophilic infiltrates, and monocytes around blood vessels. In septic patients, viscera may show abscesses and granulomas.

DIFFERENTIAL DIAGNOSIS

Neonatal listeriosis should be suspected in a meconium-stained newborn with intrauterine growth retardation who develops a papular skin eruption or subsequently failure to thrive. The differential diagnosis includes other in utero neonatal infections such as toxoplasmosis, cytomegalovirus infection, rubella, disseminated herpes simplex infection, and disseminated bacterial infections, such as those caused by group B streptococci, *Escherichia coli*, *Salmonella*, and *Pseudomonas*.

TREATMENT

Neonates with listeriosis should be treated with IV ampicillin (or penicillin) (see Table 156-1). Penicillin-allergic patients may be treated with cotrimoxazole or erythromycin. Cephalosporins are generally ineffective.[96] Primary cutaneous listeriosis appears to be self-limited in most cases, and the role for antibiotics is unclear, but nevertheless prudent to administer.[100]

PROGNOSIS, CLINICAL COURSE, AND COMPLICATIONS

In neonatal septicemia or meningitis, mortality is approximately 50%, even with treatment. In adults, prompt treatment is usually effective, unless there is a severe underlying debility. Pregnant women, even if treated, are at risk for miscarriage.

PREVENTION

Prepartum strategies to reduce neonatal group B streptococcal infections may also reduce risk of neonatal listeriosis.[104]

Farmers should not feed contaminated silage to livestock nor use untreated manure to fertilize crops. Still, it is almost impossible to guarantee *Listeria*-free foods. Therefore, people at greatest risk should avoid foods typically linked to listeriosis, such as raw (unpasteurized) dairy products, unwashed vegetables, and poorly cooked meats. Veterinarians and farmers should use gloves and protective garments when handling aborted fetuses or placentae.[103]

VIBRIO VULNIFICUS INFECTIONS

AT-A-GLANCE

- Noncholera *Vibrio* organisms are found in warm saltwater worldwide. Exposures occur via percutaneous injury, often minor (eg, while ocean fishing), or via ingestion of filter-feeding shellfish, which concentrate organisms.
- Severe illness presents with necrotizing fasciitis, hemorrhagic bullae, and hypotensive shock. Cirrhosis and other liver diseases predispose to a virulent, often fatal, course.

ETIOLOGY AND EPIDEMIOLOGY

Vibrio are facultatively anaerobic, pleomorphic, Gram-negative rods found in marine waters, estuaries, brackish lakes, and their sediments wherever the water temperature is above 20°C (68°F). The most well-known vibriosis is cholera, caused by antigenic strains of *Vibrio cholerae*. Although cholera organisms do not infect the skin, many other *Vibrio* do. The most important of these, *Vibrio vulnificus* can cause fulminant cellulitis, myositis, necrotizing fasciitis, and death.[105]

People become infected with *V. vulnificus* through oral or percutaneous exposure, which leads to 3 distinct clinical syndromes: gastroenteritis, primary sepsis (with or without secondary skin and soft-tissue infection), and primary wound infection.[106,107] After eating contaminated raw or undercooked seafood, people who have chronic liver disease (especially hemochromatosis), renal failure, diabetes mellitus, or who are otherwise immunocompromised, are at risk for primary septicemia. Percutaneous infections are acquired by handling raw seafood, by entering saltwater with an open wound, or by experiencing skin trauma while in or around saltwater. Immunocompromised individuals are again at increased risk for secondary septicemia.[108,109]

V. vulnificus lives in warm seawater, where it colonizes the skin of fish and is concentrated in filter-feeding shellfish, such as oysters. Infections are particularly common along the Gulf of Mexico and, because of global warming, are now found in increasingly higher latitudes, such as on the Baltic Sea.[110-112]

Most cases of wound infection are sporadic and depend more on host susceptibilities than environmental conditions. However, after Hurricane Katrina struck the Gulf Coast in 2005, thousands of people were exposed to brackish floodwaters. There were 18 known cases of *Vibrio* wound infections—14 caused by *V. vulnificus*, 3 caused by *Vibrio parahaemolyticus*, and 1 unspeciated case.[113] Each year in the United States, approximately 100 persons are infected with *V. vulnificus* with approximately 50% mortality.[107]

CLINICAL FINDINGS

HISTORY

There is nearly always a history of contact with saltwater, injury while ocean fishing, or consumption or handling of shellfish. After oral exposure, primary septicemia often begins with watery diarrhea, fever, chills, nausea, vomiting, and abdominal pain. People with wound infections usually recall an open skin lesion present before the saltwater exposure or a percutaneous injury during the exposure. *Vibrio* cellulitis is painful and has a rapid onset within 12 to 24 hours of exposure. Secondary bacteremia with sepsis may occur several days later.[114]

CUTANEOUS LESIONS

Infected wounds may present as pustules, lymphangitis, or cellulitis. These infections may be mild or may develop into rapidly progressive, painful cellulitis with extensive skin necrosis, myositis, and necrotizing fasciitis (Fig. 156-3). Secondary bacteremia may cause metastatic cutaneous lesions.[108,115] In septic patients, large hemorrhagic bullae commonly arise on the extremities or trunk and usually progress to necrotic ulcers and necrotizing fasciitis (see Table 156-1).

RELATED PHYSICAL FINDINGS

V. vulnificus septicemia causes high fever, tachycardia, and hypotension. One-third of patients develop Gram-negative septic shock.

LABORATORY FINDINGS

In primary septicemia, leukopenia is more common than leukocytosis. Thrombocytopenia is typical and may be part of disseminated intravascular coagulation. Usually, there is laboratory evidence for the person's predisposing condition (eg, diabetes). All *Vibrio* species can be grown in regular blood culture media and cause hemolysis on sheep blood agar, but only *V. vulnificus* ferments lactose on MacConkey agar. Histopathology shows noninflammatory bulla, epidermal necrosis, hemorrhage, and bacteria in dermal vessels. Radiographic studies show accumulations of nonspecific soft-tissue edema.

DIFFERENTIAL DIAGNOSIS

A cirrhotic or diabetic patient with fever, shock, and hemorrhagic bulla within several days of saltwater exposure or of eating raw oysters should alert the physician to possible *Vibrio* septicemia, especially if the exposure occurred along the American Gulf Coast.

Similar presentations include disseminated intravascular coagulation, clostridial myonecrosis, meningococcemia, purpura fulminans, any form of necrotizing fasciitis, and other aggressive soft-tissue infections. Wound infections sustained in fresh water suggest infection with *Aeromonas* rather than *Vibrio*. Clostridial myonecrosis may present with necrotizing fasciitis and shock, but is further suggested by local wound crepitus and the finding of Gram-positive rods.

TREATMENT

Primary or secondary septicemia caused by *V. vulnificus* (or other *Vibrio* sp.) requires prompt management of hypotensive shock, parenteral administration of antibiotics, and vigorous debridement of necrotic lesions. Amputation of the affected limb may be necessary. The antibiotics of choice are a combination of doxycycline and ceftazidime (see Table 156-1). Alternatives to doxycycline include chloramphenicol, ciprofloxacin, and minocycline. Alternatives to ceftazidime include cefotaxime. Application of compresses with modified Dakin solution (0.025% sodium hypochlorite) may help arrest the progression of the cutaneous lesions.[116]

PROGNOSIS, CLINICAL COURSE, AND COMPLICATIONS

The mortality rate for *V. vulnificus* primary septicemia is approximately 50%, about 3 times higher than the mortality for wound infections caused by the same organism.

PREVENTION

People with cirrhosis, diabetes, AIDS, and other immunocompromising illnesses should not eat raw shellfish and, if they have open skin wounds, should not enter seawater, estuaries, or brackish lakes. If an at-risk individual exposes open skin to saltwater, the site should be cleansed promptly with soap and clean water. Similarly, these individuals should not handle raw fish and shellfish. Vigilant attention to onset of illness is then required. Some authorities consider of a course of prophylactic oral doxycycline for an immunocompromised person with a high-risk exposure. In 2003, California began to require special processing of raw Gulf oysters harvested from April 1 to October 31, to eliminate *V. vulnificus*, which has reduced the number oyster-associated *Vibrio* infections.[117]

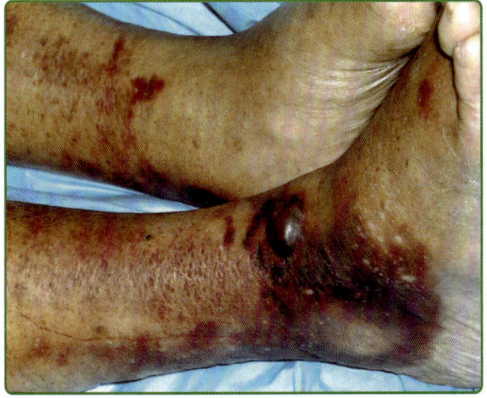

Figure 156-3 *Vibrio vulnificus* cellulitis with hemorrhagic plaque and bullae on the legs of an older diabetic patient with cirrhosis.

OTHER CUTANEOUS VIBRIO INFECTIONS

The most common other *Vibrio* to cause wound infections are *V. parahaemolyticus* and nontoxigenic *V. cholerae* (ie, antigenic strains other than 01 and 139). Usually, these *Vibrio* cause an infection after oral exposure, producing an acute but self-limited noninflammatory gastroenteritis. Wound infections may occur after open skin is exposed to saltwater. The disease course is usually less severe than that of *V. vulnificus* although in an immunocompromised host, it may cause hemorrhagic bulla, shock, and necrotizing fasciitis.

AEROMONAS HYDROPHILA INFECTIONS

AT-A-GLANCE

- Caused by a facultatively anaerobic Gram-negative bacillus found in fresh and brackish water worldwide.
- Usually presents as cellulitis after exposure to fresh or brackish water but may cause necrotizing fasciitis or myonecrosis.
- Sepsis risk in cirrhotic and immunocompromised patients.

ETIOLOGY AND EPIDEMIOLOGY

Aeromonas hydrophila is a facultatively anaerobic, Gram-negative bacillus that causes opportunistic human infections. Except for the freshwater habitat of *Aeromonas*, its taxonomic, ecologic, and epidemiologic profiles resemble those of *Vibrio* sp. Aeromonads are found in fresh and brackish water worldwide and are natural pathogens of many aquatic animals, including fish, amphibians, and reptiles. Human *Aeromonas* infections are usually associated with exposure to contaminated fresh or brackish water. The organism is typically linked with gastroenteritis,[118] but in an increasing number of cases, it has been implicated in skin, soft tissue, and muscle infections, as well as in septicemic disease.[119,120] An increasing number of soft-tissue infections are associated with the medical use of leeches (*Hirudo medicinalis*).[121-123] Medical leeches harbor the bacterium as an obligatory endosymbiont that is essential for digestion of host erythrocytes.[124] Recent reports describe a generalized folliculitis acquired after exposure to presumably contaminated waters of hot tubs or children's inflatable swimming pools.[125,126]

Fish tanks, swimming pools, and tap water have been contaminated with these organisms, leading to occasional small common-source outbreaks.[127] After the 2004 tsunami off the coast of Sumatra, approximately one-quarter of the isolates from hundreds of patients hospitalized after prolonged water exposure were from *Aeromonas* spp.[128] Other traumatic events, during occupational or recreational exposure to contaminated aquatic environments, are frequently associated with *Aeromonas* skin and soft-tissue infections.[119]

CLINICAL FINDINGS

HISTORY

The key historical feature is the contact of open skin with fresh or brackish water. In healthy individuals, *Aeromonas* infections may remain localized, but compromised hosts are at risk for severe soft-tissue and septicemic disease.[81,129]

CUTANEOUS LESIONS

The most common presentation is cellulitis associated with a laceration, often followed by abscess formation or spread to deeper subcutaneous tissues. Myonecrosis or necrotizing fasciitis may mimic clostridial gas gangrene in its rapid onset (1 to 2 days after exposure) and swift progression with severe pain, marked swelling, serosanguineous bullae, crepitation, and systemic toxicity. The exudate often has a foul or fishy odor. Occasionally, bacteremia produces ecthyma gangrenosum-like lesions.[81,130,131] The folliculitis associated with hot tubs clinically resembles *Pseudomonas*-induced hot tub folliculitis.[125]

RELATED PHYSICAL FINDINGS

Jaundice and other evidence of underlying disease may be present.

LABORATORY FINDINGS

Gram-stained aspirates from abscesses or bullae may contain Gram-negative bacilli. Wound cultures yield multiple microbes in more than 50% of cases, and specimens should be plated on both sheep blood agar and MacConkey agar. Blood cultures are rarely positive for the organism. A radiograph may detect gas in deeper soft tissues.

DIFFERENTIAL DIAGNOSIS

A history of open skin exposed to fresh or brackish water, followed by local cellulitis (often with gas formation), increasing pain, and foul discharge suggests *Aeromonas* infection. The differential diagnosis includes staphylococcal or streptococcal cellulitis (including *Streptococcus pyogenes* or *Streptococcus iniae*), clostridial myonecrosis, necrotizing fasciitis, and *V. vulnificus* infection.

PROGNOSIS AND CLINICAL COURSE

With extensive surgical intervention and appropriate antimicrobial therapy, patients improve rapidly. Prognosis is excellent except in immunocompromised individuals with bacteremia.

TREATMENT

Prompt surgical exploration and debridement are essential, guided radiographically, if possible. *A. hydrophila* produces β-lactamase and is resistant to first-generation penicillins and cephalosporins. Most isolates are susceptible to third-generation cephalosporins, fluoroquinolones, and aminoglycosides (but not streptomycin). *Aeromonas*, particularly in the developing world, are developing resistance to several antibiotics so it is essential to conduct antibiotic sensitivity tests.[120] Consideration must be given to the polymicrobial nature of these infections, so results of Gram-staining and culture should guide antimicrobial selection. Two other less-pathogenic species of *Aeromonas*, *Aeromonas caviae* and *Aeromonas sobria*, have similar antibiotic sensitivity profiles.[81,130]

There are no current recommendations for the treatment of pool water associated *Aeromonas* folliculitis. The case reports describe the condition in immunocompetent individuals who were treated with either topical gentamicin or oral fluoroquinolones.[125,126]

PREVENTION

Individuals who are immunocompromised or who have chronic liver disease should promptly clean any wounds or open skin that are exposed to fresh or brackish water. In addition, they should not undergo leech therapy.

Patients who do undergo leech therapy should consider antibiotic prophylaxis beforehand. *A. hydrophila* infection accounts for nearly all associated infectious complications. *Aeromonas* infections associated with medical leech therapy are often resistant to quinolone antibiotics.[124]

MELIOIDOSIS

AT-A-GLANCE

- Caused by *Burkholderia pseudomallei* (formerly *Pseudomonas pseudomallei*), a Gram-negative aerobic bacillus that lives as a saprophyte in freshwater and damp soil.
- Occurs in humans and animals, primarily in wet tropical areas such as Southeast Asia and

(Continued)

AT-A-GLANCE (Continued)

coastal northern Australia. People who develop melioidosis elsewhere usually had prior exposure in endemic areas.
- Rice farmers, particularly if compromised by diabetes mellitus or chronic renal disease, are most susceptible.
- The disease is acquired after exposure to contaminated soil or water, either directly via the skin or through inhalation of particulate soil or dust.
- Clinical presentation ranges from focal indolent cutaneous and subcutaneous abscesses to fulminant pneumonia with septicemia.
- On the CDC's Category B list of possible bioweapon agents.

ETIOLOGY AND EPIDEMIOLOGY

Melioidosis is caused by *Burkholderia pseudomallei* (formerly *Pseudomonas pseudomallei*), a motile, pleomorphic, Gram-negative aerobic bacillus. The organism is a natural saprophyte found in freshwater and damp soil in the humid tropics. Melioidosis infects humans, a variety of birds, and domestic and wild mammals in endemic areas, but animals are not regarded as reservoirs for human infection. Although sporadic cases occur pantropically, melioidosis has its greatest incidence in Southeast Asia, especially Singapore and northeastern Thailand, and in coastal areas of Australia's Northern Territory. Apart from rare laboratory-acquired infections, cases of melioidosis in the United States and Europe have occurred only in people previously exposed in endemic areas.[132,133]

Most cases of melioidosis are transmitted by exposure of open skin to contaminated soil or water. Cutaneous melioidosis can be a primary disease, in which infection was acquired via percutaneous inoculation and the principal manifestations of this disease appear in the skin.

In Thailand, melioidosis is most common in rice farmers and has a male-to-female ratio of 4:1, consistent with occupational exposure patterns. Serologic surveys in endemic areas of rural Thailand show that 5% to 20% of inhabitants have antibodies, suggesting prior, presumably asymptomatic, infections. The frequency of pulmonary disease suggests that melioidosis also may be acquired by inhalation of contaminated droplets, soil, or dust.[134,135] Individuals with diabetes mellitus, chronic renal disease, or alcoholic liver disease are at greater risk for infection and severe disease.

There is a marked seasonality in cases of melioidosis with peak incidence during rainy monsoon seasons. After the December 2004 tsunami, hundreds of thousands of people were exposed to flood waters and cases of severe postimmersion pneumonic melioidosis were reported throughout the region.[136-142]

During the Vietnam War, extensive immersion in rice paddies and similar conditions led to cases of melioidosis among American servicemen. Several cases were reported in Vietnam veterans whose disease appeared decades later, and the only plausible exposure was to rice paddies long before.[138]

Direct human-to-human transmission is rare. *B. pseudomallei* is infectious when aerosolized and is regarded as a Category B bioweapon for its potential use on livestock or humans. If an individual without characteristic travel or exposure history develops melioidosis, or if there is a cluster of cases, deliberate exposure may have occurred.[139]

B. pseudomallei is phylogenetically close to *B. mallei*, the cause of glanders, and the clinical presentations of both diseases are often similar. However, the organisms have different environmental niches and the diseases occur after different exposures.

CLINICAL FINDINGS

HISTORY

Melioidosis has 2 principal clinical presentations: (a) acute melioidosis with suppurative skin lesions, pneumonia, or septicemia; and (b) chronic melioidosis, the more common form of the disease, with involvement of the lungs, skin (subcutaneous abscesses and draining sinuses), bones, joints, liver, and spleen. Approximately 50% of cases involve the lungs, caused either by inhalation of pathogens or by bacteremia from a cutaneous exposure, although most patients have no obvious breaks in the skin. HIV infection does not appear to increase either the risk of acquiring the disease or its severity.[132,140]

The incubation period can be as brief as 2 or 3 days. Acute pneumonic melioidosis usually starts abruptly with fever, chills, cough, dyspnea, and chest pain. Acute septicemic melioidosis may also arise from a cutaneous focus. In 50% of patients, no source for the bacteremia can be identified, but many individuals have minor abrasions on their feet.[127]

Chronic melioidosis may follow acute disease, but more commonly starts as an indolent pulmonary infection or as a low-grade febrile illness with multiple subcutaneous abscesses. Recrudescence of latent infection years after exposure may be associated with a subsequent debility, presenting as persistent, unexplained fever.[143]

CUTANEOUS LESIONS

Approximately 15% to 20% of human melioidosis cases have cutaneous manifestations, which are largely nonspecific. The inoculation site of primary cutaneous melioidosis, seen primarily in children, is frequently an ulcer, occasionally with a purulent exudate.[144] Acute septicemia may follow minor cutaneous disease. Disseminated disease can produce multiple superficial pustules or, more rarely, ecthyma gangrenosum or necrotizing fasciitis. In chronic melioidosis, draining sinuses and subcutaneous abscesses, particularly of the scalp, are common. In children, a common presentation is acute suppurative parotitis, usually unilateral, associated with parotid pain and fever.[132,133,141,142,144-146]

RELATED PHYSICAL FINDINGS

Acute pulmonary presentations range from bronchitis to acute pneumonia, lung abscess, or empyema. Septicemia can lead to jaundice, hepatosplenomegaly, miliary pulmonary disease, myocarditis, and severe gastroenteritis. Chronic pulmonary melioidosis resembles fibrocavitary tuberculosis or lung abscesses both clinically and radiologically. The disseminated form of chronic disease may extend over many months, causing septic arthritis, osteomyelitis, suppurative lymphadenopathy, and visceral abscesses.

LABORATORY FINDINGS

B. pseudomallei grows on ordinary agar but the addition of gentamicin prevents overgrowth by other bacteria. The laboratory should be alerted of possible melioidosis so that special media can be used.[147,148] Polymerase chain reaction tests are more rapid than culture.[149,150] On histopathologic examination, sharply circumscribed abscesses are found in many organs and in the subcutaneous tissues, often with a surrounding granulomatous response.

DIFFERENTIAL DIAGNOSIS

The disease is a great imitator and diagnosis requires confirmed identification of the organism. Acute melioidosis may mimic typhoid fever, staphylococcal pneumonia, disseminated fungal infections (particularly from *Penicillium marneffei* in Thailand), glanders, or septicemia.[151] Chronic melioidosis resembles pulmonary tuberculosis, nocardiosis, deep fungal infection, and bacterial lung abscess. Chronic skin infections and draining sinuses in individuals from endemic areas should raise the possibility of melioidosis, as should an acute suppurative parotitis in a child from an endemic area.[152]

The diagnosis is supported by a recent or remote history of travel to Southeast Asia or northern Australia in a patient with unexplained sepsis. The finding of bipolar-stained Gram-negative bacilli strengthens the diagnosis. Culture of the organism establishes the etiology. Rising antibody titers also confirm the diagnosis. The indirect hemagglutination assay is the most commonly used test in Southeast Asia because it is simple to perform and cheap.[149,150,153]

TREATMENT

Antibiotic susceptibility must be determined for each isolate. In Australia's Northern Territory, where melioidosis is relatively common, treatment consists of at least 2 weeks of IV antibiotics (usually ceftazidime and carbapenem). This should be followed by several months of high-dose oral therapy with an antibiotic such as trimethoprim-sulfamethoxazole[144] or amoxicillin-clavulanic acid (or longer in the case of osteomyelitis or multiple suppurative foci) to reduce the risk of relapse.[133,154] Abscesses should be drained surgically, but only after the patient is taking appropriate antibiotics to help prevent bacteremia.

PROGNOSIS, CLINICAL COURSE, AND COMPLICATIONS

In septicemic melioidosis accompanied by shock and dissemination to skin and viscera, mortality is approximately 50%. In localized cutaneous melioidosis without bacteremia, mortality is less than 9%.

PREVENTION

There are no vaccines against melioidosis. People with diabetes or chronic renal disease should avoid exposure to fresh water when in endemic areas, particularly if they have open skin wounds. After such exposures, the skin should be cleansed thoroughly but there are no data on antibiotic prophylaxis.

ERYSIPELOID

AT-A-GLANCE

- An occupational zoonosis is caused by *Erysipelothrix rhusiopathiae* and associated with percutaneous trauma while handling raw fish or poultry.
- Classic dermatologic presentation is localized nonsuppurative purple-red plaques on the dorsal hands. Rare chronic and bacteremic forms exist.

ETIOLOGY AND EPIDEMIOLOGY

Erysipeloid, an acute infection of traumatized skin caused by *Erysipelothrix rhusiopathiae* (formerly *Erysipelothrix insidiosa*), occurs most frequently in fishermen, butchers, kitchen workers, and others who handle raw fish, poultry (especially turkey), and meat products.[149,150,155-157] The disease is especially common in pigs, where it is known as swine erysipelas. In humans, erysipeloid occurs primarily during the summer months and can be considered an occupational dermatosis.

E. rhusiopathiae is a thin, Gram-positive, microaerophilic, nonmotile bacillus that is hardy enough to survive putrefaction of tissue and exposure to saltwater or freshwater. The organism is found in rats, birds, the slime on saltwater fish, and crabs and other shellfish, and is associated with poultry, meats, hides, and bones.

In humans, organisms usually enter broken skin on the hands and takes 1 of the 4 clinical forms: (a) a local nonsuppurative cutaneous infection (erysipeloid of Rosenbach); (b) a diffuse chronic cutaneous form consisting of multiple plaques with sharply defined angular borders; (c) subacute bacterial endocarditis, particularly of the aortic valve; or (d) a bacteremic form without endocarditis, usually found only in immunocompromised patients. The disease does not seem to confer lasting immunity.[158]

CLINICAL FINDINGS

HISTORY

The patient is usually employed in the fishing or animal product industry. After inoculation, there is an incubation period of 2 to 7 days. Initially, burning pain occurs at the injured site, then a violaceous dermal plaque develops. Lymphangitis and regional adenopathy occasionally occur, as well as low-grade fever and malaise. Bacteremia and endocarditis are rare but serious sequelae. Untreated, erysipeloid usually heals on its own within 3 weeks.

CUTANEOUS LESIONS

The distinctive erysipeloid lesion is usually on a finger or the back of the hand; is violaceous, warm, and tender; and has well-defined, raised margins with an angular or polygonal border (Fig. 156-4). It often involves the web spaces but spares the terminal phalanges and does not progress beyond the wrist. The borders usually expand, whereas the central region clears without desquamation or ulceration. Rarely, multiple lesions distant from the original site of injury arise, presumably through bacteremic spread. Postinflammatory hyperpigmentation may persist after the lesion resolves.

RELATED PHYSICAL FINDINGS

Arthritis may be associated with the local lesion, and, in rare cases, distant joints are involved. Sepsis produces typical peripheral stigmata, including signs of endocarditis.[156]

LABORATORY FINDINGS

Gram stains rarely show *E. rhusiopathiae*, although culturing tissue from the advancing edge may reveal

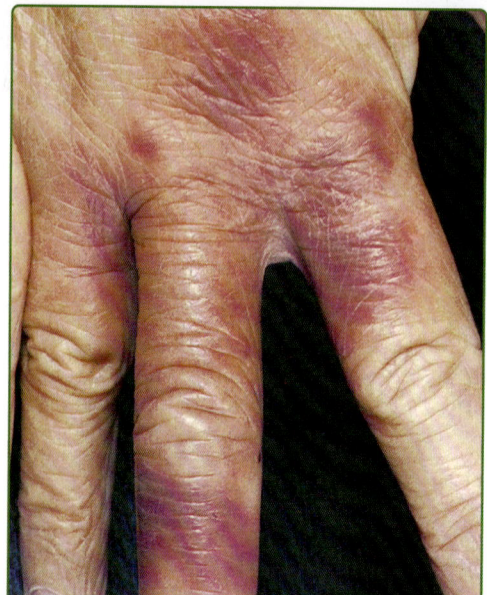

Figure 156-4 Erysipeloid. Characteristically, the violaceous, sharply marginated lesion is composed of macules and plaques and is located on the hand.

the organism. Growth occurs best on serum-fortified media between 30°C and 37°C (86°F and 98.6°F) under hypercapnic conditions. Agar-gel diffusion precipitation or fluorescent antibody techniques are helpful in establishing the diagnosis.[149,150]

HISTOPATHOLOGY

The findings are nonspecific but may include marked superficial dermal edema, vascular dilation, and mixed lymphocytic and neutrophilic perivascular infiltrates.

DIFFERENTIAL DIAGNOSIS

The character of the local lesion in a person handling fresh meat or fish products suggests the diagnosis. As its name suggests, erysipeloid resembles other forms of bacterial cellulitis or erysipelas. It may resemble a severe, acute irritant contact dermatitis. In erysipelas, the central area is most affected region compared with central clearing in erysipeloid. "Seal finger" may be mistaken for erysipeloid.

TREATMENT

The treatment of choice for erysipeloid is high-dose penicillin or ampicillin for 7 to 10 days. Patients who cannot take penicillins may be treated with a third-generation cephalosporin (such as ceftriaxone), imipenem, or ciprofloxacin (see Table 156-1). This recommendation is based primarily on in vitro studies, not clinical experience. If arthritis, septicemia, or endocarditis is present, the penicillin dosage should be increased and the drug should be administered IV for several weeks.[156]

PROGNOSIS, CLINICAL COURSE, AND COMPLICATIONS

Untreated lesions usually last for 2 to 3 weeks but may have waxing-and-waning cycles over several months. Improvement is often dramatic and recurrence is rare if penicillin is administered. The prognosis in systemic infections depends on early and appropriate treatment. The bacteremic form occasionally leads to endocarditis with its attendant morbidity and mortality.

PREVENTION

Erysipeloid can be prevented by wearing gloves when handling live animals or animal products and by washing skin wounds promptly with soap and water.

STREPTOCOCCUS INIAE INFECTIONS

AT-A-GLANCE

- Caused by a recently recognized streptococcal species that colonizes or infects freshwater fish, such as tilapia, grown in intense aquaculture.
- Most human clinical cases present as cellulitis of the hand after an accidental puncture wound during preparation of live fish for cooking.
- Bacteremia commonly occurs.

ETIOLOGY AND EPIDEMIOLOGY

S. iniae is a recently recognized Gram-positive coccus that colonizes the skin of freshwater fish, particularly those raised in intense aquaculture.

It has been found in tilapia, hybrid bass, rainbow trout, coho salmon, and other species, and can cause fatal epizootics of piscine meningoencephalitis.[159] The species name derives from the Amazonian freshwater dolphin, *Inia geoffrensis*, from which it was first isolated. In dolphins, *S. iniae* causes slow-growing nodular abscesses of the skin and subcutaneous tissues, giving it the vernacular name "golf ball disease." The condition has been noted only in captive dolphins that presumably are exposed to *S. iniae* in the fish in their diets.[160]

In humans, *S. iniae* infection usually causes hand cellulitis after the handling of live freshwater fish, particularly farm-raised tilapia (*Tilapia* sp. and *Oreochromis* sp.). Most cases have been reported in cities in China and in Asian communities in North America, particularly Toronto, where the practice of buying live fish for home preparation, rather than buying fresh fish that have already been killed and cleaned, is common.[161] Because of these cultural practices, most people who develop *S. iniae* infection are elderly (average age: >65 years) individuals of East Asian descent. Furthermore, most have underlying medical conditions, such as diabetes mellitus or cirrhosis, that predispose them to infection.[162]

CLINICAL FINDINGS

HISTORY AND CUTANEOUS LESIONS

The key element in the history is the rapid onset of hand cellulitis within 1 to 3 days after the handling of live farm-raised fish. Ascending lymphangitis and fever are early features, but neither skin necrosis nor bullae occur.[163]

RELATED PHYSICAL FINDINGS

Bacteremia frequent complicates *S. iniae* cellulitis and may lead to septic arthritis, meningitis, osteomyelitis, and endocarditis.[163]

LABORATORY FINDINGS

Cellulitis with *S. iniae* is probably underdiagnosed because many practitioners treat hand cellulitis empirically as if it were caused by *Staphylococcus aureus* or *S. pyogenes*. Furthermore, confirmation by culture of *S. iniae* is difficult because the organism exhibits variable hemolysis and cannot be placed into a Lancefield group. In culture, it resembles *Streptococcus viridans*, *Streptococcus uberis*, and *Streptococcus dysgalactiae*.

DIFFERENTIAL DIAGNOSIS

As of this writing, all reported cases have followed the culinary handling of live freshwater fish, usually tilapia. The diagnosis should be considered in individuals who develop hand cellulitis after such exposure, with or without recognized percutaneous injury. Other common causes of cellulitis (*S. pyogenes*, *S. aureus*) as well as other freshwater and fishborne pathogens (*A. hydrophila* and *V. vulnificus*) should be considered.

PROGNOSIS AND TREATMENT

The infection will respond within 2 to 4 days to penicillin, the treatment of choice. The pathogen is also susceptible to cephalosporins, macrolides, quinolones, and vancomycin, but is resistant to tetracyclines. Treatment should be maintained for 10 days or longer if there are extracutaneous complications.[163]

PREVENTION

Aquaculture farms are becoming increasingly aware of *S. iniae* infections in their produce and have an economic incentive to maintain healthy fish. Nevertheless, cooks who prepare live-bought, aquaculture-raised fish will continue to be exposed to this pathogen.

CHROMOBACTERIUM VIOLACEUM INFECTIONS

Chromobacterium violaceum is a facultatively anaerobic, Gram-negative, motile, flagellated bacillus found as a saprophyte in tropical and subtropical freshwater and soil. It is rarely pathogenic except to people with disorders of neutrophil function, especially inherited chronic granulomatous disease, who have difficulty generating an adequate host response to catalase-producing organisms, such as *C. violaceum*. Infection occurs after open skin is exposed to a contaminated source, such as stagnant or muddy water. Nearly all U.S. cases have occurred in southeastern states during summer months. After exposure, cellulitis and fevers soon develop. Pustules and nodules may appear, followed by regional adenopathy. The organisms may disseminate hematogenously, causing ecthyma gangrenosum, visceral abscesses, abdominal pain, septic shock, and death. *C. violaceum* should be cultured on a tryptophan-supplemented medium, where it will produce water-insoluble, metallic-appearing, dark-purple colonies. It is often misidentified as a *Vibrio* or *Aeromonas* or regarded as a contaminant, which delays proper treatment, possibly leading to fatal consequences in immunodeficient patients who are vulnerable to this organism. Biopsy shows a necrotizing vasculitis, bacilli in the vessels, and minimal neutrophilic infiltrate.

Treatment consists of surgical drainage of cutaneous and visceral abscesses, along with several weeks of parenteral antibiotics. Limited data show that parenteral carbapenems, chloramphenicol with gentamicin, and fluoroquinolones are effective. A prolonged course of oral doxycycline or cotrimoxazole is necessary to reduce risk of relapse. Subsequent fevers or abdominal pain may indicate need for abdominal CT or ultrasonographs to screen for abscesses. Melioidosis has a similar epidemiology, occurring in people exposed to stagnant water in tropical and subtropical environments, skin and soft-tissue lesions, sepsis and visceral abscesses, with shock and death. Anyone with *C. violaceum* infection requires evaluation for immunodeficiency, particularly chronic granulomatous disease.[164]

LEPTOSPIROSIS

AT-A-GLANCE

- Waterborne zoonosis with worldwide distribution caused by serovars of *Leptospira interrogans*, which are excreted in urine of reservoir animals, especially rodents. Outbreaks during rainy seasons or after flooding in areas with poor sanitation.
- Most human cases are mild or subclinical. In severe cases there may be fever, hepatic and renal failure, jaundice, hemorrhage, and death.
- Cutaneous findings include jaundice, conjunctival suffusion, petechiae, and nonspecific papules.

ETIOLOGY AND EPIDEMIOLOGY

Leptospirosis is a waterborne zoonosis caused by *Leptospira interrogans*. The disease is found worldwide, except in the polar regions, wherever animal urine can contaminate bodies of freshwater. Rodents are the most important reservoirs, although more than 160 species of mammals are known to harbor *Leptospira*, including wild, farm, pet, and laboratory animals. Infected humans can also serve as transient reservoirs, particularly in urban slums in the wet tropics. Reservoir animals excrete leptospires in their urine, which contaminate the environment and can survive in water sources for months to years.[165] Humans generally acquire the disease through broken skin after direct contact with an infected animal or exposure to contaminated water or soil. People are infected less commonly through mucous membranes, ingestion of contaminated water, or inhalation of fomites.[166,167]

L. interrogans thrives in warm freshwater, so leptospirosis has its highest incidence in tropical areas, particularly those with inadequate sanitation and where people go barefoot. Leptospirosis is an important cause of undifferentiated fever in the developing world, along with dengue, malaria, and typhoid. Serologic surveys in some endemic regions suggest that more than 80% of people had prior infection.[168] The disease is most prevalent among children who play or swim in contaminated water and among adults with occupational exposures (eg, sugarcane workers or rice farmers) to infected animals or to contaminated soil and water. Travelers to hyperendemic areas, particularly ecotourists or adventure travelers who are exposed to contaminated water, are at increased risk. Many outbreaks of leptospirosis have been reported after heavy rains and floods as they cause sewers to overflow.[169] Hawaii has the highest incidence in the United States.[167,169]

CLINICAL FINDINGS

HISTORY

Patients usually have had recent occupational or recreational contact with contaminated water or mud. Most human infections are asymptomatic, self-limited, and detectable only on serologic surveys. Ill patients have 1 of 2 clinical forms of the disease: (a) a mild anicteric form that resolves without complications, or (b) a severe, icteric form (Weil disease). Both forms typically have 2 phases: the acute bacteremic phase, followed by the delayed immune or convalescent phase. Incubation usually takes 5 to 14 days and then the leptospiremic phase begins suddenly with headache, fever, chills, nausea, vomiting, abdominal pain, and myalgia (particularly of the calves and thighs). This initial nonspecific phase continues for about a week, then defervescence occurs.[170]

After several relatively asymptomatic days, the second phase of illness begins with low-grade fever. In severe cases, rash, meningitis, uveitis, and hepatic and renal failure may develop.

CUTANEOUS LESIONS

In the first week of illness, the conjunctivae become suffused (red but not exudative). Skin lesions occur in fewer than 50% of cases. These consist of nonspecific macules, papules, urticaria, and petechiae, mostly on the trunk. Petechiae are a consequence of profound thrombocytopenia. Desquamation and infarcts have been observed on the hands or feet of some infected children. Weil disease has prominent hepatic (jaundice) and renal (hematuria, azotemia) components. Hemorrhages occur in a variety of organs, including the skin, and petechiae are common on the palate. A variant called *pretibial fever* or *Fort Bragg fever*, caused by *L. interrogans* serovariant *autumnalis*, has a distinctive rash that appears on the fourth or fifth day of illness, consisting of slightly raised, 1- to 5-cm, tender, erythematous papules on the shins. The rash subsides within 4 to 7 days.[171]

RELATED PHYSICAL FINDINGS

Most patients present with a fever of unknown origin without localizing signs. Other physical findings depend on the severity of the presentation, ranging nuchal rigidity in aseptic meningitis; or jaundice, hepatomegaly, and interstitial nephritis in Weil disease. Some patients have generalized hemorrhages with epistaxis, hematuria, and GI bleeding, and pretibial fever with splenomegaly.

LABORATORY FINDINGS

Laboratory tests help establish the diagnosis and the disease's severity. Direct isolation of leptospires is possible from the blood or cerebrospinal fluid during the acute phase or from urine during the convalescent phase. A recently developed serum dipstick assay rapidly detects antileptospire immunoglobulin M or immunoglobulin M antibodies. Thrombocytopenia is common but the white blood cell count is widely variable, reaching levels up to 40,000 cells/μL in Weil disease. A cerebrospinal fluid pleocytosis, with up to several hundred mononuclear cells, may be present. Liver function abnormalities and jaundice are common. Azotemia and hematuria occur in patients with renal involvement.[166]

TREATMENT

Public health authorities in endemic areas recommend starting antibiotic therapy early, perhaps presumptively, to reduce the risk of severe disease while laboratory confirmation is awaited. Doxycycline is effective and can be taken prophylactically for short-term exposure in a hyperendemic area. Penicillin also has been recommended, although controlled studies are lacking, and it may precipitate a Jarisch-Herxheimer reaction (see Table 156-1).

PROGNOSIS, CLINICAL COURSE, AND COMPLICATIONS

Perhaps 90% of patients have either asymptomatic or mild anicteric disease. Both forms resolve spontaneously without complications. In Weil disease, close attention must be given to fluid and renal status. Untreated Weil disease has a mortality rate of 5% to 40%, usually from renal failure, less often from cardiopulmonary failure or pulmonary hemorrhage. Late sequelae among survivors of untreated illness include neuropsychiatric diseases.[172]

PREVENTION

Water sanitation and rodent control measures will reduce the incidence of leptospirosis in a community. There is no vaccine against leptospirosis. Individuals who expect frequent contact with contaminated water or soils (eg, military personnel or adventure travelers) should consider protective clothing and other ways to limit exposures or they may decrease the risk of disease by taking prophylactic doxycycline 200 mg, once weekly during these periods.[166,170]

DIPHTHERIA

AT-A-GLANCE

- Classic diphtheria produces adherent gray membranous pharyngeal lesions, which may cause lethal airway obstruction. Exotoxin may cause latent peripheral neuritis or lethal cardiomyopathy.
- Cutaneous diphtheria usually affects the legs and begins as tender pustules that break down to punched-out ulcers covered by gray membranes. It is primarily found in the tropics or in travelers returning from these areas.
- Diphtheria can be prevented with toxoid immunization. It is treatable with antibiotics and antitoxin.

ETIOLOGY AND EPIDEMIOLOGY

Diphtheria is an acute febrile illness caused by *Corynebacterium diphtheriae* that in 90% of cases affects the pharynx and mucous membranes of the upper respiratory tract. The clinical manifestations of diphtheria are caused by (a) acute membranous obstruction of the airway, and (b) the tardive effects of a potent exotoxin on the myocardium and on cranial and peripheral nerves. The classic oropharyngeal lesion is a gray, leathery membrane along the tonsils and soft palate. Cutaneous diphtheria, which is far less common, can present either as a primary skin lesion or as a secondary infection of an existing break in the skin. Cutaneous diphtheria occurs most commonly in people living in or returning from tropical areas.[173,174]

Indeed, diphtheria is an underrecognized skin pathogen in travelers returning from endemic areas, and prior immunization may not prevent subsequent cutaneous infection.[174,175] Cutaneous lesions may appear after insect bites, and coinfection with other skin commensals is common, which can lead to an impetiginized appearance. Diphtheria should be in the differential in a returning traveler with a nonhealing ulcer.[176]

Although diphtheroids are widespread in nature, humans are the only natural host for *C. diphtheriae*, which colonizes the pharynx of asymptomatic individuals. Disease occurs when a nonimmune person, usually someone very young or very old, is infected by a toxigenic strain of *C. diphtheriae*. Epidemics occur when such strains become widespread among nonimmune individuals. Diphtheria has been largely controlled in

Western nations by routine childhood immunization, which is directed against diphtheria's exotoxin, not against the bacteria itself.

With the decline of the public health system in the former Soviet states, epidemic diphtheria began there in the early 1990s, infecting more than 150,000 people and causing more than 5000 deaths. In the United States, diphtheria occurs mainly in marginalized populations (such as homeless people or migrant workers) who live in crowded, unhygienic conditions and lack periodic reimmunizations. Three outbreaks among indigent alcoholics in Seattle between 1972 and 1982 involved more than 1000 cases, of which 86% were cutaneous.[177]

Because of the widespread use of toxoid immunization, the disease is rare in this country. It should be stressed, however, that this protection does not prevent the development of the carrier state and subsequent spread of organisms to susceptible nonimmunes.

CLINICAL FINDINGS

HISTORY

Classic diphtheria presents with pharyngitis and low-grade fever 2–5 days after exposure to a carrier or, much more rarely, to fomites. A thick or leathery grayish white membrane adheres to pharyngeal walls and tonsillar pillars, and usually spreads asymmetrically onto the soft palate and uvula. As the disease progresses, the patient's neck becomes painful and swollen. There is often a unilateral bloody nasal discharge. Patients appear to have a toxic process, and ensuing tracheal edema may obstruct the airway, causing lethal suffocation.

Cutaneous diphtheria typically affects the lower extremity, involves 1 or more sites, and may occur with or without concomitant pharyngeal disease. In roughly one-third of patients with cutaneous diphtheria, the same strain of *C. diphtheriae* can be recovered from the respiratory tract, which suggests inadvertent autoinoculation as the cause of the skin lesions.

CUTANEOUS LESIONS

There are 2 types of skin involvement. The first is primary cutaneous diphtheria, which starts acutely as a tender pustule and then breaks down to form an enlarging oval punched-out ulcer with a gray membrane at the base (see Table 156-1). Later, the membrane becomes dark brown, and the ulcer's border acquires edematous, rolled, bluish margins.[175,176]

Wound diphtheria is a secondary infection by *C. diphtheriae* of an existing break in the skin. This type accounts for almost all cases of cutaneous diphtheria reported in the United States. Preexisting skin lesions affected include those caused by abrasions, chronic dermatoses (eg, eczema or scabies), and common pyodermas already infected with *Staphylococcus* or *Streptococcus*. A painful ulcer is partly covered by a brownish-gray membrane, drains pus, and is surrounded by edema and erythema. In the outbreak in Seattle among indigent alcoholics, coinfection with *S. pyogenes* occurred in 73% of diphtheritic skin lesions.[177] *C. diphtheriae* has been recovered from lesions resembling impetigo, ecthyma, and infected insect bites. Whether these are truly infected or merely colonized is not clear. Mucosa of the nose, conjunctivae, or vagina can exhibit membranous diphtheria, although these cases are quite rare.

RELATED PHYSICAL FINDINGS

The most important other manifestations of diphtheria are the toxin's effects on the heart and nerves. Myocarditis and conductive heart block may develop 1 to 2 weeks after onset, whereas cranial or peripheral neuropathies may develop 2 weeks to several months after the primary lesion. Neurologic manifestations include blurred vision, diplopia, numbness of the tongue, palatal paralysis, and peripheral motor and sensory neuropathies. A Guillain-Barré–like syndrome has been reported in 3% to 5% of patients with cutaneous diphtheria.

LABORATORY FINDINGS

C. diphtheriae can be isolated from either the skin ulcer or pharyngeal membrane. It is a Gram-positive, club-shaped rod that exhibits metachromatic bipolar granules on staining with methylene blue. The organism grows well on standard culture media, but other bacteria may obscure it. Therefore, selective media such as Löffler or tellurite agar should be used. The histopathologic features of cutaneous diphtheria are nondiagnostic, and the membrane is composed of coagulation necrosis and inflammatory cells. Not all strains of *C. diphtheriae* produce diphtheria toxin, so it is recommended that the pathogen be sent to a reference laboratory to determine the toxigenicity of the particular strain.

DIFFERENTIAL DIAGNOSIS

Cutaneous diphtheria may resemble deep streptococcal or staphylococcal ecthyma, tropical ulcer, Buruli ulcer, cutaneous anthrax, cutaneous tularemia, pyoderma gangrenosum, and other entities listed on Table 156-1. Tropical ulcer, also painful, usually extends into or below the fascia. Buruli ulcer is painless. Most bacterially infected ulcers do not develop membranous coverings. Cutaneous deep fungal infections (eg, coccidioidomycosis) usually have irregular hyperkeratotic borders and lack surrounding erythema.

Diphtheria should be suspected in a patient with membranous tonsillar pharyngitis with asymmetric extension onto the soft palate and uvula. In methylene blue–stained smears from the edge of the membrane, the characteristic beaded metachromatic rods can be seen, but confirmation requires culture and demonstration of toxin production. However, the presence of a classic pharyngeal membrane is sufficient evidence to begin immediate treatment for diphtheria. Pharyngitis caused by *Streptococci*, gonococci, infectious mononucleosis, primary syphilis, Vincent's angina, or candidiasis can resemble faucial diphtheria (or can complicate the diagnosis of diphtheria).[173,178]

TREATMENT

Pharyngotonsillar diphtheria requires treatment with antibiotics (to kill the bacteria) and antitoxin (to neutralize the exotoxin). Treatment should be started on clinical suspicion without awaiting culture confirmation, because toxin produced in the interim might damage the myocardium irreversibly.

Cutaneous diphtheria must be treated with antibiotics and antitoxin (see Table 156-1). The antibiotic of choice is high-dose IV penicillin or, for those unable to take penicillin, erythromycin. Diphtheria antitoxin, available from the CDC, is administered IV after careful testing for horse serum hypersensitivity. Injection of antitoxin subcutaneously around and under the ulcer, along with superficial application to the lesion, may be beneficial, but data are incomplete. After antitoxin and antibiotics are administered, the membrane should be debrided and the ulcer kept clean. Patients with either form of the disease should be isolated for roughly 14 days.

PROGNOSIS, CLINICAL COURSE, AND COMPLICATIONS

If treatment is started early, the prognosis is excellent. Pharyngeal cultures should be repeated 2 weeks after completing treatment. In untreated, unimmunized persons with cutaneous diphtheria, ulcers may persist for as long as 6 months. Myocarditis and heart block may lead to congestive heart failure. Neurologic signs may appear 5 weeks to 5 months after the onset of illness and almost always resolve. Diphtheria deaths are usually the result of acute airway obstruction.

PREVENTION

The disease is largely preventable through routine immunizations. Many adults are unaware that they should receive a dose of tetanus and diphtheria toxoid (called Td) every 10 years. If a case of cutaneous or pharyngeal diphtheria does occur, close contacts, even if asymptomatic, should undergo cultures of their oropharynx and nasopharynx and of any skin lesions. All contacts should receive antibiotic prophylaxis with oral erythromycin or penicillin (or a single IM injection of benzathine penicillin). In addition, contacts whose diphtheria immunization status is unclear or incomplete should be immunized with diphtheria toxoid. For children, 7 years of age and older, and adults, the adult formulation of the combined Td preparation should be used rather than the pediatric diphtheria, pertussis, and tetanus (DPT) vaccine. Modern epidemics are controlled through mass immunizations.

OTHER CUTANEOUS DIPHTHEROID INFECTIONS

Corynebacterium ulcerans is a common commensal organism in cattle. Humans are rarely infected but can become ill after direct contact with cattle or by drinking raw milk. Pharyngeal disease is most common but cutaneous lesions, resembling those caused by *C. diphtheriae*, have been reported. Some strains of *C. ulcerans* produce the same diphtheria exotoxin, albeit in smaller quantities.[179] *Corynebacterium pseudotuberculosis*, which causes caseous lymphadenitis in ruminants, occasionally causes a similar necrotizing lymphadenitis in humans.

An organism closely related to corynebacteria, *Rhodococcus equi* (formerly *Corynebacterium equi*), causes pulmonary disease in AIDS patients. Rarely, this organism, which resembles *C. diphtheriae* on Gram-staining, can cause skin and soft-tissue infections in healthy individuals, especially those exposed to horse manure or after an injury contaminated with soil.

REFERENCES

1. Hart CA, Beeching NJ. A spotlight on anthrax. *Clin Dermatol*. 2002;20:365.
2. Anthrax. In: Heymann DL, ed. *Control of Communicable Diseases Manual*. 20th ed. Washington, DC: American Public Health Association; 2006:21.
3. Swartz MN. Recognition and management of anthrax—an update. *N Engl J Med*. 2001;345:1621.
4. Centers for Disease Control and Prevention (CDC). Gastrointestinal anthrax after an animal-hide drumming event—New Hampshire and Massachusetts, 2009. *MMWR Morb Mortal Wkly Rep*. 2010;59(28):872-877.
5. Centers for Disease Control and Prevention (CDC). Tularemia—Missouri, 2000-2007. *MMWR Morb Mortal Wkly Rep*. 2009;58(27):744-748.
6. Berger T, Kassirer M, Aran AA. Injectional anthrax—new presentation of an old disease. *Euro Surveill*. 2014;19(32).
7. Hicks CW, Sweeney DA, Cui X, et al. An overview of anthrax infection including the recently identified form of disease in injection drug users. *Intensive Care Med*. 2012;38(7):1092-1104.
8. Adalja AA, Toner E, Inglesby TV. Clinical management of potential bioterrorism-related conditions. *N Engl J Med*. 2015;372(10):954-962.
9. Woods CW, Ospanov K, Myrzabekov A, et al. Risk fac-

tors for human anthrax among contacts of anthrax-infected livestock in Kazakhstan. *Am J Trop Med Hyg.* 2004;71(1):48-52.
10. Shiferaw G. Anthrax in Wabessa village in the Dessie Zuria district of Ethiopia. *Rev Sci Tech.* 2004; 23(3):951-956.
11. Ichhpujani RL, Rajagopal V, Bhattacharya D, et al. An outbreak of human anthrax in Mysore (India). *J Commun Dis.* 2004;36(3):199-204.
12. Thappa DM, Karthikeyan K. Anthrax: an overview within the Indian subcontinent. *Int J Dermatol.* 2001; 40(3):216-222.
13. Karahocagil MK, Akdeniz N, Akdeniz H, et al. Cutaneous anthrax in Eastern Turkey: a review of 85 cases. *Clin Exp Dermatol.* 2008;33(4):406-411.
14. Ray TK, Hutin YJ, Murhekar MV. Cutaneous anthrax, West Bengal, India, 2007. *Emerg Infect Dis.* 2009; 15(3):497-499.
15. Siamudaala VM, Bwalya JM, Munang'andu HM, et al. Ecology and epidemiology of anthrax in cattle and humans in Zambia. *Jpn J Vet Res.* 2006;54(1):15-23.
16. Nishi JS, Ellsworth TR, Lee N, et al. An outbreak of anthrax (*Bacillus anthracis*) in free-roaming bison in the Northwest Territories, June-July 2006. *Can Vet J.* 2007;48(1):37-38.
17. Clegg SB, Turnbull PC, Foggin CM, et al. Massive outbreak of anthrax in wildlife in the Malilangwe Wildlife Reserve, Zimbabwe. *Vet Rec.* 2007;160(4):113-118.
18. Mongoh MN, Dyer NW, Stoltenow CL, et al. Risk factors associated with anthrax outbreak in animals in North Dakota, 2005: a retrospective case-control study. *Public Health Rep.* 2008;123(3):352-359.
19. Friebe S, van der Goot FG, Bürgi J. The ins and outs of anthrax toxin. *Toxins (Basel).* 2016;8(3).
20. Caksen H, Arabaci F, Abuhandan M, et al. Cutaneous anthrax in eastern Turkey. *Cutis.* 2001;67(6):488-492.
21. Smego RA Jr, Gebrian B, Desmangels G. Cutaneous manifestations of anthrax in rural Haiti. *Clin Infect Dis.* 1998;26(1):97-102.
22. Maguiña C, Flores Del Pozo J, Terashima A, et al. Cutaneous anthrax in Lima, Peru: retrospective analysis of 71 cases, including four with a meningoencephalic complication. *Rev Inst Med Trop Sao Paulo.* 2005;47(1):25-30.
23. Demirdag K, Ozden M, Saral Y, et al. Cutaneous anthrax in adults: a review of 25 cases in the eastern Anatolian region of Turkey. *Infection.* 2003;31(5):327-330.
24. Irmak H, Buzgan T, Karahocagil MK, et al. Cutaneous manifestations of anthrax in Eastern Anatolia: a review of 39 cases. *Acta Med Okayama.* 2003;57(5):235-240.
25. Shieh WJ, Guarner J, Paddock C, et al. The critical role of pathology in the investigation of bioterrorism-related cutaneous anthrax. *Am J Pathol.* 2003;163(5):1901-1910.
26. Carucci JA, McGovern TW, Norton SA, et al. Cutaneous anthrax management algorithm. *J Am Acad Dermatol.* 2002;47(5):766-769.
27. Bartlett JG, Inglesby TV Jr, Borio L. Management of anthrax. *Clin Infect Dis.* 2002;35(7):851-858.
28. Faghihi G, Siadat AH. Cutaneous anthrax associated with facial palsy: case report and literature review. *J Dermatolog Treat.* 2003;14(1):51-53.
29. Wright JG, Quinn CP, Shadomy S, et al. Use of anthrax vaccine in the United States: recommendations of the Advisory Committee on Immunization Practices (ACIP), 2009. *MMWR Recomm Rep.* 2010;59(RR-6):1-30.
30. Şenel E, Satılmış Ö, Acar B. Dermatologic manifestations of tularemia: a study of 151 cases in the mid-Anatolian region of Turkey. *Int J Dermatol.* 2015;54(1):e33-e37.
31. Jacobs RF. Tularemia. *Adv Pediatr Infect Dis.* 1996; 12:55-69.
32. Tularemia. In: Heymann DL, ed. *Control of Communicable Diseases Manual.* 18th ed. Washington DC: American Public Health Association; 2006:573.
33. Farlow J, Wagner DM, Dukerich M, et al. *Francisella tularensis* in the United States. *Emerg Infect Dis.* 2005;11(12):1835-1841.
34. Hayes EB. Tularemia. In: Goodman JL, Dennis DT, Sonenshine DE, eds. *Tick-Borne Diseases of Humans.* Washington, DC: ASM Press; 2005:207.
35. Eisen RJ, Mead PS, Meyer AM, et al. Ecoepidemiology of tularemia in the southcentral United States. *Am J Trop Med Hyg.* 2008;78(4):586-594.
36. Jounio U, Renko M, Uhari M. An outbreak of holarctica-type tularemia in pediatric patients. *Pediatr Infect Dis J.* 2010;29(2):160-162.
37. Cerný Z. Skin manifestations of tularemia. *Int J Dermatol.* 1994;33(7):468-470.
38. Maurin M, Gyuranecz M. Tularaemia: clinical aspects in Europe. *Lancet Infect Dis.* 2016;16(1):113-124.
39. Eliasson H, Bäck E. Tularaemia in an emergent area in Sweden: an analysis of 234 cases in five years. *Scand J Infect Dis.* 2007;39(10):880-889.
40. Kantardjiev T, Ivanov I, Velinov T, et al. Tularemia outbreak, Bulgaria, 1997-2005. *Emerg Infect Dis.* 2006; 12(4):678-680.
41. Feldman K, Enscore RE, Lathrop SL, et al. An outbreak of primary pneumonic tularemia on Martha's Vineyard. *N Engl J Med.* 2001;345(22):1601-1606.
42. Prentice MB, Rahalison L. Plague. *Lancet.* 2007; 369(9568):1196-1207.
43. Boisier P, Rahalison L, Rasolomaharo M, et al. Epidemiologic features of four successive annual outbreaks of bubonic plague in Mahajanga, Madagascar. *Emerg Infect Dis.* 2002;8(3):311-316.
44. Migliani R, Chanteau S, Rahalison L, et al. Epidemiological trends for human plague in Madagascar during the second half of the 20th century: a survey of 20,900 notified cases. *Trop Med Int Health.* 2006;11(8):1228-1237.
45. Stenseth NC, Atshabar BB, Begon M, et al. Plague: past, present, and future. *PLoS Med.* 2008;5(1):e3.
46. Foster CL, Mould K, Reynolds P, et al. Clinical problem-solving. Sick as a dog. *N Engl J Med.* 2015; 372(19):1845-1850.
47. Plague. In: Heymann DL, ed. *Control of Communicable Diseases Manual.* 18th ed. Washington, DC: American Public Health Association; 2006:406.
48. Centers for Disease Control and Prevention (CDC). Human plague–four states, 2006. *MMWR Morb Mortal Wkly Rep.* 2006;55(34):940-943. Accessed February 2, 2018.
49. Infectious Disease Epidemiology Section of the Louisiana Office of Public Health. Plague. Revised September 25, 2004. http://ldh.la.gov/assets/oph/Center-PHCH/Center-CH/infectious-epi/EpiManual/PlagueManual.pdf.
50. Butler T. Plague into the 21st century. *Clin Infect Dis.* 2009;49(5):736-742.
51. Chanteau S, Rahalison L, Ralafiarisoa L, et al. Development and testing of a rapid diagnostic test for bubonic and pneumonic plague. *Lancet.* 2003;361(9353):211-216.
52. Guarner J, Shieh WJ, Greer PW, et al. Immunohisto-

52. chemical detection of *Yersinia pestis* in formalin-fixed, paraffin-embedded tissue. *Am J Clin Pathol.* 2002;117(2):205-209.
53. Koirala J. Plague: disease, management, and recognition of act of terrorism. *Infect Dis Clin North Am.* 2006;20(2):273-287.
54. Brucellosis. In: Heymann DL, ed. *Control of Communicable Diseases Manual.* 18th ed. Washington, DC: American Public Health Association; 2006:82.
55. Pappas G, Akritidis N, Bosilkovski M, et al. Brucellosis. *N Engl J Med.* 2005;352(22):2325-2336.
56. Pappas G, Papadimitriou P, Akritidis N, et al. The new global map of human brucellosis. *Lancet Infect Dis.* 2006;6(2):91-99.
57. Al-Nassir W. Brucellosis. Medscape website. https://emedicine.medscape.com/article/213430-overview. Updated June 16, 2017. Accessed February 2, 2018.
58. Franco MP, Mulder M, Gilman RH, et al. Human brucellosis. *Lancet Infect Dis.* 2007;7(12):775-786.
59. Metin A, Akdeniz H, Buzgan T, Delice I. Cutaneous findings encountered in brucellosis and review of the literature. *Int J Dermatol.* 2001;40(7):434-438.
60. Milionis H, Christou L, Elisaf M. Cutaneous manifestations in brucellosis: case report and review of the literature. *Infection.* 2000;28(2):124-126.
61. Nagore E, Sánchez-Motilla JM, Navarro V, et al. Leukocytoclastic vasculitis as a cutaneous manifestation of systemic infection caused by *Brucella melitensis*. *Cutis.* 1999;63(1):25-27.
62. Perez C, Hernandez R, Murie M, et al. Relapsing leucocytoclastic vasculitis as the initial manifestation of acute brucellosis. *Br J Dermatol.* 1999;140(6):1177-1178.
63. Mazokopakis E, Christias E, Kofteridis D. Acute brucellosis presenting with erythema nodosum. *Eur J Epidemiol.* 2003;18(9):913-915.
64. Akcali C, Savas L, Baba M, et al. Cutaneous manifestations in brucellosis: a prospective study. *Adv Ther.* 2007;24(4):706-711.
65. Ashford DA, di Pietra J, Lingappa J, et al. Adverse events in humans associated with accidental exposure to the livestock brucellosis vaccine RB51. *Vaccine.* 2004;22(25-26):3435-3439.
66. Larsen JC, Johnson NH. Pathogenesis of *Burkholderia pseudomallei* and *Burkholderia mallei*. *Mil Med.* 2009;174(6):647-651.
67. Rega PP. CBRNE–Glanders and melioidosis. Medscape website. https://emedicine.medscape.com/article/830235-overview. Updated August 16, 2015. Accessed February 2, 2018.
68. Centers for Disease Control and Prevention (CDC). Glanders. https://www.cdc.gov/glanders/index.htm. Updated October 31, 2017. Accessed February 2, 2018.
69. Dvorak GD, Spickler AR. Glanders. *J Am Vet Med Assoc.* 2008;233(4):570-577.
70. Srinivasan A, Kraus CN, DeShazer D, et al. Glanders in a military research microbiologist. *N Engl J Med.* 2001;345(4):256-258.
71. Centers for Disease Control and Prevention (CDC). Laboratory-acquired human glanders–Maryland, May 2000. *MMWR Morb Mortal Wkly Rep.* 2000;49(24):532-535.
72. Bossi P, Tegnell A, Baka A, et al. Bichat guidelines for the clinical management of glanders and melioidosis and bioterrorism-related glanders and melioidosis. *Euro Surveill.* 2004;9(12):E17-E18.
73. Godey B, Morandi X, Bourdinière J, et al. Beware of dogs licking ears. *Lancet.* 1999;354(9186):1267-1268.
74. Arons MS, Fernando L, Polayes IM. *Pasteurella multocida*–the major cause of hand infections following domestic animal bites. *J Hand Surg Am.* 1982;7(1):47-52.
75. Hara H, Ochiai T, Morishima T, et al. *Pasteurella canis* osteomyelitis and cutaneous abscess after a domestic dog bite. *J Am Acad Dermatol.* 2002;46(5)(suppl):S151-S152.
76. Matsui T, Kayashima K, Kito M, et al. Three cases of Pasteurella multocida skin infection from pet cats. *J Dermatol.* 1996;23(7):502-504.
77. Talan DA, Citron DM, Abrahamian FM, et al. Bacteriologic analysis of infected dog and cat bites. *N Engl J Med.* 1999;340(2):85-92.
78. Talan DA, Abrahamian FM, Moran GJ, et al. Clinical presentation and bacteriologic analysis of infected human bites in patients presenting to emergency departments. *Clin Infect Dis.* 2003;37(11):1481-1489.
79. Migliore E, Serraino C, Brignone C, et al. Pasteurella multocida infection in a cirrhotic patient: case report, microbiological aspects and a review of literature. *Adv Med Sci.* 2009;54(1):109-112.
80. Nakwan N, Nakwan N, Atta T, et al. Neonatal pasteurellosis: a review of reported cases. *Arch Dis Child Fetal Neonatal Ed.* 2009;94(5):F373-F376.
81. Vinh DC, Embil JM. Severe skin and soft tissue infections and associated critical illness. *Curr Infect Dis Rep.* 2006;8(5):375-383.
82. Presutti RJ. Prevention and treatment of dog bites. *Am Fam Physician.* 2001;63(8):1567-1572.
83. Rat-bite fever. In: Heymann DL, ed. *Control of Communicable Diseases Manual.* 18th ed. Washington, DC: American Public Health Association; 2006:448.
84. Tandon R, Lee M, Curran E, et al. A 26-year-old woman with a rash on her extremities. *Clin Infect Dis.* 2006;43(12):1585-1586, 1616-1617.
85. Centers for Disease Control and Prevention (CDC). Fatal rat-bite fever–Florida and Washington, 2003. *MMWR Morb Mortal Wkly Rep.* 2005;53(51):1198-1202.
86. Ojukwu IC, Christy C. Rat-bite fever in children: case report and review. *Scand J Infect Dis.* 2002;34(6):474-477.
87. Freels LK, Elliott SP. Rat bite fever: Three case reports and a literature review. *Clin Pediatr (Phila).* 2004;43(3):291-295.
88. Andre JM, Freydiere AM, Benito Y, et al. Rat bite fever caused by *Streptobacillus moniliformis* in a child: human infection and rat carriage diagnosed by PCR. *J Clin Pathol.* 2005;58(11):1215-1216.
89. Elliott SP. Rat bite fever and *Streptobacillus moniliformis*. *Clin Microbiol Rev.* 2007;20(1):13-22.
90. Schachter ME, Wilcox L, Rau N, et al. Rat-bite fever, Canada. *Emerg Infect Dis.* 2006;12(8):1301-1302.
91. Gaastra W, Boot R, Ho HT, et al. Rat bite fever. *Vet Microbiol.* 2009;133(3):211-228.
92. White CP, Jewer DD. Seal finger: a case report and review of the literature. *Can J Plast Surg.* 2009;17(4):133-135.
93. Kouliev T, Cui V. Treatment and prevention of infection following bites of the Antarctic fur seal (*Arctocephalus gazella*). *Open Access Emerg Med.* 2015;7:17-20.
94. Westley BP, Horazdovsky RD, Michaels DL, et al. Identification of a novel Mycoplasma species in a patient with septic arthritis of the hip and seal finger. *Clin Infect Dis.* 2016 15;62(4):491-493.
95. Hartley JW, Pitcher D. Seal finger—tetracycline is first line. *J Infect.* 2002;45(2):71-75.

96. Allerberger F, Wagner M. Listeriosis: a resurgent foodborne infection. *Clin Microbiol Infect*. 2010;16(1):16-23.
97. Listeriosis. In: Heymann DL, ed. *Control of Communicable Diseases Manual*. 18th ed. Washington, DC: American Public Health Association; 2006:338.
98. Aureli P, Fiorucci GC, Caroli D, et al. An outbreak of febrile gastroenteritis associated with corn contaminated by *Listeria monocytogenes*. *N Engl J Med*. 2000;342(17):1236-1241.
99. Zelenik K, Avberšek J, Pate M, et al. Cutaneous listeriosis in a veterinarian with the evidence of zoonotic transmission—a case report. *Zoonoses Public Health*. 2014;61(4):238-241.
100. Godshall CE, Suh G, Lorber B. Cutaneous listeriosis. *J Clin Microbiol*. 2013;51(11):3591-3596.
101. Weinstein KB. *Listeria monocytogenes* Infection (Listeriosis). Medscape website. https://emedicine.medscape.com/article/220684-overview. Updated December 1, 2017. Accessed February 2, 2018.
102. Kelesidis T, Salhotra A, Fleisher J, et al. *Listeria endocarditis* in a patient with psoriatic arthritis on infliximab: are biologic agents as treatment for inflammatory arthritis increasing the incidence of *Listeria* infections? *J Infect*. 2010;60(5):386-396.
103. Lambotte O, Fihman V, Poyart C, et al. *Listeria monocytogenes* skin infection with cerebritis and haemophagocytosis syndrome in a bone marrow transplant recipient. *J Infect*. 2005;50(4):356-358.
104. Posfay-Barbe KM, Wald ER. Listeriosis. *Semin Fetal Neonatal Med*. 2009;14(4):228-233.
105. Cholera and other vibrioses. In: Heymann DL, ed. *Control of Communicable Diseases Manual*. 18th ed. Washington, DC: American Public Health Association; 2006:125.
106. Horseman MA, Surani S. A comprehensive review of *Vibrio vulnificus*: an important cause of severe sepsis and skin and soft-tissue infection. *Int J Infect Dis*. 2011;15(3):e157-e166.
107. Daniels NA. *Vibrio vulnificus* oysters: pearls and perils. *Clin Infect Dis*. 2011;52(6):788-792.
108. Ulusarac O, Carter E. Varied clinical presentations of *Vibrio vulnificus* infections: a report of four unusual cases and review of the literature. *South Med J*. 2004;97(2):163-168.
109. Patel VJ, Gardner E, Burton CS. *Vibrio vulnificus* septicemia and leg ulcer. *J Am Acad Dermatol*. 2002;46(5)(suppl):S144-S145.
110. Kuhnt-Lenz K, Krengel S, Fetscher S, et al. Sepsis with bullous necrotizing skin lesions due to *Vibrio vulnificus* acquired through recreational activities in the Baltic Sea. *Eur J Clin Microbiol Infect Dis*. 2004;23(1):49-52.
111. Frank C, Littman M, Alpers K, et al. *Vibrio vulnificus* wound infections after contact with the Baltic Sea, Germany. *Euro Surveill*. 2006;11(8):E060817.1.
112. Andersson Y, Ekdahl K. Wound infections due to *Vibrio cholerae* in Sweden after swimming in the Baltic Sea, summer 2006. *Euro Surveill*. 2006;11(8):E060803.2.
113. Centers for Disease Control and Prevention (CDC). *Vibrio* illnesses after Hurricane Katrina—multiple states, August-September 2005. *MMWR Morb Mortal Wkly Rep*. 2005;54(37):928-931.
114. Said R, Volpin G, Grimberg B, et al. Hand infections due to non-cholera *Vibrio* after injuries from St Peter's fish (*Tilapia zillii*). *J Hand Surg Br*. 1998;23(6):808-810.
115. Calif E, Shalom S. Hand infections caused by delayed inoculation of *Vibrio vulnificus*: does human skin serve as a potential reservoir of vibrios? *Hand Surg*. 2004;9(1):39-44.
116. Wilhelmi BJ, Calianos TA 2nd, Appelt EA, et al. Modified Dakin's solution for cutaneous vibrio infections. *Ann Plast Surg*. 1999;43(4):386-389.
117. Vugia DJ, Tabnak F, Newton AE, et al. Impact of 2003 state regulation on raw oyster-associated *Vibrio vulnificus* illnesses and deaths, California, USA. *Emerg Infect Dis*. 2013;19(8):1276-1280.
118. Ashdown LR, Koehler JM. The spectrum of *Aeromonas*-associated diarrhea in tropical Queensland, Australia. *Southeast Asian J Trop Med Public Health*. 1993;24(2):347-353.
119. Janda JM, Abbott SL. The genus *Aeromonas*: taxonomy, pathogenicity, and infection. *Clin Microbiol Rev*. 2010;23(1):35-73.
120. Ghenghesh KS, Ahmed SF, El-Khalek RA, et al. *Aeromonas*-associated infections in developing countries. *J Infect Dev Ctries*. 2008;2(2):81-98.
121. Papadakis V, Poniros N, Katsibardi K, et al. Fulminant *Aeromonas hydrophila* infection during acute lymphoblastic leukemia treatment. *J Microbiol Immunol Infect*. 2012;45(2):154-157.
122. Haycox CL, Odland PB, Coltrera MD, et al. Indications and complications of medicinal leech therapy. *J Am Acad Dermatol*. 1995;33(6):1053-1055.
123. Ouderkirk JP, Bekhor D, Turett GS, et al. *Aeromonas* meningitis complicating medicinal leech therapy. *Clin Infect Dis*. 2004;38(4):e36-e37.
124. Giltner CL, Bobenchik AM, Uslan DZ, et al. Ciprofloxacin-resistant *Aeromonas hydrophila* cellulitis following leech therapy. *J Clin Microbiol*. 2013;51(4):1324-1326.
125. Julià Manresa M, Vicente Villa A, Gené Giralt A, et al. *Aeromonas hydrophila* folliculitis associated with an inflatable swimming pool: mimicking *Pseudomonas aeruginosa* infection. *Pediatr Dermatol*. 2009;26(5):601-603.
126. Mulholland A, Yong-Gee S. A possible new cause of spa bath folliculitis: *Aeromonas hydrophila*. *Australas J Dermatol*. 2008;49(1):39-41.
127. Peacock SJ. Melioidosis. *Curr Opin Infect Dis*. 2006;19(5):421-428.
128. Kespechara K, Koysombat T, Pakamol S, et al. Infecting organisms in victims from the tsunami disaster: experiences from Bangkok Phuket Hospital, Thailand, *International Journal of Disaster Medicine*, 2005;3:1-4, 66-70. doi: 10.1080/15031430600069424.
129. Gold WL, Salit IE. *Aeromonas hydrophila* infections of skin and soft tissue: report of 11 cases and review. *Clin Infect Dis*. 1993;16(1):69-74.
130. Skoll PJ, Hudson DA, Simpson JA. *Aeromonas hydrophila* in burn patients. *Burns*. 1998;24(4):350-353.
131. Kelly KA, Koehler JM, Ashdown LR. Spectrum of extraintestinal disease due to *Aeromonas* species in tropical Queensland, Australia. *Clin Infect Dis*. 1993;16(4):574-579.
132. Cheng AC, Currie BJ. Melioidosis: epidemiology, pathophysiology, and management. *Clin Microbiol Rev*. 2005;18(2):383-416.
133. White NJ. Melioidosis. *Lancet*. 2003;361(9370):1715-1722.
134. Maharjan B, Chantratita N, Vesaratchavest M, et al. Recurrent melioidosis in patients in northeast Thailand is frequently due to reinfection rather than relapse. *J Clin Microbiol*. 2005;43(12):6032-6034.
135. Currie BJ, Fisher DA, Anstey NM, et al. Melioidosis: acute and chronic disease, relapse and re-activation. *Trans R Soc Trop Med Hyg*. 2000;94(3):301-304.
136. Cheng AC, Jacups SP, Gal D, et al. Extreme weather

events and environmental contamination are associated with case-clusters of melioidosis in the Northern Territory of Australia. *Int J Epidemiol.* 2006;35(2):323-329.
137. Currie BJ, Jacups SP. Intensity of rainfall and severity of melioidosis, Australia. *Emerg Infect Dis.* 2003; 9(12):1538-1542.
138. Ngauy V, Lemeshev Y, Sadkowski L, et al. Cutaneous melioidosis in a man who was taken as a prisoner of war by the Japanese during World War II. *J Clin Microbiol.* 2005;43(2):970-972.
139. Melioidosis. In: Heymann DL, ed. *Control of Communicable Diseases Manual.* 18th ed. Washington, DC: American Public Health Association; 2006:386.
140. Limmathurotsakul D, Chaowagul W, Chierakul W, et al. Risk factors for recurrent melioidosis in northeast Thailand. *Clin Infect Dis.* 2006;43(8):979-986.
141. Thng TG, Seow CS, Tan HH, et al. A case of nonfatal cutaneous melioidosis. *Cutis.* 2003(4);72:310-312.
142. Torrens JK, McWhinney PH, Tompkins DS. A deadly thorn: a case of imported melioidosis. *Lancet.* 1999; 353(9157):1016.
143. Currie BJ, Jacups SP, Cheng AC, et al. Melioidosis epidemiology and risk factors from a prospective whole-population study in northern Australia. *Trop Med Int Health.* 2004;9(11):1167-1174.
144. Gibney KB, Cheng AC, Currie BJ. Cutaneous melioidosis in the tropical top end of Australia: a prospective study and review of the literature. *Clin Infect Dis.* 2008;47(5):603-609.
145. Tran D, Tan HH. Cutaneous melioidosis. *Clin Exp Dermatol.* 2002;27(4):280-282.
146. Wang YS, Wong CH, Kurup A. Cutaneous melioidosis and necrotizing fasciitis caused by *Burkholderia. Emerg Infect Dis.* 2003;9(11):1484-1485.
147. Peacock SJ, Chieng G, Cheng AC, et al. Comparison of Ashdown's medium, *Burkholderia cepacia* medium, and *Burkholderia pseudomallei* selective agar for clinical isolation of *Burkholderia pseudomallei. J Clin Microbiol.* 2005;43(10):5359-5361.
148. Ulrich RL, Ulrich MP, Schell MA, et al. Development of a polymerase chain reaction assay for the specific identification of *Burkholderia mallei* and differentiation from *Burkholderia pseudomallei* and other closely related Burkholderiaceae. *Diagn Microbiol Infect Dis.* 2006;55(1):37-45.
149. Dunbar SA, Clarridge JE III. Potential errors in recognition of *Erysipelothrix rhusiopathiae. J Clin Microbiol.* 2000;38(3):1302-1304.
150. Brooke CJ, Riley TV. *Erysipelothrix rhusiopathiae*: bacteriology, epidemiology and clinical manifestations of an occupational pathogen. *J Med Microbiol.* 1999;48(9):789-799.
151. Kingsley PV, Arunkumar G, Tipre M, et al. Pitfalls and optimal approaches to diagnose melioidosis. *Asian Pac J Trop Med.* 2016;9(6):515-524.
152. Currie BJ, Fisher DA, Howard DM, et al. Endemic melioidosis in tropical northern Australia: A 10-year prospective study and review of the literature. *Clin Infect Dis.* 2000;31(4):981-986.
153. Athan E, Allworth AM, Engler C, et al. Melioidosis in tsunami survivors. *Emerg Infect Dis.* 2005;11(10): 1638-1639.
154. Cheng AC, Fisher DA, Anstey NM, et al. Outcomes of patients with melioidosis treated with meropenem. *Antimicrob Agents Chemother.* 2004;48(5): 1763-1765.
155. Barnett JH, Estes SA, Wirman JA, et al. Erysipeloid. *J Am Acad Dermatol.* 1983;9(1):116-123.
156. Gorby GL, Peacock JE Jr. *Erysipelothrix rhusiopathiae* endocarditis: microbiologic, epidemiologic, and clinical features of an occupational disease. *Rev Infect Dis.* 1988;10(2):317-325.
157. Facklam R, Elliott J, Shewmaker L, et al. Identification and characterization of sporadic isolates of *Streptococcus iniae* isolated from humans. *J Clin Microbiol.* 2005;43(2):933-937.
158. Bonar CJ, Wagner RA. A third report of golf ball disease in an Amazon River dolphin (*Inia geoffrensis*) associated with *Streptococcus iniae. J Zoo Wildl Med.* 2003;34(3):296-301.
159. de Siqueira IC, Dias J, Ruf H, et al. *Chromobacterium violaceum* in siblings, Brazil. *Emerg Infect Dis.* 2005;11(9):1443-1445.
160. Sirinavin S, Techasaensiri C, Benjaponpitak S, et al. Invasive *Chromobacterium violaceum* infection in children: case report and review. *Pediatr Infect Dis J.* 2005;24(6):559-561.
161. Lau SK, Woo PC, Tse H, et al. Invasive *Streptococcus iniae* infections outside North America. *J Clin Microbiol.* 2003;41(3):1004-1009.
162. Baiano JC, Barnes AC. Towards control of *Streptococcus iniae. Emerg Infect Dis.* 2009;15(12):1891-1896.
163. Weinstein MR, Litt M, Kertesz DA, et al. Invasive infectious due to a fish pathogen, *Streptococcus iniae. N Engl J Med.* 1997;337(9):589-594.
164. Brown KL, Stein A, Morrell DS. Ecthyma gangrenosum and septic shock syndrome secondary to *Chromobacterium violaceum. J Am Acad Dermatol.* 2006;54(5) (suppl):S224-S228.
165. Puca E, Pilaca A, Kalo T, et al. Ocular and cutaneous manifestation of leptospirosis acquired in Albania: a retrospective analysis with implications for travel medicine. *Travel Med Infect Dis.* 2016;14(2): 143-147.
166. Leptospirosis. In: Heymann DL, ed. *Control of Communicable Diseases Manual.* 18th ed. Washington, DC: American Public Health Association; 2006:384.
167. Katz AR, Ansdell VE, Effler PV, et al. Leptospirosis in Hawaii, 1974-1998: epidemiologic analysis of 353 laboratory-confirmed cases. *Am J Trop Med Hyg.* 2002;66(1):61-70.
168. Haake DA. Molecular epidemiology of leptospirosis in the Amazon. *PLoS Med.* 2006;3(8):e302.
169. Centers for Disease Control and Prevention (CDC). Brief report: leptospirosis after flooding of a university campus—Hawaii, 2004. *MMWR Morb Mortal Wkly Rep.* 2006;55(5):125-127.
170. Phraisuwan P, Whitney EA, Tharmaphornpilas P, et al. Leptospirosis: skin wounds and control strategies, Thailand, 1999. *Emerg Infect Dis.* 2002;8(12): 1455-1459.
171. Gompf SG. Leptospirosis. Medscape website. https://emedicine.medscape.com/article/220563-overview. Updated June 13, 2018. Accessed February 2, 2018.
172. Wilson MR, Naccache SN, Samayoa E, et al. Actionable diagnosis of neuroleptospirosis by next-generation sequencing. *N Engl J Med.* 2014;370(25):2408-2417.
173. Diphtheria. In: Heymann DL, ed. *Control of Communicable Diseases Manual.* 18th ed. Washington, DC: American Public Health Association; 2006:188.
174. May ML, McDougall RJ, Robson JM. *Corynebacterium diphtheriae* and the returned tropical traveler. *J Travel Med.* 2014;21(1):39-44.
175. Sánchez ME, Alvarez JB, León SH. Chronic nonhealing ulcerated nodules in a Spanish boy after traveling. *JAMA Dermatol.* 2015;151(11):1247-1248.

176. Nelson TG, Mitchell CD, Sega-Hall GM, et al. Cutaneous ulcers in a returning traveller: a rare case of imported diphtheria in the UK. *Clin Exp Dermatol.* 2016;41(1):57-59.
177. Harnisch JP, Tronca E, Nolan CM, et al. Diphtheria among alcoholic urban adults: a decade of experience in Seattle. *Ann Intern Med.* 1989;111(1):71-82.
178. Hart PE, Lee PY, Macallan DC, et al. Cutaneous and pharyngeal diphtheria imported from the Indian subcontinent. *Postgrad Med J.* 1996;72(852):619-620.
179. Wagner J, Ignatius R, Voss S, et al. Infection of the skin caused by *Corynebacterium ulcerans* and mimicking classical cutaneous diphtheria. *Clin Infect Dis.* 2001;33(9):1598-1600.

Chapter 157 :: Tuberculosis and Infections with Atypical Mycobacteria
:: Aisha Sethi

第一百五十七章
结核和非典型分枝杆菌感染

中文导读

结核病（TB）仍然是一种重要的世界性疾病。结核病目前是全世界第九大死亡原因，也是传染病的首要原因，其排名高于艾滋病。本章节常规介绍了结核病的流行病学、临床特征、危险因素、病因和发病机制、诊断、鉴别诊断、治疗等方面的内容。同时，还就一些特殊的结核感染表现，例如初次接种结核病（结核病、结核病原发性复合物）、疣状结核、寻常狼疮（狼疮样皮肤结核）等和一些非常少见特殊的结核感染形式，例如口腔结核、瘰疬性苔藓、丘疹坏死性皮结核等进行了全面的介绍。

〔汪 犇〕

AT-A-GLANCE

- Infection with *Mycobacterium tuberculosis* or other very closely related strains, as well as the inflammatory reaction of the host define, the disease (tuberculosis [TB]).
- One-third of the world's population is infected with TB.
- TB is the main cause of death of patients infected with HIV.
- TB usually affects the lung, but virtually all other organ systems may be involved.
- TB of the skin is a relatively rare manifestation with a wide spectrum of clinical findings depending on the source of infection and the immune status of the host.
- Diagnosis is based on clinical manifestations, histopathologic analysis, demonstration of the relevant mycobacteria in tissue or in culture and host reaction to *M. tuberculosis* antigen.
- Treatment is with standard multidrug regimens; cases of multidrug-resistant TB or extensively multidrug-resistant TB require special attention.
- Course and prognosis depend on the immune status of the host. Treatment is curative except for patients with a severely compromised immune system.

Tuberculosis (TB) is still an important worldwide disease. TB is currently the ninth leading cause of death worldwide and the leading cause from an infectious agent, ranking higher than HIV/AIDS. In 2016, 6.3 million new cases of TB were reported, which was up from 6.1 million in 2015. There were 476,774 reported cases of HIV-positive TB, of whom 85% were on antiretroviral therapy.[1] In 2016, there were an estimated 1.3 million TB deaths among HIV-negative people. An additional 374,000 deaths were reported among HIV-positive people. An estimated 10.4 million people fell ill with TB in 2016: The highest burden of disease was in 5 countries: India, Indonesia, China, the Philippines, and Pakistan.

In 2008, a total of 12,898 incident TB cases were reported in the United States; the TB rate declined 3.8% from 2007 to 4.2 cases per 100,000 population, the lowest rate recorded since national reporting began in 1953. In 2008, the TB rate in foreign-born persons in the United States was 10 times higher than in U.S.-born persons. TB rates among Hispanics and blacks were nearly 8 times higher than among non-Hispanic whites, and rates among Asians were nearly 23 times higher than among non-Hispanic whites. To ensure that TB rates decline further in the United States, especially among foreign-born persons and minority populations, TB prevention and control capacity should be increased. Additional capacity should be used to (a) improve case management and contact investigations; (b) intensify outreach, testing, and treatment of high-risk and hard-to-reach populations; (c) enhance treatment and diagnostic tools; (d) increase scientific research to better understand TB transmission; and (e) continue collaboration with other nations to reduce TB globally.[2]

HIV-positive people are approximately 20 times more likely than HIV-negative people to develop TB in countries with a generalized HIV epidemic, and between 26 and 37 times more likely to develop TB in countries where HIV prevalence is lower.

The so-called atypical mycobacteria (mycobacteria other than *Mycobacterium tuberculosis* [MOTT]) cause skin disease more frequently than does *M. tuberculosis*. They exist in various reservoirs in the environment. Among these organisms are obligate and facultative pathogens as well as nonpathogens. In contrast to the obligate pathogens, facultative pathogens do not cause disease by person-to-person spread.

EPIDEMIOLOGY

Tuberculosis of the skin has a worldwide distribution. Once more prevalent in regions with a cold and humid climate, it now occurs mostly in the tropics. Cutaneous TB incidence parallels that of pulmonary TB and developing countries still account for the majority of cases in the world. The emergence of resistant strains and the AIDS epidemic have led to an increase in all forms of TB (Table 157-1).

The 2 most frequent forms of skin tuberculosis are lupus vulgaris (LV) and scrofuloderma (Fig. 157-1). In the tropics, LV is rare, whereas scrofuloderma and verrucous lesions predominate. LV is more than twice as common in women than in men, whereas tuberculosis verrucosa cutis is more often found in men. Generalized miliary tuberculosis is seen in infants (and adults with severe immunosuppression or AIDS), as is primary inoculation tuberculosis. Scrofuloderma usually occurs in adolescents and the elderly, whereas LV may affect all age groups.

The pandemic of AIDS, with its profound and progressive suppression of cellular immune functions, has led to a resurgence of tuberculosis and the appearance

TABLE 157-1
Classification of Cutaneous Tuberculosis

	HOST IMMUNE STATUS	CLINICAL DISEASE
Exogenous infection	Naïve	Primary inoculation tuberculosis
	Immune	Tuberculosis verrucosa cutis
Endogenous spread	High	Lupus vulgaris
		Scrofuloderma
	Low	Acute miliary tuberculosis
		Orificial tuberculosis
		Metastatic tuberculous abscess (tuberculous gumma)
Tuberculosis caused by bacille Calmette-Guérin	Naïve	Normal primary complex-like reaction
		Perforating regional adenitis
		Postvaccination lupus vulgaris
Tuberculids	Not clear	Tuberculids: ■ Lichen scrofulosorum ■ Papulonecrotic tuberculid Facultative tuberculids: ■ Nodular vasculitis ■ Erythema nodosum

or recognition of new mycobacterial pathogens. The *Mycobacterium avium*-intracellulare complex is the most common cause of disseminated bacterial infections in patients with AIDS in the United States, but is much less frequently so in Europe. In AIDS patients, *Mycobacterium kansasii* is more common than *M. tuberculosis*. The incidence of tuberculosis in patients with AIDS is almost 500 times than that in the general population. Cutaneous disease in AIDS patients is frequently caused by MOTT.

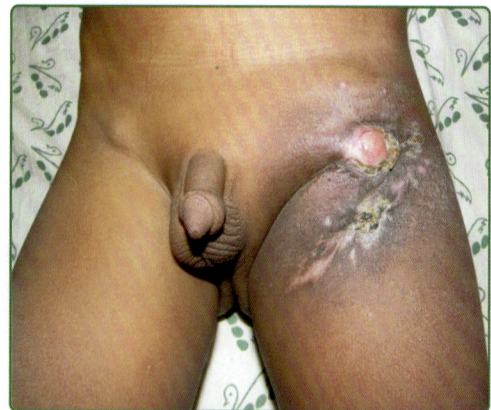

Figure 157-1 Scrofuloderma in an Ethiopian patient. (Used with permission from Dr. Kassahun Bilcha.)

ETIOLOGY AND PATHOGENESIS

THE *MYCOBACTERIUM*

Mycobacteria multiply intracellularly, and are initially found in large numbers in the tissue.

M. tuberculosis, Mycobacterium bovis, and, under certain conditions, the attenuated bacille Calmette-Guérin (BCG) organism cause all forms of skin tuberculosis.

In LV, the bacteria often have virulence as low as that of the BCG. A large number of bacteria can be found in the lesions of a primary chancre or of acute miliary tuberculosis; in the other forms, their number in the lesions is so small that it may be difficult to find them.

M. tuberculosis may become dormant in the host tissue.

New diagnostic tools are emerging,[3,4] as described below.

THE HOST

The human species is quite susceptible to infection by *M. tuberculosis*, with big differences among populations and individuals. Populations that have been in longstanding contact with tuberculosis are, in general, less susceptible than those who have come into contact with mycobacteria more recently, presumably reflecting widespread immunity from subclinical infection. Age, state of health, environmental factors, and particularly the immune system are of importance. In Africans, tuberculosis frequently takes an unfavorable course, and tuberculin sensitivity may be more pronounced than in whites.

ROUTE OF INFECTION

Cutaneous inoculation leads to a tuberculous chancre or to tuberculosis verrucosa cutis (Fig. 157-2), depending on the immunologic state of the host.

Spread of mycobacteria may occur by continuous extension of a tuberculous process in the skin (scrofuloderma) by way of the lymphatics (LV), or by hematogenous dissemination (acute miliary tuberculosis of the skin or LV).

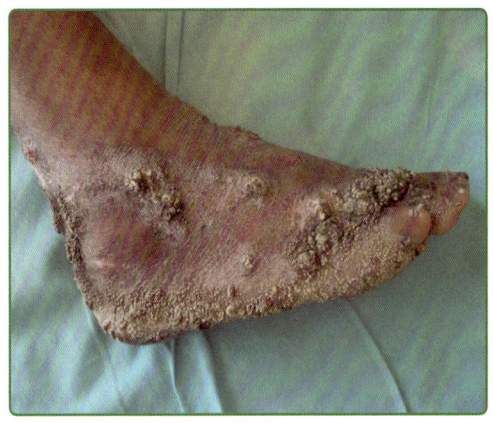

Figure 157-2 Tuberculosis verrucosa cutis on the foot of an Ethiopian patient. (Used with permission from Dr. Kassahun Bilcha.)

DIAGNOSIS

TUBERCULIN REACTION (KOCH PHENOMENON)

An extract of *M. tuberculosis* (tuberculin) was shown to produce a different skin reaction in sensitized individuals than in naïve individuals, and this difference became the basis of a widely used diagnostic test. This reaction is a delayed-type hypersensitivity reaction, induced by mycobacteria during primary infection. This "old tuberculin" has now been replaced by purified protein derivative (PPD). More recently, purified species-specific antigens have been developed.[5]

Local intradermal injection (the method most widely used) leads to the local tuberculin reaction, which usually reaches its maximum intensity after 48 hours. It consists of a sharply circumscribed area of erythema and induration, and in highly hypersensitive recipients or after large doses, a pallid central necrosis may appear.

In an attempt to quantify the tuberculin reaction, an assay known as the QuantiFERON-TB Gold test was developed to measure specific antigen-driven interferon-γ synthesis by whole blood cells and was approved by the U.S. Food and Drug Administration (FDA) in 2005.

Tuberculin sensitivity usually develops 2 to 10 weeks after infection and persists throughout life. The state of sensitivity of an individual infected with *M. tuberculosis* is of considerable significance in the pathogenesis of tuberculosis skin lesions.

In patients with clinical tuberculosis, an increase in skin sensitivity usually indicates a favorable prognosis, and in tuberculous skin disease accompanied by high levels of skin sensitivity, the number of bacteria within the lesions is small. Tuberculin sensitivity (skin reactivity) is not necessary for immunity, however, and sensitivity and immunity do not always parallel each other.

QUANTIFERON-TB GOLD TEST

In 2005, the FDA approved QuantiFERON-TB Gold (QFT-G) as an in vitro diagnostic aid. In this test, blood samples are mixed with antigens and controls. For QFT-G, the antigens include mixtures of synthetic peptides representing 2 *M. tuberculosis* proteins:

ESAT-6 and CFP-10. After incubation of the blood with antigens for 16 to 24 hours, the amount of interferon (IFN)-γ is measured.

If the patient is infected with *M. tuberculosis*, their white blood cells will release IFN-γ in response to contact with the TB antigens. The QFT-G results are based on the amount of IFN-γ that is released in response to the antigens.

Although more sensitive than the tuberculin skin test, the QFT-G may be negative in patients with early active tuberculosis and indeterminate results are more common in immunocompromised individuals and young children. Another similar assay, the T-SPOT.*TB* test, measures the number of IFN-γ–producing T cells and is currently available in Europe. QFT-G testing is indicated for diagnosing infection with *M. tuberculosis*, including both TB disease and latent TB infection. Whenever *M. tuberculosis* infection or disease is being diagnosed by any method, the optimal approach includes coordination with the local or regional public health TB control programs.

HISTOPATHOLOGY

The hallmark of tuberculosis and infections with some of the slow-growing atypical mycobacteria is the tubercle: an accumulation of epithelioid histocytes with Langhans-type giant cells among them and a varying amount of caseation necrosis in the center, surrounded by a rim of lymphocytes and monocytes. Although this tuberculoid granuloma is highly characteristic of several forms of tuberculosis, it may be mimicked by deep fungal infections, syphilis, and leprosy, as well as other diseases. As in leprosy, the histopathologic features of skin tuberculosis may be reflective of the host's immune status.

POLYMERASE CHAIN REACTION PROCEDURE

The polymerase chain reaction (PCR) procedure has been used increasingly to ascertain the presence of mycobacterial DNA in skin specimens.[6] Although the detection of specific DNA in tissues has yielded valuable information and will conceivably gain importance in the future, interpretation of the results of these tests in individual patients is still problematic.[7] In one study, samples from 16 of 20 patients with sarcoidosis contained mycobacterial DNA, both tuberculous and nontuberculous.[8] In another study of patients with confirmed or highly probable cutaneous tuberculosis or with erythema induratum, believed to indicate a host response to the infection, PCR testing showed 100% sensitivity and specificity in multibacillary disease. In paucibacillary disease, PCR testing showed 55% sensitivity and specificity, and only 80% of PCR-positive patients responded to antituberculosis therapy.[6]

TREATMENT OF CUTANEOUS TUBERCULOSIS

In general, the management of cutaneous tuberculosis is similar to that of tuberculosis of other organs.[9-12] Chemotherapy is usually the treatment of choice (Tables 157-2 and 157-3), but ancillary measures may be required. Vaccines against *M. tuberculosis* have been attempted,[9] but are still not available.

Although they are not yet established as a therapeutic option, cytokines such as interleukin-2, interferon-γ, interleukin-12, and granulocyte-macrophage colony-stimulating factor may help to control intracellular pathogens and thereby shorten the duration of therapy and overcome drug resistance.[13] The immunomodulatory drug thalidomide may prove to be useful in controlling problems related to the inflammatory response that may follow treatment of multibacillary infection and could become a useful adjunctive drug, as it is in the treatment of leprosy.

SPECIAL CONSIDERATIONS IN TREATING TUBERCULOSIS OF THE SKIN

In contrast to systemic infection, for which triple-drug therapy is recommended, tuberculosis verrucosa cutis and localized forms of LV without evidence of associated internal tuberculosis may be treated with isoniazid alone for up to 12 months. Because viable mycobacteria have been found in clinically healed lesions, treatment should be continued for at least 2 months after complete involution of the lesions. Surgical intervention is quite helpful in scrofuloderma, because it reduces morbidity and shortens the required length of chemotherapy. Small lesions of LV or tuberculosis verrucosa cutis are also best excised, but tuberculostatics should be given concomitantly. Plastic surgery is important as a corrective measure in cases of longstanding LV with mutilation.

Extensively multidrug-resistant TB is defined as resistance to at least rifampicin and isoniazid from among the first-line anti-TB drugs (which is the definition of multidrug resistant TB) in addition to resistance to any fluoroquinolone, and to at least 1 of the 3 injectable second-line anti-TB drugs used in TB treatment (capreomycin, kanamycin, and amikacin). The Centers for Disease Control and Prevention and World Health Organization have outlined that extensively drug resistant TB poses a grave global public health threat and has a higher risk of death as it renders patients virtually untreatable with currently available drugs.[14]

TABLE 157-2
Therapy Guidelines for *Mycobacterium Tuberculosis* Infections

		INITIAL PHASE		CONTINUATION PHASE			RATING (EVIDENCE)[a,b]	
REGIMEN	DRUGS	INTERVAL AND DOSES[c] (MINIMAL DURATION)	REGIMEN	DRUGS	INTERVAL AND DOSES[c,d] (MINIMAL DURATION)	RANGE OF TOTAL DOSES (MINIMAL DURATION)	HIV⁻	HIV⁺
1	INH	7 days per week for 56 doses (8 weeks) or 5 days per week for 40 doses (8 weeks)[e]	1a	INH/RIF	7 days per week for 126 doses (18 weeks) or 5 days per week for 90 doses (18 weeks)[e]	184 to 130 (26 weeks)	A (I)	A (II)
	RIF		1b	INH/RIF			A (I)	A (II)[c]
	PZA		1c[f]	INH/RPT	Twice weekly for 36 doses (18 weeks)	92 to 76 (26 weeks)	B (I)	E (I)
					Once weekly for 18 doses (18 weeks)	74 to 58 (26 weeks)		
	EMB							
2	INH	7 days per week for 14 doses (2 weeks), then twice weekly for 12 doses (6 weeks), or 5 days per week for 10 doses (2 weeks)[e], then twice weekly for 12 doses (6 weeks)	2a 2b[f]	INH/RIF	Twice weekly for 36 doses (18 weeks)	62 to 58 (26 weeks)	A (II)	B (II)[c]
					Once weekly for 18 doses (18 weeks)	44 to 40 (26 weeks)		
	RIF			INH/RPT			B (I)	E (I)
	PZA							
	EMB							
3	INH	Three times weekly for 24 doses (8 weeks)	3a	INH/RIF	Three times weekly for 54 doses (18 weeks)	78 (26 weeks)	B (I)	B (II)
	RIF							
	PZA							
	EMB							
4	INH	7 days per week for 56 doses (8 weeks) or 5 days per week for 40 doses (8 weeks)[e]	4a	INH/RIF	7 days per week for 217 doses (31 weeks) or 5 days per week for 155 doses (31 weeks)[e] Twice weekly for 62 doses (31 weeks)	273 to 195 (39 weeks)	C (I)	C (II)
	RIF		4b	INH/RIF		118 to 102 (39 weeks)	C (I)	C (II)
	EMB							

[a] Definitions of evidence ratings: A, preferred; B, acceptable alternative; C, offer when A and B cannot be given; E, should never be given.
[b] Definitions of evidence ratings: I, randomized clinical trial; II, data from clinical trials that were not randomized or were conducted in other populations; III, expert opinion.
[c] Directly Observed Therapy (DOT). Among patients with extrapulmonary tuberculosis, regimen 1 is recommended as initial therapy unless the organisms are known or strongly suspected of being resistant to the first-line drugs. If PZA cannot be used in the initial phase (ie, regimen 4), the continuation phase must be increased to 7 months. Doses of medications (maximum dose) when given daily: EMB (ethambutol) 18 mg/kg (1600 mg); INH (isoniazid), 5 mg/kg (300 mg); PZA (pyrazinamide), 25 mg/kg (2000 mg); RIF (rifampin), 10 mg/kg (600 mg); RPT (rifapentine), which is given once weekly at 10 mg/kg.
When DOT is used, drugs may be given 5 days/week and the necessary number of doses adjusted accordingly. Although there are no studies that compare 5 with 7 daily doses, extensive experience indicates this would be an effective practice.
[d] Patients with cavitation on initial chest radiograph and positive cultures at completion of 2 months of therapy should receive an 8-month (31-week; either 217 doses [daily] or 62 doses [twice weekly]) continuation phase.
[e] Five-day-a-week administration is always given by DOT. Rating for 5 day/week regimens is AIII. Not recommended for HIV-infected patients with CD4+ cell counts <100 cells/mL.
[f] Options 1c and 2b should be used only in HIV-negative patients who have negative sputum smears at the time of completion of 2 months of therapy and who do not have cavitation on initial chest radiograph. For patients started on this regimen and found to have a positive culture from the 2-month specimen, treatment should be extended an extra 3 months.
From American Thoracic Society, CDC, and Infectious Disease Society of America. Treatment of tuberculosis. *MMWR Recomm Rep.* 2003;52(RR-11):1-77.

TABLE 157-3
Antituberculosis Drugs Currently in Use in the United States

FIRST-LINE DRUGS	SECOND-LINE DRUGS
Isoniazid	Cycloserine
Rifampin	Ethionamide
Rifapentine	Levofloxacin[a]
Rifabutin[a]	Moxifloxacin[a]
Ethambutol	Gatifloxacin[a]
Pyrazinamide	p-Aminosalicylic acid
	Streptomycin
	Amikacin/kanamycin[a]
	Capreomycin

[a]Not approved by the U.S. Food and Drug Administration for use in the treatment of tuberculosis.

From American Thoracic Society, CDC, and Infectious Disease Society of America. Treatment of tuberculosis. *MMWR Recomm Rep.* 2003;52(RR-11):1-77.

SKIN DISEASES CAUSED BY *MYCOBACTERIUM TUBERCULOSIS* AND *MYCOBACTERIUM BOVIS* INFECTION

Infection with *M. tuberculosis* used to be thought to result in characteristic clinical features.[15] However, with increasing number of cases in immunocompromised individuals and improved diagnostic tools, many uncharacteristic manifestations have been discovered.

PRIMARY INOCULATION TUBERCULOSIS (TUBERCULOUS CHANCRE, TUBERCULOUS PRIMARY COMPLEX)

EPIDEMIOLOGY

Tuberculous chancre and affected regional lymph nodes constitute the tuberculous primary complex in the skin. The condition is believed rare, but its incidence may be underestimated. In some regions with a high prevalence of tuberculosis and poor living conditions, primary inoculation tuberculosis of the skin is not unusual. Children are most often affected.

ETIOLOGY AND PATHOGENESIS

Tubercle bacilli are introduced into the tissue at the site of minor wounds. Oral lesions may be caused by bovine bacilli in unpasteurized milk and occur after mucosal trauma or tooth extraction. Primary inoculation tuberculosis is initially multibacillary, but becomes paucibacillary as immunity develops.

CLINICAL FINDINGS

The chancre initially appears 2 to 4 weeks after inoculation and presents as a small papule, crust, or erosion with little tendency to heal. Sites of predilection are the face, including the conjunctivae and oral cavity, as well as the hands and lower extremities. A painless ulcer develops, which may be quite insignificant or may enlarge to a diameter of more than 5 cm (Fig. 157-3). It is shallow with a granular or hemorrhagic base studded with miliary abscesses or covered by necrotic tissue. The ragged edges are undermined and of a reddish-blue hue. As the lesions grow older, they become more indurated, with thick adherent crusts.

Wounds inoculated with tubercle bacilli may heal temporarily but break down later, giving rise to granulating ulcers. Mucosal infections result in painless ulcers or fungating granulomas. Inoculation tuberculosis of the finger may present as a painless paronychia. Inoculation of puncture wounds may result in subcutaneous abscesses.

Slowly progressive, regional lymphadenopathy develops 3 to 8 weeks after the infection (see Fig. 157-3) and may rarely be the only clinical finding. After weeks or months, cold abscesses may develop that perforate to the surface of the skin and form sinuses. The lymph nodes draining the primary glands also may be involved. Body temperature may be slightly elevated. The disease may take a more acute course, and in half of the patients, fever, pain, and swelling simulate a pyogenic infection. Early, there is an acute nonspecific inflammatory reaction in both skin and lymph nodes, and mycobacteria are easily detected by Fite stain. After 3 to 6 weeks, the infiltrate and the regional lymph nodes acquire a tuberculoid appearance and caseation may occur.

DIAGNOSIS

Any ulcer with little or no tendency to heal and unilateral regional lymphadenopathy in a child should arouse suspicion. Acid-fast organisms are found in the primary ulcer and draining nodes in the initial stages of the disease. The diagnosis is confirmed by bacterial culture. The PPD reaction is negative initially and later converts to positive (see Fig. 157-3).

DIFFERENTIAL DIAGNOSIS

The differential diagnosis encompasses all disease with a primary complex (Table 157-4).

COURSE

If untreated, the condition may last up to 12 months. Rarely, LV develops at the site of a healed tuberculous

TABLE 157-4
Differential Diagnosis of Primary Inoculation Tuberculosis

Most Likely
- Sporotrichosis
- Syphilis

Consider
- Bartonellosis
- Tularemia

Always Rule Out
- Other mycobacterioses

chancre. The regional lymph nodes usually calcify.

The primary tuberculous complex usually produces immunity, but reactivation of the disease may occur. Hematogenous spread may give rise to tuberculosis of other organs, particularly of the bones and joints. It may also lead to acute miliary disease with a fatal outcome. Erythema nodosum occurs in approximately 10% of cases.

TUBERCULOSIS VERRUCOSA CUTIS (WARTY TUBERCULOSIS, PROSECTOR'S WART, LUPUS VERRUCOSUS)

ETIOLOGY AND PATHOGENESIS

Tuberculosis verrucosa cutis is a paucibacillary disorder caused by exogenous reinfection (inoculation) in previously sensitized individuals with high immunity. Inoculation occurs at sites of minor wounds or, rarely, from the patient's own sputum. Members of professional groups handling infectious material are at risk. Children may become infected playing on contaminated ground.

CLINICAL FINDINGS

Lesions usually occur on the hands or, in children, on the lower extremities as a small asymptomatic papule or papulopustule with a purple inflammatory halo. They become hyperkeratotic and are often mistaken for a common wart. Slow growth and peripheral expansion lead to the development of a verrucous plaque with an irregular border (Fig. 157-4). Fissures discharging pus extend into the underlying brownish-red to purplish infiltrated base. The lesion usually is solitary, but multiple lesions may occur. Regional lymph nodes are rarely affected.

Lesions progress slowly and, if untreated, persist for many years. Spontaneous involution eventually occurs, leaving an atrophic scar.

HISTOPATHOLOGY

The most prominent histopathologic features are pseudoepitheliomatous hyperplasia with marked hyperkeratosis, a dense inflammatory infiltrate, and abscesses in the superficial dermis or within the pseudoepitheliomatous rete pegs. Epithelioid cells and giant cells are found in the upper and middle dermis. Typical tubercles are uncommon, and the infiltrate may be nonspecific.

DIFFERENTIAL DIAGNOSIS

Table 157-5 outlines the differential diagnosis of tuberculosis verrucosa cutis.

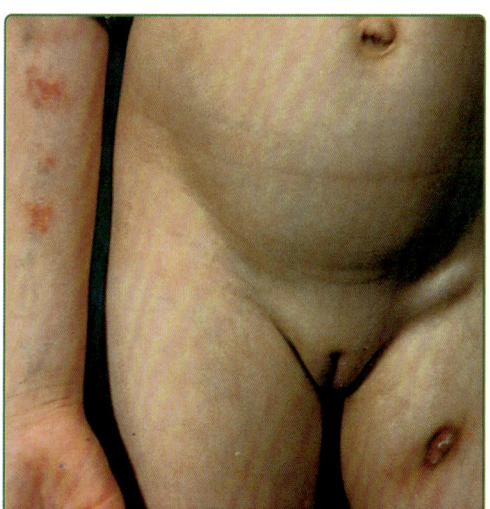

Figure 157-3 Primary inoculation tuberculosis. Note tuberculous chancre on the thigh and regional lymphadenopathy. A positive tuberculin reaction is noted on the arm.

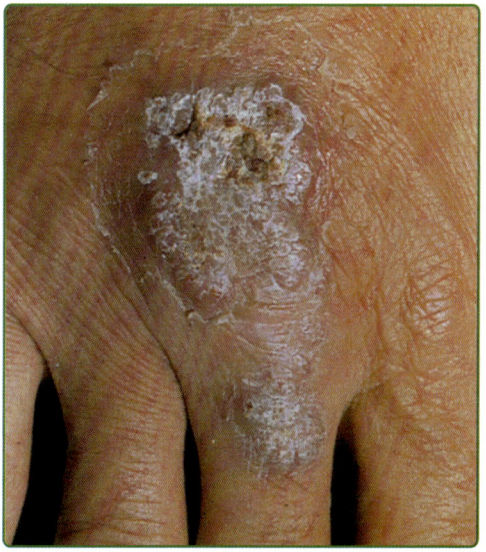

Figure 157-4 Tuberculosis verrucosa cutis on the back of the hand.

TABLE 157-5
Differential Diagnosis of Tuberculosis Verrucosa Cutis
Most Likely
Blastomycosis
Hyperkeratotic lupus vulgaris
Hypertrophic lichen planus
Warts or keratoses
Consider
Bromoderma
Chromomycosis
Tertiary syphilis
Always Rule Out
Lesions caused by other mycobacteria

ETIOLOGY AND PATHOGENESIS

LV is a postprimary, paucibacillary form of tuberculosis caused by hematogenous, lymphatic, or contiguous spread from elsewhere in the body. Spontaneous involution may occur, and new lesions may arise within old scars. Complete healing rarely occurs without therapy.

CLINICAL FINDINGS

Lesions are usually solitary, but two or more sites may be involved simultaneously. In patients with active pulmonary tuberculosis, multiple foci may develop. In approximately 90% of patients, the head and neck are involved. LV usually starts on the nose, cheek, earlobe, or scalp and slowly extends onto adjacent regions. Other areas are rarely involved.

The initial lesion is a brownish-red, soft or friable macule or papule with a smooth or hyperkeratotic surface. On diascopy, the infiltrate exhibits a typical apple jelly color. Progression is characterized by elevation, a deeper brownish color (Fig. 157-5), and formation of a plaque (Fig. 157-5). Involution in one area with expansion in another often results in a gyrate outline border. Ulceration may occur. Hypertrophic forms appear as a soft nodule or plaque with a hyperkeratotic surface. The mucosae may be primarily involved or become affected by the extension of skin lesions. Infection is manifest as small, soft, gray or pink papules, ulcers, or friable granulating masses.

After a transient impairment of immunity, particularly after measles (thus the term *lupus postexanthematicus*), multiple disseminated lesions may arise simultaneously in different regions of the body as a consequence of hematogenous spread from a latent tuberculous focus. During and after the eruption, a

LUPUS VULGARIS (TUBERCULOSIS LUPOSA)

EPIDEMIOLOGY

LV is an extremely chronic, progressive form of cutaneous tuberculosis occurring in individuals with moderate immunity and a high degree of tuberculin sensitivity. Once common, LV has declined steadily in incidence. It has always been less common in the United States than in Europe. Females appear to be affected 2 to 3 times as often as males; all age groups are affected equally.

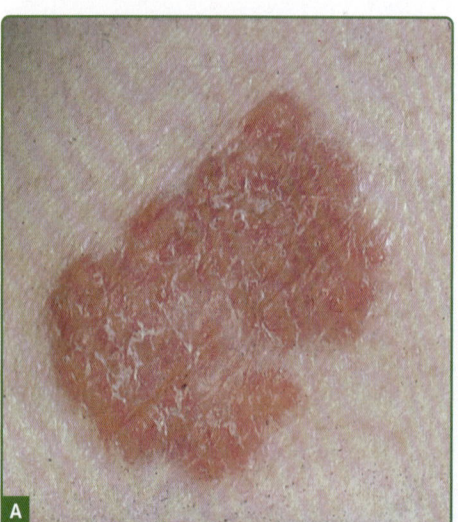 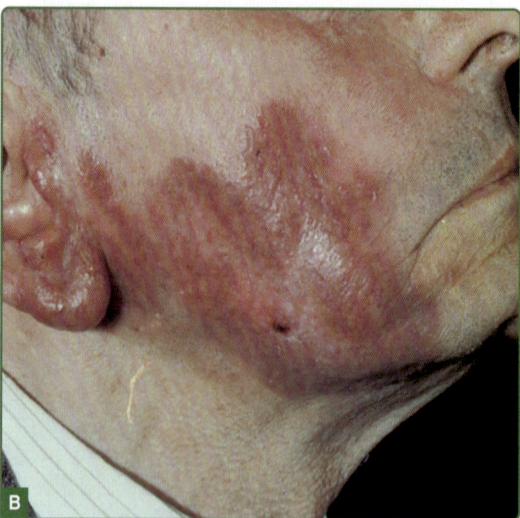

Figure 157-5 **A,** Slightly raised, brownish plaque of lupus vulgaris. **B,** Large plaque of lupus vulgaris of 10 years' duration involving the cheek, jaw, and ear.

previously positive tuberculin reaction may become negative, but will usually revert to positive as the general condition of the patient improves.

HISTOPATHOLOGY

The most prominent histopathologic feature is the formation of typical tubercles. Secondary changes may be superimposed: epidermal thinning and atrophy or acanthosis with excessive hyperkeratosis or pseudoepitheliomatous hyperplasia. Acid-fast bacilli are usually not found. Nonspecific inflammatory reactions may partially conceal the tuberculous structures. Old lesions are composed chiefly of epithelioid cells and may be impossible to distinguish from sarcoidal infiltrates.

DIAGNOSIS

Typical LV plaques may be recognized by the softness of the lesions, brownish-red color, and slow evolution. The apple jelly nodules revealed by diascopy are highly characteristic; finding them may be decisive, especially in ulcerated, crusted, or hyperkeratotic lesions. The result of the tuberculin test is strongly positive except during the early phases of postexanthematic lupus. Bacterial culture results may be negative, in which case the clinical diagnosis can usually be supported by positive PCR results for *M. tuberculosis*.

DIFFERENTIAL DIAGNOSIS

Table 157-6 outlines the differential diagnosis of LV.

COMPLICATIONS

Involvement of the nasal or auricular cartilage may result in extensive destruction and disfigurement (Fig. 157-6). Atrophic scarring, with or without prior ulceration, is characteristic, as is recurrence within a scar. Fibrosis may be pronounced and mutilating.

Dry rhinitis is often the only symptom of early nasal LV, but lesions may also destroy the cartilage of the nasal septum. Scarring of the soft palate and laryngeal stenosis also occur.

COURSE

LV is a very long-term disorder and without therapy progresses over many years to functional impairment and disfiguration (see Fig. 157-6). Longstanding LV may lead to the development of carcinoma (see Fig. 157-6). Squamous cell carcinomas outnumber basal cell carcinomas by far, and the risk of metastases is high. In 40% of patients, there is associated tuberculous lymphadenitis, and 10% to 20% have active pulmonary tuberculosis or tuberculosis of the bones and joints.[16] Pulmonary tuberculosis is 4 to 10 times more frequent in patients with LV than in the general population.

SCROFULODERMA (TUBERCULOSIS COLLIQUATIVA CUTIS)

EPIDEMIOLOGY

Prevalence is higher among children, adolescents, and the aged.

ETIOLOGY AND PATHOGENESIS

Scrofuloderma is subcutaneous tuberculosis leading to cold abscess formation and a secondary breakdown of the overlying skin. It may be either multibacillary or paucibacillary.

TABLE 157-6
Differential Diagnosis of Lupus Vulgaris

Most Likely
- Discoid lupus erythematosus
- Sarcoidosis

Consider
- Leprosy
- Lupoid leishmaniasis
- Lymphocytoma
- Tertiary syphilis

Always Rule Out
- Blastomycosis or other deep mycotic infections

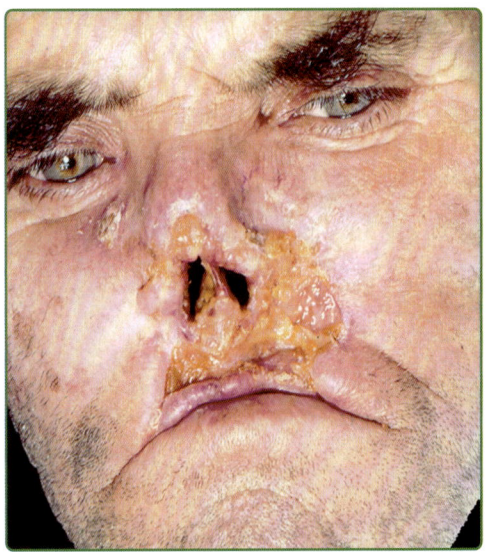

Figure 157-6 Lupus vulgaris of long duration that has led to the destruction of the nose. Ulcerating squamous cell carcinoma has developed on the upper lip.

Scrofuloderma represents contiguous involvement of the skin overlying another site of infection (eg, tuberculous lymphadenitis, tuberculosis of bones and joints, or tuberculous epididymitis).

CLINICAL FINDINGS

Scrofuloderma most often occurs in the parotideal, submandibular, and supraclavicular regions and may be bilateral. It first presents as a firm, subcutaneous nodule, usually well defined, freely movable, and asymptomatic. As the lesion enlarges, it softens. After months, liquefaction with perforation occurs, causing ulcers and sinuses (Fig. 157-7). The ulcers are linear or serpiginous with undermined, inverted, bluish edges and soft, granulating floors. Sinusoidal tracts undermine the skin. Clefts alternate with soft nodules. Scar tracts develop and bridge ulcerative areas or even stretches of normal skin. Tuberculin sensitivity is usually pronounced.

HISTOPATHOLOGY

Massive necrosis and abscess formation in the center of the lesion are nonspecific. However, the periphery of the abscesses or the margins of the sinuses contain tuberculoid granulomas.

DIAGNOSIS

If there is an underlying tuberculous lymphadenitis or bone and joint disease, the diagnosis usually presents no difficulty. Positive results on culture confirm the diagnosis.

DIFFERENTIAL DIAGNOSIS

Table 157-7 outlines the differential diagnosis of scrofuloderma.

COURSE

Spontaneous healing does occur, but the course is very protracted, and it may be years before lesions have been completely replaced by scar tissue. Presence of the typical cribriform scars permits a correct diagnosis, even after the process has become quiescent. LV may develop at or near the site of scrofuloderma.

ORIFICIAL TUBERCULOSIS (TUBERCULOSIS ULCEROSA CUTIS ET MUCOSAE, ACUTE TUBERCULOUS ULCER)

ETIOLOGY AND PATHOGENESIS

Orificial tuberculosis is a rare form of tuberculosis of the mucous membranes and orifices that is caused by autoinoculation of mycobacteria from progressive tuberculosis of internal organs.

The underlying disease is far advanced pulmonary, intestinal, or, rarely, genitourinary tuberculosis. Mycobacteria shed from these foci in large numbers are inoculated into the mucous membranes.

CLINICAL FINDINGS

A small yellowish or reddish nodule appears on the mucosa and breaks down to form a soft ulcer with a typical punched-out appearance, undermined edges, and circular or irregular border (Fig. 157-8). The ulcer floor often exhibits multiple yellowish tubercles and bleeds easily. The surrounding mucosa is edematous and inflamed. Lesions may be single or multiple and are extremely painful, resulting in dysphagia.

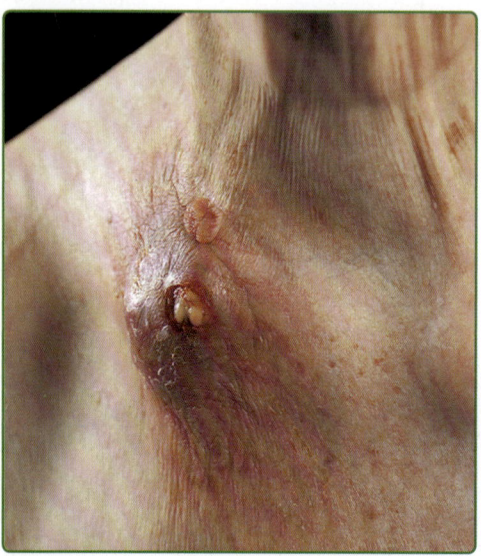

Figure 157-7 Scrofuloderma in the clavicular region. Note abscess formation, ulceration, and extrusion of purulent and caseous material.

TABLE 157-7
Differential Diagnosis of Scrofuloderma

Most Likely
- Hidradenitis suppurativa
- Sporotrichosis

Consider
- Actinomycosis
- *Mycobacterium scrofulaceum* infection
- Severe forms of acne conglobata
- Syphilitic gummas

Always Rule Out
- *Mycobacterium avium*-intracellulare lymphadenitis

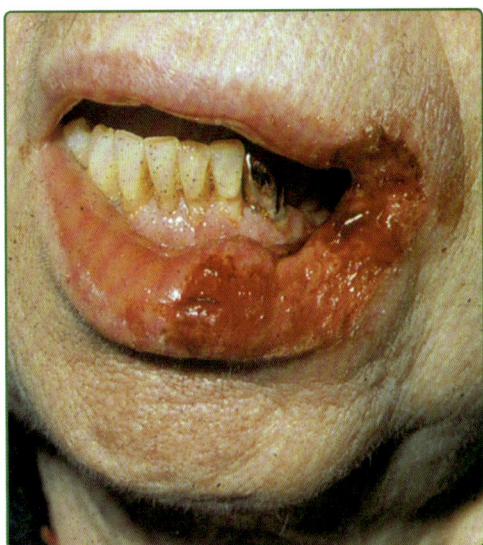

Figure 157-8 Orificial tuberculosis in advanced cavitary pulmonary tuberculosis.

The tongue is most frequently affected, particularly the tip and the lateral margins, but the soft and hard palates are also common sites. In advanced cases, the lips are involved, and the oral condition often represents an extension of ulcerative tuberculosis of the pharynx and larynx. In patients with intestinal tuberculosis, lesions develop around the anus, and in females with active genitourinary disease, the vulva is involved.

HISTOPATHOLOGY

There is a massive nonspecific inflammatory infiltrate and necrosis, but tubercles with caseation may be found deep in the dermis. Mycobacteria are easily demonstrated.

DIFFERENTIAL DIAGNOSIS

Table 157-8 outlines the differential diagnosis of orificial tuberculosis.

COURSE

Orificial tuberculosis is a symptom of advanced internal disease and usually portends a fatal outcome.

TABLE 157-8
Differential Diagnosis of Orificial Tuberculosis

Most Likely
- Aphthous ulcers

Consider
- Syphilitic lesions (not painful)

Always Rule Out
- Squamous cell carcinoma

SEQUELAE OF BACILLE CALMETTE–GUÉRIN INOCULATION

Vaccination with attenuated bovine BCG appears to protect infants and young children from the more serious forms of tuberculosis, but its ability to prevent disease in adults remains uncertain. In the United States, guidelines for BCG immunization have been developed.[17,18]

In the normal course of BCG vaccination, an infiltrated papule develops after approximately 2 weeks, attains a size of approximately 10 mm after 6 to 12 weeks, ulcerates, and then slowly heals, leaving a scar. Vaccination may provoke an accelerated reaction in a previously infected person. The regional lymph nodes may enlarge, but usually heal without breaking down. Tuberculin sensitivity appears 5 to 6 weeks after vaccination.

The true incidence of complications caused by the BCG organism is difficult to ascertain, but it is extremely low in comparison to the great number of vaccinations performed in Europe in the past 50 years.[19] Problems include the following:

- LV at or near the vaccination site (latency of months to years).
- Koch phenomenon in individuals sensitive to tuberculin (see section "Tuberculin Reaction [Koch Phenomenon]").
- Regional adenitis, sometimes severe and with systemic symptoms, more often in children.
- After deep injection, local abscesses, excessive ulceration.
- Scrofuloderma with suppuration for 6 to 12 months.
- Generalized tuberculid-like reactions (rare).
- Generalized adenitis, osteitis, organ tuberculosis (eg, in the joints) occasionally.

THE TUBERCULIDS

Lichen scrofulosorum, erythema induratum, papulonecrotic tuberculids, lupus miliaris disseminatus faciei, and other eruptions with rather exotic designations were originally included in the tuberculids (Table 157-9).

With the sharp decline in incidence and the effective treatment of tuberculosis in developed countries, the tuberculids also became rare. However, this does not apply to areas in which tuberculosis is still common, and with the recent resurgence of tuberculosis associated with AIDS in some Western countries, some tuberculids are also being observed again.

The pathogenic relationship of the tuberculids to tuberculosis is still poorly understood. Although there is no doubt that such a relationship exists for some tuberculids, in other cases it appears highly unlikely.

PCR testing revealed *M. tuberculosis* DNA in skin lesions of erythema induratum/nodular vasculitis and papulonecrotic tuberculid in one series of patients, but in another, results were uniformly negative.[20,21] Thus,

M. tuberculosis infection may be responsible directly or indirectly for some cases of these diseases but not all, and the usefulness of lesional PCR testing may vary among clinical settings. Consistent with this statement, antituberculosis drugs are beneficial in some cases but not all; spontaneous involution may occur, and some patients appear to respond well to other therapies. It should be noted that, although not considered a tuberculid, sarcoidosis has been postulated to result from an immunologic reaction to mycobacterial antigens.[22]

The following discussion includes only those conditions for which a preponderance of the evidence supports a tuberculous etiology (see Table 157-9).

LICHEN SCROFULOSORUM

EPIDEMIOLOGY AND PATHOGENESIS

Lichen scrofulosorum is an uncommon lichenoid eruption ascribed to hematogenous spread of mycobacteria in an individual strongly sensitive to *M. tuberculosis*. Usually associated with chronic tuberculosis of the lymph nodes, bones, or pleura, it also has been observed after BCG vaccination and in association with *M. avium*-intracellulare infections.[23]

CLINICAL FINDINGS

Lesions are usually confined to the trunk and occur most often in children and adolescents with active tuberculosis. The lesions are asymptomatic, firm, follicular or perifollicular flat-topped yellowish or pink papules, sometimes with fine scale. Lichenoid grouping is pronounced, and lesions may coalesce to form rough, discoid plaques. Lesions persist for months, but spontaneous involution eventually occurs. Antituberculosis therapy results in complete resolution within weeks.

HISTOPATHOLOGY

Superficial tuberculoid granulomas develop around hair follicles or independent of the adnexa. Mycobacteria are not seen in the sections and cannot be cultured from biopsy material.

DIFFERENTIAL DIAGNOSIS

Table 157-10 outlines the differential diagnosis of lichen scrofuloderma.

PAPULONECROTIC TUBERCULID

EPIDEMIOLOGY

Papulonecrotic tuberculid is a symmetric eruption of necrotizing papules, appearing in crops and healing with scar formation that occurs preferentially in children or young adults. It is rarely reported but may not be uncommon in populations with a high prevalence of tuberculosis.

ETIOLOGY AND PATHOGENESIS

As a rule, bacteria cannot be demonstrated in lesions. In most cases, the tuberculin test shows a positive reaction, and associated pulmonary or extrapulmonary tuberculosis is common. LV has been reported to evolve with papulonecrotic tuberculid. Lesions are reported to respond promptly to antituberculosis therapy whether or not a tuberculous focus is identified.

In studies of skin lesions in patients with papulonecrotic tuberculid, *M. tuberculosis* DNA was detected in approximately 50% of the skin biopsies (11 of 22 samples).[24-26] *M. kansasii* infection was documented in 1 patient.[27]

Some cases of papulonecrotic tuberculid have been associated with discoid lupus erythematosus, arthritis, or erythema nodosum. Although papulonecrotic tuberculid is classified as an id reaction and therefore, by definition, is not a result of direct involvement of the skin by the organism, some of the lesions have been positive on culture. It seems most likely that papulonecrotic tuberculid is a reaction to particulate tuberculous antigen and, in some cases, to living organisms as well.[28]

TABLE 157-9
Tuberculids

TERMINOLOGY: RELATIONSHIP TO TUBERCULOSIS	ENTITIES
Tuberculids: conditions in which *Mycobacterium tuberculosis*/ *Mycobacterium bovis* appears to play a significant role	Lichen scrofulosorum Papulonecrotic tuberculid
Facultative tuberculids: conditions in which *M. tuberculosis*/*M. bovis* may be one of several pathogenic factors	Nodular vasculitis/erythema induratum of Bazin Erythema nodosum
Nontuberculids: conditions formerly designated as tuberculids; there is no relationship to tuberculosis	Lupus miliaris disseminatus faciei Rosacea-like tuberculid Lichenoid tuberculid

TABLE 157-10
Differential Diagnosis of Lichen Scrofuloderma

Most Likely
- Lichen nitidus
- Lichen planus

Consider
- Lichenoid secondary syphilis
- Micropapular forms of sarcoidosis

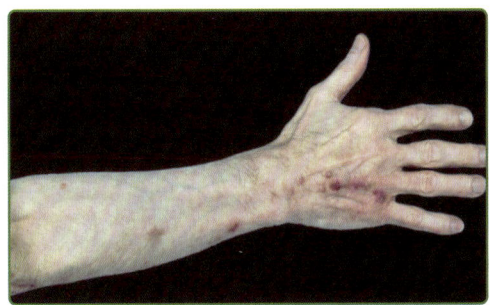

Figure 157-9 Papulonecrotic tuberculid on the forearm.

CLINICAL FINDINGS

Sites of predilection are the extensor aspects of the extremities, buttocks, and lower trunk (Fig. 157-9), but the eruption may become widespread. Distribution is symmetric, and consists of disseminated crops of livid or dusky red papules with a central depression and an adherent crust over a crater-like ulcer. There is spontaneous involution, which leaves pitted scars.

HISTOPATHOLOGY

Characteristically, a wedge-shaped necrotic area in the upper dermis extends into the epidermis. The inflammatory infiltrate surrounding this necrotic area may be nonspecific, but is usually tuberculoid. Involvement of the blood vessels is a cardinal feature and consists of an obliterative and sometimes granulomatous vasculitis leading to thrombosis and complete occlusion of the vascular channels.

DIFFERENTIAL DIAGNOSIS

Table 157-11 outlines the differential diagnosis of papulonecrotic tuberculid.

TABLE 157-11
Differential Diagnosis of Papulonecrotic Tuberculid

Most Likely
- Pityriasis lichenoides et varioliformis acuta
- Prurigo

Consider
- Lichen urticatus
- Secondary syphilis

Always Rule Out
- Leukocytoclastic necrotizing vasculitis

NODULAR VASCULITIS/ERYTHEMA INDURATUM OF BAZIN

Chapter 73 discusses nodular vasculitis in detail.

ERYTHEMA NODOSUM

Chapter 73 discusses erythema nodosum in detail.

DISEASES CAUSED BY MYCOBACTERIA OTHER THAN *MYCOBACTERIUM TUBERCULOSIS*

AT-A-GLANCE

- A heterogeneous group of diseases caused by a variety of obligate or facultatively pathogenic mycobacteria other than those of the *Mycobacterium tuberculosis* complex.
- Involvement depends on the type of *Mycobacterium*, the route of infection, and the immune status of the host.
- Various organs may be involved.
- Mycobacteria other than *M. tuberculosis* (MOTT) are more often the cause of skin disease than *M. tuberculosis*.
- Diagnosis relies on histopathologic analysis and the results of culture.
- Incidence is unknown, but endemic areas exist for certain types of MOTT.
- Treatment is unlike that of tuberculosis, and no strict international guidelines have been developed. Effective antibiotics are known for each mycobacterial species but should be checked by sensitivity testing.

MOTT were identified as human pathogens in 1938 (*Mycobacterium fortuitum*), in 1948 (*Mycobacterium ulcerans*), and in 1954 (*Mycobacterium marinum*). However, overshadowed by the infectious disease burden caused by *Mycobacterium leprae* and *M. tuberculosis*, the pathogenic potential of slow-growing MOTT species was recognized only in recent decades. Because MOTT infections usually closely mimic infections with *M. tuberculosis*, and the bacteria have strict and often unusual requirements for culture, they are still probably underdiagnosed.

ETIOLOGY AND PATHOGENESIS

MOTT are widely distributed in nature and are usually commensals or saprophytes, rather than pathogens. Atypical mycobacteria are usually acquired from environmental sources such as water or soil, and their role in disease reflects their natural distribution and, possibly, local lifestyles. These organisms are thought to cause mycobacterial skin disease more often than does *M. tuberculosis*. Cases tend to be sporadic, but certain types of exposures may lead to small community outbreaks.[29,30] Any organ or organ system may be affected (Table 157-12), but MOTT seem much less likely to disseminate than *M. tuberculosis*, and infections usually run a more benign and limited course. As a rule, MOTT are much less responsive to antituberculosis drugs but may be sensitive to other chemotherapeutic agents.

Only 2 organisms, *M. ulcerans* and *M. marinum*, produce a characteristic clinical picture. An immunosuppressed state of the host or damage to a particular organ (eg, in *M. kansasii* infection of the lung) facilitates these infections.

New mycobacterial pathogens are described from time to time, which suggests that their full pathogenic potential is not yet appreciated. Recently, an outbreak of skin disease caused by a nontuberculous mycobacteria in Pacific Islanders from Satowan was reported in the literature.[31] These patients presented with longstanding verrucous and keloidal plaques (locally known as "spam" disease; Fig. 157-10). Histopathologic and PCR data demonstrated a nontuberculous mycobacterial infection as the cause.

IDENTIFICATION OF MYCOBACTERIA OTHER THAN *MYCOBACTERIUM TUBERCULOSIS*

As with other infectious diseases, the diagnosis of mycobacterial infection depends on the identification of the microorganism isolated from the host. Specimens for culture should be sent to a special laboratory familiar with the special growth requirements of these organisms.

Antigens for intradermal skin testing (PPDs) for many of the clinically relevant mycobacterial species have been prepared in analogy to PPD from *M. tuberculosis*, but their accessibility is very limited and they are therefore little used.

Histopathologic analysis is supportive but cannot distinguish among mycobacterial species, because all share similar histopathologic features.[32]

Table 157-13 summarizes treatment for MOTT. Importantly, some MOTT organisms are resistant to standard tuberculosis therapy. PCR testing for mycobacterial DNA is not yet reliable enough to play a role in the diagnosis of disease but can sometimes be useful in distinguishing among species.

TABLE 157-12
Organ Involvement in Infections with Atypical Mycobacteria

MYCOBACTERIAL SPECIES	ORGAN INVOLVEMENT	
	SKIN, SUBCUTIS	LYMPH NODES, OTHER ORGANS
Mycobacterium tuberculosis/ Mycobacterium bovis complex (including *Mycobacterium africanum* and bacille Calmette-Guérin)	+	+
Mycobacterium marinum	+	−
Mycobacterium ulcerans	+	−
Mycobacterium gordonae	+	−
Mycobacterium haemophilum	+	−
Mycobacterium kansasii	+	+
Mycobacterium avium-intracellulare complex (including *Mycobacterium scrofulaceum*)	+	+
Fast growers: *Mycobacterium fortuitum*, *Mycobacterium chelonae*, *Mycobacterium abscessus*	+	−

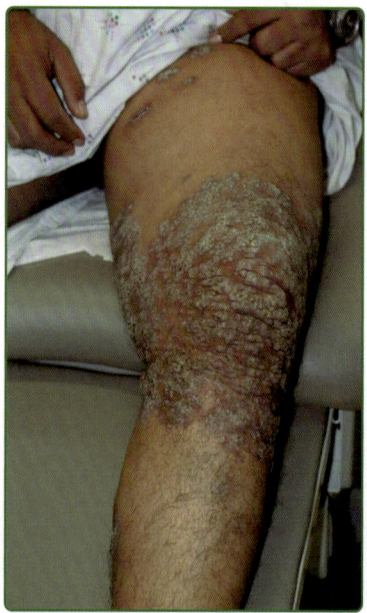

Figure 157-10 Verrucous plaque of "spam" disease on the knee of a Pacific Islander patient. (Used with permission from Dr. Joseph Lillis.)

TABLE 157-13
Treatment of Infections with Mycobacteria Other Than *Mycobacterium Tuberculosis*

TREATMENT	ULCERANS	MARINUM	KANSASII	INTRACELLULARE-AVIUM	SCROFULACEUM	HAEMOPHILUM	CHELONAE	FORTUITUM
Amikacin			+				+	+
Ansamycin				+				
Azithromycin				+				
Cefoxitin								+
Ciprofloxacin								+
Clarithromycin				+	+		+	
Clofazimine	+			+				
Cotrimoxazole	+							
Cycloserine			+					
Dapsone	+							
Doxycycline		+					+	
Erythromycin							+	
Ethambutol[a]	+		+	+				
Ethionamide			+	+				
Imipenem								+
Isoniazid			+	+	+			
Kanamycin			+					
Minocycline	+	+	+	+		+[b]		
Rifampicin	+	+	+	+	+			
Rifamycin			+	+		+		
Streptomycin[a]	+		+	+				
Tobramycin								+
Surgery	+				+		+	+

[a]Usual antituberculosis drugs.
[b]Alone or in combination with ciprofloxacin or rifampicin.

SKIN INFECTIONS WITH MYCOBACTERIA OTHER THAN *MYCOBACTERIUM TUBERCULOSIS*

MYCOBACTERIUM ULCERANS (BURULI ULCER DISEASE)

The natural habitat of *M. ulcerans* is still not known, and it has never been found outside the human body, but *M. ulcerans* infection occurs in wet, marshy, or swampy areas and seems to have to do with contaminated water. *M. ulcerans* is the third most frequent mycobacterial pathogen, after *M. tuberculosis* and *M. leprae*.

Clinical Findings: The disease is found most often in children and young adults, and affects females more often than males. A subcutaneous nodule gradually enlarges and eventually ulcerates. A blister may develop before ulceration. The ulcer is deeply undermined, and necrotic fat is exposed (Fig. 157-11). The preceding nodule, as well as the ulcer, is painless, and the patient continues to feel well. The painless nature of the ulcer has been attributed to nerve damage and tissue destruction caused by the toxin mycolactone. The lesions may occur anywhere on the body but tend to be limited to the extremities in adults. They may be large, involving a whole limb. The ulceration may persist for months and years, and healing and progression of the ulceration may occur in the same patient. This process may lead to appreciable and sometimes disabling scarring and lymphedema. Neither lymphadenopathy nor any constitutional signs appear at any time unless the disease process is complicated by bacterial superinfection.

Differential Diagnosis: Table 157-14 outlines the differential diagnosis of *M. ulcerans* lesions.

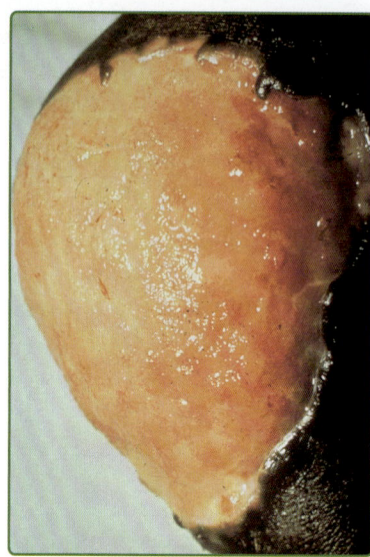

Figure 157-11 *Mycobacterium ulcerans* infection in a child in Uganda. The knee bears an ulcer with an infiltrated undermined margin and a base of necrotic adipose and connective tissue. (Used with permission from M. Dietrich, MD.)

TABLE 157-14
Differential Diagnosis of *Mycobacterium Ulcerans* Lesions

EARLY LESIONS	LATE LESIONS
Most Likely	
Foreign-body granuloma	Blastomycosis or other deep fungus infection
Sebaceous cyst	Pyoderma gangrenosum
Consider	
Phycomycosis	Suppurative panniculitis
Nodular fasciitis	
Appendageal tumor	
Always Rule Out	
Panniculitis	Necrotizing cellulitis
Nodular vasculitis	

MYCOBACTERIUM MARINUM (MYCOBACTERIUM BALNEI, FISH TANK/SWIMMING POOL GRANULOMA)

M. marinum occurs in freshwater and saltwater, including swimming pools and fish tanks.

Clinical Findings: Risk factors for *M. marinum* infection are a history of trauma and water- or fish/seafood-related hobbies and occupations. The disease begins as a violaceous papule at the site of a trauma 2 to 3 weeks after inoculation. Patients may have a nodule or a psoriasiform or verrucous plaque at the site of inoculation, usually the hands, feet, elbows, or knees (Fig. 157-12). The lesions may ulcerate. Usually, the lesions are solitary, but occasionally lymphocutaneous spread occurs. They may heal spontaneously within 1 to 2 years, with residual scarring. Occasionally, the lesions are suppurative, rather than granulomatous, and may be multiple in both normal and immunosuppressed hosts.

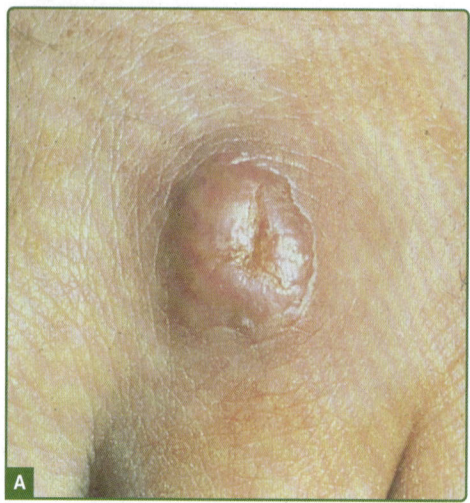 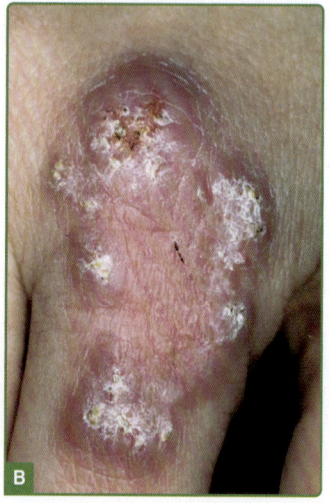

Figure 157-12 **A,** *Mycobacterium marinum* infection on the back of the hand. Granulomatous nodular lesion with central ulceration at the site of inoculation. (Used with permission from A. Kuhlwein, MD.) **B,** Verrucous, violaceous plaque with central spontaneous clearing occurring at the site of an abrasion sustained in a fish tank. The lesion was caused by *M. marinum*.

Differential Diagnosis: Table 157-15 outlines the differential diagnosis of *M. marinum* lesions.

MYCOBACTERIUM KANSASII

M. kansasii is the atypical *Mycobacterium* most closely related to *M. tuberculosis*. It is usually acquired from the environment. Endemic areas include Texas, Louisiana, the Chicago area, California, and Japan. Skin disease caused by *M. kansasii* usually occurs in adults, and is more common in individuals with underlying immunosuppression caused by Hodgkin disease, treatment for organ transplantation, or AIDS. Inoculation is usually attributable to minor trauma such as a puncture wound.

Clinical Findings: *M. kansasii* infection may present in several forms. Most frequently, there are papules in a sporotrichoid distribution. Sometimes, subcutaneous nodules extend to deeper structures and may result in a carpal tunnel syndrome or joint disease. An ulcerated plaque may also develop as a metastatic lesion. Disseminated disease caused by *M. kansasii* infection occurs in immunosuppressed patients, and such patients have cellulitis and abscesses rather than granulomatous lesions. The most commonly affected organ is the lung, usually in patients with other pulmonary conditions (silicosis, emphysema). Infection may also cause cervical lymphadenopathy. As with *M. tuberculosis*, *M. kansasii* present in nasopharyngeal secretions can lead to periorificial cutaneous infection. These infections usually progress slowly, although a chronic stable lesion or even spontaneous regression may occur. Drug therapy should be initiated as soon as the diagnosis is made.

Differential Diagnosis: Table 157-16 outlines the differential diagnosis of *M. kansasii* lesions.

MYCOBACTERIUM SCROFULACEUM

Mycobacterium scrofulaceum is widely distributed in the environment.

Clinical Findings: The usual manifestation of *M. scrofulaceum* infection is cervical lymphadenitis, frequently unilateral, in children, mainly between the ages of 1 and 3 years. Submandibular and submaxillary nodes are typically involved, rather than the tonsillar and anterior cervical nodes, as is characteristic for *M. tuberculosis* infection. There are no constitutional symptoms. Involved lymph nodes enlarge slowly over several weeks, and eventually ulcerate and develop fistulas. There is rarely an evidence of lung or other organ involvement. In most cases, the disease is benign and self-limited.

Differential Diagnosis: The differential diagnosis includes other forms of bacterial lymphadenitis; viral infections, including mumps and mononucleosis; and malignancy, including solid tumors, lymphoma, and leukemia.

MYCOBACTERIUM AVIUM-INTRACELLULARE

M. avium-intracellulare encompasses organisms with a wide variety of microbiologic and pathogenic properties. More than 20 subtypes can be separated by immunologic techniques, although this is not necessary for clinical purposes.

These organisms are usually grouped together with *M. scrofulaceum* in the so-called *M. avium*-intracellulare–scrofulaceum complex, but are separated here for clinical reasons. Whereas *M. scrofulaceum* produces only a benign, self-limited lymphadenopathy with no organ involvement, *M. avium*-intracellulare infection usually causes lung disease or, less frequently, osteomyelitis. It may also produce a cervical lymphadenitis with sinus formation that is clinically indistinguishable from tuberculous scrofuloderma.

Clinical Findings: Primary skin disease caused by *M. avium*-intracellulare has been reported in rare instances, presenting as single or multiple painless, scaly yellowish plaques, sometimes resembling LV, or as subcutaneous nodules with a tendency to ulceration and a slowly progressive, chronic course. Sometimes, skin involvement occurs secondary to disseminated infection with *M. avium*-intracellulare. Skin lesions have included generalized cutaneous ulcerations, granulomas, infiltrated erythematous lesions on the extremities, pustules, and soft-tissue swelling. *M. avium*-intracellulare infections are an important cause of morbidity in patients with AIDS (see Chap. 168).

TABLE 157-15
Differential Diagnosis of *Mycobacterium Marinum* Lesions

Most Likely
- Blastomycosis
- Coccidioidomycosis
- Sporotrichosis

Consider
- Histoplasmosis
- Nocardiosis
- Tertiary syphilis
- Yaws

Always Rule Out
- Other mycobacterial infections

TABLE 157-16
Differential Diagnosis of *Mycobacterium Kansasii* Lesions

Most Likely
- Sporotrichosis

Consider
- Tuberculosis

Always Rule Out
- Other granulomatous infections of the skin

MYCOBACTERIUM SZULGAI, MYCOBACTERIUM HAEMOPHILUM, MYCOBACTERIUM GENAVENSE

Mycobacterium szulgai, Mycobacterium haemophilum, and *Mycobacterium genavense* are rarely found to cause human disease in cases of otherwise unexplained cervical lymphadenitis, cellulitis, draining nodules and plaques, bursitis, pneumonia, and subcutaneous granulomatous eruptions.

MYCOBACTERIUM FORTUITUM, MYCOBACTERIUM CHELONAE, MYCOBACTERIUM ABSCESSUS

M. fortuitum, Mycobacterium chelonae, and *Mycobacterium abscessus*—3 species of fast-growing, facultative pathogenic mycobacteria—were previously grouped in the *M. fortuitum* complex but are now recognized as distinct species. These organisms seem to be widely distributed and can commonly be found in soil and water. Contamination of various materials, including surgical supplies, occurs but does not always result in clinical disease.

Clinical Findings: *M. fortuitum, M. chelonae,* and *M. abscessus* cause similar clinical diseases. Infection usually follows a puncture wound or a surgical procedure. The disease manifests itself as a painful red infiltrate at the site of inoculation; there are no signs of dissemination and no constitutional symptoms. Cold postinjection abscesses, especially in the tropics, also may be caused by fast-growing mycobacteria. Recent cases in the United States have followed after pedicures and water immersion in salons.

The lesion is a dark red nodule, often with abscess formation and clear fluid drainage. Healthy children and adults may become infected, but disseminated disease usually occurs in hemodialysis patients or other immunologically compromised individuals. The disease course consists of multiple recurrent episodes of abscesses on the extremities or a generalized macular and papular eruption. Internal organs may be involved.

Histopathology: There is simultaneous occurrence of polymorphonuclear leukocyte microabscesses and granuloma formation with foreign-body–type giant cells, the so-called dimorphic inflammatory response. There is usually necrosis but no caseation. Acid-fast bacilli may occasionally be found within microabscesses.

Diagnosis: Organisms of the *M. fortuitum* complex may be identified by special laboratories to permit a rational treatment.

ACKNOWLEDGMENTS

The author thanks Bernard Naafs, MD, for his work on this chapter in the previous editions of this book.

REFERENCES

1. WHO report 2009–Global Tuberculosis Control. http://apps.who.int/iris/bitstream/handle/10665/44241/9789241598866_eng.pdf;sequence=1. Last accessed March 13, 2010.
2. Centers for Disease Control and Prevention (CDC). Trends in tuberculosis—United States, 2008. *MMWR Morb Mortal Wkly Rep.* 2009;58:249.
3. Pai M, Kalantri S, Dheda K. New tools and emerging technologies for the diagnosis of tuberculosis: part II. Active tuberculosis and drug resistance. *Expert Rev Mol Diagn.* 2006;6:423.
4. Pai M, Kalantri S, Dheda K. New tools and emerging technologies for the diagnosis of tuberculosis: part I. Latent tuberculosis. *Expert Rev Mol Diagn.* 2006;6:413.
5. Tsiouris SJ, Austin J, Toro P, et al. Results of a tuberculosis-specific IFN-gamma assay in children at high risk for tuberculosis infection. *Int J Tuberc Lung Dis.* 2006;10:939.
6. Tan SH, Tan HH, Sun YJ, et al. Clinical utility of polymerase chain reaction in the detection of Mycobacterium tuberculosis in different types of cutaneous tuberculosis and tuberculids. *Ann Acad Med Singapore.* 2001;30:3.
7. Barbagallo J, Tager P, Ingleton R, et al. Cutaneous tuberculosis: diagnosis and treatment. *Am J Clin Dermatol.* 2002;3:319.
8. Li N, Bajoghli A, Kubba A, Bhawan J. Identification of mycobacterial DNA in cutaneous lesions of sarcoidosis. *J Cutan Pathol.* 1999;29:271.
9. Young DB, Stewart GR. Tuberculosis vaccines. *Br Med Bull.* 2002;62:73.
10. Myers JP. New recommendations for the treatment of tuberculosis. *Curr Opin Infect Dis.* 2005;18:133.
11. Murali MS, Sajjan BS. DOTS strategy for control of tuberculosis epidemic. *Indian J Med Sci.* 2002;56:16.
12. Iseman MD. Tuberculosis therapy: past, present and future. *Eur Respir J Suppl.* 2002;36:87s.
13. Holland SM. Cytokine therapy of mycobacterial infections. *Adv Intern Med.* 2000;45:431.
14. Centers for Disease Control and Prevention (CDC). Extensively Drug Resistant (XDR) TB Update. https://www.cdc.gov/tb/default.htm. Accessed March 14, 2010.
15. Zouhair K, Akhdari N, Nejjam F, et al. Cutaneous tuberculosis in Morocco. *Int J Infect Dis.* 2007;11:209.
16. Kivanc-Altunay I, Baysal Z, Ekmekçi TR, et al. Incidence of cutaneous tuberculosis in patients with organ tuberculosis. *Int J Dermatol.* 2003;42:197.
17. Jensen PA, Lambert LA, Iademarco MF, et al. Guidelines for preventing the transmission of Mycobacterium tuberculosis in health-care settings, 2005. *MMWR Recomm Rep.* 2005;54(RR-17):1.
18. The role of BCG vaccine in the prevention and control of tuberculosis in the United States. A joint statement

18. by the Advisory Council for the Elimination of Tuberculosis and the Advisory Committee on Immunization Practices. *MMWR Recomm Rep.* 1996;45(RR-4):1.
19. Bellet JS, Prose NS. Skin complications of bacillus Calmette-Guérin immunization. *Curr Opin Infect Dis.* 2005;18:97.
20. Degitz K. Detection of mycobacterial DNA in the skin. Etiologic insights and diagnostic perspectives. *Arch Dermatol.* 1996;132:71.
21. Tan SH, Tan BH, Goh CL, et al. Detection of Mycobacterium tuberculosis DNA using polymerase chain reaction in cutaneous tuberculosis and tuberculids. *Int J Dermatol.* 1999;38:122.
22. Drake WP, Newman LS. Mycobacterial antigens may be important in sarcoidosis pathogenesis. *Curr Opin Pulm Med.* 2006;12:359.
23. Komatsu H, Terunuma A, Tabata N, et al. Mycobacterium avium infection of the skin associated with lichen scrofulosorum: report of three cases. *Br J Dermatol.* 1999;141:554.
24. Victor T, Jordaan HF, Van Niekerk DJ, et al. Papulonecrotic tuberculid. Identification of Mycobacterium tuberculosis DNA by polymerase chain reaction. *Am J Dermatopathol.* 1992;14:491.
25. Jordan HF, Schneider JW, Abdulla EA. Nodular tuberculid: a report of four patients. *Pediatr Dermatol.* 2000;17:183.
26. Senol M, Ozcan A, Aydin A, et al. Disseminated lupus vulgaris and papulonecrotic tuberculid: case report. *Pediatr Dermatol.* 2000;17:133.
27. Callahan EF, Licata AL, Madison JF. Cutaneous Mycobacterium kansasii infection associated with a papulonecrotic tuberculid reaction. *J Am Acad Dermatol.* 1997;36:497.
28. Hay RJ. Cutaneous infection with *Mycobacterium tuberculosis*: how has this altered with the changing epidemiology of tuberculosis? *Curr Opin Infect Dis.* 2005;18:93.
29. Rastogi N, Legrand E, Sola C. The mycobacteria: an introduction to nomenclature and pathogenesis. *Rev Sci Tech.* 2001;20:21.
30. Saiman L. The mycobacteriology of non-tuberculous mycobacteria. *Paediatr Respir Rev.* 2004;5(suppl A):S221.
31. Lillis JV, Ansdell VE, Ruben K, et al. Sequelae of World War II: an outbreak of chronic cutaneous nontuberculous mycobacterial infection among Satowanese islanders. *Clin Infect Dis.* 2009;48:1541.
32. Bartralot R, Pujol RM, García-Patos V, et al. Cutaneous infections due to nontuberculous mycobacteria: histopathological review of 28 cases. Comparative study between lesions observed in immunosuppressed patients and normal hosts. *J Cutan Pathol.* 2000;27:124.

Chapter 158 :: Actinomycosis, Nocardiosis, and Actinomycetoma
:: Francisco G. Bravo, Roberto Arenas, & Daniel Asz Sigall

第一百五十八章
放线菌病、诺卡氏菌病和放线菌瘤

中文导读

　　放线菌和诺卡氏菌属于同一类放线菌，它们可引起人类疾病。长期以来，该类别的微生物被错误地归类为真菌。放线菌病是由内源放线菌属物种引起的慢性、进行性、惰性感染，内源放线菌属是人类黏膜表面（包括口腔、咽、食道远端和泌尿生殖道）的常见定植菌。皮肤诺卡氏病是环境诺卡氏菌引起的皮肤感染，这是由于外伤直接接种造成的，因此是原发性皮肤诺卡氏菌，或者是由通常来自肺源的血源性播种所致。本章节就这三种形式的细菌感染的流行病学、临床表现、诊断与治疗等方面进行了全面的讨论。

〔汪 犇〕

Actinomyces and *Nocardia* are a group of filamentous bacteria belonging to the same class, Actinobacteria, and same order, Actinomycetales. They cause human disease with prominent skin involvement. Microorganisms under this category were wrongly classified as fungi for a long time, because of their tendency to produce branching filaments, mimicking radiating hyphae (from the Greek *actino*, meaning *sun*). Their taxonomy is still evolving, resulting in continuous reclassification of different species in old and new families. Anaerobic endogenous *Actinomyces*, which are part of our normal respiratory, intestinal, and genitourinary flora, will cause localized suppurative disease with fistula formation that is analogous to the lumpy jaw of cattle. Aerobic environmental *Nocardia* sp. can cause primary cutaneous disease, ranging from cellulitis to paronychia to abscesses, with the most striking presentation being a lymphocutaneous, sporotrichoid syndrome; cutaneous nocardiosis as a consequence of hematogenous dissemination from a pulmonary source is also seen, but it is characteristically of a state of immunosuppression. In addition, other aerobic environmental species of *Nocardia* and *Actinomyces* will cause 1 of the 2 known forms of mycetoma, the actinomycetoma.

The sulfur granule or grain, a clumping of filamentous bacteria seen in infected living tissue, is considered characteristic of the infection by these microorganisms, but is not always present and is also not specific (Table 158-1). Practicing dermatologists should be aware of the various morphologic variants of these diseases and the measures that should be taken to ensure the appropriate culturing techniques required for isolation.

ACTINOMYCOSIS

AT-A-GLANCE

- Worldwide distribution, relatively uncommon.
- *Actinomyces* are part of normal upper respiratory, intestinal, and genitourinary flora.
- *Actinomyces israelii* is the most common causative agent, usually as part of a polymicrobial infection, mixed with anaerobes and Gram-positive cocci.
- Classical presentation is a chronic, localized, infiltrative, bulging process with abscess fistula formation and draining sinuses.
- Most common location is cervicofacial (related to dental pathology), followed by chest wall, abdominal, and pelvic involvement.
- Pathologic findings include a chronic inflammatory infiltrate with granulation tissue or granuloma formation.
- Grains (sulfur granules) are characteristic but neither invariably present nor pathognomonic.

DEFINITION

Actinomycosis can be defined as a chronic, progressive, indolent infection by endogenous *Actinomyces* species, which are common inhabitants of the human mucosal surfaces, including the oral cavity, pharynx, distal esophagus, and genitourinary tract. This endogenous source is the main concept used to distinguish actinomycosis from actinomycetoma; in the case of mycetomas, the infection agent is an environmental actinomyces, making the bacteria responsible for the infection of exogenous origin.

HISTORICAL PERSPECTIVE

Actinomycosis was described by Israel in 1878; its causative agent, originally named *Streptothrix israeli* (currently *Actinomyces israelii*), was described by Kruse in 1896. It remained the only described etiologic agent of the disease until 1951, where *Actinomyces naeslundii* was implicated in other human cases, while *Actinomyces odontolyticus* and *Actinomyces viscosus* were described in 1958 and 1969, respectively. Currently, 25 validly published *Actinomyces* species recovered from human material are recognized.[1]

EPIDEMIOLOGY

Actinomycosis has a worldwide distribution and is relatively rare, with a tendency to decline, especially in developed countries, because of a higher standard of oral care and the disease's susceptibility to many antibiotics. It is more commonly seen in males, ages 20 to 60 years, although females predominate in cases of genitourinary actinomycosis, because of its relationship to the use of intrauterine devices (IUDs). Nowadays, there is a tendency to see more subtle cases, restricted to the oral cavity and before the formation of fistula toward the cutaneous surface. Diagnosis in such circumstances requires a high index of suspicion.

TABLE 158-1
Diagnostic Approach to Diseases That Produce Grains

DISEASE	ACTINOMYCOSIS	NOCARDIOSIS	ACTINOMYCETOMA	EUMYCETOMA	BOTRYOMYCOSIS
Clinical pattern	Lump with draining sinuses	Sporotrichoid, cellulitis, abscesses	Lump with draining sinuses	Lump with draining sinuses	Lump with draining sinuses
Site	Cervicofacial, thorax, abdomen, pelvic	Extremities (upper > lower)	Feet, back, extremities	Feet, mainly	Hand, head, feet
Source	Endogenous flora	Environment	Environment	Environment	Endogenous and environment
Most common agent	*Actinomyces israelii*	*Nocardia brasiliensis* *Nocardia asteroides*	*Nocardia brasiliensis* *Actinomadura madurae* *Actinomadura pelletieri* *Streptomyces somaliensis*	*Madurella mycetomatis* *Madurella grisea* *Pseudallescheria boydii*	*Staphylococcus aureus* *Escherichia coli* *Pseudomonas aeruginosa*
Grains, clinically or histologically	Common	Rare (only in disseminated cases)	Always	Always	Always
Grain contents	Filamentous bacteria	Filamentous bacteria	Filamentous bacteria	Hyphae	Cocci (most common)
Staining	Gram positive	Gram positive Weak acid-fast bacillus	Gram positive Weak acid-fast bacillus (only if *Nocardia*)	Periodic acid-Schiff, Grocott	Gram positive

CLINICAL FEATURES

Actinomycosis should be suspected when dealing with 1 of 3 features: a mass-like inflammatory infiltrate of the skin and subcutaneous tissue, sinus formation with drainage, and a relapsing or refractory clinical course after short-term therapy with antibiotics. Actinomycotic granules may be seen macroscopically and is always very suggestive of the diagnosis.

CUTANEOUS FINDINGS

Cervicofacial actinomycosis is the most frequent form of disease[2,3] accounting for approximately 55% of cases. Commonly, there is a history of poor dental hygiene, dental or periodontal disease, dental procedure, surgery, or penetrating trauma through the oral mucosa. Most of the infections start as a periapical abscess. The most common location is on the jaw angle and high cervical area (60%), followed by the cheek (16%), the chin (13%), and, less commonly, the temporomandibular joint and the retromandibular area. The lesion starts as a solid mass in any of those locations, and initially may be confused with a neoplastic process (Fig. 158-1). It may progress to form recurring abscesses and later will spread to adjacent structures, not respecting anatomic planes. Propagation to lymph nodes is uncommon but eventually may involve the orbit, cranium, spine, and even vascular structures. The lesion is sometimes reported as painless, but pain may be present, as well as fever and leukocytosis. With extension to the skin surface, sinus tracts appear (Fig. 158-2). The overlying skin may have a purplish red hue. Trismus

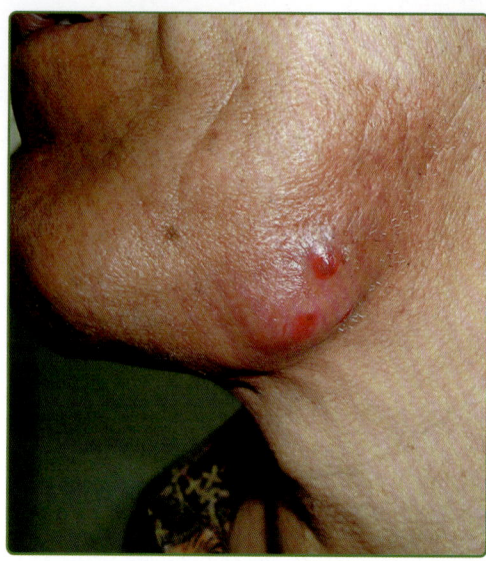

Figure 158-2 Typical cervicofacial actinomycosis: a lump with sinus formation. (Used with permission from Wilson Delgado, DDS, and Lepoldo Meneses, DDS, Universidad Peruana Cayetano Heredia, Lima, Peru.)

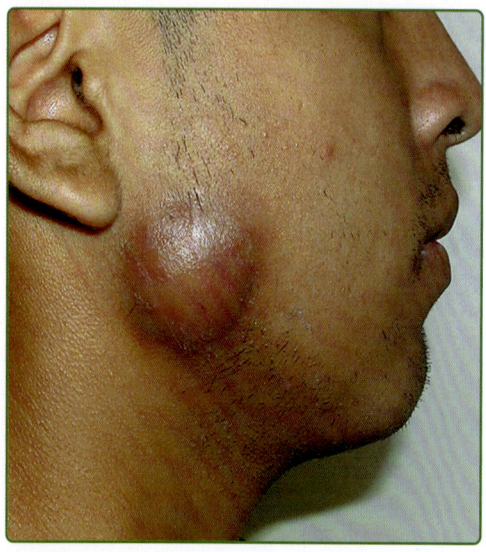

Figure 158-1 Cervicofacial actinomycosis. A solid mass on the mandibular angle that can be confused with a neoplastic process.

may develop. Bone involvement, mostly of the jaw, is present in 10% of cases. More limited disease may produce a mass or an ulcer, affecting any structure in the mouth or the nasopharyngeal region. Extension to the ear may present as chronic otitis media or mastoiditis. In addition to orbital involvement, there are reported cases of lacrimal canaliculitis and endophthalmitis. Regional lymphadenopathy is uncommon.

Thoracic actinomycosis comprises 15% to 20% of cases. The common source of infection is the aspiration of a microorganism from the oropharynx, although other routes are possible, such as propagation of cervicofacial disease to the mediastinum. The disease may involve the lung, pleura, mediastinum, and chest wall. The course is indolent, with chest pain, fever, weight loss, cough, and, less frequently, hemoptysis, mimicking tuberculosis. Radiologically, the disease will present as a mass or pneumonia, with pleural involvement by continuity. Relevant to dermatologists, up to 26% of cases will have chest wall involvement, the so-called empyema necessitans, with the development of a cutaneous abscess and sinus formation (Fig. 158-3). Parenchymal, pleural, and chest wall disease occurring together will make actinomycosis a most likely diagnosis. Mediastinal actinomycosis may show either as anterior chest wall disease (rarely sternal involvement), or paraspinal abscess. Involvement of breast tissue and breast implants also has been described.

Abdominal actinomycosis represents approximately 20% of all cases. It is usually the consequence of spreading from the GI tract or from the female genital tract. Appendicitis and diverticulitis are common precipitating events and appendicitis or diverticulitis may be present in up to 65% of cases; the clinical presentation will be of a right iliac fossa mass. Any organ in the

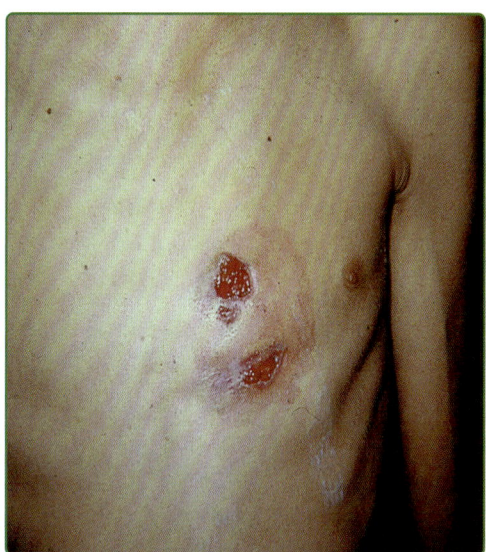

Figure 158-3 Thoracic actinomycosis from a patient who died from disseminated disease.

peritoneal cavity may be affected; by local extension, the disease may spread to the abdominal wall or perineum. An inflammatory mass may eventually appear in the skin surface of the abdominal region or the perineum, with later development of fistula. In the perianal area, multiple abscesses and fistula formation may occur. The disease may spread from the anal area to the buttocks, thighs, scrotum and groin.

Primary pelvic disease most often originates from ascending infection from the female genital tract, and less often from abdominal disease. The role of the IUD as a risk factor has been clearly established and infection is usually associated with its use for longer than 2 years. Studies show that IUD usage averages 8 years.

Punch or fist actinomycosis represents a particularly uncommon but interesting clinical presentation. It usually follows blunt trauma of a closed fist against a person's mouth; similar findings may originate from a human bite. Punch actinomycosis usually involves the proximal phalanges and metacarpal bones. The actinomycosis appears as a soft-tissue infection that eventually spreads to the bony structures. Grains are commonly seen in this particular form.[4]

NONCUTANEOUS FINDINGS

Actinomycosis of the CNS may present as brain abscess, meningitis, meningoencephalitis, subdural empyema, actinomycoma, or spinal abscess. It is usually secondary to hematogenous spread or direct extension of orocervical infection. Other sites affected include bones, muscle tissue, and prosthetic joints.

ETIOLOGY AND PATHOGENESIS

The term *actinomycosis* implies disease produced by endogenous, anaerobic, or microaerophile, Gram-positive, non–spore-forming bacteria, belonging to the families Actinomycetaceae, genus *Actinomyces*.[1] Their normal habitat is human mucosal surfaces, with considerable host specificity, from the mouth to the upper respiratory, GI, and female genital tracts. Species known to cause disease in humans include *A. israelii*, *Actinomyces gerencseriae*, *A. naeslundii*, *A. viscosus*, *A. odontolyticus*, and *Actinomyces meyeri*. In orocervical disease, the predominant species include *A. israelii*, *A. naeslundii*, *A. viscosus*, and *A. odontolyticus*, whereas in thoracic disease, *Actinomyces graevenitzii*, seems to predominate. The disease in most cases is mixed with other microorganisms sharing the same habitat, so it should be considered a synergistic infection, with the *Actinomyces* playing the role of guiding organism, defining the course, the symptoms, and the ultimate prognosis. Accompanying organisms may vary in number, from 1 to 9 different species, and may include *Fusarium* and *Bacteroides* species, microaerophile and anaerobic streptococci, *Aggregatibacter* species, and aerobic coagulase negative staphylococci.[1] This concomitant flora may be partly responsible for the disease course. In recent years, with better culturing techniques and molecular microbiology, more than 1 *Actinomyces* has been isolated from a single lesion in several patients, stressing the possibility that single bacterial isolation, common in the past, was a technical artifact.

The infection has its portal of entry at a break on a mucous membrane. Most cervical and facial cases originate from periapical abscesses or after dental procedures. *Actinomyces* bacteremia seems to occur quite often after dental procedures.

Thoracic cases represent involvement of the chest wall by local spreading either from pleural or lung disease acquired by obstruction or aspiration. The same mechanism of spreading applies to disease of the abdominal wall, secondary to gut or genital pathology, following appendicitis, diverticulitis, surgery, or trauma. Perineal disease occurs as a consequence of involvement of the internal organs of the pelvis, often secondary to use of an intravaginal device or IUD. The only exception to the endogenous origin of the infection is hand involvement that follows fist or bite trauma.[4]

In tissue, the bacteria cluster in filamentous aggregates, the so-called *sulfur granules* (grains; see Table 158-1). They are commonly surrounded by acute and chronic inflammation, usually neutrophils, granulation tissue, and fibrosis. Foamy histiocytes may be part of the infiltrate but true granuloma formation is rare. The fistula formation may give way to drainage of granules, but their presence by themselves should not be considered specific for this disease, as they also can be seen in mycetomas and botryomycosis.

RISK FACTORS

Although most patients are immunocompetent, conditions linked to immunosuppression, such as prolonged administration of steroids, bisphosphonates, leukemia with chemotherapy, HIV, lung and renal transplant receipt, alcoholism, and local tissue damage by trauma, recent surgery, or radiation, all are associated with the disease.[3]

DIAGNOSIS

LABORATORY TESTING

Most diagnoses are based on the clinical isolation of *Actinomyces* species. Laboratory tests considered useful include direct examination of draining material, culture, and biopsy. Direct examination will show the presence of filamentous *Actinomyces* on Gram stain. The isolation of *Actinomyces* in culture should be considered diagnostic, if coming from a sterile site. However, positive culture rates are as low as 35% in some series. The processing should be done in anaerobic conditions, and the laboratory should be notified of the clinical suspicion of actinomycosis. Negative culture can be the result of previous antibiotic treatment, overgrowth of concomitant microorganisms or inadequate methodology.

Best material is purulent drainage, tissue, or microscopic granules, and avoidance of any antibiotic treatment is recommended before culturing; swabs are not considered an appropriate sampling method. Appropriate culture media include thioglycolate with 0.5 sterile rabbit serum at 35°C (95°F) for 14 days. Colonies may appear within 5 to 7 days, but up to 2 weeks may be required. *A. israelii* classically will produce a "molar tooth" colony on agar and will look clumpy on broth. *A. odontolyticus* colonies are red or rusty in color. *Actinomyces* are indole-negative. The microbiologic identification of different species occurs only in a minority of cases. Tests for urease, catalase, gelatin hydrolysis, and fermentation of cellobiose, trehalose, and arabinose can be performed. New techniques that can be used include polymerase chain reaction, sequencing or restriction analysis of amplified 16S ribosomal DNA, fluorescence in situ hybridization, and mass spectrometry.[3]

PATHOLOGY

The presence of granules, either microscopically or macroscopically, is very relevant, especially if obtained from tissues not connected to mucosal surfaces. Grains are usually yellow (hence the name *sulfur granules*), but can be white, pinkish gray, gray, or brown. In tissue samples, special stains, such as Brown-Brenn, Gram, Giemsa, or Gomori, are required to demonstrate filamentous structures. The number of grains may be scanty: 25% of specimens in a study of 181 cases had a single granule in the whole sample.[3] The microscopic examination of the granules may reveal the Splendore-Hoeppli phenomena, a rim of eosinophilic material surrounding the granules in tissue cuts. The lack of staining with Fite-modified acid-fast stain separates *Actinomyces* from *Nocardia* species, which is usually acid-fast positive. Eumycetoma granules stain positive with periodic acid–Schiff and Gomori, as any other fungus, whereas granules from botryomycosis should show clumps of nonfilamentous bacteria. Direct immunofluorescent staining is available for some species, including *A. israelii*.

IMAGING

In early stages, imaging features are nonspecific and nondiagnostic. Computed tomography and magnetic resonance in advanced stages may show nonspecific findings, such as an abscess or phlegmon, but may give good anatomical references that facilitate the aspiration of pus material suitable for direct examination and cultures.

DIFFERENTIAL DIAGNOSIS

Depending on the site affected, the differential diagnosis includes infections such as tuberculosis, noninfectious inflammatory processes such as hidradenitis and inflammatory bowel disease, and neoplasia (Table 158-2).

MANAGEMENT

MEDICATIONS

Historically, the treatment of actinomycosis requires high-dose antibiotics given for a long period. The treatment of choice is penicillin G, 18 to 24 million units IV for 2 to 6 weeks, followed by oral penicillin or amoxicillin, to be given for 6 to 12 months. The risk of developing penicillin resistance is low. However, this

---

TABLE 158-2

Differential Diagnosis of Actinomycosis (Site-Specific)

Most Likely
- *Face:* tuberculosis, odontogenic abscesses, parotid tumors
- *Chest:* tuberculosis, neoplasm, pyogenic infections
- *Abdomen and pelvis:* tuberculosis, inflammatory bowel disease, hidradenitis suppurativa, neoplasm

Consider
- *Face:* lupus panniculitis, granuloma inguinale
- *Pelvis:* granuloma inguinale

prolonged therapy may not be needed in all patients. Cervicofacial disease or any limited disease can receive a shorter course of therapy. A good rule to follow is to give therapy until full resolution of clinically evident disease. Some authors recommend the initial use of a β-lactam and a β-lactam inhibitor such as clavulanate or tazobactam, which provide additional cover against potential β-lactam producers such as *Staphylococcus aureus* and Gram-negative anaerobes. Alternative treatment for those allergic to penicillin includes tetracycline, doxycycline, erythromycin, and clindamycin. Imipenem has been used successfully as short-term therapy. Chloramphenicol is the alternative to penicillin in cases of CNS involvement. Some studies show that many species of actinomyces are susceptible to new drugs, such as linezolid and tigecycline. Risk factors for relapse or death include duration of disease longer than 2 months, lack of antibiotic therapy or surgical therapy, and needle aspiration rather than open drainage or excision.

With early diagnosis and more limited disease, compared to the bulky disease of the past, treatment can be shorter: 30 days for cervicofacial disease and 3 months for pelvic or thoracic disease.[3,5] In such cases, clinical response should be closely monitored. Periapical actinomycosis can be successfully treated with curettage and 10 days of antibiotic therapy.

PROCEDURES

Surgery is indicated for bulky disease involving the chest, abdomen, pelvis, and CNS. Its aim should be resection of necrotic tissue, excision of sinus tracts, draining of empyemas and abscesses, and curettage of bone, always accompanied by antibiotic therapy.

PREVENTION

Good oral hygiene and prevention of periodontal disease may decrease colonization by *Actinomyces*. Physicians dealing with patients using an IUD should be aware of the risk of developing the disease.

NOCARDIOSIS

AT-A-GLANCE

- Aerobic Gram-positive filamentous bacteria.
- Worldwide distribution, environmentally acquired infection, results from primary traumatic inoculation.
- Pulmonary infections mostly in immunocompromised patients and skin infections mostly in immunocompetent patients.

(Continued)

AT-A-GLANCE (Continued)

- Primary skin disease mostly caused by *Nocardia brasiliensis*. If it is a consequence of hematogenous dissemination, the most likely microorganism is *Nocardia asteroides*.
- Cutaneous nocardiosis can take the form of either cellulitis or more characteristic lymphocutaneous nodules in a sporotrichoid pattern; skin lesions in the form of hemorrhagic pustules or abscesses occur in disseminated disease.
- Diagnosis is based on Gram stain of clinical specimen showing thin, Gram-positive branching bacteria, weakly positive with acid-fast staining; microbiologic isolation of *Nocardia* sp. is diagnostic, but requires keeping cultures under observation 5 to 7 days.
- Treatment: sulfonamides.

DEFINITIONS

Cutaneous nocardiosis is the infection of skin by environmental *Nocardia sp*, either as a result of direct inoculation through trauma, thus is, primary cutaneous nocardiosis, or as a consequence of hematogenous seeding, usually from a pulmonary source. Primary cutaneous nocardiosis is a disease of immunocompetent patients, whereas secondary hematogenous spreading is seen in the context of immunosuppression.

HISTORICAL PERSPECTIVE

Edward Nocard described the filamentous bacteria *Norcadia* sp. In 1888, after its clinical isolation from cattle affected by farcy. The first human case was described by Eppinger in 1890, in a patient with pulmonary and pleural involvement, under the name "pseudotuberculosis." Since then, multiple reports have emphasized the relevance of pulmonary and cutaneous nocardiosis as the most common clinical presentations, with the potential for systemic dissemination.

EPIDEMIOLOGY

By 2017, approximately 1000 cases of nocardiosis were reported annually in the United States.[6] However, considering the increasing number of transplantation patients, patients immunosuppressed by chemotherapy, patients on chronic corticosteroid therapy, HIV patients not receiving appropriated antiviral therapy, and patients with primary pulmonary diseases such as chronic obstructive pulmonary disease, the number of cases occurring annually is probably underestimated. At least 50% of patients will have some sort of immunosuppression. Nocardiosis occurs most commonly in males. The most common presentation of nocardiosis is pulmonary disease. Agricultural occupation is common in pulmonary nocardiosis, but a history of environmental exposure on a farm or in the wilderness is also common in the primary cutaneous form. Primary cutaneous involvement represents from 5% to 24% of nocardiosis cases. The higher incidence of primary cutaneous nocardiosis in Europe may be explained on the basis of more frequent isolation of *Nocardia brasiliensis* in the environment.[6]

CLINICAL FEATURES

CUTANEOUS FINDINGS

Cutaneous involvement by *Nocardia* can manifest either as an abscess, cellulitis, or more characteristically, as lymphocutaneous nodules in a sporotrichoid pattern. Disseminated disease also can be present in the skin as a consequence of hematogenous spread, from hemorrhagic pustules to ecthyma and abscesses.[7] In most series, skin disease is second in frequency after pulmonary involvement. Mycetoma caused by *Nocardia* is discussed above under "Actinomycetoma."

Predisposing factors for primary cutaneous nocardiosis include soil or sand exposure while gardening or farming; or superficial injury from domestic shrubbery, outdoor falls, or accidents. The frequent history of thorn injury or gardening may suggest, incorrectly, a diagnosis of sporotrichosis. Insect bites, cat scratches, or just barely contact with them have been reported as the portal of entry, especially in children.[8]

Most patients with primary cutaneous nocardiosis are immunocompetent, but *Nocardia* cutaneous infection may also occur in the context of immunosuppression. A series of nocardial infections in AIDS patients showed skin lesions in 11% of cases, most commonly cutaneous abscesses and suppurative adenitis.[9] Relevant to dermatologist, nocardiosis has been described in patients receiving anti–tumor necrosis factor biologic therapy for Crohn disease, and also as a complication of immunosuppressive therapy in the context of pemphigus.[10,11]

The disease has been also described in ulcerative bullous, linear/keloid, and nodulopustular forms (Fig. 158-4A) that may evolve into the more specific sporotrichoid pattern (Fig. 158-4B). This sporotrichoid or lymphocutaneous forms may account for 24% of all *Nocardia* cutaneous infections (Fig. 158-4B).[12] The first case proven to be caused by *N. brasiliensis* was described by Alarcon; the patient developed acute nodular suppurative lymphadenitis after injuring the finger with a rose thorn. Although the upper extremity is the most common location, disease of the lower extremity and cervicofacial region also have been reported. A common history is appearance of a solitary papule or nodule on the upper limbs, 2 to 4 weeks after cutaneous inoculation. Then, proximal nodules develop along lymphatic drainage. The primary lesion is initially warm and tender, then becomes fluctuant, and later ulcerates. Systemic symptoms are mild. Regional lymphadenitis is common but lymphangitis is unusual.

Patients may also present acutely with eccrine hidradenitis, or chronically with hyperkeratotic plaques. Cutaneous nocardiosis may begin suddenly, reactivate after months to years, or follow a chronic course for up to 10 years. A case of simultaneous infection in a husband and wife also has been described. Very rarely, pure cutaneous disease may lead to systemic illness. The cellulitis form most commonly affects the lower extremities, as compared to sporotrichoid form, in which the upper extremities are most often involved. The face has been reported as a rare site, with multiple draining sinuses, but no grains, which distinguishes the cutaneous form from the mycetoma form.[13] Children frequently present with cellulitis, abscesses, and lymphadenitis affecting the lower extremities and trunk; 20% of cases have lesions at multiple sites.[8]

Sternal wound infections usually develop 1 month after thoracic surgery. The symptoms include erythema, clear-to-purulent drainage, wound dehiscence, and/or fever. Diabetes mellitus seems to be the only identifiable risk factor. At least in one outbreak, the hands of an anesthesiologist were culture positive for *Nocardia farcinica*. In another case of sternal osteomyelitis and

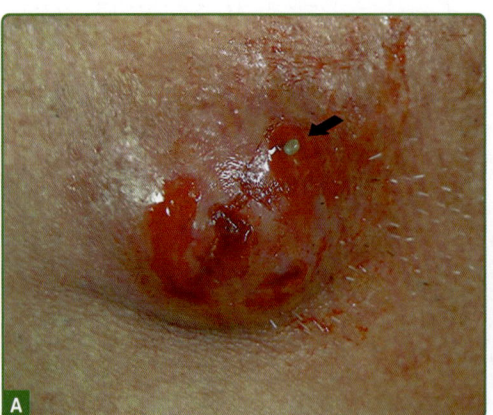
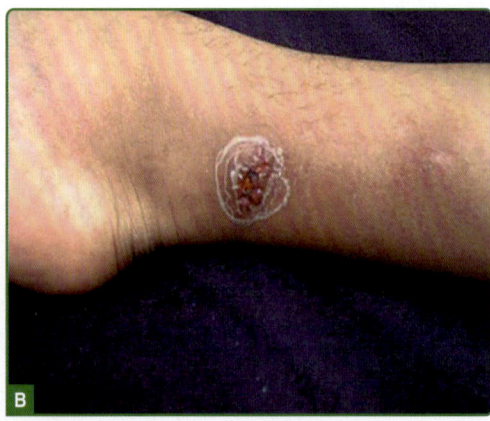

Figure 158-4 **A,** Early lesions of lymphocutaneous nocardiosis. **B,** Lymphocutaneous nocardiosis: typical sporotrichoid pattern. (Used with permission from Daniel Asz and Roberto Arenas, Hospital Manuel Gea González, Mexico City, Mexico.)

mediastinal abscess, the patient's occupation (carrying wooden crates loaded with vegetables) may have been the only risk factor for infection, in the absence of chest surgery or trauma.

NONCUTANEOUS FINDINGS

Pulmonary disease is the most common form of clinical infection, but, compared to primary cutaneous diseases, is often caused by different species (*Nocardia asteroides* predominates). The disease may take the form of an acute pneumonia or a chronic process with bronchopneumonia, abscesses, and development of cavities. In 10% of pulmonary actinomycosis there is spreading to the adjacent skin.

Bacteremia resulting from *Nocardia* is seen in patients with concomitant malignancy, and *N. asteroides* is the agent most commonly isolated. Cutaneous or subcutaneous nodules and abscesses occur in many patients, and the skin may be the portal of entry in some cases. Catheter-associated nocardemia is well documented.

ETIOLOGY AND PATHOGENESIS

The *Nocardia* genus includes more than 80 species; approximately 30 of those species have been described as cause of human disease. The *Nocardia* species of medical importance include *N. asteroides*, most commonly associated with lung and systemic disease, and *N. brasiliensis*, most commonly associated with skin infection. The most common cause of primary cutaneous nocardiosis is *N. brasiliensis*, but *N. asteroides*, *Nocardia otitidiscaviarum*, *Nocardia nova*, *N. farcinica*, and most recently, *Nocardia takedensis* also have been implicated.[14] It is only recently that many of those species have been completely separated, especially those of the *N. asteroides* group. It is interesting to note that *Nocardia* species belong to a subgroup of bacteria called the *aerobic nocardioform actinomycetes* that also include *Mycobacterium*, *Corynebacterium*, *Rhodococcus*, and *Gordona*. All these microorganisms have mycolic acid as constituent of their cell wall, which explains the varying acid fastness on appropriate staining.

The usual inflammatory response in infected tissue is neutrophilic, with branching, beading filamentous bacteria within abscesses. Sulfur granules are uncommon in primary cutaneous nocardiosis; they have been described in disseminated disease. They are more commonly seen and consider characteristic when the clinical picture is that of mycetoma (see section "Actinomycetoma").

Certain virulent strains of *Nocardia* are resistant to neutrophil-mediated killing.[15] They can inhibit phagosome-lysosome fusion in vitro, giving rise to L-forms able to survive inside macrophages. The existence of cell wall–deficient L-forms may explain the occasional late relapse. The presence of superoxide dismutase in growth media is characteristic of the more virulent strains. Complex cell wall glycolipids also contribute to virulence.[15]

The initial neutrophilic reaction is followed by a more cell-related immune response that is responsible for clearing the infection from the lung tissue and prevents dissemination. If this fails, a chronic neutrophilic response results in a more indolent course. Lack of cellular immunity predisposes transplantation and AIDS patients to infection, with transplantation patients accounting for up to 13% of cases in the United States.[6] Some species are considered more difficult to treat: *N. farcinica* has a high degree of resistance to various antibiotics, especially third-generation cephalosporins and aminoglycosides. Another recently described species, *Nocardia pseudobrasiliensis*, has a higher rate of dissemination.

RISK FACTORS

In cases of primary cutaneous nocardiosis, the classical presentation is in a immunocompetent patient. However, many cases of pulmonary nocardiosis with subsequent dissemination take place in the context of immunosuppression. Cases as such are associated with malignancy (either solid organ or hematologic) on chemotherapy or corticosteroid, transplantation (renal and heart transplantations are the most common), AIDS, IV drug abuse, systemic lupus, and nephrotic syndrome.[6,7,16] Corticosteroids, either alone or in conjunction with other drugs that cause immunosuppression, are an important risk factor for developing nocardiosis.

DIAGNOSIS

The definitive diagnosis of nocardiosis can only be made when the isolation of *Nocardia* species is accomplished in culture.

LABORATORY TESTING

Laboratory tests considered useful include direct examination of clinical specimens, culture, and biopsy. The importance of direct microscopic examination for the presence of granules, especially in disseminated cases and lesions that are suppurative, cannot be overemphasized. Organisms are detected as Gram-positive, branched, filamentous "hyphae" (in reality, they are bacteria). They characteristically branch at right angles. Acid-fast stains, including Fite-Faraco and the modified Kinyoun technique, stain the filamentous bacteria. For isolation, cultures should be kept under observation for up to 2 to 3 weeks. The microorganisms grow satisfactorily on most of the nonselective media used for isolation of bacteria, mycobacterium, and fungi. Because the slow growth of *Nocardia* colonies over 2 days to 2 weeks on routine culture media allows bacterial overgrowth, isolation of this organism from soil and nonsterile sites may be difficult. *Nocardia* do not survive the digestive procedures used routinely in mycobacterial culture. Thayer-Martin and buffered charcoal-yeast extract agar may be used, and pretreatment of specimens with a low pH potassium chloride–hydrochloric acid solution for 4 minutes is required.

After initial isolation, subcultures should be incubated at 25°C (77°F), 35°C (95°F), and 45°C (113°F). *N. asteroides* grows best at 35°C (95°F). Aerial "hyphae," giving a chalky appearance, are seen macroscopically in cultures; however, in the early stages of growth, they are only seen with the microscope. *N. asteroides* complex colonies vary from salmon pink to orange, whereas *N. brasiliensis* are usually orange, and *N. otitidiscaviarum* are usually pale. Identification of genus can be achieved by microscopic and colonial morphology, growth requirements, metabolism of glucose, arylsulfatase production, growth in lysozyme, and phenotypic molecular characteristics. Genotyping methods, including polymerase chain reaction, DNA hybridization, and sequencing of 16 ribosomal RNA, are useful, if available. The RNA sequencing on 16S ribosomal RNA is the best tool and has become the gold standard for the identification of *Nocardia* species. The identification of the species allows a more precise selection of adequate antimicrobial agents. However, it is expensive, requires sophisticated equipment, and is time consuming.[17]

PATHOLOGY

Patterns described on histology include monocytic infiltrates, fibrinopurulent exudates, granuloma formation, chronic granuloma formation, chronic nodular dermatitis, microabscess formation, and coccobacillary organisms; the presence of granules has been described in disseminated cases.[6]

IMAGING

X-ray patterns that can be seen in pulmonary nocardiosis include irregular nodular, reticulonodular or diffuse pneumonitic patterns. CT scans will also help to identify cavitary lesions.

DIAGNOSTIC ALGORITHM

In the case of sporotrichoid lesions, bacterial, mycologic, and mycobacterial cultures are indicated, as the differential diagnosis will include, in addition to nocardiosis, sporotrichosis, tuberculosis, and atypical bacteria, such as *Mycobacterium marinum*. In cases occurring in geographic areas where leishmaniasis is prevalent, direct examination, NNN (Novy-MacNeal-Nicolle) culture, and leishmanin intradermal test also should be included in the diagnostic workup. The biopsy will enable determination of whether granulomas are present in the infiltrate.

DIFFERENTIAL DIAGNOSIS

The differential diagnosis for primary cutaneous nocardiosis depends on the clinical form: abscesses have to be differentiated from suppurative processes caused by *S. aureus*, whereas in the cases of lymphocutaneous, sporotrichoid forms, the differential diagnosis includes "most likely" and "less likely" infections and other noninfectious processes (Table 158-3).

CLINICAL COURSE, MANAGEMENT, AND PROGNOSIS

In cases of primary cutaneous nocardiosis, the disease has a good prognosis when appropriate antibiotic therapy is given. Disseminated nocardiosis, especially nocardiosis associated with immunosuppression, extensive pulmonary involvement, or bacteremia, has a less-favorable prognosis. Spontaneous resolution or good clinical response despite inappropriate therapy has been described in children with *Nocardia* cellulitis or lymphadenitis.[8]

The treatment of *Nocardia* infection is appropriate antimicrobial therapy and surgical drainage and debridement. Factors to consider include site and severity of infection, the immune status of the host, potential for interactions, and the species of *Nocardia* involved.

MEDICATIONS

Sulfonamides, alone or in combination with trimethoprim, as trimethoprim-sulfamethoxazole (TMP-SMX), are the cornerstone of therapy for *Nocardia* infections, but are ineffective against *N. otitidiscaviarum*.[18] For primary cutaneous nocardiosis of mild to moderate intensity, sulfonamide (either sulfadiazine or sulfisoxazole) alone has been considered adequate therapy but other authors consider TMP-SMX the treatment of choice, despite lack of controlled trials. This recommendation is based

---

TABLE 158-3
Differential Diagnosis of Lymphocutaneous Nocardiosis

Most Likely
- Sporotrichosis
- *Mycobacterium marinum* infection
- Leishmaniasis
- Pyoderma caused by *Staphylococcus aureus*

Consider
- Cryptococcosis
- Tuberculosis
- *Mycobacterium kansasii*, *Mycobacterium chelonae*, and *Mycobacterium fortuitum*
- Cysticercosis

Rule Out
- Epithelioid sarcoma
- Metastatic disease

on synergistic activity of both drugs in vitro against *Nocardia*. The commercially available preparation has a fixed ratio of 1:5, and the dose currently recommended is 5 to 10 mg/kg TMP and 25 to 50 mg/kg SMX in 2 to 4 divided doses. For primary cutaneous nocardiosis, 5 mg/kg of TMP should be sufficient. Clinical improvement should be seen within 3 to 10 days, and 1 to 4 months of treatment should be curative for sporotrichoid nodules and cutaneous ulcers. Prolonged therapy is required for immunosuppressed patients. Minocycline 100 to 200 mg twice a day is considered the alternative treatment in cases of sulfonamide hypersensitivity or poor tolerance.

In more-severe cases or disease involving other organs, a combination of sulfonamide with a second agent is recommended. The second-line drugs most recommended are amikacin, imipenem, and ceftriaxone. Alternative second-line drugs include amoxicillin-clavulanate and linezolid. Immunosuppression is a good indication for a 2-drug regimen, including amikacin; an 88% cure rate has been reported when this drug is used.[6] Sternal infections caused by *N. asteroides* have responded to oral ofloxacin therapy. *N. farcinica* has a high degree of resistance to various antibiotics, especially third-generation cephalosporin and imipenem, and combined therapy is highly recommended. For extracutaneous nocardiosis, extended treatment with parenteral therapy followed by an oral regimen is necessary.

PROCEDURES

Surgery is indicated in cases of abscesses (drainage) or extensive necrosis (debridement).[19]

PREVENTION

The low incidence of *Nocardia* infections in immunodeficient states does not justify prophylactic use of antibiotics. AIDS patients receiving TMP-SMX for *Pneumocystis* organisms are already protected against *Nocardia*.

ACTINOMYCETOMA

AT-A-GLANCE

- Actinomycetoma is caused by bacteria, as opposed to eumycetoma, which is caused by fungi.
- More commonly seen in the tropics ("mycetoma belt").
- Several microorganisms cause the disease. Some species are specific for some geographic areas. In the Americas, *Nocardia brasiliensis* predominates.
- More common in men and in lower extremities.

- Visceral involvement has bad prognosis.
- Characteristic painless subcutaneous mass, with sinus formation and seropurulent discharge that contains grains (mycetoma triad).
- Macroscopic or microscopic grains are usually white. Gram staining shows filamentous bacteria.

DEFINITIONS

Mycetomas are chronic infections of the skin, underlying tissues, sometimes bones, and, rarely, viscera, caused by either bacteria (actinomycetomas) or fungi (eumycetomas).[20] Only actinomycetoma is discussed further in this chapter. Actinomycetomas present clinically as tumor-like swelling and sinus tracts, with discharge of grains that can be seen either microscopically or with the naked eye.

HISTORICAL PERSPECTIVE

Although the first modern description of Madura foot is attributed to Gill in 1842, in the holy city of Madurai, India, the disease was already described in ancient writings from India itself, under the name "padavalmika," meaning "foot anthill," around the fourth and fifth centuries AD.[21] The first medical case of mycetoma in Mexico was described by Cicero in 1911, but analysis of bone remains related to the Tlatilco culture, during the period from 1400 BC to 200 AD, has allowed speculation about the existence of the disease in pre-Hispanic Mexico.[22]

EPIDEMIOLOGY

Mycetoma has been included in the "top 17" list of neglected tropical diseases[13,20] and was submitted to the executive board of the World Health Organization in the World Health Assembly.[16,20,23-25]

The disease has a worldwide distribution but the endemic zone or "mycetoma belt" is placed around de Tropic of Cancer and includes African, Asian, and Latin American countries, especially India, Sudan, Somalia, Mexico, and Venezuela. In Mexico (97%), South America, and Australia, *N. brasiliensis* is the leading cause of actinomycetomas; in Africa, Saudi Arabia, and India, *Streptomyces somaliensis*, *Actinomadura pelletieri*, and *Actinomadura madurae* predominate. *A. madurae* is also identified as the etiologic agent in 10% to 15% of cases in Mexico and Venezuela.[26-28] Occasional cases are seen in the United States, particularly in the southern states. Actinomycetoma affects mainly men, with a male-to-female ratio of 3:1, and age ranges from 21 to 40 years old; frequency in patients younger than age 18 years is 4%, with similar incidence in both sexes.[29,30] The infection most commonly affects agricultural rural workers in developing countries in tropical and subtropical zones or those involved in outdoor activities.[28]

CLINICAL FEATURES

CUTANEOUS FINDINGS

Actinomycetoma is a chronic, localized, slowly progressive, painless disease of the skin and subcutaneous tissue. The pathologic process begins with a minor traumatic injury. Walking barefooted or wearing sandals may be considered a risk factor for these infections in rural communities. The lower limbs are involved in 71% of cases (Fig. 158-5), the foot being the most common site (Figs. 158-6 and 158-7). The lower leg, knee, and thigh, as well as the hand, forearm (Figs. 158-8 and 158-9), face, neck, and abdominal wall, also may be affected. In Mexico, the upper back (Figs. 158-10 and 158-11) is involved in 17% to 25% of cases in relation to occupational activity, such as firewood collection. The trunk is considered a high-risk area, because of the possibility of dissemination to the spinal cord and lungs.[28] Actinomycetoma caused by *Nocardia* species is a very inflammatory process characterized by tumefaction, a tumor-like or nodular-appearing soft-tissue swelling, deformity, and discharging sinus tracts with communicating channels that exudate pus (97%) (Fig. 158-6). Some authors consider pathognomonic a triad of a painless subcutaneous mass, sinus formation, and purulent or seropurulent discharge that contains grains. Ulceration, crusting, and scarring are also observed.[20] Mycetoma caused by *A. madurae*, *A. pelletieri*, and *S. somaliensis* are less inflammatory with smaller sinus tracts; *A. madurae* is mainly seen in women with plantar involvement (Fig. 158-7).[27] With many of these agents, the granules may be seen with the naked eye (see Table 158-1). Usually, they are creamy in color; the exception will be *A. pelletieri*, in which the granules are red.

NONCUTANEOUS FINDINGS AND COMPLICATIONS

The course is chronic and progressive, with potential involvement of bones, lung, and abdominal viscera. In women, mycetomas increase in size during pregnancy and spontaneously improve after delivery. Advanced cases may cause functional disability. Atypical clinical

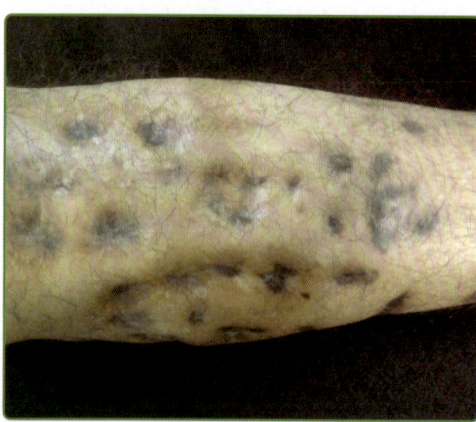

Figure 158-5 Actinomycetoma of the lower leg. Multiple, indolent, coalescing nodules.

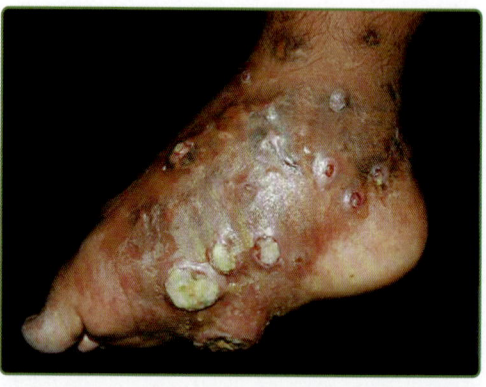

Figure 158-6 Advanced case of mycetoma of the foot produced by *Nocardia* species; typical location, with multiple draining sites.

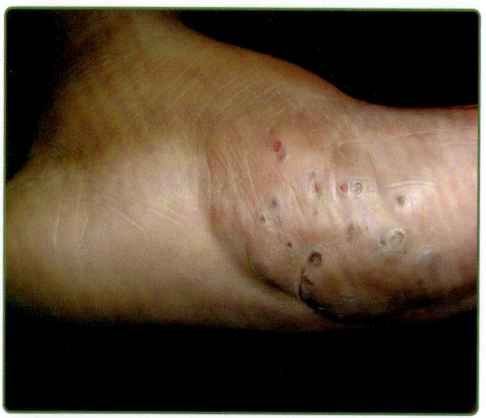

Figure 158-7 Typical mycetoma caused by *Actinomadura madurae*.

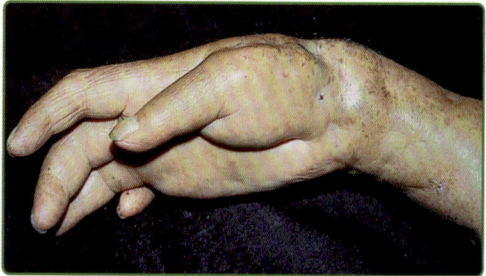

Figure 158-8 Mycetoma of the hand and wrist caused by *Nocardia brasiliensis*. Note gross deformity. (Used with permission from Roberto Arenas, MD, Hospital Manuel Gea González, Mexico City, Mexico.)

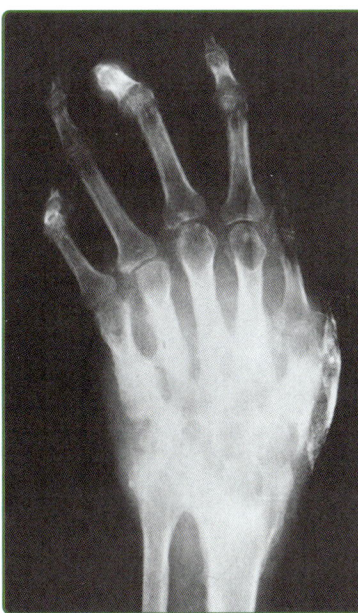

Figure 158-9 Radiograph shows associated marked destruction of bones and underlying soft tissues. (Used with permission from Roberto Arenas, MD, Hospital Manuel Gea González, Mexico City, Mexico.)

forms include the cryptic mycetoma (without sinus tracts), the so-called *minimycetoma* (single or multiple small lesions observed mainly in children and adolescents), and the occasional inguinal "metastatic" lesions from a primary mycetoma of the foot.[20]

ETIOLOGY AND PATHOGENESIS

Microorganisms reported to cause actinomycetomas include 3 genera: *Nocardia, Actinomadura,* and

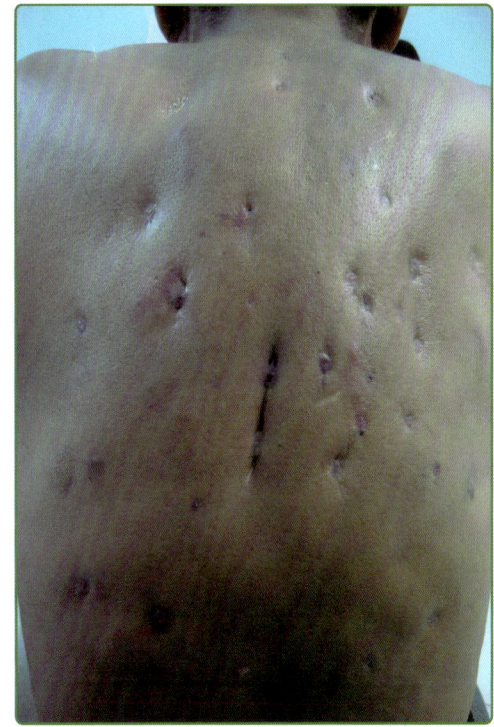

Figure 158-10 Dorsal actinomycetoma caused by *Nocardia brasiliensis.*

Streptomyces. The most frequent causes are *N. brasiliensis, A. madurae, A. pelletieri,* and *S. somaliensis.* Less frequent causes are *N. asteroides, N. otitidiscaviarum (N. caviae), Nocardiopsis dassonvillei,* and *Nocardia transvalensis. N. pseudobrasiliensis, Nocardia veterana, Nocardia mexicana, N. farcinica, Nocardia aobensis, N. takedensis, Nocardia harenae, Streptomyces sudanensis* sp. nov, and *Actinomadura latina* have been reported as new agents in human actinomycetoma.[31-35]

Recent taxonomic studies (using DNA hybridization and ribosomal RNA gene sequencing) have confirmed marked heterogeneity among

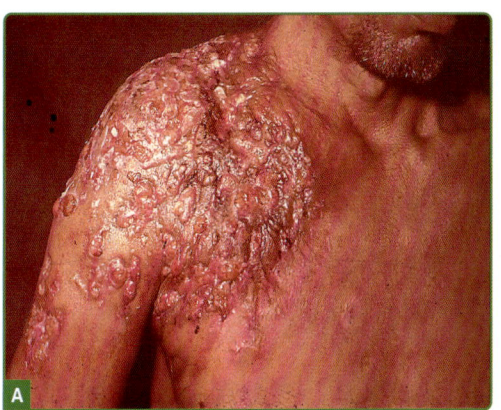
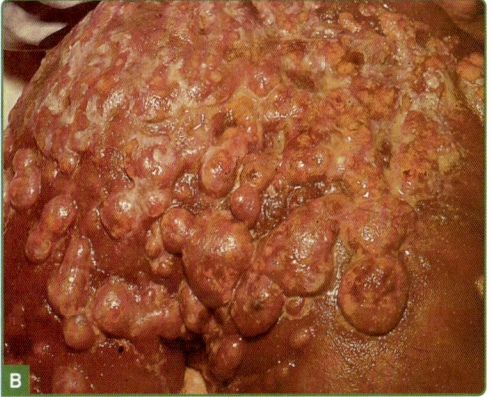

Figure 158-11 **A,** Huge scapulothoracic mycetoma caused by *Nocardia brasiliensis.* Note multiple fistulae. **B,** Closeup. Note doughnut-shaped masses and purulent drainage. (**B,** Used with permission from Maria Cecilia Albornoz, MD, Instituto de Biomedicina, Caracas, Venezuela.)

the genera of aerobic actinomycetes. Genomes of *N. brasiliensis, S. somaliensis,* and *A. madurae* have been described.[36-38]

Innate, as well as T-helper (Th)1-type and Th2-type immunity are involved in the host response against *N. brasiliensis*. CD8+ lymphocytes and macrophages are the main cells implicated. It has been shown that not only macrophages but also dendritic cells become foamy cells in either in vitro infection or an in vivo experimental actinomycetoma model by *N. brasiliensis*.[39]

N. brasiliensis as an intracellular bacterium modulates macrophage cytokine production, which helps survival of the pathogen.[40] In patients with actinomycetoma, the levels of immunoglobulin (Ig) G_1, IgG_2, IgG_3, IgG_4, and IgM are higher than in a control group. Those findings suggest that the increase or deficiency of a determined immunoglobulin class, as well as the relationship between different subclasses, play a role in the pathogenesis of actinomycetoma. In an experimental model of *N. brasiliensis* infection, hyperimmune sera with high levels of *N. brasiliensis* antigens did not protect against the infection, but IgM antibodies did.

RISK FACTORS

Walking barefoot in areas of high prevalence is consider a risk factor for the disease.

DIAGNOSIS

LABORATORY TESTING

Microbiologic diagnosis by identification of causal agent is limited to expert hands. No reliable serologic tests are available, but molecular techniques to identify relevant antigens or microorganisms have shown a real usefulness.[24]

Clinical specimens must be sent for direct examination, Gram stain, and culture. On direct examination, *Nocardia* granules are microscopic with a yellowish color (Fig. 158-12). Granules produced by other agents are macroscopic: those of *A. madurae* are white, yellow, or cream (Fig. 158-13), whereas grains from *A. pelletieri* are red and those of *S. somaliensis* are cream to brown color. Fine-needle aspiration cytology has been reported as a good diagnostic tool. The cell block technique of mycetoma aspirates can be used for cytodiagnosis, showing findings similar to histopathologic sections.[41]

The microorganisms can be cultured on Sabouraud dextrose agar or Lowenstein-Jensen at room temperature; *Nocardia* strains are white-yellow hard colonies. Microscopically, the very thin filaments are Gram-positive and acid fast with the Kinyoun stain. *A. madurae* produce slowly growing beige or pink colonies; *A. pelletieri* colonies are red. *S. somaliensis* produce beige or tanned colonies. *Actinomadura, A. israelii,* and *Streptomyces* species are acid-fast–negative.[20]

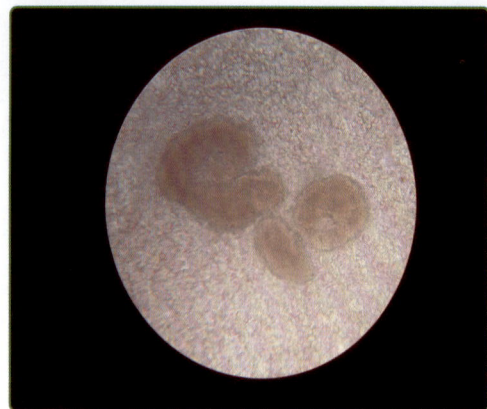

Figure 158-12 *Nocardia* species granules in direct examination (Lugol iodine stain, ×40 magnification).

Biochemistry can be used for identification. *N. brasiliensis* hydrolyzes casein and tyrosine, but not xanthine; *N. otitidiscaviarum* is negative to casein and tyrosine and positive to xanthine testing; *N. asteroides* is negative to all these tests.

The most precise diagnosis method for etiologic agents is molecular biology; the most applicable are the DNA-based identification tools such as loop-mediated isothermal amplification.

An enzyme-linked immunosorbent assay has been described for the diagnosis of mycetoma caused by *N. brasiliensis*; it has been proposed as a method to assess the response to therapy. This test detects antibodies against 2 immune-dominant antigens (24 and 26 kDa). An additional advantage of this particular assay might be its demonstrated cross-reactivity with *N. asteroides*.[42] Other diagnostic tools are latex bead agglutination assays and dipsticks, but a discriminatory antigen needs to be selected.[43]

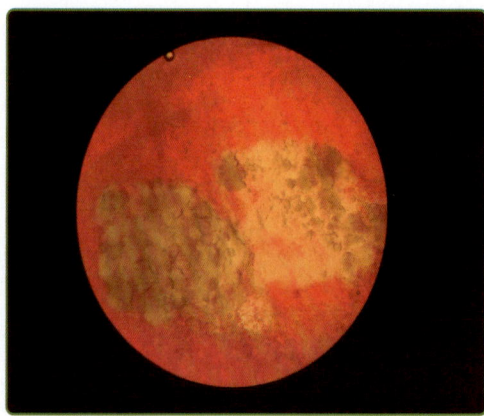

Figure 158-13 *Actinomadura madurae* granules in direct examination (Lugol iodine stain, ×10 magnification).

PATHOLOGY

Skin biopsy plays an important role in the diagnosis of actinomycetoma. Typically, in tissue sections stained with hematoxylin and eosin, there is a suppurative reaction characterized by the presence of polymorphonuclear cells, fibrosis, neovascularization, and, rarely, a granulomatous reaction with a tuberculoid granuloma.[20] *Nocardia* infection is characterized by granules 30 to 200 μm in diameter, partially basophilic to amphophilic, with an amorphous eosinophilic radially arranged material on the periphery (the so-called Splendore-Hoeppli phenomenon). Granules of *A. madurae* are soft and bigger (1 to 3 mm diameter), purple with a cartographic shape and an eosinophilic fringe (Fig. 158-14). *A. pelletieri* granules are firm and red with a diameter of 200 to 500 μm. Granules of *S. somaliensis* are rounded, hard, pale, and 1.5 to 10 mm in diameter.[20] These organisms stain in tissue with Gomori methenamine silver, periodic acid–Schiff, and the Brown-Brenn modification of the Gram stain.

IMAGING

Regarding the different imaging techniques, conventional radiographs are used to identify the limits of lesions and to determine if bone is affected.[44] The most common radiographic abnormalities are soft-tissue swelling, extrinsic pressure, bony periosteal reaction, erosion, sclerosis, joint involvement, and bone cavities ("geoda").[45] Ultrasonography is also a useful tool, showing hyperreflective echoes that help to differentiate between mycetoma (actinomycetoma and eumycetoma) and nonmycetoma. These hyperreflective echoes are observed only in mycetoma; however, when sinus tracts are present, the images may not be as clear. In eumycetoma, the grain cement produces numerous sharp bright hyperreflective echoes; in actinomycetoma, the findings are less distinct, probably because of the smaller size and the consistency of grains.[44]

Currently, MRI and CT are the most accurate diagnostic tools to determine the disease extent, especially in trunk mycetomas; they also provide evidence about the degree of visceral, muscular, and vascular invasion, and an estimate of the size of the involvement; however, those techniques do not allow to discriminate between actinomycetoma and eumycetoma.[46,47] The "dot-in-circle" sign on MRI is considered very characteristic of mycetoma, and is observed as multiple, small, round-shaped hyperintense lesions surrounded by a low-signal intensity rim (the circle), and a central, low-signal focus (the dot).[48]

DIFFERENTIAL DIAGNOSIS

The differential diagnosis includes other infections causing fistulae, such as eumycotic mycetoma, actinomycosis, botryomycosis, scrofuloderma, and atypical mycobacterial infections (Table 158-4). Botryomycosis is a condition that can mimic actinomycetoma and eumycetoma, both clinically and histologically. The disease can be caused by several organisms, most commonly *S. aureus*, *Escherichia coli*, *Pseudomonas aeruginosa*, *Proteus vulgaris*, *Actinobacillus* species, *Streptococcus* species, Gram-negative coccobacilli, *Propionibacterium acnes*, and other anaerobic bacteria. The cutaneous form accounts for 75% of the cases; visceral involvement, mainly the lung, is rare. The disease is characterized by localized areas of infiltration, with mass effect and draining sinuses. Extension to the underlying structures, including bone, is not rare. Most commonly affected areas are exposed surfaces, such as hands, head, and feet. Patients usually have a predisposing factor such as local trauma, a foreign body, diabetes or HIV. Botryomycosis is also characterized by the presence of granules, which can be seen macroscopically and microscopically. As in mycetoma, the center of the granule will show agglomeration

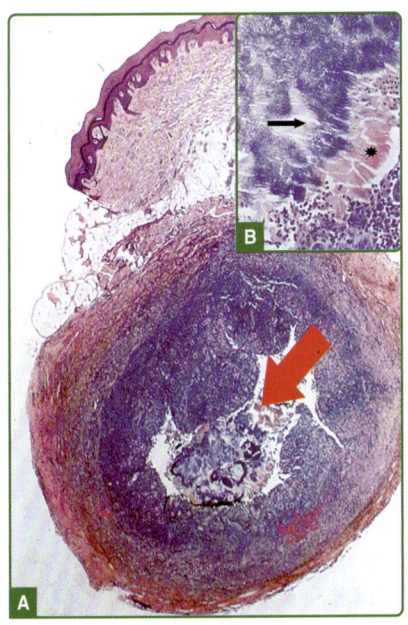

Figure 158-14 **A**, Skin biopsy of an *Actinomadura* mycetoma shows the granule (*red arrow*) inside the inflammatory reaction (hematoxylin-and-eosin stain, ×20 magnification). **B**, The contrast between the blue fibrillary material (*black arrow*), representing bacteria, and the eosinophilic proteinaceous material of the Splendore-Hoeppli phenomenon (*star*) (hematoxylin-and-eosin stain, ×100 magnification).

TABLE 158-4
Differential Diagnosis of Actinomycetoma

- Eumycotic mycetoma
- Actinomycosis
- Botryomycosis
- Atypical mycobacterial infection
- Scrofuloderma and tuberculous pseudomycetoma

of the causal agent, most commonly, Gram-positive cocci. The Splendore-Hoeppli phenomenon also may be seen around the granules. Rarely, tuberculosis may present as pseudomycetoma.[49]

MANAGEMENT

Therapy for patients with actinomycetoma should be individualized. Economic considerations may influence the choice of therapy, particularly in developing countries.

Molecular identification of the causal agents and development of genetic markers for disease can improve management. Cure can be defined by a lack of clinical activity, the absence of grains and negative cultures. The cure rates vary between 60% and 90%. Treatment periods should be prolonged, especially in those cases with bone and visceral involvement, where the prognosis is poor.[50]

MEDICATIONS

Actinomycetoma is currently treated with antibiotics, which can be used alone or, preferentially, in combination, depending on the localization, dissemination, and severity of the disease.[51] The combined therapy prevents the development of drug resistance and allows eradicating any residual infection. The treatment of choice in actinomycetoma caused by *N. brasiliensis* is diaminodiphenylsulfone (Dapsone) 100 to 200 mg/day (3 to 5 mg/kg) plus TMP-SMX 160/800 mg twice a day for several months in initial cases; the treatment should continue for up to 2 years.[20] Dapsone also can be combined with streptomycin, 1 g/day; clofazimine, 100 mg/day; rifampin, 300 mg twice/day; tetracycline, 1 g/day; or isoniazid, 300 to 600 mg/day. Some resistant cases have been treated with amoxicillin, 500 mg, plus clavulanic acid, 125 mg/day for 5 months, especially in pregnancy. The use of clindamycin, ciprofloxacin, and moxifloxacin has been suggested in *Nocardia* infections.[52]

One of the best inhibitory effects in vitro is achieved with the use of aminoglycosides. Amikacin alone or combined with imipenem are powerful antibiotics used as alternative treatments for severe or multiresistant mycetomas, especially those with bone and visceral involvement. In adults, amikacin is administered 15 mg/kg/day (500 mg IM twice a day) for 3 weeks; ototoxicity and nephrotoxicity may develop.[53] Alternative, less-effective drugs include kanamycin, fosfomycin, or streptomycin. Carbapenems, such as imipenem and meropenem, have a broad microbicidal activity refractory to hydrolysis by β-lactamases. They have demonstrated good in vitro and in vivo activity against *N. asteroides* complex, good in vitro sensitivity against *A. madurae*, and apparent low in vitro activity against *N. brasiliensis*. Imipenem has been proposed as a suitable option for severe *N. brasiliensis* infection refractory to other drug therapies.[54] Patients under therapy with IV imipenem must be hospitalized; the drug can be given as monotherapy at 500 mg 3 times daily, or in combination with intravenous amikacin in a dose of 500 mg twice daily (15 mg/kg) in cycles of 21 days, especially in patients with pulmonary or peritoneal involvement.[50]

Ramam and colleagues[55] used a 2-step regimen consisting of an intensive phase of therapy with intravenous penicillin (1,000,000 IU every 6 hours) plus intravenous gentamicin (80 mg twice a day), followed by oral TMP-SMX (80 to 400 mg twice a day) for 5 to 7 weeks.

Linezolid, an oxazolidinone, has shown in vitro antimicrobial activity against *N. brasiliensis*; it also has demonstrated efficacy in patients with nocardiosis. Its main disadvantage of this alternative is the cost. It is available as intravenous and oral preparations. The benzothiazinones are a new class of drugs that inhibit decaprenylphosphoryl-β-D-ribose oxidase (DprE1), an essential enzyme involved in the cell wall biosynthesis of Corynebacterineae. These are new antimycetoma potential drugs and could be combined with oxazolidinone molecules.[56]

Patient followup is always important, and improvement should be monitored by clinical assessment as well as by laboratory tests: hemoglobin level, white cell count, C-reactive protein, erythrocyte sedimentation rate, enzyme-linked immunosorbent assay (when available), biopsy, and culture. The use of dapsone can be associated with methemoglobinemia, hemolytic anemia, and hypersensitivity syndrome; determination of 6-glucose phosphate dehydrogenase enzyme is obligatory whenever dapsone is used. All cases receiving amikacin treatment requires close clinical observation with audiometry and renal function tests every 3 to 5 weeks to detect auditory and nephrotoxicity and adjustment dose. Carbapenems should not be prescribed in patients who are allergic to penicillin and other β-lactam antibiotics. Linezolid can cause diarrhea, headache, and nausea, but the most important adverse effect is myelosuppression. TMP-SMX is associated with many severe dermatologic reactions.[51]

PROCEDURES

Amputation is not indicated in actinomycetoma because the high risk of lymphangitic or hematogenous dissemination. Functional impairment is common with osseous, pulmonary, or abdominal visceral involvement. The disease may be fatal.

REFERENCES

1. Könönen E, Wade WG. Actinomyces and related organisms in human infections. *Clin Microbiol Rev*. 2015;28(2):419.
2. Smego RA Jr, Foglia G. Actinomycosis. *Clin Infect Dis*. 1998;26(6):1255.
3. Wong VK, Turmezei TD, Weston VC. Actinomycosis. *BMJ*. 2011;343:d6099.

4. Mert A, Bilir M, Bahar H, et al. Primary actinomycosis of the hand: a case report and literature review. *Int J Infect Dis*. 2001;5:112.
5. Sudhakar SS, Ross JJ. Short-term treatment of actinomycosis: two cases and a review. *Clin Infect Dis*. 2004;38:444.
6. Lederman ER, Crum NF. A case series and focused review of nocardiosis: clinical and microbiologic aspects. *Medicine (Baltimore)*. 2004;83:300.
7. Mosel D, Harris L, Fisher E, et al. Disseminated *Nocardia* infection presenting as hemorrhagic pustules and ecthyma in a woman with systemic lupus erythematosus and antiphospholipid antibody syndrome. *J Dermatol Case Rep*. 2013;7(2):52.
8. Fergie JE, Purcell K. Nocardiosis in South Texas children. *Pediatr Infect Dis J*. 2001;20:711.
9. Biscione F, Cecchini D, Ambrosioni J, et al. Nocardiosis in patients with human immunodeficiency virus infection [in Spanish]. *Enferm Infecc Microbiol Clin*. 2005;23:419.
10. Singh SM, Rau NV, Cohen LB, et al. Cutaneous nocardiosis complicating management of Crohn's disease with infliximab and prednisone. *CMAJ*. 2004;171(9):1063.
11. Leshem YA, Gdalevich M, Ziv M, et al. Opportunistic infections in patients with pemphigus. *J Am Acad Dermatol*. 2014;71(2):284.
12. Smego RA Jr, Castiglia M, Asperilla MO. Lymphocutaneous syndrome. A review of non-sporothrix causes. *Medicine (Baltimore)*. 1999;78:38.
13. Saoji VA, Saoji SV, Gadegone RW, et al. Primary cutaneous nocardiosis. *Indian J Dermatol*. 2012;57(5):404.
14. Chung E, Pulitzer MP, Papadopoulos EB, et al. Lymphangitic papules caused by *Nocardia takedensis*. *JAAD Case Rep*. 2015;1(3):126.
15. Lerner PI. Nocardiosis. *Clin Infect Dis*. 1996;22:891.
16. Chen B, Tang J, Lu Z, et al. Primary cutaneous nocardiosis in a patient with nephrotic syndrome: a case report and review of the literature. *Medicine (Baltimore)*. 2016;95(3):e2490.
17. Hirayama T, Takazono T, Horai Y, et al. Pulmonary nocardiosis caused by *Nocardia concava* with a literature review. *Intern Med*. 2016;55(9):1213.
18. Corti ME, Villafañe-Fioti MF. Nocardiosis: a review. *Int J Infect Dis*. 2003;7(4):243.
19. Ricci JA, Weil AA, Eberlin KR. Necrotizing cutaneous nocardiosis of the hand: a case report and review of the literature. *J Hand Microsurg*. 2015;7(1):224.
20. Arenas R, Lavalle P. Mycetoma (Madura foot). In: Arenas R, Estrada R, eds. *Tropical Dermatology*. Georgetown, Texas, US: Landes, 2001;51.
21. Schwartz E, Shpiro A. Madura foot or Philoctetes foot? *Isr Med Assoc J*. 2015;17(7):442.
22. Mansilla-Lory J, Contreras-Lopez E. Mycetoma in pre-Hispanic Mexico: study of the bone collection of the Tlatilco culture. *Rev Med Inst Mex Seguro Soc*. 2009;47(3):237.
23. World Health Organization (WHO). *The 17 Neglected Tropical Diseases*. Geneva, Switzerland: World Health Organization; 2013.
24. Zijlstra EE, van de Sande WW, Welsh O, et al. Mycetoma: a unique neglected tropical disease. *Lancet Infect Dis*. 2016;16(1):100.
25. Nenoff P, van de Sande WW, Fahal AH, et al. Eumycetoma and actinomycetoma—an update on causative agents, epidemiology, pathogenesis, diagnostics and therapy. *J Eur Acad Dermatol Venereol*. 2015;29(10):1873.
26. Dieng MT. Actinomycetomas in Senegal: study of 90 cases. *Bull Soc Pathol Exot*. 2005;98:18.
27. Davila MR, Arenas R, Asz-Sigall D et al. Epidemiologia de los micetomas en el Estado de Guanajuato, Mexico. *Monografias en Dermatologia*. 2006;19:24.
28. Bonifaz A, Tirado-Sánchez A, Calderón L, et al. Mycetoma: experience of 482 cases in a single center in Mexico. *PLoS Negl Trop Dis*. 2014;8(8):3102.
29. Bonifaz A, Ibarra G, Saul A et al. Mycetoma in children. Experience with 15 cases. *Pediatr Infect Dis J*. 2007;26:50-52.
30. Lopez-Martinez R, Mendez-Tovar LJ, Bonifaz A, et al. Actualización der la epidemiologia del micetoma en México. Revisión de 3,933 casos. *Gac Med Mex*. 2013;149:586.
31. Quintana ET, Wierzbicka K, Mackiewicz P, et al. *Streptomyces sudanensis* sp. *nov.*, a new pathogen isolated from patients with actinomycetoma. *Antonie Van Leeuwenhoek*. 2008;93(3):305.
32. Ichinomiya A, Nishimura K, Takenaka M, et al. Mycetoma caused by *Nocardia transvalensis* with repeated local recurrences for 25 years without dissemination to viscera. *J Dermatol*. 2014;41(6):556-557.
33. Kresch-Tronik NS, Carrillo-Casas EM, Arenas R, et al. *Nocardia harenae*, an uncommon causative organism of mycetoma: report on two patients. *J Med Microbiol*. 2012;61:1153.
34. Kresh-Tronik NS, Carrillo-Casas EM, Arenas R, et al. First case of mycetoma associated with *Nocardia takedensis*. *J Dermatol*. 2013;40(2):135-136.
35. Vongphoumy I, Dance DA, Dittrich S, et al. Case report: actinomycetoma caused by *Nocardia aobensis* from Lao PDR with favorable outcome after short-term antibiotic treatment. *PLoS Negl Trop Dis*. 2015;9(4).
36. Vera-Cabrera L, Ortiz R, Elizondo R, et al. Complete genome sequence of *Nocardia brasiliensis* HUJEG-1. *J Bacteriol*. 2012;194(10):2761.
37. Kirby R, Sangal V, Tucker NP, et al. Draft genome sequence of the human pathogen *Streptomyces somaliensis*, a significant cause of actinomycetoma. *J Bacteriol*. 2012;194(13):3544.
38. Vera-Cabrera L, Ortiz-Lopez R, Elizondo-Gonzalez R, et al. Draft genome sequence of *Actinomadura madurae* LIID-AJ290, isolated from a human mycetoma case. *Genome Announc*. 2014;2(2):e00201.
39. Meester I, Rosas-Taraco AG, Salinas-Carmona MC. *Nocardia brasiliensis* induces formation of foamy macrophages and dendritic cells in vitro and in vivo. *PLoS One*. 2014;9(6):e100064.
40. Salinas-Carmona MC, Zúñiga JM, Pérez-Rivera LI, et al. *Nocardia brasiliensis* modulates IFN-gamma, IL-10, and IL-12 cytokine production by macrophages from BALB/c mice. *J Interferon Cytokine Res*. 2009;29(5):263.
41. Yousif BM, Fahal AH, Shakir MY. A new technique for the diagnosis of mycetoma using fixed blocks of aspirated material. *Trans R Soc Trop Med Hyg*. 2010;104(1):6.
42. Salinas-Carmona MC, Welsh O, Casillas SM. Enzyme-linked immunosorbent assay for serological diagnosis of *Nocardia brasiliensis* and clinical correlation with mycetoma infections. *J Clin Microbiol*. 1993;31:2901.
43. Van de Sande WW, Mahgoub el S, Fahal AH, et al. The mycetoma knowledge gap: identification of research priorities. *PLoS Negl Trop Dis*. 2014;8(3):e2667.
44. Van de Sande WW, Fahal AH, Goodfellow M, et al. Merits and pitfalls of currently used diagnostic tools in mycetoma. *PLoS Negl Trop Dis*. 2014;8(7):e2918.

45. Abd El-Bagi ME, Fahal AH. Mycetoma revisited. Incidence of various radiographic signs. *Saudi Med J.* 2009;30(4):529.
46. Bonifaz A, González-Silva A, Albrandt-Salmerón A, et al. Utility of helical computed tomography to evaluate the invasion of actinomycetoma; a report of 21 cases. *Br J Dermatol.* 2008;158(4):698.
47. Fahal A, Mahgoub el S, El Hassan AM, et al. Head and neck mycetoma: the Mycetoma Research Centre experience. *PLoS Negl Trop Dis.* 2015;9(3):e0003587.
48. Laohawiriyakamol T, Tanutit P, Kanjanapradit K, et al. The "dot-in-circle" sign in musculoskeletal mycetomas on magnetic resonance imaging and ultrasonography. *Springerplus.* 2014;3:671.
49. Pizzariello G, Fernadez Pardal P, D'Atri G. Pseudomycetoma tuberculoso. Presentacion de 8 casos. *Med Cutan Ibero Lat Am.* 2013;41(6):254.
50. Ameen M, Arenas R. Developments in the management of mycetomas. *Clin Exp Dermatol.* 2008;34:1.
51. Welsh O, Al-Abdely HM, Salinas-Carmona MC, et al. Mycetoma medical therapy. *PLoS Negl Trop Dis.* 2014;8(10):e3218.
52. Chacon-Moreno BE, Welsh O, Cavazos-Rocha N, et al. Efficacy of ciprofloxacin and moxifloxacin against Nocardia brasiliensis in vitro and in an experimental model of actinomycetoma in BALB/c mice. *Antimicrob Agents Chemother.* 2009;53(1):295.
53. Welsh O, Sauceda E, Gonzalez J, et al. Amikacin alone and in combination with trimethoprim-sulfamethoxazole in the treatment of actinomycotic mycetoma. *J Am Acad Dermatol.* 1987;17(3):443.
54. Ameen M, Arenas R, Vasquez del Mercado E, et al. Efficacy of imipenem therapy for Nocardia actinomycetomas refractory to sulfonamides. *J Am Acad Dermatol.* 2010;62(2):239.
55. Ramam M, Garg T, D'Souza P, et al. A two-step schedule for the treatment of actinomycotic mycetomas. *Acta Derm Venereol.* 2000;80(5):378.
56. González-Martínez NA, Lozano-Garza HG, Castro-Garza J, et al. In vivo activity of the benzothiazinones PBTZ169 and BTZ043 against *Nocardia brasiliensis*. *PLoS Negl Trop Dis.* 2015;9(10):e0004022.

Chapter 159 :: Leprosy
:: Claudio Guedes Salgado, Arival Cardoso de Brito, Ubirajara Imbiriba Salgado, & John Stewart Spencer

第一百五十九章

麻风病

中文导读

麻风病是困扰人类的最古老的疾病之一。麻风病是一种由麻风分枝杆菌引起的慢性肉芽肿性感染，主要感染黏膜皮肤组织和周围神经，导致皮肤感觉丧失（有或没有皮肤病学病变），并在疾病发展过程中丧失能力。本章就麻风病的定义、流行病学、病因与发病机制、临床特征、诊断、鉴别诊断、临床病程和预后、临床管理进行了全面的阐释和讨论。

〔汪 犇〕

AT A GLANCE

- Definition: A chronic granulomatous disease affecting mainly the skin and nerves caused by the obligate intracellular pathogen *Mycobacterium leprae*.
- Involvement: Primarily the skin and nerves, but causing sequelae to a wide range of tissues and systems including eyes, upper respiratory tract, lymphoid tissue, testicles, muscles, and bones.
- Diagnosis: Based on clinical signs and symptoms, hallmarks include loss of sensation within skin lesions, nerve swelling or pain, or demonstration of acid-fast bacilli in skin smears or biopsies.
- Incidence: 214,783 new cases detected worldwide in 2016, essentially unchanged for the last 4 years. More than 80% of all new cases are detected in only 3 countries—India, Brazil, and Indonesia.
- Long-term morbidity: Despite the global use of multidrug therapy in use since the mid-1980s, up to 30% to 50% of all leprosy patients will experience some type of reactional episode that may result in a permanent neurologic deficit or disability.
- A clinical challenge: The long incubation time prior to the slow development of diverse symptoms (3-7 years postinfection), the very low rate of disease progression in infected individuals, and issues with misdiagnosis all create challenges to the development of ways to interrupt transmission.
- An immunologic spectrum of disease: Understanding what genetic factors and the interplay of innate and adaptive immune responses of the host that leads to resistance or susceptibility to disease are critical in developing novel treatment approaches.

INTRODUCTION

DEFINITION

Leprosy is a chronic granulomatous infection caused by *Mycobacterium leprae*, that infects mucous cutaneous tissues and peripheral nerves, leading to loss of sensation on the skin—with or without dermatologic lesions—and the development of incapacities during the progression of the disease. WHO states that any individual in endemic countries presenting skin lesions with definite sensory loss or positive skin smears may be diagnosed with leprosy.[1]

HISTORICAL PERSPECTIVE

Leprosy is one of the oldest diseases known to afflict mankind. Gerhard Armauer Hansen, a Norwegian physician, was the first to describe the *M. leprae* bacillus in 1873, identifying the first bacterial pathogen associated with human disease. The name Hansen disease is used in some countries, like Brazil, to lessen the stigma associated with the common name. The characteristic destructive changes that lead to disfigurement, deformity, and disability were among the hallmarks of the disease that allowed it to become stigmatized in ancient times.[2] Speculations about the existence of leprosy in ancient India, Egypt, and China have been proposed, with the earliest paleopathological evidence found in 4000-year-old bones from the Balathal burial site in Rajasthan, western India.[3] The first use of molecular techniques using polymerase chain reaction (PCR) to detect *M. leprae* DNA specific sequences in ancient bones dated to AD 600 was described in 1994.[4] PCR was used to identify *M. leprae* DNA in 1st century CE bones from the Tomb of the Shroud burial site in Israel, the earliest known date of existence of leprosy in this region.[5] Using paleopathological and molecular methods to analyze ancient bones from archeological sites, burial grounds, and cemeteries, evidence of the spread of leprosy has emerged, indicating the spread of the disease from Western and Central Asia from the 4th century AD into Eastern and Central Europe occurred mainly due to human migrations associated with military campaigns, expansion of territories, or migrations to effect colonization.[6] Houses were established to quarantine those with leprosy and other communicable diseases, called lazarets, in 7th-century France, but it was not until the return of the Crusaders from AD 1100 coming back from countries of the Ottoman Empire where leprosy was endemic that the disease became an increasing problem.

Leprosy in Europe and the United Kingdom peaked in the 13th and 14th centuries and then began a slow decline. Comparison of the *M. leprae* whole genome obtained from ancient European, UK, and Scandinavian gravesites show only a few dozen single nucleotide polymorphism (SNP) changes over the last 1000 years, with no mutations in any genes related to increased virulence or pathogenesis.[7] The essentially clonal nature of *M. leprae* from the ancient to modern times suggests that the precipitous decrease in leprosy prevalence was independent of features of the pathogen and were more likely related to changes in host resistance or environment. Since people with lepromatous leprosy likely had a weakened immune status, they were more likely to succumb to other infections. Events thought to have contributed to a higher death rate in those with leprosy included a serious famine in 1325, followed by the outbreak of plague, or Black Death, in 1349 that killed between one-third and two-thirds of the population in Europe and the United Kingdom. Such massive death would have severely curtailed the support networks of hospices and leprosaria whose religious clergy, patrons and physicians had cared for patients, but were likely decimated. There is also suggestive evidence that increases in population density, overcrowded living conditions, and the rise of tuberculosis after the 15th century contributed to death by coinfections with multiple diseases.[8] As those susceptible individuals succumbed to disease, the innate resistance of the surviving population to mycobacterial infection and other diseases common during that period likely improved, and coupled with improved socioeconomic conditions, sanitation, and hygiene, the lines of transmission of infection were broken. Currently, endemic cases of leprosy in Europe and the United Kingdom are extremely rare.

Comparative genomic studies of *M. leprae* isolates all over the world revealed a remarkable conservation of the genome (99.995% identity among all strain types), showing the existence of 215 polymorphic sites consisting mainly of SNPs. Four of these SNPs represented 4 main strain types that showed very strong geographical associations that were used to trace the evolution and distribution of *M. leprae* based on human migration patterns throughout history.[9] SNP Type 1 was found primarily in Southeast Asia; SNP Type 2 was found mainly in East Africa; SNP Type 3 was associated with the European/North African region, whereas SNP Type 4 was found mainly in West Africa. Leprosy did not exist in North or South America until its introduction via colonialism from Europe (SNP Type 3) and from the importation of slaves from Africa (SNP Type 4). These four main types were subdivided into 16 subtypes based on further characterization of SNPs and insertion/deletion events from modern and ancient *M. leprae* genomes from a total of 400 samples from 28 different regions of the world, namely SNP Type 1 (A-D), Type 2 (E-H), Type 3 (I-M), and Type 4 (N-P).[10] Besides humans, *M. leprae* is also found as a zoonotic infection in armadillos in the Southern United States,[11] and recently in red squirrels in the British Isles.[12] Interestingly, both armadillo and squirrel *M. leprae* have the same SNP subtype, 3I, indicating a common European ancestry.

EPIDEMIOLOGY

Leprosy is still a serious neglected disease. WHO refers the number of new cases is gradually decreasing in the last 10 years, from 265,661 in 2006 to 210,758 in 2015,[13] but different groups of researchers have demonstrated that the hidden endemics may be high,[14,15] the number of cases in children is increasing[16] or stable,[17] whereas the proportion of multibacillary patients is increasing[18] and cases with grade 2 disability seem to be stable,[19] but high,[20] indicating late diagnosis. Altogether, these factors demonstrate that instead of a true decline of new cases, delay[21] and absence of diagnosis seem to be the main problems.[15,22,23] In fact, mathematical modeling shows that in 2020 we may have 4 million cases of undiagnosed leprosy worldwide, that is, almost 20 times more than the present number of cases diagnosed annually.[24]

The definition of leprosy has changed with time. There is currently no laboratory test to diagnose leprosy. Once a patient completes multidrug therapy, the individual is usually removed from the registry and is no longer considered a case, even if disability and reactional episodes continue long after treatment. For decades, treatment of leprosy was done continuously with dapsone alone (monotherapy), and all cases that received dapsone monotherapy were registered in the system. Because of this practice, the prevalence of leprosy remained high, with more than 10 million patients on the registry during the 1980s. With the implementation of multidrug therapy in 1982, treatment was shortened to, at most, 2 years. The active registry then changed to only those being treated, while those who completed their therapy were subsequently "cleared." Thus, over the course of a decade, millions of patients who completed multidrug therapy and did not have symptoms were purged from registries.[25] The net effect was that within 20 years after the introduction of multidrug therapy, leprosy prevalence was markedly reduced by more than 85%[13] although the new case detection rate has remained relatively stable at more than 200,000 worldwide for almost 10 years (Fig. 159-1).

Currently, the most important epidemiologic indicators of leprosy burden are the new case detection rate by country, and the proportion of cases in children, those with multibacillary disease and those with grade 2 disability, indicating a late diagnosis.[13] Although India has the highest number of leprosy cases in the world, Brazil has the highest new case detection rate among all countries (Fig. 159-2). However, when we look at the other 2 most significant parameters, the percentage of cases in children (Fig. 159-3) and those with grade 2 disability (Fig. 159-4), there is a clear shift, with most of the reporting countries considered as high or very high, whereas Brazil, India, and Indonesia have medium or low percentages. Although these 3 countries collectively account for >80% of the global leprosy burden, the large number of cases reported dilutes the

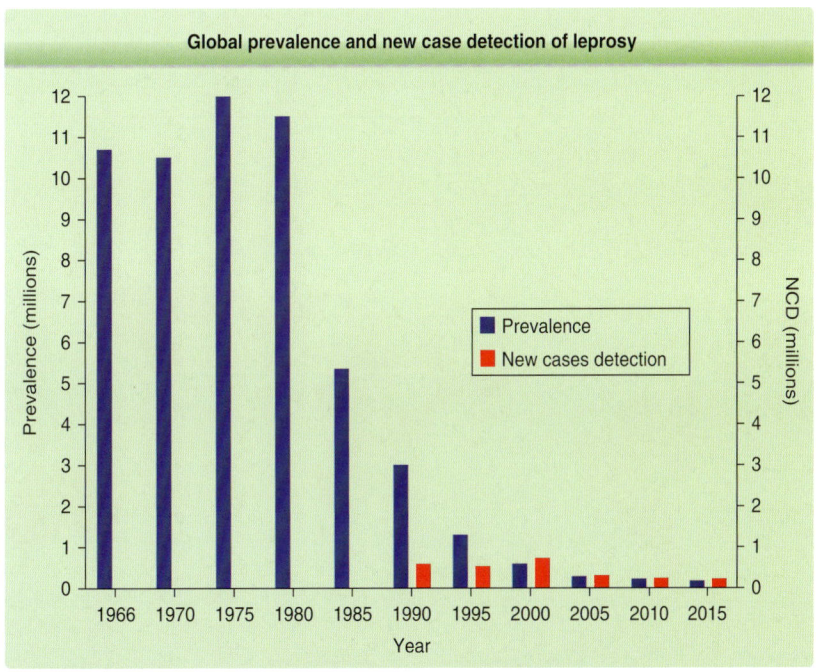

Figure 159-1 Historic evolution of global prevalence and new case detection of leprosy. The first formal attempt to estimate the global leprosy burden was made by WHO in 1966, when the case load was estimated to be 10,786,000, of whom 60% were not registered for treatment. Global detection was first reported in 1991, with 584,000 new cases detected worldwide in 1990. Currently, the new case detection is one of the most important epidemiologic indicators of leprosy burden, together with the proportion of children and proportions of grade 2 disability. (Used with permission from Prof. Josafá Barreto, Pará Federal University, Brazil.)

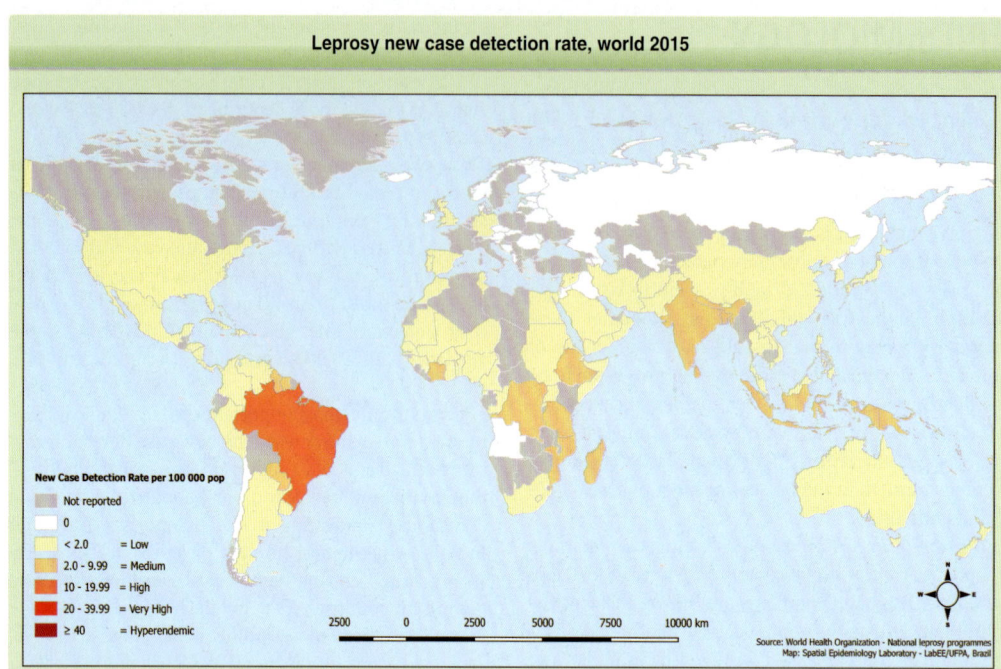

Figure 159-2 Leprosy new case detection rate per 100,000 population in the world, 2015. More than 210,000 new cases were reported in 136 countries or territories in 2015. India, Brazil, and Indonesia accounted for 81% of the global burden of leprosy. The global new case detection rate was 3.2. (Used with permission from Prof. Josafá Barreto, Pará Federal University, Brazil.)

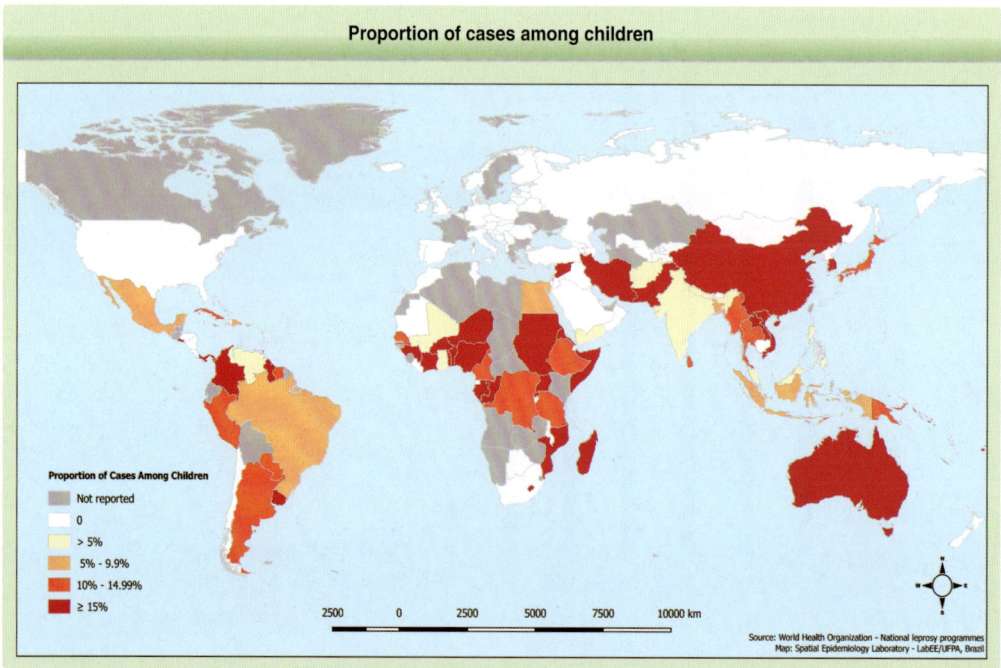

Figure 159-3 Proportion of leprosy cases among children below 15 years old, 2015. Although there is no specific classification from "low" to "high" for this indicator, it is a robust indicative of active source of infection in the community where they live. (Used with permission from Prof. Josafá Barreto, Pará Federal University, Brazil.)

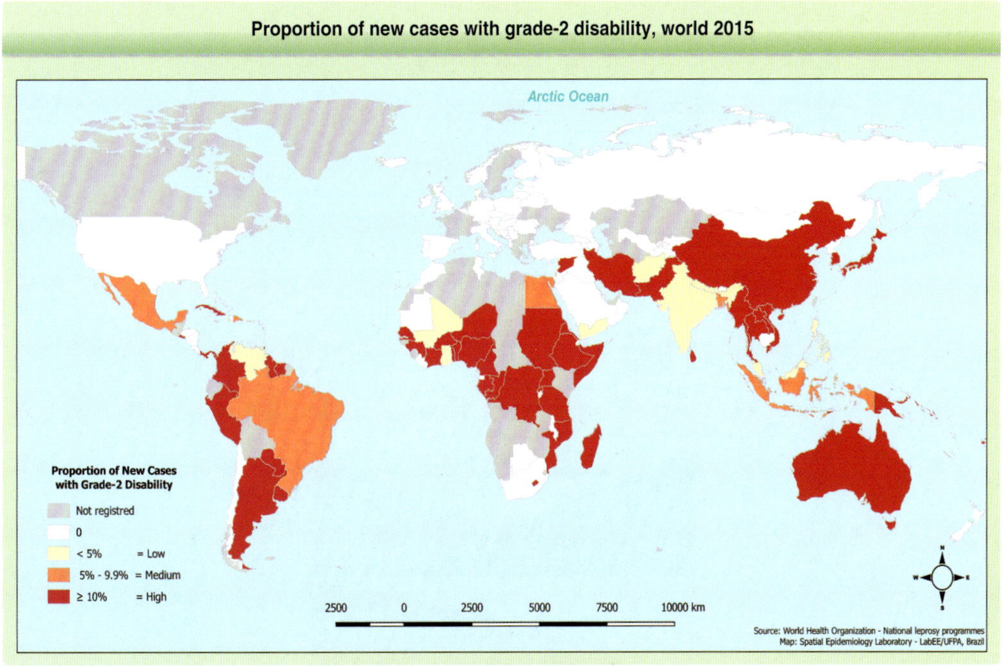

Figure 159-4 Proportion of new leprosy cases with grade 2 disability at diagnosis, 2015. It reflects long delays in the diagnosis of leprosy, highlighting a failure of the health services system and gaps in the approach to control the disease. (Used with permission from Prof. Josafá Barreto, Pará Federal University, Brazil.)

percentage of both children with leprosy and those with grade 2 disability, while countries who report less than 1000 new cases per year generally have much higher rates in both categories. A high or very high percentage of these 2 parameters likely means that children and adults are diagnosed only when presenting classical pathognomonic lesions of leprosy and/or disabilities, indicating late diagnosis.[15,21]

CLINICAL FEATURES

CUTANEOUS FINDINGS

During the IV International Leprosy Congress in Madrid, 1953, leprosy was classified in 2 stable forms, tuberculoid leprosy and lepromatous leprosy, and a borderline group between these 2 polar forms. In 1966, Ridley and Jopling proposed a 5-group classification system based on clinical, histopathologic, and immunologic criteria[26] that is still in use for classifying leprosy. The colonization of skin and invasion of peripheral nerves by the bacilli, followed by innate and adaptive immune responses by the host, results in the clinical spectrum of leprosy (Fig. 159-5). There is an overall genetic resistance toward developing leprosy, with more than 90% of people having a natural immunity, with cell-mediated immunity being most important in preventing disease progression.

All patients, except those with primary neural leprosy,[27] first present 1 or a few hypopigmented macules on the skin. Indeterminate leprosy (Fig. 159-6) may last for months or years before moving to spontaneous cure or toward one of the poles or borderline forms of the clinical spectrum, depending mainly on the cell-mediated immunity of the host against the bacilli.

At one end of the spectrum with a better cell-mediated immunity, there is polar tuberculoid leprosy, where well-defined plaques, usually a few in just one segment of the body, hypochromic and/or erythematous, sometimes atrophic, present with papules or tubercles that are mainly circinate on the periphery of the lesions (Fig. 159-7). A special self-healing type of tuberculoid leprosy, infantile nodular leprosy, can be found as a single nodular lesion, but also as papules or plaques, usually on the face of the child (Fig. 159-8).[28]

At the other end of the spectrum lies polar lepromatous leprosy, which is established by a complete lack of cell-mediated immunity, usually presenting with plentiful nodular lesions disseminated throughout the body, associated with diffuse infiltration (Fig. 159-9), including the ears (Fig. 159-10) and face, that may have facial features so marked that it gives the appearance of a lion's face, known as leonine facies (Fig. 159-11).[29] A special type of lepromatous leprosy is histoid leprosy, that has an even higher bacillary load than the usual lepromatous leprosy, with rafts of bacilli called globi, presenting diffuse shiny nodules and papules, and a variable degree of skin infiltration (Fig. 159-12).[30] Some cases of lepromatous leprosy are a challenge for less experienced health professionals to diagnose when the main skin manifestation is infiltration (Fig. 159-13). This special type is called Lucio

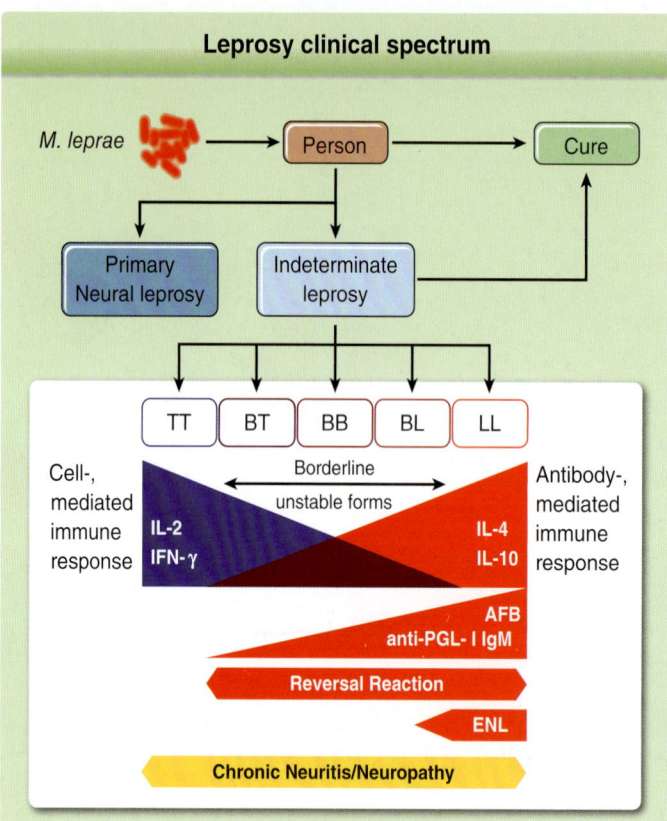

Figure 159-5 Leprosy clinical spectrum. Up to 80% of people exposed to *M. leprae* may solve the problem and get rid of the bacilli before appearance of symptoms or after subclinical leprosy. Some patients will develop primary neural leprosy, with no skin lesions. All those with skin lesions pass through an indeterminate form, and then evolve to a polar tuberculoid leprosy (TT) or lepromatous leprosy (LL) disease or to an unstable borderline form of leprosy. The paucibacillary (PB) pole toward TT has a good cellular immune response (CIR), with the presence of Th1 cytokines, while multibacillary pole toward LL present an impaired CIR and a high antibody response, with Th2 cytokines. Acid-fast bacilli and anti-PGL-I IgM are, both, low or negative on PB and increase through multibacillary pole. Reversal reaction may happen especially in borderline leprosy, whereas erythema nodosum leprosum occurs in borderline-lepromatous leprosy (BL) and LL patients. Chronic neuritis or neuropathy may happen in primary neural leprosy and in all but the indeterminate leprosy clinical form.

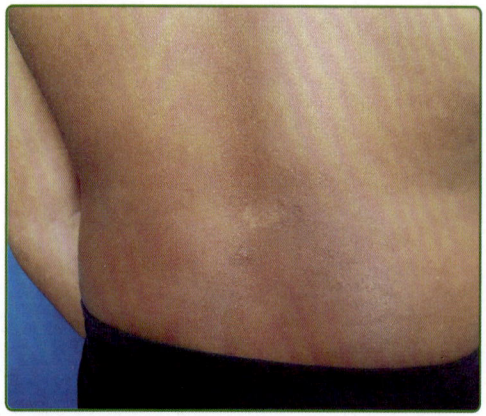

Figure 159-6 Indeterminate leprosy. Macular hypochromic lesion on the lower back.

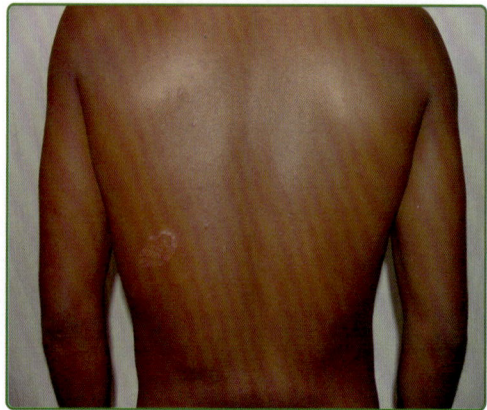

Figure 159-7 Tuberculoid leprosy. A well-circumscribed lesion, with a central macular hypochromic and atrophic appearance, and a peripheric group of papules distributed in annular pattern.

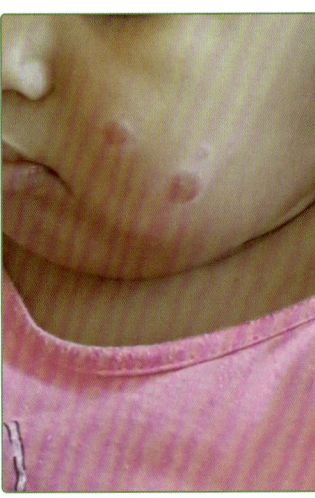

Figure 159-8 Infantile nodular leprosy. Presence of 2 tuberous lesions on the face of a child from a family where 2 adults were diagnosed with multibacillary leprosy.

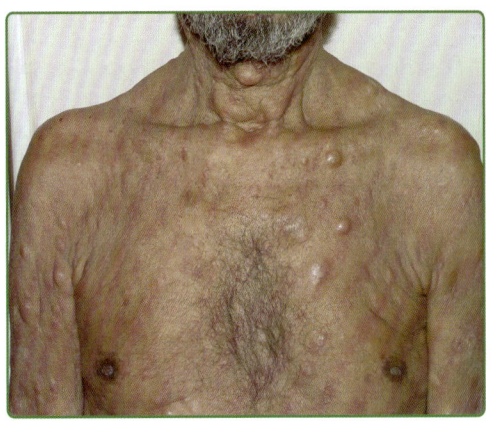

Figure 159-9 Lepromatous leprosy. Multiples nodules (hansenomes or lepromes) disseminated throughout the skin, associated to diffuse infiltration.

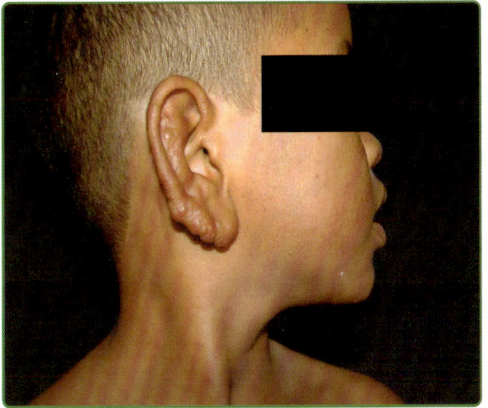

Figure 159-10 Lepromatous leprosy. Papules, nodules, and infiltration on the ear of a child. He had also many lesions on other parts of the skin.

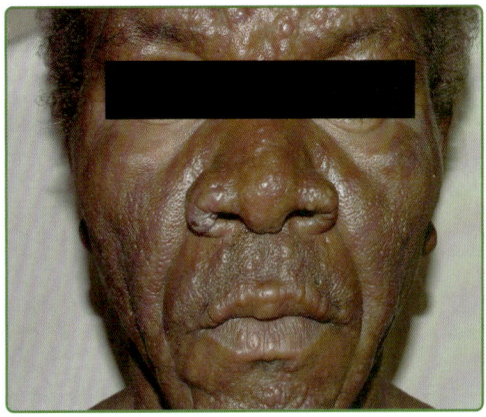

Figure 159-11 Leonine facies. Lepromatous patient with diffuse nodules and infiltration on the face, resulting in a lion's face appearance.

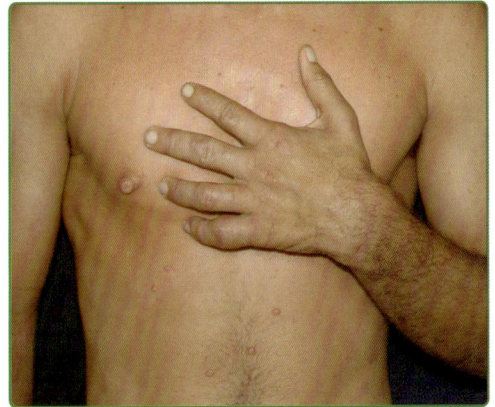

Figure 159-12 Lepromatous leprosy histoid or Wade leprosy. Presence of nodules, which may be disseminated or scattered, some resembling molluscum contagiosum lesions, as in the picture, but note the presence of a nodule on the right nipple, and also some infiltration with a claw formation on the left hand.

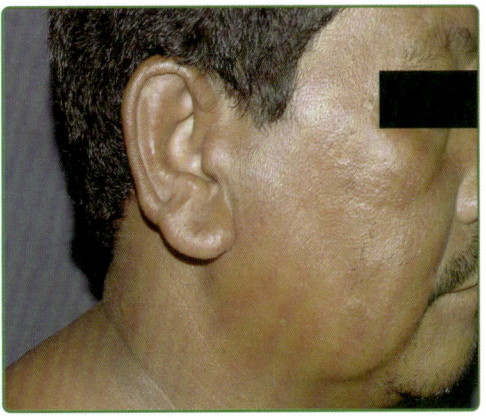

Figure 159-13 Lepromatous leprosy. Diffuse infiltration of the skin.

leprosy, first described by Lucio and Alvarado in Mexico in 1852.[31] Isolation and characterization of this new species from Lucio patients, called *Mycobacterium lepromatosis*,[32] and whole genome sequencing[33] have now firmly established that this closely related mycobacterium causes this form of leprosy found mainly in Mexico and the Caribbean.

The 3 borderline forms (borderline-tuberculoid, borderline-borderline, and borderline-lepromatous) in between are all immunologically unstable. All borderline patients have skin infiltration, varying from a few to many lesions, in one or many areas of the body. Although tuberculoid leprosy patients have just papules or tubercles with no infiltration, borderline-tuberculoid leprosy presents a clear infiltrative band around the periphery of the lesions, changing from a very sharp border in tuberculoid leprosy to a more diffuse infiltrated outer layer in borderline-tuberculoid leprosy (Fig. 159-14). As the forms progress toward the lepromatous end in borderline-borderline (Fig. 159-15) with its classical foveolar lesions, and borderline-lepromatous leprosy (Fig. 159-16), effective cell-mediated immunity decreases, allowing a progressive spread and increase in the number of bacilli, an increase in infiltration of the lesions, with the evolution to form more nodular lesions, often involving the face and ears.

The diagnosis of leprosy is based on the detection of hypo- or total anesthesia in the lesions that may be associated with hypohidrosis and alopecia. Tuberculoid leprosy patients can present both dryness of the skin and alopecia restricted to the territory of the lesions. In contrast, lepromatous leprosy patients may show extensive areas of dryness, especially on the legs, and in advanced cases may result in madarosis and hair loss in different parts of the skin. Borderline patients follow the same pattern, with more restricted features in borderline-tuberculoid leprosy and more diffuse in borderline-lepromatous leprosy.

Paresthesia is a frequent symptom associated with leprosy cases. Burning, numbness, tickling, and other sensations may be present within the lesions or following the territory innervated by the nerve trunks

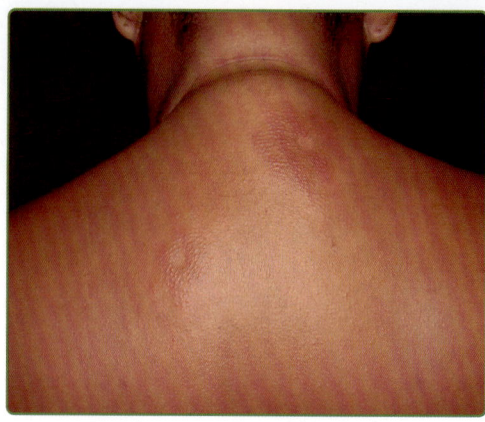

Figure 159-15 Borderline-borderline leprosy. Two foveolar lesions on the upper dorsal thorax.

in the affected area. Patients may feel these sensations in acute crisis, especially at night in cold weather, that may recur frequently, becoming increasingly common with the progression of the disease. All types of leprosy lesions must be submitted to a thorough sensitivity evaluation, including vasomotor reflex, sweating function, thermal, pain, and tactile sensitivity.

Dilation of blood capillaries as a secondary axon reflex erythema, which is dependent on nerve integrity, may be tested using a 1:1000 histamine solution, injected intradermally in normal and lesional skin. Within 5 to 10 seconds, erythema will result from the direct action of histamine on the capillaries, causing vasodilation in both areas, normal and lesional. Two minutes after this a secondary erythema caused by capillary dilation will occur only on normal skin. The last phase of triple Lewis response is exudation of liquid to the dermis, resulting in wheal formation in both areas. Therefore, the triple Lewis response is incomplete only on lesional skin, with the absence of secondary erythema.

Iodine-starch or alizarin red[34] may be used to assess sweating function of leprosy lesions. After iodine

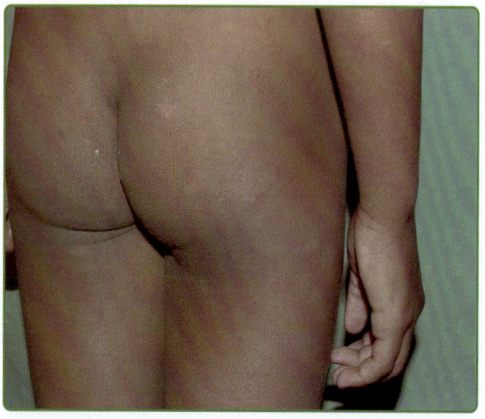

Figure 159-14 Borderline-tuberculoid leprosy. Presence of various hypochromic annular lesions, with papules and infiltration on the periphery, located on the buttocks and thighs of a child.

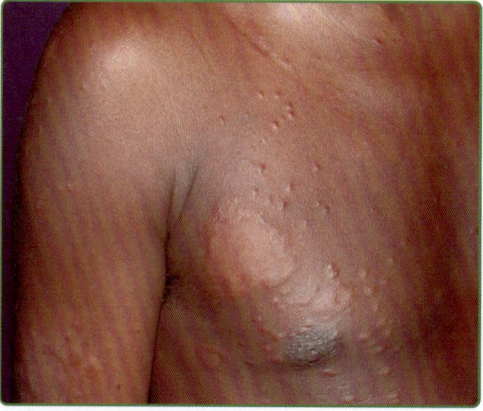

Figure 159-16 Borderline-lepromatous leprosy. Foveolar and nodular infiltrated lesions.

painting followed by starch, or after alizarin red, exercise may be required to induce sweating. When autonomic nerve function is affected sweating is impaired or completely absent and the skin remains dry. On normal skin, a bluish or dark brown (iodine-starch) or violet (alizarin red) color will appear, while there will be no reaction (anhidrosis) or irregular sweating (hypohidrosis) on leprosy lesions.

Thermal, pain and tactile, and Semmes-Weinstein Monofilaments tests are all directly dependent on correct verbal responses from the patient. Therefore, it is crucial to explain what each test is for, how to give proper feedback for the sensation elicited, and to perform the test on normal non-lesional skin sites to familiarize the individual with the sensation before testing lesion areas to measure any changes.

The thermal test is based on the capacity to discriminate between hot and cold sensitivity on touching the skin with 2 tubes containing hot (±45°C [113°F]) or cold water. The tube surface is touched on lesional and normal skin randomly, followed by recording the patients' answers. The professional must be careful to avoid touching lesional and normal skin at the same time, especially for smaller lesions.

Pain sensitivity is based on the ability to distinguish between the tip or the base of a needle, since one produces pain whereas the other does not. Also, randomly, lesional and nonlesional skin must be touched with the tip or the base of the needle, followed by recording the answers. A clear limitation of this method is the use of a perforating instrument, that may cause fear to some patients, especially children.

Tactile sensitivity is tested using a cotton wad, and the patient should answer if he/she senses the light touch of the cotton touching the skin, both normal or lesional. Semmes-Weinstein Monofilaments or esthesiometer kits are monofilament lines graded in thickness with different colors that are attached to plastic posts to apply different amounts of target pressure to the skin. The color and range of target force varies from green (range 0.008-0.07 g, normal skin sensation), the thinnest of which is like the sensation of a mosquito landing on skin, to the thickest, red (up to 300 g).[35] These devices are simple and cheap and can easily measure diminished or loss of protective sensation cause by diabetic neuropathy or neuropathy cause by leprosy nerve damage. Loss of sensation using the blue Semmes-Weinstein monofilaments indicates diminished sensation of light touch (0.16-0.4 g), purple indicates diminished protective sensation (0.6-2 g), and red indicates more profound loss of protective sensation (4-300 g). More recently, the simplicity and ease of use of Semmes-Weinstein monofilaments have supplanted all of the other tactile, thermal, and pain tests.[36] After showing the patient how the monofilament works and getting a "yes" response if he or she feels the touch, various thicknesses of Semmes-Weinstein monofilaments can test areas of skin randomly inside and outside the suspect lesion, as depicted in Video 159-1 at mhprofessional.com/fitzderm9evideos. Even children as young as 6 to 7 years old can respond very well to this kind of test, and those children who are not able to communicate well can still point to the place on the skin if they feel the device touching it (see Video 159-1 at mhprofessional.com/fitzderm9evideos).

In conclusion, the "classic" cases as defined by Ridley-Jopling classification have well-defined lesions, associated with a range of signs and symptoms, which facilitate the diagnosis of leprosy. After 35 years of multidrug therapy, the challenge now is to diagnose cases early, with the goal to eliminate disabilities.

NONCUTANEOUS FINDINGS

Although leprosy diagnosis is based primarily on the presence of skin lesions, usually when dermatologic signs are detected, at this point the peripheral nerves have been already invaded and damaged by *M. leprae* itself and/or by the response of our immune system. In fact, nerves may be the first target of *M. leprae*, and the infection itself together with immune cell infiltration and inflammation that can be clinically detected by palpation.

Palpation of the peripheral nerve trunks can establish nerve thickness and tenderness. However, even for highly trained health professionals, it is not a simple task to detect differences in thickness from one side to the other, or to decide if the nerve is soft, and therefore normal, or fibrotic. Furthermore, those differences should be considered only when it is associated to some functional harm, as (1) loss of sensation defined by hypo- or total anesthesia on the territory of the nerve; (2) motor dysfunction, as in the case of interosseous muscle hypotrophy; or (3) autonomic alteration, as with skin sweating deficit.

Although tuberculoid leprosy patients may have conspicuous alterations in just one specific peripheral nerve trunk, usually in the same segment of the skin lesion, lepromatous leprosy patients often present thickness and tenderness variations in many nerves, accompanied or not with functional alterations in different segments of the body. Borderline-tuberculoid, borderline-borderline, and borderline-lepromatous leprosy patients usually present nerve changes, varying from a few nerve trunks affected in borderline-tuberculoid leprosy to many in borderline-lepromatous leprosy. In many cases, there is some degree of pain, spontaneously reported by the patient, or mentioned during palpation.

Besides upper and lower limbs, the face also may be affected when facial or trigeminal nerves are damaged, which can result in hypo- or anesthesia, including on the cornea, and muscle hypotrophy, especially when palpebral muscles are involved, resulting in lagophthalmos (Fig. 159-17).

The presence of any of these changes in peripheral nerve trunks detected by palpation or functional loss eliminates the diagnosis of indeterminate leprosy. On the other hand, between 5% and 17% of all leprosy patients only have signs of nerve inflammation or functional deficit without any skin lesions, in which case the diagnosis may be pure neuritic, or the more

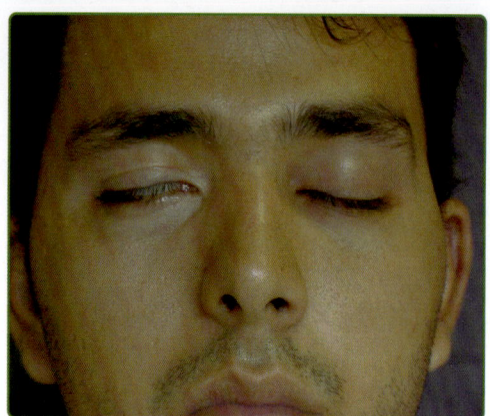

Figure 159-17 Lagophthalmos on the right eye.

common term *primary neural leprosy*,[37] because up to 35% of such cases may develop skin lesions after the diagnosis of primary neural leprosy.[38]

Primary neural leprosy accounts for about 4% to 8% of all leprosy cases, although in India it may be as high as 17%.[37] A positive acid-fast bacilli result on slit-skin smear eliminates primary neural leprosy, but a nerve biopsy can demonstrate the presence of acid-fast bacilli in 16% of these cases, whereas PCR is positive in almost half of them.[39] Definitive diagnosis of primary neural leprosy is not a simple task and may require clinical signs, nerve histopathology, electrophysiology, and ultrasonography,[37] although most of those techniques are not available in highly endemic countries.

Endocrine dysfunctions, after nerve and skin lesions, are most prominent in patients, but are not readily detected, reaching up to 25% of cases[40] leading to, among other problems, hypothyroidism, euthyroid sick syndrome, hypogonadism, sterility and osteoporosis.[41] Levels of testosterone were inversely correlated with the number of skin lesions,[40] and the level of adrenal androgen dehydroepiandrosterone sulphate had an inverse correlation with interleukin (IL)-6 and tumor necrosis factor (TNF)-α, whereas gonadotropins—luteinizing hormone and follicle-stimulating hormone—were positively correlated with proinflammatory cytokines,[42] suggesting a possible neuro-immune-endocrine correlation in leprosy.

COMPLICATIONS

The natural history of leprosy is the evolution to impairment, especially with the eyes, hands, and feet, in both soft tissues and bones, leading to disfigurement and deformity, the origin of all leprosy-related stigma. Even with bacteriological cure after multidrug therapy implementation, and assistance from social networks involved in education, training, and reintegration of those with disabilities into society, estimates of the numbers of people living with varying levels of disability, including Grade 1 (partially disabled) to Grade 2 (can be completely disabled and unable to work) caused by *M. leprae* are likely between 1 and 4 million worldwide.[43]

With the eyes, loss of corneal sensation can result in wounds, followed by infection and blindness, whereas hypotrophy of palpebral muscles may result in lagophthalmos, which can also contribute to corneal infection. Advanced cases, especially in multibacillary leprosy, mostly toward the lepromatous leprosy pole, may present characteristic facial bone malformations, resorption, and pitting, particularly involving destruction of the anterior nasal spine, resorption of the alveolar process of the maxilla, sometimes with loss of teeth, collectively characterized as rhinomaxillary syndrome.[44]

For hands and feet, complications start with a loss of sensation that may lead to wound formation (Fig. 159-18) after burns, trauma, or repetitive moderate pressure–induced skin disruption not detected by the patient, with possible evolution to fissures and ulcers, soft tissue inflammatory autolysis, muscle atrophy, bone decalcification, osteitis and resorption (Fig. 159-19), fusion and joint dislocation, osteoarthritis, and destruction.[45] At the same time, interosseous hypotrophy or amyotrophy may result in paresis or paralysis, leading to formation of claw and/or drop hand or foot (see Video 159-2 at mhprofessional.com/fitzderm9evideos), that may be mobile at first, and constitute severe impairments to leprosy patients,[46] like walking (see Video 159-3 at mhprofessional.com/fitzderm9evideos).

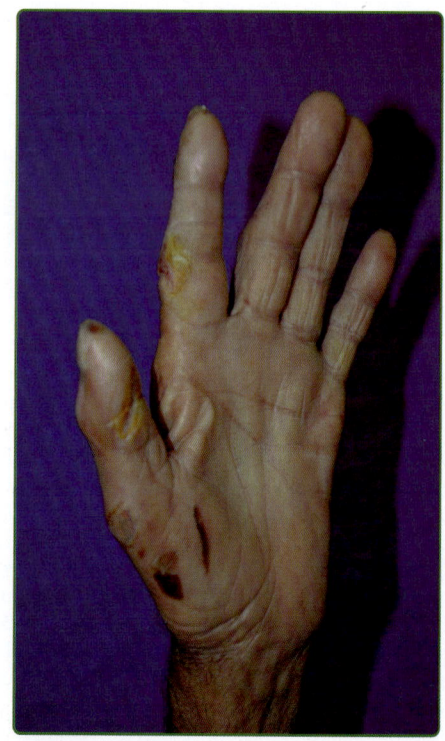

Figure 159-18 Ulcers in a hypotrophic and anhidrotic hand of a LL patient.

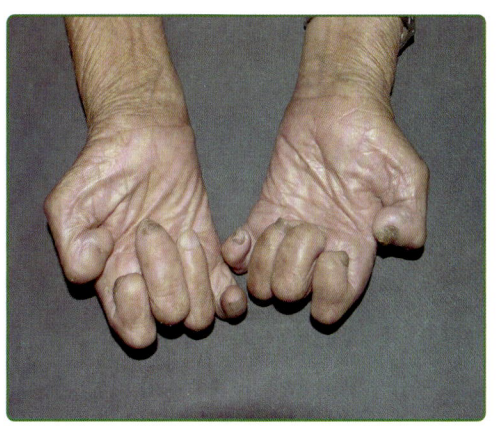

Figure 159-19 Fixed claws and bone resorption associated with anhidrosis and atrophy as sequels on the hands of a borderline-lepromatous leprosy patient.

ETIOLOGY AND PATHOGENESIS

RISK FACTORS

Mycobacterium leprae, a noncultivable obligate intracellular pathogen that mainly damages skin and peripheral nerves, is the causative agent of leprosy, resulting in a broad range of skin lesions with anesthesia, peripheral neuropathy through nerve damage, and muscle weakness and atrophy leading to bone loss by resorption, with related deformity, disfigurement, and disability along with the social stigmatization associated with this disease afflicting mankind for thousands of years. Although *M. leprae* shares roughly 1,439 gene orthologs and homologs with *M. tuberculosis*, a reductive evolutionary event that occurred between 10 and 20 million years ago resulted in massive gene deletion and decay, resulting in the transformation of nearly half of all coding genes into nonfunctional truncated gene remnants or pseudogenes.[47] This process of reductive evolution has occurred in several obligate intracellular pathogens, including Rickettsia and Chlamydia, and is thought to be a survival response to dramatic changes in ecological niche or lifestyle. The streamlining and elimination of many genes and pathways once required for survival as a free-living species would be superfluous in an intracellular habitat, resulting in deletion or inactivation of large parts of the genome. Thus, *M. tuberculosis* has 4.41 Mb, where >90% of the genome encodes 3,998 protein coding sequences, whereas *M. leprae* has 3.27 Mb, where just under 50% of the genome codes for 1614 functional genes, with the remainder coding for 1306 pseudogenes and gene remnants whose complete counterparts can be found in *M. tuberculosis*. The combined effect of gene reduction has created a minimal gene set, reducing the number of genes involved in all functional metabolic pathways, including critical pathways involved in gene regulation, detoxification, DNA repair, transport or efflux of metabolites and small molecules, while generally decreasing the frequency of genes in degradative pathways versus synthetic ones and a paucity of respiratory enzymes. Because of these deficiencies, *M. leprae* has one of the longest doubling times of any bacteria, around 13 days, possibly explaining the exceptionally long incubation time between infection and development of clinical disease, usually between 3 and 7 years, although in some cases up to 20 years. The failure to grow *M. leprae* in axenic medium despite decades of attempts is probably the result of the combined effects of gene reduction and mutations in key metabolic pathways.

One of the hallmarks of the leprosy bacillus is the ability to attach and invade Schwann cells associated with the peripheral nervous system, which leads to colonization and inflammation within nerves, causing nerve damage, demyelination, and neuropathy. Binding to the laminin-2 molecule in the basal lamina of Schwann cells is mediated by 2 bacterial cell wall components, the laminin-binding protein (encoded by ML1683c) and the terminal trisaccharide of the *M. leprae*–specific phenolic glycolipid I (PGL-I).[48] Transmission is thought to occur through the aerosol route, with the bacillus gaining entry and colonizing resident macrophages within the nasal mucosa and turbinate,[49] then disseminating to tissues and nerves through the bloodstream. Early events involved in host–pathogen interaction at the cellular level is likely mediated by host genes involved in pattern recognition receptors and mycobacterial uptake (Toll-like receptors [TLR], nucleotide-binding oligomerization domain containing 2 [NOD2], and mannose receptor C-Type 1 lectin [MRC1]), which modulate autophagy. For example, bacterial cell wall lipoproteins that recognize and bind TLR 1/2 heterodimer ligands on the host cell surface trigger an innate immune response, the outcome of which will determine whether the bacillus is contained or killed within a granuloma or grows uncontrollably. There is an overall genetic resistance toward developing leprosy, with more than 90% of people worldwide having a natural immunity.[50] Early innate immune responses to mycobacteria binding to these pattern recognition receptors and entry into the cell regulates cellular metabolism to activate NF-κB and vitamin D receptor pathways to upregulate cytokine production and genes that are critical to form and maintain granulomas required to contain the bacilli, including TNF, interferon gamma (IFN-γ) and lymphotoxin alpha. What occurs next is likely determined by the complex interplay of the adaptive immune response involving cell-mediated and humoral immune responses, with T helper 1 (Th1) cytokines and a pro-inflammatory response leading to heightened cell-mediated responses controlling bacterial growth and preventing dissemination, and a shift to T helper 2 (Th2) cytokine production downregulating the inflammatory response and leading to uncontrolled growth, high levels of ineffective antibody responses to bacterial antigens, and progressively worsening disease symptoms.

Epidemiologic studies, including twin studies, complex segregation analyses, and genomewide analyses in various genetically diverse populations from different leprosy endemic countries have indicated the probable importance of host genetics in the susceptibility or resistance to this disease. Twin studies conducted in India in the 1960s and 1970s showed that there was an overwhelming concordance (60%-80%) for monozygotic twin pairs to develop leprosy.[51,52] Genomewide analysis studies examining linkage and association of multiple gene candidates suggest that there is genetic control involved in the susceptibility of developing leprosy and a predilection to develop a particular form of disease. Evidence for the latter is seen in Mexico and the Philippines, where 90% of cases develop the lepromatous form of the disease, whereas about equal numbers of patients develop tuberculoid or lepromatous disease in many African countries and in Brazil. Extensive studies have implicated associations with human leukocyte antigen (HLA) complex genes (class I and class II) because of their primary role in the adaptive host immune response, and a number of alleles are overrepresented for leprosy susceptibility or the development of either the tuberculoid or lepromatous subtype when particular ethnic populations in different countries were examined. There is also a shared genetic background between leprosy and a number of inflammatory diseases, including Crohn disease (nucleotide-binding oligomerization domain containing 2 [NOD2]), myocardial infarction (lymphotoxin α [LTA]), Type 1 diabetes and psoriasis (vitamin D receptor [VDR]), and Parkinson disease (E3 ubiquitin-protein ligase [PARK2]).[50] More recently, genomewide association studies examining SNP differences between leprosy cases and controls in China have increased the list of genes that may be involved in regulating innate and adaptive immune response pathways associated with susceptibility or resistance to leprosy.[53] Fifteen SNPs detected among 6 genes were associated with leprosy (HLA-DR-DQ, RIPK2, TNFSF15, CCDC122, C13orf31, and NOD2), whereas pathway analysis identified a total of 35 genes involved in a single network involved in leprosy susceptibility or resistance.

Besides genetic risk factors, many studies have shown that there are a number of other factors, operational or socioeconomic, that increase the risk or predispose individuals toward developing disease. Household contacts living within a dwelling with an untreated multibacillary leprosy index case have the highest risk of eventually coming down with disease, particularly if the household contact is a blood relative to the index case.[54] Individuals who have a positive anti-PGL-I titer have up to an 8-fold higher risk of developing leprosy. Other risk factors include living in an endemic or hyperendemic area for leprosy, poverty, living in high-density households with >2 persons sleeping together in a room, poor nutritional status, poor sanitation or lack of clean water, and lack of health care availability.[55] Improving these underlying problems would greatly decrease the likelihood of those at risk of leprosy from ever developing this disease.

DIAGNOSIS

SUPPORTIVE STUDIES

PATHOLOGY

Physiopathology of Leprosy: The routes used by *M. leprae* to gain access to the target cells, mainly Schwann cells, have always been a matter of discussion. Basically, 4 different pathways have been proposed: (1) naked nerve filaments in the epidermis; (2) entrance of *M. leprae* in the epidermis, and from there to other Schwann cells; (3) phagocytosis of *M. leprae* by dermal macrophages, which then invade the perineurium, liberating bacilli to enter Schwann cells; and (4) through the blood, that is, *M. leprae* could gain access to the nerve by intraneural capillaries. Enlarged endothelial cells could facilitate bacilli entrance to the nerve system, and finally to Schwann cells.[56]

M. leprae interaction with and engulfment by endothelial cells was identified long ago.[57] Armadillo studies showed epineural thickening following *M. leprae* infection of macrophages of lymphatic and vascular endothelial cells.[58] Although this model of infection is well known, it is still not clear how *M. leprae* is then transferred from those cells to Schwann cells.

Once *M. leprae* reaches the extracellular matrix, PGL-I[48] or a histonelike 21-kDa laminin-binding protein[59] binds to the laminin α2 chain to invade Schwann cells. The presence of the G domain of α-dystroglycan (α-DG) might be necessary for the adherence of *M. leprae* to Schwann cells.[60] The matrix cytoskeleton link (α-DG, α2-laminin, β-DG) may be the route used by *M. leprae* to enter the host cell (Fig. 159-20).

M. leprae bypass neuregulin receptor (an epidermal growth factor family component) and does a direct bacterial ligation to ErbB2, signaling with no ErbB3 heterodimerization and amplifying Erk1/2 signaling that may induce myelin sheath degradation.[61] In addition, using a nonclassical pathway and MEK-independent signaling, *M. leprae* can activate Erk1/2 directly by lymphoid cell kinase (p56LcK), inducing cell proliferation and maintaining its niche of proliferation.[62] On infection, there is an increased expression of 9-*O*-acetyl GD3 ganglioside, a molecule involved in anti-apoptotic signaling and nerve regeneration (Fig. 159-20). Immunoblocking of 9-*O*-acetyl GD3 ganglioside on Schwann cells reduces Erk1/2 and cell proliferation.[63]

M. leprae can dedifferentiate and reprogram adult Schwann cells to stem cell–like cells, possibly using this to promote dissemination of infection.[64] Bacilli survival may be maintained by different mechanisms. After invasion (Fig. 159-20), *M. leprae* interferes with (1) endocytic maturation inhibiting vesicle acidification of phagosomes[65]; (2) host-cell lipid homeostasis, inducing and accumulating lipid droplets through cytoskeleton reorganization and PI3K signaling, independently of TLR-2[66]; and (3) oxidative pathways, by an intensification of glucose uptake and augmentation of glucose-6-phosphate dehydrogenase, that once inhibited can decrease *M. leprae* viability by up to 70%.[67]

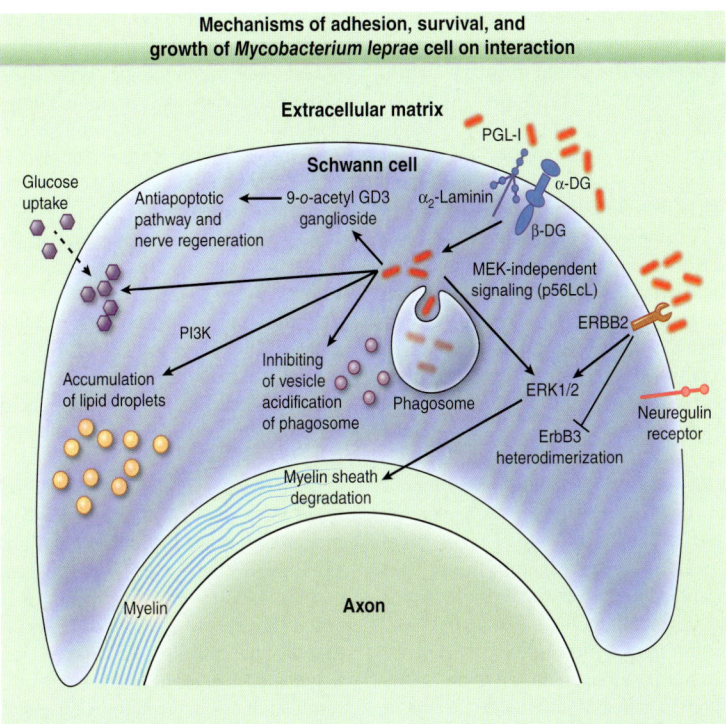

Figure 159-20 Host cell interaction of *M. leprae*. The figure shows the main mechanisms of entrance and maintenance of the bacteria inside a Schwann cell.

The immune response may initiate at any phase of the host–bacteria interaction. Epidemiologic surveys in hyperendemic areas in Brazil show a high percentage (up to 50% or more) of anti-PGL-I IgM antibodies circulating among schoolchildren, indicating infection with *M. leprae* followed by an early antibody response against the bacilli.[68] Although nerve demyelination may occur in T and B lymphocyte–depleted mice,[69] diverse immune reactions occur during infection.

There is a well-characterized dichotomy in the human immune response in leprosy, with those at the tuberculoid end of the spectrum having a strong Th1 cell–mediated response whereas those at the lepromatous end have a skewed Th2 response with T-cell anergy present. Tuberculoid leprosy cases have a strong Th1 response, with IL-2, TNF-α, IFN-γ, and IL-12 cytokine production, whereas lepromatous leprosy patients have a Th2 response, with IL-4, IL-5, IL-10 and high levels of antibody production. Those characteristics are found also in the skin, where generally the 2 situations may appear as demonstrated by the progressive disorganization of the immune cells that infiltrate the skin[70] in histochemical stained tissue sections of lesions. Tuberculoid leprosy patients present a well-organized granuloma containing epithelioid cells, CD4+ T cells, a good cell–mediated immunity, almost no antibody production, and no bacilli found by slit-skin smear bacilloscopy. On the other hand, lepromatous leprosy patients demonstrate a massive infiltration of foamy macrophages filled with large numbers of bacilli, with few lymphocytes, mostly CD8+ T cells, and a defective cell-mediated immunity with high titers of antibodies to *M. leprae* antigens, including to PGL-I.[71]

Toll-like receptors, such as TLR-1, TLR-2, and TLR-4, along with DC-SIGN (CD209) and CD163 may be involved in macrophage/dendritic cell interactions with *M. leprae*. TLR-1 and TLR-2 have a higher expression in tuberculoid leprosy in comparison with lepromatous leprosy lesions, and TLR-1/TLR-2 heterodimers mediate monocyte and dendritic cell activation, stimulating TNF-α and IL-12 production[72] (Fig. 159-19). *M. leprae* can also stimulate TNF-α, IL-6, and CXCL10 (IP-10) production through TLR-4 signaling in macrophages.[73] On the other hand, TLR-2 signaling in Schwann cells is related to apoptosis.[74]

M. leprae increases IL-10 expression in dendritic cells through DC-SIGN signaling, activating Raf-1, resulting in acetylation of the NFκB p65 subunit after TLR-induced activation of NFκB.[75] IL-10 induces phagocytosis by macrophages through DC-SIGN and differentiates monocytes into foamy macrophages by upregulation of oxidized low-density lipoprotein uptake, whereas IL-15 induces the vitamin D antimicrobial pathway, exhibiting less phagocytosis.[76] Together with upregulation of DC-SIGN and indoleamine 2,3-dioxygenase, CD163 is also increased and contributes to iron uptake and to the creation of an advantageous environment for *M. leprae* entry and survival in lepromatous leprosy macrophages[77] (Fig. 159-20). *M. leprae* can modulate NFκB activation in Schwann cells, a function that can be inhibited by thalidomide.[78] Moreover, metalloproteinases 2 and 9 and TNF-α are upregulated in Schwann cells, macrophages and endothelial cells in primary neural leprosy nerves,[79] that result in a prominent endoneurial infiltrate, with perineurial fibrosis and enlargement in comparison to non-leprosy peripheral neuropathy.[80]

Besides the Th1/Th2 cytokine profile, other factors, such as IL-17, cathelicidin LL-37, and insulinlike growth factor I also seem to be important in leprosy physiopathology. VCAM-1 is augmented in the serum of leprosy patients,[81] whereas vascular endothelial growth factor and thromboplastin expression is increased by endothelial cells of leprosy patients.[82] IL-17 is low in all leprosy patients in comparison to nonleprosy controls, but even lower in lepromatous leprosy.[83] Although IL-17-producing CD4+CD45RO+ Th17 cells were increased in peripheral blood mononuclear cells of tuberculoid leprosy patients, IL-10-producing Foxp3+ Treg cells were 5 times more prevalent in lepromatous leprosy than in tuberculoid leprosy patients, indicating a role for Tregs in multibacillary leprosy development.[84] Cathelicidin LL-37, a unique cathelicidin family member of host defense peptides found in humans that is known to modulate the immune response against *M. tuberculosis*, is low in all leprosy patients[85] (Fig. 159-21). Insulinlike growth factor I, known to decrease macrophage antimicrobial capacity, inhibiting *M. leprae* killing,[86] was also found to be low in lepromatous leprosy patients, mostly among those who did not develop Type 2 reaction or erythema nodosum leprosum (ENL).[87]

ENL, an immunologic Type III hypersensitivity response, occurs with immune complex deposition[88] with anti-PGL-I and anti-monocyte chemoattractant protein-I antibodies,[89] upregulation of Th17, IL-6, IL-1β, sIL2R, and sIL6R; a decrease of the Treg response; and an influx of neutrophils in the lesions[90] (Fig. 159-21). In addition, ENL can be initiated on IFN-γ intradermal injection in lepromatous leprosy patients,[91] there is an increase in the CD4+/CD8+ ratio, high serum levels of TNF-α are found,[92] and the use of TLR-9 agonists augments TNF-α, IL-6, and IL-1β.[93] E-selectin is expressed in a vascular pattern, higher in ENL than in nonreactional lepromatous leprosy patients,[94] and FcγRI increases in circulating neutrophils of ENL patients[95] (Fig. 159-21).

Gene expression analysis showed an increased expression of a "cell movement" biologic group, including P-selectin, E-selectin, and neutrophil adhesion to endothelial cells, with migration and inflammation. In vitro stimulation of TLR-2 induced IL-1β and FcR expression, that together with IFN-γ and granulocyte macrophage colony–stimulating factor, augmented E-selectin expression, and increased neutrophil adhesion to endothelial cells.[94] Thalidomide inhibited this neutrophil recruitment pathway, decreases neutrophil influx, FcγRI expression, and TNF-α production. C1qA, B, and C components of the classical complement pathway, and the receptors

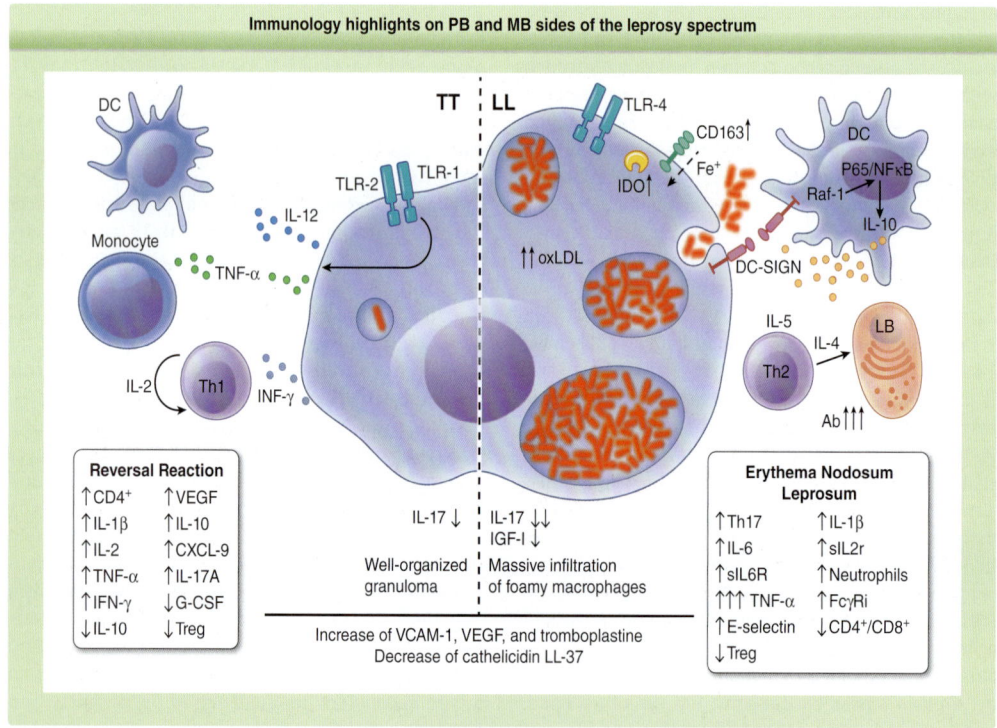

Figure 159-21 Immunology of leprosy. The main differences of tuberculoid leprosy and lepromatous leprosy poles are demonstrated, together with the key variations between reversal reaction and erythema nodosum leprosum.

C3AR1 and C5AR1, were also increased in lepromatous leprosy patients.[59]

Type 1 reaction or reversal reaction, a Type IV hypersensitivity immune response, is caused by a specific increase in cell-mediated immunity against *M. leprae*, and may rapidly evolve to nerve damage. Together with an increase of CD4⁺ T cell infiltration associated with IL-1β, IL-2, TNF-α, and IFN-γ upregulation[96] (Fig. 159-21), an augmentation of CC chemokines monocyte chemoattractant protein-I and RANTES[97] is observed.

Also, vascular endothelial growth factor, IL-10, CXCL-9, and IL-17A were demonstrated to be upregulated on the reversal reaction onset, together with downregulation of IL-10 and granulocyte colony-stimulating factor. This profile was related to a decrease of CD39⁺CCL4⁺CD25⁺⁺ regulatory T-cell subsets and an increase of *GNLY*, *GZMA/B*, and *PRF1* genes associated with cytotoxic T cell.[98]

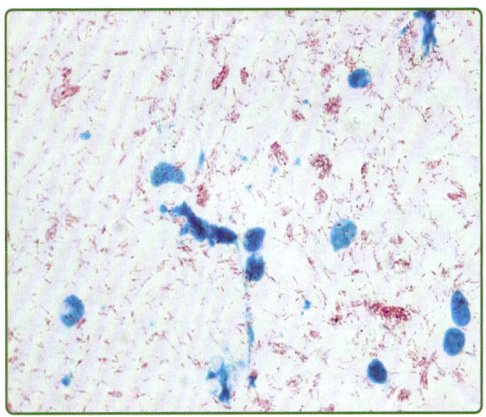

Figure 159-22 Acid-fast bacilli of a slit-skin smear of a lepromatous leprosy patient. The cells are in blue and the bacteria are in red, forming globi.

LABORATORY TESTING

Further reduction in leprosy would require the diagnosis of those in the early stages of disease to allow treatment to prevent nerve damage and impairment, but it is estimated that most patients experience up to 2 years delay in diagnosis.[99] Reasons for this are complicated, but include a reduction in the numbers of trained leprosy clinicians and laboratory technicians worldwide and the incorporation of leprosy diagnosis into the general family health delivery system, resulting in increased levels of misdiagnosis or delays in beginning treatment. When there are doubts about the clinical diagnosis, laboratory tests can be used to assist or confirm a presumptive case of leprosy.

The clinical spectrum of leprosy shows a range of pathologic manifestations in skin lesions and nerve damage that is aligned with the competence of the host's immune response, and is dependent on the strength and interaction of both cell-mediated and antibody responses.[100] The standard for laboratory diagnosis in a skin biopsy is the detection of acid-fast bacilli by the Fite-Faraco modification of the carbol fuchsin technique and characteristic cellular histologic patterns that make up the immunopathologic types of leprosy as detected by hematoxylin–eosin staining. The widely used Ridley-Jopling classification system[26] divides the disease into 5 forms based on the number of acid-fast bacilli and the degree of lymphocytic infiltration and organization, as described in pathology (above). Bacilloscopy of multiple skin biopsies or slit-skin smear can establish the bacillary index on a logarithmic scale, which can range from 0 (no acid-fast bacilli detected in tuberculoid leprosy lesions) to 6+ (>1000 acid-fast bacilli per field in lepromatous leprosy) (Fig. 159-22). For treatment purposes, detection of acid-fast bacilli in skin lesions or slit-skin smear automatically places the patient in the multibacillary category to receive 12 months of multidrug therapy.

There is currently no laboratory test capable of diagnosing leprosy or identifying asymptomatic individuals who are progressing toward developing early symptoms, so the development of a simple and cheap test that could assist health professionals to correctly diagnose the disease based on immunologic or metabolomic biomarkers of infection is desirable. A number of research groups have developed a variety of tests that partially achieve this goal, measuring antibody titers to mycobacterial antigens by rapid lateral flow devices; cell-mediated cytokine release assays (such as the detection of IFN-γ, similar to commercial whole blood assays used to detect infection by *M. tuberculosis*); amplification of mycobacterial DNA by PCR; or the use of metabolomics to detect molecular features specific to *M. leprae* infection in the blood or urine. Laboratory assays adapted to assess leprosy patient antibody titers to the *M. leprae*–specific antigen, PGL-I, have been in use for more than 30 years[101,102] and include enzyme-linked immunosorbent assays and lateral flow devices that use the soluble synthetic disaccharide of PGL-I coupled to either bovine or human albumin, called ND-O-BSA or ND-O-HSA, respectively. Another is the protein antigen LID-1, composed of the fusion of 2 well-recognized *M. leprae* proteins, ML0405 and ML2331, that is recognized by >95% of lepromatous patients.[103] Coupling the synthetic disaccharide of PGL-I to LID-1 and incorporating this NDO-LID glycoprotein in a lateral flow test resulted in enhanced sensitivity to detect leprosy patients, even those at the paucibacillary end of the spectrum.[104] Another group has combined lateral flow assays with up-converting phosphor reporter technology to assess both anti-PGL-I titers along with T cell–mediated cytokine responses (IFN-γ, IL-10, and others) in a single sample. The ability to quantitate the ratio of inflammatory Th1 cytokines versus downregulating Th2 responses provides more information about the complex interplay of cellular and humoral immunity within individuals that can be used to better predict those with asymptomatic infection or who are progressing to disease.[105,106] Another method that has been used to diagnose difficult cases is the molecular detection of the *M. leprae*–specific repetitive RLEP sequence by PCR. Because there are 37 copies of the RLEP sequence in the genome, this enables the detection of as few as 3 bacterial genomes in a sample. Recent evidence indicates that individuals who are RLEP PCR positive in biopsies of skin lesion sites, earlobe slit-skin smear, or the nasal turbinate as well as having a positive anti-PGL-I titer likely have asymptomatic infection and are at the highest risk of developing disease.[49] Our own household contact studies in hyperendemic areas in Pará, Brazil, support these findings. Initial results of multiple families living in "hot zones" indicated that in many instances >80% of household contacts had a positive anti-PGL-I titer, >70% were positive for RLEP by PCR in slit-skin smear, with up to 65% being positive for both biomarkers, demonstrating extreme rates of infection, with 1 or more individuals in each household diagnosed with leprosy based on clinical signs (Salgado et al, unpublished observations). Finally, metabolomics has been used to identify molecular features found in the serum of leprosy patients, indicating that there was an increase of circulating polyunsaturated fatty acids and phospholipids in individuals with lepromatous disease.[107] A recent report has even shown that molecular features of infection can be identified by mass spectrometry simply by pressing silica plates against patient skin lesions.[108] Moreover, the leprosy miRNome sequencing has been recently published, and revealed new markers involved on leprosy physiopathology[109]

Although advances have been made in identifying biomarkers of infection by many research groups, translating this to a rapid, cheap, point-of-care test that will aid in diagnosing all patients throughout the leprosy clinical spectrum, including asymptomatic individuals, has a long way to go. Currently, leprosy diagnosis must remain in the competent hands of well-trained leprosy clinicians and health care workers. We have shown the importance of targeting schoolchildren in school-based surveillance and followup of household contacts of those diagnosed children to detect cases early in the disease process. The use of a Geographic Information System, spatial analysis tools, and laboratory tests (anti-PGL-I enzyme-linked immunosorbent assay and RLEP PCR) has enhanced the ability to identify "hot zones" within hyperendemic cities,[110,111] which can then allow focused targeting of foci of infection by community health care agents working in local areas. Nevertheless, given the complexities of examining, diagnosing, and ensuring treatment to individuals living in hyperendemic areas,[15] developing a simple laboratory test to diagnose leprosy early is highly desirable and would facilitate breaking the lines of transmission to eventually reach the goal of leprosy elimination.

HISTOPATHOLOGY

Skin biopsies should include the dermis and, if possible, subcutis of a lesion. Hematoxylin–eosin staining is complemented using the Fite-Faraco staining method or another method to detect acid-fast bacilli.

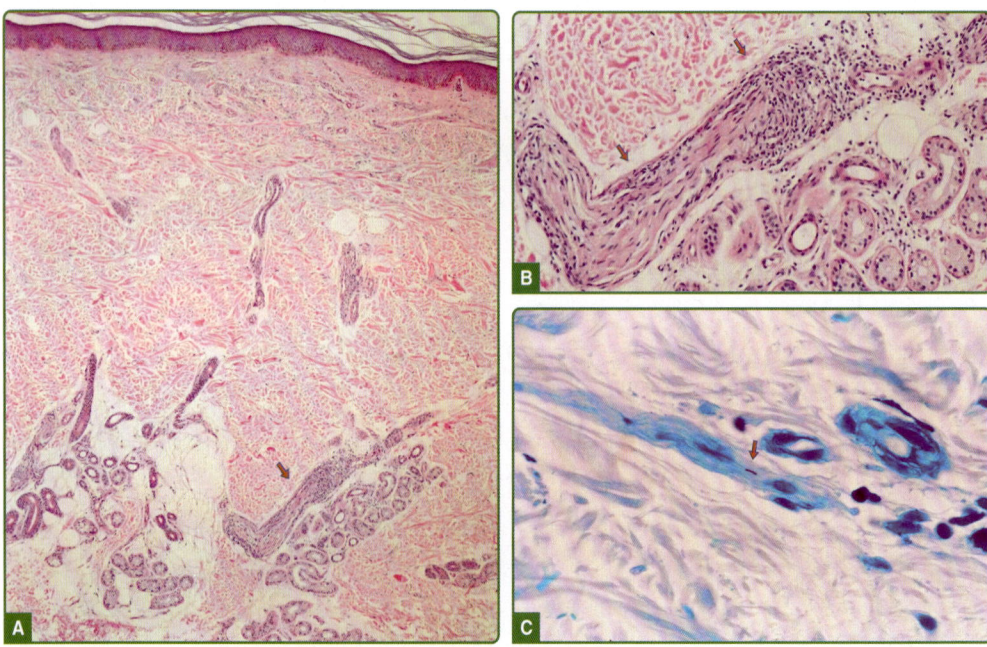

Figure 159-23 Indeterminate leprosy histopathology. Up to 70% of the indeterminate cases may have an unspecific histopathology. In 30% it is possible to observe a perineural infiltrate with nerve delamination (**A** and **B,** arrows), as demonstrated here, and if extensively searched, sometimes it is possible to find an acid-fast bacilli (**C**, arrow). (Used with permission from Dr. Jaison Barreto, Lauro de Souza Lima Institute, Brazil.)

Histopathologic findings are graded according to the Ridley and Jopling scale.[26] The tissue response in *Indeterminate* leprosy is nonspecific. The normal epidermis or basal layer of the skin show melanin reduction. Perivascular or perineural, superficial and deep dermal infiltration by few macrophages and lymphocytes are common findings. Sometimes the infiltrate surrounds skin appendages and rarely there are bacilli in nerves (Fig. 159-23).

Tuberculoid leprosy shows an epidermis that is usually normal and the subepidermal clear zone is absent. There is a noncaseating dermal granulomatous process composed chiefly of activated macrophages (epithelioid cells) with CD4+ T cells in the center of the epithelioid cells, CD8+ T cells in the mantle surrounding the granuloma, and giant cells of the Langhans type. Granulomas may contact the epidermis and are often arranged around nerves and vessels. Peripheral nerve involvement, cellular infiltration of sweat glands, and invasion of the arrectores pilorum muscle by a granulomatous infiltrate is common. There are no acid-fast bacilli or when they are present are found more frequently within peripheral nerves, arrectores pilorum muscle, or even granulomas[112,113] (Fig. 159-24).

The histopathology of the *borderline-tuberculoid* form can be distinguished from tuberculoid leprosy by the presence of a subepidermal grenz zone. In general, there is no well-defined granuloma with organized collections of epithelioid cells, and there is a reduction in the frequency of lymphocytes and scarce Langhans cells with rare acid-fast bacilli (Fig. 159-25).

In *borderline-borderline*, there are aggregates of epithelioid cells, scarce dispersed lymphocytes, no Langhans multinucleated giant cells, and increasing numbers of acid-fast bacilli (Fig. 159-26).

Borderline-lepromatous leprosy shows a subepidermal grenz zone, aggregates of macrophages, occasional epithelioid cells with abundant cytoplasm, and some foamy cells, with few lymphocytes. A great number of bacilli and some globi can be found (Fig. 159-27).[114]

In *lepromatous leprosy* there is a normal to flattened epidermis, subepidermal grenz zone, aggregates and sheets of foamy macrophages admixed with predominantly CD8+ lymphocytes and plasma cells throughout the dermis and into the subcutaneous fat. Huge numbers of acid-fast bacilli and globi are found within foamy macrophages (Virchow cells), nerves, arrectores pilorum muscle, follicular epithelium, and sweat glands (Fig. 159-28).

Histoid leprosy is characterized by epidermal atrophy, a subepidermal grenz zone, and a dermis showing sheets of predominantly spindle-shaped cells with nuclear pyknosis and foamy cytoplasm, vacuolated, and arranged in a storiform pattern. Some polygonal-shaped cells, macrophages, and inflammatory cells are present. Some cases may show a pseudocapsule. The lesion resembles a fibrohistiocytic tumor (Fig. 159-29). The Fite-Faraco stain reveals a large number of acid-fast bacilli, mostly as rafts or globi (Fig. 159-30). Bacilli can be located in nerves, Schwann cells, eccrine glands, and in the vascular endothelium. CD68-positive macrophages and spindle cells are present in histoid leprosy.[115]

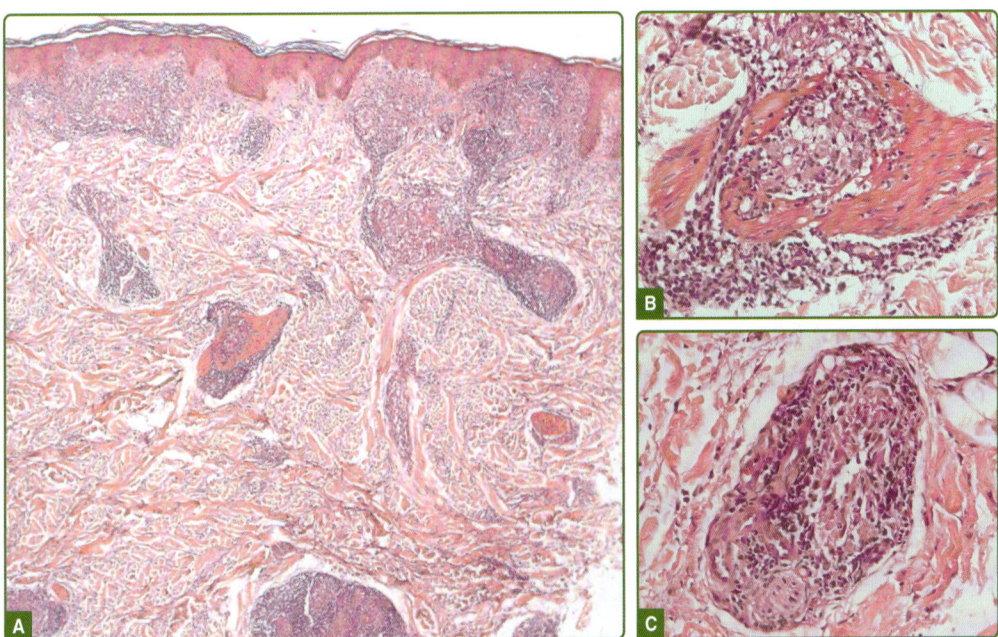

Figure 159-24 Tuberculoid leprosy histopathology. Presence of deep and superficial well-developed granuloma, that touch the epidermis (**A**), associated with lymphocyte infiltration surrounding or invading and destroying skin appendages, like nerves, erector pili muscle (**B**), or sweat gland (**C**).

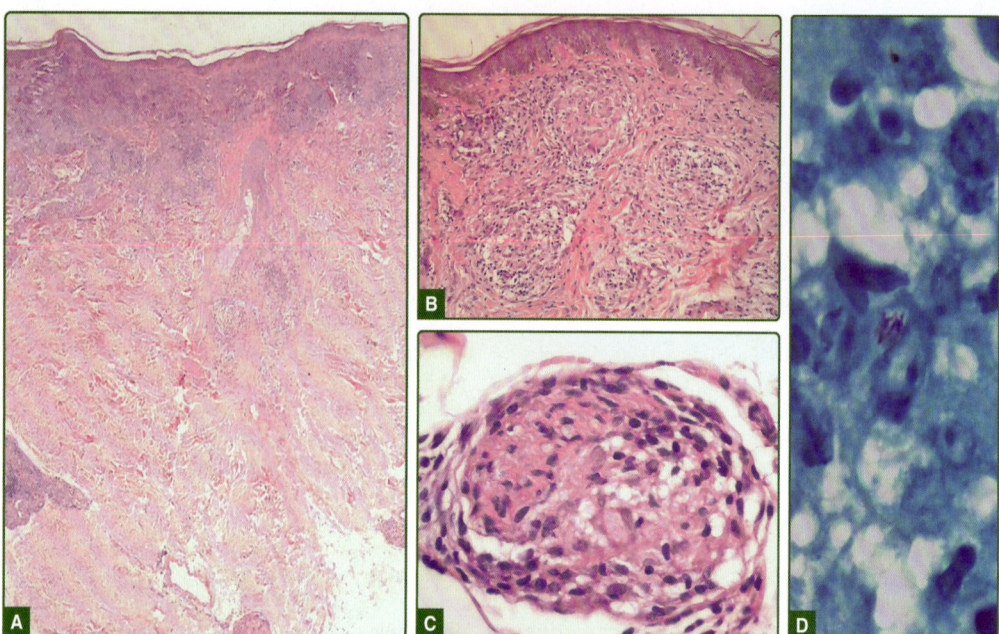

Figure 159-25 Borderline-tuberculoid leprosy histopathology. Deep and superficial tuberculoid granuloma (**A**) that does not touch the epidermis (**B**). The tuberculoid granuloma may be seen invading the nerves (**C**), and acid-fast bacilli can be found (**D**, 100×). (Used with permission from Dr. Jaison Barreto, Lauro de Souza Lima Institute, Brazil.)

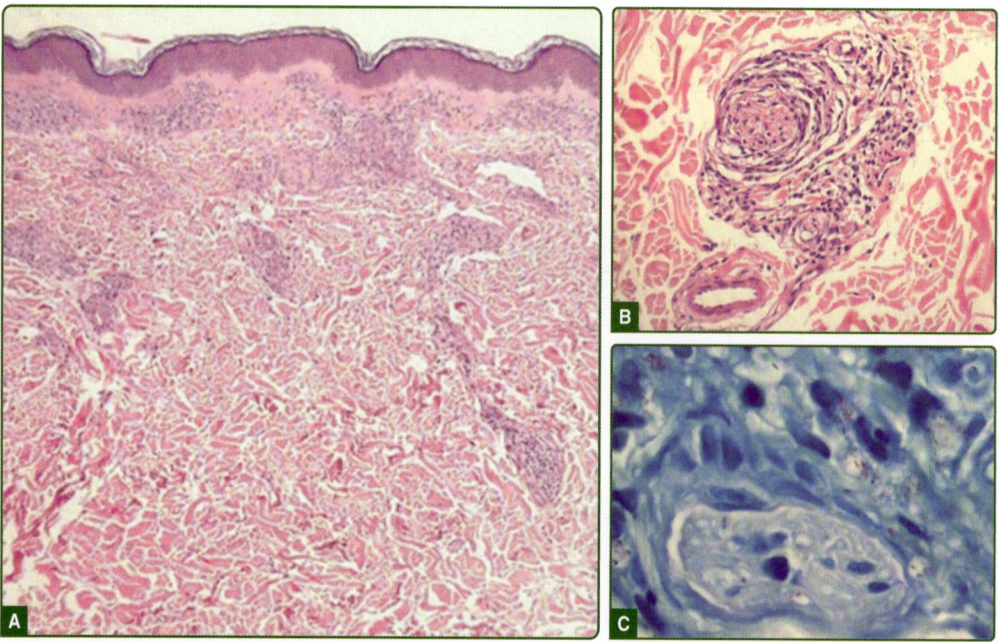

Figure 159-26 Borderline-borderline leprosy histopathology. Deep and superficial tuberculoid granuloma that does not touch the epidermis, starting to form a grenz zone (**A**). Inflammatory cells are invading cutaneous annexes and nerves, that are degenerated (**B**), and acid-fast bacilli can be found more easily, some forming globi (**C**). (Used with permission from Dr. Cleverson Soares, Lauro de Souza Lima Institute, Brazil.)

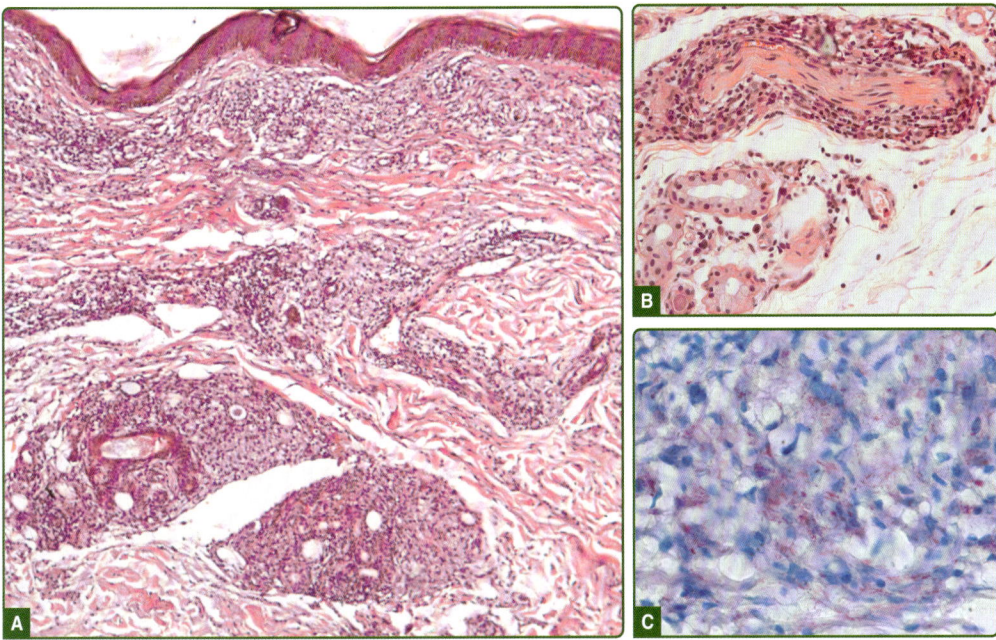

Figure 159-27 Borderline-lepromatous leprosy histopathology. There is a mixed macrophage lymphocytic inflammatory infiltrate (macrophage granuloma) on superficial and deep dermis (**A**). The mixed infiltrate does not touch the epidermis and may be seen surrounding or invading nerve bundles (**B**). A large number of acid-fast bacilli is seen (**C**).

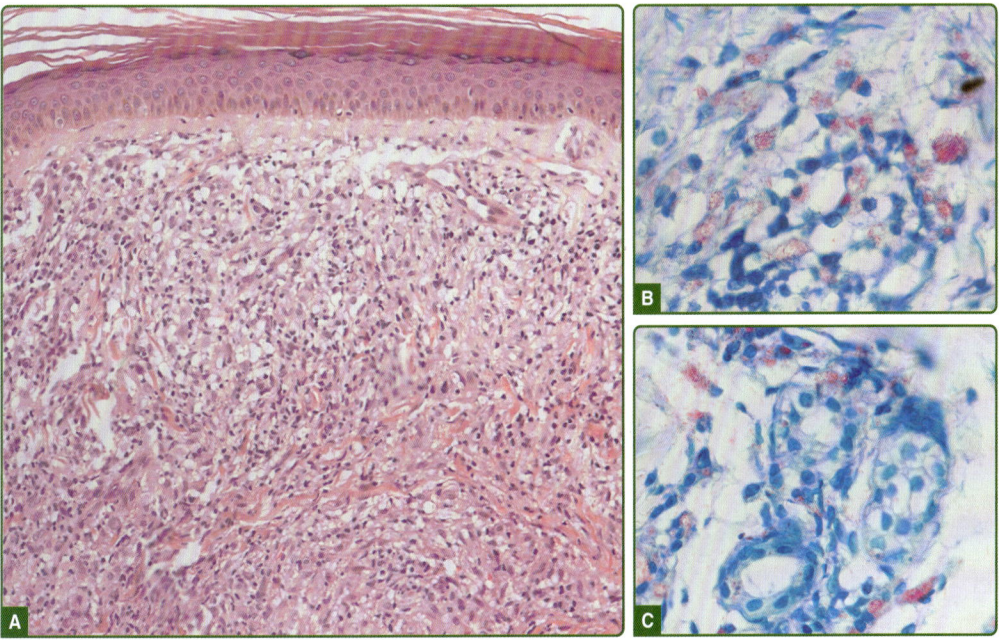

Figure 159-28 Lepromatous leprosy histopathology. An inflammatory infiltrate composed mostly by foamy macrophages is observed on the dermis. The epidermis is flattened, and there is a clear grenz zone on the dermal–epidermal interface (**A**). Fite-Faraco demonstrate acid-fast bacilli globi inside macrophages (**B**) and on sweat glands cells (**C**).

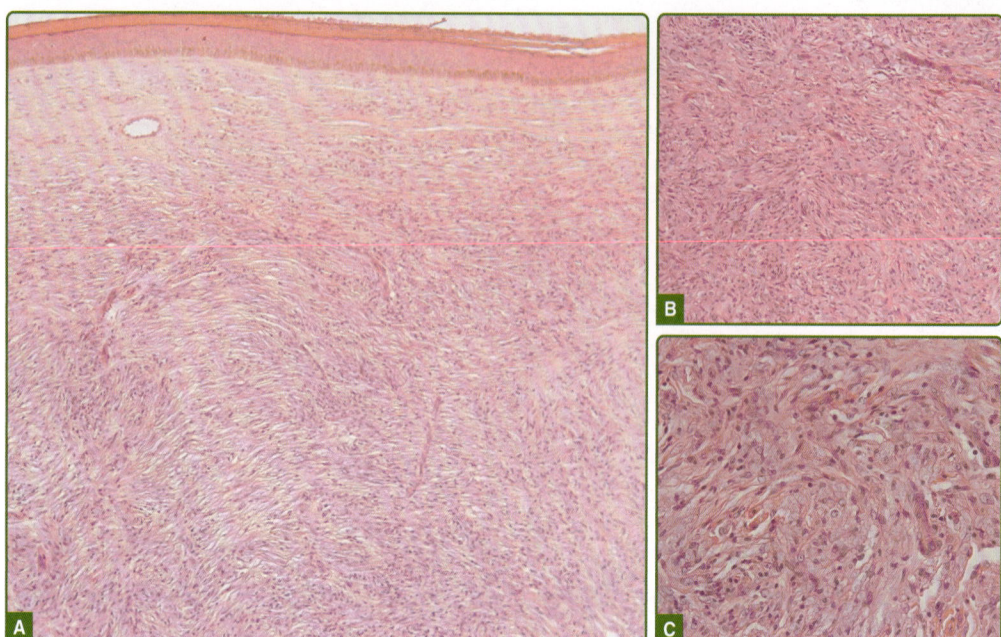

Figure 159-29 Lepromatous leprosy histoid Wade leprosy histopathology. A flattened epidermis is observed over a dense inflammatory infiltrate (**A**) of spindle and epithelioid cells arranged in a storiform or fasciculated pattern (**B**), which may have a foamy aspect on closer view (**C**).

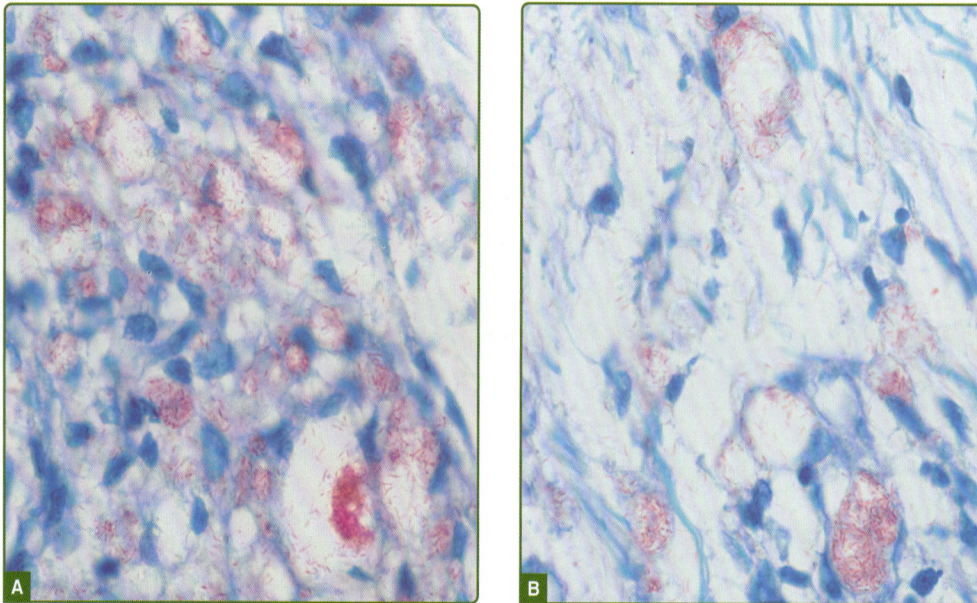

Figure 159-30 Globi. Aggregates of bacilli (globi) inside the host cells, as seen here inside macrophages (**A** and **B**), is a characteristic of *M. leprae*.

In leprosy reversal reaction, the histopathologic features are edema both extracellular as in epithelioid cell granulomas, increased number of lymphocytes and Langhans giant cells in the infiltrate, small collections of epithelioid cells, as well as a poorly organized granuloma. Fibrinoid necrosis is present in severe cases of reversal reaction. Bacilli are found in macrophages and nerves (Fig. 159-31). The downgrading reaction reveals aggregates of foamy macrophages, a remarkable reduction or complete absence in the number of lymphocytes, and acid-fast bacilli in greater numbers.[116,117]

ENL or Type 2 reaction. The characteristic histologic features are edema and a mixed inflammatory infiltrate in the dermis and in the subcutis, predominantly

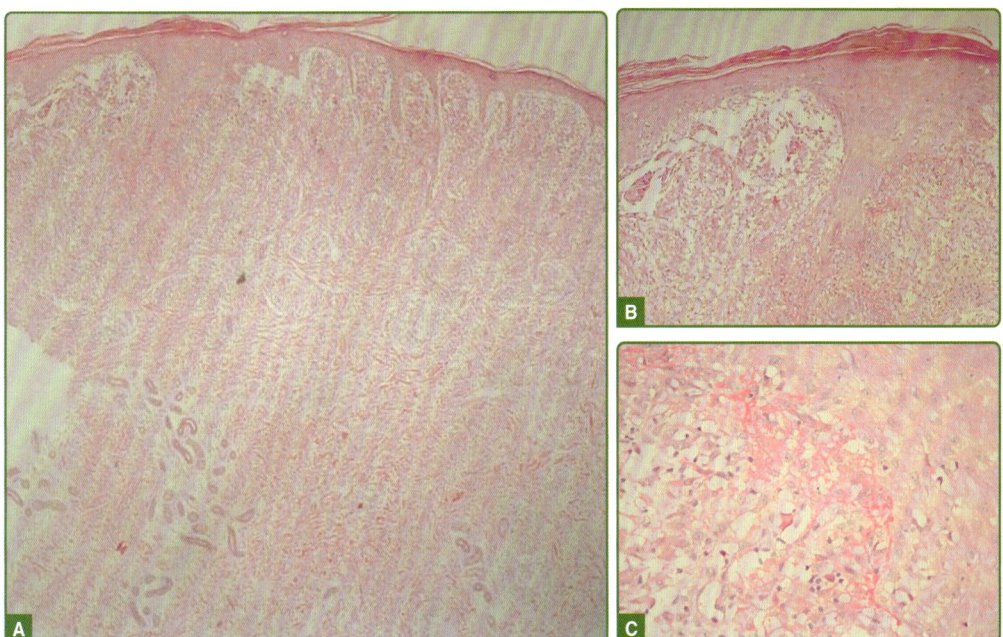

Figure 159-31 Histopathology reversal reaction. Presence of an inflammatory infiltrate, associated to epithelial hyperplasia (**A**) and foci of epidermal aggression with dermal edema (**B**) and fibrin deposit (**C**). (Used with permission from Dr. Jaison Barreto, Lauro de Souza Lima Institute, Brazil.)

neutrophils with eosinophils, lymphocytes, aggregates of foamy macrophages, plasma cells, and mast cells. Vasculitis and a mixed lobular and septal panniculitis are present in most cases (Fig. 159-32). Bacilli in large numbers, usually granular in appearance, are easily found. The predominant lymphocyte present in ENL is the T-helper cell, whereas T-suppressor cells predominate in the lepromatous leprosy.[117,118]

Lucio phenomenon or erythema necrotisans. The main microscopic features are that of a cutaneous or subcutis necrotizing vasculitis. There is fibrinoid necrosis of small and medium-sized vessels. The other histologic picture reported in *Lucio phenomenon* are necrosis of epidermis and superficial dermis, micro-abscess formation, angiogenesis, endothelial swelling, vascular occlusion caused by luminal thrombi, and deposits of fibrin in small blood vessel walls of the dermis and the subcutis. There is a mixed dermal and/or subcutis infiltrate of neutrophils, eosinophils, lymphocytes, and nuclear dust. Bacilli are found in endothelial cells, in blood vessels, nerves, arrectores pilorum muscle, follicular epithelium, sebaceous glands, and sweat glands.[119-122]

NERVE CONDUCTION STUDY— ELECTRONEUROMYOGRAPHY

Leprosy neuropathy manifests as asymmetric focal or multifocal lesions, mononeuropathy or mononeuritis multiplex, caused by the direct damage of nerves by *M. leprae* and by an inflammatory immune response of the host. There is chronic neuropathy, with acute exacerbations resulting from reversal reaction or ENL. Besides focal lesions, entrapment of the enlarged nerves is also a concern, that may require surgical intervention to decompress the nerve. Evaluation includes nerve palpation, pain evaluation, sensory assessment, muscle power measurement and autonomic examination.

Electroneuromyography is a refined tool for nerve function assessment at diagnosis, and for patient followup to detect and characterize new lesions, especially during reversal reaction or ENL, or to evaluate entrapment syndromes and neuropathic pain. Leprosy neuropathy starts with Schwann cell demyelination that may evolve to axon loss. Commonly affected sites include the elbow for the ulnar nerve, the carpal tunnel for the median nerve, the fibula head for the fibular nerve, and the tarsal tunnel for the posterior tibial nerve, all which are key areas for evaluating neuropathy.[123]

IMAGING

High-resolution ultrasound use for peripheral nerve evaluation is an established procedure. However, only recently has it seen more use in the evaluation of nerve function impairment in leprosy neuropathy. Clinical examination of nerve enlargement may be difficult to measure, even for experienced leprologists, and there are no robust parameters to be recorded to followup the leprosy patient during and after multidrug therapy.

High-resolution ultrasound can be used for evaluation of echogenicity, vascularity, and nerve thicken-

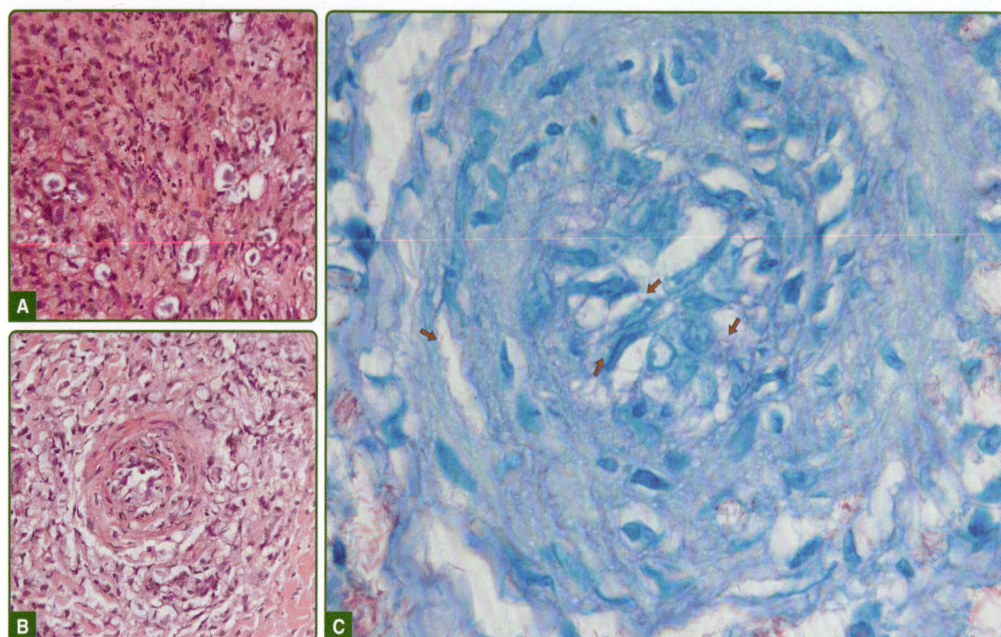

Figure 159-32 Histopathology erythema nodosum leprosum. A mixed inflammatory infiltrate, composed of foamy macrophages with large vacuoles and neutrophils (**A**) is shown. Foamy macrophages are also seen surrounding a vessel undergoing fibrinoid necrosis and presenting aggregates of inflammatory cells in its lumen and wall (**B**), where Fite-Faraco reveals the presence of large amounts of globi, and single bacilli inside a vessel and in its wall (**C**, arrows).

ing, using objective parameters and values for several neuropathies, including leprosy.[124] In addition, nerve abscesses and entrapment also can be detected early and evaluated.[123] Its utilization for leprosy neuropathy evaluation is still evolving, but very promising. Echogenicity abnormalities, intraneural Doppler and post-multidrug therapy cross-sectional areas above normal limits, with less than 30% reduction, have been linked to poor outcomes. Worsening of nerve abnormalities after multidrug therapy were found independent of leprosy classification or presence of reactions.[125]

DIAGNOSTIC ALGORITHM

See Fig. 159-33.

DIFFERENTIAL DIAGNOSIS

See Table 159-1.

CLINICAL COURSE AND PROGNOSIS

One of the most important problems during the leprosy clinical course is the appearance of acute or subacute episodes of inflammation, defined as reactions.

Leprosy reactions, caused by immune response against *M. leprae* antigens, are divided into Type 1 or reversal reaction, involving mainly peripheral nerves and skin, and Type 2 or ENL, that may have localized or systemic symptoms. Acute neuritis also may be considered as a type of reaction.

Reactions never occur in Indeterminate patients. Up to 50% of all patients on multidrug therapy may present reactions during treatment, but these reactions can also occur before and after therapy. Neuropathy present at the time of diagnosis, multibacillary leprosy, extent of the disease, and the presence of lesions overlying peripheral nerve trunks are factors that increase the risk of reactions and nerve function impairment.[126] Reversal reaction and ENL may happen together in some patients (Table 159-2).

Reversal reaction can occur in up to 30% of patients, whereas tuberculoid leprosy cases are seldom affected,[127] the majority of the reactional episodes occur in borderline forms, mainly borderline-lepromatous and borderline-borderline, followed by lepromatous leprosy.[128] It starts as a sudden worsening of skin lesions and nerve function impairment, with no apparent systemic involvement. Besides prereactional lesions presenting more infiltration and desquamation, previous and newly developing lesions may be bright red, hot, and sensitive to the touch (Fig. 159-34), sometimes ulcerated, frequently associated with peripheral nerve enlargement, and usually accompanied by pain. Reversal reaction requires immediate intervention, because it can result in nerve impairment and permanent disabilities.

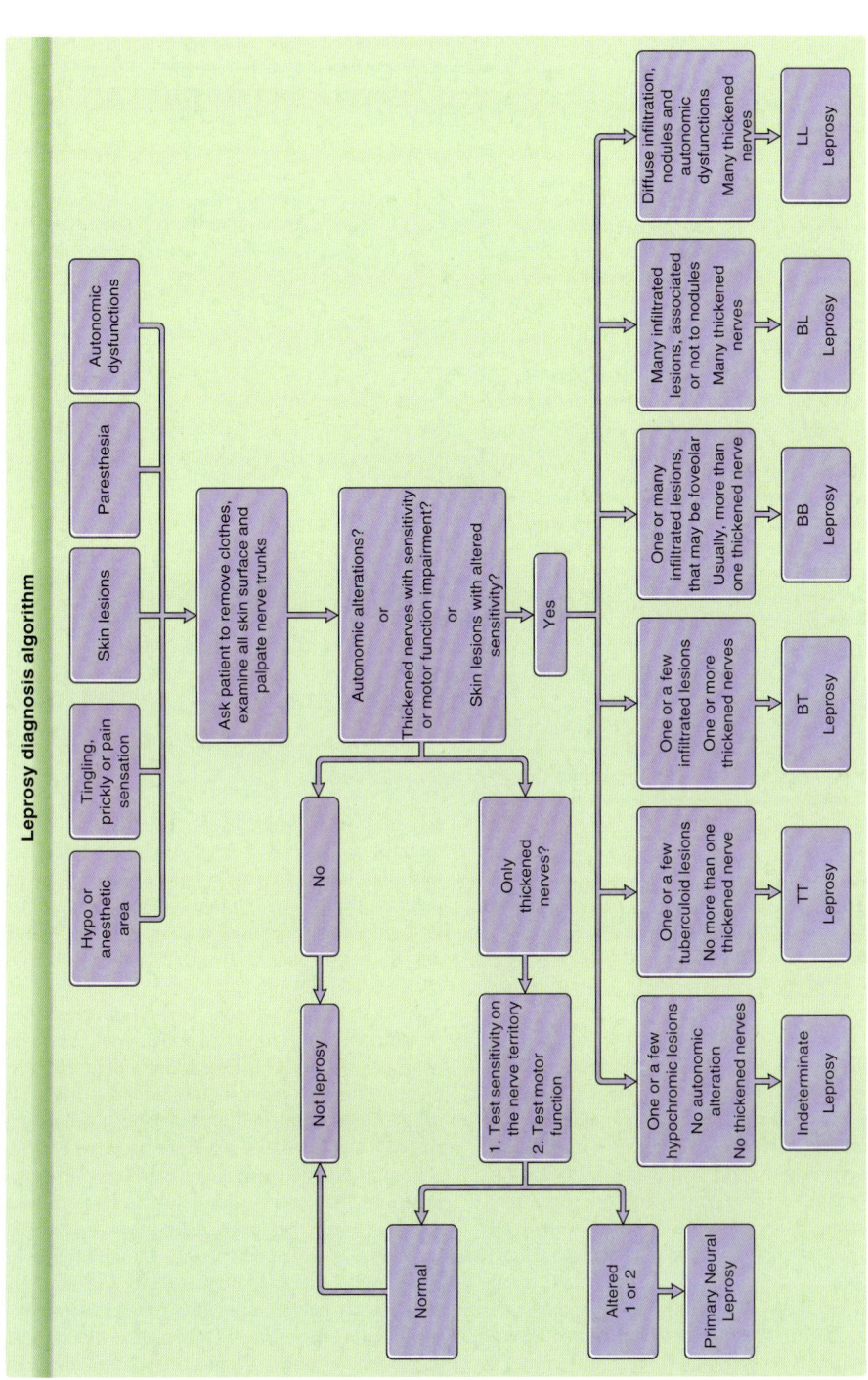

Figure 159-33 Leprosy diagnosis. At any time, it is possible to ask for laboratory examinations: slit-skin smear for acid-fast bacilli or for PCR, biopsy for histopathology, and anti-PGL-I serology.

TABLE 159-1
Differential Diagnosis

Primary Lesions
- **Macules and patches.** The hypopigmentation of pityriasis alba and indeterminate leprosy mimic each other. If the patient was born in, or had resided in, an endemic area, then the distinction between the two may be made by neurologic or histologic examination. Hypopigmented BL plaques can be so faintly indurated as to mimic patches. Telangiectasias may be eruptive or present as mats on the face and upper trunk.
- **Papular to nodular lesions.** In the dermis, leprosy may mimic, or be mimicked, by dermatofibromas, histiocytomas, lymphomas, sarcoidosis, neurofibromatosis, syphilis, anergic leishmaniasis, paracoccidioidomycosis, chromoblastomycosis, sporotrichosis, lobomycosis, tuberculosis, and other granulomas. Eruptive and recurrent inflammatory subcutaneous nodules may be ENL, erythema nodosum, erythema induratum, and vasculitis. Palpable, but not visible, subcutaneous nodules in Lucio leprosy may mimic lipomas.
- **Plaques.** Erythematous plaques may mimic mycosis fungoides. Plaques without pigmentary change may be wheal like in appearance, causing confusion with urticaria. Hypopigmented plaques may mimic papulosquamous eruptions. Islands of normal skin within a plaque may suggest psoriasis.
- **Polymorphous vesiculobullous eruption/Dermoepidermal separation.** They may occur in ENL. IgM is deposited not uncommonly at the epidermal basement membrane in LL. These antibodies are not necessarily pathogenic but may confuse diagnosis.
- **Annular lesions.** Leprosy may mimic, or be mimicked by, annular erythemas, sarcoidosis, syphilis, or tinea.

Secondary Lesions
- **Infarcts.** Lucio phenomenon lesions and necrotic ENL mimic septic infarcts.
- **Ulcers.** Ulcers occur in Lucio phenomenon and ENL secondary to vascular occlusion. In patients with nerve destruction, neurotrophic ulcers occur on the plantar surface, patients with Leg ulcers secondary to venous insufficiency are seen in Lucio leprosy.

Clinical Constellations
- **Systemic lupus erythematosus–like changes.** Fusiform fingers, swan neck deformity, false positive syphilis tests, antiphospholipid antibodies, lupus anticoagulant, hyperglobulinemia, and anemia.
- **Vasculitis.** A true vasculitis may occur in ENL, Lucio phenomenon, and Lucio leprosy. Clinically, leprosy lesions of a nodular character may be misdiagnosed as "vasculitis."

TABLE 159-2
Lepra Reactions and Management

	REVERSAL REACTION (TYPE I)	ERYTHEMA NODOSUM LEPROSUM (TYPE II)
Predominant leprosy subtype	Borderline-tuberculoid Borderline-borderline Borderline lepromatous Lepromatous leprosy	Lepromatous leprosy
Signs and symptoms	Acute worsening of skin lesions Acute worsening of nerve function impairment No apparent systemic symptoms	Erythema nodosum Erythema polymorphous Severe cutaneous necrotizing vasculitis Fever, edema, malaise
Extracutaneous involvement	Neuritis	Neuritis Panniculitis Glomerulonephritis Arthralgia Epididymitis Orchitis Eye inflammation Osteitis Lymphadenitis
Treatment	Prednisone (1-2 mg/kg/d with slow taper ~3 mo)	Thalidomide 100-400 mg/d AND prednisone (1-2 mg/kg/d) OR Pentoxifylline 400 mg thrice a day

ENL is an aggressive vasculitis with immune complex deposition affecting different organs, resulting in, among other sequelae, neuritis, panniculitis, glomerulonephritis, arthralgia, epididymitis, orchitis, eye inflammation, osteitis and lymphadenitis with systemic symptoms such as fever, edema and malaise.[129] A high bacillary index and diffuse skin infiltration are important risk factors[130] and 65% of the cases have more than one episode of ENL.[131] The main skin manifestation is erythema nodosum, more palpable than visible (Fig. 159-35), and may be accompanied by erythema polymorphous or severe cutaneous necrotizing vasculitis (Lucio phenomenon) (Fig. 159-36).

Immunologic disorders, like HIV and HTLV infections, immunosuppressive drugs, or immunobiological medications can interfere with the resolution of leprosy. The first case of leprosy occurring as a result of immune reconstitution inflammatory syndrome (IRIS) in an HIV-infected individual was described in 2003.[132] The upgrading of the cell-mediated immune response due to antiviral therapy in AIDS patients is now well recognized in IRIS,[133] and the percentage of HIV and other viral infections in leprosy patients is high, indicating that all leprosy patients should be tested for HIV, HBV, HCV and HTLV-1.[134] Viral coinfection decreases the survival of leprosy patients,[135] whereas increasing rates of neuritis, nerve function impairment, and leprosy relapses.[134] Anti-TNF therapy can result in the development of clinical leprosy in infected individuals following cessation of the immunobiological medication[136-138] regardless of whether reactional episodes are involved.

It is important to distinguish reactions from relapses. Reactions may occur before, during, and a few years after multidrug therapy. Usually, they are acute, with a rapid appearance of new lesions and infiltration of the old ones, deterioration of neural function, and/or systemic involvement, responding well to treatment with antiinflammatory drugs. On the other hand, relapses in general are slowly progressing, almost always with resurgence of primary lesions followed by the gradual appearance of new lesions, together with nerve involvement, and, in contrast, there is no response to antiinflammatory drugs. A true relapse must be defined after confirmation of completion of the first treatment by the patient. If the full course of treatment is confirmed, it

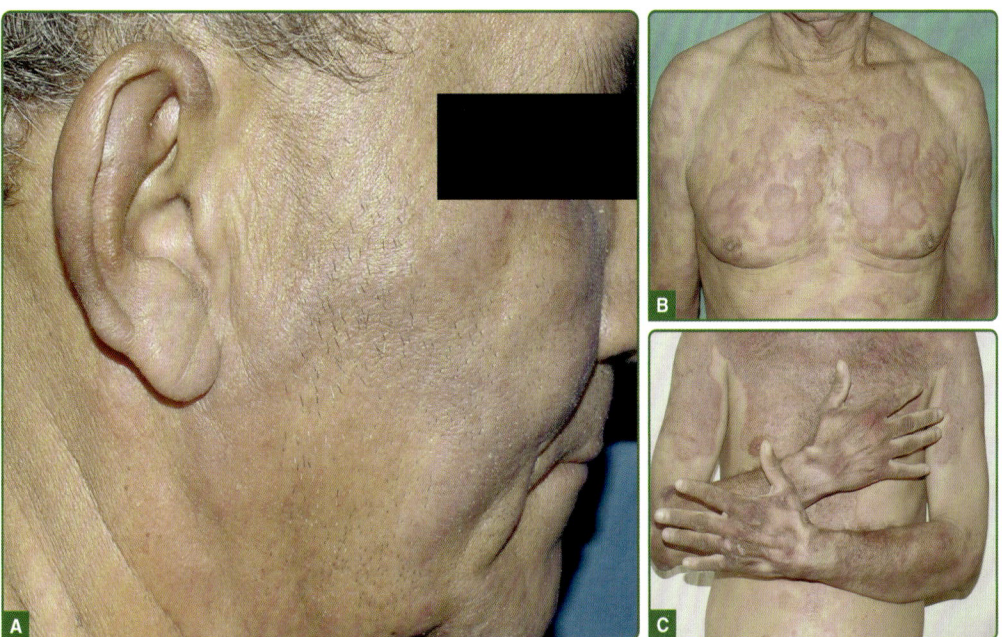

Figure 159-34 Reversal reaction. Reappearance or worsening of pre-multidrug therapy lesions, during or after treatment (**A**), usually presenting severe infiltrated lesions, that may coalesce in small, foveolar (**B**) or large scaly (**C**) plaques.

becomes necessary to test for drug resistance, although reinfection cannot be ruled out. If the patient was wrongly classified, then an insufficient length of therapy may be the case. Histopathology can be useful to distinguish a reaction from a case of relapse.[139]

Although leprosy is well known for loss of skin sensation, neuropathic pain may arise during or after multidrug therapy, due to tissue inflammation or dysfunction of the nervous system.[140] Nerve trunk pain onset may be spontaneous or appear after palpation, either abrupt or insidious, but many patients experience recurrent episodes. More than half of the patients have some pain episode during or after multidrug therapy, with a higher prevalence in lepromatous leprosy, decreasing toward the borderline and tuberculoid forms. The most affected nerves are ulnar and tibial.[140] If the pain persists during treatment, or becomes long-lasting after completing multidrug therapy, it may be defined as chronic neuritis or neuropathy.[141]

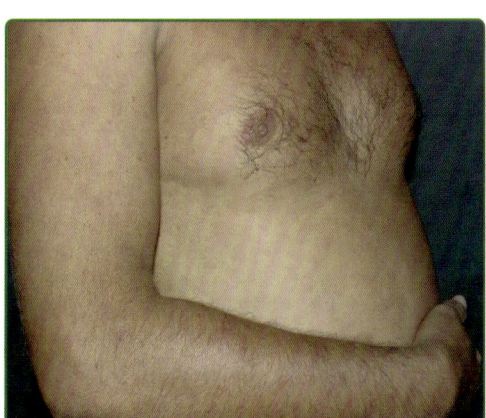

Figure 159-35 Erythema nodosum leprosum. Presence of fever and malaise with painful subcutaneous nodules that are easy to palpate, but much less apparent then reversal reactions lesions.

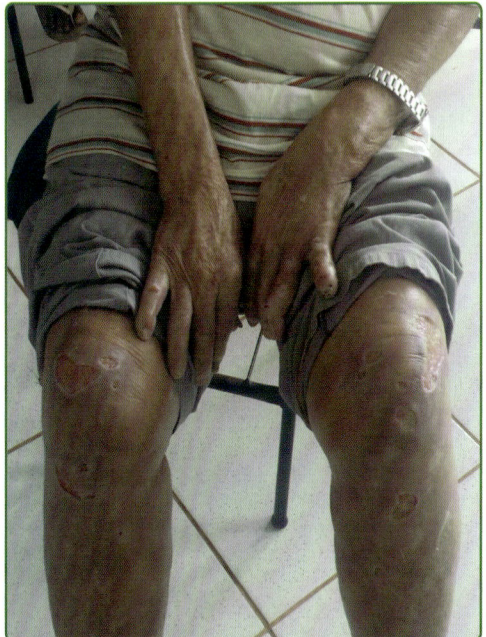

Figure 159-36 Lucio phenomenon. Small and large ulcers with infiltration in lepromatous leprosy patients. Slit-skin smear of those patients is loaded heavily with acid-fast bacilli.

MANAGEMENT

INTERVENTIONS

MEDICATIONS

There are, basically, 3 groups of medications used for treating leprosy: antibiotics, antiinflammatory or immunosuppressants and analgesic drugs. The first group, antibiotics, has a well-defined standard for treatment, the WHO Multidrug Therapy drug regimen, that contains rifampicin and dapsone, with or without clofazimine, in monthly blister packs. Antiinflammatory drugs, usually prednisone and thalidomide, are prescribed to control leprosy reactions by reducing inflammation, whereas analgesics are used to control neuropathic pain.

Before the discovery of sulfones' power to improve leprosy signs by Guy Faget in 1941,[142] chaulmoogra oil, drug used in India for decades, was the only commonly used treatment for leprosy, although its efficacy was questionable, as it generally induced only a localized inflammatory response in the skin.

Dapsone is a simple, low-cost, highly effective drug for leprosy, used in a daily dose of 100 mg or 1 to 2 mg/kg. The drug is absorbed by the GI tract and eliminated through the kidneys. It is usually well tolerated, although it is dependent on the presence of the enzyme glucose 6-phosphate dehydrogenase (G6PD), an X-chromosomally transmitted enzyme, that is lacking in 400 million people worldwide, mostly in tropical areas where malaria is present[143] and also where leprosy is prevalent. G6PD deficiency leads to serious hemolytic events by oxidative stress, including the formation of methemoglobin that is clinically detected as a violet color on sclera, lips, and the extremities of fingers together with malaise, headache, and dyspnea. In addition to a high level of hemolysis, G6PD-deficient patients using dapsone are at a greater risk of developing severe life-threatening hemolytic anemia, and must change their medication.[144] Dapsone hypersensitivity syndrome, a rare but potentially fatal event, presents with fever and cutaneous rash, eventually involving internal organs, especially the lungs, with eosinophilic infiltrates and pneumonitis. It may occur at any time during treatment, and it may be related to drug rash with eosinophilia and systemic symptoms (DRESS syndrome).[145]

Clofazimine is a pigment that, in addition to its unknown antibiotic mechanism, also has antiinflammatory properties. The main objection as far as patients are concerned is its affinity to fat tissue and macrophage deposits leading to skin hyperpigmentation, especially in the lesions. An additional side effect is skin dryness that together with pigmentation, gives the skin a highly xerodermic appearance (Fig. 159-37). It is used in a dose of 300 mg once a month, and 50 mg per day, only in multibacillary patients. Clofazimine is well-tolerated by leprosy patients.[146]

Rifampicin is highly bactericidal, and unlike the daily administration of dapsone and clofazimine, it is

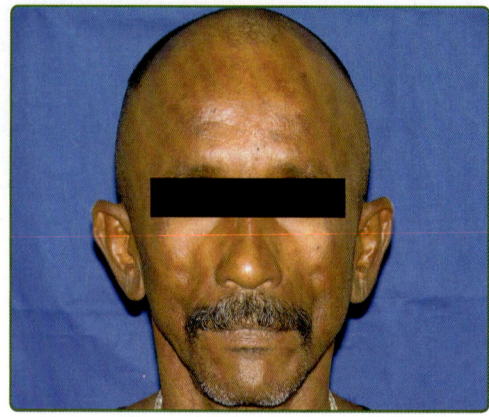

Figure 159-37. Clofazimine pigmentation. Brownish color and dry skin in a patient on multibacillary multidrug therapy.

only administered once per month with supervision, 450 mg to children and 600 mg to adults. Adverse effects include face and neck redness, pruritus and cutaneous rash, loss of appetite, nausea, vomiting, and diarrhea, malaise (which may require cessation of the drug), purpura, and epistaxis. Flulike syndrome, a not well-understood immunologic side effect occurring with the use of intermittent doses of rifampicin, is characterized by fever, asthenia, myalgia, and headache, sometimes accompanied by bone pain. Eosinophilia, nephritis, thrombocytopenia, and shock may eventually develop. Although considered rare, it was the major side effect reported in a Brazilian study with 20,667 leprosy patients on multidrug therapy.[147]

Multidrug therapy schemes used today are the same as 1982 when they were first implemented (Table 159-3), with dapsone, clofazimine, and rifampicin prescribed for multibacillary cases for up to 24 months, or dapsone and rifampicin for 6 months for paucibacillary patients. Pregnancy and breastfeeding do not contraindicate the use of multidrug therapy.[144] In the 1960s, together with the confirmation of clofazimine and rifampicin[148] efficacy against *M. leprae*, the first cases of dapsone-resistant leprosy appeared.[149] In the 1970s, WHO decided to replace dapsone monotherapy in favor of a 3-drug strategy with dapsone, rifampicin, and clofazimine combined in a new drug regimen to treat leprosy called multidrug therapy. Although drug resistance in leprosy appears to remain low,[150] reports of MDR-leprosy are increasing in the literature,[151-153] and it may be a concern for leprosy treatment in the near future.[154] The substitute drugs available, either to resistant strains or to patients with side effects on multidrug therapy, ofloxacin, minocycline, or clarithromycin (Table 159-3), appear to be safe and effective for leprosy treatment,[146] but new alternative drugs are necessary.

Although there are a few well-structured clinical trials for treating nerve damage in leprosy, with moderate-quality evidence, including one with intravenous methylprednisolone pulse therapy,[155] WHO recommends leprosy reactions must be immediately

TABLE 159-3
Antibacterial Treatment of Leprosy Recommendations

RECOMMENDING ORGANIZATION	DISEASE TYPE	RIFAMPICIN	DAPSONE	CLOFAZIMINE	DURATION	FOLLOWUP
World Health Organization	PB	600 mg/mo	100 mg/d	—	6 mo	No mandated followup. To return as needed
	MB	600 mg/mo	100 mg/d	50 mg/d 300 mg/mo	1 y	No mandated followup To return as needed
US Public Health Service	PB	600 mg/d	100 mg/d	—	1 y	At 6-mo intervals for 5 y
	MB	600 mg/d	100 mg/d	50 mg/d	2 y	At 6-mo intervals for 10 y
Other Microbicidal Agents	**Dose**					
Clarithromycin	500 mg/d					
Minocycline (substitute for dapsone or clofazimine)	100 mg/d					
Ofloxacin	400 mg/d					

PB, paucibacillary; MB, multibacillary.

treated with antiinflammatory or immunosuppressant drugs.[144] The most widely used are corticosteroids and thalidomide. Reversal reaction can be treated with prednisone at doses of 1 to 2 mg/kg/d in a regressive scheme, diminishing 10% to 15% of the dose every 15 days, with a complete cycle of treatment lasting up to 3 months. If there is a worsening of the clinical situation, it may be necessary to go back to the previous higher dose, extending this level of corticosteroid treatment for 30 to 45 days, followed by tapering off again.

Glucose levels and blood pressure must be controlled during the use of corticosteroids. Glaucoma, cataracts, moon face, striae, adrenal gland atrophy, and osteoporosis may occur with long term usage, and as with other immunosuppressive agents, other infectious diseases, such as systemic fungal infections and tuberculosis may arise. In addition, *Strongiloydes stercoralis* hyperinfection is a concern. Ivermectin 200 μg/kg/d for 2 days, repeated after 2 weeks, can be used in prevention.[156] After an equivalence conversion calculation, prednisone may be replaced by other steroids, including its metabolite prednisolone, dexamethasone, or deflazacort. Calcium intake of 1200 to 1500 mg/d and vitamin D supplements are recommended for any patient using glucocorticoids, independent of dose and duration of therapy.[157]

ENL may be treated with 100 to 400 mg/d of thalidomide. As thalidomide is a teratogenic drug, it is mandatory to test for pregnancy and prescribe 2 contraceptive methods before starting therapy in women of childbearing age. Usually, ENL appears with nerve damage, and concomitant treatment with steroids is required. Higher doses of prednisone, up to 2 mg/kg/d, are linked to improved nerve function outcome, but if therapy is initiated immediately after the first signs of reaction, lower doses of 1 mg/kg/d may have the same effect.[158] If ENL is associated with any other tissue inflammation, like orchitis or iritis, or with reactions of the hands and feet, as with osteoarthritis and soft tissue inflammation, steroids are also necessary. In cases where the use of thalidomide must be avoided, pentoxifylline 400 mg, 3 times a day, is an alternative drug, quite useful for controlling limb edema and systemic symptoms.[159]

Steroids and thalidomide may help patients with neuropathic pain by reducing edema and immunologic reactions targeting the nerve, especially in acute episodes. However, its treatment continues to be a challenge, especially for those with chronic neuritis/neuropathy. Central nerve system drugs, such as the tricyclic antidepressants amitriptyline and imipramine or the anticonvulsants carbamazepine and gabapentin have been used in an attempt to control chronic neuritis/neuropathy in those patients, but these drugs do not interfere with the nerve damage process, and therefore do not protect leprosy patients from nerve deterioration. Although some anecdotal reports show that immunosuppressive agents, like cyclosporine and azathioprine, may be useful for treating chronic neuritis/neuropathy patients, a recent trial with azathioprine did not show improvement in patients with reversal reaction.[160] More research is necessary in physiopathology and with new drugs for treating neuropathic pain.

PROCEDURES

Simple preventive techniques may be used by patients to prevent the progression of damage. Massage and hydration of the skin of hands and feet are necessary to avoid fissures, ulcers, and fixed claw formation. In addition to the use of special boot soles or customized shoes for feet with loss of sensation and with disabilities, self-examination is mandatory for early detection and immediate treatment of trauma. For hands, adduction, abduction, and opposition movements are necessary to keep trophic muscles and healthy joints. Adaptation of working instruments and household

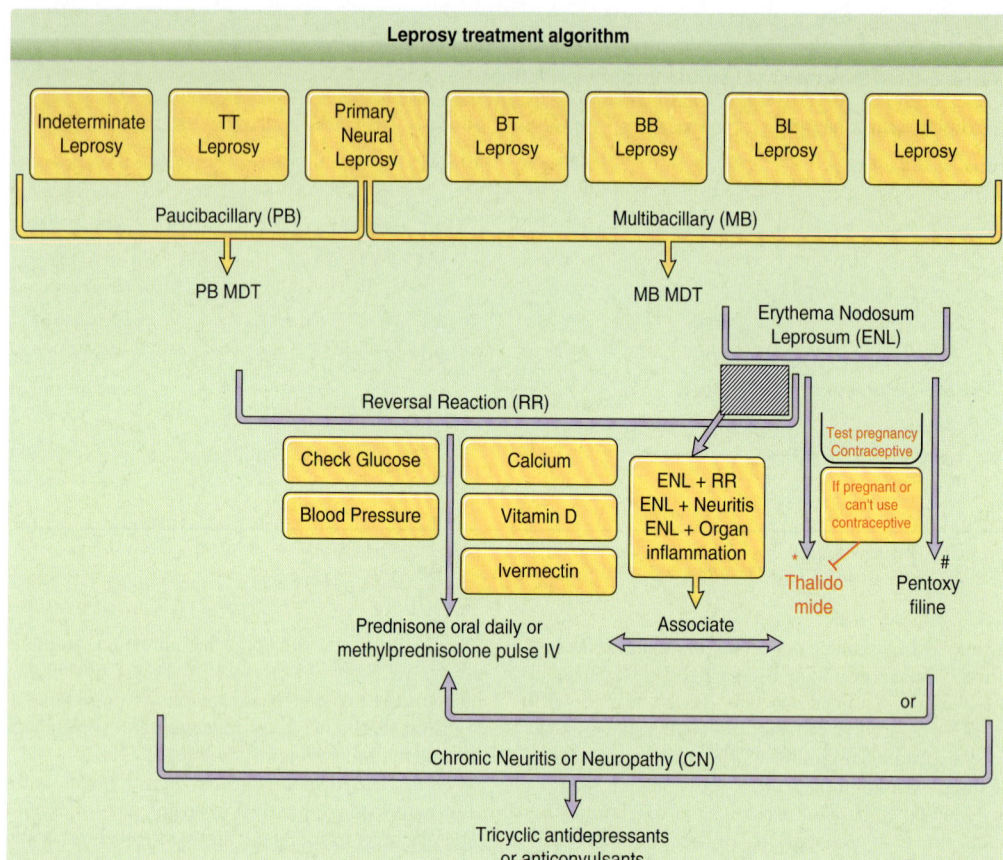

Figure 159-38 Leprosy treatment. Multidrug therapy is the choice for leprosy treatment. However, when there is intolerance to any of the drugs, available alternatives may be used, as ofloxacin, minocycline, or clarithromycin. Also, if there is no answer to multidrug therapy, drug resistance may be tested, and the same alternative drugs used in place of 1 or more multidrug therapy drugs. For reactions, thalidomide is not available in all countries, and may even be prohibited. *It is not permitted to prescribe thalidomide to pregnant women or to women of childbearing age. If it is necessary to use it, some countries have strict rules or laws that may require a pregnancy test and the use of contraceptives to prescribe thalidomide. #Pentoxyfiline is a "category C" drug for pregnancy and, therefore, it should be used only if the potential benefits justify the potential risk to the fetus.

items help to prevent trauma and burns. For eyes, the use of lubricating eye drops may prevent keratitis in cases of lagophthalmos. In more complex cases, the patients may be referred to specialized centers for more complex treatments with a multiprofessional team for physical, psychological, and social rehabilitation.

In different stages of leprosy, surgery may be necessary. Nerve abscess is infrequent, appearing more in primary neural leprosy and tuberculoid leprosy and less toward the lepromatous leprosy pole, but it may be the first clinical manifestation[161] of disease. In such cases, abscess drainage is mandatory, and the content must be sent to the laboratory for investigation. Nerve decompression may be used to improve leprosy neuropathy and muscular function, albeit there are no reliable clinical trials to definitely prove its usefulness.[162] Finally, reconstructive surgery may recover some functional aspects in the hands and feet, such as the ability to hold a glass or the capacity to raise the feet; correct eye problems, like lagophthalmos, preventing keratitis, infection, and blindness; and improve aesthetics as in the surgical correction of nose collapse, which is nowadays rare,[163] or the interosseous and first web space atrophy of the hands.[164]

COUNSELING

Counseling is a key process involved in leprosy patient management. Nerve damage and its management include counseling and harm reduction.[165] Although there was improvement in the last decades by the presence of active social movements fighting against discrimination, helping to reintegrate people into society, and banning discriminatory laws, stigma is still present in modern society. Although curable, leprosy is still a disease resulting in serious disabilities, and even patients diagnosed at the first stages of disease fear evolution through incapacities. Therefore, counseling should be available for every person diagnosed with leprosy, and their families.[166] Self-care groups are necessary, but they should not be exclusive. Leprosy-related disability care and management must be included with care for disabilities caused by other diseases in the general health services.[167]

TREATMENT ALGORITHM

See Fig. 159-38.

PREVENTION/SCREENING

There is one fundament requirement for leprosy prevention, that being contact examination. It should be a mandatory part of any leprosy program in endemic countries to examine all household contacts, and some programs expand this concept to social contacts, those who work or have closer proximity with the index case. A household contact has a 5- to 8-fold higher risk of contracting leprosy than a person without contact with a case (Fig. 159-39). However, even if there is constant vigilance, only up to 30% of the cases in a community will be detected among the household contacts; therefore, other genetic or environmental factors may be involved in the maintenance of the infection.[168]

Early detection of cases is another tool for the efficient prevention of leprosy. Besides contact examination, leprosy campaigns in the general population or in special communities, such as schoolchildren,[110] may be used to raise awareness, to diminish stigma, and to increase detection of early cases of leprosy. Although chemoprophylaxis with rifampicin has shown some degree of protection (57%) in the first 2 years, after 4 years no difference was observed in comparison between rifampicin and placebo groups[169]; therefore there is no current official recommendation to use chemoprophylaxis in leprosy contacts. For immunoprophylaxis, Brazil has been using Bacillus Calmette-Guerin (BCG) revaccination in contacts for a long time. An 18-year followup study found 56% protection for BCG-vaccinated contacts,[170] compared those who were not vaccinated; hence, Brazil guidelines for leprosy continue to include BCG vaccination for all household contacts.

REFERENCES

1. WHO | Diagnosis of leprosy. In: WHO [Internet]. World Health Organization; 2016. http://www.who.int/lep/diagnosis/en/. Accessed January 7, 2017.
2. Belcastro MG, Mariotti V, Facchini F, et al. Leprosy in a skeleton from the 7th century necropolis of Vicenne-Campochiaro (Molise, Italy). *Int J Osteoarchaeol.* 2005;15(6):431-448.
3. Robbins G, Mushrif Tripathy V, et al. Ancient skeletal evidence for leprosy in India (2000 B.C.). *PLoS One.* 2009;4(5):e5669.
4. Rafi A, Spigelman M, Stanford J, et al. DNA of *Mycobacterium leprae* detected by PCR in ancient bone. *Int J Osteoarchaeol.* 1994;4:287-290.
5. Matheson CD, Vernon KK, Lahti A, et al. Molecular exploration of the first-century tomb of the shroud in Akeldama, Jerusalem. *PLoS One.* 2009;4.
6. Donoghue HD, Michael Taylor G, Marcsik A, et al. A migration-driven model for the historical spread of leprosy in medieval Eastern and Central Europe. *Infect Genet Evol.* 2015;31:250-256.
7. Schuenemann VJ, Singh P, Mendum TA, et al. Genome-wide comparison of medieval and modern *Mycobacterium leprae. Science.* 2013;341(6142):179-183.
8. Donoghue HD, Marcsik A, Matheson C, et al. Co-infection of *Mycobacterium tuberculosis* and *Mycobacterium leprae* in human archaeological samples: a possible explanation for the historical decline of leprosy. *Proc Biol Sci.* 2005;272(1561):389-394.
9. Monot M, Honoré N, Garnier T, et al. On the origin of leprosy. *Science.* 2005;308(5724):1040-1042.
10. Monot M, Honore N, Garnier T, et al. Comparative genomic and phylogeographic analysis of *Mycobacterium leprae. Nat Genet.* 2009;41(12):1282-1289.
11. Truman RW, Singh P, Sharma R, et al. Probable zoonotic leprosy in the Southern United States. *N Engl J Med.* 2011;364(17):1626-1633.
12. Avanzi C, Del-Pozo J, Benjak A, et al. Red squirrels in the British Isles are infected with leprosy bacilli. *Science.* 2016;354:744-747.
13. Global leprosy update, 2015: time for action, accountability and inclusion. Relev épidémiologique Hebd / Sect d'hygiène du Secrétariat la Société des Nations = Wkly Epidemiol Rec / Heal Sect Secr Leag Nations. 2015;91:405-420.
14. Kumar A, Husain S, Kumar A, et al. The burden of new leprosy cases in india: a population-based survey in two states. *ISRN Trop Med.* 2013;2013:1-8.
15. Salgado CG, Barreto JG, da Silva MB, et al. What do we actually know about leprosy worldwide? *Lancet Infect Dis.* 2016;16(7):778.
16. Muthuvel T, Isaakidis P, Shewade HD, et al. Leprosy trends at a tertiary care hospital in Mumbai, India, from 2008 to 2015. *Glob Health Action.* 2016;9:32962.
17. Dogra S, Narang T, Khullar G, et al. Childhood lep-

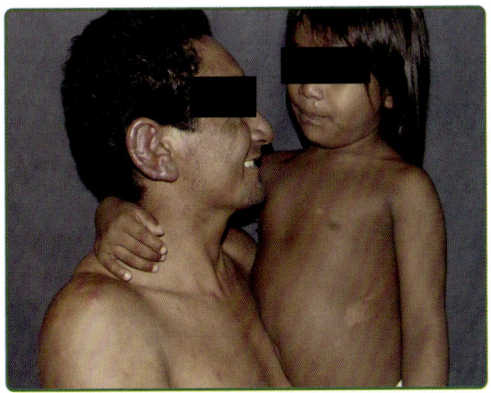

Figure 159-39 Contact examination is mandatory on leprosy programs. Note the macular hypochromic anesthetic lesion on a child that the father was diagnosed with lepromatous leprosy.

rosy through the post-leprosy-elimination era: a retrospective analysis of epidemiological and clinical characteristics of disease over eleven years from a tertiary care hospital in North India. *Lepr Rev.* 2014;85(4):296-310.
18. Kuruwa S, Joshua V, Shetty V, et al. Trends and spatial clustering of leprosy cases over a decade in a hyperendemic area of western Maharashtra, India. *Lepr Rev.* 2016;87:294-304.
19. Monteiro LD, Martins-Melo FR, Brito AL, et al. Physical disabilities at diagnosis of leprosy in a hyperendemic area of Brazil: trends and associated factors. *Lepr Rev.* 2015;86(3):240-250.
20. Shumet T, Demissie M, Bekele Y. Prevalence of disability and associated factors among registered leprosy patients in All Africa TB and Leprosy Rehabilitation and Training Centre (ALERT), Addis Ababa, Ethiopia. *Ethiop J Health Sci.* 2015;25(4):313-320.
21. Henry M, GalAn N, Teasdale K, et al. Factors contributing to the delay in diagnosis and continued transmission of leprosy in Brazil—an explorative, quantitative, questionnaire based study. *PLoS Negl Trop Dis.* 2016;10(3):e0004542.
22. Kumar A, Girdhar BK. Is increasing MB ratio a positive indicator of declining leprosy? *J Commun Dis.* 2006;38(1):24-31.
23. Salgado CG, Barreto JG, da Silva MB, et al. Are leprosy case numbers reliable? *Lancet Infect Dis.* 2018;18(2):135-137.
24. Smith WC, van Brakel W, Gillis T, et al. The missing millions: a threat to the elimination of leprosy. *PLoS Negl Trop Dis.* 2015;9(4):e0003658.
25. Bennett BH, Parker DL, Robson M. Leprosy: steps along the journey of eradication. *Public Health Rep.* 2008;123(2):198-205.
26. Ridley DS, Jopling WH. Classification of leprosy according to immunity. *Int J Lepr.* 1966;31:21.
27. Garbino JA, Marques W, Barreto JA, et al. Primary neural leprosy: systematic review. *Arq Neuropsiquiatr.* 2013;71(6):397-404.
28. Fakhouri R, Sotto MN, Manini MI, et al. Nodular leprosy of childhood and tuberculoid leprosy: a comparative, morphologic, immunopathologic and quantitative study of skin tissue reaction. *Int J Lepr Other Mycobact Dis.* 2003;71(3):218-226.
29. Salgado CG, Barreto JG. Images in clinical medicine. Leonine facies: lepromatous leprosy. *N Engl J Med.* 2012;366(15):1433.
30. Kaur I, Dogra S, De D, et al. Histoid leprosy: a retrospective study of 40 cases from India. *Br J Dermatol.* 2009;160(2):305-310.
31. Lucio R, Escuela de M de M, Alvarado I. Opúsculo sobre El Mal de San Làzaro, ó Elefanciasis de Los Griegos. Mexico; 1852.
32. Han XY, Seo YH, Sizer KC, et al. A new *Mycobacterium* species causing diffuse lepromatous leprosy. *Am J Clin Pathol.* 2008;130(6):856-864.
33. Singh P, Benjak A, Schuenemann VJ, et al. Insight into the evolution and origin of leprosy bacilli from the genome sequence of Mycobacterium lepromatosis. *Proc Natl Acad Sci U S A.* 2015;112(14):4459-4464.
34. Illigens BMW, Gibbons CH. Sweat testing to evaluate autonomic function. *Clin Auton Res.* 2009;19(2):79-87.
35. Lehman LF, Orsini MB, Nicholl AR. The development and adaptation of the Semmes-Weinstein monofilaments in Brazil. *J Hand Ther.* 1993;6(4):290-297.
36. Villarroel MF, Orsini MBP, Lima RC, et al. Comparative study of the cutaneous sensation of leprosy-suspected lesions using Semmes-Weinstein monofilaments and quantitative thermal testing. *Lepr Rev.* 2007;78(2):102-109.
37. Kumar B. Pure or Primary neuritic Leprosy (PNL). *Lepr Rev.* 2016;87:450-455.
38. Suneetha S, Sigamoni A, Kurian N, et al. The development of cutaneous lesions during follow-up of patients with primary neuritic leprosy. *Int J Dermatol.* 2005;44(3):224-229.
39. Jardim MR, Antunes SL, Santos AR, et al. Criteria for diagnosis of pure neural leprosy. *J Neurol.* 2003;250:806-809.
40. Kumar KVS, Singh R, Bhasin R, et al. Endocrine dysfunction in patients of leprosy. *Indian J Endocrinol Metab.* 2015;19:369.
41. Leal ÂM, Foss NT. Endocrine dysfunction in leprosy. *Eur J Clin Microbiol Infect Dis.* 2009;28(1):1-7.
42. Leal ÂMO, Magalhães PKR, Souza CS, et al. Pituitary-gonadal hormones and interleukin patterns in leprosy. *Trop Med Int Health.* 2006;11(9):1416-1421.
43. Richardus J, Dik J, Habbema F, et al. The impact of leprosy control on the transmission of *M. leprae*: is elimination being attained? *Lepr Rev.* 2007;78(4):330-337.
44. Andersen JG, Manchester K. The rhinomaxillary syndrome in leprosy: a clinical, radiological and palaeopathological study. *Int J Osteoarchaeol.* 1992;2(2):121-129.
45. Boulton AJM. Diabetic foot—what can we learn from leprosy? Legacy of Dr Paul W. Brand. In *Diabetes/Metabolism Research and Reviews.* Chichester: Wiley; 2012:3-7.
46. Van Brakel WH, Anderson AM. Impairment and disability in leprosy: in search of the missing link. *Indian J Lepr.* 1997;69(4):361-376.
47. Singh P, Cole ST. *Mycobacterium leprae*: genes, pseudogenes and genetic diversity. *Future Microbiol.* 2011;6:57-71.
48. Ng V, Zanazzi G, Timpl R, et al. Role of the cell wall phenolic glycolipid-1 in the peripheral nerve predilection of *Mycobacterium leprae*. *Cell.* 2000;103(3):511-524.
49. Araujo S, Freitas LO, Goulart LR, et al. Molecular evidence for the aerial route of infection of *Mycobacterium leprae* and the role of asymptomatic carriers in the persistence of leprosy. *Clin Infect Dis.* 2016;63(11):1412-1420.
50. Alter A, Grant A, Abel L, et al. Leprosy as a genetic disease. *Mamm Genome.* 2011;22(1-2):19-31.
51. Mohamed Ali P, Ramanujam K. Leprosy in twins. *Int J Lepr.* 1966;34(4):405-407.
52. Chakravartti MR, Vogel F. A twin study on leprosy [Internet]. Thieme; 1973. https://books.google.com.br/books/about/A_twin_study_on_leprosy.html?id=aXhrAAAAMAAJ&redir_esc=y.
53. Zhang FR, Huang W, Chen SM, et al. Genome-wide association study of leprosy. *N Engl J Med.* 2009;361(27):2609-2618.
54. Moet FJ, Pahan D, Schuring RP, et al. Physical distance, genetic relationship, age, and leprosy classification are independent risk factors for leprosy in contacts of patients with leprosy. *J Infect Dis.* 2006;193(3):346-353.
55. Barreto JG, Bisanzio D, Frade MAC, et al. Spatial epidemiology and serologic cohorts increase the early detection of leprosy. *BMC Infect Dis.* 2015;15:527.
56. Job CK. Nerve damage in leprosy. *Int J Lepr.* 1988;57:532-539.
57. Scollard DM. Association of *Mycobacterium leprae* with human endothelial cells in vitro. *Lab Invest.* 2000;80:663-669.

58. Scollard DM, McCormick G, Allen JL. Localization of *Mycobacterium leprae* to endothelial cells of epineurial and perineurial blood vessels and lymphatics. *Am J Pathol*. 1999;154(5):1611-1620.
59. Shimoji Y, Ng V, Matsumura K, et al. A 21-kDa surface protein of *Mycobacterium leprae* binds peripheral nerve laminin-2 and mediates Schwann cell invasion. *Proc Natl Acad Sci U S A*. 1999;96(17):9857-9862.
60. Rambukkana A, Yamada H, Zanazzi G, et al. Role of alpha-dystroglycan as a Schwann cell receptor for *Mycobacterium leprae*. *Science*. 1998;282(5396):2076-2079.
61. Tapinos N, Ohnishi M, Rambukkana A. ErbB2 receptor tyrosine kinase signaling mediates early demyelination induced by leprosy bacilli. *Nat Med*. 2006;12(8):961-966.
62. Tapinos N, Rambukkana A. Insights into regulation of human Schwann cell proliferation by Erk1/2 via a MEK-independent and p56Lck-dependent pathway from leprosy bacilli. *Proc Natl Acad Sci U S A*. 2005;102(26):9188-9193.
63. Ribeiro-Resende VT, Ribeiro-Guimarães ML, Rodrigues Lemes RM, et al. Involvement of 9-*O*-acetyl GD3 ganglioside in *Mycobacterium leprae* infection of Schwann cells. *J Biol Chem*. 2010;285(44):34086-34096.
64. Masaki T, Qu J, Cholewa-Waclaw J, et al. Reprogramming adult Schwann cells to stem cell-like cells by leprosy bacilli promotes dissemination of infection. *Cell*. 2013;152(1-2):51-67.
65. Alves L, De Mendonça Lima L, Da Silva Maeda E, et al. *Mycobacterium leprae* infection of human Schwann cells depends on selective host kinases and pathogen-modulated endocytic pathways. *FEMS Microbiol Lett*. 2004;238(2):429-437.
66. Mattos KA, Lara FA, Oliveira VG, et al. Modulation of lipid droplets by *Mycobacterium leprae* in Schwann cells: a putative mechanism for host lipid acquisition and bacterial survival in phagosomes. *Cell Microbiol*. 2011;13(2):259-273.
67. Medeiros RC, De Vasconcelos Girardi KD, Cardoso FK, et al. Subversion of Schwann cell glucose metabolism by *Mycobacterium leprae*. *J Biol Chem*. 2016;291(41):21375-21387.
68. Barreto JG, Guimarães L de S, Frade MAC, et al. High rates of undiagnosed leprosy and subclinical infection amongst school children in the Amazon Region. *Memórias do Inst Oswaldo Cruz*. 2012;107(suppl):60-67.
69. Rambukkana A, Zanazzi G, Tapinos N, et al. Contact-dependent demyelination by *Mycobacterium leprae* in the absence of immune cells. *Science*. 2002;296(5569):927-931.
70. Sieling PA, Modlin RL. Cytokine patterns at the site of mycobacterial infection. *Immunobiology*. 1994;191(4-5):378-387.
71. VanVoorhis W, Kaplan G, Sarno E, et al. The cutaneous infiltrates of leprosy: cellular characteristics and the predominant T-cell phenotypes. *N Engl J Med*. 1982;307(26):1593-1597.
72. Krutzik SR, Ochoa MT, Sieling PA, et al. Activation and regulation of Toll-like receptors 2 and 1 in human leprosy. *Nat Med*. 2003;9(5):525-532.
73. Polycarpou A, Holland MJ, Karageorgiou I, et al. *Mycobacterium leprae* activates Toll-like receptor-4 signaling and expression on macrophages depending on previous Bacillus Calmette-Guerin vaccination. *Front Cell Infect Microbiol*. 2016;6:72.
74. Oliveira RB, Ochoa MT, Sieling PA, et al. Expression of Toll-like receptor 2 on human Schwann cells: a mechanism of nerve damage in leprosy. *Infect Immun*. 2003;71(3):1427-1433.
75. Gringhuis SI, den Dunnen J, Litjens M, et al. C-type lectin DC-SIGN modulates Toll-like receptor signaling via Raf-1 kinase-dependent acetylation of transcription factor NF-??B. *Immunity*. 2007;26(5):605-616.
76. Montoya D, Cruz D, Teles RMB, et al. Divergence of macrophage phagocytic and antimicrobial programs in leprosy. *Cell Host Microbe*. 2009;6(4):343-353.
77. Moura DF, de Mattos KA, Amadeu TP, et al. CD163 favors *Mycobacterium leprae* survival and persistence by promoting anti-inflammatory pathways in lepromatous macrophages. *Eur J Immunol*. 2012;42(11):2925-2936.
78. Pereira RMS, Calegari-Silva TC, Hernandez MO, et al. *Mycobacterium leprae* induces NF-κB-dependent transcription repression in human Schwann cells. *Biochem Biophys Res Commun*. 2005;335(1):20-26.
79. Teles RMB, Antunes SLG, Jardim MR, et al. Expression of metalloproteinases (MMP-2, MMP-9, and TACE) and TNF-α in the nerves of leprosy patients. *J Peripher Nerv Syst*. 2007;12(3):195-204.
80. Antunes SLG, Chimelli L, Jardim MR, et al. Histopathological examination of nerve samples from pure neural leprosy patients: obtaining maximum information to improve diagnostic efficiency. *Mem Inst Oswaldo Cruz*. 2012;107(2):246-253.
81. Martinuzzo ME, de Larranaga GF, Forastiero RR, et al. Markers of platelet, endothelial cell and blood coagulation activation in leprosy patients with antiphospholipid antibodies. *Clin Exp Rheumatol*. 2002;20(4):477-483.
82. Nogueira MR, Latini AC, Nogueira ME. The involvement of endothelial mediators in leprosy. *Mem Inst Oswaldo Cruz*. 2016;111(10):635-641.
83. Da Motta-Passos I, Malheiro A, Gomes Naveca F, et al. Decreased RNA expression of interleukin 17A in skin of leprosy. *Eur J Dermatol*. 2012;22(4):488-494.
84. Sadhu S, Khaitan BK, Joshi B, et al. Reciprocity between regulatory T cells and Th17 cells: relevance to polarized immunity in leprosy. *PLoS Negl Trop Dis*. 2016;10(1):e0004338.
85. Matzner M, Al Samie AR, Winkler HM, et al. Low serum levels of cathelicidin LL-37 in leprosy. *Acta Trop*. 2011;117(1):56-59.
86. Batista-Silva LR, Rodrigues LS, Vivarini Ade C, et al. *Mycobacterium leprae*-induced insulin-like growth factor I attenuates antimicrobial mechanisms, promoting bacterial survival in macrophages. *Sci Rep*. 2016;6:27632.
87. Rodrigues LS, Hacker MA, Illarramendi X, et al. Circulating levels of insulin-like growth factor-I (IGF-I) correlate with disease status in leprosy. *BMC Infect Dis*. 2011;11:339.
88. Wemambu SN, Turk JL, Waters MF, et al. Erythema nodosum leprosum: a clinical manifestation of the arthus phenomenon. *Lancet*. 1969;2(7627):933-935.
89. Rojas RE, Demichelis SO, Sarno EN, et al. IgM antiphenolic glycolipid I and IgG anti-10-kDa heat shock protein antibodies in sera and immune complexes isolated from leprosy patients with or without erythema nodosum leprosum and contacts. *FEMS Immunol Med Microbiol*. 1997;19(1):65-74.
90. Polycarpou A, Walker SL, Lockwood DNJ. A systematic review of immunological studies of erythema nodosum leprosum. *Front Immunol*. 2017;8:233.

91. Sampaio EP, Moreira AL, Sarno EN, et al. Prolonged treatment with recombinant interferon gamma induces erythema nodosum leprosum in lepromatous leprosy patients. *J Exp Med*. 1992;175(6):1729-1737.
92. Sarno EN, Grau GE, Vieira LM, et al. Serum levels of tumour necrosis factor-alpha and interleukin-1 beta during leprosy reactional states. *Clin Exp Immunol*. 1991;84(1):103-108.
93. Dias AA, Silva CO, Santos JP, et al. DNA sensing via TLR-9 constitutes a major innate immunity pathway activated during erythema nodosum leprosum. *J Immunol*. 2016;197(5):1905-1913.
94. Lee DJ, Li H, Ochoa MT, et al. Integrated pathways for neutrophil recruitment and inflammation in leprosy. *J Infect Dis*. 2010;201(4):558-569.
95. Schmitz V, Prata RB, Barbosa MG, et al. Expression of CD64 on circulating neutrophils favoring systemic inflammatory status in erythema nodosum leprosum. *PLoS Negl Trop Dis*. 2016;10(8):e0004955.
96. Yamamura M, Wang XH, Ohmen JD, et al. Cytokine patterns of immunologically mediated tissue damage. *J Immunol*. 1992;149(4):1470-1475.
97. Kirkaldy AA, Musonda AC, Khanolkhar-Young S, et al. Expression of CC and CXC chemokines and chemokine receptors in human leprosy skin lesions. *Clin Exp Immunol*. 2003;134(3):447-453.
98. Geluk A, Van Meijgaarden KE, Wilson L, et al. Longitudinal immune responses and gene expression profiles in type 1 leprosy reactions. *J Clin Immunol*. 2014;34(2):245-255.
99. Henry M, GalAn N, Teasdale K, et al. Factors contributing to the delay in diagnosis and continued transmission of leprosy in Brazil—an explorative, quantitative, questionnaire based study. *PLoS Negl Trop Dis*. 2016;10(3):1-12.
100. Scollard DM, Adams LB, Gillis TP, et al. The continuing challenges of leprosy. *Clin Microbiol Rev*. 2006;19(2):338-381.
101. Cho SN, Fujiwara T, Hunter SW, et al. Use of an artificial antigen containing the 3,6-di-O-methyl-beta-D-glucopyranosyl epitope for the serodiagnosis of leprosy. *J Infect Dis*. 1984;150(3):311-322.
102. Spencer JS, Brennan PJ. The role of *Mycobacterium leprae* phenolic glycolipid I (PGL-I) in serodiagnosis and in the pathogenesis of leprosy. *Lepr Rev*. 2011;82(4):344-357.
103. Duthie MS, Hay MN, Morales CZ, et al. Rational design and evaluation of a multiepitope chimeric fusion protein with the potential for leprosy diagnosis. *Clin vaccine Immunol*. 2010;17(2):298-305.
104. Duthie MS, Raychaudhuri R, Tutterrow YL, et al. A rapid ELISA for the diagnosis of MB leprosy based on complementary detection of antibodies against a novel protein-glycolipid conjugate. *Diagn Microbiol Infect Dis*. 2014;79:233-239.
105. Corstjens PL, de Dood CJ, van der Ploeg-van Schip JJ, et al. Lateral flow assay for simultaneous detection of cellular- and humoral immune responses. *Clin Biochem*. 2011;44(14-15):1241-1246.
106. Bobosha K, Tjon Kon Fat EM, van den Eeden SJF, et al. Field-evaluation of a new lateral flow assay for detection of cellular and humoral immunity against *Mycobacterium leprae*. *PLoS Negl Trop Dis*. 2014 8;8(5):e2845.
107. Al-Mubarak R, Vander Heiden J, Broeckling CD, et al. Serum metabolomics reveals higher levels of polyunsaturated fatty acids in lepromatous leprosy: potential markers for susceptibility and pathogenesis. *PLoS Negl Trop Dis*. 2011;5(9):e1303.
108. Lima EDO, De Macedo CS, Esteves CZ, et al. Skin imprinting in silica plates: a potential diagnostic methodology for leprosy using high-resolution mass spectrometry. *Anal Chem*. 2015;87(7):3585-3592.
109. Salgado CG, Pinto P, Bouth RC, et al. miRNome expression analysis reveals new players on leprosy immune physiopathology. *Front Immunol*. 2018;9:463.
110. Barreto JG, Bisanzio D, Guimarães Lde S, et al. Spatial analysis spotlighting early childhood leprosy transmission in a hyperendemic municipality of the Brazilian Amazon region. *PLoS Negl Trop Dis*. 2014;8(2):e2665.
111. Barreto JG, Bisanzio D, Frade MAC, et al. Spatial epidemiology and serologic cohorts increase the early detection of leprosy. *BMC Infect Dis*. 2015;15:527.
112. Reddy RR, Singh G, Sacchidanand S, et al. A comparative evaluation of skin and nerve histopathology in single skin lesion leprosy. *Indian J Dermatol Venereol Leprol*. 2005;71(6):401-405.
113. Weng XM, Chen SY, Ran SP, et al. Immuno-histopathology in the diagnosis of early leprosy. *Int J Lepr Other Mycobact Dis*. 2000;68(4):426-433.
114. Massone C, Belachew WA, Schettini A. Histopathology of the lepromatous skin biopsy. *Clin Dermatol*. 2015;33(1):38-45.
115. Wade HW. The histoid variety of lepromatous leprosy. *Int J Lepr*. 1963;31:129-142.
116. Lockwood DNJ, Lucas SB, Desikan KV, et al. The histological diagnosis of leprosy type 1 reactions: identification of key variables and an analysis of the process of histological diagnosis. *J Clin Pathol*. 2008;61(5):595-600.
117. Kahawita IP, Walker SL, Lockwood DNJ. Leprosy type 1 reactions and erythema nodosum leprosum. *An Bras Dermatol*. 2008;83(1):75-82.
118. Walker SL, Saunderson P, Kahawita IP, et al. International workshop on erythema nodosum leprosum (ENL)—consensus report; the formation of ENLIST, the ENL international study group. *Lepr Rev*. 2012;83(4):396-407.
119. Rea TH, Jerskey RS. Clinical and histologic variations among thirty patients with Lucio's phenomenon and pure and primitive diffuse lepromatosis (Latapi's lepromatosis). *Int J Lepr Other Mycobact Dis*. 2005;73(3):169-188.
120. Sehgal VN. Lucio's phenomenon/erythema necroticans. *Int J Dermatol*. 2005;44(7):602-605.
121. Vargas-Ocampo F. Diffuse leprosy of Lucio and Latapí: a histologic study. *Lepr Rev*. 2007;78(3):248-260.
122. Monteiro R, Abreu MAMM de, Tiezzi MG, et al. Lucio's phenomenon: another case reported in Brazil. *An Bras Dermatol*. 2012;87(2):296-300.
123. Garbino JA, Heise CO, Marques W. Assessing nerves in leprosy. *Clin Dermatol*. 2016;34(1):51-58.
124. Goedee HS, Brekelmans GJF, van Asseldonk JTH, et al. High resolution sonography in the evaluation of the peripheral nervous system in polyneuropathy—a review of the literature. *Eur J Neurol*. 2013;20(10):1342-1351.
125. Lugão HB, Frade MAC, Marques W Jr, et al. Ultrasonography of leprosy neuropathy: a longitudinal prospective study. *PLoS Negl Trop Dis*. 2016;10(11):e0005111.
126. van Brakel WH, Nicholls PG, Das L, et al. The INFIR Cohort Study: investigating prediction, detection and pathogenesis of neuropathy and reactions in leprosy. Methods and baseline results of a cohort of

multibacillary leprosy patients in north India. *Lepr Rev.* 2005;76(1):14-34.
127. Kumar B, Dogra S, Kaur I. Epidemiological characteristics of leprosy reactions: 15 years experience from North India. *Int J Lepr Other Mycobact Dis.* 2004;72(2):125-133.
128. Nery JAC, Vieira LMM, De Matos HJ, et al. Reactional states in multibacillary Hansen disease patients during multidrug therapy. *Rev Inst Med Trop Sao Paulo.* 1998;40(6):363-370.
129. Walker SL, Balagon M, Darlong J, et al. ENLIST 1: an international multi-centre cross-sectional study of the clinical features of erythema nodosum leprosum. *PLoS Negl Trop Dis.* 2015;9(9):e0004065.
130. Pocaterra L, Jain S, Reddy R, et al. Clinical course of erythema nodosum leprosum: an 11-year cohort study in Hyderabad, India. *Am J Trop Med Hyg.* 2006;74:868-879.
131. Saunderson P, Gebre S, Byass P. ENL reactions in the multibacillary cases of the AMFES cohort in central Ethiopia: incidence and risk factors. *Lepr Rev.* 2000;71(3):318-324.
132. Lawn SD, Wood C, Lockwood DN. Borderline tuberculoid leprosy: an immune reconstitution phenomenon in a human immunodeficiency virus-infected person. *Clin Infect Dis.* 2003;36(1):e5-e6.
133. Talhari C, Mira MT, Massone C, et al. Leprosy and HIV coinfection: a clinical, pathological, immunological, and therapeutic study of a cohort from a Brazilian referral center for infectious diseases. *J Infect Dis.* 2010;202(3):345-354.
134. Machado PR, Machado LM, Shibuya M, et al. Viral coinfection and leprosy outcomes: a cohort study. *PLoS Negl Trop Dis.* 2015;9(8):e0003865.
135. Lechat MF, Shrager DI, Declercq E, et al. Decreased survival of HTLV-I carriers in leprosy patients from the Democratic Republic of the Congo: a historical prospective study. *J Acquir Immune Defic Syndr Hum Retrovirol.* 1997;15(5):387-390.
136. Scollard DM, Joyce MP, Gillis TP. Development of leprosy and type 1 leprosy reactions after treatment with infliximab: a report of 2 cases. *Clin Infect Dis.* 2006;43:e19-e22.
137. Freitas DS, Machado N, Andrigueti FV, et al. Lepromatous leprosy associated with the use of anti-TNFα therapy: case report. *Rev Bras Reumatol.* 2010;50(3):336-339.
138. Antônio JR, Soubhia RMC, Paschoal VDA, et al. Biological agents: investigation into leprosy and other infectious diseases before indication. *An Bras Dermatol.* 2013;88:23-25.
139. Pannikar V, Jesudasan K, Vijayakumaran P, et al. Relapse or late reversal reaction? *Int J Lepr Other Mycobact Dis.* 1989;57(2):526-528.
140. Stump PR, Baccarelli R, Marciano LH, et al. Neuropathic pain in leprosy patients. *Int J Lepr Other Mycobact Dis.* 2004;72(2):134-138.
141. Sena CBC De, Salgado CG, Tavares CMP, et al. Cyclosporine A treatment of leprosy patients with chronic neuritis is associated with pain control and reduction in antibodies against nerve growth factor. *Lepr Rev.* 2006;77(2):121-129.
142. Faget GH, Pogge RC, Johansen FA, et al. The promin treatment of leprosy. A progress report. *Public Health Rep.* 1943;58(48):1729.
143. Peters AL, Van Noorden CJF. Glucose-6-phosphate dehydrogenase deficiency and malaria: cytochemical detection of heterozygous G6PD deficiency in women. *J Histochem Cytochem.* 2009;57(11):1003-1011.
144. WHO. *WHO Model Prescribing Information: Drugs Used in Leprosy [Internet]*. Geneva: WHO; 1998. http://apps.who.int/medicinedocs/en/d/Jh2988e/.
145. Kosseifi SG, Guha B, Nassour DN, et al. The dapsone hypersensitivity syndrome revisited: a potentially fatal multisystem disorder with prominent hepatopulmonary manifestations. *J Occup Med Toxicol.* 2006;1:9.
146. Abinader MVM, Da Gracnulla Souza Cunha M, Cunha C. Adverse effects of alternative therapy (minocycline, ofloxacin and clofazimine) in leprosy multibacillary patients, in health care center, Manaus, Amazonas, Brazil. *J Am Acad Dermatol.* 2015;72(5):AB124.
147. Brasil MT, Opromolla DV, Marzliak ML, et al. Results of a surveillance system for adverse effects in leprosy's WHO/MDT. *Int J Lepr Other Mycobact Dis.* 1996;64(2):97-104.
148. Limalde S, Opromolla DV. First results on the treatment of leprosy with rifamycin SV. *Chemotherapia (Basel).* 1963;10:668-678.
149. Pettit JH, Rees RJ. Sulphone resistance in leprosy. An experimental and clinical study. *Lancet.* 1964;2(7361):673-674.
150. Williams DL, Gillis TP. Drug-resistant leprosy: monitoring and current status. *Lepr Rev.* 2012;83(3):269-281.
151. da Silva Rocha A, Cunha MDG, Diniz LM, et al. Drug and multidrug resistance among *Mycobacterium leprae* isolates from Brazilian relapsed leprosy patients. *J Clin Microbiol.* 2012;50(6):1912-1917.
152. Williams DL, Hagino T, Sharma R, et al. Primary multidrug-resistant leprosy, United States. *Emerg Infect Dis.* 2013;19(1):179-181.
153. Beltrán-Alzate C, López Díaz F, Romero-Montoya M, et al. Leprosy drug resistance surveillance in colombia: the experience of a sentinel country. *PLoS Negl Trop Dis.* 2016;10(10):e0005041.
154. Benjak A, Avanzi C, Singh P, et al. Phylogenomics and antimicrobial resistance of the leprosy bacillus *Mycobacterium leprae*. *Nat Commun.* 2018;9(1):352.
155. Van Veen NH, Nicholls PG, Smith WC, et al. Corticosteroids for treating nerve damage in leprosy. *Cochrane Database Syst Rev.* 2016;(5):CD005491.
156. Keiser PB, Nutman TB. *Strongyloides stercoralis* in the immunocompromised population. *Clin Microbiol Rev.* 2004;17(1):208-217.
157. Buckley L, Guyatt G, Fink HA, et al. 2017 American College of Rheumatology guideline for the prevention and treatment of glucocorticoid-induced osteoporosis. *Arthritis Care Res (Hoboken).* 2017;69(8):1095-1110.
158. Garbino JA, Virmond MDCL, Ura S, et al. A randomized clinical trial of oral steroids for ulnar neuropathy in type 1 and type 2 leprosy reactions. *Arq Neuropsiquiatr.* 2008;66(4):861-867.
159. Sales AM, de Matos HJ, Nery JAC, et al. Double-blind trial of the efficacy of pentoxifylline vs thalidomide for the treatment of type II reaction in leprosy. *Brazilian J Med Biol Res.* 2007;40(2):243-248.
160. Lockwood DNJ, Darlong J, Govindharaj P, et al. AZA-LEP: a randomized controlled trial of azathioprine to treat leprosy nerve damage and Type 1 reactions in India: main findings. *PLoS Negl Trop Dis.* 2017;11(3):e0005348.
161. Omar AE, Hussein MR. Clinically unsuspected neuritic leprosy with caseation necrosis. *Ultrastruct Pathol.*

2012;36(6):377-380.
162. Wan EL, Rivadeneira AF, Jouvin RM, et al. Treatment of peripheral neuropathy in leprosy: the case for nerve decompression. *Plast Reconstr Surg Glob Open.* 2016;4(3):e637.
163. Schwarz RJ, Macdonald M. A rational approach to nasal reconstruction in leprosy. *Plast Reconstr Surg.* 2004;114(4):876-882; discussion 883-884.
164. Duerksen F, Virmond M. Carvable silicone rubber prosthetic implant for atrophy of the first web in the hand. *Lepr Rev.* 1990;61(3):267-272.
165. White C, Franco-Paredes C. Leprosy in the 21st century. *Clin Microbiol Rev.* 2015;28(1):80-94.
166. Thakor HG, Murthy PS. Counselling of leprosy affected persons and the community. *J Indian Med Assoc.* 2004;102(12):684-687.
167. Madhavan K, Vijayakumaran P, Ramachandran L, et al. Sustainable leprosy related disability care within integrated general health services: findings from Salem District, India. *Lepr Rev.* 2007;78(4):353-361.
168. Fine PE, Sterne JS, Pönnighaus JM, et al. Household and dwelling contact as risk factors for leprosy in northern Malawi. *Am J Epidemiol.* 1997;146(1):91-102.
169. Moet FJ, Pahan D, Oskam L, et al. Effectiveness of single dose rifampicin in preventing leprosy in close contacts of patients with newly diagnosed leprosy: cluster randomised controlled trial. *BMJ.* 2008;336(7647):761-764.
170. Düppre NC, Camacho LAB, da Cunha SS, et al. Effectiveness of BCG vaccination among leprosy contacts: a cohort study. *Trans R Soc Trop Med Hyg.* 2008;102(7):631-638.

Fungal Diseases PART 24

第二十四篇　真菌性疾病

Chapter 160 :: Superficial Fungal Infection
:: Lauren N. Craddock & Stefan M. Schieke

第一百六十章
浅部真菌感染

中文导读

皮肤癣菌通过附着、入侵和使用角蛋白作为营养来源，引起皮肤、头发和指甲的浅表真菌感染，统称为皮肤癣菌病。提出浅表真菌感染是一个全球性问题，影响了超过25%的人口。本章节首先将可能引起浅部真菌感染的真菌进行了简要的分类，随后根据不同的感染部位和特征，分别就甲真菌病、孢子丝菌病、颜面癣、头癣、体癣、股癣、手足癣等各种类型的真菌感染进行了详细的阐述。

〔汪　犇〕

AT-A-GLANCE

- Mycoses are divided among 3 forms: *superficial*, *subcutaneous*, and *deep/systemic*.
- Superficial fungal infection is defined as a dermatophyte infection of keratinized tissues including skin, hair, and nails.
- Dermatophyte species are contained in 3 genera (*Epidermophyton*, *Microsporum*, and *Trichophyton*), which are further divided according to 3 natural habitats (humans, animals, and soil).
- *Trichophyton* is the most common genera isolated in the United States.
- *Trichophyton rubrum* is the most common cause of dermatophytosis of the skin.
- *Trichophyton tonsurans* is the most common cause of tinea capitis in the United States.
- Piedra, which consists of white and black forms, is an asymptomatic superficial fungal infection of the hair shaft.
- Onychomycosis is the name given to dermatophytosis of the nails.
- Microscopic examination, culture, Wood light evaluation, and histopathology may all be useful in confirming diagnosis.
- Several topical and oral antifungals are available for effective treatment of dermatophytosis.
- Infections involving hair bearing skin and nails typically require oral treatment.

MYCOSES

Mycoses are divided among 3 forms: (a) *superficial*, involving stratum corneum, hair, and nails; (b) *subcutaneous*, involving dermis and/or subcutaneous tissue; and (c) *deep/systemic*, representing hematogenous spread of organisms including opportunistic pathogens in immunocompromised hosts. This chapter focuses on the superficial mycoses and their patterns of integumentary infections (Table 160-1). Table 160-2 is a glossary of terms used in this chapter.

DERMATOPHYTES

The kingdom of fungi comprises more than 1.5 million species worldwide. Dermatophytes (the term is derived from the Greek words for "skin plant") are represented by approximately 40 species divided among the 3 genera *Trichophyton*, *Microsporum*, and *Epidermophyton*, all falling within the Arthrodermataceae family. In the United States, *Trichophyton* species, namely *Trichophyton rubrum* and *Trichophyton interdigitale*, represent the most common isolated species. Dermatophytes are classified further according to their natural habitats—humans, other animals, and soil. Their ability to attach to, invade, and use keratin as a source of nutrition underlies the pathogenesis of superficial fungal infection of skin, hair, and nails, and is termed *dermatophytosis*.[1]

TAXONOMY

Recent modifications to the taxonomical system of dermatophytes affecting clinical practice require mention. While classic taxonomy is governed by what is phenotypically observable, recent inclusion of data from genotypical analysis has necessitated regrouping of some taxa, as many of these genotypical differences are not reflected phenotypically, and vice versa.[2] Contradictions between what is phenotypically observable and found via genomic analysis make devising such a taxonomical system for dermatophytes difficult. According to the classic, yet still current, rules of taxonomy governing nomenclature, a species must be identifiable in nature, with physical specimens able to be cultured and proven to be sexually isolated

TABLE 160-1
Patterns of Integumentary Infections by Superficial Mycoses

GENERA	SKIN	HAIR	NAILS
Trichophyton	x	x	x
Microsporum	x	x	
Epidermophyton	x		x
Tinea nigra	x		
Black piedra		x	
White piedra		x	

TABLE 160-2
Glossary of Terms

- *Anthropophilic*—preferring humans over other animals as the natural habitat.
- *Arthroconidia*—asexual spore produced by segmentation of hyphae.
- *Dematiaceous*—melanin in the cell walls of its conidia, hyphae, or both results in a darkly colored fungus.
- *Ectothrix*—dermatophyte growth pattern with spores forming a sheath on the outside of the hair shaft.
- *Endothrix*—dermatophyte growth pattern with spore formation within the hair shaft.
- *Favus*—dermatophyte growth pattern with hyphae and air spaces within the hair shaft.
- *Geophilic*—preferring the soil over humans and animals as natural habitat.
- *Hyphae*—long, filamentous fungus cells forming a branching network called mycelium.
- *Macroconidia*—asexual large multinucleate spores produced by vegetative reproduction.
- *Microconidia*—asexual small spores produced by vegetative reproduction.
- *Zoophilic*—preferring animals over humans as the natural habitat.

from others, before they may be formally named. Conversely, newer molecular ecologic studies using sequencing of variable genomic regions, such as the internal transcribed spacer regions, of pooled fungal ribosomal DNA have discovered (a) more internal transcribed spacer regions than there are in known/observable species, (b) multiple species may have identical internal transcribed spacer regions, and (c) there may be multiple forms of internal transcribed spacer in one species' genome.[3] Current fungal taxonomy includes a synthesis of the new genomic data and classic phenotypical characterizations.

In the case of dermatophytes, many species overall have very little genetic diversity and may live in the same environmental niche. Phenotypically, this is reflected by similar clinical manifestations being caused by multiple taxonomically different dermatophyte species. The additional classification of superficial fungi according to natural habitat is clinically relevant, as anthropophilic, zoophilic, and geophilic dermatophytoses provide important information about the source of infection and may demonstrate varied clinical features.

ANTHROPHILIC

Anthrophilic species are typically restricted to human hosts and are transmitted via direct contact. Infected skin or hair retained in clothing, combs, caps, socks, and towels, for example, also serve as source reservoirs. Unlike the sporadic geophilic and zoophilic infections, anthropophilic infections are often epidemic in nature. These dermatophytes have adapted to humans as hosts and elicit a mild to noninflammatory host response.

ZOOPHILIC

Zoophilic species are transmitted to humans from animals. Cats, dogs, rabbits, guinea pigs, birds, horses, cattle, and other animals are common sources of infection. Transmission may occur through direct contact with the animal itself, or indirectly via infected animal hair. Exposed areas, such as the scalp, beard, face, and arms, are favored sites of infection. *Microsporum canis* is often transmitted to humans from cats and dogs, whereas guinea pigs and rabbits are a frequent source of human infection with zoophilic strains of *T. interdigitale.* Although host adaptation by zoophilic dermatophytes may lead to relatively silent infections, these dermatophytes tend to produce acute and intense inflammatory responses in humans.[1]

GEOPHILIC

Geophilic fungi cause sporadic human infection upon direct contact with the soil. *Microsporum gypseum* is the most common geophilic dermatophyte cultured from humans. There is a potential for epidemic spread as a consequence of the higher virulence of geophilic strains, as well as an ability to form long-lived spores that may reside in blankets or grooming tools. As with zoophilic infections, geophilic dermatophytes typically result in intense inflammatory responses.[4]

Table 160-3 lists the most commonly encountered dermatophyte pathogens according to their natural habitats and reservoirs. As there are still texts that use the classical names, to avoid confusion and to remain broadly reflective of the literature, this chapter uses both old and current nomenclatures.

TABLE 160-3
Habitats and Hosts of Common Dermatophytes

HABITAT	DERMATOPHYTE	HOST
Anthropophilic	Trichophyton rubrum (**syn:** Trichophyton megninii, Trichophyton gourvilii)	Humans
	Trichophyton tonsurans	
	Trichophyton interdigitale (**syn:** Trichophyton mentagrophytes **var.** interdigitale)	
	Trichophyton schoenleinii	
	Trichophyton soudanense	
	Trichophyton violaceum (**syn:** Trichophyton yaoundei)	
	Trichophyton concentricum	
	Microsporum audouinii	
	Microsporum ferrugineum	
	Epidermophyton floccosum	
Zoophilic	Trichophyton mentagrophytes (**syn:** Trichophyton mentagrophytes **var.** quinckeanum)	Rodents
	Trichophyton interdigitale (**syn:** Trichophyton mentagrophytes **var.** mentagrophytes, Trichophyton mentagrophytes **var.** granulosum)	Rodents
	Trichophyton erinacei	Hedgehogs
	Trichophyton simii	Primates
	Trichophyton verrucosum	Cattle
	Microsporum canis (**syn:** Microsporum distortum, Microsporum equinum)	Cats, dogs, horses
	Microsporum amazonicum	Rodents
	Microsporum gallinae	Poultry
	Microsporum nanum	Pigs
	Microsporum persicolor	Rodents
Geophilic	Microsporum gypseum	Soil
	Microsporum cookei	
	Microsporum persicolor	
	Trichophyton vanbreuseghemii	
	Trichophyton eboreum	
	Trichophyton terrestre	

EPIDEMIOLOGY

Superficial fungal infection is a worldwide problem that affects more than 25% of the population.[5] Some species demonstrate ubiquitous distribution, whereas others are geographically limited. Accordingly, predominant species reflect considerable geographic differences, as in the case of tinea capitis. In the United States, *Trichophyton tonsurans* replaced *Microsporum audouinii* as the most common cause of tinea capitis in the second half of the 20th century, and *M. canis* has now become the second most common cause.[6] In Europe, *M. canis* remains the most common cause of tinea capitis despite a significantly increased incidence of *T. tonsurans*.[7] The etiologic profile is quite different in Africa where *M. audouinii, Trichophyton soudanense,* and *Trichophyton violaceum* are the most prevalent pathogens.[8] However, human travel and migration results in dynamic patterns of infection. As an example, *T. soudanense* and *T. violaceum*, typically restricted to Africa, were isolated in U.S. cases of tinea capitis in 2007.[9]

Clinical presentations of dermatophytoses depend not only on the source, but also on host factors. Immunocompromised individuals are more susceptible to refractory dermatophyte infections or to deep mycoses.[10,11] Interestingly, only the severity of dermatophytosis appears to be increased with HIV infection, and not the prevalence.[12] Other host factors, such as age, sex, and race, appear to be additional epidemiologic factors for infection, although their relationship to dermatophyte susceptibility remains unclear. As an example, dermatophyte infections are 5 times more prevalent in males than females. Finally, local customs may also influence rates and patterns of dermatophytoses. The use of macerating occlusive footwear, for example, in industrialized nations has made tinea pedis and onychomycosis much more common in these regions.[13]

CLINICAL FEATURES

Clinical features of the dermatophytoses vary depending upon the causative dermatophyte (as discussed before) and the site of infection (ie, skin, hair, or nails). Skin dermatophytoses are generally named according to the following paradigm: the word *tinea* (Latin for "worm") followed by a Latin term denoting location or other descriptive factor. Diagnoses within this category include tinea barbae, tinea capitis, tinea corporis, tinea cruris, tinea favosa (derivative of Latin *favus*, meaning "honeycomb"), tinea manuum, tinea nigra, and tinea pedis. Dermatophytosis of the hair is known as *piedra*, and of the nails as *onychomycosis*. A dermatophytid or id reaction (autoeczematization) is an acute inflammatory dermatitis at sites distant from the primary inflammatory fungal infection. (See individual diagnoses listed alphabetically under the section "Dermatophytoses" for more detail.)

PATHOGENESIS

Dermatophytes exhibit a broad armamentarium of enzymes (eg, keratinolytic proteases, lipases) and other virulence factors to allow adherence, use of keratin as a source of nutrients, invasion, and growth of mycelial elements for survival in keratinized tissues. As a consequence of keratin degradation with subsequent release of proinflammatory mediators, the host develops an inflammatory response of varying degree. The degree of inflammation is dependent upon pathogen and host factors. The classic "ringworm," or annular, morphology of tinea corporis results from an inflammatory host response against a spreading dermatophyte, followed by a reduction or clearance of fungal elements from within the plaque, and (in many cases) spontaneous resolution of the infection.

ADHERENCE

Dermatophytes overcome several lines of host defense before hyphae begin to thrive in keratinized tissues. The first step is successful adherence of arthroconidia, asexual spores formed by fragmentation of hyphae, to keratin via adhesin to result in alteration of gene expression.[14,15] Dermatophytes make selective use of their proteolytic armamentarium during adherence and invasion.[16,17] Following several hours of successful adherence, the spores begin to germinate in preparation for the next step in the infective chain of events, invasion.

INVASION

Trauma and maceration facilitate penetration of dermatophytes through the skin. Invasion of germinating fungal elements is further accomplished through secretion of specific proteases, lipases, and ceramidases, the digestive products of which also serve as fungal nutrients.[18] Interestingly, components of the fungal cell wall, including β-glucan, galactomannans, and chitin, show inhibitory effects on keratinocyte proliferation (to allow invasion before desquamation) and cell-mediated immunity (discussed in the following section "Host Response").[19,20] Once dermatophytes penetrate through the epidermis to the dermis, binding of adhesin to elastin again changes gene expression.[14]

HOST RESPONSE

Dermatophytes encounter a range of host responses from the nonspecific, innate to the well-tuned, adaptive immune systems. In the line of defense mechanisms, the epithelial surface, antimicrobial peptides (defensins, cathelicidins, S100 proteins, fungistatic fatty acids in sebum), and competing bacterial flora represent the first barrier against invading fungal elements.[13,21,22] Besides acting as a passive physical barrier, epidermal keratinocytes play a more active role by expressing multiple pattern recognition receptors including C-type lectin receptors and multiple Toll-like receptors (TLRs) located either on the cell surface (TLR1, TLR2, TLR4, TLR5, and TLR6) or in the endosomes (TLR3 and TLR9).[23] The innate immune system is able to monitor for microbes via these pattern recognition receptors, which function to bridge innate and adaptive immunity upon recognition of pathogen-associated molecular patterns to result in targeted cytokine production, recruitment, and polarization of relevant T, B, and natural killer lymphocyte subsets.[21] The specific immune response generated depends upon the cell type involved.[24] Monocytes, macrophages, neutrophils, epithelial, and endothelial cells phagocytize and directly kill fungi.[24] Upon TLR binding of a fungal pathogen-associated molecular pattern, mannan, keratinocytes (a) increase proliferation to promote shedding, (b) increase secretion of antimicrobial peptides (such as human β defensins, ribonuclease 7, and Psoriasin) to inhibit growth of dermatophytes, and (c) increase secretion of proinflammatory cytokines (interferon-α, tumor necrosis factor-α, interleukin [IL]-1β, IL-8, IL-16, and IL-17) to further activate the immune system.[23,25,26] A C-type lectin receptor called Dectin-1 binds β-1,3-glucan on fungi to activate the SYK–CARD-9 signaling pathway in neutrophils, macrophages, and dendritic cells to promote IL-23 production and subsequent T-helper (Th)-17 cell induction.[21] Dendritic cells mature and promote differentiation of naïve T cells into effector Th cell subtypes after uptake of fungi.[25] Once dermatophytes are able to penetrate into deeper layers of the epidermis, new nonspecific defenses emerge, such as competition for iron by unsaturated transferrin and activation of complement to inhibit fungal growth.[20]

The next level of defense is cell-mediated immunity resulting in a specific delayed-type hypersensitivity response against invading fungi. The degree of inflammatory reaction depends on the host's immune status as well as the dermatophyte species involved. The inflammatory response associated with this hypersensitivity correlates with clinical resolution, while defective Th1 cell-mediated immunity, important for the activation of phagocytes at the site of infection, may result in chronic or recurrent dermatophytosis.[24] In patients with chronic infection, it has been reported that *T. rubrum* conidia cause macrophages to increase production of tumor necrosis factor-α and IL-10 without increased IL-12 or nitric oxide, decrease costimulatory molecules, and inhibit phagocytosis; thus, when conidia are ingested, the macrophage is unable to digest the conidia, which continue growing inside until they rupture the macrophage.[23] The Th2 response does not appear to be protective, as patients with elevated fungal antigen antibody titers are observed to have widespread dermatophyte infections.[27] A possible role for the Th17 response to dermatophyte infections is suggested by the discovery of hyphal elements binding to Dectin-2, a C-type lectin pattern recognition receptor on dendritic cells, critical for inducing Th17 responses.[28,29] Recall that many innate immune cells release proinflammatory cytokines. Some of these, such as IL-1β, transforming growth factor-β, and IL-6, promote the development of Th17 cells from naïve T cells via signal transducer and activator of transcription (STAT)-3 to induce transcription of the Th17 lineage retinoic acid-related orphan receptor gt.[21] Furthermore, cell expansion and maintenance of Th17 cells is promoted by IL-23. In return, Th17 secretion of IL-17A, IL-17F, and IL-22 activates epithelial cells, granulopoiesis, neutrophil recruitment, and production of chemokines and antimicrobial factors crucial for epithelial immunity against fungi.[21] Thus, a successful host response to dermatophyte infection is dependent upon well-orchestrated interaction and participation of both the innate, nonspecific, and adaptive, cellular immune systems.

Some fungi have evolved to evade immune surveillance. For example, anthropophilic dermatophytes induce secretion of a limited cytokine profile from keratinocytes in vitro compared to zoophilic species.[30,31] One study found the mannans from *T. rubrum* are more capable of inhibiting mitogen-induced lymphoproliferation than those of *M. canis*.[20] This difference may reflect the augmented inflammatory response generally clinically observed with zoophilic species.

In the case of the most common dermatophytic pathogen, *T. rubrum* is first recognized by keratinocytes when fungal pathogen-associated molecular patterns are sensed by pattern recognition receptors (as discussed above) to result in increased expression and transportation of TLRs (such as TLR2) to the surface of keratinocytes, with subsequent increased recognition, and secretion of proinflammatory cytokines, including interferon-inducible protein-10 and monocyte chemotactic protein-1.[32] In one study, after 24 hours of contact with *T. rubrum* conidia, surface expression of TLR2 was downregulated, resulting in decreased keratinocyte release of proinflammatory cytokines.[32] In another study, viable intact conidia inhibited TLR2 and TLR6 expression and decreased human beta defensin-1 and human beta defensin-2 production.[23] Thus, after an initial, short-lived inflammatory response resulting in clearance of active infection, *T. rubrum* is able to manipulate and evade surveillance by the epithelial innate immune system as inert conidia so as to survive until conditions are favorable for germination and recurrent infection.

GENETICS

Despite epidemiologic observation suggesting a genetic predisposition to dermatophyte infection, molecular insight confirming this hypothesis has been relatively lacking. Genetic mutations in the TLRs and their adaptors may result in increased susceptibility to bacterial and viral infection, but not to fungal infection.[21] Polymorphisms of TLR1 and TLR4 are associated with increased risk of invasive fungal disease, and polymorphisms of TLR3 are associated with cutaneous candidiasis.[21] Polymorphisms of the C-type lectin receptor Dectin-1 and mutations of CARD-9 with decreased IL-17 production are associated with chronic mucocutaneous candidiasis along with chronic dermatophyte infections.[21,33] Multiple mutations are associated with increased susceptibility to other fungi, such as IL-17 receptor and cytokine genes, *STAT1* and *STAT3*, *DOCK8*, *Tyk2*, *AIRE*, *IL-12RB1*, and *MST1/STK4*, which increase mucocutaneous fungal infections; and *CYBB*, *NCF1*, *NCF2*, *NCF4*, *CYBA*, *MAGT1*, and *RAG1*, which increase invasive fungal infections.[21]

DIAGNOSIS

Table 160-4 outlines common laboratory dermatophyte identification methods.

The clinical diagnosis of a dermatophyte infection can be confirmed by microscopic detection of fungal elements, by identification of the species through culture, or by histologic evidence of the presence of hyphae in the stratum corneum. In addition, fluorescence patterns under Wood light examination may support a clinical suspicion.

MICROSCOPIC EXAMINATION

Although microscopic evaluation of potassium hydroxide (KOH)-treated samples of scale does not allow for speciation or characterization of the susceptibility profile, it can be used as a quick and inexpensive bedside tool to provide evidence of dermatophytosis. In dermatophytosis involving the skin, hair, or nails, septate and branching hyphae without constriction (Fig. 160-1) may be visualized under microscopic examination with 10% to 20% KOH preparation. All superficial dermatophytes appear identical when visualized in this manner. Because KOH examination may yield false-negative results in up to 15% of cases, patients suspected of having dermatophytosis on clinical impression should be treated.[34] Culture confirmation should be considered whenever systemic treatment is warranted, such as in the case of onychomycosis.

To perform KOH examination of the skin, collect scale by scraping the involved area with a dull edge (eg, a no. 15 blade or edge of slide) outward from the advancing margins. This same technique may be used to scrape under affected nails (but diagnosis of onychomycosis is best confirmed with histopathology or culture as discussed further). Scrapings are then placed on a glass slide, covered with a coverslip, and

TABLE 160-4
Common Laboratory Dermatophyte Identification Methods

LABORATORY TEST	METHOD	FUNCTION	FINDINGS
Potassium hydroxide preparation (KOH)	Scales from advancing border, subungual debris, or affected hair removed and placed on a glass slide. KOH 10% dropped on specimen and covered with a cover slip. The undersurface of the glass slide may be gently heated with a low-lit flame.	KOH solution and gentle heating softens keratin and highlights the dermatophyte.	Long, narrow, septated and branching hyphae.
Culture	Sabouraud medium (4% peptone, 1% glucose, agar, water).	Facilitates growth of dermatophytes.	Microscopic morphology of microconidia and macroconidia, along with culture features including surface topography and pigmentation. The reader is referred to http://www.mycology.adelaide.edu.au/ for a comprehensive characterization of fungal colonies. Common colonies are characterized in Table 160-5.
	Modified Sabouraud medium (addition of chloramphenicol, cycloheximide, and gentamicin).	Facilitates growth of dermatophytes and inhibits growth of non–*Candida albicans*, *Cryptococcus*, *Prototheca* species, *Phaeoannellomyces werneckii*, *Scytalidium* species, and *Ochroconis gallopava*.	
Dermatophyte test medium	Scales from the advancing border, subungual debris, or affected hair embedded in the medium.	Medium contains the pH indicator phenol red. Dermatophytes use proteins, which result in excess ammonium ion and an alkaline environment.	Incubation at room temperature for 5 to 14 days results in change in medium color from yellow to bright red in the presence of a dermatophyte.
Histopathology special stains: periodic acid–Schiff (PAS) and Grocott methenamine silver (GMS)	Tissue may be obtained by skin or nail biopsy techniques.	Stains fungal cell wall to detect fungal elements in tissue sections.	Pink (PAS) or black (GMS) fungal elements noted in the stratum corneum

prepared with 10% to 20% KOH. Place several drops of KOH on the slide adjacent to the coverslip edge, allowing capillary action to wick the fluid under the coverslip. A paper towel may then be used to blot excess KOH solution from around the coverslip. Penetration of KOH into keratin may be aided by either slightly warming the slide with a low-intensity flame or by addition of dimethylsulfoxide (DMSO) in KOH solution. Some may also find the adding a drop of blue or black stain such as chlorazol black (in similar fashion as KOH solution above) helpful for better identifying fungal elements (as seen in Fig. 160-1). Hairs should be plucked (not cut), placed on a glass slide, prepared with 10% to 20% KOH, and covered with a coverslip. Slightly warming the slide with a low-intensity flame allows better penetration of the KOH solution into keratin. Low-power microscopy will reveal 3 possible patterns of infection (Fig. 160-2): (a) ectothrix—small or large arthroconidia forming a sheath around the hair shaft; (b) endothrix—arthroconidia within the hair shaft; or (c) favus—hyphae and air spaces within the hair shaft.

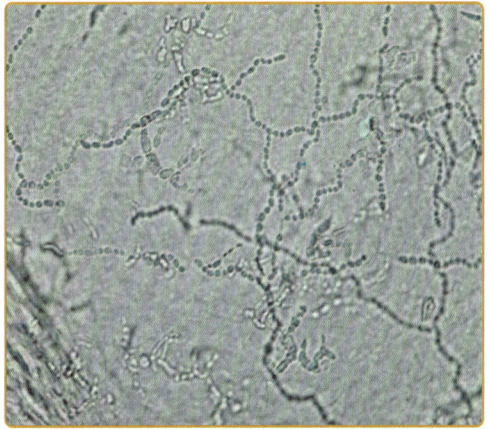

Figure 160-1 Microscopic examination of skin scrapings (scales) revealing septate, branching hyphae.

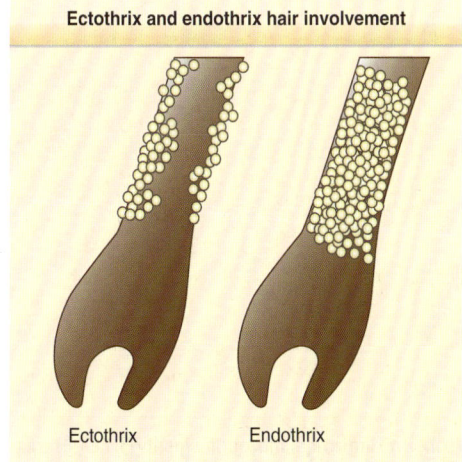

Figure 160-2 Graphic demonstration of ectothrix and endothrix hair involvement.

CULTURE

Speciation of superficial fungi is based on macroscopic, microscopic, and metabolic characteristics of the organism. Although some dermatophytes are readily identified on the basis of their primary isolation cultures, most require further differentiation through subcultures on specific media (identification culture) or through specific biochemical tests.

Sabouraud dextrose agar (SDA) is the most commonly used isolation medium for dermatophytes and it serves as the medium on which most morphologic descriptions are based. Elimination of contaminant molds, yeast, and bacteria is achieved by the addition of cycloheximide and chloramphenicol (± gentamicin) to the medium making it highly selective for the isolation of dermatophytes. The development of colonies can take 5 to 7 days in the case of *Epidermophyton floccosum* and up to 4 weeks for *Trichophyton verrucosum*. Cultures are incubated at room temperature (20°C to 25°C [68°F to 77°F]) for at least 4 weeks before being finalized as no growth. Dermatophyte test medium is an alternative isolation medium that contains the pH indicator phenol red. The medium turns red when dermatophyte proteolytic activity increases the pH to 8 or above, and it remains amber with the growth of most saprophytes. Nondermatophyte acidic byproducts turn the medium yellow. Although dermatophyte test medium serves as a good alternative for isolation of dermatophytes, it may not allow for their direct identification because of altered growth, and thus morphology, of dermatophytes in dermatophyte test medium. Table 160-5 describes general microscopic features of microconidia and macroconidia of the 3 genera of dermatophytes, and Table 160-6 describes colony and microscopic features of the most common dermatophyte species.

Identification of isolated fungi is facilitated by subculture on specific media such as potato dextrose agar or Borelli lactritmel agar that stimulate sporulation, production of pigment and development of typical morphology. Finally, dermatophytes may be differentiated further by their ability to grow on autoclaved polished rice, perforate short strands of hair in vitro, hydrolyze urea (urease test), or require nutritional supplementation for growth (Table 160-7).

TABLE 160-5 Microscopic Features of Dermatophyte Microconidia and Macroconidia		
GENERA	MICROCONIDIA	MACROCONIDIA
Trichophyton	Smooth walled; used for identification	Absent or nondiagnostic
Microsporum	Absent or nondiagnostic	Rough walled; used for identification
Epidermophyton	Absent	Smooth walled; used for identification

TABLE 160-6
Colony and Microscopic Morphology Features of the Most Common Dermatophytes

ORGANISM	COLONY MORPHOLOGY		MICROSCOPIC APPEARANCE
Epidermophyton floccosum 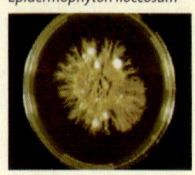	Flat feathery colonies with a central fold and yellow to dull gray-green pigment. Yellow to brown reverse pigment.	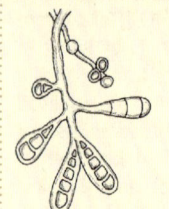	Numerous thin and thick-walled, club-shaped macroconidia.
Microsporum audouinii 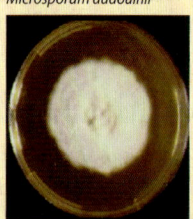	Flat and white to gray with widely spaced radial grooves. Tan to salmon reverse pigment. Salmon-pink pigment on PDA. No growth on polished rice.	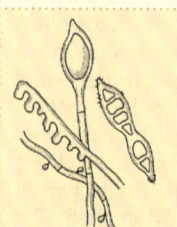	Terminal chlamydoconidia and pectinate (comb-like) hyphae.
Microsporum canis 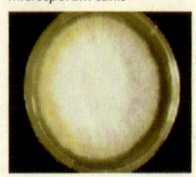	Flat, white to light yellow, coarsely hairy, with closely spaced radial grooves. Yellow to orange reverse pigment. Yellow on PDA. Growth on polished rice.	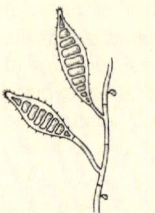	Numerous thick walled and echinulate spindle shaped macroconidia with terminal knobs and more than 6 cells.
Microsporum gypseum 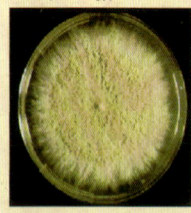	Flat and granular with tan to buff pigment, no reverse pigment.	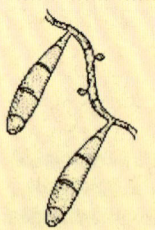	Numerous thin-walled pickle-shaped macroconidia without knobs and less than 6 cells.
Trichophyton interdigitale 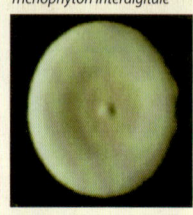	White to creamy with a cottony, mounded surface. None to light brown reverse pigment. No pigment on PDA. Urease positive, which helps to distinguish it from *Trichophyton rubrum*.	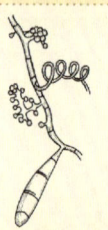	Grape-like clusters of round microconidia, rare cigar-shaped macroconidia, occasional spiral hyphae. Hair perforation positive, which helps to distinguish it from *T. rubrum*.
Trichophyton rubrum 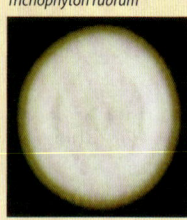	Mounded white center with maroon periphery. Maroon reverse pigment. Cherry red on PDA. Urease negative.	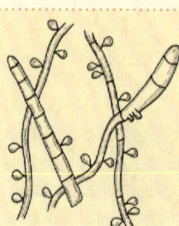	Few tear-shaped microconidia, rare pencil-shaped macroconidia. Hair perforation negative.

(Continued)

TABLE 160-6
Colony and Microscopic Morphology Features of the Most Common Dermatophytes (Continued)

ORGANISM	COLONY MORPHOLOGY	MICROSCOPIC APPEARANCE
Trichophyton schoenleinii	Heaped or folded and whitish. Colorless to yellow-tan reverse pigment.	Knobby antler-like hyphae (favic chandeliers), numerous chlamydoconidia.
Trichophyton tonsurans	Suede-like center with feathery periphery, white to yellow or maroon color. Reverse pigment usually dark maroon, sometimes none to yellow. Partial thiamine requirement.	Numerous multiform microconidia and rare cigar-shaped macroconidia.
Trichophyton verrucosum	Small and heaped, although sometimes flat, white to yellow-gray. Reverse pigment none to yellow. Requires thiamine and usually inositol for growth.	Chains of chlamydoconidia on SDA. Long and thin "rat-tail" macroconidia with thiamine.
Trichophyton violaceum	Waxy and heaped, deep purplish-red. Purple reverse pigment. Partial thiamine requirement.	Irregular hyphae with intercalary chlamydoconidia. No micro- or macroconidia on SDA, rare micro- and macroconidia with thiamine.

PDA, potato dextrose agar; SDA, Sabouraud's dextrose agar.
Used with permission from David Ellis, PhD.

TABLE 160-7
Trichophyton Nutritional Growth Requirements

Urease test	Differentiates *Trichophyton interdigitale* (positive) from *Trichophyton rubrum* (negative)		
Hair perforation test	Differentiates *T. interdigitale* (positive) from *T. rubrum* (negative)		
Nutritional requirement	Differentiates *Trichophyton* species		
	Thiamine	Trichophyton tonsurans	
		Trichophyton concentricum	
		Trichophyton violaceum	
	Thiamine + inositol	Trichophyton verrucosum	
	Nicotinic acid	Trichophyton equinum	
	Histidine	Trichophyton megninii	
Growth on polished rice	Differentiates *Microsporum* species		
	Good growth	Microsporum canis	
	Poor growth	Microsporum audouinii	
		Microsporum distortum	

HISTOPATHOLOGY

Skin biopsy is not often employed in the workup of typical dermatophytoses. Localized cutaneous eruptions suspected to represent dermatophytosis with equivocal KOH examination are often treated despite the lack of confirmation. Biopsy may confirm the diagnosis when a systemic agent is being considered for treatment of a recalcitrant or more widespread eruption. Biopsy may be used to aid in the diagnosis of Majocchi granuloma in which KOH examination of scale on the surface more often may be negative. Biopsy is also sometimes useful in confirming the presence of hyphae involving hair shafts on the scalp in tinea capitis, although culture is necessary to allow speciation of the pathogen. When present, hyphae may be appreciated in the stratum corneum on hematoxylin-and-eosin (H&E) staining. However special stains, most commonly periodic acid–Schiff (PAS) and methenamine silver stains, highlight hyphae that may otherwise be subtle in appearance on routine staining. Whereas culture is the most specific test for onychomycosis, PAS examination of nail clippings is the most sensitive and obviates the need to wait weeks for a result.[35] Full-thickness nail clippings for H&E or culture should involve the dystrophic portion, as proximal from the distal edge as possible without causing injury.

WOOD LIGHT FLUORESCENCE

Examination of involved hair bearing areas, such as the scalp or beard, with a Wood lamp (365 nm) may reveal pteridine fluorescence of hair infected with particular fungal pathogens. Hairs that fluoresce should be selected for further examination, including culture. Although ectothrix organisms *M. canis* and *M. audouinii* will fluoresce on Wood light examination, the endothrix organism *T. tonsurans* will not fluoresce. *T. tonsurans*, which is now the most common cause of tinea capitis in the United States, thus limits the use of Wood light examination. Table 160-8 lists common patterns of dermatophyte hair involvement and fluorescence.

MANAGEMENT

Table 160-9 outlines the treatment of dermatophytes, Table 160-10 lists oral antifungal agents, and Table 160-11 lists topical antifungal agents.

Multiple systemic and topical antifungal agents are available to treat dermatophytoses of skin, hair and nails.[36-38] Of note, dermatoses involving hair-bearing skin and nails typically require oral treatment. See individual diagnoses in the section "Dermatophytoses" for more information.

CLINICAL COURSE AND PROGNOSIS

The clinical course of dermatophytosis varies according to pathogen and host factors. As discussed before, some dermatophytes are able to evade or suppress host immune function, and some hosts are unable to mount an effective immune response to clear infection. As such, the severity of each infection is variable according to the combination of these factors.

DERMATOPHYTOSES

DERMATOPHYTID (ID) REACTION

A dermatophytid (or id) reaction is an inflammatory dermatitis occurring at sites distant from the primary dermatophytosis (such as tinea pedis or kerion) in 4% to 5% of patients.[39] Although the precise mechanism is unknown, the id reaction is associated with a delayed-type hypersensitivity response to the *Trichophyton* test, and so may involve a local delayed-type hypersensitivity response to systemically absorbed fungal antigen.[40] Id reactions appear polymorphic, ranging in morphology from follicular or nonfollicular papules and vesicles of the hands and feet to reactive erythemas including erythema nodosum, erythema annulare centrifugum, or urticaria.[41-44] Unlike the primary eruption, the id eruption is both KOH examination negative and culture negative. The 3 criteria for establishing the presence of an id eruption are (a) dermatophytosis on another part of body, (b) absence of fungal elements from the id eruption, and (c) resolution of the id eruption with clearing of the primary dermatophyte infection.

ONYCHOMYCOSIS

Onychomycosis describes fungal infection of the nail caused by dermatophytes, nondermatophyte molds, or yeasts. *Tinea unguium* refers strictly to dermatophyte infection of the nail. Clinically, 3 types of onychomycosis are distinguished: (a) distolateral subungual onychomycosis (DLSO), (b) proximal subungual onychomycosis (PSO), and (c) white superficial onychomycosis (WSO).

TABLE 160-8
Pattern of Hair Infection and Fluorescence

PATTERN	DERMATOPHYTE	FLUORESCENCE
Endothrix	Trichophyton soudanense Trichophyton violaceum Trichophyton tonsurans Trichophyton gourvilii Trichophyton yaoundei	None
Ectothrix	Microsporum canis Microsporum audouinii Microsporum distortum Microsporum ferrugineum	Yellow-green
	Microsporum fulvum Microsporum gypseum	None
	Trichophyton megninii Trichophyton interdigitale Trichophyton rubrum Trichophyton verrucosum	None
Favus	Trichophyton schoenleinii	Blue-gray, occasional

TABLE 160-9
Treatment of Dermatophytes

DISEASE	TOPICAL TREATMENT	SYSTEMIC TREATMENT

Tinea capitis (requires systemic treatment)	Only as adjuvant
	Selenium sulfide 1% or 2.5%
	Zinc pyrithione 1% or 2%
	Povidone-iodine 2.5%
	Ketoconazole 2%
		Adults
		■ Griseofulvin, 20 to 25 mg/kg/day × 6 to 8 weeks
		■ Terbinafine, 250 mg/day × 2 to 8 weeks
		■ Itraconazole, 5 mg/kg/day × 2 to 4 weeks
		■ Fluconazole, 6 mg/kg/day × 3 to 6 weeks
		Children
		■ Griseofulvin, daily × 6 to 8 weeks
		  ■ Age 1 month to 2 years: 10 mg/kg/day
		  ■ Age ≥2 years: 20 to 25 mg/kg/day (micro)
		  ■ Age ≥2 years: 10 to 15 mg/kg/day (ultramicro)
		■ Terbinafine daily × 2 to 4 weeks
		  ■ Weight <20 kg: 62.5 mg/day
		  ■ Weight 20 to 40 kg: 125 mg/day
		  ■ Weight >40 kg: 250 mg/day
		■ Itraconazole
		  ■ 3 to 5 mg/kg/day × 2 to 4 weeks
		  ■ 5 mg/kg/day × 1 week/month × 2 to 3 months
		■ Fluconazole (not standard therapy)
		  ■ 6 mg/kg/day × 3 to 6 weeks
		  ■ 6 mg/kg once weekly × 8 to 12 weeks

Tinea barbae (requires systemic treatment)	Only as adjuvant Zinc pyrithione 1% or 2% Povidone-iodine 2.5%	■ Griseofulvin 1 g/day × 6 weeks ■ Terbinafine 250 mg/day × 2 to 4 weeks ■ Itraconazole 200 mg/day × 2 to 4 weeks ■ Fluconazole 200 mg/day × 4 to 6 weeks
Tinea corporis/cruris	Allylamines Imidazoles Tolnaftate Butenafine Ciclopirox Gentian violet	**Adults** ■ Terbinafine 250 mg/day × 2 to 4 weeks ■ Itraconazole 100 mg/day × 1 week ■ Fluconazole 150 to 300 mg/day × 4 to 6 weeks ■ Griseofulvin 500 mg/day × 2 to 4 weeks **Children** ■ Terbinafine 3 to 6 mg/kg/day × 2 weeks ■ Itraconazole 5 mg/kg/day × 1 week ■ Griseofulvin 10 to 20 mg/kg/day × 2 to 4 weeks
Tinea pedis/manuum	Allylamine Imidazoles Ciclopirox Benzylamine Tolnaftate Undecenoic acid	**Adults** ■ Terbinafine 250 mg/day × 2 weeks ■ Itraconazole 200 mg twice daily × 1 week ■ Fluconazole 150 mg/week × 3 to 4 weeks **Children** ■ Terbinafine 3 to 6 mg/kg/day × 2 weeks ■ Itraconazole 5 mg/kg/day × 2 weeks

Onychomycosis	Ciclopirox
	Amorolfine
	Tioconazole
	Efinaconazole
		Adults
		■ Terbinafine 250 mg/day × 6 to 12 weeks
		■ Itraconazole 200 mg/day × 2 to 3 months, *or*
		■ Pulse 400 mg daily × 1 week/month × 2 to 3 months
		■ Fluconazole 150 to 300 mg/week × 3 to 12 months
		Children
		■ Terbinafine daily × 6 to 12 weeks
		  ■ Weight 10 to 20 kg: 62.5 mg/day
		  ■ Weight 20 to 40 kg: 125 mg/day
		  ■ Weight >40 kg: 250 mg/day
		■ Itraconazole 1 week/month × 2 to 3 months
		  ■ Weight <20 kg: 5 mg/kg/day
		  ■ Weight 20 to 40 kg: 100 mg/day
		  ■ Weight 40 to 50 kg: 200 mg/day
		  ■ Weight >50 kg: 200 mg twice daily
		■ Fluconazole 3 to 6 mg/kg/week × 3 to 6 months

TABLE 160-10
Oral Antifungal Agents

MEDICATION	DRUG CLASS	INDICATIONS	WARNINGS/MONITORING
Fluconazole	Triazole	Onychomycosis Tinea barbae Tinea capitis Tinea corporis/cruris Tinea pedis/manuum	*Adverse effects:* headache, GI upset *Caution:* liver and/or renal impairment *Contraindications:* pregnancy, concurrent QT-prolonging medications Monitor liver function tests, basic metabolic panel, complete blood cell count; pregnancy test prior to start in females Pregnancy category D
Griseofulvin	Inhibits fungal mitosis	Tinea barbae Tinea capitis (first-line *Microsporum*) Tinea corporis/cruris Tinea pedis/manuum	*Adverse effects:* headache, GI upset *Caution:* liver impairment *Contraindications:* porphyria, pregnancy, hepatic failure Check pregnancy test prior to start in females Pregnancy category X
Itraconazole	Triazole	Onychomycosis Tinea barbae Tinea capitis Tinea corporis/cruris Tinea pedis/manuum	*Adverse effects:* headache, GI upset *Caution/contraindication:* cardiac failure, hepatotoxicity Monitor liver function tests, basic metabolic panel, complete blood cell count baseline and at 1 month Check pregnancy test prior to start in females Pregnancy category C
Terbinafine	Allylamine	Onychomycosis (first-line) Tinea barbae Tinea capitis Tinea corporis/cruris Tinea pedis/manuum	*Adverse effects:* GI upset, taste disturbance, elevation of liver enzymes Risk of hepatotoxicity Monitor liver function tests baseline and at 1 month Pregnancy category B

TABLE 160-11
Topical Antifungal Agents

MEDICATION	CLASS/MECHANISM	FORMULATION	USE	ADMINISTRATION	WARNING/PRECAUTIONS
Amorolfine	Morpholine	Liquid, 250 mg/5 mL	Onychomycosis (dermatophyte or *Candida*) treatment and/or relapse prophylaxis	Apply 1 to 2 times/week after gentle nail filing × 6 to 12 months	Not available in the United States
Butenafine	Synthetic allylamine	Cream, 1%	Tinea corporis, cruris, pedis, versicolor	Apply 1 to 2 times daily for 1 to 4 weeks	Pregnancy category C Children ≥12 years of age
Ciclopirox	Inhibits DNA, RNA, and protein synthesis	Cream, 0.77% Suspension, 0.77% Gel, 0.77%	Tinea corporis, cruris, pedis, versicolor; cutaneous *Candida*; seborrheic dermatitis	Apply twice daily	Pregnancy category B Cream and suspension, children >10 years of age Gel and shampoo, children >16 years of age Solution, children ≥12 years of age
		Shampoo, 0.1%	Seborrheic dermatitis	Apply, wait 5 to 10 minutes prior to rinsing; use 2 to 3 times/week to treat, 1 to 2 times/week to maintain	
		Solution, 8%	Onychomycosis	Apply to nail and surrounding skin at bedtime × 7 days, then remove with rubbing alcohol and repeat	
Clotrimazole	Imidazole	Cream, 1% Ointment, 1% Solution, 1%	Tinea corporis, cruris, pedis, versicolor	Apply twice daily × 1 to 4 weeks	Pregnancy category B
Econazole	Imidazole	Cream, 1% Foam, 1%	Tinea corporis, cruris, pedis, versicolor	Apply 1 to 2 times daily × 2 to 4 weeks	Pregnancy category C Children ≥12 years of age

(Continued)

TABLE 160-11
Topical Antifungal Agents (*Continued*)

MEDICATION	CLASS/MECHANISM	FORMULATION	USE	ADMINISTRATION	WARNING/PRECAUTIONS
Efinaconazole	Triazole	Solution, 10%	Onychomycosis	Apply daily × 48 weeks	Pregnancy category C
Gentian violet	Antifungal Antibiotic	Solution, 1% and 2%	Superficial cutaneous infections, effective against some Gram+ bacteria (*Staphylococcus* sp.), fungi, some yeasts	Apply 1 to 2 times daily	Pregnancy category not classified Stains skin and clothing May tattoo open wounds
Ketoconazole	Imidazole	Cream, 2% Foam, 2% Gel, 2%	Tinea corporis, cruris, pedis, versicolor; cutaneous *Candida*; seborrheic dermatitis	Apply 1 to 2 times daily	Pregnancy category C Children ≥12 years of age
		Shampoo, 1% and 2%	Tinea capitis adjuvant, tinea versicolor, seborrheic dermatitis	Apply, wait 5 to 10 mins prior to rinsing; use 2 to 3 times/week to treat, 1 to 2 times/week as prophylaxis	
Miconazole	Imidazole	Aerosol, 2% Cream, 2% Lotion, 2% Ointment, 2% Powder, 2% Solution, 2%	Tinea corporis, cruris, pedis	Apply twice daily × 4 weeks	Pregnancy category not classified Children ≥2 years of age May increase serum concentration of vitamin K agonist
Povidine-iodine	Broad-spectrum germicidal agent	Wash, 7.5% Shampoo, 7.5%	Tinea capitis and barbae adjuvant, seborrheic dermatitis	Use twice weekly until controlled, then once weekly	Pregnancy category C Use with caution in children Hypersensitivity to iodine contraindication
Selenium sulfide	Cytostatic effects on keratinocytes	Foam, 2.25% Lotion, 2.25% Shampoo, 1% and 2.3%	Tinea capitis adjuvant, tinea versicolor, seborrheic dermatitis	Foam: twice daily Lotion: Apply, rinse after 10 minutes once daily × 1 week, then once monthly × 3 months Shampoo: Apply, wait 5 to 10 mins prior to rinsing; use 2 to 3 times/week to treat, 1 to 2 times/week as prophylaxis	Pregnancy category C Children ≥2 years of age
Terbinafine	Allylamine	Cream, 1% Gel, 1% Solution, 1%	Tinea corporis, cruris, pedis, versicolor; cutaneous candidiasis	Apply 1 to 2 times daily × 1 to 2 weeks	Pregnancy category not classified Children ≥12 years of age
Tioconazole	Imidazole	Solution, 28%	Onychomycosis	Apply twice daily × 6 to 12 months	Not available in the United States Possible allergic contact dermatitis
Tolnaftate	Distorts hyphae and mycelial growth	Aerosol, 1% Cream, 1% Lotion, 1% Powder, 1% Solution, 1%	Tinea corporis, cruris, pedis	Apply twice daily × 2 to 4 weeks	Pregnancy category not classified Children ≥2 years of age
Zinc pyrithione	Keratolytic	Bar, 2% Liquid/wash, 0.5% Shampoo, 2%	Tinea capitis and barbae adjuvant; seborrheic dermatitis	Use at least 2 times/week	Pregnancy category C

EPIDEMIOLOGY

Onychomycosis is the most prevalent nail disease and accounts for approximately 50% of all causes of onychodystrophy. It affects up to 14% of the population, with both an increasing prevalence[45] and an overall increasing incidence among older individuals.[46] Onychomycosis is also increasing in incidence among children and adolescents, and accounts for up to 20% of dermatophyte infections diagnosed in children.[47] Risk factors for nail infection include age, male sex, nail trauma, immunosuppression (including HIV infection and diabetes mellitus), and peripheral vascular insufficiency.[48] Patients with HIV and with a CD4 T-lymphocyte count of less than 400 cells/µL (reference range: 1200 to 1400 cells/µL) and who are on immunosuppressants or have defective polymorphonuclear chemotaxis have an increased risk of onychomycosis, which tends to be more widespread and involve all 20 nails.[36]

The increasing prevalence of onychomycosis may be secondary to wearing of tight shoes, increasing numbers of individuals on immunosuppressive drugs and with diabetes mellitus, and an increased use of communal locker rooms. The dermatophytosis commonly begins as tinea pedis before extending to the nail bed, where eradication is more difficult. This site serves as a reservoir for local recurrence or for infections spreading to other areas. Up to 40% of patients with toenail onychomycosis show concomitant skin infections, most commonly tinea pedis (30%).[49]

CLINICAL FEATURES

Table 160-12 summarizes the subtypes and most common causes of onychomycosis.

Distolateral Subungual Type: DLSO is the most common form of onychomycosis. It begins with invasion of the stratum corneum of the hyponychium and distal nail bed, forming a whitish to brownish–yellow opacification at the distal edge of the nail (Fig. 160-3A). The infection then spreads proximally up the nail bed to the ventral nail plate. Hyperproliferation (or altered differentiation) of the nail bed in response to the infection results in subungual hyperkeratosis, while progressive invasion of the nail plate results in an increasingly dystrophic nail.

Proximal Subungual Type: PSO (see Fig. 160-3B) results from infection of the proximal nailfold primarily with *T. rubrum* and *Trichophyton megninii* and is apparent as a white-to-beige opacity on the proximal nail plate. This opacity gradually enlarges to affect the entire nail and eventuates in subungual hyperkeratosis, leukonychia, proximal onycholysis, and/or destruction of the entire nail. Patients with PSO should be screened for HIV, as it has been identified as an a marker for this disease.[6,50]

White Superficial Type: WSO (see Fig. 160-3C) results from direct invasion of the dorsal nail plate resulting in white to dull yellow, sharply bordered patches anywhere on the surface of the toenail. It is

TABLE 160-12
Subtypes of Superficial Fungal Infections and Their Most Common Causes

Onychomycosis	
Distolateral subungual type	Trichophyton rubrum,[a] Trichophyton interdigitale
Proximal subungual type	Trichophyton rubrum, Trichophyton megninii
White superficial type	Trichophyton interdigitale (also the following nondermatophytes: *Aspergillus, Scopulariopsis, Fusarium, Candida* sp.)
Total dystrophic onychomycosis	*Candida* sp.
Tinea Barbae	
Superficial type	Trichophyton violaceum
Inflammatory type	Trichophyton interdigitale
Tinea Capitis	
Inflammatory	Microsporum audouinii, Microsporum canis, Microsporum gypseum, Microsporum nanum, Trichophyton interdigitale, Trichophyton schoenleinii, Trichophyton tonsurans, Trichophyton verrucosum
Noninflammatory	Microsporum audouinii, Microsporum canis, Microsporum ferrugineum, Trichophyton tonsurans
Black dot	Trichophyton tonsurans, Trichophyton violaceum
Favus	Trichophyton schoenleinii, Trichophyton violaceum, Trichophyton mentagrophytes
Tinea Corporis	
Tinea Corporis	Adults: *Trichophyton rubrum* Children: *Microsporum canis*
Tinea incognito	Trichophyton rubrum
Majocchi's granuloma	Trichophyton rubrum, Trichophyton interdigitale, Microsporum canis
Tinea imbricata	Trichophyton concentricum
Tinea cruris	Trichophyton rubrum, Epidermophyton floccosum, Trichophyton interdigitale, Trichophyton verrucosum
Tinea nigra	Hortaea werneckii
Tinea Pedis	
Interdigital type	Trichophyton rubrum, Trichophyton interdigitale, Epidermophyton floccosum
Chronic hyperkeratotic (moccasin) type	Trichophyton rubrum, Epidermophyton floccosum
Vesicobullous type	Trichophyton interdigitale (usually zoophilic strains)
Adult ulcerative type	Trichophyton interdigitale (zoophilic strains) with combined Gram-negative bacterial superinfection
Tinea Manuum	
Tinea manuum	Trichophyton rubrum, Trichophyton interdigitale, Epidermophyton floccosum

[a]A single dermatophyte may have more than one presentation.

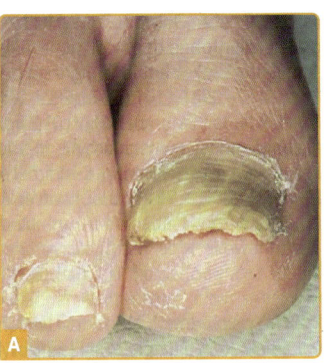
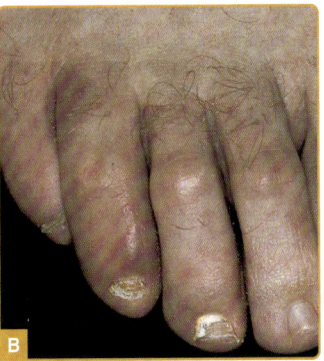
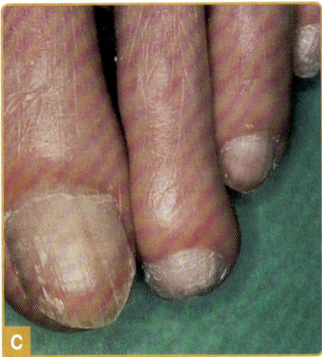

Figure 160-3 Tinea unguium. **A,** Distal subungual type. Discoloration, thickening and subungual debris of the distal aspect of the toenails. **B,** Proximal subungual type. Discoloration and thickening of the proximal nail in a patient with AIDS; Kaposi sarcoma is also seen on the fourth toe. **C,** White superficial type. Irregular opaque white patches on various parts of the nail plates.

usually caused by *T. interdigitale*, although nondermatophyte molds such as *Aspergillus, Scopulariopsis,* and *Fusarium* are also known pathogens. *Candida* species may invade the hyponychial epithelium to eventually affect the entire thickness of the nail plate.[51]

Other Clinical Presentations: Total dystrophy of the nail may result from almost complete destruction of the nail plate secondary to any of the foregoing varieties of onychomycosis; this is known as total dystrophic onychomycosis.[36] Primary total dystrophic onychomycosis is rare, usually caused by *Candida*, and typically affects immunocompromised patients.[36] Multiple patterns of onychomycosis may present in the same individual, most commonly with the combination of PSO with WSO or DLSO with WSO.[36] Secondary bacterial infection of the nail is possible. Infection with *Pseudomonas aeruginosa* presents as a green or black discoloration under the nail. It is also possible to have mixed infections with both a dermatophyte and yeast form, such as *Candida*.

ETIOLOGY AND PATHOGENESIS

In the majority of cases, onychomycosis is caused by dermatophytes, with *T. rubrum* and *T. interdigitale* responsible for approximately 90% of all cases. *T. tonsurans* and *E. floccosum* are also well-documented causative agents.[52] Yeast and nondermatophyte molds such as *Acremonium, Aspergillus, Fusarium, Scopulariopsis brevicaulis,* and *Scytalidium* are the source of approximately 10% of toenail onychomycosis. Interestingly, *Candida* species are responsible for up to 30% of fingernail cases, whereas nondermatophyte molds were not detected in diseased fingernails.[53] *Candida* (and irritant dermatitis) may also cause chronic paronychia.

Risk factors for onychomycosis include increasing age, male sex, peripheral vascular disease, trauma, hyperhidrosis, and immunosuppressed states, including HIV, diabetes mellitus, and medication-induced immunosuppression.[36] In children, onychomycosis may be responsible for up to 15% of onychodystrophies.[36] As in adults, prevalence increases with age and may be associated with occlusive footwear.

DIAGNOSIS

Table 160-4 outlines common laboratory dermatophyte identification methods and Table 160-6 outlines the colony and microscopic morphology features of the most common dermatophytes.

Although onychomycosis is responsible for 50% of dystrophic nails, laboratory diagnostic confirmation prior to treatment with potentially toxic oral antifungal treatments is judicious. KOH examination of subungual debris, culture of the nail plate and accompanying debris on SDA (with and without antimicrobials), and PAS staining of nail clippings are most useful. However, KOH examination is often negative even when clinical suspicion is high, and nails with hyphae reported on KOH examination often yield negative cultures. The simplest measure to minimize false-negatives caused by sampling error is to maximize sample size and repeat collections. The following guidelines are suggested to discern pathogens from contaminants: (a) if a dermatophyte is isolated on culture, it is considered a pathogen; (b) a nondermatophyte mold or yeast cultured is significant only if hyphae, spores, or yeast cells are seen on microscopic examination, and (c) there is repeated heavy growth of a nondermatophyte mold without concurrent isolation of a dermatophyte.[54] Whereas culture is the most specific test for onychomycosis, PAS examination of nail clippings is the most sensitive,[35] and it obviates the need to wait weeks for a result. As such, we recommend collection of nail clippings, with inclusion of full thickness of the most proximal affected areas obtainable without causing trauma, for PAS and H&E examination.

On histopathology (see Table 160-4), hyphae are seen between the nail laminae parallel to the surface and have a predilection for the ventral nail and stratum corneum of the nail bed.[55] The epidermis may show spongiosis and focal parakeratosis, and there is a minimal dermal inflammatory response. In WSO, the organisms are present superficially on the dorsal nail and display unique "perforating organs" and "eroding fronds." In candidal onychomycosis there is invasion of pseudohyphae throughout the entire nail plate, adjacent cuticle, granular layer, and stratum spinosum of the nail bed, as well as the hyponychial stratum corneum.[51]

DIFFERENTIAL DIAGNOSIS

Table 160-13 outlines the differential diagnosis of onychomycosis.

MANAGEMENT

Table 160-9 outlines the treatment of dermatophytes.

The management of onychomycosis depends on several factors, including the severity of nail involvement, presence or absence of tinea pedis, treatment efficacy, and potential adverse effects. Even though it is reasonable to not treat nail involvement, concurrent tinea pedis should always be treated to decrease risk of cellulitis, particularly in the settings of diabetes mellitus, chronic venous stasis, and other causes of chronic lower-extremity edema (see the discussion of the treatment of tinea pedis).

Systemic Therapy: An oral antifungal (see Table 160-10) is required for onychomycosis involving the matrix area, or when a shorter treatment regimen or higher chance for clearance/cure is desired. Selection of the antifungal agent should be based on the causative organism, potential adverse effects, risk of drug interactions, and comorbidities in each patient. Of note, griseofulvin is no longer considered standard treatment for onychomycosis because of its prolonged treatment course, potential for adverse effects and drug interactions, and its relatively low cure rates.

Topical Therapy: In patients with distal nail involvement, WSO, and/or contraindication for systemic treatment, topical therapy (see Table 160-11) should be considered.

Combination therapy regimens may have a higher clearance rate than either oral or topical treatments alone. Studies have been performed using combination therapy regimens with topical tioconazole, ciclopirox, and amorolfine with mixed results.[36,56,57] In vitro fungicidal activity demonstrated by thymol, camphor, menthol, and oil of *Eucalyptus citriodora* offers the potential for additional therapeutic strategies to treat onychomycosis.[58,59] Thymol 4% prepared in ethanol may be used as drops applied to the nail plate and hyponychium. The application to nails of commercially available topical preparations with thymol, such as Vicks VapoRub, has anecdotally led to success. Topical therapy may be useful as a means to prevent recurrence.

Mechanical Intervention: Trimming, debridement, nail bed curettage, and nail abrasion may speed delivery of medications to the site of action. Other options for refractory cases include laser, surgical avulsion, or chemical removal of the nail with 40% urea compounds in combination with topical or oral antifungals.

PIEDRA

Piedra is an asymptomatic superficial fungal infection of the hair shaft also known as trichomycosis nodularis. Black piedra is caused by *Piedraia hortae*, whereas white piedra is caused by pathogenic species of the *Trichosporon* genus, namely *Trichosporon asahii*, *Trichosporon ovoides*, *Trichosporon inkin*, *Trichosporon mucoides*, *Trichosporon asteroides*, and *Trichosporon cutaneum*.[60]

EPIDEMIOLOGY

Black piedra is seen commonly in humans and primates of tropical areas of South America, the Pacific Islands, and the Far East, and less commonly in Africa and Asia. *P. hortae* is present in the soil, stagnant water, and crops. Scalp hair is most often affected. In fact, infection is encouraged for religious and esthetic reasons by some indigenous cultures.[61]

White piedra is most common in temperate and semitropical climates of South America and Asia, the Middle East, India, Africa, and Japan. It occurs infrequently in the United States and Europe. White piedra affects facial, axillary, and genital hair more commonly than scalp hair. *T. ovoides* is found more commonly on scalp hair, *T. inkin* on pubic hair, and *T. asahii* on other body surfaces. Person-to-person transmission is rare, and infection is not associated with travel to endemic areas.[62]

TABLE 160-13
Differential Diagnosis of Onychomycosis

Most Likely
- Psoriasis, lichen planus, chronic trauma, onychogryphosis

Consider
- Pachyonychia congenita, acquired and congenital leukonychias, Darier-White disease, yellow nail syndrome

Rule Out
- Melanoma

CLINICAL FINDINGS

Black piedra is characterized by firmly attached, hard or gritty, brown-black–colored concretions on the hair shaft that vary in size from the microscopic range to a few millimeters in size. Concretions are most commonly noted on frontal portions of the scalp. Black piedra weakens the hair shaft and results in hair breakage.

White piedra consists of softer and less-adherent whitish to beige–colored concretions that are discrete or may coalesce into sleeve-like structures along the hair shaft. These concretions affect the outer layers of the hair shaft and may be easily detached. Broken hairs, although sometimes present, are less common than in black piedra.[60]

DIAGNOSIS

Nodules of black piedra examined by KOH preparation display a periphery of aligned hyphae and a well-organized center of thick-walled cells packed closely together, sometimes termed *pseudoparenchyma*. These nodules are mostly outside of the hair shaft. *P. hortae* grows well, albeit slowly, on most laboratory media and is uninhibited by cycloheximide. The nodules of white piedra have a less organized and more intrapilar appearance than do nodules of black piedra. Hyphae are arranged perpendicularly to the hair shaft. *T. asahii* thrives on SDA and it is inhibited by cycloheximide. Microscopy readily differentiates piedra from nits, hair casts, developmental hair shaft defects, and trichomycosis axillaris. In addition, the nodules of trichomycosis axillaris are usually smaller and may fluoresce under a Wood lamp.

DIFFERENTIAL DIAGNOSIS

Table 160-14 summarizes the differential diagnosis of piedra.

MANAGEMENT

Shaving the infected hair is curative and represents the best treatment of both black and white piedra, although this approach should be supplemented with a topical azole preparation (see Table 160-11). Because of high relapse rates, as well as evidence for intrafollicular organisms in white piedra, some advocate the use of a systemic antifungal agent such as itraconazole.[62]

TABLE 160-14
Differential Diagnosis of Piedra

Most Likely
- Pediculosis, trichomycosis axillaris, tinea capitis

Consider
- Monilethrix

TINEA BARBAE

EPIDEMIOLOGY

Tinea barbae, as its name would imply, occurs predominantly in the beard area of males. The incidence of tinea barbae has decreased as improved sanitation has reduced transmission by contaminated barbers' razors. Direct exposure to cattle, horses, or dogs is now the more common mode of acquisition, and thus accounts for a shift in prevalence toward farmers or ranchers in rural settings.

CLINICAL FINDINGS

Table 160-12 summarizes the subtypes and most common causes of tinea barbae.

Tinea barbae affects the face unilaterally and involves the beard area more often than the moustache or upper lip. Two forms exist, superficial and inflammatory types.

Superficial Type: Caused by anthropophilics such as *T. violaceum*, this form of tinea barbae is less inflammatory and resembles tinea corporis or bacterial folliculitis. The active border shows perifollicular papules and pustules accompanied by mild erythema (Fig. 160-4A). Alopecia, if present, is reversible.

Inflammatory Type: Usually caused by *T. interdigitale* (zoophilic strains) or *T. verrucosum*, inflammatory tinea barbae is the most common clinical presentation. It presents analogously to kerion formation in tinea capitis with boggy-crusted plaques and a seropurulent discharge (see Fig. 160-4B). Hairs are lusterless, brittle, and easily epilated to demonstrate a purulent mass around the root. Perifollicular pustules may coalesce and eventuate in abscess-like collections of pus, sinus tracts, and scarring alopecia.

ETIOLOGY AND PATHOGENESIS

Tinea barbae is most commonly caused by the zoophilic strains of *T. interdigitale* (formerly named *Trichophyton mentagrophytes* var. *mentagrophytes*), *T. verrucosum*, and, less commonly, *M. canis*. Among the anthropophilic organisms, *Trichophyton schoenleinii*, *T. violaceum*, and certain strains of *T. rubrum* (formerly named *T. megninii*) cause tinea barbae in endemic areas.[63]

DIAGNOSIS

Table 160-4 outlines common laboratory dermatophyte identification methods and Table 160-6 outlines the colony and microscopic morphology features of the most common dermatophytes.

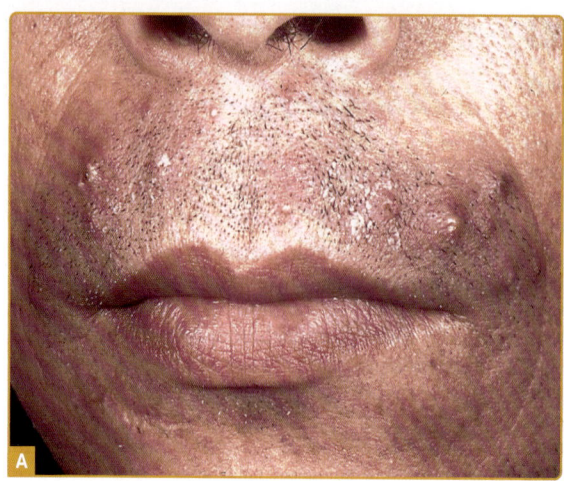
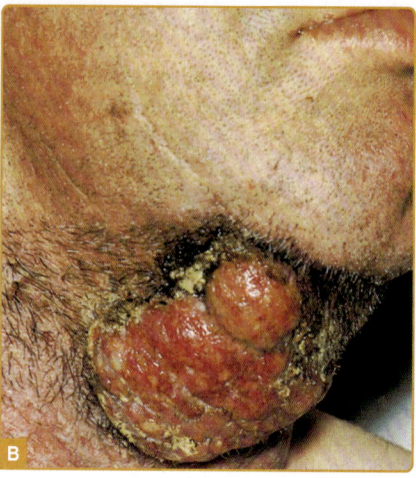

Figure 160-4 Tinea barbae. **A,** Superficial type. Scattered follicular papules, pustules, and small nodules, which may be easily mistaken for *Staphylococcus aureus* folliculitis. **B,** Kerion type. Sharply demarcated red edematous nodule studded with multiple yellowish weeping pustules. Note hairs have been lost from this nodule.

DIFFERENTIAL DIAGNOSIS

Table 160-15 summarizes the differential diagnosis of tinea barbae.

MANAGEMENT

Table 160-9 outlines the treatment of dermatophytes, Table 160-10 lists oral antifungal agents, and Table 160-11 lists topical antifungal agents.

Like tinea capitis (see below), an oral antifungal is usually necessary in the treatment of tinea barbae. Systemic glucocorticoids used for the first week of therapy are helpful in cases with severe inflammation.

TINEA CAPITIS

Tinea capitis describes a dermatophyte infection of hair and scalp typically caused by *Trichophyton* and *Microsporum* species, with the exception of *Trichophyton concentricum*.

EPIDEMIOLOGY

Tinea capitis is most commonly observed in children between the ages of 3 and 14 years.[37] The fungistatic effect of fatty acids in sebum may help to explain the sharp decrease in incidence after puberty.[64] Overall prevalence of the carrier state is approximately 4% in the United States, with a peak prevalence of approximately 13% in girls of sub-Saharan African American descent.[65] For unknown reasons, tinea capitis is generally more common among children of African descent. Transmission is increased with decreased personal hygiene, overcrowding, and low socioeconomic status. The anthropophilic dermatophyte *T. tonsurans* is the most prevalent species found in the United States and United Kingdom, while *M. canis* remains the most common cause of tinea capitis in Europe.[37,66] Organisms responsible for tinea capitis have been cultured from fomites such as combs, caps, pillowcases, toys, and theater seats. Even after shedding, hairs may harbor infectious organisms for more than 1 year.[67] The high prevalence of asymptomatic carriers thwarts eradication of the disease.

CLINICAL FINDINGS

Table 160-12 summarizes the subtypes and most common causes of tinea capitis.

The clinical appearance of tinea capitis depends on the causative species and other factors, such as the host immune response. In general, dermatophyte infection of the scalp results in hair loss and scaling with varying degrees of an inflammatory response.

Noninflammatory Type: Also called the seborrheic form of tinea capitis (because scale is the predominant feature),[68] noninflammatory tinea capitis is seen most commonly with anthropophilic organisms such as *M. audouinii* or *Microsporum ferrugineum*. Arthroconidia may form a sheath around affected hairs, turning them gray and causing them to break off just above the level of the scalp. Alopecia may be imperceptible or, in more inflammatory cases, may have circumscribed erythematous scaly patches of nonscarring alopecia

TABLE 160-15
Differential Diagnosis of Tinea Barbae

Most Likely
- Bacterial folliculitis (sycosis vulgaris), pseudofolliculitis barbae, acne vulgaris, rosacea, contact dermatitis, perioral dermatitis, candidal folliculitis

Rule Out
- Herpes simplex, halogenoderma

with breakage of hairs ("gray patch" type; Fig. 160-5). Patches often occur on the occiput.[67] When involving an ectothrix pattern, infected hairs may exhibit green fluorescence under Wood light (see Table 160-8).

"Black Dot" Tinea Capitis: The "black dot" form of tinea capitis (Fig. 160-6) is typically caused by the anthropophilic endothrix organisms *T. tonsurans* and *T. violaceum*. Hairs broken off at the level of the scalp leave behind grouped black dots within patches of polygonal-shaped alopecia with finger-like margins. Normal hairs also remain within patches of broken hairs. Diffuse scaling is also often present. Even though "black dot" tinea capitis tends to be minimally inflammatory, some patients may develop follicular pustules, furuncle-like nodules, or, in rare cases, kerion—a boggy, inflammatory mass studded with broken hairs and follicular orifices oozing with pus.[69]

Inflammatory Type: Zoophilic or geophilic pathogens, such as *M. canis*, *M. gypseum*, and *T. verrucosum*, are more likely to cause an inflammatory type of tinea capitis via a hypersensitivity reaction. Resultant inflammation ranges from follicular pustules to furunculosis (Fig. 160-7) or kerion (Fig. 160-8). Intense inflammation may also result in scarring alopecia. The

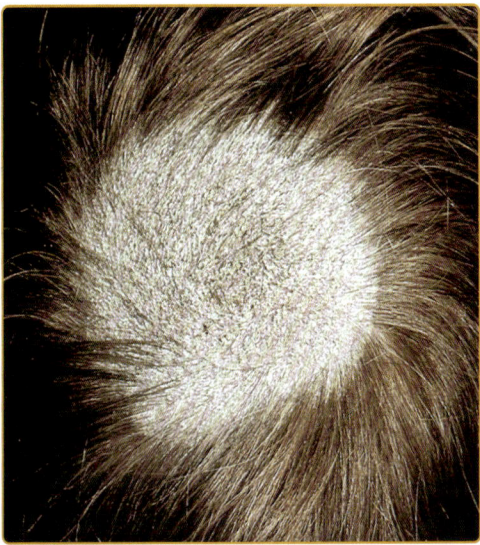

Figure 160-5 Tinea capitis "gray patch" type. A large, round, hyperkeratotic plaque of alopecia, a result of breaking off of hair shafts close to the surface, gives the appearance of a mowed wheat field on the scalp of a child. Remaining hair shafts and scales exhibit a green fluorescence when examined with a Wood lamp. *Microsporum canis* was isolated on culture.

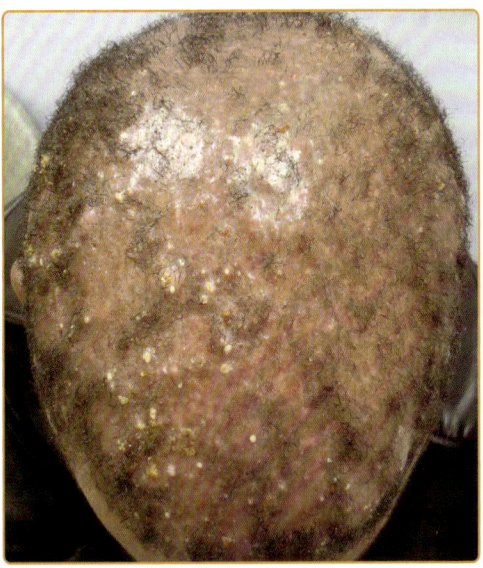

Figure 160-7 Inflammatory tinea capitis caused by *Microsporum canis*. Along with alopecia, there are inflammatory papules, pustules, and nodules. This patient also had posterior cervical lymphadenopathy.

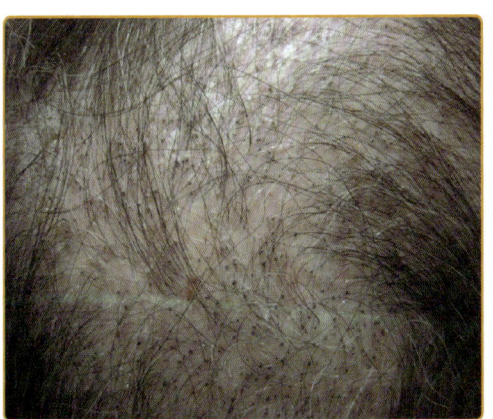

Figure 160-6 "Black dot" tinea capitis caused by *Trichophyton tonsurans*.

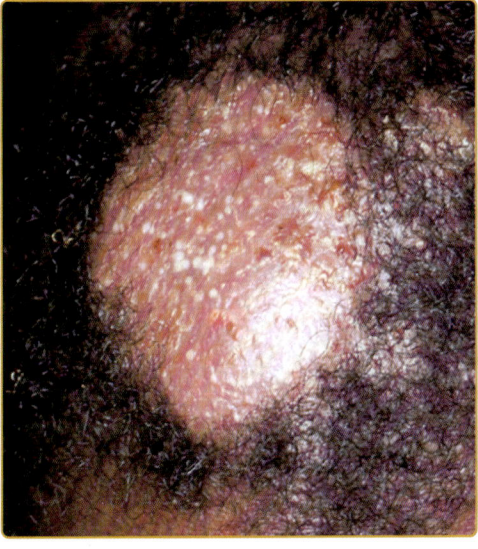

Figure 160-8 Kerion of the scalp.

scalp is usually pruritic or tender. Posterior cervical lymphadenopathy is often present, and may serve as a clinical pearl in differentiating tinea capitis from other inflammatory disorders involving the scalp.

DIAGNOSIS

Table 160-4 outlines common laboratory dermatophyte identification methods and Table 160-6 outlines the colony and microscopic morphology features of the most common dermatophytes.

Infection of hair by dermatophytes follows 3 main patterns—ectothrix, endothrix, and favus. Dermatophytes establish infection in the perifollicular stratum corneum and spread around and into the hair shaft of mid- to late-anagen hairs before descending into the follicle to penetrate the cortex. With hair growth, the infected part of the hair rises above the surface of the scalp where it may break because of its increased fragility.

In *ectothrix* infections (see Fig. 160-2), although hyphae are also present within the hair shaft, only the arthroconidia on the surface of the hair shaft may be visualized and the cuticle is destroyed. On Wood lamp examination, a yellow-green fluorescence may be detected, depending on the causative organism. In *endothrix* infections (see Fig. 160-2), arthroconidia and hyphae remain within the hair shaft and leave the cortex and cuticle intact. This pattern of tinea capitis is associated with the appearance of "black dots," which represent broken hairs at the surface of the scalp. *Endothrix* organisms do not show fluorescence on Wood lamp examination. *Favus* is characterized by longitudinally arranged hyphae and air spaces within the hair shaft. Arthroconidia are not usually noted in infected hairs of favus.

On histopathology of tinea capitis, PAS and methenamine silver stains readily reveal hyphae around and within hair shafts. The dermis demonstrates a perifollicular mixed cell infiltrate with lymphocytes, histiocytes, plasma cells, and eosinophils. Follicular disruption leads to an adjacent foreign-body giant cell reaction. Markedly inflammatory lesions, such as a kerion, demonstrate an acute infiltrate of polymorphonuclear leukocytes within the dermis and follicle.[70] Organisms may not be visualized in kerion because the intense host response destroys many of the fungal organisms. However, fungal antigens may be detectable with immunofluorescent techniques.[71]

DIFFERENTIAL DIAGNOSIS

Table 160-16 summarizes the differential diagnosis of tinea capitis.

MANAGEMENT

Table 160-9 outlines the treatment of tinea capitis, Table 160-10 lists oral antifungal agents, and Table 160-11 lists topical antifungal agents.

Infections involving hair-bearing skin usually necessitate oral antifungal treatment, as dermatophytes penetrating the follicle are typically "out of reach" for topically applied agents. As such, topical therapy alone is not recommended for the management of tinea capitis.[37] It is reasonable to begin empiric oral treatment reflecting local epidemiology and the most likely culprit organism while awaiting confirmatory mycology.[37]

Adjuvant Therapy: Selenium sulfide (1% and 2.5%), zinc pyrithione (1% and 2%), povidone-iodine (2.5%), and ketoconazole (2%) are shampoo preparations that help eradicate dermatophytes from the scalp. Adjunctive use of these shampoos is recommended 2 to 4 times weekly for 2 to 4 weeks.[72] The thrice weekly use of ketoconazole 2% shampoo or selenium sulfide 2.5% by all household members also reduces transmission by decreasing the shedding of spores.[73] Oral glucocorticoids may reduce the incidence of scarring associated with markedly inflammatory varieties of tinea capitis. Although there is no consistent evidence for improved cure rates with use of oral glucocorticoids, they appear to relieve pain and swelling associated with infections. The usual regimen is prednisone 1 to 2 mg/kg each morning during the first week of therapy.

TABLE 160-16
Differential Diagnosis of Tinea Capitis

Most Likely
- Seborrheic dermatitis, contact dermatitis, pustular or plaque psoriasis, atopic dermatitis, bacterial pyodermas, folliculitis decalvans, lichen planopilaris, and dissecting cellulitis of the scalp

Consider
- Alopecia areata, trichotillomania, pseudopelade, psoriasiform reaction to tumor necrosis factor-α inhibitor

Rule Out
- Discoid lupus erythematosus, syphilis

TINEA CORPORIS

Tinea corporis refers to any dermatophytosis of glabrous skin except palms, soles, and the groin.

EPIDEMIOLOGY

Tinea corporis may be transmitted directly from infected humans or animals, via fomites, or it may occur via autoinoculation from reservoirs of dermatophyte colonization on the feet.[74] Children are more likely to contract zoophilic pathogens, especially *M. canis*, from dogs or cats. Occlusive clothing and a humid climate are associated with more frequent and severe eruptions.[75] Wearing of occlusive clothing, frequent skin-to-skin contact, and minor traumas, such as the mat burns in competitive wrestling, create an environment in which dermatophytes flourish. "Tinea corporis gladiatorum" is caused most commonly by *T. tonsurans*, and it occurs most frequently on the head, neck, and arms.[76]

CLINICAL FINDINGS

Table 160-12 summarizes the subtypes and most common causes of tinea corporis.

The classic presentation is that of an annular ("ringworm"-like; Fig. 160-9A) or serpiginous plaque with scale across the entire active erythematous border. The border, which may be vesicular, advances centrifugally. The center of the plaque is usually scaly but may exhibit complete clearance. Whereas concentric vesicular rings suggest tinea incognito (often caused by *T. rubrum*), the erythematous concentric rings of tinea imbricata demonstrate little to no vesiculation. *T. rubrum* infections may also present as large, confluent, polycyclic (Fig. 160-9B) or psoriasiform (Fig. 160-9C) plaques, especially in immunosuppressed individuals.

Majocchi granuloma is a superficial and subcutaneous dermatophytic infection involving deeper portions of the hair follicles, presenting as scaly, follicular papules and nodules that coalesce in an annular arrangement (Fig. 160-10). It is most commonly caused by *T. rubrum*, *T. interdigitale*, and *M. canis*. Majocchi granuloma is observed on the legs of women who become inoculated after shaving or who apply topical corticosteroids to the involved area, thereby facilitating infection. It also has been increasingly observed among immunocompromised patients.[77]

ETIOLOGY AND PATHOGENESIS

Although any dermatophyte can cause tinea corporis, it is caused most commonly caused by *T. rubrum*, which is also the most likely candidate in cases with concomitant follicular involvement.[69] *E. floccosum*, *T. interdigitale* (anthropophilic and zoophilic strains), *M. canis*, and *T. tonsurans* are also common pathogens.[1] Tinea imbricata, caused by *T. concentricum*, is limited geographically to areas of the Far East, South Pacific, and South and Central America.

DIAGNOSIS

Table 160-4 outlines common laboratory dermatophyte identification methods and Table 160-6 outlines the colony and microscopic morphology features of the most common dermatophytes.

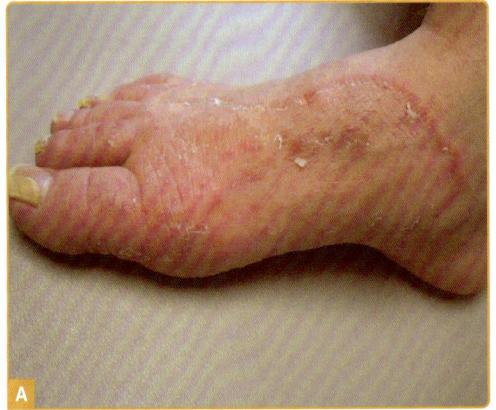
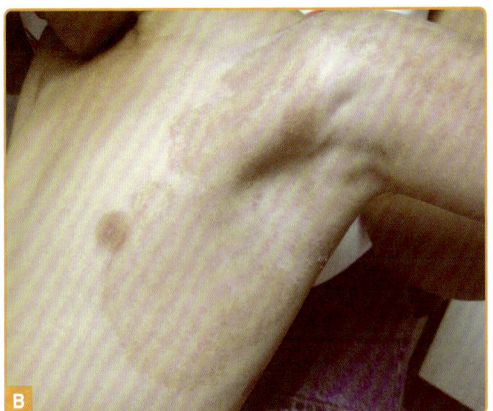
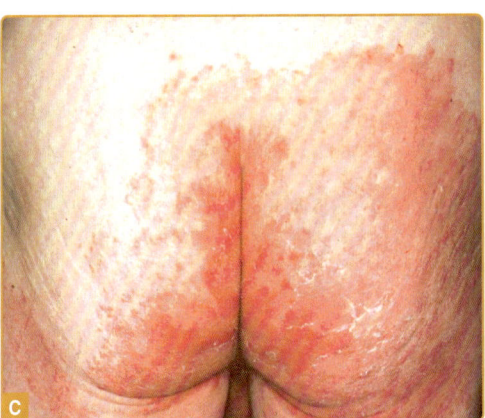

Figure 160-9 Tinea corporis. **A,** Annular. Tinea corporis demonstrating the classic annular or "ringworm"-like configuration and advancing raised erythematous and scaly border. Note that because the dorsum of the foot is predominantly involved, this eruption is considered tinea corporis and not tinea pedis. **B,** Polycyclic. Tinea corporis demonstrating multiple polycyclic red erythematous plaques with a raised scaly border. **C,** Psoriasiform. Tinea corporis resembling psoriasis.

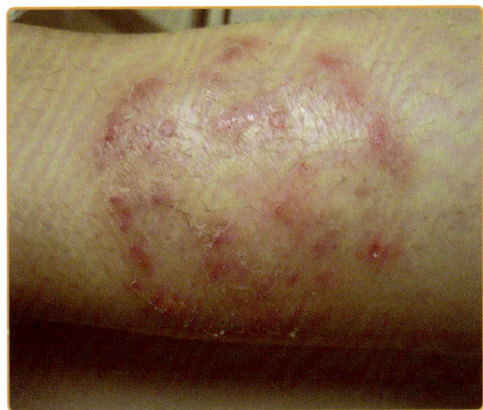

Figure 160-10 Majocchi granuloma. Follicular papules and nodules with scale coalescing to form an annular-shaped plaque on the leg of a woman applying topical corticosteroids to the area.

DIFFERENTIAL DIAGNOSIS

Table 160-17 summarizes the differential diagnosis of tinea corporis.

MANAGEMENT

Table 160-9 outlines the treatment of tinea corporis, Table 160-10 lists oral antifungal agents, and Table 160-11 lists topical antifungal agents.

For isolated plaques on the glabrous skin, topical allylamines (eg, terbinafine), imidazoles (eg, clotrimazole), tolnaftate, butenafine, and ciclopirox are effective. Most are applied twice daily for 2 to 4 weeks. Oral antifungal agents are reserved for widespread or more inflammatory eruptions.

TINEA CRURIS

Tinea cruris is a dermatophytosis of the groin, genitalia, pubic area, and perineal and perianal skin. The designation is a misnomer, because in Latin, "cruris" means "of the leg." It is the second-most common type of dermatophytosis worldwide.

EPIDEMIOLOGY

Much like tinea corporis, tinea cruris spreads via direct contact or fomites, and is exacerbated by occlusion and humidity. Autoinfection from distant reservoirs of *T. rubrum* or *T. interdigitale* on the feet, for example, is common.[74] Tinea cruris is 3 times more common in men, and adults are affected more often than children.

CLINICAL FINDINGS

Tinea cruris presents classically as a well-marginated annular plaque with a scaly raised border that extends from the inguinal fold to the inner thigh, often bilaterally. Presentation with erythematous, scaly patches with papules and vesicles involving the inner thighs is also common but perhaps less obvious. Pruritus is common, as is pain when plaques are macerated or secondarily infected. Plaques in tinea cruris caused by *E. floccosum* are more likely to demonstrate central clearing with involvement of the genitocrural crease and medial upper thigh. In contrast, plaques in tinea cruris caused by *T. rubrum* coalesce with extension to the pubic, perianal, buttock, and lower abdominal areas (Fig. 160-11). Genitalia (including the scrotum) are infrequently affected and may be useful to distinguish from other conditions such as inverse psoriasis.[63]

ETIOLOGY AND PATHOGENESIS

Most tinea cruris is caused by *T. rubrum* and *E. floccosum*, the latter being most often responsible for epidemics.[63] *T. interdigitale* and *T. verrucosum* are implicated less often.

DIAGNOSIS

Table 160-4 outlines common laboratory dermatophyte identification methods and Table 160-6 outlines the colony and microscopic morphology features of the most common dermatophytes.

DIFFERENTIAL DIAGNOSIS

Table 160-18 summarizes the differential diagnosis of tine cruris.

MANAGEMENT

Medical treatment of tinea cruris is the same as that for tinea corporis, which is discussed earlier.

In addition to medical treatment, it also may be helpful to correct any underlying moisture issues in the affected area (with use of loose-fitted clothing and regular application of barrier-protective zinc-containing cream) or other areas of infection (eg, tinea pedis). If tinea pedis is present, in addition to medical treatment targeting the feet, one might also recommend the patient apply socks before underwear so as to prevent autoinoculation of the area.

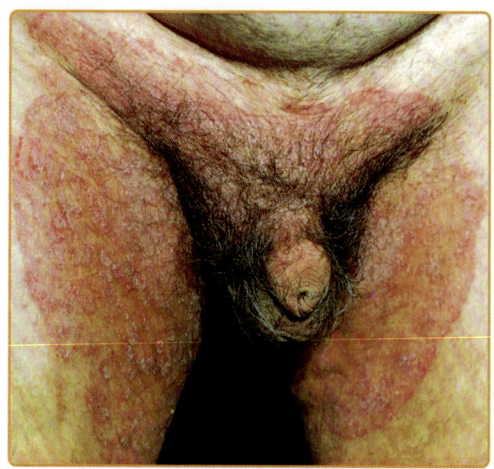

Figure 160-11 Tinea cruris. Annular erythematous plaques with a raised scaling border expanding from the inguinal on the inner thighs and pubic region.

TABLE 160-17
Differential Diagnosis of Tinea Corporis

Most Likely
- Erythema annulare centrifugum, nummular eczema, psoriasis, tinea versicolor, subacute cutaneous lupus erythematosus, cutaneous candidiasis

Consider
- Contact dermatitis, atopic dermatitis, pityriasis rosea, seborrheic dermatitis

Rule Out
- Mycosis fungoides, parapsoriasis, secondary syphilis

TABLE 160-18
Differential Diagnosis of Tinea Cruris

Most Likely
- Erythrasma, cutaneous candidiasis, intertrigo, contact dermatitis, inverse psoriasis, seborrheic dermatitis, lichen simplex chronicus, folliculitis

Consider
- Familial benign pemphigus, Darier-White disease, histiocytosis

TINEA FAVOSA

Tinea favosa or favus (Latin for "honeycomb") is a chronic dermatophyte infection of the scalp that rarely involves glabrous skin and/or nails, and is characterized by thick yellow crusts (scutula) within the hair follicles that lead to scarring alopecia.

EPIDEMIOLOGY

Favus is usually acquired before adolescence, but may extend into adulthood.[78] It is associated with malnutrition and poor hygiene. Over the last century, favus has become geographically limited and is now seen almost exclusively in Africa, the Middle East, and parts of South America. Even these regions have had a dramatic decrease in incidence with studies from South Africa, Libya, and Arabia suggesting disappearance of favus over the last few decades.[79-81]

CLINICAL FINDINGS

During the first 3 weeks of infection, early favus is characterized by patchy perifollicular erythema with slight scaling and matting of the hair. Progressive hyphal invasion distends the follicle, first producing a yellow-red follicular papule, then a yellow concave crust (scutulum) around a single dry hair (Fig. 160-12) that is less brittle than hair of endothrix infections. The scutulum may reach 1 cm in diameter, engulfing surrounding hairs, and coalescing with other scutula to form large, adherent mats with an unpleasant cheese-like or musky odor. Over several years, the plaques advance peripherally leaving behind central, atrophic areas of alopecia.[63]

ETIOLOGY AND PATHOGENESIS

T. schoenleinii is the most common cause of human favus, with *T. violaceum* and *M. gypseum* also as rare isolates.[63] Although favus occurs in animals including domesticated birds (*Microsporum gallinae*) and mice (*T. mentagrophytes* formerly named *T. mentagrophytes* var. *quinckeanum*), there exist only a few reports of human infection by the same pathogens responsible for animal favus.[82]

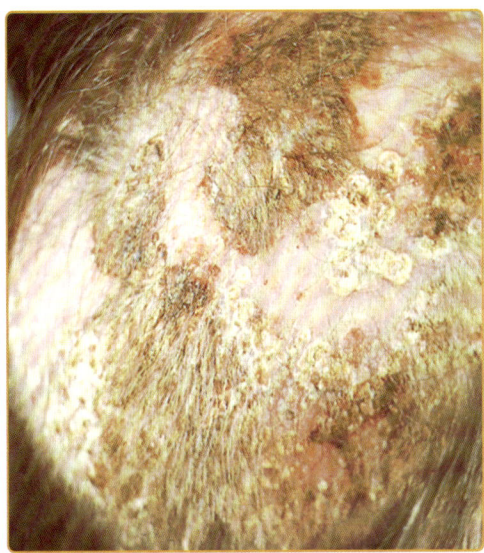

Figure 160-12 Favus caused by *Trichophyton schoenleinii*. Note the numerous yellow scutula.

DIAGNOSIS

Table 160-4 outlines common laboratory dermatophyte identification methods and Table 160-6 outlines the colony and microscopic morphology features of the most common dermatophytes.

T. schoenleinii exhibits subtle, blue-gray fluorescence along the entire hair with Wood lamp examination. Microscopy with KOH preparation reveals hyphae arranged lengthwise around and within the hair shaft, rare arthroconidia, and vacant air spaces.[63]

DIFFERENTIAL DIAGNOSIS

Table 160-13 outlines the differential diagnosis of onychomycosis.

MANAGEMENT

Treatment is the same as for tinea capitis.

TINEA MANUUM

Tinea manuum is discussed with tinea pedis under the section "Tinea Pedis and Tinea Manuum."

TINEA NIGRA

Tinea nigra is a superficial dermatomycosis caused by dematiaceous, darkly pigmented, *Hortaea werneckii* (formerly named *Phaeoannellomyces werneckii* and *Exophiala werneckii*).[83]

EPIDEMIOLOGY

Tinea nigra occurs in tropical or subtropical areas, including Central and South America, Africa, and Asia. Its incidence is low in the United States and Europe. Although the majority of the approximately 150 North American cases reported since 1950 were associated with tropical travel,[63] endemic foci exist in the coastal southeastern United States and in Texas. Person-to-person transmission is rare.[84] Tinea nigra has a female-to-male predilection of 3:1.

CLINICAL FINDINGS

Tinea nigra is found on otherwise healthy people and presents typically as an asymptomatic, mottled brown to greenish-black macule or patch with minimal to no scale on the palms or soles (Fig. 160-13). The macule is often darkest at the advancing border. Because of its coloration and location on palms and soles, tinea nigra is frequently misdiagnosed as acral lentiginous melanoma.

ETIOLOGY AND PATHOGENESIS

Tinea nigra is almost always caused by *H. werneckii*, although other dematiaceous fungi such as *Stenella araguata* may produce the same clinical picture. Dematiaceous fungi are commonly found in soil, sewage, and decaying vegetation.[84] Tinea nigra arises after trauma to the skin with subsequent inoculation, and a typical incubation period of 2 to 7 weeks.

DIAGNOSIS

KOH examination of scrapings from the macule reveals brown to olive-colored, thick branching hyphae, along with oval to spindle-shaped yeast cells that occur singly or in pairs with a central transverse septum. Cultures performed on SDA with cycloheximide and chloramphenicol grow within 1 week. The colony is initially yeast-like with a brown to shiny black color and appears as typical 2-celled yeast forms under microscopic examination. With time, mycelial growth predominates creating a fuzzy grayish-black colony.

DIFFERENTIAL DIAGNOSIS

Table 160-19 outlines the differential diagnosis of tinea nigra.

MANAGEMENT

Table 160-9 outlines the treatment of dermatophytes and Table 160-11 lists topical antifungal agents.

Tinea nigra responds readily to topical therapy with a keratolytic (Whitfield ointment, 2% salicylic acid), tincture of iodine, or topical antifungal.[85,86] Treatment should be continued for 2 to 4 weeks after clinical resolution to prevent relapse. Although oral ketoconazole, itraconazole, and terbinafine are also effective, systemic therapies are rarely indicated.[83]

TINEA PEDIS AND TINEA MANUUM

Tinea pedis denotes dermatophytosis of the feet, whereas tinea manuum involves the palmar and interdigital areas of the hands. Infection of the dorsal aspects of feet and hands is considered to be tinea corporis.

EPIDEMIOLOGY

Occurring worldwide, tinea pedis and tinea manuum are the most common dermatophytoses. Estimated to be approximately 10%, the high prevalence is attributed primarily to modern occlusive footwear, although increased worldwide travel also has been implicated.[63] Incidence of tinea pedis is higher among those using communal baths, showers, or pools. With the

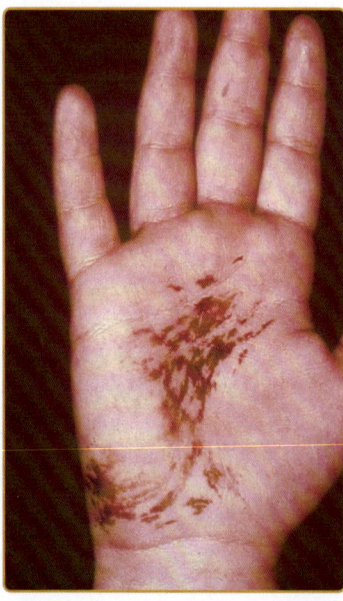

Figure 160-13 Tinea nigra palmaris. An irregular, brownish-black patch on the palm caused by *Hortaea werneckii*.

TABLE 160-19
Differential Diagnosis of Tinea Nigra

Most Likely
- Junctional nevus, dysplastic nevus, melanoma

Consider
- Chemical exposure

Rule Out
- Addison disease, syphilis, yaws

ubiquitous presence of dermatophytes in the environment, however, it may be that host factors, such as an individual's immune response to dermatophytes, play a determining role in the development of tinea pedis.

Tinea manuum is acquired through direct contact with an infected person or animal, the soil, or via autoinoculation. Most commonly only 1 hand (*singular*: tinea manus) is involved, concomitant with infection of feet and toenails for which the term *two feet–one hand* syndrome has been coined. This classic presentation of tinea manus represents a secondary infection of the hand acquired from excoriating and picking infected feet and toenails.[87] Tinea manuum should be suspected in individuals who have fine dry scaling of the palm or palms, often accentuated in the creases.

CLINICAL FINDINGS

Table 160-12 summarizes the subtypes and most common causes of tinea pedis and tinea manuum.

Tinea pedis may present as any of the following forms, or combinations thereof.

Interdigital Type: The interdigital type, the most common presentation of tinea pedis, begins as scaling, erythema, and maceration of the interdigital and subdigital skin of the feet, particularly between the lateral third and fourth and fourth and fifth toes (Fig. 160-14A). Under appropriate conditions, the infection will spread to the adjacent sole or instep, but it rarely involves the dorsum. Occlusion and bacterial coinfection (*Pseudomonas*, *Proteus*, and *Staphylococcus aureus*) soon produce the interdigital erosions with pruritus and malodor that are characteristic of the dermatophytosis complex, or "athlete's foot."

Chronic Hyperkeratotic (Moccasin) Type: Chronic hyperkeratotic (moccasin) type tinea pedis, is characterized by patchy or diffuse scaling on the soles and the lateral and medial aspects of the feet, in a distribution similar to a moccasin on a foot (see Fig. 160-14B). The degree of erythema is variable, and there may also exist a few minute vesicles that heal with collarets of scale less than 2 mm in diameter. The most common pathogen is *T. rubrum* followed by *E. floccosum* and anthropophilic strains of *T. interdigitale*.

Vesiculobullous Type: Vesiculobullous type of tinea pedis, typically caused by zoophilic strains of *T. interdigitale* (formerly named *T. mentagrophytes* var. *mentagrophytes*), features tense vesicles larger than 3 mm in diameter, vesiculopustules, or bullae on the soles and periplantar areas (see Fig. 160-14C). This type of tinea pedis is uncommon in childhood but has been caused by *T. rubrum*.[88]

Acute Ulcerative Type: Acute ulcerative type tinea pedis caused by zoophilic *T. interdigitale* in combination with Gram-negative bacterial superinfection produces vesicles, pustules, and purulent ulcers on the plantar surface. Cellulitis, lymphangitis, lymphadenopathy, and fever are frequently associated.

Vesicular Id Reaction: Vesiculobullous and acute ulcerative types commonly produce a vesicular id reaction, either on the lateral foot or toes, or on the lateral aspects of the fingers.

Tinea Manuum: Dermatophyte infection of the hand usually has a noninflammatory presentation with diffuse dry scaling and accentuation in the creases (Fig. 160-15). However, vesicles, pustules, and exfoliation may be present, especially when zoophilic dermatophytes are involved. Tinea manuum commonly occurs in association with moccasin-type tinea pedis and onychomycosis, all of which should be treated to minimize relapse.[89]

ETIOLOGY AND PATHOGENESIS

Tinea pedis and tinea manuum are caused predominantly by *T. rubrum* (most common), *T. interdigitale*, and *E. floccosum*.

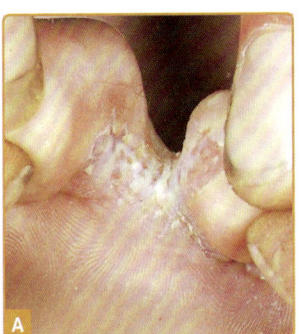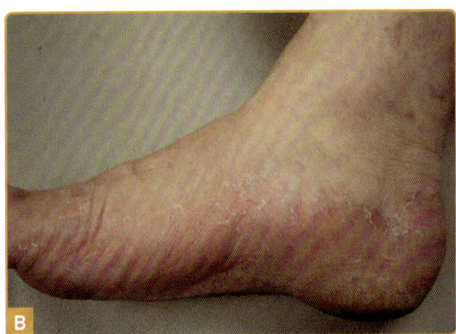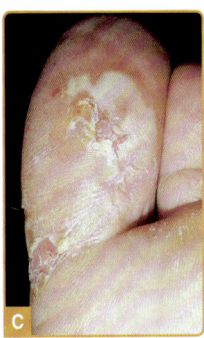

Figure 160-14 Tinea pedis. **A,** Interdigital type. The interdigital space is macerated with opaque white scales and has erosions. **B,** Moccasin type. Patchy erythema and scaling in a moccasin distribution on the foot. The arciform pattern of scales is characteristic. **C,** Bullous type. Ruptured bullae, erosions and erythema on the plantar aspect of the great toe. Hyphae were detected on KOH 10% preparation obtained from epithelial cell on the roof of the inner aspect of the bulla.

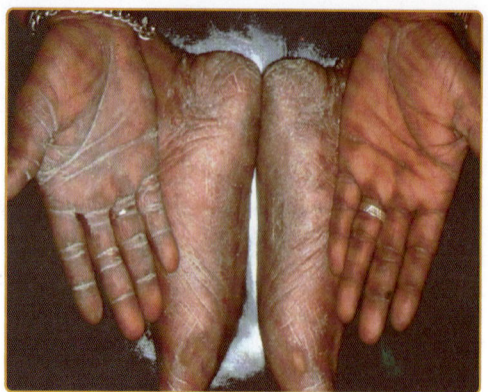

Figure 160-15 Tinea pedis and manus. "Two feet–one hand" presentation of *Trichophyton rubrum*. Scaling in the involved (*right*) hand is accentuated in the creases.

TABLE 160-20
Differential Diagnosis of Tinea Pedis

Most Likely
- *Interdigital:* erosio interdigitalis blastomycetica, erythrasma, bacterial coinfection
- *Hyperkeratotic:* dyshidrosis, psoriasis, contact dermatitis, atopic dermatitis, hereditary or acquired keratodermas
- *Vesiculobullous:* dyshidrosis, contact dermatitis, pustular psoriasis, bacterid or other autoeczematization, palmoplantar pustulosis, bacterial pyodermas, scabies

Consider
- Pityriasis rubra pilaris

Rule Out
- Reactive arthritis

DIAGNOSIS

Table 160-4 outlines common laboratory dermatophyte identification methods and Table 160-6 outlines the colony and microscopic morphology features of the most common dermatophytes.

KOH examination of blister roofs (vesicles or bullae) yields the highest rate of positive findings. Histopathologic evaluation of tinea pedis reveals fungal organisms highlighted in the stratum corneum by PAS or methenamine silver stains, sometimes accompanied by foci of neutrophils. There also may be a sparse, chronic, superficial perivascular infiltrate in the dermis. Subcorneal or spongiotic intraepithelial vesiculation may be seen in the vesiculobullous type of tinea pedis.

DIFFERENTIAL DIAGNOSIS

Table 160-20 outlines the differential diagnosis of tinea pedis.

MANAGEMENT

Table 160-9 outlines the treatment of dermatophytes, Table 160-10 lists oral antifungal agents, and Table 160-11 lists topical antifungal agents.

Mild interdigital tinea pedis without bacterial involvement is treated topically with allylamine, imidazole, ciclopirox, benzylamine, tolnaftate, or undecenoic acid–based creams. Terbinafine cream applied twice daily for 1 week is effective in 66% of cases.[90] Topical or systemic corticosteroids may be helpful for symptomatic relief during the initial period of antifungal treatment of vesiculobullous tinea pedis. Associated onychomycosis is common, and if present, requires a more durable oral treatment of the onychomycosis to prevent recurrence of tinea pedis. Maceration, denudation, pruritus, and malodor obligate a search for bacterial coinfection by Gram stain and culture, the results of which most often demonstrate the presence of Gram-negative organisms including *Pseudomonas* and *Proteus*. Patients suspected of having Gram-negative coinfections should be treated with a topical or systemic antibacterial agent based on the culture and sensitivity report. Another useful treatment of both cutaneous fungal and bacterial (including pseudomonas) infection is the use of dilute acetoacetic acid soaks; this may be of particular benefit to reduce the risk of cellulitis in patients with diabetes mellitus, chronic venous stasis or other causes of lower-extremity edema.

ACKNOWLEDGMENTS

Many thanks, to Dr. Amit Garg who served as senior author of previous editions and provided the great majority of clinical images in this chapter.

REFERENCES

1. Aly R. Ecology and epidemiology of dermatophyte infections. *J Am Acad Dermatol*. 1994;31:S21.
2. Graser Y, Scott J, Summerbell R. The new species concept in dermatophytes—a polyphasic approach. *Mycopathologia*. 2008;166:239.
3. Hibbett D. The invisible dimension of fungal diversity. *Science*. 2016;351:1150-1151.
4. Greer DL. An overview of common dermatophytes. *J Am Acad Dermatol*. 1994;31:S112.
5. Havlickova B, Czaika VA, Friedrich M. Epidemiological trends in skin mycoses worldwide. *Mycoses*. 2008;51(suppl 4):2.
6. Foster KW, Ghannoum MA, Elewski BE. Epidemiologic surveillance of cutaneous fungal infection in the United States from 1999 to 2002. *J Am Acad Dermatol*. 2004;50:748.
7. Ginter-Hanselmayer G, Weger W, Ilkit M, et al. Epidemiology of tinea capitis in Europe: current state and changing patterns. *Mycoses*. 2007;50(suppl 2):6.
8. Seebacher C, Bouchara JP, Mignon B. Updates on the epidemiology of dermatophyte infections. *Mycopathologia*. 2008;166:335.
9. Magill SS, Manfredi L, Swiderski A, et al. Isolation of *Trichophyton violaceum* and *Trichophyton soudanense* in Baltimore, Maryland. *J Clin Microbiol*. 2007; 45:461.
10. Chastain MA, Reed RJ, Pankey GA. Deep dermatophytosis: report of 2 cases and review of the literature.

Cutis. 2001;67:457.
11. Tsang P, Hopkins T, Jimenez-Lucho V. Deep dermatophytosis caused by *Trichophyton rubrum* in a patient with AIDS. *J Am Acad Dermatol.* 1996;34:1090.
12. Johnson RA. Dermatophyte infections in human immune deficiency virus (HIV) disease. *J Am Acad Dermatol.* 2000;43:S135.
13. Garg AP, Muller J. Fungitoxicity of fatty acids against dermatophytes. *Mycoses.* 1993;36:51.
14. Bitencourt TA, Macedo C, Franco ME, et al. Transcription profile of *Trichophyton rubrum conidia* grown on keratin reveals the induction of an adhesin-like protein gene with a tandem repeat pattern. *BMC Genomics.* 2016;17:249.
15. Baeza LC, Bailao AM, Borges CL, et al. cDNA representational difference analysis used in the identification of genes expressed by *Trichophyton rubrum* during contact with keratin. *Microbes Infect.* 2007;9:1415.
16. Staib P, Zaugg C, Mignon B, et al. Differential gene expression in the pathogenic dermatophyte *Arthroderma benhamiae* in vitro versus infection. *Microbiology.* 2010;156(pt 3):884-895.
17. Baldo A, Mathy A, Tabart J, et al. Secreted subtilisin Sub3 from *Microsporum canis* is required for adherence to but not for invasion of the epidermis. *Br J Dermatol.* 2010;162(5):990-997.
18. Monod M, Capoccia S, Lechenne B, et al. Secreted proteases from pathogenic fungi. *Int J Med Microbiol.* 2002;292:405.
19. Blake JS, Dahl MV, Herron MJ, et al. An immunoinhibitory cell wall glycoprotein (mannan) from *Trichophyton rubrum. J Invest Dermatol.* 1991;96:657.
20. Dahl MV. Dermatophytosis and the immune response. *J Am Acad Dermatol.* 1994;31:S34.
21. Lilic D. Unravelling fungal immunity through primary immune deficiencies. *Curr Opin Microbiol.* 2012;15:420-426.
22. Treat J, James WD, Nachamkin I, et al. Growth inhibition of *Trichophyton* species by *Pseudomonas aeruginosa. Arch Dermatol.* 2007;143:61.
23. García-Madrid LA, Huizar-López M del R, Flores-Romo L, et al. *Trichophyton rubrum* manipulates the innate immune functions of human keratinocytes. *Cent Eur J Biol.* 2011;6:902-910.
24. Romani L. Immunity to fungal infections. *Nat Rev Immunol.* 2011;11:275-288.
25. Firat YH, Simanski M, Rademacher F, et al. Infection of keratinocytes with *Trichophytum rubrum* induces epidermal growth factor-dependent RNase 7 and human beta-defensin-3 expression. *PLoS One.* 2014;9:e93941.
26. Jensen JM, Pfeiffer S, Akaki T, et al. Barrier function, epidermal differentiation, and human beta-defensin 2 expression in tinea corporis. *J Invest Dermatol.* 2007;127:1720.
27. Leibovici V, Evron R, Axelrod O, et al. Imbalance of immune responses in patients with chronic and widespread fungal skin infection. *Clin Exp Dermatol.* 1995;20:390.
28. Sato K, Yang XL, Yudate T, et al. Dectin-2 is a pattern recognition receptor for fungi that couples with the Fc receptor gamma chain to induce innate immune responses. *J Biol Chem.* 2006;281:38854.
29. Robinson MJ, Osorio F, Rosas M, et al. Dectin-2 is a Syk-coupled pattern recognition receptor crucial for Th17 responses to fungal infection. *J Exp Med.* 2009;206:2037.
30. Shiraki Y, Ishibashi Y, Hiruma M, et al. Cytokine secretion profiles of human keratinocytes during *Trichophyton tonsurans* and *Arthroderma benhamiae* infections. *J Med Microbiol.* 2006;55:1175.
31. Tani K, Adachi M, Nakamura Y, et al. The effect of dermatophytes on cytokine production by human keratinocytes. *Arch Dermatol Res.* 2007;299:381.
32. Huang X, Yi J, Yin S, et al. Trichophyton rubrum conidia modulate the expression and transport of Toll-like receptor 2 in HaCaT cell. *Microb Pathog.* 2015;83-84:1-5.
33. Glocker EO, Hennigs A, Nabavi M, et al. A homozygous CARD9 mutation in a family with susceptibility to fungal infections. *N Engl J Med.* 2009;361:1727.
34. Panasiti V, Borroni RG, Devirgiliis V, et al. Comparison of diagnostic methods in the diagnosis of dermatomycoses and onychomycoses. *Mycoses.* 2006;49:26.
35. Weinberg JM, Koestenblatt EK, Tutrone WD, et al. Comparison of diagnostic methods in the evaluation of onychomycosis. *J Am Acad Dermatol.* 2003;49:193.
36. Ameen M, Lear JT, Madan V, et al. British Association of Dermatologists' guidelines for the management of onychomycosis 2014. *Br J Dermatol.* 2014;171:937-958.
37. Fuller LC, Barton RC, Mohd Mustapa MF, et al. British Association of Dermatologists' guidelines for the management of tinea capitis 2014. *Br J Dermatol.* 2014;171(3):454-463.
38. Hawkins DM, Smidt AC. Superficial fungal infections in children. *Pediatr Clin North Am.* 2014;61(2):443-455.
39. Grappel SF, Bishop CT, Blank F. Immunology of dermatophytes and dermatophytosis. *Bacteriol Rev.* 1974;38:222.
40. Kaaman T, Torssander J. Dermatophytid—a misdiagnosed entity? *Acta Derm Venereol.* 1983;63:404.
41. Veien NK, Hattel T, Laurberg G. Plantar *Trichophyton rubrum* infections may cause dermatophytids on the hands. *Acta Derm Venereol.* 1994;74:403.
42. Gianni C, Betti R, Crosti C. Psoriasiform id reaction in tinea corporis. *Mycoses.* 1996;39:307.
43. Calista D, Schianchi S, Morri M. Erythema nodosum induced by kerion celsi of the scalp. *Pediatr Dermatol.* 2001;18:114.
44. Weary PE, Guerrant JL. Chronic urticaria in association with dermatophytosis. Response to the administration of griseofulvin. *Arch Dermatol.* 1967;95:400.
45. Gupta AK, Jain HC, Lynde CW, et al. Prevalence and epidemiology of unsuspected onychomycosis in patients visiting dermatologists' offices in Ontario, Canada—a multicenter survey of 2001 patients. *Int J Dermatol.* 1997;36:783.
46. Ghannoum MA, Hajjeh RA, Scher R, et al. A large-scale North American study of fungal isolates from nails: the frequency of onychomycosis, fungal distribution, and antifungal susceptibility patterns. *J Am Acad Dermatol.* 2000;43:641.
47. Lange M, Roszkiewicz J, Szczerkowska-Dobosz A, et al. Onychomycosis is no longer a rare finding in children. *Mycoses.* 2006;49:55.
48. Svejgaard EL, Nilsson J. Onychomycosis in Denmark: prevalence of fungal nail infection in general practice. *Mycoses.* 2004;47:131.
49. Szepietowski JC, Reich A, Garlowska E, et al. Factors influencing coexistence of toenail onychomycosis with tinea pedis and other dermatomycoses: a survey of 2761 patients. *Arch Dermatol.* 2006;142:1279.
50. Prose NS, Abson KG, Scher RK. Disorders of the nails and hair associated with human immunodeficiency virus infection. *Int J Dermatol.* 1992;31:453.
51. Zaias N. Onychomycosis. *Arch Dermatol.* 1972;105:263.
52. Effendy I, Lecha M, Feuilhade de Chauvin M, et al.

Epidemiology and clinical classification of onychomycosis. *J Eur Acad Dermatol Venereol.* 2005;19(suppl 1):8.
53. Gupta AK, Jain HC, Lynde CW, et al. Prevalence and epidemiology of onychomycosis in patients visiting physicians' offices: a multicenter Canadian survey of 15,000 patients. *J Am Acad Dermatol.* 2000;43:244.
54. Summerbell RC, Cooper E, Bunn U, et al. Onychomycosis: a critical study of techniques and criteria for confirming the etiologic significance of nondermatophytes. *Med Mycol.* 2005;43:39.
55. Scher RK, Daniel CR. *Nails: Therapy, Diagnosis, Surgery.* Philadelphia, PA: Saunders; 1997.
56. Baran R. Topical amorolfine for 15 months combined with 12 weeks of oral terbinafine, a cost-effective treatment for onychomycosis. *Br J Dermatol.* 2001;145(suppl 60):15.
57. Gupta AK. Ciclopirox topical solution, 8% combined with oral terbinafine to treat onychomycosis: a randomized, evaluator-blinded study. *J Drugs Dermatol.* 2005;4:481.
58. Ramsewak RS, Nair MG, Stommel M, et al. In vitro antagonistic activity of monoterpenes and their mixtures against "toe nail fungus" pathogens. *Phytother Res.* 2003;17:376.
59. Pinto E, Pina-Vaz C, Salgueiro L, et al. Antifungal activity of the essential oil of *Thymus pulegioides* on *Candida, Aspergillus* and dermatophyte species. *J Med Microbiol.* 2006;55:1367.
60. Schwartz RA. Superficial fungal infections. *Lancet.* 2004;364:1173.
61. Coimbra Junior CE, Santos RV. Black piedra among the Zoró Indians from Amazonia (Brazil). *Mycopathologia.* 1989;107:57.
62. Kalter DC, Tschen JA, Cernoch PL, et al. Genital white piedra: epidemiology, microbiology, and therapy. *J Am Acad Dermatol.* 1986;14:982.
63. Rippon JW. Dermatophytosis and dermatomycosis. In: Rippon JW, ed. *Medical Mycology: Pathogenic Fungi and the Pathogenic Actinomycetes* . Philadelphia, PA: Saunders; 1988:169.
64. Shy R. Tinea corporis and tinea capitis. *Pediatr Rev.* 2007;28:164.
65. Sharma V, Hall JC, Knapp JF, et al. Scalp colonization by *Trichophyton tonsurans* in an urban pediatric clinic-asymptomatic carrier state. *Arch Dermatol.* 1988;124:1511.
66. Patel GA, Schwartz RA. Tinea capitis: still an unsolved problem? *Mycoses.* 2011;54(3):183-188.
67. Howard R, Frieden IJ. Tinea capitis: new perspectives on an old disease. *Semin Dermatol.* 1995;14:2.
68. Arenas R, Toussaint S, Isa-Isa R. Kerion and dermatophytic granuloma. Mycological and histopathological findings in 19 children with inflammatory tinea capitis of the scalp. *Int J Dermatol.* 2006;45:215.
69. Smith ML. Tinea capitis. *Pediatr Ann.* 1996;25:101.
70. Langley JB. Fungal diseases. In: Elder D, ed. *Lever's Histopathology of the Skin*. Philadelphia, PA: Lippincott; 1997:517.
71. Imamura S, Tanaka M, Watanabe S. Use of immunofluorescence staining in kerion. *Arch Dermatol.* 1975;111:906.
72. Pomeranz AJ, Sabnis SS. Tinea capitis: epidemiology, diagnosis and management strategies. *Paediatr Drugs.* 2002;4:779.
73. Elewski BE. Treatment of tinea capitis: beyond griseofulvin. *J Am Acad Dermatol.* 1999;40:S27.
74. Rebell G, Zaias N. Introducing the syndromes of human dermatophytosis. *Cutis.* 2001;67:6.
75. Taplin D. Dermatophytosis in Vietnam. *Cutis.* 2001;67:19.
76. Adams BB. Tinea corporis gladiatorum. *J Am Acad Dermatol.* 2002;47:286.
77. Elgart ML. Tinea incognito: an update on Majocchi granuloma. *Dermatol Clin.* 1996;14:51.
78. Khan KA, Anwar AA. Study of 73 cases of tinea capitis and tinea favosa in adults and adolescents. *J Invest Dermatol.* 1968;51:474.
79. Morar N, Dlova NC, Gupta AK, et al. Tinea capitis in Kwa-Zulu Natal, South Africa. *Pediatr Dermatol.* 2004;21:444.
80. Gargoom AM, Elyazachi MB, Al-Ani SM, et al. Tinea capitis in Benghazi, Libya. *Int J Dermatol.* 2000;39:263.
81. Venugopal PV, Venugopal TV. Tinea capitis in Saudi Arabia. *Int J Dermatol.* 1993;32:39.
82. Besbes M, Cheikhrouhou F, Sellami H, et al. Favus due to *Trichophyton mentagrophytes* var. *quinckeanum*. *Mycoses.* 2003;46:358.
83. Schwartz RA. Superficial fungal infections. *Lancet.* 2004;364:1173.
84. Vanvelsor H, Singletary H. Tinea nigra palmaris. A report of 15 cases from coastal North Carolina. *Arch Dermatol.* 1964;90:59.
85. Burke WA. Tinea nigra: treatment with topical ketoconazole. *Cutis.* 1993;52:209.
86. Shannon PL, Ramos-Caro FA, Cosgrove BF, et al. Treatment of tinea nigra with terbinafine. *Cutis.* 1999;64:199.
87. Daniel CR 3rd, Gupta AK, Daniel MP, et al. Two feet-one hand syndrome: a retrospective multicenter survey. *Int J Dermatol.* 1997;36:658.
88. Neri I, Piraccini BM, Guareschi E, et al. Bullous tinea pedis in two children. *Mycoses.* 2004;47:475.
89. Seeburger J, Scher RK. Long-term remission of two feet-one hand syndrome. *Cutis.* 1998;61:149.
90. Lebwohl M, Elewski B, Eisen D, et al. Efficacy and safety of terbinafine 1% solution in the treatment of interdigital tinea pedis and tinea corporis or tinea cruris. *Cutis.* 2001;67:261.

Chapter 161 :: Yeast Infections
:: Iris Ahronowitz & Kieron Leslie

第一百六十一章

酵母菌感染

中文导读

本章重点介绍了由念珠菌和马拉色氏酵母这两类真菌引起的皮肤酵母菌感染,它们都是人类常见的共生生物。念珠菌表现为机会病原体,可造成具有特征性的炎症性皮肤、黏膜和指甲感染,有可能产生侵袭性甚至威胁生命的传播性疾病。本章节分别就这两类疾病的流行病学、临床特征、危险因素、病因和发病机制、诊断、鉴别诊断、临床病程和预后、临床管理进行了全面的阐释和讨论。

〔汪 犇〕

This chapter reviews the spectrum of cutaneous yeast infections caused by *Candida* and *Malassezia* yeasts, both of which are frequent commensal organisms on human hosts. *Candida* behaves as an opportunistic pathogen, producing fairly characteristic patterns of inflammatory skin, mucosal, and nail infection, with the potential to produce invasive and sometimes life-threatening disseminated disease. *Malassezia*, by contrast, produces several superficial cutaneous patterns is rarely a culprit in systemic disease.

CANDIDIASIS

AT-A-GLANCE

- *Candida* species produce a variety of inflammatory mucosal and cutaneous manifestations.
- Favored areas of involvement include the oral mucosa and lips, fingers and nails, intertriginous zones, and genitalia.
- A variety of conditions can predispose patients to chronic mucocutaneous candidiasis with diffuse skin, mucosal, and nail involvement.
- *Candida* can cause invasive disease, including bloodstream infection, and is the most common culprit in fatal fungal sepsis.
- Risk factors for infection include extremes of age, malnutrition, obesity, diabetes, and immune deficiency.
- In mucocutaneous disease, morphology can be very helpful in making a clinical diagnosis, although confirmatory testing with potassium hydroxide preparations, culture, and histopathology (and in invasive disease, serology and polymerase chain reaction) also may be helpful.
- Treatment includes topical imidazoles and nystatin, and in more-severe disease, systemic agents, including oral azoles and echinocandins.

EPIDEMIOLOGY

Candida yeasts are found throughout the environment and are also common commensals of the human skin, oropharyngeal, respiratory, GI, and genital mucosa.

Candidal colonization has been reported in the oral mucosa of more than 40% of healthy adults, with higher rates of carriage in women and smokers.[1] At least 15 of the more than 200 *Candida* species have been implicated in human disease. Although *Candida albicans* is the most commonly implicated *Candida* species in localized mucocutaneous candidiasis, an increasing number of other species have been implicated in mucocutaneous disease, including *Candida glabrata, Candida tropicalis, Candida krusei, Candida parapsilosis,* and *Candida dubliniensis*. Additionally, while *albicans* is still the single most common species, non-*albicans* species collectively now account for the majority of invasive candidiasis and candidemia.[2] Other specific risk factors for infection are described below (see section "Risk Factors").

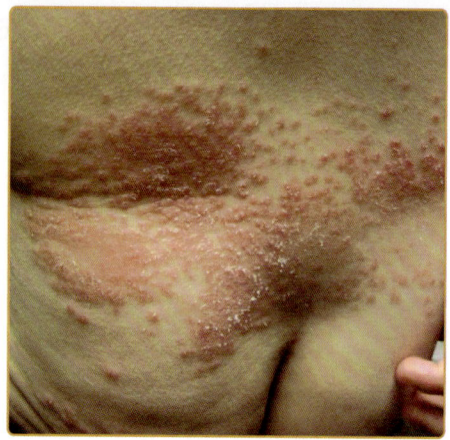

Figure 161-1 Typical morphology of cutaneous candidiasis demonstrating erythematous papules coalescing into plaques, with satellite papules and vesiculopustules.

CLINICAL FEATURES

CUTANEOUS FINDINGS

Localized *Candida* infection in the skin classically presents as beefy-red patches and plaques with satellite papules and pustules at the periphery (Fig. 161-1).

Intertriginous areas, particularly the axillae, inframammary folds, groin folds, and infrapannus area, are frequently affected, and maceration may be an additional feature in these sites (Fig. 161-2A, B). *Candida* also may

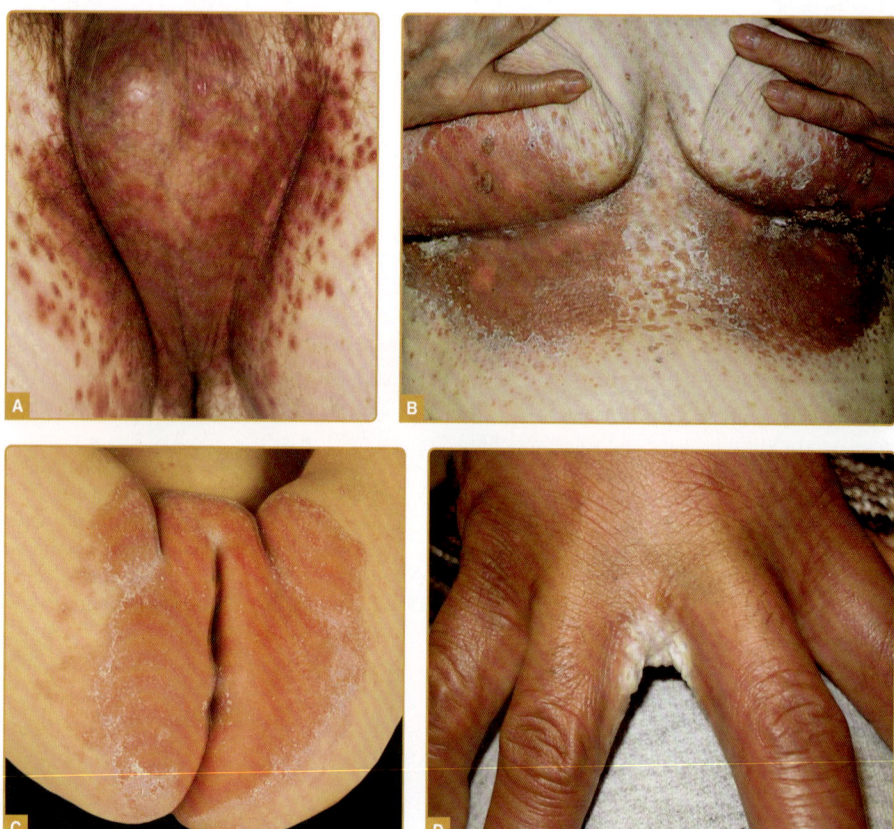

Figure 161-2 Examples of *Candida* intertrigo. **A,** Erythematous papules becoming confluent over the inguinal area with prominent satellite papules (with scrotal involvement, in contrast to tinea cruris). **B,** Erythematous plaques with erosion and satellite papules. **C,** Diaper candidiasis demonstrated erythematous, partially eroded plaques, and satellite papules. **D,** Erosio interdigitalis blastomycetica demonstrating an erythematous plaque with prominent maceration in the interdigital webspace.

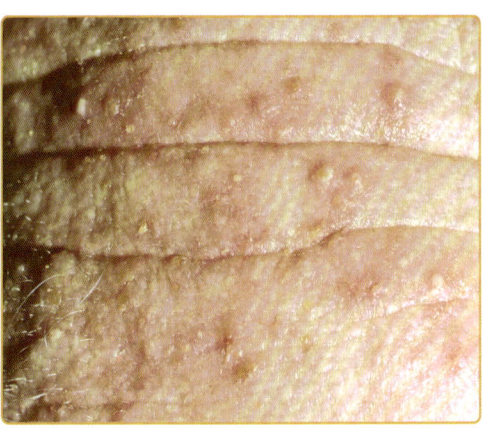

Figure 161-3 Miliaria caused by *Candida* seen on the forehead of a diabetic patient who had applied a partially occlusive dressing for headache symptoms.

be implicated in miliaria arising on occluded skin surfaces, manifesting as small monomorphous vesicles (Fig. 161-3). On oropharyngeal mucosal surfaces, background erythema with adherent whitish material may be seen, as in the pseudomembranous form of oropharyngeal candidiasis (thrush) (Fig. 161-4A, D), however an erythematous form, characterized by a shiny depapillated lingual surface, as in median rhomboid glossitis, also occurs, and may be seen in those who wear dentures (Fig. 161-4B). Additionally, fissuring and crusting at the oral commissures may be seen in angular cheilitis (also known as perleche; Fig. 161-4C). In breastfeeding women, nipple candidiasis may present with shiny erythema of the areola and nipple, which may be associated with flaking of the skin, and thrush may concurrently be apparent in the infant's mouth.[3] On genital skin and mucosa, including the vulva, glans penis, and prepuce, *Candida* may present with patchy erythema or erythematous plaques with associated itching and burning sensation. In patients with vulvovaginitis, a thick, white, curd-like discharge is typical. Pustules are seen more frequently in balanitis and balanoposthitis than in vulvitis (Fig. 161-5). In the diaper area, the classic presentation is beefy-red erythematous plaques with satellite papules and pustules (Fig. 161-2C). In the interdigital spaces, particularly the third webspace of the hands, a macerated whitish plaque on erythematous background (erosio interdigitalis blastomycetica) may be

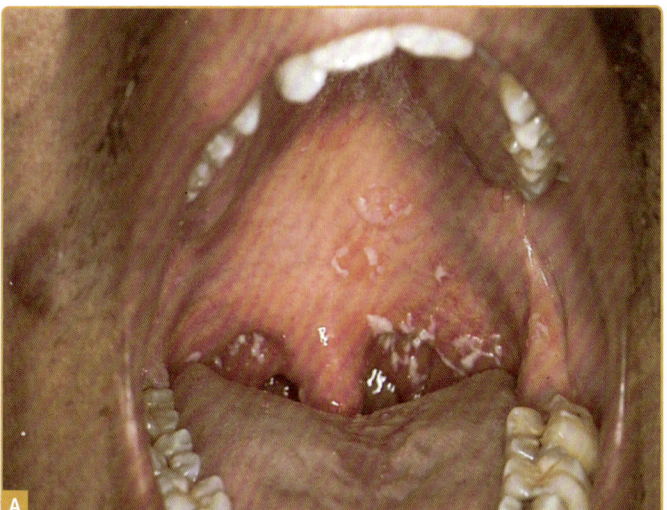
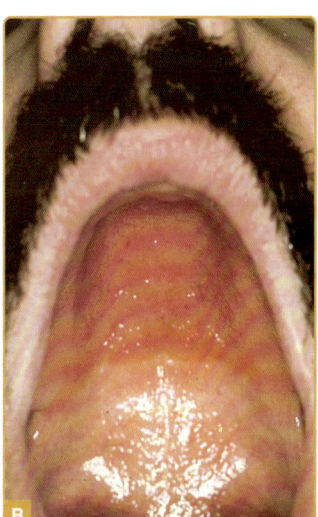
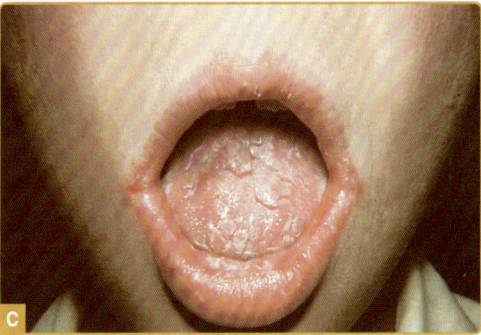
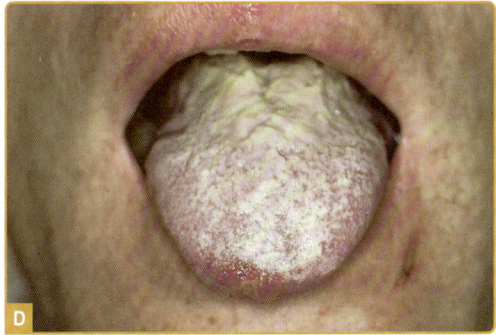

Figure 161-4 A, Oral candidiasis (pseudomembranous form, thrush). Typical white palatal patches and plaques. **B,** Atrophic candidiasis demonstrating a shiny erythematous depapillated areas under areas in contact with dentures. **C,** Angular cheilitis (perleche) demonstrating fissured erythematous plaques at the bilateral oral commissures. **D,** Hyperplastic candidiasis on the dorsal lingual surface.

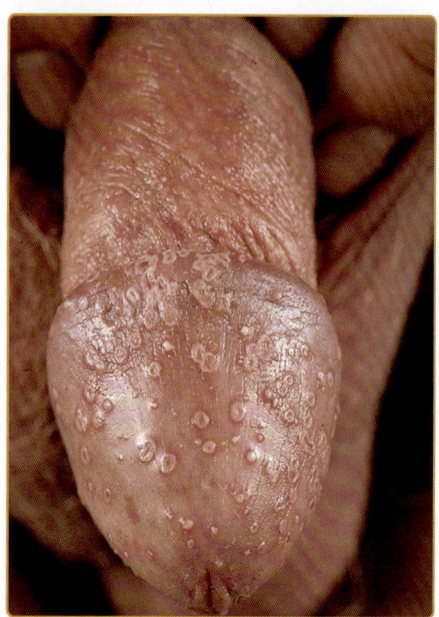

Figure 161-5 Balanoposthitis caused by *Candida* demonstrating pustules on the glans penis and foreskin.

seen, especially in patients with chronic exposure to moisture from wet work (Fig. 161-2D).

Candida also has been implicated in chronic paronychia, which presents with erythema of the proximal nailfold area with loss of the cuticle and skin breakdown (sometimes with associated onycholysis and nail dystrophy; Fig. 161-6A). More recently, however, the *Candida* has been hypothesized to play a secondary role as a colonizer with either chronic wet work leading to skin barrier breakdown or chronic contact dermatitis being the primary insult.[4] *Candida*, usually starting as paronychia, can also directly invade the nail plate and produce onychomycosis (5% to 10% of onychomycosis overall is caused by *Candida*; Fig. 161-6B), and is implicated in several presentations, including a distal subungual presentation and total dystrophic onychomycosis.[5,6] *Candida* onychomycosis is more often seen in the fingernails than in the toenails, and is often associated with pain on pressure or movement of the nail plate (both of these features are in contrast to dermatophytes), and more often affects the dominant hand.[6] Exposure to moisture and occupational wet work are important risk factors.

Patients with chronic mucocutaneous candidiasis may present with erythematous plaques with overlying scale reminiscent of plaque psoriasis (Fig. 161-7). In patients with candidemia, the presence of skin lesions, most typically discrete sparse lesions ranging from erythematous papules with central pallor or necrosis to erythematous nodules to (less commonly) plaques, may be an important clue to the diagnosis (Fig. 161-8).[7] The distribution favors the trunk and proximal extremities although the head and face may be involved. These classic skin lesions are reported to appear approximately 10% to 30% of the time in candidemia, and are most commonly seen in *C. tropicalis* infection.[8]

NONCUTANEOUS FINDINGS

In patients with candidemia, the classic clinical triad of fever, rash, and myalgia has been described as a sufficient basis for initiation of empiric treatment for presumptive invasive candidiasis in a hospitalized patient.[9] The myalgia is the result of hematogenous dissemination of *Candida* to muscle (usually in the lower extremities) causing muscle abscesses, clinically presenting with a warm, sore muscle and seen in up to 25% of patients with candidemia.[10] Additionally,

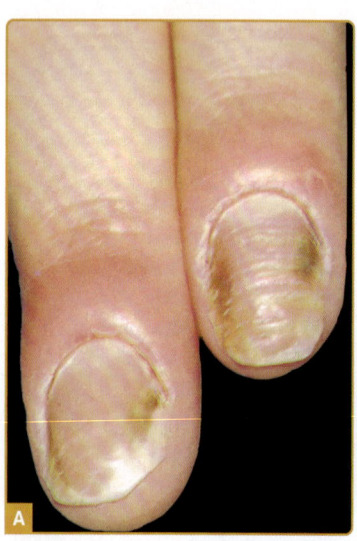
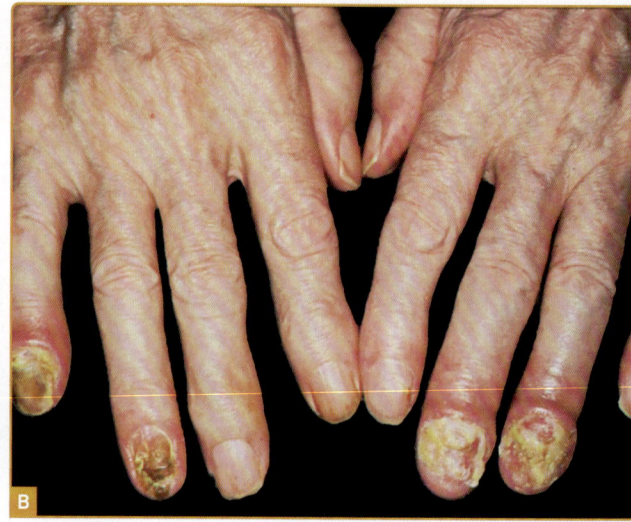

Figure 161-6 **A**, Chronic paronychia caused by *Candida albicans* demonstrating erythematous, edematous proximal nailfold with onycholysis and mild dystrophy. **B**, Severely inflammatory candidal paronychia that has spread to the nail plate to produce onychomycosis.

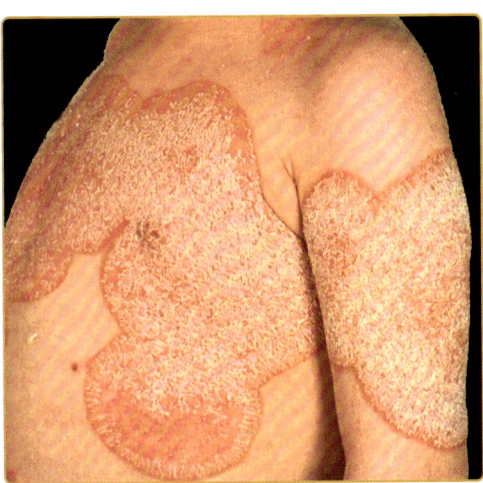

Figure 161-7 Patient with chronic mucocutaneous candidiasis. Sharply marginated erythematous plaques with prominent scaling, reminiscent of plaque psoriasis.

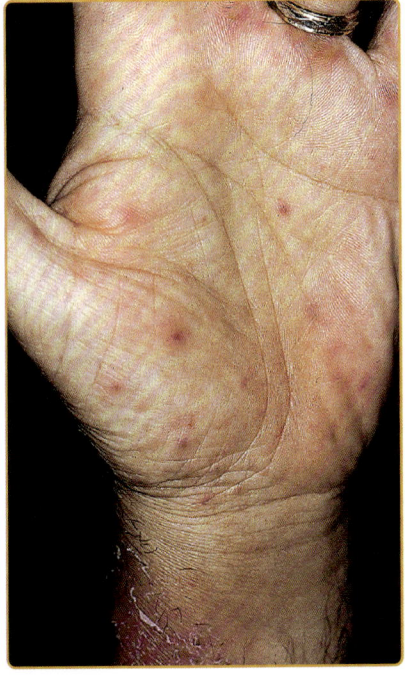

Figure 161-8 Disseminated candidiasis with candidemia. Neutropenic febrile patient with acute myeloid leukemia demonstrating erythematous papules and nodules on the hand, some with central pustulation. Biopsy demonstrated *Candida* organisms and blood cultures were positive for *Candida tropicalis*.

chorioretinitis, vitritis, and endophthalmitis may result from hematogenous spread in roughly 4% to 7% of patients with candidemia.[11,12] Although a majority of patients do complain of symptoms that include visual changes (if able to articulate symptoms), ocular *Candida* is also detected in asymptomatic patients.[11]

COMPLICATIONS

Candida may cause multiorgan failure as a manifestation of septic shock, or may hematogenously disseminate to any organ in the setting of candidemia, with the liver, spleen, kidneys, heart (and heart valves), and meninges among the more common. Retinal involvement may be painless and result in permanent visual loss.

ETIOLOGY AND PATHOGENESIS

Although typically a commensal organism, *Candida* does act as an opportunistic pathogen under favorable circumstances, including alteration in normal flora or immune function, a breach of skin, or a breach of mucosal integrity. A variety of virulence factors assist it in establishing infection, including, importantly, the ability to adhere to human epithelial cells.[13] *Candida* infection elicits both innate and adaptive host immune responses largely through the interleukin-17 (IL-17) pathway, and defects in this pathway, including in genes such as *STAT1*, *STAT3*, *IL17F*, *IL17RA*, among many others, are associated with susceptibility to chronic mucocutaneous candidiasis.[14,15] Recent research also has identified that mutations in caspase recruitment domain-containing protein 9 (*CARD9*), a molecule necessary for the induction of T-helper-17 cells, result in a specific defect in the ability of neutrophils to kill *Candida*, resulting in vulnerability to invasive *Candida* infections.[16] Interestingly, the importance of the IL-17 pathway to *Candida* susceptibility is borne out in patients taking the increasingly prevalent IL-17–blocking medications, with early evidence suggesting an increase in *Candida* infections in psoriasis and psoriatic arthritis patients taking the new anti–IL-17 medications brodalumab, secukinumab, and ixekizumab.[17]

RISK FACTORS

Risk factors for localized/superficial *Candida* infections include extremes of age; diabetes; obesity; pregnancy; HIV/AIDS (although prevalence has decreased significantly in the era of highly active antiretroviral therapy)[18]; and use of broad-spectrum antibiotics, corticosteroids, or immunosuppressive medications, specifically anti–IL-17-blocking medications as discussed above. Risk factors for oral candidiasis include xerostomia; wearing of dentures or other oral hardware; inhaled and systemic corticosteroids; vitamin deficiencies; radiation therapy to the head/neck; and hypothyroidism.[1] Risk factors for invasive candidiasis/candidemia include neutropenia and neutrophil dysfunction (including *CARD9* mutations); hematologic malignancy; stem cell transplantation; indwelling intravascular catheters (including patients on hemodialysis); intensive care unit placement; and immunosuppressive medications.[19]

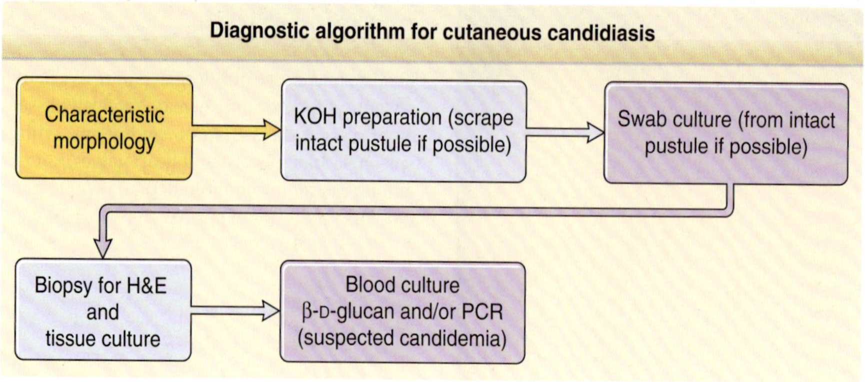

Figure 161-9 Diagnostic algorithm for cutaneous candidiasis. H&E, hematoxylin and eosin; KOH, potassium hydroxide; PCR, polymerase chain reaction.

DIAGNOSIS

Figure 161-9 is an algorithm summarizing current recommendations for diagnosing cutaneous candidiasis.

SUPPORTIVE STUDIES

The morphology may be distinctive and sufficient to make a clinical diagnosis in many cases of superficial *Candida* skin infection. Rapid confirmation may be achieved with bedside potassium hydroxide (KOH) preparation (either from a scraping from an intact pustule, or a touch preparation from a punch biopsy specimen) demonstrating pseudohyphae and budding yeast (Fig. 161-10).

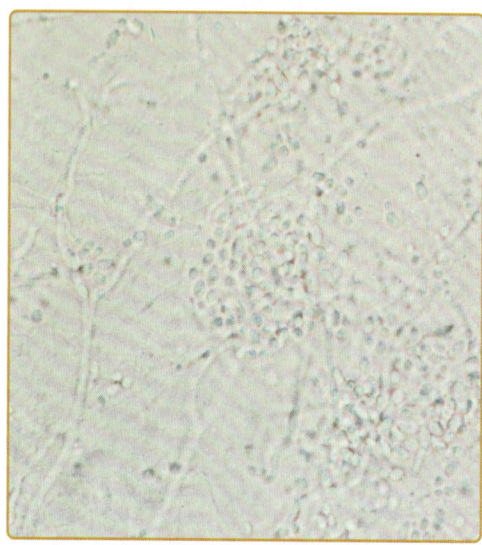

Figure 161-10 Potassium hydroxide (KOH) preparation demonstrating *Candida* forms including pseudohyphae and budding yeasts.

LABORATORY TESTING

Definitive diagnosis and speciation can be achieved via either swab culture (taken from an intact pustule if possible) or tissue culture from biopsy specimens taken from affected areas. In patients suspected of having candidemia, positive blood cultures are still considered the "gold standard" however with poor sensitivity (approximately 50%), adjunctive techniques such as β-D-glucan assay and polymerase chain reaction may be helpful.[20]

PATHOLOGY

Skin biopsies are of variable yield in making the diagnosis. While in localized mucocutaneous candidiasis, organisms may sometimes be readily seen in the epithelium with Grocott methenamine silver or periodic acid–Schiff staining, in patients with disseminated candidiasis, organisms (sometimes forming microabscesses) are more likely to be found in and around the dermal blood vessels, although sometimes only a mononuclear inflammatory infiltrate is seen.[21]

DIFFERENTIAL DIAGNOSIS

Table 161-1 summarizes the differential diagnosis for cutaneous candidiasis.

CLINICAL COURSE AND PROGNOSIS

While most localized mucocutaneous *Candida* infections cause minor symptoms and respond readily to treatment, in patients with underlying risk factors (see "Risk Factors" before) infection may be recurrent and chronic, contributing to varying degrees of morbidity although not life-threatening. By contrast, mortality in

TABLE 161-1
Differential Diagnosis for Cutaneous Candidiasis

For Cutaneous Candidiasis
- Seborrheic dermatitis
- Tinea corporis/dermatophytosis
- Impetigo
- Erythrasma
- Intertrigo
- Irritant contact dermatitis
- Allergic contact dermatitis
- Atopic dermatitis
- Bacterial folliculitis
- Herpes simplex or herpes zoster (localized or folliculitis)

For Oral Mucosal Candidiasis/Thrush
- Herpes simplex virus infection
- Oral hairy leukoplakia
- Morsicatio buccarum (chronic cheek chewing)
- Lichen planus white sponge nevus

For Paronychia and Onychomycosis
- Tinea unguium (dermatophyte nail infection)
- Nondermatophyte mold infections (eg, *Acremonium*, *Alternaria*)
- Acute bacterial paronychia
- Herpetic whitlow
- Squamous cell carcinoma

For Disseminated Candidiasis
- Disseminated fungal infections: *Fusarium*, *Aspergillus*, zygomycosis
- Bacterial sepsis including meningococcemia, gonococcemia, and ecthyma gangrenosum
- Disseminated herpes simplex, primary varicella, or disseminated herpes zoster

patients with candidemia is significant, at 35% over 12 weeks in one larger study[2]; in some case series, the mortality exceeds 80%.[8]

MANAGEMENT

Table 161-2 summarizes the management of cutaneous candidiasis. The Infectious Diseases Society of America guidelines were most recently updated in 2016 (as of this writing) and provide clinicians with comprehensive guidance in the treatment of localized and disseminated *Candida* infections,[22] as summarized below, and may be consulted for further detailed recommendations. Areas not covered by these guidelines include the treatment of localized cutaneous candidiasis, chronic mucocutaneous candidiasis, paronychia, and onychomycosis, for which other relevant sources are provided.

CUTANEOUS CANDIDIASIS

First-line treatment of localized disease includes topical formulations of imidazoles (ketoconazole, clotrimazole, miconazole, econazole) in various formulations, which may include creams or powders. Nystatin topical is also effective. More severe cases typically require short courses of oral antifungals such as fluconazole 150 mg for several doses.

ORAL CANDIDIASIS

Clotrimazole 10-mg troches 5 times daily or miconazole 50-mg buccal tablets for 1 to 2 weeks is first-line treatment, with nystatin suspension 100,000 units/mL, 4 to 6 mL 4 times daily for 1 to 2 weeks as an alternative. Moderate and severe cases may require fluconazole 100 to 200 mg oral daily for 1 to 2 weeks. Itraconazole, posaconazole, voriconazole, and amphotericin B solutions and suspensions are alternatives for refractory or resistant disease. For denture wearers, disinfection of dentures is an important adjunctive step to prevent reinfection; the most effective methods for removal of *Candida* include soaking with commercially available effervescent denture tablets or a dilute bleach concentration of 1:32 or higher.[23,24] For HIV-positive patients, initiation of highly active antiretroviral therapy is recommended to decrease chances of recurrence. For patients with recurrent disease, chronic suppressive dosing of fluconazole 150 mg orally 3 times weekly can be helpful.

PARONYCHIA AND ONYCHOMYCOSIS

First-line treatment of *Candida* onychomycosis is itraconazole given orally as pulsed dosing at 400 mg daily for 1 week monthly or 200 mg daily continuous dosing, for a total minimum duration of 4 weeks for fingernail and 12 weeks for toenail disease. Fluconazole is considered equally effective and can be given at 50 mg daily or 300 mg weekly dosing for similar durations. Although terbinafine has lower efficacy, cure rates are improved by longer courses of 250 mg daily for 4 months or longer, which makes compliance a potential concern.[6]

For chronic paronychia, avoidance of wet work or wearing of gloves to keep the skin dry is recommended. Given recent evidence that *Candida* colonization may play a secondary role, with the primary insult being skin barrier breakdown resulting from wet work and possible contact dermatitis,[4] a role for topical corticosteroids has been demonstrated. In a randomized trial, topical corticosteroids were shown to yield a higher cure rate than systemic antifungals.[25] Topical tacrolimus also is effective.[26] Topical imidazole solutions, as well as thymol 40% compounded in ethanol or dilute acetic acid soaks, also have been used adjunctively in the treatment of chronic paronychia.

VULVOVAGINITIS AND BALANITIS

Topical antifungals such miconazole and clotrimazole are first-line treatment for *Candida* vulvovaginitis. Oral fluconazole (usually 150 mg in a single dose) is an alternative. Two to 3 doses 72 hours apart are recommended for more-severe cases, and even longer courses for recurrent cases. For balanitis and balanoposthitis, topical antifungal creams, in some cases in conjunction with low- to mid-potency topical corticosteroids, are employed.

TABLE 161-2
Candidiasis Treatment Algorithm

	FIRST LINE	SECOND LINE
Cutaneous	Topical imidazoles Topical nystatin	Oral fluconazole
Paronychia	Avoid wet work/use of gloves Topical corticosteroids Topical tacrolimus	Topical imidazole solutions Thymol 40% in ethanol Dilute acetic acid soaks
Onychomycosis	Oral itraconazole Oral fluconazole	Oral terbinafine
Oral (thrush)	Mild: • Clotrimazole troches • Miconazole buccal tablets • Disinfect dentures Severe or immunosuppressed: • Oral fluconazole	Nystatin suspension Itraconazole, posaconazole, voriconazole, or amphotericin B solutions/suspensions
Vulvovaginitis	Topical miconazole, clotrimazole, terconazole	Oral fluconazole
Balanoposthitis	Topical antifungal creams	Low- to mid-potency topical corticosteroids (adjunctive)
Chronic mucocutaneous	Oral imidazoles Oral triazoles (voriconazole and posaconazole) Long courses often required	Resistant disease: • Echinocandins • Liposomal amphotericin • Flucytosine
Disseminated (candidemia) **Infectious disease consultation is required**	Hemodynamically stable immunocompetent patients: • Echinocandin (caspofungin, micafungin, or anidulafungin) • Fluconazole Neutropenic patients: • Empiric echinocandin • Switch to fluconazole once stable	Liposomal amphotericin

CHRONIC MUCOCUTANEOUS CANDIDIASIS

Given the high likelihood of recurrence, prolonged courses of oral imidazoles or newer triazoles (including voriconazole and posaconazole) are first-line treatment. Because of the development of resistance, echinocandins, liposomal amphotericin, or flucytosine is sometimes required.[27]

DISSEMINATED CANDIDIASIS

Treatment of patients with invasive candidiasis should be undertaken with the assistance of an infectious disease specialist. Either an echinocandin (caspofungin, micafungin, or anidulafungin) or fluconazole is a first-line treatment recommended in hemodynamically stable immunocompetent patients.

Neutropenic patients should be started on empiric echinocandin and switched to fluconazole once stable.[22] Resistance to azoles and echinocandins is a potential concern, particularly in non–*Candida albicans* species disease and in patients with prior exposure to these medications. Lipid formulation amphotericin B is an alternative in situations of resistance to first-line agents. Followup blood cultures and ophthalmologic examination are recommended for all patients with candidemia.

MALASSEZIA

AT-A-GLANCE

- *Malassezia* species are normal flora of human skin.
- *Malassezia* species can produce a variety of clinical presentations including pityriasis (tinea) versicolor, *Malassezia* folliculitis, seborrheic dermatitis, and neonatal cephalic pustulosis. Rarely, *Malassezia* species have been implicated in systemic infections, including catheter-related fungemia.
- The diagnosis can be made via potassium hydroxide (KOH) preparation or skin biopsy. The organism is not typically cultured for this purpose as it requires special growing conditions (additional lipid).
- *Malassezia* skin infections generally respond readily to topical treatments, including azole antifungals and selenium sulfide–based preparations. More extensive cases or those with folliculitis may require systemic antifungals.
- *Malassezia* infections tend to have high recurrence rates and may require prophylactic treatment to prevent further episodes.

EPIDEMIOLOGY

Malassezia (formerly known as *Pityrosporum*) are lipophilic dimorphic fungi that have been implicated in several skin conditions: pityriasis (tinea) versicolor, and *Malassezia* folliculitis. These organisms also have been identified at increased rates in inflammatory conditions including seborrheic dermatitis and atopic dermatitis, although their role in these conditions is less clear and thought to be more an exacerbating factor rather than a true infection.[28] There are currently 14 species in the genus *Malassezia*, of which 11 have been detected as commensals on human skin.[29] Colonization tends to occur by the age of 3 to 6 months, with earlier colonization in the neonatal phase associated with length of neonatal intensive care unit stays.[30] Higher rates of *Malassezia* skin infections are seen in tropical climates and at the ages of peak sebum production (adolescence to young adulthood).[31] In pityriasis versicolor and *Malassezia* folliculitis, *Malassezia globosa* is the most commonly isolated species,[32,33] with *Malassezia restricta* and *Malassezia sympodialis* also frequently isolated from *Malassezia* folliculitis.[34]

These fungi also have been found to play a role in internal infections, with *Malassezia* (most frequently *M. restricta* and *M. globosa*) isolated from the sinuses of both healthy controls and patients with chronic rhinosinusitis.[35] *Malassezia* species also are implicated in urinary tract infections, meningitis, pneumonia, and nosocomial bloodstream infections.[36,37] Cather-related fungemia has been reported in neonates (most commonly by *Malassezia pachydermatis*, particularly preterm infants receiving parenteral lipid infusions and those with prolonged vascular catheterization.[38] *Malassezia* fungemias also have been described in a series of immunocompromised older children and adults (with leukemias, solid tumors, diabetes, and severe combined immunodeficiency) with indwelling catheters, none of whom were receiving lipid infusions.[39]

CLINICAL FEATURES

CUTANEOUS FINDINGS

Pityriasis versicolor is a superficial *Malassezia* infection most commonly seen in adolescents and young adults. This condition is also known as tinea versicolor, but this nomenclature may be misleading as other tinea presentations are caused by dermatophytes rather than yeast. This condition manifests with asymptomatic to mildly pruritic patches and thin plaques with overlying fine scale favoring the neck, chest and back, upper arms, and, less commonly, the scalp, abdomen, and groin areas (Fig. 161-11). The name "versicolor" alludes to the spectrum of skin color changes that may be seen including hypopigmentation and hyperpigmentation, as well as erythematous to salmon-colored skin lesions (Fig. 161-12).

Malassezia folliculitis presents as follicularly based erythematous monomorphic papules and pustules on the face, trunk, and upper arms (Fig. 161-13A). In contrast to acne vulgaris, comedones are a not a feature, and *Malassezia* folliculitis tends to spare the centrofacial areas.[33] The lesions are often, but not always, pruritic. The condition is frequently diagnosed as misdiagnosed as acne vulgaris, and may even appear concurrently with acne.

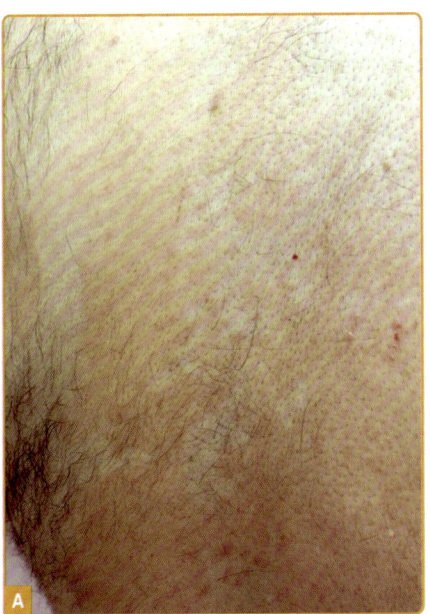 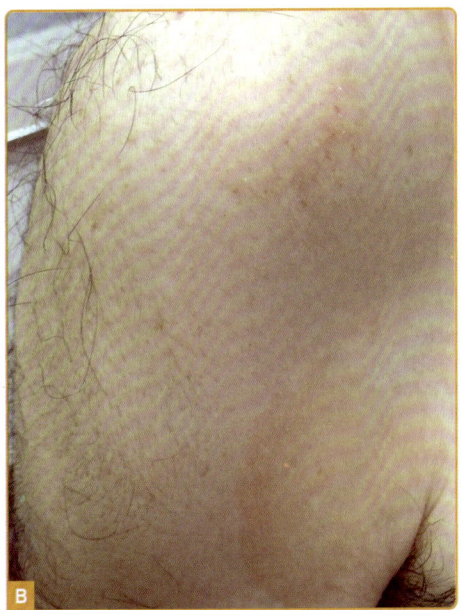

Figure 161-11 Pityriasis (tinea) versicolor. **A,** Multiple round to oval salmon-colored patches over the trunk. **B,** Salmon-colored patches and thin plaques on the shoulder and upper arm with fine overlying scale.

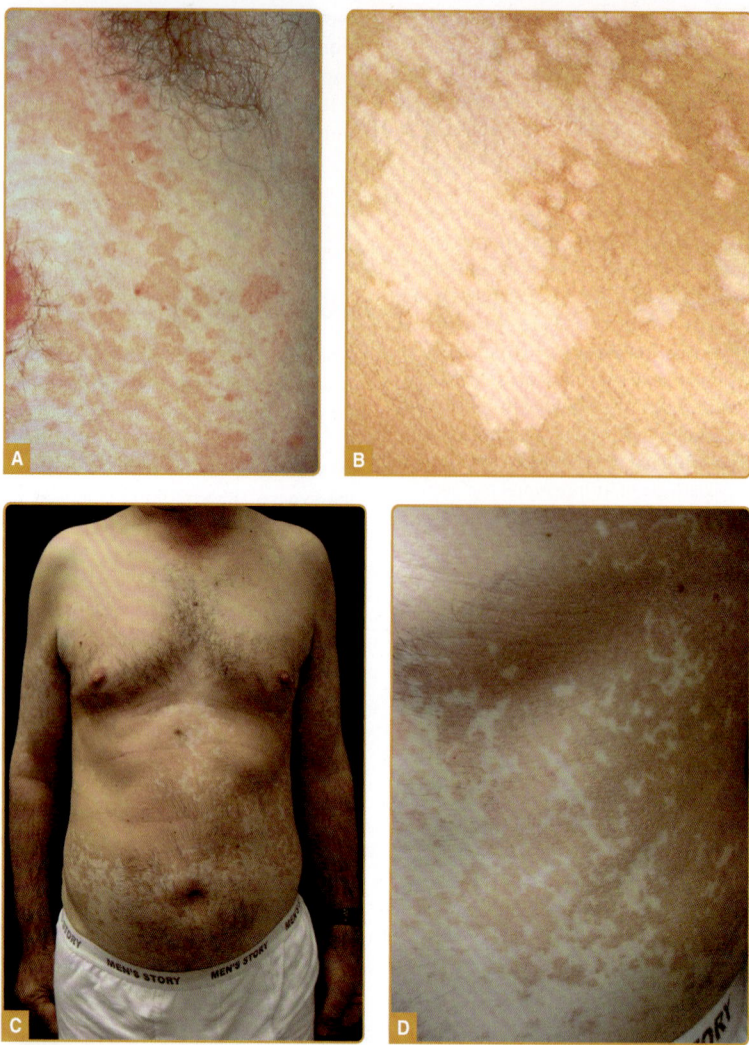

Figure 161-12 Pityriasis (tinea) versicolor. **A,** Erythematous macules and patches. **B,** Hypopigmented macules and patches that can be mistaken for vitiligo. **C,** Salmon-pink macules coalescing into patches. **D,** Characteristic fine overlying scale seen close up.

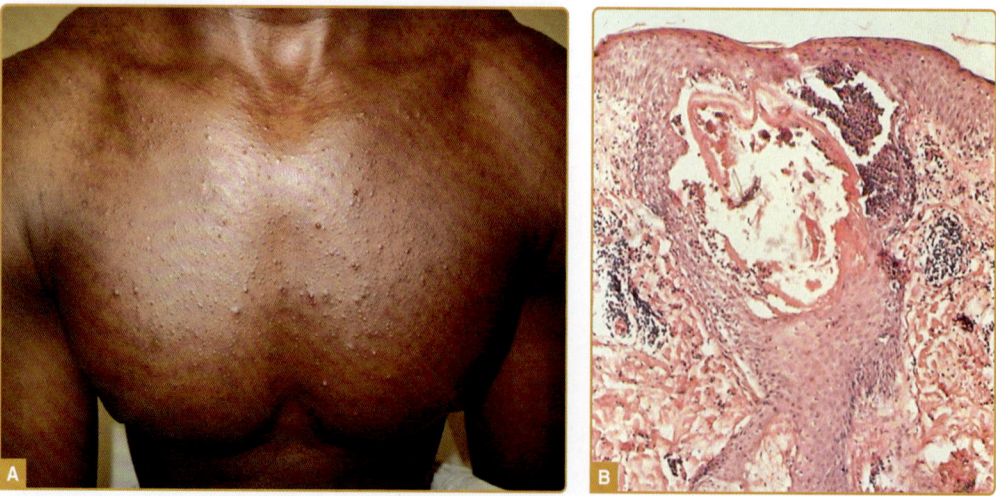

Figure 161-13 **A,** *Malassezia* folliculitis on the chest. **B,** Histopathology demonstrating yeast forms in the follicular infundibulum on hematoxylin-and-eosin (H&E) staining.

ETIOLOGY AND PATHOGENESIS

Malassezia are normal flora of human skin, and rely upon hydrolysis of their human host sebum triglycerides as they lack a fatty acid synthase to allow endogenous production of C14-C16 saturated fatty acids.[28,40] The free fatty acids thereby produced are believed to provoke inflammation in the skin of the host, as evidenced by the presence of a perivascular inflammatory infiltrate on histopathology.[31] In pityriasis versicolor, the organism is able to transition to its pathogenic mycelial form and invade the stratum corneum. The pigmentary alterations produced in the skin are believed to be achieved via several mechanisms. The hypopigmentation seen especially in darker-skinned patients is thought to be a result of the production of azelaic acid, a dicarboxylic acid that inhibits of tyrosinase (an enzyme that catalyzes a key step in melanin synthesis) and also may be directly cytotoxic to melanocytes,[41] while hyperpigmented lesions have been attributed to increased melanosomes and thickening of the stratum corneum.[42]

RISK FACTORS

Tropical climates and heavy sweating are associated with increased rates of both pityriasis versicolor and *Malassezia* folliculitis. In addition, immunosuppression, oral antibiotics, and corticosteroids also are reported risk factors for *Malassezia* folliculitis.[43] There has not been a consistent gender predilection reported.

DIAGNOSIS

Figure 161-14 summarizes the diagnostic recommendations for cutaneous *Malassezia* infections.

SUPPORTIVE STUDIES

Pityriasis versicolor is often diagnosed visually based on its fairly distinctive morphology. Dermoscopy has been recommended as an ancillary tool in making the diagnosis of pityriasis versicolor as it highlights the fine scaling that may not always be readily visible to the naked eye.[44] In both pityriasis versicolor and *Malassezia* folliculitis, illumination with a Wood lamp may reveal yellow-green fluorescence.

KOH preparation can be a particularly useful in-clinic diagnostic test for pityriasis versicolor or *Malassezia* folliculitis and it will reveal short hyphae and yeast forms (the "ziti and meatballs" sign; Fig. 161-15). Although a superficial scraping of skin scales is adequate in pityriasis versicolor, the use of a comedone extractor or a needle to puncture an intact pustule is recommended to obtain a specimen in cases of *Malassezia* folliculitis where the yeast is situated deeper within the follicle.[34,45] Staining with calcofluor white or May-Grunwald-Giemsa stain may improve visualization.[43]

LABORATORY TESTING

Culture is not generally used to confirm *Malassezia* infection because of the organism's lipid requirement, which makes culture more logistically challenging—a layer of olive oil must be added or special growth media such as modified Dixon are required—and this is complicated further by slightly different growth requirements among different species.[31]

PATHOLOGY

Histopathology demonstrates *Malassezia* yeast forms; in pityriasis versicolor, they may be seen within the stratum corneum, while in *Malassezia* folliculitis they are found within dilated infundibula of plugged follicles in association with keratin debris (see Fig. 161-13B).[46] A perivascular inflammatory infiltrate of lymphocytes,

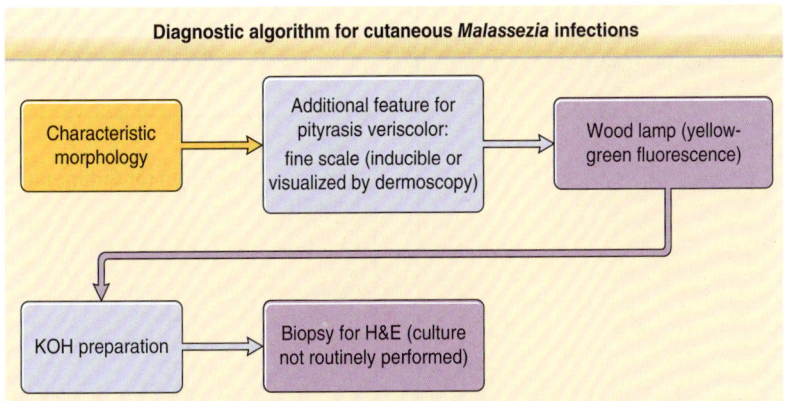

Figure 161-14 Diagnostic algorithm for cutaneous *Malassezia* infections. H&E, hematoxylin and eosin; KOH, potassium hydroxide.

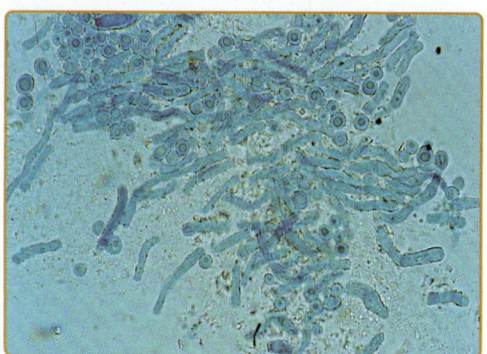

Figure 161-15 Potassium hydroxide (KOH) preparation of *Malassezia* demonstrating "ziti and meatballs" appearance of hyphae and yeast forms.

histiocytes, and neutrophils may be seen, which is typically mild unless the follicle has ruptured. A periodic acid–Schiff stain will highlight the organism.

DIFFERENTIAL DIAGNOSIS

Table 161-3 summarizes the differential diagnosis for cutaneous *Malassezia* infections.

CLINICAL COURSE AND PROGNOSIS

Superficial *Malassezia* infections are generally innocuous, and although most will respond readily to appropriate antifungal therapy, recurrence is common, particularly in those individuals with strong risk factors. Preterm neonates, immunosuppressed patients, and patients on parenteral lipid infusions are at higher risk of disseminated infection, as discussed above.

MANAGEMENT

Table 161-4 summarizes the management of cutaneous *Malassezia* infections. For pityriasis versicolor, first-line treatments are topical and include shampoos (pyrithione zinc or selenium sulfide), propylene glycol in aqueous solution, and azole antifungal creams (ketoconazole is the most studied).[45] For particularly extensive involvement or disease refractory to topicals, oral antifungal medications, including fluconazole (300 mg for 2 doses 7 days apart) or itraconazole (200 mg daily for 7 days), are effective; however, fluconazole may be preferable because of its more variable bioavailability.[45,47] Ketoconazole, once a mainstay of treatment, is no longer recommended as on May 19, 2016, the U.S. Food and Drug Administration issued a statement warning against the use of oral ketoconazole for skin and nail fungal infections because of risk of liver damage and adrenal dysfunction.[48] Despite a complete mycologic cure, pigmentary changes (particularly hypopigmented patches) may take many months to resolve and patients should be counseled about appropriate expectations.

Given the high propensity for recurrence, prophylactic long-term treatment may be warranted in some patients; options include either periodic use of topical selenium sulfide shampoo or ketoconazole 2% shampoo, or itraconazole 200 mg twice daily 1 day per month for 6 months.[49]

For *Malassezia* folliculitis, given the presence of the fungus deep within the hair follicle, monotherapy with topical antifungals is of less reliable efficacy. The addition of a keratolytic such as propylene glycol may improve the efficacy of topical antifungal treatment.[45] Ultimately, many patients may require systemic treatment, with itraconazole being the best-studied treatment (200 mg daily for 1 to 3 weeks).[45]

TABLE 161-3
Differential Diagnosis for Cutaneous *Malassezia* Infections

For Pityriasis Versicolor:
- Seborrheic dermatitis
- Pityriasis rosea
- Pityriasis alba
- Confluent and reticulated papillomatosis of Gougerot and Carteaud
- Tinea corporis/dermatophytosis
- Impetigo
- Secondary syphilis
- Mycosis fungoides
- Erythrasma
- Irritant contact dermatitis
- Allergic contact dermatitis
- Atopic dermatitis
- Epidermodysplasia verruciformis

For *Malassezia* Folliculitis:
- Acne vulgaris
- Bacterial folliculitis
- Steroid folliculitis
- Eosinophilic folliculitis
- Rosacea
- *Demodex* folliculitis

TABLE 161-4
Treatment Algorithm for Cutaneous *Malassezia* Infections

	FIRST LINE	SECOND LINE
Pityriasis versicolor	Shampoos (pyrithione zinc or selenium sulfide) Propylene glycol in aqueous solution Topical imidazoles (ketoconazole)	Oral fluconazole Oral itraconazole
Malassezia folliculitis	Topical antifungal ± keratolytic (propylene glycol)	Oral itraconazole

REFERENCES

1. Arendorf TM, Walker DM. The prevalence and intraoral distribution of *Candida albicans* in man. *Arch Oral Biol.* 1980;25:1-10.
2. Horn DL, Neofytos D, Anaissie EJ, et al. Epidemiology and outcomes of candidemia in 2019 patients: data from the prospective antifungal therapy alliance registry. *Clin Infect Dis.* 2009;48:1695-1703.
3. Barrett ME, Heller MM, Fullerton Stone H, et al. Dermatoses of the breast in lactation. *Dermatol Ther.* 2013;26:331-336.
4. Bahunuthula RK, Thappa DM, Kumari R, et al. Evaluation of role of Candida in patients with chronic paronychia. *Indian J Dermatol Venereol Leprol.* 2015;81:485-490.
5. Elewski BE. Onychomycosis: pathogenesis, diagnosis, and management. *Clin Microbiol Rev.* 1998;11:415-429.
6. Ameen M, Lear JT, Madan V, et al. British Association of Dermatologists' guidelines for the management of onychomycosis 2014. *Br J Dermatol.* 2014;171:937-958.
7. Grossman ME, Fox LP, Kovarik C, et al. *Cutaneous Manifestations of Infection in the Immunocompromised Host.* Berlin, Germany: Springer Science & Business Media; 2012.
8. Bae GY, Lee HW, Chang SE, et al. Clinicopathologic review of 19 patients with systemic candidiasis with skin lesions. *Int J Dermatol.* 2005;44:550-555.
9. Jarowski CI, Fialk MA, Murray HW, et al. Fever, rash, and muscle tenderness. A distinctive clinical presentation of disseminated candidiasis. *Arch Intern Med.* 1978;138:544-546.
10. Crum-Cianflone NF. Nonbacterial myositis. *Curr Infect Dis Rep.* 2010;12:374-382.
11. Adam MK, Vahedi S, Nichols MM, et al. Inpatient ophthalmology consultation for fungemia: prevalence of ocular involvement and necessity of funduscopic screening. *Am J Ophthalmol.* 2015;160:1078-1083.e2.
12. Shah CP, McKey J, Spirn MJ, et al. Ocular candidiasis: a review. *Br J Ophthalmol.* 2008;92:466-468.
13. Munro CA, Bates S, Buurman ET, et al. Mnt1p and Mnt2p of *Candida albicans* are partially redundant alpha-1,2-mannosyltransferases that participate in O-linked mannosylation and are required for adhesion and virulence. *J Biol Chem.* 2005;280:1051-1060.
14. Kashem SW, Kaplan DH. Skin immunity to *Candida albicans*. *Trends Immunol.* 2016;37:440-450.
15. Pichard DC, Freeman AF, Cowen EW. Primary immunodeficiency update: part II. Syndromes associated with mucocutaneous candidiasis and noninfectious cutaneous manifestations. *J Am Acad Dermatol.* 2015;73:367-381; quiz 381-382.
16. Drewniak A, Gazendam RP, Tool AT, et al. Invasive fungal infection and impaired neutrophil killing in human CARD9 deficiency. *Blood.* 2013;121:2385-2392.
17. Saunte DM, Mrowietz U, Puig L, et al. *Candida* infections in psoriasis and psoriatic arthritis patients treated with IL-17 inhibitors and their practical management. *Br J Dermatol.* 2017;177(1):47-62.
18. Patuwo C, Young K, Lin M, et al. The changing role of HIV-associated oral candidiasis in the era of HAART. *J Calif Dent Assoc.* 2015;43:87-92.
19. Alangaden GJ. Nosocomial fungal infections: epidemiology, infection control, and prevention. *Infect Dis Clin North Am.* 2011;25:201-225.
20. Clancy CJ, Nguyen MH. Finding the "missing 50%" of invasive candidiasis: how nonculture diagnostics will improve understanding of disease spectrum and transform patient care. *Clin Infect Dis.* 2013;56(9):1284-1292.
21. Jacobs MI, Magid MS, Jarowski CI. Disseminated candidiasis. Newer approaches to early recognition and treatment. *Arch Dermatol.* 1980;116:1277-1279.
22. Pappas PG, Kauffman CA, Andes DR, et al. Clinical practice guideline for the management of candidiasis: 2016 update by the Infectious Diseases Society of America. *Clin Infect Dis.* 2016;62:e1-e50.
23. Buergers R, Rosentritt M, Schneider-Brachert W, et al. Efficacy of denture disinfection methods in controlling *Candida albicans* colonization in vitro. *Acta Odontol Scand.* 2008;66:174-180.
24. Dahlan AA, Haveman CW, Ramage G, et al. Sodium hypochlorite, chlorhexidine gluconate, and commercial denture cleansers as disinfecting agents against *Candida albicans*: an in vitro comparison study. *Gen Dent.* 2011;59:e224-e229.
25. Tosti A, Piraccini BM, Ghetti E, et al. Topical steroids versus systemic antifungals in the treatment of chronic paronychia: an open, randomized double-blind and double dummy study. *J Am Acad Dermatol.* 2002;47:73-76.
26. Rigopoulos D, Gregoriou S, Belyayeva E, et al. Efficacy and safety of tacrolimus ointment 0.1% vs. betamethasone 17-valerate 0.1% in the treatment of chronic paronychia: an unblinded randomized study. *Br J Dermatol.* 2009;160:858-860.
27. Firinu D, Massidda O, Lorrai MM, et al. Successful treatment of chronic mucocutaneous candidiasis caused by azole-resistant *Candida albicans* with posaconazole. *Clin Dev Immunol.* 2011;2011:283239.
28. Harada K, Saito M, Sugita T, et al. *Malassezia* species and their associated skin diseases. *J. Dermatology.* 2015;42:250-257.
29. Findley K, Oh J, Yang J, et al. Topographic diversity of fungal and bacterial communities in human skin. *Nature.* 2013;498:367-370.
30. Ashbee HR, Leck AK, Puntis JW, et al. Skin colonization by *Malassezia* in neonates and infants. *Infect Control Hosp Epidemiol.* 2002;23:212-216.
31. Gupta AK, Bluhm R, Summerbell R. Pityriasis versicolor. *J Eur Acad Dermatol Venereol.* 2002;16:19-33.
32. Morishita N, Sei Y, Sugita T. Molecular analysis of *Malassezia* microflora from patients with pityriasis versicolor. *Mycopathologia.* 2006;161:61-65.
33. Durdu M, Güran M, Ilkit M. Epidemiological characteristics of *Malassezia* folliculitis and use of the May-Grünwald-Giemsa stain to diagnose the infection. *Diagn Microbiol Infect Dis.* 2013;76:450-457.
34. Akaza N, Akamatsu H, Sasaki Y, et al. *Malassezia* folliculitis is caused by cutaneous resident *Malassezia* species. *Med Mycol.* 2009;47:618-624.
35. Gelber JT, Cope EK, Goldberg AN, et al. Evaluation of *Malassezia* and common fungal pathogens in subtypes of chronic rhinosinusitis. *Int Forum Allergy Rhinol.* 2016;6:950-955.
36. Chang HJ, Miller HL, Watkins N, et al. An epidemic of *Malassezia pachydermatis* in an intensive care nursery associated with colonization of health care workers' pet dogs. *N Engl J Med.* 1998;338:706-711.
37. Baker RM, Stegink RJ, Manaloor JJ, et al. *Malassezia* pneumonia: a rare complication of parenteral nutrition therapy. *JPEN J Parenter Enteral Nutr.* 2016;40(8):1194-1196.
38. Chryssanthou E, Broberger U, Petrini B. *Malassezia pachydermatis* fungaemia in a neonatal intensive care

38. ... unit. *Acta Paediatr.* 2001;90:323-327.
39. Barber GR, Brown AE, Kiehn TE, et al. Catheter-related *Malassezia furfur* fungemia in immunocompromised patients. *Am J Med.* 1993;95:365-370.
40. Saunders CW, Scheynius A, Heitman J. *Malassezia* fungi are specialized to live on skin and associated with dandruff, eczema, and other skin diseases. *PLoS Pathog.* 2012;8:e1002701.
41. Nazzaro-Porro M, Passi S. Identification of tyrosinase inhibitors in cultures of *Pityrosporum. J Invest Dermatol.* 1978;71:205-208.
42. Galadari I, el Komy M, Mousa A, et al. Tinea versicolor: histologic and ultrastructural investigation of pigmentary changes. *Int J Dermatol.* 1992;31:253-256.
43. Rubenstein RM, Malerich SA. *Malassezia (Pityrosporum)* folliculitis. *J Clin Aesthet Dermatol.* 2014;7:37-41.
44. Zhou H, Tang XH, De Han J, et al. Dermoscopy as an ancillary tool for the diagnosis of pityriasis versicolor. *J Am Acad Dermatol.* 2015;73, e205–206.
45. Hald M, Arendrup MC, Svejgaard EL, et al. Evidence-based Danish guidelines for the treatment of *Malassezia*-related skin diseases. *Acta Derm Venereol.* 2015; 95:12-19.
46. Mittal RR, Prasad D, Singh P. Comparative histopathology of pityriasis versicolor and *Pityrosporum* folliculitis. *Indian J Dermatol Venereol Leprol.* 1992;58:262.
47. Hu SW, Bigby M. Pityriasis versicolor: a systematic review of interventions. *Arch Dermatol.* 2010;146:1132-1140.
48. U.S. Food and Drug Administration (FDA). FDA drug safety communication: FDA warns that prescribing of Nizoral (ketoconazole) oral tablets for unapproved uses including skin and nail infections continues; linked to patient death. http://www.fda.gov/Drugs/DrugSafety/ucm500597.htm. Updated July 26, 2013. Accessed September 11, 2016.
49. Faergemann J, Gupta AK, Al Mofadi A, et al. Efficacy of itraconazole in the prophylactic treatment of pityriasis (tinea) versicolor. *Arch Dermatol.* 2002;138:69-73.

Chapter 162 :: Deep Fungal Infections
:: Roderick J. Hay

第一百六十二章

深部真菌感染

中文导读

深部真菌感染包括两种不同的病症：皮下真菌病和全身性真菌病。两者都不常见，皮下真菌病主要局限于热带和亚热带。近年来，全身性真菌病已成为免疫功能低下患者（包括艾滋病患者和接受恶性肿瘤治疗的患者）中重要的机会性感染并发症。皮下真菌感染患者经常会呈现出皮肤受累迹象，而相比之下，全身性真菌病患者仅偶尔会出现皮肤病变。皮下真菌病部分，主要就孢子丝菌病、足菌肿和着色芽生菌病三种疾病进行介绍；全身性真菌感染部分，详细介绍了深部真菌病发病不同部位的一些临床特点和病理组织特点。对组织胞浆菌病、非洲组织胞浆菌病、酿母菌病、球孢子菌病、巴西副球孢子菌、隐球菌病等多种系统感染的真菌疾病进行了临床表现、诊断、治疗等多方面的介绍。

〔汪 犇〕

Deep fungal infections comprise 2 distinct groups of conditions: subcutaneous mycoses and systemic mycoses. Neither are common, and the subcutaneous mycoses, with some exceptions, are largely confined to the tropics and subtropics. In recent years, the systemic mycoses have become important opportunistic infectious complications in immunocompromised patients, including those with AIDS and patients receiving treatment for malignancies. They also include a group of primary respiratory tract infections, such as histoplasmosis and coccidioidomycosis, which may affect otherwise healthy individuals and those with underlying illness. The fungi that cause these respiratory tract infections are usually dimorphic or exist in a different morphologic phase (eg, yeast or mold) at different stages of their life cycle.

Patients with subcutaneous fungal infections often present to a physician with signs of skin involvement. By contrast, patients with systemic mycoses only occasionally have skin lesions, either following direct involvement of the skin as a portal of entry or after dissemination from a deep focus of infection. There are a number of excellent texts about fungi and the diseases they cause.[1-4]

Treatment of these conditions remains difficult in many cases, although there is now a wide range of antifungal drugs with different modes of action.

SUBCUTANEOUS MYCOSES

AT-A-GLANCE

Subcutaneous mycoses:
- Are usually sporadic.
- Are contracted in the tropics and subtropics.
- May cause chronic disability.
- Are best diagnosed by histopathology, except for sporotrichosis.
- Often require months of successful antifungal treatment.

The subcutaneous mycoses (Table 162-1), or mycoses of implantation, are infections caused by fungi that

TABLE 162-1
Summary of Subcutaneous Mycoses

SUBCUTANEOUS MYCOSES	CAUSATIVE AGENTS	EPIDEMIOLOGY	CLINICAL FEATURES	HISTOPATHOLOGY	TREATMENT
Sporotrichosis	*Sporothrix schenckii* *S. brasiliensis* *Sporothrix brasiliensis* *Sporothrix globosa* *Sporothrix luriei* *Sporothrix mexicana*	North, South, Central Americas, including southern United States and Mexico, Africa, Egypt, Japan, Australia	Lymphangitic: dermal nodule that breaks down into a small ulcer Fixed: localized to one site, with granuloma formation and ulceration	Mixed granulomatous reaction with neutrophilic microabscesses Fungus is 3 to 5 μm, cigar-shaped or oval Distinctive asteroid body	Itraconazole 200 mg once daily Terbinafine 200 mg once daily treatment continued until 1 week after clinical resolution Saturated solution of potassium iodide (SSKI), 4 to 6 mL thrice daily × 3 to 4 weeks
Mycetoma (maduromycosis, Madura foot)	Fungal (eumycetoma) Filamentous bacteria (actinomycetoma): *Nocardia sp.* *Madurella mycetomatis* *Streptomyces somaliensis* *Scedosporium apiospermum*	Usually in dry tropical areas, such as Central America, Mexico, Sudan, and the Middle East	The foot, lower leg, or hand is commonly involved; may affect head or back Characterized by a firm, painless nodule that spreads slowly with development of papules and draining sinus tracts; later signs include local swelling, chronic sinus formation, and bone involvement	Chronic inflammatory reaction with neutrophil abscesses and scattered giant cells and fibrosis Grains found at center	*Eumycetoma:* Ketoconazole 200 mg Itraconazole 200 mg Voriconazole 200 to 400 mg daily × several months *Actinomycetoma:* Dapsone + streptomycin Sulfamethoxazole-trimethoprim + rifampin or streptomycin Surgery, either local dissection or (in severe cases) amputation
Chromoblastomycosis (chromomycosis)	*Phialophora verrucosa* *Fosecaea pedrosoi* *Fonsecaea compactum* *Wangiella dermatitidis* *Cladophialophora carrionii*	Central and South America, Caribbean, Africa, South Asia, Australasia, Japan	The feet, legs, arms, or upper trunk are commonly involved Begins as a slowly expanding warty papule; may be a plaque-like lesion with an atrophic center. May develop satellite lesions from autoinoculation	Mixed granulomatous response, with small neutrophilic abscesses and exuberant epidermal hyperplasia The organism may appear singly or in small groups of brown-pigmented cells	Itraconazole 200 mg once daily or Terbinafine 250 mg once daily or IV amphotericin B (up to 1 mg/kg/day) Treatment continued for several months, until clinical resolution Surgery only as an adjunct to medical treatment; lesions can be spread by surgery

Phaeohyphomycosis (phaeomycotic cyst, cystic chromomycosis)	Exophiala jeanselmei Wangiella dermatitidis	More common in the tropics	Lesions present as cysts.	Cyst wall consists of palisades of macrophages and other inflammatory cells surrounded by a fibrous capsule; fungal hyphae may be found in the macrophage zone	Surgical excision advised, but relapse may occur
Lobomycosis (keloidal blastomycosis, Lobo disease)	Lacazia loboi	Central and tropical South America	Usually exposed areas such as legs, arms, and face; may spread by autoinoculation Characterized by keloid-like lesions	Large, pop-bead organisms within histiocytes and multinucleated giant cells	Antifungal therapy is not effective Surgical removal is the main treatment
Subcutaneous mucormycosis	Basidiobolus ranarum (Basidiobolus haptosporus)	South America, Africa, Indonesia	Develop around limb-girdle sites A firm, slowly spreading woody cellulitis	Chronic granulomatous response with many eosinophils; fungi are present as large, strap-like hyphae without cross walls or septa Splendore-Hoeppli phenomenon	Ketoconazole 400 mg daily Itraconazole 100 to 200 mg daily Treatment with SSKI (similar to sporotrichosis treatment)
	Conidiobolus coronatus		Facial involvement, beginning in the inferior nasal turbinates and spreading to the central part of the face; swelling is hard and painless		
Rhinosporidiosis	Rhinosporidium seeberi	Southern India, Sri Lanka, South America, the Caribbean, and South Africa	The nasal mucosa is the main affected site; conjunctival mucosa also may be susceptible Characterized by polyps studded with white flecks	Large sporangia or spore sacs in different phases of development	Surgical excision is the only treatment

have been introduced directly into the dermis or subcutaneous tissue through a penetrating injury, such as a thorn prick. Although many are tropical infections, others, such as sporotrichosis, are also prevalent in temperate climates; any of these infections may present as an imported disease in a patient who has originated from an endemic area, sometimes after a lapse of many years. The most common subcutaneous mycoses are sporotrichosis, mycetoma, and chromoblastomycosis. Rarer infections include lobomycosis and subcutaneous mucormycosis.

SPOROTRICHOSIS

DEFINITIONS

Sporotrichosis is a subcutaneous or systemic fungal infection caused by the dimorphic fungus *Sporothrix*. Based on molecular techniques, there are now known to be at least 5 different species that vary in geographic distribution: *Sporothrix schenckii, Sporothrix brasiliensis, Sporothrix globosa, Sporothrix luriei,* and *Sporothrix mexicana*.[5,6]

HISTORICAL PERSPECTIVE

The fungus occurs in the natural environment, presumably in mold (cells growing in a chain) form, but develops as a yeast (cells growing as single cells) in infections. The most frequent site of this infection is the dermis or subcutis. There is also a systemic form of sporotrichosis whose clinical features range from pulmonary infection to arthritis or meningitis. One important characteristic of the diagnosis of cutaneous lesions is the scarcity of organisms in tissue, making confirmation of the diagnosis by microscopy potentially difficult.[6] Sometimes in tissue, fungal cells are surrounded by an eosinophilic refractile fringe, the asteroid body, that is a characteristic of the organism, although a similar phenomenon may occur with other infectious organisms (eg, *Schistosome* eggs).

EPIDEMIOLOGY

Infections occur in both temperate and tropical countries. They are seen in North, South, and Central America, including the southern United States and Mexico, as well as in Africa, Egypt, Japan, and Australia.[6] The countries where the highest rates of infection occur are Mexico, Brazil, and South Africa. However, sometimes hyperendemic areas are found where large numbers of cases occur.[7] In the United States, infections are most common in the midwestern river valleys. Infections are now rare in much of Europe. In nature, the fungus grows on decaying vegetable matter such as plant debris, leaves, and wood. Although it is usually a cause of sporadic infection, *Sporothrix* also may affect groups of workers exposed to the organism, such as those using straw as a packing material, gardeners, forestry workers, and those whose recreational activities bring them into contact with plant debris. A recent outbreak of sporotrichosis in Brazil (mainly caused by *S. brasiliensis*) has accentuated the role of exposure to other sources of infection, in this domestic or feral cats. The organism is thought to be introduced into the skin through a local injury.

CLINICAL FEATURES

Cutaneous Findings: The 2 clinical varieties of sporotrichosis are the subcutaneous and systemic forms of disease.[5,8,9] Subcutaneous sporotrichosis is by far the more common and includes 2 main forms: (a) lymphangitic and (b) fixed infections. The lymphangitic form is the more common and usually develops on exposed skin sites such as hands or feet. The first sign of infection is the appearance of a dermal nodule that breaks down into a small ulcer. Draining lymphatics become inflamed and swollen, and a chain of soft secondary nodules develops along the course of the lymphatic (Fig. 162-1); these also may break down and ulcerate. In the fixed variety, which accounts for approximately 15% of cases, the infection remains localized to 1 site, such as the face, and a granuloma develops that subsequently may ulcerate. Satellite nodules or ulcers may form around the rim of the primary lesion. Other clinical variants of subcutaneous sporotrichosis may mimic mycetoma, lupus vulgaris, and chronic venous ulceration. In some cases, deep extension of the infection may affect joints or tendon sheaths. Patients with AIDS who develop sporotrichosis often have multiple cutaneous lesions[9] without prominent lymphatic involvement, but deep infections, such as arthritis, are also reported.

Noncutaneous Findings: In the much rarer systemic form of sporotrichosis, lesions can develop almost anywhere, although chronic lung nodules, with cavitation, arthritis, and meningitis have been described most frequently. These may coexist with cutaneous lesions of sporotrichosis.

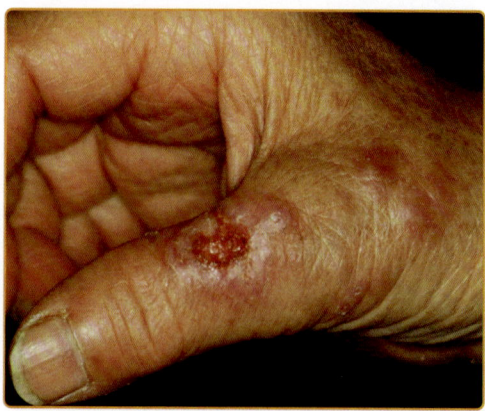

Figure 162-1 Sporotrichosis. An ulcerated nodule is seen on the thumb, with proximal lymphangitic spread represented by subcutaneous nodules. (Used with permission from Takeji Nishikawa, MD.)

DIAGNOSIS

Laboratory Testing: The best sources of diagnostic material are smears, exudates, and biopsies. *Sporothrix* is seen very rarely in direct microscopic examination because yeasts are usually present only in small numbers; the organism can be isolated readily on Sabouraud agar. In primary culture, the fungus grows as a mold, with compact, white colonies that darken with age. Microscopically, the hyphae produce small oval or triangular conidia either on specialized hyphae or elsewhere on the mycelium. Ideally, the organism should be converted to yeast phase on enriched media such as brain-heart infusion agar at 37°C (98.6°F) to complete the identification.

Pathology: Pathologically, sporotrichosis causes a mixed granulomatous reaction with neutrophil microabscesses. The fungus, if present, is usually in the form of small (3 to 5 μm) cigar-shaped or oval yeasts that may, on occasion, be surrounded by a thick, radiating eosinophilic fringe forming the distinctive asteroid body. Organisms are usually sparsely distributed in lesions, and it may be necessary to scan several sections to identify a single yeast. An intradermal sporotrichin skin test is available in some countries and may have a role to play in allowing the physician to identify the most appropriate laboratory investigations to instigate.

DIFFERENTIAL DIAGNOSIS

Conditions commonly confused with sporotrichosis are mycobacterial (see Chap. 157) and primary cutaneous *Nocardia* infections (see Chap. 158) and leishmaniasis (see Chap. 178). The nontuberculous mycobacterial infection caused by *Mycobacterium marinum* (fish-tank granuloma), in particular, closely resembles lymphangitic sporotrichosis.

CLINICAL COURSE AND PROGNOSIS

With the correct treatment, cases of sporotrichosis resolve readily, but untreated they can persist for more than 3 years.

MANAGEMENT

Interventions: Although spontaneous remissions may occur, most patients are treated with antifungal chemotherapy.[10] Treatments include itraconazole (200 mg daily) and terbinafine (250 mg daily), which are better tolerated, and intravenous amphotericin B for deep infection; as of this writing there has been little experience with voriconazole or posaconazole. In all cases, treatment is continued for at least 1 week after clinical resolution. A cheaper alternative is potassium iodide (saturated solution), 4 to 6 mL thrice daily, which is effective in the cutaneous types of sporotrichosis and should be continued for 3 to 4 weeks after clinical cure. The daily dose is built up slowly from 1 mL thrice daily over 2 to 3 weeks to avoid side effects such as hypersalivation and nausea. This is an inexpensive form of therapy, but it is unpalatable.

Prevention: There is no preventive management.

MYCETOMA (MADUROMYCOSIS, MADURA FOOT)

DEFINITIONS

Mycetoma is a chronic localized infection caused by different species of fungi or actinomycetes. It is characterized by the formation of aggregates of the causative organisms, known as *grains* that are found within abscesses. These either drain via sinuses onto the skin surface or involve adjacent bone, causing a form of osteomyelitis. Grains are discharged onto the skin surface via these sinuses. The disease advances by direct spread, and distant metastatic sites of infection are very rare. Mycetomas caused by species of fungi are known as *eumycetomas*, and those caused by aerobic actinomycetes or filamentous bacteria are known as *actinomycetomas* (see Chap. 158). The organisms are usually soil or plant saprophytes[11] that are only incidental human pathogens.

HISTORICAL PERSPECTIVE

Mycetoma has been designated a neglected tropical disease by the World Health Organization.[12]

EPIDEMIOLOGY

Mycetomas are mainly, but not exclusively, found in the dry tropics where there is low annual rainfall.[11,12] They are sporadic infections that are seldom common, even in endemic areas.[13] Occasionally, nonimported cases are reported from temperate climates, although in these cases, the most common organism is *Scedosporium apiospermum*. Actinomycetomas caused by *Nocardia* sp. are most common in Central America and Mexico. In other parts of the world, the most common organism is a fungus, *Madurella mycetomatis*. The actinomycete *Streptomyces somaliensis* is isolated most often from patients originating from Sudan and the Middle East. The causative organisms of mycetoma have been isolated or detected by molecular methods from either soil or plant material, including Acacia thorns, in endemic areas.

The organisms are implanted subcutaneously, usually after a penetrating injury. It is unusual to find any underlying predisposition in patients with mycetoma, and the persistence of the organism after the initial inoculation appears to be related to its ability to evade host defenses through a variety of adaptations, such as cell-wall thickening and melanin deposition.[14]

CLINICAL FEATURES

Cutaneous Features: The clinical features of both fungal and actinomycete mycetomas are very similar.[12] They are most common on the foot, lower leg, or hand, although head or back involvement also may occur. Infection of the chest wall is most characteristic of *Nocardia* infections (see Chap. 158). The earliest stage of infection is a firm, painless nodule that spreads slowly with the development of papules and draining sinus tracts over the surface (Fig. 162-2).

Complications: Local tissue swelling, chronic sinus formation, and later bone involvement distort and deform the original site of infection (Figs. 162-3 and 162-4). Lesions are seldom painful except in the late stages and where sinus tracts are about to emerge onto the skin surface.

Noncutaneous Findings: Dissemination from the initial site is exceptionally rare, although local lymphadenopathy may occur.

DIAGNOSIS

Laboratory Testing: Finding the mycetoma grains is the key to establishing the diagnosis, and these are generally discharged from the openings of sinus tracts. However, they also may be obtained by removing the surface crust from a pustule or sinus tract with a sterile needle and gently squeezing the edges. Grains are 250- to 1000-μm white, black, or red particles that can be seen with the naked eye (Table 162-2). Direct microscopy of grains is important because it will show whether the grain is composed of the small actinomycete or broader fungal filaments. In general, it is not possible to distinguish

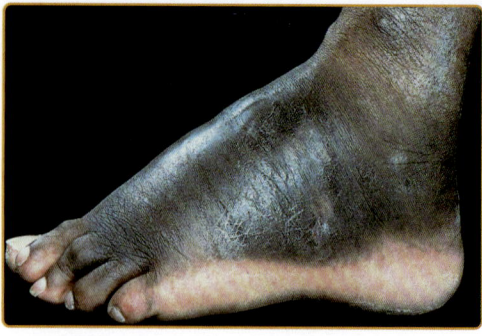

Figure 162-3 Eumycetoma caused by *Scedosporium* leading to significant distortion of the forefoot.

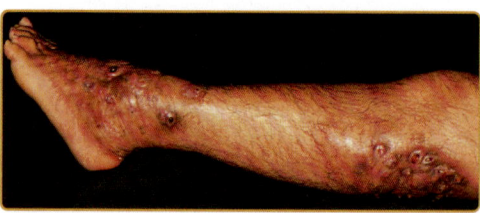

Figure 162-4 Mycetoma. Chronic fibrotic involvement of the foot with lymphatic spread to the popliteal fossa.

TABLE 162-2
Macroscopic and Histopathologic Features of Mycetoma Grains[a]

ORGANISMS	HEMATOXYLIN AND EOSIN SECTION APPEARANCES
Eumycetoma	
Dark grains	
Madurella mycetomatis, Madurella fahalii, M. sudanensis	Cement present, vesicles sometimes prominent
Trematosphaeria grisea	Cement absent, compact outer layer
Falciformispora senegalensis	Cement in outer zone, dark periphery with vesicular center
Exophiala jeanselmei	Cement absent, often hollow
Medicopsis romeroi	Cement lacking, compact outer layer
Pale grains	
Fusarium sp., Acremonium, Scedosporium apiospermum, Aspergillus nidulans, Neotestudina rosati	Compact, pigment lacking, interwoven fungal filaments (*Scedosporium apiospermum* may have prominent vesicles)
Actinomycetoma	
Pale (white to yellow) grains	
Actinomadura madurae	Basophilic-stained fringe in layers
Nocardia brasiliensis	Small, pale blue, eosinophilic fringe
Yellow to brown grains	
Streptomyces somaliensis	Grains fractured, basophilic, or pink
Red to pink grains	
Actinomadura pelletieri	Small, basophilic layers

[a]Helpful rules of thumb:
- Black or dark grains are always produced by fungi;
- Red grains are always produced actinomycetes;
- But pale (white) grains may be produced by either fungi or actinomycetes.

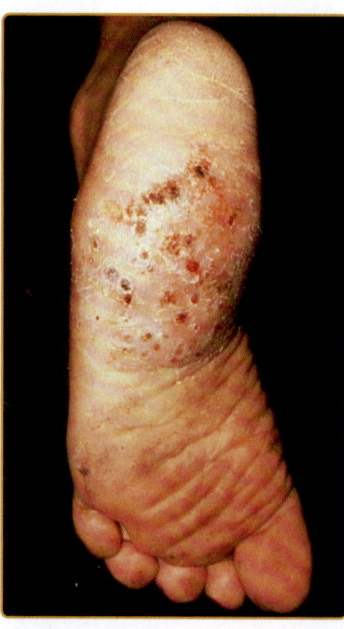

Figure 162-2 Mycetoma. Brawny edema and crusted papules on the plantar surface.

the fine actinomycete filaments in potassium hydroxide (KOH) mounts or, for that matter, in hematoxylin-and-eosin–stained material. In addition, black grains are always caused by fungi; red grains, by actinomycetes (Table 162-2).

Final identification requires isolation of the causal agent in culture. In view of the number of possible species, a series of different culture media and conditions of incubation should be used. Morphologic and physiologic characteristics are used to distinguish between the genera and species. There are now a few examples where the organism has been identified using specific primers through use of the polymerase chain reaction (PCR). Serology is diagnostically helpful only in some cases (eg, in *S. somaliensis*), and even then, more as a guide to therapeutic response. In a few centers, molecular tools are used to identify organisms and this has resulted in changes in their nomenclature (see Table 162-2).

Pathology: Histologically, there is a chronic inflammatory reaction with neutrophil abscesses and scattered giant cells and fibrosis.[11] Grains are found in the center of the inflammation. Their size and shape may help in the identification, although with nonpigmented (pale or white grain) eumycetomas, this is seldom sufficient (Fig. 162-5).

Imaging: X-ray changes include periosteal erosion and proliferation, as well as the development of lytic lesions in the bone. Bone scans or MRI may identify bone lesions and soft-tissue changes at an earlier stage.

DIFFERENTIAL DIAGNOSIS

Chronic bacterial or tuberculous osteomyelitis may resemble mycetoma. Actinomycosis (see Chap. 158) is also similar but usually develops close to certain sites, such as the mouth or the cecum, where the causative organisms are sometimes commensal.

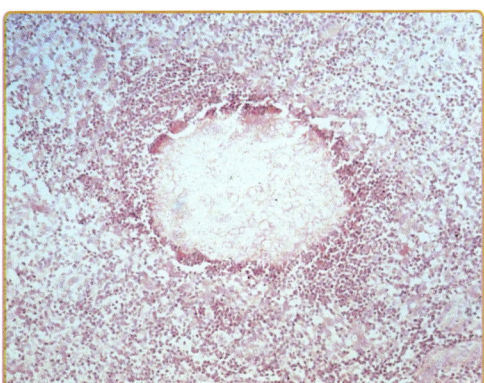

Figure 162-5 Pale eumycetoma grain (hematoxylin-and-eosin stain).

CLINICAL COURSE AND PROGNOSIS

There is no spontaneous remission.

MANAGEMENT

Medications: Of the fungal causes of mycetoma, some cases of *M. mycetomatis* infection respond to ketoconazole 200 mg, itraconazole 200 mg, or voriconazole 200 to 400 mg daily over several months. For the others, a trial of therapy with griseofulvin or terbinafine is worth attempting. However, responses to chemotherapy are unpredictable, although antifungals may slow the course of infection.

Actinomycetomas (see Chap. 158) generally respond to antibiotics such as a combination of dapsone with streptomycin or sulfamethoxazole-trimethoprim plus rifampin or streptomycin. Amikacin, moxifloxacin, or imipenem also may be used in recalcitrant *Nocardia* infections. The responses in all but a few cases are good.[15]

Procedures: Surgery, usually amputation, is the definitive procedure and may have to be used in advanced cases. However, in defined lesions surgical dissection following antifungal therapy can produce excellent results.[15]

Prevention: Diagnosis of early lesions will form part of a new targeted strategy for mycetoma.

CHROMOBLASTOMYCOSIS (CHROMOMYCOSIS)

DEFINITIONS

Chromoblastomycosis is a chronic fungal infection of the skin and subcutaneous tissues caused by pigmented (dematiaceous) fungi that are implanted into the dermis from the environment. In the ensuing inflammation, they form thick-walled single cells or cell clusters (sclerotic or muriform bodies), and these may elicit a marked form of pseudoepitheliomatous hyperplasia, which is often accompanied by transepidermal elimination of organisms.

HISTORICAL PERSPECTIVE

The infection can be caused by a number of different pigmented fungi, the most common being *Phialophora verrucosa*, *Fonsecaea pedrosoi*, *Fonsecaea compactum*, *Wangiella dermatitidis*, and *Cladophialophora carrionii*.[16]

EPIDEMIOLOGY

The fungi that cause chromoblastomycosis can be isolated in the environment from wood, plant debris, or soil.[17] The majority of infections are caused by *F. pedrosoi* and *C. carrionii*. As with other subcutaneous mycoses, infection follows implantation through a tissue injury. The infection is found as a sporadic condition in Central and South America, and rarely in North America. It occurs in the Caribbean region, Africa (particularly Madagascar), South Asia, Australasia, and Japan. It also may occur as an imported infection outside the usual endemic areas. The disease is most frequent in male rural workers.

CLINICAL FEATURES

Cutaneous Findings: The initial site of the infection is usually on the feet, legs, arms, or upper trunk. The clinical features vary.[17] The initial lesion is often a warty papule that expands slowly over months or years (Figs. 162-6 and 162-7). Alternatively, lesions may be plaque-like with an atrophic center. The more common verrucous form spreads slowly and locally. Individual lesions may be very thick and often develop secondary bacterial infection. Satellite lesions around the initial site of infection are local extensions of the infection and usually are produced by scratching.

Complications: Complications of chromoblastomycosis include local lymphedema, leading to elephantiasis and squamous cell carcinomas in some chronic lesions.

DIAGNOSIS

Laboratory Testing: The typical sclerotic or muriform fungal cells can be seen in skin scrapings taken from the surface of lesions, particularly areas where there is a small, dark spot on the skin surface, using KOH mounts.

In culture, these fungi are very similar in gross macroscopic appearance, producing black colonies with a downy surface. Their cultural identification depends on demonstrating the presence of different but specific types of sporulation, and either single or multiple sporulation mechanisms may be seen in each organism. Accurate differentiation between the different fungi may be difficult. At this stage, the choice of treatment does not depend critically on correct identification of the organisms, although there may be differences in the speed of response to azole drugs (see section "Management (mycetoma)").

Pathology: The lesions also should be biopsied because the pathologic changes and presence of muriform cells are typical. The histology shows a mixed granulomatous response, with small neutrophil abscesses and often exuberant epidermal hyperplasia.[18] The organisms, which are often seen either in giant cells or in neutrophil abscesses, appear singly or in small groups of brown pigmented cells, often with a single or double septum and thick cell wall.

DIFFERENTIAL DIAGNOSIS

The disease must be differentiated from podoconiosis or chronic tropical lymphedema with hyperplasia (mossy foot), which is a result of a reaction to soil microparticles. Other chronic verrucous lesions, such as tuberculosis, sporotrichosis, and blastomycosis, should also be considered. The identification of organisms in the lesions of chromoblastomycosis is essential.

CLINICAL COURSE AND PROGNOSIS

There is no spontaneous remission.

MANAGEMENT

Medications: The main treatments for chromoblastomycosis are itraconazole, 200 mg daily[19];

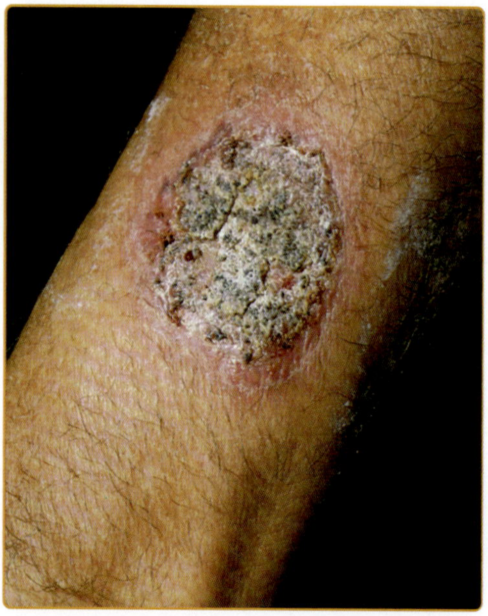

Figure 162-6 Chromoblastomycosis. A solitary, large, verrucous plaque surrounded by a halo of erythema is seen on the calf. (Used with permission from Ted Rosen, MD, and Howard Rubin, MD.)

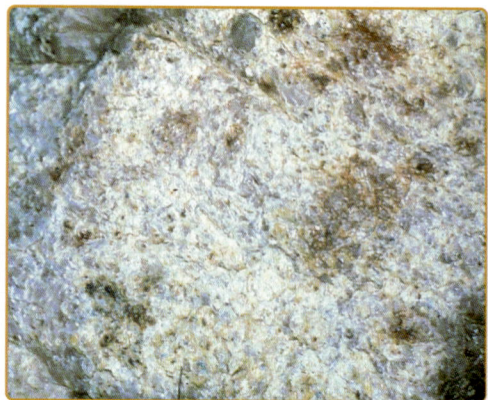

Figure 162-7 Closeup view of chromoblastomycosis. Note hyperkeratosis with pigmentation.

terbinafine, 250 mg daily[20]; and, in extensive cases, IV amphotericin B (up to 1 mg/kg daily). The responses of these fungi to different antifungal agents do not appear to differ significantly, although there is some evidence that *C. carrionii* responds more rapidly to terbinafine and itraconazole. In any event, treatment is continued until there is clinical resolution of lesions, which usually takes several months. Extensive lesions often respond poorly to conventional treatment and combinations of antifungal drugs, for example, amphotericin B and flucytosine or itraconazole and terbinafine, have been used.

Procedures: Lesions can be spread by surgery, which should be used only as an adjunctive therapy after drug treatment. The local application of heat might be helpful in some instances.

PHAEOHYPHOMYCOSIS (PHAEOMYCOTIC CYST, CYSTIC CHROMOMYCOSIS)

Phaeohyphomycosis is a rare infection characterized by the formation of subcutaneous inflammatory cysts or plaques. It is caused by dematiaceous fungi, the most common of which are *Exophiala jeanselmei* and *W. dermatitidis*, but some 103 species have been described as causal agents.[21] However, unlike in chromoblastomycosis, these organisms form short, irregular, pigmented hyphae in tissue. The infection may occur in any climatic area, although it is more common in the tropics. It also may appear in immunosuppressed patients, particularly those receiving long-term glucocorticoid therapy. The lesions present as cysts and may be mistaken for other similar structures, such as synovial or Baker cysts. The diagnosis is usually made after surgical excision. Histologically, the cyst wall consists of palisades of macrophages and other inflammatory cells surrounded by a fibrous capsule, and the fungal hyphae are found in the macrophage zone. Although the fungi in tissue lesions are usually pigmented, this is not always the case; cystic lesions caused by nonpigmented fungi are called *hyalohyphomycotic cysts*. The treatment is surgical excision, although relapse can occur, particularly in immunocompromised patients.

LOBOMYCOSIS (KELOIDAL BLASTOMYCOSIS, LOBO DISEASE)

Lobomycosis is an uncommon infection seen in Central and tropical South America, often in remote rural areas. The source of the organism is unknown, although similar lesions have been found on freshwater dolphins. Lobomycosis is characterized by the appearance of keloid-like skin lesions on exposed sites.[22] Although it cannot be cultured in vitro, it is caused by a fungus, *Lacazia loboi*, that forms chains of rounded cells in tissue, each joined by a small tubule. Lesions may occur anywhere on the body but usually are found on exposed parts such as the legs, arms, and face. They can spread from site to site by autoinoculation. Antifungal drugs are not effective, and surgical removal is the main treatment.

SUBCUTANEOUS MUCORMYCOSIS (BASIDIOBOLOMYCOSIS, SUBCUTANEOUS PHYCOMYCOSIS, AND CONIDIOBOLOMYCOSIS, [RHINO]-ENTOMOPHTHOROMYCOSIS]

Subcutaneous mucormycosis is a rare tropical subcutaneous mycosis characterized by the development and spread of a chronic, firm, swelling involving subcutaneous tissue. There are 2 main varieties caused by different organisms.[23] The first, most often caused by *Basidiobolus ranarum* (*Basidiobolus haptosporus*), is more common in children. It occurs in a wide variety of countries and environments from South America to Africa and Indonesia. The organism can be found in plant debris and in the intestinal tracts of reptiles and amphibians. Lesions usually develop around limb girdle sites and present with a firm, slowly spreading, woody cellulitis. The second form, caused by *Conidiobolus coronatus*, is seen in adults. The organism can be isolated from soil, plant debris, and some insects. The early infection starts in the region of the inferior turbinates of the nose. Spread involves the central part of the face, and once again, the swelling is hard and painless. It may cause very severe deformity of the nose, lips, and cheeks. These infections are distinct to those caused by related fungi.

Histopathologically, a chronic granulomatous response with large numbers of eosinophils can be seen. The fungi are present as large, strap-like hyphae without cross walls or septa. They are also often surrounded by refractile eosinophilic material (Splendore-Hoeppli phenomenon). The organisms can be cultured readily on Sabouraud agar. Ketoconazole (400 mg daily) and itraconazole (100 to 200 mg daily) also may be useful in this condition, although experience as of this writing is limited to a few cases. Lesions also respond to oral treatment with potassium iodide, given in similar doses to those used in sporotrichosis (see "Management" under "Sporotrichosis").

RHINOSPORIDIOSIS

Rhinosporidiosis is a chronic infection caused by the organism *Rhinosporidium seeberi*, which causes the development of polyps affecting the mucous membranes. The organism has never been cultured, and it is now thought to be an aquatic protist and a member of the Mesomycetozoea. Rhinosporidiosis is seen most often in Southern India and Sri Lanka. Cases also have been described in South America, the Caribbean, and South Africa. Exposure to water (lakes, pools) is associated with the infection. The main site affected is the nasal mucosa, but the conjunctival mucosa also may be affected.[24] The infection causes the development of polyps that are studded with white flecks; these are small cysts or sporangia containing small spores. These are best seen in histopathologic sections, where the large sporangia or spore sacs in different phases of development are readily seen. The only treatment is surgical excision.

SYSTEMIC MYCOSES

AT-A-GLANCE

- Where the patient has lived or visited is important for diagnosis of systemic mycoses.
- History of underlying disease states and their treatment is critical.
- Erythema nodosum may be caused by some endemic mycoses (eg, coccidioidomycosis).
- Skin biopsy is important in making the diagnosis.
- Positive fungal culture must be interpreted with caution, as the organism identified may simply be colonizing the site.
- Warn the laboratory if you are sending material from a suspected endemic mycosis case for culture, as these are dangerous pathogens and require containment facilities.
- Treatment may require prolonged therapy with IV drugs such as amphotericin B, voriconazole, and caspofungin.

The systemic mycoses are fungal infections whose initial portal of entry into the body is usually a deep site such as the lung, GI tract, or paranasal sinuses. They have the capacity to spread via the bloodstream to produce a generalized infection. In practice, there are 2 main varieties of systemic mycosis: (a) the opportunistic mycoses and (b) the endemic respiratory mycoses.

The chief opportunistic systemic mycoses seen in humans are systemic or deep candidiasis, aspergillosis, and systemic zygomycosis. These affect patients with severe underlying disease states, such as AIDS, or with neutropenia associated with malignancy, as well as recipients of solid-organ transplantations, immunomodulating biologic therapies, or extensive surgery. With the use of combination antiretroviral therapy, the incidence of systemic mycoses in patients infected with HIV has dropped considerably. In the neutropenic patient in particular, other fungi also may cause infection occasionally. Different underlying conditions predispose to different mycoses; Table 162-3 outlines a scheme for this. Generally, skin involvement is not common with most of these opportunistic infections, which can occur in any climate and environment. The clinical manifestations of the opportunistic mycoses are also variable because they depend on the site of entry of organism and the underlying disease.

The endemic respiratory mycoses are histoplasmosis (classic and African types), blastomycosis, coccidioidomycosis, paracoccidioidomycosis, and infections due to *Talaromyces marneffei*. The clinical manifestations of these infections are affected by the underlying state of the patient, and many develop in the presence of particular immunodeficiency states, notably AIDS. However, they follow similar clinical patterns in all infections. These infections also may affect otherwise healthy individuals. They have well-defined endemic areas determined by factors that favor the survival of the causative organisms in the environment, such as climate. The usual route of infection is via the lung (Fig. 162-8).

In practice, because of the tendency for both groups of infections to develop in predisposed patients, the distinction between opportunistic and endemic mycoses is blurred. This is particularly the case with cryptococcosis, which shares clinical and pathologic features of the 2 main types of respiratory systemic mycoses but is mainly seen now in untreated AIDS patients.

TABLE 162-3
Underlying Predisposition and Opportunistic Systemic Mycoses

PREDISPOSITION	INFECTION
Neutropenia (whatever cause) functional neutrophil defects	Aspergillosis, oropharyngeal, and/or systemic candidiasis, mucormycosis, infections caused by rare organisms
CD4 lymphopenia (eg, AIDS)	Oropharyngeal candidiasis, cryptococcosis, and endemic respiratory mycoses such as histoplasmosis, nocardiosis
Biologic therapy (eg, anti–tumor necrosis factor or anti–interferon-γ)	Endemic mycoses (eg, histoplasmosis, coccidioidomycosis, *Talaromyces* infection)
Diabetes mellitus	Mucormycosis
Heart valve surgery	Various but mainly *Candida albicans* and non-*albicans* Candida sp.
Abdominal surgery	Candidiasis

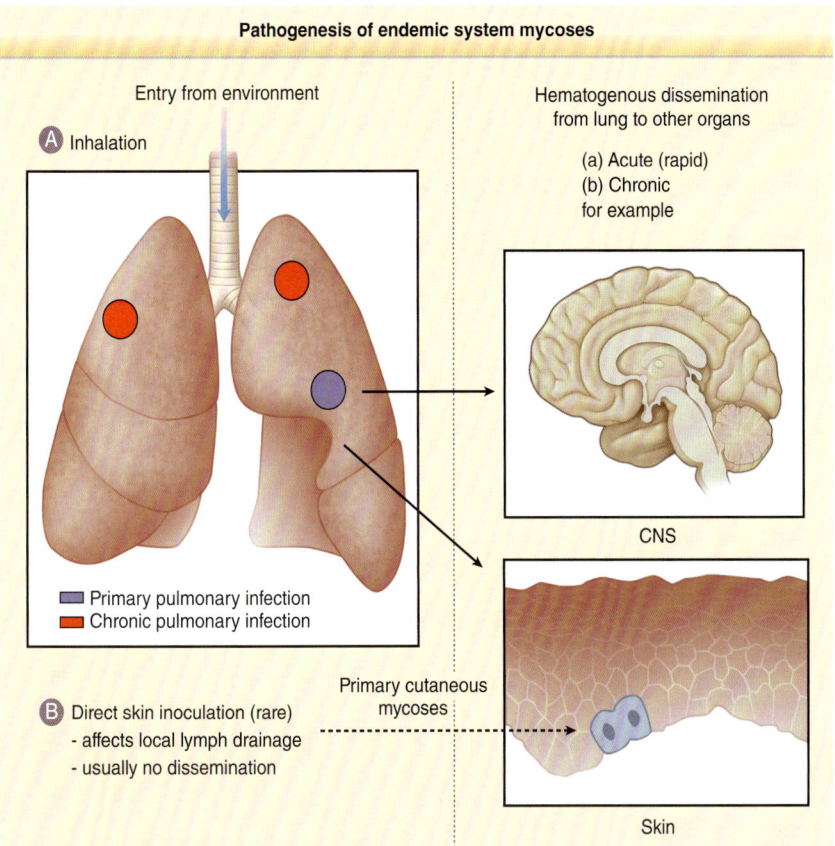

Figure 162-8 The route of infection and dissemination to the skin of the endemic (respiratory) mycoses.

HISTOPLASMOSIS

DEFINITION

Fungi of the dimorphic genus *Histoplasma* cause a number of different infections in animals and humans. These range from equine farcy, or equine histoplasmosis, a disseminated infection of horses caused by *Histoplasma farciminosum* to 2 human infections known as (a) classic or small-form histoplasmosis and (b) African histoplasmosis. These are caused, respectively, by 2 variants of *Histoplasma capsulatum*: (1) *H. capsulatum* var. *capsulatum* and (2) *H. capsulatum* var. *duboisii*. They can be distinguished because their respective yeast phases differ in size, the *capsulatum* variety producing cells from 2 to 5 μm in diameter and the *duboisii* form producing cells of 10 to 15 μm in diameter. The other important differences are in their epidemiology and clinical manifestations. They also show minor antigenic differences that are apparent in serodiagnosis but their mycelial phases are identical.

HISTORICAL PERSPECTIVE

The 2 types of human infections are referred to here as histoplasmosis and African histoplasmosis because this nomenclature is used most widely.

SMALL-FORM OR CLASSIC HISTOPLASMOSIS OR HISTOPLASMOSIS CAPSULATI

DEFINITIONS

Histoplasmosis results from infection with the dimorphic fungus *H. capsulatum* var. *capsulatum*. A sexual state of this fungus, *Ajellomyces capsulatus*, also has been described. The infection starts as a pulmonary infection that, in most individuals, is asymptomatic and heals spontaneously, the only evidence of exposure being the development of a positive intradermal skin test reaction to a fungal antigenic extract, histoplasmin.[25] However, there is, in addition, a symptomatic disease that includes respiratory tract infections and acute or chronic pulmonary histoplasmosis, as well as a disseminated infection that may spread to affect the skin or mucous membranes. Direct inoculation into the skin may occur as a result of a laboratory accident.

EPIDEMIOLOGY

Histoplasmosis occurs in many countries from the Americas to Africa, India, and the Far East. In the United States, it is endemic in the Mississippi and Ohio River valleys, where often more than 80% of the population may have acquired the infection asymptomatically. Exposure rates are usually lower in all other endemic areas, although high rates are also found in northern South America and some Caribbean islands. Histoplasmosis is not found in Europe. *H. capsulatum* is an environmental organism that can be isolated from soil, particularly when it is contaminated with bird or bat excreta. The disease is acquired by inhalation of spores, and epidemics of respiratory tract infection may occur in persons exposed to a spore-laden environment when exploring caves or cleaning sites heavily contaminated with bird droppings, such as bird roosts or barns. Although any person can acquire histoplasmosis through inhalation, it causes a distinctive disseminated infection in patients with disease affecting cellular immune capacity, such as AIDS or lymphoma.[26,27]

CLINICAL FEATURES

The spectrum of histoplasmosis includes both asymptomatic and benign symptomatic infections, and a progressive disseminated variety with bloodstream spread to multiple organs.[25] Skin lesions may develop as a result of immune-complex formation in the primary infection (erythema multiforme) or from direct spread after dissemination from the lungs; rarely, infections may develop at a point of inoculation into the skin.

Asymptomatic forms of histoplasmosis are, by definition, without signs or symptoms, but those exposed usually have a positive histoplasmin skin test. The percentage of skin test reactors in the community indicates the chances of exposure, and, in endemic areas, this may range from 5% to 90%. Occasionally, asymptomatic pulmonary nodules removed at surgical exploration or autopsy are found to contain *Histoplasma*.

Acute Pulmonary Histoplasmosis: In acute pulmonary histoplasmosis, patients are often exposed to large quantities of spores such as may be encountered in a cave or after cleaning a bird-infested area. Patients present with cough, chest pain, and fever, often with accompanying joint pains and rash—toxic erythema, erythema multiforme, or erythema nodosum. These skin rashes are not common, occurring in fewer than 15% of patients, but they may be precipitated by treatment of the acute infection. On chest radiography, there is often diffuse mottling, which may calcify with time.

Chronic Pulmonary Histoplasmosis: Chronic pulmonary histoplasmosis usually occurs in adults and presents with pulmonary consolidation and cavitation, closely resembling tuberculosis. Skin involvement is not seen.

Acute Progressive Disseminated Histoplasmosis: In patients with acute disseminated histoplasmosis, there is widespread dissemination to other organs, such as the liver and spleen, lymphoreticular system, and bone marrow. Patients present with progressive weight loss and fever. This form is the type that is most likely to occur in untreated AIDS patients, who often develop skin lesions as a manifestation of disseminated infection (Fig. 162-9).[28] There are papules, small nodules, or small molluscum-like lesions that subsequently may develop into shallow ulcers. These skin lesions are more common in HIV-positive patients than in others with disseminated histoplasmosis. Diffuse micronodular pulmonary infiltrates also may develop. Patients have progressive and severe weight loss, fever, anemia, and hepatosplenomegaly.

The distinction between acute and chronic dissemination in histoplasmosis is somewhat artificial because these merely represent extremes of behavior, with progression occurring over a few months, on the one hand, and over several years, on the other. Intermediate forms occur, and other organs such as the meninges and heart may be affected.

Chronic Progressive Disseminated Histoplasmosis: Chronic disseminated histoplasmosis may appear months or years after a patient has left an endemic area. The most common clinical presenting features are oral or pharyngeal ulceration, hepatosplenomegaly, or adrenal insufficiency (Addison disease) resulting from adrenal infiltration. The mouth ulcers are often large, irregular, and persistent, and may affect the tongue as well as the buccal mucosa. The patients otherwise may appear well, but it is important to investigate for evidence of infection elsewhere (eg,

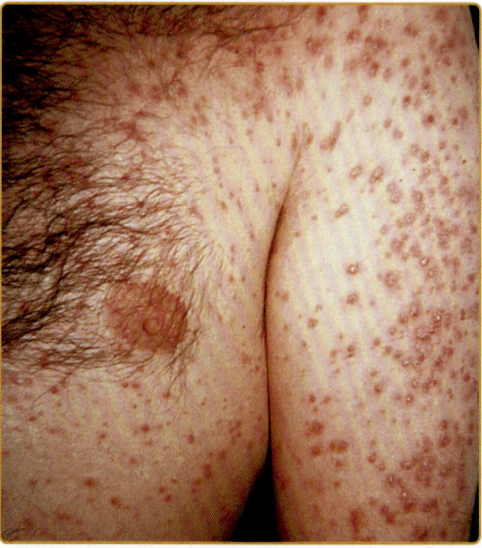

Figure 162-9 Histoplasmosis, disseminated. Multiple erythematous keratotic papules and small plaques resembling guttate pattern psoriasis are seen on the chest and arm of a man with advanced HIV disease. (Used with permission from J. D. Fallon, MD.)

by abdominal CT scan). Adrenal infection in particular should be excluded.

Primary Cutaneous Histoplasmosis: Primary cutaneous histoplasmosis is rare and follows inoculation of the organism into the skin, for instance, after accidental laboratory-acquired or postmortem room-acquired infection. The primary lesion is a nodule or indurated ulcer, and there is often local lymphadenopathy.

DIAGNOSIS

Laboratory Testing: The diagnosis of histoplasmosis is established by identifying the small intracellular yeast-like cells of *Histoplasma* in sputum, peripheral blood, bone marrow, or biopsy specimens. *Histoplasma* must be separated from *T. marneffei* because the 2 organisms are of a similar size, although the latter shows characteristic septa formation. The identity of the organism should be confirmed by culture; it grows as a mold at room temperature. The white, cottony colonies develop at room temperature on Sabouraud glucose agar to produce 2 types of spores, the larger (8 to 15 µm in diameter), rounded, tuberculate macroconidia being typical; the smaller microconidia are infectious. Confirmation of the identity should be obtained by demonstrating ribosomal RNA using a DNA probe. Mycelial-phase cultures of *H. capsulatum* are very infectious, and laboratories receiving specimens should be warned about the suspected diagnosis.

The intradermal histoplasmin skin test is an epidemiologic tool that is of no help in diagnosis. In patients with disseminated histoplasmosis, it is often negative. By contrast, serology is often useful in diagnosis. A rising complement-fixation titer indicates dissemination. Precipitins detected by immunodiffusion are also valuable because the presence of antibodies to specific H and M antigens correlates well with active or recent infection.[28] A new development, particularly helpful in AIDS patients, has been serologic or urine tests for the detection of circulating *Histoplasma* antigens.[29] PCR-based molecular diagnostic methods are available in some centers.

Pathology: In histopathologic sections, *H. capsulatum* is an intracellular parasite often seen in macrophages. The cells are small (2 to 4 µm in diameter) and oval in shape with small buds (Fig. 162-10). Mycelial forms are seen rarely in tissue.

DIFFERENTIAL DIAGNOSIS

The organism is the same size as a number of others causing deep mycoses such as *T. marneffei* and small forms of *Blastomyces* and *Cryptococcus* (see "Laboratory Testing" above). It is also similar in size to *Leishmania* sp., and in the tropics, kala azar is an important part of the differential diagnosis. These observations emphasize the importance of carrying out appropriate laboratory tests to confirm the diagnosis.

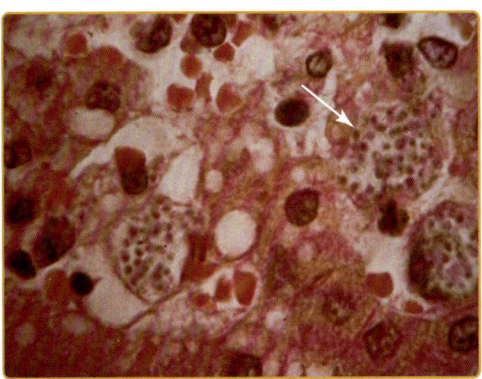

Figure 162-10 Histoplasmosis, disseminated. Lesional biopsy specimen shows dermal macrophages packed with dozens of tiny yeast forms of *Histoplasma capsulatum* (arrow).

AFRICAN HISTOPLASMOSIS (LARGE-FORM HISTOPLASMOSIS OR HISTOPLASMOSIS DUBOISII)

African histoplasmosis is sporadic and uncommon even in AIDS patients.[30] It is seen in patients from areas south of the Sahara and north of the Zambezi River in Africa. Infections seen outside Africa are all imported. The most common clinically involved sites are the skin and bone, although lymph nodes and other organs, including the lungs, may be affected. Skin lesions range from small papules resembling molluscum contagiosum to cold abscesses, draining sinuses, or ulcers. It is not clear if there is an asymptomatic form of African histoplasmosis as in classic histoplasmosis. The diagnosis is confirmed by culture and microscopy (direct microscopy or histopathology). The organisms of *H. capsulatum* var. *duboisii* are different from the smaller *capsulatum* forms. They are usually 10 to 15 µm in diameter, slightly pear-shaped, and clustered in giant cells. *Histoplasma* serology, using conventional tests, is often negative in African histoplasmosis.

CLINICAL COURSE AND PROGNOSIS

Prognosis depends on the site and type of infection. But the choice of therapy for histoplasmosis generally depends on the severity of the illness.

MANAGEMENT

Medications: For patients with some disseminated or localized forms of the disease, oral itraconazole (200 to 400 mg daily) is highly effective. It also has been used for long-term suppressive treatment of the disease in AIDS patients after primary therapy either with itraconazole or amphotericin B.[31] However, there is now evidence that provided CD4 counts do not fall in patients on highly active antiretroviral therapy (HAART) therapy (see Chap. 173), suppressive treatment can be discontinued. In AIDS, some patients receiving treatment of histoplasmosis, an immune reconstitution syndrome has been reported after commencing HAART therapy with intestinal obstruction, uveitis, and arthralgia. Intravenous amphotericin B (up to 1 mg/kg daily) is given to patients with widespread and severe infections and is the main alternative used. Posaconazole and voriconazole are effective in some cases. In African histoplasmosis, itraconazole is also the treatment of choice, but once again, in severe cases amphotericin B may be used.[30]

BLASTOMYCOSIS (NORTH AMERICAN BLASTOMYCOSIS)

Blastomycosis is a chronic mycosis caused by the dimorphic pathogen *Blastomyces dermatitidis*.[32] Its chief sites of involvement are the lungs, but disseminated forms of the infection may affect skin, bones, CNS, and other sites.

EPIDEMIOLOGY

Blastomycosis is found in North America and Canada.[33] Most cases, though, come from the Great Lakes region and southern states of the United States. It also occurs sporadically in Africa, with the largest numbers of cases coming from Zimbabwe,[34] and cases also have been reported from the Middle East and India.

It is thought that the natural habitat of *Blastomyces* is in some way related to wood debris and is close to rivers or lakes or in areas subjected to periodic flooding. However, it is difficult to isolate *Blastomyces* from the natural environment.[35] Blastomycosis also may affect domestic animals such as dogs.

CLINICAL FEATURES

As with histoplasmosis, there is a subclinical form of the infection; its prevalence has not been defined in detail because of lack of a commercial *Blastomyces* skin-test antigen and the extent of antigenic crossreactivity with fungi such as *Histoplasma*. Primary cutaneous blastomycosis is also very rare and follows trauma to the skin and the subsequent introduction of fungus, for instance, in laboratory workers or pathologists.[36] After inoculation, an erythematous, indurated area with a chancre appears in 1 to 2 weeks with associated lymphangitis and lymphadenopathy.

Pulmonary blastomycosis is very similar in clinical presentation to pulmonary tuberculosis.[33,36,37] There may be no symptoms, or there may be low-grade fever, chest pain, cough, and hemoptysis, and unlike histoplasmosis, it often coexists with disseminated disease. Skin lesions are a common presenting feature of disseminated blastomycosis.[36,38] They are often symmetric and usually affect the face and extremities. The early lesion is a papule or nodule, which may ulcerate and discharge pus. With time, this enlarges to form a hyperkeratotic lesion, often with central ulceration and/or scarring (Figs. 162-11 and 162-12). Oral lesions are less common. Multiple skin lesions are often found in disseminated infection. Other patients may present with nodules and abscesses, and in many patients lesions of different morphologies are present. African patients with blastomycosis have a higher frequency

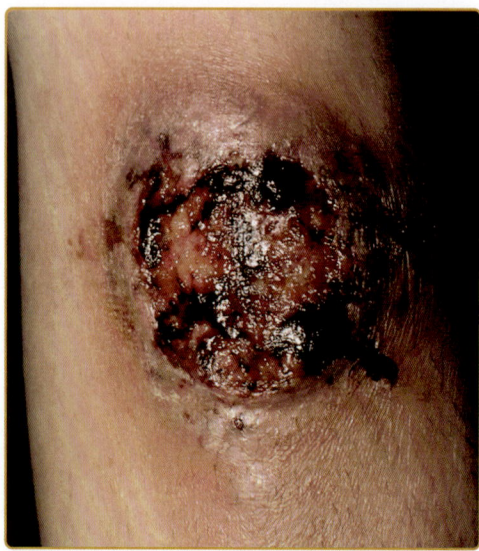

Figure 162-11 Blastomycosis. Inflammatory plaque with ulceration resembling pyoderma gangrenosum on the calf. (Used with permission from Elizabeth M. Spiers, MD.)

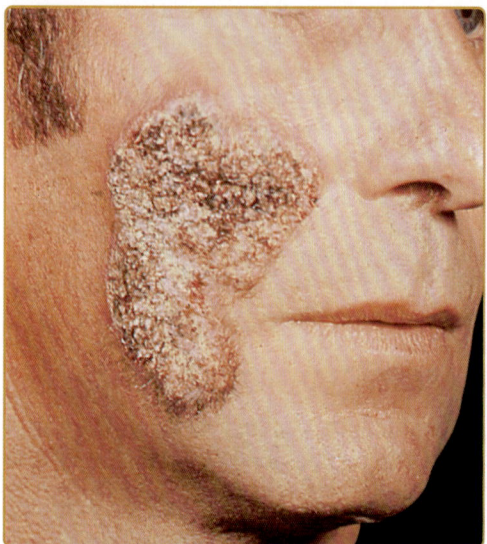

Figure 162-12 Blastomycosis. Chronic verrucous plaque on the cheek.

of skin and bone involvement.[34] Although blastomycosis can affect almost any organ, other common sites for dissemination include the bone, the epididymis, and the adrenal gland. Less commonly, there is widespread rapid dissemination with multiple organ involvement, and *B. dermatitidis* can produce a form of adult respiratory distress syndrome. Skin lesions in widespread disseminated disease are usually papules, abscesses, or small ulcers. Widespread blastomycosis has been described in AIDS patients, but it is not common.[39]

DIAGNOSIS

Laboratory Testing: The fungus can be found in KOH mounts of pus, skin scrapings, or sputum as thick-walled, rounded, refractile, spherical cells with broad-based buds (Fig. 162-13). In culture, the fungus grows as a mycelial fungus at room temperature. It produces small, rounded, or pear-shaped conidia. At higher temperature (37°C [98.6°F]) and on enriched media, it produces yeast forms with the characteristic buds. Molecular probes will confirm the identity. These are often found in giant cells or surrounded by neutrophils (Fig. 162-14). Precipitating antibodies to *B. dermatitidis* are often present in the sera of infected patients, and a characteristic precipitin line, the E band, has been described in a high proportion of proven cases; there is also an enzyme-linked immunosorbent assay for blastomycosis. There is also an antigen detection system that is most accurate in urine samples.

Pathology: In tissue sections, the typical organisms with broad buds may be found, although it may be necessary to search several fields to find the characteristic cells.

DIFFERENTIAL DIAGNOSIS

The chronic skin granulomas must be differentiated from those caused by tuberculosis, other deep mycoses, nonmelanoma skin cancers, pyoderma gangrenosum, and drug reactions caused by bromides and iodides.

CLINICAL COURSE AND PROGNOSIS

As with histoplasmosis, the course depends on the site of infection and the presence of any underlying disease.

MANAGEMENT

Medications: Treatment is similar to that used for histoplasmosis; itraconazole (200 to 400 mg daily) is used in the less-severe forms of the infection or when there is only localized spread. Voriconazole is also active against this infection. Treatment is usually given for at least 6 months. Followup surveillance is necessary because relapse can occur, particularly where there are deep sites of infection or the patient is immunosuppressed. Amphotericin B (up to 1 mg/kg daily) is generally used for the treatment of widespread disseminated forms of blastomycosis.

COCCIDIOIDOMYCOSIS (COCCIDIOIDAL GRANULOMA, VALLEY FEVER, SAN JOAQUIN VALLEY FEVER, DESERT RHEUMATISM)

DEFINITIONS

Coccidioidomycosis is the infection caused by the fungal species *Coccidioides immitis* and *Coccidioides posadasii*; *C. posadasii* is phenotypically identical to *C. immitis* and produces identical disease, but is mainly found outside California. Both show an unusual form of dimorphism, with a mold form at room temperature and the development of spherules, large spore-containing structures, in infected tissue. As with other endemic mycoses, there are asymptomatic, acute and chronic

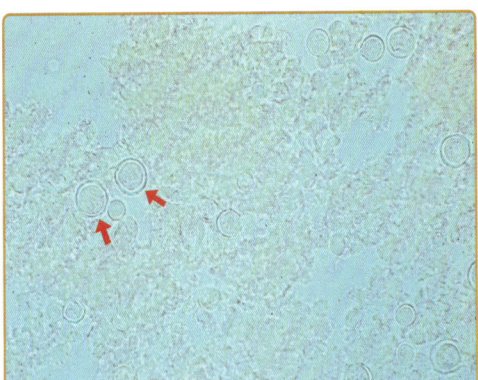

Figure 162-13 Direct preparation (potassium hydroxide) of *Blastomyces* (arrows).

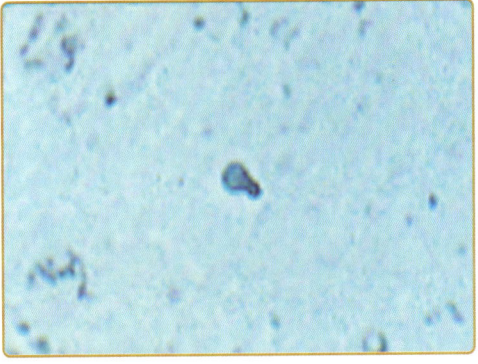

Figure 162-14 Blastomycosis. Lesional biopsy specimen shows a budding yeast form (Gomori methenamine silver stain).

pulmonary, and disseminated forms. The disease can affect otherwise healthy individuals or predisposed patients, including those with AIDS.

EPIDEMIOLOGY

C. immitis is endemic in some semidesert areas of South and Southwest of the United States, and *C. posadasii* elsewhere (Arizona, New Mexico, and Texas) and in parts of Mexico and Central and South America. The climate of the endemic areas is marked by very high summer temperatures and low annual rainfall, demonstrated by a characteristic vegetation with cacti and mesquite bushes. Skin tests with coccidioidin show that the incidence of exposure in endemic areas may be as high as 95%. The fungus is found in soil and can affect other animals as well as humans. Exposure may result from a brief visit to an endemic area, and local weather can determine exposure rates.[40] For instance, dust storms may cause infection in large numbers of individuals. The usual route of infection is respiratory, although direct implantation into the skin can occur rarely.

CLINICAL FEATURES

As with other systemic mycoses, there is an asymptomatic or subclinical form of coccidioidomycosis that is common in endemic areas, judging by the percentages of skin test reactors to coccidioidin in the healthy population. The primary pulmonary form, which is the most common clinical type, presents as a chest infection with fever, cough, and chest pain. Complications such as pleural effusion may occur. Erythema multiforme or erythema nodosum,[40] often accompanied by arthralgia or anterior uveitis, occurs from the third to the seventh week in approximately 10% to 15% of patients, and is more common in females. Sometimes an early, generalized, macular and erythematous rash is seen in some patients.

The chronic pulmonary form of the disease presents with chronic cough and resembles tuberculosis. Skin lesions normally do not occur in this phase.

In the rare primary skin infection,[41] after inoculation, there is an indurated nodule that develops 1 to 3 weeks after local trauma. This is followed by regional lymphadenopathy.

Disseminated coccidioidomycosis develops in fewer than 0.5% of infected individuals. It is mainly seen in patients from certain ethnic backgrounds (African Americans, Filipinos, and Mexicans),[40] apparently independent of occupational exposure or socioeconomic class, in pregnant women, and in immunosuppressed patients, including those with AIDS.[42,43] In disseminated disease, lesions may develop in the skin, subcutaneous tissues, bones, joints, and all organs. The skin lesions (Fig. 162-15) are papules, nodules, abscesses, granulomas, ulcers, or discharging sinuses in which there is underlying bone or joint disease. Some lesions appear as flat plaques with central atrophy. Meningitis is an important complication of dissemination and is usually not associated with signs of infection in other sites. In

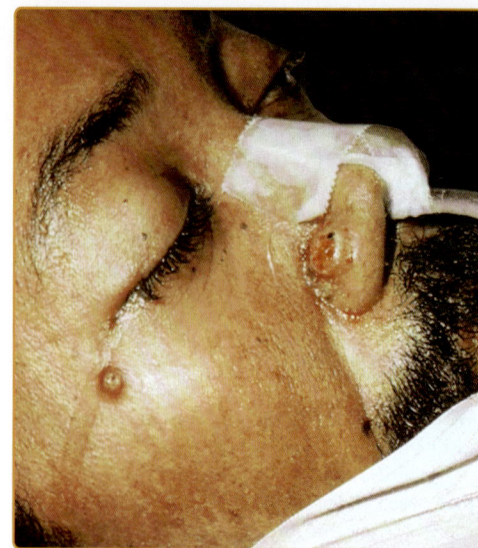

Figure 162-15 Coccidioidomycosis, disseminated. Two intact and ulcerated papules/nodules are seen on the cheek and nose of this comatose patient with coccidioidomycotic meningitis. (Used with permission from Francis Renna, MD.)

AIDS patients, persistent pneumonia, skin lesions, and widespread dissemination can all occur.

DIAGNOSIS

Laboratory Testing: A characteristic of the laboratory findings is the ability of *Coccidioides* to form spore-containing spherules. These are large (up to 250 μm in diameter) and can be seen in KOH mounts of sputum, cerebrospinal fluid, or pus. In culture, colonies of *Coccidioides* are mycelial, fast growing, white, and cottony. On microscopy, there are chains of arthrospores at intervals on the older mycelium. *Coccidioides* in the mold phase is highly infectious, and cultures should be handled carefully. There is, as yet, no commercial molecular test for coccidioidomycosis.

A variety of serologic tests are of value in the diagnosis and prognosis of coccidioidomycosis.[44] Precipitins develop in approximately 90% of infected individuals within 2 to 6 weeks but are short-lived; complement-fixing antibodies are characteristic of more-severe infections and, in active infection, increase to a maximum after 6 months. Skin tests with coccidioidin are of little value in diagnosing infections. Spherulin is an antigen obtained from spherules of *C. immitis* and may be better than coccidioidin for detecting sensitization. However, in severe infections, cutaneous anergy to both is common.

Pathology: Spherules containing large endospores can be seen in tissue sections, although there are a variety of less-distinct intermediate stages in spherule formation that also can be seen. Before endospores form, the cytoplasm of the immature spherule is basophilic and subsequently breaks up into spores. Mycelium is seen rarely in histopathologic sections.

DIFFERENTIAL DIAGNOSIS

Physicians in endemic areas should be aware of the connection between erythema nodosum and coccidioidomycosis. It also may occur in visitors to endemic areas after only a short stay.

CLINICAL COURSE AND PROGNOSIS

As with histoplasmosis, the course depends on the site of infection and the presence of any underlying disease.

MANAGEMENT

Medications: No specific therapy apart from rest is necessary in the primary pulmonary infection, and there is little evidence that the symptoms are either improved or shortened by giving an oral azole drug, even though it is widespread practice. For disseminated disease, the results of treatment are still variably, but amphotericin B (1 mg/kg daily), itraconazole (200 to 400 mg daily), or fluconazole (200 to 600 mg daily) can all be given.[45] Experience with the newer antifungal agents, such as voriconazole and posaconazole, is limited at present. It is important to follow patients carefully, given the frequency of relapse. Meningitis and progressive disseminated infection involving multiple sites are all particularly refractory to therapy. Generally, soft-tissue coccidioidomycosis (skin and joint) has a better prognosis, and the mortality in patients who present with such lesions is low.

Prevention: A vaccine, Spherulin, for coccidioidomycosis has been studied, but the results were inconclusive and at present there is no immunization against this infection.[45]

PARACOCCIDIOIDOMYCOSIS (SOUTH AMERICAN BLASTOMYCOSIS, PARACOCCIDIOIDAL GRANULOMA)

DEFINITIONS

Paracoccidioides brasiliensis is a dimorphic fungus that causes a respiratory tract infection with a tendency to disseminate to the mucous membranes and lymph nodes. It is confined to Central and South America.[46]

EPIDEMIOLOGY

Paracoccidioidomycosis has been reported from most Latin American countries, but the infection is found most commonly in parts of Brazil, Colombia, and Argentina. The infection does not occur in the United States, although it has been reported in Mexico. Exposure rates can be estimated by skin test reactivity and appear to be equal in both males and females, although the prevalence of positive reactors in endemic areas seldom exceeds 25%; work with a skin test derived from purified glycoprotein 43 antigen generally demonstrates that exposure rates are higher than previously believed. The active infection is seen predominantly in males. The mechanism is thought to be connected to the presence of a cytoplasmic estrogen receptor on the fungus, and, in vitro, estradiol suppresses the conversion of mycelium to yeast.[47] The ecologic niche of the organisms is unknown, but the condition is much more frequent in rural areas; exposure is associated with proximity to water or areas of high atmospheric humidity.[48]

CLINICAL FEATURES

There are a number of different clinical patterns of paracoccidioidomycosis infection that depend on the predominant site of clinical involvement. These include the lung (pulmonary form), the mucous membranes (mucocutaneous form), and the lymph nodes (lymphatic form). Many patients have a mixed type of infection with involvement of different organ groups.[46]

Patients rarely present with an acute form of pulmonary infection, although this has been observed rarely and reported to subside while dissemination occurs. More usually, pulmonary infection tends to be chronic and slowly progressive with weight loss and chronic cough. The lesions may be bilateral and nodular on chest radiography, and there is often extensive fibrosis. Other sites of involvement include mucocutaneous areas. Oral or circumoral lesions are common in the mucocutaneous forms of paracoccidioidomycosis; lesions also occur in the nose, conjunctivae, or around the anus. These lesions may be small granulomas or ulcers. They heal with scarring, which may cause considerable deformity.

The cervical lymph nodes are sometimes enlarged, tender, and tethered to the overlying skin; they rarely suppurate. Other systemic sites of involvement include the spleen, intestines, lungs, and liver. Paracoccidioidomycosis is uncommon in AIDS patients, although there is a widespread variety that is a more rapidly progressive form of disseminated infection occurring in young adults or older children without recognizable predisposition.[49]

DIAGNOSIS

Laboratory Testing: Sputum, exudates, and scrapings can be screened using KOH. They show numbers of round yeasts with a characteristic form of multiple budding in which a parent cell is surrounded by large numbers of smaller buds. The organism is dimorphic and produces a cottony mycelial-phase growth on primary isolation at room temperature. Once again, the characteristic yeast phase can be induced on enriched media such as brain–heart infusion agar at 37°C (98.6°F). Serology is very helpful in confirming the diagnosis, the main tests being the immunodiffusion assay and a complement-fixation test. Antibodies to pb27 and 87-kDa antigens have been found to be highly specific for this infection in immunoblotting. There are also antigen-detection tests useful for monitoring patients with disseminated disease.

Pathology: Histopathologically, there is a mixed granulomatous response with fibrosis. The organisms can be seen with special fungal stains such as methenamine silver (Grocott modification). In tissue, the characteristic budding pattern can be seen, although it may be necessary to search several fields to find the most typical structures (Fig. 162-16). In widespread infections, masses of small yeast forms may be mistaken for *Histoplasma*.

DIFFERENTIAL DIAGNOSIS

Differential diagnosis includes tuberculosis, leishmaniasis, and other deep mycoses.

CLINICAL COURSE AND PROGNOSIS

As with histoplasmosis, the course depends on the site of infection and the presence of any underlying disease.

MANAGEMENT

Medications: The treatment of choice in most cases is itraconazole, which can produce remissions in 3 to 6 months.[50] Voriconazole produces similar responses. Relapses can occur, and, where possible, patients should be reviewed periodically after primary therapy. In very extensive infections and in severely ill patients, such as those with the progressive disseminated type of infection, intravenous amphotericin B may be necessary. Severe pulmonary or intraoral fibrosis may remain after treatment.

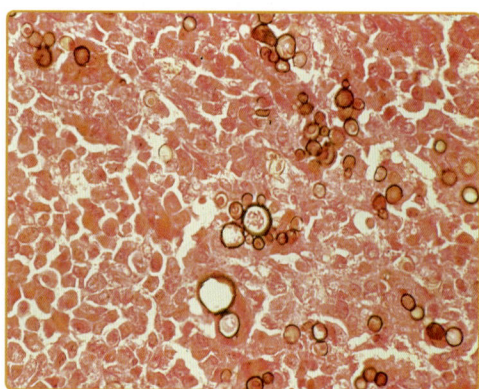

Figure 162-16 Biopsy of oral mucosal lesion showing multiple budding *Paracoccidioides brasiliensis*.

INFECTIONS CAUSED BY *TALAROMYCES MARNEFFEI* (PENICILLIOSIS, PENICILLIOSIS MARNEFFEI)

DEFINITIONS

T. marneffei infection is a more recently recognized disease found in Southeast Asia. *T. marneffei* was originally thought to be a member of the common genus *Penicillium*.[51] It shows an unusual pattern of dimorphism in that it develops yeast-like cells that reproduce with septal formation, dividing the cells into two. It is inhaled via the lungs, and it is not known whether there is a primary cutaneous form of the infection.

EPIDEMIOLOGY

The natural source of *T. marneffei* is unknown. Infections are confined to Southeast Asia, particularly Thailand, South China, and Vietnam. However, there are reports in other Asian countries, including Northeast India, and imported cases are seen in Europe and the United States. Natural infections are known to occur in bamboo rats of the genus *Cannomys*, which are large burrowing rodents. The infection affects otherwise healthy individuals as well as those with immune defects and is most common after the rainy season.[52] Patients with AIDS, as well as those receiving rituximab biologic therapy, appear to be particularly susceptible to this infection.

CLINICAL FEATURES

There has been no work to demonstrate that there is a subclinical form of *Talaromyces* infection, even though this is likely. Patients usually present with localized pulmonary or disseminated disease. The chest signs are those of chronic pulmonary disease.[53,54] More than 50% of AIDS patients with this infection have multiple skin lesions, which are umbilicated papules that may enlarge and ulcerate. They are usually widely scattered on the face and trunk. Other organs, including the liver, GI tract, spleen, and bone marrow, may be affected.

DIAGNOSIS

Laboratory Testing: *T. marneffei* forms characteristic yeast-like cells that are divided by a septum in tissue and are best seen in histopathologic sections stained with methenamine silver. These cells are small (2 to 4 μm in diameter) and difficult to see in blood films or skin or bone marrow smears, but they may be highlighted with stains such as leishmanin. In culture, *T. marneffei* is a green or grayish mold that produces typical conidiophores and a diffusible red pigment. There is no commercial serologic test as yet, although both antigen detection systems and PCR have been used in diagnosis, the PCR for identification of cultures.

DIFFERENTIAL DIAGNOSIS

The main differential diagnosis is with other disseminated mycoses, such as histoplasmosis and cryptococcosis, which also can be found in the endemic area in AIDS patients. Biopsy and, when necessary, culture will distinguish between the different causes.

CLINICAL COURSE AND PROGNOSIS

As with histoplasmosis, the course depends on the site of infection and the presence of any underlying disease.

MANAGEMENT

Medications: In severe cases, amphotericin B is necessary. In many cases, however, there is a good response to itraconazole (200 to 400 mg daily). In AIDS patients, this is continued after initial therapy to prevent relapse.[54]

CRYPTOCOCCOSIS

DEFINITIONS

Cryptococcosis is the infection caused by the encapsulated yeasts *Cryptococcus neoformans* and *Cryptococcus gattii*. Although the main portal of entry is through inhalation into the lungs, the disease usually presents with signs of extrapulmonary dissemination such as meningitis. Cutaneous lesions can develop as a result of dissemination or, rarely, through inoculation. It is associated with HIV infection.[55]

EPIDEMIOLOGY

Cryptococcosis has a worldwide distribution although exposure rates probably differ markedly in different countries. *C. neoformans* has 2 variants: (a) *C. neoformans* var. *neoformans* and (b) *C. neoformans* var. *grubii*.

These correspond to 3 clusters of serotypes: (a) D, (b) A, and (c) B or C.[56] The *neoformans* and *grubii* varieties can be isolated from pigeon excreta and are more common in AIDS patients; the *gattii* form is found in the debris of certain eucalyptus trees in Australia, and California as well as some tropical areas, but it is less often isolated from AIDS patients. Two sexual varieties called *Filobasidiella neoformans* and *Filobasidiella bacillispora* correspond to the *neoformans/grubii* and *gattii* species, respectively. Clinically the main differences to be seen are those between the *neoformans* and *gattii* species, for example, a higher prevalence of symptomatic pulmonary disease with the *gattii* species. Patients with certain immunodeficiency states caused by AIDS, malignant lymphomas, sarcoidosis, collagen disease, carcinoma, and those receiving systemic glucocorticoid therapy are particularly susceptible. The incidence of cryptococcosis in patients with established untreated AIDS varied in different countries, from 3% to 6% in the United States, to 3% in the United Kingdom, to more than 12% in parts of Africa (eg, Democratic Republic of the Congo). However, with the widespread use of HAART therapy the incidence has declined. Strains of serotype D are more likely to be found in skin lesions, which occur in 10% to 15% of cases of disseminated cryptococcosis.

CLINICAL FEATURES

The advent of the AIDS epidemic affected the epidemiology of cryptococcosis considerably, and in areas such as northern Thailand, it is one of the main secondary complications of HIV infection.[55] There is probably a subclinical form of cryptococcosis because unaffected individuals may have positive skin tests. However, the most common clinical manifestation of disease is meningoencephalitis. This presents with classic signs of meningitis, changes in consciousness, mental changes, and nerve palsies. In AIDS patients, these signs may be only weakly expressed. Pulmonary infection can be found in approximately 10% of those with meningitis. Chest signs include the appearance of nodular shadows, cavitation, and pleural effusion. Patients with AIDS often present with fever and mild headache, and few other features of infection.[55] Cutaneous lesions may develop in approximately 10% of cases, but are seldom pathognomonic.[57-60] Acneiform papules or pustules progressing to warty or vegetating, crusted plaques, ulcers, and hard infiltrated plaques or nodules are characteristic of widespread systemic infection (Fig. 162-17). Cold abscesses, cellulitis, and nodular lesions also occur. In otherwise healthy patients and in those with sarcoidosis, lesions may be solitary, and in such patients, they may be the only clinical manifestation of infection.

In primary cutaneous cryptococcosis with direct inoculation of organisms into the skin, the skin lesions are usually solitary nodules that break down and ulcerate. Local lymphadenopathy also develops. The term *primary cutaneous cryptococcosis* is also used loosely to describe solitary lesions of cryptococcosis, but in many such cases there is also evidence of dissemination to other internal organs. It is important to investigate all patients who present with cutaneous lesions for evidence of dissemination to other sites.[58]

DIAGNOSIS

Laboratory Testing: Cryptococci are large (5 to 15 μm in diameter), budding cells with capsules that are best observed by direct microscopy of India ink or Nigrosin mounts (Fig. 162-18). The organism is not

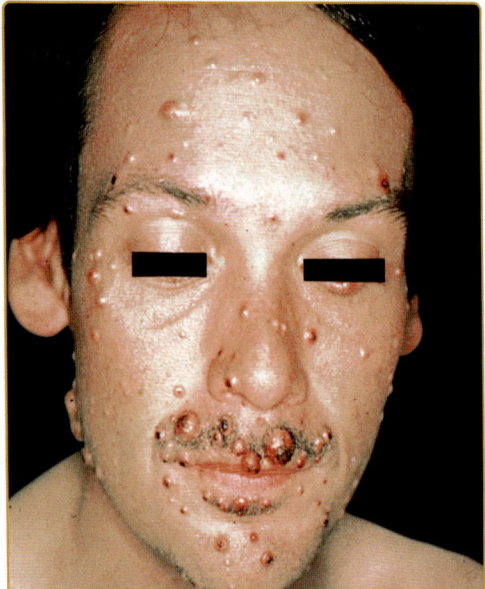

Figure 162-17 Cryptococcosis, disseminated. Multiple, discrete, skin-colored papules, and nodules resembling molluscum contagiosum are seen on the face of a male with advanced HIV disease. (Used with permission from Loïc Vaillant, MD.)

or very little inflammation. The capsules of the cells can be stained using the mucicarmine or Alcian blue stains.

DIFFERENTIAL DIAGNOSIS

Cryptococcal skin lesions may mimic a range of other conditions, particularly other systemic mycoses in AIDS patients. It is important to biopsy and culture suspicious lesions in immunocompromised patients.

MANAGEMENT

Medications: The most frequently used drug regimen in the non-AIDS patient is IV amphotericin B combined with flucytosine. In patients with single skin lesions and no other signs of infection, alternatives such as fluconazole or itraconazole can be used. Because there is a very high relapse rate in AIDS patients, the usual policy is to give a 10- to 14-day course of amphotericin B with or without flucytosine, followed by long-term fluconazole.[61] However, it is possible to stop long-term suppressive therapy in patients receiving HAART. High-dose fluconazole given on its own is an alternative approach.

difficult to grow in culture. Various biochemical features, such as the production of urease and the ability to pigment on *Guizotia* seed medium, are characteristic; molecular probes can be used to confirm the identity. Serologic tests are rapid and specific. The main test is an antigen-detection assay using latex agglutination or enzyme-linked immunosorbent assay, and this is simple and very rapid to perform on blood or cerebrospinal fluid. Very high titers are found in serum and cerebrospinal fluid from AIDS patients. Non-AIDS patients with single, localized skin lesions are often antigen negative.

Pathology: In tissue sections, the large pleomorphic yeasts stimulate either a granulomatous reaction

CUTANEOUS ASPECTS OF SYSTEMIC OPPORTUNISTIC MYCOSES

Skin lesions are not common with the opportunistic fungal infections, but they can occur in some patients, particularly in certain predisposed groups. When they occur, their presence may be very helpful because it is possible to biopsy easily accessible lesions to establish the diagnosis.

SYSTEMIC CANDIDIASIS

Systemic candidiasis follows dissemination of *Candida* sp. from the GI tract or via the bloodstream. Skin lesions can occur, especially in 2 situations: (a) in neutropenic patients, there is often a severe disseminated disease with widespread skin nodules and associated muscle pains,[62] and (b) in IV drug abusers, candidiasis may present with a follicular, pustular rash in the beard area and scalp. Other lesions include retinal and vitreal deposits and abscesses around the costochondral junctions.

Systemic candidiasis is usually treated with IV amphotericin B (conventional or lipid-associated), caspofungin, or fluconazole. Resistance to some azole drugs, such as fluconazole and ketoconazole, is more common with certain non-*albicans Candida* sp., and these antifungal agents should be avoided in infections caused by these species. Newly recognized species, such as *Candida auris,* have been found to cause

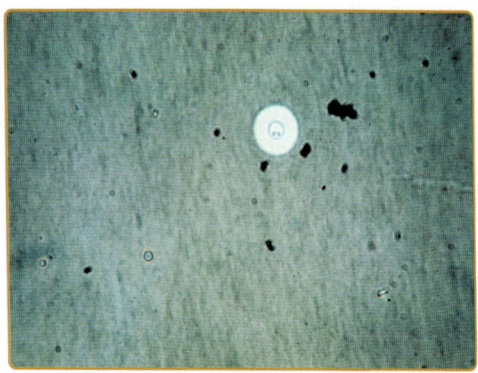

Figure 162-18 Cryptococcosis. India ink preparation of cerebrospinal fluid.

systemic infection resistant to common therapeutic drugs such as fluconazole and amphotericin B.[63]

MUCORMYCOSIS (PHYCOMYCOSIS, ZYGOMYCOSIS)

Mucormycosis is a rare disease caused by Mucoromycetes fungi such as *Mucor, Lichtheimia,* and *Rhizopus. Cunninghamella bertholletiae* and *Saksenaea vasiformis* are less-common causes. These fungi cause disease in patients with poorly controlled diabetes, neutropenia, or renal disease. Direct invasion through abrasions has been reported following trauma from a natural disaster (eg, during a mudslide or tsunami).[64] They can invade necrotic burned areas or involve the facial skin secondary to invasive infection of the paranasal sinuses (Fig. 162-19). Mucormycosis also has been caused by close apposition of the skin with contaminated dressing materials in the case of *Rhizopus rhizopodiformis*[65] or with wooden tongue depressors in the case of *Rhizopus microsporus*.[66] These fungi have a tendency to invade blood vessels, causing widespread infarction. Infections may respond to IV amphotericin, and recent results with lipid-associated amphotericin B formulations have been encouraging.

OTHER OPPORTUNISTIC MYCOSES

Other fungi causing systemic infections also may produce skin lesions in the process of bloodstream dissemination. The best known of these organisms are *Aspergillus, Scedosporium, Trichosporon,* and *Fusarium*. Skin infection is seen mainly in severely immunocompromised patients such as those with neutropenia.

Aspergillus may produce large necrotic lesions such as ecthyma gangrenosum, but smaller papules and cold abscesses also can occur.[67] *Fusarium* infections may produce widely distributed target-like lesions that may undergo central necrosis and, in some cases, digital cellulitis and superficial white onychomycosis precede dissemination.[68] Treatment for all these infections is usually amphotericin B, although voriconazole is increasingly used with aspergillosis.

DIAGNOSIS

Laboratory Testing: Laboratory confirmation of the diagnosis is fraught with difficulties chiefly because many of the organisms are also commensals in human sites; because they occur in severely ill patients, the capacity to produce diagnostic antibody titers is compromised. The interpretation of laboratory data is consequently difficult and has to be related to the

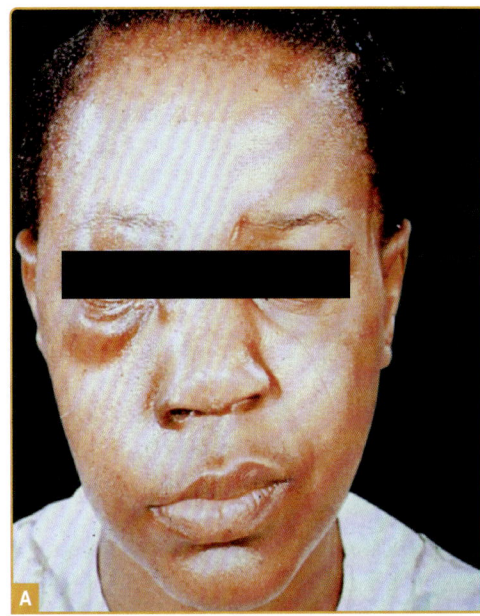
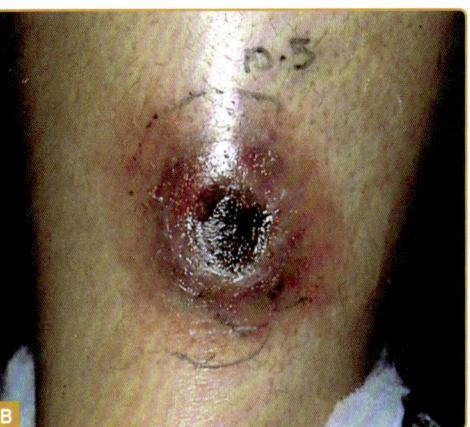
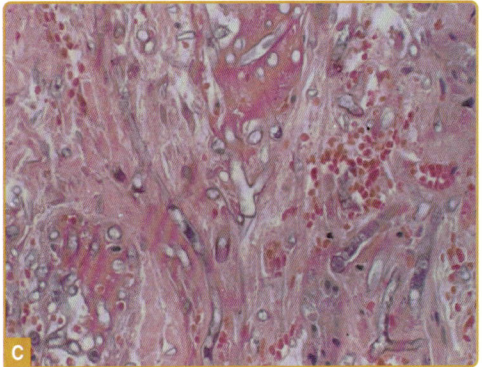

Figure 162-19 Mucormycosis. **A,** The face of this young woman with diabetes mellitus shows proptosis, unilateral facial edema, and a right-sided facial palsy associated with infection beginning in the right maxillary sinus. **B,** Ulcer. **C,** Hyphae in tissue.

clinical state of the patient. Newer tests for aspergillosis and candidiasis, such as detection of galactomannan (aspergillosis) or PCR-based molecular assays, are proving helpful in some cases.

Pathology: Ideally, a histologic diagnosis should be made, although biopsy may be impossible because of the risk of bleeding.

MANAGEMENT

In many cases, the diagnosis of a systemic mycosis is presumptive, and treatment is given empirically.

ACTINOMYCOSIS AND NOCARDIOSIS

Actinomycosis is an infection caused by filamentous bacteria that form large granules (sulfur granules) in abscess cavities. Draining sinuses communicate from the center of the abscess to the skin or mucosal surface. Nocardiosis is an acute and chronic infection also caused by filamentous bacteria. These lead to localized skin, subcutaneous, and systemic infections. Actinomycosis and nocardiosis are discussed in detail in Chap. 158.

REFERENCES

1. Chandler FW, Ajello L, Kaplan W. *A Colour Atlas and Textbook of the Histopathology of Mycotic Diseases.* London, UK: Wolfe Medical; 1980:92, 98.
2. Merz WG, Hay RJ. *Topley and Wilson's Microbiology and Microbial Infections: Medical Mycology.* London, UK: Hodder Arnold; 2005.
3. Kibbler CC, Mackenzie DWR, Odds FC, et al. *Principles and Practice of Clinical Mycology.* Chichester, UK: Wiley; 1996.
4. Dismukes WE, Pappas PG, Sobel JD. *Clinical Mycology.* New York, NY: Oxford University Press; 2003.
5. Rodrigues AM, de Hoog G, Zhang Y, et al. Emerging sporotrichosis is driven by clonal and recombinant *Sporothrix* species. *Emerg Microbes Infect.* 2014;3(5):e32.
6. Ramos-e-Silva M, Vasconcelos C, Carneiro S, et al. Sporotrichosis. *Clin Dermatol.* 2007;25:181.
7. Pappas PG, Tellez I, Deep AE, et al. Sporotrichosis in Peru: description of an area of hyperendemicity. *Clin Infect Dis.* 2000;30:65.
8. da Rosa AC, Scroferneker ML, Vettorato R, et al. Epidemiology of sporotrichosis: a study of 304 cases in Brazil. *J Am Acad Dermatol.* 2005;52:451.
9. Bibler MR, Luber HJ, Glueck HI, et al. Disseminated sporotrichosis in a patient with HIV infection after treatment for acquired factor VIII inhibitor. *JAMA.* 1986;256:3125.
10. Kauffman CA, Hajjeh R, Chapman SW. Practice guidelines for the management of patients with sporotrichosis. For the Mycoses Study Group. Infectious Diseases Society of America. *Clin Infect Dis.* 2000; 30:684.
11. Fahal AH. Mycetoma: a thorn in the flesh. *Trans R Soc Trop Med Hyg.* 2004;98:3.
12. Zijlstra EE, van de Sande WWJ, Welsh O, et al. Mycetoma: a unique neglected tropical disease. *Lancet Infect Dis.* 2016;16:100.
13. Ahmed AO, van Leeuwen W, Fahal A, et al. Mycetoma caused by *Madurella mycetomatis*: a neglected infectious burden. *Lancet Infect Dis.* 2004;4:566.
14. Wethered DB, Markey MA, Hay RJ, et al. Ultrastructural and immunogenic changes in the formation of mycetoma grains. *J Med Vet Mycol.* 1986;25:39.
15. Welsh O, Al-Abdely HM, Salinas-Carmona MC, et al. Mycetoma medical therapy. *PLoS Negl Trop Dis.* 2014;8:e3218.
16. Esterre P. Chromoblastomycosis. In: Merz WG, Hay RJ, eds. *Topley and Wilson's Microbiology and Microbial Infections: Medical Mycology.* London, UK: Hodder Arnold; 2004:356.
17. López Martínez R, Méndez Tovar LJ. Chromoblastomycosis. *Clin Dermatol.* 2007;25:188.
18. Goette DK, Robertson D. Transepithelial elimination in chromomycosis. *Arch Dermatol.* 1984;120:400.
19. Restrepo A. Treatment of tropical mycoses. *J Am Acad Dermatol.* 1994;31:S91.
20. Bonifaz A, Saúl A, Paredes-Solis V, et al. Treatment of chromoblastomycosis with terbinafine: experience with four cases. *J Dermatolog Treat.* 2004;16:47.
21. Matsumoto T, Ajello L, Matsuda T, et al. Developments in hyalohyphomycosis and phaeohyphomycosis. *J Med Vet Mycol.* 1994;32:329.
22. Brun AM. Lobomycosis in three Venezuelan patients. *Int J Dermatol.* 1999;38:302.
23. Yang X, Li Y, Zhou X, et al. Rhinofacial conidiobolomycosis caused by *Conidiobolus coronatus* in a Chinese rice farmer. *Mycoses.* 2010;53:369-373.
24. Arseculeratne SN. Rhinosporidiosis: what is the cause? *Curr Opin Infect Dis.* 2005;18:113.
25. Ali T. Clinical use of anti-TNF therapy and increased risk of infections. *Drug Healthc Patient Saf.* 2013;5:79.
26. Cano MV, Hajjeh RA. The epidemiology of histoplasmosis: a review. *Semin Respir Infect.* 2001;16:109.
27. Kauffman CA. Histoplasmosis: a clinical and laboratory update. *Clin Microbiol Rev.* 2010;20:115.
28. Gutierrez ME, Canton A, Sosa N, et al. Disseminated histoplasmosis in patients with AIDS in Panama: a review of 104 cases. *Clin Infect Dis.* 2005;40:1199.
29. Wheat LJ, Kohler RB, Tewari RP. Diagnosis of disseminated histoplasmosis by detection of *Histoplasma capsulatum* antigen in serum and urine specimen. *N Engl J Med.* 1986;314:83.
30. Khalil MA, Hassan AW, Gugnani HC. African histoplasmosis: report of four cases from north-eastern Nigeria. *Mycoses.* 1998;41:293.
31. Wheat J. Endemic mycoses in AIDS: a clinical review. *Clin Microbiol Rev.* 1995;8:149.
32. Lemos LB, Guo M, Baliga M. Blastomycosis: organ involvement and etiologic diagnosis. A review of 123 patients from Mississippi. *Ann Diagn Pathol.* 2000; 4:391.
33. Bradsher RW, Chapman SW, Pappas PG. Blastomycosis. *Infect Dis Clin North Am.* 2003;17:21.
34. Emerson PA, Higgins E, Branfoot A. North American blastomycosis in Africans. *Br J Dis Chest.* 1984;78:286.
35. Baumgardner DJ, Steber D, Glazier R, et al. Geographic information system analysis of blastomycosis in northern Wisconsin, USA: waterways and soil. *Med Mycol.* 2005;43:117.
36. Bradsher RW. A clinician's view of blastomycosis. *Curr Top Med Mycol.* 1994;5:181.
37. McAdams HP, Rosado-de-Christenson ML, Lesar M, et al. Thoracic mycoses from endemic fungi: radiologic-pathologic correlation. *Radiographics.* 1995;15:255.

38. Weil M, Mercurio MG, Brodell RT, et al. Cutaneous lesions provide a clue to mysterious pulmonary process: pulmonary and cutaneous North American blastomycosis infection. *Arch Dermatol.* 1996;132:822.
39. Herd AM, Greenfield SB, Thompson GW, et al. Miliary blastomycosis and HIV infection. *CMAJ.* 1990;143:1329.
40. Rosenstein NE, Emery KW, Werner SB, et al. Risk factors for severe pulmonary and disseminated coccidioidomycosis: Kern County, California, 1995-1996. *Clin Infect Dis.* 2001;32:708.
41. Chang A, Tung RC, McGillis TS, et al. Primary cutaneous coccidioidomycosis. *J Am Acad Dermatol.* 2003;49:944.
42. Crum NF, Lederman ER, Stafford CM, et al. Coccidioidomycosis: a descriptive survey of a reemerging disease. Clinical characteristics and current controversies. *Medicine (Baltimore).* 2004;83:149.
43. Ampel NM. Coccidioidomycosis in persons infected with HIV-1. *Ann N Y Acad Sci.* 2007;1111:336.
44. Martins TB, Jaskowski TD, Mouritsen CL, et al. Comparison of commercially available enzyme immunoassay with traditional serological tests for detection of antibodies to *Coccidioides immitis*. *J Clin Microbiol.* 1995;33:940.
45. Galgiani JN. Coccidioidomycosis. *Clin Infect Dis.* 2005;41:1217.
46. Ramos-E-Silva M, Saraiva Ldo E. Paracoccidioidomycosis. *Dermatol Clin.* 2008;26:257.
47. Restrepo A, Salazar ME, Cano LE, et al. Estrogens inhibit mycelium to yeast transformation in the fungus *Paracoccidioides brasiliensis*: implications for resistance of females to paracoccidioidomycosis. *Infect Immun.* 1984;46:346.
48. Simões LB, Marques SA, Bagagli E. Distribution of paracoccidioidomycosis: determination of ecologic correlates through spatial analyses. *Med Mycol.* 2004;42:517.
49. Caseiro MM, Etzel A, Soares MC, et al. Septicemia caused by Paracoccidioides brasiliensis (Lutz, 1908) as the cause of death of an AIDS patient from Santos, São Paulo State, Brazil—a nonendemic area. *Rev Inst Med Trop Sao Paulo.* 2005;47:209.
50. Negroni R, Palmieri O, Koren F, et al. Oral treatment of paracoccidioidomycosis and histoplasmosis with itraconazole in humans. *Rev Infect Dis.* 1987;9:S47.
51. Segretain G. Description d'une nouvelle espece de penicillium: *Penicillium marneffei* n. sp. *Bull Soc Mycol Fr.* 1959;75:412.
52. Chariyalertsak S, Sirisanthana T, Supparatpinyo K, et al. Seasonal variation of disseminated *Penicillium marneffei* infections in northern Thailand: a clue to the reservoir? *J Infect Dis.* 1996;173:1490.
53. Lu PX, Zhu WK, Liu Y, et al. Acquired immunodeficiency syndrome associated disseminated Penicillium marneffei infection: report of 8 cases. *Chin Med J.* 2005;118:1395.
54. Supparatpinyo K, Khamwan C, Baosoung V, et al. Disseminated *Penicillium marneffei* infection in southeast Asia. *Lancet.* 1994;344:110.
55. Mitchell TG, Perfect JR. Cryptococcosis in the era of AIDS: 100 years after the discovery of *Cryptococcus neoformans*. *Clin Microbiol Rev.* 1995;8:515.
56. Bennett JE, Kwon-Chung KJ, Howard DH. Epidemiologic differences among serotypes of *Cryptococcus neoformans*. *Am J Epidemiol.* 1984;120:582.
57. Manrique P, Mayo J, Alvarez JA, et al. Polymorphous cutaneous cryptococcosis: nodular, herpes-like, and molluscum-like lesions in a patient with the acquired immunodeficiency syndrome. *J Am Acad Dermatol.* 1992;26:122.
58. Murakawa GJ, Kerschmann R, Berger T. Cutaneous cryptococcus infection and AIDS: report of 12 cases and review of the literature. *Arch Dermatol.* 1996;132:545.
59. Manfredi R, Mazzoni A, Nanetti A, et al. Morphologic features and clinical significance of skin involvement in patients with AIDS-related cryptococcosis. *Acta Derm Venereol.* 1996;76:72.
60. Pomar V, Carrera G, Paredes R, et al. Disseminated cryptococcosis resembling milliary tuberculosis in an HIV-1-infected patient. *Lancet Infect Dis.* 2005;5:189.
61. Pappas PG, Perfect JR, Cloud GA, et al. Cryptococcosis in human immunodeficiency virus–negative patients in the era of effective azole therapy. *Clin Infect Dis.* 2001;33:690.
62. Bae GY, Lee HW, Chang SE, et al. Clinicopathologic review of 19 patients with systemic candidiasis with skin lesions. *Int J Dermatol.* 2005;44:550.
63. Lee WG, Shin JH, Uh Y, et al. First three reported cases of nosocomial fungemia caused by *Candida auris*. *J Clin Microbiol.* 2011;49:3139.
64. Hay RJ. Mucormycosis: an infectious complication of traumatic injury. *Lancet.* 2005;365:830.
65. Gartenberg G, Bottone EJ, Keusch GT, et al. Hospital-acquired mucormycosis (*Rhizopus rhizopodiformis*) of skin and subcutaneous tissue: epidemiology, mycology and treatment. *N Engl J Med.* 1978;299:1115.
66. Mitchell SJ, Gray J, Morgan ME, et al. Nosocomial infection with *Rhizopus microsporus* in preterm infants associated with wooden tongue depressors. *Lancet.* 1996;348:441.
67. Wong J, McCracken G, Ronan S, et al. Coexistent cutaneous *Aspergillus* and cytomegalovirus infection in a liver transplant recipient. *J Am Acad Dermatol.* 2001;44:370.
68. Marcoux D, Jafarian F, Joncas V, et al. Deep cutaneous fungal infections in immunocompromised children. *J Am Acad Dermatol.* 2009;61:857.

Viral Diseases PART 25

第二十五篇 病毒性疾病

Chapter 163 :: Exanthematous Viral Diseases :: Vikash S. Oza & Erin F. D. Mathes

第一百六十三章
病毒疹性疾病

中文导读

病毒疹性疾病指由病毒感染所致的以发疹为主要皮肤损害的一大类疾病。本章共分为13节：①麻疹；②风疹；③传染性红斑和微小病毒B19感染；④EB病毒；⑤Gianotti-Crosti综合征；⑥人巨细胞病毒；⑦人疱疹病毒6型；⑧人疱疹病毒7型；⑨肠病毒；⑩手足口病；⑪柯萨奇病毒A6型相关性非典型手足口病；⑫发疹性假性血管瘤；⑬单侧胸外测疹。分别介绍了这些病毒疹性疾病的流行病学、临床特征、危险因素、病因和发病机制、诊断、鉴别诊断、临床病程和预后及临床管理。

第一节介绍了具有高度传染性的病毒性疾病麻疹，至今为止其仍然是世界范围内发病率和死亡率高的重要原因。人类是其唯一宿主，通过呼吸道黏膜或结膜进入宿主。Koplik斑是麻疹的典型早期特征，同时可伴有高热、鼻炎或结膜炎等前驱症状，麻疹活疫苗接种后麻疹的发病率可被明显控制。

第二节介绍了最常发生在冬末春初的风疹病毒，人类同样是唯一宿主。风疹前驱症状的特征是低热、肌痛、头痛及结膜炎等，是一种典型的自限性疾病，治疗以对症支持治疗为主，三联疫苗可预防。

第三节介绍了能感染人类的最小的DNA单链病毒B19病毒，特征性皮疹为开始于颧骨处汇合的红斑水肿斑块，似"拍打脸颊"样，后逐渐累积四肢，并发展为网状。血清抗病毒B19 IgM可确诊，但目前尚无疫苗，也没有特定的抗病毒治疗，治疗以对症支持治疗为主。

第四节介绍了EB病毒，又称人类疱疹病毒4型。其呈全球分布，90%以上的成人潜伏感染。通过近期原发性感染患者的唾液传播，又被称为"接吻病"。其治疗独具特点，不推荐使用常规以阿昔洛韦为主导的抗病毒治疗，而是以支持治疗为主，具体见表163-8。

第五节介绍了Gianotti-Crosti综合征，也称婴儿丘疹性肢端炎和儿童丘疹性肢端炎，是一种常见的自限性皮疹，被认为是对感染的病毒、细菌或疫苗的免疫反应，发病之前多有疫苗接种史，与皮肤直接感染无关。多发于3月～15岁儿童，发病高峰为1～6岁，成人病例不常见。

第六节介绍了最常见的人类先天性病毒（HCMV）人巨细胞病毒。据调查，有10%～20%的儿童在进入青春期前感染HCMV，血清阳性率随年龄增长而增加。在美国有0.5%～2%的患病率，10%～15%的先天性感染伴随后遗症。

第七节介绍了婴儿常感染的人疱疹病毒6型，高达80%的人群在2岁时感染，通常发生在6月～2岁，其中春季发病率最高。但目前尚无任何药物被正式批准用于治疗HHV-6感染，只能使用HCMV治疗和预防的药物。

第八节介绍了和人疱疹病毒6型具有同源性的人疱疹病毒7型，但其感染率远低于HHV-6病毒。两者在血清学和生物学上的截然不同造就了两者不同的临床特性。

第九节介绍了人类单链RNA肠病毒，包括埃可病毒、柯萨奇病毒以及脊髓灰质炎病毒，绝大多数肠病毒感染预后良好。

第十节介绍了手足口病，其是一种肠病毒感染性疾病，标志性皮损是手掌和足底出现水疱，临床诊断甚至不需要实验室辅助检查，以对症支持治疗为主，预后良好。

第十一节介绍了柯萨奇病毒A6型相关性非典型手足口病，柯萨奇病毒A6型是手足口病的致病病毒。其导致的非典型手足口病与典型的手足口病相比皮损分布更为广泛，形态也更为多样。

第十二节介绍了发疹性假性血管瘤，现在初步认为和埃可病毒有关，但尚未确认。

第十三节介绍了单侧胸外侧疹，虽然病因尚不清楚，但其临床表现十分符合病毒感染的情形。好发于冬末春初1～5岁儿童中，也可能在8个月～10岁出现，又被称为儿童非对称屈侧周疹。

〔张江林〕

MEASLES

AT-A-GLANCE

- Prodrome of fever, cough, coryza, and conjunctivitis
- Koplik spots on the buccal mucosa are pathognomonic
- Morbilliform eruption lasts 3 to 5 days
- Severe complications include pneumonia and post-measles encephalomyelitis
- Vitamin A treatment may reduce morbidity and mortality

Measles, or rubeola, is a highly contagious, viral disease that remains an important cause of morbidity and mortality worldwide. The incidence and mortality rates are highest in developing countries, particularly in Africa and Asia where large populations are unvaccinated.

EPIDEMIOLOGY

A measles vaccine was first licensed in the United States in 1968. Prior to the introduction of the vaccine, approximately 90% of Americans were infected with measles prior to 15 years old.[1] By 2000, endemic transmission of measles within the United States ceased and measles was declared eliminated.[2] However, measles outbreaks continue to occur in the United States partly because of travel to countries with higher rates of measles and the spread of the virus in U.S. communities with pockets of unvaccinated people.[3] For instance, a multistate outbreak in late 2014 as a consequence of transmission at Disneyland in Anaheim, California, was responsible for 111 of the total 189 cases of measles in the United States in 2015.[4]

Worldwide, measles rates have also precipitously declined as the result of the implementation of measles vaccine programs. As of 2014, 85% of children across the globe had received at least 1 dose of the measles vaccine.[5] Despite this improvement, measles is still a leading cause of childhood mortality with 114,900 deaths in 2014.[5] The epidemiology of measles in the developing world is highly dependent on funding resources, public health infrastructure and political stability.

ETIOLOGY AND PATHOGENESIS

Measles virus is a highly contagious, single-stranded, enveloped RNA virus that is a member of the Paramyxoviridae family. Humans are the only natural hosts. Transmission occurs via person-to-person contact or airborne respiratory secretions. Infectious droplets have been reported to remain airborne for up to 2 hours, allowing for easy transmission in public spaces.[6]

The measles virus enters the host via the respiratory mucosa or conjunctiva where it can replicate, spread locally to lymphatic nodes and later disseminate into the bloodstream. The humoral immune system controls viral replication and confers antibody protection, whereas the cell-mediated response eliminates infected cells. A transient immunosuppression occurs during measles virus infection, causing depressed delayed-type hypersensitivity and T-cell counts, as well as an increased risk of bacterial infections.[7]

CLINICAL FEATURES

Measles infection is characterized by an incubation period, prodrome and exanthem. The incubation period from acquiring the virus to developing fever ranges between 7 and 21 days.

The prodrome consists of fever (as high as 40.5°C [104.9°F]), malaise, conjunctivitis (palpebral, extending to lid margin), coryza, and cough (brassy or barking) and can last up to 4 days. Koplik spots are the pathognomonic enanthem of measles and develop during the prodrome. The spots begin as small, bright red macules that have a 1- to 2-mm blue-white speck within them and are typically found on the buccal mucosa near the second molars (Fig. 163-1). Koplik spots typically occur 48 hours prior to the onset of the rash and only last 12 to 72 hours. Koplik' spots may be absent if a patient presents several days into the patient's rash.[8]

The measles exanthem consists of nonpruritic, erythematous macules and papules progressing in a cranial-to-caudal direction. The exanthem begins on the forehead and behind the ears (Fig. 163-2) and spreads to involve the neck, trunk, and extremities (Fig. 163-3). The hands and feet are involved. Lesions may coalesce, especially on the face and neck. The rash usually peaks within 3 days and begins to disappear in 4 to 5 days in the order that it appeared. Desquamation and brownish dyspigmentation in fair patients can occur as the rash resolves.[8]

DIAGNOSIS

The laboratory diagnosis of measles is based on virus detection or positive serologic findings. The measles virus can be isolated using real-time reverse transcription polymerase chain reaction (PCR) from nasopharyngeal aspirates, throat swabs, blood or urine. Viral detection is most successful when collection occurs within 3 days of the rash's onset.

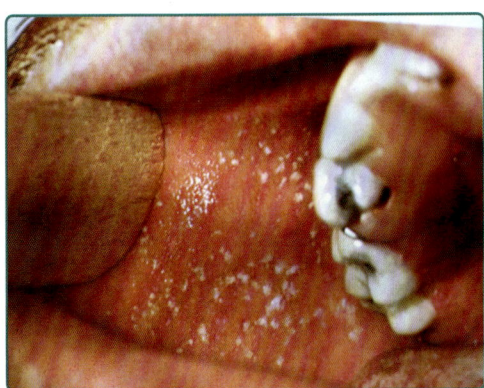

Figure 163-1 Measles. The pathognomonic Koplik spots of measles appear as tiny white lesions—"grains of sand"—surrounded by an erythematous halo. They precede the generalized rash by 1 to 2 days. (Image used with permission from the Fitzsimmons Army Medical Center Dermatology Archive.)

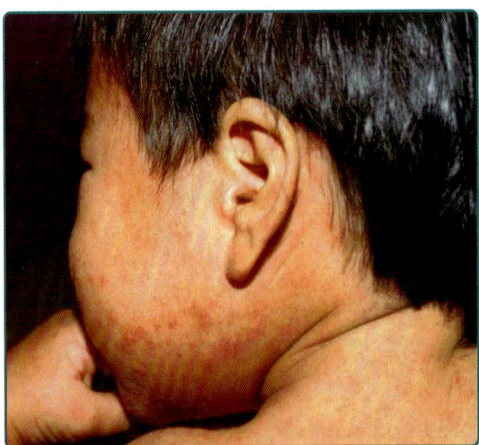

Figure 163-2 The morbilliform eruption of measles in a toddler.

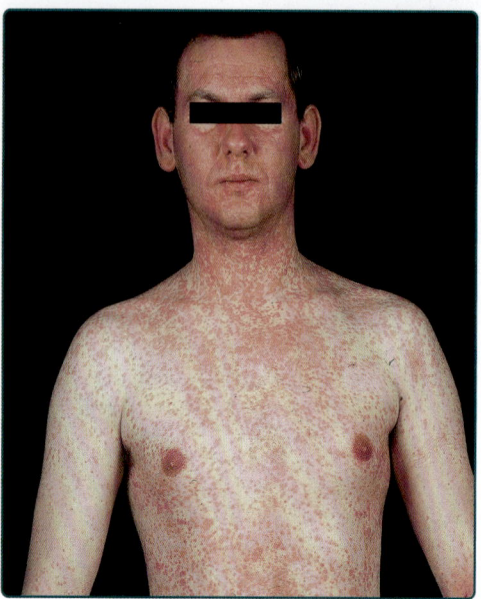

Figure 163-3 Measles. Classic morbilliform exanthem with red papules spreading from forehead and postauricular area to neck, trunk and then extremities. (Used with permission from Wolff K, Johnson R, Saavedra AP, et al. *Fitzpatrick's Color Atlas and Synopsis of Clinical Dermatology*, 8th ed. New York, NY: McGraw-Hill; 2017.)

5 days prior to the onset of the rash until 4 days after the onset of the rash.

Complications from measles infection occur in approximately 40% of cases.[8] Complications include severe diarrhea; pneumonia (either viral or superimposed bacterial infection); otitis media; transient immunosuppression with lymphopenia and decreased cell-mediated immunity; encephalitis, and a rare form of a progressive neurodegenerative disease termed *subacute sclerosing panencephalitis*. Most deaths are attributed to either respiratory illness or encephalitis. In developing nations, measles remains a major cause of infant mortality. Patient groups at risk for complications include infants, the elderly, pregnant women, the immunocompromised, and the malnourished.

MANAGEMENT

The management of measles is supportive as there are no specific antiviral therapies approved Table 163-2). Treatment focuses on antipyretics, fluids, and managing complications related to bacterial superinfection, respiratory compromise, and neurologic sequela. In the hospitalized setting, patients should be on standard and airborne transmission precautions for 4 days after the rash onset (entire duration of illness in

Serologic studies are also very useful in confirming the diagnosis of measles. Enzyme-linked immunoassays are commonly used. A positive serum immunoglobulin (Ig) M antibody for measles confirms the diagnosis. IgM testing is typically positive on the first day of the rash and remains positive for at least 30 days afterward. Within the first 72 hours of the rash, the IgM assay may be falsely negative, so repeat testing should be considered if there is a high clinical suspicion.[9] IgG confirmation of a measles diagnosis requires documentation of a fourfold increase in titers, therefore serum samples should be drawn during the rash and weeks later during the convalescent stage. In the United States, measles should be reported to the local or state health department which can also help with selecting and processing laboratory tests.

TABLE 163-1
Differential Diagnosis of Measles

Most Likely
- Drug hypersensitivity reaction
- Rubella

Consider
- Henoch-Schönlein purpura (atypical cases)
- Other viral infection (parvovirus, enterovirus, adenovirus, human herpesvirus-6, Epstein-Barr virus)
- Rocky Mountain spotted fever (atypical cases)

Always Rule Out
- Graft-versus-host disease (recent bone marrow transplantation)
- Kawasaki disease

DIFFERENTIAL DIAGNOSIS

Table 163-1 outlines the differential diagnosis of measles.

CLINICAL COURSE AND PROGNOSIS

Uncomplicated measles is self-limited, lasting 10 to 12 days. An infected patient is considered to be contagious

TABLE 163-2
Treatments for Measles

- First-line
  - Immunoglobulin, IM[a]
  - Measles vaccine
  - Supportive care
  - Treat secondary infections
  - Vitamin A[a]
- Second-line
  - Ribavirin[a]

[a]In select cases; please see text.

immunocompromised patients).[10] The World Health Organization recommends that vitamin A should be administered to all children with measles regardless of their country of residence.[8] Vitamin A deficiency is associated with increased disease severity and risk for complications, likely through depressing cell-mediated immunity. A 2005 Cochrane review of vitamin A supplementation to treat measles in children found an association between using vitamin A (200,000 international units per day or 100,000 international units per day for infants) on 2 consecutive days and a reduced risk of measles mortality in children younger than 2 years old.[11]

Ribavirin is a medication that has been used in children with severe disease or an immunocompromised state. A randomized trial of 100 children found decreased duration of symptoms, hospital stay, and risk of complications in children receiving ribavirin compared to supportive therapy.[12] However, larger studies are needed prior to recommending this therapy as part of routine practice.

Postexposure prophylaxis plays an important role in curtailing outbreaks and decreasing morbidity of the virus. Individuals at risk for severe illness and complications (infants younger than 1 year of age, pregnant women, unimmunized, and immunocompromised) should be given measles immunoglobulin if presenting within 6 days of exposure. Measles immunoglobulin can be given either via an IM (0.5 mL/kg; maximum dose: 15 mL) or IV route (400 mg/kg). In healthy individuals, the measles-mumps-rubella (MMR) vaccine should be given to boost immunity if it can be administered within 72 hours of measles exposure.[10]

PREVENTION (IMMUNIZATIONS)

The incidence of measles has decreased worldwide as a direct result of immunization. Two doses of the live-attenuated measles vaccine (with the first dose at or after 12 months of age) produces detectable levels of antibody in 99% of individuals, conferring lifelong immunity.[10] The measles vaccine is typically administered in the form of combination vaccines: MMR vaccine or MMR and varicella vaccine. The second dose of the vaccine should be administered no sooner than 28 days later. The American Academy of Pediatrics, recommends MMR at age 12 to 15 months and then again prior to school entry, between 4 and 6 years old.

Measles vaccine administration is contraindicated in individuals who have a moderate to severe illness, as well as in those who have had an immediate anaphylactic reaction to a previous measles vaccine. It is also contraindicated in pregnant women and those with impaired immune systems (HIV infection, immunosuppressive therapy). Hypersensitivity reactions can occur to components of the vaccine, such as gelatin, neomycin, or egg white cross-reacting proteins.[10]

RUBELLA

AT-A-GLANCE

- Also called German measles and 3-day measles.
- Epidemic disease; worldwide distribution.
- Short prodrome; rash duration of 2 to 3 days.
- Enlargement of cervical, suboccipital, and postauricular glands.
- High risk of fetal malformations with congenital infection (microcephaly, congenital heart disease, and deafness), particularly in the first trimester.

EPIDEMIOLOGY

Rubella virus has a worldwide distribution with outbreaks occurring most frequently in late winter and early spring months. Humans are the only hosts for infection.[13] School-age children, adolescents, and young adults most often develop the disease. Epidemics occasionally occur in developing countries, especially where vaccines are unavailable.

Since introduction of the rubella vaccine in the United States in 1969, the incidences of rubella and congenital rubella syndrome have drastically declined with no widespread epidemics occurring in the United States. Since 2003, fewer than 20 cases are reported annually in the United States.[14] Occasional outbreaks have largely been attributed to failure to vaccinate susceptible individuals. Yet, recent serologic surveys indicate that approximately 10% of the United States–born population older than age 5 years is susceptible to rubella.[13,14] Epidemiologic studies have identified that individuals born outside the country or in a vaccine-poor area have an increased risk of rubella.[13]

ETIOLOGY AND PATHOGENESIS

Rubella is an enveloped positive-stranded RNA virus in the Togaviridae family that is spread through direct or droplet contact from nasopharyngeal secretions.[13] Infected individuals shed virus for 5 to 7 days before and up to 14 days after onset of rash,[15] with viremia unlikely after the rash occurs. In most individuals, infection leads to lifelong immunity.

Congenital rubella occurs when a nonimmunized, susceptible, pregnant woman is exposed to the virus. Transplacental infection of the fetus occurs during the viremic stage. The risk is greatest to a fetus exposed to the virus in the first trimester. Congenitally infected infants may shed the virus through urine, blood, and nasopharyngeal secretions for up to 12 months after birth, thus being a potential source of viral exposure to other susceptible individuals.[13,15]

CLINICAL FINDINGS

HISTORY

Primary rubella infection is typically a mild, subclinical disease, particularly in adults.[13,15] The prodrome is characterized by low-grade fever, myalgia, headache, conjunctivitis, rhinitis, cough, sore throat, and lymphadenopathy; symptoms that may last up to 4 days and often resolve with appearance of rash. Up to 50% of children with primary rubella infection may have a subclinical infection or present only with lymphadenopathy or rash (no prodrome).[15] Conversely, older adults may have more-severe and persistent prodromal symptoms that may make distinction from rubeola difficult in some situations. The presence of Koplik spots in the mouth favors rubeola. As the prodrome resolves and the rash begins to appear, some patients develop an enanthem consisting of tiny red macules on the soft palate and uvula (Forchheimer spots).[16] This enanthem is not diagnostic for rubella.

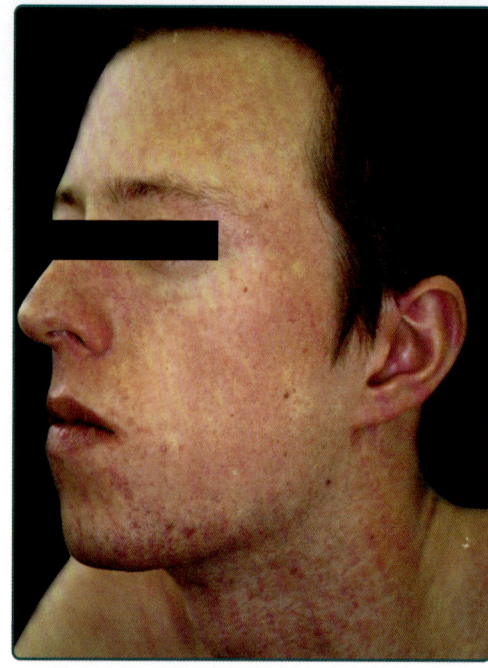

Figure 163-4 Rubella. Erythematous macules and papules appearing initially on the face and spreading to trunk, arms, legs within 24 hours.

CUTANEOUS LESIONS

The exanthem, occurring 14 to 17 days after exposure, is characterized by pruritic pink to red macules and papules that begin on the face, quickly progressing to involve neck, trunk, and extremities (Fig. 163-4).[15] Lesions on the trunk may coalesce, whereas those on the extremities often remain more discrete. The rash usually begins to disappear in 2 to 3 days, unlike rubeola, which can be more persistent and clears the head and neck first. Desquamation may follow resolution of the rash.

RELATED PHYSICAL FINDINGS

Lymphadenopathy is usually most severe in the posterior cervical, suboccipital, and postauricular lymph nodes, and is noted up to 7 days before the rash appears.[13] Enlargement of the nodes may persist for several weeks.

Adults, particularly women (up to 70%), may develop arthritis of small and large joints with rubella infection.[13] Joint symptoms often first appear as the rash fades and can last several weeks. In some individuals, the symptoms may become persistent or recurrent, and joint swelling may progress to joint effusion.

DIAGNOSIS

Diagnosis is typically made using serology to detect rubella-specific IgM antibody (up to 8 weeks after infection) or to document a fourfold rise in antibody titer in acute and convalescent-phase serum.[16] As with measles, rubella cases should be reported to local or state health departments.

Viral culture (nose, throat, blood, urine, cerebrospinal fluid [CSF], and synovial fluid) is sensitive but often difficult because of the influence of timing, collection procedure, and transport on the specimen.[17] Reverse transcription PCR may be used to detect rubella virus from throat swab or oral fluid with subsequent genotyping of strains to identify a source during outbreaks.[17] Complete blood cell count usually shows leukopenia with relative neutropenia. Increased numbers of atypical lymphocytes or abundant plasma cells may be noted as well. Patients with meningeal involvement have lymphocytes in the CSF.

CONGENITAL RUBELLA SYNDROME

Women who are infected with rubella during pregnancy may only exhibit minor clinical symptoms, however the effects of rubella infection on the fetus can be profound.[15] The greatest risk of fetal malformation is in the early stages of pregnancy. Up to 85% of fetuses exposed to rubella within the first 12 weeks of gestation develop serious sequelae such as microcephaly with mental retardation; congenital heart disease (ventricular septal defect, patent ductus arteriosus, pulmonary artery stenosis); sensorineural deafness; cataracts; glaucoma; low birthweight; and fetal death.[14-16] Neonatal manifestations of congenital infection include growth retardation, interstitial pneumonitis, radiolucent bone disease, hepatosplenomegaly, thrombocytopenia, and dermal erythropoiesis ("blueberry muffin lesions").[13]

Diagnosis of congenital rubella infection is obtained by isolating rubella virus in the throat, cataracts, urine, or CSF of the affected neonate. Serologic testing is not as sensitive, but is easily available for confirmatory testing. IgM antibody can be detected from birth to 1 month of age; IgG antibody titers may be stable or increase over several months. Laboratory confirmation of congenital infection in children older than age 1 year is difficult as viral isolation is rare.[13,15]

DIFFERENTIAL DIAGNOSIS

Table 163-3 outlines the differential diagnosis of rubella.

CLINICAL COURSE AND PROGNOSIS

Rubella is typically a self-limited disease. Infants who have congenital rubella are infectious until viral shedding from the nasopharynx and urinary tract ends. The majority of infants (85%) infected in utero excrete virus in the first month of life; 1% to 3% of infants infected in utero continue to excrete virus in the second year of life.[13,16] Pregnant women caring for these infants are at risk for developing rubella. Clinical course depends on how severely affected the fetus is from intrauterine infection.

Rarely, rubella infection may lead to encephalitis (1 in 6000 cases), with mortality rates varying from 0% to 50%.[16] Other rare complications include peripheral neuritis, optic neuritis, encephalitis, myocarditis, pericarditis, hepatitis, orchitis, hemolytic anemia, thrombocytopenia, and hemophagocytic syndrome.[15]

MANAGEMENT

Treatment of primary, uncomplicated rubella is supportive. Standard and droplet precautions are recommended for patients with rubella for 7 days after rash onset.[13] In nonpregnant individuals, rubella vaccine administration within 3 days of exposure theoretically may prevent illness, although this is yet to be proven.[13] Limited data indicate that IM immunoglobulin (0.55 mL/kg) as postexposure prophylaxis for rubella-susceptible patients may decrease infection, viral shedding, and rate of viremia.[13,18]

Neonates with congenital rubella syndrome require supportive care as well as appropriate attention to significant health issues. These infants are contagious and should be isolated to prevent transmission to susceptible individuals.[13,15] Contact isolation is recommended for these infants until they are at least 12 months old or repeated cultures are negative after 3 months of age.[13]

PREVENTION (IMMUNIZATIONS)

Rubella vaccine is typically administered as part of a threefold vaccine (MMR) or fourfold vaccine (MMR and varicella) at 12 to 15 months of age and again at 4 to 6 years of age. Seroconversion after a single dose of MMR vaccine occurs in 95% of individuals.[13,14] It is imperative that individuals at risk for rubella infection are immunized, such as health care workers, military recruits, college students, and recent immigrants.[13]

Potential adverse reactions to rubella vaccine occur in susceptible individuals and include fever (6 to 12 days after vaccine), morbilliform rash, lymphadenopathy, and arthralgia. Febrile seizures occur more frequently in children 1 to 2 years old when receiving the first MMR vaccine.[13]

Pregnant women should not receive the rubella vaccine because of the theoretical risk to the fetus.[19] Any woman receiving the rubella vaccine should not become pregnant for 28 days. Infants of vaccinated breastfeeding mothers may become infected with rubella via breastmilk. Typically, they develop a mild erythematous exanthem of macules and papules with no serious effects.[16]

Certain immunosuppressed and immunodeficient patients should not be vaccinated with live-attenuated virus vaccines, including rubella. Vaccine strain rubella virus has been found in cutaneous granulomas in immunodeficient hosts.[20]

TABLE 163-3
Differential Diagnosis of Rubella

Most Likely
- Drug hypersensitivity reaction
- Rubeola (measles)

Consider
- Other viral infection (enterovirus, adenovirus, parvovirus, human herpesvirus-6)

Always Rule Out
- Streptococcal scarlet fever

For the differential diagnosis of congenital rubella syndrome with blueberry muffin lesions, see Table 163-10.

ERYTHEMA INFECTIOSUM AND PARVOVIRUS B19 INFECTION

AT-A-GLANCE

- Erythema infectiosum (fifth disease): childhood illness with "slapped cheeks" followed by an erythematous, lacy eruption on the trunk and extremities.
- Symmetric polyarthritis, particularly of the small joints in adults.
- Papular purpuric gloves-and-socks syndrome: pruritic erythema, edema, and petechiae of the hands and feet, fever, and oral erosions in adolescents.
- Aplastic crisis in patients with increased red blood cell turnover, chronic anemia in immunocompromised persons, and fetal hydrops.

EPIDEMIOLOGY

Erythema infectiosum (fifth disease) is worldwide in distribution, can occur throughout the year, and can affect all ages. It tends to occur in epidemics, especially associated with school outbreaks in the late winter and early spring. Serologic studies show increasing prevalence of antibodies with age—from 15% to 60% of children 5 to 19 years of age to more than 90% in the elderly.[21] Previous infection with B19 seems to confer lifelong immunity.

The incubation period for erythema infectiosum is from 4 to 14 days. Low-grade fever and nonspecific complaints occur at the time of viremia, 6 to 14 days after inoculation, followed by rash at day 17 or 18.[22] Parvovirus B19 is thought to be transmitted primarily by the respiratory route via aerosolized droplets during the viremic phase.[22] After the rash of erythema infectiosum appears, B19 is usually not found in respiratory secretions or serum, suggesting that persons with erythema infectiosum are infectious only before the onset of the rash.

The virus seems to be effectively spread after close contact. The secondary attack rate among susceptible household contacts is approximately 50%. Transmission may occur via blood transfusion, from blood products, and vertically from mother to fetus.[23]

ETIOLOGY AND PATHOGENESIS

The B19 virus belongs to the family Parvoviridae and the genus *Erythrovirus*. B19 lacks an envelope and contains single-stranded DNA. It is the smallest single-stranded DNA-containing virus known to infect humans, measuring 18 to 26 μm in diameter. Parvoviruses are widespread in veterinary medicine, but animal parvoviruses are not thought to be transmissible to humans.[24]

The more serious manifestations of parvovirus infection relate to the fact that the virus infects and lyses erythroid progenitor cells. The blood group P antigen (globoside) is a receptor of parvovirus. Because some individuals lack P antigen, they are not susceptible to infection with B19.[25] In patients with increased red blood cell destruction or loss who depend on compensatory increases in red cell production to maintain stable red cell indices, B19 infection may lead to transient aplastic crisis. Such patients include those with anemia associated with acute or chronic blood loss. When parvovirus infects the erythroblasts in a developing fetus with decreased red cell survival, the result may be hemolysis and anemia. Anemia may trigger congestive heart failure, edema (fetal hydrops), and possibly fetal death. Additionally, parvovirus B19 DNA can be detected in nonerythroid tissues and is associated with increased inflammatory gene expression in these tissues.[26] Immune complex deposition also has been implicated in some of the manifestations of B19 infection, including erythema infectiosum.

CLINICAL FEATURES

PARVOVIRUS B19 IN CHILDREN

Most infections caused by B19 are asymptomatic and unrecognized. Fifth disease, the most common clinical picture associated with the virus, usually begins with nonspecific symptoms such as headache, coryza, and low-grade fever approximately 2 days before the onset of the rash.[27] Patients may have headache, pharyngitis, fever, malaise, myalgia, coryza, diarrhea, nausea, cough, and conjunctivitis coinciding with the rash. Approximately 10% of children with erythema infectiosum develop arthralgia or arthritis. Large joints are affected more often than small joints.[28] Occasionally, children may present with chronic joint complaints suggestive of juvenile idiopathic arthritis.

The characteristic rash begins with confluent, erythematous, edematous plaques on the malar eminences, the "slapped cheeks" (Fig. 163-5). As the facial rash fades over 1 to 4 days, pink to erythematous macules or papules appear on the trunk, neck, and extensor surfaces of the extremities. These lesions have some central fading, giving them a lacy or reticulated appearance (Fig. 163-6).[27] The rash can be morbilliform, confluent, circinate, or annular, and there are reports of palmar and plantar involvement.[28] The eruption typically lasts 5 to 9 days, but can recur for weeks or months with triggers such as sunlight, exercise, temperature change, bathing, and emotional stress. In some outbreaks, pruritus is a major feature of the rash in children.[28]

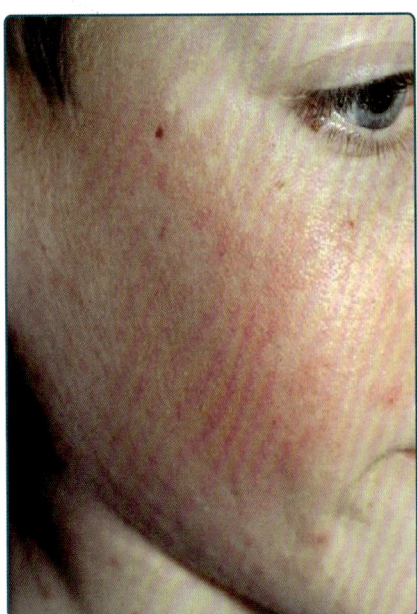

Figure 163-5 Erythema infectiosum. Child with the characteristic "slapped cheeks."

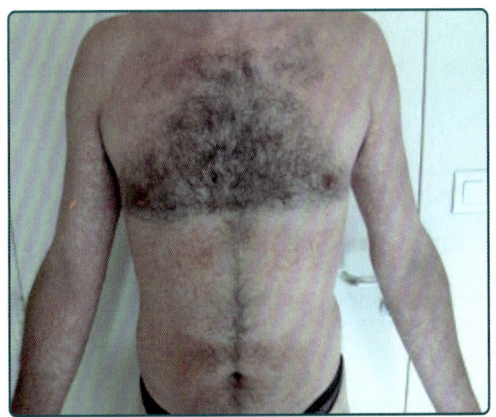

Figure 163-6 Reticulate and annular erythema of the torso and upper limbs in acute parvovirus B19 infection. (Image from Mage V, Lipsker D, Barbarot S, et al. Different patterns of skin manifestations associated with parvovirus B19 primary infection in adults. *J Am Acad Dermatol.* 2014;71(1):62-69, with permission. Copyright © American Academy of Dermatology.)

There have been occasional reports of parvovirus B19 associated with generalized petechiae, and vascular purpura, including Henoch–Schönlein purpura.[29,30] A microvesicular eruption also has been reported.[31] An enanthem consisting of erythema of the tongue and pharynx and red macules on the buccal mucosa and palate can occur.

PARVOVIRUS B19 IN ADULTS

Acute arthropathy is the primary manifestation of B19 viral infection in adults.[32] It occurs mainly in women and affects the knees and the small joints of the hands. Other joints, such as the spine and costochondral joints, are occasionally involved. This symmetric polyarthritis is usually of sudden onset and is self-limited but can be persistent or recurrent for months. It may mimic Lyme arthritis or rheumatoid arthritis.

The constitutional symptoms are usually more severe in adults than in children. Fever, adenopathy, and a mild arthritis without a rash is the usual course. Women are more likely than men to have joint complaints and rash, whereas men often present with only a flu-like illness.[32] Some adults may have fatigue, malaise, and depression for weeks after the infection. Asymptomatic infection can certainly occur in adults as well as in children. Numbness and tingling of the fingers and pruritus have been reported with or without a rash.[33] It has been suggested that if pruritus is a complaint in a patient with acute-onset arthritis, parvovirus should be considered as a possible cause.

The rash in adults, if present at all, is usually macular and blotchy or lacy, often on the extremities, and rarely demonstrates the characteristic slapped-cheek appearance.[32] Other cutaneous manifestations associated with B19 infection in adults include purpura, vesicles and pustules, palmoplantar desquamation, a morbilliform exanthema, occasional oral petechiae and small erosions, and livedo reticularis.

PAPULAR PURPURIC GLOVES-AND-SOCKS SYNDROME

In 1990, a unique syndrome of pruritic erythema and edema of the hands and feet with petechiae, fever, and oral erosions was described.[34] This rare exanthem, now known as *papular purpuric gloves-and-socks syndrome*, seems to affect teenagers and adults. However, it also can affect children.[35] Patients usually have mild prodromal symptoms of fatigue and low-grade fever, myalgia, and arthralgia. Subsequently, itchy, painful, symmetric edema and erythema of the distal hands and feet occurs. Purpuric papules appear on the hands and feet with abrupt demarcation at the wrists and ankles. The enanthem, if present, arises on the lips, soft palate, and buccal mucosa. The syndrome resolves spontaneously within 2 weeks. Importantly, papular purpuric gloves-and-socks syndrome is contagious when the eruption is present, in contrast to erythema infectiosum.

DIAGNOSIS

LABORATORY TESTING

In patients with erythema infectiosum, laboratory results are usually normal. Patients with aplastic crisis have reticulocytopenia and anemia, the severity of which depends on the degree of underlying anemia. Reticulocytopenia, anemia, lymphopenia, neutropenia, and thrombocytopenia can occur in healthy individuals with B19 infection, although these are usually not significant enough to cause clinical symptoms. The erythrocyte sedimentation rate is rarely elevated, and in some cases of parvovirus-associated arthritis, rheumatoid factor has been positive.

Detection of recent infection is usually performed with assays for IgM antibody. IgM can be detected within a few days after onset of illness and is present for up to 6 months in many cases, although there is a decline in titer in the second month after onset. The sensitivity of IgM ranges from 62% to 70%. IgG can be identified by the seventh day of illness and lasts for years and is therefore best for documenting past infection. Parvovirus antibody is often not detectable in immunodeficient persons.

PCR is used to detect B19 DNA. This technique is considered one of the most sensitive approaches for detection of the virus within a number of different specimens including serum or plasma, amniotic fluid, placental or fetal tissue, or bone marrow. It is considered the test of choice in an immunocompromised patient, and to confirm fetal infection. One caveat is that parvovirus DNA fragments may be present for more than a year after infection, however this does not always indicate that the viable virus is present.[36] PCR should be used along with IgM and IgG in pregnant patients.[37]

PATHOLOGY

The histopathologic changes in the skin of patients with erythema infectiosum include a sparse superficial perivascular lymphocytic infiltrate that is not considered diagnostic. Immunohistochemical techniques can be used to detect B19 parvovirus antigen in a number of different tissues.

DIFFERENTIAL DIAGNOSIS

Table 163-4 outlines the differential diagnosis of parvovirus B19 infection.

PROGNOSIS AND CLINICAL COURSE

Parvovirus B19 infection in healthy individuals is self-limited. The eruption of erythema infectiosum and the parvovirus arthropathy usually resolve in 1 to 2 weeks, but can recur or persist for months. If untreated, transient aplastic crisis can be fatal, but most patients recover in 1 week. Chronic anemia from B19 usually resolves if treated with γ-globulin. Fetal hydrops can lead to fetal death if not treated.

TABLE 163-4
Differential Diagnosis of Parvovirus B19 Infection

Most Likely
- Drug reaction
- Enteroviral infection
- Erysipelas on the cheek
- Erythema infectiosum
- Hand-foot-mouth disease
- Papular purpuric gloves-and-socks syndrome

Consider
- Atypical measles
- Collagen vascular disease (systemic lupus erythematosus, dermatomyositis)
- Erythema infectiosum
- Measles
- Papular purpuric gloves-and-socks syndrome
- Roseola
- Rubella

Always Rule Out
- Kawasaki disease
- Rocky Mountain spotted fever
- Scarlet fever

COMPLICATIONS

An increasing number of complications from parvovirus B19 are now recognized. Subclinical infection is quite common. However, this virus can be responsible for a variety of hematologic, rheumatologic, and neurologic abnormalities.

TRANSIENT APLASTIC CRISIS

Parvovirus B19 is the most common cause of transient aplastic crisis in patients with chronic hemolytic anemias,[38] as well as in other conditions of decreased red cell production or increased red cell destruction. The aplastic crisis may be the initial manifestation of the underlying hematologic disease. Patients typically have fever and constitutional complaints, followed 1 week later by fatigue, pallor, and worsening anemia.[38] Cutaneous manifestations are rarely seen with the aplastic crisis. The hemoglobin may fall below 4 μg/dL and is not associated with reticulocyte production. Bone marrow examination shows hypoplasia or aplasia of the erythroid series. Red blood cell transfusion may be necessary, and most patients recover in 1 week, although the problem can be fatal if untreated. Transient red cell aplasia can occur in healthy persons without underlying hematologic abnormalities.[38] It is likely that the aplasia is missed in individuals without disorders of shortened erythrocyte survival because the hemoglobin does not drop low enough to cause symptoms.

CHRONIC B19 INFECTION

In immunocompromised patients, B19 infection can cause a serious, prolonged anemia from persistent lysis of red blood cell precursors.[39] Parvovirus-related chronic anemia has been reported in HIV-infected patients, as well as in transplantation recipients and those with congenital immunodeficiencies, acute leukemias, lupus erythematosus, and during the first year of life without immunodeficiency. These patients respond dramatically to IV γ-globulin, suggesting that antibody is the main defense to human parvovirus infection.[39]

FETAL B19 INFECTION

Fetal infection with B19 may result in either an unaffected fetus or spontaneous abortion (especially in the first half of pregnancy), hydrops fetalis in the second half of pregnancy, congenital anemia, and even late fetal death.[37] Nonimmune fetal hydrops is the most common complication of intrauterine infection with B19. Because B19 virus can infect erythroid precursors, extensive hemolysis can occur in the fetus, leading to severe anemia, tissue anoxia, high-output heart failure, and generalized edema. The fetus may show ultrasonographic evidence of subcutaneous edema, ascites, pleural effusion, pericardial effusion, placental edema, and polyhydramnios. The overall risk of fetal death is not clearly known, but recent studies suggest that this risk is approximately 6.5% with maternal infection.[37] The risk of fetal death for a woman with unknown serologic status is estimated to be less than 2.5% after a household exposure and less than 1.5% after a significant work exposure. It seems that in B19-infected pregnant women, 33% to 50% of fetuses are infected, with an adverse outcome in 10% of infected fetuses.[37,40] Furthermore, approximately 50% of women of childbearing age are immune to parvovirus infection because of prior infection.

Because parvoviruses are known teratogens in animals, there has been much concern about whether they cause birth defects in humans, but it appears that parvovirus B19 is not a common cause of birth defects.

OTHER COMPLICATIONS

There are reports of B19 infection causing encephalitis, meningitis, brachial neuritis, a myasthenia-like syndrome, and motor weakness. Parvovirus infection has been blamed for a granulomatosis with polyangiitis (Wegener) illness, polyarteritis nodosa, Kawasaki disease, and a systemic lupus erythematosus-like picture.[41-43] In addition, there are reports of other hematologic complications, including idiopathic thrombocytopenic purpura, transient neutropenia, myocarditis, a hemophagocytic syndrome, and the Blackfan-Diamond syndrome.

TREATMENT

There is no specific treatment available for parvovirus B19 infection. Erythema infectiosum is a benign condition, and usually no treatment is necessary. Supportive therapy for relief of fatigue, malaise, pruritus, and arthralgia may be needed. The chronic anemia of persistent B19 infection may be treated successfully with commercially available IV immunoglobulin,, which contains neutralizing anti-B19 antibodies. Transient aplastic crisis, which can be life-threatening, may require oxygen therapy and blood transfusion.

Serologic testing for B19 IgG and IgM should be offered to pregnant women who are exposed to parvovirus B19. Infected pregnant women are followed by frequent ultrasonograms. Evidence of hydrops fetalis warrants umbilical cordocentesis to check for anemia, viral DNA, IgG, and IgM. The management of infected fetuses is controversial. Some physicians advocate observation because spontaneous resolution is common. Fetuses with severe anemia and compromise are usually managed with intrauterine exchange transfusion, but this procedure does carry risk Table 163-5).

PREVENTION

There is currently no vaccine to prevent parvovirus B19 infection. Vaccine development has been problematic; however, Phase II clinical trials have been completed.[44] It is not known whether immunoglobulin given around the time of exposure prevents infection or alters the course of the disease.

Because patients with erythema infectiosum are no longer infectious by the time they develop the illness, control measures directed toward these individuals are not likely to be effective. If these persons are hospitalized, no special precautions need to be taken. Because the virus is transmitted before the rash appears, the disease is easily spread in situations of close prolonged contact such as schools, day care centers, workplaces, and homes.

Patients with aplastic crisis or immunosuppression with chronic B19 anemia may have high-titer viremia and are particularly infectious. These individuals should be placed in respiratory and contact isolation if hospitalized, and pregnant health care providers should not care for them directly. Hospital workers are at risk of contracting nosocomial infections from these patients and could spread the virus to patients if adequate precautions are not taken.

TABLE 163-5
Treatments for Parvovirus B19 Infections

▪ Erythema infectiosum	Supportive treatment of fatigue, malaise, pruritus, arthralgia
▪ Chronic anemia	IV immunoglobulin
▪ Transient aplastic crisis	Oxygen and/or blood transfusion may be necessary
▪ Hydrops fetalis	Possible intrauterine exchange transfusion

EPSTEIN-BARR VIRUS

AT-A-GLANCE

- Epstein-Barr virus is also known as human herpesvirus 4.
- In developed countries, primary infection most often occurs during adolescence/early adulthood.
- Infectious mononucleosis is characterized by the triad of fever, lymphadenopathy, and pharyngitis.
- Morbilliform exanthem with primary infection; most common after administration of ampicillin or amoxicillin.
- Oral hairy leukoplakia, nasopharyngeal carcinoma, Burkitt lymphoma, Hodgkin disease, Kikuchi histiocytic necrotizing lymphadenitis, and certain types of cutaneous T-cell lymphoma are associated with Epstein-Barr virus infection.

Ebstein-Barr virus (EBV), also known as human herpesvirus 4, is a ubiquitous viral infection. Primary infection occurs early in life followed by lifelong, latent infection. EBV has been implicated in a diverse set of inflammatory dermatologic disorders and neoplasms. The manifestations of EBV infection are strongly influenced by the patient's age and immunologic status.

EPIDEMIOLOGY

EBV is a worldwide pathogen with more than 90% of adults latently infected.[45] The age of onset of primary EBV infection is in part dependent on geographic location and socioeconomic status. Patients from developing countries or of lower socioeconomic status are more likely to acquire EBV during early childhood. Early childhood EBV infection is frequently asymptomatic or nonspecific in presentation and does not present with infectious mononucleosis, a manifestation characteristic of EBV infection during adolescence and young adulthood. Within in the United States, 50% of 6- to 8-year-old children are seropositive for EBV.[46] The rest of the population acquires EBV infection later in life with 89% of the population becoming seropositive by 18 to 19 years old.[46] Risk factors for early seropositivity include lower household income, parental education level, uninsured status, and being Mexican American or Black (non-Hispanic).[46]

ETIOLOGY AND PATHOGENESIS

EBV is an enveloped, double-stranded DNA virus with a genome that encodes approximately 100 proteins. EBV exists as 2 distinct types, EBV-1 and EBV-2, but no specific differences in symptoms or disease associations have been identified between the two. EBV-1 is found worldwide and EBV-2 infection occurs most often in Africa.[47]

EBV is typically transmitted via saliva from patients with recent primary infection or from low-grade viral shedding in patients with latent EBV infection. After infectious mononucleosis, viral shedding continues for a median duration of 6 months.[48] The virus also has been isolated from breastmilk, cervical epithelial cells, and semen.[49]

EBV often first infects oropharyngeal epithelial cells with subsequent infection of B-lymphocytes in the oropharynx.[50] EBV infects B lymphocytes through the binding of the EBV glycoprotein gp350 with CD21 on the surface of B cells. The infected B cells are then activated, and their population is expanded.[51] These B lymphocytes allow dissemination of the virus throughout the lymphoreticular system. A clonal expansion of cytotoxic T lymphocytes allows recovery from primary and reactivation infection and is the source of the atypical lymphocytes associated with EBV infection.[52] Symptoms occur after a 4- to 8-week incubation period and likely result from this immunologic response.

EBV establishes an indefinite latent infection within B cells. EBV can periodically reactivate and be shed in oral secretions. An impaired cellular immune system can result in poorly controlled primary EBV infection, EBV reactivation, and promote EBV-induced malignancy. Both X-linked lymphoproliferative disease and GATA2 deficiency are inherited immunodeficiencies particularly associated with impaired immune responses to EBV infection.[53]

CLINICAL FEATURES

INFECTIOUS MONONUCLEOSIS

EBV is transmitted through bodily fluids, especially saliva, and then infects the oropharyngeal epithelium. An incubation period of 30 to 50 days occurs prior to symptoms.[54] The most common manifestation of EBV infection in adolescents and adults is infectious mononucleosis, also referred to as the "kissing disease." Infectious mononucleosis presents with the classic triad of fever, lymphadenopathy, and pharyngitis in approximately 50% of cases.[55] Fevers can last 1 to 3 weeks and lymphadenopathy can be tender and frequently found in the posterior cervical chain. Accompanying pharyngitis can vary in intensity from mild erythema to grossly enlarged tonsils with white exudate that can impact breathing. Other systemic features include fatigue, headache, mild transaminitis, cytopenias, and atypical lymphocytosis.

EBV can infect nearly every organ. Complications of infectious mononucleosis occur in approximately 20% of patients and include airway obstruction, autoimmune hemolytic anemia or thrombocytopenia, neutropenia, myocarditis, and hepatitis. Splenomegaly occurs in 50% of patients and typically resolves by the fourth to sixth week of illness.[56] Splenic rupture is a rare, potentially life-threatening complication more common in young men. The risk of splenic rupture is estimated at 0.1% and is spontaneous in greater than 50% of cases.[57] EBV also is associated with various neurologic complications that typically occur within 1 month of illness including aseptic meningitis, transverse myelitis, peripheral neuritis, Guillain-Barré syndrome, and cranial nerve palsies.[55] EBV infection during pregnancy is not thought to be teratogenic.[58]

Cutaneous eruptions with infectious mononucleosis occur in up to 25% of cases and can adopt a morbilliform, scarlatiniform, urticarial, erythema multiforme-like, or petechial morphology.[59] Eruptions also frequently occur when patients with infectious mononucleosis are treated with antibiotics, classically ampicillin. This association was first described in the 1960s and coined the *ampicillin rash*.[60] Beginning 7 to 10 days after the initiation of ampicillin, patients develop a generalized, pruritic, morbilliform rash with an erythematous or copper color that resolves in a week (Fig. 163-7). This eruption also has been reported with other antibiotics, such as amoxicillin, cephalexin, erythromycin, and levofloxacin. *Ampicillin rash* was originally cited as occurring in up to 100% of antibiotic-exposed patients, but the current literature indicates a much lower rate of only 30%.[59] The rash is thought to be a result of EBV-induced antibodies that are produced in response to the administered drug and form complement-fixing immune complexes.[61] The exanthem does not usually indicate a permanent allergy to the medication.[62]

NON–SEXUALLY RELATED ACUTE GENITAL ULCERS

EBV infection also has been implicated in the development of non–sexually related acute genital ulcers or Lipschütz ulcers.[63] Lipschütz ulcers frequently occur in prepubertal or adolescent females and present as painful, multiple ulcers with red-purple ragged edges on the medial or outer surface of the labia minora. The ulcers are often deep with a necrotic or fibrinous base and can adopt a "kissing" pattern if symmetric.[49] Inguinal lymphadenopathy can also be frequently found on exam. Less common locations for Lipschütz ulcers include the labia majora and inner thighs. Ulcers can also occur in males with involvement of the scrotum (Fig. 163-8). EBV-associated genital ulcers are not recurrent and self-resolve in 2 to 6 weeks. Patients may be misdiagnosed as having herpes simplex infections, Behçet disease, or as victims of sexual abuse. The role of EBV in these ulcers has been confirmed by the detection of EBV DNA via PCR from ulcers and serology confirming acute infection.[64] Other infectious implicated in causing Lipschütz ulcers include cytomegalovirus (CMV), group A *Streptococcus*, mumps, *Salmonella*, toxoplasmosis, influenza A virus, and *Mycoplasma pneumoniae*.[49]

OTHER NONNEOPLASTIC ASSOCIATIONS WITH EPSTEIN-BARR VIRUS

EBV infection also is associated with multiple inflammatory dermatologic conditions, including

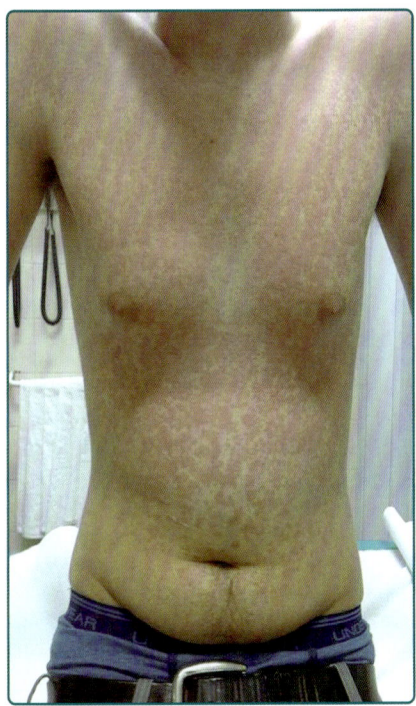

Figure 163-7 Morbilliform rash in Epstein-Barr virus infection. (From Rabach I, Berti I, Bibalo C, Longo G. A curious rash. *J Pediatr.* 2013;162(5):1071-1072, with permission.)

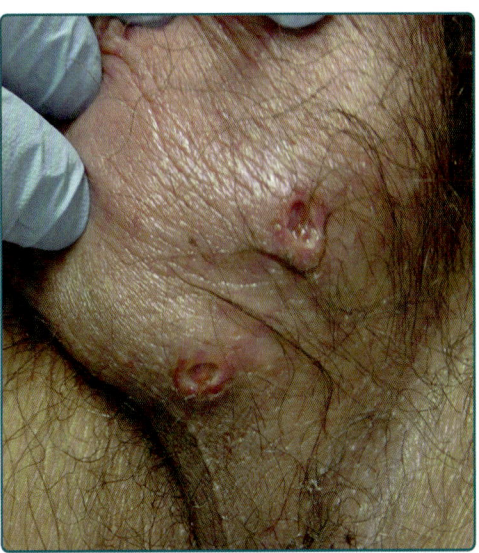

Figure 163-8 Two scrotal ulcers in a patient with documented Epstein-Barr virus infection.

Gianotti-Crosti syndrome when the infection occurs in young children, erythema multiforme, leukocytoclastic vasculitis, erythema nodosum, erythema annulare centrifugum, pityriasis lichenoides, granuloma annulare, and cold urticaria.[49]

NEOPLASTIC CONDITIONS

The latent infection established by EBV is linked to the development of several malignancies, including nasopharyngeal carcinoma, Burkitt lymphoma, and Hodgkin lymphoma Table 163-6).[65] EBV-associated malignancies occur mainly in patients who are immunocompromised because of HIV infection or congenital immunodeficiency, and those who receive immunosuppressant therapy, such as organ transplant recipients. Latent EBV infection of lymphocytes may allow for their transformation, immortalization, and eventual malignant transformation.[66] Different EBV genes are expressed in each type of malignancy and the biology is quite complex.

Nasal-type extranodal natural killer/T cell lymphoma (ENK/T) is strongly associated with EBV.[67] Hallmarks of this aggressive, non-Hodgkin lymphoma include a natural killer–cell phenotype (expression of CD2, CD56, and cytoplasmic CD3 but a lack of surface CD3), angioinvasion and necrosis.[68] ENK/T is rare in the United States, Europe, and Africa, but is endemic in Asia, especially Southern China, and among native populations of Central and South America. Males are more commonly affected than females in a 2:1 ratio, and the tumor typically presents around 50 years of age.[69] The nasal type presents with an ulcerated midfacial tumor, previously termed *lethal midline granuloma*, that can lead to nasal obstruction, facial swelling, sinusitis, and destruction of the underlying sinuses and palate. Extranasal ENK/T can also occur and involve the skin, soft tissue, GI tract, and testes. Radiation therapy is typically used for localized disease and combined with chemotherapy for advanced stages.

Another rare EBV-driven T-cell disorder is hydroa vacciniforme–like lymphoproliferative (HVLL) disease. HVLL disease affects children from Asia and Central and South America. Patients present similarly to photoinduced, self-resolving hydroa vacciniforme with the development of vesicles, crusting, and varicelliform scarring.[70] However, HVLL is distinguished by systemic symptoms (fever, weight loss, hepatosplenomegaly, and lymphadenopathy), extensive facial edema, ulcerations and scarring, and lesions located in photoprotected sites.[70] Histopathology reveals a monoclonal proliferation of T cells with a CD8 phenotype and less often a natural killer–cell phenotype.[71] The clinical course is variable and patients can have prolonged periods of relapsing fevers and skin eruptions. Severe cases can progress to develop hematophagocytic syndrome and natural killer/T-cell lymphoma.[70] GATA2 deficiency has been implicated in some cases of HVLL.[53]

Lymphomatoid granulomatosis is a rare, angioinvasive proliferation of EBV-infected B cells and a reactive, polyclonal T-cell population.[72] Pulmonary involvement is seen in almost all patients presenting with cough, fever, and cavitary lung nodules that at times can mimic Wegner granulomatosis.[66] Cutaneous involvement may be a presenting feature and is documented in up to 40% of cases.[73] As a result of the angiocentric and destructive proliferation, patients may present with stellate ulceration and subcutaneous nodules for which the differential may include medium-vessel vasculitis/vasculopathy and angioinvasive opportunistic infections.[74] A diagnosis of lymphomatoid granulomatosis should prompt a workup of an underlying immunodeficiency, as it has been described in the setting of immunosuppressive medications, congenital immunodeficiency, and autoimmune disease.[75] Lymphomatoid granulomatosis most often presents in the fourth to sixth decade of life and requires the initiation of chemotherapy.

EBV is also strongly associated with other B-cell neoplasms, including Burkitt lymphoma, Hodgkin lymphoma, and EBV+ diffuse large B-cell lymphoma of the elderly.

TABLE 163-6
Epstein-Barr Virus–Associated Lymphoproliferative Diseases and Malignancy

B-cell neoplasms
- EBV+ diffuse large B-cell lymphoma of the elderly
- Endemic Burkitt lymphoma
- Hodgkin lymphoma

T-cell and natural killer cell neoplasms
- Angioimmunoblastic T-cell lymphoma
- Extranodal natural killer/T-cell lymphoma
- Hydroa vacciniforme–like lymphoproliferative disease
- Subcutaneous panniculitis-like T-cell lymphoma[a]

Hemophagocytic syndrome
Leiomyosarcoma[b]
Posttransplantation lymphoproliferative disorder

[a]Most cases of subcutaneous panniculitis T-cell lymphoma are sporadic but Epstein-Barr virus (EBV) positivity has been reported in Asian patients.
[b]EBV-associated smooth muscle tumors have been reported in immunocompromised children.

DIAGNOSIS

The diagnosis of infectious mononucleosis should be considered in adolescents and young adults who present with fever, fatigue, pharyngitis, and lymphadenopathy. Suggestive features of primary EBV infection include splenomegaly, posterior, as opposed to anterior, cervical lymphadenopathy and lymphocytosis with a predominance of atypical lymphocytes (defined as more than 10% of total lymphocytes). Other nonspecific laboratory abnormalities include mild neutropenia, thrombocytopenia, and transaminitis.

Heterophile antibody and EBV-specific antibodies can be used to confirm an EBV infection. The monospot test is a heterophile antibody test frequently used to confirm infectious mononucleosis in adolescents and adults with classic symptoms because of its rapid turnaround time and high specificity in the appropriate clinical setting. A heterophile antibody is an antibody that recognizes antigens on erythrocytes from a different specifies; in the case of the monospot test, it is antibodies against horse red blood cells produced in a person with an EBV infection. The sensitivity of rapid diagnosis heterophile antibody tests is approximately 85%.[76] The monospot test may be negative in the first week of infection and is not a sensitive test for children younger than 4 years old.[77]

EBV-specific antibodies are often employed to confirm EBV infection in young children and when a suspicion for EBV infection remains high despite a negative heterophile antibody test. Host IgM and IgG antibodies form against viral capsid antigen (VCA) and are positive during acute infection. IgM VCA wanes 3 months after clinical illness and IgG VCA remains positive for life. EBV nuclear antigen (EBNA) is expressed when the virus establishes latency; consequently, IgG to EBNA becomes positive usually 6 to 12 weeks after symptoms develop. A positive IgM VCA and negative IgG EBNA confirms acute infection, whereas a positive IgG EBNA argues against an acute EBV infection. Lastly, antibodies to early antigen also can be tested and are present at the onset of the illness. IgG to early antigen exists as 2 subsets, anti-D and anti-R. Anti-D antibodies occur during recent infection and resolve with recovery. The clinical significance of anti-R antibodies is not clear.[78]

PCR-based assays to detect EBV viral load can be useful in detecting infection in immunocompromised states where a host's antibody production may be compromised. EBV serum PCR studies are also frequently used to monitor for posttransplantation lymphoproliferative disease as trending high viral loads serve as a marker for impending posttransplantation lymphoproliferative disease.[79] PCR testing on tissue also may be used to identify EBV-induced neoplasms.

The histopathology of the morbilliform exanthem associated with EBV is nonspecific with a mild perivascular infiltrate of inflammatory cells. Specific cutaneous manifestations of EBV may show their own characteristic histopathologic features.

TABLE 163-7
Differential Diagnosis of Infectious Mononucleosis

Most Likely
- Cytomegalovirus mononucleosis
- Group A streptococcal infection
- Toxoplasmosis

Consider
- Adenovirus
- Enterovirus
- Measles
- Rubella
- Viral hepatitis

Always Rule Out
- Drug rash with eosinophilia and systemic symptoms syndrome
- Primary exanthem of HIV

EBV infection and persists for more than 6 months with severe illness and histologic evidence for organ disease. EBV DNA or antigens can be demonstrated from tissue, and usually EBV antibody titers are significantly elevated.

MANAGEMENT

Treatment for uncomplicated infectious mononucleosis is symptomatic Table 163-8). Acetaminophen or nonsteroidal antiinflammatory agents may be useful in treating the fever or throat discomfort. Because splenomegaly is often an associated finding, contact sports should be avoided until the spleen has returned to its normal size to avoid splenic rupture.

Systemic corticosteroids have been used to reduce the duration of fever or pharyngeal symptoms in infectious mononucleosis. However, a large metaanalysis failed to show any clinical benefit and therefore systemic steroids should not be used to treat typical cases of infectious mononucleosis.[80] Acyclovir has some activity against EBV through the inhibition of the EBV DNA polymerase. A reduction of viral shedding has been documented with acyclovir treatment,

DIFFERENTIAL DIAGNOSIS

Table 163-7 outlines the differential diagnosis of infectious mononucleosis.

CLINICAL COURSE AND PROGNOSIS

Recovery from infectious mononucleosis is typically over 2 to 3 weeks without specific treatment.[65] Disease may be more protracted in older adults. Chronic active EBV infection occurs rarely. It begins as a primary

TABLE 163-8
Treatment for Epstein-Barr Virus Infectious Mononucleosis

First-line therapy	Fever, throat discomfort, myalgia, headache	Acetaminophen/ nonsteroidal antiinflammatory drugs
	Splenomegaly	Avoid contact sports until spleen size normalizes to prevent splenic rupture
Second-line therapy	Impending airway obstruction, thrombocytopenia, hemolytic anemia	Systemic corticosteroids

but clinical benefit has not; as a result, acyclovir is not routinely used in the management of EBV infection.[81]

A commercial vaccine against EBV is not currently available, but investigations are underway with the goal of reducing EBV infection burden, particularly in high-risk patients.[82]

GIANOTTI-CROSTI SYNDROME

AT-A-GLANCE

- Papular acrodermatitis of childhood.
- Common, self-limited dermatosis.
- Monomorphic dome-shaped or flat-topped papules symmetrically distributed on face and extensor extremities.
- Associated with multiple viral triggers and immunizations.
- Historically associated with hepatitis B infection, but now more often triggered by Epstein-Barr virus.

Gianotti-Crosti syndrome (GCS), also known as *infantile papular acrodermatitis* and *papular acrodermatitis of childhood*, is a common, self-limited exanthem. GCS typically affects children between the ages of 3 months and 15 years, with the peak age of onset being 1 to 6 years.[83] Adult cases are uncommon and almost exclusively occur in women. GCS was first described in 1953 by one of Italy's first pediatric dermatologists, Fernandino Gianotti, and his chairman, Professor Agostino Crosti, in Milan.[84] Since this time, GCS is widely known to dermatologists and pediatricians alike as a distinct childhood exanthem with varying infectious triggers.

ETIOLOGY AND PATHOGENESIS

GCS is believed to be an immune reaction to a preceding virus, bacterium, or vaccine, and not related to direct infection of the skin. In cases of EBV-associated GCS, EBV antigen was unable to be isolated from involved skin.[85] The likelihood of developing GCS is likely dependent upon how a host immunologically responds to a preceding infection. Both young age and a history of atopic dermatitis are host risk factors associated with GCS.[86]

Viral infections are the most common trigger of GCS. An association between GCS and hepatitis B was first published in the 1970s, and, for some time thereafter, hepatitis B was thought to be the exclusive cause of GCS. More recent studies implicate numerous other infections agents. In most developed countries, EBV is frequently cited as the most common cause of GCS.[87] Other important viral causes include molluscum pox virus, CMV, echovirus, poxvirus, poliovirus, coxsackievirus (A6, A16, B4, and B5), parvovirus B19, HIV, hepatitis A, hepatitis C, mumps virus, human herpesvirus-6, vaccinia virus, rubella virus and parainfluenza virus.[83] Often overlooked, GCS complicates approximately 5% of cases of molluscum contagiosum, and therefore a recent history or concurrent molluscum should be explored in children with GCS.[88] Bacterial pathogens include *M. pneumoniae*, *Borrelia burgdorferi*, *Bartonella henselae*, and group A β-hemolytic *Streptococcus*.[83] Lastly, a number of vaccines have been documented as preceding the onset of GCS, including influenza, diphtheria-pertussis-tetanus (DPT), bacillus Calmette-Guérin, *Haemophilus influenzae* type b, MMR, hepatitis B, Japanese encephalitis, and oral polio vaccine. Despite these varied infectious triggers, the clinical morphology of GCS remains consistent.

CLINICAL FEATURES

GCS presents with an abrupt onset of symmetrically distributed, monomorphous papules or papulovesicles on the face, extensor surface of extremities, and buttocks (Fig 163-9). Papules range between 1 and 5 mm in size, are pink to red-brown in color, often are dome shaped or flat-topped, and can coalesce to form large plaques. Infrequently, lesions may be hemorrhagic or have scale. Involvement of the trunk, palms, soles, or mucosal surfaces makes a diagnosis of GCS unlikely. Pruritus is the most common accompanying symptom.

Patients with GCS are typically well appearing. GCS can be preceded by malaise, pharyngitis, low-grade fever, and lymphadenopathy (typically cervical, axillary, or inguinal). Noncutaneous findings may also reflect the underlying infectious process triggering GCS, such as hepatomegaly and lymphadenopathy in the setting of hepatitis B infection or splenomegaly in the setting of EBV.

DIAGNOSIS

GCS is a clinical diagnosis. Usually, no further workup is needed. A skin biopsy is rarely needed owing to the characteristic features of GCS. In the setting of hepatomegaly, splenomegaly, or hepatitis, a laboratory workup for viral hepatitis (hepatitides A, B, and C, EBV, and CMV) should be performed.

DIFFERENTIAL DIAGNOSIS

Table 163-9 outlines the differential diagnosis of GCS.

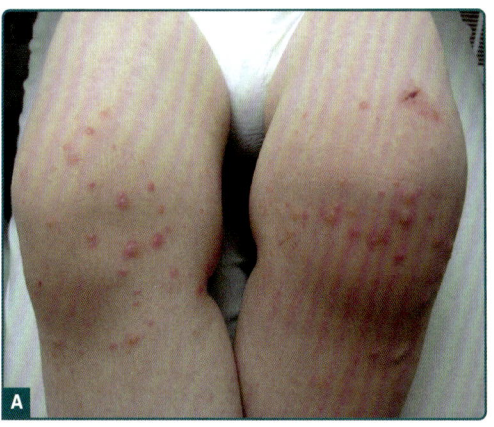 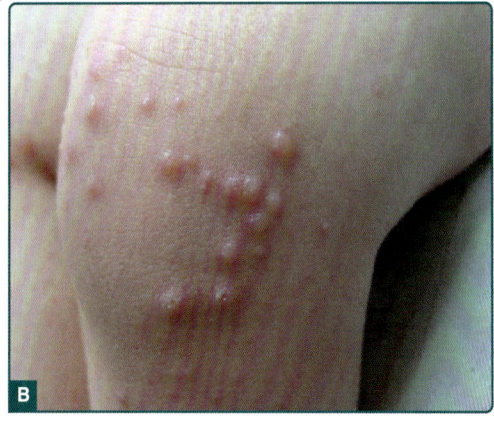

Figure 163-9 **A** and **B,** Erythematous edematous monomorphous dome-shaped papules on the extensor extremities in a toddler with Gianotti-Crosti syndrome.

CLINICAL COURSE AND PROGNOSIS

GCS is self-limited; however, families should be counseled that it might last longer than most rashes associated with viruses. GCS gradually fades over 10 to 60 days. GCS resolves without scarring but can resolve with temporary, postinflammatory hyperpigmentation or hypopigmentation. Reactive lymphadenopathy associated with GCS may take months to fully resolve.

MANAGEMENT

No treatment is necessary in the majority of cases. In some patients, medium-potency topical steroids may decrease the duration of lesions when applied once daily for 1 to 2 weeks. However, patients should be monitored closely because worsening of findings with topical steroid use has been documented.[89] Oral antihistamines or topical antiitch lotions may diminish severe pruritus.

HUMAN CYTOMEGALOVIRUS

AT-A-GLANCE

- Cytomegalovirus is also known as human herpesvirus 5.
- High prevalence in the population.
- Establishes latent infection and is capable of reactivation in immunosuppressed states.
- Primary infection is mainly asymptomatic; it is the cause of severe morbidity and mortality in utero and in immunocompromised patients.
- Petechiae and blueberry muffin syndrome occur with congenital infection.
- Congenital infection is major cause of hearing loss.
- Infected cells are cytomegalic with intranuclear inclusions.

TABLE 163-9
Differential Diagnosis of Gianotti-Crosti Syndrome

Most Likely
- Id reaction
- Papular urticaria

Consider
- Erythema infectiosum
- Erythema multiforme
- Follicular eczema
- Hand-foot-mouth disease
- Lichen planus
- Lichenoid drug eruption
- Molluscum contagiosum
- Pityriasis lichenoides et varioliformis acuta
- Pityriasis rosea

Always Rule Out
- Henoch-Schönlein purpura
- Infectious mononucleosis
- Scabies

EPIDEMIOLOGY

Human cytomegalovirus (HCMV) is ubiquitous around the world. The seroprevalence in the population increases with age, with 10% to 20% of children infected before they reach puberty. By adulthood, the prevalence of HCMV is 40% to 100%. For unclear reasons, there is a higher prevalence in developing countries and areas of low socioeconomic status. HCMV is the most common congenital viral infection in humans, with an incidence of 0.5% to 2% of live births in the United States.[90] Ten percent to 15% of congenital infections exhibit sequelae.[90] Nearly all HIV-infected patients are infected with HCMV.[91] It is a significant cause of morbidity in bone marrow transplant and solid-organ transplant patients.

CLINICAL FEATURES

CONGENITAL HUMAN CYTOMEGALOVIRUS INFECTION

History: Congenital HCMV (cytomegalic inclusion disease of the newborn) occurs mostly in children of primiparous women with primary infection during pregnancy. Fifty-five percent of maternal primary HCMV infections result in intrauterine HCMV infection of the fetus, and approximately one-third of those are symptomatic. Reactivation or secondary HCMV infection of a HCMV-immune woman during pregnancy rarely results in symptomatic HCMV infection for the baby.[90]

Cutaneous Lesions: Cutaneous findings in the newborn include a petechial rash secondary to thrombocytopenia, jaundice caused by hepatitis and blueberry muffin lesions from dermal erythropoiesis. In one study, approximately 70% of children with symptomatic congenital HCMV infections had petechiae and jaundice.[92] Dermal erythropoiesis, also known as *thrombocytopenic purpura* or *blueberry muffin syndrome*, also can be seen with congenital rubella, toxoplasmosis, and blood dyscrasias. These purpuric lesions are present at birth and evolve during the first 24 to 48 hours of life. They are papular and range from 2 to 10 mm in diameter. Lesions are initially dark-blue to violaceous and fade to red or copper-brown. They regress during the first 6 weeks of life despite continued presence of the virus. Histology shows plaque-like aggregates of nucleated cells and nonnucleated erythrocytes in the reticular dermis.[93]

Related Physical Findings: Related findings include hepatosplenomegaly in virtually all newborns, microcephaly, periventricular calcifications, ventriculomegaly, encephalitis, chorioretinitis, hearing loss or neurodevelopmental sequelae, intrauterine growth retardation, and postnatal failure to thrive. After congenital HCMV infection, approximately 50% of symptomatic and 10% of asymptomatic children have hearing loss.[90,94]

PERINATAL HUMAN CYTOMEGALOVIRUS INFECTIONS

History: Perinatal infection with HCMV is very different from congenital HCMV infection, and is without diffuse visceral or CNS involvement. Transmission of the virus occurs via cervical secretions, breastmilk, or blood transfusions between 4 and 16 weeks of age. It is usually asymptomatic, although it may be manifested by self-limited lymphadenopathy, hepatosplenomegaly, or afebrile pneumonitis.[90]

Cutaneous Lesions: There are usually no cutaneous findings with perinatal HCMV infection. Uncommon presentations for HCMV infection in infants and children include GCS, gray pallor, hepatosplenomegaly with self-limited respiratory deterioration in preterm infants, and cutaneous vasculitis.[95,96] Perineal ulcers have been reported in an immunocompetent preterm infant.[97]

HUMAN CYTOMEGALOVIRUS INFECTION IN IMMUNOCOMPETENT ADULTS AND CHILDREN

History: Although primary HCMV infection in the immunocompetent patient is usually asymptomatic, some can present with an infectious mononucleosis–like picture. Approximately 10% of infectious mononucleosis cases are caused by HCMV. Symptoms and signs are indistinguishable from EBV-induced mononucleosis, including fever, malaise, splenomegaly, hepatitis, and peripheral and atypical lymphocytosis. Unlike EBV mononucleosis, HCMV-induced mononucleosis patients do not typically have pharyngitis and lymphadenopathy.[98] Given the lack of heterophile antibodies, HCMV mononucleosis is also known as heterophile-negative mononucleosis. HCMV mononucleosis can occur between 3 and 6 weeks after exposure to CMV-positive blood products.[98]

Reactivation of various herpesviruses, including HCMV, EBV, human herpesvirus (HHV)-6, and HHV-7, has been reported in the setting of drug-induced hypersensitivity syndrome (see Chap. 45) and other severe cutaneous adverse drug reactions, which, in some cases, might lead to multiorgan failure after the causative drug is discontinued.[99]

Cutaneous Lesions: A few patients with HCMV mononucleosis develop a rubelliform or morbilliform eruption; if given ampicillin, 80% to 100% of patients develop a morbilliform rash within 1 week.[100] There are reports of erythema nodosum and urticaria associated with acute HCMV mononucleosis.[101] Cutaneous ulcers caused by CMV have been reported in patients with severe cases of drug-induced hypersensitivity syndrome.[102]

HUMAN CYTOMEGALOVIRUS AND THE IMMUNOCOMPROMISED

History: Immunocompromised patients are at risk for both HCMV primary infection and reactivation, resulting in persistent viremia and disseminated systemic disease. Immunosuppressive agents, such as azathioprine and cyclophosphamide alone, can reactivate HCMV disease, as can systemic corticosteroids in conjunction with other immunosuppressive agents. CMV infection in this setting is defined as evidence of CMV replication with or without disease symptoms. CMV disease is defined as CMV infection with these symptoms: viral syndrome with fever, malaise, leukopenia, and thrombocytopenia; or tissue invasive disease with variable pneumonitis, enteritis, hepatitis, retinitis, and CNS disease.[103]

Solid-Organ Transplantation Recipients: Solid-organ transplantation recipients who are not infected with HCMV but who receive an organ from an HCMV-positive individual are at highest risk of developing HCMV disease posttransplantation. Additional risk factors include higher levels of immunosuppression and allograft rejection.

Bone Marrow Transplantation Patients: The risk of HCMV disease in bone marrow transplantation patients is lower with the use of seronegative donors and of leukocyte-depleted blood products.[104] Risk factors for both first and subsequent CMV infection in seropositive patients include myeloablative conditioning, graft-versus-host disease, lymphoma/myeloma, and low CD3 graft content.[105]

HIV-Infected Patients: HCMV retinitis was seen in up to 25% of HIV-infected patients before the use of highly active antiretroviral therapy.[106] Other clinical manifestations of HCMV infection include immune recovery vitreitis, encephalopathy, peripheral polyradiculopathy, pneumonitis, and colitis.[107] Asymptomatic CMV coinfection in HIV-infected patients on highly active antiretroviral therapy may impair CD4:CD8 ratio normalization.[108]

Cutaneous Lesions: Cutaneous manifestations of HCMV disease in immunocompromised patients are rare compared with involvement of other organs. Perianal and rectal ulceration are most common.[109] Also seen are indurated hyperpigmented nodules or plaques, papular and purpuric eruptions, vesiculobullous lesions, purpura, petechiae, indurated plaques, and, occasionally, verrucous and necrotic nodules.[110-112] Some of these cutaneous manifestations may be caused by infection of the endothelium of cutaneous blood vessels.[109]

DIAGNOSIS

The gold standard for diagnosis of HCMV infection is viral culture from blood using human fibroblasts. Because it takes days to several weeks to see the cytopathic effect in culture, culture has been supplanted by PCR for the diagnosis of active HCMV infection.[103,113] The diagnosis of congenital HCMV infection can be made by detection of virus in urine or saliva via PCR.[113] HCMV PCR also can be used to identify primary infection in children younger than 12 months of age as they shed the virus for long periods of time.

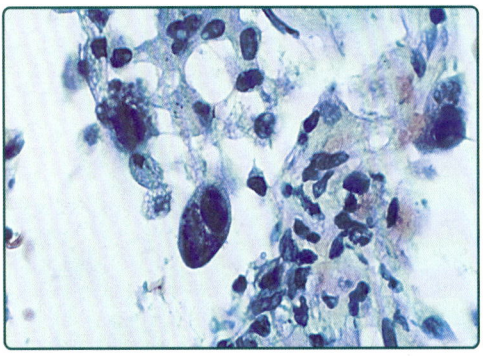

Figure 163-10 Intracellular inclusions in a cell infected by human cytomegalovirus. (From Konstadt JW, Gatusso P, Eng A, et al. Disseminated cytomegalovirus infection with cutaneous involvement in a heart transplant patient. *Clin Cases Dermatol.* 1990;2:3.)

HCMV serology (IgG) is the most reliable method to determine past infection and is used as part of pretransplantation screening. In immunocompetent individuals, IgM is usually positive during primary infection, although the reported sensitivity of IgM varies. Rheumatoid factor and EBV IgM may yield false-positive results.[114] IgG may be negative during active infection, but a subsequent fourfold rise in IgG titer is indicative of infection. In immunocompromised patients, quantitative nucleic acid amplification testing for CMV is the most widely used test for diagnosis, and monitoring response to treatment.[103]

The characteristic histologic feature of CMV infection is cytomegalic cells with nuclear inclusions. In the skin, enlarged endothelial cells with large intranuclear inclusions and a clear halo (owl's eye cells) are seen in small dermal vessels.[115] Cytopathic changes seen in the vascular lumen vary according to the stage of infection of each cell, including intranuclear and intracytoplasmic inclusions (Fig. 163-10). Histologic diagnosis is specific but sensitivity is low.

The diagnosis of invasive CMV disease can be challenging because the presence of the virus does not mean causality given that the virus establishes latency after primary infection.

DIFFERENTIAL DIAGNOSIS

Tables 163-10 and 163-11 outline the differential diagnosis of HCMV blueberry muffin syndrome and mononucleosis infection, respectively.

PROGNOSIS AND CLINICAL COURSE

HCMV disease in immunocompetent individuals is usually self-limited. Immunocompromised patients with systemic HCMV disease have a poor prognosis

TABLE 163-10

Differential Diagnosis of Congenital Human Cytomegalovirus (Blueberry Muffin Syndrome)

Most Likely
- Causes of dermal (extramedullary) hematopoiesis
  - Congenital infection
    - Enterovirus
    - Herpes simplex virus infection
    - Rubella
    - Toxoplasmosis
  - Hereditary spherocytosis
  - Rhesus and ABO incompatibility
  - Twin–twin transfusion syndrome

Consider
- Langerhans cell histiocytosis
- Neonatal lupus erythematosus

Always Rule Out
- Congenital leukemia
- Neuroblastoma with skin metastases

and suffer direct effects of CMV disease in addition to indirect effects such as allograft rejection, higher risk of other infections, graft-versus-host disease, and secondary malignancies.[103]

COMPLICATIONS

Possible complications of postnatal HCMV infection include interstitial pneumonia, hemolytic anemia, splenic infarction, thrombocytopenia and hemolytic anemia, hepatitis, Guillain-Barré syndrome, meningoencephalitis, myocarditis, arthritis, and GI/genitourinary syndromes (colitis, esophagitis, cervicitis, and urethral syndromes).

MANAGEMENT

HCMV infection in immunocompetent hosts is usually asymptomatic or self-limited, not requiring treatment with antiviral drugs. Ganciclovir, valacyclovir, foscarnet, and cidofovir have been approved for systemic treatment of HCMV disease. Ganciclovir and valacyclovir are also used for HCMV prophylaxis.[103] Oral valganciclovir for 6 months improves hearing and neurodevelopmental outcomes in patients with symptomatic congenital HCMV infection.[116]

PREVENTION

Prevention of HCMV infection in HCMV-negative transplanted patients can be achieved with use of blood and tissues from HCMV-negative donors. Preemptive (at time of high risk for disease but before symptoms) or prophylactic treatment with ganciclovir, valganciclovir, or valacyclovir can be used for immunocompromised individuals who are at risk of infection from blood transfusions or organ transplantation with ganciclovir. Risk stratification for preemptive versus prophylactic treatment depends on various risk factors, including type of transplant, immunosuppression, and other host factors.[103] There are currently no candidate vaccines that are near licensure.[116]

HUMAN HERPESVIRUS 6

AT-A-GLANCE

- Causes exanthem subitum (roseola infantum, sixth disease).
- Febrile seizures often without rash in children.
- High seroprevalence in general population by 1 year of age.
- Reactivation in immunocompromised individuals is a cause of morbidity.

Consistent with other herpesviruses, HHV-6 infection is chronic, existing in a latent stage with the ability to reactivate. HHV-6 primary infection often presents either as an acute febrile illness or as the distinct illness exanthem subitum (ES), also known as *roseola infantum* and *sixth disease*.

EPIDEMIOLOGY

HHV-6 is a common viral infection with up to 80% of the population acquiring the infection by 2 year of age.[117] Primary infection typically occurs between the ages of 6 months and 2 years when maternal passive immunity wanes.[117] Primary infection exhibits seasonal variation with the highest incidence in spring; summer and fall epidemics also have been reported.

TABLE 163-11

Differential Diagnosis of Human Cytomegalovirus Mononucleosis

Most Likely
- Epstein-Barr virus mononucleosis

Consider
- Toxoplasmosis
- Viral hepatitis

Always Rule Out
- Lymphoma

ETIOLOGY AND PATHOGENESIS

HHV-6 is a member of the β-Herpesviridae subfamily and exists as 2 distinct species: HHV-6a and HHV-6b. HHV-6b causes ES and reactivates in immunocompromised hosts. It is unclear what diseases, if any, are caused by HHV-6a.[118]

HHV-6 infects a wide range of human cells, including monocytes/macrophages, natural killer cells, and neuronal cells, such as astrocytes, and preferentially infects activated CD4+ T lymphocytes. The immune regulatory protein CD46 is the cellular receptor for HHV-6 infection.[119] HHV-6 viral DNA may also integrate into host cell chromosomes in up to 1% of the general population, thereby serving as an alternative means of HHV-6 persistence.[120]

As the salivary glands are an important site of viral replication, HHV-6 transmission occurs via shared saliva and can readily be detected in the saliva of adults and children.[117] In transplantation recipients, most cases of HHV-6 infection constitute reactivation of latent infection; however, transmission of HHV-6 from the donor organ has been infrequently described.[121]

The incubation period for HHV-6 infection is 5 to 15 days, with an average of 10 days. Viremia in immunocompetent children lasts 3 to 4 days in ES, whereas viremia from HHV-6 reactivation in allogeneic bone marrow transplantation patients lasts weeks.[120]

CLINICAL FEATURES

HHV-6 primary infection in early childhood may be subclinical or can present with nonspecific symptoms, including high fever, irritability, rhinorrhea, and diarrhea. The fever lasts approximately 3 to 7 days and is followed by the characteristic rash of roseola in only 23% of cases.[122,123]

HHV-6 infection can also occur when the virus reactivates in the setting of immunosuppression. HHV-6 reactivation is particularly common in stem cell transplantation patients where reactivation occurs in 50% of patients and peaks 2 to 4 weeks posttransplantation.[124] HHV-6 reactivation is thought to occur less frequently in solid-organ transplantation patients. Reactivation may be asymptomatic or result in fever, diarrhea, morbilliform rash, and transient myelosuppression.

EXANTHEM SUBITUM

HHV-6 is the cause of ES, also known as *roseola*, which was first described in 1910.[125] The hallmark of ES is the development of "rose"-colored macules and papules measuring 2 to 5 mm and surrounded by a white halo (Fig. 163-11). The exanthem lasts 3 to 5 days and is widespread spread on the neck and trunk, and occasionally occurs on the face and proximal extremities. A unique feature of ES is that it presents 1 day before to 1 to 2 days after the fever resolves, as opposed to most viral exanthems where eruptions occur at the onset of the illness. Children with ES may also have palpebral edema resulting in a "sleepy" appearance and erythematous papules on the soft palate (Nagayama spots) that may precede the viral exanthem.

PITYRIASIS ROSEA

See Chap. 31 and "Human Herpesvirus 7" below.

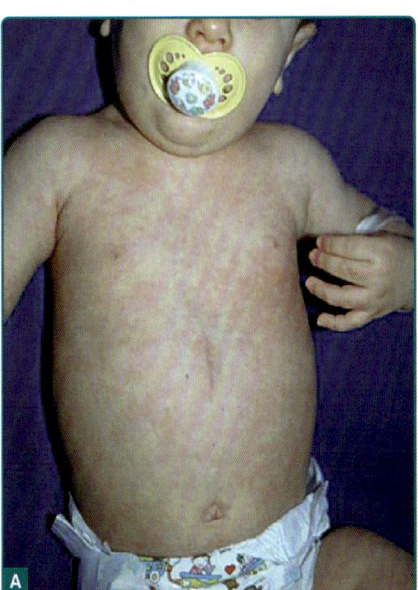
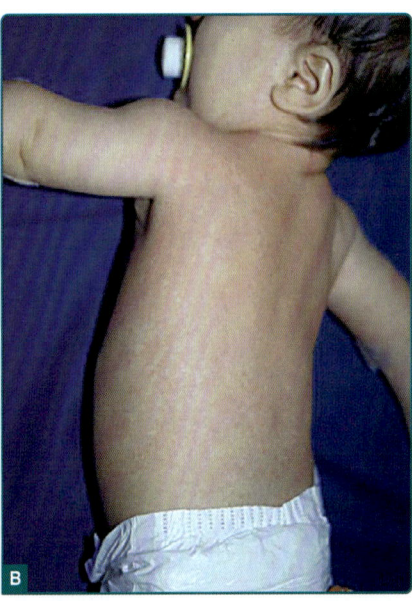

Figure 163-11 **A** and **B,** Exanthem subitum in an infant showing truncal pink macules and some papules that appeared 1 day after defervescence.

ROSAI-DORFMAN DISEASE

The HHV-6 genome has been detected in tissue from patients with sinus histiocytosis with massive lymphadenopathy or Rosai-Dorfman disease (see Chap. 117), and immunohistochemical studies suggest a possible pathogenic involvement.[126,127]

DRUG-INDUCED HYPERSENSITIVITY SYNDROME

Although HHV-6 reactivation is well-described in drug hypersensitivity reactions (see Chap. 45), its role in driving systemic inflammation in this setting is unclear.

DIAGNOSIS

HHV-6 primary infection in childhood and in the setting of ES is typically a clinical diagnosis and laboratory testing is rarely needed. A challenge in the laboratory testing of HHV-6 is distinguishing between latent versus active replicating infection. Most patients older than 2 years of age are seropositive for HHV-6 and approximately 5% of healthy adults are IgM-positive at any given time.[128] A fourfold increase of HHV-6 IgG during the convalescent stage is suggestive of HHV-6 infection.

Quantitative real-time PCR is increasingly being used to detect HHV-6 infection with intermediate and high levels of HHV-6 DNA suggestive of active, as opposed to latent, infection. Real-time PCR testing also can be performed on any tissue. Qualitative real-time PCR does not distinguish latent from active infection. Because of the low sensitivity and longer turnaround time, viral culture is rarely employed.

CLINICAL COURSE AND PROGNOSIS

HHV-6 primary infection and ES in childhood is generally benign and self-limited. Fever typically resolves in 1 week and the rash over 3 to 5 days. The most common complication of a primary infection is the development of a febrile seizure. Febrile seizures occur in 8% of children with primary infection.[102] Rare complications of primary infection also include hepatitis, mononucleosis-like syndrome, meningoencephalitis, hemophagocytic syndrome, pneumonitis, and thrombocytopenia.[122] Treatment is not typically needed for the immunocompetent patient.

Although HHV-6 in transplantation recipients is linked to various complications, establishing pathogenicity is challenging given that these hosts are frequently coinfected by other viral infections and the limitations of PCR technology to distinguish between latent and active infection. In bone marrow transplantation recipients, complications include subacute encephalitis, bone marrow suppression, pneumonitis, and thrombotic microangiopathy. The role of HHV-6 in triggering or increasing the severity of acute graft-versus-host disease is controversial.[129]

MANAGEMENT

There are no controlled clinical trials, and no compounds have been formally approved for treatment of HHV-6 infection. The same drugs used for HCMV treatment and prophylaxis have been used for HHV-6. The activities of various antiviral compounds against HHV-6 have been tested in vitro.[130] Several case reports support the clinical effectiveness of ganciclovir in HHV-6 treatment and prophylaxis.[131] Foscarnet and cidofovir might also prove to be useful.[131]

PREVENTION

Prophylaxis with ganciclovir may prevent HHV-6 reactivation in bone marrow transplantation and stem cell transplantation recipients, but low-dose prophylaxis may facilitate the development of resistance.[132] Preemptive therapy (treatment after systemic detection of virus but before clinical symptoms of disease) has been proposed instead.

HUMAN HERPESVIRUS 7

AT-A-GLANCE

- Human herpesvirus 7 causes a small subset of cases of exanthem subitum.
- Primary infection typically occurs later in life than human herpesvirus 6 infection.

EPIDEMIOLOGY

In seroconversion studies, 10% of ES cases are caused by HHV-7.[133] Primary infection occurs during childhood, but later than, and at a slower rate than, infection with HHV-6. Both viruses are ubiquitous in adulthood and have a worldwide distribution. HHV-7 can be isolated from saliva samples of healthy seropositive adults.[134]

ETIOLOGY AND PATHOGENESIS

HHV-7 is a member of the β-Herpesviridae family. Even though it has significant homology to HHV-6, it is serologically and biologically distinct. HHV-7 establishes persistent infection in salivary glands, and transmission is likely through saliva.[134] Latent virus can be activated in vitro from peripheral blood mononuclear cells, and its DNA can be found in CD4+ T cells. Similar to many other herpesviruses, HHV-7 can downregulate expression of CD4 and major histocompatibility complex class I, which may play a role in establishment of latency or pathogenesis.[134,135] Reactivation of HHV-7 occurs more often than reactivation of HHV-6.[136]

CLINICAL FEATURES

EXANTHEM SUBITUM

HHV-7 causes a small subset of ES cases. When HHV-7 is associated, ES tends to occur later in life than when HHV-6 is associated.[134] The rash associated with HHV-7 is lighter in color and occurs later in the course of the disease than HHV-6–associated ES.[134]

PITYRIASIS ROSEA

HHV-7 DNA has been isolated from skin biopsy specimens, peripheral blood mononuclear cells, and plasma of patients with pityriasis rosea (see Chap. 31) and not controls.[137] However, these findings have not been confirmed by other studies. It is possible that the inflammatory milieu in pityriasis rosea activates HHV-7 and HHV-6 within the lesions, but there is no evidence for causality.

LICHEN PLANUS

HHV-7 DNA and virion-like structures have been found in lesional lichen planus skin samples compared to nonlesional skin and psoriatic skin samples.[89] Although suggestive, further studies are needed to establish a causal relationship.

DIAGNOSIS

There is limited cross-reactivity between HHV-7 and HHV-6 in serologic studies. Because of high prevalence, a single positive IgG is not sufficient to establish a diagnosis. PCR is widely available and is useful for timely diagnosis. Diagnosis of active infection by PCR can only be made from acellular material such as CSF, serum, or plasma, because the virus is latent in peripheral blood mononuclear cells and tissue.

Immunohistochemical studies for viral antigens in biopsy specimens can be performed.

DIFFERENTIAL DIAGNOSIS

Table 163-12 outlines the differential diagnosis of HHV-6– and HHV-7–associated ES.

CLINICAL COURSE AND PROGNOSIS

ES is a self-limiting disease that does not require specific antiviral treatment. Disease in immunocompromised patients can be more serious and require treatment.

Complications of HHV-7–associated ES include acute hemiplegia and febrile seizures with CSF findings consistent with encephalitis and hepatitis.[138]

MANAGEMENT

Treatment for HHV-7 has not been evaluated in clinical trials but can be guided by treatment recommendations for HHV-6.

ENTEROVIRUSES

Human enteroviruses cause a variety of exanthems and clinical syndromes. They are small, single-stranded RNA picornaviruses and include echovirus, coxsackieviruses A and B, and poliovirus.[139] Most enterovirus infections are benign. However, nonpolio enteroviruses are also the most common cause of aseptic (viral) meningitis and, rarely, can cause life-threatening infections involving encephalitis, myocarditis, or sepsis.[139]

TABLE 163-12

Differential Diagnosis for Human Herpesvirus 6– and Human Herpesvirus 7–Associated Exanthem Subitum

Most Likely
- Drug hypersensitivity reaction
- Enterovirus (including coxsackie, echovirus)
- Human herpesvirus–associated exanthem subitum

Consider
- Adenovirus
- Epstein–Barr virus
- Fifth disease (erythema infectiosum, parvovirus)
- Measles/rubeola
- Rubella (German measles)

Always Rule Out
- Kawasaki disease
- Scarlet fever

Severe infections are more common in neonates and immunocompromised individuals.

Enteroviruses are one of the most common causes of nonspecific exanthems. Infected patients present with scattered, pink, small macules and papules that fade within 1 week. Exanthems may also include petechiae and purpuric macules and therefore may be confused with more life-threatening infections such as Rocky Mountain spotted fever or meningococcemia. Well-described exanthems caused by enteroviruses include hand-foot-mouth disease; coxsackievirus A6–associated atypical hand-foot-mouth disease; herpangina; eruptive pseudoangiomatosis; and the Boston exanthem.

HAND-FOOT-MOUTH DISEASE

AT-A-GLANCE

- Hand-foot-mouth disease is a viral exanthem seen mostly commonly in children in summer and fall.
- Erosions in the mouth and papulovesicles on the palms and soles.
- Caused by enteroviruses including coxsackievirus A16 and enterovirus 71.
- Self-resolving without serious sequelae in the majority of cases, but may have serious complications when caused by enterovirus 71.

Hand-foot-mouth disease (HFMD) is the best-recognized enteroviral exanthem with a worldwide distribution.

EPIDEMIOLOGY

Children younger than 10 years of age are most frequently affected, and infected adults rarely show signs of infection. In temperate climates, HFMD is most common in the summer and fall.

ETIOLOGY AND PATHOGENESIS

Traditionally, HFMD has been caused by coxsackievirus A16 and enterovirus 71. Other causes of often HFMD include coxsackieviruses A5, A6, A7, A9, A10, A16, B1, B2, B3, and B5, echoviruses, and other enteroviruses.[140]

Viral transmission is via the fecal–oral route and, less commonly, respiratory inhalation. Once inhaled or ingested, virus replication ensues in the oropharynx and/or GI tract with subsequent viremia. The incubation period of HFMD is believed to be short, lasting 3 to 6 days, with viral shedding lasting up to 5 weeks.[141]

CLINICAL FEATURES

HFMD usually begins with a nonspecific prodrome involving low-grade fever (38°C to 39°C [100.4°F to 102.2°F]) that lasts 1 to 2 days, malaise, and, occasionally, abdominal pain or upper respiratory tract symptoms. Sore throat or a sore mouth is common and can lead to poor oral intake and dehydration.

The hallmark of HFMD is the development of a vesicular eruption on the palms and soles. The lesions start as bright pink macules and papules that progress to small 4- to 8-mm vesicles with surrounding erythema. Vesicles quickly erode and form yellow to gray, oval or "football-shaped" erosions surrounded by an erythematous halo. Cutaneous vesicles are found on the palms, soles (Figs. 163-12B and 163-12C), sides of hands and feet, buttocks and, occasionally, external genitalia. In classic HFMD, nearly all patients also develop an enanthem consisting of similarly appearing oral erosions involving the tongue (Fig. 163-12A) buccal mucosa, hard palate, and, less frequently, the oropharynx.

DIAGNOSIS

HFMD is a clinical diagnosis and laboratory tests are typically not needed. If laboratory confirmation is required, viral culture or PCR based assays can be performed. The virus can be recovered from skin vesicles as well as throat and stool swabs. PCR is frequently performed on the CSF and serum when working up systemic viral infection.[142]

Skin biopsies are not typically performed. Nonspecific findings, such as intraepidermal blister formation from vacuolar and degeneration of keratinocytes, are seen as in other viral blisters.[143]

CLINICAL COURSE AND PROGNOSIS

The cutaneous vesicles in HFMD typically crust over and fade in in 7 to 10 days. Onychomadesis has occasionally been reported as a consequence of coxsackievirus A16 and enterovirus 71 infections.

Patients with HFMD rarely experience complications. The most common serious complication associated with HFMD is aseptic meningitis. Aseptic meningitis is rarely life threatening, and patients typically do not develop permanent sequela. However, enterovirus 71, an important cause of HFMD outbreaks in Asia, is associated with severe illness. Epidemics of enterovirus 71 are associated with severe neurologic disease, including encephalitis, encephalomyelitis, and polio-like syndromes. Enterovirus 71 infection may also lead to myocarditis, pulmonary edema, pulmonary hemorrhage, and death.[144]

COXSACKIEVIRUS A6–ASSOCIATED ATYPICAL HAND-FOOT-MOUTH DISEASE

AT-A-GLANCE

- Papulovesicles, vesicles and erosions on the palms, soles, extremities and perioral area.
- Oral erosions occur less frequently than in classic hand-foot-mouth disease.
- Large bullae and purpuric macules may occur.
- Self-resolving without serious sequela in the majority of cases.

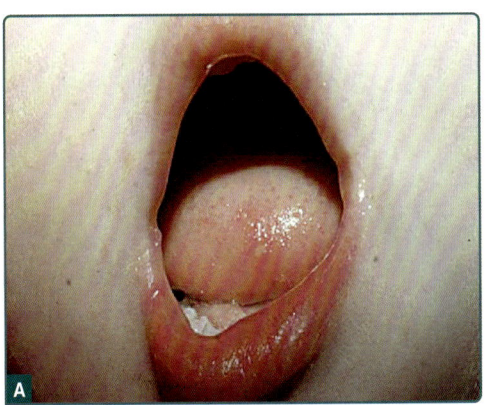
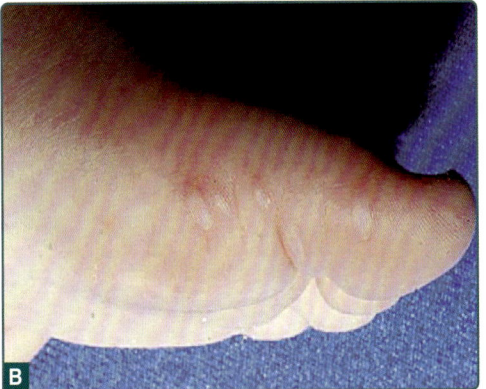
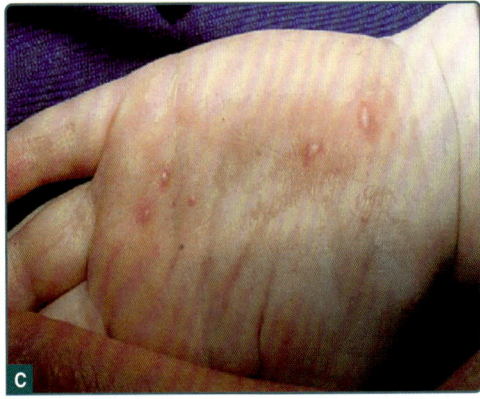

Figure 163-12 Classic hand-foot-mouth disease in a toddler. **A,** Vesicles and surrounding erythema on the tongue. **B** and **C,** Elliptical, "football-shaped" vesicles with halo of erythema on the palms and soles.

An emerging cause of HFMD disease in many countries around the world is coxsackievirus A6 (CVA6).[146] Within the United States, CVA6 was first isolated as the cause of clinically atypical HFMD disease in 2011, and is now commonly identified in HFMD outbreaks.[147] Compared to classic HFMD, CVA6 infection frequently results in a cutaneous presentation that is more varied and extensive in distribution. Presumably because of a lack of previous immunity, adults may also present with CVA6-associated HFMD.[148]

ETIOLOGY AND PATHOGENESIS

Similar to other enteroviruses, CVA6 is transmitted via a fecal–oral route and less often via respiratory secretions.

CLINICAL FEATURES

In keeping with classic HFMD, CVA6-associated HFMD frequently presents with erythematous macules and vesicles on the palmoplantar surfaces and buttocks. However, the exanthem is not limited to those sites. Papulovesicles, rounded vesicles, and erosions commonly involve the upper and lower extremities and the perioral area, occasionally leading to a misdiagnosis of bullous impetigo (Fig. 163-13). Diffuse involvement with the exanthem extending onto the trunk may also occur.[149] In a review of 81 patients with CVA6 disease, the exanthem involved greater than 10% body surface area in 61% of patients.[147] CVA6 infection can result in the development of large bullae measuring greater than 2 cm, typically in children younger than 1 year of age (Fig. 163-14) and acrally distributed petechiae and purpura, often in children older than 5 years of age, which may be confused for leukocytoclastic vasculitis.[147] Localization of vesicles and erosions of atopic dermatitis is also well described and has been termed *eczema coxsackium*, highlighting that this presentation may mimic eczema

MANAGEMENT

Treatment is typically supportive with attempts to reduce discomfort and dehydration. Novel antiviral agents and vaccine development targeting enterovirus 71 is an active area of investigation because of the strain's virulence, geographic spread, rising prevalence, and risk for devastating brainstem encephalitis.[145]

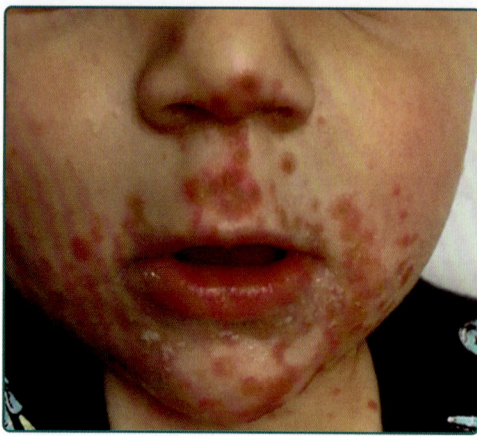

Figure 163-13 Coxsackievirus A6–associated hand-foot-mouth disease with perioral distribution.

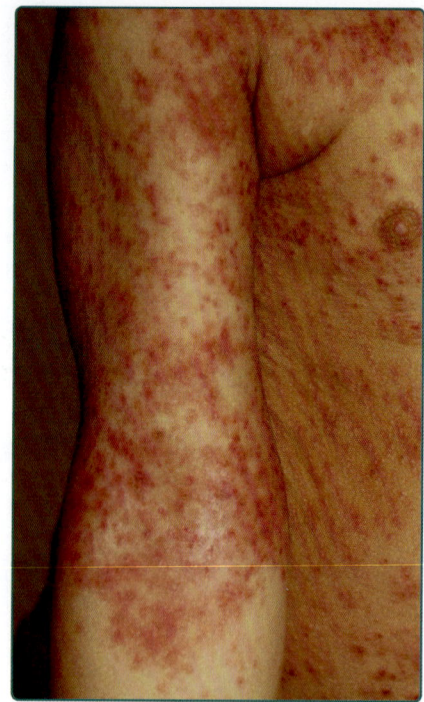

Figure 163-15 Eczema coxsackium. Localization of vesicles and erosions to affected areas of atopic dermatitis in a coxsackievirus A6–infected patient.

herpeticum (Fig. 163-15). Clinical features more suggestive of eczema coxsackium include concurrent oral aphthae, palmoplantar macules and vesicles, perioral involvement, the lack of herpetiform grouping of vesicles, and the onset occurring the context of family or community outbreak. The CVA6 exanthem generally resolves in 1 to 2 weeks.

Oral ulcerations, a defining feature in classic HFMD, found in nearly 100% of patients, are seen less frequently in CVA6 infection and are documented in CVA6-associated HFMD in only 50% of cases.[147] Viral prodrome symptoms associated with CVA6 infection include fever, sore throat, headache, cough, and diarrhea.

DIAGNOSIS

In complicated cases, CVA6 infection can be confirmed by performing enterovirus reverse-transcriptase PCR on samples collected by swabs from stool, throat, the base of skin vesicles, or serum samples.[150] PCR is more sensitive in the detection of CVA6 than enterovirus culture.

Skin biopsies of this exanthem have revealed intraepidermal vesiculation with a predilection for the stratum granulosum and upper stratum spinulosum and a neutrophil rich infiltrate.[151]

DIFFERENTIAL DIAGNOSIS

Table 163-13 outlines the differential diagnosis of HFMD.

CLINICAL COURSE AND PROGNOSIS

Despite the occasionally extensive cutaneous presentation, CVA6 is not generally associated with severe systemic illness. Therefore, CVA6 infections appear to be more in keeping with CVA16 than enterovirus

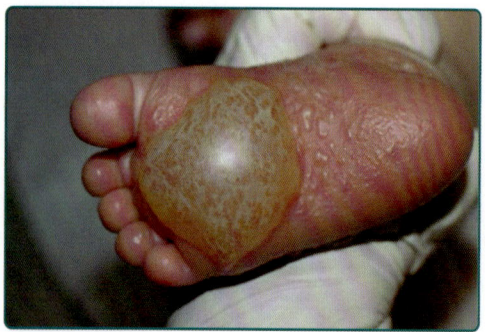

Figure 163-14 Coxsackievirus A6–associated hand-foot-mouth disease with large bullae on the sole of an infant. (Image used with permission from Dr. Ilona Frieden.)

TABLE 163-13 Differential Diagnosis of Hand-Foot-Mouth Disease
Most Likely
▪ Eczema herpeticum
Consider
▪ Autoimmune blistering disorder (eg, liner immunoglobulin A bullous dermatosis)
▪ Disseminated herpes zoster
▪ Drug eruption
▪ Stevens-Johnson syndrome
▪ Erythema multiforme
▪ Leukocytoclastic vasculitis
▪ Varicella
Always Rule Out
▪ Herpes simplex virus infection

71. The 2 most common complications of CVA6 are desquamation of the hands and feet, which often occurs weeks after the exanthem resolves, and onychomadesis, which occurs 1 to 2 months later. Onychomadesis may occur in the absence of any history of the HFMD exanthema, and all patients with CVA6-associated HFMD should be made aware of this complication.[152] Patients with onychomadesis can be expected to have normal nail growth after the shedding is complete.

MANAGEMENT

The management of CVA6 HFMD is supportive and focuses on managing pain, and local wound care for larger vesicles and bullae.

ERUPTIVE PSEUDOANGIOMATOSIS

Cherry and colleagues first described a syndrome in 1969 in which 4 children with acute echovirus infection (2 with echovirus 25 and 2 with echovirus 32) developed small, 2- to 4-mm, red papules that resembled angiomas on the face and extremities.[153] The papules blanched on pressure and were surrounded by a small, 1- to 2-mm, halo. The eruption was short lived and typically resolved within 10 days.[154] Patients often had associated fever, malaise, headache, diarrhea, and respiratory complaints.

While echovirus was first linked to eruptive pseudoangiomatosis, the etiology in most cases cannot be identified. Adenovirus, CMV, arthropod bites, and immunocompromised states also have been identified in eruptive pseudoangiomatosis cases.

Other children and adults have been described with similar outbreaks. Although a virus is likely to cause eruptive pseudoangiomatosis, echoviruses have not been consistently confirmed as the causative agent.[155-158]

UNILATERAL LATEROTHORACIC EXANTHEM

AT-A-GLANCE

- Unilateral laterothoracic exanthem is also called *asymmetric periflexural exanthem of childhood*.
- Typically affects children 1 to 5 years of age.
- Pink papules that start in a large flexural region, become bilateral, but remain asymmetric.
- Probably viral etiology.

Unilateral laterothoracic exanthem (ULE), also known as *asymmetric periflexural exanthem of childhood*, has a seasonal variation and occurs most frequently in late winter and early spring. It typically occurs in children between 1 and 5 years of age, but may be seen from 8 months to 10 years of age.[159] Rare cases in adults have been reported.[160] There is a slight female predominance, and it is more common in whites.

ETIOLOGY AND PATHOGENESIS

The etiology of ULE is unknown, but because of its seasonality, associated viral symptoms and lack of response to antibiotics, a viral trigger is suspected. The pathogenesis is also unknown.

CLINICAL FEATURES

ULE typically presents with 1- to 2-mm, pinpoint, pruritic, pink papules with a surrounding pale halo localized to a large flexural region like the axillae or groin. The papules then spread centrifugally (Fig. 163-16). ULE can become bilateral and more widespread within 5 to 15 days, but a unilateral and asymmetric distribution remains. A variety of morphologies also have been described, including macules, papules, morbilliform, annular, scarlatiniform, and annular.[159] Pruritus may be severe.

In cases of ULE, a preceding viral syndrome consisting of mild upper respiratory tract, low-grade fever, or GI tract symptoms can often be elicited. In the area of the eruption, enlargement of regional lymph nodes are frequently identified.

DIAGNOSIS

ULE is a clinical diagnosis and no laboratory tests are indicated.

DIFFERENTIAL DIAGNOSIS

Table 163-14 outlines the differential diagnosis of ULE.

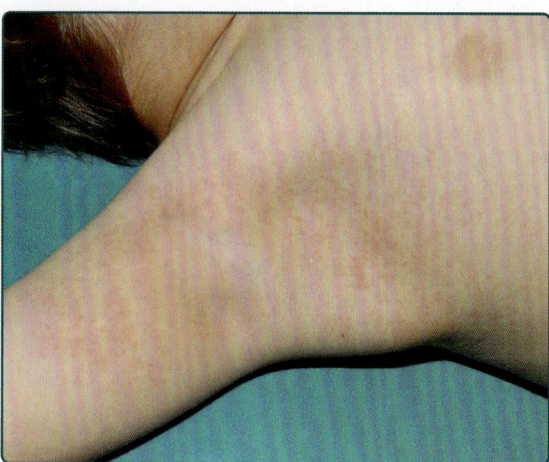

Figure 163-16 Rough pink papules in the right axilla, characteristic of unilateral laterothoracic exanthem. (Used with permission from Antonio Torrelo, MD.)

TABLE 163-14
Differential Diagnosis of Unilateral Laterothoracic Exanthem

Most Likely
- Allergic or irritant contact dermatitis
- Scarlet fever

Consider
- Other viral exanthems

Always Rule Out
- Atopic dermatitis
- Herpes zoster

CLINICAL COURSE AND PROGNOSIS

The rash typically lasts from 2 to 6 weeks but may last as long as 2 months. Resolution is spontaneous and without scarring. During the healing stage, desquamation and postinflammatory pigment change also may be present as the exanthem resolves.

MANAGEMENT

Treatment for ULE is typically focused on controlling pruritus. This can be done with topical corticosteroids, antiitch lotions, and oral antihistamines.

SUMMARY

Table 163-15 summarizes viral infections with characteristic exanthems.

REFERENCES

1. Langmuir AD, Henderson DA, Serfling RE, et al. The importance of measles as a health problem. *Am J Public Health Nations Health*. 1962; 52(2)Suppl:1-4. PMID: 14462171.
2. Papania MJ, Wallace GS, Rota PA, et al. Elimination of endemic measles, rubella, and congenital rubella syndrome from the Western hemisphere: the US experience. *JAMA Pediatr*. 2014;168(2):148-155.
3. Fiebelkorn AP, Redd SB, Gallagher K, et al. Measles in the United States during the postelimination era. *J Infect Dis*. 2010;202(10):1520-1528.
4. Zipprich J, Winter K, Hacker J, et al. Measles outbreak—California, December 2014-February 2015. *MMWR Morb Mortal Wkly Rep*. 2015;60(6):153-154.
5. World Health Organization (WHO). Measles. http://www.who.int/en/news-room/fact-sheets/detail/measles. Updated February 19, 2018. Accessed October 4, 2016.
6. Chen RT, Goldbaum GM, Wassilak SG, et al. An explosive point-source measles outbreak in a highly vaccinated population. Modes of transmission and risk factors for disease. *Am J Epidemiol*. 1989;129(1):173-182.
7. Hirsch RL, Griffin DE, Johnson RT, et al. Cellular immune responses during complicated and uncomplicated measles virus infections of man. *Clin Immunol Immunopathol*. 1984;31(1):1-12.
8. Moss WJ, Griffin DE. Measles. *Lancet*. 2012;379(9811):153-164.
9. Helfand RF, Kebede S, Mercader S, et al. The effect of timing of sample collection on the detection of measles-specific IgM in serum and oral fluid samples after primary measles vaccination. *Epidemiol Infect*. 1999;123(3):451-455.
10. Committee on Infectious Diseases, American Academy of Pediatrics. Measles. In: Kimberlin DW, Brady MT, Jackson MA, Long SS, eds. *Red Book: 2015 Report of the Committee on Infectious Diseases*. 30th ed. Elk Grove Village, IL: American Academy of Pediatrics; 2015: 535-547. (Available at: https://redbook.solutions.aap.org/DocumentLibrary/9781581109276.pdf.)
11. Yang HM, Mao M, Wan CM. Vitamin A for treating measles in children. *Cochrane Database Syst Rev*.

TABLE 163-15
Viral Infections with Characteristic Exanthems

	ETIOLOGIC AGENT	CHARACTERISTIC EXANTHEM OR ASSOCIATED RASH	EXTRACUTANEOUS MANIFESTATIONS, ENANTHEMS
Measles (Rubeola)	Paramyxoviridae	Nonpruritic, erythematous macules and papules with craniocaudal spread	Fever, malaise, conjunctivitis, coryza, cough, Koplik spots
Rubella (3-day measles; German measles)	Togaviridae	Pruritic pink to red macules and papules on the face, progressing to neck, trunk, and extremities	Low-grade fever, myalgia, headache, conjunctivitis, rhinitis, cough, sore throat, lymphadenopathy; Forchheimer spots
Erythema Infectiosum (fifth disease)	Parvovirus (B19)	Confluent, erythematous, edematous plaques on malar eminence (slapped cheek); lesions may recur for weeks or months	Erythema of the tongue, pharynx and red macules on the buccal mucosa and palate; acute arthropathy in adults
Papular purpuric gloves-and-socks syndrome		Itchy, painful, symmetric edema and erythema of the distal hands and feet with abrupt demarcation at the wrists and ankles	Fatigue, low-grade fever, myalgia and arthralgia; enanthem on the lips, soft palate and buccal mucosa
Epstein-Barr virus	Epstein-Barr viruses 1 and 2 (human herpesvirus 4)	"Ampicillin rash" in individuals treated with antibiotics; Gianotti-Crosti syndrome; erythema multiforme, leukocytoclastic vasculitis, erythema nodosum, erythema annulare centrifugum, pityriasis lichenoides, granuloma annulare, cold urticaria	Fever, lymphadenopathy and pharyngitis (Infectious mononucleosis); acute genital ulcers (Lipschütz ulcers) with associated inguinal lymphadenopathy; neoplastic conditions (see Table 163-6)
Gianotti-Crosti syndrome (popular acrodermatitis of childhood; infantile popular acrodermatitis)	Various viral and bacterial pathogens	Symmetrical monomorphic papules or papulovesicles on the face, extensors, and buttocks	Malaise, pharyngitis, low-grade fever, and lymphadenopathy
Human cytomegalovirus[a]	Cytomegalovirus (human herpesvirus-5)	Erythema nodosum, morbilliform eruption similar to ampicillin rash of Epstein-Barr virus infection; urticaria	Infectious mononucleosis–like symptoms
Exanthem subitum (roseola infantum, sixth disease)	Human herpesvirus-6	Rose-colored macules and papules surrounded by a white halo over the neck and trunk	High fever, irritability, rhinorrhea, and diarrhea; palpebral edema; Nagayama spots
Hand-foot-mouth disease	Coxsackievirus A16 and Enterovirus 71	Vesicular eruption of the palms and soles, with "football-shaped" erosions surrounded by an erythematous halo	Low-grade fever, malaise, abdominal pain or upper respiratory tract symptoms, sore throat or sore mouth; oral erosions of the tongue, buccal mucosa, hard palate, and oropharynx
Atypical hand-foot-mouth disease	Coxsackievirus A6	Papulovesicles, vesicles, and erosions of the palms, soles, extremities, and perioral; oral mucosa less frequently involved	Fever, sore throat, headache, cough, and diarrhea
Eruptive pseudoangiomatosis	Echovirus 25, echovirus 32	Small papules resembling angiomas on the face and extremities	Fever, malaise, headache, diarrhea, and respiratory complaints
Unilateral thoracic exanthema (symmetric periflexural exanthema of childhood)	Unknown, likely viral trigger	Pinpoint pink papules with pale halo localized to large flexural region; unilateral and asymmetric distribution; pruritus	Mild upper respiratory tract, low-grade fever or GI symptoms

[a]Congenital infections, infections in neonates, and immunocompromised individuals are discussed in the text.

2005;(4):CD001479.
12. Pal G. Effects of ribavirin on measles. *J Indian Med Assoc.* 2011;109(9):666-667.
13. Committee on Infectious Diseases, American Academy of Pediatrics. Rubella. In: Kimberlin DW, Brady MT, Jackson MA, Long SS, eds. *Red Book: 2015 Report of the Committee on Infectious Diseases*. 30th ed. Elk Grove Village, IL: American Academy of Pediatrics; 2015: 730-737. (Available at: https://redbook.solutions.aap.org/DocumentLibrary/9781581109276.pdf.)
14. Louie JK, Shaikh-Laskos R, Preas C, et al. Re-emergence of another vaccine-preventable disease?-Two cases of rubella in older adults. *J Clin Virol.* 2009;46(1):98-100.
15. Vander Straten MR, Tyring SK. Rubella. *Dermatol Clin.* 2002;20(2):225-231.
16. Control and prevention of rubella: evaluation and management of suspected outbreaks, rubella in pregnant women, and surveillance for congenital rubella syndrome. *MMWR Morb Mortal Wkly Rep.* 2001;50(RR-12):1-23.
17. Nakayama T. Laboratory diagnosis of measles and rubella infection. *Vaccine.* 2009;27(24):3228-3229.
18. Young MK, Cripps AW, Nimmo GR, et al. Post-exposure passive immunisation for preventing rubella and congenital rubella syndrome. *Cochrane Database Syst Rev.* 2015;(9):CD010586.

19. Badilla X, Morice A, Avila-Aguero ML, et al. Fetal risk associated with rubella vaccination during pregnancy. *Pediatr Infect Dis J*. 2007;26(9):830-835.
20. Perelygina L, Plotkin S, Russo P, et al. Rubella persistence in epidermal keratinocytes and granuloma M2 macrophages in patients with primary immunodeficiencies. *J Allergy Clin Immunol*. 2016;138(5):1436-1439.e11.
21. Cohen BJ, Buckley MM. The prevalence of antibody to human parvovirus B19 in England and Wales. *J Med Microbiol*. 1988;25(2):151-153.
22. Anderson MJ, Higgins PG, Davis LR, et al. Experimental parvoviral infection in humans. *J Infect Dis*. 1985;152(2):257-265.
23. McCarter-Spaulding D. Parvovirus B19 in pregnancy. *J Obstet Gynecol Neonatal Nurs*. 31(1):107-112.
24. Cohen B. Parvovirus B19: an expanding spectrum of disease. *BMJ*. 1995;311(7019):1549-1552.
25. Brown KE, Hibbs JR, Gallinella G, et al. Resistance to parvovirus B19 infection due to lack of virus receptor (erythrocyte P antigen). *N Engl J Med*. 1994;330(17):1192-1196.
26. Adamson-Small LA, Ignatovich IV, Laemmerhirt MG, et al. Persistent parvovirus B19 infection in non-erythroid tissues: possible role in the inflammatory and disease process. *Virus Res*. 2014;190:8-16.
27. Feder HM, Anderson I. Fifth disease. A brief review of infections in childhood, in adulthood, and pregnancy. *Arch Intern Med*. 1989;149(10):2176-2178.
28. Plummer FA, Hammond GW, Forward K, et al. An erythema infectiosum—like illness caused by human parvovirus infection. *N Engl J Med*. 1985;313(2):74-79.
29. Edmonson MB, Riedesel EL, Williams GP, et al. Generalized petechial rashes in children during a parvovirus B19 outbreak. *Pediatrics*. 2010;125(4):e787-e792.
30. Lefrère JJ, Couroucé AM, Soulier JP, et al. Henoch-Schönlein purpura and human parvovirus infection. *Pediatrics*. 1986;78(1):183-184.
31. Martín JM, Beteta G, Allende A, et al. Parvovirus B19-associated microvesicular eruption. *Pediatr Dermatol*. 2015;32(6):e303-e304.
32. Woolf AD, Campion G V, Chishick A, et al. Clinical manifestations of human parvovirus B19 in adults. *Arch Intern Med*. 1989;149(5):1153-1156.
33. Faden H, Gary GW, Korman M. Numbness and tingling of fingers associated with parvovirus B19 infection. *J Infect Dis*. 1990;161(2):354-355.
34. Harms M, Feldmann R, Saurat JH. Papular-purpuric "gloves and socks" syndrome. *J Am Acad Dermatol*. 1990;23(5, pt 1):850-854.
35. Petter G, Rytter M, Haustein UF. Juvenile papular-purpuric gloves and socks syndrome. *J Eur Acad Dermatol Venereol*. 2001;15(4):340-342.
36. Molenaar-de Backer MW, de Waal M, Sjerps MC, et al. Validation of new real-time polymerase chain reaction assays for detection of hepatitis A virus RNA and parvovirus B19 DNA. *Transfusion*. 2016;56(2):440-448.
37. Dijkmans AC, de Jong EP, Dijkmans BA, et al. Parvovirus B19 in pregnancy: prenatal diagnosis and management of fetal complications. *Curr Opin Obstet Gynecol*. 2012;24(2):95-101.
38. Kerr JR. A review of blood diseases and cytopenias associated with human parvovirus B19 infection. *Rev Med Virol*. 2015;25(4):224-240.
39. Kurtzman G, Frickhofen N, Kimball J, et al. Pure red-cell aplasia of 10 years' duration due to persistent parvovirus B19 infection and its cure with immunoglobulin therapy. *N Engl J Med*. 1989;321(8):519-523.
40. Prospective study of human parvovirus (B19) infection in pregnancy. Public Health Laboratory Service Working Party on Fifth Disease. *BMJ*. 1990;300(6733):1166-1170.
41. Kerr JR. The role of parvovirus B19 in the pathogenesis of autoimmunity and autoimmune disease. *J Clin Pathol*. 2016;69(4):279-291.
42. Nigro G, Pisano P, Krzysztofiak A. Recurrent Kawasaki disease associated with co-infection with parvovirus B19 and HIV-1. *AIDS*. 1993;7(2):288-290.
43. Corman LC, Dolson DJ. Polyarteritis nodosa and parvovirus B19 infection. *Lancet*. 1992;339(8791):491.
44. Rogo LD, Mokhtari-Azad T, Kabir MH, et al. Human parvovirus B19: a review. *Acta Virol*. 2014;58(3):199-213.
45. Levin LI, Munger KL, Rubertone MV, et al. Temporal relationship between elevation of Epstein-Barr virus antibody titers and initial onset of neurological symptoms in multiple sclerosis. *JAMA*. 2005;293(20):2496.
46. Dowd JB, Palermo T, Brite J, et al. Seroprevalence of Epstein-Barr virus infection in U.S. children ages 6-19, 2003-2010. *PLoS One*. 2013;8(5):e64921.
47. Farrell PJ. Epstein-Barr virus strain variation. *Curr Top Microbiol Immunol*. 2015;390(pt 1):45-69.
48. Fafi-Kremer S, Morand P, Brion J-P, et al. Long-term shedding of infectious Epstein-Barr virus after infectious mononucleosis. *J Infect Dis*. 2005;191(6):985-989.
49. Hall LD, Eminger LA, Hesterman KS, et al. Epstein-Barr virus: dermatologic associations and implications: part I. Mucocutaneous manifestations of Epstein-Barr virus and nonmalignant disorders. *J Am Acad Dermatol*. 2015;72(1):1-19.
50. Sixbey JW, Nedrud JG, Raab-Traub N, et al. Epstein-Barr virus replication in oropharyngeal epithelial cells. *N Engl J Med*. 1984;310(19):1225-1230.
51. Fingeroth JD, Weis JJ, Tedder TF, et al. Epstein-Barr virus receptor of human B lymphocytes is the C3d receptor CR2. *Proc Natl Acad Sci U S A*. 1984;81(14):4510-4514.
52. Callan MF, Steven N, Krausa P, et al. Large clonal expansions of CD8+ T cells in acute infectious mononucleosis. *Nat Med*. 1996;2(8):906-911.
53. Cohen JI, Dropulic L, Hsu AP, et al. Association of GATA2 deficiency with severe primary Epstein-Barr virus (EBV) infection and EBV-associated cancers. *Clin Infect Dis*. 2016;63(1):41-47.
54. Dunmire SK, Grimm JM, Schmeling DO, et al. The incubation period of primary Epstein-Barr virus infection: viral dynamics and immunologic events. *PLoS Pathog*. 2015;11(12):e1005286.
55. Cohen JI. Epstein-Barr virus infection. *N Engl J Med*. 2000;343(7):481-492.
56. Hosey RG, Kriss V, Uhl TL, et al. Ultrasonographic evaluation of splenic enlargement in athletes with acute infectious mononucleosis. *Br J Sports Med*. 2008;42(12):974-977.
57. Farley DR, Zietlow SP, Bannon MP, et al. Spontaneous rupture of the spleen due to infectious mononucleosis. *Mayo Clin Proc*. 1992;67(9):846-853.
58. Avgil M, Diav-Citrin O, Shechtman S, et al. Epstein-Barr virus infection in pregnancy—a prospective controlled study. *Reprod Toxicol*. 2008;25(4):468-471.
59. Chovel-Sella A, Ben Tov A, Lahav E, et al. Incidence of rash after amoxicillin treatment in children with infectious mononucleosis. *Pediatrics*. 2013;131(5):e1424-e1427.
60. Patel BM. Skin rash with infectious mononucleosis and ampicillin. *Pediatrics*. 1967;40(5):910-911.
61. Ikediobi NI, Tyring SK. Cutaneous manifestations

of Epstein-Barr virus infection. *Dermatol Clin.* 2002;20(2):283-289.
62. Weary PE, Cole JW, Hickam LH. Eruptions from ampicillin in patients with infectious mononucleosis. *Arch Dermatol.* 1970;101(1):86-91.
63. Farhi D, Wendling J, Molinari E, et al. Non-sexually related acute genital ulcers in 13 pubertal girls: a clinical and microbiological study. *Arch Dermatol.* 2009;145(1):38-45.
64. Sárdy M, Wollenberg A, Niedermeier A, et al. Genital ulcers associated with Epstein-Barr virus infection (ulcus vulvae acutum). *Acta Derm Venereol.* 2011;91(1):55-59.
65. Cohen JI. Epstein-Barr virus infection. *N Engl J Med.* 2000;343(7):481-492.
66. Ok CY, Li L, Young KH. EBV-driven B-cell lymphoproliferative disorders: from biology, classification and differential diagnosis to clinical management. *Exp Mol Med.* 2015;47:e132.
67. Harabuchi CY, Yamanaka N, Kataura A, et al. Epstein-Barr virus in nasal T-cell lymphomas in patients with lethal midline granuloma. *Lancet.* 1990;20(335):128-130.
68. Choi Y-L, Park J-H, Namkung J-H, et al. Extranodal NK/T-cell lymphoma with cutaneous involvement: "nasal" vs. "nasal-type" subgroups—a retrospective study of 18 patients. *Br J Dermatol.* 2009;160(2):333-337.
69. Au W, Weisenburger DD, Intragumtornchai T, et al. Clinical differences between nasal and extranasal natural killer/T-cell lymphoma: a study of 136 cases from the International Peripheral T-Cell Lymphoma Project. *Blood.* 2009;113(17):3931-3937.
70. Quintanilla-Martinez L, Ridaura C, Nagl F, et al. Hydroa vacciniforme-like lymphoma: a chronic EBV+ lymphoproliferative disorder with risk to develop a systemic lymphoma. *Blood.* 2013;122(18):3101-3110.
71. Xu Z, Lian S. Epstein-Barr virus-associated hydroa vacciniforme-like cutaneous lymphoma in seven Chinese children. *Pediatr Dermatol.* 2010;27(5):463-469.
72. Myers JL, Kurtin PJ, Katzenstein AL, et al. Lymphomatoid granulomatosis. Evidence of immunophenotypic diversity and relationship to Epstein-Barr virus infection. *Am J Surg Pathol.* 1995;19(11):1300-1312.
73. Eminger LA, Hall LD, Hesterman KS, et al. Epstein-Barr virus: dermatologic associations and implications: part II. Associated lymphoproliferative disorders and solid tumors. *J Am Acad Dermatol.* 2015;72(1):21-34.
74. McNiff JM, Cooper D, Howe G, et al. Lymphomatoid granulomatosis of the skin and lung. An angiocentric T-cell-rich B-cell lymphoproliferative disorder. *Arch Dermatol.* 1996;132(12):1464-1470.
75. Roschewski M, Wilson WH. Lymphomatoid granulomatosis. *Cancer J.* 2012;18(5):469-474.
76. Linderholm M, Boman J, Juto P, et al. Comparative evaluation of nine kits for rapid diagnosis of infectious mononucleosis and Epstein-Barr virus-specific serology. *J Clin Microbiol.* 1994;32(1):259-261.
77. Pitetti RD, Laus S, Wadowsky RM. Clinical evaluation of a quantitative real time polymerase chain reaction assay for diagnosis of primary Epstein-Barr virus infection in children. *Pediatr Infect Dis J.* 2003;22(8):736-739.
78. Hess RD. Routine Epstein-Barr virus diagnostics from the laboratory perspective: still challenging after 35 years. *J Clin Microbiol.* 2004;42(8):3381-3387.
79. Holman CJ, Karger AB, Mullan BD, et al. Quantitative Epstein-Barr virus shedding and its correlation with the risk of post-transplant lymphoproliferative disorder. *Clin Transplant.* 2012;26(5):741-747.
80. Rezk E, Nofal YH, Hamzeh A, et al. Steroids for symptom control in infectious mononucleosis. *Cochrane Database Syst Rev.* 2015;(11):CD004402.
81. van der Horst C, Joncas J, Ahronheim G, et al. Lack of effect of peroral acyclovir for the treatment of acute infectious mononucleosis. *J Infect Dis.* 1991;164(4):788-792.
82. Smith C, Khanna R. The development of prophylactic and therapeutic EBV vaccines. *Curr Top Microbiol Immunol.* 2015;391:455-473.
83. Brandt O, Abeck D, Gianotti R, et al. Gianotti-Crosti syndrome. *J Am Acad Dermatol.* 2006;54(1):136-145.
84. Crosti A, Gianotti F. Eruptive dermatosis of probable viral origin situated on the acra [in French]. *Dermatologica.* 1957;115(5):671-677.
85. Smith KJ, Skelton H. Histopathologic features seen in Gianotti-Crosti syndrome secondary to Epstein-Barr virus. *J Am Acad Dermatol.* 2000;43(6):1076-1079.
86. Chuh A, Zawar V, Lee A, et al. Is Gianotti-Crosti syndrome associated with atopy? A case-control study and a postulation on the intrinsic host factors in Gianotti-Crosti syndrome. *Pediatr Dermatol.* 2016;33(5):488-492.
87. Hofmann B, Schuppe HC, Adams O, et al. Gianotti-Crosti syndrome associated with Epstein-Barr virus infection. *Pediatr Dermatol.* 14(4):273-277.
88. Berger EM, Orlow SJ, Patel RR, et al. Experience with molluscum contagiosum and associated inflammatory reactions in a pediatric dermatology practice: the bump that rashes. *Arch Dermatol.* 2012;148(11):1257-1264.
89. De Vries HJ, van Marle J, Teunissen MB, et al. Lichen planus is associated with human herpesvirus type 7 replication and infiltration of plasmacytoid dendritic cells. *Br J Dermatol.* 2006;154(2):361-364.
90. Bialas KM, Swamy GK, Permar SR. Perinatal cytomegalovirus and varicella zoster virus infections: epidemiology, prevention, and treatment. *Clin Perinatol.* 2015;42(1):61-75, viii.
91. Gallant JE, Moore RD, Richman DD, et al. Incidence and natural history of cytomegalovirus disease in patients with advanced human immunodeficiency virus disease treated with zidovudine. The Zidovudine Epidemiology Study Group. *J Infect Dis.* 1992;166(6):1223-1227.
92. Boppana SB, Pass RF, Britt WJ, et al. Symptomatic congenital cytomegalovirus infection: neonatal morbidity and mortality. *Pediatr Infect Dis J.* 1992;11(2):93-99.
93. Brough AJ, Jones D, Page RH, et al. Dermal erythropoiesis in neonatal infants. A manifestation of intrauterine viral disease. *Pediatrics.* 1967;40(4):627-635.
94. Fowler KB, Boppana SB. Congenital cytomegalovirus (CMV) infection and hearing deficit. *J Clin Virol.* 2006;35(2):226-231.
95. Heilbron B, Saxe N. Scleredema in an infant. *Arch Dermatol.* 1986;122(12):1417-1419.
96. Ballard RA, Drew WL, Hufnagle KG, et al. Acquired cytomegalovirus infection in preterm infants. *Am J Dis Child.* 1979;133(5):482-485.
97. Hancox JG, Shetty AK, Sangueza OP, et al. Perineal ulcers in an infant: an unusual presentation of postnatal cytomegalovirus infection. *J Am Acad Dermatol.* 2006;54(3):536-539.
98. Horwitz CA, Henle W, Henle G, et al. Clinical and laboratory evaluation of cytomegalovirus-induced mononucleosis in previously healthy individuals.

99. Chen Y-C, Chiang H-H, Cho Y-T, et al. Human herpes virus reactivations and dynamic cytokine profiles in patients with cutaneous adverse drug reactions-a prospective comparative study. *Allergy.* 2015;70(5):568-575.
100. Klemola E. Hypersensitivity reactions to ampicillin in cytomegalovirus mononucleosis. *Scand J Infect Dis.* 1970;2(1):29-31.
101. Spear JB, Kessler HA, Dworin A, et al. Erythema nodosum associated with acute cytomegalovirus mononucleosis in an adult. *Arch Intern Med.* 1988;148(2):323-324.
102. Asano Y, Yoshikawa T, Suga S, et al. Clinical features of infants with primary human herpesvirus 6 infection (exanthem subitum, roseola infantum). *Pediatrics.* 1994;93(1):104-108.
103. Kotton CN, Kumar D, Caliendo AM, et al. Updated international consensus guidelines on the management of cytomegalovirus in solid-organ transplantation. *Transplantation.* 2013;96(4):333-360.
104. Strauss RG. Optimal prevention of transfusion-transmitted cytomegalovirus (TTCMV) infection by modern leukocyte reduction alone: CMV sero/antibody-negative donors needed only for leukocyte products. *Transfusion.* 2016;56(8):1921-1924.
105. Cohen L, Yeshurun M, Shpilberg O, et al. Risk factors and prognostic scale for cytomegalovirus (CMV) infection in CMV-seropositive patients after allogeneic hematopoietic cell transplantation. *Transpl Infect Dis.* 2015;17(4):510-517.
106. Wood AJJ, Jacobson MA. Treatment of cytomegalovirus retinitis in patients with the acquired immunodeficiency syndrome. *N Engl J Med.* 1997;337(2):105-114.
107. Karavellas MP, Plummer DJ, Macdonald JC, et al. Incidence of immune recovery vitreitis in cytomegalovirus retinitis patients following institution of successful highly active antiretroviral therapy. *J Infect Dis.* 1999;179(3):697-700.
108. Poizot-Martin I, Allavena C, Duvivier C, et al. CMV+ serostatus associates negatively with CD4:CD8 ratio normalization in controlled HIV-infected patients on cART. *PLoS One.* 2016;11(11):e0165774.
109. Choi Y-L, Kim J-A, Jang K-T, et al. Characteristics of cutaneous cytomegalovirus infection in non-acquired immune deficiency syndrome, immunocompromised patients. *Br J Dermatol.* 2006;155(5):977-982.
110. Bhawan J, Gellis S, Ucci A, et al. Vesiculobullous lesions caused by cytomegalovirus infection in an immunocompromised adult. *J Am Acad Dermatol.* 1984;11(4, pt 2):743-747.
111. Feldman PS, Walker AN, Baker R. Cutaneous lesions heralding disseminated cytomegalovirus infection. *J Am Acad Dermatol.* 1982;7(4):545-548.
112. Lesher JL. Cytomegalovirus infections and the skin. *J Am Acad Dermatol.* 1988;18(6):1333-1338.
113. Shah T, Luck S, Sharland M, et al. Fifteen-minute consultation: diagnosis and management of congenital CMV. *Arch Dis Child Educ Pract Ed.* 2016;101(5):232-235.
114. Genser B, Truschnig-Wilders M, Stünzner D, et al. Evaluation of five commercial enzyme immunoassays for the detection of human cytomegalovirus-specific IgM antibodies in the absence of a commercially available gold standard. *Clin Chem Lab Med.* 2001;39(1):62-70.
115. Walker JD, Chesney TM. Cytomegalovirus infection of the skin. *Am J Dermatopathol.* 1982;4(3):263-265.
116. James SH, Kimberlin DW. Advances in the prevention and treatment of congenital cytomegalovirus infection. *Curr Opin Pediatr.* 2016;28(1):81-85.
117. Zerr DM, Meier AS, Selke SS, et al. A population-based study of primary human herpesvirus 6 infection. *N Engl J Med.* 2005;352(8):768-776.
118. Krueger GR, Wassermann K, De Clerck LS, et al. Latent herpesvirus-6 in salivary and bronchial glands. *Lancet.* 1990;336(8725):1255-1256.
119. Santoro F, Kennedy PE, Locatelli G, et al. CD46 is a cellular receptor for human herpesvirus 6. *Cell.* 1999;99(7):817-827.
120. Frenkel N, Katsafanas GC, Wyatt LS, et al. Bone marrow transplant recipients harbor the B variant of human herpesvirus 6. *Bone Marrow Transplant.* 1994;14(5):839-843.
121. Le J, Gantt S. AST Infectious Diseases Community of Practice. Human herpesvirus 6, 7 and 8 in solid organ transplantation. *Am J Transplant.* 2013;13(suppl 4):128-137.
122. De Bolle L, Naesens L, De Clercq E. Update on human herpesvirus 6 biology, clinical features, and therapy. *Clin Microbiol Rev.* 2005;18(1):217-245.
123. Pruksananonda P, Hall CB, Insel RA, et al. Primary human herpesvirus 6 infection in young children. *N Engl J Med.* 1992;326(22):1445-1450.
124. Dulery R, Salleron J, Dewilde A, et al. Early human herpesvirus type 6 reactivation after allogeneic stem cell transplantation: a large-scale clinical study. *Biol Blood Marrow Transplant.* 2012;18(7):1080-1089.
125. Zahorsky J. Roseola infantum. *Arch Pediatr.* 1954;71(4):124-128.
126. Levine PH, Jahan N, Murari P, et al. Detection of human herpesvirus 6 in tissues involved by sinus histiocytosis with massive lymphadenopathy (Rosai-Dorfman disease). *J Infect Dis.* 1992;166(2):291-295.
127. Luppi M, Barozzi P, Garber R, et al. Expression of human herpesvirus-6 antigens in benign and malignant lymphoproliferative diseases. *Am J Pathol.* 1998;153(3):815-823.
128. Suga S, Yoshikawa T, Asano Y, et al. IgM neutralizing antibody responses to human herpesvirus-6 in patients with exanthem subitum or organ transplantation. *Microbiol Immunol.* 1992;36(5):495-506.
129. Zerr DM, Corey L, Kim HW, et al. Clinical outcomes of human herpesvirus 6 reactivation after hematopoietic stem cell transplantation. *Clin Infect Dis.* 2005;40(7):932-940.
130. Yoshida M, Yamada M, Tsukazaki T, et al. Comparison of antiviral compounds against human herpesvirus 6 and 7. *Antiviral Res.* 1998;40(1-2):73-84.
131. Prichard MN, Whitley RJ. The development of new therapies for human herpesvirus 6. *Curr Opin Virol.* 2014;9:148-153.
132. Rapaport D, Engelhard D, Tagger G, et al. Antiviral prophylaxis may prevent human herpesvirus-6 reactivation in bone marrow transplant recipients. *Transpl Infect Dis.* 2002;4(1):10-16.
133. Hidaka Y, Okada K, Kusuhara K, et al. Exanthem subitum and human herpesvirus 7 infection. *Pediatr Infect Dis J.* 1994;13(11):1010-1011.
134. Emery VC, Clark DA. HHV-6A, 6B, and 7: persistence in the population, epidemiology and transmission. In: Arvin A, Campadelli-Fiume G, Mocarski E, et al, eds. *Human Herpesviruses: Biology, Therapy, and Immunoprophylaxis.* Cambridge, UK: Cambridge

135. Smith C, Khanna R. Immune regulation of human herpesviruses and its implications for human transplantation. *Am J Transplant.* 2013;13(s3):9-23.
136. Hall CB, Caserta MT, Schnabel KC, et al. Characteristics and acquisition of human herpesvirus (HHV) 7 infections in relation to infection with HHV-6. *J Infect Dis.* 2006;193(8):1063-1069.
137. Drago F, Ranieri E, Malaguti F, et al. Human herpesvirus 7 in pityriasis rosea. *Lancet.* 1997;349(9062):1367-1368.
138. Torigoe S, Koide W, Yamada M, et al. Human herpesvirus 7 infection associated with central nervous system manifestations. *J Pediatr.* 1996;129(2):301-305.
139. Sawyer MH. Enterovirus infections: diagnosis and treatment. *Semin Pediatr Infect Dis.* 2002;13(1):40-47.
140. Nassef C, Ziemer C, Morrell DS. Hand-foot-and-mouth disease: a new look at a classic viral rash. *Curr Opin Pediatr.* 2015;27(4):486-491.
141. Chang L-Y, Tsao K-C, Hsia S-H, et al. Transmission and clinical features of enterovirus 71 infections in household contacts in Taiwan. *JAMA.* 2004;291(2):222-227.
142. Ramers C, Billman G, Hartin M, et al. Impact of a diagnostic cerebrospinal fluid enterovirus polymerase chain reaction test on patient management. *JAMA.* 2000;283(20):2680-2685.
143. Kimura A, Abe M, Nakao T. Light and electron microscopic study of skin lesions of patients with the hand, foot and mouth disease. *Tohoku J Exp Med.* 1977;122(3):237-247.
144. Chang P-C, Chen S-C, Chen K-T. The current status of the disease caused by enterovirus 71 infections: epidemiology, pathogenesis, molecular epidemiology, and vaccine development. *Int J Environ Res Public Health.* 2016;13(9).
145. Bek EJ, McMinn PC. The pathogenesis and prevention of encephalitis due to human enterovirus 71. *Curr Infect Dis Rep.* 2012;14(4):397-407.
146. Puenpa J, Vongpunsawad S, Osterback R, et al. Molecular epidemiology and the evolution of human coxsackievirus A6. *J Gen Virol.* 2016;97(12):3225-3231.
147. Mathes EF, Oza V, Frieden IJ, et al. "Eczema coxsackium" and unusual cutaneous findings in an enterovirus outbreak. *Pediatrics.* 2013;132(1):e149-e157.
148. Downing C, Ramirez-Fort MK, Doan HQ, et al. Coxsackievirus A6 associated hand, foot and mouth disease in adults: clinical presentation and review of the literature. *J Clin Virol.* 2014;60(4):381-386.
149. Neri I, Dondi A, Wollenberg A, et al. Atypical forms of hand, foot, and mouth disease: a prospective study of 47 Italian children. *Pediatr Dermatol.* 2016;33(4):429-437.
150. Zeng H, Lu J, Zheng H, et al. The epidemiological study of coxsackievirus a6 revealing hand, foot and mouth disease epidemic patterns in Guangdong, China. *Sci Rep.* 2015;5:10550.
151. Laga AC, Shroba SM, Hanna J. Atypical hand, foot and mouth disease in adults associated with coxsackievirus A6: a clinico-pathologic study. *J Cutan Pathol.* 2016;43(11):940-945.
152. Miyamoto A, Hirata R, Ishimoto K, et al. An outbreak of hand-foot-and-mouth disease mimicking chicken pox, with a frequent association of onychomadesis in Japan in 2009: a new phenotype caused by coxsackievirus A6. *Eur J Dermatol.* 2014;24(1):103-104.
153. Cherry JD, Bobinski JE, Horvath FL, et al. Acute hemangioma-like lesions associated with ECHO viral infections. *Pediatrics.* 1969;44(4):498-502.
154. Prose NS, Tope W, Miller SE, et al. Eruptive pseudoangiomatosis: a unique childhood exanthem? *J Am Acad Dermatol.* 1993;29(5, pt 2):857-859.
155. Chuh A, Panzer R, Rosenthal A-C, et al. Annular eruptive pseudoangiomatosis and adenovirus infection: a novel clinical variant of paraviral exanthems and a novel virus association. *Acta Derm Venereol.* 2017;97(3):354-357.
156. Henry M, Savaşan S. Eruptive pseudoangiomatosis in a child undergoing chemotherapy for Hodgkin lymphoma. *Pediatr Blood Cancer.* 2012;59(2):342-343.
157. Oka K, Ohtaki N, Kasai S, et al. Two cases of eruptive pseudoangiomatosis induced by mosquito bites. *J Dermatol.* 2012;39(3):301-305.
158. Pitarch G, Torrijos A, García-Escrivá D, et al. Eruptive pseudoangiomatosis associated to cytomegalovirus infection. *Eur J Dermatol.* 17(5):455-456.
159. McCuaig CC, Russo P, Powell J, et al. Unilateral laterothoracic exanthem. A clinicopathologic study of forty-eight patients. *J Am Acad Dermatol.* 1996;34(6):979-984.
160. Gutzmer R, Herbst RA, Kiehl P, et al. Unilateral laterothoracic exanthem (asymmetrical periflexural exanthem of childhood): report of an adult patient. *J Am Acad Dermatol.* 1997;37(3, pt 1):484-485.

Chapter 164 :: Herpes Simplex
Jeffrey I. Cohen

第一百六十四章
单纯疱疹

中文导读

单纯疱疹病毒感染在世界范围内非常常见，由2种密切相关的HSV类型引起。它们的主要临床表现均为黏膜皮肤感染，但也略有不同。其中1型HSV（HSV-1）多与口腔及颌面部的感染有关，感染常表现为累及硬腭、软腭、颊黏膜、舌部及邻近面部区域的溃疡性皮损，是大多数复发性唇疱疹的原因，儿童时期感染率最高，约为人群的30%~60%。临床2型HSV（HSV-2）的获得则与性行为以及潜在的性伴侣中的感染相关，好发在生殖器部位，感染常表现为水疱、脓疱、红斑及溃疡。单纯疱疹的鉴别诊断十分关键，已将鉴别要点列于表164-1和表164-2。本章分别介绍了单纯疱疹的流行病学、临床特征、危险因素、病因和发病机制、诊断、鉴别诊断、临床病程和预后及临床管理。

〔张江林〕

AT-A-GLANCE

- Herpes simplex viruses (HSVs) are common human DNA viral pathogens that intermittently reactivate. After replication in the skin or mucosa, the virus infects the local nerve endings and ascends to the ganglia where it becomes latent until reactivation.

- There are two types of HSV: HSV-1 and HSV-2. HSV-1 is mostly associated with orofacial disease, whereas HSV-2 usually causes genital infection, but both can infect oral and genital areas and cause acute and recurrent infections.

- Most of the adult population is seropositive for HSV-1, and the majority of infections are acquired in childhood. About one-fourth of adults are infected with HSV-2 in the United States. Acquisition of HSV-2 correlates with sexual behavior.

- Most primary HSV infections are asymptomatic or not recognized, but they can also cause severe disease. Most recurrences are not symptomatic and most transmissions occur during asymptomatic shedding.

- Genital herpes is the most prevalent sexually transmitted disease worldwide and is the most common cause of ulcerative genital disease; it is an important risk factor for acquisition and transmission of HIV.

- HSV can cause diseases involving the eye, CNS, and neonatal infection. Cellular immunity defects are a risk factor for severe and disseminated disease.

- Diagnosis is made by polymerase chain reaction, viral culture, or serology, depending on the clinical presentation.

- Treatment is with acyclovir, valacyclovir, or famciclovir. Regimens and dosages vary with the clinical setting. Resistance is rare, other than in immunocompromised patients.

Herpes simplex virus (HSV) infections are common worldwide and are caused by 2 closely related types of HSV. Their main clinical manifestations are mucocutaneous infections, with HSV Type 1 (HSV-1) being mostly associated with orofacial disease, and HSV Type 2 (HSV-2) usually being associated with genital infection. HSV-1 is increasingly becoming a more common cause of genital mucosal infections in young women in the United States than HSV-2.[1]

EPIDEMIOLOGY

The incidence of primary infection with HSV-1, which is responsible for the vast majority of recurring labial herpes, is greatest during childhood, when 30% to 60% of children are exposed to the virus. Rates of infection with HSV-1 increase with age and reduced socioeconomic status. From 20% to 40% of the population has had episodes of herpes labialis. The frequency of recurrent episodes is extremely variable, and, in some studies, averages approximately once per year. From 2005 to 2010 the seroprevalence of HSV-1 in the United States was 30% in persons 14 to 19 years of age, 50% in persons 20 to 29 years of age, and 62% in persons 30 to 39 years of age.[2] The rate of HSV-1 declined by 7% from 1999-2004 to 2005-2010.

Acquisition of HSV-2 correlates with sexual behavior and the prevalence of infection in one's potential sexual partners. Antibodies to HSV-2 are rare in people before the onset of intimate sexual activity and rise steadily thereafter. From 2005 to 2010 the seroprevalence of HSV-2 in the United States was 1.2% in persons 14 to 19 years of age, 9.9% in persons 20 to 29 years of age, and 19% in persons 30 to 39 years of age.[2] The rate of HSV-2 seropositivity did not change significantly from 1999-2004 to 2005-2010. Although most persons infected with HSV-1 or HSV-2 are asymptomatic, they still can transmit the virus.[3] Even though HSV-2–asymptomatic persons shed virus less frequently than symptomatic persons, the amount of HSV-2 shed during asymptomatic shedding is similar in symptomatic and asymptomatic groups.[4] In one study, 21% of genital swabs were positive for HSV by polymerase chain reaction (PCR) in persons who were HSV-2 seropositive, and 12% of oral swabs were positive for HSV by PCR in persons who were HSV-1 seropositive.[5] It is estimated that more than 70% of HSV-2 transmission is associated with asymptomatic shedding. The rate of transmission is no higher in persons with frequent symptomatic recurrences than it is in persons with infrequent recurrences. The average risk of transmission for couples discordant for genital herpes (ie, one partner has genital herpes and the other does not) varies from 5% to 10% per year.[6] As with other sexually-transmitted infections, the rate of acquisition of HSV-2 infection is higher for women than for men. Asymptomatic HSV-2 infection is more common among men and persons who are also seropositive for HSV-1, suggesting that prior infection with HSV-1 reduces one's likelihood of experiencing symptomatic HSV-2 infection.[7] Studies show that genital HSV infections significantly increase the risk for acquisition and transmission of HIV. Randomized trials with acyclovir reduced the frequency of genital ulcers and slightly reduced HIV viral loads, but did not reduce transmission of HIV.[8]

CLINICAL FINDINGS

CUTANEOUS FINDINGS

The clinical manifestations of HSV infection depend on the site of infection and the immune status of the host. Primary infections with HSV, namely those that develop in persons without preexisting immunity to either HSV-1 or HSV-2, are usually more severe, frequently involve systemic signs and symptoms, and have a higher rate of complications, compared to episodes associated with reactivation of HSV.

OROFACIAL INFECTIONS

Herpetic gingivostomatitis (Fig. 164-1) and pharyngitis are most commonly associated with a primary HSV-1 infection. The symptoms of primary oral herpes may resemble those of aphthous stomatitis and include ulcerative lesions involving the hard and soft palate, tongue, and buccal mucosa, as well as neighboring facial areas. Patients with pharyngitis exhibit ulcerative and exudative lesions of the posterior pharynx that can be difficult to differentiate from streptococcal pharyngitis. Other common symptoms include fever, malaise, myalgias, pain on swallowing, irritability, and cervical adenopathy.

Reactivation of virus from these primary infections involves the perioral facial area, mainly the lips, with the outer one-third of the lower lip being the most commonly affected area (Fig. 164-2). Other facial locations include the nose, chin, and cheek, and account for fewer than 10% of cases (Fig. 164-3). Two-thirds

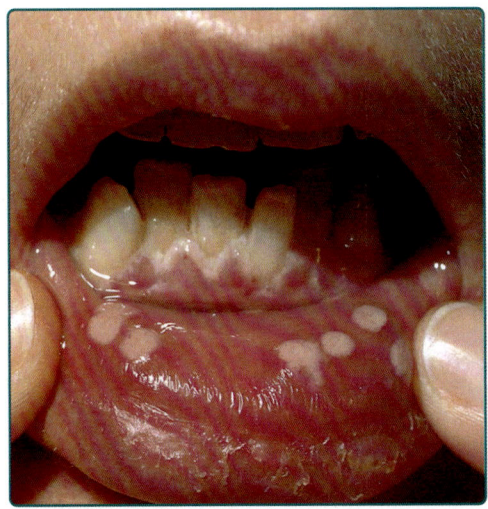

Figure 164-1 Primary herpetic gingivostomatitis. (Used with permission from Clyde S. Crumpacker, MD.)

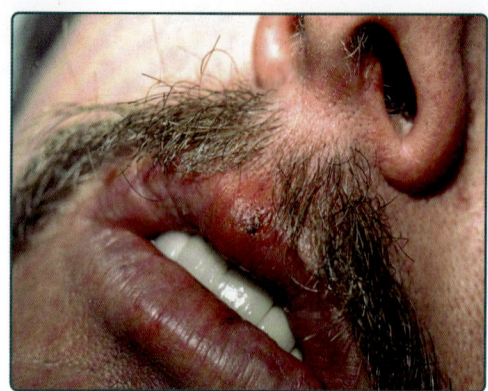

Figure 164-2 Herpes simplex virus infection. Erythema and early vesicles caused by recurrent herpes labialis of the upper lip. (Used with permission of the William Weston Collection.)

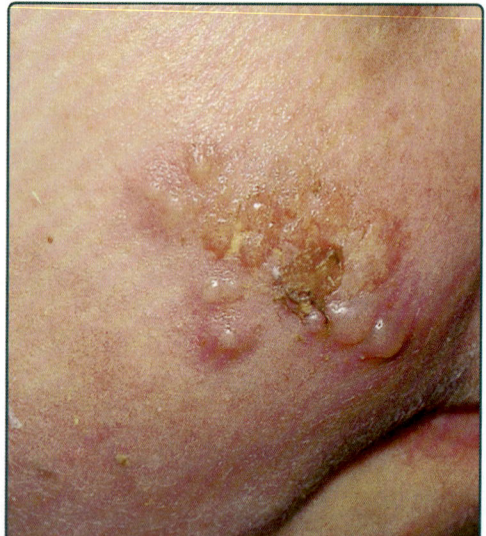

Figure 164-3 Recurrent facial herpes simplex with grouped vesicles and crusting. (Used with permission from Clyde S. Crumpacker, MD.)

The progression of classical herpes lesions has been divided according to the following stages based on their features: prodromal, erythema, and papule (the developmental stage); vesicle, ulcer, and hard crust (disease stage); followed by dry flaking and residual swelling (resolution stage). The lesions usually resolve within 5 to 15 days.

Triggers for oral herpes recurrences include emotional stress, illness, exposure to sun, trauma, fatigue, menses, chapped lips, and the season of the year. Other well-documented triggers include exposure to ultraviolet irradiation, trigeminal nerve surgery, oral trauma, epidural administration of morphine, and abrasive, laser, and chemical facial cosmetic procedures. The exact mechanism by which these diverse factors trigger HSV reactivation is unknown.

HSV-2 causes a primary orofacial infection that is indistinguishable from that associated with HSV-1, except that it is usually in adolescents and young adults, following genital–oral contact. HSV-2 orolabial infections are 120 times less likely to reactivate than orolabial HSV-1 disease.

GENITAL INFECTIONS

Genital herpes is the major clinical presentation of HSV-2 infection, but HSV-1 is becoming a more common cause of genital herpes in young women.[9,10] Because of their epidemiology, acquisition of HSV-1 in a person with prior HSV-2 infection is unusual, but HSV-2 acquisition in the presence of previous HSV-1 infection is common, and infection of the genital tract with both HSV-1 and HSV-2 has been described. Patients with previously known HSV-1 genital infection who develop frequent genital herpes recurrences should be tested for HSV-2 infection. Viremia occurs in approximately 25% of persons during primary genital herpes.

The clinical course of acute first-episode genital herpes among patients with HSV-1 and HSV-2 infections is similar. These infections are associated with extensive genital lesions in different stages of evolution, including vesicles, pustules, and erythematous ulcers that may require 2 to 3 weeks to resolve (Fig. 164-4). In males, lesions commonly occur on the glans penis or the penile shaft; in females, lesions may involve the vulva, perineum, buttocks, vagina, or cervix. There is accompanying pain, itching, dysuria, vaginal and urethral discharge, and tender inguinal lymphadenopathy. Systemic signs and symptoms are common and include fever, headache, malaise, and myalgias. Herpetic sacral radiculomyelitis with urinary retention, neuralgias, and constipation, can occur. HSV cervicitis occurs in more than 80% of women with primary infection. It can present as purulent or bloody vaginal discharge; examination reveals areas of diffuse or focal friability and redness, extensive ulcerative lesions of the exocervix, or, rarely, necrotic cervicitis. Cervical discharge is usually mucoid, but it is occasionally mucopurulent.

The rates of recurrence for genital HSV-2 infections vary greatly among individuals and over time within the same individual. Infections caused by HSV-2 reactivate approximately 16 times more frequently than

of labial lesions involve the vermilion border, and the rest occur at the junction of the border with the skin. In patients with frequent recurrences, lesions may differ slightly in location with each episode. Immunocompetent patients tend not to experience recurrent intraoral lesions, but can present with clusters of tiny vesicles and ulcers, or linear fissures on the gingivae and anterior hard palate that are mildly symptomatic. Prodromal symptoms precede herpes labialis in 45% to 60% of episodes. Patients experience pain, burning, or itching at the site of the subsequent eruption. Even in the immunocompetent patient, the severity of recurrent herpes labialis is extremely variable and may vary from that of prodromal symptoms alone without the subsequent development of lesions (aborted episodes) to extensive disease induced by severe local sunburn.

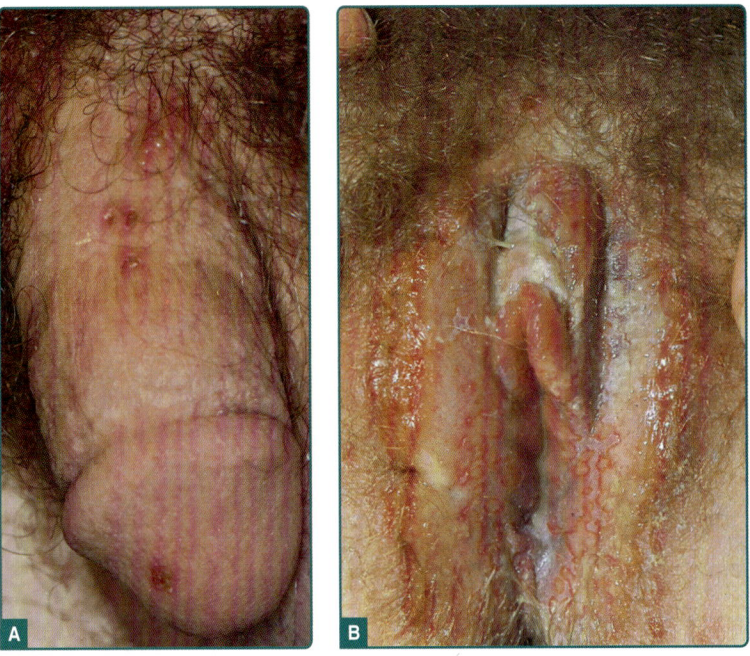

Figure 164-4 **A,** Primary genital herpes with vesicles. (Used with permission from Clyde S. Crumpacker, MD.) **B,** Primary herpetic vulvitis.

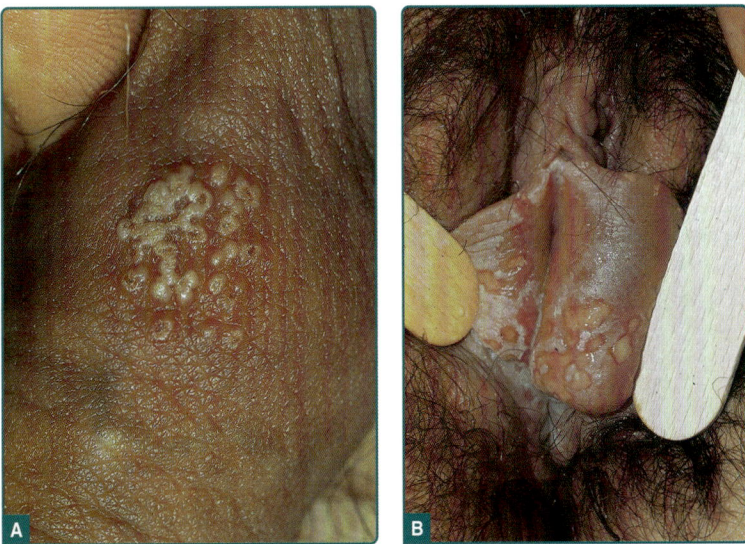

Figure 164-5 **A,** Genital herpes. Recurrent infection of the penis. Group of vesicles with early central crusting on a red base arising on the shaft of the penis. This "textbook" presentation, however, is much less common than small asymptomatic erosions or fissures. **B,** Genital herpes. Recurrent vulvar infection. Large, painful erosions on the labia. Extensive lesions such as these are uncommon in recurrent genital herpes in an otherwise healthy individual.

HSV-1 genital infections, and average 3 to 4 times per year, but may appear virtually weekly. Recurrences tend to be more frequent in the first months to years after initial infection. The classical clinical manifestations of recurrent HSV-2 infection include multiple small, grouped, vesicular lesions in the genital area (Fig. 164-5), but which can occur anywhere in the perigenital region, including the groin, buttocks, and thighs; the lesions may recur at the same site or change location. The recurrence of genital lesions may be heralded by a prodrome of tenderness, itching, burning, or tingling, and the outbreaks are less severe than primary infection. Without treatment, the lesions usually heal in 6 to 10 days. Herpetic cervicitis is less common in recurrent disease, occurring in 12% of patients. It may present without external lesions.

Signs and symptoms that are less classical for genital HSV infection and that can divert one from the correct diagnosis include small erythematous lesions, fissures, pruritus, and urinary symptoms. HSV can cause urethritis, usually manifested only as a clear mucoid discharge, dysuria, and frequency. Occasionally, HSV can be associated with endometritis, salpingitis, or prostatitis. Symptomatic or asymptomatic rectal and perianal infections are common. Herpetic proctitis presents with anorectal pain, anorectal discharge, tenesmus, and constipation, with ulcerative lesions of the distal rectal mucosa. Genital herpes can recur at nongenital sites as well.

OTHER CUTANEOUS FINDINGS

HSV can infect any skin site (Fig. 164-6). The common theme among virtually all of these cutaneous presentations is the requirement that virus have penetrated otherwise normal and well-keratinized tissues. Herpetic whitlow (Fig. 164-7) is infection of the fingers by HSV acquired by direct inoculation or by direct spread from mucosal sites at the time of primary infection. Whitlow occurs in children who suck their fingers during a primary gingivostomatitis outbreak. It is also a well documented occupational hazard for medical personnel. It is usually caused by HSV-1, but HSV-2 whitlow may develop as a manifestation of primary inoculation following manual–genital contact with an infected partner. The infected region becomes erythematous and edematous. Lesions are usually present at the fingertip and can be pustular and very painful. Fever and local lymphadenopathy are common. Whitlow is often misdiagnosed as a bacterial paronychial infection, but surgical drainage, often needed for a bacterial infection, is unnecessary and potentially harmful, while antiviral therapy speeds healing. Whitlow may recur.

Cutaneous herpes can be transmitted between athletes involved in contact sports, such as wrestling (herpes gladiatorum) and rugby (herpes rugbiorum or scrum pox), and may occur as outbreaks or small epidemics among team members. In these instances, multiple herpetic lesions may appear across the thorax, ears, face, arms, and hands, in which infection is facilitated by trauma to the normally-keratinized skin during sport activities (Fig. 164-8). Concomitant ocular herpes can occur.

Eczema herpeticum (Kaposi varicelliform eruption; Fig. 164-9) results from widespread infection following inoculation of virus to skin damaged by eczema. It is usually a manifestation of primary HSV-1 infection in a child with atopic dermatitis; the expression of antimicrobial peptides in the skin may be a factor in controlling susceptibility to eczema herpeticum in these patients. Cathelicidin and beta-defensins are antimicrobial peptides that inhibit HSV replication. Skin lesions from patients with eczema herpeticum have lower levels of cathelicidin and beta-defensins than do skin lesions from persons with atopic dermatitis or psoriasis.[11] Mycosis fungoides, Sézary syndrome, Darier disease, various bullous diseases of the skin (particularly if patients are receiving immunosuppressive therapy), and second-degree and third-degree burns also can be complicated by cutaneous dissemination of HSV. The severity of eczema herpeticum ranges from mild to fatal, with mortality rates of up to 10% being reported before antiviral therapy was available. Mortality was primarily caused by bacterial superinfection and bacteremia. Common pathogens include *Staphylococcus aureus*, beta-hemolytiic *Streptococcus*, and *Pseudomomas aerugionosa*. In a typical severe primary attack, vesicles develop in large numbers over areas of active or recently healed atopic dermatitis, particularly the face, several days after exposure and continue to appear in crops for several more days. The vesicles become pustular and markedly umbilicated

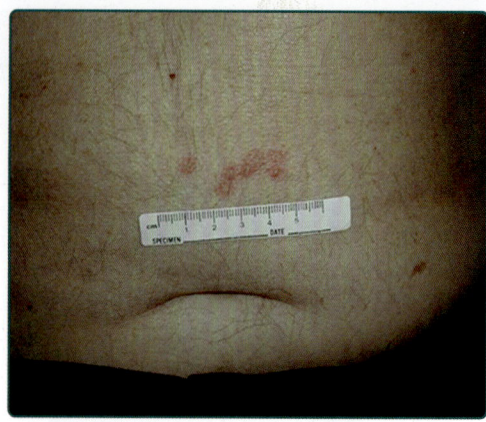

Figure 164-6 Recurrent genital herpes on the abdomen (zosteriform herpes simplex).

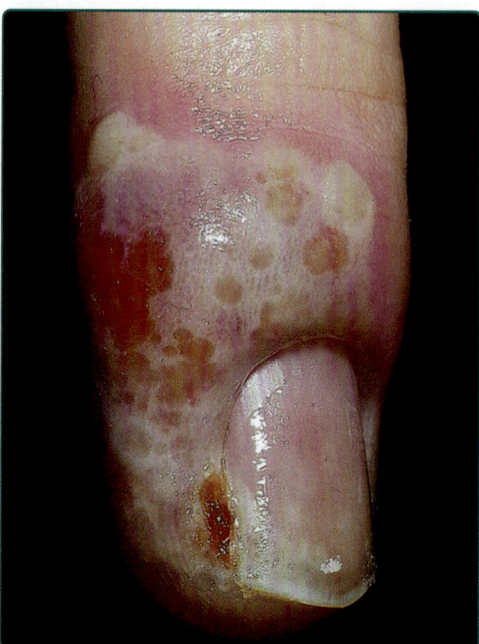

Figure 164-7 Herpes simplex virus infection. Herpetic whitlow. Painful, grouped, confluent vesicles on an erythematous, edematous base at the distal finger where the first (and presumed primary) symptomatic infection occurred.

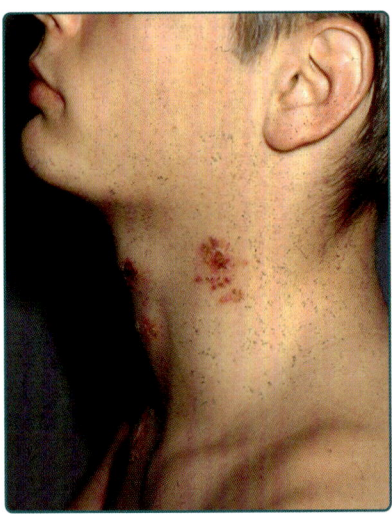

Figure 164-8 Herpes simplex gladiatorum with lesions on the neck.

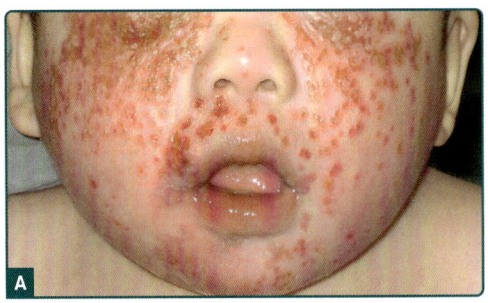

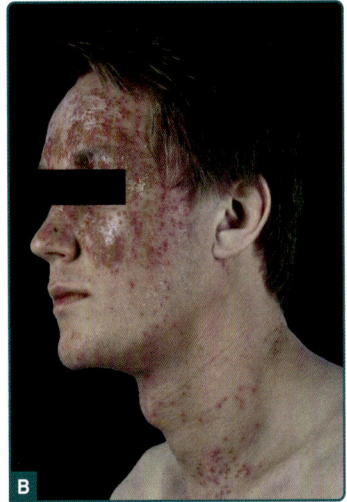

Figure 164-9 Two examples of eczema herpeticum. Confluent and discrete crusted erosions associated with erythema and edema of the face of a child (**A**) and man (**B**) with atopic dermatitis. Note the monomorphic vesicles and punched out erosions. (Image **A**, Used with permission from Anna L. Bruckner, MD.)

and quickly progress to monomorphic erosions. Patients commonly have high fever and adenopathy. Viremia with infection of internal organs can be fatal. Recurrences are usually far milder than the first infection. Arriving at the correct diagnosis can be delayed because of secondary impetigo involving the lesions, but it should be considered in children with infected eczema, particularly if the child is more systemically ill than one might anticipate with impetigo. Eczema herpeticum of the young infant is a medical emergency, and early treatment with acyclovir can prove lifesaving.

Recurrent HSV infection is the most common precipitating event in cases of recurrent erythema multiforme (see Chap. 43). HSV-associated erythema multiforme is usually an acute, self-limited, recurrent disease, that lasts approximately 3 weeks. The lesions are usually symmetric, occurring on acral extremities and the face, and there is grouping of lesions over the elbow and knees as well as nailfold involvement. Mucosal involvement is usually mild and restricted to the mouth. Constitutional symptoms are rare, and the skin lesions heal without scarring.

NEONATAL HERPES

The neonate is a special category of immunodeficient host. The prevalence of neonatal herpes varies from 1 case per 12500 to 1700 live births.[12] Primary maternal genital herpes is associated with a risk of neonatal infection of 25% to 50% for vaginally-delivered babies, and accounts for 50% to 80% of cases of neonatal HSV infection. In contrast, recurrent maternal infection is associated with a risk of transmission of less than 3%, and transplacental antibodies likely play a role in decreasing the risk of infection.[13] Other risk factors for development of neonatal herpes include vaginal delivery, presence of cervical HSV infection, use of invasive monitors, isolation of HSV from the genital tract, and prolonged rupture of membranes.

Neonatal herpes infections manifest in 1 of 3 forms: skin, eye, and mouth involvement; encephalitis; or disseminated disease (Fig. 164-10). The encephalitic and disseminated disease forms account for more than 50% of cases of neonatal herpes. It is important to remember that more than 20% of neonates with neurologic and disseminated disease do not develop cutaneous vesicles. Without therapy, the overall mortality of neonatal herpes is 65%, and fewer than 10% of untreated neonates with CNS infection will develop normally. With current therapeutic modalities, most babies with skin, eye, and mouth disease survive and have normal development at age 1 year. For treated babies with encephalitis, mortality is 64%, with approximately 30% developing normally within 2 years after infection. Suppressive oral acyclovir for 6 months in neonates who survive CNS disease results in improved neurologic outcomes.[14] For treated babies with disseminated disease, mortality is 30%, with approximately 80% of the survivors apparently developing normally within 2 years after infection.[12]

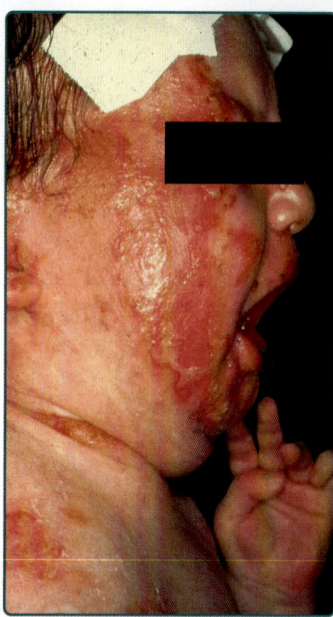

Figure 164-10 Neonatal herpes simplex virus Type-2.

NONCUTANEOUS FINDINGS

OCULAR INFECTIONS

HSV is a leading cause of recurrent keratoconjunctivitis and its associated corneal opacification and visual loss. It is usually caused by HSV-1, except in neonates in whom HSV-2 is more prevalent. The majority of HSV eye disease is caused by reactivation of the virus in the trigeminal ganglia, but primary infections of the eye can also occur. Usually, the initial manifestation of herpetic eye disease is a superficial infection of the eyelids and conjunctiva (blepharoconjunctivitis), or corneal surface (dendritic or geographic epithelial ulcer with pain and blurred vision). Deeper involvement of the cornea (stromal keratitis) or anterior uvea (iritis) represents more serious forms of the disease and can cause permanent visual loss. Acute retinal necrosis is a rare but rapidly progressive disease characterized by retinal arteriolar sheathing, uveitis, and peripheral retinal opacification with variable pain and visual loss. Retinal detachment is common and it is usually associated with HSV-1 infection.

NEUROLOGIC DISORDERS

All HSV infections involve the nervous system, as neurons are the sole proven site of virus latency. HSV meningitis is manifested by headache, fever, stiff neck, and mild photophobia with lymphocytic pleocytosis in the cerebrospinal fluid. Most cases result from HSV-2 infection, which resolve spontaneously in 2 to 7 days. HSV infection may involve the sacral nerves with autonomic nervous system dysfunction, numbness, pelvic pain, tingling, urinary retention, constipation, and cerebrospinal fluid pleocytosis. Symptoms usually resolve in a few days, but in some cases, the neurologic residua take weeks to months to disappear, occasionally becoming permanent. Reactivation of HSV or varicella-zoster virus is associated with Bell's palsy with acute, peripheral facial paresis caused by compression of the facial nerve in the temporal bone. HSV encephalitis is the most commonly identified acute, sporadic viral encephalitis in the United States, accounting for 10% to 20% of all cases. Nearly all of the cases arising after the neonatal period are caused by HSV-1. HSV encephalitis usually presents with acute focal neurologic symptoms, fever, and involvement of the temporal lobe. PCR of the cerebrospinal fluid for HSV DNA is the most common diagnostic technique.

COMPLICATIONS

All manifestations of HSV infection seen in the immunocompetent host also can be seen in immunocompromised patients, but they are usually more severe, more extensive, and more difficult to treat; for many of them, recurrences are more frequent. Patients with defects in T-cell immunity, such as those with AIDS or transplantation recipients, are at particular risk for progressive mucocutaneous or visceral infections, but the degree of dissemination depends on the level of immunodeficiency of the host. Recurrent and persistent ulcerative HSV lesions are among the most common and defining opportunistic infections in patients with AIDS.[15] Genital herpes is very common in patients with HIV and can be persistent and severe. Oropharyngeal HSV in immunocompromised patients can present with widespread involvement of skin (Fig. 164-11), the mucosa, and extremely painful, friable, hemorrhagic, and necrotic lesions, similar to mucositis caused by cytotoxic agents. The lesions can spread locally to involve the esophagus. Esophagitis presents with odynophagia, dysphagia, substernal pain, and multiple ulcerative lesions. Esophagitis can also arise directly by reactivation of HSV and its spread to the esophagus via the vagus nerve. Tracheobronchitis and pneumonitis can also occur by spreading of the virus from oropharyngeal HSV.

HSV can reactivate from visceral ganglia of the autonomic nervous system or disseminate hematogenously to other visceral organs (causing pneumonitis, hepatitis, pancreatitis, or meningitis) and the GI tract. Most of these severe infections are caused by HSV-1, but HSV-2 can cause them as well.

ETIOLOGY AND PATHOGENESIS

RISK FACTORS

The risk of severe HSV disease and the recurrence rate correlate with the level of cellular immune competence

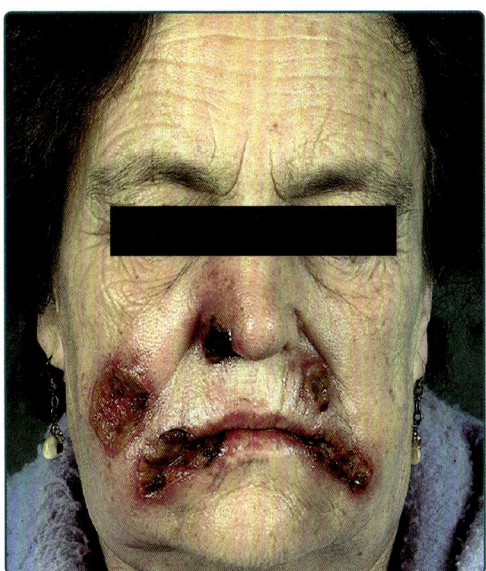

Figure 164-11 Herpes simplex virus infection. Chronic ulcer in an immunocompromised host. Multiple, slowly spreading, deep ulcers with central necrosis and hemorrhagic crusts on the lips, cheeks, and nose of a woman with leukemia.

of the host. Patients with mild decreases in cellular immunity may experience only an increased number of recurrences and a slower resolution of lesions, while severely compromised patients are more likely to develop disseminated, chronic, or drug-resistant infections. CD8+ and CD4+ T-lymphocyte subsets, natural killer cells, and inflammatory cytokines like interferon-γ are important in mediating protection against HSV. Innate immunity is also important and polymorphisms in TLR2 are associated with increased rates of genital lesions in seropositive persons.[16] Mutations in proteins important for interferon responses, including STAT1, TYK2, and UNC-93B, are associated with herpes simplex encephalitis.[17] Constant immune surveillance and engagement are required to maintain latency, mainly by HSV-specific CD8+ lymphocytes. T-cells reactive to HSV-1 are clustered around latently infected neurons in ganglia from HSV-1 seropositive persons. Dendritic cells and HSV-2–specific CD8+ lymphocytes localize to sites of reactivation, rapidly contain virus-infected cells,[18] and persist in the skin for weeks after lesions are cleared.[19] These virus-specific CD8 cells are oligoclonal CD8αα+ cells that persist in the dermal–epidermal junction, and produce cytotoxic granules.[20]

Patients with defects in humoral immunity have no increase in HSV disease severity, but the humoral immune response is important in reducing virus titers at the site of inoculation and in regional neural tissues during primary infection. The transfer of HSV-specific antibodies from mother to child is a key factor in protecting against neonatal herpes.

DIAGNOSIS

LABORATORY TESTING

The method of choice for diagnosis of HSV infection depends on the clinical presentation. In many instances, the history and clinical findings may be sufficient, but the social, emotional, and therapeutic implications of a diagnosis dictate that it be confirmed by laboratory testing when possible. For patients with active lesions, virus can be isolated in cell culture. In culture, HSV causes typical cytopathic effects, and most specimens will prove positive within 48 to 96 hours after inoculation. The sensitivity of culture depends on the quantity of virus in the specimen. Even in the most experienced centers, only approximately 60% to 70% of fresh genital lesions are culture positive. Isolation of virus is most successful when lesions are cultured during the vesicular stage and when specimens are taken from immunocompromised patients or from patients suffering from a primary infection.

PCR is more sensitive than viral isolation and has become the preferred method for diagnosis. PCR has been extensively used for the diagnosis of CNS infections and neonatal herpes. It is also useful for the detection of HSV in late-stage ulcerative lesions. Both viral culture and PCR assays enable typing of the isolate as HSV-1 or HSV-2. This information helps to predict the frequency of reactivation after a first episode of HSV infection.

Serologic detection of IgG antibodies to HSV can be helpful in certain settings, but the results are often misinterpreted. The main function of serologic testing is to differentiate a primary episode from a recurrent infection (Table 164-1). A positive serologic test result can be useful in patients with recurrent, genital lesions that are not present at the time of examination, thereby making a positive culture unobtainable. Serologic testing also can be helpful for counseling patients with initial episodes of disease and their partners, especially during pregnancy, and in counseling partners of patients with genital herpes about their risk of acquiring HSV.

Type-specific serologic assays are based on antigenic differences between HSV-1 and HSV-2 glycoprotein G. These tests are often used to counsel patients about the meaning of the test results in terms of the natural history of the disease, disease transmission, and the emotional and social implications of the diagnosis.

PATHOLOGY

Direct fluorescent antibody staining of lesion scrapings also can be used, but its sensitivity is lower than that of viral culture. The Tzanck test is helpful in rapid diagnosis of herpesvirus infections, but it is less sensitive than culture and staining with fluorescent antibody, with positive results in fewer than 40%

TABLE 164-1
Classification of Herpes Simplex Infections According to Viral Isolation and Paired Serologic Test Results

CLASSIFICATION	VIRUS ISOLATED	SEROLOGY (ACUTE)		SEROLOGY (CONVALESCENT)	
		HSV-1 IgG	HSV-2 IgG	HSV-1 IgG	HSV-2 IgG
Primary HSV-1	HSV-1	–	–	+	–
Primary HSV-2	HSV-2	–	–	–	+
Primary HSV-1 plus previous HSV-2 infection (rare)	HSV-1	–	+	+	+
Primary HSV-2 plus previous HSV-1 infection	HSV-2	+	–	+	+
Recurrent HSV-1	HSV-1	+	– or +	+	– or +
Recurrent HSV-2	HSV-2	– or +	+	– or +	+

–, Negative; +, positive; HSV, herpes simplex virus.

of culture-proven cases. It is performed by scraping the base of a freshly-ruptured vesicle and staining the slides with Giemsa or Wright stain (the Papanicolaou staining method also can be used), followed by examination for multinucleated giant cells that are diagnostic of herpetic infection (Fig. 164-12). Both HSV and varicella-zoster virus will cause these changes. In skin biopsy specimens, epithelial cells are enlarged, swollen, and often separated. Multinucleated cells with intranuclear eosinophilic inclusion bodies can be seen.

DIFFERENTIAL DIAGNOSIS

The differential diagnosis of orolabial herpes includes aphthous ulcers, syphilis, and herpangina. Diseases that can mimic genital herpes include chancroid, syphilis, and lymphogranuloma venereum (Table 164-2).

CLINICAL COURSE AND PROGNOSIS

Although most patients with HSV infections are asymptomatic, primary infections can be severe. Most recurrences are asymptomatic, but symptomatic recurrences are milder than symptomatic primary infections. The frequency and severity of recurrent HSV-1 and HSV-2 disease decrease over time; therefore, the need for continued suppressive therapy should be reevaluated.

MANAGEMENT

INTERVENTIONS

COUNSELING

All sexually-active persons should be educated regarding the nature and risks of acquiring and transmitting sexually-transmitted infections, including HSV.

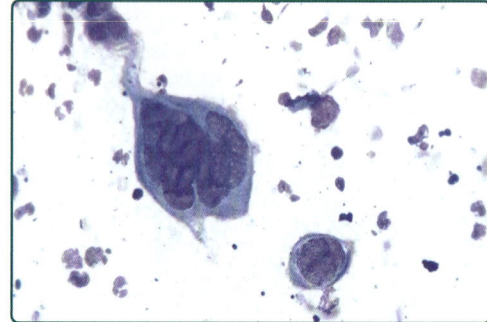

Figure 164-12 Herpes simplex virus: Positive Giemsa smear for Tzanck cells. A giant, multinucleated keratinocyte on a Giemsa-stained smear obtained from a vesicle base. Compare size of the giant cell to that of neutrophils also seen in this smear.

Studies show that approximately one-half of patients with asymptomatic HSV-2 infection have mild, unrecognized disease and can be taught to recognize the symptoms and signs of genital herpes. Also, patients should be counseled regarding safer sex practices. It must be emphasized that the majority of transmission occurs in asymptomatic phases and from people who have no classical lesions. Patients with genital herpes should be counseled to refrain from sexual intercourse during outbreaks and for 1 to 2 days after, and to use condoms between outbreaks. Suppressive antiviral therapy is also an option for individuals concerned about transmission to a partner.

Pregnant women who are known to have genital herpes should be reassured that the risk of transmitting herpes to the baby during childbirth is extremely low. Recommendations for the management of pregnant women with recurrent genital herpes include clinical evaluation at delivery, with delivery by cesarean section indicated if there are signs and symptoms of active infection (including prodrome). But cesarean section delivery may not reliably prevent neonatal HSV infection when membranes are ruptured for long

TABLE 164-2
Differential Diagnosis of Orolabial and Genital Herpes

	DISEASE OR CONDITION	DIFFERENCES FROM HERPES
Orolabial	Aphthous ulcers	Not preceded by vesicles, located only on mucosa
	Syphilis	Painless, not preceded by vesicles
	Herpangina	Posterior portion of mouth (soft palate, tonsils)
	Erythema multiforme	Partial involvement of oral mucosa with targetoid plaques with vesicular or erosive centers; lesions may be confluent
	Stevens-Johnson syndrome	Diffuse erosive mucositis plus generalized skin lesions
Genital	Chancroid	Deep ulceration with exudate
	Syphilis	Painless, not preceded by vesicles
	Lymphogranuloma venereum	Painless ulcer, unimpressive primary lesions
	Granuloma inguinale	Painless ulcer, exuberant lesions

periods (≥24 hours). Women with primary HSV infection during pregnancy should be treated with antiviral therapy. For women at or beyond 36 weeks of gestation who are at risk for recurrent HSV infection, suppressive antiviral therapy has been recommended, as this decreases viral shedding, the incidence of active lesions near term, and the need for cesarean delivery because of HSV.[21] Close followup; sequential PCR or cultures for HSV of infants born to seropositive mothers who are shedding virus at the time of delivery; prophylactic therapy with intravenous acyclovir for infants born to mothers with primary infection; and intravenous acyclovir, if HSV is detected in infants of seropositive mothers, all have been suggested.[12]

Women who are known by history and serologic tests not to have genital herpes should be counseled about signs and symptoms of HSV and how to avoid acquiring the infection during pregnancy. Serology is helpful in counseling a couple in which the male partner has recurrent genital herpes and the pregnant wife is susceptible.

MEDICATIONS (SEE CHAP. 191)

Many HSV infections require no specific treatment. Keeping lesions clean and dry while they heal by themselves may be all that is required. Treatment is warranted for infections that are likely to prove protracted, highly symptomatic, or complicated. Acyclovir has a highly favorable therapeutic index because of its preferential activation in infected cells and preferential inhibition of the viral DNA polymerase. It must be phosphorylated to be active, and it requires the viral thymidine kinase for phosphorylation. Acyclovir inhibits HSV-1 and HSV-2 replication by 50% at a concentration of 0.1 and 0.3 μg/mL (range: 0.01 to 9.9 μg/mL), respectively, but is toxic at concentrations of greater than 30 μg/mL. Any strain that requires more than 3 μg/mL of acyclovir to be inhibited is said to be relatively drug resistant.

Valacyclovir, the L-valyl ester of acyclovir, is an oral prodrug of acyclovir that achieves 3- to 5-fold higher bioavailability after oral administration, and can be used in a more convenient dosage regimen. Famciclovir is the well absorbed oral form of penciclovir. Similar to acyclovir, famciclovir is converted by phosphorylation to its active metabolite penciclovir triphosphate. The efficacy and adverse effect profile of famciclovir is comparable to that of acyclovir. Penciclovir 1% cream is approved by the U.S. Food and Drug Administration (FDA) for the treatment of herpes simplex labialis. Docosanol 10% cream is approved by the FDA for nonprescription treatment of recurrent herpes labialis. Docosanol is a long-chain saturated alcohol that inhibits entry of lipid-enveloped virus into the cell. It decreases healing time by 18 hours when compared with placebo.

The current recommendations for antiviral treatment depend on the clinical disease, on host immune status, and whether one is treating a primary or recurrent episode or considering suppressive therapy (Tables 164-3 to 164-5).[22] For disseminated or severe herpes infections, the treatment of choice remains intravenous acyclovir 10 to 15 mg/kg every 8 hours. The dose of intravenous acyclovir for neonatal herpes is 20 mg/kg per dose given every 8 hours.

For first episodes of genital HSV-2 infections, oral acyclovir, famciclovir, or valacyclovir all speed healing and resolution of symptoms, and decrease viral shedding. When compared with placebo, acyclovir decreases time to healing from 16 to 12 days, the duration of pain from 7 to 5 days, and the duration of constitutional symptoms from 6 to 3 days. Valacyclovir was compared with acyclovir in the treatment of primary episodes and shown to be equivalent. Antiviral treatment of initial herpes episodes does not decrease subsequent recurrences, probably because HSV establishes latent infection within hours after infection and days before symptoms evolve.

Treatment of recurrent episodes of genital herpes with famciclovir, acyclovir, or valacyclovir reduces the time of healing from approximately 7 to 5 days, time of cessation of viral shedding from 4 to 2 days, and duration of symptoms from 4 to 3 days when compared with placebo. Valacyclovir and acyclovir are equivalent; valacyclovir was similar to famciclovir in one study, but slightly superior to famciclovir to suppress genital herpes in another study. For persons with frequent or complicated genital recurrences, long-term suppressive therapy with acyclovir or its analogs is the most effective management strategy. Suppressive therapy was effective during the first year after acquisition of genital herpes. Suppressive therapy reduces the rate of shedding in healthy persons and those with HIV. Suppressive therapy with valacyclovir was more effective to reduce the burden of genital herpes

TABLE 164-3

Recommended Regimens for the Treatment of Orofacial Herpes Simplex Infections

DISEASE	ACCEPTABLE REGIMEN ALTERNATIVES		DURATION	COMMENTS
	ADULTS	PEDIATRIC[a]		
Primary infection	Acyclovir, 200 mg orally 5 times a day Acyclovir, 400 mg orally 3 times a day Valacyclovir, 1 g orally twice a day Famciclovir, 250 mg orally 3 times a day	Acyclovir 15 mg/kg orally 5 times a day	7-10 days or until resolution of symptoms	IV acyclovir for severely ill individuals No studies have been done in adults; regimens are extrapolated from their effectiveness in primary genital herpes
Recurrent infection: episodic treatment	Topical penciclovir, 1% cream q2h while awake Topical docosanol, 10% cream 5 times a day Acyclovir, 400 mg orally 5 times a day Famciclovir, 500 mg orally 2 or 3 times a day Valacyclovir, 2 g orally twice a day for 1 day Famciclovir, 1500 mg single dose or 750 mg twice a day for 1 day		4-5 days or until lesions are healed	Treatment is generally not warranted
Recurrent infection: prophylaxis	Acyclovir, 400 mg orally twice a day			Start just before and during precipitating event, such as intensive ultraviolet light exposure
Recurrent infection: suppression of confirmed frequent recurrences	Acyclovir, 400 mg orally twice a day Valacyclovir, 500 mg once a day Valacyclovir, 1 g once a day	There are no pediatric studies, but children with confirmed frequent recurrences may benefit from suppressive oral acyclovir therapy		

[a]Oral dosage of acyclovir in children should not exceed 80 mg/kg/day. Children who weigh 40 kg or more should receive the adult dose.

Note: The doses are for patients with normal renal function. Neither valacyclovir nor famciclovir is approved by the U.S. Food and Drug Administration for use in children.

disease than episodic therapy. Because genital herpes is not progressive in the normal host and because the rate of recurrences varies over time and may decrease after some years, it is wise to recommend a "holiday" from treatment every year or so to reassess the continuing need for treatment. Sunscreen has shown benefit in some, but not all trials, but there is no evidence for lysine or gammaglobulin.[23] Novel antivirals that inhibit the HSV helicase–primase complex[24,25] were effective for treatment of recurrent genital herpes in Phase II trials, but are not licensed.

The use of antiviral suppressive therapy during the late phase of pregnancy to avoid neonatal herpes also has been advocated, but a formal study of the approach would require a very large number of participants because of the rare incidence of neonatal herpes. A more achievable goal is to decrease the need for cesarean deliveries caused by herpes recurrences during labor. Studies show that antiviral therapy in late pregnancy (beginning at 36 weeks) prevents clinical recurrences, cesarean sections associated with genital herpes, and the risk of HSV-viral shedding at delivery.

Orolabial HSV infections warrant antiviral treatment less often than do genital infections. Primary HSV gingivostomatitis should be treated with oral acyclovir. The pediatric dose is 15 mg/kg of acyclovir suspension orally 5 times a day for 7 days. When it is started within 3 days of onset of the disease, this regimen decreases the duration of oral and extraoral lesions, fever, and eating and drinking difficulties. Valacyclovir and famciclovir may be equally effective, but they have not been studied in this setting and are not currently approved for use in children. Severely ill children may need to be hospitalized for hydration, and IV acyclovir may be necessary.

Treatment of recurrent herpes labialis with antiviral drugs in immunocompetent hosts has shown only modest benefits.[23] Oral infections are inherently briefer and less symptomatic than genital herpes. Treatment is only effective if used very early in the disease, especially in the prodromal or erythema lesion stages. Patients who wish treatment should have the medication available and be vigilant for the earliest signs and symptoms of a recurrence. When treatment is thought to be required, penciclovir 1% cream every 2

TABLE 164-4
Recommended Regimens for the Treatment of Genital Herpes Simplex Infections

DISEASE	ACCEPTABLE REGIMEN ALTERNATIVES		DURATION	COMMENTS
	ADULTS	PEDIATRIC[a]		
Primary infection	Acyclovir, 200 mg orally 5 times a day Acyclovir, 400 mg orally 3 times a day Valacyclovir, 1 g orally twice a day Famciclovir, 250 mg orally 3 times a day	Acyclovir, 40-80 mg/kg/day orally divided in 3 to 4 doses (maximum 1 g/day)	7–10 days or until clinical resolution occurs.	
Recurrent infection	Acyclovir, 400 mg orally 3 times a day Acyclovir, 200 mg orally 5 times a day Acyclovir, 800 mg orally twice a day Valacyclovir, 500 mg orally twice a day Valacyclovir, 1 g orally once a day Valacyclovir, 1 g orally twice a day[b] Famciclovir, 500 mg,[b] 250 mg, 125 mg orally twice a day Famciclovir, 1 g orally twice a day for 1 day (patient initiated) Famciclovir, 500 mg, then 250 mg twice daily for 2 days	For children ≥12 years of age: Acyclovir, 200 mg orally 5 times a day for 5 days Acyclovir, 800 mg orally twice a day for 5 days Acyclovir, 800 mg 3 times a day for 2 days		
Suppression of recurrences	Acyclovir, 400 mg orally twice a day Acyclovir, 800 mg orally once a day Valacyclovir, 500 mg, 1000 mg orally once a day[c] Valacyclovir, 250 mg orally twice a day[c] Valacyclovir, 500 mg twice a day or 1000 mg orally once a day[b] Famciclovir, 250 mg orally twice a day Famciclovir, 125 mg, 250 mg orally 3 times a day	For children ≥12 years of age: Acyclovir, 400 mg orally twice a day		Duration of the therapy is controversial; some authorities will offer treatment for 1 year and then reassess the need to resume it
Reduction of transmission	Valacyclovir, 500 mg orally once a day			Safer sex practices should continue to be used

[a]Oral dosage of acyclovir in children should not exceed 80 mg/kg/day. Children who weigh 40 kg or more should receive the adult dose.
[b]HIV patients.
[c]The high once-a-day and twice-daily doses of valacyclovir are more effective in patients who present with more than 10 recurrences per year.
Note: The doses are for patients with normal renal function. Neither valacyclovir nor famciclovir is approved by the U.S. Food and Drug Administration for use in children.

hours while awake, for 4 days can be used. Treatment should be initiated as early as possible. When initiated within 1 hour of first symptoms of recurrence, penciclovir sped the healing of lesions (4.8 days vs 5.5 days) and decreased the duration of pain (3.5 days vs 4.1 days). This regimen is approved by the FDA. Docosanol 10% cream is approved by the FDA for nonprescription treatment of herpes simplex labialis. It is applied 5 times a day at the first sign of recurrence of herpes simplex labialis. There has been no direct comparison with topical penciclovir. Oral acyclovir, 400 mg 5 times a day for 5 days, affords marginal benefit if begun in the earliest hour or two of the outbreak. Famciclovir, 500 mg 3 times a day for 5 days, when started within 48 hours after experimental ultraviolet radiation, decreased the median time to healing from 6 to 4 days, but is not useful for the more usual sporadic cases of herpes labialis. Valacyclovir (2 g twice daily for 1 day) decreased the mean duration of cold sore episodes by 1 day when compared with placebo, if started in the prodrome period. Similarly, a single dose of famciclovir (1500 mg) reduced time to healing of herpes labialis lesions by approximately 2 days compared with placebo. Creams and ointments containing 5% and 10% acyclovir are not beneficial in recurrent herpes labialis.

The use of suppressive acyclovir for herpes labialis is controversial. In one small study, oral acyclovir, 400 mg twice a day, was effective in decreasing recurrences of herpes labialis. In another study, suppressive therapy with valacyclovir was more effective than episodic therapy with valacyclovir for herpes labialis. In studies with skiers (who have significant sun exposures), acyclovir 400 mg twice a day, was shown to reduce recurrences in one study, whereas acyclovir, 800 mg twice daily, failed to prevent recurrences in another study. Both perioperative famciclovir (125 or 250 mg orally twice daily given 1 to 2 days before to 5 days after the procedure) and valacyclovir (500 mg twice daily for 14 days, starting either a day before or the day of the procedure) appeared to reduce the recurrence of orofacial HSV in patients undergoing facial laser resurfacing. Valacyclovir also suppresses recurrences of herpes gladiatorum.

TABLE 164-5
Recommended Regimens for Other Herpes Cutaneous Diseases

DISEASE	ACCEPTABLE REGIMEN ALTERNATIVES		DURATION	COMMENTS
	ADULTS	PEDIATRIC[a]		
Neonatal herpes		IV acyclovir, 20 mg/kg every 8 h	14-21 days	For infants with CNS disease, 6 months of acyclovir suppression is effective (see text)
Disseminated infection	IV acyclovir, 10-15 mg/kg 3 times a day	IV acyclovir, 10 mg/kg 3 times a day	14-21 days	
Herpes gladiatorum, herpetic whitlow	Acyclovir, 200 mg orally 5 times per day; Acyclovir, 400 mg orally 3 times a day; Valacyclovir, 1 g orally twice a day; Famciclovir, 250 mg orally 3 times a day	Acyclovir, 40-80 mg/kg/day orally divided into 3 to 4 doses (maximum: 1 g/day)	7-10 days or until resolution of symptoms	No studies have been done; regimens are extrapolated from the treatment of genital herpes. Consider suppressive antiviral therapy for patients with frequent recurrences
Eczema herpeticum	Acyclovir, 200 mg orally 5 times a day; Acyclovir, 400 mg orally 3 times a day; Valacyclovir, 1 g orally twice a day; IV acyclovir, 10-15 mg/kg 3 times a day	Acyclovir, 40-80 mg/kg/day orally divided into 3 to 4 doses (maximum: 1 g/day); IV acyclovir 10-15 mg/kg 3 times daily	14-21 days	No studies have been done. Use IV acyclovir in severely ill individuals. Consider suppressive antiviral therapy for patients with recurrences. Ocular involvement should be treated in consultation with an ophthalmologist

[a]Oral dosage of acyclovir in children should not exceed 80 mg/kg/day. Children who weigh 40 kg or more should receive the adult dose.
Note: The doses are for patients with normal renal function. Neither valacyclovir nor famciclovir is approved by the U.S. Food and Drug Administration for use in children.

Herpetic eye disease should always be treated in consultation with an ophthalmologist. Options usually involve topical antivirals, including vidarabine, trifluridine, acyclovir, or ganciclovir. Topical antivirals are effective in shortening the duration of dendritic and geographic keratitis, and are used to prevent corneal epithelial disease in patients with blepharitis and conjunctivitis, as well as patients on topical steroid therapy for corneal stromal inflammation and iridocyclitis. Oral acyclovir is also effective for dendritic and geographical epithelial keratitis. Suppressive antiviral therapy reduces the rates of all types of recurrent ocular HSV disease, and it is most important for patients with a history of HSV stromal keratitis because it can prevent additional episodes and potential loss of vision.

Antiviral Resistance: Virtually all clinically relevant drug resistance has been seen in immunocompromised patients. The primary mechanism of acyclovir resistance is selection of viral mutants defective or deficient in thymidine kinase expression. Most mutants that are thymidine kinase deficient are somewhat attenuated for virulence in vivo.

The treatment of resistant HSV infection is complicated. Very few people who claim to be "resistant" to one of the antiviral drugs actually harbor resistant virus. There is a common misconception that treatment prevents all recurrences. One should suspect resistance only in people who continue to have culture-proven or PCR-proven outbreaks of unaltered frequency and severity, especially if the lesions do not heal by themselves. When resistance is suspected, virus should be cultured and tested for sensitivity to acyclovir. These tests are expensive but are available through commercial reference laboratories. Foscarnet does not require activation by HSV thymidine kinase and is usually effective in the treatment of acyclovir-resistant HSV. The drug requires IV therapy and can cause numerous adverse reactions, including nephrotoxicity, electrolyte disturbances, anemia, and seizures. Rare foscarnet-resistant HSV strains have been reported.

Cidofovir also does not require activation by HSV thymidine kinase. Cidofovir has been used in cases of acyclovir-resistant HSV and topical cidofovir has been used with success to treat progressive herpetic lesions. Intravenous cidofovir is associated with considerable nephrotoxicity and requires the coadministration of saline hydration and probenecid. A few patients with acyclovir-resistant genital herpes have responded to imiquimod 5% cream. Imiquimod causes severe inflammation in some patients with recurrent herpes labialis. Resiquimod reduced the rate of new lesions in 1 study of persons without drug-resistant virus, but had no effect on genital herpes in 4 other studies. Continuous intravenous acyclovir also has been used to treat acyclovir-resistant HSV. Long-term suppressive acyclovir therapy reduced the rate of drug-resistant HSV disease in hematopoietic stem cell transplant recipients.

PREVENTION

Strategies to prevent HSV infection have proved inadequate. HSV infection can be prevented by total abstinence, as indicated by very low seroprevalence rates in cloistered nuns. Condoms reduce rates of transmission if used routinely. Male circumcision reduced the rate of HSV-2 infection in one study, but not in another study. Other than these public health approaches, most efforts involve antiviral therapy and vaccines directed at genital herpes.

Antiviral Therapy: Acyclovir, famciclovir, and valacyclovir all decrease both symptomatic and subclinical shedding of HSV-2, from approximately 8% of the days in the placebo group to 0.3% to 0.6% of the days in the treatment group, when assessed by culture. Once-daily valacyclovir reduced shedding by PCR from 14% to 3% in patients with newly diagnosed genital herpes. Valacyclovir 500 mg once daily was effective in reducing the transmission of HSV-2 between partners by 48%, and reduced clinical disease in the susceptible partner by 7% in a randomized, placebo-controlled trial involving immunocompetent, heterosexual couples in stable relationships.[6] This therapy can be recommended for individuals concerned about transmission to a partner, in conjunction with the use of condoms. Frequency of HSV-2 shedding was reduced with high-dose acyclovir (800 mg 3 times daily) or high-dose valacyclovir (1 g 3 times daily) compared with standard dose valacyclovir (500 mg daily); however, the high-dose therapies did not reduce recurrence rates compared with standard dose valacyclovir.[26] Tenofovir gel applied vaginally within 12 hours before and 12 hours after coitus reduced the incidence of HSV-2 by approximately 50%.[27] Oral tenofovir and emtricitabine-tenofovir had a modest effect on reducing acquisition of HSV-2.[28] Vaginal microbicides are also being studied, mostly focusing on decreasing HIV transmission, but some of the compounds also have anti-HSV activity and may also affect HSV transmission.

Vaccines: No vaccine is licensed to protect against acquisition of HSV (prophylactic) or to reduce the number of recurrent episodes (therapeutic).[29] A recombinant HSV-2 glycoprotein D vaccine was ineffective at preventing genital herpes disease, infection, or HSV shedding.[30] Several candidate vaccines are under development to prevent recurrent genital HSV.[31] A replication-defective mutant, deleted for 2 essential viral proteins, is currently in a clinical trial. Initial results with a subunit vaccine containing HSV-2 gD2 and ICP4 protein showed a 50% reduction in HSV-2 genital shedding after vaccination. A Phase II study of a vaccine consisting of HSV-2 peptides linked to heat shock protein with an adjuvant, showed a 15% reduction in HSV-2 genital shedding.

ACKNOWLEDGMENTS

The author recognizes the contribution of Adriana Marques, who was a coauthor of this chapter in the previous edition. Much of the text is based on the chapter from the prior edition.

REFERENCES

1. Bernstein DI, Bellamy AR, Hook EW 3rd, et al. Epidemiology, clinical presentation, and antibody response to primary infection with herpes simplex virus type 1 and type 2 in young women. *Clin Infect Dis*. 2013;56:344-351.
2. Bradley H, Markowitz LE, Gibson T, et al. Seroprevalence of herpes simplex virus types 1 and 2—United States, 1999-2010. *J Infect Dis*. 2014;209:325-333.
3. Johnston C, Corey L. Current concepts for genital herpes simplex virus infection: diagnostics and pathogenesis of genital tract shedding. *Clin Microbiol Rev*. 2016;29:149-161.
4. Tronstein E, Johnston C, Huang ML, et al. Genital shedding of herpes simplex virus among symptomatic and asymptomatic persons with HSV-2 infection. *JAMA*. 2011;305:1441-1449.
5. Mark KE, Wald A, Magaret AS, et al. Rapidly cleared episodes of herpes simplex virus reactivation in immunocompetent adults. *J Infect Dis*. 2008;198:1141-1149.
6. Corey L, Wald A, Patel R, et al. Once-daily valacyclovir to reduce the risk of transmission of genital herpes. *N Engl J Med*. 2004;350:11-20.
7. Langenberg AG, Corey L, Ashley RL, et al. A prospective study of new infections with herpes simplex virus type 1 and type 2. Chiron HSV Vaccine Study Group. *N Engl J Med*. 1999;341:1432-1438.
8. Mujugira A, Magaret AS, Celum C, et al; Partners in Prevention HSV/HIV Transmission Study Team. Daily acyclovir to decrease herpes simplex virus type 2 (HSV-2) transmission from HSV-2/HIV-1 coinfected persons: a randomized controlled trial. *J Infect Dis*. 2013;208:1366-1374.
9. Horowitz R, Aierstuck S, Williams EA, et al. Herpes simplex virus infection in a university health population: clinical manifestations, epidemiology, and implications. *J Am Coll Health*. 2010;59:69-74.
10. Gupta R, Warren T, Wald A. Genital herpes. *Lancet*. 2007;370:2127-2137.
11. Hata TR, Kotol P, Boguniewicz M, et al. History of eczema herpeticum is associated with the inability to induce human β-defensin (HBD)-2, HBD-3 and cathelicidin in the skin of patients with atopic dermatitis. *Br J Dermatol*. 2010;163:659-661.
12. Corey L, Wald A. Maternal and neonatal herpes simplex virus infections. *N Engl J Med*. 2009;361:1376-1385.
13. James SH, Kimberlin DW. Neonatal herpes simplex virus infection: epidemiology and treatment. *Clin Perinatol*. 2015;42:47-59.
14. Kimberlin DW, Whitley RJ, Wan W, et al. Oral acyclovir suppression and neurodevelopment after neonatal herpes. *N Engl J Med*. 2011;365:1284-1292.
15. Wauters O, Lebas E, Nikkels AF. Chronic mucocutaneous herpes simplex virus and varicella zoster virus infections. *J Am Acad Dermatol*. 2012;66:e217-e227.
16. Bochud PY, Magaret AS, Koelle DM, et al. Polymorphisms in TLR2 are associated with increased viral shedding and lesional rate in patients with genital herpes simplex virus type 2 infection. *J Infect Dis*. 2007;196:505-509.
17. Sancho-Shimizu V, Perez de Diego R, Jouanguy E, et al. Inborn errors of anti-viral interferon immunity in humans. *Curr Opin Virol*. 2011;1:487-496.
18. Schiffer JT, Corey L. Rapid host immune response and viral dynamics in herpes simplex virus-2 infection. *Nat Med*. 2013;19:280-290.

19. Zhu J, Koelle DM, Cao J, et al. Virus-specific CD8+ T cells accumulate near sensory nerve endings in genital skin during subclinical HSV-2 reactivation. *J Exp Med*. 2007;204:595-603.
20. Zhu J, Peng T, Johnston C, et al. Immune surveillance by CD8αα+ skin-resident T cells in human herpes virus infection. *Nature*. 2013;497:494-497.
21. Money D, Steben M; Society of Obstetricians and Gynaecologists of Canada. SOGC clinical practice guidelines: guidelines for the management of herpes simplex virus in pregnancy. Number 208, June 2008. *Int J Gynaecol Obstet*. 2009;104:167-171.
22. Cernik C, Gallina K, Brodell RT. The treatment of herpes simplex infections: an evidence-based review. *Arch Intern Med*. 2008;168:1137-1144.
23. Chi CC, Wang SH, Delamere FM, et al. Interventions for prevention of herpes simplex labialis (cold sores on the lips). *Cochrane Database Syst Rev*. 2015;8:CD010095.
24. Tyring S, Wald A, Zadeikis N, et al. ASP2151 for the treatment of genital herpes: a randomized, double-blind, placebo- and valacyclovir-controlled, dose-finding study. *J Infect Dis*. 2012;205:1100-1110.
25. Wald A, Corey L, Timmler B, et al. Helicase-primase inhibitor pritelivir for HSV-2 infection. *N Engl J Med*. 2014;370:201-210.
26. Johnston C, Saracino M, Kuntz S, et al. Standard-dose and high-dose daily antiviral therapy for short episodes of genital HSV-2 reactivation: three randomised, open-label, cross-over trials. *Lancet*. 2012;379:641-647.
27. Abdool Karim SS, Abdool Karim Q, Kharsany AB, et al; CAPRISA 004 Trial Group. Tenofovir gel for the prevention of herpes simplex virus type 2 infection. *N Engl J Med*. 2015;373:530-539.
28. Celum C, Morrow RA, Donnell D, et al. Daily oral tenofovir and emtricitabine-tenofovir preexposure prophylaxis reduces herpes simplex virus type 2 acquisition among heterosexual HIV-1-uninfected men and women: a subgroup analysis of a randomized trial. *Ann Intern Med*. 2014;161:11-19.
29. Dropulic LK, Cohen JI. The challenge of developing a herpes simplex virus 2 vaccine. *Expert Rev Vaccines*. 2012;11:1429-1440.
30. Belshe RB, Leone PA, Bernstein DI, et al; Herpevac Trial for Women. Efficacy results of a trial of a herpes simplex vaccine. *N Engl J Med*. 2012;366:34-43.
31. Johnston C, Gottlieb SL, Wald A. Status of vaccine research and development of vaccines for herpes simplex virus. *Vaccine*. 2016;34:2948-2952.

Chapter 165 :: Varicella and Herpes Zoster :: Myron J. Levin, Kenneth E. Schmader, & Michael N. Oxman

第一百六十五章

水痘-带状疱疹

中文导读

水痘-带状疱疹病毒（VZV）全球分布广泛，98%的成人血清学阳性，可引起水痘和带状疱疹两种不同的病毒性皮肤病。水痘是具有高度传染性的水疱型皮肤病，儿童多见。带状疱疹是一种局部皮肤以单侧放射状疼痛和水疱性皮疹为主要特征的皮肤病，老年人多见。造成这种区别的原因在于水痘是VZV的原发性感染，大多数人被感染后并不呈现临床症状或症状很轻微而被忽视，少数感染者出现皮疹。但所有感染者感染后病毒持续潜伏在神经节细胞中，在各种诱发刺激下被再次激活，造成带状疱疹。水痘和带状疱疹的临床诊断具有迷惑性，需要与许多病毒疹性疾病相鉴别，鉴别要点列于表165-2中。本章分别介绍了水痘-带状疱疹的流行病学、临床特征、危险因素、病因和发病机制、诊断、鉴别诊断、临床病程和预后及临床管理。

〔张江林〕

AT A GLANCE

VARICELLA

- Varicella (chickenpox) and herpes zoster (shingles) are distinct clinical entities caused by a single member of the herpesvirus family, varicella-zoster virus (VZV).
- Varicella, a highly contagious exanthem that occurs most often in childhood, is the result of primary VZV infection of a susceptible individual.
- The rash of varicella usually begins on the face and scalp and spreads rapidly to the trunk, with relative sparing of the extremities. Lesions are scattered, rather than clustered, reflecting viremic spread to the skin, and they progress sequentially from rose-colored macules to papules, vesicles, pustules, and crusts. Lesions in all stages are usually present at the same time.
- In immunocompetent children, systemic symptoms are usually mild and serious complications are rare. In adults and immunocompromised persons of any age, varicella is more likely to be severe and can be associated with life-threatening complications.
- Varicella results in lifelong latent VZV infection of sensory and autonomic neurons, and host immunity to VZV.
- Live attenuated Oka VZV varicella vaccines have virtually eliminated varicella in countries where they have been deployed.

HERPES ZOSTER

- Herpes zoster is characterized by unilateral dermatomal pain and rash that results from reactivation and multiplication of latent VZV that persisted within neurons following varicella.
- The erythematous maculopapular and vesicular lesions of herpes zoster are clustered within a single dermatome, because VZV reaches the skin via the sensory nerve from the single ganglion in which latent VZV reactivates, and not by viremia.
- Herpes zoster is most common in older adults and in immunocompromised individuals.
- Pain is an important manifestation of herpes zoster. The most common debilitating complication is chronic neuropathic pain that persists long after the rash resolves, a complication known as postherpetic neuralgia (PHN).
- Antiviral therapy and analgesics reduce the acute pain of herpes zoster. Lidocaine patch (5%), high-dose capsaicin patch, gabapentin, pregabalin, opioids, and tricyclic antidepressants may reduce the pain of PHN.
- A live attenuated Oka/Merck strain VZV herpes zoster vaccine (ZVL; Zostavax®) reduces the incidence of herpes zoster by one-half and the incidence of PHN by two-thirds. An adjuvanted recombinant glycoprotein E subunit herpes zoster vaccine (RZV; Shingrix®) has substantially greater efficacy for herpes zoster and PHN, but it requires 2 doses and is more reactogenic.

INTRODUCTION

Varicella (chickenpox) and herpes zoster (shingles, zoster) are distinct clinical entities caused by a single member of the herpesvirus family, varicella-zoster virus (VZV). The different clinical manifestations of these 2 diseases are the result of differences in the host immune response and in the pathogenesis of the VZV infection, and not due to differences in the etiologic agent. Varicella, a highly contagious vesicular exanthem that occurs most often in childhood, is the result of exogenous primary infection of a susceptible individual. In contrast, herpes zoster results from reactivation of endogenous virus that persists in latent form within ganglionic neurons following an earlier attack of varicella. Herpes zoster is a localized dermatomal disease characterized by unilateral radicular pain and a vesicular dermatomal eruption.

HISTORICAL PERSPECTIVE

There was a report in 1892 of 5 instances in which varicella occurred in children exposed to adults with herpes zoster, and in the ensuing half century, clinical and histologic evidence lent support to the suggestion that susceptible individuals could develop varicella after exposure to someone with herpes zoster.[1-5] This included the development of varicella by children without a prior history of varicella who were inoculated with vesicle fluid from herpes zoster. In the 1950s, viruses isolated from varicella and herpes zoster were shown to have similar properties in tissue culture, and when compared by complement fixation and immunofluorescence techniques.[6] Nucleic acid identification methods subsequently demonstrated that the viruses isolated from a case of varicella and from a later case of herpes zoster in the same patient were identical.[7]

EPIDEMIOLOGY

EPIDEMIOLOGY OF VARICELLA

Varicella is distributed worldwide, but its age-specific incidence differs in temperate versus tropical climates, and in populations that have received varicella vaccine. In temperate climates, in the absence of varicella vaccination, varicella is endemic, with a regularly recurring seasonal prevalence in winter and spring, and periodic epidemics that reflect the accumulation of susceptible persons. In Europe and North America in the prevaccination era, 90% of cases occurred in children younger than 10 years of age and fewer than 5% in individuals older than the age of 15.[8] From 1988 to 1995, before varicella vaccine was introduced, there were approximately 11,000 hospitalizations and 100 deaths caused by varicella each year in the United States.[9,10] The risk of hospitalization and death was much higher in infants and adults than in children, and most varicella-related deaths occurred in previously healthy people. In tropical and semitropical countries, the mean age of varicella is higher, and susceptibility among adults is significantly greater, than in temperate climates. High levels of susceptibility to varicella among adult immigrants from tropical climates are well documented in the US military, for example, among recruits from Puerto Rico.[11] This geographical variation is important for hospitals, where susceptible health care workers from semitropical areas, such as the Philippines and Mexico, may pose a significant risk of nosocomial varicella.

Widespread use of varicella vaccine has markedly altered the epidemiology of varicella in the United States. Two-dose varicella vaccine coverage now exceeds 90% in young children.[12] This has resulted in a marked reduction in varicella-related morbidity. Varicella incidence and outpatient visits have declined by >85%, and hospitalizations have declined by ≥93%.[13-18] The decline is greatest among children aged 1 to 4 years who were targeted for vaccination, but cases have declined in all age groups, including unvaccinated infants and adults, reflecting herd immunity. Varicella-related mortality also declined substantially after the introduction of the varicella vaccine, and is now rare.[19] Varicella vaccine effectiveness has been demonstrated in a number of countries.[20]

Varicella is highly contagious. Attack rates of 87% among susceptible siblings in households and nearly 70% among susceptible patients on hospital wards have been reported.[21] More than 95% of cases of varicella are clinically apparent, although occasionally the exanthem may be so sparse and transient as to pass unnoticed. A typical patient is infectious for 1 to 2 days before the exanthem appears, and for 4 or 5 days thereafter, until the last crop of vesicles has crusted. Immunocompromised patients, who may experience successive crops of lesions for a week or more, are infectious longer. The mean incubation period of varicella is 14 to 17 days, with a range of 10 to 23 days, but it may be prolonged in patients who develop varicella after passive immunization with varicella-zoster immune globulin, or after postexposure immunization with varicella vaccine.[22]

The major route by which varicella is acquired and transmitted is from the respiratory tract by airborne droplets or aerosols, but infection also may be spread by direct contact. Varicella crusts are not infectious, and the duration of infectivity of droplets containing virus is probably quite limited. Although the infectiousness of patients with varicella is thought to depend largely on virus shed from the mucous membranes of the upper respiratory tract, VZV has rarely been cultured from pharyngeal secretions. However, VZV DNA can be detected in the oropharynx of most patients using polymerase chain reaction (PCR)–based assays.[23]

Varicella generally confers lifelong immunity, although subsequent exposure to VZV boosts humoral and cell-mediated immune responses, indicating subclinical reinfection.[24] Most reported second episodes of varicella represent incorrect diagnoses. Second episodes of varicella reported in immunocompromised patients usually represent cutaneous dissemination of herpes zoster.[25] Even severely immunocompromised patients very rarely develop second episodes of varicella after reexposure. Modified and breakthrough varicella now account for a significant proportion of the varicella occurring in the USA. Modified varicella occurs in individuals who develop varicella early in infancy in the presence of maternal antibody or following postexposure prophylaxis with varicella-zoster immune globulin or varicella vaccine. Breakthrough varicella occurs when vaccinated individuals are reinfected following exposure to wildtype VZV. Breakthrough varicella is frequently mild. However, both modified and breakthrough varicella are infectious for susceptible contacts.

EPIDEMIOLOGY OF HERPES ZOSTER

Herpes zoster occurs sporadically throughout the year without seasonal prevalence and independent of the prevalence of varicella. There is no convincing evidence that herpes zoster can be acquired by contact with persons with varicella or herpes zoster.[1] Rather, the incidence of herpes zoster is determined by factors that influence the host–virus relationship and the presence of immune responses necessary to prevent reactivation of latent VZV. The incidence of herpes zoster in community-dwelling populations ranges from 2 to 5 per 1000 person-years.[26,27]

A major risk factor for herpes zoster is age (Fig. 165-1A). The incidence of herpes zoster increases with increasing age; in older adults, it ranges from 8 to 12 per 1000 person-years in population-based and health care records–based studies on 4 continents.[1,27-34] We estimate that there are at least 1.5 million new cases of herpes zoster in the United States each year, more than half of which occur in persons ≥60 years of age; this number will increase dramatically as the population ages.[1,27-29,33,35-38]

Another major risk factor for herpes zoster is decreased VZV-specific cell-mediated immunity.[29,34,39] Immunocompromised patients have a significantly greater risk of herpes zoster (depending on their underlying condition) than immunocompetent individuals of the same age.[40-43] Ten percent of herpes zoster cases occur in immunocompromised patients.[33] Immunocompromising conditions associated with increased risk of herpes zoster include bone marrow and solid organ transplants, hematologic and solid tumor malignancies, and immune-mediated diseases

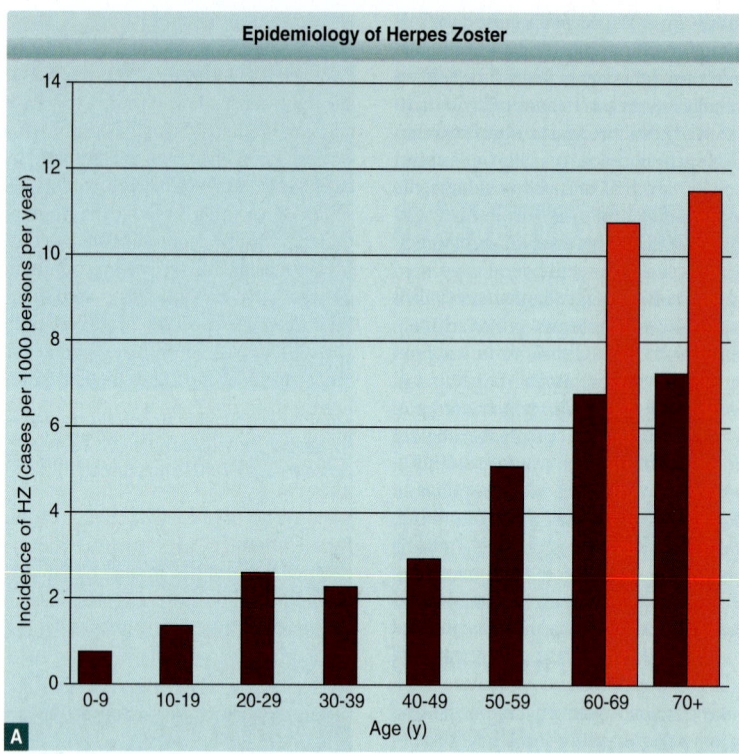

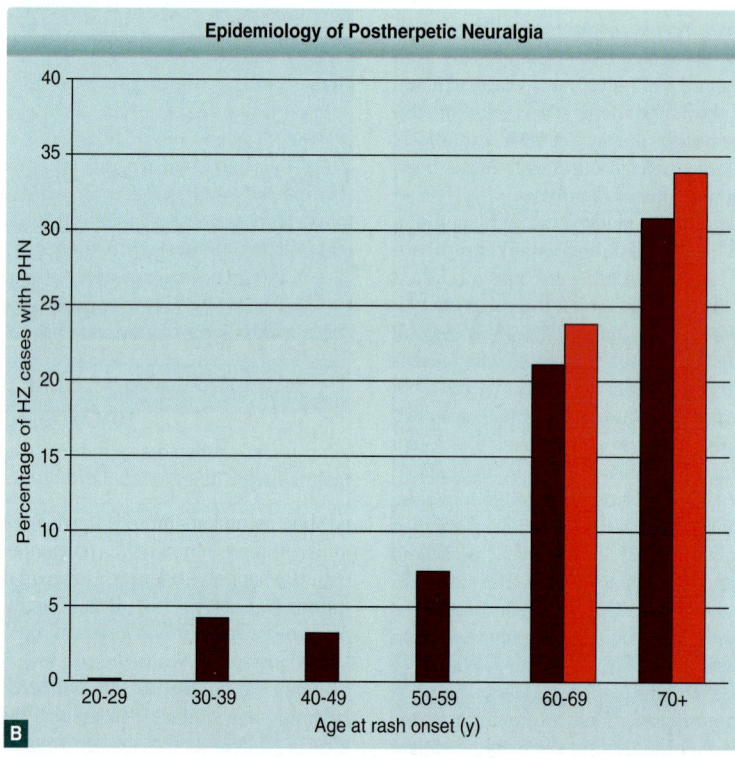

Figure 165-1 Epidemiology of Herpes Zoster (HZ) and Postherpetic Neuralgia (PHN). **A,** Incidence of herpes zoster (cases per 1000 persons per year) versus age. Dark red = data from Hope-Simpson RE. *Proc R Soc Med.* 1965;58:9.[1] Bright red = data for persons ≥60 years of age from the Shingles Prevention Study placebo recipients; Oxman MN et al. *N Engl J Med.* 1995;352:2271.[28] **B,** Percentage of cases of herpes zoster with postherpetic neuralgia. Postherpetic neuralgia is defined as clinically significant pain or discomfort due to herpes zoster persisting for ≥30 days after rash onset. Dark red = data from Hope-Simpson RE. Postherpetic neuralgia. *J R Coll Gen Pract.* 1975;25:571-575. Bright red = data for persons ≥60 years of age from the Shingles Prevention Study placebo recipients; Oxman MN et al: *N Engl J Med.* 1995;352:2271.[28]

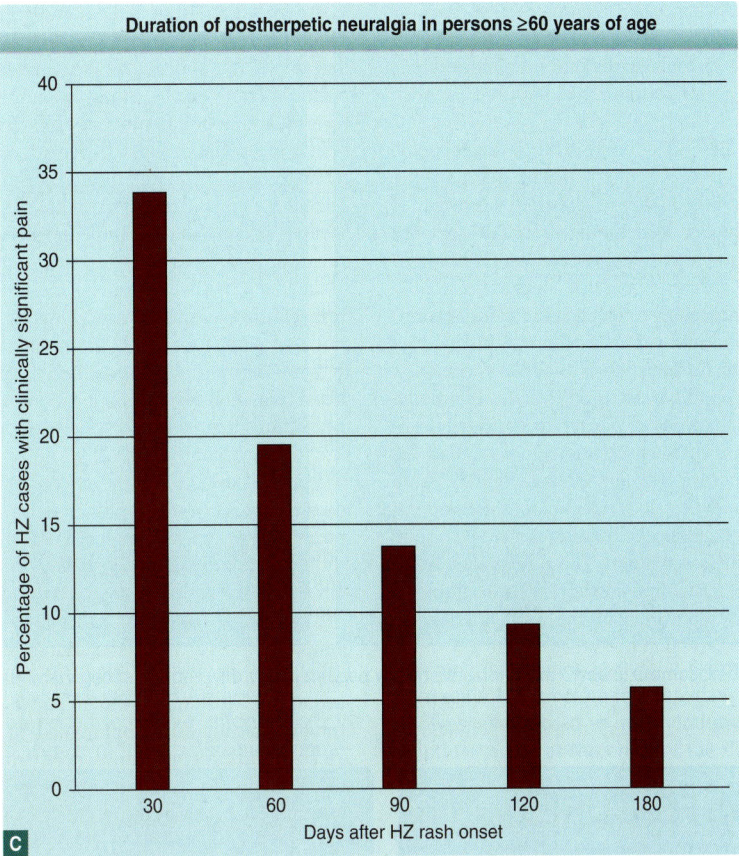

Figure 165-1 (*Continued*) **C,** Duration of postherpetic neuralgia in persons ≥60 years of age. Bright red = duration of clinically significant pain or discomfort due to herpes zoster among Shingles Prevention Study placebo recipients with confirmed herpes zoster; calculated from data in Oxman MN et al. *N Engl J Med.* 1995;352:2271.[28]

(eg, systemic lupus erythematous, rheumatoid arthritis). Many cases of herpes zoster that occur in patients with immune-mediated diseases are the result of the use of chemotherapy or therapy with immune modulators or corticosteroids.[40-43] Herpes zoster is a prominent and early "opportunistic infection" in persons infected with HIV, in whom it is often the first sign of immune deficiency.[44,45] Thus, HIV infection should be considered in young individuals who develop herpes zoster.

Other factors reported to correlate with the risk of herpes zoster include female sex,[32] physical trauma in the affected dermatome,[46] IL-10 gene polymorphisms,[47] family history of herpes zoster,[48-50] and white race.[31,32,51] The likelihood of recurrent herpes zoster is reported to range from 1% to 6%.[1,27,30,32] Much of this variation is dependent on the observation interval after the first episode of herpes zoster, as well as the accuracy of the diagnosis; not all of the cases reported may have actually been herpes zoster. Among the 19,276 placebo recipients in the Shingles Prevention Study followed for a median of 3.12 years,[28] the incidence of second episodes of documented herpes zoster was less than 1/10th the incidence of documented first episodes.

A large retrospective effectiveness study also indicated that the recurrence rate of herpes zoster in immunocompetent persons is low.[53] Recurrent herpes zoster is more common in patients who are immunocompromised, and they are more likely to have multidermatomal or bilateral disease.[52,54] Immunocompetent patients thought to be suffering multiple episodes of herpes zoster, especially when they occur in the same dermatome, are more likely to have recurrent zosteriform herpes simplex.[55] Second episodes of herpes zoster in immunocompetent persons almost always involve a different dermatome than that involved in the first episode.

Patients with herpes zoster are less contagious than patients with varicella. The rate at which susceptible household contacts develop varicella after exposure to herpes zoster appears to be about one-third of the rate observed following exposure to varicella.[1,56] Virus can be isolated from vesicles and pustules in uncomplicated herpes zoster for up to 7 days after the appearance of the rash, and for much longer periods in immunocompromised individuals. Patients with uncomplicated herpes zoster appear to spread the infection by means of direct contact with their lesions, although airborne transmission also has been documented.[57,58] Patients with disseminated herpes zoster may also transmit the infection via aerosols, so that airborne precautions, as well as contact precautions, are required for such patients.

The effect on the epidemiology of herpes zoster of the marked reduction in endemic varicella, due to widespread varicella vaccination of children, is unclear. A recent study showed that the age-specific incidence of HZ has increased >4-fold over the last 6 decades.[59] However, this temporal increase began before the availability of varicella vaccine; has occurred in countries without varicella vaccination programs[60-62]; was not altered by the introduction of varicella vaccination programs[13,59,63,64]; and has occurred in states that had a relatively low inclusion of children in varicella vaccination programs. These observations indicate that the reduction in exposure of adults to exogenous VZV due to varicella vaccination does not explain the temporal increase in the incidence of herpes zoster.[13,65,66] They also suggest that reactivations of endogenous latent VZV, in which rapid mobilization of host immune responses limits replication of the reactivated virus and prevents progression to herpes zoster ("neutralized reversions"[1,67]), is the major factor slowing the age-related decline in VZV-specific cell-mediated immunity observed in immunocompetent persons.

CLINICAL FEATURES

VARICELLA

PRODROME

In young children, prodromal symptoms are uncommon. In older children and adults, the rash is often preceded by 2 to 3 days of mild fever, chills, malaise, headache, anorexia, backache and, in some patients, sore throat and dry cough.

RASH

In unvaccinated persons, the rash usually begins on the face and scalp and spreads rapidly to the trunk, with relative sparing of the extremities.[1,68,69] New lesions appear in successive crops, and are mainly distributed centrally (Fig. 165-2A,B). The rash tends to be denser on the back between the shoulder blades than on the scapulae and buttocks, and more profuse on the medial than on the lateral aspects of the limbs. It is not uncommon to have a few lesions on the palms and soles, and vesicles often appear earlier and in larger numbers in areas of inflammation, such as diaper rash or sunburn.

A characteristic feature of varicella lesions is their rapid progression, over as little as 12 hours, from rose-colored macules to papules, and then to vesicles, pustules, and crusts (Fig. 165-2A-D). The typical vesicle is 2 to 3 mm in diameter and elliptical, with its long axis parallel to the folds of the skin. The early vesicle is superficial and thin-walled, and surrounded by an irregular area of erythema (Fig. 165-2C), which gives the lesions the appearance of a "dewdrop on a rose petal."[70] The vesicular fluid soon becomes cloudy with the influx of inflammatory cells that converts the vesicle to a pustule, which then dries, beginning in the center, producing an umbilicated pustule (Fig. 165-2E) and then a crust. Crusts fall off spontaneously in 1 to 3 weeks, leaving shallow pink depressions that gradually disappear. Scarring is rare unless the lesions were traumatized by the patient or superinfected with bacteria. Healing lesions may leave hypopigmented macules that persist for weeks to months; if scars occur, they are depressed and poxlike. In immunocompromised patients, lesions may lack surrounding erythema, and progression of vesicles to pustules may be delayed or absent (Fig. 165-2F).

Vesicles also develop in the mucous membranes of the mouth, nose, pharynx, larynx, trachea, esophagus, GI tract, urinary tract, and vagina. These mucosal vesicles rupture so rapidly that only shallow 2- to 3-mm ulcers remain and the vesicular stage is typically missed.

A distinctive feature of varicella is the simultaneous presence, in any one area of the skin, of lesions in all stages of development (Fig. 165-2A and B). Careful prospective studies have shown that the average number of lesions in healthy children is 250 to 500; secondary cases resulting from household exposure are more severe than cases resulting from exposure at school, presumably because more intense and prolonged exposure at home results in a higher virus inoculum.[21]

FEVER

Fever usually persists as long as new lesions continue to appear, and its height is generally proportional to the severity of the rash. It may be absent in mild cases or rise to 40.5°C (105°F) in severe cases with extensive rash. Prolonged fever or recurrence of fever after defervescence may signify a secondary bacterial infection or another complication.

PRURITUS

The most distressing symptom is pruritus, which is usually present until all lesions are crusted.

BREAKTHROUGH DISEASE

Approximately 10% to 15% of vaccinees immunized with a single dose of varicella vaccine develop "breakthrough" varicella after exposure to active VZV infections. Breakthrough varicella is usually atypical. The rash is predominantly maculopapular, with fewer lesions (less than 60) and fewer vesicles than the rash of unmodified varicella. These patients shed VZV, but are generally less contagious than patients who have not been immunized. The incidence and severity of fever is also less than that in natural varicella.[71] The routine administration of a second dose of varicella

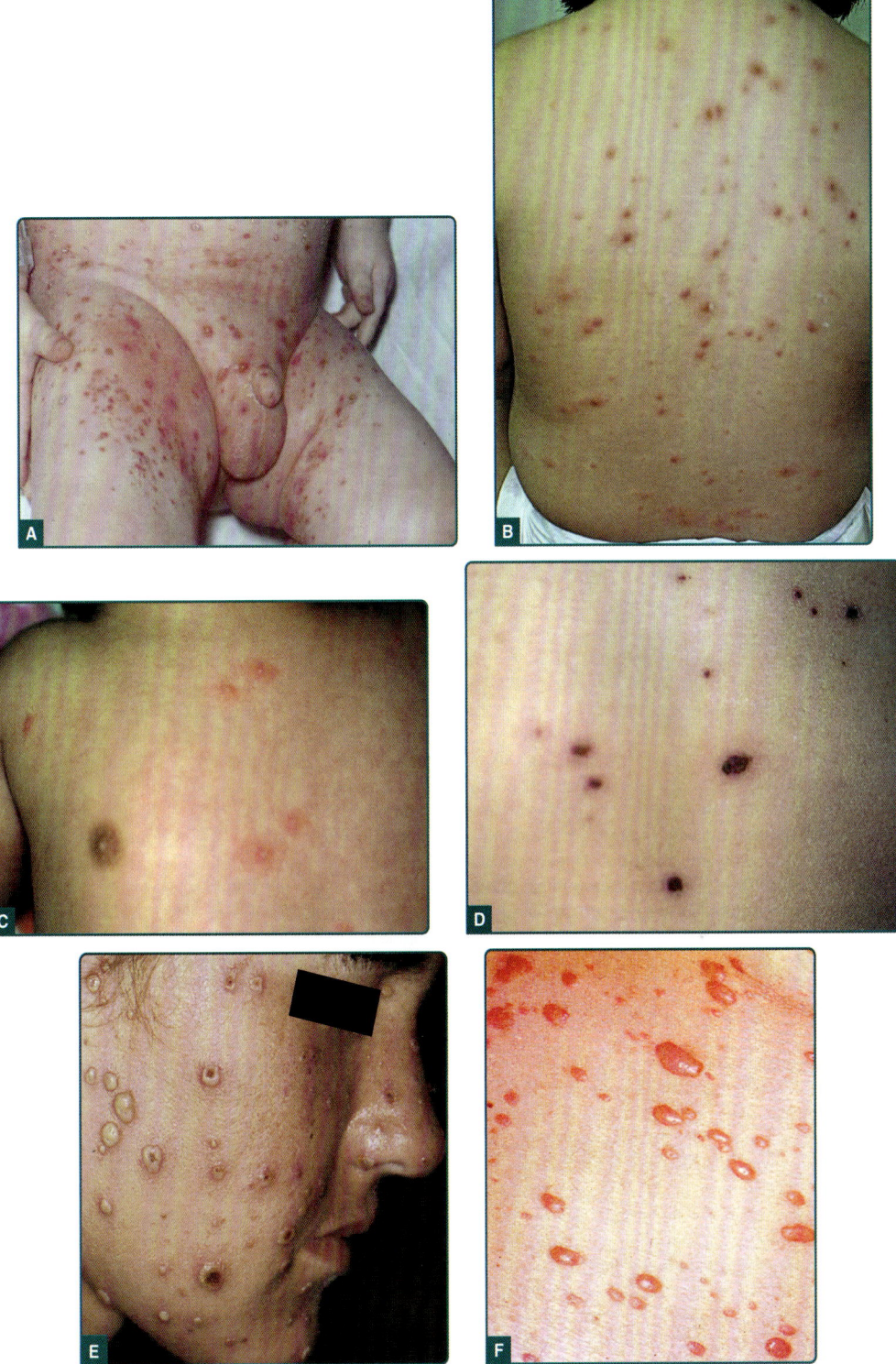

Figure 165-2 Varicella. **A** and **B,** Typical cases of varicella in two 4-year-old children. Note the presence of lesions in all stages of development and erosions at sites of excoriation. **C,** Early vesicles with surrounding erythema ("dewdrops on rose petals") in an immunocompetent child with varicella. **D,** Crusted lesions in the same child on rash day 3. **E,** Many large pustules and umbilicated pustules in a 21-year-old woman who was febrile and "toxic" and had varicella pneumonia. **F,** Varicella in an immunocompromised bone marrow transplant recipient. There are large numbers of vesicles, many of which have fused to form larger vesicles; none have progressed to pustules and none are surrounded by erythema. (Images **A-D,** Used with permission from Dr. M.G. Myers.)

vaccine has further reduced the incidence of varicella and greatly reduced the incidence of breakthrough disease.[18,66]

COMPLICATIONS OF VARICELLA

In the normal child, varicella is rarely complicated. The most common complication is secondary bacterial infection of skin lesions, usually by *Staphylococci* or *Streptococci*, which may produce impetigo, cellulitis, erysipelas, and, rarely, necrotizing fasciitis.[72] These local infections often lead to scarring and, rarely, to septicemia and metastatic infection. Bullous lesions may develop when vesicles are superinfected by *Staphylococci* that produce exfoliative toxins. Varicella is frequently complicated by invasive group A streptococcal infections, which usually occur within 2 weeks of the onset of the varicella rash and are particularly virulent.[73] In the prevaccine era, 15% to 30% of invasive group A streptococcal infections were associated with varicella. Widespread varicella vaccination has reduced the proportion of invasive group A streptococcal hospitalizations associated with varicella in the United States to 2%.[74]

In adults, fever and constitutional symptoms are more prominent and prolonged, the rash of varicella is more profuse, and complications are more frequent. A small number of patients develop varicella pneumonia, which is the major severe complication of varicella in adults. Varicella pneumonia is characterized by cough, dyspnea, tachypnea, high fever, pleuritic chest pain, cyanosis, and hemoptysis beginning 1 to 6 days after rash onset. The severity of the symptoms usually exceeds the physical findings, but imaging typically reveals diffuse, peribronchial nodular densities throughout both lung fields with a tendency to concentrate in the perihilar regions and at the bases. The mortality in adults with frank varicella pneumonia is estimated to be between 10% and 30%, but it is less than 10% if immunocompromised patients are excluded and patients receive prompt antiviral therapy.[75]

Varicella during pregnancy is a threat to both mother and fetus.[76] Disseminated infection and varicella pneumonia may result in maternal death, but neither the incidence nor the severity of varicella pneumonia appear to be significantly increased by pregnancy.[77] The fetus may die as a consequence of premature labor or maternal death caused by severe varicella pneumonia, but varicella during pregnancy does not, otherwise, substantially increase fetal mortality. However, even in uncomplicated varicella, maternal viremia can result in intrauterine (congenital) VZV infection that results in a characteristic constellation of congenital abnormalities.[76] The overall risk of congenital varicella syndrome is about 1% when maternal varicella occurs during the first 20 weeks of gestation, with the highest risk (2%) when maternal varicella occurs between 13 and 20 weeks.[76] Perinatal varicella (occurring within 10 days of birth) is much more serious than varicella in infants infected even a few weeks later.[78]

The morbidity and mortality of varicella are markedly increased in immunocompromised patients. In these patients, continued virus replication and dissemination result in a prolonged high-level viremia, more extensive rash, prolongation of new vesicle formation, and clinically significant visceral involvement. Severe abdominal and back pain are common prodromal symptoms of severe varicella with visceral dissemination in immunocompromised patients.[79] Immunocompromised patients may also develop pneumonia, hepatitis, encephalitis, and hemorrhagic complications of varicella, which range in severity from mild febrile purpura to severe and often fatal purpura fulminans with disseminated intravascular coagulation.

CNS complications of varicella include several distinct syndromes. Formerly common, varicella-associated Reye syndrome (acute encephalopathy with fatty degeneration of the liver) is now very rare since the etiologic role of salicylates was recognized and their use in children with fever contraindicated.[80] Acute cerebellar ataxia is more common than other neurologic complications of varicella, occurring in 1 in 4000 cases, but it has an excellent prognosis.[81] Encephalitis is much less common (1 per 33,000 cases), but frequently causes death or permanent neurologic sequelae. The pathogenesis of cerebellar ataxia and encephalitis remains obscure, but in many cases it is possible to detect VZV antigens, VZV antibodies, and VZV DNA in the cerebrospinal fluid of patients, suggesting direct infection of the CNS.

Although mildly elevated aminotransferase levels are common during varicella, clinical hepatitis is rare, except as a complication in immunocompromised patients. Other rare complications of varicella include myocarditis, glomerulonephritis, orchitis, pancreatitis, gastritis and ulcerative lesions of the bowel, arthritis, Henoch-Schönlein vasculitis, optic neuritis, keratitis, and iritis. Most are likely due to parenchymal or endovascular VZV infection.

HERPES ZOSTER

PRODROME

Pain and paresthesia in the involved dermatome often precede the eruption by 1 to 3 days, but occasionally by a week or longer. Abnormal sensations vary from superficial itching, tingling, or burning to severe, deep, boring, or lancinating pain. The pain may be constant or intermittent, and it is often accompanied by tenderness and hyperesthesia of the skin in the involved dermatome. The prodromal pain of herpes zoster may be confused with pain from disease in a visceral organ (such as myocardial infarction, cholecystitis, renal colic, prolapsed intervertebral disk), and this may lead to misdiagnosis and misdirected investigations and interventions.[68] Prodromal pain is uncommon in immunocompetent persons younger than 30 years, but it occurs in the majority of persons with herpes zoster over the age of 60 years. A few patients experience acute segmental neuralgia without ever developing a cutaneous eruption—a condition known as *zoster sine herpete*.[83]

RASH

The most distinctive feature of herpes zoster is the localization and distribution of the rash, which is unilateral and is generally limited to the area of skin innervated by a single sensory ganglion (Fig. 165-3A,B). The skin supplied by the trigeminal nerve, particularly the ophthalmic division (10%-15%), and the trunk from T3 to L2 (>50%), are most frequently affected; herpes zoster lesions are uncommon distal to the elbows or knees.[1,30,68,69]

Although the individual lesions of herpes zoster and varicella are histologically indistinguishable, those of herpes zoster tend to evolve more slowly and usually consist of closely grouped vesicles on an erythematous base, rather than the more discrete, randomly distributed vesicles of varicella (Fig. 165-3C,D). This difference reflects intraneural (axonal) spread of virus to the skin in herpes zoster, as opposed to viremic spread in varicella. Herpes zoster lesions begin as erythematous macules and papules in a dermatomal distribution. Vesicles form within 12 to 24 hours and evolve into pustules by the third day (Fig. 165-3E). These dry and crust in 7 to 10 days. The crusts generally persist for 2 to 3 weeks. In normal individuals, new lesions continue to appear for 1 to 4 days (occasionally for as long as 7 days). The rash is most severe and lasts longest in older people, and is least severe and of shortest duration in children.

Between 10% and 15% of cases of herpes zoster involve the ophthalmic division of the trigeminal nerve (Fig. 165-4A,B).[84] The rash of ophthalmic zoster may extend from the level of the eye to the vertex of the skull, but it terminates sharply at the midline of the forehead. When only the supratrochlear and supraorbital branches are involved, the eye is usually spared. Involvement of the nasociliary branch, which innervates the eye, as well as the tip and side of the nose, provides VZV with direct access to intraocular structures. Thus, when ophthalmic zoster involves the tip and the side of the nose (Hutchinson sign), careful attention must be given to the condition of the eye. Involvement of the nasociliary branch is frequently accompanied by unilateral conjunctivitis and impaired corneal sensation, which can lead to corneal ulceration and sight-threatening bacterial infection. The eye is involved in 20% to 70% of patients with ophthalmic zoster.

Herpes zoster affecting the second and third divisions of the trigeminal nerve (Fig. 165-4C,D), as well as other cranial nerves, may produce symptoms and lesions in the mouth (Fig. 165-4E,F), ears, pharynx, or larynx. The Ramsay Hunt syndrome (facial palsy in combination with herpes zoster of the external ear, ear canal, or tympanic membrane, with or without tinnitus, vertigo, and deafness) results from involvement of the facial and auditory nerves. The ear and external auditory canal are innervated by the 5th, 7th, 9th, and 10th cranial nerves and by the upper cervical nerves, and the facial nerve anastomoses with all of them. Thus, when herpes zoster involves the ganglia of any of these nerves it may cause facial paralysis and cutaneous lesions on or around the ear[68] (Fig. 165-4G,H).

PAIN

Although the rash is important, pain is the cardinal symptom of herpes zoster, especially in the elderly. Some patients with herpes zoster do not experience pain, but most (>85% over age 50) have dermatomal pain or discomfort during the acute phase (the first 30 days following rash onset) that ranges from mild to severe. Patients describe their pain or discomfort as "burning," "deep aching," "tingling," or "stabbing." In some patients, itching may be the predominant symptom. For some patients, the pain intensity is so great that words like "horrible" or "excruciating" are used to describe the experience. Acute herpes zoster pain is associated with decreased physical functioning, emotional distress, and decreased social functioning.[85,86]

PRURITUS

Itching is often a prominent and distressing symptom throughout the acute phase of herpes zoster. It frequently persists until all crusts have fallen off.

COMPLICATIONS OF HERPES ZOSTER

See Table 165-1.

The sequelae of herpes zoster include cutaneous, ocular, neurologic, and visceral complications.[68] Most are associated with the spread of VZV from the initially involved sensory ganglion, nerve, or skin, either via the bloodstream or by direct neural extension, including involvement of the spinal cord. The rash may disseminate after the initial dermatomal eruption has become apparent. When immunocompetent patients are carefully examined, it is not uncommon to identify a few vesicles in areas distant from the involved and immediately adjacent dermatomes, especially as age increases. The disseminated lesions usually appear within a week of the onset of the segmental eruption and, if few in number, are easily overlooked and are not problematic. More extensive dissemination (with 25-50 lesions or more), producing a varicella-like eruption (disseminated herpes zoster, Fig. 165-5), may occur in immunocompromised patients. If the rash spreads widely from a small, painless area of herpes zoster, the initial dermatomal presentation may go unnoticed, and the ensuing disseminated eruption may be mistaken for varicella.[25,68]

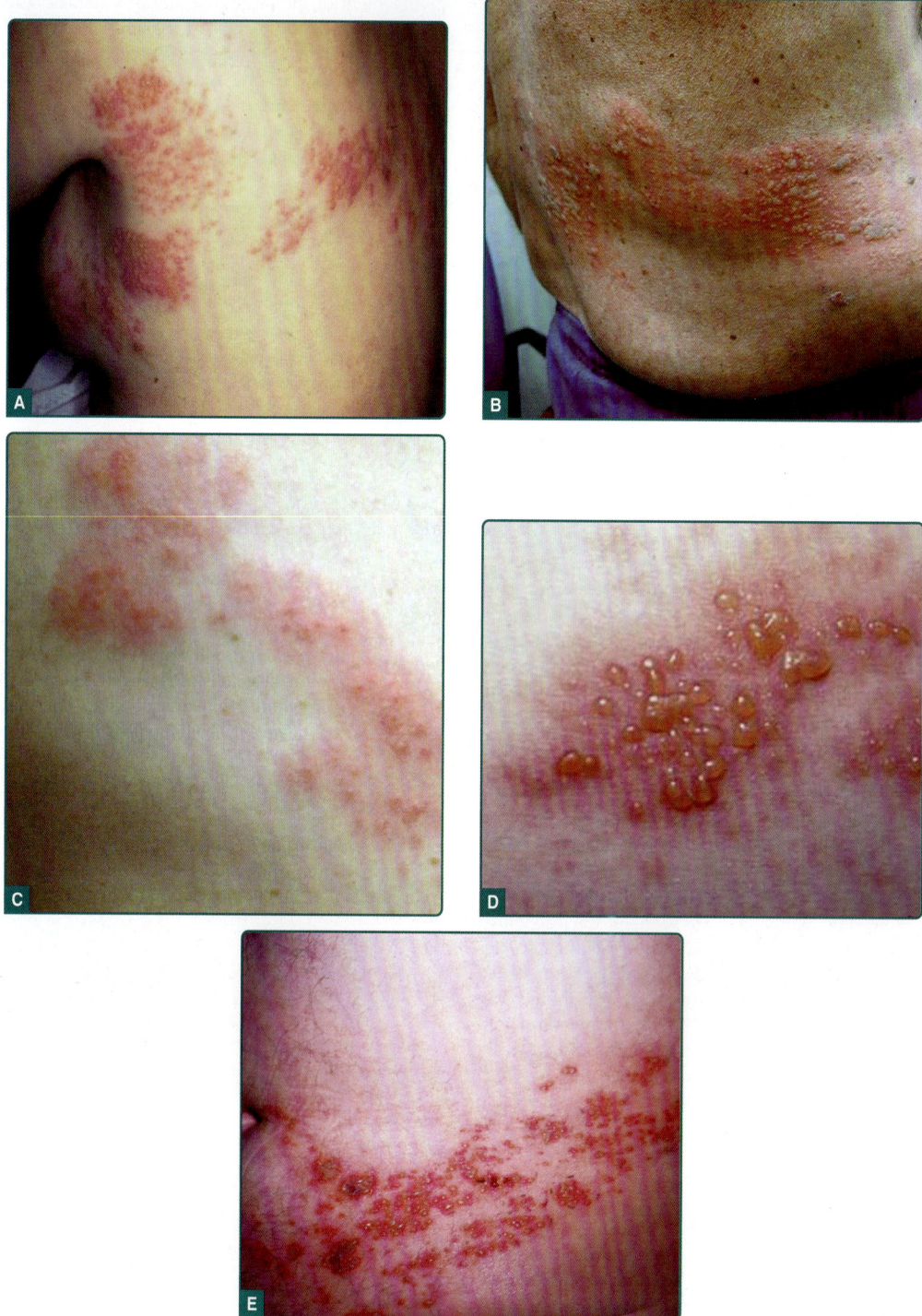

Figure 165-3 Herpes zoster. **A,** Classical herpes zoster in the left T4 dermatome. Note the concentration of lesions in areas of the dermatome innervated by the posterior primary division and the lateral branch of the anterior primary division of the left T4 spinal nerve. **B,** Right T10 herpes zoster with numerous pustular lesions. **C,** Early lesions of herpes zoster. Note the closely grouped vesicles on a confluent erythematous base, in contrast to the discrete randomly distributed vesicles of varicella (Fig. 165-2). **D,** Clustered vesicular lesions of herpes zoster. **E,** Left T8 herpes zoster with numerous pustular lesions and early crusting.

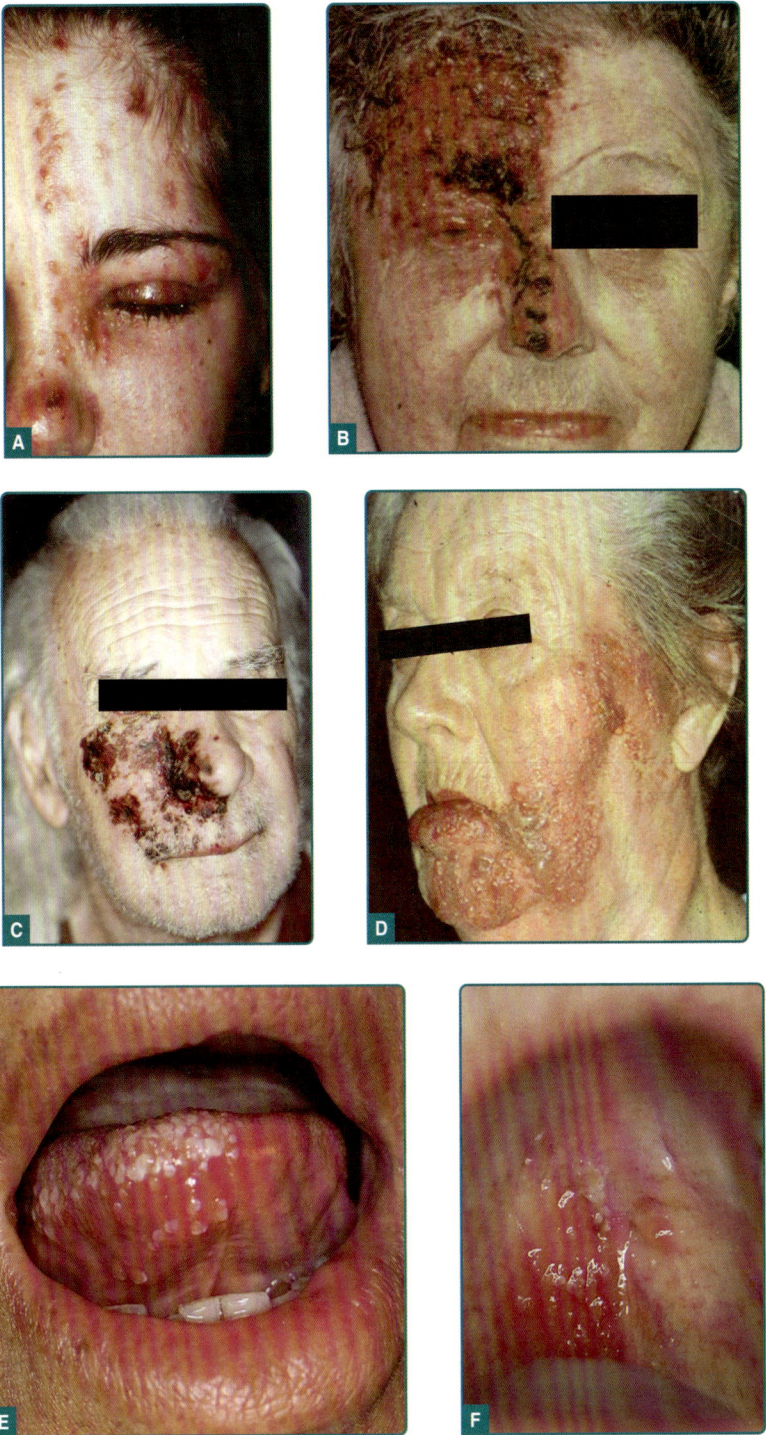

Figure 165-4 Herpes zoster involving cranial nerves. **A** and **B,** Ophthalmic herpes zoster involving the first (ophthalmic) division of the fifth cranial nerve (V1). Involvement of the nasociliary branch, as evidenced by lesions on the tip and side of the nose (Hutchinson sign), provides VZV with direct access to the eye. This is frequently accompanied by unilateral conjunctivitis and impaired corneal sensation, which can lead to corneal ulceration and sight-threatening bacterial infection. **A,** Left ophthalmic herpes zoster with involvement of the nasociliary branch, as evidenced by lesions on the tip and side of the nose (Hutchinson sign). **B,** Severe right ophthalmic herpes zoster with involvement of the nasociliary nerve and eye, as well as superficial gangrene. **C,** Herpes zoster involving the second division of the right fifth cranial nerve (V2). **D,** Herpes zoster involving the third division of the left fifth cranial nerve (V3). **E** and **F,** Cranial nerve herpes zoster in a 60-year-old woman with right-sided facial palsy (Hunt syndrome) and vesicles on her tongue (**E**) and palate (**F**). **G** & **H,** Ramsey Hunt Syndrome: An 83-year-old woman developed left ear pain and fever followed by an erythematous vesicular rash involving her left ear

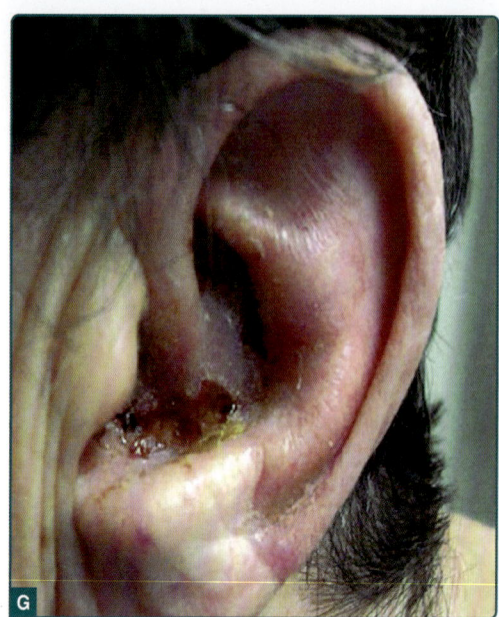 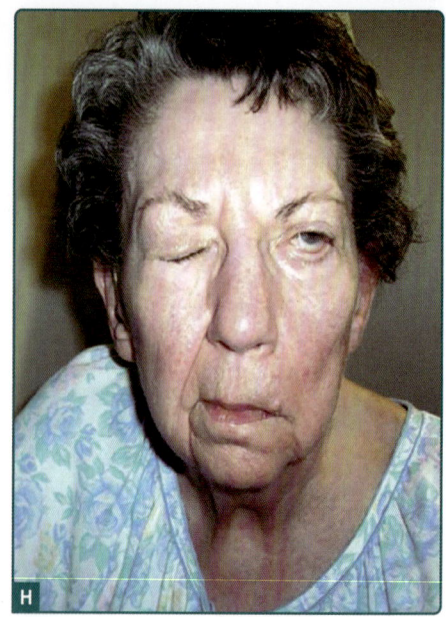

Figure 165-4 (*Continued*) (**G**) with left-sided hearing loss and left facial paresis (**H**). She also had evidence of involvement of the other cranial nerves as indicated by difficulty swallowing, leftward tongue protrusion, hoarse dysphonia and absent palatal elevation on the left. Despite treatment with oral acyclovir, 800 mg 5 times daily for 10 days, she had no resolution of her left-sided hearing loss and facial paresis 4 months later. (Images G and H, Reproduced with permission from Espay AJ, Bull RL: *Arch Neurol*. 2005;62(11):1774-1775. Copyright © 2005 American Medical Association. All rights reserved.)

TABLE 165-1
Complications of Herpes Zoster

CUTANEOUS	VISCERAL	NEUROLOGIC
▪ Bacterial superinfection	▪ Pneumonitis	▪ Postherpetic neuralgia
▪ Scarring	▪ Hepatitis	▪ Meningoencephalitis
▪ Zoster gangrenosum	▪ Esophagitis	▪ Transverse myelitis
▪ Cutaneous dissemination	▪ Gastritis	
	▪ Pericarditis	▪ Peripheral nerve palsies
	▪ Cystitis	Motor
	▪ Arthritis	Autonomic
		▪ Cranial nerve palsies
		▪ Sensory loss
		▪ Deafness
		▪ Ocular complications
		▪ Granulomatous angiitis (causing contralateral hemiparesis)

When the dermatomal rash is particularly extensive, as it often is in severely immunocompromised patients, there may be superficial gangrene with delayed healing and subsequent scarring (Fig. 165-3B). Secondary bacterial infection (usually with *Staphylococci* or *Streptococci*) may delay healing and cause scarring in both immunocompetent and immunocompromised patients.

Ophthalmic zoster may be accompanied by a wide range of complications.[84] Corneal sensation is generally impaired and, when that impairment is severe, it may lead to neurotrophic keratitis with chronic ulceration and bacterial infection.

Herpes zoster may be attended by a variety of neurologic complications, of which postherpetic neuralgia (PHN) is the most common and important.[87] PHN has been variably defined as pain after rash healing, or any pain 1 month, 3 months, 4 months, or 6 months after rash onset.[88-91] The prevalence of PHN was reported to be 5% to 30% in a systematic review of 49 studies published between 1945 and 2012 that encompassed a wide variety of PHN definitions and patient ages.[27] Age is the most significant risk factor for PHN (Fig. 165-1B). Clinically significant pain lasting 3 months or more is rare in immunocompetent persons younger than 50 years of age. In a large UK general practice database study, PHN defined as any pain ≥3 months from rash onset was 11%, 13%, 15%, 18%, and 21% in patients ages 60-64, 65-69, 70-74, 75-79, and 80-84 years, respectively.[92] A meta-analysis of 18 cohort studies found that the incidence of PHN increased by 1.22% to 3.11% for each 10-year increase in age.[93] Other risk factors for PHN include the presence of prodromal pain, severe pain during the acute phase of herpes zoster, extensive rash, and significant sensory abnormalities in the affected dermatome.

PHN usually remits gradually over several months (Figs. 165-1C) but, as with the incidence of PHN, its duration increases with increasing age.

Patients with PHN may suffer from constant pain (described as "burning," "aching," or "throbbing"), intermittent lancinating pain ("stabbing," "shooting"), and/or stimulus-evoked pain, including allodynia ("tender," "burning," "stabbing"). Allodynia, which is pain elicited by stimuli that are normally not painful, is a particularly disabling component of the disease that is present in approximately 90% of patients with PHN.[94] Patients with allodynia may suffer severe pain after even the lightest touch to the affected skin, such as by a breeze or by contact with clothing. PHN often results in disordered sleep, depression, anorexia, weight loss, chronic fatigue, and social isolation, and it may interfere with dressing, bathing, general activity, traveling, shopping, cooking, and housework.[93]

Dorsal root ganglia contain visceral, as well as cutaneous, afferent neurons, which likely explains the occurrence of visceral as well as cutaneous lesions in patients with herpes zoster. The affected viscera usually have afferent innervation corresponding to the infected dermatome. Thus, herpes zoster lesions in the gastric mucosa are observed in patients with thoracic herpes zoster, hemicystitis is observed in patients with sacral herpes zoster, and herpes zoster in other dermatomes can result in mucosal lesions causing esophagitis, pleuritis, and peritonitis. Infection via visceral afferents originating in mechanoreceptors involved with GI and bladder motility and sphincter function can result in ileus, symptoms of GI obstruction, and dysfunction of the bladder and anus. Transmission of ganglionic infection via proprioceptive afferents can also result in myositis.[68] Latent VZV in enteric neurons provides another potential source of virus causing visceral complications, which may explain episodes of visceral herpes zoster in the absence of skin lesions.[95] Innervation of cerebral blood vessels by neurons in cranial and dorsal root ganglia accounts for a syndrome of ophthalmic herpes zoster and delayed contralateral hemiplegia.[96-98] VZV from infected neurons in the involved ganglion infects these cerebral arteries, causing segmental granulomatous angiitis that results in a contralateral stroke, which may occur weeks to months after the episode of ophthalmic herpes zoster (average interval = 7-8 weeks); the delayed onset of the contralateral stroke may obscure its relationship to the episode of ophthalmic herpes zoster.[96-98] Although most cases have followed ophthalmic herpes zoster and involved the ipsilateral middle and anterior cerebral arteries, some have followed herpes zoster in other cranial and cervical dermatomes. Evidence also has been presented associating temporal arteritis, myocardial infarction, and aortic aneurysms due to granulomatous angiitis with reactivation of latent VZV.[99,100] Other studies of this relationship have not always been confirmatory, and these associations remain controversial.[101-104]

Most serious complications of herpes zoster are more common in immunocompromised persons. These include necrosis of skin and scarring, and cutaneous dissemination (Fig. 165-5). Patients with cutaneous dissemination

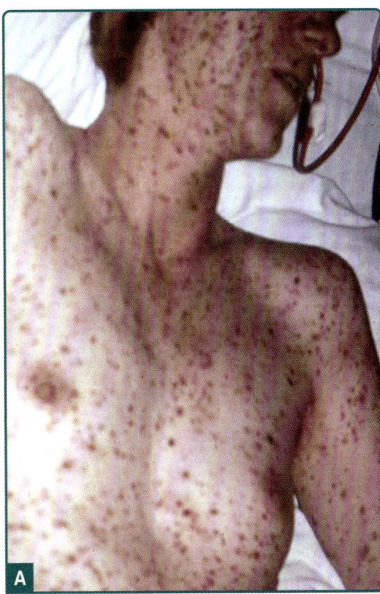
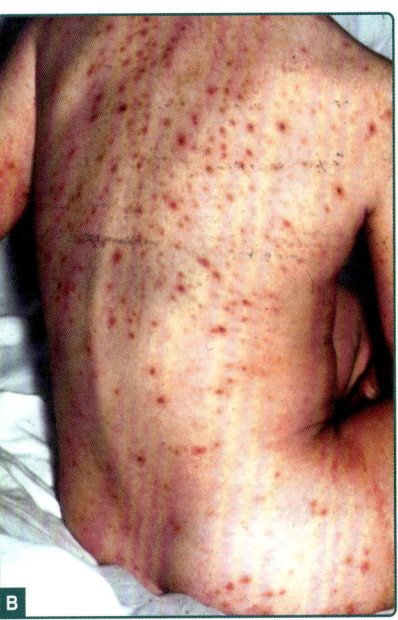

Figure 165-5 Disseminated herpes zoster. **A** and **B**, An immunocompromised adult with leukemia on treatment with disseminated herpes zoster and varicella-zoster virus pneumonia.

may also have widespread, often fatal, visceral dissemination, particularly to the lungs, liver, and brain.

HIV-infected patients who are not treated with combination antiretroviral therapy often suffer multiple recurrences of herpes zoster as their HIV infection progresses. Recurrences may be in the same or different dermatomes or in several contiguous or noncontiguous dermatomes. Cutaneous and visceral dissemination may also occur in patients with untreated HIV infection. In addition, patients with AIDS may develop chronic verrucous, hyperkeratotic, or ecthymatous cutaneous lesions caused

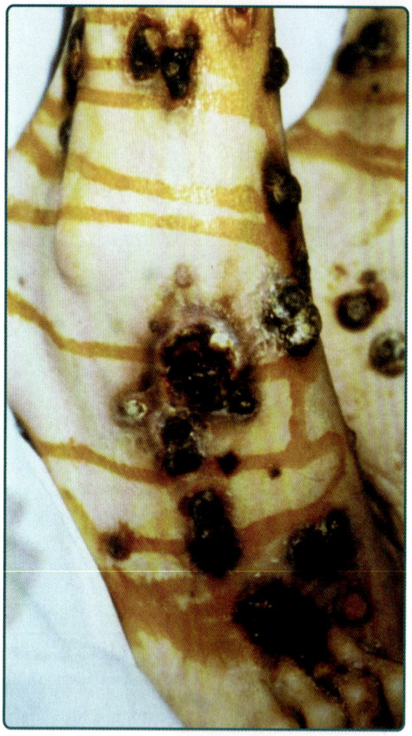

Figure 165-6 Chronic disseminated herpes zoster caused by acyclovir-resistant varicella-zoster virus in an immunocompromised patient. Chronic verrucous lesions disseminated herpes zoster caused by acyclovir-resistant varicella-zoster virus in an immunocompromised patient with AIDS. (Used with permission from Dr. V. Asensi.)

by acyclovir-resistant VZV (Fig. 165-6) (see also Chap. 168). These manifestations of severe HIV infection are rare in the current era of effective antiretroviral therapy for HIV infection.

ETIOLOGY AND PATHOGENESIS

VZV is a member of the herpesvirus family. All herpesviruses are morphologically indistinguishable and share a number of properties, including the capacity to establish latent infections that persist for life. VZV and herpes simplex virus (Types I and II) are further classified as α-herpesviruses because they become latent in sensory neurons after primary infection.

The VZV genome contains at least 71 genes, most of which have functional and DNA-sequence homology to genes of other herpesviruses.[105] Immediate early gene products regulate VZV replication. Early gene products, such as VZV thymidine kinase and VZV DNA polymerase, support virus replication, whereas late genes encode virus structural proteins. There is only 1 VZV serotype. However, there are 7 or 8 VZV genotypes (clades) that display geographic segregation and recombination.[106,107] Variations in nucleotide sequences allow one to distinguish wildtype from vaccine virus strains, and to "fingerprint" viruses isolated from individual patients.[105,108-110]

PATHOGENESIS OF VARICELLA

Entry of VZV is through the mucosa of the upper respiratory tract and oropharynx, where VZV infects tonsillar T cells that disseminate virus via the blood and lymphatics (the primary viremia). Infected T cells carry virus to the reticuloendothelial system, the major site of virus replication during the remainder of the incubation period, and to the skin. Viremia occurs early in the incubation period, but VZV replication and rash formation are delayed by innate immune responses, for example, by interferon and natural killer cells, and by developing VZV-specific immune responses.[105,111,112]

Virus replication eventually overcomes these host defenses, so that some 10 to 14 days after infection a much larger (secondary) viremia occurs, resulting in systemic symptoms and skin lesions. In addition, immunopathology contributes to rash development. Skin lesions appear in successive crops, reflecting a cyclic viremia that in the normal host is terminated after about 3 to 5 days by VZV-specific immune responses, primarily VZV-specific T cell–mediated immune responses. Virus circulates in mononuclear leukocytes, primarily lymphocytes. Even in uncomplicated varicella, viremia results in subclinical infection of many organs in addition to the skin. T cell–mediated immunity to VZV is required for recovery from varicella. The immunologic memory that develops during varicella persists for life and is essential to protect against second episodes of varicella and against herpes zoster.[1,29,111,112]

PATHOGENESIS OF HERPES ZOSTER

During varicella, VZV passes from lesions in the skin and mucosal surfaces into contiguous endings of sensory nerves and is transported up the sensory fibers to the sensory ganglia. In the ganglia, the virus establishes latent infections in neurons that persist for life. The density of latent VZV is greatest in ganglia innervating areas of skin with the greatest density of varicella lesions. Consequently, herpes zoster occurs most often in dermatomes where the rash of varicella is most dense-skin innervated by the first (ophthalmic) division of the trigeminal ganglion and by spinal sensory ganglia from T1 to L2.[1,68,69] The viremia that occurs during varicella may provide VZV with another means to access sensory neurons.

Latent VZV in ganglia produces a latency-associated transcript (LAT) homologous to that produced by latent HSV, but no infectious virus.[113] However, latent

VZV may reactivate sporadically, producing infectious virus. The frequency and mechanism of these reactivations are unknown, but VZV reactivation and replication resulting in HZ has been associated most clearly with immunosuppression. VZV may also reactivate without producing overt disease; presumably, because replication and spread of the reactivated virus is terminated by preexisting or rapidly mobilized VZV-specific immunity. The small quantity of viral antigen released during such "contained reactivations" is postulated to stimulate and sustain host immunity to VZV.[1,67,114]

When VZV-specific T cell–mediated immunity falls below some critical level, reactivated virus can no longer be contained.[1,29] Virus multiplies and spreads within the ganglion, causing neuronal necrosis and intense inflammation, processes that are often accompanied by severe neuropathic pain.[115,116] VZV then spreads antidromically down the sensory nerve, and is released from the sensory nerve endings in the skin, where it produces the characteristic cluster of zoster vesicles. Spread of the ganglionic infection proximally along the posterior nerve root to the meninges and spinal cord may result in local leptomeningitis, cerebrospinal fluid pleocytosis, and segmental myelitis. Infection and destruction of neurons in the dorsal horn may play a role in persistent neuropathic pain (see section "Pathogenesis of Pain in Herpes Zoster and Postherpetic Neuralgia" below); infection of motor neurons in the anterior horn and inflammation of the anterior nerve root account for the local palsies that may accompany the cutaneous eruption.[115] Extension of infection within the CNS may result in rare complications of herpes zoster, such as meningoencephalitis or transverse myelitis. Viremia also occurs during herpes zoster.[23]

PATHOGENESIS OF PAIN IN HERPES ZOSTER AND POSTHERPETIC NEURALGIA

A number of different but overlapping mechanisms, which vary from patient to patient and over time in any individual patient, appear to be involved in the pathogenesis of pain in herpes zoster and in PHN.[91,117-119] Injury to the peripheral nerve and to neurons in the ganglion trigger afferent pain signals (neuropathic pain). Inflammation in the skin triggers nociceptive pain signals that further amplify this pain. Damage to neurons in the spinal cord and ganglion, and to the peripheral nerve, is important in the pathogenesis of PHN. Postmortem examination of patients with herpes zoster and severe PHN compared with patients with herpes zoster and no persistent pain demonstrated dorsal horn atrophy and cell, axon, and myelin loss with fibrosis in sensory ganglia only in patients with persistent pain.[115] Damaged primary afferent nerves may become spontaneously active and hypersensitive to peripheral stimuli, and also to sympathetic stimulation. Excessive nociceptor activity and ectopic impulse generation may, in turn, sensitize CNS neurons, augmenting and prolonging central responses to innocuous as well as noxious stimuli.[91,118-121] Clinically, these mechanisms result in allodynia.

DIAGNOSIS

CLINICAL DIAGNOSIS

VARICELLA

Varicella can usually be diagnosed by the appearance and evolution of the rash (see Fig. 165-2), particularly when there is a history of exposure within the preceding 2 to 3 weeks. The rapid evolution of lesions from macules to papules, to vesicles, to pustules and crusts, and the simultaneous presence of lesions at all stages of development, distinguish varicella from most other generalized rashes.

Disseminated herpes zoster may be mistaken for varicella, especially when there is widespread dissemination of VZV from a small, painless area of herpes zoster or from the affected sensory ganglion in the absence of an obvious dermatomal eruption. Although disseminated HSV infections may resemble varicella, this is a rare disease that is limited to severely immunocompromised patients. There is usually an obvious concentration of lesions at and surrounding the site of the primary or recurrent infection, for example, the mouth or external genitalia, and there is often marked toxicity and visceral involvement.

The remaining differential diagnoses of varicelliform rashes are listed in Table 165-2. The character, distribution, and evolution of the lesions, together with a careful epidemiologic history, usually differentiate these diseases from varicella. When any doubt exists, the clinical impression should be confirmed by laboratory testing.

HERPES ZOSTER

In the preeruptive stage, the prodromal pain of herpes zoster is often confused with other causes of localized pain. Once the eruption appears, the character and dermatomal location of the rash, coupled with dermatomal pain and localized sensory abnormalities, usually makes the diagnosis obvious (Figs. 165-3 and 165-4).[68]

A cluster of vesicles, particularly near the mouth or genitals, may represent herpes zoster, but it also may be recurrent HSV infection (Fig. 165-7).[55] Zosteriform herpes simplex is often impossible to distinguish from herpes zoster on clinical grounds. In the absence of profound and clinically obvious immune deficiency, a history of multiple recurrences in the same dermatome distinguishes zosteriform herpes simplex from herpes zoster. Table 165-2 lists other considerations in the differential diagnosis of herpes zoster.

TABLE 165-2
Differential Diagnosis of Varicella and Herpes Zoster

VARICELLA	HERPES ZOSTER
Most Likely	**Most Likely**
▪ Vesicular exanthems of Coxsackieviruses and echoviruses ▪ Eczema herpeticum ▪ Disseminated herpes zoster ▪ Impetigo ▪ Insect bites ▪ Contact dermatitis ▪ Rickettsialpox ▪ Disseminated herpes simplex[a]	▪ Zosteriform herpes simplex ▪ Contact dermatitis ▪ Insect bites ▪ Burns
Consider	**Consider**
▪ Papular urticaria ▪ Erythema multiforme ▪ Drug eruptions ▪ Disseminated herpes simplex ▪ Molluscum contagiosum ▪ PLEVA[b] ▪ Scabies ▪ Secondary syphilis ▪ Dermatitis herpetiformis ▪ Bullous pemphigoid ▪ Pemphigus vulgaris	▪ Papular urticaria ▪ Erythema multiforme[a] ▪ Drug eruptions[a] ▪ Scabies ▪ Molluscum contagiosum ▪ Bullous pemphigoid (isotopic response)

[a]May resemble disseminated herpes zoster.
[b]Pityriasis lichenoides et varioliformis acuta.

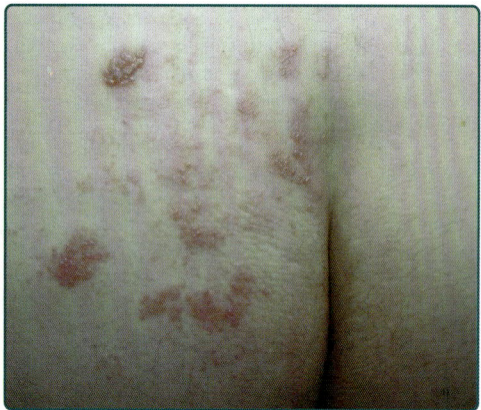

Figure 165-7 Zosteriform herpes simplex. This immunocompetent adult with no history of genital herpes or prior herpetic lesions presented with a 1-day history of mild tenderness of her left buttock, followed by the onset of the clustered vesicular lesions in her left S2/S3 dermatomes. They were mildly tender and pruritic. PCR assay and viral culture both revealed HSV-2.

LABORATORY DIAGNOSIS

The lesions of varicella and herpes zoster are indistinguishable by histopathology (Fig. 165-8). VZV infection of the skin is initiated by infection of epithelial cells in the basal layer (stratum germinativum) and the stratum spinosum. The resulting papular lesions evolve into intraepithelial vesicles within 12 to 24 hours as a result of infection of increasing numbers of epithelial cells, which show acanthosis, "ballooning degeneration," eosinophilic (acidophilic) intranuclear inclusion bodies, and multinucleated giant cell formation. An influx of edema fluid elevates the uninvolved stratum corneum to form a delicate clear vesicle containing large amounts of cell-free infectious virus and multinucleated giant cells with eosinophilic intranuclear inclusion bodies (Fig. 165-8A,B). The multinucleated giant cells form by fusion of infected epithelial cells with adjacent infected and uninfected cells at the base and periphery of the vesicle. The underlying dermis shows edema and mononuclear cell infiltration. The presence of multinucleated giant cells and epithelial cells containing acidophilic intranuclear inclusion bodies distinguishes the cutaneous lesions produced by VZV from all other vesicular eruptions, such as those caused by poxviruses, Coxsackieviruses, and echoviruses, except for those produced by HSV. These cells can be demonstrated in Tzanck smears prepared at the bedside from material scraped from the base of vesicular lesions and stained with hematoxylin and eosin, Giemsa, or similar stains (Fig. 165-8C). When virus-containing vesicle fluid is inoculated into human fibroblast tissue cultures, similar multinucleated giant cells containing acidophilic intranuclear inclusion bodies form by fusion of infected cells with adjacent infected and uninfected cells (Fig. 165-8D).

The best diagnostic test for detection of VZV is polymerase chain reaction (PCR) because of its very high sensitivity and specificity, ready availability, and relatively quick (1 day or less) turnaround time.[110,122,123] Vesicle fluid is the best specimen for PCR analysis, but lesion scrapings, crusts, tissue biopsy, or cerebrospinal fluid are equally useful. PCR can distinguish VZV from HSV, and wildtype VZV from Oka vaccine strains of VZV.[110] Isolation of virus is less sensitive and may take a week or more, but it is the only technique that yields infectious VZV for further analysis, such as determination of sensitivity to antiviral drugs. VZV is extremely labile, and only 30% to 60% of cultures from proven cases are generally positive. To maximize virus recovery, specimens should be inoculated into cell culture immediately. It is important to select new vesicles containing clear fluid for aspiration, because the probability of isolating VZV diminishes rapidly as lesions become pustular. VZV is almost never isolated from crusts.

Immunofluorescent or immunoperoxidase staining of cellular material from fresh vesicles or prevesicular lesions can detect VZV significantly more often and faster than virus culture.[124] Enzyme immunoassays provide another rapid and sensitive method for antigen detection. These techniques have a somewhat faster turnaround time than PCR, but lack the excellent sensitivity and specificity of PCR, which remains the diagnostic method of choice.[122,123]

Serologic tests permit the retrospective diagnosis of varicella and herpes zoster when acute and convalescent sera are available for comparison, but this is rarely

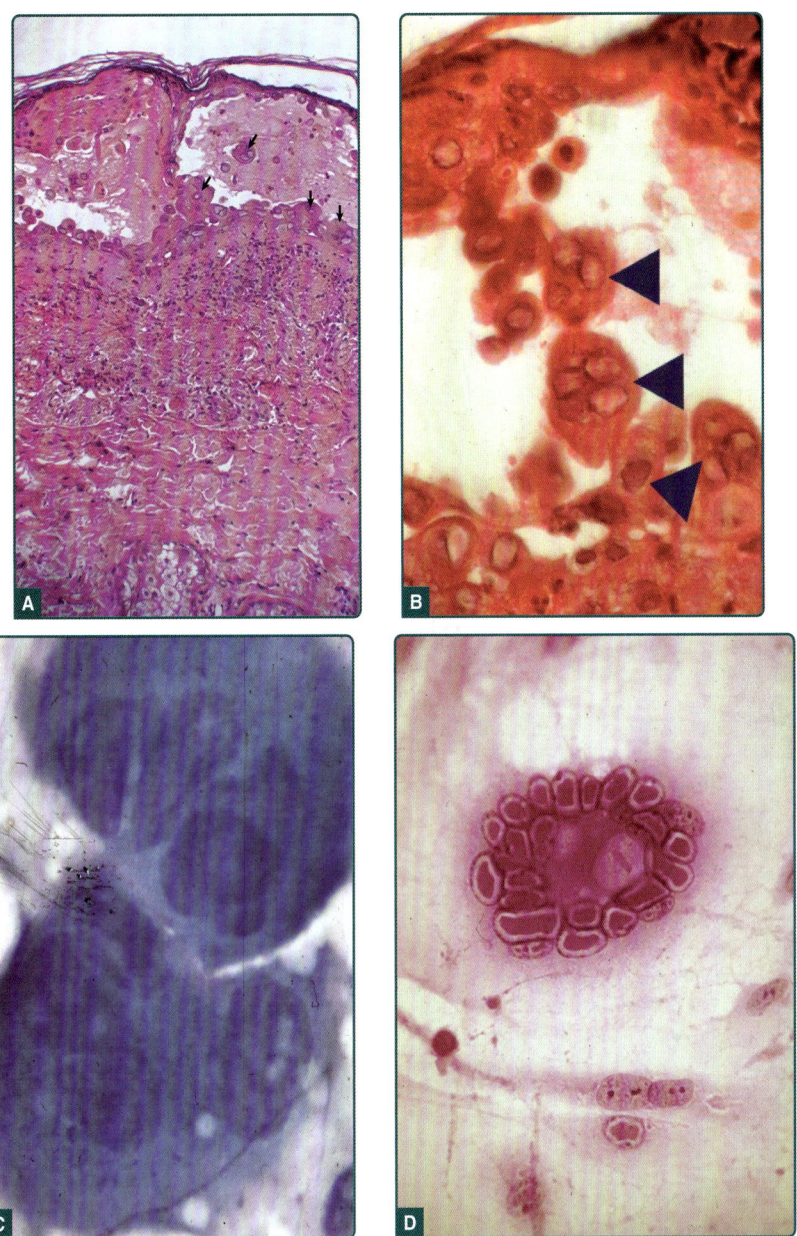

Figure 165-8. Varicella zoster histopathology. **A** and **B,** Papular lesions of varicella evolve into intraepithelial vesicles within 12 to 24 hours. An influx of edema fluid elevates the uninvolved stratum corneum to form a delicate clear vesicle containing large amounts of cell-free infectious virus and multinucleated giant cells, containing eosinophilic intranuclear inclusion bodies, formed by fusion of infected epithelial cells with adjacent infected and uninfected cells. The underlying dermis shows edema and mononuclear cell infiltration (**A,** H&E ×100; **B,** H&E ×400). **C,** The multinucleated giant cells are readily identified in Tzanck smears prepared from material scraped from the base of vesicular lesions and stained with H&E, Giemsa, or similar stains. Giemsa ×1000. **D,** Infected human fibroblast tissue cultures show similar multinucleated giant cells containing eosinophilic intranuclear inclusion bodies that are formed by fusion of infected cells with adjacent infected and uninfected cells. H&E ×1000. (Images **A** and **B,** Used with permission from Dr. R. J. Barr.)

done.[122,123] Serologic tests are more important to identify susceptible individuals who may be candidates for isolation or prophylaxis. The technique most commonly used is a solid-phase enzyme-linked immunosorbent assay (ELISA). However, these assays (there are many commercial sources) often lack sensitivity, failing to detect antibody in a significant number of persons who are immune, especially those who received varicella vaccine. False-positive results in susceptible individuals are less common, but problematic, especially in health care workers in whom susceptibility to VZV is a risk for nosocomial varicella.

DIFFERENTIAL DIAGNOSIS

See Table 165-2.

MANAGEMENT

ANTIVIRAL AGENTS

Chapter 191 provides a detailed description of the treatment of varicella and herpes zoster. The nucleoside analogs acyclovir, famciclovir, valacyclovir, and brivudin, and the pyrophosphate analog foscarnet, are efficacious in treating VZV infections. Acyclovir and penciclovir are guanosine analogs that are selectively phosphorylated by VZV thymidine kinase; they are poor substrates for cellular thymidine kinase and thus are not activated in, and are not toxic for, uninfected cells. Cellular enzymes then convert acyclovir monophosphate and penciclovir monophosphate to the corresponding triphosphates, which interfere with viral DNA synthesis by inhibiting viral DNA polymerase. VZV is approximately tenfold less sensitive than HSV to acyclovir and penciclovir.

Two prodrugs, valacyclovir (for acyclovir) and famciclovir (for penciclovir), are better and more reliably absorbed than acyclovir following oral administration.[125] Thus, they produce much higher blood levels of antiviral activity and permit less frequent dosing than acyclovir. Valacyclovir is a valine ester of acyclovir that is converted enzymatically to acyclovir after absorption. Famciclovir is a prodrug of penciclovir, a nucleoside analog similar to acyclovir in mechanism of action and antiviral activity against VZV and HSV. Famciclovir is converted enzymatically to penciclovir after absorption. Brivudin is a thymidine analog, also activated by viral thymidine kinase, with very high activity against VZV. Although effective in the treatment of herpes zoster, it is not licensed in the United States, in part because of a potentially lethal interaction with 5-fluorouracil.[126]

Foscarnet, a second-line drug that is an analog of inorganic pyrophosphate, inhibits the replication of all known herpesviruses in vitro. It exerts its antiviral activity by selective inhibition at the pyrophosphate-binding site of virus-specific DNA polymerases at concentrations that do not greatly inhibit cellular DNA polymerases. Foscarnet does not require phosphorylation by thymidine kinase to be activated and is therefore active against nucleoside-resistant VZV mutants that have reduced or altered thymidine kinase activity, but it is more toxic than the nucleoside analogs. Cidofovir is another drug that directly inhibits viral DNA polymerase but, because of its toxicity, is considered a third-line drug. A new antiviral agent, amenamevir, is a potent helicase-primase inhibitor that is active against acyclovir-resistant VZV and HSV. A single dose of 400 mg daily was as effective and as well tolerated as valacyclovir 1 g 3 times daily in Japanese patients with proven herpes zoster.[127]

Topical antiviral therapy has no role in the treatment of varicella. It has limited efficacy against herpes zoster and is not recommended. Systemic therapy, either oral or parenteral, is the standard of care. Because of their superior pharmacokinetics and the reduced sensitivity of VZV compared to HSV to acyclovir and penciclovir, famciclovir, or valacyclovir are preferred over acyclovir for oral therapy of VZV infections. Acyclovir-resistant VZV has been documented in varicella and herpes zoster in severely immunosuppressed patients, such as patients with advanced AIDS. Because of the usual mechanism of acyclovir resistance (mutations in the viral thymidine kinase gene), these acyclovir-resistant mutants are cross-resistant to ganciclovir, valacyclovir, famciclovir, and penciclovir. They usually respond to foscarnet and are sensitive to amenamevir, an investigational helicase-primase inhibitor.

TREATMENT OF VARICELLA

TOPICAL THERAPY

In healthy children, varicella is generally benign and self-limited. Cool compresses, calamine lotion or Caladryl Clear (zinc acetate 0.1% + pramoxine 1%) locally, tepid baths with baking soda or colloidal oatmeal (3 cups per tub of water), and oral antihistamines may relieve itching. Creams and lotions containing glucocorticoids and occlusive ointments should not be used. Antipyretics may be needed, but salicylates must be avoided because of their association with Reye syndrome. Minor bacterial infections are treated with warm soaks. Bacterial cellulitis requires systemic antimicrobial therapy that is effective against *Staphylococcus aureus* and group A β-hemolytic streptococcus.

ANTIVIRAL THERAPY

Immunocompetent Children: See Table 165-3. A large randomized, controlled trial of acyclovir treatment of otherwise healthy children 2 to 12 years of age found that treatment with oral acyclovir (20 mg/kg 4 times per day for 5 days) initiated within 24 hours of rash onset modestly reduced the maximum number of lesions, the time to cessation of new lesion formation, and the duration of the rash, fever, and constitutional symptoms when compared to placebo.[128] Treatment initiated more than 24 hours after rash onset was not effective. Because varicella is a relatively benign infection in children and the clinical benefits of treatment are modest, routine antiviral treatment is not recommended in immunocompetent children.[66,129,130] Some experts favor its use where cost is not a concern; when it can be begun in time to benefit the patient (within 24 hours of rash onset); and where there is a perceived need to speed resolution of the infection. Because secondary cases among susceptible children in the household are generally more severe than the index cases,[21]

TABLE 165-3
Antiviral Treatment of Varicella in the Normal and Immunocompromised Host

PATIENT GROUP	REGIMEN
Normal[a]	
Neonate	Acyclovir 10 mg/kg or 500 mg/m² every 8 h for 10 d
Child (2 to <18 y of age)	Symptomatic treatment alone, or Valacyclovir 20 mg/kg every 8 h for 5 d[b] (not to exceed 3 g/d) or Acyclovir 20 mg/kg orally 4 times a day × 5 d (not to exceed 3200 mg/d)
Adolescent (≥40 kg) or adult, especially with mild immunocompromise (eg, use of inhaled glucocorticoids)	Valacyclovir 1 g orally every 8 h for 7 d or Famciclovir 500 mg orally every 8 h for 7 d or Acyclovir 800 mg orally 5 times a day for 7 d
Pneumonia	Acyclovir 10 mg/kg IV every 8 h × 7–10 d[b]
Pregnancy	Routine use of acyclovir is not recommended. If there are complications (eg, pneumonia) treat pneumonia as per recommendation above.
Immunocompromised	
Mild varicella or mild immunocompromise	Valacyclovir 1 g orally every 8 h for 7-10 d or Famciclovir 500 mg orally every 8 h for 7-10 d or Acyclovir 800 mg orally 5 times a day for 7-10 d
Severe varicella or severe immunocompromise	Acyclovir 10 mg/kg IV every 8 h for 7–10 d
Acyclovir resistant (advanced AIDS)	Foscarnet 40 mg/kg IV every 8 h until healed

[a]Oral acyclovir or preferably, famciclovir or valacyclovir, should be considered for otherwise healthy persons at increased risk for moderate-to-severe varicella (eg, persons aged >12 y, persons with chronic cutaneous or pulmonary disorders, persons receiving long-term salicylate therapy, and persons receiving short, intermittent, or aerosolized courses of corticosteroids). (From Marin M et al. Prevention of varicella: Recommendations of the Advisory Committee on Immunization Practices [ACIP]. MMWR Recomm Rep. 2007;56:1-40.)

[b]Must prepare suspension by grinding 500-mg valacyclovir caplets and suspending in cherry-flavored Suspension Structural Vehicle USP-NF (SSV) at 25 mg/mL or 50 mg/mL in lots of 100 mL at time of dispensing.

and because early initiation of treatment is more readily accomplished in that setting, treatment with acyclovir is an option for such secondary cases.

We recommend oral antiviral therapy, preferably valacyclovir or famciclovir, for persons >12 years of age, persons with chronic cutaneous or pulmonary disorders or other debilitating diseases, persons receiving long-term salicylate therapy, and persons receiving short, intermittent, or aerosolized courses of corticosteroids because these individuals are at increased risk for moderate-to-severe varicella.[130]

Immunocompetent Adolescents and Adults: A randomized, controlled trial of acyclovir treatment of healthy adolescents 13 to 18 years of age found that early treatment with oral acyclovir (800 mg 5 times a day for 5 days) reduced the maximum number of lesions and time to cessation of new lesion formation compared to placebo.[131] A randomized, placebo-controlled trial of oral acyclovir in healthy young adults with varicella showed that early treatment (within 24 hours of rash onset) with oral acyclovir (800 mg 5 times a day for 7 days) significantly reduced the time to crusting of lesions, the extent of disease, and duration of symptoms and fever.[75] Thus, routine treatment of varicella in adults seems reasonable, especially because varicella complications are more frequent in adults. Although not tested, famciclovir 500 mg orally every 8 hours or valacyclovir 1000 mg orally every 8 hours would be more convenient and appropriate substitutes for acyclovir in normal adolescents and adults. Many physicians do not prescribe oral acyclovir in uncomplicated varicella during pregnancy because the risk of treatment to the fetus is unknown. Other physicians recommend oral antiviral therapy for infections in the third trimester when organogenesis is complete, because of the risk of varicella pneumonia, and of spread of the infection to the newborn. Intravenous acyclovir is often considered for pregnant women with varicella who have extensive cutaneous and/or systemic disease. Though limited in size, registries of pregnant women treated with acyclovir did not reveal any toxicity for pregnant women or their fetuses,[132-134] and extensive, though unrecorded, clinical experience also confirms its safety in pregnant women. Consequently, we recommend treatment for pregnant women with varicella who have extensive rash, toxicity, any signs of systemic infection, or any risk factors such as the use of immunosuppressive medications.

Uncontrolled trials in immunocompetent adults with varicella pneumonia suggest that early treatment (within 36 hours of hospitalization) with IV acyclovir (10 mg/kg every 8 hours) reduces fever and tachypnea and improves oxygenation.[135] Other serious complications of varicella in the immunocompetent host, such as encephalitis, meningoencephalitis, myelitis, and ocular complications, should be treated with IV acyclovir.

Immunocompromised Patients: Controlled trials in immunocompromised patients with varicella demonstrated that treatment with IV acyclovir decreased the incidence of life-threatening visceral complications when treatment was initiated within 72 hours of rash onset.[136] Intravenous acyclovir has been the standard of care for varicella in patients with substantial immunodeficiency. Although oral therapy with famciclovir or valacyclovir should suffice for patients with mild degrees of immunologic impairment, there are no controlled clinical trials to guide the decision. Patients who are started on IV therapy may be switched to oral therapy when new lesions cease to appear and the patient is stable.

TREATMENT OF HERPES ZOSTER

TOPICAL THERAPY

During the acute phase of herpes zoster, the application of cool compresses, calamine lotion or Caladryl Clear, cornstarch, or baking soda may lessen local symptoms and hasten the drying of vesicular lesions. Occlusive ointments and creams or lotions containing glucocorticoids should not be used. Topical treatment with antiviral agents is not effective. Bacterial superinfection of herpes zoster lesions is uncommon and should be treated with warm soaks; bacterial cellulitis requires systemic antibiotic therapy.

ANTIVIRAL THERAPY

The major goals of antiviral therapy in patients with herpes zoster are to limit the extent, duration, and severity of pain and rash in the primary dermatome and to prevent disease elsewhere.

Except for PHN, most complications of herpes zoster, including vasculopathy, result from continuing replication and spread of VZV from the affected ganglion, and may thus be prevented by early initiation of effective antiviral therapy.

Immunocompetent Adolescents and Adults: Table 165-4 lists current evidence-based recommendations for treatment of herpes zoster based on the results of randomized controlled trials. Recommended antivirals reduce the time to rash healing, and the duration and severity of acute pain in older adults with herpes zoster who are treated within 72 hours of rash onset.[137] In some studies, the duration of chronic pain was also reduced, but the FDA has not approved these agents for the prevention of PHN.[138] Randomized controlled trials comparing antivirals demonstrated equivalent results in rash healing, acute pain, and the duration of chronic pain.[139-141] Oral acyclovir, famciclovir, and valacyclovir are all acceptable antivirals for older adults. However, famciclovir or valacyclovir are preferred because of their thrice-daily dosing schedule, their greater oral bioavailability, and the higher and more reliable blood levels of antiviral activity achieved. This is important because of the reduced sensitivity to acyclovir of VZV compared with HSV, and the potential existence of barriers to the entry of antiviral agents into tissues that are sites of VZV replication.

The utility of antiviral agents is unproven if treatment is initiated more than 72 hours after rash onset. Nevertheless, we believe that it is prudent to initiate antiviral therapy even if more than 72 hours have elapsed after rash onset in patients with herpes zoster involving cranial nerves (eg, ophthalmic zoster), in patients who continue to have new vesicle formation, or in patients who are of advanced age and may thus have a delay in development of effective immune responses.[135]

TABLE 165-4
Antiviral Treatment of Herpes Zoster in the Normal and Immunocompromised Host

PATIENT GROUP	REGIMEN
Normal	
Age <50 y	Symptomatic treatment alone, or
	Famciclovir 500 mg orally every 8 h for 7 d or
	Valacyclovir 1 g orally every 8 h for 7 d or
	Acyclovir 800 mg orally 5 times a day for 7 d[a]
Age ≥50 y, and patients of any age with cranial nerve involvement (eg, ophthalmic zoster)	Famciclovir 500 mg orally every 8 h for 7 d or
	Valacyclovir 1 g orally every 8 h for 7 d or
	Acyclovir 800 mg orally 5 times a day for 7 d[a]
Immunocompromised	
Mild immunocompromise, including HIV-1 infection	Famciclovir 500 mg orally every 8 h for 7-10 d or
	Valacyclovir 1 g orally every 8 h for 7-10 d or
	Acyclovir 800 mg orally 5 times a day for 7-10 d[a]
Severe immunocompromise	Acyclovir 10 mg/kg IV every 8 h for 7-10 d
Acyclovir resistant (eg, advanced AIDS)	Foscarnet 40 mg/kg IV every 8 h until healed

[a]Famciclovir or valacyclovir are preferred because their greater and more reliable oral bioavailability result in higher blood levels of antiviral activity, the lower susceptibility of VZV (compared to HSV) to acyclovir and penciclovir, and the existence of barriers to the entry of antiviral agents into tissues that are sites of VZV replication.

Ophthalmic zoster represents a special therapeutic challenge because of the risk of ocular complications. Examination by an ophthalmologist should be sought in most cases, for example, when there is any evidence of involvement of the eye and when the nasociliary nerve is involved. Oral acyclovir was effective in preventing ocular complications of ophthalmic zoster in a randomized, controlled trial.[142] Famciclovir and valacyclovir appear to have efficacy comparable to that of acyclovir in the treatment of ophthalmic zoster, and are preferred for the reasons cited above.[143,144]

Immunocompromised Patients: A randomized, double-blind, placebo-controlled trial in immunocompromised patients with herpes zoster showed that IV acyclovir (500 mg/m^2 every 8 hours for 7 days) halted progression of the disease, both in patients with localized herpes zoster and in patients with cutaneous dissemination.[145] Acyclovir accelerated the rate of clearance of virus from vesicles and markedly reduced the incidence of subsequent visceral and progressive cutaneous dissemination. Pain subsided faster in acyclovir recipients, and fewer reported PHN, but these differences were not statistically significant. In patients with mild immunocompromise and localized herpes zoster, oral famciclovir or valacyclovir will usually suffice.[146,147] A randomized, controlled trial of oral famciclovir versus oral acyclovir in patients with localized herpes zoster following bone marrow or organ transplantation or cancer chemotherapy showed that both treatments were equivalent in rash healing and loss of acute pain, and were well tolerated.[147] However, oral famciclovir or valacyclovir are preferable to oral acyclovir.

ANTIINFLAMMATORY THERAPY

The possibility that inflammation within the sensory ganglion and contiguous neural structures contributes to PHN provided the rationale for the use of glucocorticoids during the acute phase of herpes zoster. Randomized controlled trials, however, showed that the addition of glucocorticoids to acyclovir did not change the incidence of chronic pain.[148-150] However, glucocorticoids did reduce acute pain in most trials, and in one trial of acyclovir and prednisone, the time to uninterrupted sleep, return to baseline daily activity, and cessation of analgesic therapy was reduced in patients who received glucocorticoids.[149] Consequently, some experts advocate oral glucocorticoids for otherwise healthy older adults whose rash is complicated by moderate-to-severe pain and who have no contraindications to glucocorticoids.[137] Others believe that the common adverse effects of glucocorticoids outweigh their benefits, and argue against their routine use in older patients with herpes zoster. We agree and do not recommend the use of glucocorticoids in this setting.

ANALGESICS

Greater severity of acute pain is a risk factor for PHN, and acute pain may contribute to central sensitization and the genesis of chronic pain. Therefore, aggressive pain control is both reasonable and humane.[137] The severity of acute herpes zoster pain should be determined using standardized pain scales. Clinicians should prescribe analgesics with the goal of limiting the severity of pain to less than 3 on a 0-to-10 scale, and to a level of pain that does not interfere with sleep. The choice, dosage, and schedule of drugs are governed by the patient's pain severity, underlying conditions, and response to and side effects of specific drugs. A randomized controlled trial of oxycodone, gabapentin, or placebo in older adults during the early phase of herpes zoster showed that oxycodone, but not gabapentin, provided significantly greater pain relief than placebo in patients with moderate-to-severe pain.[151] This trial was not powered to analyze PHN, and there are no other controlled trials of the effect of treatment with opioids or gabapentin during the acute phase of herpes zoster on the subsequent development of PHN. A crossover study of a single dose of 900 mg of gabapentin during the acute phase of herpes zoster showed greater pain relief than placebo.[152] If pain control remains inadequate, regional or local anesthetic nerve blocks should be considered for acute pain control.[137,153]

A randomized controlled trial demonstrated that a single epidural injection of corticosteroids and local anesthetics in the acute phase of herpes zoster reduced acute pain but did not prevent the subsequent development of PHN.[153]

TREATMENT OF POSTHERPETIC NEURALGIA

PHN is difficult to treat. Fortunately, it resolves spontaneously in most patients, although this often requires several months (Fig. 165-1C). Severity and duration of PHN are a function of age. Clinicians have advocated a wide range of treatments, including many oral and topical medications, epidural injection of local anesthetic and glucocorticoids, acupuncture, biofeedback, subcutaneous injections of triamcinolone, transepidermal electrical nerve stimulation, spinal cord stimulators, and systemic administration of a variety of compounds, but most have not been validated by controlled trials. The results of randomized controlled trials demonstrated efficacy for pain relief in PHN for the following drugs: gabapentin, pregabalin, tricyclic antidepressants, opioid analgesics, tramadol, 5% lidocaine patch, and high-concentration capsaicin patch.[154-157] The choice among these medications should be guided by the adverse event profiles, potential for drug interactions, patient comorbidities, and treatment preferences. On average, these agents provide adequate pain relief (defined as reduction of pain to below 3 on a 0- to 10-point scale or by 50% on a visual analog scale) in 30% to 60% of patients. These modalities are now recommended as evidence-based pharmacotherapy for PHN as described in more detail in practice management guidelines.[154,155,158-160]

PREVENTION

PREVENTION OF VARICELLA

VARICELLA VACCINE

Live attenuated Oka VZV varicella vaccines are immunogenic and efficacious in protecting susceptible children against varicella. Similar results were obtained in susceptible adults when 2 doses were given 4 to 8 weeks apart. Vaccinated children and adults developed breakthrough varicella caused by wildtype VZV at a rate of 1% to 3% per year (cumulative ~15%) compared to an attack rate of 8% to 13% per year in unvaccinated children.[161] Breakthrough varicella is relatively mild, with fewer lesions and milder constitutional symptoms. The FDA licensed the Oka/Merck varicella vaccine in the United States in 1995. In 2005, the FDA approved a combined measles, mumps, rubella, and varicella (MMRV) vaccine for routine immunization of children 12 months to 12 years of age.

Because of the frequency of breakthrough varicella, the CDC Advisory Committee on Immunization Practices (ACIP) now recommends two 0.5-mL doses of varicella vaccine for healthy children aged ≥12 months, and for all adolescents and adults without evidence of immunity.[162] Because of the increased severity of varicella in adults, all susceptible adults should be identified and vaccinated. Particular effort should be devoted to identifying and vaccinating susceptible adults who may be at increased risk for exposure or transmission, including (1) health care providers, (2) household contacts who might infect immunocompromised persons, or susceptible pregnant women, (3) persons who live or work in environments in which transmission of VZV is likely (eg, teachers, day care employees, residents, and staff in institutional settings), (4) persons who live or work in environments in which transmission has been reported (eg, college students, inmates and staff members of correctional institutions, and military personnel), (5) nonpregnant women of childbearing age, (6) adolescents and adults living in households with children, and (7) international travelers. Second-dose catch-up varicella vaccination is recommended for children, adolescents, and adults who previously received only 1 dose.[66,163]

The immunity to varicella induced by varicella vaccine is not as solid as that induced by wildtype VZV infection, and the duration of vaccine-induced immunity is not yet known. However, a high percentage of children followed long-term have remained seropositive.[164] Recent experience in clinical practice indicates that vaccine effectiveness in children is modestly lower than vaccine efficacy in clinical trials, and outbreaks of breakthrough varicella in schools and day care centers still occur.[163,165-167] Several studies have indicated that vaccine effectiveness declines over 10 years.[168] A CDC analysis of 10 years of surveillance data for varicella (1995-2004) showed that the annual rate of breakthrough varicella increased with time since vaccination, from 1.6 cases per 1000 person-years within 1 year after vaccination to 9.0 cases per 1000 person-years at 5 years and 58.2 cases per 1000 person-years at 9 years.[168] Although most breakthrough varicella in children is characterized by mild disease, more recent reports indicate that 25% to 30% of breakthrough cases are not mild, are clinically similar to varicella in unvaccinated children,[169] and are often as contagious as cases in unvaccinated persons.

Varicella vaccine is remarkably safe and well tolerated, causing mainly minor rashes and injection site reactions.[169] Serious adverse events have been rare (2.6/100,000 doses distributed) and, in the majority of cases, a causal relationship between the serious adverse event and varicella vaccine could not be established.

Herpes zoster occurs in vaccinees, but at a lower rate than herpes zoster following varicella caused by wildtype VZV. Cases of laboratory-confirmed herpes zoster in vaccinees include cases caused by reactivation of vaccine virus and many cases caused by reactivation of wildtype VZV that established latent infection during unrecognized varicella acquired prior to or after vaccination.[82]

Among children <18 years of age in a managed care plan, the incidence of herpes zoster was 79% lower among recipients of varicella vaccine than among unvaccinated children. Half of the cases of herpes zoster in vaccinated children were caused by Oka vaccine VZV and half were caused by wildtype VZV, whereas all cases of herpes zoster in unvaccinated children were caused by wildtype VZV.[82]

POSTEXPOSURE PROPHYLAXIS AND INFECTION CONTROL

Patients with varicella and herpes zoster often transmit VZV to susceptible individuals. When exposure is recognized (risk period of 1-2 days before rash until crusting is well under way), preventive measures include varicella vaccine, high-titer varicella-zoster immune globulin (VARIZIG), and postexposure chemoprophylaxis with acyclovir.

Active immunization with varicella vaccine is effective in preventing illness or modifying varicella severity in immunocompetent children if administered within 3 days after exposure.[170] Comparable information is not available for immunocompromised patients. An alternative for these patients is VARIZIG, a purified human immune globulin prepared from plasma containing high levels of immunoglobulin G antibody to VZV. This product may be considered for patients who have been exposed to varicella and are at increased risk for severe disease and complications.[171] It is dosed on a weight basis and should be given as soon as possible, preferably with 96 hours of exposure, although current recommendations permit an interval of up to 10 days.[172]

Whereas protection afforded by VARIZIG is transient, varicella vaccine induces long-lasting VZV immunity and protection against subsequent exposures. Therefore, the ACIP recommends varicella vaccine for postexposure prophylaxis in unvaccinated susceptible immunocompetent persons.[162] Varicella vaccine is also much less expensive than VARIZIG.

Chemoprophylaxis with acyclovir also has been studied in susceptible children following household exposure to varicella. Children who received postexposure treatment with acyclovir had either no varicella or experienced fewer and less severe cases of varicella than children in the control group.[173] However, appropriate timing is critical, and immunity to varicella may not be achieved, especially with early postexposure treatment. Reported experience with postexposure treatment with acyclovir is lacking in immunocompromised patients. Oral famciclovir or valacyclovir are preferable to oral acyclovir for postexposure chemoprophylaxis.

The importance of infection control practices for VZV varies with the age and immune status of the exposed susceptible individual. It is not imperative to prevent exposure of susceptible normal children to VZV, but exposure of immunocompromised patients, newborn infants, and adults, particularly women of childbearing age, should be avoided. Exposure of susceptible immunocompromised patients to VZV warrants reduction in the dosage of glucocorticoids and other immunosuppressive drugs, and administration of VariZIG. Hospital and long-term care facility personnel without a clear history of varicella or herpes zoster should be tested for antibody to VZV prior to employment, and susceptible personnel vaccinated against varicella. Appropriate leave from work should be instituted following VZV exposure of any susceptible personnel who are not vaccinated. In hospitals, airborne and contact precautions are recommended for patients with varicella, immunocompromised patients with localized herpes zoster, and any patient with disseminated herpes zoster until all lesions are crusted.[174] Contact precautions are recommended for immunocompetent patients with localized herpes zoster.

PREVENTION OF HERPES ZOSTER

Until universal varicella vaccination greatly reduces the number of people latently infected with wildtype VZV, prevention of herpes zoster must be aimed at preventing reactivation of latent VZV that results in clinical disease. Long-term suppressive acyclovir treatment is only practical in immunocompromised patients at proven risk of developing herpes zoster within a defined time period, for example, in the year following bone marrow or solid organ transplantation.

LIVE ATTENUATED ZOSTER VACCINE

Live attenuated Oka VZV zoster vaccines (ZVL) boost VZV-specific cellular immunity in older adults sufficiently to prevent or attenuate herpes zoster.[108] The clinical rationale for zoster vaccine is the substantial morbidity of herpes zoster in older adults and the need to initiate antiviral therapy within 72 hours of rash onset for maximum benefit; even then, antiviral therapy does not prevent PHN. In addition, treatment of PHN is often ineffective and poorly tolerated by older adults.

In 2006, the ACIP recommended routine administration of live attenuated Oka/Merck strain VZV zoster vaccine (ZVL; Zostavax®) to adults 60 years of age and older for the prevention of herpes zoster and its complications, particularly PHN.[37] This recommendation is based on the results of the Shingles Prevention Study, a randomized, double-blind, placebo controlled VA Cooperative Study conducted in 38,546 community-dwelling adults ≥60 years of age at 22 study sites across the continental United States.[28] ZVL reduced the burden of illness due to herpes zoster (a clinically relevant measure of the adverse impact of herpes zoster) by 61.1%; reduced the incidence of clinically significant PHN by 66.5%; and reduced the incidence of herpes zoster by 51.3%. Clinically significant PHN is defined as pain and discomfort (eg, allodynia, severe pruritus) due to herpes zoster scored as ≥3 on a 0-10 scale that persists for more than 90 days after rash onset. ZVL also decreased the adverse impact of herpes zoster on capacity to perform activities of daily living and health-related quality of life.[175] Reactions at the injection site were more frequent among vaccine recipients but were generally mild. The proportion of subjects reporting serious adverse events, and rates of hospitalization and death were comparable in vaccine and placebo recipients.[28,176]

Long-term followup studies of Shingles Prevention Study participants demonstrated that ZVL efficacy for herpes zoster burden of illness and incidence of herpes zoster declined over time, but persisted through 5 to 7 years postvaccination, declining markedly thereafter.[177,178] ZVL efficacy for herpes zoster burden of illness was 61.1% from 0.0 to 4.9 years postvaccination, 50.1% from 3.3 to 7.8 years postvaccination, and 58.6% from 0.0 to 7.8 years postvaccination. Comparable figures for incidence of herpes zoster were 51.3%, 39.6%, and 48.7%, and for incidence of PHN were 66.5%, 60.1%, and 64.9%.

A number of retrospective reviews of the use of ZVL in "real world" practice settings using electronic records from large integrated health care organizations and administrative medical claims databases showed very similar results for vaccine effectiveness for the incidence of herpes zoster.[179-185] These studies confirmed declines in effectiveness of ZVL for incidence of herpes zoster similar to those demonstrated in the Shingles Prevention Study and its Persistence Substudies.[28,177,178] However, ZVL effectiveness in persons vaccinated when they were ≥70 years of age was similar to vaccine effectiveness in younger vaccinees; furthermore, ZVL effectiveness for PHN was higher and better preserved over time than for incidence of herpes zoster.[181-184] In addition, ZVL reduced the duration and severity of pain in vaccinees who developed herpes zoster, reduced the incidence of ophthalmic zoster, and reduced the incidence and severity of prodromal pain.[179,185] Although these data suggest that a second dose of ZVL may be needed, and a second dose of ZVL administered ≥10 years after the initial dose did significantly boost VZV-specific immune responses,[186] there is currently no recommendation for revaccination from the ACIP.[187] In a large, randomized, placebo-controlled trial, the efficacy of ZVL for incidence of herpes zoster in 50- to 59-year-old individuals was 69.8%, which led to expansion of FDA licensure to include this age group.[188] However, the ACIP did not modify the recommendation to administer ZVL at ≥60 years of age. Neither the FDA nor the ACIP have set an upper age limit for the use of ZVL. Older individuals are at highest risk for herpes zoster and PHN, and reduction in herpes zoster pain, severity, and duration occurs in very old recipients of ZVL even when herpes zoster is not prevented.[28,181]

Although highly attenuated, ZVL is contraindicated in immunocompromised persons.

Nevertheless, it has been administered to a number of immunocompromised patients, with very rare adverse events.[180,189-199] With more than 30 million doses administered to persons ≥60 years of age in the United States since 2006, more than 10 million doses administered to persons ≥70 years of age in the United Kingdom since 2010, and additional doses in Japan and other countries, ZVL has proven to have a remarkable safety profile.[184,200]

ZVL may be administered without screening for a history of varicella or herpes zoster, or serologic testing for varicella immunity.[37] Persons known to be VZV seronegative should be vaccinated against varicella according to current recommendations.[162] Older adults who have PHN or who have a current episode of herpes zoster may ask to be vaccinated, but ZVL is not indicated to treat acute herpes zoster or PHN. Some patients may want to receive ZVL after a recent episode of herpes zoster has resolved. The optimal time to immunize an individual after a recent episode of herpes zoster is unknown, and the clinical diagnosis of herpes zoster is not always correct. The authors believe that an interval of 2 to 3 years after onset of a well-documented case of herpes zoster is reasonable. Administration of ZVL to Shingles Prevention Study placebo recipients 5 to 85 months after documented herpes zoster was safe and well tolerated.[201]

When considering ZVL, older adults may express concerns about transmission of vaccine virus to other individuals, but transmission of vaccine virus from recipients of ZVL to susceptible household contacts has not been documented. Thus, immunocompetent older adults in contact with immunocompromised patients should receive ZVL to reduce the risk that they will develop herpes zoster and transmit wild-type VZV to their susceptible immunocompromised contacts.[37,108] For the same reasons, older adult contacts of susceptible pregnant women and infants should receive zoster vaccine. ZVL recipients with susceptible pregnant or immunocompromised contacts need not take any special precautions following vaccination, except in the rare situation that a vesicular rash develops, in which case standard contact precautions are adequate.[37] In the very unlikely event that an immunocompromised contact develops a significant illness caused by vaccine virus, he or she can be treated with antiviral agents.

ADJUVANTED GLYCOPROTEIN E SUBUNIT ZOSTER VACCINE

A new adjuvanted recombinant VZV subunit zoster vaccine (RZV; Shingrix®) consisting of recombinant VZV glycoprotein E (gE) and a powerful $AS01_B$ adjuvant system was approved in October 2017 by the US FDA for the prevention of herpes zoster in adults ≥50 years of age. RZV is administered intramuscularly on a 2-dose schedule with a 2- to 6-month interval.[202] The ACIP has recommended RZV for prevention of herpes zoster in immunocompetent adults ≥50 years of age, with preference for RZV over ZVL for initial immunization and for administration to older adults who have already received ZVL.[203] VZV gE is a major component of the virus envelope that is essential for virus replication and cell-to-cell spread and is a major target for VZV-specific CD4+ T-cell responses. $AS01_B$ is a liposome-based adjuvant system that contains monophosphoryl lipid A (a Toll-like receptor 4 agonist) and the saponin QS21 (a purified extract from the *Quillaja saponaria* tree). QS21 stimulates strong humoral and CD4+ T-cell responses to gE.[204] A number of Phase I, I/II, and II studies established that 2 doses of RZV formulated with 50 µg of gE and $AS01_B$ containing 50 µg monophosphoryl lipid A and 50 µg QS21 administered 2 months apart induced strong immune responses to gE that, on the basis of a small followup study, appear to decline significantly over the first 3 years postvaccination and then persist above baseline levels for at least 9 years.[205,206] The VZV/gE-specific CD4+ T-cell and humoral responses induced by RZV were much more robust and long-lasting than those induced by ZVL, and addition of an Oka varicella vaccine did not increase the magnitude or durability of the immune responses to RZV.[204]

Two large blinded randomized placebo-controlled Phase III trials conducted concurrently at the same sites in 18 countries assessed the safety and efficacy of 2 doses of RZV administered intramuscularly 2 months apart in adults ≥50 years of age (ZOE-50; 15,411 participants) and ≥70 years of age (ZOE-70; 13,900 participants).[207,208] In ZOE-50 and ZOE-70, subjects were stratified into decades (50-59, 60-69, and ≥70 years) and (70-79 and ≥80 years), respectively; the study design was similar to that of the Shingles Prevention Study, except that T cell–mediated immune responses were measured by enumerating T cells expressing ≥2 of 4 activation markers: interferon-γ, interleukin-2, tumor necrosis factor-α, and CD40 ligand[207,208] rather than by responder cell frequency and ELISPOT.[28,209,210] In ZOE-50, during a mean followup of 3.2 years, RZV had an overall efficacy for incidence of herpes zoster of 97.2%, with no decrement in the ≥70-year age group.[207] Solicited and unsolicited adverse events were reported in 84.4% of RZV recipients and 37.8% of placebo recipients. Most were mild to moderate intensity, but 17.0% in RZV recipients and 3.2% in placebo recipients prevented normal everyday activities (grade 3). These were mostly injection-site reactions (pain, redness, swelling) in 81.5% of RZV recipients (9.5% grade 3) and 11.9% of placebo recipients (0.4% grade 3), and systemic reactions (myalgia, fatigue, headache, shivering, fever, and GI symptoms) in 66.1% of RZV recipients (11.4% grade 3) and 29.5% of placebo recipients (2.4% grade 3).[207]

In ZOE-70, during a mean followup of 3.7 years, RZV efficacy for incidence of herpes zoster was 89.8%; 90.0% in 70- to 79-year-olds and 89.1% in those ≥80 years of age.[208] In a pooled analysis of data from subjects ≥70 years of age in ZOE-50 and ZOE-70 (15,596 subjects), RZV efficacy for incidence of herpes zoster was 91.3% and for PHN was 88.8%. Adverse reactions were similar to those reported in ZOE-50, but tended to be less frequent among subjects ≥80 years of age than among younger subjects. Incidence of serious adverse events and potential immune-mediated diseases were similar in the RZV and placebo recipients.[208] Most were mild to moderate intensity, but 11.9% in RZV recipients and 2.0% in placebo recipients prevented normal everyday activities (grade 3). These were mostly injection-site reactions (pain, redness, swelling) in 74.1% of RZV recipients (8.5% grade 3) and 9.9% of placebo recipients (0.2% grade 3), and systemic reactions (myalgia, fatigue, headache, shivering, fever, and GI symptoms) in 53.0% of RZV recipients (6.0% grade 3) and 25.1% of placebo recipients (2.0% grade 3).[208]

Because RZV contains only the gE subunit of VZV, it is incapable of replication, and there is no danger of vaccine virus replication causing disease. A number of Phase I, I/II, and small Phase III studies have demonstrated that RZV is safe and immunogenic in persons with various immunosuppressive conditions, including HIV infection and hematopoietic cell transplant recipients.[211,212] RZV can be safely coadministered with other vaccines,[213] to persons previously vaccinated with ZVL,[214] and to persons with previous herpes zoster.[215] Although no results are available from head-to-head studies, RZV appears to be substantially more immunogenic in persons previously immunized with ZVL than a booster dose of ZVL.[186,214] Table 165-5 summarizes the current ACIP recommendations.

The development and clinical evaluation of RZV are summarized in an excellent review by Cunningham and Heineman,[217] in which pooled data from ZOE-50 and ZOE-70 indicate that overall RZV efficacy for incidence of herpes zoster declines from 97.6% in year 1 to 87.9% in year 4 postvaccination. If that rate of decline continues, persons vaccinated with RZV at 50 years of age, as recommended by the ACIP may require additional immunization to ensure an adequate level of protection later in life when the incidence and severity of herpes zoster and PHN are markedly increased.

Although the absence of recognized autoimmune diseases in RZV recipients followed for approximately 4 years postvaccination is encouraging, it does not eliminate the theoretical concern that the powerful $AS01_B$ adjuvant system might induce or aggravate autoimmune diseases, especially because the interval between their initiation and clinical recognition may be many years. At this point, it is incumbent on the US FDA, to ensure that large, well-designed, and relevant Phase IV postmarketing studies are expeditiously completed.[218,219]

ACKNOWLEDGMENTS

Dedicated to the memory of Stephen E. Straus, a coauthor of this chapter in previous editions and to Michiaki Takahashi who developed the attenuated Oka strain of VZV used in all live attenuated zoster and varicella vaccines.

MNO is grateful to M. Ashbaugh and W. Buchanan for assistance with the figures, to R. Harbecke and D. Mussatto for useful discussion and invaluable assistance with manuscript preparation, and for the support of the Veterans Medical Research Foundation and the James R. and Jesse V. Scott Fund for Shingles Research.

REFERENCES

1. Hope-Simpson RE. The nature of herpes zoster: a long-term study and a new hypothesis. *Proc R Soc Med.* 1965;58:9-20.
2. Garland J. Varicella following exposure to herpes zoster. *N Engl J Med.* 1943;228:336-337.
3. Kundratitz K. Experimentelle Übertragung von Herpes zoster auf den Menschen und die Beziehungen von Herpes zoster zu Varicellen. *Monatsschrift für Kinderheilkunde.* 1925;129:516-22.
4. Lipschütz B, Kundratitz K. Über die Ätiologie des Zoster und über seine Beziehungen zu Varicellen. *Wien klin Wochenschr.* 1925;38:499-503.
5. Bruusgaard E. The mutual relation between zoster and varicella. *Br J Dermatol.* 1932;44:1-24.
6. Weller TH, Witton HM. The etiologic agents of varicella and herpes zoster; serologic studies with the viruses as propagated in vitro. *J Exp Med.* 1958;108(6):869-890.
7. Straus SE, Reinhold W, Smith HA, et al. Endonuclease analysis of viral DNA from varicella and subsequent zoster infections in the same patient. *N Engl J Med.* 1984;311(21):1362-1364.
8. Choo PW, Donahue JG, Manson JE, et al. The epidemiology of varicella and its complications. *J Infect Dis.* 1995;172(3):706-712.
9. Seward J, Galil K, Wharton M. Epidemiology of varicella. In: Arvin AM, Gershon AA, eds. *Varicella-Zoster Virus Virology and Clinical Management*. Cambridge, UK: Cambridge University Press; 2000:187.
10. Kilgore PE, Kruszon-Moran D, Seward JF, et al. Varicella in Americans from NHANES III: implications for control through routine immunization. *J Med Virol.* 2003;70(suppl 1):S111-S118.
11. Longfield JN, Winn RE, Gibson RL, et al. Varicella outbreaks in Army recruits from Puerto Rico. Varicella susceptibility in a population from the tropics. *Arch Intern Med.* 1990;150(5):970-973.
12. Seither R, Calhoun K, Street EJ, et al. Vaccination coverage for selected vaccines, exemption rates, and provisional enrollment among children in

TABLE 165-5
Recommendations for the Use of Herpes Zoster Vaccines (2018 ACIP Recommendations)[203]

1. Recombinant zoster vaccine (RZV) is recommended for the prevention of herpes zoster and related complications for immunocompetent adults aged ≥50 y. RZV is administered in 2 doses 2-6 mo apart.
2. RZV is recommended for the prevention of herpes zoster and related complications for immunocompetent adults who previously received live attenuated zoster vaccine (ZVL). RZV should not be administered <2 mo after receipt of ZVL.
3. RZV is preferred over ZVL for the prevention of herpes zoster and related complications.

Note: These recommendations serve as a supplement to the existing recommendations for the use of ZVL in immunocompetent adults aged ≥60 y. RZV can be administered concomitantly, at different anatomic sites, with other adult vaccines.[216]

13. Jumaan AO, Yu O, Jackson LA, et al. Incidence of herpes zoster, before and after varicella-vaccination-associated decreases in the incidence of varicella, 1992-2002. *J Infect Dis*. 2005;191(12):2002-2007.
14. Davis MM, Patel MS, Gebremariam A. Decline in varicella-related hospitalizations and expenditures for children and adults after introduction of varicella vaccine in the United States. *Pediatrics*. 2004;114(3):786-792.
15. Bialek SR, Perella D, Zhang J, et al. Impact of a routine two-dose varicella vaccination program on varicella epidemiology. *Pediatrics*. 2013;132(5):e1134-e1140.
16. Leung J, Harpaz R. Impact of the maturing varicella vaccination program on varicella and related outcomes in the United States: 1994-2012. *J Pediatric Infect Dis Soc*. 2016;5(4):395-402.
17. Marin M, Zhang JX, Seward JF. Near elimination of varicella deaths in the US after implementation of the vaccination program. *Pediatrics*. 2011;128(2):214-220.
18. Lopez AS, Zhang J, Marin M. Epidemiology of varicella during the 2-dose varicella vaccination program—United States, 2005-2014. *MMWR Morb Mortal Wkly Rep*. 2016;65(34):902-905.
19. Nguyen HQ, Jumaan AO, Seward JF. Decline in mortality due to varicella after implementation of varicella vaccination in the United States. *N Engl J Med*. 2005;352(5):450-458.
20. Marin M, Marti M, Kambhampati A, et al. Global varicella vaccine effectiveness: a meta-analysis. *Pediatrics*. 2016;137(3):e20153741.
21. Ross AH. Modification of chicken pox in family contacts by administration of gamma globulin. *N Engl J Med*. 1962;267:369-376.
22. White CJ, Kuter BJ, Hildebrand CS, et al. Varicella vaccine (VARIVAX) in healthy children and adolescents: results from clinical trials, 1987 to 1989. *Pediatrics*. 1991;87(5):604-610.
23. Levin MJ. Varicella-zoster virus and virus DNA in the blood and oropharynx of people with latent or active varicella-zoster virus infections. *J Clin Virol*. 2014;61(4):487-495.
24. Arvin AM, Korpchak CM, Wittek AE. Immunologic evidence of reinfection with varicella-zoster virus. *J Infect Dis*. 1983;148(2):200-205.
25. Schimpff S, Serpick A, Stoler B, et al. Varicella-Zoster infection in patients with cancer. *Ann Intern Med*. 1972;76(2):241-254.
26. Yawn BP, Gilden D. The global epidemiology of herpes zoster. *Neurology*. 2013;81(10):928-930.
27. Kawai K, Gebremeskel BG, Acosta CJ. Systematic review of incidence and complications of herpes zoster: towards a global perspective. *BMJ Open*. 2014;4(6):e004833.
28. Oxman MN, Levin MJ, Johnson GR, et al. A vaccine to prevent herpes zoster and postherpetic neuralgia in older adults. *N Engl J Med*. 2005;352(22):2271-2284.
29. Oxman MN. Immunization to reduce the frequency and severity of herpes zoster and its complications. *Neurology*. 1995;45:S41-S46.
30. Ragozzino MW, Melton LJ 3rd, Kurland LT, et al. Population-based study of herpes zoster and its sequelae. *Medicine (Baltimore)*. 1982;61(5):310-316.
31. Schmader K, George LK, Burchett BM, et al. Racial differences in the occurrence of herpes zoster. *J Infect Dis*. 1995;171(3):701-704.
32. Thomas SL, Hall AJ. What does epidemiology tell us about risk factors for herpes zoster? *Lancet Infect Dis*. 2004;4(1):26-33.
33. Yawn BP, Saddier P, Wollan PC, et al. A population-based study of the incidence and complication rates of herpes zoster before zoster vaccine introduction. *Mayo Clin Proc*. 2007;82(11):1341-1349.
34. Schmader K, Gnann JW Jr, Watson CP. The epidemiological, clinical, and pathological rationale for the herpes zoster vaccine. *J Infect Dis*. 2008;197(suppl 2):S207-S215.
35. Insinga RP, Itzler RF, Pellissier JM, et al. The incidence of herpes zoster in a United States administrative database. *J Gen Intern Med*. 2005;20(8):748-753.
36. Donahue JG, Choo PW, Manson JE, et al. The incidence of herpes zoster. *Arch Intern Med*. 1995;155(15):1605-1609.
37. Harpaz R, Ortega-Sanchez IR, Seward JF. Prevention of herpes zoster: recommendations of the Advisory Committee on Immunization Practices (ACIP). *MMWR Recomm Rep*. 2008;57(RR-5):1-30; quiz CE2-CE4.
38. Cohen JI. Herpes zoster. *N Engl J Med*. 2013;369(3):255-263.
39. Cohen JI. A new vaccine to prevent herpes zoster. *N Engl J Med*. 2015;372(22):2149-2150.
40. Forbes HJ, Bhaskaran K, Thomas SL, et al. Quantification of risk factors for herpes zoster: population based case-control study. *BMJ*. 2014;348:g2911.
41. Yun H, Yang S, Chen L, et al. Risk of herpes zoster in autoimmune and inflammatory diseases: implications for vaccination. *Arthritis Rheumatol*. 2016;68(9):2328-2337.
42. Kawai K, Yawn BP. Risk factors for herpes zoster: a systematic review and meta-analysis. *Mayo Clin Proc*. 2017;92(12):1806-1821.
43. Strangfeld A, Listing J, Herzer P, et al. Risk of herpes zoster in patients with rheumatoid arthritis treated with anti-TNF-alpha agents. *JAMA*. 2009;301(7):737-744.
44. Buchbinder SP, Katz MH, Hessol NA, et al. Herpes zoster and human immunodeficiency virus infection. *J Infect Dis*. 1992;166(5):1153-1156.
45. Engels EA, Rosenberg PS, Biggar RJ. Zoster incidence in human immunodeficiency virus-infected hemophiliacs and homosexual men, 1984-1997. District of Columbia Gay Cohort Study. Multicenter Hemophilia Cohort Study. *J Infect Dis*. 1999;180(6):1784-1789.
46. Thomas SL, Wheeler JG, Hall AJ. Case-control study of the effect of mechanical trauma on the risk of herpes zoster. *BMJ*. 2004;328(7437):439.
47. Haanpaa M, Nurmikko T, Hurme M. Polymorphism of the IL-10 gene is associated with susceptibility to herpes zoster. *Scand J Infect Dis*. 2002;34(2):112-114.
48. Hicks LD, Cook-Norris RH, Mendoza N, et al. Family history as a risk factor for herpes zoster: a case-control study. *Arch Dermatol*. 2008;144(5):603-608.
49. Hernandez PO, Javed S, Mendoza N, et al. Family history and herpes zoster risk in the era of shingles vaccination. *J Clin Virol*. 2011;52(4):344-348.
50. Lai YC, Yew YW. Risk of herpes zoster and family history: a meta-analysis of case-control studies. *Indian J Dermatol*. 2016;61(2):157-162.
51. Joon Lee T, Hayes S, Cummings DM, et al. Herpes zoster knowledge, prevalence, and vaccination rate by race. *J Am Board Fam Med*. 2013;26(1):45-51.
52. Yawn BP, Wollan PC, Kurland MJ, et al. Herpes zoster recurrences more frequent than previously reported. *Mayo Clin Proc*. 2011;86(2):88-93.

53. Tseng HF, Chi M, Smith N, et al. Herpes zoster vaccine and the incidence of recurrent herpes zoster in an immunocompetent elderly population. *J Infect Dis.* 2012;206(2):190-196.
54. Sundriyal D, Kapoor R, Kumar N, et al. Multidermatomal herpes zoster. *BMJ Case Rep.* 2014;2014.
55. Kalman CM, Laskin OL. Herpes zoster and zosteriform herpes simplex virus infections in immunocompetent adults. *Am J Med.* 1986;81(5):775-778.
56. Viner K, Perella D, Lopez A, et al. Transmission of varicella zoster virus from individuals with herpes zoster or varicella in school and day care settings. *J Infect Dis.* 2012;205(9):1336-1341.
57. Lopez AS, Burnett-Hartman A, Nambiar R, et al. Transmission of a newly characterized strain of varicella-zoster virus from a patient with herpes zoster in a long-term-care facility, West Virginia, 2004. *J Infect Dis.* 2008;197(5):646-653.
58. Leclair JM, Zaia JA, Levin MJ, et al. Airborne transmission of chickenpox in a hospital. *N Engl J Med.* 1980;302(8):450-453.
59. Kawai K, Yawn BP, Wollan P, et al. Increasing incidence of herpes zoster over a 60-year period from a population-based study. *Clin Infect Dis.* 2016;63(2):221-226.
60. Brisson M, Edmunds WJ, Law B, et al. Epidemiology of varicella zoster virus infection in Canada and the United Kingdom. *Epidemiol Infect.* 2001;127(2):305-314.
61. Russell ML, Schopflocher DP, Svenson L, et al. Secular trends in the epidemiology of shingles in Alberta. *Epidemiol Infect.* 2007;135(6):908-913.
62. Toyama N, Shiraki K. Epidemiology of herpes zoster and its relationship to varicella in Japan: a 10-year survey of 48,388 herpes zoster cases in Miyazaki prefecture. *J Med Virol.* 2009;81(12):2053-2058.
63. Leung J, Harpaz R, Molinari NA, et al. Herpes zoster incidence among insured persons in the United States, 1993-2006: evaluation of impact of varicella vaccination. *Clin Infect Dis.* 2011;52(3):332-340.
64. Hales CM, Harpaz R, Joesoef MR, et al. Examination of links between herpes zoster incidence and childhood varicella vaccination. *Ann Intern Med.* 2013;159(11):739-745.
65. Mullooly JP, Riedlinger K, Chun C, et al. Incidence of herpes zoster, 1997-2002. *Epidemiol Infect.* 2005;133(2):245-253.
66. Marin M, Guris D, Chaves SS, et al. Prevention of varicella: recommendations of the Advisory Committee on Immunization Practices (ACIP). *MMWR Recomm Rep.* 2007;56(RR-4):1-40.
67. Malavige GN, Jones L, Black AP, et al. Varicella zoster virus glycoprotein E-specific CD4+ T cells show evidence of recent activation and effector differentiation, consistent with frequent exposure to replicative cycle antigens in healthy immune donors. *Clin Exp Immunol.* 2008;152(3):522-531.
68. Oxman MN. Clinical manifestations of herpes zoster. In: Arvin AM, Gershon AA, eds. *Varicella-Zoster Virus: Virology and Clinical Management.* Cambridge, UK: Cambridge University Press; 2000:246.
69. Stern ES. The mechanism of herpes zoster and its relation to chickenpox. *Br J Dermatol Syphylol.* 1937;49:263-271.
70. Wesselhoeft C. The differential diagnosis of chicken pox and smallpox. *N Engl J Med.* 1944;230(1):15-19.
71. Johnson CE, Stancin T, Fattlar D, et al. A long-term prospective study of varicella vaccine in healthy children. *Pediatrics.* 1997;100(5):761-766.
72. Aebi C, Ahmed A, Ramilo O. Bacterial complications of primary varicella in children. *Clin Infect Dis.* 1996;23(4):698-705.
73. Kiska DL, Thiede B, Caracciolo J, et al. Invasive group A streptococcal infections in North Carolina: epidemiology, clinical features, and genetic and serotype analysis of causative organisms. *J Infect Dis.* 1997;176(4):992-1000.
74. Patel RA, Binns HJ, Shulman ST. Reduction in pediatric hospitalizations for varicella-related invasive group A streptococcal infections in the varicella vaccine era. *J Pediatr.* 2004;144(1):68-74.
75. Wallace MR, Bowler WA, Murray NB, et al. Treatment of adult varicella with oral acyclovir. A randomized, placebo-controlled trial. *Ann Intern Med.* 1992;117(5):358-363.
76. Enders G, Miller E, Cradock-Watson J, et al. Consequences of varicella and herpes zoster in pregnancy: prospective study of 1739 cases. *Lancet.* 1994;343(8912):1548-1551.
77. Zhang HJ, Patenaude V, Abenhaim HA. Maternal outcomes in pregnancies affected by varicella zoster virus infections: population-based study on 7.7 million pregnancy admissions. *J Obstet Gynaecol Res.* 2015;41(1):62-68.
78. Meyers JD. Congenital varicella in term infants: risk reconsidered. *J Infect Dis.* 1974;129(2):215-217.
79. Morgan ER, Smalley LA. Varicella in immunocompromised children. Incidence of abdominal pain and organ involvement. *Am J Dis Child.* 1983;137(9):883-885.
80. CDC. Reye syndrome—United States, 1984. *MMWR Morb Mortal Wkly Rep.* 1985;34(1):13-16.
81. Liu GT, Urion DK. Pre-eruptive varicella encephalitis and cerebellar ataxia. *Pediatr Neurol.* 1992;8(1):69-70.
82. Weinmann S, Chun C, Schmid DS, et al. Incidence and clinical characteristics of herpes zoster among children in the varicella vaccine era, 2005-2009. *J Infect Dis.* 2013;208(11):1859-1868.
83. Lewis GW. Zoster sine herpete. *Br Med J.* 1958;2(5093):418-421.
84. Liesegang TJ. Herpes zoster ophthalmicus natural history, risk factors, clinical presentation, and morbidity. *Ophthalmology.* 2008;115(2)(suppl):S3-S12.
85. Katz J, Cooper EM, Walther RR, et al. Acute pain in herpes zoster and its impact on health-related quality of life. *Clin Infect Dis.* 2004;39(3):342-348.
86. Schmader KE, Sloane R, Pieper C, et al. The impact of acute herpes zoster pain and discomfort on functional status and quality of life in older adults. *Clin J Pain.* 2007;23(6):490-496.
87. Gilden DH, Kleinschmidt-DeMasters BK, LaGuardia JJ, et al. Neurologic complications of the reactivation of varicella-zoster virus. *N Engl J Med.* 2000;342(9):635-645.
88. Jung BF, Johnson RW, Griffin DR, et al. Risk factors for postherpetic neuralgia in patients with herpes zoster. *Neurology.* 2004;62(9):1545-1551.
89. Drolet M, Brisson M, Schmader KE, et al. The impact of herpes zoster and postherpetic neuralgia on health-related quality of life: a prospective study. *CMAJ.* 2010;182(16):1731-1736.
90. Johnson RW, Bouhassira D, Kassianos G, et al. The impact of herpes zoster and post-herpetic neuralgia on quality-of-life. *BMC Med.* 2010;8:37.
91. Baron R, Binder A, Wasner G. Neuropathic pain: diagnosis, pathophysiological mechanisms, and treatment. *Lancet Neurol.* 2010;9(8):807-819.
92. Gauthier A, Breuer J, Carrington D, et al. Epidemiology and cost of herpes zoster and post-herpetic

92. neuralgia in the United Kingdom. *Epidemiol Infect.* 2009;137(1):38-47.
93. Forbes HJ, Thomas SL, Smeeth L, et al. A systematic review and meta-analysis of risk factors for postherpetic neuralgia. *Pain.* 2016;157(1):30-54.
94. Wood MJ. Herpes zoster and pain. *Scand J Infect Dis Suppl.* 1991;80:53-61.
95. Chen JJ, Gershon AA, Li Z, et al. Varicella zoster virus (VZV) infects and establishes latency in enteric neurons. *J Neurovirol.* 2011;17(6):578-589.
96. Rosenblum WI, Hadfield MG. Granulomatous angiitis of the nervous system in cases of herpes zoster and lymphosarcoma. *Neurology.* 1972;22(4):348-354.
97. Bourdette DN, Rosenberg NL, Yatsu FM. Herpes zoster ophthalmicus and delayed ipsilateral cerebral infarction. *Neurology.* 1983;33(11):1428-1432.
98. Hilt DC, Buchholz D, Krumholz A, et al. Herpes zoster ophthalmicus and delayed contralateral hemiparesis caused by cerebral angiitis: diagnosis and management approaches. *Ann Neurol.* 1983;14(5):543-553.
99. Nagel MA, Gilden D. Developments in varicella zoster virus vasculopathy. *Curr Neurol Neurosci Rep.* 2016;16(2):12.
100. Gilden D, Cohrs RJ, Mahalingam R, et al. Neurological disease produced by varicella zoster virus reactivation without rash. *Curr Top Microbiol Immunol.* 2010;342:243-253.
101. Kennedy PG, Grinfeld E, Esiri MM. Absence of detection of varicella-zoster virus DNA in temporal artery biopsies obtained from patients with giant cell arteritis. *J Neurol Sci.* 2003;215(1-2):27-29.
102. Muratore F, Croci S, Tamagnini I, et al. No detection of varicella-zoster virus in temporal arteries of patients with giant cell arteritis. *Semin Arthritis Rheum.* 2017;47(2):235-240.
103. Ing EB, Ing R, Liu X, et al. Does herpes zoster predispose to giant cell arteritis: a geo-epidemiologic study. *Clin Ophthalmol.* 2018;12:113-118.
104. Buckingham EM, Foley MA, Grose C, et al. Identification of herpes zoster-associated temporal arteritis among cases of giant cell arteritis. *Am J Ophthalmol.* 2018;187:51-60.
105. Arvin AM, Gilden D. Varicella-zoster virus. In: Knipe DM, Howley PM, eds. *Fields Virology.* 6th ed. Philadelphia, PA: Lippincott Williams & Wilkins; 2013:2015-2057.
106. Breuer J, Grose C, Norberg P, et al. A proposal for a common nomenclature for viral clades that form the species varicella-zoster virus: summary of VZV Nomenclature Meeting 2008, Barts and the London School of Medicine and Dentistry, 24-25 July 2008. *J Gen Virol.* 2010;91(pt 4):821-828.
107. Jensen NJ, Rivailler P, Tseng HF, et al. Revisiting the genotyping scheme for varicella-zoster viruses based on whole-genome comparisons. *J Gen Virol.* 2017;98(6):1434-1438.
108. Oxman MN. Zoster vaccine: current status and future prospects. *Clin Infect Dis.* 2010;51(2):197-213.
109. Depledge DP, Yamanishi K, Gomi Y, et al. Deep sequencing of distinct preparations of the live attenuated varicella-zoster virus vaccine reveals a conserved core of attenuating single-nucleotide polymorphisms. *J Virol.* 2016;90(19):8698-8704.
110. Harbecke R, Oxman MN, Arnold BA, et al. A real-time PCR assay to identify and discriminate among wild-type and vaccine strains of varicella-zoster virus and herpes simplex virus in clinical specimens, and comparison with the clinical diagnoses. *J Med Virol.* 2009;81(7):1310-1322.
111. Ku CC, Besser J, Abendroth A, et al. Varicella-Zoster virus pathogenesis and immunobiology: new concepts emerging from investigations with the SCIDhu mouse model. *J Virol.* 2005;79(5):2651-2658.
112. Arvin AM. Humoral and cellular immunity to varicella-zoster virus: an overview. *J Infect Dis.* 2008;197(suppl 2):S58-S60.
113. Depledge DP, Ouwendijk WJD, Sadaoka T, et al. A spliced latency-associated VZV transcript maps antisense to the viral transactivator gene 61. *Nature Communications.* 2018;9:1167. doi: 10.1038/s41467-018-03569-2
114. Krause PR, Klinman DM. Varicella vaccination: evidence for frequent reactivation of the vaccine strain in healthy children. *Nat Med.* 2000;6(4):451-454.
115. Watson CP, Deck JH, Morshead C, et al. Post-herpetic neuralgia: further post-mortem studies of cases with and without pain. *Pain.* 1991;44(2):105-117.
116. Head H, Campbell AW. The pathology of herpes zoster and its bearing on sensory localisation. *Brain.* 1900;23(3):353-523.
117. Kost RG, Straus SE. Postherpetic neuralgia—pathogenesis, treatment, and prevention. *N Engl J Med.* 1996;335(1):32-42.
118. Rowbotham M, Baron R, Petersen KI, et al. Spectrum of pain mechanisms contributing to PHN. In: Watson CP, Gershon AA, eds. *Herpes Zoster and Postherpetic Neuralgia.* 2nd ed. Amsterdam: Elsevier; 2001:167.
119. Wallace MS, Oxman MN. Acute herpes zoster and postherpetic neuralgia. *Anesthesiol Clin North America.* 1997;15:371-405.
120. Fields HL, Rowbotham M, Baron R. Postherpetic neuralgia: irritable nociceptors and deafferentation. *Neurobiol Dis.* 1998;5(4):209-227.
121. Rowbotham MC, Petersen KL, Fields HL. Is postherpetic neuralgia more than one disorder? *Pain Forum.* 1998;7(4):231-237.
122. Levin MJ, Weinberg A, Schmid DS. Herpes simplex virus and varicella-zoster virus. In: Hayden RT, Wolk DM, Carroll KC, et al, eds. *Diagnostic Microbiology of the Immunocompromised Host.* 2nd ed. Washington, DC: American Society for Microbiology; 2016:135-156.
123. Boivin G, Mazzulli T, Petric M, et al. Diagnosis of viral infections. In: Richman DD, Whitley RJ, Hayden FG, eds. *Clinical Virology.* 3rd ed. Washington, DC: ASM Press; 2009:265.
124. Schmidt NJ, Gallo D, Devlin V, et al. Direct immunofluorescence staining for detection of herpes simplex and varicella-zoster virus antigens in vesicular lesions and certain tissue specimens. *J Clin Microbiol.* 1980;12(5):651-655.
125. Stein GE. Pharmacology of new antiherpes agents: famciclovir and valacyclovir. *J Am Pharm Assoc (Wash).* 1997;NS37(2):157-163.
126. Keizer HJ, De Bruijn EA, Tjaden UR, et al. Inhibition of fluorouracil catabolism in cancer patients by the antiviral agent (E)-5-(2-bromovinyl)-2′-deoxyuridine. *J Cancer Res Clin Oncol.* 1994;120(9):545-549.
127. Kawashima M, Nemoto O, Honda M, et al. Amenamevir, a novel helicase-primase inhibitor, for treatment of herpes zoster: a randomized, double-blind, valaciclovir-controlled phase 3 study. *J Dermatol.* 2017;44(11):1219-1227.
128. Dunkle LM, Arvin AM, Whitley RJ, et al. A controlled trial of acyclovir for chickenpox in normal children. *N Engl J Med.* 1991;325(22):1539-1544.

129. Klassen TP, Hartling L, Wiebe N, et al. Acyclovir for treating varicella in otherwise healthy children and adolescents. Cochrane Database Syst Rev. 2005;(4):CD002980.
130. Non-HIV Antiviral Drugs (Table 4.9) in Red Book; 2015 Report of the Committee on Infectious Diseases 30th ed. In: Kimberlin DW, Brady MT, Jackson MA, et al, eds. Elk Grove Village, IL: American Academy of Pediatrics; 2015.
131. Balfour HH Jr, Rotbart HA, Feldman S, et al. Acyclovir treatment of varicella in otherwise healthy adolescents. The Collaborative Acyclovir Varicella Study Group. *J Pediatr.* 1992;120(4, pt 1):627-633.
132. Ratanajamit C, Vinther Skriver M, Jepsen P, et al. Adverse pregnancy outcome in women exposed to acyclovir during pregnancy: a population-based observational study. *Scand J Infect Dis.* 2003;35(4):255-259.
133. Pasternak B, Hviid A. Use of acyclovir, valacyclovir, and famciclovir in the first trimester of pregnancy and the risk of birth defects. *JAMA.* 2010;304(8):859-866.
134. Stone KM, Reiff-Eldridge R, White AD, et al. Pregnancy outcomes following systemic prenatal acyclovir exposure: conclusions from the international acyclovir pregnancy registry, 1984-1999. *Birth Defects Res A Clin Mol Teratol.* 2004;70(4):201-207.
135. Haake DA, Zakowski PC, Haake DL, et al. Early treatment with acyclovir for varicella pneumonia in otherwise healthy adults: retrospective controlled study and review. *Rev Infect Dis.* 1990;12(5):788-798.
136. Nyerges G, Meszner Z, Gyarmati E, et al. Acyclovir prevents dissemination of varicella in immunocompromised children. *J Infect Dis.* 1988;157(2):309-313.
137. Dworkin RH, Johnson RW, Breuer J, et al. Recommendations for the management of herpes zoster. *Clin Infect Dis.* 2007;44(suppl 1):S1-S26.
138. Tyring S, Barbarash RA, Nahlik JE, et al. Famciclovir for the treatment of acute herpes zoster: effects on acute disease and postherpetic neuralgia. A randomized, double-blind, placebo-controlled trial. Collaborative Famciclovir Herpes Zoster Study Group. *Ann Intern Med.* 1995;123(2):89-96.
139. Beutner KR, Friedman DJ, Forszpaniak C, et al. Valaciclovir compared with acyclovir for improved therapy for herpes zoster in immunocompetent adults. *Antimicrob Agents Chemother.* 1995;39(7):1546-1553.
140. Tyring SK, Beutner KR, Tucker BA, et al. Antiviral therapy for herpes zoster: randomized, controlled clinical trial of valacyclovir and famciclovir therapy in immunocompetent patients 50 years and older. *Arch Fam Med.* 2000;9(9):863-869.
141. Degreef H. Famciclovir, a new oral antiherpes drug: results of the first controlled clinical study demonstrating its efficacy and safety in the treatment of uncomplicated herpes zoster in immunocompetent patients. *Int J Antimicrob Agents.* 1994;4(4):241-246.
142. Cobo LM, Foulks GN, Liesegang T, et al. Oral acyclovir in the treatment of acute herpes zoster ophthalmicus. *Ophthalmology.* 1986;93(6):763-770.
143. Colin J, Prisant O, Cochener B, et al. Comparison of the efficacy and safety of valaciclovir and acyclovir for the treatment of herpes zoster ophthalmicus. *Ophthalmology.* 2000;107(8):1507-1511.
144. Tyring S, Engst R, Corriveau C, et al. Famciclovir for ophthalmic zoster: a randomised aciclovir controlled study. *Br J Ophthalmol.* 2001;85(5):576-581.
145. Balfour HH Jr, Bean B, Laskin OL, et al. Acyclovir halts progression of herpes zoster in immunocompromised patients. *N Engl J Med.* 1983;308(24):1448-1453.
146. Gnann JW Jr, Crumpacker CS, Lalezari JP, et al. Sorivudine versus acyclovir for treatment of dermatomal herpes zoster in human immunodeficiency virus-infected patients: results from a randomized, controlled clinical trial. Collaborative Antiviral Study Group/AIDS Clinical Trials Group, Herpes Zoster Study Group. *Antimicrob Agents Chemother.* 1998;42(5):1139-1145.
147. Tyring S, Belanger R, Bezwoda W, et al. A randomized, double-blind trial of famciclovir versus acyclovir for the treatment of localized dermatomal herpes zoster in immunocompromised patients. *Cancer Invest.* 2001;19(1):13-22.
148. Wood MJ, Johnson RW, McKendrick MW, et al. A randomized trial of acyclovir for 7 days or 21 days with and without prednisolone for treatment of acute herpes zoster. *N Engl J Med.* 1994;330(13):896-900.
149. Whitley RJ, Weiss H, Gnann JW Jr, et al. Acyclovir with and without prednisone for the treatment of herpes zoster. A randomized, placebo-controlled trial. The National Institute of Allergy and Infectious Diseases Collaborative Antiviral Study Group. *Ann Intern Med.* 1996;125(5):376-383.
150. He L, Zhang D, Zhou M, et al. Corticosteroids for preventing postherpetic neuralgia. *Cochrane Database Syst Rev.* 2008;(1):CD005582.
151. Dworkin RH, Barbano RL, Tyring SK, et al. A randomized, placebo-controlled trial of oxycodone and of gabapentin for acute pain in herpes zoster. *Pain.* 2009;142(3):209-217.
152. Berry JD, Petersen KL. A single dose of gabapentin reduces acute pain and allodynia in patients with herpes zoster. *Neurology.* 2005;65(3):444-447.
153. van Wijck AJ, Opstelten W, Moons KG, et al. The PINE study of epidural steroids and local anaesthetics to prevent postherpetic neuralgia: a randomised controlled trial. *Lancet.* 2006;367(9506):219-224.
154. Dworkin RH, O'Connor AB, Backonja M, et al. Pharmacologic management of neuropathic pain: evidence-based recommendations. *Pain.* 2007;132(3):237-251.
155. Attal N, Cruccu G, Haanpaa M, et al. EFNS guidelines on pharmacological treatment of neuropathic pain. *Eur J Neurol.* 2006;13(11):1153-1169.
156. Backonja M, Wallace MS, Blonsky ER, et al. NGX-4010, a high-concentration capsaicin patch, for the treatment of postherpetic neuralgia: a randomised, double-blind study. *Lancet Neurol.* 2008;7(12):1106-1112.
157. Moulin DE, Clark AJ, Gilron I, et al. Pharmacological management of chronic neuropathic pain-consensus statement and guidelines from the Canadian Pain Society. *Pain Res Manag.* 2007;12(1):13-21.
158. Dubinsky RM, Kabbani H, El-Chami Z, et al. Practice parameter: treatment of postherpetic neuralgia: an evidence-based report of the Quality Standards Subcommittee of the American Academy of Neurology. *Neurology.* 2004;63(6):959-965.
159. Johnson RW, Rice AS. Clinical practice. Postherpetic neuralgia. *N Engl J Med.* 2014;371(16):1526-1533.
160. Finnerup NB, Attal N, Haroutounian S, et al. Pharmacotherapy for neuropathic pain in adults: a systematic review and meta-analysis. *Lancet Neurol.* 2015;14(2):162-173.
161. Baxter R, Ray P, Tran TN, et al. Long-term effectiveness of varicella vaccine: a 14-year, prospective cohort study. *Pediatrics.* 2013;131:e1389.

162. Marin M, Guris D, Chaves SS, et al. Prevention of varicella. Recommendations of the Advisory Committee on Immunization Practices (ACIP). June 22, 2007. Contract No. RR04.
163. Marin M, Nguyen HQ, Keen J, et al. Importance of catch-up vaccination: experience from a varicella outbreak, Maine, 2002-2003. *Pediatrics*. 2005;115(4):900-905.
164. Asano Y, Suga S, Yoshikawa T, et al. Experience and reason: twenty-year follow-up of protective immunity of the Oka strain live varicella vaccine. *Pediatrics*. 1994;94(4, Pt 1):524-526.
165. Galil K, Lee B, Strine T, et al. Outbreak of varicella at a day-care center despite vaccination. *N Engl J Med*. 2002;347(24):1909-1915.
166. Vazquez M, LaRussa PS, Gershon AA, et al. Effectiveness over time of varicella vaccine. *JAMA*. 2004;291(7):851-855.
167. Seward JF, Zhang JX, Maupin TJ, et al. Contagiousness of varicella in vaccinated cases: a household contact study. *JAMA*. 2004;292(6):704-708.
168. Chaves SS, Gargiullo P, Zhang JX, et al. Loss of vaccine-induced immunity to varicella over time. *N Engl J Med*. 2007;356(11):1121-1129.
169. Chaves SS, Zhang J, Civen R, et al. Varicella disease among vaccinated persons: clinical and epidemiological characteristics, 1997-2005. *J Infect Dis*. 2008;197 Suppl 2:S127-S131.
170. Watson B, Seward J, Yang A, et al. Postexposure effectiveness of varicella vaccine. *Pediatrics*. 2000;105(1, pt 1):84-88.
171. CDC. A new product (VariZIG) for postexposure prophylaxis of varicella available under an investigational new drug application expanded access protocol. *MMWR Morb Mortal Wkly Rep*. 2006;55(8):209-210.
172. CDC. FDA approval of an extended period for administering VariZIG for postexposure prophylaxis of varicella. *MMWR Morb Mortal Wkly Rep*. 2012;61(12):212.
173. Asano Y, Yoshikawa T, Suga S, et al. Postexposure prophylaxis of varicella in family contact by oral acyclovir. *Pediatrics*. 1993;92(2):219-222.
174. Bolyard EA, Tablan OC, Williams WW, et al. Guideline for infection control in healthcare personnel, 1998. Hospital Infection Control Practices Advisory Committee. *Infect Control Hosp Epidemiol*. 1998;19(6):407-463.
175. Schmader KE, Johnson GR, Saddier P, et al. Effect of a zoster vaccine on herpes zoster-related interference with functional status and health-related quality-of-life measures in older adults. *J Am Geriatr Soc*. 2010;58(9):1634-1641.
176. Simberkoff MS, Arbeit RD, Johnson GR, et al. Safety of herpes zoster vaccine in the shingles prevention study: a randomized trial. *Ann Intern Med*. 2010;152(9):545-554.
177. Morrison VA, Johnson GR, Schmader KE, et al. Long-term persistence of zoster vaccine efficacy. *Clin Infect Dis*. 2015;60(6):900-909.
178. Schmader KE, Oxman MN, Levin MJ, et al. Persistence of the efficacy of zoster vaccine in the shingles prevention study and the short-term persistence substudy. *Clin Infect Dis*. 2012;55(10):1320-1328.
179. Tseng HF, Smith N, Harpaz R, et al. Herpes zoster vaccine in older adults and the risk of subsequent herpes zoster disease. *JAMA*. 2011;305(2):160-166.
180. Langan SM, Smeeth L, Margolis DJ, et al. Herpes zoster vaccine effectiveness against incident herpes zoster and post-herpetic neuralgia in an older US population: a cohort study. *PLoS Med*. 2013;10(4):e1001420.
181. Baxter R, Bartlett J, Fireman B, et al. Long-term effectiveness of the live zoster vaccine in preventing shingles: a cohort study. *Am J Epidemiol*. 2018;187(1):161-169.
182. Tseng HF, Harpaz R, Luo Y, et al. Declining effectiveness of herpes zoster vaccine in adults aged ≥60 years. *J Infect Dis*. 2016;213(12):1872-1875.
183. Izurieta HS, Wernecke M, Kelman J, et al. Effectiveness and duration of protection provided by the live-attenuated herpes zoster vaccine in the Medicare population ages 65 years and older. *Clin Infect Dis*. 2017;64(6):785-793.
184. Amirthalingam G, Andrews N, Keel P, et al. Evaluation of the effect of the herpes zoster vaccination programme 3 years after its introduction in England: a population-based study. *Lancet Public Health*. 2018;3(2):e82-e90.
185. Marin M, Yawn BP, Hales CM, et al. Herpes zoster vaccine effectiveness and manifestations of herpes zoster and associated pain by vaccination status. *Hum Vaccin Immunother*. 2015;11(5):1157-1164.
186. Levin MJ, Schmader KE, Pang L, et al. Cellular and humoral responses to a second dose of herpes zoster vaccine administered 10 years after the first dose among older adults. *J Infect Dis*. 2016;213(1):14-22.
187. Hales CM, Harpaz R, Ortega-Sanchez I, et al. Update on recommendations for use of herpes zoster vaccine. *MMWR Morb Mortal Wkly Rep*. 2014;63(33):729-731.
188. Schmader KE, Levin MJ, Gnann JW Jr, et al. Efficacy, safety, and tolerability of herpes zoster vaccine in persons aged 50-59 years. *Clin Infect Dis*. 2012;54(7):922-928.
189. Tseng HF, Tartof S, Harpaz R, et al. Vaccination against zoster remains effective in older adults who later undergo chemotherapy. *Clin Infect Dis*. 2014;59(7):913-919.
190. Tseng HF, Luo Y, Shi J, et al. Effectiveness of herpes zoster vaccine in patients 60 years and older with end-stage renal disease. *Clin Infect Dis*. 2016;62(4):462-467.
191. Shafran SD. Live attenuated herpes zoster vaccine for HIV-infected adults. *HIV Med*. 2016;17(4):305-310.
192. Bombatch C, Pallotta A, Neuner EA, et al. Evaluation of herpes zoster vaccination in HIV-infected patients 50 years of age and older. *Ann Pharmacother*. 2016;50(4):326-327.
193. Benson C, Hua L, Andersen J, et al. ZOSTAVAX is generally safe and immunogenic in HIV+ adults virologically suppressed on ART: results of a Phase 2, randomized, double-blind, placebo-controlled trial. Paper presented at the 19th Conference on Retroviruses and Opportunistic Infections, Seattle, WA, 5-8 March 2012.
194. Issa NC, Marty FM, Leblebjian H, et al. Live attenuated varicella-zoster vaccine in hematopoietic stem cell transplantation recipients. *Biol Blood Marrow Transplant*. 2014;20(2):285-287.
195. Naidus E, Damon L, Schwartz BS, et al. Experience with use of Zostavax(®) in patients with hematologic malignancy and hematopoietic cell transplant recipients. *Am J Hematol*. 2012;87(1):123-125.
196. Perry LM, Winthrop KL, Curtis JR. Vaccinations for rheumatoid arthritis. *Curr Rheumatol Rep*. 2014;16(8):431.
197. Tsigrelis C, Ljungman P. Vaccinations in patients with hematological malignancies. *Blood Rev*. 2016;30(2):139-147.

198. Zhang J, Delzell E, Xie F, et al. The use, safety, and effectiveness of herpes zoster vaccination in individuals with inflammatory and autoimmune diseases: a longitudinal observational study. *Arthritis Res Ther.* 2011;13(5):R174.
199. Zhang J, Xie F, Delzell E, et al. Association between vaccination for herpes zoster and risk of herpes zoster infection among older patients with selected immune-mediated diseases. *JAMA.* 2012;308(1):43-49.
200. Willis ED, Woodward M, Brown E, et al. Herpes zoster vaccine live: a 10 year review of post-marketing safety experience. *Vaccine.* 2017;35(52):7231-7239.
201. Morrison VA, Oxman MN, Levin MJ, et al. Safety of zoster vaccine in elderly adults following documented herpes zoster. *J Infect Dis.* 2013;208(4):559-563.
202. GlaxoSmithKline. Shingrix® Package Insert. https://www.fda.gov/downloads/biologicsbloodvaccines/vaccines/approvedproducts/ucm581605.pdf. Accessed March 8-, 2018.
203. Dooling KL, Guo A, Patel M, et al. Recommendations of the Advisory Committee on Immunization Practices for Use of Herpes Zoster Vaccines. *MMWR Morb Mortal Wkly Rep.* 2018;67(3):103-108.
204. Leroux-Roels I, Leroux-Roels G, Clement F, et al. A phase 1/2 clinical trial evaluating safety and immunogenicity of a varicella zoster glycoprotein e subunit vaccine candidate in young and older adults. *J Infect Dis.* 2012;206(8):1280-1290.
205. Chlibek R, Pauksens K, Rombo L, et al. Long-term immunogenicity and safety of an investigational herpes zoster subunit vaccine in older adults. *Vaccine.* 2016;34(6):863-868.
206. Schwarz TF, Volpe S, Catteau G, et al. Persistence of immune response to an adjuvanted varicella-zoster virus subunit vaccine for up to year nine in older adults. *Hum Vaccin Immunother.* 201;14(6):1370-1377.
207. Lal H, Cunningham AL, Godeaux O, et al. Efficacy of an adjuvanted herpes zoster subunit vaccine in older adults. *N Engl J Med.* 2015;372(22):2087-2096.
208. Cunningham AL, Lal H, Kovac M, et al. Efficacy of the herpes zoster subunit vaccine in adults 70 years of age or older. *N Engl J Med.* 2016;375(11):1019-1032.
209. Levin MJ, Oxman MN, Zhang JH, et al. Varicella-zoster virus-specific immune responses in elderly recipients of a herpes zoster vaccine. *J Infect Dis.* 2008;197(6):825-835.
210. Weinberg A, Zhang JH, Oxman MN, et al. Varicella-zoster virus-specific immune responses to herpes zoster in elderly participants in a trial of a clinically effective zoster vaccine. *J Infect Dis.* 2009;200(7):1068-1077.
211. Berkowitz EM, Moyle G, Stellbrink HJ, et al. Safety and immunogenicity of an adjuvanted herpes zoster subunit candidate vaccine in HIV-infected adults: a phase 1/2a randomized, placebo-controlled study. *J Infect Dis.* 2015;211(8):1279-1287.
212. Stadtmauer EA, Sullivan KM, Marty FM, et al. A phase 1/2 study of an adjuvanted varicella-zoster virus subunit vaccine in autologous hematopoietic cell transplant recipients. *Blood.* 2014;124(19):2921-2929.
213. Schwarz TF, Aggarwal N, Moeckesch B, et al. Immunogenicity and safety of an adjuvanted herpes zoster subunit vaccine coadministered with seasonal influenza vaccine in adults aged 50 years or older. *J Infect Dis.* 2017;216(11):1352-1361.
214. Grupping K, Campora L, Douha M, et al. Immunogenicity and safety of the HZ/su adjuvanted herpes zoster subunit vaccine in adults previously vaccinated with a live attenuated herpes zoster vaccine. *J Infect Dis.* 2017;216(11):1343-1351.
215. Godeaux O, Kovac M, Shu D, et al. Immunogenicity and safety of an adjuvanted herpes zoster subunit candidate vaccine in adults ≥ 50 years of age with a prior history of herpes zoster: a phase III, non-randomized, open-label clinical trial. *Hum Vaccin Immunother.* 2017;13(5):1051-1058.
216. Kroger AT, Duchin J, Vázquez M. General Best Practice Guidelines for Immunization. Best Practices Guidance of the Advisory Committee on Immunization Practices (ACIP). www.cdc.gov/vaccines/hcp/acip-recs/general-recs/downloads/general-recs.pdf. Accessed March 9, 2018.
217. Cunningham AL, Heineman T. Vaccine profile of herpes zoster (HZ/su) subunit vaccine. *Expert Rev Vaccines.* 2017;16(7):1-10.
218. Oxman MN, Harbecke R, Koelle DM. Clinical usage of the adjuvanted herpes zoster subunit vaccine (HZ/su): revaccination of recipients of live attenuated zoster vaccine and coadministration with a seasonal influenza vaccine. *J Infect Dis.* 2017;216(11):1329-1333.
219. Woloshin S, Schwartz LM, White B, et al. The Fate of FDA Postapproval Studies. *N Engl J Med.* 2017;377(12):1114-1117.

Chapter 166 :: Poxvirus Infections
:: Ellen S. Haddock & Sheila Fallon Friedlander

第一百六十六章
痘病毒感染

中文导读

痘病毒是目前已知最大的双链DNA动物病毒，其感染人体可引起不同程度的局部或系统性病变。本章共分为3节：①正痘病毒感染（包括天花、牛痘和天花接种免疫和猴痘）；②副痘病毒感染（包括挤奶工结节和Orf）；③软疣痘病毒属感染：传染性软疣。分别介绍了这些痘病毒感染的流行病学、临床特征、危险因素、病因和发病机制、诊断、鉴别诊断、临床病程和预后及临床管理。

第一节介绍了正痘病毒感染。其中天花已经灭绝，但病毒株仍存在，希望读者了解相关知识，关注可能存在的使用天花病毒的生物恐怖主义；同时，报道了一些牛痘（天花疫苗）接种免疫引发的严重皮疹案例；猴痘则为在非洲较为流行的人畜共患病，其特征性的临床症状为感染者淋巴结肿大。

第二节介绍了副痘病毒感染。本节介绍了副痘病毒属包括的2种在人类中引起疾病的病毒：挤奶工结节和orf病毒。这2种副痘病毒感染在临床表现和组织学上是难以区分的，鉴别诊断需要借助临床病史和PCR分析。在表166-5中列举了挤奶工结节和Orf病毒的鉴别要点。

第三节介绍了软疣痘病毒属感染所致的传染性软疣，好发于儿童，炎症反应严重的病变部位有时被误认为继发性细菌感染或蜂窝组织炎。

〔张江林〕

AT-A-GLANCE

- Poxviruses are the largest animal viruses; they can cause disease of varying severity in humans.
- Smallpox is the only poxvirus whose sole reservoir is humans, which allowed its eradication.
- The virus used in smallpox vaccines, vaccinia, has its own adverse effects.
- Monkeypox is a zoonotic infection endemic in Africa.
- Milker's nodule and orf mainly cause localized cutaneous infections.
- Molluscum contagiosum is generally a benign cutaneous disease most frequently seen in children and immunocompromised individuals.
- Histopathologic features of poxviral cutaneous lesions include the presence of intracytoplasmic eosinophilic inclusion bodies.

Poxviruses are a family of double-stranded DNA viruses that replicate in the cytoplasm of host cells (Table 166-1). They are the largest known animal viruses and can be seen with light microscopy.[1] The poxvirus family is divided into multiple genera. Four genera affect humans: *Orthopoxvirus*, *Parapoxvirus*, *Molluscipoxvirus*, and *Yatapoxvirus*. The poxviruses that cause significant disease in humans are reviewed here. Their effects on humans range from systemic disease to localized infection to epithelial cell proliferation without other findings.

ORTHOPOXVIRUS INFECTIONS

Members of the *Orthopoxvirus* genus that cause disease in humans include variola (smallpox), vaccinia, cowpox, and monkeypox. Variola, vaccinia, and monkeypox are discussed in detail below. Cowpox, whose major reservoir is thought to be cats and small rodents rather than cows, rarely infects humans.

SMALLPOX (VARIOLA)

AT-A-GLANCE

- Mortality from the major form of smallpox is approximately 30%.
- Smallpox is transmitted mainly by the respiratory route; viremia leads to cutaneous and visceral involvement.
- The eruption consists of multiple papules in a centrifugal distribution that progress en masse through vesicular and pustular stages.
- The disease has not been seen since 1978, but concern exists about the potential use of variola virus for bioterrorism.
- Smallpox vaccination has been reinstituted on a selective basis for response in the case of an outbreak.

Variola virus is the pathogen responsible for smallpox, a disease that devastated humankind in catastrophic epidemics for more than 3000 years. This poxvirus scarred and killed millions of people in both the Old and New Worlds, affecting entire populations on every continent. It is estimated to have killed approximately 500 million people in the 20th century alone.[2] The practice of variolation, the intentional introduction of smallpox virus from a pustule of an infected person into a healthy nonimmune person to induce a mild form of the disease as prophylaxis against a full-scale infection, gained popularity in the 18th century.[3] This practice reduced mortality significantly but caused full-scale disease in a subset of individuals, resulting in 1% to 2% mortality.[3] Edward Jenner altered the course of history in 1796 when he created the first vaccine by inoculating patients with cowpox virus to protect them against the related smallpox virus. Later, vaccinia virus was used for vaccination, and smallpox was eradicated in the United States in 1949. The World Health Organization (WHO) launched a global campaign to eradicate smallpox in 1959,[3] and an intensive effort culminated in global eradication by 1980.[3,4]

After eradication, the WHO directed all laboratories other than the Centers for Disease Control and Prevention (CDC) in the United States and the Vector laboratory in Russia to destroy their smallpox samples. However, a misplaced vial of variola virus was discovered at the National Institutes of Health facility in Bethesda, Maryland in 2014,[5] raising the theoretical possibility that other unreported stocks of virus may exist and could be used as a biologic weapon. Concerns about bioterrorism have renewed the need for knowledge about smallpox and the development of improved vaccines and treatments in case the disease reemerges.

EPIDEMIOLOGY

Unlike other members of the poxvirus family, smallpox only affects humans and cannot be acquired from other species. Transmission is generally via respiratory droplets and requires close contact but aerosol spread also has been reported. Outbreaks occur in the winter and early spring seasons when conditions of low humidity and low temperature favor survival of the aerosolized virus.[6] Smallpox is less infectious than other diseases spread by the respiratory route, including measles, varicella, and influenza. The estimated rate of secondary infection of unvaccinated contacts is 37% to 88%.[7] Secondary cases are often limited to family members or health care workers. Spread of smallpox is facilitated by the large quantity of virus in the aerosolized droplets, high population density, and extensive contact between the infected individual and others. The very young, the elderly, and pregnant women are more susceptible to infection.[8] Individuals with more-severe clinical disease are reported to be more infectious, but these same people also tend to be toxemic and confined to bed.

There are 2 main strains of variola virus: (a) variola major, the more common, severe, and often lethal form, and (b) variola minor, a milder less-lethal form.

Today, the majority of the world's population is susceptible to smallpox disease, as routine vaccination of civilians was discontinued in the United States in 1971 and worldwide in the 1980s. Those vaccinated before 1972 have uncertain levels of immunity remaining. Until 2002, only laboratory workers handling non–highly attenuated orthopoxviruses still were advised to receive routine vaccination. Since that time, military

TABLE 166-1
Poxviruses with Humans as Hosts

GENUS	SPECIES	HOSTS	MAIN PORTAL OF ENTRY	CLINICAL FEATURES	TREATMENT
Orthopoxvirus	Variola virus (smallpox)	Humans	Respiratory tract	High fever and myalgia precede oropharyngeal enanthem and centrifugal exanthem. Simultaneous progression of skin lesions from macules to papulovesicles, pustules, and crusts, resulting in significant scars. Last reported case in 1978; concern for use in bioterrorism.	Postexposure vaccination to reduce severity and disease occurrence (prior to onset of clinical symptoms) Tecovirimat (SIGA Technologies) Brincidofovir (CMX001, Chimerix)
	Vaccinia virus	Humans	Skin	Used as vaccine for smallpox. Also protects against monkeypox. Vaccination site progresses from papule to vesicle, pustule, and crust, leaving scar. Adverse events occur when virus spreads locally or in a generalized manner, more severe in individuals with disruption of the skin barrier or immune compromise.	Symptomatic treatment for minor local reactions, or for typical systemic symptoms Vaccinia immune globulin or cidofovir for extensive lesions distant from vaccination site Skin care Fluid and electrolyte repletion
	Monkeypox virus	Rodents, humans, monkeys, anteaters	Skin	Clinical presentation similar to that of smallpox but with more prominent lymphadenopathy and lower mortality.	Postexposure prophylaxis with vaccinia virus (4-14 days after exposure) Tecovirimat Cidofovir Brincidofovir
	Cowpox virus	Rodents, cats, humans, cattle	Skin	Contact with infected animal host gives rise to papule that becomes vesicular, hemorrhagic, pustular, and ulcerative; resulting eschar heals over 3-4 weeks with scarring. Constitutional symptoms and lymphangitis common. Can be extensive or severe if skin barrier is disrupted.	No known treatment
Parapoxvirus	Orf virus	Sheep, goats, humans	Skin	Contact with infected animal or fomite leads to 1 or more papules, usually on hand. Papule progresses into pustule or nodule with central umbilication and surrounding gray-white or violaceous ring and outer zone of erythema. Becomes weepy, then dries and crusts. Healing occurs over 4-8 weeks, usually without scarring. Constitutional symptoms are uncommon.	Resolves within 4-6 weeks Debridement, topical cidofovir, or topical imiquimod may speed resolution
	Pseudocowpox virus (paravaccinia virus)	Cattle, humans	Skin	Transmission by contact with infected teats/mouths of cattle. Causes milker's nodule. Clinical findings and course similar to orf; differentiated by animal hosts.	Disease is self-limited; symptomatic treatment only Curettage of large lesions may speed resolution
	Bovine papular stomatitis virus	Cattle, humans	Skin	Transmitted by contact with infected mouths of cattle. Clinical findings and course similar to orf and paravaccinia.	Similar to above

(Continued)

TABLE 166-1
Poxviruses with Humans as Hosts (Continued)

GENUS	SPECIES	HOSTS	MAIN PORTAL OF ENTRY	CLINICAL FEATURES	TREATMENT
Molluscipoxvirus	Molluscum contagiosum virus	Humans	Skin	Discrete firm, dome-shaped papules; may have central umbilication. Can be extensive in individuals with atopic dermatitis or immune compromise. Most cases resolve spontaneously in months to years, but lesions often are treated to reduce symptoms and minimize autoinoculation. Can be persistent/refractory in immunocompromised individuals.	Cantharidin 0.7% topically for 2-6 hours, before rinsing. Imiquimod cream. Intralesional candida antigen. Oral cimetidine. Podophyllotoxin. Cidofovir. Physically destructive therapies (curettage, cryotherapy, CO_2 laser, pulsed-dye laser, electrodessication)
Yatapoxvirus	Tanapox virus	Humans, monkeys	Possibly skin	Uncertain mode of transmission; possible mosquito vector from infected monkeys to humans. Short fever precedes eruption of 1 or more pruritic, indurated papules with surrounding edema. Become necrotic and/or ulcerative, then heal within 6 weeks with scarring.	Self-resolving within 6 weeks, with resulting lifelong immunity

personnel and a small group of U.S. civilians who would serve as first-line responders in a bioterrorism attack have been vaccinated.[9] The risk of adverse effects from the vaccine, particularly in immunocompromised patients and individuals with atopic dermatitis or other skin barrier defects, has prevented mass vaccination policies.

CLINICAL FEATURES

Prodrome: An infected individual is asymptomatic during the incubation period of viral replication. A prodrome of high fever (39°C to 41°C [102.2°F to 105.8°F]), chills, myalgia, and severe headache develops within 7 to 17 days of exposure, with an average incubation of 10 to 12 days.[7] The prodrome usually lasts 2 to 3 days, during which the affected individual is severely ill and often bedridden.

Cutaneous Findings: Approximately 1 day after the onset of fever, an enanthem of red macules develops on the mouth, tongue, and oropharynx and subsequently vesiculates and ulcerates, releasing high concentrations of transmissible virus particles in respiratory secretions. A skin rash (exanthem) usually follows a day later.[7] The fever usually declines with appearance of the rash.[10]

The classic smallpox rash begins as macules on the face and extremities but quickly spreads to cover the body. Involvement of all parts of the body, including palms and soles, occurs within 24 to 48 hours. Smallpox tends to have a centrifugal distribution, meaning that lesions are most concentrated on the face and distal extremities. A key characteristic of smallpox is that all lesions progress synchronously through macular, papular, vesicular, and pustular stages. Each stage lasts 1 to 2 days. Macules become raised papules 2 to 3 mm in diameter within 1 or 2 days and then form vesicles 2 to 5 mm in diameter (Fig. 166-1) within another 1 or 2 days. Firm, deep-seated pustules 4 to 6 mm in diameter (Fig. 166-2) develop 4 to 7 days after the onset of the rash and may umbilicate or become confluent. After 8 to 10 days, the lesions begin to crust (Fig. 166-3). Fever may reoccur during the pustular stage, especially if a secondary bacterial infection has developed. Scabs begin separating 2 weeks after the

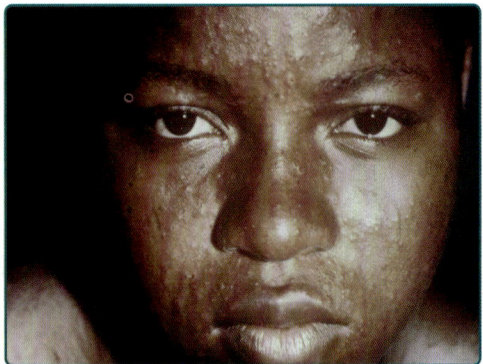

Figure 166-1 Day 3 of rash in a young woman with smallpox, with fluid accumulating in several vesicles. (From the Centers for Disease Control and Prevention [CDC] Public Health Image Library, Atlanta, GA, USA.)

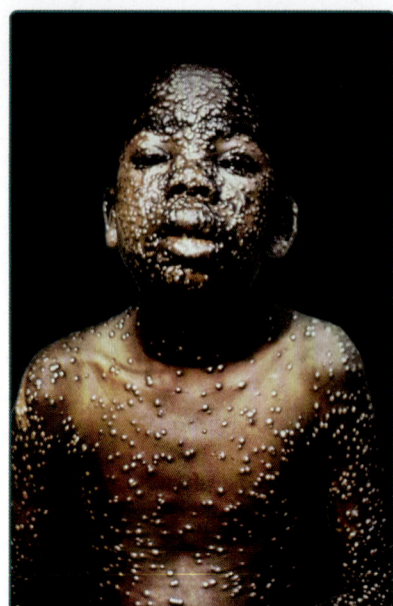

Figure 166-2 Pustular smallpox lesions with characteristic highest density on the face and extremities. (From the Centers for Disease Control and Prevention [CDC] Public Health Image Library, Atlanta, GA, USA.)

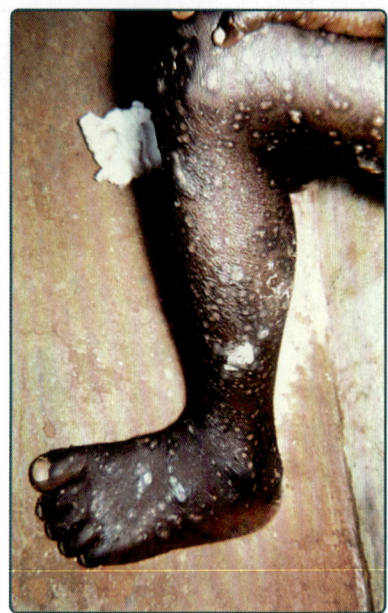

Figure 166-4 Scars and pockmarks remain after the crusts have fallen off. (From the Centers for Disease Control and Prevention [CDC] Public Health Image Library, Atlanta, GA, USA, and contributed by J. Noble, Jr., MD.)

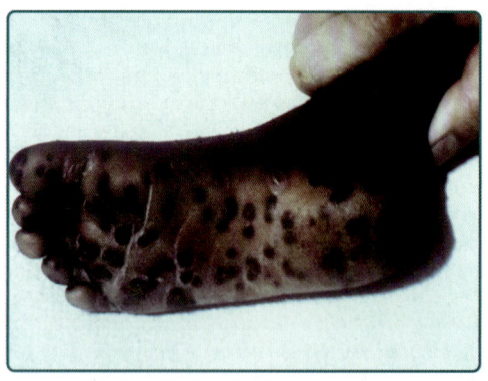

Figure 166-3 Crusted lesions on the foot at day 21 of the rash of smallpox. (From the Centers for Disease Control and Prevention [CDC] Public Health Image Library, Atlanta, GA, USA, and contributed by Paul B. Dean, MD.)

onset of the rash and typically have all separated by 4 weeks. After their resolution, pitted scars ("pockmarks") remain on 65% to 80% of survivors and can be disfiguring (Fig. 166-4).[7] Scarring is most common on the face, where there are larger and more numerous sebaceous glands, which are particularly susceptible to infection and destruction by variola virus.[4]

Classic or ordinary smallpox, described above, is the most common type, accounting for 85% of smallpox outbreaks.[2,4]

In addition to ordinary smallpox, the WHO recognizes 3 other clinically recognizable forms of variola major, which differ in disease presentation and rash burden.[2,10] These are modified smallpox, flat smallpox, and hemorrhagic smallpox.

Modified smallpox (approximately 5% to 7% of all cases) is a mild, nonfatal form of variola major infection that occurs in previously vaccinated individuals. It has a milder prodrome, fewer lesions, and an accelerated and abbreviated course because the disease has been "modified" or attenuated by previous vaccination.[2] Lesions tend not to progress to vesicles or pustules, crusting by day 10.

Flat smallpox (also called *malignant smallpox*) is an uncommon form of variola major infection (approximately 5% of cases) in which lesions develop slowly and persist as soft, velvety vesicles that coalesce into confluent, edematous plaques with a flat appearance.[2] It usually occurs in children and unvaccinated individuals lacking cellular immunity. Affected individuals become severely ill with toxic fever, and most die with hemorrhagic lesions and pneumonia.[7]

Hemorrhagic smallpox, also known as *fulminant smallpox*, involves hemorrhage into the skin or mucous membranes and is the rarest (<1% of cases) and deadliest form of smallpox.[2] It is equally common in unvaccinated and vaccinated persons and is almost always fatal.[2] In the early hemorrhagic form, massive hemorrhage from mucosal surfaces occurs before any rash develops and leads to death before the sixth day of illness.[11] This form is more common in adults, and pregnant women are especially susceptible. In the late hemorrhagic form, hemorrhage occurs after onset of the typical rash and death occurs within 12 days.[11] This form affects women and men equally.[4]

Variola sine eruption, is a brief febrile illness (48 hours or less) without a rash that can occur when a vaccinated individual is exposed to someone infected with variola major. This brief illness can be confirmed by serologic studies showing a rise in antibody titers against smallpox virus.[7]

Infections with the variola minor strain, the milder strain of smallpox, are clinically indistinguishable from cases of modified smallpox and mild cases of ordinary smallpox. Historically, outbreaks were diagnosed retrospectively as variola minor if the fatality rate was low (1% or less). Minor and major strains can now be differentiated by polymerase chain reaction (PCR).[4]

Noncutaneous Findings: Variola virus spreads by the blood to noncutaneous systems. It can infect the metaphyses of growing bones and lead to arthritis in up to 2% of affected children. Osteomyelitis variolosa is less frequent but may also cause bone deformities.[12] Swelling of the eyelids and a mild conjunctivitis are common findings. Cough and bronchitis may be seen in some cases of smallpox. A degree of encephalopathy often occurs, with symptoms ranging from headache and hallucinations to delirium and psychosis.[4] Gross hematuria can occur with the hemorrhagic type of variola major.[13]

Complications: Secondary bacterial infection occurs commonly in skin lesions, as well as at regional lymph nodes, affecting 5% of individuals. Keratitis and corneal ulceration, common in malnourished individuals, result in blindness in 1% of cases. Variola virus or bacterial superinfection can lead to respiratory complications, including pneumonia, at days 8 to 10 of illness. Both arthritis and osteomyelitis can lead to limb deformities, including bone shortening, subluxation, and flail joints. Orchitis is less common and usually unilateral. Encephalitis is reported in 0.2% of cases.[4]

ETIOLOGY AND PATHOGENESIS

Smallpox is caused by the variola virus, a linear, double-stranded DNA virus of the genus *Orthopoxvirus*. Variola virus measures approximately 300 × 250 × 200 nm and has a brick-shaped appearance on electron microscopy (Fig. 166-5).

Although the 2 major forms, variola major and variola minor, have approximately 98% genetic homology, variola major is markedly more virulent, with significantly higher mortality.[14]

Humans are the only natural reservoir of the variola virus. Smallpox usually spreads by implantation of droplets containing virus on to nasal, oral, or pharyngeal mucous membranes or alveoli of the lung.[4] Household contacts of an infected individual and others with prolonged face-to-face exposure are at greatest risk of infection.[9] Variola virus is less commonly spread by accidental inoculation into the skin, through the conjunctiva, and through contact with infected body fluids or highly contaminated fomites. Rarely, it is transmitted transplacentally, by long-range airborne viral particles, or by viral particles suspended in enclosed areas.[15]

The virus attaches to respiratory epithelial cells, travels to regional lymph nodes, and replicates at these sites. Transient primary viremia with uptake of the virus by macrophages occurs, and the virus spreads to the reticuloendothelial organs, where asymptomatic replication continues. A massive secondary viremia follows and causes the onset of symptoms (the prodromal period). The virus spreads to the skin and mucosa, along with other organs and tissues such as the liver and kidneys.[7,16]

Variola virus is transmissible beginning in the late prodromal phase by aerosolization of viral particles from the oropharynx. It is most infectious during the first week of the rash, which is when enanthem lesions have ulcerated and are releasing virus into mouth and pharynx secretions.[4] The virus remains transmissible until all scabs have fallen off of skin lesions.[16]

DIAGNOSIS

An acute, generalized rash with characteristic well-circumscribed, firm, deep-seated vesicles or pustules should raise concern for smallpox.

The CDC protocol for evaluation of acute, generalized vesicular or pustular rashes, available on the CDC website (cdc.gov), should be consulted and followed whenever suspicion arises.[17] Airborne and contact precautions should be implemented immediately. The next step is defining the suspicion for smallpox as high, moderate, or low, based on the CDC's major and minor smallpox criteria.

Major criteria include (a) febrile prodrome 1 to 4 days before rash onset; (b) classic smallpox lesions, defined as deep-seated, firm/hard, round, well-circumscribed vesicles or pustules; and (c) lesions in the same stage of development (ie, all vesicles or all pustules) on any one part of the body.

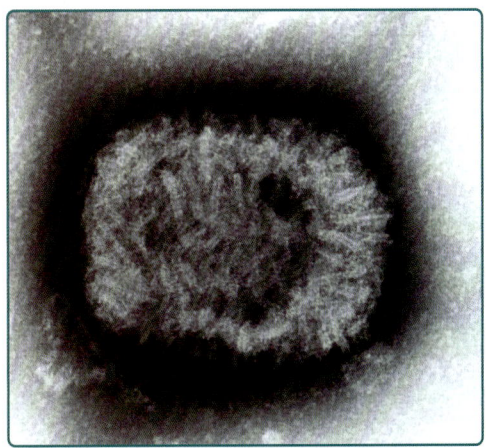

Figure 166-5 Electron micrograph of the variola virus. (From the Centers for Disease Control and Prevention [CDC] Public Health Image Library, Atlanta, GA, USA, and contributed by J. Nakano.)

Minor criteria include (a) centrifugal distribution, meaning that lesions are most concentrated on the face and distal extremities; (b) lesions first occurred on the oral mucosa/palate, face, or forearms; (c) patient appears toxic or moribund; (d) slow evolution of lesions, meaning that they evolve from macules to papules to pustules, with each stage lasting 1 to 2 days; and (e) lesions on palms and soles.

Risk for smallpox is considered to be high if patients meet all major criteria. Patients with febrile prodrome plus 1 other major criteria or 4 or more minor criteria are considered to have a moderate risk for smallpox. Patients with febrile prodrome but fewer than 4 minor criteria or no febrile prodrome are considered to have a low risk for smallpox.

The recommended workup depends on smallpox risk status. When the risk of smallpox is determined to be high, local and state health departments should be contacted immediately; they will lead diagnosis and management efforts, in coordination with the CDC. High-risk specimens should be tested only at laboratories with appropriate expertise and biosafety levels.

Moderate- and low-risk cases should be worked up for more common causes of febrile exanthema, such as varicella zoster virus (VZV), herpes simplex virus (HSV), and enterovirus. The CDC recommends Tzanck smear to evaluate for HSV as well as direct fluorescent antibody assay to evaluate for HSV and VZV. PCR for VZV, HSV, and enterovirus should be performed. If possible, electron microscopy to distinguish between poxvirus and VZV should be performed, and the virus can be cultured. Biopsy to evaluate for erythema multiforme also can be considered. PCR for nonvariola *Orthopoxvirus* should be conducted and can be coordinated by the CDC. PCR for all orthopoxviruses, including variola, also can be performed. Multiple diagnostic methods are used to improve diagnostic certainty.

For high-risk cases, the focus is on ruling out variola before any additional testing is performed. All testing should be performed by a biosafety level 3 laboratory. Electron microscopy can be performed under biosafety level 3 conditions at a local facility. All other testing should be performed by a Laboratory Research Network facility or by the CDC. These laboratories will perform variola-specific PCR, nonvariola *Orthopoxvirus* PCR, and PCR that tests for all orthopoxviruses. In high-risk cases, testing for VZV, HSV, and enterovirus will only be pursued once variola has been ruled out.[18]

Special Tests: Since the eradication of smallpox the positive predictive value of any one test is very low, so multiple methods of testing are used to confirm a diagnosis of smallpox.

Real-time PCR (RT-PCR) is the quickest and most sensitive assay for detecting and differentiating between orthopoxviruses. As mentioned above, 3 different assays are used to evaluate a possible smallpox infection: (a) *Orthopoxvirus* RT-PCR, which detects all *Orthopoxvirus* including variola; (b) nonvariola *Orthopoxvirus* RT-PCR, which detects all *Orthopoxvirus* except for variola; and (c) RT-PCR assay that detects only variola. PCR is very useful for distinguishing viral species but cannot determine whether a virus is viable.

Viral culture for virus isolation has the benefit of providing additional material for testing, but should only be performed by the CDC. Historically, orthopoxviruses could be differentiated by the morphology of the pocks they produced on the chorioallantoic membranes of chicken embryos, but this is not commonly performed today.[16]

Electron microscopy is most useful for confirming the presence of a virus and differentiating between poxvirus and varicella. It can distinguish between brick-shaped orthopoxviruses and icosahedral varicella viruses, but cannot distinguish among orthopoxviruses (ie, cannot distinguish variola from vaccinia, monkeypox, or cowpox).[19]

Serologic testing, including immunofluorescence and enzyme-linked immunosorbent assay, has limited usefulness in diagnosis of smallpox because orthopoxviruses are closely related and there is significant antibody cross-reactivity. Serologic testing cannot reliably distinguish between variola, vaccinia, and monkeypox infection. However, it can be useful for confirming past exposure to *Orthopoxvirus*.[19]

As with serologic testing, current immunohistochemistry assays can identify *Orthopoxvirus* but cannot differentiate among species of *Orthopoxvirus*. However, immunohistochemistry can be helpful in identifying other microorganisms such as HSV, VZV, enterovirus, syphilis, and rickettsia.[19]

Laboratory Abnormalities: The white blood cell count may increase as the skin lesions of smallpox become pustular. Severe thrombocytopenia occurs in hemorrhagic smallpox, both early and late types. A marked decrease in the level of factor V (accelerator globulin) and increase in thrombin time are noted in the early hemorrhagic form, likely from disseminated intravascular coagulation. The late hemorrhagic form has a smaller degree of these coagulation disturbances.[4]

Pathology: Skin biopsy specimens from early papules show edema and dilation of the capillaries of the papillary dermis with a perivascular infiltrate of lymphocytes, histiocytes, and plasma cells. With progression, the cells of the epidermis become vacuolated and swollen and undergo ballooning degeneration. These vesicles have characteristic intracytoplasmic inclusion bodies called *Guarnieri bodies*. Pustules form with migration of polymorphonuclear cells into the vesicles. Eventually, the pustule becomes a crust, with new epithelium growing to repair the surface. Mucous membrane lesions show similar changes but also have extensive necrosis of the epithelial cells leading to rapid ulceration rather than vesiculation.[20]

The CDC algorithm recommends histopathologic and immunohistochemical analysis only after workup for VZV, HSV, and enterovirus and *Orthopoxvirus* PCR analysis are negative.[18]

DIFFERENTIAL DIAGNOSIS

Table 166-2 outlines the differential diagnosis of smallpox.

The exanthem of smallpox is most often confused with that of chickenpox (varicella). Smallpox lesions are deep-seated and firm, whereas chickenpox vesicles are more superficial ("dewdrops on a rose petal"). Smallpox lesions progress simultaneously, so all lesions on any one part of the body are in the same stage (eg, all papules or all vesicles), whereas chicken pox lesions appear in crops, so multiple different stages (a mix of papules, vesicles, pustules, and crusts) are seen at once. Chickenpox lesions progress more quickly than smallpox lesions, evolving from macule to papule to vesicle to crust in less than 24 hours. In contrast, each stage of smallpox lasts 1 to 2 days. Overall, chickenpox has a shorter disease course, with all lesions crusting within 4 to 6 days from initial appearance.[16] In contrast to smallpox, which is preceded by a severe febrile prodrome with prostration, headache, backache, chills, vomiting, or abdominal pain, chickenpox is not preceded by a significant prodrome, and patients do not appear toxic. Smallpox has a centrifugal distribution, with lesions most concentrated on the face and distal extremities. In contrast, chickenpox has a centripetal distribution, with lesions most concentrated on the trunk. Palms and soles may be affected in smallpox, but are rarely involved in chickenpox.[17]

Disseminated herpes zoster can appear similar to varicella but usually begins in a dermatomal distribution. The morbilliform prodromal rash of smallpox can be confused with coxsackievirus or measles infections.

Human monkeypox clinically resembles smallpox but often manifests with lymphadenopathy. It is a zoonotic disease and is not spread as easily between persons.

Secondary syphilis should be considered, especially when there are lesions on the palms and soles, but these lesions do not progress.

Table 166-2 lists other eruptions in the differential diagnosis.

The lesions of hemorrhagic smallpox can be similar to those of meningococcemia, viral hemorrhagic fevers such as Ebola, dengue or rift valley fever, severe acute leukemia, and other acute hemorrhagic eruptions, such as those associated with coagulopathies.

CLINICAL COURSE AND PROGNOSIS

Death from smallpox typically occurs during the second week of illness and is thought to be caused by toxemia associated with immune complexes with variola antigens, which induce hypotension/shock and multiorgan failure. Underlying host immune deficiencies likely play a role in the most severe flat and hemorrhagic forms of the disease.[2] Encephalitis is an important factor in death from variola minor but not from variola major.[4,7]

The overall mortality rate for variola major is 30%, compared to less than 1% for variola minor.[3,4] Mortality

TABLE 166-2
Differential Diagnosis of Smallpox and Monkeypox

Most Likely
- Papulovesicular eruption
  - Coxsackievirus infection
  - Extensive arthropod or mite infestation
  - Varicella
  - Disseminated zoster
  - Generalized vaccinia
  - Prodromal morbilliform eruption
  - Erythema multiforme
  - Drug eruption
- Hemorrhagic lesions (smallpox only)
  - Meningococcemia
  - Disseminated intravascular coagulation
- Mucosal lesions
  - Hand-foot-and-mouth disease
  - Stevens-Johnson syndrome

Consider
- Papulovesicular eruption
  - Kaposi varicelliform eruption
  - Eczema vaccinatum
  - Extensive molluscum contagiosum (in immunosuppressed patients)
  - Bullous impetigo
  - Pityriasis lichenoides et varioliformis acuta
  - Rickettsialpox
- Prodromal morbilliform eruption
  - Measles
  - Other viral infections
- Hemorrhagic lesions (smallpox only)
  - Acute leukemia
  - Viral hemorrhagic fevers
- Mucosal lesions
  - Oral herpes simplex

Always Rule Out
- Papulovesicular eruption
  - Secondary syphilis
- Hemorrhagic lesions (smallpox only)
  - Acquired coagulopathy
- Mucosal lesions
  - Stevens-Johnson syndrome

from ordinary smallpox ranges from less than 10% when lesions are discrete to 50% to 75% when lesions are confluent. Modified smallpox is associated with less than 10% mortality. In contrast, flat smallpox has a case fatality rate of more than 90%, and hemorrhagic forms have nearly 100% mortality. Those who survive the disease will have lifetime immunity.

MANAGEMENT

A patient suspected of having smallpox should be isolated in a negative-pressure room.

Postexposure vaccination before the development of clinical symptoms can reduce disease occurrence and severity, as discussed below; however, vaccination after the development of clinical symptoms does not appear to provide any benefit.[21]

Treatments for smallpox infection have not been studied in humans but have been investigated under the Animal Efficacy Rule, which allows the U.S. Food and Drug Administration (FDA) to grant approval based on animal model studies when studies in humans are not ethical or feasible.[22]

Tecovirimat (SIGA Technologies, New York, NY), an *Orthopoxvirus*-specific antiviral medication, was added to the U.S. Strategic National Stockpile in 2013 for treatment of smallpox.[23,24] In the event of a smallpox outbreak, it would be used under the Emergency Use Authorization. It works by targeting the *F13L* vaccinia gene that is highly conserved among orthopoxviruses and preventing viral egress from infected cells.[21] It reduces morbidity and mortality of variola infection in nonhuman primates in both prelesional and postlesional settings.[25]

Brincidofovir (CMX001; Chimerix, Durham, NC), a lipid conjugate of cidofovir with broad-spectrum in vitro activity against double-stranded DNA viruses, is being studied as a potential smallpox therapy under the Animal Efficacy Rule. Initial studies in a rabbit model of smallpox were promising, with a significant reduction in mortality when treated after the first sign of clinical disease.[25A]

A National Institutes of Health strategy for developing smallpox treatments is to identify broad-spectrum antivirals that have obtained regular FDA approval for other viral indications and then seek approval for use against orthopoxviruses under the Animal Efficacy Rule.[23]

Prevention: Vaccination with vaccinia virus (Table 166-3) is 90% to 96% effective in preventing smallpox disease when given before exposure to variola virus. For postexposure prophylaxis, vaccination within 2 to 3 days of exposure can protect against severe disease. Vaccination within 4 to 5 days may protect against death.[3]

Vaccination with vaccinia virus is not currently available to the general public, as the risk of smallpox outbreak is thought to be low, the risk of adverse effects is significant, particularly in the immunosuppressed and those with skin barrier defects, and postexposure prophylaxis is effective. However, vaccination is indicated for laboratory workers handling non–highly attenuated orthopoxviruses as well as individuals designated to respond to a suspected smallpox outbreak.[9]

In the event of an outbreak, the U.S. government has stockpiled enough smallpox vaccine to vaccinate the entire U.S. population.[2] The 3 currently stockpiled vaccines are: ACAM2000 (Emergent, Gaithersburg, MD), Aventis Pasteur Smallpox Vaccine (APSV; Sanofi Pasteur, Lyon, France), and Imvamune (Bavarian Nordic, Zealand, Denmark). ACAM2000 and APSV contain replication-competent virus, meaning that they can replicate in mammalian cells. ACAM2000 vaccine, grown in cell culture, was licensed by the FDA in 2007 and replaced the previously licensed Dryvax vaccine, made in calf skin, which was destroyed.[2,3,26] APSV, a calf-lymph-origin vaccine manufactured the 1950s, contains the same strain of virus used to produce Dryvax and ACAM2000. Imvamune contains a replication-deficient strain of vaccinia virus, which was attenuated by multiple passages through tissue culture and cannot replicate in mammalian cells. It was designed for individuals at high risk for complications from vaccination with replication-competent virus. In the event of an outbreak, APSV and Imvamune would be used under Investigational New Drug or Emergency Use Authorization regulatory mechanisms.[2]

The primary strategy for postexposure protection in an outbreak is vaccination with replication-competent ACAM2000 and APSV. These are derived from the strain used during the eradication campaign, so confidence in their efficacy is high. ACAM2000 will be used first, and the older APSV will be used after supplies of ACAM2000 run out. The viral strain used in the Imvamune vaccine was not used in the eradication campaign, so its efficacy is less certain, and it requires 2 doses (a primary–booster sequence), so it is not optimal for emergency treatment.[2]

In the event of an outbreak of smallpox, individuals with known exposure to smallpox should be vaccinated with replication-competent smallpox vaccine unless they are severely immunodeficient and not expected to benefit from vaccine, such as those who have received bone marrow transplants within the past 3 months, individuals infected with HIV with CD4 cell counts <50 cells/μL (or age-adjusted equivalent levels in children), and individuals with severe combined immunodeficiency or complete DiGeorge syndrome. When minimal benefit from vaccination is expected, treatment with antiviral therapy is preferred, but there is no absolute contraindication to vaccination during an outbreak, and Imvamune is a reasonable option if antivirals are not available. Pregnant and breastfeeding women should be vaccinated with replication-competent vaccine.[2]

Vaccination with replication-competent vaccine also may be advised for individuals with no known

---

TABLE 166-3

Vaccination Against Smallpox Using Vaccinia Virus[a]

Indications
- Preexposure prevention of smallpox for laboratory workers, first responders, and some military personnel.
- Postexposure prophylaxis against severe disease and death.

Contraindications
- Contraindications in the preexposure setting:
  - History of atopic dermatitis or current disruption of the skin barrier in self or close contact.
  - Immunosuppression in self or close contact.
  - Heart disease or significant cardiac risk factors.
  - Serious allergy to vaccine component.
  - Age younger than 12 months.
  - Pregnancy, breastfeeding, or pregnant close contact.
- Contraindications in the postexposure setting:
  - No absolute contraindications in the case of an actual smallpox outbreak.

[a]Current (as of this writing) Centers for Disease Control and Prevention (CDC) recommendations were issued in 2016.[38]

exposure but high risk for infection. However, in the absence of known exposure, vaccination with replication-competent vaccine is relatively contraindicated for individuals with atopic dermatitis and individuals with HIV infection with CD4 counts 50 to 199 cells/μL (or age-adjusted equivalent levels in children). Instead, these individuals should be vaccinated with Imvamune if availability and time allow.[2]

Vaccination does not provide lifelong immunity. Most estimates suggest that primary vaccination gives full protection for 3 to 5 years and waning immunity for at least another 10 years. Revaccination may give significant protection for at least 30 years.[27]

VACCINIA AND SMALLPOX VACCINATION

AT-A-GLANCE

- The smallpox vaccine contains live vaccinia virus.
- Smallpox vaccination is not currently available to the public.
- Smallpox vaccination can cause serious adverse effects in some individuals.
- Vaccination soon after exposure to smallpox can prevent severe disease and death.
- The U.S. government has stockpiled enough smallpox vaccine to immunize all U.S. citizens in case of an outbreak.

Discussion here focuses on the features of vaccinia virus used as a smallpox vaccine; vaccinia virus is not known to cause natural infection. The discussion pertains specifically to replication-competent vaccinia used in ACAM2000 and APSV, and Dryvax vaccines. The Imvamune vaccine, which contains highly attenuated vaccinia incapable of replicating in human cells, is not discussed here because it produces no skin reaction and has no risk of secondary transmission.[2]

EPIDEMIOLOGY

Vaccinia is member of the *Orthopoxvirus* genus with similarities to cowpox. Although the original smallpox vaccination contained cowpox, over time vaccination strains became contaminated with vaccinia, which was similarly effective and eventually replaced cowpox as the main vaccination agent during the 19th century.[3]

Routine smallpox vaccination was discontinued in the United States in 1972 and globally after 1980. Vaccination of the military and a small group of voluntary public health and health care workers who would be first-line responders in a possible outbreak was reinitiated in the United States in 2002.[2,9,28]

Vaccination with the replication-competent vaccinia virus causes a major local skin reaction, which indicates that the vaccination has been effective. It carries risk of more severe adverse effects in some individuals, including young children and individuals with atopic dermatitis.

Because of significant homology with other poxviruses, vaccination with vaccinia virus provides protection not only against smallpox but also against closely related orthopoxviruses including monkeypox and cowpox.[4]

CLINICAL FEATURES

Cutaneous Findings: The normal local skin reaction to vaccination begins 3 to 5 days after administration, starting with a papule that develops into a vesicle (Jennerian vesicle) and then a pustule around days 7 to 9. It crusts and scabs over during days 10 to 14, with the scab detaching at days 17 to 21 and leaving a residual scar (Fig. 166-6). A robust local cutaneous reaction 7.5 cm or larger in diameter occurs in up to 16% of vaccinations (Fig. 166-7). This can be mistaken for bacterial cellulitis, but it peaks 6 to 12 days after vaccination and improves spontaneously without antibiotic therapy in 24 to 72 hours.[29] In contrast, secondary bacterial infections usually occur within the first 5 days or 30 days after vaccination.

Minor local reactions that can occur near the primary site include intense surrounding erythema or edema and nearby satellite lesions.[27]

Noncutaneous Findings: Soreness almost universally occurs at the vaccination site, and lymphadenopathy/lymphangitis also may be seen. Systemic symptoms can occur and are considered normal reactions. Systemic symptoms include fever (greater than 37.7°C [99.9°F] and more common in children), chills, headache, myalgias, and malaise. They generally peak at days 8 to 10 and last 1 to 3 days. Approximately 30% of vaccine recipients feel too ill to carry out normal activities.[30]

Cutaneous Complications: Adverse effects from vaccinia vaccinations were studied most extensively for the first-generation vaccine (Dryvax), which is no longer used. Fewer individuals have been vaccinated with the newer second-generation vaccines (ACAM2000, APSV, and Imvamune), so their adverse effects are less-well studied. However, because ACAM2000 is derived from the same viral strain used in manufacturing Dryvax, its safety profile is expected to be similar, if not identical.[2,3] With a larger population of immunosuppressed individuals and rising prevalence of atopic dermatitis, the potential for adverse effects from replication-competent vaccines is higher than it was historically.[3] Replication-competent vaccines are relatively contraindicated in these populations, and highly attenuated vaccinia vaccines like Imvamune have been developed for use in these populations.

Adverse cutaneous reactions associated with replication-competent smallpox vaccination can be localized or generalized. Adverse events can occur at any age, but infants and children younger than the age of

Primary Vaccination Site Reaction

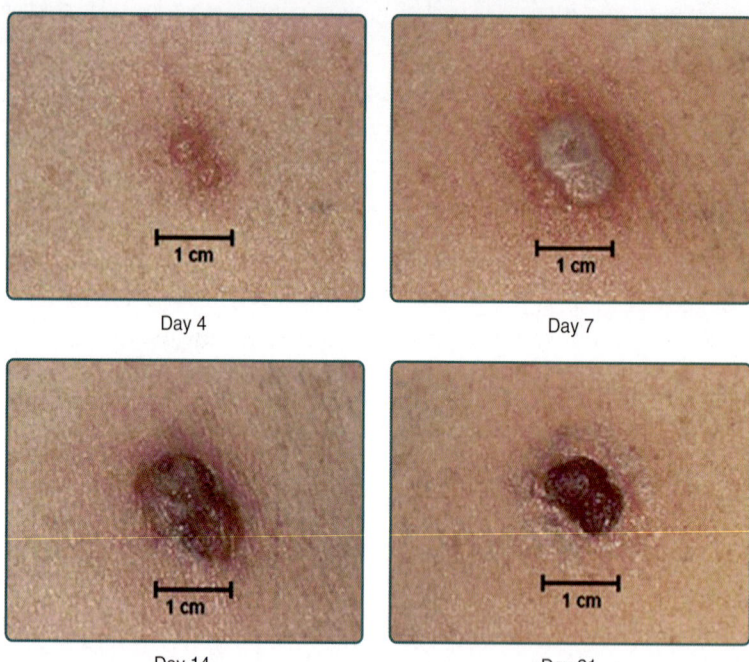

Figure 166-6 Normal progression seen at the smallpox vaccination site. (From the Centers for Disease Control and Prevention [CDC], Atlanta, GA, USA.)

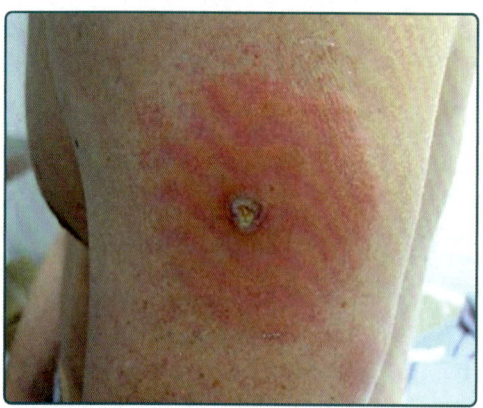

Figure 166-7 A robust take after smallpox vaccination. (From the Centers for Disease Control and Prevention [CDC], Atlanta, GA, USA.)

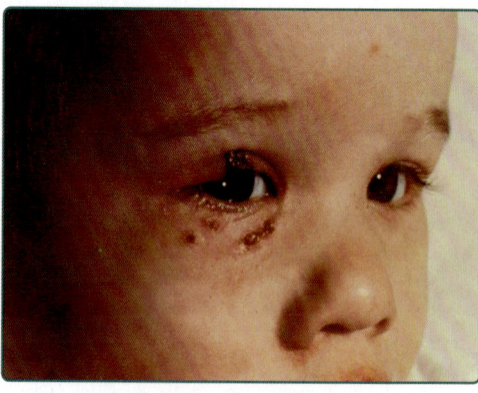

Figure 166-8 Inadvertent inoculation of vaccinia to the eyelid. (From the Centers for Disease Control and Prevention [CDC] Public Health Image Library, Atlanta, GA, USA, and contributed by Michael Lane, MD.)

5 years tend to be particularly affected. Adverse reactions are 10 times more common with primary vaccination than revaccination. Secondary bacterial infection, usually by staphylococci or group A streptococci, can occur at the primary site.

Accidental vaccinia is the autoinoculation of vaccinia virus from the vaccination site to another area. It is the most common adverse event seen and accounts for about half of all adverse events. The most common sites of transfer are the eyelids (Fig. 166-8), nose, mouth, and genitalia. Lesions are seen at these areas 7 to 10 days after vaccination, and they usually follow the time course of the original primary lesion. The lesions may be more attenuated if autoinoculation occurs more than 5 days after vaccination as the host immune response is developing.[28] Accidental inoculation to the eyes can lead to conjunctivitis, keratitis, or iritis. Vaccinia keratitis can cause corneal ulceration with scarring and visual loss.

Generalized, nonspecific, immune-mediated reactions, including morbilliform and roseola-like rashes, may develop. Vaccination can lead to generalized

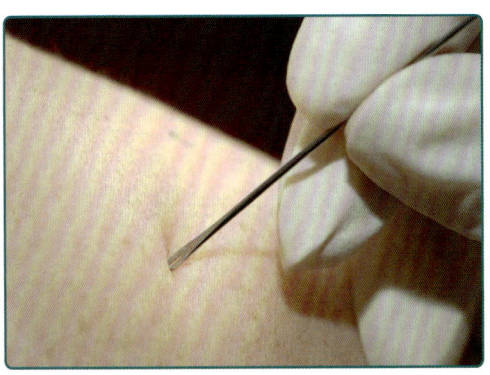

Figure 166-14 Bifurcated needle used for smallpox vaccination. (From the Centers for Disease Control and Prevention [CDC] Public Health Image Library, Atlanta, GA, USA, and contributed by James Gathany.)

is administered, viable, transmissible vaccinia virus is present at the resulting skin lesion until the lesion scabs and separates. A major cutaneous reaction is expected and is the primary indication of an effective immune response. The area heals with scarring at the injection site. Infection is usually limited by the host response with the development of antibody-mediated and cell-mediated immunity.[16] Adverse events and complications occur when the virus spreads outside of the local area, either by transfer or because of host inability to contain the response.

Studies suggest that immunoglobulin M antibodies, detected as early as day 4 of vaccination, may play a role in preventing potentially deadly early viral spread.[36] Neutralizing immunoglobulin G antibodies and cellular immunity start to become detectable around day 7 of vaccination and are responsible for maintaining the long-term host-immune response to the virus.

DIAGNOSIS

Recent personal history of vaccinia vaccination supports the diagnosis. History of recent vaccinia vaccination of a close contact should raise suspicion for secondary transmission.

CLINICAL COURSE AND PROGNOSIS

Typically a papule develops at the inoculation site several days after administration and evolves into a vesicle and then a pustule. A scab typically forms within 2 weeks and falls off within 3 weeks, leaving a scar (see Fig. 166-6).

Potentially fatal adverse reactions from smallpox vaccination are eczema vaccinatum, progressive vaccinia, and postvaccinial CNS disease, described above. The mortality rate for eczema vaccinatum is 30% to 40%.[3] Progressive vaccinia is universally fatal if untreated. CNS complications have a 15% to 25% fatality rate. Individuals with postvaccinial encephalopathy, encephalitis, or encephalomyelitis may recover in approximately 2 weeks, but 25% of survivors are left with residual sequelae (eg, mental impairment, paralysis).[34]

Most fatalities from secondary transmission occur in infants younger than 1 year of age who develop eczema vaccinatum after contact with a recently vaccinated individual. Fetal vaccinia often results in fetal or neonatal death.[31,34]

Management: Symptomatic treatment alone is needed for minor local events (robust take, lymphangitis, intense erythema, or edema) and typical systemic symptoms (headache, malaise, myalgia, fever) occurring after vaccination. Secondary bacterial infections should be treated with appropriate antimicrobial therapy. Uncomplicated cases of accidental secondary transmission of vaccinia do not require therapy.

Extensive vaccinial lesions distant from the vaccination site and secondary transmission of vaccinia can be treated by IV administration of vaccinia immune globulin (VIG) or cidofovir to speed recovery. VIG is an FDA-approved sterile solution of the immunoglobulin fraction of plasma from persons vaccinated with vaccinia. The Strategic National Stockpile contains limited quantities of both VIG and cidofovir. Cidofovir is used under an Investigational New Drug protocol.

Generalized vaccinia usually requires only symptomatic treatment, but if severe, such as in those with immunodeficiency, VIG may be beneficial.

With severe eczema vaccinatum in which there is significant loss of the skin barrier, meticulous skin care and fluid and electrolyte repletion are needed. Early treatment with VIG has been shown to reduce mortality from eczema vaccinatum (from 30% to 40% down to 7%, based on preeradication era data).[33] VIG administration and care in an intensive care unit also reduces the case fatality rate of progressive vaccinia from 100% to 20% to 30%.[34]

Treatment of neurologic complications is supportive care; there is no evidence that VIG is effective in these cases.

Given the rarity of fetal vaccinia, inadvertent vaccination during pregnancy is not ordinarily a reason for termination. There is no indication for prophylactic administration of VIG to the pregnant woman, but it might be considered for a viable infant born with vaccinial lesions.[27,37]

Prevention: Vaccinia virus can be isolated from the vaccination site as soon as a papule forms and until the scab separates, approximately two week after vaccination.[9] To prevent inadvertent transmission of the live, replication-competent virus to other sites on the body or to unvaccinated individuals, the vaccination site should be covered with gauze and an overlying semipermeable membrane bandage until scabs have shed. Contact precautions and frequent hand washing are important when caring for the vaccination site.

As a consequence of elevated risks of adverse events, preevent vaccination is contraindicated for individuals who have a history of atopic dermatitis or a currently disrupted skin barrier, are immunosuppressed, are allergic to any component of the vaccine, or are pregnant or breastfeeding. Vaccination is also contraindicated for individuals with household contacts who have a history of atopic dermatitis or a currently disrupted skin barrier, are immunosuppressed, or are pregnant. Preevent vaccination of individuals younger than 18 years of age is not recommended, and preevent vaccination of children younger than 1 year of age is contraindicated. The CDC also recommends against vaccination of individuals with known cardiac disease.[38]

> **AT-A-GLANCE**
>
> - Monkeypox is a member of the *Orthopoxvirus* genus, along with variola and vaccinia.
> - Since the eradication of smallpox, monkeypox is the main *Orthopoxvirus* affecting human populations.[39]
> - Its clinical presentation is similar to that of smallpox, with a key difference being that lymphadenopathy is more common in monkeypox.[39]

MONKEYPOX

In contrast to smallpox, which was described in writings as far back as 340 AD, monkeypox is a relatively recently recognized disease. It was first identified in 1958 as an illness of cynomolgus monkeys, hence its name. Monkeypox was first documented to cause human illness in 1970 in Zaire (the present Democratic Republic of the Congo), when it was isolated from a patient with suspected smallpox infection.[39]

EPIDEMIOLOGY

Human monkeypox is a disease acquired mainly from infected animals. The disease is endemic to the Congo Basin of Central Africa, with the majority of human monkeypox infections occurring in the Democratic Republic of Congo, but cases are also reported in the Central African Republic, the Republic of Congo, and Sudan.[39] The majority of cases are in children. Transmission occurs mainly during handling of infected animals or contact with their body fluids. Person-to-person spread via respiratory droplets and close contact can occur as with smallpox, but usually in a more limited manner. Outbreaks in the Democratic Republic of Congo in 1996-1997 showed sustained human-to-human transmission for the first time, and the incidence of human monkeypox infection has been rising. This may reflect decreased immunity after the discontinuation of routine smallpox vaccination which is protective against monkeypox.[4,39] In spring 2003, the first cases of human monkeypox in the Western Hemisphere were identified in the Midwest region of the United States (72 reported cases, 37 laboratory confirmed). All cases were associated with contact with infected pet prairie dogs previously housed with rodents imported from Ghana.[40,41]

CLINICAL FEATURES

Prodrome: Similar to smallpox, symptoms of monkeypox manifest after a 7- to 17-day incubation period. A prodrome of fever, chills, malaise, headache, myalgias, and back pain occurs, lasting 1 to 4 days.[39] Some individuals experience sore throat, cough, or shortness of breath. Diarrhea and abdominal pain also may be reported.[4,42]

Cutaneous Findings: As with ordinary smallpox, a rash generally develops 1 to 3 days after the onset of fever, initially consisting of monomorphic macules and papules. Most commonly, the eruption begins on the face and/or trunk, with the lesions spreading in a centrifugal pattern to become generalized. They then progress over 14 to 21 days to vesicles and pustules that umbilicate, crust, and desquamate (Figs. 166-15 and 166-16). Dyspigmented and pitted scars result. Monkeypox lesions can involve the oral and genital mucous membranes.[43]

In the outbreak in the United States, only 1 patient (a child) had a generalized rash as extensive as those

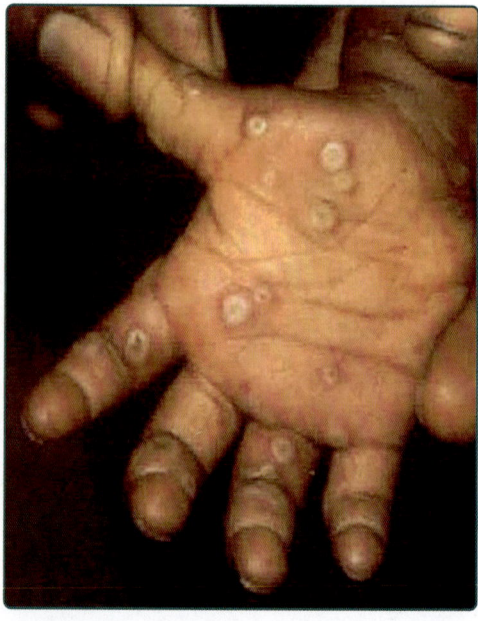

Figure 166-15 Umbilicated pustular lesions on the palm from monkeypox. (Used with permission from the Joint Pathology Center, Silver Spring, MD, USA.)

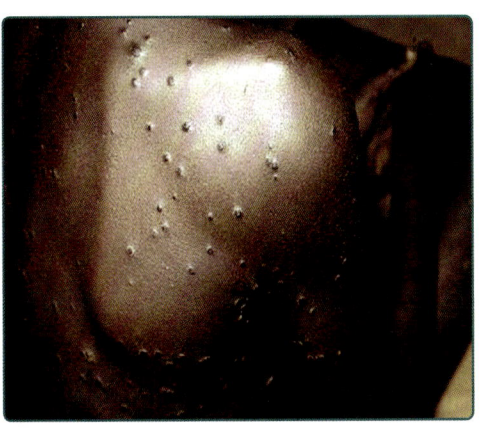

Figure 166-16 A 5-year-old male from the Democratic Republic of Congo with late desquamative monkeypox lesions. (Used with permission from the Joint Pathology Center, Silver Spring, MD, USA.)

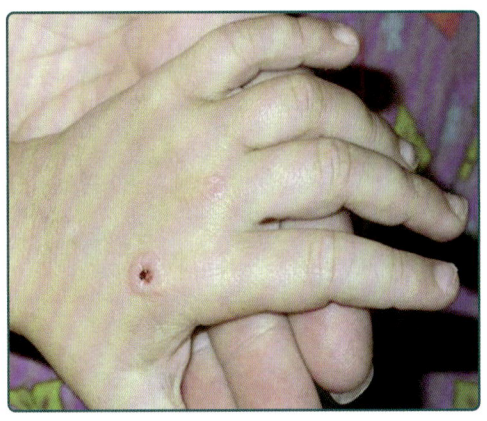

Figure 166-18 Monkeypox lesions resolving in the same 3-year-old child. (Copyright © Marshfield Clinic, Inc. All rights reserved. Reprinted with permission from Marshfield Clinic, Inc., Marshfield, WI, USA.)

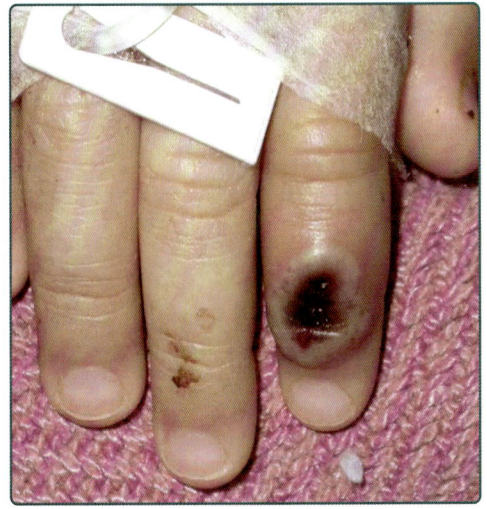

Figure 166-17 The primary inoculation site of monkeypox virus in a 3-year-old child, 14 days after being bitten by a prairie dog. (Copyright © Marshfield Clinic, Inc. All rights reserved. Reprinted with permission from Marshfield Clinic, Inc., Marshfield, WI, USA.)

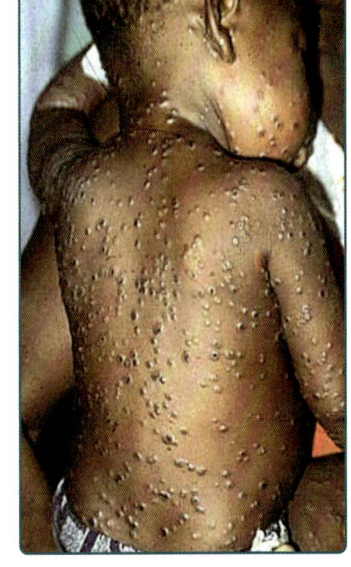

Figure 166-19 Significant postauricular lymphadenopathy with pustular skin lesions in a 2-year-old female with monkeypox. (Used with permission from the Joint Pathology Center, Silver Spring, MD, USA.)

seen in cases in Africa. The other affected individuals had only localized lesions, mostly on the hands, that were associated with direct contact with the infected animals from Ghana (Figs. 166-17 and 166-18). This may indicate that West African strains of monkeypox virus are less virulent than those of Central Africa.[40,42]

Noncutaneous Findings: Significant lymphadenopathy develops 1 to 2 days before the onset of the rash, usually in submandibular, cervical, or inguinal areas (Fig. 166-19). Conjunctivitis and keratitis may occur. Confusion and seizures are rare.[44,45]

Complications: Secondary skin and soft-tissue infections may occur (approximately 20% of cases). Affected individuals may also develop pneumonitis (12%), encephalitis (less than 1%), and ocular complications, including scarring with corneal lesions.[43]

ETIOLOGY AND PATHOGENESIS

Monkeypox is caused by the monkeypox virus, a zoonotic virus. Like variola and vaccinia viruses, it is a type of *Orthopoxvirus* with a brick shape on electron microscopy. The monkeypox viral genome is 96% identical to that of the variola virus at the central region, which encodes essential enzymes and structural proteins. The end regions that encode virulence and host-range factors are substantially different, and the range of hosts for the monkeypox virus is much wider than that for variola virus.[46] In addition to humans, hosts for monkeypox include cynomolgus and other monkeys, other primates (apes, gorillas, chimpanzees, orangutans), and nonprimate animals such as rabbits, mice, guinea pigs, rats, squirrels, and giant anteaters.

Monkeypox is mainly transmitted through abraded skin after a bite or scratch from an infected animal or by contact with its infected bodily fluids. The virus multiplies locally at the site of injury and is rapidly transported to regional lymph nodes, where multiplication continues. Invasion of the bloodstream disseminates the virus to distant sites. The monkeypox virus is also transmissible from person to person via aerosolization of the virus or contact with lesions or body fluids during the first week of the rash, although its transmissibility is significantly lower than that of smallpox.[39] Monkeypox rarely may be transmitted by contaminated fomites.[47]

The longest documented chain of person-to-person spread is believed to have affected 6 individuals, which suggests that monkeypox has less potential for the type of epidemic spread seen with smallpox.[39]

DIAGNOSIS

Laboratory Testing: Leukocytosis, elevated transaminase levels, and low blood urea nitrogen levels are often seen. Lymphocytosis and thrombocytopenia occur less often.[48]

Pathology: On examination of skin biopsy specimens, features of monkeypox are indistinguishable from those of smallpox. There is similar dermal papillary edema, acute inflammation, and ballooning degeneration of keratinocytes (Fig. 166-20). Cytoplasmic eosinophilic inclusion bodies (Guarnieri bodies) are also seen. Focal necrosis may occur.[45]

Special Tests: PCR analysis of a swab, crust, or other material can confirm monkeypox virus infection. Electron microscopy and serologic tests can confirm *Orthopoxvirus* infection, but cannot distinguish monkeypox from variola or vaccinia.

DIFFERENTIAL DIAGNOSIS

Table 166-2 outlines the differential diagnosis of monkeypox virus infection.

The clinical features of monkeypox are similar to but less severe than those of ordinary smallpox. Lymphadenopathy is a distinctive hallmark of monkeypox not usually seen in smallpox. It is observed in 90% of unvaccinated individuals and 53% of vaccinated individuals.[4]

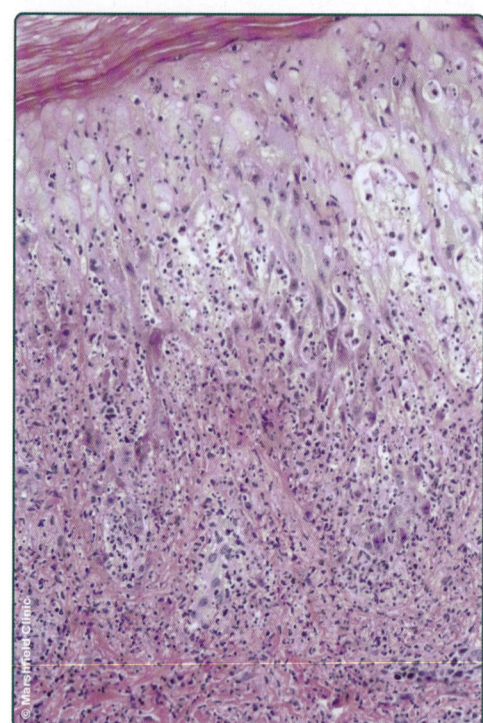

Figure 166-20 Histopathology of a monkeypox lesion with dermal papillary edema, acute inflammation, and ballooning degeneration of keratinocytes. (hematoxylin and eosin [H&E]. (Copyright © Marshfield Clinic, Inc. All rights reserved. Reprinted with permission from Marshfield Clinic, Inc., Marshfield, WI, USA.)

Varicella causes a milder and shorter/absent viral prodrome, has a centripetal distribution, and is not associated with lymphadenopathy.

Orf and bovine stomatitis, caused by poxviruses of the *Parapoxvirus* genus, can produce similar but more localized skin lesions.

Also in the differential diagnosis are drug eruptions, eczema herpeticum, and rickettsialpox (see Table 166-2). Immunocompromised individuals may develop extensive molluscum lesions that can look similar.

CLINICAL COURSE AND PROGNOSIS

In Africa, mortality ranges from 1% to 10% and mainly occurs in children. Death usually occurs during the second week of disease and is secondary to bacterial superinfection, GI complications, or pulmonary complications. These are likely compounded by poor nutrition and inaccessibility of medical care.[4,40] All individuals affected by the 2003 outbreak in the United States survived.[49]

Scars left by the rash may improve over time.

MANAGEMENT

Contact and droplet precautions should be instituted, and suspected cases should be isolated in a negative air pressure room if possible.

Postexposure prophylaxis with vaccinia virus is the preferred treatment strategy.[46] It is recommended for those within 4 days of direct exposure to monkeypox virus and should be considered up to 14 days after exposure, including in children younger than 12 months of age, pregnant women, and people with skin conditions, as the risk of contracting monkeypox is considered greater for most individuals than the risk of developing complications from vaccination.[46]

However, vaccination is contraindicated in individuals with severe immunodeficiency in T-cell function, even if they have been directly exposed, as their risk of severe complications from vaccination approaches or exceeds their risk from monkeypox exposure.

Other treatment options include tecovirimat, which can be used under an Investigational New Drug protocol to treat monkeypox infection and is maintained in the U.S. Strategic National Stockpile.[50] Tecovirimat prevents death and reduces severity of monkeypox infection in nonhuman primate models, even when administered after the appearance of clinical symptoms.[21,51] Cidofovir and brincidofovir also can be used.[52] However, the efficacy of these drugs against monkeypox infection in humans has not been studied and is uncertain.

Prevention: Global eradication of monkeypox is more difficult than smallpox eradication, because of the wide range of animal hosts. Vaccination with the Dryvax smallpox vaccine containing vaccinia was found to be effective in preventing human monkeypox. Observation of cases in Africa showed that vaccination was 85% protective against monkeypox, and those who were not fully protected developed only mild disease.[45] The newer ACAM2000 vaccine has similar immunogenicity to Dryvax and showed equal protection against monkeypox virus in a nonhuman primate model.[53,54] However, vaccination with vaccinia virus is not currently in use in monkeypox-endemic areas because the risk of severe adverse events is thought to outweigh the potential benefit.[39]

The CDC currently recommends preexposure vaccination for laboratory workers, investigators of monkeypox cases, and health care providers who may care for patients with monkeypox, provided they have no contraindication to smallpox vaccination (Table 166-4).[46]

PARAPOXVIRUS INFECTIONS

The *Parapoxvirus* genus includes 3 viruses that produce disease in humans: pseudocowpox virus (the cause of milker's nodule), orf virus, and bovine papular stomatitis virus. These entities, sometimes grouped together as "barnyard pox," are clinically and histologically indistinguishable.[13] They are distinguished primarily by clinical history and PCR assay. Unlike the orthopoxviruses, parapoxviruses tend to cause localized rather than systemic disease in healthy individuals. Milker's nodule and orf are reviewed here.

MILKER'S NODULE

AT-A-GLANCE

- Milker's nodules are caused by pseudocowpox, also known as paravaccinia, a virus transmitted by cows.
- Lesions are clinically indistinguishable from orf and bovine papular stomatitis.
- Unlike the *Orthopoxvirus* cowpox, pseudocowpox does not immunize against smallpox.[1,55]

TABLE 166-4

Vaccination against Human Monkeypox Using Vaccinia Virus[a]

Indications
- Preexposure vaccination for laboratory workers, investigators of monkeypox cases, and health care providers who may care for patients with monkeypox.
- Postexposure vaccination for those within 4 days of direct exposure to monkeypox virus; should be considered up to 14 days after exposure.

Contraindications
- Contraindications in the preexposure setting:
  - Same as for vaccination against smallpox with vaccinia virus (see Table 166-3).
- Contraindications in the postexposure setting:
  - Severe immunodeficiency in T-cell function, defined as HIV-infected individuals with CD4 count <200 cells/µL (or age-adjusted equivalent level in children), recipients of high-dose immunosuppressive therapy, and people with lymphosarcoma, hematologic malignancies, or primary T-cell congenital immunodeficiencies.[46]

[a]Current Centers for Disease Control and Prevention (CDC) recommendations issued in 2003 and 2016.[38,36]

EPIDEMIOLOGY

Pseudocowpox is present worldwide, but disease develops only in individuals in close contact with cattle. It is an occupational disease of milkers, veterinarians, and meat industry workers. Most cases are in newly employed milkers who have not developed immunity.[1] Cases are mostly sporadic, but small epidemics have been reported. No natural cases of human-to-human transmission have been reported.

CLINICAL FEATURES

Paravaccinia inoculation usually occurs on the hands or, less commonly, the face. The incubation period for

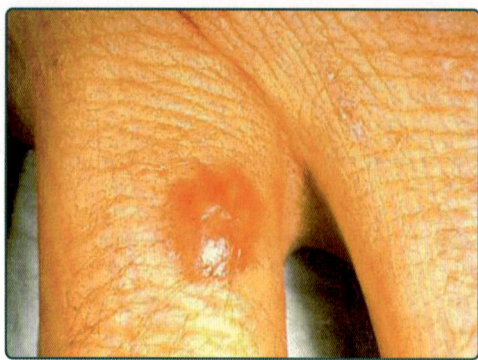

Figure 166-21 A milker's nodule on the hand. (From the National Institute for Occupational Safety and Health [NIOSH], Atlanta, GA, USA, with permission.)

milker's nodule is 4 to 7 days. In a minority of cases, the infected individual develops mild systemic symptoms, such as a transient low-grade fever.[56]

Cutaneous Findings: After the incubation period, 1 to several lesions usually develop. In rare cases, numerous lesions may develop. Lesions progress through 6 typical stages, each lasting approximately a week. A lesion begins as a red, and occasionally pruritic, macule that develops into a raised papule (Fig. 166-21). It evolves into a papulovesicle with a target-like appearance—a red center surrounded by a white or gray ring and outer red halo. The lesions then develop into bluish or violaceous tender nodules. Some ulcerate or have a central depression (Fig. 166-22A), which results in formation of eschars with crust. Lesions usually heal in 4 to 8 weeks and typically resolve without scarring.[56]

The clinical presentation of milker's nodule is virtually identical to that of orf and bovine papular stomatitis.[13,57]

Noncutaneous Findings: Lymphangitis is often present in the skin surrounding the primary lesion(s). Lymphadenopathy is not common.

Complications: Secondary bacterial infection can occur but is rare. Erythema multiforme, morbilliform eruptions, and erythema nodosum have been reported in cases of milker's nodule.

ETIOLOGY AND PATHOGENESIS

Milker's nodule is caused by the pseudocowpox virus, also known as paravaccinia, which is a member of the *Parapoxvirus* genus. Although historically pseudocowpox and bovine papular stomatitis sometimes were considered to be the same entity, they are genetically distinct.[57] Pseudocowpox most commonly causes lesions on the teats of cows while bovine papular stomatitis most commonly causes lesions in the oral cavity.[13]

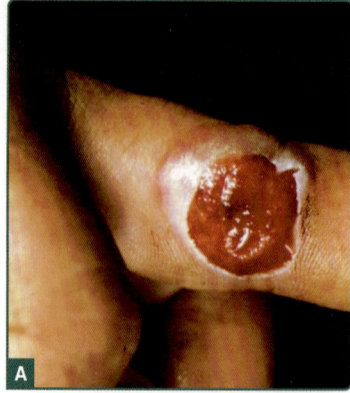

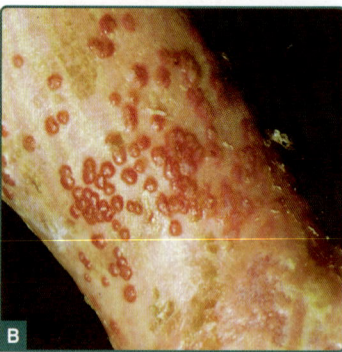

Figure 166-22 **A,** Firm, eroded milker's nodule. **B,** Multiple lesions at the site of a second-degree scalding burn sustained in a milking barn.

Humans can become accidental hosts for pseudocowpox after contacting infected animals or contaminated fresh meat. Pseudocowpox virus is transferred by direct inoculation into the skin, often through a break in the skin barrier.[58] Cases of transmission from contaminated fomites to individuals with burn injury have been reported (see Fig. 166-22B).[59]

DIAGNOSIS

Pathology: Histopathologic findings depend on the stage of the lesion. Early lesions show vacuolization and ballooning of cells in the upper third of the epidermis, which sometimes leads to multilocular vesicles. Intracytoplasmic inclusion bodies may be seen. Epidermal necrosis may be observed focally with ulceration and crust as the lesion progresses. Neutrophils are seen in the epidermis and superficial papillary dermis with epidermal necrosis. Mature lesions have finger-like epidermal projections, papillary dermal edema, and a mixed inflammatory infiltrate that includes lymphocytes, histiocytes, and eosinophils. Regressing lesions have decreasing acanthosis and inflammation.[58,60]

Special Tests: When blister fluid or crusts are viewed with electron microscopy, *Parapoxvirus* virions typically are smaller than orthopoxviruses and have an ovoid (as opposed to brick-like) shape with a crisscross filament pattern.[57] Electron microscopy cannot differentiate among *Parapoxvirus* species. RT-PCR can confirm *Parapoxvirus* genus and distinguish between pseudocowpox, orf, and bovine papular stomatitis.[13,57]

DIFFERENTIAL DIAGNOSIS

Milker's nodules are clinically indistinguishable from orf and bovine papular stomatitis, but clinical history helps with differentiation: cattle are the source of infection for milker's nodules and bovine papular stomatitis while sheep or goats are the source of infection for orf. PCR can distinguish among the 3 viruses.

Milker's nodules must also be differentiated from the *Orthopoxvirus* cowpox. Cowpox is very rare in humans and, contrary to its name, is rarely transmitted from cows. It has a longer incubation period and causes more pain and lymphadenopathy. It is a more-severe infection that may cause death in individuals who have atopic dermatitis or are immunocompromised. Large lesions of milker's nodule also can be confused with anthrax, pyogenic granuloma, giant herpetic lesions, and keratoacanthoma (Table 166-5).

CLINICAL COURSE AND PROGNOSIS

Milker's nodule is a self-limited illness. Most cases heal without scarring. Infection does not produce lifelong immunity; up to 12% of individuals have second infections.[57]

TABLE 166-5
Differential Diagnosis of Milker's Nodule and Orf

Most Likely
- Few to multiple lesions
  - Bovine papular stomatitis
  - Cowpox
  - Herpetic whitlow
- Solitary lesion
  - Pyogenic granuloma
  - Pyoderma

Consider
- Few to multiple lesions
  - Atypical mycobacterial infection
  - Sporotrichosis
- Solitary lesion
  - Tularemia
  - Giant herpetic lesion
  - Giant molluscum
  - Erysipeloid

Always Rule Out
- Few to multiple lesions
  - Anthrax
  - Primary inoculation tuberculosis
- Solitary lesion
  - Keratoacanthoma
  - Syphilitic chancre

MANAGEMENT

Because the disease is self-limited, treatment, if needed, is symptomatic. Surgical curettage of large lesions may help speed healing.[61]

Prevention: As discussed above, there is no cross-immunity between orthopoxviruses and parapoxviruses, so smallpox vaccination does not prevent milker's nodules. Prevention mainly consists of isolation of infected animals and contact precautions.

ORF

AT-A-GLANCE

- Orf virus is usually transmitted to humans from sheep or goats.
- Orf infection looks similar to milker's nodule and progresses through similar clinical stages before resolving spontaneously.

Orf, also known as contagious pustular dermatosis, infectious pustular dermatitis, scabby mouth disease, and sore mouth disease, is a self-limited zoonotic viral infection that usually affects the hands of people handling infected animals. The disease is endemic in sheep and goats, and it is transmitted to humans through contact with infected tissue or fomites. Orf shares clinical characteristics with milker's nodule and bovine papular stomatitis. It may be mistaken for more serious and life-threatening disorders such as tularemia, anthrax, and erysipeloid (see Table 166-5).

The name *orf* is derived from the Nordic word *Hrufa*, meaning boil or scab.[59] Walley first identified orf as a contagious disease in sheep in 1890, and Newson and Cross first described the disease in humans in 1934.[59]

EPIDEMIOLOGY

Orf virus is a member of the *Parapoxvirus* genus, which also includes pseudocowpox and bovine papular stomatitis. Although sheep and goats are the most common sources of infection, the virus also has been found in mountain goats, gazelles, musk oxen, and reindeer. The nostrils and lips of infected animals are affected, as well as the teats of ewes suckling young. Human disease is most often seen in farmers, shepherds, veterinarians, and butchers, but anyone who has contact with small ruminants is at risk.[62] The disease has been reported in children with exposure to farms or petting zoos.[63] Humans develop disease after contact with animals or fomites such as barn doors, feeding troughs, wire fencing, bottles, and harnesses.

Multiple cases of orf infection following the Muslim feast of the sacrifice (Eid al-Adha), during which lambs are slaughtered, have been reported.[64] According to the CDC, the disease is not transmitted from human to human.

CLINICAL FEATURES

Cutaneous Findings: Orf lesions usually develop on the hands but can occur anywhere, including the face and perianal area.[61,65] A solitary lesion is the most common presentation, but multiple lesions are possible.[65]

As with milker's nodule lesions, orf lesions evolve through 6 clinical stages, each lasting roughly 1 week (Table 166-6).[65,66] A red macule appears a few days after inoculation and develops into a red papule by 1 week after the inoculation. During the second week, the lesion evolves into a targetoid nodule with a red papule surrounded by a white ring and enclosed by a peripheral halo of erythema (Fig. 166-23). During the third week, considered the acute stage, the lesion becomes weepy (Fig. 166-24). It may appear as a flat-topped, crusted, hemorrhagic pustule 2 to 3 cm in diameter (Fig. 166-25A).[59] During the fourth week, the lesion enters the regenerative stage, during which it dries out and black dots composed of pyknotic cells form on its surface (Fig. 166-25B). During the fifth week, papillomas develop on the surface of the lesion. In the final, regressive stage, a dry crust forms at the periphery of the lesion and gradually extends centrally. The crust may shed and reform several times before the lesion flattens and heals.[65] Lesions are typically painless.[59]

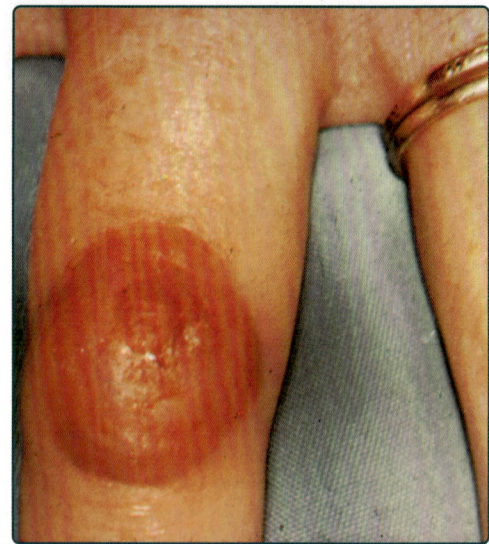

Figure 166-23 The target phase of orf shows a white circle with central and peripheral erythema.

Noncutaneous Findings: Systemic findings are uncommon in immunocompetent individuals but can include lymphadenopathy and lymphangitis. Rarely, fever and malaise may occur.[65]

Complications: Orf lesions can become secondarily infected.[67] An estimated 7% to 18% of individuals with orf infections develop erythema multiforme.[68] Vesiculopapular, papular (see Fig. 166-25A), and bullous-pemphigoid like eruptions also may develop.[69,70] Additionally, secondary spread within active atopic dermatitis skin lesions has been reported.[71] Rare complications include giant orf lesions and Stevens-Johnson syndrome.[62,72]

TABLE 166-6
Clinical Manifestation of Orf

TIME AFTER EXPOSURE	CLINICAL MANIFESTATIONS
3-7 days	1-4 papules on hand (typically only 1 lesion): begin as a red maculopapular lesion ↓ Vesicle ↓
10-14 days	Target lesion with red center, white middle ring, and red halo ↓
14-21 days	Acute weeping stage ↓
21-28 days	Regenerative dry stage with black dots ↓
28-35 days	Papillomatous stage ↓
35 days	Regressive stage with dry crust and eventual shedding of the scab

Adapted from Clark J, Diven D. Poxviruses. In: Tyring SK, Moore AY, Lupi O, eds. *Mucocutaneous Manifestations of Viral Diseases*. 2nd ed. London, UK: Informa Healthcare; 2010:51, with permission.

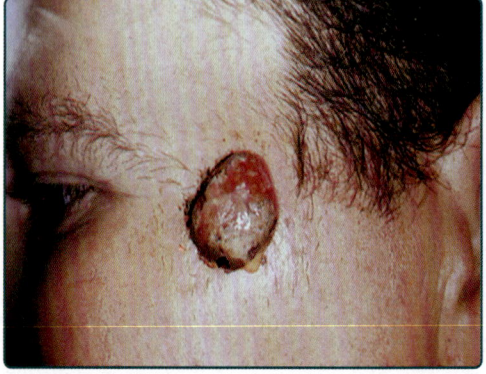

Figure 166-24 In the acute phase, there is weeping of the surface overlying an elevated tumor.

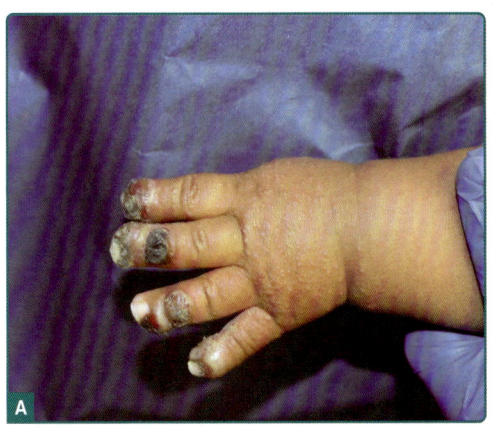

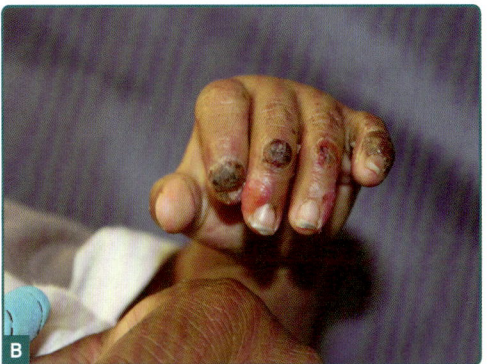

Figure 166-25 A, Multiple orf papulonodules with unusually extensive hemorrhagic crust during the acute weeping stage, 16 days after a goat bite to multiple fingers. A diffuse papular eruption that developed after the primary orf lesions is also visible. **B,** Twenty-two days after the goat bite, the primary orf lesions have begun to dry out and flatten, and the secondary eruption is resolving. (Used with permission from Victoria R. Barrio, MD.)

ETIOLOGY AND PATHOGENESIS

Orf is an ovoid crosshatched particle approximately 250 nm long × 150 nm wide.[64] The virus is very stable and can survive heating, drying, and solvents. It is transmitted to humans from animals or fomites through a crack in the skin and replicates within the epidermis.

Orf virus encodes immunomodulatory genes that interfere with host response and allow time for viral replication within epidermal cells. Orf virus interferon resistance protein and virus interleukin-10 inhibit interferon and inflammatory cytokine production. Additionally, granulocyte-macrophage colony-stimulating factor inhibitory factor inhibits the biologic activity of granulocyte-macrophage colony-stimulating factor and interleukin-2.[73] Clearance of the infection occurs when host immune response eventually overcomes orf's immunomodulatory proteins.

Risk Factors: Exposure to infected animals is the greatest risk factor for orf infection. Infections tend to occur most often during the spring and summer months, which is lambing season, as young animals are most susceptible to infection.[63] Vaccination of sheep with a commercially available unattenuated, live orf vaccine with the intent of conferring immunity is a risk factor for humans.[63]

Immunocompromised individuals have an increased risk of developing giant (greater than 3 cm in diameter) orf lesions and may have difficulty clearing them.[63,74]

DIAGNOSIS

Clinical appearance and history of ungulate exposure are usually diagnostic. Dermoscopy of orf lesions shows central ulceration surrounded by white structureless areas, white shiny streaks, dotted and hairpin vessels, and fine peripheral scale.[75]

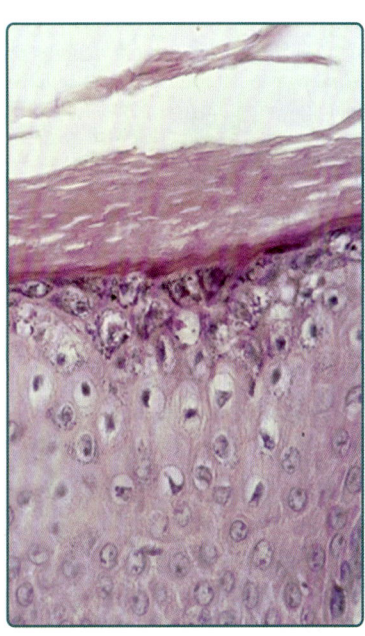

Figure 166-26 Orf histopathology. In the target phase, there are superficial vacuolated epidermal cells with inclusion bodies.

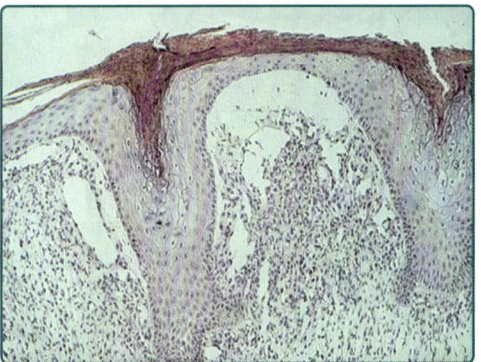

Figure 166-27 Orf histopathology. Later in the target stage, there are finger-like projections of the epidermis and a dense inflammatory infiltrate accompanied by massive edema in the papillary body.

Pathology: In the maculopapular and target stages, intranuclear and intracytoplasmic inclusions are present in vacuolated epidermal cells, with an accumulation of neutrophils, basophils, dendritic cells, and lymphocytes (Fig. 166-26). During the acute stage, multilocular vesicles form and the epidermis degenerates. Papillomatosis and acanthosis subsequently develop, and marked finger-like downward projections of the epidermis may be seen (Fig. 166-27).[65]

Special Tests: RT-PCR testing, which is available through the CDC, is the most rapid and accurate way to make the diagnosis when clinical uncertainty exists. Electron microscopy cannot definitively distinguish between *Orthopoxvirus* and *Parapoxvirus*.

DIFFERENTIAL DIAGNOSIS

A variety of bacterial and infectious diseases can present with findings similar to those of orf (see Table 166-5). Milker's nodule and bovine papular stomatitis are clinically and histologically indistinguishable from orf, but are associated with different animal exposure. The lesion of anthrax is more hemorrhagic with rapid progression to an eschar. Herpetic whitlow may resemble orf but tends to be more painful. Tularemia and syphilis are associated with chancres. Sporotrichosis begins as a single necrotic nodule but is followed by multiple nodules arising in a linear fashion along the lymphatics. Primary inoculation tuberculosis and atypical mycobacterial infection can give rise to ulcerative lesions that may take months to years to heal.

CLINICAL COURSE AND PROGNOSIS

Orf usually resolves within 4 to 6 weeks without treatment. Typically, scarring does not occur. Immunocompromised individuals can develop progressive, destructive lesions that may require interventions such as debridement, antiviral therapy such as cidofovir cream, or imiquimod topical immunomodulatory therapy.[63,74,76] Recurrence is uncommon but has been reported.[74]

MANAGEMENT

Supportive care is the most appropriate intervention for immunocompetent patients. Application of compresses, culture of lesion specimens, and antibiotic coverage may be appropriate if secondary bacterial infection is suspected. Immunocompromised patients may require medical intervention, as described above.

Prevention: Barrier precautions, such as use of gloves and good hand hygiene, help prevent orf infection. Individuals with an impaired skin barrier from either abrasions or intrinsic skin disease (eg, atopic dermatitis) should be particularly vigilant about avoiding contact with infected animals or potential fomites.

MOLLUSCIPOXVIRUS INFECTION: MOLLUSCUM CONTAGIOSUM

AT-A-GLANCE

- Molluscum contagiosum is a common benign cutaneous infection with associated signs isolated to the skin.
- Children are most commonly affected.
- Severe inflammatory responses can occur at the site of the lesions, which are sometimes mistaken for secondary bacterial infection or cellulitis.
- A number of associated skin findings, including eczematous reactions surrounding the lesions, more diffuse autoeczematization-type reactions, or lichenoid, Gianotti-Crosti type lesions may develop.

Molluscum contagiosum (MC) is a common benign cutaneous viral infection specific to humans that occurs worldwide and is transmitted by skin-to-skin-contact. Since the eradication of smallpox, MC virus is the primary poxvirus affecting humans.[77]

MC infection was first described clinically by Bateman in 1817. Henderson and Paterson identified its characteristic intracytoplasmic viral inclusion bodies in 1841.[78]

EPIDEMIOLOGY

MC infection most commonly affects children, sexually active adults, athletes participating in contact sports, and individuals with impaired cellular immunity.[77] The infection is most prevalent before the age of 14 years, with a median age of 5 years in a retrospective study of 170 children at Johns Hopkins.[79,80] A metaanalysis estimates that 5.1% to 11.5% of children ages 0 to 16 years are affected at any given time, but true prevalence is likely higher, as some infections may be subclinical.[79] Seropositivity to MC virion surface protein in unaffected individuals ranges from 6% in Japan to approximately 30% in the United Kingdom.[81,82]

MC lesions are mainly limited to the skin, but rarely develop on mucosal surfaces, including the eye.[77] In children, lesions are usually on exposed areas, whereas in adults, many cases are limited to the genital area, suggesting sexual transmission.[83] Genital and perianal lesions can also develop in children, but are rarely associated with sexual transmission in this age group.[84] The prevalence of sexually transmitted MC infections in adults has risen over the past several decades, with a large Spanish study noting a threefold increase in the yearly incidence (from 1.3% to 4%) in a sexually transmitted disease unit between 1988 and 2007.[85] An earlier study showed an 11-fold increase in patient visits for MC in the United States between 1966 and 1983. One theorized explanation is that reduced transmission in childhood may result in more adults who are immunologically naïve and vulnerable to sexual transmission.[85]

MC infections are more common in individuals infected with HIV. Data from the 1980s and early 1990s suggested a prevalence of 5% to 18% in this population, but with the increased use of antiretroviral therapy, the rate may now be lower.[86]

Transmission may occur via direct skin or mucous membrane contact, or via fomites. Bath towels, swimming pools, and public or shared baths are reported as sources of infection.[87] Autoinoculation and koebnerization also play a role in the spread of lesions. Vertical transmission from mother to neonate during the intrapartum period has been reported.[88,89]

MC lives in the epidermis and does not remain latent in the body after the cutaneous lesions have cleared.[77]

CLINICAL FEATURES

Cutaneous Findings: MC often presents as small pink, pearly, or skin-colored papules that enlarge to 2 to 5 mm in size. As they enlarge they may become flat-topped, dome-shaped, and opalescent. Lesions may have a central dell or umbilication (Fig. 166-28A), from which a white curd-like substance containing the virus can be expressed with pressure. Children usually develop multiple papules, often in exposed sites like the face and extremities or intertriginous sites, such as the axillae and popliteal fossae. Lesions may be grouped in clusters or appear in a linear array. The latter often results from koebnerization or development of lesions at sites of trauma. In adults, lesions typically develop in the genital area.

Immunosuppressed patients typically have more-severe and extensive disease, and may develop giant molluscum as large as 2.5 cm in diameter.[90,91]

Noncutaneous Findings: MC is not associated with systemic complications.

Complications: Although many patients are asymptomatic, pruritus may be a significant problem, particularly in those patients with underlying atopic dermatitis. Chronic conjunctivitis and punctate keratitis may develop in patients with eyelid lesions. Secondary bacterial infection can occur, particularly if patients scratch their lesions.

Approximately 19% to 39% of children with MC develop an erythematous, eczematous dermatitis surrounding their molluscum lesions, known as *molluscum dermatitis*.[87,92] This is more common in children with atopic dermatitis; roughly half of children with both atopic dermatitis and MC develop molluscum dermatitis.[92]

In approximately 20% of patients, molluscum lesions may become inflamed, with erythema and swelling (see Fig. 166-28B), and these inflamed lesions may become pustular or fluctuant.[87,92] The development of inflamed MC lesions suggests a robust immune response and tends to be associated with a subsequent decline in the number of lesions.[92]

A small subset of individuals with MC develop a Gianotti-Crosti–like reaction consisting of pruritic monomorphous, edematous, erythematous papules or papulovesicles, centered on the elbows and

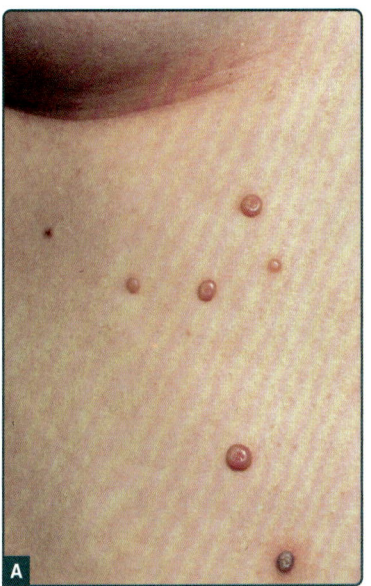 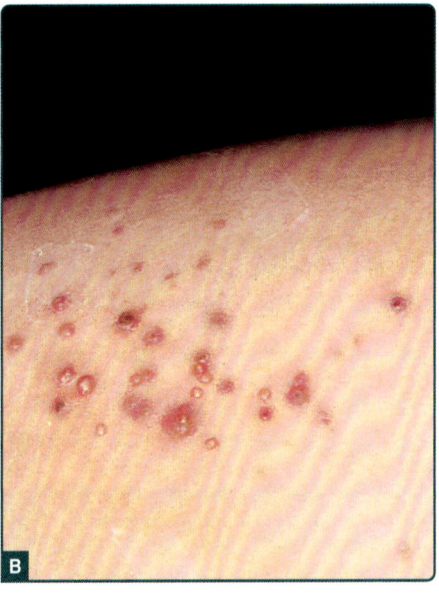

Figure 166-28 Molluscum contagiosum. **A,** Discrete, solid, skin-colored papules, 1 to 2 mm in diameter with central umbilication. **B,** Multiple, scattered, and discrete lesions, some of which are inflamed.

knees, which lasts for several weeks. This eruption also tends to be followed by reduction in the number of MC lesions and may be considered a favorable prognostic sign.[92]

ETIOLOGY AND PATHOGENESIS

MC virus is a large, brick-shaped double-stranded DNA poxvirus with genomic similarities to other poxviruses. It shares two-thirds of the viral genes of vaccinia and variola viruses.[80] There are 4 clinically indistinguishable subtypes of MC virus. MC virus genotype 1 is responsible for 98% of disease in the United States.[93,94] MC virus genotype 2 is primarily seen in adults and immunocompromised individuals and is most commonly transmitted by sexual contact. The incubation period of the virus estimated to be approximately 2 to 6 weeks.[95]

MC virus replicates in the cytoplasm of epithelial cells. Viral inclusion bodies known as Henderson-Paterson bodies develop in the basal layer of the epidermis and enlarge as cells rise through the epidermis, pushing cellular organelles against the sides of the cell.[90] Proliferation and enlargement of the virion-packed cells causes disintegration of the stratum corneum and the formation of a dimple-like ostium through which the virions are released when the inclusion bodies rupture.[90]

Molluscum lesions can persist for a long time without significant inflammatory cell infiltration because the MC virus possesses multiple genes that impede host immune response.[90] These include genes coding for (a) a homolog of a major histocompatibility class 1 heavy chain, which may interfere with antigen presentation; (b) a chemokine homolog that inhibits chemotaxis; (c) a protein that inhibits apoptosis by preventing activation of the death effector domain of caspase 8; and (d) a glutathione peroxidase homolog that prevents apoptosis in cells damaged by ultraviolet radiation and hydrogen peroxide.[77,90,96] Eventually the immune system detects the virus and mounts a localized response involving plasmacytoid dendritic cells, interferon-induced dendritic cells, natural killer cells, and cytotoxic T lymphocytes, ultimately clearing the infection.[97]

Risk Factors: A 2014 metaanalysis of risk factors found an association between recent history of swimming and development of MC, with the relative risk of MC among swimmers approximately twice that of nonswimmers.[98]

Altered skin barrier function and immunity in atopic dermatitis may be a risk factor for MC, with 18% to 47% of MC patients having a history of atopic dermatitis.[80,92,99-101] Atopic dermatitis may be somewhat overrepresented because children with atopic dermatitis may be assessed by physicians more often than those without, in whom molluscum may go undiagnosed.[99] Individuals with atopic dermatitis may have more widespread involvement and pruritus, as well as increased risk of developing molluscum dermatitis.[80,101]

HIV is a risk factor for MC infection, and affected individuals are at higher risk for extensive prolonged disease.[102] MC infection is associated with a CD4+ count of <200 cells/μL.[103] Additionally, MC eruption can occur in association with immune reconstitution inflammatory syndrome after initiation of antiretroviral therapy.[104]

Individuals with a *DOCK8* (dedicator of cytokinesis 8) mutation, which results in T-cell and B-cell deficiency, are at risk for extensive molluscum infections.[90,105]

Patients receiving immunosuppressive medications for organ transplants or other indications also have increased risk. MC infections have been reported in patients taking methotrexate, alone or in combination with a tumor necrosis factor-α inhibitor or cyclosporine, for treatment of Crohn disease, mycosis fungoides, mixed connective tissue disease, psoriasis, and exfoliative dermatitis.[106] Additionally, treatment with Janus kinase inhibitors and fingolimod also are implicated in the development of MC virus infections.[107,108]

DIAGNOSIS

Clinical diagnosis is usually straightforward and can be aided by dermoscopic examination where MC lesions typically have a central polylobular white-yellow amorphous structure surrounded by a peripheral crown of blood vessels (red corona).[109,110] The appearance corresponds to hyperplastic squamous epithelium expanding into the dermis, separated by septae of compressed dermis.[109] Punctiform, radial, and mixed patterns also may be seen.[111]

Pathology: Evaluation of the central contents of the lesion using a crush preparation and Wright or Giemsa staining can be carried out when necessary (Fig. 166-29). Histopathologic examination reveals a hypertrophied and hyperplastic epidermis. Above the

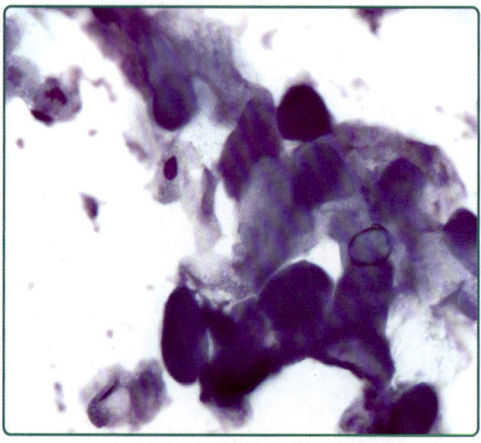

Figure 166-29 Microscopic examination (Giemsa stain) of cellular material from the area of central umbilication shows intracytoplasmic molluscum inclusion bodies.

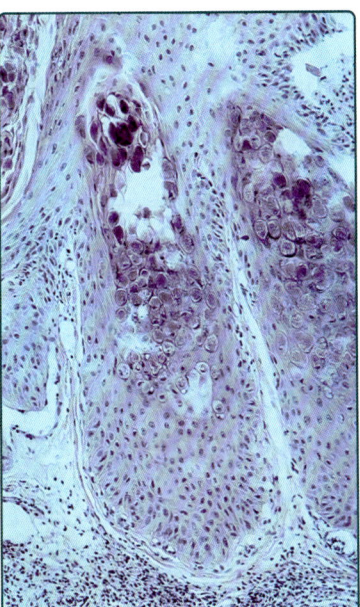

Figure 166-30 Molluscum contagiosum. Histopathology (skin biopsy, hematoxylin and eosin [H&E]) shows downgrowth of infected epidermal cells bearing large eosinophilic cytoplasmic inclusion bodies (Henderson-Paterson bodies).

basal layer, enlarged cells containing large, intracytoplasmic inclusions (Henderson-Paterson bodies) can be seen (Fig. 166-30).

Special Tests: PCR confirmation can be performed but is usually not necessary.

DIFFERENTIAL DIAGNOSIS

The differential diagnosis includes verrucae, pyogenic granulomas, amelanotic melanoma, basal cell carcinomas, and appendageal tumors. Fungal infections caused by *Cryptococcus*, histoplasmosis, and *Penicillium* must be considered in immunocompromised hosts (Table 166-7).

TABLE 166-7
Differential Diagnosis of Molluscum Contagiosum

Most Likely
- Verrucae

Consider
- Pyogenic granuloma
- Papular granuloma annulare
- Epidermal inclusion cyst
- Sebaceous hyperplasia

Always Rule Out
- Appendageal tumors
- Basal cell carcinoma
- Amelanotic melanoma
- Cryptococcosis/histoplasmosis/penicilliosis

CLINICAL COURSE AND PROGNOSIS

MC infections typically resolve spontaneously within months to years. Each individual lesion lasts approximately 2 months, but the total duration of infection is longer because lesions spread by autoinoculation.[90] In the largest prospective cohort of children with MC infection, the average duration was 13.3 months.[112] A retrospective review of 170 children with MC evaluated in the Division of Pediatric Dermatology at the Johns Hopkins Children's Center found that treatment did not shorten time to resolution.[80] Lesions typically resolve without scarring, but scratching or destructive treatments may result in scarring.

In patients infected with HIV, MC may resolve with initiation of antiretroviral therapy and improvement in CD4 cell counts.[102]

MANAGEMENT

It is important to discuss the risks and benefits of individual therapies with families before embarking on treatment of this essentially benign condition, which typically resolves without complication in the immunocompetent individual. For some children, no treatment is the best option as the child's native immune response may clear the MC without additional intervention. Nevertheless, treatment may be warranted for persistent, pruritic, spreading, or cosmetically undesirable lesions, as well as to prevent autoinoculation or transmission to others.[113] However, robust analysis of the comparative efficacy of treatments is lacking. A 2017 Cochrane Database analysis of treatments for MC identified only 22 randomized controlled trials of MC treatments and concluded that no single intervention is convincingly effective for the treatment of MC.[114] The analysis did not include several therapies commonly used by pediatric dermatologists because of insufficient data.[113,115]

In the absence of compelling evidence for the superiority of any particular treatment, multiple therapies are used, including destructive, immunomodulatory, cytotoxic, and antiviral therapies.[113]

Physically destructive therapies include curettage, cryotherapy, CO_2 laser, pulsed-dye laser, and electrodessication.[116] They may work by rupturing the intracytoplasmic sacs containing MC viral proteins and triggering an immunologic response that clears the infection.[77]

Chemically destructive therapies include potassium hydroxide, silver nitrate, trichloracetic acid, phenol, and the blistering agent cantharidin, which is likely the most commonly used therapy.[77,115,117] Cantharidin 0.7% in a collodion base is applied to the lesions and washed off after 2 to 6 hours.[118] This substance, which was originally extracted from the blister beetle, causes dissolution of desmosomal plaques, resulting in acantholysis and intraepidermal blistering, with extrusion of the molluscum bodies.[118,119] Cantharidin is the preferred treatment for children because it is painless at time of application, in contrast with curettage and cryotherapy, which are painful and may be traumatic for children. However, families must be counseled regarding the small risk of extreme reaction or scarring, and cantharidin should not be used on the thin skin of the face and genital areas. MC typically resolves after an average of 2.1 treatments with cantharidin.[120] A randomized controlled trial of cantharidin treatment versus placebo for treatment of MC that was published in 2014 found no significant difference, but was limited by sample size and short duration of follow up.[117,121] Parent and physician satisfaction with the therapy is high; 78% to 95% of parents say they would use cantharidin treatment again for molluscum reoccurrence.[120,122,123]

Immunomodulatory therapies include intralesional interferon-α or interferon-β, intralesional *Candida* antigen injection, cimetidine, and imiquimod.[77,90] Oral cimetidine has been used with some success, although evidence is contradictory.[124,125] Although imiquimod cream is favored by some physicians and may be effective for genital lesions, randomized controlled trials have found it ineffective in children.[115,126-129]

The cytotoxic therapy podophyllotoxin and antiviral therapy cidofovir, which can be administered topically or IV, are also used.

For genital molluscum, the 2014 United Kingdom national guidelines recommend either nontreatment or treatment with podophyllotoxin 0.5%, imiquimod 5% cream, or liquid nitrogen therapy.[130] Podophyllotoxin and imiquimod should be avoided during pregnancy and breastfeeding.[130]

Immunosuppressed patients may be unresponsive to traditional therapies. Treatment of the underlying disease is thought to be the most effective therapy for resolving MC infection. In HIV patients, MC infection may improve as CD4 count rises. A recent systematic review of 13 studies found little evidence to support any particular intervention for MC in HIV.[102] Combination therapies may be tried.[77] Some clinicians recommend that adolescents and adults with new-onset MC infection undergo evaluation for HIV infection and/or other causes of an immunocompromised state.[83]

Medium-strength topical steroids sometimes are used to treat molluscum dermatitis and Gianotti-Crosti–like reactions. Data on whether treating these secondary eruptions raises the risk of MC recurrence are contradictory, and this issue needs further study.[87,92]

Prevention/Screening: Spread through autoinoculation can be reduced by treating existing lesions, avoiding scratching, and using antipruritics as necessary. As mentioned above, treating molluscum dermatitis with topical steroids may reduce autoinoculation via scratching but potentially raises the risk of relapse by dampening the immune response to molluscum, and should be considered on a case-by-case basis until studied further.[87,92]

MC infection should not prevent children from attending school or playing sports.[131] To prevent spread to others, the CDC advises covering lesions that could contact other individuals with clothing or bandages. This is especially important when participating in contact sports and sharing equipment like helmets and baseball gloves. The CDC recommends avoiding swimming unless all lesions can be covered by watertight bandages.

ACKNOWLEDGMENTS

The authors acknowledge the contributions of Drs. Caroline Piggott and Wynnis Tom, former authors of this chapter.

REFERENCES

1. Diven DG. An overview of poxviruses. *J Am Acad Dermatol*. 2001;44(1):1-16.
2. Petersen BW, Damon IK, Pertowski CA, et al. Clinical guidance for smallpox vaccine use in a postevent vaccination program. *MMWR Recomm Rep*. 2015;64(2):1-32.
3. Voigt EA, Kennedy RB, Poland GA. Defending against smallpox: a focus on vaccines. *Expert Rev Vaccines*. 2016:1-15.
4. Fenner F, Henderson DA, Arita I, et al. *Smallpox and Its Eradication*. Geneva, Switzerland: World Health Organization; 1988.
5. Arita I. Discovery of forgotten variola specimens at the National Institutes of Health in the USA. *Expert Rev Anti Infect Ther*. 2014;12(12):1419-1421.
6. Huq F. Effect of temperature and relative humidity on variola virus in crusts. *Bull World Health Organ*. 1976;54(6):710-712.
7. Breman JG, Henderson DA. Diagnosis and management of smallpox. *N Engl J Med*. 2002;346(17):1300-1308.
8. Kiang KM, Krathwohl MD. Rates and risks of transmission of smallpox and mechanisms of prevention. *J Lab Clin Med*. 2003;142(4):229-238.
9. Wharton M, Strikas RA, Harpaz R, et al. Recommendations for using smallpox vaccine in a pre-event vaccination program. Supplemental recommendations of the Advisory Committee on Immunization Practices (ACIP) and the Healthcare Infection Control Practices Advisory Committee (HICPAC). *MMWR Recomm Rep*. 2003;52(RR-7):1-16.
10. WHO Expert Committee on Smallpox Eradication. WHO Expert Committee on Smallpox Eradication. Second report. *World Health Organ Tech Rep Ser*. 1972;493:1-64.
11. McKenzie PJ, Githens JH, Harwood ME, et al. Haemorrhagic smallpox. 2. Specific bleeding and coagulation studies. *Bull World Health Organ*. 1965;33(6):773-782.
12. Arora A, Agarwal A, Kumar S. Osteomyelitis variolosa: a report of two cases. *J Orthop Surg (Hong Kong)*. 2008;16(3):355-358.
13. MacNeil A, Lederman E, Reynolds MG, et al. Diagnosis of bovine-associated parapoxvirus infections in humans: molecular and epidemiological evidence. *Zoonoses Public Health*. 2010;57(7-8):e161-e164.
14. Slifka MK, Hanifin JM. Smallpox: the basics. *Dermatol Clin*. 2004;22(3):263-274.
15. Henderson DA, Inglesby TV, Bartlett JG, et al. Smallpox as a biological weapon: medical and public health management. Working Group on Civilian Biodefense. *JAMA*. 1999;281(22):2127-2137.
16. Moore ZS, Seward JF, Lane JM. Smallpox. *Lancet*. 2006;367(9508):425-435.
17. Centers for Disease Control and Prevention (CDC). *Acute, Generalized Vesicular or Pustular Rash Illness Protocol*. https://www.cdc.gov/smallpox/clinicians/

algorithm-protocol.html. Published December 5, 2016. Accessed September 29, 2018.
18. Centers for Disease Control and Prevention (CDC). *Acute, Generalized Vesicular or Pustular Rash Illness Testing Protocol in the United States*. https://www.cdc.gov/smallpox/pdfs/rash-illness-protocol.pdf. Accessed September 29, 2018.
19. Centers for Disease Control and Prevention (CDC), Association of Public Health Laboratories. *Laboratory Approach to the Diagnosis of Smallpox*. July 2011. https://www.aphl.org/programs/preparedness/Smallpox/index.html.
20. Fenner F, Wittek R, Dumbell KR. *The Orthopoxviruses*. San Diego, CA: Academic Press; 1989.
21. Berhanu A, Prigge JT, Silvera PM, et al. Treatment with the smallpox antiviral tecovirimat (ST-246) alone or in combination with ACAM2000 vaccination is effective as a postsymptomatic therapy for monkeypox virus infection. *Antimicrob Agents Chemother*. 2015;59(7):4296-4300.
22. U.S. Department of Health and Human Services, Food and Drug Administration, Center for Drug Evaluation and Research (CDER), et al. *Product Development Under the Animal Rule—Guidance for Industry*. October 2015. https://www.fda.gov/downloads/Drugs/GuidanceComplianceRegulatoryInformation/Guidances/UCM399217.pdf. Accessed September 29, 2018.
23. U.S. Department of Health and Human Services. *2014 Public Health Emergency Medical Countermeasures Enterprise (PHEMCE) Strategy and Implementation Plan*. February 2015. http://www.phe.gov/Preparedness/mcm/phemce/Documents/2014-phemce-sip.pdf. Accessed September 29, 2018.
24. U.S. Department of Health and Human Services. *2015 Public Health Emergency Medical Countermeasures Enterprise (PHEMCE) Strategy and Implementation Plan*. December 2015. https://www.phe.gov/Preparedness/mcm/phemce/Documents/2015-PHEMCE-SIP.pdf. Accessed September 29, 2018.
25. Mucker EM, Goff AJ, Shamblin JD, et al. Efficacy of tecovirimat (ST-246) in nonhuman primates infected with variola virus (smallpox). *Antimicrob Agents Chemother*. 2013;57(12):6246-6253.
25A. Trost LC, Rose ML, Khouri J, et al. The efficacy and pharmacokinetics of brincidofovir for the treatment of lethal rabbitpox virus infection: a model of smallpox disease. *Antiviral Res*. 2015;117:115-121.
26. Centers for Disease Control and Prevention (CDC). Notice to readers: newly licensed smallpox vaccine to replace old smallpox vaccine. *MMWR Morb Mortal Wkly Rep*. 2008;57(08);207-208. Available at https://www.cdc.gov/mmwr/preview/mmwrhtml/mm5708a6.htm
27. Fulginiti VA, Papier A, Lane JM, et al. Smallpox vaccination: a review, part I. Background, vaccination technique, normal vaccination and revaccination, and expected normal reactions. *Clin Infect Dis*. 2003; 37(2):241-250.
28. Rotz LD, Dotson DA, Damon IK, et al; Advisory Committee on Immunization Practices. Vaccinia (smallpox) vaccine: recommendations of the Advisory Committee on Immunization Practices (ACIP), 2001. *MMWR Recomm Rep*. 2001;50(RR-10):1-25.
29. Casey C, Vellozzi C, Mootrey GT, et al. Surveillance guidelines for smallpox vaccine (vaccinia) adverse reactions. *MMWR Recomm Rep*. 2006;55(RR-1):1-16.
30. Frey SE, Couch RB, Tacket CO, et al. Clinical responses to undiluted and diluted smallpox vaccine. *N Engl J Med*. 2002;346(17):1265-1274.
31. Lupatkin H, Lupatkin JF, Rosenberg AD. Smallpox in the 21st century. *Anesthesiol Clin North America*. 2004;22(3):541-561.
32. Neff JM. Contact vaccinia—transmission of vaccinia from smallpox vaccination. *JAMA*. 2002;288(15): 1901-1905.
33. Cono J, Casey CG, Bell DM; Centers for Disease Control and Prevention. Smallpox vaccination and adverse reactions. Guidance for clinicians. *MMWR Recomm Rep*. 2003;52(RR-4):1-28.
34. Tom WL, Kenner JR, Friedlander SF. Smallpox: vaccine reactions and contraindications. *Dermatol Clin*. 2004; 22(3):275-289.
35. Bartlett J, Borio L, Radonovich L, et al. Smallpox vaccination in 2003: key information for clinicians. *Clin Infect Dis*. 2003;36(7):883-902.
36. Moyron-Quiroz JE, McCausland MM, Kageyama R, et al. The smallpox vaccine induces an early neutralizing IgM response. *Vaccine*. 2009;28(1):140-147.
37. Maurer DM, Harrington B, Lane JM. Smallpox vaccine: contraindications, administration, and adverse reactions. *Am Fam Physician*. 2003;68(5):889-896.
38. Petersen BW, Harms TJ, Reynolds MG, et al. Use of vaccinia virus smallpox vaccine in laboratory and health care personnel at risk for occupational exposure to orthopoxviruses—recommendations of the Advisory Committee on Immunization Practices (ACIP), 2015. *MMWR Morb Mortal Wkly Rep*. 2016;65(10):257-262.
39. McCollum AM, Damon IK. Human monkeypox. *Clin Infect Dis*. 2014;58(2):260-267.
40. Reed KD, Melski JW, Graham MB, et al. The detection of monkeypox in humans in the western hemisphere. *N Engl J Med*. 2004;350(4):342-350.
41. Reynolds MG, Carroll DS, Olson VA, et al. A silent enzootic of an orthopoxvirus in Ghana, West Africa: evidence for multi-species involvement in the absence of widespread human disease. *Am J Trop Med Hyg*. 2010; 82(4):746-754.
42. Ligon BL. Monkeypox: a review of the history and emergence in the western hemisphere. *Semin Pediatr Infect Dis*. 2004;15(4):280-287.
43. Nalca A, Rimoin AW, Bavari S, et al. Reemergence of monkeypox: prevalence, diagnostics, and countermeasures. *Clin Infect Dis*. 2005;41(12):1765-1771.
44. Breman JG. Monkeypox: an emerging infection for humans? In: Scheld WM, Craig WA, Hughes JM, eds. Emerging infections. 4th ed. Washington DC: ASM Press; 2000:45-67.
45. Pattyn SR. Monkeypoxvirus infections. *Rev Sci Tech*. 2000;19(1):92-97.
46. Centers for Disease Control and Prevention (CDC). *Interim Centers for Disease Control and Prevention (CDC) Guidance for Use of Smallpox Vaccine, Cidofovir, and Vaccinia Immune Globulin (VIG) for Prevention and Treatment in the Setting of an Outbreak Monkeypox Infections*. June 11, 2003. CDC Stacks. https://www.cdc.gov/poxvirus/monkeypox/clinicians/smallpox-vaccine.html. Accessed September 29, 2018.
47. Cho CT, Wenner HA. Monkeypox virus. *Bacteriol Rev*. 1973;37(1):1-18.
48. Huhn GD, Bauer AM, Yorita K, et al. Clinical characteristics of human monkeypox, and risk factors for severe disease. *Clin Infect Dis*. 2005;41(12): 1742-1751.

49. Centers for Disease Control and Prevention (CDC). Update: multistate outbreak of monkeypox—Illinois, Indiana, Kansas, Missouri, Ohio, and Wisconsin, 2003. *MMWR Morb Mortal Wkly Rep*. 2003;52(27):642-646.
50. Centers for Disease Control and Prevention (CDC). *Receiving, Distributing, and Dispensing Strategic National Stockpile Assets: A Guide to Preparedness, Version 11*. February 2014. http://ema.ohio.gov/Documents/Plans/ReceivingDistributingand DispensingStrategicNationalStockpileAssets_%20 AGuidetoPreparedness_Version11.pdf. Accessed September 29, 2018.
51. Jordan R, Goff A, Frimm A, et al. ST-246 antiviral efficacy in a nonhuman primate monkeypox model: determination of the minimal effective dose and human dose justification. *Antimicrob Agents Chemother*. 2009;53(5):1817-1822.
52. Centers for Disease Control and Prevention (CDC). Monkeypox: treatment. http://www.cdc.gov/poxvirus/monkeypox/clinicians/treatment.html. Accessed August 14, 2016.
53. Marriott KA, Parkinson CV, Morefield SI, et al. Clonal vaccinia virus grown in cell culture fully protects monkeys from lethal monkeypox challenge. *Vaccine*. 2008;26(4):581-588.
54. Handley L, Buller RM, Frey SE, et al. The new ACAM2000 vaccine and other therapies to control orthopoxvirus outbreaks and bioterror attacks. *Expert Rev Vaccines*. 2009;8(7):841-850.
55. Wheeler CE, Cawley EP. The etiology of milker's nodules. *AMA Arch Derm*. 1957;75(2):249-259.
56. Adriano AR, Quiroz CD, Acosta ML, et al. Milker's nodule—case report. *An Bras Dermatol*. 2015; 90(3):407-410.
57. Zhao H, Wilkins K, Damon IK, et al. Specific qPCR assays for the detection of orf virus, pseudocowpox virus and bovine papular stomatitis virus. *J Virol Methods*. 2013;194(1-2):229-234.
58. Groves RW, Wilson-Jones E, MacDonald DM. Human orf and milkers' nodule: a clinicopathologic study. *J Am Acad Dermatol*. 1991;25(4):706-711.
59. Tan ST, Blake GB, Chambers S. Recurrent orf in an immunocompromised host. *Br J Plast Surg*. 1991;44(6):465-467.
60. Barraviera SRCS. Diseases caused by poxvirus-orf and milker's nodules: a review. *J Venom Anim Toxins Incl Trop Dis*. 2005;11(2):1-7.
61. Kennedy C, Lyell A. Perianal orf. *J Am Acad Dermatol*. 1984;11(1):72-74.
62. Key SJ, Catania J, Mustafa SF, et al. Unusual presentation of human giant orf (ecthyma contagiosum). *J Craniofac Surg*. 2007;18(5):1076-1078.
63. Lederman ER, Austin C, Trevino I, et al. Orf virus infection in children: clinical characteristics, transmission, diagnostic methods, and future therapeutics. *Pediatr Infect Dis J*. 2007;26(8):740-744.
64. Nougairede A, Fossati C, Salez N, et al. Sheep-to-human transmission of orf virus during Eid al-Adha religious practices, France. *Emerg Infect Dis*. 2013; 19(1):102-105.
65. Leavell UW, McNamara MJ, Muelling R, et al. Orf. Report of 19 human cases with clinical and pathological observations. *JAMA*. 1968;204(8):657-664.
66. Clark J, Diven D. Poxviruses. In: Tyring SK, Moore AY, Lupi O, eds. *Mucocutaneous Manifestations of Viral Diseases*. 2nd ed. London, UK: Informa; 2016:51.
67. Midilli K, Erkiliç A, Kuşkucu M, et al. Nosocomial outbreak of disseminated orf infection in a burn unit, Gaziantep, Turkey, October to December 2012. *Euro Surveill*. 2013;18(11):20425.
68. Joseph RH, Haddad FA, Matthews AL, et al. Erythema multiforme after orf virus infection: a report of two cases and literature review. *Epidemiol Infect*. 2014; 143(2):385-390.
69. White KP, Zedek DC, White WL, et al. Orf-induced immunobullous disease: a distinct autoimmune blistering disorder. *J Am Acad Dermatol*. 2008;58(1): 49-55.
70. Stewart AC. Epidemiology of orf. *N Z Med J*. 1983; 96:100-101.
71. Dupre A, Christol B, Bonafe JL, et al. Orf and atopic dermatitis. *Br J Dermatol*. 1981;105:103-104.
72. Yirrell DL, Vestey JP, Norval M. Immune responses of patients to orf virus infection. *Br J Dermatol*. 1994; 130(4):438-443.
73. Haig DM, Thomson J, McInnes C, et al. Orf virus immuno-modulation and the host immune response. *Vet Immunol Immunopathol*. 2002;87:395-399.
74. Geerinck K, Lukito G, Snoeck R, et al. A case of human orf in an immunocompromised patient treated successfully with cidofovir cream. *J Med Virol*. 2001;64(4):543-549.
75. Chavez-Alvarez S, Barbosa-Moreno L, Villarreal-Martinez A, et al. Dermoscopy of contagious ecthyma (orf nodule). *J Am Acad Dermatol*. 2016;74(5):e95-e96.
76. Lederman ER, Green GM, DeGroot HE, et al. Progressive orf virus infection in a patient with lymphoma: successful treatment using imiquimod. *Clin Infect Dis*. 2007; 44(11):e100-e103.
77. Smith KJ, Skelton H. Molluscum contagiosum: recent advances in pathogenic mechanisms, and new therapies. *Am J Clin Dermatol*. 2002;3(8):535-545.
78. Meirowsky E, Keys S, Behr G. The cytology of molluscum contagiosum, with special regard to the significance of the so-called vacuoles. *J Invest Dermatol*. 1946;7(4):165-169.
79. Olsen JR, Gallacher J, Piguet V, et al. Development and validation of the Molluscum Contagiosum Diagnostic Tool for Parents: diagnostic accuracy study in primary care. *Br J Gen Pract*. 2014;64(625): e471-e476.
80. Basdag H, Rainer BM, Cohen BA. Molluscum contagiosum: to treat or not to treat? Experience with 170 children in an outpatient clinic setting in the northeastern United States. *Pediatr Dermatol*. 2015;32(3):353-357.
81. Sherwani S, Farleigh L, Agarwal N, et al. Seroprevalence of molluscum contagiosum virus in German and UK populations. *PLoS One*. 2014;9(2):e88734-e88711.
82. Konya J, Thompson CH. Molluscum contagiosum virus: antibody responses in persons with clinical lesions and seroepidemiology in a representative Australian population. *J Infect Dis*. 1999;179(3): 701-704.
83. Gur I. The epidemiology of molluscum contagiosum in HIV-seropositive patients: a unique entity or insignificant finding? *Int J STD AIDS*. 2008;19(8): 503-506.
84. Becker TM, Blount JH, Douglas J, et al. Trends in molluscum contagiosum in the United States, 1966-1983. *Sex Transm Dis*. 1986;13(2):88-92.
85. Villa L, Varela JA, Otero L, et al. Molluscum contagiosum: a 20-year study in a sexually transmitted infections unit. *Sex Transm Dis*. 2010;37(7):423-424.
86. Gottlieb SL, Myskowski PL. Molluscum contagiosum. *Int J Dermatol*. 1994;33(7):453-461.

87. Osio A, Deslandes E, Saada V, et al. Clinical characteristics of molluscum contagiosum in children in a private dermatology practice in the greater Paris area, France: a prospective study in 661 patients. *Dermatology.* 2011;222(4):314-320.
88. Luke JD, Silverberg NB. Vertically transmitted molluscum contagiosum infection. *Pediatrics.* 2010;125(2):e423-e425.
89. Berbegal-DeGracia L, Betlloch-Mas I, DeLeon-Marrero F-J, et al. Neonatal molluscum contagiosum: five new cases and a literature review. *Australas J Dermatol.* 2015;56(2):e35-e38.
90. Chen X, Anstey AV, Bugert JJ. Review molluscum contagiosum virus infection. *Lancet Infect Dis.* 2013;13(10):877-888.
91. Petersen CS, Gerstoft J. Molluscum contagiosum in HIV-infected patients. *Dermatology.* 1992;184(1):19-21.
92. Berger EM, Orlow SJ, Patel RR, et al. Experience with molluscum contagiosum and associated inflammatory reactions in a pediatric dermatology practice. *Arch Dermatol.* 2012;148(11):1257-1258.
93. Smith KJ, Col, Usa MC, et al. Molluscum contagiosum: its clinical, histopathologic, and immunohistochemical spectrum. *Int J Dermatol.* 1999;38(9):664-672.
94. Senkevich TG, Koonin EV, Bugert JJ, et al. The genome of molluscum contagiosum virus: analysis and comparison with other poxviruses. *Virology.* 1997;233(1):19-42.
95. Braue A, Ross G, Varigos G, et al. Epidemiology and impact of childhood molluscum contagiosum: a case series and critical review of the literature. *Pediatr Dermatol.* 2005;22(4):287-294.
96. Shisler JL. Immune evasion strategies of molluscum contagiosum virus. *Adv Virus Res.* 2015;92:201-252.
97. Vermi W, Fisogni S, Salogni L, et al. Spontaneous regression of highly immunogenic molluscum contagiosum virus (MCV)-induced skin lesions Is associated with plasmacytoid dendritic cells and IFN-DC infiltration. *J Invest Dermatol.* 2011;131(2):426-434.
98. Olsen JR, Gallacher J, Piguet V, et al. Epidemiology of molluscum contagiosum in children: a systematic review. *Fam Pract.* 2014;31(2):130-136.
99. Dohil MA, Lin P, Lee J, et al. The epidemiology of molluscum contagiosum in children. *J Am Acad Dermatol.* 2006;54(1):47-54.
100. Olsen JR, Piguet V, Gallacher J, et al. Molluscum contagiosum and associations with atopic eczema in children: a retrospective longitudinal study in primary care. *Br J Gen Pract.* 2015;66(642):e53-e58.
101. Seize MB, Ianhez M, Cestari Sda C. A study of the correlation between molluscum contagiosum and atopic dermatitis in children. *An Bras Dermatol.* 2011;86(4):663-668.
102. Martin P. Interventions for molluscum contagiosum in people infected with human immunodeficiency virus: a systematic review. *Int J Dermatol.* 2016;55(9):956-966.
103. Maurer T, Rodrigues LK, Ameli N, et al. The effect of highly active antiretroviral therapy on dermatologic disease in a longitudinal study of HIV type 1-infected women. *Clin Infect Dis.* 2004;38(4):579-584.
104. Drain PK, Mosam A, Gounder L, et al. Recurrent giant molluscum contagiosum immune reconstitution inflammatory syndrome (IRIS) after initiation of antiretroviral therapy in an HIV-infected man. *Int J STD AIDS.* 2014;25(3):235-238.
105. Chu EY. Cutaneous manifestations of DOCK8 deficiency syndrome. *Arch Dermatol.* 2012;148(1):79-15.
106. Beutler BD, Cohen PR. Molluscum contagiosum of the eyelid: case report in a man receiving methotrexate and literature review of molluscum contagiosum in patients who are immunosuppressed secondary to methotrexate or HIV infection. *Dermatol Online J.* 2016;22(3).
107. Kinoshita M, Ogawa Y, Kawamura T, et al. Case of disseminated molluscum contagiosum caused by ruxolitinib, a Janus kinase 1 and 2 inhibitor. *J Dermatol.* 2016;43(11):1387-1388.
108. Behle V, Wobser M, Goebeler M, et al. Extensive molluscum contagiosum virus infection in a young adult receiving fingolimod. *Mult Scler.* 2016;22(7):969-971.
109. Morales A, Puig S, Malvehy J, et al. Dermoscopy of molluscum contagiosum. *Arch Dermatol.* 2005;141(12):1644-1644.
110. Vazquez-Lopez F, Kreusch J, Marghoob AA. Dermoscopic semiology: further insights into vascular features by screening a large spectrum of nontumoral skin lesions. *Br J Dermatol.* 2004;150(2):226-231.
111. Ianhez M, Cestari Sda C, Enokihara MY, et al. Dermoscopic patterns of molluscum contagiosum: a study of 211 lesions confirmed by histopathology. *An Bras Dermatol.* 2011;86(1):74-79.
112. Olsen JR, Gallacher J, Finlay AY, et al. Time to resolution and effect on quality of life of molluscum contagiosum in children in the UK: a prospective community cohort study. *Lancet Infect Dis.* 2015;15(2):190-195.
113. McCuaig C, Silverberg N, Santer M. Commentaries on "Interventions for cutaneous molluscum contagiosum." *Evid Based Child Health.* 2011;6(5):1602-1605.
114. van der Wouden JC, van der Sande R, Kruithof EJ, et al. Interventions for cutaneous molluscum contagiosum. *Cochrane Database Syst Rev.* 2017; (5):CD004767.
115. Coloe J, Morrell DS. Cantharidin use among pediatric dermatologists in the treatment of molluscum contagiosum. *Pediatr Dermatol.* 2009;26(4):405-408.
116. Griffith RD, Yazdani Abyaneh M-A, Falto-Aizpurua L, et al. Pulsed dye laser therapy for molluscum contagiosum: a systematic review. *J Drugs Dermatol.* 2014;13(11):1349-1352.
117. Coloe Dosal J, Stewart PW, Lin J-A, et al. Cantharidin for the treatment of molluscum contagiosum: a prospective, double-blinded, placebo-controlled trial. *Pediatr Dermatol.* 2014;31(4):440-449.
118. Mathes EF, Frieden IJ. Treatment of molluscum contagiosum with cantharidin: a practical approach. *Pediatr Ann.* 2010;39(3):124-128, 130.
119. Moed L, Shwayder TA, Chang MW. Cantharidin revisited: a blistering defense of an ancient medicine. *Arch Dermatol.* 2001;137(10):1357-1360.
120. Silverberg NB, Sidbury R, Mancini AJ. Childhood molluscum contagiosum: experience with cantharidin therapy in 300 patients. *J Am Acad Dermatol.* 2000;43(3):503-507.
121. Osier E, Eichenfield LF. The utility of cantharidin for the treatment of molluscum contagiosum. *Pediatr Dermatol.* 2015;32(2):295-296.
122. Moye VA, Cathcart S, Morrell DS. Safety of cantharidin: a retrospective review of cantharidin treatment in 405 children with molluscum contagiosum. *Pediatr Dermatol.* 2014;31(4):450-454.
123. Cathcart S, Coloe J, Morrell DS. Parental satisfaction, efficacy, and adverse events in 54 patients treated with cantharidin for molluscum contagiosum infection. *Clin Pediatr (Phila).* 2008;48(2):161-165.

124. Dohil M, Prendiville JS. Treatment of molluscum contagiosum with oral cimetidine: clinical experience in 13 patients. *Pediatr Dermatol*. 1996;13(4):310-312.
125. Cunningham BB, Paller AS, Garzon M. Inefficacy of oral cimetidine for nonatopic children with molluscum contagiosum. *Pediatr Dermatol*. 1998;15(1):71-72.
126. Farhangian ME, Huang KE, Feldman SR, et al. Treatment of molluscum contagiosum with imiquimod in the United States: a retrospective cross-sectional study. *Pediatr Dermatol*. 2015;33(2):227-228.
127. Syed TA, Goswami J, Ahmadpour OA, et al. Treatment of molluscum contagiosum in males with an analog of imiquimod 1% in cream: a placebo-controlled, double-blind study. *J Dermatol*. 1998;25(5):309-313.
128. Katz KA. Dermatologists, imiquimod, and treatment of molluscum contagiosum in children. *JAMA Dermatol*. 2015;151(2):125-122.
129. Medicis Pharmaceutical Corp. Aldara Drug Label. 2010. https://www.accessdata.fda.gov/drugsatfda_docs/label/2010/020723s022lbl.pdf. Accessed September 29, 2018.
130. Fernando I, Pritchard J, Edwards SK, et al. UK national guideline for the management of genital molluscum in adults, 2014 Clinical Effectiveness Group, British Association for Sexual Health and HIV. *Int J STD AIDS*. 2015;26(10):687-695.
131. Kimberlin DW, Brady MT, Jackson MA, et al, eds. *Red Book:2015 Report of the Committee on Infectious Diseases*. 30th ed. 2015. http://ebooks.aappublications.org/content/red-book-30th-edition-2015. Accessed September 29, 2018.

Chapter 167 :: Human Papillomavirus Infections :: Jane C. Sterling

第一百六十七章
人乳头瘤病毒感染

中文导读

人乳头瘤病毒（HPV）感染在世界范围内非常常见，可以影响皮肤的任何部位，可感染所有年龄和种族的人。本章共分为5节：①简介；②病毒学；③流行病学；④皮肤人乳头瘤病毒感染；⑤黏膜和黏膜周围人乳头瘤病毒感染。

第一节介绍了HPV感染的概况，作者将肛门-生殖器区域或口咽部的前恶性肿瘤和侵袭性癌症与其他所谓的高危HPV类型列于表167-1中。

第二节介绍了HPV的病毒特性，图167-1展示了乳头瘤病毒颗粒，图167-2展示了乳头瘤病毒的遗传结构。已有的研究表明病毒颗粒可以通过皮肤黏膜微擦伤等其他皮肤屏障功能受损情况致感染，侵入细胞则依赖于病毒粒子同硫酸肝素和a6-整合素与细胞的初始黏附，但具体过程尚未明确。

第三节介绍了HPV感染的地域分布特点和年龄分布特点，值得注意的是近年来报道的儿童出现与肛门-生殖器HPV感染相关的性虐待。

第四节介绍了HPV感染后的皮肤疣、疣状表皮发育不全和疣状表皮发育不全综合征的临床特征、病因和发病机制、诊断及组织学、病程和预后及管理等方面的详细情况。

第五节介绍了黏膜和黏膜周围HPV感染后的肛门-生殖器疣、口腔疣、肛门-生殖器上皮内瘤变和癌症。分别从临床特征、病因和发病机制、诊断及组织学、病程和管理及预后四个方面进行了详细描述。

〔张江林〕

AT-A-GLANCE

- Human papillomavirus (HPV) has a worldwide occurrence, affecting people of all ages and all races. It is most common in children and young adults.
- There are more than 150 genotypes of HPV, with some regional specificity. Low-risk types cause warts; high-risk types are associated with intraepithelial neoplasia and malignancy.
- The lesions are well-defined, raised papules or plaques with a rough or hard surface, usually without inflammation.
- The lesions are most common on the hands or feet, but any skin site may be affected, including the lower genital or oral mucosa.
- Treatments include destructive, antiviral, antiproliferative, and immunologic modalities.

INTRODUCTION

Human papillomavirus (HPV) infections are very common, occurring in a worldwide distribution, affecting all ages and lasting months or years. The majority of individuals will have at least one infection with the virus during the course of a lifetime, although the severity and duration of the disease will depend, to a large extent, on the immune response raised against the virus-infected cells.

The clinical disease caused by the virus is also dependent on the viral genotype and the body site. Whereas skin and mucosal warts are benign and induced by one of several different types according to body site, premalignancies and invasive cancer of the anogenital area or oropharynx are associated with other, so-called high-risk, HPV types (Table 167-1).

VIROLOGY

The papillomaviruses form a large group of closely related viruses, defined by their host range. HPVs only infect humans and, in particular, epithelial keratinocytes. In experimental systems, the virus does not infect keratinocytes in monolayer tissue culture.

Papillomaviruses are DNA viruses with each virus particle or virion consisting of a nonenveloped icosahedral capsid containing the double-stranded genetic material as a circular genome (Fig. 167-1). The virus is much smaller, both in particle size and length of genetic material, than other common viruses that infect skin such as herpes simplex virus and molluscum contagiosum virus. The genes are all transcribed in one direction from one DNA strand, leading to the production of 5 to 6 early (E) proteins involved in DNA replication, cell cycle control and immune evasion; and 2 late (L) proteins, L1 and L2, that form the outer shell or capsid (Fig. 167-2).

The virus is shed from the surface of the skin or mucosa within sloughed, dead keratinocytes. New infection occurs when the virus particle contacts the basal epidermal keratinocyte, presumed to be via small microabrasions in the skin or mucosa. Maceration of skin can increase the chance of infection because of impairment of barrier function. Cell entry depends on

TABLE 167-1
Diseases Caused by or Associated with Human Papillomavirus Infection

DISEASE	CLINICAL	MOST COMMONLY ASSOCIATED HPV TYPES[a]	PV GENUS
Cutaneous warts	Common warts,	2, 27, 57 (7)	Alpha
	filiform warts,	4, (60)	Mu
	mosaic warts	(48)	Gamma
	Palmar and plantar warts	1, (63)	Nu
	Butchers' warts	2, 7	Alpha
	Plane warts	3, 10 (28)	Alpha
Anogenital warts	Vulval warts, vaginal warts, penile warts, perianal warts	6, 11 (and others)	Alpha
Oral warts		6, 11 (and others)	Alpha
EV and EV-like syndromes	Benign scaly or flaky lesions;	9, 12, 15, 19, 22-25, 36-38, 80	Beta
	Plane warts	3, 10	Alpha
	Skin SCC	5, 8, 14, 17, 20, 21, 47, 93, 96	Beta
Skin SCC	Periungual SCC	16	Alpha
	Carcinoma cuniculatum or verrucous carcinoma	(11, 6)	Alpha
AGIN	VIN, VaIN, CIN, PIN, AIN	16, (18, 31, 33, 35, 45, 52, 58 and others)	Alpha
Anogenital SCC	SCC of vulva, vagina, cervix, penis, anal area	16, 18, 31, 33, 35, 42 (and others)	Alpha
Oropharyngeal SCC	SCC of mouth, pharynx	16 (18, 31, 33 35 and others)	Alpha

[a]Human papillomavirus (HPV) types in parentheses are found less commonly.
AGIN, anogenital intraepithelial neoplasia; AIN, anal and perianal intraepithelial neoplasia; CIN, cervical intraepithelial neoplasia; EV, epidermodysplasia verruciformis; PIN, penile intraepithelial neoplasia; PV, papilloma virus; SCC, squamous cell carcinoma; VaIN, vaginal intraepithelial neoplasia; VIN, vulval intraepithelial neoplasia.

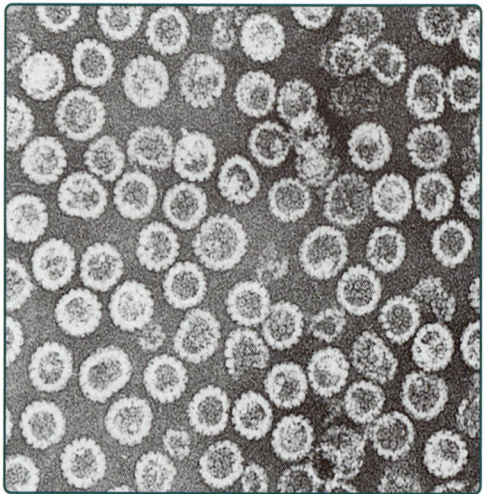

Figure 167-1 Papillomavirus virus–like particles. Transmission electron micrograph of human papillomavirus type 16 virus–like particles composed of the L1 and L2 proteins. These proteins were synthesized in cell culture and self-assembled into 55-nm particles that are morphologically similar to natural infectious virus except that they do not contain the viral DNA. The particles in the electron micrograph were purified from the cells. (Micrograph used with permission from Heather Greenstone. Courtesy of Prof. Elliot Androphy.)

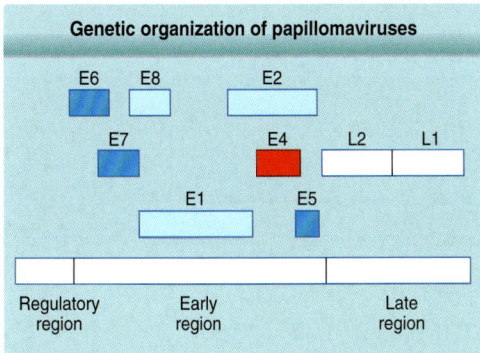

Figure 167-2 Genetic organization of papillomaviruses. The circular human papillomavirus genome of approximately 8000 nucleotide base pairs is represented here as a linear strand. (Used with permission from Prof. Elliot Androphy.)

an initial adherence of the virion to the cell via heparin sulphate and α6-integrins,[1,2] although the full process of receptor binding leading to internalization by endocytosis has not yet been clarified. Within a stem cell or transit amplifying cell of the basal layer, the virus is maintained in low copy number. It is carried to the surface in daughter cells, producing, as it goes, the early viral proteins. High-volume viral DNA amplification and L1 and L2 protein production occurs in the upper layers, with formation of completely new virus particles in the granular layer. The switch to capsid protein production depends on a change in splice site usage in the early genes.[3] The E6 and E7 proteins are pivotal to the process of viral genome amplification, which also depends on the E1 and E2 proteins. The viral E1^E4 protein can interact with keratin filaments, weakening cytoplasmic structure and potentially facilitating virus particle release at the surface.[4]

There are more than 150 HPV types, defined according to the DNA sequence within the *L1* gene.[5] A virus is defined as a distinct type if there is greater than 10% dissimilarity from other known HPVs in the DNA of this region. The HPVs have been grouped, according to phylogeny, into five genera: alpha, beta, gamma, mu, and nu (see Table 167-1). HPVs that are not found in malignancies or premalignancies are termed *low-risk types*, and those found in invasive or preinvasive disease are called *high-risk types*. The high-risk anogenital HPVs fall into the large alpha genus. High-risk genital HPV types can integrate within the host cell genome, and the maintained expression of their E6 and E7 proteins has oncogenic effects on cell division and cell function. These E6 and E7 proteins affect cell cycle control and apoptosis via interaction with ubiquitin ligases, telomerase, and several other cellular pathways.[6] In the process of integration, the E2, E4, L2, and to a lesser extent the L1 regions of the genome are frequently disrupted. In malignant lesions, late proteins and virus particles are rarely, if ever found, although episomal (nonintegrated) viral DNA may be maintained in preinvasive disease.

EPIDEMIOLOGY

Infection with HPV occurs throughout the world and in all ages. Benign cutaneous warts are most common in childhood and into the 20s, with 30% to 70% of school-age children having skin warts,[7,8] but anogenital warts, which are usually spread via sexual contact, are most common in early adult life. In children, anogenital warts should raise consideration of sexual abuse, although HPV types that cause common warts may often be found in warts of prepubertal children.[9] Squamous cell malignancy, associated most strongly with the high-risk anogenital HPV types, usually only develops after an infection has persisted for several years.

Spread of infection can be via direct contact, but the virus particles, released from epithelial surfaces as keratinocytes are shed, can remain present in the environment for an unknown duration and may later lead to infection in another individual.[10] Even after infection, it can take months before a visible wart appears.[11] After being established, infection can spread on the surface to adjacent skin.

Protection against a new infection is via neutralizing antibodies. The anti-HPV vaccines, produced as the L1 capsid protein assembled into virus-like particles, lead to a humoral response against the virus particle. In natural infection, seroconversion also occurs, but in this situation, anti-HPV antibodies are not effective in the resolution of established infection. Clearance of the virus from infected tissue is dependent on a cell-mediated immune response, and as yet there is no available, effective therapeutic vaccine. Most warts in children will clear within 2 years,[8] but in a minority of otherwise well individuals, warts can spread and persist longer.[12]

In individuals with long-term immune compromise, especially those with inherited immunodeficiency and transplant recipients receiving high-dose immune suppression, warts and malignancy caused by HPVs can be a major problem. Five years after renal transplant, it is estimated that approximately 90% of patients have warts[13] caused by the HPV types that cause warts in healthy people.[14] Many other HPV types, mainly from the beta papilloma viruses (PVs), can be detected by polymerase chain reaction (PCR) on the skin (normal or lesional) of transplant recipients.[15-17] Using such sensitive methods, these virus types are also found on the skin and in the hair follicles of healthy individuals.[18])

SKIN HUMAN PAPILLOMAVIRUS INFECTIONS

CUTANEOUS WARTS

CLINICAL FEATURES

Viral warts are initially asymptomatic and often unnoticed but grow to form well-defined, thickened, hyperkeratotic lesions (Fig. 167-3). These are often unsightly and may cause pain if sited at pressure points or if they crack and bleed. Walking and use of the hands can be affected according to the site of the warts (Fig. 167-4). Common sites are the hands and feet, especially at areas of minor trauma, such as knuckles or around nails (Fig. 167-5). On the dorsal aspects of hands or feet or on the limbs, warts are exophytic or "cauliflower shaped" (Fig. 167-6), but on soles or palms, they are often relatively flat to the surface with a more endophytic growth pattern. The term *mosaic warts* is applied to a group of small adjacent but relatively flat warts on the sole (Fig. 167-7). Smaller and flatter warts, often on the backs of the hands or face, may be *plane warts* (also called *verruca plana*; see Fig. 167-8). On the face and limbs, warts can sometimes have a small base and longer, fingerlike projections, a morphological type called *filiform warts* (Fig. 167-9).

Warts are most common in children and young adults[19] but can occur at any age.

ETIOLOGY AND PATHOGENESIS

Common warts are caused most frequently by HPV-2/27/57, HPV-4, and HPV-1 (soles and palms) and less frequently by HPV-7 (called *butcher's warts*). Flat warts are usually caused by type 3 or 10 or very occasionally type 28.

Butchers' warts were originally described in meat workers, whose hands were in direct contact with wet meat. The finding of HPV-7 is not limited to these warts but has been reported rarely in hand warts, face warts, and HIV infection.

HPV-1 warts are found only on the palms and soles and may be called *myrmecia*. They produce higher amounts of new particles compared to other cutaneous types. Some unusual HPV types, HPV-57 and -60, have been found in epidermoid plantar cysts of Japanese patients.[20]

DIAGNOSIS AND HISTOLOGY

Warts can usually be diagnosed clinically without the need for histologic confirmation. Paring the surface of a

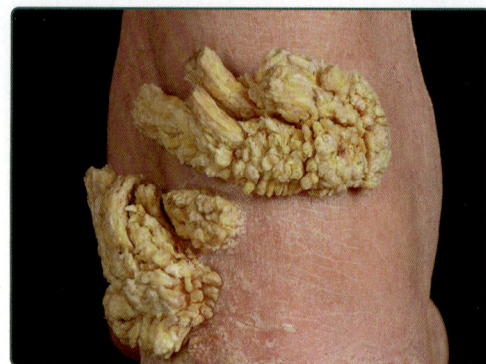

Figure 167-4 Very hyperkeratotic warts over the Achilles tendon.

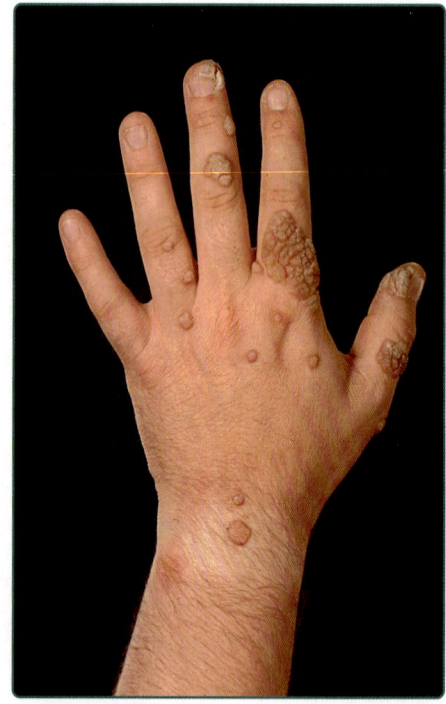

Figure 167-5 Multiple warts on the hand with periungual warts affecting nail growth.

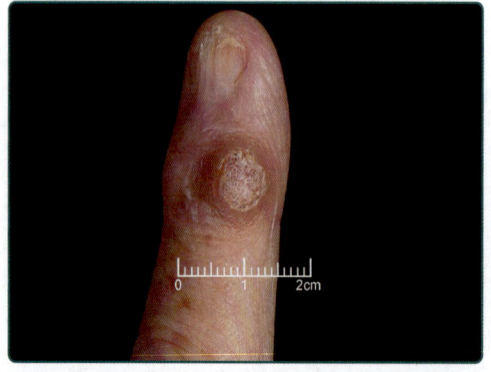

Figure 167-3 Well-defined wart on the finger. Small thrombosed capillaries are visible as black dots. (The nail had been damaged previously from trauma.)

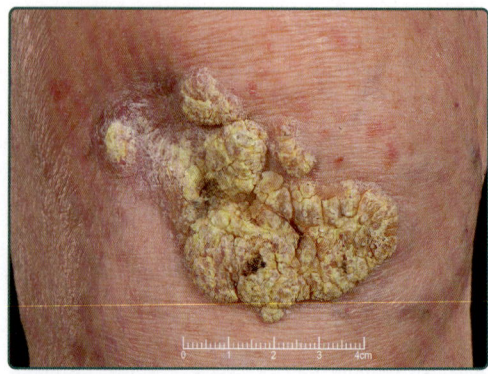

Figure 167-6 Warts on the knee.

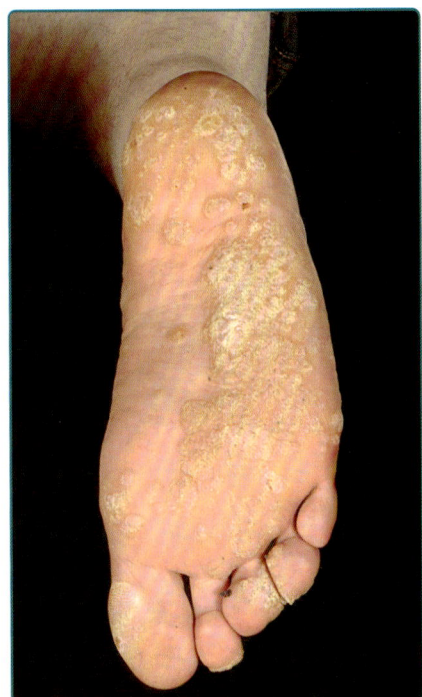

Figure 167-7 Mosaic warts on the sole.

wart will reveal capillary loops close to the surface and often causes bleeding. These capillaries often thrombose and then appear as black dots (see Fig. 167-3).

The histology is of acanthosis, hypergranulosis, and hyperkeratosis of the epidermis. The keratinocytes of the upper granular layer may show koilocytosis with clear cytoplasm and a dense twisted nucleus (Fig. 167-10). Detection of HPV DNA by PCR or in situ hybridization will confirm the diagnosis but is not in use for standard clinical care.

The differential diagnoses are listed in Table 167-2.

CLINICAL COURSE, PROGNOSIS, AND MANAGEMENT

Untreated, warts in young people usually clear spontaneously within about 2 years, and only a few remain at 4 years.[21] In adults, clearance can often be very slow, with warts persisting for years. Large and widespread warts (Fig. 167-11) are common in immunosuppressed individuals such as transplant recipients and in children or adults with genetic immunodeficiency (Table 167-3). In these cases, large areas of skin may be affected as well as mucous membranes, and the condition may be called *generalized verrucosis*.[22]

Treatment can speed clearance in warts but often fails in immunosuppressed individuals.

There is no virus-specific anti-viral therapy for warts, so available treatments aim to (1) damage the infected epithelium and debulk the lesions, (2) have some effect on the virus life cycle, or (3) to stimulate an immune response (Table 167-4). It is possible that most treatments may have more than one effect. Recent

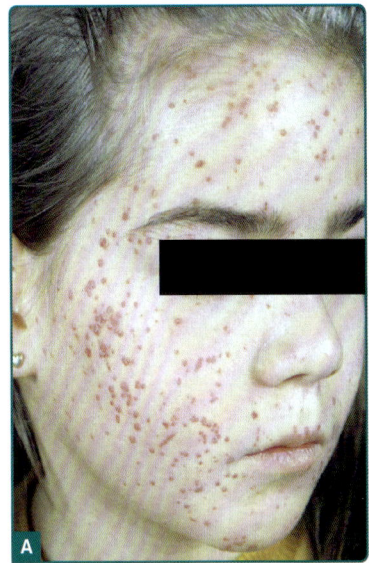

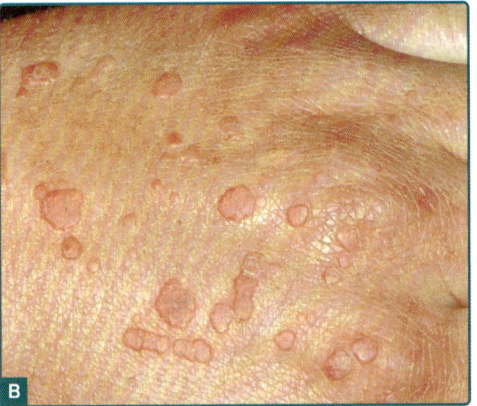

Figure 167-8 Plane warts (verruca plana). **A,** Multiple pink flat warts on the face of an 11-year-old girl. **B,** Many flat-topped papules occur in a linear configuration resulting from self-inoculation. (Used with permission from Prof. Elliot Androphy.)

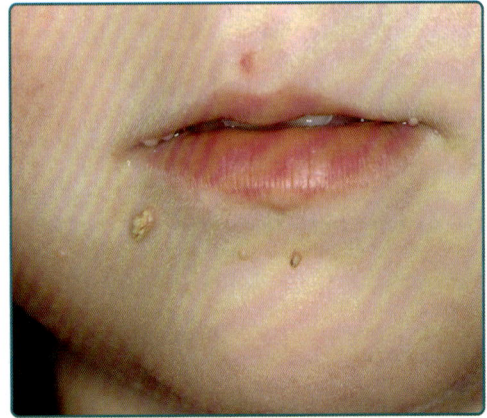

Figure 167-9 Common warts. Filiform warts on the chin and lips of a child. (Used with permission from Prof. Elliot Androphy.)

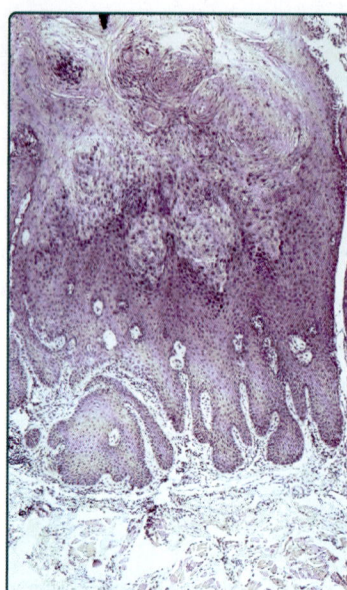

Figure 167-10 Verruca vulgaris. The process is one of extensive hyperplasia, and the hyperplastic cells contain both intranuclear and intracytoplasmic inclusion bodies. (Used with permission from Prof. Elliot Androphy.)

reviews of treatments for warts give more detail of the spectrum and potential efficacy of the range of treatments used today.[38–40]

The most commonly used treatments for warts are destructive and include topical applications with salicylic acid and physical treatment with cryotherapy. For the greatest effect, treatment needs to be repeated and of long duration. It is worth informing patients that regular treatment for at least 3 months or longer is likely to be required. Even with assiduous treatment, the clearance rate for most common treatments is 60% to 70% compared with 30% clearing with placebo.[41]

Salicylic acid (12%–17% in a paint or up to 50% in plasters or an ointment) is applied to the wart, which can be rubbed down or pared gently beforehand. Occlusion with an adhesive dressing after application may improve clearance. Daily treatment is recommended, but as the salicylic acid gradually destroys and so removes the keratin layer, the wart or more likely surrounding tissue can become sore, and treatment may need to be reduced in frequency. For this reason, salicylic acid in these strengths is not recommended for facial or anogenital warts.

Cryotherapy (see Chap. 206) with liquid nitrogen is best used as a double freeze, repeated every 3 weeks for at least 3 months. This is a painful treatment and often not tolerated to warts around nails, on the soles, or by children.

Other treatments that damage or destroy the infected epithelium include caustics such as silver nitrate, phenol, mono- or trichloroacetic acid, and surgical approaches with laser or excisional surgery.

Plane warts require less keratolysis, and treatment with other topical applications such as the immune modulator imiquimod can be effective.

TABLE 167-2 Differential Diagnosis of Warts

COMMON WARTS	PLANE WARTS	GENITAL WARTS
Seborrheic keratosis	Seborrheic keratosis	Seborrheic keratosis
Actinic keratosis	Actinic keratosis	Vulval or penile papillomatosis
Bowen disease	Lichen planus	Lichen planus
SCC, keratoacanthoma	Adenoma sebaceum	VIN, PIN, AIN
Acrokeratosis verruciformis	Syringomas	Verrucous carcinoma
Epidermal naevus	Trichoepitheliomas	Condyloma acuminatum (secondary syphilis)
Pyogenic granuloma	Disseminated superficial actinic porokeratosis	Sebaceous gland hyperplasia
Fish tank granuloma		
Verrucous tuberculosis		
Callus		
Soles and Palms Only		
Palmoplantar keratoderma		
Corn		
Inclusion cyst		
Palmar pits (Darier disease, Gorlin syndrome)		
Carcinoma cuniculatum		

AIN, anal and perianal intraepithelial neoplasia; PIN, penile intraepithelial neoplasia; SCC, squamous cell carcinoma; VIN, vulval intraepithelial neoplasia.

Severe proliferative warts may be helped but sometimes only for the duration of the treatment by treatments that reduce or slow epidermal growth, such as podophyllotoxin or retinoids.

In immune compromise, clearance of warts, either spontaneously or with treatment, is rare and treatment is usually aimed at measures to reduce wart bulk, maintain function, and avoid pain.

EPIDERMODYSPLASIA VERRUCIFORMIS AND EPIDERMODYSPLASIA VERRUCIFORMIS–LIKE SYNDROMES

CLINICAL FEATURES

Epidermodysplasia verruciformis (EV) is a rare, heritable skin disorder with a mild underlying primary

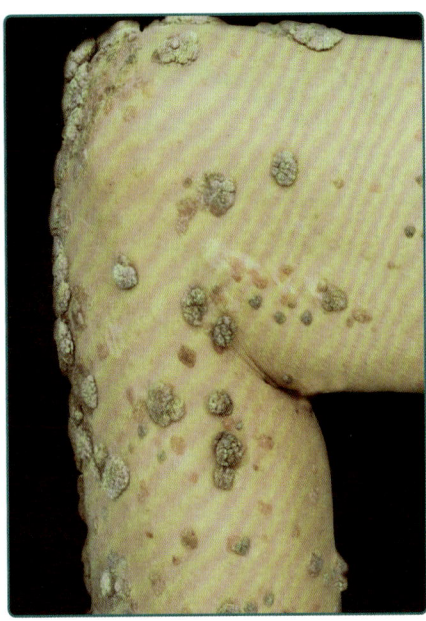

Figure 167-11 Leg with numerous warts. The large, scaly, and horny warts contain human papillomavirus (HPV)-2. The smaller, flatter, less scaly papules are warts that contain HPV-3. With extensive warts such as these, an assessment of immune function is indicated. (Used with permission from Prof. Elliot Androphy.)

immunodeficiency. The signs of EV become apparent in late childhood or adolescence, but in the absence of a family history, diagnosis may be delayed until a decade or two later. Widespread flaky, scaly, or flat warty lesions are seen on the face, hands, and forearms and other sun-exposed sites (Fig. 167-12). There is often erythema, hyperpigmentation, or more rarely hypopigmentation of lesions, and there can be confusion with pityriasis versicolor and plane warts. In early adult life, actinic keratoses, Bowen disease, and invasive squamous cell carcinoma (SCC) can develop at affected sites (Fig. 167-13). Metastatic disease can follow.

Patients with EV have a mild cell-mediated immune impairment.[42] This is often not obvious on clinical grounds because widespread susceptibility to other infections is not a feature but can reduce susceptibility to contact allergy.

A clinical appearance very similar to EV, called acquired EV, may be seen after long-term immunocompromise from several causes[43,44] (Table 167-5).

ETIOLOGY AND PATHOGENESIS

EV can be inherited, usually with an autosomal recessive pattern. The genes implicated most commonly are *EVER-1* and *-2*, which produce the transmembrane, zinc-containing proteins TMC6 and TMC8.[45]

A large number of HPV types are associated with EV lesions and the clinically unaffected skin of patients.[46] These include HPV-3 and -10, the cause of plane warts, as well as the beta PVs, some of which are found in SCCs and some of which are only found in benign lesions (see Table 167-1). Patients may also have warts harboring the usual HPV types found in common warts.

DIAGNOSIS AND HISTOLOGY

Diagnosis may be made on a combination of clinical features and family history. Skin biopsy shows mild acanthosis and hyperkeratosis. In some lesions, there may also be pallor or clearing of the cytoplasm of the upper spinous layer keratinocytes, called ballooning, with small dense nuclei (so-called clear cells; see Fig. 167-14). With sensitive HPV detection, the beta PVs are found most commonly.

TABLE 167-3
Syndromes of Immune Compromise in Which Warts May Be a Prominent Clinical Feature

ONSET	SYNDROME	FEATURES	REFERENCES
Infancy	SCID, both pre or post bone marrow transplant	Warts	23
Infancy	Wiskott Aldrich	Warts	24
Early childhood	Common variable immunodeficiency	Warts	25
Early childhood	Ataxia-telangiectasia	Warts	26
Childhood	Bittner syndrome	Warts of palms and soles, Bowen disease	27
Childhood or adult	GATA-2 deficiency (also called WILD syndrome)	Warts, anogenital SCC	28-30
Childhood or adult	DOCK-8 deficiency	Warts; atopic disease, bacterial and viral infections	31
Childhood or adult	Selective IgA deficiency	Warts	32
Childhood or adult	Intestinal lymphangiectasia, Waldman disease	Lymphedema and rarely warts of hands and feet	33
Adult	Idiopathic CD4 lymphocytopenia	Cutaneous warts, anogenital warts, AGIN, EV-like	34,35
Adult	IL-7 deficiency	Warts; Cryptococcus meningitis	36
Adult	WHIM syndrome	Warts, anogenital SCC	37

AGIN, anogenital intraepithelial neoplasia; EV, epidermodysplasia verruciformis; IgA, immunoglobulin A; SCC, squamous cell carcinoma; SCID, severe combined immunodeficiency; WHIM, warts, hypogammaglobulinemia, immunodeficiency, and myelokathexis.

TABLE 167-4
Commonly Used Treatments for Cutaneous and Anogenital Warts

Treatments Damaging or Destroying the Epithelium[a]
Topical
Salicylic acid
Cantharidin
Phenol
Monochloroacetic or trichloroacetic acid
Silver nitrate
5-Fluorouracil
Zinc oxide
Retinoid
Bleomycin (IL)

Physical
Cryotherapy
Cautery
Photodynamic therapy
Laser (pulsed dye)
Surgical removal

Reduction of Proliferation
Retinoid (topical or oral)
Podophyllotoxin
Cidofovir

Virucidal
Formalin
Glutaraldehyde

Immune Modulation
Imiquimod
Diphencyprone or squaric acid topical immunotherapy
Immunotherapy with *Candida* or mumps antigen (IL)
Interferon (IL)
Zinc sulphate (oral)
Cimetidine (oral)

Further details in References 37 to 39.
IL, intralesional.

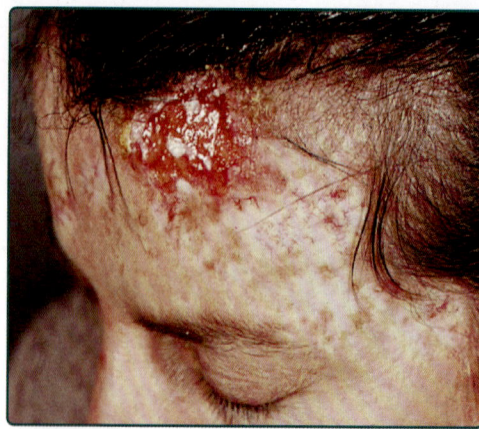

Figure 167-13 Invasive cancer in an epidermodysplasia verruciformis patient infected with numerous human papillomavirus (HPV) types, including HPV-5, -8, -9, -14, and others. In the tumor cells, HPV-5 DNA was detected in a high copy number. This large squamous cell carcinoma did not metastasize and did not recur after surgery. There are numerous actinic keratoses on the forehead. (Used with permission from Prof. Elliot Androphy.)

TABLE 167-5
Conditions That May Lead to Acquired Epidermodysplasia Verruciformis

Transplantation (organ or bone marrow)
HIV infection

Less Common Causes
Common variable immunodeficiency
Coronin-1-A deficiency
Connective tissue disease (eg, SLE treated with long-term immunosuppression)
Graft-versus-host disease
IgM deficiency
Leprosy
Lymphoma
Myasthenia gravis

IgM, immunoglobulin M; SLE, systemic lupus erythematosus.

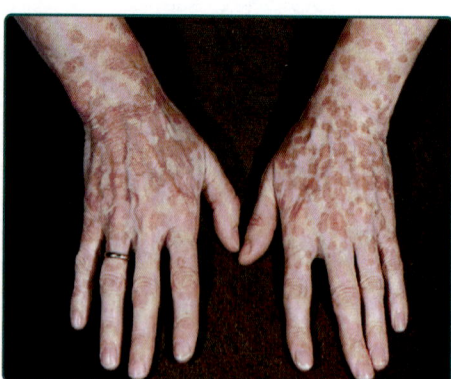

Figure 167-12 Epidermodysplasia verruciformis. Plane wart–like lesions on the dorsa of the hands and forearms associated with human papillomavirus-5 and -8. The lesions are numerous, flat, reddish, and partly confluent. (Used with permission from Prof. Elliot Androphy.)

CLINICAL COURSE, PROGNOSIS, AND TREATMENT

Treatments usually make little lasting difference, but short-term, cosmetic improvement can be obtained

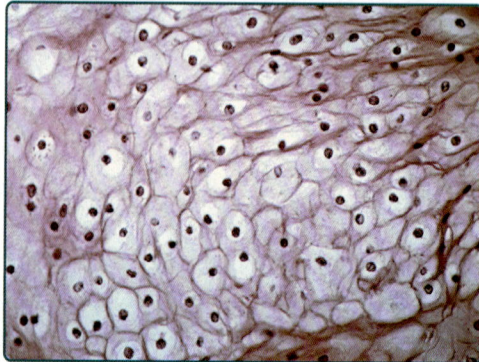

Figure 167-14 Characteristic cytopathic effect of epidermodysplasia verruciformis–specific human papillomavirus (HPV) in a patient found to be infected with HPV-5, -8, and -9. Very abundant clear large cells with small pyknotic nuclei replace almost the entire epidermis. (Used with permission from Prof. Elliot Androphy.)

by a number of approaches that remove the hyperkeratosis.[42,43] Cryotherapy, topical salicylic acid, 5-fluorourcil, and imiquimod have all been used with varying results.[47,48] Photodynamic therapy (PDT)[49] or an oral retinoid, such as acitretin,[50] can produce a useful improvement in lesions.

To reduce the risk of skin cancers, sun protection is important. Regular surveillance for SCC and early treatment of suspicious lesions may avoid metastatic disease.

SQUAMOUS CELL CARCINOMA AND HUMAN PAPILLOMAVIRUS

Common warts in immunocompetent individuals are not forerunners of skin cancer. However, there are a very few reports, usually in the setting of immunosuppression, of long-standing periungual warts progressing into Bowen disease (full-thickness dysplasia) or invasive SCC.[51] In such cases, the high-risk anogenital HPV type, HPV-16, is usually present. Long-standing and slowly enlarging warty areas on the soles, fingers, or anogenital skin can be a feature of carcinoma cuniculatum or verrucous carcinoma (Buschke-Löwenstein tumour), in which the HPV types usually associated with anogenital warts, HPV-6 or -11, are occasionally detected.[52,53]

Skin SCCs on sun exposed skin are also found to contain a number of EV-related beta HPV types, with a higher yield in the cancers of immunosuppressed individuals. These HPVs are often found in normal skin of both immunocompetent and immunocompromised individuals,[16,18] and the exact role they play in the steps of carcinogenesis is still under debate.[54]

MUCOSAL AND PERI-MUCOSAL HUMAN PAPILLOMAVIRUS INFECTIONS

ANOGENITAL WARTS

CLINICAL FEATURES

Warts can affect the vulva, vagina, cervix, penis, scrotum, perianal skin, and anal canal. They may present singly but are usually found as multiple, well-defined papules or as flat or filiform lesions and may grow into larger protuberant lesions (Fig. 167-15). The moist fold beneath an abdominal apron of an obese patient is another site for these warts.[55] On mucosal surfaces, they are often macerated and appear pale, but on drier skin, they can become more obviously hyperkeratotic and hard. They may be asymptomatic but can be itchy and uncomfortable and may be traumatized with movement or sexual activity.

DIAGNOSIS

HPV-6 or -11 are the most common causative agents, but other HPV types are found with PCR analysis. Anogenital warts produce less virus particles than cutaneous warts.

For differential diagnosis, see Table 167-2.

CLINICAL COURSE, PROGNOSIS, AND TREATMENT

Anogenital warts are usually treated with a topical application as first-line therapy.[56] Podophyllotoxin or imiquimod are both self-applied treatments with a 50% to 70% clearance rate.[57] Recurrence rates after imiquimod treatment are slightly less than after podophyllotoxin.[58]

Other treatments in use include topical trichloroacetic acid,[59] sinecatechins from green tea,[60] and physical therapies with cryotherapy, PDT, laser, electrocautery, or surgery.

Since the introduction of the quadrivalent anti-HPV vaccine in 2007, there has been a recorded decrease in presentation of genital warts or prevalence of HPV-6 and -11.[61,62]

ORAL WARTS

Warts can develop on the lips, in the oral cavity, and in upper respiratory tract and are usually regarded as a sexually transmitted disease. Because of the moist site, they are usually macerated and can be flat or cauliflower shaped (Fig. 167-16). The low-risk genital HPV types are the usual cause. Laryngeal warts (laryngeal papillomatosis) can develop in childhood, probably caused by infection from the mother at birth, and can affect speech and breathing.

Oral warts are common in HIV infection and may worsen, rather than improve, during antiretroviral therapy.[63]

ANOGENITAL INTRAEPITHELIAL NEOPLASIA AND CANCER

CLINICAL FEATURES

Anogenital intraepithelial neoplasia (AGIN) includes dysplasia of the vulva (vulvar intraepithelial neoplasia; see Fig. 167-17), vagina (vaginal intraepithelial

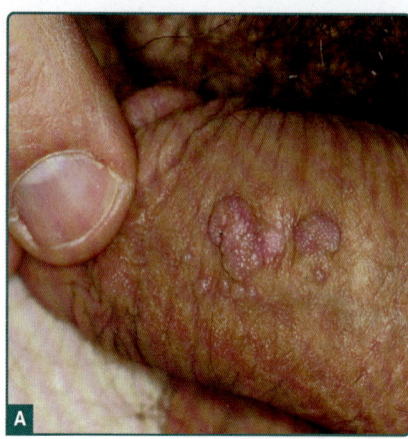
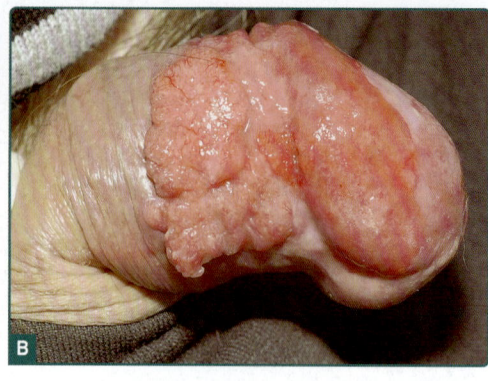
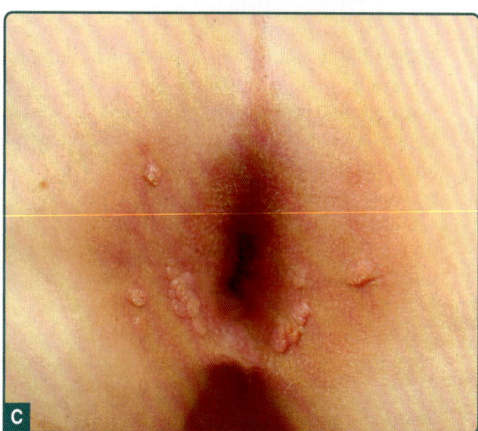
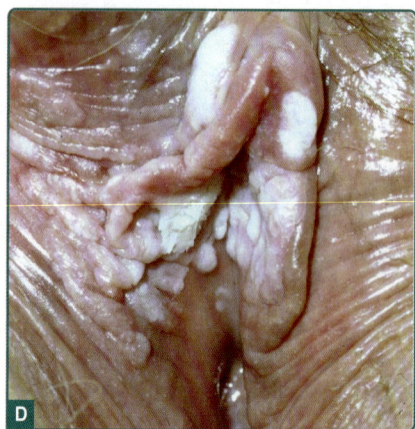

Figure 167-15 Mucosal warts. **A,** Multiple condylomata acuminata on the shaft of the penis. **B,** Erythroplasia of the glans with exophytic squamous cell carcinoma extending onto prepuce. **C,** Multiple perianal condylomata in a child. Sexual abuse must be considered. **D,** Multiple confluent condylomata on the labia minora, majora, and fourchette. (Images **A, C,** Used with permission from Prof. Elliot Androphy. Image **B,** Used with permission from Reinhard Kirnbauer, MD.)

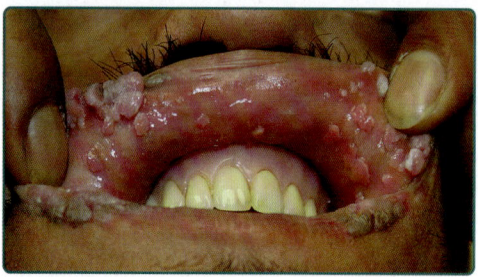

Figure 167-16 Multiple mucosal warts extending to the vermillion border, where they become highly keratinized. (Used with permission from Prof. Elliot Androphy.)

neoplasia), cervix (cervical intraepithelial neoplasia), penis (penile intraepithelial neoplasia), perianal skin, and anal canal (anal intraepithelial neoplasia). The term *Bowenoid papulosis* has been used to describe the disorder, especially when the lesions are pigmented and resemble seborrheic keratosis. AGIN may also present with velvety plaques, white macerated, warty lesions or less distinct erythematous areas.[64]

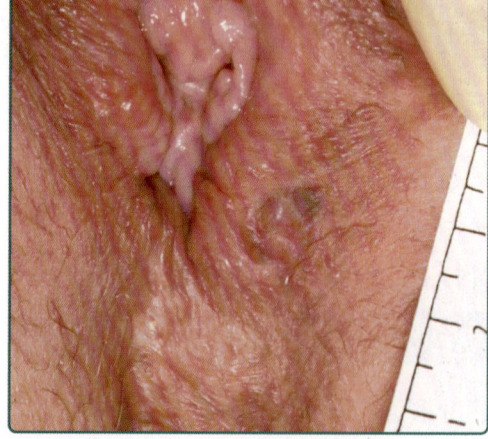

Figure 167-17 Vulval intraepithelial neoplasia, grade III. Small area of raised and minimally pigmented skin near the posterior fourchette.

ETIOLOGY

The high risk HPV types, especially HPV-16, are associated with these disorders.

Biopsy is essential for diagnosis with the histology showing full-thickness epidermal dysplasia, classified as undifferentiated intraepithelial neoplasia. Differentiated intraepithelial neoplasia occurs in association with chronic inflammatory genital disease, such as lichen sclerosus, and histologically is a subtler basal dysplasia, often with acanthosis and hyperkeratosis, and is not associated with HPV infection (see Chap. 64).

CLINICAL COURSE, PROGNOSIS, AND MANAGEMENT

Surgery is the treatment of choice for single lesions if the site is easily operable but may not be best for multifocal or multicentric disease. Laser or topical immunotherapy with imiquimod offers an alternative approach.[65] Both the patient and physician need to be aware of the changes that could indicate malignant change, and these include a persistent area of discomfort, an ulcer, or a frank tumor. It is estimated that an individual with AGIN has an approximate 5% lifetime risk of developing cancer. Cancer can be the presenting feature.

ORAL AND OROPHARYNGEAL SQUAMOUS CELL CARCINOMA

Silent infection with high risk HPVs within the mouth or throat can present later in life with oropharyngeal SCC. The traditional association of this malignancy with smoking and alcohol is being replaced with a stronger association with HPV infection, especially in younger male patients. The incidence of this malignancy is rising but should be reduced following the introduction of the anti-HPV vaccine to male patients.[66]

REFERENCES

1. Johnson KM, Kines RC, Roberts JN, et al. Role of heparan sulfate in attachment to and infection of the murine female genital tract by human papillomavirus. *J Virol.* 2009;83(5):2067-2074.
2. Raff AB, Woodham AW, Raff LM, et al. The evolving field of human papillomavirus receptor research: a review of binding and entry. *J Virol.* 2013;87(11):6062-6072.
3. Doorbar J, Egawa N, Griffin H, et al. Human papillomavirus molecular biology and disease association. *Rev Med Virol.* 2016;25(suppl 1):2-13.
4. Doorbar J. The E4 protein; structure, function and patterns of expression. *Virology.* 2013;445(1-2):80-98.
5. Bernard H-U, Burk RD, Chen Z, et al. Classification of papillomaviruses (PVs) based on 189 PV types and proposal of taxonomic amendments. *Virology.* 2010;401(1):70-79.
6. McLaughlin-Drubin ME, Meyers J, Munger K. Cancer associated human papillomaviruses. *Curr Opin Virol.* 2012;2(4):459-466.
7. van Haalen FM, Bruggink SC, Gusseklo J, et al. Warts in primary schoolchildren: prevalence and relation with environmental factors. *Br J Dermatol.* 2009;161(1):148-152.
8. Bruggink SC, Eekhof JAH, Egberts PF, et al. Natural course of cutaneous warts among primary schoolchildren: a prospective cohort study. *Ann Fam Med.* 2013;11(5):437-441.
9. Padel AF, Venning VA, Evans MF, et al. Human papillomaviruses in anogenital warts in children: typing by in situ hybridisation. *Br Med J.* 1990;300(6738):1491-1494.
10. Strauss S, Sastry P, Sonnex C, et al. Contamination of environmental surfaces by genital human papillomaviruses. *Sex Transm Infect.* 2002;78(2):135-138.
11. Bunney MH. *Viral Warts: Their Biology and Treatment.* Oxford: Oxford University Press; 1982.
12. Tomson N, Sterling J, Ahmed I, et al. Human papillomavirus typing of warts and response to cryotherapy. *J Eur Acad Derm Verereol.* 2010;25(9):1108-1111.
13. Leigh IM, Glover MT. Skin cancer and warts in immunosuppressed renal transplant recipients. *Recent Results Cancer Res.* Vol 139, *Skin Cancer: Basic Science, Clinical Research and Treatment.* Springer-Verlag; Berlin, Heidelberg; 1995:69-86.
14. Rüdlinger R, Smith IW, Bunney MH, et al. Human papillomavirus infections in a group of renal transplant recipients. *Br J Dermatol.* 1986;115(6):681-692.
15. Shamanin V, zur Hausen H, Lavergne D, et al. Human papillomavirus infections in nonmelanoma skin cancers from renal transplant recipients and nonimmunosuppressed patients. *J Natl Cancer Inst.* 1996;88(12):802-811.
16. Boxman IL, Berkhout RJ, Mulder LH, et al. Detection of human papillomavirus DNA in plucked hairs from renal transplant recipients and healthy volunteers. *J Invest Dermatol.* 1997;108(5):712-715.
17. de Villiers EM, Lavergne D, McLaren K, et al. Prevailing papillomavirus types in non-melanoma carcinomas of the skin in renal allograft recipients. *Int J Cancer.* 1997;73(3):356-361.
18. de Koning MN, Struijk L, Bavinck JN, et al. Betapapillomaviruses frequently persist in the skin of healthy individuals. *J Gen Virol.* 2007;88(Pt 5):1489-1495.
19. Kyriakis K, Pagana G, Michailides C, et al. Lifetime prevalence fluctuations of common and plane viral warts. *J Eur Acad Dermatol Venereol.* 2007;21(2):260-262.
20. Egawa K, Kitasato H, Honda Y, et al. Human papillomavirus 57 identified in a plantar epidermoid cyst. *Br J Dermatol.* 1998;138(3):510-514.
21. Williams HC, Pottier A, Strachan D. The descriptive epidemiology of warts in British schoolchildren. *Br J Dermatol.* 1993;128(5):504-511.
22. Sri JC, Dubina MI, Kao GF, et al. Generalized verrucosis: a review of the associated diseases, evaluation, and treatments. *J Am Acad Dermatol.* 2012;66(2):292-311.
23. Laffort C, Le Deist F, Favre M, et al. Severe cutaneous papillomavirus disease after haemopoietic stem cell transplantation in patients with severe combined immune deficiency caused by common γc cytokine receptor subunit or JAK-3 deficiency. *Lancet.* 2004;363(9426):2051-2054.
24. Zinn KH, Belohradsky BH. Wiskott-Aldrich-Syndrom mit Verrucae vulgares. *Hautarzt.* 1977;28(12):664-667.

25. Reid TM, Fraser NG, Kernohan IR. Generalized warts and immune deficiency. *Br J Dermatol*. 1976;95(5):559-564.
26. Barnett N, Mak H, Winkelstein JA. Extensive verrucosis in primary immunodeficiency diseases. *Arch Dermatol*. 1983;119(1):5-7.
27. Stritzler C, Sawitsky A, Stritzler R. Bittner's syndrome. *Arch Dermatol*. 1971;103(5):548-549.
28. Kreuter A, Hochdorfer B, Brockmeyer NH, et al. A human papillomavirus-associated disease with disseminated warts, depressed cell-mediated immunity, primary lymphedema, and anogenital dysplasia: WILD syndrome. *Arch Dermatol*. 2008;144(3):366-372.
29. Hsu AP, Sampaio EP, Khan J, et al. Mutations in GATA2 are associated with the autosomal dominant and sporadic monocytopenia and mycobacterial infection (MonoMAC) syndrome. *Blood*. 2011;118(10):2653-2655.
30. Dorn JM, Patnaik MS, Van Hee M, et al. WILD syndrome is GATA2 deficiency: a novel deletion in the GATA2 gene. *J Allergy Clin Immunol Pract*. 2017;5(4):1149-1152;e1.
31. Chu EY, Freeman AF, Jing H, et al. Cutaneous manifestations of *DOCK8* deficiency syndrome. *Arch Dermatol*. 2012;148(1):79-84.
32. Jorgensen GH, Gardulf A, Sigurdsson MI, et al. Clinical symptoms in adults with selective IgA deficiency: a case-control study. *J Clin Immunol*. 2013;33(4):742-747.
33. Lee SJ, Song HJ, Boo S-J, et al. Primary intestinal lymphangiestasia with generalized warts. *World J Gastrenterol*. 2015;21(27):8467-8472.
34. Stetson CL, Rapini RP, Tyring SK, et al. CD4[+] T lymphocytopenia with disseminated HPV. *J Cutan Pathol*. 2002;29(8):502-505.
35. Fischer LA, Norgaard A, Permin H, et al. Multiple flat warts associated with idiopathic CD4-positive T lymphocytopenia. *J Am Acad Dermatol*. 2008;58(suppl 2):S37-S38.
36. Horev L, Unger S, Molho-Pessach V, et al. Generalized verrucosis and HPV-3 susceptibility associated with CD4 T-cell lymphopenia caused by inherited human interleukin-7 deficiency. *J Am Acad Dermatol*. 2015;72(6):1082-1084.
37. Tarzi MD, Jenner M, Hattotuwa K, et al. Sporadic case of warts, hypogammaglobulinemia, immunodeficiency, and myelokathexis syndrome. *J Allergy Clin Immunol*. 2005;116(5):1101-1105.
38. Mulhem E, Pinelis S. Treatment of nongenital cutaneous warts. *Am Fam Physician*. 2011;84(3):288-293.
39. Kwok CS, Gibbs S, Bennett C, et al. Topical treatments for cutaneous warts. *Cochrane Database Syst Rev*. 2013;9:CD001781.
40. Sterling JC, Gibbs S, Haque Hussain S, et al. British Association of Dermatologists' Guidelines for the management of cutaneous warts 2014. *Br J Dermatol*. 2014;171(4):696-712.
41. Kwok CS, Holland R, Gibbs S. Efficacy of topical treatments for cutaneous warts: a meta-analysis and pooled analysis of randomized controlled trials. *Br J Dermatol*. 2011;165(2):233-246.
42. Patel T, Morrison K, Rady P, et al. Epidermodysplasia verruciformis and susceptibility to HPV. *Dis Mark*. 2010;29(3-4):199-206.
43. Rogers HD, Macgregor JL, Nord KM, et al. Acquired epidermodysplasia verruciformis. *J Am Acad Dermatol*. 2009;60(2):315-320.
44. Zampetti A, Giurdanella F, Manco S, et al. Acquired epidermodysplasia verruciformis: a comprehensive review and a proposal for treatment. *Dermatol Surg*. 2013;39(7):974-980.
45. Ramoz N, Rueda LA, Bouadjar B, et al. Mutations in two adjacent novel genes are associated with epidermodysplasia verruciformis. *Nat Genet*. 2002;32(4):579-581.
46. Dell'Oste V, Azzimonti B, De Andrea M, et al. High β-HPV DNA loads and strong seroreactivity are present in epidermodysplasia verruciformis. *J Invest Dermatol*. 2009;129(4):1026-1034.
47. Berthelot C, Dickerson MC, Rady P, et al. Treatment of a patient with epidermodysplasia verruciformis carrying a novel EVER2 mutation with imiquimod. *J Am Acad Dermatol*. 2007;56(5):882-886.
48. Janssen K, Lucker GP, Houwing RH, et al. Epidermodysplasia verruciformis: unsuccessful therapeutic approach with imiquimod. *Int J Dermatol*. 2007;46(suppl 3):45-47.
49. Karrer S, Szeimies R, Abels C, et al. Epidermodysplasia verruciformis treated using topical 5-aminolaevulinic acid photodynamic therapy. *Br J Dermatol*. 1999;140(5):935-938.
50. Nijhawan RI, Osei-Tutu A, Hugh JM. Sustained clinical resolution of acquired epidermodysplasia verruciformis in an immunocompromised patient after discontinuation of oral acitretin with topical imiquimod. *J Drugs Dermatol*. 2013;12(3):348-349.
51. Riddell C, Rashid R, Thomas V. Ungual and periungual human papillomavirus-associated squamous cell carcinoma: a review. *J Am Acad Dermatol*. 2011;64(6):1147-1153.
52. Schwartz RA. Verrucous carcinoma of the skin and mucosa. *J Am Acad Dermatol*. 1995;32(1):1-21.
53. del Pino M, Bleeker MC, Quint WG, et al. Comprehensive analysis of human papillomavirus prevalence and the potential role of low-risk types in verrucous carcinoma. *Mod Pathol*. 2012;25(10):1354-1363.
54. Quint KD, Genders RE, de Koning MNC, et al. Human *beta-papillomavirus* infection and keratinocyte carcinomas. *J Pathol*. 2015;235(2):342-354.
55. Staples CG, Henderson H, Tsongalis GJ. Condylomata of the pannus in 3 obese patients: a new location for a common disease. *Arch Dermatol*. 2012;146(5):572-574.
56. Park IU, Introcaso C, Dunne EF. Human papillomavirus and genital warts: a review of the evidence for the 2015 Centers for Disease Control and Prevention Sexually Transmitted Diseases Treatment Guidelines. *Clin Infect Dis*. 2015;61(suppl 8):S849-S855.
57. Werner RN, Westfechtel L, Dressler C, et al. Self-administered interventions for anogenital warts in immunocompetent patients: a systematic review and meta-analysis. *Sex Transm Infect*. 2017;93(3):155-161.
58. Moore RA, Edwards JE, Hopwood J, et al. Imiquimod for the treatment of genital warts: a quantitative systematic review. *BMC Infect Dis*. 2001;1:3.
59. Scheinfeld N. Update on the treatment of genital warts. *Dermatol Online J*. 2013;19(6):18559.
60. Stockfleth E, Meyer T. Sinecatechins (Polyphenon E) ointment for treatment of external genital warts and possible future indications. *Expert Opin Biol Ther*. 2014;14(7):1033-1043.
61. Ali H, Donovan B, Wand H, et al. Genital warts in young Australians five years into national human papillomavirus vaccination programme: national surveillance data. *Br Med J*. 2013;346:f2032.
62. Markowitz LE, Hariri S, Lin C, et al. Reduction in human papillomavirus (HPV) prevalence among young women following HPV vaccine introduction in the United States, National Health and Nutrition Examination Surveys, 2003-2010. *J Infect Dis*.

63. Shiboski CH, Lee A, Chen H, et al. Human papillomavirus infection in the oral cavity of HIV patients is not reduced by initiating antiretroviral therapy. *AIDS.* 2016;30(10):1573-1582.
64. Cararach M, Dexeus D. Preinvasive lesions of the vulva. *CME J Gynecol Oncol.* 2007;12:1466-1473.
65. van Seters M, van Beurden M, ten Kate FJ, et al. Treatment of vulvar intraepithelial neoplasia with topical imiquimod. *N Engl J Med.* 2008;358(14):1465-1473.
66. Gooi Z, Chan JY, Fakhry C. The epidemiology of the human papillomavirus related to oropharyngeal head and neck cancer. *Laryngoscope.* 2016;126(4):894-900.

Chapter 168 :: Cutaneous Manifestations of HIV and Human T-Lymphotropic Virus
:: Adam D. Lipworth, Esther E. Freeman, & Arturo P. Saavedra

第一百六十八章
HIV和人类嗜T细胞病毒感染的皮肤表现

中文导读

本章共分为2节：①HIV感染黏膜和皮肤表现；②人类嗜T细胞病毒感染黏膜和皮肤表现。第一节分为HIV感染概述、HIV感染的药物相互作用、HIV感染的黏膜表现、HIV皮肤恶性肿瘤、HIV的皮肤和黏膜炎症相关疾病及免疫重建炎症综合征。分别介绍了这些疾病的流行病学、临床特征、危险因素、病因和发病机制、诊断、鉴别诊断、临床病程和预后及临床管理。

第一节介绍了HIV感染黏膜及其皮肤表现。首先指出，现在HIV感染在全世界范围内仍未得到控制，随着HIV感染者生存期延长，感染者会出现各种并发症，然而每年有超过3000万人因接受抗逆转录病毒治疗（ART）受益，HIV感染相关诊断在全世界范围内具有重要意义。

在HIV感染的过程中，由于后天免疫缺陷或治疗，几乎每个病人都有皮肤损害。而且，据估计，在未经治疗的HIV患者中，药物不良反应出疹的发生率比一般人群高出100倍，而且可能随着免疫缺陷进展而进一步上升。麻疹样爆发是目前最常见的表现，约占75%至95%的病例。荨麻疹、多形性红斑、苔藓样疹、血管炎和固定药疹也有报道。

在HIV感染晚期，严重的免疫抑制使患者容易受到机会性感染。即使在免疫重建后，HIV患者仍然比血清阴性的个体患各种皮肤感染的风险更高（如葡萄球菌脓皮病、带状疱疹再激活以及各种人乳头瘤病毒感染等）。本章详细介绍了晚期HIV/AIDS的黏膜皮肤感染，以及那些在稳定HIV疾病中具有独特特征的感染。

HIV相关的皮肤恶性肿瘤列举了卡波西肉瘤、人乳头瘤病毒引起的异常增生和鳞状细胞癌、HIV的皮肤淋巴瘤和其他非角化细胞癌。其中肛门HPV感染在感染HIV患者中更为普遍，相比之下感染HIV的女性除了患肛门癌风险更高，浸润性宫颈癌的风险也有所增加。HIV相关淋巴瘤的发病率通常与免疫抑制的程度相关。

HIV的皮肤和黏膜炎症相关疾病列举了银屑病、脂溢性皮炎、瘙痒性丘疹性皮炎和嗜酸性毛囊炎。银屑病和HIV感染的联系尚存在争议；研究者观察到在HIV患者中，脂溢性皮炎的患病率可高达83%，而且随着免疫抑制的恶化患病率和严重程度往往会增加；瘙痒性丘疹性皮炎（PPE）是一种常见的HIV相关皮肤病，成人和儿童的患病率可能高达46%和42%。

随着HIV免疫功能的恢复，以前未被识别或耐受的抗原可能引发强烈的免疫反应，这种反应被称为免疫重建炎症综合征（IRIS），在接受抗逆转录病毒治疗的患者中出现率甚至高达20%。这种综合征大多数是自限性的，以对症支持治疗为主。

第二节介绍了人类发现的第一个逆转录病毒嗜T细胞病毒感染的黏膜和皮肤表现，这种病无法治愈，而且长期复发预后非常差。提倡通过阻断其母婴、性接触、血液和静脉注射药物及器官移植传播途径予以预防。

〔张江林〕

MUCOCUTANEOUS MANIFESTATIONS OF HIV

AT-A-GLANCE

- HIV is a retrovirus that causes immune suppression and dysregulation primarily via depletion of CD4+ lymphocytes and CD4+ cells of monocytic lineage.
- In spite of better screening programs, availability of antiretroviral therapy (ART), and improved side-effect profiles, new infections continue to be documented.
- The range of dermatologic complications seen in HIV/AIDS relates to the evolving immunologic state of the patient, specific viral characteristics of the serotype causing infection, the period of time from infection to dermatologic complication, and the length of antiretroviral treatment.
- Acute HIV infection presents as a mononucleosis-like syndrome that can include a morbilliform exanthem 3 to 6 weeks after infection with HIV.
- In resource-limited areas, untreated infection may lead to progressive dermatologic disease.
- In reconstituted individuals and long-term viral suppression, sun-induced neoplasia and viral-induced neoplasia are significant burdens.

AN OVERVIEW OF HIV INFECTION

According to the World Health Organization (WHO), by the end of 2015, 36.7 million people worldwide were living with the HIV, lymphotropic human retrovirus. Approximately 2.1 million of those were newly diagnosed that year, and approximately 1.1 million died from complications of AIDS. CD4 count parameters that serve as guidelines for the initiation of treatment have increased from less than 200 cells/μL in 2003 to 500 cells/μL in 2011. As of 2015, all newly diagnosed HIV patients are candidates for antiretroviral therapy (ART); upwards of 30 million people will be eligible for treatment.[1] Nevertheless, infections continue to occur both locally and abroad despite prevention programs and newly developed recommendations from the Centers for Disease Control and Prevention for optout screening in all health care settings in the absence of written consent for screening.[2] These figures suggest that whereas progress has been made, a significant number of infections continue to occur, and the burden of disease will continue to exist as infected individuals live longer. Consequently, identification of HIV infection-associated diagnoses is relevant in both resource-limited settings and in resource-abundant zones. The field of HIV medicine continues to rapidly evolve, and excellent internet resources that are frequently updated include the U.S. Department of Health and Human Services' AIDS*info* (https://aidsinfo.nih.gov) and the Centers for Disease Control and Prevention's National Prevention Information Network (https://npin.cdc.gov/).

ETIOLOGY AND PATHOGENESIS

HIV is predominantly transmitted through sexual contact. Other important means of transmission include exposure to infected blood (including needles shared by injecting drug users and "skin popping") and transmission from an infected mother to her fetus during pregnancy, delivery, or breastfeeding. HIV-1 is the most common cause of HIV infection globally, while HIV-2 infection has been detected mainly in West Africa. Although both HIV subtypes cause clinically similar disease, HIV-2 is associated with slower progression of immunosuppression, decreased infectivity, and resistance to nonnucleoside reverse transcriptase inhibitors.[3]

The profound immunosuppression that defines HIV disease results from progressive depletion of CD4+ T lymphocytes. Efficient infection of a target cell by HIV requires not only expression of a CD4 molecule on that cell's surface, but also the presence of a coreceptor (such as chemokine receptor 5 [CCR5] or chemokine-related receptor 4 [CXCR4]). Although HIV infects primarily CD4+ T lymphocytes and CD4+ cells of monocytic lineage, any cell that expresses CD4 and an appropriate coreceptor may be infected by HIV.[4]

CLINICAL FEATURES

Cutaneous disorders occur in nearly every patient during the course of HIV disease, either as a result of acquired immunodeficiency or from treatment. HIV disease is a continuum that progresses from primary infection to death via a sequence of opportunistic infections and neoplasms that mark the gradual deterioration of the immune system. *Acute HIV infection* or *acute retroviral syndrome* presents approximately 3 to 6 weeks following primary infection, with the majority of individuals developing an acute mononucleosis-like syndrome. Clinical manifestations include fever, lethargy, rash, myalgia/arthralgia, cervical and axillary lymphadenopathy, pharyngitis, mucosal ulcers, night sweats, nausea/vomiting/diarrhea, weight loss, and laboratory abnormalities including leukopenia, thrombocytopenia, and transaminitis.[5] The rash typically manifests as asymptomatic macules and papules on the face and upper trunk, although the eruption may be more diffuse and pruritic.[6] Urticaria and pustules also have been reported.[6,7] Symptoms generally last an average of 2 to 3 weeks and resolve gradually as levels of plasma viremia decrease. The presentation of acute retroviral syndrome provides a valuable opportunity for early diagnosis of HIV disease, during a particularly critical time when levels of viremia, and therefore the degree of infectivity, are at extremely high levels.[8]

Unfortunately, this diagnostic opportunity may be missed if clinical suspicion is not sufficiently high; recent estimates place the proportion of HIV patients in the United States who are currently undiagnosed at 14%,[9] and the diagnosis is often missed despite the suggestive symptoms of acute retroviral syndrome,[10] in part because the protean manifestations are easily mistaken for other infections such as Epstein-Barr virus.[11] Even when acute HIV infection is suspected, the diagnosis can be missed because patients may present prior to seroconversion, resulting in false-negative HIV antibody tests. When acute HIV infection is considered, clinicians should perform more sensitive direct tests for HIV viral RNA or for the p24 core structural protein (see section "Diagnosis").[5,10]

Individuals who have access to combination ART have a markedly altered course of disease if immune restoration is successfully achieved. In most cases, there is a marked reduction in the incidence of opportunistic infections, but certain neoplasms, particularly those induced by sun exposure or arising as a result of virus-induced dysplasia, now amount to a significant dermatologic burden. Globally, however, the majority of HIV-infected individuals lack access to ART and, consequently, many of the cutaneous manifestations associated with HIV disease become chronic and progressive.

TABLE 168-1
Correlation of Mucocutaneous Manifestations of HIV Infection with CD4 T-Cell Counts

CD4 T-CELL COUNT >500 CELLS/µL	CD4 T-CELL COUNT 250–500 CELLS/µL	CD4 T-CELL COUNT <200 CELLS/µL
Acute retroviral syndrome	Dermatophyte infections, recurrent or persistent	Bacillary angiomatosis
Herpes zoster infection (nondisseminated)	Oral candidiasis	Hyperkeratotic scabies
Seborrheic dermatitis	Oral hairy leukoplakia Herpes zoster infection, disseminated	Cutaneous military tuberculosis Eosinophilic folliculitis Herpes simplex virus infection (>1 month's duration) Idiopathic pruritus Invasive fungal infections Kaposi sarcoma Molluscum contagiosum, large facial lesions Papular pruritic eruption of HIV

"window period." However, core structural protein p24 antigen may be detected several weeks prior to seroconversion. The viral-RNA assay detects infection up to 5 days earlier than the p24 assay, and appears to be more sensitive.[12]

AIDS is now designated by the Centers for Disease Control and Prevention as HIV stage 3. In this new staging system, an HIV-seropositive individual older than 6 years of age with a CD4+ T-cell count <200 cells/µL, a CD4+ T-cell percentage <14%, or with any of several diseases considered to be indicative of a severe defect in cell-mediated immunity is considered to have AIDS.[14] Table 168-2 lists the conditions deemed to be AIDS-defining in a patient with a confirmed HIV infection.

DIAGNOSIS

Studies have documented that in the past, up to 25% of those with HIV infection were not tested, despite suggestive symptoms.[12] In fact, 2% of individuals thought to have Epstein-Barr virus were found to have HIV when tested retrospectively in one study, and approximately half of those had acute primary HIV infection.[13] The laboratory diagnosis of HIV-1 infection is typically made by either identification of antibodies to HIV or direct detection of HIV antigens or nucleic acids (Table 168-1). A delay of 3 to 4 weeks typically occurs between newly acquired HIV-1 infection and development of antibodies, which is referred to as the

CLINICAL COURSE, PROGNOSIS, AND MANAGEMENT

The length of time between initial infection and the development of symptomatic disease varies significantly. This period of clinical latency does not necessarily imply disease latency. Viral replication may persist, and CD4+ T-cell levels progressively decline. Thus, between 2013 and 2015, after the completion of 3 randomized controlled trials, guidelines recommended therapy with ART upon diagnosis regardless of CD4 count.[15] The more severe and life-threatening complications of HIV disease typically occur when

TABLE 168-2
AIDS (HIV Stage 3)—Defining Illnesses

- Candidiasis of bronchi, trachea, or lungs
- Candidiasis of esophagus
- Cervical cancer, invasive
- Coccidioidomycosis, disseminated or extrapulmonary
- Cryptococcosis, extrapulmonary
- Cryptosporidiosis, chronic intestinal (>1 month's duration)
- Cytomegalovirus disease (other than liver, spleen, or nodes), onset at age >1 month
- Cytomegalovirus retinitis (with loss of vision)
- Encephalopathy attributed to HIV
- Herpes simplex: chronic ulcers (>1 month's duration) or bronchitis, pneumonitis, or esophagitis (onset at age >1 month)
- Histoplasmosis, disseminated or extrapulmonary
- Isosporiasis, chronic intestinal (>1 month's duration)
- Kaposi sarcoma
- Lymphoma, Burkitt (or equivalent term) or immunoblastic (or equivalent term)
- Lymphoma, primary, of brain
- *Mycobacterium avium* complex or *Mycobacterium kansasii*, disseminated or extrapulmonary
- *Mycobacterium tuberculosis* of any site, pulmonary, disseminated, or extrapulmonary
- *Mycobacterium*, other species or unidentified species, disseminated or extrapulmonary
- *Pneumocystis jirovecii* (previously known as *Pneumocystis carinii*) pneumonia
- Pneumonia, recurrent
- Progressive multifocal leukoencephalopathy
- *Salmonella* septicemia, recurrent
- Toxoplasmosis of brain, onset at age >1 month
- Wasting syndrome attributed to HIV

Adapted from Centers for Disease Control and Prevention (CDC). Appendix A: AIDS-defining conditions. *MMWR Recomm Rep.* 2008;57 (RR-10):9. Available at https://www.cdc.gov/mmwr/preview/mmwrhtml/rr5710a2.htm.

CD4+ T-cell counts fall below 200 cells/μL. As a consequence of accessibility to ART, patients with HIV are living longer. As a result, dermatologic complications from long-term well-controlled HIV disease, such as virus-induced and sun-induced neoplasias, are now increasingly recognized.

MEDICATIONS AND MEDICATION-RELATED EFFECTS IN THE SETTING OF HIV

AT-A-GLANCE

- There is nearly a 100-fold increase in adverse cutaneous drug reactions in the setting of HIV/AIDS.
- Sulfonamides and penicillins are common causes of these reactions.

- Antiretroviral medications themselves also frequently cause adverse reactions, including morbilliform, urticarial, retinoid-like, vasculitic or bullous eruptions. Chronically, they may cause alopecia, hirsutism, dyspigmentation, and lipodystrophy/lipoatrophy.
- Treatment includes supportive care, cessation of the etiologic agent when necessary, topical and oral corticosteroid use, and, less commonly, advanced immunosuppressants.

The incidence of adverse cutaneous drug eruptions is estimated to be as much as 100 times higher in individuals with untreated HIV disease than in the general population, and may rise further with advancing immunodeficiency.[16] Adverse reactions can complicate upwards of 20% of prescriptions. Sulfonamide drugs and penicillins are common causative agents of cutaneous drug eruptions, accounting for 75% of cases in one study.[17] Of note, individuals that are sulfa-allergic are at increased risk of more-severe reactions to sulfa drugs in the setting of immune reconstitution. Given the high incidence of sulfa-induced reactions, it is important to note that darunavir, tipranavir, amprenavir (no longer marketed in the United States), and fosamprenavir contain sulfa moieties. Drug reactions may present in the setting of immune restoration, and in the midst of immune reconstitution inflammatory syndrome (IRIS). In such cases, drug reactions are likely to be more severe than at other points in the HIV disease course.[17]

Drug interactions should also be considered when patients with HIV are treated for other dermatologic concerns. For instance, reports exist documenting iatrogenic Cushing syndrome in patients treated with topical, intranasal, and intramuscular steroids as a result of ritonavir-induced and atazanavir-induced inhibition of cytochrome P450.[18,19] (Refer to Table 168-3 for the various classes of ARTs and their most significant dermatologic manifestations.)

CLINICAL FEATURES

Morbilliform eruptions are by far the most common manifestation, accounting for approximately 75% to 95% of cases.[20] Urticaria, erythema multiforme (major and minor), lichenoid eruption, vasculitis, and fixed drug eruption are also reported. Approximately 20% of cases are associated with systemic symptoms, such as fever, headache, myalgia, and arthralgia.[17] In patients who are positive for HLA-B5701, drug reaction with eosinophilia and systemic syndrome may develop in patients treated with abacavir. Cardiovascular collapse has been reported in these cases. Severe bullous eruptions and desquamatory reactions appear to be more common in HIV disease (Fig. 168-1). In one study, the incidence of toxic epidermal necrolysis (TEN) in HIV-infected individuals was found to be 375 times greater than that in the general population.[21]

TABLE 168-3
Adverse Effects of Antiretroviral Drugs

DRUGS	SYSTEMIC SIDE EFFECTS	DERMATOLOGIC SIDE EFFECTS
Nucleoside Reverse Transcription Inhibitors (NRTIs)		
Abacavir (ABC) Didanosine (ddI) Emtricitabine (FTC) Lamivudine (3TC) Stavudine (d4T) Tenofovir (TDF) Tenofovir alafenamide fumarate (TAF) Zidovudine (AZT) Zalcitabine (ddC)*	Pancreatitis, peripheral neuropathy, lactic acidosis and hepatotoxicity (didanosine, stavudine, zalcitabine) Hepatotoxicity (emtricitabine, lamivudine) Renal toxicity (tenofovir) Anemia, granulocytopenia, myopathy, lactic acidosis, hepatotoxicity, and nausea (zidovudine) Oropharyngeal and esophageal ulcerations (zalcitabine)	Hypersensitivity, with rare instances of Stevens-Johnson syndrome/toxic epidermal necrolysis (SJS/TEN) Systemic hypersensitivity reactions in up to 8% of patients is associated with HLA-B5701/HLA-DR7/HLA-DQ3; incidence reduced by prescreening for HLA-B5701 (abacavir) Leukocytoclastic vasculitis (didanosine) Hyperpigmentation of the nail bed, palms, and soles (emtricitabine) Hyperpigmentation of the nails (including multiple longitudinal and transverse bands), diffuse hyperpigmentation of the skin and oral mucosa, leukocytoclastic vasculitis, and hypertrichosis (zidovudine) Lipohypotrophy with (stavudine, zidovudine) Paronychia with nailfold pyogenic granuloma (lamivudine, zidovudine)
Nonnucleoside Reverse Transcription Inhibitors (NNRTIs)		
Delavirdine Efavirenz Etravirine Nevirapine Rilpivirine	Hepatotoxicity (all) Depression and mood changes (efavirenz, rilpivirine)	Hypersensitivity reactions are common within the first 6 weeks of therapy, with rare progression to systemic hypersensitivity or SJS/TEN (highest incidence with nevirapine) Lipodystrophies with rilpivirine
Protease Inhibitors (PIs)[a]		
Amprenavir[b] Atazanavir Darunavir Fosamprenavir Indinavir Lopinavir Nelfinavir Ritonavir Saquinavir Tipranavir	Nausea, vomiting, diarrhea, headaches, lipid anomalies, and hyperglycemia PR prolongation and hyperbilirubinemia (atazanavir) Hepatotoxicity and intracranial hemorrhage (tipranavir) Nephrolithiasis and hyperbilirubinemia (indinavir) Ritonavir may affect levels of many other medications, including saquinavir and intralesional steroids (leading to the development of Cushing syndrome)[c]	Hypersensitivity reactions with rare progression to SJS (amprenavir, fosamprenavir, tipranavir) Acute exanthematous pustulosis Lipohypertrophy (indinavir) Dose-dependent retinoid-like effects (xerosis, cheilitis, alopecia, lateral nailfold pyogenic granuloma, curly hair, and recurrent paronychia), acute porphyria, "frozen shoulder," and venous thrombosis (indinavir) Spontaneous bleeding and hematomas (ritonavir) Rare cases of fixed drug eruptions (saquinavir) Darunavir, tipranavir, fosamprenavir, and amprenavir contain sulfa moieties and should be used with caution in sulfa-allergic patients
Fusion Inhibitors		
Enfuvirtide	Increased frequency of bacterial pneumonia	Systemic hypersensitivity reactions in <1% of patients Injection-site reactions in up to 98% of patients, requiring discontinuation in only 3%
Integrase Inhibitors		
Raltegravir Dolutegravir Elvitegravir	Well tolerated: nausea, diarrhea, headache, insomnia Hepatotoxicity	Pruritus Rare cases of skin hypersensitivity (dolutegravir)
Chemokine Receptor 5 (CCR5) Antagonist		
Maraviroc	Hepatotoxicity, nasopharyngitis, cough, abdominal pain, dizziness, musculoskeletal symptoms	

[a]Simeprevir, boceprevir, and ombitasvir/paritaprevir/dasabuvir are not included in this table even though they are protease inhibitors with activity against HIV because they are U.S. Food and Drug Administration–approved only for treatment of hepatitis C.

[b]Denotes that this medication is no longer marketed or has been discontinued by the manufacturer. Please note that in the case of amprenavir, a prodrug (fosamprenavir) is available.

[c]Cobicistat, a pharmacokinetic enhancer ("boosting agent") is used for its ability to increase the blood levels of agents such as atazanavir and darunavir. It does not have antiviral activity against HIV. Because this agent inhibits cytochrome P450, the risk of Cushing syndrome exists when corticosteroids are used concurrently.

Retinoid-like effects such as cheilitis, paronychia, and eruption of pyogenic granuloma are seen with some nucleoside reverse transcriptase inhibitors and protease inhibitors (Fig. 168-2). These effects are generally dose-dependent and can be managed if alternative regimens are not the best option for an individual patient. Other dermatologic manifestations that are specific to individual antiretroviral medications

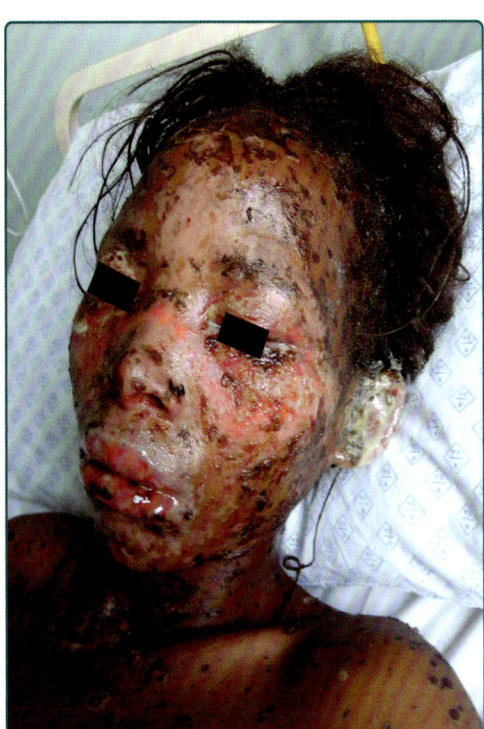

Figure 168-1 Toxic epidermal necrolysis in an HIV-infected patient. (Used with permission from Dr. Anisa Mosam.)

include melanonychia (zidovudine), leukocytoclastic vasculitis (didanosine), and infection-site reactions (enfuvirtide) (see Table 168-3).

The lipodystrophy syndrome and its accompanying metabolic syndrome warrants specific mention (see Chap. 74). HIV-related lipodystrophy is characterized by abnormal fat distribution, which may include lipohypertrophy, lipoatrophy, or both. It generally arises from ART, but HIV infection itself may also cause lipodystrophy.[22] Lipohypertrophy is most commonly associated with protease inhibitor therapy, while lipoatrophy is frequently associated with nuclease reverse transcription inhibitors, particularly the thymidine analogs stavudine and zidovudine. Lipohypertrophy presents with central obesity, cushingoid habitus ("buffalo hump"), increased neck girth, increased abdominal girth from intraabdominal fat ("protease pouch" or "crix belly"), and breast enlargement (Fig. 168-3A). Lipoatrophy most commonly presents with flattening of convex contours of the face (Fig. 168-3B). Abnormal fat distribution is often accompanied by metabolic abnormalities, such as fasting glucose levels, fasting insulin levels, hypertriglyceridemia, hypercholesterolemia, and decreased high-density lipoprotein.

ETIOLOGY AND PATHOGENESIS

Factors associated with increased risk of drug eruptions include female gender, peripheral CD4+ T-cell count <200 cells/μL, CD8+ T-cell count >460 cells/μL, and a history of drug eruptions in the past.[23] Recently, the role of skin-directed lymphocytes has been studied as the skin-directed lymphocytes relate to the pathogenesis of TEN. In HIV-infected individuals, a relative decrease in tissue-specific CD4+ cells, with decreased CD4+/CD8+ ratio was noted in comparison to uninfected hosts. Specifically, a decrease in dermal CD3+ CD4+ CD25+ (and FoxP3+) regulatory T cells was noted, suggesting a role for regulatory T cells in prevention of adverse cutaneous drug reactions.[24]

DIAGNOSIS

Diagnosis of adverse cutaneous drug reactions remains largely clinical, and is often a diagnosis of exclusion. The most significant consideration is whether the correct culprit has been identified, understanding that some reactions can occur even 2 weeks after drug discontinuation. HIV-infection may itself lead to new-onset hypersensitivity to medications not previously noted by the patient. Identification of culprit medications prevents repeat exposures and is a determinant of morbidity, most notably in the case of Stevens-Johnson syndrome/TEN where drugs with longer half-life, such as nevirapine, have been correlated to more severe disease and duration.[25] Individuals commencing therapy with abacavir are now frequently prescreened for HLA-B5701 and other HLA subtypes to prevent hypersensitivity reactions. Significant controversy exists in the literature regarding the value of peripheral eosinophilia in evaluating drug reactions, and its absence does not exclude the diagnosis.[26]

DIFFERENTIAL DIAGNOSIS

The most difficult entity to exclude when a patient presents with a morbilliform exanthem is viral infection. Often, drug-induced vasculitis is difficult to differentiate from other causes of leukocytoclastic vasculitis, including infection, autoimmune disorders, and HIV itself, or from idiopathic subtypes.

CLINICAL COURSE, PROGNOSIS, AND MANAGEMENT

In the absence of mucosal involvement and systemic symptoms, a causative medication may often be continued with close clinical monitoring. However, if early symptoms of urticaria/angioedema or Stevens-Johnson syndrome/TEN are present, the drug should be immediately discontinued.

Short-term corticosteroid therapy appears to be safe in most HIV-infected individuals.[23] Desensitization is an option for individuals with a history of uncomplicated cutaneous drug eruptions.[27] The management of Stevens-Johnson syndrome and TEN remain controversial. Supportive care should be initiated in a supervised setting where hydration, followup of electrolyte abnormalities, wound care, and early recognition of infection can be delivered. Treatment with IV immunoglobulin, cyclosporine, and anti–tumor necrosis

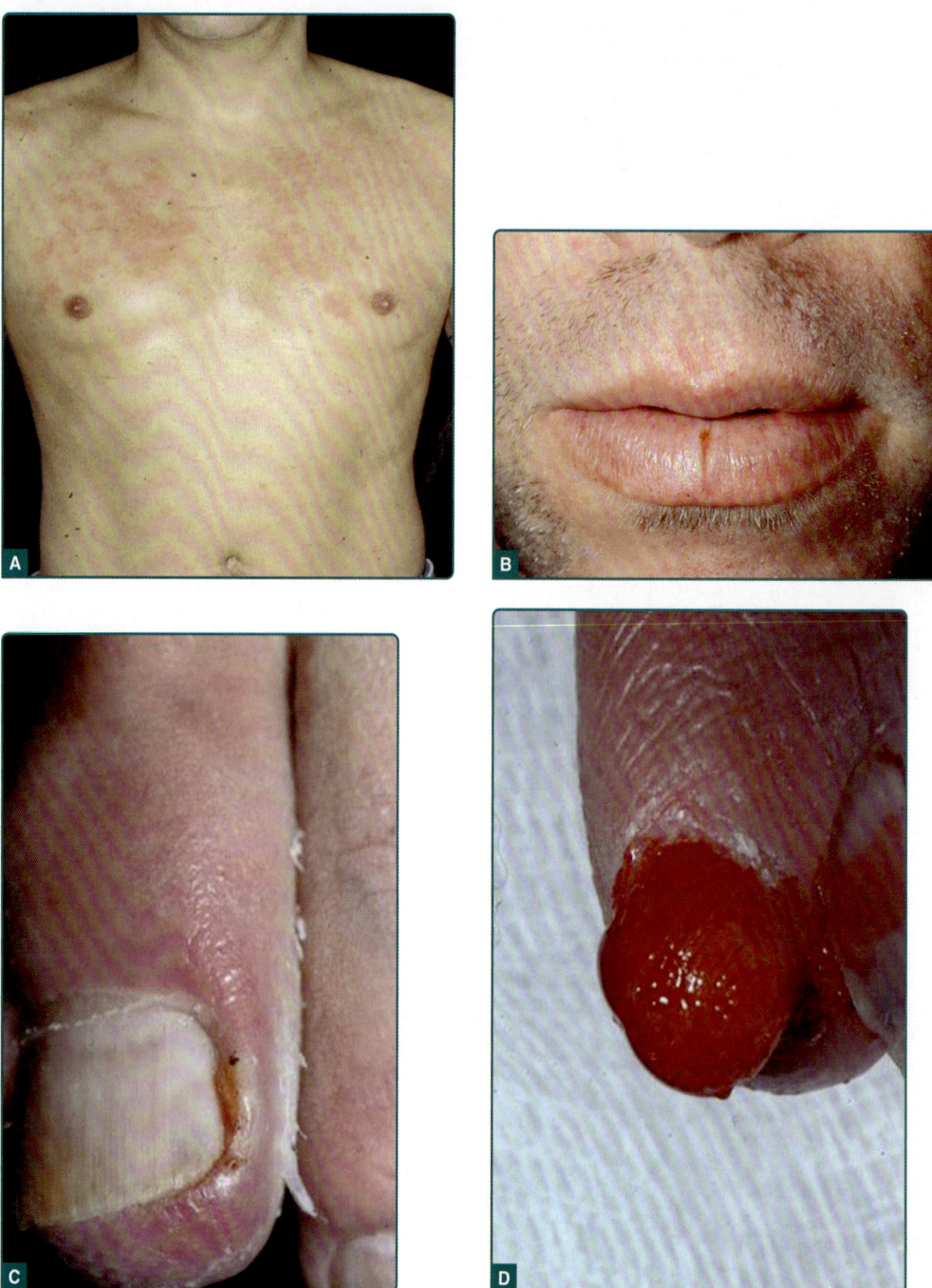

Figure 168-2 Retinoid-like effects in a patient with HIV disease treated with indinavir. **A,** Eczematous dermatitis superimposed on severe asteatosis; **B,** cheilitis; **C,** paronychia; **D,** pyogenic granuloma. Pruritus and scalp defluvium are also commonly seen.

agents, among others has been reported, but large-scale, definitive trials are lacking.[28]

Management of lipodystrophy remains challenging. Substitution of ART regimens containing stavudine and zidovudine are of partial benefit for lipoatrophy.[29] Although switching individuals to nuclease reverse transcription inhibitor–sparing regimens have produced modest results in lipoatrophy, the improvement in fat distribution may come at the expense of lipid anomalies if patients are switched to protease inhibitors.[30] Facial lipoatrophy has been treated with soft-tissue fillers, such as poly-L-lactic acid or calcium hydroxylapatite, with varying degrees of success.[31] Liposuction has been used to treat the dorsocervical lipomatosis, but results are often unsatisfactory.

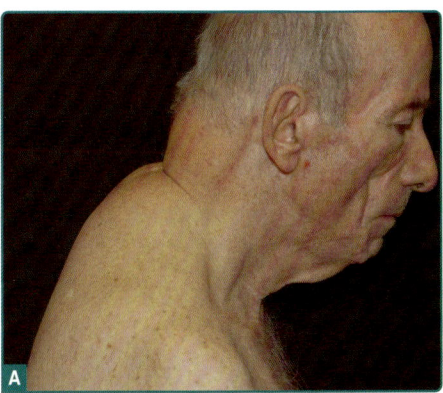

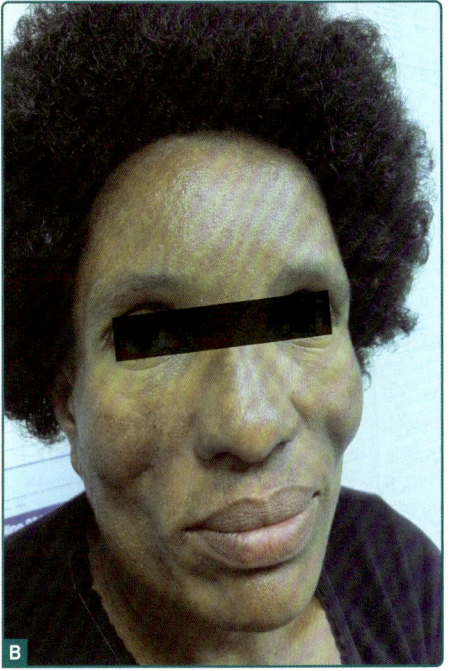

Figure 168-3 Antiretroviral therapy–induced lipodystrophy. **A**, Protease inhibitor–induced lipodystrophy; **B**, facial lipoatrophy. (Used with permission from Dr. Anisa Mosam.)

MUCOCUTANEOUS INFECTIONS IN HIV DISEASE

AT-A-GLANCE

- HIV patients are at elevated risk for a wide variety of infections, many of which affect the skin and mucous membranes. Coinfecting pathogens often interact with HIV in complex and potentially symbiotic ways that alter the course of both diseases.

- In well-controlled HIV with normal CD4+ T-cell counts, patients remain at risk for several specific persistent or newly acquired infections, such as staphylococcal pyodermas, herpes simplex and herpes zoster reactivation, syphilis, and a variety of human papillomavirus–related diseases.

- In advanced HIV disease, severe immunocompromise predisposes patients to opportunistic infections, often with high morbidity and potentially high mortality. Opportunistic infections include oral hairy leukoplakia, bacillary angiomatosis, cutaneous miliary tuberculosis, and invasive mycoses.

- AIDS patients are also at risk for infection with more typical human pathogens, but with unusually severe or atypical presentations, including severe dermatophytoses, giant molluscum contagiosum, crusted scabies, and atypical leishmaniasis.

- AIDS-defining infections should raise suspicion for HIV in patients whose HIV status is unknown.

In advanced HIV disease, the profoundly immunosuppressed state predisposes patients to opportunistic infections from organisms that are rarely pathogenic to immunocompetent individuals. Even after immune reconstitution, HIV patients remain at higher risk than seronegative individuals for a variety of cutaneous infections, such as staphylococcal pyodermas, herpes zoster reactivation, and various human papillomavirus (HPV)-related diseases. This section examines the mucocutaneous infections of advanced HIV/AIDS and then those infections with unique features in stable HIV disease. It focuses on those features of each infection that are specific to HIV disease, as general characteristics are presented elsewhere in this text. Nearly all of the infections presented can flare or manifest as part of the IRIS, discussed later in this chapter (see section "Immune Reconstitution Inflammatory Syndrome").

INFECTIONS IN ADVANCED HIV DISEASE (OPPORTUNISTIC INFECTIONS)

With the rise in access to effective ART, highly morbid opportunistic infections are becoming increasingly rare, but they remain quite common in the developing world. In developed countries, they pose outsized diagnostic and therapeutic challenges, because clinical familiarity with AIDS-associated infections has declined in step with their incidence.

Oral Hairy Leukoplakia and Other Epstein-Barr Virus–Related Disease: Chapter 163 discusses viral diseases like oral hairy leukoplakia in greater detail.

Oral hairy leukoplakia is a benign Epstein-Barr virus infection of oral mucosal epithelium in immunosuppressed patients. Clinically, oral hairy leukoplakia presents on one or both lateral aspects of the tongue with asymptomatic, corrugated white plaques that cannot be removed by scraping with a tongue depressor.[32] Treatment is not required, but the lesions may resolve with antiretroviral drugs. Local therapies with reported efficacy include podophyllin,[33,34] gentian violet,[35] and cryotherapy.[36] HIV patients are also more susceptible to Epstein-Barr virus–associated malignancies with cutaneous manifestations including Burkitt lymphoma, diffuse large B-cell lymphoma, and leiomyosarcoma.[37,38]

Bacillary Angiomatosis: Chapter 154 discusses bacterial infections in greater detail.

Bacillary angiomatosis, caused by *Bartonella henselae* and *Bartonella quintana*, occurs most commonly in HIV patients with a CD4+ T-cell count <200 cells/μL.[39] Clinically, the cutaneous lesions of bacillary angiomatosis are red-to-violaceous, dome-shaped papules, nodules, or plaques that may resemble cherry angiomas, pyogenic granulomas, or Kaposi sarcoma,[40] although many atypical appearances have been reported.[41] Nearly any cutaneous site may be involved, but the palms, soles, and oral cavity are usually spared. Hematogenous or lymphatic dissemination of *B. henselae* and *B. quintana* can result in soft-tissue masses, osseous lesions, lymphadenopathy, splenomegaly, and hepatomegaly.[42,43]

The organism can be seen on tissue biopsy using a silver stain such as Warthin-Starry stain. The antibiotics of choice for bacillary angiomatosis are erythromycin (500 mg 4 times daily) or doxycycline (100 mg twice daily), for at least 4 weeks or until the lesions resolve.[44] Lifelong secondary prevention may be indicated in patients with recurrent bacillary angiomatosis. Bacillary angiomatosis has become rare in developed countries because of the widespread use of ART and macrolide prophylaxis for *Mycobacterium avium* complex.

Mycobacterial Infections: Tuberculosis is the most common opportunistic infection in HIV, but cutaneous manifestations are relatively rare even in this immunocompromised population.[45] Not surprisingly, of the many forms of cutaneous tuberculosis (see Chap. 157), the most commonly reported in AIDS are those associated with low levels of cell-mediated immunity to *Mycobacterium tuberculosis* or *Mycobacterium bovis*. These multibacillary presentations include scrofuloderma, gummatous tuberculosis, and, especially, cutaneous miliary tuberculosis.[46-49] Miliary tuberculosis was only rarely reported in adults prior to the AIDS epidemic. It presents with disseminated but asymmetric red-brown pinpoint macules, papules, and papulovesicles that may crust over.[49] Miliary tuberculosis is treated with multidrug antituberculosis therapy, but mortality rates are high (>50%), particularly in the case of multidrug-resistant organisms.[48]

Non-tuberculous mycobacterial infections (see Chap. 157), especially *M. avium* complex, may rarely disseminate to the skin in profoundly immunocompromised individuals. A wide variety of lesions have been described, including papules, plaques, nodules, abscesses, pustules, ulcers, and more. Cutaneous and blood cultures are key to diagnosis, as they are more sensitive than acid-fast stains of tissue alone, and in vitro susceptibility testing can guide selection of antibiotics.[50]

Most data, including a large 2015 cohort study, suggest that HIV infection does not substantially impact the prevalence or clinical course of concomitant leprosy infection (see Chap. 159).[51] However, a 13-year Brazilian longitudinal case series of coinfected patients made several provocative observations to the contrary.[52] These authors argue that an elevated prevalence of leprosy among HIV-infected individuals has been obscured by various diagnostic challenges, including atypical morphology of leprosy lesions on coinfected patients, conflation of HIV-related and leprosy-related neuropathy, and the limited window for diagnosis in patients with concomitant lepromatous leprosy and AIDS, which they observed to be rapidly fatal, as well as associated with other confounding severe comorbidities.[52] Both the 2015 cohort study and the Brazilian longitudinal case series observed upgrading reactions when coinfected patients began antiretroviral and antileprosy therapy.[51,52]

Invasive Mycoses: Chapter 162 discusses fungal infections in greater detail.

Disseminated fungal infections in advanced HIV disease may arise either by (a) local invasion of the skin or mucosa with secondary lymphatic or hematogenous dissemination or (b) reactivation of a latent pulmonary focus of infection. Cutaneous dissemination usually occurs in patients with a CD4+ T-cell count <50 cells/μL,[53-55] and may present with a wide variety of skin lesions shared by most of the opportunistic fungi, including cellulitis-like plaques, pink or skin-colored nodules, deep ulcerations, acneiform papules and pustules, and umbilicated papules that resemble molluscum.[56-62] These papules tend to favor the face and upper trunk, and they lack the white core of molluscum-infected keratinocytes at the base of a molluscum papule's dell. Fungal pathogens with potential for angioinvasion, such as *Aspergillus* species, may also present with purpuric papules and plaques of septic vasculitis.

Mortality is high for AIDS patients with systemic mycoses that have disseminated to the skin. Because the cutaneous lesions may develop prior to manifestations of internal organ involvement, they provide an opportunity for early diagnosis and intervention if the clinician maintains a sufficiently high index of suspicion. Cryptococcosis, histoplasmosis, and penicilliosis are a subset of deep fungal infections for which AIDS is the primary risk factor for cutaneous infection.

The yeast species *Cryptococcus neoformans* and *Cryptococcus gatti* are common worldwide, resulting in widespread pulmonary exposures that are rarely problematic for immunocompetent people.[63] However, the yeast may invade and disseminate in AIDS patients, most commonly to the CNS.[45] Skin lesions occur only in approximately 10% of AIDS patients with

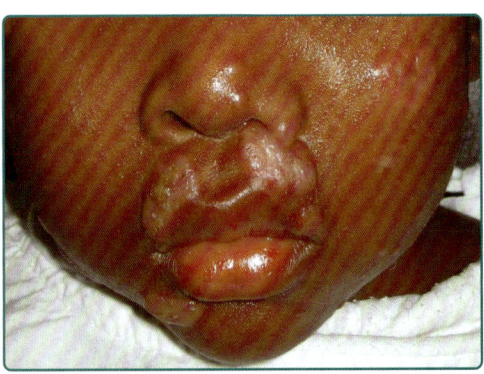

Figure 168-4 Cryptococcosis in a child with congenital HIV and AIDS: pink plaques with crusted erosions on the face.

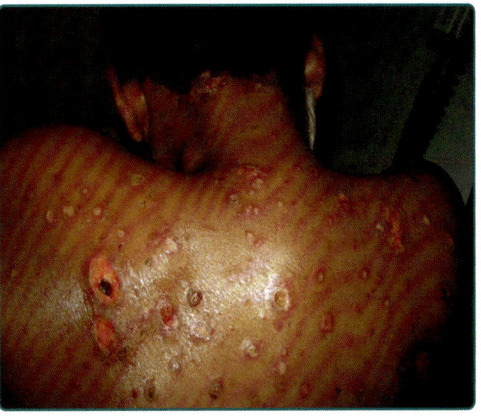

Figure 168-5 Disseminated histoplasmosis in AIDS. A young woman from South Africa with advanced untreated HIV/AIDS presented with cervical adenopathy and disseminated skin-colored papules (some umbilicated), pustules, and ulcerated nodules of varying sizes.

disseminated cryptococcosis, presenting with any of the various lesions described above, including umbilicated papules (Fig. 168-4). Diagnosis can be secured by a latex agglutination test for capsular antigen, culture, or staining with India ink or periodic acid–Schiff stains.[55,63] Treatment is typically with amphotericin-B and flucytosine in combination, followed by a long course of an oral azole antifungal medication.[64]

Histoplasma capsulatum var. *capsulatum* is a dimorphic soil fungus endemic to river valleys of the midwestern and southeastern United States, southeastern South America, and southern and eastern Africa. However, it may be found worldwide, especially in caves and other areas with bat and bird droppings.[65] Like the other fungal infections discussed in this section, pulmonary histoplasmosis is relatively common in exposed populations, but disseminated histoplasmosis is limited to profoundly immunosuppressed patients. Disseminated disease presents with fevers, weight loss, pulmonary symptoms, lymphadenopathy, hepatosplenomegaly, and the polymorphic mucocutaneous lesions common to all the invasive mycoses discussed in this section, again including umbilicated papules, nodules, and necrotic ulcers (Fig. 168-5).[58,59] Heavy involvement of the face, including nasal and oropharyngeal mucosa, is common.

Histopathologic examination demonstrates 2- to 4-μm intracellular yeast forms within parasitized macrophages; in central and western sub-Saharan Africa, some histoplasmosis patients will demonstrate larger, 8- to 15-μm intracellular pathogens, signaling infection with the related species *H. capsulatum* var. *duboisii*.[65] The African histoplasmosis variant *duboisii* appears far less prevalent among AIDS patients than the *capsulatum* variant, even in southern Africa. However, dermatologists should be familiar with it because disseminated African histoplasmosis favors cutaneous sites, along with lymph nodes and bone. Both forms are treated with long courses of itraconazole, sometimes after an initial course of amphotericin B.[66]

The dimorphic fungus *Penicillium marneffei* is a leading cause of mortality among AIDS patients in Southeast Asia.[62] Unlike cryptococcosis, disseminated penicilliosis involves the skin in the great majority of patients—more than 80% in a recent Vietnamese study.[62] Skin lesions, including umbilicated papules, often precede the dyspnea, fever, weight loss, anemia, and lymphadenopathy common to those with more advanced disease.[62] Like *Histoplasma* species, *P. marneffei* parasitizes macrophages, and is observed as 2- to 5-μm intracellular oval yeast forms with transverse septae.[65] Treatment with amphotericin or itraconazole is often effective, although relapse is common.[67]

Superficial Mycoses: Chapter 160 discusses superficial fungal infection in greater detail.

Unlike the opportunistic infections discussed thus far, superficial mycoses and the remaining infections discussed in this section are common in *both* AIDS *and* in well-controlled HIV. However, in immunocompromised patients, these common infections often present with atypical manifestations not seen in patients with stable HIV disease.

Candida colonization of the oropharynx is common in HIV-infected individuals, and has been reported in up to 90% of individuals with advanced disease.[68] Oropharyngeal candidiasis typically presents in 4 different clinical patterns: pseudomembranous (thrush), hyperplastic, erythematous (atrophic), and angular cheilitis. Pseudomembranous candidiasis typically involves the tongue, and presents with yellow-white plaques that are removable by scraping. Hyperplastic candidiasis usually involves the buccal mucosa, and consists of white plaques that are not removable by scraping. Erythematous candidiasis commonly presents with erythematous patches of the palate and the dorsal tongue with associated depapillation. Angular cheilitis manifests as erythema with curd-like flecks or painful fissures at the angles of the lips. Other forms of superficial mucocutaneous candidiasis also occur with greater incidence in advanced HIV disease, including vulvovaginal candidiasis in women,[69] and candida intertrigo in children.[70]

Fungal nail infections are particularly common in HIV disease, caused not only by dermatophytes,

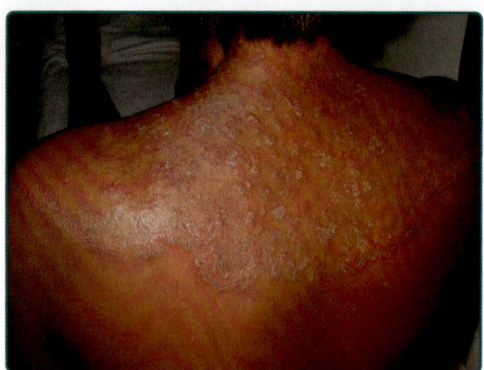

Figure 168-6 Extensive tinea corporis in AIDS. This plaque extended to the chest and face as well.

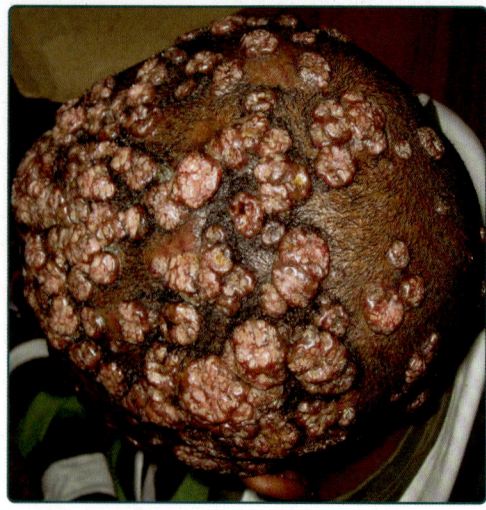

Figure 168-7 Giant molluscum on the scalp in of a patient with AIDS.

but also by *Candida* and nondermatophyte molds.[71,72] Infection of the undersurface of the proximal nail plate is termed *proximal subungual onychomycosis*, and while relatively uncommon even in AIDS patients, it is highly *specific* for advanced immunocompromised patients and should prompt an HIV test in patients whose HIV status is unknown.[73] Antiretrovirals are sometimes effective in clearing onychomycosis,[74] although oral terbinafine or triazole antifungals often are required; drug–drug interactions should be checked carefully before commencing systemic antifungal therapy.

In HIV disease, dermatophyte infections of the epidermis, commonly caused by *Trichophyton rubrum* may be asymptomatic and extensive (Fig. 168-6). The morphology also may be atypical, often lacking the raised erythematous border and annular shape.[75] *Malassezia*-related diseases, including pityriasis versicolor, *Pityrosporum* folliculitis, and seborrheic dermatitis, are all far more prevalent, and often more severe, in HIV patients, particularly at low CD4 counts.[76]

Severe Molluscum Contagiosum:
Chapter 166 discusses poxvirus infections in greater detail.

Approximately 33% of advanced HIV patients with CD4+ T-cell counts of <100 cells/μL have molluscum contagiosum.[77] In this population, the characteristic umbilicated papules with yellow-white cores often coalesce into large confluent plaques and nodules, particularly on the face (Fig. 168-7).[39,77] Whereas most molluscum papules resolve with effective immune reconstitution,[78,79] these giant molluscum lesions may persist for many months or years, and may worsen as part of IRIS.[80] In addition to commonly used treatments such as cantharidin, electrofulguration and curettage, extrusion of the papule cores, and imiquimod 5% cream,[81,82] severe cases can be treated with topical cidofovir, a nucleotide analog with activity against several DNA viruses.[83,84]

Scabies:
Chapter 178 discusses scabies in greater detail.

Scabies usually presents in the typical manner in HIV patients, with pruritus, interdigital burrows, and excoriated papules favoring the genital region, finger webs, and axillae. However, individuals with advanced HIV disease are more likely to have severe hypersensitivities to the *Sarcoptes scabiei* mites, resulting in widespread scabetic nodules, as well as vesicles and pustules.[85] Advanced AIDS patients who are not able to control mite replication are at risk for developing crusted scabies, a highly infectious variant in which the presence of thousands or millions of mites (as opposed to the 10 to 15 typically harbored by immunocompetent hosts) produces extensive thick hyperkeratotic plaques with gray-brown scale, involving atypical locations such as the scalp, beard area, palms, and soles. The plaques may be nonpruritic or minimally pruritic.[86,87] For crusted scabies, multiple doses of ivermectin (200 μg/kg weekly for up to 7 weeks) may be and should be combined with a topical scabicide and a keratolytic cream to improve penetration.[88]

Atypical Leishmaniasis:
Chapter 176 discusses leishmaniasis in greater detail.

HIV and *Leishmania* species are both intracellular pathogens in many of the same myeloid cells, including macrophages and dendritic cells. In coinfected patients, the 2 pathogens interact in complex and often symbiotic ways, substantially altering the course of both diseases.[89] Among the many pathophysiologic mechanisms, the HIV-induced shift in cytokines toward a TH2-dominant milieu impairs the TH1 response critical to controlling leishmaniasis. In turn, the *Leishmania*-induced activation of immune cells creates an abundance of target cells for HIV infection.[89] The result in coinfected patients is a more rapid progression to AIDS, higher HIV viral loads, and increased infectivity.[89,90] These patients also suffer more severe and persistent *Leishmania* infections; atypical and disseminated forms of cutaneous and mucocutaneous leishmaniasis are common, with widespread ulcers that are highly refractory to therapy.[89,91,92] Visceral leishmaniasis is of particular concern in HIV-infected patients, who are at 100 to 2320 times the risk of this often deadly variant.[90]

INFECTIONS IN WELL-CONTROLLED HIV

With access and adherence to ART, most patients can avoid or recover from the profound immunosuppressed state of advanced AIDS. These patients with chronic, stable, well-controlled HIV disease are, of course, susceptible to all typical infections that can affect any seronegative individual. In addition, certain infections remain more prevalent among these patients relative to the seronegative population, despite undetectable viral loads and normal CD4 counts. As patients live with stable HIV disease for decades, these conditions account for an increasing proportion of the care HIV patients receive from dermatologists.

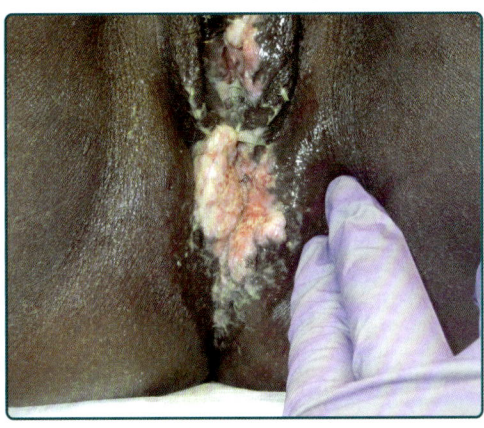

Figure 168-8 Herpes vegetans in well-controlled HIV. The verrucous weeping plaques and nodules had been present for longer than 5 years, despite continual adherence to antiretroviral therapy and a CD4+ T-cell count higher than 600 cells/μL.

Staphylococcal Infections:
Chapters 150 to 152 discuss staphylococcal infections in greater detail.

HIV-infected individuals tend to present with the same wide range of primary *Staphylococcus aureus* skin and soft-tissue infections that are normally seen in seronegative individuals, as well as secondary *S. aureus* infection of molluscum, herpetic ulcers, atopic dermatitis, and other primary dermatoses. Despite normal CD4+ T-cell counts, even patients with well-controlled HIV remain at elevated risk for a number of clinically relevant *S. aureus*–related mucocutaneous complications.

At all stages of HIV, the prevalence of *S. aureus* nasal carriage exceeds that of the general population, with estimates as high as 30% to 50% colonization of HIV-infected individuals.[93,94] Colonization with methicillin-resistant *S. aureus* (MRSA) specifically is approximately 3 times more prevalent among even well-controlled HIV patients than among seronegative patients (16.8% vs 5.8% in a large, prospective, cohort study from 2009).[95] The relative risk of actual infection with community-associated MRSA among HIV patients is even higher, 6 times that of HIV-negative controls in a large 2010 population analysis.[96] Of those HIV patients who develop MRSA skin or soft-tissue infections, recurrences are extremely common, with estimates as high as 50% over the 9 months following the initial infection, and 71% over a 3-year period.[97]

Management of staphylococcal infections should be directed at treatment the acute infection, and treatment of any underlying dermatoses. Well-controlled HIV is not an indication for systemic antibiotics for pyodermas that could otherwise be treated adequately with local therapy, such as incision and drainage for most abscesses, or topical antibiotics for impetigo. The role of eradication of *S. aureus* nasal carriage, more extensive decolonization regimens, and chronic oral prophylaxis for recurrent *S. aureus* infections all remain controversial.

Herpes Simplex Viruses 1 and 2 Infections:
Chapter 164 discusses herpes simplex in greater detail.

In advanced HIV disease, primary and recurrent herpes simplex virus (HSV) 1 and HSV-2 infections are often more severe, longer lasting and refractory to therapy, and recurrences are more frequent than in immunocompetent patients. A chronic herpetic ulcer lasting more than 1 month is a marker of profound immunosuppression and has been designated an AIDS-defining condition.[98] However, one uncommon form of chronic HSV, called *verrucous HSV* or *herpes vegetans*, occurs in patients with advanced AIDS and in patients with well-controlled HIV. In this variant, thick, proliferative, vegetative plaques and nodules may persist for months or years (Fig. 168-8). Most reported cases are resistant to thymidine kinase–dependent antivirals such as acyclovir and valacyclovir.[99] High doses of thymidine kinase–dependent antivirals can sometimes overcome this resistance mechanism, but when that fails, thymidine kinase–independent options include topical imiquimod, IV foscarnet, and cidofovir in topical, intralesional, or IV form.[100-102]

The synergy between HSV and HIV also critically impacts the pathogenicity of HIV infection. HSV-2 imparts a twofold to threefold increased risk of HIV acquisition, which in areas of high HSV-2 prevalence might be responsible for up to 25% of HIV infections.[103] The pathophysiology of this increased HIV risk goes well beyond enhanced HIV entry through epithelium disrupted by HSV ulcers; local HSV-2 viral shedding occurs more frequently than recurrences of actual ulcers, and the resultant near continual subclinical inflammation increases the number of target cells for HIV to infect, even with the use of low-dose prophylactic acyclovir or valacyclovir. In people who are already coinfected, HSV-2 enhances HIV viral replication, thereby increasing HIV plasma viral load and HIV shedding in genital mucosa, further increasing the transmissibility of HIV.[103]

Varicella Zoster Virus Infection:
Chapter 165 discusses varicella-zoster virus in greater detail.

In advanced HIV disease, atypical presentations of varicella-zoster virus reactivation are common, including recurrent dermatomal herpes zoster (HZ), disseminated HZ, and chronic HZ.[104,105] Individual lesions may exhibit unusual morphology, such as ecthymatous ulcers, hyperkeratotic papules, or vegetative plaques.[106,107] Complications such as postherpetic neuralgia are common, despite the younger age of most HIV patients who develop HZ.[108,109]

The risk of HZ correlates inversely with CD4+ T-cell counts, except during the 6-month period after ART initiation, when the risk of HZ is actually highest, possibly because of IRIS.[110-112] At least for treated HIV patients younger than 65 years old, the risk of HZ never decreases to the level of the age-matched general population, even long after CD4+ T-cell count recovery. The risk is higher among those who ever experienced a low CD4+ T-cell count nadir.[110]

The HZ live vaccine can be safely administered to HIV patients who are not severely or moderately immunosuppressed.[113,114] Prophylactic oral acyclovir (400 mg twice daily) can also reduce the HZ risk in HIV patients—by 62% in one randomized controlled trial.[115] Acyclovir resistance has been reported but appears to be rare.[116,117] AIDS patients who develop dermatomal HZ or mild primary varicella may be treated with oral valacyclovir or famciclovir, but any evidence of disseminated disease, visceral involvement, or other severe complications should prompt initiation of IV acyclovir 10 mg/kg 3 times daily.

Human Papillomavirus Infections: Chapter 167 discusses HPV infections in greater detail.

While the introduction of effective ART has reduced the incidence of AIDS-defining malignancies including HPV-induced cervical cancer (see section "Human Papillomavirus–induced Dysplasia and Squamous Cell Carcinoma"), the incidence and burden of HPV disease overall may actually be increasing with the improving life expectancy of HIV patients.[118-121] HPV infections are far more prevalent in HIV-infected individuals than in the general population,[122,123] in part because both can be sexually transmitted, but also because HIV at all stages is associated with more-extensive and more-severe HPV lesions, lower clearance rates, and slower response to therapy.[124]

HIV patients are also at high risk for simultaneous infection with multiple HPV types, including high-risk oncogenic types, and the malignancies they cause may clinically resemble benign HPV lesions.[124,125] Even in the absence of malignancy, extensive and refractory warts can substantially impact the lives of patients with otherwise well-controlled HIV disease. The adverse medical and social impact is perhaps most pronounced from oral and anogenital condyloma, typically caused by HPV-6 and HPV-11. Oral florid papillomatosis and anogenital giant condyloma of Buschke and Lowenstein can be locally destructive and deforming, and are considered by some to be variants of verrucous carcinoma.

Cases of verruca and condyloma resolution with ART alone have been reported,[126,127] but many patients require therapy specifically targeting their warts. Immune-mediated treatments, such as imiquimod[128-133] and intralesional candida antigen,[134] appear to be safe and potentially effective in HIV patients.

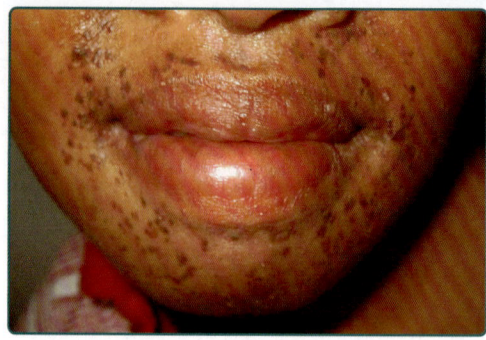

Figure 168-9 Acquired epidermodysplasia verruciformis in a child with congenital HIV disease.

Other therapies with reported success for refractory warts include topical podophyllotoxin,[135] intralesional cidofovir,[136-138] intralesional bleomycin,[139] intralesional and systemic interferon,[140,141] CO_2 laser,[142] and photodynamic therapy,[142] potentially in combinations.

Another form of extensive HPV disease, acquired epidermodysplasia verruciformis, has been described in children with congenital HIV, and also reported in adults with well-controlled HIV. As in hereditary epidermodysplasia verruciformis, children with the acquired form develop extensive, thin, flat-topped papules resembling verruca plana or tinea versicolor from unusual susceptibility to the beta subtypes of HPV, including types HPV-5, HPV-8, and HPV-9 (Fig. 168-9).[143] Treatment of this stigmatizing disease is challenging; mixed success has been reported with topical cidofovir, topical imiquimod, oral retinoids, and interferon-α in combination with ribavirin.[144-147]

Syphilis: Chapter 170 discusses syphilis in greater detail.

Given that the vast majority of HIV infections are sexually transmitted, individuals with HIV infection should also be screened for other sexually transmitted diseases such as chlamydia, gonorrhea, and genital ulcerative diseases, including syphilis and chancroid.

Syphilis is a particularly important disease to consider in HIV-infected patients, because asymptomatic coinfections are curable if caught early and are more morbid than in seronegative patients if not adequately treated. Syphilis patients with HIV are at higher risk for multiple primary chancres, longer-lasting chancres, more-severe manifestations of secondary syphilis such as lues maligna and condyloma lata,[148] and early progression to neurosyphilis[149,150]; this heightened risk of neurosyphilis should prompt consideration of a lumbar puncture for any new diagnosis of syphilis in a patient with advanced HIV disease, or in a patient with well-controlled HIV disease who has syphilis of unknown stage, or a rapid plasma reagin titer of at least 1:32.[150]

HIV coinfection increases the risk of treatment failure from a single dose of intramuscular penicillin for primary and secondary syphilis, but treatment guidelines are the same for HIV seronegative and seropositive patients as alternative treatment regimens have not been found to be more effective.[151] Adverse reactions to syphilis therapy, including drug eruptions and the Jarisch-Herxheimer reaction, are more common in HIV patients.[150]

Further complicating matters, testing for syphilis is less reliable in HIV patients. HIV patients with secondary syphilis may have falsely negative nontreponemal antibody (ie, rapid plasma reagin and Venereal Disease Research Laboratory) titers either from delayed antibody formation, or from the prozone phenomenon, in which HIV-related immune dysregulation causes massively elevated titers, high enough impair the assay.[152,153]

As in many other coinfections, the clinical impact of HIV and syphilis coinfection is bidirectional; just as HIV alters the course of syphilis infection, syphilis also appears to adversely impact HIV disease progression and transmissibility, and is associated with decreased CD4+ T-cell counts and increased HIV viral loads.[154]

CUTANEOUS MALIGNANCY IN HIV

AT-A-GLANCE

- Kaposi sarcoma remains one of the most common HIV-associated malignancies worldwide, even with reduction in incidence because of ART. Recently, a novel group of HIV-infected patients has been identified that develop new-onset Kaposi sarcoma while already virologically suppressed on ART.
- HPV-induced dysplasia and squamous cell carcinoma are more common in HIV-infected men and women than in the general population, with a high burden in men who have sex with men. Screening for anal and cervical dysplasia is particularly important for HIV-positive patients.
- Cutaneous lymphomas and other nonkeratinocyte cancers are also more prevalent in HIV-positive patients. Primary cutaneous lymphomas in HIV patients tend to be aggressive rather than indolent, with survival often less than 1 year.

KAPOSI SARCOMA

Kaposi sarcoma (KS) is vascular and lymphatic neoplasm caused by human herpesvirus-8. There are several subtypes of KS, including AIDS-related KS, classic/Mediterranean KS, endemic African KS, and transplant-associated KS. AIDS-related KS is an AIDS-defining malignancy. At the beginning of the HIV epidemic, KS was one of the first opportunistic sequela noted in what would later be defined as AIDS[155] and was a frequent presenting sign of HIV/AIDS.

Even though incidence of HIV-related KS in the United States and Europe has decreased with the advent of ART,[156-158] KS remains one of the most common HIV-associated cancers in sub-Saharan Africa, with an incidence among HIV-infected persons of 164 to 334 per 100,000 person-years.[159,160] This incidence is on par with the incidence of prostate cancer in the United States.[156,161]

Despite the successes of ART, ART is not tantamount to cure and not all ART-adherent patients have their health fully restored. In addition to KS that does not respond completely to ART, we are now faced with a new group of patients who develop KS for the first time while on ART, separate from unmasking IRIS. Dermatologists were at the forefront of identifying that a novel group of HIV-infected patients on ART with no prior KS were developing new-onset cutaneous KS despite virologic supression.[162] ART decreases KS incidence,[156] but does not bring it down to zero, even with ART adherence. Understanding why new KS develops despite ART is an area of active investigation in several research sites in Africa.

Diagnosis: KS diagnosis is made based on clinical appearance and biopsy. Tissue confirmation is strongly recommended, even in resource-poor settings.[163] When routine histology is indeterminate, or to confirm histologic findings, anti–latency-associated nuclear antigen staining can be used to establish the presence of human herpesvirus-8.

Differential Diagnosis: Differential diagnosis for KS includes other vascular lesions, postinflammatory hyperpigmentation, and scar, among others.[163] Oval plaques could be mistaken for lichen planus, pityriasis rosea, syphilis, or psoriasis. Violaceous or vascular lesions can mimic lichen planus, psoriasis, lichen simplex chronicus, acroangiodermatitis, and stasis dermatitis. Of particular importance, bacillary angiomatosis can mimic KS (Fig. 168-10), and mistaking bacillary angiomatosis for KS, without performing a biopsy, could lead to unnecessary chemotherapy with poor outcome.[40]

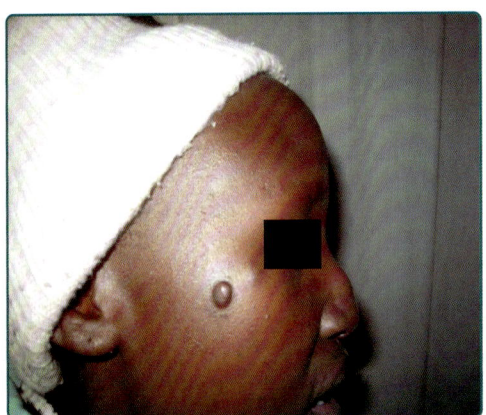

Figure 168-10 Bacillary angiomatosis mimicking Kaposi sarcoma in a Kenyan patient. Note the subcutaneous nodule of bacillary angiomatosis on the nose. (Used with permission from Toby Maurer.)

Clinical Course, Prognosis, and Management: Survival following diagnosis of KS remains poor in the areas hardest hit, such as sub-Saharan Africa, even in the era of available ART.[164] This poor survival despite ART has been speculated to be, at least in part, a consequence of late presentation and delayed diagnosis of the disease in resource-poor settings. For example, newer studies have found that 69% to 86% of KS patients in Africa are diagnosed only at an advanced stage of the disease.[165,166] Dermatologists can have a role in early diagnosis both in identifying cutaneous lesions and in asking about potentially dangerous symptoms that could be suggestive of systemic involvement worthy of further workup, such as unexplained GI bleeding or a persistent cough in the absence of tuberculosis.

Treatment of HIV-related KS in mild to moderate cases consists of ART; in more-severe cases, chemotherapy is also required. The distinction of what constitutes "mild" versus "severe" KS requiring chemotherapy is an area of debate. The 2014 WHO guidelines (Table 168-4) go beyond the AIDS Clinical Trials Group staging[167] and incorporate functional status, such as difficulty swallowing or difficulty walking, into the criteria for chemotherapy.[168]

In addition to ART and possibly systemic chemotherapy, local therapies such as radiation,[169] direct injections of chemotherapy agents such as bleomycin, vincristine, and vinblastine,[170-172] and topicals such as imiquimod[173] and alitretinoin gel[174] can be useful adjuvants for lesion control, localized edema, and cosmesis.

TABLE 168-4
HIV-Associated Kaposi Sarcoma Treatment According to World Health Organization Guidelines

MILD/MODERATE KS DISEASE	SEVERE/SYMPTOMATIC KS DISEASE
Immediate ART initiation is recommended	Immediate ART initiation in combination with systemic chemotherapy
WHO definition of mild/moderate:	WHO definition of severe:
• Confined to skin and/or lymph nodes • No symptomatic visceral disease • No significant oral disease (ie, does not interfere with chewing or swallowing) • No significant edema affecting function • Not functionally disabling or immediately life-threatening	• Symptomatic visceral disease (pulmonary or GI) • Extensive oral KS lesions which interfere with chewing or swallowing • Painful or disabling tumor-associated facial/genital/peripheral edema or ulcerated tumors • Life-threatening or functionally disabling disease • Progressive or persistent disease despite ART

ART, antiretroviral therapy; KS, Kaposi sarcoma; WHO, World Health Organization.

HUMAN PAPILLOMAVIRUS-INDUCED DYSPLASIA AND SQUAMOUS CELL CARCINOMA

Anal HPV infection is more prevalent in HIV-infected men and women than in the general population. In men who have sex with men (MSM), anal HPV infection is present in 40% to 60% of HIV-negative individuals, but in up to 94% of HIV-positive MSM.[175-178] Similarly, in HIV-negative women, HPV DNA can be detected anally in 42%, but in as many as 76% of HIV-positive women.[179] The relative risk of HPV-related invasive anal cancer is also much higher in HIV patients, with an age-, sex-, and race-standardized relative risk of invasive anal cancer in HIV-infected men compared to HIV-uninfected men of 37.9, and in HIV-infected women compared to uninfected women of 6.8.[180] In addition to higher levels of anal cancer in HIV-infected women, invasive cervical cancer is also increased in HIV infection, with a relative risk of 5.8.[180]

Clinical Features: The presence of anal or genital condyloma is suggestive of HPV infection, and warrants further screening for invasive disease. Perianal squamous cell carcinoma in situ (also known as Bowen disease) or invasive squamous cell carcinoma can present as pruritus, mass, bleeding, or pain.

Prevention, Screening, and Diagnosis: The quadrivalent or nonavalent HPV vaccine is recommended for all HIV-positive females 9 to 26 years of age and all males 9 to 21 years of age. Males 22 to 26 years of age should also be vaccinated if not vaccinated at younger ages.[181] Vaccination does not replace screening.

Screening for anal and cervical dysplasia is particularly important for HIV-positive patients. For anal dysplasia and cancer, at baseline and followup visits, both men and women should be asked about anal symptoms such as itching, bleeding, diarrhea, and pain. Dermatologists can also assist by performing a visual inspection of the perianal region.[182] There are no universally accepted guidelines on anal Papanicolaou tests for HIV patients. New York State Department of Health AIDS Institute recommends that anal cytology be obtained at baseline and annually in all HIV-positive MSM, any HIV patient with a history of anogenital condyloma/warts (men and women), and HIV-positive women with abnormal cervical and/or vulvar histology.[182] The Infectious Disease Society of America guidelines for HIV patients are similar, adding that women with a history of receptive anal intercourse should also be screened.[181] However, there also have been arguments for a more inclusive screening policy, that all HIV-positive patients, men and women, should receive cytologic screening starting at age 30 years.[183]

Clinical Course, Prognosis, and Management: HIV-positive patients with anal cancer treated with chemotherapy and radiation appear to have similar rates of tumor response and local control to HIV-negative counterparts.[184-186] However, overall survival of HIV patients after a diagnosis of anal cancer is lower than in the general population with anal cancer, possibly because of coinfections and morbidities.[184,187]

CUTANEOUS LYMPHOMAS IN HIV

Epidemiology: In the ART era, the risk of lymphoma in HIV patients is at least 11 to 15 times that of the general population[23,188]; pre-ART it may have been as high as 352-fold.[189] Incidence of HIV-associated lymphomas is generally correlated with the degree of immunosuppression, however, with increasingly widespread and early initiation of ART, the incidence of non-Hodgkin lymphoma is declining and is increasingly noted at higher CD4+ counts.[190]

Cutaneous lymphomas, in particular, differ in their epidemiology in HIV-infected individuals as compared to uninfected individuals.[189,191,192] Infected individuals are at increased risk of developing CD30+ anaplastic large-cell lymphoma, diffuse B-cell lymphoma, and plasmablastic lymphoma, a malignancy that is virtually unseen outside of AIDS. Mycosis fungoides, however, has a similar presentation, clinical course, and management paradigm to that for uninfected individuals.[193]

Clinical Features: Cutaneous manifestations can vary widely. Primary cutaneous lymphomas have been described as singular nodules or tumors that can have ulceration.[38,189] Plasmablastic lymphomas may present in the oral mucosa.[194]

Diagnosis and Differential Diagnosis: Skin biopsy with histologic examination and immunohistochemical staining are the mainstays of diagnosis of cutaneous lesions suspicious for malignancy in the HIV patient.[189,195] Diagnosis on clinical grounds alone is difficult because of the diversity of presentations. In the clinical context of HIV, primary cutaneous lymphoma may be especially difficult to differentiate from systemic lymphoma because of the presence of systemic symptoms such as lymphadenopathy.[195] However, this distinction is of interest because of the differences in prognosis, clinical course, and management between primary cutaneous and systemic lymphoma.

Clinical Course, Prognosis, and Management: In HIV-negative individuals, primary cutaneous lymphomas typically have a more indolent course and better prognosis when compared to systemic lymphomas. In contrast, primary cutaneous lymphomas in HIV patients tend to be aggressive, with survival often less than 1 year.[189,192,194,195] Patients often die because of complications of immunosuppression, such as sepsis, rather than the lymphoma itself, although metastasis has been noted, especially with CD30+ anaplastic large-cell lymphoma.[189,192,196]

No guidelines exist for management of cutaneous lymphomas and other nonkeratinocytic malignancies in the setting of HIV. If amenable, lesions of some subtypes may be managed with excision and local radiotherapy.[38,195] Because of the high risk of sepsis and complications of immunosuppression, the literature suggests that chemotherapy is used best when in combination with ART and adequate HIV control. This is true in both resource-abundant as well as resource-poor settings.[196,197] Cyclophosphamide, hydroxydaunorubicin, vincristine, and prednisone (CHOP), and Adriamycin and vincristine monotherapy have been tried.[194] Reports of spontaneous clearance of lymphoma following HIV control exist.[195]

OTHER NONKERATINOCYTE CANCERS

HIV predisposes patients to other nonkeratinocytic cutaneous cancers as well. Merkel cell carcinoma and appendageal carcinoma have an increased incidence in this population.[198] Melanoma incidence is also slightly increased in HIV, with a recent metaanalysis showing a relative risk of 1.50 (95% confidence interval, 1.12 to 2.01) among studies in the ART era that accounted for ethnicity.[199] In pediatric patients, smooth muscle tumors are the second most common malignancy in patients with HIV and cutaneous variants have been observed.[38]

CUTANEOUS AND MUCOCUTANEOUS INFLAMMATORY CONDITIONS IN HIV

AT-A-GLANCE

- Plaque psoriasis is the most common variant of psoriasis in HIV patients, but unusual presentations of psoriasis should prompt HIV testing.
- Seborrheic dermatitis can be severe and extensive in HIV patients, with prevalence and severity increasing with worsening immunosuppression. Prolonged treatment may be required.
- Papular pruritic eruption (PPE) is characterized by pruritic, symmetric papules of the distal extremities, and is more commonly found in tropical and subtropical zones. Eosinophilic folliculitis (EF), in contrast, favors the midline. The mainstay of therapy for both PPE and EF is antiretroviral therapy.

PSORIASIS

While there has been debate regarding whether HIV infection may increase or decrease the prevalence of psoriasis, a recent large study of U.S. data found no association.[200,201] Plaque psoriasis is still the most prevalent variant in HIV-associated psoriasis in U.S. studies, but the presence of rupioid psoriasis, sebopsoriasis, reactive arthritis with keratoderma blenorrhagica with palmoplantar manifestations, acute onset of severe psoriasis, severe exacerbation of existing psoriasis, or psoriasis with multiple morphologies in a single patient should raise concern for concomitant HIV infection.[200,202-204] Erythroderma has been reported as the most prevalent variant in small studies of the sub-Saharan African population.[205]

Although typical psoriasis presentations are diagnosed clinically, biopsy plays a greater role in diagnosing HIV-associated psoriasis because of the higher proportion of severe or atypical presentations, and because HIV confers a higher risk of clinical mimickers, such as lymphoma, tinea, and secondary syphilis.[200,206] In the pediatric population, HIV-associated psoriasis has been noted in infancy and may mimic, or complicate, a diaper rash.[207]

The pathogenesis of psoriasis in HIV infection is poorly understood, and generates several apparent paradoxes. Psoriasis is a disease of T-cell–mediated inflammation, and yet HIV, which destroys T cells, has been noted to worsen it.[208] Psoriasis sometimes emerges late in the course of HIV disease, when the patient is severely immunosuppressed,[200,203] although it also has been noted to regress before death in severe AIDS.[200,209]

As in HIV-negative patients, treatment of HIV-associated psoriasis depends on severity of disease and degree of skin involvement.[200,210] Guidelines for treatment are based on case series, reports, and small reviews. Topical therapies, including emollients, vitamin D analogs, and corticosteroids are recommended for mild disease, although as mentioned earlier, high-potency topical steroid use requires caution in the setting of ART regimens that include ritonavir or cobicistat. Phototherapy may be used for moderate-to-severe disease, after carefully weighing its benefits against the HIV-related increased risks of photosensitive eruptions and of skin cancer.[198-200] Acitretin may be used alone as a second-line therapy for moderate-to-severe disease or in combination with phototherapy.[200,210]

Given that psoriasis can be exacerbated by severity of concomitant HIV infection, ART is also first-line therapy for moderate-to-severe disease, and may be used as monotherapy.[210] Care must be taken to watch for severe exacerbations in the setting of IRIS.[211]

Refractory cases of psoriasis may respond to methotrexate, cyclosporine (especially when needing rapid response), and hydroxyurea. Tumor necrosis factor-α inhibitors, which are often a mainstay of treatment in HIV-negative patients, need to be approached very cautiously in HIV-positive patients.[200,210,212] Treatment with these agents may be complicated by worsening immunosuppression. In addition, HIV patients on biologic therapy are at higher risk for progressive multifocal leukoencephalopathy caused by reactivation of the John Cunningham (JC) virus.[213]

SEBORRHEIC DERMATITIS

In the general population, the prevalence of seborrheic dermatitis hovers around 3% to 5%. In HIV, the prevalence of seborrheic dermatitis can be as high as 83%, and both the prevalence and severity tend to increase with worsening immunosuppression.[214,215]

A case series of 20 HIV patients with seborrheic dermatitis from the United States, Botswana, and South Africa demonstrated that seborrheic dermatitis can be severe and extensive in HIV patients. The case series described extensive involvement of the scalp (Fig. 168-11), axillae, groin, and flexural extremities, with frequent bacterial superinfection, and with markedly thick and greasy yellow scaling of the scalp. Patients also exhibited extension beyond the typical seborrheic distribution, sometimes progressing to erythroderma.[216]

HIV patients are often refractory to standard seborrheic dermatitis treatments, and they experience frequent treatment failure and recurrence.[216,217] ART itself may improve seborrheic dermatitis, or may help its response to other treatments.[216,218,219] The mainstays of treatment are topical and systemic antifungals, topical or oral corticosteroids, and oral antibiotics when needed to address bacterial superinfection.[216] Ketoconazole may have more activity against *Malassezia furfur*, thought to be an underlying pathogen in seborrheic dermatitis, over other azoles such as fluconazole and itraconazole, although this has

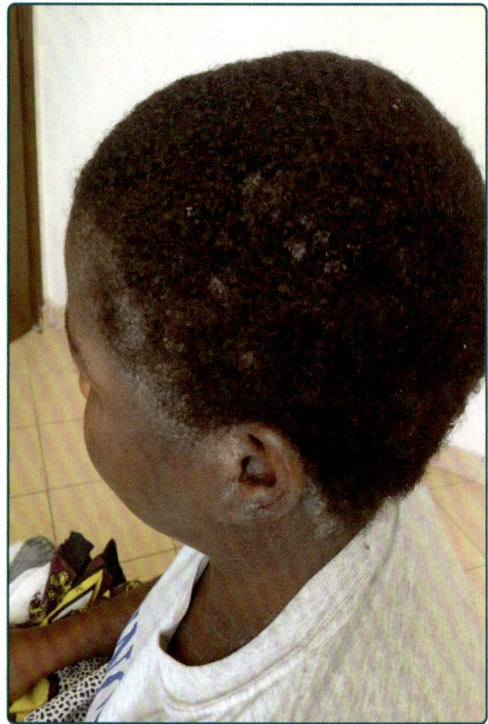

Figure 168-11 Seborrheic dermatitis in HIV with extensive scalp involvement. This patient from Kenya was compliant with her antiretroviral therapy and had already failed topical antifungals.

primarily been demonstrated in the laboratory rather than in human studies.[220,221] The current WHO guidelines recommend topical ketoconazole as first-line therapy, with the addition of topical corticosteroids in severe or unresponsive cases.[168] Prolonged treatment courses are often required.

PAPULAR PRURITIC ERUPTION

Papular pruritic eruption (PPE) is a common HIV-associated skin condition, particularly in tropical and subtropical regions. Prevalence may be as high as 46% in adults and 42% in children, depending on geography.[222-228] PPE is characterized by pruritic, symmetric papules. The eruption favors the distal extremities (Fig. 168-12), but can also appear on the face and trunk. It generally spares the palms, soles, and mucous membranes.[168] Scabies, eosinophilic folliculitis, papulonecrotic tuberculid, and drug eruptions should be considered in the differential diagnosis of PPE.

The pathophysiology is poorly understood, but is proposed to be a hypersensitivity and/or recall reaction to arthropod assault in the setting of HIV.[229] Patients with PPE have significantly lower CD4+ T-cell counts than patients without PPE.[230] Independent of the CD4+ T-cell count, the development of PPE is also associated with greater HIV viral loads at ART commencement.[231]

PPE resolves with ART,[232] which is considered the mainstay of treatment. Initial worsening after ART initiation may occur as part of IRIS; one study found exacerbation of the dermatitis in 13% of patients after starting ART.[232] For symptomatic control, the current WHO recommendations include oral antihistamines and topical corticosteroids.[168] Other therapies that have been tried with some success include pentoxifylline[233,234] and oral promethazine.[235] Given the concern that PPE may represent a reaction to arthropod assault, mosquito repellant and other protective measures also have been suggested.[230]

EOSINOPHILIC FOLLICULITIS

Eosinophilic folliculitis (EF) comes in several forms, including HIV-associated, infancy-associated, and classic. With regard to HIV-associated EF specifically, prevalence varies widely in different studies from the United States and Asia, ranging from 4% to 19%.[236,237] Low CD4+ T-cell count and advanced immunosuppression are associated with the development of EF.[168,238]

EF is characterized by follicular pruritic papules and pustules, favoring the midline, of the face, neck, scalp, trunk, and proximal extremities (Fig. 168-13). This distribution stands in contrast to PPE, which favors the distal extremities, although the 2 entities can appear clinically similar. Both the distribution and morphology of EF lesions mimic those of acne; although sometimes challenging to distinguish, pruritus and sudden emergence at low CD4+ T-cell counts or after commencing ART are suggestive of EF over acne.

Similar to PPE, the mainstay of treatment is ART. Patients who develop EF IRIS should continue to be treated with ART.[168] Other therapeutic options include oral itraconazole,[239] oral isotretinoin,[240] and phototherapy.[241] Current WHO recommendations suggest, in addition to evaluating the patient for ART, (a) starting an oral antihistamine, followed by additional symptomatic control with (b) topical steroids, (c) oral itraconazole, and, finally, if no response to the above, trying (d) permethrin 5% applied above the waist.[168]

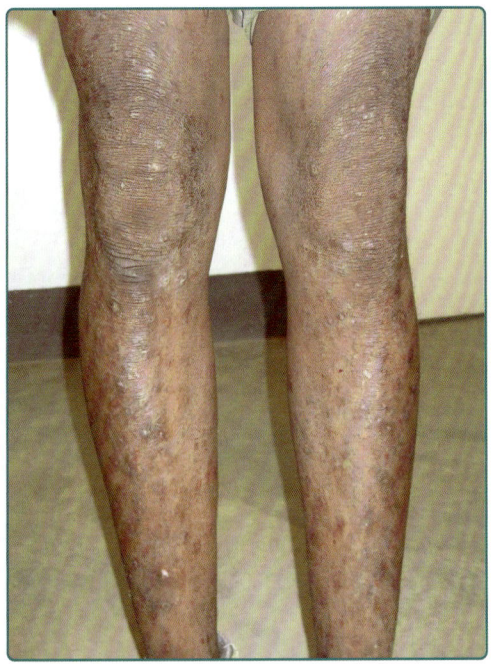

Figure 168-12 Papular pruritic eruption in HIV. The eruption favors the distal extremities. (Used with permission from Serling Chua.)

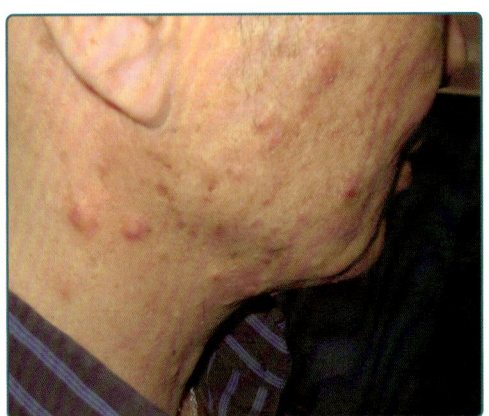

Figure 168-13 HIV-associated eosinophilic folliculitis, favoring the face. The eruption can appear acne-like, but is severely pruritic. (Used with permission from Toby Maurer.)

IMMUNE RECONSTITUTION INFLAMMATORY SYNDROME

AT-A-GLANCE

- Previously tolerated antigens may lead to robust inflammatory reactions in the setting of immune reconstitution following treatment with antiretroviral therapy (ART).
- Both inflammatory conditions and infections can flare in this setting.
- High viral load and low CD4 counts at the time of initiation of ART are risk factors.
- Most reactions eventually subside so treatment may range from supportive care to oral steroids in significant reactions; life-threatening reactions may require ART interruption.

TABLE 168-5

Immune Reconstitution Inflammatory Syndrome

Major Criteria
1. Atypical presentation of opportunistic infections or tumors in patients responding to antiretroviral therapy (ART).
2. Decrease in plasma HIV RNA level by at least 1 $\log^{10}$ copies/mL.

Minor Criteria
1. Increased blood CD4+ T-cell count after ART.
2. Increase in immune response specific to the relevant pathogen.
3. Spontaneous resolution of disease without specific antimicrobial therapy or tumor chemotherapy with continuation of ART.

As immune function is restored in HIV, previously unrecognized or tolerated antigens may lead to strong stimulation of the immune response. Commonly referred to as IRIS, this reaction has been reported in up to 20% of patients receiving ART and usually occurs in the first 2 to 3 months following the initiation of ART.[242] When a clinically unrecognized disease is noted after the initiation of ART, the term *unmasking IRIS* is used. In turn, when a previously recognized clinical entity flares, the term *paradoxical IRIS* applies.

CLINICAL FEATURES

Inflammatory disorders such as EF, adverse cutaneous drug reactions, sarcoid, connective tissue disorders, AIDS-related lymphoma, non-Hodgkin lymphoma, and neurologic disease may flare in the setting of IRIS. Other systemic symptoms may include fever and lymphadenopathy. Minor cognitive disorders are not uncommon. Infectious agents previously tolerated also can be increasingly recognized by the immune response. Mycobacteria (both tuberculous and nontuberculous), HSV, varicella zoster virus, *Cryptococcus*, hepatitides B and C viruses, molluscum virus, the progressive multifocal leukoencephalopathy (progressive multifocal leukoencephalopathy) virus, and cytomegalovirus are common agents known to "flare" in the setting of IRIS.[243]

ETIOLOGY AND PATHOGENESIS

The pathogenesis of IRIS is multifactorial and immunologic mechanisms suggest that 2 main factors are related to the likelihood of disease: (a) lower CD4+ count and/or percentage and (b) higher HIV RNA, prior to initiation of ART. Younger patients and male patients are disproportionately affected. Other risk factors include shorter interval between initiating treatment of an opportunistic infection and starting ART, and rapidly falling viral load.

DIAGNOSIS

IRIS is diagnosed clinically. Serologic tests, skin biopsy and radiographic studies may be helpful in uncovering culprits, but these do not diagnose IRIS. Case definition relies on a previous diagnosis of AIDS with low pretreatment count, a positive virology and immunologic response to ART, and a temporal association between the initiation of ART and disease development. In the case of unmasking IRIS, there must be solid reason to believe that the pathogen or antigen was present before it became manifest and before ART initiation. Table 168-5 reviews one published set of diagnostic criteria. This syndrome must be differentiated from patient nonadherence to ART (and progression of HIV), antimicrobial resistance, and tachyphylaxis.

CLINICAL COURSE, PROGNOSIS, AND MANAGEMENT

Most IRIS reactions are self-limited. Clinically significant dermatologic reactions that may lead to patient nonadherence may be treated with prednisone up to 1 mg/kg, rapidly tapered. One notable exception is KS, where systemic corticosteroids may lead to worse outcomes. Infectious agents are treated based on the extent of involvement and systemic disease (WHO guidelines for dermatologic disease). Rarely, the syndrome may be fatal if central neurologic structures are affected. Perhaps the most important aspect of treatment entails continuation of ART and educating the patient to understand that as the immune system recovers, most of these reactions improve. Notably, molluscum, PPE, and EF in the setting of IRIS are best treated in this fashion. Some physicians advocate for "slowing down" immune recovery in an effort to lessen the acute inflammatory responses, and to stop it only if life-threatening to the patient.[244] The AIDSinfo website (https://aidsinfo.nih.gov/guidelines/search/4/IRIS/0) has up-to-date information on each entity that flares with IRIS.

MUCOCUTANEOUS MANIFESTATIONS OF THE HUMAN T-LYMPHOTROPHIC VIRUS

AT-A-GLANCE

- Human T-cell lymphotropic virus (HTLV)-1 was the first retrovirus discovered.
- Seroprevalence is highest in Japan, the Caribbean, equatorial Africa, and South America.
- Because most infected hosts are asymptomatic carriers, screening protocols are necessary to prevent further transmission and disease development.
- Time from infection to development of disease can be up to 60 years.
- Transmission is mostly via breastfeeding, sexual intercourse, drug use and blood transfusion.
- Important dermatologic manifestations include infective dermatitis and cutaneous manifestations of acute T-cell leukemia/lymphoma.
- HTLV-1–associated diseases often respond poorly to treatment.

Human T-lymphotropic virus-1 (HTLV-1) was the first retrovirus discovered. Currently, more than 20 million people are thought to be infected worldwide, with highest prevalence in southern Japan (up to 37%), but it also has been reported in equatorial Africa, the Caribbean (prevalence of 5% in Jamaica), and in virtually every country in South America.[245] In Brazil, more than 2.5 million people are infected.[246] Although 3 more related viruses also have been reported in Central Africa (HTLV-2, HTLV-3, and HTLV-4), only HTLV-1 has been definitively linked to human disease.[247]

HTLV-1 is transmitted from mother-to-child with 20% efficiency, primarily through breastfeeding, although 5% of transmissions occur in the intrauterine or perinatal period. Transmission also has been documented via sexual intercourse (most commonly from male to female partner), blood transfusion, and IV drug use. More recently, transmission also has been documented after organ transplantation.[246] IV transmission is considered to be the most efficient route of infection. The period of seroconversion can be up to 65 days. Although infection with HTLV-1 is persistent in human CD4+ lymphocytes, more than 90% of hosts remain asymptomatic carriers. It is unclear how infected individuals develop disease.[247] The rate of coinfection with HIV among HTLV-1 patients is not clear but is estimated to be approximately 12.5%. Interestingly, HTLV-1 coinfected HIV patients have been observed to exhibit higher CD4+ T-cell counts than matched HTLV-1–negative patients infected by HIV, but have clinically more advanced HIV disease at any given CD4+ T-cell count.[248]

CLINICAL FEATURES

The most significant dermatologic manifestations of HTLV-1 infection include infective dermatitis and cutaneous adult T-cell leukemia (ATL). Other dermatologic conditions have been noted in asymptomatic carriers, particularly atopic dermatitis, seborrheic dermatitis, crusted scabies, dermatophytosis, and ichthyosis. These dermatologic diseases are considered important in the future development of systemic manifestations of HTLV-1.

Infective dermatitis is most common in tropical areas of high HTLV-1 seroprevalence such as Jamaica and Brazil, often among patients with high HTLV-1 viral loads.[246,249] The disease resembles seborrheic dermatitis and presents as recalcitrant, relapsing eczematous dermatitis, and blepharoconjunctivitis, usually in children and adolescents. The scalp and neck, as well as intertriginous areas, are particularly involved. Periorbital papules with seborrheic scale may be commonly seen near the eyebrows as well as retroauricular fissuring in a minority of patients (Fig. 168-14). Patients may also develop rhinorrhea, bacterial pustulosis, and a high nasal carrier rate of *Staphylococcus* and *Streptococcus* spp. The resulting exudative discharge is often foul smelling. Infective dermatitis is associated with a marked TH1 response, and can be severely pruritic.[246,249]

ATL develops in less than 5% of infected hosts, but in its acute form carries a poor prognosis. ATL can present in 4 systemic subtypes, some with cutaneous manifestations. The acute systemic fulminant type can present dermatologically as infiltration of skin by neoplastic cells, most commonly as papules and nodules. The chronic and smoldering subtypes are less common and show lesions similar to mycosis fungoides (Fig. 168-15). Lesions may be papulosquamous and nodular, but erythrodermic variants also have been described. The fourth subtype is a systemic lymphomatous presentation. HTLV-1 can also cause a progressive myeloneuropathy called HTLV-1–associated myelopathy/tropical spastic paraparesis. Whereas ATL has been associated with infection via breastfeeding, HTLV-1–associated myelopathy/tropical spastic paraparesis has been associated with transmission via blood transfusions.[247]

DIAGNOSIS

Infective dermatitis is usually diagnosed with serologic confirmation of HTLV-1 in at-risk patients with clinical manifestations of the disease, such as recalcitrant eczema in endemic zones. Histopathology is rarely necessary, and when obtained, it is nonspecific. ATL is diagnosed mostly by showing anti–HTLV-1 antibodies in patient's serum, initially with enzyme-linked immunosorbent assay testing, but Western blot is often used for confirmation. Proviral DNA insertion can be shown via polymerase chain reaction testing. The presence of ATL cells (flower cells), which in skin may be CD25+ or CD25–, is also helpful.

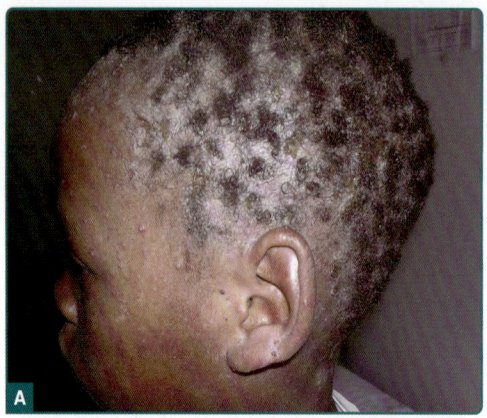
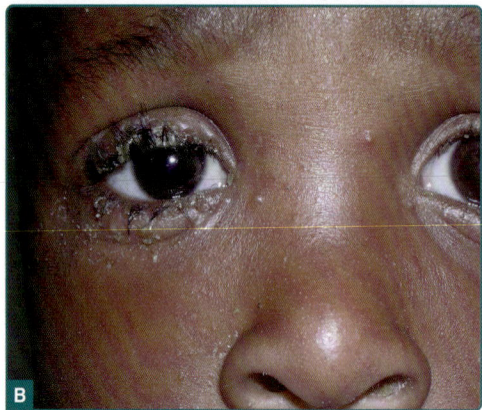
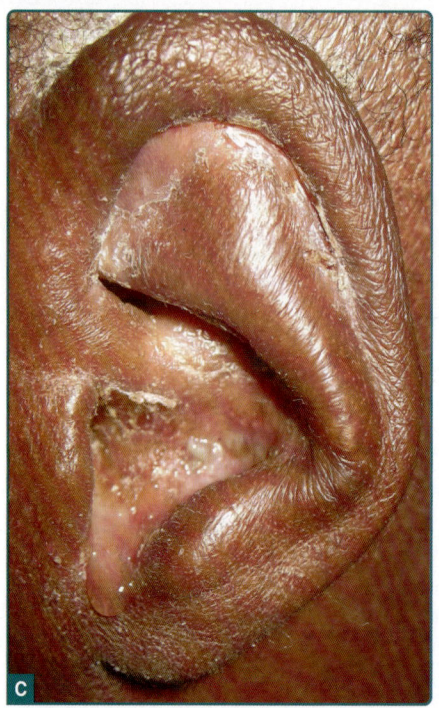

Figure 168-14 Infective dermatitis. **A,** Note atopic/seborrheic dermatitis-like eruption with notable areas of exudate and pyoderma, (**B**) blepharoconjunctivitis, and (**C**) retroauricular fissuring. (Images **A** and **B,** Used with permission from Dr. Anisa Mosam.)

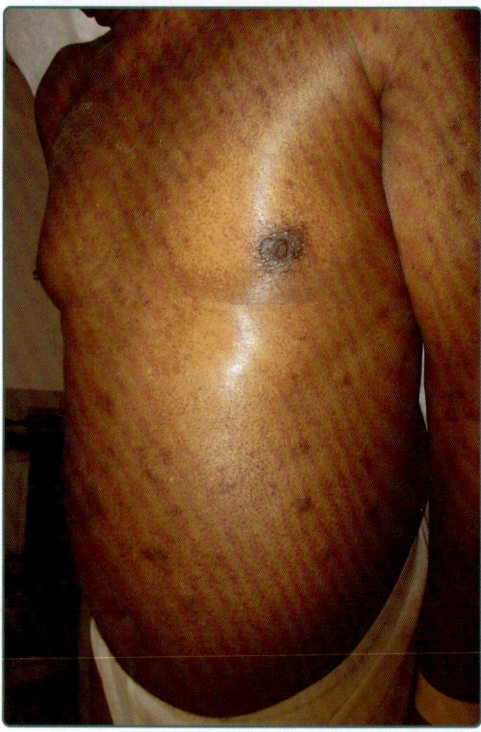

Figure 168-15 Cutaneous adult T-cell leukemia/lymphoma, smoldering type. Note the mixture of disseminated papules, plaques, and violaceous nodules in this patient from Jamaica. (Used with permission from Dr. Thomas Kupper and Maryanne Tawa, NP.)

DIFFERENTIAL DIAGNOSIS

The most important considerations in infective dermatitis include seborrheic dermatitis, atopic dermatitis, folliculitis, contact dermatitis, ichthyosis, xerosis, and impetigo. Cutaneous ATL involvement is histopathologically differentiated from other forms of cutaneous T-cell lymphoma, psoriasis, nummular eczema, and, in rare instances, infiltrative disease such as sarcoid.

CLINICAL COURSE, PROGNOSIS, AND MANAGEMENT

Infective dermatitis is often treated with antibiotics. The disease is not curable and is chronically relapsing. Trimethoprim-sulfamethoxazole is the agent of choice and treats symptomatic staphylococcal infection and improves the eczematous dermatitis. In fact, it is often used as a diagnostic maneuver when the disease is in question. High-potency topical steroids and immunomodulators have been used for symptomatic control.

Prognosis of ATL is very poor, particularly in the acute form, where resistance to multiple chemotherapeutic agents is rapidly demonstrated. Symptomatic control of cutaneous lesions in chronic and smoldering subtypes has been obtained with superpotent topical steroids, intralesional steroids and intralesional chemotherapy.

Because no vaccines are yet available for HTLV-1, screening programs are of paramount importance. In the case of HTLV-1 seropositivity, the use of cesarean section is recommended to prevent vertical transmission. Avoidance of breastfeeding and cross-feeding is also recommended, particularly if the serological status of the milk mother is unknown. Safe sexual intercourse methods are also recommended, as is counseling of IV drug users.[247]

REFERENCES

1. World Health Organization, 2016. Accessed August 29, 2016, at http://www.who.int/hiv/en/.
2. Centers for Disease Control and Prevention (CDC). HIV/AIDS: HIV Testing: Guidelines. http://www.cdc.gov/hiv/guidelines/testing.html
3. Campbell-Yesufu OT, Gandhi RT. Update on human immunodeficiency virus (HIV)-2 infection. *Clin Infect Dis*. 2010;52(6):780-787.
4. Fevrier M, Dorgham K, Rebollo A. CD4+ T cell depletion in human immunodeficiency (HIV) infection: role of apoptosis. *Viruses*. 2011;3(5):586-612.
5. Cohen MS, Shaw GM, McMichael AJ, et al. Acute HIV-1 infection. *N Engl J Med*. 2011;364:1943-1954.
6. Macneal RJ, Dinulos JG. Acute retroviral syndrome. *Dermatol Clin*. 2006;24:431-438, v.
7. Vanhems P, Dassa C, Lambert J, et al. Comprehensive classification of symptoms and signs reported among 218 patients with acute HIV-1 infection. *J Acquir Immune Defic Syndr*. 1999;21:99-106.
8. Quinn TC, Wawer MJ, Sewankambo N, et al. Viral load and heterosexual transmission of human immunodeficiency virus type 1. Rakai Project Study Group. *N Engl J Med*. 2000;342:921-929.
9. Hall HI, An Q, Tang T, et al. Prevalence of diagnosed and undiagnosed HIV infection—United States, 2008-2012. *MMWR Morb Mortal Wkly Rep*. 2015;64:657-662.
10. Kahn JO, Walker BD. Acute human immunodeficiency virus type 1 infection. *N Engl J Med*. 1998;339:33-39.
11. Rosenberg ES, Caliendo AM, Walker BD. Acute HIV infection among patients tested for mononucleosis. *N Engl J Med*. 1999;340:969.
12. Kahn JO, Walker BD. Acute human immunodeficiency virus type 1 infection. *N Engl J Med*. 1998;339(1):33-39.
13. Rosenberg ES, Caliendo AM, Walker BD. Acute HIV infection among patients tested for mononucleosis. *N Engl J Med*. 1999;340(12):969.
14. Centers for Disease Control and Prevention (CDC). About HIV/AIDS. http://www.cdc.gov/hiv/basics/whatishiv.html. Accessed August 29, 2016.
15. Eholie SP, Badje A, Kouame GM, et al. Antiretroviral treatment regardless of CD4 count: the universal answer to a contextual question. *AIDS Res Ther*. 2016;(13):27.
16. Roujeau JC, Stern RS. Severe adverse cutaneous reactions to drugs. *N Engl J Med*. 1994;331:1272-1285.
17. Smith KJ, Skelton HG, Yeager J, et al. Increased drug reactions in HIV-1-positive patients: a possible explanation based on patterns of immune dysregulation seen in HIV-1 disease. The Military Medical Consortium for the Advancement of Retroviral Research (MMCARR). *Clin Exp Dermatol*. 1997;22(3):118-123.
18. Levine D, Ananthakrishnan S, Garg A. Iatrogenic Cushing syndrome after a single intramuscular corticosteroid injection and concomitant protease inhibitor therapy. *J Am Acad Dermatol*. 2011;65(4):877.
19. Tempark T, Phatarakijnirund V, Chatproedprai S, et al. Exogenous Cushing's syndrome due to topical corticosteroid application: case report and review literature. *Endocrine*. 2010;38:328-334.
20. Coopman SA, Johnson RA, Platt R, et al. Cutaneous disease and drug reactions in HIV infection. *N Engl J Med*. 1993;328(23):1670-1674.
21. Saiag P, Caumes E, Chosidow O, et al. Drug-induced toxic epidermal necrolysis (Lyell syndrome) in patients infected with the human immunodeficiency virus. *J Am Acad Dermatol*. 1992;26(4):567-574.
22. Miller J, Carr A, Emery S, et al. HIV lipodystrophy: prevalence, severity and correlates of risk in Australia. *HIV Med*. 2003;4(3):293-301.
23. Eliaszewicz M, Flahault A, Roujeau JC, et al. Prospective evaluation of risk factors of cutaneous drug reactions to sulfonamides in patients with AIDS. *J Am Acad Dermatol*. 2002;47(1):40-46.
24. Yang C, Mosam A, Mankahala A, et al. HIV Infection predisposes skin to toxic epidermal necrolysis via depletion of skin-directed CD4+ cells. *J Am Acad Dermatol*. 2014;70(6):1096-1102.
25. Garcia-Doval I, LeCleach L, Bocquet H, et al. Toxic epidermal necrolysis and Stevens-Johnson syndrome: does early withdrawal of causative drugs decrease the risk of death? *Arch Dermatol*. 2010;136(3):323-327.
26. Romagosa R, Kapoor S, Sanders J, et al. Inpatient adverse cutaneous drug eruptions and eosinophilia. *Arch Dermatol*. 2001;137(4):511-512.
27. Yoshizawa S, Yasuoka A, Kikuchi Y, et al. A 5-day course of oral desensitization to trimethoprim/sulfamethoxazole (T/S) in patients with human immunodeficiency virus type-1 infection who were previously intolerant to T/S. *Ann Allergy Asthma Immunol*. 2000;85(3):241-244.
28. Dodiuk-Gad RP, Olteanu C, Jeschke MG, et al. Treatment of toxic epidermal necrolysis in North America. *J Am Acad Dermatol*. 2015;73(5):876-877.
29. Carr A, Workman C, Smith DE, et al. Abacavir substitution for nucleoside analogs in patients with HIV lipoatrophy: a randomized trial. *JAMA*. 2002;288(2):207-215.
30. Tebas P, Zhang J, Yarasheski K, et al. Switching to a protease inhibitor-containing, nucleoside-sparing regimen (lopinavir/ritonavir plus efavirenz) increases limb fat but raises serum lipid levels: results of a prospective randomized trial (AIDS clinical trial group 5125s). *J Acquir Immune Defic Syndr*. 2007;45(2):193-200.
31. Silvers SL, Eviatar JA, Echavez MI, et al. Prospective, open-label, 18-month trial of calcium hydroxylapatite (Radiesse) for facial soft-tissue augmentation in patients with human immunodeficiency virus-associated lipoatrophy: one-year durability. *Plast Reconstr Surg*. 2006;118:34S-45S.
32. Hall LD, Eminger LA, Hesterman KS, et al. Epstein-Barr virus: dermatologic associations and implications: part I. Mucocutaneous manifestations of Epstein-Barr virus and nonmalignant disorders. *J Am Acad Dermatol*. 2015;72:1-19; quiz 19-20.
33. Lozada-Nur F, Costa C. Retrospective findings of the clinical benefits of podophyllum resin 25% sol on hairy leukoplakia. Clinical results in nine patients. *Oral Surg Oral Med Oral Pathol*. 1992;73:555-558.

34. Moura MD, Guimaraes TR, Fonseca LM, et al. A random clinical trial study to assess the efficiency of topical applications of podophyllin resin (25%) versus podophyllin resin (25%) together with acyclovir cream (5%) in the treatment of oral hairy leukoplakia. *Oral Surg Oral Med Oral Pathol Oral Radiol Endod.* 2007;103:64-71.
35. Bhandarkar SS, MacKelfresh J, Fried L, et al. Targeted therapy of oral hairy leukoplakia with gentian violet. *J Am Acad Dermatol.* 2008;58:711-712.
36. Goh BT, Lau RK. Treatment of AIDS-associated oral hairy leukoplakia with cryotherapy. *J Infect Dis.* 1994;5:60-62.
37. Eminger LA, Hall LD, Hesterman KS, et al. Epstein-Barr virus: dermatologic associations and implications: part II. Associated lymphoproliferative disorders and solid tumors. *J Am Acad Dermatol.* 2015;72:21-34; quiz 35-36.
38. Tetzlaff MT, Nosek C, Kovarik CL. Epstein-Barr virus-associated leiomyosarcoma with cutaneous involvement in an African child with human immunodeficiency virus: a case report and review of the literature. *J Cutan Pathol.* 2011;38:731-739.
39. Jung AC, Paauw DS. Diagnosing HIV-related disease: using the CD4 count as a guide. *J Gen Intern Med.* 1998;13:131-136.
40. Forrestel AK, Naujokas A, Martin JN, et al. Bacillary angiomatosis masquerading as Kaposi's sarcoma in East Africa. *J Int Assoc Provid AIDS Care.* 2015;14:21-25.
41. Schwartz RA, Nychay SG, Janniger CK, et al. Bacillary angiomatosis: presentation of six patients, some with unusual features. *Br J Dermatol.* 1997;136:60-65.
42. Plettenberg A, Lorenzen T, Burtsche BT, et al. Bacillary angiomatosis in HIV-infected patients—an epidemiological and clinical study. *Dermatology.* 2000;201:326-331.
43. Perkocha LA, Geaghan SM, Yen TS, et al. Clinical and pathological features of bacillary peliosis hepatis in association with human immunodeficiency virus infection. *N Engl J Med.* 1990;323:1581-1586.
44. Stevens DL, Bisno AL, Chambers HF, et al. Practice guidelines for the diagnosis and management of skin and soft tissue infections: 2014 update by the Infectious Diseases Society of America. *Clin Infect Dis.* 2014;59:e10-e52.
45. Chang CC, Crane M, Zhou J, et al. HIV and co-infections. *Immunol Rev.* 2013;254:114-142.
46. Santos JB, Figueiredo AR, Ferraz CE, et al. Cutaneous tuberculosis: epidemiologic, etiopathogenic and clinical aspects-part I. *An Bras Dermatol.* 2014;89:219-228.
47. Regnier S, Ouagari Z, Perez ZL, et al. Cutaneous miliary resistant tuberculosis in a patient infected with human immunodeficiency virus: case report and literature review. *Clin Exp Dermatol.* 2009;34:e690-e692.
48. High WA, Evans CC, Hoang MP. Cutaneous miliary tuberculosis in two patients with HIV infection. *J Am Acad Dermatol.* 2004;50:S110-S113.
49. Libraty DH, Byrd TF. Cutaneous miliary tuberculosis in the AIDS era: case report and review. *Clin Infect Dis.* 1996;23:706-710.
50. Endly DC, Ackerman LS. Disseminated cutaneous mycobacterium avium complex in a person with AIDS. *Dermatol Online J.* 2014;20:22616.
51. Pires CA, Juca Neto FO, de Albuquerque NC, et al. Leprosy reactions in patients coinfected with HIV: clinical aspects and outcomes in two comparative cohorts in the Amazon region, Brazil. *PLoS Negl Trop Dis.* 2015;9:e0003818.
52. Talhari C, Mira MT, Massone C, et al. Leprosy and HIV coinfection: a clinical, pathological, immunological, and therapeutic study of a cohort from a Brazilian referral center for infectious diseases. *J Infect Dis.* 2010;202:345-354.
53. Murakawa GJ, Kerschmann R, Berger T. Cutaneous *Cryptococcus* infection and AIDS. Report of 12 cases and review of the literature. *Arch Dermatol.* 1996;132:545-548.
54. Nnoruka EN, Chukwuka JC, Anisuiba B. Correlation of mucocutaneous manifestations of HIV/AIDS infection with CD4 counts and disease progression. *Int J Dermatol.* 2007;46(suppl 2):14-18.
55. Warkentien T, Crum-Cianflone NF. An update on *Cryptococcus* among HIV-infected patients. *Int J STD AIDS.* 2010;21:679-684.
56. Supparatpinyo K, Khamwan C, Baosoung V, et al. Disseminated *Penicillium marneffei* infection in southeast Asia. *Lancet.* 1994;344:110-113.
57. Duong TA. Infection due to *Penicillium marneffei*, an emerging pathogen: review of 155 reported cases. *Clin Infect Dis.* 1996;23:125-130.
58. Angius AG, Viviani MA, Muratori S, et al. Disseminated histoplasmosis presenting with cutaneous lesions in a patient with acquired immunodeficiency syndrome. *J Eur Acad Dermatol Venereol.* 1998;10:182-185.
59. Laochumroonvorapong P, DiCostanzo DP, Wu H, et al. Disseminated histoplasmosis presenting as pyoderma gangrenosum-like lesions in a patient with acquired immunodeficiency syndrome. *Int J Dermatol.* 2001;40:518-521.
60. Ramos-e-Silva M, Lima CM, Schechtman RC, et al. Systemic mycoses in immunodepressed patients (AIDS). *Clin Dermatol.* 2012;30:616-627.
61. Crum-Cianflone N, Hullsiek KH, Satter E, et al. Cutaneous malignancies among HIV-infected persons. *Arch Intern Med.* 2009;169:1130-1138.
62. Larsson M, Nguyen LH, Wertheim HF, et al. Clinical characteristics and outcome of Penicillium marneffei infection among HIV-infected patients in northern Vietnam. *AIDS Res Ther.* 2012;9:24.
63. Antinori S. New insights into HIV/AIDS-associated cryptococcosis. *ISRN AIDS.* 2013;2013:471363.
64. Perfect JR, Dismukes WE, Dromer F, et al. Clinical practice guidelines for the management of cryptococcal disease:2010 update by the infectious diseases society of America. *Clin Infect Dis.* 2010;50:291-322.
65. Guarner J, Brandt ME. Histopathologic diagnosis of fungal infections in the 21st century. *Clin Microbiol Rev.* 2011;24:247-280.
66. Loulergue P, Bastides F, Baudouin V, et al. Literature review and case histories of *Histoplasma capsulatum* var. *duboisii* infections in HIV-infected patients. *Emerg Infect Dis.* 2007;13:1647-1652.
67. Supparatpinyo K, Perriens J, Nelson KE, et al. A controlled trial of itraconazole to prevent relapse of *Penicillium marneffei* infection in patients infected with the human immunodeficiency virus. *N Engl J Med.* 1998;339:1739-1743.
68. Laskaris G, Hadjivassiliou M, Stratigos J. Oral signs and symptoms in 160 Greek HIV-infected patients. *J Oral Pathol Med.* 1992;21:120-123.
69. Duerr A, Sierra MF, Feldman J, et al. Immune compromise and prevalence of *Candida* vulvovaginitis in human immunodeficiency virus-infected women. *Obstet Gynecol.* 1997;90:252-256.
70. Prose NS. HIV infection in children. *J Am Acad Dermatol.* 1990;22:1223-1231.

71. Gupta AK, Daigle D, Foley KA. The prevalence of culture-confirmed toenail onychomycosis in at-risk patient populations. *J Eur Acad Dermatol Venereol.* 2015;29:1039-1044.
72. Surjushe A, Kamath R, Oberai C, et al. A clinical and mycological study of onychomycosis in HIV infection. *Indian J Dermatol Venereol Leprol.* 2007;73:397-401.
73. Johnson RA. Dermatophyte infections in human immune deficiency virus (HIV) disease. *J Am Acad Dermatol.* 2000;43:S135-S142.
74. Moreno-Coutino G, Arenas R, Reyes-Teran G. Improvement in onychomycosis after initiation of combined antiretroviral therapy. *Int J Dermatol.* 2013;52:311-313.
75. Aly R, Berger T. Common superficial fungal infections in patients with AIDS. *Clin Infect Dis.* 1996;22(suppl 2):S128-S132.
76. Di Silverio A, Brazzelli V, Brandozzi G, et al. Prevalence of dermatophytes and yeasts (*Candida* spp., *Malassezia furfur*) in HIV patients. A study of former drug addicts. *Mycopathologia.* 1991;114:103-107.
77. Koopman RJ, van Merrienboer FC, Vreden SG, et al. Molluscum contagiosum; a marker for advanced HIV infection. *Br J Dermatol.* 1992;126:528-529.
78. Hicks CB, Myers SA, Giner J. Resolution of intractable molluscum contagiosum in a human immunodeficiency virus-infected patient after institution of antiretroviral therapy with ritonavir. *Clin Infect Dis.* 1997;24:1023-1025.
79. Sen S, Bhaumik P. Resolution of giant molluscum contagiosum with antiretroviral therapy. *Indian J Dermatol Venereol Leprol.* 2008;74:267-268.
80. Drain PK, Mosam A, Gounder L, et al. Recurrent giant molluscum contagiosum immune reconstitution inflammatory syndrome (IRIS) after initiation of antiretroviral therapy in an HIV-infected man. *Int J STD AIDS.* 2014;25:235-238.
81. Strauss RM, Doyle EL, Mohsen AH, et al. Successful treatment of molluscum contagiosum with topical imiquimod in a severely immunocompromised HIV-positive patient. *Int J STD AIDS.* 2001;12:264-266.
82. Buckley R, Smith K. Topical imiquimod therapy for chronic giant molluscum contagiosum in a patient with advanced human immunodeficiency virus 1 disease. *Arch Dermatol.* 1999;135:1167-1169.
83. Toro JR, Wood LV, Patel NK, et al. Topical cidofovir: a novel treatment for recalcitrant molluscum contagiosum in children infected with human immunodeficiency virus 1. *Arch Dermatol.* 2000;136:983-985.
84. Calista D. Topical cidofovir for severe cutaneous human papillomavirus and molluscum contagiosum infections in patients with HIV/AIDS. A pilot study. *J Eur Acad Dermatol Venereol.* 2000;14:484-488.
85. Thappa DM, Karthikeyan K. Exaggerated scabies: a marker of HIV infection. *Indian Pediatr.* 2002;39:875-876.
86. Roberts LJ, Huffam SE, Walton SF, et al. Crusted scabies: clinical and immunological findings in seventy-eight patients and a review of the literature. *J Infect.* 2005;50:375-381.
87. Hengge UR, Currie BJ, Jager G, et al. Scabies: a ubiquitous neglected skin disease. *Lancet Infect Dis.* 2006;6:769-779.
88. Currie BJ, McCarthy JS. Permethrin and ivermectin for scabies. *N Engl J Med.* 2010;362:717-725.
89. Okwor I, Uzonna JE. The immunology of Leishmania/HIV co-infection. *Immunol Res.* 2013;56:163-171.
90. Alvar J, Aparicio P, Aseffa A, et al. The relationship between leishmaniasis and AIDS: the second 10 years. *Clin Microbiol Rev.* 2008;21:334-359.
91. Couppie P, Clyti E, Sobesky M, et al. Comparative study of cutaneous leishmaniasis in human immunodeficiency virus (HIV)-infected patients and non-HIV-infected patients in French Guiana. *Br J Dermatol.* 2004;151:1165-1171.
92. Lindoso JA, Barbosa RN, Posada-Vergara MP, et al. Unusual manifestations of tegumentary leishmaniasis in AIDS patients from the New World. *Br J Dermatol.* 2009;160:311-318.
93. Nguyen MH, Kauffman CA, Goodman RP, et al. Nasal carriage of and infection with *Staphylococcus aureus* in HIV-infected patients. *Ann Intern Med.* 1999;130:221-225.
94. Ganesh R, Castle D, McGibbon D, et al. Staphylococcal carriage and HIV infection. *Lancet.* 1989;2:558.
95. Shet A, Mathema B, Mediavilla JR, et al. Colonization and subsequent skin and soft tissue infection due to methicillin-resistant *Staphylococcus aureus* in a cohort of otherwise healthy adults infected with HIV type 1. *J Infect Dis.* 2009;200:88-93.
96. Popovich KJ, Weinstein RA, Aroutcheva A, et al. Community-associated methicillin-resistant *Staphylococcus aureus* and HIV: intersecting epidemics. *Clin Infect Dis.* 2010;50:979-987.
97. Graber CJ, Jacobson MA, Perdreau-Remington F, et al. Recurrence of skin and soft tissue infection caused by methicillin-resistant *Staphylococcus aureus* in a HIV primary care clinic. *J Acquir Immune Defic Syndr.* 2008;49:231-233.
98. From the Centers for Disease Control and Prevention. 1993 revised classification system for HIV infection and expanded surveillance case definition for AIDS among adolescents and adults. *JAMA.* 1993;269:729-730.
99. Patel AB, Rosen T. Herpes vegetans as a sign of HIV infection. *Dermatol Online J.* 2008;14:6.
100. Gilbert J, Drehs MM, Weinberg JM. Topical imiquimod for acyclovir-unresponsive herpes simplex virus 2 infection. *Arch Dermatol.* 2001;137:1015-1017.
101. Lalezari J, Schacker T, Feinberg J, et al. A randomized, double-blind, placebo-controlled trial of cidofovir gel for the treatment of acyclovir-unresponsive mucocutaneous herpes simplex virus infection in patients with AIDS. *J Infect Dis.* 1997;176:892-898.
102. Wanat KA, Gormley RH, Rosenbach M, et al. Intralesional cidofovir for treating extensive genital verrucous herpes simplex virus infection. *JAMA Dermatol.* 2013;149:881-883.
103. Barnabas RV, Celum C. Infectious co-factors in HIV-1 transmission herpes simplex virus type-2 and HIV-1: new insights and interventions. *Curr HIV Res.* 2012;10:228-237.
104. Onunu AN, Uhunmwangho A. Clinical spectrum of herpes zoster in HIV-infected versus non-HIV infected patients in Benin City, Nigeria. *West Afr J Med.* 2004;23:300-304.
105. Nikkels AF, Snoeck R, Rentier B, et al. Chronic verrucous varicella zoster virus skin lesions: clinical, histological, molecular and therapeutic aspects. *Clin Exp Dermatol.* 1999;24:346-353.
106. Gilson IH, Barnett JH, Conant MA, et al. Disseminated ecthymatous herpes varicella-zoster virus infection in patients with acquired immunodeficiency syndrome. *J Am Acad Dermatol.* 1989;20:637-642.

107. Lokke Jensen B, Weismann K, Mathiesen L, et al. Atypical varicella-zoster infection in AIDS. *Acta Derm Venereol.* 1993;73:123-125.
108. Blank LJ, Polydefkis MJ, Moore RD, et al. Herpes zoster among persons living with HIV in the current antiretroviral therapy era. *J Acquir Immune Defic Syndr.* 2012;61:203-207.
109. Gebo KA, Kalyani R, Moore RD, et al. The incidence of, risk factors for, and sequelae of herpes zoster among HIV patients in the highly active antiretroviral therapy era. *J Acquir Immune Defic Syndr.* 2005;40:169-174.
110. Grabar S, Tattevin P, Selinger-Leneman H, et al. Incidence of herpes zoster in HIV-infected adults in the combined antiretroviral therapy era: results from the FHDH-ANRS CO4 cohort. *Clin Infect Dis.* 2015;60:1269-1277.
111. Wood SM, Shah SS, Steenhoff AP, et al. Primary varicella and herpes zoster among HIV-infected children from 1989 to 2006. *Pediatrics.* 2008;121:e150-e156.
112. Shearer K, Maskew M, Ajayi T, et al. Incidence and predictors of herpes zoster among antiretroviral therapy-naive patients initiating HIV treatment in Johannesburg, South Africa. *Int J Infect Dis.* 2014;23:56-62.
113. Shafran SD. Live attenuated herpes zoster vaccine for HIV-infected adults. *HIV Med.* 2016;17:305-310.
114. Weinberg A, Levin MJ, Macgregor RR. Safety and immunogenicity of a live attenuated varicella vaccine in VZV-seropositive HIV-infected adults. *Hum Vaccin.* 2010;6:318-321.
115. Barnabas RV, Baeten JM, Lingappa JR, et al. Acyclovir prophylaxis reduces the incidence of herpes zoster among HIV-infected individuals: results of a randomized clinical trial. *J Infect Dis.* 2016;213:551-555.
116. Bernhard P, Obel N. Chronic ulcerating acyclovir-resistant varicella zoster lesions in an AIDS patient. *Scand J Infect Dis.* 1995;27:623-625.
117. Saint-Leger E, Caumes E, Breton G, et al. Clinical and virologic characterization of acyclovir-resistant varicella-zoster viruses isolated from 11 patients with acquired immunodeficiency syndrome. *Clin Infect Dis.* 2001;33:2061-2067.
118. Greenspan D, Canchola AJ, MacPhail LA, et al. Effect of highly active antiretroviral therapy on frequency of oral warts. *Lancet.* 2001;357:1411-1412.
119. Meys R, Gotch FM, Bunker CB. Human papillomavirus in the era of highly active antiretroviral therapy for human immunodeficiency virus: an immune reconstitution-associated disease? *Br J Dermatol.* 2010;162:6-11.
120. Maurer T, Rodrigues LK, Ameli N, et al. The effect of highly active antiretroviral therapy on dermatologic disease in a longitudinal study of HIV type 1-infected women. *Clin Infect Dis.* 2004;38:579-584.
121. Palefsky J. Human papillomavirus infection in HIV-infected persons. *Top HIV Med.* 2007;15:130-133.
122. Kojic EM, Cu-Uvin S. Update: human papillomavirus infection remains highly prevalent and persistent among HIV-infected individuals. *Curr Opin Oncol.* 2007;19:464-469.
123. Palefsky JM, Holly EA, Efirdc JT, et al. Anal intraepithelial neoplasia in the highly active antiretroviral therapy era among HIV-positive men who have sex with men. *AIDS.* 2005;19:1407-1414.
124. Gormley RH, Kovarik CL. Dermatologic manifestations of HPV in HIV-infected individuals. *Curr HIV/AIDS Rep.* 2009;6:130-138.
125. Lissouba P, Van de Perre P, Auvert B. Association of genital human papillomavirus infection with HIV acquisition: a systematic review and meta-analysis. *Sex Transm Infect.* 2013;89:350-356.
126. Spach DH, Colven R. Resolution of recalcitrant hand warts in an HIV-infected patient treated with potent antiretroviral therapy. *J Am Acad Dermatol.* 1999;40:818-821.
127. Roark TR, Pandya AG. Combination therapy of resistant warts in a patient with AIDS. *Dermatol Surg.* 1998;24:1387-1389.
128. Cusini M, Salmaso F, Zerboni R, et al. 5% Imiquimod cream for external anogenital warts in HIV-infected patients under HAART therapy. *Int J STD AIDS.* 2004;15:17-20.
129. Gilson RJ, Shupack JL, Friedman-Kien AE, et al. A randomized, controlled, safety study using imiquimod for the topical treatment of anogenital warts in HIV-infected patients. Imiquimod Study Group. *AIDS.* 1999;13:2397-2404.
130. Juschka U, Hartmann M. Topical treatment of common warts in an HIV-positive patient with imiquimod 5% cream. *Clin Exp Dermatol.* 2003;28(suppl 1):48-50.
131. Kreuter A, Potthoff A, Brockmeyer NH, et al. Imiquimod leads to a decrease of human papillomavirus DNA and to a sustained clearance of anal intraepithelial neoplasia in HIV-infected men. *J Invest Dermatol.* 2008;128:2078-2083.
132. Saiag P, Bauhofer A, Bouscarat F, et al. Imiquimod 5% cream for external genital or perianal warts in human immunodeficiency virus-positive patients treated with highly active antiretroviral therapy: an open-label, noncomparative study. *Br J Dermatol.* 2009;161:904-909.
133. Walzman M. Successful treatment of profuse recalcitrant extra-genital warts in an HIV-positive patient using 5% imiquimod cream. *Int J STD AIDS.* 2009;20:657-658.
134. Wong A, Crawford RI. Intralesional *Candida* antigen for common warts in people with HIV. *J Cutan Med Surg.* 2013;17:313-315.
135. Kilewo CD, Urassa WK, Pallangyo K, et al. Response to podophyllotoxin treatment of genital warts in relation to HIV-1 infection among patients in Dar es Salaam, Tanzania. *Int J STD AIDS.* 1995;6:114-116.
136. Matteelli A, Beltrame A, Graifemberghi S, et al. Efficacy and tolerability of topical 1% cidofovir cream for the treatment of external anogenital warts in HIV-infected persons. *Sex Transm Dis.* 2001;28:343-346.
137. Orlando G, Fasolo MM, Beretta R, et al. Combined surgery and cidofovir is an effective treatment for genital warts in HIV-infected patients. *AIDS.* 2002;16:447-450.
138. Orlando G, Fasolo MM, Beretta R, et al. Intralesional or topical cidofovir (HPMPC, VISTIDE) for the treatment of recurrent genital warts in HIV-1-infected patients. *AIDS.* 1999;13:1978-1980.
139. Shah M, Murphy M, Price JD, et al. Intralesional bleomycin for the treatment of non-genital warts in HIV-infected patients. *Acta Derm Venereol.* 1996;76:81-82.
140. Frega A, di Renzi F, Stentella P, et al. Management of human papilloma virus vulvo-perineal infection with systemic beta-interferon and thymostimulin in HIV-positive patients. *Int J Gynaecol Obstet.* 1994;44:255-258.

141. Lozada-Nur F, Glick M, Schubert M, et al. Use of intralesional interferon-alpha for the treatment of recalcitrant oral warts in patients with AIDS: a report of 4 cases. *Oral Surg Oral Med Oral Pathol Oral Radiol Endod.* 2001;92:617-622.
142. Xu J, Xiang L, Chen J, et al. The combination treatment using CO(2) laser and photodynamic therapy for HIV seropositive men with intraanal warts. *Photodiagnosis Photodyn Ther.* 2013;10:186-193.
143. Moore RL, de Schaetzen V, Joseph M, et al. Acquired epidermodysplasia verruciformis syndrome in HIV-infected pediatric patients: prospective treatment trial with topical glycolic acid and human papillomavirus genotype characterization. *Arch Dermatol.* 2012;148:128-130.
144. Javelle E, Lightburne E, Dukan P, et al. Human immunodeficiency virus (HIV)-associated epidermodysplasia verruciformis eradicated after interferon-alpha and ribavirin treatment. *Int J Dermatol.* 2014;53:487-489.
145. Haas N, Fuchs PG, Hermes B, et al. Remission of epidermodysplasia verruciformis-like skin eruption after highly active antiretroviral therapy in a human immunodeficiency virus-positive patient. *Br J Dermatol.* 2001;145:669-670.
146. Darwich E, Darwich L, Canadas MP, et al. New human papillomavirus (HPV) types involved in epidermodysplasia verruciformis (EV) in 3 HIV-infected patients: response to topical cidofovir. *J Am Acad Dermatol.* 2011;65:e43-e45.
147. Lee KC, Risser J, Bercovitch L. What is the evidence for effective treatments of acquired epidermodysplasia verruciformis in HIV-infected patients? *Arch Dermatol.* 2010;146:903-905.
148. Stevenson J, Heath M. Syphilis and HIV infection: an update. *Dermatol Clin.* 2006;24:497-507, vi.
149. Centers for Disease Control and Prevention (CDC). Symptomatic early neurosyphilis among HIV-positive men who have sex with men—four cities, United States, January 2002-June 2004. *MMWR Morb Mortal Wkly Rep.* 2007;56:625-628.
150. Kassutto S, Sax PE. HIV and syphilis coinfection: trends and interactions. *AIDS Clin Care.* 2003;15:9-15.
151. Workowski KA, Bolan GA; Centers for Disease Control and Prevention. Sexually transmitted diseases treatment guidelines, 2015. *MMWR Recomm Rep.* 2015;64(RR-03):1-137.
152. Jurado RL, Campbell J, Martin PD. Prozone phenomenon in secondary syphilis. Has its time arrived? *Arch Intern Med.* 1993;153:2496-2498.
153. Kingston AA, Vujevich J, Shapiro M, et al. Seronegative secondary syphilis in 2 patients coinfected with human immunodeficiency virus. *Arch Dermatol.* 2005;141:431-433.
154. Kofoed K, Gerstoft J, Mathiesen LR, et al. Syphilis and human immunodeficiency virus (HIV)-1 coinfection: influence on CD4 T-cell count, HIV-1 viral load, and treatment response. *Sex Transm Dis.* 2006;33:143-148.
155. Centers for Disease Control (CDC). Kaposi's sarcoma and Pneumocystis pneumonia among homosexual men—New York City and California. *MMWR Morb Mortal Wkly Rep.* 1981;30:305-308.
156. Semeere AS, Busakhala N, Martin JN. Impact of antiretroviral therapy on the incidence of Kaposi's sarcoma in resource-rich and resource-limited settings. *Curr Opin Oncol.* 2012;24:522-530.
157. Lodi S, Guiguet M, Costagliola D, et al. Kaposi sarcoma incidence and survival among HIV-infected homosexual men after HIV seroconversion. *J Natl Cancer Inst.* 2010;102:784-792.
158. Clifford GM, Polesel J, Rickenbach M, et al. Cancer risk in the Swiss HIV Cohort Study: associations with immunodeficiency, smoking, and highly active antiretroviral therapy. *J Natl Cancer Inst.* 2005;97:425-432.
159. Rohner E, Valeri F, Maskew M, et al. Incidence rate of Kaposi sarcoma in HIV-infected patients on antiretroviral therapy in Southern Africa: a prospective multicohort study. *J Acquir Immune Defic Syndr.* 2014;67:547-554.
160. Semeere A, Wenger M, Busakhala N, et al. A prospective ascertainment of cancer incidence in sub-Saharan Africa: the case of Kaposi sarcoma. *Cancer Med.* 2016;5:914-928.
161. Howlader N, Noone AM, Krapcho M, et al, eds. SEER Cancer Statistics Review, 1975-2011. Bethesda, MD: National Cancer Institute; 2014. https://seer.cancer.gov/csr/1975_2011/
162. Maurer T, Ponte M, Leslie K. HIV-associated Kaposi's sarcoma with a high CD4 count and a low viral load. *N Engl J Med.* 2007;357:1352-1353.
163. Amerson E BN, Buziba, N, Wabinga H, et al. Diagnosing Kaposi's Sarcoma (KS) in East Africa: how accurate are clinicians and pathologists? *Infect Agent Cancer.* 2012;7(suppl 1):P6.
164. Semeere AS, Freeman EE, Wenger M, et al. A more representative and less biased approach to estimating mortality after diagnosis of Kaposi's sarcoma among HIV-infected adults in sub-Saharan Africa in the era of antiretroviral therapy. Paper presented at: 15th International Conference on Malignancies in AIDS and Other Acquired Immunodeficiencies; October 26-27, 2015; Bethesda, MD.
165. Chu KM, Mahlangeni G, Swannet S, et al. Determinants of mortality and disease progression of Kaposi's sarcoma in the ART programme of Khayelitsha, South Africa. Paper presented at: 16th Conference on Retroviruses and Opportunistic Infections; 2009; Montreal, Canada.
166. Uldrick TS, Mosam A, Shaik F, et al. Prognosis of patients with AIDS-associated Kaposi's sarcoma receiving antiretroviral therapy +/− chemotherapy in Kwazulu-Natal, South Africa: an analysis of 1-yr survival data from NCT00380770. Paper presented at: 11th International Conference on Malignancies in AIDS and Other Acquired Immunodeficiencies; 2008; Bethesda, MD.
167. Krown SE, Metroka C, Wernz JC. Kaposi's sarcoma in the acquired immune deficiency syndrome: a proposal for uniform evaluation, response, and staging criteria. AIDS Clinical Trials Group Oncology Committee. *J Clin Oncol.* 1989;7:1201-1207.
168. World Health Organization. *Guidelines on the Treatment of Skin and Oral HIV-Associated Conditions in Children and Adults.* Geneva, Switzerland: World Health Organization;2014.Availableat:http://apps.who.int/iris/bitstream/handle/10665/136863/9789241548915_eng.pdf;jsessionid=AB011C11883345F328CD821A271B8608?sequence=1
169. Swift PS. The role of radiation therapy in the management of HIV-related Kaposi's sarcoma. *Hematol Oncol Clin North Am.* 1996;10:1069-1080.
170. Brambilla L, Boneschi V, Beretta G, et al. Intralesional chemotherapy for Kaposi's sarcoma. *Dermatologica.* 1984;169:150-155.

171. Brambilla L, Bellinvia M, Tourlaki A, et al. Intralesional vincristine as first-line therapy for nodular lesions in classic Kaposi sarcoma: a prospective study in 151 patients. *Br J Dermatol*. 2010;162:854-859.
172. Flaitz CM, Nichols CM, Hicks MJ. Role of intralesional vinblastine administration in treatment of intraoral Kaposi's sarcoma in AIDS. *Eur J Cancer B Oral Oncol*. 1995;31B:280-285.
173. Rosen T. Limited extent AIDS-related cutaneous Kaposi's sarcoma responsive to imiquimod 5% cream. *Int J Dermatol*. 2006;45:854-856.
174. Bodsworth NJ, Bloch M, Bower M, et al; International Panretin Gel KS Study Group. Phase III vehicle-controlled, multi-centered study of topical alitretinoin gel 0.1% in cutaneous AIDS-related Kaposi's sarcoma. *Am J Clin Dermatol*. 2001;2:77-87.
175. Goldstone S, Palefsky JM, Giuliano AR, et al. Prevalence of and risk factors for human papillomavirus (HPV) infection among HIV-seronegative men who have sex with men. *J Infect Dis*. 2011;203:66-74.
176. Chin-Hong PV, Vittinghoff E, Cranston RD, et al. Age-specific prevalence of anal human papillomavirus infection in HIV-negative sexually active men who have sex with men: the EXPLORE study. *J Infect Dis*. 2004;190:2070-2076.
177. Schofield AM, Sadler L, Nelson L, et al. A prospective study of anal cancer screening in HIV-positive and negative MSM. *AIDS*. 2016;30:1375-1383.
178. Blas MM, Brown B, Menacho L, et al. HPV prevalence in multiple anatomical sites among men who have sex with men in Peru. *PLoS One*. 2015;10:e0139524.
179. Palefsky JM, Holly EA, Ralston ML, et al. Prevalence and risk factors for anal human papillomavirus infection in human immunodeficiency virus (HIV)-positive and high-risk HIV-negative women. *J Infect Dis*. 2001;183:383-391.
180. Frisch M, Biggar RJ, Goedert JJ. Human papillomavirus-associated cancers in patients with human immunodeficiency virus infection and acquired immunodeficiency syndrome. *J Natl Cancer Inst*. 2000;92:1500-1510.
181. Aberg JA, Gallant JE, Ghanem KG, et al. Primary care guidelines for the management of persons infected with HIV: 2013 update by the HIV Medicine Association of the Infectious Diseases Society of America. *Clin Infect Dis*. 2014;58:1-10.
182. Clinical Guidelines: Adult HIV Care—Anal Dysplasia and Cancer. 2007.
183. Panther L. *HPV-Related Complications. HIV Update Course*. Boston, MA: Beth Israel Deaconess Medical Center; 2016.
184. Edelman S, Johnstone PA. Combined modality therapy for HIV-infected patients with squamous cell carcinoma of the anus: outcomes and toxicities. *Int J Radiat Oncol Biol Phys*. 2006;66:206-211.
185. Blazy A, Hennequin C, Gornet JM, et al. Anal carcinomas in HIV-positive patients: high-dose chemoradiotherapy is feasible in the era of highly active antiretroviral therapy. *Dis Colon Rectum*. 2005;48:1176-1181.
186. Das P, Crane CH, Eng C, et al. Prognostic factors for squamous cell cancer of the anal canal. *Gastrointest Cancer Res*. 2008;2:10-14.
187. Das P, Bhatia S, Eng C, et al. Predictors and patterns of recurrence after definitive chemoradiation for anal cancer. *Int J Radiat Oncol Biol Phys*. 2007;68:794-800.
188. Gibson TM, Morton LM, Shiels MS, et al. Risk of non-Hodgkin lymphoma subtypes in HIV-infected people during the HAART era: a population-based study. *AIDS*. 2014;28:2313-2318.
189. Wilkins K, Turner R, Dolev JC, et al. Cutaneous malignancy and human immunodeficiency virus disease. *J Am Acad Dermatol*. 2006;54:189-206; quiz 207-210.
190. Yanik EL, Achenbach CJ, Gopal S, et al. Changes in clinical context for Kaposi's Sarcoma and non-Hodgkin lymphoma among people with HIV infection in the United States. *J Clin Oncol*. 2016;34(27):3276-3283.
191. Cerroni L. Cutaneous lymphomas in HIV-infected individuals. In: *Skin Lymphoma: The Illustrated Guide*. 4th ed. Hoboken, NJ: Wiley-Blackwell; 2014:275-280.
192. Beylot-Barry M, Vergier B, Masquelier B, et al. The spectrum of cutaneous lymphomas in HIV infection: a study of 21 cases. *Am J Surg Pathol*. 1999;23:1208-1216.
193. Wilkins K, Dolev JC, Turner R, et al. Approach to the treatment of cutaneous malignancy in HIV-infected patients. *Dermatol Ther*. 2005;18:77-86.
194. Jambusaria A, Shafer D, Wu H, et al. Cutaneous plasmablastic lymphoma. *J Am Acad Dermatol*. 2008;58:676-678.
195. Saggini A, Anemona L, Chimenti S, et al. HIV-associated primary cutaneous anaplastic large cell lymphoma: a clinicopathological subset with more aggressive behavior? Case report and review of the literature. *J Cutan Pathol*. 2012;39:1100-1109.
196. Baptista MJ, Garcia O, Morgades M, et al. HIV-infection impact on clinical-biological features and outcome of diffuse large B-cell lymphoma treated with R-CHOP in the combination antiretroviral therapy era. *AIDS*. 2015;29:811-818.
197. Bateganya MH, Stanaway J, Brentlinger PE, et al. Predictors of survival after a diagnosis of non-Hodgkin lymphoma in a resource-limited setting: a retrospective study on the impact of HIV infection and its treatment. *J Acquir Immune Defic Syndr*. 2011;56:312-319.
198. Lanoy E, Dores GM, Madeleine MM, et al. Epidemiology of nonkeratinocytic skin cancers among persons with AIDS in the United States. *AIDS*. 2009;23:385-393.
199. Olsen CM, Knight LL, Green AC. Risk of melanoma in people with HIV/AIDS in the pre- and post-HAART eras: a systematic review and meta-analysis of cohort studies. *PLoS One*. 2014;9:e95096.
200. Morar N, Willis-Owen SA, Maurer T, et al. HIV-associated psoriasis: pathogenesis, clinical features, and management. *Lancet Infect Dis*. 2010;10:470-478.
201. Kanada KN, Schupp CW, Armstrong AW. Association between psoriasis and viral infections in the United States: focusing on hepatitis B, hepatitis C and human immunodeficiency virus. *J Eur Acad Dermatol Venereol*. 2013;27:1312-1316.
202. Obuch ML, Maurer TA, Becker B, et al. Psoriasis and human immunodeficiency virus infection. *J Am Acad Dermatol*. 1992;27:667-673.
203. Fernandes S, Pinto GM, Cardoso J. Particular clinical presentations of psoriasis in HIV patients. *Int J STD AIDS*. 2011;22:653-654.
204. Tull TJ, Noy M, Bunker CB, et al. Sebopsoriasis in HIV positive patients: a case series of twenty patients. *Br J Dermatol*. 2017;176(3):813-815.
205. Kassi K, Mienwoley OA, Kouyate M, et al. Severe skin forms of psoriasis in black Africans: epidemiological, clinical, and histological aspects related to 56 cases. *Autoimmune Dis*. 2013;2013:561032.

206. Bittencourt Mde J, Brito AC, Nascimento BA, et al. A case of secondary syphilis mimicking palmoplantar psoriasis in HIV infected patient. *An Bras Dermatol.* 2015;90:216-219.
207. Carnero L, Betlloch I, Ramon R, et al. Psoriasis in a 5-month-old girl with HIV infection. *Pediatr Dermatol.* 2001;18:87-89.
208. Fife DJ, Waller JM, Jeffes EW, et al. Unraveling the paradoxes of HIV-associated psoriasis: a review of T-cell subsets and cytokine profiles. *Dermatol Online J.* 2007;13:4.
209. Colebunders R, Blot K, Mertens V, et al. Psoriasis regression in terminal AIDS. *Lancet.* 1992;339:1110.
210. Menon K, Van Voorhees AS, Bebo BF, et al. Psoriasis in patients with HIV infection: from the medical board of the National Psoriasis Foundation. *J Am Acad Dermatol.* 2010;62:291-299.
211. Tripathi SV, Leslie KS, Maurer TA, et al. Psoriasis as a manifestation of HIV-related immune reconstitution inflammatory syndrome. *J Am Acad Dermatol.* 2015;72:e35-e36.
212. Lee ES, Heller MM, Kamangar F, et al. Hydroxyurea for the treatment of psoriasis including in HIV-infected individuals: a review. *Psoriasis Forum.* 2011;17:180-187.
213. Di Lernia V. Progressive multifocal leukoencephalopathy and antipsoriatic drugs: assessing the risk of immunosuppressive treatments. *Int J Dermatol.* 2010;49:631-635.
214. Mathes BM, Douglass MC. Seborrheic dermatitis in patients with acquired immunodeficiency syndrome. *J Am Acad Dermatol.* 1985;13:947-951.
215. Wiwanitkit V. Prevalence of dermatological disorders in Thai HIV-infected patients correlated with different CD4 lymphocyte count statuses: a note on 120 cases. *Int J Dermatol.* 2004;43:265-268.
216. Forrestel AK, Kovarik CL, Mosam A, et al. Diffuse HIV-associated seborrheic dermatitis—a case series. *Int J STD AIDS.* 2016;27(14):1342-1345.
217. Buchness MR. Treatment of skin diseases in HIV-infected patients. *Dermatol Clin.* 1995;13:231-238.
218. Dunic I, Vesic S, Jevtovic DJ. Oral candidiasis and seborrheic dermatitis in HIV-infected patients on highly active antiretroviral therapy. *HIV Med.* 2004;5:50-54.
219. Hengge UR, Franz B, Goos M. Decline of infectious skin manifestations in the era of highly active antiretroviral therapy. *AIDS.* 2000;14:1069-1070.
220. Zissova LG, Kantarjiev TB, Kuzmanov AH. Drug susceptibility testing of *Malassezia furfur* strains to antifungal agents. *Folia Med (Plovdiv).* 2001;43:10-12.
221. Miranda KC, de Araujo CR, Costa CR, et al. Antifungal activities of azole agents against the *Malassezia* species. *Int J Antimicrob Agents.* 2007;29:281-284.
222. Bason MM, Berger TG, Nesbitt LT Jr. Pruritic papular eruption of HIV-disease. *Int J Dermatol.* 1993;32:784-789.
223. Boonchai W, Laohasrisakul R, Manonukul J, et al. Pruritic papular eruption in HIV seropositive patients: a cutaneous marker for immunosuppression. *Int J Dermatol.* 1999;38:348-350.
224. Rosatelli JB, Machado AA, Roselino AM. Dermatoses among Brazilian HIV-positive patients: correlation with the evolutionary phases of AIDS. *Int J Dermatol.* 1997;36:729-734.
225. Sivayathorn A, Srihra B, Leesanguankul W. Prevalence of skin disease in patients infected with human immunodeficiency virus in Bangkok, Thailand. *Ann Acad Med Singapore.* 1995;24:528-533.
226. Smith KJ, Skelton HG 3rd, James WD, et al. Papular eruption of human immunodeficiency virus disease. A review of the clinical, histologic, and immunohistochemical findings in 48 cases. The Military Medical Consortium for Applied Retroviral Research. *Am J Dermatopathol.* 1991;13:445-451.
227. Panya MF, Mgonda YM, Massawe AW. The pattern of mucocutaneous disorders in HIV-infected children attending care and treatment centres in Dar es Salaam, Tanzania. *BMC Public Health.* 2009;9:234.
228. Lowe S, Ferrand RA, Morris-Jones R, et al. Skin disease among human immunodeficiency virus-infected adolescents in Zimbabwe: a strong indicator of underlying HIV infection. *Pediatr Infect Dis J.* 2010;29:346-351.
229. Penneys NS, Nayar JK, Bernstein H, et al. Chronic pruritic eruption in patients with acquired immunodeficiency syndrome associated with increased antibody titers to mosquito salivary gland antigens. *J Am Acad Dermatol.* 1989;21:421-425.
230. Farsani TT, Kore S, Nadol P, et al. Etiology and risk factors associated with a pruritic papular eruption in people living with HIV in India. *J Int AIDS Soc.* 2013;16:17325.
231. Chua SL, Amerson EH, Leslie KS, et al. Factors associated with pruritic papular eruption of human immunodeficiency virus infection in the antiretroviral therapy era. *Br J Dermatol.* 2014;170:832-839.
232. Colebunders R, Moses KR, Laurence J, et al. A new model to monitor the virological efficacy of antiretroviral treatment in resource-poor countries. *Lancet Infect Dis.* 2006;6:53-59.
233. Lakshmi SJ, Rao GR, Ramalakshmi, et al. Pruritic papular eruptions of HIV: a clinicopathologic and therapeutic study. *Indian J Dermatol Venereol Leprol.* 2008;74:501-503.
234. Berman B, Flores F, Burke G 3rd. Efficacy of pentoxifylline in the treatment of pruritic papular eruption of HIV-infected persons. *J Am Acad Dermatol.* 1998;38:955-959.
235. Navarini AA, Stoeckle M, Navarini S, et al. Antihistamines are superior to topical steroids in managing human immunodeficiency virus (HIV)-associated papular pruritic eruption. *Int J Dermatol.* 2010;49:83-86.
236. Goldstein B, Berman B, Sukenik E, et al. Correlation of skin disorders with CD4 lymphocyte counts in patients with HIV/AIDS. *J Am Acad Dermatol.* 1997;36:262-264.
237. Kim TG, Lee KH, Oh SH. Skin disorders in Korean patients infected with human immunodeficiency virus and their association with a CD4 lymphocyte count: a preliminary study. *J Eur Acad Dermatol Venereol.* 2010;24:1476-1480.
238. Rajendran PM, Dolev JC, Heaphy MR Jr, et al. Eosinophilic folliculitis: before and after the introduction of antiretroviral therapy. *Arch Dermatol.* 2005;141:1227-1231.
239. Berger TG, Heon V, King C, et al. Itraconazole therapy for human immunodeficiency virus-associated eosinophilic folliculitis. *Arch Dermatol.* 1995;131:358-360.
240. Otley CC, Avram MR, Johnson RA. Isotretinoin treatment of human immunodeficiency virus-associated eosinophilic folliculitis. Results of an open, pilot trial. *Arch Dermatol.* 1995;131:1047-1050.

241. Lim HW, Vallurupalli S, Meola T, et al. UVB phototherapy is an effective treatment for pruritus in patients infected with HIV. *J Am Acad Dermatol.* 1997;37:414-417.
242. French MA, Lenzo N, John M, et al. Immune restoration disease after the treatment of immunodeficient HIV-infected patients with highly active antiretroviral therapy. *HIV Med.* 2000;1(2):107-115.
243. French MA. Immune reconstitution inflammatory syndrome: a reappraisal. *Clin Infect Dis.* 2009; 48(1):101-107.
244. French MA, Price P, Stone SF. Immune restoration after antiretroviral therapy. *AIDS.* 2004;18(12):1615-1627.
245. Cook LB, Elemans M, Rowan AG, et al. HTLV-1: persistence and pathogenesis. *Virology.* 2013;435: 131-140.
246. Ferreira LC, Caramelli P, Carneiro-Proietti AB. Human T-cell lymphotropic virus type 1 (HTLV-1): when to suspect infection? *Rev Assoc Med Bras.* 2010;56(3):340-347.
247. Goncalves DU, Proietti FA, Ribas JG, et al. Epidemiology, treatment and prevention of human T-cell leukemia virus type 1-associated diseases. *Clin Microbiol Rev.* 2010;23(3):577-589.
248. Schechter M, Harrison LH, Halsey NA, et al. Coinfection with human T-cell lymphotropic virus type I and HIV in Brazil. Impact on markers of HIV disease progression. *JAMA.* 1994;271(5):353-357.
249. Oliveria MF, Brites C, Ferraz N, et al. Infective dermatitis associated with the human T-cell lymphotropic virus type 1 in Salvador, Bahia, Brazil. *Clin Infect Dis.* 2005;40(11):90-96.

Chapter 169 :: Mosquito-Borne Viral Diseases
:: Edwin J. Asturias & J. David Beckham

第一百六十九章

蚊媒病毒性疾病

中文导读

蚊媒病毒性疾病是一种由节肢动物传播的人畜共患病，病毒通过蚊虫从灵长类动物传染给人类，或在人类之间相互传播。表169-1介绍了各种蚊媒疾病的概况。本章共分为2节：①黄病毒感染；②甲病毒属。文中对此作了详尽的阐述，更是将第一节分为登革病毒、寨卡病毒、黄热病毒和西尼罗病毒，将第二节分为基孔肯雅热和Mayaro、O'nyong-nyong、Ross River和Sindbis病毒组，分别介绍了这些疾病的流行病学、临床特征、危险因素、病因和发病机制、诊断、鉴别诊断、临床病程和预后及临床管理。

第一节介绍了黄病毒感染。作者首先指出，黄病毒科是一群具有包膜的正单链RNA病毒，也是全球最常见的蚊媒病毒。皮肤通常首先受累，造成以皮疹和结膜炎为主要临床症状的发热性疾病。出血和神经系统疾病则为常见的并发症。

登革热流行广泛，在东南亚、美洲、西太平洋、非洲和地中海东部地区的100多个国家均有报道。其由四种登革热病毒（DENV 1-4）引起，并由伊蚊传播，在急性感染和病毒血症高峰期后，炎性介质的释放可导致严重的血管内皮功能障碍从而造成出血。多数登革热病是有自限性的，大多数患者可以康复且无明显后遗症，现已有包含四种登革热血清型的减毒活重组疫苗。

寨卡病毒的RNA在精液中存活的时间比在血液、唾液，甚至发病后6个月的尿液中还长，以至于其独特之处在于可通过体液完成性传播和母婴垂直传播。与其他黄病毒相比，寨卡病毒的临床症状相对较轻，而小儿先天性感染可表现为特征性的小头畸形、脉络膜视网膜炎、听力下降、烦躁不安、高渗以及食管功能障碍，需要对感染孕妇进行管理。

黄热病毒是非洲和南美地区的特有病，病毒在肝脏、肾脏及胃肠道等器官的内质网中繁殖，黄疸是其感染的特有症状，重病患者可因肾衰竭、消化道出血和休克死亡。疫苗已使疫情的爆发大大减少。

西尼罗病毒感染的病例约80%是无症状的，约5%~22%的患者可出现全身躯干及四肢广泛爆发的玫瑰花状非瘙痒性粉红色斑疹，不到1%的患者会并发神经侵袭性疾病。目前尚无疫苗及特异性抗病毒药物。

第二节介绍了甲病毒属。甲病毒也是一群具有包膜的正单链RNA病毒，关节痛和关节炎是常见的并发症。基孔肯雅热病毒可直接感染成骨细胞，炎症反应过程中免疫细胞浸入周围的关节和组织从而引发关节炎，40%~50%的感染患者会出现多种黏膜及皮肤病变。Mayaro、O'nyong-nyong、Ross River和Sindbis病毒组感染患者除了发热和皮疹，多数还可出现头痛、肌痛和关节痛，症状可持续数周或数月，需与基孔肯雅热病毒感染相鉴别。

〔张江林〕

INTRODUCTION

DEFINITIONS

Mosquito-borne viral diseases are also called arbovirus (**ar**thropod-**bo**rne) infections. They are considered zoonotic diseases that are transmitted to humans indirectly via mosquitos or ticks from primates to humans, or humans to humans. An overview of mosquito-borne diseases is shown in Table 169-1.

HISTORICAL PERSPECTIVE

Since the arrival of the Spanish into the Americas in 1495, the "Black Death" or "Blood Vomit" (Xekik in Mayan) was a feared disease that affected people in the Caribbean and on the American continent. Outbreaks along the Mediterranean coast were suspected to have been brought from Africa.[1] However, the connection between arthropods and disease was not postulated until 1881 when Cuban doctor and scientist Carlos Finlay proposed that yellow fever (YF) may be transmitted by mosquitoes instead of human contact, a reality that was verified by Major Walter Reed in 1901.[2] By 1930, besides YF, dengue was the other important arbovirus infection that had been described.[3] From 1950 on, the use of vertebrate tissue culture and mosquito cell lines led to the discovery of many more arbovirus pathogens that are important in humans.[4]

FLAVIVIRUS INFECTIONS

AT-A-GLANCE

- Most common mosquito-borne infections worldwide
- Febrile illness associated with rash, conjunctivitis, or both
- Hemorrhagic or neurologic disease as complications
- Zika virus is transmitted from a mother to her child and through human secretions.

INTRODUCTION

The *Flaviviridae* (Latin, *flavus*, yellow) are a family of positive sense, single-stranded, enveloped RNA viruses, commonly found in mosquitos and ticks that can infect primates and humans. As transmission occurs via mosquitos, the skin is the primary site of infection. Flavivirus of human importance include dengue virus (DENV), Japanese encephalitis virus (JEV), Murray Valley encephalitis virus (MVEV), St. Louis encephalitis virus (SLEV), West Nile virus (WNV), Spondweni virus (SPOV), Zika virus (ZIKV), Wesselsbron virus (WESSV), and yellow fever virus (YFV). Of these, only DENV, WNV, SPOV, ZIKV, and YFV have demonstrated skin tropism with cutaneous manifestations. Epidermal Langerhans cells (LCs) along with dermal dendritic cells (DCs), macrophages, and T cells provide the first line of defense against these viruses.[5] The local trauma and inflammation resulting from the mosquito bite might enhance the recruitment of many of these cells.

DENGUE VIRUS

ETIOLOGY AND PATHOGENESIS

Dengue is a flaviviral disease caused by the four dengue virus serotypes (DENV 1–4) and transmitted by *Aedes* mosquitoes. Dengue is endemic in more than 100 countries in southeast Asia, the Americas, the western Pacific, Africa, and the eastern Mediterranean regions. It is estimated to cause an estimated 390 million human infections per year globally, of which 96 million manifests with symptoms.[6] After the initial acute infection and peak viremia, release of inflammatory mediators leads to endothelial dysfunction and vascular leak in severe dengue. Vascular leak is typically evident 3 to 6 days after the onset of illness, lasts for 24 to 48 hours, and usually shows rapid and complete reversal.[7]

CLINICAL FEATURES

After an incubation period of 3 to 10 days, infection by any dengue virus can produce a wide spectrum of illness, most being asymptomatic or subclinical. Around 10% to 15% will manifest as a self-limited febrile illness classically characterized by elevated temperature (≤40°C), severe headache, retro-orbital pain, malaise, severe joint and muscle pain, nausea, and vomiting, with a rash appearing after 3 to 4 days of fever onset.[8] In about 5% of symptomatic patients, especially after a second infection with dengue, severe dengue will be complicated by plasma leakage with or without bleeding. This critical phase occurs around defervescence from the initial fever and can lead to hypovolemic shock, organ failure, metabolic acidosis, disseminated intravascular coagulation (DIC), and severe hemorrhage.[9,10]

CUTANEOUS FINDINGS

A skin exanthem is present in 50% to 80% of patients who have symptomatic dengue. In the first 24 to 48 hours of the febrile episode, erythematous flushing of the face, neck, and chest is common, likely caused by capillary dilation. By day 3 to 5 of illness, a generalized morbilliform dark erythematous eruption with areas of clearing described as "islands of white in a sea of red" is

TABLE 169-1
An Overview of Mosquito-Borne Viral Diseases

CONDITION	VIRAL FAMILY	INCUBATION PERIOD (DAYS)	PRODROMAL SYMPTOMS	DERMATOLOGIC MANIFESTATIONS	LABORATORY TESTS	COMMENTS AND OTHER DIAGNOSTIC FEATURES
Dengue virus	Flavivirus	3–10	Usually none; 70% asymptomatic	Erythema early on ("islands of white in a sea of red"), maculopapular or urticarial exanthem in febrile phase (50%–80%)	Leukopenia, thrombocytopenia, elevated transaminases; Dengue PCR or NS1 Ag positive in first 7 days of illness; dengue IgM positive after 5 days of illness in 80%	Second infections carry 5% risk of hospitalization and severe dengue (hemorrhagic or third spacing); infants at high risk of severe dengue because of maternal antibodies
Zika virus	Flavivirus	3–7	Variable; 80% asymptomatic	Common (70%–85%); erythema, macular, or maculopapular and very pruritic	Leukocytosis, thrombocytopenia, elevated transaminases; Zika blood PCR diagnostic in first 5–10 days; Zika IgM positive in 5–15 days; false-positives occur in dengue endemic areas	Nonpurulent conjunctivitis (60%), facial and neck edema (70%)
Yellow Fever virus	Flavivirus	3–6	Fever, muscle pain, backache, headache, shivers, vomiting in acute phase	Acute phase: facial flushing, conjunctival hyperemia; Toxic phase (15%): jaundice, petechiae, hemorrhage	Leukopenia, thrombocytopenia, elevated transaminases and bilirubin; blood PCR positive in first 5–7 days, IgM positive in 5–15 days	40%–50% mortality rate in those progressing to "toxic" stage; Vaccine confers lifelong immunity
West Nile virus	Flavivirus	3–14 (≤28)	70% symptomatic; high fever (>39°C), headache, severe polyarthralgia, myalgia	Affects ~20%; small pink to red macules and papules on the torso and proximal extremities	Mild leukocytosis and hyponatremia; PCR positive in first 3–5 days of illness but usually negative when presenting; IgM and IgG serology most helpful	Hospitalization in 30%; fatigue for 1 mo in 95%; neuroinvasive disease in 1%
Chikungunya virus	Alphavirus	2–6	Fever, headache, flulike symptoms, myalgia, GI symptoms	Variable: morbilliform, vesiculobullous, and psoriatic-like presentations; postinflammatory hyperpigmentation	Leukopenia and lymphopenia; PCR positive first in 3 days of illness; IgM and IgG serology after 1 week of illness	Symmetric arthralgia and arthritis in 70% (can last 6–12 mo)
Mayaro virus	Alphavirus	Unknown	Acute febrile illness with headache, malaise; red eyes in 45%	Rash with pruritus in 30%–50%	Leukopenia; IgM and IgG ELISA	Endemic in South America and the Caribbean; Arthralgia and arthritis in 50%–90% (can last 6–12 months)
O'nyong-nyong virus	Alphavirus	Unknown	Acute febrile illness in 80%–100%, headache, myalgia	Rash in 70%–90%	Leukopenia; IgM and IgG ELISA	Outbreaks in Africa; Arthralgia and arthritis in 60%–100% (can last 6–12 mo)
Ross River virus	Alphavirus	7–9	Acute febrile illness in 20%–60%, headache, photophobia	Rash in 40%–50%	Leukopenia; IgM and IgG ELISA	Endemic in Australia; Arthralgia and arthritis in 80%–100% (can last 6–12 mo)
Sindbis virus	Alphavirus	2–10	Acute febrile illness in 15%–40%, headache, malaise, and arthralgia	Rash in 80%–90%	Leukopenia; IgM and IgG ELISA	Endemic in Eurasia, Africa, and Oceania; Arthralgia and arthritis in 90% (can last 6–12 mo)

Ag, antigen; ELISA, enzyme-linked immunosorbent assay; GI, gastrointestinal; IgG, immunoglobulin G; IgM, immunoglobulin M; NS1, nonstructural protein 1; PCR, polymerase chain reaction.

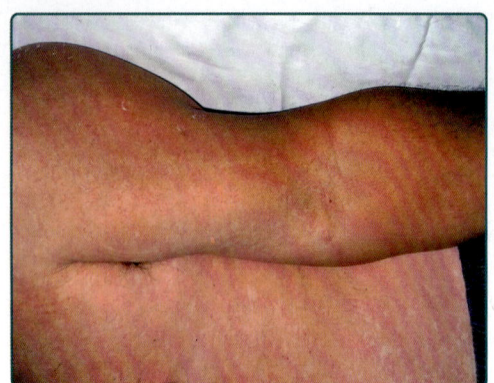

Figure 169-1 Rash of classical dengue. (Reproduced from Carod-Artal FJ, Wichmann O, Farrar J, et al. Neurological complications of dengue virus infection. *Lancet Neurol.* 2013;12(9):906-919; with permission. Copyright © Elsevier.)

seen in 70% of patients presenting with rash (Fig. 169-1). This rash frequently involves the palms and soles and commonly is associated with mild edema of the hands and feet. Other less common presentations include maculopapular eruptions, petechiae, purpura, and in 15% to 30% mucosal involvement with oral or genital bleeding, which signals dengue hemorrhagic fever. The typical cutaneous maculopapular eruption lasts up to 5 days. Involvement of the palms and soles may be followed by desquamation. There may be cutaneous hyperesthesia with alteration of the sense of touch.

NONCUTANEOUS FINDINGS

Only one of every 7 to 14 dengue infections is symptomatic. Clinical manifestations vary from self-limited fever to severe hemorrhagic fever and shock syndrome. Although rare, oral mucosal manifestations of dengue include acute gingival and palate bleeding, dryness of the mouth, taste changes, and erythematous plaques and vesicles on the tongue and palate.[11]

COMPLICATIONS

Between 10% and 20% of children confirmed with dengue will be hospitalized.[12] Besides dengue hemorrhagic fever and plasma leakage, severe dengue can also lead to hepatitis, neurologic disorders, and myocarditis. If untreated, the mortality rate can be as high as 20%.

DIAGNOSIS

Acute dengue infection can be confirmed by virus isolation in culture, detection of viral genomic RNA, viral products (capture and detection of the secreted NS1 protein), or the host immune response to virus infection (immunoglobulin [Ig] M). Reverse transcriptase polymerase chain reaction (RT-PCR) is the preferred method of virologic confirmation and can detect 69% to 82% of cases in the first 3 days of illness. NS1 antigen parallels viremia, and testing can detect 84% to 90% of cases in the first 5 to 7 days of illness.[13] Dengue IgM is positive in 10% to 20% of dengue cases by day 5 of illness but becomes progressively positive up to 80% to 90% of cases after 10 days of illness onset.[8]

Supportive Studies: Laboratory abnormalities include leukopenia, thrombocytopenia (platelets <100,000 × mm³), elevated transaminases, elevated hematocrit, and hyponatremia.

DIFFERENTIAL DIAGNOSIS

In endemic areas, approximately 10% of the febrile episodes in children are caused by dengue.[12] The fever and rash of dengue must be differentiated from other flavivirus infections as well as other conditions, including typhoid fever, rickettsiosis, secondary syphilis, chikungunya, primary HIV infection, drug reactions, and other common viral exanthems (enterovirus, measles, rubella, human herpesvirus 6 [HHV6], and parvovirus B19 infections).

CLINICAL COURSE, PROGNOSIS, MANAGEMENT, AND PREVENTION

Most cases of dengue are self-limited, and most patients recover without sequelae. Fatigue can last for several weeks, leading to absenteeism and loss of productivity. No specific antiviral therapy is available for dengue. Treatment of patients with dengue with warning signs and severe dengue includes rehydration, supportive care, avoidance of nonsteroidal and steroidal antiinflammatory therapy, and transfusion if needed. A recently licensed live attenuated recombinant vaccine containing the four dengue serotypes has been shown to reduce severe dengue by 90%, hospitalization by 80%, and clinical dengue by 50% to 60%.[14]

ZIKA VIRUS

ETIOLOGY AND PATHOGENESIS

ZIKV is an emerging mosquito-borne virus belonging to the genus *Flavivirus* and initially discovered in the Zika Forest of Uganda in 1947 in rhesus monkeys and in humans in 1952. Primarily transmitted by the *Aedes* mosquito, ZIKV became a pandemic of emergency proportions after its spread to Brazil in 2015. Since 2013, 84 countries have been affected. Unique to ZIKV is its ability to be transmitted from human to human through body fluids, sexual contact, and vertically from mother to fetus. ZIKV RNA persists in semen longer than in blood, saliva, or urine for up to 6 months after the onset of illness. Tissue pathology in congenital Zika syndrome is caused by direct viral infection of neural structures but in Guillain-Barré syndrome (GBS) is likely caused by postinfectious host-directed immune response.[15]

CLINICAL FEATURES

Most ZIKV infections in humans are asymptomatic (~80%). In 20% of infected patients, a mild febrile illness is associated with nonpurulent conjunctivitis, rash, malaise, and arthralgia, which will resolve within 2 to 7 days, and rarely requires hospitalization.

CUTANEOUS FINDINGS

The classic ZIKV exanthema appears within 1 to 2 days of illness and is associated with low-grade fever in 55% of patients. Distributed mainly on the trunk and extremities, it affects the palms and soles rarely. The rash is described as micropapular, descending, and pruritic in adults and children (Fig. 169-2B). Itching is the main reason for consultation due to severity associated with insomnia in 20% of cases.[16] Biopsies of the skin demonstrate a nonspecific perivascular lymphocytic infiltrate in the upper dermis.

NONCUTANEOUS FINDINGS

Associated mucous lesions include conjunctival hyperemia without purulence in 56% (Fig. 169-2A), facial and neck edema (60%–70%) (Fig. 169-2A), and acral edema that affects adults (50%) more than children (15%).

COMPLICATIONS

ZIKV congenital syndrome is characterized by microcephaly, chorioretinitis, hearing loss, irritability, hypertonia, and esophageal dysfunction.[17-20] GBS can occur 2 to 6 weeks after a ZIKV infection.[21,22]

DIAGNOSIS

Symptomatic patients infected with ZIKV are viremic for a mean of 3 days, and the virus can be detected in blood or serum samples using RT-PCR assays for at least 1 week. Serologic diagnosis using ZIKV IgM and IgG production with paired acute and convalescent serum can be used after 5 days of illness. However, given its commonality with other flaviviruses such as dengue or Japanese encephalitis, a high degree of serologic cross-reactivity to ZIKV serology is usually observed. More specific tests such as the plaque reduction neutralization test can improve differentiation between flaviviruses in endemic areas.[23,24]

Supportive Studies: Head ultrasonography, magnetic resonance imaging, and hearing and ophthalmologic examinations should be considered in any child exposed to ZIKV during pregnancy.

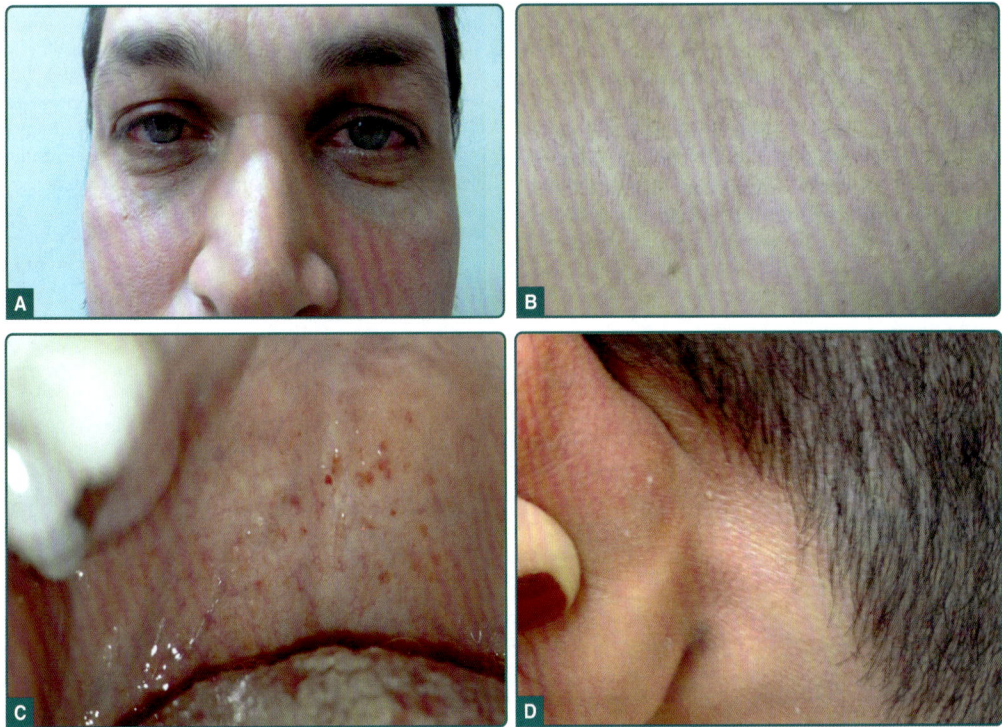

Figure 169-2 Presentation of Zika virus infection. **A,** Edema and erythema of the malar region of the face and conjunctival injection. **B,** Macular rash on the abdomen. **C,** Hyperemia and petechiae in the hard palate. **D,** Tender, mobile, soft lymph node, about 15 mm in diameter, behind the left ear. (Reproduced from Brasil P, Calvet GA, de Souza RV, et al. Exanthema associated with Zika virus infection. *Lancet Infect Dis.* 2016;16(7):866; with permission. Copyright © Elsevier.)

DIFFERENTIAL DIAGNOSIS

The clinical manifestations of ZIKV infection resemble other mosquito-transmitted diseases such as Chikungunya (CHIKV) and Dengue, but in comparison, ZIKV-related symptoms are usually milder and shorter and rarely lead to hospitalization.[25] The rare Spowendi virus infection in Africa can present with a rash similar to Zika but is characterized by a sunburn-like appearance.[26]

CLINICAL COURSE, PROGNOSIS, MANAGEMENT, AND PREVENTION

In pregnant women with laboratory evidence of recent ZIKV infection, approximately 5% of their fetuses or infants will demonstrate birth defects potentially associated with ZIKV infection.[27] No specific antiviral therapy is available for ZIKV, and several ZIKV vaccines are under development.[28]

YELLOW FEVER VIRUS

ETIOLOGY AND PATHOGENESIS

Endemic in Africa and South America, YF is caused by a RNA virus member of the family Flaviviridae. YF virus is maintained in nature by transmission between nonhuman primates and blood-feeding mosquitoes mainly belonging to the genera *Haemagogus* in Africa and *Aedes* in South America.[29] After inoculation by the vector, YF virus replicates within the endoplasmic reticulum of hepatocytes and other organs such as the kidneys, heart, and the gastrointestinal (GI) tract. Jaundice, the hallmark of this infection, arises from hepatocellular necrosis and the formation of intracellular hyaline deposits within the hepatic lobules.

CLINICAL FEATURES

YF incubates in humans for 3 to 6 days followed by infection that can occur in one or two phases. The first "acute" phase usually causes fever, muscle pain with prominent backache, headache, shivers, loss of appetite, and nausea or vomiting. Most patients improve after 3 to 4 days of illness. In 15% of patients, a second "toxic" phase ensues within 24 hours of the initial remission with high fever, jaundice, abdominal pain, vomiting, mucosal bleeding, and GI hemorrhage. Renal failure and shock can lead to death.

CUTANEOUS FINDINGS

In the mild acute phase of the disease, facial flushing and conjunctival hyperemia are common. In severe "toxic" forms of disease, jaundice can be accompanied by petechiae, and skin hemorrhage from thrombocytopenia and DIC is common.[30]

DIAGNOSIS

YF should be suspected in any person from or returning from an endemic area with acute onset of fever and jaundice appearing within 14 days of onset of the first symptoms.

Supportive Studies: Laboratory diagnosis of YF is generally accomplished by serologic testing for virus-specific IgM and neutralizing antibodies.[31] Sometimes the virus can be detected by RT-PCR in blood samples taken early in the illness.[32,33] In severe or fatal cases, RT-PCR, histopathology with immunohistochemistry and virus culture of biopsy or autopsy tissues can also be positive.

DIFFERENTIAL DIAGNOSIS

Mild YF infections may mimic any of the acute febrile illnesses in the tropics, including dengue, Zika, chikungunya, influenza, and other viral infections. Severe YF hemorrhagic fever should be differentiated from Lassa, Crimean-Congo, Ebola, and other South American hemorrhagic fevers.

CLINICAL COURSE, PROGNOSIS, MANAGEMENT, AND PREVENTION

The majority of individuals recover fully from the acute phase of illness, with no consequences and life-long immunity to YF. Of the 15% who will progress to severe disease, half will recover fully with lifelong immunity, and 40% to 50% will die. No antivirals are approved for treatment of YF, yet nitazoxanide has been shown to interfere with its replication.[34] A very effective vaccine against YF exists, and only one dose is required to protect thru life.[35] Since 2006, more than 105 million people have been vaccinated in mass campaigns in West Africa with dramatic reduction in outbreaks.

WEST NILE VIRUS

First isolated in 1937 from a woman in Uganda, WNV disease caused sporadic outbreaks in Africa, Asia, and Europe. In the summer of 1999, it emerged in North America and by 2003 caused the largest outbreak of WNV ever reported with 9862 confirmed cases, of which 2866 (29%) were neuroinvasive.[36] WNV is now considered endemic in most of the United States and is maintained in an enzootic cycle between birds and mosquitoes. It is known to infect more than 300 species of birds, but in the Western Hemisphere, American crows and robins as well as sparrows, finches, grackles, jays, and magpies are the most common reservoirs.[37]

CLINICAL FEATURES

Transmission of WNV to humans occurs predominantly through the bite of the Culex family of mosquitos. Rare cases occur as a consequence of blood transfusion or organ transplantation, and infection can occur in utero or postnatally from breastfeeding.[38] After a typical incubation period of 3 to 14 days but as long as 28 days after infection, systemic symptoms can develop. WNV infection is asymptomatic in about 80% of cases, and many additional patients with mild infection never seek medical attention.

CUTANEOUS FINDINGS

A maculopapular rash appears in 5% to 22% of patients as a roseola-like, nonpruritic eruption, characterized by pink macules or papules, 5 to 10 mm in diameter, frequently affecting the torso and proximal extremities but sparing the palms and soles and lasting 5 to 7 days (Fig. 169-3). Younger patients, as well as those without neuroinvasive disease, are frequently affected.[39-41] Other skin manifestations may include roseola-like eruptions, a punctate exanthem, and rarely purpura fulminans.[42]

NONCUTANEOUS FINDINGS

One in five WNV-infected patients have symptoms characterized as nonspecific "flulike" symptoms consisting of fever, headache, malaise, anorexia, abdominal pain, sore throat, back pain, or diarrhea.[38,43,44] In one series of patients, it was noted that the most commonly reported symptoms were fever (100%), generalized fatigue (74%), nausea or vomiting (44%), headache (48%), and back or limb pain (35%).[45]

COMPLICATIONS

Fatigue is a common complication reported in 96% of patients for a median of 36 days. Hospitalization occurs in 30% for a median stay of 5 days, and 57 of 72 (79%) patients who normally attended school or work could not do so with a mean absence of 10 days. Fewer than 1% of patients develop neuroinvasive disease, classified as meningitis, encephalitis, or acute flaccid paralysis.[46] Older age, chronic medical conditions, and immunosuppression increase the likelihood of complications. Cranial nerve palsies are found in about 10% of patients and most commonly involve the second and seventh cranial nerves, causing optic neuritis (see later) or peripheral facial palsy, respectively. Involvement of lower cranial nerves can result in vertigo, dysphagia, or dysarthria. Brainstem involvement can be extensive enough that some patients develop bulbar dysfunction, leading to subsequent respiratory failure.[43] Aside from optic neuritis, other neuroophthalmologic manifestations of WNV infection include chorioretinitis, uveitis, and vitreitis.[47,48]

DIAGNOSIS

Specific testing for WNV usually involves RT-PCR and serologies. RT-PCR testing from serum is generally not as helpful as serologic testing because the majority of patients will no longer have detectable viremia by the time they develop neuroinvasive symptoms. WNV-specific immunoglobulin (IgM) in cerebrospinal fluid (CSF) with confirmatory plaque reduction neutralization is the test of choice for neuroinvasive disease.[49] CSF IgM can persist for up to 199 days. WNV IgM or IgG can cross-react with other flaviviruses and results in patients with other flavivirus exposure are only indicative of recent or previous flavivirus infection (eg, West Nile, dengue, Japanese encephalitis, or ZIKV) or vaccination (eg, Japanese encephalitis or YF vaccine).

Supportive Studies: Patients with WNV typically have a normal complete blood cunt or a mild leukocytosis. Hyponatremia can be seen, as well as elevation of liver enzymes. Neuroinvasive WNV shows a lymphocytic pleocytosis of less than 500 cells/mm³ in the CSF.

DIFFERENTIAL DIAGNOSIS

The rash of WNV must be differentiated from primary HIV infection, drug reactions, and other common viral exanthems (enterovirus, measles, rubella, HHV6, and parvovirus B19 infections). In returning travelers, other flavivirus (dengue) and alphavirus infections (CHIKV), as well as other conditions, including typhoid fever, rickettsiosis, and secondary syphilis, should be thought of.

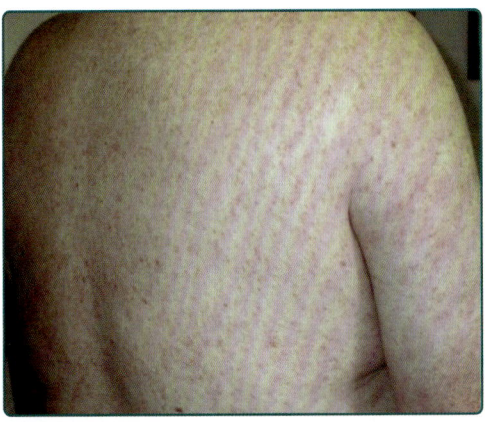

Figure 169-3 Diffuse maculopapular rash associated with West Nile virus infection. (Reproduced from Sejvar JJ. Clinical manifestations and outcomes of West Nile virus infection. *Viruses*. 2014;6(2):606-623. Licensed under CC BY 3.0.)

CLINICAL COURSE, PROGNOSIS, MANAGEMENT, AND PREVENTION

Most WNV infections are asymptomatic or mildly symptomatic. Hospitalization and death are rare but are more frequent in older adults and those affected by chronic conditions or immunosuppression. The mortality rate in neuroinvasive disease has been 9% from 1999 and 2015.

The mainstay of prevention revolves around avoiding mosquito bites with insect repellants that contain DEET, picaridin, IR3535, or oil of lemon eucalyptus. It is recommended to wear long clothing and to make home modifications to prevent mosquito accessibility and breeding by installing screens on windows or using air conditioning. It is important to eliminate sources of standing water, including pots, bowls, and rubber tires. If sleeping outside, the use of a mosquito bed net is recommended. No antiviral treatments for WNV infection are available, and there are not yet vaccines approved for human use.[50]

ALPHAVIRUSES

AT-A-GLANCE

- Mosquito-borne infections causing rheumatologic and neurologic diseases
- Chikungunya, Mayaro, Ross River, Sindbis and O'nyong-nyong viruses manifest as febrile illness associated with rash, conjunctivitis, or both.
- Arthralgia and arthritis are common complications.

INTRODUCTION

Alphaviruses are a genus of enveloped, positive-sense, single-stranded RNA viruses, usually transmitted by mosquitoes, and together with the genus Rubivirus belong to the Togaviridae family. Alphaviruses are commonly referred to as "Old World" and "New World" viruses, with Old World viruses generally associated with dermatologic and rheumatic disease in humans (CHIKV and Mayaro virus [MAYV]) and "New World" viruses (Venezuelan, Eastern, Western, and Venezuelan equine encephalitis) primarily associated with potentially fatal encephalitic disease in the Americas.[51]

CHIKUNGUNYA

ETIOLOGY AND PATHOGENESIS

Chikungunya fever is caused by CHIKV, an alphavirus from the Togaviridae family transmitted by the *Aedes aegypti* and *albopictus* mosquitos. First described in Tanzania in 1952, epidemics subsequently occurred in Africa, Asia, and India and in 2013 to 2014 emerged in the Caribbean and Latin America.[52] Since 2000, the virus has been reemerging, causing several outbreaks of more severe forms of the disease in southeast Asia, the Caribbean, and Latin America. Most of the manifestations of chikungunya infection are caused by high levels of viremia present in the blood during early stages of infection. This high viremia correlates with an intense inflammatory response that results in infiltration of immune cells into infected joints and surrounding tissues, producing arthritis. Direct infection of osteoblasts may explain the arthritis and arthralgia during infection.

CLINICAL FEATURES

After the bite of an infectious mosquito, the incubation period is 2 to 4 (≤10) days. Chikungunya means "that which bends up" in Swahili or Makonde for the posture assumed by affected patients. Approximately 70% of acute CHIKV infections are symptomatic, presenting with abrupt onset of high fever (>39°C), headache, severe polyarthralgia and myalgia, and an erythematous maculopapular rash (Fig. 147-4B), which varies in severity from mild and localized to generalized.[52]

CUTANEOUS FINDINGS

A variety of mucocutaneous lesions occur in 40% to 50% of patients with CHIKV infection. Morbilliform exanthem is the most common presentation, but pigmented, vesiculobullous, and psoriatic-like lesion are also described in children.[53,54] Postinflammatory hyperpigmentation may appear soon after the evanescence of the rash. Facial flushing, xerosis of skin with scaling, desquamation of palms, acute intertrigo-like lesions with genital or perianal ulceration, aphthous-like ulcers, and lymphedema in an acral distribution have also been reported. Hemorrhagic skin lesions and purpura are more typical of dengue but are occasionally reported with CHIKV infection. Rarely, CHIKV infection can mimic atypical Kawasaki syndrome in young children.[54-59]

NONCUTANEOUS FINDINGS

Most patients have joint pain and swelling with severe morning stiffness, consistent with in inflammatory arthritis (Fig. 147-4A). The joint pain is typically symmetrical, and almost any joint can be affected, especially during the acute phase, although the distal extremities are affected more frequently.

COMPLICATIONS

CHIKV antigen and RNA has been shown to persist in macrophages for up to 90 days, and in one patient, CHIKV RNA and protein was found in synovial macrophages 18 months after infection. Chronic, episodic, often debilitating, polyarthralgia or polyarthritis associated with fatigue is the most common and feared

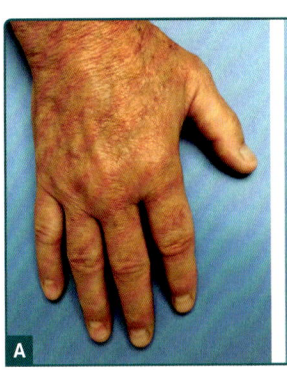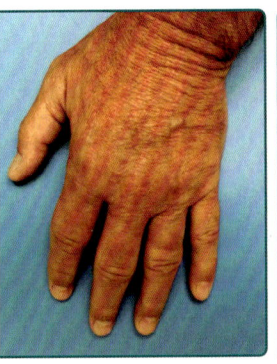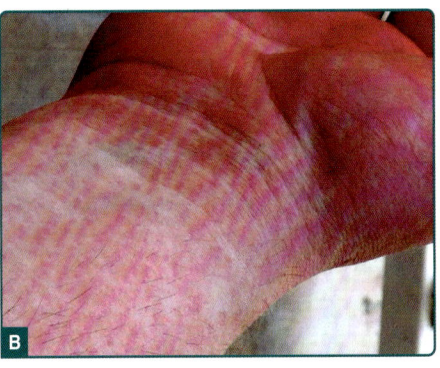

Figure 169-4 Clinical features of disease in patients with chikungunya virus infection. **A,** Active symmetric synovitis in the metacarpophalangeal and proximal interphalangeal joints during the chronic phase of chikungunya-associated arthritis. The patient was a white man aged 57 years. The patient developed high fever, a diffuse maculopapular rash, joint pain, stiffness, and swelling consistent with an acute pattern. **B,** Maculopapular rash during the acute infectious phase. The rash was distributed over the entire body, resolved after a few days and was followed by desquamation. The patient was a white woman aged 33 years. The patient developed fever, diffuse arthritis, and an erythematous, maculopapular rash over her entire body. Both individuals traveled to Haiti during a chikungunya virus outbreak. (Reproduced from Miner JJ, Aw-Yeang HX, Fox JM, et al. Chikungunya viral arthritis in the United States: a mimic of seronegative rheumatoid arthritis. *Arthritis Rheumatol.* 2015;67:1214-1220; with permission. Copyright © 2015 John Wiley & Sons.)

complication. Currently, no strong evidence exists that CHIKV arthritis can predispose to autoimmune disease.[60]

DIAGNOSIS

CHIKV infection should be considered in patients with acute onset of fever and polyarthralgia, especially travelers returning from endemic or outbreak areas. Laboratory diagnosis is best accomplished by testing serum or plasma to detect virus, viral nucleic acid, or virus-specific IgM and neutralizing antibodies. Viral culture may detect virus in the first 3 days of illness; however, CHIKV should be handled under biosafety level conditions. In the first week of illness, RNA detection using RT-PCR is preferable. IgM antibodies normally develop toward the end of the first week of illness.

Supportive Studies: Leucopenia and lymphopenia are common during CHIKV infection but less pronounced than with dengue. Thrombocytopenia and hemorrhagic manifestations are rare.

DIFFERENTIAL DIAGNOSIS

Pruritus, although rarely pronounced, can help distinguish CHIKV from ZIKV infection because this symptom is more common in the later. Petechiae and purpura are rare with CHIKV and more common with dengue. Mayaro, Sindbis, O'nyong-nyong, and rubella virus infections can mimic CHIKV, especially in female patients.

CLINICAL COURSE, PROGNOSIS, MANAGEMENT, AND PREVENTION

No licensed vaccine or antiviral drug is available against CHIKV. Current treatment mainly involves the use of antiinflammatory drugs for symptomatic relief. No specific treatment or vaccine is currently available to prevent infection.

MAYARO, O'NYONG-NYONG, ROSS RIVER, AND SINDBIS GROUP VIRUSES

ETIOLOGY AND PATHOGENESIS

MAYV was first isolated from sick forest workers in Trinidad in 1954, and it is now endemic in South America, where is causes periodic outbreaks, most recently Haiti. O'nyong-nyong virus first emerged in Uganda in 1959 and so far has caused at least three outbreaks in Africa. Ross River virus (RRV) was first isolated in 1959 from mosquitoes trapped in Queensland, Australia, where it is endemic, causing an average of 4000 cases per year. Sindbis virus was first isolated from mosquitoes in 1952 in Egypt and is the most widely distributed arbovirus found in Eurasia, Africa, and Oceania.[51,61]

CLINICAL FEATURES

Illnesses caused by MAYV, RRV, O'nyong-nyong, and the Sindbis virus group commonly present with an acute febrile illness of 3 to 5 days' duration after a 2- to 7-day incubation period. Most patients present with headache, myalgia, rash, and arthralgia that may last for weeks or months.

CUTANEOUS FINDINGS

Rash occurs in 30% to 50% of cases in MAYV and RRV infections but is almost universal (≤90%) with Sindbis and O'nyong-nyong viruses. The morphology is either maculopapular or micropapular, and the exanthema usually appears by the fifth day and fades within 3 to 4 days. The incidence of rash is higher in children than in adults.

NONCUTANEOUS FINDINGS

Arthralgia, accompanied by joint edema in 20% of cases, is a very prominent sign that causes temporary incapacity in many patients. Arthralgia is present in virtually all confirmed cases and persists in some for at least 2 months but with decreasing severity.

COMPLICATIONS

Arthritis, similar to CHIKV, is the most common complication. Protracted disease—primarily arthralgia—is well documented for Sindbis virus, RRV, and MAYV disease and can be persistent and incapacitating for up to 12 months. Fatalities are rare.

DIAGNOSIS

Serologies, including IgM and IgG enzyme-linked immunosorbent tests, are used as standard for laboratory-based diagnoses of arthritogenic alphavirus disease. MAYV, RRV, Sindbis, and O'nyong-nyong infection can be confirmed by RT-PCR or virus isolation, but the viremic phase is short.

Supportive Studies: Leucopenia is a constant finding in all cases. Mild albuminuria and slight thrombocytopenia are occasionally seen.

DIFFERENTIAL DIAGNOSIS

Rubella virus and CHIKV infection should be considered in the differential diagnosis of these viruses. The geographical location and travel exposure of the patient should help differentiate these viruses.

MANAGEMENT AND PREVENTION

No antiviral therapy or vaccines are available for these infections. Avoiding mosquito bites by wearing protective clothing and ng repellents and insecticide-impregnated mosquito nets is important for prevention.

REFERENCES

1. Holbrook MR. Historical perspectives on flavivirus research. *Viruses*. 2017;9(5).
2. Reed W, Carroll J, Agramonte A, et al. The etiology of yellow fever—a preliminary note. *Public Health Pap Rep*. 1900;26:37-53.
3. Cleland JB, Bradley B. Dengue fever in Australia: its history and clinical course, its experimental transmission by Stegomyia fasciata, and the results of inoculation and other experiments. *J Hyg (Lond)*. 1918;16(4):317-418.
4. Shope RE. The discovery of arbovirus diseases. *Ann N Y Acad Sci*. 1994;740:138-145.
5. Briant L, Despres P, Choumet V, et al. Role of skin immune cells on the host susceptibility to mosquito-borne viruses. *Virology*. 2014;464-465:26-32.
6. Bhatt S, Gething PW, Brady OJ, et al. The global distribution and burden of dengue. *Nature*. 2013;496(7446):504-507.
7. Malavige GN, Ogg GS. Pathogenesis of vascular leak in dengue virus infection. *Immunology*. 2017;151(3):261-269.
8. Muller DA, Depelsenaire AC, Young PR. Clinical and laboratory diagnosis of dengue virus infection. *J Infect Dis*. 2017;215(suppl 2):S89-S95.
9. Guzman MG, Harris E. Dengue. *Lancet*. 2015;385(9966):453-465.
10. Carod-Artal FJ, Wichmann O, Farrar J, et al. Neurological complications of dengue virus infection. *Lancet Neurol*. 2013;12(9):906-919.
11. Pedrosa MS, de Paiva M, Oliveira L, et al. Oral manifestations related to dengue fever: a systematic review of the literature. *Aust Dent J*. 2017;62(4):404-411.
12. L'Azou M, Moureau A, Sarti E, et al. Symptomatic dengue in children in 10 Asian and Latin American countries. *N Engl J Med*. 2016;374(12):1155-1166.
13. Hunsperger EA, Munoz-Jordan J, Beltran M, et al. Performance of dengue diagnostic tests in a single-specimen diagnostic algorithm. *J Infect Dis*. 2016;214(6):836-844.
14. Malisheni M, Khaiboullina SF, Rizvanov AA, et al. Clinical efficacy, safety, and immunogenicity of a live attenuated tetravalent dengue vaccine (CYD-TDV) in children: a systematic review with meta-analysis. *Front Immunol*. 2017;8:863.
15. Ritter JM, Martines RB, Zaki SR. Zika virus: pathology from the pandemic. *Arch Pathol Lab Med*. 2017;141(1):49-59.
16. Cordel N, Birembaux X, Chaumont H, et al. Main characteristics of zika virus exanthema in Guadeloupe. *JAMA Dermatol*. 2017;153(4):326-328.
17. Krauer F, Riesen M, Reveiz L, et al. Zika virus infection as a cause of congenital brain abnormalities and Guillain-Barré syndrome: systematic review. *PLoS Med*. 2017;14(1):e1002203.
18. de Paula Freitas B, de Oliveira Dias JR, Prazeres J, et al. Ocular findings in infants with microcephaly associated with presumed zika virus congenital infection in Salvador, Brazil. *JAMA Ophthalmol*. 2016 Feb 9. doi: 10.1001/jamaophthalmol.2016.0267. [Epub ahead of print].
19. Ventura CV, Maia M, Ventura BV, et al. Ophthalmological findings in infants with microcephaly and presumable intra-uterus Zika virus infection. *Arq Bras Oftalmol*. 2016;79(1):1-3.
20. Miranda-Filho Dde B, Martelli CM, Ximenes RA, et al. Initial description of the presumed congenital Zika syndrome. *Am J Public Health*. 2016;106(4):598-600.
21. Oehler E, Watrin L, Larre P, et al. Zika virus infection complicated by Guillain-Barre syndrome—case report, French Polynesia, December 2013. *Euro Surveill*. 2014;19(9).
22. Araujo LM, Ferreira ML, Nascimento OJ. Guillain-Barre syndrome associated with the Zika virus outbreak in Brazil. *Arq Neuropsiquiatr*. 2016;74(3):253-255.
23. Eppes C, Rac M, Dunn J, et al. Testing for Zika virus infection in pregnancy: key concepts to deal

with an emerging epidemic. *Am J Obstet Gynecol*. 2017;216(3):209-225.
24. Landry ML, St George K. Laboratory diagnosis of Zika virus infection. *Arch Pathol Lab Med*. 2017;141(1):60-67.
25. Waggoner JJ, Gresh L, Vargas MJ, et al. Viremia and clinical presentation in nicaraguan patients infected with Zika Virus, chikungunya virus, and dengue virus. *Clin Infect Dis*. 2016;63(12):1584-1590.
26. Wolfe MS, Calisher CH, McGuire K. Spondweni virus infection in a foreign resident of Upper Volta. *Lancet*. 1982;2(8311):1306-1308.
27. Shapiro-Mendoza CK, Rice ME, Galang RR, et al. Pregnancy outcomes after maternal Zika Virus infection during pregnancy—U.S. territories, January 1, 2016-April 25, 2017. *MMWR Morb Mortal Wkly Rep*. 2017;66(23):615-621.
28. Focosi D, Maggi F, Pistello M. Zika virus: implications for public health. *Clin Infect Dis*. 2016;63(2):227-233.
29. Monath TP, Vasconcelos PF. Yellow fever. *J Clin Virol*. 2015;64:160-173.
30. Carneiro SC, Cestari T, Allen SH, et al. Viral exanthems in the tropics. *Clin Dermatol*. 2007;25(2):212-220.
31. Niedrig M, Kursteiner O, Herzog C, et al. Evaluation of an indirect immunofluorescence assay for detection of immunoglobulin M (IgM) and IgG antibodies against yellow fever virus. *Clin Vaccine Immunol*. 2008;15(2):177-181.
32. Domingo C, Escadafal C, Rumer L, et al. First international external quality assessment study on molecular and serological methods for yellow fever diagnosis. *PLoS One*. 2012;7(5):e36291.
33. Domingo C, Patel P, Yillah J, et al. Advanced yellow fever virus genome detection in point-of-care facilities and reference laboratories. *J Clin Microbiol*. 2012;50(12):4054-4060.
34. Boldescu V, Behnam MAM, Vasilakis N, et al. Broad-spectrum agents for flaviviral infections: dengue, Zika and beyond. *Nat Rev Drug Discov*. 2017;16(8):565-586.
35. Barrett ADT. Yellow fever live attenuated vaccine: a very successful live attenuated vaccine but still we have problems controlling the disease. *Vaccine*. 2017;35(44):5951-5955.
36. Tyler KL. Current developments in understanding of West Nile virus central nervous system disease. *Curr Opin Neurol*. 2014;27(3):342-348.
37. Hollidge BS, Gonzalez-Scarano F, Soldan SS. Arboviral encephalitides: transmission, emergence, and pathogenesis. *J Neuroimmune Pharmacol*. 2010;5(3):428-442.
38. Debiasi RL, Tyler KL. West Nile virus meningoencephalitis. *Nat Clin Pract Neurol*. 2006;2(5):264-275.
39. Sejvar JJ, Marfin AA. Manifestations of West Nile neuroinvasive disease. *Rev Med Virol*. 2006;16(4):209-224.
40. Ferguson DD, Gershman K, LeBailly A, et al. Characteristics of the rash associated with West Nile virus fever. *Clin Infect Dis*. 2005;41(8):1204-1207.
41. Del Giudice P, Schuffenecker I, Zeller H, et al. Skin manifestations of West Nile virus infection. *Dermatology*. 2005;211(4):348-350.
42. Shah S, Fite LP, Lane N, et al. Purpura fulminans associated with acute West Nile virus encephalitis. *J Clin Virol*. 2016;75:1-4.
43. Davis LE, DeBiasi R, Goade DE, et al. West Nile virus neuroinvasive disease. *Ann Neurol*. 2006;60(3):286-300.
44. Hayes EB, Sejvar JJ, Zaki SR, et al. Virology, pathology, and clinical manifestations of West Nile virus disease. *Emerg Infect Dis*. 2005;11(8):1174-1179.
45. Jeha LE, Sila CA, Lederman RJ, et al. West Nile virus infection: a new acute paralytic illness. *Neurology*. 2003;61(1):55-59.
46. Patel H, Sander B, Nelder MP. Long-term sequelae of West Nile virus-related illness: a systematic review. *Lancet Infect Dis*. 2015;15(8):951-959.
47. Davis LE, Beckham JD, Tyler KL. North American encephalitic arboviruses. *Neurol Clin*. 2008;26(3):727-757, ix.
48. Khairallah M, Ben Yahia S, Ladjimi A, et al. Chorioretinal involvement in patients with West Nile virus infection. *Ophthalmology*. 2004;111(11):2065-2070.
49. Tardei G, Ruta S, Chitu V, et al. Evaluation of immunoglobulin M (IgM) and IgG enzyme immunoassays in serologic diagnosis of West Nile Virus infection. *J Clin Microbiol*. 2000;38(6):2232-2239.
50. Biedenbender R, Bevilacqua J, Gregg AM, et al. Phase II, randomized, double-blind, placebo-controlled, multicenter study to investigate the immunogenicity and safety of a West Nile virus vaccine in healthy adults. *J Infect Dis*. 2011;203(1):75-84.
51. Suhrbier A, Jaffar-Bandjee MC, Gasque P. Arthritogenic alphaviruses—an overview. *Nat Rev Rheumatol*. 2012;8(7):420-429.
52. Burt FJ, Chen W, Miner JJ, et al. Chikungunya virus: an update on the biology and pathogenesis of this emerging pathogen. *Lancet Infect Dis*. 2017;17(4):e107-e117.
53. Nawas ZY, Tong Y, Kollipara R, et al. Emerging infectious diseases with cutaneous manifestations: viral and bacterial infections. *J Am Acad Dermatol*. 2016;75(1):1-16.
54. Seetharam KA, Sridevi K, Vidyasagar P. Cutaneous manifestations of chikungunya fever. *Indian Pediatr*. 2012;49(1):51-53.
55. Bandyopadhyay D, Ghosh SK. Mucocutaneous manifestations of Chikungunya fever. *Indian J Dermatol*. 2010;55(1):64-67.
56. Bandyopadhyay D, Ghosh SK. Mucocutaneous features of Chikungunya fever: a study from an outbreak in West Bengal, India. *Int J Dermatol*. 2008;47(11):1148-1152.
57. Bhat RM, Rai Y, Ramesh A, et al. Mucocutaneous manifestations of chikungunya fever: a study from an epidemic in coastal karnataka. *Indian J Dermatol*. 2011;56(3):290-294.
58. Kumar V, Jain R, Kumar A, et al. Chikungunya fever presenting as life threatening thrombotic thrombocytopenic purpura. *J Assoc Physicians India*. 2017;65(7):96-100.
59. Lee YS, Quek SC, Koay ES, et al. Chikungunya mimicking atypical Kawasaki disease in an infant. *Pediatr Infect Dis J*. 2010;29(3):275-277.
60. Goupil BA, Mores CN. A Review of Chikungunya Virus-induced arthralgia: clinical manifestations, therapeutics, and pathogenesis. *Open Rheumatol J*. 2016;10:129-140.
61. Tesh RB, Watts DM, Russell KL, et al. Mayaro virus disease: an emerging mosquito-borne zoonosis in tropical South America. *Clin Infect Dis*. 1999;28(1):67-73.

Sexually Transmitted Diseases

PART 26

第二十六篇　　性传播疾病

Chapter 170 :: Syphilis
:: Susan A. Tuddenham & Jonathan M. Zenilman

第一百七十章

梅毒

中文导读

　　本章主要介绍了苍白密螺旋体引起的性传播感染——梅毒。并从历史背景、流行病学、临床表现（皮肤系统及皮肤系统外）、发病机理、诊断与鉴别诊断、病程与预后、疾病的管理和预防等几个方面进行了介绍。概览如下：

　　梅毒是苍白密螺旋体所引起的一种慢性性传播感染。它很多的临床表现都与皮肤相关。而且近年来，它的发病率在发展中国家并未出现下降，在发达国家有回升的趋势。因此对于皮肤科医生来说，掌握这种疾病是非常重要的。

　　梅毒第一次在全球范围内的流行起源于1494年的意大利那不勒斯，即哥伦布从美洲回到欧洲后的第一年。到了20世纪30年代，估算有大约10%的美国人感染梅毒，每年有50万例新发感染和6万例新发先天梅毒。由于梅毒的皮肤相关临床表现，梅毒的治疗和研究一直主要由皮肤科医生领导。1943年，盘尼西林第一次被用于梅毒治疗，并且在第二次世界大战后被广泛运用。梅毒发病率在20世纪50年代出现大幅下降，到了20世纪80年代，梅毒发病率有小幅度的回弹。20世纪80年代末到20世纪90年代初期，梅毒又重新在美国南部和大城市中出现，而且在黑人、可卡因使用者和性服务者中发病比例更高。20世纪90年代后期至二十一世纪初，可卡因流行度下降，而且美国疾病控制中心在全国范围内开展根除梅毒计划，梅毒在异性恋者中发病率下降。但是从20世纪90年代后期起，在美国和其他发达国家，梅毒在有同性性行为的男性中发病率上升。自梅毒病例开始上报以来（1941年），在2000年和2001年，美国一期和二期梅毒新发病例达到最低点，每10万人中仅有2.1例。但是进入21世纪，美国梅毒发病率却开始逐渐上升，2014年美国一期和二期梅毒新发病例达到每10万人6.3例，为自1994年起的最高发病率。这主要是因为梅毒在有同性性行为的男性中发病率上升所致，而且，一期梅毒与二期梅毒发病率与该人群中HIV感染率密切相关。在世界其他国家，梅毒发病率仍较高。每年有大约一千二百万新增梅毒病例，约一百万次妊娠受到梅毒影响。

梅毒主要通过性接触传播（接触另外一个梅毒感染者身上的有感染性的皮损）。非性传播梅毒十分罕见，通常由输注未筛查的血液、职业暴露（如检验人员或医护人员）或非职业暴露（如纹身）或子宫内感染。母亲在感染的任意阶段都可能将梅毒传染给胎儿，但在疾病早期感染概率大很多。

未经治疗的后天梅毒可分为四个典型临床分期：

一期梅毒特点为硬下疳，表现为在感染后10~90天（平均3周）感染部位出现硬下疳，典型皮损为单发无痛性硬性溃疡。硬下疳开始为暗红色斑疹，然后变成丘疹，很快中央形成圆形至椭圆形溃疡。典型的硬下疳直径为数毫米至2厘米，境界清楚，疮面质硬，稍隆起于皮面，类软骨变化。皮损底部通常是清洁的，偶有渗出，内含大量梅毒螺旋体。一期梅毒的鉴别诊断总结于表170-2。

二期梅毒，典型皮损被称为梅毒疹，特点为局部或弥漫性的多形皮肤黏膜损害，通常伴随全身淋巴结肿大，而且有血清或组织的实验室证据提示梅毒螺旋体存在。皮肤和黏膜损害是最常见的，通常在硬下疳出现后3~12周出现（最晚可到感染后6个月出现）。几乎所有二期梅毒均发疹，但发疹类型可能有变化。40%~70%的二期梅毒患者通常出现躯干、四肢对称分布的红肿性斑疹（梅毒玫瑰疹）或斑丘疹。丘疹、鳞屑性丘疹及苔藓样变皮损少见。其他皮肤改变包括虫蚀状脱发（弥漫性头皮脱发较少见）、外三分之一眉毛脱落、口周鼻周环形丘疹斑块、黏膜斑和扁平湿疣。另外也可发生蛎壳样溃疡、甲损害以及其他少见皮损。黏膜斑和扁平湿疣皮损含有大量梅毒螺旋体，因此传染性较强，其他皮肤病损的传染性较小。二期梅毒通常在4~12周自主消退，不形成瘢痕，但可能产生色素改变和皮肤萎缩。二期梅毒也可累及皮肤外系统（包括神经梅毒）。

潜伏期梅毒，特点为症状消失，仅有血清学感染证据，它是排他性诊断。需要排除一到三期梅毒以及神经梅毒后方可确诊。可分为早期潜伏期梅毒和晚期潜伏期梅毒。感染梅毒1年内的潜伏梅毒被称为早期潜伏梅毒，治疗同一期和二期梅毒，反之为晚期潜伏期梅毒，需要更长疗程的治疗。

三期梅毒，特点为有皮肤、神经或心血管等多系统病变。有研究表明，大约1/3的未经治疗的潜伏期梅毒患者进展至三期梅毒，尤其是在感染后15至40年，另2/3患者终身保持潜伏期梅毒状态。最常见的改变是梅毒树胶肿（肉芽肿性、侵蚀性的结节型损害，主要导致皮肤和骨改变）和心血管梅毒，也包括晚期神经梅毒。未涉及心血管、神经等重要脏器的三期梅毒被称为晚期良性梅毒。

神经梅毒和眼梅毒可发生于疾病的任何一个时期。

胎传梅毒可分为早期、晚期与胎传潜伏梅毒三类。它不发生硬下疳，类似于后天二期梅毒，常伴有较严重的内脏病变，严重影响胎儿健康。

梅毒的病程长，症状多变。需结合病史（暴露史）、体格检查以及实验室检查方可确诊。不同的梅毒血清学检查的敏感性及特异性总结见表170-6。在临床上运用"逆向检测流程"，即首先行特异性梅毒螺旋体血清学实验，再行非特异性梅毒螺旋体血清学实验，可以提高检出率（图170-39）。

许多种类梅毒的推荐治疗均为苄星青霉

素G，疗程与剂量根据梅毒分期而有所不同（表170-5）。治疗时要注意吉海反应以及预防药物过敏事件发生。所有梅毒阳性的患者均需要检测是否有其他性传播感染，包括HIV。临床医生要对梅毒病例进行上报，对患者进行性安全教育以及积极鼓励梅毒确诊患者的性伴侣共同治疗。

〔张江林〕

AT-A-GLANCE

- A disease caused by the spirochete *Treponema pallidum* subspecies *pallidum* that is almost exclusively sexually transmitted.

- In the United States, syphilis disproportionately affects men who have sex with men and African American heterosexual communities.

- The most common and recognizable manifestations are usually cutaneous.

- Syphilis passes through 4 distinct clinical phases:
  - Primary stage, characterized by a chancre.
  - Secondary stage, characterized typically by skin eruption(s) with or without lymphadenopathy and organ disease.
  - A latent period of varied duration, characterized by the absence of signs or symptoms of disease, with only reactive serologic tests as evidence of infection.
  - Tertiary stage, with cutaneous, neurologic, or cardiovascular manifestations.

- Neurosyphilis and ophthalmic syphilis can occur at any stage.

- The recommended treatment for most types of syphilis is benzathine penicillin G, with dose and administration schedule determined by disease stage.

- Any patient diagnosed with syphilis should be tested for other sexually transmitted infections, including HIV.

DEFINITIONS

Syphilis is a sexually transmitted infection caused by *Treponema pallidum* subspecies *pallidum*. Many of its manifestations are cutaneous, making it of interest and importance to dermatologists, especially as morbidity from syphilis rises in the developed world and continues in the developing world.

HISTORICAL PERSPECTIVE

Whether syphilis arose in the New World, the Old World, or both remains a controversial subject.[1-3] Pandemics of syphilis began in the Old World in Naples, Italy, 1 year after Columbus returned from the New World.[2,4,5] Syphilis earned the moniker "great pox,"[5] to distinguish it from another virulent disease with cutaneous manifestations, smallpox. The disease takes its name from a poem, called *Syphilis, Sive Morbus Gallicus* (*Syphilis*, or *the French Disease*), written in 1530 by Giralomo Fracastoro, a physician and poet of Verona. Part of the poem recounts the story of a shepherd, named Syphilus, who, as punishment for angering Apollo, was afflicted with the disease known as syphilis.[4] Other names besides Morbus Gallicus and the Great Pox by which the disease has been known include lues, the Great Mimic, the Great Masquerader, the Great Imitator, and the Neapolitan disease.[4] The cause of syphilis, the bacterium *T. pallidum*, was discovered by Schaudinn and Hoffman in 1905.[6] Darkfield microscopy was pioneered in 1906 by Landsteiner, and serologic testing for syphilis was pioneered in 1910 by Wasserman.[5]

Because of the skin manifestations, syphilis historically has been of major interest to dermatologists, who were leaders in syphilis research and treatment in Europe and the United States, especially in the prepenicillin era.[7-12] One of the leading American dermatology journals, currently called *Archives of Dermatology*, was before 1955 called *Archives of Dermatology and Syphilology*. An editorial explaining the jettisoning of "Syphilology" from the journal's title stated:

> The diagnosis and treatment of patients with syphilis is no longer an important part of dermatologic practice. The papers on syphilis that are now submitted to the Archives are few and far between. Few dermatologists now have patients with syphilis; in fact, there are decidedly fewer patients with syphilis, and so continuance of the old label, "Syphilology," on this publication seems no longer warranted.

Elsewhere in the world, however, the link between dermatology and syphilology (and other sexually transmitted diseases) remains stronger.[13,14]

Treatments for syphilis in the prepenicillin era included burning sores with hot irons, rubbing mercury-containing ointments (calomel) on lesions, administering mercury orally, and treating with arsenicals, including salvarsan (also called "606" or arsphenamine), which was the first systemic treatment and was discovered by Ehrlich and Hata in 1909.[5] Arsenical and other heavy metal-based therapies required multiple injections for at least a year, and were highly toxic. Recognition that *T. pallidum* was heat sensitive led the Viennese psychiatrist Julius Wagner von Jauregg to develop syphilis malariotherapy in 1917,[15] an accomplishment for which he received the Nobel Prize in Medicine in 1927.[16] That therapy involved inoculating syphilis patients with malaria, allowing them to experience, optimally, between 10 and 12 febrile episodes, and then treating them with quinine.[10,16-18] The treatment reportedly led to complete or partial remission of neurosyphilis (general paresis) in a substantial proportion of patients, although it killed an estimated 10% of those receiving the therapy.[17]

Two studies have provided the most insight into the natural history of syphilis. The first was a retrospective study of approximately 2000 persons with syphilis in Oslo, where mercury treatments standard in other places were not used.[18] The second was the infamous Tuskegee syphilis study, in which 399 black men from Alabama who had late syphilis were prospectively followed from 1932 to 1972.[19] The men were denied treatment for syphilis, even after the discovery of the effectiveness of penicillin for the disease. There were multiple other serious ethical lapses in the study. The aftermath of the study led to major changes in ethical requirements for conducting clinical research in the United States.[20]

Of historical interest, persons said to have suffered from syphilis include Ivan the Terrible, Henry VIII, Henri de Toulouse-Lautrec, and Al Capone,[5] among many others.[21] Osler, aware of the high prevalence and protean manifestations of syphilis, has been quoted as saying, "He who knows syphilis knows medicine."[5] By the early 1930s, it was estimated that approximately 10% of Americans had syphilis, with 500,000 new infections and 60,000 cases of congenital syphilis per year.[22] In 1937, Surgeon General Thomas Parran, keenly interested in syphilis, published a book, titled *Shadow on the Land*,[23] that focused on the substantial public health harms of the then-prevalent disease.[22] Parran developed and implemented a national program for syphilis prevention and control, emphasizing screening, treatment, community involvement, and education.[22,24] Penicillin was first used to treat syphilis in 1943, and became widely available in the postwar era.[5] As a result of effective treatment, syphilis incidence then declined sharply in the 1950s, followed by a modest rebound through the mid-1980s. In the late 1980s and early 1990s syphilis reemerged in the United States in the South and in large cities, disproportionately affecting black Americans, and associated with crack cocaine and commercial sex workers.[2,25] The waning of the crack epidemic and development of the National Plan to Eliminate Syphilis from the United States, released in 1999 by the Centers for Disease Control and Prevention (CDC), resulted in declining rates in heterosexuals.[26] However, since the late 1990s, there has been a dramatic increase in incidence in men who have sex with men in the United States and other developed countries.

EPIDEMIOLOGY

In 2000 and 2001, the rate of reported primary and secondary syphilis in the United States was the lowest it had been since reporting began in 1941, at 2.1 cases per 100,000 population. Unfortunately, syphilis incidence in the United States has been increasing steadily since 2001; the rate of primary and secondary syphilis (which is indicative of incident infection) was 6.3 cases per 100,000 population in 2014, the highest rate reported since 1994.[27] The current syphilis epidemic in the United States has been primarily driven by increasing cases among gay, bisexual, and other men who have sex with men (MSM). Of 19,999 reported cases of primary and secondary syphilis in 2014, 12,226 (61.1%) were among MSM and 3,407 (17.0%) were among men without information about the gender of the sex partner. Among male cases with information on gender of sex partner, 82.9% occurred in MSM.[27] Incidence of syphilis and other sexually transmitted infections among MSM had declined during the AIDS epidemic, and the subsequent increased incidence among MSM has been attributed to a number of factors, including a decrease in safe sex practices resulting from successful HIV treatments, use of the internet to meet sex partners, serosorting (ie, attempting to choose sex partners who share the same HIV status), and an increase in use of recreational drugs, including methamphetamine and erectile dysfunction medicines.[2,28,29] Studies that led to the approval, in 2012, for the use of oral antiretroviral medications for pre-exposure prophylaxis to prevent HIV acquisition in high-risk individuals generally did not report increased sexual risk behavior or acquisition of sexually transmitted infections.[30] However, how widespread rollout of preexposure prophylaxis may affect syphilis rates, particularly in MSM, remains to be seen.[31] The epidemics of HIV and syphilis in the United States MSM population have been intimately linked. Not only are a high proportion of patients coinfected (in 2014, 51.2% of cases of reported primary and secondary syphilis among MSM were also HIV-positive),[27] but incident syphilis infection also is associated with a significantly increased risk of HIV acquisition.[32-34] All patients diagnosed with syphilis should be tested for the other sexually transmitted infections, including HIV. Conversely, all patients diagnosed with HIV should also be tested for the other sexually transmitted infections, including syphilis.[35]

Although rising syphilis incidence in the United States is primarily attributable to cases in MSM, the general male and female populations are affected as well. During 2013-2014, the primary and secondary syphilis rate increased 14.4% in men and 22.7% in women.[27] The increase in women has been particularly concerning because of a concomitant rise in reported cases of congenital syphilis. In 2015, the CDC released a report warning of a 38% increase in reported cases of congenital syphilis between 2012 and 2014. Although rates in all ethnic groups increased, the rate of congenital syphilis in blacks remained approximately 10 times the rate among whites in 2014.[36]

Rates of primary and secondary syphilis nationwide are highest in persons 20 to 29 years old. There is a major health disparity; blacks are disproportionately affected by primary and secondary syphilis, with rates in 2014 more than 5 times higher than rates among non–Hispanic whites overall.[27]

Recently, there has been an increase in reported cases of ocular syphilis. Between December 2014 and March 2015, 12 cases of ocular syphilis were reported from San Francisco, California, and Seattle, Washington. Several of these patients suffered severe sequelae, including permanent vision loss. Subsequent case finding indicated more than 200 cases reported over the past 2 years from 20 states. As a result, in October 2015, the CDC released a clinical advisory calling for vigilance and careful screening for visual complaints in any patient at risk for syphilis.[37,38]

Internationally, morbidity from syphilis remains substantial. Each year an estimated 12 million new cases of syphilis occur, and 1 million pregnancies are complicated by syphilis.[2]

TABLE 170-1
Stages of Syphilis

Contact (one-third become infected)
↓ (10-90 days)
Primary (chancre)
↓ (3-12 weeks)
Secondary (mucocutaneous lesions, organ involvement)
↓ (4-12 weeks)
Early latent → Relapsing (1/4) (1 year from contact)
↓
Late latent (more than 1 year)

| Continue late latent (two-thirds) | Tertiary (one-third)
• Late benign (16%)
• Cardiovascular (10%)
• Neurosyphilis (5% to 10%) |

Neurosyphilis can occur (including ocular syphilis)

CLINICAL FEATURES

When considering syphilis in the differential diagnosis in a patient, clinicians should take into account the epidemiology and routes of transmission of the disease. This requires taking a complete sexual history. Patients should be asked about partners (including gender and number of recent sexual partners), sexual practices (including anatomic exposure site and use of condoms), and past history of sexually transmitted infections. Effective interviewing skills characterized by respect and a nonjudgmental attitude are critical to obtaining an accurate assessment of behavioral risk.[35]

Untreated syphilis is characterized by multiple distinct stages of disease, each of which is associated with different clinical (including cutaneous) manifestations. Table 170-1 outlines the natural history of syphilis.

EXPOSURE AND INCUBATING SYPHILIS

Syphilis in adults is almost exclusively sexually acquired, when a person comes in contact with infectious lesions of syphilis on another person. Of note, these lesions are only present during primary or secondary syphilis, so the infection is considered sexually transmissible solely in these stages. Importantly, patients with early latent syphilis (within the first year of infection) can relapse into secondary syphilis and become infectious again.[16] Infectious lesions of syphilis in adults, which include chancres, condyloma lata, and mucous patches, can be present anywhere on the body but are typically located in or around the genital, anal, or oral area. Direct contact with infectious lesions during oral, vaginal, or anal sex, or during other sexual activities, can result in inoculation and infection. Lesions on keratinized skin (eg, secondary syphilis palmoplantar lesions and maculopapular rash on the trunk) typically do not contain sufficient treponemes to be infectious, and prophylaxis for persons exposed to noninfectious lesions such as those is neither necessary nor indicated. Infectious lesions of congenital syphilis include discharge from rhinitis ("snuffles") and bullous lesions on the skin.

Nonsexually acquired syphilis rarely occurs[39] and when it does, it is usually via blood transfusion (of unscreened blood),[40] accidental inoculation in an occupational setting (eg, laboratory or health care worker)[41] or nonoccupational setting (eg, tattooing),[42] or through exposure in utero.[43] Transmission to the fetus may occur at any stage of maternal infection, although it is far more likely in the early stages of disease.[16,44]

Estimates of the risk of acquisition ("transmission efficiency") of syphilis following sexual exposure to a person with infectious syphilis are varied and have been derived in 2 types of sources.[45] The first source are data from 3 prospective placebo-controlled trials of prophylactic treatment, in which 9%,[46] 28%,[47] or 63%[48] of sexual contacts to syphilis acquired syphilis. The second source is from studies of persons identified as sex contacts in contact-tracing interviews of persons diagnosed with syphilis, in which 18% to 88% of contacts acquired syphilis.[45] Nevertheless, the relatively high estimates of syphilis acquisition following exposure underscores the importance of prompt treatment and testing of sexual contacts, as discussed 'Disease Reporting and Management of Persons Exposed to Syphilis' section. Persons recently exposed to and infected with syphilis who have yet to manifest signs or symptoms of the disease are said to have incubating syphilis.

PRIMARY SYPHILIS

Primary syphilis is the first stage of syphilis, and is characterized by the appearance of 1 or more chancres. Treponemes in the cerebrospinal fluid (CSF) can be demonstrated in up to 30% of primary and secondary syphilis cases.[49] There may be overlap of secondary syphilis or even neurosyphilis manifestations with primary syphilis.

CUTANEOUS FINDINGS

At the inoculation site, a chancre develops after an incubation period that ranges from 10 to 90 days (average: 3 weeks). The chancre starts as a dusky red macule that evolves into a papule and then a round-to-oval ulcer (Figs. 170-1 to 170-4). The typical chancre, also called a *Hunterian chancre* or *ulcus durum* (hard ulcer), ranges in diameter from a few millimeters to 2 cm and is sharply demarcated with regular, raised borders that are indurated, giving the lesion a cartilaginous feel. The base is usually clean, and the chancre is classically painless. Pain can be reported,[50] and multiple chancres have been reported in 32% to 47% of cases.[51] The absence of any of the typical features of a chancre does not rule out syphilis, however. Variations in clinical presentation can result from the number of spirochetes inoculated, the patient's immune status, concurrent antibiotic therapy, and impetiginization.[52-54] Because they are typically painless, patients might not be aware of chancres, especially if painless and located in areas that are not visible, such as the ventral uncircumcised penis, anus, vagina, cervix, or oral cavity.[55,56]

Common genital locations for a chancre in men include the glans, the coronal sulcus, and the foreskin.[57,58] Retraction of the foreskin when a chancre is present on the underside causes the foreskin to flip suddenly, a sign known as the *dory flop*, after the movement of a dory, a small wooden fishing boat, which flips suddenly when overturned.[57] The dory flop sign can help distinguish chancres from other nonindurated causes of genital ulcer disease, such as herpes simplex virus infection and chancroid, that present without the induration that leads to the sudden flip of the foreskin. Uncommon presentations include giant necrotic chancre, phagedenic chancre (a deep, bright-red, necrotic ulcer with a soft base and exudate, resulting from secondary bacterial infection associated with immunosuppression), phimosis resulting from adherence of a chancre on the foreskin to the glans, endourethral ulcers leading to swelling or serosanguinous discharge, and balanitis.[56,58]

Common genital locations in women include the cervix, labia majora, labia minora, fourchette, urethra and perineum (see Fig. 170-4).[58,59] Chancres in women, especially labial ones, can be more edematous than indurated.[58] *Edema indurativum* is a unilateral labial swelling with rubbery consistency and intact surface, indicative of a deep-seated chancre.

Extragenital chancres occur where there may be exposure, and are most frequent in the oropharyngeal cavity.[60,61] Syphilis can be transmitted via either receptive or active oral sexual exposure, and is seen in both heterosexual and MSM.[62,63] Oral lesions are often larger and may lack the indurated borders that are more typical in keratinized tissues (Fig. 170-5). Anal sex can lead

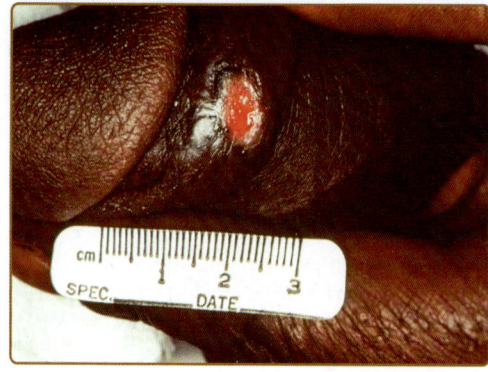

Figure 170-2 Early chancre on the penile shaft, demonstrating a clean base.

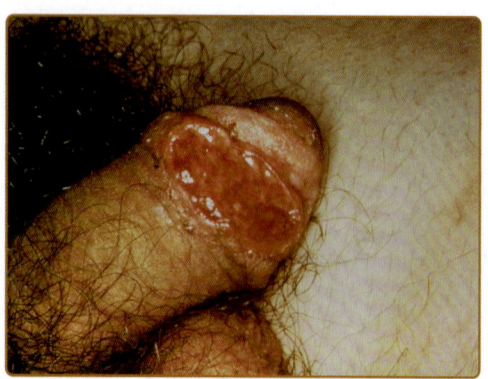

Figure 170-1 Early chancre presenting as a large oval ulcer with elevated borders on the shaft of the penis.

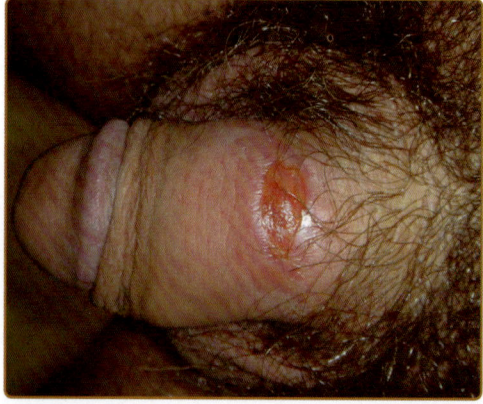

Figure 170-3 Chancre on the penile shaft, demonstrating a clean base and elevated borders

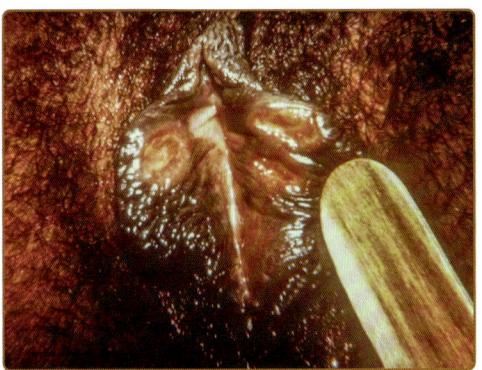

Figure 170-4 Chancres on the labia in a female.

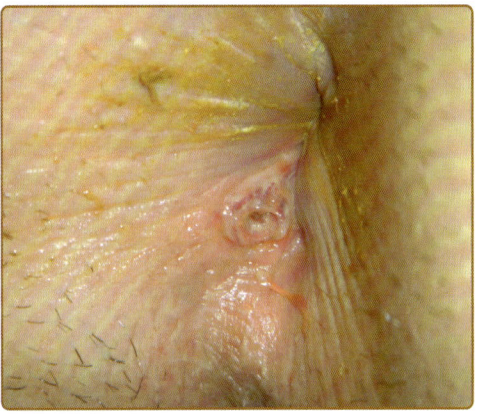

Figure 170-6 Chancre in the perianal area. Fecal material is also present in the area.

to development of chancres in the perianal (Fig. 170-6) or anal areas that can be difficult to detect on routine physical examination.[50,64] Digital or other[65,66] contact with the oral, genital, or anal areas, or receiving a bite (eg, on the nipple during sex)[67] can also lead to infection and chancre on the exposed area.

The chancre heals in 3 to 6 weeks without treatment and 1 to 2 weeks with treatment. Scarring typically does not occur, although thin atrophic scars may occur.[55] Coinfection with herpes simplex virus or *Haemophilus ducreyi*, the causative organism of chancroid, can be present in rare cases.[68-70] Relapses of primary syphilis, called *monorecidive syphilis* or *chancre redux*, arise in the setting of untreated or inadequately treated syphilis and are rare.[71]

Table 170-2 outlines the differential diagnosis of chancres.

NONCUTANEOUS FINDINGS

In 60% to 70% of cases of primary syphilis, painless regional lymphadenopathy arises 7 to 10 days after the chancre appears, especially when the chancre's location is genital. Unilateral lymphadenopathy is more common earlier in the course of disease, with bilateral involvement later in the course.[71]

SECONDARY SYPHILIS

Secondary syphilis is essentially an infectious vasculitis, characterized by localized or diffuse mucocutaneous lesions, often with generalized lymphadenopathy, in the presence of laboratory evidence from tissues or sera consistent with syphilis.[72] Cutaneous and mucosal locations are most common.[73]

CUTANEOUS FINDINGS

Lesions of secondary syphilis, classically called *syphilids* or, when affecting the skin, *syphiloderms*,[58] typically erupt 3 to 12 weeks after the chancre appears (up to 6 months after exposure). In some cases lesions of the secondary syphilis develop while the chancre is still present,[51,53] with overlap more common among HIV-infected persons.[53] Rash is present in nearly all cases of secondary syphilis, although the specific type of rash varies.[51,52,74] Erythematous macules (*roseola syphilitica*) or maculopapules are commonly present

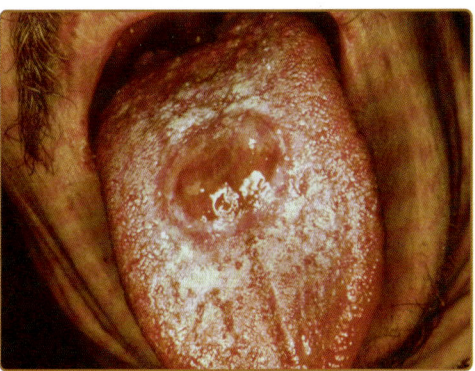

Figure 170-5 Chancre on the tongue.

TABLE 170-2
Differential Diagnosis of Primary Syphilis

Infectious
- Aphthous ulcer
- Chancroid
- Erosive candidal vulvitis or balanitis
- Granuloma inguinale
- Herpes simplex
- Lymphogranuloma venereum
- Vaccinia

Noninfectious
- Basal cell carcinoma
- Behçet disease
- Fixed-drug eruption
- Squamous cell carcinoma
- Traumatic erosion or ulcer

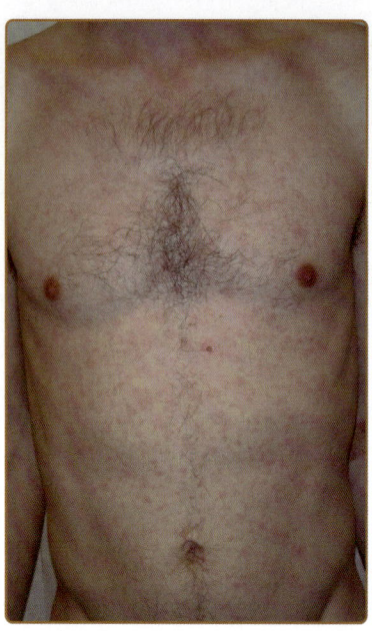

Figure 170-7 Rash of secondary syphilis with nonscaling, oval pink, ill-defined macules and patches on the trunk.

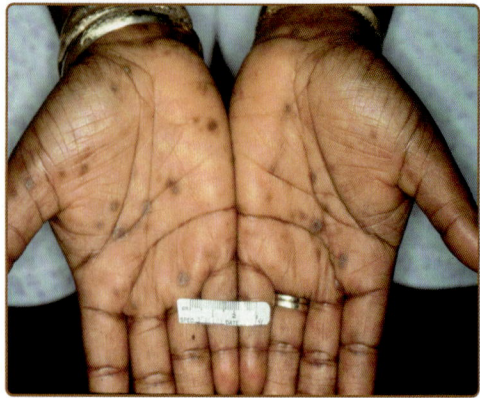

Figure 170-9 Secondary syphilis lesions: multiple, hyperpigmented scaly papules on the palms.

symmetrically on the trunk and extremities in 40% to 70% of cases (Fig. 170-7), with papular, papulosquamous, or lichenoid presentations less common.[51,74] A white scaly ring on the surface of papulosquamous lesions, called the *Biett collarette* (Fig. 170-8), is characteristic of, but not pathognomonic for, syphilis. The face is typically spared in these generalized syphilids, although seborrheic dermatitis–like lesions around the hairline, termed the *Crown of Venus* or *corona veneris*, can form a crown-like pattern.[55] Lesions are not usually pruritic,[58] although pruritus was reported in up to 40% of patients in one study.[58] The presentation of the rash overall can be subtle or florid, or can develop from subtle macules to more florid papules over time.[75] Erythematous to copper-colored round papules or macules, well demarcated and sometimes with an annular scale, are present on the palms and soles in nearly 75% of cases (Figs. 170-9 to 170-12) and classically cross the palmar creases.[51] Plantar lesions can be variously mistaken for calluses (*clavi syphilitici*). Plantar lesions can also extend to the lateral and posterior aspects of the foot (Fig. 170-13).

Other dermatologic manifestations include a patchy nonscarring alopecia, described as *moth-eaten* (see Fig. 170-11) or, less commonly, a diffuse alopecia of the scalp. Loss of lateral third of the eyebrows can occur. Annular papules and plaques can be present around the mouth and nose, in a presentation colloquially referred to as "nickels and dimes" (Fig. 170-14).[58] Papules and plaques, sometimes annular and occasionally papulosquamous, also can be present on the penis and scrotum (Fig. 170-15). Mucous patches are white-to-yellow erosions on the tongue that efface lingual papillae (Fig. 170-16).[58] Confluence of mucous patches on the tongue has been termed *plaques fauchée*

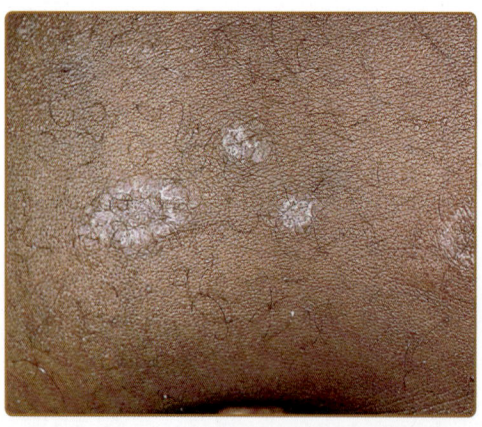

Figure 170-8 Papulosquamous syphilitic eruption with erythematous, well-demarcated, flattened plaques covered with scales (Biett collarette).

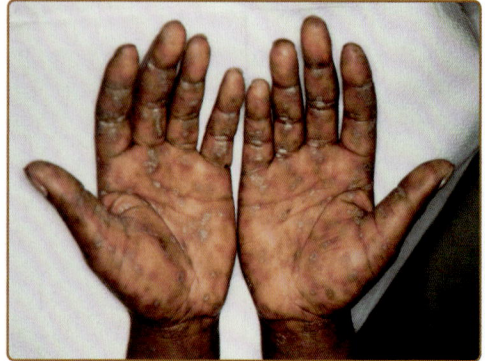

Figure 170-10 Secondary syphilis lesions: multiple, hyperpigmented papules with more pronounced scale on the palms.

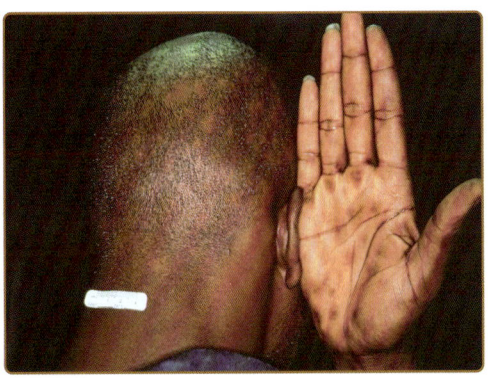

Figure 170-11 Secondary syphilis lesions on palm and moth-eaten alopecia of secondary syphilis.

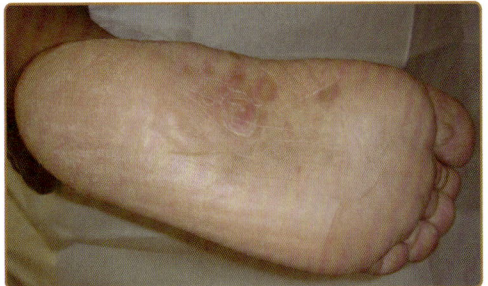

Figure 170-12 Secondary syphilis lesions on sole of foot.

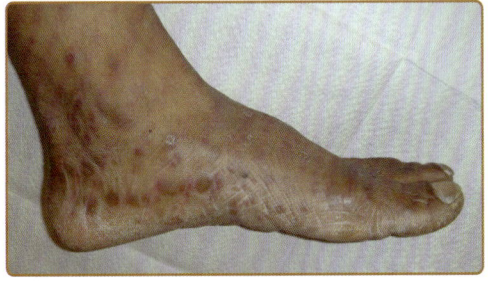

Figure 170-13 Plantar lesions of secondary syphilis extending to the lateral aspect of the foot.

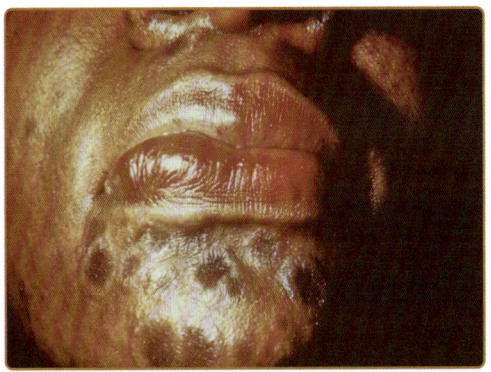

Figure 170-14 Annular plaques of secondary syphilis on the face, colloquially referred to as "nickels and dimes."

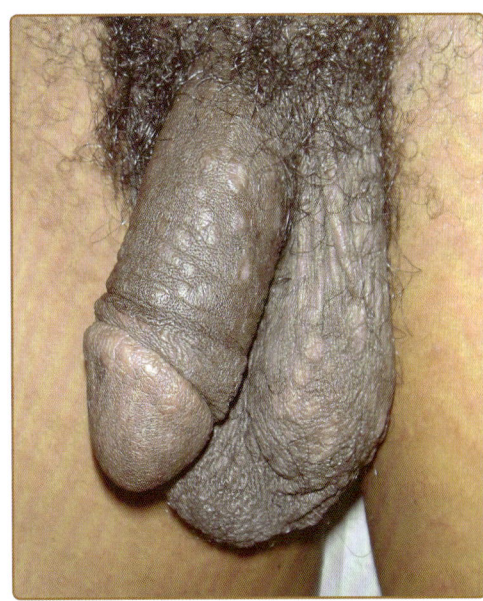

Figure 170-15 Papules of secondary syphilis on the penis.

en prairie. Mucous patches can be present elsewhere in the oral cavity (Fig. 170-17), on other mucous membranes (such as on the genitalia), or at the corners of the mouth, where they appear as "split papules," with an erosion traversing the center (Fig. 170-18). Mucous patches are teeming with spirochetes and, hence, highly infectious. Also highly infectious are condyloma lata, which present as moist, flat, well-demarcated papules or plaques with macerated or eroded surfaces in intertriginous areas, commonly in

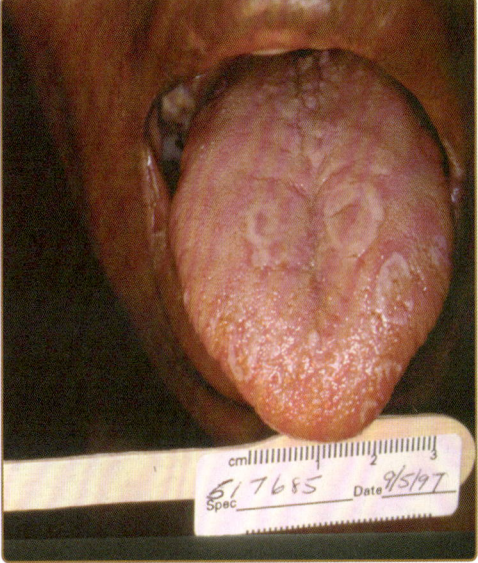

Figure 170-16 Mucous patches of the tongue in secondary syphilis. Note lack of typical lingual papillae in affected areas.

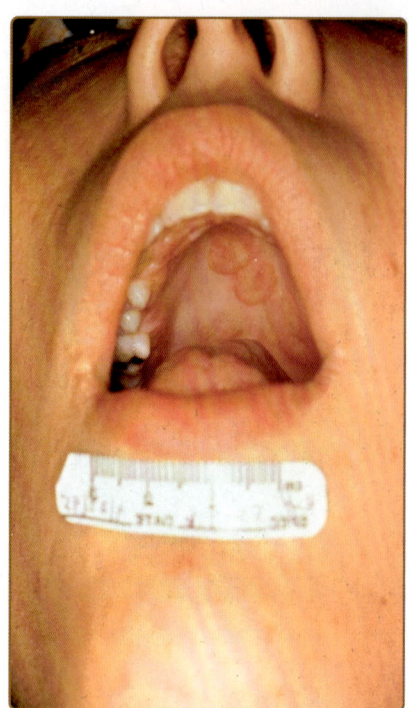

Figure 170-17 Mucous patches on hard palate.

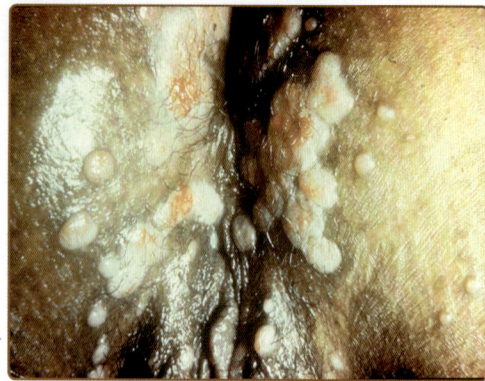

Figure 170-19 Condyloma lata, presenting as moist papules in the perineum.

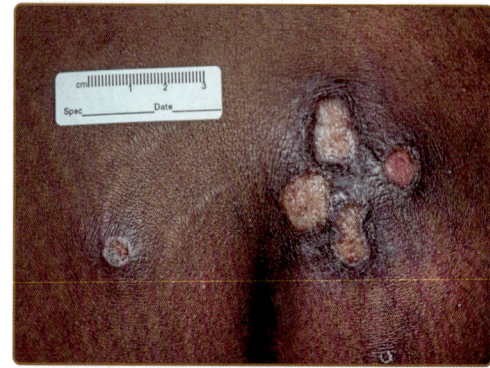

Figure 170-20 Condyloma lata, presenting as moist, flat-topped plaques on the buttocks.

the labial folds in females or in the perianal region in all patients (Figs. 170-19 to 170-21).[58] However, any moist intertriginous area of the body can harbor condyloma lata, including the axillae, web spaces between toes, and the folds under breasts, umbilicus (Fig. 170-22) or an abdominal panniculus. Mucous patches and condyloma lata have been reported in 8% and 17% of patients with secondary syphilis, respectively.[51] Malignant lues is a rare manifestation that presents as crusted or scaly papules and plaques that

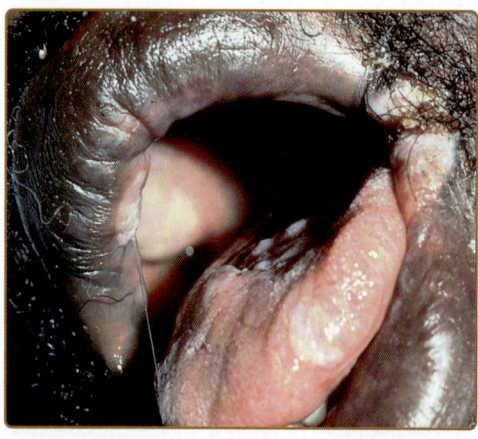

Figure 170-18 Split papule, a type of mucous patch of secondary syphilis that can be present at the angle of the mouth, with a characteristic slit traversing its center.

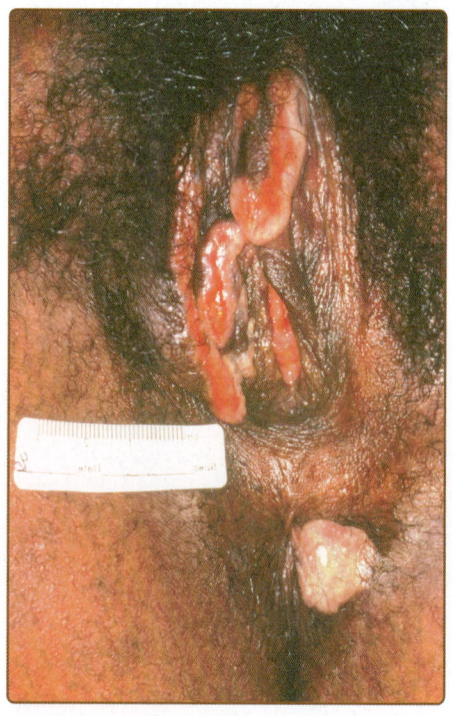

Figure 170-21 Condyloma lata in a female.

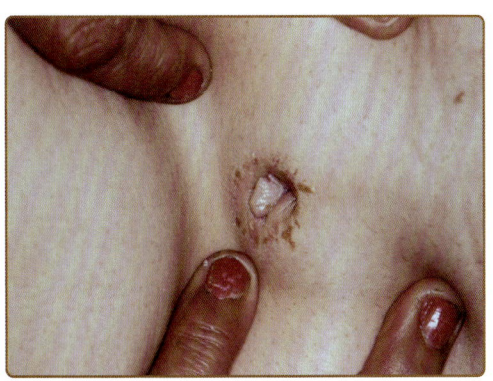

Figure 170-22 Moist papule in the umbilicus in secondary syphilis.

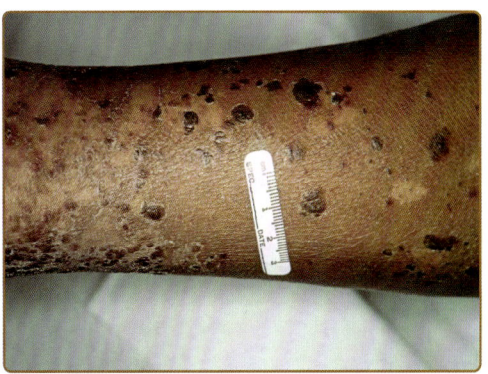

Figure 170-24 Multiple hyperpigmented papules of secondary syphilis on the arm.

can ulcerate or become necrotic, with an oyster shell-like surface (Fig. 170-23). These lesions, described as rupioid, are often seen in association with high nontreponemal titers and systemic symptoms.[76] Nail changes including fissuring, onycholysis, Beau lines, and onychomadesis have been reported.[55] Less-common presentations of secondary syphilis include hyperkeratotic, lichenoid, nodular, follicular, pustular, frambesiform, and corymbose eruptions and palmoplantar keratodermas (Figs. 170-24 to 170-26).[56,77-80] With the exception of mucous patches and condyloma lata, cutaneous manifestations of secondary syphilis do not contain a substantial number of treponemes and, therefore, are not typically infectious.

The maculopapular rash of secondary syphilis can resemble almost any generalized or localized maculopapular eruption (Table 170-3); mucous membrane lesions resemble mucosal manifestations of other dermatoses, and syphilitic hair loss has to be separated from other etiologies of alopecias.

Without treatment, the secondary stage typically recedes 4 to 12 weeks after it appears. Scarring typically does not occur, although pigmentary changes (leukoderma colli syphiliticum or, if on the neck, "necklace of Venus") can result[55] from inhibition of melanogenesis. Dermal atrophy, possibly related to elastin degradation, may occur. Absence of syphilids in cinnabar-containing red tattoos has been reported as well, possibly resulting from the antitreponemal effect of mercury in cinnabar.[81]

NONCUTANEOUS FINDINGS

In addition to neurosyphilis (including ocular syphilis),[82] discussed in section "Neurosyphilis" patients with secondary syphilis may experience systemic symptoms that include sore throat, malaise, headache, weight loss, fever, musculoskeletal aches, pruritus, and hoarseness.[74] Pharyngitis and tonsillitis,[83] laryngitis,[84] gastritis,[85] hepatitis,[85] renal disease (membranous glomerulopathy),[86] and periostitis[87] have all been reported in secondary syphilis, as have hematologic abnormalities including lymphopenia, anemia, and elevated erythrocyte sedimentation rate.[88] Lymphadenopathy is common, and is often bilateral and symmetric in distribution.[58]

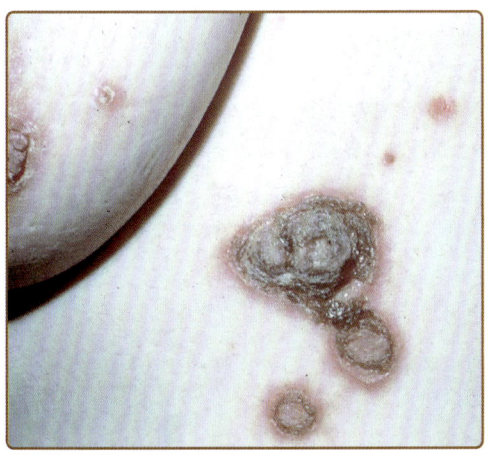

Figure 170-23 Sharply marginated, necrotic ulcers of secondary syphilis described as "rupioid," covered by thick, dirty crusts (like oyster shells).

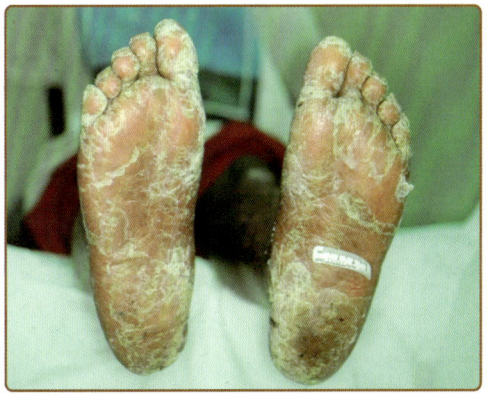

Figure 170-25 Hyperkeratotic lesions of secondary syphilis on the soles.

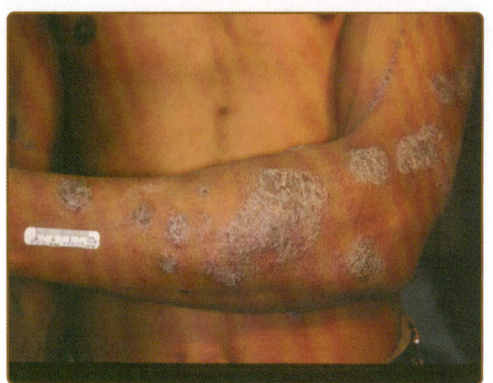

Figure 170-26 Psoriaform lesions of secondary syphilis on the arm.

LATENT SYPHILIS

The secondary stage is followed by an asymptomatic stage with no clinical findings, with seroreactivity by definition the only evidence of infection. So-called latent syphilis is a diagnosis of exclusion, after primary, secondary, and tertiary syphilis (including neurosyphilis) have been ruled out. Asymptomatic patients who have acquired syphilis within the last year are classified as having "early latent" infection.[35] The distinction between *early latent* and asymptomatic syphilis acquired more than 1 year ago (often termed *late latent syphilis*), is important for 2 reasons. First, up to 25% of patients with early latent syphilis may relapse into secondary syphilis, leading to possible sexual transmission.[16] Second, clinical management of patients with early latent syphilis differs from management of patients with late latent syphilis.[16,35] The treatment of early latent syphilis is the same as that of primary and secondary (collectively termed *early syphilis*), whereas late syphilis requires an extended therapeutic course.[35]

Persons who acquired syphilis during the preceding year can be diagnosed with *early* latent syphilis. A patient can be classified as having early latent syphilis if, within the year preceding discovery of the reactive serologic test, the patient had 1 of the following:

1. Documented seroconversion or a sustained (longer than 2 weeks) fourfold or greater increase in nontreponemal test titers;
2. Unequivocal symptoms of primary or secondary syphilis;
3. A sex partner documented to have primary, secondary, or early latent syphilis; or
4. Reactive nontreponemal and treponemal tests if the patient's only possible exposure occurred within the previous 12 months.[35]

To make a diagnosis of early latent syphilis based on the first or third criterion above, clinicians often need, and should seek, the assistance of the local health department. Because syphilis diagnoses and results of reactive serologic tests for syphilis are reportable in every state and territory of the United States, local or state health departments compile (or attempt to compile) records of all syphilis diagnoses and reactive serologic titers for persons residing in the jurisdiction. Clinicians can contact the "reactor desk" of their local or state health jurisdiction, where syphilis diagnostic and titer histories are maintained, to inquire about a patient's titer history and prior diagnoses and treatments, so that a patient can be staged as having early latent syphilis according to the first criterion above. Public health workers can also search diagnostic and titer histories in their databases for the names of sex partners identified by seroreactive patients, to enable staging patients with early latent syphilis under the third criteria above.

Patients in whom the duration of infection cannot be established based on the criteria reference above should be assumed to have late latent syphilis and must be managed accordingly. Latent syphilis may remain indefinitely or progress to the tertiary stage.

TABLE 170-3
Differential Diagnosis of the Maculopapular Rash of Secondary Syphilis

Most Likely
- Drug eruption
- Pityriasis rosea
- Psoriasis
- Viral eruption
- Differential for condyloma lata: Condyloma acuminata

Consider
- Balanitis
- Cutaneous T-cell lymphoma
- Dermatophytosis
- Eczema
- Erythema multiforme
- Granuloma annulare
- Lichen planus
- Lupus erythematosus
- Sarcoid
- Vasculitis
- Vulvitis

TERTIARY SYPHILIS

Late manifestations of syphilis are rarely seen. However, historically, on the basis of information from the Oslo and Tuskegee studies, approximately one-third of patients with untreated latent syphilis progress to tertiary syphilis, typically after 15 to 40 years, while the other two-thirds remain in latency.[16] Tertiary syphilis manifestations may include gummas (granulomatous, erosive, nodular lesions which most commonly affect the skin and bones), and cardiovascular syphilis.[35] Although neurosyphilis can occur at any stage of disease (see "Neurosyphilis" later), late manifestations of neurosyphilis are also considered to be a manifestation of tertiary syphilis.

CUTANEOUS FINDINGS

The signs and symptoms of syphilis that occur after secondary syphilis that do not involve the cardiovascular or nervous systems have historically been referred to as *late benign syphilis*. Lesions of late benign syphilis are caused by delayed-type hypersensitivity responses to the small number of treponemes present in the involved tissue or organ.[54] The hallmark of late benign syphilis is the *gumma*, a granulomatous nodular lesion with variable central necrosis, which most commonly affect the skin or mucous membranes (80% of gummas).[54] Gummas are nontender pink to dusky-red nodules or plaques that vary in size from millimeters to many centimeters in diameter. They favor sites of previous trauma and may arise anywhere on the body, but are more common on the scalp, forehead (Fig. 170-27), buttocks, and presternal, supraclavicular, or pretibial areas. The nodule is initially firm but develops a gummy consistency from accumulation of necrotic tissue. Gummas may grow both horizontally and vertically, and many assume geometric configurations. Small ulcers and abscesses may be present within the lesions. As the central gumma heals, new lesions may develop on the periphery, forming scalloped borders. In contrast to noduloulcerative lesions, gummas are deeper and more destructive (Fig. 170-28). Tissue necrosis eventuates in cylindrical, punched-out ulcers with clean granulomatous bases covered with adherent yellow-white slough (Fig. 170-29). The ulcer may enlarge, remain unchanged, or heal spontaneously, even as the gumma enlarges. Superficial gummas heal with atrophic scars, whereas deeper lesions

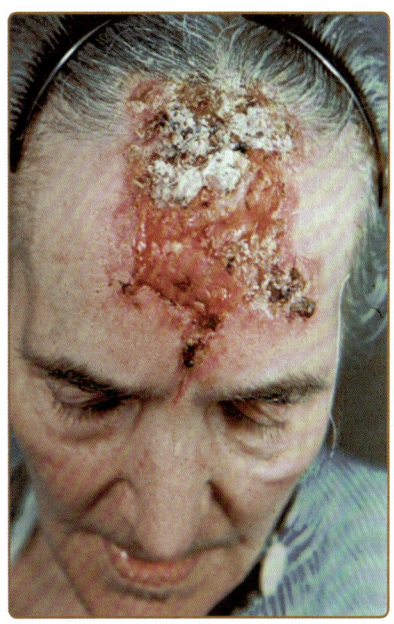

Figure 170-28 Aggressive gumma of the forehead causing destruction of the calvarium, mimicking advanced, destructive basal cell carcinoma.

leave thickened, pitted, ridged scars. Pseudochancre redux refers to a solitary gumma of the penis.

Gummas involving the mucous membranes typically affect the palate, nasal mucosa, tongue, tonsils, and pharynx. The lesions ulcerate and can be disfiguring, as when they cause a saddle-nose deformity from destruction of nasal cartilage and bone, or perforation

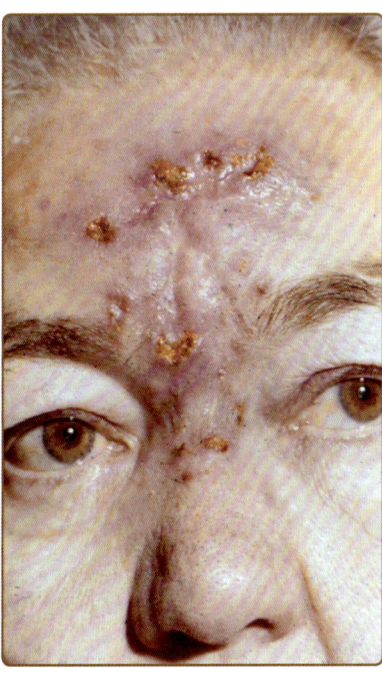

Figure 170-27 Disfiguring gummatous infiltration of the glabella and forehead with scattered ulcerations in a 60-year-old woman with late benign syphilis.

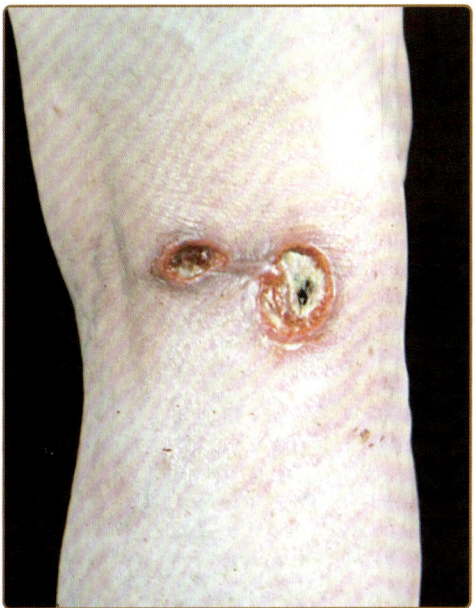

Figure 170-29 Two deep, punched-out ulcers in the popliteal fossa covered with an adherent yellow slough at the base. This is the classical appearance of nodular gummas.

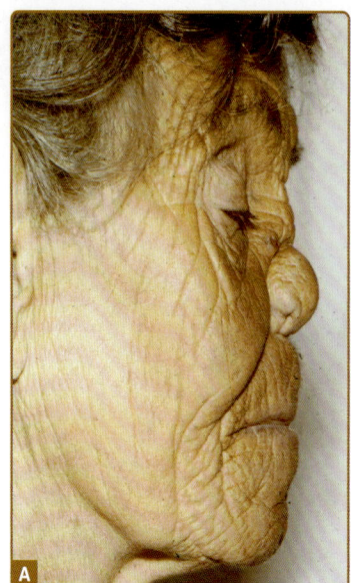 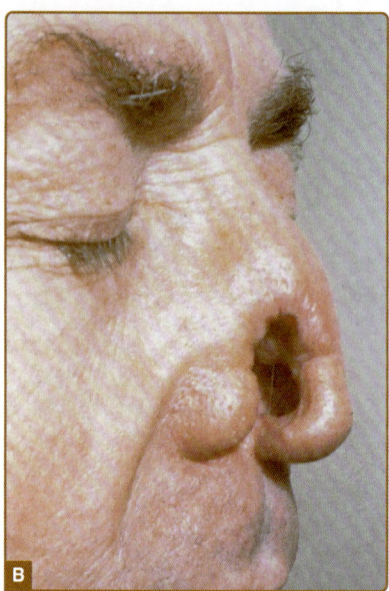

Figure 170-30 Destruction of the nasal cartilage and bone by a gumma leads to a saddle nose (**A**) and to the perforation of the nasal cartilage and skin and thus to considerable mutilation (**B**).

of the nose or palate (Fig. 170-30).[54] Gummas do not heal without appropriate antibiotic therapy, but in the setting of appropriate therapy respond briskly, leaving scars.[16] Chronic interstitial glossitis can develop even after penicillin treatment and may undergo malignant degeneration (Fig. 170-31).

Other manifestations of late benign syphilis affecting the skin include granulomatous nodular and noduloulcerative lesions and psoriasiform plaques.[55] Nodular and noduloulcerative lesions are superficial, firm, painless, dull-red, shiny, flat nodules that range in size from several millimeters to 2 cm. They appear in a grouped configuration, can coalesce into large plaques or ulcerate, and can resemble granuloma annulare.[89,90] Psoriasiform plaques are most commonly seen on the arms, back, and face.

Table 170-4 outlines the differential diagnosis of dermatologic manifestations of tertiary syphilis.

NONCUTANEOUS FINDINGS

Besides the skin and mucous membranes, gummas can affect practically any organ, but especially the bones, as well as the liver, heart, brain, stomach, and upper respiratory tract.[16] When they involve critical organs such as the brain, gummas can have serious complications.[91]

Historically, cardiovascular manifestations of tertiary syphilis affected 10% to 40% of those infected and were thought to be responsible for most deaths caused by syphilis.[16] Syphilis typically causes syphilitic aortitis, leading to aortic regurgitation in 10% of individuals with untreated disease,[92] and can also cause coronary ostial stenosis and saccular aneurysm.[93] T. pallidum DNA has been detected in an aortic aneurysm, demonstrating that infection of the aorta leads to direct damage to the tissue.[94]

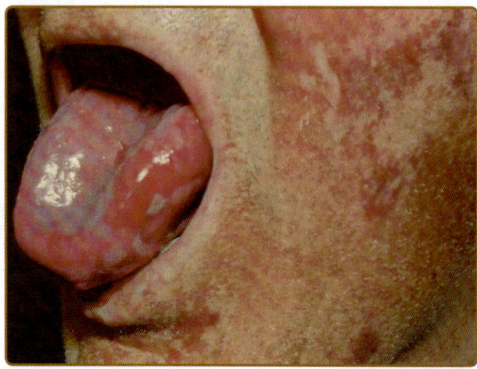

Figure 170-31 Premalignant, chronic, interstitial glossitis secondary to gummatous infiltration of the tongue.

TABLE 170-4
Differential Diagnosis of Tertiary Syphilis

Consider
- Deep fungal infections
- Granulomatosis with polyangiitis (Wegener polyangiitis)
- Leishmaniasis
- Lupus vulgaris
- Lymphomas
- Metastatic carcinoma
- Psoriasis
- Sarcoid
- Sarcomas
- Vasculitis

NEUROSYPHILIS

Infection of the CNS by *T. pallidum* can occur during any stage of infection. "Neuroinvasion," in which *T. pallidum* disseminates to CSF and meninges, occurs very early in syphilis.[95] Neuroinvasion can be transient, with the body clearing the infection, or more sustained, in which case it is called asymptomatic neurosyphilis, defined by CSF abnormalities. Asymptomatic neurosyphilis, if discovered, is usually treated to prevent progression to symptomatic neurosyphilis, although benefits of treatment for asymptomatic neurosyphilis are not well documented.

Early symptomatic neurosyphilis typically manifests as meningitis, resulting in meningismus, fever, or cranial nerve abnormalities (especially cranial nerves II, III, IV, VI, VII, and VIII), or meningovasculitis, resulting in meningitis with stroke, usually affecting the portion of the brain supplied by the middle cerebral artery.[95] Uveitis is the most common ophthalmic manifestation of early neurosyphilis (see "Ocular Syphilis" below), presenting as eye pain, redness, and photophobia, and sensorineural hearing loss is the most common manifestation of otologic syphilis. Ophthalmic and otologic manifestations of early neurosyphilis are managed in the same way as neurologic manifestations.[35,95]

Early symptomatic neurosyphilis is not uncommon. A review of syphilis cases among HIV-infected men in 4 large U.S. cities during 2002 to 2004 showed that almost 2%, including persons at each stage of infection, had symptomatic early neurosyphilis. Ocular abnormalities were most common among those affected, followed by other cranial nerve involvement, acute meningitis, other syndromes (headache, altered mental status, or both), and cerebrovascular accidents. Of those with symptomatic early neurosyphilis, nearly one-third had persistent neurologic deficits 6 months after receiving appropriate treatment.[96]

The 2 syndromes commonly associated with late neurosyphilis are general paresis of the insane, also known as dementia paralytica, and tabes dorsalis.[95] General paresis presents as a rapidly progressive dementia, accompanied by personality changes. Tabes dorsalis presents with sensory ataxia and bowel and bladder dysfunction, resulting from damage to the posterior columns of the spinal cord. Tabes dorsalis can be accompanied by an Argyll Robertson pupil (which accommodates, but does not react to, light) and optic atrophy. These syndromes are now very rare in the developed world.

Clinicians diagnosing a person with syphilis should perform a neurologic review of systems and perform a neurologic examination. According to CDC recommendations, indications for CSF examination in persons with syphilis include neurologic, ophthalmic, or otologic signs or symptoms; evidence of active tertiary syphilis; or treatment failure. HIV infection in-and-of-itself is not an indication for CSF examination.[35]

OCULAR SYPHILIS

Although the syndromes may not always overlap, ocular syphilis has generally been considered to be a subset of neurosyphilis, and as per CDC recommendations should be clinically managed as such.[35] Given the recent increase in reported cases, clinicians should be careful to ask about eye symptoms in evaluating any patient suspected to have syphilis. Ocular syphilis may occur during any stage of infection, and may involve almost any portion of the eye. Chancres or gummas of the conjunctiva, conjunctivitis, and scleroconjunctivitis; syphilitic interstitial keratitis; anterior, posterior, and pan uveitis; multiple retinal complications including retinal detachment, cataracts, and glaucoma, as well as optic nerve involvement (including papillitis, retrobulbar neuritis, optic atrophy, optic nerve gumma, and various stroke syndromes) are among the clinical syndromes that have been described. Furthermore, multiple manifestations of syphilis can be observed in the eye, such as pupillary abnormalities (including the Argyll Robertson pupil), palsies of the third, fourth and sixth nerve, usually from syphilitic basilar meningitis, and focal gummas along the nerves, brainstem infarction, or syphilitic aneurysmal compression or hemorrhage that may involve the optic and oculomotor nerves. Syphilitic basilar meningitis or gummas may cause a chiasmal syndrome with bitemporal hemianopia. Finally, eyelid chancres or condyloma lata of the eyelids have been described, although these do not directly involve the eye.[37,97-99]

CONGENITAL SYPHILIS

Congenital syphilis results from infection in utero with *T. pallidum*. Transplacental fetal infection can occur at any time during pregnancy and at any stage of maternal infection.[100] Probability of transmission of infection depends on the stage of infection in an untreated mother, ranging from 70% to 100% in primary syphilis, 40% for early latent syphilis, and 10% for late latent syphilis.[101] Because infection is spread hematogenously, a chancre is not present on the fetus or infant.[100] In 30% to 40% of cases, congenital syphilis results in stillbirth.[43] Of infants who survive, two-thirds are asymptomatic at delivery and only later develop symptoms.[100]

Clinical findings in symptomatic infants are similar to congenital infections caused by cytomegalovirus, toxoplasmosis, herpes simplex virus, rubella, and other infections.[43] The most prominent manifestations of early congenital syphilis, defined as syphilis in a child younger than 2 years of age, include fever, rash, hepatosplenomegaly, and persistent rhinitis ("snuffles").[100] Hydrops fetalis (edema), lymphadenopathy, neurosyphilis, leukocytosis, thrombocytopenia, periostitis, and osteochondritis also may be present, with the pain associated with osteochondrotic lesions causing the infant to refuse to move the affected anatomic area ("pseudoparalysis of

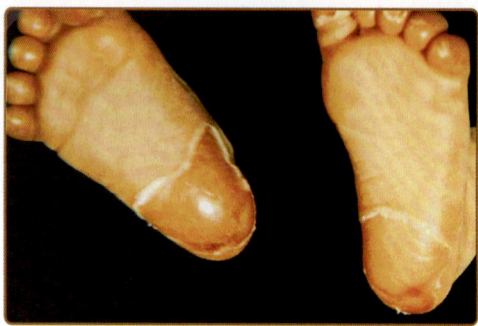

Figure 170-32 Bullous eruptions on the soles of a newborn with early prenatal syphilis. Bullae have ruptured and now present as erosions ("syphilitic pemphigus").

Parrot").[43,100] If present at delivery, the rash is usually bullous ("syphilitic pemphigus"; Fig. 170-32) and very infectious.[100] Rash that presents at 2 weeks or more after birth, however, is typically maculopapular, with small copper-red lesions similar to lesions of secondary syphilis most commonly affecting the hands and feet.[43] Desquamation and crusting can then occur.[102] Other cutaneous lesions present can include condyloma lata (Fig. 170-33), mucous patches, fissures around the lips, nares, or anus, and petechiae from thrombocytopenia.[43] The skin of the syphilitic neonate is often dry and wrinkled and, in newborns with fair skin, may have a café-au-lait hue (Fig. 170-34).

Late congenital syphilis is defined as disease occurring in a child who is at least 2 years old that typically manifests over the first 2 decades of life.[43] Many manifestations of late congenital syphilis result from damage caused during early infection and are not reversible with treatment. Those manifestations include scars (*rhagades*; Fig. 170-35) resulting from cutaneous fissures; a saddle-nose deformity, resulting from destruction of nasal cartilage; frontal bossing (Olympian brow), thickening of the sternoclavicular portion of the clavicle (Higoumenakia sign), anterior bowing of the midtibia (saber shins), and scaphoid scapula, all resulting from chronic periostitis; and

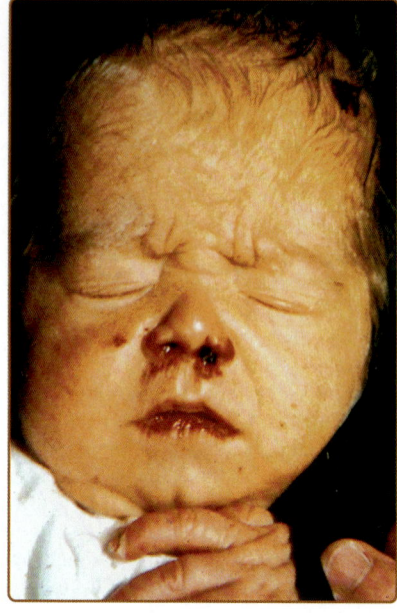

Figure 170-34 Early prenatal syphilis in a newborn. The skin is dry and wrinkled, with a yellowish-brownish hue. There is hemorrhagic rhinitis. This is what Diday described as "a little wrinkled potbellied *(not seen here)* old man with a cold in his head." Note also the aged appearance of the fingers in this newborn.

peg-shaped notched central incisors (Hutchinson teeth; Fig. 170-36) and mulberry molars, resulting from syphilis vasculitis in developing tooth buds. Other manifestations include eighth nerve deafness and eye abnormalities, including interstitial keratitis, glaucoma, or corneal scarring. The Hutchinson triad refers to Hutchinson teeth, interstitial keratitis, and eighth nerve deafness.[43]

Of note, as with any sexually transmitted disease, the diagnosis of syphilis in a child beyond the neonatal period should raise the question of child abuse.[35]

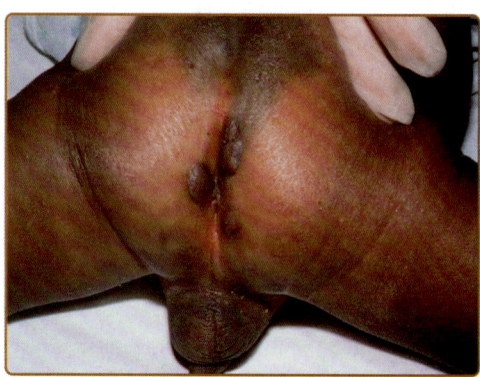

Figure 170-33 Hyperpigmented papules of syphilis in a neonate.

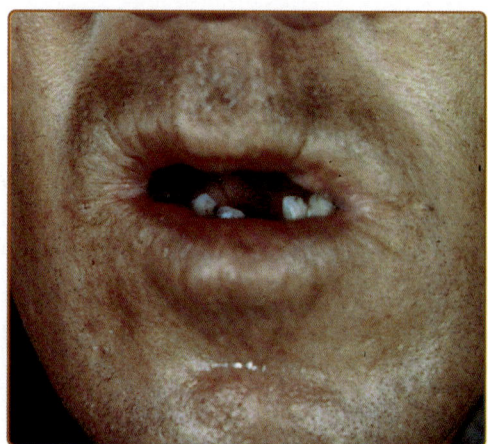

Figure 170-35 Perioral rhagades are linear scars that result from ulcerations that appear during early congenital syphilis and persist to adulthood.

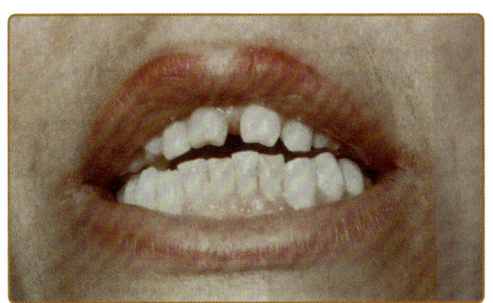

Figure 170-36 The presence of small, notched, peg-shaped upper incisors (Hutchinson teeth) is also part of the late congenital syphilis triad.

SYPHILIS AND HIV INFECTION

Chap. 168 discusses cutaneous manifestations of the HIV.

The interaction of syphilis and HIV infection is complex.[29] The clinical presentation of syphilis varies in minor ways between HIV-infected and HIV-uninfected persons.[29] HIV-infected persons are more likely to present with more than 1 chancre and with larger and deeper chancres in primary syphilis,[53,103] and are more likely to manifest signs of secondary syphilis while at least 1 chancre is present.[53,104] Atypical and aggressive presentations of syphilis in HIV-infected persons might also be more common, although those presentations are not thought to be unique to HIV coinfection.[29,103]

Some studies have shown syphilis to transiently increase HIV viral load and decrease CD4+ T-cell count during infection, with resolution following treatment.[105-111] Those changes might facilitate HIV transmission by HIV-infected patients coinfected with syphilis.[29,109] An effect of syphilis on progression to AIDS or mortality has not been found.[112] Syphilis also is associated with HIV acquisition,[113] and all persons presenting with syphilis who are not known to be infected with HIV should be tested for HIV.[35] The disruption of epidermal or mucosal barriers caused by syphilis ulcers, and the migration to these lesions of inflammatory cells that are targets for HIV are 2 biologic mechanisms that might account for the synergy between the 2 infections. Common behavioral factors (eg, lack of condom use) also likely contribute to risk of coinfection. All HIV-infected persons entering HIV care should have a serologic test for syphilis, which should be repeated yearly thereafter in all those who are sexually active, or more frequently (every 3 to 6 months) if indicated (depending on risk behaviors).[114] HIV infection also is associated with repeat syphilis infection.[115]

Because of its effect on the immune system, HIV infection is thought to increase risk of neurosyphilis.[29,95] This is based on studies correlating abnormal CSF findings with advanced HIV disease[116] and failure to normalize CSF–VDRL (Venereal Disease Research Laboratory) test results in the presence of HIV infection,[117] especially with lower CD4 cell counts. Additionally, HIV-infected persons with syphilis can experience "neurorelapse," meaning the development of neurosyphilis following appropriate treatment for primary, secondary, or early latent syphilis, and declines in nontreponemal titers consistent with cure.[95]

HIV infection can sometimes complicate serologic diagnosis of syphilis and subsequent followup, as unusual serologic responses have been observed in HIV-infected persons with syphilis.[35] False-negative serologic test results in the setting of the prozone phenomenon[118] and seronegative syphilis[119] have been reported. Also, serofast reactions (ie, persistently reactive nontreponemal test results, even following appropriate treatment) can occur.[120] When syphilis is suspected clinically and serology is nonreactive, skin biopsy can be useful diagnostically, as can darkfield microscopy[35,121] or polymerase chain reaction (PCR)-based assays for T. pallidum,[68] if available.

CDC treatment recommendations for syphilis do not depend on HIV infection status, and are supported by limited data indicating that outcomes are not improved with more intense or prolonged treatment.[29,35,122] Titers might decline more slowly in appropriately treated HIV-infected persons,[29,35,123] particularly in those who have lower titers on initial diagnosis.[124] Compared with HIV-uninfected persons, HIV-infected persons with primary or secondary syphilis should have more frequent followup (Table 170-5).[35]

ETIOLOGY AND PATHOGENESIS

T. pallidum subspecies *pallidum* is a motile, spiral-shaped bacterium for which humans are the only natural host.[16] *T. pallidum* ranges in size from 5 to 16 μm in length and is 0.2 to 0.3 μm in diameter.[121] The bacterium is surrounded by a cytoplasmic membrane, which is itself enclosed by a loosely associated outer membrane. Between those membranes lies a thin layer of peptidoglycan, which provides structural stability and houses endoflagella, organelles that are responsible for *T. pallidum*'s characteristic corkscrew motility. Microscopically the bacterium is indistinguishable from other pathogenic treponemes that cause nonvenereal diseases, including *T. pallidum* subspecies *endemicum* (bejel), *T. pallidum* subspecies *pertenue* (yaws), and *T. pallidum* subspecies *carateum* (pinta). The *T. pallidum* genome, sequenced in 1998,[125] is 1.14 Mb in length, relatively small for a bacterium.[16]

The bacterium has very limited metabolic capabilities, making it reliant on host pathways for many of its metabolic needs.[16,73] *T. pallidum* does not survive more than a few hours to days outside its host and cannot be cultured easily in vitro for sustained periods, complicating efforts to understand the organism.[16,73] Instead, it must be propagated in mammals, with rabbits the preferred species because, following testis inoculation, rabbits, unlike mice, experience disease

TABLE 170-5
Centers for Disease Control and Prevention Recommendations for Treatment and Followup of Adults with Primary, Secondary, Early Latent, or Late Latent Syphilis.[35]

STAGE OF DISEASE	HIV STATUS OF PERSON	RECOMMENDED TREATMENT[a]	ALTERNATIVE TREATMENT FOR PENICILLIN-ALLERGIC PERSONS (NONPREGNANT WOMEN ONLY)[b]	SCHEDULE FOR FOLLOWUP AFTER TREATMENT[c]	TIME FRAME TO EXPECT FOURFOLD DECLINE IN TITER[d]
Primary or secondary	HIV-uninfected	Benzathine penicillin G, 2.4 million units, administered IM in a single dose	Doxycycline 100 mg orally twice daily for 14 days	6 and 12 months	6 to 12 months
	HIV-infected	Benzathine penicillin G, 2.4 million units, administered IM in a single dose	Doxycycline 100 mg orally twice daily for 14 days	3, 6, 9, 12, and 24 months	6 to 12 months
Early latent	HIV-uninfected	Benzathine penicillin G, 2.4 million units, administered IM in a single dose	Doxycycline 100 mg orally twice daily for 14 days	6, 12, and 24 months after treatment	12 to 24 months
	HIV-infected	Benzathine penicillin G, 2.4 million units, administered IM in a single dose	Doxycycline 100 mg orally twice daily for 14 days	6, 12, 18, and 24 months	12 to 24 months
Late latent (>1 year), or latent of unknown duration	HIV-uninfected	Benzathine penicillin G: 3 doses of 2.4 million units IM given at 1 week intervals	Doxycycline 100 mg orally twice daily for 28 days	6, 12, and 24 months after treatment	12 to 24 months
	HIV-infected	Benzathine penicillin G: 3 doses of 2.4 million units IM given at 1 week intervals	Doxycycline 100 mg orally twice daily for 28 days	6, 12, 18, and 24 months	12 to 24 months

[a]Initial treatment is the same for HIV-uninfected and HIV-infected persons.
[b]Pregnant women must not be treated with doxycycline. If allergic to penicillin, pregnant women must be desensitized and then treated with benzathine penicillin G.
[c]Some persons (eg, men who have sex with men or women who become pregnant) should be screened appropriately in addition to being followed at the recommended intervals to assess clinical and serologic response to treatment.
[d]If titers have not declined fourfold after the stated time frame, consider reinfection or treatment failure (including treatment failure because of neurosyphilis). If at any time after treatment signs or symptoms of syphilis appear, also consider those same possibilities.

manifestations.[16,73] *T. pallidum* divides slowly, taking from 30 to 50 hours in vitro. That slow reproduction rate has important implications for treatment, which must be present in the body for a long period to assure effectiveness against the bacterium.[16]

Following inoculation, *T. pallidum* attaches to host cells, including epithelial, fibroblast-like, and endothelial cells, likely by binding to fibronectin, laminin, or other components of host serum, cell membranes, and the extracellular matrix.[16] It can invade rapidly into the bloodstream—within minutes of inoculation, based on rabbit models—and can cross many barriers in the body, such as the blood–brain barrier and the placental barrier, to infect many tissues and organs. That dissemination leads ultimately to manifestations of syphilis distant from the site of the initial chancre(s) in an infected person and in a developing fetus.[16]

T. pallidum lacks virulence factors common to many other bacteria, including lipopolysaccharide endotoxin.[16] It does, however, produce a brisk immune response, mediated by membrane lipoproteins,[126] that begins shortly after infection. Infection at all stages leads to infiltration by lymphocytes, macrophages, and plasma cells.[73] CD4+ T cells predominate in chancres, and CD8+ T cells predominate in lesions of secondary syphilis.[73] Infection leads also to elaboration of T-helper (Th)-1 cytokines, including interleukin-2 and interferon-γ, although downregulation of the Th1 response during secondary syphilis, coincident with the peaking of antibody titers,[73] might contribute to the organism's ability to evade the host immune response.[54,127] Subtyping studies of *T. pallidum* have linked certain strains of the organism to neurosyphilis.[128]

The humoral immune response begins with production of immunoglobulin (Ig) M antibodies approximately 2 weeks after exposure, followed 2 weeks thereafter by IgG antibodies.[126] IgM, in addition to IgG, continues to be produced during infection and can lead to immune-complex formation.[126] Antibody titers peak during bacterial dissemination in secondary syphilis.[73] Some antibodies cross-react with other treponemal species, and some are specific for *T. pallidum* subspecies *pallidum*. The immune response is somewhat active against the organism, helping block attachment of the organism to host cells, conferring passive immunity in rabbit models, and enhancing phagocytosis in vitro.[73]

The immune response is sufficient to prevent syphilis reinfection in persons who have untreated syphilis.

In other words, in what is called the *law of Colles* or *chancre immunity*, persons with untreated syphilis will not experience another episode of primary syphilis as long as they remain untreated.[73] However, the immune response is insufficient to eradicate *T. pallidum* from the host. In addition to suppressing the Th1 response, the organism is thought to evade those host defenses by taking harbor in immune-privileged tissues (eg, CNS, eye, and placenta), failing to be present in sufficient quantities (eg, during latent infection) to trigger a host response, varying its surface proteins during infection through gene conversion, and overcoming host attempts to prevent bacterial access to iron, which is necessary for bacterial growth.[16,73] The immune response is also inadequate to prevent reinfection after a person is cured of syphilis, although it might modify the course of reinfection. Compared with persons with syphilis for the first time, for example, reinfected persons may be more likely to be asymptomatic.[129]

The immune response is also likely responsible for the tissue damage caused in syphilis.[16] Damage to axons located near the site of a chancre might explain why that lesion, although ulcerative, is typically painless.[130]

Interest in a vaccine for syphilis continues, with focus on using outer membrane protein antigens to elicit an immunoprotective response.[131] However, a number of barriers to vaccine development exist. Those include variability in outer membrane protein antigens, the limited number of antigens on *T. pallidum* to which immunoprotective antibodies could bind, the possibility that the formation of a host protein coat around *T. pallidum* might prevent antibody binding, and a potential lack of commercial incentive to produce a vaccine.[131]

DIAGNOSIS

Diagnosis of syphilis depends on clinical suspicion combined with laboratory testing to directly or indirectly detect infection with *T. pallidum*. Of note, in cases where clinical suspicion for syphilis is high, clinicians should not wait for the results of laboratory testing before administering appropriate treatment. Clinicians should also remember that serologies can be negative in up to 30% of patients with primary syphilis.[132]

DIRECT DETECTION OF *T. PALLIDUM*

Direct detection of *T. pallidum*, provides definitive evidence of infection, and is particularly important in primary syphilis, given that serologies may be negative. However, these tests, including darkfield microscopy, which has been a mainstay of diagnosis for decades, are rarely available outside of specialized settings.[133]

DARKFIELD MICROSCOPY

When available, darkfield microscopic examination is the diagnostic test of choice in chancres, moist lesions

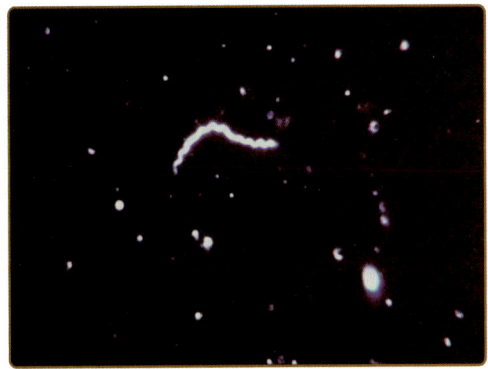

Figure 170-37 Darkfield microscopy showing a treponeme.

of secondary syphilis (condylomata lata and mucous patches), and the discharge from rhinitis in congenital syphilis. Darkfield examination (Fig. 170-37) will often be positive before serologic tests become reactive.[134] Importantly, because nonpathogenic treponemes are normally present in the oral cavity and can be mistaken for *T. pallidum*, darkfield microscopy cannot be used to test oral lesions.[135] The number of *T. pallidum* organisms in secondary syphilis lesions except for mucous patches and condyloma lata is generally not sufficient to allow darkfield diagnosis.

Universal precautions must be used when collecting and handling darkfield specimens, as lesions of syphilis suitable for darkfield examination are very infectious. Darkfield specimens are prepared by removing crusts from the surface of the lesion, cleaning the surface of the lesion with a sterile saline-soaked gauze, squeezing the base of the lesion with 2 gloved fingers to induce the presence of a serous exudate on the surface, and collecting the exudate with a glass slide, cover slip, or bacteriologic loop. Only if the amount of exudate is insufficient to prevent the slide from drying out prior to microscopic examination should a drop of nonbacteriostatic normal saline be added before covering the slide with a cover slip. The slide is examined within 5 to 20 minutes by a trained microscopist, using a darkfield microscope, for the presence of organisms with the characteristic morphology and motility of *T. pallidum*.[121] Sensitivity is approximately 74% to 79%, but declines as minutes elapse, as dead treponemes cannot exhibit the motility required for diagnosis.[121] Of note, prior application of a topical antibiotic to a lesion can yield a false-negative darkfield specimen.

DIRECT FLUORESCENCE ANTIBODY TEST

The lesional exudate is smeared on a glass slide and stained with fluorescein-labeled anti–*T. pallidum* immunoglobulin. In contrast to darkfield microscopic examination, the smear can be held for later evaluation and oral or anal lesions can be examined because only *T. pallidum* is stained. The sensitivity of the test is 73% to 100%.[121]

MOLECULAR TESTS

In research settings, PCR-based methods have been used to detect T. pallidum DNA from lesions.[68]

HISTOPATHOLOGIC EXAMINATION

Histopathologic examination is not essential for a diagnosis of syphilis, which can in many cases be made on the basis of clinical findings, serologic testing, and, for appropriate lesions, and if available, darkfield microscopy. In unusual or questionable cases, however, histopathologic examination can be useful.

PRIMARY SYPHILIS

At the edge of a chancre, the epidermis shows changes similar to those of secondary syphilis, discussed later.[136] The papillary dermis shows edema and a perivascular and interstitial infiltrates characterized by lymphocytes (predominantly CD4+ T cells), histiocytes, and plasma cells, with neutrophils admixed. T. pallidum organisms can be visualized along the dermal–epidermal junction and in and around blood vessels, using Livaditis or Warthin-Starry stains or by immunofluorescent techniques.[136]

SECONDARY SYPHILIS

Although clinically different in appearance, lesions of primary and secondary syphilis share many histologic features, with changes more marked in papular lesions and less so in macular lesions.[136] In the epidermis those changes include psoriasiform hyperplasia, exocytosis of lymphocytes, spongiform pustulation, and parakeratosis; in the dermis those changes include marked papillary dermal edema and perivascular and/or perianexal infiltrate composed of lymphocytes and/or histiocytes, sometimes granulomatous, and most intense in the papillary dermis. Plasma cells are present in three-fourths of cases, and T. pallidum organisms can be seen on appropriately stained sections in one-third of cases, usually in the epidermis and less commonly around superficial dermal blood vessels.[136]

TERTIARY SYPHILIS

Histopathologically, gummatous lesions are characterized by granulomas with central zones of acellular necrosis. Endarteritis obliterans and angiocentric plasma cell infiltrates of dermal blood vessels also can be present. Nodular lesions show small granulomas in the dermis, accompanied by islands of epithelioid cells, multinucleated giant cells, lymphocytes, and plasma cells.[136]

SEROLOGY

Serologic tests for syphilis include nontreponemal tests, which detect IgG and IgM antibodies to lipoidal material released from damaged host cells and possibly from T. pallidum, and treponemal tests, which detect antibodies to T. pallidum itself. Accurate serologic diagnosis of syphilis requires both types of test. Table 170-6 outlines the sensitivity and specificity of selected serologic tests for syphilis.[121,126,137-139]

NONTREPONEMAL SEROLOGIC TESTS

The 2 most widely used nontreponemal tests are the VDRL and rapid plasma reagin (RPR) tests. These

TABLE 170-6
Sensitivity and Specificity of Selected Serologic Tests for Syphilis[121,137-139]

TEST	SENSITIVITY (%)				SPECIFICITY (%)
	PRIMARY SYPHILIS	SECONDARY SYPHILIS	LATENT SYPHILIS	TERTIARY SYPHILIS	
Nontreponemal Tests					
RPR	86 (77-99)	100	98 (95-100)	73	98 (93-99)
VDRL	78 (74-87)	100	96 (88-100)	71 (37-94)	98 (96-99)
Treponemal Tests					
TPPA	88 (86-100)	100	97 (97-100)	94	96 (95-100)
MHA-TP	76 (69-90)	100	97 (97-100)	94	99 (98-100)
FTA-ABS	84 (70-100)	100	100	96	97 (94-100)
TPHA	77 (53-86)	100	99 (99-100)	100	96-99
EIA[a]	85-97	97-100	100 (early latent) 75-100 (late latent)	NA	99-100

[a]Various EIAs from different manufacturers were tested. See Ref. 137 for details.
EIA, enzyme immunoassay; FTA-ABS, fluorescent treponemal antibody absorption assay; MHA-TP, microhemagglutination assay for *Treponema pallidum*; RPR, rapid plasma reagin; TPHA, *T. pallidum* hemagglutination; TPPA, *T. pallidum* particle agglutination; VDRL, Venereal Disease Research Laboratory.

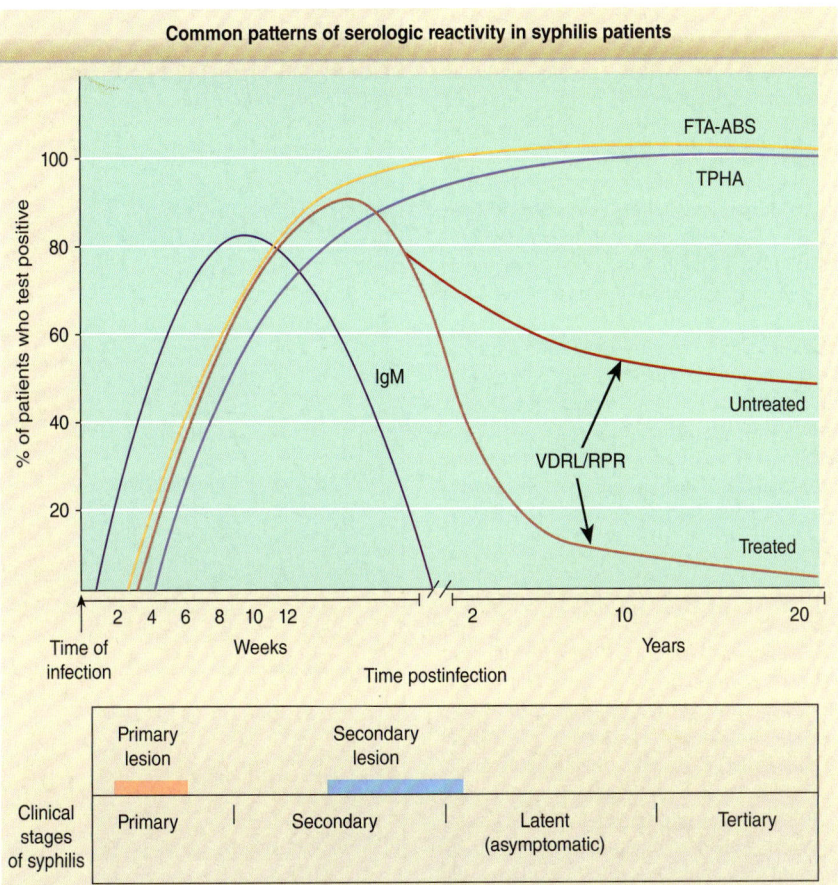

Figure 170-38 Common patterns of serologic reactivity in syphilis patients. FTA-ABS, Fluorescent treponemal antibody absorption assay; IgM, immunoglobulin M; RPR, rapid plasma reagin; TPHA, *Treponema pallidum* hemagglutination test; VDRL, Venereal Disease Research Laboratory. (From Peeling RW, Ye H. Diagnostic tools for preventing and managing maternal and congenital syphilis: an overview. *Bull World Health Organ*. 2004;82(6):439-446. By permission of World Health Organization.)

tests are used both to diagnose syphilis, and to monitor response to treatment. The VDRL and RPR begin to become reactive 4 to 5 weeks after infection, with 100% sensitivity by approximately 12 weeks, and revert to nonreactive in 25% to 30% of cases during late latent syphilis (Fig. 170-38).[140] Cases of seronegative secondary syphilis in HIV-infected persons have been reported.[119] Results can be qualitative (reactive/nonreactive) or quantitative. Quantitative results are reported as titer, which refers to serial dilutions of serum by a factor of 2 (1:2, 1:4, 1:8, and so on). The reported titer represents the most dilute sample that gives a reactive result. RPR and VDRL titers cannot be directly compared, and even for the same test, reported titers may differ slightly between laboratorians and laboratories. Because of the importance of using nontreponemal titers to assess response to treatment, a titer for each person diagnosed with syphilis must be obtained on the day-of-treatment. Without a day-of-treatment titer, it is very difficult to interpret subsequent titers to determine whether the person has responded to treatment appropriately.

Treatment success is defined serologically as a fourfold (two-dilution) decline in nontreponemal test titer (see section "Management"), although in many persons, following appropriate treatment nontreponemal titers will revert to nonreactive. In persons treated for primary syphilis, nontreponemal tests become nonreactive in 60% by 4 months, and in nearly all patients by 12 months.[141] In persons treated for secondary syphilis, the tests usually become nonreactive 12 to 24 months after treatment. However, in some cases, more frequently if therapy is administered in the latent stage, nontreponemal tests may remain reactive in low titers for up to 5 years or longer. In some persons nontreponemal antibodies can persist at a low titer for long periods, and sometimes for life.[142] Both patients who fail to achieve a fourfold decline in titer, as well as those who have adequate serologic decline but whose nontreponemal test titers do not become undetectable, have been referred to as *serofast*. However, current CDC guidelines recommend additional followup and testing only for the group of serofast patients who do not achieve a fourfold decline in titer (see section "Management").[35,133]

False-negative results occur during very early infection or in latent and late syphilis. In a small percent of secondary syphilis cases, very high antibody titers inhibit test reactivity, producing a false-negative result, called the prozone phenomenon. To exclude the prozone phenomenon, the test must be repeated with diluted serum. Many laboratories do not routinely check for the prozone phenomenon, so clinicians must request a ruling out of the prozone phenomenon in the appropriate setting (eg, a patient with a suspicious rash and a negative nontreponemal test result). Importantly, nontreponemal titers may decline over time even in the absence of treatment, so persons with late latent syphilis who have never been treated may have nonreactive nontreponemal test results (see "The Reverse Sequence Algorithm" below).[133]

Biologic false-positive results constitute approximately 1% of reactive nontreponemal tests and usually have low titers (<1:8). Table 170-7 outlines the causes of biologic false-positive results.

In the traditional algorithm for diagnosis of syphilis, the nontreponemal test is performed first, followed by a treponemal test for confirmation if the nontreponemal test is positive.

TREPONEMAL SEROLOGIC TESTS

Examples of treponemal serologic tests include the *T. pallidum* particle agglutination (TPPA) test, the microhemagglutination assay for *T. pallidum* (MHA-TP), the fluorescent treponemal antibody absorption assay (FTA-ABS), the *T. pallidum* hemagglutination test (TPHA), and various treponemal enzyme immunoassays (EIAs) and immunochemiluminescence assays. These tests, which use whole or fragments of *T. pallidum* as antigen, detect the presence of antibodies to *T. pallidum*. Compared with nontreponemal tests, they are more cumbersome to perform—except for treponemal EIAs—but have greater sensitivity in the primary and late stages and slightly higher specificity. They have historically been used, and in many settings are still used, to confirm syphilis, because a reactive treponemal test result essentially rules out the possibility of a biologic false-positive reaction on a nontreponemal test. Consequently, a reactive nontreponemal test result followed by a reactive treponemal test result confirms a diagnosis of syphilis. The test results must be interpreted in light of clinical findings and prior serologic test results to determine whether the case of syphilis is new or old, and if old, previously treated successfully or unsuccessfully.

Persons who have had syphilis usually will have reactive treponemal test results for life, even after successful treatment, making a reactive treponemal test in a person with a history of syphilis generally not useful clinically. However, 15% to 25% of treponemal tests become nonreactive between 2 and 3 years after treatment of primary syphilis.[143] The tests are highly specific and sensitive during the secondary and the late phases of the disease. Treponemal test titers do not correlate with, and are not used to monitor, disease activity. Sensitivity is low in the weeks after infection, but is nearly 100% by 12 weeks (see Fig. 170-38). False-positive results in treponemal tests are also rare, but are associated with infections, autoimmune or connective tissue disease, and narcotic addiction.[126,143,144]

TABLE 170-7
Causes of Biologic False-Positive Nontreponemal Tests

	ACUTE	CHRONIC
Physiologic	Pregnancy[a]	Advanced age
Spirochete	Leptospirosis	Endemic syphilis
Infection	Lyme disease Rat-bite fever Relapsing fever	Pinta Yaws
Viral infection	Cytomegalovirus Infectious mononucleosis Hepatitis Herpes simplex Herpes zoster-varicella infection Measles Mumps *Mycoplasma pneumonia* Toxoplasmosis Viral sepsis	Human T-cell leukemia/lymphoma virus 1 HIV infection
Bacterial infection	Pneumonia	Lepromatous leprosy Lymphogranuloma venereum Tuberculosis
Protozoan infection	Malaria	Kala azar Trypanosomiasis
Autoimmune		Autoimmune hemolytic syndrome
Disease		Autoimmune thyroiditis Idiopathic thrombocytopenic purpura Mixed connective tissue disease Polyarteritis nodosa Primary biliary cirrhosis Rheumatoid arthritis Sjögren syndrome Systemic lupus erythematosus
Other		Drug abuse Dysproteinemias Hepatic cirrhosis Malnutrition Malignancy Lymphoproliferative disorders

[a]Evidence for pregnancy as a cause of biologic false-positive reactions is limited and concern persists for clinicians failing to diagnosis syphilis in pregnancy.

THE REVERSE SEQUENCE ALGORITHM

The automation of EIA tests, a form of treponemal test, has made EIAs less expensive for large-volume laboratories to perform.[126,145] As a result, many large-volume laboratories have begun to use EIAs rather than nontreponemal tests as the first step of the algorithm for laboratory diagnosis of syphilis.[39] In this "reverse sequence" algorithm, a treponemal EIA is performed first. If and only if the EIA result is reactive, is a nontreponemal test performed. Reactive results on both tests confirm a diagnosis of syphilis. In approximately 3% of cases, a reactive treponemal EIA result is followed by a nonreactive nontreponemal test result. In those cases, a tie-breaker test, consisting of an alternate treponemal test, can be performed, with data combined with clinical suspicion to determine diagnosis and treatment.[145]

The use of the reverse sequence algorithm does lead to the identification of a number of serodiscordant patients in whom both the initial and "tie-breaker" treponemal tests are positive, but the nontreponemal test is negative. This can occur in the setting of the prozone phenomenon, early primary syphilis, adequately treated past syphilis, or untreated syphilis of long duration. Patients with a history of treatment will require no further management unless the sexual history suggests recent reexposure. Those without a history of treatment should be treated. Knowledge of sexual history, clinical findings and results of prior serologic tests for syphilis is therefore necessary to appropriately interpret the results of serologic testing.[35,133] Figure 170-39 illustrates the interpretation of reverse sequence algorithm results.

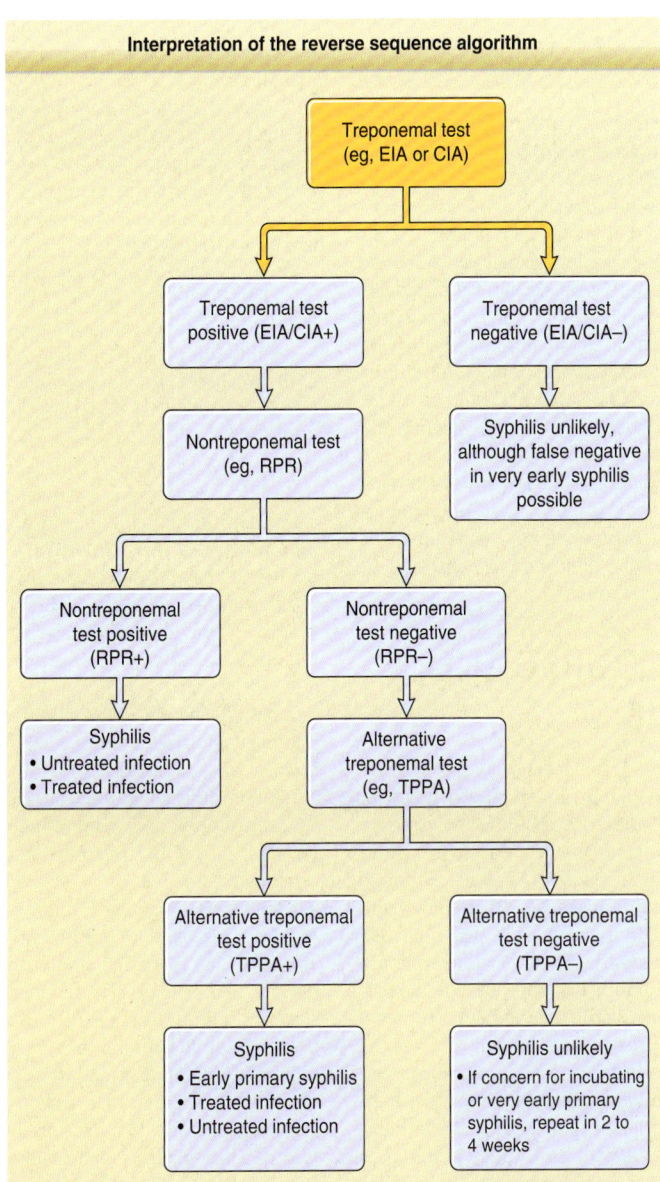

Figure 170-39 Interpretation of the reverse sequence algorithm.[133,145] CIA, Chemiluminescent immunoassay; EIA, enzyme immunoassay; RPR, rapid plasma reagin; TPPA, *Treponema pallidum* particle agglutination.

RAPID SEROLOGIC TESTS

Of note, several rapid, point-of-care serologic tests for syphilis are in use or under development internationally. One has been cleared for use outside of laboratory settings in the United States, and others are under development.[146]

CONGENITAL SYPHILIS

Transplacental transfer of maternal nontreponemal and treponemal IgG antibodies to the fetus complicates serologic diagnosis of congenital syphilis.[35] Infants born to mothers with reactive nontreponemal and treponemal tests should be evaluated with a quantitative nontreponemal serologic test performed on infant serum, as umbilical cord blood might be contaminated with maternal blood, yielding a false-positive result. Treponemal tests are difficult to interpret in this setting and are not recommended by the CDC. All infants whose mothers have reactive serologic tests should be examined carefully for evidence of congenital syphilis. If possible, suspicious lesions or body fluids (eg, nasal discharge) should be tested using darkfield microscopy or PCR testing. Pathologic examination of the placenta using specific staining or a *T. pallidum* PCR test should be considered.[35] Any neonate with proven, highly probable or possible congenital syphilis (based on assessment of physical examination, serologic tests, darkfield microscopy or PCR of lesions or body fluid, and adequacy of maternal treatment) should have CSF tested for VDRL reactivity, white blood cell count, and protein level, as well as other tests that would suggest other diseases in the differential diagnosis. Other tests, such as long-bone radiographs, chest radiographs, liver function tests, neuroimaging, ophthalmologic examination, and auditory brainstem response may be necessary as clinically indicated.[35]

CLINICAL COURSE AND PROGNOSIS

Despite decades of use, *T. pallidum* has remained sensitive to penicillin. Although treatment failures do occur, and may be more common in HIV-infected patients, penicillin treatment is generally very effective at eradicating the infection in all stages of syphilis. Although severe, and in a few rare cases, life-threatening complications of secondary syphilis can occur,[147] the vast majority of patients with primary and secondary syphilis will have resolution of symptoms with no permanent sequelae (even without treatment). The goal of antibiotic therapy, then, is not only to address the immediate syndrome, but also to prevent transmission to sexual partners, and progression to tertiary syphilis. Unfortunately, in tertiary syphilis, irreversible damage to vital structures may occur through gummas or cardiovascular or CNS involvement. Neurosyphilis, which can occur at any stage, can be life-threatening. Of note, several patients in the recently reported cluster of 12 ocular syphilis cases developed permanent sequelae despite appropriate treatment; 2 of the 12 became legally blind.[37]

MANAGEMENT

Based on data from case series and clinical trials and long clinical experience,[148] penicillin is the recommended treatment for all stages of syphilis, with the preparation, dose, and length of treatment dependent on the clinical manifestations, stage of disease, and age of the patient.[35] Benzathine penicillin G, the recommended preparation of penicillin for most stages of syphilis, has a long half-life, which is critical therapeutically because of the slow dividing time of *T. pallidum*. The choice of penicillin formulation is important in assuring adequate treatment. In the United States, the only penicillin product that is appropriate for treatment of primary, secondary, or latent syphilis is Bicillin L-A, which contains only benzathine penicillin G. Another similarly packaged product, Bicillin C-R, contains procaine penicillin G in addition to benzathine penicillin G and is not an appropriate treatment. Substantial confusion and errors relating to those 2 products have been reported.[149,150]

Penicillin-allergic persons with syphilis who are not pregnant and do not have neurosyphilis may be treated with doxycycline. Pregnant women who are penicillin-allergic must be desensitized to and treated with penicillin, which is the only drug that is known to prevent maternal transmission and to treat infection in the fetus.[35] Reports of treatment failures and emergence in *T. pallidum* of resistance to macrolides, including azithromycin, at one point a convenient alternative to penicillin because of its oral formulation, now precludes use of that class of drug in the United States and much of the world,[151-153] although it may still be used with caution in some areas.[137] As discussed previously, CDC-recommended treatment regimens do not differ on the basis of a person's HIV infection status.[35]

Table 170-5 outlines the CDC recommendations for treatment and followup of adults with primary, secondary, early latent or late latent syphilis. For information on children and for congenital syphilis, as well as neurosyphilis and ocular syphilis (which require IV penicillin), CDC treatment guidelines should be consulted.[35]

Clinical and serologic followup is important to monitor response to treatment (see Table 170-5). Treatment success is generally defined as a fourfold decline in serologic nontreponemal titer (or reversion to nonreactive result) following appropriate treatment, in the absence of persistent signs or symptoms of syphilis, and within a specified time frame depending on stage of infection and HIV infection status of the infected person.[35] An example of a fourfold decline in titer is a 1:64 titer declining to 1:16, or a 1:16 titer declining to 1:4. The CDC recommends followup at 6-month intervals until a fourfold decline is documented, except for HIV-infected persons with primary or secondary syphilis, for whom followup at 3, 6, 9, 12, and 24 months is recommended, and congenital syphilis, for whom followup every 2 to 3 months is recommended.[35] Approximately 15% to 20% of persons with primary and secondary syphilis who are treated appropriately will remain serofast and will not achieve the fourfold decline in titer. The CDC guidelines recommend additional clinical followup, and in some cases, retreatment or CSF evaluation to rule out CNS infection.[35]

A fourfold titer increase following appropriate treatment indicates reinfection or treatment failure—the latter in some cases associated with neurosyphilis—with treatment depending on which of those is believed to have caused the increase. Reinfection must be assessed by clinical history and physical examination. If treatment failure cannot be ruled out, the patient should be treated with 7.2 million units of benzathine penicillin G (divided into 3 weekly doses); CSF examination should be performed to determine whether neurosyphilis is present, and, if it is, the patient also should be treated for neurosyphilis.[35]

COMPLICATIONS OF TREATMENT

The Jarisch-Herxheimer reaction is a self-limited clinical syndrome consisting of fever, headache, flare of mucocutaneous lesions, tender lymphadenopathy, pharyngitis, malaise, myalgia, and leukocytosis. It occurs within the first 24 hours after initiating therapy. The fever peaks 6 to 8 hours after the onset, usually around 39°C (102.2°F), but it can be as high as 42°C (107.6°F). Patients should be warned about the possibility of developing this reaction before receiving treatment. Acetaminophen can be used to attempt to diminish the reaction, although very little evidence of its effectiveness exists.[35] The patient should be encouraged to rest, maintain fluid intake, and seek medical attention if symptoms are severe. The pathogenesis of the Jarisch-Herxheimer reaction is unknown, but is thought to result from cytokine release mediated by the release of lipoproteins from dying *T. pallidum* organisms.[154] In pregnant patients, the Jarisch-Herxheimer reaction may lead to premature labor or fetal distress, events that should prompt the patient to seek evaluation. However, given the potentially devastating effects of congenital syphilis, prompt treatment of maternal syphilis is critical.[35]

Anaphylaxis from administration of penicillin injection is a life-threatening emergency that is managed by epinephrine and other medications, such as antihistamines, along with emergent transfer to a monitored setting.[155]

At the time of initial treatment, patients should be educated to distinguish an allergic reaction, which precludes further treatment with penicillin or related drugs, from a Jarisch-Herxheimer reaction, which does not.

DISEASE REPORTING AND MANAGEMENT OF PERSONS EXPOSED TO SYPHILIS

As reflected by the efforts to eliminate syphilis in the United States, prevention and control of syphilis are of substantial public health interest in the United States and worldwide.[2,35] Syphilis is a nationally notifiable disease in the United States, meaning that both clinicians and laboratories are mandated by law to report cases or laboratory results diagnostic of or suspicious for syphilis to their local or state public health authorities. Clinicians should contact their local or state health department to familiarize themselves with local reporting requirements, including required forms and need for paper-based or electronic reports, for syphilis and other reportable diseases.[35]

Local or state public health authorities maintain databases of syphilis diagnoses, laboratory results, and treatments for persons diagnosed with syphilis. That information is available to clinicians taking care of persons with suspected syphilis and can be helpful in staging infections (eg, determining if criteria for early latent syphilis are met) and assuring appropriate treatment. Clinicians should routinely encourage persons diagnosed with syphilis to inform their sex partners of exposure to syphilis and followup with patients to assure that disclosure has occurred. Identifying which sex partners are at risk of infection depends both on the elapsed time since last exposure and stage of infection in the source patient. This risk period is 3 months plus duration of symptoms for primary syphilis, 6 months plus duration of symptoms for secondary syphilis, and 1 year for early latent syphilis and latent syphilis of unknown duration. Clinicians should also inform persons they diagnose with syphilis that the case will be reported to the public health authority and that, in many cases, health department workers (sometimes called Communicable Disease Investigators or Disease Intervention Specialists) will contact the person to ensure that treatment was adequate, provide education about syphilis, solicit contact information for sex partners, and inquire about sexual behaviors so that prevention and control resources can be targeted to affected populations. It is a principle of public health practice, including in syphilis contact-tracing investigations, to protect the confidentiality of the source partner.[35]

Management of at-risk sex partners of persons diagnosed with syphilis also depends on elapsed time since exposure. Sex partners exposed during the 90 days preceding the diagnosis of primary, secondary, or early latent syphilis should be examined and tested for syphilis. However, regardless of results of the physical examination and laboratory tests, those partners should be treated presumptively because of the high efficacy of prophylactic treatment and the likelihood (up to 63%) that they been infected but have yet to show clinical or laboratory evidence of disease. Persons exposed more than 90 days before the diagnosis of primary, secondary, or early latent syphilis should also be examined and tested and treated presumptively if serologic test results are not available immediately and the opportunity for followup is uncertain. Sex partners of persons with late latent syphilis should be evaluated and tested, and then managed on the basis of those findings.[35]

PREVENTION AND SCREENING

Safer sex practices are critical for prevention of syphilis transmission. Screening also may be important in identifying asymptomatic patients who should be treated. The CDC recommends that all pregnant women be screened at the first prenatal visit, with retesting early in the third trimester and at delivery if at high risk for syphilis. Sexually active MSM should be screened at least annually, and every 3 to 6 months if at increased risk (eg, patient or sexual partner has multiple partners). Persons with HIV who are sexually active should be screened at first HIV evaluation and then at least annually thereafter, with more frequent screening depending on individual risk behaviors and the local epidemiology.[35]

ACKNOWLEDGMENTS

We appreciate the significant contributions of Dr. Kenneth Katz to this chapter. We also thank Dr. Gerald Lazarus for his help in reviewing and selecting the images for this chapter.

REFERENCES

1. de Melo FL, de Mello JC, Fraga AM, et al. Syphilis at the crossroad of phylogenetics and paleopathology. *PLoS Negl Trop Dis.* 2010;4(1):e575.
2. Fenton KA, Breban R, Vardavas R, et al. Infectious syphilis in high-income settings in the 21st century. *Lancet Infect Dis.* 2008;8(4):244-253.
3. Rothschild BM. History of syphilis. *Clin Infect Dis.* 2005;40(10):1454-1463.
4. Glickman FS. Syphilus. *J Am Acad Dermatol.* 1985;12(3):593-596.
5. Sefton AM. The great pox that was...syphilis. *J Appl Microbiol.* 2001;91(4):592-596.
6. Waugh M. The centenary of *Treponema pallidum*: on the discovery of *Spirochaeta pallida*. *Int J STD AIDS.* 2005;16(9):594-595.
7. Arnold HL Jr. Dermatology, 50 years ago. *JAMA.* 1989;262(6):824-825.
8. Dunst KM, Gurunluoglu R, Aubock J, et al. Adolf Jarisch (1850-1902): an important contributor to Austrian dermatology. *Arch Dermatol Res.* 2006;297(9):383-388.
9. Leslie KS, Levell NJ. Dermatologists, beacons of epidemics; past, present and future! *Int J Dermatol.* 2004;43(6):468-470.
10. Sartin JS, Perry HO. From mercury to malaria to penicillin: the history of the treatment of syphilis at the Mayo Clinic—1916-1955. *J Am Acad Dermatol.* 1995;32(2, pt 1):255-261.
11. Steffen C. Why a historical approach has clinical benefits: John Hinchman Stokes and George Miller MacKee. *Skinmed.* 2006;5(1):31-36.
12. Wallach D, Tilles G. First International Congress of Dermatology and Syphilology, Paris, Aug. 5-10, 1889. *J Am Acad Dermatol.* 1992;26(6):995-1001.
13. Gruber F. History of venereology in Croatia. *Acta Dermatovenerol Croat.* 2009;17(4):247-262.
14. Thappa DM. Evolution of venereology in India. *Indian J Dermatol Venereol Leprol.* 2006;72(3):187-196; quiz 197.
15. Albert MR. Fever therapy for general paresis. *Int J Dermatol.* 1999;38(8):633-637.
16. Lafond RE, Lukehart SA. Biological basis for syphilis. *Clin Microbiol Rev.* 2006;19(1):29-49.
17. Whitrow M. Wagner-Jauregg and fever therapy. *Med Hist.* 1990;34(3):294-310.
18. Harrison LW. The Oslo study of untreated syphilis, review and commentary. *Br J Vener Dis.* 1956;32(2):70-78.
19. Jones JH, Tuskegee Institute. *Bad Blood: The Tuskegee Syphilis Experiment.* New and expanded ed. New York, NY: Free Press; 1993.
20. The National Commission for the Protection of Human Subjects of Biomedical and Behavioral Research. *The Belmont Report: Ethical Principles and Guidelines for the Protection of Human Subjects of Research.* Bethesda, MD: U.S. Department of Health, Education, and Welfare; 1978. Available at https://videocast.nih.gov/pdf/ohrp_belmont_report.pdf
21. Hayden D. *Pox: Genius, Madness, and the Mysteries of Syphilis.* New York, NY: Basic Books; 2003.
22. Brandt AM. *No Magic Bullet: A Social History of Venereal Disease in the United States Since 1880.* New York, NY: Oxford University Press; 1985.
23. Parran T. *Shadow on the Land: Syphilis.* New York, NY: Reynal & Hitchcock; 1937.
24. Hook EW 3rd. Elimination of syphilis transmission in the United States: historic perspectives and practical considerations. *Trans Am Clin Climatol Assoc.* 1999;110:195-203; discussion 203-204.
25. Nakashima AK, Rolfs RT, Flock ML, et al. Epidemiology of syphilis in the United States, 1941-1993. *Sex Transm Dis.* 1996;23(1):16-23.
26. Division of STD Prevention, National Center for HIV, STD and TB Prevention, Centers for Disease Control and Prevention, Department of Health and Human Services. *The National Plan to Eliminate Syphilis From the United States.* Atlanta, GA: Division of STD Prevention, National Center for HIV, STD, and TB Prevention, Centers for Disease Control and Prevention; 2006. Available at https://www.cdc.gov/stopsyphilis/SEEPlan2006.pdf.
27. Centers for Disease Control and Prevention (CDC). *2014 Sexually Transmitted Diseases Surveillance.* Archived at http://www.cdc.gov/std/stats14/syphilis.htm. Last accessed September 18, 2018.
28. Peterman TA, Furness BW. The resurgence of syphilis among men who have sex with men. *Curr Opin Infect Dis.* 2007;20(1):54-59.

29. Zetola NM, Klausner JD. Syphilis and HIV infection: an update. *Clin Infect Dis.* 2007;44(9):1222-1228.
30. Fonner VA, Dalglish SL, Kennedy CE, et al. Effectiveness and safety of oral HIV pre-exposure prophylaxis (PrEP) for all populations: a systematic review and meta-analysis. *AIDS.* 2016;30(12):1973-1983.
31. Chen YH, Snowden JM, McFarland W, et al. Pre-exposure prophylaxis (PrEP) Use, seroadaptation, and sexual behavior among men who have sex with men, San Francisco, 2004-2014. *AIDS Behav.* 2016;20(12):2791-2797.
32. Solomon MM, Mayer KH, Glidden DV, et al. Syphilis predicts HIV incidence among men and transgender women who have sex with men in a preexposure prophylaxis trial. *Clin Infect Dis.* 2014;59(7):1020-1026.
33. Pathela P, Braunstein SL, Blank S, et al. The high risk of an HIV diagnosis following a diagnosis of syphilis: a population-level analysis of New York City men. *Clin Infect Dis.* 2015;61(2):281-287.
34. Peterman TA, Newman DR, Maddox L, et al. High risk for HIV following syphilis diagnosis among men in Florida, 2000-2011. *Public Health Rep.* 2014;129(2):164-169.
35. Workowski KA, Bolan GA. Centers for Disease Control and Prevention. Sexually transmitted diseases treatment guidelines, 2015. *MMWR Recomm Rep.* 2015;64(RR-03):1-137.
36. Bowen V, Su J, Torrone E, et al. Increase in incidence of congenital syphilis—United States, 2012-2014. *MMWR Morb Mortal Wkly Rep.* 2015;64(44):1241-1245.
37. Woolston S, Cohen SE, Fanfair RN, et al. A cluster of ocular syphilis cases—Seattle, Washington, and San Francisco, California, 2014-2015. *MMWR Morb Mortal Wkly Rep.* 2015;64(40):1150-1151.
38. Centers for Disease Control and Prevention (CDC). Clinical Advisory: Ocular Syphilis in the United States. Updated March 24, 2016. https://www.cdc.gov/std/syphilis/clinicaladvisoryos2015.htm. Last accessed October 6, 2016.
39. Ozturk F, Gurses N, Sancak R, et al. Acquired secondary syphilis in a 6-year-old girl with no history of sexual abuse. *Cutis.* 1998;62(3):150-151.
40. Orton S. Syphilis and blood donors: what we know, what we do not know, and what we need to know. *Transfus Med Rev.* 2001;15(4):282-291.
41. Meyer GS. Occupational infection in health care. The century-old lessons from syphilis. *Arch Intern Med.* 1993;153(21):2439-2447.
42. Kazandjieva J, Tsankov N. Tattoos: dermatological complications. *Clin Dermatol.* 2007;25(4):375-382.
43. Woods CR. Syphilis in children: congenital and acquired. *Semin Pediatr Infect Dis.* 2005;16(4):245-257.
44. Wicher V, Wicher K. Pathogenesis of maternal-fetal syphilis revisited. *Clin Infect Dis.* 2001;33(3):354-363.
45. Garnett GP, Aral SO, Hoyle DV, et al. The natural history of syphilis. Implications for the transmission dynamics and control of infection. *Sex Transm Dis.* 1997;24(4):185-200.
46. Moore MB Jr, Price EV, Knox JM, et al. Epidemiologic treatment of contacts to infectious syphilis. *Public Health Rep.* 1963;78:966-970.
47. Schroeter AL, Turner RH, Lucas JB, et al. Therapy for incubating syphilis. Effectiveness of gonorrhea treatment. *JAMA.* 1971;218(5):711-713.
48. Alexander LJ, Schoch AG. Prevention of syphilis; penicillin calcium in oil and white wax, U.S. P., bismuth ethylcamphorate and oxophenarsine hydrochloride in treatment, during incubation stage, of persons exposed to syphilis. *Arch Derm Syphilol.* 1949;59(1):1-10.
49. Lukehart SA, Hook EW 3rd, Baker-Zander SA, et al. Invasion of the central nervous system by *Treponema pallidum*: implications for diagnosis and treatment. *Ann Intern Med.* 1988;109(11):855-862.
50. Hourihan M, Wheeler H, Houghton R, et al. Lessons from the syphilis outbreak in homosexual men in east London. *Sex Transm Infect.* 2004;80(6):509-511.
51. Rompalo AM, Joesoef MR, O'Donnell JA, et al. Clinical manifestations of early syphilis by HIV status and gender: results of the syphilis and HIV study. *Sex Transm Dis.* 2001;28(3):158-165.
52. Golden MR, Marra CM, Holmes KK. Update on syphilis: resurgence of an old problem. *JAMA.* 2003;290(11):1510-1514.
53. Rompalo AM, Lawlor J, Seaman P, et al. Modification of syphilitic genital ulcer manifestations by coexistent HIV infection. *Sex Transm Dis.* 2001;28(8):448-454.
54. Zeltser R, Kurban AK. Syphilis. *Clin Dermatol.* 2004;22(6):461-468.
55. Lautenschlager S. Cutaneous manifestations of syphilis: recognition and management. *Am J Clin Dermatol.* 2006;7(5):291-304.
56. Dourmishev LA, Dourmishev AL. Syphilis: uncommon presentations in adults. *Clin Dermatol.* 2005;23(6):555-564.
57. Katz KA. Dory flop sign of syphilis. *Arch Dermatol.* 2010;146(5):572.
58. Crissey JT, Denenholz DA. Syphilis. *Clin Dermatol.* 1984;2(1):1-166.
59. Davies T. *Primary Syphilis in the Female [thesis (MD)]*. London, UK: Oxford University Press; 1931.
60. Ramoni S, Cusini M, Gaiani F, et al. Syphilitic chancres of the mouth: three cases. *Acta Derm Venereol.* 2009;89(6):648-649.
61. Allison SD. Extragenital syphilitic chancres. *J Am Acad Dermatol.* 1986;14(6):1094-1095.
62. Emerson CR, Lynch A, Fox R, et al. The syphilis outbreak in Northern Ireland. *Int J STD AIDS.* 2007;18(6):413-417.
63. Centers for Disease Control and Prevention (CDC). Transmission of primary and secondary syphilis by oral sex—Chicago, Illinois, 1998-2002. *MMWR Morb Mortal Wkly Rep.* 2004;53(41):966-968.
64. Gunn RA. Expedited intervention services for possible occult primary syphilis among MSM with asymptomatic incident syphilis. *Sex Transm Dis.* 2009;36(9):594-595.
65. Ramoni S, Cusini M, Boneschi V, et al. Primary syphilis of the finger. *Sex Transm Dis.* 2010;37(7):468.
66. Bernabeu-Wittel J, Rodriguez-Canas T, Conejo-Mir J. Primary syphilitic chancre on the hand with regional adenopathy. *Sex Transm Dis.* 2010;37(7):467.
67. Oh Y, Ahn SY, Hong SP, et al. A case of extragenital chancre on a nipple from a human bite during sexual intercourse. *Int J Dermatol.* 2008;47(9):978-980.
68. Scott LJ, Gunson RN, Carman WF, et al. A new multiplex real-time PCR test for HSV1/2 and syphilis: an evaluation of its impact in the laboratory and clinical setting. *Sex Transm Infect.* 2010;86(7):537-539.
69. Lai W, Chen CY, Morse SA, et al. Increasing relative prevalence of HSV-2 infection among men with genital ulcers from a mining community in South Africa. *Sex Transm Infect.* 2003;79(3):202-207.
70. Hope-Rapp E, Anyfantakis V, Fouere S, et al. Etiology of genital ulcer disease. A prospective study of 278 cases seen in an STD clinic in Paris. *Sex Transm Dis.* 2010;37(3):153-158.

71. Eccleston K, Collins L, Higgins SP. Primary syphilis. *Int J STD AIDS*. 2008;19(3):145-151.
72. Centers for Disease Control and Prevention (CDC). 2014 Sexually Transmitted Diseases Surveillance. Appendix C1. Case Definitions for Nationally Notifiable Infectious Diseases. 2014. Archived at https://www.cdc.gov/std/stats14/appendixc.htm. Last accessed October 16, 2016.
73. Peeling RW, Hook EW 3rd. The pathogenesis of syphilis: the Great Mimicker, revisited. *J Pathol*. 2006;208(2):224-232.
74. Chapel TA. The signs and symptoms of secondary syphilis. *Sex Transm Dis*. 1980;7(4):161-164.
75. Baughn RE, Musher DM. Secondary syphilitic lesions. *Clin Microbiol Rev*. 2005;18(1):205-216.
76. Watson KM, White JM, Salisbury JR, et al. Lues maligna. *Clin Exp Dermatol*. 2004;29(6):625-627.
77. Lejman K, Starzycki Z. Keratopustular variety of framboesiform syphilis: a case report. *Br J Vener Dis*. 1977;53(3):195-199.
78. Kirby JS, Goreshi R, Mahoney N. Syphilitic palmoplantar keratoderma and ocular disease: a rare combination in an HIV-positive patient. *Cutis*. 2009;84(6):305-310.
79. Tham SN, Ng SK. Secondary syphilis with framboesiform lesions. *Genitourin Med*. 1990;66(2):99-100.
80. Beck MH, Hubbard HC, Dave VK, et al. Secondary syphilis with framboesiform facial lesions: a case report. *Br J Vener Dis*. 1981;57(2):103-105.
81. Goldman L. Macular syphilides absent in red tattoo. *Cutis*. 1989;44(4):313.
82. Fonollosa A, Giralt J, Pelegrin L, et al. Ocular syphilis—back again: understanding recent increases in the incidence of ocular syphilitic disease. *Ocul Immunol Inflamm*. 2009;17(3):207-212.
83. Kolios AG, Weber A, Sporri S, et al. Syphilitic pharyngitis. *Arch Dermatol*. 2010;146(5):570-572.
84. Brass LS, White JA. Granulomatous disease of the larynx. *J La State Med Soc*. 1991;143(1):11-14.
85. Mylona EE, Baraboutis IG, Papastamopoulos V, et al. Gastric syphilis: a systematic review of published cases of the last 50 years. *Sex Transm Dis*. 2010;37(3):177-183.
86. Hunte W, al-Ghraoui F, Cohen RJ. Secondary syphilis and the nephrotic syndrome. *J Am Soc Nephrol*. 1993;3(7):1351-1355.
87. Middleton S, Rowntree C, Rudge S. Bone pain as the presenting manifestation of secondary syphilis. *Ann Rheum Dis*. 1990;49(8):641-642.
88. Cruz AR, Pillay A, Zuluaga AV, et al. Secondary syphilis in Cali, Colombia: new concepts in disease pathogenesis. *PLoS Negl Trop Dis*. 2010;4(5):e690.
89. Wu SJ, Nguyen EQ, Nielsen TA, et al. Nodular tertiary syphilis mimicking granuloma annulare. *J Am Acad Dermatol*. 2000;42(2, pt 2):378-380.
90. Sule RR, Deshpande SG, Dharmadhikari NJ, et al. Late cutaneous syphilis. *Cutis*. 1997;59(3):135-137.
91. Horowitz HW, Valsamis MP, Wicher V, et al. Brief report: cerebral syphilitic gumma confirmed by the polymerase chain reaction in a man with human immunodeficiency virus infection. *N Engl J Med*. 1994;331(22):1488-1491.
92. Roberts WC, Ko JM, Vowels TJ. Natural history of syphilitic aortitis. *Am J Cardiol*. 2009;104(11):1578-1587.
93. Jackman JD Jr, Radolf JD. Cardiovascular syphilis. *Am J Med*. 1989;87(4):425-433.
94. O'Regan AW, Castro C, Lukehart SA, et al. Barking up the wrong tree? Use of polymerase chain reaction to diagnose syphilitic aortitis. *Thorax*. 2002;57(10):917-918.
95. Marra CM. Update on neurosyphilis. *Curr Infect Dis Rep*. 2009;11(2):127-134.
96. Centers for Disease Control and Prevention (CDC). Symptomatic early neurosyphilis among HIV-positive men who have sex with men—four cities, United States, January 2002-June 2004. *MMWR Morb Mortal Wkly Rep*. 2007;56(25):625-628.
97. Moradi A, Salek S, Daniel E, et al. Clinical features and incidence rates of ocular complications in patients with ocular syphilis. *Am J Ophthalmol*. 2015;159(2):334-343;e1.
98. Li JZ, Tucker JD, Lobo AM, et al. Ocular syphilis among HIV-infected individuals. *Clin Infect Dis*. 2010;51(4):468-471.
99. Margo CE, Hamed LM. Ocular syphilis. *Surv Ophthalmol*. 1992;37(3):203-220.
100. Jenson HB. Congenital syphilis. *Semin Pediatr Infect Dis*. 1999;10(3):183-194.
101. Doroshenko A, Sherrard J, Pollard AJ. Syphilis in pregnancy and the neonatal period. *Int J STD AIDS*. 2006;17(4):221-227; quiz 228.
102. Lugo A, Sanchez S, Sanchez JL. Congenital syphilis. *Pediatr Dermatol*. 2006;23(2):121-123.
103. Schofer H, Imhof M, Thoma-Greber E, et al. Active syphilis in HIV infection: a multicentre retrospective survey. The German AIDS Study Group (GASG). *Genitourin Med*. 1996;72(3):176-181.
104. Hutchinson CM, Hook EW 3rd, Shepherd M, et al. Altered clinical presentation of early syphilis in patients with human immunodeficiency virus infection. *Ann Intern Med*. 1994;121(2):94-100.
105. Buchacz K, Patel P, Taylor M, et al. Syphilis increases HIV viral load and decreases CD4 cell counts in HIV-infected patients with new syphilis infections. *AIDS*. 2004;18(15):2075-2079.
106. Dyer JR, Eron JJ, Hoffman IF, et al. Association of CD4 cell depletion and elevated blood and seminal plasma human immunodeficiency virus type 1 (HIV-1) RNA concentrations with genital ulcer disease in HIV-1-infected men in Malawi. *J Infect Dis*. 1998;177(1):224-227.
107. Kofoed K, Gerstoft J, Mathiesen LR, et al. Syphilis and human immunodeficiency virus (HIV)-1 coinfection: influence on CD4 T-cell count, HIV-1 viral load, and treatment response. *Sex Transm Dis*. 2006;33(3):143-148.
108. Manfredi R, Sabbatani S, Pocaterra D, et al. Syphilis does not seem to involve virological and immunological course of concurrent HIV disease. *AIDS*. 2006;20(2):305-306.
109. Modjarrad K, Vermund SH. Effect of treating co-infections on HIV-1 viral load: a systematic review. *Lancet Infect Dis*. 2010;10(7):455-463.
110. Palacios R, Jimenez-Onate F, Aguilar M, et al. Impact of syphilis infection on HIV viral load and CD4 cell counts in HIV-infected patients. *J Acquir Immune Defic Syndr*. 2007;44(3):356-359.
111. Sadiq ST, McSorley J, Copas AJ, et al. The effects of early syphilis on CD4 counts and HIV-1 RNA viral loads in blood and semen. *Sex Transm Infect*. 2005;81(5):380-385.
112. Weintrob AC, Gu W, Qin J, et al. Syphilis co-infection does not affect HIV disease progression. *Int J STD AIDS*. 2010;21(1):57-59.
113. Tobian AA, Quinn TC. Herpes simplex virus type 2 and syphilis infections with HIV: an evolving synergy in transmission and prevention. *Curr Opin HIV AIDS*. 2009;4(4):294-299.

114. Aberg JA, Gallant JE, Ghanem KG, et al. Primary care guidelines for the management of persons infected with HIV: 2013 update by the HIV Medicine Association of the Infectious Diseases Society of America. *Clin Infect Dis*. 2014;58(1):1-10.
115. Katz KA, Lee MA, Gray T, et al. Repeat syphilis among men who have sex with men—San Diego County, 2004-2009. *Sex Transm Dis*. 2011;38(4):349-352.
116. Marra CM, Maxwell CL, Smith SL, et al. Cerebrospinal fluid abnormalities in patients with syphilis: association with clinical and laboratory features. *J Infect Dis*. 2004;189(3):369-376.
117. Marra CM, Maxwell CL, Tantalo L, et al. Normalization of cerebrospinal fluid abnormalities after neurosyphilis therapy: does HIV status matter? *Clin Infect Dis*. 2004;38(7):1001-1006.
118. Smith G, Holman RP. The prozone phenomenon with syphilis and HIV-1 co-infection. *South Med J*. 2004;97(4):379-382.
119. Kingston AA, Vujevich J, Shapiro M, et al. Seronegative secondary syphilis in 2 patients coinfected with human immunodeficiency virus. *Arch Dermatol*. 2005;141(4):431-433.
120. Agmon-Levin N, Elbirt D, Asher I, et al. Syphilis and HIV co-infection in an Israeli HIV clinic: incidence and outcome. *Int J STD AIDS*. 2010;21(4):249-252.
121. Larsen SA, Pope V, Johnson RE, et al, eds. *A Manual of Tests for Syphilis*. 9th ed. Washington, DC: American Public Health Association; 1998.
122. Rolfs RT, Joesoef MR, Hendershot EF, et al. A randomized trial of enhanced therapy for early syphilis in patients with and without human immunodeficiency virus infection. The Syphilis and HIV Study Group. *N Engl J Med*. 1997;337(5):307-314.
123. Gonzalez-Lopez JJ, Guerrero ML, Lujan R, et al. Factors determining serologic response to treatment in patients with syphilis. *Clin Infect Dis*. 2009;49(10):1505-1511.
124. Yinnon AM, Coury-Doniger P, Polito R, et al. Serologic response to treatment of syphilis in patients with HIV infection. *Arch Intern Med*. 1996;156(3):321-325.
125. Fraser CM, Norris SJ, Weinstock GM, et al. Complete genome sequence of *Treponema pallidum*, the syphilis spirochete. *Science*. 1998;281(5375):375-388.
126. Sena AC, White BL, Sparling PF. Novel *Treponema pallidum* serologic tests: a paradigm shift in syphilis screening for the 21st century. *Clin Infect Dis*. 2010;51(6):700-708.
127. Fitzgerald TJ. The Th1/Th2-like switch in syphilitic infection: is it detrimental? *Infect Immun*. 1992;60(9):3475-3479.
128. Marra C, Sahi S, Tantalo L, et al. Enhanced molecular typing of *Treponema pallidum*: geographical distribution of strain types and association with neurosyphilis. *J Infect Dis*. 2010;202(9):1380-1388.
129. Kenyon C, Lynen L, Florence E, et al. Syphilis reinfections pose problems for syphilis diagnosis in Antwerp, Belgium—1992 to 2012. *Euro Surveill*. 2014;19(45):20958.
130. Wrzolkowa T, Kozakiewicz J. Ultrastructure of vascular and connective tissue changes in primary syphilis. *Br J Vener Dis*. 1980;56(3):137-143.
131. Cullen PA, Cameron CE. Progress towards an effective syphilis vaccine: the past, present and future. *Expert Rev Vaccines*. 2006;5(1):67-80.
132. Huber TW, Storms S, Young P, et al. Reactivity of microhemagglutination, fluorescent treponemal antibody absorption, Venereal Disease Research Laboratory, and rapid plasma reagin tests in primary syphilis. *J Clin Microbiol*. 1983;17(3):405-409.
133. Tuddenham S, Ghanem KG. Emerging trends and persistent challenges in the management of adult syphilis. *BMC Infect Dis*. 2015;15:351.
134. Wheeler HL, Agarwal S, Goh BT. Dark ground microscopy and treponemal serological tests in the diagnosis of early syphilis. *Sex Transm Infect*. 2004;80(5):411-414.
135. Tsang RS, Morshed M, Chernesky MA, et al. Canadian Public Health Laboratory Network laboratory guidelines for the use of direct tests to detect syphilis in Canada. *Can J Infect Dis Med Microbiol*. 2015;26 (suppl A):13A-17A.
136. Crowson AN, Magro C, Martin M Jr., Treponemal diseases. In: Elder DE, Elenitsas R, Johnson B Jr, et al, eds. *Lever's Histopathology of the Skin*. 10th ed. Philadelphia, PA: Lippincott Williams & Wilkins; 2009: 579-591.
137. Cole MJ, Perry KR, Parry JV. Comparative evaluation of 15 serological assays for the detection of syphilis infection. *Eur J Clin Microbiol Infect Dis*. 2007;26(10):705-713.
138. Lesinski J, Krach J, Kadziewicz E. Specificity, sensitivity, and diagnostic value of the TPHA test. *Br J Vener Dis*. 1974;50(5):334-340.
139. Cantor AG, Pappas M, Daeges M, et al. Screening for syphilis: updated evidence report and systematic review for the US Preventive Services Task Force. *JAMA*. 2016;315(21):2328-2337.
140. Peeling RW, Ye H. Diagnostic tools for preventing and managing maternal and congenital syphilis: an overview. *Bull World Health Organ*. 2004;82(6):439-446.
141. Baker-Zander SA, Roddy RE, Handsfield HH, et al. IgG and IgM antibody reactivity to antigens of *Treponema pallidum* after treatment of syphilis. *Sex Transm Dis*. 1986;13(4):214-220.
142. Clement ME, Okeke NL, Hicks CB. Treatment of syphilis: a systematic review. *JAMA*. 2014;312(18):1905-1917.
143. Romanowski B, Sutherland R, Fick GH, et al. Serologic response to treatment of infectious syphilis. *Ann Intern Med*. 1991;114(12):1005-1009.
144. Larsen SA, Hambie EA, Pettit DE, et al. Specificity, sensitivity, and reproducibility among the fluorescent treponemal antibody-absorption test, the microhemagglutination assay for *Treponema pallidum* antibodies, and the hemagglutination treponemal test for syphilis. *J Clin Microbiol*. 1981;14(4):441-445.
145. Centers for Disease Control and Prevention (CDC). Syphilis testing algorithms using treponemal tests for initial screening—four laboratories, New York City, 2005-2006. *MMWR Morb Mortal Wkly Rep*. 2008;57(32):872-875.
146. Peterman TA, Fakile YF. What is the use of rapid syphilis tests in the United States? *Sex Transm Dis*. 2016;43(3):201-203.
147. Ridruejo E, Mordoh A, Herrera F, et al. Severe cholestatic hepatitis as the first symptom of secondary syphilis. *Dig Dis Sci*. 2004;49(9):1401-1404.
148. Kampmeier RH. The introduction of penicillin for the treatment of syphilis. *Sex Transm Dis*. 1981;8(4):260-265.
149. Centers for Disease Control and Prevention (CDC). Inadvertent use of Bicillin C-R for treatment of syphilis—Maryland, 1998. *MMWR Morb Mortal Wkly Rep*. 1999;48(35):777-779.

150. Centers for Disease Control and Prevention (CDC). Inadvertent use of Bicillin C-R to treat syphilis infection—Los Angeles, California, 1999-2004. *MMWR Morb Mortal Wkly Rep.* 2005;54(9):217-219.
151. Zhou P, Qian Y, Xu J, et al. Occurrence of congenital syphilis after maternal treatment with azithromycin during pregnancy. *Sex Transm Dis.* 2007;34(7):472-474.
152. Zhou P, Li K, Lu H, et al. Azithromycin treatment failure among primary and secondary syphilis patients in Shanghai. *Sex Transm Dis.* 2010;37(11):726-729.
153. Katz KA, Klausner JD. Azithromycin resistance in *Treponema pallidum*. *Curr Opin Infect Dis.* 2008;21(1):83-91.
154. Pound MW, May DB. Proposed mechanisms and preventative options of Jarisch-Herxheimer reactions. *J Clin Pharm Ther.* 2005;30(3):291-295.
155. Zilberstein J, McCurdy MT, Winters ME. Anaphylaxis. *J Emerg Med.* 2014;47(2):182-187.

Chapter 171 :: Endemic (Nonvenereal) Treponematoses
:: Francisco G. Bravo, Carolina Talhari, & Khaled Ezzedine

第一百七十一章

地方性（非性病性）密螺旋体病

中文导读

地方性密螺旋体病的病原体与引起梅毒的病原体苍白密螺旋体同属密螺旋体科。此类疾病包括由品他密螺旋体引起的品他，细密螺旋体引起的雅司以及地方性苍白密螺旋体引起的贝杰（又称地方性梅毒）。本章从历史背景、流行病学、临床表现（皮肤系统及皮肤系统外）、发病机理、诊断与鉴别诊断、病程与预后和疾病的管理等几个方面对这几种地方性密螺旋体病进行了介绍。

地方性密螺旋体病主要流行于热带地区，被WHO定义为被忽视的热带疾病。与梅毒相似，每一种地方性密螺旋体病都会经历早期（一期与二期）、潜伏期和晚期（三期）。它们在流行地区的发病率高，疾病进展主要涉及皮肤、骨和软骨组织的病变，引起严重的畸形、疼痛、残疾以及社交隔离，给流行地区本就贫困的人民带来更大的伤害。表171-1比较了3种地方性密螺旋体病的临床特点。

品他是一种慢性地方性流行病，流行于中美洲及南美洲北部的热带雨林地区，可累及各年龄段人群。品他是最早在人类中发病的密螺旋体病，也是最为良性的地方性密螺旋体病，仅累及皮肤系统。本病发展阶段分为两期，即早期与晚期。早期又分为一期（初疹）与二期（泛发性皮疹）。初疹发生于品他螺旋体侵入皮肤后7-20天，表现为局部出现一个至数个红色鳞屑性丘疹，主要累及面部、四肢或其他暴露部位。皮损有蔓延倾向，可形成大小不一、形态各异的红斑鳞屑性或红斑性的色素沉着斑块（弓形的、环形的、多环形和匐行性的）。一般来说无明显症状，但随着疾病进展常有瘙痒症状。常见局部淋巴结肿大。早期感染时非特异性梅毒螺旋体（心磷脂）以及特异性梅毒螺旋体血清学试验结果可能是阴性的。二期皮疹发生于感染后6个月至3年，表现为色素减退、色素沉着及红斑鳞屑疹，为品他皮肤扩散阶段。多数皮损有不同程度的角化过度表现。它们通常小而圆，逐渐增大、融合，累及大面积皮肤，而皮损中部表现类似正常皮肤。这些皮损被称为品他疹。皮损刚发生时呈红色至暗红色，之后变成蓝灰色、褐色、灰色或黑色。不同临床分期的皮损可能同时出现在一个患者身上，导致临床表现多形性。晚期（三期）在感染后2~5年出现，表现为色素沉着、色素减退、过度角化和皮肤萎缩，尤其是在身体的暴露部位，如手背、手腕、手肘、胫前、踝部和足背、足底。在这个时期，上肢、躯干和双大腿常出现大面积色素减退。二期和三期均可出现淋巴结肿大表现。多数患者特异性梅毒血清学检查呈阳性。典型的临床表现、流行地区、感染史以及梅毒血清学试验阳性可诊断此病。品他的推荐治疗为苄星青霉素G 120万单位，单次肌注，小于10岁的儿童剂量减半。

雅司主要流行于西太平洋的热带、亚热带国家以及非洲中东部，如巴布亚新几内亚、所罗门群岛、瓦努阿图和加纳。主要累及生活在平均气温超过27℃、降雨量大、卫生条件差、生活条件差的人群。它是最为常见的地方性密螺旋体病，通常累及儿童，6~10岁儿童最常受累，由皮肤接触传染。本病潜伏期9~90天（通常为21天），可分为三期。一期又称母雅司期。感染后经过潜伏期在感染部位发生单个皮疹，为扁平或半球形隆起性丘疹，逐渐增大，进展为2~5cm痂皮附着的质硬溃疡，最常见于腿部，极少累及外生殖器部位。它即为雅司的原发疹，被称为"母雅司"。即使未治疗，母雅司在出现3~6月后自行消退，留下色素沉着性瘢痕。患者可同时出现一期、二期皮损。二期皮损在原发疹1~2月后出现（最长可达24个月），二期皮损与一期相似，但较小，数量较多，好发于颜面及四肢。代表着雅司随着血行或淋巴播散至皮肤组织和骨组织。对于皮肤症状来说，皮损可表现为渗出性的、增生性以及乳头状瘤性的，或者干燥无渗出的丘疹鳞屑型。无论是否治疗，二期皮损均可自行消退。大约10%的未经治疗的二期雅司可进入三期，表现为皮下组织树胶样肿，大面积组织损害、坏死及无痛性溃疡。三期最常见的表现为皮肤和骨组织同时受累。鼻软骨破坏和鼻三角塌陷可导致毁形性鼻咽炎。品他型色素减退和掌跖色素沉着也可出现在这一时期。雅司的皮肤外表现主要为关节痛、淋巴结肿大、头痛等，亦常累及骨关节部位，导致骨膜炎或指（趾）炎。根据本病的流行地区、感染史、典型皮损与渗出液暗视野显微镜下观察到细密螺旋体即可诊断。但在某些热带医疗条件较差的地区，非特异性梅毒螺旋体以及特异性梅毒螺旋体血清学检查也是诊断该疾病的有力工具。雅司的推荐治疗为苄星青霉素G 120万单位，单次肌注，小于10岁的儿童剂量减半。

贝杰最常见于15岁以下的儿童，通过皮肤接触以及使用被污染过的水容器传播。本病在非洲撒哈拉沙漠以及沙特阿拉伯地区最为流行（气候炎热干旱的地区）。一期皮损在临床上少见，典型者为口或鼻咽部黏膜下疳，二期皮损类似后天梅毒黏膜损害（累及口黏膜、扁桃体、舌、嘴唇以及鼻咽部）、扁平湿疣以及全身广泛发疹，三期皮损出现较早（6个月至数年），呈树胶样肿或损毁性溃疡。贝杰也可能产生骨损害，但神经系统、心血管系统受累以及母婴传播罕见。贝杰早期损害中可以检查出大量的地方性苍白密螺旋体，特异性及非特异性梅毒螺旋体血清学实验均为阳性，但晚期可能呈弱阳性或阴性。生活在流行区或据临床特征及梅毒血清学试验阳性即可确诊。贝杰的推荐治疗亦为苄星青霉素G 120万单位，单次肌注，小于10岁的儿童剂量减半。

〔张江林〕

INTRODUCTION

The endemic treponematoses are infectious diseases caused by microorganisms that are closely related to *Treponema pallidum*, the causative agent of syphilis. This group of entities includes (1) pinta, caused by *Treponema carateum*; (2) yaws, caused by *T. pallidum* ssp. *pertenue*; and (3) bejel, caused by *T. pallidum* ssp. *endemicum*. Although all these entities are caused by *Treponema* species, there are important differences between the endemic treponematoses and syphilis, including a nonvenereal form of transmission, an endemic occurrence in very specific geographic areas, a tendency to affect children rather than sexually active adults, and a less likely risk for congenital transmission to occur. In common with syphilis, every endemic treponematosis goes through an early stage (including primary and secondary), a period of latency, and a late stage. Significant morbidity is associated with progression of the disease, mainly affecting the skin, bone, and cartilage, leading to significant disfigurement, pain, disability, and social isolation, causing more suffering to already disadvantaged populations living in poverty.

From an epidemiologic point of view, global efforts commanded by the World Health Organization (WHO) from 1952 through 1964 resulted in more than 50 million individuals who were treated for endemic treponematosis, with special attention to yaws. The global incidence of endemic treponematoses was reduced significantly, by 95%, from 50 million cases worldwide to a merely 2.5 million cases.[1] However, after all the efforts of such campaign, the sustainability of the control program was transferred to local primary care systems in endemic areas. Because of waning and poor commitment in such surveillance programs, there has been a resurgence in the incidence of the endemic treponematoses. A recent study estimates that at least 89 million people are living in yaws-endemic areas.[2] The WHO now recognizes all endemic treponematosis as neglected tropical diseases.[3] The current WHO goal is to eliminate yaws by 2020; stricter and more sensitive surveillance programs are required to reach such goal. Table 171-1 shows a quick comparison among the three diseases.

PINTA

AT-A-GLANCE

- Pinta is a chronic infectious and contagious disease recognized by the World Health Organization as a neglected tropical disease.
- It is the most benign form of endemic treponematosis, with clinical manifestations limited to the skin, including vitiligo-like achromic lesions as well as hyperpigmented lesions.
- It affects people of all ages.
- It is neither sexually transmitted nor congenitally acquired.
- Treatment includes single or divided dose of long-acting benzathine penicillin (1.2 MU for adults; 0.6 MU for children).

INTRODUCTION

DEFINITIONS

Pinta, also known as azula (blue), carate, and mal de pinto (pinto sickness), is the most benign of the endemic treponematosis because it affects only the skin. The word pinta comes from Spanish for painted, spot, or mark.[4]

The etiologic agent of pinta, *Treponema carateum*, cannot be distinguished morphologically or serologically from the not-yet-cultivable *T. pallidum* subspecies that cause venereal syphilis, yaws, and bejel.[1,2]

TABLE 171-1
Clinical Aspect of the Endemic Treponematosis

FEATURE	PINTA	YAWS	BEJEL
Etiology	*Treponema carateum*	*Treponema pallidum* ssp. *pertenue*	*Treponema pallidum* ssp. *endemicum*
World distribution, main areas	Probably present focally in Brazilian and Venezuelan green forest	Papua New Guinea, Solomon Islands, and Ghana	African Sahel and Saudi Arabia
Climate conditions	Tropical green forest	Tropical humid	Hot and dry climate
Population affected	Children and adults	Mostly children	Mostly children
Transmission	Close contact	Close contact	Close contact and fomites
Primary lesion	Evident, can be multiple, several locations	One to several, lower extremities	Rarely evident
Predominant lesion	Vitiligo-like and hyperchromic lesions	Exudative, papillomatous or papulo-squamous lesions	Moist lesions near mucosal surface or intertriginous areas
Nonskin involvement	None	Periositis, osteitis	Periositis, osteitis

HISTORICAL PERSPECTIVE

Pinta is considered the first treponematosis to occur in humans. It was described in Aztec and Caribbean Amerindians in the early years of the 16th century.[5,6] Initially, it was thought that a pathogenic fungus caused pinta. However, two observations suggested otherwise. First, laboratory studies of pinta patients' sera showed that result for the Wassermann test, an early serology test for syphilis (STS), was positive in the majority of cases. Second, treatments that were effective against syphilis (ie, mercury and arsenicals) were also effective against pinta.[7] In 1938, Armenteros and Triana (Cuba)[6] recognized *Treponema carateum* as the causative agent of pinta. Leon Blanco, in Mexico, reproduced the disease by inoculating exudates on himself and human volunteers in 1942. The same author also demonstrated that patients with late-stage pinta could not be reinfected, but patients whose early-stage pinta had been cured could be reinfected.[8,9] Padilha-Gonçalves established that pinta was a different treponematosis from syphilis or yaws.[10,11]

EPIDEMIOLOGY

Most patients acquire the infection during childhood. There is no difference between the two sexes. The indigenous population is the most affected.[3]

In the 1950s, pinta existed in Mexico, Central America, and the northern countries of South America. The WHO then considered the disease endemic in 15 Latin American countries, including Brazil, Colombia, Ecuador, Peru, and Venezuela. Lower numbers of cases were seen in Bolivia, Dominican Republic, El Salvador, Guatemala, Haiti, Honduras, and Nicaragua. The disease was occasionally seen in Cuba, Guadeloupe, Panama, Puerto Rico, and the Virgin Islands.[12] The last report of cases from Colombia was in 1977.[12] Although Cuba had reported its last case in 1975, in 1998, a patient who had lived in Cuba for 7 years was diagnosed with pinta in Austria.[13] In 1982 and 1983, clinical evidence of pinta was discovered in 20% of the examined inhabitants of a remote village of Panama.[14]

In Brazil, the disease was supposed to be extinct until 1975, when 265 new cases of pinta were diagnosed among Indians from Baniwas, Canamari, Paumari, and Tikuna ethnic groups.[4,5,15] These Indians lived in small communities on the banks of the Amazon river, including the Içana, Juruá, Purus, and upper Negro rivers as well as in some tributaries of the western Amazon river. Since 1979, no further cases of pinta have been reported to the WHO from previously Brazilian endemic areas.[5,15]

Because of the lack of surveillance data, the current prevalence of pinta is unknown; it is believed that the disease still exists in very isolated communities in remote rural areas of Mexico and South America, especially in a few scattered areas in the Brazilian Amazon rainforest. Nonpublished cases have been reported affecting the Yaruro community in Venezuela by R. Hernandez-Perez (FB, personal communication), near the border with Brazil.

There is no proof of a spontaneous cure for the disease; because cell-mediated immunity is not completely effective, the infection persists indefinitely. Patients may harbor subclinical disease and be contagious for a long time. It has been said that pinta was man's best friend: it follows him to the grave.[12]

CLINICAL FEATURES

CUTANEOUS FINDINGS

The disease is classified into two different clinical stages, the primary and late stages.

The primary stage is characterized by two phases, an early phase or initial period, and a secondary phase or period of cutaneous dissemination. According to Padilha-Gonçalves,[10,11] the initial period appears 7 to 20 days after the treponema inoculation. The primary lesions consist of one to several erythematous scaly papules (Fig. 171-1) affecting most commonly the face, upper and lower extremities, or other exposed areas. These lesions tend to grow in extension, producing erythematosquamous or erythematous, hyperpigmented plaques, varying in size and shape (arciform, circinate, polycyclic, and serpiginous) (Fig. 171-2). Generally, the lesions are asymptomatic, but eventually patients may complain of pruritus (Fig. 171-3).

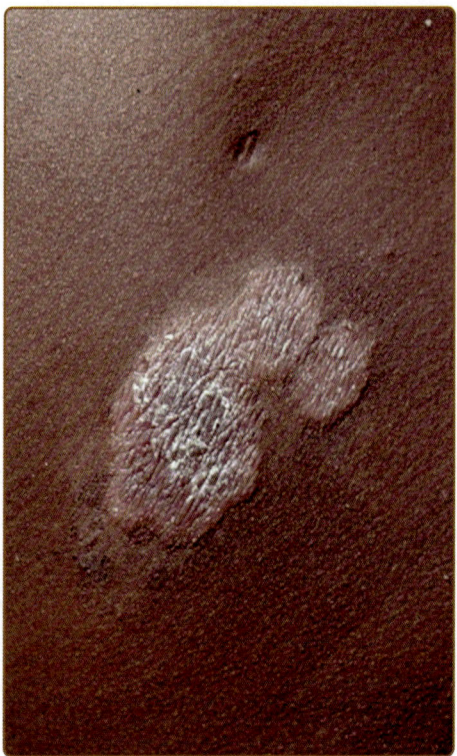

Figure 171-1 Pinta. Early phase in a Tikuna Indian presenting with an erythematous scaly plaque on the abdomen.

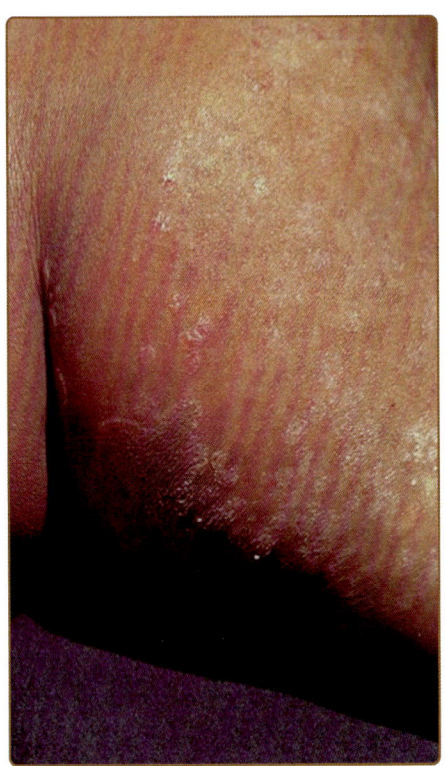

Figure 171-2 Pinta. Early phase in a Tikuna Indian presenting with multiple erythematosquamous papules.

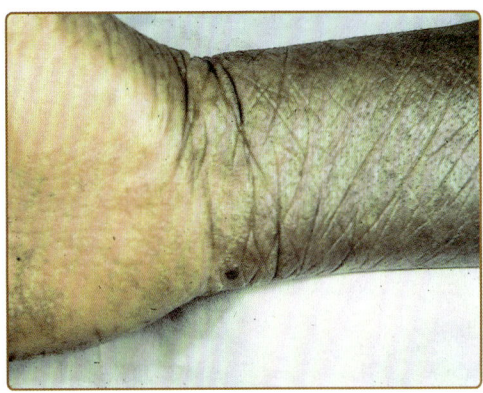

Figure 171-3 Lichenification and dyschromic changes in early pinta.

area, and the inner and upper parts of the thighs are often spared. Another very important aspect of the late phase of pinta is the appearance of hyperchromic and hyperkeratotic patches most commonly on exposed areas of the upper and lower extremities. On the palmar surfaces, hyperpigmented and achromic patches associated with hyperkeratosis are usually observed (Fig. 171-5). Plantar hyperkeratosis is quite frequent. In some patients, even with a prolonged history of the disease, the cutaneous lesions may be confined to a limited area of the body.[5,12]

Regional lymphadenopathy is common. During early infection, the STS result may be negative for antibodies to nontreponemal (cardiolipin) and treponemal antigens. Within 6 months to 2 to 3 years of the first lesions' appearance, hypochromic, erythematous, or erythematohypochromic patches appear, initiating the period of cutaneous dissemination (secondary phase). Those lesions present variable degrees of hyperkeratosis.[5,12] The lesions are small and occasionally nummular in morphology. They gradually enlarge and coalesce, affecting large areas of the body; the centers of the lesions look like normal skin. These lesions are referred to as pintides and are initially red to violaceous and later become slate-blue, brown, gray, or black. Lesions from different periods may be present in a single patient, giving a polymorphic clinical picture.[1,3,4]

The late or tertiary stage, which appears 2 to 5 years after the first lesion, is characterized by the appearance of achromic patches, especially over body prominences, such as the dorsum of the hands, wrist, elbows, anterior aspect of the tibia, ankles, and dorsal and plantar areas of the foot. In this period, large hypochromic areas commonly appear on the upper extremities, trunk, and thighs. One may observe cutaneous atrophy, achromic dotlike lesions, and multiple hyperchromic lesions, producing a mottled pattern. The presence of hypochromic patches with irregular borders and hypochromic macules is quite frequent on buttocks (Fig. 171-4). Curiously, the groin, genital

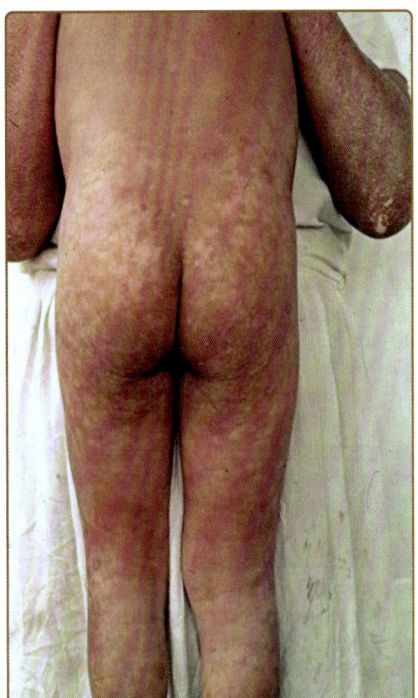

Figure 171-4 Dissemination period in a Tikuna child and his mother. The child (the pictures shows his back, held by the mother) presents with hypochromic scaly patches, and the mother shows achromic lesions on the elbows (late pinta).

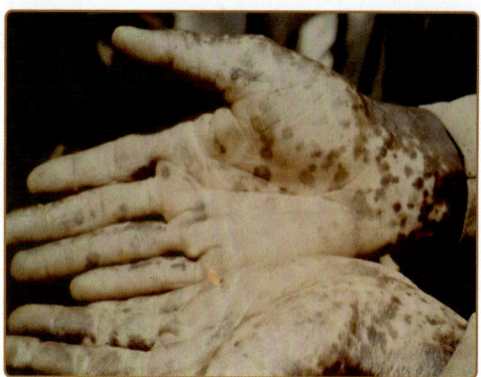

Figure 171-5 Vitiligoid and hyperchromic changes in late pinta.

NONCUTANEOUS FINDINGS

There is no evidence of involvement of other organs, even after many years of evolution.[2,5,8]

COMPLICATIONS

Although early pinta lesions heal within several months after specific treatment, the therapy cannot reverse the skin changes of late pinta that can stigmatize those who were infected.[8] Unlike the other treponematoses, neither destructive skin and bone lesions nor cardiovascular and neurologic manifestations are seen in patients with pinta.[3]

ETIOLOGY AND PATHOGENESIS

The disease is caused by *T. carateum*, an organism that is morphologically and antigenically identical to the etiologic agents of syphilis and yaws.[3,12,15] However, *T. carateum* has not been propagated in experimentally infected animals and has not been characterized genetically.[16]

The disease is found in warm and humid environments and is usually acquired during early childhood. Pinta is thought to spread mostly via direct contact with an infected person, although it is said that transmission may occur via fomites. The treponema enters the skin through small cuts, scratches, or other skin damage. The only known reservoir is human beings.[3,12,15]

DIAGNOSIS

LABORATORY TESTING

Dark-field microscopy can be used to identify viable spirochetes from lesion swabs; however, in most settings where pinta is still prevalent, this technique is not routinely available. Therefore, serology remains the cornerstone of diagnosis. The *T. pallidum* particle agglutination (TPPA) and hemagglutination (TPHA) assays are used to detect *Treponema*-specific antibodies; when the result is positive, it usually remains positive for life. The venereal disease research laboratory (VDRL) and rapid plasma reagin (RPR) tests are nonspecific tests. Although these tests are less specific, they are more accurate to reflect disease activity than TPPA or TPHA, with titers falling rapidly after successful treatment.[3] However, serologic techniques cannot distinguish pinta from syphilis or any of the other nonvenereal treponematoses.

PATHOLOGY

The histopathologic examination is important for the diagnosis of pinta. The primary lesions are characterized by mild acanthosis and spongiosis, with lymphocyte migration and vacuolar degeneration of the basal cell layer, but in the dermis, the changes consist of a slight lymphohistiocytic and plasmocytic infiltrate and mild vascular reaction.[5,15] The hypochromic lesions from the secondary phase present with moderate hyperkeratosis, acanthosis, and spongiosis, plus a superficial infiltrate around the thickened vessels. In the erythematous and squamous lesions, acanthosis, hyperkeratosis, and spongiosis are seen in the epidermis plus a lymphohistiocytic infiltrate in the dermis with edema and vascular proliferation in the papillary dermis. In the achromic lesions, there are hyperkeratosis, atrophy of the epidermis, and complete absence of melanin in the basal layer but some perivascular inflammatory infiltrate. It is possible to demonstrate the presence of treponema in the epidermis through special stains such as Warthin-Starry, in all lesions, except for those that are already achromic.[4,6,12]

DIFFERENTIAL DIAGNOSIS

See Table 171-2.

TABLE 171-2
Differential Diagnosis of Pinta

Primary Stage
- Tinea
- Psoriasis
- Erythema dyschromicum perstans
- Tinea versicolor
- Eczema
- Leprosy
- Cutaneous tuberculosis

Late Stage
- Vitiligo

CLINICAL COURSE AND PROGNOSIS

Primary and secondary lesions of pinta may resolve spontaneously. However, despite treatment, patients may present with lifelong late lesions.[3,12,15]

MANAGEMENT

MEDICATIONS

The recommended treatment for pinta, irrespective of the stage of the disease, is a single or divided dose of long-acting benzathine penicillin (1.2 MU for adults; 0.6 MU for children), which renders the lesions noninfectious in less than 24 hours. Within a few days, the hypochromic and erythematosquamous lesions disappear. Later, the hyperpigmented and recent achromic lesions disappear. The old achromic patches do not usually respond to the treatment and persist for life, giving a vitiligo-like clinical aspect in some patients.[5,12,17]

PREVENTION AND SCREENING

At present, the WHO has not developed a specific strategy for the control or eradication of pinta. However, it has launched a campaign to eradicate yaws by 2020. The strategy is based on mass treatment of endemic communities with an oral dose of azithromycin, a macrolide antibiotic with demonstrated efficacy against yaws.[1,2,7,18] If *T. carateum* is sensitive to azithromycin, this treatment strategy could have a concomitant effect on pinta in areas of Latin America where yaws and pinta may be coendemic.[7]

YAWS

AT-A-GLANCE

- Yaws is the most prevalent of the endemic treponematosis.
- It is most commonly seen in children.
- Countries with the largest number of cases are Papua New Guinea, the Solomon Islands, and Ghana.
- Primary lesions are either papillomatous or ulcerated lesion on the lower extremities.
- Secondary lesions are multiple, bilateral, and symmetrical. They are either moist and papillomatous (raspberry-like) or dry and papulosquamous.
- Eroded or hyperkeratotic palmoplantar lesions with fissuring induce a crablike gait (crab yaws).
- Periostitis and dactylitis are common.
- Penicillin and azithromycin are both effective in the treatment of patients with yaws.

INTRODUCTION

DEFINITION

Yaws is an infectious disease caused by *T. pallidum* ssp. *pertenue*. The term *yaws* probably originates either from the Carib word *yaya* (sore) or from the African word *yaw* (berry). The clinical appearance of a typical lesion of yaws, resembling a raspberry, explains also one of the names given to the disease, *framboesia tropica* (*framboesia* is the French word for raspberry). Other names used to refer to the same disease include pian, buba, bouba, parangui, and paru.

HISTORICAL PERSPECTIVE

Yaws was the 17th century term used by the Dutch physician Willen Piso when he wrote one of the first clinical descriptions of the disease in South America. In 1679, Thomas Sydenham described classical yaws in African slaves and thought it was the same disease as syphilis. In 1905, Castellani found spirochetes in the ulcers of patients with yaws from Ceylon.[18]

Some phylogenetic analyses identify yaws as the oldest of the treponemal diseases and suggest that syphilis and bejel evolved subsequently. The Unitarian hypothesis proposed by Hudson stated that syphilis, as a venereal disease, arose from yaws brought to Europe by the slave trade. However, recent genetic studies by Gray and Mulligan[19] support the idea of a parallel evolution of the three subspecies of *T. pallidum* responsible for yaws, syphilis, and bejel.

EPIDEMIOLOGY

The geographical distribution of yaws has changed dramatically since the 1950s following the very successful programs developed by the WHO and UNICEF to eradicate the disease. Those programs were directed to identify active disease as well as latent disease and to treat them with long-acting penicillin. Furthermore, the programs were also intended to establish alert systems for early detection of any new cases. In 1950, yaws was still present in tropical and subtropical areas around the world, including Central and South America, most of Central Africa, India, Southeast Asia, and the Western Pacific region. Since then, the map has changed drastically; the disease has almost disappeared from the Americas. Ecuador was the last country reporting elimination of the disease; Guyana reported residual cases in 2003. India also reported elimination of the disease by the year 2003.

The number of affected African countries has diminished, and the disease is now confined to few countries of East Central Africa. On the contrary, yaws is still clearly present in Western Pacific countries, such as Papua New Guinea, the Solomon Islands, and Vanuatu. A recent systematic review published in 2015 identified 256,343 cases reported to the WHO in 13 endemic countries in the 2010 to 2013 period.[2,3] The prevalence of active disease in such endemic areas ranged from 0.31% to 14%, and the prevalence of latent disease ranged from 2.4% to 31%. Near 84% of reported cases came from three countries, Papua New Guinea, the Solomon Islands, and Ghana.

CLINICAL FEATURES

CUTANEOUS FINDINGS

Yaws is transmitted by direct skin contact with an infectious lesion and facilitated by abrasion or erosion of the skin. Children are most commonly affected, up to 15 years of age, with a peak incidence between 6 and 10 years. The disease affects people living in rural communities under poor sanitary condition in tropical areas of the world with an average temperature over 27°C (80°F) and heavy rainfall.

The primary lesion of yaws is usually a papule that develops 21 days (range, 9 to 90 day) after initial contact. The papule evolves into a proliferative, exudative, papillomatous lesion 2 to 5 cm in diameter or evolves into a crusted, nontender ulcer, most commonly located on the legs. Genital location is extremely uncommon. This primary lesion is known under different names, including "mother yaws," "maman pian," or "buba madre" (Fig. 171-6A). Even if left untreated, the lesion resolves spontaneously over a 3- to 6-month period, leaving a pigmented scar. A patient may have primary and secondary lesions simultaneously.[20]

Secondary lesions appear after 1 to 2 months (up to 24 months). They represent hematogenous and lymphatic spreading to the skin and bone. In the skin, the lesions can be exudative, proliferative, and papillomatous (Fig. 171-6B) (*pianomes* in French) or dry and papulosquamous (*pianides* in French). The exudative papules (*pianomes* or *frambresiomas*) are usually generalized, bilateral, and symmetrical, from a few millimeters to 2 cm in diameter, soft, wet, red yellowish in color, with either a moist surface or a crust. By resembling raspberries, they are the most representative lesions of yaws. They can affect scalp and folds; in the latter location, they may resemble condyloma lata of syphilis. Mucosal lesions tend to be located around natural orifices, presenting as a bilateral exudative, angular cheilitis (Fig. 171-6C). The dry, papulosquamous papules (*pianides*) are multiple and generalized, and they can have annular or discoid morphology, with a squamous collaret (tinea yaws), grouped in a corymbose pattern. On the face, lesions may resemble psoriasis or seborrheic dermatitis. Multiple, florid lesions are associated with the wet seasons; they become scarce and restricted to intertriginous areas in dry climate.

On the palms and soles, the lesions can be also exudative papules or papulosquamous plaques, keratodermic, with a tendency to form fissures (Fig. 171-7). Because the acral lesions are tender or painful, patients develop a peculiar gait, known as crab yaws. Pianic

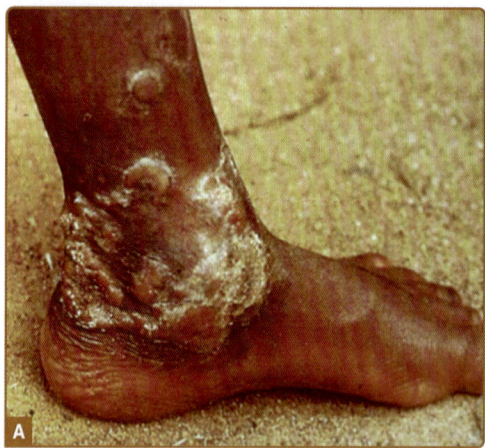

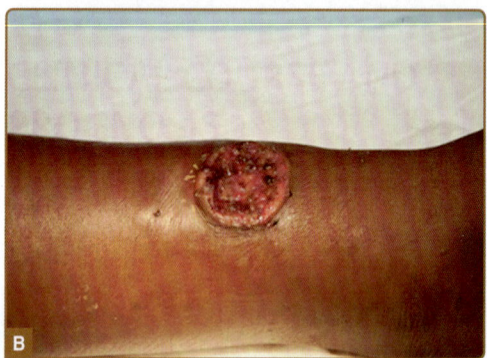

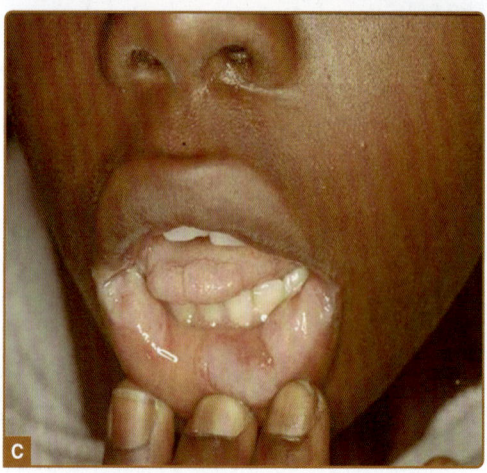

Figure 171-6 **A,** Primary lesion in yaws, also known as maman pian. **B,** The secondary, exudative lesion, known as pianome. **C,** Mucosal and perioral lesion of yaws, quite similar to the mucosal condylomas of syphilis.

onychia is a paronychia that originates from hyperkeratotic lesions in the nail folds.[21]

All secondary yaws resolves, either spontaneously or after treatment, healing with or without scarring. If left untreated, the patient will enter the latent phase and remain as such for the rest of her or his life. Relapsing yaws tend to localize in perioral, perianal, and axillary areas. Relapses may occur for as long as 5 years after the initial infection.

About 10% of untreated patients progress to the tertiary sate. Late-stage lesions are subcutaneous gummatous nodules with massive tissue destruction and necrosis, sometimes resulting in large serpiginous ulcerations, followed by debilitating deformity and contractures. The most common manifestations associated with this state are a result of simultaneous involvement of the skin and bone structures .The complete destruction of the nasal cartilage and the collapse of the nasal pyramid results in a deformity known as gangosa (Fig. 171-8). Pintoid dyschromia and palmoplantar hyperkeratosis have been described at this late stage (Fig. 171-9).

In areas of reduced transmission, because of climate condition or after mass treatment, a milder form of disease can be seen, associated with few lesions (attenuated yaws).

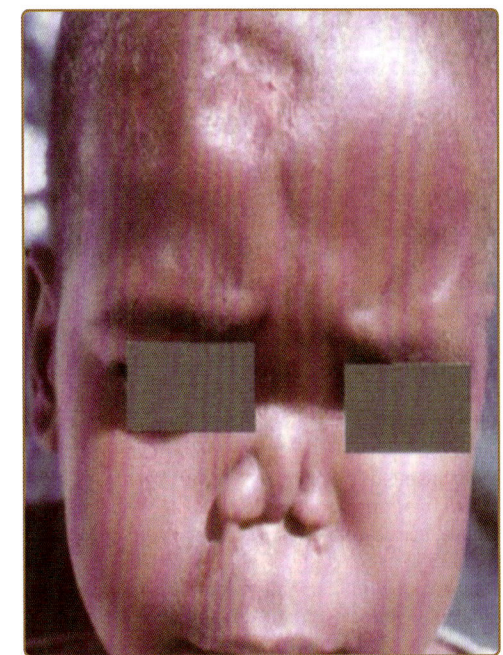

Figure 171-8 Gangosa seen in yaws. See the significant destruction of nasal cartilage.

NONCUTANEOUS FINDINGS

Arthralgia, generalized lymphadenopathy, headaches, and malaise are common, as well as asymptomatic cerebrospinal fluid changes.

The most important noncutaneous findings refer to the involvement of osteoarticular structures. In secondary yaws, early osteoperiostitis of fingers (dactylitis) or long bones (forearm, fibula, and tibia) might result in nocturnal bone pain swelling. Early bone changes can be visualized on radiography, and the thickened periosteum can be palpated clinically; a fusiform swelling of a finger affecting the two proximal phalanges is a common expression of this dactylitis (ghoul hand). The average number of bones involved is three, with common involvement of hand and feet. A specific hypertrophic bone exostosis of the paranasal area known as goundou is rarely seen nowadays.

In late yaws, besides the destructive central face involvement known as rhinopharyngitis obliterans or gangosa, patients may also develop a saddle-nose deformity, bowing of the tibia, or sabre shins. Another manifestation includes the presence of juxtaarticular nodes. Opposite of tertiary syphilis, late yaws is not associated with cardiovascular or neurologic disease. Optic atrophy, however, has been reported in the tertiary stage.[21] *T. pallidum* spp. *pertenue* is not associated with congenital transmission.

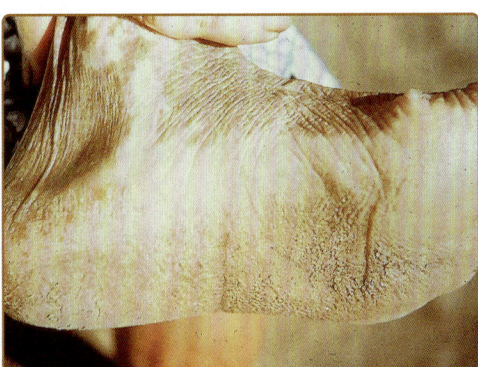

Figure 171-7 Crab yaws: plantar keratoderma with fissuring.

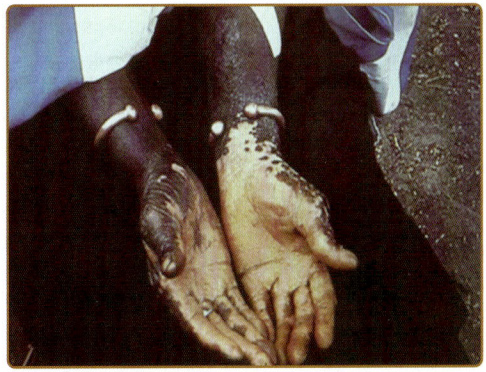

Figure 171-9 Pintoid dyschromia and hyperkeratosis seen in late yaws.

ETIOLOGY AND PATHOGENESIS

T. pallidum ssp. *pertenue* is a spiral-shaped, gram-negative bacteria that belongs to the family Spirochaetaceae, closely related to other subspecies of *T. pallidum*, from which it is morphologically and serologically identical. *T. pallidum* ssp. *pertenue* is 10 to 15 μm long and has a diameter of 0.2 μm; it is not seen on regular microscopy but can be seen on dark-light microscopy. A cytoplasmic membrane enclosed by a loosely associated outer membrane surrounds the bacterium. Some proteins of this outer membrane are able to induce opsonic activity.[18] *Treponema* has a characteristic corkscrew motility and can swim efficiently in gel-like media or environment, such as the connective tissue, a factor that contributes to its virulence. The microorganism multiplies very slowly, at a rate of 1 every 30 to 33 hours. It does not grow on culture media but can be isolated and reproduced in experimental animals, such as rabbits and golden hamsters. In vitro assays based on *Treponema* protein synthesis have demonstrated that *T. pallidum* ssp. *pertenue* is sensitive to penicillin, tetracycline, and erythromycin.

T. pallidum ssp. *pertenue* is 99.8% identical in its genomic sequence to *T. pallidum* ssp. *pallidum*. Established differences between the two microorganisms include a one pair base difference in the *tpp15* gene, one nucleotide difference in the *gpd* gene, a base pair deletion in the *tpr* gene, sequence variation in the *arp* gene, and sequence variation of the intergenic spacer IGR19.[18]

The microorganism enters the skin by small abrasions. After penetrating the epidermis, it reaches the extracellular matrix and attaches to fibronectin-coated surfaces. After minutes, the spirochetes reach lymph nodes and disseminate extensively in hours. The lymph node enlarges and teems with treponemas for several weeks. In the skin, the initial reaction is mainly neutrophilic and later composed mainly of plasma cell. *T. pallidum* ssp. *pertenue* is seen as extracellular clusters in upper regions of the epidermis on immunohistochemistry staining. The immune response to the microorganism is both humoral and cellular. The organism, because of its low metabolic rate, is able to maintain infection with few viable cells, avoiding the stimulation of the immune system in the latent state. Adults rarely develop new skin lesions, suggesting that untreated individuals can develop immunity to reinfection.

DIAGNOSIS

The diagnosis is easy in the endemic areas, although attenuated yaws may be more challenging. Health care workers not familiar with the disease may need laboratory methods to confirm the diagnosis

LABORATORY TESTING

Treponemas can be detected in a wet preparation using dark-field microscopy. However, the scarce availability of the method in rural setting makes it unpractical. The best diagnostic aid is serology testing using the same techniques as in syphilis. Nontreponemal agglutination tests, such as the RPR and the VDRL, can be used for diagnosis and follow-up after treatment, as they are used in syphilis. False positives can be seen in patients with other tropical diseases such as malaria and leprosy, as well as in rheumatic diseases. Results of treponemal tests, such as TPHA, TPPA, and fluorescent treponemal antibody absorption (FTA-ABS) are also positive, but as in syphilis, they remain positive forever and are not useful for follow-up.

The new rapid diagnostic test, including the immunochromatographic strips developed for syphilis, are also very useful and easy to use in the primary care setting. Differential diagnosis with syphilis itself might be tricky; real-time polymerase chain reaction remains, in such cases, the technique of choice, although it is expensive and limited to research centers. In such cases, epidemiologic and clinical data need to be carefully evaluated to establish the correct diagnosis.

PATHOLOGY

The histologic findings of yaws is quite similar to those of syphilis and include epidermal hyperplasia, focal spongiosis, and a dermal infiltrate. Some authors describe an early accumulation of neutrophils in the epidermis,[18] but others state that is mainly plasmocytic from the beginning.[1] Plasma cells predominate in all evolved lesions. An important difference with syphilis is that yaws does not induce vascular changes or endothelial proliferation. The same immunohistochemistry staining used in syphilis is quite useful in yaws by demonstrating the spirochetes in large numbers at the epidermal level.

IMAGING

Radiographic studies are particularly valuable in cases of periostitis and bone involvement; onion layering periosteal reaction and loss of clarity of the cortex are seen on plain radiographs (Fig. 171-10). Bowing of the tibia, destructive osteitis of facial bones (such as seen in gangosa), and the hypertrophic periostitis and exostosis seen in gondou are quite evident on radiology studies.

DIFFERENTIAL DIAGNOSIS

See Table 171-3.

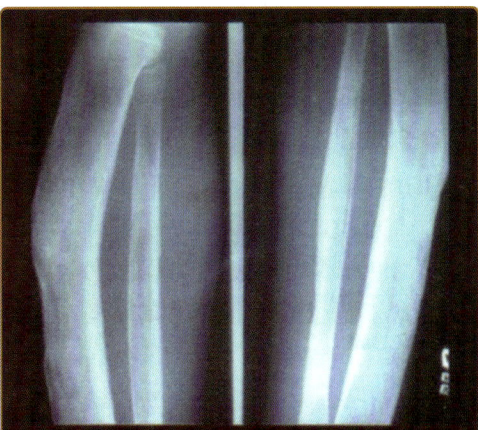

Figure 171-10 Radiographic evidence of periosteitis of yaws.

TABLE 171-3
Differential Diagnosis of Yaws

Primary Lesion
- Leishmaniasis
- Tropical phagedenic ulcer
- Ecthyma
- Tuberculosis
- Buruli ulcer
- Sickle cell anemia

Secondary Lesions
- Eczema
- Psoriasis
- Syphilis
- Disseminated leishmaniasis
- Superficial mycosis
- Infective dermatitis of HTLV-1
- Leprosy
- Impetigo
- Pyoderma vegetans

Facial Lesions
- Leishmaniasis
- Lupus vulgaris
- Leprosy
- Paracoccidioidomycosis
- Rhinoscleroma
- Rhinosporidiosis
- Rhinoentomophthoromycosis
- T-NK lymphomas

Pintoid Lesions
- Vitiligo
- Pinta

HTLV, human T-lymphotropic virus; T-NK, it is a type of extranodal lymphoma caused by a proliferation of Natural Killer cells or T lymphocytes.

CLINICAL COURSE AND PROGNOSIS

Primary and secondary lesions may resolve spontaneously. Up to 10% of patients in a latent stage may evolve into the most disfiguring, disabling late stage after 5 years of an untreated infection.

MANAGEMENT

MEDICATIONS

Single-dose, long-acting penicillin has been the treatment of choice for yaws and the base of the successful eradication program. A dose of 1.2 million units for patients older than 10 years and a dose of 0.6 million units for those younger than 10 years is still the recommended regimen. Cure rates are above 95% for early active yaws.

One oral dose of azithromycin (30 mg/kg, to a maximal dose of 2 g) is considered as effective as penicillin. Since 2012, the WHO considers the one single dose of azithromycin equivalent to the standard penicillin regimen. Oral tetracyclines, doxycycline, and erythromycin are considered alternative drugs for adults who are allergic to penicillin; erythromycin is the choice for children younger than 12 years of age.

Oral therapy with azithromycin has many advantages over intramuscular penicillin therapy. When it is used in massive control programs, it can be administrated by less skilled health workers, and there is a reduced risk of anaphylaxis. However, a higher potential risk of developing resistance does exist when macrolides are used. In such cases, follow-up is recommended, allowing early retreatment with penicillin when needed.

The effectiveness of therapy is expressed by several facts. Yaws lesions become noninfectious in 24 hours after therapy. Joint pain disappears in 24 to 48 hours. All clinical lesions resolve within 2 to 4 weeks after therapy. However, therapy will not resolve the destruction and deformities seen in the tertiary stage, thus justifying the importance of early intervention. RPR and VDRL testing titers decrease to a minimum within 6 to 12 months and become negative or remain at low titers in the next 2 years.

PREVENTION AND SCREENING

The success of the WHO eradication effort in the 1950s was followed by a loss of continuity of such a program. The responsibility of maintaining the program was rapidly transferred to primary care systems that were either too weak or nonexistent in many endemic areas; this lack of continuity translated into a resurge of yaws in the past decades. Of note, the success of this program in India and Ecuador remain an exception because both countries have now been declared free of yaws. One of the conclusions of the

1950s efforts was the importance of subclinical or latent cases as a source of reinfection. The initial program was directed to treat active disease cases; resurveys of the treated communities showed that all new cases were individuals in the latent stage who did not receive treatment.

In 2012, the WHO endorsed the commitment to eradicate yaws by the year 2020. This time, the strategy includes some variations. Surveys are directed to detect precisely the villages and communities affected by yaws. Oral azithromycin instead of intramuscular penicillin is the treatment of choice. The aim of the program is the treatment of the whole community, which will be repeated if the first attempt did not cover 90% of the population. The follow-up surveillance program will include passive and active search of new cases, tracing and treating contacts, intensive information and educational efforts, and monthly reporting of case (including no new cases) and yearly serologic surveys in children younger than 5 years. Indeed, improvement of education and sanitary conditions in affected communities are important factors that will facilitate the success of the eradication program.[18]

BEJEL

AT-A-GLANCE

- Bejel is most commonly seen in children.
- Transmission routes include direct contact and fomites by sharing utensils.
- Countries and regions with the largest number of cases are the African Sahelian countries and Saudi Arabia (dry, hot climates).
- Primary lesions are not easily identified or seen.
- Secondary lesions are represented by moist plaques on mucosal and perioral areas, mimicking condyloma lata or angular stomatitis.
- Gummas and gangosa represent tertiary lesions.
- Involvement of the nasopharynx and larynx is common.
- Periostitis and saber shins may be seen.
- The treatment of choice is penicillin.

INTRODUCTION

DEFINITIONS

The name *bejel* has been coined from Arabic and is the term used for nonvenereal (endemic) treponematoses. Other names have been used to designate the disease, including *njovera* in Zimbabwe, *belesch* or *bishel* in Saudi Arabia, and *dichuchwa* in Botswana. The causative agent is the spirochete *T. pallidum* ssp. *endemicum*. Bejel is a disease of countries of dry and arid climate and is often found in isolated communities with poor hygiene. The disease mainly involves children from 2 to 15 years of age, but it can also be seen in adults belonging to nomadic people. This treponematosis is likely transmitted not only by nonvenereal direct mucosal or skin contact but also by sharing utensils and drinking vessels. Bejel is therefore often considered as a "familial" disease.

HISTORICAL PERSPECTIVE

Endemic syphilis or bejel has been described in many European countries since the 16th century. The first description appeared in 1575 in Brno, Czech Republic, where it was called *morbus Brunogallicus*. It was associated with the use of communal bath and bloodletting. A similar disease was described in southwest Scotland and received the name of *sibbens* or *sivvens*. In Croatia in the 1800s, an entity named *morbus Skrljevo* sharing similar clinical features with nonvenereal syphilis was commonly seen and clearly associated with poverty and poor hygiene. The republic of Bosnia and Herzegovina were a site of endemic syphilis for centuries. By the 20th century, additional cases were seen in Russia and Bulgaria. Europe was able to eliminate the disease basically by improving sanitary conditions, and the few persistent endemic areas disappeared with the massive use of penicillin in the 1950s.[22]

EPIDEMIOLOGY

As with the other endemic treponematosis, bejel was once described as endemic in many areas of the world, such as Northern Europe, the Balkans, Russia, Mongolia, the near East, the eastern Mediterranean, and southern and northern Africa, affecting mainly those living in poverty. Improvements in the social and economic status in many of these populations have led to a marked reduction in the prevalence of the infection, even preceding the massive campaigns efforts of the 1950s by the WHO. However, there are still areas of the world where the disease is yet prevalent, mostly in the Near East (rural areas of Saudi Arabia) and the African Sahel, the geographic area between the southern border of the Sahara desert and the Sudanese sabana. In the 1980s, bejel was reported in Burkina Faso and Mali. In the 1990s, cases were reported in Niger and Mauritania. It is an interesting observation that bejel predominates in countries with dry climate, but in the nearby countries with more humid climates, yaws is the predominant disease.[1]

Few additional cases have been reported in Turkey, Mozambique, and, most recently, Iran but only as isolated cases.[23]

CLINICAL FEATURES

CUTANEOUS FINDINGS

The main population affected are children younger than 15 years of age. Overcrowding, poor sanitary conditions, and poor personal hygiene seem to facilitate the infection. Distinctly in bejel, the primary lesion is infrequently observed. When the lesion has been noted, it is described as a painless and superficial mucosal ulceration in the mouth or the nasopharynx. An anecdotal report of a primary lesion in the nipple of a nursing woman has been reported that tended to simulate the genital primary chancre of syphilis.

The secondary lesions are quite similar also to what is seen in syphilis in the oral mucosae, tonsils, tongue, lips, and nasopharynx. They are oval, almost painless patches, with a whitish, slightly elevated cap. Lesions of angular stomatitis can be part of bejel, similar to what is seen in yaws. Patients also may have generalized, nonitchy skin eruptions, generalized lymphadenopathy, and laryngitis. Condylomata lata-like lesions (Fig. 171-11) may also be present in mucosal and intertriginous areas. On hairless skin, circinate papules may appear (Fig. 171-12). The secondary lesions take 6 to 9 months to heal, and then the disease enters the latency period.

The tertiary stage may develop earlier than in yaws, as early as 6 months or taking several years to show. The lesions are gummas that can progress to very destructive ulcerations. They may heal spontaneously, but leave significant scars, surrounded by hyperpigmentation. Involvement of central face and nasal cartilage and bone may result in the picture of gangosa, as described in yaws.

NONCUTANEOUS FINDINGS

Patients with bejel may develop the same osteitis and periostitis of long bones and hands seen in patients with yaws. Such patients will complain of nocturnal

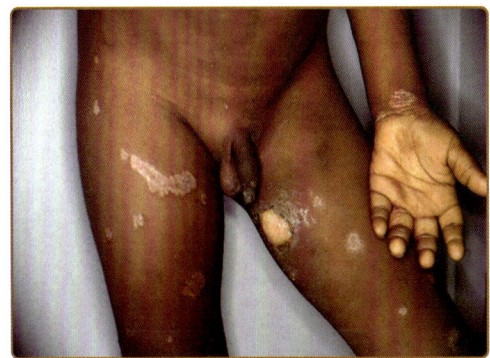

Figure 171-12 Dry and exudative lesions of bejel.

pain. The bone changes may evolve into saber tibias, although it is said that such involvement is less severe than in yaws.

Neurologic and cardiovascular involvement, as well as congenital transmission are all said to be rare in bejel, but there is a report that mentioned uveitis, optic atrophy, and choroidal atrophic scar. An attenuated form of bejel, manifested mainly as leg pain and radiographic evidence of periostitis, has been described in Saudi Arabia.[1]

ETIOLOGY AND PATHOGENESIS

The disease is caused by *T. pallidum* ssp. *endemicum*. The microorganism is morphologically identical to all spirochetes of the genus *Treponema*. There is a 99.7 genome sequence identity with the genome of *T. pallidum* ssp *pallidum*[24]; its genome size is 1137.7 kbp.

As the other endemic treponematosis, acquiring the disease during childhood and a direct transmission through the skin seem to be the classical scenario. However, bejel is the disease in which more emphasis should be put on the risk of transmission by fomites transported in utensils and drinking vessels.

DIAGNOSIS

Most cases of bejel are diagnosed on the basis of clinical findings. Among all the nonvenereal treponematosis, bejel is the one with which the differential diagnosis with venereal syphilis might be tricky.

LABORATORY TESTING

Results of the nontreponemal agglutination tests, such as the RPR and VDRL, as well as the most specific treponemal tests, TPHA, TPPA and FTA-ABS, are

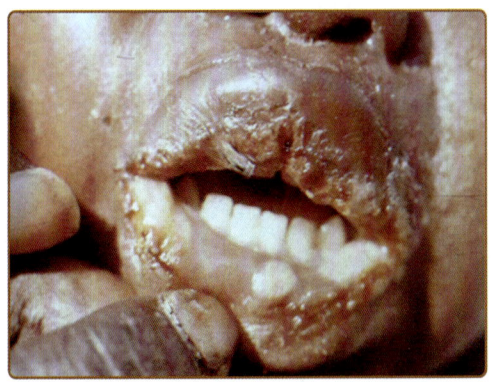

Figure 171-11 Cheilitis and angular stomatitis, representing secondary lesions of bejel.

positive, as in yaws. Clear distinction with venereal syphilis is most difficult and should be based on a careful history and evaluation of the mother and siblings, as illustrated by a recent case seen in Canada.[25] In a small number of cases, the final diagnosis may require molecular studies that, unfortunately, are only available in research centers.

PATHOLOGY

The cutaneous lesions show a superficial dermal lymphoplasmacytic infiltrate. In early lesions, epidermal changes such hyperplasia and spongiosis are expected. Treponemas can be then visualized with the aid of immunohistochemistry. Additional findings that may be seen include a lichenoid pattern of the infiltrate and endothelial swelling in superficial capillary plexus, as in venereal syphilis. Tuberculoid granulomas are described occasionally.[20]

IMAGING

Periostitis as well as bone involvement can be seen on radiographs, very much as they are seen in yaws.

DIFFERENTIAL DIAGNOSIS

See Table 171-4.

MANAGEMENT

MEDICATIONS

Penicillin remains the treatment of choice for bejel. As in yaws, the WHO recommends 1.2 million units of benzathine penicillin for treatment of all stages in adults; half the dose is used in children younger than 10 years.

Strategies for eradication are the same as proposed by the WHO in the case of yaws. Accessibility to health care for deprived populations is an important part of any future effort to control and elimination of bejel.

ACKNOWLEDGMENTS

Figures 171-6A to C and 171-8 to 171-12 were obtained by one of the authors (KE) while working at the NGOs Centre René Labusquière and the Réseau Dermatrop, from patients from Mali, Senegal, and Ghana.

REFERENCES

1. Giacani L, Lukehart SA. The endemic treponematoses. *Clin Microbiol Rev.* 2014;27(1):89-115.
2. Mitjà O, Marks M, Konan DJ, et al. Global epidemiology of yaws: a systematic review. *Lancet Glob Health.* 2015; 3(6):e324-e331.
3. Marks M, Solomon AW, Mabey DC. Endemic treponemal diseases. *Trans R Soc Trop Med Hyg.* 2014; 108(10):601-607.
4. Talhari S, Dourado HV, Alecrim WD, et al. Pinta em população nativa do estado do Amazonas. *Acta Amazônica.* 1975;5:199-202.
5. Talhari S. Pinta. In: Talhari S, Neves RG, eds. *Dermatologia Tropical.* Rio de Janeiro: Medsi; 1995:291-300.
6. Engelkens HJ, Vuzevski VD, Stolz E. Nonvenereal treponematoses in tropical countries. *Clin Dermatol.* 1999; 17:143-152.
7. Stamm LV. Pinta: Latin America's forgotten disease? *Am J Trop Med Hyg.* 2015;93(5):901-903.
8. Carrillo AM. From badge of pride to cause of stigma: combating mal del pinto in Mexico. *Endeavor.* 2013;37: 13-20.
9. Pardo-Castello V, Ferrer I. Pinta. Mal del pinto; carate. *Arch Dermatol Syph.* 1942;45:843-864.
10. Gonçalves AP. Pinta: presentation of 2 patients. *An Bras Derm Sifilogr.* 1950;25:185-186.
11. Gonçalves AP. Immunologic aspects of pinta. *Dermatologica.* 1967;135:199-204.
12. Medina R. Pinta: an endemic treponematoses in the Americas. *Bol Oficina Sanit Panam.* 1979;86:242-255
13. Woltsche-Kahr I, Schmidt B, Aberer W, et al. Pinta in Austria (or Cuba?). Import of an extinct disease? *Arch Dermatol.* 1999;135(6):685-688.
14. Fohn MJ, Wignall S, Baker-Zander SA, et al. Specificity of antibodies from patients with pinta for antigens of Treponema pallidum subspecies pallidum. *J Infect Dis.* 1988;157(1):32-37.
15. Talhari S. Pinta: aspectos clínicos, laboratoriais e situação epidemiológica no estado do Amazonas (Brasil). PhD thesis. São Paulo, Brazil: Escola Paulista de Medicina; 1988.
16. Čejková D, Strouhal M, Norris SJ, et al. A retrospective study on genetic heterogeneity within Treponema Strains: subpopulations are genetically distinct in a limited number of positions. *PLoS Negl Trop Dis.* 2015; 9(10):e0004110.

TABLE 171-4
Differential Diagnosis of Bejel

Primary and Secondary Cutaneous Lesions
- Syphilis
- Condyloma acuminatum
- Molluscum contagiosum
- Seborrheic dermatitis
- Psoriasis dermatophytosis

Tertiary Gummatous Lesions
- Syphilis
- Gummas of tuberculosis
- Deep fungal infections
- Rhinosporidiosis
- Rhinoscleroma

Mucosal and Perioral Lesions
- Syphilis
- Angular cheilitis
- Herpes simplex
- Aphthous disease

17. Carrillo AM. From badge of pride to cause of stigma: combating mal del pinto in Mexico. *Endeavor.* 2013; 37:13-20.
18. Mitjà O, Asiedu K, Mabey D. Yaws. *Lancet.* 2013; 381(9868):763-773.
19. Gray RR, Mulligan CJ, Molini BJ, et al. Molecular evolution of the tprC, D, I, K, G, and J genes in the pathogenic genus Treponema. *Mol Biol Evol.* 2006; 23(11):2220-2233.
20. Padilha-Goncalves A, Basset A, Maleville J. Tropical treponematosis. In: Canizares O, Harman RM, eds. *Clinical Tropical Dermatology.* 2nd ed. Boston: Blackwell Scientific Publications; 1992:129-150.
21. Farnsworth N, Rosen T. Endemic treponematosis: review and update. *Clin Dermatol.* 2006;24(3):181-190.
22. Lipozencic J, Marinovic B, Gruber F. Endemic syphilis in Europe. *Clin Dermatol.* 2014;32(2):219-226.
23. Abdolrasouli A, Croucher A, Hemmati Y, et al. A case of endemic syphilis, Iran. *Emerg Infect Dis.* 2013; 19(1):162-163.
24. Mitja O, Smajs D, Bassat Q. Advances in the diagnosis of endemic treponematosis: yaws, bejel and pinta. *PLoS Negl Trop Dis.* 2013;7(10):e2283.
25. Fanella S, Kadkhoda K, Tsang R. Local transmission of imported endemic syphilis, Canada, 2011. *Emerg Infect Dis.* 2012;18(6):1002-1004.

Chapter 172 :: Chancroid
:: Stephan Lautenschlager & Norbert H. Brockmeyer

第一百七十二章

软下疳

中文导读

软下疳是由杜克勒嗜血杆菌感染所致的局部急性溃疡性疾病，通过性传播途径致病。本章从历史背景、流行病学、临床表现（皮肤系统及皮肤系统外）、发病机理、诊断与鉴别诊断、病程与预后和疾病的管理等几个方面对软下疳进行了介绍。

直至19世纪90年代，软下疳常见于发展中国家，尤其是非洲和亚洲，这些地区超过50%的生殖器溃疡中可分离出杜克勒嗜血杆菌。一篇纳入49项研究（其中35个研究发表于1980年至1999年，14个研究发表于2000年至2014年）的系统性综述显示，在1980年至1999年间，由杜克勒嗜血杆菌导致的生殖器溃疡占生殖器溃疡的0%（泰国）至69%（中国）。在2000年至2014年间，由杜克勒嗜血杆菌导致的生殖器溃疡占生殖器溃疡的百分比明显降低（低于10%），但除外马拉维（占生殖器溃疡性疾病的15%）和北印度（占生殖器溃疡性疾病的24%）。而在美国，2015年仅有11例软下疳报道，在欧洲，软下疳局限于罕见的散发病例，通常首诊被误诊为生殖器溃疡。近年发病率明显下降是由于WHO在世界各地引入的生殖器溃疡治疗的综合征管理。然而，由于微生物学确诊难度较大，全球的杜克勒嗜血杆菌流行记录是不充分的。因此，杜克勒嗜血杆菌感染可能是严重诊断不足的。在非洲进行的数项研究表明，软下疳是异性之间HIV传播的高危因素。在西非，有2%的女性性工作者是杜克勒嗜血杆菌的无症状携带者。在女性中，未治疗的情况下传染性约可持续45天。女性至男性的传染率至今不明，相反的是，有研究报道1次性行为男性传染女性的概率为70%。包皮环切术有助于减少软下疳的感染率。近来，在亚洲太平洋区域，杜克勒嗜血杆菌非性传播导致的非生殖器区域皮肤溃疡报道大多出现在儿童人群中。通过全基因组测序和已确定的基因位点，证据显示皮肤杜克勒嗜血杆菌菌株（Ⅱ型）在相对近期的时间由生殖器杜克勒嗜血杆菌菌株（Ⅰ型）演变而来。

软下疳皮损局限于外生殖器部位，通常可合并腹股沟淋巴结炎。潜伏期为3~7天，很少超过10天。没有前驱症状。感染部位最初出现一个小的质软炎性丘疹，24~48小时后迅速加重（图172-1），形成疼痛剧烈的深溃疡，边缘粗糙不整齐（图172-2）。溃疡表面通常覆盖坏死性黄灰色的渗出物，溃疡底部由易出血的肉芽组织组成。与梅毒相反，软下疳溃疡通常是软的和/或疼痛的，而不是质硬的。溃疡直径为0.01~2cm。半数的男性皮损为单发，多位于包皮的外表面或内表面、阴茎带或龟头（图172-4）。皮损可增大或自体接种，导致"对吻式溃疡"（图172-5）或者巨大的累及腹股沟区域或大腿的匍行性溃疡。尿道口、阴茎体和肛门较少受累（图172-6）。常见包皮水肿。如果杜克勒嗜血杆菌累及尿道，可导致化脓性尿道炎。男性患者临床症状常较严重。女性患者皮损常发生于阴唇，尤其是阴唇系带、小阴唇和前庭。曾有阴道、宫颈和肛周溃疡报道。外伤和摩擦可能是导致这些生殖器外表现的重要因素。发生于乳房、手指、大腿和口腔内等生殖器外软下疳皮损也曾被报道。50%的患者的初始皮损在数天至2周间（平均1周）出现。在多数患者中，淋巴结炎发生于单侧，淋巴结周围皮肤红肿为典型症状。炎性淋巴结可能变得有波动感，而且可能自行破溃。淋巴结渗出物通常是浓稠质地。淋巴结炎在女性中较少见。临床上也可能出现一些不典型的软下疳，如巨大软下疳、毛囊性软下疳、大匍行性溃疡、崩蚀性软下疳、一过性软下疳以及丘疹型软下疳。在极少数的情况下，软下疳可能伴随轻度全身症状。在未治疗的患者中，约半数可自行消退，而且没有后遗症。但延迟治疗可能导致多种合并症（见表172-3）。本病通常是自限性的，在偶发情况下，未经治疗的患者可有持续多年的生殖器溃疡和腹股沟脓肿。患者常诉局部疼痛。如果在治疗1周后没有临床症状的改善，需考虑另一种性传播疾病共患病、伴随HIV感染、依从性不佳或杜克勒嗜血杆菌耐药菌种感染。杜克勒嗜血杆菌感染患者对其不能形成免疫力，有可能再次感染。为了预防再次感染，需对患者进行性安全教育。

诊断需结合临床表现、流行病学史及实验室检查。杜克勒嗜血杆菌在显微镜下表现为小的革兰阴性杆菌，但直接涂片镜检的敏感性和特异性均不佳，因此不推荐用作常规诊断工具。杜克勒嗜血杆菌确诊要求细菌培养阳性，但该检查检出率仅达75%。不过，当需要鉴定抗生素药物敏感模式以防治疗失败时，细菌培养是必要的。杜克勒嗜血杆菌仅可在拭子上存活几个小时，因此床旁接种（使用2种不同的选择强化培养基）后马上进行培养可以减少标本运输过程中的细菌损失。细菌培养标本也可使用核酸检测技术进行鉴定。它可在临床样本中很好地检测出杜克勒嗜血杆菌，检出率较细菌培养高。现在已经有数种院内检测杜克勒嗜血杆菌的多聚酶链式反应方法，其中有一些还可以同时检测其他相关的病原体，尤其是苍白密螺旋体和单纯疱疹病毒。软下疳在临床上需要与其他感染性和非感染性疾病相鉴别。最有可能误诊的疾病为生殖器疱疹（病原体为单纯疱疹病毒I型及II型）、梅毒（病原体为苍白密螺旋体）和性病性淋巴肉芽肿（病原体为沙眼衣原体的性病性淋巴肉芽肿变种L1、L2、L3）。其他可能的鉴别诊断见表172-2。在诊断软下疳时需要同时排除生殖器疱疹、梅毒和HIV感染。

软下疳的推荐治疗方案为大环内酯类抗生素：阿奇霉素1g，单次口服。其他备选方案见表172-4。

〔张江林〕

AT-A-GLANCE

- Chancroid is a sexually transmitted acute ulcerative disease usually localized at the anogenital area and often associated with inguinal adenitis or bubo.
- *Haemophilus ducreyi*—a Gram-negative, facultative anaerobic coccobacillus—is the causative agent.
- Chancroid is disappearing even from most countries where *H. ducreyi* was previously epidemic, with the exception of North India and Malawi. Nevertheless, recent sporadic case reports from Western Europe have been described, often initially misdiagnosed as genital herpes.
- Painful, soft ulcers with ragged undermined margins develop 1 to 2 weeks after inoculation (usually prepuce and frenulum in men and vulva, cervix, and perianal areas in women).
- *H. ducreyi* facilitates the transmission of HIV.
- In contrast to a sustained reduction in the proportion of genital ulcer disease caused by *H. ducreyi*, the bacterium is increasingly found in the South Pacific region and in Africa as a common cause of nongenital cutaneous ulcers especially in children.
- Laboratory culture of *H. ducreyi* is problematic, but greater sensitivity can be expected by nucleic acid amplification methods, which are not routinely available.
- Azithromycin and ceftriaxone are recommended as single-dose treatment, enhancing compliance.

EPIDEMIOLOGY

Until the 1990s chancroid was seen most commonly in developing countries, especially in Africa and Asia, where it was isolated from more than 50% of patients with genital ulcers.[1-3] A systematic review analyzed 49 studies (35 were published during 1980-1999 and 14 during 2000-2014) on chancroid.[4] During 1980-1999, the percentage of genital ulcers caused by *Haemophilus ducreyi* ranged from 0% in Thailand and China to 69% in South Africa. During 2000-2014, the percentage of genital ulcers caused by H. ducreyi was low (<10%) except for Malawi with 15% of genital ulcer disease[5] and North India with 24% of genital ulcer disease.[6] A recent report from Cuba described no infection with *H. ducreyi* in genital ulcer disease patients.[7] In the United States, only 11 cases of chancroid were reported in 2015.[8] In Europe, chancroid is restricted to rare sporadic cases, often misdiagnosed as genital herpes.[9,10] The distinct decrease in prevalence has followed the introduction by the World Health Organization (WHO) of syndromic management for treating genital ulcer disease.[4] Nevertheless, the global epidemiology of *H. ducreyi* is poorly documented because of difficulties in confirming a microbiologic diagnosis. As a result, this condition may be substantially underdiagnosed.[8]

Lower-class prostitutes appeared to be a reservoir in all previously reported outbreaks of this disease where men had a markedly higher incidence than women. Male circumcision is associated with a reduced risk of contracting chancroid.[11] Several studies in Africa show that chancroid ulcer was an important risk factor for the heterosexual spread of HIV.[12,13] In West Africa, it has been shown that 2% of female sex workers carry the organism asymptomatically.[14] The duration of infectivity in the absence of treatment is estimated to be 45 days for women. The transmission rate from females to males is not known, in contrast to a reported transmission rate from males to females of 70% per sex act.[15] Nonsexual transmission leading to nongenital skin ulcers mostly in children in the Asia Pacific region has been recently reported.[16,17] Based on sequencing of whole genomes and defined genetic loci, it appears that the cutaneous *H. ducreyi* strains (Class II) diverged from the class I genital strains relatively recently.[18]

CLINICAL FINDINGS

The incubation period is between 3 and 7 days, rarely more than 10 days. No prodromal symptoms are known. The chancre begins as a soft papule surrounded by erythema. After 24 to 48 hours it becomes pustular, then eroded and ulcerated (Fig. 172-1); vesicles are not seen. The edges of the ulcers are often ragged and undermined (Fig. 172-2). The ulcer is usually covered by a necrotic, yellowish-gray exudate (Fig. 172-3), and its base is composed of granulation tissue that bleeds readily on manipulation. In contrast to syphilis, chancroid ulcers are usually tender and/or painful, not indurated (soft chancre). The diameter varies from 1 mm to 2 cm. Half of the males present with a single ulcer, and most lesions are found on the external or internal surface of the prepuce, on the frenulum, or on the glans (Fig. 172-4). Lesions may spread by extension and autoinoculation, leading to "kissing ulcers" (Fig.172-5) or large serpiginous ulcers involving the groin or thigh. Meatus and shaft of the penis and the anus (Fig. 172-6) are involved less frequently. Edema of the prepuce is often seen. Rarely, if the chancre is localized in the urethra, *H. ducreyi* causes purulent urethritis.[19]

In females, the lesions are mostly localized on the vulva (Fig. 172-7), especially on the fourchette, the labia minora, and the vestibule. Vaginal, cervical, and perianal ulcers also have been described. Extragenital lesions of chancroid have been reported on the breasts, fingers, thighs, and inside the mouth. Trauma and abrasion may be important for such extragenital manifestations.

Painful inguinal adenitis (bubo) occurs in up to 50% of patients within a few days to 2 weeks (average: 1 week) after onset of the primary lesion (Fig. 172-8). The adenitis is unilateral in most patients, and erythema of the overlying skin is typical. Buboes can become fluctuant and may rupture spontaneously. The pus of bubo is usually thick and creamy. Buboes

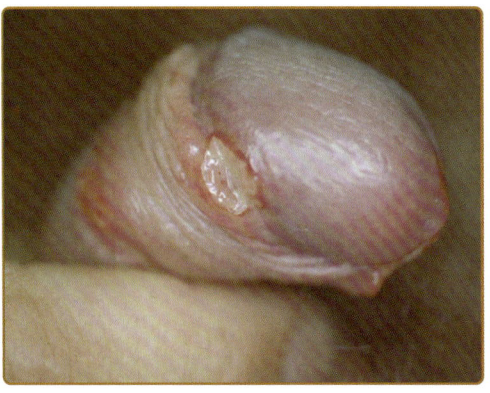

Figure 172-1 Early sharply circumscribed ulcer in the coronal sulcus.

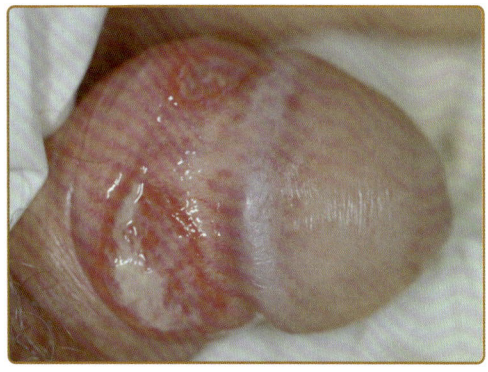

Figure 172-3 Chancroid with necrotic, yellowish-gray exudates.

are less common in female patients. Besides the common types of chancroid described above, a number of clinical variants have been reported (Table 172-1). Mild systemic symptoms can rarely accompany chancroid, but systemic infection by *H. ducreyi* has never been observed. The significance of the recent detection of genetic material of *H. ducreyi* in oesophageal lesions of HIV patients[20] is not yet clear.

DIFFERENTIAL DIAGNOSIS

The 3 classic etiologic agents for genital ulceration are (a) *H. ducreyi*, (b) *Treponema pallidum*, and (c) herpes simplex. The clinical appearance of the diseases caused by these 3 organisms can be extremely variable in both men and women, making clinical diagnosis of genital ulcer disease with reasonable certainty possible only for a minority of patients.[21] The etiology of genital ulcers (Table 172-2)[22] also differs considerably by geographic region. In industrialized countries, isolated painful chancres are most likely caused by herpes simplex

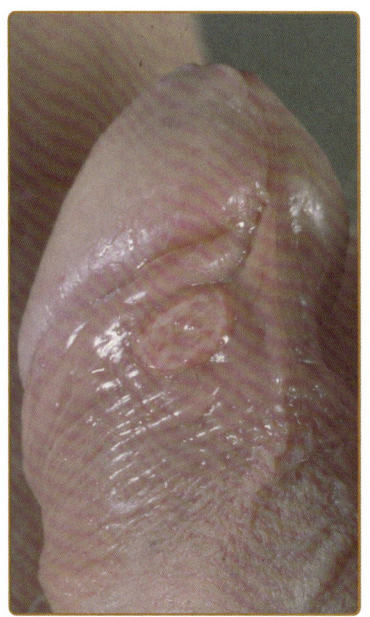

Figure 172-4 Isolated small soft chancre on the glans.

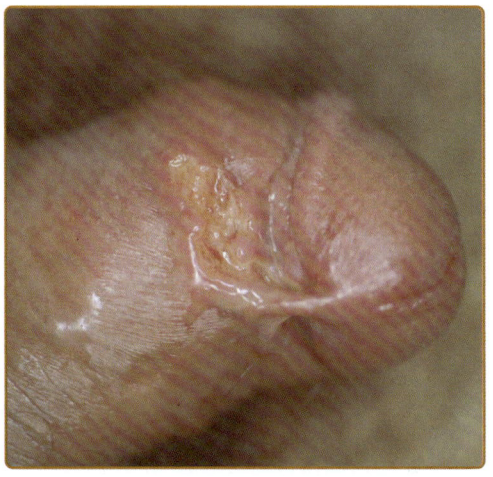

Figure 172-2 Ragged edges of a soft ulcer.

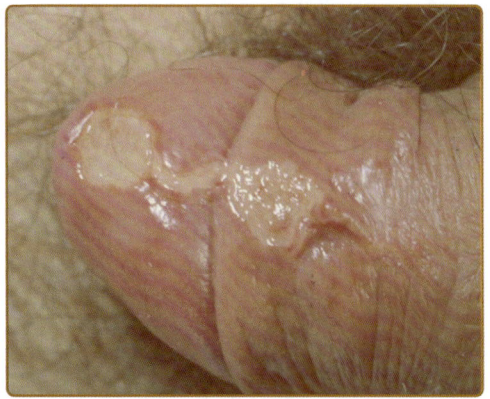

Figure 172-5 Spreading of *Haemophilus ducreyi* by autoinoculation ("kissing ulcer") from the frenulum to the glans.

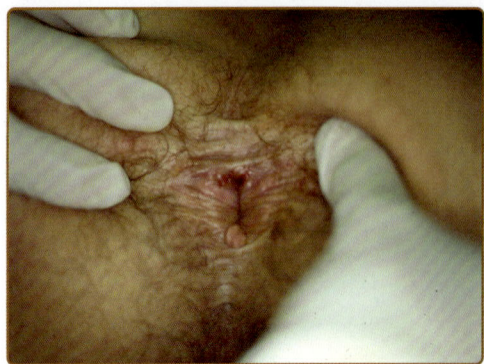

Figure 172-6 Anal chancroid.

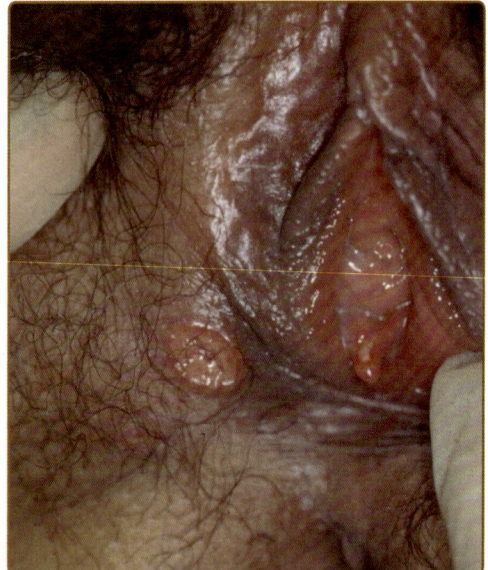

Figure 172-7 Vulvar chancroid with undermined edges.

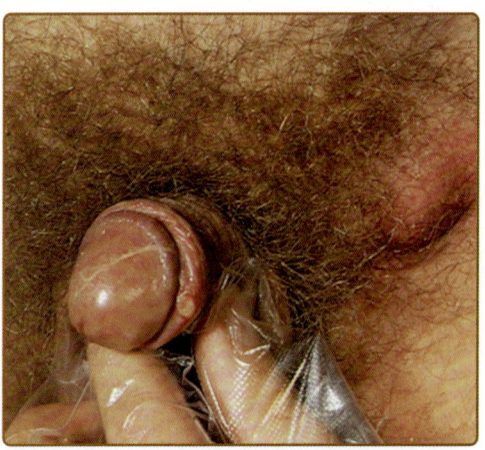

Figure 172-8 Small soft ulcer on the internal surface of the prepuce with painful, fluctuant inguinal adenitis (bubo).

TABLE 172-1 Clinical Variants of Chancroid	
Giant chancroid	Single lesion extends peripherally and shows extensive ulceration.
Large serpiginous ulcer	Lesion that becomes confluent, spreading by extension and autoinoculation. The groin or thigh may be involved (*Ulcus molle serpiginosum*).
Phagedenic chancroid	Variant caused by superinfection with fusospirochetes. Rapid and profound destruction of tissue can occur (*Ulcus molle gangrenosum*).
Transient chancroid	Small ulcer that resolves spontaneously in a few days may be followed 2 to 3 weeks later by acute regional lymphadenitis (French: *chancre mou volant*).
Follicular chancroid	Multiple small ulcers in a follicular distribution.
Papular chancroid	Granulomatous ulcerated papule may resemble donovanosis or condylomata lata (*Ulcus molle elevatum*).

virus.[23] In a high percentage of genital ulcers, no pathogen can be isolated but coinfections with syphilis (*Ulcus mixtum*) or herpes simplex are not uncommon.[24,25]

DIAGNOSIS

H. ducreyi appears as small Gram-negative rods. Microscopy may be done on ulcer swabs, but because of low sensitivity and specificity, microscopy is not routinely recommended for diagnosis. A definitive diagnosis of chancroid requires the identification of *H. ducreyi* on culture media; however, the advent of more-sensitive DNA amplification techniques has demonstrated that the sensitivity of culture of *H. ducreyi* reaches only 75% at best. Culture is particularly important when testing of antimicrobial susceptibility pattern is needed, such as in cases of therapeutic failure. *H. ducreyi* will only survive a few hours on the swab, and bedside inoculation of culture plates (2 different selective, enriched culture media) followed by immediate incubation can be done to reduce loss of viable bacteria during transportation.[26]

Specimens taken for culture also may be used for nucleic acid amplification techniques. These are excellent for demonstrating *H. ducreyi* in clinical sample material with higher detection rates than culture. Various different in-house polymerase chain reaction methods have been described, some of which have the advantage of simultaneously testing for other relevant pathogens, in particular *T. pallidum* and herpes simplex virus.[26]

COMPLICATIONS

In about half of the untreated patients, the course is that of spontaneous resolution without complications. As a consequence of delay in treatment, various complications may occur (Table 172-3).

TABLE 172-2
Differential Diagnosis of Chancroid

	DISEASE	ETIOLOGIC AGENT
Most Likely	Genital herpes	Herpes simplex virus Type 1 and Type 2
	Syphilis	*Treponema pallidum*
	Lymphogranuloma venereum	*Chlamydia trachomatis* serovars L1 to L3
Consider	Other bacterial sexually transmitted infection:	
	Donovanosis (formerly granuloma inguinale)	*Klebsiella granulomatis* (formerly *Calymmatobacterium granulomatis*)
	Other bacterial infections	*Streptococcus* species, staphylococcal and fusospirillary infections, *Mycobacterium tuberculosis*, *Corynebacterium diphtheriae* (very rare)
	Viral infections:	
	Acute HIV infection	HIV
	Chronic anogenital ulcers in HIV-positive patients	Cytomegalovirus
	Ulcus vulvae acutum	Epstein-Barr virus, cytomegalovirus, adenovirus, and others
	Genital herpes zoster	Varicella-zoster virus
	Parasitic infections:	
	Amebiasis	*Entamoeba histolytica*
	Leishmaniasis	*Leishmania* species
	Scabies	*Sarcoptes scabiei*
	Inflammatory diseases:	
	Behçet disease	
	Aphthosis	
	Crohn disease	
	Pyoderma gangraenosum	
	Drug induced:	
	Fixed drug eruption	For example, Trimethoprim-sulfamethoxazole
	Toxic	For example, Foscarnet
	Traumatic and self-induced genital ulcers and neoplasms	
Always Rule Out	Genital herpes	Herpes simplex virus Type 1 and Type 2
	Syphilis	*T. pallidum*
	HIV infection	

TABLE 172-3
Complications of Chancroid

- Painful inguinal adenitis (up to 50%)[27] (see Fig. 172-8)
- Spontaneous ruptures of inguinal buboes with occurrence of large abscesses and fistula formation (rare)
- Spreading of *Haemophilus ducreyi* to distant sites ("kissing ulcers" [see Fig. 172-5] and/or extragenital lesions resulting from autoinoculation; the phenomenon of spreading of Hd through autoinoculation occurs in 50% of male patients)
- Esophageal lesions in HIV patients[20]
- Acute conjunctivitis (very rare)[28]
- Bacterial superinfection (including anaerobes) leading to extensive destruction (rare)
- Scarring leading to phimosis (rare)
- Erythema nodosum (very rare)[29]
- Enhanced HIV transmission (3-fold to 10-fold increased risk)

PROGNOSIS AND CLINICAL COURSE

The disease is usually self-limited. Occasionally, without treatment, genital ulcer and inguinal abscess have been reported to persist for years. Local pain is the most frequent complaint. If no clinical improvement is evident 1 week after the start of therapy, incorrect diagnosis, coinfection with another sexually transmitted infection, concomitant HIV infection, poor compliance, or a resistant strain of *H. ducreyi* must be considered.

Infections do not confer immunity and reinfections are possible. To avoid reinfections, patients must be instructed to use condoms properly.

TREATMENT

Beginning in the 1970s with the emergence of β-lactamase–producing strains of *H. ducreyi* treatment failures became common. Plasmid-mediated resistance to tetracycline, sulfonamides, chloramphenicol, and aminoglycosides also has been reported.[30,31] Little is known about chromosomally mediated resistance in *H. ducreyi*, but decreased susceptibilities to various antibiotics in the absence of identifiable resistant plasmids suggests such mechanisms.[30] Based on in vitro susceptibility, the most active drugs against *H. ducreyi* are azithromycin, ceftriaxone, ciprofloxacin, and erythromycin. Worldwide, several isolates with intermediate resistance to either ciprofloxacin or erythromycin have been reported.[31] Although no antimicrobial susceptibility data for *H. ducreyi* have been published for 2 decades, it is still assumed that the infection will respond successfully to treatment with recommended cephalosporin-, macrolide-, or fluoroquinolone-based regimens.[32] Table 172-4 lists the regimens recommended by the Centers for Disease Control and Prevention, the WHO, and the *European STI Guidelines* (2017).[26,33,34] Antibiotic combinations (eg, ceftriaxone and streptomycin) showed synergy

TABLE 172-4
Regimens Recommended by the Centers for Disease Control and Prevention, the World Health Organization,[a] and the *European STI Guidelines* (2017)[b]

ANTIBIOTICS	DOSAGE	LIMITATIONS
Azithromycin	1 g orally in a single dose	High cost, limited availability
or		
Ceftriaxone[a]	250 mg IM in a single dose	Parenterally, may perform less well in HIV-positive patients
or		
Ciprofloxacin	500 mg orally twice daily for 3 days	High cost, compliance, pregnancy
or		
Erythromycin base	500 mg orally q.i.d. for 7 days	Compliance, GI intolerance, QT interval prolongation

[a]WHO recommends as alternative therapy only.
[b]Lautenschlager S, Kemp M, Christensen JJ, et al. 2017 European guideline for the management of chancroid. *Int J STD AIDS.* 2017;28(4):324-329.
Q.i.d., quarter in die sumendus (which is same as q.d.s.)

in an animal model and may be promising to improve single-dose treatment, but clinical evaluation is needed.[35] Local treatment consists of antiseptic dressings (eg, povidone-iodine). Suppurative nodes should not be incised; if necessary, they can be punctured to prevent spontaneous rupture and sinus tract formation. A large syringe should be used and the fluctuant buboes entered laterally through normal skin. In patients with phimosis, a circumcision may be necessary when all active lesions have healed. In pregnancy, ceftriaxone is the preferred drug, but azithromycin also can be used.[36]

Even after correct treatment, relapses occur in approximately 5% of patients and retreatment with the original regimen is recommended. Usually reinfection by an untreated sexual partner is the suspected cause of relapse.

HIV infection and lack of circumcision appear to be associated with increased likelihood of infection with *H. ducreyi* and treatment failure.[11] In resource-poor areas of the world, syndromic management can be recommended, but local epidemiology must be considered.[18,34] Flow charts for the management of genital ulcers have been developed that do not require laboratory identification of the causative pathogen.[37] If a patient complains of one or more small blisters or an ulcer with a history of recent blisters, then herpes management should be followed. If an isolated small ulcer and painful matted gland is present, lymphogranuloma venereum, chancroid, and syphilis should be treated, and if only an ulcer is present, syphilis and chancroid should be treated.[37]

RELATION BETWEEN HIV INFECTION AND CHANCROID

During the 1990s, renewed interest in chancroid led to evidence that genital ulcers promote the heterosexual transmission and acquisition of HIV.[38-42] During this time it was shown that effective treatment of genital ulcers reduced the incidence of HIV.[43]

Furthermore, it was shown that concomitant HIV infection has clinically significant effects on the course of the chancroid disease, and failure of single-dose[12] or short-course[40] therapy for chancroid in men is associated with HIV-1 seropositivity. A wide variation of the clinical picture of chancroid has been observed in HIV-infected patients.[40] As in every patient with a sexually transmitted infection, patients with chancroid should also be tested for HIV antibodies and HIV-seropositive patients with chancroid should be monitored closely and treated with a multiday regimen.

PREVENTION

The augmentation of the HIV epidemic by *H. ducreyi*, especially in Africa, has made chancroid control an urgent priority. As a result of the widespread syndromic treatment of genital ulcers combined with behavioral change within communities in response to the global HIV epidemic, chancroid has been nearly eliminated in many countries where it was previously endemic. In the rare case of diagnosis of chancroid nowadays,[4,9,10] patients should be advised to abstain from sexual activity until all clinical lesions have cleared. Sexual contacts of the patient (within 10 days of symptom presentation) should be examined and treated regardless of whether symptoms of the disease are present, as asymptomatic carriage of *H. ducreyi* is possible.[14] Antibiotics may provide some protection from reinfection; a single dose of azithromycin lasted as long as 2 months after treatment.[44] Chancroid survives in populations in which many men are having sex with a few women. As a result of the dramatic decrease of the incidence of chancroid with only a few exceptions,[4] eradication seems to be a feasible public health objective.[45] Nevertheless, *H. ducreyi* should be considered as a cause of chronic limb ulcers in adults, and especially in children, in the Pacific region and Africa.[16-18] The reservoir for *H. ducreyi* cutaneous infection remains to be elucidated.

REFERENCES

1. Behets FM, Liomba G, Lule G, et al. Sexually transmitted diseases and human immunodeficiency virus control in Malawi: a field study of genital ulcer disease. *J Infect Dis*. 1995;171:451-455.
2. D'Costa LJ, Plummer FA, Bowmer I, et al. Prostitutes are a major reservoir of sexually transmitted diseases in Nairobi, Kenya. *Sex Transm Dis*. 1985;12:64-67.
3. Totten PA, Kuypers JM, Chen CY, et al. Etiology of genital ulcer disease in Dakar, Senegal, and comparison of PCR and serologic assays for detection of *Haemophilus ducreyi*. *J Clin Microbiol*. 2000;38:268-273.
4. Gonzalez-Beiras C, Marks M, Chen CY, et al. Epidemiology of *Haemophilus ducreyi* infections. *Emerg Infect Dis*. 2016;22:1-8.
5. Phiri S, Zadrozny S, Weiss HA, et al. Etiology of genital ulcer disease and association with HIV infection in Malawi. *Sex Transm Dis*. 2013;40:923-928.
6. Hassan I, Anwar P, Rather S, et al. Pattern of sexually transmitted infections in a Muslim majority region of North India. *Indian J Sex Transm Dis*. 2015;36:30-34.
7. Noda AA, Blanco O, Correa C, et al. Etiology of genital ulcer disease in male patients attending a sexually transmitted diseases clinic: first assessment in Cuba. *Sex Transm Dis*. 2016;43:494-497.
8. Centers for Disease Control and Prevention, National Center for HIV/AIDS, Viral Hepatitis, STD, and TB Prevention, Division of STD Prevention. *Sexually Transmitted Disease Surveillance 2016*. Atlanta, GA: U.S Department of Health and Human Services; 2017. https://www.cdc.gov/std/stats16/CDC_2016_STDS_Report-for508WebSep21_2017_1644.pdf.
9. Fouéré S, Lassau F, Rousseau C, et al. First case of chancroid in 14 years at the largest STI clinic in Paris, France. *Int J STD AIDS*. 2016;27:805-807.
10. Barnes P, Chauhan M. Chancroid-desperate patient makes own diagnosis. *Int J STD AIDS*. 2014;25:768-770.
11. Weiss HA, Thomas SL, Munabi SK, et al. Male circumcision and risk of syphilis, chancroid, and genital herpes: a systematic review and meta-analysis. *Sex Transm Infect*. 2006;82:101-109.
12. Jessamine PG, Plummer FA, Ndinya Achola JO, et al. Human immunodeficiency virus, genital ulcers and the male foreskin: synergism in HIV-1 transmission. *Scand J Infect Dis Suppl*. 1990;69:181-186.
13. Mohammed TT, Olumide YM. Chancroid and human immunodeficiency virus infection—a review. *Int J Dermatol*. 2008;47:1-8.
14. Hawkes S, West B, Wilson S, et al. Asymptomatic carriage of *Haemophilus ducreyi* confirmed by the polymerase chain reaction. *Genitourin Med*. 1995;71:224-227.
15. Plummer FA, D'Costa LJ, Nsanze H, et al. Epidemiology of chancroid and *Haemophilus ducreyi* in Nairobi, Kenya. *Lancet*. 1983;2:1293-1295.
16. Ussher JE, Wilson E, Campanella S, et al. *Haemophilus ducreyi* causing chronic skin ulceration in children visiting Samoa. *Clin Infect Dis*. 2007;44:e85-e87.
17. McBride WJ, Hannah RC, Le Cornec GM, et al. Cutaneous chancroid in a visitor from Vanuatu. *Australas J Dermatol*. 2008;49:98-99.
18. Lewis DA, Mitja O. *Haemophilus ducreyi*: from sexually transmitted infection to skin ulcer pathogen. *Curr Opin Infect Dis*. 2016;29:52-57.
19. Kunimoto DY, Plummer FA, Namaara W, et al. Urethral infection with *Haemophilus ducreyi* in men. *Sex Transm Dis*. 1988;15:37-39.
20. Borges MC, Colares JK, Lima DM, et al. *Haemophilus ducreyi* detection by polymerase chain reaction in oesophageal lesions of HIV patients. *Int J STD AIDS*. 2009;20:238-240.
21. DiCarlo RP, Martin DH. The clinical diagnosis of genital ulcer disease in men. *Clin Infect Dis*. 1997;25:292-298.
22. Lautenschlager S. Cutaneous manifestations of syphilis: recognition and management. *Am J Clin Dermatol*. 2006;7:291-304.
23. Lautenschlager S, Eichmann A. The heterogeneous clinical spectrum of genital herpes. *Dermatology*. 2001;202:211-219.
24. Chen CY, Ballard RC, Beck-Sague CM, et al. Human immunodeficiency virus infection and genital ulcer disease in South Africa: the herpetic connection. *Sex Transm Dis*. 2000;27:21-29.
25. O'Farrell N. Increasing prevalence of genital herpes in developing countries: implications for heterosexual HIV transmission and STI control programmes. *Sex Transm Infect*. 1999;75:377-384.
26. Lautenschlager S, Kemp M, Christensen JJ, et al. 2017 European guideline for the management of chancroid. *Int J STD AIDS*. 2017;28:324-329.
27. Lagergard T. *Haemophilus ducreyi*: pathogenesis and protective immunity. *Trends Microbiol*. 1995;3:87-92.
28. Gregory JE, Henderson RW, Smith R. Conjunctivitis due to *Haemophilus ducreyi* infection. *Br J Vener Dis*. 1980;56:414.
29. Kaur C, Thami GP. Erythema nodosum induced by chancroid. *Sex Transm Infect*. 2002;78:388-389.
30. Erbelding E, Quinn TC. The impact of antimicrobial resistance on the treatment of sexually transmitted diseases. *Infect Dis Clin North Am*. 1997;11:889-903.
31. Dangor Y, Ballard RC, Miller SD, et al. Antimicrobial susceptibility of *Haemophilus ducreyi*. *Antimicrob Agents Chemother*. 1990;34:1303-1307.
32. Lewis DA. Epidemiology, clinical features, diagnosis and treatment of *Haemophilus ducreyi*-a disappearing pathogen? *Expert Rev Anti Infect Ther*. 2014;12:687-696.
33. Centers for Disease Control and Prevention: Sexually Transmitted Treatment Guidelines, 2015. *MMWR Recomm Rep*. 2015;64:26-27.
34. World Health Organisation. *Guidelines for the Management of Sexually Transmitted Infections*. 2003. http://apps.who.int/iris/bitstream/handle/10665/42782/9241546263_eng.pdf;jsessionid=71C39D6930AA74D06292B34123ACC5DD?sequence=1.
35. Roy-Leon JE, Lauzon WD, Toye B, et al. In vitro and in vivo activity of combination antimicrobial agents on *Haemophilus ducreyi*. *J Antimicrob Chemother*. 2005;56:552-558.
36. Geisler WM. Diagnosis and management of uncomplicated *Chlamydia trachomatis* infections in adolescents and adults: summary of evidence reviewed for the 2015 Centers for Disease Control and Prevention Sexually Transmitted Diseases Treatment Guidelines. *Clin Infect Dis*. 2015;61(suppl 8):S774-S784.
37. Lewis DA. Chancroid: clinical manifestations, diagnosis, and management. *Sex Transm Infect*. 2003;79:68-71.
38. Wasserheit JN. Epidemiological synergy. Interrelationships between human immunodeficiency virus infection and other sexually transmitted diseases. *Sex Transm Dis*. 1992;19:61-77.

39. Telzak EE, Chiasson MA, Bevier PJ, et al. HIV-1 seroconversion in patients with and without genital ulcer disease. A prospective study. *Ann Intern Med*. 1993;119:1181-1186.
40. Abeck D, Ballard RC. Chancroid. *Curr Probl Dermatol*. 1996;24:90-96.
41. Royce RA, Sena A, Cates W Jr, et al. Sexual transmission of HIV. *N Engl J Med*. 1997;336:1072-1078.
42. Fleming DT, Wasserheit JN. From epidemiological synergy to public health policy and practice: the contribution of other sexually transmitted diseases to sexual transmission of HIV infection. *Sex Transm Infect*. 1999;75:3-17.
43. Grosskurth H, Mosha F, Todd J, et al. Impact of improved treatment of sexually transmitted diseases on HIV infection in rural Tanzania: randomised controlled trial. *Lancet*. 1995;346:530-536.
44. Thornton AC, O'Mara EM Jr, Sorensen SJ, et al. Prevention of experimental *Haemophilus ducreyi* infection: a randomized, controlled clinical trial. *J Infect Dis*. 1998;177:1608-1613.
45. Steen R. Eradicating chancroid. *Bull World Health Organ*. 2001;79:818-826.

Chapter 173 :: Lymphogranuloma Venereum
:: Norbert H. Brockmeyer & Stephan Lautenschlager

第一百七十三章

性病性淋巴肉芽肿

中文导读

性病性淋巴肉芽肿是由沙眼衣原体的性病性淋巴肉芽肿变种L1、L2、L3引起的性传播疾病。本章从历史背景、流行病学、临床表现（皮肤系统及皮肤系统外）、发病机理、诊断与鉴别诊断、病程与预后和疾病的管理等几个方面对性病性淋巴肉芽肿进行了介绍。

性病性淋巴肉芽肿流行于非洲、东南亚和南美洲、中美洲，发达国家罕见。在非洲和印度的部分地区，性病性淋巴肉芽肿占生殖器溃疡性疾病的7%~19%。它好发于15~40岁的性活跃人群，以生活在城市且社会经济状态较低下的人群居多。男性比女性出现临床症状的可能性大6倍。在发达国家，本病发病率低，且常局限于从流行地区回国的旅行者和军人。但自从2003年起，在欧洲、澳大利亚和北美洲，有同性性行为的HIV阳性的男性群体中曾出现小规模暴发性病性淋巴肉芽肿的报道，尤其是以结肠炎的形式。而且从2015年8月至2016年4月，美国芝加哥报道38例有同性性行为的男性性病性淋巴肉芽肿群集发病，然而美国性病性淋巴肉芽肿的真实发病率并不可知，因为国家强制性性病性淋巴肉芽肿上报在1995年就结束了。

性病性淋巴肉芽肿由直接接触性分泌物感染，通常任何形式的无保护性交均可致病，如口交、经阴道性交和肛交。传染率未知。无症状的直肠感染和/或阴道和口腔感染可能是传染源。边缘性行为，如拳交和共用性玩具可能是其他的传播途径。由于诊断率和上报率低下，人们对性病性淋巴肉芽肿的流行病学特点仍然了解得很少。常见的实验室诊断方法并非特异性的，而且流行地区缺乏这些诊断手段。就算在发达国家，仅有少数实验室有性病性淋巴肉芽肿血清型特异性检查。当缺少这些检查方法时，很多性病性淋巴肉芽肿案例被误诊为常见的沙眼衣原体泌尿生殖系统感染。导致性病性淋巴肉芽肿诊断率低下的另一大原因是无症状携带者。与其他泌尿生殖道感染（如沙眼衣原体感染或淋病）类似，女性尤其可能有子宫颈上皮的持续无症状感染，从而成为性病性淋巴肉芽肿的传染源。

性病性淋巴肉芽肿又名热带或气候性腹股沟淋巴结炎、性病性淋巴结病或Nicolas-Favre病。近年暴发的大多数均由沙眼衣原体性病性淋巴肉芽肿血清变异型L2的数个菌株（L2b）引起，意味着这些暴发很可能代表本病逐渐演变的流行病学特征和对其日渐增长的疾病认识。西班牙、芬兰、捷克和荷兰均报道新发病例（荷兰报道首例由L2b菌株引起的女性腹股沟淋巴结炎性的性病性淋巴肉芽肿）。在法国，自2013年起，由L2b菌株感染引起的性病性淋巴肉芽肿数量下降，而L2菌株引起的感染数量上升。L2c菌株的侵袭力更强，其感染可导致严重的直肠炎。

沙眼衣原体是革兰阴性菌，细胞内寄生。它分为两个区别明显的形态学形式，即为小的新陈代谢不活跃的有感染性的原体和大的新陈代谢活跃的无感染性的网状体。沙眼衣原体因细胞膜外蛋白不同被分为数个血清型，这些不同血清型的菌株导致不同的疾病。血清型A、B、C是沙眼的病原体。沙眼在北美和欧洲罕见，但在非洲和亚洲较为常见。血清型D至K可导致眼部、生殖器部位和呼吸道感染。与A~K血清型不同，性病性淋巴肉芽肿血清型侵袭性更强，且与巨噬细胞亲和力更强。在黏膜接种性病性淋巴肉芽肿血清型菌株后，细菌在巨噬细胞中增殖，并回流至淋巴结，导致淋巴结炎。

性病性淋巴肉芽肿的临床表现是千变万化的，与患者性别、感染方式和感染分期有关。其潜伏期达3~30天，临床可分为3期。无特异性的皮肤损害如结节性红斑、多形红斑、荨麻疹和猩红热样皮疹可发生于本病的任意分期。在性病性淋巴肉芽肿一期，最初表现为感染部位出现5~8mm无痛性红肿性丘疹或小的疱疹样溃疡，常单发。痛性溃疡和非特异性尿道炎少见。因此，初疮可通过缺乏疼痛症状与生殖器疱疹相鉴别。初疮为一过性的，通常在数日内痊愈，患者可能无自觉症状。初疮发生数周后进入二期，出现典型腹股沟淋巴结肿大和血行播散。继而出现多变的发热、头痛、关节痛、乏力、皮肤发疹等全身症状。在腹股沟淋巴结炎发生后1~2个月，约35%患者出现光敏感。也有少数患者出现脑膜炎、肝脾肿大、关节痛和虹膜炎。淋巴结炎通常在8~12周后自行消退。根据传播途径不同，临床主要可见2个综合征：急性生殖综合征或腹股沟综合征，急性肛门直肠综合征。前者特点为腹股沟和/或股骨淋巴结受累，是发展中国家男性的主要临床表现。最初受累淋巴结上的皮肤是红肿质硬的（图173.3），在随后的1~2周，淋巴结继续增大、融合，形成活动度差的团块，最后团块软化、波动、破溃，通过瘘管流出脓液。腹股沟韧带将肿大淋巴结上下分开，形成"槽形征"，是性病性淋巴肉芽肿的特征性表现，但仅10%~20%患者呈阳性，且极少双侧受累。急性肛门直肠综合征特点为直肠旁结节性受累、急性出血性直肠炎和显著的全身症状。这是女性和进行肛交的男性中最常见的临床表现。女性直肠播散主要来源是阴道下1/3淋巴回流。晚期患者多为淋巴腺炎未治疗女性，也可为男性，最常见表现为直肠狭窄，也可能出现会阴部窦道、直肠阴道瘘等后遗症。

本病衣原体血清学试验是阳性的，但不能排除其他类型衣原体感染。核酸扩增试验，如多聚酶链式反应，是针对沙眼衣原体的性病性淋巴肉芽肿变种（L1、L2、L3）的特异性试验。最常用的非特异性试验是补体结合试验，滴度达到或超过1:64即可确诊。另外微量免疫荧光法也可用于本病诊断。

本病推荐治疗为多西环素100 mg口服，每天2次，疗程3周，其他治疗见表173-2。

〔张江林〕

AT-A-GLANCE

- Lymphogranuloma venereum is a sexually transmitted infection caused by L serovars (serologic variants) of *Chlamydia trachomatis*.
- Endemic in Africa, Southeast Asia, and South and Central America, and rare in developed countries.
- Outbreaks have occurred among men who have sex with men in Europe, Australia, and North America.
- Clinically manifests as inguinal and anorectal syndromes, in 3 stages.
- Hematogenous spread with manifestations of systemic infection.
- Diagnosis is by identification of organism and by serology or genotyping.
- Doxycycline or azithromycin (second-line) treatment is curative if given early in the infection course.

EPIDEMIOLOGY

Lymphogranuloma venereum (LGV) is a sexually transmitted infection caused by specific *Chlamydia* variants that is rare in developed countries. It is endemic in East and West Africa, India, Southeast Asia, South and Central America, and some Caribbean Islands; LGV accounts for 7% to 19% of genital ulcer diseases in areas of Africa and India.[1,2] The peak incidence occurs in sexually active persons 15 to 40 years of age, in urban areas, and in individuals of lower socioeconomic status. Men are 6 times more likely than women to manifest clinical infection.[3] The incidence of LGV is low in the developed world where cases are usually limited to travelers or military personnel returning from endemic areas. Since 2003, however, outbreaks of LGV have appeared in Europe, Australia, and North America, particularly in the form of proctitis, among HIV-positive men who have sex with men (MSM).[4-8] In 2013, more than 1000 cases were reported to the European Centre for Disease Prevention and Control, approximately 50% of them from the United Kingdom[9]; however, the real number is likely to be higher, as LGV is not routinely recorded in many European countries. In addition, a cluster of 38 LGV cases among MSM was reported in the United States in Michigan for the period August 2015 thru April 2016[10]; the true incidence of LGV in the United States, however, is unknown because national reporting of LGV ended in 1995.

LGV is contracted by direct contact with infectious secretions, usually through any type of unprotected intercourse, whether oral, vaginal, or anal. Transmission efficiency is unknown.[11] Asymptomatic rectal infection and/or penile and oral infection is the likely source of onward transmission.[12] Sexual practices, such as fisting and sex-toy sharing, may be other routes of transmission. In a study that compared sexual behaviors in men with LGV and men with non-LGV chlamydial proctitis, fisting was a major predisposing factor.[13] An epidemic of LGV has been reported among "crack" cocaine users in the Bahamas.[14]

As a consequence of underdiagnosis and underreporting, the epidemiology of LGV remains poorly understood. Common diagnostic laboratory methods are nonspecific and not readily available in endemic areas. Even in industrialized countries, only a few laboratories offer specific assays to LGV serovars (serologic variants).[15] Without such assays, many LGV cases are misdiagnosed as common chlamydial urogenital infection. Underdiagnosis of LGV is also largely a result of the presence of an asymptomatic carrier state. Women, in particular, may harbor asymptomatic persistent infection in the cervical epithelium, thus serving as reservoirs of the infection as they do for other urogenital chlamydial infections and gonorrhea. A large study conducted in the United Kingdom found that only 6% of MSM were asymptomatic carriers of LGV *Chlamydia* serovars; the majority of cases of LGV in the rectum and urethra were symptomatic,[16] whereas a recent study reported a prevalence of asymptomatic rectal infection of 19%.[17] Infectivity in men usually ceases after healing of the primary mucosal lesion. Interestingly, most of the detected cases in the recent outbreaks are in men who practice receptive anal sex, suggesting that a high proportion of men who practice insertive anal sex are misdiagnosed or undiagnosed. The reasons behind this are unclear but may be organism-related, host-related (eg, sexual practices such as fisting and the use of sex toys, IV drug use, HIV status) or physician-related (failure to diagnose genital LGV). The resurgence of LGV as a health problem may simply reflect increased awareness rather than increased incidence.

ETIOLOGY AND PATHOGENESIS

LGV (tropical or climatic bubo, lymphopathia venerea, Nicolas-Favre disease) is caused by *Chlamydia trachomatis* serovars L1, L2, and L3.[18] Most of the recent outbreaks are caused by a number of strains of *C. trachomatis* L2 serovar (L2b), suggesting that these outbreaks most likely represent increased awareness of a slowly evolving endemic.[5,6,16,19] There are new cases in Spain, Finland, Czech Republic, and The Netherlands (where the first case of a female patient with bubonic LGV caused by a serovar L2b was reported).[20-23] In France, a change in epidemiology since 2013 has been reported with declining infections of the L2b type and increasing numbers of the L2 type.[24] Case reports with infection of the L2c variant suggest a more aggressive clinical course, causing severe proctitis.[25]

Chlamydiae are obligate intracellular bacteria characterized by 2 distinct morphologic forms: (a) the small metabolically inactive and infectious elementary body, and (b) the larger metabolically active and noninfectious reticulate body (Fig. 173-1). *C. trachomatis* has been subdivided into several serovars that differ

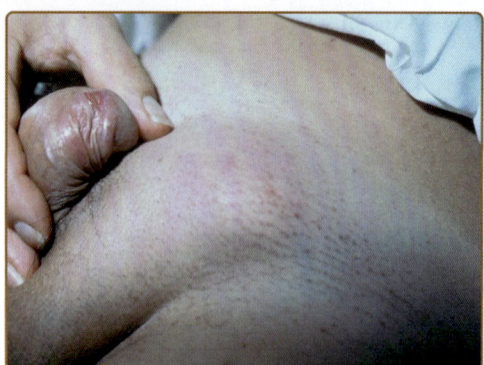

Figure 173-1 Lymphogranuloma venereum.

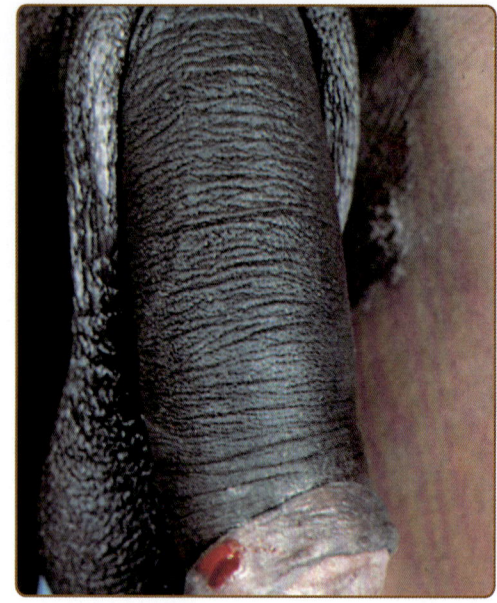

Figure 173-2 Lymphogranuloma venereum: soft painless erosion on the prepuce.

in their major outer membrane proteins, and which are associated with several diseases. Serovars A, B, and C are the causes of trachoma ocular infections. These infections are rarely seen in North America and Europe, but are quite frequently seen in Africa and Asia, where they represent an important cause of blindness.[26] Serovars D to K are responsible for ocular, genital, and respiratory tract infections.[15,27,28] In contrast to the A-to-K serovars that remain confined to the mucosa, LGV serovars are more invasive and have a high affinity for macrophages.[18] After being inoculated onto the mucosal surface, the organisms replicate within macrophages, and find their way to the draining lymph nodes, and cause lymphadenitis.

CLINICAL FINDINGS

CUTANEOUS LESIONS AND RELATED PHYSICAL FINDINGS

Clinical manifestations are protean, depending on the sex of the patient, acquisition mode, and the infection stage. Three clinical stages characterize LGV. Nonspecific cutaneous lesions such as erythema nodosum, erythema multiforme, urticaria, and scarlatiniform exanthema may occur with any of these stages.[29]

PRIMARY STAGE

Three to 30 days after infection, 5- to 8-mm painless erythematous papule(s) or small herpetiform ulcers appear at the site of inoculation (Fig. 173-2). Painful ulcerations[30] and nonspecific urethritis are less common. Thus, the initial lesions may be differentiated from the more common herpetic lesions by the lack of pain associated with the lesions. In males, the lesion is usually found on the coronal sulcus, prepuce, or glans penis, and in females, on the posterior wall of the vagina, vulva, or, occasionally, the cervix. Inoculation also may be rectal, at the lip, or pharyngeal.[15,31]

The primary lesion is transient, often heals within a few days, and may go unnoticed.[25]

SECONDARY STAGE

A few weeks after the primary lesion appears, marked lymph node involvement and hematogenous dissemination occur, manifested by variable signs and symptoms, including fever, myalgia, decreased appetite, and vomiting. Photosensitivity may develop in up to 35% of the patients, often 1 to 2 months after bubo formation (painful inflammation of lymph node, characterized by a unilateral enlargement, suppuration, and abscesses, also firm and tender immovable mass).[32] Less commonly, patients may develop meningoencephalitis, hepatosplenomegaly, arthralgia, and iritis.[33,34] The lymphadenitis episodes often resolve spontaneously in 8 to 12 weeks. Depending on the mode of transmission, 2 major syndromes are seen.

The acute genital syndrome or inguinal syndrome is characterized by inguinal and/or femoral lymph node involvement and is the major presentation in men in developing countries. Initially, the skin overlying the affected lymph node is erythematous and indurated (Fig. 173-3). Over the subsequent 1 to 2 weeks, the lymph node enlarges and coalesces to form a firm and tender immovable mass (bubo; Fig. 173-4), which may rupture and drain through the skin, forming sinus tracts. Bilateral involvement occurs in one-third of the cases (Fig. 173-5). Nodal enlargement on either side of the inguinal ligament, the "groove sign," is pathognomonic of LGV, but only presents in 10% to 20% of cases[35] and is rarely bilateral.[15] In women, inguinal lymphadenitis is unusual because the lymphatic drainage of the vagina and cervix is to the deep pelvic/

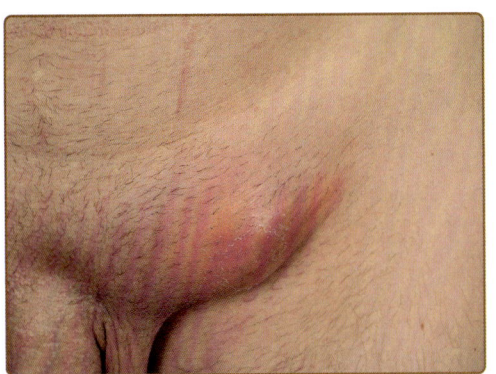

Figure 173-3 Lymphogranuloma venereum: lymph node involvement. Initially, the overlying skin is erythematous and indurated.

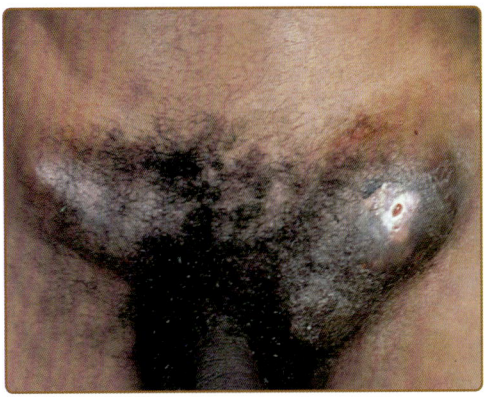

Figure 173-5 Lymphogranuloma venereum: bilateral, firm, immovable masses above the Poupart ligament.

retroperitoneal lymph nodes. When these nodes are involved, low abdominal/back pain that exacerbates upon lying supine and pelvic adhesions may ensue.

The acute anorectal syndrome is characterized by perirectal nodal involvement, acute hemorrhagic proctitis, and pronounced systemic symptoms. It is the most common presentation in women and in homosexual men who practice anal sex. The major source of rectal spread in women is the internal lymphatic drainage of the lower two-thirds of the vagina. Patients may complain of anal pruritus, bloody and/or purulent rectal discharge, tenesmus, diarrhea, constipation, and lower abdominal pain.[36] In a recent outbreak of LGV in Western Europe, 96% of MSM patients presented with signs and symptoms of proctitis.[37] LGV proctitis mimics chronic inflammatory bowel disease, both clinically and in pathologic substrate. These cases may present with an incomplete or undisclosed history of proctosigmoiditis, without the characteristic adenopathy syndrome.[38] Reactive arthritis in MSM following LGV proctitis has been reported in several cases in recent years.[34] Despite affecting mostly HIV-positive MSM, LGV has not behaved as an opportunistic infection in the recent outbreak, and clinical features have not differed between HIV-positive and HIV-negative cases.[39]

TERTIARY STAGE

This stage is seen more often in women with untreated anorectal syndrome than in men, although it is also seen in homosexual men, because of the location of the involved lymphatics. It includes rectal strictures (most common) and abscesses, perineal sinuses, rectovaginal fistulae (leading to "watering can perineum"), and "lymphorrhoids" (perianal outgrowths of lymphatic tissue). Esthiomene (Greek for "eating away") is a rare primary infection of the external genitalia (mostly in women), leading to progressive lymphangitis and genital destruction. Infertility and "frozen pelvis" are potential sequelae of ruptured deep pelvic nodes in women. Late sequelae of the genital syndrome are less common and include urethral strictures and genital elephantiasis with ulcers and fistulas (in 4% of patients).[40] Penile deformities, such as the saxophone penis, may also occur.[41]

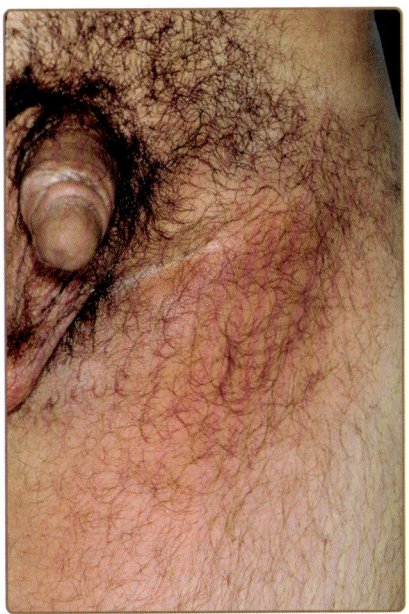

Figure 173-4 Early bubo consisting of unilateral enlargement and coalescence of inguinal lymph nodes. Note the absence of the primary lesion in this case. (Used with permission of Shukrallah Zaynoun, MD.)

OTHER UNUSUAL MANIFESTATIONS

Extragenital-anal inoculation of LGV is rare. Oropharyngeal infection may manifest initially as pinhead-sized vesicles on the lip, and later on as cervical lymphadenopathy with constitutional symptoms, closely mimicking lymphoma. Tonsillitis, supraclavicular and mediastinal lymphadenopathy, and pericarditis rarely occur.[42-44] Ocular autoinoculation of infected discharges may lead to conjunctivitis with marginal corneal perforation, often with preauricular lymphadenopathy.[45] Although most rectal LGV among MSM appears to be symptomatic, some investigators have noted that asymptomatic infections can occur.[46]

LABORATORY TESTS

Diagnosis of LGV may be difficult, but LGV should be suspected in any patient with infected sexual contacts, genital ulcer, perianal fistula, or bubo. The accuracy of clinical diagnosis has been reported to be as low as 20%.[47] Consequently, laboratory tests are important to establish the diagnosis and are usually divided into 2 broad categories: (a) nonspecific tests that do not distinguish between LGV and non-LGV serovars, and (b) specific LGV tests. In practice, a positive test on lymph node aspirate is considered diagnostic of LGV, in contrast to a positive test on a primary genital or anorectal lesion where further specific testing is required to rule out common chlamydial urogenital infections.

Another assay described by Twin et al.[56] targets a 61-bp PCR fragment of the omp1 gene, where LGV and non LGV serovars deviate from each other by one nucleotide that allows differentiation by high resolution melting analysis (HRMA). The assay correctly identifies LGV and non LGV types in 44/47 (93,6%) specimens previously analyzed by a multiplex real time PCR assay published from the same group.[54]

A dual target PCR assay based on the cryptic plasmid for highly sensitive detection of C. trachomatis and pmpH to differentiate between LGV and non LGV strains in a single reaction has been shown to distinguish LGV and non LGV infection in 95% of 156 analyzed C. trachomatis positive samples, including 65/67 (97%) anorectal smears.[57] The advantage of this test is to use a second target recommended to prevent missed infections due to target sequence variation[49] and to differentiate LGV and non-LGV genotypes simultaneously in a single reaction.

All these assays are commercially unavailable inhouse developments that are not FDA approved. Nevertheless, these tests may be used for laboratory testing after evaluation of test performance characteristics according to quality assurance of microbiological diagnostics, such as CLIA (Clinical Laboratory Improvement Amendments).[15]

SPECIFIC TESTS FOR LYMPHOGRANULOMA VENEREUM

Confirmation of LGV requires identification of the genotype L1, L2 or L3. Typing is important because the recommended antibiotic treatment for LGV is longer than for non-LGV cases.[25,48] Nucleic acid amplification tests (NAAT), like polymerase chain reaction (PCR), may be performed on all specimens, and has been the diagnostic method of choice in recent outbreaks. Several currently available commercial NAATs allow sensitive and specific detection of C. trachomatis, but do not provide any information about the underlying genotype(s).[49,50] Using these tests identification of LGV in positive specimens would require a separate analysis.

Methods for typing include genotype-specific PCRs, multiplex-nested PCR and RFLP- or sequence analysis of appropriate omp1 gene regions.[51-54] LGV- and non LGV strains can also be differentiated by real time PCR tests based on pmpH or omp1 gene regions that contain specific deletions or single nucleotide polymorphisms.[53,55,56]

A real-time quadriplex PCR assay has been developed that is capable of detecting LGV, non-LGV, or mixed infections simultaneously in rectal specimens. The assay also contains a supplemental amplification target for the confirmation of C. trachomatis infection as well as a human DNA control for monitoring sample adequacy and PCR inhibition.[55]

NONSPECIFIC CHLAMYDIAL TESTS

The complement fixation test is the most commonly used test. Titers greater than 1:64 are considered diagnostic, titers greater than 1:256 are highly suggestive of LGV, and titers below 1:32 exclude the diagnosis unless the infection is in its early stages.[58] The microimmunofluorescence test for the L-type serovar is more sensitive and specific, but less readily available.[59] The use of species-specific proteins and peptides in immunoblots or line assays further improves the specificity of serologic testing,[60] but as of this writing no LGV-specific serologic marker has been identified.

In addition, direct fluorescence microscopy using conjugated monoclonal antibody against C. trachomatis on smears from bubo material or genital swab can be done.[61] Serology assays are sensitive but nonspecific because of cross-reactivity with other chlamydial infections. In addition, the assays do not differentiate current from prior infection. The Frei test, the earliest diagnostic modality to identify LGV, consists of an intradermal skin test assessing delayed hypersensitivity to chlamydial antigens. It is no longer used because of its low sensitivity and limited specificity, a consequence of cross-reaction with C. trachomatis serovars D to K.[17] Finally, other nonspecific laboratory findings include mild leukocytosis, false-positive Venereal Disease Research Laboratory, cryoprecipitates, rheumatoid factor, and high serum levels of immunoglobulin A and immunoglobulin G.[62]

DIAGNOSTIC PROCEDURES

Proctoscopic examination reveals, in the setting of the anorectal syndrome, multiple discrete and irregular superficial ulcerations and friable granulation tissue, usually confined to the distal 10 cm of the anorectal canal.[63,64]

To confirm clinically suspected LGV the detection of *C. trachomatis* genotypes specific for LGV by laboratory methods is required. Today PCR-based assays, as described above, are preferred over culture because of their higher sensitivity. Clinical material suitable for testing includes anorectal swabs and genital swabs from suspicious epithelial lesions or bubo aspirates. According to the European guideline, anorectal swabs from mucosal lining taken during proctoscopy are recommended, but blind swabs are also acceptable. Commercial *C. trachomatis* nucleic acid amplification tests are not approved for testing anorectal sample types, but several studies have shown that nucleic acid amplification test–based testing of such specimens is superior to other direct detection procedures.[65,66] When the test is positive for *C. trachomatis* a second assay to identify the presence of an LGV genotype or detection of *C. trachomatis* and differentiation of LGV/non-LGV genotypes in a single assay (as described above) is required. If no epithelial lesion is present and lymph node aspirates cannot be obtained, serology may be applied for evaluation. A high complement fixation titer or detection of immunoglobulin A against *C. trachomatis* support LGV diagnosis, but represent no definite proof. On the other hand, serology has a high negative predictive value. Antibody-negative results largely rule out LGV, as the inguinal stage usually takes several weeks to appear.

HISTOPATHOLOGIC EXAMINATION

Primary lesions reveal nonspecific ulceration with granulation tissue, and endothelial swelling. Organisms are rarely demonstrated using Giemsa stain. Biopsy of affected lymph nodes reveals suppurative granulomatous inflammation. Necrotic foci may enlarge into stellate abscesses, which, in turn, may coalesce into discharging sinuses. These histopathologic findings are not specific to LGV and can be found in chancroid, cat-scratch disease, tularemia, and some deep fungal infections. The pathology of LGV-proctocolitis is similar to that of Crohn disease and includes crypt distortion, submucosal fibrosis, and follicular inflammation with occasional granuloma formation.[63] The LGV-proctocolitis will be also similar to syphilitic proctocolitis.[67]

DIFFERENTIAL DIAGNOSIS

Table 173-1 outlines the differential diagnosis of LGV.

In contrast to LGV primary stage, chancroid ulcers are usually larger and more painful, and donovanosis (granuloma inguinale) ulcers have abundant friable granulation tissue without associated lymphadenitis. Acute genital syndrome may be hard to differentiate from chancroid. Buboes containing little or no pus are, however, more likely to be caused by LGV. Suspecting LGV proctitis in HIV-positive MSM who present with signs and symptoms of Crohn disease (Fig. 173-6) or malignancy (Fig. 173-7) is important, even in the absence of LGV pathognomonic findings.[68] Both conditions have similar proctoscopic findings; however, Crohn disease is more proximally localized. Studies from The Netherlands, the United Kingdom, and Australia show that 7% to 23% of patients with rectal chlamydial infection and signs or symptoms of proctitis have LGV.[46,69,70]

COMPLICATIONS

In addition to the complications seen in the tertiary stage, the ulcerative nature of LGV may facilitate the acquisition and transmission of bloodborne pathogens such as HIV[71] and hepatitis C.[18] In addition, several

---

TABLE 173-1

Differential Diagnosis of Lymphogranuloma Venereum (Stage Specific)

- Primary stage
  - Ulcerogenital diseases (herpes simplex virus, syphilis, chancroid, donovanosis)
  - *Neisseria gonorrhoeae* and/or common chlamydial urogenital infection
  - Noninfectious causes: trauma, balanitis, fixed drug eruption
- Secondary stage
  - Acute genital syndrome
  - Ulcerogenital diseases with lymphadenopathy (syphilis, chancroid, herpes simplex virus)
  - Incarcerated inguinal hernia
  - Reactive inguinal lymphadenitis to a lower-extremity focus of infection
  - Bubonic plague (in endemic areas)
  - AIDS
  - Kaposi sarcoma
  - Tularemia
  - Mycobacterial infections
  - Acute anorectal syndrome
  - Inflammatory bowel disease
  - Oropharyngeal lymphogranuloma venereum
  - Lymphoma
  - Infectious mononucleosis
  - Cat-scratch disease
- Tertiary stage
  - Malignancy
  - Filariasis and other parasitic infections
  - Pseudoelephantiasis (no lymphadenitis) of tuberculosis and donovanosis
  - Deep fungal infection
  - Hidradenitis suppurativa
  - Trauma

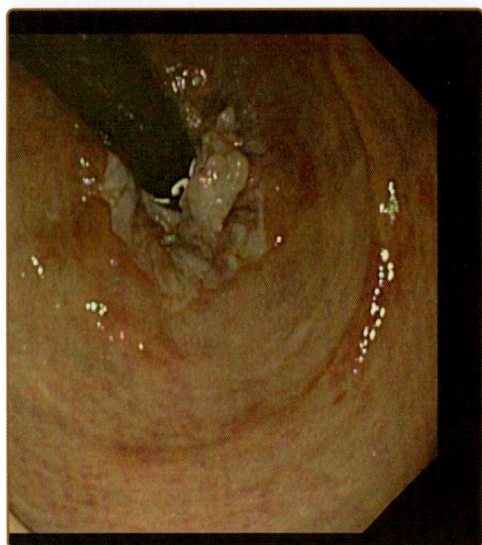

Figure 173-6 Lymphogranuloma venereum imitating Crohn disease.

case reports have described an association between LGV and sexually acquired reactive arthritis in HLA-B27–positive individuals.[34,72]

PROGNOSIS AND CLINICAL COURSE

Antibiotic treatment, if given early, is curative, with acute anorectal syndrome responding more dramatically than acute genital syndrome.

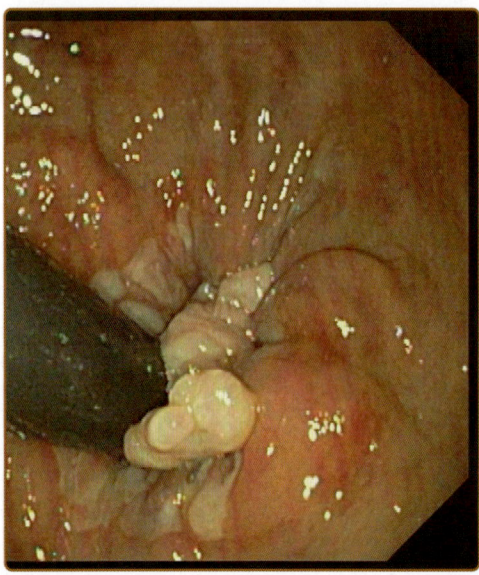

Figure 173-7 Exophytic tumor caused by lymphogranuloma venereum.

TREATMENT

Oral doxycycline, 100 mg twice daily for 3 weeks, is the treatment of choice.[73] When contraindicated, oral azithromycin, 1 to 1.5 g once weekly for 3 weeks or as a third-line erythromycin base, at a dose of 500 mg 4 times a day for 3 weeks, may be given.[15,48,74] Pregnant and lactating women can be treated with azithromycin or erythromycin. Doxycycline should be avoided in the second and third trimester of pregnancy because of the risk for discoloration of teeth and bones; doxycycline is, however, compatible with breastfeeding.[75] It should be noted that the duration of treatment needed to eradicate *C. trachomatis* is longer for the LGV serovars compared with the other less-invasive serovars of *C. trachomatis*. Therefore, when in doubt about the *Chlamydia* serovar, a 3-week course of antibiotics is advised.[76] Therapy may be prolonged in HIV-positive patients and, in general, should not be stopped until the complete resolution of all signs and symptoms (Table 173-2).

Surgery is often required in the late stages of LGV and includes lateral aspiration of buboes through intact skin (direct incision has a high risk of fistula formation), rectal stricture dilation, abscess drainage, rectovaginal fistula repair, genital reconstruction, and colostomy. Avoidance of sexual activity until complete resolution of signs and symptoms is important.[48,74]

PREVENTION

LGV seems to be a rapidly spreading universal problem. Effective control should include periodic evaluation of high-risk individuals, reinforcement of health education aiming at early recognition and counseling, improving community and clinician awareness of LGV, and increasing the availability of specific diagnostic tests. All sexual contacts should be traced and treated. Persons who have had sexual contacts with a patient who has LGV within the 60 days before onset of the patient's symptoms should be examined and tested for urethral, cervical, or rectal chlamydial infection, depending on a anatomic site of exposure. They should be presumptively treated with a *Chlamydia* regimen.[74] The role of screening in asymptomatic

TABLE 173-2
Treatment of Lymphogranuloma Venereum

	DRUG	DOSE	LENGTH OF TREATMENT
First-line	Oral doxycycline	100 mg twice daily	3 weeks
Second-line	Oral azithromycin	1 to 1.5 g once weekly	3 weeks
Third-line	Oral erythromycin	500 mg 4 times daily	3 weeks

patients is not yet clear and cannot be recommended. LGV case reporting should be mandatory by law for more reliable monitoring of prevalence trends. To exclude reinfections, retesting by nuclear amplification tests (also including HIV, syphilis, and hepatitis C) during a followup test 3 months after an LGV diagnosis should be offered.[25] It is assumed that in a reasonable period of time a *Chlamydia*-vault vaccine will be available to eradicate infections.[77,78]

REFERENCES

1. Memish ZA, Osoba AO. International travel and sexually transmitted diseases. *Travel Med Infect Dis.* 2006;4(2):86-93.
2. Goeman J, Piot P. The epidemiology of sexually transmitted diseases in Africa and Latin America. *Semin Dermatol.* 1990;9(2):105-108.
3. Simms I, Ward H, Martin I, et al. Lymphogranuloma venereum in Australia. *Sex Health.* 2006;3(3):131-133.
4. Sethi G, Allason-Jones E, Richens J, et al. Lymphogranuloma venereum presenting as genital ulceration and inguinal syndrome in men who have sex with men in London, UK. *Sex Transm Infect.* 2009;85(3):165-170.
5. Stark D, van Hal S, Hillman R, et al. Lymphogranuloma venereum in Australia: anorectal *Chlamydia trachomatis* serovar L2b in men who have sex with men. *J Clin Microbiol.* 2007;45(3):1029-1031.
6. Meyer T, Arndt R, von Krosigk A, et al. Repeated detection of lymphogranuloma venereum caused by *Chlamydia trachomatis* L2 in homosexual men in Hamburg. *Sex Transm Infect.* 2005;81(1):91-92.
7. Kropp RY, Wong T. Emergence of lymphogranuloma venereum in Canada. *CMAJ.* 2005;172(13):1674-1676.
8. Rönn MW, Ward H. The association between LGV and HIV among MSM: systematic review and metaanalysis. *BMC Infect Dis.* 2011;11:70.
9. European Centre for Disease Prevention and Control. *Sexually Transmitted Infections in Europe 2013.* Stockholm, Sweden: ECDC; 2015.
10. de Voux A, Kent JB, Macomber K, et al. Notes from the field: cluster of lymphogranuloma venereum cases among men who have sex with men—Michigan, August 2015-April 2016. *MMWR Morb Mortal Wkly Rep.* 2016;65(34):920-921.
11. Stein RO. Conjugal lymphogranulomatosis inguinalis. *Z Haut Geschlechtskr.* 1950;9(5):208-215.
12. Haar K, Dudareva-Vizule S, Wisplinghoff H, et al. Lymphogranuloma venereum in men screened for pharyngeal and rectal infection, Germany. *Emerg Infect Dis.* 2013;19(3):488-492.
13. Hamill M, Benn P, Carder C, et al. The clinical manifestations of anorectal infection with lymphogranuloma venereum (LGV) versus non-LGV strains of *Chlamydia trachomatis*: a case-control study in homosexual men. *Int J STD AIDS.* 2007;18(7):472-475.
14. Bauwens JE, Orlander H, Gomez MP, et al. Epidemic lymphogranuloma venereum during epidemics of crack cocaine use and HIV infection in the Bahamas. *Sex Transm Dis.* 2002;29(5):253-259.
15. Stoner BP, Cohen SE. Lymphogranuloma venereum 2015: clinical presentation, diagnosis, and treatment. *Clin Infect Dis.* 2015;61(8):865-873.
16. Ward H, Alexander S, Carder C, et al. The prevalence of lymphogranuloma venereum infection in men who have sex with men: results of a multicentre case finding study. *Sex Transm Infect.* 2009;85(3):173-175.
17. Pallawela S, Bradshaw D, Hodson L, et al. Screening for asymptomatic lymphogranuloma venereum co-infection in men who have sex with men newly diagnosed with HIV, hepatitis C or syphilis. *Int J STD AIDS.* 2015;27(8):625-627.
18. Kapoor S. Re-emergence of lymphogranuloma venereum. *J Eur Acad Dermatol Venereol.* 2008;22(4):409-416.
19. Wang SP, Kuo CC, Barnes RC, et al. Immunotyping of *Chlamydia trachomatis* with monoclonal antibodies. *J Infect Dis.* 1985;152(4):791-800.
20. Korhonen S, Hiltunen-Back E, Puolakkainen M. Genotyping of *Chlamydia trachomatis* in rectal and pharyngeal specimens: identification of LGV genotypes in Finland. *Sex Transm Infect.* 2012;88:465-469.
21. Cabello Úbeda A, Fernández Roblas R, García Delgado R, et al. Anorectal lymphogranuloma venereum in Madrid: a persistent emerging problem in men who have sex with men. *Sex Transm Dis.* 2016;43(7):414-419.
22. Vanousova D, Zakoucka H, Jilich D, et al. First detection of *Chlamydia trachomatis* LGV biovar in the Czech Republic, 2010-2011. *Euro Surveill.* 2012;17(2):20055.
23. Verweij SP, Ouburg S, de Vries H, et al. The first case record of a female patient with bubonic lymphogranuloma venereum (LGV), serovariant L2b. *Sex Transm Infect.* 2012;88(5):219-220.
24. Peuchant O, Touati A, Sperandio C, et al. Changing pattern of *Chlamydia trachomatis* strains in lymphogranuloma venereum outbreak, France, 2010-2015. *Emerg Infect Dis.* 2016;22(11):1945-1947.
25. De Vries HJ, Zingoni A, Kreuter A, et al. 2013 European guideline on the management of LGV. *J Eur Acad Dermatol Venereol.* 2015;29:1-6.
26. Taylor HR, Burton MJ, Haddad D, et al. Trachoma. *Lancet.* 2014;384(9960):2142-2152.
27. Lanjouw E, Ouburg S, de Vries HJ, et al. 2015 European guideline on the management of *Chlamydia trachomatis* infections. *Int J STD AIDS.* 2016;27:333-348.
28. Geisler WM, Suchland RJ, Whittington WL, et al. The relationship of serovar to clinical manifestations of urogenital *Chlamydia trachomatis* infection. *Sex Transm Dis.* 2003;30(2):160-165.
29. Marchand C, Granier F, Cetre JC, et al. Anal lymphogranuloma venereum with erythema nodosa. Apropos of a case [in French]. *Ann Dermatol Venereol.* 1987;114(1):65-69.
30. Sturm PD, Moodley P, Govender K, et al. Molecular diagnosis of lymphogranuloma venereum in patients with genital ulcer disease. *J Clin Microbiol.* 2005;43(6):2973-2975.
31. Dosekun O, Edmonds S, Stockwell S, et al. Lymphogranuloma venereum detected from pharynx in four London men who have sex with men. *Int J STD AIDS.* 2013;24(6):495-496.
32. Sonck C. On the occurrence of solar dermatitis in lymphogranuloma inguinale. *Acta Derm Venereol.* 1939;20:529.
33. Myhre EB, Mardh PA. Unusual manifestations of *Chlamydia trachomatis* infections. *Scand J Infect Dis Suppl.* 1982;32:122-126.
34. Perry ME, White SA. Three causes of reactive arthritis secondary to LGV. *J Clin Rheumatol.* 2015;21:33-34.
35. Schachter J, Osoba AO. Lymphogranuloma venereum. *Br Med Bull.* 1983;39(2):151-154.
36. Van der Bij AK, Spaargaren J, Morré SA, et al. Diagnostic and clinical implications of anorectal lymphogranuloma venereum in men who have sex with men: a

retrospective case-control study. *Clin Infect Dis.* 2006; 42(2):186-194.
37. Ward H, Martin I, Macdonald N, et al. Lymphogranuloma venereum in the United Kingdom. *Clin Infect Dis.* 2007;44(1):26-32.
38. Høie S, Knudsen LS, Gerstoft J. Lymphogranuloma venereum proctitis: a differential diagnose to inflammatory bowel disease. *Scand J Gastroenterol.* 2011; 46(4):503-510.
39. White JA. Manifestations and management of lymphogranuloma venereum. *Curr Opin Infect Dis.* 2009; 22(1):57-66.
40. Hopsu-Havu VK, Sonck CE. Infiltrative, ulcerative, and fistular lesions of the penis due to lymphogranuloma venereum. *Br J Vener Dis.* 1973;49(2):193-202.
41. Kumaran MS, Gupta S, Ajith C, et al. Saxophone penis revisited. *Int J STD AIDS.* 2006;17(1):65-66.
42. Trebing D, Brunner M, Kröning Y, et al. Tumorous extragenital manifestation of lymphogranuloma venereum [in German]. *J Dtsch Dermatol Ges.* 2005;3(6):445-447.
43. Andrada MT, Dhar JK, Wilde H. Oral lymphogranuloma venereum and cervical lymphadenopathy. Case report. *Mil Med.* 1974;139(2):99-101.
44. Albay DT, Mathisen GE. Head and neck manifestations of lymphogranuloma venereum. *Ear Nose Throat J.* 2008;87(8):478-480.
45. Buus DR, Pflugfelder SC, Schachter J, et al. Lymphogranuloma venereum conjunctivitis with a marginal corneal perforation. *Ophthalmology.* 1988;95(6):799-802.
46. de Vrieze NH, van Rooijen M, Schim van der Loeff MF, et al. Anorectal and inguinal lymphogranuloma venereum among men who have sex with men in Amsterdam, The Netherlands: trends over time, symptomatology and concurrent infections. *Sex Transm Infect.* 2013;89:548-552.
47. Dangor Y, Ballard RC, da L Exposto F, et al. Accuracy of clinical diagnosis of genital ulcer disease. *Sex Transm Dis.* 1990;17(4):184-189.
48. Bremer V, Brockmeyer NH, Frobenius W et al. S2k-Leitlinie: Infektionen mit *Chlamydia trachomatis*. AWMF-Register Nr. 2016;059/005. https://www.awmf.org/uploads/tx_szleitlinien/059-005l_S2k_Chlamydia-trachomatis_Infektionen_2016-12.pdf. Accessed Aug, 2016.
49. Papp JR, Schachter J, Gaydos CA, et al. Recommendations for the laboratory-based detection of Chlamydia trachomatis and Neisseria gonorrhoeae. *MMWR Recomm Rep.* 2014;63:1-19.
50. Meyer T. Diagnostic procedures to detect Chlamydia trachomatis infections. *Microorganisms.* 2016;4,pii:E25. doi: 10.3390/microorganisms4030025.
51. White JA. Manifestations and management of lymphogranuloma venereum. *Curr Opin Infect Dis.* 2009;22:57-66.
52. Meyer T, Arndt R, von Krosigk A, et al. Repeated detection of lymphogranuloma venereum caused by Chlamydia trachomatis L2 in homosexual men in Hamburg. *Sex Transm Infect.* 2005;81:91-92.
53. Morre SA, Spaargaren J, Fennema JS, et al. Real-time polymerase chain reaction to diagnose lymphogranuloma venereum. *Emerg Infect Dis* 11: 2005;1311-1312.
54. Stevens MP, Twin J, Fairley CK, et al. Development and evaluation of an ompA quantitative real-time PCR assay for Chlamydia trachomatis serovar determination. *J Clin Microbiol.* 2010;48: 2060-2065.
55. Chen CY, Chi KH, Alexander S, et al. The molecular diagnosis of lymphogranuloma venereum: evaluation of a real time multiplex polymerase chain reaction test using rectal and urethral specimens. *Sex Transm Dis.* 2007;34:451-455.
56. Twin J, Stevens MP, Garland SM. et al. Rapid determination of lymphogranuloma venereum serovars of Chlamydia trachomatis by quantitative high-resolution melt analysis (HRMA). *J Clin Microbiol.* 2012;50:3751-3753.
57. Meyer T, Brockmeyer NH. Implementation of Lymphgranuloma venereum identification in Chlamydia trachomatis testing by nucleic acid amplification. *Clin Microbiol.* 2017;6:1. DOI: 10.4172/2327-5073.1000274.
58. van Dyck E, Piot P. Laboratory techniques in the investigation of chancroid, lymphogranuloma venereum and donovanosis. *Genitourin Med.* 1992;68(2): 130-133.
59. Clad A, Freidank HM, Kunze M, et al. Detection of seroconversion and persistence of *Chlamydia trachomatis* antibodies in five different serological tests. *Eur J Clin Microbiol Infect Dis.* 2000;19(12):932-937.
60. Forsbach-Birk V, Simnacher U, Pfrepper KI, et al. Identification and evaluation of a combination of chlamydial antigens to support diagnosis of severe and invasive *Chlamydia trachomatis* infections. *Clin Microbiol Infect.* 2009;16:1237-1244.
61. Viravan C, Dance DA, Ariyarit C, et al. A prospective clinical and bacteriologic study of inguinal buboes in Thai men. *Clin Infect Dis.* 1996;22(2):233-239.
62. Sonck CE, Räsänen JA, Mustakallio KK, et al. Autoimmune serum factors in active and inactive lymphogranuloma venereum. *Br J Vener Dis.* 1973;49(1):67-68.
63. Greaves AB. The frequency of lymphogranuloma venereum in persons with perirectal abscesses, fistulae in ano, or both. With particular reference to the relationship between perirectal abscesses of lymphogranuloma origin in the male and inversion. *Bull World Health Organ.* 1963;29:797-801.
64. Quinn TC, Goodell SE, Mkrtichian E, et al. *Chlamydia trachomatis* proctitis. *N Engl J Med.* 1981;305(4):195-200.
65. Schachter J, Moncada J, Liska S, et al. Nucleic acid amplifications tests in the diagnosis of chlamydial and gonococcal infections of the oropharynx and rectum of men who have sex with men. *Sex Transm Dis.* 2008;35(7):637-642.
66. Ota KV, Tamari IE, Smieja M, et al. Detection of *Neisseria gonorrhoeae* and *Chlamydia trachomatis* in pharyngeal and rectal specimens using the BD Probetec ET system, the Gen-Probe Aptima Combo 2 assay and culture. *Sex Transm Infect.* 2009;85(3): 182-18.
67. Arnold CA, Limketkai BN, Illei PB, et al. Syphilitic and lymphogranuloma venereum (LGV) proctocolitis: clues to a frequently missed diagnosis. *Am J Surg Pathol.* 2013;37(1):38-46.
68. Rob F, Kašpírková J, Jůzlová K, et al. Lymphogranuloma venereum with only proximal rectal involvement mimicking inflammatory bowel disease: a potential diagnostic pitfall. *J Eur Acad Dermatol Venereol.* 2017;31(5):e264-e265.
69. Hill SC, Hodson L, Smith A. An audit on the management of lymphogranuloma venereum in a sexual health clinic in London, UK. *Int J STD AIDS.* 2010;21: 772-776.
70. Bissesor M. Characteristics of LGV infection among homosexual men in Melbourne. Abstracts of the 19th Biennial Conference of the International Society for Sexually Transmitted Diseases Research, Quebec City, Canada, 2011. *Sex Transm Infect.* 2011;87(1):A139.
71. Fleming DT, Wasserheit JN. From epidemiological synergy to public health policy and practice: the

71. [continued] contribution of other sexually transmitted diseases to sexual transmission of HIV infection. *Sex Transm Infect.* 1999;75(1):3-17.
72. El Karoui K, Méchaï F, Ribadeau-Dumas F, et al. Reactive arthritis associated with L2b lymphogranuloma venereum proctitis. *Sex Transm Infect.* 2009;85(3):180-181.
73. Leeyaphan C, Ong JJ, Chow EP, et al. Systematic review and meta-analysis of doxycycline efficacy for rectal lymphogranuloma venereum in men who have sex with men. *Emerg Infect Dis.* 2016;22(10):1778-1784.
74. Workowski KA, Bolan GA; Centers for Disease Control and Prevention. Sexually transmitted diseases treatment guidelines, 2015. *MMWR Recomm Rep.* 2015;64(RR-03):1-137.
75. Briggs GC, Freeman RK, Yaffe SJ. *Drugs in Pregnancy and Lactation.* 9th ed. Philadelphia, PA: Lippincott Williams & Wilkins; 2011.
76. Mohrmann G, Noah C, Sabranski M, et al. Ongoing epidemic of lymphogranuloma venereum in HIV-positive men who have sex with men: how symptoms should guide treatment. *J Int AIDS Soc.* 2014;17(4)(suppl 3):19657.
77. Poston TB, Gottlieb SL, Darville T. Status of vaccine research and development of vaccines for *Chlamydia trachomatis* infection. *Vaccine.* 2017 [Epub ahead of print].
78. Jiang J, Liu G, Kickhoefer VA, et al. A protective vaccine against *Chlamydia* genital infection using vault nanoparticles without an added adjuvant. *Vaccines (Basel).* 2017;5(1):3.

Chapter 174 :: Granuloma Inguinale
:: Melissa B. Hoffman & Rita O. Pichardo

第一百七十四章

腹股沟肉芽肿

中文导读

　　腹股沟肉芽肿是一种罕见的由肉芽肿荚膜杆菌引起的主要通过性传播的慢行进行性溃疡性疾病，主要影响外生殖器及周围皮肤。本章从历史背景、流行病学、临床表现（皮肤系统及皮肤系统外）、发病机理、诊断与鉴别诊断、病程与预后和疾病的管理等几个方面对腹股沟肉芽肿进行了介绍。

　　近年来，腹股沟肉芽肿发病率显著下降，如今被认为是散发疾病。虽然此病目前罕见，但它临床病程发展迅速，因此及时诊断和治疗是必要的。腹股沟肉芽肿主要在温暖、中度潮湿的热带和亚热带气候中传播。该病的典型流行地区包括巴布亚新几内亚、南非、印度部分地区、巴西和澳大利亚土著社区。非洲南部、西印度和南美洲的其他地区也有散发的腹股沟肉芽肿案例报道。但这种疾病在欧洲和北美洲是十分罕见的。自1989年起，美国每年的新报道病例少于10例。虽然近年的流行病学数据有限，但总体来说，尤其在原先的流行地区，如巴布亚新几内亚和澳大利亚，腹股沟肉芽肿的发病率呈下降趋势。该病在澳大利亚基本被消灭，2004年仅有5例新报道病例。腹股沟肉芽肿好发于20到40岁的社会经济地位低下和性生活活跃的成年人，没有种族或性别差异。虽然普遍认为性传播是该病的主要传播形式，但这是有争议的。大多数腹股沟肉芽肿发生于有性生活史的人群，而且性行为越活跃的年龄段发病率越高。通常，该病患者曾与性工作者发生性接触，且与其他性传播感染共患病。然而，儿童和无性生活成年人中也曾有腹股沟肉芽肿案例报道，而且，与其他性传播感染相比，腹股沟肉芽肿的传播率相对较低。在非常罕见的情况下，也曾出现分娩时经阴道传染腹股沟肉芽肿的案例。

　　腹股沟肉芽肿又名杜诺凡病。其病原菌为兼性革兰阴性球杆菌，不能运动，在大的单核细胞胞浆中生长繁殖，菌体呈多形性。虽然该菌成熟形式是有荚膜的，但在未成熟期不包被荚膜，呈闭合安全别针样结构。其感染导致肉芽肿性炎症反应，引起局部组织损毁和皮肤溃疡。腹股沟肉芽肿的潜伏期是不确定的，但通常被认为是2~3周。首先表现为单发质硬丘疹或皮下结节，随后发生溃疡并逐渐增大。可分为4型：溃疡肉芽肿型、增生型、坏死型以及硬化型。其中溃疡肉芽肿型最为常见，表现为血管增生、牛肉红色的质硬溃疡，触之出血（图174-1）。未经治疗的话，溃疡可能自体接种，发展至周围组织，形成多个溃疡。这些溃疡通常模拟对方的外型，形成"对吻式溃疡"（图174-2）。腹股沟肉芽肿边缘可能呈光滑、增生或疣状改变，后者类似增生型尖锐湿疣（图174-3）。坏死型通常在长期病程中出现，表现为有异味的深在溃疡，伴大量灰色脓性渗出及周围组织广泛损伤（图174-4）。在罕见的干性坏死型中，皮损表现为无出血溃疡，形成纤维性条状瘢痕。90%的腹股沟肉芽肿累及生殖器部位，10%累及腹股沟部位。男性最常见的受累部位包括冠状沟、包皮和龟头。女性最常见的受累部位为小阴唇、阴唇系带和会阴部。在某些情况下，腹股沟肉芽肿表现为类似腺癌的阴道或宫颈肿物。而且尤其在男同性恋人群中，腹股沟肉芽肿可能累及肛门和结肠。腹股沟肉芽肿可能扩散至区域淋巴结之上的组织，表现为脓肿或皮下肉芽肿，被称为假性腹股沟淋巴结炎，随后破溃。在未合并超级细菌感染的情况下，淋巴结极少受累。罕见由淋巴管瘢痕和阻塞导致的生殖器象皮肿。虽然较为罕见，约6%的病例有生殖器外受累。累及部位包括嘴唇、牙龈、颊部、上颚、咽部、颈部、鼻部、喉部和胸部。扩散至骨（导致骨髓炎）或肝脏的播散性病例更为少见。在妊娠期，腹股沟肉芽肿的侵袭性更强，高危地区孕妇的非典型皮损也需要考虑本病。虽然尚无先天性感染的报道，有阴道分娩时经产道感染的案例。本病的婴儿表现多样，包括中耳炎、淋巴结炎、乳突炎及脑膜炎。和其他性传播感染相同，腹股沟肉芽肿患者也需要考虑HIV共同感染。HIV/AIDS相关免疫改变可能导致腹股沟肉芽肿临床表现的变异。当合并HIV感染时，本病发展可能更为迅速，生殖系统外扩散更加常见，而且原发溃疡可能持续更长时间，导致更大程度的组织损伤。合并HIV感染的患者一线治疗成功率亦下降。

生殖器皮损涂片或组织病理中出现多诺万小体即可确诊腹股沟肉芽肿。通过组织涂片和活检切片吉姆萨染色、莱特染色、银染色或革兰染色均可证明多诺万小体的存在。与活检切片相比，合格涂片中更容易找到多诺万小体。涂片最好使用最先取样标本，且取样前不要用抗菌溶液或生理盐水清洁，以提高取样浓度和检出率。从组织学上来说，多诺万小体群在大的单核细胞中空泡状胞浆中找到。细菌配套或血清学检查在诊断中作用不大。多聚酶链式反应诊断方法暂时仅在研究中运用。腹股沟肉芽肿的临床鉴别诊断包括其他几种导致生殖器溃疡的疾病。腹股沟肉芽肿的特征性表现为无痛、牛肉红外观和"对吻式溃疡"的出现。表174-1依据生殖器溃疡、坏死性皮损或生殖器外受累情况的临床表现总结了腹股沟肉芽肿最常见的一些鉴别诊断。

通过治疗，可使皮损停止发展，溃疡由周缘至中央愈合。腹股沟肉芽肿无自发愈合的倾向。未经治疗的话，腹股沟肉芽肿可扩散至内脏器官，包括肝脏、卵巢、子宫或骨。若诊断有误，本病系统性扩散可能致命。本病推荐治疗为阿奇霉素1g口服，每周1次，或500mg口服，每天1次，至少三周，直至症状完全消退，其他治疗选择见表174-2。

〔张江林〕

AT-A-GLANCE

- Granuloma inguinale (GI) is a rare, chronic, progressive ulcerative disease that mainly affects the genital and perigenital skin.
- GI is primarily contracted through sexual transmission.
- GI is caused by infection with *Klebsiella granulomatis*, a gram-negative bacteria.
- It affects mostly people of lower socioeconomic status living in tropical or subtropical areas.
- Diagnosis confirmed by demonstrating intracellular Donovan bodies on histology.

INTRODUCTION

Granuloma inguinale (GI), or donovanosis, is a rare chronic ulcerative disease affecting mainly genital and perigenital skin. The microorganism was first identified in 1905 by Donovan, who noted the characteristic Donovan bodies in macrophages. In 1955, the name "donovanosis" was proposed.[1] The prevalence of GI has decreased markedly in recent times, and it can now be considered a sporadic disease. Despite its rarity, GI can have an aggressive clinical course so prompt recognition and treatment are necessary.

EPIDEMIOLOGY

GI is typically found in warm, moderately humid tropical and subtropical climates. GI has characteristically been reported in specific endemic areas, including Papua New Guinea, South Africa, parts of India and Brazil, and among the Aboriginal community of Australia.[2]

Sporadic cases have been reported elsewhere in southern Africa, the West Indies, and South America.[3] The disease is very rare in Europe and North America. Since 1989, fewer than 10 cases per year have been reported in the United States.[4] Recent epidemiologic data is limited, but overall, the incidence of GI is decreasing, especially in previously endemic areas such as Papua New Guinea and Australia.[3,5] The disease has nearly been eradicated from Australia, with only five cases reported in 2004.[5] GI is most commonly seen in individuals with lower socioeconomic status and sexually active adults between ages 20 and 40 years. No true race or gender predilection has been determined.

MODE OF TRANSMISSION

Although the mode of transmission is generally thought to be sexual, this is controversial. The consensus that donovanosis is transmitted sexually has been predominant since the middle of the 20th century. The majority of cases of GI occur in patients who have a history of sexual activity, and there is an increased incidence of the disease in age groups with the highest sexual activity. Often individuals with GI have history of sexual contact with sex professionals and concurrent sexually transmitted infections (STIs).[6] The predominance of genital lesions and lesions on the cervix only or on the anus in men involved with receptive anal intercourse all favor venereal origin. However, GI has occurred in young children and sexually inactive adults, challenging the idea that all cases are sexually transmitted. Furthermore, transmission rate between sexual partners is lower compared with other STIs.[2] The incidence of GI is also relatively low among sex workers and their conjugal partners. In rare cases, transvaginal transmission of GI during delivery can occur.[7]

CLINICAL FEATURES

The incubation period is uncertain, with estimates ranging between 1 and 360 days.[8] Most often the incubation period is stated to be about 2 to 3 weeks, which is based on human experimental data in which lesions appeared on average 50 days after exposure in a group of volunteers.[9] GI usually first presents as a single firm papule or subcutaneous nodule that later ulcerates and gradually increases in size. Four clinical types have been described—ulcerogranulomatous, hypertrophic, necrotic, and sclerotic. The most common presentation is the ulcerogranulomatous type, which presents as highly vascular, beefy-red ulcers that are nontender but bleed to the touch (Fig. 174-1). If untreated, the ulcers may extend to adjacent tissues via self-inoculation and form multiple ulcers. These ulcers are often mirror images of each other and have been described as "kissing lesions" (Fig. 174-2). The ulcers of GI may have a smooth border or a hypertrophic or verrucous border resembling condyloma acuminatum in the hypertrophic type (Fig. 174-3). The necrotic type often occurs in long-standing donovanosis and presents as a foul-smelling, deep ulcer with copious gray exudate and extensive destruction to surrounding tissues (Fig. 174-4). In the rare dry sclerotic type, lesions are nonbleeding ulcers that form fibrous band–like scars.

The genital region is affected in 90% of cases and the inguinal area in 10%. The most common locations involved in men are the coronal sulcus, prepuce, and glans penis and in women are the labia minora, fourchette, and perineum.[10] Occasionally, GI presents as a mass in the vagina or cervix and can mimic a carcinoma.[11] The anus and colon may be involved, especially in homosexual men. GI may spread to the tissue overlying the regional lymph nodes and present as abscess or subcutaneous granuloma called a pseudobubo that later ulcerates.[10] The lymph nodes themselves are rarely involved unless there is an overlying bacterial superinfection. Rarely, pseudoelephantiasis of the genitals has occurred because of cicatrization and blockage of the lymph channels.[12]

Although rare, extragenital lesions account for about 6% of cases. Sites of involvement include the lips, gums, cheek, palate, pharynx, neck, nose, larynx, and chest.[6,8,13] Even more rare is disseminated donovanosis with spread to bone (causing osteomyelitis) or liver.[14,15]

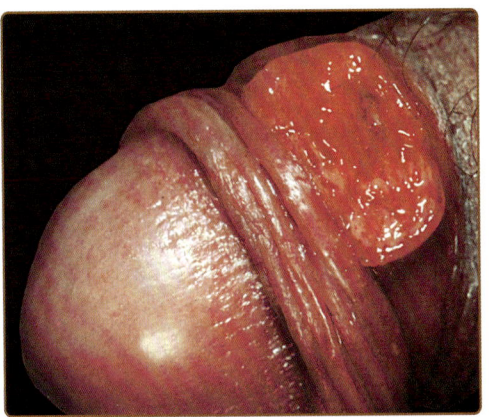

Figure 174-1 Granuloma inguinale, ulcerogranulomatous type. Beefy red, ulcerated plaque that bleeds easily. (Used with permission from A. Eichmann, MD.)

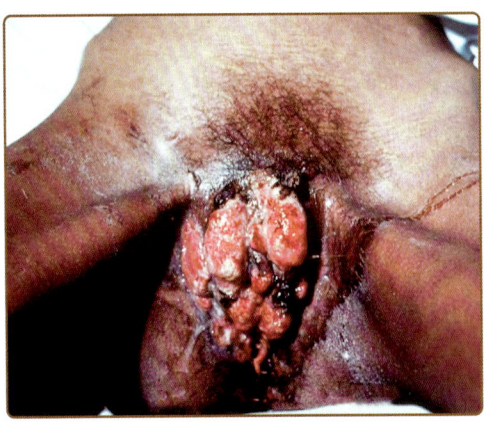

Figure 174-3 Granuloma inguinale. Long-standing hypertrophic lesion causing significant destruction to surrounding tissue. (Reproduced with permission from the Graham Library of Wake Forest Department of Dermatology.)

GI takes on an aggressive course during gestation and should be considered in women with atypical lesions living in high-risk areas.[16] Although no congenital infections have been reported, there are cases in which the infection was passed to the infant during vaginal delivery. The presentation of exposed infants has varied from otitis media and lymphadenitis to mastoiditis and meningitis.[7,17]

As with other STIs, patients with GI may be coinfected with HIV. HIV/AIDS-related immune alteration may alter the clinical manifestations of GI.[18] The natural history is usually more rapid, extragenital dissemination may occur more frequently, and ulcers may persist for prolonged periods, leading to more tissue destruction. HIV-infected patients with GI also have high failure rates to first-line therapy.[19]

ETIOLOGY AND PATHOGENESIS

GI is caused by the organism *Klebsiella granulomatis*, previously called *Calymmatobacterium granulomatis*. The name was changed after sequencing the phoE and 16S ribosomal RNA genes and demonstrating close homology with *Klebsiella pneumoniae* and *Klebsiella rhinoscleromatis*.[20] *K. granulomatis* is a facultative gram-negative, nonmotile, pleomorphic bacteria that resides

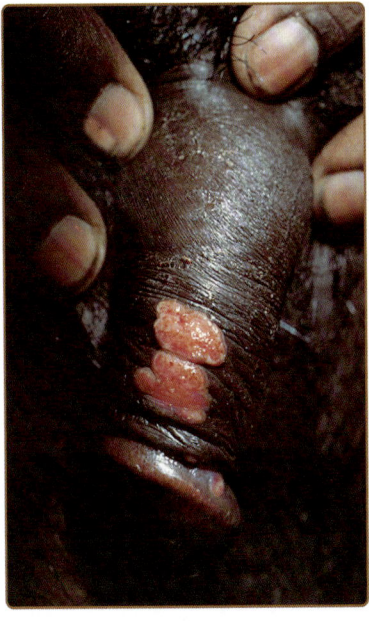

Figure 174-2 Granuloma inguinale, kissing lesions. Two adjacent ulcers that are essentially mirror images of each other. (Used with permission from Shukrallah Zaynoun, MD.)

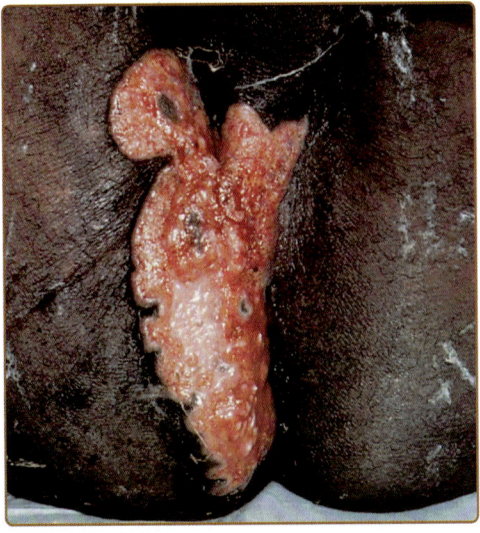

Figure 174-4 Granuloma inguinale. Large ulcerative lesion with destruction to surrounding tissues.

in the cytoplasm of large mononuclear cells. Although the mature form is encapsulated, it can be unencapsulated and demonstrates a closed safety pin appearance in its immature form.[2] Infection leads to a granulomatous inflammatory response, causing local tissue destruction and cutaneous ulceration.

DIAGNOSIS

Clinical suspicion of GI can be confirmed by the demonstration of the characteristic inclusion bodies called Donovan bodies within large mononuclear cells either in smears obtained directly from tissue or biopsy samples (Fig. 174-5). Whereas the cells are 25 to 90 μm in diameter, the Donovan bodies are 0.5 to 0.7 μm by 1 to 1.5 μm and may or may not be encapsulated.[3] Rarely, the Donovan bodies are found extracellularly or within neutrophils.[21] Both tissue smears and biopsies can be stained with Giemsa, Wright, silver or Gram stains to demonstrate the Donovan bodies. The bodies are more easily visualized with properly done smears than with biopsy. If GI is suspected and multiple swabs are being taken from an ulcer for detection of other organisms, the swab for GI should be taken first so that an adequate amount of cellular material can be obtained. It is also recommended that the ulcer not be cleaned with topical antimicrobials or saline because this may lead to negative smears.[18] The ulcer should be gentle wiped with a cotton swab only before taking the smear. Tissue smears should be prepared by rolling a swab firmly across lesion and then rolling this swab evenly across glass slide to deposit the material. A rapid Giemsa method such as Rapi-Diff can then be used to stain tissue smears for rapid diagnosis. Tissue for biopsy should be taken from the advancing edge of the ulcer.

Histologically, the epidermis may exhibit pseudoepitheliomatous hyperplasia or ulcerations (or both) depending on the site biopsied. The dermis often contains a dense mixed inflammatory infiltrate composed of histiocytes, plasma cells, and rare lymphocytes. The hypertrophic and cicatricial forms of GI may exhibit fibrosis. The clusters of Donovan bodies appear as safety pin–like structures inside vacuolated cytoplasms of large mononuclear cells.

Neither cultures nor serology play a major role in diagnosis. *K. granulomatis* is difficult to culture and store; however, successful culture has been accomplished by two laboratories using human peripheral blood mononuclear cells and in HEp-2 cells.[22,23] A polymerase chain reaction (PCR) test using a colorimetric detection system has been developed but is currently only in use for research purposes.[24] No commercial PCR test for GI is available currently. Serologic tests have been developed but are not reliable.

DIFFERENTIAL DIAGNOSIS

The clinical differential diagnosis of GI includes several other disorders that cause genital ulcers. Distinguishing features of GI ulcers include the lack of pain, beefy-red appearance, and presence of "kissing lesions." Table 174-1 reviews the most common differential diagnoses (organized by clinical presentation of genital ulcers, necrotic lesions, or extragenital involvement).

CLINICAL COURSE AND PROGNOSIS

Treatment has been shown to halt progression of lesions, and healing typically proceeds inward from the ulcer margins. GI shows no tendency for spontaneous healing. If left untreated, GI may disseminate to internal organs, including the liver, ovaries, and uterus or to bone. If not correctly diagnosed, systemic dissemination can be fatal.[20] If left untreated, genital complications include genital swelling that may progress to

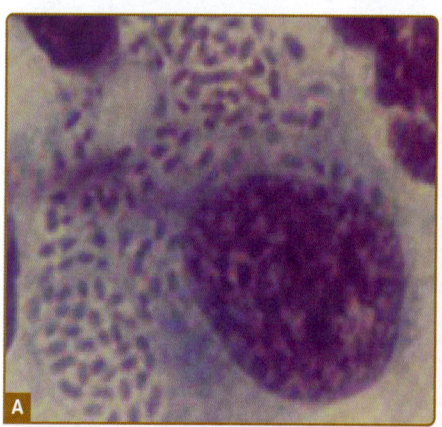
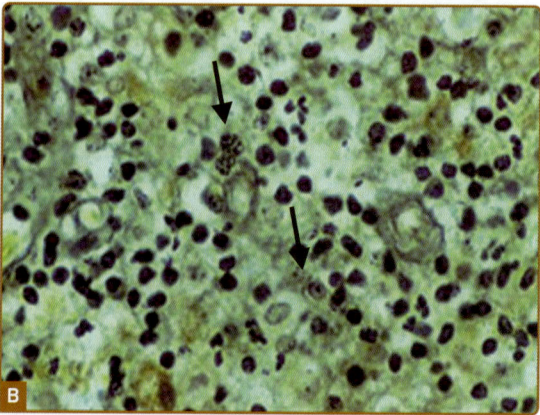

Figure 174-5 Granuloma inguinale. **A,** Large, mononuclear cell demonstrating multiple Donovan bodies. **B,** Donovan bodies (arrows) readily stained with Giemsa stain (Image **A,** From O'Farrell N. Donovanosis. In: Longo, DL, Fauci AS, Kasper DL, et al, eds. *Harrison's Principles of Internal Medicine.* 18th ed. New York: McGraw-Hill; 2012:1321; with permission.)

TABLE 174-1
Differential Diagnosis of Granuloma Inguinale

DISORDER	CONSIDERATIONS
Genital Ulcers	
Primary syphilis	Chancre: painless, punched-out, pink ulcer with nonpurulent clean base and indurated raised border; usually hard and firm
Secondary syphilis	Condyloma lata: present as pale, white, moist warty plaque but may rarely ulcerate
Lymphogranuloma venereum	Initially presents as an asymptomatic, genital papule or pustule or a symptomatic ulceration; later inguinal buboes form
Chancroid	Painful ulcers, often yellow in color, with surrounding erythema and painful lymphadenopathy
Condyloma acuminatum	White, gray, or skin-colored warty papules or may be giant cauliflower-like lesions
Malacoplakia	Solitary or multiple soft papules and nodules, often in urinary tract
Long-Standing Necrotic Lesions	
Squamous cell carcinoma	Important to rule out malignancy in long-standing necrotic lesions, especially those that do not respond to conventional therapy
Genital amebiasis	Painful genital ulcers with or without genitourinary discharge
Chronic herpes simplex in immunosuppressed	May present with chronic nonhealing genital ulcers with exuberant granulation tissue or with more verrucous growth
Extragenital Involvement	
Leishmaniasis	Often starts as nonhealing papule or nodule that enlarges slowly and may develop central ulceration or raised, indurated border
Paracoccidiomycosis	Red painful plaques and nodules on oral and nasal mucosa
Pyoderma gangrenosum	Painful solitary nodule or pustule than transforms into ulcer with dusky, undermined border
Cutaneous tuberculosis	Tuberculous chancres: firm shallow ulcer with granular base; may also have dissemination to organs such as liver or bone

pseudoelephantiasis, phimosis, paraphimosis, and progressive tissue destruction that may lead to destruction of the whole penis or other involved organs.[25] Another major risk of untreated GI is the presence of painless ulcers that bleed easily upon contact greatly increases the risk of HIV transmission. Development of carcinoma is another serious but rare complication that is predicted to occur in 0.25% of cases. A recent case report demonstrated coexisting squamous cell carcinoma and GI in an HIV-infected patient.[25] Malignancies should always be ruled out in cases of long-standing ulcers not responsive to treatment. Despite these complications, if proper treatment is initiated early in the course of disease, the prognosis is generally good.

MANAGEMENT

The optimal way to manage a possible case of GI is to establish diagnosis as soon as possible so appropriate antibiotics and specific patient education can be given. The patient should be educated about the complications of untreated GI and the risk for acquiring other STIs, including HIV. Several antimicrobial regimens have proven effective, but only a limited number of controlled trials have been published. Prolonged therapy is usually required to permit granulation and reepithelialization of the ulcers. It should be noted that standard treatment regimens used for other STIs such as chancroid may not be adequate in both dose and duration for GI, highlighting the importance of appropriate diagnosis. Table 174-2 outlines the most current treatment recommendations by both the Centers for Disease Control and World Health Organization.[26,27] Duration of treatment should be for at least 3 weeks and until complete healing is achieved. The addition of another antibiotic to these regimens, specifically an aminoglycoside (gentamicin 1 mg/kg IV every 8 hours), can be considered if improvement is not evident within the first few days of therapy. The addition of aminoglycosides is particularly important in patients who are pregnant or HIV positive, given the aggressive clinical course in these subsets of patients. Children with GI should receive a short course of azithromycin 20 mg/kg. Children born to mothers with GI should receive prophylaxis with a 3-day course of azithromycin 20 mg/kg once daily.[28]

Relapse may occur 6 to 18 months after apparently effective therapy, thus requiring follow-up by the physician. Long-standing cases may be complicated by secondary bacterial infections or by fistula and abscess formation, which require surgical intervention and render antibiotic treatment alone ineffective.[29] Patients with GI should be screened for other STIs, notably HIV and syphilis. Although donovanosis is uncommon in partners of index cases, all sexual contacts in the previous 6 months should be examined. Treatment of sexual partners is not necessary unless they develop signs and symptoms of GI.

ACKNOWLEDGMENTS

The authors acknowledge the contributions of Abdul-Ghani Kibbi, Ruba F. Bahhady, and Myrna El-Shareef, the former authors of this chapter.

REFERENCES

1. Marmell M, Santora E. Donovanosis; granuloma inguinale; incidence, nomenclature, and diagnosis. *Am J Syph Gonorrhea Vener Dis*. 1950;34(1):83-90.
2. Basta-Juzbasic A, Ceovic R. Chancroid, lymphogranuloma venereum, granuloma inguinale, genital herpes simplex infection, and molluscum contagiosum. *Clin Dermatol*. 2014;32(2):290-298.

TABLE 174-2
Treatment of Granuloma Inguinale

	CDC (2015)	WHO (2003)
Recommendations[a]	Azithromycin 1 g orally once weekly or 500 mg/day	Azithromycin 1 g orally once; then 500 mg/day or Doxycycline 100 mg orally twice daily
Alternatives	Doxycycline 100 mg orally twice daily or Ciprofloxacin 750 mg orally twice daily or Erythromycin base 500 mg orally four times daily or Trimethoprim-sulfamethoxazole one double-strength (160 mg/800 mg) tablet orally twice daily	Erythromycin 500 mg four times daily or Tetracycline 500 mg four times daily or Trimethoprim 80 mg/sulfamethoxazole 400 mg, 2 tablets, twice daily for a minimum of 14 days
Pregnancy	Macrolide antibiotic (azithromycin or erythromycin) as dosed above	

[a]Duration of treatment with any regimen is for at least 3 weeks and until all lesions have completely epithelialized.
CDC, Centers for Disease Control and Prevention; WHO, World Health Organization.

3. O'Farrell N. Donovanosis. *Sex Transm Infect*. 2002;78(6): 452-457.
4. Lupi O, Madkan V, Tyring SK. Tropical dermatology: bacterial tropical diseases. *J Am Acad Dermatol*. 2006;54(4):559-578; quiz 578-580.
5. Bowden FJ. Donovanosis in Australia: going, going. *Sex Transm Infect*. 2005;81(5):365-366.
6. Veeranna S, Raghu TY. A clinical and investigational study of donovanosis. *Indian J Dermatol Venereol Leprol*. 2003;69(2):159-162.
7. Ahmed N, Pillay A, Lawler M, et al. Donovanosis causing lymphadenitis, mastoiditis, and meningitis in a child. *Lancet*. 2015;385(9987):2644.
8. O'Farrell N. Donovanosis: an update. *Int J STD AIDS*. 2001;12(7):423-427.
9. Greenblatt RB, Dienst RB, Pund ER, et al. Experimental and clinical granuloma inguinale. *JAMA*. 1939;113(12): 1109-1116.
10. Velho PE, Souza EM, Belda Junior W. Donovanosis. *Braz J Infect Dis*. 2008;12(6):521-525.
11. Taneja S, Jena A, Tangri R, et al. Case report. MR appearance of cervical donovanosis mimicking carcinoma of the cervix. *Br J Radiol*. 2008;81(966):e170-e172.
12. Narang T, Kanwar AJ. Genital elephantiasis due to donovanosis: forgotten but not gone yet. *Int J STD AIDS*. 2012;23(11):835-836.
13. Veeranna S, Raghu TY. Oral donovanosis. *Int J STD AIDS*. 2002;13(12):855-856.
14. Fletcher HM, Rattray CA, Hanchard B, et al. Disseminated donovanosis (granuloma inguinale) with osteomyelitis of both wrists. *West Indian Med J*. 2002;51(3):194-196.
15. Paterson DL. Disseminated donovanosis (granuloma inguinale) causing spinal cord compression: case report and review of donovanosis involving bone. *Clin Infect Dis*. 1998;26(2):379-383.
16. Liverani CA, Lattuada D, Mangano S, et al. Hypertrophic donavanosis in a young pregnant woman. *J Pediatr Adolesc Gynecol*. 2012;25(4):e81-e83.
17. Govender D, Naidoo K, Chetty R. Granuloma inguinale (donovanosis): an unusual cause of otitis media and mastoiditis in children. *Am J Clin Pathol*. 1997;108(5):510-514.
18. Marfatia YS, Menon DS, Jose S, et al. Nonhealing genital ulcer in AIDS: a diagnostic dilemma! *Indian J Sex Transm Dis*. 2016;37(2):197-200.
19. Jamkhedkar PP, Hira SK, Shroff HJ, et al. Clinico-epidemiologic features of granuloma inguinale in the era of acquired immune deficiency syndrome. *Sex Transm Dis*. 1998;25(4):196-200.
20. Hart G. Donovanosis. *Clin Infect Dis*. 1997;25(1):24-30; quiz 31-22.
21. Richens J. The diagnosis and treatment of donovanosis (granuloma inguinale). *Genitourin Med*. 1991;67(6): 441-452.
22. Carter J, Hutton S, Sriprakash KS, et al. Culture of the causative organism of donovanosis (Calymmatobacterium granulomatis) in HEp-2 cells. *J Clin Microbiol*. 1997;35(11):2915-2917.
23. Kharsany AB, Hoosen AA, Kiepiela P, et al. Growth and cultural characteristics of Calymmatobacterium granulomatis—the aetiological agent of granuloma inguinale (Donovanosis). *J Med Microbiol*. 1997;46(7):579-585.
24. Carter JS, Kemp DJ. A colorimetric detection system for Calymmatobacterium granulomatis. *Sex Transm Infect*. 2000;76(2):134-136.
25. Sardana K, Garg VK, Arora P, et al. Malignant transformation of donovanosis (granuloma inguinale) in a HIV-positive patient. *Dermatol Online J*. 2008;14(9):8.
26. Centers for Disease Control and Prevention. 2015 sexually transmitted diseases treatment guidelines, granuloma inguinale (donovanosis). 2015. https://www.cdc.gov/std/tg2015/donovanosis.htm.
27. World Health Organization. Guidelines for the management of sexually transmitted infections 2001:44. http://www.who.int/hiv/hiv_aids_2001_01.pdf.
28. Bowden FJ, Bright A, Rode JW, et al. Donovanosis causing cervical lymphadenopathy in a five-month-old boy. *Pediatr Infect Dis J*. 2000;19(2):167-169.
29. Bozbora A, Erbil Y, Berber E, et al. Surgical treatment of granuloma inguinale. *Br J Dermatol*. 1998;138(6): 1079-1081.

Chapter 175 :: Gonorrhea, Mycoplasma, and Vaginosis
:: Lindsay C. Strowd, Sean McGregor, & Rita O. Pichardo

第一百七十五章
淋病、支原体感染和细菌性阴道病

中文导读

美国每年新发超过两千万例性传播疾病患者。尿道炎在男性和女性中均是性传播疾病常见的表现症状。高危患者常有数种性传播疾病共患病。性传播疾病通常可通过直接镜检、病原体培养或更先进的诊断方法如核酸扩增试验诊断。性传播疾病早期且适当的抗菌治疗通常预后较好。本章从历史背景、流行病学、临床表现（皮肤系统及皮肤系统外）、发病机理、诊断与鉴别诊断、病程与预后和疾病的管理等几个方面对几种最常见的性传播疾病进行了介绍。

淋病是由淋病奈瑟菌引起的细菌感染，人类是其唯一的天然宿主，常通过性活动传播。淋病奈瑟菌是革兰阴性的需氧双球菌，多位于多核型白细胞内部。淋病是一种常见的性传播疾病，男性和女性均受累，尤其好发于少年和青年人。根据美国疾病控制预防中心的数据，在美国，每年约有82万人新发淋病奈瑟菌感染，但仅有约半数经公共健康系统上报。因此，淋病是美国第二常见的感染性疾病，仅次于衣原体感染。就皮肤感染而言，在男性中，淋病潜伏期为2~8天，常见临床表现为尿道炎，特征为自发的、自阴茎分泌混浊或脓性分泌物（图175-2）。前尿道黏膜炎症可导致排尿特痛或烧灼感，以及尿道红肿（图175-3）。男性感染者中仅10%无症状。在女性中，50%的淋病感染无症状。但合理筛查、早期诊断和治疗非常重要。因为淋病的严重并发症可导致不育。子宫颈内膜是常见的局部感染部位。女性中尿道炎表现为黏脓性分泌物、阴道瘙痒和排尿困难。然而，性成熟女性的阴道上皮不支持淋病奈瑟菌生长，因此阴道炎仅发生于青春期前女童和绝经后女性。其他皮肤感染部位包括前庭大腺和斯基恩氏腺，引起局部肿胀和压痛。发生无保护性行为被动肛交的人群可能感染本病引起直肠炎。因此，淋病性直肠炎最常见于有同性性行为的男性。由于肛门直肠内膜完整性破坏以及局部HIV靶向细胞局部募集效应，这类男性感染HIV的可能性更大。女性也可能通过宫颈分泌物的自体接种或被动肛交引起直肠炎。淋病的皮肤系统外表现可能有咽炎及盆腔炎性疾病。直肠炎症状包括直肠黏脓性分泌物、排便疼痛、便秘和里急后重。淋病奈瑟菌亦可通过血行播散引起全身症状，被称为播散性淋病或淋球菌血症。新生儿也可能经产道感染，引起新生儿眼炎。淋病的诊断需结合病史、临床表现和实验室检查。淋病的实验室检查有直接涂片检查与淋球菌培养，后者是诊断的金标准。局部淋病的推荐治疗为头孢曲松250mg，单次肌注合并阿奇霉素1g，单次口服，其他治疗选择见表175-2。扩散性淋病的推荐治疗为头孢曲松1g，静脉注射，每日1次，连续七天合并阿奇霉素1g，单次口服，其他治疗选择见表175-3。

生殖道支原体感染：支原体是最小的能在无生命培养基中生长、增殖的细菌。在人类呼吸道以及泌尿生殖道中定植。性活跃人群的支原体生殖道分离率高于儿童和无性经历的成年人，女性高于男性。生殖道支原体感染在男性中最常见的临床表现为尿道炎，特征为排尿困难、尿痛和尿道瘙痒，以及黏脓性分泌物，发生概率较淋病性尿道炎和衣原体性尿道炎低。也可仅有分泌物而无尿道刺激症状。本病的体征和症状与衣原体性非淋菌性尿道炎无法区分。在女性中，最常见的皮肤感染为宫颈炎，发生率也比淋病性宫颈炎和衣原体性宫颈炎低。表现为子宫颈内膜黏脓性分泌物、宫颈口易破裂出血、异常性阴道分泌物以及经期间阴道出血。生殖道支原体感染也可导致盆腔炎性疾病或血行播散引起全身症状。支原体是缓慢生长的微生物，培养时间最长可达6个月，且分离培养十分困难，因此核酸扩增试验，如多聚酶链式反应是更合适的诊断工具。本病推荐治疗为阿奇霉素1g，单次口服，其他治疗选择见表175-5。

沙眼衣原体感染：在美国，沙眼衣原体感染是最常见的生殖系统感染，它也是女性盆腔炎性疾病的首要致病因素。沙眼衣原体感染的临床表现根据感染部位、性别、年龄以及血清型不同有所不同。最常见的为泌尿生殖系统感染。男性中尿道最常受累，表现为排尿困难、稀薄或黏液样分泌物。可能仅有少量分泌物，一些患者仅诉内裤上有异常污渍。与之相比，淋菌性尿道炎的分泌物更偏向于化脓性的，且量更多。然而临床症状上这几种性传播感染有显著的重叠，因此分泌物性质和伴随排尿困难的严重程度均不能用作特异性诊断。沙眼衣原体也可能在男性中引起附睾炎，在两性中均可引起直肠炎。在女性中，最常受累部位为尿道和宫颈，宫颈炎表现为经宫颈口排出黏脓性分泌物。然而女性中大多数尿道沙眼衣原体感染为无症状的。宫颈炎患者可能主诉阴道分泌物、出血或腹痛。如果有排尿困难表现，可能提示合并尿道炎。围产期感染可能导致新生儿结膜炎和肺炎。虽然临床症状可以为本病诊断提供线索，但其确诊需要实验室证据。本病可通过细胞培养确诊，但随着技术的进步，核酸扩增试验，如多聚酶链反应逐渐取代了细胞培养。本病推荐治疗为阿奇霉素1g，单次口服，或多西环素100mg口服，每天2次，疗程7天，其他治疗选择总结于表175-7。

细菌性阴道病是15~44岁女性中最常见的阴道感染，是由多种微生物参与协同发生的疾病。其中无症状感染可达84%。临床表现主要为阴道分泌物异常，分泌量增多，颜色呈灰白色，带有鱼腥味。外阴阴道瘙痒和炎症常不显著。通常通过分泌物外观、气味，分泌物pH增高（>4.5），氨试验阳性及分泌物涂片可见超过20%线索细胞即可诊断。细菌性阴道病是早产或新生儿低体重的危险因素，也可能导致盆腔炎性疾病。本病推荐治疗为甲硝唑500mg口服，每天2次，疗程7天，其他治疗方案见表175-8。

〔张江林〕

AT-A-GLANCE

- More than 20 million new sexually transmitted diseases (STDs) occur annually in the United States.
- In the United States, chlamydia is currently the most common reported STD. It is also the most common cause of pelvic inflammatory disease in women.
- Urethritis is a common presenting symptom of STDs in both men and women.
- High-risk patients often have coinfection with multiple STDs.
- Diagnosis can usually be made through direct microscopy, culture, or newer diagnostic methods such as nucleic acid amplification tests.
- Early and appropriate antimicrobial therapy of STDs results in good prognosis.

GONORRHEA

INTRODUCTION

Gonorrhea is a bacterial infection by *Neisseria gonorrhoeae*, a gram-negative, aerobic coccus-shaped bacterium found in pairs. The organisms are usually visualized intracellularly, located within polymorphonuclear leukocytes (Fig. 175-1). Gonorrhea is a common sexually transmitted disease (STD) affecting both men and women, particularly teenagers and young adults. In adult patients, gonococcal infection can affect the genitals, anus, or pharynx and can be acquired through vaginal, anal, or oral intercourse. It can also be transmitted vertically from mother to child during vaginal birth, manifesting as an inflammatory eye infection (ophthalmia neonatorum).

Albert Ludwig Sigismund Neisser first discovered the causative agent of gonorrhea in 1879. The origins of gonococcal infections are unknown, but references to gonorrhea, or "the clap" as it has been termed, go back to the 16th century in Europe.[1] Before the advent of antibiotics, silver preparations including silver nitrate and silver proteinate (Protargol) were used to treat gonorrhea in the 19th and 20th centuries.

EPIDEMIOLOGY

More than 820,000 people are estimated to acquire new gonococcal infections in the United States yearly according to the Centers for Disease Control and Prevention (CDC), although only about half are actually reported through the public health system. This makes gonorrhea the second most commonly reported infectious disease in the United States, second only to chlamydia. Higher endemic areas of the country include the southern United States and Alaska, with the lowest prevalence being in the northwestern states.[2] The rate of new infections declined after the implementation of a national gonorrhea control program in the United States during the mid-1970s and continued to decrease through the late 1990s. The yearly prevalence of gonococcal infections reached an all-time low in 2009. It has risen every year since 2009, with the exception of 2013, when it decreased slightly.[2] Newer epidemiologic data from the CDC and state registries indicates that there is increasing heterosexual transmission that may explain the increasing prevalence. The highest rate of reported gonococcal infections is among sexually active teenagers and young adults, aged 15 to 24 years. There is notable ethnic disparity, with the reported gonorrhea rate in African Americans being twenty times higher and in Hispanics twice as high compared with whites.[2] Such racial disparity is multifactorial and may be attributable to differences in accessibility to health care, lack of use of available resources, and sexual partner preferences. Risk factors for acquisition of gonorrheal infection include new or multiple sex partners, younger age, unmarried status, commercial sex work, minority ethnicity, substance and alcohol abuse, lower socioeconomic and educational levels, inconsistent condom use, and any previous STD infection. Prior gonorrhea is an especially important risk factor for acquisition of a new gonococcal infection because recidivism is particularly common.[3] As is true of most STDs, alcohol ingestion to the point of inebriation is associated with risky sexual behavior, including unprotected intercourse and sex with multiple partners, and is thus a major factor in acquisition of gonorrhea.[4]

Since the 1980s, prevalence rates among men and women have been similar in all age categories, although for any given age range, the prevalence will be slightly higher in women. Recent data indicate larger increases in infection among women compared with men. Although men having sex with men (MSM) is traditionally thought to be a high-risk group for gonorrhea, heterosexual women and men show an increasing prevalence of infection.[5] A relatively high divorce rate and the wide availability of drugs to treat erectile dysfunction have both contributed to a resurgence of STDs (including gonorrhea) among middle-aged and older individuals living in industrialized countries.[6]

CLINICAL FEATURES

CUTANEOUS FINDINGS

Cutaneous Disease (Men): The incubation period in men is typically from 2 to 8 days, although it may rarely be longer because most infections are symptomatic by 2 weeks after exposure. Only about 10% of infections are asymptomatic in men. The most common manifestation of gonococcal infection in men

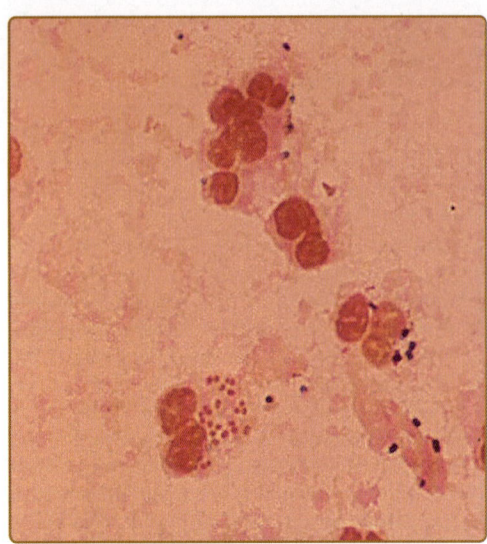

Figure 175-1 Diagnostic Gram-stained smear of urethral discharge of a man with acute gonorrhea. Gonococci (*red*) within a polymorphonuclear leukocyte. There are also some gram-positive cocci in this smear (*dark blue*). (Used with permission from Angelika Stary, MD.)

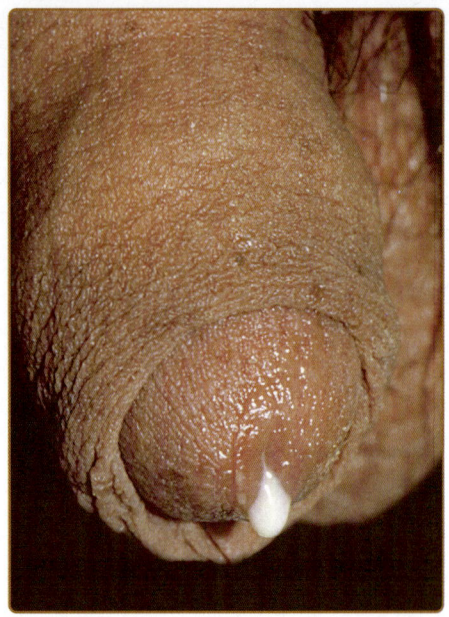

Figure 175-2 Acute gonorrhea in a male manifesting as creamy purulent discharge from the urethra. (Used with permission from Dr. Ted Rosen.)

is urethritis, characterized by a spontaneous, often profuse, cloudy or purulent discharge from the penile meatus (Fig. 175-2). Mucosal membrane inflammation in the anterior urethra leads to pain or burning upon urination and meatal erythema and swelling (Fig. 175-3). In some cases, there is so much soft tissue inflammation that the entire distal penis becomes swollen, so-called "bull head clap" (Fig. 175-4). Testicular pain and swelling may indicate epididymitis or orchitis and may be the only presenting symptom. However, epididymitis is more commonly caused by *Chlamydia trachomatis* or by combined infection with *N. gonorrhoeae*. There have been rare instances of genital skin furuncles caused by gonorrhea.[7]

Cutaneous Disease (Women): Fifty percent of women infected with *N. gonorrhoeae* are asymptomatic. Appropriate screening, prompt diagnosis, and treatment are crucial in women because of serious complications that can result in sterility. The endocervix is a common site of local infection. Symptoms of urethritis include mucopurulent discharge, vaginal pruritus, and dysuria. However, vaginitis does not occur except in prepuberal girls and postmenopausal women because the vaginal epithelium of sexually mature women does not support growth of *N. gonorrhoeae*. Other sites of infection include the Bartholin and Skene glands, which results in swelling and tenderness.[7]

Proctitis: Proctitis is a manifestation of gonococcal infection manifesting in those who practice unprotected anoreceptive intercourse. Thus, it is most common in MSM. As a result of gonococcal proctitis, MSM are at a higher risk of acquiring HIV infection because of both damaged anorectal epithelial integrity and local recruitment of HIV-target cell types (CCR5/CD4+ T cells and DC-SIGN [DC-specific intercellular adhesion molecule 3 grabbing nonintegrin] + dendritic cells).[8] Women may also develop proctitis through autoinoculation from cervical discharge or from anoreceptive intercourse. Proctitis symptoms include rectal mucopurulent discharge, pain on defecation, constipation, and tenesmus.

Disseminated Disease: Spread of infection from the primary site of inoculation to other parts of

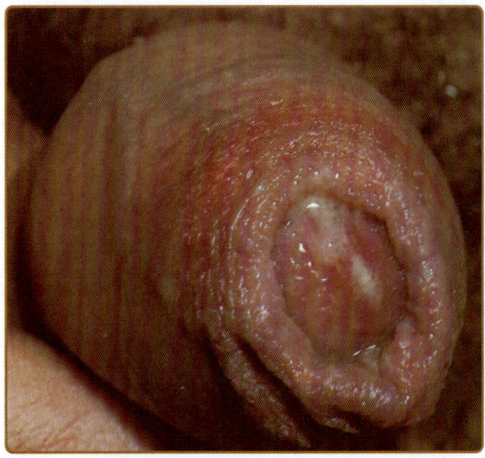

Figure 175-3 Acute gonorrhea in an uncircumcised male. There is a purulent discharge from the urethra and concomitant inflammation of the prepuce and glans. (Used with permission from Dr. Ted Rosen.)

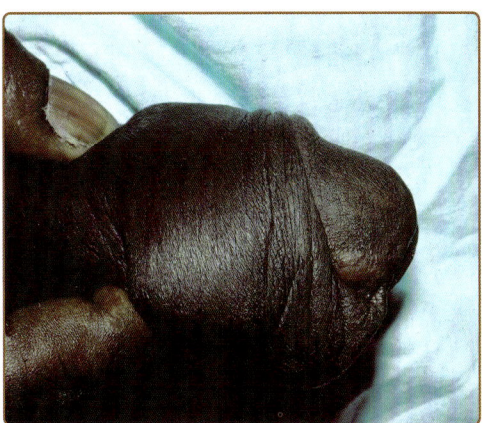

Figure 175-4 Swelling of the distal shaft characterizes "bull head clap," which is actually a manifestation of urethral gonococcal infection. (Used with permission from Dr. Ted Rosen.)

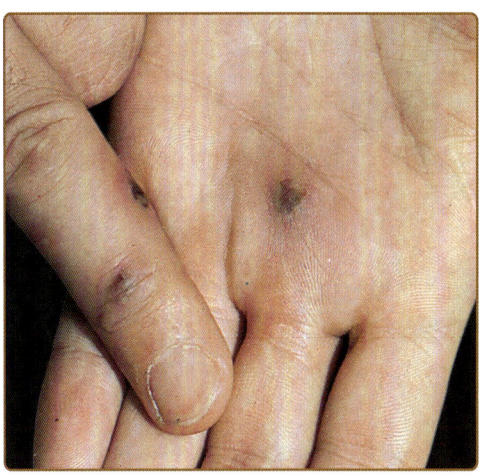

Figure 175-5 Disseminated gonococcal infection. Tender, hemorrhagic, and necrotic pustules on the fingers and palms. (Used with permission from Dr. Ted Rosen.)

the body through the bloodstream leads to disseminated gonococcal infection (DGI), also known as gonococcemia. Disseminated disease occurs in 0.5% to 3% of cases and is associated with a classic triad of dermatitis, migratory polyarthritis, and tenosynovitis. Skin findings consist of small- to medium-sized macules or, most typically, hemorrhagic vesicopustules on an erythematous base located on palms and soles (Fig. 175-5) or on the trunk and elsewhere on the extremities. Skin lesions may develop necrotic centers. The concurrence of some degree of hemorrhage and necrosis led to the term "gun metal gray" to describe the cutaneous lesions of DGI. On the palms and soles, lesions may be tender, but in other sites, they tend to be both nonpruritic and painless. Skin lesions disappear after appropriate treatment has been administered. Cutaneous lesions may be present in 40% to 70% of cases of disseminated disease. Histologically, perivascular neutrophilia, dermal vasculitis, and epidermal neutrophil infiltration may be seen.

NONCUTANEOUS FINDINGS

Pharyngitis: Pharyngitis caused by N. gonorrhoeae was once thought to be rare. However, the common practice of fellatio among heterosexual adolescents and young adults, as well as among MSM, often in lieu of penetrative intercourse, has made pharyngeal gonorrhea much more common.[9] It is estimated that in adolescent women, 11% to 26% of cases of gonorrhea are composed solely of asymptomatic pharyngeal infection.[9] Although it may be asymptomatic, pharyngeal disease may serve as a source for disseminated gonococcal disease. When present, symptoms range from cervical lymphadenopathy and mild to moderate pharyngeal erythema to severe ulceration with pseudomembrane formation.[10]

Pelvic Inflammatory Disease: Organisms may invade the upper genital tract, including the uterus, fallopian tubes, and ovaries, resulting in pelvic inflammatory disease (PID). PID occurs in about 10% to 40% of uncomplicated gonorrheal infections in women and is characterized by fever, lower abdominal pain, back pain, vomiting, vaginal bleeding, dyspareunia, and adnexal or cervical tenderness during movement associated with a pelvic examination. Sequelae of untreated infection include tubo-ovarian abscesses, subsequent ectopic pregnancies, chronic pelvic pain, and infertility caused by chronic inflammation with resultant scarring. Symptoms tend to occur or worsen at the time of menses and cannot be distinguished from nongonococcal causes.[11,12] Fitz-Hugh–Curtis syndrome, involving inflammation of the liver capsule, is associated with genitourinary tract infection and may be present in up to one fourth of women with PID caused by either N. gonorrhoeae or C. trachomatis. Presenting symptoms include right upper quadrant pain and tenderness with abnormal liver function test results.[13] This syndrome must be distinguished from acute viral hepatitis.

Disseminated Disease: Tenosynovitis is defined as pain and swelling of the synovium, or a fluid-filled capsule that surrounds a tendon. With regards to the arthritis seen in disseminated disease, pain and swelling may occur in a single joint or in multiple joints asymmetrically. Whereas true septic arthritis caused by gonorrhea is more typically monoarticular or pauciarticular, polyarticular disease is most often associated with active bacteremia.[14] Neisseria meningitidis infection is highly associated with meningitis, but N. gonorrhoeae infection can also rarely lead to meningitis in disseminated disease. Gonococcal meningitis tends to be less severe than meningococcal meningitis because several cases in the literature describe patients who spontaneously recovered without treatment.[15] Gonococcal endocarditis represents a rare complication of disseminated disease, affecting 1% to 2% of those with disseminated gonococcus. Vegetations preferentially affect the aortic valve in young male patients with no prior history of cardiac or valvular disease. Gonococcal endocarditis is a serious complication that often fails antimicrobial therapy and requires surgical intervention in approximately 50% of cases and carries a mortality rate of up to 19%.[16]

Newborns and Children: Neonates may acquire *N. gonorrhoeae* during passage through the birth canal from contact with infected secretions. Such ocular infections are known as ophthalmia neonatorum and are characterized by profuse, purulent ocular discharge[17] and can lead to severe corneal perforation or scarring. Most states, by law, require the prophylactic use of silver nitrate drops, erythromycin, or tetracycline ophthalmic ointment for prevention of ophthalmia neonatorum (Table 175-1). However, the efficacy of prophylactic ocular antibiotics has been recently questioned, and its use in low-risk patient populations may someday be discontinued.[18] Pharyngeal or genital gonococcal infection in children is often a sign of sexual abuse and warrants further investigation.[17]

COMPLICATIONS

Permanent sequelae of gonococcal infection in women may be infertility and increased risk of ectopic pregnancy as a result of untreated PID. Untreated DGI can lead to septic arthritis, yielding permanent joint damage. Meningitis and endocarditis are rare manifestations of DGI, which can lead to death or permanent disability caused by central nervous system or cardiac damage. Neonatal infection can lead to growth retardation, low birth weight, prematurity, blindness, and sometimes even infant death.[19]

ETIOLOGY AND PATHOGENESIS

Gonorrhea is a bacterial infection caused by *N. gonorrhoeae*, a gram-negative, aerobic coccus-shaped bacterium transmitted via mucosal secretions. Pathogenesis involves bacterial attachment to columnar epithelial cells via pili or fimbriae. The most common sites of attachment include the mucosal cells of the male and female urogenital tracts.

TABLE 175-1
Prophylaxis for Gonococcal Infection in Neonates

- Erythromycin 0.5% ophthalmic ointment to both eyes immediately after birth
  Or
- Ceftriaxone 25–50 mg/kg IV or IM in a single dose, not to exceed 125 mg

IM, intramuscular; IV, intravenous.

Outer membrane proteins, PilC and Opa, on the bacteria aid in attachment and local invasion. Invasion is mediated by bacterial adhesins and sphingomyelinase, which contribute to the process of endocytosis. Gonococci also induce upregulated target cell integrins, which prevent mucosal cell shedding, a natural defense mechanism. Certain gonococcal strains produce immunoglobulin A proteases that cleave the heavy chain of the human immunoglobulin and block the host's normal bactericidal immune response. When inside the cell, the organism undergoes replication and can grow in both aerobic and anaerobic environments. After cellular invasion, the organism replicates and proliferates locally, inducing an inflammatory response. Outside the cell, the bacteria are susceptible to temperature changes, ultraviolet light, drying, and other environmental factors. The outer membrane contains lipooligosaccharide endotoxin, which is released by the bacteria during periods of rapid growth and contributes to its pathogenesis in disseminated infection. Delays in proper antibiotic treatment, physiologic changes in host defenses, resistance to immune responses, and highly virulent strains of bacteria contribute to hematogenous spread and disseminated infection. Humans are the only natural hosts of *N. gonorrhoeae*.[20]

RISK FACTORS

The prevalence of gonococcal infection amongst patient populations considered high risk varies by geographic location within the United States. Risk factors of infection include having multiple sex partners; sex partners with known sexually transmitted infections (STIs); engaging in unprotected oral, vaginal, or anal intercourse; and engaging in other risky sexual practices such as exchanging sex for money or drugs.[5] With respect to other STIs being a risk factor, there is frequent coinfection of patients with both *N. gonorrhoeae* and *C. trachomatis*. Patients with HIV are also at increased risk for other STIs, including gonorrhea. Studies have examined factors that may facilitate spread of asymptomatic gonococcal infection, including pregnancy, viral hepatitis, menstruation, and alcoholism.[21]

DIAGNOSIS

LABORATORY TESTING

Syndromic treatment is widely regarded as unacceptable practice because a majority of gonococcal infections are asymptomatic.[19] Because of high specificity (>99%) and sensitivity (>95%), a Gram stain of a urethral specimen that demonstrates polymorphonuclear leukocytes with intracellular gram-negative diplococci can be considered diagnostic for infection with *N. gonorrhoeae* in symptomatic men.[18] However, because of lower sensitivity, a negative Gram stain result cannot be considered sufficient for ruling out gonococcal infection in asymptomatic men at high risk for infection. In contrast to urethral Gram stains, the sensitivity of Gram stain in endocervical swabs is less than 35% and should not be used a screening tool in women.[18] Vaginal specimens are never recommended for diagnostic purposes because the vaginal mucosa resists gonococcal invasion.

Bacterial culture has been the "gold standard" diagnostic test for years, although newer and more specific tests are now being widely used. Culturing *N. gonorrhoeae* requires media containing heme, nicotinamide adenine dinucleotide, yeast extract, carbon dioxide, and other supplements required for isolation. Culture can be performed on modified Thayer-Martin medium. In men, culture is performed on secretions or urethral swabs. Endocervical and endourethral specimens for culture yield accurate results in women. Cultures on pharyngeal and rectal swabs may also be performed if infection is suspected in these areas.

There is a growing trend among health departments and STI clinics to use nucleic acid amplification tests (NAATs) to provide more rapid diagnosis. These tests use methods such as polymerase chain reaction (PCR); transcription-mediated amplification; and strand displacement amplification on urine, urethral, pharyngeal, or rectal samples. Overall, NAATs are highly sensitive and specific and may be able to detect even the presence of one organism, and some can provide point of care testing with rapid turnaround time in 30 to 60 minutes.[19] However, there is much variability in the cost, sensitivity, and indicated anatomic testing sites, so these tests are subject to ongoing controversy.[20] In addition, diagnosis via any nonculture method does not allow for antibiotic sensitivity testing.

In DGI, cultures, and if available, NAAT, should be done on blood, joint fluid, and skin lesions. Synovial fluid from affected joints must be analyzed for cell count, Gram stain, and culture. Of necessity, diagnosis may rely on clinical suspicion and pertinent findings because tests for DGI yield positive results only in a small number of cases.

inform CDC recommendations regarding treating for gonococcal infections. Strains of *N. gonorrhoeae* with increasing resistance to cefixime increased in 2009 and 2010 and subsequently decreased in 2012 and 2013 after the CDC changed its treatment recommendations to dual therapy. The most current CDC guidelines for first-line treatment of patients with *N. gonorrhoeae* are a combination of ceftriaxone and azithromycin.[22] Of concern are more recent studies that show emerging gonococcal isolates resistant to azithromycin in some areas of Europe.[23] About 10% to 30% of people with gonococcal infection are coinfected with *Chlamydia*. Table 175-2 shows current CDC recommendations, as revised in 2015, for uncomplicated cervical, urethral, pharyngeal, and rectal gonococcal infections.[5] Because of the increased prevalence of antimicrobial resistance of tetracyclines, fluoroquinolones, and penicillin, these antibiotics are not recommended for the routine treatment of any gonococcal infections.[24]

Studies show that provider adherence to current CDC treatment recommendations varies between 76% and 88%, with two main areas of nonadherence identified as lack of dual therapy and incorrect dosing. Only about one third of patients had appropriate posttreatment follow-up, and there is large variation in the percentage of partners who receive treatment.[25]

Patients with DGI may require hospitalization caused by septic arthritis, meningitis, or endocarditis. The recommended regimen for DGI affecting the joints is ceftriaxone, 1 g intramuscularly (IM) or intravenously (IV) every 24 hours, continuing for 7 days. The CDC also recommends a single dose of azithromycin 1 g by mouth. The treatment is similar for gonococcal meningitis and endocarditis, but the ceftriaxone is dosed as 1 to 2 g IV every 12 to 24 hours for 10 to 14 days, as well as the single 1 g of azithromycin orally (Table 175-3). Therapy for gonococcal infections in neonates is shown in Table 175-4. Gonococcal ophthalmia neonatorum should be treated with ceftriaxone, 25 to 50 mg/kg IV or IM, not to exceed 125 mg in a single dose. For treatment regimens for

PROGNOSIS AND CLINICAL COURSE

The prognosis is excellent if infection is treated early with appropriate antibiotics. Previously treated gonococcal infection does not reduce the risk of reinfection. DGI has a good prognosis if treated appropriately and before permanent damage to joints or organs occurs.

TREATMENT

The Gonococcal Isolate Surveillance Project was established in 1986 by the CDC with the purpose of tracking antimicrobial susceptibilities to *N. gonorrhoeae* strains in the United States. These data have been used to help

TABLE 175-2
Treatment of Localized, Uncomplicated Gonococcal Infection of the Cervix, Rectum, Pharynx, or Urethra (2015 CDC Guidelines)

First-Line Treatment
- Ceftriaxone 250 mg IM single dose *plus*
- Azithromycin 1 g PO single dose

Alternative Therapy
- Cefixime 400 mg PO single dose *plus*
- Azithromycin 1 g PO single dose

Single-dose injectable cephalosporin regimens (other than ceftriaxone 250 mg IM) that are safe and generally effective against uncomplicated urogenital and anorectal gonococcal infections include ceftizoxime (500 mg IM), cefoxitin (2 g IM with probenecid 1 g PO), and cefotaxime (500 mg IM)

IM, intramuscular; IV, intravenous; PO, oral.

TABLE 175-3
Treatment of Disseminated Gonococcal Infection

Treatment of Arthritis and Arthritis-Dermatitis Syndrome
- Ceftriaxone 1 g IV every 24 hours for 7 days *plus*
- Azithromycin 1 g PO single dose

Treatment of Meningitis and Endocarditis
- Ceftriaxone 1–2 g IV every 12–24 hours for 10–14 days *plus*
- Azithromycin 1 g PO single dose

IV, intravenous; PO, oral.

PID and epididymitis, readers are referred to the CDC's website.[5]

Sexual partners of those found to have gonococcal infections should be evaluated. However, because this is not always feasible, empiric treatment may be advisable. In general, treatment of partners of female or heterosexual male patients diagnosed with gonorrhea empirically is as or more effective than the traditional reliance on referral, testing, and as-needed treatment.[21] One way of doing this is via expedited partner therapy (having the index patient deliver therapy to the partner); such expedited therapy decreases the risk of persistent or recurrent infection in the index patient.[26] No studies have evaluated empiric treatment of gonorrhea (or chlamydia) in MSM. State laws vary with regard to expedited partner therapy and must be considered. Moreover, this type of empiric therapy misses the opportunity to counsel partners and treat comorbid disease when detected.

CONTRAINDICATIONS

Allergic reactions are uncommon with third-generation cephalosporins. Use of ceftriaxone or cefixime is contraindicated in persons with a history of an immunoglobulin (Ig) E–mediated penicillin allergy. Other regimens include dual treatment with single doses of oral gemifloxacin 320 mg plus oral azithromycin 2 g or dual treatment with single doses of intramuscular gentamicin 240 mg plus oral azithromycin 2 g. Providers treating persons with cephalosporin or IgE-mediated penicillin allergy should consult an infectious disease specialist.

TABLE 175-4
Treatment of Gonococcal Infection in Neonates

- Ceftriaxone, 25–50 mg/kg/day IV or IM in a single daily dose for 7 days or for 10–14 days if meningitis is documented
  Or
- Cefotaxime, 25 mg/kg IV or IM every 12 hours for 7 days, or for 10–14 days if meningitis is documented

IM, intramuscular; IV, intravenous.

SCREENING RECOMMENDATIONS

The CDC currently recommends yearly screening of men who engage in receptive anal intercourse, all sexually active women younger than 25 years old, any woman with a new sex partner, multiple sex partners, or a sex partner with a known STI. Other at-risk populations include those who are not in monogamous relationships, have a current or past history of STIs, or who exchange sex for money or drugs.[5]

Epidemiologic studies have indicated most providers screen for gonococcal infection with pharyngeal or urethral swabs, but far fewer providers do anal screening. One study looking at gonococcal screening results of more than 52,000 men in the United States between January 2013 and May 2015 showed that only about 4% of patients had a rectal screen, but of those who underwent rectal screening, 17% had a positive test result.[27] Other studies have shown that there is a percentage of patients who only have extragenital infection and therefore would be missed if they did not receive pharyngeal or anal testing. Any patient who is being tested for gonococcal infection should also undergo testing for other STIs, especially chlamydia, given it high rate of coinfection and for HIV.[28]

GENITAL MYCOPLASMAS

INTRODUCTION

Mycoplasma are the smallest free-living, self-replicating bacteria. These organisms developed by degenerative evolution from lactobacilli and lack a cell wall (Fig. 175-6). These organisms routinely colonize the respiratory and urogenital tracts of humans. *Mycoplasma* spp. and other *Ureaplasma* spp. are referred to as the genital mycoplasmal organisms and may be found in the lower urogenital tracts of sexually active adults. Seven mycoplasmal strains have

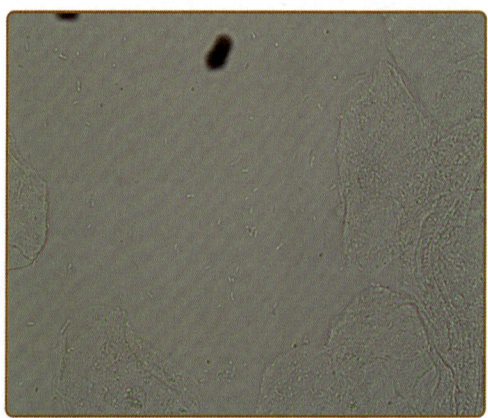

Figure 175-6 Lactobacilli from genital mycoplasma infection. (Used with permission from Dr. Libby Edwards.)

been isolated from the genital tract. The most common strains include *Mycoplasma hominis* and *Mycoplasma genitalium*. *M. genitalium* was identified first in the 1980s and is now thought to be responsible for 30% of persistent urethritis.[29] Less common strains include *Mycoplasma fermentans*, *Mycoplasma penetrans*, *Mycoplasma pneumoniae*, *Mycoplasma primatum*, and *Mycoplasma spermatophilum*.[30]

EPIDEMIOLOGY

The global prevalence of *M. genitalium* among all sexually active women ranges from 1% to 6.4%. About 40% to 80% of sexually active women in the United States have urogenital colonization with *Ureaplasma* organisms. *M. hominis* has also been isolated in 20% to 50% of sexually active women. Rates of colonization tend to be lower in men, except in the setting of HIV coinfection. The rates of colonization in children and nonsexually active adults are even lower. Newborns may be infected by passage through the birth canal of an infected mother. Although the most common cause of symptomatic non-gonococcal urethritis (NGU) remains *Chlamydia* spp., the genital mycoplasmas also cause this disorder. *Ureaplasma* organisms have been found to be the cause of more than 20% of nonchlamydial NGU, and *M. genitalium* accounts for 10% to 20% of cases of nonchlamydial NGU.[31] The detection of *M. hominis* in a urethral smear is irrelevant to NGU because numerous studies have isolated *M. hominis* independently of symptoms and in most cases is thought to be a commensal organism with low virulence.[32]

CLINICAL FEATURES

CUTANEOUS FINDINGS

Cutaneous Disease (Men): The most common cutaneous disease in men with mycoplasma infection is urethritis, although is less commonly implicated than gonococcal and chlamydial urethritis. Urethritis presents with dysuria, urethral pain and pruritus, and a mucopurulent discharge. Occasionally, men have urethral discharge but are otherwise asymptomatic. Physical findings and symptomatology are indistinguishable from those seen with chlamydial NGU.

Cutaneous Disease (Women): The most common cutaneous disease in women with mycoplasma infection is cervicitis, although is less commonly implicated than gonococcal and chlamydial cervicitis. Cervicitis presents with mucopurulent exudate visible in the endocervical canal, a friable cervical os that bleeds with minimal manipulation, abnormal vaginal discharge, and intermenstrual vaginal bleeding.[29]

NONCUTANEOUS FINDINGS

As with gonorrhea and chlamydia, various genital mycoplasmas infections can result in noncutaneous disease such as urethritis, cervicitis, PID, endometritis, salpingitis, and chorioamnionitis. Other species can cause respiratory infection, septic arthritis, surgical wound infections, neonatal pneumonia, and meningitis. Infection with these organisms needs to be considered if workup results for the more commonly isolated organisms are negative. There is no clear relationship between genital mycoplasma and epididymitis or prostatitis. In cases of bacterial vaginitis, coinfection with *Mycoplasma* spp. (particularly *M. hominis*) may worsen the condition.

COMPLICATIONS

Invasion by different species of *Mycoplasma* and *Ureaplasma* spp. can cause disseminated disease, especially in immunocompromised hosts who have deficiencies in antibody production. Disseminated disease may result in respiratory tract invasion, osteomyelitis, or infectious arthritis. Bacteremia as a result of *M. hominis* has been shown after renal transplantation. *M. hominis* has also been found in surgical wound infections, pericardial effusions, prosthetic heart valves, and subcutaneous abscesses, as well as in synovial fluid of people with rheumatoid arthritis.

There is an increased frequency of *M. hominis* and *Ureaplasma* spp. in cervical cultures from women who are unable to conceive, suggesting a causative role in infertility. The role of *M. genitalium* in infertility is not well studied in this regard. Although this may represent an overinterpretation, for some cases of premature rupture of the fetal membranes, preterm labor, intraamniotic infection, and chorioamnionitis, the presence of genital mycoplasmas suggests that these organisms may play a role in the pathogenesis of these complications of pregnancy.[33] *Ureaplasma* spp. and *M. hominis* have been isolated from the blood of febrile women postpartum and postabortion. Some studies have suggested infection with *M. genitalium* may facilitate coinfection with another sexually transmitted pathogen.[34] It is not currently known if infection with *M. genitalium* leads to male infertility or can be responsible for proctitis from anal infection.

ETIOLOGY AND PATHOGENESIS

The bacteria can attach to and penetrate epithelial cells by adhesion proteins on the back of the cell body. The structure and function of adhesion proteins for *M. genitalium* (P110 and P140) and *M. hominis* (P100) are well characterized. The abundance of urea to metabolize predisposes *Ureaplasma* spp. to the urinary tract. The specific adhesion proteins for *Ureaplasma* spp. are still unknown. All genital mycoplasmas multiply as parasites because they are unable to complete various metabolic reactions. Cholesterol is required for growth and is taken from the epithelial cell; *Ureaplasma* spp. need urea as well. Because of their parasitic nature and specific nutritional requirements, *Mycoplasma* spp. tend to remain localized to mucosal surfaces. Disseminated infection is rare and tends to occur only in immunocompromised hosts or in cases of epithelium severely traumatized by instrumentation.

RISK FACTORS

Risk factors for genital mycoplasmas include multiple partners, younger age, ethnic minority, presence of other STIs, and past or present bacterial vaginosis (BV).

DIAGNOSIS

LABORATORY TESTING

Mycoplasmas are slow-growing organisms, and culture can take up to 6 months to speciate. Culture specimens should be obtained from the urethra or first voided urine in men and from the cervix, urethra, and vagina in women. *M. hominis* and *U. urealyticum* can be cultured on special media, which is enriched with horse serum as a nutrient source. Because of this, the preferred method of testing involves NAAT. First-voided urine is actually the preferred specimen to submit when the reference laboratory plans to use NAAT.[30] There is currently no Food and Drug Administration (FDA)–approved diagnostic laboratory test for detection of Mycoplasma spp. The standard of care is empiric treatment for mycoplasma infection in cases of persistent or recurrent urethritis, cervicitis, and PID.[29]

Laboratory tests for genital mycoplasmas may be limited because most specimens must be sent to reference laboratories. PCR assay is required to detect *M. genitalium* and may also optionally be used by laboratories to identify other *Mycoplasma* spp. Although various commercial tests are available for antibodies (complement-binding reaction [CBR], hemagglutination, immunofluorescence), the mere detection of *Mycoplasma* antibodies is not sufficient to verify infection because of the possibility of prior colonization and cross reactions. Increased titer levels may be a sign of acute infection. Because *Mycoplasma* spp. do not possess a cell wall, Gram stain will not detect these organisms.

PROGNOSIS AND CLINICAL COURSE

The prognosis in immunocompetent hosts is excellent with prompt diagnosis and appropriate treatment.

TABLE 175-5
Treatment of Mycoplasma Urethritis

- Azithromycin 1 g PO single dose *or*
- Azithromycin 500 mg PO on day 1 + 250 mg PO for 4 days Or
- Moxifloxacin 400 mg/day for 7–14 days

PO, oral.

TREATMENT

Because these organisms lack a cell wall, they are inherently resistant to β-lactam and cephalosporin antibiotics because these drugs target cell wall synthesis. Urethritis is often treated with 7 days of doxycycline, but this only provides effective treatment in about one third of mycoplasma infections. A single high dose of azithromycin or a 5-day course of azithromycin provides significantly higher cure rates than doxycycline. Patients who fail azithromycin usually have a macrolide-resistant strain of mycoplasma, and in some areas of the world, these emerging resistant strains can represent up to 50% of isolates. In macrolide-resistant mycoplasma infection, consider a course of oral moxifloxacin and retesting of patients 3 to 4 weeks after therapy completion to assess for clearance (Table 175-5).[35]

Current CDC guidelines for empiric treatment of PID do not recommend antibiotics that are effective against mycoplasma, particularly *M. genitalium*. If *M. genitalium* is isolated or if the patient does not respond to treatment on standard PID regimens, the CDC recommends consideration of treatment with moxifloxacin 400 mg/day for 14 days.[34]

SCREENING RECOMMENDATIONS

The CDC does not currently recommend routine screening for mycoplasma infection, and there are no FDA-approved diagnostic screening tests available in the United States.

CHLAMYDIA

INTRODUCTION

Chlamydia is a common STI that has implications in a variety of organ systems. The disease primary affects the mucous membranes of the ophthalmic, genitourinary, and respiratory systems. Depending on the organ system affected, there are clinically distinct manifestations that occur. However, common themes, including an enduring nature and inflammatory sequelae, are noted throughout each infection.[36] This chapter highlights some of those manifestations but focuses mainly on genitourinary infections.

EPIDEMIOLOGY

In the United States, C. trachomatis remains the most frequently reported STI, with more than 1.4 million cases reported in 2012.[37] The National Health and Nutrition Examination Survey (NHANES) is used by the CDC to monitor the population prevalence of chlamydial infections.[37] According to NHANES data, the overall prevalence of chlamydia infections between 2007 and 2012 was 1.7% (95% confidence interval [CI], 1.4%–2.0%), and the highest prevalence was seen in non-Hispanic blacks (5.2%).[37] Prevalence among US patients with at least two sexual partners was 3.2% (CI, 2.2%–4.2%).[37] In comparison, the prevalence of chlamydia infections in patients with one sexual partner was 1.4% (CI, 1.1%–1.7%).[37] The prevalence of chlamydia in sexually active women is inversely proportional to age, with the highest rates of infection occurring between the ages of 14 and 24 years.[37] Additionally, 1 in 7 non-Hispanic black women and 1 in 22 Mexican American women between the ages of 14 to 24 years were infected with chlamydia compared with 1 in 55 non-Hispanic white women.[37] The reason for such racial disparities is unknown but may be due to differences in sexual networks, decreased access to care, and untimely partner treatment.

CLINICAL FEATURES

CUTANEOUS FINDINGS

The clinical manifestations of C. trachomatis infections vary based on the site of involvement, the sex and age of the patient, and the serovar responsible for infection. Urogenital infections are the most common manifestations of C. trachomatis infections. The most common site of infection in men is the urethra. In comparison, the urethra and cervix are the most common sites in women.[37] In men, urethritis is the most common manifestation of infection and is characterized by dysuria and a watery or mucoid discharge from the urethra. The discharge may be scant, and some patients may only complain of stained underwear. In comparison, the discharge in gonococcal urethritis is more purulent and profuse. However, there is considerable clinical overlap, and neither the nature of the discharge nor the severity of accompanying dysuria can be reliably used to make a specific diagnosis. C. trachomatis may also cause epididymitis in males and proctitis in both sexes. C. trachomatis and N. gonorrhoeae are the most common causes of epididymitis in male patients younger than 35 years of age.[36] Epididymitis presents as unilateral testicular pain and swelling accompanied by dysuria and fever. Proctitis is caused by direct inoculation of serovars D to K and presents as pruritus, pain, and a mucopurulent discharge. The infection is limited to the rectum and not as severe as proctitis due to serovars L1 to L3 in lymphogranuloma venereum. Cervicitis caused by C. trachomatis is the female counterpart to urethritis in men. The classic presentation is mucopurulent cervicitis with discharge from the cervical os. However, the majority of women with urogenital C. trachomatis infections are asymptomatic. Patients may complain of vaginal discharge, bleeding, or abdominal pain. If dysuria is present, it may indicate concomitant urethritis.

COMPLICATIONS

PID is a complication of C. trachomatis infection as well as gonococcal infections. PID is the overarching clinical presentation encompassing combinations of endometritis, salpingitis, and peritonitis. The diagnosis of acute PID is typically clinical, and patients present with fever; lower abdominal pain; vomiting; and cervical, uterine, and adnexal motion tenderness. Patients may also have an indolent or "silent" form of the disease with similar degrees of inflammation. The sequelae of both forms of PID include infertility, ectopic pregnancy, and chronic pelvic pain resulting from inflammation and scarring.

Perinatal infections may result in conjunctivitis and pneumonia. Neonatal conjunctivitis or ophthalmia neonatorum is acquired during birth from an infected birth canal. It may result from either gonorrhea or chlamydia infections. It typically presents 1 to 2 weeks after birth and is characterized by a purulent ocular discharge with erythema and swelling of the eyelids. Neonatal chlamydial pneumonia typically presents within 8 weeks of birth and is characterized by nasal symptoms, tachypnea, and cough. The cough is staccato in nature, and patients are typically symptomatic for at least 3 weeks before presentation. Cultures positive for C. trachomatis can be obtained from nasopharyngeal specimens. Wheezing is typically absent. However, a peripheral eosinophilia may be observed, and patients may be prone to developing asthma later in life.

Genital infections with C. trachomatis may also result in reactive arthritis. Reactive arthritis is an immune-mediated arthritis resulting from a mucosal infection, urethritis in the case of chlamydia, with concomitant conjunctivitis and cutaneous lesions involving the genitals. Individuals with the histocompatibility marker HLA-B27 are at increased risk of developing reactive arthritis.

ETIOLOGY AND PATHOGENESIS

RISK FACTORS

C. trachomatis is a nonmotile, gram-negative, obligate intracellular bacteria that replicates within human cells. Its replication is characterized by a two-phase life cycle that begins with an infectious form known as the elementary body (EB). The EB enters the host epithelial cell via endocytosis, resulting in the formation of a chlamydial inclusion. The Greek-derived word *chlamys* means "cloak draped around the shoulder." This refers to the draping of intracytoplasmic inclusions containing *C. trachomatis* around the nucleus of an infected cell. Six to 8 hours after entry, the EB converts into the reticulate body (RB), which replicates via binary fission. The RBs are then converted back into EBs and released from the cell to infect other cells. Recently, extrusion of chlamydial inclusions with subsequent phagocytosis by macrophages has been implicated as a means of immune evasion and ultimately dissemination of infectious particles.[38]

C. trachomatis strains are classified into 15 serovars with different clinical presentations. Serovars A through C cause chronic conjunctivitis and trachoma and are endemic in Africa and Asia, D through K cause urogenital tract infections, and L1 though L3 cause lymphogranuloma venereum. The target cells of *C. trachomatis* include the epithelial cells of the endocervix, conjunctiva, urethra, rectum, and epididymis. Infected cells release interleukin-8 and other proinflammatory cytokines that recruit neutrophils to the site of infection. This is followed by lymphocytes, macrophages, plasma cells, and eosinophils. Upon resolution, fibrosis and scarring ensue, which are increased in response to repeated infections. Transmission is through oral, anal, or vaginal intercourse with symptoms occurring 1 to 3 weeks after exposure. Coinfection with other STDs occurs frequently, most commonly with gonorrhea. Additionally, there is an association between positive *C. trachomatis* testing and the presence of high-risk human papilloma virus (HPV).[39] Various serotypes have been associated with an increased risk of cervical squamous cell carcinoma, suggesting that *Chlamydia* spp. may act as a cofactor with oncogenic, high-risk HPV in neoplastic transformation.[40,41]

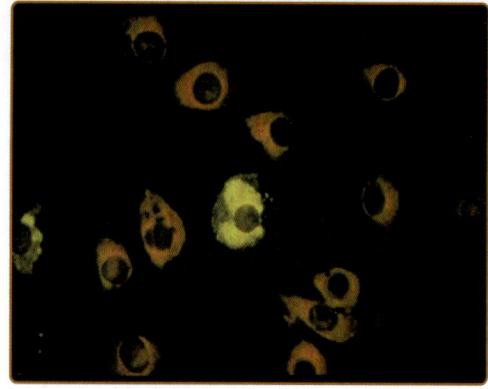

Figure 175-7 Detection of *Chlamydia trachomatis* by direct immunofluorescence with monoclonal antibodies. (Used with permission from Dr. Ted Rosen.)

DIAGNOSIS

Traditionally, chlamydial infection was diagnosed by cell culture with specimens obtained from the endocervix, urethra, rectum, or conjunctiva, as indicated. Modern techniques have largely replaced this method of diagnosis. Specifically, the nucleic acid amplification test (NAAT) is the preferred method of testing (Fig. 175-7). Although specific symptoms may suggest infection with *C. trachomatis*, laboratory confirmation is necessary for diagnosis. Urogenital infections may be diagnosed by collecting endocervical or vagina specimens in women, urethral specimens in men, or a first-catch urine specimen in either sex. NAATs are the most sensitive tests available and are almost as specific as culture. They are approved by the FDA for the diagnosis of urogenital infections caused by *C. trachomatis*. Although rectal and oropharyngeal specimens may be obtained, NAATs are not FDA approved for the diagnosis of infection at such sites. NAATs offer some advantages over prior diagnostic strategies in that they are relatively noninvasive and easy to perform. However, they are expensive and unable to differentiate among different serovars of *C. trachomatis*. Additionally, they only detect the DNA or RNA of chlamydial species and may remain positive up to 3 weeks after treatment.[42]

DIFFERENTIAL DIAGNOSIS

Table 175-6 shows the differential diagnosis for all mucosal-oriented venereal diseases.

TABLE 175-6
Differential Diagnosis for All Mucosal-Based Venereal Diseases

LOCALIZED	SYSTEMIC	ALWAYS RULE OUT
- Urinary tract infection	- Septic arthritis	- Tubo-ovarian abscess
- Chlamydia	- Rheumatoid arthritis	- Ectopic pregnancy
- Gonorrhea	- Psoriatic arthritis	- Pregnancy
- Pelvic inflammatory disease	- Bowel-bypass syndrome	- Appendicitis
- Trichomoniasis	- Hepatitis B and C	- Meningococcemia
- Herpes simplex virus	- Behçet disease	- Coinfection with syphilis and HIV
- Bacterial vaginosis	- Reiter syndrome	- Sexual abuse (in children)
- Vaginitis	- Lyme disease	
- Endometriosis	- Rheumatic fever	
- Mycoplasmal infection		
- Orchitis and epididymitis		
- Lymphatic occlusion caused by pelvic neoplasm		

CLINICAL COURSE, PROGNOSIS, AND MANAGEMENT

The treatment of infection due to *C. trachomatis* is summarized in Table 175-7. The first-line treatment of chlamydial infections are doxycycline 100 mg orally twice daily for 7 days or azithromycin given orally as a single 1-g dose.[37] Single-dose therapy with azithromycin is advantageous because it can be administered as directly observed therapy minimizing issues with adherence and follow-up. In comparison with doxycycline, single-dose therapy with azithromycin appears to be equally effective. This was demonstrated in a meta-analysis of the treatment of chlamydial infections in which azithromycin provided a 97% cure rate compared with a 98% cure rate with doxycycline.[43] There are studies that question the efficacy of azithromycin, particularly when rectal infection is present.[44,45] In a recent study of men who had sex with women, the failure rate of single-dose azithromycin was 12.8%.[46] The failure rate was 6.2% when adjusted for false positives and reinfection.[46]

PREVENTION AND SCREENING

If the symptoms persist or there is concern for reinfection, repeat testing can be indicated. However, it should be performed at least 3 weeks after therapy if NAAT is used to prevent false-positive results. In a study comparing pregnant and nonpregnant women with chlamydial infections, NAAT test results after single-dose treatment were negative in all women at 4 weeks.[47] Additionally, routine testing for cure is not recommended in the early treatment period unless the aforementioned criteria are met, lack of adherence to therapy is suspected, or the patient is pregnant. It is recommended that both men and women should be retested at 3 months or within at least 1 year of treatment. Notably, most recurrences are the result of reinfection rather than treatment failure. As a result, the CDC recommends abstinence from sexual activity until the patient and all partners are treated.[37] Additionally, patients are often coinfected with other STIs and should be tested for gonorrhea, HIV, and syphilis.

Early treatment with appropriate antibiotic therapy results in excellent prognosis and reduces the risk of long-term complications such as infertility from PID. The CDC recommends annual screening of all sexually active women younger than the age of 25 years and for older women with risk factors (eg, those who have a new sex partner or multiple sex partners).[37] The primary goals of screening are to detect infection and prevent complications. Similar to early treatment, screening has been shown to decrease the chance of developing PID.[48,49] Additionally, the CDC recommends annual screening at areas of contact for MSM.[37] A large study of male patients between 15 and 60 years of age indicated that 17.1% of rectal specimens were positive for *N. gonorrhea*, *C. trachomatis*, or both and provides support of these recommendations.[50] Evidence is insufficient to recommend routine screening for *C. trachomatis* in sexually active young men, based on feasibility, efficacy, and cost-effectiveness. However, screening in young men should be considered in high-prevalence clinical settings.[37]

BACTERIAL VAGINOSIS

EPIDEMIOLOGY

Bacterial vaginosis (BV) is the most common vaginal infection in women ages 15 to 44 years. BV occurs in one third of adult women in the United States. It is an unpleasant, mild infection of the vagina caused by bacteria. It is sometimes asymptomatic and self-resolving but can lead to more serious problems. It is estimated that approximately 10% to 30% of pregnant women in the United States may have BV during their pregnancy because of the hormonal changes that occur during this period. BV is twice as common in African American women as in white women.[51] The reasons are not entirely clear. Incidence rates are difficult to determine because of the high prevalence of asymptomatic infection but it is approximately 10% to 25% in patients attending obstetric clinics and as high as 30% to 65% in patients attending STD clinics. Having sex at an early age and new or multiple sex partners are the most common risk factors for BV infection. Others include smoking, pregnancy, use of intrauterine devices, douching, tub bathing (bubble bath), and use of bidet toilets.[52-54] These factors may contribute to the development of BV because of the disruption of normal bacterial flora.

BV may rarely occur in prepubertal or virginal girls and boys. Most of the cases are related to vaginal, oral, and anal sex. Some studies have shown an increased prevalence among women who have sex with women,

TABLE 175-7
Treatment of *Chlamydia* Infection

- Azithromycin, 1 g PO in a single dose
  Or
- Doxycycline, 100 mg PO twice a day for 7 days

Alternative regimens:
- Erythromycin base 500 mg PO, four times daily for 7 days
  Or
- Erythromycin ethylsuccinate 800 mg PO, four times daily for 7 days
  Or
- Ofloxacin 300 mg PO, twice daily for 7 days
  Or
- Levofloxacin 500 mg/day for 7 days

Recommended treatment for pregnant women:
- Azithromycin 1 g PO as a single dose

Recommended treatment for ophthalmia neonatorum:
- Erythromycin base or ethylsuccinate 50 mg/kg/day PO, divided into four doses daily, for 14 days

PO, oral.

perhaps based on transfer of pathogenic vaginal flora related to frequent use of lubricant and shared vaginal sex toys.[55] There is evidence that shows that hormonal contraception (both combined estrogen–progestin and progestin only) is protective against development of BV.

ETIOLOGY AND PATHOGENESIS

BV is a synergistic polymicrobial infection caused by an imbalance of the bacterial flora normally present in the vagina. Although the exact causative pathogen has not been established, it has been observed that there is a corresponding decrease in the population of the lactobacilli species. Lactobacilli are large rod-shaped organisms that help maintain the acidic pH of healthy vaginas and inhibit other anaerobic microorganisms. Normally, lactobacilli are found in high concentrations in healthy vaginas. This change in the population of lactobacilli results in the increase in the pH of the vaginal lumen because of the reduction in the lactic acid production. Apart from the lactic acid, the production of Lactocin and H_2O_2 also contributes to the disease state. In general, the lactobacilli is replaced with the increased population of pathogenic gram-negative anaerobic bacteria such as *Gardnerella vaginalis*; *M. hominis*; *Mycoplasma curtisii*; anaerobic gram-negative rods belonging to the genera *Prevotella*, *Porphyromonas*, and *Bacteroides*; and *Peptostreptococcus* spp.[56,67]

CLINICAL PRESENTATION

The number of asymptomatic infections is as high as 84%.[58] Women with BV report an increased volume of white or gray vaginal discharge and a fishy odor, especially after contact with alkaline semen during intercourse.[59] Vulvovaginal pruritus and inflammation are generally absent or mild. On physical examination, a milky, homogenous vaginal coating may be seen adherent to the vaginal wall. This infection is not common in men; however, the urethras of men whose sexual partners have symptoms of BV are frequently colonized with the same strain of *G. vaginalis*.

DIAGNOSIS

According to the Amsel criteria for diagnosing BV, three of the following four findings must be present:

1. Profuse milky vaginal discharge
2. A positive whiff test result (presence of a fishy odor when secretions are exposed to 10% or 20% potassium hydroxide)
3. A vaginal fluid pH greater than 4.5
4. Presence of clue cells greater than 20% on microscopic examination (Fig. 175-8)

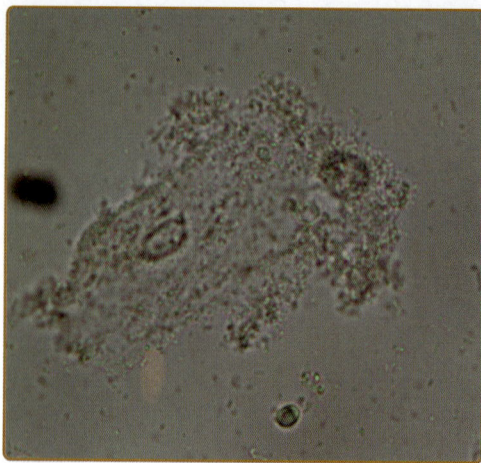

Figure 175-8 Bacterial vaginosis. Clue cells are large epithelial cells covered with bacteria. (Used with permission from Dr. Libby Edwards.)

Clue cells are squamous epithelial cells covered by coccobacilli that give the cytoplasm a ground-glass appearance and obscure the crisp margins of the cell, leaving ragged borders.[38] The presence of clue cells representing at least 20% of the epithelial cells on saline wet mount is the most reliable indicator of BV. Other important considerations are the absence of lactobacilli and no increase in white blood cells.

In the Nugent method, the swab was obtained from the lateral vaginal wall and rolled on a glass slide. This method involves the use of Gram staining to distinguish between the normal bacterial flora of gram-positive rods and lactobacilli from the gram-negative morphotypes seen in BV. Because of the variety of bacterial species, culture is not a reliable diagnostic test. A DNA probe-based test (16SrRNA gene) has a sensitivity of 92.8% and a specificity of 85.7% on a study comparing the utility of microscopic techniques.[60] The AmpliSens Florocenosis/Bacterial vaginosis-FRT multiplex real-time PCR (Florocenosis-BV) assay results in 100% sensitivity compared with Amsel's criteria.[61] The immunochromatographic test, OSOM BVBlue, showed a sensitivity of 100.0%, specificity of 98.3%, positive predictive value of 94.4%, and negative predictive value of 100.0% compared with Gram stain (Nugent's method).[62]

COMPLICATIONS

BV has been shown to be a risk factor in pregnancy for premature deliveries and babies with low birth weight.[63] Having BV makes women more susceptible to acquiring HIV, as well as other STDs such as herpes simplex virus, chlamydia, and gonorrhea.[64] BV may increase the risk of developing a postsurgical infection after procedures such as hysterectomy or dilation and curettage. BV can sometimes cause PID, increasing the risk of infertility.

Studies have produced conflicting data as to whether BV is associated with a higher risk of acquiring cervical intraepithelial neoplasia.[65] There are some studies that have linked BV to postpartum fever, postpartum endometritis, and postabortal infections; however, further studies are needed to investigate the relationship between BV and these complications.[66]

PROGNOSIS AND CLINICAL COURSE

Uncomplicated cases of BV resolve after appropriate treatment. There are reports of cases that may resolve on their own without therapy. Complications are rare, but long-standing or untreated BV may lead to more serious sequelae. Recurrent infections have been reported. Providers should suspect concomitant infections such as candidiasis if symptoms do not resolve after treatment.

TREATMENT

Treatment of patients with BV is summarized in Table 175-8. Treatment in asymptomatic BV is not necessary in women who are not pregnant. The established benefits of therapy for BV in symptomatic nonpregnant women are to (1) relieve vaginal symptoms and signs of infection and (2) reduce the risk for infectious complications after a variety of gynecologic procedures (endometrial biopsy, hysterectomy, hysterosalpingography, placement of an IUD, cesarean section, uterine curettage, and abortion). In pregnant women, treatment of BV also reduces the risk of postpartum infectious complications as well as the risk of preterm labor.[67,78]

Probiotics sometimes are used for BV, mainly to help with repopulation of normal lactobacilli to prevent recurrence.[69] Although the optimal treatment for recurrent disease is not yet established, the recommendation is to use longer courses of medications.

PREVENTION

Given the prevalence of the STIs discussed in this chapter, it is important for clinicians to discuss safe sex practices with all patients, especially patients who fall into one of the high-risk demographic groups. Educating patients on transmission methods, STD complications, and treatment options is critical in raising awareness of these disease entities. The CDC provides comprehensive and unbiased information for both providers and patients. Physicians should be aware of the available screening tests for each STD and the limitations of these tests. Routine screening and empiric treatment in high-risk groups or when there is a high clinical suspicion will aid in reducing transmission rates and disease burden.

ACKNOWLEDGMENTS

The authors thank Dr. Ted Rosen, who was the author of this chapter in the eighth edition.

REFERENCES

1. Higgins J. *The Mirror for Magistrates* as cited in the *Oxford English Dictionary* entry for "clap." 1587.
2. Centers for Disease Control and Prevention. Sexually transmitted diseases in the United States, 2009. http://www.cdc.gov/std/stats09/trends.pdf.
3. Fowler T, Caley M, Johal R, et al. Previous history of gonococcal infection as a risk factor in patients presenting with gonorrhea. *Int J STD AIDS*. 2010;21:277.
4. Nicoletti A. The STD/alcohol connection. *J Pediatr Adolesc Gynecol*. 2010;23:53.
5. Workowski KA, Bolan GA. Sexually transmitted diseases treatment guidelines. *MMWR Recommend Rep*. 2015;64(RR3):1-137.
6. Fang L, Oliver A, Jayaraman GC, et al. Trends in gender disparities between younger and middle-age adults among reported rates of Chlamydia, gonorrhea and infectious syphilis in Canada: findings from 1997dispari *Sex Transm Dis*. 2010;37:18.
7. Rosen T. Unusual presentations of gonorrhea. *J Am Acad Dermatol*. 1982;6:369.
8. Kaul R, Pettengell C, Sheth PM, et al. The genital tract immune milieu: an important determinant of HIV susceptibility and secondary transmission. *J Reprod Immunol*. 2008;77:32.
9. Giannini CM, Kim HK, Mortensen J, et al. Culture of non-genital sites increases the detection of gonorrhea in women. *J Pediatr Adolesc Gynecol*. 2010;23:246.

TABLE 175-8
Treatment of Bacterial Vaginosis

- Metronidazole 500 mg PO twice daily for 7 days
  Or
- Tinidazole 2 g PO once daily for 3 days
  Or
- Metronidazole gel, 075%, 5 g intravaginally once daily for 5 days
  Or
- Clindamycin cream, 5%, 5 g intravaginally once a day for 7 days

In pregnant women:
- Metronidazole 250 mg PO three times daily for 7 days
  Or
- Metronidazole 500 mg PO twice daily for 7 days
  Or
- Clindamycin 300 mg twice daily for 7 days

Alternative regimen:
- Tinidazole 1 g PO once daily for 5 days
  Or
- Metronidazole 2 g PO in a single dose
  Or
- Clindamycin ovules 100 g intravaginally once a day for 3 days

PO, oral.

10. Little JW. Gonorrhea: update. *Oral Surg Oral Med Oral Pathol Oral Radiol Endod*. 2006;101:137.
11. Crossman SH. The challenge of pelvic inflammatory disease. *Am Fam Physician*. 2006;73:859.
12. Judlin P. Current concepts in managing pelvic inflammatory disease. *Curr Opin Infect Dis*. 2010;23:83.
13. Peter NG, Clark LR, Jaeger JR. Fitz-Hugh-Curtis syndrome: a diagnosis to consider in women with right upper quadrant pain. *Cleve Clin J Med*. 2004;71:233.
14. Rice PA. Gonococcal arthritis (disseminated gonococcal infection). *Infect Dis Clin North Am*. 2005;19:853.
15. Knapp JS, Holmes KK. Disseminated gonococcal infections caused by Neisseria gonorrhoeae with unique nutritional requirements. *J Infect Dis*. 1975;132(2):204-208.
16. Shetty A, Ribeiro D, Evans A, et al. Gonococcal endocarditis: a rare complication of a common disease. *J Clin Pathol*. 2004;57(7):780-781.
17. Woods CR. Gonococcal infections in neonates and young children. *Semin Pediatr Infect Dis*. 2005;16:258.
18. Darling EK, McDonald H. A meta-analysis of the efficacy of ocular prophylactic agents used for the prevention of gonococcal and chlamydial ophthalmia neonatorum. *J Midwifery Womens Health*. 2010;55:319.
19. Herbst de Cortina S, Bristow CC, Joseph Davey D, et al. A systematic review of point of care testing for Chlamydia trachomatis, Neisseria gonorrhoeae, and Trichomonas vaginalis. *Infect Dis Obstet Gynecol*. 2016;2016:4386127.
20. Todar K. The pathogenic Neisseriae. In: *Todarer Online Textbook of Bacteriology*. Madison, WI: University of Wisconsin-Madison Department of Bacteriology; 2008.
21. Martin MC, Pérez F, Moreno A, et al. Neisseria gonorrhoeae meningitis in pregnant adolescent. *Emerg Infect Dis*. 2008;14(10):1672-1674.
22. Watson J, Carlile J, Dunn A, et al. Increased gonorrhea cases—Utah, 2009-2014. *MMWR Morb Mortal Wkly Rep*. 2016;65:889-893.
23. Brunner A, Nemes-Nikodem E, Jeney C, et al. Emerging azithromycin-resistance among the Neisseria gonorrhoeae strains isolated in Hungary. *Ann Clin Microbiol Antimicrob*. 2016;15(1):53.
24. Skinner JM, Distefano J, Warrington J, et al. Trends in reported syphilis and gonorrhea among HIV-infected people in Arizona: implications for prevention and control. *Public Health Reports*. 2014;129 (suppl 1):85-94.
25. Boyajian AJ, Murray M, Tucker M, et al. Identifying variations in adherence to the CDC sexually transmitted disease treatment guidelines of Neisseria gonorrhoeae. *Public Health*. 2016;136:161-165.
26. Tabrizi SN, Chen S, Tapsall J, et al. Evaluation of opa-based real-time PCR for detection of Neisseria gonorrhoeae. *Sex Transm Dis*. 2005;32:199.
27. Tao G, Hoover KW, Nye MB, et al. Rectal infections with Neisseria gonorrhoeae and Chlamydia trachomatis in men in the United States. *Clin Infect Dis*. 2016;63(10):1325-1331.
28. Nall J, Barr B, McNeil CJ, et al. Implementation of oral and rectal gonococcal and chlamydial nucleic acid amplification-based testing as a component of local health department activities. *Sex Transm Dis*. 2016;43(10):605-607.
29. Centers for Disease Control and Prevention. Sexually transmitted diseases treatment guidelines 2006; diseases characterized by urethritis and cervicitis. http://www.cdc.gov/std/treatment/2006/ urethritis-and-cervicitis.htm#uc6.
30. Hartmann J. Genital mycoplasmas. *J Dtsch Dermatol Ges*. 2009;7:371.
31. Martin DH. Nongonococcal urethritis: new views through the prism of modern molecular microbiology. *Curr Infect Dis Rep*. 2008;10:128.
32. Stirling KM, Hussain N, Sanders MM, et al. Association between maternal genital mycoplasma colonization and histologic chorioamnionitis in preterm births. *J Neonatal Perinatal Med*. 2016;9(2):201-209.
33. Larsen B, Hwang J. Mycoplasma, ureaplasma, and adverse pregnancy outcomes: a fresh look. *Infect Dis Obstet Gynecol*. 2010;2010. pii: 521921.
34. Ona S, Molina RL, Diouf K. Mycoplasma genitalium: an overlooked sexually transmitted pathogen in women? *Infect Dis Obstet Gynecol*. 2016;2016:4513089.
35. Bjornelius E, Magnusson C, Jensen JS. Mycoplasma genitalium macrolide resistance in Stockholm, Sweden. *Sex Transm Infect*. 2017;93(3):167-168.
36. Batteiger BE, Tan M. Chlamydia trachomatis (trachoma, genital infections, perinatal infections, and lymphogranuloma venereum). In: *Mandell, Douglas, and Bennett's Principles and Practice of Infectious Diseases*. 8th ed. Philadelphia: Elsevier Saunders; 2015:2154-2170.
37. Workowski KA, Bolan GA, Centers for Disease Control and Prevention. Sexually transmitted diseases treatment guidelines, 2015. *MMWR Recomm Rep*. 2015;64(RR-03):1-137. Erratum in: *MMWR Recomm Rep*. 2015;64(33):924.
38. Zuck M, Ellis T, Venida A, et al. Extrusions are phagocytosed and promote Chlamydia survival within macrophages. *Cell Microbiol*. 2017 Apr;19(4). doi: 10.1111/cmi.12683. Epub 2016 Nov 21.
39. Bianchi S, Boveri S, Igidbashian S, et al. Chlamydia trachomatis infection and HPV/Chlamydia trachomatis co-infection among HPV-vaccinated young women at the beginning of their sexual activity. *Arch Gynecol Obstet*. 2016;294(6):1227-1233.
40. Anttila T, Saikku P, Koskela P, et al. Serotypes of Chlamydia trachomatis and risk for development of cervical squamous cell carcinoma. *JAMA*. 2001;285(1):47-51.
41. Madeleine MM, Anttila T, Schwartz SM, et al. Risk of cervical cancer associated with Chlamydia trachomatis antibodies by histology, HPV type and HPV cofactors. *Int J Cancer*. 2007;120(3):650-655.
42. Dukers-Muijrers NH, Morr Schwartz SM, et al. Risk of cervical cancer associated with Chlamydia trachomatis antibodies by histology, HPV type and Ht taken at least 3 weeks after treatment. *PLoS One*. 2012;7(3):e34108.
43. Lau CY, Qureshi AK. Azithromycin versus doxycycline for genital chlamydial infections: a meta-analysis of randomized clinical trials. *Sex Transm Dis*. 2002;29(9):497-502.
44. Kong FY, Tabrizi SN, Fairley CK, et al. The efficacy of azithromycin and doxycycline for the treatment of rectal chlamydia infection: a systematic review and meta-analysis. *J Antimicrob Chemother*. 2015;70(5):1290-1297.
45. Geisler WM, Uniyal A, Lee JY, et al. Azithromycin versus doxycycline for urogenital chlamydia trachomatis infection. *N Engl J Med*. 2015;373(26):2512-2521.
46. Kissinger PJ, White S, Manhart LE, et al. Azithromycin treatment failure for chlamydia trachomatis among heterosexual men with nongonococcal urethritis. *Sex Transm Dis*. 2016;43(10):599-602.
47. Lazenby GB, Korte JE, Tillman S, et al. A recommendation for timing of repeat Chlamydia trachomatis test following infection and treatment in

pregnant and nonpregnant women. *Int J STD AIDS*. 2017;28(9):902-909.
48. Scholes D, Stergachis A, Heidrich FE, et al. Prevention of pelvic inflammatory disease by screening for cervical chlamydial infection. *N Engl J Med*. 1996;334(21):1362-1366.
49. Kamwendo F, Forslin L, Bodin L, et al. Decreasing incidences of gonorrhea- and chlamydia-associated acute pelvic inflammatory disease. A 25-year study from an urban area of central Sweden. *Sex Transm Dis*. 1996;23(5):384-391.
50. Tao G, Hoover KW, Nye MB, et al. Rectal infection with Neisseria gonorrhoeae and Chlamydia trachomatis in men in the United States. *Clin Infect Dis*. 2016;63(10):1325-1331.
51. Ness RB, Hillier S, Richter HE, et al. Can known risk factors explain racial differences in the occurrence of bacterial vaginosis? *J Natl Med Assoc*. 2003 Mar;95(3):201-212.
52. Madden T, Grentzer JM, Secura GM, et al. Risk of bacterial vaginosis in users of the intrauterine device: a longitudinal study. *Sex Transm Dis*. 2012;39(3):217-222.
53. Ogino M, Iino K, Minoura S. Habitual use of warm water cleaning toilets is related to aggravation of the vaginal microflora. *J Obstet Gynaecol*. 2010;36(5):1071-1074.
54. Ness RB, Hillier SL, Richter HE, et al. Douching in relation to bacterial vaginosis, lactobacilli, and facultative bacteria in the vagina. *Obstet Gynecol*. 2002 Oct;100(4):765.
55. Marrazzo JM, Thomas KK, Agnew K, et al. Prevalence and risks for bacterial vaginosis in women who have sex with women. *Sex Transm Dis*. 2010;37:335.
56. Hillier S. The complexity of microbial diversity in bacterial vaginosis. *N Eng J Med*. 2005;353:1886-1887.
57. Hill GB. The microbiology of bacterial vaginosis. *Am J Obstet Gynecol*. 1993;169:450-454.
58. Centers for Disease Control and Prevention. Sexually Transmitted diseases treatment guidelines 2006; bacterial vaginosis. http://www.cdc.gov/mwr/preview/mmwrhtml/rr5511a1.
59. Edwards L, Lynch PJ. *Genital Dermatology Atlas*. 2nd ed. St. Louis: Lippincott Williams & Wilkins; 2011:268-288.
60. Rumyantseva TA, Bellen G, Romanuk TN, et al. Utility of microscopic techniques and quantitative real-time polymerase chain reaction for the diagnosis of vaginal microflora alterations. *J Low Genit Tract Dis*. 2015;19(2):124-128.
61. Rumyantseva T, Shipitsvna E, Guschin A, et al. Evaluation and subsequent optimizations of the quantitative AmpliSens Florocenosis/Bacterial vaginosis-FRT multiplex real-time PCR assay for diagnosis of bacterial vaginosis. *APMIS*. 2016;124(12):1099-1108.
62. Kampan NC, Suffian SS, Ithnin NS, et al. Evaluation of BV(SZ, Jamil MS, in A, Unemo M. Evaluation and subsequent opt *Sex Reprod Healthc*. 2011;2(1):1-5.
63. Klebanoff MA, Hillier SL, Nugent RP, et al. Is bacterial vaginosis a stronger risk factor for preterm birth when it is diagnosed earlier in gestation? *Am J Obstet Gynecol*. 2005;192:470.
64. Myer L, Denny L, Telerant R, et al. Bacterial vaginosis and susceptibility to HIV infection in South African women: a nested case-control study. *J Infect Dis*. 2005; 192:1372.
65. Boyle DC, Barton SE, Uthayakumar S, et al. Is bacterial vaginosis associated with cervical intraepithelial neoplasia? *Int J Gynecol Cancer*. 2003;13:159.
66. Uthayakumar S, Boyle DC, Barton SE, et al. Bacterial vaginosis and cervical intraepithelial neoplasiaecause or coincidence? *J Obstet Gynecol*. 1998;18:572.
67. Hay P, Ugwumadu AHN, Manyonda IT. Oral clindamycin prevents spontaneous preterm birth and mid trimester miscarriage in pregnant women with bacterial vaginosis. *Int J STD AIDS*. 2001;12(suppl 2):70.
68. Ugwumadu A, Reid F, Hay P, et al. Natural history of bacterial vaginosis and intermediate flora in pregnancy and effect of oral clindamycin. *Obstet Gynecol*. 2004;104:114.
69. Larsson PG, Stray-Pedersen B, Ryttig KR, et al. Human lactobacilli as supplementation of clindamycin to patients with bacterial vaginosis reduce the recurrence rate; a 6-month, double-blind, randomized, placebo-controlled study. *BMC Womens Health*. 2008 Jan 15;8:3.

Infestations, Bites, and Stings

PART 27

第二十七篇　虫媒叮咬和感染性疾病

Chapter 176 :: Leishmaniasis and Other Protozoan Infections :: Esther von Stebut

第一百七十六章
利什曼病和其他原虫感染

中文导读

原生动物被认为是人畜共患病的真核单细胞生物。本章主要介绍了临床表现在皮肤的原生动物感染，包括利什曼病、锥虫病、阿米巴病以及鼻孢子虫病，简要介绍了其他一过性皮肤感染的原生动物感染。

第一节利什曼病，介绍了其流行病学、病因及发病机制、临床表现、诊断、治疗、预防和疫苗。主要讲述了利什曼病是通过媒介传播的第三种最常见的传染病。临床感染范围从皮肤到黏膜或内脏，以及隐匿性感染，皮肤临床表现中"火山"结节溃疡性形态具有特征性。在感染第一周采集标本，诊断敏感度接近90%。葡萄糖酸锑钠和锑酸葡甲胺是系统治疗的主要药物。

第二节非洲锥虫病（昏睡病），介绍了其流行病学、病因及发病机制、临床表现、诊断、治疗、预防。主要讲述了非洲锥虫病是由布氏锥虫感染引起的，未经治疗的患者死亡率接近100%。发病分为两个阶段，第一个阶段是血淋巴阶段；第二个阶段是脑膜脑炎阶段。皮肤表现常被误认为是昆虫叮咬或毛囊炎。其诊断是通过在血片或Giemsa染色的厚涂片、淋巴结、骨髓或脑脊液中检测出锥虫。目前治疗药物有喷他脒、苏拉明、美拉胂醇、依氟鸟啡、硝呋替莫等。

第三节恰加斯病（美洲锥虫病），介绍了恰加斯病是由克氏锥虫引起的人畜共患病，临床表现分为三个阶段。诊断和治疗都有难度，早期诊断包括血液标本的薄涂片、血培养，晚期诊断较难。治疗适用于急性感染、先天性感染、免疫抑制患者和患有慢性病的儿童，药物为苯硝唑和硝呋莫司。

第四节疟疾，介绍了其是由感染疟原虫属原生动物引起的，通过被感染的雌性按蚊叮咬传播的。人类疟疾由5种疟原虫引起。临床表现中皮肤表现很少报道。抗疟系统治疗对皮肤效果佳，但针对疟疾的疫苗尚未上市。

第五节至第十二节，简要概述了滴虫病、鼻孢子虫病、隐孢子虫病、贾第鞭毛虫病、阿米巴病、机会致病性阿米巴病、棘阿米巴性角膜炎、弓形虫病的流行病学、病因及发病机制、临床表现、诊断、治疗、预防。

〔粟 娟〕

Protozoa are considered to be zoonotic, eukaryotic, single-celled organisms. They possess a cellular membrane and, in contrast to bacteria, a nucleus. Many protozoa have different proliferative stages and undergo substantial changes during their life cycle. As a consequence of their size, which ranges from 10 μm to greater than 50 μm, they can very often easily be found in various tissues (eg, stool, other body fluids). Protozoa are widely distributed throughout the world.

A number of protozoan pathogens are human parasites and can induce severe courses of disease, especially as inducers of opportunistic disease (eg, in patients with HIV/AIDS). Treatment of protozoan infections is often difficult and prophylaxis through vaccination, for example, does not exist yet.

Among the protozoan infections (Table 176-1), leishmaniasis, trichomoniasis, and (rarely) amebiasis, as well as rhinosporidiosis, primarily manifest in the skin. The other protozoan infections are associated with (transient) skin affection and are only briefly mentioned in this chapter.

LEISHMANIASIS

AT-A-GLANCE

- Leishmaniasis is a complex of diseases caused by the protozoa *Leishmania* and transmitted by the bite of infected phlebotomine sandflies.
- Four major human diseases: (a) localized cutaneous leishmaniasis, (b) diffuse cutaneous leishmaniasis, (c) mucocutaneous leishmaniasis, and (d) visceral leishmaniasis.
- Which of the 4 diseases results depends mainly on the interaction between *Leishmania* species and the immunologic status of the host.
- Diagnosis is by organism isolation or serology, but species identification is only possible with isoenzyme analysis and new molecular techniques.
- Management ranges from observation to systemic therapy, primarily with antimonials, and vaccines in development.

EPIDEMIOLOGY

Together with malaria and dengue, leishmaniasis is the third most frequent infectious disease transmitted by a vector. Annually, approximately 1.6 million new cases are reported; among these, it is estimated that approximately 200,000 to 400,000 cases represent visceral leishmaniasis, and 700,000 to 1.2 million cases represent cutaneous leishmaniasis. Around 12 million individuals are currently infected worldwide.[1-3]

The World Health Organization (WHO) considers leishmaniasis to belong among the so-called neglected tropical diseases. Neglected tropical diseases are poverty-associated infectious diseases that are primarily prevalent in subtropical and tropical regions, and for which there is little to no public interest, little research activity, high morbidity and mortality, and no safe and long-lasting therapies (as of this writing).

Leishmaniasis is endemic in 90 countries around the world, mainly in tropical and subtropical regions (excluding Australia and Southeast Asia). The different clinical presentations, cutaneous, mucocutaneous and visceral disease, have a distinct distribution as shown in Figs. 176-1 (cutaneous leishmaniasis) and 176-2 (visceral leishmaniasis):

- Cutaneous leishmaniasis (CL) is widely distributed, with approximately one-third of cases occurring in each of 3 epidemiologic regions: the Americas, the Mediterranean basin, and western Asia from the Middle East to Central Asia. The 10 countries with the highest case counts are Afghanistan, Algeria, Brazil, Colombia, Costa Rica, Ethiopia, Iran, Peru, Sudan, and Syria. Together these 10 countries account for 70% to 75% of all CL cases.[4]

TABLE 176-1
Protozoan Infections Important for Humans

MODE OF TRANSMISSION	PATHOGEN	DISEASE	MAIN ORGAN INVOLVED
Insect bite	*Leishmania* spp.	(Muco-)cutaneous, and visceral leishmaniasis	Skin, lymph nodes, mucous membranes, visceral organs
	Trypanosoma brucei	African trypanosomiasis (sleeping sickness)	Blood, lymph nodes, liquor
	Trypanosoma cruzi	American trypanosomiasis (Chagas disease)	
	Plasmodium spp.	Malaria	Liver, blood
Sexually transmitted	*Trichomonas vaginalis*	Trichomoniasis	Genital tract
Water	*Rhinosporidium seeberi*	Rhinosporidiosis	Nasal/oral mucosa, rarely skin
Food/water ingestion	*Cryptosporidium* spp.	Cryptosporidiosis	Intestine
	Giardia lamblia	Giardiasis	Intestine
	Entamoeba histolytica	Amebiasis	Intestine, (skin)
	Toxoplasma gondii	Toxoplasmosis	Intestine Cysts in various organs

- More than 90% of global visceral leishmaniasis (VL) cases occur in 6 countries: Bangladesh, Brazil, Ethiopia, India, South Sudan, and Sudan.
- Close to 90% of mucocutaneous leishmaniasis (MCL) cases occur in Bolivia, Brazil, and Peru.

The distribution of disease is strongly associated with the distribution of its vector, the sand fly. Outside of endemic regions, the disease is very often only recognized by travelers after their return home.

In recent years, coinfections of *Leishmania* with HIV have become a major concern. Because HIV-infected individuals have longer periods of parasitemia, humans potentially become reservoirs for the parasite as well. This is one possible explanation for the increased rate of leishmaniasis cases in some regions

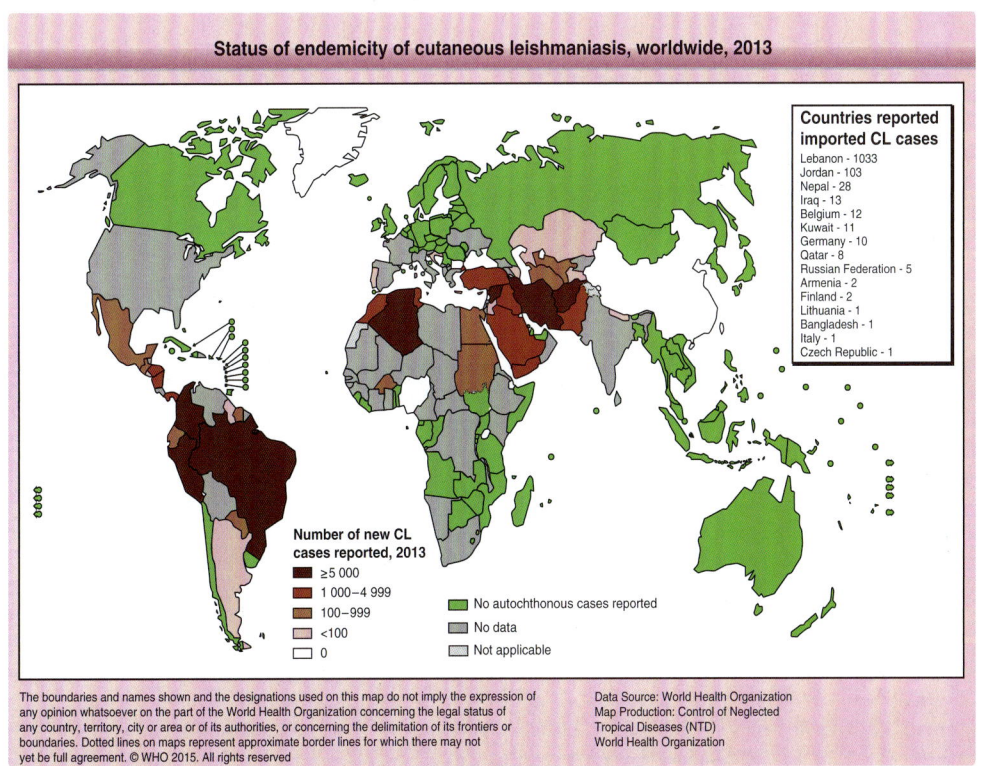

Figure 176-1 Geographic distribution of cutaneous leishmaniasis according to the World Health Organization. (Copyright 2015 by the World Health Organization [WHO]. All rights reserved. Used with permission.)

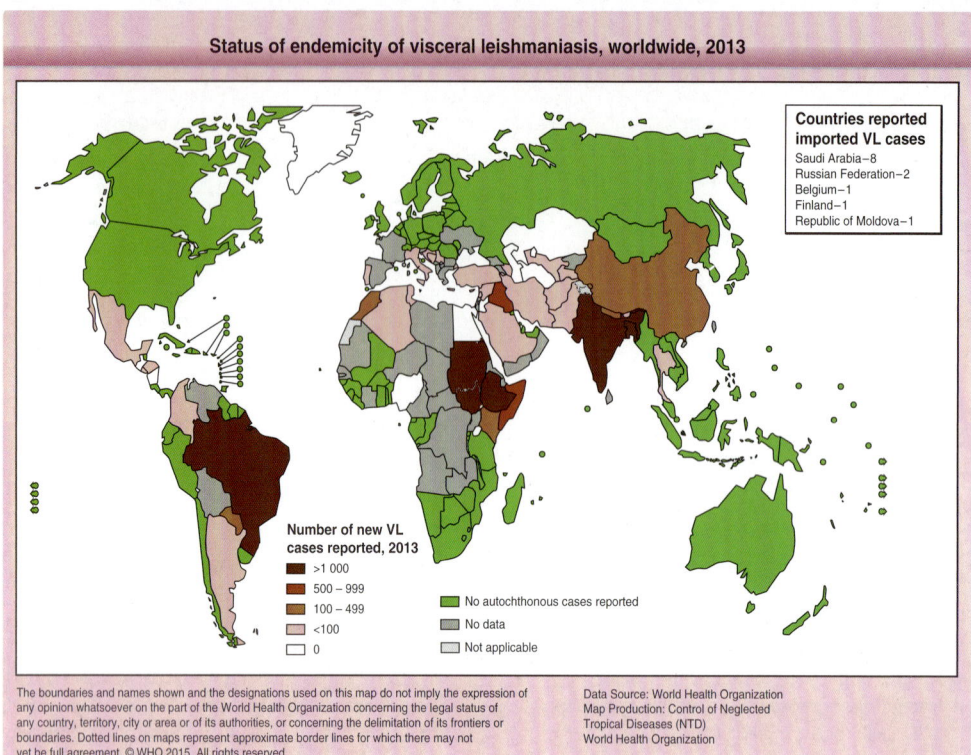

Figure 176-2 Geographic distribution of visceral leishmaniasis. (Copyright 2015 by the World Health Organization [WHO]. All rights reserved. Used with permission.)

that reportedly have high numbers of HIV/*Leishmania* coinfected patients (eg, Southern Europe; Fig. 176-3).

ETIOLOGY

PARASITE AND LIFE CYCLE

The genus *Leishmania* consists of parasitic protozoa of the phylum *Sarcomastigophora*, order Kinetoplastida, and family Trypanosomatidae. Two subgenera, *Leishmania* and *Viannia*, exist.[5-7] For clinical purposes, a nomenclature omitting the subgenus is often used. More than 20 species are pathogenic for humans, which are transmitted by the bite of an infected female phlebotomine sand fly (Table 176-2). Cases of venereal and vertical transmission, as well as transmission from infected blood transfusion or needles have, however, been reported.

Leishmania are dimorphic parasites (Fig. 176-4). In the gut of the sand fly or in culture, they exist in a spindle-shaped motile (single anterior flagellum) promastigote form (10 to 20 μm). Upon transmission to the host, *Leishmania* parasites are ingested by macrophages and neutrophil granulocytes and—as a consequence of the shift toward a low pH in phagolysosomes—transform into the obligate intracellular, oval, nonmotile amastigote form (2 to 6 μm) that has a relatively large basophilic nucleus and a smaller rod-shaped kinetoplast at the base of the lost flagellum.

After ingestion during a blood meal of a sand fly, infected macrophages are ruptured and the amastigotes are released into the stomach of the insect where they immediately transform into the promastigote form. The promastigotes subsequently migrate to the alimentary tract of the fly, multiply extracellularly by binary fission, and, in a few days, reach the esophagus and the salivary glands of the fly, where they change into infective metacyclic promastigotes, which will be released into the skin at next bite. Promastigotes are then phagocytosed by resident host (skin) macrophages and neutrophils, where they transform into amastigotes that multiply by binary fission and get released following cellular burst to infect other cells of the host.

RESERVOIR HOST

Leishmaniasis is mostly zoonotic, being incidentally transmitted to humans from wild and domestic animals (primary reservoir hosts) (see Table 176-2). The main reservoir hosts are the great gerbil, the fat

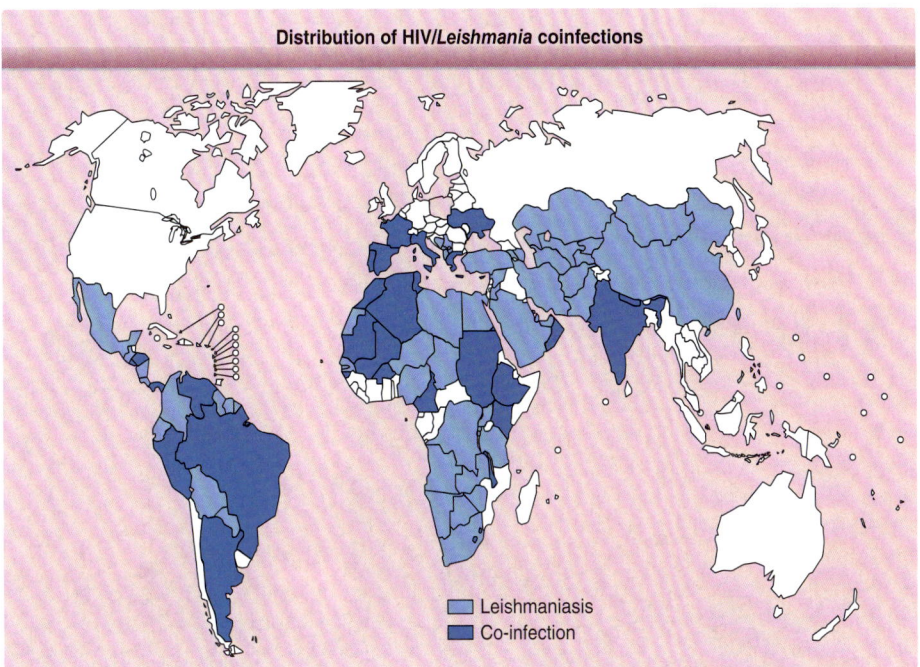

Figure 176-3 Distribution of HIV/*Leishmania* coinfections.

sand rat, *Meriones* spp., and other rodents, as well as dogs, the opossum, sloths, and others. In several regions, however, the zoonotic host is not even fully characterized, leading to difficulties in reservoir and vector control strategies.

VL caused by *Leishmania donovani* and Old Word CL caused by some *Leishmania tropica* strains are anthroponotic diseases (ie, humans are the primary reservoir hosts). Additional factors that may contribute to the increasing relevance of humans as reservoir hosts are alterations in the natural habitats (eg, human settlements in close proximity to forests, restrictions in the diversity and distribution of mammals available for sand fly feeding).

TABLE 176-2
Leishmania Species and Geographic Distribution

LEISHMANIA SPECIES	VECTOR	TRANSMISSION	GEOGRAPHIC LOCATION
Old World			
L. (L.) major	Phlebotomus	Zoonotic	Central Asia, West Asia, North Africa
L. (L.) tropica		Anthroponotic	
L. (L.) infantum		Zoonotic	Mediterranean basin, North Africa
L. (L.) aethiopica			Ethiopia, Kenya, Yemen, Sudan
L. (L.) chagasi			Brazil
L. (L.) donovani		Anthroponotic	India, Bangladesh, Nepal, Sudan
New World			
L. (V.) braziliensis	Lutzomyia	Zoonotic	Central and South America
L. (L.) mexicana	Psychodopygus		
L. (L.) amazonesis			
L. (V.) panamensis			
L. (V.) peruviana			
L. (V.) venezuelensis			
L. (V.) guyanensis			

L., *Leishmania*; (L.), subgenus *Leishmania*, (V.) subgenus *Viannia*.

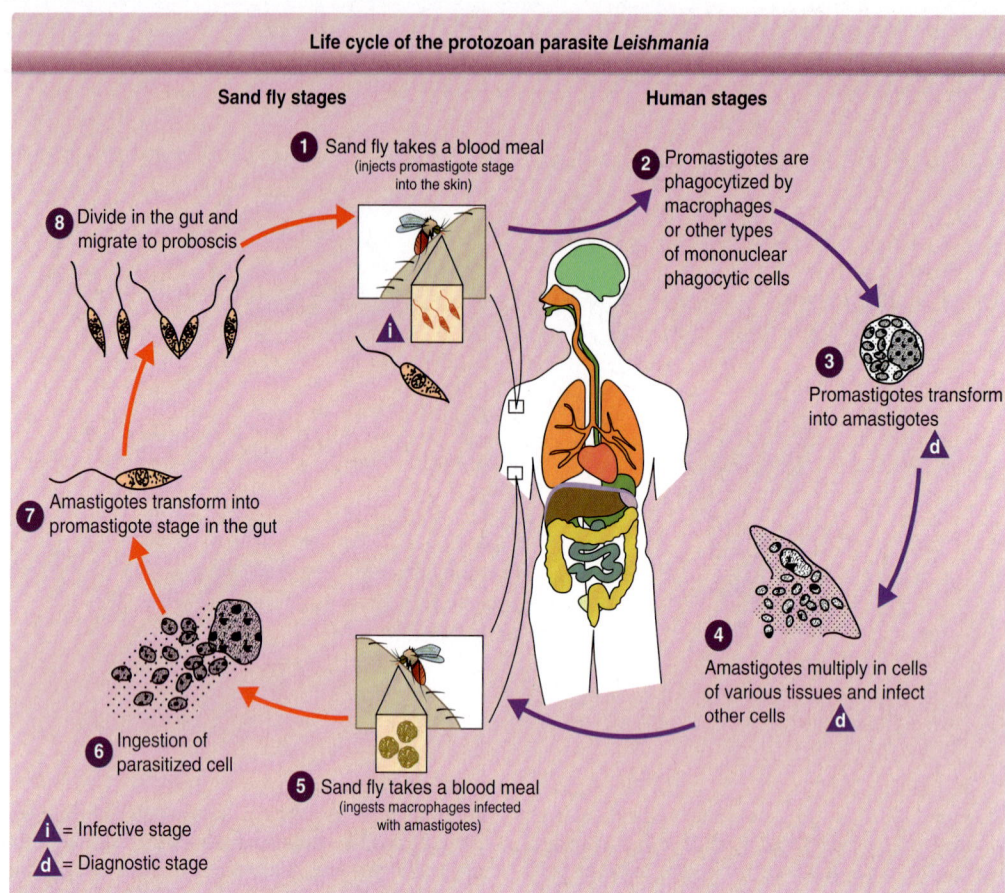

Figure 176-4 Life cycle of the protozoan parasite *Leishmania*. (From the Centers for Disease Control and Prevention [CDC].)

INSECT VECTOR

The insect vector of leishmaniasis, the female phlebotomine sand fly, is grouped under the suborder *Nematocera* of the order Diptera.[1] Three genera (*Phlebotomus* in the Old World, and *Lutzomyia* and *Psychodopygus* in the New World), and approximately 70 species are implicated as vectors (see Table 176-2). They are widely distributed and have predilection to intertropical and warm temperate zones. Presumably as a consequence of globalization and global warming, Phlebotominae have been spreading into, for example, northern European regions in recent years.

Only the female sand fly is hematophagus. They live for approximately 40 days and are known as pool feeders, because they tear open the skin with their wide mouthparts and suck the blood as it collects.

Phlebotomine sandflies are small (<3 mm), and do not fly far from their breeding site. Their activity is mostly crepuscular or nocturnal while the host is asleep. They rest during the day and lay their eggs in dark, cool, humid, and organic matter-rich places, such as rodent burrows, bird's nests, and house wall fissures. Being exophilic and exophagic, they prefer to rest and to have their meal outdoors, which limits their control through house spraying.

PATHOGENESIS

The resulting disease depends on the fate of the phagocytosed amastigotes. This, in turn, is a function of numerous parasite-related and host-related factors, as well as other factors that may account for geographical differences. In general, parasites interfere with the signaling pathways, intracellular kinases, transcription factors, and gene expression of macrophages, compromising their ability to generate leishmanicidal substances. In addition, they impair dendritic cell activation, migration, and the ability to secrete T-helper 1 (Th1) cytokines.

PARASITE-RELATED FACTORS[7]

Sand fly saliva is increasingly recognized as an essential element in the pathogenesis of the disease. Besides containing vasodilators, anticoagulants, and immunomodulators, it may also increase the inoculum size and the diameter of the lesion in previously unexposed individuals. Intraspecific variations of sand fly saliva may even affect the overall clinical outcome of *Leishmania infantum*–induced disease by shifting the adaptive immunity from a Th1 to a Th2 immune response. The development of antisaliva antibodies after exposure may account for the decline with age of susceptibility to the infection in endemic areas.

Other parasite-related factors include infectivity, pathogenicity, virulence, and tissue tropism. These differ from one species to the other. For example, lipophosphoglycan and gp63 are 2 important promastigote virulence factors that impair the overall functions of infected cells, with lipophosphoglycan being clearly involved in *Leishmania major* disease, but absent in *Leishmania mexicana*. Although viscerotropic species tend to spread to the reticuloendothelial system, they may become dermotropic as a consequence of treatment such as seen in post–kala-azar dermal leishmaniasis (PKDL). Similarly, *L. tropica*, classically dermotropic, may cause visceral disease.

HOST-RELATED FACTORS[7]

Malnutrition, immunosuppression, and the host genetic background influence host susceptibility as well as resistance to disease.

The output of acquired T-cell immunity, which depends on the net effect of the opposing Th1 and Th2 responses, largely determines the course and the therapeutic response of the infection. A dominant Th1/cytotoxic T-cell Type 1 response resulting in the production of interferon-γ and nitric oxide leads to a leishmanicidal state of macrophages, and accounts for subclinical infection or self-healing LCL and the positive Montenegro skin test (that assesses delayed-type hypersensitivity to leishmanial antigen). A dominant Th2 response accounts for progressive disease such as diffuse cutaneous leishmaniasis (DCL), and is characterized by anergy to leishmanial antigen (negative Montenegro skin test). In addition, regulatory T cells, as well as the so-called Th17 cells producing interleukin-17A, contribute to disease susceptibility. The majority of parasite-specific T cells home to the site of infection, thus, cytokine profiles of T cells in peripheral blood may not reflect the actual immune status well. Mucosal leishmaniasis patients will have both Th1 and Th2 responses, with slight predominance of Th2 immunity, explaining persistence of the disease. To summarize, T-cell immunity would be intact in localized cutaneous leishmaniasis (LCL), defective in DCL, and pathologically exuberant in MCL. Humoral immunity seems to play a role during parasite opsonization, but little or no role in determining the course of the infection. High titers of antileishmanial immunoglobulin (Ig) G correlate more with chronic, non-healing, and visceral disease.

HIV coinfection of individuals both leads to a more-severe course of infection with *Leishmania*, but also worsens disease outcome of the HIV infection. Other coinfections prevalent in endemic countries, such as malaria, also are known to have an effect on the course of disease.

TABLE 176-3
Leishmaniasis Disease Forms and Causative *Leishmania* Species

DISEASE PRESENTATION	LEISHMANIA SPP. OLD WORLD	LEISHMANIA SPP. NEW WORLD
Localized cutaneous leishmaniasis	L. (L.) major L. (L.) tropica L. (L.) infantum L. (L.) aethiopica	L. (V.) braziliensis L. (L.) mexicana L. (L.) amazonensis L. (V.) panamensis L. (V.) guyanensis
Diffuse cutaneous leishmaniasis (rare)	L. (L.) aethiopica L. (L.) major[a]	L. (L.) mexicana L. (L.) amazonensis L. (V.) braziliensis[a]
Mucocutaneous leishmaniasis (rare)		L. (V.) braziliensis L. (V.) guyanesis (rare) L. (V.) panamensis (rare)
Visceral leishmaniasis	L. (L.) donovani L. (L.) infantum	L. (L.) chagasi
Post–kala-azar dermal leishmaniasis	L. (L.) donovani	

[a]Upon immunosuppression of the human host.
L., *Leishmania*; (L.), subgenus *Leishmania*, (V.) subgenus *Viannia*.

CLINICAL FINDINGS

Depending on host factors and the parasites species, leishmaniasis primarily presents as CL, whereas other (sub-)species have the tendency to spread across mucosal membranes to induce MCL or spread into visceral organs (VL) (Table 176-3).[2-7]

The clinical spectrum ranges from CL to MCL or VL, and cryptic infections.

CUTANEOUS LEISHMANIASIS

Localized Cutaneous Leishmaniasis: LCL constitutes 50% to 75% of all incident cases. It is the mildest form of *Leishmania* diseases and the one that prevails in the Old World. It can be caused by all *Leishmania* species.

Old World LCL (Aleppo boil, Baghdad boil, Oriental sore, leishmaniasis tropica, Biskra button, Delhi boil, Bouton d'Orient, Lahore sore, Rose of Jericho, Kandahar sore, the little sister) is caused mainly by *L. major*, *L. tropica*, *Leishmania aethiopica*, and to a lesser extent *L. infantum* (see Table 176-3). The morphologic spectrum of Old World LCL is wide. Lesions start as erythematous papules that enlarge over a few weeks to form nodules/plaques and often ulcerate and become crusted (Figs. 176-5 to 176-9). The "volcanic" nodulo-ulcerative morphology is characteristic and consists of a painless crateriform ulcer with a rolled margin and a necrotic base that is often covered with an adherent crust (Fig. 176-5). Two major types, (a) the moist type (mainly caused by *L. major*) (Fig. 176-5) and (b) the dry

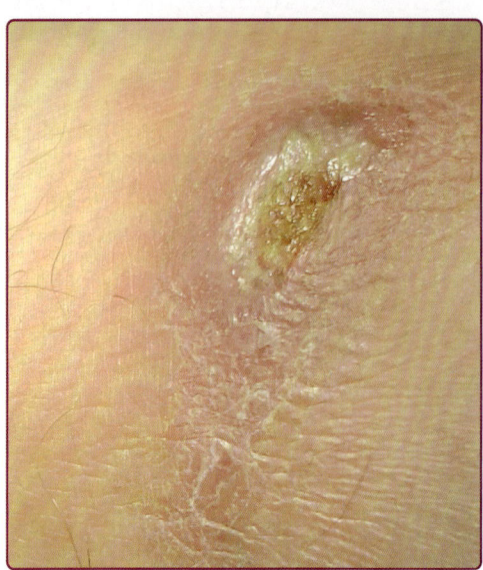

Figure 176-5 Old World localized cutaneous leishmaniasis on the arm ("moist type").

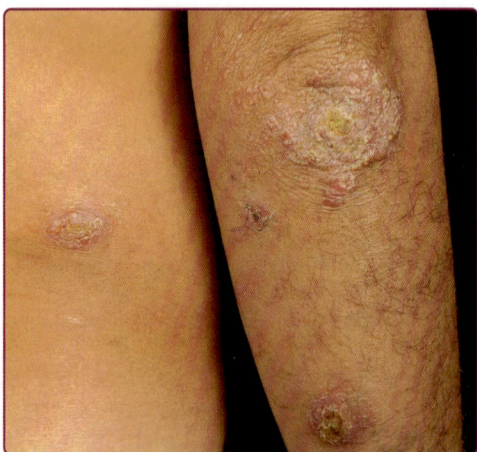

Figure 176-6 Acute Old World localized cutaneous leishmaniasis: multiple nodules on the arm and trunk caused by *Leishmania major*.

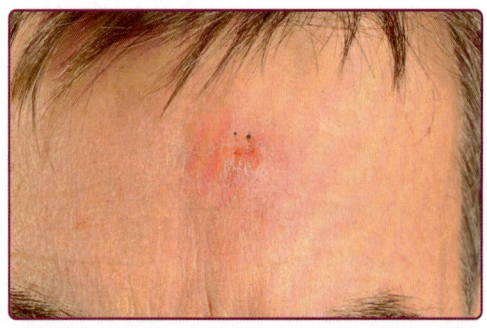

Figure 176-7 Acute Old World localized cutaneous leishmaniasis. Single crusted erythematous plaque on the forehead.

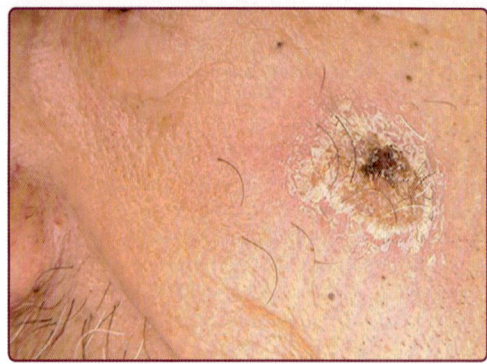

Figure 176-8 Old World localized cutaneous leishmaniasis of the left cheek.

type (primarily caused by *L. tropica*) (Fig. 176-6), are identified. Both types may coexist in the same patient. Other presentations include "iceberg nodules," and eczematoid, psoriasiform, erysipeloid, zosteriform, paronychial, chancriform, annular, palmoplantar, verrucous, and keloidal lesions.

Depending on the causing subspecies, the following characteristics also may be noted:

- *L. major* tends to cause multiple, moist ulcerations resembling furuncles with lymphadenopathy.
- *L. tropica*–associated lesions are fewer, mainly in the face, without lymph node involvement. Recurrences are found in approximately 10% of patients close to the original lesions.
- *L. infantum*, the causative agent of Mediterranean VL in children, may cause a self-limited skin disease in adults with rare ulceration.
- *L. aethiopica* may cause a similar cutaneous disease to *L. tropica*, but carries a higher risk of evolving into DCL in up to 20% of affected individuals.

Species identification cannot be made clinically and requires biochemical/molecular techniques.

Satellitosis, regional lymphadenopathy, localized lymphadenitis, sporotrichoid lymphatic spread, subcutaneous lymphatic nodules, and localized hypoesthesia may occur. Mature lesions may be elongated and oriented parallel to skin creases.

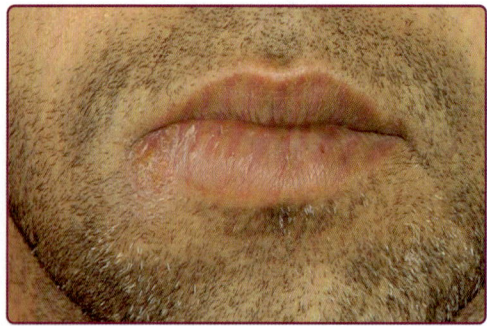

Figure 176-9 Acute Old World localized cutaneous leishmaniasis. Crusted erythematous nodule underneath the right perioral area.

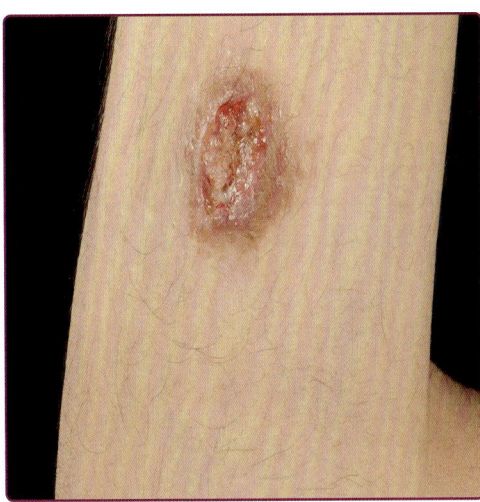

Figure 176-10 Acute Old World localized cutaneous leishmaniasis ("moist type") on the forearm.

New World LCL (Valley sickness, Andean sickness, white leprosy, chiclero ulcer, uta, pian bois, and bay sore) is caused by *L. mexicana* and *Leishmania (Viannia) braziliensis* complexes mainly (see Table 176-3). Pure cutaneous disease is very similar to Old Word LCL and isolated ulcers in exposed areas are the most common presentations (Figs. 176-10 to 176-14). The progression of the lesions gives rise to a characteristic scar consisting of thin pale skin at the ulcer site with a hyperpigmented border.

Infection with *L. mexicana* or *L. (V.) Leishmania (Viannia) guyanensis* causes only cutaneous disease in contrast to infection with *L. (V) braziliensis* and *Leishmania (Viannia) panamensis*, which may, in 40% to 80% of cases, progress to MCL. Approximately 50% of the lesions caused by *L. mexicana* heal within 3 months, whereas those caused by *L. braziliensis* persist much longer and are often associated with lymphadenopathy. Sporotrichoid lymphatic spread (see Fig. 176-12C)

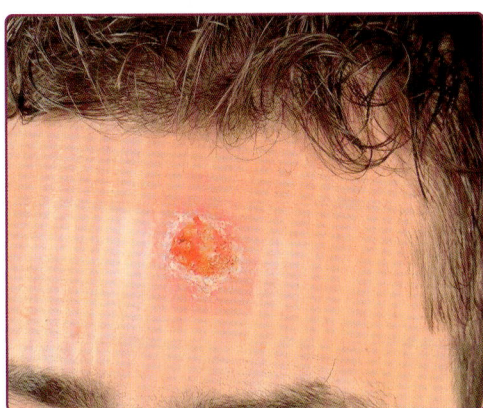

Figure 176-11 Acute New World localized cutaneous leishmaniasis acquired in Costa Rica. Classical noduloulcerative lesion on the forehead. Note that the ulcerated nodules look similar to volcanoes seen from above ("volcano sign").

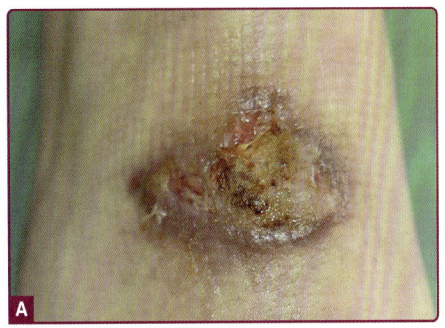

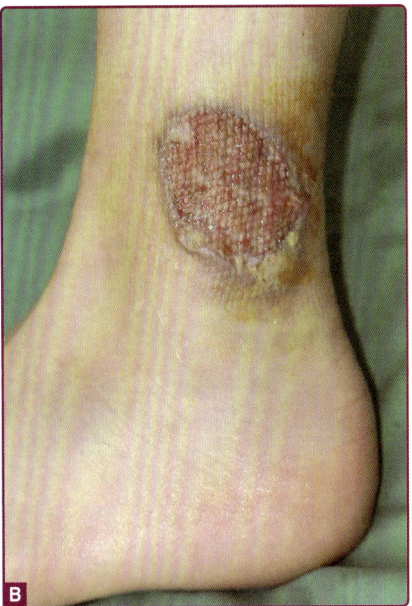

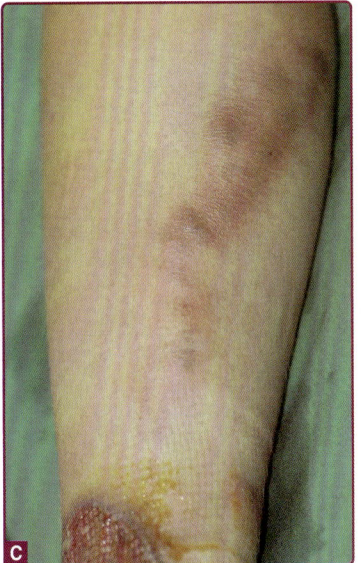

Figure 176-12 Acute New World localized cutaneous leishmaniasis with large volcaniform lesions on the dorsum of the right foot (**A**) and the ankle of the left foot (**B**) caused by *Leishmania guyanensis* infection of a young boy. **C,** Sporotrichoid extension of the lesion into the lymphatic system with erythematous papules on the outside of the left lower leg.

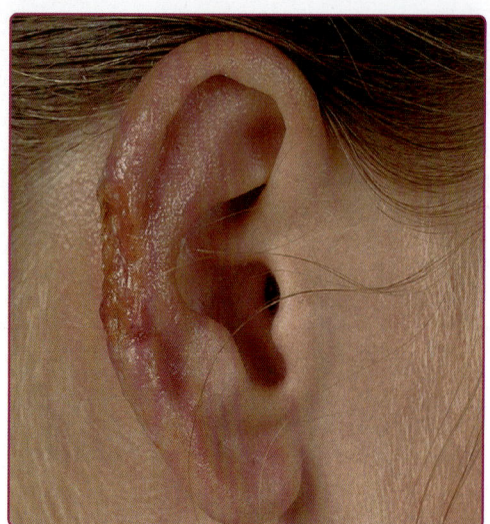

Figure 176-13 New World localized cutaneous leishmaniasis chiclero ulcer. A deep ulcer on the helix at the site of a sand fly bite. (From Wolff K, Johnson R, Saavedra AP, et al. *Fitzpatrick's Color Atlas and Synopsis of Clinical Dermatology*, 8th ed. New York, NY: McGraw-Hill; 2017, with permission.)

can be found more frequently, especially in children and immunosuppressed patients. Mature lesions may be elongated and oriented parallel to skin creases.

Disease caused by certain subspecies has the following specific presentations:

- *L. mexicana* is the causative organism of chiclero ulcer, a chronic mutilating infection of the pinna of the ear of forest workers in Mexico and Central America (see Fig. 176-13). *Lutzomyia flaviscutellata* is the major vector.
- In Brazil, the lower limbs are commonly affected, causing the typical Bauru ulcers.

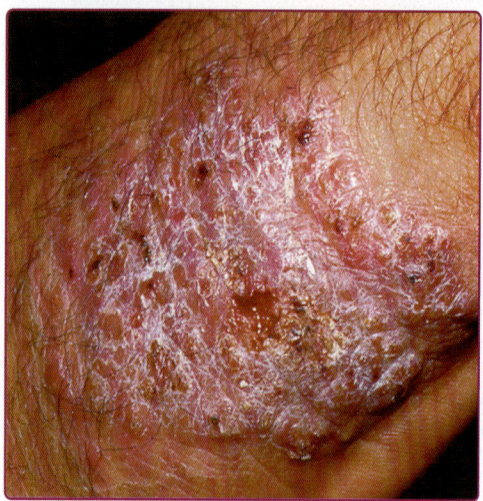

Figure 176-14 Chronic-localized cutaneous leishmaniasis. Verrucous, scaly, erythematous plaque with focal ulceration and crusting. (Used with permission from Raj Kubba, MD.)

- Uta, the Andean cutaneous form of leishmaniasis, is caused by *L. braziliensis* and predominantly affects exposed areas in children. Its principal vector is *Lutzomyia peruensis*.

An atypical nodular form of New World CL caused by *Leishmania donovani chagasi* has been reported from Honduras and Nicaragua. Unusual clinical pictures have been reported, especially in immunosuppressed patients.

Complications of Localized Cutaneous Leishmaniasis: Secondary bacterial infection is common. Additional complications include permanent scarring, disfigurement, and social stigma. Autoinoculation or koebnerization following trauma, tattooing, or surgery has been reported. Major complications of LCL include chronic LCL, DCL, and MCL (in New World LCL). AIDS and other immunosuppressive conditions increase the risk of mucocutaneous and visceral dissemination, and of recurrence following therapy. Disseminated CL, defined as more than 10 pleomorphic lesions in noncontiguous areas of the body, has been reported in increasing frequency, complicating New World LCL and HIV-associated Old World LCL.

Other Forms of Localized Cutaneous Leishmaniasis: Most cases of LCL heal spontaneously within 1 year and are characterized as acute LCL. Disease lasting more than 1 year is termed *chronic LCL*. Typically, the lesions evolve from papules to chronic disfiguring indurated nodules/plaques that are larger than average acute LCL lesions and may exhibit variable degrees of scaling, ulceration, verrucosity, and scarring (see Fig. 176-14). The diagnosis may be challenging because of the paucity of organisms seen on histologic examination.

Leishmaniasis recidivans is a rare form of chronic LCL and accounts for 3% to 10% of all LCL cases. It is caused mostly by *L. tropica* in the Old World, and less commonly by *L. (V) braziliensis* in the New World as well as by *Leishmania amazonensis, L. (V) panamensis*, and *L. (V) guyanensis*. Erythematous scaly papules, often with an apple jelly appearance, at the borders of a completely or partially healed CL lesion, are characteristic. It may complicate vaccination with a live strain of *Leishmania* and usually occurs in the setting of hyperactive T-cell immunity and low antibody titers.

Reactivation of dormant infection (up to 15 years after apparent resolution) after an unknown stimulus such as trauma or topical corticosteroids, rather than reinfection with different strains, is believed to account for most of the cases. In fact, several studies have demonstrated persistence of the intracellular living organisms in "healed" *Leishmania* lesions, this being more likely to occur if therapy was incomplete or deficient. Approximately 6% of all untreated, primary LCL cases develop leishmaniasis recidivans.

Lupoid leishmaniasis shares a similar etiology and clinical picture with leishmaniasis recidivans; lupoid leishmaniasis, however, is not a recurrent lesion. The lesion characteristically occurs over the face and may clinically resemble lupus vulgaris or discoid lupus

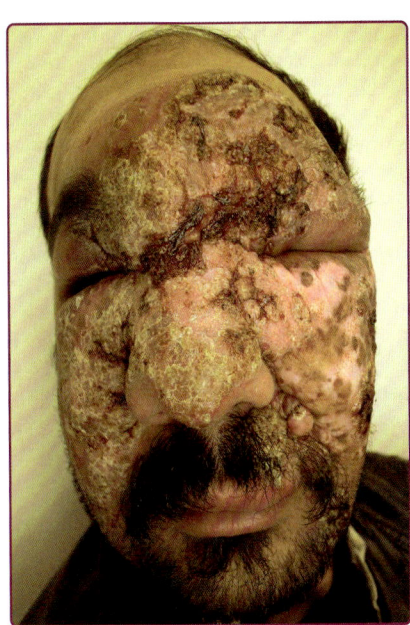

Figure 176-15 Disfiguring lupoid leishmaniasis of several years duration in a Middle Eastern man.

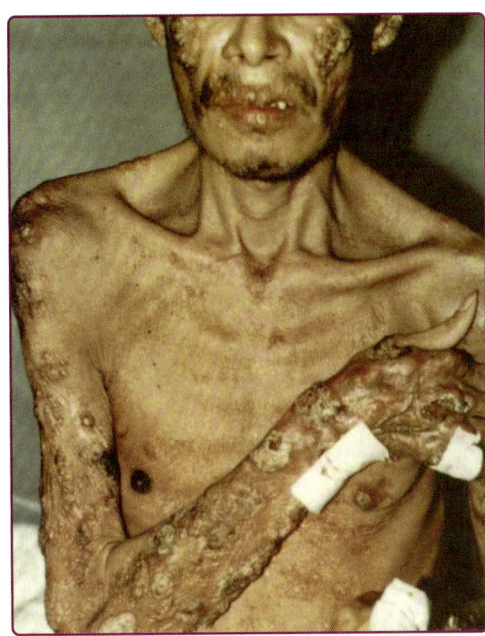

Figure 176-16 Diffuse cutaneous leishmaniasis with multiple, nodular lesions on the arms, trunk, and face of a patient from Mexico. (Used with permission from Dr. Sven Krengel, Lübeck, Germany.)

erythematosus. In the absence of molecular identification of parasites, the diagnosis may be delayed for several years leading to mutilation (Fig. 176-15).

DCL, also called *pseudolepromatous leishmaniasis*, is an anergic rare form of CL that occurs in the setting of deficient cell-mediated immunity, and clinically and histologically mimics lepromatous leprosy. It is usually caused by L. aethiopica in the Old World and by L. amazonensis, L. braziliensis, L. guyanensis, and L. mexicana in the New World. In North Brazil, DCL develops in approximately 0.2% of L. braziliensis infections. In Sudan and Ethiopia, 20% of cases develop DCL. Immunosuppressed patients, especially HIV-infected individuals, may develop a severe form of DCL (>200 lesions) with no species-specific relation.

Following a classical LCL lesion, dissemination occurs (immediately in 30% of cases, but up to 11 years in others) in the form of nonulcerated and parasite-laden nodules (Fig. 176-16) with a predilection for exposed areas of the body such as the face, where lesions may coalesce leading to leonine facies. Viscera are not involved. A progressive/chronic course with relapse after therapy is classical.

MUCOCUTANEOUS LEISHMANIASIS

MCL may complicate up to 10% of LCL patients and is characterized by the chronic and progressive spread of lesions to the nasal, pharyngeal, and buccal mucosa. Lesions appear 1 to 5 years after resolution of the primary lesion(s), or, less commonly, while they are still present. It is often a complication of New World LCL caused by L. (V) braziliensis, L. (V) panamensis, L. amazonensis, and L. (V) guyanensis. Ninety percent of cases occur in Bolivia, Brazil, and Peru. In the Old World, similar mucosal lesions caused by L. aethiopica may be seen but have a better prognosis.

MCL results from direct extension or hematogenous/lymphatic spread to the upper respiratory tract, and, rarely, ocular and genital mucosa, and liver. Bony structures are usually spared. Stuffy nose, epistaxis, coryza, hyperemia, and nasal septum crusting and ulceration are frequent presenting symptoms and signs. If untreated, the disease evolves into either septal perforation with resulting collapse of the nasal bridge and free hanging nose (tapir nose or parrot beak) or partial/total nasooropharyngeal mutilating ulceration (espundia; Fig. 176-17). In rare cases, the lips, cheeks, soft palate, or larynx is involved. Lymphadenopathy is common in L. braziliensis–induced disease and may be associated with hepatomegaly and systemic symptoms.

The major causes of mortality are secondary infection, pharyngeal obstruction, and respiratory failure. Cure rates decrease with advanced disease.

VISCERAL LEISHMANIASIS

VL (Sikari disease, Burdwan fever, Shahib disease, tropical splenomegaly, kala-azar, death fever, dumdum fever) is endemic in the tropical and subtropical parts of the world. Ninety percent of cases occur in Bangladesh, Ethiopia, India, Nepal, Brazil, and Sudan. The causative agents are L. donovani and Leishmania chagasi/L. infantum and to a lesser extent L. amazonensis, and Leishmania (Viannia) colombiensis. Infection with L. donovani occurs in the Old World (India and Sudan), is anthroponotic and highly

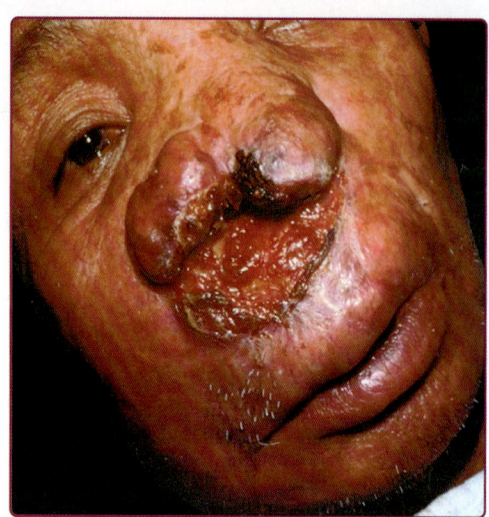

Figure 176-17 Mucocutaneous leishmaniasis, South American. Painful, mutilating ulceration with destruction of portion of the nose. (Used with permission from Eric Kraus, MD.)

endemic, and involves *Phlebotomus argentipes* as a vector. Other infections are zoonotic, and dogs are the major reservoir hosts. *L. infantum* afflicts mainly malnourished children in China, Africa, the Middle East, and the Mediterranean basin.

Hematogenous dissemination of the parasite to the reticuloendothelial system follows skin inoculation. However, congenital (transplacental) transmission may occur. Most infections remain subclinical. The incubation period and the duration of the disease are variable. The cardinal features of VL are persistent, high, undulating fever; leucopenia; anemia; splenomegaly; and hypergammaglobulinemia. Other findings include emaciation, burning feet (peripheral neuropathy), hepatogastrointestinal disturbances, epistaxis, thrombocytopenia, and lymphadenopathy.

Skin lesions develop later in the course of the disease and consist of ashy hyperpigmented patches on the temple, around the mouth, and on the abdomen, hands, and feet in light skin persons; hence, the name kala-azar (*black sickness* in Hindi). Other findings include hair and skin depigmentation (in Kenyan patients), cutaneous nodules and mucosal ulcers (in Sudanese patients), trichomegaly (Pitalugo sign), petechiae, and jaundice.

Without treatment, the fatality rate in developing countries approaches 100% in 2 years with the major complications being cachexia, secondary infections, enteritis, and pneumonia. Hemolytic anemia, acute renal damage, and severe mucosal hemorrhage are less common.

Visceral Leishmaniasis/HIV Coinfection:
Most coinfection cases have IV drug use as a common denominator and represent diagnostic and therapeutic challenges, as VL precipitates the onset of AIDS and HIV increases the risk of VL. The problem is mostly described in Spain, Italy, France, and Portugal. *L. infantum* is the major causative agent; however, other *Leishmania* species that do not normally visceralize have been isolated.

MCL-like, PKDL-like, and DCL-like pictures may result and cutaneous lesions are highly variable. Multiple dermatofibroma-like and Kaposi sarcoma–like papulonodular lesions may occur, and should be differentiated from parasitic colonization of Kaposi sarcoma. The presence of amastigotes in atypical locations tends to correlate with the degree of immunosuppression.

People with both conditions have a worse prognosis, shortened survival time, higher relapse rate, and inferior response to treatment compared with HIV-negative patients. VL is now being proposed to be integrated into the Centers for Disease Control and Prevention clinical category C as an AIDS-defining illness.

OTHER FORMS OF LEISHMANIASIS

Post–Kala-Azar Dermal Leishmaniasis:
PKDL is extremely rare in the New World and is mostly seen, in 2 major forms, in Sudan and India. As the name implies, it is a cutaneous manifestation of VL that usually develops months to years after resolution of VL, and rarely during its treatment. In India, PKDL is the most common skin manifestation of leishmaniasis presenting as polymorphic or macular lesions (Fig. 176-18).

Affected patients are the major reservoirs of the infection. High blood concentration of the immunosuppressive cytokine interleukin-10 in VL patients is predictive of PKDL development. The parasite count is low and detection of organisms is not always possible. With polymerase chain reaction (PCR) technique, however, *Leishmania* parasites are recovered in skin lesions in up to 83% and 94% of Sudanese and Indian PKDL patients, respectively. The development of skin lesions in PKDL is closely linked to *Leishmania*-specific lymphocyte reactivity, or in HIV patients, to immune reconstitution during highly active antiretroviral therapy treatment. The reason behind the 2 major clinical forms of PKDL remains essentially unclear.

Viscerotropic Leishmaniasis:
Caused by *L. tropica*, viscerotropic leishmaniasis has been described among American veterans of Operation Desert Storm. Visceral infection manifests as fever, malaise, and variable hematologic and hepatogastrointestinal findings. Classic signs of VL are absent and the skin is usually not involved; however, a recent report in a young Afghani refugee living in the United States demonstrated cutaneous lesions. Positive culture from bone marrow aspirates and good response to antimonials are typical.

Leishmanid:
Leishmanid refers to an id reaction consisting of a diffuse, asymptomatic, and symmetric papular eruption in the setting of acute LCL or leishmaniasis recidivans. It typically resolves within 8 weeks of its appearance. Leishmanid may develop during treatment and is not an indication to withhold therapy.

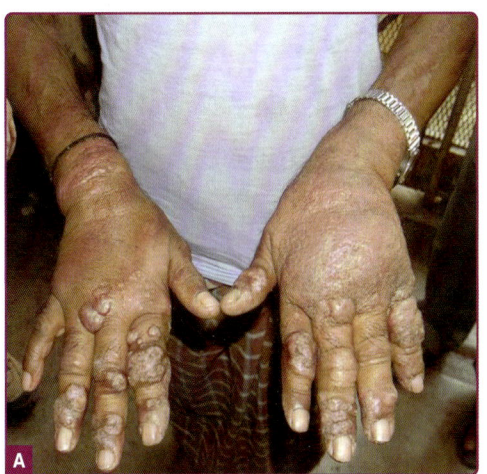

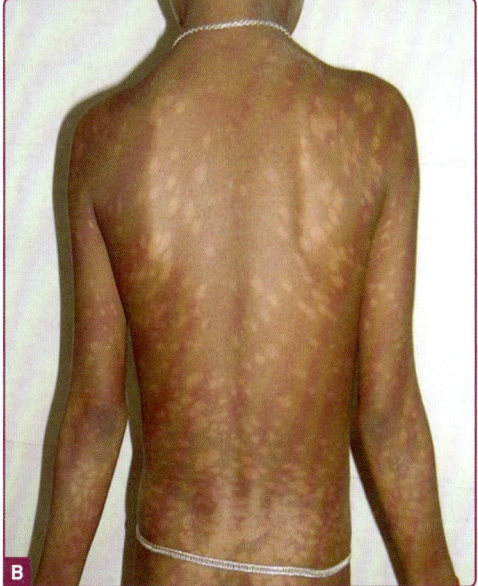

Figure 176-18 A, Polymorphic and (**B**) macular post–kala-azar dermal leishmaniasis. (Used with permission from Prof. Mitali Chatterjee, Calcutta, India.)

Cryptic Leishmaniasis: Both cutaneous and visceral infection can remain subclinical or manifest with mild, nonspecific, and transient symptoms.

DIAGNOSIS

Given the potential treatment toxicity, confirmation of the diagnosis is always mandatory. Parasite subspecies determination is important for treatment decisions.[7-14] Even when smear, histology, and culture results are combined, the parasite may not be detected in 10% to 20% of cases. The diagnostic challenge is often greater in New World disease and in chronic lesions. The sensitivity of both tissue smear and culture approaches 90% when specimens are taken during the first weeks of infection. The best approach is to use several diagnostic methods.

Taken from the infiltrated margin, a skin biopsy may be divided into 3 parts: one for an impression smear, one for histologic examination, and another for culture.

IMPRESSION SMEAR

Several smear techniques may be used with a success rate ranging between 50% and 80%. They are obtainable from fine-needle aspirates or tissue scrapings, air-dried, fixed with methyl alcohol, stained with Giemsa stain, and viewed under oil-immersion microscopy. Impression smears, made by gently pressing the skin biopsy against a glass slide 2 to 5 times, provide better sensitivity than hematoxylin-and-eosin examination.

HISTOLOGY

The histopathologic examination of early lesions of LCL reveals a dense and diffuse mixed inflammatory cell infiltrate composed predominantly of histiocytes, and scattered multinucleated giant cells, lymphocytes, and plasma cells (sometimes with intracytoplasmic homogenous eosinophilic immunoglobulin material called *Russell bodies*). The hallmark of the disease (in approximately 70% of the cases) is the presence of numerous extracellular and intracellular (within histiocytes) amastigotes (also known as *Leishman-Donovan bodies*) (Fig. 176-19A). Giemsa stain stains the parasite nonmetachromatically and the kinetoplast bright red (Fig. 176-19B). The organisms also may be highlighted by the Wright and Feulgen stains. Monoclonal antibodies can identify amastigotes and promastigotes in smear, biopsy, or culture specimens, constituting a rapid screening test for leishmaniasis; however, they are not commercially available.

The histologic differential diagnosis includes diseases characterized by parasitized macrophages. The presence of halo surrounding the yeasts in histoplasmosis, safety pin-like encapsulated Donovan bodies in granuloma inguinale, and Mikulicz cells in rhinoscleroma distinguishes these conditions from leishmaniasis. Other considerations are blastomycosis, paracoccidiomycosis, toxoplasmosis, and trypanosomiasis. As the lesion evolves, the number of amastigotes per section decreases and the histology approaches that of a chronic LCL, where the predominant histologic pattern is nodular/diffuse noncaseating tuberculoid granulomatous dermatitis. Epidermal hyperplasia and ulceration are variable. Scarring with marked loss of elastic fibers may be seen.

In DCL, a diffuse infiltrate composed of vacuolated macrophages with numerous intracellular and extracellular amastigotes is characteristic. The major differential diagnosis is lepromatous leprosy.

In MCL, the histopathologic findings are similar to those of LCL but organisms are usually sparse.

In PKDL, Pautrier-like epidermal microabscesses and a dense lymphoplasmacytic infiltrate with papillary dermal edema (in early lesions) are characteristic.

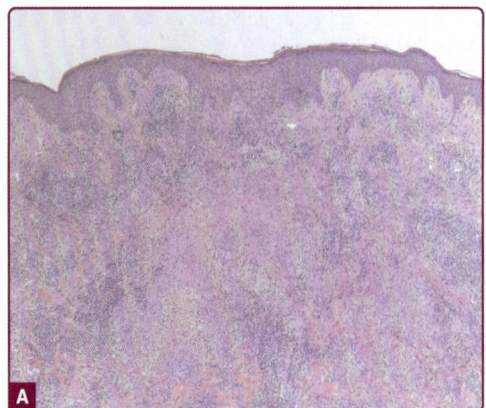
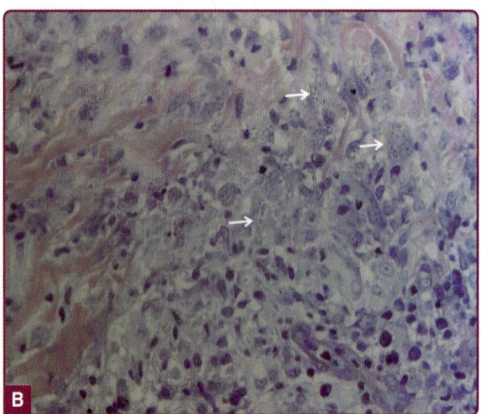

Figure 176-19 A Histologic examination (hematoxylin and eosin). Cutaneous leishmaniasis with tuberculoid granulomatous dermatitis. Note the presence of multinucleated giant cells and the surrounding lymphoplasmacytic infiltrate.

CULTURE

Culture (at room temperature), by means of a biphasic medium such as Novy-MacNeal-Nicolle or chick embryo medium, is the gold standard of diagnosis, but with a sensitivity of only approximately 50%, depending on the experience of the laboratory. It can be performed using aspirates, scrapings, or fresh skin biopsies. Promastigotes often appear after several days, but occasionally may take few weeks. Species identification is not possible based on their morphology.

MOLECULAR ANALYSES

Molecular techniques using species-specific oligonucleotide probes for kinetoplast DNA may be used on all specimens. PCR methods are particularly useful and offer superior specificity and sensitivity in the diagnosis of CL, MCL, and VL, especially in cases where organisms are scarce. False-positive reactions and species identification in New World CL can be problematic.

Together with PCR, isoenzyme analysis is currently considered to be the gold standard for *Leishmania* specification. It consists of enzyme electrophoresis of cultured promastigotes and is based on the fact that morphologically similar promastigotes of different species have different enzyme profiles; however, it is lengthy and costly.

DIAGNOSIS IN VISCERAL LEISHMANIASIS

In VL, microscopic detection and/or culture of parasites in tissue aspirates from spleen (sensitivity >97%), lymph nodes (sensitivity 60%), or bone marrow (sensitivity 55% to 97%) is diagnostic. However, as these techniques are invasive, several serologic and molecular methods have been developed. Anti-K39 antibody based on a recombinant antigen from *L. chagasi* has high sensitivity and specificity. It is an immunochromatographic strip test using fingerprick blood and is helpful in resource-poor regions. As a last resort, PCR of peripheral blood or tissue aspirate can be done, and it is extremely sensitive.

MONTENEGRO SKIN TEST (LEISHMANIN)

The Montenegro skin test is analogous to the tuberculin test and consists of phenol-killed promastigotes injected in the dermis. This allows the detection of exposure to *Leishmania* without distinguishing between past and active infection. Up to 50% of people living in endemic areas may test positive without a history of previous or active disease. The test is positive once crusting has developed, and negative in anergic states such as DCL and PKDL or often in lesions (less than 3 months old). In most countries, the antigen for the test is not available.

TECHNIQUES WITH LIMITED VALUE

Serology is not useful because of its low sensitivity (antibodies present in low titer) and specificity (because of cross-reaction with leprosy, malaria, and other trypanosomal infections). Laboratory animal inoculation (xenodiagnosis) is useful when the parasite load is low. Electron microscopy offers no advantage over light microscopy and its use is limited.

DIFFERENTIAL DIAGNOSIS

Depending on the form of leishmaniasis, different disease entities need to be considered (Table 176-4).

TREATMENT

Given the clinical diversity of leishmaniasis and the lack of adequately controlled therapeutic trials, each case needs to be individualized based on the parasite species, extent of the disease, host immune and nutritional status, presence of intercurrent diseases, geographic region, and cost, availability, and toxicity of the various therapeutic options.[7-14]

TABLE 176-4
Differential Diagnosis for Cutaneous and Visceral Leishmaniasis

LEISHMANIASIS FORM	DIFFERENTIAL DIAGNOSIS
Localized cutaneous leishmaniasis	Arthropod bite
	Infections: pyoderma, Majocchi granuloma, tuberculosis, atypical mycobacterial and deep fungal infections), lupus, leprosy
	Sarcoidosis, foreign-body granulomas, discoid lupus
	Pyoderma gangrenosum
	Malignancy: basal cell/squamous cell carcinoma, keratoacanthoma, lymphoma, pseudolymphoma
Diffuse cutaneous leishmaniasis	Infections: lepromatous leprosy, deep fungal infections
	Xanthomas
	Lymphoma
Mucocutaneous leishmaniasis	Infections: leprosy, syphilitic gumma, yaws, tuberculosis, deep fungal infections (eg, paracoccidioidomycosis)
	Granulomatosis with polyangiitis (Wegener)
	Malignancy: nasopharyngeal carcinoma, squamous cell carcinoma and lymphoma
Visceral leishmaniasis	Infections: malaria, syphilis, tuberculosis, typhoid fever, brucellosis, histoplasmosis, schistosomiasis
	Systemic lupus erythematosus
	Leukemia/lymphoma
	Tropical splenomegaly syndrome
Post-kala-azar dermal leishmaniasis	Infections: syphilis, yaws, leprosy

THERAPEUTIC OPTIONS

Local Therapy: Various regimens have shown some efficacy (Table 176-5). Long-term experience exists regarding intralesional application of antimony. Excision of single lesions can be considered. The combination of paromomycin with methylbenzethonium chloride was shown to be effective mainly against Old World CL. Application of photodynamic therapy resulted in the ablation of affected tissue leading to good clinical results. Moist wound treatment with sodium chloride is low priced and effective.

Systemic Therapy: Table 176-6 summarizes the systemic therapies used for leishmaniasis. Sodium stibogluconate and meglumine antimoniate are pentavalent antimony derivatives with slightly differing antimony concentrations and comparable efficacy and safety profiles. They are the mainstay of systemic treatment. Indian VL is treated with 20 mg/kg/day IM or IV once daily for 40 days versus 28 days if the disease is contracted elsewhere. Antimony resistance is a serious issue in India and Iran. Resistant cases may benefit from combining antimonials with pentoxifylline, allopurinol, paromomycin, azithromycin, interferon-γ, granulocyte-macrophage colony-stimulating factor, and topical imiquimod.

Recently, treatment with liposomal amphotericin B or miltefosine has proven to be efficacious for many CL and VL cases. Side effects are less severe and transient.

Other reported systemic therapies include terbinafine, metronidazole, dapsone, interferon-γ, allopurinol, trimethoprim-sulfamethoxazole, rifampin, nifurtimox, quinolones, pyrimethamine, anti–interleukin-10 (experimentally lead to sterile cure), and azithromycin.

CHOICE OF TREATMENT

Species determination is important for the choice of the systemic drug. Resistance and drug ineffectiveness for distinct subspecies is an increasing problem. None of the drugs has universal anti-*Leishmania* activity. Current guidelines aid the decision about the choice of drug. Table 176-7 summarizes current recommendations about the treatment of CL, MCL, and VL caused by different subspecies.

In general, New World CL tends to be more severe and progressive than Old World CL. In addition, New World CL caused by *L. braziliensis* may progress into MCL ("espundia"), thus necessitating systemic therapy. As a rule, patients should be monitored until the lesions have completely healed. Follow up at 6 months is appropriate.

Because many lesions caused by *L. major* and *L. mexicana* heal spontaneously within 4 months, a less-aggressive approach can be favored. Local therapy (see Table 176-5) is appropriate for small, noninflamed and localized lesions that are not at risk to progress to MCL. Patients with uncomplicated CL can be treated with local therapy. Pregnancy may favor local treatment because of the toxicity of the drugs.

Patients exhibiting "complex" lesions should receive systemic therapy. *Complex lesions* have more than 3 lesions or at least one larger than 4 cm and localized on cosmetically or functionally important sites such as the joints or face. In addition, patients with persistent, diffuse, progressive, recurrent, satellite, and sporotrichoid lesions and/or MCL and VL should receive systemic treatment. Patients with immunosuppression (eg, as a result of HIV infection or medication) have an increased risk for parasite persistence and recurrences and should thus be treated systemically. In general, Old World CL requires shorter courses compared to New World CL.

TABLE 176-5
Local Therapy Against Cutaneous Leishmaniasis

- Excision/curettage or laser ablation
- Cryotherapy, thermotherapy, electrotherapy, photodynamic therapy
- Intralesional antimonial, combined with cryotherapy
- Paromomycin ointment alone or combined with 12% methylbenzethonium chloride
- Sodium chloride (moist wound treatment)

Others:
Topical azoles, topical amphotericin B, topical glyceryl trinitrate or nitric oxide donor, intralesional metronidazole, intralesional interferon-γ

TABLE 176-6
Systemic Drugs Available Against Leishmaniasis

DRUG/DOSE	MECHANISM OF ACTION	ADVERSE EVENTS
Pentavalent antimonials: • sodium stibogluconate (Pentostam) IV • meglumine antimoniate (Glucantime) IM/IV 20 mg/kg/day for 20 to 30 days	Inhibition of glycolysis and oxidation of fatty acids of the parasite	Dose dependent and resolve after discontinuation of drug Pain at injection site, myalgia (68%), pancreatitis (18%), hepatitis, marrow suppression, QT prolongation, fatigue, headache, rash, and nausea
Pentoxifylline (with pentavalent antimony) 400 mg orally 2 to 3 times/day	Inhibits tumor necrosis factor-α	No significant side effects related to pentoxifylline
Pentamidine 2 to 4 mg/kg/day IM or IV every other day for 4 to 7 days	Not established yet	Risk of diabetes mellitus in high-dose course, nephrotoxicity, hypotension, arrhythmias, nausea, vomiting, diarrhea, pancytopenia, cough, bronchospasm, confusion, and hallucinations
Amphotericin B 1 mg/kg every other day for up to 30 days IV (15 mg/kg total dose)	Binding to sterols present in parasite's membrane causing a change in permeability	Hyperpyrexia, hypotension, thrombophlebitis, renal complications, anemia, and hepatitis
Liposomal amphotericin 2 to 3 mg/kg/day IV for 5 to 14 days		Less renal toxicity than amphotericin B
Miltefosine 1.5 to 2.5 mg/kg/day for 28 days orally	Inhibits phosphatidylcholine biosynthesis in parasites	Diarrhea, vomiting, reproductive toxicity in animals
Imidazoles	Inhibition of demethylation of lanosterol, blocking ergosterol synthesis	No significant side effects, hepatotoxicity
Paromomycin sulfate 15 mg/kg daily IM for 21 days	Inhibition of protein synthesis	Rarely: nephrogenic, ototoxic, hepatotoxic
Zinc sulfate 2.5 to 10 mg/kg/day orally for 30 to 40 days	Boosting of Th1 reaction as well as phagocytosis of parasites	Necrosis at injection site

TABLE 176-7
Systemic Treatment Recommendations for Leishmaniasis

PATHOGEN	RECOMMENDED DRUGS (ORDER OF CHOICE)
Old World	
Leishmania major	1. Miltefosine, fluconazole, ketoconazole 2. Liposomal amphotericin B 3. Antimony IV (+ pentoxifylline)
Leishmania tropica	1. Azoles (oral) 2. Liposomal amphotericin B 3. Antimony IV (± allopurinol)
Leishmania infantum	1. Liposomal amphotericin B 2. Miltefosine or antimony IV (± pentoxifylline)
Leishmania aethiopica	Liposomal amphotericin B, miltefosine, Antimony IV (+ pentoxifylline)
New World	
Leishmania braziliensis	1. Antimony IV (+ pentoxifylline) 2. Miltefosine 3. Liposomal amphotericin B
Leishmania guyanensis	1. Miltefosine 2. Pentamidine 3. Antimony IV (+ pentoxifylline)
Leishmania mexicana	1. Ketoconazole 2. Miltefosine 3. Antimony IV (+ pentoxifylline)

PREVENTION AND VACCINE

Essential to prevention is the promotion of personal protective measures through the use of protective clothing, insect repellents containing 30% to 35% N,N-diethyl-3-methylbenzamide (DEET), and permethrin-treated bed nets; the avoidance of endemic areas; and staying on higher floors of buildings in the evening.

One method of reservoir control of L. major was achieved by destroying burrows made by the rodent host. In endemic areas where dogs could be hosts of parasites, a dog collar coated with deltamethrin could be a useful way to control transmission. Targeting anthroponotic foci that are at the origin of deadly epidemics, suspecting leishmaniasis in persons with skin lesions or febrile illnesses returning from endemic areas, and deferring prospective blood donors from donating blood for at least 1 year after their return are other measures. Control of HIV in southern Europe where leishmaniasis is closely associated with HIV has generated positive outcome.

New diagnostic tests, drugs, and vaccines are in development. Vaccine development for tropical diseases is often limited by the lack of financial return. "Leishmanization," the self-inoculation of the live parasite in inconspicuous areas of the body, has been practiced in endemic areas to prevent disfiguring facial lesions, but was later abandoned because of its complications. Killed promastigotes vaccines with and without adjuvant bacille Calmette-Guérin seem to be useful in some endemic areas. Adjuvants such as bacille Calmette-Guérin are important to prime a Th1 response. Attenuated live parasites–based and plasmid DNA–based vaccines using leishmanial antigens have shown efficacy in mouse models. Experimental vaccines containing a component of sand fly saliva proteins appear to be promising. Despite being experimentally successful, a safe nonliving prophylactic vaccine has not yet been able to confer significant protection in humans. A vaccine for dogs has been approved. The sequencing of the *Leishmania* genome in 2007 might lead the way to new ways for prevention, control, and treatment of the condition.

AFRICAN TRYPANOSOMIASIS (SLEEPING SICKNESS)

EPIDEMIOLOGY

African trypanosomiasis afflicts humans (sleeping sickness) and cattle (nagana), and affects up to half a million people every year in the middle latitudes of Africa, where the vector is found.[2] The fatality rate is close to 100% in untreated patients. The disease is very rare in the United States.

African trypanosomiasis is caused by infections with *Trypanosoma brucei*. Depending on the species involved, African trypanosomiasis presents in 2 distinct forms:

- West African or Gambian trypanosomiasis (caused by *Trypanosoma brucei gambiense*) is a chronic predominantly anthroponotic disease present in rural areas west of the Rift Valley.
- East African or Rhodesian trypanosomiasis (caused by *Trypanosoma brucei rhodesiense*) is an acute fatal disease (within weeks, if untreated) that infects mainly livestock/game animals east of the Rift Valley, and sporadically herdsmen, hunters, photographers, and tourists.

Water requirements of the *Glossina palpalis* group of tsetse flies and the savannah habitat of *Glossina morsitans* determine the geographic distribution of Gambian trypanosomiasis and Rhodesian trypanosomiasis, respectively. This ecologic separation, however, is not as strict as it was in the past, with an overlap of the 2 forms of the disease in Uganda.

ETIOLOGY AND PATHOGENESIS

T. brucei, a unicellular organism, enters the bloodstream of a mammalian host via the bite of a blood-feeding infected male or female tsetse fly of the genus

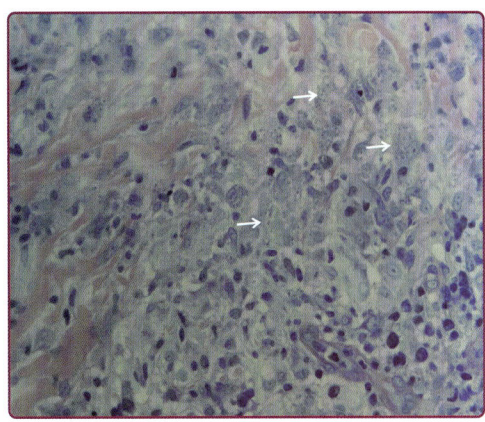

Figure 176-20 Giemsa stain of skin biopsy with cutaneous leishmaniasis. Moderately dense lymphohistiocytic infiltrate with numerous parasitized macrophages containing amastigotes (Leishman bodies, marked with white arrows).

Glossina.[15] Other uncommon ways to contract the disease include placental transmission, blood transfusion, and sexual contact.

The tsetse flies are attracted by dust clouds of moving objects and animals, as well as black and blue colors. They bite most during early daylight and at dusk, and ingest trypomastigotes from infected blood meals (Fig. 176-20).

Trypomastigotes have a glycoprotein-coated surface that is protective against lytic factors in human plasma. Furthermore, the extensive antigenic variation of the glycoprotein present on the parasite's surface allows evasion from humoral immunity,[16] which explains why a vaccine targeting trypanosomes is extremely difficult to develop.[17]

CLINICAL FINDINGS

In Rhodesian trypanosomiasis, a painful chancre develops at the site of the tsetse bite and resolves within 1 to 3 weeks leaving no scar. It consists of a circumscribed, rubbery, indurated, 2- to 5-cm dusky red nodule, often with a central eschar (Fig. 176-21).[17-19] In Gambian trypanosomiasis, however, the initial lesion consists of a single, nonspecific nodule that is often mistaken for an insect bite or a folliculitis.

Afterward, African trypanosomiasis will evolve in 2 stages: the hemolymphatic or early stage and the meningoencephalitic or late stage. In contrast to the late stage, when the skin is not involved, cutaneous changes may be seen in the early stage and are more commonly observed in Rhodesian trypanosomiasis and in light-skin patients. Perhaps for this reason, skin lesions are rarely reported in native Africans.

EARLY STAGE

The hemolymphatic stage occurs 3 to 10 days after the initial bite, with the parasites entering the

LATE STAGE

The late stage is characterized by CNS involvement weeks to months after exposure in Rhodesian trypanosomiasis, and months to years after exposure in Gambian trypanosomiasis, and occurs when parasites cross the blood–brain barrier. Severe headache develops followed by chronic meningoencephalitis, somnolence, coma, and death. Delayed bilateral pain disproportionate to a sharp squeeze applied to soft tissues, known as the Kerandel sign (deep, delayed hyperesthesia), is characteristically found in European patients, but is uncommon in African patients.[20] Patients may also develop behavioral changes, psychosis, and focal neurologic symptoms. Marked weight loss can ensue.

DIAGNOSIS

Diagnosis of African trypanosomiasis is via detection of trypanosomes in blood film or Giemsa-stained thick smears, chancre/lymph node aspirate, buffy coat, bone marrow, or cerebrospinal fluid. Histologically, long, thin trypanosomes are best seen using Giemsa stain, in the midst of a perivascular lymphoplasmacytic infiltrate.[20] Because of antigenic variability, serologic tests lack sensitivity and specificity. Differentiation of Rhodesian trypanosomiasis from Gambian trypanosomiasis is usually based on epidemiology. PCR is the method of choice, but cost limits its use in African countries. New diagnostic tools are being developed.

TREATMENT

A lumbar puncture is essential for the differentiation between the early and late stages because treatment varies based on stage. Four registered drugs are currently provided free of charge by the WHO. Table 176-8 outlines the drugs and the stages for which the drugs

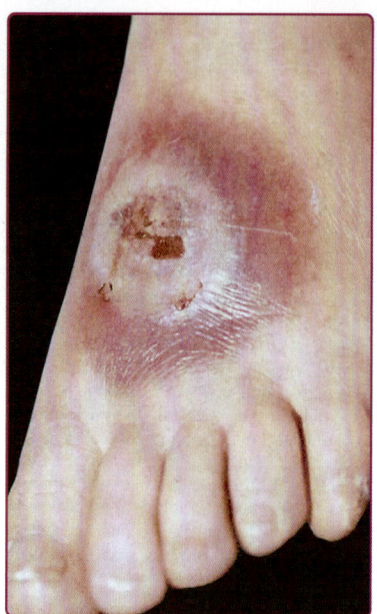

Figure 176-21 East African trypanosomiasis. The trypanosome chancre consists of erythematous nodule with central bulla and ulceration. This patient was treated with suramin and survived. (From Moore AC, Ryan ET, Waldron MA. Case Records of the Massachusetts General Hospital. Weekly clinicopathological exercises. Case 20-2002. A 37-year-old man with fever, hepatosplenomegaly, and a cutaneous foot lesion after a trip to Africa. *N Engl J Med.* 2002;346[26]:2069-2076, with permission of the Massachusetts Medical Society. Copyright © 2002 Massachusetts Medical Society.)

circulation and causing irregularly spiking fever. Hepatosplenomegaly, constitutional symptoms, normocytic anemia, thrombocytopenia, and pruritus (especially presternal) develop, and may be related to circulating immune complexes. Local lymphadenopathy progresses to generalized lymphadenopathy in virtually all African natives and in about half of European patients. Involvement of the posterior cervical (Winterbottom sign) and supraclavicular lymph node is characteristic only of Gambian trypanosomiasis. The disease is more severe in Rhodesian trypanosomiasis where severe parasitemia, myocarditis, and, rarely, fatal disseminated intravascular coagulopathy develop.[18] Trypanids are distinctive eruptions that develop 6 to 8 weeks after the onset of fever in approximately half the light-skin patients, and consist of poorly defined, centrally pale, evanescent, annular, targetoid, or blotchy erythematous macular, hemorrhagic, urticarial, or erythema nodosum-like lesions, commonly on the trunk.[19] These lesions might be the result of a Type III hypersensitivity reaction.[2] A sensation of formication may be associated. The eruption waxes and wanes over weeks with accentuation upon exposure to cold, heat, or sweat. Painless swelling of the face (imparting a sad look), and of the hands and feet may occur. Other findings include ichthyosis, acroparesthesias, icterus, petechiae, and generalized flushing.

TABLE 176-8
Treatment Options against African Trypanosomiasis

DRUG	EARLY STAGE	LATE STAGE
Pentamidine	Rhodesian trypanosomiasis (RT), Gambian trypanosomiasis (GT)	
Suramin	RT, GT	
Melarsoprol	RT, GT	RT, GT Effective against CNS life forms, neurotoxic
Eflornithine	GT	GT Effective against CNS life forms, neurotoxic
Nifurtimox		RT, GT

are given. Of concern, HIV-positive patients receiving treatment for Rhodesian trypanosomiasis may succumb to full-blown AIDS.

Combination therapy using the available drugs was investigated and all trials showed better results than monotherapy.[21,22] Of note, combination therapy containing melarsoprol leads to severe drug reactions. A multicountry study comparing nifurtimox (registered for the treatment of Chagas disease) and eflornithine to eflornithine alone was undertaken for late-stage Gambian trypanosomiasis. The combination therapy resulted in fewer infusions, shorter treatment duration, and fewer adverse effects.

Various small molecules of diverse chemical nature are currently being investigated in clinical trials.

PREVENTION

Control of African trypanosomiasis in endemic areas is highly cost-effective and entails case detection and treatment, keeping tsetse populations at low levels,[2,21] and mass screening of at-risk populations.

CHAGAS DISEASE (AMERICAN TRYPANOSOMIASIS)

EPIDEMIOLOGY

American trypanosomiasis is a zoonotic disease caused by *Trypanosoma cruzi* and transmitted to humans by blood-sucking triatomine bugs (kissing bugs, assassin bugs, reduviid bugs).[1,2] It is endemic in many rural areas of Central and South America and Mexico. In the United States, as many as 300,000 individuals are affected and as many as 45,000 individuals have the clinical disease.

ETIOLOGY AND PATHOGENESIS

Triatomine bugs are large (3 to 4 cm), "cone-nosed" bedbugs that thrive in poor housing conditions and become infected with *T. cruzi* by feeding on contaminated blood. An infected triatomine bug takes a blood meal usually at night, and releases trypomastigotes in its feces near the site of the bite wound, usually a mucocutaneous junction. Human infection occurs when mucous membranes, especially the conjunctiva, or skin breaks are contaminated with the feces upon rubbing/scratching (Fig. 176-22). Other reported ways of transmission of the disease seem to be via the intake of reduviid feces–contaminated fruits and fruit products. Congenital (transplacental) transmission and transmission by blood transfusion and organ transplantation may also occur.

CLINICAL FINDINGS

American trypanosomiasis progresses in 3 stages.[23-25]

ACUTE PHASE (FIRST STAGE)

Transient parasitemia is usually asymptomatic or associated with fever, lymphadenopathy, mild hepatosplenomegaly, and morbilliform/urticarial rash; it can last for as long as 8 weeks. This stage may be fatal in young children or immunosuppressed individuals.

Other dermatologic manifestations seen in the first stage include:

- *Chagoma*, a painful inflammatory reaction at the site of inoculation, approximately 1- to 3-cm in size, erythematous, often ulcerated nodule with a surrounding pale halo. Local lymphadenopathy often present.
- *Schizotrypanides*, a generalized morbilliform eruption, or transient skin rash resembling measles.
- *Romaña sign* (or ophthalmoganglionar complex), which manifests as unilateral conjunctivitis with palpebral edema (from conjunctival inoculation).

INDETERMINATE PHASE (SECOND STAGE)

During this chronic, asymptomatic, but infectious stage, low levels of the parasite are found in blood. Reactivation of the infection may occur following organ transplantation (disseminated, painful, subcutaneous and/or ulcerated nodules).

SYMPTOMATIC CHRONIC PHASE (THIRD STAGE)

The third stage is characterized by lethal, dilated cardiomyopathy, arrhythmias, megaesophagus, and megacolon. It occurs in 10% to 30% of patients, often many years after initial infection. Genetic variability of *T. cruzi* might determine the clinical presentation of chronic disease. The pathogenesis was thought to be mediated by molecular mimicry; however, parasites persistence in tissues were recently demonstrated by PCR and in situ hybridization.

DIAGNOSIS

Diagnosis and treatment are problematic. In the first stage, diagnosis involves microscopic demonstration of trypomastigotes in blood specimens, especially thin smears, hemoculture, or xenodiagnosis. Thereafter,

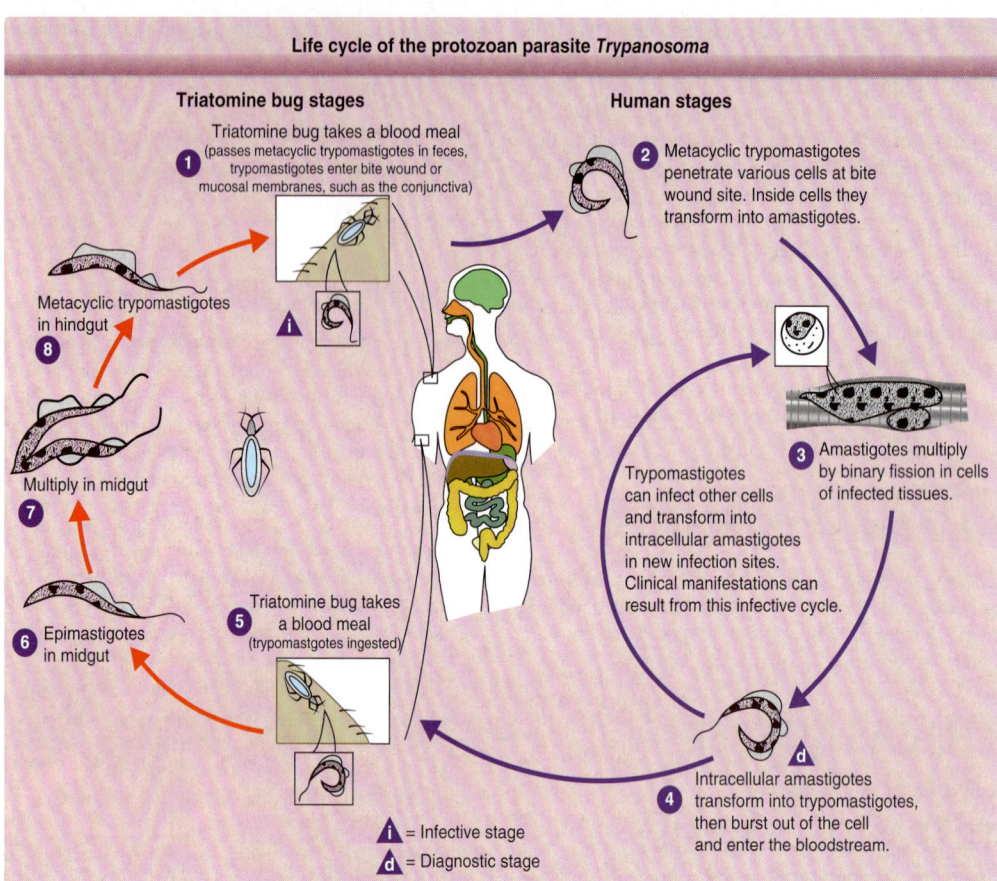

Figure 176-22 Life cycle of the protozoan parasite *Trypanosoma*. (From the Centers for Disease Control and Prevention [CDC].)

detection of organisms becomes difficult, and diagnosis relies more on serologic testing or PCR. The WHO recommends using at least 2 antigen detection tests for confirmation of the disease.[2,26]

chemotherapeutic intervention at any stage of the disease is currently recommended.

Allopurinol and itraconazole also have been tried for chronic disease.

TREATMENT

Treatment is indicated for acute infections, congenital infections, patients who are immunosuppressed, and children with chronic disease.[2,27-29] Both drugs that are available, benznidazole and nifurtimox, are toxic and most effective when given during the first stage of the infection or in congenital infections.

Because of their toxicity, potential carcinogenic risk, decreased efficacy in chronic disease, and the presumably autoimmune nature of the latter, treatment of chronic disease has long been considered controversial. Later studies, however, revealed the persistence of the parasite in heart muscle as well as digestive tissue in patients with the chronic condition. In addition, patients with chronic cardiomyopathy who were given benznidazole had less clinical deterioration a decade later as well as lower serologic titers. Consequently,

PREVENTION

Preventive measures are aimed at eradicating the vectors, improving diagnostic tests, developing less toxic and more efficient drugs, and implementing serologic screening of organ donors and recipients. Control programs have reduced the incidence of American trypanosomiasis by 70% in some countries of South America.[2]

MALARIA

EPIDEMIOLOGY

Malaria transmission occurs in 95 countries/territories; 3.2 billion people (half of the world's population) are at risk of acquiring malaria. Sub-Saharan Africa carries the largest burden with 88% of malaria cases and 90% of malaria-associated deaths. However, Asia, Latin America and, to a lesser extent, the Middle East also are at risk.[30]

According to the WHO, in 2015, 214 million patients with malaria were reported together with approximately 450,000 fatal cases. Between 2000 and 2015, the global burden has fallen by approximately 40% as a result of efficient control programs; however, in sub-Saharan Africa the decline has lagged behind.

The exact incidence of cutaneous lesions in malaria is not known, but it appears to be rare.

ETIOLOGY AND PATHOGENESIS

Malaria is caused by infection with the protozoan parasite of the genus *Plasmodium*. Malaria is spread by the bite of infected, female *Anopheles* mosquitoes (Fig. 176-23). The mosquitos bite between dusk and dawn. Transmission efficacy depends on parasite, vector, environmental (temperature, humidity and habitat conditions), and host factors.

Human malaria is caused by 5 species of *Plasmodium*, among which *Plasmodium falciparum* and *Plasmodium vivax* are most threatening. *P. falciparum* is the most prevalent species on the African continent with the most malaria-related deaths globally. *P. vivax* is the dominant parasite outside of sub-Saharan Africa.

Patients at higher risk to develop malaria are mainly infants, children ages 5 years and younger, pregnant women, patients with immunosuppression (eg, HIV/AIDS), and nonimmune immigrants and travelers. Partial immunity after years of exposure does not provide complete protection, but it reduces the risk for severe disease.

Skin manifestations in malaria are rare[31]; their type appears to depend on the immunopathologic mechanism:

1. IgE antibodies against the parasite are found in individuals from endemic areas. Mast cell activation in malaria plays a central role in the pathophysiology. The precise mechanism for mast cell activation is unknown; clinically, it presents as urticaria.
2. IgG antimalarial antibodies are known to be protective against infection. IgG and IgE containing immune complexes are elevated in malaria. Purpura and petechiae may result from cytoadherence, vasculitis, and immune-complex–associated vessel damage.

CLINICAL FINDINGS

Malaria is characterized by an acute febrile disease. Symptoms appear, starting with fever, headache, chills and vomiting, 7 to 14 days after the infective mosquito bite. The initial symptoms may be mild and nonspecific, leaving it difficult to recognize as malaria. If not treated early, *P. falciparum* can progress to severe illness that is often associated with death. Severe malaria (mainly seen in children) is characterized by severe anemia, respiratory distress with metabolic acidosis, and cerebral malaria. Multiorgan involvement in adults is frequent. Asymptomatic infections in endemic areas in individuals with partial immunity may occur.

Cutaneous manifestations are rarely reported and are not specific for malaria.[31] Their onset appears to occur at the time systemic symptoms develop. If reported, they are described as urticaria/angioedema, petechiae/purpura, or disseminated intravascular coagulopathy.

DIAGNOSIS

The diagnosis is made by investigation, blood count, hemogram, and liver function assessment.

TREATMENT

Symptomatic treatment can be initiated to mitigate skin symptoms (eg, antihistamines, corticosteroids). However, upon initiation of antimalarial systemic treatment, skin lesions appear to resolve within a few days.

A vaccine against malaria is under development, but not available yet.

Prevention methods can be highly effective, ranging from utilization of vector-control measures (insecticide-treated mosquito nets, indoor spraying with insecticides) to chemoprophylaxis for travelers. However, malaria-endemic areas such as sub-Saharan Africa and India are causing significant concern because of high levels of malaria transmission and widespread reports of insecticide resistance.

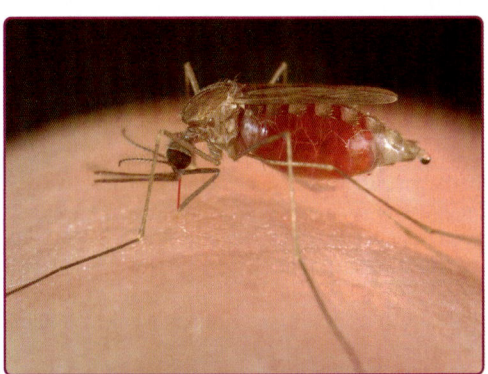

Figure 176-23 *Anopheles* mosquito. (Image from Centers for Disease Control and Prevention [CDC] and James Gathany.)

TRICHOMONIASIS

EPIDEMIOLOGY

Trichomoniasis is considered the most prevalent nonviral sexually transmitted disease worldwide. It appears that millions of *Trichomonas vaginalis* infections remain undiagnosed and untreated.[32] *T. vaginalis* infections affect approximately 3% of all females (ages 14 to 49 years), and are mostly asymptomatic. Approximately 20% of all females between 16 and 35 years of age suffer at least 1 *T. vaginalis* infection.

T. vaginalis is most often transmitted during sexual contact. It remains viable for 24 hours in a humid and warm milieu, and transmission through contaminated objects is possible. Females are more often affected and symptomatic than males. Female sex workers have the highest incidence at 50% to 70%. Approximately 70% of all females with gonorrhea suffer from trichomoniasis.

Spontaneous remission is frequent (about one-third of cases). Only approximately 5% of male patients in a sexually transmitted disease outpatient clinic are positive for *T. vaginalis*. Approximately 15% of nongonorrhea urethritis in males is caused by *T. vaginalis*, however.

ETIOLOGY AND PATHOGENESIS

Three species of *Trichomonas* are pathogenic for humans exhibiting specific localizations. The most common, *T. vaginalis*, prefers cornified mucosa such as the urethra. Other species, such as *Trichomonas tenax*, are found in the oral cavity and can cause gingivitis and other infections. *Pentatrichomonas hominis* is associated with GI symptoms.

T. vaginalis is 4 to 45 μm in length and 2 to 14 μm wide. It contains 4 frontal and 1 larger back flagella, which is embedded into an undulating membrane. Because of its characteristic twitching movements, the pathogen is easy to recognize under the microscope.

CLINICAL FINDINGS

T. vaginalis prefers the epithelia of the vagina and the urethra, and less of the cervix. Rarely, bladder and ureter are affected.[32] Only 15% to 20% of all infected females are symptomatic and suffer from diffuse, malodorous, yellow-green vaginal discharge with or without vulvar involvement. Sexual intercourse may be painful. An untreated trichomoniasis of a female can be associated with inflammatory pelvic disease, neoplasia of the cervix and premature labor. *T. vaginalis* carriers are more prone to acquire HIV, human papillomavirus, and herpes virus infections.

Infection of the prostate, ureter, and foreskin of males is most often asymptomatic. Dysuria and ureter discharge with balanoposthitis are possible. Ascending infections of the prostate and epididymis are very rare.

DIAGNOSIS

WET-MOUNT MICROSCOPY

Swabs of vagina, cervix, or ureter can be examined for the typically large, moving pathogen. This is the most commonly used method, and it has a relatively low cost. The sensitivity is low (51% to 65% in vagina secretions; even lower in male specimens). The sensitivity declines dramatically with a delayed evaluation of the sample.

CULTURE

Before molecular testing methods became available, culture was considered the gold standard for diagnosing *T. vaginalis* infections. It has a sensitivity of 75% to 95% and a high specificity. Several culture media are available.

MOLECULAR TESTS

Nucleic acid amplification tests are available for detection of *T. vaginalis* in vaginal, endocervical, and urine specimens of women. The specificity is very high; the sensitivity is 95% to 100%.[33]

SEROLOGY

The antibody response is variable and not reliable; a routine test for antibodies against *T. vaginalis* is not recommended.

TREATMENT

Treatment reduces both symptoms and transmission.[34]

Systemic treatment consists of metronidazole, 2 g orally in a single dose, or tinidazole 2 g can be given in a single dose. The cure rates after metronidazole regimens were 84% to 98%, those after tinidazole 92% to 100%. An alternative regimen, metronidazole 500 mg orally twice a day for 7 days, can be administered. The response rate is considered to be 90% to 95%. One study showed that topical metronidazole 750 mg combined with 200 mg miconazole twice daily for 7 days was as effective as systemic treatment with metronidazole alone.

Long-term treatment with metronidazole should be avoided. During pregnancy, treatment options are limited. Topical metronidazole can be considered.

RHINOSPORIDIOSIS

EPIDEMIOLOGY

Rhinosporidium seeberi is an aquatic pathogen; it is still unclear if it can be classified as protozoan or a fungus.[35,36] It can be found in America, Europe, Africa, and Asia, mainly in tropical regions (predominantly in South India, Sri Lanka, and South America).

ETIOLOGY AND PATHOGENESIS

The mode of transmission is largely unknown, but appears to be associated with spore transmission during fresh water contact (eg, during bathing). Within the inoculated tissue, the organisms replicate locally with hyperplasia, followed by a localized immune response resulting in a granulomatous disease.

CLINICAL FINDINGS

Rhinosporidiosis is mainly seen in males at the nasal, nasopharyngeal, and oral mucosa. Symptoms present as painless nodules that slowly grow to large, hyperplastic polyps with irregular, erythematous surfaces.

The external skin is only rarely affected. Conjunctiva, rectum and external genitalia can be involved.

DIAGNOSIS

The protozoan cannot be cultured yet, thus the diagnosis is based on biopsy specimen followed by histology. A large sporangium (mature form of the pathogen, 100 to 400 μm in size) is seen with thousands of endospores inside.

TREATMENT

Removal of the affected tissue is the main therapy; however, recurrences are frequent. Injection of amphotericin B appears to minimize development of recurrences. Long-term treatment with dapsone has been reported.

CRYPTOSPORIDIOSIS

EPIDEMIOLOGY

Cryptosporidiosis is a disease caused by the protozoan parasite *Cryptosporidium*. Both giardiasis and cryptosporidiosis belong to the most common intestinal parasitic infections worldwide.[37,38]

Children and people taking care of infected individuals have an increased risk of acquiring the infection. In addition, travelers (especially backpackers, campers), swimmers, people who handle infected cattle, and individuals exposed to human feces during sexual contact are more likely to get infected.

ETIOLOGY AND PATHOGENESIS

The life cycle of *Cryptosporidium* can be completed in humans and many animals. *Cryptosporidium parvum* infects humans and animals, whereas *Cryptosporidium hominis* is only found in humans.

Oral infection is established through uptake of *Cryptosporidium* oocysts via contaminated earth, water, uncooked food or after contact with feces of an infected individual or animal. Oocysts are highly resistant to disinfectants; they remain viable and infective for long periods.

After ingestion, oocysts exist in the small intestine and release sporozoites that attach to the microvilli of the intestinal epithelial cells. Then then develop into trophozoites, reproduce by multiple fission, and become merozoites. Released merozoites attach to epithelial cells and become macrogamonts (female sexual form) or microgamonts (male form). Finally, zygotes form after the microgamont penetrates the macrogamont. Zygotes then develop into oocysts, which are then released with the feces.

CLINICAL FINDINGS

After 2 to 10 days of parasite ingestion, watery diarrhea, abdominal cramps/pain, dehydration, nausea and vomiting, fever, weight loss, and lack of appetite develop. The symptoms last for about a week with cycles of transient improvement. Extraintestinal symptoms are arthralgia, headache, and drowsiness. Pulmonary involvement shows unspecific symptoms such as coughing.

Some individuals may be asymptomatic. However, young children and severely immunosuppressed patients (eg, those with HIV/AIDS) have a higher risk for developing severe disease forms.

Spontaneous (chronic) urticaria and angioedema are associated with *Cryptosporidium*-associated diarrhea.[37,38]

DIAGNOSIS

Stool specimens can be investigated for the presence of oocysts. At least 3 different stool samples should be inspected. Antibody detection in serum and molecular methods are available.[39]

TREATMENT

A specific treatment is not available. Paromomycin and other drugs reduce the symptoms of cryptosporidiosis.

GIARDIASIS

EPIDEMIOLOGY

Giardia lamblia (synonyms: *Giardia intestinalis* and *Giardia duodenalis*) is a flagellated protozoan parasite. Infections with *G. lamblia* are the most common intestinal infection in the United States, especially in children.[38,40] In the United States, 5 to 6 cases per 100,000 population are reported. Annually, 1.2 million cases are estimated for the United States.

ETIOLOGY AND PATHOGENESIS

G. lamblia cysts are highly infectious; approximately 10 cysts are sufficient to cause an infection. Transmission occurs mainly by consumption of contaminated water (pools, lakes, inadequately purified drinking water, seasonal), but less frequently also via contaminated food, or fecal–oral transmission (nonseasonal) (Fig. 176-24).

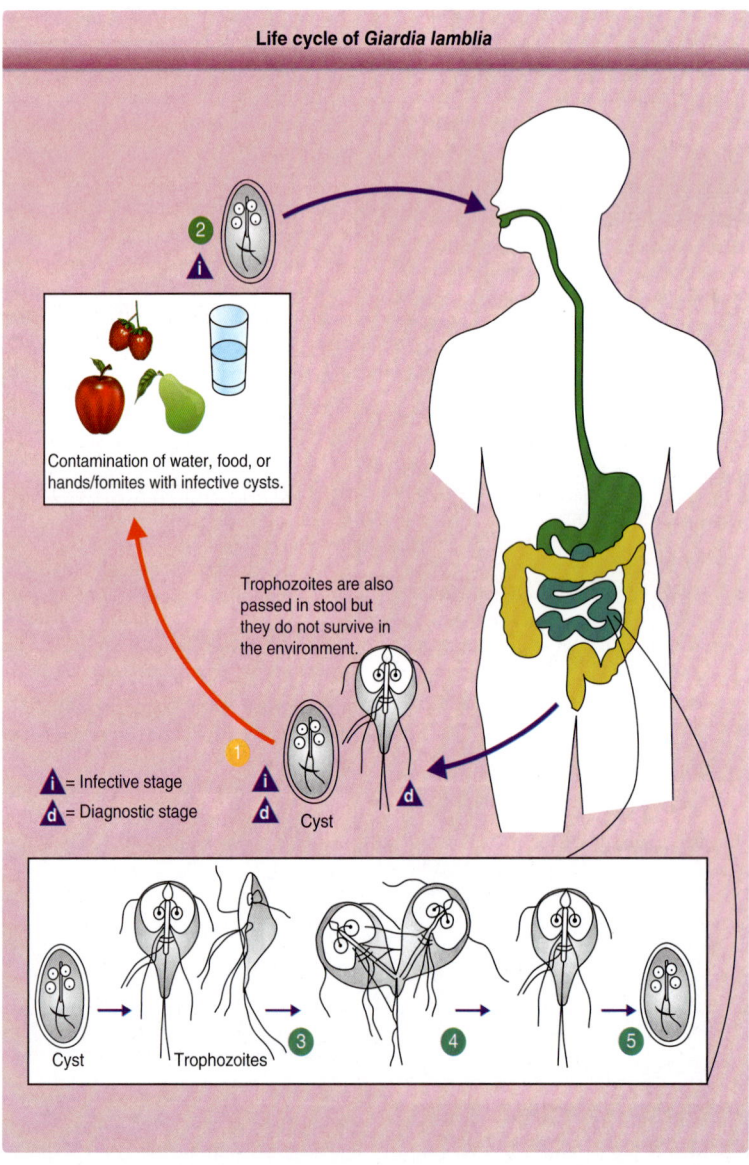

Figure 176-24 Life cycle of *Giardia lamblia*. (From the Centers for Disease Control and Prevention [CDC].)

CLINICAL FINDINGS

Giardiasis is a self-limited disease characterized by diarrhea, abdominal cramps, bloating, dehydration, weight loss, and malabsorption. Symptoms vary and can last for up to 2 weeks; asymptomatic cases are reported.

Skin symptoms of giardiasis are less common and most often present as acute urticaria and/or as angioedema. Giardiasis is also known as pathogen causing chronic urticaria.[41]

DIAGNOSIS

The diagnosis is made by microscopic identification of *Giardia* cysts in stool.

TREATMENT

Systemic treatment with metronidazole, tinidazole, and nitazoxanide is effective.[42] Alternative drugs that can be used to treat giardiasis are paromomycin, quinacrine, albendazole, and furazolidone.

AMEBIASIS

EPIDEMIOLOGY

Amebiasis is the second leading cause of death from parasitic diseases. Annually, 50 million individuals are affected by the infection, and approximately 100,000 deaths are reported. A higher incidence is reported in Mexico and in developing tropical countries.[2,43]

In developed countries, risk groups include male homosexuals, travelers, immigrants, and institutionalized patients. In Europe, asymptomatic intestinal infections are seen in 1% of the population; in homosexuals, asymptomatic intestinal infections are seen in approximately 20% of individuals.

ETIOLOGY AND PATHOGENESIS

Only a few ameba are pathogenic for humans. Within the genus *Entamoeba*, *Entamoeba histolytica* is a pathogenic ameba that can cause intestinal and extraintestinal diseases. Nonpathogenic ameba can be found in the colon. Within the genus *Acanthamoeba*, some facultatively pathogenic species are relevant as inducers of opportunistic infections.

E. histolytica exists in 2 forms: (a) the capsuled cyst (10 to 15 μm) or infective stage, and (b) the mobile trophozoite or tissue-invasive stage. Cysts are known to remain viable for several months in a cold, humid milieu, but they are labile to heat and dryness.

Both forms are passed in the feces. Human beings are the only natural hosts and asymptomatic carriers are the main risk for infection. Infection generally occurs by ingestion of mature cysts in fecally contaminated food, water, or hands. In industrial countries, anal sex and contaminated enema equipment are the main modes of transmission.[2,43]

Trophozoites have marked phagocytic, proteolytic, and cytolytic capabilities, releasing proteases, collagenase, hyaluronidase, *N*-acetylglucosaminidase, phospholipase A, and secretagogues.[2,44] Consequently, they can invade human colonic mucosa and occasionally penetrate through to the portal circulation, reaching the liver and other organs, causing fatal lesions. Some mammalian cells are resistant to trophozoite adherence.

Most cases of asymptomatic noninvasive "luminal amebiasis" are caused by *Entamoeba dispar*, rather than *E. histolytica*.

CLINICAL FINDINGS

Depending on the extent of invasion and the transmission mode, the clinical spectrum includes 3 major presentations[2,43-45]:

1. Invasive intestinal disease (dysentery, colitis, and amebomas).
2. Invasive extraintestinal disease (liver abscess, peritonitis, and pleuropulmonary abscess).
3. Cutaneous disease is rare and can be either primary or secondary:
   - In primary cutaneous amebiasis, an extremely rare condition, the skin is affected without underlying intestinal or extraintestinal disease. It is thought to be secondary to direct inoculation from scratching with contaminated fingers in areas with poor hygiene. Penile lesions are often acquired through anal intercourse with infected individuals.
   - In secondary cutaneous amebiasis, the skin can be infected following extension from an underlying/contiguous intestinal or extraintestinal abscess, draining catheter, fistula, colostomy or laparotomy incision. Trophozoites can also spread through contaminated stool to the anogenital skin. This is often seen in children with diarrhea following direct and prolonged contact with infected feces in their diapers. Autoinoculation via contaminated hands may account for more distal lesions.

   Both types of cutaneous transmissions are rare and result in rapidly progressive, foul smelling, and painful punched-out ulcers with a hemopurulent, raw beef-like base; necrotic, cord-like, and undermined borders; and surrounding erythema (Fig. 176-25). Lesions may reach up to 20 cm in diameter and are often destructive if untreated. Chronic urticaria may be associated and local lymphadenopathy is common. Without prompt diagnosis and treatment, the prognosis is poor. In rare cases, even primary cutaneous amebiasis has a fatal outcome.

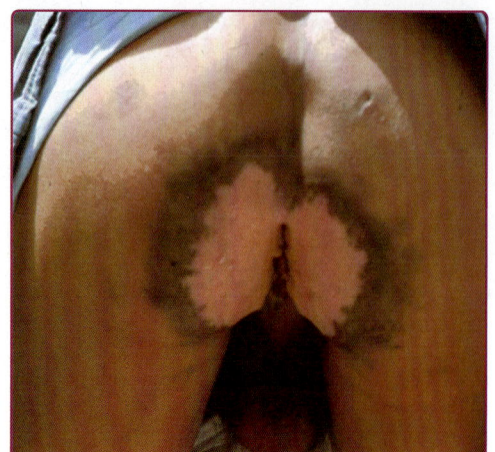

Figure 176-25 Cutaneous amebiasis. (From Kristal L, Prose NS: *Color Atlas of Pediatric Dermatology*, 5th ed. New York, NY: McGraw-Hill; 2017, with permission.)

DIAGNOSIS

The diagnosis relies on identification of cysts and/or trophozoites in infected stool, mucosa, or skin. This method cannot distinguish between *E. histolytica* and *E. dispar*. For this, enzyme-linked immunosorbent assays are useful. Stool culture and PCR are only available as research tools. Serology may be helpful, but false-negativity may occur in early infection.

Skin biopsy reveals ulceration, mixed inflammatory cell infiltrate, and areas of necrosis where trophozoites may be identified as round or oval cells (20 to 50 μm) with basophilic cytoplasm, an eccentric nucleus with central karyosome, and often displaying erythrophagocytosis (sign of pathogenicity).

TREATMENT

For symptomatic intestinal or extraintestinal disease, the drug of choice is oral or IV metronidazole (250 to 800 mg every 8 to 12 hours for 10 days), followed by treatment with one of the luminal agents: iodoquinol, paromomycin, diloxanide furoate, dehydroemetine, or chloroquine.

OPPORTUNISTIC AMEBAS

EPIDEMIOLOGY AND ETIOLOGY

The free-living amebas belonging to the genera *Naegleria*, *Acanthamoeba*, *Balamuthia*, and lately described *Sappinia* are ubiquitous in air, soil, and water; they rarely cause disease in immunocompetent patients; reported presentations include acanthamebic keratitis (in contact lens wearers) and primary amebic meningoencephalitis (caused by *Naegleria fowleri*). Immunocompromised AIDS and organ transplantation patients are at risk of disseminated disease, as well as at risk of developing granulomatous amebic encephalitis, a rare, gradually progressive, fatal neurologic disease caused by *Acanthamoeba* species. Free-living amebas can also harbor bacteria, such as *Legionella*, *Mycobacterium avium*, *Burkholderia* spp., *Escherichia coli*, and *Vibrio cholerae*, possibly serving as vectors of bacterial infections in humans.

The portal of entry of the amebas is usually the nasal mucosa, from which they can reach the CNS. They can also enter through a skin break or through the respiratory tract with subsequent hematogenous dissemination to the CNS.

CLINICAL FINDINGS

Cutaneous lesions have been mainly reported in *Acanthamoeba*-induced disease, mostly in HIV-positive patients.[43-45] *Balamuthia mandrillaris*–related skin involvement, however, is being increasingly reported. In HIV-positive patients, skin lesions are the most common (75% to 90% of the cases) and sometimes the sole manifestation of disseminated disease. The extremities (lower more than upper) and the face are commonly involved. Numerous widely distributed papules, plaques, nodules, and pustules, as well as cellulitis, nonhealing ulcers with rolled borders, eschars, and palatal ulceration have been described. Lymphadenopathy may be present. An asymptomatic plaque over the central face with possible satellite lesions along with neurologic symptoms is a characteristic presentation of *B. mandrillaris* disease.

One study suggested that the immunologic state of the patient determines the clinical outcome of cutaneous acanthamebiasis. On the one hand, immunocompromised patients were unexpectedly found to develop multiple subacute skin lesions without CNS involvement and to respond better to therapy. On the other hand, immunocompetent patients had a worse prognosis with slowly progressive cutaneous lesions and more CNS involvement.

DIAGNOSIS

Histopathologically, a dermal and/or subcutaneous predominantly neutrophilic infiltrate is present, sometimes with vasculitic, and granulomatous changes. The identification of 20- to 30-μm trophozoites with abundant vacuolated cytoplasm, and central nuclear karyosome is diagnostic but may be difficult because of their macrophage-like appearance. Gomori methenamine silver and periodic acid–Schiff stains may highlight the organisms. *B. mandrillaris* may occasionally exhibit more than 1 nucleolus, distinguishing it from *Acanthamoeba*. Definite diagnosis and speciation is possible using indirect immunofluorescence, culture or PCR.

TREATMENT

The disease is often fatal, but early treatment using a combination of IV pentamidine and oral fluconazole, sulfadiazine, isethionate, or 5-fluorocytosine may improve the outcome. HIV patients may benefit from antiretroviral therapy.

ACANTHAMOEBA KERATITIS

EPIDEMIOLOGY AND ETIOLOGY

Acanthamoeba is a ubiquitous protozoan parasite among which 8 species can cause keratitis.[46] Main risk factors are contact lens wear, poor hygiene, and contact with contaminated water.

CLINICAL FINDINGS

The keratitis has can acute onset showing a painful keratitis with destruction of the epithelial layer of the cornea. Secondary scleritis can occur. Typically, only 1 eye is affected. The course can be potentially sight-threatening.

DIAGNOSIS

A corneal scraping can be analyzed by histology, tissue culture, and/or PCR. In scraping material, *Acanthamoeba* can be detected after addition of 10% potassium hydroxide.

TREATMENT

Various local treatments using topical antiseptics, neomycin, paromomycin, polymyxin B, azole antimycotics, and antiinflammatory steroids are effective.

The prognosis is poor because of an often delayed diagnosis, and frequently a lack of effective medical management.

TOXOPLASMOSIS

EPIDEMIOLOGY

Toxoplasmosis, caused by the parasitic protozoan *Toxoplasma gondii* (class Sporozoa), is one of the most common human infections worldwide[47]; approximately 50% of the world's population is infected without symptoms (in United States, it is approximately 23% of the population; in some areas it is as much as 95%).

ETIOLOGY

The main reservoirs of *T. gondii* infection are members of the cat family (Felidae), which become infected by carnivorism; dogs and rabbits can also host the parasite. Viable organisms invade the feline intestinal epithelium, where they undergo an asexual cycle followed by a sexual cycle and then form oocysts, which are excreted in large numbers and are resistant to harsh environmental conditions and disinfectants. Human infection results mainly from ingestion of cyst-containing undercooked meat or milk, but can also result from ingestion of the oocytes from fecally contaminated hands or food, organ transplantation, blood transfusion, or transplacental transmission.

The parasites become tachyzoites and form tissue cysts, mostly in skeletal muscle, myocardium, brain, eye, and placenta, and may remain asymptomatic. Invasion of the reticuloendothelial/endothelial systems results in suppuration and granuloma formation.

CLINICAL DIAGNOSIS

The 3 major clinical forms are congenital, acquired, and disseminated.[2,48-50]

CONGENITAL TOXOPLASMOSIS

It occurs in 1 per 1000 live births in the United States. The risk of transmission is highest in the third trimester; however, the disease is more severe if transmitted in early pregnancy. Approximately 10% of affected newborns will have chorioretinitis and blindness, and 20% will have generalized or CNS disease. Infection may manifest as abortion, stillbirth, microcephaly, tramtrack intracerebral calcifications, deafness, hydrocephalus, mental retardation, or seizures.

Skin lesions include purpura, jaundice, blueberry muffin lesions (dermal erythropoiesis), and erythroderma. Untreated subclinical infection may reactivate during the second to third decade of life, mostly in the form of retinochoroiditis.

ACQUIRED TOXOPLASMOSIS

In immunocompetent persons, it is often asymptomatic in 80% to 90% of cases. However, 10% to 20% of patients, preferentially including pregnant women, develop cervical or occipital lymphadenopathy and a flu-like illness. Rarely, myocarditis, pneumonitis, encephalitis, and polymyositis may occur.

TABLE 176-9

Spectrum of Cutaneous Lesions Seen in Acquired Toxoplasmosis in Immunocompetent Persons[48-50]

- Dermatomyositis-like syndrome.
- Pityriasis lichenoides
- Cellulitis
- Others: Sweet syndrome; cold urticaria; erythroderma; palmoplantar maculopapular rash; morphea; mastocytosis; lichen planus pilaris; pityriasis rubra pilaris; capillaritis; papular acantholytic dermatosis; keratosis lichenoides chronica; chronic prurigo; scarlatiniform eruption; panniculitis; erythema multiforme; roseola; papular urticaria

Cutaneous manifestations are protean reflecting the heterogeneous immune responses to the organism, and include among others dermatomyositis-like syndrome and pityriasis lichenoides (Table 176-9). Toxoplasmosis should be sought in patients with an acute dermatomyositis-like picture. Both conditions share a common underlying pathogenic mechanism related to the expression on muscle fibers of human leukocyte antigen class I, as well as production of certain cytokines.[3]

TOXOPLASMOSIS IN IMMUNODEFICIENT PATIENTS

This is often secondary to reactivation of latent infection and presents as disseminated disease. Toxoplasmic encephalitis is the most common cause of intracerebral lesions in AIDS patients.

Disseminated papular/nodular eruption may occur. Rare cases of graft-versus-host disease–like rash have been reported in patients who underwent hematopoietic stem cell transplantation. Histology may not be helpful in differentiating between the 2 conditions. A high degree of suspicion of toxoplasmosis and molecular confirmation are important to distinguish between the 2 conditions.

DIAGNOSIS

Diagnosis is routinely made by serology.

Protozoa may be identified in bronchoalveolar lavage, lymph node specimens, or skin biopsies. Tachyzoites, visualized with Wright or Giemsa stains, are crescent-shaped and have a prominent, centrally placed nucleus. The most common histologic finding is subacute histiolymphocytic vasculitis with demonstration of trophozoites within macrophages. Epidermotropic infection and neural infiltration may occur. Immunoperoxidase stains are specific and are particularly helpful when small tissue specimens are submitted.

PCR-based testing has a high diagnostic value in acute disease and has become the preferred method of diagnosis, particularly in prenatal diagnosis of toxoplasmosis and in immunocompromised patients with disseminated toxoplasmosis. PCR detection of the parasite in fluid specimens (blood, amniotic fluid, cerebrospinal fluid, urine, vitreous, and aqueous fluid), as well as fetal and brain tissues, is indicative of active infection.

TREATMENT

Treatment should be initiated in all patients with acute or active disease or congenital infection, and in immunosuppressed individuals.[3] Sulfadiazine and pyrimethamine act synergistically and together provide effective therapy. Clindamycin can be used in sulfonamide-allergic patients. Cotrimoxazole was recently reported to be effective in the treatment of toxoplasmic lymphadenitis.

ACKNOWLEDGMENTS

The author acknowledges the contributions of Joelle M. Malek and Samer H. Ghosn, the previous authors of this chapter.

REFERENCES

1. Esch KJ, Petersen CA. Transmission and epidemiology of zoonotic protozoal diseases of companion animals. *Clin Microbiol Rev.* 2013;26(1):58-85.
2. Lupi O, Bartlett BL, Haugen RN, et al. Tropical dermatology: tropical diseases caused by protozoa. *J Am Acad Dermatol.* 2009;60(6):897-925.
3. Kollipara R, Peranteau AJ, Nawas ZY, et al. Emerging infectious diseases with cutaneous manifestations: fungal, helminthic, protozoan and ectoparasitic infections. *J Am Acad Dermatol.* 2016;75(1):19-30.
4. David CV, Craft N. Cutaneous and mucocutaneous leishmaniasis. *Dermatol Ther (Heidelb).* 2009;22(6):491-502.
5. Reithinger R, Dujardin JC, Louzir H, et al. Cutaneous leishmaniasis. *Lancet Infect Dis.* 2007;7(9):581-596.
6. Bailey MS, Lockwood DN. Cutaneous leishmaniasis. *Clin Dermatol.* 2007;25(2):203-211.
7. von Stebut E. Leishmaniasis. *J Dtsch Dermatol Ges.* 2015;13(3):191-200.
8. González U, Pinart M, Reveiz L, et al. Interventions for Old World cutaneous leishmaniasis. *Cochrane Database Syst Rev.* 2008;(4):CD005067.
9. Khatami A, Firooz A, Gorouhi F, et al. Treatment of acute Old World cutaneous leishmaniasis: a systematic review of the randomized controlled trials. *J Am Acad Dermatol.* 2007;57(2):335.e1-e29.
10. Palumbo E. Current treatment for cutaneous leishmaniasis: a review. *Am J Ther.* 2009;16(2):178-182.
11. Barrett MP, Croft SL. Management of trypanosomiasis and leishmaniasis. *Br Med Bull.* 2012;104:175-196.
12. Aronson N, Herwaldt BL, Libman M, et al. Diagnosis and treatment of leishmaniasis: clinical practice guidelines by the Infectious Diseases Society of America (IDSA) and the American Society of Tropical Medicine and Hygiene (ASTMH). *Am J Trop Med Hyg.* 2016;63(12):e202-e264.

13. Copeland NK, Aronson NE. Leishmaniasis: treatment updates and clinical practice guidelines review. *Curr Opin Infect Dis*. 2015;28(5):426-437.
14. Blum J, Buffet P, Visser L, et al. LeishMan recommendations for treatment of cutaneous and mucosal leishmaniasis in travelers, 2014. *J Travel Med*. 2014;21(2):116-129.
15. Wamwiri FN, Changasi RE. Tsetse flies (*Glossina*) as vectors of human African trypanosomiasis: a review. *Biomed Res Int*. 2016;2016:6201350.
16. Geiger A, Bossard G, Sereno D, et al. Escaping deleterious immune response in their hosts: lessons from trypanosomatids. *Front Immunol*. 2016;7:212.
17. Brun R, Blum J. Human African trypanosomiasis. *Infect Dis Clin North Am*. 2012;26(2):261-273.
18. Moore AC, Ryan ET, Waldron MA. Case records of the Massachusetts General Hospital. Weekly clinicopathological exercises. Case 20-2002. A 37-year-old man with fever, hepatosplenomegaly, and a cutaneous foot lesion after a trip to Africa. *N Engl J Med*. 2002;346(26):2069-2076.
19. Ezzedine K, Darie H, Le Bras M, et al. Skin features accompanying imported human African trypanosomiasis: hemolymphatic *Trypanosoma gambiense* infection among two French expatriates with dermatologic manifestations. *J Travel Med*. 2007;14(3):192-196.
20. Kennedy PG. The continuing problem of human African trypanosomiasis (sleeping sickness). *Ann Neurol*. 2008;64(2):116-126.
21. Singh Grewal A, Pandita D, Bhardwaj S, et al. Recent updates on development of drug molecules for human African trypanosomiasis. *Curr Top Med Chem*. 2016;16(20):2245-2265.
22. Priotto G, Kasparian S, Mutombo W, et al. Nifurtimox-eflornithine combination therapy for second-stage African *Trypanosoma brucei* gambiense trypanosomiasis: a multicentre, randomised, phase III, non-inferiority trial. *Lancet*. 2009;374(9683):56-64.
23. Benziger CP, do Carmo GA, Ribeiro AL. Chagas cardiomyopathy: clinical presentation and management in the Americas. *Cardiol Clin*. 2017;35(1):31-47.
24. Andrade DV, Gollob KJ, Dutra WO. Acute Chagas disease: new global challenges for an old neglected disease. *PLoS Negl Trop Dis*. 2014;8(7):e3010.
25. Kransdorf EP, Zakowski PC, Kobashigawa JA. Chagas disease in solid organ and heart transplantation. *Curr Opin Infect Dis*. 2014;27(5):418-424.
26. Rodriguez JB, Falcone BN, Szajnman SH. Detection and treatment of *Trypanosoma cruzi*: a patent review (2011-2015). *Expert Opin Ther Pat*. 2016;26(9):993-1015.
27. Nabavi SF, Sureda A, Daglia M, et al. Flavonoids and Chagas' disease: the story so far! *Curr Top Med Chem*. 2017;17(4):460-466.
28. Wiens MO, Kanters S, Mills E, et al. Systematic review and meta-analysis of the pharmacokinetics of benznidazole in the treatment of Chagas disease. *Antimicrob Agents Chemother*. 2016;60(12):7035-7042.
29. Salomao K, Menna-Barreto RF, de Castro SL. Stairway to heaven or hell? Perspectives and limitations of Chagas disease chemotherapy. *Curr Top Med Chem*. 2016;16(20):2266-2289.
30. Cullen KA, Mace KE, Arguin PM; Centers for Disease Control and Prevention (CDC). Malaria surveillance—United States, 2013. *MMWR Surveill Summ*. 2016;65(2):1-22.
31. Vaishnani JB. Cutaneous findings in five cases of malaria. *Indian J Dermatol Venereol Leprol*. 2011;77(1):110.
32. Leitsch D. Recent advances in the *Trichomonas vaginalis* field. *F1000Res*. 2016;5.
33. Hollman D, Coupey SM, Fox AS, et al. Screening for *Trichomonas vaginalis* in high-risk adolescent females with a new transcription-mediated nucleic acid amplification test (NAAT): associations with ethnicity, symptoms, and prior and current STIs. *J Pediatr Adolesc Gynecol*. 2010;23:312-316.
34. de Brum Vieira P, Tasca T, Secor WE. Challenges and persistent questions in treatment of trichomoniasis. *Curr Top Med Chem*. 2017;17(11):1249-1265.
35. Das S, Kashyap B, Barua M, et al. Nasal rhinosporidiosis in humans: new interpretations and a review of the literature of this enigmatic disease. *Med Mycol*. 2011;49(3):311-315.
36. Lupi O, Tyring SK, McGinnis MR. Tropical dermatology: fungal tropical diseases. *J Am Acad Dermatol*. 2005;53(6):931-951.
37. Cacciò SM, Chalmers RM. Human cryptosporidiosis in Europe. *Clin Microbiol Infect*. 2016;22(6):471-480.
38. Huang DB, White AC. An updated review on *Cryptosporidium* and *Giardia*. *Gastroenterol Clin North Am*. 2006;35(2):291-314, viii.
39. Chalmers RM, Katzer F. Looking for *Cryptosporidium*: the application of advances in detection and diagnosis. *Trends Parasitol*. 2013;29(5):237-251.
40. Painter JE, Gargano JW, Collier SA, et al; Centers for Disease Control and Prevention. Giardiasis surveillance—United States, 2011-2012. *MMWR Suppl*. 2015;64(3):15-25.
41. McKnight JT, Tietze PE. Dermatologic manifestations of giardiasis. *J Am Board Fam Pract*. 1992;5(4):425-428.
42. Escobedo AA, Lalle M, Hrastnik NI, et al. Combination therapy in the management of giardiasis: what laboratory and clinical studies tell us, so far. *Acta Trop*. 2016;162:196-205.
43. Stanley SL Jr. Amoebiasis. *Lancet*. 2003;361(9362):1025-1034.
44. Parshad S, Grover PS, Sharma A, et al. Primary cutaneous amoebiasis: case report with review of the literature. *Int J Dermatol*. 2002;41(10):676-680.
45. Fernández-Díez J, Magaña M, Magaña ML. Cutaneous amebiasis: 50 years of experience. *Cutis*. 2012;90(6):310-314.
46. Maycock NJ, Jayaswal R. Update on *Acanthamoeba* keratitis: diagnosis, treatment, and outcomes. *Cornea*. 2016;35(5):713-720.
47. Flegr J, Prandota J, Sovičková M, et al. Toxoplasmosis—a global threat. Correlation of latent toxoplasmosis with specific disease burden in a set of 88 countries. *PLoS One*. 2014;9(3):e90203.
48. Rand AJ, Buck AB, Love PB, et al. Cutaneous acquired toxoplasmosis in a child: a case report and review of the literature. *Am J Dermatopathol*. 2015;37(4):305-310.
49. Mawhorter SD, Effron D, Blinkhorn R, et al. Cutaneous manifestations of toxoplasmosis. *Clin Infect Dis*. 1992;14(5):1084-1088.
50. Leyva WH, Santa Cruz DJ. Cutaneous toxoplasmosis. *J Am Acad Dermatol*. 1986;14(4):600-605.

Chapter 177 :: Helminthic Infections
:: Kathryn N. Suh & Jay S. Keystone

第一百七十七章
蠕虫感染

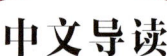

中文导读

蠕虫是多细胞寄生虫，可感染多种哺乳动物，包括人类。引起人类疾病的有3类：线虫、吸虫和绦虫。本章分6节：①流行病学；②临床特征；③病因和发病机制；④诊断；⑤临床管理；⑥重要的特殊蠕虫感染疾病。其中重点介绍了引起皮肤病的蠕虫感染。

第一节介绍了蠕虫感染的流行病学，其是人类最常见的疾病之一，在温带和北部气候中较少流行，在发达国家和气候较冷的地方，更多地是由来自流行地区的旅行者或移民输入的。

第二节临床特征介绍了旅行史询问的重要性，蠕虫感染引起的皮肤损伤呈现多种形态，最常见的为皮肤幼虫移行症，同时也影响呼吸系统、胃肠道、神经系统和眼睛。

第三节介绍了病因和发病机制包含了多种可能机制，包括直接穿透皮肤导致的局部免疫反应，蠕虫迁徙引起的全身免疫反应，淋巴水肿导致正常皮肤结构的破坏，以及不明确的全身免疫反应。

第四节介绍了诊断蠕虫感染依赖组织标本、血液或排泄物，疾病的穿透期和急性期诊断往往很困难；慢性感染中，可以根据识别寄生虫卵或幼虫或偶尔识别成虫来确定诊断，但粪便检查的敏感度也可能因寄生虫而异。

第五节介绍了引起皮肤表现的蠕虫感染的推荐和替代治疗方法。

第六节介绍了重要的特殊蠕虫感染疾病，包括皮肤幼虫移行综合征、蛔虫病、丝虫病、血吸虫感染、类圆线虫病的流行病学、临床特点、诊断与鉴别诊断与临床管理。

〔粟　娟〕

AT-A-GLANCE

- Helminthic infections are a major cause of morbidity and mortality, particularly in tropical and developing countries.
- The majority of infected individuals has a low worm burden and is asymptomatic.
- Dermatologic symptoms and cutaneous findings may be associated with or present features of many helminthic infections.
- Returned travelers and immigrants from endemic areas may differ in the dermatologic manifestations of helminthic infection.
- Migratory lesions, subcutaneous masses, papular eruptions, urticaria, and pruritus are the most common presenting symptoms of helminthic infections.
- Cutaneous larva migrans is the most common helminthic dermatosis identified.
- Recognition of skin findings or helminthic infections and an appropriate epidemiologic history can guide appropriate investigations and effective therapy.

Helminths (worms) are variably sized multicellular parasites that can infect a wide range of mammals, including humans. Those causing human disease belong to 3 groups: nematodes (roundworms), trematodes (flukes), and cestodes (tapeworms); trematodes and cestodes are collectively referred to as platyhelminths (flatworms). A variety of helminths can infect humans and cause cutaneous findings (Table 177-1).[1,2] This chapter focuses on those helminths that are notable for causing dermatologic disease.

EPIDEMIOLOGY

Globally, helminthic infections are among the most common diseases of humans. However, the true prevalence of helminthiases is difficult to determine, particularly as the majority of infected individuals harbor relatively few worms and are asymptomatic. Large worm burdens and symptomatic disease affect a relatively small proportion of those who are infected.

While some helminths such as *Enterobius vermicularis* and *Toxocara canis* are found worldwide, others are more geographically restricted. Most infections occur in developing tropical or subtropical countries, where environmental conditions are conducive to the completion of the life cycle of many helminths, and the requisite animal hosts and vectors for ongoing transmission exist. In addition, the high population density, poverty, and poor sanitation commonly found in these areas further facilitate the transmission of these diseases. Knowledge of the geographic distribution of specific helminths is important for the clinician, and will help to direct appropriate investigations and management.

Helminthic infections are less prevalent in temperate and northern climates, although some diseases are endemic even in these regions. In developed countries and colder climates, helminthic diseases are more often imported by travelers to or immigrants from endemic areas. Less frequently, helminthic infections in developed nations can be locally acquired (eg, trichinellosis resulting from improperly prepared food) or transmitted via person-to-person spread (eg, enterobiasis).

SKIN DISEASES IN TRAVELERS

Dermatologic disorders are the third most common illness in travelers.[3] Observational studies over the past decade have consistently demonstrated that between 10% and 23% of travelers develop a dermatologic condition during or after travel.[4-11] These figures cannot be generalized to all travelers, however, as studies included only individuals assessed in specialty (travel and tropical medicine) clinics and may also have been subject to geographic biases (because of the specific populations studied and/or the destinations of these individuals).

Infections, including tropical skin diseases, are common causes of dermatoses among travelers. Insect bites, allergic reactions, and other rashes are among the most prevalent noninfectious dermatologic diagnoses in travelers. Of the helminthic skin infections, cutaneous larva migrans (CLM) is by far the most commonly reported in travelers and accounts for up to 25% of all skin diseases in this group.[7-11] Most other helminthic infections that may be associated with dermatologic findings are relatively rare in travelers.

SKIN DISEASES IN IMMIGRANTS AND REFUGEES

The prevalence of dermatologic conditions in immigrants and refugees has not been exhaustively studied,[5,6,9,10] but in general they appear to occur no more frequently than in travelers. These observations are subject to the same biases noted above. The helminths that cause skin findings in this population, and the clinical presentations, may differ from those in travelers, however. For example, filarial infections are more commonly encountered in individuals who have resided in endemic areas for prolonged periods rather than in travelers, because they usually require repeated exposures to insect vectors for effective transmission to occur. Strongyloidiasis is also more prevalent in immigrants from endemic areas, particularly southeast Asia, and often presents with eosinophilia and few, if any, abdominal symptoms; most are asymptomatic. Onchocerciasis rarely occurs in short-term (at least 1 month) visitors to endemic areas and characteristically presents as an acute dermatitis

TABLE 177-1
Helminths Causing Cutaneous Disease: Common Dermatologic Findings

SPECIES	LOCALIZED EDEMA	MIGRATORY SKIN LESIONS	NODULES OR MASSES	PAPULES	PETECHIAE	PRURITUS	URTICARIA	ULCER	VESICLE/BULLA
Nematodes (Roundworms)									
Ancylostoma braziliense, Ancylostoma caninum		X		X		X	X		X
Ancylostoma duodenale, Necator americanus (human hookworm)		X				X	X		X
Ascaris lumbricoides						X	X		
Dirofilaria spp.		Rare	X						
Dracunculus medinensis	X[a]	X						X	X
Enterobius vermicularis						X			
Filariae									
Brugia malayi, Brugia timori	X[b]		X						
Loa loa	X[a]	X	X			X	X		
Mansonella ozzardi, Mansonella perstans, Mansonella streptocerca	X[b]			X		X			
Onchocerca volvulus	Rare[a]		X	X		X	X		
Wuchereria bancrofti	X[b]		X						
Gnathostoma spinigerum, others	X[a]	X	X			X	X		
Strongyloides stercoralis		X		X	X[c]	X	X		
Toxocara canis, Toxocara cati						X	X		
Trichinella spiralis	X[a]		X		X	X	X		
Trematodes (Flukes)									
Fasciola hepatica		X				X	X		
Paragonimus westermani		X	X			X	X		
Schistosoma spp. (human and avian)			X	X		X	X		
Cestodes (Tapeworms)									
Echinococcus granulosis, Echinococcus multilocularis			X						
Spirometra mansonoides, others (sparganosis)		X	X						
Taenia multiceps, others (coenurosis)			X						
Taenia solium (cysticercosis)			X						

[a]Focal or localized edema.
[b]Lymphedema with filarial infections.
[c]Disseminated strongyloidiasis.

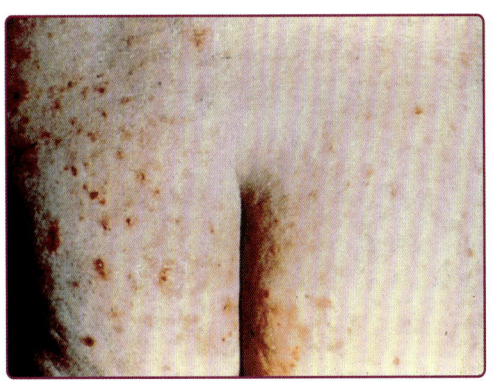

Figure 177-1 Onchocercal dermatitis. (Used with permission from Herman Zaiman, MD.)

with a hyperimmune response manifested by pruritus and rash (Fig. 177-1), despite low parasite loads. In contrast, infected immigrants more commonly have chronic onchodermatitis, with chronic skin changes, including atrophy, hypopigmentation, and lichenification, and onchocercal nodules (Fig. 177-2).

LIFE CYCLE AND TRANSMISSION OF HELMINTHS

All helminths have complex life cycles that include maturation from eggs (or other infective forms) to larvae (or other immature forms) to adults. Human disease results from ingestion of eggs or other infective forms, or, alternatively, exposure of the skin to infective forms (larvae or cercariae) by direct contact or via the bite of an insect vector. Humans may be the primary hosts for some helminths (eg, *Strongyloides stercoralis*), or may be incidental or accidental hosts (eg, avian schistosomes, animal hookworm, and *T. canis*). Helminths that are well adapted to humans can mature from the infective stage into adult forms in the human host; infection generally persists for the life span of the adult worm, which in some cases can be for many years. In contrast, animal helminths cannot mature into adult forms in humans (who in this setting are therefore "dead-end" hosts), although infection can still cause tissue damage and clinical findings.

In general, helminths do not multiply in the human host. Most helminths (with the notable exception of *S. stercoralis*) are incapable of completing an entire life cycle in the human host, and depend on the environment (eg, soil, water), plants, or other animal hosts or insects, for their survival. Consequently, transmission of infection requires the presence of appropriate environmental conditions, specific intermediate hosts (in whom only the asexual reproductive cycle occurs), and/or specific insect vectors, explaining in large part the localized geographic distributions of many helminthic diseases.

Examples of helminthic diseases acquired by ingestion of infective forms (eggs or metacercariae) in contaminated food or water include *Ascaris lumbricoides* and *Fasciola hepatica*. In ascariasis, swallowed eggs are consumed, larvae are released within the GI tract, and migrate through the portal–systemic circulation to the lungs, from which they are swallowed. Skin disease, such as urticaria, may occur during the larval migration phase. Once in the GI tract, larvae mature into adult worms where sexual reproduction may take place; either eggs or adult worms can be shed in stool. Eggs must mature in soil before releasing infective larvae. In fascioliasis, infective metacercariae ingested on watercress excyst in the small intestine and migrate through the intestinal wall and peritoneum to their target tissue, the biliary tract, where they become adults. Again, skin findings typically occur as immature forms migrate. Eggs produced by adult flukes are passed in feces and become infective for humans only after maturation in a suitable (intermediate) snail host.

Schistosomiasis results from penetration of intact skin by infective cercariae. Dermatologic findings in early disease manifest either at the time of cercarial penetration (swimmer's itch or cercarial dermatitis), or during migration of immature forms (schistosomulae) from the skin and through tissue to the venous systems of their target organs (bladder or bowel, depending on the infecting species), where they mature into adults. Sexual reproduction leads to the release of eggs into the local circulation. En route to the bladder or bowel, eggs may sometimes become trapped in ectopic tissues, including skin, where they cause a granulomatous reaction. Eggs hatch in fresh water, releasing cercariae that must undergo further maturation in one

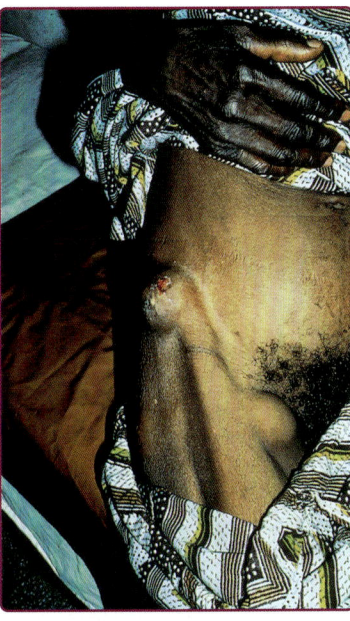

Figure 177-2 Onchocercal nodule over iliac crest. (Used with permission from Jay S. Keystone, MD, FRCPC.)

of several intermediate snail hosts in order to infect humans.

Infection can also result from penetration of intact skin by larvae, as exemplified by human hookworm infection. Larvae then migrate to the circulatory system where they are carried to the lungs, penetrate the alveoli and ascend the bronchial tree, are swallowed, and enter the GI tract. Skin findings may occur during larval migration to the lungs. Maturation into adult worms occurs in the small intestine, where they reproduce and release eggs into stool. Under the appropriate environmental conditions, eggs mature into infective larvae in soil. In contrast, larvae of animal hookworms (eg, *Ancylostoma braziliense*) cannot mature beyond the larval stage in humans and tunnel aimlessly in the skin before the infection eventually extinguishes itself.

Larvae also can be introduced through intact skin by insect bites (eg, in filarial infections). The insect vector and the target tissue both vary according to the infecting species; cutaneous disease may be seen during either migration of larval forms through tissue, or as a result of adult worms in tissue. Microfilariae (larvae) released from mature adult worms are taken up by an insect during a subsequent blood meal, and then undergo maturation to infective forms within the insect before being introduced into another human host.

CLINICAL FEATURES

APPROACH TO THE PATIENT

With the exception of CLM, most travelers and immigrants who present with dermatologic complaints will not have a diagnosis attributable to a helminthic infection. However, clearly these must be considered if the epidemiologic and exposure history and clinical findings are consistent with a helminthic infection, as these are treatable infections that have important clinical implications, such as disseminated strongyloidiasis in an immunocompromised host.

As with all diseases of travelers and immigrants, a thorough history is essential in order to direct the clinician toward the correct diagnosis. The history should focus on aspects related to travel (or residence in endemic areas), general medical conditions, and medications. In addition, specific details of the dermatologic complaints must also be obtained. Finally, the clinician should be knowledgeable about (or know how to find out about) outbreaks of disease that may have been ongoing during an individual's travel or residence in a given area.

EXPOSURE HISTORY: TRAVEL AND AREAS OF RESIDENCE

The travel history (or history of residence in endemic areas) must be thorough in order to elucidate likely exposures to helminths. Specific details may be more readily obtained in recently returned travelers than immigrants, although immigrants are much more likely to be aware of local and endemic diseases (albeit often by local names). Details to be obtained include the exact dates, durations, and locations of travel or residence; purpose of travel; activities or occupations, inquiring specifically about those that would increase exposure to specific helminths; dietary intake; a history of similar signs and symptoms in other family members or fellow travelers; and the use of preventive measures.

The exact destinations of travel (urban versus rural), not only the country or countries visited, are important to obtain. While some diseases may be endemic throughout a world region or area, the prevalence of others may vary greatly, sometimes within a given country. For example, onchocerciasis and loaisis are endemic in Central and West Africa, but generally not in other parts of Africa; and both infections are found only in rural areas, unlike bancroftian filariasis (*Wuchereria bancrofti*) that is often transmitted in urban centers. The risk of disease may not be present in all areas of a country in which a disease is considered to be endemic; for example, schistosomiasis is found in Brazil, but predominantly in the eastern and northeastern regions. Duration of travel or residence in an endemic area (and hence duration of exposure) is relevant for some diseases; schistosomiasis can be acquired after a single exposure to infective cercariae in freshwater, whereas filariasis is often acquired only after numerous bites, and therefore is rare among short-term travelers to endemic areas.

The purpose of travel is also correlated with the likelihood of exposure to specific pathogens. Rural and adventure travelers are more likely to be exposed to helminthic infections than are business travelers, travelers whose itineraries are limited to urban areas, and those whose travels are of shorter durations.

Certain activities and occupations will place individuals at greater risks of helminthic infections while abroad. Examples of common exposures and associated diseases include barefoot walking or walking in open shoes (sandals) (eg, CLM; strongyloidiasis); freshwater swimming in Africa (eg, schistosomiasis); and dietary indiscretions such as consumption of salads or undercooked or contaminated meat or fish (eg, ascariasis, echinococcosis, fascioliasis, gnathostomiasis). Although direct exposure to animals is not a risk factor for helminthic infections, the risk of CLM is greater in areas with a higher prevalence of stray dogs and cats. For those infections that are vector borne, such as filarial infections transmitted by mosquitoes, black flies and deer flies, the use of preventive measures such as appropriate clothing, insect repellent and bed nets can reduce the risk of infection.

GENERAL MEDICAL HISTORY

In addition to the travel history, a general medical history should be obtained. Skin findings may be related to underlying medical conditions, or to any associated treatment for these. The differential diagnosis of skin lesions in a returned traveler or immigrant also includes noninfectious disorders such as contact dermatitis (including to jewelry), drug eruptions, and photosensitivity reactions (that may be precipitated by travel-related medications such as doxycycline). A list of prescription and nonprescription medications or supplements should be obtained, in particular those that may have been started recently and/or prescribed abroad, as well as any recent use of topical medications or products.

DERMATOLOGIC HISTORY

The dermatologic history should include details regarding the initial presentation, morphology, and anatomic distribution of skin lesions; the progression and duration of lesions; time of onset relative to potential exposures; and any associated local and systemic signs and symptoms. While some manifestations of helminthic infections, such as urticaria or maculopapular eruptions, are nonspecific, the differential diagnosis of helminthic dermatoses can often be narrowed based on the description and morphology of the lesion(s) present. For some diseases such as CLM, skin findings are virtually pathognomonic and the diagnosis can be established by history and careful examination of skin lesions, often without the need for additional investigations.

CUTANEOUS FINDINGS OF HELMINTHIC INFECTIONS

Skin lesions caused by helminthic infections can assume a variety of morphologies. The most commonly encountered problem is that of migratory skin lesions. CLM is the most common cause of migratory lesions in general. Subcutaneous nodules, papular eruptions, and urticaria and pruritus are also common manifestations of helminthic infections.

MIGRATORY SKIN LESIONS

Migratory lesions can be caused by multiple helminths. Migratory lesions can be linear (serpiginous) or may be more ill-defined areas of erythema and swelling, and may be painless, painful, or pruritic. Table 177-2 lists the most common helminthic causes of migratory lesions, as well as characteristic features of these lesions.

Serpiginous and linear lesions are most commonly caused by CLM (most frequently caused by *A. braziliense* and *Ancylostoma caninum*; see also "Cutaneous Larva Migrans Syndrome"). Usually 1 to 3 (or more) erythematous, serpiginous, and intensely pruritic lesions

TABLE 177-2
Differential Diagnosis of Migratory Skin Lesions

HELMINTH	MORPHOLOGY OF LESION	DESCRIPTION	MOST COMMON LOCATION
Ancylostoma braziliense, Ancylostoma caninum	Serpiginous (cutaneous larva migrans [CLM])	Typically 1 to 3 serpiginous lesions, 3 mm wide and up to 20 cm in length; intensely pruritic, may be vesicobullous; movement up to several cm per day	Feet, buttocks
Ancylostoma duodenale, Necator americanus (human hookworm)	Serpiginous	Pruritic tracks from larval migration	Feet
Dracunculus medinensis	Localized area of edema or swelling with movement beneath	Moving mass may be seen just before emergence of adult worm through skin	Feet
Fasciola hepatica	Migratory subcutaneous swellings	Erythematous, painful, pruritic subcutaneous nodules may have a migratory component; larval track marks also may be seen	Abdomen, back, extremities
Loa loa	Migratory subcutaneous swelling or serpiginous	Migration of adult worm across conjunctivae or under skin	Skin, eye
Gnathostoma spinigerum	Serpiginous (CLM)	Migration of larvae can cause creeping eruption; movement 1 cm per hour	Trunk, upper body
	Migratory subcutaneous swellings (eosinophilic panniculitis)	Intermittent single or multiple erythematous swellings; may be migratory, pruritic or painful; last 1 to 4 weeks, with recurrences in different anatomic areas after variable asymptomatic periods	Thighs
Paragonimus westermani	Migratory subcutaneous swellings or nodules	Firm migratory swellings or nodules, may be migratory; slightly tender and slightly mobile, up to 6 cm in diameter; swellings contain immature flukes	Lower abdomen, inguinal region
Spirometra mansonoides, others (sparganosis)	Migratory subcutaneous swellings	Slow growing, typically painful swellings that may be migratory; may be pruritic	Abdomen, lower extremities
Strongyloides stercoralis (larva currens)	Serpiginous (larva currens)	Movement at 5 to 10 cm per hour; intensely pruritic, transient, but recurrent	Buttocks, groin, trunk, thighs

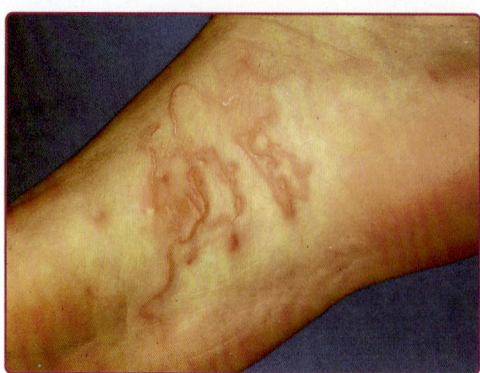

Figure 177-3 Cutaneous larva migrans. (Used with permission from Jay S. Keystone, MD, FRCPC.)

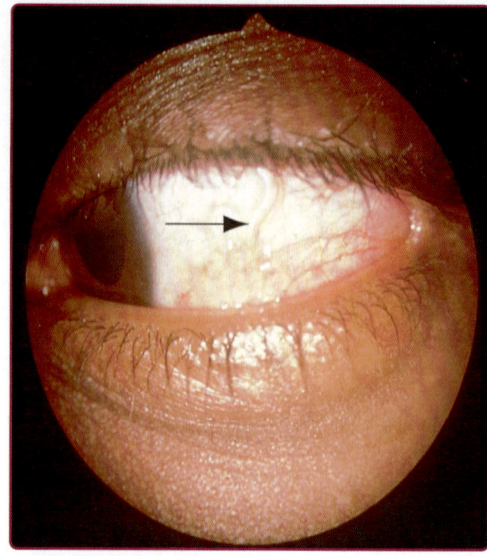

Figure 177-5 Loiasis. Adult worm crossing bulbar conjunctiva of the eye (*arrow*). (Used with permission from Murray Wittner, MD, PhD.)

caused by intradermal larval migration are present (Fig. 177-3). Serpiginous skin lesions in *S. stercoralis* infection, a pathognomonic manifestation of strongyloidiasis known as larva currens, typically present as recurrent, transient, and rapidly moving skin lesions (Fig. 177-4). Larval migration may occur at rates of 5 to 10 cm per hour, and the lesions usually disappear within hours only to recur over subsequent weeks to years. Linear migratory lesions also can be seen occasionally in human hookworm infection (*Ancylostoma duodenale* and *Necator americanus*) at the site of larval penetration, and in gnathostomiasis (usually relatively slow migration at 1 cm per hour). Linear migratory lesions also can be seen in loaiasis, and result from movement of the adult worm (not larvae) in tissue, typically under the skin or also across the bulbar conjunctivae (Fig. 177-5).

Migratory subcutaneous swellings and nodules are characteristic of infections caused by *Loa loa*, *Fasciola*, *Gnathostoma*, and *Paragonimus*, and in sparganosis (*Spirometra* spp.). Lesions may be painful or pruritic. Migratory swelling resulting from the movement of adult worms is also seen in dracunculiasis, in which movement within a bullous, vesicular, or edematous lesion on the foot is often noted prior to eruption of the skin lesion and egress of the adult worm (Fig. 177-6). Since the implementation of a global eradication and drinking water monitoring program in endemic countries, cases of dracunculiasis have decreased dramatically and the disease has almost been eliminated.

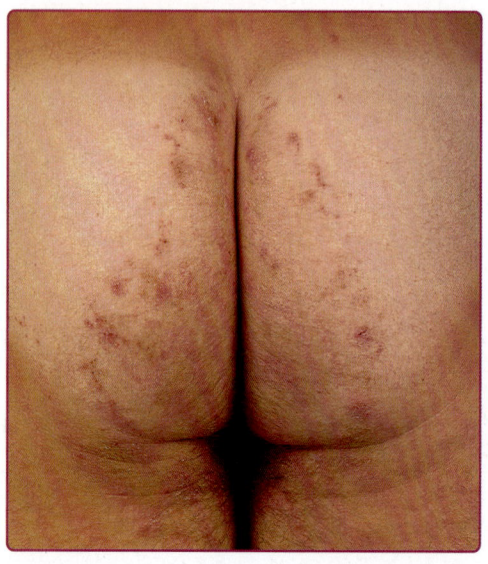

Figure 177-4 Larva currens in chronic strongyloidiasis. Multiple serpiginous, inflammatory lesions are visible on the buttocks.

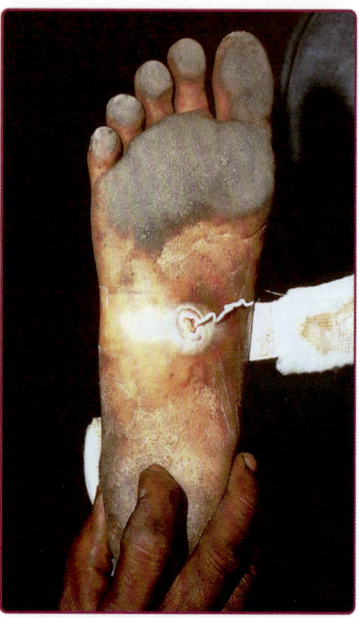

Figure 177-6 Dracunculiasis. (Used with permission from Jay S. Keystone, MD, FRCPC.)

SUBCUTANEOUS NODULES AND MASSES

Subcutaneous and soft-tissue masses may have variable characteristics, including overlying erythema, pain or tenderness, and pruritus. They may be single or multiple, and fixed or mobile. Table 177-3 lists the more common etiologies of nodular lesions.

Solitary nodules or masses are found in echinococcosis, filariasis caused by *Brugia malayi* and *W. bancroftii* (both of which may cause scrotal masses in men from lymphatic obstruction), dirofilariasis, and coenurosis (*Taenia multiceps*). *Multiple nodules* are typical of cysticercosis (*Taenia solium* infection), in which small, painless subcutaneous or intramuscular nodules are present, although single nodules can also occur. Subcutaneous cysticercosis, reported commonly in infected individuals in older case series, currently occurs in less than 10% of cases. Most other helminths that manifest as subcutaneous nodules or masses may present with single or multiple lesions. *Painless nodules* are most characteristic of coenurosis, cysticercosis, dirofilariasis, echinococcus, and onchocerciasis. *Painful nodules* are seen in paragonimiasis and sparganosis. Transient painful lesions that resolve and subsequently recur in different anatomic areas are characteristic of *Gnathostoma* infection and loiasis. *Fixed lesions* are typical of cysticercosis, echinococcosis, and onchocerciasis.

PAPULAR AND MACULAR LESIONS

Papules and macules occur in relatively few helminthic infections (Table 177-4). Papular lesions may occur at sites of skin penetration by infective larvae or cercariae in CLM and schistosomiasis. In CLM, papules are typically in the feet or buttocks, similar to the distribution of migratory lesions. In schistosomiasis, exposure to infected freshwater (for avian or human schistosomes) or salt water (avian schistosomes) may cause pruritus, which is followed rapidly by a papular eruption in previously sensitized individuals. Chronic

TABLE 177-3
Differential Diagnosis of Nodular Skin and Subcutaneous Lesions

HELMINTH	DESCRIPTION OF NODULAR LESION	MOST COMMON LOCATION
Brugia malayi	Hydrocele/scrotal mass caused by lymphatic obstruction	Scrotum
Dirofilaria spp.	Single erythematous, well-defined, firm nodule or mass, usually 1 to 5 cm in diameter; usually asymptomatic but may be tender; rarely may be migratory	Head and neck, breasts, extremities, scrotum
Dracunculus medinensis	Edematous lesion/mass may be seen just before emergence of adult worm through skin; movement underneath lesion due to movement of adult worm	Feet
Echinococcus spp.	Firm subcutaneous (or muscular) nodules or masses; usually single but may be multiple; may feel fluctuant; nontender. Rarely with fistulization and inflammation of skin (*Echinococcus multilocularis*). True cutaneous lesions are rare	Abdomen
Gnathostoma spinigerum	Intermittent single or multiple erythematous swellings; may be migratory, pruritic or painful; last 1 to 4 weeks, with recurrences in different anatomic areas after variable asymptomatic periods	Trunk, upper body, thighs
Loa loa	Calabar swellings–localized angioedema, 5 to 20 cm in diameter, usually lasting 2 to 4 days but recurrent; caused by migration of adult worms	Eyelid, upper extremities, periarticular regions (especially knee, wrist)
Mansonella perstans	Calabar swellings–localized swellings lasting 1 to 4 days, recurrent	Face, upper extremities (especially forearms), hands
Onchocerca volvulus	Well-defined, fixed, painless nodules containing adult worms in deep dermis and subcutaneous tissue	Over bony prominences including skull (South America), ribs, iliac crest (Africa), others
Paragonimus westermani	Firm swellings or nodules, may be migratory; slightly tender and slightly mobile, up to 6 cm in diameter; swellings contain immature flukes	Lower abdomen, inguinal region
Spirometra mansonoides, others (sparganosis)	Slow growing, typically painful swellings that may be migratory; may be pruritic	Abdomen, lower extremities
Taenia multiceps, others (coenurosis)	Solitary subcutaneous (or muscular) nodule, usually 2 to 6 cm in diameter; painless	Trunk (especially intercostal regions), anterior abdominal wall; head, neck, extremities less commonly
Taenia solium (cysticercosis)	Painless, fixed, well-circumscribed rubbery subcutaneous nodules in 50% of patients with cysticercosis; may be single or multiple; average size 2 cm in diameter	Trunk, extremities
Wuchereria bancrofti	Hydrocele/scrotal mass caused by lymphatic obstruction	Scrotum

TABLE 177-4
Differential Diagnosis of Papular and Macular Lesions

HELMINTH	DESCRIPTION	MOST COMMON LOCATION
Ancylostoma braziliense, Ancylostoma caninum (CLM)	Pruritic erythematous papule(s) within days of larval penetration; may be vesicular; also papular larva migrans	Feet, buttocks
Ancylostoma duodenale, Necator americanus (human hookworm)	Ground itch: in sensitized individuals, pruritic papular lesions at sites of larval entry; may be vesicular	Feet, hands
perstans, Mansonella streptocerca	Multiple pruritic papules; hypopigmented and hyperpigmented macules and lichenification may be present	Upper chest (M. streptocerca)
Onchocerca volvulus	*Acute:* multiple pruritic papules, may become vesicular or pustular; may be erythematous and edema may be present	Face, trunk, extremities
	Chronic: intensely pruritic, flat papules (3 to 9 mm) or macules, may be hyperpigmented or lichenified	Shoulders, buttocks, waist, extremities
Schistosoma spp. (avian)	Erythematous papular or maculopapular lesions, may be vesicular or urticarial; intensely pruritic; onset within 24 hours of saltwater or freshwater exposure, lasts 1 to 3 weeks	Any surface exposed to water
Schistosoma spp. (human)	*Acute:* erythematous papular and urticarial lesions in previously sensitized individuals; onset within hours of freshwater exposure, lasting 1 week	Any surface exposed to water
	Chronic: bilharziasis cutanea tarda; slightly pigmented, 2- to 4-mm, firm, pruritic, oval papules or papulonodular lesions, may be verrucous or polypoid; may appear in crops; caused by granulomatous reaction to eggs in skin	Trunk, especially periumbilical region; buttocks, genitalia

papular lesions (bilharziasis cutanea tarda) may be present in chronic schistosomiasis. Papular lesions also may be manifestations of acute or chronic infection with *Onchocerca volvulus*, and have been reported in disseminated and chronic strongyloidiasis.

URTICARIA AND PRURITUS

Pruritus (Table 177-5) may be present in the absence of skin findings, either as a primary symptom of infection (eg, filariasis caused by *Mansonella perstans* or *O. volvulus*),

TABLE 177-5
Helminthic Infections Causing Urticaria and Pruritus

HELMINTH	COMMENTS
Nematodes (Roundworms)	
Ancylostoma braziliense, Ancylostoma caninum	Pruritus and urticaria after skin penetration and during larval migration
Ancylostoma duodenale, Necator americanus (human hookworm)	Pruritus and urticaria after skin penetration and during larval migration
Ascaris lumbricoides	Pruritus and urticaria during larval migration (with Loeffler syndrome)
Enterobius vermicularis	Pruritus ani
Filariae	
Loa loa	Pruritus and urticaria
Mansonella ozzardi, Mansonella perstans, Mansonella streptocerca	Pruritus occurs early, may be only symptom
Onchocerca volvulus	Pruritus and urticaria in acute or chronic disease
Gnathostoma spinigerum, others	Pruritus and urticaria during larval migration
Strongyloides stercoralis	Pruritus and urticaria after skin penetration and during larval migration, including chronic infection; pruritus ani
Toxocara canis, Toxocara cati	Pruritus and urticaria during larval migration
Trichinella spiralis	Pruritus and urticaria during larval migration
Trematodes (Flukes)	
Fasciola hepatica	Urticaria during migration of adult flukes
Paragonimus westermani	Urticaria during larval migration
Schistosoma spp. (human and avian)	Transient urticaria with pruritus within 24 hours of exposure to cercariae; urticaria with Katayama fever (acute schistosomiasis)

or before the onset of skin lesions (eg, schistosomiasis). Pruritus is a common feature of many helminthic infections, with the noteworthy exceptions of lymphatic filariasis (eg, caused by *Brugia* spp. and *W. bancrofti*) and tapeworm infections. *Pruritus ani* is characteristic of strongyloidiasis and enterobiasis (pinworm infection).

Urticaria are often present in the acute phase of infection, during which larvae or other immature forms actively invade human tissues. Helminths that infect humans by penetration of skin may cause a local urticarial rash at the sites of penetration. Migration of immature forms in the circulation may cause a generalized hypersensitivity reaction; urticaria is common during this phase of infection by many helminths (see Table 177-5). Chronic spontaneous urticaria, recurrent episodes of wheals, and/or angioedema lasting 6 weeks or longer, is associated with parasitic infections, including *T. canis* and *Anisakis simplex*.[12]

LOCALIZED EDEMA

Although edema or swelling may be an associated feature of many helminthic skin lesions, localized edema may is highly suggestive of the presence of certain infections.

Eyelid edema in particular may be seen in gnathostomiasis and loiasis (Calabar swelling), and violaceous periorbital edema is characteristic of trichinosis. *Limb edema* is highly suggestive of lymphatic filariasis (caused by *Brugia* spp. and *W. bancrofti*). Rarely, limb edema ("gros bras camerounais") may occur with acute onchocerciasis.[13]

CHANGES IN SKIN TEXTURE OR PIGMENTATION

Hypopigmentation of skin can be a feature of chronic infection caused by *O. volvulus* ("leopard skin"), *M. perstans*, and *Mansonella streptocerca*. Hypopigmented macules are the most common cutaneous findings in streptocerciasis. In onchocerciasis, depigmentation is characterized by perifollicular pigmentation within macular or minimally depressed areas, with yellow-brown hypopigmentation, and is particularly noticeable in dark-skinned individuals. *Hyperpigmentation* can also occur with mansonellosis caused by *M. streptocerca*, as well as in chronic schistosomiasis and onchocerciasis. *Lichenification* is a feature of onchocerciasis ("sowda" in Arabic), and to a lesser extent mansonellosis; hyperpigmented plaques eventually coalesce and become lichenified over time, particularly over the lower extremities and in young adults in Yemen and Sudan. *Verrucous lesions* may be seen in chronic schistosomiasis (bilharziasis cutanea tarda). *Ichthyosis* also may be present in chronic onchocerciasis.

OTHER CUTANEOUS MANIFESTATIONS

Petechiae may be present with trichinellosis and are frequently seen in disseminated strongyloidiasis, in which they are particularly prominent on the trunk. *Vesicles* or *bullae* may be seen at the site of larval skin penetration in up to 15% of patients with CLM, in human hookworm infection, and occasionally in dracunculiasis, onchocerciasis, and strongyloidiasis. *Ulcers* are uncommon findings in most helminthiases, with the exception of dracunculiasis; multiple ulcers are common. Ulcerative genital lesions, particularly in women, may occasionally be present in schistosomiasis and tend to occur more often with acute disease (eg, in travelers).

Erythema nodosum is rare in helminthic infections, but has been described as a clinical finding with hookworm infection, visceral larva migrans, sparganosis, and lymphatic filariasis. It also has been reported in 1 patient in conjunction with ascariasis,[14] although erythema nodosum in this patient may also have been caused by concomitant *Chlamydia pneumoniae* pneumonia. *Erythema multiforme* has been reported in CLM. *Eosinophilic panniculitis* has been documented in gnathostomiasis and toxocariasis. *Eosinophilic cellulitis* (Wells syndrome) may occur in ascariasis, onchocerciasis, and toxocariasis. *Eosinophilic folliculitis* has been rarely described in CLM and in toxocariasis. *Exfoliative dermatitis* of the affected limb may occur during the resolution phase of acute adenolymphangitis or following secondary bacterial-mediated cellulitis in *W. bancrofti* infection.

INTERVAL BETWEEN EXPOSURE AND ONSET OF SYMPTOMS

The time of onset of skin disease (and other key symptoms) relative to travel and likely exposures can be helpful in establishing a diagnosis (Table 177-6). Some infections, such as cercarial dermatitis in schistosomiasis or CLM, become evident within hours to days of exposure, whereas others may not present until months to years after infection.

PROGRESSION AND DURATION OF SKIN LESIONS

Skin lesions resulting from helminthic infections can persist for variable durations (see Table 177-6). For helminths that cause infection by penetration of skin, local dermatologic findings last only for a short time during infection by human helminths, but may persist longer with animal helminths (eg, CLM). During the chronic phase of infection, however, the duration of cutaneous manifestations varies depending on the infecting helminth. For infections in which skin findings are the result of inflammatory reactions to larvae (eg, onchocerciasis) or eggs (eg, schistosomiasis) in tissues, clinical manifestations can persist for the life span of the adult worms, which in some cases may be years. Even with appropriate therapy for chronic infections, chronic skin changes may not resolve completely.

TABLE 177-6
Interval from Exposure to Onset, and Duration, of Cutaneous Symptoms

SPECIES	TYPICAL INTERVAL BETWEEN EXPOSURE AND ONSET OF CUTANEOUS SYMPTOMS (RANGE)	TYPICAL DURATION OF SYMPTOMS (RANGE)
Nematodes (Roundworms)		
Ancylostoma braziliense, Ancylostoma caninum	Usually 1 to 5 days, typically within 1 month	2 to 14 weeks, rarely longer (up to 2 years)
Ancylostoma duodenale, Necator americanus (human hookworm)	Ground itch: 1 to 2 days Urticaria: 1 to 3 weeks	1 to 2 weeks
Ascaris lumbricoides	Urticaria: 10 to 14 days	Several weeks
Dirofilaria spp.	Subcutaneous nodules: several months	
Dracunculus medinensis	Edema, vesicle or bulla formation, ulceration with worm protrusion: 1 year	Several weeks
Enterobius vermicularis	Pruritus ani: weeks to months	30 to 45 days (self-limited) or until treated
Filariae		
Brugia malayi, Brugia timori	Hydrocele: years	Years
Loa loa	Calabar swelling, urticaria: >6 months to years Adult worm migration: years	Several days to weeks Years
Mansonella ozzardi, Mansonella perstans, Mansonella streptocerca	Pruritus, dermatitis, hypopigmentation: unknown	Years
Onchocerca volvulus	Onchodermatitis: months to years Onchocercoma: years	Years Years
Wuchereria bancrofti	Hydrocele: years	Years
Gnathostoma spinigerum, others	Creeping eruption: 1 to 2 days Migratory masses: 3 to 4 weeks	Up to 3 months 1 to 2 weeks, but recur for years
Strongyloides stercoralis	Larva currens: months to years Chronic urticaria, larva currens: years Petechiae, purpura (in disseminated disease): variable	Hours, but recur for years Years —
Toxocara canis, Toxocara cati	Urticaria: weeks to months	Years
Trichinella spiralis	Eyelid edema, petechiae: 1 to 3 weeks	2 to 3 weeks
Trematodes (Flukes)		
Fasciola hepatica	Urticaria: 6 to 12 weeks (with abdominal pain, fever, weight loss)	Several weeks to months
Paragonimus westermani	Urticaria: 2 days to 2 weeks Subcutaneous nodules: 2 to 3 weeks	Several weeks Years
Schistosoma spp. (human and avian)	Swimmer's itch: <24 hours Urticaria: 2 weeks to months Bilharzia cutanea tarda: years	Days to 3 weeks 2 to 10 weeks Years
Cestodes (Tapeworms)		
Echinococcus granulosis, Echinococcus multilocularis	Years	Years
Spirometra mansonoides, others (sparganosis)	20 days to 3 years	Years
Taenia multiceps, others (coenurosis)	Months to years	Years
Taenia solium (cysticercosis)	Variable—months to years	Years

NONCUTANEOUS FINDINGS

Apart from the skin, symptoms of helminthic infections tend to most frequently involve the respiratory, GI, and neurologic systems, and the eye. Disease may also occur in many other tissues as a consequence of aberrant migration of larvae and adult worms.

Because the skin lesions of many helminthic infections tend to occur in acute (larval) infection, and nondermatologic symptoms often result from the presence of adult helminths or their products of reproduction, it is important to appreciate that skin findings often precede other manifestations of disease. However, dermatologic and nondermatologic symptoms may coexist in some acute infections, as well as in chronic infections.

PULMONARY DISEASE

Loeffler syndrome, a hypersensitivity syndrome consisting of dyspnea, wheezing, cough, and fever, typically results from larval migration through lung tissue and may be seen in infection caused by human hookworms, *Ascaris*, and *Strongyloides*. Because these symptoms are a result of larval migration, they begin shortly after infection and may occur coincidentally with an urticarial rash. Loeffler syndrome typically lasts for 1 to 2 weeks. Diffuse pulmonary infiltrates and nodules may be seen during larval migration in acute schistosomiasis (Katayama syndrome) that occurs several weeks after exposure.[15]

Other pulmonary symptoms are generally not simultaneous with dermatologic symptoms, occurring after larvae have matured into adult forms. *Hemoptysis* is uncommon; among helminthic infections it is most frequently a feature of paragonimiasis, but also can be a symptom of echinococcal disease and disseminated strongyloidiasis. *Pulmonary nodules* may be seen in dirofilariasis, a zoonotic filariasis transmitted by mosquitoes, in conjunction with subcutaneous swellings and ocular lesions. *Pleural effusions* also occur rarely, and in helminthic infections are more likely to be eosinophilic. The most common parasitic etiology is *Paragonimus*, but effusions also can be caused by a variety of other helminths.[16]

GASTROINTESTINAL DISEASE

Abdominal pain is most commonly seen in ascariasis and human hookworm infection, after dermatologic manifestations have resolved, and in strongyloidiasis. Abdominal pain in strongyloidiasis is typically epigastric. Because *S. stercoralis* can complete its entire life cycle within the human host, larvae and adult worms may coexist simultaneously, and thus abdominal symptoms may be coincident with larva currens and pruritus ani. Right-upper-quadrant abdominal pain also may be a manifestation of acute fascioliasis, caused by larval penetration of the hepatic capsule; urticaria also may be present during this phase. *Diarrhea* can be a symptom with heavy *Strongyloides* or *Schistosoma* infections, and rarely hookworm infection. *Hepatitis* may be seen in acute fascioliasis. *Liver masses* or abdominal masses may be the presenting symptom of echinococcosis; hypodense liver lesions are commonly seen in fascioliasis as well. *Hepatomegaly* is one of the classic findings of visceral larva migrans (toxocariasis), typically occurring in children and usually in conjunction with fever, respiratory symptoms (wheezing) and occasionally urticaria. Hepatomegaly also has been reported as a finding of several other helminthiases including fascioliasis. *Granulomatous hepatitis* may also cause hepatomegaly, and is most commonly encountered in schistosomiasis (the result of granuloma formation around eggs in the periportal circulation), but also can be a feature of ascariasis (eggs), strongyloidiasis (larvae), and toxocariasis (larvae). *Biliary disease* may be a result of either occlusion of the biliary tract by adult worms or flukes (eg, ascariasis, fascioliasis) or from compression of the biliary tract by a mass lesion (eg, echinococcosis). *Hepatic fibrosis* can be a complication of chronic schistosomiasis.

NEUROLOGIC DISEASE

Helminthic infections most commonly affecting the CNS include neurocysticercosis and strongyloidiasis. *Seizures*, typically focal but sometimes generalized, are the most common presentation of neurocysticercosis. Neurocysticercosis should be considered in the presence of subcutaneous cysticercosis. The clinical presentation of neurocysticercosis is determined by the number, size, and location of intracranial lesions, as well as the viability of cysts (dying cysts produce more inflammation and are more likely to be associated with seizures). Globally, neurocysticercosis is among the most common causes of seizure disorders. Seizures may also occur with infection caused by *Schistosoma* spp. and *Paragonimus*, and in sparganosis. *Meningitis* can be seen in strongyloidiasis. *S. stercoralis* larvae may be visualized in cerebrospinal fluid, but more commonly meningitis is a result of Gram-negative bacteremia caused by enteric organisms that are carried across the bowel mucosa during larval penetration in disseminated disease; abdominal petechiae or purpura are often present. *Eosinophilic meningitis* or *meningoencephalitis* may be a feature of cysticercosis, gnathostomiasis, paragonimiasis, schistosomiasis, toxocariasis, angiostrongyliasis, baylisascariasis, and, less commonly, strongyloidiasis, among others.[17] *Mass lesions* or *cysts* can be caused by *Echinococcus* spp., *Paragonimus*, *Taenia* spp. causing coenurosis, and *Toxocara*. In schistosomiasis, intracranial infection is most commonly associated with *Schistosoma japonicum* infection and may result from the development of granulomas around ectopic eggs. Other CNS manifestations of helminthic infections, including brain abscesses, transverse myelitis and myelopathy, and intracranial hemorrhage, may occasionally be seen.

OCULAR DISEASE

Although ocular involvement is most frequently associated with infections caused by *Loa loa* and *O. volvulus* (river blindness), disease involving the conjunctiva, sclera, and all chambers of the eye can be occasional features of many helminthic infections. Onchocerciasis is a major cause of blindness worldwide. Ocular symptoms and findings are often related to the presence of larvae or microfilariae migrating through and causing inflammatory reactions in various chambers of the eye and the retina. Onchodermatitis is common in chronic infection, and skin findings and eye disease may be present simultaneously. Ocular disease is also one of the most frequent presentations of sparganosis.

Conjunctivitis is the typical ocular manifestation of gnathostomiasis and sparganosis, but also has been reported in a variety of other infections. *Keratitis* is most commonly present in onchocerciasis and coenurosis. *Uveitis* is characteristic of onchocerciasis and schistosomiasis. *Retinitis* or *chorioretinitis* may be present in onchocerciasis and toxocariasis. *Migration of adult worms* through the eye may be seen in loiasis and dirofilariasis, and less commonly in fascioliasis and gnathostomiasis, and gives rise to a foreign-body sensation in the eye. *Granulomatous nodules* in the eye or conjunctivae may be present in toxocariasis, schistosomiasis and *M. perstans* infection. *Eyelid swelling* (Calabar swelling) may be the result of infection by *Loa loa* and *M. perstans*.

LYMPHADENOPATHY

Lymphadenopathy is an uncommon finding in helminthic infections, with the exception of filarial infections. *Regional lymphadenopathy* can be present with lymphatic filariasis (caused by infection with *Brugia* spp. and *W. bancrofti*), as well in loiasis, *M. streptocerca* infection, and onchocerciasis. *Generalized lymphadenopathy* may be present in lymphatic filariasis, and in acute schistosomiasis (Katayama fever).

OTHER SYMPTOMS

Fever and urticaria can be features of Loeffler syndrome, which may be the initial manifestation of infection due to *A. lumbricoides*, human hookworm, *S. stercoralis*, and in toxocariasis. Fever in acute trichinellosis usually occurs in conjunction with other symptoms including myalgias, cough, facial edema, and splinter hemorrhages in the nails. Fever is also a finding in acute schistosomiasis (Katayama fever) and fascioliasis, and also may be present in other helminthiases, typically during larval migration. *Gram-negative sepsis* may occur in disseminated strongyloidiasis, a result of translocation of enteric bacteria as *Strongyloides* larvae penetrate the intestinal lumen; a petechial or purpuric eruption, particularly on the trunk, has been well reported in disseminated strongyloidiasis (see section "Strongyloidiasis").

COMPLICATIONS

Secondary complications including excoriation and secondary superinfection are not uncommon, especially when pruritic lesions are present. Skin changes, such as lichenification and pigment changes, as noted above, may be persistent. Other significant complications of specific cutaneous helminthic diseases are discussed below.

ETIOLOGY AND PATHOGENESIS

Cutaneous manifestations can be seen at every phase of the helminth life cycle in humans: by larvae or cercariae during skin penetration; during larval migration and tissue invasion; and because of the presence of eggs and adult worms in skin and soft tissues. Skin lesions also may occur during either early (acute) or chronic infection.

The pathogenesis of skin lesions in helminthic infections is varied. Direct penetration of skin may lead to a localized immune response, as seen in CLM or cercarial dermatitis. Migration of helminths can cause a generalized immune response (urticaria, maculopapular eruptions), particularly from migration of larvae or immature forms (eg, with *Ascaris* or *Toxocara* infection); a local inflammatory reaction to adult worms or eggs may also develop, as occurs with cutaneous nodules caused by *O. volvulus* and in schistosomiasis and cysticercosis, or subcutaneous swellings caused by *Loa loa* and *Gnathostoma*. Skin changes can also result from disruption of the normal skin structures because of lymphedema, as with filarial infections. Finally, ill-defined systemic immune reactions, such as erythema nodosum or erythema marginatum, rarely reported manifestations of several helminthic infections, also may be present. Skin findings of helminthic infections do not generally result from hematogenous spread of parasites, in contrast to many bacterial and viral infections.

Helminths induce a dramatic expansion of the T helper 2 (Th2) lymphocyte subset, with elevated levels of immunoglobulin E (IgE), peripheral eosinophilia, and an increase in tissue mast cells. It is unclear whether these Th2-derived responses are important in the protective immune response against the parasite or are responsible for immune-mediated pathology, or both.[12] Despite high levels of IgE and other features of Th2 cell activation, allergic responses are rarely observed in infected individuals except during the invasive phase of infection, when pruritus and/or urticaria may occur. Infected hosts have evolved elaborate immune evasion strategies to permit long-lived helminthic infections, including the induction of tolerance to parasite antigens.

DIAGNOSIS

The definitive diagnosis of most helminthic infections rests on identification of 1 or more of the various stages of the helminth (eg, larvae, eggs, adult worms) in tissue specimens, blood, or excretions (stool or urine). Occasionally, adult worms may be observed during medical procedures (eg, endoscopy or surgery). In many helminthic infections causing skin disease, however, cutaneous findings occur during the larval migration phase, and hence precede the presence of adult worms and the production of eggs or larvae that may not be detectable for weeks or months. The diagnosis of a helminthic infection is therefore often difficult during the penetration and acute phase of the disease; the diagnosis may be suspected because of associated epidemiologic and clinical findings. In chronic infection, the diagnosis can be established based on the identification of parasite eggs or larvae, or occasionally adult worms, but the sensitivity of stool examination can also vary depending on the parasite.

SUPPORTIVE STUDIES

Results of routine blood tests, including eosinophilia, are neither sensitive nor specific for diagnosing helminthic infections. While most hematologic and biochemical tests are nonspecific, the presence of eosinophilia can suggest specific diseases when combined with clinical findings and/or the exposure history, and should prompt additional investigations.[18,19] Diagnosis of helminthic infections also may be aided by results of ancillary investigations (eg, chest radiography; abdominal imaging).

LABORATORY TESTING

Eosinophilia: Eosinophilia, defined as an absolute eosinophil count of greater than 500 eosinophils per mm^3, is not typical of infections caused by most pathogens other than helminths; helminth antigens are effective stimuli for inducing eosinophilia. Levels of eosinophils in the blood can be affected by host factors, including the response to other bacterial, viral, or fungal coinfections (which lower eosinophil counts), the use of systemic steroids (which lower eosinophil counts), and an immunosuppressed state. In helminthic infection, eosinophil counts vary according to the stage of infection and the infecting helminth. Tissue invasion is the key factor in the development of eosinophilia. For example, eosinophilia is not a feature of intestinal lumen-dwelling helminths, except during the larval migration phase for those helminths in which this occurs; in contrast, helminthic infections in which adults, larvae, or eggs persist in tissues are typically associated with eosinophilia. Eosinophil counts are usually normal during the penetration phase and reach their highest levels (often markedly elevated) during the invasive phase of the cycle. Eosinophilia often accompanies the urticarial rash during the invasive stage of infection; thereafter, the eosinophil count often decreases slowly and may fluctuate more or less above the normal value during the chronic phase of infection. However, the detection of helminthic infection in returned travelers who present with asymptomatic eosinophilia is often very low. A transient hypereosinophilia may be also observed approximately 10 days after the start of effective antihelminthic treatment, and eosinophilia may persist for one to two months after successful helminth eradication.

Table 177-7 lists the helminths that typically cause eosinophilia. Severe or high-grade eosinophilia (an eosinophil count of >3000/mm^3) is suggestive of infection caused by relatively few of these parasites (Table 177-7).

Additional Laboratory Tests: Other laboratory tests may be abnormal but may not aid with establishing a specific diagnosis. Other than leukocytosis, which may reflect only the presence of eosinophilia, hematologic studies obtained when skin lesions are present are unlikely to be helpful. Evidence of disseminated intravascular coagulation may be present in disseminated strongyloidiasis. Iron-deficiency anemia is a feature of established hookworm infection, but occurs well after the resolution of cutaneous disease.

Biochemical testing may reveal abnormal liver function tests and enzymes in acute fascioliasis and toxocariasis, when urticaria may be present. Granulomatous hepatitis may be associated with a disproportionately elevated alkaline phosphatase. Most biochemical tests are otherwise nonspecific and are of limited use in determining the correct diagnosis.

Serology: Serologic assays are available for many helminthic infections, but vary greatly in their sensitivity and specificity. Their utility is also limited by cross-reactivity of tests among the various helminths, especially with filarial antibodies. Another significant limitation to serologic testing relates to the delayed appearance of antibodies after acute infection. Antibody production typically begins during the invasive (acute) phase of disease, when skin lesions are clinically apparent, but titers may be negative at this time. Serologic tests may not become positive for 2 months or more after the onset of infection. Although the presence of antibodies often supports or establishes the clinical diagnosis, antibodies may reflect prior infection and do not necessarily imply active or acute disease, and titers often remain positive for years after helminthic infections have been eradicated. The exception is strongyloidiasis, where a decrease in antibody titer is often used as a test of cure.

Molecular Testing: Molecular testing by polymerase chain reaction is highly sensitive and specific, and may be especially useful in the diagnosis of mixed infections.[20,21] However, its use is limited by the technical requirements of testing and cost, and it is not readily available in many diagnostic laboratories in North America.

Pathology: Additional diagnostic tests may include pathologic examination of tissue specimens or blood (for microfilariae), or microscopic examination of other specimens (eg, bronchoscopy specimens in disseminated strongyloidiasis).

TABLE 177-7

Helminthic Infections That May Be Associated with Eosinophilia

DISEASE	COMMENTS
Ascariasis[a]	Marked eosinophilia in early infection
Cysticercosis	
Dirofilariasis	
Dracunculiasis	
Fascioliasis[a]	Marked eosinophilia in early infection
Filariasis[a]	Eosinophilia may be marked especially in loiasis and with pulmonary symptoms
Gnathostomiasis[a]	
Hookworm infection (CLM)[a]	Can be marked during larval migration
Paragonimiasis[a]	Marked eosinophilia in early infection
Schistosomiasis[a]	Especially during early infection (Katayama fever)
Sparganosis	
Strongyloidiasis[a]	Eosinophilia may be moderate in chronic infection
Toxocariasis (VLM)[a]	

[a]Marked eosinophilia (eosinophil count >3000/mm^3) may be present.
CLM, cutaneous larva migrans; VLM, visceral larva migrans.

RADIOLOGIC INVESTIGATIONS

Symptomatic patients with Loeffler syndrome and acute schistosomiasis will typically have diffuse patchy infiltrates or nodules on chest radiographs; urticaria may be present at this time. Radiologic findings consistent with acute respiratory distress syndrome may be present in disseminated strongyloidiasis. Chest radiographs also may be abnormal in paragonimiasis (cystic lesions, pleural effusion). Pleural effusions may be present in infection caused by other helminths, as previously noted. A solitary pulmonary nodule may be noted in dirofilariasis.

Abdominal imaging (ultrasonography, CT, or MRI) should be directed by abdominal symptoms and is suggestive of a diagnosis in relatively few helminthic infections. Septated hepatic cysts are characteristic of cystic echinococcosis, whereas in alveolar hydatid disease hepatic lesions are usually solid. Hepatic masses or nodules (hypodense lesions up to 10 mm in size) may be visualized on ultrasonography or CT scan in fascioliasis. Tracts or tunnels representing migration of immature flukes through the liver also may be noted in fascioliasis.

Imaging studies of the CNS are diagnostic in neurocysticercosis, in which CT or MRI usually reveals parenchymal cysts and occasionally intraventricular or subarachnoid cysts. In cerebral gnathostomiasis, worm-like tracts have been noted.

MANAGEMENT

Treatment varies depending on the specific diagnosis. Recommended and alternate therapies for treatment of helminthic infections causing cutaneous findings can be found in recent reviews and guidelines.[22] Table 177-8 lists treatment of selected infections that are discussed in detail below.

SPECIFIC HELMINTHIC DISEASES OF MAJOR IMPORTANCE

The sections that follow describe key features of the most important helminthic infections. CLM syndrome and enterobiasis (pinworm infection) are encountered relatively frequently by clinicians in developed countries. In comparison, filariasis and schistosomiasis are uncommon, but may lead to chronic dermatologic complications. Strongyloidiasis, also seen relatively infrequently, must be considered in the appropriate clinical context; failure to diagnose and treat the infection may have significant clinical consequences for immunocompromised patients in particular, in whom disseminated strongyloidiasis carries a significant mortality risk. For these reasons, these 5 infections are described below.

CUTANEOUS LARVA MIGRANS SYNDROME

The terms *CLM* and *creeping eruption* are often used interchangeably when referring to disease caused by animal hookworms. Even though CLM is the most common cause of creeping eruption,[23] technically CLM refers to a syndrome in which the larvae of any animal nematode infect humans *and* in which the infected human is a dead-end host. These nematodes include animal hookworms (mostly from dogs and cats), *Gnathostoma* species, and agents of zoonotic filariases including Spirurina type X, *Pelodera strongyloides*, and zoonotic *Strongyloides* species. By definition, CLM syndrome does *not* include diseases in which creeping eruption is the result of: (a) nonlarval forms of parasites (eg, dracunculiasis, loiasis); (b) larval forms of human nematodes such as *S. stercoralis* (larva currens); or (c) larval forms of trematodes such as *Fasciola gigantica*. Creeping eruption refers to the clinical finding (sign) of a migratory serpiginous lesion, but does not denote the etiology of the lesion.

Hookworm-related CLM (creeping verminous dermatitis, sand-worm eruption, plumber's itch, duck hunter's itch), is most commonly caused by animal hookworms, and in particular *A. braziliense*. Other skin-penetrating hookworm larvae that produce similar disease include *A. caninum*, *Uncinaria stenocephala* (hookworm of European dogs), and *Bunostomum phlebotomum* (hookworm of cattle). *A. caninum* causes eosinophilic enteritis as well as cutaneous disease. Cats and dogs are hosts for *Ancylostoma ceylanicum* and *A. caninum*.

Clinically, the hallmark of CLM is a creeping eruption. The different helminthic diseases causing creeping eruption can often be distinguished based on the epidemiologic and exposure history, the characteristics of the cutaneous trail(s) (location, number, width and length, rate of movement) (see Table 177-2), and the duration of symptoms (see Table 177-6), in addition to other clinical and laboratory findings. The correct diagnosis is required for appropriate treatment.

EPIDEMIOLOGY

Hookworm-related CLM is widely distributed but is most commonly found in tropical and subtropical areas, especially the southeastern United States, Caribbean, Africa, Central and South America, India, and Southeast Asia. Contact with sand or soil contaminated with animal feces is required for infection to occur; infection can be prevented by avoiding skin contact with fecally contaminated soil.

CLINICAL FEATURES

Infection results from direct skin penetration by infective larvae of animal hookworms. Larvae migrate up to several centimeters a day, usually between the stratum germinativum and stratum corneum, and induce a localized eosinophilic inflammatory reaction.

TABLE 177-8
Treatment of Selected Helminthic Infections Causing Cutaneous Diseases

DISEASE	PRIMARY THERAPY (ADULT DOSES)	ALTERNATE THERAPY (ADULT DOSES)	COMMENTS
Cutaneous larva migrans	Albendazole 400 mg by mouth daily × 3 days	Ivermectin 200 μg/kg daily × 1 to 2 days Thiabendazole, topical 10% Albendazole, topical	
Enterobiasis	Albendazole 400 mg by mouth once	Mebendazole 100 mg once Pyrantel pamoate 11 mg/kg (maximum: 1 g) once	Treatment should be repeated 2 weeks after the first treatment, regardless of the agent used. Treatment of household contacts recommended
Filariasis	Endosymbiotic *Wolbachia* bacteria may play a role in filarial development and host response for all filariasis except loiasis. Doxycycline 100 to 200 mg by mouth daily × 6 to 8 weeks can reduce *Wolbachia* and block microfilariae production Antihistamines or glucocorticoids may be required to reduce the allergic reaction secondary to microfilariae disintegration during the treatment of filarial infections In patients with microfilariae in the blood, diethylcarbamazine (DEC) may cause severe allergic or febrile reactions. When microfilariae are present, it is advisable to start with a low dose and escalate (eg, 50 mg on day 1; 50 mg thrice daily on day 2; 100 mg by mouth thrice daily on day 3; then full dose)		
Brugia malayi, Brugia timori	DEC 2 mg/kg by mouth thrice daily × 12 days		In chronic disease, elevation of the affected limb, compression stockings, good skin care, treatment of superficial fungal and bacterial infections are important. Surgical treatment can sometimes be considered
Loa loa	DEC 3 mg/kg by mouth thrice daily × 21 days		Surgical removal of adult worm may be required
Mansonella ozzardi	Ivermectin 200 μg/kg by mouth once		Ivermectin reduces microfilarial burden. DEC is ineffective. Doxycycline may be effective
Mansonella perstans	Doxycycline 100 to 200 mg daily × 6 to 8 weeks		DEC, mebendazole, and ivermectin are ineffective
Mansonella streptocerca	DEC 2 mg/kg by mouth thrice daily × 12 days	Ivermectin 150 μg/kg by mouth once	
Onchocerca volvulus	Ivermectin 150 μg/kg by mouth once, then every 6 months until asymptomatic		DEC must not be used as rapid killing of worms can cause ocular side effects
Wuchereria bancrofti	DEC 2 mg/kg by mouth thrice daily × 12 days		Single-dose combination of albendazole 400 mg plus either ivermectin 200 μg/kg or diethylcarbamazine 6 mg/kg is effective in suppressing *W. bancrofti* microfilaremia. Chronic disease: see *Brugia* spp.
Schistosomiasis			Systemic steroids (eg, prednisone) may be helpful during acute disease
Schistosoma haematobium, Schistosoma intercalatum, Schistosoma mansoni	Praziquantel 40 mg/kg/day in 1 or 2 doses × 1 day	Oxamniquine 15 mg/kg by mouth once (**S. mansoni only**)	Oxamniquine unavailable in the United States, and is generally not as effective as praziquantel, but has been effective in some areas when praziquantel is less effective. In East Africa, increase oxamniquine dose to 30 mg/kg. In Egypt and South Africa, increase oxamniquine dose to 30 mg/kg/day × 2 days. Oxamniquine is contraindicated in pregnancy
Schistosoma japonicum, Schistosoma mekongi	Praziquantel 60 mg/kg/day in 2 or 3 doses × 1 day		
Strongyloidiasis	Ivermectin 200 μg/kg/day × 2 days	Albendazole 400 mg by mouth twice daily × 7 days	In immunocompromised patients or disseminated disease, it may be necessary to prolong or repeat therapy. Combination therapy (ivermectin plus albendazole) may be indicated in disseminated disease

DEC, diethylcarbamazine.

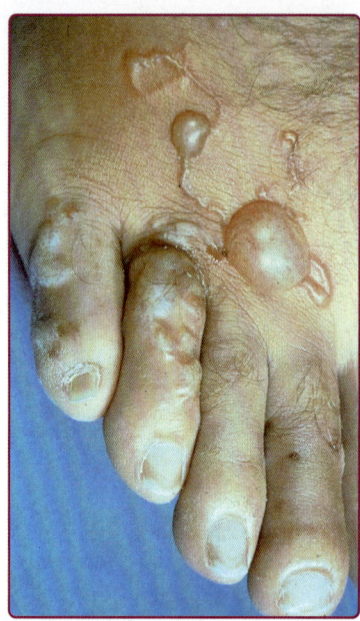

Figure 177-7 Cutaneous larva migrans with vesicular and bullous lesions. (Used with permission from Jay S. Keystone, MD, FRCPC.)

In contrast to human hookworm infection, animal hookworm larvae cannot mature beyond the larval stage in humans; they are unable to invade deeper tissues and die after days to months.

Typical skin lesions appear 1 to 5 days after exposure. The characteristic lesion of hookworm-related CLM is an erythematous, raised, and vesicular, linear, or serpentine cutaneous trail that progresses at a rate of 2 to 3 cm per day (see Fig. 177-6). Vesicular, papular or bullous lesions may be seen at the site of larval skin penetration in up to 15% of patients with CLM (Fig. 177-7). Lesions are approximately 3 mm wide and may reach 15 to 20 cm in length. They can be single or multiple, are intensely pruritic, and may be painful. The hookworm larvae advance a few millimeters to a few centimeters daily. The most common anatomic sites (usually 3 to 4 cm from the penetration site) include the feet (see Fig. 177-3) and buttocks (Fig. 177-8), although other sites may be affected. Excoriation and impetiginization are uncommon (10% of cases). Skin lesions usually last between 2 and 8 weeks, but have been reported to last for as long as 2 years. Systemic signs and symptoms (wheezing, dry cough, urticaria) are rare.

A less frequent but well-reported clinical presentation is that of hookworm folliculitis, consisting of 20 to 100 eosinophilic follicular papules and pustules confined to a particular area of the body, usually the buttocks. Patients with folliculitis usually also have creeping eruption. Papular lesions without CLM (papular larva migrans) are a less-common presentation. Other cutaneous signs related to the subcutaneous migration of helminth larvae have been occasionally described, such as urticaria and panniculitis.

DIAGNOSIS

The diagnosis of hookworm-related CLM is based on clinical findings. Hookworm folliculitis also can be diagnosed clinically when creeping eruption is also present; if not, skin biopsy may be required. Histopathologic findings include larvae trapped within the follicular canal, the stratum corneum, or the dermis, together with an inflammatory eosinophilic infiltrate.[24] Skin scrapings in patients with folliculitis may reveal live and dead larvae when examined by light microscopy with mineral oil.

MANAGEMENT

Both albendazole (400 mg by mouth daily for 3 days) and ivermectin (200 μg/kg daily for 1 or 2 days) are effective therapies for hookworm-related CLM[25,26] (see Table 177-8). Treatment of hookworm folliculitis may require repeated treatments. Topical therapy with thiabendazole, 10% albendazole, or ivermectin also may be used, but may be less effective than oral therapy. Thiabendazole is often not readily available. Because larvae have usually migrated beyond the end of the visible skin lesion and their location cannot be reliably determined, surgical excision or cryotherapy is not recommended.

ENTEROBIASIS (PINWORM INFECTION)

EPIDEMIOLOGY

Enterobiasis (threadworm, pinworm, or seatworm infection; oxyuriasis) is caused by *E. vermicularis*. It is among the most widely distributed helminthic infections and is found worldwide. Transmission is by the fecal–oral route; infection results from ingestion of *E. vermicularis* eggs (eg, by contact with contaminated fomites or via contaminated fingers) and rarely by inhalation and ingestion of aerosolized eggs in dust. The highest rates of infection are among children. Infection can be prevented by treatment of infected cases and good personal hygiene.

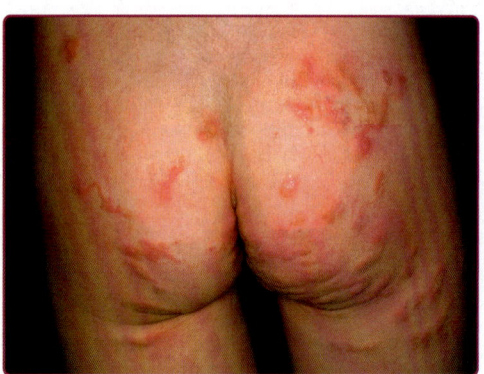

Figure 177-8 Cutaneous larva migrans of the buttocks. (Used with permission from Jay S. Keystone, MD, FRCPC.)

CLINICAL FEATURES

Nocturnal anal and perianal pruritus is the primary clinical feature. The worm may be seen around the anus. The skin may become impetiginized, and cellulitis may occur as a complication.

Women may rarely develop vulvovaginitis; vulvar granuloma and an association with Bartholin cysts also have been described. Nondermatologic extraintestinal manifestations are rare but have been reported. Epidemiologically, enterobiasis is often associated with an intestinal protozoan, *Dientamoeba fragilis*, which may produce GI upset. A recent study detected *D. fragilis* DNA on washed pinworm ova.[27]

DIAGNOSIS

The diagnosis is established by identification of *E. vermicularis* eggs in the perianal area, most effectively by the sticky-tape method. A piece of tape, sticky side out, can be attached to a wooden tongue depressor and firmly pressed against the perianal skin immediately on waking in the morning, before defecation or bathing. The tape is removed and placed sticky side down on a slide, and examined under a microscope. Sensitivity of this method is 70% with 3 specimens and increases to almost 100% with 7 specimens. Eggs are found in stool in only 10% to 15% of infections. Occasionally, the adult worm (white, up to 4 mm in length) is found in the perianal area, vulva, vagina, or underclothes. When ectopic sites are involved, the parasite may be identified in tissue sections.

DIFFERENTIAL DIAGNOSIS

The differential diagnosis includes strongyloidiasis, atopic dermatitis, contact dermatitis, and neurodermatitis.

MANAGEMENT

Enterobiasis is self-limited if reinfection does not occur. Treatment with 1 dose of albendazole 400 mg, mebendazole 100 mg, or pyrantel pamoate 11 mg/kg, is effective (see Table 177-8). Treatment of household members is also recommended, as household transmission is common. Treatment should be repeated once, 2 weeks after the first course of therapy, as medications are relatively ineffective against developing larvae and newly ingested eggs. Specific personal hygiene measures are also important for eradication of infection; these include wearing underwear and pajamas to sleep, bathing in the morning, keeping fingernails short, changing underwear daily and bedsheets weekly, and dusting the environment to remove eggs.

FILARIASIS

Filarial infections have been broadly grouped into 3 categories of disease based on the location of disease: lymphatic, cutaneous, and body cavity. Morbidity is almost entirely attributable to those species that cause lymphatic disease, and to a lesser extent cutaneous disease. Body cavity infection, caused by *Mansonella ozzardi*, is usually asymptomatic and is not discussed further.

EPIDEMIOLOGY

Lymphatic filariasis is caused mainly by *W. bancrofti* (bancroftian filariasis), which causes 90% of disease, and *B. malayi* (Malayan filariasis), which accounts for only 10% of all cases.[28] Infection caused by *Brugia timori* is rare. Lymphatic filariasis is widely distributed in both urban and rural areas of tropical and subtropical areas, with the largest number of infections occurring in India, South Asia, East Asia, and the Pacific Islands, and sub-Saharan Africa. *W. bancrofti* is also endemic in northern parts of South America (Guyana, Surinam, and some coastal regions of Brazil). In developed countries, infections are seen primarily in immigrants and persons with prolonged visits to endemic areas. Infection is transmitted to humans by mosquitoes, and can be prevented by avoidance of mosquito bites. The incubation period is usually 5 to 18 months, during which time microfilariae migrate to the lymphatic system, mature into adults, mate, and release microfilariae (larvae); occasionally symptoms develop within 3 months of exposure. Lymphatic filariasis is first acquired in childhood, often with as many as one-third of children in endemic areas infected before the age of 5 years.[29] The characteristic symptoms typically occur years after infection and the prevalence of clinical disease increases after age 20 years in endemic areas. Adult worms live an average of 10 to 15 years, and microfilariae probably 6 to 12 months.

Cutaneous filariasis is caused by *Loa loa*, *M. perstans*, *M. streptocerca*, and *O. volvulus*. Loiasis is endemic in rural areas of Central and West Africa, affecting an estimated 3 to 13 million residents. *Loa loa* is transmitted by the day-biting *Chrysops* fly; infection can be prevented by avoiding bites from *Chrysops* in endemic areas, diethylcarbamazine chemoprophylaxis, and treatment of infected humans to reduce the source of parasites. Symptoms usually begin an average of 24 months after exposure, but can begin as early as 4 months or as late as a decade or more after infection. The adult worm can live longer than 20 years in the human host.

Infection caused by both *M. perstans* and *M. streptocerca* is often asymptomatic. *M. perstans* is endemic in sub-Saharan Africa, as well as parts of Central and South America, where it is transmitted by *Culicoides* midges. Like lymphatic filariasis, infection during childhood is common, and reinfection may occur.[30] In highly endemic areas, the prevalence of infection may be as high as 80%. *M. streptocerca* is endemic in forested areas of West and Central Africa. Transmission is also by infected midges.

Onchocercosis (river blindness; erysipelas de la costa in Mexico and Guatemala; sowda in Arabic speaking areas; craw-craw in West Africa) is concentrated in rural areas of equatorial Africa and the Arabian peninsula, and in Latin America. Onchocerciasis is transmitted by black-flies of the genus *Simulium*. In the human, infective larvae mature to adult worms that are encapsulated in fibrous tissue and reside in nodules in the subcutaneous tissue and deep fascia. The incubation period is usually 1 to 2 years with a range of months to several years, although microfilariae may first appear 3 to 15 months after exposure; symptoms may precede microfilaremia but often develop only after months or years of infection. Microfilariae can survive in humans for up to 2 to 3 years, and adult worms for 10 to 15 years. The primary means of preventing onchocerciasis are through vector control and mass treatment with ivermectin of the population in endemic areas.

CLINICAL FEATURES

Lymphatic Filariasis (*Brugia malayi, Brugia timori; Wuchereria bancrofti*): Clinical manifestations may be acute, chronic, or recurrent. Initial infection may be subclinical but may also cause recurrent lymphangitis with characteristic retrograde progression (beginning in the affected lymph node and moving distally), lymphadenitis, orchitis, epididymitis, or, occasionally, fever. Lymphangitis typically recurs 6 to 10 times per year, with each episode lasting 3 to 7 days. The affected body part clinically appears normal between early episodes, although during the resolution of the acute phase of *W. bancrofti* filariasis, there may be extensive exfoliation of the skin of the affected limb. Intermittent fevers and adenolymphangitis can recur for the lifetime of the adult worm. Travelers (>1 month) to endemic areas less frequently acquire infection but may present with more intense inflammatory reactions to filarial parasites. The findings may include lymphangitis, lymphadenitis, groin pain from the associated lymphatic inflammation, urticaria, and peripheral eosinophilia.

Chronic disease with sequelae of lymphatic obstruction (lymphedema, elephantiasis, hydrocele, and chyluria) becomes evident 10 to 15 years after infection. The skin over the involved area can become hypertrophic, verrucous, and fibrotic with redundant skin folds (Fig. 177-9). Fissures, ulceration, secondary bacterial infection, and gangrene may occur. The lower extremity, scrotum, and penis are most commonly affected, and less frequently the upper extremity, breast, and vulva are involved. Although antiparasitic treatment does not reverse the late findings of scarring and lymphatic obstruction, a 6-week course of doxycycline can reduce mild-to-moderate lymphedema independent of active filarial infection by reducing vascular endothelial growth factor.[31]

The differential diagnosis for lymphatic filariasis includes acute infection that can resemble bacterial lymphangitis and other causes of nodular lymphangitis (eg, sporotrichosis, leishmaniasis). Other causes of lymphedema and elephantiasis must also be considered during evaluation of chronic disease.

Cutaneous Filariasis: Loaisis (*Loa loa*): The characteristic finding of loiasis is the Calabar swelling (Fig. 177-10), a localized area of angioedema caused by migration of adult worms through subcutaneous tissues. Calabar swellings usually begin years after infection, typically around joints of the upper extremities, generally last 2 to 4 days, and may be associated with pruritus or pain. They range in size from 5 to 20 cm in diameter and may recur in different locations. Fatigue, myalgias, arthralgias, and fever are rare. Adult worms may be seen moving across the bulbar conjunctiva of the eye (see Fig. 177-5) and eyelid. Pruritus may also occur. High-grade peripheral eosinophilia, leukocytosis, and elevated IgE levels are often present.

The differential diagnosis includes other causes of migratory and nodular skin lesions (see Tables 177-2 and 177-3).

Cutaneous Filariasis: Mansonelliasis (*Mansonella perstans, Mansonella streptocerca*): Cutaneous manifestations of *M. perstans* infection include Calabar-like swellings, typically in the

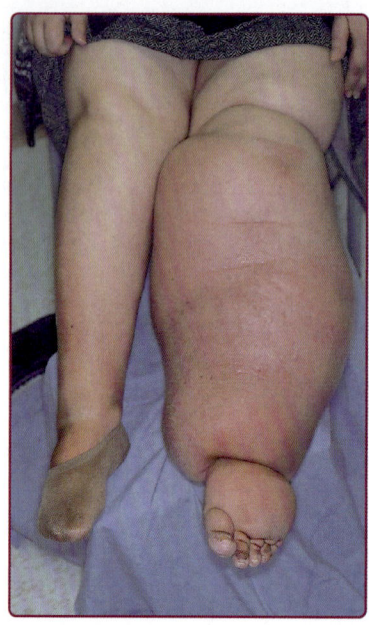

Figure 177-9 Lymphatic filariasis. (Used with permission from Jay S. Keystone, MD, FRCPC.)

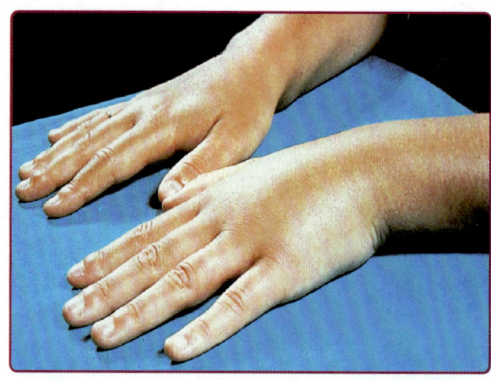

Figure 177-10 Calabar swelling in loiasis. (Used with permission from Jay S. Keystone, MD, FRCPC.)

forearms, hands and face, and pruritus with or without a papular rash. The exact interval between infection and onset of symptoms is unclear. Pruritus, papular lesions, and hypopigmented, hyperpigmented, or lichenified macules, typically found on the upper chest, are seen with *M. streptocerca* infection. Eosinophilia is often present in *Mansonella* infections, but also may be from the high prevalence of coinfection with other filarial or helminthic infections.

Cutaneous Filariasis: Onchocerciasis (*Onchocerca volvulus*): Individuals with onchocerciasis may be asymptomatic. Clinical manifestations most commonly involve the skin and eye. Heavy infections can result in blindness from chronic keratitis or retinitis. Six different patterns of skin changes have been described in onchocerciasis: acute and chronic papular onchodermatitis (see Fig. 177-1), lichenified onchodermatitis, atrophy, depigmentation, and onchocercal nodules (see Fig. 177-2). More than one pattern of skin involvement may be present simultaneously, or one pattern of skin involvement may evolve into another pattern.

Pruritus is the most prominent and persistent symptom of infection. Acute papular onchodermatitis most often involves the face, extremities, and trunk, and includes widespread small pruritic papules, vesicles and pustules, sometimes with associated erythema and edema. Short-term visitors to endemic regions typically present with acute pruritus and rash (see Fig. 177-1),[32] and demonstrate immune hyperresponsiveness despite low levels of parasites[33]; skin nodules and eye involvement are usually absent. After exposures in forested areas of West and Central Africa, travelers and expatriates may have an acute form of onchocerciasis characterized by acute pruritic and erythematous swelling of a limb known as *gros bras camerounais*[13] or onchocerciasis-associated limb swelling.[34]

The skin lesions of chronic papular onchodermatitis are macules and lichenoid papules varying in size from 3 to 9 mm in diameter. Pruritus is common, and postinflammatory hyperpigmentation may be present. The most commonly affected anatomic areas are the buttocks, shoulders, and waist (see Fig. 177-1). Palpable asymptomatic onchocercal nodules containing the adult worm involve the deep dermis and subcutaneous tissue (see Fig. 177-2), and occur over bony prominences such as the skull, iliac crest, knee, rib, sacrum, scapula, and trochanter.

Diagnosis is made by finding microfilariae in the skin by biopsy or skin snips (superficial 2- to 4-mm snips of the upper dermis placed in saline and incubated for 24 hours; the fluid is then examined for microfilariae). Peripheral eosinophilia and elevated IgE levels are common findings.

The differential diagnosis for onchocercal nodules includes other parasitic causes of nodules (see Table 177-3) and epidermal inclusion cysts. Acute onchodermatitis may resemble miliaria, insect bites, scabies or eczema. Chronic onchodermatitis may resemble a chronic or lichenoid eczema or atopic dermatitis. Skin changes resembling lichenified onchodermatitis can be the result of conditions causing significant pruritus or rubbing. Atrophic changes resemble those associated with aging. Onchocercal depigmentation may be confused with postinflammatory hypopigmentation or depigmentation.

DIAGNOSIS

Eosinophilia, sometimes high-grade, and elevated IgE levels are common in filarial infections. Diagnosis rests primarily on demonstration of microfilariae in blood (for lymphatic filariasis, loiasis, and cutaneous filariasis caused by *Mansonella* species; note that daytime blood specimens are appropriate for all except bancroftian filariasis, which requires nocturnal specimens for diagnosis) or in skin snips (for *Mansonella* and *Onchocerca* infections). However, persons with active filarial infection may not be microfilaremic. Microfilariae may not appear in blood until 5 to 6 months after infection in loiasis. Diagnosis also can be established through identification of the adult worm.

Filarial serology is often very sensitive but is nonspecific because of cross-reaction with other helminthiases. A positive serologic test for bloodborne species should be followed by both a blood examination for larvae and test for filarial antigen, to confirm whether serology represents an active infection or a previous one.

Infiltrates may be present on chest radiography in individuals with lymphatic filariasis and tropical pulmonary eosinophilia, an aberrant immune response to the infection. Inguinal lymph node ultrasonography may show active adult worms ("filarial dance sign"), more commonly seen in men than in women. Lymph node biopsy is contraindicated.

MANAGEMENT

Management of filariasis depends on the infecting species. Table 177-8 summarizes treatment of filariasis.

SCHISTOSOMAL INFECTIONS

EPIDEMIOLOGY

Cercarial dermatitis (swimmer's itch) occurs worldwide and may be acquired by contact with infective cercariae of many species of nonhuman schistosomal parasites in both freshwater and salt water. Attack rates during outbreaks usually range from 55% to 100% of those exposed, with highest attack rates in those with a history of previous cercarial dermatitis.

An estimated 200 million people worldwide have schistosomiasis (bilharziasis) and over half a billion live in endemic areas. Infection can be caused by *Schistosoma haematobium*, *Schistosoma intercalatum*, *Schistosoma japonicum*, *Schistosoma mansoni*, and *Schistosoma mekongi*. Humans are the only important reservoir for *S. haematobium*, which is prevalent in Africa and the Middle East. *Schistosoma mansoni* is endemic in the same areas, as well as parts of the Caribbean and South America; *S. intercalatum* in central Africa; *S. japonicum* in China, Indonesia, and the Philippines; and *S. mekongi* primarily in Cambodia and Laos.

Infection can be acquired after a brief exposure in an endemic area, often in travelers,[35-37] typically after swimming, wading, rafting, or bathing in slow-moving freshwater in endemic areas. Attack rates in nonimmune, exposed persons (eg, travelers) can be as high as 100%. Cutaneous manifestations can be seen at every phase of the infection.

CLINICAL FEATURES

Clinical findings of cercarial dermatitis are confined to the skin and are usually distributed on skin surfaces exposed directly to water. Pruritus may begin while swimming, followed rapidly by the appearance of an erythematous macular rash that persists for several hours. Ten to 15 hours after exposure, papules, vesicles, and urticaria develop. Marked pruritus is characteristic. Symptoms peak 48 to 72 hours after exposure, and gradually resolve spontaneously over the next several weeks.

Cercariae of *S. haematobium*, *S. intercalatum*, *S. japonicum*, *S. mansoni*, and *S. mekongi* can penetrate intact skin within 30 seconds to 10 minutes and may elicit a local inflammatory response (penetration phase). The first exposure to cercariae typically results in erythema and pruritus that resolve within hours. In those previously sensitized, a pruritic, erythematous, papular, and urticarial rash develops, usually lasting 1 week. Migration of the larvae (schistosomulae) usually occurs 2 to 6 weeks after exposure and leads to an acute parasitic hypersensitivity reaction with circulating immune complexes. This invasive phase (Katayama fever or acute schistosomiasis) has historically been described with *S. japonicum* (Katayama fever, sensu stricto), *S. mansoni*, and, to a lesser extent, with *S. haematobium*. Symptoms of acute schistosomiasis are most prominent in primary infection in nonimmune persons and include fever, fatigue, myalgia, cough, and headache that may persist for several weeks. Abdominal symptoms and diarrhea also may be present. Urticaria, purpura, subungual hemorrhages, and edema of the face, the extremities, genitals, and trunk may be seen during the invasive phase.

Chronic infection may be asymptomatic, or associated with abdominal pain (*S. mansoni*, *S. japonicum*) or hematuria (*S. haematobium*). Chronic dermal schistosomiasis (bilharziasis cutanea tarda) may begin after years of infection and result from a granulomatous inflammatory reaction to the deposition of eggs in the dermis (Fig. 177-11), which may continue for the life span of the adult worm (10 years or more). It is seen primarily in persons who have lived in endemic regions. Lesions are skin-colored or slightly pigmented, 2- to 4-mm firm, pruritic, oval papules that appear in crops and clusters, typically on the trunk and especially the periumbilical region, and remain unchanged without treatment. Lesions also appear in the genital and buttocks areas, especially on the vulva in women and the scrotum and penis in men. Chronic lesions may also include painless, skin-colored, pink, or brown eroded papules and warty, vegetative, polypoid lesions that may be ulcerated and necrotic, with fistulous tracts. Chronic skin disease can be complicated by lymphedema and elephantiasis, secondary bacterial infection, and squamous cell carcinoma.

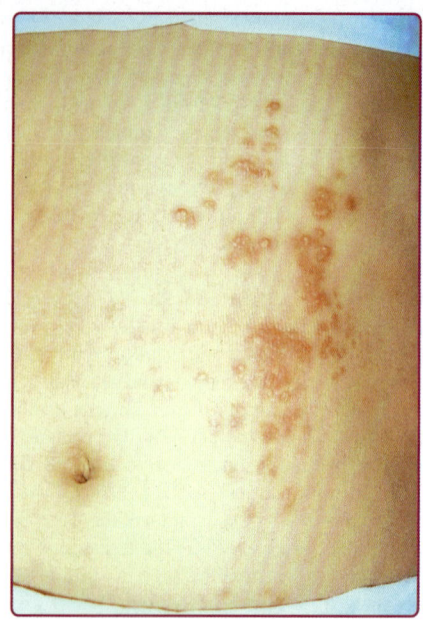

Figure 177-11 Ectopic deposition of *Schistosoma mansoni* eggs.

DIFFERENTIAL DIAGNOSIS

The differential diagnosis of acute schistosomiasis includes other causes of urticaria. Bilharziasis cutanea tarda of the genitals and buttocks must be differentiated from syphilis, condyloma latum, condyloma acuminatum, other granulomatous diseases, malignancy, and hemorrhoids.

DIAGNOSIS

Cercarial dermatitis is largely a clinical and epidemiologic diagnosis. In schistosomiasis, prominent eosinophilia may be present in early infection, especially during the invasive phase, and subsequently fluctuates more or less above the normal value during the chronic phase. Onset of eosinophilia may lag behind appearance of clinical symptoms. Acute disease can be suspected based on the history of exposure and cercarial dermatitis, although many patients do not develop the dermatitis. Identification of eggs in the stool or urine occurs only after the acute phase of infection, generally 2 to 3 months after the onset of infection. Similarly, serology does not become positive until approximately 2 months after infection.

MANAGEMENT

Cercarial dermatitis is self-limited and does not require specific therapy. Table 177-8 outlines management of schistosomiasis.

STRONGYLOIDIASIS

EPIDEMIOLOGY

Strongyloidiasis is caused by *S. stercoralis*, which is endemic to Africa, Asia, Southeast Asia, and Central and South America. Disease is also found in the Caribbean, and to a much lesser extent in Europe, Japan, Australia, and parts of the southern United States. Humans are the only hosts. Infection caused by *Strongyloides fuelleborni*, found sporadically in Africa and Papua New Guinea, is relatively rare. The prevalence of infection can be high in endemic areas, as well as among institutionalized mentally impaired persons, in former prisoners of war, and in refugees and immigrants from endemic areas. Most infected persons have low worm burdens and are persistently infected for life, often with minimal or no symptoms.

The life cycle of *Strongyloides* helminths differs from that of most other helminths in that an entire parasite life cycle may be completed within the human host. Infection typically results from penetration of skin or mucous membranes by infective larvae, usually from soil; the risk of infection is high for persons with frequent soil contact (eg, walking barefoot) in warm, moist areas contaminated by human feces. Filariform larvae travel via the circulatory system to the lungs where they penetrate the alveoli, ascend the trachea, are swallowed, and then mature into adult worms in the small intestine. Although sexual reproduction does take place within the intestine, adult females are also parthenogenetic (capable of reproduction without males). Eggs are deposited in the intestinal mucosa, hatch, and release rhabditiform larvae, which are excreted in the stool to begin another "free-living" cycle, developing into adults in soil where they reproduce sexually and give rise to infective filariform larvae. However, rhabditiform larvae in the bowel may also transform directly into filariform larvae (the "parasitic cycle") that penetrate the perianal skin and/or intestinal mucosa and enter the circulation, and begin another cycle of infection (autoinfection). In the appropriate clinical setting this may lead to disseminated disease (hyperinfection syndrome).

Appropriate sanitation and avoidance of soil contact by skin in endemic areas reduce the risk of infection. Persons with a history of prior residence or activities that place them at an increased risk for strongyloidiasis should be evaluated for presence of the infection, and should be treated even if asymptomatic. This is especially important in persons who receive or will receive immune suppressing therapy.

CLINICAL FEATURES

Cutaneous manifestations may be seen at any phase of infection. Following skin penetration, an urticarial eruption or larva currens may develop. Larva currens, a migratory serpiginous and intensely pruritic lesion caused by intradermal migration of larvae, can be differentiated from CLM by the high rate of movement (up to 5 to 10 cm per hour). Larva currens typically disappears within a few hours, only to recur over the course of weeks to years. Perianal larva currens may be present (see Fig. 177-4) and is pathognomonic of chronic infection. Lesions on the buttocks and in the perianal region result from larvae exiting the GI tract and reinfecting the host by penetrating the perianal skin. Persons chronically infected with *Strongyloides* may also experience pruritus ani and chronic urticaria, which may be complicated by prurigo nodularis or lichen simplex chronicus. The dermatologic manifestation of hyperinfection and disseminated strongyloidiasis is a rapidly and progressively diffuse petechial and purpuric eruption, often with a reticular pattern, typically involving the trunk and proximal extremities (Fig. 177-12).[38,39] The "thumbprint sign," a unique pattern of periumbilical purpura resembling multiple thumbprints,[40] also may be seen.

During the invasive phase of the infection, transient pulmonary manifestations (cough, wheezing, infiltrates) are manifestations of pulmonary migration and may be associated with urticaria. Chronic strongyloidiasis gives rise to nonspecific GI complaints (epigastric pain, nausea, vomiting, diarrhea, constipation, malabsorption, weight loss).

COMPLICATIONS

Hyperinfection syndrome is the most severe complication, typically occurring in the presence of impaired cellular immunity as seen with use of systemic steroids but also with other immunocompromised states, including human T-cell lymphotropic virus (HTLV)-1

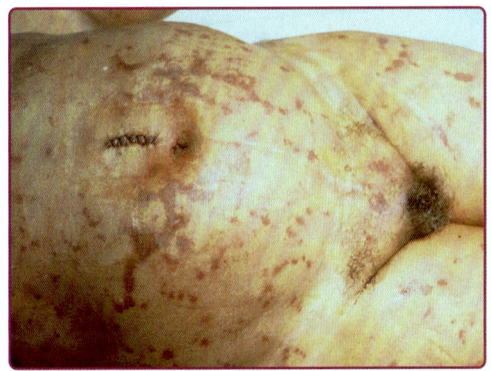

Figure 177-12 Disseminated strongyloidiasis, with non-palpable purpura on the abdominal wall. (Reprinted with permission from Grossman ME, Roth J. *Cutaneous Manifestations of Infection in the Immunocompromised Host*. Baltimore, MD: Lippincott, Williams & Wilkins; 1995.)

infection. Interestingly, HIV infection is not associated with an increased risk of disseminated disease.

Insidious GI symptoms may be present in hyperinfection syndrome. Pulmonary disease is the most common extraintestinal manifestation of hyperinfection syndrome and is characterized by diffuse pulmonary infiltrates with dyspnea, cough, wheezing, or hemoptysis. Diarrhea and abdominal pain occur frequently, with inflammation leading to small-bowel-wall edema; ileus may develop in late stages. In uncontrolled hyperinfection, filariform larvae also penetrate organs not normally involved in the life cycle, including the urinary tract, liver, brain, and skin. The finding of filariform larvae in stool may be an early sign of hyperinfection even in those with minimal symptoms. Gram-negative bacillary infections including bacteremia, peritonitis, meningitis and sepsis may result from the concurrent migration of bacteria and larvae across the bowel wall. The mortality rate for disseminated disease is approximately 50%.

DIAGNOSIS

Peripheral eosinophilia is present in up to 80% of patients with intestinal disease. Eosinophilia may be high grade during larval migration, but is rarely a feature of disseminated infection (although pulmonary eosinophilia may be noted in the latter), and may be absent in patients on systemic steroids and who are otherwise severely immunocompromised. In chronic disease, the eosinophil level fluctuates and is often mildly elevated (mild to moderate increase) but may be normal. Hence, the absence of eosinophilia does not rule out strongyloidiasis.

The diagnosis of larva currens is based on its characteristic clinical features. The identification of larvae in the stool, small bowel contents, and, rarely, in other body fluids confirms the diagnosis. Larvae first appear in the stool 2 to 4 weeks after exposure. Multiple stool examinations are often necessary to make the diagnosis; a single stool specimen may fail to detect larvae in up to 70% of cases, although sensitivity approaches 100% with 7 consecutive stool samples. Although the agar plate method is a very good test that has a sensitivity of 90%,[41] it is not readily available. A stool sample is placed on solid bacterial medium, incubated, and subsequently examined for bacterial tracks created by larvae dragging enteric bacteria as they migrate across the plate. Serology has become the test of choice, with a sensitivity of approximately 90%, but lacks specificity and may cross-react with other helminthic infections (in particular filariasis, ascariasis, and acute schistosomiasis). However, because strongyloidiasis is potentially fatal, and most individuals are not infected with other helminths, except in the tropics, the lack of sensitivity is not clinically relevant. Because studies show that antibody levels drop significantly over the first year following successful therapy, serology is often used as a test of cure.[42] Skin biopsy of the larva currens eruption often fails to reveal larvae, whereas they may be visualized in biopsy specimens of purpuric and petechial lesions with hyperinfection.

MANAGEMENT

Treatment of strongyloidiasis in asymptomatic individuals is often successful. Ivermectin 200 µg/kg daily for 2 days is the recommended therapy (see Table 177-8). Albendazole 400 mg twice daily for 7 days appears to be a less-effective alternative, although data are more limited; the drug is not approved by the U.S. Food and Drug Administration for this indication.

In contrast, patients with disseminated disease may require prolonged or repeated courses of therapy; some experts also suggest that combination therapy with ivermectin and albendazole be used in this setting. Patients with concurrent HTLV-1 infection may require lifetime therapy, given intermittently, owing to the inability of the host to eliminate the parasite. If possible, immunosuppressant therapy should be discontinued in those with hyperinfection.

For patients in whom strongyloidiasis is suspected epidemiologically or clinically and who require immunosuppression therapy, *Strongyloides* therapy should be given "on spec" if the diagnosis cannot be ruled out in a timely manner prior to initiating immunosuppressants.

REFERENCES

1. Lupi O, Downing C, Lee M, et al. Mucocutaneous manifestations of helminth infections: nematodes. *J Am Acad Dermatol*. 2015;73:929.
2. Lupi O, Downing C, Lee M, et al. Mucocutaneous manifestations of helminth infections: trematodes and cestodes. *J Am Acad Dermatol*. 2015;73:947.
3. Caumes E. Skin diseases. In: Keystone JS, Freedman DO, Kozarsky PE, eds, et al. *Travel Medicine, Third Edition*. e Philadelphia, PA: Elsevier; 2013:487-500.
4. Ansart S, Perez L, Vergely O, et al. Illness in travelers returning from the tropics: a prospective study of 622 patients. *J Travel Med*. 2005;12:312.
5. Freedman DO, Weld LH, Kozarsky PE, et al. Spectrum of disease and relation to place of exposure among ill returned travelers. *N Engl J Med*. 2006;354:119.
6. O'Brien DP, Leder K, Matchett E, et al. Illness in returned travelers and immigrants/refugees: the 6 year experience of two Australian infectious diseases units. *J Travel Med*. 2006;13:145.
7. Ansart S, Perez L, Jaureguiberry S, et al. Spectrum of dermatoses in 165 travelers returning from the tropics with skin diseases. *Am J Trop Med Hyg*. 2007;76:184.
8. Lederman ER, Weld LH, Elyazar IR, et al. Dermatologic conditions of the ill returned traveler: an analysis from the GeoSentinel Surveillance Network. *Int J Infect Dis*. 2008;12:593.
9. Herbinger KH, Seiss C, Nothdurft HD, et al. Skin disorders among travellers returning from tropical and non-tropical countries consulting a travel medicine clinic. *Trop Med Int Health*. 2011;16:1457.
10. Stevens MS, Geduld J, Libman M, et al. Dermatoses among returned Canadian travellers and immigrants: surveillance report based on CanTravNet data, 2009-2012. *CMAJ Open*. 2015;3:E119-E126.

11. Herbinger KH, Alberer M, Berens-Riha N, et al. Spectrum of imported infectious diseases: a comparative prevalence study of 16,817 German travelers and 977 immigrants from the tropics and subtropics. *Am J Trop Med Hyg*. 2016;94:757.
12. Kohlkir P, Balakirski G, Merk HF, et al. Chronic spontaneous urticaria and internal parasites—a systematic review. *Allergy*. 2016;71:308.
13. Nozais JP, Caumes E, Datry A, et al. Apropos of 5 new cases of onchocerciasis edema [in French]. *Bull Soc Pathol Exot*. 1997;90:335.
14. Bergler-Czop B, Lis-Swiety A, Kamińska-Winciorek G, et al. Erythema nodosum caused by ascariasis and *Chlamydophila pneumoniae* pulmonary infection—a case report. *FEMS Immunol Med Microbiol*. 2009;57:236.
15. Pavlin BI, Kozarsky P, Cetron MS. Acute pulmonary schistosomiasis: case report and review of the literature. *Travel Med Infect Dis*. 2012;10:209.
16. Martin GJ. Approach to the patient in the tropics with pulmonary disease. In: Guerrant RL, Walker DH, Weller PF, eds. *Tropical Infectious Diseases: Principles, Pathogens and Practice, Third Edition*. Philadelphia, PA: Elsevier; 2011:982-990.
17. Graeff-Teixiera C, Ara'mburu da Silva AC, Yoshimura K. Update on eosinophilic meningoencephalitis and its clinical relevance. *Clin Microbiol Rev*. 2009;22:322.
18. Schulte C, Krebs B, Jelinek T, et al. Diagnostic significance of blood eosinophilia in returning travelers. *Clin Infect Dis*. 2007;34:407.
19. O'Connell EM, Nutman TB. Eosinophilia in infectious diseases. *Immunol Allergy Clin North Am*. 2015;35:493.
20. Llewellyn S, Inpankaew T, Nery SV, et al. Application of a multiplex quantitative PCR to assess prevalence and intensity of intestinal parasite infections in a controlled clinical trial. *PLoS Negl Trop Dis*. 2016;10::e0004380.
21. Utzinger J, Becker SL, van Lieshout L, et al. New diagnostic tools in schistosomiasis. *Clin Microbiol Infect*. 2015;21:529.
22. Drugs for parasitic infections. *Med Lett Drugs Ther*. 2013;11(suppl):e1.
23. Vanhaecke C, Perignon A, Monsel G, et al. Aetiologies of creeping eruption: 78 cases. *Br J Dermatol*. 2014;170:1166.
24. Caumes E, Ly F, Bricaire F. Cutaneous larva migrans with folliculitis: report of seven cases and review of the literature. *Br J Dermatol*. 2002;146:1.
25. Hochedez P, Caumes E. Hookworm-related cutaneous larva migrans. *J Travel Med*. 2007;14:326.
26. Kincaid L, Klowak M, Klowak S, et al. Management of imported cutaneous larva migrans: a case series and mini-review. *Travel Med Infect Dis*. 2015;13:382.
27. Ögren J, Dienus O, Löfgren S, et al. *Dientamoeba fragilis* DNA detection in *Enterobius vermicularis* eggs. *Pathog Dis*. 2013;69:157.
28. Mendoza N, Li A, Gill A, et al. Filariasis: diagnosis and treatment. *Dermatol Ther*. 2009;22:475.
29. Witt C, Ottesen EA. Lymphatic filariasis: an infection of childhood. *Trop Med Int Health*. 2001;6:582.
30. Asio SM, Simonsen PE, Onapa AW. *Mansonella perstans* filariasis in Uganda: patterns of microfilaraemia and clinical manifestations in two endemic communities. *Trans R Soc Trop Med Hyg*. 2009;103:266.
31. Mand S, Debrah AY, Klarmann U, et al. Doxycycline improves filarial lymphedema independent of active filarial infection: a randomized controlled clinical trial. *Clin Infect Dis*. 2012;55:621.
32. Nguyen JC, Murphy ME, Nutman TB, et al. Cutaneous onchocerciasis in an America traveler. *Int J Dermatol*. 2004;4;125.
33. Henry NL, Law M, Nutman TB, et al. Onchocerciasis in a nonendemic population: clinical and immunologic assessment before treatment and at the time of presumed care. *J Infect Dis*. 2001;183:512.
34. Chakvetadze C, Bani-Sadr F, Develoux M, et al. Limb swelling and hypereosinophilia. *Lancet*. 2006;368:1126.
35. Leshem E, Maor Y, Meltzer E, et al. Acute schistosomiasis outbreak: clinical features and economic impact. *Clin Infect Dis*. 2008;47:1499.
36. Clerinx J, Van Gompel A. Schistosomiasis in travellers and migrants. *Travel Med Infect Dis*. 2011;9:6.
37. Coltart CE, Chew A, Storrar N, et al. Schistosomiasis presenting in travellers: a 15 year observational study at the Hospital for Tropical Diseases, London. *Trans R Soc Trop Med Hyg*. 2015;109:214.
38. von Kuster LC, Genta RM. Cutaneous manifestations of strongyloidiasis. *Arch Dermatol*. 1988;124:1826.
39. Basile A, Simzar S, Bentow J, et al. Disseminated *Strongyloides stercoralis* hyperinfection during medical immunosuppression. *J Am Acad Dermatol*. 2010;63:896.
40. Bank DE, Grossman ME, Kohn SR, et al. The thumbprint sign: rapid diagnosis of disseminated strongyloidiasis. *J Am Acad Dermatol*. 1990;23:324.
41. Sato Y, Kobayashi J, Toma H, et al. Efficacy of stool examination for detection of *Strongyloides* infection. *Am J Trop Med Hyg*. 1996;53:248.
42. Loutfy MR, Wilson M, Keystone JS, et al. Serology and eosinophil count in the diagnosis and management of strongyloidiasis in a non-endemic area. *Am J Trop Med Hyg*. 2002;66:749.

Chapter 178 :: Scabies, Other Mites, and Pediculosis
Chikoti M. Wheat, Craig N. Burkhart, Craig G. Burkhart, & Bernard A. Cohen

第一百七十八章
疥疮、其他螨类和虱病

中文导读

本章分3节：①疥疮；②除疥疮外的其他螨类；③虱病。介绍了这些疾病的流行病学、病因和发病机制、临床表现、鉴别诊断、治疗和随访。

第一节疥疮，介绍了其为一个影响各个年龄、种族和社会经济水平的世界性问题。若皮肤瘙痒与皮损分布和流行病史特征相关，均要考虑疥疮的诊断，重要临床特征为夜间剧烈瘙痒，治疗上需要除螨与媒介管理相结合。

第二节介绍了一些可能影响人类的除疥疮外的其他螨类疾病。主要提到人蠕形螨和短蠕形螨是仅有的常规生活在人类身上的螨类；毛囊蠕形螨存在于毛囊中，短蠕形螨存在于皮脂腺的漏斗中，它们的存在可能与玫瑰痤疮、口周皮炎和化脓性毛囊炎有关。屋尘螨是哮喘、过敏性呼吸道症状的常见诱因，特应性皮炎的加重因素。

第三节介绍了虱分类：头虱、体虱和阴虱。头虱病局限于头皮，最容易被发现在枕部和耳后区域。体虱的特点为背部、颈部、肩部和腰部线状抓痕伴瘙痒，衣物内缝可见到虱子。阴虱病需要检查所有有毛发的区域，包括睫毛、眉毛和阴阜区域。

〔粟 娟〕

SCABIES

AT-A-GLANCE

- Human infestation caused by the *Sarcoptes scabiei* var. *hominis* mite that lives its entire life cycle within the epidermis.
- Causes a diffuse, pruritic eruption after an incubation period of 4 to 6 weeks.
- Is transmitted by close physical contact or by fomites.
- Topical therapy with permethrin 5% cream is most effective topical therapy, but oral ivermectin, although off-label, is also effective.
- Because of the common occurrence of asymptomatic mite carriers in the household, all family members and close contacts should be treated simultaneously.

EPIDEMIOLOGY

Scabies is a worldwide issue that affects all ages, races, and socioeconomic levels. Prevalence varies considerably with some underdeveloped countries having rates from 4% to 100% of the general population.[1] In the developing world the populations affected include children, the elderly, and immunosuppressed individuals. An infested host usually harbors between 3 and 50 oviparous female mites,[2] but the number may vary considerably among individuals. For example, patients with crusted, formerly "Norwegian," scabies (Fig. 178-1) who have a defective immunologic or sensory response (ie, leprosy, paraplegic, or HIV-infected patients) harbor millions of mites on their skin surface, with minimal pruritus. Infants and the elderly may not be effective scratchers and harbor intermediate numbers between 50 and 250 mites.

It is well established that close personal contact is a prime route of transmission. Although sometimes considered a sexually transmitted disease, the equally high prevalence in children attests that close nonsexual contact among children and other family members is also sufficient to transmit the infestation. Transmission via inanimate objects has been best demonstrated with crusted scabies but is much less likely to occur in normal hosts. Crusted scabies is notoriously contagious, and anyone roaming within the general vicinity of these patients risks acquiring the infestation. Indeed, 6000 mites/g of debris from sheets, floor, screening curtains, and nearby chairs have been detected.[3] Mites are also prevalent in the personal environment of normal scabies patients.[4,5] In one study, live mites were recovered from dust samples taken from bedroom floors, overstuffed chairs, and couches in every patient's dwelling.[5]

ETIOLOGY AND PATHOGENESIS

Scabies is an infestation by the highly host-specific mite, *Sarcoptes scabiei* var. *homini*, family Sarcoptidae, class Arachnida. The mite is pearl-like, translucent, white, eyeless, and oval in shape with 4 pairs of short stubby legs. The adult female mite is 0.4×0.3 mm with the male being slightly smaller—just slightly too small to be seen by the naked eye. The scabies mite is able to live for 3 days away from the host in a sterile test tube, and for 7 days if placed in mineral oil mounts.[4,6] Mites cannot fly or jump.

The life cycle of mites is completed entirely on human skin. The female mite, by a combination of chewing and body motions, is able to excavate a sloping burrow of 0.5 to 5 mm/day in the stratum corneum to the boundary of the stratum granulosum.[7,8] Along this path, which can be 1 cm long, she lays anywhere from 0 to 4 eggs a day, or up to 50 eggs during her life span of 30 days. Eggs hatch in 10 to 12 days and larvae leave the burrow to mature on the skin surface. After the larvae molt, they become nymphs which can only survive 2 to 5 days off host. The male mite lives on the surface of the skin and enters burrows to procreate.

CLINICAL FINDINGS

The diagnosis of scabies is suspected by pruritus associated with a characteristic distribution of lesions and epidemiologic history. Onset is typically insidious, with the patient complaining of intense nocturnal pruritus. Pruritus typically appears 4 to 6 weeks after initial infestation, although many patients may not develop symptoms for 3 months and some patients are never sensitized. With subsequent reinfestations, symptoms develop within 2 to 3 days.[9] Similar to the human response to other insects such as fleas, yellow jackets, and mosquitoes, there is a wide range of clinical responses to an infestation with scabies and some individuals remain asymptomatic despite being infested. These individuals are considered "carriers."

On physical examination, patients display excoriations and eczematous dermatitis that favors the interdigital webs (see Fig. 178-1), sides of fingers, volar aspects of the wrists and lateral palms (Fig. 178-2), elbows, axillae, scrotum, penis (Fig. 178-3), labia, and areolae in women. The head and neck are usually spared in healthy adults, but in infants, elderly, and immunocompromised individuals, all skin surfaces are susceptible. Indurated, crusted nodules can be seen in infants and young children on intertriginous areas as well as on the trunk. In crusted scabies (see Fig. 178-1), hyperkeratotic plaques develop diffusely on the palmar and plantar regions, with thickening and dystrophy of the toenails and fingernails. Although, patients with crusted type have an enormous mite burden they have few or no symptoms.

The pathognomonic lesion is a burrow, which is a thin, thread-like, linear, or often J-shaped structure (see Figs. 178-2 and 178-4) 1 to 10 mm in length. It is a tunnel caused by the movement of the mite in the stratum corneum. When present, the burrow is best seen in the interdigital webs and wrists; however, it can be difficult to find in early stages of the condition, or after the patient has extensively excoriated the lesions. In infants and young children who are less-effective scratchers, burrows can be identified on palms and soles as well as intertriginous areas and the trunk. Identification of a burrow can be facilitated by rubbing a black felt-tip marker across an affected area. After the excess ink is wiped away with an alcohol pad, the burrow appears darker than the surrounding skin because of ink accumulation in the burrow.

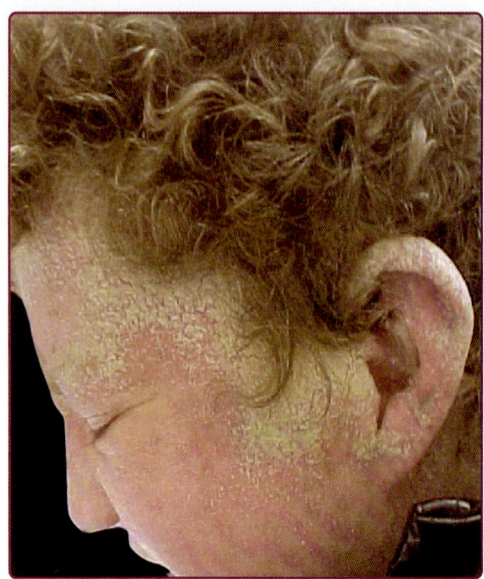

Figure 178-1 Crusted scabies. Hyperkeratotic plaques populated with thousands of mites.

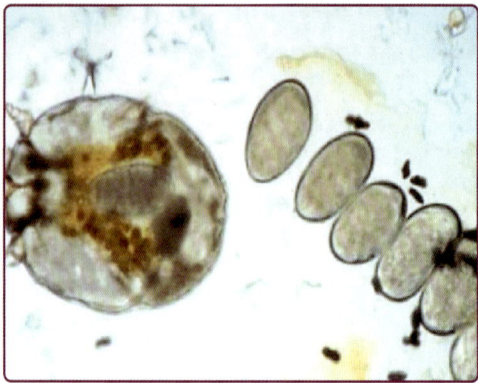

Figure 178-3 Scabies. Microscopic examination of a mineral oil preparation after scraping a burrow reveals a gravid female mite with oval, gray eggs and fecal pellets.

A definitive diagnosis is made by microscopic identification of the scabies mites, eggs, or fecal pellets (scybala). This is accomplished by placing a drop of mineral oil over a burrow and then scraping longitudinally with a number 15 scalpel blade along the length of the burrow or a suspicious skin area, being careful not to cause bleeding. Scrapings are best taken from a burrow, papule, or vesicle that is not excoriated. The scrapings are then applied to a glass slide and examined under low power (see Fig. 178-3). Confocal microscopy and dermoscopy also can be used to examine the mite in vivo.[10,11] The classic dermoscopic finding is the "delta-wing jet" sign of dense scabies head parts and body, eggs, and a burrow (see Fig. 178-4). A skin biopsy can be diagnostic, if the mite happens to be transected in the stratum corneum (Fig. 178-5).

An enzyme-linked immunosorbent assay has been developed for serologic testing of other mite infestations in animals; however, no serologic tests for scabies exist for humans.[12] Despite the possibility of confirming the presence of mites via multiple methods of testing, the diagnosis usually is based on clinical impression, and solidified by response to treatment.

DIFFERENTIAL DIAGNOSIS

Table 178-1 outlines the differential diagnosis of scabies.

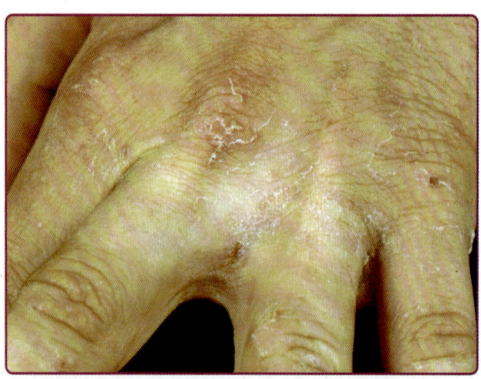

Figure 178-2 Scabies. Several thread-like burrows are present in the web spaces of the fingers and on the knuckles, a common location for these lesions in scabies. Longitudinal scraping of a burrow will often reveal the mite or mite products under microscopic examination.

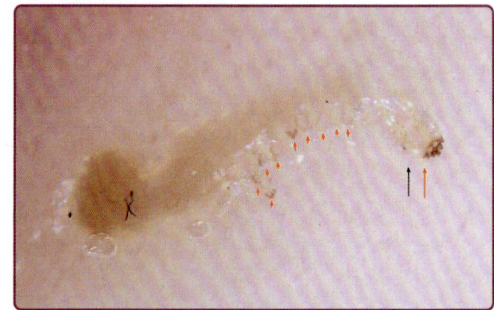

Figure 178-4 A dermoscopic image of triangle or "delta-wing jet" sign of dense scabies head parts (*long red arrow*), relatively translucent scabies body (*long black arrow*), scabies eggs (*short red arrows*), and classic S-shaped burrow. Heine Delta 20× dermatoscope with Nikon Coolpix 4500 camera. (From Fox G. Diagnosis of scabies by dermoscopy. *BMJ Case Rep*. 2009;2009. Reproduced by permission from BMJ Publishing Group Ltd.)

COMPLICATIONS

Secondary impetiginization may occur and poststreptococcal glomerulonephritis has resulted from scabies-induced pyodermas caused by *Streptococcus pyogenes*. Lymphangitis and septicemia also have been reported in crusted scabies. Finally, scabies infestation can also trigger bullous pemphigoid.[13,14]

TREATMENT

Scabies is treated by a combination of a scabicide and fomite control. With all insecticidal therapies, a second application, usually a week after the initial treatment, is required to reduce the potential for reinfestation from fomites as well as to kill any nymphs that may have hatched after treatment as a result of a semiprotective environment within the egg. All household and close contacts must be simultaneously treated to prevent reinfestation from mildly symptomatic and asymptomatic carriers.

Topical scabicides are applied overnight to the entire skin surface with special attention to finger and toe creases, cleft of the buttocks, belly button, and beneath the fingernails and toenails. In adults, one can exclude treating the scalp and face. Most treated individuals experience relief from symptoms within 3 days, but patients must be informed that even after adequate scabicidal therapy, the rash and pruritus may persist for up to 4 weeks. The itching experienced during this time period is commonly referred to as "postscabetic itch." Patients should be educated that excessive washing of the skin with harsh soaps will aggravate their skin irritation. Instead, oral antihistamines and emollients can be beneficial. Table 178-2 summarizes the treatments for scabies, but a few comments are warranted:

- Lindane has received a "black box" warning as well as restrictive labeling changes from the U.S. Food and Drug Administration (FDA) to greatly restrict its usage.[15,16] Moreover, it is banned in California.[17] A physician should write a prescription for lindane only when cognizant of all the caveats noted by the FDA (see the footnote to Table 178-2).[18]
- There are no documented cases of scabies resistance to permethrin, but tolerance is beginning to develop.[19] Pregnant females, breastfeeding mothers, and children younger than age 2 years should limit their 2 applications (1 week apart) to 2 hours only when using permethrin.
- Crotamiton is considerably less effective than all other options offered.
- Five percent to 10% sulfur is messy, malodorous, tends to stain, and can produce irritant dermatitis, but is inexpensive and may be the only choice in areas of the world in which a lack of funds dictates therapy.[20] The efficacy and toxicity of sulfur has not been critically evaluated in recent years, but many believe that it is the safest choice for neonates and pregnant females.[21]

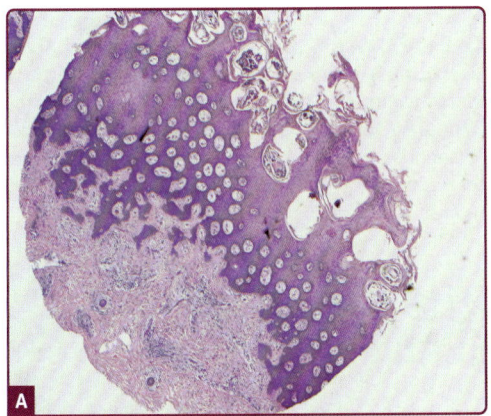
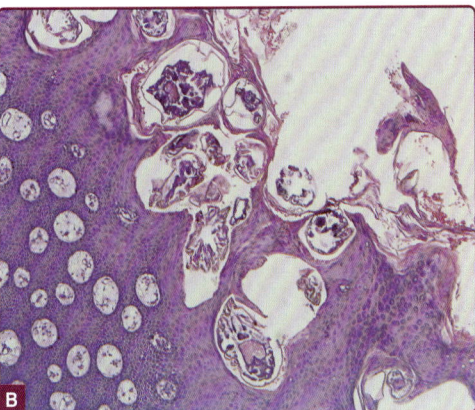

Figure 178-5 A skin biopsy can be diagnostic, if the mite happens to be transected in the stratum corneum. Images show (**A**) ×4 magnification and (**B**) ×10 magnification of scabies mite within the stratum corneum.

TABLE 178-1
Differential Diagnosis of Scabies

Most Likely
- Atopic dermatitis
- Dyshidrotic eczema
- Pyoderma
- Contact dermatitis
- Insect bite reaction
- Id reaction
- Varicella
- Miliaria

Consider
- Dermatitis herpetiformis
- Psoriasis
- Bullous pemphigoid
- Linear immunoglobulin A bullous dermatosis
- Drug eruption
- Systemic causes of pruritus
- Delusions of parasitosis

TABLE 178-2
Treatment of Scabies

DRUG	DOSE	COMMENTS
Permethrin 5% cream	Apply to entire body (neck down) for 8 to 14 hours then wash off, repeat in 7 days; if crusted scabies use daily for 7 days then twice weekly until cured	Most common treatment presently; pregnancy category B, tolerance seems to be developing
Lindane 1% lotion	Apply for 8 hours, repeat in 7 days	U.S. Food and Drug Administration "black box" warning now in effect[a]; banned in California
Crotamiton 10% cream	Apply for 8 hours on days 1, 2, 3, and 8	Has antipruritic qualities; effectiveness is marginal
Precipitated sulfur 5% to 10%	Apply for 8 hours on days 1, 2, and 3	Considered safe in neonates and during pregnancy; limited efficacy data; inexpensive
Benzyl benzoate 10% lotion	Apply for 24 hours	Not available in United States
Ivermectin 200 μg/kg	Taken orally on days 1 and 8; if crusted scabies take on days 1, 2, 8, 9, and 15	Highly effective with good safety profile; not recommended for children who weigh less than 15 kg (33 lb) or for pregnant or lactating women; wash sheets and clothing at 60°C (140°F) and dry in a hot dryer; items that cannot be placed in a washer can be placed in a sealed plastic bag in a warm area for 2 weeks

[a]"Black box" warning warns against usage in premature infants and individuals with known uncontrolled seizure disorders, as well as cautious usage in infants, children, and the elderly including people who weigh less than 50 kg (110 pounds) and over 65 years old may be at risk of serious neurotoxicity.

Ivermectin is an anthelmintic agent derived from a class of compounds known as avermectins. It has been used in veterinary medicine since 1981, and has excellent antiparasitic properties.[22-24] Ivermectin has been approved since 1996 by the FDA for treatment of 2 diseases, namely onchocerciasis and strongyloides. Clinical efficacy for scabies has been impressive at a dosage of 200 μg/kg given twice 1 week apart.[25,26] Given that millions of people have been treated for onchocerciasis worldwide without significant side effects including pregnant women, it appears to be extremely safe. Nevertheless, because the drug acts on nerve synapses that utilize glutamate or γ-aminobutyric acid, and because the blood–brain barrier is not fully developed in young children, it is not recommended for use in children who weigh less than 15 kg (33 lbs) or in pregnant or lactating women. Success rates approach 100% in studies where entire households and close contacts of infested individuals are treated while maintaining strict fomite controls.[24,27]

In crusted scabies, the combination of oral ivermectin and a topical scabicide is recommended as the oral medication will not penetrate into the thickness of the keratinous debris under the nails.

PREVENTION

Several measures should be considered to reduce the potential of reinfestation by fomite transmission. Because of the common occurrence of asymptomatic mite carriers in the household, all family members and close contacts should be treated simultaneously. After treatment, treated individuals should wear clean clothing, and all clothing, pillow cases, towels and bedding used during the previous week should be washed in hot water and dried at high heat. Nonwashables should be dry-cleaned, ironed, put in the clothes dryer without washing, or stored in a sealed plastic bag in a warm area for 2 weeks. Floors, carpets, upholstery (in both home and car) play areas, and furniture should be carefully vacuumed. Fumigation of living spaces is not recommended. Pets also do not need to be treated because they do not harbor the human scabies mite.

OTHER MITES BESIDES SCABIES

AT-A-GLANCE

- Scabies and *Demodex* live in the skin, most other mites drop off human host after feeding.
- Some species are vectors of human disease.
- Chiggers can cause pruritic vesicular, papular, or granulomatous lesions.

There are 45,000 described species of mites that belong to the subclass Acarina and the class Arachnida. Table 178-3 lists some of the mites that can affect humans. Human infestation by these mites occurs only accidentally (save for *Demodex* species).

Demodex folliculorum hominis and *Demodex brevis* are the only mites that routinely live on humans; *D. folliculorum* resides in the hair follicle and *D. brevis* resides in the infundibulum of the sebaceous gland. Their presence has been linked with rosacea, perioral dermatitis, and suppurative folliculitis; however, a causal role for mites in these diseases has not been established.

Although animal and fowl mites are not primary parasites of humans, *Pyemotes* sp. can cause straw itch, oak leaf eruption, or itch mite eruptions. These mites can cause epidemics of dermatitis with outbreaks in the last decade occurring in several Midwestern States. *Pyemotes ventricosus* and *Pyemotes tritici* occur in animal handlers, farmers participating in harvesting of grain, and those exposed to decorative grain.[28,29] *Pyemotes herfsi*'s normal host is the leaf galls on oak trees, and therefore this eruption characteristically occurs in people who spend time outdoors in or near wooded areas. Typical bites appear on exposed skin as red macules with a small blister center 10 to 16 hours after contact.

Harvest mites (also called berry bugs, red bugs, scrub-itch mites, and chiggers) are in the family Trombiculidae and are distributed worldwide.[30] In the United States, they inhabit mostly the southeast, south, and midwest, in areas of grasslands and forest, and damp areas along lakes and streams. Humans are susceptible to the larvae from April until the first frost. The minute, reddish larvae of *Trombicula* are less than 0.5 mm long and feed on skin cells of animals, including humans. Rather than sucking blood, these mites inject digestive enzymes into the skin breaking down cells, which can subsequently cause severe reactions and swelling. Each bite has a characteristic red papule with a white, hard central area. After feeding, they drop off their hosts and mature into adults, which are harmless to humans. Rarely does a victim realize when the bite is occurring, as itching from a chigger bite does not develop until 1 to 2 days after the bite. Chiggers prefer warm, covered areas of the body, and thus the bites are often clustered behind the knees, or beneath tight undergarments such as socks, underwear, and brassieres.

The house dust mite is a cosmopolitan guest in human habitation and feeds off flakes of shed human skin. The mites are harmless, but their bodies and excreta are believed to play a role in human disease. They are a common precipitant of asthma, hay fever, and allergic respiratory symptoms worldwide. In addition, atopic dermatitis may be exacerbated in some patients by dust mite allergens.[31,32]

PEDICULOSIS

Pediculosis, the infestation of humans by lice, has been a human affliction since antiquity. Three species of lice infest humans: (a) *Pediculus humanus capitis*, the head louse, (b) *Pediculus humanus humanus*, the body or clothing louse, and (c) *Phthirus pubis*, the pubic, or crab, louse. Patients present with pruritus secondary to a delayed hypersensitivity reaction. After the initial exposure, it may take 2 to 6 weeks for the pruritus to occur. Subsequent exposure results in symptoms within 1 to 2 days of exposure.[33]

PEDICULOSIS CAPITIS (HEAD LICE)

AT-A-GLANCE

- Infestation occurs worldwide affecting hairs of the scalp most commonly in children between the ages of 3 and 12 years.
- Presence of 0.8-mm eggs (nits) firmly attached to scalp hairs is most common sign of infestation.
- Spread by close physical contact and sharing of headgear, combs, brushes, and pillows.
- Resistance to traditional nonprescription preparations is growing; topical malathion and ivermectin should be considered in resistant cases.

EPIDEMIOLOGY

Head lice infestations occur worldwide and are most common in children between the ages of 3 and 12 years.[34] Based on pediculicide sales in the United States, an estimated 10 to 12 million children are

TABLE 178-3
Mites Other Than Scabies

TYPE OF MITE	SCIENTIFIC NAME	CLINICAL FEATURES/DISEASE ASSOCIATION
Follicle	*Demodex folliculorum hominis* and *Demodex brevis*	Associated with rosacea, idiopathic facial burning
Fowl	*Dermanyssus gallinae* and *Demodex avium*	Pruritic papules, sometimes with a hemorrhagic center
Straw itch	*Pyemotes tritici, Pyemotes ventricosus,* and *Pyemotes herfsi*	Patchy dermatitis on trunk and arms during and after harvesting
Harvest or red (chiggers)	Genus *Trombicula*: *Eurotrombicula alfreddugesi* and *Eurotrombicula splendens*	Scrub typhus vector; papular to vesicular lesions found on ankles, waist, or warm skinfolds; most common in United States
Animal	*Ornithonyssus bacoti, Liponyssoides sanguineus, Cheyletiella* sp. (Cheyletielosis)	Endemic/murine typhus vector; rickettsialpox vector; nonspecific pruritic eruption on body parts in close contact with infested pets
House dust	*Dermatophagoides* sp.	Atopic dermatitis, allergies

infected each year. Head lice affect all levels of society, and all ethnic groups; however, the incidence is low among African Americans in the United States, possibly as a consequence of an anatomic inability of female lice in America to deposit eggs on coarse curly hair.[35] A recent study by Koch and associates showed an increase in trend in the number of prescriptions suggesting either an increase in the number of infestations or increased failure rates of nonprescription home regimens.[36]

Transmission occurs primarily by means of direct head-to-head contact and less commonly by indirect (fomite) transmission through combs, brushes, blow-dryers, hair accessories, upholstery, pillows, bedding, helmets, or other headgear.[37-42] Lice can be dislodged by air movement, blow-dryers, combs, and towels, and passively transferred to fabric, facilitating new infestations.[30-32,34,35]

ETIOLOGY AND PATHOGENESIS

Head lice are blood-sucking, wingless, highly host-specific insects belonging to the order Anoplura. They are almost 2 mm long with 3 pairs of claw-like legs that are well adapted for grasping hair. Their entire life cycle is on the scalp (Fig. 178-6). More than 95% of infested individuals have fewer than 100 adult lice in their scalps. The female louse lays 5 to 10 eggs per day during her 30-day life span. After 10 days, the eggs hatch producing larvae, which are referred to as nymphs or "instars." Instars look like miniature adult louse and go through 3 stages of development that take 14 days for full maturation. The eggs are laid approximately 1 cm from the scalp surface, firmly attached to individual hairs with a proteinaceous glue secreted by the female louse and that closely resembles the amino acid composition of the human hair shaft itself.[43,44]

Lice typically survive less than 2 days away from the scalp, although under favorable conditions of heat and humidity, survival has been reported at 4 days. Nits can survive for 10 days away from the scalp.

CLINICAL FINDINGS

Pediculosis capitis is confined to the scalp with nits (Fig. 178-7) found most readily in the occipital and retroauricular regions. Most patients experience pruritus. The average incubation before symptoms is 4 to 6 weeks. Some individuals remain asymptomatic despite infestation, and can be considered "carriers."

Mite bites may produce 2-mm erythematous macules or papules, but usually an examiner only finds excoriations, erythema, and scaling. Other findings may include a low-grade fever, regional lymphadenopathy, and irritability.

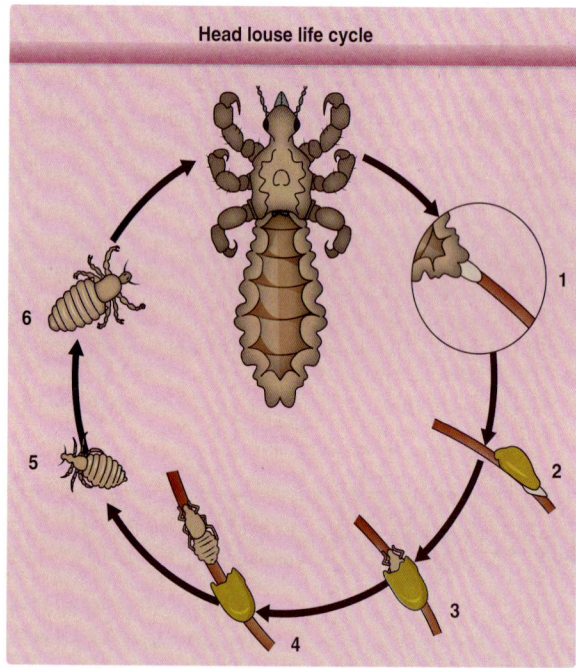

Figure 178-6 Head louse life cycle. During egg laying, the female louse secretes a proteinaceous cement that flows from the genital opening to adhere the egg tightly onto the hair shaft (*1* and *2*). The hatch-ready louse uses its mouthparts to cut a circular hole in the operculum and sucks in air, which is expelled from its posterior, causing it to be quickly ejected from the egg, typically 5 to 10 days after the egg was first laid (*3* and *4*). The emerged instar requires a blood meal soon after hatching, and completes 3 molts, taking a blood meal between each, before developing into an adult 9 to 12 days after hatching (*4*, *5*, and *6*). (Adapted from Figure 1 in Koch E, Clark JM, Cohen B, et al. Management of head louse infestations in the United States—a literature review. *Pediatr Dermatol.* 2016;33:466-472, with permission. Copyright © 2016, John Wiley and Sons.)

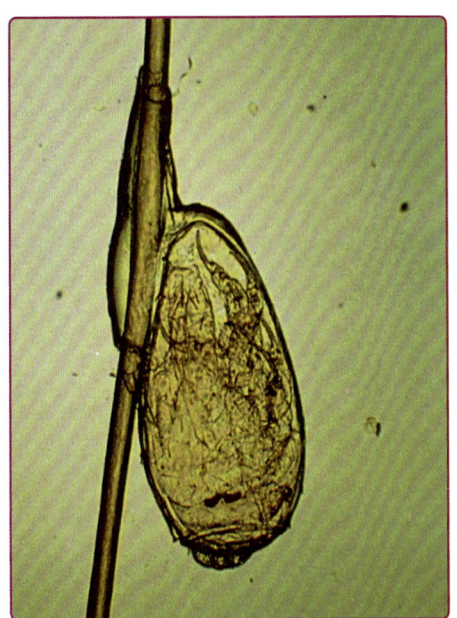

Figure 178-7 Nit sheath. Microscopic view of an egg, containing an unhatched louse, attached to a hair shaft.

Infestations are diagnosed by demonstrating egg capsules (nits) and live lice. Nits are readily seen by the naked eye and are an efficient marker of past or present infestation. They can be differentiated from dandruff, hair casts, and the like, as nits are not easily removed from the hair shaft.[45] The color of newly laid or viable eggs is tan to brown; the remains of eggs that have hatched are clear, white, or light in color. Moreover, newly laid eggs are usually identified within a few millimeters of the scalp and lice embryos can be seen on dermoscopy, while hatched nits are usually further from the scalp. The presence of adult lice confirms active infestation. However, lice are fast, avoid light, and blend in with the hair, making them difficult to find. Finding live adult lice or immature nymphs is best achieved with fine combing the hair with a nit comb. Wet combing, in which water and conditioner are applied to the hair prior to using the nit comb, increases the yield by prying the adult lice from the hair follicles.[44,45]

DIFFERENTIAL DIAGNOSIS

Table 178-4 outlines the differential diagnosis of head lice.

COMPLICATIONS

Although head lice have never been identified as a source of transmission of infection, secondary bacterial infections can occur with pediculosis capitis. In fact, head lice are thought to be the most common cause of pyodermas of the scalp in the developed world.[46]

Head lice and body lice are closely related, so it is not surprising that head lice can serve as host for rickettsiae and have the potential of transmitting diseases.[47,48] Head lice in laboratory experiments have been readily infected with *Rickettsia prowazekii*.[49] *Bartonella quintana*, which causes trench fever, also has been isolated in head lice.[50-53] Transmission of these infections to humans by pediculosus capitis, however, has never been described and it is highly unlikely to occur outside of experimental conditions.

TREATMENT

Standard treatment recommendations for pediculosis capitis utilize a 2-step process of confirming active infestation with live lice and then treating the infestation with a nonprescription or prescription pediculicidal therapy. Pediculicide choice is typically based on local resistance patterns and access of patients to a physician for prescription medications.[54] However, with increasing resistance to pediculicides, a multimodal approach, similar to *Staphylococcus aureus* therapy, is warranted to prevent widespread resistance to currently available products.[55] This is especially important when treating with prescription pediculicides.

Physical methods to treat infestations, including shaving one's head to avoid infestation, dates back to the 6th century BC, when priests and wealthy Egyptians removed scalp hair and wore wigs. The routine of head shaving for military services today was founded on the same principle. While a buzz haircut may be a solution for boys, such an approach would be traumatic psychologically for girls. Another method is to comb the nits out after application of a hair moisturizer such as Cetaphil. The moisturizer is applied, left in for 2 minutes, then all the lotion is combed out. The hair is then dried with a hair dryer. This can be done every few days, with the best results showing cure rates of 95% if done over a 24-day period.[56] However, combing out nits is difficult, tedious, time-consuming, and somewhat painful. Although wet combing can be an adjuvant to topical insecticidal therapy, it is not, by itself, sufficient in most situations.[47]

Pediculicides remain the most effective treatment for head lice.[57-64] Given (a) variable ovicidal activity,

TABLE 178-4
Differential Diagnosis of Head Lice

- Seborrheic dermatitis (dandruff)
- Insect bites
- Eczema
- Psoriasis
- Hair gel hair spray
- Piedra (a fungal infection)
- Pseudonits (desquamated epithelial cells with sebaceous plugs encircling the hair)
- Delusions of parasitosis

(b) possible lack of patient compliance, (c) growing resistance to pediculicides, and (d) the potential of fomite reinfestation, it is recommended to repeat treatment with all insecticidal treatments in 1 week.

Table 178-5 summarizes the array of treatments for head lice. One of the leading factors for the increasing number of infestations is resistance of lice to topical therapies.[65-70] Since the introduction of insecticides years ago, the louse has adapted by several genetic alterations. The agents with the highest success rates, namely malathion and ivermectin, are prescription products. One trial has shown oral ivermectin given twice at a 7-day interval to be more effective than topical malathion lotion.[71] However, both pediculicides are highly effective and treatment decisions should be based on local resistance patterns and individual patient characteristics.

There are a number of anecdotal and market-driven reports with occlusive and suffocation methods (such as with application of petrolatum, mayonnaise, dimethicone, vegetable oil, mineral oil, hair pomade, and olive oil).[72,73] However, there are no studies establishing the safety and efficacy.[36] To accurately evaluate pediculicidal activity of any compound, one must appreciate that head lice have the ability to "resurrect" from a state of seeming death, in which respiratory and motor function appear to have ceased.[74,75] These insects are less dependent than mammals for continuous nervous control of respiration and circulation, and the exact point of death is not readily defined. Indeed, the World Health Organization recommends pediculicidal testing to be read 24 hours after application of insecticide because doing otherwise results in overestimation of mortality rates.[52] Not following these guidelines has led to overestimates of the efficacy of several alternative treatments with occlusive agents and essential oils from health food stores. Such products slow the movements of adult lice and may allow them to be more easily combed out of the scalp, but these substances are usually not lethal to lice.

Patients should be counseled in at least some effective measures to prevent reinfestation by fomite transmission. After treatment, treated individuals should wear clean clothing, and all clothing, hats, pillow cases, towels, and bedding used during the previous week should be washed in hot water and dried at high heat. Nonwashables should be dry-cleaned, ironed, put in the clothes dryer without washing, or stored in a sealed plastic bag in a warm area for 2 weeks. Combs and brushes may be washed in very hot water (65°C [149°F]) or may be coated with the pediculicide for 15 minutes. Floors, carpets, upholstery (in both

TABLE 178-5
Treatment of Head Lice and Crab Lice

	ADMINISTRATION	RISK FACTORS
Pyrethrins synergized (RID, Pronto, etc.)[a]	Topically for 10 minutes[b]	Allergy to chrysanthemums, ragweed, or related plants; increased resistance with steep decline in effectiveness
Permethrin 1%[a] lotion (Nix)	Topically to damp hair for 10 minutes, rinse then repeat in 7 days[b]	First-choice treatment except in places with known resistance; approved for patients older than age 2 months
Permethrin 5% cream	Topically overnight[b]	None; if used for "resistant" head lice, no evidence that it is more effective than permethrin 1% lotion
Malathion 0.5% (Ovide) shampoo	Topically to dry hair and leave on for 8 to 12 hours allowing to dry naturally; then shampoo and use a lice comb	High flammability so avoid hair dryer or open flame while wet; burning/stinging at sites of eroded skin; approved for patients older than age 6 years
Carbaryl 0.5%	Topically overnight	Not available in United States
Lindane 1%	Topically for 4 minutes[b]	U.S. Food and Drug Administration (FDA) "black box" warning now in effect[c]; banned in California
Benzyl alcohol 5% lotion	Topically to dry hair for 10 minutes, rinse then repeat in 7 days	Dosed by hair length so can be costly; can be used in pregnant and lactating women; approved for children older than age 6 months; minor side effects
Topical ivermectin 0.5% lotion	Topically to hair once although most experts recommend reapplication a week later	Approved for patients older than age 6 months
Ivermectin (Stromectol), oral 200 µg/kg	Orally on days 1, 8, and 15	Very good efficacy on adult lice although inferior to permethrin; not ovicidal, hence nits are safe until they hatch; not recommended for pregnant females or children weighing less than 15 kg (33 lbs); not FDA approved for pediculosis
Spinosad 0.9% suspension	Topically to dry hair for 10 minutes then rinse; repeat in 7 days	Do not use in infants younger than age 6 months because of benzyl alcohol content; minor side effects

[a]Available in nonprescription form.
[b]Apply to dry scalp and hair followed by adequate washing out with nonmedicated shampoo (head lice).
[c]See footnote to Table 178-2. "Black box" warning: Lindane is still available for patients weighing more than 50 kg (110 lbs) and younger than age 65 years, but is cautioned against use because of neurotoxicity.

home and car), play areas, and furniture should be carefully vacuumed to remove any hairs with viable eggs attached. Fumigation of living spaces is not recommended and pets do not need to be treated because they do not harbor the human head louse. Despite treatment, nits can remain on the hair for months. Therefore a strict "no nit" policy will only result in significant absence from school.[76] As a result, the American Academy of Pediatrics does not recommend a "no nit" policy.

PEDICULOSIS CORPORIS (BODY LICE)

AT-A-GLANCE

- Infestations most commonly found in homeless individuals, refugees, and victims of war and natural disasters.
- Diagnosis made by presence of nits in lining of clothing, particularly the seams.
- Infections transmitted by body lice include epidemic typhus, trench fever, and relapsing fever.

ETIOLOGY AND PATHOGENESIS

P. humanus humanus, body lice, have a very similar morphology to head lice, except they are 30% larger. The body louse's life span is 20 days during which the female may lay up to 300 eggs. The lice lay their eggs in the seams of clothing, while obtaining their blood meals from the host. The body louse can survive without a blood meal for up to 3 days.

EPIDEMIOLOGY

Pediculosis corporis requires exposure to the louse and favors an inability to wash and change clothing. Consequently, it is most commonly found on homeless individuals, refugees, victims of war and natural disasters, or those forced into crowded living conditions with poor hygiene. The infestation is usually transmitted by contaminated clothing or bedding. After exposure, the inability to wash or change clothes allows the infestation to persist.

CLINICAL FINDINGS

Symptomatically, patients complain of pruritus. Most commonly, the only sign of body lice is excoriations, often linear and primarily on the back, neck, shoulders, and waist. Postinflammatory pigmentation is seen in chronic cases. Adult lice are not easily seen except in heavy infestations. Diagnosis is made by closely examining the lining of the clothing, particularly at the seams, for the presence of nits. The clothing also may be shaken over a sheet of white paper, at which time the lice may be seen moving about on the paper.

DIFFERENTIAL DIAGNOSIS

Table 178-6 outlines the differential diagnosis of body lice.

COMPLICATIONS

Several important human diseases are transmitted by the body louse. The major diseases include epidemic typhus (caused by a rickettsiae, *R. prowazekii*), murine typhus (caused by *Rickettsia typhi*), trench fever (caused by *B. quintana*), and relapsing fever (caused by a spirochete, *Borrelia recurrentis*).[77-81] Lice obtain organisms, such as rickettsiae and spirochetes, from ingestion of blood meals from infested hosts. Transmission of microorganisms from body lice is not from the louse bite, but rather by (a) contaminated fecal material being scratched into excoriated skin of bite sites, (b) inhalation of dry, powdery louse feces from handling typhus-contaminated bedding or clothing, or (c) an infected louse having its gut ruptured, allowing an infective blood meal to enter excoriations on the skin. In addition, excoriation can lead to secondary infection with *S. aureus*, *S. pyogenes*, and other bacteria.

TREATMENT

The most important treatment for body lice is disinfestation of all clothing and bedding. Beds should be burned or sprayed with lice sprays, because the body louse may lay eggs on the seams of the mattress or couch. Clothing is best treated like biohazardous waste, bagged, and tightly sealed in specially marked, plastic, biohazard bags. The waste is handled separately from other trash until it can be incinerated, maintaining a temperature of 65°C (149°F) for 30 minutes. If this is not possible, clothing and bedding should be fumigated, machine washed in hot water, and dried on high heat or dry-cleaned. Hot ironing of the seams of upholstered furniture should also be performed and exposure to infested items should

TABLE 178-6
Differential Diagnosis of Body Lice

- Scabies
- Atopic dermatitis
- Contact dermatitis
- Drug reaction
- Viral exanthem
- Other animal parasites
- Systemic causes of pruritus
- Delusions of parasitosis

be strictly avoided for 2 weeks. The patient should be treated from head to toe with a topical insecticide or given oral ivermectin.

PEDICULOSIS PUBIS (CRAB LICE)

AT-A-GLANCE

- Best to call "crab lice" (rather than "pubic lice") as infestations may involve other hair-bearing sites such as mustache, beard, axillae, eyelashes, eyebrows, and scalp hair.
- Transmitted by sexual or close contact, as well as via fomites (contaminated clothing, towels, and bedding).
- Topical therapy options similar to pediculosis capitis, but oral ivermectin is the preferred treatment for this infestation.

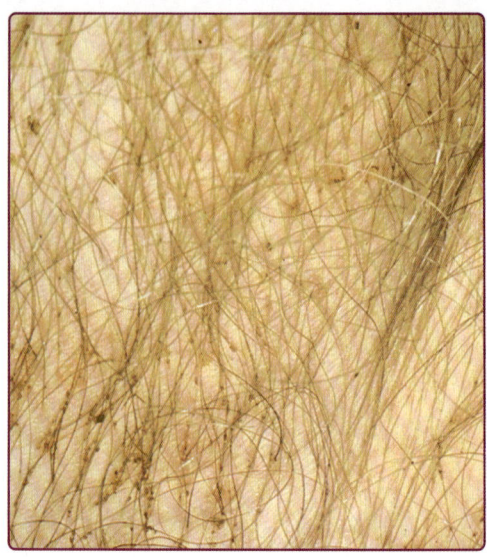

Figure 178-8 Pediculosis pubis. Several lice and their dot-like nits attached to the hair shafts can be seen in the pubic area of this patient. (Used with permission from D.A. Burns, MD.)

ETIOLOGY AND PATHOGENESIS

Pediculosis pubis is caused by infestation of the body with *P. pubis*. Crab lice range from 0.8 to 1.2 mm in length and have wide, short bodies resembling tiny crabs. They have a serrated edge on their first claw, which gives them traction on flat, hairless, surfaces; thus, they can navigate across the entire body surface. They most commonly are found in the pubic and perianal region, but occasionally they also reside in mustache, beard, axillae, eyelashes, eyebrows, and scalp hair. In hirsute individuals, they are also found on the short hairs of the thighs and trunk. The louse has a life span of less than 3 weeks, during which time the female will lay approximately 25 eggs on human hairs. The adult crab louse can survive for 36 hours off the human host, and the eggs are viable for up to 10 days.

EPIDEMIOLOGY

Crab lice can be found in all levels of society and all ethnic groups. Patients with crab lice often have another concurrent sexually transmitted disease. Although pediculosis pubis is considered a sexually transmitted disease, transmission has been documented to occur from contaminated clothing, towels, and bedding.

CLINICAL FINDINGS

In the case of crab lice, all hairy parts of the body should be examined, especially the eyelashes, eyebrows, and perianal area. Many individuals have 2 different hair-bearing sites infested.[82] These lice can be mistaken for scabs or moles, or can blend in with skin color, making them difficult to detect. Infested patients have an average of 10 to 25 adult organisms on their body. Nits also can be identified near the base of hairs (Fig. 178-8). The diagnosis can be confirmed by microscopic examination of the plucked hair to identify the nits and/or adult lice. Although rare, skin lesions named maculae caerulea, representing hemorrhage, can be seen with pubic lice, with slate gray to bluish, irregular-shaped macules approximately 1 cm in diameter. Pediculosis palpebrarum, or phthiriasis palpebrarum, is the infestation of the eyelashes with crab lice.

DIFFERENTIAL DIAGNOSIS

Table 178-7 outlines the differential diagnosis of crab lice.

TREATMENT

Shaving is not curative as the louse will seek another hairy area of the body to reside. Crab lice are treated with the same topical therapy as that for pediculosis

TABLE 178-7
Differential Diagnosis of Crab Lice

- Excoriations
- Scabies
- Contact dermatitis
- Piedra
- Trichomycosis pubis
- Hair casts
- Nevi

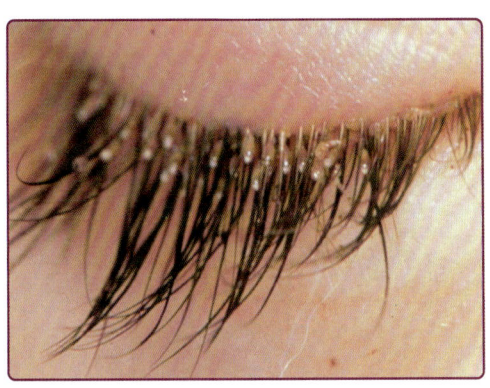

Figure 178-9 Pediculosis pubis. Eyelash infestation with *Pthirus pubis*. Nits can be seen attached to the eyelashes. (Used with permission from D.A. Burns, MD.)

capitis (see Table 178-5).[83] In vitro and in vivo resistance to pyrethrins have been shown.[84] There is a lack of appreciation for their tendency to inhabit rectal hair.[82] Unless the physician is certain that only one body area is involved, all hairy areas of the body should be treated because (a) it is not uncommon to have other areas infested, and (b) lice can migrate away from a treated areas to other hair-bearing locations. For this reason, oral ivermectin is recommended for this entity.[52] However, as ivermectin treatment relies on the insect obtaining a blood meal, so the nits are not affected and the patient requires repeat oral ivermectin on day 8 and day 15.

Phthiriasis palpebrarum (Fig. 178-9) has traditionally been treated with petrolatum (Vaseline), but this treatment is slow and needs to be applied at least 5 times a day for weeks. Ivermectin is the first-line therapy for this condition.[85]

Fomite precautions mirror those discussed previously for pediculosis capitis. Treatment failure is usually a result of failure to treat all hairy areas (especially perirectally) or reinfestation from neglecting to treat sexual contacts. Other household members are also infested occasionally and should be carefully questioned for symptoms and/or examined.

REFERENCES

1. Burkhart CG. Scabies: an epidemiologic reassessment. *Ann Intern Med*. 1983;98:498-503.
2. Mellanby K. *Scabies*. 2nd ed. Hampton, England: E.W. Classey Ltd; 1972.
3. Carslaw RW, Dobson RM, Hood AJ. Mites in the environment of cases of Norwegian scabies. *Br J Dermatol*. 1975;92:333-337.
4. Estes SA, Arlian L. Survival of *Sarcoptes scabiei*. *J Am Acad Dermatol*. 1981;5:343-345.
5. Arlian LG, Estes SA, Vyszenski-Moher DL. Prevalence of *Sarcoptes scabiei* in the environment of scabietic patients. *J Am Acad Dermatol*. 1988;1:806-811.
6. Arlian LG, Runyan RA, Achar S. Survival and infectivity of *Sarcoptes scabiei* var. *canis* and var. *hominis*. *J Am Acad Dermatol*. 1984;11:210-215.
7. Burgess I. *Sarcoptes scabiei* and scabies. *Adv Parasitol*. 1994;33:235-293.
8. Fimiani M, Mazzatenta C, Alessandrini C, et al. The behaviour of Sarcoptes scabiei var. hominis in human skin: an ultrastructural study. *J Submicrosc Cytol Pathol*. 1997;29(1):105-113.
9. Bergström FC, Reynolds S, Johnstone M, et al. Scabies mite inactivated serine protease paralogs inhibit the human complement system. *J Immunol*. 2009;182:7809-7817.
10. Prins C, Stucki L, French L. Dermoscopy for the in vivo detection of *Sarcoptes scabiei*. *Dermatology*. 2004;208:241-243.
11. Argenziano G, Fabbrocini G, Delfino M. Epiluminescence microscopy. A new approach to in vivo detection of *Sarcoptes scabiei*. *Arch Dermatol*. 1997;133:751-753.
12. van der Heijden HM, Rambags PG, Elbers AR. Validation of ELISAs for the detection of antibodies to *Sarcoptes scabiei* in pigs. *Vet Parasitol*. 2000;89:95-107.
13. Chung SD, Lin HC, Wang KH. Increased risk of pemphigoid following scabies: a population-based matched-cohort study. *J Eur Acad Dermatol Venereol*. 2014;28:558-564.
14. Bornhövd E, Partscht K, Flaig MJ, et al. Bullous scabies and scabies triggered bullous pemphigoid [in German]. *Hautarzt*. 2001;52:56-61.
15. Labeling changes for Lindane. *FDA Consum*. 2003;37:6.
16. Center for Drug Evaluation and Research. *FDA Public Health Advisory. Safety of Topical Lindane Products for the Treatment of Scabies and Lice*. http://www.fda.gov/cder/drug/infopage/lindane/default.htm. Accessed Jun 5, 2003.
17. California Department of Health Services. State Health Director Offers Tips for Protecting Children From Head Lice. Sacramento, CA: California Department of Health Services; October 10, 2000. News Release No. 54-00.
18. Burkhart CG, Burkhart CN. Safety and efficacy of pediculicides for head lice. *Expert Opin Drug Saf*. 2006;5:169-176.
19. Pasay C, Arlian L, Morgan M, et al. The effect of insecticide synergists on the response of scabies mites to pyrethroid acaricides. *PLoS Negl Trop Dis*. 2009;3:e354.
20. Pruksachatkunakorn C, Damrongsak M, Sinthupuan S. Sulfur for scabies outbreaks in orphanages. *Pediatr Dermatol*. 2002;19:448-453.
21. Diaz M, Cazorla D, Acosta M. Efficacy, safety, and acceptability of precipitated sulphur petrolatum for topical treatment of scabies at the city of Coro, Falcon State, Venezuela. *Rev Invest Clin*. 2004;56:615-622.
22. Pulliam JD, Preston JM. Safety of ivermectin in target animals. In: Campbell WC, ed. *Ivermectin and Abamectin*. New York, NY: Springer-Verlag; 1989:149-161.
23. Benz GW, Roncalli RA, Gross SJ. Use of ivermectin in cattle, sheep, goats, and swine. In: Campbell WC, ed. *Ivermectin and Abamectin*. New York, NY: Springer-Verlag; 1989:215-229.
24. Burkhart CN. Ivermectin: an assessment of its pharmacology, microbiology, and safety. *Vet Hum Toxicol*. 2000;42:30-35.
25. Meinking TL, Taplin D, Hermida JL. The treatment of scabies with ivermectin. *N Engl J Med*. 1996;333:26-30.
26. Aubin F, Humbert P. Ivermectin for crusted (Norwegian) scabies. *N Engl J Med*. 1995;332:1995.

27. Marty P, Gari-Toussaint M, LeFichoux Y. Efficacy of ivermectin in the treatment of an epidemic of *Sarcoptes scabiei*. *Ann Trop Med Parasitol*. 1994;88:433.
28. Grob M, Dorn K, Lautenschlager S. Grain mites: a small epidemic caused by *Pyemotes* species [in German]. *Hautarzt*. 1998;49:838-843.
29. Kunkle GA, Greiner EC. Dermatitis in horses and man caused by the straw itch mite. *J Am Vet Med Assoc*. 1982;181:467-469.
30. Elston DM. What's eating you? Chiggers. *Cutis*. 2006;77:350-352.
31. Jeong SK, Kim HJ, Youm JK. Mite and cockroach allergens activate protease-activated receptor 2 and delay epidermal permeability barrier recovery. *J Invest Dermatol*. 2008;128:1930-1939.
32. Bussmann C, Böckenhoff A, Henke H, et al. Does allergen-specific immunotherapy represent a therapeutic option for patients with atopic dermatitis? *J Allergy Clin Immunol*. 2006;118:1292-1298.
33. Gunning K, Pippitt K, Kiraly B, et al. Pediculosis and scabies: treatment update. *Am Fam Physician*. 2012;15;86(6):535-541.
34. Mumcuoglu KY, Klaus S, Kafka D. Clinical observation related to head lice infestation. *J Am Acad Dermatol*. 1991;25:248-251.
35. Carter D. *Insect egg glue* [doctoral thesis]. Cambridge, UK: Department of Applied Biology, Cambridge University; 1990.
36. Koch E, Clark JM, Cohen B, et al. Management of head louse infestations in the United States—a literature review. *Pediatr Dermatol*. 2016;33(5):466-472.
37. Burkhart CN. Fomite transmission with head lice: a continuing controversy. *Lancet*. 2003;361:99-100.
38. Takano-Lee M, Edman JD, Mullens BA, et al. Transmission potential of the human head louse, *Pediculus capitis* (Anoplura: Pediculidae). *Int J Dermatol*. 2005;44:811-816.
39. Burkhart CN, Burkhart CG. Fomite transmission in head lice. *J Am Acad Dermatol*. 2007;56:1044-1047.
40. Burgess IF. Human lice and their management. *Adv Parasitol*. 1995;36:271-342.
41. Mauder JW. An update on head lice. *Health Visit*. 1993;66:317-318.
42. Speare R, Cahill C, Thomas G. Head lice on pillows, and strategies to make a small risk even less. *Int J Dermatol*. 2003;42:626-629.
43. Burkhart CN, Stankiewicz BA, Pchalek I, et al. Molecular composition of the louse sheath. *J Parasitol*. 1999;85:559-561.
44. Burkhart CN. *Nit Sheath and Bacterial Symbiotes of the Human Head Louse (Pediculus Humanus Capitis)* [master's thesis]. Toledo, OH: Medical College of Ohio; 2003.
45. Burkhart CN, Burkhart CG, Pchalak I. The adherent cylindrical nit structure and its chemical denaturation in vitro: an assessment with therapeutic implication for head lice. *Arch Pediatr Adolesc Med*. 1998;1152:711-712.
46. Dodd C. Treatment of head lice: choice of treatment will depend on local patterns of resistance. *BMJ*. 2001;323(7321):1084.
47. Roberts RJ, Casey D, Morgan DA, et al. Comparison of wet combing with malathion for treatment of head lice in the UK: a pragmatic randomized controlled trial. *Lancet*. 2000;356:540-544.
48. Jahnke C, Bauer E, Hengge UR, et al. Accuracy of diagnosis of pediculosis capitis: visual inspection vs wet combing. *Arch Dermatol*. 2009;145:309-313.
49. Fournier A. Human pathogens in body and head lice. *Emerg Infect Dis*. 2002;8:1515-1518.
50. Robinson B. Potential role of head lice, *Pediculus humanus capitis*, as vectors of *Rickettsia prowazekii*. *Parasitol Res*. 2003;90:209-211.
51. Weyer KF. Biological relationships between lice and microbial agents. *Annu Rev Entomol*. 1960;5:405-420.
52. World Health Organization. *Instructions for Determining the Susceptibility or Resistance of Body Lice and Head Lice to Insecticides*. Geneva, Switzerland: WHO;1981. Available at http://apps.who.int/iris/bitstream/handle/10665/70733/WHO_VBC_81.808_eng.pdf?sequence=1&isAllowed=y
53. Sasaki T, Poudel SK, Isawa H, et al. First molecular evidence of *Bartonella quintana* in *Pediculus humanus capitis* (Phthiraptera: Pediculidae) collected from Nepalese children. *J Med Entomol*. 2006;43:110-112.
54. Frankowski BL, Weiner LB; Committee on School Health the Committee on Infectious Diseases, American Academy of Pediatrics. Head lice. *Pediatrics*. 2002;110(3):638-643.
55. Grayson ML. The treatment triangle for staphylococcal infections. *N Engl J Med*. 2006;355(7):724-727.
56. Tebrueggge M, Runnuacles J. Is wet combing effective in children with pediculosis capitis infestation? *Arch Dis Child*. 2007;92(9):818-820.
57. Meinking TL, Serrano L, Hard B, et al. Comparative in vitro pediculicidal efficacy of treatments in a resistant head lice population in the United States. *Arch Dermatol*. 2002;138:220-224.
58. Meinking TL, Taplin D, Kalter DC, et al. Comparative efficacy of treatments for pediculosis capitis infestations. *Arch Dermatol*. 1986;122:267-271.
59. Meinking TL, Entzel P, Villar ME, et al. Comparative efficacy of treatments for pediculosis capitis infestations: update 2000. *Arch Dermatol*. 2001;137(3):287-292.
60. Downs AM, Stafford KA, Hunt LP, et al. Widespread insecticide resistance in head lice to over-the-counter pediculocides in England, and the emergence of carbaryl resistance. *Br J Dermatol*. 2002;146:88-89.
61. Burkhart CN, Burkhart CG. Topical pyrethroids: assessment of function and efficacy in head lice. *Int J Pediatr*. 2002;17:209-212.
62. Chosidow O, Chastang C, Brue C. Controlled study of malathion and d-phenothrin lotions for *Pediculus humanus* var *capitis*-infested school children. *Lancet*. 1994;344:1724-1727.
63. Meinking TL, Serrano L, Hard B. Comparative in vitro pediculocidal efficacy of treatments in a resistant head lice population. *Arch Dermatol*. 2002;138:220-224.
64. Meinking TL, Vicaria M, Eyerdam DH, et al. Efficacy of a reduced application time of Ovide lotion (0.5% malathion) compared to Nix crème rinse (1% permethrin) for the treatment of head lice. *Pediatr Dermatol*. 2004;21:670-674.
65. Burgess IF, Brown CM, Peck S. Head lice resistant to pyrethroid insecticides in Britain. *Br Med J*. 1995;311:752.
66. Downs AM, Stafford KA, Coles GC. Head lice: prevalence in school children and insecticide resistance. *Parasitol Today*. 1999;15:1-5.
67. Bailey AM, Prociv P. Persistent head lice following multiple treatments: evidence for insecticide resistance in *Pediculus humanus capitis*. *Australas J Dermatol*. 2001;42:146-149.
68. Mumcuoglu KY, Hemingway J, Miller J. Permethrin resistance in the head louse *Pediculus capitis* from Israel. *Med Vet Entomol*. 1995;9:427-432.

69. Rupes V, Moravek J, Shmela J. A resistance of head lice, *Pediculus capitis*, to permethrin in the Czech Republic. *Cent Eur J Public Health*. 1995;3:30-32.
70. Gellatly KJ, Krim S, Palenchar DJ, et al. EXpansion of the knockdown resistance frequency map for human head lice (Phthiraptera: Pediculidae) in the United States using quantitative sequencing. *J Med Entomol*. 2016; 53:653-659.
71. Chosidow O, Giraudeau B, Cottrell J, et al. Oral ivermectin versus malathion lotion for difficult-to-treat head lice. *N Engl J Med*. 2010;362:896-905.
72. Burkhart CN, Burkhart CG. Recommendation to standardize pediculicidal and ovicidal testing for head lice (Anoplura: Pediculidae). *J Med Entomol*. 2001; 38(2):127-129.
73. Burkhart CG, Burkhart CN. Asphyxiation of lice with topical agents, not a reality…yet. *J Am Acad Dermatol*. 2006;54:721-722.
74. Narahashi T. Neuronal ion channels as the target sites of insecticides. *Pharmacol Toxicol*. 1996;79:1-14.
75. Adams ME, Miller TA. Neural and behavioral correlates of pyrethroid and DDT type poisoning in the house fly *Musca domestica*. *Pestic Biochem Physiol*. 1980;13:137-147.
76. Frankowski BL, Bocchini JA Jr; Council on School Health and Committee on Infectious Diseases. Head lice. *Pediatrics*. 2010;126(2):392-403.
77. Bonilla DL, Kabeya H, Henn J, et al. *Bartonella quintana* in body lice and head lice from homeless persons, San Francisco, California, USA. *Emerg Infect Dis*. 2009; 15:912-915.
78. Fang R, Houhamdi L, Raoult D. Detection of *Rickettsia prowazekii* in body lice and their feces by using monoclonal antibodies. *J Clin Microbiol*. 2002;40: 3358-3363.
79. Houhamdi L, Fournier PE, Fang R, et al. An experimental model of human body louse infection with *Rickettsia prowazekii*. *J Infect Dis*. 2002;186:1639-1646.
80. Raoult D, Roux V. The body louse as a vector of reemerging human diseases. *Clin Infect Dis*. 1999;29: 888-911.
81. Alcantara V, Rolain JM, Eduardo AG, et al. Molecular detection of *Bartonella quintana* in human body lice from Mexico City. *Clin Microbiol Infect*. 2009;15: 93-94.
82. Burkhart CG, Burkhart CN. Oral ivermectin for *Phthirus pubis*. *J Am Acad Dermatol*. 2004;51:1038.
83. Kalter DC, Sperber J, Rosen T. Treatment of pediculosis pubis: clinical comparison of efficacy and tolerance of 1% lindane shampoo vs. 1% permethrin crème rinse. *Arch Dermatol*. 1987;123:1315-1319.
84. Speare R, Koehler JM. A case of pubic lice resistant to pyrethrins. *Aust Fam Physician*. 2001;30:572-574.
85. Burkhart CG, Burkhart CN. Oral ivermectin therapy for phthiriasis palpebrum. *Arch Ophthal*. 2000; 118:134-135.

Chapter 179 :: Lyme Borreliosis
:: Roger Clark & Linden Hu

第一百七十九章
莱姆病

中文导读

本章介绍了莱姆病的流行病学、临床特征、病因与发病机制、诊断、临床管理。莱姆病是美国和欧洲最常见的节肢动物传播疾病，得名于20世纪70年代对康涅狄格州莱姆镇及其周围儿童少关节型关节炎病例的调查。蜱虫、小鼠、田鼠等是主要传播媒介。皮肤表现中移行性红斑通常是感染后出现的第一个症状，晚期可出现慢性萎缩性肢端皮炎、皮肤硬化、皮肤萎缩及皮肤淋巴水肿。皮肤外表现常引起中枢和外周神经系统、心脏和关节等特定部位的表现。根据体格检查、潜在接触史、已知蜱虫叮咬或与莱姆病典型的多系统表现相一致的症状都有助于作出诊断。抗生素治疗适用于莱姆病的所有阶段，多西环素被认为是一线治疗药物。

〔粟 娟〕

AT-A-GLANCE

- Lyme disease is caused by *Borrelia burgdorferi*, a tickborne spirochete.
- Clinical course can be prolonged and may involve multiple organ systems.
- The most common cutaneous finding is the erythema migrans rash. Other cutaneous manifestations include lymphocytoma and acrodermatitis chronica atrophicans, which are only seen in European disease.
- Diagnosis is typically made on clinical identification of the erythema migrans rash and/or serologic testing.
- Early treatment with antibiotics (doxycycline, amoxicillin, or cefuroxime) is highly successful.

HISTORICAL PERSPECTIVE

Lyme borreliosis, or Lyme disease, is the most commonly reported arthropod-borne illness in both the United States and Europe.[1] The disease acquired its name from epidemiologic investigations in the 1970s of cases of oligoarticular arthritis among children in and around the town of Lyme, Connecticut.[2] Certain features, including the tight clustering of cases in a heavily wooded area, and a rash that preceded arthritis that occurred predominantly in the summer, were suggestive that this was an arthropod-borne infectious disease.

In 1981, Burgdorfer isolated a new spirochetal bacterium, *Borrelia burgdorferi*, from the midgut of the *Ixodes dammini* tick (now *Ixodes scapularis*).[3] Recovery of the organism from cutaneous lesions, cerebrospinal fluid, and blood specimens of patients with Lyme disease in both the United States[4,5] and Europe[6-8] definitively linked the disease with *B. burgdorferi*. Subsequently, additional genospecies causing Lyme disease were recognized. The original North American genospecies was designated *B. burgdorferi* sensu stricto and other species (including the 2 most prominent genospecies in other parts of the world, *Borrelia garinii* and *Borrelia afzelii*) were considered part of the *B. burgdorferi* sensu lato group. Recently, a change in the genus of Lyme disease causing *Borrelia* to *Borreliella* has been proposed to recognize significant differences with relapsing fever *Borrelia*. *Borreliella* encompasses all the genospecies that were originally designated as part of the sensu lato group. However, this has not been fully accepted so we will continue to use the *Borrelia* designation conventions.

EPIDEMIOLOGY

Lyme disease occurs in the northern hemisphere in North America, Europe and Asia. The prevalence of strains differs between the continents, with *B. burgdorferi* being the predominant species in North America, *B. garinii* and *B. afzelii* being predominant in Asia, and all three present in Europe. Disease is often focal with high rates in some countries/states but not others. In Europe, the incidence is highest in the Austria, Belgium, Estonia, Lithuania, The Netherlands, Slovenia, and Sweden, with approximately 120,000 reported cases per year in Europe. The disease is less common in Asia, but has been reported in Russia, China, Korea, and Japan. In the United States, the majority of the cases are reported from the Northeast and mid-Atlantic areas and the North Central part of the country. There is also a smaller foci of disease in the Northwestern United States.

Lyme disease *Borrelia* are transmitted by ticks in the *Ixodes ricinus* group. In the United States, the major tick vector is *I. scapularis*. *Ixodes pacificus* serves as the vector in the western United States. The white-footed mouse is the primary amplifying host of *B. burgdorferi*, with other small mammals, such as voles, shrews, chipmunks, and birds, playing a lesser role. *B. burgdorferi* sensu stricto is by far the dominant genospecies in the United States, although there have been recent reports of other species causing human disease (*Borrelia bissettii*, *Borrelia mayonii*).[9-11]

In Europe, the disease is transmitted by the *I. ricinus* tick, which feeds on more than 300 species of animals. Birds, shrews, voles, and other small mammals serve as the major amplifying hosts of *Borrelia* species in Europe.[12] Three genospecies constitute the majority of human-infecting organisms in Europe: *B. burgdorferi* sensu stricto, *B. afzelii*, and *B. garinii*.

Ixodes persulcatus is the main vector of *B. burgdorferi* in Asia. Human infections are less common throughout most of Asia and correspondingly, less is understood about the epidemiology. *I. persulcatus* is only known to transmit *B. garinii* and *B. afzelii*.

B. burgdorferi has an enzootic cycle that involves the *Ixodes* ticks and small mammals and birds, as noted above. *Ixodes* ticks undergo 4 stages during a 2-year cycle: egg, larva, nymph, and adult. There is no transovarial (ie, transmission of disease from the adult tick to the larva via the eggs) passage of *B. burgdorferi*. Ticks must acquire the bacterium by taking a blood meal from an animal that can maintain the living organism. Once acquired, there is transstadial transmission (passage from one stage in the tick lifecycle to the next). The majority of human transmission is from infected nymphal stage ticks, although infected adult ticks are also able to transmit disease.

In the United States, the incidence and range of the organism has steadily grown over the last several decades. Deer, which do not get infected with *B. burgdorferi* but can transport infected ticks, and birds are thought to be the primary drivers in dispersal of infected ticks into new areas. In the United States, the Centers for Disease Control and Prevention initiated surveillance for Lyme disease in 1982, and the Council of State and Territorial Epidemiologists made Lyme disease a nationally notifiable disease in 1991. From 1992 to 2006 the number of cases reported annually doubled, from 9908 cases to 19,931 cases.[13] By 2015, the number of new cases reported annually in the United States was 34,390.[12] In 2015, accounting for unreported cases, the Centers for disease control and prevention estimated that the incidence of Lyme disease in the U.S. was approximately 300,000 cases per year.[14,15] During the period 2005 to 2014, approximately 96% of reported cases occurred in 14 states located in the Northeastern, mid-Atlantic, and North Central regions: Connecticut, Delaware, Maine, Maryland, Massachusetts, Minnesota, New Hampshire, New Jersey, New York, Pennsylvania, Rhode Island, Vermont, Virginia, and Wisconsin (Fig. 179-1).[16] Disease in many of the states with low incidence represents travelers infected during travel to more endemic regions.

In the United States, Lyme disease is slightly more prevalent in males (53.1%) than in females, and whites are disproportionately represented at 94.1% of cases. Two-thirds of cases of have onset in the summer months of June, July, and August. There is a bimodal age distribution of Lyme disease in the United States, with peaks at ages 5 to 9 years (8.6 cases per 100,000 population) and 55 to 59 years (7.8 cases per 100,000 population).[13]

CLINICAL FEATURES

CUTANEOUS FINDINGS

EARLY CUTANEOUS FINDINGS

Erythema Migrans: Lyme disease initiates with movement of bacteria from the tick to the patient during tick attachment. Bacteria first multiply locally in the skin. The erythema migrans (EM) rash, which is typically the first symptom to develop with infection, begins 3 to 30 days (average: 7 days)[17] after completion of tick feeding.

EM is thought to be present in 70% to 80% of those individuals infected, with estimates reported to be as high as 90% in patients diagnosed with Lyme disease.[5,17,18] EM rash is a result of the host inflammatory response to the nascent infection. The histopathologic description of EM is a superficial and deep perivascular infiltrate of eosinophils at the center of the lesion and plasma cells, lymphocytes, and histiocytes peripherally (Fig. 179-2).[19] Immunohistochemical studies indicate the infiltrate to be composed of CD4+ T lymphocytes, with the exception of those seen in association with HIV infection in which the infiltrate is mainly CD8+ T lymphocytes, reflective of the CD4 lymphopenia of HIV infection.[20] The organism can be readily cultured from biopsy of the EM lesion and can be seen in tissue samples by immunofluorescence.[21]

Solitary EM rash typically occurs at the site of the tick bite, although in many cases, a definite history of a tick bite at the site of the lesion is not obtained.[22] Certain areas on the body are more likely to sustain tick bites long enough to allow for transmission of the spirochete, which is typically thought to require a minimum of 36 hours. Ticks may go unnoticed in the popliteal fossa, the groin, axilla, back, and on the head; likewise EM rash may also go unobserved in these areas. In small children, solitary EM rash occurs more often on the head and neck than in older children or adults, where these areas are seldom affected.[18]

EM rash is classically described as a large (>5 cm), expanding, erythematous, round or oval lesion, with the longer axis along the lines of least skin tension (Langer lines) and central clearing, often with a darker punctate center at the site of the tick bite (so-called Bull's-eye rash) (Figs. 179-3 and 179-4). However, this classic appearance only occurs in a minority of cases. In one observational study of 118 microbiologically proven cases of Lyme disease, only 9% of EM rash had this appearance, whereas 59% had a homogeneous appearance.[23] In another study of 14 patients with microbiologically proven Lyme disease, 10 (71%) of 14 EM rashes lacked the classic central clearing (Fig. 179-5).[24] Central clearing may be more common in *B. garinii* than with *B. burgdorferi*. Strle and others compared characteristics of culture-proven EM rash from *B. garinii* in Slovenia and *B. burgdorferi* in the United States. Central clearing was found in 71% of those with *B. garinii* versus 35.3% with *B. burgdorferi* (p = 0.0002) (Table 179-1).[25]

The lesion in itself is usually asymptomatic, but approximately 30% to 50% of patients report mild tingling, itching, or burning.[25,26] Systemic manifestations, reported in approximately 50% of patients, may appear before, during, or after the classic lesion.[27,28] Uncommon presentations of EM rash include forms with marked central necrosis, EM of minimal size (size of the ring less than 5 cm at initial presentation) (2%), and the vesicular variant (5%).[29-31]

The bacteria can disseminate from the inoculation site as early as 3 days after the presence of the original EM lesion. The most common manifestation of

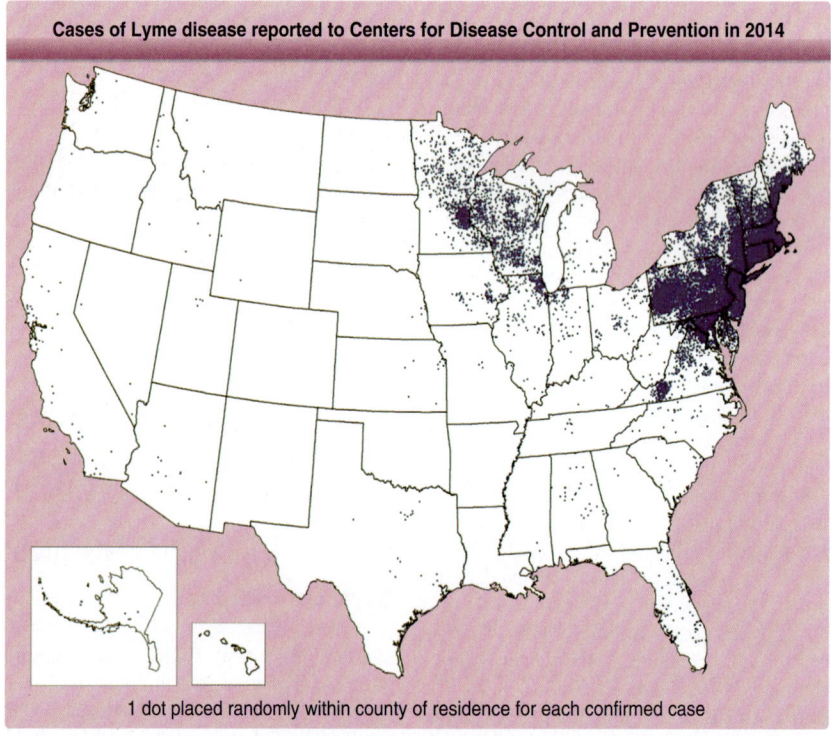

Figure 179-1 Cases of Lyme disease reported to Centers for Disease Control and Prevention in 2014. Cases shown indicate the county or residence of the infected individuals, and do not necessarily indicate where the infection occurred.

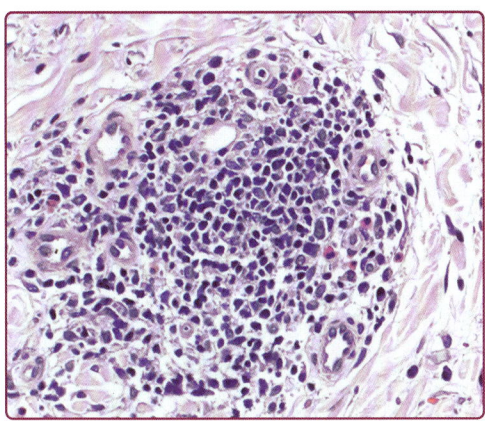

Figure 179-2 Histopathology of erythema migrans. Dense nodular perivascular lymphoid cell infiltrate with many plasma cells and few eosinophils in a biopsy from a later stage of erythema migrans. (Hematoxylin and eosin stain, ×40 magnification.)

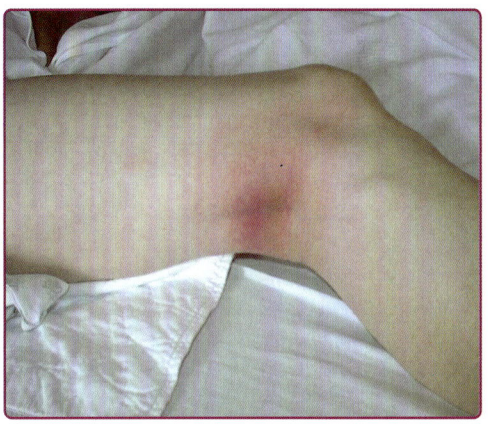

Figure 179-3 Erythema migrans with the classic "bull's-eye" appearance with a dark center, surrounding area of clearance, and a darker, advancing border. While this represents the classic appearance, it occurs only in a minority of cases.

hematogenous dissemination of the spirochete are multiple EM rashes, which are scattered over the body. These are randomly distributed and do not represent multiple localized infections at individual tick bite sites. The appearance of multiple EM lesions appears to have become less common, as Lyme disease is more widely recognized and treated early in the disease process. As of this writing, it is estimated that multiple EM lesions occur approximately 10% to 18% of the time in those infected with *B. burgdorferi*.[5,32,33] Secondary EM lesions are generally smaller than the primary EM lesions, but are otherwise indistinguishable, either visually or histologically (Figs. 179-6 to 179-8).

LATE CUTANEOUS FINDINGS

There are several dermatologic findings of Lyme disease that occur months to years after the initial infection. The majority of these are reported only in European infections and have not been seen in North American or Asian cases of disease.

Acrodermatitis Chronica Atrophicans:
Observed mainly in elderly patients in Europe, acrodermatitis chronica atrophicans (ACA) has an insidious onset and appears to have a predilection for females.[34] Rare cases of ACA have been reported in children.[35] The time interval from the spirochete inoculation to the onset of symptoms of ACA is extremely difficult to evaluate. Most patients do not recall the specific tick bite that initiated the disease.[8,36] That the spirochete can survive for decades is favored by reports indicating recovery of the spirochete from biopsies of skin from ACA patients even after 20 years.[8]

An inflammatory phase characterizes the early clinical stages of this biphasic disease.[37] The inflammatory phase presents as a bluish-red discoloration on the extensor aspect of fingers, hands, joints, and lower extremities (Fig. 179-9). Joints usually involved include the elbows and knees. Infiltrated purple bands of varying widths may be observed adjacent to involved joint(s). Associated findings include a cushion-like ("doughy") swelling of the dorsum of the hands and feet.[37] The extremities are most commonly involved, although extensive lesions on the trunk also have been documented. Lesions typically extend from the distal to the proximal portion of the extremity involved. Although the erythema and swelling initially vary in intensity ("waxes and wanes"), swelling of the posterior aspect of the lower extremities is believed by some to be particularly indicative of Lyme disease.[38]

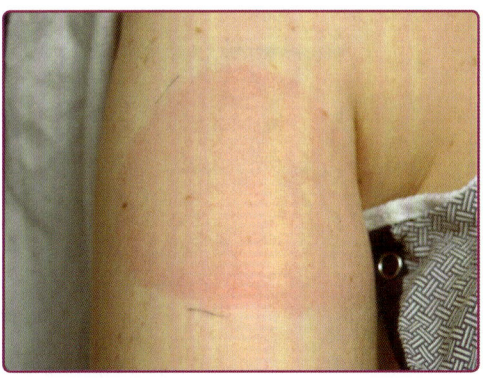

Figure 179-4 Erythema migrans lesion. Note the relative central clearing. This lesion lacks the darker punctate center sometimes found in the classic "bull's-eye" lesion. (From Clark RP. Tickborne infections. In: McKean S, Ross J, Dressler D, et al, eds. *Principles and Practice of Hospital Medicine*. 2nd ed. New York NY: McGraw-Hill; 2017, with permission.)

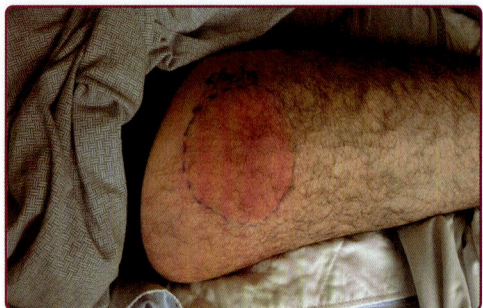

Figure 179-5 Erythema migrans. Note the lack of central clearance. This is the most common form of EM rash in the United States, appearing as an expanding, homogeneous, round or oval erythematous rash.

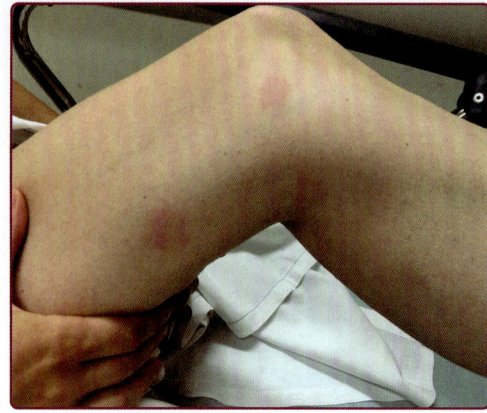

Figure 179-6 Disseminated erythema migrans. These are often smaller than the primary EM rash noted at the site of the tick bite.

Cutaneous atrophy characteristic of the later clinical stage is not an obligatory sequel to the inflammatory phase of ACA.[37] Rarely, coexistence of both kinds of lesions at different sites in the same patient has been documented. The atrophic phase is characterized by lesions with a "cigarette paper-like" appearance and a prominence of superficial veins (Fig. 179-10).

CNS and peripheral nervous system involvement also have been documented in approximately 45% of patients with ACA. Thirty percent to 45% of patients suffer from a polyneuropathy, often most pronounced in the limb with cutaneous involvement.[39] Chronic joint and bone involvement, attributed to persistence of spirochetes in cutaneous lesions, is most often seen in patients with longstanding ACA or an untreated lesion of EM or ACA and is typically restricted to the extremity involved. The characteristic symptom, exhibited in approximately one-third of patients in one study, was a swollen or painful foot and heel.[39] Other symptoms include subluxation of small joints, bursitis, arthritis, and cortical thickening of bone. Solitary or multiple fibrotic lesions near joints, particularly in the olecranon area, may develop in some patients.[37]

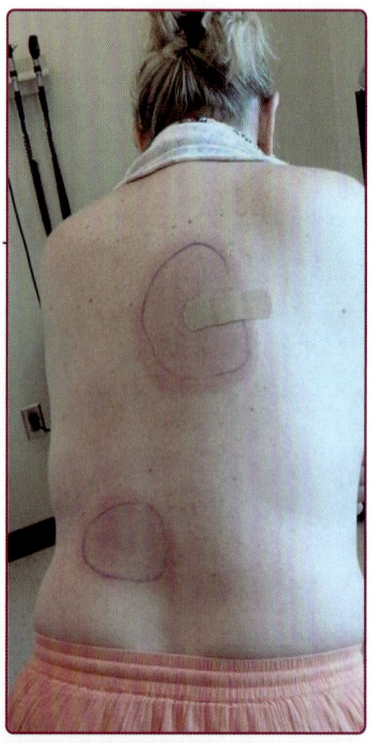

Figure 179-7 Disseminated erythema migrans lesions with uniformly erythematous, round, or oval morphology. This does not represent multiple tick bites; rather, it represents hematogenous spread of the spirochete in a random distribution on the skin. This patient also had lesions present in multiple other locations. (From Clark RP. Tickborne infections. In: McKean S, Ross J, Dressler D, et al, eds. *Principles and Practice of Hospital Medicine*. 2nd ed. New York NY: McGraw-Hill; 2017, with permission.)

TABLE 179-1
Characteristics of Erythema Migrans

CHARACTERISTICS	FREQUENCY (%) LYME—U.S. (N = 79)	FREQUENCY (%) LYME—EUROPE (N = 231)
Patients:		
Median Age (years)	38	46.7
(range in years)	(16-76)	(15-83)
Male	62%	43%
Female	38%	57%
Median diameter at presentation	13 cm	26 cm
Multiple EM lesions	18%	6%
"Bull's-eye" or central clearing	37%	71%

Data from Nadelman RB, Nowakowski J, Forseter G, et al. The clinical spectrum of early Lyme borreliosis in patients with culture-confirmed erythema migrans. *Am J Med*. 1996;100(5):502-508; and Strle F, Nelson JA, Ruzic-Sabljic E, et al. European Lyme borreliosis: 231 culture-confirmed cases involving patients with erythema migrans. *Clin Infect Dis*. 1996; 23(1):61-65.

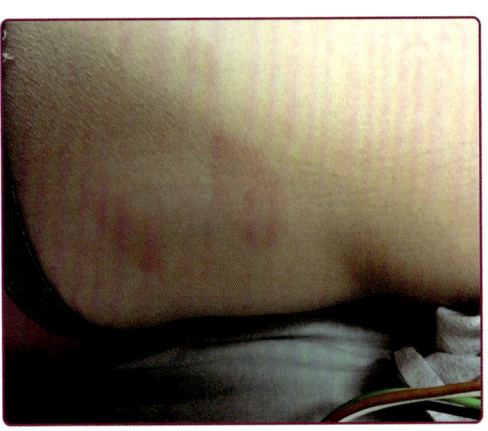

Figure 179-8 Disseminated erythema migrans. The lesion on the left is elongated, almost linear in appearance, whereas the one on the right is almost elliptical, with a "bull's-eye" morphology.

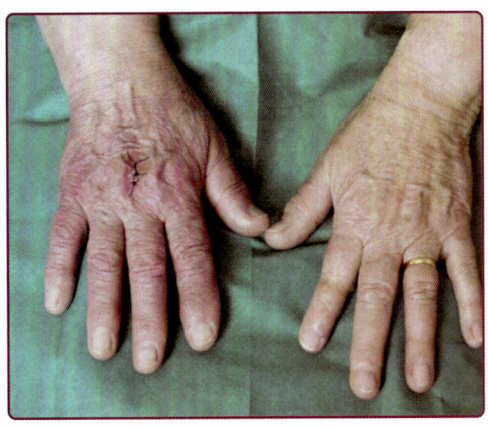

Figure 179-10 Acrodermatitis chronica atrophicans with bluish-red discoloration and cutaneous atrophy as evidenced by the "tissue paper" appearance of the dorsum of the right hand. (Image used with permission of Franc Strle, MD.)

All 3 species of *B. burgdorferi* that infect humans have been found in ACA lesions.[40] Histopathologic features of biopsied lesions vary with the clinical phase of ACA. In inflammatory lesions, 3 layers are typically described: an atrophic epidermis, a zone of uninvolved papillary dermis, and a layer of inflammatory cells composed of lymphocytes and plasma cells.[41] The presence of plasma cells in the infiltrate is documented mainly from studies from Europe, as American reports indicate that few or no plasma cells are found.[36] The infiltrate may be deep with extension into the subcutis.[38] Occasionally, interface dermatitis has been reported. Unusual findings include the presence of vacuoles, either singly or in groups, at different levels of the dermis.[42] Although some believe these represent mature adipocytes, others believe them to be an expression of lymphedema, given that they are mainly observed from biopsies of markedly edematous sites. In favor of the expression-of-lymphedema hypothesis is the absence of such vacuoles from the same site after treatment.

Phenotypic studies indicate the lymphocytes in the infiltrate are mainly of the CD4 phenotype, favoring the concept that ACA is a T-cell–mediated immune response.[43] Further in support of this theory is the expression of adhesion molecules, such as intracellular adhesion molecule-1, on endothelial cells, lymphocytes, and basal keratinocytes in the inflammatory infiltrate.[44] Chronicity of the lesions may be partially explained by downregulation of major histocompatibility complex class II molecules on Langerhans cells.[45]

Cutaneous Scleroborrelioses: Sclerotic skin lesions clinically indistinguishable from primary lichen sclerosus et atrophicus or morphea develop not only in association with other dermatoborrelioses (approximately 10% of patients with ACA and borrelial lymphocytoma [see below]) but also in the absence of other cutaneous manifestations of Lyme disease.[29,46,47]

Periarticular ("ulnar") fibrous nodules described in association ACA, may also occur in the absence of dermatoborrelioses.[48] They usually present as hard nodules on the elbows and knees, and on the lateral aspect of the digits near joints, and have been reported to be provoked by trauma, surgery, and electromagnetic radiation.[49]

Uncommon sclerotic disorders associated with Lyme disease include progressive facial hemiatrophy (Parry-Romberg syndrome) and eosinophilic fasciitis (Shulman syndrome) (see Chap. 64).[50] In support of an infectious etiology is the clinical similarity of the cutaneous lesions, positive history of tick bite, and, in rare cases, antiborrelial serologic evidence and positive culture and polymerase chain reaction (PCR) from lesions.[51,52] Eosinophilic fasciitis associated with borrelial infection has been termed *borrelial fasciitis*, reflective of the

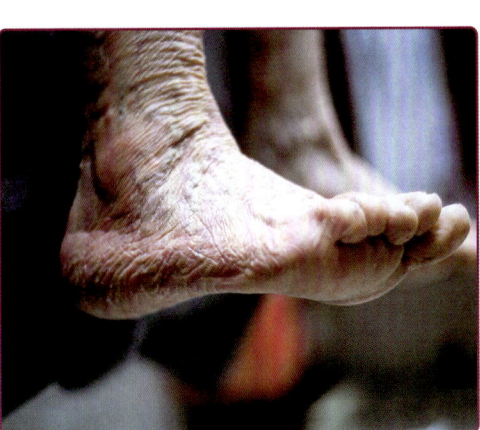

Figure 179-9 Acrodermatitis chronica atrophicans. Note the classical "tissue paper–like" cutaneous atrophy. (Image used with permission of Franc Strle, MD.)

infectious nature of these lesions.[52] However, patients with borrelial fasciitis lack the peripheral blood eosinophilia typical of patients with Shulman disease.

A unifying feature of lichen sclerosus et atrophicus–like and morphea-like scleroborrelioses is the abundance of plasma cells in the inflammatory infiltrate.[37] Unusual histologic findings include a scleromyxedema-like picture with increased dermal mucin and fibroblast proliferation.[48]

Histopathologic examination of a periarticular fibrous nodule reveals relatively well-circumscribed nodules of broad hyalinized bundles of collagen with macrophages and plasma cells.[49,53] Adjacent capillaries may be occluded by similar deposits.

Progressive facial hemiatrophy and eosinophilic fasciitis show variable dermal sclerosis, loss of appendages, and a perivascular infiltrate composed predominantly of lymphocytes and plasma cells with scattered histiocytes.[38] In borrelial fasciitis, eosinophilic infiltration of the fascial planes is not as impressive as in "idiopathic" Shulman disease.[50]

Cutaneous Atrophoborrelioses: Atrophic lesions indistinguishable from primary anetoderma (see Chap. 70) may also occur in the absence of other dermatoborrelioses.[37,54] When associated with ACA, these lesions are usually seen at the periphery of an extensive lesion.[55]

Biopsy specimens from atrophic or anetoderma-like skin lesions show abnormal elastic tissue fibers in association with a perivascular infiltrate of lymphocytes with occasional histiocytes, neutrophils, or eosinophils.[37] Spirochetes are found with difficulty in histologic sections.

Cutaneous Lymphoborrelioses (B-Cell and T-Cell Lymphoid Hyperplasias): Lymphocytic infiltrates associated with *Borrelia* are the least common of the cutaneous hallmarks of Lyme disease (1%) and may present either as single borrelial lymphocytoma (lymphadenosis benigna cutis) or as multiple lesions.[38] The coexistence of lymphocytoma with other dermatoborrelioses led to the suggestion of a unifying causative organism, favored by the development of EM-like lesions following passive inoculation of an infiltrate from a lesion of lymphadenosis benigna cutis.[8,56] Lymphocytoma has been reported solely in Europe. However, all 3 species of *B. burgdorferi* sensu lato are associated with lymphocytoma, so it is unclear whether the lack of U.S. cases is related to strain differences.[40]

More common in children than in adults, lymphocytoma clinically presents as a nodulopapular lesion in the ear lobes (Fig. 179-11) and scrotum in children and the nipple-areolar area (Fig. 179-12) in adults.[29] The precise reason for this predilection is not known but is believed to be tissue temperature related.[38] As with the other dermatoborrelioses, most patients are not aware of a preceding tick bite. The incubation period varies anywhere from a few weeks to 10 months. The duration of an untreated solitary lesion can vary from months to years (average: 5 years). Spontaneous resolution may occur, but typically lesions resolve

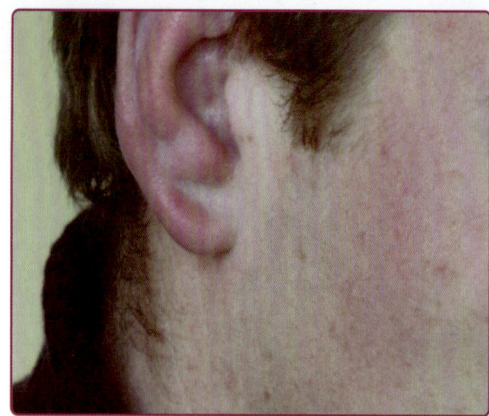

Figure 179-11 Borrelial lymphocytoma in a young adult with an erythematous nodulopapular lesion of the ear lobe. (Image used with permission of Franc Strle, MD.)

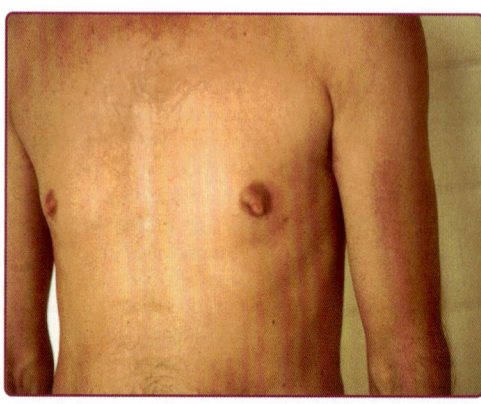

Figure 179-12 Borrelial lymphocytoma involving the left nipple. (Photograph used with permission of Franc Strle, MD.)

more rapidly with antibiotic therapy.[39] Lesions of multiple lymphocytomas can be entirely subcutaneous, may last for decades, and typically have no specific site predilection or associations with other dermatoborrelioses.

Direct evidence of an infective etiology has been provided from studies demonstrating the presence of fragmented spiral forms suggestive of *B. burgdorferi* in lesions of benign lymphocytic infiltrates,[57] and has been confirmed by immunofluorescence using species-specific monoclonal antibodies. Spirochetes may be cultured directly from biopsy specimens or *B. burgdorferi* DNA may be detected by PCR. High titers of antiborrelial antibodies have been reported in more than 50% of patients with lymphadenosis benigna cutis solitaria.[56] The common denominator in patients with *Borrelia*-associated lymphoma appears to be a high titer of antibodies, typical of the chronic stage of the infection, against *B. burgdorferi*.[56]

Discoid lesions "starting as small papules and expanding peripherally with central clearance" that wax and wane also have been described in association with borrelial infection.[57] The name given for these lesions is *benign lymphocytic infiltrates* of the skin (Jessner-Kanof) (see Chap. 120). More common in men, they tend to be located on the face, neck, and upper trunk. Annular lesions clinically resembling EM also have been described.

Several reports suggest an association of low-grade cutaneous B-cell lymphoma with *B. burgdorferi* infection.[58,59] Clinical presentation of *Borrelia*-ssociated B-cell lymphoproliferative disease is varied and consists of multiple ill-defined, slowly progressive plaques and nodules presenting on the trunk, extremities, or both, of usually older patients. The highest frequency of infection with *Borrelia* has been found in marginal zone lymphoma (20% to 52%), followed by follicular center lymphoma (15% to 26%) and diffuse large B-cell lymphoma (15% to 16%; see Chaps. 119 and 120).[58,60] That antigenic drive by *Borrelia* may be a pathogenic factor in more than 1 subtype is supported by the association of *B. burgdorferi* with multiple subtypes of cutaneous B-cell lymphoma. Demonstration of the organism in the skin before development of overt cutaneous B-cell lymphoma serves to confirm the temporal progression of *B. burgdorferi*–associated B-cell lymphoproliferative disease. Clinical regression of marginal zone lymphoma after eradication of *B. burgdorferi* argues in favor of a benign process.[59,61,62]

Histopathologic findings of benign B-cell– and T-cell–dominant hyperplasias are essentially similar to benign lymphoid hyperplasias secondary to an arthropod bite, vaccination, or other causes (see Chap. 120). Definitive classification of *Borrelia*-associated B-cell lymphoma is confounded by the immunohistochemical profile: expression of CD5 and CD10 (common acute lymphoblastic leukemia antigen), antigens typically associated with centrocytic lymphoma, are absent in *Borrelia*-associated B-cell lymphoma.[58]

Other Cutaneous Lesions: Other cutaneous lesions reported in patients with documented Lyme disease include panniculitis, vasculitis, granuloma annulare, erythema multiforme, and a syphilis-like papulosquamous eruption, but *B. burgdorferi* has not been directly recovered from any of these lesions (Table 179-2).

NONCUTANEOUS FINDINGS

After the initial inoculation into skin and resultant EM lesion, *B. burgdorferi* quickly disseminates to other parts of the body causing site-specific manifestations. Common areas for dissemination include the central and peripheral nervous system, the heart and the joints. Often in early Lyme disease there are multiple, nonspecific symptoms in addition to rash. The frequency of these symptoms appears to vary depending on the genospecies is involved (Table 179-3).

NERVOUS SYSTEM MANIFESTATIONS

B. burgdorferi can cause neurologic disease in 10% to 15% of patients in the United States who have not received antibiotics. Meningitis, cranial neuropathy, and radiculopathy are the most common neurologic manifestations and can manifest as soon as 1 week after EM.[63] Facial palsy is the most characteristic neuropathy of early Lyme disease in the United States, occurring in 40% to 50% of patients with borrelial neurologic involvement, usually within 4 weeks after onset of EM. Bilateral facial palsy should immediately raise suspicion for Lyme disease, as it is uncommon in most other causes of facial palsy. Involvement of other cranial nerves has been reported, but is relatively rare.[63] The triad of lymphocytic meningitis, cranial palsy (often facial), and radiculoneuritis, known as Bannwarth syndrome, is pathognomonic for Lyme disease. It is frequently reported in Europe but is rare in the United States.[64,65] It is thought that *B. garinii* causes meningitis and radiculopathy more frequently than *B. burgdorferi*.[66] Acute or subacute myelitis leading to spastic paraparesis and cerebrospinal fluid pleocytosis, mononeuritis, and a Guillain-Barré–like syndrome may also occur in early disseminated disease.[67,68] Late neurologic manifestations include encephalomyelitis, encephalopathy, and chronic polyneuropathies.[69,70]

CARDIAC MANIFESTATIONS

Cardiac involvement occurs in anywhere from 1% to 10% of untreated patients in the United States[71,72] and in 0.3% to 4% of European patients.[73,74] The wide ranges probably reflect the fact that in recent years, Lyme disease is recognized and treated sooner, resulting in lower incidence than in the past. It usually occurs within several weeks after the onset of infection, although it can occur as early as 1 week and as late as 7 months into the infection.[71,75] Within the heart, *B. burgdorferi* has a predilection for the atrioventricular node, resulting in atrioventricular block. Acute myopericarditis and left ventricular dysfunction can also occur, but are usually self-limited and mild, only sometimes resulting in transient cardiomegaly or pericardial effusion.[76] *B. burgdorferi* has been isolated from endomyocardial biopsy samples from several European patients with chronic dilated cardiomyopathy, a complication observed less frequently in the United States.[77,78] In the United States, there have been cases of cardiac sudden death where autopsies have revealed myocarditis caused by undiagnosed Lyme disease.[72]

MUSCULOSKELETAL MANIFESTATIONS

Early musculoskeletal manifestations of *B. burgdorferi* infection are typically nonspecific. Inflammatory arthritis is the most frequent clinical sign of late-disseminated Lyme disease in the United States, occurring

TABLE 179-2
Cutaneous Manifestations of Lyme Disease

	ONSET	DIAGNOSIS/DIFFERENTIAL DIAGNOSIS
Common Manifestations		
Erythema migrans	Weeks to months (early)	Arthropod bite, erythema multiforme granuloma annulare, urticaria, erysipelas, brown recluse spider bite, fixed drug eruption
Acrodermatitis chronica atrophicans	Months to years (late)	Venous insufficiency, lichen sclerosus, scleroderma, physiologic age-related atrophy, corticosteroid-induced atrophy
Uncommon Manifestations		
Cutaneous scleroborrelioses	Months to years (late)	
▪ Morphea		▪ Primary morphea
▪ Lichen sclerosus et atrophicus		▪ Primary lichen sclerosus et atrophicus
▪ Periarticular fibrous nodules		▪ Rheumatoid nodule, gouty tophi
▪ Progressive facial hemiatrophy		▪ Primary progressive facial hemiatrophy/Parry-Romberg syndrome
▪ Eosinophilic fasciitis		▪ Primary eosinophilic fasciitis/Shulman syndrome
Cutaneous atrophoborrelioses	Months to years (late)	
▪ Anetoderma		▪ Primary anetoderma
Cutaneous lymphoborrelioses	Months to years (late)	
▪ B-cell dominant (including B-cell lymphoma)		▪ Arthropod bite reaction, response to vaccination, granulomas, neoplasm
▪ T-cell dominant		▪ Pityriasis lichenoides, polymorphous light eruption
Other cutaneous lesions	Weeks to months to years (early or late)	
▪ Panniculitis		▪ Erythema nodosum
▪ Granuloma annulare		▪ Insect bite reaction
▪ Erythema multiforme		▪ Drug eruption
▪ Syphilis-like papulosquamous eruption		▪ Secondary syphilis

in approximately 60% of patients with untreated or incompletely treated infection.[62,79] It usually presents 1 or more months after the onset of Lyme disease as asymmetric monoarthritis or oligoarthritis of large joints, most often of the knee. Migratory arthralgia is also relatively common, especially during disseminated Lyme disease. Bouts of arthritis are generally frequent and short at first, becoming longer and less frequent with time, each lasting from several days to 1 year.[79]

OTHER MANIFESTATIONS OF LYME DISEASE

Ophthalmic complications in the form of conjunctivitis, keratitis, iridocyclitis, retinal vasculitis, chorioiditis, and optic neuropathy are rare manifestations of Lyme disease. They are thought to be the direct result of tissue inflammation by *B. burgdorferi* and are usually associated with other signs and symptoms of disease. The eye also may be affected by extraocular manifestations of Lyme disease, such as cranial nerve pareses and orbital myositis. Findings in other organ systems (GI, lymphatic, respiratory, urinary, and genital) have been reported, but the associations with borrelial infection are loose.

PERINATAL LYME DISEASE

Studies in both human and animal models indicate that *B. burgdorferi* can cross the placenta during the

TABLE 179-3
Clinical Manifestations of Early Lyme Disease

SYMPTOM OR LABORATORY ABNORMALITY	FREQUENCY (%) LYME U.S. (N = 79)	FREQUENCY (%) LYME EUROPE (N = 231)	FREQUENCY (%) *B. MAYONII* (N = 6)
Fatigue	54	10	67
Arthralgia	44	25	17
Myalgia	44	11	67
Headache	42	20	83
Neck stiffness/meningeal signs	35	1	50
GI symptoms	26	0.4	67
Regional lymphadenopathy	23	7	N/A
Fever	16	4	83

initial spirochetemia, but evidence of a fetal immune response or an adverse neonatal outcome are not definitively established. Several studies have found no link between maternal infection with Lyme and subsequent birth defects.[80-84]

LYME DISEASE IN CHILDREN

Other than differences in localization of EM lesions (more typically in the head and neck), pediatric Lyme disease is similar to that of adults. Of note, however, optic nerve involvement may lead to blindness in children.[85]

COMPLICATIONS

All manifestations of Lyme disease resolve over time, even in the absence of antibiotic therapy. Antibiotic therapy can hasten resolution of some (EM, arthritis), but not all (facial palsy, radiculitis) manifestations, and antibiotic therapy can clearly abort late manifestations.

Coinfection with *B. burgdorferi* and either (or both) of *Babesia microti* or *Anaplasma phagocytophilum* occurs at different frequencies depending on the geographic location, and may alter the clinical presentation of Lyme disease in some patients. Some studies suggest more-severe disease in patients who are coinfected, but this remains uncertain.[86-89]

A small number of patients have symptoms that persist for years despite appropriate antibiotic therapy. Up to 10% of patients with Lyme arthritis who are treated with appropriate antibiotics may have continued arthritis that persists for years.[90,91] Arthritis in these patients does typically respond to immunosuppressive agents (methotrexate, anti–tumor necrosis factor therapies), which has led to suggestions that these patients may have an autoimmune syndrome. Molecular mimicry of borrelial antigens with host proteins has been proposed as one possible mechanism, but this remains unproven.[92,93]

There are many reports of patients who continue to have symptoms beyond a standard treatment course for Lyme disease of 2 to 4 weeks, including profound fatigue, depression, myalgia, polyarthralgias without arthritis, and paresthesias, as well as neurocognitive difficulties involving memory, concentration (particularly auditory), and decreased mental flexibility (ie, impaired verbal fluency) after infection with *B. burgdorferi*.[92] This syndrome is often referred to as posttreatment Lyme disease syndrome. The linkage of these symptoms with *B. burgdorferi* infection remains controversial and several large epidemiologic studies have shown that patients who have contracted Lyme disease are no more likely to suffer from these symptoms than persons in the general population.[94-96] There are numerous studies demonstrating that longer-than-standard courses of antibiotics for Lyme disease do not improve long-term symptoms.[97-99] However, prolonged courses of antibiotics for Lyme disease do have serious adverse effects.[100,101] At this time, courses of antibiotics exceeding the standard duration are not recommended.

ETIOLOGY AND PATHOGENESIS

RISK FACTORS

The risk of acquiring Lyme disease is almost completely dependent on exposure to the tick vector in areas where Lyme disease is prevalent. These areas are detailed in section "Epidemiology". Avoidance of environments where ticks are likely to be found is an effective strategy to prevent disease. Other methods to reduce the risk of acquiring Lyme disease and coinfecting organisms are found in section "Prevention".

PATHOGENESIS

B. burgdorferi sensu lato, the agent of Lyme borreliosis, belongs to the eubacterial phylum of *Spirochaetales*, which are vigorously motile, corkscrew-shaped bacteria. Recently, it has been proposed that *B. burgdorferi* sensu lato be renamed as *Borreliella burgdorferi* to distinguish it from relapsing fever *Borrelia*. Here we will continue to use the *Borrelia* designation. The borrelial genome is made up of a linear chromosome and more than 20 circular and linear plasmids, the largest number known for any bacteria.[102,103] Some of the plasmids can be considered minichromosomes, as they are required for survival of the organism. Among the interesting characteristics of the organism are the large number of lipoproteins (more than 150) encoded by the genome. *Borrelia* lack biosynthetic machinery to produce many essential nutrients (eg, amino acids, fatty acids), suggesting that *B. burgdorferi* is highly dependent on its hosts for obtaining crucial nutrients.[102,103]

Ixodes ticks have a 2-year, 3-stage (larval, nymphal, and adult) life cycle. Larval ticks acquire *B. burgdorferi* organisms by taking a blood meal from an infected animal and maintain the infection during the subsequent molting to the nymphal and adult stages. *B. burgdorferi* remain dormant in the tick's midgut between feedings.[104] Each tick life stage takes 1 blood meal: larval ticks feed in late summer, nymphal ticks feed the subsequent spring and early summer, and adult ticks feed in the fall and early winter.[104] The major reservoirs for *B. burgdorferi* are small rodents and birds that are fed on by larval and nymphal ticks. Adult ticks feed on larger mammals (eg, deer) that are not important reservoirs for *B. burgdorferi* but are an important feeding source for adult ticks. Reductions in deer populations can lead to significant decreases in the tick population.[105] Humans are incidental hosts not important in maintaining *B. burgdorferi* in the wild. Most cases of human illness occur in the late spring and summer months when the nymphs are most active and human outdoor activity is greatest.

Of clinical relevance, certain *Ixodes* ticks are vectors of other tick-borne illnesses in addition to Lyme disease: *I. scapularis* ticks in the United States and *I. ricinus* ticks in Europe may transmit *B. microti* (a red blood cell parasite), *A. phagocytophilum* (formerly referred to as the agent of human granulocytic ehrlichiosis) and *Borrelia miyamotoi* (a relapsing fever type *Borrelia*).[86,102,103] *I. ricinus* in Europe and *I. persulcatus* in Asia are also vectors of tick-borne encephalitis virus, whereas *I. scapularis* transmits a related Powassan family virus (deer tick virus).[106,107] Patients who have been bitten by *Ixodes* ticks may be coinfected with multiple organisms.

B. burgdorferi rapidly adapt to different host environments by changing protein expression.[104] There are multiple levels of control of gene expression but 2 of the major regulators of borrelial gene expression are the histidine kinase-1 (HK1)/response regulator-1 (Rrp1) pathway and the Response regulator-2 (Rrp2)/RNA polymerase, sigma S (RpoS)/RNA polymerase, sigma N (RpoN) pathway. The HK1/Rrp1 pathway becomes activated as bacteria exit a mammalian host and enter a tick host. The Rrp2/RpoS/RpoN system becomes activated as the bacteria readies itself for entry into a mammalian host. Other regulatory factors such as BosR, a Fur-like transcription factor, and RpoD, a sigma factor, also help to control expression of genes upon tick feeding and transition to the mammalian host. Genes upregulated by Rrp2/RpoS/RpoN include those that may assist with immune evasion and cellular adhesion, as well as genes identified as essential for establishment of initial infection whose functions are unknown.

At the tick bite site, the spirochete is injected along with tick saliva into the skin. The presence of the tick salivary protein, Salp15, on the surface of the spirochete is instrumental in helping the organism evade the mammalian immune system during early infection.[108] After a latency period of 3 days to 1 month, the organism spreads through the skin. The immune response to the bacteria causes the characteristic EM rash. The bacteria enter the blood circulation and disseminate hematogenously. This generally occurs within days to weeks after infection. This dissemination is caused by both host and pathogen factors. For instance, it has been found that in North America, infection with certain strains of *B. burgdorferi,* such as OspC type A (RST 1), are particularly likely to result in hematogenous spread of the organism.[109] Host proteases, such as plasmin and matrix metalloproteinases, may assist the bacteria as it moves through tissues.

With its ability to establish long-term infection in mammalian hosts, several important factors in escaping immune defenses have been identified. Motility is a critical element of *B. burgdorferi* survival.[110] *B. burgdorferi* move very quickly within tissues and have been clocked at up to 4 µM/s which is faster than neutrophils or macrophages can travel. Another important element is antigenic variation. *B. burgdorferi* have the ability to change the antigenic composition of a dominant protein expressed during mammalian infection, VlsE, through recombination into a portion of the gene from silent cassettes.[106,107] Finally, *B. burgdorferi* have been shown to express proteins that bind a host complement inhibitory protein, factor H. Binding of factor H by specific *B. burgdorferi* has been shown in vitro to help it evade complement mediated killing.[111-113] However, the importance of individual factor H–binding proteins in vivo is not known, possibly a consequence of redundancy among the proteins.

DIAGNOSIS

Physical findings, a history of potential exposure, known tick bites, or symptoms consistent with the typical multisystem presentation of Lyme disease can all be helpful in making a diagnosis. In the presence of classic EM or of Bannwarth syndrome, the diagnosis of Lyme disease can be made on clinical grounds alone. Diagnostic conundrums arise in presentations that involve other compatible skin, cardiac, neurologic, or musculoskeletal symptoms in the absence of a history of EM or tick exposure. In these cases, laboratory testing can aid in making the diagnosis.

DIRECT DETECTION OF *BORRELIA BURGDORFERI*

The gold standard for diagnosis of most infectious diseases is culture. However, the need for specialized media and the slow growth of the organism make it impractical in most clinical settings. *B. burgdorferi* can be readily cultured from biopsies of EM and ACA,[21] but rarely grows in synovial fluid in patients with Lyme arthritis or cerebrospinal fluid samples in patients with meningitis.[7,114] Studies also have demonstrated that the organism can be recovered from the blood in up to 50% of untreated adult patients with multiple EM.[115] However, cultures are generally insensitive in patients with extracutaneous manifestations of Lyme borreliosis, particularly in later-stage disease.

PCR assays are very sensitive in detecting *B. burgdorferi* DNA in skin biopsy and synovial fluid specimens from patients with EM and Lyme arthritis, respectively.[116] PCR testing for *B. burgdorferi* DNA has not been approved by the U.S. Food and Drug Administration (FDA), and its main use is in detecting *B. burgdorferi* in synovial fluid where Lyme arthritis is suspected. In this setting its sensitivity is between 70% and 85%,[116-118] but a positive test does not necessarily mean there are living organisms.

SEROLOGIC DIAGNOSIS OF LYME DISEASE

Immunologic diagnosis is the main laboratory modality used to support a clinical diagnosis of Lyme disease.

In the United States, the FDA has approved more than 70 different immunoassays for Lyme disease—mainly enzyme-linked immunoabsorbent (ELISA) and Western immunoblot assays.[119] ELISA tests use whole-cell lysates of *B. burgdorferi* sensu lato or purified *B. burgdorferi* antigens to capture either anti-*B. burgdorferi* immunoglobulin (Ig) G and/or IgM antibodies present in a given sample. Although relatively sensitive, ELISA tests are associated with a high rate of false-positive results.[120,121] Patients with autoimmune diseases (lupus, rheumatoid arthritis), Epstein-Barr virus, bacterial endocarditis, and other tick-borne diseases appear to be at an increased risk for false-positive IgM serologic testing; syphilis, *Helicobacter pylori*, systemic lupus erythematosus, ehrlichiosis, and babesiosis cause false-positive IgG serologic testing.[120,121] A newer ELISA test that uses only a small peptide of the constant region of *B. burgdorferi* VlsE protein appears to have greater specificity than traditional whole-cell ELISA testing. This test, also known as the *C6 peptide test*, measures only IgG antibody, but IgG antibody to the C6 peptide develops early in the course of disease and the sensitivity of the assay in patients with early disease has been equivalent to that seen with IgM whole-cell ELISA tests.[121,122] Western immunoblot assays are more specific because they enable detection of antibodies to individual components of *B. burgdorferi*. Currently, there are no widely accepted standard tests or criteria for serodiagnosis of Lyme disease in either Europe or Asia, in part because of the presence of multiple strains of *B. burgdorferi* that have only partial antigen cross-reactivity.

Because of its limitations, particularly high false-positive results within the general population, serologic testing should be initiated based on the pretest probability of disease and serve only to support a clinical diagnosis.[7] It is most helpful in patients with an intermediate pretest probability of Lyme disease—namely those who reside in endemic areas and who present with signs and symptoms consistent with, but not diagnostic of, Lyme disease (eg, facial palsy, arthritis, or atrioventricular nodal conduction abnormalities in the absence of an EM lesion). Patients who reside in areas of high endemicity and have clear EM lesions should be diagnosed on clinical grounds alone without laboratory testing. Testing should be avoided in patients with low suspicion for disease (patients not living in endemic areas, or with nonspecific systemic symptoms, or after a tick bite) as the rates of false-positive tests greatly outnumber true positive tests in this setting. Figure 179-13 shows one algorithm for the workup of patients presenting with an eruption suspicious for EM.

Once the decision is made to obtain serologic testing, current recommendations are for 2-stage testing, starting with a highly sensitive ELISA test first.[123] If the ELISA is negative, the likelihood of Lyme disease is low, and further testing is not generally recommended. However, if the test is positive or indeterminate, a Western immunoblot assay with high specificity should be used to confirm the results. The specificity of this 2-step approach is thought to be 99% to 100% in late-stage Lyme disease.[119] If testing is negative early in the course of disease, the tests can be repeated in 3 to 4 weeks (antibiotic therapy, if given very early, may abort antibody development). It is important to note that in patients with disease untreated for longer than 1 month, IgM testing should not be performed. A positive IgM Western blot with a negative IgG Western blot in this setting is considered a negative result owing to the high false-positivity rate of IgM testing. Misuse or misinterpretation of the IgM tests is a major factor in over diagnosis of Lyme disease. Seronegativity in patients suspected of having late Lyme disease practically excludes the diagnosis.[124] Finally, because IgG and IgM antibody titers may persist for years despite antibiotic therapy, persistent seropositivity is not in itself an indication of treatment failure, nor is it proof of recent infection or reinfection. Currently, there is no test that allows confirmation of successful clearance of the organism after treatment.

Some recent studies suggest that the use of 2-step testing for Lyme disease may result in underdiagnosis of Lyme disease. The performance of traditional ELISA tests against nonisogenic genotypes of *B. burgdorferi* is reduced and results in lower sensitivity in patients infected with these strains early in the course of disease.[119] The C6 antibody test appears to function better across genotypes of *B. burgdorferi* sensu stricto and with the European strains *B. garinii* and *B. afzelii*. Newer strategies using the C6 ELISA as the second step (dual enzyme immunoassay), replacing Western blot testing[125] or using a C6 band in the second step Western blot IgG test[126] show promising results but require further confirmation before they can be recommended.

DIFFERENTIAL DIAGNOSIS

The differential diagnosis of Lyme disease is dependent upon the specific manifestation. Early, nonspecific systemic symptoms (fevers, myalgia, headache, lymphadenopathy) have often been described as "viral-like" and cannot be distinguished from many infectious and noninfectious causes of these types of symptoms.

EM is the most distinctive clinical manifestation of infection. The differential diagnosis for EM includes cellulitis or erysipelas, tinea, insect bites, fixed drug eruptions, and erythema multiforme. EM can usually be distinguished from other conditions by its size, onset, duration, local symptoms (eg, itching, pain at site) or presence of systemic symptoms. A newer inclusion in the differential diagnosis is another tick-associated disease called southern tick-associated rash illness (STARI). STARI is associated with the bite of a different tick, *Amblyomma americanum*, but the causative agent has not been identified. Most cases of STARI have occurred in the southern United States where Lyme disease is uncommon. However, as *A. americanum* has spread northward and Lyme disease has expanded southward, there is now overlap in the geographic regions where STARI and Lyme occur.

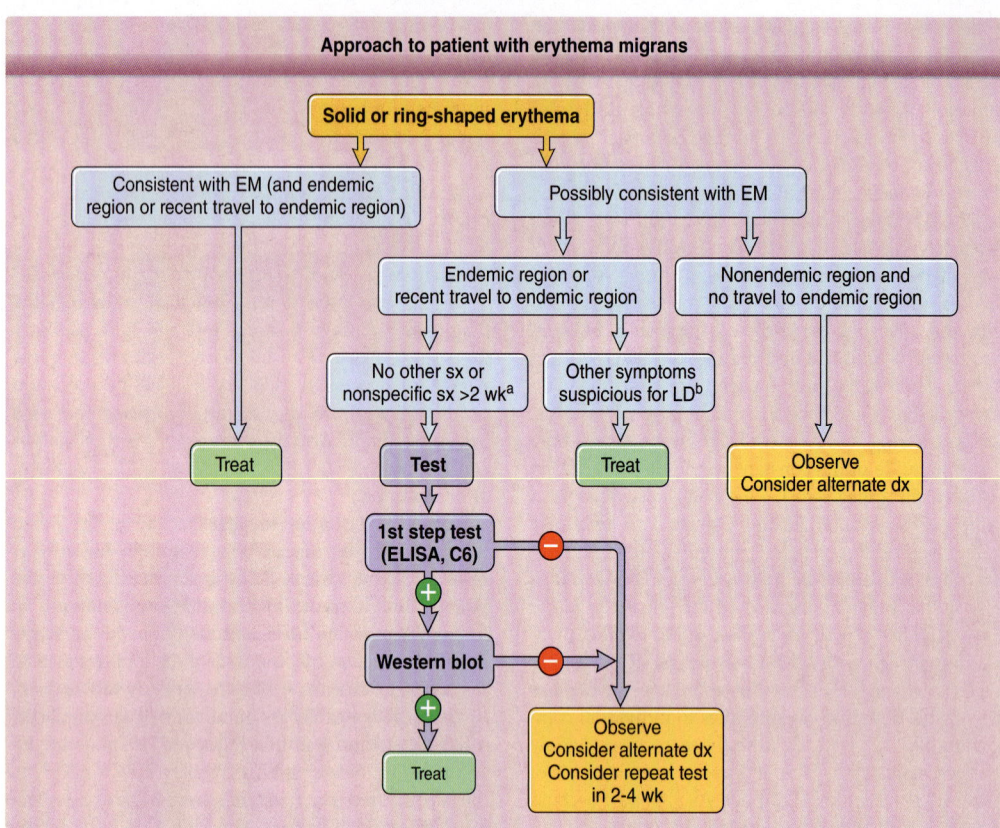

Figure 179-13 Approach to patient with erythema migrans (EM). [a]Fever, chills, fatigue. [b]Bell palsy, radiculoneuritis, meningitis, arthritis. dx, Diagnosis; ELISA, enzyme-linked immunosorbent assay; LD, Lyme disease; sx, symptoms.

STARI is typically a self-limited disease that does not require treatment.

Table 179-4 lists the differential diagnoses for other cutaneous manifestations of Lyme disease. For many of the cutaneous manifestations of borreliosis, the clinical and histologic appearances are insufficient to make a definitive diagnosis. Obtaining a good clinical history is important. Lesions of ACA are notoriously overlooked or misinterpreted. In those with a relevant clinical history, the onset appears to be related to an untreated lesion of EM and/or neurologic manifestations. In one study, a history of EM months to years earlier on the same side was found in approximately 18% of patients.[45] Serologic testing is typically positive in patients with ACA, but are more variable with other cutaneous manifestations.[47] Direct identification of the spirochete in the affected skin by immunofluorescence, culture or PCR is often necessary to make a definitive diagnosis.

MANAGEMENT

Antibiotic treatment is indicated for all stages of Lyme disease, even though most manifestations resolve over time without therapy. Patients may not be asymptomatic at the time of completion of the antibiotic course but this is not an indication for extending length of therapy; symptoms generally continue to improve steadily over time. Of note, Jarisch-Herxheimer reactions (fevers, chills, and worsening arthralgia and myalgia) are sometimes reported after the initial dose of antibiotics; the reaction is thought to be caused by host reaction to the dying organisms.

The Infectious Disease Society of America has published guidelines for the treatment of all manifestations of Lyme disease,[127] although many of the recommendations are based on expert opinion and not on rigorously controlled clinical trials. Treatment patterns differ in different countries, but no data suggest differences in either the efficacy of specific antibiotics or in the optimal duration of therapy between patients in North America and Europe.

Treatment of all of the cutaneous manifestations of Lyme disease should initially be with oral antibiotics. Doxycycline is generally considered as first-line therapy, because it has excellent penetration into the CNS and is also effective against *A. phagocytophilum*, the agent of human granulocytic ehrlichiosis. Doxycycline should be used in children and pregnant women.[128] Cefuroxime is an alternative first-line agent. These 3

TABLE 179-4
Differential Diagnosis of Erythema Migrans

DIAGNOSTIC ENTITY	DESCRIPTION	DISTINGUISHING FEATURES TO DIFFERENTIATE FROM ERYTHEMA MIGRANS
Single Lesions		
Cellulitis, erysipelas	Erythematous painful, spreading rash, often with associated edema, most commonly on lower extremity	Generally painful, seldom round or ovoid
Hypersensitivity to tick bite	Red papule at bite site with surrounding pruritic erythema, edema, urticaria	Typically pruritic, seldom exceeds 5 cm
Tinea corporis	Erythematous, annular lesions	Scaly, often with tiny vesicles at the border
Contact dermatitis	Acute erythematous rash which may form papules, vesicles, scale; in chronic cases lichenification, fissuring and erosions may occur	Generally in areas exposed to jewelry, clothing, often with unusual patterns; often pruritic
Southern tick-associated rash illness (STARI)	Clinically indistinguishable from erythema migrans rash	Generally occurs in the South and Southwestern United States, but the geographic range is spreading to overlap with Lyme disease
Multiple Lesions		
Urticaria	Multiple, small, localized cutaneous edema with blanching erythema, generally pruritic	Usually presents as a pruritic, erythematous wheal; lesions generally last for minutes to hours
Tinea corporis	Erythematous, annular lesions	Scaly, often with tiny vesicles at the border
Pityriasis rosea	Multiple, small 2- to 4-cm oval lesions, often preceded by a larger "Herald patch"	Scaly, often appear in a classic "Christmas tree" pattern, generally on the trunk
Erythema annulare centrifugum	Expanding erythematous, annular, migrating lesions	Generally chronic, with waxing/waning course
Erythema multiforme	Circular, erythematous plaques, generally not exceeding 3 cm, sometimes with wheal with dark center; lesions often become confluent	Acral distribution, may involve mucous membranes; sometimes follows herpes simplex virus or *Mycoplasma pneumoniae* infection

agents have been found to be equally effective.[129-131] Macrolides are second-line agents and should only be used in those who cannot tolerate the other agents. If macrolides are used to treat Lyme disease, close monitoring and follow up should take place.[127] Duration of therapy for EM is generally recommended to be 10 to 14 days; a randomized, double-blinded, placebo-controlled study showed similar outcomes in patients with EM treated with either a 10-day or a 20-day course of oral doxycycline.[131-133]

IV antibiotics (ceftriaxone, cefotaxime, or penicillin G) may be recommended for patients with cutaneous manifestations that are accompanied by neurologic disease (meningitis, encephalopathy) or high-degree heart block. However, multiple recent studies suggest that outcomes for treatment of neurologic disease with either oral doxycycline or IV ceftriaxone are similar. IV antibiotics are also sometimes used for patients with refractory ACA or arthritis.

Table 179-5 outlines the choice of antibiotics and duration of treatment of the major cutaneous and noncutaneous manifestations of Lyme disease.

Treatment of patients with nonspecific fibromyalgia-like disease after infection with *B. burgdorferi* is controversial. There are multiple controlled trials showing no benefit to prolonging therapy with currently recommended oral or IV antibiotics.[127,134]

PREVENTION

Prevention of Lyme disease on a personal level can be approached in many ways, including avoidance of environments where ticks which can carry *B. burgdorferi* are likely to reside. However, in some areas of the United States with a high prevalence of Lyme disease, avoidance may not be possible, as ticks are found in and around human habitations.

REPELLANTS AND ACARICIDES

The evidence for performing tick checks and bathing after engaging in activities where exposure to ticks is expected is mixed.[135,136] However, these are simple and reasonable measures and removal of crawling or even attached ticks can prevent disease as it is thought that there is minimal transmission of spirochetes before 36 hours of attachment and feeding.[127] Under certain conditions (see footnote for Table 179-5) if an attached tick is found, a single dose of oral doxycycline may be recommended as prophylaxis against the development of Lyme disease.[137]

There are several commercially available products marketed as insect repellants that have activity in preventing tick bites. The active ingredients, DEET

(N,N-diethyl-meta-toluamide), IR3535, paramenthane-3,8-diol (PMD, which is refined from the oil of lemon eucalyptus), and picaridin are generally considered to have the greatest efficacy. However, because the duration of efficacy of each of these agents for repelling ticks is less than 2 hours, they require frequent reapplication. DEET has been in use for 70 years and has a strong safety record. DEET-treated clothing has been demonstrated to provide up to 92% protection against tick bites when applied to military clothing.[138]

Acaricides have potent acaricidal and insecticidal properties. The efficacy in actually reducing human infection with Lyme disease and other tick-borne illnesses through applying pyrethrins to the environment (such

TABLE 179-5
Treatment Recommendations for Adults in the United States with Lyme Disease, by Clinical Findings

CLINICAL FINDING	ANTIBIOTIC	DURATION	ALTERNATIVE	REFERENCES
Prophylaxis[a]	Doxycycline 200 mg × 1 dose		Watchful waiting	127,137
Skin Manifestations				
Erythema migrans	Doxycycline 100 mg by mouth twice daily Amoxicillin 500 mg by mouth three times daily Cefuroxime axetil 500 mg by mouth twice daily	10 days 14 days 14 days	Azithromycin 500 mg by mouth daily for 7-10 days	131-133
Acrodermatitis chronica atrophicans	See regimen for erythema migrans	21 days		127
Borrelial lymphocytoma	See regimen for erythema migrans	14-21 days	Azithromycin 500 mg by mouth daily for 7 to 10 days	127
Musculoskeletal Manifestations				
Lyme arthritis	Doxycycline 100 mg by mouth twice daily	28 days	Amoxicillin 500 mg by mouth 3 times daily × 28 days Cefuroxime axetil 500 mg by mouth twice daily × 28 days	127
Failure/recurrence after initial treatment	Doxycycline 100 mg by mouth twice daily or Ceftriaxone 2 g IV daily	28 days 14-28 days	Amoxicillin 500 mg by mouth 3 times daily × 28 days Cefuroxime axetil 500 mg by mouth twice daily × 28 days	127
Cardiac Manifestations				
Lyme carditis	**Nonhospitalized** Doxycycline 100 mg by mouth twice daily Amoxicillin 500 mg by mouth 3 times daily Cefuroxime axetil 500 mg by mouth twice daily **Hospitalized**[b] Ceftriaxone 2 g IV daily until stable/discharge, then complete course with antibiotics listed above for nonhospitalized	14-21 days 14-21 days		127
Neurologic Manifestations				
Cranial neuropathy/radiculopathy	Doxycycline 100 mg by mouth twice daily or 200 mg by mouth daily	14 days	Amoxicillin 500 mg by mouth three × daily for 14 days Cefuroxime axetil 500 mg by mouth twice daily for 14 days	127, 144-148
Meningitis	**Nonhospitalized** Doxycycline 100 mg by mouth twice daily **Hospitalized**[c] Ceftriaxone 2 g IV daily[d]	14 days 14 days	Penicillin G 18 to 24 million units IV divided in 6 daily doses (every 4 hours)	127, 144-149

[a]Prophylaxis should only be offered when all of the following conditions are met[114]:
The attached tick can be reliably identified as an adult or nymphal *Ixodes scapularis*
Tick that is estimated to have been attached for >36 hours
Prophylaxis can be started within 72 hours
[b]Ecologic information indicates that the local rate of infection of these ticks with *Borrelia burgdorferi* is >20%; *and*
Doxycycline treatment is not contraindicated.
[c]Hospitalization recommended for patients who are symptomatic, who have first-degree atrioventricular block with PR interval exceeding 30 msec, or with second- or third-degree atrioventricular block
[d]Many European studies have shown that oral doxycycline is as efficacious as IV beta-lactam therapy in treating Lyme meningitis. Some U.S. experts are similarly using oral doxycycline for this indication, although no U.S. studies have been reported at the time of the preparation of this manuscript.
Consider deescalation to oral doxycycline upon discharge from the hospital to complete therapy.

as spraying residential lawns) has been unclear. Recently, however, a large, randomized, double-blinded, placebo-controlled trial was conducted over 2 years in 3 states in the Northeast. The trial showed a 63% decrease in the number of ticks found, but no difference in tick-borne infections, based on both self-report and medical record review, by applying pyrethrins to the environment.[139] Certain pyrethrins, such as permethrin, can be applied to clothing as an effective acaricide against some species of ticks which carry Lyme disease.[140]

VACCINATION

An effective human vaccine against Lyme disease was developed against the outer-surface protein A antigen and introduced in the United States in 1998. This was shown to reduce the risk of infection by approximately 76% in those who were vaccinated.[141] However, a series of factors lead to its voluntary withdrawal from the market in 2002, a result of low demand.[142,143] There is currently no human vaccine available against Lyme disease. Vaccination for dogs is currently available.

ACKNOWLEDGMENTS

This chapter is based on a previous version of the chapter written by Drs. Meera Mahalingam, Jag Bhawan, Daniel Eisen, and Linden Hu.

REFERENCES

1. Centers for Disease Control and Prevention. Lyme disease—United States, 2001-2002. *MMWR Morb Mortal Wkly Rep.* 2004;53(17):365-369.
2. Steere AC, Malawista SE, Snydman DR, et al. Lyme arthritis: an epidemic of oligoarticular arthritis in children and adults in three Connecticut communities. *Arthritis Rheum.* 1977;20(1):7-17.
3. Burgdorfer W, Barbour AG, Hayes SF, et al. Lyme disease-a tick-borne spirochetosis? *Science.* 1982;216(4552):1317-1319.
4. Benach JL, Bosler EM, Hanrahan JP, et al. Spirochetes isolated from the blood of two patients with Lyme disease. *N Engl J Med.* 1983;308(13):740-742.
5. Steere AC, Bartenhagen NH, Craft JE, et al. The early clinical manifestations of Lyme disease. *Ann Intern Med.* 1983;99(1):76-82.
6. Ackermann R, Kabatzki J, Boisten HP, et al. *Ixodes ricinus* spirochete and European erythema chronicum migrans disease. *Yale J Biol Med.* 1984;57(4):573-580.
7. Aguero-Rosenfeld ME, Wang G, Schwartz I, et al. Diagnosis of lyme borreliosis. *Clin Microbiol Rev.* 2005;18(3):484-509.
8. Asbrink E. Erythema chronicum migrans Afzelius and acrodermatitis chronica atrophicans. Early and late manifestations of *Ixodes ricinus*-borne *Borrelia* spirochetes. *Acta Derm Venereol Suppl (Stockh).* 1985;118:1-63.
9. Golovchenko M, Vancova M, Clark K, et al. A divergent spirochete strain isolated from a resident of the southeastern United States was identified by multilocus sequence typing as *Borrelia bissettii*. *Parasit Vectors.* 2016;9:68.
10. Rudenko N, Golovchenko M, Vancova M, et al. Isolation of live *Borrelia burgdorferi sensu lato spirochaetes* from patients with undefined disorders and symptoms not typical for Lyme borreliosis. *Clin Microbiol Infect.* 2016;22(3):267.e9-267.e15.
11. Pritt BS, Mead PS, Johnson DK, et al. Identification of a novel pathogenic *Borrelia* species causing Lyme borreliosis with unusually high spirochaetaemia: a descriptive study. *Lancet Infect Dis.* 2016;16(5):556-564.
12. Gern L, Estrada-Pena A, Frandsen F, et al. European reservoir hosts of *Borrelia burgdorferi sensu lato*. *Zentralbl Bakteriol.* 1998;287(3):196-204.
13. Bacon RM, Kugeler KJ, Mead PS; Centers for Disease Control and Prevention (CDC). Surveillance for Lyme disease—United States, 1992-2006. *MMWR Surveill Summ.* 2008;57(10):1-9.
14. Nelson CA, Saha S, Kugeler KJ, et al. Incidence of clinician-diagnosed Lyme disease, United States, 2005-2010. *Emerg Infect Dis.* 2015;21(9):1625-1631.
15. Hinckley AF, Connally NP, Meek JI, et al. Lyme disease testing by large commercial laboratories in the United States. *Clin Infect Dis.* 2014;59(5):676-681.
16. Centers for Disease Control and Prevention (CDC). Lyme Disease Data Tables. 2006-2016. http://www.cdc.gov/lyme/stats/tables.html. Accessed October 5, 2016.
17. Steere AC, Sikand VK. The presenting manifestations of Lyme disease and the outcomes of treatment. *N Engl J Med.* 2003;348(24):2472-2474.
18. Gerber MA, Shapiro ED, Burke GS, et al. Lyme disease in children in southeastern Connecticut. Pediatric Lyme Disease Study Group. *N Engl J Med.* 1996;335(17):1270-1274.
19. Wilson TC, Legler A, Madison KC, et al. Erythema migrans: a spectrum of histopathologic changes. *Am J Dermatopathol.* 2012;34(8):834-837.
20. Berger BW. Erythema migrans in Lyme disease: a correction. *JAMA.* 1992;268(7):874.
21. Berger BW, Johnson RC, Kodner C, et al. Cultivation of *Borrelia burgdorferi* from erythema migrans lesions and perilesional skin. *J Clin Microbiol.* 1992;30(2):359-361.
22. Shapiro ED, Gerber MA. Lyme disease. *Clin Infect Dis.* 2000;31(2):533-542.
23. Smith RP, Schoen RT, Rahn DW, et al. Clinical characteristics and treatment outcome of early Lyme disease in patients with microbiologically confirmed erythema migrans. *Ann Intern Med.* 2002;136(6):421-428.
24. Schutzer SE, Berger BW, Krueger JG, et al. Atypical erythema migrans in patients with PCR-positive Lyme disease. *Emerg Infect Dis.* 2013;19(5):815-817.
25. Strle F, Ruzic-Sabljic E, Logar M, et al. Comparison of erythema migrans caused by *Borrelia burgdorferi* and *Borrelia garinii*. *Vector Borne Zoonotic Dis.* 2011;11(9):1253-1258.
26. Duray PH, Asbrink E, Weber K. The cutaneous manifestations of human Lyme disease: a widening spectrum. *Adv Dermatol.* 1989;4:255-275; discussion 276.
27. Berger BW. Cutaneous manifestations of Lyme borreliosis. *Rheum Dis Clin North Am.* 1989;15(4):627-634.
28. Berger BW, Clemmensen OJ, Ackerman AB. Lyme disease is a spirochetosis. A review of the disease and evidence for its cause. *Am J Dermatopathol.* 1983;5(2):111-124.

29. Goldberg NS, Forseter G, Nadelman RB, et al. Vesicular erythema migrans. *Arch Dermatol*. 1992;128(11):1495-1498.
30. Malane MS, Grant-Kels JM, Feder HM Jr, et al. Diagnosis of Lyme disease based on dermatologic manifestations. *Ann Intern Med*. 1991;114(6):490-498.
31. Wu YS, Zhang WF, Feng FP, et al. Atypical cutaneous lesions of Lyme disease. *Clin Exp Dermatol*. 1993;18(5):434-436.
32. Strle F, Nadelman RB, Cimperman J, et al. Comparison of culture-confirmed erythema migrans caused by *Borrelia burgdorferi sensu stricto* in New York State and by *Borrelia afzelii* in Slovenia. *Ann Intern Med*. 1999;130(1):32-36.
33. Nadelman RB, Nowakowski J, Forseter G, et al. The clinical spectrum of early Lyme borreliosis in patients with culture-confirmed erythema migrans. *Am J Med*. 1996;100(5):502-508.
34. Kaufman LD, Gruber BL, Phillips ME, et al. Late cutaneous Lyme disease: acrodermatitis chronica atrophicans. *Am J Med*. 1989;86(6, pt 2):828-830.
35. Gellis SE, Stadecker MJ, Steere AC. Spirochetes in atrophic skin lesions accompanied by minimal host response in a child with Lyme disease. *J Am Acad Dermatol*. 1991;25(2, pt 2):395-397.
36. DiCaudo DJ, Su WP, Marshall WF, et al. Acrodermatitis chronica atrophicans in the United States: clinical and histopathologic features of six cases. *Cutis*. 1994;54(2):81-84.
37. Burgdorf WH, Worret WI, Schultka O. Acrodermatitis chronica atrophicans. *Int J Dermatol*. 1979;18(8):595-601.
38. Mullegger RR, McHugh G, Ruthazer R, et al. Differential expression of cytokine mRNA in skin specimens from patients with erythema migrans or acrodermatitis chronica atrophicans. *J Invest Dermatol*. 2000;115(6):1115-1123.
39. Duray PH. Clinical pathologic correlations of Lyme disease. *Rev Infect Dis*. 1989;11(suppl 6):S1487-S1493.
40. Duray PH. The surgical pathology of human Lyme disease. An enlarging picture. *Am J Surg Pathol*. 1987;11(suppl 1):47-60.
41. Asbrink E, Brehmer-Andersson E, Hovmark A. Acrodermatitis chronica atrophicans—a spirochetosis. Clinical and histopathological picture based on 32 patients; course and relationship to erythema chronicum migrans Afzelius. *Am J Dermatopathol*. 1986;8(3):209-219.
42. Buechner SA, Rufli T, Erb P. Acrodermatitis chronic atrophicans: a chronic T-cell-mediated immune reaction against *Borrelia burgdorferi*? Clinical, histologic, and immunohistochemical study of five cases. *J Am Acad Dermatol*. 1993;28(3):399-405.
43. Ilowite NT. Muscle, reticuloendothelial, and late skin manifestations of Lyme disease. *Am J Med*. 1995;98(4A):63S-68S.
44. Silberer M, Koszik F, Stingl G, et al. Downregulation of class II molecules on epidermal Langerhans cells in Lyme borreliosis. *Br J Dermatol*. 2000;143(4):786-794.
45. Kaya G, Berset M, Prins C, et al. Chronic borreliosis presenting with morphea- and lichen sclerosus et atrophicus-like cutaneous lesions. a case report. *Dermatology*. 2001;202(4):373-375.
46. Tuffanelli D. Do some patients with morphea and lichen sclerosis et atrophicans have a *Borrelia* infection? *Am J Dermatopathol*. 1987;9(5):371-373.
47. Espana A, Torrelo A, Guerrero A, et al. Periarticular fibrous nodules in Lyme borreliosis. *Br J Dermatol*. 1991;125(1):68-70.
48. Marsch WC, Mayet A, Wolter M. Cutaneous fibroses induced by *Borrelia burgdorferi*. *Br J Dermatol*. 1993;128(6):674-678.
49. Granter SR, Barnhill RL, Duray PH. Borrelial fasciitis: diffuse fasciitis and peripheral eosinophilia associated with *Borrelia* infection. *Am J Dermatopathol*. 1996;18(5):465-473.
50. Stanek G, Konrad K, Jung M, et al. Shulman syndrome, a scleroderma subtype caused by *Borrelia burgdorferi*? *Lancet*. 1987;1(8548):1490.
51. Abele DC, Anders KH. The many faces and phases of borreliosis. I. Lyme disease. *J Am Acad Dermatol*. 1990;23(2, pt 1):167-186.
52. Marsch WC, Wolter M, Mayet A. Juxta-articular fibrotic nodules in *Borrelia* infection—ultrastructural details of therapy-induced regression. *Clin Exp Dermatol*. 1994;19(5):394-398.
53. Hofer T, Goldenberger D, Itin PH. Anetoderma and borreliosis: is there a pathogenetic relationship? *Eur J Dermatol*. 2003;13(4):399-401.
54. Aberer E, Stanek G. Histological evidence for spirochetal origin of morphea and lichen sclerosus et atrophicans. *Am J Dermatopathol*. 1987;9(5):374-379.
55. Hovmark A, Asbrink E, Olsson I. The spirochetal etiology of lymphadenosis benigna cutis solitaria. *Acta Derm Venereol*. 1986;66(6):479-484.
56. Abele DC, Anders KH, Chandler FW. Benign lymphocytic infiltration (Jessner-Kanof): another manifestation of borreliosis? *J Am Acad Dermatol*. 1989;21(4, pt 1):795-797.
57. Garbe C, Stein H, Dienemann D, et al. *Borrelia burgdorferi*-associated cutaneous B cell lymphoma: clinical and immunohistologic characterization of four cases. *J Am Acad Dermatol*. 1991;24(4):584-590.
58. Goodlad JR, Davidson MM, Hollowood K, et al. *Borrelia burgdorferi*-associated cutaneous marginal zone lymphoma: a clinicopathological study of two cases illustrating the temporal progression of *B. burgdorferi*-associated B-cell proliferation in the skin. *Histopathology*. 2000;37(6):501-508.
59. Slater DN. *Borrelia burgdorferi*-associated primary cutaneous B-cell lymphoma. *Histopathology*. 2001;38(1):73-77.
60. Roggero E, Zucca E, Mainetti C, et al. Eradication of *Borrelia burgdorferi* infection in primary marginal zone B-cell lymphoma of the skin. *Hum Pathol*. 2000;31(2):263-268.
61. Kutting B, Bonsmann G, Metze D, et al. *Borrelia burgdorferi*-associated primary cutaneous B cell lymphoma: complete clearing of skin lesions after antibiotic pulse therapy or intralesional injection of interferon alfa-2a. *J Am Acad Dermatol*. 1997;36(2, pt 2):311-314.
62. Steere AC. Lyme disease. *N Engl J Med*. 1989;321(9):586-596.
63. Pachner AR, Steere AC. The triad of neurologic manifestations of Lyme disease: meningitis, cranial neuritis, and radiculoneuritis. *Neurology*. 1985;35(1):47-53.
64. Bannwarth A. Chronische lymphocytare Meningitis, entzundliche Polyneuritis und "Rheumatismus." Ein beitrag zum Problem "Allergie und Nervensystem. *Arch Psychiatr Nervenkr*. 1941;113:284.
65. Oschmann P, Dorndorf W, Hornig C, et al. Stages and syndromes of neuroborreliosis. *J Neurol*. 1998;245(5):262-272.
66. Stanek G, Strle F. Lyme disease: European perspective. *Infect Dis Clin North Am*. 2008;22(2):327-339, vii.
67. Garin C, Bujadoux A. Paralysis by ticks. 1922. *Clin*

Infect Dis. 1993;16(1):168-169.
68. Logigian EL, Steere AC. Clinical and electrophysiologic findings in chronic neuropathy of Lyme disease. *Neurology.* 1992;42(2):303-311.
69. Kaplan RF, Meadows ME, Vincent LC, et al. Memory impairment and depression in patients with Lyme encephalopathy: comparison with fibromyalgia and nonpsychotically depressed patients. *Neurology.* 1992;42(7):1263-1267.
70. Cox J, Krajden M. Cardiovascular manifestations of Lyme disease. *Am Heart J.* 1991;122(5):1449-1455.
71. Steere AC, Batsford WP, Weinberg M, et al. Lyme carditis: cardiac abnormalities of Lyme disease. *Ann Intern Med.* 1980;93(1):8-16.
72. Forrester JD, Meiman J, Mullins J, et al. Notes from the field: update on Lyme carditis, groups at high risk, and frequency of associated sudden cardiac death—United States. *MMWR Morb Mortal Wkly Rep.* 2014;63(43):982-983.
73. Grzesik P, Oczko-Grzesik B, Kepa L. Cardiac manifestations of Lyme borreliosis [in Polish]. *Przegl Epidemiol.* 2004;58(4):589-596.
74. Mayer W, Kleber FX, Wilske B, et al. Persistent atrioventricular block in Lyme borreliosis. *Klin Wochenschr.* 1990;68(8):431-435.
75. van der Linde MR, Crijns HJ, Lie KI. Transient complete AV block in Lyme disease. Electrophysiologic observations. *Chest.* 1989;96(1):219-221.
76. Stanek G, Klein J, Bittner R, et al. Isolation of *Borrelia burgdorferi* from the myocardium of a patient with longstanding cardiomyopathy. *N Engl J Med.* 1990;322(4):249-252.
77. Sonnesyn SW, Diehl SC, Johnson RC, et al. A prospective study of the seroprevalence of *Borrelia burgdorferi* infection in patients with severe heart failure. *Am J Cardiol.* 1995;76(1):97-100.
78. Mikkila HO, Seppala IJ, Viljanen MK, et al. The expanding clinical spectrum of ocular lyme borreliosis. *Ophthalmology.* 2000;107(3):581-587.
79. Steere AC, Schoen RT, Taylor E. The clinical evolution of Lyme arthritis. *Ann Intern Med.* 1987;107(5):725-731.
80. Walsh CA, Mayer EW, Baxi LV. Lyme disease in pregnancy: case report and review of the literature. *Obstet Gynecol Surv.* 2007;62(1):41-50.
81. Strobino BA, Williams CL, Abid S, et al. Lyme disease and pregnancy outcome: a prospective study of two thousand prenatal patients. *Am J Obstet Gynecol.* 1993;169(2, pt 1):367-374.
82. Maraspin V, Cimperman J, Lotric-Furlan S, et al. Treatment of erythema migrans in pregnancy. *Clin Infect Dis.* 1996;22(5):788-793.
83. Strobino B, Abid S, Gewitz M. Maternal Lyme disease and congenital heart disease: a case-control study in an endemic area. *Am J Obstet Gynecol.* 1999;180(3, pt 1):711-716.
84. Gerber MA, Zalneraitis EL. Childhood neurologic disorders and Lyme disease during pregnancy. *Pediatr Neurol.* 1994;11(1):41-43.
85. Rothermel H, Hedges TR 3rd, Steere AC. Optic neuropathy in children with Lyme disease. *Pediatrics.* 2001;108(2):477-481.
86. Krause PJ, Telford SR 3rd, Spielman A, et al. Concurrent Lyme disease and babesiosis. Evidence for increased severity and duration of illness. *JAMA.* 1996;275(21):1657-1660.
87. Horowitz HW, Aguero-Rosenfeld ME, Holmgren D, et al. Lyme disease and human granulocytic anaplasmosis coinfection: impact of case definition on coinfection rates and illness severity. *Clin Infect Dis.* 2013;56(1):93-99.
88. Krause PJ, McKay K, Thompson CA, et al. Disease-specific diagnosis of coinfecting tickborne zoonoses: babesiosis, human granulocytic ehrlichiosis, and Lyme disease. *Clin Infect Dis.* 2002;34(9):1184-1191.
89. Diuk-Wasser MA, Vannier E, Krause PJ. Coinfection by *Ixodes* tick-borne pathogens: ecological, epidemiological, and clinical consequences. *Trends Parasitol.* 2016;32(1):30-42.
90. Steere AC, Levin RE, Molloy PJ, et al. Treatment of Lyme arthritis. *Arthritis Rheum.* 1994;37(6):878-888.
91. Gross DM, Forsthuber T, Tary-Lehmann M, et al. Identification of LFA-1 as a candidate autoantigen in treatment-resistant Lyme arthritis. *Science.* 1998;281(5377):703-706.
92. Weinstein A, Britchkov M. Lyme arthritis and post-Lyme disease syndrome. *Curr Opin Rheumatol.* 2002;14(4):383-387.
93. Brown CR, Reiner SL. Clearance of *Borrelia burgdorferi* may not be required for resistance to experimental lyme arthritis. *Infect Immun.* 1998;66(5):2065-2071.
94. Wormser GP, Weitzner E, McKenna D, et al. Long-term assessment of fatigue in patients with culture-confirmed Lyme disease. *Am J Med.* 2015;128(2):181-184.
95. Kalish RA, Kaplan RF, Taylor E, et al. Evaluation of study patients with Lyme disease, 10-20-year follow-up. *J Infect Dis.* 2001;183(3):453-460.
96. Seltzer EG, Gerber MA, Cartter ML, et al. Long-term outcomes of persons with Lyme disease. *JAMA.* 2000;283(5):609-616.
97. Klempner MS, Hu LT, Evans J, et al. Two controlled trials of antibiotic treatment in patients with persistent symptoms and a history of Lyme disease. *N Engl J Med.* 2001;345(2):85-92.
98. Krupp LB, Hyman LG, Grimson R, et al. Study and treatment of post Lyme disease (STOP-LD): a randomized double masked clinical trial. *Neurology.* 2003;60(12):1923-1930.
99. Fallon BA, Keilp JG, Corbera KM, et al. A randomized, placebo-controlled trial of repeated IV antibiotic therapy for Lyme encephalopathy. *Neurology.* 2008;70(13):992-1003.
100. Patel R, Grogg KL, Edwards WD, et al. Death from inappropriate therapy for Lyme disease. *Clin Infect Dis.* 2000;31(4):1107-1109.
101. Ettestad PJ, Campbell GL, Welbel SF, et al. Biliary complications in the treatment of unsubstantiated Lyme disease. *J Infect Dis.* 1995;171(2):356-361.
102. Casjens S, Palmer N, van Vugt R, et al. A bacterial genome in flux: the twelve linear and nine circular extrachromosomal DNAs in an infectious isolate of the Lyme disease spirochete *Borrelia burgdorferi*. *Mol Microbiol.* 2000;35(3):490-516.
103. Fraser CM, Casjens S, Huang WM, et al. Genomic sequence of a Lyme disease spirochaete, *Borrelia burgdorferi*. *Nature.* 1997;390(6660):580-586.
104. Radolf JD, Caimano MJ, Stevenson B, et al. Of ticks, mice and men: understanding the dual-host lifestyle of Lyme disease spirochaetes. *Nat Rev Microbiol.* 2012;10(2):87-99.
105. Telford SR 3rd, Mather TN, Moore SI, et al. Incompetence of deer as reservoirs of the Lyme disease spirochete. *Am J Trop Med Hyg.* 1988;39(1):105-109.
106. El Khoury MY, Camargo JF, White JL, et al. Potential role of deer tick virus in *Powassan* encephalitis cases in Lyme disease-endemic areas of New York, U.S.A.

Emerg Infect Dis. 2013;19(12):1926-1933.

107. Henningsson AJ, Lindqvist R, Norberg P, et al. Human tick-borne encephalitis and characterization of virus from biting tick. *Emerg Infect Dis.* 2016;22(8):1485-1487.
108. Dai J, Wang P, Adusumilli S, et al. Antibodies against a tick protein, Salp15, protect mice from the Lyme disease agent. *Cell Host Microbe.* 2009;6(5):482-492.
109. Wormser GP, Brisson D, Liveris D, et al. *Borrelia burgdorferi* genotype predicts the capacity for hematogenous dissemination during early Lyme disease. *J Infect Dis.* 2008;198(9):1358-1364.
110. Sultan SZ, Manne A, Stewart PE, et al. Motility is crucial for the infectious life cycle of *Borrelia burgdorferi*. *Infect Immun.* 2013;81(6):2012-2021.
111. Kraiczy P, Skerka C, Kirschfink M, et al. Immune evasion of *Borrelia burgdorferi* by acquisition of human complement regulators FHL-1/reconectin and factor H. *Eur J Immunol.* 2001;31(6):1674-1684.
112. Stevenson B, El-Hage N, Hines MA, et al. Differential binding of host complement inhibitor factor H by *Borrelia burgdorferi* Erp surface proteins: a possible mechanism underlying the expansive host range of Lyme disease spirochetes. *Infect Immun.* 2002;70(2):491-497.
113. McDowell JV, Wolfgang J, Tran E, et al. Comprehensive analysis of the factor h binding capabilities of *Borrelia* species associated with lyme disease: delineation of two distinct classes of factor h binding proteins. *Infect Immun.* 2003;71(6):3597-3602.
114. Wormser GP, Bittker S, Cooper D, et al. Comparison of the yields of blood cultures using serum or plasma from patients with early Lyme disease. *J Clin Microbiol.* 2000;38(4):1648-1650.
115. Wormser GP, Nowakowski J, Nadelman RB, et al. Improving the yield of blood cultures for patients with early Lyme disease. *J Clin Microbiol.* 1998;36(1):296-298.
116. Nocton JJ, Dressler F, Rutledge BJ, et al. Detection of *Borrelia burgdorferi* DNA by polymerase chain reaction in synovial fluid from patients with Lyme arthritis. *N Engl J Med.* 1994;330(4):229-234.
117. Li X, McHugh GA, Damle N, et al. Burden and viability of *Borrelia burgdorferi* in skin and joints of patients with erythema migrans or lyme arthritis. *Arthritis Rheum.* 2011;63(8):2238-2247.
118. Persing DH, Rutledge BJ, Rys PN, et al. Target imbalance: disparity of *Borrelia burgdorferi* genetic material in synovial fluid from Lyme arthritis patients. *J Infect Dis.* 1994;169(3):668-672.
119. Wormser GP, Liveris D, Hanincova K, et al. Effect of *Borrelia burgdorferi* genotype on the sensitivity of C6 and 2-tier testing in North American patients with culture-confirmed Lyme disease. *Clin Infect Dis.* 2008;47(7):910-914.
120. Magnarelli LA, Miller JN, Anderson JF, et al. Cross-reactivity of nonspecific treponemal antibody in serologic tests for Lyme disease. *J Clin Microbiol.* 1990;28(6):1276-1279.
121. Nocton JJ, Steere AC. Lyme disease. *Adv Intern Med.* 1995;40:69-117.
122. Goettner G, Schulte-Spechtel U, Hillermann R, et al. Improvement of Lyme borreliosis serodiagnosis by a newly developed recombinant immunoglobulin G (IgG) and IgM line immunoblot assay and addition of VlsE and DbpA homologues. *J Clin Microbiol.* 2005;43(8):3602-3609.
123. Sanchez E, Vannier E, Wormser GP, et al. Diagnosis, treatment, and prevention of Lyme disease, human granulocytic anaplasmosis, and babesiosis: a review. *JAMA.* 2016;315(16):1767-1777.
124. Avery RA, Frank G, Eppes SC. Diagnostic utility of *Borrelia burgdorferi* cerebrospinal fluid polymerase chain reaction in children with Lyme meningitis. *Pediatr Infect Dis J.* 2005;24(8):705-708.
125. Branda JA, Linskey K, Kim YA, et al. Two-tiered antibody testing for Lyme disease with use of 2 enzyme immunoassays, a whole-cell sonicate enzyme immunoassay followed by a VlsE C6 peptide enzyme immunoassay. *Clin Infect Dis.* 2011;53(6):541-547.
126. Branda JA, Aguero-Rosenfeld ME, Ferraro MJ, et al. 2-Tiered antibody testing for early and late Lyme disease using only an immunoglobulin G blot with the addition of a VlsE band as the second-tier test. *Clin Infect Dis.* 2010;50(1):20-26.
127. Wormser GP, Dattwyler RJ, Shapiro ED, et al. The clinical assessment, treatment, and prevention of lyme disease, human granulocytic anaplasmosis, and babesiosis: clinical practice guidelines by the Infectious Diseases Society of America. *Clin Infect Dis.* 2006;43(9):1089-1134.
128. Steere AC. Lyme disease. *N Engl J Med.* 2001;345(2):115-125.
129. Nadelman RB, Luger SW, Frank E, et al. Comparison of cefuroxime axetil and doxycycline in the treatment of early Lyme disease. *Ann Intern Med.* 1992;117(4):273-280.
130. Dattwyler RJ, Volkman DJ, Conaty SM, et al. Amoxycillin plus probenecid versus doxycycline for treatment of erythema migrans borreliosis. *Lancet.* 1990;336(8728):1404-1406.
131. Wormser GP, Ramanathan R, Nowakowski J, et al. Duration of antibiotic therapy for early Lyme disease. A randomized, double-blind, placebo-controlled trial. *Ann Intern Med.* 2003;138(9):697-704.
132. Stupica D, Lusa L, Ruzic-Sabljic E, et al. Treatment of erythema migrans with doxycycline for 10 days versus 15 days. *Clin Infect Dis.* 2012;55(3):343-350.
133. Kowalski TJ, Tata S, Berth W, et al. Antibiotic treatment duration and long-term outcomes of patients with early lyme disease from a lyme disease-hyperendemic area. *Clin Infect Dis.* 2010;50(4):512-520.
134. Auwaerter PG, Bakken JS, Dattwyler RJ, et al. Scientific evidence and best patient care practices should guide the ethics of Lyme disease activism. *J Med Ethics.* 2011;37(2):68-73.
135. Connally NP, Durante AJ, Yousey-Hindes KM, et al. Peridomestic Lyme disease prevention: results of a population-based case-control study. *Am J Prev Med.* 2009;37(3):201-206.
136. Vazquez M, Muehlenbein C, Cartter M, et al. Effectiveness of personal protective measures to prevent Lyme disease. *Emerg Infect Dis.* 2008;14(2):210-216.
137. Nadelman RB, Nowakowski J, Fish D, et al. Prophylaxis with single-dose doxycycline for the prevention of Lyme disease after an *Ixodes scapularis* tick bite. *N Engl J Med.* 2001;345(2):79-84.
138. Schreck CE, Snoddy EL, Spielman A. Pressurized sprays of permethrin or DEET on military clothing for personal protection against *Ixodes dammini* (Acari: Ixodidae). *J Med Entomol.* 1986;23(4):396-399.
139. Hinckley AF, Meek JI, Ray JA, et al. Effectiveness of residential acaricides to prevent Lyme and other tick-borne diseases in humans. *J Infect Dis.* 2016;214(2):182-188.

140. Lane RS. Treatment of clothing with a permethrin spray for personal protection against the western black-legged tick, Ixodes pacificus (Acari: Ixodidae). *Exp Appl Acarol.* 1989;6(4):343-352.
141. Steere AC, Sikand VK, Meurice F, et al. Vaccination against Lyme disease with recombinant *Borrelia burgdorferi* outer-surface lipoprotein A with adjuvant. Lyme Disease Vaccine Study Group. *N Engl J Med.* 1998;339(4):209-215.
142. Poland GA. Vaccines against Lyme disease: What happened and what lessons can we learn? *Clin Infect Dis.* 2011;52(suppl 3):s253-s258.
143. Nigrovic LE, Thompson KM. The Lyme vaccine: a cautionary tale. *Epidemiol Infect.* 2007;135(1):1-8.
144. Karlsson M, Hammers-Berggren S, Lindquist L, et al. Comparison of intravenous penicillin G and oral doxycycline for treatment of Lyme neuroborreliosis. *Neurology.* 1994;44(7):1203-1207.
145. Dotevall L, Hagberg L. Successful oral doxycycline treatment of Lyme disease-associated facial palsy and meningitis. *Clin Infect Dis.* 1999;28(3):569-574.
146. Borg R, Dotevall L, Hagberg L, et al. Intravenous ceftriaxone compared with oral doxycycline for the treatment of Lyme neuroborreliosis. *Scand J Infect Dis.* 2005; 37(6-7):449-454.
147. Ljostad U, Skogvoll E, Eikeland R, et al. Oral doxycycline versus intravenous ceftriaxone for European Lyme neuroborreliosis: a multicentre, non-inferiority, double-blind, randomised trial. *Lancet Neurol.* 2008; 7(8):690-695.
148. Bremell D, Dotevall L. Oral doxycycline for Lyme neuroborreliosis with symptoms of encephalitis, myelitis, vasculitis or intracranial hypertension. *Eur J Neurol.* 2014;21(9):1162-1167.
149. Ljostad U, Henriksen TH. Management of neuroborreliosis in European adult patients. *Acta Neurol Scand Suppl.* 2008;188:22-28.

Chapter 180 :: The Rickettsioses, Ehrlichioses, and Anaplasmoses
:: Maryam Liaqat, Analisa V. Halpern, Justin J. Green, & Warren R. Heymann

第一百八十章
立克次体病、埃氏立克次体病和无浆体病

中文导读

本章首先介绍了"立克次体"类型，将几种非立克次体病原体也纳入本章对立克次体疾病的讨论中。根据共同的遗传学、免疫学模式和细胞内生长特征，立克次体分为斑点热群和斑疹伤寒群。斑点热群立克次体完全生活在细胞质内，可引起洛山矶斑疹热、地中海斑点热和非洲蜱叮咬热、立克次体痘；斑疹伤寒组生活在细胞质或细胞核内，可引起地方性伤寒、流行性斑疹伤寒、恙虫病、埃氏立克次体病等。随后介绍了这些疾病的流行病学、病因与发病机制、临床特征、实验室检查、诊断与鉴别诊断、治疗与预防。重点提到了立克次体主要通过蜱虫叮咬传播，在哺乳动物宿主中引起发热性疾病和皮疹。发热、头痛、肌痛和不适是立克次体、埃氏立克次体和无浆体感染的常见症状；皮疹在立克次体疾病中常见，在埃氏立克次体感染中偶见，在无浆体病中很少见。感染的早期迹象和症状通常是非特异性的，可以模仿自限性病毒疾病或其他危及生命的疾病。高度可疑病例应考虑早期经验性使用多西环素，直到明确排除立克次体感染为止，因为延迟治疗会导致严重的后遗症和高死亡率。

〔粟 娟〕

AT-A-GLANCE

- *Rickettsiae* primarily target vascular endothelial cells, causing febrile illness and rash in the mammalian host.
- Transmission is predominantly via tick bites, with certain pathogens transmitted by human body lice and mites.
- Fever, headache, myalgia, and malaise are common to rickettsial, ehrlichial, and *Anaplasma* infections; rash is common in rickettsial disease, occasional in ehrlichial infection, and rare in anaplasmosis.
- The early signs and symptoms of infection are often nonspecific and can mimic self-limited viral illnesses or other life-threatening illnesses.
- Early empiric treatment with doxycycline should be considered in highly suspicious cases until rickettsial infection is definitively ruled out, as delayed treatment can lead to severe sequelae and high mortality rates.

Rickettsial diseases are curable infections that, if unrecognized, can be readily lethal. Early nonspecific symptoms can mimic benign viral illnesses and should be considered in any patient who presents with constitutional symptoms, fever, headache, and a characteristic petechial rash. The advent of modern molecular technologies, including genetic analysis, has allowed for significant taxonomic reclassification of the rickettsiae, including moving the family *Bartonella* (see Chap. 154) and the genus *Coxiella* out of the order Rickettsiales to the orders Rhizobiales (*Bartonella*) and Legionellales (*Coxiella*). "Rickettsiae" now includes a polyphyletic group of microorganisms in the class Proteobacteria, comprising species belonging to the genera *Rickettsia, Orientia, Ehrlichia, Anaplasma,* and *Neorickettsia*. Several nonrickettsial agents that were historically included in the group of infections loosely termed the *rickettsioses* remain incorporated in the discussion of rickettsial disease herein to reflect that precedent.[1]

Historically rickettsiae and *Rickettsia*-like organisms (eg, *Coxiella burnetii*) were endemic pathogens; the rise of international travel, however, has allowed for the spread of rickettsial infections to nonendemic areas.

ETIOLOGY AND PATHOGENESIS OF SPOTTED FEVER AND TYPHUS GROUPS

Rickettsiae are obligate, intracellular, Gram-negative bacteria. They are pleomorphic 0.3 to 1 μm coccobacilli composed of DNA and RNA and reproduce through binary fission. Rickettsiae are propagated by arthropod vectors that use mammals (and sometimes the arthropods themselves) as reservoirs of infection. Rickettsiae are separated into the spotted fever group and the typhus group on the basis of common genetics, immunologic patterns, and intracellular growth characteristics. The typhus group lives entirely within the cell cytoplasm, whereas the spotted fever group can reside within the cytoplasm or nucleus. Rickettsiae are differentiated by unique antigenic structures on cell surface proteins. *Rickettsia rickettsii* has 2 major surface proteins, outer membrane protein A (OmpA) and outer membrane protein B (OmpB), which are the main targets for serologic testing. Additionally, Sca1 and Sca2 are autotransporter proteins that play a role in actin-based mobility and induction of phagocytosis of host cells.

Infection occurs through arthropod-induced breaks in the skin allowing access of the pathogen to the blood and lymph. Spotted fever rickettsiae are injected into the host through the saliva of the feeding tick, whereas typhus group rickettsiae enter through the feces of infected human body lice or fleas. Manipulation of the bite site, a long attachment of the arthropod, and exposure to arthropod hemolymph during tick removal aid in the transmission of pathogenic organisms. The rickettsial organisms then spread via the hematogenous and lymphatic systems, attach to endothelial cell membranes, and are phagocytosed. Spotted fever group rickettsiae stimulate host cells to produce reactive oxygen species and cause actin polymerization that aid in bacterial extrusion. In contrast, typhus group rickettsiae replicate intracellularly until the host cell bursts.[2] The severe clinical manifestations of rickettsial infection (eg, hypovolemia, purpura, pulmonary and cerebral edema) are caused by proliferation of bacteria within the vascular endothelium resulting in a multifocal, systemic vasculitis and microvascular leakage.[3]

SPOTTED FEVER GROUP

ROCKY MOUNTAIN SPOTTED FEVER

Rocky Mountain Spotted Fever (RMSF) was first recognized in 1896 in the Snake River Valley of Idaho and was originally called *black measles* because of the characteristic appearance of the rash. Caused by the tick-borne *R. rickettsii*, it is the most frequently reported rickettsial infection in the United States. Incidence has increased from less than 2 cases per million persons in 2000 to over 11 cases per million in 2014.[4] However, according to the Centers for Disease Control and Prevention, associated mortality has declined to less than 0.5%.[5]

EPIDEMIOLOGY

The vector largely responsible for RMSF in the eastern two-thirds of the United States is the American dog tick, *Dermacentor variabilis*. Rocky Mountain wood tick, *Dermacentor andersoni*, is prevalent in the Western United States and *Rhipicephalus sanguineus*, in Mexico and Arizona (Fig. 180-1). RMSF is most prevalent in the Southeastern and South Central states, during spring and early summer. Surveillance data in the United States during 2008-2012 demonstrates highest incidence in persons 60 to 69 years of age; the highest case-fatality rate, however, is among children younger than age 10 years.[6] Table 180-1 outlines the principal epidemiologic characteristics of RMSF.

CLINICAL AND LABORATORY FINDINGS

A high index of suspicion is important to the diagnosis of RMSF. One or 2 classic symptoms, as outlined

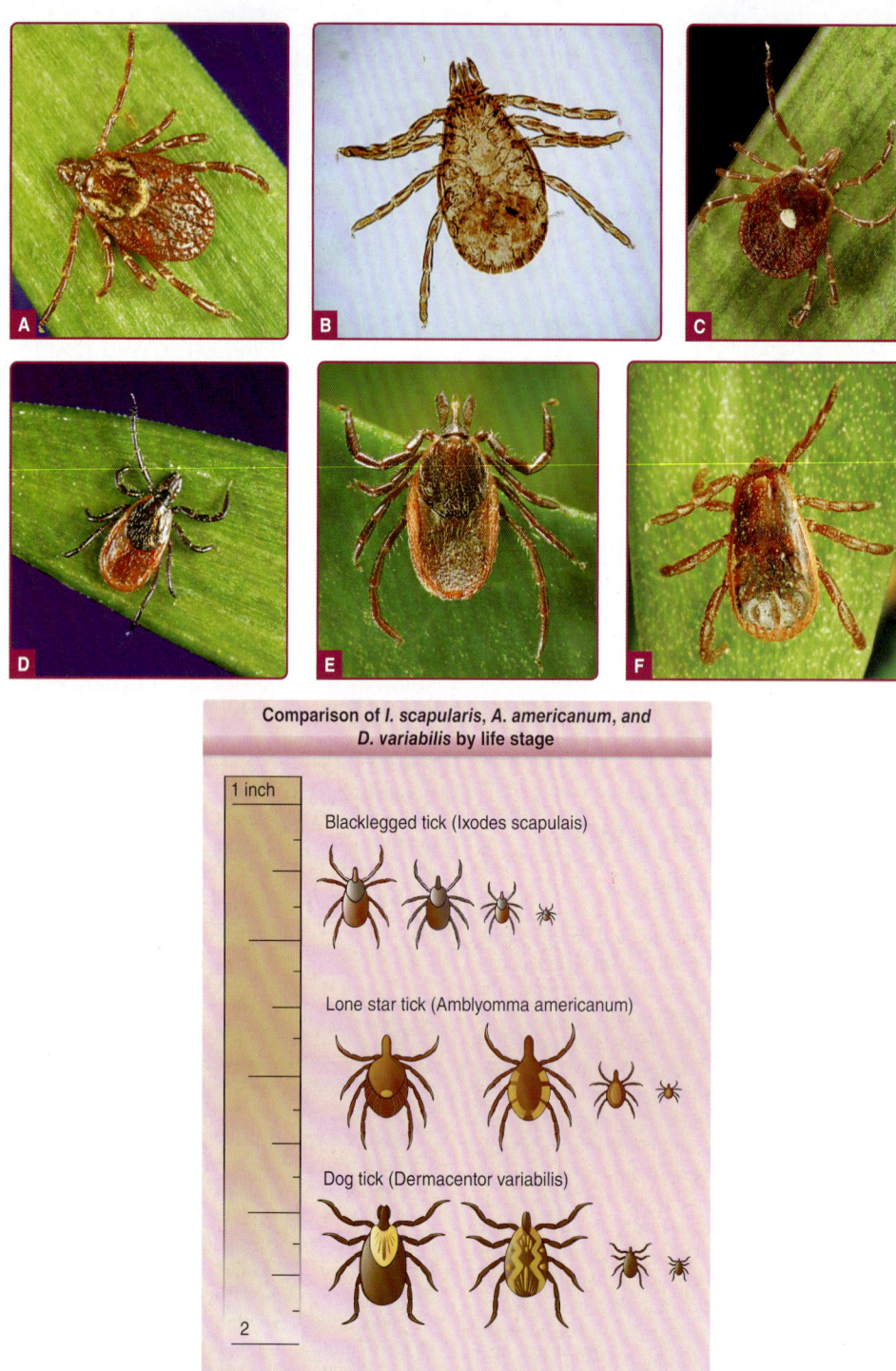

Figure 180-1 Tick species responsible for transmission of rickettsia, ehrlichia, and anaplasma. **A,** *Dermacentor variabilis*. **B,** *Dermacentor andersoni*. **C,** *Amblyomma americanum*. **D,** *Ixodes scapularis*. **E,** *Ixodes pacificus*. **F,** *Rhipicephalus sanguineus*. **G,** Comparison of *I. scapularis*, *A. americanum*, and *D. variabilis* by life stage. (From the Centers for Disease Control and Prevention. https://www.cdc.gov/ticks/tickbornediseases/tickID.html.)

TABLE 180-1
Epidemiologic Features, Prognosis, and Treatment of *Rickettsia*, *Ehrlichia*, and *Anaplasma* Infection

DISEASE (AGENT)	PRIMARY VECTOR(S)	EPIDEMIOLOGY	INCUBATION PERIOD	RISK FACTORS[a]	PROGNOSIS	FIRST-LINE TREATMENT	SECOND-LINE TREATMENTS
Rocky Mountain spotted fever (*Rickettsia rickettsii*)	*Dermacentor variabilis* (American dog tick), *Dermacentor andersoni* (Rocky Mountain wood tick), *Amblyomma americanum* (lone star tick), *Rhipicephalus sanguineus* (brown dog tick), *Amblyomma cajennense* (Central and South America), *Haemaphysalis leporispalustris* ticks	Widespread in the United States, concentrated in South Atlantic and South-Central states; Argentina, Brazil, Columbia, Costa Rica, Mexico, Panama, Canada Spring–Summer	2 to 14 days	Males; adults 40 to 64 years of age, children <10 years of age; rural dwelling	Severe disease: glucose-6-phosphate dehydrogenase (G6PD) deficiency (rapid decompensation, fulminant disease with higher incidence of necrosis), males, elderly, neurologic disease, hepatitis, jaundice, thrombocytopenia, acute renal failure, sulfa medications, delayed diagnosis and treatment	Adults[b]: doxycycline 100 mg by mouth q12h × 5 to 10 days Children[c]: doxycycline 2.2 mg/kg by mouth q12h × 5 to 10 days Pregnancy[c]: doxycycline 100 mg by mouth q12h for 5 to 10 days	Adults: chloramphenicol, 50 to 75 mg/kg by mouth q6h × 5 to 10 days or tetracycline 500 mg by mouth q6h × 5 to 10 days Children: chloramphenicol, 12.5 to 25 mg/kg by mouth q6h × 5 to 10 days Pregnancy[d]: chloramphenicol
Mediterranean spotted fever (*Rickettsia conorii*)	*Rhipicephalus sanguineus* (brown dog tick)	Endemic to Southern Europe, Middle East, Southwest Asia, India, and Africa Summer	5 to 7 days	Exposure to dogs	Mild disease (mainly in children) has good prognosis. Severe disease "malignant Mediterranean spotted fever: alcoholics, elderly, G6PD deficiency, diabetes mellitus, heart disease, delayed diagnosis and treatment	Adults: doxycycline 200 mg by mouth q12h × 1 day or 100 mg by mouth q12h for 2 to 5 days Children[c]: doxycycline 2.2 mg/kg by mouth q12h × 5 to 10 days Pregnancy: azithromycin 500 mg by mouth daily × 3 days	Adults: tetracycline 500 mg by mouth q6h × 10 days or ciprofloxacin 750 mg q12h for 8 days Children: clarithromycin, 15 mg/kg/day divided q12h for 7 days or azithromycin, 10 mg/kg/day daily × 3 days Pregnancy[d]: chloramphenicol
Rickettsialpox (*Rickettsia akari*)	*Liponyssoides sanguineus* (*Allodermanyssus sanguineus*) (house mouse, *Mus musculus*, mite)	United States (mainly eastern seaboard), South Africa, Korea, Ukraine, Croatia Sporadic	~7 days (eschar), ~7 to 24 days (systemic symptoms and rash)	Males; urban dwellers (likely from mice exposure); IV drug users	Excellent	Self-limiting	Doxycycline can be used for severe cases

TABLE 180-1
Epidemiologic Features, Prognosis, and Treatment of *Rickettsia*, *Ehrlichia*, and *Anaplasma* Infection (Continued)

DISEASE (AGENT)	PRIMARY VECTOR(S)	EPIDEMIOLOGY	INCUBATION PERIOD	RISK FACTORS[a]	PROGNOSIS	FIRST-LINE TREATMENT	SECOND-LINE TREATMENTS
Endemic typhus (*Rickettsia typhi*; *Rickettsia felis*)	*Xenopsylla cheopis* (rat flea), *Ctenocephalides felis* (cat flea)	Southeast United States, Gulf region, Southern California; worldwide most cases in Africa (reported on all continents except Antarctica) Summer	1 to 2 weeks (~12 days)	Exposure to fleas, poverty, poor hygiene	Excellent prognosis with treatment. Complicated disease occurs with alcoholism, elderly, hematologic disorders, and exposure to sulfa-containing drugs	Adults: doxycycline 100 mg by mouth q12h for 7 to 14 days Children[c]: doxycycline 2.2 mg/kg by mouth q12h × 5 to 10 days Pregnancy[c,d]: chloramphenicol or doxycycline	Adults: chloramphenicol, 80 to 100 mg/kg/day by mouth divided q6h Children: chloramphenicol, 12.5 to 25 mg/kg by mouth q6h for 5 to 10 days Pregnancy: azithromycin
Epidemic typhus (*Rickettsia prowazekii*)	*Pediculus humanus* var. *corporis* (human body louse), *Neohaematopinus sciuropteri* lice, *Orchopeas howardi* fleas	United States, Eastern Europe, Africa, Central and South America, China, Himalayan region Sporadic (increased in winter)	~1 to 2 weeks (average: 8 days)	Wartime, poor hygiene, natural disasters, cold weather	Good prognosis with treatment. Fever abates in 2 weeks without treatment and in 48 hours with treatment. Recovery of strength in 2 to 3 months	Adults[e]: doxycycline 200 mg single dose (or until afebrile for 24 hours) Children[c]: doxycycline 2.2 mg/kg by mouth q12h × 5 to 10 days Pregnancy[c,d]: chloramphenicol or doxycycline	Adults: chloramphenicol, 80 to 100 mg/kg/day by mouth divided q6h Children: chloramphenicol, 12.5 to 25 mg/kg by mouth q6h for 5 to 10 days Pregnancy: azithromycin
Human monocytic ehrlichiosis (*Ehrlichia chaffeensis*)	*Amblyomma americanum* (lone star tick), *Dermacentor variabilis* (American dog tick), *Ixodes pacificus* ticks	South and Mid-Atlantic, North-/South-Central United States, isolated areas of New England[f] Spring and summer (peak in May to July)	5 to 14 days	Males; adults older than age 70 years	Poor prognosis: immunosuppression (HIV, transplantation, glucocorticoids); cough, lymphadenopathy, diarrhea; use of trimethoprim-sulfamethoxazole	Adults: doxycycline 100 mg by mouth q12h for 5 to 14 days Children[c]: doxycycline 2.2 mg/kg by mouth q12h × 5 to 14 days Pregnancy[c]: doxycycline 100 mg by mouth q12h for 5 to 14 days	Adults: tetracycline 500 mg by mouth q6h × 5 to 14 days or Rifampin 300 mg by mouth q12h × 7 to 10 days Children: tetracycline 25 to 50 mg/kg/day by mouth divided q6h × 5 to 14 days or Rifampin 10 mg/kg by mouth q12h × 7 to 10 days Pregnancy: rifampin 300 mg by mouth q12h × 7 to 10 days

(Continued)

| Human granulocytic anaplasmosis (*Anaplasma phagocytophilum*) | *Ixodes scapularis* (Eastern United States) and *Ixodes pacificus* (Western United States), *Ixodes ricinus* (Europe) (black-legged ticks) | New England, upper Midwest Mid-Atlantic, and northern California in United States and Europe[g] Spring and summer (peaks in July and November) | 5 to 21 days | Males; adults 60 to 69 years of age | Poor prognosis: elderly, marked lymphopenia, anemia, immunosuppression (HIV, transplantation, glucocorticoids); development of opportunistic infections (eg, aspergillosis, disseminated candidiasis) | Adults[b]: doxycycline 100 mg by mouth q12h for 5 to 14 days Children[c,h]: doxycycline 2.2 mg/kg by mouth q12h × 5 to 14 days Pregnancy[c,h]: doxycycline 100 mg by mouth q12h for 5 to 14 days | Adults: tetracycline 500 mg by mouth q6h × 5 to 14 days *or* rifampin 300 mg by mouth q12h × 7 to 10 days Children: tetracycline 25 to 50 mg/kg/day by mouth divided q6h × 5 to 14 days *or* rifampin 10 mg/kg by mouth q12h × 7 to 10 days Pregnancy: rifampin 300 mg by mouth q12h × 7 to 10 days |

Children are defined as persons who weigh less than 45 kg (99 lbs). The maximum daily dose for tetracycline is 2 g and for chloramphenicol it is 4 g.

[a]Males appear to be at higher risk of all tick-borne rickettsial diseases, presumably because of greater recreational and occupational exposure. Disease occurs in all age groups; numbers reflect highest age-specific incidence.
[b]Treat for 3 days after fever subsides and until clinical improvement is noted, typically for a minimum of 5 to 7 days. More-severe illness may require longer duration of therapy.
[c]In severe, life-threatening cases, or when Rocky Mountain spotted fever cannot be ruled out, doxycycline should be considered first-line therapy for individuals of any age and during pregnancy.
[d]Use with caution in the third trimester of pregnancy as chloramphenicol may cause gray baby syndrome in neonates (abdominal distension, pallor, cyanosis, vasomotor collapse). Doxycycline should be considered in near-term gravidas.
[e]For recrudescent disease (Brill-Zinsser), a second course of antibiotics is usually curative.
[f]In 2016, four states (Missouri, Arkansas, New York, and Virginia) accounted for 50% of all reported cases of ehrlichiosis.
[g]In 2016, eight states (Vermont, Maine, Rhode Island, Minnesota, Massachusetts, Wisconsin, New Hampshire, and New York) account for 90% of all reported cases of anaplasmosis.
[h]Treatment is extended to treat potential coinfection with Lyme disease.

Data from Parola P, Paddock CD, Raoult D. Tick-borne rickettsioses around the world: emerging diseases challenging old concepts. *Clin Microbiol Rev.* 2005;18:719; and Dana AN. Diagnosis and treatment of tick infestation and tick-borne diseases with cutaneous manifestations. *Dermatol Ther.* 2009;22:293-326.

TABLE 180-2
Clinical and Diagnostic Findings in Rocky Mountain Spotted Fever, Human Monocytic Ehrlichiosis, and Human Granulocytic Anaplasmosis

	ROCKY MOUNTAIN SPOTTED FEVER	HUMAN MONOCYTIC EHRLICHIOSIS	HUMAN GRANULOCYTIC ANAPLASMOSIS
Tropism	- Endothelial cells	- Monocytes	- Granulocytes
Common initial signs and symptoms	- Fever to 38.9°C (102°F), chills, malaise, myalgia, nausea, vomiting, anorexia, headache - Periorbital edema, abdominal pain mimicking appendicitis (children > adults), conjunctival injection, palatal petechiae, edema of dorsal hands, calf pain	- Fever, chills, headache, malaise, myalgia, nausea, vomiting, anorexia, photophobia - Abdominal pain mimicking appendicitis (children > adults), conjunctival injection, palatal petechiae, edema of dorsal hands, calf pain	- Malaise, fever, myalgia, headache - Less common: arthralgia, nausea, vomiting, diarrhea, cough
Rash	- Erythematous blanching macules and/or papules 2 to 4 days after fever onset; starts at wrists/ankles and spreads centripetally; may involve palms, soles; rash evolves over a few days to petechial and purpuric lesions	- Erythematous macules and/or papules, petechiae, or diffuse erythema approximately 5 days after onset of systemic symptoms	- Rare
Common laboratory abnormalities	- Common: thrombocytopenia, anemia, mild hyponatremia - Variably elevated: liver transaminases, lactate dehydrogenase, creatine kinase, bilirubin, alkaline phosphatase, blood urea nitrogen, creatinine - Cerebrospinal fluid: leukocytosis, moderately elevated protein, and a normal glucose level	- Leukopenia, lymphopenia, thrombocytopenia, transaminitis, and anemia	- Thrombocytopenia, transaminitis, leukopenia, anemia, elevated creatinine - Neutropenia is more common than lymphopenia
Systemic sequelae	- Cardiovascular: hypotension, hypovolemia, peripheral edema, inappropriate tachycardia, myocarditis, arrhythmias - GI: bleeding, perforation, hepatomegaly, jaundice - Neurologic: confusion, delirium, stupor, meningismus, coma, motor deficits, cranial nerve palsy, deafness, photophobia, hallucinations, seizures, Guillain-Barré syndrome - Other: conjunctivitis, acute renal failure, adult respiratory distress syndrome	- Respiratory: cough, dyspnea, respiratory insufficiency/adult respiratory distress syndrome - Neurologic: Meningoencephalitis, altered mental status, cranial or peripheral motor nerve paralysis, sudden transient deafness - Other: acute renal failure, disseminated intravascular coagulation, and pericarditis	- General: septic or toxic shock–like syndrome (see Chap. 172), coagulopathy, disseminated intravascular coagulation (see Chap. 140), rhabdomyolysis, pancreatitis - Respiratory: adult respiratory distress syndrome - Neurologic: brachial plexopathy, demyelinating polyneuropathy, cranial nerve paralysis - Other: acute abdominal syndrome, myocarditis, acute renal failure, hemorrhage, opportunistic infections

in Table 180-2, may be seen at presentation, but only approximately 60% of patients will have the complete clinical triad of fever (>39.5°C [102°F]), headache, and rash. Fever usually presents within the first 3 days of the illness, followed by a characteristic rash 2 to 4 days after the onset of fever. The rash usually starts on the wrists and ankles, spreading centripetally over the next 6 to 18 hours. Palms and soles are typically involved with relative sparing of the face.[6] Cutaneous lesions are initially blanchable red macules that become papular and display evidence of petechiae or purpura (Fig. 180-2). Atypical "spotless" fever, seen in approximately 20% of cases does not imply milder disease, and is more common in the elderly and darker-skinned individuals.[3] Periorbital edema, confusion, abdominal pain mimicking an acute abdomen, conjunctival injection, palatal petechiae, edema of dorsal hands, and calf pain are sometimes appreciated. Necrosis from overwhelming vasculitis is rare and preferentially occurs in peripheral locations such as the digits, penis, and scrotum (Fig. 180-3).[7] Such episodes of gangrene may ultimately require amputation.

Thrombocytopenia, anemia, mild hyponatremia, and mild transaminitis may be present. Even though the white blood cell count is typically normal, an increase in bands may be observed.[6] Severe and life-threatening cardiac, GI, hepatic, neurologic, ophthalmologic, renal, and pulmonary manifestations can occur with delayed or inadequate treatment. In patients with severe RMSF who survive the acute illness, long-term sequelae are usually the result of neurologic deficits or acral necrosis. In a case series by Buckingham and colleagues of 92 children diagnosed with RMSF, the median delay between seeking medical attention and antibiotic therapy was 6 days, with only 49% reporting a tick bite.[8] Table 180-2 outlines the cutaneous and systemic manifestations of RMSF, as well as common laboratory abnormalities.

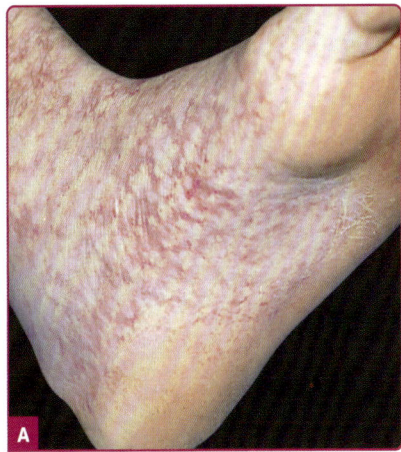
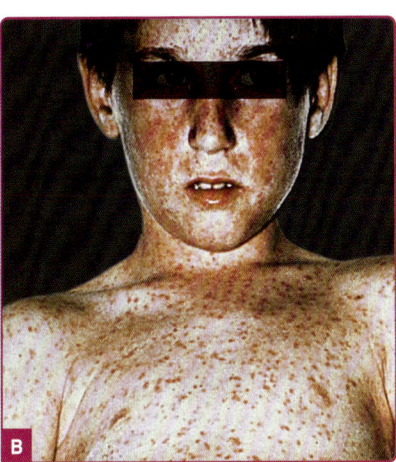
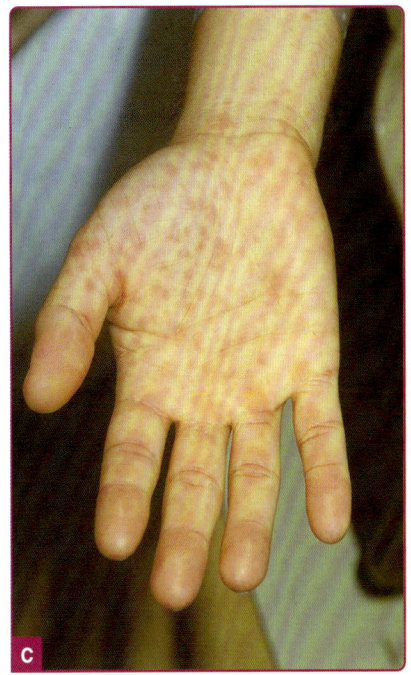
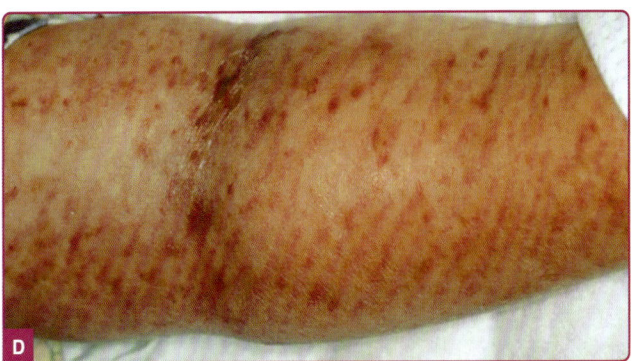

Figure 180-2 **A,** Early macular blanchable macules and papules on the ankle and sole. No truncal lesions were present at this time. **B,** Truncal and facial hemorrhagic macules and papules 7 days after the onset of the rash. **C,** Erythematous macular lesions on the palm may develop into a petechial rash that spreads centrally. **D,** Petechial lesions on the arm of a child with fulminant Rocky Mountain spotted fever. (Image C, Used with permission from Daniel Noltkamper, MD. Reprinted from Hardin JM. Cutaneous conditions. In: Knoop KJ, Stack LB, Storrow AB, et al, eds. *The Atlas of Emergency Medicine*, 4th ed. New York, NY: McGraw-Hill, 2016; Image D, Used with permission from Chapman AS, Bakken JS, Folk SM, et al; Tickborne Rickettsial Diseases Working Group; CDC. Diagnosis and management of tickborne rickettsial diseases: Rocky Mountain spotted fever, ehrlichioses, and anaplasmosis—United States: a practical guide for physicians and other health-care and public health professionals. *MMWR Recomm Rep*. 2006;55(RR-4):1-27, available at http://www.cdc.gov/mmwr/preview/mmwrhtml/rr5504a1.htm.)

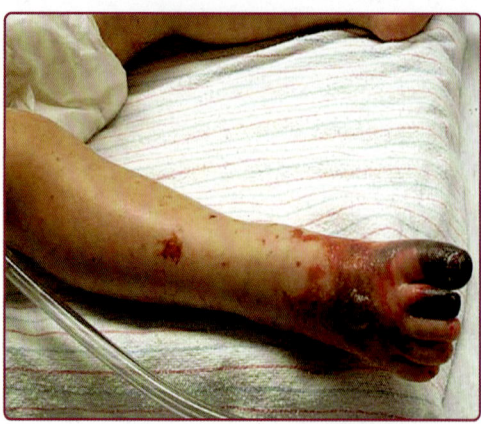

Figure 180-3 Gangrene of the toes in Rocky Mountain spotted fever. (From Chapman AS, Bakken JS, Folk SM, et al; Tickborne Rickettsial Diseases Working Group; CDC. Diagnosis and management of tickborne rickettsial diseases: Rocky Mountain spotted fever, ehrlichioses, and anaplasmosis—United States: a practical guide for physicians and other health-care and public health professionals. *MMWR Recomm Rep.* 2006;55(RR-4):1-27, Figure 18, available at http://www.cdc.gov/mmwr/preview/mmwrhtml/rr5504a1.htm. Used with permission from Gary Marshall, MD).

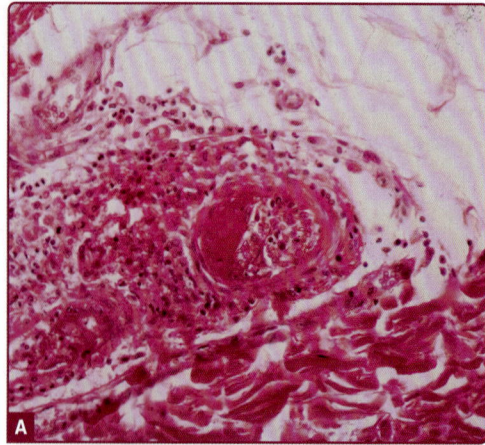

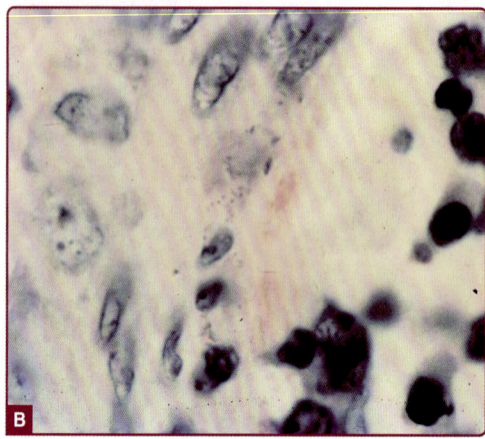

Figure 180-4 A, Vascular lesion of Rocky Mountain spotted fever as seen in an arteriole in the skin. An early thrombus is present. **B,** Rickettsiae are seen in endothelial cells from a biopsy of a cutaneous lesion.

PATHOLOGY

Histopathologic examination shows a septic vasculitis (Fig. 180-4). Early lesions demonstrate dermal edema with a predominantly perivascular lymphohistiocytic infiltrate and extravasated erythrocytes. Lymphohistiocytic vasculitis can progress to leukocytoclastic vasculitis. Basal cell vacuolization, lymphocytic exocytosis, fibrin thrombi, and capillary wall necrosis also can be appreciated. Immunohistology reveals positive staining for *R. rickettsii* in infected endothelial cells and tick hemolymph (Fig. 180-5). Most rickettsial diseases share a similar histology.

DIAGNOSIS AND DIFFERENTIAL DIAGNOSIS

Serologic examination using the indirect immunofluorescence assay (IFA) is the gold standard for diagnosis of RMSF. It detects convalescent antibodies (at a diagnostic titer of ≥64 immunoglobulin [Ig] G and ≥32 IgM) but is seldom diagnostic before the seventh day of disease, and often not until far into the second week. An effective treatment of RMSF should begin by the fifth day of illness. The causative *Rickettsia* species is not determined unless Western immunoblotting and cross-absorption with appropriately selected antigens are performed. It is vital to begin empiric therapy while awaiting serologies. Because of inferior sensitivity and specificity, the Weil-Felix test (agglutination of certain *Proteus* sp.) and complement fixation tests have been largely supplanted by newer diagnostic methods. Immunohistochemical staining of skin or organ tissue biopsy and polymerase chain reaction (PCR) may also confirm the diagnosis.[9]

When a patient presents without a rash, the differential diagnosis for RMSF is broad (Tables 180-3 and 180-4). Macules and papules, petechiae, or purpuric

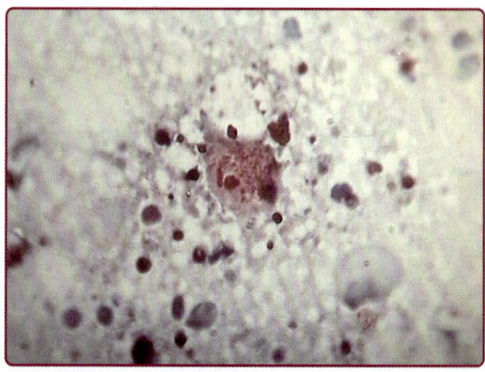

Figure 180-5 Giemsa stain of Rocky Mountain spotted fever in tick lymph cells. (From the Centers for Disease Control and Prevention. http://www.cdc.gov/ncidod/dvrd/rmsf/organism.htm.)

TABLE 180-3
Differential Diagnosis of Rickettsial and Ehrlichial Diseases
Most Likely
▪ Enteroviral infection (eg, coxsackievirus, echovirus)
▪ Roseola infantum (human herpesvirus 6)
▪ Drug eruption
▪ Group A streptococcal pharyngitis
▪ Vasculitis
▪ Kawasaki disease
▪ Measles (coryza, Koplik spots, cough)
▪ Epstein-Barr virus/infectious mononucleosis
Consider
▪ Viral meningoencephalitis
▪ *Mycoplasma pneumoniae* infection
▪ Parvovirus B19
▪ Tularemia
▪ Leptospirosis
▪ Immune complex–mediated illness
▪ Atypical erythema multiforme
▪ Typhoid fever
▪ Dengue
▪ Viral hemorrhagic fevers (Ebola, Marburg, Lassa)
Always Rule Out
▪ Meningococcemia (more rapid-onset rash and leukocytosis, but both may show gangrenous lesions)
▪ Disseminated gonococcal infection
▪ Lyme disease
▪ Tick-borne viral fevers (eg, Colorado tick fever)
▪ Thrombotic thrombocytopenic purpura and immune thrombocytopenic purpura
▪ Toxic shock syndrome
▪ Stevens-Johnson syndrome
▪ Secondary syphilis

lesions may sometimes develop in these diseases as well, further precluding the ability to distinguish them from RMSF on clinical grounds alone.

TREATMENT

Tetracyclines, specifically doxycycline, are the drugs of choice for all rickettsial diseases in patients of all ages, even during pregnancy. Although repeated exposure to tetracycline increases the risk of tooth staining, studies suggest that limited use of this antibiotic in children during the first 6 to 7 years of life has a negligible effect on the color of permanent incisors.[10] Sulfa-based medications are not recommended, as they may result in a more complicated disease course.[11]

Chloramphenicol may be used if tetracyclines are contraindicated because of allergies. Side effects include aplastic anemia, reversible bone marrow suppression, and gray baby syndrome in near-term gravidae.[12] Aggressive supportive care is crucial, with particular attention to electrolyte and fluid balance. Treatment and management strategies for RMSF are listed in Tables 180-1 and 180-5.

Fulminant RMSF leading to more rapid decompensation has characteristically been reported in chronic alcoholics and black males with glucose-6-phosphate dehydrogenase deficiency. These patients have a higher risk of cutaneous necrosis.[3] Prompt empiric administration of appropriate antibiotic therapy is recommended, as it is the most important factor affecting survival.

PREVENTION

Avoiding tick exposure, wearing protective clothing, performing tick checks regularly while in tick-infested areas, and proper tick extractions are important for lowering the risk of infection. Chemical repellants, such as diethyltoluamide (DEET) in concentrations up to 35%, are safe for use in adults and children. Prophylactic antibiotics after tick exposure are not recommended.

TICK-BITE ASSOCIATED: MEDITERRANEAN SPOTTED FEVER AND AFRICAN TICK BITE FEVER

Several other tick-borne rickettsial species are pathogenic to humans. Mediterranean spotted fever (MSF), also known as *Boutonneuse fever* or *Marseille fever*, caused by *Rickettsia conorii*, was first documented as a cause of human rickettsial disease is 1932. MSF is the prototypical illness of the non-RMSF spotted fever group. African tick bite fever (ATBF), caused by *Rickettsia africae*, is a distinct clinical entity.

EPIDEMIOLOGY

R. conorii is transmitted by an infected *R. sanguineus* tick (see Fig. 180-1) and is endemic throughout Africa, the Middle East, South Asia, and Eastern Europe. Contact with dogs is reported in up to 90% of cases of MSF. Table 180-1 summarizes the epidemiologic characteristics of MSF. *R. africae* is transmitted by an infected *Amblyomma* tick endemic to sub-Saharan Africa.

CLINICAL AND LABORATORY FINDINGS

The constitutional symptoms, systemic complications, and laboratory abnormalities of the tick-bite–associated spotted fevers are similar to those of RMSF. The classic cutaneous hallmark of this group is the tache noir, occurring in approximately 13% to 68% of patients with *R. conorii* infection (Fig. 180-6A).[13] The tache noir occurs at the site of inoculation as an erythematous, indurated papule with a central necrotic eschar that represents locally aggressive endothelial invasion by rickettsiae. Temporal and morphologic pattern of the rash in this group of spotted fevers is similar to RMSF;

TABLE 180-4
Selected Differential Diagnosis of Fever and Erythematous or Petechial Rash

DISEASE	AGENT	SEASON	ONSET	CLINICAL FEATURES
Rocky Mountain spotted fever	Rickettsia rickettsii	Spring to summer	Fever, headache, malaise, GI symptoms, rash after 2 to 4 days; rapid progression to severe systemic illness	Rash starting on ankles/wrists, spreads centripetally, may involve palms/soles, progresses from erythematous macules to petechiae
Endemic (murine) typhus	Rickettsia typhi	Sporadic	Fever, malaise, headache, rash after 4 to 5 days	Erythematous macules and/or papules involving trunk > extremities
Human monocytic ehrlichiosis	Ehrlichia chaffeensis	Spring to summer	Fever malaise, headache, rash in ~30% of patients	Erythematous macules and/or papules, or petechial rash; more common in children > adults
Meningococcal disease	Neisseria meningitidis	Year-round, but more common late winter to early spring	Fever and rash within 24 h, rapid progression to severe systemic illness	Erythematous macules and/or papules, petechiae usually beginning on lower extremities and spreading centripetally; toxic appearing
Group A streptococcal pharyngitis	Streptococcus pyogenes	Fall to winter	Abrupt onset of fever and sore throat, malaise; rash follows acute illness	May cause petechial rash in children who appear well
Fifth disease (erythema infectiosum)	Human parvovirus B19	Late winter to early summer	Low fever and mild constitutional signs before rash onset	"Slapped cheek"–appearing erythematous rash on face, lacy erythematous rash on trunk; papular-purpuric gloves-and-socks syndrome—young adults
Roseola infantum	Human herpesvirus 6	Year-round	Fever for 3 to 5 days, then rash; commonly in children <2 years of age	Morbilliform rash begins on trunk, spreads and fades rapidly
Enteroviral infection	Echovirus, coxsackie viruses, other non-polio enteroviruses	Summer to early fall most commonly, but occurs year-round	Nonspecific febrile illness, with or without rash	Fine morbilliform rash at fever onset; begins on face and spreads caudally; occasionally petechial

Adapted from Chapman AS, Bakken JS, Folk SM, et al; Tickborne Rickettsial Diseases Working Group; CDC. Diagnosis and management of tickborne rickettsial diseases: Rocky Mountain spotted fever, ehrlichioses, and anaplasmosis—United States: a practical guide for physicians and other health-care and public health professionals. *MMWR Recomm Rep.* 2006;55(RR-4):1-27, available at http://www.cdc.gov/mmwr/preview/mmwrhtml/rr5504a1.htm.

however, the eruption may be more diffuse and is less frequently petechial or purpuric (Fig. 180-6B). The presence of multiple tick bites, multiple eschars (seen in 50% of patients with ATBF), and lymphadenitis, distinguish ATBF from MSF,[1] although children with MSF may have cervical lymphadenopathy.[13]

TABLE 180-5
Management of Rickettsial, Ehrlichial, and *Anaplasma* Infections

- Delays in treatment can lead to severe sequelae and fatal outcome.
- Clinical history, symptoms, physical examination, and laboratory findings should guide approach to management and treatment.
- Clinicians may consider a "watch-and-wait" approach for 24 to 48 hours for patients early in the course of illness who have nonsupporting history, nonspecific clinical signs, and normal laboratory findings.
- Doxycycline is the drug of choice for the treatment of presumptive or confirmed rickettsial disease in both adults and children.
- Limited courses of tetracycline-class antibiotics (eg, doxycycline) do not pose a substantial threat of tooth staining in children.
- Tetracyclines are typically contraindicated in pregnancy but are warranted in life-threatening cases of Rocky Mountain spotted fever when clinical suspicion arises.
- When early invasive meningococcal infection cannot be ruled out, antibiotics for *Neisseria meningitides* must be started.
- Prophylactic use of antibiotics after a tick bite is not recommended, as atypical presentations may result, delaying adequate diagnosis and treatment. If prophylaxis is given, a full 10-day course should be administered.
- In patients for whom tetracyclines are absolutely contraindicated, chloramphenicol can be used for rickettsial disease; rifampin or rifabutin may be considered for the ehrlichioses/anaplasmosis.
- When treating ehrlichial infections, consider continuation for 14 to 21 days to allow for adequate treatment of concomitant Lyme disease in areas endemic for *Borrelia burgdorferi*.

Adapted from Chapman AS, Bakken JS, Folk SM, et al; Tickborne Rickettsial Diseases Working Group; CDC. Diagnosis and management of tickborne rickettsial diseases: Rocky Mountain spotted fever, ehrlichioses, and anaplasmosis—United States: a practical guide for physicians and other health-care and public health professionals. *MMWR Recomm Rep.* 2006;55(RR-4):1-27, available at http://www.cdc.gov/mmwr/preview/mmwrhtml/rr5504a1.htm.

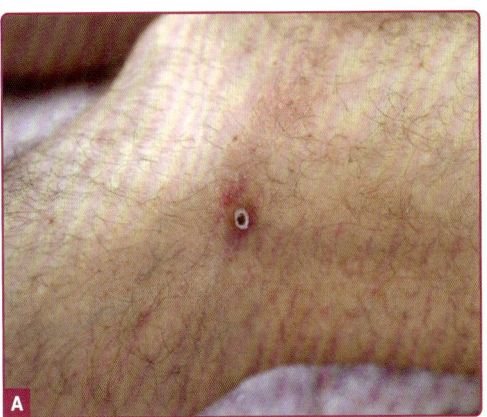 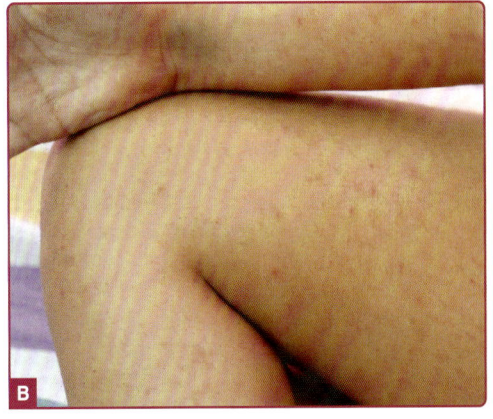

Figure 180-6 **A,** Mediterranean spotted fever. Tache noire with eschar at the site of the mite bite. **B,** Multiple disseminated red papules in the same patient. (Used with permission from VisualDx. Copyright Logical Images, Inc.)

DIAGNOSIS AND DIFFERENTIAL DIAGNOSIS

Like RMSF, diagnosis of MSF or ATBF is by IFA. Biopsy from an eschar for immunohistochemistry is particularly sensitive in MSF. PCR or Western blot analysis can be used to differentiate between *R. conorii* and *R. africae*. The addition of shell-vial culture along with real-time PCR is purported to improve diagnosis of MSF.[14] Newer serologic assays and PCR have been useful in identifying the numerous emerging agents of spotted fever around the globe, including *Rickettsia japonica* (Japanese spotted fever) and *Rickettsia slovaca*.[1] *R. slovaca*, along with *Rickettsia raoultii* are associated with TIBOLA/DEBONEL (tick-borne lymphadenopathy/*Dermacentor*-borne necrosis erythema and lymphadenopathy), a recently recognized rickettsial disease associated with eschar formation at the tick-bite site and painful lymphadenopathy. TIBOLA/DEBONEL is usually seen in the pediatric population with tick-bites involving the scalp.[15]

The rash of MSF generates a similar differential diagnosis as that of RMSF. If a tache noir is seen, one must also consider brown recluse spider bite, cutaneous anthrax, scrub typhus, rickettsialpox, aspergillosis, or mucormycosis.

TREATMENT

Table 180-1 outlines the guidelines for treatment of MSF. Overall, non-RMSF spotted fevers run a less-aggressive course than RMSF. However, MSF has been reported to cause severe cardiac, renal, and neurologic complications, as well as death in approximately 1% of cases.[13] In general, all non-RMSF spotted fevers are treated similarly to MSF. Even though macrolide antibiotics may offer a better risk-to-benefit ratio than tetracyclines in the pediatric age group, doxycycline is still first-line therapy.[16]

MITE-BITE ASSOCIATED: RICKETTSIALPOX

Rickettsialpox is an acute, self-limited, febrile disease so named because of its clinical resemblance to varicella (chickenpox). Its etiologic agent is *Rickettsia akari*. *Mus musculus*, the house mouse, is the reservoir, and the vector is the rodent mite, *Liponyssoides sanguineus* (formerly *Allodermanyssus sanguineus*).[17] The colorless rodent mite inflicts a painless bite and is too small to be readily recognized by the victim.

EPIDEMIOLOGY

Most cases of rickettsialpox in the United States have occurred in large metropolitan areas of the Northeastern United States. Anthrax attacked raised attention of physicians to skin eschars and rash and allowed the identification of 34 cases of rickettsialpox in New York City between 2001 and 2002.[18] Table 180-1 describes the salient epidemiologic features of rickettsialpox.

CLINICAL AND LABORATORY FINDINGS

A primary lesion occurs at the site of the mite bite as early as 1 to 2 days after transmission. It consists of a painless, erythematous, indurated papule ranging in size from 0.5 to 3 cm. Vesicle formation is followed by desiccation, which produces an eschar to form the characteristic tache noir (Fig. 180-7). Regional lymphadenopathy is common. Resolution of the primary lesion occurs within 1 month.

Approximately 7 days after the primary lesion appears, fever, chills, diaphoresis, myalgia (often manifesting as backache), malaise, and headache begin. The fever persists with remissions for approximately 1 week before abating. Two to 3 days after the onset of systemic symptoms, a generalized papulovesicular eruption occurs (see Fig. 180-7B). Small vesicles or pustules appear with subsequent central crust formation. Roughly 5 to 40 lesions may be found, typically resolving in 1 week. Less frequently, an enanthem characterized by small erosions on the tongue, palate and pharynx, photophobia, generalized lymphadenopathy, and GI symptoms may be noted. Thrombocytopenia is common during the acute febrile illness, and a mild leukopenia with a relative lymphocytosis may be seen.

PATHOLOGY

In contrast to RMSF, MSF, ATBF, and typhus group Rickettsioses, the perivascular macrophage, not the endothelial cell, appears to be the target of *R. akari*. Primary lesions are characterized by extensive necrosis and an acute inflammatory infiltrate. Secondary papulovesicular lesions display a subepidermal split with superficial edema, and a perivascular lymphohistiocytic infiltrate that can become vasculitic.

DIAGNOSIS AND DIFFERENTIAL DIAGNOSIS

Antibody titers peak after 3 to 4 weeks and could be delayed for up to 8 weeks with antibiotic use. Biopsy for direct immunofluorescence with anti–*R. rickettsii* immunoglobulin is highly sensitive; however, because of cross-reactivity among the spotted fever group rickettsiae, confirmatory cross-adsorption testing may be considered with *R. akari* and *R. rickettsii* antigens. The preferred method to identify the organism is by swabbing eschar or vesicles of patients with rickettsioses allowing DNA detection by PCR. The use of multiplex real-time PCR offers greater sensitivity than nested PCR assays to distinguish various rickettsial species.[19]

The differential diagnosis includes varicella, smallpox, gonococcemia, infectious mononucleosis, echovirus (Types 9 and 16), and coxsackievirus infection (A9, A16, and B5), in addition to those diseases discussed under the differential diagnosis of MSF. In varicella, one observes a "dewdrop on a rose petal," referring to a primarily vesicular lesion surrounded by macular erythema. This is distinct from the erythematous papule surmounted by a vesicle seen with rickettsialpox.[17] Fever occurs with the rash of varicella but precedes the eruption of rickettsialpox.

TREATMENT

Rickettsialpox is self-limited. Even without antibiotics, it will resolve within 2 weeks. In the rare severe case, tetracycline antibiotics continued for up to 5 days are the most effective therapy; defervescence is typical within 48 hours.[17]

TYPHUS GROUP

ENDEMIC TYPHUS (MURINE OR FLEA-BORNE TYPHUS)

Endemic typhus is caused mainly by *Rickettsia typhi*, and is classically transmitted to humans by the rat flea (*Xenopsylla cheopis*), with rats serving as the reservoir. *Rickettsia felis* has emerged as an important agent of endemic typhus with characteristics of both the typhus and spotted fever group rickettsiae. *R. felis* has been identified in peridomestic cats, dogs, opossums, and their fleas (eg, cat flea, *Ctenocephalides felis*) in parts of southern Texas, southern California, and Mexico.[20,21]

EPIDEMIOLOGY

Murine typhus has been reported from all continents except Antarctica, although most cases today occur in

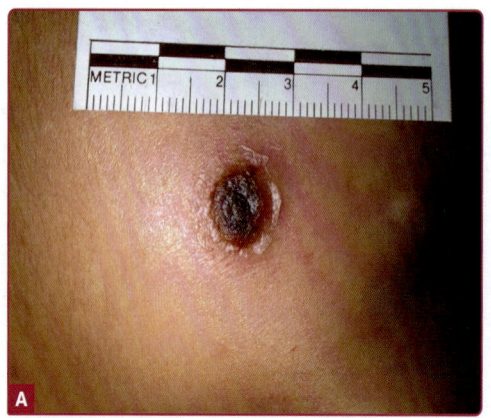 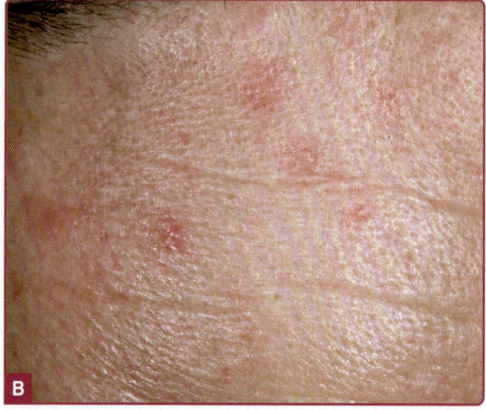

Figure 180-7 **A,** Rickettsialpox: tache noir. A crusted, ulcerated lesion with eschar and a faint red halo at the site of the mite bite. **B,** Mediterranean spotted fever: 32-year-old white male with eschar on thigh, followed by fever, and erythematous papules and small pustules. (Used with permission from VisualDx. Copyright Logical Images, Inc.)

Africa. It is most likely underdiagnosed and mistaken for a viral illness because flea bites are not usually recalled and most cases are self-limited.[22] Table 180-1 outlines the epidemiologic characteristics of murine typhus.

CLINICAL AND LABORATORY FINDINGS

Most infected persons experience fever, headache, backache, and joint pain 6 to 14 days after contact with an infected flea. Nonspecific GI symptoms may be present, especially in children.[23] Extremely high fever, 41.1°C (106°F), may last up to 2 weeks. Commonly, a rash begins on the chest and spreads to the sides and back. The palms and soles are rarely involved. The rash may last only a few hours and consists of erythematous macules and/or papules. Petechiae are found infrequently. Rash is seen in less than 20% of patients at presentation. Fifty percent to 60% of patients will develop a rash over the course of the illness, with a median onset of 6 days after the onset of fever.[20] More-severe complications are uncommon but may include seizures, meningoencephalitis, retinitis, acute hepatitis, splenic rupture, endocarditis, renal insufficiency, pneumonia, and respiratory failure. Thrombocytopenia, transaminitis, and hyponatremia are common, although usually mild.

DIAGNOSIS AND DIFFERENTIAL DIAGNOSIS

Diagnostic IFA titers are present in 50% of patients by day 7, and in virtually 100% of patients by day 15; however, these may not distinguish between endemic and epidemic typhus. Although Western blot and cross-adsorption studies can differentiate the 2 diseases, they require expensive, specialized laboratories.[23] The differential diagnosis of endemic typhus is broad as a result of the nonspecific nature of the cutaneous eruption (see Table 180-3).

TREATMENT

Treatment of endemic typhus is similar to that of RMSF (see Table 180-1). With institution of appropriate antibiotics, fever typically resolves in 2 to 3 days. Spontaneous recovery often occurs within 2 weeks in untreated patients. Prior infection with *R. typhi* provides lifelong immunity to subsequent infection.

EPIDEMIC (LOUSE-BORNE) TYPHUS

Epidemic typhus (also called *prison fever*, *famine fever*, and *ship fever*) is caused by *Rickettsia prowazekii*, and is transmitted to humans primarily via the body louse (*Pediculus humanus* var. *corporis*). Epidemic typhus may result in long-term latent asymptomatic infection. A reemergence of the illness known as Brill–Zinsser disease (BZD) can occur in survivors who may suffer recrudescent infection, even decades after the initial infection.

EPIDEMIOLOGY

Louse infestation occurs when cold weather, poor hygiene, crowding, and poverty are prevalent. These conditions are most commonly found today in refugee camps, and among the homeless and imprisoned. The most recent outbreak of epidemic typhus occurred during the mid-1990s in rural highlands of Central and South America (especially Peru) and Africa (including Burundi), with smaller outbreaks in Russia and Kazakhstan.[24] Table 180-1 details the epidemiologic characteristics of epidemic typhus.

The major reservoir for disease is humans, with lice acquiring the infection by feeding on persons with primary illness or BZD. The lice are spread through close personal contact or infested clothing. The infected louse will defecate while taking a blood meal, and the organisms in the feces are then scratched into the skin, enabling transmission. Lice die of infection within 3 weeks, however, their feces can be infectious for up to 100 days, thereby allowing human-to-human transmission through clothes or close contact. Contact with southern flying squirrels (*Glaucomys volans*) is associated with outbreaks of epidemic typhus in the Eastern United States, where the fleas or lice from these rodents can be important vectors.[25]

CLINICAL AND LABORATORY FINDINGS

After an incubation period of 1 to 2 weeks, abrupt onset of intractable headache, fever (to 40°C [104°F]), chills, and myalgia occurs. If left untreated, prostration resulting from overwhelming hypotension and vascular collapse may ensue. Typically, a rash begins in the axillary folds and upper trunk on the fifth day of illness. Initial lesions consist of erythematous macules that become papular and petechial over several days. In contrast with most rickettsial diseases, the eruption spreads centrifugally but spares the face, palms, and soles. Complications include acral gangrene, cerebral thrombosis, and other neurologic sequelae, multiorgan system failure, and death. Laboratory abnormalities include thrombocytopenia, elevated transaminases, and elevated lactate dehydrogenase. Leukocytosis is seen in a minority of patients.

BZD occurs as a recrudescence of previous infection with *R. prowazekii*. Provocation by immunologic stress induced by poor living conditions may play a role. The illness is usually milder than the primary disease. In the United States it was most commonly seen in those who were exposed to epidemic typhus in World War II.

DIAGNOSIS AND DIFFERENTIAL DIAGNOSIS

Techniques for diagnosis are identical to those used for other rickettsial diseases, with the IFA test the most widely used method. The differential diagnosis is similar to that of endemic typhus. The diagnosis of epidemic typhus should be considered when the appropriate clinical characteristics are seen in the setting of known or suspected louse infestation, or, in the United States, when a history of an exposure to flying squirrels is elicited. The centrifugal spread, lack of eschar, and predilection for colder months helps differentiate epidemic typhus from other rickettsial infections. Endemic typhus is typically less severe than epidemic typhus. When lice and rats are both prevalent (eg, poor hygienic conditions, prison), a risk exists for both diseases. In such situations, it is critical to discriminate between *R. typhi* and *R. prowazekii* infections, as *R. prowazekii* has markedly greater epidemic potential.

TREATMENT

Fatal illness is rare if proper therapy is initiated early (see Table 180-1). Although a single dose of doxycycline may be curative, optimal therapy should be continued for 2 to 3 days after defervescence. BZD is treated identically to primary epidemic typhus. Therapy failures have been documented with azithromycin for BZD.[26]

PREVENTION

Prevention begins with regular bathing and clothes washing. Delousing with appropriate agents, such as permethrin, malathion, lindane or dichlorodiphenyltrichloroethane (DDT), is effective.

SCRUB TYPHUS

Scrub typhus (*tsutsugamushi fever* or *chigger fever*), is a mite-transmitted zoonosis caused by *Orientia tsutsugamushi*. The vector is the larval stage (chigger) of the trombiculid mite (*Leptotrombidium deliense* and other *Leptotrombidium* sp.). The mites and the rodents that carry them serve as the major reservoirs.

EPIDEMIOLOGY

Named for the type of vegetation that harbors the mite vector, scrub typhus is endemic to a region spanning the Indian subcontinent to Eastern Asia and the Western Pacific Rim (Japan, Korea, India, Pakistan, Taiwan, Southeast Asia, and Australia). Scrub vegetation is a transitional terrain between tall forests and cleared land, composed of plantations, fields, groves, and tall grass. Accordingly, the illness is more common in rural settings and is a common occupational disease. Because of the long incubation period, scrub typhus can present in travelers returning to nonepidemic areas.

CLINICAL AND LABORATORY FINDINGS

An erythematous papule appears within 2 days of the chigger bite and undergoes ulceration and eschar formation in one-half to two-thirds of patients. The eschar may be absent in intertriginous areas. Regional lymphadenopathy is followed by generalized lymphadenopathy. One to 2 weeks after the bite, there is a sudden onset of high fever (40°C to 40.6°C [104°F to 105°F]). Chills, headache, cough, myalgia, anorexia, nausea, diarrhea, dyspnea, ocular pain, and conjunctival injection are variably present. Approximately 4 to 5 days after the fever begins a centrifugal macular followed by papular eruption occurs in approximately 35% of cases. The eruption starts on the trunk, spreads to the extremities, and fades within a few days. Hepatosplenomegaly and a relative bradycardia may be appreciated. Severe complications include adult respiratory distress syndrome, myocarditis, pericarditis, disseminated intravascular coagulation, hemophagocytic syndrome, retinal vein occlusion, renal failure, and hepatitis. Nuchal rigidity, meningoencephalitis, tremors, slurred speech, deafness, and tinnitus are seen rarely. Examination of the cerebrospinal fluid in these cases reveals only a slight monocytosis.

DIAGNOSIS AND DIFFERENTIAL DIAGNOSIS

The differential diagnosis is similar to that for endemic typhus. Enzyme-linked immunosorbent assay, dot blot urine immunoassay, rapid immunochromatographic flow assay, and PCR have the greatest sensitivity and specificity but are limited by their availability in endemic areas. Diagnostically, IFA remains the gold standard. Conclusive diagnosis is based on a fourfold increase in titer of paired samples drawn at least 2 weeks apart. A single acute titer of greater than 1:50 can be used as a preliminary diagnostic cutoff in travelers returning from endemic areas.[27] In 2009, an association was reported between high *O. tsutsugamushi* DNA loads determined by PCR and disease severity.[28] However, newer evidence suggests IgM enzyme-linked immunosorbent assay has higher diagnostic accuracy and may be used as alternative reference to the IgM IFA.[29]

TREATMENT

Although single dose or short courses (3 days) of doxycycline may prove to be efficacious, treatment is recommended for 14 days. Naturally occurring doxycycline-resistant and chloramphenicol-resistant strains of *O. tsutsugamushi* have been found in northern Thailand; azithromycin, rifampin, and ciprofloxacin are alternatives in this setting.[30] With the institution of proper antibiotics, defervescence occurs abruptly, usually within 24 hours. In untreated patients, fever lasts for approximately 2 weeks. While vaccine development has yielded disappointing results further research is crucial as prevention given increasing resistance to available antibiotic therapies.[31]

PREVENTION

DEET applied to the skin or impregnated into clothing is effective at preventing transmission. Chemoprophylaxis with weekly doxycycline may be efficacious when traveling to endemic areas. Paradoxically, rodent control may increase the risk of human disease as chiggers lose their natural host and target humans.

THE EHRLICHIOSES

The ehrlichial pathogens were reclassified in 1994 based on distinct phylogenetic and pathogenic characteristics. Disease previously known as Human granulocytic ehrlichiosis is now called Anaplasmosis or Human granulocytic Anaplasmosis (HGA) and is caused by organism in the Anaplasma genus. In contrast, Human monocytic ehrlichiosis (HME) is attributed to the Ehrlichia species.[6]

EPIDEMIOLOGY

Human disease attributed to ehrlichial organisms has been reported in the United States since 1986. The causative agent of HME is *Ehrlichia chaffeensis*, and the main reservoirs are deer, dogs, and coyote. The white-footed mouse (*Peromyscus leucopus*) and white-tailed deer (*Odocoileus virginianus*) are the principal reservoirs for *Anaplasma phagocytophilum*, the causative agent of HGA. Table 180-1 describes the principal epidemiologic characteristics of HME and HGA.

HGA infection occurs in a geographic pattern identical to that of Lyme disease (*Borrelia burgdorferi*; see Chap. 179), namely in the Northeast, parts of the Pacific Northwest, and the upper Midwest United States. The vector for both HGA and Lyme is the *Ixodes* tick (see Fig. 180-1D and E). In addition to *A. phagocytophilum* and *B. burgdorferi*, *Ixodes* ticks can transmit *Babesia microti*, *Borrelia afzelii*, and *Borrelia garinii*. Not surprisingly, most cases of HGA are found in areas with high incidences of Lyme disease and babesiosis.

The lone star tick (*Amblyomma americanum*) and the American dog tick (*D. variabilis*), the vectors of *E. chaffeensis*, also transmit *R. rickettsii* and *Francisella tularensis*, the causative agents of RMSF and tularemia (see Chap. 156), respectively (see Fig. 180-1). It is essential to consider possible coinfection with these potentially life-threatening organisms in patients with known or suspected ehrlichial disease. Although mainly a tick-borne disease, HGA has been reported after blood transfusions, as well as after contact with contaminated animal tissue.[32,33]

ETIOLOGY AND PATHOGENESIS

Ehrlichiae and Anaplasmodiae are small, obligate intracellular bacteria. *E. chaffeensis* is trophic for monocytic cells, whereas *A. phagocytophilum* prefer myeloid or granulocytic cells. The organisms grow within membrane-bound vacuoles, and form intracytoplasmic microcolonies called morulae, which may be seen in peripheral blood smears.[6,34]

CLINICAL AND LABORATORY FINDINGS

There is substantial overlap in the clinical presentation and laboratory evaluation of patients with HME, HGA, and RMSF (see Table 180-2). Patients give a history of a tick bite in only approximately 68% of cases of ehrlichiosis. The clinical course ranges from asymptomatic seroconversion to multisystem organ failure and death (see Table 180-2) The rash of HME is often indistinguishable from that of RMSF, and can present as erythematous macules and papules, petechiae, or as a diffuse erythema. It is observed in approximately 33% of adults and 66% of children with HME. Rash is rare in HGA; the absence of a rash in a patient with systemic findings suggestive of RMSF should prompt consideration of anaplasmosis. Conversely, if a rash is present in a patient with anaplasmosis, coinfection with meningococcus, *R. rickettsii*, or *B. burgdorferi* should be considered. Laboratory abnormalities include leukopenia (often with a left shift), thrombocytopenia, and elevated transaminases. Despite similar presentations, HME usually has a more-severe progression and higher case fatality ratio, where as HGA has a high prevalence of opportunistic infections.[35]

PATHOLOGY

In contrast to the rickettsioses, neither endothelial cell injury nor frank vasculitis is a typical feature. A single retrospective case study suggests HME rarely may be associated with cutaneous vasculitis such as polyarteritis nodosa.[36]

DIAGNOSIS AND DIFFERENTIAL DIAGNOSIS

Clinical illness nearly always precedes laboratory diagnosis by any method. Morulae stained with Wright or Giemsa stains are occasionally observed inside the leukocytes in peripheral blood smears, buffy coat preparations, or cerebrospinal fluid, usually during the first week of infection (Fig. 180-8). Smear sensitivities are low and variably dependent upon the experience of the microscopist.[34] Consequently, a negative smear should not delay treatment. False-positives can occur with toxic granulation, superimposed platelets, and Döhle bodies.

Confirmatory testing should be performed with serologic assays available through commercial and state public health laboratories. The sensitivity of the IFA is dependent on the timing of collection and is estimated to be 94% to 100% sensitive after 14 days. Antibody titers are typically as high as 1:640 during acute infection.[37] Paired serum samples taken 2 to 3 weeks apart should demonstrate a fourfold rise in titers. PCR of whole blood may be more useful than tissue biopsy in HME and HGA, as these pathogens are trophic for circulating leukocytes. Immunohistochemical staining of formalin-fixed, paraffin-embedded tissue may be useful for documenting infection in the first 48 hours of disease.[6]

The differential diagnosis is extensive and similar to RMSF (see Tables 180-3 and 180-4). The presence of a rash, normal white blood cell count, lack of morulae, and pathologic evidence of vasculitis is more consistent with RMSF.

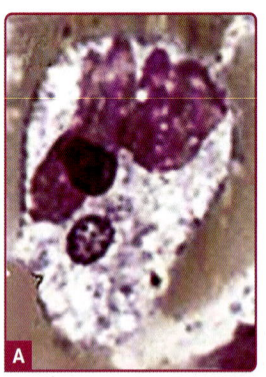
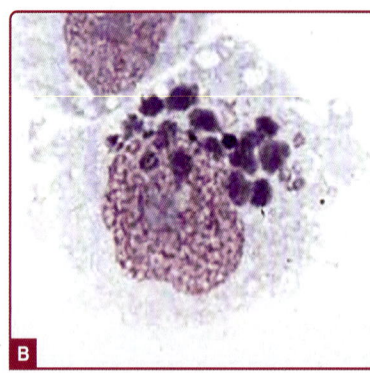
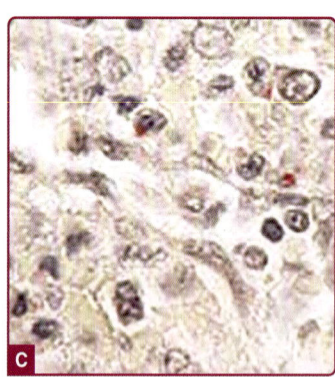
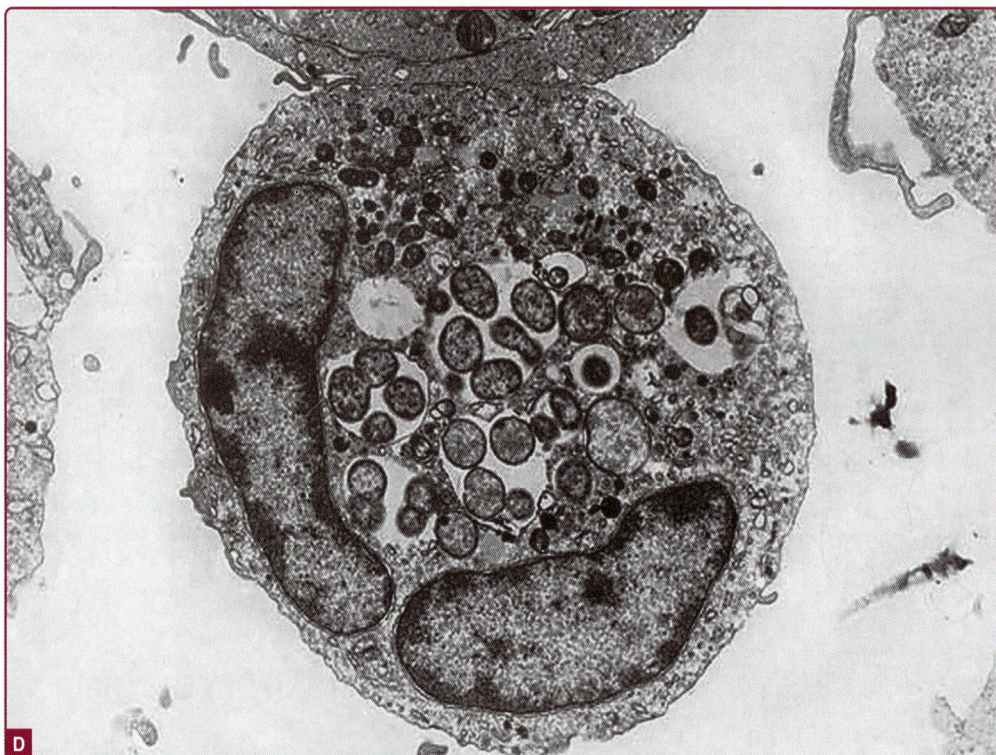

Figure 180-8 **A,** *Anaplasma phagocytophilum* in human peripheral blood band neutrophil (Wright stain, original magnification ×1000). **B,** *A. phagocytophilum* in THP-1 myelomonocytic cell culture (Leukostat stain, original magnification ×400). **C,** *A. phagocytophilum* in neutrophils infiltrating human spleen (immunohistochemistry with hematoxylin counterstain; original magnification ×100). **D,** *A. phagocytophilum* ultrastructure by transmission electron microscopy in HL-60 cell culture (original magnification ×21,960). (Used with permission from Dumler JS, Choi KS, Garcia-Garcia JC, et al. Human granulocytic anaplasmosis and *Anaplasma phagocytophilum*. Emerg Infect Dis. 2005;11(12):1828-1834, Fig. 1. Available at https://wwwnc.cdc.gov/eid/article/11/12/05-0898_article.)

TREATMENT

The median duration of disease is 1 to 2 weeks with treatment. Defervescence usually occurs within 1 to 2 days. Tables 180-1 and 180-5 detail appropriate therapy. Treatment with doxycycline for 5 to 14 days is generally effective, but continued therapy for 14 to 21 days is indicated if coinfection with *B. burgdorferi* is suspected.[6,34] Rifampin has been successfully used to treat HGA in pregnant women and young children.

PREVENTION

Preventive measures include avoidance of tick exposure, use of chemical repellants such as DEET, light-colored clothing (to visualize ticks), and careful removal of attached ticks.

ACKNOWLEDGMENTS

We would like to thank Sandra A. Kopp, who contributed to this chapter in the previous edition of *Fitzpatrick's Dermatology in General Medicine*.

REFERENCES

1. Parola P, Paddock CD, Raoult D. Tick-borne rickettsioses around the world: emerging diseases challenging old concepts. *Clin Microbiol Rev*. 2005;18:719.
2. Todar K. Rickettsial diseases, including typhus and rocky mountain spotted fever. *Todar's Online Textbook of Bacteriology*. 2008-2012:2-6. http://textbookofbacteriology.net/Rickettsia.html. Accessed July 20, 2018.
3. Walker DH, Raoult D. *Rickettsia rickettsii* and other spotted fever group rickettsiae (Rocky Mountain spotted fever and other spotted fever). In: Mandell GL, Bennett JE, Dolin R, eds. *Principles and Practice of Infectious Diseases*. Vol 2. 8th ed. Philadelphia, PA: Churchill Livingstone; 2015:2198.
4. Chapman AS, Bakken JS, Folk SM, et al; Tickborne Rickettsial Diseases Working Group; CDC. Diagnosis and management of tickborne rickettsial diseases: Rocky Mountain spotted fever, ehrlichioses, and anaplasmosis—United States: a practical guide for physicians and other health-care and public health professionals. *MMWR Recomm Rep*. 2006;55(RR-4):1-27.
5. Centers for Disease Control and Prevention (CDC). Rocky Mountain Spotted Fever (RMSF). Statistics and Epidemiology. https://www.cdc.gov/rmsf/stats/index.html. Accessed July 31, 2018.
6. Biggs HM, Behravesh CB, Bradley KK, et al. Diagnosis and management of tickborne rickettsial diseases: Rocky Mountain spotted fever and other spotted fever group rickettsioses, ehrlichioses, and anaplasmosis—United States. *MMWR Recomm Rep*. 2016;65(RR-2):1-44.
7. Kirkland KB, Marcom KP, Sexton DJ, et al. Rocky Mountain spotted fever complicated by gangrene: report of six cases and review. *Clin Infect Dis*. 1993;16:629.
8. Buckingham SC, Marshall GS, Gordon ES, et al. Clinical and laboratory features, hospital course, and outcome of Rocky Mountain spotted fever in children. *J Pediatr*. 2007;150:180-184.
9. Dana AN. Diagnosis and treatment of tick infestation and tick-borne diseases with cutaneous manifestations. *Dermatol Ther*. 2009;22:293-326.
10. Lochary ME, Lockhart PB, Williams WT Jr. Doxycycline and staining of permanent teeth. *Pediatr Infect Dis J*. 1998;17:429.
11. Elston DM. Rickettsial skin disease: uncommon presentations. *Clin Dermatol*. 2005;23:541.
12. Stallings SP. Rocky Mountain spotted fever and pregnancy: a case report and review of the literature. *Obstet Gynecol Surv*. 2001;155:37.
13. Rovery C, Raoult D. Mediterranean spotted fever. *Infect Dis Clin North Am*. 2008;22:515-530.
14. Segura F, Pons I, Sanfeliu I, et al. Shell-vial culture, coupled with real-time PCR, applied to *Rickettsia conorii* and *Rickettsia massiliae*-Bar29 detection, improving the diagnosis of the Mediterranean spotted fever. *Ticks Tick Borne Dis*. 2016;7(3):457-461.
15. Parola P, Rovery C, Rolain J, et al. *Rickettsia slovaca* and *R. raoultii* in tick-bourne Rickettsioses. *Emerg Infect Dis*. 2009;15:105-108.
16. Cascio A, Colomba C, Di Rosa D, et al. Efficacy and safety of clarithromycin as treatment for Mediterranean spotted fever in children: a randomized controlled trial. *Clin Infect Dis*. 2001;33:409.
17. Heymann WR. Rickettsialpox. *Clin Dermatol*. 1996;14:279.
18. Didier R. Rickettsialpox. In: Mandell GL, Bennett JE, Dolin R, eds. *Principles and Practice of Infectious Diseases*. Vol 2. 8th ed. Philadelphia, PA: Churchill Livingstone; 2015:2206.
19. Denison A, Amin B, Nicholson W, et al. Detection of *Rickettsia rickettsii*, *Rickettsia parkeri*, and *Rickettsia akari* in skin biopsy specimens using multiplex real-time polymerase chain reaction assay. *Clin Infect Dis*. 2014;59:635.
20. Dumler JS. *Rickettsia typhi* (murine typhus). In: Mandell GL, Bennett JE, Dolin R, eds. *Principles and Practice of Infectious Diseases*. Vol 2. 8th ed. Philadelphia, PA: Churchill Livingstone; 2015: 2221.
21. Zavala-Velazquez JE, Zavala-Castro JE, Vado-Solís I, et al. Identification of *Ctenocephalides felis* fleas as a host of *Rickettsia felis*, the agent of a spotted fever rickettsiosis in Yucatan, Mexico. *Vector Borne Zoonotic Dis*. 2002;2:69.
22. Purcell K, Fergie J, Richman K, et al. Murine typhus in children, South Texas. *Emerg Infect Dis*. 2007;13:926-927.
23. Whiteford SF, Taylor JP, Dumler JS. Clinical, laboratory and epidemiologic features of murine typhus in 97 Texas children. *Arch Pediatr Adolesc Med*. 2001;155:396.
24. Raoult DA, Roux V, Ndihokubwayo JB, et al. Jail fever (epidemic typhus) outbreak in Burundi. *Emerg Infect Dis*. 1997;3(3):357-360.
25. Walker DH. *Rickettsia prowazekii* (epidemic or louse-borne typhus). In: Mandell GL, Bennett JE, Dolin R, eds. *Principles and Practice of Infectious Diseases*. Vol 2. 8th ed. Philadelphia, PA: Churchill Livingstone; 2015:2217.
26. Turcinov D, Kuzman I, Herendic B. Failure of azithromycin in treatment of Brill-Zinsser disease. *Antimicrob Agents Chemother*. 2000;44:1737.
27. Blacksell SD, Bryant N, Paris D, et al. Scrub typhus serologic testing with the indirect immunofluorescence method as a diagnostic gold standard: a lack of consensus leads to a lot of confusion. *Clin Infect Dis*. 2007;44:391.
28. Sonthayanon P, Chierakul W, Wuthiekanun V, et al. Association of high *Orientia tsutsugamushi* DNA loads

with disease of greater severity in adults with scrub typhus. *J Clin Microbiol*. 2009;47:430-434.
29. Blacksell SD, Lim C, Tanganuchitcharnchai A, et al. Optimal cutoff and accuracy of an IgM enzyme-linked immunosorbent assay for diagnosis of acute scrub typhus in northern Thailand: an alternative reference method to the IgM immunofluorescence assay. *J Clin Microbiol*. 2016;54(6):1472-1478.
30. Watt G, Kantipong P, Jongsakul K, et al. Doxycycline and rifampicin for mild scrub-typhus infections in northern Thailand: a randomised trial. *Lancet*. 2000; 356:1057.
31. Chattopadhyay S, Richards AL. Scrub typhus vaccines: past history and recent developments. *Hum Vaccin*. 2007;3(3):73-80.
32. Bakken JS, Krueth J, Lund T, et al. Exposure to deer blood may be a cause of human granulocytic ehrlichiosis. *Clin Infect Dis*. 1996;23:198.
33. Centers for Disease Control and Prevention (CDC). *Anaplasma phagocytophilum* transmitted through blood transfusion—Minnesota. *MMWR Morb Mortal Wkly Rep*. 2008;57:1145-1148.
34. Dumler JS, Choi KS, Garcia-Garcia JC, et al. Human granulocytic anaplasmosis and *Anaplasma phagocytophilum*. *Emerg Infect Dis*. 2005;11(12):1828-1834.
35. Dumler SJ, Madigan JE, Pusterla N, et al. Ehrlichioses in humans: epidemiology, clinical presentation, diagnosis, and treatment. *Clin Infect Dis*. 2007;45(suppl 1): S45-S51.
36. Pick N, Potasman I, Strenger C, et al. Ehrlichiosis associated vasculitis. *J Intern Med*. 2000;247:674.
37. Sanchez E, Vannier E, Wormser GP, et al. Diagnosis, treatment and prevention of lyme disease, human granulocytic anaplasmosis, and babesiosis: a review. *JAMA*. 2016;315:1767.

Chapter 181 :: Arthropod Bites and Stings
:: Robert A. Schwartz & Christopher J. Steen

第一百八十一章

节肢动物咬伤和蛰伤

中文导读

节肢动物咬伤和蛰伤是影响世界范围内发病率的重要原因。虽然许多节肢动物的攻击只会产生轻微的、短暂的皮肤变化，但可能会出现更严重的局部和全身后遗症，包括潜在的致命毒性和过敏反应，而且节肢动物也是许多系统性疾病的传播媒介。本章分为6节：①组织病理学；②治疗原则；③蛛行纲；④唇足纲和双足纲；⑤昆虫纲；⑥预防。介绍了节肢动物咬伤和蛰伤的相关知识。

第一节组织病理学，介绍大多数节肢动物咬伤都会产生相似的组织反应模式，急性期有血管周围和间质的楔形炎性浸润，慢性期可能具有假性淋巴瘤特征。

第二节介绍了治疗原则，包括局部伤口护理，必要时应制定全身毒性和过敏反应的支持性措施。继发感染应该用适当的抗生素治疗，部分需要预防破伤风或使用抗蛇毒血清。

第三节介绍了蛛行纲包含3个具有医学意义的目：蜘蛛纲（蜘蛛）、蜱螨纲（蜱螨）、蝎子纲（蝎子）。分别介绍了这些动物咬伤的临床特征及管理。

第四节介绍了唇足纲和倍足纲分别由蜈蚣和千足虫组成，蜈蚣叮咬可出现剧烈疼痛和红肿，同时可合并严重的器官损伤，千足虫释放出有毒物质，除皮肤外，需要注意各种眼部损伤。

第五节介绍了昆虫纲包含无翅目（虱子）、双翅目（苍蝇、蚊子）、鞘翅目（甲虫）、半翅目（臭虫）、蚤目（蚤）、膜翅目（蚂蚁、蜜蜂、黄蜂）和鳞翅目（蝴蝶和飞蛾），分别简单介绍了它们咬伤的临床表现和临床管理。

第六节介绍了预防措施来最大限度地减少节肢动物咬伤的发生，包括衣物的穿戴、使用化学驱避剂等。

〔粟 娟〕

AT-A-GLANCE

- Many arthropod species are capable of inflicting bites and stings on humans.
- Reactions to arthropod assaults can range from mild to life threatening.
- Arthropods also serve as vectors for systemic diseases.
- The terrestrial arthropods of medical importance include the orders Arachnida (arachnids), Chilopoda (centipedes), Diplopoda (millipedes), and Insecta (insects).

Arthropod bites and stings are a significant cause of morbidity worldwide. Although many arthropod attacks produce only mild, transient cutaneous changes, more severe local and systemic sequelae can occur, including potentially fatal toxic and anaphylactic reactions. Arthropods also serve as vectors for numerous systemic diseases. The medically significant classes of nonaquatic arthropods are Arachnida, Chilopoda, Diplopoda, and Insecta (Fig. 181-1).[1]

HISTOPATHOLOGY

Many arthropod bites produce a similar histologic reaction pattern. In the acute phase, there is a superficial and deep, perivascular, and interstitial inflammatory infiltrate, which is characteristically wedge shaped. The infiltrate is usually mixed in composition with an abundance of lymphocytes and eosinophils, although neutrophils and histiocytes also can be seen. Neutrophils may predominate in reactions to fleas, mosquitoes, fire ants, and brown recluse spiders. Over the most prominent superficial infiltrates, spongiosis can be seen, sometimes with progression to vesicle formation or epidermal necrosis. Older, excoriated areas are usually altered by the effects of scratching, with the development of parakeratosis, serum exudates, and a dermal infiltrate with neutrophils and more abundant lymphocytes. Although not commonly seen on histology, insects or insect parts, including burrowed scabies mites, eggs, feces, or the retained mouthparts of ticks, may be visible. Chronic lesions, which most often result when arthropod parts are retained in the skin, may have a pseudolymphomatous appearance (Chap. 120).

TREATMENT PRINCIPLES

The morbidity from arthropod bites and stings varies with the species inflicting the injury. Although species-specific clinical findings and treatment will be discussed in further detail, there are several applicable general treatment principles (Table 181-1). Local wound care is essential following arthropod assault. Wounds should be cleansed; any remaining arthropod parts, including stingers, should be removed expeditiously. Patient discomfort should be addressed and can involve a variety of treatment modalities, including the use of ice packs, application of topical corticosteroids and antipruritics, injection of local anesthetics, and, less frequently, the use of systemic analgesics. Supportive measures for systemic toxic and allergic reactions, including anaphylaxis, should be instituted when necessary. Secondary infection should be treated with appropriate antibiotics. Bites from several terrestrial arthropods species may require tetanus prophylaxis. Severe envenomation from particular species, such as the black widow spider, may require antivenom administration. Documented hypersensitivity to some species can be treated with desensitization immunotherapy. Awareness of the potential arthropod-borne illnesses spread by each species is also important.

DIFFERENTIAL DIAGNOSIS

See Table 181-2.

ARACHNIDA

The class Arachnida contains 3 orders of medical significance: (1) Araneae (spiders), (2) Acarina (ticks and mites), and (3) Scorpiones (scorpions). Arachnids are distinguished anatomically from other arthropods by a lack of wings or antennae and the presence of 4 pairs of legs and 2 body segments. Larval ticks, which only have 3 pairs of legs, are an exception to this rule (Fig. 181-1).

ARANEAE

Spiders are carnivorous members of the animal kingdom that use webs and venom to capture and kill prey. Within the United States, 3 genera contain species whose bites are toxic to man: (1) *Latrodectus*, (2) *Loxosceles*, and (3) *Tegenaria*. The American Association of Poison Control Centers reported more than 15,000 spider bites in the United States in 2004.[2] In the same year, only 1 death was attributed to spider envenomation in the United States.

LATRODECTUS

Members of the *Latrodectus* genus, or widow spiders, are often black in color and have a red, hourglass-shaped marking on their abdomens (Fig. 181-2). Although there are more than 20 species of widow spiders, *Latrodectus mactans*, the Southern black widow spider, is the most common and notorious in the United States and can be found in all but the most northern parts of the country. Other widow spiders encountered in the United States include *Latrodectus various* (Northern black widow), *Latrodectus hesperus* (Western black widow), *Latrodectus bishopi* (red-legged widow), and *Latrodectus geometricus* (brown widow). Members of the *Latrodectus* genus are nonaggressive, trapping spiders that spin webs in protected areas and await their prey. Human bites are often the result of accidental or deliberate provocation. Webs are

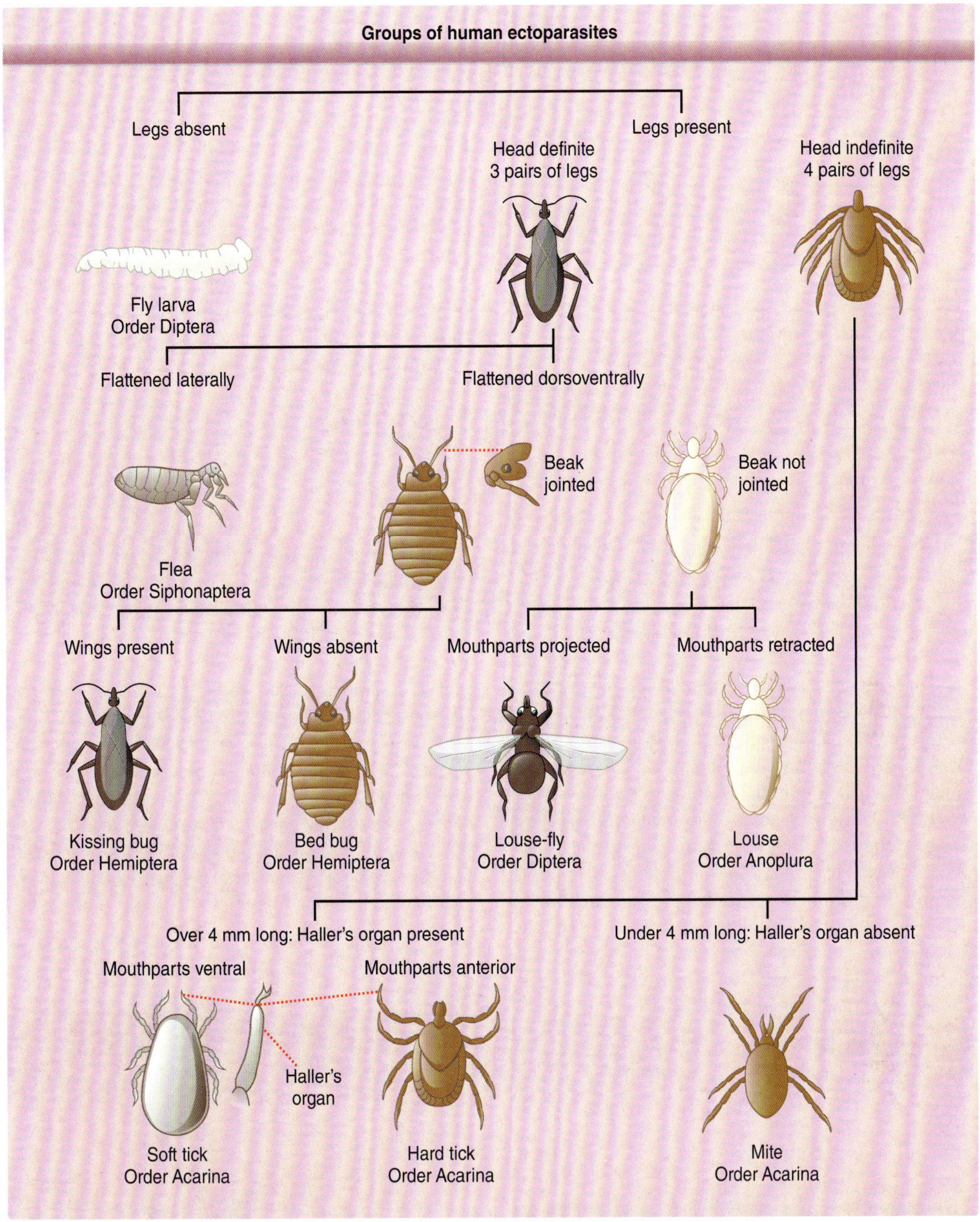

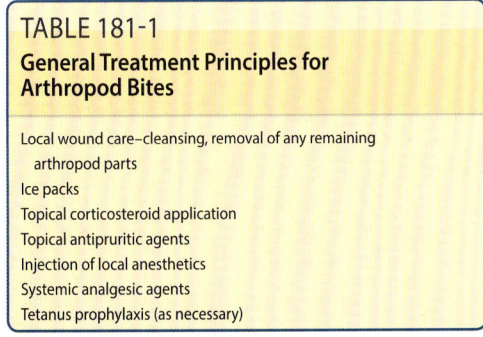

Figure 181-1 Pictorial key to groups of human ectoparasites. (Used with permission from C. J. Stojanovich and H. G. Scott, US Department of Health, Education, and Welfare, Public Health Service.)

TABLE 181-1
General Treatment Principles for Arthropod Bites

Local wound care–cleansing, removal of any remaining arthropod parts
Ice packs
Topical corticosteroid application
Topical antipruritic agents
Injection of local anesthetics
Systemic analgesic agents
Tetanus prophylaxis (as necessary)

typically found on the corners of doors and windows, underneath woodpiles, in garages and sheds, and on the undersides of eaves. Webs also can be found around outdoor toilet seats, a location that has led to bites on or near the genitalia.[3]

Clinical Findings: Bites of the black widow spider (*L. mactans*), which are often painful, usually only result in mild dermatologic manifestations. Within the first 30 minutes, localized erythema, piloerection, and sweating may appear at the wound site. A sensation of numbness or aching pain may develop shortly

> **TABLE 181-2**
> **Differential Diagnosis of Arthropod Bites and Stings**
>
> - Black widow bite: acute abdomen (appendicitis, etc.), meningitis, tetanus, drug withdrawal, acute renal failure, acute myocarditis, acute coronary syndrome, other arthropod bite
> - Brown recluse bite: hobo spider bite, chemical burn, Lyme disease, cutaneous anthrax infection, pyoderma gangrenosum, ecthyma, trauma, vasculitis, neoplasm, other arthropod bite
> - Scorpion sting: other arthropod bite, tetanus, botulism, Guillain–Barré, organophosphate toxicity, medication overdose
> - Centipede bite: other arthropod bite, cellulitis
> - Millipede "burn": contact dermatitis, conjunctivitis
> - Insect bites (flies, fleas, bedbugs, kissing bugs): other arthropod bites (scabies, lice), atopic dermatitis, contact dermatitis, papular urticaria, delusions of parasitosis
> - Hymenoptera bite/sting: other arthropod bite, anaphylaxis
> - Lepidopterism: other arthropod bite, contact dermatitis, atopic dermatitis, phytodermatitis

after the bite. Urticaria and cyanosis may occur at the bite site. Black widow venom contains the neurotoxin α-latrotoxin, which acts by opening ion channels at presynaptic nerve terminals, thereby causing an irreversible release of acetylcholine at motor nerve endings and catecholamines at adrenergic nerve endings.[4] Consequently, black widow bites may produce agonizing crampy abdominal pain and muscle spasm that may mimic an acute abdomen.[4] Other signs and symptoms include headache, paresthesias, nausea, vomiting, hypertension, lacrimation, salivation, seizures, tremors, acute renal failure, and sometimes, paralysis; fortunately, death is uncommon. Based on the spectrum of symptoms, black widow bite may be misdiagnosed as drug withdrawal, appendicitis, meningitis, or tetanus, to name a few.[4]

Management: Although many widow spider bites require only local wound care, more serious reactions may necessitate hospitalization. Those patients at increased risk for serious complications include the very young, very old, and those with underlying cardiovascular disease. Current treatments for black widow envenomation include intravenous calcium gluconate (10%), narcotic analgesics, muscle relaxants, and benzodiazepines.[5] *L. mactans* antivenom prepared from equine serum is also available. Additionally, there appears to be an effective cross-reactivity among antivenom for a number of other *Latrodectus* species.[6-8] The benefits of the antivenom in treating complications of widow bites should be weighed against the potential for allergic reaction to the antivenom. Patients should also be up to date on tetanus immunization.

LOXOSCELES

Members of the *Loxosceles* genus, also called *recluse spiders* or *fiddle-back spiders*, are nonaggressive spiders characterized by a dark brown marking on their cephalothorax in the shape of a fiddle or violin (Fig. 181-3). The brown recluse spider, *Loxosceles reclusa*, is the most well-known member of this genus and is most abundant in the American Midwest and Southeast. Other medically significant members of this genus include *Loxosceles deserta* (desert recluse), *Loxosceles rufescens* (Mediterranean recluse), *Loxosceles kaiba* (Grand Canyon recluse), and *Loxosceles arizonica* (Arizona recluse). Recluse spiders are so named because they will often seek out shelter in undisturbed places such as closets, attics, and storage areas for bedding and clothing. Bites usually occur when the spider feels threatened or provoked, such as when someone tries to put on clothing that contains the spider.[1]

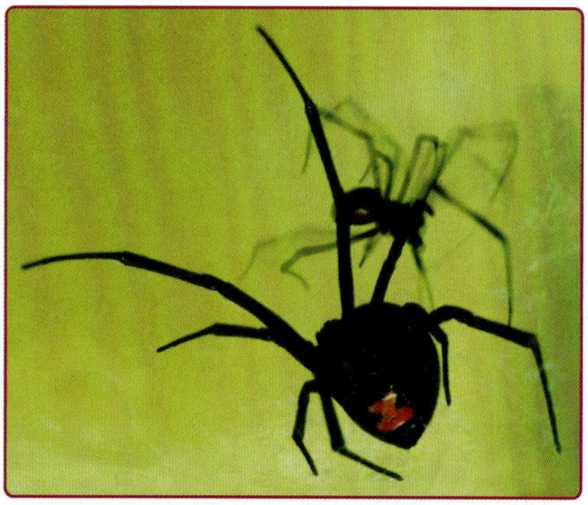

Figure 181-2 Black widow spider with characteristic red hourglass marking on the underside of its abdomen.

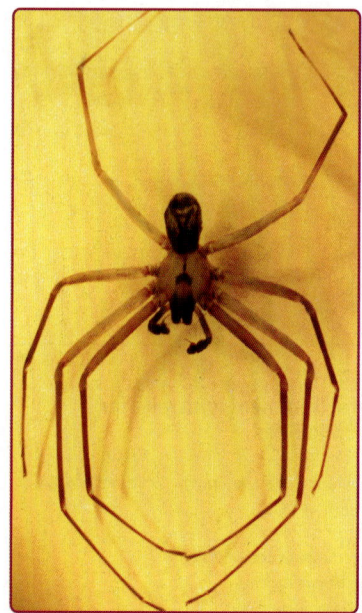

Figure 181-3 Brown recluse spider with characteristic fiddle-shaped marking on cephalothorax.

Clinical Findings: Bites of the brown recluse spider (*L. reclusa*) vary from mild, local reactions to severe ulcerative necrosis, a reaction known as *necrotic arachnidism*. After a bite, transient erythema may develop, with the formation of a central vesicle or papule. The hallmark "red, white, and blue" sign of a brown recluse bite is characterized by a central violaceous area surrounded by a rim of blanched skin that is further surrounded by a large asymmetric erythematous area (Fig. 181-4A). In a small percentage of cases, the initial wound may progress to necrosis (Fig. 181-4B), which usually begins 2 to 3 days after the bite, with eschar formation occurring between the fifth and seventh days.[9] Eventually deep ulcers develop. The bite reaction may mimic pyoderma gangrenosum or erythema migrans of Lyme disease.[10] Cutaneous anthrax and chemical burns have been mistaken for a brown recluse spider bite.[11,12] The potential for misdiagnosis has led to the development of a sensitive enzyme-linked immunosorbent assay for *Loxosceles* species venom that may eventually be available for clinical application.[13]

Brown recluse venom contains a number of proteins, including sphingomyelinase D, esterase, hyaluronidase, and alkaline phosphatase, which all contribute to tissue destruction. Sphingomyelinase D, the major component of the venom, cleaves sphingomyelin to form cermade-1-phosphate and choline and also hydrolyzes lysophosphatidylcholine to produce lysophosphatidic acid.[14] Lysophosphatidic acid then triggers a proinflammatory response and causes platelet aggregation and increased vascular permeability.[14] Sphingomyelinase D is also capable of inducing complement-mediated hemolysis.[15] Systemic symptoms may develop within 1 to 2 days after envenomation and include nausea, vomiting, headache, fever, and chills. Rare but serious sequelae of brown recluse bites include renal failure, hemolytic anemia, hypotension, and disseminated intravascular coagulation.[16,17]

Management: General treatment measures for recluse bites include cleansing the bite site and the application of cold compresses. Patients may also require analgesics to control pain. Antibiotics may be useful in reducing secondary bacterial infection of the wound site. Warm compresses and strenuous exercise should be avoided. Although *Loxosceles* antivenoms have been developed and are frequently used in South America, there is little evidence to support their effectiveness, particularly against local cutaneous effects.[8] A number of treatment modalities have been suggested, including hyperbaric oxygen, dapsone, intralesional and systemic corticosteroids, colchicine, and diphenhydramine.[18,19] However, one study that used a rabbit model to compare dapsone, colchicine, intralesional triamcinolone, and diphenhydramine showed no effect on eschar size from any of these medications.[18] Necrotic wounds heal slowly, sometimes over many months, and may require surgical excision and reconstruction to close the resulting defect. Surgical interventions should be delayed until the wound has stabilized.

TEGENARIA

Tegenaria agrestis, the hobo spider or "aggressive house spider," is the predominant cause of necrotic arachnidism in the Pacific Northwest of the United States and can be found in an area ranging from Alaska to Utah.[20] Although *Loxosceles* species are not typically found in the same geographic distribution, bites from hobo spiders are often mistaken for brown recluse bites. These spiders are brown in color with a gray herringbone pattern on the abdomen.[21] The hobo spider typically builds funnel-shaped webs in crawl spaces, basements, wood piles, and bushes. Most hobo spider bites occur from July to September when the more venomous male spiders are seeking mates.

Clinical Findings: The local cutaneous effects after envenomation by the hobo spider, which can range from mild to serious, are similar to those caused by the brown recluse.[22] The initial bite is often painless. Induration and paresthesia of the bite site may develop

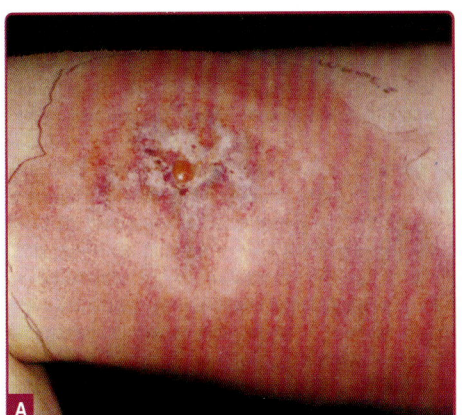
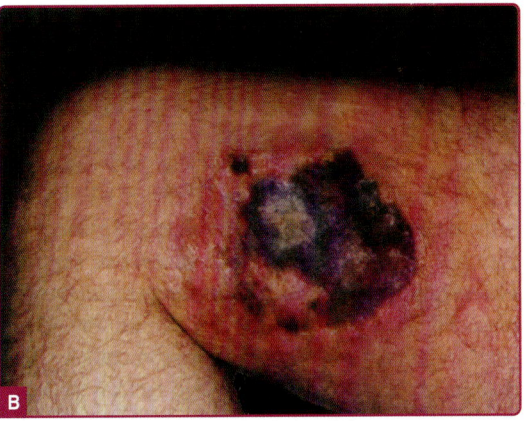

Figure 181-4 **A**, Clinically typical brown recluse spider bite showing the "red, white, and blue" sign. **B**, Late brown recluse spider bite with overlying eschar.

within 30 minutes, and a large erythematous area may form around the site. Vesicle formation often occurs during the first 36 hours. Eschar formation may follow in severe cases, with necrosis and sloughing of the underlying tissue.

Management: Wounds usually heal within several weeks. The most common systemic symptom after a hobo spider bite is a severe headache, which can persist for up to 1 week.[23] Other symptoms may include fatigue, nausea, vomiting, diarrhea, paresthesias, and memory impairment. Although rare, death may ensue due to severe systemic effects, including aplastic anemia.[23]

TARANTULA

Tarantulas are indigenous to certain regions of the United States and are also kept as exotic pets. Tarantulas are members of the family Theraphosidae and are hair covered and larger than many other types of spider, with leg spans of up to 12 inches reported in certain species. Unlike the other venomous spiders discussed, tarantula bites generally only produce mild local symptoms. However, more serious reactions can be caused by urticating hairs on the spider's abdomen. When threatened, tarantulas may rub their back legs together in a motion that flicks these hairs off. These hairs may become embedded in the skin or eyes. Cutaneous responses to the hairs range from mild, local pruritus to granulomatous reactions. Ocular sequelae from hairs embedded in the cornea range from conjunctivitis and keratouveitis to corneal granulomas and chorioretinitis.[24-27] Although cutaneous reactions can be treated with topical corticosteroids, ocular involvement requires ophthalmologic evaluation.

SCORPIONES

The order Scorpiones (scorpions) comprises terrestrial arachnids most commonly encountered in tropical or arid regions, including the southwestern United States, northern Africa, Mexico, and the Middle East. These nocturnal creatures seek shelter under stones and tree barks during the day. As with other arachnids, scorpions are generally shy and sting humans only when provoked. Although capable of producing significant local wounds, the potential for serious, even lethal, cardiovascular complications following a scorpion sting remains of primary concern.[1] The scorpion of principal interest in the United States is *Centruroides exilicauda* (formerly *Centruroides sculpturatus*), whose sting is potentially fatal (Fig. 181-5). *Centruroides* species possess a small spine at the base of the stinger, a feature that may help distinguish them from other species of scorpion.[28,29]

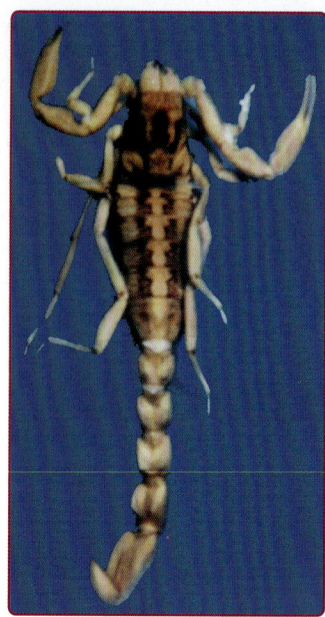

Figure 181-5 *Centruroides* scorpion.

CLINICAL FINDINGS

Scorpion stings usually produce an immediate, sharp, burning pain. This may be followed by numbness extending beyond the sting site. Regional lymph node swelling, and, less commonly, ecchymosis and lymphangitis, may develop. *C. exilicauda* venom contains a powerful neurotoxin, capable of producing muscle spasticity, nystagmus, blurred vision, slurred speech, excessive salivation, respiratory distress, pulmonary edema, and myocarditis.[30-35] Infants and young children are at the greatest risk for serious complications.[29]

MANAGEMENT

Mild scorpion envenomations may only require symptomatic treatment, including analgesics and local ice compresses. Any child stung by a scorpion, especially if identified as *C. exilicauda*, should be hospitalized for close monitoring of respiratory, cardiac, and neurologic status.[36] Specific antivenom is the treatment of choice for severe envenomation. Critically ill children with neurotoxic effects of scorpion envenomation can benefit greatly and promptly with intravenous administration of scorpion-specific F(ab')(2) antivenom.[29] Lack of it may have serious consequences. Studies indicate that *C. exilicauda* antivenom is safe, with a low incidence of anaphylactic reaction following infusion and a rapid onset of symptom relief.[34,37] Although serum sickness is common after antivenom infusion, it is usually self-limited and can be managed with antihistamines and corticosteroids.[34,37]

ACARINA

The order Acarina contains ticks and mites (Fig. 181-1). Ticks are the most numerous members of this order, with approximately 800 known species. They are important worldwide as vectors of systemic disease, capable of transmitting viruses, rickettsia, spirochetes, bacteria, and parasites to humans.

MITES

See Chap. 178.

TICKS

Ticks are divided into 2 families: (1) Ixodidae (hard ticks) and (2) Argasidae (soft ticks). Hard ticks are responsible for the majority of tick-related disease. Ticks pass through multiple stages during their life cycle, including egg, larva, nymph, and adult, and require blood meals for transition between the latter 3 stages. Ticks are distinguished from other mites by the presence of a barbed hypostome, which is inserted into the skin for feeding (Fig. 181-6). Ticks ingest blood from a diversity of vertebrate hosts, including birds, reptiles, and mammals.[38] Adult hard ticks are capable of ingesting several hundred times their unfed body weight when taking a blood meal and may survive for months without feeding. When searching for a suitable host, hard ticks exhibit a unique behavior called "questing" during which the tick crawls to the edge of a leaf or blade of grass and holds its front pair of legs stretched out to grab onto a passing host.[39-41] Humans often become infested by contact with tall grass or brush that harbors the unfed ticks or by their association with domestic animals like cats or dogs. Ticks are attracted to the smell of sweat, the color white, and body heat. Once on a host, a tick may spend up to 24 hours in search of a protected site to feed, such as a skin fold or the hairline. Tick feeding time ranges from 2 hours to 7 days, with the tick dropping off of the host once fully engorged.

Many different tick species are responsible for local tick bite reactions and transmission of disease in human hosts. In the United States, *Ixodes scapularis* (deer tick or black-legged tick), *Dermacentor andersoni* (American wood tick), *Dermacentor variabilis* (American dog tick), *Ixodes pacificus* (Western black-legged tick), and *Amblyomma americanum* (Lone Star tick) are among the most common. In the Eastern Hemisphere, important tick species include *Ixodes ricinus* (castor bean tick or sheep tick) and *Ixodes persulcatus* (Taiga tick). Among the diseases transmitted by ticks are Lyme disease (Chap. 179), ehrlichiosis, babesiosis, Rocky Mountain spotted fever (Chap. 180), Colorado tick fever, Q fever, and tularemia (Chap. 156).

Clinical Findings: The majority of tick bites occur in the spring and summer, coinciding with the life cycle of the tick. Tick bites are usually painless, as the tick introduces an anesthetic and anticoagulant substance when biting. Often, a person will not even know he or she has been bitten, but will see or feel an attached tick while scratching or bathing. Tick bites may incite foreign body granuloma formation, reactions to injected toxins and salivary secretions, and other hypersensitivity responses. Rarely, delayed hypersensitivity reactions occur with fever, pruritus, and urticaria.[42] A red papule is usually seen at the bite site, and may progress to localized swelling and erythema.[42,43] A cellular response to the bite can lead to induration and nodularity after a few days. Foreign-body reactions may occur when mouthparts are retained in skin after incomplete removal of the tick. Chronic tick bite granulomas may present diagnostic problems and persist for months to years.

Tick paralysis is a potentially lethal complication of tick infestation and is thought to be caused by a neurotoxin contained within tick salivary secretions. The illness may start with headache and malaise and rapidly progress to an acute ascending lower motor neuron paralysis, similar to that of Guillain–Barré syndrome, which may result in respiratory failure and death.[44,45] Several species of tick are capable of causing tick paralysis, including *D. andersoni*, *D. variabilis*, and *A. americanum*. Typically, the onset of symptoms occurs 4 to 6 days after attachment of the tick. Symptoms resolve once the tick is removed from the patient. Supportive measures, including mechanical ventilation, may be required until symptoms resolve.

Management: After potential exposure, the skin should be inspected for ticks to remove them before they begin feeding and risk transmitting disease. Once a tick has inserted its hypostome into the skin, it must be forcibly removed. Although many methods have

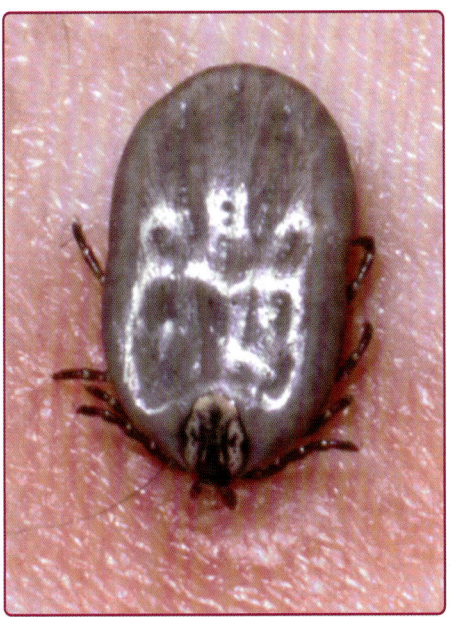

Figure 181-6 *Dermatocentor variabilis* feeding. The tick has been attached for 24 hours.

been suggested for removing ticks, physical methods, such as slow, steady pulling on the tick, are probably the safest and most useful. Retained tick parts should be removed surgically if necessary to prevent development of foreign body granulomas. Antibiotic prophylaxis after tick bites is controversial. Although there is some evidence that prophylaxis may help prevent acquisition of Lyme disease and other vector-borne illnesses, the risks of antibiotic therapy must be weighed against the risks and prevalence of vector-borne illnesses in a particular region. In areas highly endemic for Lyme disease, the benefits of prophylactic treatment may outweigh the risks, especially in cases in which the tick has been attached to the host for an extended period of time and can accurately be identified as a vector for Lyme borreliosis. In these cases, the authors suggest a course of oral doxycycline (Chap. 179).

CHILOPODA AND DIPLOPODA

The arthropod classes Chilopoda and Diplopoda are composed of centipedes and millipedes, respectively. Centipedes and millipedes are terrestrial arthropods with multiple body segments.

CENTIPEDES

Centipedes, which have one pair of legs per body segment, are nocturnal carnivores that may produce extremely painful bites with a pair of poisonous claws. The *Scolopendra* species is found throughout the southwestern United States and may attack when its habitat is disturbed. In addition to severe pain and erythema following a bite, localized sweating, edema, secondary infection, and ulceration may be seen. There are also case reports of proteinuria, acute coronary ischemia, and myocardial infarction following centipede bite.[46-50] Treatment consists of analgesia, including injection of local anesthetics, antihistamines, and tetanus prophylaxis. Antibiotics may be required to treat secondary infection.

MILLIPEDES

Millipedes, which have 2 pairs of legs per body segment, usually feed on living and dead plant matter. They lack poison claws and neither bite nor sting. However, millipedes possess repugnatorial glands on either side of each segment and may emit a toxic substance if threatened. The oily, viscous liquid can cause a brownish discoloration of the skin that can persist for months and may produce burning and blistering.[51-53] Severe reactions are mainly seen in tropical species. Some species are capable of squirting the toxin several inches. This can result in various eye lesions, including periorbital edema, periorbital discoloration, conjunctivitis, and keratitis.[54] Although ophthalmologic evaluation should be considered for eye exposures, thorough immediate cleansing with soap and water is usually adequate for skin contact.

INSECTA

The class Insecta contains several orders of medical importance: Anoplura (lice; Chap. 178), Diptera (flies, mosquitoes), Coleoptera (beetles), Hemiptera (bedbugs, kissing bugs), Siphonaptera (fleas), Hymenoptera (ants, bees, wasps), and Lepidoptera (butterflies and moths). Insects can be distinguished from other arthropods by the presence of 3 body segments, a pair of compound eyes, paired antennae, and 6 legs.

DIPTERA

The order Diptera, or true flies, contains several important families: Culicidae (mosquitoes), Simuliidae (black flies), Ceratopogonidae (biting midges), Tabanidae (horse flies and deer flies), Psychodidae subfamily Phlebotominae (sandflies), and Glossinidae (tsetse flies). Not only do members of this order inflict cutaneous injury with their bites, they are also, collectively, responsible for the transmission of more disease worldwide than any other arthropod order.

The family Culicidae contains more than 2000 species of mosquito, many of which transmit disease. Several genera of mosquito, including *Anopheles*, *Culex*, and *Aedes*, serve as vectors for malaria, yellow fever, dengue fever, filariasis, and encephalitis viruses, including West Nile virus, which caused the largest arboviral meningoencephalitis outbreak ever recorded in North America.[55] *Aedes aegypti* mosquitoes, which are most active during daylight hours, are linked with infections by both dengue and zika viruses. Personal protection technologies such as insecticide-treated clothing using permethrin provides some individual protection. The efficacy of permethrin-treated clothing on personal protection has been assessed in the laboratory setting.[56] Because male mosquitoes lack piercing mouthparts, female mosquitoes inflict all human bites. Mosquito bites incite the formation of pruritic wheals and papular lesions, which form in response to irritating salivary secretions that are injected by the mosquito to prevent coagulation. Mosquito bites may have an urticarial, vesicular, eczematous, or granulomatous appearance. Bite reactions usually subside over several days.

Other biting flies include midges, black flies, horseflies, tsetse flies, and sandflies. Black flies of the family Simuliidae are vectors for onchocerciasis (African river blindness; Chap. 177) and tularemia (Chap. 156). Within the Tabanidae family, *Tabanus* species (horse flies) also serve as vectors for tularemia, and *Chrysops* species (deer flies or mango flies) are responsible for transmission of *Loa loa* filariasis (Chap. 177) and tularemia.

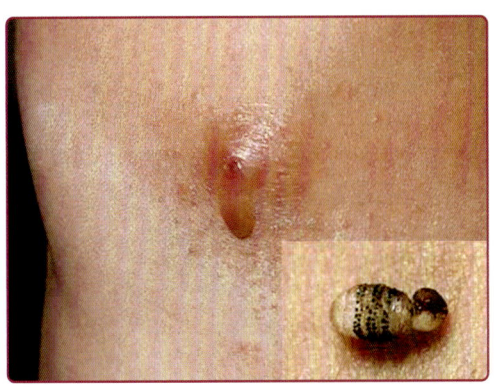

Figure 181-7 Cutaneous myiasis: a domed nodule resembling a furuncle at the site of deposition of a botfly larva. The lesion has a central pore through which the posterior end of the larva intermittently protrudes. The inset shows the larva that has been extracted.

Cutaneous myiasis (Fig. 181-7) may be caused by the deposition of fly larvae into intact skin or open wounds by several species, including *Dermatobia hominis* (human botfly).[57] Numerous species of sandflies also spread disease, with *Phlebotomus* species transmitting Old World leishmaniasis (Chap. 176) and *Lutzomyia* species transmitting New World leishmaniasis and Carrión disease/verruca peruana (bartonellosis; Chap. 176). *Glossina* species (tsetse flies) serve as vectors for African trypanosomiasis (Chap. 176).

Diptera bites should be cleansed thoroughly with soap and water to avoid secondary infection. A short course of topical steroids and systemic antihistamines may be used to control pruritus. Rare allergic reactions should be treated aggressively. Cutaneous myiasis is often best treated with local surgical excision of the larva and involved surrounding tissue. The antihistamines cetirizine or ebastine taken prophylactically as a single 10-mg dose have been demonstrated in studies to decrease wheal formation and subsequent pruritus following mosquito bites.[58,59]

COLEOPTERA

The Coleoptera order is the largest order in the animal kingdom, containing more than 300,000 species of beetles. Although beetles generally do not bite or sting humans, many species of beetle contain chemicals that can cause blistering of human skin.[60] Although some beetles are capable of emitting these chemicals, most cases of blister beetle dermatosis are the result of a beetle being crushed against the skin. The most well-known beetle to cause blister beetle dermatosis is *Lytta vesicatoria*, the Spanish fly, which is found in Southern Europe and contains the chemical cantharidin. Cantharidin, which causes vesiculation of the skin, is used in the treatment of warts and molluscum contagiosum. Several other species of beetle found in different regions of the world, including the central and southeastern United States, contain similar chemicals and can cause blistering.[61,62] *Paederus* species (rove beetles) contain the vesicant pederin and are another cause of beetle dermatitis.[62] Washing of affected areas immediately after exposure may help prevent vesication. Blisters should be treated with local wound care until resolved.

Another beetle with dermatologic significance is the carpet beetle. The most common species found in the United States are *Attagenus megatoma* (black carpet beetle) and *Anthrenus scrophulariae* (common carpet beetle). Although adult carpet beetles are of little clinical importance, cutaneous exposure to carpet beetle larvae, which feed on wool, carpets, clothing, and other organic material, can cause an allergic papulovesicular dermatitis.[63]

HEMIPTERA

The Hemiptera order encompasses 2 families of clinical significance: (1) the Cimicidae, which includes *Cimex lectularius* (bedbugs), and (2) the Reduviidae, which includes *Triatoma* species (kissing bugs). Although most members of this order are herbivores, these 2 families are frequent human parasites.

CIMICIDAE

The common bedbug (*C. lectularius*; see Fig. 181-1) has been a scourge of mankind for centuries. The bedbug is a nocturnal feeder that stays hidden during the day in cracks and crevices of headboards, in picture frames, behind loose wallpaper, or any other dark place that accommodates its flattened body.[1] After a potential victim has gone to bed, the insects come out of hiding for a blood meal. They are attracted to the warmth and carbon dioxide production of their victim. Bedbugs usually complete their meal in a matter of minutes and then return to hiding. Although bedbugs can survive for 1 year or more without feeding, they usually seek a blood meal every 5 to 10 days.[1] Bedbugs are common and are distributed worldwide. They can be spread in clothing and baggage of travelers and visitors, on secondhand mattresses, and via laundry.

Along with other blood-sucking arthropods, the role of bedbugs in infectious disease transmission has gained increasing interest in recent years. Although laboratory studies have shown that these insects are capable of incubating and shedding pathogens such as hepatitis B virus for several weeks after feeding on an infected bloodmeal, there is currently no convincing evidence that *Cimex* species act as vectors in their natural state.[64]

Bedbug bites are usually painless and may be overlooked unless large numbers of bites are present. Bites are usually multiple and may be grouped in a linear fashion. A row of 3 bedbug bites is sometimes referred to as *breakfast, lunch, and dinner*[65] (Fig. 181-8). Reactions to the bites consist of wheals and papules, often with a small hemorrhagic punctum at the center. Bullous reactions to bites are also possible in sensitized

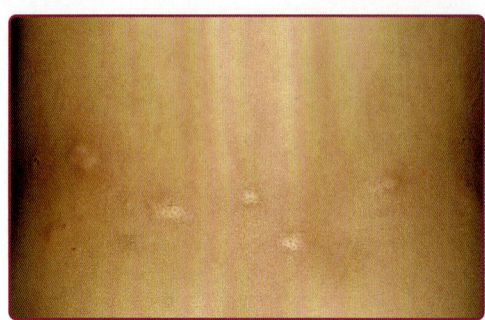

Figure 181-8 Papular urticaria: bedbug bites. These are pruritic urticarial papules, arranged in a row (breakfast, lunch, and dinner).

individuals, and hypersensitivity reactions have been reported.[65-67] Flecks of blood also may be found on bed linens. Minimal symptomatic treatment of bites and good local wound care to prevent pruritus and secondary infection are sufficient in most cases.[67] In the presence of a secondary infection, topical antiseptic lotion or antibiotic cream should be applied.[66] Topical corticosteroids and oral antihistamines may be used for pruritus. Once a bedbug infestation has been diagnosed, a professional exterminator is often necessary to eradicate the insects. Evidence for disease transmission is lacking.

REDUVIIDAE

The kissing bug, or assassin bug, belongs to the family Reduviidae and is distinguished by a triangular shape on its back formed by the meeting of the membranous wings. All reduviid bugs possess piercing mouthparts used to feed on blood. Most species of Reduviidae are found in the Americas, with a few species located in Africa, Asia, and Europe. Within the United States, these insects are found in the Southwest from Texas to California.[68] Reduviidae are of great clinical significance because they act as vectors for *Trypanosoma cruzi*, the causative agent of Chagas disease, which affects an estimated 15 to 20 million people living in South America and Central America (Chap. 176). Kissing bugs earned their name for their predilection to bite on or near the lips. After taking a blood meal, reduviids characteristically turn around and defecate immediately. The trypanosomes are inoculated when the victim subsequently scratches the infected feces into the wound.[1]

Although they are nocturnal feeders and usually prey on rodents, during periodic flights they move toward the lights of desert homes. Defensive bites of reduviids are extremely painful. The painless bite of a feeding reduviid occurs only while the host is sleeping, because the blood meal takes several minutes to complete. Bites have been associated with papular, urticarial, and bullous reactions. A small proportion of victims may develop generalized, acute allergic reactions that cause the victim to awaken with sudden-onset anaphylactic signs and symptoms.[69] Defensive bites may incite more severe local cutaneous reactions, including necrosis and ulceration.

SIPHONAPTERA

Fleas belong to the insect order Siphonaptera (Fig. 181-1). These small bloodsucking insects are wingless and are capable of jumping to a height of 18 cm. Members of the family Pulicidae, most notably the rat fleas (*Xenopsylla cheopis* and *Xenopsylla brasiliensis*), transmit bubonic plague (*Yersinia pestis*) (Chap. 154). Other members of this family are also capable of transmitting disease, including the cat flea (*Ctenocephalides felis*), which is a vector for bubonic plaque and endemic typhus (*Rickettsia prowazekii*).

Fleabites produce minimal irritation in nonsensitized individuals, typically resulting in linear or clustered urticarial papules, frequently found on the lower legs (Fig. 181-9). In sensitized individuals, most often young children, the antigenic saliva is capable of producing papular urticaria, an eruption characterized by recurrent or chronic pruritic papules occurring on exposed skin areas.[1,70] Bullous reactions to fleabites may also develop in patients with hypersensitivity. Conservative topical therapy with corticosteroids and antipruritics, along with oral antihistamines, is usually sufficient for most fleabites. Antibiotics may be necessary should secondary bacterial infection develop. Once a flea infestation occurs, complete eradication of the insects is necessary to prevent additional bites.

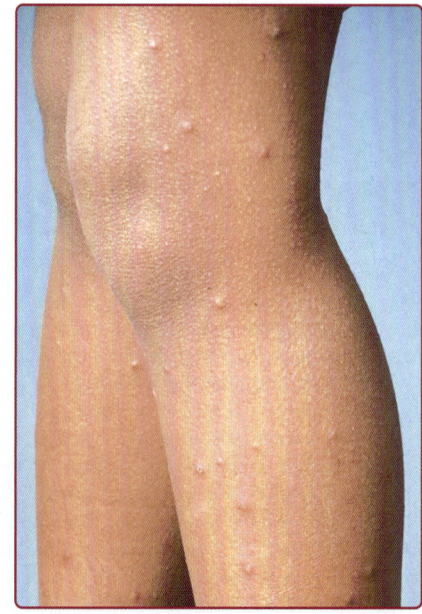

Figure 181-9 Papular urticaria: fleabites. Multiple, pruritic urticarial papules, usually <1 cm in diameter; they may be topped by a vesicle. Here, they occur on the legs of a child.

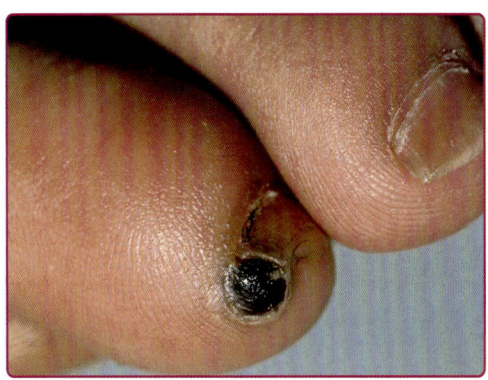

Figure 181-10 Tungiasis: a necrotic periungual papule on the fifth toe. The larva can be visualized by removing the overlying crust.

The Tungidae family contains a tropical flea species called *Tunga penetrans* (the sand flea, chigoe flea, or jigger) that is the etiologic agent of tungiasis, an infestation caused by penetration of the adult female flea into human skin to lay eggs.[71] The usual sites of attachment are feet, particularly plantar surface, subungual or periungual skin or web spaces, and legs, but any body surface in contact with the ground can be affected. Solitary or multiple erythematous papules slowly enlarge over a few weeks to 4 to 10 mm in diameter (Fig. 181-10). A fully developed white or yellowish, firm, somewhat translucent nodule may be painful, especially if subungual, or the pain may reflect secondary impetigo and rarely lymphangitis and septicemia. Dermoscopy facilitates visualization of ovoid eggs, and thus the diagnosis of tungiasis.[72] Tungiasis may be also be associated with pain, pruritus, and, sometimes, autoamputation of toes.[73] Death from tetanus also has been reported. One need elicit a history of travel or residence in an endemic area. Treatment options include surgical excision of the affected area or killing the adult female flea with cryotherapy or topical agents. Tetanus prophylaxis is recommended, and systemic antibiotics should be used when necessary. Prevention can be enhanced in endemic areas by avoiding walking along beaches barefoot or in sandals and not sitting or lying in the sand in parts of Nigeria, the Caribbean, India, and Brazil.

HYMENOPTERA

The order Hymenoptera contains the families Apidae and Bombidae (bees), Vespidae (wasps), and Formicidae (ants). Many members of this order have evolved poison glands used for defense and/or hunting. Aside from local cutaneous reactions, Hymenoptera stings are an important problem because of their high incidence and ability to produce fatal anaphylactic reactions.[74]

All Hymenoptera stings are inflicted by female insects via a modified ovipositor or egg-laying apparatus. Most Hymenoptera stings occur when the nest or individual insects are threatened. The honeybee stings with a barbed ovipositor, which it leaves impaled into the skin. The honeybee dies after stinging because it eviscerates itself to expel its paired venom sacs. The stinger should be removed as swiftly as possible after a sting because the musculature attached to the stinger can continue to pump venom into the skin. If possible, the stinger should not be squeezed during removal with fingers or tweezers as additional venom can be injected into the victim. One method for removal is to scrape the edge of a credit card or the dull blade of a butter knife along the skin at an angle almost parallel to the surface. This will dislodge the stinger while minimizing the injection of additional venom. Other Hymenoptera species lack a barbed stinger and may sting repeatedly.

Imported fire ants (*Solenopsis invicta*), originally from Brazil, are an aggressive species that has become well established in the southeastern United States. *Solenopsis* venom contains a nonproteinaceous, hemolytic factor identified as a dialkylpiperidine, solenopsin D, which induces mast cell degranulation.[75] Imported fire ants often attack in groups. Their sting results in an intense inflammatory, wheal-and-flare reaction that becomes a sterile pustule and may progress to localized necrosis and scarring. Sensitized individuals may experience significant bullous reactions following a sting. When attacking, the ants tend to bite the flesh with their powerful jaws and then pivot and sting in a circular pattern, resulting in ring-shaped lesions.

CLINICAL MANIFESTATIONS

Hymenoptera stings typically produce immediate burning and pain, followed by the development of an intense, local, erythematous reaction with swelling and urticaria. This "typical" reaction to hymenoptera stings usually subsides within several hours. However, more severe local reactions can occur, including extensive swelling at the sting site and prolonged induration lasting for up to 1 week. A cell-mediated immune response also has been implicated in these reactions.[76] Generalized systemic reactions to hymenoptera stings occur in approximately 0.4% to 3.0% of patients. Anaphylactic reactions may be evident as generalized urticaria, angioedema, and bronchospasm.

MANAGEMENT

Treatment of a Hymenoptera sting is governed by the severity of the reaction. Mild local cutaneous reactions may only require local cleansing, application of ice, and possible injection of local anesthetic to control pain. Oral or parenteral diphenhydramine may help control urticaria and pruritus. Anaphylaxis must be treated vigorously with subcutaneous epinephrine (0.5 mL of 1:1000 dilution) and the institution of intramuscular epinephrine, exit to an emergency room, and the supportive measures. Individuals with known Hymenoptera hypersensitivity should always carry a preloaded epinephrine-filled syringe for emergency self-administration. Desensitization therapy should be considered for any patient with a positive intradermal skin test to Hymenoptera venom and a history of sting-induced anaphylaxis. Fire ant hypersensitivity is a potentially deadly condition for which rush immunotherapy may be a good option to achieve protection quickly.

LEPIDOPTERA

The Lepidoptera order is the second largest order of insects and contains more than 100,000 species of caterpillars, moths, and butterflies. An estimated 100 to 150 species within this order are thought to produce *lepidopterism*, the term used to describe the aggregate of medical effects caused by caterpillars, moths, and butterflies.[77,78] Multiple theories regarding the mechanisms of lepidopterism have been proposed, including mechanical irritation by pointed hairs (setae), toxin injection through hollow setae, and cell-mediated hypersensitivity to the hairs. One well-known cause of erucism or caterpillar dermatitis is *Lymantria dispar* (gypsy moth caterpillar).[79,80] Cutaneous contact with hairs from this caterpillar may produce a pruritic dermatitis characterized by multiple erythematous papules often arranged in linear streaks. Urticaria, angioedema, and anaphylaxis may occur with processionary caterpillars (genus *Thaumetopoea*). Wind-borne hairs may produce keratoconjunctivitis and respiratory symptoms. *Megalopyge opercularis* (asp or puss caterpillar), which can inject venom through its hollow syringe-like hairs, is capable of inflicting an intensely painful sting, and may produce a characteristic train-track pattern of purpura at the sting site (Fig. 181-11).[81,82] Other species that cause lepidopterism in the Americas include *Automeris io* (io moth), *Euproctis chrysorrhoea* (brown-tailed moth), *Sibine stimulate* (saddleback moth), and *Hemerocampa pseudotsugata* (Douglas-fir tussock moth).

Treatment for lepidopterism is largely symptomatic. Systemic antihistamines, topical preparations containing menthol and camphor, and moderate- to high-potency topical corticosteroids can be used to control pruritus. Systemic steroids may be beneficial for severe reactions. The intractable pain caused by the sting of the puss caterpillar may require oral or parenteral narcotic analgesics. Embedded setae can be removed from the skin by "stripping" with adhesive tape. There is an antivenom available that should be employed for potentially fatal Lonomia genus caterpillar envenomation, still responsible for deaths in southern Brazil.[83]

PREVENTION

Several relatively simple steps can be taken to minimize the occurrence of arthropod bites. Spider bites can be reduced by wearing gloves while working in crawl spaces, garages, or basements or when manipulating woodpiles or rubbish piles. In scorpion-endemic areas, shaking out clothing and footwear before putting them on is advisable. Wearing appropriate clothing with good coverage and avoiding rubbing against high brush and grass may help avoid tick bites. Bright colors and artificial scents like perfume, which are attractants for mosquitoes and other flying insects, are best avoided on warm summer nights. In tropical regions, proper footwear is essential to preventing tungiasis. Infestations of living areas by arthropods, including fleas and bedbugs, are difficult to eliminate and may require the assistance of a professional exterminator.

Chemical repellents are also useful in preventing arthropod bites. Several different chemical compounds have been studied, including *N,N*-diethyl-3-methylbenzamide (DEET, previously diethyltoluamide), picaridin (KBR 3203), and *p*-menthane-3,8-diol (Eucalyptus oil). The most effective repellent for all biting flies, including mosquitoes, is DEET, which is available in many products in concentrations up to 100%. Generally, a product containing 10% to 30% DEET provides adequate protection for

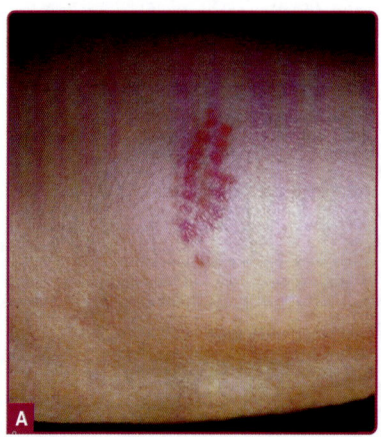
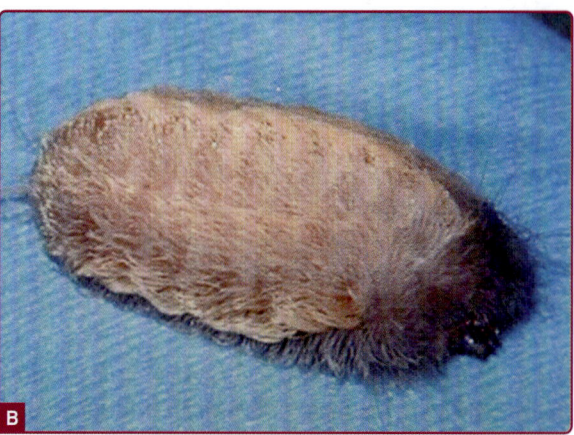

Figure 181-11 **A,** Cutaneous reaction from contact with a puss caterpillar showing the typical grid-like pattern. **B,** Puss caterpillar (*Megalopyge opercularis*) demonstrating the corresponding gridlike pattern of its hairs.

most outdoor activities, with higher concentrations of DEET providing longer protection times. Although DEET has an excellent safety record, there are reports of encephalopathy developing, particularly in children, after exposure to this chemical.[84,85] For this reason, only products with DEET concentrations of less than 10% should be used on children. Permethrin, an insecticide often used to treat pediculosis and scabies, is available as a tick repellent that can be sprayed on or impregnated into clothing and fabrics, including tents, bed nets, and sleeping bags, and remains effective through several wash cycles.[86] Combined use of permethrin-treated clothing and DEET applied to the skin provides the maximum protection. Long-lasting insecticidal nets and indoor residual spraying can be effective indoors, but significant exposure occurs outdoors. Accordingly, an outdoor mosquito control device, a synthetic human odor–baited mosquito device with multiple electrocuting grids, has been devised to attract and kill outdoor host-seeking mosquitoes, including important malaria vectors *An. arabiensis* and *An. funestus* sensu stricto, and shows considerable promise.[87] Rapid, noninvasive mass screening and posttherapeutic followup for scabies and selected other cutaneous infestations can be facilitated by use of videodermatoscopy, dermatoscopy, reflectance confocal microscopy, and optical coherence tomography.[88]

REFERENCES

1. Steen CJ, Carbonaro PA, Schwartz RA. Arthropods in dermatology. *J Am Acad Dermatol.* 2004;50(6):819-842; quiz 842-844.
2. Mowry JB, Spyker DA, Brooks DE, et al. 2014 Annual Report of the American Association of Poison Control Centers' National Poison Data System (NPDS): 32nd Annual Report. *Clin Toxicol (Phila).* 2015;53(10):962-1147.
3. Kang J, Bhate C, Schwartz RA. Spiders in dermatology. *Semin Cutan Med Surg.* 2014;33(3):123-127.
4. Elston DM. What's eating you? *Latrodectus mactans* (the black widow spider). *Cutis.* 2002;69(4):257-258.
5. Monte AA. Black widow spider (*Latrodectus mactans*) antivenom in clinical practice. *Curr Pharm Biotechnol.* 2012;13(10):1935-1939.
6. Daly FF, Hill RE, Bogdan GM, et al. Neutralization of *Latrodectus mactans* and *L. hesperus* venom by redback spider (*L. hasseltii*) antivenom. *J Toxicol Clin Toxicol.* 2001;39(2):119-123.
7. Graudins A, Padula M, Broady K, et al. Red-back spider (*Latrodectus hasselti*) antivenom prevents the toxicity of widow spider venoms. *Ann Emerg Med.* 2001;37(2):154-160.
8. Isbister GK, Graudins A, White J, et al. Antivenom treatment in arachnidism. *J Toxicol Clin Toxicol.* 2003;41(3):291-300.
9. Sams HH, Dunnick CA, Smith ML, et al. Necrotic arachnidism. *J Am Acad Dermatol.* 2001;44(4):561-573; quiz 573-576.
10. Hoover EL, Williams W, Koger L, et al. Pseudoepitheliomatous hyperplasia and pyoderma gangrenosum after a brown recluse spider bite. *South Med J.* 1990;83(2):243-246.
11. Roche KJ, Chang MW, Lazarus H. Images in clinical medicine. Cutaneous anthrax infection. *N Engl J Med.* 2001;345(22):1611.
12. Vetter RS, Bush SP. Chemical burn misdiagnosed as brown recluse spider bite. *Am J Emerg Med.* 2002;20(1):68-69.
13. Gomez HF, Krywko DM, Stoecker WV. A new assay for the detection of *Loxosceles* species (brown recluse) spider venom. *Ann Emerg Med.* 2002;39(5):469-474.
14. van Meeteren LA, Frederiks F, Giepmans BN, et al. Spider and bacterial sphingomyelinases D target cellular lysophosphatidic acid receptors by hydrolyzing lysophosphatidylcholine. *J Biol Chem.* 2004;279(12):10833-10836.
15. Tambourgi DV, Pedrosa MF, de Andrade RM, et al. Sphingomyelinases D induce direct association of C1q to the erythrocyte membrane causing complement mediated autologous haemolysis. *Mol Immunol.* 2007;44(4):576-582.
16. da Silva PH, da Silveira RB, Appel MH, et al. Brown spiders and loxoscelism. *Toxicon.* 2004;44(7):693-709.
17. Elbahlawan LM, Stidham GL, Bugnitz MC, et al. Severe systemic reaction to *Loxosceles reclusa* spider bites in a pediatric population. *Pediatr Emerg Care.* 2005;21(3):177-180.
18. Elston DM, Miller SD, Young RJ 3rd, et al. Comparison of colchicine, dapsone, triamcinolone, and diphenhydramine therapy for the treatment of brown recluse spider envenomation: a double-blind, controlled study in a rabbit model. *Arch Dermatol.* 2005;141(5):595-597.
19. Wilson JR, Hagood CO Jr, Prather ID. Brown recluse spider bites: a complex problem wound. A brief review and case study. *Ostomy Wound Manage.* 2005;51(3):59-66.
20. Centers for Disease Control and Prevention (CDC). Necrotic arachnidism—Pacific Northwest, 1988–1996. *MMWR Morb Mortal Wkly Rep.* 1996;45(21):433-436.
21. Sadler MA, Force RW, Solbrig RM, et al. Suspected *Tegenaria agrestis* envenomation. *Ann Pharmacother.* 2001;35(11):1490-1491.
22. Wasserman GS, Anderson PC. Loxoscelism and necrotic arachnidism. *J Toxicol Clin Toxicol.* 1983;21(4-5):451-472.
23. Vest DK. Necrotic arachnidism in the northwest United States and its probable relationship to *Tegenaria agrestis* (Walckenaer) spiders. *Toxicon.* 1987;25(2):175-184.
24. Bernardino CR, Rapuano C. Ophthalmia nodosa caused by casual handling of a tarantula. *Clao J.* 2000;26(2):111-112.
25. Choi JT, Rauf A. Ophthalmia nodosa secondary to tarantula hairs. *Eye (Lond).* 2003;17(3):433-434.
26. Sandboe FD. Spider keratouveitis. A case report. *Acta Ophthalmol Scand.* 2001;79(5):531-532.
27. Watts P, McPherson R, Hawksworth NR. Tarantula keratouveitis. *Cornea.* 2000;19(3):393-394.
28. Skolnik AB, Ewald MB. Pediatric scorpion envenomation in the United States: morbidity, mortality, and therapeutic innovations. *Pediatr Emerg Care.* 2013;29(1):98-103.
29. Coorg V, Levitan RD, Gerkin RD, et al. Clinical presentation and outcomes associated with different treatment modalities for pediatric bark scorpion envenomation. *J Med Toxicol.* 2017;13(1):66-70.
30. Amitai Y. Clinical manifestations and management of scorpion envenomation. *Public Health Rev.* 1998;26(3):257-263.

31. Amitai Y, Mines Y, Aker M, et al. Scorpion sting in children. A review of 51 cases. *Clin Pediatr (Phila)*. 1985;24(3):136-140.
32. Bhadani UK, Tripathi M, Sharma S, et al. Scorpion sting envenomation presenting with pulmonary edema in adults: a report of seven cases from Nepal. *Indian J Med Sci*. 2006;60(1):19-23.
33. Elston DM, Stockwell S. What's eating you? *Centruroides exilicauda*. *Cutis*. 2002;69(1):16, 20.
34. LoVecchio F, McBride C. Scorpion envenomations in young children in central Arizona. *J Toxicol Clin Toxicol*. 2003;41(7):937-940.
35. Carbonaro PA, Janniger CK, Schwartz RA. Scorpion sting reactions. *Cutis*. 1996;57(3):139-141.
36. Shah N, Martens MG. Scorpion envenomation in pregnancy. *South Med J*. 2016;109(6):338-341.
37. LoVecchio F, Welch S, Klemens J, et al. Incidence of immediate and delayed hypersensitivity to Centruroides antivenom. *Ann Emerg Med*. 1999;34(5):615-619.
38. Eisen L, Eisen RJ, Lane RS. The roles of birds, lizards, and rodents as hosts for the western blacklegged tick *Ixodes pacificus*. *J Vector Ecol*. 2004;29(2):295-308.
39. Daniel M, Zitek K, Danielová V, et al. Risk assessment and prediction of *Ixodes ricinus* tick questing activity and human tick-borne encephalitis infection in space and time in the Czech Republic. *Int J Med Microbiol*. 2006;296(suppl 40):41-47.
40. Mays SE, Houston AE, Trout Fryxell RT, et al. Comparison of novel and conventional methods of trapping ixodid ticks in the southeastern U.S.A. *Med Vet Entomol*. 2016;30(2):123-134.
41. Tsunoda T, Tatsuzawa S. Questing height of nymphs of the bush tick, *Haemaphysalis longicornis*, and its closely related species, *H. mageshimaensis*: Correlation with body size of the host. *Parasitology*. 2004;128(pt 5):503-509.
42. Krinsky WL. Dermatoses associated with the bites of mites and ticks (Arthropoda: Acari). *Int J Dermatol*. 1983;22(2):75-91.
43. Bhate C, Schwartz RA. Lyme disease: part I. Advances and perspectives. *J Am Acad Dermatol*. 2011;64(4):619-636; quiz 637-638.
44. Li Z, Turner RP. Pediatric tick paralysis: Discussion of two cases and literature review. *Pediatr Neurol*. 2004;31(4):304-307.
45. Pek CH, Cheong CS, Yap YL, et al. Rare cause of facial palsy: case report of tick paralysis by *Ixodes holocyclus* imported by a patient travelling into Singapore from Australia. *J Emerg Med*. 2016;51(5):e109-e114.
46. Bouchard NC, Chan GM, Hoffman RS. Vietnamese centipede envenomation. *Vet Hum Toxicol*. 2004;46(6):312-313.
47. Hasan S, Hassan K. Proteinuria associated with centipede bite. *Pediatr Nephrol*. 2005;20(4):550-551.
48. Ozsarac M, Karcioglu O, Ayrik C, et al. Acute coronary ischemia following centipede envenomation: case report and review of the literature. *Wilderness Environ Med*. 2004;15(2):109-112.
49. Yildiz A, Biçeroglu S, Yakut N, et al. Acute myocardial infarction in a young man caused by centipede sting. *Emerg Med J*. 2006;23(4):e30.
50. Elston DM. What's eating you? Centipedes (Chilopoda). *Cutis*. 1999;64(2):83.
51. Hendrickson RG. Millipede exposure. *Clin Toxicol (Phila)*. 2005;43(3):211-212.
52. De Capitani EM, Vieira RJ, Bucaretchi F, et al. Human accidents involving *Rhinocricus* spp., a common millipede genus observed in urban areas of Brazil. *Clin Toxicol (Phila)*. 2011;49(3):187-190.
53. Elston DM. What's eating you? Millipedes (Diplopoda). *Cutis*. 2001;67(6):452.
54. Hudson BJ, Parsons GA. Giant millipede "burns" and the eye. *Trans R Soc Trop Med Hyg*. 1997;91(2):183-185.
55. Petersen LR, Marfin AA, Gubler DJ. West Nile virus. *JAMA*. 2003;290(4):524-528.
56. Orsborne J, DeRaedt Banks S, Hendy A, et al. Personal protection of permethrin-treated clothing against *Aedes aegypti*, the vector of dengue and zika virus, in the laboratory. *PLoS One*. 2016;11(5):e0152805.
57. Hohenstein EJ, Buechner SA. Cutaneous myiasis due to *Dermatobia hominis*. *Dermatology*. 2004;208(3):268-270.
58. Karppinen A, Kautiainen H, Petman L, et al. Comparison of cetirizine, ebastine and loratadine in the treatment of immediate mosquito-bite allergy. *Allergy*. 2002;57(6):534-537.
59. Karppinen A, Petman L, Jekunen A, et al. Treatment of mosquito bites with ebastine: a field trial. *Acta Derm Venereol*. 2000;80(2):114-116.
60. Elston DM. What's eating you? Blister beetles. *Cutis*. 2004;74(5):285-286.
61. Brazzelli V, Martinoli S, Prestinari F, et al. Staphylinid blister beetle dermatitis. *Contact Dermatitis*. 2002;46(3):183-184.
62. Claborn DM, Polo JM, Olson PE, et al. Staphylinid (rove) beetle dermatitis outbreak in the American southwest? *Mil Med*. 1999;164(3):209-213.
63. Ahmed AR, Moy R, Barr AR, et al. Carpet beetle dermatitis. *J Am Acad Dermatol*. 1981;5(4):428-432.
64. Silverman AL, Qu LH, Blow J, et al. Assessment of hepatitis B virus DNA and hepatitis C virus RNA in the common bedbug (*Cimex lectularius* L.) and kissing bug (*Rodnius prolixus*). *Am J Gastroenterol*. 2001;96(7):2194-2198.
65. Elston DM, Stockwell S. What's eating you? Bedbugs. *Cutis*. 2000;65(5):262-264.
66. Leverkus M, Jochim RC, Schäd S, et al. Bullous allergic hypersensitivity to bed bug bites mediated by IgE against salivary nitrophorin. *J Invest Dermatol*. 2006;126(1):91-96.
67. Thomas I, Kihiczak GG, Schwartz RA. Bedbug bites: A review. *Int J Dermatol*. 2004;43(6):430-433.
68. Lynch PJ, Pinnas JL. "Kissing bug" bites. Triatoma species as an important cause of insect bites in the southwest. *Cutis*. 1978;22(5):585-591.
69. Anderson C, Belnap C. The kiss of death: a rare case of anaphylaxis to the bite of the "red margined kissing bug." *Hawaii J Med Public Health*. 2015;74(9)(suppl 2):33-35.
70. Stibich AS, Schwartz RA. Papular urticaria. *Cutis*. 2001;68(2):89-91.
71. Heukelbach J. Tungiasis. *Rev Inst Med Trop Sao Paulo*. 2005;47(6):307-313.
72. Cabrera R, Daza F. Dermoscopy in the diagnosis of tungiasis. *Br J Dermatol*. 2009;160(5):1136-1137.
73. Sunenshine PJ, Janniger CK, Schwartz RA. Tungiasis. In: Demis DJ, ed. *Clinical Dermatology*. Philadelphia, PA: Lippincott & Williams Wilkins; 1999, Unit 18-33:1-10.
74. Steen CJ, Janniger CK, Schutzer SE, et al. Insect sting reactions to bees, wasps, and ants. *Int J Dermatol*. 2005;44(2):91-94.
75. Yi GB, McClendon D, Desaiah D, et al. Fire ant venom alkaloid, isosolenopsin A, a potent and selective inhibitor of neuronal nitric oxide synthase. *Int J Toxicol*. 2003;22(2):81-86.
76. Case RL, Altman LC, VanArsdel PP Jr. Role of cell-mediated immunity in Hymenoptera allergy. *J Allergy Clin Immunol*. 1981;68(5):399-405.

77. Diaz JH. The epidemiology, diagnosis, and management of caterpillar envenoming in the southern US. *J La State Med Soc*. 2005;157(3):153-157.
78. Dunlop K, Freeman S. Caterpillar dermatitis. *Australas J Dermatol*. 1997;38(4):193-195.
79. Allen VT, Miller OF 3rd, Tyler WB. Gypsy moth caterpillar dermatitis—revisited. *J Am Acad Dermatol*. 1991; 24(6, pt 1):979-981.
80. Wills PJ, Anjana M, Nitin M, et al. Population explosions of tiger moth lead to lepidopterism mimicking infectious fever outbreaks. *PLoS One*. 2016;11(4):e0152787.
81. Gardner TL, Elston DM. Painful papulovesicles produced by the puss caterpillar. *Cutis*. 1997;60(3):125-126.
82. Pinson RT, Morgan JA. Envenomation by the puss caterpillar (*Megalopyge opercularis*). *Ann Emerg Med*. 1991; 20(5):562-564.
83. Hossler EW. Caterpillars and moths. Part II. Dermatologic manifestations of encounters with Lepidoptera. *J Am Acad Dermatol*. 2010;62(1):13-28.
84. Hampers LC, Oker E, Leikin JB. Topical use of DEET insect repellent as a cause of severe encephalopathy in a healthy adult male. *Acad Emerg Med*. 1999; 6(12):1295-1297.
85. Sudakin DL, Trevathan WR. DEET: a review and update of safety and risk in the general population. *J Toxicol Clin Toxicol*. 2003;41(6):831-839.
86. Alpern JD, Dunlop SJ, Dolan BJ, et al. Personal protection measures against mosquitoes, ticks, and other arthropods. *Med Clin North Am*. 2016;100(2):303-316.
87. Matowo NS, Koekemoer LL, Moore SJ, et al. Combining synthetic human odours and low-cost electrocuting grids to attract and kill outdoor-biting mosquitoes: field and semi-field evaluation of an improved mosquito landing box. *PLoS One*. 2016; 11(1):e0145653.
88. Micali G, Lacarrubba F, Verzì AE, et al. Scabies: advances in noninvasive diagnosis. *PLoS Negl Trop Dis*. 2016;10(6):e0004691.

Chapter 182 :: Bites and Stings of Terrestrial and Aquatic Life
:: Camila K. Janniger, Robert A. Schwartz, Jennifer S. Daly, & Mark Jordan Scharf

第一百八十二章
陆生和水生生物的叮咬和蜇伤

中文导读

本章分为4节：①陆生动物咬伤；②水生生物叮咬和蜇伤；③水媒感染；④海产品摄入与中毒的皮肤表现。主要介绍了陆上动物咬伤的有害影响，以及它们可能传播的细菌和病毒感染，同时回顾了海洋生物可能造成的咬伤、蜇伤和其他形式的伤害。

第一节介绍了狗咬是最常见的陆生动物咬伤。所有咬伤的评估和治疗应该包括仔细记录事件的历史、动物的类型、咬伤的地点和地理环境，根据评估给予相应的治疗和处理。同时详细介绍了动物咬伤引起的特殊细菌感染和特定病毒感染，包括狂犬病、猴疱疹病毒(B病毒)感染等，最后介绍了蛇咬伤的相关知识。

第二节水生生物叮咬和蜇伤，介绍了各类水生生物咬伤引起的伤害和处理，包括海豹、水母、海葵、珊瑚、海绵、海胆、海星、海参以及海洋蠕虫、软体动物、有毒鱼等。

第三节水媒感染介绍了海洋生物造成的伤口可能会引起病原体感染，表182-8列出了通常与水传播感染有关的生物体。

第四节简单介绍了鱼类和甲壳类动物、鲭鱼食物中毒、雪卡毒素等海产品摄入与中毒的皮肤表现。

〔栗 娟〕

AT-A-GLANCE

- Dog bites account for 80% to 90% of all mammalian bites involving humans, but cat bites are more likely to become infected.

- Whether or not postexposure prophylaxis with rabies immunoglobulin and human diploid cell rabies vaccine is needed depends on the circumstances surrounding the bite.

- In the United States, there are approximately 5 to 6 deaths from snakebites and probably 6000 to 7000 snakebite envenomations each year.

- Most stingray injuries occur when bathers, waders, or fishermen accidentally step on rays as they lie partially covered with sand in shallow waters. The extreme pain caused by the venom may be relieved by soaking the affected body part in very warm water.

- Cnidarian envenomations cause more annual deaths than do shark attacks.

Humans are a part of the environment and ideally live peacefully with other animals and plants. However, sometimes the interactions between man and the environment prove harmful to one or the other. The first 2 sections of this chapter consider the harmful effects of land-borne animal bites, as well as the bacterial and viral infections they may transmit. The last section reviews bites and stings and other forms of injury that may be inflicted by marine life.

BITES OF LAND ANIMALS

EPIDEMIOLOGY

Dog bites account for 80% to 90% of all mammalian bites involving humans. Four to 5 million dog bites are estimated to occur each year in the United States. In 2001, it was estimated that 368,245 persons were treated for dog bite–related injuries.[1] The human victim is often a 5- to 9-year-old boy who may have been teasing or playing with a dog. Sometimes the bite occurs when a person is trying to break up a pair of fighting dogs or trying to aid an animal. In the United States, 4% to 5% of dog bites are work related and include bites sustained by postal carriers. Overseas, a higher percentage are produced by untamed animals.[2-4] Most dog bite injuries involve the upper extremities, especially the hands. Cat bites are the second most common type of mammalian bite after dog bites, but the wounds following a cat's bite are nearly twice as likely to become infected as wounds from dog bites.[5] In addition, millions of exotic pets are transported legally and illegally into the United States and Europe annually. The approximately 1 million iguanas in America today may bite.[6]

CLINICAL APPROACH (PATHOGENESIS AND TREATMENT)

The evaluation and treatment of all bite wounds should include taking a careful history of the incident, the type of animal, the site of the bite, and the geographic setting. Hand wounds, puncture wounds, and crush injuries are likely to become infected. Specimens from infected bites should be cultured and a Gram-stained smear prepared; the wound should then be washed, well irrigated, and left open. Most patients with bites on the hands, deep cat bites (Table 182-1), deep cat scratches, and sutured wounds should be treated with amoxicillin/clavulanic acid or ceftriaxone because of the risk of *Pasteurella multocida* infection; if the patient is allergic to these agents, a quinolone or a tetracycline should be used. Evidence that the use of prophylactic antibiotics is of benefit exists only for bites of the hand. However, once the patient has an infection, intravenous antibiotics and surgical drainage are often required.[4,6-8] Tetanus immune status should be evaluated, and rabies prophylaxis should be considered, depending on the type of animal, local epidemiologic factors, and ability to quarantine the animal for 10 days.[9]

Human bites and monkey bites deserve special mention, because 30% become infected with aerobic or anaerobic mouth organisms. Infection caused by anaerobes may spread through the metacarpal–phalangeal space and causes severe damage. The same procedure should be followed as for other animal bites, that is, culture and Gram stain, thorough washing, and debridement. Wounds, especially hand wounds, should be left open if possible. Evidence suggests that patients with human bites that penetrate the epidermis should be treated prophylactically with amoxicillin/clavulanic acid for 7 to 10 days or, if the patient is allergic to penicillins, with a fluoroquinolone plus an antianaerobic agent such as clindamycin.[7,10] Clenched-fist injuries should be evaluated by a hand surgeon because of the high likelihood of infectious complications, including septic arthritis and osteomyelitis.[2]

TABLE 182-1
Standard Management for Dog/Cat Bites

Culture and Gram stain
Wash wound and irrigate well
Ideally, wounds should be left open
Amoxicillin/clavulanic acid *or* ceftriaxone for prophylaxis* for 7-10 d
Intravenous antibiotics and surgical drainage for active infections
Evaluate tetanus immune status
Consider rabies prophylaxis or treatment

*Quinolone or tetracycline, if patient is allergic.

SPECIFIC BACTERIAL INFECTIONS CAUSED BY ANIMAL BITES

PASTEURELLA MULTOCIDA INFECTION

(See Chap. 156). An organism commonly infecting bite wounds is *P. multocida*, a bacterium present in the nasopharynx in 50% to 66% of dogs and 70% to 90% of cats. The most common pattern is that of local infection with adenitis after a dog or cat bite or scratch. *P. multocida* is the most common pathogen in cat bite infections and may also complicate 26% of dog bite wounds.[5] The infection usually presents within 24 to 48 hours, often within several hours. In patients with a cat bite, the infection may be followed by tenosynovitis or osteomyelitis as a result of inoculation of the organism into the periosteum by the long, sharp tooth of the animal. *Pasteurella* infections also have been reported after bites of large cats such as lions and tigers.

Systemic infection may also occur as bacteria may enter the respiratory tract through the inspiration of contaminated barn dust, or by inhalation of infectious droplets sprayed by the sneeze of an animal. In such cases, the bacteria probably colonize the respiratory tract and in some patients cause active infection. Bronchiectasis, emphysema, peritonsillar abscess, and sinusitis have all been described with this organism. Finally, systemic infection with bacteremia or meningitis may occur.

P. multocida is a small, gram-negative, ovoid bacillus that grows well on blood agar but does not grow on selective gram-negative media such as MacConkey agar. Because of the superficial resemblance of *P. multocida* to *Haemophilus influenzae* and *Neisseria* organisms, infections of the respiratory tract and CNS with this bacillus may be misdiagnosed initially.

Treatment of the patient with presumptive *P. multocida* infection should consist of careful washing of the wound and an attempt to leave it open. The empiric antibiotic of choice is amoxicillin/clavulanic acid orally for 7 to 10 days, with careful followup examination of the wound. *P. multocida* is susceptible to penicillin alone, and patients may be switched to penicillin if they have a pure infection with this organism. A fluoroquinolone, a tetracycline, and a trimethoprim-sulfamethoxazole are alternatives. In most patients, the antibiotic is aimed at both the patient's skin flora (such as *Staphylococcus aureus*) and organisms from the animal's mouth. Given the increasing prevalence of community acquired methicillin-resistant *S. aureus* (MRSA), patients should be treated with vancomycin, clindamycin, tetracycline, or trimethoprim-sulfamethoxazole if MRSA is suspected (Chaps. 154 and 156).[11]

STAPHYLOCOCCUS INTERMEDIUS INFECTION

S. intermedius is an organism associated with dogs weighing more than 40 lb. It is more commonly found in canine gingival flora than is *S. aureus* (39% vs 10%).[12] It is a gram-positive, coagulase-positive coccus that can be differentiated from *S. aureus* in the laboratory by biochemical testing. In comparison with *S. aureus*, *S. intermedius* does not produce acetoin from glucose and has β-galactosidase activity. If these tests are not performed (ie, if only a latex assay is used to identify *Staphylococci*), the laboratory may incorrectly report an isolate as *S. aureus* or unspecified *Staphylococcus*. Antibiotic treatment is the same as that for infections with *S. aureus*, although resistance to oxacillin is uncommon in *S. intermedius* and is growing in importance for *S. aureus*.[11]

CAPNOCYTOPHAGA CANIMORSUS INFECTION

C. canimorsus is a capnophilic ("carbon dioxide–loving"), facultatively anaerobic, slow-growing, gram-negative rod associated with dog bites.[13-16] The organism has been found in the oral cavity of 17% of cats and 24% of dogs. Most infections occur in splenectomized or immunocompromised hosts, although fatal infections including meningitis have been reported in immunocompetent hosts and present as overwhelming sepsis.

INFECTION BY PORPHYROMONAS SPECIES

Porphyromonas sp. are slow-growing anaerobic bacteria found in the deep gingival pockets of animal and humans. The organism is difficult to culture, requiring 4 to 6 days for colony formation as well as vitamin K and hemin in the media.[17,18] Citron and coworkers[19] found *Porphyromonas* sp. in 28% of culture specimens from patients with infected dog and cat bite wounds.

CAT SCRATCH DISEASE

Bartonella henselae is the most common etiologic agent of cat scratch disease. *Afipia felis* and other *Bartonella* species may cause some cases (Chap. 154).

Serratia marcescens may induce an unpleasant cellulitis in iguana bites in pet owners.[6] The treatment is trimethoprim-sulfamethoxazole or a quinolone antibiotic.

PLAGUE

(See Chap. 156).

TULAREMIA

(See Chap. 156).

RAT-BITE FEVER

(See Chap. 156).

SPECIFIC VIRAL INFECTIONS CAUSED BY ANIMAL BITES

RABIES

Epidemiology: The most notorious viral disease to occur after an animal bite is rabies, which is caused by a Rhabdovirus. Its epidemiology has changed in the past few years as a result of improved control of rabies in the domestic animal population. Now, nonimmune dogs and domestic animals account for only 8% of cases, whereas sylvatic animals, such as skunks, raccoons, red and gray foxes, and bats, represent the greatest potential danger. Rodents, such as squirrels and hamsters, are probably inconsequential as sources of rabies. However, cases of rabies in cattle are increasing.[20] Postexposure prophylaxis, which is nearly 100% effective, has reduced the number of cases of human rabies from more than 100/year a century ago to an average of 1 to 4 cases a year in the United States today. In 2004, of the 8 cases in the 49 states and Puerto Rico, 4 were acquired as a result of patients' receiving transplanted organs from an infected donor.[20,21] Although in the United States death in humans from rabies is rare, WHO estimates that 55,000 deaths occur each year in developing countries, half in children under 15 years.[22]

Live virus is introduced into nerve tissue at the time of the bite, multiplies at the site, and then spreads to the CNS. It replicates in gray matter and then spreads along autonomic nerves to the salivary glands, adrenal glands, and heart. The incubation period varies with the site of the bite from 5 days to as long as several years. Clinical features include a prodromal period of 1 to 4 days, followed by high fever, headache, and malaise. Paresthesia at the site of inoculation occurs in 80% of patients. The next sequence of events is familiar: agitation, hyperesthesia, dysphagia, excessive thirst, paralysis, and death.

Diagnosis: The diagnosis of clinical rabies is difficult and is often not made until after the death of the patient. Viral isolation methods may yield positive results for specimens of saliva or cerebral spinal fluid during the first 2 weeks of the illness, and saliva is infectious, so isolation precautions are needed. Serum antibodies may be detected as early as day 6 and usually by day 13. The fluorescent antibody method for detection of the viral antigen is the most rapid and sensitive means of making the diagnosis, and no matter where the actual bite site is, once patients have CNS disease, the diagnosis can be made from a biopsy of skin from the highly innervated hair-covered area of the neck or from brain tissue.

Prevention and Treatment: The most effective prevention for rabies is to avoid contact with any wild animal or any unfamiliar domestic animal. Persons at risk of unavoidable contact with rabies, such as spelunkers, veterinarians, virologists, and travelers spending time in countries where rabies is enzootic, should receive preexposure prophylaxis with the human diploid cell rabies vaccine (HDRV) series (3 intramuscular injections on days 0, 7, and 21 or 28) given in the deltoid muscle and repeated every 2 years. In persons vaccinated intradermally (using a lower intradermal dose), the neutralizing antibody titer should be performed, because the immune response may not be fully protective.[23]

The need for postexposure prophylaxis can be determined by the answers to the following questions: (1) What is the status of animal rabies in the locale where the exposure took place? (2) Was the attack provoked or unprovoked? (3) Of what species and size was the animal? (4) What was the state of health and vaccination record of the animal? (5) Will the brain of the animal be examined within 48 hours? (6) Can the animal be effectively quarantined? Most animals transmit rabies virus in saliva only a few days before becoming ill themselves; bats, however, may harbor the virus for many months.

Bites by Household Pets: If the dog or cat responsible for the bite is healthy and available for observation for 10 days, the patient should not be treated unless the animal develops rabies. At the first sign of rabies in the animal, the patient should be treated with rabies immunoglobulin (RIG) and the vaccine HDRV. The symptomatic animal should be killed and tested as soon as possible. If the animal is rabid or suspected of being rabid, or if it does not have up-to-date vaccination records, the patient should be treated with RIG and HDRV (see section "Specifics of Treatment").[24]

Bites by Wild Animals: All skunks, bats, groundhogs, foxes, coyotes, raccoons, bobcats, and other carnivores should be regarded as rabid unless laboratory test results prove negative. The patient should be treated with RIG and HDRV.

Bites by Other Animals: Bites by other animals (livestock, rodents, lagomorphs such as rabbits and hares, and ferrets) should be considered individually.[23] Local and state public health officials should be consulted about the need for prophylaxis. Bites by squirrels, hamsters, guinea pigs, gerbils, chipmunks, rats, mice, and other small rodents almost never call for anti-rabies prophylaxis.

Specifics of Treatment: The most important step is to cleanse the wound immediately with a brush and soap to remove as much virus as possible. The wound should be rinsed well and then scrubbed a second time with green soap or 70% alcohol, which is rabicidal. If vaccine treatment is indicated, both RIG and HDRV should be given as soon as possible, regardless of the interval after exposure, unless the patient has been previously vaccinated and a serologic assay shows current immunity. In this case, only HDRV is needed and should be given on day 0 and day 3. For nonimmune hosts, administration of RIG is the most urgent. If HDRV is not immediately available, RIG should be started and HDRV given as soon as it is obtained. RIG (20 IU/kg) should be given immediately—50% around the site of the bite and 50% in the thigh or the arm. This passive immunization not only will result in the early appearance of antibody but will also inhibit development of the active antibody from HDRV, hence the need for a 28-day series. Active immunization is accomplished using HDRV, given intramuscularly for a total of 5 doses on days 0, 3, 7, 14, and 28. Serum for rabies antibody testing should be collected 2 weeks after the fifth dose. If there is no antibody response, an additional booster should be given.

Management of the Patient with Clinical Rabies: In the rare cases in which a patient is admitted with the clinical diagnosis of rabies, several steps should be taken immediately. First, the diagnosis must be suspected and the patient placed on isolation precautions while the diagnosis is made rapidly by fluorescent antibody staining of specimens from various tissues, as well as immunofluorescence staining of the source animal's brain tissue. Elevated antibody titers in the absence of immunization are clear evidence of infection. The first signs of clinical rabies are usually nonspecific, such as malaise, anorexia, fatigue, headache, and fever. The acute neurologic illness that follows is most commonly characterized by intermittent episodes of hyperactivity. In some cases, however, a progressive paralysis occurs. The usual period from onset of symptoms to onset of coma is 10 days. Risk of exposure for hospital staff includes contact with open wounds or mucous membranes with saliva or other potentially infectious material such as neurologic tissue, spinal fluid, or urine. Blood, serum, and stool are not considered infectious.

Basic clinical management consists of anticipating and preventing all treatable complications of the rabies infection and induction of coma to manage the patient until the patient generates an immune response.[25] Pulmonary hypoxia should be prevented by tracheostomy at the first sign of respiratory difficulty, monitoring of actual partial pressure of oxygen, and use of supplemental oxygen. There are no specific antiviral treatments for rabies, although ribavirin has been tried.[25] Anticonvulsant therapy should also be instituted. Extreme increases in intracranial pressure may be prevented by insertion of a cerebrospinal fluid reservoir that allows withdrawal of the intraventricular fluid and measurement of intracranial pressure. Cardiac arrhythmias may be anticipated with careful monitoring. Rabies had been regarded as uniformly fatal, but there have been patients who have survived with prolonged cardiorespiratory support, and there is serologic evidence that some animals have survived. An aggressive approach to treatment of the patient with known rabies infection is worthwhile. In 2004, a 15-year-old girl without a history of prior rabies vaccination survived after her physicians used a treatment based on induced coma as well as other supportive measures and antiviral agents.[20,25] The World Health Organization has complied information regarding treatment and prevention accessible on their website.[22]

HERPESVIRUS SIMIAE (B VIRUS) INFECTION

Herpesvirus simiae (B virus) is enzootic in Old World monkeys, especially rhesus, cynomolgus, and other macaques. The illness in monkeys is similar to that caused by herpes simplex in humans, and asymptomatic monkeys may shed the virus in saliva. Most cases in humans have occurred after direct exposure to macaque monkeys or monkey tissue through bites, scratches, or cuts.[26] A vesicular lesion develops at the wound site with progressive lymphadenitis and fever. Over the next few days to weeks, patients develop a severe illness, which is characterized by rapidly progressive ascending neuropathy and encephalitis. The illness is rare and before the availability of antiviral therapy, 72% of cases were fatal. A cluster of 4 cases occurring in 1987 in Pensacola, Florida, were treated with acyclovir. The 2 patients who received acyclovir when their infections were localized responded well to therapy and were maintained on oral acyclovir. All macaques should be presumed to be shedding B virus and should be handled accordingly. All monkey-inflicted injuries should be cleansed, specimens should be collected for viral culture, and a physician should evaluate the patient. Clinical and serologic monitoring is critical, and high-risk or infected patients should be treated according to established guidelines. The use of acyclovir or ganciclovir initially and acyclovir for years has led to improved survival in infected patients.

SNAKEBITES

In the United States, there are approximately 5 to 6 deaths from snakebites and probably 6000 to 7000 snakebite envenomations each year.[26] The largest number of venomous snakebites occur in the Southwestern States. Worldwide as many as 125,000 fatal snakebites may occur each year.[27] Because of regional differences in varieties of snakes, management recommendations including specific antivenom recommendations differ by geographic area. The World Health Organization has published guidelines to help ensure the quality and availability of antivenom immunoglobulins worldwide, and has an online database that can be used to explore the global distributions of venomous snake species, and access information on antivenom products and their manufacturers.[28]

The 2 major poisonous snakes in the Americas are the pit viper (family Viperidae, subfamily Crotalinae, which includes the rattlesnake, water moccasin, and copperhead) and the coral snake (family Elapidae). Poisonous snakes are found in all states of the United

States except Maine, Hawaii, and Alaska.[29] The northern copperhead, also called the highland moccasin, is pink or reddish brown and is marked with large chestnut brown barrels resembling dumbbells or hourglasses (Fig. 182-1). The bite is painful but rarely fatal. The timber rattler is dark brown with chevrons of black and brown (Fig. 182-2).

The degree of toxicity of a snakebite depends on the potency of the venom, the amount injected, the size and condition of the snake, and the size of the person bitten. Pain occurs at the site of the bite (usually within 5 minutes). Signs and symptoms at the bite site include wheal with local edema, numbness, and, within moments, ecchymosis and painful lymphadenopathy (Fig. 182-3).

Nausea, vomiting, sweating, fever, drowsiness, and slurred speech may develop. Bleeding of the gums and hematemesis are common hemorrhagic manifestations. If edema and erythema have not developed within 8 hours after the bite, it can be assumed that significant envenomation did not occur. Estimated mortality rates for victims who receive antivenom in a health care facility are less than 1% and probably less than 0.1%.

For proper treatment, it is extremely important to establish that the bite is from a poisonous snake. Many patients experience symptoms related to fear that may mimic symptoms from venom. The patient should have distinct fang punctures and immediate local pain, followed by edema and discoloration within 30 minutes. It is helpful to inspect the snake, because those that are poisonous may be differentiated from those that are not by the presence of fangs and the shape of the pupils (Fig. 182-4). Availability of a photograph of snakes common to a specific geographic area is important for all hospital emergency wards to aid practitioners in deciding if the patient has been bitten by a poisonous snake.

Although there are still insufficient evidence-based criteria for first aid and out-of-hospital treatment for snakebite envenomations, a rational approach is outlined in Table 182-2.[30] In summary, the patient should be stabilized and transported as rapidly as possible to a health care facility capable of administering antivenom, and the affected site should be immobilized

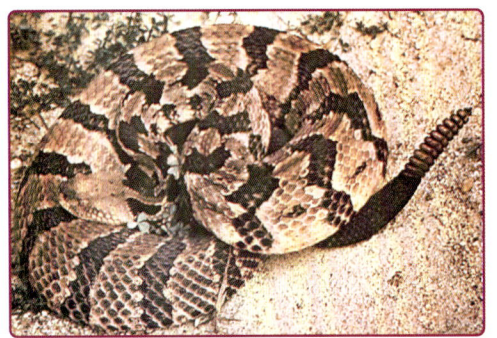

Figure 182-2 Timber rattlesnake.

below the level of the heart. Constricting bands such as watches or jewelry should be removed; the routine use of venous compression bands is not recommended.[29] The patient should be kept as immobilized as possible.[29] Venous compression techniques are designed to impede the return of venous and lymphatic flow from the bite site without sacrificing blood flow to the extremity. In cases in which there is likely to be a significant delay in transport and the victim is developing systemic signs of envenomation such as hypotension, these techniques may be of value.[30] Arguments against the use of venous compression techniques include the time that it takes to apply the treatments, which may further delay transport time. Additional arguments against the use of these techniques include the potential for concentrating the venom in the affected limb, which may worsen local necrosis, along with the possibility of a bolus effect when the compression is released.[30] Another possible disadvantage of the use of these compression techniques is the potential for them to cause arterial compression if the affected limb swells in reaction to the toxin. If a decision is made to use a venous compression band in the field, arterial pulses should be palpable distal to the ligature, and the dressing should be checked frequently to make sure that it is has not become too tight. If a venous compression dressing has been applied in the field and is not causing vascular compromise, it should be left in place until the patient reaches a health care facility and antivenom is at the bedside.[30]

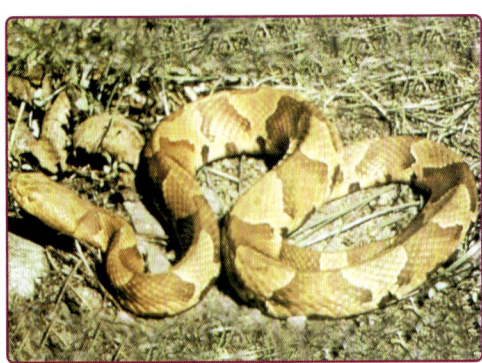

Figure 182-1 Northern copperhead.

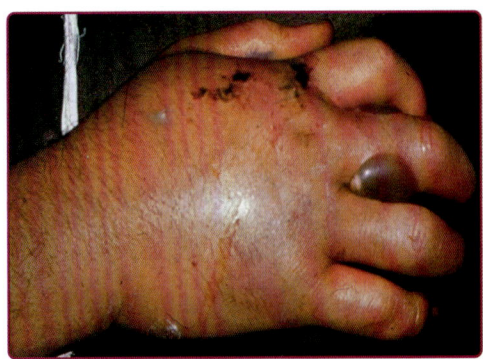

Figure 182-3 Copperhead snakebite.

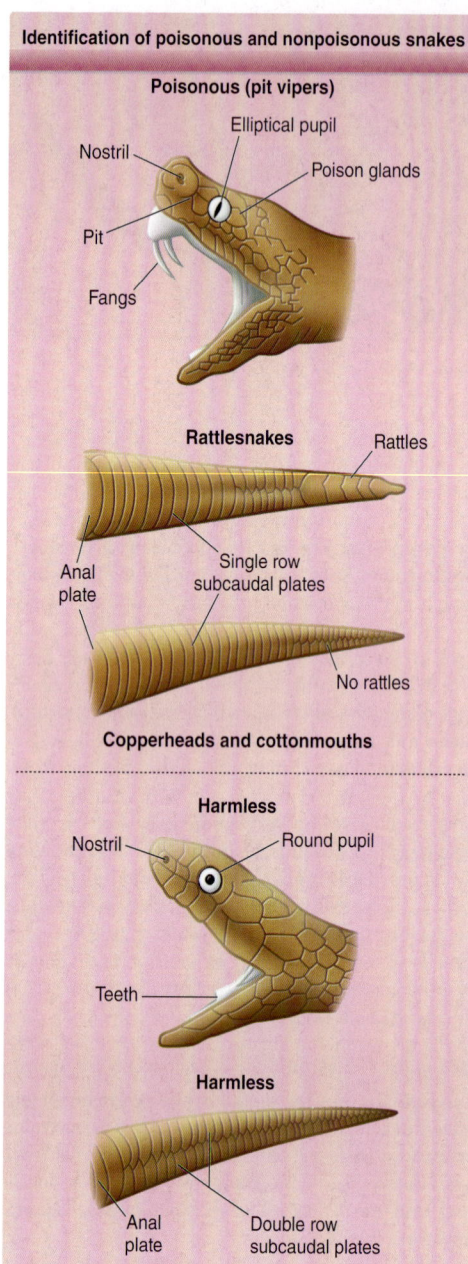

Figure 182-4 Identification of poisonous and nonpoisonous snakes. (From Wingert WA, Wainschel J: A quick handbook on snake bites. *Resid Staff Physician*, 1977, p. 56, with permission.)

TABLE 182-2
First Aid and Out-of-Hospital Treatment for Snakebite Envenomation

1. The patient should be stabilized and transported as rapidly as possible to a health care facility capable of administering antivenom. Consult the CDC and WHO websites for updated information on antivenom availability and use.[28]
2. The affected site should be immobilized below the level of the heart, constricting bands such as watches or jewelry should be removed, and the patient should be kept as immobile as possible.[29]
3. The use of venous compression bands or pressure immobilization is not recommended,[29] although there is controversy surrounding their use if there is likely to be a significant delay in transport and the victim is developing systemic signs of envenomation such as hypotension, and in such a case these techniques may be of value.[30]
4. The value of using a suction device to extract venom is debated in the literature.[29] If such a device is applied in the field and fluid is accumulating in the suction cup, it can be left in place until the patient reaches a medical facility.[30]
5. The use of cryotherapy, incision, or excision of the bite site, arterial tourniquets, and electroshock therapy as part of emergency field therapy should be discouraged.

CDC, Centers of Disease Control and Prevention; WHO, World Health Organization.

bites to a digit, if there is severe swelling and the finger is tense, blue, or pale, a digit dermotomy may be of use. True compartment syndrome involving an extremity is a rare complication of snakebite envenomation. Fasciotomy should be used only in cases of increased compartment pressure that has not responded to prompt and sufficient treatment with antivenom.[31]

The primary treatment for crotaline snake venom poisoning is prompt and adequate dosing with antivenom. Antivenom is most effective if given within 4 hours of the snakebite (Table 182-3).

FabAV should be used for all severe American crotaline snakebites, but not those of the coral snake. The dosage should be guided by the severity and progression of local changes and systemic clinical signs. Because some patients develop recurrent manifestations of envenomation after initial treatment, both a loading dose of 4 to 6 vials of FabAV and then, once initial control has been achieved, 3 maintenance doses 6, 12, and 18 hours later are recommended.[29]

The role of surgical intervention in the treatment of snakebite envenomations is limited in most cases. Surgery is appropriate only if medical treatment fails. This includes elevation of the bitten body part in conjunction with the administration of 4 to 6 vials of Crotalidae polyvalent immune Fab (ovine) (FabAV) over the course of 1 hour.[29] Debridement of truly necrotic skin and subcutaneous tissues is recommended 4 to 5 days after envenomation. In cases of

TABLE 182-3
Antivenom for Crotaline Snake Bites

- Emergency information and antivenom are available in the United States through the New Jersey Poison Control Center Network, which can be reached 24 hours a day by calling 800-222-1222.[29]
- The World Health Organization website has a database with information and pictures to aid providers in finding the correct antivenom[28]: http://apps.who.int/bloodproducts/snakeantivenoms/database/.

Supportive treatment is indicated, including hospitalization with careful evaluation of baseline hematocrit, platelet count, and prothrombin time. Coagulopathy should be corrected by using antivenin, because fresh-frozen plasma is ineffective.[29] The wound should be cleansed and covered. Antitetanus therapy and antibiotic prophylaxis with penicillin, ampicillin/sulbactam, or tetracycline should be initiated for severe bites.

BITES AND STINGS OF AQUATIC ORGANISMS

SEAL BITE

Normally, a seal bite occurs on the finger of a trainer or a seal hunter—thus the term *seal finger* or *spaek finger*.[32,33] Bites and contact abrasions also occur in in open-water swimmers from harbor seals, are uncommon, and usually involve the lower extremities.[33] An infection may ensue, the etiologic agent of which may be unclear. One study suggests that a virus similar to that causing Orf may be the culprit,[33] although *Mycoplasma* sp. have been isolated, and some patients respond to tetracycline (Chap. 156). The incubation period of 4 to 8 days is followed by throbbing pain, erythema at the site, and swelling of the joint proximal to the bite. Untreated, seal finger progresses to cellulitis, tenosynovitis, and arthritis Tetracycline, 500 mg orally 4 times a day for 10 days, remains the antibiotic of choice.[30,32] It is also helpful to immobilize and elevate the finger as well as soak it several times a day (Chap. 156).

INJURIES CAUSED BY JELLYFISH, PORTUGUESE MAN-OF-WAR, SEA ANEMONES, AND CORALS

Stings caused by jellyfish, Portuguese man-of-war, sea anemones, and corals are the most common envenomations experienced by humans in marine environments. All of these creatures are members of the phylum Cnidaria, formerly known as *Coelenterata*. They are divided into 3 major classes. The first class, Hydrozoa, includes the Portuguese man-of-war, fire corals, and hydroids. Jellyfish belong to the second class, Scyphozoa. The third class, Anthozoa, encompasses sea anemones and true corals. Approximately 100 of the 9000 species of Cnidaria that have been identified may cause injury to humans.[34]

Cnidarians are radially symmetric animals with body walls formed by an inner and outer layer of cells enclosing a jellylike substance. They may be either free floating in the water like jellyfish or sessile like corals.[34] Almost all cnidarians possess nematocysts, or stinging capsules, which are usually concentrated on some form of tentacle. Each nematocyst contains a toxin or group of toxins and a coiled thread-like apparatus with a barbed end that functions like a flexible hypodermic syringe (Fig. 182-5). When the nematocyst comes into contact with a victim, the barbed end is discharged, and the toxin is injected into the skin.

Cnidarian stings range from mild, self-limited irritations to extremely painful and serious injuries,

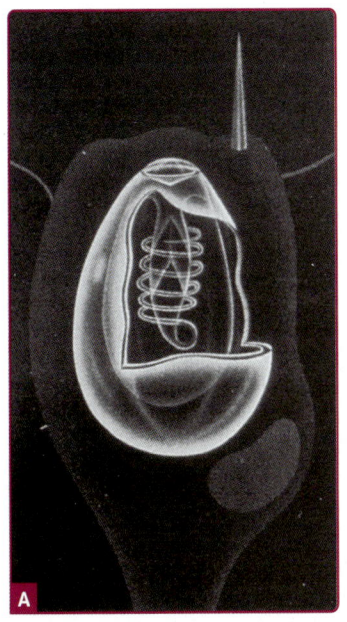 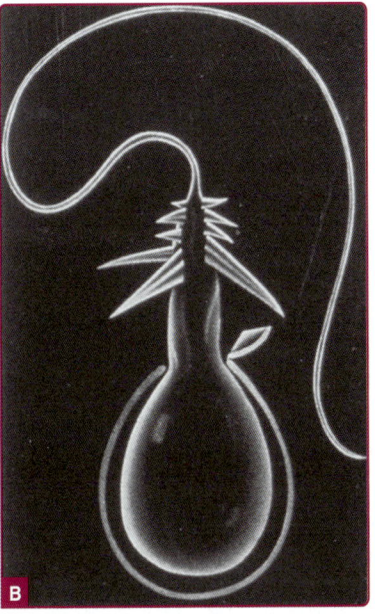

Figure 182-5 From left to right, a diagrammatic view of an intact and discharged coelenterate nematocyst. (R. Kreuzinger, used with permission from World Life Research Institute.)

depending on the toxin of the species involved and the magnitude of the envenomation. Stings from certain species such as the cubomedusae, or box jellyfish, can be fatal.

In most cases, jellyfish stings elicit toxic reactions that may be localized and/or systemic. Although immediate-type hypersensitivity reactions, including urticaria, angioedema, and anaphylaxis, occur less frequently, they require prompt medical intervention, because shock and death may ensue in highly sensitized individuals. Allergic contact dermatitis, delayed and persistent hypersensitivity reactions, granuloma annulare, and erythema nodosum are other possible cutaneous reactions to jellyfish stings.[35]

INJURIES CAUSED BY JELLYFISH

Sea Nettles: Among the organisms most commonly causing jellyfish stings are the sea nettles, which comprise 2 different species, both of which inhabit Atlantic as well as Indo-Pacific waters. *Cyanea capillata* and its relatives are the larger of the 2 species, with a bell measuring up to 1 m and numerous tentacles reaching 30 m in length (Fig. 182-6).[36] *Chrysaora fuscescens* (Fig. 182-7) is found in the Pacific waters off the coast of California. *Chrysaora quinquecirrha* is smaller, with a white or rusty bell that may reach 30 cm with 4 digestive tentacles hanging from it. Although sea nettle stings are seldom lethal, they can be quite painful.[37] Initially the victim experiences a sharp burning pain in the area contacted by the tentacles. Within minutes, the sting area develops a zigzag, whip-like pattern of raised red welts 2 to 3 mm wide (Fig. 182-8). The duration of acute pain may vary, but the pain often begins to abate in 30 minutes. The wheals usually subside by 1 hour, but purplish brown petechial and postinflammatory pigmentation may persist for several days.

Portuguese Man-of-War: *Physalia physalis* is the species name for the Portuguese man-of-war, which is a member of the class Hydrozoa and is therefore not a true jellyfish. *P. physalis* is encountered in both Atlantic and Mediterranean waters, and is easily recognized by its translucent blue to pink or purple bladderlike float with multiple tentacles (Fig. 182-9). *P. physalis* is distinguished from its Pacific ocean relative *Physalia utriculus*, commonly known as the *blue bottle*, by its larger bell, which ranges in size from 10 to 30 cm, and multiple fishing tentacles extending up to 30 m; in contrast, *P. utriculus* has only a single tentacle that rarely exceeds 5 m.[38] These tentacles are armed along their entire length with hundreds of thousands of nematocysts arranged in stinging batteries, with each battery containing hundreds of nematocysts. The nematocysts remain active even after portions of the tentacles are broken off in storms or when these animals are stranded on the shoreline by high winds or waves. A beached Portuguese man-of-war can cause a severe sting when stepped on or touched. Children who are stung after handling these animals and then cry and rub their eyes may develop an acute conjunctivitis.

Stings of *P. physalis* are more painful and severe than those caused by sea nettles and are more extensive and serious than those caused by *P. utriculus*. At the moment of contact with the tentacles of *P. physalis*,

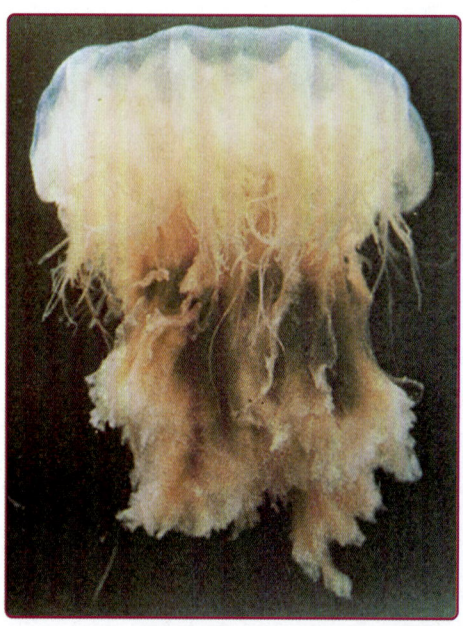

Figure 182-6 *Cyanea capillata*, also known as *sea nettle* or *lion's mane*, is a common cause of jellyfish stings. (B.W. Halstead, used with permission from World Life Research Institute.)

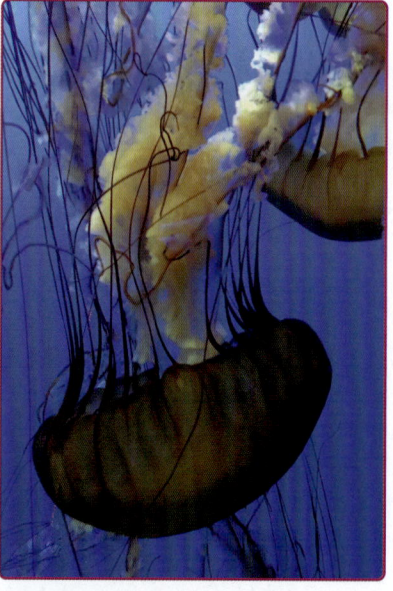

Figure 182-7 *Chrysaora achlyos*, commonly known as the black sea nettle, ranges from Monterey Bay to southern Baja California. This giant jelly sting causes consternation and painful stings that rarely need medical attention. (Used with permission from Jeffery Lee, D.D.S., Monte Sereno, CA.)

Figure 182-8 Whiplike sting pattern caused by *Cyanea capillata* in a young boy. (J.H. Barnes, used with permission from World Life Research Institute.)

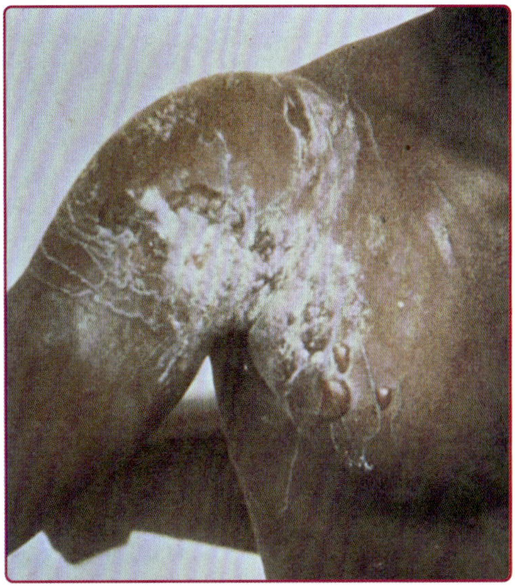

Figure 182-10 This diver surfaced directly under a large Portuguese man-of-war and suffered a severe sting with bulla formation and tissue necrosis. (S. Anderson, used with permission from World Life Research Institute.)

the victim experiences a sharp, shocklike, burning pain. There may be painful paresthesias or numbness in the sting area. Initially, the sting area appears as an irregular single line or multiple lines composed of red papules, beaded streaks, or erythematous welts that correspond to the areas of tentacle contact. The wheals resolve in hours but may progress to vesicular, hemorrhagic, necrotic, or ulcerative stages before healing (Fig. 182-10).[39]

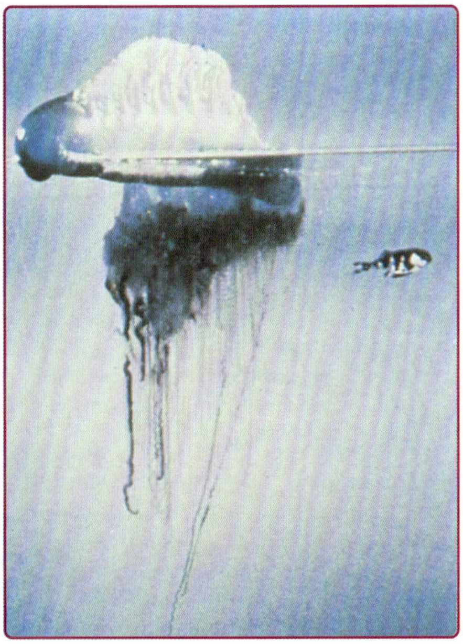

Postinflammatory striae may persist for weeks to months. Severe localized complications of *P. physalis* stings may also include arterial spasm in the sting site that can result in distal digital gangrene.[40,41]

Within 10 to 15 minutes of a *Physalia* sting, the victim may develop symptoms of an envenomation reaction characterized by nausea, abdominal cramps, muscular pains, backache, irritability, dyspnea, and chest tightness. Intravascular hemolysis and acute renal failure were reported in a 4-year-old girl after a severe sting by *P. physalis*.[42] Most reports of death due to stings of *P. physalis* are not well documented, but well-substantiated case reports of human fatalities do exist.[43-45]

Cubomedusae (Class Cubozoa): Box Jellyfish:

Of all the species of jellyfish that cause painful stings and distress to swimmers, the species with the most established record of lethality are the cubozoans. *Chironex fleckeri* or box jellyfish causes at least one death each year in Australia.[46] The fatality is usually a child, presumably because the size of the victim and the total area of the sting determine the likelihood of death. Until recently, most of the published cases of *C. fleckeri* stings involved fatal or nearly fatal envenomations, but less serious stings do occur in endemic areas.[47-49]

C. fleckeri (commonly known as the *sea wasp*) is an advanced species of jellyfish, with a semitransparent cubic bell that may grow to a volume of 9 L and weigh

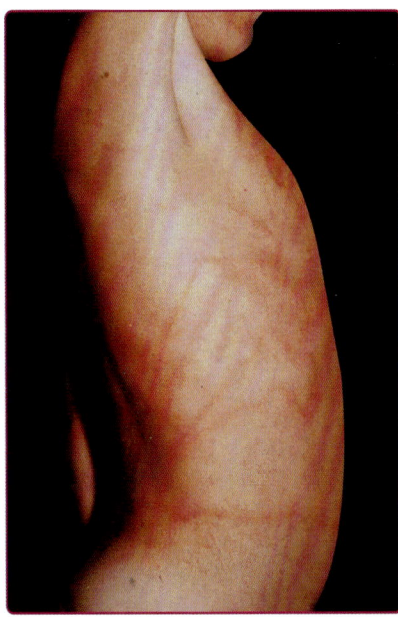

Figure 182-9 *Physalia physalis*, the Portuguese man-of-war, is distinguished by its bladder-like float and numerous trailing tentacles. (B.W. Halstead, used with permission from World Life Research Institute.)

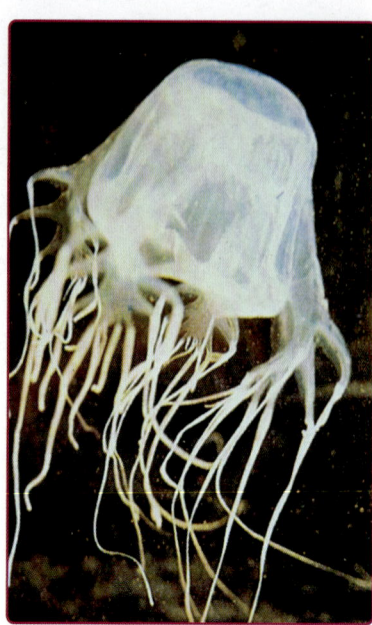

Figure 182-11 The deadly box jellyfish, *Chironex fleckeri*, is found in Indo-Pacific waters off the coast of Northern Australia. (Used with permission from R. Hartwick.)

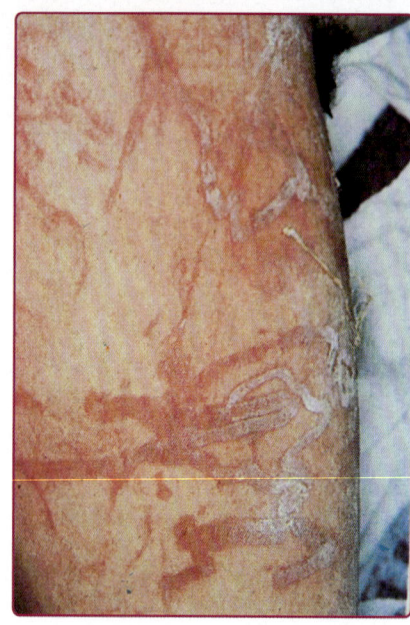

Figure 182-12 Characteristic frosted cross-hatched tentacle marks diagnostic of a sting caused by *Chironex fleckeri*. (Used with permission from Townsville General Hospital, Department of Medical Illustration, Townsville, Queensland, Australia.)

more than 6 kg (Fig. 182-11).[46] Trailing from the bell are up to 60 stinging tentacles, which may reach 2 to 3 m in length. When a human comes into contact with a box jellyfish, some of the tentacles are torn off and adhere to the skin. Rescuers of *C. fleckeri* sting victims must exercise caution, because they also are at risk of envenomation until the tentacles have been neutralized and removed.

The stings appear initially as linear welts that give the patient the appearance of having been whipped.[46] Fresh stings of *C. fleckeri* are easily recognized because they have a diagnostic, frosted, cross-hatched, or ladderlike appearance (Fig. 182-12). Microscopic diagnosis is also possible from blade scrapings or tape-strippings from the sting site. The intense pain may persist for many hours. Severely stung areas of skin take on a dusky cyanotic appearance, and blister formation and necrosis may occur. The healing process is slow and may be complicated by bacterial superinfection and scarring.

Death may ensue within minutes due to cardiotoxic and neurotoxic agents in the venom that can produce ventricular arrhythmias and cardiac arrest, and respiratory failure, respectively.[48] Intravascular hemolysis caused by the toxin can precipitate acute renal failure. First aid for these victims frequently involves cardiopulmonary resuscitation. Intravenous verapamil has been proposed for both treatment and prophylaxis of ventricular arrhythmias.[50,51] Antivenom is available for *C. fleckeri* stings, and its early use in severe envenomations may be lifesaving and significantly reduces the pain and inflammation at the sting site.[47]

Irukandji syndrome is a severe and delayed response (usually 30 minutes but between 5 and 40 minutes) to the sting of a small box jellyfish, termed the *Irukandji jellyfish*, that has resulted in the death of 2 tourists in the Cairns–Port Douglas region of Australia.[52] The classic syndrome consists of local signs of inflammation together with severe back pain, excruciating muscle cramps, piloerection, sweating, nausea, vomiting, headache, and palpitations. The most severe cases may progress to include extreme hypertension and cardiac failure. Only one species, *Carukia barnesi*, has been clearly linked to this syndrome, but it is thought that at least 6 different species of small jellyfish, each with only 1 tentacle arising from each corner of the bell (carybdeids), may be etiologic agents. The stings most often occur in deep water. Treatment includes application of vinegar to discharge nematocysts and victim transport for medical attention including pain control and α-blockade, because the venom is thought to act as a presynaptic neuronal sodium agonist and to stimulate norepinephrine release.

Prevention and Treatment of Jellyfish Stings: Cnidarian envenomations cause more deaths than shark attacks annually.[53] Tables 182-4 through 182-6 give details on the prevention of jellyfish stings and first aid for and treatment of the stings. Systemic reactions may occur, and the treatment for these includes support of vital functions with cardiopulmonary resuscitation, oxygen, and intravenous fluids.[54] Application of a venous-lymphatic constriction bandage proximal to the wound site should be considered

TABLE 182-4
Prevention of Jellyfish Stings

1. Swim only at patrolled beaches with properly trained lifeguards and adequate treatment facilities.
2. Avoid swimming in infested waters, especially after a storm, because stings may result from remnants of floating damaged tentacles.
3. Beware of apparently dead or beached jellyfish.
4. When snorkeling or scuba diving, wear protective clothing such as a wet suit, long-sleeved shirt, pants, or long woolen underwear, and gloves. In areas where Irukandji syndrome occurs, wear a Lycra stinger suit.
5. Use sunblock containing jellyfish and "sea lice" repellent.
6. Bathing beaches should be closed during periods of high jellyfish infestation.

TABLE 182-6
Organism-Specific and Followup Treatment of Jellyfish Stings

1. If *Chironex fleckeri* or other box jellyfish species that cause the Irukandji syndrome are suspected, douse or spray dilute acetic acid (3%-10%) or household vinegar over all areas of tentacle contact for at least 30 s.
2. For sea nettles, mix sodium bicarbonate (baking soda) with water to form a slurry and pour over the affected area or apply the powder directly to the tentacles.
3. For *Physalia physalis* stings, a slurry of baking soda is indicated. Vinegar had been reported to neutralize nematocysts of *P. physalis*, but work with species from Australia indicate that it may cause a discharge of nematocysts in some cases.
4. If vinegar or baking soda is unavailable, papain, available as a powdered meat tenderizer, may be applied directly as a powder or mixed in water as a slurry to sting areas and tentacles of both sea nettles and Portuguese man-of-war.
5. If nothing else is available, the tentacles can be rinsed off with seawater.
6. Do not use fresh water, methylated spirits, or alcohol in any form to deactivate tentacles, because these all may cause a rapid massive discharge of nematocysts.
7. After the tentacles have been disarmed, they may be carefully removed with a forceps or gently scraped away from the skin with shaving cream and a razor or a plastic card, shell, or knife.
8. Consider use of hot-water immersion rather than ice packs as first aid to enhance pain relief.

in the case of severe stings when systemic reactions are present or likely to occur, when topical deactivation of tentacles is not possible, and when transport to receive specific antivenin for *C. fleckeri* stings is available. The antivenin is prepared from sheep serum and may therefore pose a risk of allergic reaction in sensitive individuals.[35,37] The preferred route of administration is intravenous, but the antivenin may be given intramuscularly. In severe stinging, it has proved lifesaving. It is also the only treatment that can alleviate the intense pain and may reduce inflammation at the sting site and decrease the chance of scarring. Intravenous administration of verapamil has been advocated for both treatment and prophylaxis of arrhythmias.[50,51] For pain in severe stinging, parenteral narcotic analgesics and ice packs, as well as antivenin, should be considered. Local reactions may be treated with topical anesthetic ointments, creams, lotions, or sprays to relieve itching or burning pain.[34] Hot-water immersion as first aid enhances pain relief and has been judged better than ice packs.[53] For delayed-type hypersensitivity reactions, which may occur days to weeks after the stinging (Fig. 182-13), topical glucocorticoids, topical tacrolimus, antihistamines, and systemic glucocorticoids should be used as necessary.[36]

Secondary infections should be treated with the appropriate parenteral antibiotics, and antitetanus therapy should be considered. Application of ice or cold packs can relieve the pain of mild to moderate stings of many types of jellyfish, and aspirin or acetaminophen, alone or in combination with codeine, can be used to relieve persistent pain.

TABLE 182-5
First-Aid Treatment of Jellyfish Stings

1. Remove or rescue the victim from the water.
2. Stabilize vital functions: Airway, breathing, circulation.
3. Immobilize the affected part to prevent further envenomation by adherent tentacles.
4. Identify the type of jellyfish sting by considering locale, time of year, and indigenous species and by observing the sting pattern. Preserve a portion of the tentacle for future identification. Tape-strip or scrape the sting site for microscopic analysis of the nematocysts if no tentacles are available.
5. To prevent further envenomation of the victim and to reduce the chance of a sting to the rescuer, disarm the nematocysts before removing the adherent tentacles.

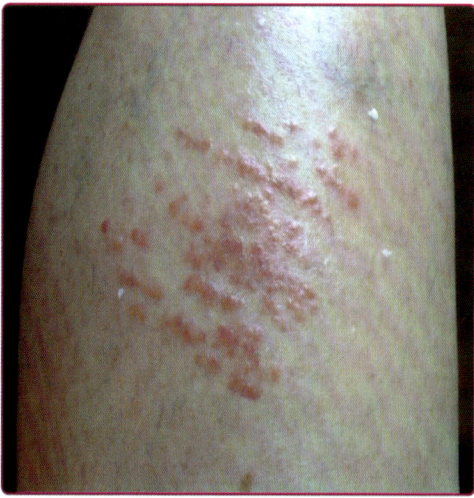

Figure 182-13 Delayed-type hypersensitivity reaction occurring about 2 weeks after jellyfish stings on the leg.

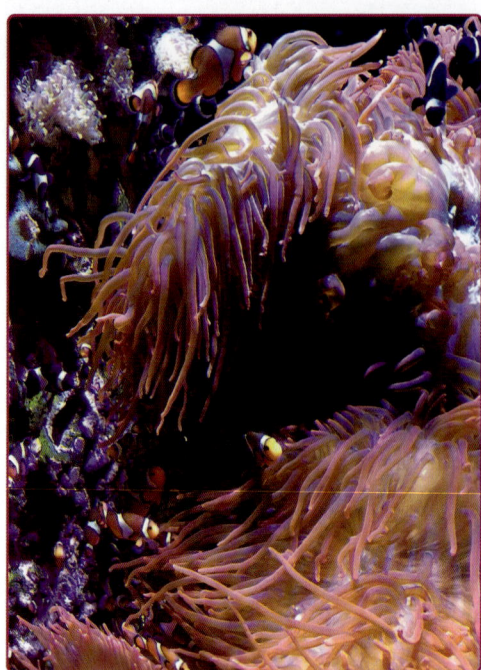

Figure 182-14 The elongated tentacles of the sea anemone cause can envenomations similar to shellfish stings. (Used with permission from Jeffery Lee, D.D.S., Monte Sereno, CA.)

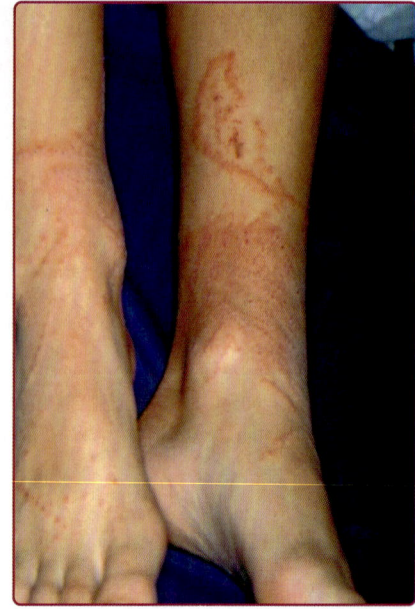

Figure 182-15 Delayed-type hypersensitivity reaction to a presumed sea anemone sting. This 11-year-old girl stepped into a hole while wading in shallow waters on the South Carolina coast. She experienced an immediate burning pain with erythema and swelling of both lower legs that subsided within a day. Several days later, she developed a pruritic linear eruption. A diagnosis was made of a delayed-type hypersensitivity reaction that developed in the sting site and corresponded with the tentacle marks from what was presumed to be a sea anemone envenomation.

SEA ANEMONE DERMATITIS

Sea anemones are members of the phylum Cnidaria, class Anthozoa. They are sessile creatures with flowery tentacles armed with nematocysts (Fig. 182-14). The stings of sea anemones may cause dermatitis in sponge fishermen, sponge divers, and beachcombers who gather snails and crabs from rocky hollows along the shore. Their toxicity to humans depends on the species. After the immediate reaction has subsided, delayed-type hypersensitivity reactions can develop at the site of a sting from a sea anemone (Fig. 182-15).

The genus *Sagartia* is the cause of sponge fisherman's disease.[34] This anemone lives at the base of sponges sought by commercial fishermen. When they harvest or sort the sponges with their bare hands or forearms, they are likely to come into contact with the tentacles of *Sagartia*. Itching and burning occur at the sting site within minutes, accompanied by erythema, edema, and vesicles.[34]

Treatment of sea anemone stings is similar to that of jellyfish envenomations (see section "Prevention and Treatment of Jellyfish Stings").[55] The tentacles should be removed carefully.[34] Both vinegar and Stingose (an aqueous solution of 20% aluminum sulfate and 11% surfactant) have been suggested for application to neutralize the sites of anemone stings.[56] Sea anemone sting sites often heal slowly and may require treatment with antibiotics.

INJURIES CAUSED BY FIRE CORAL AND CORAL CUTS

Corals are colonial organisms belonging to the phylum Cnidaria. Coral injuries may be caused by nematocyst stings or lacerations. Both injuries may occur at the same time and may be complicated by foreign-body reactions, bacterial infections, and localized eczematous reactions. For most true corals, nematocyst envenomation is a relatively innocuous experience, resulting in mild pruritic erythema that requires little if any treatment. Calamine lotion or antipruritic lotions may bring relief.[57]

In contrast to the stings of true corals, the sting of the fire coral, *Millepora alcicornis*, is quite painful, as many scuba divers and snorkelers from the Florida Keys to the Caribbean will attest (Fig. 182-16). The wet mucous membrane or slime surrounding the organism contains numerous nematocysts that readily discharge on contact with the skin, causing immediate burning and stinging pain. Within 1 to several hours a pruritic erythematous papular eruption appears, which in severe cases may become pustular and, in rare cases, may progress to necrosis and eschar formation.[57] Lesions heal in 1 to 2 weeks, often with postinflammatory hyperpigmentation. A delayed and persistent allergic

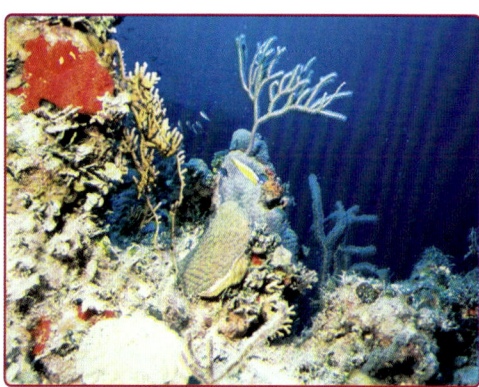

Figure 182-16 The mustard-colored finger-like outcropping in the upper left quadrant of this formation of coral and hydroids is a typical example of fire coral.

contact dermatitis also has been reported to occur from a fire coral sting in the Red Sea.[58]

Fire coral stings should be rinsed with seawater to remove undischarged nematocysts. The sting area can then be compressed with either 5% acetic acid (vinegar) or 40% to 70% isopropyl alcohol for 15 to 30 minutes or until the pain is relieved.[37,59] Seawater compresses, hot to the point of tolerance, are also reported to inactivate the toxin. A topical steroid cream or ointment may relieve pruritus and promote healing.

Coral cuts—lacerations caused by the razor-sharp exoskeletons of coral—are notorious for their slow healing and propensity for secondary infection. Factors that complicate healing include the following: (1) wounds often involve the lower extremities and these generally heal more slowly because of decreased tissue blood supply; (2) wound edges are often irregular, contused, crushed, and abraded; (3) contamination of wounds is likely because of pathogenic bacteria in shore waters; and (4) foreign bodies, including marine algae growing on the coral or portions of the coral itself, may be implanted in the wound.

Treatment of coral cuts should begin with vigorous cleansing of the wound with soap and water with a soft brush or rough towel, followed by copious irrigation with saline to remove foreign bodies. If the wound is extensive, local anesthesia may be required to allow adequate cleansing, exploration, and debridement and to achieve good hemostasis. Hydrogen peroxide washing of the wound before dressing it is recommended.

The decision whether to perform primary closure of a coral cut wound or to allow it to heal by secondary intention depends on the location of the wound, the degree of tissue trauma at the wound margins, and the likelihood of subsequent infection. Tape-stripping is preferable to suturing of leg wounds, because sutured leg wounds have a high chance of abscess formation. Once the wound is closed, antibiotic ointment and rest are advisable. Tetanus prophylaxis should be given according to immunization history.

DERMATITIS FROM SPONGES

Sponges are members of the phylum Porifera, class Desmospongiae. They are simple multicellular animals that live attached to the sea bottom. Sponges grow by forming a series of hollow-centered branching tubes composed of a fibrous material called *spongin*, which contains spicules of calcium carbonate or silica.[34,60,61] Spicules of certain species of sponges are capable of penetrating the skin, causing a localized irritant or foreign-body reaction. Treatment of sponge spicule dermatitis involves tape-stripping of the affected area.

At least 13 species of sponges can cause a toxic dermatitis. Of these, the most commonly encountered are the West Indian and Hawaiian fire sponge, *Tedania ignis*; the poison bun sponge, *Fibula nolitangere* (Fig. 182-17); and the red sponge, *Microciona prolifera*, found in the northeastern United States.[62] These creatures are covered by a surface secretion, or slime, that produces an irritant or toxin-induced dermatitis when contacted by bare skin.[61]

Symptoms of itching, prickling, stinging, or burning appear within minutes of exposure and are followed within a few hours by pain, swelling, and stiffness. If the fingers are involved, they often become immobile within 24 hours. The first cutaneous sign of sponge poisoning is local erythema, which progresses to a papular, vesicular, or bullous eruption with weeping of a serous or purulent fluid.[61,62] Desquamation of the site occurs within several days. Erythema multiforme and anaphylactoid reactions have been reported in highly sensitized individuals. Treatment of sponge dermatitis is similar to that of severe poison ivy.[62]

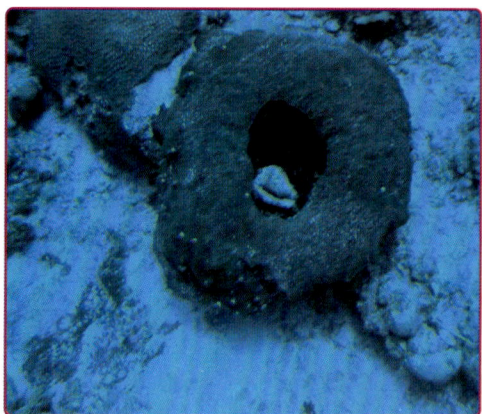

Figure 182-17 The poison bun sponge, *Fibula nolitangere*, can cause a severe irritant or toxin-induced contact dermatitis.

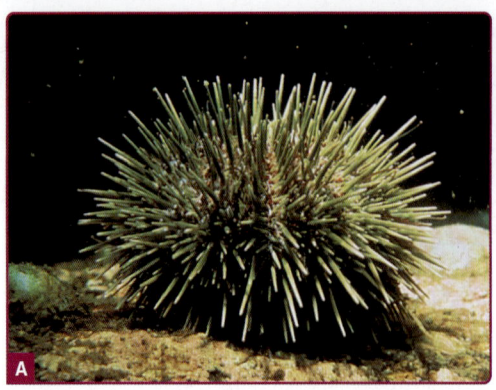
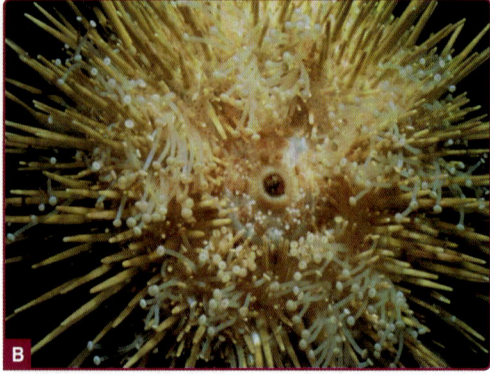

Figure 182-18 Lateral (**A**) and ventral (**B**) views of a sea urchin demonstrate this animal's protective spines and venomous pedicellaria underneath. (Used with permission from Marty Gilman, Worcester, MA.)

INJURIES CAUSED BY ECHINODERMS: SEA URCHINS, STARFISH, AND SEA CUCUMBERS

SEA URCHINS

Sea urchins are spiny creatures that belong to the phylum Echinodermata, class Echinoidea. They are encased in a fragile, roughly spherical, calcareous shell, which is protected by a formidable array of mobile spines and pincer-like organs known as *pedicellariae* (Fig. 182-18).[63,64]

Bathers, surfers, divers, and fishermen are all at risk for sea urchin injuries. These creatures, such as the purple sea urchin, hide in rocks in low-tide zones along the Pacific coast between Alaska and Mexico (Fig. 182-19). Injuries may occur when the victim steps on an urchin, driving the spines into an unprotected foot, or as a result of loss of balance or wave action, in which case the hands or other body parts may be impaled. Sea urchin spines are composed of calcium carbonate and are covered with a proteinaceous membrane.[61] Injuries from sea urchins may be inflicted either by penetrating wounds from the animals' spines, which often break off and become imbedded in the wound, or by bites from the pedicellaria. In certain species, the spines or pedicellaria are venomous. This fact may explain why the pain of some sea urchin wounds is so excruciating and disproportionate to the apparent injury.

Encounters with sea urchins can result in both immediate and delayed reactions. Immediate reactions are usually localized and are initially manifested by a severe burning pain at the wound site, which quickly becomes red and swollen and may bleed profusely. There may be a black or purple discoloration at the site of the spine penetration due to either retained spines in the wound or to a tattoolike effect from dye released by spines that have exited intact, but this discoloration will likely disappear within 48 to 72 hours.[59] Paresthesias may develop at the wound area. Systemic symptoms are not common but can occur in injuries due to particularly venomous species. Symptoms may include nausea, syncope, paresthesias, ataxia, muscle cramps, paralysis, and respiratory distress.[62]

Delayed-type hypersensitivity reactions may occur with erythema and intense pruritus days after the initial injury.[65] In one of these cases, the diagnosis was confirmed by patch testing with extracts of the ground sea urchin spines.[66] Nodular reactions are localized to the area of spine penetration and are not usually painful. Nodules may take on colors from the dye in the spines[63] and may have a central umbilication or a keratotic surface[63] (Fig. 182-20).

The diffuse form more commonly involves the fingers or toes and is manifested by a fusiform swelling of the affected digit with accompanying pain and loss of function.[62,63] In addition to joint synovitis and arthritis, osteoarticular complications of sea urchin spine penetration may include tenosynovitis with or without destruction of the underlying bone, fasciitis, and bursitis.[67] Sea urchin spine wounds may also cause

Figure 182-19 Purple sea urchin, *Strongylocentrotus purpuratus*, commonly found along the Pacific coast of the United States.

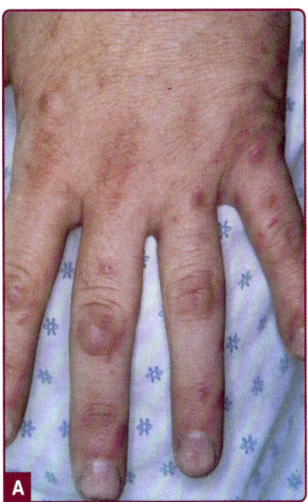 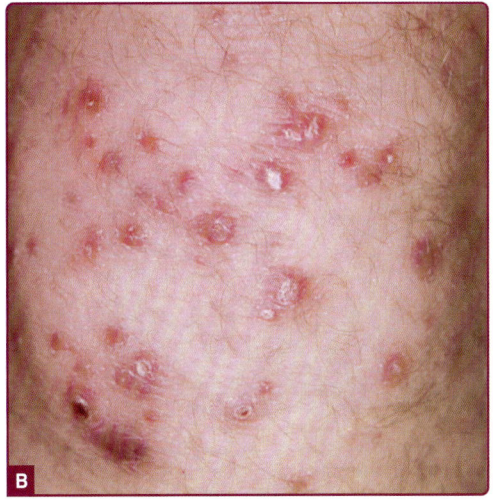

Figure 182-20 **A** and **B,** Nodular reactions to imbedded sea urchin spines. (Used with permission from Karen Rothman, MD.)

direct mechanical injuries to nerves and may be complicated by secondary infection.[68]

Initial first aid for the pain from immediate reactions is to soak the affected area in hot water (43°C-46°C [110°F-115°F]) for 30 to 90 minutes until maximal relief is obtained. Infiltration of the wound site with 1% to 2% lidocaine without epinephrine may be required in some cases to produce significant pain relief.[69] Spines protruding from the wound may be carefully removed. They are very fragile; therefore, it is difficult to extract the entire spine intact. Tumescence of the skin with a local anesthetic may allow superficially imbedded spines to be extracted when radiographs demonstrate no evidence of joint or bony impingement.[64] More invasive attempts at spine removal should not be made without the benefit of aseptic surgical facilities and radiographs to confirm the spine locations. Removal of the spines may be aided by the use of an operating microscope. Antibiotics are indicated for secondary infections, and tetanus prophylaxis should be given if indicated.

STARFISH

Certain species of starfish may produce puncture wound injuries similar to those caused by sea urchins. The crown-of-thorns starfish, *Acanthaster planci*, accounts for most severe starfish envenomations.[62] The ice pick–like spines of *A. planci*, which may reach 4 to 6 cm in length, are covered with a thin skin and glandular tissue that produce a poisonous slime.[69] The resulting wound is quite painful and may be accompanied by numbness and paresthesias. Systemic symptoms including nausea, vomiting, and muscle weakness are infrequent and short-lived.[62] Fragments of spines and their surrounding integument may become imbedded in the wounded area, resulting in granulomatous reactions.

Treatment is similar to that of sea urchin wounds.

SEA CUCUMBERS

Sea cucumbers are sausage-shaped, bottom-feeding echinoderms that can produce a papular contact dermatitis by means of a toxic liquid substance, known as *holothurin*, that is secreted from their body walls.[34] Conjunctivitis, even blindness, can result from corneal involvement if the toxin comes in contact with the eyes.[62] Prevention of sea cucumber dermatitis involves protecting the skin and eyes from contact with these creatures and educating children and curious divers about the risk of handling them. Treatment consists of washing the affected area with soap and water to remove the toxin and then treating as for a mild contact dermatitis.

DERMATITIS AND BITES FROM MARINE WORMS

BRISTLEWORM DERMATITIS

Bristleworms are multisegmented marine worms of the phylum Annelida, class Polychaeta (which means "many bristles"; Fig. 182-21). Each segment of the worm is armed with rows of silky or bristle-like, hollow, venom-filled setae that can easily penetrate and break off in the unprotected skin of a victim as do cactus spines.[69] Contact with the bristleworm results in an erythematous papular or urticarial eruption at the site, accompanied by symptoms of paresthesias, intense itching, or burning pain.[34,69] The bristles are too small and fragile in most cases

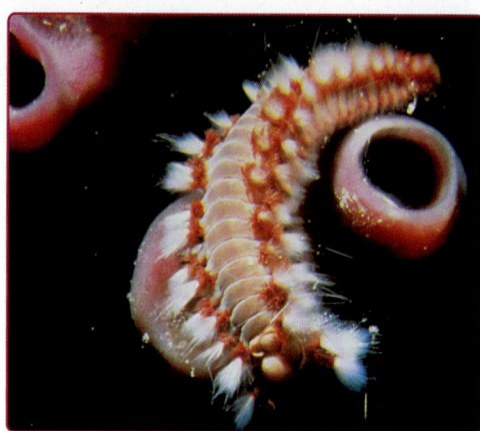

Figure 182-21 *Hermodice carunculata*, the West Indian bristleworm, can inflict a painful wound with its hollow, venom-filled bristle-like setae. (Used with permission from Marty Gilman, Worcester, MA.)

to be removed with a forceps; however, tape-stripping with cellophane adhesive tape can be effective. After the setae have been removed, the application of ammonia soaks or alcohol or water compresses may bring symptomatic relief.

LEECH BITES

Leeches are another class of segmental worms whose bites may be encountered in freshwater or saltwater as well as on land. Although freshwater leeches are capable of attaching painlessly to their human hosts, saltwater leeches produce bites with pain similar to that of a bee sting. Leeches inject a powerful anticoagulant, hirudin, into the wound, as well as other antigenic substances that are capable of eliciting allergic reactions (including anaphylaxis) in sensitized individuals. Local symptoms of leech bites include bleeding from the puncture marks, pain, swelling, redness, and severe pruritus; urticarial, bullous, or necrotic reactions may occur in sensitized persons.[34] Leech bites and medical leech therapy result in infection by *Aeromonas hydrophila*.

Severe ulcerations may result if the leech is removed forcibly and its mouth parts are left behind in the bite site. Leeches must be induced to fall off by applying a noxious agent (such as alcohol, vinegar, brine, or a match flame) to their site of attachment.

CERCARIAL DERMATITIS (CLAM DIGGER'S ITCH)

Cercarial dermatitis, also known as *schistosome dermatitis* or *swimmer's* or *clam digger's itch*, is an acute pruritic eruption resulting from penetration of the skin by the cercarial forms of certain parasitic flatworms of the family Schistosomatidae.

Symptoms of cercarial dermatitis begin with urticaria-like lesions and a prickling sensation of the skin, which lasts about half an hour after exposure to cercaria-infested waters. Severe pruritus of the affected area occurs 10 to 12 hours later. Within 24 hours, erythematous papules appear that may progress to vesicles and later to pustules. Pain and swelling of the area accompanies the intense itching, which usually peaks in 48 to 72 hours. Headache, fever, and superinfection with lymphangitis are occasionally present.

In the Great Lakes region, several species of *Schistosoma cercariae* that cause swimmer's itch have been reported, and many other such species have been discovered throughout the world in both freshwater and saltwater.[70,71] A severely disabling form of cercarial dermatitis affects the paddy workers and rice farmers of the Far East. Cercarial dermatitis also has been described in individuals exposed to shallow coastal waters, notably on Long Island Sound where the condition affects clam diggers, giving rise to the name, *clam digger's itch* (Fig. 182-22). There is one reported case of cercarial dermatitis occurring on the hands and arms of a patient after he cleaned the aquarium in which he kept native water snails.[72]

Humans are accidental hosts in the life cycle of dermatitis-producing schistosomes. The cycle begins when the primary host, a waterfowl, marsh bird, finch, muskrat, mouse, or deer, passes schistosomal eggs in its feces into a body of water. Each egg hatches in 10 to 15 minutes, releasing a secondary stage miracidium. The miracidia are free-swimming and must locate and infect their definitive snail host within 12 hours or they will die. The miracidia migrate to the snail's digestive

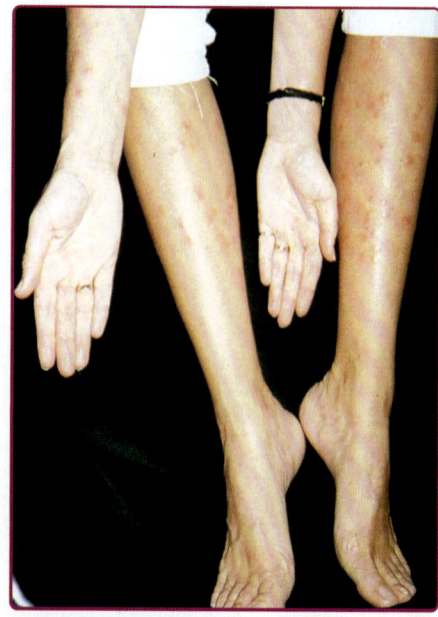

Figure 182-22 Intensely pruritic papulovesicles suggestive of a severe reaction to flea bites in a patient with clam digger's itch. The left hand, which was not in the water and was holding the pail for collecting the clams, was spared.

gland, where they develop into multiple sporocysts. In about 5 weeks, the sporocysts give rise to hundreds of fork-tailed cercariae that measure 0.75 mm in length. The cercariae are released from the snail under favorable conditions of light and heat, and are carried toward the shore by prevailing winds and currents.[71] When an appropriate host is encountered, the cercaria attach to the skin with their oral suckers and penetrate the epidermis and dermis by means of histolytic enzymes. They lose their tails in this process and are now called schistosomula. The schistosomula migrate via the blood vessels through the heart and lungs to the intrahepatic veins, where they mature into adult male and female trematode flukes. When the worms mate, they pass in pairs through the mesenteric venules of the intestinal wall where the female lays hundreds of eggs.[71] The eggs then penetrate the gut wall and are discharged in the feces, and the cycle is repeated.

When cercariae that do not cause schistosomiasis in humans accidentally attach to the skin, they may penetrate the epidermis but are unable to reach the bloodstream. The organisms die in the superficial papillary dermis and undergo total histolysis within 3 to 4 days. The cercarial protein residua stimulate a delayed-type hypersensitivity response, which may increase in severity with repeated exposures. Skin biopsies taken at 3 to 4 days reveal an amorphous eosinophilic mass at the site of the dissolved cercaria, with an intense lymphocytic infiltrate. Later, histiocytes appear in the middle and deep papillary dermis.

The differential diagnosis of cercarial dermatitis includes insect bites from chiggers, mosquitoes, and fleas; contact dermatitis from poison ivy; and the stings of other marine coelenterates. In Africa, Asia, South America, and Puerto Rico, swimmer's itch must be distinguished from the dermatitis associated with human schistosomiasis, which produces an eruption with very similar but milder and more transient symptoms.[73] Swimmer's itch must also be distinguished from sea bather's eruption (SE), which is discussed in the next section.

Prevention of cercarial dermatitis in waters where swimmer's itch is known to be a problem is difficult. Coating the skin with petrolatum and various chemical repellents has been tried, but the effectiveness of these methods remains unproven. Clothing barriers may be of some help.

Treatment of cercarial dermatitis is largely symptomatic. In mild cases, antipruritic or drying lotions, oatmeal or starch baths, and antihistamines may alleviate pruritus. Aspirin may be helpful for the pain and swelling, and a bedtime sedative may be required to allow the patient much-needed sleep. Proper washing and hygiene should be maintained to prevent bacterial superinfection. In severe cases, potent topical glucocorticoids and occasionally systemic glucocorticoids may be required.

SEA BATHER'S ERUPTION

SE, also known as *marine dermatitis* and often misnamed *sea lice infestation*, is an acute dermatitis that begins shortly after bathing in seawater. SE is often confused with swimmer's itch (cercarial dermatitis, see previous section), not only because they both occur after exposure to water but also because the common names of these 2 conditions are easily confused. For many years, the cause of SE remained a mystery, but it is now known that the responsible agents in at least 2 types of SE are the larval forms of marine coelenterates. In waters off the coast of Florida and in the Caribbean, the tiny larvae of the thimble jellyfish, *Linuche unguiculata*, are to blame.[74] Off the coast of Long Island, New York, researchers found that the larval forms of the sea anemone *Edwardsiella lineata* were responsible for the eruption.

In addition to having a different etiology, SE can be distinguished from cercarial dermatitis by several other characteristics: SE primarily involves areas of the body covered by bathing suits from which water evaporates slowly, as opposed to uncovered areas as is typical of swimmer's itch. Most symptoms are not noted until the bather has left the water (although some of those affected have complained of a prickling sensation while still in the water).

The eruption is caused by minute stings from the nematocysts of the coelenterate larvae, which become trapped underneath swimwear or may adhere to hairy areas of the body. In addition to SE after contact with the larvae, which are most abundant in May and June, swimmers and bathers may also develop SE after contact with the other 2 free-swimming stages of *L. unguiculata*, the ephyrae and medusae stages.[75]

The lesions begin within 4 to 24 hours after exposure as erythematous macules, papules, or wheals that may itch or burn (Fig. 182-23).[34] These lesions may progress to vesiculopapules, which crust over and heal in 7 to 10 days. Associated systemic symptoms may include

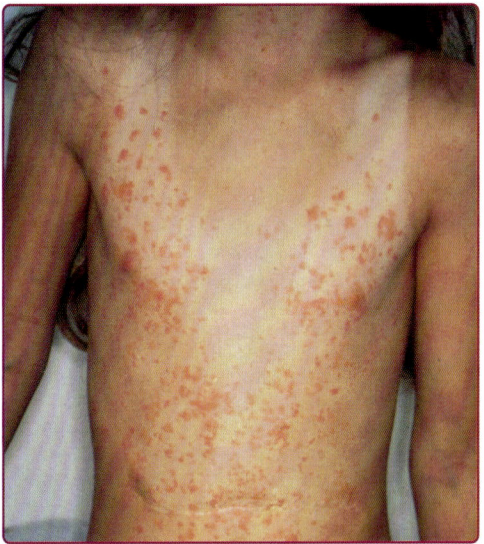

Figure 182-23 Sea bather's eruption in a young girl after a swim at a Florida beach. (Used with permission from Karen Rothman, MD.)

chills and a low-grade fever as well as nausea, vomiting, diarrhea, headache, weakness, muscle spasms, and malaise. Febrile and systemic symptoms are more common in children and adolescents.[76] In the presence of such constitutional symptoms, caregivers who fail to recognize the pattern of the eruption or who fail to take a history of exposure to saltwater may mistakenly make the diagnosis of a viral syndrome.

In waters along the coast of South Florida, the season for SE is between March and August with a peak in May. The incidence among bathers during May and June 1993 in Palm Beach County was reported to be 16%.[76] The strongest risk factor for developing SE is a previous history of the condition, which is consistent with the theory that SE represents a hypersensitivity response to the nematocyst stings. Other risk factors include age younger than 16 years and surfing. Showering with swimwear removed was found to be a protective measure.[76]

Prevention of SE includes the measures listed in Table 182-7. Treatment of SE is symptomatic and includes the use of antipruritic lotions, colloidal baths with starch or oatmeal, antihistamines, and topical glucocorticoids. Severe unremitting cases may warrant systemic glucocorticoid therapy.[74] Secondary bacterial infections may complicate the condition and should be diagnosed and treated appropriately.

INJURIES CAUSED BY MOLLUSKS

CONE SNAIL ENVENOMATIONS

Venomous marine snails are univalvular gastropods whose ornate cone-shaped shells (Fig. 182-24) are highly prized by shell collectors and divers. A number of species have a highly developed venom apparatus that can inflict a lethal sting. Most of the dangerous cone shell species are found in the shallow waters of the Indo-Pacific. Cone shells are carnivorous. They live on the ocean bottom and, depending on the species, may hunt worms, other mollusks, or fish. Cone shells kill their prey by means of a spear-like venomous radular tooth that is thrust out from the animal's proboscis. Cone shell venom contains several different kinds of neurotoxins; death may result from respiratory paralysis. There is so far no antivenin for cone shell toxin; mortality rates after envenomations from the more dangerous species (*Conus geographicus* and *C. magus*) may be as high as 15% to 20%.[34]

Injuries from cone shells are of the puncture wound variety. The degree of pain is variable, ranging from a mild stinging sensation, similar to that of an insect bite, to excruciating pain. Early symptoms may include edema, ischemia, numbness, and paresthesias of the wound site. Paresthesias may become widespread, with the lips and mouth commonly affected.[34,62] Localized muscular paralysis may progress to generalized weakness or paralysis with eventual respiratory distress and cardiopulmonary failure.[77] Neurotoxic symptoms that indicate severe envenomation include diplopia, blurred vision, aphonia, dysphagia, and coma. Rare cases of disseminated intravascular coagulation have been reported after cone shell envenomation.

Great care must be exercised in handling live cone shells. Thick protective gloves should be worn, and the soft underportion of the animal should be avoided. Cone shells should never be placed in pockets of clothing or swimwear, because they have been known to sting through clothing.[78]

Treatment of cone shell envenomations is supportive. The victim should be kept at rest and the sting area kept dependent and immobilized. A compression dressing should be applied to occlude lymphatic-venous, but not arterial, flow.[78] Local suction may be helpful if it can be applied immediately to the wound site with a plunger device, such as the Extractor Vacuum Pump (Sawyer Products, Safety Harbor, Florida).

TABLE 182-7
Prevention of Seabather's Eruption

1. Bathers should remove their swimwear and shower as soon as possible after leaving the water. Because fresh water may cause discharge of the nematocysts, it is important that the suits be removed before showering begins.
2. Bathing suits should be rinsed with soap and water and heat dried, because the eruption can recur when the suit is air-dried.
3. T-shirts should not be worn in the water. Women may consider wearing a 2-piece suit to reduce the surface area under which larvae may be trapped.
4. Whole-body Lycra swimsuits or wet suits with snug-fitting collars and cuffs may be protective, but the eruption may still occur along the collar or cuff edges.
5. Highly sensitized individuals should avoid swimming in infested waters during outbreaks of seabather's eruption.

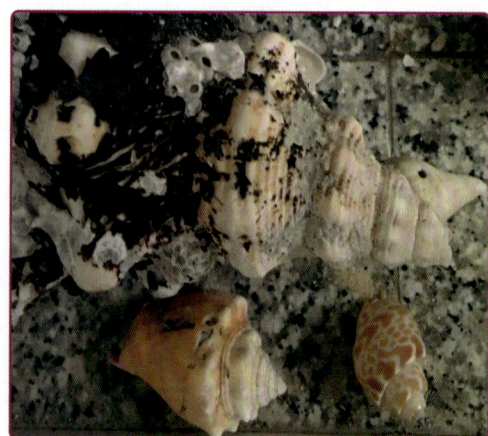

Figure 182-24 Cone shells collected digging in sand by one of the authors (R.A.S.) on Naples, Florida, beach.

OCTOPUS BITES

Octopuses are an advanced group of mollusks belonging to the class Cephalopoda. The octopus bites with a parrotlike chitinous beak located on the ventral side of the head in the middle of its 8 tentacles (Fig. 182-25). Species of octopi range in size from a few centimeters to 1 to 2 m in diameter.[79] They are shy and reclusive creatures that tend to avoid encounters with humans; however, bites can occur when curious divers, fishermen, or beachgoers encounter these animals and handle them carelessly. Most octopus bites are not life-threatening to humans. The bite site may be immediately painful, as after a bee sting, and is recognized by the presence of 2 small puncture wounds, which may bleed profusely.[78] Symptoms from octopus bites are usually mild and transient and consist of redness, swelling, and itching.[79]

The most dangerous species of octopus, the Australian blue-ringed octopus, *Hapalochlaena maculosa*, is found in Australian coastal waters. Mortality rates after bites from *H. maculosa* may be as high as 25%. *H. maculosa* produces a toxin in its salivary glands that is introduced into the bite site by the animal's powerful beak and contains a fraction identical to tetrodotoxin; this toxin blocks peripheral nerve conduction and results in paralysis of the victim with subsequent respiratory failure. The bite of the blue-ringed octopus may or may not be painful, so that victims may not realize they have been bitten until neurologic symptoms develop.[62]

There is no antivenin for bites of *H. maculosa*. Treatment is supportive and similar to that recommended in the previous section for severe cone shell envenomations.

INJURIES CAUSED BY VENOMOUS FISH SPINES

Ichthyoacanthotoxicosis is the proper term for envenomations as a result of puncture wounds or lacerations inflicted by the spines of venomous fish. There are more than 200 species of venomous fish in the world that can cause injury to humans.[62] The most notorious of these species are the stingrays, catfish, lionfish, scorpionfish, stonefish, weevers, toadfish, and spiny dogfish. All of these fish have in common a venom apparatus consisting of a single spine or multiple spines, in various locations, which are covered by an integumentary sheath enclosing various forms of venom glands. When the spine of the animal penetrates the victim, the sheath is torn and the venom glands release their toxins into the wound. The toxins from some of these fish may remain potent for 24 to 48 hours after the death of the fish.[80]

STINGRAYS

Stingrays are one of the most common causes of venomous fish stings confronting humans, with as many as 1500 to 2000 stingray attacks reported each year in the United States alone.[69,81] Rays are grouped into one of 4 categories: (1) gymnurid (butterfly rays), (2) urolophid (round stingrays), (3) myliobatid (bat or eagle rays), and (4) dasyatid (proper stingrays). The groupings are based on their relative stinging ability, which depends on the size, number, and location of the caudal stinging appendages. The most dangerous group, the dasyatid or true stingrays, have the largest spines located further out on their tails, which makes them the most potent striking weapons. The spines have retroserrated teeth, so that removal is difficult (Fig. 182-26).

Most stingray injuries occur when bathers, waders, or fishermen accidentally step on rays as they lie partially covered with sand in shallow waters.[82,83] Severe lacerations and puncture wounds are inflicted by the ray as it defensively whips its tail upward and forward when stepped on or threatened (Fig. 182-27).[82,83]

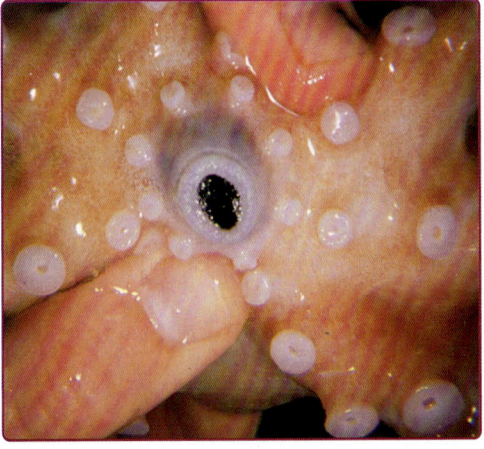

Figure 182-25 Ventral view of the underside of an octopus exposing the animal's centrally located mouth and parrotlike beak. (From Fulghum DD. Octopus bite resulting in granuloma annulare. *South Med J.* 1986;79:1434, with permission.)

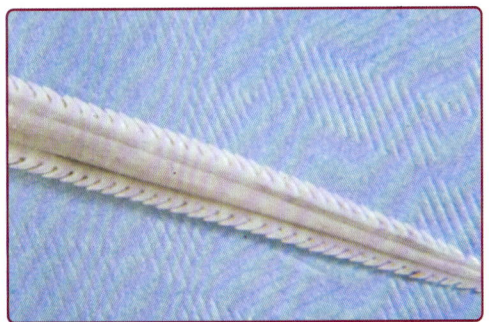

Figure 182-26 A close-up view of a stingray stinger without its outer membrane and venom glands, demonstrating the retroserrated spine. (Used with permission from David Fulghum, MD.)

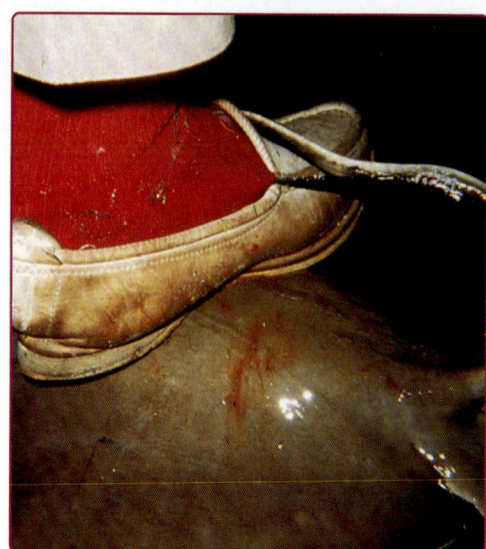

Figure 182-27 Stingrays reflexively swing their barbed tails up when stepped on, causing painful lacerations and puncture wounds. (The leg used for this photograph was a prosthesis; the stingray was alive.) (Used with permission from David Fulghum, MD.)

The majority of wounds, therefore, are located on the dorsum of the foot or lower leg. Penetrating wounds to other locations have occurred to fishermen stung while attempting to remove rays from their lines or nets. Rarely these injuries are fatal. Soaking in warm water relieves the pain.

CATFISH

Both freshwater and saltwater catfish are armed with stout, sharp spines located immediately in front of the soft rays of their dorsal and pectoral fins. Catfish defensively lock these spines into an extended position when they are handled or threatened. Bathers may sustain stings on their feet or legs if they step on a catfish, but most catfish stings involve the hand or upper extremity of fishermen or seafood processors.[84] To prevent these injuries, it has been suggested that the offending spines be removed with a pair of pliers before cleaning of the fish is attempted. Empiric intravenous antibiotics may be required to cover common aquatic bacteria.

Swimmers and bathers in the Amazon River are at risk for urologic injuries if they encounter a very small species of catfish called the *candiru*, which has the ability to enter the human urethra. Barbs on the head of this fish prevent it from swimming backward out of the orifice, and surgical intervention is often required to extract the fish.

SCORPIONFISH

Scorpionfish, family Scorpaenidae, are divided into 3 main groups on the basis of their stinging apparatus.

All have venomous spines of varying sizes and toxicity, which may be found in dorsal, pelvic, and anal locations, depending on the species.

Scorpionfish, genus *Scorpaena*, have stings that are of intermediate severity. They are bottom dwellers with superior camouflage abilities that allow them to blend in almost invisibly with their surroundings (Fig. 182-28). Their spines are long and heavy and have moderate-sized venom glands.

Stonefish, genus *Synanceja*, are the most dangerous members of the scorpionfish family. They live in shallow waters, sometimes partially buried in sand or mud, or in holes of rocky shoals, reef areas, or tidal pools.[69] Injuries occur when a wader steps on the erect venomous dorsal spine that the stonefish raises in defense. Stonefish spines are short and thick and have very large and well-developed venom glands. The wounds caused by stonefish are quite severe and may be fatal. A stonefish antivenin is available.

WEEVERFISH

In European coastal waters, the weeverfish is one of the most common and serious causes of venomous fish spine injuries.[85] These fish are equipped with between 5 and 8 venomous dorsal spines and 2 venomous opercular spines (one on each side of the head near the gill plate).[86] Waders and bathers are at risk when they step on weeverfish that lie partly buried in mud or sand in shallow waters.

LOCAL AND SYSTEMIC SYMPTOMS OF FISH SPINE ENVENOMATIONS

The toxicity of a given venomous fish sting depends on a number of factors, including the species of fish involved, the location and severity of the wound, the amount of venom released, and the first aid and subsequent medical care provided to the victim. In general, these wounds produce pain disproportionate to the

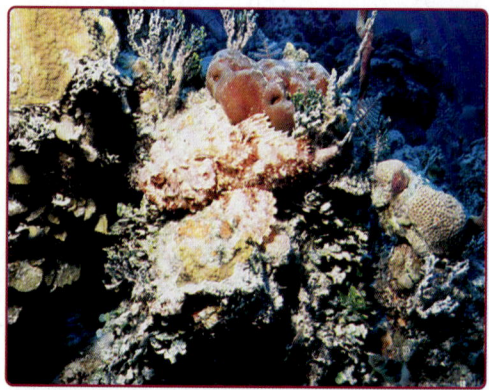

Figure 182-28 *Scorpaena plumieri*, a species of scorpionfish, is found in the waters of the West Indies. Its camouflage abilities are exceeded only by its painful sting.

apparent severity of the injury. The pain is immediate and intense. In the case of scorpionfish stings, the pain may be so severe as to cause the victim to thrash about wildly, scream, and finally lose consciousness.

Initially, the sting site may appear pale or cyanotic. The area around the wound may be anesthetic or hyperesthetic. Erythema and edema soon develop, giving the appearance of a cellulitis. Vesicles may form. In severe stinging, especially those caused by stonefish, the wounded area may become indurated and develop areas of ischemic necrosis with subsequent sloughing and ulcer formation.

Systemic effects from toxic fish spine envenomations may range from mild to severe, depending on the species involved and the amount of venom entering the wound. They can include headache, nausea, vomiting, diarrhea, abdominal cramps and pain, fever, local lymphangitis and lymphadenitis, joint aches, muscle weakness, diaphoresis, peripheral neuropathy, limb paralysis, restlessness, delirium, seizures, cardiac arrhythmias, myocardial ischemia, pericarditis, hypotension, and respiratory distress, and can lead to death.[84,87,88]

PREVENTION

Prevention of toxic fish spine wounds begins with knowledge of and appreciation for the various venomous species that may be encountered in a given area. Waders and bathers should shuffle their feet to scare away and avoid stepping on rays or scorpionfish. Fishermen must exercise care when removing rays or catfish from their fishing lines or when cleaning fish with venomous spines. Fish hobbyists and divers should wear protective clothing and avoid handling venomous species.

TREATMENT

Puncture wounds and lacerations from venomous fish spines should be irrigated immediately with sterile saline or water, if available, and with seawater as a last resort.[78] The wounded area should then be soaked as quickly as possible in hot (not scalding) water of approximately 43°C to 46°C (110°F-115°F) for 30 to 90 minutes or until maximal pain relief is achieved. Hot soaks may be repeated if the pain returns. Because the wound or extremity may be partially anesthetic, the person administering first aid must test the water's temperature for the victim.[53,89] One source of hot water that is often overlooked and may be useful in an emergency is hot seawater from a boat motor's cooling system.

Local infiltration of the wound with 1% to 2% lidocaine without epinephrine may bring about significant pain relief and allow exploration of the wound after radiographs have been obtained to locate retained portions of spines.[59,69] Longer-acting anesthetics such as procaine and bupivacaine may be chosen to provide a longer period of pain relief. The wound should be thoroughly cleaned to remove any remnants of integumentary sheath. Abdominal and thoracic wounds and deep wounds to the hands, feet, or fascial compartments of the legs should be explored in the operating room.[69] Debridement of necrotic tissues may be required at the time of exploration, and sequential debridement may be necessary. In general, these wounds should be left open or closed loosely with tape or suture to allow for adequate drainage and to prevent abscess formation.

Tetanus prophylaxis should be administered if indicated, and antibiotics are recommended if the wound is more than 6 hours old, is extensive, or involves deep puncture injuries to the hand or foot. The choice of antibiotic should be based on the bacteriology of the marine environment in which the wound occurred and, subsequently, on results of deep wound or tissue cultures. Empiric antibiotic therapy for infections of wounds occurring in saltwater should include coverage for *Vibrio* species. Before final wound culture results are known, initial choices of parenteral antibiotics include intravenous ciprofloxacin, imipenem-cilastatin, a third-generation cephalosporin, gentamicin, tobramycin, or trimethoprim-sulfamethoxazole.

Stonefish stings complicated by severe reactions may be treated with antivenin by slow intravenous infusion. Antivenom is not usually required for the stings of lionfish and other species of scorpionfish except for stonefish.[69] Stonefish antivenom is available from the Australian Commonwealth Serum Laboratory, Melbourne, Australia.

FISH BITES

There are many species of fish whose bites are dangerous to humans. Among the best known are the sharks and barracudas, whose bites may cause severe injuries.

Although they are well publicized by the news media, shark attacks are relatively rare events. The average number of unprovoked shark attacks worldwide in 2012-2016 was 83 incidents annually.[90] Only 32 of the 400 known species of sharks have been reported to attack humans. Most shark attacks involve surfers, scuba divers, and swimmers. Because sharks are attracted to bright or shiny objects, as well as to those with contrasting colors, these items should not be worn in the water. Sharks are also attracted by any sort of blood in the water; therefore, women who are menstruating should refrain from water sports in areas in which sharks may be prevalent, and no one should swim with an open bleeding wound. Spear fishermen should never tie their catch to themselves, and should place their catch in the dive boat as soon as possible. Although most shark bites are not life-threatening, more severe attacks may cause extensive soft-tissue loss with massive hemorrhage, which, in the worst cases, can result in amputation of a limb or death.[91,92]

Barracuda attacks are even rarer than shark bites. They tend to occur in turbid waters where these predators may mistake jewelry or other brightly colored objects worn by bathers for the baitfish on which they feed. Barracuda bites typically produce straight or V-shaped lacerations.

Divers and aquarium hobbyists must be careful when feeding or handling moray eels, which have powerful jaws and knife-like teeth. Although they are not considered venomous by most sources, they can produce deep puncture wounds and lacerations (Fig. 182-29).[78] When biting, moray eels tend to lock onto their prey; decapitation of the eel or disarticulation of its jaw may be required to release the victim.[93] As with all deep puncture wounds or lacerations, victims of moray eel bites should receive tetanus prophylaxis. Empiric antibiotic therapy for prophylaxis or treatment can include ciprofloxacin or cefuroxime for coverage of *Vibrio* or *Pseudomonas* species.[93]

WATERBORNE INFECTIONS

A variety of infections may result from exposures to aquatic environments. Pathogenic organisms may be actively introduced into the bite, sting, or laceration wounds caused by marine life; preexisting wounds may be passively infected when exposed to contaminated waters. *V. carchariae*, a halophilic (saltwater-loving) gram-negative bacillus, was reported as the cause of a wound infection after a shark bite.[94] Table 182-8 lists those organisms commonly associated with waterborne infections (see also Chap. 156). A host of other agents, such as *Streptococcus* and *Staphylococcus* sp., *Bacteroides fragilis*, *Clostridium perfringens*, *Escherichia coli*, *Salmonella enteritidis*, marine *Vibrio* sp., *Chromobacterium violaceum*, and *Chlorella*, also require consideration when dealing with infections associated with aquatic settings.[69] Life-threatening saltwater necrotizing fasciitis may result from a minor skin wound infected with a *Vibrio* species.[95]

CUTANEOUS MANIFESTATIONS OF SEAFOOD INGESTION AND SEAFOOD POISONING

Allergy to fish and crustaceans, such as shrimp, lobster, crab, and crawfish, is common, with most seafood allergies being lifelong.[96] Dermatologic reactions may appear after the ingestion of seafood. Urticaria, angioedema, and, rarely, leukocytoclastic vasculitis may occur in individuals sensitized to fish or shellfish. Many seafoods, such as kelp, contain large amounts of iodine, which may cause acneiform eruptions.

Scombroid food poisoning involves the ingestion of spoiled fish from the Scombridae family of fish, such as tuna, mackerel, and Bonita.[97] If these fish are not kept cold enough after being caught, their flesh

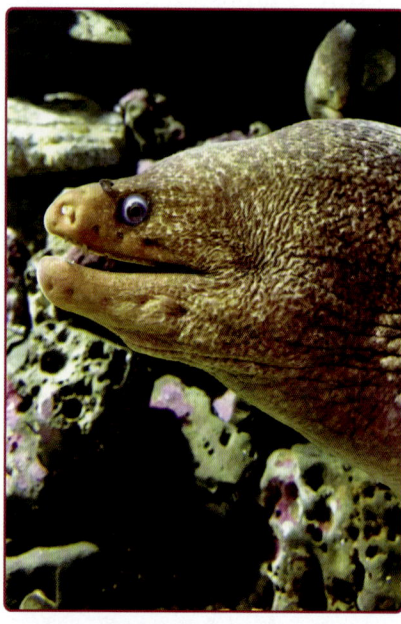

Figure 182-29 California Moray eel (*Gymnothorax mordax*), ranging from Point Conception to southern Baja California, with bites uncommon, but their incidence is rising because divers feed them at popular dive sites. (Used with permission from Jeffery Lee, D.D.S., Monte Sereno, CA.)

TABLE 182-8	
Wound Infections Associated with Waterborne Organisms	
ORGANISM	CLINICAL FEATURES
Aeromonas hydrophilia	Cellulitis (may be bullous), fasciitis, myonecrosis, bacteremia.
Edwardsiella tarda	Cellulitis, abscess, osteomyelitis, bacteremia.
Erysipelothrix rhusiopathiae	Slowly progressive cellulitis without adenopathy or lymphangitis, almost always involving the hand; septic arthritis; subacute bacterial endocarditis.
Mycobacterium balnei or *Mycobacterium marinum*	Swimming pool granuloma; fish fancier's finger; chronic cellulitis and culture-negative ulcers; often the primary lesion is on the hand and then a series of lesions develop in draining lymphatics.
Pfiesteria piscicida	Raw, red pock-marked lesions in fish in polluted waterways; in humans, rashes, respiratory problems, and memory deficits.
Prototheocosis	Papular or eczematoid dermatitis in immunosuppressed patients; localized infection of the olecranon bursa.
Pseudomonas species	Trench foot; gram-negative toe web space infections; swimmer's ear; hot tub folliculitis.
Streptococcus iniae	Cellulitis and bacteremia after skin injuries during the handling of fresh fish raised by aquaculture.
Vibrio vulnificus, other *Vibrio* sp.	Cellulitis, sometimes with bulla formation; may progress to septicemia, especially in alcoholics, diabetics, and immunosuppressed patients; metastatic cellulitis, meningitis, and death may result from fulminant infections.

develops scombrotoxins as a consequence of the bacterial breakdown of histidine into histamine, saurine, and possibly other toxic by-products. These can cause striking erythema and flushing of the face, neck, and upper trunk, as well as pruritus and urticarial and angioedematous eruptions. Oral antihistamines are the usual therapeutic option.

Ciguatera toxin, which is produced during blooms of toxic dinoflagellates, is incorporated into the marine food chain and concentrated in the flesh of a variety of fish. It is heat stable. Symptoms may occur after eating cooked or raw fish containing the toxin. Dermatologic symptoms of ingesting these fish may include generalized pruritus and diffuse erythematous macular and papular exanthems, which may progress to blister formation and desquamation.

ACKNOWLEDGMENTS

We thank Dr Bruce Halstead of the World Life Research Institute, Colton, California, for allowing us to reprint the photographs from the first and second editions of *Poisonous and Venomous Marine Animals of the World*. We also thank the legendary Professor Rajendra Kapila, who is in his 52nd year at Rutgers New Jersey Medical School, for his assistance.

REFERENCES

1. CDC. Nonfatal dog bite–related injuries treated in hospital emergency departments—United States, 2001. *MMWR Morb Mortal Wkly Rep*. 2003;52(26):605-610.
2. Aziz H, Rhee P, Pandit V, et al. The current concepts in management of animal (dog, cat, snake, scorpion) and human bite wounds. *J Trauma Acute Care Surg*. 2015;78(3):641-648.
3. Tuncali D, Bingul F, Terzioglu A, et al. Animal bites. *Saudi Med J*. 2005;26(5):772-776.
4. Benson LS, Edwards SL, Schiff AP, et al. Dog and cat bites to the hand: treatment and cost assessment. *J Hand Surg Am*. 2006;31(3):468-473.
5. Garcia VF. Animal bites and Pasteurella infections. *Pediatr Rev*. 1997;18(4):127-130.
6. Grim KD, Doherty C, Rosen T. Serratia marcescens bullous cellulitis after iguana bites. *J Am Acad Dermatol*. 2010;62(6):1075-1076.
7. Rittner AV, Fitzpatrick K, Corfield A. Best evidence topic report. Are antibiotics indicated following human bites? *Emerg Med J*. 2005;22(9):654.
8. Chaudhry MA, MacNamara AF, Clark S. Is the management of dog bite wounds evidence based? A postal survey and review of the literature. *Eur J Emerg Med*. 2004;11(6):313-317.
9. Mansfield KL, Andrews N, Goharriz H, et al. Rabies pre-exposure prophylaxis elicits long-lasting immunity in humans. *Vaccine*. 2016;34(48):5959-5967.
10. Talan DA et al. Clinical presentation and bacteriologic analysis of infected human bites in patients presenting to emergency departments. *Clin Infect Dis*. 2003;37(11):1481-1489.
11. Suchard JR. "Spider bite" lesions are usually diagnosed as skin and soft-tissue infections. *J Emerg Med*. 2011;41(5):473-481.
12. Barnham M, Holmes B. Isolation of CDC group M-5 and *Staphylococcus intermedius* from infected dog bites. *J Infect*. 1992;25(3):332-334.
13. Blanche P, Meyniard O, Ratovohery D, et al. *Capnocytophaga canimorsus* lymphocytic meningitis in an immunocompetent man who was bitten by a dog. *Clin Infect Dis*. 1994;18(4):654-655.
14. Linton DM, Potgieter PD, Roditi D, et al. Fatal *Capnocytophaga canimorsus* (DF-2) septicaemia. A case report. *S Afr Med J*. 1994;84(12):857-860.
15. Deshmukh PM, Camp CJ, Rose FB, et al. *Capnocytophaga canimorsus* sepsis with purpura fulminans and symmetrical gangrene following a dog bite in a shelter employee. *Am J Med Sci*. 2004;327(6):369-372.
16. van de Ven AR, van Vliet AC, Maraha B, et al. Fibrinolytic therapy in *Capnocytophaga canimorsus* sepsis after dog bite. *Intensive Care Med*. 2004;30(10):1980.
17. Elliott DR, Wilson M, Buckley CM, et al. Cultivable oral microbiota of domestic dogs. *J Clin Microbiol*. 2005;43(11):5470-5476.
18. Summanen PH, Durmaz B, Väisänen ML, et al. *Porphyromonas somerae* sp. nov., a pathogen isolated from humans and distinct from *Porphyromonas levii*. *J Clin Microbiol*. 2005;43(9):4455-4459.
19. Citron DM, Hunt Gerardo S, Claros MC, et al. Frequency of isolation of *Porphyromonas* species from infected dog and cat bite wounds in humans and their characterization by biochemical tests and arbitrarily primed-polymerase chain reaction fingerprinting. *Clin Infect Dis*. 1996;23(suppl 1):S78-S82.
20. Krebs JW, Mandel EJ, Swerdlow DL, et al. Rabies surveillance in the United States during 2004. *J Am Vet Med Assoc*. 2005;227(12):1912-1925.
21. Burton EC, Burns DK, Opatowsky MJ, et al. Rabies encephalomyelitis: clinical, neuroradiological, and pathological findings in 4 transplant recipients. *Arch Neurol*. 2005;62(6):873-882.
22. World Health Organization (WHO). *Rabies and Envenomings: A Neglected Public Health Issue: Report of a Consultative Meeting*, 2007. http://www.who.int/bloodproducts/animal_sera/Rabies.pdf. Accessed July 25, 2018.
23. Kositprapa C, Limsuwun K, Wilde H, et al. Immune response to simulated postexposure rabies booster vaccinations in volunteers who received preexposure vaccinations. *Clin Infect Dis*. 1997;25(3):614-616.
24. Fishbein DB, Robinson LE. Rabies. *N Engl J Med*. 1993;329(22):1632-1638.
25. Willoughby RE Jr, Tieves KS, Hoffman GM, et al. Survival after treatment of rabies with induction of coma. *N Engl J Med*. 2005;352(24):2508-2514.
26. Holmes GP, Chapman LE, Stewart JA, et al. Guidelines for the prevention and treatment of B-virus infections in exposed persons. The B virus Working Group. *Clin Infect Dis*. 1995;20(2):421-439.
27. WHO Guidelines for the Production, Control and Regulation of Snake Antivenom Immunoglobulins, 2018. http://www.who.int/bloodproducts/snake_antivenoms/snakeantivenomguide/en/. Accessed July 25, 2018.
28. World Health Organization (WHO). *Venomous snakes and antivenoms search interface*, 2018. http://apps.who.int/bloodproducts/snakeantivenoms/database/default.htm. Accessed 2018.
29. Gold BS, Dart RC, Barish RA. Bites of venomous snakes. *N Engl J Med*. 2002;347(5):347-356.
30. McKinney PE. Out-of-hospital and interhospital management of crotaline snakebite. *Ann Emerg Med*. 2001;37(2):168-174.

31. Hall EL. Role of surgical intervention in the management of crotaline snake envenomation. *Ann Emerg Med.* 2001;37(2):175-180.
32. Eadie PA, Lee TC, Niazi Z, et al. Seal finger in a wildlife ranger. *Ir Med J.* 1990;83(3):117-118.
33. Nuckton TJ, Simeone CA, Phelps RT. California sea lion (*Zalophus californianus*) and Harbor seal (*Phoca vitulina richardii*) bites and contact abrasions in open-water swimmers: a series of 11 cases. *Wilderness Environ Med.* 2015;26(4):497-508.
34. Fisher AA. Aquatic dermatitis, Part I. Dermatitis caused by coelenterates. *Cutis.* 1999;64(2):84-86.
35. Auerbach PS, Hays, JT. Erythema nodosum following a jellyfish sting. *J Emerg Med.* 1987;5(6):487.
36. Lakkis NA, Maalouf GJ, Mahmassani DM. Jellyfish stings: a practical approach. *Wilderness Environ Med.* 2015; 26(3):422-429.
37. Auerbach PS. Envenomations from jellyfish and related species. *J Emerg Nurs.* 1997;23(6):555-565; quiz 566-567.
38. Burnett JW, Calton GJ. Jellyfish envenomation syndromes updated. *Ann Emerg Med.* 1987;16(9):1000-1005.
39. Halstead BW. Coelenterate (cnidarian) stings and wounds. *Clin Dermatol.* 1987;5(3):8-13.
40. Williamson JA, Burnett JW, Fenner PJ, et al. Acute regional vascular insufficiency after jellyfish envenomation. *Med J Aust.* 1988;149(11-12):698-701.
41. Giordano AR, Vito L, Sardella PJ. Complication of a Portuguese man-of-war envenomation to the foot: a case report. *J Foot Ankle Surg.* 2005;44(4):297-300.
42. Guess HA, Saviteer PL, Morris CR. Hemolysis and acute renal failure following a Portuguese man-of-war sting. *Pediatrics.* 1982;70(6):979-981.
43. Burnett JW, Gable WD. A fatal jellyfish envenomation by the Portuguese man-o'war. *Toxicon.* 1989;27(7):823-824.
44. Stein MR, Marraccini JV, Rothschild NE, et al. Fatal Portuguese man-o'-war (*Physalia physalis*) envenomation. *Ann Emerg Med.* 1989;18(3):312-315.
45. Bengtson K, Nichols MM, Schnadig V, et al. Sudden death in a child following jellyfish envenomation by *Chiropsalmus quadrumanus*. Case report and autopsy findings. *JAMA.* 1991;266(10):1404-1406.
46. Sutherland S. Lethal jellyfish. *Med J Aust.* 1985; 143(12-13):536.
47. Fenner PJ, Harrison SL. Irukandji and *Chironex fleckeri* jellyfish envenomation in tropical Australia. *Wilderness Environ Med.* 2000;11(4):233-240.
48. Bailey PM, Little M, Jelinek GA, et al. Jellyfish envenoming syndromes: unknown toxic mechanisms and unproven therapies. *Med J Aust.* 2003;178(1):34-37.
49. O'Reilly GM, Isbister GK, Lawrie PM, et al. Prospective study of jellyfish stings from tropical Australia, including the major box jellyfish *Chironex fleckeri*. *Med J Aust.* 2001; 175(11-12):652-655.
50. Burnett JW, Calton GJ. The case for verapamil use in alarming jellyfish stings remains. *Toxicon.* 2004;44(8):817-818; author reply 819-820.
51. Burnett JW. The case for the use of verapamil in alarming Chironex stings. *Anaesth Intensive Care.* 1998; 26(4):461-464.
52. Collated by CRC Reef on behalf of the Queensland Government Irukandji Jellyfish Response Task Force, current status of knowledge and action on Irukandji, v.8.3. 6/1/2006:6/1/2006. http://www.reef.crc.org.au/iscover/plantsanimals/pdf/StatusofKnowledgeandActionPaperSep2002.pdf. Accessed November 22, 2011.
53. Wilcox CL, Yanagihara AA. Heated debates: hot-water immersion or ice packs as first aid for cnidarian envenomations? *Toxins (Basel).* 2016;8(4):97.
54. Fenner PJ, Williamson JA. Worldwide deaths and severe envenomation from jellyfish stings. *Med J Aust.* 1996;165(11-12):658-661.
55. Garcia PJ, Schein RM, Burnett JW. Fulminant hepatic failure from a sea anemone sting. *Ann Intern Med.* 1994; 120(8):665-666.
56. Nicholls D. Sea anemone sting while SCUBA diving. *N Z Med J.* 1992;105(936):245.
57. Sagi A, Rosenberg L, Ben-Meir P, et al. "The fire coral" (*Millepora dichotoma*) as a cause of burns: a case report. *Burns Incl Therm Inj.* 1987;13(4):325-326.
58. Camarasa JG, Nogues Antich E, Serra-Baldrich E. Red Sea coral contact dermatitis. *Contact Dermatitis.* 1993; 29(5):285-286.
59. Auerbach PS. *Diving Medicine Articles: I Have Been Stung: What Should I Do?* [updated 2004], 2004, Divers Alert Network. Accessed July 26, 2018.
60. Isbister GK, Hooper JN. Clinical effects of stings by sponges of the genus Tedania and a review of sponge stings worldwide. *Toxicon.* 2005;46(7):782-785.
61. Burnett JW, Calton GJ, Morgan RJ. Dermatitis due to stinging sponges. *Cutis.* 1987;39(6):476.
62. Kizer KW. Marine envenomations. *J Toxicol Clin Toxicol.* 1983;21(4-5):527-555.
63. Baden HP. Injuries from sea urchins. *Clin Dermatol.* 1987;5(13):112-117.
64. Burnett JW, Burnett MG. Sea urchins. *Cutis.* 1999; 64(1):21-22.
65. Burke WA, Steinbaugh JR, O'Keefe EJ. Delayed hypersensitivity reaction following a sea urchin sting. *Int J Dermatol.* 1986;25(10):649-650.
66. Asada M, Komura J, Hosokawa H, et al. A case of delayed hypersensitivity reaction following a sea urchin sting. *Dermatologica.* 1990;180(2):99-101.
67. Guyot-Drouot MH, Rouneau D, Rolland JM, et al. Arthritis, tenosynovitis, fasciitis, and bursitis due to sea urchin spines. A series of 12 cases in Reunion Island. *Joint Bone Spine.* 2000;67(2):94-100.
68. De La Torre C, Toribio J. Sea-urchin granuloma: histologic profile. A pathologic study of 50 biopsies. *J Cutan Pathol.* 2001;28(5):223-228.
69. Auerbach PS. Marine envenomations. *N Engl J Med.* 1991;325(7):486-493.
70. Verbrugge LM, Rainey JJ, Reimink RL, et al. Prospective study of swimmer's itch incidence and severity. *J Parasitol.* 2004;90(4):697-704.
71. Hoeffler DF. "Swimmers' itch" (cercarial dermatitis). *Cutis.* 1977;19(4):461-465, 467.
72. Folster-Holst R, Disko R, Röwert J, et al. Cercarial dermatitis contracted via contact with an aquarium: case report and review. *Br J Dermatol.* 2001;145(4):638-640.
73. Gonzalez E. Schistosomiasis, cercarial dermatitis, and marine dermatitis. *Dermatol Clin.* 1989;7(2):291-300.
74. Rossetto AL, Da Silveira FL, Morandini AC, et al. Seabather's eruption: report of fourteen cases. *An Acad Bras Cienc.* 2015;87(1):431-436.
75. Segura-Puertas L, Ramos ME, Aramburo C, et al. One Linuche mystery solved: All 3 stages of the coronate scyphomedusa *Linuche unguiculata* cause seabather's eruption. *J Am Acad Dermatol.* 2001;44(4):624-628.
76. Kumar S, Hlady WG, Malecki JM. Risk factors for seabather's eruption: a prospective cohort study. *Public Health Rep.* 1997;112(1):59-62.
77. Halford ZA, Yu PY, Likeman RK, et al. Cone shell

envenomation: epidemiology, pharmacology and medical care. Diving Hyperb Med 2015;45(3):200-207.
78. Halstead BW, Auerbach PS, eds. *Dangerous Aquatic Animal of the World: A Color Guide, With Prevention, First Aid, and Emergency Treatment Procedures*. Princeton, NJ: Darwin Press; 1990.
79. Burnett JW. Aquatic adversaries: human injuries induced by octopi. *Cutis.* 1998;62(3):124.
80. Soppe GG. Marine envenomations and aquatic dermatology. *Am Fam Physician.* 1989;40(2):97-106.
81. Germain M, Smith KJ, Skelton H. The cutaneous cellular infiltrate to stingray envenomization contains increased TIA+ cells. *Br J Dermatol.* 2000;143(5):1074-1077.
82. Meyer PK. Stingray injuries. *Wilderness Environ Med.* 1997;8(1):24-28.
83. Fenner PJ, Williamson JA, Skinner RA. Fatal and non-fatal stingray envenomation. *Med J Aust.* 1989;151(11-12):621-625.
84. Das SK, Johnson MB, Cohly HH. Catfish stings in Mississippi. *South Med J.* 1995;88(8):809-812.
85. Davies RS, Evans RJ. Weever fish stings: a report of two cases presenting to an accident and emergency department. *J Accid Emerg Med.* 1996;13(2):139-141.
86. Borondo JC, Sanz P, Nogué S, et al. Fatal weeverfish sting. *Hum Exp Toxicol.* 2001;20(2):118-119.
87. Trestrail JH III, Al-Mahasneh QM. Lionfish string experiences of an inland poison center: a retrospective study of 23 cases. *Vet Hum Toxicol.* 1989;31(2):173-175.
88. Perkins RA, Morgan SS. Poisoning, envenomation, and trauma from marine creatures. *Am Fam Physician.* 2004;69(4):885-890.
89. Atkinson PR, Boyle A, Hartin D, et al. Is hot water immersion an effective treatment for marine envenomation? *Emerg Med J.* 2006;23(7):503-508.
90. Burgess GH, Piercy A. International Shark Attack File: 2018 Worldwide Shark Attack Summary, Florida Museum of Natural History, University of Florida. http://www.flmnh.ufl.edu/fish/sharks/isaf/graphs.htm#trends. Accessed June 2018.
91. Woolgar JD, Cliff G, Nair R, et al. Shark attack: review of 86 consecutive cases. *J Trauma.* 2001;50(5):887-891.
92. Byard RW, Gilbert JD, Brown K. Pathologic features of fatal shark attacks. *Am J Forensic Med Pathol.* 2000;21(3):225-229.
93. Erickson T, Vanden Hoek TL, Kuritza A, et al. The emergency management of Moray eel bites. *Ann Emerg Med.* 1992;21(2):212-216.
94. Pavia AT, Bryan JA, Maher KL, et al. *Vibrio carchariae* infection after a shark bite. *Ann Intern Med.* 1989;111(1):85-86.
95. Schwartz RA, Kapila R. Dermatologic manifestations of necrotizing Fasciitis Medscape Reference. http://emedicine.medscape.com/article/1054438-overview. Updated June 21, 2018.
96. Husain Z, Schwartz RA. Food allergy update: more than a peanut of a problem. *Int J Dermatol.* 2013;52(3):286-294.
97. Guergué-Díaz de Cerio O, Barrutia-Borque A, Gardeazabal-García J. Scombroid poisoning: a practical approach. *Actas Dermosifiliogr.* 2016;107(7):567-571.

Topical and Systemic Treatments

PART 28

第二十八篇 外用和系统药物治疗

Chapter 183 :: Principles of Topical Therapy
:: Mohammed D. Saleem, Howard I. Maibach, & Steven R. Feldman

第一百八十三章
外用药物的治疗原则

中文导读

皮肤科外用药物的有效性取决于三个因素：药物的涂抹，活性分子通过载体的传递，以及活性分子的内在效力。本章分为12节：①前言；②经皮给药；③扩散；④三室模型；⑤皮肤代谢；⑥吸收；⑦病理过程对皮肤屏障功能的影响；⑧其他影响吸收的因素；⑨外用制剂的分类和临床应用；⑩外用制剂；⑪副作用及预防措施；⑫总结。

第一节前言，重点提到了外用药物使用过程中容易忽略的依从性问题，依从性差与疾病的不良结局有关，并提到了提高原发性不依从和继发性不依从的可能方法。

第二节经皮给药，介绍了外用药物的治疗效果与其固有的药效和药物穿透皮肤的能力有关，但吸收只是功效的一个因素，低吸收并不一定就会低疗效。

第三节介绍了外用于皮肤表面的化合物的扩散定律，沿着浓度梯度迁移，不带电化合物在膜或任何均质屏障上的扩散遵循菲克第一定律和第二定律。

第四节介绍了外用药物的药代动力学分析，与皮肤表面、皮肤屏障角质层及活体组织三个部分相关，组成了一个三室模型，在每个隔间内，化合物可能沿着浓度梯度向下扩散，与特定成分结合或被代谢。

第五节皮肤代谢，介绍了皮肤含有广泛的酶活性，包括第一阶段氧化、还原、水解，第二阶段结合反应，以及一个完整的药物代谢酶的补充。皮肤组织的新陈代谢在决定外用活性化合物的命运方面起着重要作用。

第六节介绍了皮肤微血管对化合物的吸收，与交换毛细血管的表面积及其血流直接相关。

第七节介绍了病理过程对皮肤屏障功能的影响，这可能是与潜在活组织中缺乏酶或结构蛋白、角质形成细胞增殖增加导致角质层形成不当、负责屏障活动恢复的稳态机制等有关。

第八节介绍了其他影响吸收的因素，包括角质层、封包疗法、药物的使用频率、使用量，以及按摩、毛发等因素。

第九节外用制剂的分类和临床应用，介绍了外用制剂中的许多常用成分，外用制剂通常具有冷却、保护、润肤、封闭或收敛的特性，具有非特异性效果。

第十节外用制剂，介绍了各种剂型的成分、特征及功能。

第十一节外用药物的副作用及预防措施，包括外用药物效应引起的皮肤过敏、皮肤萎缩、皮肤瘙痒、刺激性接触性皮炎、过敏性接触性皮炎以及可能出现恶性肿瘤等，此外外用药物可引起全身效应，如免疫性接触性荨麻疹、恶性肿瘤，还有对内分泌系统的影响。

第十二节总结了外用药物治疗是皮肤科医生的主要治疗方法，医生需要了解药物的浓度、渗透性、有效性和皮肤病治疗之间的相互作用，以及外用和全身毒性，可以最大限度地提高外用治疗的疗效和耐受性。

〔粟　娟〕

AT-A-GLANCE

- Efficacy of a topically applied drug depends on three things: whether the drug is applied, the delivery of the active molecule by its vehicle, and the inherent potency of the active molecule.
- Adherence to topical treatment is often poor and decreases over time.
- Factors that affect penetration of applied drug include soluble medication concentration, regional variations in skin barrier properties, application frequency, and effects of the vehicle on barrier function.
- The primary barrier that limits the percutaneous absorption of compounds is the stratum corneum.
- The delivery of a topical agent is highly dependent on the physicochemical properties of the vehicle; this influences the kinetics of release and absorption and the onset, duration, and extent of a biologic response.
- Either the vehicle or its active ingredient(s) may cause local toxicity, systemic toxicity, or both.

INTRODUCTION

Topical therapy involves three key steps: topical application, percutaneous absorption, and binding of the active molecule to its target site. Sensible topical drug therapy involves selection of an appropriate agent that patients are able and willing to procure and apply (which may depend on the areas of the body affected), a vehicle that will effectively deliver the active molecule without irritation, and an active drug of the appropriate potency, along with a defined duration of use that maximizes efficacy and minimizes adverse side effects. Behind each of these considerations are basic principles that help guide the practitioner toward a rational plan of therapy.

ADHERENCE

The first principle of topical treatment is the ubiquity of poor adherence. Adherence is an often-ignored aspect of medication efficacy. Nonadherence to prescribed medicines in chronic conditions is between 30% and 50%.[1,2] Poor adherence to topical treatment is a common cause of poor response to drugs and is linked with poor outcomes in diseases such as psoriasis, atopic dermatitis, and acne.[3]

Poor adherence may be intentional or unintentional. Intentional nonadherence is driven by the patient's perception of the need for treatment weighed against their concern for toxicities and other costs. Unintentional nonadherence results from forgetfulness or lack of knowledge on prescribed regimens. Depression, socioeconomic status, single marital status, complicated treatment regimens, and high prescription costs are associated with nonadherence.[1,4-6]

There are varying patterns of poor adherence. Primary nonadherence refers to when patients do not fill their prescription or initiate treatment. Secondary nonadherence occurs when patients initiate treatment but use the medication poorly. Secondary nonadherence includes both poor execution (using the medication intermittently) and early discontinuation of treatment.

A variety of approaches have been promoted and tested as means to promote better adherence to topical treatment. Written instructions, discussing treatment expectations, and early follow-up visits after receiving a prescription can improve adherence and decrease the overall required visits. Simplifying treatment regimens, prescribing patient preferred vehicles, treatment reminders, and support groups also improve adherence.[1,4] Last, a trusting and supportive doctor–patient relationship is critical to achieving adequate adherence.[7]

Nonadherence is often mistaken for treatment resistant disease. Adherence to topical therapies is often overestimated, resulting in switches to more costly and riskier alternative therapies.[8] Tachyphylaxis, defined as the decrease in drug response over time, is often a result of nonadherence rather than loss of corticosteroid receptor function.[9,10]

CUTANEOUS DELIVERY OF APPLIED DRUGS

Therapeutic efficacy of a topical drug relates to its inherent potency and the ability of the drug to penetrate the skin.[11] Many potent agents, such as hydrocortisone and fluocinolone acetonide, are poorly absorbed after topical application. Conversely, many well-absorbed agents with weak potency have negligible therapeutic use.

In contrast to many orally administered drugs that are nearly completely absorbed within a few hours, topical medicines generally have a poor total absorption and a slow absorption rate. For example, less than 1% of a topically applied corticosteroid such as hydrocortisone is absorbed after a single application left on the skin for more than 1 day. Furthermore, peak rates of absorption are reached up to 12 to 24 hours after application. Fortunately, low absorption does not necessarily translate into low efficacy. Drugs such as topical corticosteroids are effective because of their inherent potency and can exert clinically significant effects despite low absorption. In this light, absorption represents only one of many facets of efficacy.

DIFFUSION

LAWS OF DIFFUSION

Compounds applied topically to the skin surface migrate along concentration gradients according to well-described laws governing diffusion of solutes in solutions or their diffusion across membranes. For a detailed discussion of relevant equations, readers are referred to comprehensive reviews.[12]

FICK'S LAWS

Diffusion of uncharged compounds across a membrane or any homogeneous barrier is described by Fick's first and second laws. The first law

$$J = -D\,(\Delta C/\Delta \delta)$$

states that the steady-state flux of a compound (J = moles/cm/s) per unit path length (δ, cm) is proportional to the concentration gradient (ΔC) and the diffusion coefficient (D, cm^2/s). The negative sign indicates that the net flux is in the direction of the lower concentration. This equation applies to diffusion-mediated processes in isotropic solutions under steady-state conditions. Fick's second law predicts the flux of compounds under non–steady-state conditions. Diffusion is an effective transport mechanism over very short distances but not over long ones. The relationship between the time (Δt) it takes for a molecule to migrate along a path length (x) and its diffusion coefficient is governed by the equation:

$$\Delta t = x^2/2D.$$

For example, diffusion coefficient for water in an aqueous solution is: 2.5×10^{-5} cm^2/s, suggesting that a water molecule would migrate over a 10-μm path (the equivalent of the width of the stratum corneum) in 0.4 ms. However, because diffusion depends on the square of the distance, longer distances are not efficiently covered; a 100-μm path would take 40 ms.

THREE-COMPARTMENT MODEL

Although pharmacokinetic analysis of topical preparations may require the description of a relatively large number of compartments, this discussion is confined to the three outlined in Fig. 183-1: (1) skin surface, (2) stratum corneum, and (3) viable tissue. The formulation itself forms a reservoir, from which the compound must be released; to undergo percutaneous absorption, the compound then must penetrate the stratum corneum; diffuse into and through the viable epidermis into the dermis; and, finally, gain access to the systemic compartment through the vascular system. In addition, the substance may diffuse through the dermal and hypodermal layers to reach underlying tissues. As summarized in Table 183-1, within each compartment, the compound may diffuse down along its concentration gradient, bind to specific components, or be metabolized. The size or characteristics of each compartment may alter with time, and the factors determining diffusion within each compartment may be affected by disease state as well as the nature or the

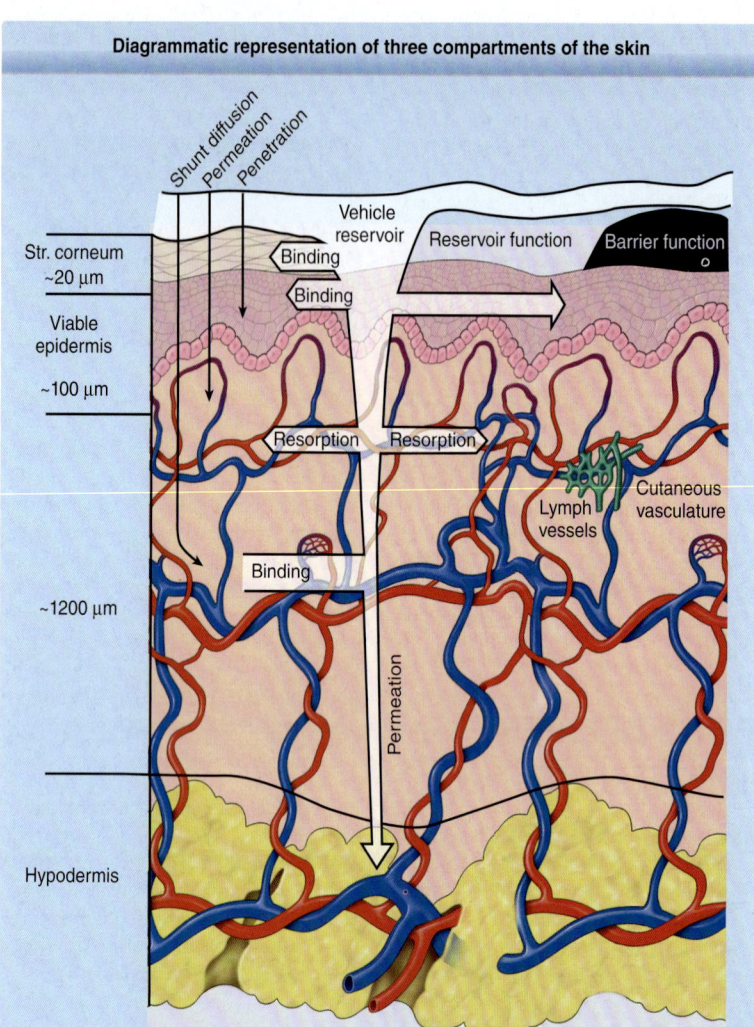

Figure 183-1 Diagrammatic representation of three compartments of the skin: surface, stratum (Str.) corneum, and viable tissues. Topical medication efficacy is a multifactorial process that involves the selection of a medication, adequate adherence, and drug delivery to the skin. Adequate adherence is a prerequest for successful drug delivery and can be classified as primary (filling a prescription and initiating treatment) or secondary (correct administration and continuation after initiation). Drug delivery can be simplified to three compartments of the skin: surface, stratum corneum, and viable tissues. After surface applications, evaporation and structural or compositional alterations in the applied formulation may play important roles in determining the bioavailability of drugs. Stratum corneum, the outermost layer, plays the most significant role in determining the diffusion of compounds into the body. After absorption, compounds may bind or diffuse within the viable tissues or become resorbed by the cutaneous vasculature.

pharmacologic or biologic activity of the drug or its excipients. Table 183-2 lists the parameters that affect the amount of drug in the skin compartments.

SKIN SURFACE

SURFACE APPLICATIONS OF FORMULATIONS

Formulations differ in their physicochemical properties, and, as discussed in section "Formulations", this influences the kinetics of release, absorption, or both. However, the principal consideration is that topically applied drug products represent a physically small compartment, which limits the amount of compound that can be applied to the skin surface. When a patient applies a dermatologic preparation, the layer of a formulation covering the skin is thin (~0.5 to 2.0 mg/cm^2). Thicker layers are felt as "unpleasant" and are consciously or subconsciously rubbed off or spread to larger surfaces. This restricts the amount of an active compound that can effectively come in contact with the skin surface to approximately 5 to 20 µg/cm^2 for a 1% (wt/wt) topical formulation.

TABLE 183-1
Compartments Encountered by Substances Undergoing Percutaneous Absorption: General Relevance of Processes to Bioavailability

COMPARTMENT	PROCESSES	GENERAL RELEVANCE TO BIOAVAILABILITY
Vehicle	Diffusion	++
	Thermodynamic activity	++
	Evaporation	+
	Precipitation	±
Stratum corneum	Reservoir function	+++
	Diffusion	+++
	Binding	+
	Metabolism	−
Epidermis	Diffusion	±
Cutaneous vasculature	Metabolism	±
	Binding	++
	Resorption	+
Underlying tissues including dermis	Diffusion	±
	Metabolism	±
	Binding	−

−, although theoretically possible, this process is probably not of general relevance; ±, this process is of direct relevance but only in a restricted number of cases; +, the process is in general relevant but not as important as ++ or +++.

However, even after being rubbed in, formulations do not remain homogeneous over the time course of penetration. For example, topical applications containing water, alcohol, or similar solvents undergo rapid evaporation.[13] This phenomenon, readily recognized by patients as a cooling sensation, results in rapidly increasing concentrations of nonvolatile substances on the skin surface, which may result in the formation of supersaturated "solutions" or, alternatively, precipitation of active ingredients. Formulations may also mix with skin-surface lipids or undergo time-dependent changes in their composition as excipients and drugs undergo absorption. Altogether, these considerations suggest that dramatic changes in the composition and structure of formulations may occur after surface application, all of which may determine the subsequent bioavailability of active ingredients.

RESERVOIR

The reservoir function, first described by Vickers,[14] describes that simple occlusion leads to the renewed onset of a glucocorticoid-mediated vasoconstriction several hours after it had declined. He interpreted this effect as renewed liberation of the glucocorticoid from a "reservoir" stored in the upper skin layers.

We define as *reservoir* the amount of an active ingredient that is still in contact with the nonvolatile constituents of its formulation after the latter had been massaged into the skin surface. The compound has not yet penetrated, but it cannot be removed by simple rubbing or contact with clothing or other tissues. The reservoir thus adheres to the skin surface and resides in the wrinkles and layers of the stratum corneum. Reservoirs on eczematous skin may become even more prominent because of the scaliness of the skin. The upper volume of the follicular channels also serves as a reservoir, which may result in a relative increase in absorption through appendages. In vivo laser scanning microscopy measurements found that the hair follicles represent an efficient reservoir for topically applied formulations, which can be compared with the reservoir of the stratum corneum on several body sites.[15,16] This phenomenon may be increased in formulations that contain particles or precipitates, given the evidence that appropriately sized particles can rapidly penetrate along the shafts of hair follicles to a depth of up to 100 to 500 μm.[17-19]

Optimum size of the particles for penetration into hair follicles is between 300 and 600 nm, which corresponds to the cuticular structure of the hairs.[20,21] The rigid hair shaft acts as a geared pump because this effect could only be observed in the case of moving hairs.[20] The follicular reservoir may result in a relative increase in the absorption of topically applied substances. No evidence has been found that topically applied substances penetrate efficiently into the sweat glands. This may be caused by sweat outflow or other, unknown reasons.

TABLE 183-2
Parameters That Affect Drug Amounts in Skin Compartments

- As applied products dry on the skin, the formulations may undergo drastic changes in composition and structure. Increasing concentration of drug may result in greater drug delivery or, if the active drug precipitates at high concentration, a reduction in drug delivery.
- Drug or formulation may affect the skin barrier, resulting in time-dependent changes of the barrier function.
- Skin barrier may be affected by the type and progression of a disease.
- There may be regional variations in the barrier properties of the skin.
- The therapeutic response to a topical drug can enhance or retard percutaneous absorption.
- Metabolic capacity of skin may lead to exposure of skin or systemically to both parent drug and pharmacologically active metabolite(s).

FORMULATIONS

Formulations can be differentiated on the basis of whether they are designed to remain on the skin surface (sunscreen products and cosmetics), to be delivered to compartments in the skin (topical formulations), or to migrate across the skin into the central compartment (transdermal formulations).

Formulations may affect the kinetics and the degree of percutaneous absorption and, subsequently, the onset, duration, and extent of a biologic response. In the context of percutaneous absorption, several parameters should be considered when selecting a formulation:[22] the thermodynamic activity of the active ingredient,[23] amount of compound that can be incorporated into the formulation,[24] stability of the formulation on the skin surface (eg, emulsions may break easily),[25] partition coefficient of the active ingredient between the vehicle and the stratum corneum,[26] and enhancer activity.

In general, percutaneous absorption is proportional to the thermodynamic activity of the compound. Thus, the greatest flux is observed at the active ingredient's maximum solubility in a vehicle.

The physical chemical properties of the formation have critical importance when considering compounding medications. Drug compounding is the process of combining or altering ingredients to create tailored medication and are widely used by dermatologists. Dermatologists may tailor therapies to patients' specific needs; for example, they can be designed with less irritating vehicles or excluding specific allergenic components. Compounded drugs are not approved by the U.S. Food and Drug Administration (FDA), and their safety, effectiveness, or quality are not verified by the FDA. When a topical product is mixed with another product—for example, mixing 0.1% triamcinolone cream with a moisturizing cream or other product—the activity of the resulting product is not predictable. Although a 1:1 mixture would reduce the concentration of triamcinolone from 0.1% to 0.05%, the physical chemical properties of the vehicle will have changed. The resulting compounded product could be more effective, equally effective, or less effective than the original 0.1% triamcinolone cream depending on how well the modified vehicle delivers triamcinolone past the cutaneous barrier.

SKIN BARRIER

See Chap. 14.

The primary compartment that limits percutaneous absorption of compounds is the stratum corneum. This thin (10 to 20 μm) layer effectively surrounds the body and represents a highly differentiated structure that determines the diffusion of compounds across the skin. The physical description of the stratum corneum is well documented,[27] and it can be accurately described as "bricks" of bundled, water-insoluble proteins, embedded in a "mortar" of intercellular lipid, and water.

Stratum corneum is a highly organized, differentiated structure. To participate fully in forming an effective barrier to diffusion, the biogenesis of the corneocytes as well as the synthesis and processing of the intercellular lipid must proceed in an orderly manner. Disruption in the kinetics of skin barrier formation by accelerating the division of the keratinocytes in the underlying layers will lead to a disruption in its barrier properties.[28] Thus, the concept of dead or dying skin forming a passive barrier to diffusion is now replaced by a model of the stratum corneum as a highly differentiated structure with unique properties that are particularly suited for its role in forming the skin barrier.[29]

APPENDAGES

Appendages penetrate stratum corneum and epidermis, facilitating thermal control and providing a protective covering. Appendages are potential sites of discontinuity in the integrity of the skin barrier. The density of the hair follicles varies on different body sites. Hair follicles represent a reservoir that may store topically applied substances. A detailed analysis of the reservoir of the hair follicles showed that the highest reservoir is on the scalp followed by the forehead and the calf.[30] On the forehead, there are a high number of small follicles; the calf contains fewer but larger hair follicles. These reservoirs are comparable to the reservoir of the stratum corneum on these body sites. The percentage of the hair follicles on the total skin surface varies between 0.2% and 1.3%, depending on body site.[30] Differences in the follicular penetration were observed in different ethnic groups.[31] Hair follicles present an important pathway for percutaneous absorption in nondiseased skin.[26,32] This can be explained by the fact that only the upper wall of the follicular apparatus (the acroinfundibulum) is protected by a coherent stratum corneum, but in the lower part (infrainfundibulum), the corneocytes appear undifferentiated, and protection is incomplete, if not absent. Even solid particles may enter deep into the follicular orifice,[17,27,33] a phenomenon that lends itself to the concept of follicular targeting of drugs.[27]

It follows that in relationship to the integral protection against the passage of xenobiotics in general, and drugs specifically, the barrier function of the interfollicular stratum corneum is even more potent than previously believed, but more research is needed relative to the follicular pathway. Recent investigations hint to the presence of active follicles (open to penetration) and passive ones.[18]

PENETRATION PATHWAYS

In principle, three penetration pathways are possible: (1) intercellular penetration, inside the lipid layers around the corneocytes; (2) follicular penetration; and (3) intracellular penetration. Although in the past, the transcorneal penetration was assumed to be the only penetration pathway, recent investigations, as cited earlier in section "Appendages", demonstrate that penetration via the hair follicles should be taken into consideration.[30,31]

Up to the present time, no evidence is available that topically applied substances pass the skin barriers by means of the intracellular route.

Pathways Across the Stratum Corneum: Studies have directly visualized penetration pathways across the stratum corneum by electron microscopy. For example, osmium vapor can be used to precipitate n-butanol that has penetrated stratum corneum.[34] After a brief (5 to 60 s) exposure of murine or human stratum corneum, the alcohol was found to be enriched in the intercellular spaces (threefold), although significant levels were also found in the corneocytes. By using a different approach that involved rapid freezing, water, ethanol, and cholesterol were also found preferentially concentrated in the intercellular lipid spaces.[35] Similarly, the penetration of mercury chloride through the intercellular lipid can be detected after precipitation with ammonium sulfide vapor.

However, in most of these investigations, there was also significant localization of compounds in the corneocytes, more prevalent in the upper layers (stratum disjunctum). Thus, corneocytes undergoing desquamation appear to be relatively permeable, even to rather bulky ions such as mercury. There is additional evidence that other compounds can and do penetrate corneocytes. It is well established, for example, that occlusion or immersion of skin in a bath leads to swelling of the corneocytes, consistent with the entry of water. Other compounds have also been localized in corneocytes, such as the anionic surfactants that are bound to keratins. Low-molecular-weight moisturizers such as glycerol are likely to partition into the corneocytes and alter their water-binding capacity. Thus, the penetration of compounds into corneocytes cannot be excluded from considerations of percutaneous absorption pathways. Relevance of this step relates to whether it is rate determining (ie, whether the diffusion of compounds within the intercellular lipid is restricted by the corneocytes).

Pathways Across Hair Follicles: Using the method of differential stripping—a combination of tape stripping with cyanoacrylate surface biopsies—the amount of formulation stored in the hair follicles can be quantified.[36] Nanoparticles are stored 10 times longer in hair follicles than in the stratum corneum.[20] Note that when topically applied substances penetrate into hair follicles, they do not necessarily penetrate through the skin barrier into the living tissue because hair follicles also have barrier properties.

On the other hand, the particles can be used as efficient carrier systems for drug delivery into hair follicles. The hair follicles represent an important target structure because they are surrounded by a close network of blood capillaries. Additionally, they host stem and dendritic cells, which are important for regenerative medicine and immunomodulation.

For optimal action, drug should be released from the particles after having penetrated deep into the hair follicles. The pharmacokinetics is determined mainly by the process of the drug release from the particles in this case.

There have been attempts to detect follicular penetration.[37-39] Experiments were performed on animal and human skin, with different densities of the hair follicles. Unfortunately, in all cases, the properties of the stratum corneum had also changed.

Analysis of follicular penetration became possible after the development of a method that artificially closes the hair follicles in vivo.[40] Using this method, it was demonstrated that the small molecules, such as caffeine, may penetrate through the skin barrier not only by the transcorneal but also by follicular routes.[41]

INTER- AND INTRAINDIVIDUAL VARIATION IN SKIN BARRIER FUNCTION

Finally, it is worthwhile to consider the level of inter- and intraindividual variation in skin barrier activity, including that of follicles. An accurate and reproducible measurement of skin barrier activity is transepidermal water loss.[42] The extent of variation of this parameter for the same individual is estimated to be 8% by site and 21% according to the day of measurement. Variations among individuals are reported to be somewhat larger, ranging from 35% to 48%.[43] There appear to be no significant gender- or ethnic-dependent differences in skin barrier activity. Skin barrier activity of premature babies[44] is markedly impaired, although skin barrier function appears normal for full-term infants. Differences in skin barrier activity among different sites have been observed; barrier function can be ranked as arm ~ abdomen > postauricular > forehead.[42]

VIABLE TISSUE

Although the primary barrier to percutaneous absorption lies within the stratum corneum, diffusion within the viable tissue, as well as metabolism and resorption, also influence the bioavailability of compounds in specific skin compartments. These processes are interrelated, and factors that increase the rate of one of these processes inevitably influence the others. Because the development of dermatologic formulations is often focused on "targeted" delivery to living tissues, manipulation of these processes offers a clear-cut rationale for increasing the therapeutic efficacy of dermatologic drugs.

The passage of compounds from the stratum corneum into the viable epidermis results in a substantial dilution. This is not only the relatively larger volume of the epidermis compared with that of the stratum corneum but also the lower resistance to diffusion within viable tissues, approximately corresponding to that of an aqueous protein gel.[43] Drug concentrations of 10^{-4} to

10^{-6} M may be attained in the epidermis and dermis for substances that permeate readily. Although the actual concentration gradient of a compound is affected by the physicochemical properties of the compounds as well as by the duration of application, a concentration gradient is present at all times. In other words, strategies to enhance percutaneous absorption generally result in a relatively uniform and parallel increase in the concentration of compounds in all compartments.

SKIN METABOLISM

Skin contains a wide range of enzymatic activities, including phase I oxidative, reductive, hydrolytic, and phase II conjugation reactions, as well as a full complement of drug-metabolizing enzymes.[45,46] Metabolic activity is a primary consideration in the design of prodrugs and may influence the bioavailability of drugs delivered via dermatologic or transdermal formulations. Alterations in skin metabolism have been implicated in a range of diseases, including hirsutism and acne, and they may be relevant to the risk of topical exposure to carcinogens. Metabolic processing of antigens by Langerhans cells is involved in the presentation of allergens to the immune system. Thus, metabolism in skin compartments plays a significant role in determining the fate of a topically applied active compound.

A variety of compounds of differing physicochemical properties—including estrone, estradiol, and estriol, as well as glucocorticoids, prostaglandins, retinoids, benzoyl peroxide, aldrin, anthralin, 5-fluorouracil, nitroglycerin, theophylline, and propranolol—are metabolized in the skin.[47] Arylamine-type hair dye ingredients are also subject to metabolism in human and animal skin, resulting in N-acetylated metabolites.[48-50] The enzyme responsible is believed to be epidermal N-acetyltransferase-1.[48] For example, cutaneous metabolism reduces the systemic bioavailability of nitroglycerin administered in a transdermal drug formulation in rhesus monkeys by 16% to 21% and hydrolyzes virtually 100% of a salicylate diester.[51] It is convenient to classify metabolic reactions in terms of their cofactor dependence.[52] Processes that require cofactors are likely to be energy dependent, and these are located within viable tissues. Among the best-studied examples are the interconversion of steroids (eg, estrone and estradiol) and oxidation of polycyclic aromatic hydrocarbons with mixed-function monooxygenases. In contrast, cofactor-independent processes involve catabolism and may be located outside of viable tissues (ie, in the transition region between the stratum corneum and stratum granulosum). The best characterized of these involve hydrolytic reactions such as nonspecific ester hydrolysis.

Metabolic activity is found in (1) skin-surface microorganisms, (2) appendages, (3) stratum corneum, (4) viable epidermis, and (5) dermis. In considering the site of the most significant metabolism, one has to consider the relevant enzymes and their specific activity, as well as their capacity relative to the size of the compartment.

Thus, although the level of many enzymes is highest in the epidermis, the relatively large size of the dermal compartment may result in a significant role in the metabolism of topically applied substances. A further consideration is that enzymes involved in cutaneous metabolism may be induced upon exposure to xenobiotics. This has been well described for various mixed-function monooxygenases.[53] Finally, the qualitative and quantitative extrapolation of results from animal models to humans is uncertain, owing to the significant species differences in the metabolism of compounds.

Percutaneous absorption and metabolism of compounds can be viewed as two events in kinetic competition with each other. Generally, compounds that remain in the skin for longer periods of time undergo significantly more metabolism. Furthermore, the type of metabolism of a substance may also be influenced by the nature of its formulation, as illustrated by investigations on the metabolism of several transdermal nitroglycerin formulations.[54] The inclusion of enhancers in the formulation not only increased the bioavailability of the nitroglycerin but also the ratio of one metabolic compound (1,2-glyceryl dinitrate) in relation to another (1,3-glyceryl dinitrate). This may limit suitability of in vitro experiments for estimating the significance of cutaneous metabolism because the vasculature is not functional in vitro. It is difficult to extrapolate quantitatively the level of metabolism obtained for different formulations. This has significant implications for the estimation of bioequivalence.

However, despite the variety of skin-associated metabolic processes, the extent of metabolism is normally modest (ie, 2% to 5% of the absorbed compounds), although for N-acetylation of arylamines, metabolism may be quantitative.[50] Metabolism is limited not only by the relatively short period that a compound spends in the viable layers of the skin but also by the overall low level of enzyme activity. Thus, under many circumstances, the available enzymes are saturated by the level of compound undergoing percutaneous absorption.[45]

RESORPTION

Resorption, defined as the uptake of compounds by the cutaneous microvasculature, is directly related to the surface area of the exchanging capillaries as well as their blood flow. Total blood flow to the skin may vary up to 100-fold, a process primarily regulated by vascular shunts, but also by recruitment of new capillary beds. It is estimated that under resting conditions, only 40% of the blood flow passes via exchanging capillaries capable of acting as a sink for absorbed compounds. However, this value demonstrates considerable variation among body sites, individuals, and species and is influenced by disease states and environmental conditions. In particular, changes in temperature and humidity as well as the presence of vasoactive compounds may directly influence skin blood flow.[55]

For most compounds and situations, resorption does

not change the rate of diffusion to the central compartment after topical applications. This is a result of the relatively high resistance to diffusion within the stratum corneum compared with uptake by the vasculature. However, for compounds or situations in which diffusion across the stratum corneum is rapid, resorption limits the maximum rate of absorption.[55] Evidence that resorption can limit the delivery of compounds to the central compartment comes primarily from studies that examined the influence of blood flow on this process. The percutaneous absorption of methyl salicylate is increased by elevated ambient temperature or strenuous exercise, an observation consistent with increased resorption as a result of cutaneous blood flow.[56] Moreover, intravenously administered nicotine (a vasoconstrictor) reduces the percutaneous absorption of topically applied nicotine.[50] Regional differences in the percutaneous absorption of piroxicam, a nonsteroidal antiinflammatory drug, depend on the local vasculature rather than on skin barrier function.[57]

An additional consideration is that the rate of resorption may indirectly influence the diffusion of compounds to the underlying musculature, tissues, and joints.[58] The principle of locally enhanced delivery to underlying musculature has been demonstrated for piroxicam as well as several local anesthetic preparations.[59]

INFLUENCE OF PATHOLOGIC PROCESSES ON SKIN BARRIER FUNCTION

Reduced skin barrier function has been observed in pathologic conditions, including the ichthyoses,[60] psoriasis,[27] atopic dermatitis,[61] and contact dermatitis.[61] It is generally accepted that this is attributable to structural alterations in the stratum corneum. These structural deficiencies may arise from an absence of an enzyme or structural protein in the underlying viable tissues or may be related to the improper formation of the stratum corneum resulting from an increase in keratinocyte proliferation. Thus, in individuals predisposed to a defective barrier, a minor perturbation may become amplified as the skin "attempts to compensate" by increasing keratinocyte proliferation.[62] A further consideration is that the homeostatic mechanisms responsible for recovery of barrier activity after perturbation may be altered in some diseases or physiologic states.

For example, whereas the skin of aged people exhibits normal barrier function, the recovery of barrier activity after perturbation is markedly reduced.[63] This kinetic basis for reduced barrier function may also account for interindividual variation in barrier function or the apparently increased susceptibility of certain individuals to contact dermatitis.[64]

OTHER FACTORS THAT AFFECT ABSORPTION

STRATUM CORNEUM

Stratum corneum, the rate-limiting barrier to percutaneous drug delivery, is composed of ceramides, free fatty acids, and cholesterol in a 1:1:1 molar ratio. By weight, the stratum corneum consists of 50% ceramides (acylceramides being the most abundant), 35% cholesterol, and 15% free fatty acids. Stratum corneum thickness and thus drug penetration vary depending on body site (Fig. 183-2).[65]

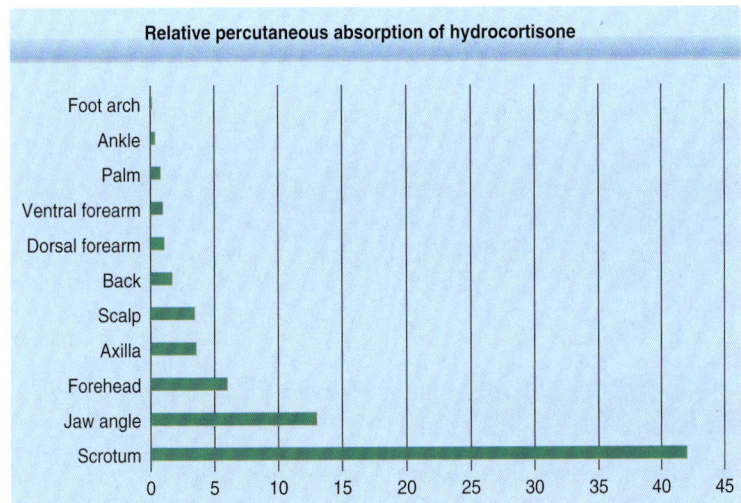

Figure 183-2 Relative percutaneous absorption of hydrocortisone. Regional variation was measured in males using carbon[14]-labeled hydrocortisone dissolved in acetone solvent. Values depicted are relative to the percutaneous absorption of topical applied to the ventral forearm. (Adapted from Feldman RJ, Maibach HI. Regional variation in percutaneous penetration of 14C cortisol in man. *J Invest Dermatol*. 1967;48(2):181-83.)

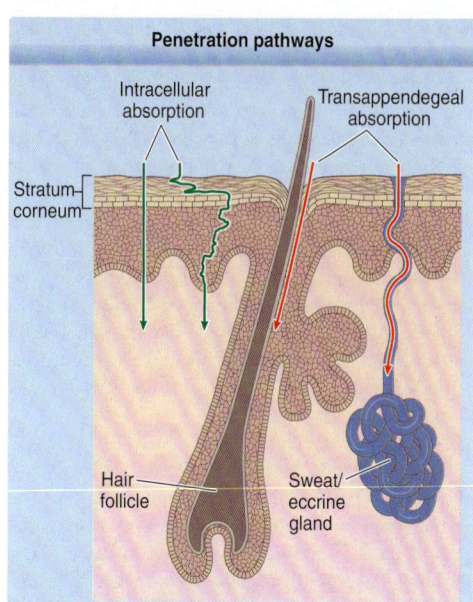

Figure 183-3 Penetration pathways.

There are two main routes for permeation through the stratum corneum: the (1) transepidermal and (2) transappendageal pathways (Fig. 183-3). The transappendageal, or shunt, route involves the flow of molecules through eccrine glands and hair follicles via the associated sebaceous glands.[66] In the transepidermal route, molecules pass between the corneocytes via the intercellular micropathway or through the cytoplasm of dead keratinocytes and intercellular lipids, defined as the *transcellular micropathway*.[66,67] The intercellular pathway is considered the most important route for cutaneous drug delivery.

An important consideration in topical therapy is that diseased skin may have an altered (increased, decreased, or absent) stratum corneum, thus changing the body site's barrier function.[68] Abraded or eczematized skin presents less of a barrier. Solvents, surfactants, and alcohols can denature the cornified layer and increase penetration; as a result, topical medications with these components may enhance absorption.[69] Importantly, simple hydration of the stratum corneum enhances the absorption of topically applied steroids by four to five times.[10] Abnormal epidermal proliferation disrupts the skin barrier architecture, enhancing percutaneous absorption.

OCCLUSION

Occlusion via closed, airtight dressings or greasy ointment bases increases stratum corneum hydration; limits rub-off and wash-off of the drug; and, consequently, enhances penetration. Occlusion techniques range from application under an airtight dressing such as vinyl gloves, plastic wrap, and hydrocolloid dressings to occlusion at night for treatment of hands and feet, to application of a medication already impregnated into an airtight dressing, as seen in flurandrenolide tape. With many drugs, occlusion increases drug delivery by 10 times the amount of drug delivered when not occluded.[70] This approach can lead to more rapid onset times and increased efficacy when compared with topical application alone. On the other hand, occlusion may also lead to a more rapid appearance of the drug's adverse effects, such as the ability of topical corticosteroids to induce local skin atrophy or suppression of the hypothalamus–pituitary–adrenal axis. Occlusion may promote infection, folliculitis, or miliaria. In the case of topical anesthetics such as lidocaine and prilocaine, occlusion hastens absorption into both the skin and the bloodstream, which has led in rare cases to cardiac complications from lidocaine toxicity or methemoglobinemia from prilocaine toxicity.

APPLICATION FREQUENCY

The frequency of topical application for some drugs, such as corticosteroids, appear to saturate the stratum corneum so that multiple daily application yields minimum penetration increases compared with once-daily application.[71,72] Clinical studies support the same conclusion, so many topical package inserts are labeled for once-daily use.

QUANTITY OF APPLICATION

The quantity of the drug applied likely has a negligible effect on drug absorption. Obviously, enough drug must be dispensed and spread to cover the affected areas. Furthermore, the quantity of drug applied might affect patient adherence to the prescribed regimen. For example, too much applied drug might negatively alter the subjective experience of having a medication on the skin, that is, the drug may feel "wrong" (greasy, caked, chalky, and so on) or is cosmetically unattractive (shiny, white color). Regardless, the amount prescribed must be adequate to treat the affected body surface area (BSA) for the necessary length of time. In this regard, patient education is critical to prevent wasteful overuse or ineffective underuse of the medication. The amounts of topical medications to dispense is based on the estimated BSA, frequency of application, and duration of therapy. For topical medications such as sunscreens that are used over large areas, underapplication is a problem for most patients. However, for smaller areas, patients may apply a large amount of an ointment, for example, leading to complaints of greasiness or rubbing off on clothing, which can be minimized by using an appropriate amount. The finger-tip unit (FTU) is a measurement that allows health care providers and patients to easily communicate about treatment application. An FTU is the amount of topical dispensed from a 5-mm-diameter nozzle onto the tip of the palmar aspect of the index finger to the distal interphalangeal joint skin crease. One FTU is equivalent to approximately 500 mg of the topical agent, which can cover about 2% of the BSA.

MISCELLANEOUS FACTORS

Vigorous rubbing or massaging of the drug into the skin not only increases the surface area of skin covered but also increases blood supply to the area locally, augmenting systemic absorption. It may cause a local exfoliative effect that also enhances penetration. The presence of hair follicles on a particular body site also enhances drug delivery, with the scalp and beard areas presenting less of a barrier compared with the relatively hairless body sites.

Reducing the particle size of the active ingredient increases its surface area–volume ratio, allowing for a greater solubility of the drug in its vehicle. This forms the basis for the increased absorption of certain micronized drugs.[73]

CLASSIFICATION AND CLINICAL APPLICATION OF TOPICAL FORMULATIONS

The vehicle is the inactive part of a topical preparation that brings a drug into contact with the skin. Before the mid-1970s, pharmaceutical companies performed limited testing of the impact of vehicle on the potency of a given formulation. Lack of a scientific analysis of the vehicle led to the marketing of topical drugs that, although having different concentrations of the same active ingredient, nevertheless exhibited similar bioavailability and potency. For example, older preparations of triamcinolone acetonide showed no real differences in potency among the 0.025%, 0.1%, and 0.5% concentrations. By contrast, modern drug development attempts to maximize drug bioavailability by optimizing vehicle formulation. Additionally, during the current drug development process, dose–response studies determine the maximal effective concentration within a given vehicle, above which any further increase in concentration serves no therapeutic benefit.

Vehicle of a topical formulation often has beneficial nonspecific effects by possessing cooling, protective, emollient, occlusive, or astringent properties. Rational topical therapy matches an appropriate vehicle that contains an effective concentration of the drug. The vehicle functions optimally when it is stable both chemically and physically and does not inactivate the drug. The vehicle also should be nonirritating, nonallergenic, cosmetically acceptable, and easy to use. Additionally, the vehicle must release the drug into the pharmacologically important compartment of the skin. Finally, the patient must accept using the vehicle or else compliance will be poor. For example, although ointments are often pharmacodynamically more effective than creams, patients generally prefer creams to ointments, and thus, more prescriptions are written for cream-based formulations. Table 183-3 lists many commonly used ingredients in topical preparations. Many of these compounds serve more than one function in a particular formulation.

TOPICAL FORMULATIONS

See Table 183-4.

POWDERS

Powders absorb moisture and decrease friction. Because they adhere poorly to skin, their use is mainly limited to cosmetic and hygienic purposes. Generally, powders are used in the intertriginous areas and on the feet. Adverse effects of powders include caking (especially if used on weeping skin), crusting, irritation, and granuloma formation. Furthermore, powders may be inhaled by the user. Most powders contain zinc oxide for antiseptic and covering properties, talc (primarily composed of magnesium silicate) for lubricating and drying properties, and a stearate for improved adherence to the skin. Calamine is a popular skin-colored powder composed of 98% zinc oxide and 1% ferric oxide and acts as an astringent to relieve pruritus. Other drugs formulated as powders include some over-the-counter antifungals.[73]

POULTICES

A poultice, also referred to as a *cataplasm*, is a wet solid mass of particles, sometimes heated, that is applied to diseased skin. Historically, poultices contained meal, herbs, plants, and seeds. The modern poultice often consists of porous beads of dextranomer. Poultices are used as wound cleansers and absorptive agents in exudative lesions such as decubiti and leg ulcers.[73]

OINTMENTS

Ointments, semisolid preparations that spread easily, are petrolatum-based vehicles capable of providing occlusion, hydration, and lubrication. Drug potency often is increased by an ointment vehicle because of its ability to enhance permeability.[5] Ointment bases used in dermatology can be classified into five categories: (1) hydrocarbon bases, (2) absorption bases, (3) emulsions of water-in-oil, (4) emulsions of oil-in-water, and (5) water-soluble bases. Dermatologists commonly refer to the hydrocarbon bases and absorption bases as

TABLE 183-3
Vehicle Ingredients Commonly Used In Topical Preparations

Emulsifying Agents
- Cholesterol
- Disodium mono-oleamidosulfosuccinate
- Emulsifying wax
- Polyoxyl 40 stearate
- Polysorbates
- Sodium laureth sulfate
- Sodium lauryl sulfate

Auxiliary Emulsifying Agents or Emulsion Stabilizers
- Carbomer
- Catearyl alcohol
- Cetyl alcohol
- Glyceryl monostearate
- Lanolin and lanolin derivatives
- Polyethylene glycol
- Stearyl alcohol

Stabilizers
- Benzyl alcohol
- Butylated hydroxyanisole
- Butylated hydroxytoluene
- Chlorocresol
- Citric acid
- Edetate disodium
- Glycerin
- Parabens
- Propyl gallate
- Propylene glycol
- Sodium bisulfite
- Sorbic acid or potassium sorbate

Solvents
- Alcohol
- Diisopropyl adipate
- Glycerin
- 1,2,6-Hexanetriol
- Isopropyl myristate
- Propylene carbonate
- Propylene glycol
- Water

Thickening Agents
- Beeswax
- Carbomer
- Petrolatum
- Polyethylene
- Xanthan gum

Emollients
- Caprylic or capric triglycerides
- Cetyl alcohol
- Glycerin
- Isopropyl myristate
- Isopropyl palmitate
- Lanolin and lanolin derivatives
- Mineral oil
- Petrolatum
- Squalene
- Stearic acid
- Stearyl alcohol

Humectants
- Glycerin
- Propylene glycol
- Sorbitol solution

ointments and the water-in-oil and oil-in-water emulsion bases as *creams*. In pharmaceutical terms, all of these preparations are ointments and are specifically indicated for conditions affecting the glabrous skin (palms and soles) and lichenified areas.[10]

HYDROCARBON BASES

Also called *oleaginous bases*, hydrocarbon bases are often referred to as *emollients* because they prevent the evaporation of moisture from skin, are composed of a mixture of hydrocarbons of varying molecular weights, with petrolatum being the most commonly used (white petrolatum, except for being bleached, is identical to yellow petrolatum). They are greasy and can stain clothing. Silicon ointments are composed of alternating oxygen and silicon atoms bonded to organic groups, such as phenyl or methyl, and are excellent skin protectants. They can be used for diaper rash, incontinence, bedsores, and colostomy sites. Hydrocarbon bases are generally stable and do not contain preservatives. They cannot absorb aqueous solutions and thus are not used for water-soluble drugs.[73]

ABSORPTION BASES

Absorption bases contain hydrophilic substances that allow for the absorption of water-soluble drugs. The hydrophilic (polar) compounds may include lanolin and its derivatives, cholesterol and its derivatives, and partial esters of polyhydric alcohols such as sorbitan monostearate. These ointments are lubricating and hydrophilic, and they can form emulsions. They function well as emollients and protectants. They are greasy to apply but are easier to remove than hydrocarbon bases. They do not contain water. Examples include anhydrous lanolin and hydrophilic petrolatum.[73]

WATER-IN-OIL EMULSIONS (CREAMS)

Emulsions are two-phase systems involving one or more immiscible liquids dispersed in another, with the assistance of one or more emulsifying agents. A water-in-oil emulsion, by definition, contains less than 25% water, with oil being the dispersion medium. The two phases may separate unless shaken. The emulsifier (or surfactant) is soluble in both phases and surrounds the dispersed drops to prevent their coalescence. Examples of surfactants used include sodium lauryl sulfate, quaternary ammonium compounds, Spans (sorbitan fatty acid esters), and Tweens (polyoxyethylene sorbitan fatty acid esters). Preservatives are frequently added to increase emulsion's shelf life. Water-in-oil emulsions are less greasy, spread easily on the skin, and provide a protective film of oil that remains on the skin as an emollient, and the slow evaporation of the water phase provides a cooling effect.[5]

TABLE 183-4
Summary of Topical Formulations

FORMULATION	COMMON COMPONENTS	DESCRIPTION
Powders	Zinc oxide, talc (magnesium silicate)	Cosmetic, hygienic purposes; ideal for intertriginous areas and feet
Poultice	Dextranomer beads	Wound cleansers, absorptive agents; applied on decubiti or leg ulcers
Ointments		
Hydrocarbon base (ointments; oleaginous bases; emollients)	Petrolatum most commonly used Silicon ointments	Prevent evaporation of moisture from the skin; contain no preservatives; not for water-soluble drug use; ideal for diaper rash, incontinence, bedsores, colostomy sites
Absorption base	Lanolin and lanolin derivatives Cholesterol and cholesterol derivatives Sorbitan monostearate	Lubricating and hydrophilic substances; can form emulsions; emollients and protectants; easier to remove than hydrocarbon bases
Emulsions (water in oil; <25% water) (creams)	Sodium lauryl sulfate, quaternary ammonium compounds, spans, tweens	Less greasy; easy to spread on film; provide a protective film of oil as an emollient with a cooling effect
Emulsions (oil in water; >31% water) (creams)	Glycerin, propylene glycol, PEG, paraffin alcohols	Most commonly used to deliver a drug; easily spread, water washable and less greasy; easily removed from the skin; preservative containing (parabens)
Water-soluble bases	PEGs (liquid or solid)	No preservatives or additives; less occlusive, nonstaining, greaseless, easily washed off from the skin; poor absorption into the skin but maintains a high surface concentration; ideal for topical antifungals and topical antibiotics
Gels	Water, propylene glycol, PEGS with a cellulose derivative or Carbopol	Organic molecules uniformly distributed in a lattice throughout the liquid; deposits drug in concentrated form; ideal for use in facial or hair bearing areas; lack protective or emollient effects; may cause drying or stinging
Pastes (up to 50% powder in ointment base)	Zinc oxide, starch, calcium carbonate, talc	Less greasy than ointments; more drying and less occlusive; used as protectants, sunblocks, or for localizing a drug that may be staining or irritating
Liquids		
Solutions	Liquid vehicle may be aqueous, hydroalcoholic, or nonaqueous - Tincture: hydroalcoholic solution with 50% alcohol; collodion: nonaqueous solution of pyroxylin with ether and ethanol - Liniments: nonaqueous solutions or drugs in oil or alcoholic soap solutions	Function as astringents, counterirritants, antipruritics, emollients
Suspensions	Biphasic solution: insoluble drug in up to 20% concentration dispersed in liquid	Cooling effect; easier to apply and allows for uniform coating of larger affected areas; more drying than ointments
Shake lotions	Solutions with added powder; zinc oxide, talc, calamine, glycerol, alcohol, and water	Used to dry and cool wet and weeping skin
Foams	Triphasic solution with oil, organic solvents, and water, formulated with a hydrocarbon propellant	Deliver a greater amount of drug at an increased rate; especially useful for scalp application
Aerosols	Drug in a solution mixed with a pure propellant (nonpolar hydrocarbons)	Deliver drugs formulated as solutions, suspensions, emulsions, powders, and semisolids; ease of application to hair-bearing areas

PEG, polyethylene glycol.

OIL-IN-WATER EMULSIONS

An oil-in-water emulsion contains greater than 31% water. In fact, the aqueous phase may constitute up to 80% of the formulation. This type of formulation is most commonly chosen to deliver a dermatologic drug. Clinically, oil-in-water emulsions spread easily, are water washable and less greasy, and are easily removed from the skin and clothing. Invariably, they contain preservatives, such as the parabens, to inhibit mold growth. Additionally, oil-in-water emulsions contain a humectant (an agent that draws moisture into the skin), such as glycerin, propylene glycol, or polyethylene glycol (PEG), to prevent the cream from drying out. The oil phase may contain either cetyl or stearyl alcohol (paraffin alcohols) to impart a stability and velvety smooth feel upon application to the skin. After application, the aqueous phase evaporates, leaving behind a small hydrating oil layer and a concentrated drug deposit.[73]

WATER-SOLUBLE BASES

Water-soluble bases consist either primarily or completely of various PEGs. Depending on their molecular weight, PEGs are either liquid (PEG 400) or solid (PEG 4000). These formulations are water soluble, do not decompose, and do not support mold growth and therefore require no preservative additives. They are much less occlusive than water-in-oil emulsions and are nonstaining, greaseless, and easily washed off of the skin. Without water, the ointment poorly delivers its coformulated drug. Therefore, it is useful in scenarios when the practitioner desires a high surface concentration and low percutaneous absorption of drug. For example, topical antifungal drugs and topical antibiotics (eg, mupirocin) are formulated in this base.

Gels are made from water-soluble bases by formulating water, propylene glycol, and/or PEGs with a cellulose derivative or Carbopol. A gel consists of organic macromolecules uniformly distributed in a lattice throughout the liquid. After application, the aqueous or alcoholic component evaporates, and the drug is deposited in a concentrated form. This provides a faster release of the drug independent of its water solubility. Gels are popular because of their clarity and ease of both application and removal. They are suitable for facial or hairy areas because after application, little residue remains.[10] Nevertheless, they lack protective or emollient properties. If they contain high concentrations of alcohol or propylene glycol, they tend to be drying or cause stinging. Gels require preservatives.[12] Newer gel formulations may contain the humectant glycerin, the emollient dimethicone, or the viscoelastic polysaccharide hyaluronic acid, which can mitigate some of the associated irritation. Nonaqueous gels, with bases such as glycerol, may be used for poorly solubilized therapeutics such as 5-aminolevulonic acid.[74]

Microspheres, or microsponges, are formulated in an aqueous gel. Medication, in this case tretinoin, is combined into porous beads 10 to 25 μm in diameter. The beads are made up of methyl methacrylate and glycol dimethacrylate.

PASTES

Pastes are simply the incorporation of high concentrations of powders (up to 50%) into an ointment such as a hydrocarbon base or a water-in-oil emulsion. The powder must be insoluble in the ointment. Invariably, they are "stiffer" than the original ointment. Powders commonly used are zinc oxide, starch, calcium carbonate, and talc. Pastes function to localize the effect of a drug that may be staining or irritating (ie, anthralin). They also function as impermeable barriers that serve as protectants or sunblocks. Pastes are less greasy than ointments, more drying, and less occlusive.[73]

LIQUIDS

Liquids can be subdivided into solutions, suspensions, emulsions (discussed in section "Ointments"), and foams.

SOLUTIONS

A solution involves the dissolution of two or more substances into homogenous clarity. The liquid vehicle may be aqueous, hydroalcoholic, or nonaqueous (alcohol, oils, or propylene glycol). An example of an aqueous solution is aluminum acetate or Burow solution. A hydroalcoholic solution with a concentration of alcohol of approximately 50% is called a *tincture*. A collodion is a nonaqueous solution of pyroxylin in a mixture with ether and ethanol and is applied to the skin with a soft brush. Flexible collodions have added castor oil and camphor and are used, for example, to deliver 10% salicylic acid as a keratolytic agent. Liniments are nonaqueous solutions of drugs in oil or alcoholic solutions of soap. The base of oil or soap facilitates application to the skin with rubbing or massage. Liniments can be used as counterirritants, astringents, antipruritics, emollients, and analgesics.[73]

SUSPENSIONS (LOTIONS)

A suspension, or lotion, is a two-phase system consisting of a finely divided, insoluble drug dispersed into a liquid in a concentration of up to 20%. Nonuniform dosing can result if the suspended particles coalesce and separate out of a homogeneous mixture, therefore shaking of the lotion before application may be required. Examples include calamine lotion, steroid lotions, and emollients containing urea or lactic acid. The applied lotion leaves skin feeling cooler via evaporation of the aqueous component. Lotions are easier to apply and allow for uniform coating of the affected area and are often the favorite preparation in treating children. Lotions are more drying than ointments, and preparations with alcohol tend to sting eczematized or abraded skin. Lotions are suitable for application to large surface areas because of their ability to spread easily.[73]

SHAKE LOTIONS

Shake lotions are lotions to which a powder is added to increase the surface area of evaporation. As a result of increased evaporation, application of shake lotions effectively dries and cools wet and weeping skin. Generally, shake lotions consist of zinc oxide, talc, calamine, glycerol, alcohol, and water, to which specific drugs and stabilizers may be added. Shake lotions tend to sediment and derive their name from the need to shake the preparation before each use to obtain a homogeneous suspension. In addition, after water has evaporated from the lotion, the powder component may clump together and become abrasive. Therefore, patients should be instructed to remove the residual particles before the reapplication of shake lotions.[73]

FOAMS

Foams are triphasic liquids composed of oil, organic solvents, and water, kept under pressure in aluminum cans. Foams are formulated with a hydrocarbon propellant, either butane or propane.[75] The foam lattice is formed when the valve is activated. When in contact with skin, the lattice breaks down, the alcohol evaporates within 30 seconds and leaves minimal residue in the skin. The alcohol component of the foam is thought to act as a penetration enhancer, momentarily altering the barrier properties of the stratum corneum and increasing drug delivery through the intercellular route.[75] Foam vehicles are highly effective in delivering greater amount of active drug at an increased rate compared with other vehicles that traditionally depend on hydration of the intercellular spaces within the stratum corneum. Foams have not been associated with an increase in the adverse events, and compliance seems to be better with this formulation, especially for localized conditions affecting the scalp.[75]

AEROSOLS

Topical aerosols may be used to deliver drugs formulated as solutions, suspensions, emulsions, powders, and semisolids. Aerosols involve formulating the drug in a solution within a pure propellant. Usually, the propellant is a blend of nonpolar hydrocarbons. When applied to abraded or eczematized skin, aerosols lack the irritation of other formulations, especially when the quality of the skin makes direct application painful or difficult. Furthermore, aerosols dispense a drug as a thin layer with minimal waste, and the unused portion cannot be contaminated. Aerosol foams, a relatively new vehicle for drug delivery, are commonly used to deliver corticosteroids such as betamethasone valerate and clobetasol propionate. The foam contains the drug within an emulsion formulated with a foaming agent (a surfactant), a solvent system (eg, water and ethanol), and a propellant. On application, a foam lattice forms transiently until it is broken by both the heat of the skin and the heat of rubbing the foam onto skin. Foams that are alcohol based leave little residue within seconds of application. Furthermore, a given corticosteroid formulated in a foam vehicle demonstrates comparable potency compared with the same corticosteroid in other vehicles.[11,76]

Although aerosols allow for the ease of application (especially to hair-bearing areas) and high patient satisfaction, they suffer from the disadvantages of being expensive and potentially ecologically damaging.[73]

LIPOSOMES AS TRANSDERMAL DELIVERY SYSTEMS

Liposomes are microscopic spheres consisting of a bilayer that encloses an inner aqueous core. A wide variety of cosmetics contain liposomes. Liposome-based formulations are safe, cosmetically attractive, and well accepted. There is considerable evidence that, at least for some preparations, application of liposomes is mildly occlusive and improves stratum corneum hydration. Interest in the use of liposomes to enhance the delivery of drugs across the skin has been spurred by observations in animal models: liposome formulations were believed to enhance the penetration of compounds across the skin or to optimize the retention of bioactive compounds in target tissues.[32] However, these early studies, which relied largely on animal models, were followed by relatively few in vivo studies for humans conducted under standard conditions.[69]

Action mechanism of liposomes is based on a partly damaged liquid layer of the stratum corneum, so that the liposomes can penetrate efficiently into the skin barrier. Deep in the stratum corneum, the liposomes get damaged and release their drug, which has to pass through the last cell layers of the stratum corneum by itself to reach the living cells.

There is no clear evidence that liposomes can pass the skin barrier as intact structures, but intact liposomes can penetrate along the hair shaft, and this route may be appropriate for delivery of bioactive compounds into sebaceous glands or hair follicles.[16,66] Rigid liposomes penetrate better into the hair follicles than flexible liposomes, which supports the assumption that the moving hairs act as a geared pump.[52,66]

PENETRATION ENHANCERS

CHEMICAL ENHANCERS

A penetration enhancer is a compound that is able to promote drug transport through skin. Skin hydration and interaction with the polar head group of the lipids are mechanisms for increasing penetration. Water, alcohols (mainly ethanol), sulphoxides (dimethylsulphoxide), decylmethylsulphoxide, azones (laurocapram), and urea are some commonly used compounds.[67] Urea is thought to act as a penetration enhancer because of its keratolytic properties and by increasing the water content in the stratum corneum. Other substances that may also act as enhancers include propylene glycol, surfactants, fatty acids, and esters.[69]

Vesicular systems are widely used in dermatologic and cosmetic fields to enhance drug transport into the skin through the transcellular and follicular pathways. Examples of vesicular systems include liposomes (phospholipid-based vesicles), niosomes (nonionic surfactant vesicles), proliposomes, and proniosomes, which, respectively, are converted to liposomes and niosomes upon hydration.[77]

PHYSICAL ENHANCERS

Physical methods such as the application of a small electric current (iontophoresis), ultrasound energy (phono- or sonophoresis), and the use of microneedles increase cutaneous drug penetration.[67] Microdermoabrasion is the application of crystals (generally aluminum oxide) on the skin and the collection of such crystals and skin debris under vacuum suction. This technique enhances drug permeation and facilitates drug absorption by altering the architecture of the stratum corneum.[78]

STABILIZERS

Stabilizers are nontherapeutic ingredients and include the preservatives, antioxidants, and chelating agents. Preservatives protect the formulation from microbial growth. The ideal preservative is effective at a low concentration against a broad spectrum of organisms, nonsensitizing, odor free, color free, stable, and inexpensive. Unfortunately, the ideal preservative does not exist. The parabens are the most frequently added preservatives and are active against molds, fungi, and yeasts but less effective against bacteria. Alternative agents include the halogenated phenols, benzoic acid, sodium benzoate, formaldehyde-releasing agents, and previously, thimerosal. Most commonly used preservatives may act as contact sensitizers.

Antioxidants or preservatives prevent the drug or vehicle from degrading via oxidation. Examples include butylated hydroxyanisole and butylated hydroxytoluene, used in oils and fats. Ascorbic acid, sulfites, and sulfur-containing amino acids are used in water-soluble phases. Chelating agents, such as sodium EDTA (ethylenediaminetetraacetic acid) and citric acid, work synergistically with antioxidants by complexing heavy metals in aqueous phases.

THICKENING AGENTS

Thickening agents increase the viscosity of products or suspend ingredients in a formulation. Examples include beeswax and carbomers. In addition to functioning as an ointment vehicle, petrolatum may be added to an emulsion to increase its viscosity. As in this example, an ingredient may have a therapeutic effect as well as acting as part of a vehicle.

SIDE EFFECTS AND PRECAUTIONS

LOCAL EFFECTS

Either the vehicle or its active ingredients may cause local toxicity to the applied site. Local adverse effects are usually minor and reversible. Major cutaneous side effects include irritation, allergenicity, atrophy, comedogenicity, formation of telangiectases, pruritus, stinging, and pain. The mechanism of toxicity may be as simple as the desiccation of the stratum corneum (eg, the removal of sebum and oils by the preparation's emulsifiers) or involve a more complex effect on either the cells of the epidermis or dermis and the structures these cells comprise (ie, epidermis, adnexae). Local damage may occur either directly at or within close proximity to the treated site. Furthermore, irritation and damage may appear even after a drug has been discontinued. Often the therapeutic effects of the active ingredient mask or immediately treat the toxic effects of the formulation so that acutely toxic effects are transient.[79] For example, allergic contact dermatitis to a preservative in a topical steroid may be masked by the effects of the glucocorticoid itself.

IRRITANT CONTACT DERMATITIS

Irritation is driven less by drug penetration and more by drug concentration. Thus, lowering the concentration of an irritating drug may lower the risk of side effects. However, a change in formulation may reduce the preparation's efficacy. Nevertheless, often using a less concentrated preparation over a greater period of time is as therapeutically efficacious while minimizing adverse effects (eg, the use of benzoyl peroxide 2% to 5% preparations in contrast to 10% preparations).[79] In some instances, though, skin irritancy might be central to drug efficacy. For example, although not conclusively shown, the power of immunomodulating agents such as imiquimod might rely on an increased innate (inflammatory or irritant) immune response.

SUBJECTIVE OR SENSORY IRRITANT CONTACT DERMATITIS

Patients may detect burning or stinging sensations without any signs of cutaneous irritation after applying a topical medication. Several compounds, such as tacrolimus, sorbic acid, propylene glycol, benzoyl peroxide hydroxy acids, mequinol, ethanol, lactic acid, azelaic acid, benzoic acid, and tretinoin, may induce sensory irritant contact dermatitis in predisposed individuals.[80,81]

ALLERGIC CONTACT DERMATITIS

Contact allergy development depends on local penetration. Allergy is driven by antigen recognition and presentation, so percutaneous absorption of the drug must be at a level that guarantees interaction with the immune effector cells of the skin. Therefore, the contact allergenicity of a drug relates significantly to percutaneous absorption. In some instances, cutaneous allergy may be therapeutic, for example, the treatment of patients with cutaneous T-cell lymphoma with topical nitrogen mustard. The shift in malignant T cells from T helper (Th) 2 to Th1-type cytokine expression is believed to lead to apoptosis of the malignant T cells and tumor regression.[82]

MALIGNANCIES

Rarely, topical therapy may result in neoplasia. For example, the risk of secondary malignancies, such as keratoacanthomas, basal and squamous cell carcinomas, lentigo maligna, and primary melanoma, have been reported with the long-term use of nitrogen mustard.[82]

OTHERS

The application of topical corticosteroids to the periorbital skin has been suggested to induce cataracts and increase intraocular pressure.[10]

SYSTEMIC EFFECTS

One should be aware of the potential systemic toxicities of topical drugs. Although generally safer than the other administration routes, topical application can result in systemic toxicities ranging from end-organ toxicity (central nervous system, cardiac, renal, and so on), teratogenicity, and carcinogenicity to drug interactions. These outcomes may relate to the drug itself, its metabolites, or even a component of the vehicle.

The kinetics of topically applied drugs differ significantly from those administered by other routes. An important consideration is the lack of hepatic first-pass metabolism of a topical drug. This is especially relevant to drugs such as salicylic acid that are relatively innocuous when given enterally but may manifest central nervous system toxicity when applied topically. Additionally, acting as a reservoir, the stratum corneum may store large amounts of a topical drug, and a subsequently long diffusion period of many days may ensue, delivering a steady supply of drug to the systemic circulation.

Percutaneous toxicity directly relates to percutaneous absorption. Therefore, factors that modulate absorption also influence toxicity: concentration of drug, its vehicle, use of occlusion, body site and area treated, frequency of use, duration of therapy, and nature of the diseased skin. For example, 6% salicylic acid in Eucerin used for 11 days in the treatment of psoriasis has been associated with epistaxis and deafness, and the same concentration of salicylic acid in hydrophilic cream under occlusion for 4 days for the treatment of dermatitis (involving the same amount of BSA) may result in hallucination.[79] Similar to their effect on systemically administered drugs, renal and hepatic diseases, by influencing drug clearance, also contribute to an increased potential for drug toxicity.

Infants and young children have a greater surface area–volume ratio and thus are at greater risk of percutaneous toxicity than adults. This phenomenon necessitates alternative drugs, formulations, and dosing schedules for children with widespread cutaneous disease. Patients with acute flares of cutaneous illness (eg, psoriasis or atopic dermatitis) may require treatment of a larger BSA in a relatively abbreviated period. These patients may also increase their dose and frequency of application during such flares. Coupled with the likely increased percutaneous absorption of the diseased skin, these scenarios exponentially increase the possibility of systemic toxicity, and patient education is vital to prevent adverse outcomes.[73] To reduce the risk of toxicity from topical drugs and to increase treatment efficacy, many practitioners will rationally advocate systemic approaches (ie, methotrexate, cyclosporine, injectable or infusable biologics, or ultraviolet radiotherapy) to patients whose disease involves an extensive BSA. Nonimmunologic acute toxicity results from substances such as pesticides and chemical warfare agents that rapidly diffuse through the skin and reach target organs.

IMMUNOLOGIC CONTACT URTICARIA

In rare instances, anaphylactic shock can be precipitated by topical drug application. For example, when applied to diseased or abraded skin, bacitracin ointment can induce an immediate-type (Type I) hypersensitivity reaction in susceptible individuals. Such reactions might be represented by a local and then subsequently generalized pruritus, leading to cardiopulmonary arrest.[73]

MALIGNANCIES

Systemic calcineurin inhibitors have been associated with increased risk of lymphoma and nonmelanoma skin cancer. But the topical use of such drugs does not yet appear to induce cancer.[83] In fact, the risk for lymphoma with the use of topical calcineurin inhibitors was assessed in animal studies that demonstrated an increased risk only when blood levels were 30 times higher than those measured after topical application in human subjects.[83] More than 50 cases of lymphoma have been reported, although the topical calcineurin inhibitor use may be coincidental. Nevertheless, there is a need for additional follow-up information to establish the long-term safety profile of these drugs.[83]

ENDOCRINE SYSTEM

Topical corticosteroids can rarely cause hypothalamic–pituitary–adrenal axis suppression, growth retardation, hyperglycemia, iatrogenic Cushing syndrome, and femoral head osteonecrosis.[10] Factors that enhance drug absorption are directly related to an increase in these side effects; therefore, careful monitoring must be ensured when prescribing usage in large surfaces areas, prolonged use of potent corticosteroids, usage under occlusion, high-potency corticosteroids, or use for the pediatric age group (because of their increased surface–body mass ratio).

TRANSDERMAL DRUGS

Transdermal drug delivery, in contrast to topical drug delivery, uses topical application of therapeutic drug as a delivery system for systemic therapy. Transdermal patches have been approved by the FDA since 1981 (scopolamine being the first) for the delivery of numerous medications, with more seeking approval. Advantages of this approach include controlled release, a steady blood-level profile with zero-order kinetics, lack of a plasma peak, and, in some cases, improved patient compliance. These patches remain on the skin for 12 hours to 1 week. A patch consists of a plastic backing, a reservoir of medication, and either a rate-controlling membrane or a polymer matrix system for controlled diffusion followed by an adhesive facing the skin. The most common adhesives used are acrylates, silicones, and polyisobutylenes. These patches have been tested and are approved for use on the thighs, buttocks, lower abdomen, upper arms, and chest; application to other sites can lead to either sub- or supratherapeutic blood levels. Adverse effects of patches include local irritation and allergic contact dermatitis to either an adhesive or to the drug itself and may necessitate discontinuation.

CONCLUSIONS

Topical therapies are a mainstay of treatment for the dermatologist. An understanding of the interactions between a drug's concentration, penetration, availability, and treatment of diseased skin allows physicians to maximize both efficacy and tolerability of topical therapy. An understanding of local and systemic toxicities allows selection of appropriate, safe therapy for patients and minimizes unwanted effects. Appropriate selection of topical agents and patient education on proper use can optimize therapeutic outcomes.

ACKNOWLEDGMENTS

Previous authors were Aieska De Souza, Bruce E. Strober, Hans Schaefer, Thomas E. Redelmeier, Gerhard J. Nohynek, and Jürgen Lademann.

REFERENCES

1. Feldman SR, Vrijens B, Gieler U, et al. Treatment adherence intervention studies in dermatology and guidance on how to support adherence. *Am J Clin Dermatol.* 2017;18(2):253-271.
2. Foley P, Stockfleth E, Peris K, et al. Adherence to topical therapies in actinic keratosis: a literature review. *J Dermatolog Treat.* 2016;27(6):538-545.
3. Lee IA, Maibach HI. Pharmionics in dermatology: a review of topical medication adherence. *Am J Clin Dermatol.* 2006;7(4):231-236.
4. Anderson KL, Dothard EH, Huang KE, et al. Frequency of primary nonadherence to acne treatment. *JAMA Dermatol.* 2015;151(6):623.
5. Zaghloul SS, Goodfield MJD. Objective assessment of compliance with psoriasis treatment. *Arch Dermatol.* 2004;140(4):408-414.
6. Kulkarni AS, Balkrishnan R, Camacho FT, et al. Medication and health care service utilization related to depressive symptoms in older adults with psoriasis. *J Drugs Dermatol.* 3(6):661-666.
7. Molassiotis A, Morris K, Trueman I. The importance of the patient–clinician relationship in adherence to antiretroviral medication. *Int J Nurs Pract.* 2007;13(6):370-376.
8. Snyder A, Farhangian M, Feldman SR. A review of patient adherence to topical therapies for treatment of atopic dermatitis. *Cutis.* 2015;96(6):397-401.
9. Feldman SR. Tachyphylaxis to topical corticosteroids: the more you use them, the less they work? *Clin Dermatol.* 2006;24(3):229-230; discussion 230.
10. Tadicherla S, Ross K, Shenefelt PD, et al. Topical corticosteroids in dermatology. *J Drugs Dermatol.* 2009;8(12):1093-1105.
11. Franz TJ. Kinetics of cutaneous drug penetration. *Int J Dermatol.* 1983;22(9):499-505.
12. Bronaugh RL, Maibach HI, eds. *Percutaneous Absorption: Drugs, Cosmetics, Mechanisms, Methodology (Drugs and the Pharmaceutical Sciences).* 4th ed. Abingdon, UK: Taylor & Francis; 2005.
13. Flynn G. General introduction and conceptual differentiation of topical and transdermal drug delivery systems. In: Shah VP, Maibach HI, eds. *Topical Drug Bioavailability: Bioequivalence and Penetration.* New York: Plenum: Springer; 1993:369.
14. Vickers CF. Existence of reservoir in the stratum corneum. Experimental proof. *Arch Dermatol.* 1963;88:20-23.
15. Lademann J, Lange-Asschenfeldt S, Ulrich M, et al. Application of laser scanning microscopy in dermatology and cutaneous physiology. In: *Non Invasive Diagnostic Techniques in Clinical Dermatology.* Berlin: Springer Berlin Heidelberg; 2014:101-113.
16. Otberg N, Richter H, Schaefer H, et al. Visualization of topically applied fluorescent dyes in hair follicles by laser scanning microscopy. *Laser Phys.* 2003;13(5):761-764.
17. Rolland A. Particulate carriers in dermal and transdermal drug delivery: myth or reality. In: Walters K, Hadgraft J, eds. *Pharmaceutical Particulate Carriers: Therapeutic Applications.* New York: Marcel Dekker; 1993:367.
18. Lademann J, Otberg N, Richter H, et al. Investigation of follicular penetration of topically applied substances. *Skin Pharmacol Appl Skin Physiol.* 2001;14(suppl 1):17-22.
19. Schaefer H, Lademann J. The role of follicular penetration. A differential view. *Skin Pharmacol Appl Skin Physiol.* 2001;14(suppl 1):23-27.
20. Toll R, Jacobi U, Richter H, et al. Penetration profile of microspheres in follicular targeting of terminal hair

follicles. *J Invest Dermatol.* 2004;123(1):168-176.
21. Lademann J, Richter H, Schaefer UF, et al. Hair follicles—a long-term reservoir for drug delivery. *Skin Pharmacol Physiol.* 2006;19(4):232-236.
22. Higuchi T. Physical chemical analysis of percutaneous absorption process from creams and ointments. *J Soc Cosmet Chem.* 1960;11(85).
23. Guy R, Hadgraft J, Maibach H. A pharmacokinetic model for percutaneous absorption. *Int J Pharm.* 1982;11(119).
24. Gupta SK, Bashaw E, Hwang S. Pharmacokinetic and pharmacodynamic modeling of transdermal products: in vivo methods, problems, and pitfalls. In: Shah V, Maibach H, eds. *Topical Drug Bioavailability: Bioequivalence and Penetration.* New York, Plenum; 1993.
25. Kubota K, Sznitowska M, Maibach HI. Percutaneous absorption: a single-layer model. *J Pharm Sci.* 1993; 82(5):450-456.
26. Williams PL, Riviere JE. A biophysically based dermatopharmacokinetic compartment model for quantifying percutaneous penetration and absorption of topically applied agents. I. Theory. *J Pharm Sci.* 1995;84(5): 599-608.
27. Schaefer H (Hans), Redelmeier TE. *Skin Barrier: Principles of Percutaneous Absorption.* Basel, Switzerland: Karger; 1996.
28. Elias PM, Menon GK. Structural and lipid biochemical correlates of the epidermal permeability barrier. *Adv Lipid Res.* 1991;24:1-26.
29. Elias PM, Feingold KR. Coordinate regulation of epidermal differentiation and barrier homeostasis. *Skin Pharmacol Appl Skin Physiol.* 2001;14(suppl 1):28-34.
30. Otberg N, Richter H, Schaefer H, et al. Variations of hair follicle size and distribution in different body sites. *J Invest Dermatol.* 2004;122(1):14-19.
31. Mangelsdorf S, Otberg N, Maibach HI, et al. Ethnic variation in vellus hair follicle size and distribution. *Skin Pharmacol Physiol.* 2006;19(3):159-167.
32. Egbaria K, Weiner N. Liposomes as a drug delivery system. *Adv Drug Deliv Rev.* 1990;(5):287-300.
33. Rolland A, Wagner N, Chatelus A, et al. Site-specific drug delivery to pilosebaceous structures using polymeric microspheres. *Pharm Res.* 1993;10(12):1738-1744.
34. Nemanic MK, Elias PM. In situ precipitation: a novel cytochemical technique for visualization of permeability pathways in mammalian stratum corneum. *J Histochem Cytochem.* 1980;28(6):573-578.
35. Squier CA, Lesch CA. Penetration pathways of different compounds through epidermis and oral epithelia. *J Oral Pathol.* 1988;17(9-10):512-516.
36. Teichmann A, Jacobi U, Ossadnik M, et al. Differential stripping: determination of the amount of topically applied substances penetrated into the hair follicles. *J Invest Dermatol.* 2005;125(2):264-269.
37. Maibach HI, Feldman RJ, Milby TH, et al. Regional variation in percutaneous penetration in man. Pesticides. *Arch Environ Health.* 1971;23(3):208-211.
38. Hueber F, Besnard M, Schaefer H, et al. Percutaneous absorption of estradiol and progesterone in normal and appendage-free skin of the hairless rat: lack of importance of nutritional blood flow. *Skin Pharmacol.* 1994;7(5):245-256.
39. Hueber F, Schaefer H, Wepierre J. Role of transepidermal and transfollicular routes in percutaneous absorption of steroids: in vitro studies on human skin. *Skin Pharmacol.* 1994;7(5):237-244.
40. Teichmann A, Otberg N, Jacobi U, et al. Follicular penetration: development of a method to block the follicles selectively against the penetration of topically applied substances. *Skin Pharmacol Physiol.* 2006;19(4):216-223.
41. Otberg N, Teichmann A, Rasuljev U, et al. Follicular penetration of topically applied caffeine via a shampoo formulation. *Skin Pharmacol Physiol.* 2007;20(4):195-198.
42. Pinnagoda J, Tupker RA, Agner T, et al. Guidelines for transepidermal water loss (TEWL) measurement. A report from the Standardization Group of the European Society of Contact Dermatitis. *Contact Dermatitis.* 1990; 22(3):164-178.
43. Scheuplein RJ. Mechanism of percutaneous absorption. II. Transient diffusion and the relative importance of various routes of skin penetration. *J Invest Dermatol.* 1967;48(1):79-88.
44. Rutter N. Clinical consequences of an immature barrier. *Semin Neonatol.* 2000;5(4):281-287.
45. Kao J, Carver MP. Cutaneous metabolism of xenobiotics. *Drug Metab Rev.* 1990;22(4):363-410.
46. Rolsted K, Benfeldt E, Kissmeyer A-M, et al. Cutaneous in vivo metabolism of topical lidocaine formulation in human skin. *Skin Pharmacol Physiol.* 2009;22(3):124-127.
47. Jacobi U, Toll R, Sterry W, et al. Do follicles play a role as penetration pathways in in vitro studies on porcine skin? An optical study. *Las Phys.* 2005;15:1594.
48. Nohynek GJ, Skare JA, Meuling WJA, et al. Urinary acetylated metabolites and N-acetyltransferase-2 genotype in human subjects treated with a para-phenylenediamine-containing oxidative hair dye. *Food Chem Toxicol.* 2004;42(11):1885-1891.
49. Dressler WE, Appelqvist T. Plasma/blood pharmacokinetics and metabolism after dermal exposure to para-aminophenol or para-phenylenediamine. *Food Chem Toxicol.* 2006;44(3):371-379.
50. Nohynek GJ, Duche D, Garrigues A, et al. Under the skin: biotransformation of para-aminophenol and para-phenylenediamine in reconstructed human epidermis and human hepatocytes. *Toxicol Lett.* 2005; 158(3):196-212.
51. Guzek DB, Kennedy AH, McNeill SC, et al. Transdermal drug transport and metabolism. I. Comparison of in vitro and in vivo results. *Pharm Res.* 1989;6(1):33-39.
52. Novotný J, Kovaríková P, Novotný M, et al. Dimethylaminoacid esters as biodegradable and reversible transdermal permeation enhancers: effects of linking chain length, chirality and polyfluorination. *Pharm Res.* 2009; 26(4):811-821.
53. Mukhtar H, Khan WA. Cutaneous cytochrome P-450. *Drug Metab Rev.* 1989;20(2-4):657-673.
54. Higo N, Hinz RS, Lau DT, et al. Cutaneous metabolism of nitroglycerin in vitro. II. Effects of skin condition and penetration enhancement. *Pharm Res.* 1992;9(3):303-306.
55. Riviere JE, Sage B, Williams PL. Effects of vasoactive drugs on transdermal lidocaine iontophoresis. *J Pharm Sci.* 1991;80(7):615-620.
56. Danon A, Ben-Shimon S, Ben-Zvi Z. Effect of exercise and heat exposure on percutaneous absorption of methyl salicylate. *Eur J Clin Pharmacol.* 1986; 31(1):49-52.
57. Monteiro-Riviere NA, Inman AO, Riviere JE, et al. Topical penetration of piroxicam is dependent on the distribution of the local cutaneous vasculature. *Pharm Res.* 1993;10(9):1326-1331.
58. Singh P, Roberts MS. Blood flow measurements in skin and underlying tissues by microsphere method: application to dermal pharmacokinetics of polar nonelectrolytes. *J Pharm Sci.* 1993;82(9):873-879.
59. Kushla GP, Zatz JL, Mills OH, et al. Noninvasive assessment of anesthetic activity of topical lidocaine

formulations. *J Pharm Sci*. 1993;82(11):1118-1122.
60. Williams ML. Ichthyosis: mechanisms of disease. *Pediatr Dermatol*. 1992;9(4):365-368.
61. Werner Y, Lindberg M. Transepidermal water loss in dry and clinically normal skin in patients with atopic dermatitis. *Acta Derm Venereol*. 1985;65(2):102-105.
62. Ghadially R, Brown BE, Sequeira-Martin SM, et al. The aged epidermal permeability barrier. Structural, functional, and lipid biochemical abnormalities in humans and a senescent murine model. *J Clin Invest*. 1995;95(5):2281-2290.
63. Lavrijsen AP, Bouwstra JA, Gooris GS, et al. Reduced skin barrier function parallels abnormal stratum corneum lipid organization in patients with lamellar ichthyosis. *J Invest Dermatol*. 1995;105(4):619-624.
64. Wilhelm KP, Surber C, Maibach HI. Effect of sodium lauryl sulfate-induced skin irritation on in vivo percutaneous penetration of four drugs. *J Invest Dermatol*. 1991;97(5):927-932.
65. Feldman RJ, Maibach HI. Regional variation in percutaneous penetration of 14C cortisol in man. *J Invest Dermatol*. 1967;48(2):181-183.
66. El Maghraby GM, Barry BW, Williams AC. Liposomes and skin: from drug delivery to model membranes. *Eur J Pharm Sci*. 2008;34(4-5):203-222.
67. Trommer H, Neubert RHH. Overcoming the stratum corneum: the modulation of skin penetration. A review. *Skin Pharmacol Physiol*. 2006;19(2):106-121.
68. Chiang A, Tudela E, Maibach HI. Percutaneous absorption in diseased skin: an overview. *J Appl Toxicol*. 2012;32(8):537-563.
69. Dragicevic N, Maibach HI, eds. *Percutaneous Penetration Enhancers Chemical Methods in Penetration Enhancement: Modification of the Stratum Corneum*. Springer-Verlag: Berlin Heidelberg; 2016.
70. Ryan T, ed. Beyond occlusion: dermatology proceedings. In: *No. 137 of International Congress Symposium Series*. London: Royal Society of Medicine Services; 1988.
71. Wester RC, Noonan PK, Maibach HI. Frequency of application on percutaneous absorption of hydrocortisone. *Arch Dermatol*. 1977;113(5):620-622.
72. Eaglstein WH, Farzad A, Capland L. Editorial: topical corticosteroid therapy: efficacy of frequent application. *Arch Dermatol*. 1974;110(6):955-956.
73. Ricciatti-Sibbald D, Sibbald RG. Dermatologic vehicles. *Clin Dermatol*. 7(3):11-24.
74. McCarron PA, Donnelly RF, Andrews GP, et al. Stability of 5-aminolevulinic acid in novel non-aqueous gel and patch-type systems intended for topical application. *J Pharm Sci*. 2005;94(8):1756-1771.
75. Huang X, Tanojo H, Lenn J, et al. A novel foam vehicle for delivery of topical corticosteroids. *J Am Acad Dermatol*. 2005;53(1 suppl 1):S26-S38.
76. Franz TJ, Parsell DA, Halualani RM, et al. Betamethasone valerate foam 0.12%: a novel vehicle with enhanced delivery and efficacy. *Int J Dermatol*. 1999;38(8):628-632.
77. Choi MJ, Maibach HI. Liposomes and niosomes as topical drug delivery systems. *Skin Pharmacol Physiol*. 2005;18(5):209-219.
78. Karimipour DJ, Karimipour G, Orringer JS. Microdermabrasion: an evidence-based review. *Plast Reconstr Surg*. 2010;125(1):372-377.
79. Zesch A. Short and long-term risks of topical drugs. *Br J Dermatol*. 1986;115 suppl:63-70.
80. Farage MA, Katsarou A, Maibach HI. Sensory, clinical and physiological factors in sensitive skin: a review. *Contact Dermatitis*. 2006;55(1):1-14.
81. Kligman AM, Sadiq I, Zhen Y, et al. Experimental studies on the nature of sensitive skin. *Skin Res Technol*. 2006;12(4):217-222.
82. Kim YH. Management with topical nitrogen mustard in mycosis fungoides. *Dermatol Ther*. 2003;16(4):288-298.
83. Thaçi D, Salgo R. Malignancy concerns of topical calcineurin inhibitors for atopic dermatitis: facts and controversies. *Clin Dermatol*. 28(1):52-56.

Chapter 184 :: Glucocorticoids
:: Avrom Caplan, Nicole Fett, & Victoria Werth

第一百八十四章

糖皮质激素

中文导读

　　本章分为2节，主要介绍了系统使用糖皮质激素和外用糖皮质激素的相关内容。

　　系统使用糖皮质激素分为6个方面。①药理作用机制主要有三种：第一是通过糖皮质激素受体与糖皮质激素反应元件的结合对基因表达产生直接影响；第二是通过糖皮质激素受体与其他转录因子的相互作用间接影响基因表达；第三是糖皮质激素受体介导的第二信使级联效应。此外，具有一定的细胞效应，影响细胞的复制和运动，诱导单核细胞减少、嗜酸性粒细胞减少和淋巴细胞减少，对T细胞的影响大于对B细胞的影响；②在表184-1中列举皮肤疾病的适应症；③给药方案：全身性糖皮质激素可经皮损内、肌肉注射和静脉注射或口服，治疗的途径和方法取决于所治疗疾病的性质和程度；④初始治疗，基本原则为在开始使用前，应权衡实际预期的益处，防止潜在的副作用，进行治疗前评估，糖皮质激素的选择必须要考虑众多因素；⑤表184-3概述了全身性糖皮质激素治疗的副作用预防措施，需要注意饮食、感染、免疫接种、肾上腺功能抑制等；⑥副作用：与全身性糖皮质激素治疗相关的并发症，随着剂量的增加、治疗持续时间的延长和用药频率的增加而增加。

　　外用糖皮质激素分为5个方面。①作用机制：抗增殖作用和对真皮毛细血管的血管收缩作用显著；②适应症：用于炎症性皮肤病的抗炎活性、抗有丝分裂作用以及减少结缔组织分子合成的能力，同时介绍了外用糖皮质激素在儿科、老年患者及孕妇中的应用；③给药方案：外用皮质类固醇的频率是以经验的方式发展的，大多数教科书和医生建议每天使用两次；④副作用预防措施：表184-7概述了在开始外用皮质类固醇时的一般原则。预防副作用的外用药物的注意事项在表184-8中列出；⑤副作用：外用糖皮质类固醇的不良反应比全身反应更为普遍，包括萎缩性改变、痤疮样反应、感染、过敏反应以及全身不良反应。

〔粟　娟〕

SYSTEMIC GLUCOCORTICOIDS

> **AT-A-GLANCE**
>
> - Systemic glucocorticoids are potent immunosuppressive and antiinflammatory agents that are frequently used for severe dermatologic diseases.
> - Complications are increased with fluorinated compounds, higher doses, longer duration of therapy, and more frequent administration.
> - Intralesional, IM, IV, topical, and oral routes of administration can be used.
> - Careful monitoring of systemic and cutaneous side effects is an essential component of therapy.
> - Glucocorticoid-induced osteoporosis begins early in treatment and should be aggressively managed in all patients on long-term therapy.

Glucocorticoids are a mainstay of dermatologic therapy because of their potent immunosuppressive and antiinflammatory properties. By understanding the properties and mechanisms of action of glucocorticoids, one can maximize their efficacy and safety as therapeutic agents.

PHARMACOLOGY AND MECHANISM OF ACTION

The major naturally occurring glucocorticoid is cortisol (hydrocortisone). It is synthesized from cholesterol by the adrenal cortex. Normally, less than 5% of circulating cortisol is unbound; this free cortisol is the active therapeutic molecule. The remainder is inactive because it is bound to cortisol-binding globulin (also called transcortin) or to albumin. Daily cortisol production is 5 to 7 mg/m^2, with a diurnal peak around 8:00 AM.[1] Cortisol has a plasma half-life of 90 minutes. It is metabolized primarily by the liver, although it exerts hormonal effects on virtually every tissue in the body. The metabolites are excreted by the kidney and the liver.

The mechanism of glucocorticoid action involves passive diffusion of the glucocorticoids through the cell membrane, followed by binding to soluble receptor proteins in the cytoplasm.[2] This hormone-receptor complex then moves to the nucleus and regulates the transcription of a limited number of target genes. There are 3 main mechanisms of glucocorticoid action. The first is direct effects on gene expression by the binding of glucocorticoid receptors to glucocorticoid-responsive elements, leading to the induction of proteins like annexin I and MAPK (mitogen-activated protein kinase) phosphatase 1. Annexins reduce phospholipase A$_2$ activity, which reduces the release of arachidonic acid from membrane phospholipids, limiting the formation of prostaglandins and leukotrienes.[3-5] The second mechanism is indirect effects on gene expression through the interactions of glucocorticoid receptors with other transcription factors. For example, inhibitory effects on AP-1 and nuclear factor κB, coupled with increased inhibitor of nuclear factor κB (IκB), decreases the synthesis of a number of proinflammatory molecules, including cytokines, interleukins, adhesion molecules, and proteases.[6] The third is glucocorticoid receptor–mediated effects on second messenger cascades through nongenomic pathways such as the phosphatidylinositol 3′-kinase (PI3K)-Akt-endothelial nitric oxide synthase (eNOS) pathway.[7,8]

There is usually a delay in the onset of pharmacologic activity of glucocorticoids relative to their peak blood concentrations, which is probably consequent to altering the transcription of genes,[7] although some actions appear to be independent of transcription. Some effects of glucocorticoids are too rapid to be mediated by genomic glucocorticoid action,[9] which might explain the additive benefits of very-high-pulse glucocorticoids.

CELLULAR EFFECTS OF CORTICOSTEROIDS

Glucocorticoids profoundly affect the replication and movement of cells. They induce monocytopenia, eosinopenia, and lymphocytopenia, and have a greater effect on T cells than on B cells.[10] The lymphocytopenia appears to be caused by a redistribution of cells as they migrate from the circulation to other lymphoid tissues. The increase in circulating polymorphonuclear leukocytes is related to demargination of cells from the bone marrow and a diminished rate of removal from the circulation, at least partially mediated by the increase in annexin 1[11]; there also appears to be inhibition of neutrophil apoptosis.[12]

Glucocorticoids affect cell activation, proliferation, and differentiation. They modulate the levels of mediators of inflammation and immune reactions, as seen with the inhibition of cytokines and tumor necrosis factor synthesis or release.[13,14] Additionally, macrophage functions, including phagocytosis, antigen processing, and cell killing, are decreased by cortisol, and this decrease affects immediate and delayed hypersensitivity.[15,16]

Glucocorticoids suppress monocyte and lymphocyte function (both Th1 and Th2 cells) more than polymorphonuclear leukocyte function.[17] This effect is clinically important because granulomatous infectious diseases, such as tuberculosis, are prone to exacerbation and relapse during prolonged glucocorticoid therapy. The antibody-forming cells, B lymphocytes and plasma cells, are relatively resistant to the suppressive effects of glucocorticoids.

INDICATIONS

There is a long list of indications for skin disorders (Table 184-1). In addition, short courses of glucocorticoids may be used for a variety of forms of severe dermatitis, including contact dermatitis, atopic dermatitis, photodermatitis, exfoliative dermatitis, and erythrodermas. The use of glucocorticoids is controversial in the treatment of erythema nodosum, lichen planus, cutaneous T-cell lymphoma, and discoid lupus erythematosus.

DOSING REGIMEN

Systemic glucocorticoids can be administered intralesionally, orally, intramuscularly, and intravenously. The route and regimen are determined by the nature and extent of the disease being treated.

Intralesional glucocorticoid administration allows direct access to either a relatively few lesions or a particularly resistant lesion. The concentration depends on the site of injection and the nature of the lesion. Lower concentrations are used on the face to prevent atrophy of the skin. In conditions requiring sustained effects, such as keloids and alopecia areata, longer-acting glucocorticoids, such as triamcinolone diacetate (Aristospan), can be administered alone or mixed with the more typically used triamcinolone acetonide (Kenalog). It is best to limit the total monthly dose of Kenalog to 20 mg to ensure that the hypothalamic–pituitary–adrenal (HPA) axis will not be suppressed.[18]

IM administration of glucocorticoids is associated with variable benefits and challenges. Although IM administration removes concerns for compliance and is not affected by nausea, vomiting, or inability to achieve intravenous access, potential drawbacks include erratic absorption and lack of daily control of the dose. Furthermore, IM injections may result in lipoatrophy or sterile abscesses.[19] Long-acting formulations such as triamcinolone acetonide have increased side effects over short-acting formulations, including increased potential of HPA axis suppression. Because this medication produces effects lasting up to 3 weeks, IM administration of triamcinolone acetonide should not be given more than a few times per year to avoid adrenal suppression.[19]

Intravenous glucocorticoids are used in 2 situations: The first is to provide stress coverage for patients who are acutely ill or are undergoing surgery (see below in section on Adrenal Suppression for discussion on glucocorticoids and surgery) and who have adrenal suppression from daily glucocorticoid therapy. The second is for patients with certain diseases—such as resistant pyoderma gangrenosum, severe pemphigus or bullous pemphigoid, serious systemic lupus erythematosus, or dermatomyositis—so as to gain rapid control of the disease and minimize the need for long-term, high-dose, oral steroid therapy.[20] Methylprednisolone is used at a dose of 500 mg to 1 g daily because of its high potency and low sodium-retaining activity. Serious side effects associated with IV administration include anaphylactic reactions, seizures, arrhythmias, and sudden death. Other, less serious adverse reactions include hypotension, hypertension, hyperglycemia, electrolyte shifts, and acute psychosis. Slower administration over 2 to 3 hours minimizes many of the serious side effects. Patients without underlying renal or cardiac disease do not need to be treated in a monitored bed, although vital signs should be monitored regularly during administration.[19] It is important to monitor serum electrolytes before and after pulse therapy, particularly when patients are on concomitant diuretic therapy.

Prednisone is the most commonly prescribed oral glucocorticoid. The initial dose is most often daily to control the disease process and can range from 2.5 mg to several hundred milligrams daily.

INITIATING THERAPY

FUNDAMENTAL PRINCIPLES

Before therapy with glucocorticoids is begun, the benefit that can realistically be expected should be weighed against the potential side effects. Alternative or adjunctive therapies should be considered, especially if long-term treatment is contemplated. Coexisting illnesses such as diabetes, hypertension, and osteoporosis need to be considered. The predisposition of the patient to side effects should be included in an assessment of risk.

CHOOSING AMONG GLUCOCORTICOIDS

A number of considerations bear on the choice of glucocorticoids (Table 184-2). First, a preparation with minimal mineralocorticoid effect is usually picked to decrease sodium retention. Second, the

---

TABLE 184-1
Most Common Indications of Systemic Steroids

- Serious blistering diseases (pemphigus, bullous pemphigoid, cicatricial pemphigoid, linear immunoglobulin A bullous dermatoses, epidermolysis bullosa acquisita, herpes gestationis, erythema multiforme, toxic epidermal necrolysis)
- Connective tissue diseases (dermatomyositis, systemic lupus erythematosus, mixed connective tissue disease, eosinophilic fasciitis, relapsing polychondritis)
- Vasculitis
- Neutrophilic dermatoses (pyoderma gangrenosum, acute febrile neutrophilic dermatosis, Behçet disease)
- Sarcoidosis
- Type I reactive leprosy
- Hemangioma of infancy
- Panniculitis
- Urticaria/angioedema

TABLE 184-2
Glucocorticoid Equivalencies

	EQUIVALENT DOSE (mg)	GLUCOCORTICOID POTENCY	HPA SUPPRESSION	MINERALOCORTICOID POTENCY	PLASMA HALF-LIFE (min)	BIOLOGIC HALF-LIFE (h)
Short-acting Glucocorticoids						
Cortisol	20	1.0	1.0	1.0	90	8-12
Cortisone	25	0.8		0.8	80-118	8-12
Intermediate-acting Glucocorticoids						
Prednisone	5	4.0	4.0	0.3	60	18-36
Prednisolone	5	5.0		0.3	115-200	18-36
Triamcinolone	4	5.0	4.0	0	30	18-36
Methylprednisolone	4	5.0	4.0	0	180	18-36
Long-acting Glucocorticoids						
Dexamethasone	0.75	30	17	0	200	36-54
Betamethasone	0.6	25-40		0	300	36-54
Mineralocorticoids						
Fludrocortisone	2	10	12.0	250	200	18-36
Desoxycorticosterone acetate		0		20	70	

HPA, hypothalamic–pituitary–adrenal axis.
From Chrousos G, Pavlaki AN, Magiakou MA. Glucocorticoid therapy and adrenal suppression. [Updated January 11, 2011.] In: De Groot LJ, Chrousos G, Dungan K, et al., eds. Endotext [Internet]. South Dartmouth, MA: MDText.com, Inc; 2000. https://www.ncbi.nlm.nih.gov/books/NBK279156/, with permission. Copyright © 2000-2018, MDText.com, Inc.

long-term oral use of prednisone or a similar drug, with an intermediate half-life and relatively weak steroid-receptor affinity, may reduce side effects. Long-term use of drugs like dexamethasone, which has a longer half-life and high glucocorticoid-receptor affinity, may produce more side effects without additional therapeutic effects. Third, if a patient does not respond to cortisone or prednisone, the substitution of the biologically active form, cortisol or prednisolone, should be considered. However, even in severe liver disease, substitution has not proved to be very important.

EVALUATION BEFORE TREATMENT

To minimize potential problems, the baseline evaluation should include a personal and family history, with special attention to predisposition to diabetes, hypertension, hyperlipidemia, glaucoma, and associated diseases that could be affected by steroid therapy. Side-effect-specific evaluation and monitoring recommendations during glucocorticoid therapy are discussed below in the section "Adverse Effects".

SIDE EFFECTS AND PRECAUTIONS

Table 184-3 outlines side effect preventive measures for systemic glucocorticoid therapy.

DIET

Diet should be low in calories, fat, and sodium, and high in protein, potassium, and calcium as tolerated, also considering any associated comorbidities. Protein intake is important to reduce steroid-induced nitrogen wasting.[21] Use of alcohol, coffee, and nicotine should be minimized. Exercise should be encouraged.

INFECTIONS

Glucocorticoid therapy increases the risk to patients for common and uncommon infections.[22] All patients anticipated to be on glucocorticoid doses of 15 mg or greater for 1 month or longer should be screened for tuberculosis with either a tuberculin skin test by injecting a purified protein derivative or an interferon-gamma release assay (QuantiFERON-TB Gold In-Tube Test or T-SPOT.TB). Patients with a positive screening test should have chest radiography to evaluate for active tuberculosis. Patients with a negative chest radiograph require treatment for latent tuberculosis. Anergic patients should have a baseline chest radiograph to search for evidence of previous tuberculosis. Of note, glucocorticoids downregulate delayed-type hypersensitivity and may suppress the purified protein derivative response. A positive purified protein derivative in this population is considered 5 mm or more of induration. Attention must also be paid to patients on high doses of glucocorticoids with underlying lung

TABLE 184-3
Side Effects and Preventive Measures for Systemic Glucocorticoid Therapy

SIDE EFFECT	PREVENTIVE MEASURES
Hypertension	Blood pressure (baseline; repeat with each visit)
Weight gain	Weight (baseline; repeat with each visit)
Reactivation of infection	Purified protein derivative or interferon-gamma release assay; hepatitis screen; consider *Pneumocystis jiroveci* pneumonia prophylaxis
Metabolic abnormalities	Electrolytes, lipids, glucose (baseline; repeat early after starting therapy; repeat annually; more frequent monitoring with known factors [eg, diabetes, hyperlipidemia])
Osteoporosis	Bone density (baseline; repeat annually); instruct about diet, exercise; initiate calcium and vitamin D supplementation; start bisphosphonate for men, postmenopausal women based on bone mineral density evaluation
Eyes	Refer for ophthalmologic evaluation and consider more frequent screening if history of cataracts or glaucoma
Peptic ulcer	In patients on concomitant nonsteroidal antiinflammatory drugs, initiate prophylaxis with a proton pump inhibitor; with 2 or more risk factors, consider prophylaxis with proton pump inhibitor
Suppression of hypothalamic–pituitary–adrenal axis	Single, early morning doses, preferably every other day

disease, low lymphocyte counts, underlying conditions further contributing to immunosuppression, and/or patients on concomitant cytotoxic therapies, as these patients are at increased risk for development of *Pneumocystis* pneumonia. Some advocate use of trimethoprim-sulfamethoxazole prophylaxis against *Pneumocystis jiroveci* for high-risk patients who are on high doses of glucocorticoids. Examination for other covert infections should be based on history and physical examination. For instance, a stool culture for *Strongyloides* should be performed for those who have lived in tropical countries and for Vietnam veterans.[23]

IMMUNIZATIONS

Immunization with live vaccines can be done if the duration of glucocorticoid use is less than 2 weeks at any dose, if the dose of glucocorticoid is less than 20 mg/day of any duration or less than 2 mg/kg in patients who weigh less than 10 kg, and if long-term alternate-day treatment with short-acting preparations is used. Immunization with live vaccines should not be done for at least 1 month after receiving high doses of glucocorticoids (>20 mg/day) for more than 2 weeks.[24]

ADRENAL SUPPRESSION

Patients receiving daily glucocorticoid therapy for longer than 3 to 4 weeks must be assumed to have adrenal suppression that requires tapering of the glucocorticoids to allow for recovery of the HPA axis. Prescribers may choose from among a variety of tapering algorithms and may choose to test the HPA axis to guide the need for short-term maintenance therapy at the low end of the taper.

If a prescriber chooses to test the HPA axis, it should be done with an 8 AM cortisol (to time the test when physiologic cortisol production peaks) prior to taking the daily steroid dose and after tapering that daily dose to a dose less than or equal to the daily physiologic cortisol level (<5 mg prednisone/day; or 15 to 20 mg hydrocortisone/day). If the 8 AM plasma cortisol levels are 5 μg/dL or less, then continued glucocorticoid therapy and rechecking of the serum cortisol every 3 to 6 months until levels are higher than 10 μg/dL is required. If levels are 5 μg/dL or higher but 20 μg/dL or less, prescribers may choose to perform further testing, such as a corticotropin-releasing hormone stimulation test; it is reasonable, however, to continue maintenance therapy with a very gradual taper.[25] At any point during tapering or within a year of stopping glucocorticoids, a stress caused, for example, by trauma, surgery, diarrhea, or fever can precipitate adrenal insufficiency related to an inadequate stress response. During such situations, it may be necessary to give higher doses of glucocorticoids in divided doses. Patients must be educated about the need for stress coverage and should wear bracelets or carry cards indicating that they are receiving glucocorticoids.

Most patients can be maintained on their regular dose of glucocorticoids in preparation for surgery. Prior guidelines for preoperative and perioperative management were based on cortisol response to severity of surgery.[26] However, expert opinion demonstrates a shifting paradigm.[27,28] Consideration may be given to high-dose glucocorticoids (50 mg hydrocortisone every 8 hours until tolerating oral intake) for patients undergoing major surgical procedures or patients with primary adrenal failure, congenital adrenal hyperplasia, or hypopituitarism.[28] Few randomized controlled trials have been done, and data is sparse. Clinicians must remain vigilant for intraoperative hypotension or other signs of adrenal insufficiency for at-risk patients undergoing surgical procedures and treat appropriately if acute adrenal insufficiency is the etiology.

ADVERSE EFFECTS

Complications associated with systemic glucocorticoid therapy (Table 184-4) increase with higher doses, longer duration of therapy, and more frequent administration.[19,29] However, osteoporosis and cataracts develop with alternate-day dosing, and avascular necrosis (AVN) can be seen after only short courses of glucocorticoids.

OSTEOPOROSIS

Osteoporosis occurs in 40% of individuals treated long-term with systemic glucocorticoids.[30,31] Bone loss occurs most rapidly in the first few months of glucocorticoid use, but continues at a slower rate after that.[30,32] Even low doses of prednisone (2.5 mg per day) adversely affect bone and increase vertebral and hip fractures.[33]

Glucocorticoids have both direct and indirect effects on bone. They decrease bone formation and increase resorption by inhibiting osteoblasts and increasing activity of osteoclasts.[30] Indirectly, glucocorticoids increase calcium excretion by the kidney, decrease intestinal calcium absorption, and reduce estrogen and testosterone levels.

Any patient anticipated to be on glucocorticoid therapy for 3 months or longer should receive calcium 1200 mg/day and vitamin D 800 International Units/day through diet and supplement.[34] Patients with comorbidities, such as patients with sarcoidosis or renal stones, may require close monitoring or adjustment of this recommendation. Clinicians may consider checking vitamin D levels and repleting prior to initiating maintenance therapy. Patients anticipated to be on prednisone 5 mg or more per day for 3 months or longer and all patients considered at high risk for osteoporosis should be evaluated with dual-energy x-ray absorptiometry or by the World Health Organization (WHO)'s fracture risk assessment tool, the FRAX equation (http://www.shef.ac.uk/FRAX/), for consideration of initiation of bisphosphonates. Rare side effects of bisphosphonates include osteonecrosis of the jaw and atypical femoral fractures. Additionally, bisphosphonates are contraindicated in patients with creatinine clearance below 30 mL/min. Oral bisphosphonates are contraindicated for patients who cannot sit upright for 30 minutes after swallowing a pill and for patients with esophageal disorders that impact swallowing, such as achalasia, strictures, reflux, or varices. Initiating bisphosphonates in women of childbearing potential should be considered case-by-case. In general, these women should avoid bisphosphonates in the absence of fragility fractures or ongoing bone loss.[35] Long-term use of glucocorticoids and/or high-risk patients may be evaluated for initiation of teriparatide. Secondary causes for osteoporosis should be considered and evaluated in all patients.

AVASCULAR NECROSIS

AVN is manifest by pain and limitation of motion in one or more joints. Various mechanisms have been postulated to explain AVN. Early detection is important because early intervention may prevent progression to degenerative joint disease requiring joint replacement. Patients should be regularly questioned about pain and limitation of motion of joints. If abnormalities develop, a radiograph, bone scan, or MRI should be ordered. Because radiographs can be normal in AVN, if suspicion for this side effect is high, clinicians should consider evaluation by MRI. If multiple joints may be involved, then a bone scan may be needed. If imaging shows AVN, an orthopedic surgeon skilled in early intervention with core decompression may be able to halt progression of the disease.

TABLE 184-4

Complications Associated with Systemic Glucocorticoid Therapy

Bone health
- Avascular necrosis of bone
- Osteoporosis

Cardiovascular
- Atherosclerosis
- Dislipidemia
- Hypertension
- Sodium and fluid retention

Cutaneous
- Fibroblast inhibition
- Inhibition of wound healing
- Subcutaneous tissue atrophy (striae, purpura, ecchymoses)

Endocrine/Metabolic
- Alterations of fat distribution (typical cushingoid appearance)
- Fatty infiltration of the liver
- Growth failure
- Hyperglycemia and unmasking genetic predisposition to diabetes mellitus
- Secondary amenorrhea
- Suppression of hypothalamic–pituitary–adrenal axis

Gastrointestinal
- GI bleeding
- Intestinal perforation
- Pancreatitis
- Peptic ulcer

Immunity
- Effects on phagocyte kinetics and function
- Immunosuppression, anergy
- Increased incidence of infections
- Suppression of host defenses

Miscellaneous
- Anaphylaxis
- Drug interactions (for example, increased INR on patients on both prednisone and coumadin)
- Hypersensitivity reactions
- Myopathy
- Urticaria

Ophthalmologic
- Cataracts
- Glaucoma

Psychiatric/Mood disturbances
- Depression, mania
- Sleep disturbances
- Thoughts of self-harm

CARDIOVASCULAR DISEASE

Glucocorticoid use is associated with an increased risk for ischemic heart disease and heart failure,[36,37] although these risks appear to be greatest in patients with iatrogenic Cushing syndrome.[38,39] Various mechanisms may contribute to this increased risk for cardiovascular events among patients with hypercortisolism, including hypercortisolism-induced hypertension, increased atherosclerosis, structural changes such as ventricular hypertrophy and myocardial fibrosis, and electrocardiographic changes. However, data is limited. Many studies excluded patients with iatrogenic Cushing syndrome, and comorbidities such as glucose intolerance, weight gain, and dyslipidemia may have resulted in confounding of study results.[40-43]

Increased cardiovascular risk may persist for years after normalization of the serum cortisol level in Cushing disease.[44,45] Although studies primarily address Cushing disease, it is prudent to remain aware of this increased risk for patients on glucocorticoids or with iatrogenic Cushing syndrome, as metabolic syndrome may persist after removal of glucocorticoids contributing to ongoing risk for cardiovascular disease.

Cardiovascular risk factors should be aggressively managed. Blood pressure, diet, serum lipids, and glucose levels should be measured serially. Abnormalities should be treated with dietary manipulation and medication as necessary and according to current guidelines.

GASTROINTESTINAL COMPLICATIONS

There is a significantly increased risk for peptic ulcer disease and GI bleeding in patients taking both glucocorticoids and nonsteroidal antiinflammatory agents, although it is unclear whether glucocorticoids independently increase this risk.[46-48] In patients on combined therapy with a nonsteroidal antiinflammatory agent and glucocorticoid, prophylaxis with a proton pump inhibitor should be initiated. Prophylaxis should be highly considered in patients with 2 or more risk factors (such as those with a previous history of peptic ulceration or advanced malignant disease).

SUPPRESSION OF THE HYPOTHALAMIC–PITUITARY–ADRENAL AXIS AND THE STEROID WITHDRAWAL SYNDROME

The HPA axis is rapidly suppressed after the onset of glucocorticoid therapy. However, if therapy is limited to 1 to 3 weeks, the recovery of the HPA axis is rapid. As noted above, longer daily glucocorticoid therapy is associated with suppression of the HPA axis. Symptoms of adrenal insufficiency include lethargy, weakness, nausea, anorexia, fever, orthostatic hypotension, hypoglycemia, and weight loss.

There also exists a steroid withdrawal syndrome, in which patients experience symptoms of adrenal insufficiency despite having an apparently normal cortisol response to adrenocorticotropic hormone. Symptoms most commonly include anorexia, lethargy, malaise, nausea, weight loss, desquamation of the skin, headache, and fever. Less commonly, vomiting, myalgia, and arthralgia occur.[49] These patients have adjusted to high levels of glucocorticoids, and symptoms disappear after the glucocorticoids are restarted. This problem can be treated by slower tapering of the glucocorticoids or by temporarily increasing the dose.[25,49]

PSYCHIATRIC EFFECTS

Mood and cognitive changes are dose dependent and can appear shortly after the start of glucocorticoids. Age and gender appear to be risk factors for specific side effects. Women may be more likely to develop depression, whereas men may be more likely to develop mania.[50] The risk of depression, mania, delirium, confusion, and disorientation increases with age, but the opposite is true of suicidal behavior and panic disorder. The incidence of neuropsychiatric events is highest in the first 3 months of therapy. Prednisone doses greater than 80 mg/day place patients at increased risk for steroid psychosis.[50]

CONCERNS DURING LACTATION AND PREGNANCY

Glucocorticoids cross the placenta, but they are not teratogenic. Even though glucocorticoids are secreted into breastmilk, no adverse effect has been reported among breastfed infants of mothers taking glucocorticoids. Prednisolone instead of prednisone and avoiding breastfeeding for 4 hours after a dose may decrease the amount of drug transferred during breastfeeding.[51]

ISSUES SPECIFIC TO PEDIATRICS

In the pediatric population, glucocorticoids cause growth suppression and early osteoporosis.[52] Glucocorticoids inhibit bone formation, affect calcium and phosphorus metabolism, and interfere with growth hormone via affects on growth hormone secretion, growth hormone receptor expression and signal transduction from growth hormone to target tissues.[52] These effects can be reversed by treatment with growth hormone. Osteoporosis can reverse after glucocorticosteroids are stopped.

TOPICAL GLUCOCORTICOIDS

AT-A-GLANCE

- Topical glucocorticoids are the most frequently prescribed of all dermatologic drug products.
- They are effective at reducing the symptoms of inflammation, but do not address the underlying cause of the disease.
- Topical glucocorticoid research has focused on strategies to optimize potency while minimizing side effects.
- As with systemic glucocorticoids, careful monitoring of side effects is an essential component of therapy.

MECHANISM OF ACTION

The mechanism of action, antiinflammatory effects, and immunosuppressive effects are as described in "Systemic Glucocorticoids" above. Topical steroids are also notable for their antiproliferative effect and their vasoconstrictive effect on dermal capillaries.

ANTIPROLIFERATIVE EFFECTS

This effect of topical corticosteroids is mediated by inhibition of DNA synthesis and mitosis, partly explaining the therapeutic action of these drugs in scaling dermatoses.[53] They are known to reduce the keratinocyte size and proliferation. Fibroblast activity and collagen formation are also inhibited by topical corticosteroids.[54]

VASOCONSTRICTION

Topical steroids cause capillaries in the superficial dermis to constrict, thus reducing erythema. The mechanism by which corticosteroids induce vasoconstriction is not yet completely clear. It is thought to be related to inhibition of natural vasodilators such as histamine, bradykinins, and prostaglandins, and possibly via augmentation of vascular tone.[55-58] Vasoconstriction assays are used to predict the clinical activity of an agent. These assays have been used to separate the topical corticosteroids into 7 classes based on potency according to the United States' classification system and 4 classes according to the United Kingdom and France's classification systems. In the U.S. system, Class 1 includes the most potent, while Class 7 contains the least potent topical corticosteroids. Table 184-5 lists many of the available topical corticosteroids according to this classification.

PHARMACOKINETICS

Before choosing a topical glucocorticoid preparation, one must consider patient-related factors such as age,

TABLE 184-5
Potency Ranking of Selected Topical Corticosteroid Preparations

Class 1—Superpotent
- Betamethasone dipropionate 0.05% optimized vehicle
- Clobetasol propionate 0.05%
- Diflorasone diacetate 0.05%
- Fluocinonide 0.1% optimized vehicle
- Flurandrenolide 4 μg/cm^2
- Halobetasol propionate 0.05%

Class 2—Potent
- Amcinonide 0.1%
- Betamethasone dipropionate 0.05%
- Desoximetasone 0.25%
- Desoximetasone 0.05%
- Diflorasone diacetate 0.05%
- Fluocinonide 0.05%
- Halcinonide 0.1%
- Mometasone furoate 0.1%

Class 3—Potent, Upper Midstrength
- Amcinonide 0.1%
- Betamethasone dipropionate 0.05%
- Betamethasone valerate 0.1%
- Diflorasone diacetate 0.05%
- Fluocinonide 0.05%
- Fluticasone propionate 0.005%
- Triamcinolone acetonide 0.5%

Class 4—Midstrength
- Betamethasone valerate 0.12%
- Clocortolone pivalate 0.1%
- Desoximetasone 0.05%
- Fluocinolone acetonide 0.025%
- Flurandrenolide 0.05%
- Hydrocortisone probutate 0.1%
- Hydrocortisone valerate 0.2%
- Mometasone furoate 0.1%
- Prednicarbate 0.1%
- Triamcinolone acetonide 0.1%

Class 5—Lower Midstrength
- Betamethasone dipropionate 0.05%
- Betamethasone valerate 0.1%
- Fluocinolone acetonide 0.025%
- Fluocinolone acetonide 0.01%
- Flurandrenolide 0.05%
- Fluticasone propionate 0.05%
- Hydrocortisone butyrate 0.1%
- Hydrocortisone valerate 0.2%
- Prednicarbate 0.1%
- Triamcinolone acetonide 0.1%
- Triamcinolone acetonide 0.025%

Class 6—Mild Strength
- Alclometasone dipropionate 0.05%
- Desonide 0.05%
- Fluocinolone acetonide 0.01%
- Triamcinolone acetonide 0.025%

Class 7—Least Potent
- Topicals with dexamethasone, flumethasone, hydrocortisone, methylprednisolone, prednisolone

extent and location of body surface area, and presence or absence of inflammation, as well as drug-related factors such as concentration, duration, vehicle, and intrinsic characteristics of the agent.

Penetration of the glucocorticoid varies according to the skin site, which, in turn, is related to the thickness of the stratum corneum and the vascular supply to the area. For example, penetration of topical steroids through the eyelids and scrotum is greater than through the forehead and significantly greater than through the palms and soles. Inflamed, moist, and denuded skin also shows increased penetration. Potent topical steroids (Classes 1 and 2) should rarely, if ever, be used in the areas with the highest level of penetration.

The target site for topical corticosteroids is the viable epidermis or dermis, and clinical response to a formulation is directly proportional to the concentration of corticosteroid achieved at the target site.

Topical corticosteroids are compounded in several formulations and with varying strengths. Treatment adherence in the management of skin conditions is vital, as such, formulations including spray, foam, lotion, hydrogel, and shampoo have been developed to improve patient convenience and acceptance.

Both increasing hydration of the stratum corneum and using occlusive dressings may enhance absorption of topical corticosteroids. Expert consensus recommends soak and smear methods for treating atopic dermatitis, which consists of a warm bath followed by a generous application of topical corticosteroids, though evidence from studies remains limited.

INDICATIONS

Topical corticosteroids are used for an antiinflammatory activity in inflammatory skin diseases, antimitotic effects, and for their capacity to decrease the synthesis of connective tissue molecules.[55] The responsiveness of diseases to topical glucocorticoids varies and thus must be considered when prescribing topical corticosteroids. Diseases can be divided into the 3 categories shown in Table 184-6: (a) highly responsive, (b) moderately responsive, and (c) least responsive.

PEDIATRIC USES

Children and, in particular, infants, are at an increased risk of absorbing topical corticosteroids for several reasons. They have a higher body-surface-area-to-weight ratio, and thus have a higher degree of absorption for the same amount applied as an adult,[59] and they also have thinner skin. Infants also may be less able to metabolize potent glucocorticoids rapidly.[60] Application of topical steroids to the diaper area results in occlusion of the steroid by the diaper, and increased penetration occurs. As with other skin conditions, selecting the appropriate strength according to the body site, the extent of involvement, and the flare intensity is essential for treatment success.

TABLE 184-6
Responsiveness of Dermatoses to Topical Application of Corticosteroids

Highly responsive	- Atopic dermatitis (children) - Intertrigo - Psoriasis (intertriginous) - Seborrheic dermatitis
Moderately responsive	- Atopic dermatitis (adults) - Lichen simplex chronicus - Nummular eczema - Papular urticaria - Parapsoriasis - Primary irritant dermatitis - Psoriasis
Least responsive	- Allergic contact dermatitis, acute phase - Dyshidrotic eczema - Granuloma annulare - Insect bites - Lichen planus - Lupus erythematosus - Necrobiosis lipoidica diabeticorum - Palmoplantar psoriasis - Pemphigus - Psoriasis of nails - Sarcoidosis

Concerns for atrophy, hypopigmentation, osteoporosis, and telangiectasias are minimized when topical steroids are used in accordance with guidelines.[61] High-potency newer formulations of corticosteroids are effective in pediatric atopic dermatitis and may be considered for short courses, although the highest potency steroids may not be recommended by all experts for pediatric use.[59,62,63] Rarely, high-potency applications can result in systemic absorption and cutaneous side effects. The low risk for side effects and highly effective treatment modality should be carefully explained to parents to maximize compliance and understanding and minimize undertreatment. Results from numerous surveys demonstrate a "corticosteroid phobia" among patients/caregivers that leads to treatment noncompliance.[64-67]

GERIATRIC USES

Elderly patients may have thin skin, which allows for increased penetration of topical glucocorticoids. They are also more likely to have preexisting skin atrophy secondary to aging and may be diaper dependent. Similar precautions used in the treatment of infants should be used when treating elderly patients.

USES IN PREGNANCY

Most topical steroids are rated by the U.S. Food and Drug Administration as category C drugs. Best available evidence suggests no significant effects for pregnant women who use mild or moderate topical corticosteroids during pregnancy. A risk for low birth weight is associated with high-potency topical steroids, although the risk is small if used in the short term and increases with heavier use of strong topical corticosteroids.[68] However, studies are observational and imprecision was noted in regard to the outcome of low birth weight.[69] Topical corticosteroids have not been studied during breastfeeding; however, based on National Institutes of Health recommendations, it is recommended to limit long-term exposure to high-potency corticosteroids while breastfeeding. In addition, use only water-miscible cream or gel products to limit exposure of infants to mineral paraffins while breastfeeding. Topical corticosteroids should be wiped off prior to breastfeeding.[51]

DOSING REGIMEN

The frequency of topical application of corticosteroids was developed in an empirical manner, with most textbooks and physicians recommending twice-daily use. For superpotent corticosteroids once-daily application is considered as beneficial as twice-daily application. Observations suggest once-daily dosing also may be beneficial when using lesser-potency corticosteroids.

Tachyphylaxis has been demonstrated in experimental conditions by diminished vasoconstriction, rebound of DNA synthesis, and recovery of histamine wheals after application of topical steroids in patients with a history of long-term topical steroid usage.[70] Whether this tachyphylaxis is clinically relevant remains unclear. For example, patient adherence to therapy may explain what could be seen clinically as tachyphylaxis in pediatric eczema treated with appropriate topical corticoisteroids.[61]

SIDE EFFECTS AND PRECAUTIONS

Both local and systemic side effects have been documented with the use of topical corticosteroids. Application of corticosteroids to large surface areas, occlusion, higher concentrations, or more potent derivatives directly increases the risk of systemic absorption and subsequent side effects. Side effect–specific monitoring parameters are discussed below.

Under normal conditions, up to 99% of the applied topical corticosteroid is cleared from the skin, and only 1% is therapeutically active. Cutaneous adverse effects can result from the small percentage of percutaneously absorbed corticosteroid or also may result from its transient presence onto the skin. Continued use of topical corticosteroids also may lead to tachyphylaxis, as noted above.

Table 184-7 outlines some general principles that should be remembered when initiating topical corticosteroids.[55] Considerations for prescribing topical corticosteroids to prevent side effects should be followed (Table 184-8).[54,71]

TABLE 184-7
Principles When Initiating Topical Steroid Therapy

- Initiate lowest potency to sufficiently control disease.
- Topical corticosteroids should be avoided on ulcerated or atrophic skin, and on skin with coexistent infectious dermatoses.
- Prolonged use of insufficiently potent agent should be avoided.
- Treatment with low to medium potency preparations is recommended for large surface areas.
- Highly responsive diseases will usually respond to weak steroid preparations, whereas less-responsive diseases require medium-potency or high-potency topical steroids.
- Low-potency, ideally nonhalogenated, preparations should be used on the face and intertriginous areas.
- Very potent steroid therapy, frequently under occlusion, is usually required for hyperkeratotic or lichenified dermatoses and for involvement of palms and soles.
- Because of the increased body-surface-area-to-body-mass-index ratio and increased risk of systemic absorption, high-potency preparations and halogenated–medium-potency preparations, should be avoided in infants and young children, other than for short-term application.

ADVERSE EFFECTS

Local adverse effects of topical corticosteroid use are more prevalent than systemic reactions.

ATROPHIC CHANGES

Skin atrophy is a prominent and potential cutaneous adverse effect, and involves both the epidermis and dermis. Dermal atrophy develops from the direct antiproliferative effects of topical corticosteroids on fibroblasts, with inhibition of collagen and mucopolysaccharide synthesis, resulting in loss of dermal support. Reduction of glycosaminoglycan production and changes to structure and proportion has

TABLE 184-8
Continuing Use of Topical Steroids

- Highly potent formulations should be used for short periods (2 to 3 weeks) or intermittently.
- Once disease control is partially achieved, the use of a less-potent compound should be initiated.
- Reduce frequency of application (eg, application only in the morning, alternate-day therapy, weekend use) once disease control is partially achieved.
- Sudden discontinuation should be avoided after prolonged use to prevent rebound phenomena.
- Special guidelines should be followed when treating certain body areas (eg, intertriginous areas) or certain populations (eg, children or the elderly) to prevent the occurrence of local or systemic adverse effects.
- Close monitoring and further evaluation is recommended if systemic absorption of corticosteroids is suspected.
- Use combination therapy when clinically indicated (eg, addition of topical calcineurin inhibitor, tretinoin or calcipotriene).

been described, though of note, low-potency therapy may have a lesser effect.[72] Levels of hyaluronan, the major glycosaminoglycan in the skin, are also rapidly decreased after short-term glucocorticoid treatment.[73,74] Fragmentation and thinning of elastic fibers develop in the upper layers of the dermis, whereas deeper fibers form a compact and dense network. As a result of these atrophic changes, there is vascular dilation, purpura, easy bruising, stellate pseudoscars (purpuric, irregularly shaped, and hypopigmented atrophic scars), and ulceration. Atrophy is more likely to occur with high-potency topical corticosteroids, but this effect has been clinically reversed by reduction of potency.[75] Clinicians must consider these findings when prescribing corticosteroids and use appropriate doses, formulations, and durations to minimize risk for skin atrophy and reverse this side effect if it develops.

ACNEIFORM REACTIONS

The development or exacerbation of dermatoses of the face, including steroid rosacea, acne, and perioral dermatitis, is a well-known side effect of topical corticosteroids.[76] Although steroids initially lead to the suppression of inflammatory papules and pustules, patients may flare when treatment is withdrawn, thus leading to continued use of greater potency topical corticosteroids. For these reasons, steroid use should be discouraged in the treatment of rosacea and perioral and periocular dermatitis.

OTHER CUTANEOUS EFFECTS

Decreased pigmentation and hypertrichosis are reported with use of topical corticosteroid therapy.[76] Patients may also experience a burning sensation primarily on the face after withdrawal from continuous high dose steroid therapy.[77] Even though data regarding this reaction is limited, clinicians may consider this in the differential for such reactions.

DEVELOPMENT OF INFECTIONS

Topical corticosteroids may exacerbate and/or mask cutaneous infectious diseases including tinea versicolor, disseminated *Alternaria* infection, and dermatophytosis. Granuloma gluteale infantum, characterized by reddish-purplish granulomatous lesions on the diaper area, is a well-known complication of diaper dermatitis during treatment with corticosteroids.[76]

ALLERGIC REACTIONS

Allergic contact dermatitis from steroids should be suspected when dermatitis worsens with corticosteroid therapy, does not lead to improvement, or changes the clinical pattern of disease. In a 6-year retrospective study, 127 patients (10.69%) had an allergic reaction to at least one corticosteroid. Among the 1188 patients, 71 (5.98%) reacted to 1 corticosteroid, 28 (2.36%) to 2 corticosteroids, 6 (0.51%) to 3 corticosteroids, 6 (0.51%) to 4 corticosteroids, and 16 (1.35%) to more than 4 corticosteroids.[78] Patients suspected of having an allergy to a topical corticosteroid should undergo patch testing to determine whether the vehicle or the steroid is causing the contact dermatitis.[79] If patch testing is unavailable, the clinician should prescribe a Class C steroid (from a classification A through D of steroids according to cross-reactivity in association with allergic contact dermatitis; Table 184-9 outlines the classification of corticosteroids by cross-reactivity). Table 184-10 outlines potential allergens in topical corticosteroids.

TABLE 184-9
Classification of Corticosteroids by Cross-reactivity

STRUCTURAL CLASS	A	B	C	D1	D2
Type	Hydrocortisone	Triamcinolone Acetonide	Betamethasone	Betamethasone dipropionate	Methylprednisolone aceponate
Structure	C16—no methyl substitution		C16 methyl substitution	C16 methyl substitution	C16—no methyl substitution, no halogenation
	Probable C21—short-chain ester			C17/21 long-chain ester	
Cross-reactions	Cross-reacts with D2	Budesonide specifically cross-reacts with D2			Cross-reacts with A and budesonide
Patch-test substance	Tixocortol-21-pivalate	Budesonide		Clobetasol-17-propionate	Hydrocortisone-17-butyrate
		Triamcinolone acetonide			

Adapted from Jacob SE, Steele T. Corticosteroid classes: a quick reference guide including patch test substances and cross-reactivity. *J Am Acad Dermatol.* 2006;54(4):723-27.

TABLE 184-10
Potential Allergens in Topical Corticosteroids Vehicles

- Formaldehyde-releasing preservatives (imidazolidinylurea/diazolidinylurea)
- Fragrance
- Lanolin
- Methylchloroisothiazolinone/methylisothiazolinone
- Parabens
- Propylene glycol
- Sorbitan sesquioleate

SYSTEMIC ADVERSE EFFECTS

Topical glucocorticoids, especially high-potency Class 1 agents, may result in HPA axis suppression and, rarely, other systemic adverse effects. Clinicians should be aware of this possibility when using high-potency topical corticosteroids or when patients report inappropriate use of high-potency corticosteroids.

ACKNOWLEDGMENTS

We would like to thank Isabel C. Valencia and Francisco A. Kerdel, who contributed to the previous version of this chapter in the 8th edition.

REFERENCES

1. Esteban NV, Loughlin T, Yergey AL, et al. Daily cortisol production rate in man determined by stable isotope dilution/mass spectrometry. *J Clin Endocrinol Metab*. 1991;72(1):39-45.
2. Bloom E, Matulich DT, Lan NC, et al. Nuclear binding of glucocorticoid receptors: Relations between cytosol binding, activation and the biological response. *J Steroid Biochem*. 1980;12:175-184.
3. Flower RJ, Rothwell NJ. Lipocortin-1: cellular mechanisms and clinical relevance. *Trends Pharmacol Sci*. 1994;15(3):71-76.
4. Pepinsky RB, Tizard R, Mattaliano RJ, et al. Five distinct calcium and phospholipid binding proteins share homology with lipocortin I. *J Biol Chem*. 1988;263(22):10799-10811.
5. Wallner BP, Mattaliano RJ, Hession C, et al. Cloning and expression of human lipocortin, a phospholipase A2 inhibitor with potential anti-inflammatory activity. *Nature*. 1986;320(6057):77-81.
6. Adcock IM, Caramori G, Ito K. New insights into the molecular mechanisms of corticosteroids actions. *Curr Drug Targets*. 2006;7(6):649-660.
7. Rhen T, Cidlowski JA. Antiinflammatory action of glucocorticoids—new mechanisms for old drugs. *N Engl J Med*. 2005;353(16):1711-1723.
8. Buttgereit F, Saag KG, Cutolo M, et al. The molecular basis for the effectiveness, toxicity, and resistance to glucocorticoids: Focus on the treatment of rheumatoid arthritis. *Scand J Rheumatol*. 2005;34(1):14-21.
9. Groner B, Hynes NE, Rahmsdorf U, et al. Transcription initiation of transfected mouse mammary tumor virus LTR DNA is regulated by glucocorticoid hormones. *Nucleic Acids Res*. 1983;11(14):4713-4725.
10. Cupps TR, Fauci AS. Corticosteroid-mediated immunoregulation in man. *Immunol Rev*. 1982;65:133-155.
11. Goulding NJ, Euzger HS, Butt SK, et al. Novel pathways for glucocorticoid effects on neutrophils in chronic inflammation. *Inflamm Res*. 1998;47(suppl 3):S158-S165.
12. Liles WC, Dale DC, Klebanoff SJ. Glucocorticoids inhibit apoptosis of human neutrophils. *Blood*. 1995;86(8):3181-3188.
13. Amano Y, Lee SW, Allison AC. Inhibition by glucocorticoids of the formation of interleukin-1 alpha, interleukin-1 beta, and interleukin-6: Mediation by decreased mRNA stability. *Mol Pharmacol*. 1993;43(2):176-182.
14. Kitajima T, Ariizumi K, Bergstresser PR, et al. A novel mechanism of glucocorticoid-induced immune suppression: the inhibition of T cell-mediated terminal maturation of a murine dendritic cell line. *J Clin Invest*. 1996;98(1):142-147.
15. Balow JE, Rosenthal AS. Glucocorticoid suppression of macrophage migration inhibitory factor. *J Exp Med*. 1973;137(4):1031-1041.
16. Hogan MM, Vogel SN. Inhibition of macrophage tumoricidal activity by glucocorticoids. *J Immunol*. 1988;140(2):513-519.
17. Parrillo JE, Fauci AS. Mechanisms of glucocorticoid action on immune processes. *Annu Rev Pharmacol Toxicol*. 1979;19:179-201.
18. Franchin G, Diamond B. Pulse steroids: how much is enough? *Autoimmun Rev*. 2006;5(2):111-113.
19. Jackson S, Gilchrist H, Nesbitt LT Jr. Update on the dermatologic use of systemic glucocorticosteroids. *Dermatol Ther*. 2007;20(4):187-205.
20. Sabir S, Werth VP. Pulse glucocorticoids. *Dermatol Clin*. 2000;18(3):437-446, viii-ix.
21. Cogan MG, Sargent JA, Yarbrough SG, et al. Prevention of prednisone-induced negative nitrogen balance. Effect of dietary modification on urea generation rate in patients on hemodialysis receiving high-dose glucocorticoids. *Ann Intern Med*. 1981;95(2):158-161.
22. Youssef J, Novosad SA, Winthrop KL. Infection risk and safety of corticosteroid use. *Rheum Dis Clin North Am*. 2016;42(1):157-176, ix-x.
23. Genta RM. Global prevalence of strongyloidiasis: critical review with epidemiologic insights into the prevention of disseminated disease. *Rev Infect Dis*. 1989;11(5):755-767.
24. National Center for Immunization and Respiratory Diseases. General recommendations on immunization—recommendations of the Advisory Committee on Immunization Practices (ACIP). *MMWR Recomm Rep*. 2011;60(2):1-64.
25. Nieman LK, Biller BM, Findling JW, et al. Treatment of Cushing's syndrome: an Endocrine Society clinical practice guideline. *J Clin Endocrinol Metab*. 2015;100(8):2807-2831.
26. Salem M, Tainsh RE Jr, Bromberg J, et al. Perioperative glucocorticoid coverage. A reassessment 42 years after emergence of a problem. *Ann Surg*. 1994;219(4):416-425.
27. Axelrod L. Perioperative management of patients treated with glucocorticoids. *Endocrinol Metab Clin North Am*. 2003;32(2):367-383.
28. MacKenzie CR, Goodman SM. Stress dose steroids: myths and perioperative medicine. *Curr Rheumatol Rep*. 2016;18(7):47.
29. Vittorio CC, Werth VP. Preventive techniques to limit glucocorticoid-induced side effects. *Adv Dermatol*. 2000;16:273-297; discussion 298.

30. Whittier X, Saag KG. Glucocorticoid-induced osteoporosis. *Rheum Dis Clin North Am*. 2016;42(1):177-189, x.
31. Dykman TR, Gluck OS, Murphy WA, et al. Evaluation of factors associated with glucocorticoid-induced osteopenia in patients with rheumatic diseases. *Arthritis Rheum*. 1985;28(4):361-368.
32. LoCascio V, Bonucci E, Imbimbo B, et al. Bone loss in response to long-term glucocorticoid therapy. *Bone Miner*. 1990;8(1):39-51.
33. Van Staa TP, Leufkens HG, Abenhaim L, et al. Use of oral corticosteroids in the United Kingdom. *Q J Med*. 2000;93(2):105-111.
34. Grossman JM, Gordon R, Ranganath VK, et al. American college of rheumatology 2010 recommendations for the prevention and treatment of glucocorticoid-induced osteoporosis. *Arthritis Care Res (Hoboken)*. 2010;62(11):1515-1526.
35. Abraham A, Cohen A, Shane E. Premenopausal bone health: osteoporosis in premenopausal women. *Clin Obstet Gynecol*. 2013;56(4):722-729.
36. Souverein PC, Berard A, Van Staa TP, et al. Use of oral glucocorticoids and risk of cardiovascular and cerebrovascular disease in a population based case-control study. *Heart*. 2004;90(8):859-865.
37. Wei L, MacDonald TM, Walker BR. Taking glucocorticoids by prescription is associated with subsequent cardiovascular disease. *Ann Intern Med*. 2004;141(10):764-770.
38. Fardet L, Petersen I, Nazareth I. Risk of cardiovascular events in people prescribed glucocorticoids with iatrogenic Cushing's syndrome: cohort study. *BMJ*. 2012;345:e4928.
39. Etxabe J, Vazquez JA. Morbidity and mortality in Cushing's disease: an epidemiological approach. *Clin Endocrinol (Oxf)*. 1994;40(4):479-484.
40. Alexandraki KI, Kaltsas GA, Vouliotis AI, et al. Specific electrocardiographic features associated with Cushing's disease. *Clin Endocrinol (Oxf)*. 2011;74(5):558-564.
41. Muiesan ML, Lupia M, Salvetti M, et al. Left ventricular structural and functional characteristics in Cushing's syndrome. *J Am Coll Cardiol*. 2003;41(12):2275-2279.
42. Yiu KH, Marsan NA, Delgado V, et al. Increased myocardial fibrosis and left ventricular dysfunction in Cushing's syndrome. *Eur J Endocrinol*. 2012;166(1):27-34.
43. Neary NM, Booker OJ, Abel BS, et al. Hypercortisolism is associated with increased coronary arterial atherosclerosis: analysis of noninvasive coronary angiography using multidetector computerized tomography. *J Clin Endocrinol Metab*. 2013;98(5):2045-2052.
44. Colao A, Pivonello R, Spiezia S, et al. Persistence of increased cardiovascular risk in patients with Cushing's disease after five years of successful cure. *J Clin Endocrinol Metab*. 1999;84(8):2664-2672.
45. Dekkers OM, Horvath-Puho E, Jorgensen JO, et al. Multisystem morbidity and mortality in Cushing's syndrome: a cohort study. *J Clin Endocrinol Metab*. 2013;98(6):2277-2284.
46. Hernandez-Diaz S, Rodriguez LA. Steroids and risk of upper gastrointestinal complications. *Am J Epidemiol*. 2001;153(11):1089-1093.
47. Piper JM, Ray WA, Daugherty JR, et al. Corticosteroid use and peptic ulcer disease: role of nonsteroidal anti-inflammatory drugs. *Ann Intern Med*. 1991;114(9):735-740.
48. Luo JC, Chang FY, Chen TS, et al. Gastric mucosal injury in systemic lupus erythematosus patients receiving pulse methylprednisolone therapy. *Br J Clin Pharmacol*. 2009;68(2):252-259.
49. Dixon RB, Christy NP. On the various forms of corticosteroid withdrawal syndrome. *Am J Med*. 1980;68(2):224-230.
50. Fardet L, Petersen I, Nazareth I. Suicidal behavior and severe neuropsychiatric disorders following glucocorticoid therapy in primary care. *Am J Psychiatry*. 2012;169(5):491-497.
51. Sammaritano LR, Bermas BL. Rheumatoid arthritis medications and lactation. *Curr Opin Rheumatol*. 2014;26(3):354-360.
52. Allen DB. Growth suppression by glucocorticoid therapy. *Endocrinol Metab Clin North Am*. 1996;25(3):699-717.
53. Almawi WY, Saouda MS, Stevens AC, et al. Partial mediation of glucocorticoid antiproliferative effects by lipocortins. *J Immunol*. 1996;157(12):5231-5239.
54. Smith EW. Do we need new and different glucocorticoids? A re-appraisal of the various congeners and potential alternatives. *Curr Probl Dermatol*. 1993;21:1-10.
55. Brazzini B, Pimpinelli N. New and established topical corticosteroids in dermatology: clinical pharmacology and therapeutic use. *Am J Clin Dermatol*. 2002;3(1):47-58.
56. Altura BM. Role of glucocorticoids in local regulation of blood flow. *Am J Physiol*. 1966;211(6):1393-1397.
57. Juhlin L, Michaelsson G. Cutaneous vascular reactions to prostaglandins in healthy subjects and in patients with urticaria and atopic dermatitis. *Acta Derm Venereol*. 1969;49(3):251-261.
58. Ullian ME. The role of corticosteroids in the regulation of vascular tone. *Cardiovasc Res*. 1999;41(1):55-64.
59. Eichenfield LF, Tom WL, Berger TG, et al. Guidelines of care for the management of atopic dermatitis: section 2. Management and treatment of atopic dermatitis with topical therapies. *J Am Acad Dermatol*. 2014;71(1):116-132.
60. West DP, Worobec S, Solomon LM. Pharmacology and toxicology of infant skin. *J Invest Dermatol*. 1981;76(3):147-150.
61. Mooney E, Rademaker M, Dailey R, et al. Adverse effects of topical corticosteroids in paediatric eczema: Australasian consensus statement. *Australas J Dermatol*. 2015;56(4):241-251.
62. Woods MT, Brown PA, Baig-Lewis SF, et al. Effects of a novel formulation of fluocinonide 0.1% cream on skin barrier function in atopic dermatitis. *J Drugs Dermatol*. 2011;10(2):171-176.
63. Wollenberg A, Oranje A, Deleuran M, et al. ETFAD/EADV eczema task force 2015 position paper on diagnosis and treatment of atopic dermatitis in adult and paediatric patients. *J Eur Acad Dermatol Venereol*. 2016;30(5):729-747.
64. Zuberbier T, Orlow SJ, Paller AS, et al. Patient perspectives on the management of atopic dermatitis. *J Allergy Clin Immunol*. 2006;118(1):226-232.
65. Charman CR, Morris AD, Williams HC. Topical corticosteroid phobia in patients with atopic eczema. *Br J Dermatol*. 2000;142(5):931-936.
66. Lee JY, Her Y, Kim CW, et al. Topical corticosteroid phobia among parents of children with atopic eczema in Korea. *Ann Dermatol*. 2015;27(5):499-506.
67. Aubert-Wastiaux H, Moret L, Le Rhun A, et al. Topical corticosteroid phobia in atopic dermatitis: a study of its nature, origins and frequency. *Br J Dermatol*. 2011;165(4):808-814.
68. Chi CC, Wang SH, Mayon-White R, et al. Pregnancy outcomes after maternal exposure to topical corticosteroids: a UK population-based cohort study. *JAMA Dermatol*. 2013;149(11):1274-1280.

69. Chi CC, Wang SH, Wojnarowska F, et al. Safety of topical corticosteroids in pregnancy. *Cochrane Database Syst Rev*. 2015;(10):CD007346.
70. Singh G, Singh PK. Tachyphylaxis to topical steroid measured by histamine-induced wheal suppression. *Int J Dermatol*. 1986;25(5):324-326.
71. Fusaro RM, Kingsley DN. Topical glucocorticoids. how they are used and misused. *Postgrad Med*. 1986;79(1):283-291.
72. Sarnstrand B, Brattsand R, Malmstrom A. Effect of glucocorticoids on glycosaminoglycan metabolism in cultured human skin fibroblasts. *J Invest Dermatol*. 1982;79(6):412-417.
73. Gebhardt C, Averbeck M, Diedenhofen N, et al. Dermal hyaluronan is rapidly reduced by topical treatment with glucocorticoids. *J Invest Dermatol*. 2010;130(1):141-149.
74. Zhang W, Watson CE, Liu C, et al. Glucocorticoids induce a near-total suppression of hyaluronan synthase mRNA in dermal fibroblasts and in osteoblasts: a molecular mechanism contributing to organ atrophy. *Biochem J*. 2000;349(pt 1):91-97.
75. Lee A, Bradford J, Fischer G. Long-term management of adult vulvar lichen sclerosus: a prospective cohort study of 507 women. *JAMA Dermatol*. 2015;151(10):1061-1067.
76. Hengge UR, Ruzicka T, Schwartz RA, et al. Adverse effects of topical glucocorticosteroids. *J Am Acad Dermatol*. 2006;54(1):1-15; quiz 16-18.
77. Hajar T, Leshem YA, Hanifin JM, et al. A systematic review of topical corticosteroid withdrawal ("steroid addiction") in patients with atopic dermatitis and other dermatoses. *J Am Acad Dermatol*. 2015;72(3):541-549.e2.
78. Davis MD, el-Azhary RA, Farmer SA. Results of patch testing to a corticosteroid series: a retrospective review of 1188 patients during 6 years at Mayo Clinic. *J Am Acad Dermatol*. 2007;56(6):921-927.
79. Coloe J, Zirwas MJ. Allergens in corticosteroid vehicles. *Dermatitis*. 2008;19(1):38-42.

Chapter 185 :: Retinoids
:: Anna L. Chien, Anders Vahlquist, Jean-Hilaire Saurat, John J. Voorhees, & Sewon Kang

第一百八十五章
维甲酸类药物

中文导读

维甲酸是一种通过自身或代谢转化与维甲酸受体结合并激活的分子。本章分为5节：①导言和背景；②药理作用机制；③适应证和禁忌证；④给药方案；⑤副作用及预防措施。

第一节介绍了维甲酸的概念，其由具有维生素A活性的天然化合物和视黄醇的合成类似物，拓展到通过自身或代谢转化，与维甲酸受体（RAR）结合并激活的分子。

第二节药理作用机制，介绍了RAR的发现和鉴定是具有里程碑意义的。维甲酸类药物的代谢包括视黄醇的酯化与氧化、全反式维甲酸羟基化反应，维甲酸类药物的口服生物利用度在脂肪餐中显著提高，维甲酸的代谢主要是通过氧化和链缩短亲水性代谢物而失去生物活性。

第三节适应证和禁忌证，介绍了外用维甲酸的临床应用仅限于全反式维甲酸，被批准用于治疗痤疮、光老化皮肤和黄褐斑。外用阿达帕林和他扎罗汀也被批准用于痤疮；他扎罗汀也被批准用于银屑病和光老化。贝沙罗汀被批准用于治疗皮肤T细胞淋巴瘤，阿利维甲酸被批准用于卡波西肉瘤。但不推荐新生儿和孕妇外用维甲酸类药物。维甲酸类药物口服主要应用包括异维甲酸在治疗痤疮方面非常有效；阿维A用于治疗银屑病；贝沙罗汀作为口服疗法，用于治疗至少一种全身治疗无效的CTCL；阿维A对癌前病变，包括人乳头瘤病毒诱发的肿瘤和光化性角化病有效；低剂量口服维甲酸改善光老化；口服维甲酸治疗也被用于各种形式的鱼鳞病。

第四节给药方案中介绍了维甲酸是唯一可用于临床的外用维甲酸，应根据皮肤反应进行个体化和滴定给药方案的确定。口服维甲酸类药物应根据药物种类及适应证不一而不一样。

第五节副作用及预防措施，介绍了外用维甲酸最常见的不良反应是皮肤刺激，可通过减少使用频率或数量以及通过润肤剂的使用而减轻症状；口服维甲酸最严重的不良反应是致畸，同时可出现嘴唇、皮肤和黏膜干燥等症状。最后提到了口服维甲酸类药物与其他具有类似副作用的疗法同时使用可能会增加这些不良事件的风险，应避免使用。

〔栗　娟〕

AT-A-GLANCE

- A retinoid is any molecule that by itself or through metabolic conversion binds to and activates retinoic acid receptors.
- Retinoid receptors are ligand-dependent transcription factors.
- The predominant retinoid receptors in human skin are retinoic acid receptor α (RAR-α), RAR-γ, retinoid X receptor α (RXR-α), and RXR-β. RAR-γ/RXR-α heterodimers bind to retinoic acid–responsive elements and are responsible for retinoid signaling.
- Clinical use of topical retinoids:
  - Approved indications: acne, psoriasis, cutaneous T-cell lymphoma, Kaposi sarcoma, melasma, photoaged skin
  - Unapproved indications with clinical studies supporting benefit: postinflammatory hyperpigmentation, and early stretch marks
- Clinical use of oral retinoids:
  - Approved indications: acne, chronic hand eczema, psoriasis, and cutaneous T-cell lymphoma
  - Unapproved indications with clinical studies supporting benefit: pityriasis rubra pilaris, premalignancies, photoaging, ichthyosis, and Darier White disease
- Teratogenicity is the most concerning side effect. Mucocutaneous (cheilitis, xerosis, skin peeling, conjunctivitis) involvements are common, as are reversible abnormal results on laboratory tests (hyperlipidemia, increased liver enzyme levels, and hypothyroidism [bexarotene/alitretinoin]). Musculoskeletal and central nervous system side effects are rare.

INTRODUCTION AND BACKGROUND

Retinoids are widely used as prescription drugs as well as cosmeceuticals. They are able to elicit skin responses by mediating their effects through their intranuclear retinoid receptors, acting as transcription factors. Indeed, the discovery of retinoic acid receptors (RARs) and retinoid X receptors (RXRs) have been pivotal to our understanding of the retinoid action mechanism.[1,2] In 1976, Michael Sporn and his colleagues originally defined retinoids as both the naturally occurring compounds with vitamin A activity and the synthetic analogs of retinol. This concept is no longer adequate. Now, retinoid is defined as any molecule that, by itself or through metabolic conversion, binds to and activates the RARs, thereby eliciting transcriptional activation of retinoic acid–responsive genes, resulting in specific biologic responses. Our understanding of retinoid mechanism, as highlighted in this chapter, is primarily based on action of topical natural retinoids in vivo. Mechanism for oral retinoids is less clear, and further elucidation is needed.

PHARMACOLOGY AND MECHANISM OF ACTION

STRUCTURE

NOMENCLATURE

All-*trans*-retinoic acid (tretinoin), which binds to and activates RARs, is derived from sequential oxidation of all-*trans*-retinol (or vitamin A) and all-*trans*-retinaldehyde. It is a 20-carbon molecule that consists of a cyclohexenyl ring, a side chain with four double bonds (all arranged in *trans*-configuration), and a carboxylic-acid end group (Fig. 185-1). The numbering of the carbon atoms is as shown in Fig. 185-1. The terms *9-cis-* (alitretinoin) and *13-cis-retinoic acid* (isotretinoin) refer to stereoisomers of all-*trans*-retinoic acid in which the double bond that begins with the 9th and 13th carbon atoms, respectively, is in the *cis-* rather than *trans-*configuration. The fourth carbon atom is located in the cyclohexenyl ring of retinoic acid and is involved in a hydroxylation reaction to generate 4-hydroxy-retinoic acid (see Fig. 185-1). The addition of a hydroxyl group to the cyclohexenyl ring renders the molecule more polar, making it more amenable to excretion/elimination.[3,4]

A group of compounds referred to as *retinyl esters* functions as the molecular storage form of retinol. The compounds are formed by esterification of retinol with fatty acids (see Fig. 185-1), which specify the ester. Hydrolysis of retinyl esters regenerates retinol (see Fig. 185-1).

Retinoids are also classified into first, second, and third generations. First-generation retinoids include all-*trans*-retinoic acid (tretinoin), 13-*cis*-retinoic acid (isotretinoin), and 9-*cis*-retinoic acid (alitretinoin). Through replacement of the β-ionone ring in all-*trans*-retinoic acid with an aromatic structure, newer retinoids, also known as second-generation of retinoids, were synthesized in the 1970s. These include etretinate, which is an ethyl ester, and its free acid metabolite, acitretin. With the discovery of retinoic acid receptors, receptor-specific, third-generation retinoids adapalene, tazarotene, and bexarotene were developed (Fig. 185-2). In fact, the second- and third-generation retinoids are also known as synthetic retinoids. They bear no structural similarities to all-*trans*-retinol or retinoic acid yet are still considered retinoids by virtue of their ability to activate the receptor(s), therefore mediating the retinoid effect.

RETINOID RECEPTORS

The discovery and characterization of RARs as having molecular features that are similar to steroid and thyroid hormone receptors were landmark findings.[1,2] A

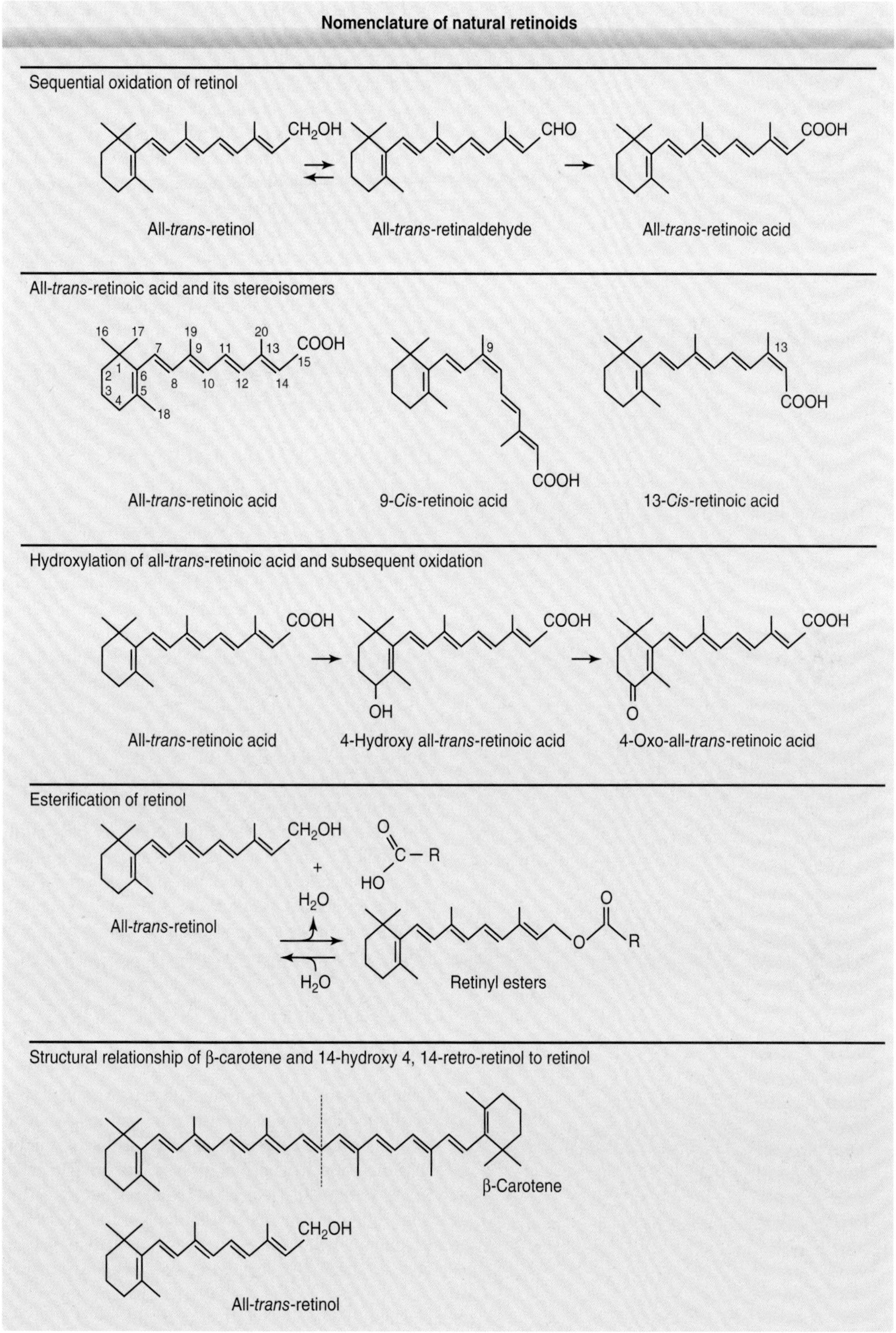

Nomenclature of natural retinoids

Figure 185-1 Nomenclature of natural retinoids.

characteristic common to these receptors is that they bind to regulatory regions in DNA called *hormone response elements*, or *target sequences*, and activate gene transcription in a ligand-dependent manner. These receptors bind to specific DNA sequences as dimers. The critical partner for heterodimerization and functioning of RAR is the RXR,[5] whose physiologic ligand is 9-*cis*-retinoic acid.[3] There are three different members of RAR (α, β, and γ) and RXR (α, β, and γ), each encoded by different genes. When the heterodimer binds to the hormone response element, specifically the retinoic acid–responsive element (RARE) in the gene promoter, the basal transcriptional machinery is stimulated. In skin, cellular retinoic acid binding protein (CRABP) II, cellular retinol binding protein (CRBP), retinoic acid 4-hydroxylase (CYP26), and keratin 6—all of which contain RAREs—are regulated by all-*trans*-retinoic acid.[6-9] These protein products, in turn, activate other non–RARE-containing genes in a cascading reaction to produce the clinical features of retinoid action in skin (Fig. 185-3). Please see Table 185-1 for additional genes regulated by topical retinoids.

METABOLISM

ESTERIFICATION AND OXIDATION OF RETINOL

Treatment of human skin with all-*trans*-retinol or retinaldehyde increases retinyl ester levels in the epidermal layer by more than 10-fold.[6] This reaction is catalyzed by two enzymes: (1) lecithin/retinol acyltransferase and (2) acyl-coenzyme A/retinol acyltransferase. In human keratinocytes, lecithin/retinol acyltransferase has the predominant retinol-esterifying activity.[10]

Sequential oxidation of all-*trans*-retinol forms all-*trans*-retinoic acid, with all-*trans*-retinaldehyde as the intermediate metabolite. The first step (oxidation of all-*trans*-retinol to all-*trans*-retinaldehyde) is rate limiting for all-*trans*-retinoic acid formation. Application of all-*trans*-retinol or retinaldehyde to human skin results in histologic and molecular alterations that mimic those after all-*trans*-retinoic acid treatment.[6] These include epidermal hyperplasia; epidermal spongiosis; compaction of the stratum corneum; and induction of CRBP, CRABP-II, and CYP26.[10,11]

HYDROXYLATION OF ALL-*TRANS*-RETINOIC ACID

In human skin, all-*trans*-retinoic acid is catabolized primarily to the more polar 4-hydroxy-all-*trans*-retinoic acid, which is further metabolized to 4-oxo-retinoic acid. In untreated normal human skin, CYP26 activity is minimally detectable. Administration of all-*trans*-retinoic acid, all-*trans*-retinol or retinaldehyde to human skin, however, increases its activity several fold.[11,12] The CYP26 activity can be effectively inhibited by ketoconazole and a related azole, liarozole.[12,13] By blocking this major inactivation pathway of all-*trans*-retinoic acid, topical liarozole can serve as a retinoic acid mimetic amplifying human skin responses to all-*trans*-retinol and all-*trans*-retinoic acid.[13] This approach of targeting CYP26 has given rise to a novel class of new chemical entities referred to as *retinoic acid metabolism blocking agents* (RAMBAs). The drug development progress for RAMBA, however, has been slow.

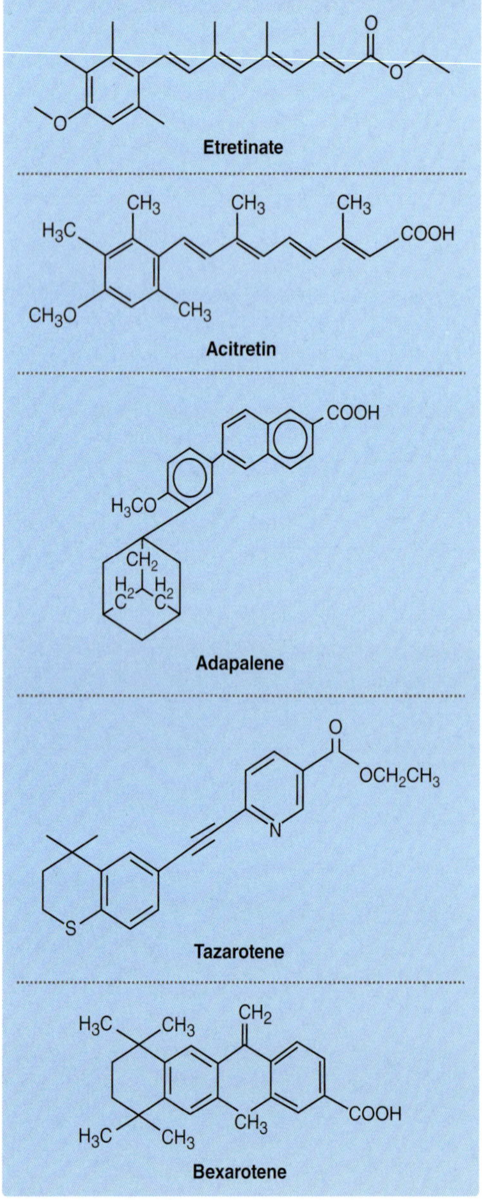

Figure 185-2 Chemical structures of the synthetic retinoids etretinate, acitretin, adapalene, tazarotene, and bexarotene.

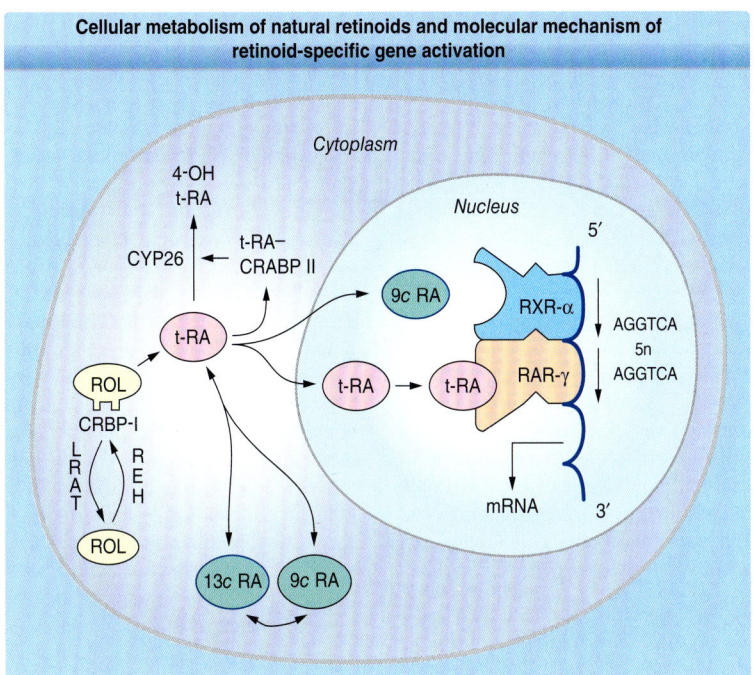

Figure 185-3 Cellular metabolism of natural retinoids and molecular mechanism of retinoid-specific gene activation. Retinol (ROL) delivered to a cell is bound to cellular retinol binding protein-I (CRBP-I). ROL can be esterified, via lecithin:retinol acyltransferase (LRAT), and stored as ROL esters. Hydrolysis of ROL ester by its hydrolase (REH) yields free ROL. Sequential oxidation of ROL generates retinoic acid (RA), which is bound to cellular retinoic acid binding protein (CRABP). All-*trans*-RA (*t*-RA) can be isomerized to 9-*cis*-RA (9*c* RA). Hydroxylation of *t* RA by cytochrome-P$_{450}$ enzyme CYP26 generates 4-OH RA, which is relatively inactive. Retinoic acid receptors (RARs) and retinoid X receptors (RXRs) are intranuclear receptors for retinoids. In human skin, RAR-γ and RXR-α heterodimers bound to RA-response elements (such as AGGTCA direct repeats) transduce retinoid effects in the presence of RAR ligands. mRNA, messenger RNA.

TABLE 185-1
Retinoid Target Genes

GENE[a]	ROLE
Cellular retinol binding protein (CRBP)	Intracellular transport protein for retinol
Cellular retinoic acid binding protein (CRABP) II	Intracellular transport protein for retinoic acid
Retinoic acid 4-hydroxylase (CYP26)	Cytochrome P450 enzyme that inactivates all-*trans*-retinoic acid by hydroxylation at the fourth carbon molecule; this CYP26 is inducible by retinoic acid
Keratin 6	An intermediate filament; pairs with keratin 16 or 17
Heparin-binding (HB)-EGF	Induced by retinoic acid; stimulates basal cell growth via EGF receptor activation; neither HB-EGF nor AR possesses RARE; thus, RAR/RXR is likely regulating other transcription factor(s) that would, in turn, regulate AR and HB-EGF gene expression
Amphiregulin (AR)	

[a]Genes known to be regulated by topical retinoids.
(HB)-EGF, heparin binding-epidermal growth factor; RARE, retinoic acid–responsive element; RXR, retinoid X receptor.

ORAL RETINOIDS

Metabolism and pharmacokinetics for oral retinoids share similarities as topical retinoids but also exhibit differences. Because of their lipophilicity, the oral bioavailability of all retinoids is markedly enhanced when they are administrated with food, especially with fatty meals. Retinoids are metabolized mainly by oxidation and chain shortening to biologically inactive and hydrophilic metabolites, which facilitate biliary or renal elimination (or both).

Isotretinoin and Other First-Generation Retinoids: Isotretinoin and alitretinoin are partially interconvertible isomers that differ in their elimination half-lives. Isotretinoin undergoes first-pass metabolism in the liver and subsequent enterohepatic recycling. The major metabolite is 4-oxoisotretinoin, which has reduced bioactivity; both compounds are excreted in urine and feces. After the end of treatment, endogenous concentrations of isotretinoin and its major metabolite are reached within 2 weeks. Therefore, a 1-month posttherapy period of contraception provides an adequate safety margin.[14]

Acitretin and Etretinate: Etretinate is a prodrug of acitretin that undergoes extensive hydrolysis in the body to yield the corresponding acid metabolite. Acitretin has a great pharmacokinetic advantage because it is eliminated more rapidly than etretinate.[15] Whereas etretinate is approximately 50 times more lipophilic than acitretin and binds strongly to plasma lipoproteins, acitretin binds to albumin. Thus, after etretinate is taken, it is stored in adipose tissue from which it is released slowly; it has a half-life of up to 120 days. In contrast, acitretin has a half-life of only 2 days.[15] However, small amounts of etretinate can be formed in patients receiving acitretin if it is taken simultaneously with alcohol.[16] This has prompted the manufacturer to extend the time of compulsory contraception in patients taking acitretin to 2 years (3 years in the United States).[17] Acitretin still has a pharmacokinetic advantage over etretinate; however, all women must strictly avoid alcohol consumption during treatment and for 2 months thereafter.[16] Acitretin metabolism primarily involves isomerization instead of oxidation. The major metabolite of acitretin is its 13-cis-isomer, which is inactive.

Bexarotene: Bexarotene is approximately 100-fold more potent in activating retinoid X receptors than RARs. The half-life for this drug is between 7 and 9 hours.[18] Bexarotene is metabolized by CYP 3A4 and generates its own inactive oxidative metabolites via hepatic CYP 3A4 induction. Neither bexarotene nor its metabolites are excreted in urine; thus, elimination is believed to occur primarily via the hepatobiliary system.[19]

INDICATIONS AND CONTRAINDICATIONS

TOPICAL RETINOIDS

Until recently, clinical use of topical retinoids has been limited to all-*trans*-retinoic acid, which is approved in the United States for the treatment of acne, photoaged skin, and melasma. Topical adapalene and tazarotene have also received approval for acne; tazarotene has received approval for psoriasis and photoaging. Bexarotene is approved for management of cutaneous T-cell lymphoma, and alitretinoin is approved for patients with Kaposi sarcoma (KS).

It is widely accepted that topical retinoids are extremely effective for acne therapy, especially for comedonal lesions. Of the different antiacne medications, retinoids are thought to be the best, if not the only, agents to normalize the abnormal follicular epithelial differentiation and desquamation that occur in acne. Therefore, the use of retinoids can also provide protection against the development of new lesions. This prophylactic property is the basis for including topical retinoid in almost all antiacne regimens. Moreover, in an era in which antibiotic stewardship has come to the forefront, retinoid is playing an even more important role in acne treatment in place of antibiotics.

Fine wrinkles and dyspigmentation are two features of photoaged skin that are improved by topical tretinoin or tazarotene. Several weeks of treatment are required before clinical improvement is appreciated.[20-22] For the effacement of fine wrinkles by topical tretinoin, partial restoration of markedly reduced levels of collagen in sun-exposed skin toward those seen in sun-protected skin appears to be responsible.[21,23]

Primary cutaneous T-cell lymphoma (CTCL) is characterized by clonal proliferation of skin-homing malignant T lymphocytes. As an RXR-selective retinoid, topical bexarotene inhibits tumor cell growth, encourages terminal differentiation, and induces apoptosis.[24] It may also play a role in chemoprophylaxis.[25,26]

Alitretinoin gel was approved in 1999 for the management of cutaneous KS, which is caused by human herpes virus 8 (HHV-8). Alitretinoin's mechanism of action in KS is not entirely clear, but it presumably relates to inhibition of cellular proliferation as well as induction of apoptosis seen with other retinoids. Furthermore, alitretinoin and tretinoin have been reported to inhibit herpes simplex virus replication; thus, alitretinoin may have an antiviral role against HHV-8.[27] In clinical trials, most patients saw improvement after 4 to 8 weeks of treatment with the most significant response occurring after 14 weeks of therapy.[28]

Besides the approved indications, topical retinoids have been demonstrated to be effective in the treatment of several other conditions. These include, but are not limited to, postinflammatory hyperpigmentation in blacks,[29] actinic dyspigmentation in Chinese and Japanese individuals,[30] and early stretch marks.[31] The controlled studies show more than therapeutic efficacies. They also provide valuable information to dispel some of the myths about retinoid use in humans. For example, African Americans and Asians tolerate topical tretinoin as well as, if not better than,[29,30,32] whites.[21,33] Furthermore, the often observed retinoid dermatitis does not usually lead to postinflammatory hyperpigmentation in those with greater constitutive pigmentation.

Many other skin disorders have been reported to be improved by topical retinoids, but most of them have not been rigorously studied; thus, their therapeutic claims should be interpreted with caution. Molluscum contagiosum, warts, and various forms of ichthyosis may be improved by topical retinoids to a variable degree. In psoriasis, especially, irritation of treated skin has limited the use. Topical tazarotene, which is approved for psoriasis, does not appear to have fully overcome the irritation problem[34]; thus, it is typically used in combination with topical steroids.

With such a wide variety of skin conditions treatable by topical retinoids, their use has included all age groups, perhaps with the exception of neonates. The use of topical retinoids in pregnancy is an emotional issue. As discussed later, teratogenicity is not caused by topical retinoids. However, because none of the dermatologic conditions seen in pregnancy that may respond to topical retinoids (ie, acne, melasma, stretch marks) is life threatening to the mother or the fetus, it seems prudent to delay the treatment until after delivery.

ORAL RETINOIDS

Isotretinoin is remarkably effective in treating acne, possibly because it affects majority of etiologic factors implicated in the pathogenesis of acne: sebum production (caused by atrophy of sebaceous glands not achievable by topical retinoids or other systemic retinoids), comedogenesis, and colonization with *Propionibacterium acnes*.[35] In the early 1980s, isotretinoin treatment was restricted to patients with severe nodulocystic acne. Its use now has extended to patients with less severe disease who respond unsatisfactorily to conventional therapies or who have extensive scarring.[36,37] Lastly, in the age of antibiotic stewardship, isotretinoin has also been explored for the treatment of rosacea in an off-label manner.[38,39]

In addition to acne, oral retinoid is also used to manage psoriasis and the retinoid of choice is acitretin. The best results have been obtained in pustular psoriasis of the palmoplantar or generalized (von Zumbusch) type.[40-42] Rebound does not usually occur after cessation of treatment, and reintroduction of the drug produces a beneficial response.[43] Although complete clearing of plaque-type psoriasis is achieved in only approximately 30% of treated patients, significant improvement is obtained in a further 50%.[44-46] The decrease in the psoriasis area and severity index is approximately 60% to 70%, depending on the dosage.[44,47] Combination of acitretin with other antipsoriatic agents may be required.

Oral retinoid can also be used to manage chronic hand eczema. Alitretinoin is approved in Europe and Canada for treatment-resistant chronic hand eczema. Between 3 and 6 months of therapy is usually required to fully appreciate the effect.[48] This medication is not yet available in the United States.

In 1999, the U.S. Food and Drug Administration (FDA) approved bexarotene as oral therapy for the treatment of CTCL that is refractory to at least one systemic therapy. In early (IA–IIA) and advanced (IIB–IVB) stages of CTCL, oral bexarotene monotherapy produced approximately 60% and 50% response rates, respectively, at a dosage of 300 mg/m² or more per day within the first 2 months in most patients.[49,50]

Multiple other skin disorders respond to oral retinoids but for only a few of them is the effect established in controlled studies.[51] In pityriasis rubra pilaris, early treatment with acitretin appears to offer the best chance for clearing of this eruption. In extensive cases, concomitant use of methotrexate may be advantageous, but this combination carries an increased risk for toxicity.[52]

Acitretin is effective in the treatment of premalignancies, including human papillomavirus–induced tumors and actinic keratoses. In basal cell nevus syndrome and xeroderma pigmentosum, these drugs dramatically reduce the incidence of malignant degeneration of the precancers. A double-blind study demonstrated that acitretin at a dosage of 30 mg/day for 6 months prevented the development of premalignant and malignant skin lesions in renal transplant recipients.[53]

More recently, there is an increase in usage of low-dose oral retinoids for photoaging, especially outside of the United States. However, data regarding this indication are mixed. In one study, isotretinoin significantly improved the clinical features of photoaging and increased collagen as well as elastic fiber density.[54] In contrast, other studies found no significant differences in clinical and histologic improvement of photoaging when comparing isotretinoin to topical retinoic acid 0.05%. No significant differences were also seen when comparing isotretinoin to daily sunscreen use.[55,56] More rigorous studies are needed to further elucidate these effects. Furthermore, one must also consider the potential adverse effects of oral retinoids when choosing this treatment modality for skin aging.

Oral retinoid therapy has also been used in various forms of ichthyosis. The best results are obtained with acitretin for autosomal recessive congenital ichthyoses such as lamellar ichthyosis. Moderate to severe forms of Darier-White disease have also been shown to respond to retinoid therapy. Care should be taken to initiate therapy with a low dosage, such as 10 mg/day of acitretin, to prevent initial exacerbation of the disease; usually 20 mg/day is sufficient for significant improvement. Long-term treatment is usually needed to prevent relapse.

DOSING REGIMEN

TOPICAL RETINOIDS

For decades, tretinoin was the only topical retinoid available for clinical use sold under the trade name Retin-A. Now, tretinoin is also available in other formulations (Table 185-2). Adapalene is also available in varying formulations, and more recently, combination medications have been introduced (see Table 185-2). For acne and psoriasis, topical tazarotene is available and for photoaging treatment, tretinoin and tazarotene are approved for use. Tretinoin 0.05%/hydroquinone 4%–fluocinolone 0.1% is a topical combination approved for the treatment of melasma. Different formulations allow some flexibility in terms of tailoring the therapy to an individual's skin dryness or oiliness. Finally, more recently approved topical retinoids, including bexarotene and alitretinoin, are sold in gel formulations.

The most important element in topical retinoid therapy is patient education. It must be explained to each patient that local skin irritation, characterized by redness and peeling, can be expected. The concept that clinical improvement correlates with the degree of irritation has been erased through a large, controlled clinical study in which 0.025% and 0.1% tretinoin were shown to be equally efficacious, but the former was significantly less irritating than the latter.[22] Therefore, unlike most medications for which the dosing schedule may be set as once or twice daily, administration of a topical retinoid should be individualized and titrated

TABLE 185-2
Dosing Regimen of Topical Retinoids

TOPICAL RETINOID	DOSAGE SCHEDULES AND EXAMPLE FORMS
Tretinoin	Avita (0.025% cream and gel)
	Atralin (0.05% gel)
	Refissa (0.05% cream)
	Renova (0.02% cream)
	Retin-A (0.025%, 0.05%, 0.1% cream; 0.01%, 0.025% gel)
	Retin-A Micro (0.04% and 0.1% microsphere gel)
	Tretin-X (0.025%, 0.05%, 0.1% cream; 0.01%, 0.025% gel)
	TriLuma (tretinoin 0.05%/hydroquinone 4%–fluocinolone 0.1% cream)
	Ziana (tretinoin 0.025%/clindamycin 1.2% gel)
Adapalene	Differin 0.1% cream; 0.1%, 0.3% gel)
	Epiduo (adapalene 0.1%/benzoyl peroxide 2.5% gel)[a]
Tazarotene	Tazorac 0.05%, 0.1% gel and cream
	Avage (0.1% cream)
Bexarotene	Targretin gel
Alitretinoin	Panretin gel

[a]The chemical structure of adapalene renders it more resistant to oxidation (thus permitting its combination with benzoyl peroxide) and ultraviolet degradation frequently seen with retinoids.

depending on the skin reaction.

Under the nonprescription category, there are countless "natural retinoid" preparations with various claims (mostly antiaging). Most of these contain retinyl esters, which are less active than retinol and retinaldehyde. Whether any of these products can deliver retinoid activity to human skin should be established in every case and formulation. Current experts' views are that, with appropriate dosing and formulation, some preparations do induce biological effects that may reverse and partially prevent skin aging.

ORAL RETINOIDS

The consensus is that optimal benefit in acne would be achieved with a daily dose of isotretinoin, approximately 0.5 to 1 mg/kg of body weight per day (Table 185-3).[35] Posttherapy relapse is minimized by administering a cumulative dose of at least 120 mg/kg.[57] This implies 6 to 8 months of therapy. A lag period of 1 to 3 months may occur before the onset of the therapeutic effect, and a flare-up of disease during the first few weeks may be observed. Continued healing of acne after the discontinuation of therapy regularly occurs. Approximately one third of patients with acne require a second course of therapy for either persistent disease or relapse.

The recommended alitretinoin dose in treatment of chronic hand eczema is 10 to 30 mg/day. Treatment periods of up to 6 months are often needed before a full evaluation of the therapeutic effects can be made.

In psoriasis, patients are typically given an initial low dose of 10 to 25 mg/day of acitretin followed by progressively increasing doses.[58] Total clearing of the lesions may require a combination of treatments, such as retinoids plus topical glucocorticoids, topical vitamin D derivatives, dithranol (anthralin), ultraviolet B irradiation, or photochemotherapy (psoralen and ultraviolet A light [PUVA] treatment).[59-63]

The recommended initial dosage of bexarotene is 300 mg/m²/day, administered as a single oral dose with meals. Based on the severity of adverse effects, the dosage may be adjusted down to 100 or 200 mg/m²/day, or administration may be suspended temporarily. If CTCL does not respond after 8 weeks of therapy, the dosage may be increased to 400 mg/m²/day with careful monitoring.[49,50]

SIDE EFFECTS AND PRECAUTIONS

ADVERSE EFFECTS

TOPICAL RETINOIDS

The most common adverse effect associated with topical retinoid use is local skin irritation. This predictable skin response is temporary, but troubling, for many patients. It tends to peak within the first month of treatment and diminishes thereafter. It responds to a

TABLE 185-3
Dosing Regimens of Retinoids in Major Indications

DRUG	INDICATION	INITIALLY (mg/kg/day)	SUSTAINED (mg/kg/day)	LENGTH OF THERAPY (months)
Isotretinoin	Acne	0.3–0.5	0.5–1.0	4–6
Acitretin	Psoriasis	0.2–0.5	0.3–0.8	>3
	DOK[a]	0.3–0.6	0.5–1.0	>3
Alitretinoin	Hand eczema	10–30[b]	10–30[b]	>6
Bexarotene	CTCL	4–8	2–4 (8)	>2

[a]Lower dosing is recommended for Darier-White disease and epidermolytic ichthyosis.
[b]Daily dose in milligrams.
CTCL, cutaneous T-cell lymphoma; DOK, disorders of keratinization (genetic).

temporary reduction in the frequency or amount of retinoid application and to liberal use of emollients.

For bexarotene and alitretinoin, local irritation is also the most common side effect. With alitretinoin, the local erythema can increase to edema and vesiculation with continued use. However, most reactions are mild to moderate with only 7% of patients requiring treatment withdrawal in clinical trials.[28] Finally, the central hypothyroidism seen with systemic bexarotene is not observed when used in the gel formulation.[64,65]

Systemic retinoid exposure, as discussed later, has been well established as a cause of embryonic death and congenital malformation, and understandably, there is concern about potential teratogenicity from long-term topical retinoid use. Systemic absorption of retinoids from topical application is negligible, and the levels of endogenous retinoic acid in the blood are not increased by twice-daily application of 0.025% tretinoin to more than 40% of body area over 1 month. Furthermore, controlled topical administration of tretinoin at doses used for acne therapy (2 g of 0.025% gel applied daily to the face, neck, and upper part of the chest for 14 days) has less influence on plasma levels of endogenous retinoids than diurnal and nutritional factors.[66] Indeed, a large, population-based study demonstrated no excess risk of birth defects in offspring born to mothers who were exposed to topical tretinoin during pregnancy.[67] Therefore, no evidence exists for teratogenicity of topical tretinoin in humans.

ORAL RETINOIDS

See Table 185-4.

Teratogenesis as alluded to earlier is the most serious adverse effect of oral retinoids. Retinoid-induced birth defects include auditory, cardiovascular, craniofacial, ocular, axial and acral skeletal, central nervous system (hydrocephalus, microcephaly), and thymus gland abnormalities.[68] In men, retinoid therapy does not appear to produce abnormalities in spermatogenesis, sperm morphology, or sperm motility.[69] However, it is usually recommended that men who are actively trying to father children avoid systemic retinoid therapy.

Most patients receiving oral retinoids will also develop dryness of the lips, skin, and mucous membranes. More severe cases can lead to significant retinoid dermatitis, which can be misdiagnosed as an allergic reaction to the drug with resulting inappropriate discontinuation of the retinoid medication. Bexarotene appears to induce fewer mucocutaneous and ocular side effects than other classes of retinoids; localized or extensive exfoliative dermatitis is the most common cutaneous side effect with bexarotene.[18] *Staphylococcus aureus* colonization tends to correlate with isotretinoin-induced reduction in sebum production and may lead to overt cutaneous infections.[70] Various ill-defined skin eruptions, called *retinoid dermatitis*, are also observed frequently.

Blepharoconjunctivitis occurs with varying severity in about one third of patients treated with isotretinoin, likely related to its effects on meibomian glands. If artificial tears fail to alleviate the conjunctivitis, ophthalmologic consultation should be sought. Alterations in visual function, mainly poor night vision, excessive glare sensitivity, and changes in color perception, also have been reported.[71]

Diffuse or localized hair loss (telogen effluvium), which is more severe during treatment with acitretin than with isotretinoin, is a common complaint, although objective alopecia tends to occur only at higher dosage levels and after several months of therapy. Nail thinning and paronychia-like changes with periungual granulation tissue may occur.

Bone pain without objective evidence of any abnormalities and without sequelae is frequent in retinoid-treated patients. Several reports with conflicting results have implicated synthetic retinoids in the formation of diffuse idiopathic skeletal hyperostosis (DISH) syndrome–like bone changes and calcification of tendons and ligaments.[72-74] Prospective studies have shown that the hyperostotic effects of retinoids are mostly asymptomatic and likely involve worsening of preexisting skeletal overgrowth rather than de novo changes.[75,76] No baseline radiographs are required, although monitoring patients at high risk who receive prolonged high-dose retinoid treatment may be useful.

TABLE 185-4
Adverse Effects of Systemic Retinoids: A Summary

	ISOTRETINOIN	ALITRETINOIN	ACITRETIN	BEXAROTENE
Teratogenicity	+	+	+	+
Mucocutaneous	+	+	+	+
Ocular	++	+	+	+
Alopecia	(+)	+	+	+
Headache	+	++	+	+
Musculoskeletal	++	+	+	+
Hepatotoxicity	(+)	(+)	+	+
Neutropenia	−	−	−	+
Hyperlipidemia	++	+	+	++
Hypothyroidism	−	+	−	+

Muscle pain and cramps rarely occur in patients taking etretinate or acitretin; however, these muscle effects are frequent with isotretinoin, particularly in individuals involved in vigorous physical activity. Increased muscle tone, axial muscle rigidity, and myopathy were reported to be related to etretinate and acitretin therapy.[77]

Central nervous system side effects are rare. Although signs of increased intracranial pressure are observed occasionally, the complete syndrome with papilledema (pseudotumor cerebri) and impaired vision is exceptional.[78] Concomitant use of isotretinoin and tetracyclines, which rarely produce increased intracranial hypertension, is the major risk factor for development of pseudotumor cerebri.

Anecdotal reports suggest a causal association between isotretinoin therapy and severe depression with suicide attempts.[79] However, large-scale epidemiologic studies provide no evidence that isotretinoin exposure is associated with any greater risk of psychiatric disorders than is antibiotic use in patients with acne.[80]

Clinical and biochemical central hypothyroidism occurred in 40% of patients in the trials of bexarotene therapy for CTCL. It was rapidly and completely reversible with cessation of therapy without any clinical sequelae.[49,81] The same adverse effect has been noted with alitretinoin, which is expected because both drugs bind to RXR that dimerizes with the nuclear thyroid receptor.

In very rare cases, isotretinoin has been linked to exacerbation of inflammatory bowel disease. A 5-year prospective study did not demonstrate an increased risk of inflammatory bowel disease or of cancer, diabetes, or cardiovascular disease in association with long-term etretinate use for psoriasis[82]; similar safety of long-term acitretin, bexarotene, or alitretinoin therapy has not been established.

Serum lipid changes are the most frequent abnormalities in laboratory test results seen with retinoid therapy. Interestingly, retinoid-induced hyperlipidemia is not associated with accelerated atherosclerosis or increased risk of cardiovascular disease with prolonged therapy. Depending on the type and dosage of retinoid, triglyceride levels are elevated in 50% to 80% and cholesterol levels in 30% to 50% of treated patients.[49,73,83] Disturbance of blood lipid levels is generally higher with isotretinoin and bexarotene than with acitretin. In cases of severe retinoid-induced hypertriglyceridemia, eruptive xanthomas and acute pancreatitis may occur. Discontinuation of therapy is required if the triglyceride level reaches 800 mg/dL. A less severe increase may be treated by dosage reduction or lifestyle changes. In some instances, use of lipid-lowering agents may be indicated.[84] Coadministration of atorvastatin with bexarotene is recommended.[18]

Transient abnormal elevations in serum transaminase levels have been reported in approximately 20% of patients treated with etretinate or acitretin and occur much less frequently with other retinoids. Increases in serum alkaline phosphatase levels have been reported infrequently with isotretinoin and are clinically insignificant. Transaminase elevations of more than three times the upper normal range should lead to discontinuation of retinoid therapy. It is believed that in patients with hepatic insufficiency, there is impaired retinoid drug elimination.[85]

A high incidence (28%) of dose-related neutropenia has been reported with the use of bexarotene therapy for CTCL, occurring as early as 2 to 4 weeks after initiation of treatment.[49] Hematologic abnormalities are much less common with other retinoids. Bleeding complications caused by isotretinoin-induced fibrinolysis has been reported.[86]

MONITORING OF THERAPY

Most adverse effects associated with retinoids are preventable and manageable with proper patient selection, dosage adjustments, discontinuation of treatment, and routine monitoring for potential toxicity. With isotretinoin, women with childbearing potential must have two negative results on a pregnancy test spaced 30 days apart and must practice effective contraception during treatment and for 1 month (2 months in some countries) after the completion of therapy.[87] The iPLEDGE program (http://www.ipledgeprogram.com) has been put into effect by the FDA and the manufacturer to minimize the risk of isotretinoin teratogenicity. Similar but less strict programs exist in Europe and elsewhere.

Ensuring that the patient avoids pregnancy during therapy is as imperative when prescribing acitretin and etretinate as when prescribing isotretinoin. However, because of the frequent prospect of long-term treatment of more chronic diseases (eg, psoriasis and ichthyosis) and the slow elimination of aromatic retinoids from the body after interruption of therapy, acitretin (or etretinate) therapy is usually not recommended for female patients with childbearing potential. Additional precautions before oral retinoid therapy include measurement of baseline serum lipid, complete blood count, thyroid function (bexarotene, alitretinoin), and liver enzyme levels. Laboratory studies are also performed during therapy. Providers should also assess for any history of skeletal abnormalities.

DRUG INTERACTIONS

The major avenue of tretinoin inactivation is through CYP26. Ketoconazole and liarozole are effective inhibitors of CYP26 and thus concurrent use of these azoles and topical tretinoin can prolong the half-life of tretinoin locally in the skin, thereby aggravating local side effect. Other than retinoids, no other compounds have been shown to induce CYP26.

The concurrent use of oral retinoids with other therapies having similar side effects may increase the risk of these adverse events. Tetracyclines (increased intracranial pressure, phototoxicity), alcohol (increased conversion of acitretin to etretinate, hepatotoxicity), methotrexate (hepatotoxicity), and vitamin A supplements (hypervitaminosis A) should be avoided. The concomitant administration of bexarotene and gemfibrozil may result in increased plasma concentrations of bexarotene.

ACKNOWLEDGMENTS

We would like to acknowledge the contributions of Laura Vangoor, BFA, for the graphic illustrations.

REFERENCES

1. Petkovich M, Brand NJ, Krust A, et al. A human retinoic acid receptor which belongs to the family of nuclear receptors. *Nature.* 1987;330(6147):444-450.
2. Giguere V, Ong ES, Segui P, et al. Identification of a receptor for the morphogen retinoic acid. *Nature.* 1987;330(6149):624-629.
3. Levin AA, Sturzenbecker LJ, Kazmer S, et al. 9-cis retinoic acid stereoisomer binds and activates the nuclear receptor RXRa. *Nature.* 1992;355(6358):359-361.
4. Heyman RA, Mangelsdorf DJ, Dyck JA, et al. 9-cis retinoic acid is a high affinity ligand for the retinoid X receptor. *Cell.* 1992;68(2):397-406.
5. Yu VC, Delsert C, Andersen B, et al. RXR beta: a co-regulator that enhances binding of retinoic acid, thyroid hormone, and vitamin D receptors to their cognate response element. *Cell.* 1991;67(6):1251-1266.
6. Kang S, Duell EA, Fisher GJ, et al. Application of retinol to human skin in vivo induces epidermal hyperplasia and cellular retinoid binding proteins characteristic of retinoic acid but without measurable retinoic acid levels or irritation. *J Invest Dermatol.* 1995;105(4):549-556.
7. Aström A, Pettersson U, Chambon P, et al. Retinoic acid induction of human cellular retinoic acid-binding protein-II gene transcription is mediated by retinoic acid receptor retinoid X receptor heterodimers bound to one far upstream retinoic acid-responsive element with 5-base pair spacing. *J Biol Chem.* 1994;269(35):22334-22339.
8. Fisher GJ, Reddy AP, Datta SC, et al. All-trans retinoic acid induces cellular retinol-binding protein in vivo. *J Invest Dermatol.* 1995;105(1):80-86.
9. Rosenthal DS, Griffiths CE, Yuspa SH, et al. Acute or chronic topical retinoic acid treatment of human skin in vivo alters the expression of epidermal transglutaminase, loricrin, involucrin, filaggrin, and keratins 6 and 13 but not keratins 1, 10, and 14. *J Invest Dermatol.* 1992;98(3):343-350.
10. Kurlandsky SB, Duell EA, Kang S, et al. Auto-regulation of retinoic acid biosynthesis through regulation of retinol esterification in human keratinocytes. *J Biol Chem.* 1996;28;271(26):15346-15352.
11. Duell EA, Kang S, Voorhees JJ. Retinoic acid isomers applied to human skin in vivo each induce a4-hydroxylase that inactivates only trans retinoic acid. *J Invest Dermatol.* 1996;106(2):316-320.
12. Duell EA, Aström A, Griffiths CE, et al. Human skin levels of retinoic acid and cytochrome P-450-derived 4-hydroxyretinoicacid after topical application of retinoic acid in vivo compared to concentrations required to stimulate retinoic acid receptor-mediated transcription in vitro. *J Clin Invest.* 1992;90(4):1269-1274.
13. Kang S, Duell EA, Kim KJ, et al. Liarozole inhibits human epidermal retinoic acid 4-hydroxylase activity and differentially augments human skin responses to retinoic acid and retinol in vivo. *J Invest Dermatol.* 1996;107(2):183-187.
14. Wiegand UW, Chou RC. Pharmacokinetics of oral isotretinoin. *J Am Acad Dermatol.* 1998;39(2 Pt 3):S8-S12.
15. Wiegand UW, Chou RC. Pharmacokinetics of acitretin and etretinate. *J Am Acad Dermatol.* 1998;39(2 Pt 3):S25-S33.
16. Gronhoj Larsen F, Steinkjer B, Jakobsen P, et al. Acitretin is converted to etretinate only during concomitant alcohol intake. *Br J Dermatol.* 2000;143(6):1164-1169.
17. Saurat JH. Systemic retinoids. What's new? *Dermatol Clin.* 1998;16(2):331-340.
18. Nguyen E-QH, Wolverton SE. Systemic retinoids. In: Wolverton SE, ed. *Comprehensive Dermatologic Drug Therapy.* Philadelphia: WB Saunders; 2001:269.
19. Howell SR, Shirley MA, Grese TA, et al. Bexarotene metabolism in rat, dog, and human, synthesis of oxidative metabolites, and in vitro activity at retinoid receptors. *Drug Metab Dispos.* 2001;29(7):990-998.
20. Kang S, Leyden JJ, Lowe NJ, et al. Tazarotene cream for the treatment of facial photodamage: a multicenter, investigator-masked, randomized, vehicle-controlled, parallel comparison of 0.01%, 0.025%, 0.05%, and 0.1% tazarotene creams with tretinoin emollient cream applied once daily for 24 weeks. *Arch Dermatol.* 2001;137(12):1597-1604.
21. Cho S, Loew L, Hamilton TA, et al. Long term treatment of photoaged human skin with topical retinoic acid improves epidermal cell atypia and thickens collagen band in the papillary dermis. *J Am Acad Dermatol.* 2005;53(5):769-774.
22. Griffiths CE, Kang S, Ellis CN, et al. Two concentrations of topical tretinoin (retinoic acid) cause similar improvement of photoaging but different degrees of irritation: a double-blind, vehicle controlled comparison of 0.1% and 0.025% tretinoin creams. *Arch Dermatol.* 1995;131(9):1037-1044.
23. Griffiths CE, Russman AN, Majmudar G, et al. Restoration of collagen formation in photodamaged human skin by tretinoin (retinoic acid). *N Engl J Med.* 1993;329(8):530-535.
24. Querfeld C, Nagelli LV, Rosen ST, et al. Bexarotene in the treatment of cutaneous T-cell lymphoma. *Expert Opin Pharmacother.* 2006;7(7):907-915.
25. Wu K, Kim HT, Rodriguez JL, et al. Suppression of mammary tumorigenesis in transgenic mice by RXR-selective retinoid, LGD 1069. *Cancer Epidemiol Biomarkers Prev.* 2002;11(5):467-474.
26. Rizvi NA, Marshall JL, Dahut W, et al. Phase I study of LGD 1069 in adults with advanced cancer. *Clin Cancer Res.* 1999;5(7):1658-1664.
27. Issacs CE, Kascsak R, Pullarkat RK, et al. Inhibition of herpes simplex virus replication by retinoic acid. *Antiviral Res.* 1997;33(2):117-127.
28. Cheer SM, Foster RH. Alitretinoin. *Am J Clin Dermatol.* 2000;1(5):307-314.
29. Bulengo-Ransby SM, Griffiths CE, Kimbrough-Green CK, et al. Topical tretinoin (retinoic acid) therapy for hyperpigmented lesions caused by inflammation of the skin in black patients. *N Engl J Med.* 1993;328(20):1438-1443.
30. Griffiths CE, Goldfarb MT, Finkel LJ, et al. Topical tretinoin (retinoic acid) treatment of hyperpigmented lesions associated with photoaging in Chinese and Japanese patients: a vehicle-controlled trial. *J Am Acad Dermatol.* 1994;30(1):76-84.
31. Kimbrough-Green CK, Griffiths CE, Finkel LJ, et al. Topical retinoic acid (tretinoin) for melasma in black patients: a vehicle-controlled clinical trial. *Arch Dermatol.* 1994;130(6):727-733.
32. Kang S, Kim KJ, Griffiths CE, et al. Topical tretinoin (retinoic acid) improves early stretch marks. *Arch Dermatol.*

1996;132(5):519-526.
33. Griffiths CE, Finkel LJ, Ditre CM, et al. Topical tretinoin (retinoic acid) improves melasma: a vehicle-controlled clinical trial. *Br J Dermatol.* 1993;129(4):415-421.
34. Esgleyes-Ribot T, Chandraratna RA, Lew-Kaya DA, et al. Response of psoriasis to a new topical retinoid, AGN 190168. *J Am Acad Dermatol.* 1994;30(4):581-590.
35. Layton AM, Knaggs H, Taylor J, et al. Isotretinoin for acne vulgaris: 10 years later: a safe and successful treatment. *Br J Dermatol.* 1993;129(3):292-296.
36. Eady EA, Jones CE, Tipper JL, et al. Antibiotic resistant propionibacteria in acne: need for policies to modify antibiotic usage. *Br Med J.* 1993;306(6877):555-556.
37. Cunliffe WJ, van de Kerkhof PC, Caputo R, et al. Roaccutane treatment guidelines: results of an international survey. *Dermatology.* 1997;194(4):351-357.
38. Park H, Del Rosso JQ. Use of oral isotretinoin in the management of rosacea. *J Clin Aesthet Dermatol.* 2011 Sep;4(9):54-61.
39. Asai Y, Tan J, Baibergenova A, et al. Canadian Clinical Practice Guidelines for Rosacea. *J Cutan Med Surg.* 2016 Sep;20(5):432-445.
40. Lassus A, Geiger JM. Acitretin and etretinate in the treatment of palmoplantar pustulosis: a double-blind comparative trial. *Br J Dermatol.* 1988;119(6):755-759.
41. Ozawa A, Ohkido M, Haruki Y, et al. Treatments of generalized pustular psoriasis: a multicenter study in Japan. *J Dermatol.* 1999;26(3):141-149.
42. Wolska H, Jablonska S, Langner A, et al. Etretinate therapy in generalized pustular psoriasis (Zumbusch type). Immediate and long-term results. *Dermatologica.* 1985;171(5):297-304.
43. Dubertret L, Chastang C, Beylot C, et al. Maintenance treatment of psoriasis by Tigason: a double-blind randomized clinical trial. *Br J Dermatol.* 1985;113(3):323-330.
44. van de Kerkhof P, Verfaille C. Retinoids and retinoic acid metabolism blocking agents in psoriasis. In: Vahlquist A, Duvic, eds. *Retinoids and Carotenoids in Dermatology.* New York: Informa Healthcare; 2007:125.
45. Ellis CN, Voorhees JJ. Etretinate therapy. *J Am Acad Dermatol.* 1987;16(2 Pt 1):267-291.
46. Lowe NL. When systemic retinoids fail to work in psoriasis. In: Saurat JH, eds. *Retinoids: 10 Years On.* Basel, Switzerland: Karger; 1991:341.
47. Geiger JM, Czarnetzki BM. Acitretin (Ro 10-1670, etretin): overall evaluation of clinical studies. *Dermatologica.* 1988;176(4):182-190.
48. Ruzika T, Larsen FG, Galewicz D, et al. Oral alitretinoin (9-cis retinoic acid) therapy for chronic hand dermatitis in patients refractory to standard therapy: results of a randomized, double-blind, placebo-controlled, multicenter trial. *Arch Dermatol.* 2004;140(12):1453-1459.
49. Duvic M, Martin AG, Kim Y, et al. Phase 2 and 3 clinical trial of oral bexarotene (Targretin capsules) for the treatment of refractory or persistent early-stage cutaneous T-cell lymphoma. *Arch Dermatol.* 2001;137(5):581-593.
50. Duvic M, Hymes K, Heald P, et al. Bexarotene is effective and safe for treatment of refractory advanced-stage cutaneous T-cell lymphoma: multinational phase II-III trial results. *J Clin Oncol.* 2001;19(9):2456-2471.
51. Arechalde A, Saurat JH. Retinoids: unapproved uses or indications. *Clin Dermatol.* 2000;18(1):63-76.
52. Clayton BD, Jorizzo JL, Hitchcock MG, et al. Adult pityriasis rubra pilaris: a 10-year case series. *J Am Acad Dermatol.* 1997;36(6 Pt 1):959-964.
53. Bavinck JN, Tieben LM, Van der Woude FJ, et al. Prevention of skin cancer and reduction of keratotic skin lesions during acitretin therapy in renal transplant recipients: a double-blind, placebo-controlled study. *J Clin Oncol.* 1995;13(8):1933-1938.
54. Bravo BS, Azulay DR, Luiz RR, et al. Oral isotretinoin in photoaging: objective histological evidence of efficacy and durability. *An Bras Dermatol.* 2015;90(4):479-486.
55. Bagatin E, Guadanhim LR, Enokihara MM, et al. Low-dose oral isotretinoin versus topical retinoic acid for photoaging: a randomized, comparative study. *Int J Dermatol.* 2014;53(1):114-122.
56. Bagatin E, Parada MO, Miot HA, et al. A randomized and controlled trial about the use of oral isotretinoin for photoaging. *Int J Dermatol.* 2010;49(2):207-214.
57. Lehucher-Ceyrac D, Weber-Buisset MJ. Isotretinoin and acne: a prospective analysis of 188 cases over 9 years. *Dermatology.* 1993;186(2):123-128.
58. Geiger JM, Saurat JH. Acitretin and etretinate. How and when they should be used. *Dermatol Clin.* 1993;11(1):117-129.
59. Lauharanta J, Juvakoski T, Lassus A. A clinical evaluation of the effects of an aromatic retinoid (Tigason), combination of retinoid and PUVA and PUVA alone in severe psoriasis. *Br J Dermatol.* 1981;104(3):325-332.
60. Saurat JH, Geiger JM, Amblard P, et al. Randomized double-blind multicenter study comparing acitretin-PUVA, etretinate-PUVA and placebo-PUVA in the treatment of severe psoriasis. *Dermatologica.* 1988;177(4):218-224.
61. Tanew A, Guggenbichler A, Hönigsmann H, et al. Photochemotherapy for severe psoriasis without or in combination with acitretin: a randomized, double-blind comparison study. *J Am Acad Dermatol.* 1991;25(4):682-684.
62. Roenigk HH Jr. Acitretin combination therapy. *J Am Acad Dermatol.* 1999;41(3 Pt 2):S18-S21.
63. Lebwohl M. Acitretin in combination with UVB or PUVA. *J Am Acad Dermatol.* 1999;41(3 Pt 2):S22-S24.
64. Breneman D, Duvic M, Kuzel T, et al. Phase 1 and 2 trial of bexarotene gel for skin-directed treatment of patients with cutaneous T-cell lymphoma. *Arch Dermatol.* 2002;138(3):325-332.
65. Heald P, Mehlmauer M, Martin AG, et al. Worldwide Bexarotene Study Group. Topical bexarotene therapy for patients with refractory or persistent early-stage cutaneous T-cell lymphomas: results of the phase III clinical trial. *J Am Acad Dermatol.* 2003;49(5):801-815.
66. Buchan P, Eckhoff C, Caron D, et al. Repeated topical administration of all-trans-retinoic acid and plasma levels of retinoic acids in humans. *J Am Acad Dermatol.* 1994;30(3):428-434.
67. Jick SS, Terris BZ, Jick H. First trimester topical tretinoin and congenital disorders. *Lancet.* 1993;341(8854):1181-1182.
68. Lammer EJ, chen DT, Hoar RM, et al. Retinoic acid embryopathy. *N Engl J Med.* 1985;313(14):837-841.
69. Koo J, Nguyen Q, Gambla C. Advances in psoriasis therapy. *Adv Dermatol.* 1997;12:47-72.
70. Williams RE, Doherty VR, Perkins W, et al. Staphylococcus aureus and intranasal mupirocin in patients receiving isotretinoin for acne. *Br J Dermatol.* 1992;126(4):362-366.
71. Safran AB, Halioua B, Roth A, et al. Ocular side-effects of oral treatment with retinoids. In: Saurat JH, eds. *Retinoids: 10 Years On.* Basel, Switzerland: Karger; 1991:315.
72. Carey BM, Parkin GJ, Cunliffe WJ, et al. Skeletal toxicity with isotretinoin therapy: a clinico-radiological evaluation. *Br J Dermatol.* 1988;119(5):609-614.
73. Tfelt-Hansen P, Knudsen B, Petersen E, et al. Spinal cord compression after long-term etretinate. *Lancet.* 1989;2(8658):325-326.

74. Kilcoyne RF. Effects of retinoids in bone. *J Am Acad Dermatol*. 1988;19(1 Pt 2):212-216.
75. van Dooren-Greebe RJ, Lemmens JA, De Boo T, et al. Prolonged treatment with oral retinoids in adults: no influence on the frequency and severity of spinal abnormalities. *Br J Dermatol*. 1996;134(1):71-76.
76. Ling TC, Parkin G, Islam J, et al. What is the cumulative effect of long-term, low-dose isotretinoin on the development of DISH? *Br J Dermatol*. 2001;144(3):630-632.
77. Lister RK, Lecky BR, Lewis-Jones MS, et al. Acitretin-induced myopathy. *Br J Dermatol*. 1996;134(5):989-990.
78. Bonnetblanc JM, Hugon J, Dumas M, et al. Intracranial hypertension with etretinate. *Lancet*. 1983;2(8356):974.
79. Chu A, Cunliffe WJ. The inter-relationship between isotretinoin/acne and depression. *J Eur Acad Dermatol Venereol*. 1999;12(3):263.
80. Jick SS, Kremers HM, Vasilakis-Scaramozza C. Isotretinoin use and risk of depression, psychotic symptoms, suicide, and attempted suicide. *Arch Dermatol*. 2000;136(10):1231-1236.
81. Sherman SI, Gopal J, Haugen BR, et al. Central hypothyroidism associated with retinoid X receptor-selective ligands. *N Engl J Med*. 1999;340(14):1075-1079.
82. Katz HL, Waalen J, Leach EE. Acitretin in psoriasis: an overview of adverse effects. *J Am Acad Dermatol*. 1999;41(3 Pt 2):S7-S12.
83. David M, et al. Adverse effects of retinoids. *Med Toxicol*. 1998;3:273.
84. Vahlquist C, Olsson AG, Lindholm, et al. Effects of gemfibrozil (Lopid) on hyperlipidemia in acitretin-treated patients. Results of a double-blind cross-over study. *Acta Derm Venereol*. 1995;75(5):377-380.
85. Vahlquist A, Lööf L, Nordlinder H, et al. Differential hepatotoxicity of two oral retinoids (etretinate and isotretinoin) in a patient with palmoplantar psoriasis. *Acta Derm Venereol*. 1985;65(4):359-362.
86. Bäck O, Nilsson TK. Retinoids and fibrinolysis. *Acta Derm Venereol*. 1995;75(4):290-292.
87. Leyden JL, Del Rosso JQ, Baum EW. The Use of Isotretinoin in the Treatment of Acne Vulgaris: Clinical Considerations and Future Directions. *J Clin Aesthet Dermatol*. 2014 Feb;7(2 Suppl):S3–S21.

Chapter 186 :: Systemic and Topical Antibiotics
:: Sean C. Condon, Carlos M. Isada, & Kenneth J. Tomecki

第一百八十六章
系统使用和外用抗生素

中文导读

　　皮肤和软组织感染的经验性治疗通常是成功的，不同的皮肤疾病选择的抗生素不一样。本章首先介绍了背景，指出大多数皮肤和软组织感染（SSTIs）是由革兰氏菌引起的，其中大多数对抗菌活性谱相对较窄的药物敏感，β-内酰胺类抗生素已成为治疗SSTIs的主要方法。但由于近年来社区获得性耐药病原体如耐甲氧西林金黄色葡萄球菌（MRSA）不断增加，治疗方法应以SSTIs的类型和临床严重程度为指导，在中重度化脓性SSTIs的经验性治疗中应覆盖MRSA。

　　接下来分别介绍了系统使用抗生素的药物作用机制、适应证和禁忌证、给药方案、副作用及预防措施，这些抗生素包括了青霉素、头孢菌素、四环素、克林霉素、大环内酯类、氟喹诺酮、复方磺胺甲恶唑及其他抗生素如万古霉素、达托霉素等。

　　最后介绍了外用抗生素在许多常见皮肤病的治疗中起着重要作用。对于局限性浅表感染外用抗生素可以消除全身治疗的需要，而对烧伤者外用抗生素进行预防性治疗通常是合理的，并介绍了克林霉素、莫匹罗星、杆菌肽、瑞他帕林、氨基糖苷类（新霉素和庆大霉素）、多粘菌素B、磺胺嘧啶银、夫西地酸的作用机制、适用疾病及注意事项等。

〔粟　娟〕

AT-A-GLANCE

- Empiric therapy for skin and soft-tissue infections (SSTIs) is usually successful.
- β-Lactam antibiotics (penicillins and cephalosporins) and clindamycin are first line options for empiric therapy for mild and moderate nonpurulent SSTIs.
- Antibiotic resistance is a growing concern. Culture and sensitivity help to define better management.
- Empiric therapy for moderate and severe purulent SSTIs should cover methicillin-resistant *Staphylococcus aureus* (MRSA).
- β-Lactam antibiotics and vancomycin inhibit bacterial cell wall synthesis.
- Several antibiotic classes interfere with bacterial protein synthesis by binding ribosomal subunits: tetracyclines at 30S; lincosamides (clindamycin), macrolides, streptogramins, and oxazolidinones (linezolid) at 50S.
- New agents for SSTIs include ceftaroline, lipoglycopeptides (dalbavancin, oritavancin, and televancin), and oxazolidinones (tedizolid).
- Topical antibiotics may negate the need for systemic antibiotics in the treatment of impetigo; they are unnecessary as postsurgical prophylaxis to prevent wound infection.

BACKGROUND

Antibiotics are soluble compounds usually produced by organisms that inhibit bacterial growth, and also include synthetic compounds. The majority of skin and soft tissue infections (SSTIs) are caused by Gram-positive organisms, most of which are susceptible to agents with a relatively narrow spectrum of antimicrobial activity. β-Lactams have been the mainstay of therapy for SSTIs.[1] Increased use and misuse of antibiotics have led to selection and propagation of resistant bacteria. Community-acquired resistant pathogens such as methicillin-resistant *Staphylococcus aureus* (MRSA) have increased in recent years and MRSA now accounts for 50% of all SSTIs with significant morbidity, mortality, and health-care cost.[2-5] The therapeutic approach should be guided by the type of SSTI (purulent or nonpurulent) and clinical severity (mild, moderate, or severe). Empiric therapy for moderate or severe purulent SSTIs should include coverage for MRSA.[6] β-Lactams remain the recommended empiric therapy for mild or moderate nonpurulent SSTIs. The emergence of complicated SSTIs with resistant pathogens, for example, MRSA and vancomycin-resistant *Enterococcus* (VRE) are even more ominous; such complicated infections involve deeper tissues or occur in patients with underlying disease, and may necessitate surgical intervention.

Most SSTIs respond to antibiotic monotherapy (Table 186-1). Combination therapy may be necessary in severe situations such as necrotizing fasciitis. Increasing pathogen resistance and the relative paucity of new antimicrobials may pose therapeutic challenges for physicians. Understanding the pharmacologic properties of antibiotics ensures judicious use of these agents, and familiarity with antibiotic dosing schedules and adverse events will lead to therapeutic choices that achieve the highest degree of patient compliance.

PENICILLINS

PHARMACOLOGY AND MECHANISM OF ACTION

STRUCTURE

Penicillins are members of the β-lactam family, one of the oldest and largest groups of antibiotics widely used throughout medical practice. Antibiotic activity originates with the thiazolidine ring nucleus and β-lactam ring; different side chains alter activity and resistance to degradation.[7] However, all β-lactams share a similar mechanism of action: they bind to specific penicillin-binding proteins; inhibit cell wall peptidoglycan synthesis; and inactivate an inhibitor of autolytic enzymes present on bacterial cell walls.

Penicillins are grouped by their chemical structure and resistance to bacterial degradation and can be broadly classified as natural or semisynthetic. In common practice, they are classified as natural, aminopenicillins, anti-staphylococcal, or extended-spectrum penicillins.

Natural penicillins are susceptible to β-lactamases and thus have a narrow spectrum of activity. Penicillin G is the best example in this group. Administered parenterally, penicillin G is active against *Streptococcus* spp., *Clostridium* spp., spirochetes, *Pasteurella multocida*, *Eikenella corrodens*, *Erysipelothrix rhusiopathiae*, and non–β-lactamase producing staphylococci. It is the treatment of choice for all *Treponema pallidum* infections. Penicillin V is adminstered orally, is less potent than penicillin G, and is indicated for minor infections.

Aminopenicillins (ampicillin, amoxicillin) are oral agents with a broad spectrum of activity. However, they are still susceptible to β-lactamase, have limited activity against staphylococci and enteric organisms, and lack activity against *Pseudomonas*. Aminopenicillins are commonly used for community-acquired infections of the upper airway and head and neck (bronchitis, sinusitis, otitis).

Extended-spectrum penicillins include carboxypenicillins (carbenicillin, ticarcillin) and ureidopenicillins (piperacillin), which also have a broad spectrum and susceptibility to β-lactamase. Carboxypenicillins have some activity against *Pseudomonas* spp. and *Proteus* spp., and are often administered concomitantly with aminoglycosides for serious pseudomonal infections. The ureidopenicillins, derived from ampicillin with similar Gram-positive coverage, have greater activity against Gram-negative organisms including *Pseudomonas*. Amoxicillin, ticarcillin, and piperacillin are often combined with β-lactamase inhibitors (tazobactam, clavulanic acid, sulbactam) to increase activity against *Staphylococcus aureus*.

Lastly, the antistaphylococcal penicillins (oxacillin, dicloxacillin, nafcillin) are β-lactamase resistant with good activity against *S. aureus*, but without activity against enterococci or Gram-negative organisms. β-Lactamase–resistant penicillins remain the drug of choice for methicillin-sensitive *S. aureus* SSTIs and are a good empiric therapeutic choice for mild nonpurulent SSTIs such as cellulitis where community-acquired MRSA is not suspected.

METABOLISM, ABSORPTION, AND DISTRIBUTION

Penicillin absorption is variable and depends on each compound's stability in an acidic environment and presence of food in the stomach. Most oral penicillins should be taken at least 1 hour before or after meals to avoid food binding. Amoxicillin absorption is unaffected by food. Penicillin G, nafcillin, carbenicillin, ticarcillin, and piperacillin are unstable at low pH and poorly absorbed; as such they are given parenterally. Once absorbed, penicillins are widely distributed in body fluids except for cerebrospinal fluid, prostate, and intraocular fluid where concentration is lower. Penicillins typically do not cross the blood–brain barrier, but meningitis can enhance permeability, allowing for therapeutic drug levels. Natural penicillins form low-solubility salts with amines (procaine, benzathine) that are added to penicil-

TABLE 186-1
Recommended Therapies

ORGANISM	DISEASE	FIRST-LINE THERAPY	ALTERNATIVE THERAPY
Actinomyces israelii	Actinomycosis	Penicillin or amoxicillin	Doxycycline, clindamycin, erythromycin
Bacillus anthracis	Cutaneous anthrax	Doxycycline, ciprofloxacin, levofloxacin, or moxifloxacin	Penicillin or amoxicillin (if sensitive)
Bartonella spp.	Cat-scratch disease, bacillary angiomatosis, Carrion disease, trench fever	Azithromycin (cat-scratch) Aminoglycosides (other Bartonella)	Clarithromycin, rifampin, ciprofloxacin, TMP-SMX Erythromycin or doxycycline (BA)
Borrelia burgdorferi	Lyme disease	Doxycycline or amoxicillin	Ceftriaxone, cefuroxime axetil, cefotaxime
Borrelia recurrentis	Relapsing fever	Doxycycline	Penicillin, erythromycin
Chlamydia trachomatis	Chlamydia	Doxycycline or azithromycin	Erythromycin, ofloxacin, levofloxacin
Clostridium perfringens	Gas gangrene	Penicillin G ± clindamycin	Doxycycline, chloramphenicol, metronidazole
Coxiella burnetii	Q fever	Doxycycline	Clarithromycin, TMP-SMX (pregnancy)
Ehrlichia spp.	Ehrlichiosis	Doxycycline	Tetracycline, rifampin, ciprofloxacin
Eikenella corrodens	Human bite infection	Penicillin or ampicillin	Amoxicillin-clavulanate (empiric), TMP-SMX, cefuroxime, doxycycline
Erysipelothrix rhusiopathiae	Erysipeloid	Penicillin	Cephalosporins, clindamycin, fluoroquinolones
Francisella tularensis	Tularemia	Streptomycin	Gentamicin, doxycycline, ciprofloxacin, chloramphenicol
Haemophilus ducreyi	Chancroid	Azithromycin or ceftriaxone	Erythromycin, ciprofloxacin
Klebsiella granulomatis	Granuloma inguinale	Azithromycin	Doxycycline, ciprofloxacin, erythromycin, TMP-SMX
Klebsiella rhinoscleromatis	Rhinoscleroma	Fluoroquinolones	Rifampin[a] + TMP-SMX
Neisseria gonorrhoeae	Gonorrhea	Ceftriaxone + azithromycin	Ceftriaxone + doxycycline, cefixime + azithromycin
Nocardia spp.	Nocardiosis	TMP-SMX	Susceptibility recommended
Pasteurella multocida	Animal bite infections	Penicillin, ampicillin, or amoxicillin	Doxycycline, TMP-SMX
Pseudomonas aeruginosa	Pseudomonas	Ciprofloxacin	Antipseudomonal penicillin or cephalosporin
Rickettsia spp.	Typhus, Rickettsialpox, RMSF	Doxycycline	Chloramphenicol, fluoroquinolone
Staphylococcus aureus	MSSA	Oxacillin or nafcillin	Clindamycin, macrolides
Staphylococcus aureus	HA-MRSA	Vancomycin, ceftaroline, oritavancin, dalbavancin, linezolid, tedizolid, quinupristin/dalfopristin, tigecycline	
Staphylococcus aureus	CA-MRSA	TMP-SMX, doxycycline, clindamycin	Minocycline, rifampin[a]
Streptococcus pyogenes	Erysipelas	Penicillin	Other β-lactams, clindamycin, macrolides
Treponema pallidum	Syphilis	Penicillin	Doxycycline, tetracycline
Vibrio vulnificus	Necrotizing wound infection	Doxycycline + ceftazidime	Cefotaxime, fluoroquinolones

[a]Rifampin is not recommended as monotherapy because of significant development of resistance.
BA, bacillary angiomatosis; CA-MRSA, community-acquired methicillin-resistant *Staphylococcus aureus*; HA-MRSA, healthcare–acquired methicillin-resistant *S. aureus*; MSSA, methicillin-sensitive *S. aureus*; RMSF, Rocky Mountain spotted fever; TMP-SMZ, trimethoprim-sulfamethoxazole.

lin and administered intramuscularly to allow for slower release and prolonged drug delivery. Unabsorbed penicillin is degraded by colonic bacteria, and the majority of free penicillin is excreted renally. Nafcillin, oxacillin, and ureidopenicillins are excreted via the hepatobiliary system and dose adjustment is not required in patients with renal failure. Penicillins are pregnancy category B; although excreted in breastmilk in low quantity, they are considered safe to use during breastfeeding.

INDICATIONS AND CONTRAINDICATIONS

Table 186-2 outlines the indications for penicillin therapy.

Table 186-3 outlines the contraindications and precautions for penicillin therapy.

TABLE 186-2
Indications for Penicillin Therapy

- Syphilis and nonvenereal treponematoses
- Skin and soft tissue infections (SSTIs) caused by *Streptococcus* spp. (erysipelas, scarlet fever, impetigo, etc.)
- Empiric treatment of mild or moderate nonpurulent SSTIs
- Infected human and animal bites
- Erysipeloid (*Erysipelothrix rhusiopathiae*)
- Listeriosis
- Actinomycosis
- Lyme disease (when tetracyclines are contraindicated)
- Leptospirosis (alternative to tetracyclines; pregnant woman and children <9 years old)
- Anthrax (alternative, if sensitive)

TABLE 186-3
Contraindications and Precautions of Penicillin Therapy

- Known hypersensitivity to penicillin
- Increased penicillin levels with probenecid and disulfiram
- Enhanced effect of methotrexate and warfarin
- Use with caution in patients with renal impairment

DOSING REGIMEN

Table 186-4 outlines the dosing regimens of commonly prescribed antibiotics for the treatment of SSTIs.

SIDE EFFECTS AND PRECAUTIONS

Hypersensitivity reactions are the most common adverse events reported with penicillins with manifestations ranging from mild to severe (Table 186-5).[8] Reported incidence varies and prevalence is unknown because of a lack of prospective studies. However, penicillin is the leading cause of drug-induced anaphylaxis, accounting for approximately 1% to 10% of all cases of anaphylaxis.[9] Approximately 5% to 10% of the general population reports an allergy to penicillin, but such hypersensitivity is probably overreported. If penicillin allergy is uncertain and if penicillin treatment is required, skin prick testing can detect Type I hypersensitivity, followed by intradermal testing if negative. Negative testing may allow a challenge dose of oral penicillin under observation. Approximately 10% to 20% of patients with a reported history of penicillin allergy have a positive skin test, and approximately 3% of those with a negative skin and history of allergy have an allergic response after a challenge dose of penicillin. The majority of these reactions tend to be mild. If a β-lactam is necessary for a patient with a positive skin test, desensitization is recommended.

CEPHALOSPORINS

PHARMACOLOGY AND MECHANISM OF ACTION

STRUCTURE

Cephalosporins, like penicillins, are β-lactams and inhibit bacterial cell wall synthesis by blocking peptidoglycan incorporation.[10] However, cephalosporins differ from penicillins in their structural nucleus, which has a dihydrothiazine and not a thiazolidine ring like penicillins. The dihydrothiazine ring provides resistance to some, but not all, β-lactamases. Most cephalosporins have some activity against both Gram-positive (excluding enterococci) and Gram-negative organisms, but the spectrum of activity varies widely within the group. The cephalosporins have 5 "generations" based on spectrum of activity and evolution of development. The first generation includes cephalexin, cefadroxil, and the parenteral agent cefazolin; all of which have good activity against methicillin-sensitive *S. aureus* and *Streptococcus* spp. with limited activity against Gram-negative organisms such as *Escherichia coli* and *Klebsiella* spp. Second-generation cephalosporins include cefprozil, cefaclor, cefuroxime axetil, and the parenteral agents cefotetan, cefoxitin, and cefuroxime, offering expanded Gram-negative activity over the first-generation agents, namely *Haemophilus influenzae* and *Moraxella catarrhalis*. Third-generation agents include cefdinir and the parenteral agents cefotaxime, ceftriaxone, and ceftazidime. Gram-negative coverage is expanded with the third generation but less effective against Gram-positive organisms. Thus, third-generation cephalosporins are effective in treating Gram-negative nosocomial infections. Cefotaxime and ceftriaxone cross the blood–brain barrier; as such, they are effective treatment for meningitis caused by *H. influenzae*, *Neisseria meningitidis*, and penicillin-sensitive *Streptococcus pneumoniae*. Ceftazidime is active against *Pseudomonas aeruginosa*, and cefdinir is useful in the treatment of SSTIs because of its activity against *S. aureus* and *Streptococcus* spp. Fourth-generation cephalosporins include cefepime, which has increased activity against Gram-positive bacteria compared to third-generation cephalosporins. Cefepime is active against Gram-negative bacteria such as *Pseudomonas*, *Enterobacteriaceae*, *Neisseria*, and *H. influenzae* but has greater activity against Gram-negative organisms that produce extended-spectrum β-lactamase.[11] Fifth-generation agents, or advanced-generation cephalosporins, are relatively new and include only ceftaroline. Ceftaroline is given parenterally with broad-spectrum activity against Gram-positive organisms, including MRSA, resistant *S. pneumoniae*, and Gram-negative organisms such as *H. influenzae* and *M. catarrhalis*, but not *P. aeruginosa*. Ceftaroline is indicated for the use of complicated SSTIs, including those caused by MRSA and is an option for empiric therapy for severe purulent SSTIs.[12]

TABLE 186-4
Dosing Regimens of Commonly Prescribed Antibiotics for the Treatment of Skin and Soft Tissue Infections[6]

CLASS	GENERIC NAME	ROUTE	ADULT DOSING
β-Lactam	Penicillin G	IV	1 to 4 million units q4-6h[a]
			(18 to 24 million units daily for neurosyphilis)
	Benzathine penicillin G	IM	2.4 million units × 1 dose (primary, secondary, and early latent [<1 year] syphilis)[a]
			2.4 million units weekly × 3 doses (late latent [<1 year]/unknown duration syphilis)
	Dicloxacillin	By mouth	250 to 500 mg q6h
	Nafcillin or oxacillin	IV	1 to 2 g q4-6h
	Amoxicillin	By mouth	500 mg q8h[a]
	Amoxicillin-clavulanate	By mouth	875 mg q12h[a]
	Cephalexin	By mouth	250 to 500 mg q6h
	Cefdinir	By mouth	300 mg q12h
	Cefprozil	By mouth	250 mg q12h or 500 mg q24h
	Cefazolin	IV	1 g q8h
Tetracycline	Tetracycline	By mouth	500 mg q6h (twice daily for acne)[a]
	Doxycycline	By mouth	100 mg q12-24h
	Minocycline	By mouth	100 mg q12h[a]
Macrolide	Erythromycin base	By mouth	250 to 500 mg q6 or 12h
		IV	500 mg to 1 g q6h[a]
	Clarithromycin	By mouth	250 to 500 mg q12h
	Azithromycin	By mouth	500 mg on day 1, then 250 mg daily × 2 to 5 days
			Chlamydia: 1 g single dose
		IV	500 mg q24h
Fluoroquinolone	Ciprofloxacin	By mouth, IV	Chancroid: 500 mg q12h × 3 days
			Cutaneous anthrax: 500 mg q12h × 60 days
	Levofloxacin	By mouth, IV	Uncomplicated SSTI: 500 mg q24h[a]
			Complicated SSTI: 750 mg q24 h[a]
Lincosamide	Clindamycin	By mouth	300 to 450 mg q6h
		IV	600 to 900 mg q8h
Trimethoprim-sulfamethoxazole		By mouth	1 to 2 double-strength tablets (180 mg/800 mg) q12-24h[a]

[a]Adjustments in dose or frequency of administration may be required in patients with renal impairment.
[b]Centers for Disease Control and Prevention recommendations for the treatment of gonococcal urethritis/cervicitis include concomitant therapy with azithromycin or doxycycline.
[c]Following a single dose of ceftriaxone 1 g IM or IV.

METABOLISM, ABSORPTION, AND DISTRIBUTION

Cephalosporins are a chemically diverse class of antibiotics with unique pharmacokinetic and pharmacodynamic properties. Most oral cephalosporins can be taken without food, but the esterified cephalosporins (cefuroxime, cefpodoxime) require food to extend mucosal contact time and allow enzymatic cleavage. Medications that lower the gastric pH may reduce absorption of these 2 cephalosporins. Cefaclor is an extended release formulation and requires food. Most cephalosporins are renally excreted. Cephalosporins are pregnancy category B and excreted in breastmilk to varying degrees.

INDICATIONS AND CONTRAINDICATIONS

Table 186-6 outlines the indications for cephalosporin therapy.
Table 186-7 outlines the contraindications and precautions of cephalosporin therapy.

DOSING REGIMEN

Table 186-4 outlines the dosing regimens of commonly prescribed antibiotics for the treatment of SSTIs.

TABLE 186-5
Adverse Effects

ANTIBIOTIC CLASS	PREGNANCY CLASS	COMMON ADVERSE EFFECTS	UNCOMMON ADVERSE EFFECTS
Penicillins	B	Hypersensitivity reactions: - Exanthem, urticaria - Diarrhea	Hypersensitivity reactions: - Exfoliative dermatitis, SJS, vasculitis, AGEP - Angioedema, anaphylaxis, serum sickness - Anaphylactoid reaction - Hepatitis, interstitial nephritis - Neurotoxicity (high dose) - Pulmonary infiltrate with eosinophilia (PIE) - Immune-mediated hematologic reactions - Pseudomembranous colitis
Cephalosporins	B	- Hypersensitivity as above - Diarrhea	- Hypersensitivity as above - Renal tubular necrosis - Disulfiram-like reaction (specific) - Thrombophlebitis (IV site) - Serum sickness-like reaction (cefaclor, cefprozil) - Pseudocholelithiasis (ceftriaxone)
Tetracyclines	D	- Skin and nail hyperpigmentation (minocycline) - Dental hyperpigmentation (infants, children) - GI irritation	- Photosensitivity (doxycycline) - Photoonycholysis - Fixed drug eruption - Pseudotumor cerebri - Esophageal erosion/stricture - Skeletal hypoplasia - Serum sickness - Renal toxicity - Vestibular toxicity (minocycline) - Fanconi syndrome (outdated tetracycline) - Thyroid discoloration - SJS, TEN - Pancreatitis - Blood dyscrasias (long-term use) - Hypersensitivity reactions (various) - Pseudomembranous colitis
Fluoroquinolones	C	- Nausea, vomiting - Cephalgia, dizziness	- Exanthem, photosensitivity - Delirium, seizure - Tendon rupture, arthropathy (in the immature) - QT prolongation - Hepatitis (trovafloxacin–withdrawn from United States)
Trimethoprim-sulfamethoxazole	D	- Exanthem, photosensitivity - Nausea, vomiting, anorexia - Glossitis, stomatitis - (Rare/severe reactions are more common in HIV/AIDS patients)	- SJS, TEN, vasculitis, urticaria - Pustular eruption, Sweet syndrome - Cholestatic hepatitis, hepatic necrosis - Blood dyscrasias - Severe hypersensitivity reaction - Cephalgia, hallucination, tremor - Nephrolithiasis, interstitial nephritis

(Continued)

TABLE 186-5
Adverse Effects (*Continued*)

ANTIBIOTIC CLASS	PREGNANCY CLASS	COMMON ADVERSE EFFECTS	UNCOMMON ADVERSE EFFECTS
Lincosamides (clindamycin)	B	- Diarrhea - Exanthem, urticaria	- Pseudomembranous colitis - Erythema multiforme, SJS, TEN - Elevated hepatic transaminases (reversible) - Blood dyscrasias - Neuromuscular blockade
Macrolides	B/C	- Nausea, diarrhea, abdominal pain - Dysgeusia (clarithromycin)	- Cholestatic hepatitis - Pseudomembranous colitis - Prolonged QT/torsades de pointes - Anaphylaxis - SJS

AGEP, acute generalized exanthematous pustulosis; SJS, Stevens-Johnson syndrome; TEN, toxic epidermal necrolysis.

SIDE EFFECTS AND PRECAUTIONS

Table 186-5 outlines the adverse events.

First- and second-generation cephalosporins cross-react with penicillin in approximately 10% of penicillin-allergic patients, whereas third-generation cephalosporins cross-react in 2% to 3% of penicillin-allergic patients.[9] Although penicillins and cephalosporins share a common β-lactam ring, the side chains tend to predict cross-reactivity. For example, cefoxitin, cefamandole, and cephaloridine have side chains similar to penicillin, while cefaclor, cephalexin, and cefadroxil have structural side chains similar to amoxicillin. Some oral agents lack side chain similarity to penicillin, ampicillin, or amoxicillin, including cefdinir, cefpodoxime, and cefuroxime, and may be safer for use in patients with a penicillin allergy. Patients reporting a penicillin allergy with a negative penicillin allergy skin test have no greater risk of allergic reaction to β-lactams than the general population. Cephalosporins are also able to elicit cephalosporin-specific allergic reactions as a result of their metabolite profile.

TETRACYCLINES

PHARMACOLOGY AND MECHANISM OF ACTION

STRUCTURE

Tetracyclines inhibit bacterial protein synthesis by binding to the 30S ribosomal subunit and blocking transfer RNA binding to the messenger RNA–ribosome complex.[13] Doxycycline and minocycline are semisynthetic second-generation tetracyclines that are more lipophilic and thus have greater activity than tetracycline, especially against *S. aureus* and community-acquired strains of MRSA; they may be used as empiric therapy for moderate purulent SSTIs.[6,14] As a class, tetracyclines have a broad spectrum of activity, including many Gram-positive and Gram-negative bacteria, spirochetes, *Mycoplasma*, *Rickettsia*, *Chlamydia*, and even some protozoa. Doxycycline is the preferred therapy for infections caused by *Borrelia* spp., *Chlamydia* spp., *Ehrlichia* spp. (monocytic and granulocytic ehrlichiosis), *Coxiella burnetii* (Q fever), *Leptospira* spp., *Mycoplasma* spp., and *Rickettsia* spp. Doxycycline is also used to treat infections caused by *Actinomyces* spp., *Bacillus anthracis*, *Mycobacterium marinum*, *Klebsiella granulomatis* (granuloma inguinale), and *Vibrio vulnificus*. In patients allergic to

TABLE 186-6
Indications of Cephalosporin Therapy

- Uncomplicated skin and soft tissue infections (SSTIs) caused by *Staphylococcus aureus* and *Streptococcus pyogenes* (first- and second-generation agents, plus cefdinir)
- Empiric therapy for mild or moderate nonpurulent SSTIs
- Empiric therapy for severe purulent SSTIs (ceftaroline)
- Complicated SSTIs caused by *S. aureus* (including methicillin-resistant *S. aureus*) and *S. pyogenes* (ceftaroline)
- Gonorrhea
- Lyme disease (ceftriaxone: meningitis and late disease; cefuroxime: early disease)
- Bacterial meningitis (ceftriaxone, cefotaxime)

TABLE 186-7
Contraindications and Precautions of Cephalosporin Therapy

- Known hypersensitivity to cephalosporin or penicillin (see the section "Side Effects and Precautions")
- Reduced absorption of cefdinir with antacids and iron salts
- Increased cyclosporine levels with ceftriaxone and ceftazidime
- Altered effect of warfarin with cefotetan, cefamandole, cefoperazone, cefixime, and cefaclor
- Impaired renal excretion of most cephalosporins with probenecid

penicillin, doxycycline is an acceptable treatment for animal bites and syphilis. The activity is variable for *Streptococcus pyogenes*. For nonpurulent SSTIs, among which *S. pyogenes* is common, tetracyclines are not recommended as empiric monotherapy. A tetracycline combined with a β-lactam such as amoxicillin or doxycycline can be used for empiric treatment of SSTIs when both *S. pyogenes* and MRSA are considered. Tetracyclines can be helpful for many inflammatory diseases, for example, acne, rosacea, perioral dermatitis, some autoimmune blistering diseases (bullous pemphigoid, linear immunoglobulin A bullous dermatosis, and dermatitis herpetiformis), and confluent and reticulated papillomatosis.

METABOLISM, ABSORPTION, AND DISTRIBUTION

Tetracycline is absorbed incompletely, primarily in the stomach and small intestine, necessitating its ingestion on an empty stomach. Doxycycline and minocycline are unaffected by the presence or absence of food and have longer half-lives than tetracycline, requiring less-frequent dosing. They also have much greater lipid solubility than tetracycline, allowing for good tissue penetration with rapid availability in secretions in the prostate, respiratory tract, female reproductive tract, and bile. However, patients should avoid concurrent ingestion of iron preparations, aluminum hydroxide gels, calcium and magnesium salts, or milk products, as these significantly lower absorption of all tetracyclines. Tetracycline is excreted primarily by the kidneys, and therefore dosing should be adjusted in patients with renal failure. Doxycycline is excreted in the feces and does not require adjustments in patients with hepatic or renal failure. Minocycline is largely metabolized before excretion, and does not accumulate in patients with hepatic failure. Tetracyclines can accumulate in developing bone and teeth, cross the placenta, and appear in high concentrations in breastmilk. They are pregnancy category D and should be avoided during pregnancy, while nursing, and throughout childhood.

INDICATIONS AND CONTRAINDICATIONS

Table 186-8 outlines the indications for for tetracycline therapy.

Table 186-9 outlines the contraindications and precautions of tetracycline therapy.

DOSING REGIMEN

Table 186-4 outlines the dosing regimens of commonly prescribed antibiotics for the treatment of SSTIs.

SIDE EFFECTS AND PRECAUTIONS

Table 186-5 outlines the adverse events of tetracycline therapy and Table 186-9 outlines the contraindications and precautions of tetracycline therapy.

CLINDAMYCIN

PHARMACOLOGY AND MECHANISM OF ACTION

STRUCTURE

Clindamycin is a lincosamide antibiotic derived through chemical modification of lincomycin.[15] Its absorption and spectrum are much better than lincomycin, a now obsolete medication. Clindamycin binds to the bacterial 50S ribosomal subunit and inhibits protein synthesis through blockade of peptide chain initiation. The binding site overlaps the sites of other antibiotics that bind the 50S subunit such as macrolides (erythromycin), accounting for antagonism between the drugs. Clindamycin facilitates opsonization and phagocytosis and decreases bacterial adhesion to host cells and production of staphylococcal exotoxin. Clindamycin has antiparasitic activity by targeting protein synthesis of the apicoplast, an organelle essential for parasite survival.[16]

Clindamycin is effective against most Gram-positive cocci, anaerobes, and some protozoa. In dermatologic practice, it is active against most *Streptococcus* species

TABLE 186-8
Indications for Tetracycline Therapy

First-Line Therapy
- *Borrelia* spp. infections
- *Chlamydia* spp. infections
- Ehrlichiosis
- Empiric treatment of moderate purulent skin and soft-tissue infections
- Methicillin-resistant *Staphylococcus aureus* infections
- Lyme disease
- Rickettsial diseases
- Mild to moderate tularemia
- *Mycobacterium marinum*
- Lymphogranuloma venereum
- Alternative therapy

Actinomycosis (Penicillin Allergic)
- Animal bites (*Pasteurella multocida*)
- Granuloma inguinale
- Syphilis (penicillin allergic)
- Bacillary angiomatosis
- Anthrax (*Bacillus anthracis*)
- *Yersinia pestis* infections
- Rhinoscleroma

> **TABLE 186-9**
> **Contraindications and Precautions of Tetracycline Therapy**
>
> - Patients with renal failure (impaired excretion and antianabolic properties)
> - Photosensitivity (doxycycline)
> - Nursing, pregnancy, and childhood years (<9 years of age)
> - Impaired absorption by calcium, magnesium, aluminum (other cations), iron, sodium bicarbonate, and cimetidine
> - Increased metabolism of doxycycline with the use of phenytoin, carbamazepine, barbiturates, and alcohol
> - Reduced insulin requirements in diabetic patients
> - Increased serum levels of digoxin, lithium, and warfarin
> - Methoxyflurane anesthesia (renal failure)

(including *Streptococcus viridans*), *S. aureus*, *Staphylococcus epidermidis*, *B. anthracis*, and *Nocardia* spp., but is ineffective against *Enterococcus*, Gram-negative aerobes, *Clostridium difficile*, and *T. pallidum*. Its anaerobic spectrum includes *Bacteroides fragilis*, fusobacterium, *Peptostreptococcus*, and *Clostridium perfringens*. Its protozoal spectrum includes *Toxoplasma gondii*, *Babesia* spp., and *Plasmodium falciparum*. Clindamycin is an option for mild and moderate nonpurulent SSTIs, but is not recommended as empiric therapy for purulent SSTIs because of the possibility of clindamycin resistance in MRSA.

METABOLISM, ABSORPTION, AND DISTRIBUTION

Clindamycin reaches therapeutic levels in most tissues except cerebrospinal fluid, and preferentially accumulates in polymorphonuclear leukocytes, which may explain its impact on abscesses. Clindamycin is not inhibited by food intake and is primarily metabolized by the liver and excreted in the bile with some (~10%) excretion in the urine. Dosing adjustments are necessary for patients with hepatic failure or combined hepatic and renal failure. Clindamycin is not effectively removed by dialysis.

INDICATIONS AND CONTRAINDICATIONS

Table 186-10 outlines the indications clindamycin therapy.

Table 186-11 outlines the contraindications and precautions of clindamycin therapy.

DOSING REGIMEN

Table 186-4 outlines the dosing regimens of commonly prescribed antibiotics for the treatment of SSTIs.

SIDE EFFECTS AND PRECAUTIONS

Table 186-5 outlines the adverse events.

Clindamycin frequently causes GI upset and diarrhea, the latter in 20% to 35% of patients. *C. difficile*-associated diarrhea and pseudomembranous colitis are life threatening complications that may occur in clindamycin therapy, albeit infrequently. Despite the well-known association with clindamycin, comparative studies have shown equivalent or even higher risk of *C. difficile*-associated diarrhea with other antibiotics.[16]

MACROLIDES

PHARMACOLOGY AND MECHANISM OF ACTION

STRUCTURE

Macrolide antibiotics are a diverse family with a large macrolactam ring.[17] Erythromycin is the prototypical macrolide with newer derivatives that include clarithromycin and azithromycin. Macrolides reversibly bind to the 50S ribosomal subunit and inhibit RNA-dependent protein synthesis as well as inhibit neutrophil chemotaxis and interleukin-8 secretion.[18] Macrolides have good but varied activity against Gram-positive pathogens: clarithromycin > erythromycin > azithromycin. *S. aureus* has variable susceptibility to erythromycin and resistance to *Streptococcus* species is increasing—approximately 50% of group A streptococci isolates were resistant to erythromycin in a recent pediatric population study.[18] Streptococcal resistance to macrolides is not drug specific; it occurs throughout the class. Erythromycin has poor Gram-negative coverage and its systemic use has largely been replaced by clarithromycin and azithromycin, which have good activity against *H. influenzae*, *Neisseria gonorrhoeae*, *M. catarrhalis*, *Chlamydia*, *Mycoplasma pneumoniae*, *Helicobacter pylori*, *T. gondii*, *T. pallidum*, *Borrelia burgdor-*

> **TABLE 186-10**
> **Indications for Clindamycin Therapy**
>
> - Uncomplicated skin and soft-tissue infections (SSTIs) caused by susceptible bacteria and protozoa
> - Empiric treatment of mild and moderate nonpurulent SSTIs
> - Deep tissue infections: streptococcal myositis, necrotizing fasciitis, or infections with *Clostridium perfringens* in conjunction with penicillin and surgical debridement
> - Surgical prophylaxis in penicillin-allergic patients
> - Prophylaxis for recurrent staphylococcal infection
> - Foot ulcers (in combination with agents for Gram-negative infection) in diabetic patients
> - Hidradenitis suppurativa
> - Bacterial vaginosis

> **TABLE 186-11**
> **Contraindications and Precautions of Clindamycin Therapy**
>
> - Hepatic failure
> - Colitis
> - Enhancement of neuromuscular blockade with tubocurarine and pancuronium
> - Possible antagonism with erythromycin

feri, and nontuberculous mycobacteria. Azithromycin has good activity against *P. multocida* and *E. corrodens*, making it a useful alternative in the treatment of infected animal bites. Clarithromycin is the most active macrolide against *Mycobacterium leprae* and is widely used for skin infections with several other nontuberculous mycobacteria, notable *Mycobacterium chelonae*, *Mycobacterium abscessus*, and *Mycobacterium fortuitum*.

METABOLISM, ABSORPTION, AND DISTRIBUTION

Macrolides accumulate intracellularly in polymorphonuclear leukocytes and macrophages, which accounts for their activity against intracellular pathogens. Erythromycin base is absorbed in the small intestine and inactivated by gastric acidity, hence the need for enteric-coated tablets or capsules. Erythromycin esters (erythromycin estolate, stearate, and ethylsuccinate) are less acid labile than the base form and can be taken without food. Structural modifications of clarithromycin and azithromycin confer increased acid stability, tissue penetration and spectrum of activity compared to erythromycin. Food decreases the absorption of azithromycin and has no effect on clarithromycin. Tissue concentrations of macrolides typically exceed plasma levels. Clarithromycin and azithromycin have longer half-lives than erythromycin, which allows for less-frequent dosing (see Table 186-4). Azithromycin remains in tissue longer and accumulates at high levels intracellularly allowing for daily short-term dosing after a loading dose. Erythromycin and azithromycin are metabolized by the liver, whereas clarithromycin is metabolized by the kidneys, thus requiring dose adjustment in patients with renal failure. Erythromycin and clarithromycin interact with the cytochrome P450 system, which poses numerous potential drug interactions (see Table 186-13). Clarithromycin is pregnancy category C, whereas erythromycin and azithromycin are category B.

INDICATIONS AND CONTRAINDICATIONS

Table 186-12 outlines the indications for macrolide therapy.

Table 186-13 outlines the contraindications and precautions of macrolide therapy.

DOSING REGIMEN

Table 186-4 outlines the dosing regimens of commonly prescribed antibiotics for the treatment of SSTIs.

SIDE EFFECTS AND PRECAUTIONS

Table 186-5 outlines the adverse events.

The most common side effects are abdominal pain, nausea, vomiting, and diarrhea as well as drug interactions. Macrolides may produce cardiac conduction defects and arrhythmias. A recent metaanalysis determined that macrolide therapy may be associated with increased risk of sudden cardiac death or ventricular tachyarrhythmias and cardiovascular death, but without increased all-cause mortality.[19] At present, there is no significant difference related to all-cause mortality with the use of macrolide antibiotics.

FLUOROQUINOLONES

PHARMACOLOGY AND MECHANISM OF ACTION

STRUCTURE

Fluoroquinolones are fluorinated derivatives of the first quinolone, nalidixic acid, which was originally isolated from the antimalarial agent chloroquine.[20] Fluoroquinolones inhibit the action of bacterial topoisomerase II (DNA gyrase) and topoisomerase IV, leading to disruption of DNA replication, transcription, and repair. In Gram-positive organisms, the primary target is topoisomerase IV; in Gram-negative organisms, the primary target is topoisomerase II. Fluoroquinolones in the United States include cipro-

> **TABLE 186-12**
> **Indications for Macrolide Therapy**
>
> - Granuloma inguinale
> - Chlamydia
> - Uncomplicated nonpurulent skin and soft tissue infections (folliculitis, erysipelas, cellulitis, etc)
> - Bites—animal and human (*Pasteurella multocida*, *Eikenella corrodens*—azithromycin)
> - Lyme disease
> - *Bartonella* infections (except Oroya fever—*Bartonella bacilliformis*)
> - Nontuberculous mycobacterial skin disease (clarithromycin)
> - Lymphogranuloma venereum (alternative)

TABLE 186-13

Contraindications and Precautions of Macrolide Therapy

- CYP3A4 inhibition:
  - Increased drug toxicity (increased serum levels)
  - Warfarin, carbamazepine, buspirone, benzodiazepines, corticosteroids (methylprednisolone), HMG-CoA reductase inhibitors, oral contraceptives, cyclosporine, tacrolimus, disopyramide, felodipine, ergot alkaloids
- CYP1A2 inhibition:
  - Increased drug toxicity (increased serum levels)
  - Theophylline, omeprazole
- Other:
  - Digoxin (levels elevate because of change in drug metabolism by gut flora)
  - Fluconazole (increased clarithromycin levels)

floxacin, levofloxacin, moxifloxacin, ofloxacin, and gemifloxacin. All have a broad-spectrum of activity with appreciable bacteriocidal activity against many Gram-negative organisms, including *Salmonella, Shigella, Enterobacter,* and *Campylobacter.* Ciprofloxacin is most active against *P. aeruginosa.* As a class, the fluoroquinolones have limited anaerobic activity, but gemifloxacin and moxifloxacin exhibit lower minimum inhibitory concentrations against anaerobic organisms and have better activity against Gram-positive organisms. Moxifloxacin is approved therapy for uncomplicated SSTIs. Levofloxacin and moxifloxacin have good activity against *Streptococcus.* Levofloxacin is better than moxifloxacin for *S. aureus* infections, but resistance may develop. Neither should be first line therapy for uncomplicated SSTIs, but each is helpful in the treatment of complicated, polymicrobial, and/or Gram-negative infections, such as diabetic ulcers and severe nosocomial infections. Ciprofloxacin and levofloxacin are effective agents for *Chlamydia,* erysipeloid, granuloma inguinale, and chancroid (see Table 186-14 below). Fluoroquinolones are no longer recommended as treatment of gonococcal disease. Fluoroquinolones also can be effective against some *Mycobacterium* species including *M. tuberculosis, M. chelonae, M. fortuitum,* and *M. kansasii.*[21-23]

METABOLISM, ABSORPTION, AND DISTRIBUTION

Fluoroquinolones are rapidly absorbed after ingestion with a large volume of distribution. Food does not inhibit absorption, but antacids or products containing divalent cations, such as milk, may reduce absorption. Unlike β-lactams, fluoroquinolones act in a concentration-dependent manner and can be administered once or twice daily. Except for moxifloxacin, which is eliminated by the liver, most fluoroquinolones are excreted by the kidneys with adjustment needed in patients with renal failure. None of the fluoroquinolones are removed by dialysis. Most are excreted in breastmilk in small, almost negligible quantities.

INDICATIONS AND CONTRAINDICATIONS

Table 186-14 outlines the indications for fluoroquinolone therapy.

Table 186-15 outlines the contraindications and precautions of fluoroquinolone therapy.

DOSING REGIMEN

Table 186-4 outlines the dosing regimens of commonly prescribed antibiotics for the treatment of SSTIs.

SIDE EFFECTS AND PRECAUTIONS

Table 186-5 outlines the adverse events.

TRIMETHOPRIM-SULFAMETHOXAZOLE

PHARMACOLOGY AND MECHANISM OF ACTION

STRUCTURE

Trimethoprim-sulfamethoxazole (cotrimoxazole, TMP-SMX) is a combination of trimethoprim and a sulfamethoxazole in a 1:5 ratio, which work synergistically to inhibit bacterial nucleic acid synthesis by inhibiting dihydrofolate reductase (trimethoprim) and dihydropteroate synthetase (sulfamethoxazole). These 2 enzymes are involved in the synthesis of tetrahydrofolic acid.[24]

TMP-SMX is a broad spectrum antibiotic with good activity against many aerobic Gram-positive

TABLE 186-14

Indications for Fluoroquinolone Therapy

First-Line Therapy
- Skin and soft tissue infections (SSTIs) caused by Gram-negative pathogens (see section "Mechanism of Action")
- *Pseudomonas aeruginosa* infections (otitis externa, ecthyma gangrenosum, SSTI) (ciprofloxacin)
- Rhinoscleroma
- Chancroid
- Anthrax

Alternative Therapy
- *Bartonella* spp. infections
- *Chlamydia* (levofloxacin, ofloxacin)
- Granuloma inguinale
- Erysipeloid (*Erysipelothrix rhusiopathiae*)

TABLE 186-15
Contraindications and Precautions of Fluoroquinolone Therapy

- Decreased bioavailability with antacids (aluminum, magnesium, alum), iron, zinc, and sucralfate
- Inhibited theophylline and aminophylline metabolism (ciprofloxacin)
- Tendon rupture (in patients with renal disease, hemodialysis, or steroid use)
- Decreased seizure threshold
- Decreased warfarin and cyclosporine metabolism

cocci including *S. aureus*, *S. viridans*, and community-acquired MRSA.[14] It is also effective against: *H. influenzae*, *E. coli*, *Proteus mirabilis*, *Klebsiella pneumoniae*, *Shigella*, *Yersinia*, *Vibrio cholera*, *Nocardia* spp., *M. marinum*, *M. fortuitum*, and *Brucella*. The use of TMP-SMX for SSTIs caused by *S. pyogenes* is controversial because of concern for resistance, which may result from laboratory testing techniques.[25] Nonetheless, TMP-SMX is not recommended for nonpurulent SSTIs. However, TMP-SMX is active against most community-acquired MRSA and can be used for empiric therapy for moderate purulent SSTIs. The following organisms are resistant to TMP-SMX: *Mycoplasma* spp., *Rickettsia* spp., *M. tuberculosis*, and *T. pallidum*. *P. aeruginosa* is not sensitive to TMP-SMX, but other pseudomonal species are susceptible. TMP-SMX is occasionally effective for *Nocardia* infections and nontuberculous mycobacteria infections. TMP-SMX is not active against anaerobes.

METABOLISM, ABSORPTION, AND DISTRIBUTION

TMP and SMX are well absorbed, but achieve different serum concentrations following administration of equal quantities of drug. A serum ratio of 1:20 (TMP:SMX) is necessary for optimal synergy against most pathogens, which can be achieved by administration of the compound in a fixed 1:5 ratio. Both drugs are rapidly distributed to tissues including cerebrospinal fluid and sputum. Excretion is via the kidneys.

INDICATIONS AND CONTRAINDICATIONS

Table 186-16 outlines the indications for TMP-SMX therapy.

Table 186-17 outlines the contraindications and precautions of TMP-SMX therapy.

DOSING REGIMEN

Table 186-4 outlines the dosing regimens of commonly prescribed antibiotics for the treatment of SSTIs.

SIDE EFFECTS AND PRECAUTIONS

Table 186-5 outlines the adverse events.

TMP-SMX is pregnancy category D and should be avoided for breastfeeding women, especially during the first 6 weeks of the newborn's life.[24]

OTHER AGENTS

Even though the aforementioned drugs are most of the antibiotics used in dermatologic practice, several new or infrequently used medications deserve attention for the treatment of complicated SSTIs or systemic infections caused by resistant pathogens. Most have restricted use, predicated on approval by an infectious disease specialist.

VANCOMYCIN

Vancomycin is a glycopeptide antibiotic effective against Gram-positive bacteria; specifically, Gram-positive infections resistant to β-lactams or when β-lactam use is contraindicated. Vancomycin is a first line therapy for complicated and/or severe SSTIs caused by hospital-acquired MRSA. Vancomycin is an option for empiric therapy for severe purulent and nonpurulent (plus piperacillin and tazobactam) SSTIs. Vancomycin inhibits bacterial cell wall peptidoglycan synthesis. Dosing is determined by the patient's weight (15 to 20 mg/kg), and frequency of administration by the patient's creatinine clearance, which necessitates renal function monitoring during therapy. Potential adverse reactions include nephrotoxicity, ototoxicity, phlebitis at the injection site, hypersensitivity reactions,

TABLE 186-16
Indications for Trimethoprim-Sulfamethoxazole Therapy

- Community-acquired methicillin-resistant *S. aureus*
- *Nocardia asteroides* infections
- Empiric therapy for moderate purulent skin and soft tissue infections (SSTIs)
- Uncomplicated SSTIs caused by susceptible pathogens (see section "Mechanism of Action")
- Granuloma inguinale (alternative)

TABLE 186-17
Contraindications and Precautions of Trimethoprim-Sulfamethoxazole Therapy

- Severe reactions in patients with HIV/AIDS
- Prolonged prothrombin time in patients on warfarin
- Contraindicated for patients on methotrexate

and leukopenia. "Red man syndrome," secondary to histamine release, is an uncommon reaction thought to be caused by drug impurities; it can be minimized by more refined preparations and slower infusions. Drug-induced linear immunoglobulin A disease is a rare cutaneous side effect. There are isolated reports of vancomycin-resistant *S. aureus* and *Enterococcus faecium*.

LIPOGLYCOPEPTIDES: DALBAVANCIN, ORITAVANCIN, AND TELAVANCIN

The lipoglycopeptides, semisynthetic derivatives of glycopeptides (vancomycin), disrupt bacterial cell wall integrity and/or inhibit bacterial cell wall synthesis.[26] They are recommended for treatment of complicated SSTIs, especially infections with Gram-positive organisms, including *S. aureus*, streptococci, and clostridia, as well as MRSA, VRE, and multidrug-resistant pneumocci. Telavancin is an option for empiric therapy for severe purulent SSTIs. Lipoglycopeptides are administered intravenously. Long half-lives for oritavancin and dalbavancin allow infrequent dosing, for example, a single-dose (oritavancin) or two-dose (dalbavancin) regimen, which is useful in outpatient therapy. Telavancin and dalbavancin require dose adjustment in patients with renal failure, whereas oritavancin does not. Lipoglycopeptides are pregnancy category C and should not be administered to breastfeeding mothers. As a class, these drugs can induce a hypersensitivity reaction similar to vancomycin-related "red man syndrome," suggesting a possible cross-allergy. Oritavancin may lead to an increased risk of osteomyelitis. Patients treated with telavancin have an increased risk of taste disturbances, nephrotoxicity, and QT prolongation. Transaminitis may occur with dalbavancin and oritavancin, while oritavancin and telavancin can interfere with coagulation studies. Oritavancin inhibits CYP2C9 and 2C19 and induces CYP3A4 and 2D6, which suggests that caution should be exercised when coadministering oritavancin and warfarin.[26]

OXAZOLIDINONES: LINEZOLID, TEDIZOLID

Until recently, linezolid was the only available oxazolidinone approved for the treatment of complicated SSTIs caused by MRSA, VRE, and vancomycin-resistant *S. aureus*. Tedizolid was approved in 2014 and early experience has shown advantages compared to linezolid.[27] Oxazolidinones inhibit protein synthesis by binding to the 23S portion of the 50S ribosomal subunit, a unique mechanism that minimizes cross-resistance to other antibiotics. Oxazolidinones are active against Gram-positive organisms (including anaerobes) and nontuberculous mycobacteria such as *M. chelonae* and *M. fortuitum*. Tedizolid and linezolid have a similar spectrum of activity, but tedizolid is 2-fold to 8-fold more potent against Gram-positive bacteria. Linezolid is generally well tolerated and side effects are infrequent. Reversible thrombocytopenia and leukopenia occur in 2% of patients and correlates with duration of therapy, which necessitates complete blood cell count monitoring during therapy. High oral bioavailability allows identical oxazolidinone dosing intravenously or orally; Linezolid dosing is 600 mg twice daily and tedizolid is 200 mg once daily. GI side effects and thrombocytopenia tend to occur less frequently in tedizolid-treated patients. Given its broader spectrum of coverage and better safety profile, tedizolid may be more efficacious than linezolid. The ability to convert to oral administration is an attractive component of oxazolidinone treatment. Linezolid is recommended as a first-line option as empiric treatment of severe purulent SSTIs.

QUINUPRISTIN-DALFOPRISTIN

Quinupristin and dalfopristin are streptogramin antibiotics combined in a fixed ratio of 3:7.[28] Both quinupristin and dalfopristin irreversibly inhibit bacterial protein translation by binding to different sites of the 50S ribosomal subunit. They exhibit synergistic activity against a variety of multidrug-resistant Gram-positive organisms, including MRSA, VRE, and vancomycin-resistant *S. aureus*. The recommended dose is 7.5 mg/kg IV twice daily for at least 7 days, with lower dosing for patients with hepatic insufficiency. Patient tolerability can be a problem, especially if phlebitis (75%), arthralgia, or myalgia occurs. Quinupristin-dalfopristin is metabolized by the liver and excreted in the bile. Elevation of hepatic transaminases and bilirubin can occur. Concomitant administration with drugs metabolized by the CYP3A4 system is contraindicated. Quinupristin-dalfopristin should be used in caution in patients taking cyclosporine or agents that prolong the QT interval.

DAPTOMYCIN

Daptomycin, a member of the lipopeptide antibiotic class derived from the fermentation of *Streptomyces roseosporus*, exerts its activity via a multistep process involving the disruption of bacterial cell wall function.[29] It is approved for the treatment of complicated SSTIs caused by *S. aureus* (including MRSA), penicillin-resistant *S. pneumoniae*, and VRE. Dosing is typically 4 mg/kg IV every 24 hours for 7 to 14 days, with excretion primarily by the kidneys, which requires dosage adjustments for patients with renal impairment. The drug is generally well tolerated, with headache and GI complaints reported most commonly. The primary serious adverse event is myopathy, which is usually transient and reversible, without progression to rhabdomyolysis.

ERTAPENEM

Ertapenem is a β-lactam member of the carbapenem family, which also includes imipenem and meropenem. Carbapenems are unique among β-lactams in their stability and resistance to extended-spectrum β-lactamases. Ertapenem is long acting with a broad spectrum of antimicrobial activity similar to the older carbapenems, but with poor activity against *Pseudomonas, Acinetobacter*, and enterococci. Although comparable to piperacillin-tazobactam in the treatment of complicated SSTIs, and active against both Gram-positive and Gram-negative aerobes and anaerobes, ertapenem use should be reserved for polymicrobial infections not otherwise sensitive to agents with more narrow spectra of activity. Compared to other carbapenems, ertapenem has a long half-life, which allows for once daily intravenous administration (1 g/day for 7 to 14 days) but should be used cautiously in patients with renal impairment. CNS effects and hypersensitivity reactions may occur.[30]

TIGECYCLINE

Tigecycline is a glycylcycline antibiotic with broad-spectrum activity indicated for the treatment of complicated SSTIs caused by susceptible organisms, including MRSA, VRE, *Acinetobacter*, and Gram-negatives that produce extended-spectrum β-lactamase.[31] A derivative of minocycline, tigecycline shares the same 30S ribosomal binding site and has a spectrum of activity similar to the classic tetracyclines. Compared to tetracyclines, tigecycline has a greater volume of distribution, better activity against organisms with tetracycline resistance, and better activity against *Streptococcus* spp. Tigecycline dosing is 50 mg IV twice daily following a 100-mg loading dose. Lower dosing is necessary for patients with hepatic disease. Tigecycline has a similar side effect profile to the tetracycline family and the same precautions should be taken.

TOPICAL ANTIBIOTICS

Topical antibiotics (Table 186-18) play an important role in the management of many common dermatologic conditions. For localized superficial infections, such as impetigo, a topical antibiotic may eliminate the need for systemic therapy. Extensive impetigo, infection on the legs, or infection in immunocompromised individuals deserve treatment with systemic antibiotics. Topical antibiotics are still prescribed as prophylactic therapy after minor surgical or cosmetic procedures to decrease postoperative wound infections and speed wound healing. But such use is unnecessary and perhaps counterproductive, given the expense and the risk of inducing allergy. For most surgical procedures, petrolatum is adequate postsurgical care.[32] Burns are unique in that they produce a fertile ground for secondary infection and prophylactic treatment with topical antibiotics is often reasonable.

CLINDAMYCIN

Clindamycin is primarily used for the treatment of acne and is available as a 1% gel, solution, lotion, foam, and swab. It is also available in a preparation with benzoyl peroxide. The addition of benzoyl peroxide may slow development of antibiotic resistance to clindamycin. Pseudomembranous colitis rarely has been reported to occur with the topical use of clindamycin.[33] Clindamycin is safe to use during pregnancy.

MUPIROCIN

Mupirocin, formerly known as *pseudomonic acid A*, a topical agent derived from *Pseudomonas fluorescens*, reversibly binds to isoleucyl-transfer RNA synthetase and inhibits protein synthesis. Activity is limited to Gram-positive bacteria, particularly staphylococci and most streptococci. Activity is enhanced with an acid pH (5.5), the normal pH of skin. Mupirocin may lose efficacy when exposed to high temperatures. Treatment with mupirocin ointment 2% is 3 times daily, principally for localized impetigo caused by *S. aureus* and *S. pyogenes*. Prolonged use can lead to resistance.[34] Formulations with calcium salts (to aid in stability) are available. The ointment can be used intranasally twice daily in each nostril for 5 days to eradicate MRSA colonization.

RETAPAMULIN

Retapamulin, a semisynthetic pleuromutilin antibiotic isolated from *Clitopilus scyphoides*, inhibits protein synthesis via 50S bacterial ribosomes at protein L3, near the peptidyl transferase center.[35] Retapamulin binding inhibits peptidyl transferase and partial inhibition of binding of initiator transfer RNA to the P-site of the ribosome. It is approved for the topical treatment of impetigo caused by *S. aureus* (excluding MRSA) and *S. pyogenes* in patients older than 9 months of age. Allergic contact dermatitis to the active ingredient may occur, but is uncommon.

TABLE 186-18
Topical Antibiotics

TOPICAL AGENT (FORMULATION)	MECHANISM OF ACTION	ANTIBACTERIAL COVERAGE AND INDICATION	APPLICATION	SAFETY	ADVERSE EFFECTS
Clindamycin (1% gel, solution, lotion, foam, swab)	Binds to bacterial 50S ribosomal subunit; inhibits protein synthesis	Gram-positive cocci, anaerobes; *Propionibacterium acnes* (acne vulgaris)	Once per day	Category B	Pseudomembranous colitis (rare)
Mupirocin (2% ointment)	Reversibly binds to isoleucyl-transfer RNA synthetase; inhibits protein synthesis	Gram-positive bacteria: staphylococci, most streptococci (impetigo); also for eradication of methicillin-resistant *Staphylococcus aureus* (MRSA) from colonized sites	3 times per day	Category B	Avoid application with polyethylene glycol-based preparations to large open wounds to prevent toxic absorption
Retapamulin	Inhibits peptidyl transferase via 50S bacterial ribosomes at protein L3; inhibits protein synthesis	*S. aureus*, excluding MRSA; *Streptococcus pyogenes* (impetigo)	Twice per day × 5 days	For use in children >9 months of age only; Category B	Allergic contact dermatitis (rare)
Bacitracin	Interferes with bacterial cell-wall synthesis	Gram-positive cocci (staphylococci, streptococci)	1 to 3 times per day	Category C	Allergic contact sensitization; anaphylactic shock (rare)
Polymyxin B (ointment)	Cationic detergent; disrupts bacterial membrane integrity	Gram-negative organisms (*Pseudomonas aeruginosa*, *Enterobacter*, *Escherichia coli*)	1 to 3 times per day	Category C	Allergic contact dermatitis
Aminoglycosides (neomycin, gentamicin)	Binds to 30S ribosomal subunit; inhibits protein synthesis	Neomycin: aerobic, Gram-negative bacteria Gentamicin: prophylactic for *P. aeruginosa*	Neomycin: 1 to 3 times per day Gentamicin: 3 to 4 times per day	Neomycin: Category D Gentamicin: Category C	Allergic contact dermatitis (neomycin)
Silver sulfadiazine	Targets bacterial cell wall and membrane integrity	Broad spectrum; useful in the treatment of burns	1 to 2 times per day	Category B	Transient leukopenia
Fusidic acid (2% cream, ointment)	Interrupts elongation factor G; inhibits protein synthesis	*S. aureus* (including MRSA), *Staphylococcus epidermidis*, *Corynebacterium minutissimum*, *S. pyogenes*, *P. acnes*	2 to 3 times per day for up to 2 weeks	Safe to use during pregnancy	Allergic contact dermatitis

BACITRACIN

Bacitracin, a polypeptide antibiotic originally isolated from the Tracy-I strain of *Bacillus subtilis*, is a cyclic polypeptide with multiple components (A, B, and C). Bacitracin A is the major component of commercial products and often used as the zinc salt. It interferes with bacterial cell-wall synthesis by binding to the well and inhibiting the dephosphorylation of a membrane-bound lipid pyrophosphate; is active against Gram-positive cocci such as staphylococci and streptococci, but inactive against most Gram-negative organisms and yeasts. Available as bacitracin ointment and zinc bacitracin, with 400 to 500 units/g, topical bacitracin is effective treatment of impetigo, furunculosis and pyodermas. It is often combined with polymyxin B and neomycin as a triple antibiotic. Unfortunately, the topical application carries the risk of allergic contact sensitization and, rarely, anaphylactic shock.[36]

POLYMYXIN B

Polymyxin B, a topical antibiotic derived from a spore-forming soil aerobe *Bacillus polymyxa*, is a mixture of cyclic polypeptides (polymyxin B1 and polymyxin B2) that functions as a cationic detergent to disrupt the integrity of the membrane. Polymyxin B is active against a wide range of Gram-negative organisms including *P. aeruginosa*, *Enterobacter*, and *E. coli*. It is available in ointment form (5000 to 10,000 units/g) in combination with bacitracin or as a triple antibiotic ointment with bacitracin and neomycin. Recommended use is 1 to 3 times per day.

AMINOGLYCOSIDES: NEOMYCIN AND GENTAMICIN

Aminoglycosides exert their antibacterial effects by binding to the 30S ribosomal subunit and interfering with protein synthesis. Neomycin, isolated from *Streptomyces fradiae*, has activity against aerobic Gram-negative bacteria, and is commonly packaged in combination with other antibiotics. The risk of allergic contact dermatitis is high—9% of patients who undergo patch testing.[37]

Gentamicin, isolated from *Micromonospora purpurea*, is available as a 0.1% cream or ointment and used by some surgeons for operations on the ear, especially in diabetic or immunocompromised patients, to provide prophylaxis against malignant otitis externa caused by *P. aeruginosa*. The ophthalmic formulation can be used for operative wounds in the periorbital area.

SILVER SULFADIAZINE

Silver sulfadiazine is a topical product that releases silver slowly and exerts its effect on the bacterial cell wall and membranes. It has broad-spectrum activity and is useful in the treatment of burns.

FUSIDIC ACID

Fusidic acid, a fusidate antibiotic that inhibits bacterial protein synthesis translocation by interrupting elongation factor G, is active against *S. aureus* (including MRSA), *S. epidermidis*, *Corynebacterium minutissimum*, *S. pyogenes*, and *Propionibacterium acnes*.[38] Typically applied 2 to 3 times per day for up to 2 weeks, fusidic acid is available at 2% in a cream or ointment; it is unavailable in the United States. Allergic contact dermatitis is uncommon (<1%) and cross-resistance with other antibiotics is uncommon. In some locales, fusidic acid is combined with steroids for the treatment of atopic dermatitis.

ACKNOWLEDGMENTS

The authors thank Drs. Gasbarre, Schmitt, Bonner, and James for their work on this chapter in previous editions.

REFERENCES

1. Rosen T. Update on treating uncomplicated skin and skin structure infections. *J Drugs Dermatol*. 2005;4(6)(suppl):s9-s14.
2. Esposito S, Noviello S, Leone S. Epidemiology and microbiology of skin and soft tissue infections. *Curr Opin Infect Dis*. 2016;29(2):109-115.
3. Fritsche TR, Jones RN. Importance of understanding pharmacokinetic/pharmacodynamic principles in the emergence of resistances, including community-associated staphylococcus aureus. *J Drugs Dermatol*. 2005;4(6)(suppl):s4-s8.
4. Moran GJ, Krishnadasan A, Gorwitz RJ, et al. Methicillin-resistant *S. aureus* infections among patients in the emergency department. *N Engl J Med*. 2006;355(7):666-674.
5. Guillamet CV, Kollef MH. How to stratify patients at risk for resistant bugs in skin and soft tissue infections? *Curr Opin Infect Dis*. 2016;29(2):116-123.
6. Stevens DL, Bisno AL, Chambers HF, et al. Practice guidelines for the diagnosis and management of skin and soft tissue infections: 2014 update by the Infectious Diseases Society of America. *Clin Infect Dis*. 2014;59(2):e10-e52.
7. Kadurina M, Bocheva G, Tonev S. Penicillin and semisynthetic penicillins in dermatology. *Clin Dermatol*. 2003;21(1):12-23.
8. Thethi AK, Van Dellen RG. Dilemmas and controversies in penicillin allergy. *Immunol Allergy Clin North Am*. 2004;24(3):445-461, vi.
9. Mirakian R, Leech SC, Krishna MT, et al. Management of allergy to penicillins and other beta-lactams. *Clin Exp Allergy*. 2015;45(2):300-327.
10. Del Rosso JQ. Cephalosporins in dermatology. *Clin Dermatol*. 2003;21(1):24-32.
11. Yahav D, Paul M, Fraser A, et al. Efficacy and safety of cefepime: a systematic review and meta-analysis. *Lancet Infect Dis*. 2007;7(5):338-348.
12. Frampton JE. Ceftaroline fosamil: a review of its use in the treatment of complicated skin and soft tissue infections and community-acquired pneumonia. *Drugs*. 2013;73(10):1067-1094.
13. Klein NC, Cunha BA. Tetracyclines. *Med Clin North Am*. 1995;79(4):789-801.
14. Klein NC, Cunha BA. New uses of older antibiotics. *Med Clin North Am*. 2001;85(1):125-132.
15. Falagas ME, Gorbach SL. Clindamycin and metronidazole. *Med Clin North Am*. 1995;79(4):845-867.
16. Guay D. Update on clindamycin in the management of bacterial, fungal and protozoal infections. *Expert Opin Pharmacother*. 2007;8(14):2401-2444.
17. Alzolibani AA, Zedan K. Macrolides in chronic inflammatory skin disorders. *Mediators Inflamm*. 2012;2012:159354.
18. Scheinfeld NS, Tutrone WD, Torres O, et al. Macrolides in dermatology. *Dis Mon*. 2004;50(7):350-368.
19. Cheng YJ, Nie XY, Chen XM, et al. The role of macrolide antibiotics in increasing cardiovascular risk. *J Am Coll Cardiol*. 2015;66(20):2173-2184.
20. Sable D, Murakawa GJ. Quinolones in dermatology. *Clin Dermatol*. 2003;21(1):56-63.
21. Saravolatz LD, Leggett J. Gatifloxacin, gemifloxacin, and moxifloxacin: the role of 3 newer fluoroquinolones. *Clin Infect Dis*. 2003;37(9):1210-1215.
22. Suh B, Lorber B. Quinolones. *Med Clin North Am*.

1995;79(4):869-894.
23. Blondeau JM. The role of fluoroquinolones in skin and skin structure infections. *Am J Clin Dermatol*. 2002;3(1):37-46.
24. Michalek K, Lechowicz M, Pastuszczak M, et al. The use of trimethoprim and sulfamethoxazole (TMP-SMX) in dermatology. *Folia Med Cracov*. 2015;55(1):35-41.
25. Bowen AC, Lilliebridge RA, Tong SY, et al. Is *Streptococcus pyogenes* resistant or susceptible to trimethoprim-sulfamethoxazole? *J Clin Microbiol*. 2012;50(12):4067-4072.
26. Van Bambeke F. Lipoglycopeptide antibacterial agents in Gram-positive infections: a comparative review. *Drugs*. 2015;75(18):2073-2095.
27. Rybak JM, Roberts K. Tedizolid phosphate: a next-generation oxazolidinone. *Infect Dis Ther*. 2015 [Epub ahead of print].
28. Allington DR, Rivey MP. Quinupristin/dalfopristin: a therapeutic review. *Clin Ther*. 2001;23(1):24-44.
29. Lee SY, Fan HW, Kuti JL, et al. Update on daptomycin: the first approved lipopeptide antibiotic. *Expert Opin Pharmacother*. 2006;7(10):1381-1397.
30. Congeni BL. Ertapenem. *Expert Opin Pharmacother*. 2010;11(4):669-672.
31. Stein GE, Babinchak T. Tigecycline: an update. *Diagn Microbiol Infect Dis*. 2013;75(4):331-336.
32. Smack DP, Harrington AC, Dunn C, et al. Infection and allergy incidence in ambulatory surgery patients using white petrolatum vs bacitracin ointment. A randomized controlled trial. *JAMA*. 1996;276(12):972-977.
33. Parry MF, Rha CK. Pseudomembranous colitis caused by topical clindamycin phosphate. *Arch Dermatol*. 1986;122(5):583-584.
34. Vasquez JE, Walker ES, Franzus BW, et al. The epidemiology of mupirocin resistance among methicillin-resistant *Staphylococcus aureus* at a veterans' affairs hospital. *Infect Control Hosp Epidemiol*. 2000;21(7):459-464.
35. Yang LP, Keam SJ. Retapamulin: a review of its use in the management of impetigo and other uncomplicated superficial skin infections. *Drugs*. 2008;68(6):855-873.
36. Sood A, Taylor JS. Bacitracin: allergen of the year. *Am J Contact Dermat*. 2003;14(1):3-4.
37. Warshaw EM, Belsito DV, Taylor JS, et al. North American Contact Dermatitis Group patch test results: 2009 to 2010. *Dermatitis*. 2013;24(2):50-59.
38. Schofer H, Simonsen L. Fusidic acid in dermatology: an updated review. *Eur J Dermatol*. 2010;20(1):6-15.

Chapter 187 :: Dapsone
:: Chee Leok Goh & Jiun Yit Pan

第一百八十七章
氨苯砜

中文导读

氨苯砜（4,4′-二氨基二苯砜）是一种具有独特药理作用的磺胺类药物，目前被用作抗感染药，并常用作皮质类固醇保留剂。本章分为9节：①引言；②作用机制；③化学与药理学；④医学适应证；⑤使用剂量；⑥不良反应；⑦氨苯砜严重不良反应；⑧氨苯砜治疗的启动和监测；⑨药物过量治疗。

第一节引言，介绍了氨苯砜是1908年合成的，但作为抗菌药的研究始于1937年。随着认识的增加，发现氨苯砜具有双重功能，结合了抗菌、抗疟原虫和抗感染作用。

第二节作用机制，介绍了氨苯砜作为一种抑菌抗生素，通过干扰生物合成途径起作用，同时可能通过抑制中性粒细胞向趋化信号和白三烯B4的趋化性来抑制中性粒细胞向炎症区域的迁移而发挥其抗感染作用。

第三节介绍了氨苯砜的溶解度变化很大，取决于所使用的溶剂，口服氨苯砜几乎完全从肠道吸收，生物利用度超过86%。氨苯砜吸收后进行肝肠循环，被肝脏代谢，约20%的氨苯砜通过尿液以未改变的药物形式排出，70%~85%在结合后作为水溶性代谢物被消除。丙磺舒和甲氧苄啶会升高氨苯砜血药浓度，利福平会降低DSS血药浓度。

第四节医学适应证，介绍了其抗菌方面最常用于联合利福平和氯法齐明治疗麻风病，利用其抗炎作用，主要治疗疱疹样皮炎、隆起性红斑、线状IgA大疱性皮病等。

第五节使用剂量，介绍了氨苯砜的治疗剂量从25~200 mg/d不等，通常是一次性给药。少部分患者可能需要300 mg/d才能看到疗效。建议的起始剂量为50~100 mg/d，以尽量减少潜在的药物不良反应，特别是溶血。

第六节不良反应，介绍了氨苯砜最常见的副作用是剂量相关性溶血，此外还有高铁血红蛋白血症、氨苯砜中毒性肝炎和胆汁淤积性黄疸、皮疹，以及其他恶心、头痛、疲劳、失眠、精神病和周围神经病变等不良反应。

第七节介绍了氨苯砜严重不良反应包括氨苯砜过敏综合征、溶血和高铁血红蛋白血症、粒细胞缺乏症、再生障碍性贫血。

第八节氨苯砜治疗的启动和监测，介绍了在开始使用氨苯砜之前，应进行有针对性的病史和体格检查，以筛选是否存在明显的贫血、心肺疾病和周围神经病变，并加强治疗过程中的监测。

第九节药物过量治疗，介绍了过量服用氨苯砜，需应对严重的溶血和高铁血红蛋白血症，其中重复透析有助于治疗过量；活性炭将通过清除肠道内的药物来降低药物浓度；1%亚甲蓝溶液静脉滴注，可降低高铁血红蛋白血症程度；亚甲基蓝、抗坏血酸也被用于治疗过量的情况。

〔粟 娟〕

AT-A-GLANCE

- Dapsone (4,4'-diaminodiphenylsulfone) is a sulfonamide with unique pharmacologic action.
- It is used as an antiinfective in particular against Hensen disease and selected fungal infections such as actinomycetoma and rhinosporidiosis. It is also used for the treatment of malaria and as a prophylaxis for toxoplasmosis.
- It is also an antiinflammatory agents and is effective against dermatitis herpetiformis, erythema elevatum diutinum, linear immunoglobulin A dermatosis and chronic bullous disease of childhood, and bullous eruption of systemic lupus erythematosus.
- It has antineutrophilic effect and used against collagen vascular and autoimmune diseases and recently topically for acne.
- It is often used as corticosteroid-sparing agent.
- Significant side effects to watch for include hemolysis and methemoglobinemia, which are frequently observed in patient with glucose-6-phosphate dehydrogenase (G6PD) deficiency. Dapsone should only be given with great caution and in very special circumstances to patients with G6PD deficiency when the benefits outweigh the risks when constant hemoglobin and monitoring of reticulocyte counts is essential.
- Other serious side effects include drug hypersensitivity syndrome (sulphone syndrome), Stevens-Johnson syndrome, and agranulocytosis.
- Dapsone is classified as C Pregnancy Category (ie, risk not ruled out).

INTRODUCTION

Dapsone is 4,4'-diaminodiphenylsulfone,[1,2] an aniline derivative belonging to the group of synthetic sulfones. Although dapsone is classified as a sulfonamide, cross-reactions occur in only 7% to 22% of sulfa-allergic patients. They are usually mild.[3,4]

The molecule was synthesized in 1908, but research into dapsone as an antimicrobial agent started only in 1937.[5,6] Later it was recognized to possess antiinflammatory effects, and it was investigated predominantly by in vitro studies aiming to get more information on the effect of dapsone on inflammatory effector cells, cytokines, and mediators, such as cellular toxic oxygen metabolism, myeloperoxidase-halogenid system, adhesion molecules, chemotaxis, membrane-associated phospholipids, prostaglandins, leukotrienes, interleukin-8, tumor necrosis factor-α (TNF-α), lymphocyte functions, and tumor growth. The latter capabilities primarily were used in treating chronic inflammatory disorders.

Hence, dapsone has dual functions, combining antimicrobial, antiprotozoal, and antiinflammatory effects resembling those of the nonsteroidal antiinflammatory drugs (NSAIDs).

MECHANISM OF ACTION

DAPSONE AS A BACTERIOSTATIC ANTIBIOTIC AGENT

Dapsone acts by interfering in the folate biosynthetic pathway. It inhibits the synthesis of dihydrofolic acid by competing with para-aminobenzoic acid for the active site of dihydropteroate synthetase.[7,8] It has been used for the treatment of Hensen disease since 1945 (often in combination with other antibiotics, eg, rifampicin and clofazimine). It is also used to treat toxoplasmosis and is used for pneumocystis pneumonia (PCP) prophylaxis in immunocompromised patients in whom it is often prescribed in combination with pyrimethamine and leucovorin. It is also used as chemoprophylaxis for Plasmodium falciparum malaria.

In the early 2000s, a topical 5% dapsone gel was reported to be effective against acne without causing clinically significant declines in hemoglobin levels, even in patients with glucose-6-phosphate dehydrogenase (G6PD) deficiency.[9] In February 2016, the U.S. Food and Drug Administration (FDA) approved a 7.5% dapsone gel for once-daily application versus twice-daily application of the 5% formulation for acne vulgaris.[10] The mechanism of action of topical dapsone here is likely to result from its combined antiinflammatory and antimicrobial activities.

DAPSONE AS AN ANTIINFLAMMATORY AGENT

The antiinflammatory effects of dapsone was studied in animals in the 1970s. Studies showed wide variations in dapsone antiinflammatory properties. The conclusion then was that dapsone can be attributed as an antiinflammatory potential comparable to the NSAIDs. But its exact antiinflammatory mechanism remains unknown. Since then it has been used for its antiinflammatory action on selected dermatologic disorders, especially in those with neutrophilic chemotaxis (eg, dermatitis herpetiformis and leukocytoclastic vasculitis).

Dapsone inhibits migration of neutrophils to areas of inflammation by inhibiting neutrophil chemotaxis to the chemoattractant signals F-met-leu-phe[6,11] and leukotriene B_4 (LTB$_4$).[12-14] Dapsone also inhibits the adherence of neutrophils to skin-localized immunoglobulin A (IgA)[15] and endothelium.[16] Additionally, dapsone inhibits the release of inflammatory mediators, including interleukin (IL)-8,[17] prostaglandin D_2, and TNF-α.[18] Dapsone also inhibit the myeloperoxidase H_2O_2-halide–mediated cytotoxic system,[19,20] likely via the inhibition of the calcium flux necessary for these events.[21] Myeloperoxidase is the enzyme in the azurophilic granules of neutrophils and in the lysosomes of monocytes that catalyzes the conversion of hydrogen peroxide and chloride ions into hypochlorous acid, a potent oxidant that causes cell damage.[22]

The dual antimicrobial and antiinflammatory functions and the long-term usage safety profile of dapsone place it in a unique position as a therapeutic agent different from other drugs. First, its antimicrobial effects can be used in immunocompromised conditions to prevent and treat opportunistic infections in patients (eg, against bacterial and protozoal infection). Second, it is safe for use in long-term treatment (eg, lifelong use in leprosy, long-term intermittent therapy in inflammatory dermatoses). Third, it has unique powerful disease-specific antiinflammatory activities (eg, prompt decrease of pruritus and control of skin lesions in dermatitis herpetiformis to the extent that the disease rapid and dramatic response to dapsone is sometime used as a diagnostic test of the disease).

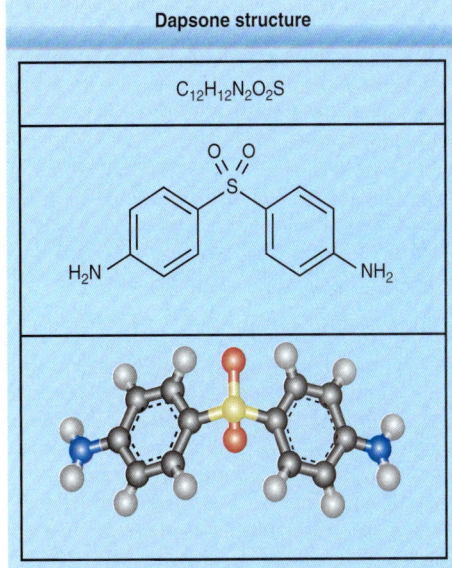

Figure 187-1 Dapsone structure.

CHEMISTRY AND PHARMACOLOGY OF DAPSONE

Chemically, dapsone is an aniline derivative. As a sulfone, it shows the structure of a sulphur atom linking to two carbon atoms (Fig. 187-1). The solubility of dapsone varies over a wide range depending on the solvent used (eg, water, 0.2 mg/mL vs methanol, 52 mg/mL). After oral administration, dapsone is almost completely absorbed from the gut with bioavailability exceeding 86%. Peak serum concentrations are attained within 2 to 8 hours. After ingestion of a single 50- to 300-mg dose of dapsone, maximum serum concentrations range from 0.63 to 4.82 mg/L.[23,24] Under steady-state conditions, 100 mg/day (the dose most frequently used) results in serum concentrations of 3.26 mg/L (maximum) and 1.95 mg/L (after 24 hours).[8,23,24] These dapsone serum concentrations attained in vivo must be kept in mind when interpreting the results of in vitro investigations.

After absorption, dapsone undergoes enterohepatic circulation. It is metabolized by the liver but also by activated polymorphonuclear leukocytes (PMNs) and mononuclear cells.[25] In the liver, dapsone is metabolized primarily through acetylation by N-acetyltransferase to monacetyl-dapsone (MADDS) and through hydroxylation by cytochrome P-450 enzymes, resulting in the generation of dapsone hydroxylamine (DDS-NOH). In fact, administration of dapsone has been used to determine the acetylation phenotype (rapid vs slow acetylator). In terms of both efficacy and induction of adverse effects, the most important issue is the generation of DDS-NOH. This metabolic pathway also occurs in lesional skin of inflammatory dermatoses and is thought to be mediated by activated PMN.[25] Dapsone is distributed to virtually all organs and retained in the skin, muscle, kidneys, and liver. Trace concentrations of the drug may be presented in these tissues up to 3 weeks after discontinuation of dapsone treatment. The drug is also distributed into sweat, saliva, sputum, tears, and bile. Dapsone is 50% to 90% bound to plasma proteins, but MADDS is almost completely bound to plasma proteins. It crosses the blood–brain barrier and placenta and is detectable in breast milk.[26,27] Cases have been reported in which dapsone therapy of the mother resulted in neonatal hemolysis and cyanosis.[28]

Approximately 20% of dapsone is excreted as unchanged drug via urine, and 70% to 85% is eliminated as water-soluble metabolites after conjugation with glucuronic acid. This step is mediated by uridine diphosphate glucuronosyltransferase. Additionally, a small amount might be excreted in faeces, including some yet unidentified metabolites. The complex metabolic pathway of dapsone has been reviewed.[24,25,29]

When dapsone is administered, there is equilibrium between acetylation and deacetylation. Thus, there is the possibility that PMNs in peripheral blood are exposed both to dapsone and its metabolites. These metabolites, such as DDS-NOH, have been shown to be pharmacologically active. However, they are believed to be responsible for its antiinflammatory mechanisms (eg, inhibition of chemotaxis) but also for a number of side effects. This has been clearly documented for DDS-NOH. Interestingly, Khan and coworkers[30] recently demonstrated that human keratinocytes that had been stimulated by various cytokines such as TNF-α, IL-1β, and interferon γ (INF-γ) can produce DDS-NOH as well.

Dapsone tablets are available in 25- and 100-mg sizes; therapeutic doses for various conditions range from 25 mg to approximately 400 mg. Dapsone is well absorbed from the gut with peak levels being reached 2 to 6 hours after a single dose. The half-life, approximately 30 hours because of enterohepatic recirculation.[24] This allows for once-daily dosing and explains the utility of activated charcoal in reducing drug levels during accidental or intentional overdose.[31] Dapsone and its metabolites may be transmitted through human milk, and hemolysis has occurred in nursing infants.[27,32,33] No teratogenicity has been observed, but no controlled studies have been performed in humans, and it is classified as Pregnancy Category C.[34,35]

Topical dapsone in a 5% gel formulation was approved in 2005 for the treatment of acne vulgaris.[36,37] Twice-daily application on up to 22% of patients' body surface area resulted in systemic levels of dapsone and its metabolites that were 100-fold less than oral dapsone at a therapeutic dose. There was no hemolytic anemia or methemoglobinemia, even in patients who were G6PD deficient.[9,38-40] Therefore, in 2008, the FDA removed the requirement for pretreatment G6PD testing. Overall, topical dapsone gel has a favorable short- and long-term safety profile.

A higher concentration of 7.5% dapsone gel as a once-daily application has shown to be effective in multiple subgroups of patients.[41-44] It was well tolerated, with a low incidence of treatment-related adverse events, with the majority of adverse events being administration site related and mild or moderate in severity.[42,45] Topical dapsone has also been shown in a case report to be effective in the treatment of leukocytoclastic vasculitis.[46,47]

Dapsone is metabolized in the liver. The two major metabolic pathways involve acetylation[48,49] and N-hydroxylation.[43-45] Dapsone is acetylated polymorphically; that is, some patients rapidly acetylate dapsone to MADDS, but others acetylate dapsone slowly. However, in all patients, MADDS is rapidly deacetylated. Thus, equilibrium between MADDS and dapsone is quickly reached and sustained. Dapsone's efficacy, half-life, and toxicities appear unrelated to the rate of acetylation, and checking the acetylator phenotype is unnecessary before use of dapsone.

The most clinically significant metabolic pathway of dapsone involves hydroxylation of one of the amino groups by cytochrome 2C19,[43] 3A4, and 2C9 and 2C8[44] to form dapsone hydroxylamine. Dapsone hydroxylamine is a potent oxidant that is responsible for development of methemoglobinemia, hemolysis, and liver damage.[45,47,50,51] Dapsone hydroxylamine is reduced back to dapsone by methemoglobin reductase in erythrocytes and cytochrome b_5 reductase and cytochrome P2D in hepatocytes. Reduced levels of these enzymes have been detected in dapsone-treated patients who developed symptomatic methemoglobinemia. Genetic variability in detoxifying enzymes may therefore explain patients' differential development of methemoglobinemia.[52] Recent studies have also shown that dapsone can be hydroxylated by keratinocytes themselves. These hydroxylated metabolites then form drug–protein adducts that generate stress signals, which are delivered to draining lymph nodes. This may be responsible for the pathogenesis of some of the cutaneous side effects of dapsone.[53-55]

Dapsone is predominantly metabolized by the hepatocytes, but a small study indicated that there is no need to adjust dapsone doses in patients with cirrhosis.[56] However, it is prudent to exercise caution when prescribing dapsone in patients with hepatic disease.

Probenecid[57] and trimethoprim[58] have been shown to lead to higher blood levels of dapsone (Table 187-1), hence the need to exercise caution when prescribing them concurrently. Conversely, rifampicin reduces dapsone blood levels by upregulating the P_{450} system.[59] Cimetidine and omeprazole, which block N-hydroxylation of dapsone, have been used to mitigate some of the side effects of dapsone. Cimetidine dosed 400 mg three times a day has reduced methemoglobin levels in reported patients by 27% to 60%.[60-63]

Dapsone and its metabolites are excreted by the kidneys; therefore, it is important to check renal functions before prescribing dapsone to patients. Dapsone should be avoided in patients with significant renal dysfunction.

MEDICAL INDICATIONS OF DAPSONE

Since its introduction, dapsone has had therapeutic trials and anecdotal successes in a multitude of diseases (Table 187-2). However, there are only a few conditions for which dapsone is considered the drug of choice.

ANTIMICROBIAL ACTION

Dapsone is most commonly used in combination with rifampicin and clofazimine for the treatment of leprosy.[64] It is also used to both treat and prevent PCP,[65] especially in immunocompromised hosts. It is also used for toxoplasmosis in people who are unable to tolerate trimethoprim with sulfamethoxazole.[65]

ANTIINFLAMMATORY ACTION

Other indications include dermatitis herpetiformis (in combination with a gluten-free diet),[66,67] erythema

TABLE 187-1
Common Drug Interactions

Increase Blood Levels of Dapsone (Greater Chance of Adverse Events)
- Probenecid
- Trimethoprim

Reduces Blood Levels of Dapsone (Lowers Effectiveness)
- Rifampicin

Block N-Hydroxylation of Dapsone (Lessening Side Effects)
- Cimetidine
- Omeprazole

TABLE 187-2
Therapeutic Indications for Dapsone[1,22,226]

As an Antiinfective Drug
Infections diseases: Hensen disease, malaria, leishmaniasis, nocardiosis, *Pneumocystis* prophylaxis

As an Antiinflammatory Drug
Consistently responsive: dermatitis herpetiformis, erythema elevatum diutinum, linear IgA dermatosis and chronic bullous dermatosis of childhood (idiopathic or drug induced), bullous SLE, prurigo pigmentosa, acropustulosis infantalis

Used as an Adjunctive Combination Treatment
Autoimmune blistering diseases: pemphigus (foliaceus, vulgaris and IgA variants), bullous pemphigoid, epidermolysis bullosa acquisita, mucous membrane pemphigoid
Neutrophilic dermatosis: subcorneal pustular dermatosis (idiopathic and drug induced), acute febrile neutrophilic dermatosis (Sweet syndrome), pyoderma gangrenosum
Autoimmune diseases: rheumatoid papules, relapsing polychondritis, subacute lupus erythematosus, chronic cutaneous lupus erythematosus, lupus panniculitis, vasculitides, cutaneous polyarteritis nodosa, urticarial vasculitis, Henoch-Schönlein purpura, chronic leukocytoclastic vasculitis
Others: Behçet disease, acne and related disorders, hidradenitis suppurativa, granuloma faciale, perifolliculitis capitis abscedens et suffodiens, brown recluse spider bites that becomes necrotic, generalized granuloma annulare, chronic idiopathic thrombocytopenia purpura, chronic urticaria, aphthous stomatitis, psoriasis, Melkersson-Rosenthal syndrome, eosinophilic fasciitis, α_1-antitrypsin deficiency–related panniculitis, neutrophilic eccrine hidradenitis, insect bite–like reactions in patients with leukemia, erythema multiforme, Rosai-Dorfman disease, idiopathic angioedema, eosinophilic folliculitis (Ofuji disease)

Used in Nondermatologic Disorders
Rheumatoid arthritis, eosinophilic fasciitis, immune thrombocytopenia, stroke, asthma, seizure disorders, glioblastoma

---

elevatum diutinum (effective in 80% of early cases of the disease),[68,69] linear IgA dermatosis and chronic bullous dermatosis of childhood,[70-73] and the bullous eruption of systemic lupus erythematosus.[74,75] Patients with these disorders achieve a clinical response within 24 to 48 hours, and their conditions flare over the same time course with drug withdrawal. In 2015, dapsone was reported to be effective against generalized granuloma annulare.[76]

Other noninfectious conditions in which dapsone has found sporadic success span the spectrum of dermatologic disease (see Table 187-2).[75,77-147] As a unifying feature, most of these diseases have granulocytes (neutrophils or eosinophils) as the predominant infiltrating cell, especially early in the pathologic process. The response to dapsone therapy is not as rapid, regular, or predictable in these diseases. However, dapsone may have a role as a second-line or steroid-sparing agent.

DOSAGES

A therapeutic dose of dapsone varies from 25 mg to 200 mg/day, usually in a single dose. Rarely, patients may require 300 mg/day before a response is seen. The recommended starting dose is between 50 and 100 mg/day to minimize potential pharmacologic adverse effects, in particular hemolysis. If a therapeutic trial of dapsone is successful, the dose of dapsone should be decreased to a point at which lesions recur to be sure that the improvement was indeed caused by dapsone and that there is a continuing need for the drug. Reducing the dose of dapsone to the lowest effective dose is an important means to minimize potential side effects.

TOPICAL DAPSONE

Topical dapsone (5% gel) is FDA approved for acne vulgaris in adults[9,36-40] and adolescents[77] up to 12 years old. It has not been reported to cause hemolysis even in patients with G6PD deficiency.[9] Clinical trials showed that it can reduce the mean total lesion count by 39% and 49%.[9,36,40,77] It can be used in conjunction with other acne medications, including adapalene and benzoyl peroxide gel.[78]

Topical dapsone, when applied together with benzoyl peroxide, may cause yellow-orange discoloration of the skin; it is washable from skin but may stain clothing.[79] Dapsone 7.5% gel has been FDA approved for the treatment of mild to moderate acne vulgaris as a single daily application since 2016.[80]

ADVERSE REACTIONS FROM DAPSONE (TABLE 187-3)

HEMATOLOGY

HEMOLYSIS

The commonest side effects of dapsone is dose-related hemolysis. Hemolysis may lead to hemolytic anemia and methemoglobinemia. About 20% of patients receiving dapsone treatment develop hemolysis.[22] The side effect is more common and severe in those with G6PD deficiency. G6PD deficiency should be ruled out before initiating therapy in all patients.[148] Hemolysis is more profound at the initiation of therapy and is often accompanied by a compensatory reticulocytosis. However, G6PD-deficient patients are less susceptible to methemoglobinemia production, but more susceptible to hemolysis.[22] A case of hemolysis in a neonate from dapsone in breast milk has been reported.[27,32]

METHEMOGLOBINEMIA

Methemoglobinemia is a predictable consequence of dapsone therapy caused by dapsone hydroxylamine's

TABLE 187-3
Adverse Effects of Dapsone[a]

Hematology
- Hemolysis
- Methemoglobinemia

Liver
- Toxic hepatitis
- Cholestatic jaundice
- Transaminitis
- Hypoalbuminemia

Skin
- Exfoliative dermatitis
- Erythema multiforme
- Urticaria
- Erythema nodosum
- Morbilliform exanthem
- Scarlatiniform exanthem
- Photosensitivity

Others
- Gastrointestinal upset (nausea)
- Headache
- Fatigue
- Insomnia
- *Psychosis*
- Peripheral neuropathy
- Motor neuropathy

Life-Threatening Side Effects
- Dapsone hypersensitivity syndrome
- Hemolysis
- Methemoglobinemia
- *Agranulocytosis*
- *Aplastic anemia*
- Hemophagocytic syndrome
- *Toxic epidermal necrolysis, Stevens-Johnson syndrome*[194]

[a]Italicized adverse effects are idiosyncratic and not dose dependent.

generation of reactive oxygen species (ROS).[149-156] Methemoglobinemia usually occurs only with the intake of oral dapsone; however, a single case of methemoglobinemia has been reported in a patient using topical 5% dapsone.[49] Methemoglobin is the form of hemoglobin in which the iron molecule is in the oxidized ferric (Fe^{3+}) state rather than in the ferrous state (Fe^{2+}). As such, the molecule itself is unable to carry oxygen or carbon dioxide.[151] The signs and symptoms of methemoglobinemia are those of poor oxygenation, including cyanosis, headache, shortness of breath, chest pain, and fatigue. And although some degree of methemoglobinemia occurs in most patients, symptomatic methemoglobinemia is rare. Symptoms usually occur with methemoglobin levels of 20% to 30%.[155,156] Pulse oximetry is a reasonable screening test for methemoglobinemia because a normal value excludes significant methemoglobin levels. However, an abnormal value must be followed up with a direct methemoglobin determination.[152-157] Cimetidine, which blocks the hydroxylation of dapsone, has been used intentionally to lower methemoglobin levels in dapsone-treated patients by 27% to 60%.[60-63,158] Lipoic acid, a dietary supplement with antioxidant properties, has also been shown in vitro to decrease methemoglobin formation, and 90 mg/day of lipoic acid daily has been suggested for dapsone-treated patients.[159]

Although G6PD-deficient individuals are at greater risk for hemolytic anemia and methemoglobinemia, the clinician should remember that these events are also seen in patients without G6PD deficiency.[160]

LIVER

Toxic hepatitis and cholestatic jaundice from dapsone have been reported. Hepatitis and jaundice may also occur as part of the dapsone hypersensitivity reaction or syndrome. Dapsone is metabolized by the cytochrome P450 system. Dapsone metabolites produced by the cytochrome P450 2C19 isozyme are associated with the methemoglobinemia side effect of the drug.

SKIN

Various skin eruptions from dapsone have been described.[161] They include exfoliative dermatitis, erythema multiforme, urticaria, erythema nodosum, morbilliform and scarlatiniform exanthema, and Stevens-Johnson syndrome or toxic epidermal necrolysis. Dapsone-induced photosensitivity is quite rare but usually not dose dependent. When used topically, dapsone can cause mild skin irritation, redness, dry skin, burning, and itching.

OTHER ADVERSE EFFECTS

These include nausea, headache, fatigue, insomnia, psychosis, and peripheral neuropathy. Also reported are varied neurologic side effects, including a distal motor neuropathy, most often without a sensory component.[162-164] These are usually reversible with dose decrease or discontinuation of dapsone. Checking a patient's distal motor strength at follow-up visits may alert the clinician to such side effects.

Effects on the lung occur rarely and may be serious, although they are generally reversible.[165]

SERIOUS ADVERSE REACTIONS TO DAPSONE

DAPSONE HYPERSENSITIVITY SYNDROME

Hypersensitivity reactions to dapsone occur in some patients. This reaction may be more frequent in patients receiving multiple-drug therapy.[166-168] The reaction manifests with a rash and may also present with fever, jaundice, and eosinophilia.[169-173] In general, these symptoms occur within the first 6 weeks of therapy and may be ameliorated by corticosteroid therapy.

This reaction appears to be more frequent in patients receiving multiple-drug therapy.[168] Latencies of the hypersensitivity syndrome after initiation of dapsone treatment were less than 20 days, 24.5%; 21 to 28 days, 35.0%; 29 to 35 days, 20.9%; and more than 36 days, 19.6%. Maximum latency was 20 weeks; 91% and 97% of patients presented with a rash and fever respectively, and 73.7% had lymphadenopathy. Hepatic dysfunction could be detected in the majority of cases, its severity ranging from abnormal liver test results over hepatosplenomegaly and jaundice to hepatic coma. About half of the patients demonstrated hematologic changes (leucocytosis in 56.6%, eosinophilia in 43.8%). After withdrawal of dapsone (and in most cases, steroid therapy), the majority of patients (82.3%) recovered, but nearly 10% had a fatal outcome, hepatic coma being the most frequent cause of death. Early discontinuation of dapsone was associated with a better prognosis.[22,174] Corticosteroids have proved helpful, but dosages up to 1g/day of methylprednisolone for 3 days may be required followed by a prednisone taper over 4 to 6 weeks.

Clinicians should be alert for rashes that present with fever and other systemic symptoms because these may be manifestations of the dapsone hypersensitivity syndrome.[175-190] The incidence of this syndrome ranges from 0.2% to 5% of treated patients.[175-178] It is similar to hypersensitivity syndrome seen with some anticonvulsants and other medications.[179,180] These syndromes are postulated to be due to drug-allergy-induced immunosuppression[53,54,178,179] leading to a reactivation of human herpesvirus 6 (HHV6) or other latent viruses such as cytomegalovirus and Epstein-Barr virus. They develop between 2 and 7 weeks after initiating the medication and inevitably include the triad of fever, rash, and hepatitis. The rash is most often an exfoliative dermatitis,[180] but maculopapular and Stevens-Johnson–like lesions have occurred. It is the reactivation of HHV6 that is thought to cause the late flaring of rash, fever, and hepatitis characteristically seen in this class of drug reactions, necessitating such a long steroid taper.[178] The hepatitis has a mixed hepatocellular and cholestatic picture with elevations in both transaminases[181-186] and alkaline phosphatase.[187] Additionally, any other end-organ damage must be managed supportively.[175,176] Plasma exchange has also been successfully used in a patient in whom tapering of steroids led to recrudescence of symptoms.[190]

HEMOLYSIS AND METHEMOGLOBINEMIA

Dapsone therapy is often associated with hemolysis and sometimes methemoglobinemia in a dose-dependent fashion.[191] These adverse effects are caused by the hydroxylated metabolite, dapsone hydroxylamine, a potent oxidant.[45,47,192-197] Within the erythrocytes, dapsone hydroxylamine generates ROS, which oxidize oxyhemoglobin into methemoglobin. Acute methemoglobinemia occurs rarely but may result in dyspnea, anemia, and vascular collapse; in serious cases, it may result in death. The oxidized hemoglobin becomes microscopically visible as Heinz bodies. These Heinz bodies and hydroxylated metabolite/cellular protein adducts may label the red blood cells (RBCs) as senescent, targeting them for removal by the spleen. Glutathione within the erythrocytes is responsible for reversing oxidative damage; however, production of glutathione depends on G6PD. Patients with G6PD deficiency are less tolerant of pharmacologic oxidative stress and are at risk for substantial hemolysis. There are two types of G6PD deficiency that are screened for with the same laboratory assay: "A-type" G6PD deficiency occurs in African Americans and is milder than the type seen in patients of Mediterranean heritage.[198] G6PD deficiency should be ruled out before initiating dapsone therapy in all patients.[148] Baseline anemias should be worked up before starting patients on dapsone. The frequency of symptomatic anemia is 10%,[199] but it might be higher in certain populations such as solid organ allograft recipients (23%).[200,201] This higher rate of hemolysis may be attributable to the greater frequency of renal insufficiency in this patient population or a potential interaction with medicines such as sirolimus. If dapsone therapy is efficacious but hemolysis is limiting therapy, coadministration of darbepoetin may allow continuation of drug at therapeutic doses.[202,203]

AGRANULOCYTOSIS

Agranulocytosis is another rare, idiosyncratic side effect and has been estimated to occur in 0.2% to 0.4% of treated patients.[148,159,191,204-209] It usually occurs during the first 3 months of therapy. Although usually reversible within days when patients stop therapy, it may be fatal because of superseding infection. Symptoms of agranulocytosis include fever, pharyngitis, dysphagia, and oral ulcerations.[148,191] Patients should be warned to seek medical care immediately if these symptoms develop. Recombinant granulocyte colony-stimulating factor has been used to produce a more rapid resolution of agranulocytosis.[210]

APLASTIC ANEMIA

Individual case reports of other hematologic sequelae of dapsone include two cases of pure RBC aplasia[211] and a single case of hemophagocytic syndrome induced by dapsone.[212] Abnormalities in white blood cell formation, including aplastic anemia, are rare yet are the cause of the majority of deaths attributable to dapsone therapy.[213-215]

INITIATING AND MONITORING OF DAPSONE THERAPY

Before starting patients on dapsone, a targeted history and physical examination to screen for significant preexisting anaemia, cardiopulmonary disease, and peripheral neuropathy should be performed. Laboratory tests (Table 187-4) should include a complete blood cell count and reticulocytes counts to determine baseline white blood cell count, hemoglobin, and reticulocytes. G6PD deficiency should be ruled out, as should significant hepatic or renal dysfunction. After therapy has begun, a white blood cell count with differential and hemoglobin levels and reticulocytes count should be obtained weekly for the first month and then twice a month during the next 2 months.[148,191] A drop in hemoglobin of 1 to 2 g/dL should be anticipated and, in the absence of symptoms, should not prompt drug discontinuation. Monitoring reticulocyte counts also provide an estimation of the adequacy of compensation for hemolysis. A profoundly elevated reticulocyte count suggests that erythropoiesis is at its maximum and that further dose increases are not likely to be well tolerated. Even during long-term therapy, complete blood cell counts should be obtained periodically. Checking methemoglobin levels is unnecessary in the absence of symptoms. Patients should also be told to carry a medication card so that in an emergency, treating physicians will know they are taking a drug with hemolytic and methemoglobin-generating potential. It is important that all patients be made aware of the potential clinical manifestations of adverse events. Especially during the first 3 months of therapy when the risk of agranulocytosis and the dapsone hypersensitivity syndrome is highest, patients should be reminded to seek medical attention immediately for significant fever, pharyngitis, dysphagia, swollen lymph nodes, oral ulcerations, and rash.[148,191] Patients with diabetes should also be made aware that dapsone causes falsely low hemoglobin A1c values because of the accelerated RBC turnover; monitoring fructosamine levels avoids this potential confounder.[216]

It might be suggested to patients who have mild symptoms of anemia or methemoglobinemia to take cimetidine 400 mg three times daily and lipoic acid 90 mg/day to see if these might ameliorate symptoms enough for dapsone administration to continue.[60-63,169]

Dapsone is contraindicated in patients who are allergic to the drug. It should not be administered to patients with severe anaemia. Dapsone must be used with caution in the following conditions: G6PD deficiency, methemoglobinemia reductase deficiency, severe hepatopathy, cardiac insufficiency or heart failure, and pulmonary diseases as well as comedication with methemoglobinemia-inducing drugs or compounds.

TREATING OVERDOSE

In the case of accidental or intentional dapsone overdose, the clinician should be prepared for significant hemolysis (which may be delayed by up to 9 days because of enterohepatic recirculation) and methemoglobinemia.[217-219] Massive intravascular hemolysis seen in dapsone overdose has been linked to optic ischemic injury.[220-222] Although dapsone is 50% to 80% protein bound in the circulation, the unbound portion can be dialyzed off, and repeated dialysis has been helpful in the case of overdose.[223] Because of dapsone's enterohepatic recirculation, administration of activated charcoal will reduce drug levels by removing drug from the gut. Methylene blue, 1% solution given 1 to 2 mg/kg slowly intravenously,[224,225] can be used to decrease the degree of methemoglobinemia. Methylene blue is a cofactor for methemoglobin reductase after first being reduced by cellular stores of NADPH (nicotinamide adenine dinucleotide phosphate hydrogen) to leukomethylene blue. G6PD-deficient patients should not be given methylene blue because they may have insufficient NADPH, and unreduced methylene blue is its own direct hemolytic agent. Ascorbic acid 1000 mg intravenously every 12 hours has also been used in a case of overdose and certainly could be used until G6PD status is reviewed so that methylene blue can be administered. Ascorbic acid's effect is caused by its ability to increase methemoglobin reductase activity.[218]

ACKNOWLEDGMENTS

We acknowledge Joni G. Sago and Russell P. Hall III, who wrote the previous version of this chapter. The new version is adapted from the previous version.

TABLE 187-4
Laboratory Monitoring

Before Initiation of Therapy
- Glucose-6-phosphate dehydrogenase
- CBC
- Reticulocyte count
- Hepatic function tests
- Renal function tests

During Therapy
- CBC (with WBC differential) weekly for the first month and twice a month for the next 2 months; periodically thereafter
- Reticulocyte count weekly for the first month and twice a month for the next 2 months; periodically thereafter

CBC, complete blood count; G6PD, glucose-6-phosphate dehydrogenase; WBC, white blood cell.

REFERENCES

1. Lang PG. Sulfones and sulfonamides in dermatology today. *J Am Acad Dermatol*. 1979;1:479.
2. Zhu YI, Stiller MJ. Dapsone and sulfones in dermatology: overview and update. *J Am Acad Dermatol* 2001;45:420.
3. Holtzer CD, Flaherty JFJ, Coleman RL. Crossreactivity

3. in HIV-infected patients switched from trimethoprim-sulfamethoxazole to dapsone. *Pharmacotherapy*. 1998;18:831.
4. Beumont MG, Graziani A, Ubel PA, et al. Safety of dapsone as Pneumocystis carinii pneumonia prophylaxis in human immunodeficiency virus-infected patients with allergy to trimethoprim/sulfamethoxazole. *Am J Med*. 1996;100:611.
5. Buttle GAH, Stephenson D, Smith T, et al. The treatment of streptococcal infections in mice with 4:20diamino-diphenylsulfone. *Lancet*. 1937;229:1331-1334.
6. Debol SM, Herron MJ, Nelson RD. Anti-inflammatory action of dapsone: inhibition of neutrophil adherence is associated with inhibition of chemoattractant-induced signal transduction. *J Leukoc Biol*. 1997;62:827-836.
7. Coleman MD. Dapsone: modes of action, toxicity and possible strategies for increasing patient tolerance. *Br J Dermatol*. 1993;129:507-513.
8. Dapsone In: McEvoy GK (ed). *AHFS Drug Information*. Bethesda, MD: American Society of Health-System Pharmacists; 2011:622-626.
9. Stotland M, Shalita AR, Kissling RF. Dapsone 5% gel: a review of its efficacy and safety in the treatment of acne vulgaris. *Am J Clin Dermatol*. 2009;10(4):1594-1602.
10. Allergan. Aczone (dapsone) 7.5% Gel prescribing information (PDF). Allergan USA, Inc.; Madison, NJ: February 2016.
11. Harvath L, Yancey KB, Katz SI. Selective inhibition of human neutrophil chemotaxis to N-formylmethionyl-leucyl-phenylalanine by sulfones. *J Immunol*. 1986;137:1305.
12. Maloff BL, Fox D, Bruin E, et al. Dapsone inhibits LTB4 binding and bioresponse at the cellular and physiologic levels. *Eur J Pharmacol*. 1988;158:85.
13. Wozel G, Blasum C, Winter C, et al. Dapsone hydroxylamine inhibits the LTB4-induced chemotaxis of polymorphonuclear leukocytes into human skin: results of a pilot study. *Inflamm Res*. 1997;46:420.
14. Wozel G, Lehmann B. Dapsone inhibits the generation of 5-lipoxygenase products in human polymorphonuclear leukocytes. *Skin Pharmacol*. 1995;8:196.
15. Thuong-Nguyen V, Kadunce DP, Hendrix JD, et al. Inhibition of neutrophil adherence to antibody by dapsone: a possible therapeutic mechanism of dapsone in the treatment of IgA dermatoses. *J Invest Dermatol*. 1993;100:349.
16. Coleman MD, Smith JK, Perris AD, et al. Studies on the inhibitory effects of analogues of dapsone on neutrophil function in-vitro. *J Pharm Pharmacol*. 1997;49:53.
17. Schmidt E, Reimer S, Kruse N, et al. The IL-8 release from cultured human keratinocytes, mediated by antibodies to bullous pemphigoid autoantigen 180, is inhibited by dapsone. *Clin Exp Immunol*. 2001;124:157.
18. Abe M, Shimizu A, Yokoyama Y, et al. A possible inhibitory action of diaminodiphenyl sulfone on tumour necrosis factor-alpha production from activated mononuclear cells on cutaneous lupus erythematosus. *Clin Exp Dermatol*. 2008;33(6):759-763.
19. Stendahl O, Dahlgren C. The inhibition of polymorphonuclear leukocyte cytotoxicity by dapsone; a possible mechanism in the treatment of dermatitis herpetiformis. *J Clin Invest*. 1977;62:214.
20. Kazmierowski JA, Ross JE, Peizner DS, et al. Dermatitis herpetiformis: effects of sulfones and sulfonamides on neutrophil myeloperoxidase-mediated iodination and cytotoxicity. *J Clin Immunol*. 1984;4:55.
21. Suda T, Suzuki Y, Matsui T, et al. Dapsone suppresses human neutrophil superoxide production and elastase release in a calcium-dependent manner. *Br J Dermatol*. 2005;152:887.
22. Wozel G, Blasu C. Dapsone in dermatology and beyond. *Arch Dermatol Res*. 2014;306:103-124.
23. Ahmad RA, Rogers HJ. Pharmacokinetics and protein binding interactions of dapsone and pyrimethamine. *Br J Clin Pharmacol*. 1980;10:519-524.
24. Zuidema J, Hilbers-Modderman ES, Merkus FW. Clinical pharmacokinetics of dapsone. *Clin Pharmacokinet*. 1986;11:299-315.
25. Uetrecht J, Zahid N, Shear NH, et al. Metabolism of dapsone to a hydroxylamine by human neutrophils and mononuclear cells. *J Pharmacol Exp Ther*. 1988;245:274-279.
26. Branski D, Kerem E, Gross-Kieselstein E, et al. A Bloody diarrhea—a possible complication of sulfasalazine transferred through human breast milk. *J Pediatr Gastroenterol Nutr*. 1986;5:316-317.
27. Sanders SW, Zone JJ, Foltz RL, et al. Hemolytic anemia induced by dapsone transmitted through breast milk. *Ann Intern Med*. 1982;96:465-466.
28. Lowe J. Studies in sulphone therapy. *Lepr Rev*. 1952;23:4-29.
29. Wolf R, Tuzun B, Tuzun Y. Dapsone: unapproved uses or indications. *Clin Dermatol*. 2000;18:37-53.
30. Khan FD, Roychowdhury S, Nemes R, et al. Effect of pro-inflammatory cytokines on the toxicity of the arylhydroxylamine metabolites of sulpha-methoxazole and dapsone in normal human keratinocytes. *Toxicology*. 2006;218:90-99.
31. Endre ZH, Charlesworth JA, Macdonald GJ, et al. Successful treatment of acute dapsone intoxication using charcoal hemoperfusion. *Aust N Z J Med*. 1983;13:509.
32. Edstein MD, Veenendaal JR, Newman K, et al. Excretion of chloroquine, dapsone and pyrimethamine in human milk. *Br J Clin Pharmacol*. 1986;22:733.
33. Hocking DR. Neonatal haemolytic disease due to dapsone. *Med J Aust*. 1968;1:1130.
34. Maurus JN. Hansen's disease in pregnancy. *Obstet Gynecol*. 1978;52:22.
35. Collier PM, Kelly SE, Wojnarowska F. Linear IgA disease and pregnancy. *J Am Acad Dermatol*. 1994;30:407.
36. Draelos Z, Carter E, Maloney J, et al. Two randomized studies demonstrate the efficacy and safety of dapsone gel 5% for the treatment of acne vulgaris. *J Am Acad Dermatol*. 2007;56:439.e1-e10.
37. Scheinfeld N. Aczone, a topical gel formulation of the antibacterial, anti-inflammatory dapsone for the treatment of acne. *Curr Opin Investig Drugs*. 2009;10(5):474-481.
38. Thiboutot D, Willmer J, Sharata H, et al. Pharmacokinetics of dapsone gel, 5% for the treatment of acne vulgaris. *Clin Pharmaokinet*. 2007;46(8):697-712.
39. Piette W, Taylor S, Pariser D, et al. Hematologic safety of dapsone gel 5% for topical treatment of acne vulgaris. *Arch Dermatol*. 2008;144(12):1564-1570.
40. Lucky A, Maloney JM, Roberts J, et al. Dapsone gel 5% for the treatment of acne vulgaris: safety and efficacy of long-term (1 year) treatment. *J Drugs Dermatol*. 2007;6(10):981-987.
41. Al-Salama ZT, Deeks ED. Dapsone 7.5% gel: a review in acne vulgaris. *Am J Clin Dermatol*. 2017;18(1):139-145.

42. Draelos ZD, Rodriguez DA, Kempers SE, et al. Treatment response with once-daily topical dapsone gel, 7.5% for acne vulgaris: subgroup analysis of pooled data from two randomized, Double-blind studies. *J Drugs Dermatol*. 2017;16(6):591-598.
43. Caraco Y, Wilkinson GR, Wood AJ. Differences between white subjects and Chinese subjects in the in vivo inhibition of cytochrome P450s 2C19, 2D6 and 3A by omeprazole. *Clin Pharmacol Ther*. 1996;60:396.
44. Gill JP, Gil Berglund E. CYP2C8 and antimalaria drug efficacy. *Pharmacogenomics*. 2007;8(2):187-198.
45. Cucinell SA, Israili ZH, Dayton PG. Microsomal N-oxidation of dapsone as a cause of methemoglobin formation in human red cells. *Am J Trop Med Hygiene*. 1972;21:322.
46. Pate DA, Johnson LS, Tarbox MB. Leukocytoclastic vasculitis resolution with topical dapsone. *Cutis*. 2017;99(6):426-428.
47. Hjelm M, DeVerdier CH. Biochemical effects of aromatic amines-I. Methaemoglobinaemia, haemolysis and Heinz-body formation induced by 4,4′-diaminodiphenylsulphone. *Biochem Pharmacol*. 1965;14:1119.
48. Ellard GA, Gammon PT, Savin JA, et al. Dapsone acetylation in dermatitis herpetiformis. *Br J Dermatol*. 1974;90:441.
49. Ellard GA, Gammon PT, Helmy HS, et al. Dapsone acetylation and the treatment of leprosy. *Nature*. 1972;239:159.
50. Clement B, Helmy HS, Rees RJ. et al. Reduction of sulfamethoxazole and dapsone hydroxylamines by a microsomal enzyme system purified from pig liver and pig and human liver microsomes. *Life Sci*. 2005;77:205.
51. Ganesan S, Sahu R, Walker LA, et al. Cytochrome P450-dependent toxicity of dapsone in human erythrocytes. *J Appl Toxicol*. 2010;30(3):271-275.
52. Eichelbaum M, Evert B. Influence of pharmacogenetics on drug disposition and response. *Clin Exp Pharmacol Physiol*. 1996;23:983.
53. Roychowdhury S, Vyas PM, Reilly TP, et al. Characterization of the formation and localization of sulfamethoxazole and dapsone-associated drug-protein adducts in human epidermal keratinocytes. *J Pharmacol Exp Ther*. 2005;314:43.
54. Roychowdhury S, Cram AE, Aly A, et al. Detection of haptenated proteins in organotypic human skin explant cultures exposed to dapsone. *Drug Metab Dispos*. 2007;35:1463-1465.
55. Khan F, Vyas PM, Gaspari AA, et al. Effect of arylhydroxylamine metabolites of sulfamethoxazole and dapsone on stress signal expression in human keratinocytes. *J Pharm Exp Ther*. 2007;323(3):771-777.
56. May DG, Arns PA, Richards WO, et al. The disposition of dapsone in cirrhosis. *Clin Pharmacol Ther*. 1992;51:689.
57. Goodwin CS, Sparell G. Inhibition of dapsone excretion by probenecid. *Lancet*. 1969;294:884.
58. Lee BL, Medina I, Benowitz NL, et al. Dapsone, trimethoprim, and sulfamethoxazole plasma levels during treatment of Pneumocystis pneumonia in patients with the acquired immunodeficiency syndrome (AIDS). Evidence of drug interactions. *Ann Intern Med*. 1989;110:606.
59. Balakrishnan SPS. Drug interactions—The influence of rifampicin and clofazimine on the urinary excretion of DDS. *Lepr India*. 1981;53:17.
60. Rhodes LE, Tingle MD, Park BK, et al. Cimetidine improves the therapeutic/toxic ratio of dapsone in patients on chronic dapsone therapy. *Br J Dermatol*. 1995;132:257.
61. Coleman M. Improvement of patient tolerance to dapsone: current and future developments. *Dermatol Online J*. 2007;13(4):18.
62. Mehta M. Cimetidine and dapsone-mediated methaemoglobinaemia. *Anaesthesia*. 2007;62:1188.
63. Goolamali S, Macfarlane C. The use of cimetidine to reduce dapsone-dependent haematological side-effects in a patient with mucous membrane pemphigoid. *Clin Exp Dermatol*. 2009;34:e1025-e1026.
64. Grunwald MH, Amichai B. Dapsone—the treatment of infectious and inflammatory diseases in dermatology. *Int J Antimicrob Agents*. 1996;7:187-192.
65. Rossi S, ed. *Australian Medicines Handbook*. Adelaide, Australian Medicines Handbook; 2006.
66. Kruizinga EE, Hamminga H. Treatment of dermatitis herpetiformis with diaminodiphenylsulphone (DDS). *Dermatologica*. 1953;106:386.
67. Katz SI. Treatment: drugs and diet, in dermatitis herpetiformis: the skin and the gut. *Ann Intern Med*. 1980;93:857.
68. Katz SI, Gallin JI, Hertz KC, et al. Erythema elevatum diutinum: skin and systemic manifestations, immunologic studies, and successful treatment with dapsone. *Medicine (Baltimore)*. 1977;56:443.
69. Farley-Loftus R, Dadlani C, Wang N, et al. Erythema elevatum diutinum. *Dermatol Online J*. 2008;14(10):13.
70. Leonard JN, Haffenden GP, Ring NP, et al. Linear IgA disease in adults. *Br J Dermatol*. 1982;107:301.
71. Jablonska S, Chorzelski TP, Rosinska D, et al. Linear IgA bullous dermatosis of childhood (chronic bullous dermatosis of childhood). *Clin Dermatol*. 1992;9:393.
72. Wojnarowska F, Marsden RA, Bhogal B, et al. Chronic bullous disease of childhood, childhood cicatricial pemphigoid and linear IgA disease of adults: a comparative study demonstrating clinical and immunopathologic overlap. *J Am Acad Dermatol*. 1988;19:792.
73. Nanda A, Dvorak R, Al-Sabah H, et al. Linear IgA bullous disease of childhood: an experience from Kuwait. *Pediatr Dermatol*. 2006;23(5):442-447.
74. Hall RP, Lawley TJ, Smith HR, et al. Bullous eruption of systemic lupus erythematosus. Dramatic response to dapsone therapy. *Ann Intern Med*. 1982;97:165.
75. Callen JP. Treatment of cutaneous lesions in patients with lupus erythematosus. *Dermatol Clin* 1994;12:201.
76. Lukács J, Schliemann S, Elsner P. Treatment of generalized granuloma annulare—a systematic review. *J Eur Acad Dermatol Venereol*. 2015;29(8):1467-1480.
77. Raimer S, Maloney JM, Bourcier M, et al. Efficacy and safety of dapsone gel 5% for the treatment of acne vulgaris in adolescents. *Cutis*. 2008;81:171-178.
78. Fleischer A, Shalita A, Eichenfield LF, et al. Dapsone gel 5% in combination with Dapalene Gel 0.1%, benzoyl peroxide gel 4% or moisturizer for the treatment of acne vulgaris: a 12-week, randomized, double-blind study. *J Drugs Dermatol*. 2010;9(1):33-40.
79. Dubina M, Fleischer A. Interaction of topical sulfacetamide and topical dapsone with benzoyl peroxide. *Arch Dermatol*. 2009;145(9):1027-1029.
80. Marcus KA. Office of Drug Evaluation III Center for Drug Evaluation and Research FDA. Federal Food, Drug, and Cosmetic Act (FDCA) for ACZONE (dapsone) Gel, 7.5%. 2016.
81. Yasuda H, Kobayashi H, Hashimoto T, et al. Subcorneal pustular dermatosis type of IgA pemphigus: demon-

stration of autoantibodies to desmocollin-1 and clinical review [review]. *Br J Dermatol*. 2000;143:144.

82. Heaphy MR, Kobayashi H, Hashimoto T, et al. Dapsone as a glucocorticoid-sparing agent in maintenance-phase pemphigus vulgaris. *Arch Dermatol*. 2005;141:699.

83. Martin LK, Agero AL, Werth V, et al. Interventions for pemphigus vulgaris and pemphigus foliaceus. Cochrane Database of Systematic Reviews 2009, Issue 1. Art. No.: CD006263. doi: 10.1002/14651858. CD006263.pub2.

84. Gurcan H, Ahmed R. Efficacy of dapsone in the treatment of pemphigus and pemphigoid: analysis of current data. *Am J Clin Dermatol*. 2009;10(6):383-396.

85. Person JR, Rogers RS. Bullous pemphigoid responding to sulfapyridine and the sulfones. *Arch Dermatol*. 1977;113:610.

86. Venning VA, Millard PR, Wojnarowska F. Dapsone as first line therapy for bullous pemphigoid. *Br J Dermatol*. 1989;120:83.

87. Bouscarat F, Chosidow O, Picard-Dahan C, et al. Treatment of bullous pemphigoid with dapsone: retrospective study of thirty-six cases. *J Am Acad Dermatol*. 1996;34:683.

88. Schmidt E, Kraensel R, Goebeler M, et al. Treatment of bullous pemphigoid with dapsone, methylprednisolone, and topical clobetasol propionate: a retrospective study of 62 cases. *Cutis*. 2005;76:205.

89. Motegi S, Abe M, Tamura A, et al. Childhood bullous pemphigoid successfully treated with diaminodiphenyl sulfone. *J Dermatol*. 2005;32:809-812.

90. Kirtschig G, Murrell D, Wojnarowska F, et al. Interventions for mucous membrane pemphigoid/cicatricial pemphigoid and epidermolysis bullosa acquisita: a systematic literature review. *Arch Dermatol*. 2002;138:380.

91. Rogers RS, Mehregan DA. Dapsone therapy of cicatricial pemphigoid. *Semin Dermatol*. 1998;7:201.

92. Miserocchi E, Baltatzis S, Roque MR, et al. The effect of treatment and its related side effects in patients with severe ocular cicatricial pemphigoid. *Ophthalmology*. 2002;109:111.

93. Cohen D, Ben-Amitai D, Feinmesser M, et al. Childhood lichen planus pemphigoides: a case report and review of the literature. *Pediatr Dermatol*. 2009;26(5):569-574.

94. Cheng S, Edmonds E, Ben-Gashir M, et al. Subcorneal pustular dermatosis: 50 years on. *Clin Dermatol*. 2007; 33:229-233.

95. Aram H. Acute febrile neutrophilic dermatosis (Sweet's syndrome). Response to dapsone. *Arch Dermatol*. 1984;120:245.

96. Walling HW, Snipes CJ, Gerami P, et al. The relationship between neutrophilic dermatosis of the dorsal hands and Sweet syndrome: report of 9 cases and comparison to atypical pyoderma gangrenosum. *Arch Dermatol*. 2006;142:57.

97. Cohen P. Neutrophilic dermatoses: a review of current treatment options. *Am J Clin Dermatol*. 2009;10(5):301-312.

98. Callen JP, Taylor WB. Pyoderma gangrenosum—a literature review. *Cutis*. 1978;21:61.

99. Teasley L, Foster C, Baltatzis S. Sclerokeratitis and facial skin lesions: a case report of pyoderma gangrenosum and its response to dapsone therapy. *Cornea*. 2007;26:215-219.

100. Chang DJ, Lamothe M, Stevens RM, et al. Dapsone in rheumatoid arthritis [review]. *Semin Arthritis Rheum*. 1996;25:390.

101. Martin JA, Jarrett P. Rheumatoid papules treated with dapsone. *Clin Exp Dermatol*. 2004;29:387.

102. Barranco VP, Minor DB, Soloman H. Treatment of relapsing polychondritis with dapsone. *Arch Dermatol*. 1976;112:1286.

103. Damiani JM, Levine HL. Relapsing polychondritis—report of ten cases. *Laryngoscope*. 1979;89(6 Pt 1): 929-946.

104. Walling H, Sontheimer R. Cutaneous lupus erythematosus: issues in diagnosis and treatment. *Am J Clin Dermatol*. 2009;10(6):365-381.

105. Ujiie H, Shimizu T, Ito M, et al. Lupus erythematosus profundus successfully treated with dapsone: review of the literature. *Arch Dermatol*. 2006;142:399.

106. Guillevin L. Treatment of polyarteritis nodosa with dapsone. *Scand J Rheumatol*. 1986;15(1):95-96.

107. Fortson JS, Zone JJ, Hammond ME, et al. Hypocomplementemic urticarial vasculitis syndrome responsive to dapsone. *J Am Acad Dermatol*. 1986;15:1137.

108. Iqbal H, Evans A. Dapsone therapy for Henoch-Schönlein purpura: a case series. *Arch Dis Child*. 2005; 90:985.

109. Shin J, Lee J, Chung K. Dapsone therapy for Henoch-Schonlein purpura. *Arch Dis Child*. 2006;91(8):714.

110. Fredenberg MF, Malkinson FD. Sulfone therapy in the treatment of leukocytoclastic vasculitis. Report of three cases. *J Am Acad Dermatol*. 1987;16:772.

111. Sunderkötter C, Pappelbaum KI, Ehrchen J. Management of leukocytoclastic vasculitis. *J Dermatol Treat*. 2005;16:193.

112. Chen K, Carlson J. Clinical approach to cutaneous vasculitis. *Am J Clin Dermatol*. 2008;9(2):71-92.

113. Sharquie KE. Suppression of Behçet's disease with dapsone. *Br J Dermatol*. 1984;110:493.

114. Sharquie KE, Najim RA, Abu-Raghif AR. Dapsone in Behçet's disease: a double-blind, placebo-controlled, cross-over study. *J Dermatol*. 2002;29:267.

115. Prendiville JS, Logan RA, Russell-Jones R. A comparison of dapsone with 13-cis retinoic acid in the treatment of nodular cystic acne. *Clin Exp Dermatol*. 1988;13:67.

116. Kaur M, Lewis H. Hidradenitis suppurativa treated with dapsone: a case series of five patients. *J Dermatol Treat*. 2006;17:211-213.

117. van de Kerkhof P. On the efficacy of dapsone in granuloma faciale. *Acta Derm Venereol*. 1994;74:61.

118. Bolz S, Jappe U, Hartschuh W. Successful treatment of perifolliculitis capitis abscedens et suffodiens with combined isotretinoin and dapsone. *J German Soc Dermatol*. 2007;6(1):44-47.

119. Godeau B, Durand JM, Roudot-Thoraval F, et al. Dapsone for chronic autoimmune thrombocytopenic purpura: a report of 66 cases. *Br J Haematol*. 1997;97:336.

120. Damodar S, Viswabandya A, George B, et al. Dapsone for chronic idiopathic thrombocytopenic purpura in children and adults—a report on 90 patients. *Eur J Haematol*. 2005;75:328-331.

121. Cassano N, D'Argento V, Filotico R, et al. Low-dose dapsone in chronic idiopathic urticaria: preliminary results of an open study. *Acta Dermato Venereol*. 2005;85:254.

122. Criado R, Criado PR, Martins JE, et al. Urticaria unresponsive to antihistaminic treatment: an open study of therapeutic options based on histopathologic features. *J Dermatol Treat*. 2008;19(2):92-96.

123. Engin B, Ozdemir M. Prospective randomized non-

blinded clinical trial on the use of dapsone plus antihistamine vs. antihistamine in patients with chronic idiopathic urticaria. *J Eur Acad Dermatol Venereol.* 2007;22(4):481-486.
124. Letsinger JA, McCarty MA, Jorizzo JL. Complex aphthosis: a large case series with evaluation algorithm and therapeutic ladder from topicals to thalidomide. *J Am Acad Dermatol.* 2005;52:500.
125. Mimura M, Hirota SK, Sugaya NN, et al. Systemic treatment in severe cases of recurrent aphthous stomatitis: an open trial. *Clinics.* 2009;64(3):193-198.
126. Lynde C, Bruce A, Rogers R. Successful treatment of complex aphthosis with colchicine and dapsone. *Arch Dermatol.* 2009;145(3):273-276.
127. Steiner A, Pehamberger H, Wolff K. Sulfone treatment of granuloma annulare. *J Am Acad Dermatol* 1985;13:1004.
128. Cyr P. Diagnosis and management of granuloma annulare. *Am Fam Physician.* 2006;74(10):1729-1734.
129. Halverstam C, Lebwohl M. Nonstandard and off-label therapies for psoriasis. *Clin Dermatol.* 2009;26(5):546-553.
130. Rees R, Campbell D, Rieger E, et al. The diagnosis and treatment of brown recluse spider bites. *Ann Emerg Med.* 1987;16:945.
131. Rees RS, Altenbern DP, Lynch JB, et al. Brown recluse spider bites. A comparison of early surgical excision versus dapsone and delayed surgical excision. *Ann Surg.* 1985;202:659.
132. Cole HP, Wesley RE, King LEJ. Brown recluse spider envenomation of the eyelid: an animal model. *Ophthalmol Plast Reconstr Surg.* 1994;11:153.
133. Elston DM, Miller SD, Young RJ, et al. Comparison of colchicine, dapsone, triamcinolone, and diphenhydramine therapy for the treatment of brown recluse spider envenomation: a double-blind, controlled study in a rabbit model. *Arch Dermatol.* 2005;141:595.
134. Mold JW, Thompson DM. Management of brown recluse spider bites in primary care. *J Am Board Fam Pract.* 2004;17:347.
135. Peterson MD. Brown spider envenomation. *Clin Tech Small Anim Pract.* 2006;21(4):191-193.
136. Tan J, Rao B. Mesotherapy-induced panniculitis treated with dapsone: case report and review of reported adverse effects of mesotherapy. *J Cut Med Surg.* 2006;10(2):92-95.
137. Gokdemir G, Kucukunal A, Sakiz D. Cutaneous granulomatous reaction from mesotherapy. *Dermatol Surg.* 2009;35(2):291-293.
138. Sobjanek M, Włodarkiewicz A, Zelazny I, et al. Successful treatment of Melkersson-Rosenthal syndrome with dapsone and triamcinolone injections. *J Eur Acad Dermatol Venereol.* 2008;22(8):1029.
139. Smith L, Cox N. Dapsone treatment for eosinophilic fasciitis. *Arch Dermatol.* 2008;144(7):845-847.
140. Pittelkow MR, Smith KC, Su WP. Alpha-1-antitrypsin deficiency and panniculitis. Perspectives on disease relationship and replacement therapy. *Am J Med.* 1988;84:80.
141. Korver G, Liu C, Peterson M. Alpha-1-antitrypsin deficiency presenting with panniculitis and incidental discovery of chronic obstructive pulmonary disease. *Int J Dermatol.* 2007;46(10):1078-1090.
142. Lee S, In SG, Shin JH, et al. Neutrophilic eccrine hidradenitis in non-small cell lung cancer. *Int J Dermatol.* 2007;46(1):59-60.
143. Ulmer A, Metzler G, Schanz S, et al. Dapsone in the management of "insect bite-like reaction" in a patient with chronic lymphocytic leukemia. *Br J Dermatol.* 2007;156:163.
144. Mahendran R, Grant JW, Norris PG. Dapsone-responsive persistent erythema multiforme. *Dermatology.* 2000;200:281-282.
145. Hoffman L, Hoffman M. Dapsone in the treatment of persistent erythema multiforme. *J Drugs Dermatol.* 2006;5(4):375-377.
146. Chan CC, Chu CY. Dapsone as a potential treatment for cutaneous Rosai-Dorfman disease with neutrophilic predominance. *Arch Dermatol.* 2006;142:428-430.
147. González P, Soriano V, Caballero T, et al. Idiopathic angioedema treated with dapsone. *Allergol Immunopathol (Madr).* 2005;33:54.
148. Wolverton S, Remlinger K. Suggested guidelines for patient monitoring: hepatic and hematologic toxicity attributable to systemic dermatologic drugs. *Dermatol Clin.* 2007;25(2):195-205.
149. Coleman MD, Coleman NA. Drug-induced methaemoglobinaemia. Treatment issues. *Drug Safe.* 1996;14:394.
150. Williams S, MacDonald P, Hoyer JD, et al. Methemoglobinemia in children with acute lymphoblastic leukemia (ALL) receiving dapsone for Pneumocystis carinii pneumonia (PCP) prophylaxis: a correlation with cytochrome b5 reductase (CB5R) enzyme levels. *Pediatr Blood Cancer.* 2005;44:55.
151. Zosel A, Rychter K, Leikin J. Dapsone-induced methemoglobinemia: case report and literature review. *Am J Ther.* 2007;14:585-587.
152. Salamat A, Watson HG. Drug-induced methaemoglobinaemia presenting with angina following the use of dapsone. *Clin Lab Haem.* 2003;25:327.
153. Groeper K, Katcher K, Tobias JD. Anesthetic management of a patient with methemoglobinemia. *South Med J.* 2003;96:504.
154. Ashurst J, Wasson MN, Hauger W, et al. Pathophysiologic mechanisms, diagnosis, and management of dapsone-induced methemoglobinemia. *J Am Osteopath Assoc.* 2010;110(1):18-20.
155. Choi A, Sarang A. Drug-induced methaemoglobinaemia following elective coronary artery bypass grafting. *Anaesthesia.* 2007;62:737-740.
156. Orion E, Matz H, Wolf R. The life-threatening complications of dermatologic therapies. *Clin Dermatol.* 2005;23:182-192.
157. Rausch-Madison S, Mohsenifar Z. Methodologic problems encountered with cooximetry in methemoglobinemia. *Am J Med Sci.* 1997;314:203-206.
158. Coleman MD, Rhodes LE, Scott AK, et al. The use of cimetidine to reduce dapsone-dependent methaemoglobinaemia in dermatitis herpetiformis patients. *Br J Clin Pharmacol.* 1992;34:244.
159. Coleman M, Taylor C. Effects of dihydrolipoic acid (DHLA), α-lipoic acid. N-acetyl cysteine and ascorbate on xenobiotic-mediated methaemoglobin formation in human erythrocytes in vitro. *Environ Toxicol Pharmacol.* 2003;14(3):121-127.
160. Ranawaka R, Mendis S, Weerakoon HS. Dapsone-induced haemolytic anaemia, hepatitis and agranulocytosis in a leprosy patient with normal glucose-6-phosphatedehydrogenase activity. *Lepr Rev.* 2008;79:436-440.
161. Kar BR. Dapsone-induced photosensitivity: a rare clinical presentation. *Photodermatol Photoimmunol Photomed.* 2008;24:270-271.
162. Saqueton AC, Lorincz AL, Vick NA, et al. Dapsone

and peripheral motor neuropathy. *Arch Dermatol*. 1969;100:214.
163. Daneshmend TK, Homeida M. Dapsone-induced optic atrophy and motor neuropathy. *Br Med J (Clin Res Ed)*. 1981;283:311.
164. Daneshmend TK. The neurotoxicity of dapsone. *Adv Drug React Ac Pois Rev*. 1984;3:43.
165. Jaffuel D, Lebel B, Hillaire-Buys D, et al. Eosinophilic pneumonia induced by dapsone. *BMJ*. 1998; 317(7152):181.
166. Richardus JH, Smith TC. Increased incidence in leprosy of hypersensitivity reactions to dapsone after introduction of multidrug therapy. *Lepr Rev*. 1989;60(4):267-273.
167. Kumar RH, Kumar MV, Thappa DM. Dapsone syndrome—a five year retrospective analysis. *Indian J Lepr*. 1998;70(3):271-276.
168. Rao PN, Lakshmi TS. Increase in the incidence of dapsone hypersensitivity syndrome—an appraisal. *Lepr Rev*. 2001;72(1):57-62.
169. Joseph MS. Hypersensitivity reaction to dapsone. Four case reports. *Lepr Rev*. 1985;56(4):315-320.
170. Jamrozik K. Dapsone syndrome occurring in two brothers. *Lepr Rev*. 1986;57(1):57-62.
171. Hortaleza AR, Salta-Ramos NG, Barcelona-Tan J, et al. Dapsone syndrome in a Filipino man. *Lepr Rev*. 1995;66(4):307-313.
172. Tomecki KJ, Catalano CJ. Dapsone hypersensitivity. The sulfone syndrome revisited. *Arch Dermatol*. 1981;117(1):38-39.
173. Zhang F-R, Liu H, Irwanto A, et al. *HLA-B*13:01* and the dapsone hypersensitivity syndrome. *N Eng J Med*. 2013;369(17):1620-1628.
174. Lorenz M, Wozel G, Schmitt J. Hypersensitivity reactions to dapsone: a systematic review. *Acta Derm Venereol*. 2012;92:194-199.
175. Teo R, Tay YK, Tan CH, et al. Presumed dapsone-induced hypersensitivity syndrome causing reversible hypersensitivity myocarditis and thyrotoxicosis. *Ann Acad Med Singapore*. 2006;35:833-836.
176. Alves-Rodrigues E, Ribero LC, Silva MD, et al. Dapsone syndrome with acute renal failure during leprosy treatment: case report. *Braz J Infect Dis*. 2005;9(1):84-86.
177. Alves-Rodrigues EN, Ribeiro LC, Silva MD, et al. Renal hypersensitivity vasculitis associated with dapsone. *Am J Kidney Dis*. 2005;46:E51.
178. Tohyama M, Hashimoto K, Yasukawa M, et al. Association of human herpesvirus 6 reactivation with the flaring and severity of drug-induced hypersensitivity syndrome. *Br J Dermatol*. 2007;157:934-940.
179. Takahashi H, Tanaka M, Tanikawa A, et al. A case of drug-induced hypersensitivity syndrome showing transient immunosuppression before viral reactivation during treatment for pemphigus foliaceus. *Clin Exp Dermatol*. 2006;31:33.
180. Agrawal S, Agrawal A. Dapsone hypersensitivity syndrome: a clinico-epidemiological review. *J Dermatol*. 2005;32:883.
181. Frey HM, Gershon AA, Borkowsky W, et al. Fatal reaction to dapsone during treatment of leprosy. *Ann Intern Med*. 1981;94:777.
182. Prussick R, Shear NH. Dapsone hypersensitivity syndrome. *J Am Acad Dermatol*. 1996;35:346.
183. McKenna KE, Robinson J. The dapsone hypersensitivity syndrome occurring in a patient with dermatitis herpetiformis [letter]. *Br J Dermatol*. 1997;137:657.
184. Leslie K, Gaffney K, Ross CN, et al. A near fatal case of the dapsone hypersensitivity syndrome in a patient with urticarial vasculitis. *Clin Exp Dermatol*. 2003;28:496-498.
185. Kosseifi S, Guha B, Nassour DN, et al. The dapsone hypersensitivity syndrome revisited: a potentially fatal multisystem disorder with prominent hepatopulmonary manifestations. *J Occup Med Toxicol*. 2006;1:9.
186. Johnson DA, Cattau EL Jr, Kuritsky JN. Liver involvement in the sulfone syndrome. *Arch Intern Med*. 1986;46:875.
187. Itha S, Kumar A, Dhingra S, et al. Dapsone induced cholangitis as a part of dapsone syndrome: a case report. *BMC Gastroenterol*. 2003;3:21.
188. Dhanya N, Shanmuga Sundaram V, Rai R, et al. Dapsone syndrome with leukemoid reaction. *Indian J Lepr*. 2006;78(4):359-363.
189. Zhu K, He FT, Jin N, et al. Complete atrioventricular block associated with dapsone therapy: a rare complication of dapsone-induced hypersensitivity syndrome. *J Clin Pharm Ther*. 2009;34:489-492.
190. Higuchi M, Agatsuma T, Iizima M, et al. A case of drug-induced hypersensitivity syndrome with multiple organ involvement treated with plasma exchange. *Ther Apheresis Dialysis*. 2005;9(5):412-416.
191. Hall RP. Dapsone. In: Wolverton SE, ed. *Comprehensive Dermatologic Drug Therapy*. Philadelphia: WB Saunders; 2001:230.
192. DeGowin RL. A review of the therapeutic and hemolytic effects of dapsone. *Arch Intern Med*. 1967;120:242-248.
193. Graham WR. Adverse effects of dapsone. *Int J Dermatol*. 1975;14:494-500.
194. Stroupe J, Stephens JR, Reust R, et al. Adverse reactions associated with dapsone therapy in HIV-positive patients: a case presentation and review. *The AIDS Reader*. 2006;16:47-48, 53-55.
195. McMillan DC, Simson JV, Budinsky RA, et al. Dapsone-induced hemolytic anemia: effect of dapsone hydroxylamine on sulfhydryl status, membrane skeletal proteins and morphology of human and rat erythrocytes. *J Pharmacol Exp Ther*. 1995;274:540.
196. Jollow DJ, Bradshaw TP, McMillan DC. Dapsone-induced hemolytic anemia. *Drug Metab Rev*. 1995; 27:107.
197. McMillan DC, Powell CL, Bowman ZS, et al. Lipids versus proteins as major targets of pro-oxidant, direct-acting hemolytic agents. *Toxicol Sci*. 2005;88:274.
198. Motulsky AG, Yoshida A. Stametoyannopoulos G. Variants of glucose-6-phosphate dehydrogenase. *Ann N Y Acad Sci*. 1971;179:636.
199. Wertheim M, Males JJ, Cook SD, et al. Dapsone induced haemolytic anaemia in patients treated for ocular cicatricial pemphigoid. *Br J Ophthalmol*. 2006;90(4):516.
200. Lee I, Barton TD, Goral S, et al. Complications related to dapsone use for pneumocystis jirovecii pneumonia prophylaxis in solid organ transplant patients. *Am J Transplant*. 2005;5:2791-2795.
201. Naik P, Lyon GM 3rd, Ramirez A, et al. Dapsone-induced hemolytic anemia in lung allograft recipients. *J Heart Lung Transplant*. 2008;27:1198-1202.
202. Flosadottir E, Bjarnason B. Full dapsone dose made possible by control of anaemia with darbepoetin-alpha. *Acta Derm Venereol*. 2008;88:540-541.
203. Mobacken H. Commentary to a paper by Flosadottir & Bjarnason on full dapsone dose made possible by control of anaemia with darbepoetin alpha. *Acta*

204. Hornsten P, Keisu M, Wiholm BE. The incidence of agranulocytosis during treatment of dermatitis herpetiformis with dapsone as reported in Sweden, 1972 through 1988. *Arch Dermatol*. 1990;126:919.
205. Andersohn F, Konzen C, Garbe E. Systematic review: agranulocytosis induced by nonchemotherapy drugs. *Ann Intern Med*. 2007;146(9):657-665.
206. Ognibene AJ. Agranulocytosis due to dapsone. *Ann Intern Med*. 1970;72:521.
207. Potter MN, Yates P, Slade R, et al. Agranulocytosis caused by dapsone therapy for granuloma annulare. *J Am Acad Dermatol*. 1989;20:87.
208. Cockburn EM, Wood SM, Waller PC, et al. Dapsone-induced agranulocytosis: spontaneous reporting data [letter]. *Br J Dermatol*. 1993;128:702.
209. Coleman MD. Dapsone-mediated agranulocytosis: risks, possible mechanisms and prevention. *Toxicology*. 2001;162:53.
210. Miyagawa S, Shiomi Y, Fukumoto T, et al. Recombinant granulocyte colony-stimulating factor for dapsone-induced agranulocytosis in leukocytoclastic vasculitis. *J Am Acad Dermatol*. 1993;28:659.
211. Borrás-Blasco J, Conesa-García V, Navarro-Ruiz A, et al. Pure red cell aplasia associated with dapsone therapy. *Ann Pharmacother*. 2005;39:1137.
212. Hiura Y, Kawabata H, Kanekura T, et al. Hemophagocytic syndrome induced by diaminodiphenylsulfone. *J Dermatol*. 2007;34:730-731.
213. Foucauld J, Uphouse W, Berenberg J. Dapsone and aplastic anemia. *Ann Intern Med*. 1985;102(1):139.
214. Meyerson MA, Cohen PR. Dapsone-induced aplastic anemia in a woman with bullous systemic lupus erythematosus. *Mayo Clin Proc*. 1994;69(12):1159-1162.
215. Björkman A, Phillips-Howard PA. Adverse reactions to sulfa drugs: implications for malaria chemotherapy. *Bull World Health Organ*. 1991;69(3):297-304.
216. Froud T, Faradji RN, Gorn L, et al. Dapsone-induced artifactual A1c reduction in islet transplant recipients. *Transplantation*. 2007;83(6):824-825.
217. Dawson AH, Whyte IM. Management of dapsone poisoning complicated by methaemoglobinaemia. *Med Toxicol Adverse Drug Exp*. 1989;4:387.
218. Shadnia S, Rahimi M, Moeinsadat M, et al. Acute methemoglobinemia following attempted suicide by dapsone. *Arch Med Res*. 2006;37:410-414.
219. Ferguson J, Lavery G. Deliberate self-poisoning with dapsone—a case report and summary of relevant pharmacology and treatment. *Anaesthesia*. 1997;52:359-363.
220. Kenner DJ, Holt K, Agnello R, et al. Permanent retinal damage following massive dapsone overdose. *Br J Ophthalmol*. 1980;64:741.
221. Leonard JN, Tucker WF, Fry L, et al. Dapsone and the retina [letter]. *Lancet*. 1982;1:453.
222. Hussain N, Agrawal S. Optical coherence tomographic evaluation of macular infarction following dapsone overdose. *Indian J Ophthalmol*. 2006;54(4):271-272.
223. Thunga G, Sam KG, Patel D, et al. Effectiveness of hemodialysis in acute dapsone overdose—a case report. *Am J Emerg Med*. 2008;26:1070.e1-1070.e4.
224. Clifton J, Leikin JB. Methylene blue. *Am J Ther*. 2003;10:289.
225. Prasad R, Singh R, Mishra OP, et al. Dapsone induced methemoglobinemia: intermittent vs continuous intravenous methylene blue therapy. *Indian J Pediatr*. 2008;75(3):245-247.
226. Wozel G. Innovative use of dapsone. *Dermatol Clin*. 2010;28(3):599-610.

Chapter 188 :: Antifungals
:: Mahmoud Ghannoum, Iman Salem, & Luisa Christensen

第一百八十八章
抗真菌药

中文导读

外用抗真菌药物主要应用在局限于皮肤表面的真菌感染，包括咪唑类、烯丙基胺类、苄胺类、多烯类和环吡咯。治疗甲真菌病和头癣或大面积浅表真菌感染需要系统使用抗真菌药。本章首先介绍了背景，指出浅部真菌病，主要由皮肤癣菌和酵母菌引起，是世界上最常见的感染之一，外用抗真菌药物是治疗的首选方法。全身和外用抗真菌药物的主要靶点是麦角甾醇，麦角甾醇是真菌细胞膜的基本甾醇。主要抗真菌药物是烯丙基胺和苄胺类、咪唑类和多烯类。接下来分别介绍了目前临床使用的主要外用和系统用抗真菌药物的作用机制、药代动力学、适应证、剂量和配方及副作用等。

〔粟　娟〕

AT-A-GLANCE

- Topical agents should be used for superficial fungal infections of limited extent.
- Topical agents have the advantage of low cost, nonprescription availability, ease of use, and high patient compliance.
- Topical antifungals include imidazoles, allylamines, benzylamines, polyenes, and ciclopirox.
- A number of new carrier vehicles have been investigated to improve the bioavaliabilty of topical antifungals.
- Systemic agents should be used to treat onychomycosis and tinea capitis, or when superficial fungal infection affects a large surface area.
- Attention should be paid to drug–drug interactions when prescribing systemic antifungals.
- Combination therapy with topical and systemic drugs presents several advantages.

INTRODUCTION/BACKGROUND

Superficial mycoses, caused mainly by dermatophytes and yeast, are among the most frequent infections worldwide, affecting approximately 20% to 25% of the world's population.[1] Topical antifungals are the preferred option for the treatment of most of these infections, achieving high patient compliance. Moreover, many topical drugs have additional antibacterial action, which is beneficial in cases of superimposed bacterial infections. Further, many also possess anti-inflammatory properties, which are advantageous in minimizing the effects of the host local inflammatory reactions to mycotic infection.[2] Systemic antifungals are the mainstay treatment of tinea capitis and onychomycosis; also, dermatologists tend to reserve them for extensive, recurrent, or recalcitrant dermatomycosis.[3,4] Despite the diversity in the structure of the fungal cell membrane and the unique existence of the mycotic cell wall compared to mammalian cells, the similarities in the metabolic profile between both kingdoms allow for limited numbers of organism-specific targets. Overall, the main target of both systemic and topical antifungals is ergosterol (Fig. 188-1), the fundamental mycotic cell membrane sterol. As of this writing, the 3 main antifungal categories targeting ergosterol are (1) allylamines and benzylamines, (2) azoles (imidazole and triazoles), and (3) polyenes. Whereas allylamines, benzylamines, and azoles block the biosynthesis of ergosterol, polyenes bind the molecule with high affinity, creating cell membrane pores. Other systemic antifungal agents (griseofulvin and flucytosine) act on intracellular structures via mechanisms similar to cancer chemotherapeutic agents.[5,6] Although both are clinically effective, azoles exhibit superior activity against yeasts compared to allylamines, but less activity against dermatophytes.[7] Although the most common adverse effects associated with topical therapy are mild, transient, and localized hypersensitivity skin reactions, systemic antifungals demonstrate various degrees of organ toxicity and possible serious drug interactions.[3] This chapter aims to discuss the main topical and systemic antifungal agents currently in clinical use (Tables 188-1 through 188-4).

ALLYLAMINES

Two agents represent this family: terbinafine, available in both topical and oral forms, and naftifine, available only for topical application.[8]

MECHANISM OF ACTION

Allylamines exhibit differential antifungal activity against *Candida* species (fungistatic), and dermatophytes (fungicidal). They act through the suppression of ergosterol synthesis by inhibiting the action of squalene epoxidase enzyme, the enzyme that catalyzes the conversion of squalene precursors into ergosterol. The resultant deficiency of ergosterol is responsible for the fungistatic effect, while the buildup of squalene accounts for fungicidal activity.[8]

NAFTIFINE

Naftifine is a broad-spectrum topical allylamine.

MECHANISM OF ACTION

In addition to its antifungal activity, naftifine has antibacterial activity (gram-positive and gram-negative) as well as antiinflammatory properties secondary to its ability to suppress the synthesis of leukotrienes and prostaglandins.[9]

PHARMACOKINETICS

The lipophilic properties of naftifine account for its efficient penetration through the stratum corneum. Therapeutic drug levels can persist in stratum corneum up to 5 days following a single application. Only 3% to 6% of the applied drug can be systemically absorbed.[9-11]

CLINICAL INDICATIONS

Naftifine is indicated for the treatment of interdigital tinea pedis, tinea cruris, tinea corporis, tinea versicolor, and *Candida* infections.[8]

DOSAGE AND FORMULATIONS

Naftifine is commercially available as 1% gel and cream. A single daily application of naftifine is usually recommended for 2 to 4 weeks according to the indication (Table 188-1).[12]

SIDE EFFECTS

The side effects of naftifine are generally minor and include dryness, pruritus, local irritation, and erythema.[8]

TERBINAFINE

MECHANISM OF ACTION

Terbinafine works through the suppression of squalene epoxidase enzyme, blocking the formation of ergosterol.[13]

PHARMACOKINETICS

The systemic absorption of topical terbinafine is inconsequential (3%-5%).[8] The oral absorption of the drug is not influenced by food intake and, owing to its lipophilic properties, tends to rapidly distribute and accumulate in hair follicles, nails, and skin with minimal concentrations in plasma. It has a long half-life of 17 hours. The oxidative biotransformation of the drug takes place in the liver by the means of CYP2D6 enzyme. Most of the drug is eliminated in urine. A dose adjustment is necessary in patients with advanced renal or liver diseases.[8,13-15]

INDICATIONS

Topical terbinafine is efficacious in the treatment of all superficial mycoses, including tinea versicolor.[8,13] Unless contraindicated, terbinafine is the first line of treatment of dermatophytosis owing to its fungicidal activity, high efficacy, tolerability, single daily dose, better pharmacokinetic profile, and high affinity to stratum corneum.[16] Oral terbinafine exhibits a potent fungicidal action, superior to griseofulvin and itraconazole, against *Trichophyton rubrum* and *T. mentagrophytes*. Although considered the first treatment option in dermatophyte onychomycosis, terbinafine does not demonstrate efficacy against nondermatophyte and *Candida* onychomycosis.[15]

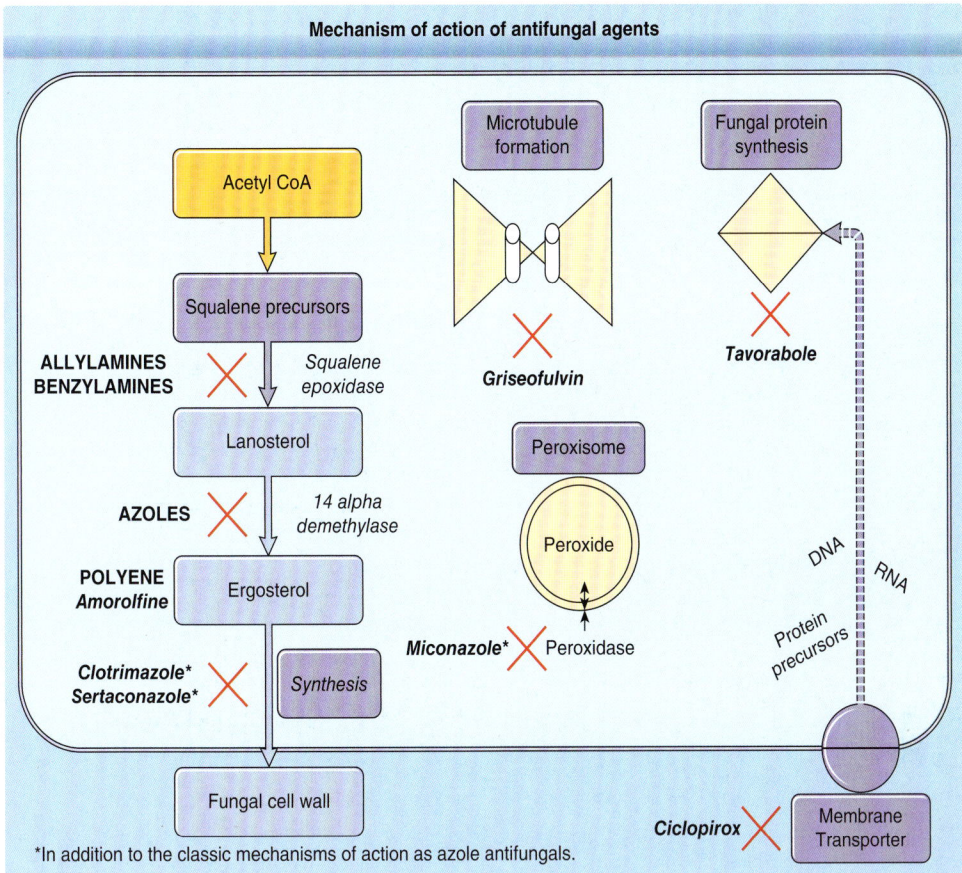

Figure 188-1 Mechanism of action of antifungal agents.

Terbinafine and griseofulvin are the only FDA-approved drugs for the treatment of tinea capitis in children. However, terbinafine is less effective than griseofulvin in eradicating ectothrix tinea capitis in the pediatric population, particularly, that caused by *Microsporum canis* and *Trichophyton tonsurans*, because of its high tendency to accumulate in sebum. Immature preadolescent sebaceous glands produce less sebum, thus resulting in lower drug concentrations.[17-19] Many clinical studies have shown efficacy of terbinafine in the treatment of cutaneous and lymphocutaneous sporotrichosis at a dose of 500 mg twice daily for 2 to 4 weeks beyond the clinical resolution. Terbinafine has also shown efficacy in the treatment of phaeohyphomycosis, chromoblastomycosis, mucormycosis, and maduromycosis.[17]

DOSAGE AND FORMULATIONS

The following terbinafine formulations are available for topical use—cream, powder, solution, spray, and gel 1% (Table 188-1). Oral terbinafine formulations include 250-mg tablets and oral granules. Because terbinafine can persist in keratinized tissue up to 6 months after the last dose,[19] a pulse regimen could represent an alternate treatment strategy for onychomycosis. A daily dose of 250 mg for 1 week monthly continued for 1 year has shown a mycological cure rate of 90% compared to 75% achieved with itraconazole pulse dosage.[17] Terbinafine at a daily dose of 250 mg for a period ranging from 2 to 4 weeks is effective in the management of tinea barbae, tinea corporis, tinea cruris, tinea faciei, and moccasin-type tinea pedis (Table 188-2).[12]

SIDE EFFECTS

The side effects of the topical application are not common (6%) and are typically limited to mild localized cutaneous reaction. In general, the oral route is well tolerated, with fewer side events reported with the pulse regimen compared to continuous dosing. Minimal GI tract upset (eg, abdominal pain, nausea, vomiting, diarrhea), appetite changes, and weight gain are the most common terbinafine adverse effects. A unique side effect is altered taste, which can last up to 6 weeks with or without loss of smell and tongue discoloration. Severe but rare adverse events are hepatotoxicity leading to possible organ failure and hematologic disorders including pancytopenia; these are usually reversible after drug stoppage. Cutaneous hypersensitivity eruptions as severe as

TABLE 188-1
Trade Names and Formulations of Representative Topical Antifungals

DRUG/CLASS	TRADE NAMES	USUAL FORMULATION	INDICATIONS	DOSING REGIME	PREGNANCY CATEGORY
Polyenes					
Nystatin	Mycostatin, Nystop, Pedi-Dri (Rx)	Cream, powder, ointment	Mucosal and cutaneous candidiasis	Twice daily	B
Azoles					
Imidazoles					
Clotrimazole	Clotrim, Cruex, Lotrimin, Mycelex (OTC)	Cream, solution, lotion	Tinea corporis/cruris/pedis	Twice daily for 2-4 wk	B
Econazole	Spectazole, Ecoza (Rx)	Cream, powder, foam, solution	Dermatophytoses, tinea versicolor, cutaneous candidiasis	Once daily (twice for candidiasis) for 2 wk	C
Oxiconazole	Oxistat (Rx)	Cream, lotion	Dermatophytoses, tinea versicolor	Once-twice daily for 2 wk	B
Miconazole	Miconazole OTC	Cream, ointment, powder or spray	Dermatophytoses	Twice daily for 2-4 wk	C
Sertaconazole	Ertaczo (Rx)	Cream, lotion, gel, powder, solution	Interdigital tinea pedis	Twice daily for 4 wk	C
Ketoconazole	Ketoconazole (Rx)	Cream, shampoo	Dermatophytoses, tinea versicolor, cutaneous candidiasis	Once daily for 2-6 wk	C
Triazoles					
Efinaconazole	Jublia (Rx)	Solution	Onychomycosis	Once daily for 48 wk	C
Allylamines					
Terbinafine	Lamisil (OTC)	Cream, powder, solution, spray, gel	Dermatophytoses, tinea versicolor	Once or twice daily for 2-4 wk	B
Naftifine	Naftin (Rx)	Cream, gel	Dermatophytoses	Once-twice daily for 2-6 wk	B
Benzylamines					
Butenafine	Lotrimin Ultra (OTC), Mentax (Rx)	Cream, spray, powder	Dermatophytoses, tinea versicolor	Once-twice daily for 2 wk	C
Hydroxypyridones					
Ciclopirox olamine	Loprox (Rx)	Cream, suspension, gel, nail lacquer solution	Dermatophytoses, onychomycosis	Twice daily for 2-4 wk; nail lacquer—apply once daily for 48 wk	B
Morolphines					
Amorolfine	Loceryl (Rx) Not available in the USA	Nail lacquer solution	Onychomycosis	Apply once daily for 48 wk	D
Oxaborole					
Tavaborole	Kerydin (Rx)	Nail lacquer solution	Onychomycosis	Apply once daily for 48 wk	C

Stevens–Johnson syndrome and toxic epidermal necrolysis have been reported, mainly within 4 to 5 weeks of treatment. Drug discontinuation may result in GI and cutaneous adverse events, and headaches, vertigo, and transient optic neuropathy may also occur (Table 188-3).[20]

DRUG–DRUG INTERACTIONS

Terbinafine exhibits a potent inhibitory effect on CYP2D6, and therefore increases the potential toxicity of drugs metabolized by this enzyme, including nortriptyline, amitriptyline, venlafaxine, and

TABLE 188-2
Trade Names and Formulations of Representative Systemic Antifungals

DRUG/CLASS	TRADE NAMES	USUAL FORMULATION	INDICATIONS	DOSING REGIME ADULT	DOSING REGIME PEDIATRIC	PREGNANCY CATEGORY
Allylamines						
Terbinafine	Lamisil, Terbinex	1. Tablets 250 mg 2. Oral granules	Tinea unguium[a]	Continuous 250 mg/d >20 kg Fingernail for 6 wk Toenail for 9-12 wk Pulse 500 mg/d for 1 wk/m for same duration	Continuous >20 kg 62.5 mg/d 20-40 kg 125 mg/d for same duration	B
			T. capitis[a]	250 mg/d for 2-8 wk	5 mg/kg/d[c] for 2-4 wk	
			T. pedis, cruris, corporis[b]	250 mg/d 2-4 wk		
			Seborrheic dermatitis[b]	250 mg/d 4-6 wk		
Azoles						
Triazoles						
Fluconazole	Diflucan	1. Capsule 150 mg 2. Tablets 150 mg 3. Solution for IV infusion	1. Esophageal candidiasis[a]	150 mg/d for 2-3 wk after clinical improvement	6 mg/kg/d until clinical improvement, then 3 mg/kg/d for 2 wk	C
			2. Vaginal candidiasis[a]	150 mg once Recurrence 150 mg/wk for 6 mo		
			3. Cutaneous, mucocutaneous candidiasis[a]	300 mg/wk for 2 wk		
			4. T. capitis[b]		6 mg/kg/d *Trichophyton tonsurans* for 20 d *Microsporum canis* 2 wk	
			5. Onychomycosis[b]	150-300 mg/wk Fingernail for 6-9 mo Toenail for 9-15 mo	3-6 mg/kg/d Fingernail 12-16 wk Toenail 18-26 wk	
			6. Tinea pedis, cruris, corporis, barbae[b]	150 mg/wk for 2-6 wk		
			7. Tinea versicolor[b]	300 mg/wk for 2 wk		
Itraconazole	Sporanox Sporanox pluspak Onmel	1. Capsules 100 mg 2. Cyclodextrin oral solution	1. Onychomycosis[a]	**Continuous** 200 mg/d Fingernail for 6 wk Toenail for 12 wk **Pulse** 400 mg/d for 1 wk/mo Fingernail 2 pulses Toenail 3 pulses	**Pulse** 5 mg/kg/d for 1 wk/mo Fingernail 2 pulses Toenail 3 pulses	C
			2. Oropharyngeal candidiasis[a]	Oral solution 100-200 mg/d for 1-2 wk after clinical improvement	>15 kg 100 mg/d 15-30 kg 100 mg/d alternating with 200 mg/d 30-45 kg 200 mg/d same duration as adults	

(Continued)

TABLE 188-2
Trade Names and Formulations of Representative Systemic Antifungals (Continued)

DRUG/CLASS	TRADE NAMES	USUAL FORMULATION	INDICATIONS	DOSING REGIME ADULT	DOSING REGIME PEDIATRIC	PREGNANCY CATEGORY
			3. T. capitis[b]	200 mg/d for 2-8 wk	5 mg/kg/d T. tonsurans for 2-4 wk M. canis for 4-8 wk	
			4. T. pedis, cruris, corporis[b]	200 mg/d for 1 wk		
			5. Pityriasis versicolor[b]	TTT 200 mg/d for 1 wk Prophylaxis 400 mg once every month		
Other						
Griseofulvin	Griseofulicin Griseofulvic Gris-PEG Grifulvin V	1. Tablets Microsize 250, 500 mg Ultramicrosize 125, 165, 250 mg 2. Oral suspension 125 mg/5 mL	1. T. capitis[a]	Microsize 500 mg/d or ultramicrosize 300-375 mg/d for 4-8 wk	Microsize 15-20 mg/kg/d or ultramicrosize 5-10 mg/kg/d for 6-12 wk	C
			2. T. cruris,[a] corporis	Same doses as above for 2-4 wk	Same doses as above for 2-4 wk	
			3. T. pedis[a]	Microsize 750-1000 mg/d or ultramicrosize 660-750 mg/d for 4-8 wk	Microsize 10-20 mg/kg/d or ultramicrosize 5-10 mg/kg/d for 4-8 wk	

[a]FDA-approved indications.
[b]Off-label indications.
[c]Indicated for children older than 4 years.

desipramine. In addition, terbinafine reduces the elimination of caffeine and cyclosporine. The concomitant administration of terbinafine with rifampicin or cimetidine should be avoided as well, as they are known to increase its toxicity and decrease its efficacy, respectively (Table 188-4).[8,13,20]

BENZYLAMINES

Benzylamines are structurally and functionally related to allylamines.[8]

BUTENAFINE

Butenafine is the only available antifungal derivative of benzylamine, and has a chemical formula N-(4-tert-butylbenzyl)-N-methyl-1-naphthalenemethylamine hydrochloride.[8]

MECHANISM OF ACTION

Similar to allylamines, butenafine inhibits the synthesis of ergosterol, with subsequent enhancement in membrane permeability and leakage of important cellular components, resulting in mycotic cell death.[8]

INDICATIONS

Butenafine is indicated for the treatment of dermatophyte infections, with efficacy superior to that of the allylamines; additionally, it can be used in cases of pityriasis versicolor (PV) and candidiasis (Table 188-1).[8,13]

DOSAGE AND FORMULATIONS

The only available commercial formulation is a 1% cream,[9] applied once daily for 2 to 4 weeks.[8]

SIDE EFFECTS

Side effects of butenafine are minimal and include itching, burning, erythema, and contact dermatitis.

AZOLES

The azoles are group of antifungals characterized by 1 or more azole rings. They can be further subclassified into imidazoles, which include ketoconazole, butoconazole, clotrimazole, econazole, luliconazole,

TABLE 188-3
Side Effects, Contraindications, and Monitoring of Representative Systemic Antifungals

DRUG	SIDE EFFECTS	PRECAUTIONS/CONTRAINDICATIONS	MONITORING
Terbinafine	1. Ageusia (altered taste), loss of smell, and tongue discoloration+ 2. Hepatotoxicity, hematologic disorders ++ 3. GIT upset, aggravate psoriasis, lupus erythematosus	1. Hepatic disease (chronic or active) 2. Renal impairment (creatinine clearance <50 mL/min)	1. Baseline LFTs 2. Full CBC 3. BUN, creatinine 4. Plasma level of CYP2D6-metabolized drugs
Fluconazole	1. Cardiac abnormalities (torsade de pointes), exfoliative skin reactions, anaphylactic reactions++ 2. Headache, myalgia, dizziness, GIT upset+++ 3. Hepatic, renal functions abnormalities	1. Hepatic and renal impairment 2. In patients with risk for arrhythmias 3. Coadministration with astemizole, terfenadine, cisapride (increased risk of developing torsade de pointes) 4. Coadministration with statins (increased myopathy)	1. Baseline LFTs 2. Full CBC 3. Regular LFTs 4. Close monitor of oral hypoglycemic, and blood glucose
Itraconazole	1. Triad of hypertension, hypokalemia, &edema in elderly+ 2. Negative inotropic fulminant hepatitis, Stevens–Johnson syndrome; Anaphylaxis++ 3. GIT upset, esp. odious taste with cyclo-dextrin solution+++ 4. Headache, rhinitis, sinusitis, hepatic, renal impairment	1. Heart failure 2. Liver disease 3. Patients with hypersensitivity to other azoles (use with caution)	1. Patients with risk factors for CHF for developing signs or symptoms of CHF 2. Baseline LFTs 3. Regular LFTs 4. Blood glucose in patients using oral hypoglycemic 5. Plasma level of drugs metabolized with by CYP3A4
Griseofulvin	1. Hetaotoxicity, pancytopenia++ 2. Hypersensitivity skin eruptions, Photosensitivity, 3. GIT upset+++ 4. Neurologic problems	1. Porphyria 2. LCF 3. Patients with penicillin sensitivity (use with cautious) 4. Females using OCP should change the contraceptive method or add another form	1. Liver enzymes after 8 wk of continuous use 2. BUN, creatinine after 8 wk of continuous use

+, Most unique; ++, most serious; +++, most common; LFTs, liver function tests; BUN, blood urea nitrogen; CBC, complete blood picture; CHF, chronic heart failure; CYP, cytochrome P; GIT, gastrointestinal tract; LCF, liver cell failure; OCP, oral contraceptive pills.

miconazole, and sertaconazole, and triazoles, which include fluconazole, itraconazole, efinaconazole, and isavuconazole.[5]

MECHANISM OF ACTION

Azoles act through the inhibition of lanosterol demethylase enzyme (14α-demethylase), a fungal cytochrome P450 (CYP)–dependent enzyme that catalyzes the conversion step of lanosterol into ergosterol, thereby blocking the biosynthesis of ergosterol. Subsequently, the reduced level of ergosterol disrupts the membrane permeability. Additionally, the buildup of the 14α-methylated sterols precursors will interfere with cell growth, leading eventually to cell death. Azoles in normal concentrations are typically fungistatic agents; however, high concentrations of azoles can be fungicidal. The heme-containing pocket is the binding site of azoles on the lanosterol demethylase enzyme and variations in its conformation, together with variation in the drug structure, are the determinants of the azole binding affinity and cross resistance.[21]

IMIDAZOLES

CLOTRIMAZOLE

Mechanism of Action: Clotrimazole is the first developed topical imidazole that can disrupt mycotic phospholipids, resulting in leakage of intracellular iron, degradation of nucleic acids, and suppression of cell respiration.[8]

Pharmacokinetics: Application of clotrimazole is associated with negligible systemic absorption (0.5%).[13]

Indications: Clotrimazole can be used for all superficial mycoses, achieving mycological cure rates ranging from 60% to 100% in dermatophytosis, and 80% to 100% in cutaneous candidiasis.[13]

Dosage and Formulations: Clotrimazole is available as cream, lotion, spray, powder, lozenge, suppository, and 1% solution (Table 188-1). As with most azoles, clotrimazole is applied twice daily for 2 to 4 weeks according to the indication.[8]

TABLE 188-4
Drug–Drug Interactions of Representative Systemic Antifungals

ANTIFUNGAL AGENT	INTERACTING DRUG/CLASS	MECHANISM OF INTERACTION	RESULTING EFFECTS	RECOMMENDATION
Terbinafine	1. CYP2D6 metabolizing agents (TCAs, SSRI haloperidol, some BB)	Terbinafine is a CYP2D6 isoenzyme inhibitor ++	Inhibition of their breakdown, and increase their toxicity	Cautious coadministration
	2. Warfarin	Terbinafine is a potential *CYP*-450 2C9 inducer	Decrease the anticoagulant activity and increase the risk of thrombosis	Close monitoring of anticoagulation parameters (ie, INR, PT)
	3. Rifampicin, phenytoin	CYP-450 enzyme inducer	Induce the metabolism of terbinafine, decrease its level	Avoid combination, or increase the dose of terbinafine
	4. Cimetidine	CYP2D6 enzyme inhibitor	Inhibit the metabolism of terbinafine, decrease its clearance	Avoid combination, or decrease the dose of terbinafine
Fluconazole	1. Terfenadine, astemizole, cisapride	Synergism (prolongation of QT interval)	Serious arrhythmias (torsades de pointes)	Coadministration is contraindicated
	2. CYP3A4-metabolizing agents (eg, CCBs, benzodiazepines, SSRIs, TCA, phenytoin, carbamazepine, cyclosporine, PDIs, warfarin)	Fluconazole is CYP3A4 inhibitor +	Increase the plasma level and decrease the clearance of coadministered drug	Monitor the level of coadministrated drug or their effects, or consider terbinafine as alternative
	3. CYP2C9 metabolizing agents, phenytoin, oral hypoglycemic agents, (eg, sulfonylurea, rosiglitazone, and nateglinide)	Fluconazole is a CYP2C9 isoenzyme inhibitor	Clinically evident phenytoin toxicity, hypoglycemia respectively	Consider other alternatives (terbinafine, itraconazole, griseofulvin)
	4. CYP3A4 inducers (eg, phenytoin, carbamazepine, phenobarbital, rifampin, rifabutin, INH, nevirapine)	Induce the metabolism of fluconazole	Decrease its therapeutic effects	Avoid combination, or increase the dose of fluconazole
	5. CYP3A4 inhibitors (clarithromycin, indinavir, ritonavir)	Decrease the metabolism of fluconazole	Increase its therapeutic and side effects	Avoid combination, or decrease the dose of fluconazole
Itraconazole	1. H2 blocker antihistamines (eg, cimetidine, ranitidine) antacids, proton pump inhibitors (eg, omeprazole pantoprazole), oral didanosine	Decrease gastric acidity	Decrease itraconazole absorption and bioavailability	Itraconazole capsules can be taken 2 h after the concurrent drug, or consider alternatives not affected by gastric acidity (eg, itraconazole solution, terbinafine or fluconazole)
	2. Drug metabolized by cytochrome 3A4 (CYP3A4) isoenzyme (eg, statins, darunavir, CCBs, benzodiazepines, warfarin)	Itraconazole is a CYP3A4 inhibitor ++	Decrease the metabolism of these drugs; hence increase their therapeutic and side effects	Monitor the level of coadministrated drug or their effects (eg, close. monitoring of the level of myopathy and myoglobinuria in case of statins), or consider terbinafine as alternative
	3. Digoxin, quinidine	Itraconazole is a P gp and CYP3A4 inhibitor	Digoxin toxicity	Terbinafine, fluconazole, or griseofulvin can be safely administered
	4. CYP3A4 inducers	Increases the hepatic metabolism of itraconazole	Accelerate the clearance of itraconazole	Avoid combination, or increase the dose of itraconazole
	5. CYP3A4 inhibitors (clarithromycin, indinavir, ritonavir)	Decreases the hepatic metabolism of itraconazole	Decrease the clearance of itraconazole	Avoid combination, or decrease the dose of itraconazole

(Continued)

TABLE 188-4
Drug–Drug Interactions of Representative Systemic Antifungals (Continued)

ANTIFUNGAL AGENT	INTERACTING DRUG/CLASS	MECHANISM OF INTERACTION	RESULTING EFFECTS	RECOMMENDATION
Griseofulvin	1. Warfarin, phenobarbital, and estrogens	Griseofulvin is an enzymatic inducer	Increase the metabolism of these drugs	Dose adjustment of the concurrent drugs
	2. Phenobarbitone	Decrease the oral absorption and induces metabolism of Griseofulvin.	Failure in griseofulvin therapy	Avoid coadministration

+, mild potency or needs high doses; ++, high potency; CYP, cytochrome P; BB, beta blockers; CCBs, calcium channel blockers; INH, isoniazid; INR, International Normalized Ratio; PDIs, phosphodiesterase inhibitors; PT, prothrombin time; SSRI, selective serotonin-reuptake inhibitors; TCAs, tricyclic antidepressants.

Side Effects: Similar to other topical antifungals, clotrimazole can result in local skin reaction in the form of itching, erythema, and rash.[8,13]

Pregnancy Category: B.

KETOCONAZOLE

Ketoconazole was the first marketed oral broad-spectrum antifungal agent.[13]

Mechanism of Action: Ketoconazole inhibits 14α-demethylase, blocking the conversion of lanosterol into ergosterol. It has fungicidal activity at high concentrations.[3] Possible antiinflammatory activity of topical ketoconazole has been postulated.[22]

Pharmacokinetics: Systemic absorption of topical ketoconazole is negligible, whereas 5% of the drug reaches the hair keratin 12 hours from the first shampoo application.[8] The absorption of oral ketoconazole is enhanced by acidic beverages, and decreases with the increase in gastric pH.[13]

Indications: Ketoconazole is used topically for the treatment of all dermatomycoses and its shampoo formulation is effective in the treatment of seborrheic dermatitis (Table 188-1). However, the prescription of oral preparations has now been markedly restricted by the FDA and other health organizations due to drug interaction and serious side effects on the liver and adrenal glands.[23-25]

Dosage and Formulations: The commercial formulations in the United States include 5% shampoo, 2% cream, and 200-mg tablets. Ketoconazole shampoo is applied once daily (left for 5-10 minutes) for 1 to 4 weeks in the treatment of PV, and once weekly for prophylaxis (Table 188-1).[26] In cases of scalp seborrheic dermatitis, the shampoo is used twice a week for 4 weeks. Oral ketoconazole is used once daily for 10 to 20 days in cases of superficial mycosis.[13]

Side Effects: The adverse effects of the topical drug are generally minimal and uncommon, including itching, allergic reactions, and contact dermatitis. Serious side effects have been recorded with the oral formulation, encompassing liver toxicity, anaphylactic reactions, and marked depression. More common but less serious side effects include nausea, vomiting, diarrhea, abdominal pain, headache, sleeping disturbances, dizziness, and pancytopenia, as well as impotence, gynecomastia, and decreased libido owing to its androgen-opposing properties at both the adrenal and testicular levels.[8]

Drug–Drug Interactions: Ketoconazole is a strong inhibitor of CYP3A4 and can increase the serum concentrations of coadministered drugs foremost metabolized by this enzyme, leading to a decrease in therapeutic efficacy and increase in adverse effects.[8]

MICONAZOLE

Mechanism of Action: In addition to the mechanism inherent to azoles, miconazole is capable of blocking the mycotic peroxidase enzyme, leading to the accumulation of toxic peroxide and subsequent cell death.[8]

Pharmacokinetics: Miconazole efficiently penetrates the stratum corneum, with <1% absorbed to systemic circulation.[8]

Indications: Miconazole cream is an efficacious treatment for tinea cruris, tinea corporis, and tinea pedis, in addition to its efficacy in treating PV and cutaneous candidiasis (Table 188-1).

Dosage and Formulations: The commercial preparations of miconazole include vaginal suppositories (100 mg, 200 mg), gel (2%), cream (2%), ointment, lotion, and powder.[8,13]

Side Effects: Miconazole side effects include those inherent to topical azoles, with cross-sensitivity recorded with the majority.[8]

LULICONAZOLE

Luliconazole and sertaconazole are the most recently developed imidazoles.

Mechanism of Action: Luliconazole mechanism of action is the same as azoles, though the modification of its structure renders it less liable to keratin binding and more available for penetration into deeper nail layers. Therefore, many studies are now investigating the use of luliconazole for treating onychomycosis.[27]

Pharmacokinetics: Luliconazole is characterized by second meta-replaced chlorine on its benzene ring, which is responsible for its superior potency over lanoconazole.[28]

Indications: Luliconazole is FDA approved for the treatment tinea cruris, tinea pedis, and tinea corporis (Table 188-1).[12]

Dosage and Formulations: Luliconazole 1% cream is the only available formulation in the United States.[29]

Side Effects: Mild cutaneous irritation is uncommonly reported with luliconazole.[29]

SERTACONAZOLE

Sertaconazole is a benzothiophene imidazole derivative.[28]

Mechanism of Action: Sertaconazole, in addition to the typical action of azoles, is capable of exhibiting fungicidal action at high concentration through binding to nonsterol lipids in the mycotic cell wall, increasing its permeability and resulting in cell lysis. In addition, sertaconazole has antiinflammatory, antibacterial, and antipruritic properties.[28]

Pharmacokinetics: Insignificant amounts of sertaconazole may reach the systemic circulation after topical application; additionally, sertaconazole forms a drug depot that can persist in the stratum corneum up to 48 hours after the last dose.[28]

Indications: In the EU, sertaconazole is approved for all dermatomycoses (PV, seborrheic dermatitis, cutaneous candidiasis, and dermatophytosis), whereas in the United States, its license is limited to tinea pedis.[28]

Dosage and Formulations: Sertaconazole is available as 2% cream and solution (Table 188-1).[28]

Side Effects: Topical application can result in mild local dryness, burning sensation, and dermatitis.[28]

Pregnancy Category: C.

EFINACONAZOLE

Mechanism of Action: Efinaconazole reduces the ergosterol synthesis in a dose-dependent manner.[30] It inhibits lanosterol 14-alphademethylase, which prevents transformation of lanosterol into ergosterol.

Pharmacokinetics: Less efinaconazole is bound to keratin compared to amorolfine and ciclopirox, which allows more drug to penetrate the nail plate. In addition, its lipophilic ester component reduces the surface tension, allowing more nail penetration.[28]

Indications: Efinaconazole is FDA licensed for the topical treatment of onychomycosis.[28]

Dosage and Formulations: Efinaconazole 10% solution is applied as a single daily application for 48 weeks (Table 188-1).[27,28]

Side Effects: Local eczema and ingrown nails have been reported with efinaconazole use.[27,28]

Pregnancy Category: C.

TRIAZOLES

Both triazoles and imidazoles are 5-membered ring heterocycles. Imidazoles have 2-ring nitrogen atoms, whereas triazoles contain 3 and are less prone to metabolic degradation.

FLUCONAZOLE

Fluconazole is a water-soluble *bis*-triazole that became FDA approved in the early 1990s.[8]

Mechanism of Action: Fluconazole inhibits lanosterol 14-demethylase and prevents conversion of lanosterol to ergosterol.[27,31]

Pharmacokinetics: Fluconazole has an excellent oral bioavailability, attaining nearly 90% (comparable to that achieved by intravenous route). Its pharmacokinetics are linear, predictable, and independent of gastric acidity, food intake, or disease activity. Unlike most other antifungal agents, only a small percentage of fluconazole is bound to plasma protein, resulting in greater amounts of free drug for therapeutic activity.[6,32] The drug is also characterized by a long half-life of 25 to 30 hours.[4] In addition, the wide distribution in various tissues including skin, nail, vitreous chamber of the eye, and cerebral spinal fluid (CSF), together with a good safety profile especially in immunocompromised patients, have qualified the use of fluconazole for the treatment of invasive fungal infections for almost 3 decades. The drug is poorly metabolized by the liver, and hence the kidney is the main route of drug elimination; therefore, dose adjustment is required with renal insufficiency.[6,32]

Indications: Fluconazole is one of the most commonly used antifungals in the treatment of esophageal, vaginal, and oropharyngeal candidiasis, and cryptococcal meningitis. It is efficacious against all *Candida* except *C. krusei*. Additionally, fluconazole is used as an off-label treatment for onychomycosis, tinea infections, PV, and chronic mucocutaneous candidiasis when itraconazole and terbinafine are contraindicated (Table 188-2).[8,13]

Dosage and Formulation: Fluconazole is available in the following formulations: 150 mg capsules, tablet, liquid, and solution for intravenous infusion. Fluconazole is used in the treatment of onychomycosis in adults at a weekly dose of 150 to 450 mg for 3 and 6 months for finger and toe nail onychomycosis, respectively. In children, the dose is calculated based on body weight, 3-6 mg/kg/wk for 6 to 12 weeks in cases of finger onychomycosis extended to 9 to 15 weeks in cases of toe nail involvement. The recommended dose in cases of dermatophytosis is 150 mg once a week for 2 to 4 weeks in cases of tinea barbae, tinea pedis, and tinea corporis, and 4 to 6 weeks in tinea cruris and tinea capitis. Fluconazole is effective in the treatment of cutaneous and chronic mucocutaneous candidiasis and PV at a dose of 300 mg/wk for 2 weeks and once monthly for prophylaxis (Table 188-2).[3,26,33]

Side Effects: In general, fluconazole has fewer side effects than other antifungals. The most frequent drug side effects are headache, myalgia, dizziness, nausea, dyspepsia, diarrhea, and abdominal pain. In addition, cardiac abnormalities such as prolonged QT intervals and torsade de pointes are uncommonly reported with fluconazole. Exfoliative cutaneous reactions including Stevens–Johnson syndrome and toxic epidermal necrolysis were rarely described with the drug. Other adverse events include anaphylactic reactions, angioedema, acneform eruption, eye hemorrhage, and neutropenia (Table 188-3).[8]

Drug–Drug Interactions: Fluconazole is a substrate of the CYP3A hepatic isoenzyme. In addition, it has a moderate suppressing effect on CYP3A and CYP2C9, and a weak inhibitory effect on CYP2C19; therefore, the concurrent administration with drugs metabolized by any of these enzymes could result in deleterious drug interactions. An example would be fatal arrhythmias with the concomitant administration of astemizole, cisapride, pimozide, and terfenadine (Table 188-4).[3,8,32]

Pregnancy Category: C

ITRACONAZOLE

Itraconazole is a broad-spectrum fungistatic triazole, synthetically derived from ketoconazole through the prolongation of its hydrophobic side chains, promoting the binding of the drug to the apoprotein of the 14α-demethylase enzyme.[3]

Mechanism of Action: Like other azoles, itraconazole acts through the inhibition of 14-α-demethylase, suppressing the conversion of lanosterol to ergosterol.[3]

Pharmacokinetics: Itraconazole is a highly lipophilic agent. The capsule formulation requires gastric acidity for optimum absorption, as it delays the gastric emptying and increases the drug dissolution; therefore, it is best administered after a meal. In contrast, a cyclodextrin oral solution of itraconazole is not influenced by gastric acidity, and is best absorbed when taken on an empty stomach. Like terbinafine, itraconazole has a high affinity to nail and can accumulate there, forming a drug reservoir for 6 to 9 months after discontinuation of the drug. The half-life of itraconazole is typically 21 hours, and it has been postulated that its efficacy as a prophylactic agent is directly proportional to its plasma level, but should not, however, exceed 17 μg/mL by bioassay measurement to avoid drug toxicity. A twice-daily scheduling of doses is required in children because of drug lower plasma concentrations compared to adults.[3] Itraconazole undergoes an extensive hepatic metabolism by cytochrome CYP3A4 enzyme; as a result, a dose adjustment is required in patients with progressive liver disease. Renal insufficiency and renal dialysis have no influence on the drug plasma concentration. An exception is the intravenous formulation, which should be avoided when the creatinine clearance is less than 30 mL/min.[13]

Indications: Itraconazole is considered the best choice in treatment of *Candida* and nondermatophyte onychomycosis; its short course of treatment and good tolerability make it an especially good treatment choice for children.[15] Itraconazole is also used as an off-label treatment for many dermatophytoses, including tinea corporis, tinea capitis, tinea pedis, tinea cruris, tinea manuum, and PV (Table 188-2).

Dosage and Formulations: The recommended dose for tinea infections and PV is 100 mg twice daily for 5 days (Table 188-2). For the treatment of onychomycosis, itraconazole is prescribed as a continuous regimen (a daily dose of 200 mg for 6 weeks) or a monthly pulse dose (400 mg/d for 1 week). The dosage of the drug in children is calculated based on body weight (5 mg/kg/d) and both continuous or pulse regimens can be followed (Table 188-2).[8,13]

Side Effects: The most frequent side effects of itraconazole are GI disorders, especially the characteristic unpleasant taste associated with the hydroxypropyl-b-cyclodextrin vehicle, which can lead to patient noncompliance. Elderly patients on itraconazole often experience a triad of edema, hypertension, and hyperkalemia. In addition, itraconazole has a negative inotropic effect that can predispose to complete heart failure; therefore, it should be avoided in patients with a history of heart disease. Side effects such as hepatitis, jaundice, Stevens–Johnson syndrome, peripheral neuropathy, and adrenal suppression have been infrequently reported (Table 188-3).[3]

Drug–Drug Interactions: Itraconazole is a hepatic CYP3A4 enzyme substrate and inhibitor, and thus can affect the serum level, efficacy, and toxicity of drugs metabolized by the same enzyme. Similarly, CYP3A4 enzyme inducers and other inhibitors can increase or decrease the metabolism of the drug, respectively, and special considerations should be taken when combining itraconazole with one or more of these drugs. Given the necessity of gastric acidity for the optimum absorption of itraconazole, drugs such as H2 receptor blockers and proton pump blockers will decrease the drug absorption and subsequently its therapeutic effect (Table 188-4).[8]

Pregnancy Category: C.

POLYENES

NYSTATIN

Nystatin is a topical polyene derived from *Streptomyces* spp.[8]

MECHANISM OF ACTION

Nystatin has both fungistatic and fungicidal activity. It acts through binding to the mycotic ergosterol, for which its affinity is higher than that of the cholesterol found in mammalian cells. This binding will result in creation of pores in the cell membrane with subsequent leakage of essential fungal intracellular components, resulting in cell death.[34]

PHARMACOKINETICS

Because of the high toxicity associated with its intravenous administration, nystatin is confined to topical use only. Systemic absorption after cutaneous or mucous membrane application is insignificant.[8]

INDICATIONS

Nystatin is commonly used in the treatment of cutaneous, oropharyngeal, and vaginal candidiasis. The drug is not effective against dermatophytes or *Malassezia* spp. (Table 188-1).[8,34,35]

DOSAGE AND FORMULATIONS

Nystatin is available in cream, ointment, liquid, suspension, powder, and lozenge formulations. A twice-daily application for 4 to 5 days is the recommended dose for cutaneous infections, while the regimen for the treatment of oral candidiasis is a rinse 4 times daily for 14 days (Table 188-1).[8,35,36]

SIDE EFFECTS

Few side effects were reported with all formulations of nystatin; these include localized hypersensitivity reactions associated with the cutaneous application and manifested as allergic contact dermatitis, erythema, itching, and edema. Nausea, vomiting, and diarrhea have been reported with large doses of oral formulations.[8,25]

Pregnancy Category: B.

OTHER ANTIFUNGALS

CICLOPIROX

Ciclopirox olamine is a synthetic ethanolamine salt derivative of hydroxypyridone.[37]

MECHANISM OF ACTION

Ciclopirox exhibits broad-spectrum fungicidal and fungistatic, antibacterial, and antiinflammatory activities. It acts through the inhibition of the transmembrane uptake of RNA, DNA, and protein precursors. High drug concentrations (>50 μg/mL) alter the integrity of the cell membrane, leading to leakage of K ions, peptides, and amino acids. Ciclopirox also suppresses aerobic glycolysis in the yeast cell, and subinhibitory concentrations decrease the adherence of *Candida albicans* to both vaginal and buccal epithelial cells. The drug is capable of chelating trivalent molecules as Al^{3+} and Fe^{3+}, cofactors for the enzymes involved in detoxification of hazardous metabolites, mitochondrial electron transport chain, and energy production. The antiinflammatory effect of ciclopirox is attributed to its ability to reduce the synthesis and release of the proinflammatory prostaglandin E_2.[38]

PHARMACOKINETICS

The vaginal application of ciclopirox was associated with 15% to 20% systemic absorption, whereas the systemic absorption from other routes was insignificant.[38] Compared to efinaconazole and luliconazole, ciclopirox exhibits the least nail permeation. Ciclopirox is metabolized by glucuronidation and its metabolites are eliminated mainly by the kidney.[39]

INDICATIONS

Ciclopirox is used in the treatment of various dermatophytoses.[11] A ciclopirox monotherapy of onychomycosis has been associated with a cure rate of 5.5% to 8.5% after 48 weeks,[40] whereas a combination with oral terbinafine increased the cure rate to 88.2% compared to 64.7% achieved by terbinafine alone.[41] Ciclopirox also can be used in the treatment of cutaneous candidiasis, tinea versicolor, and scalp seborrheic dermatitis (Table 188-1).[38]

DOSAGE AND FORMULATIONS

Ciclopirox can be incorporated in one of the following formulations with either isopropyl or benzyl alcohol as a vehicle: 0.77% cream, gel, 1% shampoo, and 8% nail lacquer solution. For most indications, twice-daily application is required and should be continued for 4 weeks, regardless of clinical improvement. The ciclopirox shampoo should be left for 3 minutes before rinsing. The nail lacquer, on the other hand, should be applied on a daily basis and removed with alcohol once a week before reapplication (Table 188-1).[38,42]

SIDE EFFECTS

Side effects include mild erythema and itching of the skin adjacent to the application site and infrequent nail alterations.[42]

AMOROLFINE

MECHANISM OF ACTION

Amorolfine interrupts the ergosterol synthesis at the 14-reduction and the 7-8 isomerization in the ergosterol pathway, resulting in the depletion of ergosterol as well as the accumulation of 24-methylene ignosterol.[43]

PHARMACOKINETICS

The nail lacquer tends to build a reservoir that continues to release the drug to the nail plate in an exponential pattern. Negligible systemic absorption is associated with topical application. The drug is generally eliminated in urine and stool at a very slow rate.[43]

INDICATIONS

Amorolfine has both fungistatic and concentration- and time-dependent fungicidal action against yeasts, and exhibits fungicidal activity against most dermatophytes and other filamentous fungi. Amorolfine nail lacquer is approved for the treatment of onychomycosis in the absence of matrix involvement in Europe but not in the United States. The use of amorolfine vaginal tablets has been associated with high clinical cure rates of vulvovaginal candidiasis (90%-95%), though with a high recurrence rate (Table 188-1).

DOSAGE AND FORMULATIONS

Amorolfine is available as a 0.25% cream and 5% nail lacquer. For superficial dermatomycosis, cream is applied once daily for 2 to 4 weeks, whereas the regimen for onychomycosis is a weekly application of nail lacquer until the regeneration of nail (approximately 6 or 12 months in finger- and toenail onychomycosis, respectively) (Table 188-1).[44]

SIDE EFFECTS

Side effects include mild allergic reaction of adjacent skin.[43]

Pregnancy Category: D.

TAVABOROLE

Tavaborole is a novel oxaborole antifungal drug that encloses a fluorine atom, decreasing the pH of the boronic center, which inhibits fungal peptide synthesis. Tavaborole exhibits broad-spectrum activity against a variety of fungi, including the dermatophytes (*Trichophyton rubrum*, *Trichophyton mentagrophytes*, *T. tonsurans*, and *Epidermophyton floccosum*), some *Microsporum* species, and *C. albicans*.[45]

MECHANISM OF ACTION

Tavaborole acts through inhibiting a new target, aminoacyl transfer RNA synthetase (AARS), for which its affinity is a thousand times that of the mammalian cell and thereby selectively inhibits the mycotic protein synthesis.[27]

PHARMACOKINETICS

Tavaborole is incorporated in an alcohol-based solution and is therefore not suitable for ophthalmic, oral, or intravaginal use. It is characterized by low molecular weight, which accounts for enhanced nail penetration. Tavaborole usually undergoes extensive metabolism before finally being eliminated in the urine.[27]

INDICATIONS

Tavaborole is approved for the topical treatment of onychomycosis (Table 188-1).[27]

DOSAGE AND FORMULATIONS

Tavaborole is available as a 5% topical solution, applied once daily for 48 weeks (Table 188-1).[46]

SIDE EFFECTS

The most common side effects are exfoliation, erythema, and dermatitis.[47]

Pregnancy Category: C.

GRISEOFULVIN

Griseofulvin is a metabolic derivative of *Penicillium griseofulvum*, classically used for the treatment of dermatophytes. It has no activity against yeast and molds.[8]

MECHANISM OF ACTION

Griseofulvin is a fungistatic drug, blocking the growth and proliferation of the fungal cell. Griseofulvin binds tubulin- and microtubule-associated proteins (MAPs) along the polymerized microtubules, suppressing the formation of the mitotic spindle at the G2/M phase of the cell cycle. This inhibits cell division and forces the cell to undergo apoptosis.[48]

PHARMACOKINETICS

Griseofulvin is a water-insoluble drug, known for its low bioavailability profile. Most of the drug absorption occurs in the duodenum, and better absorption of griseofulvin can occur either when coated with polyethylene glycol or on coadministration with fatty meals.[49,50] Griseofulvin is characterized by its accumulation in the keratin-producing tissues, where it is adherently bound to newly formed keratin, rendering it resistant to fungal penetration. The 6-desmethyl enzyme is responsible for the metabolism of griseofulvin in the liver. The cutaneous elimination of the drug is slower than its elimination from plasma, allowing for extended drug activity even after its discontinuation. Griseofulvin is eliminated from the body mainly through the kidney in the form of metabolites.[3]

INDICATIONS

Griseofulvin remains the first line of treatment for tinea capitis caused by *Microsporum* species owing to its higher efficacy compared to terbinafine, and similar efficiency yet lower cost compared to itraconazole and fluconazole.[19] It is also the only FDA-approved treatment for pediatric onychomycosis, though its efficacy is limited to dermatophytes only (Table 188-2).[15]

DOSAGE AND FORMULATIONS

Griseofulvin is available in the following formulations: 250- and 500-mg microsize and 125-, 165-, and 250-mg ultramicrosize tablets, and 125-mg/5-mL oral suspensions.[8] Griseofulvin is recommended at a daily dose of 1-g microsize, or 660- to 750-mg ultramicrosize for 4 to 8 weeks in the treatment of tinea pedis and half of these doses for the treatment of tinea cruris and corporis. The recommended daily dosing of griseofulvin for the treatment of tinea capitis in children is dependent on their body weight and is as follows: ultramicrosize 10 to 15 mg/kg, oral suspension 15 to 25 mg/kg, microsize 20 to 25 mg/kg, continued for 1 to 2 months (Table 188-2).[3]

SIDE EFFECTS

The main side effects associated with griseofulvin are related to hypersensitivity, which ranges from mild urticaria, serum sickness, acute generalized exanthematous pustulosis, subacute cutaneous lupus erythematous, Stevens–Johnson syndrome, and toxic epidermal necrolysis. Photosensitivity, including photo-toxic and photo-allergic reactions, also has been commonly reported with griseofulvin.[51] Other cutaneous eruptions include lichenoid eruption, porphyria, and pityriasis rosea.[12,13] Rare but serious side effects include hepatotoxicity, leukopenia, thrombocytopenia, and anemia.[51] Neurologic problems such as peripheral neuritis, memory loss, confusion, and insomnia were uncommonly recorded in some patients (Table 188-3).[52,53]

DRUG–DRUG INTERACTIONS

Griseofulvin should not be prescribed concurrently with phenobarbitone because it decreases the absorption and increases the metabolism of griseofulvin.[44] Interactions with alcohol, cyclosporine, oral contraceptives, aspirin, and warfarin also have been reported (Table 188-4).[54-56]

Pregnancy Category: C.

NEW CARRIER VEHICLES AND FORMULATIONS

A number of new carrier vehicles have been investigated to improve the bioavailability of topical antifungals and enhance their therapeutic effects. Different mechanisms include incorporation of the drug in a lipid core matrix to achieve a maintained drug release up to 24 hours and to prevent light degradation of the drug. New carriers include micelles, solid lipid nanoparticles and nanostructured lipid carriers, and drug microemulsions. Vesicular carrier systems include liposomes, niosomes, transferosomes, ethosomes, and penetration enhancer vesicles.[57,58]

COMBINATION THERAPY

For the treatment of onychomycosis, combination therapy of a topical agent with a systemic antifungal provides several advantages, including higher rates of fungal killing, prevention of drug resistance, and expansion of spectrum activity.[3,15,59] Further, because the duration of therapy is shorter and oral medications can be used at lower doses, combination therapy decreases drug-related toxicity.[15,59,60] A case in which combination therapy can be of particular use is in onycholysis secondary to onychomycosis, as the separation of the nail plate from the subungual tissue interrupts the transport of drug from the nail plate to the nail bed and vice-versa. Using topical as well as oral therapy would ensure the nail plate and nail bed both are in contact with the antifungal agent.[3,59-61]

In the case of superficial skin infections, the addition of topical steroids to antifungal therapy, either in the same formulation or separately, is controversial. Because of the concern about the side effects associated with the abuse of topical steroids, many studies have discouraged this combination and suggested the use of topical antifungals with antiinflammatory properties instead.[12]

REFERENCES

1. Havlickova B, Czaika VA, Friedrich M. Epidemiological trends in skin mycoses worldwide. *Mycoses.* 2008;51(suppl 4):2-15.
2. Weinstein A, Berman B. Topical treatment of common superficial tinea infections. *Am Fam Physician.* 2002; 65(10):2095-2102.
3. Gupta AK, Cooper EA. Update in antifungal therapy of dermatophytosis. *Mycopathologia.* 2008;166(5-6): 353-367.
4. Gupta AK, Foley KA, Versteeg SG. New antifungal agents and new formulations against dermatophytes. *Mycopathologia.* 2017;182(1-2):127-141.
5. Dismukes WE. Antifungal therapy: lessons learned over the past 27 years. *Clin Infect Dis.* 2006;42(9):1289-1296.
6. Lewis RE. Current concepts in antifungal pharmacology. *Mayo Clin Proc.* 2011;86(8):805-817.
7. Del Rosso JQ, Kircik LH. Optimizing topical antifungal therapy for superficial cutaneous fungal infections: Focus on topical naftifine for cutaneous dermatophytosis. *J Drugs Dermatol.* 2013;12(11)(suppl):s165-s171.
8. Zhang A, Camp W, Elewski B. Advances in topical and systemic antifungals. *Dermatol Clin.* 2007;25(2): 165-183.
9. Gupta AK, Ryder JE, Cooper EA. Naftifine: a review. *J Cutan Med Surg.* 2008;12(2):51-58.
10. Nigam PK. Antifungal drugs and resistance: current concepts. *Our Dermatol Online.* 2015;6(2):212-221.
11. High WA, Fitzpatrick JE. Topical antifungal agents. In: Fitzpatrick TB, Wolff K, eds. *Fitzpatrick's Dermatology in General Medicine.* 7th ed. New York, NY: McGraw-Hill; 2008.
12. Sahoo AK, Mahajan R. Management of tinea corporis, tinea cruris, and tinea pedis: a comprehensive review. *Ind Dermatol Online J.* 2016;7(2):77-86.
13. Dias MFRG, Bernardes-Filho F, Quaresma-Santos MVP, et al. Treatment of superficial mycoses: review—part II. *An Bras Dermatol.* 2013;88(6):937-944.
14. Leyden J. Pharmacokinetics and pharmacology of terbinafine and itraconazole. *J Am Acad Dermatol.* 1998; 38(5):S42-S47.
15. Ameen M, Lear JT, Madan V, et al. British association of dermatologists' guidelines for the management of onychomycosis 2014. *Br J Dermatol.* 2014; 171(5):937-958.
16. Van Duyn Graham L, Elewski BE. Recent updates in oral terbinafine: its use in onychomycosis and tinea capitis in the US. *Mycoses.* 2011;54(6):e679-e685.
17. Hossain MA, Ghannoum MA. New developments in chemotherapy for non-invasive fungal infections. *Exp Opin Invest Drugs.* 2001;10(8):1501-1511.
18. Kakourou T, Uksal U. Guidelines for the management of tinea capitis in children. *Pediatr Dermatol.* 2010; 27(3):226-228.
19. Michaels BD, Del Rosso JQ. Tinea capitis in infants: recognition, evaluation, and management suggestions. *J Clin Aesthet Dermatol.* 2012;5(2):49-59.
20. Newland JG, Abdel-Rahman SM. Update on terbinafine with a focus on dermatophytoses. *Clin Cosmet Investig Dermatol.* 2009;2:49-63.
21. Mast N, Zheng W, Stout C, et al. Antifungal azoles: structural insights into undesired tight binding to cholesterol-metabolizing CYP46A1. *Mol Pharmacol.* 2013;84(1):86-94.
22. Del Rosso JQ. Adult seborrheic dermatitis. *J Clin Aesthet Dermatol.* 2011;4(5):32-38.
23. Greenblatt HK, Greenblatt DJ. Liver injury associated with ketoconazole: review of the published evidence. *J Clin Pharmacol.* 2014;54(12):1321-1329.
24. Banankhah PS, Garnick KA, Greenblatt DJ. Ketoconazole. Associated liver injury in drug-drug interaction studies in healthy volunteers. *J Clin Pharmacol.* 2016; 56(10):1196-1202.
25. Gupta AK, Daigle D, Foley KA. Drug safety assessment of oral formulations of ketoconazole. *Expert Opin Drug Saf.* 2015;14(2):325.
26. Renati S, Cukras A, Bigby M. Pityriasis versicolor. *BMJ.* 2015;350:h1394.
27. Saunders J, Maki K, Koski R, et al. Tavaborole, efinaconazole, and luliconazole: three new antimycotic agents for the treatment of dermatophytic fungi. *J Pharm Pract.* 2017;30(6):621-630.
28. Del Rosso JQ. The role of topical antifungal therapy for onychomycosis and the emergence of newer agents. *J Clin Aesthet Dermatol.* 2014;1;7(7):10-18.
29. Scher RK, Nakamura N, Tavakkol A. Luliconazole: a review of a new antifungal agent for the topical treatment of onychomycosis. *Mycoses.* 2014;57(7): 389.
30. Tatsumi Y, Nagashima M, Shibanushi T, et al. Mechanism of action of efinaconazole, a novel triazole antifungal agent. *Antimicrob Agents Chemother.* 2013;57(5): 2405-2409.
31. Lyon JP, Carvalho CR, Rezende RR, et al. Synergism between fluconazole and methylene blue-photodynamic therapy against fluconazole-resistant candida strains. *Ind J Med Microbiol.* 2016;34(4):506-508.
32. Ashley ES, Lewis R, Lewis JS, et al. Pharmacology of systemic antifungal agents. *Clin Infect Dis.* 2006;43(suppl 1): S28-S39.
33. Cornely OA, Bassetti M, Calandra T, et al. ESCMID* Guideline for the diagnosis and management of Candida diseases 2012: non-neutropenic adult patients. *Clin Microbiol Infect.* 2012;18(suppl 7):19-37.
34. Vandeputte P, Ferrari S, Coste A. Antifungal resistance and new strategies to control fungal infections. *Int J Microbiol.* 2012;2012:713687.
35. Darwazeh AM, Darwazeh TA. What makes oral candidiasis recurrent infection? A clinical view. *J Mycology.* 2014;2014:758394.
36. Akpan A, Morgan R. Oral candidiasis. *Postgrad Med J.* 2002;78(922):455-459.
37. Gupta AK. Ciclopirox: an overview. *Int J Derm.* 2001;40(5): 305-310.
38. Subissi A, Monti D, Togni G, et al. Ciclopirox. *Drugs.* 2010;70(16):2133-2152.
39. Matsuda Y, Sugiura K, Hashimoto T, et al. Efficacy coefficients determined using nail permeability and antifungal activity in keratin-containing media are useful for predicting clinical efficacies of topical drugs for onychomycosis. *PLoS One.* 2016;21;11(7):e0159661.
40. Gupta AK, Skinner AR. Ciclopirox for the treatment of superficial fungal infections: a review. *Int J Dermatol.* 2003;42(suppl 1):3-9.
41. Avner S, Nir N, Henri T. Combination of oral terbinafine and topical ciclopirox compared to oral terbinafine for the treatment of onychomycosis. *J Dermatol Treat.* 2005;16(5-6):327-330.
42. Gupta AK, Bluhm R. Ciclopirox (Loprox) gel for superficial fungal infections. *Skin Therapy Lett.* 2004;9(7):4-5, 9.
43. Rotta I, Sanchez A, Gonçalves PR, et al. Efficacy and safety of topical antifungals in the treatment of dermatomycosis: a systematic review. *Br J Dermatol.* 2012; 166(5):927-933.

44. Polak AM. Preclinical data and mode of action of amorolfine. *Clin Exp Dermatol.* 1992;17(suppl 1):8-12.
45. Gupta AK, Daigle D, Foley KA. Topical therapy for toenail onychomycosis: an evidence-based review. *Am J Clin Dermatol.* 2014;15(6):489-502.
46. Gupta G, Foley KA, Gupta AK. Tavaborole 5% solution: a novel topical treatment for toenail onychomycosis. *Skin Therapy Lett.* 2015;20(6):6-9.
47. Markham A. Tavaborole: first global approval. *Drugs.* 2014;74(13):1555-1558.
48. Rathinasamy K, Jindal B, Asthana J, et al. Griseofulvin stabilizes microtubule dynamics, activates p53 and inhibits the proliferation of MCF-7 cells synergistically with vinblastine. *BMC Cancer.* 2010;10(1):213.
49. Debruyne D, Coquerel A. Pharmacokinetics of antifungal agents in onychomycoses. *Clin Pharmacokinet.* 2001;40(6):441-472.
50. Elewski B, Tavakkol A. Safety and tolerability of oral antifungal agents in the treatment of fungal nail disease: a proven reality. *Ther Clin Risk Manag.* 2005;1(4):299-306.
51. Iorizzo M, Piraccini BM, Tosti A. Today's treatments options for onychomycosis. *J Dtsch Dermatol Ges.* 2010;8(11):875-879.
52. Moossavi M, Bagheri B, Scher RK. Systemic antifungal therapy. *Dermatol Clin.* 2001;19(1):35-52.
53. Zuber TJ, Baddam K. Superficial fungal infection of the skin: where and how it appears help determine therapy. *Postgrad Med.* 2001;109(1):117-120, 123-126, 131-132.
54. Himanshu B, Shyam M, Yatin M. Drug-drug interactions in medical ICU. *Ind J Pharm.* 2015;2(1):62-69.
55. Katz HI. Possible drug interactions in oral treatment of onychomycosis. *J Am Pod Med Assoc.* 1997;87(12):571-574.
56. Brodell RT, Elewski B. Antifungal drug interactions. Avoidance requires more than memorization. *Postgrad Med.* 2000;107(1):41-43.
57. Güngör S, Erdal M, Aksu B. New formulation strategies in topical antifungal therapy. *J Cosmetics Dermatol Sci Appl.* 2013;3(1):56-65.
58. Bseiso E, Nasr M, Abd El Gawad N, et al. Recent advances in topical formulation carriers of antifungal agents. *Ind J Dermatol Venereol Leprol.* 2015;81(5):457-463.
59. Baran R, Kaoukhov A. Topical antifungal drugs for the treatment of onychomycosis: an overview of current strategies for monotherapy and combination therapy. *J Eur Acad Dermatol Venereol.* 2005;19(1):21-29.
60. Hay RJ. The future of onychomycosis therapy may involve a combination of approaches. *Br J Dermatol.* 2001;145(suppl 60):3-8.
61. Lecha M, Effendy I, Feuilhade de Chauvin M, et al. Treatment options—development of consensus guidelines. *J Eur Acad Dermatol Venereol.* 2005;19(suppl 1):25-33.

Chapter 189 :: Antihistamines
:: Michael D. Tharp

第一百八十九章
抗组胺药

中文导读

组胺是一种低分子量的胺，由组氨酸脱羧酶合成。组氨酸脱羧酶是一种全身许多细胞表达的酶。组胺通过4种不同的受体发挥作用，H1受体和H2受体广泛表达于神经元、平滑肌、上皮细胞、内皮细胞和多种免疫细胞上。本章重点介绍了H1受体拮抗剂和H2受体拮抗剂的作用机制、药代动力学、适应证、给药方案、风险及防范措施、药物相互作用及特殊患者群体的用药。并提到了H1抗组胺药是治疗慢性特发性荨麻疹和物理性荨麻疹的首选药物，在使用抗组胺药时，某些特殊患者群体包括儿童、老年人和肾或肝损伤患者，可能需要调整剂量。而在慢性特发性荨麻疹/血管性水肿的难治性病例中，H2抗组胺药可能是H1抗组胺治疗的有效辅助药物。

〔粟 娟〕

AT-A-GLANCE

- H_1 antihistamines are first-line therapy for chronic idiopathic and physical urticarials.
- H_1 agents may be useful in treating conditions with histamine-associated pruritus.
- Limited evidence supports the use of H_1 in the treatment of atopic dermatitis.
- Certain special patient populations, including children, the elderly, and patients with renal or hepatic impairment, may require dosage adjustments when using antihistamines.
- H_2 antihistamines may be a useful adjunct to H_1 antihistamine therapy in refractory cases of chronic idiopathic urticaria/angioedema.

Histamine is a low-molecular-weight amine that is synthesized from L-histidine by histidine decarboxylase, an enzyme expressed by numerous cells throughout the body. Histamine exerts its effects through 4 different receptors that play a role in embryonic development, cellular growth and proliferation, hematopoiesis and immunity, inflammation, and wound healing. This amine is an important neurotransmitter in the CNS and is produced in neurons located in the tuberomammillary nucleus of the posterior hypothalamus. Nerves arising from this area regulate the sleep–wake cycle, endocrine homeostasis, cognition and memory. Histamine also exerts anticonvulsant effects. Histamine is metabolized by 2 major pathways: diamine oxidase and histamine methyl transferase.[1,2]

Histamine receptors are heptahelical transmembrane molecules that transmit extracellular signals to intracellular second messengers via G proteins. These receptors have constitutive activity, and thus are able to trigger downstream events in the absence of ligand stimulation. Active and inactive states of histamine receptors exist in equilibrium and can be shifted to a greater proportion of active or inactive states by histamine and antihistamines, respectively.[3,4] Both H_1 and H_2 histamine receptors are widely expressed on neurons, smooth muscle, epithelium, endothelium, and multiple immune cells. H_2 receptors also exist on gastric mucosal parietal cells; consequently, occupation by specific H_2 antihistamines inhibits gastric acid secretion. H_3 and H_4 receptors have more limited expression in the body with H_3 receptors occurring primarily on histaminergic neurons and immune cells, whereas H_4 receptors are highly expressed in the bone marrow and on peripheral hematopoietic cells.[2,5]

H_1 ANTIHISTAMINES

The first H_1 antihistamines were introduced in the 1940s after groundbreaking work by Bovet in the 1930s. The H_1 antihistamines—diphenhydramine, chlorpheniramine, and promethazine—all became available for clinical use during this time, and these and other agents were the primary source of antihistamine therapy until the 1980s when less-sedating, second-generation antihistamines were developed. First-generation antihistamines are divided into 6 groups on the basis of chemical structure: (a) ethylenediamines, (b) ethanolamines, (c) alkylamines, (d) phenothiazines, (e) piperazines, and (f) piperidines. The presence of multiple aromatic or heterocyclic rings and alkyl substituents enhances the lipophilicity of these compounds, permitting penetration of the blood–brain barrier, thereby leading to sedation. Second-generation antihistamines are less capable of accumulating in the CNS, and thus are less sedating. Compared to first-generation antihistamines, these second-generation agents also have the added advantage of longer half-lives, thus requiring for less-frequent dosing. Today, more than 45 H_1 antihistamines exist worldwide as prescription and nonprescription medications, and are used for the treatment of allergic reactions, urticaria, pruritus, nausea, vertigo, sleep, and anxiety.[4,6]

MECHANISM OF ACTION

H_1 antihistamines are inverse agonists that reversibly bind and stabilize the inactive form of the H_1 receptor, thereby favoring the inactive state (Table 189-1). By means of the H_1 receptor, H_1 antihistamines decrease the production of proinflammatory cytokines, the expression of cell-adhesion molecules, and chemotaxis of eosinophils and other immune cells (Fig. 189-1).[1,4] H_1 antihistamines may also decrease mediator release from mast cells and basophils through inhibition of calcium ion channels. In addition to binding to histamine receptors, first-generation H_1 antihistamines also act on muscarinic, α-adrenergic, and serotonin receptors, as well as cardiac ion channels. Some of the more significant side effects associated with first-generation H_1 antihistamines, such as urinary retention, hypotension, and cardiac arrhythmias, are mediated through these nonhistamine receptors.

Many of the low-sedating, second-generation H_1 antihistamines are chemically derived from first-generation agents.[1,2] For example, cetirizine is a metabolite of hydroxyzine and loratadine is related to azatadine. The second-generation H_1 antihistamines bind noncompetitively to the H_1 receptor, and thus are not easily displaced by histamine. They dissociate slowly, and have a longer duration of action than first-generation H_1 antihistamines. As a result of the selectivity of second-generation antihistamines for the H_1 receptor and their reduced lipophilicity, these agents are far less likely to cause sedation and have fewer side effects than the first-generation antihistamines.[1,3,6]

Some low-sedating H_1 antihistamines affect cell trafficking in the skin and other tissues, presumably by modulating the release of inflammatory mediators and the expression of adhesion molecules. In a skin chamber model, cetirizine administration reduced eosinophil influx after allergen challenge; however, similar effects have not been seen in the nasal mucosa following allergen exposure. In vitro studies demonstrate that cetirizine inhibits eosinophil, monocyte, and T-lymphocyte chemotaxis to N-formyl-methionyl-leucyl-phenylalanine and platelet-activating factor.[7] H_1 antihistamines may also modulate the expression of cellular adhesion molecules such as antigen-induced intercellular adhesion molecule 1 that exists on keratinocytes, Langerhans cells, and endothelial cells These antihistamines also may influence the release of inflammatory mediators from leukocytes.[8] In vitro, desloratadine and emedastine inhibit platelet-activating factor–induced eosinophil chemotaxis, tumor necrosis factor-α–induced eosinophil adhesion, and spontaneous and phorbol myristate–induced superoxide generation.[9,10]

PHARMACOKINETICS

FIRST-GENERATION H_1 ANTIHISTAMINES

After oral administration, the sedating effects of first-generation H_1 antihistamines can be observed within 30 minutes to 1 hour and generally persist for 4 to

TABLE 189-1
Basic Pharmacology of Antihistamines

- Both H_1 and H_2 antihistamines are inverse agonists that reversibly bind and stabilize the inactive form of the histamine receptor, thereby favoring the inactive state.
- First-generation H_1 agents are relatively lipophilic, which enhances penetration of the blood–brain barrier and leads to sedation.
- First-generation H_1 antihistamines may interact with other drugs metabolized by the hepatic cytochrome P450 system leading to drug–drug interactions.
- Second-generation H_1 antihistamines have poor penetration of the blood–brain barrier and thus are less sedating.
- Second-generation H_1 antihistamines bind selectively to peripheral H_1 receptors and have fewer CNS effects.
- Second-generation H_1 antihistamines require less hepatic metabolism and thus are less likely to interact with other medications.
- There is no evidence of tolerance or tachyphylaxis to first-generation or second-generation antihistamines.

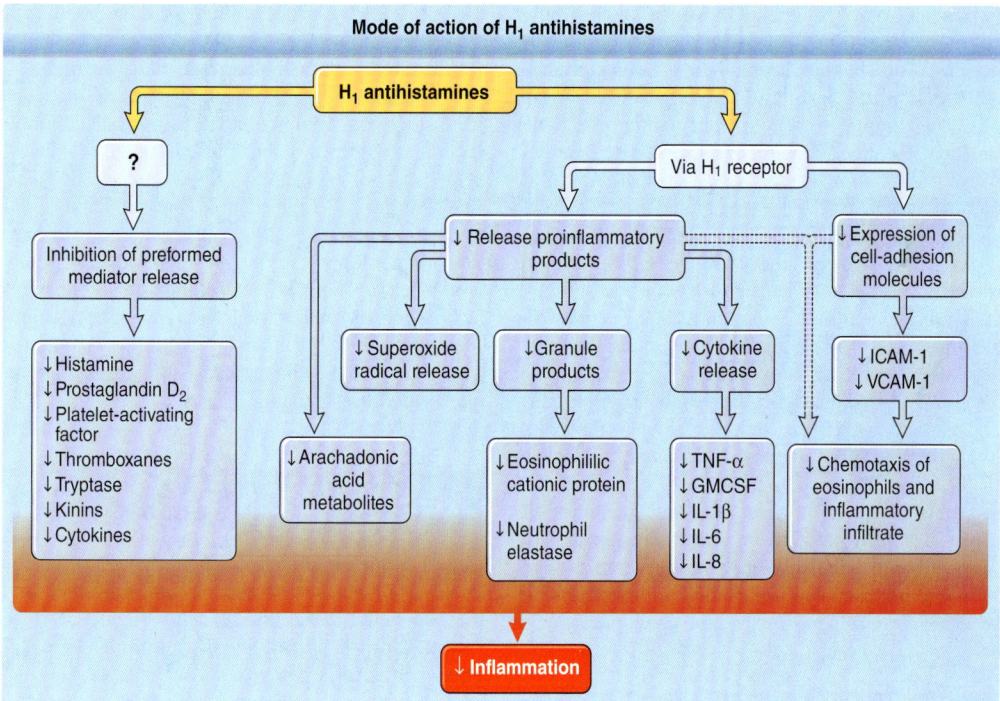

Figure 189-1 Mode of action of H_1 antihistamines. By means of the H_1 receptor, H_1 antihistamines inhibit the release of preformed mediators and decrease the production of proinflammatory cytokines, the expression of cell-adhesion molecules, and chemotaxis of eosinophils and other cells. ↓, Decreased; GMCSF, granulocyte-macrophage colony-stimulating factor; ICAM-1, intercellular adhesion molecule 1; IL, interleukin; TNF-α, tumor necrosis factor-α; VCAM-1, vascular cellular adhesion molecule 1.

6 hours. However, sedation may last for 24 hours or longer for some agents in some individuals. For example, after the oral administration of a single dose, the serum half-lives of brompheniramine, chlorpheniramine, and hydroxyzine exceed 20 hours in adults. First-generation H_1 antihistamines are metabolized by hepatic cytochrome P450 (CYP) enzyme 3A4, forming glucuronides before excretion in urine.[1,4]

The potency and relative concentration of H_1 antihistamines in the skin can be compared by their inhibition of the cutaneous wheal-and-flare response induced by intradermal histamine. First-generation H_1 antihistamines are typically administered in divided doses at intervals of 4 to 8 hours (see section "Dosing Regimens"), although once-daily dosing may suffice for agents with longer serum half-lives. In placebo-controlled, double-blind studies, there is no evidence of tolerance or tachyphylaxis to these antihistamines over a 3-month period. Interestingly, despite the relatively short half-lives of first-generation antihistamines, suppression of allergen-induced wheal-and-flare reactions may persist for up to 7 days after discontinuation.[1,4]

Topical H_1 antihistamine formulations for dermatologic use are available, although these preparations tend to be less effective and are associated with the potential for delayed allergic contact reactions.

SECOND-GENERATION H_1 ANTIHISTAMINES

Most second-generation, H_1 antihistamines are low sedating. They are administered once or twice daily and generally achieve peak plasma concentrations within 1 to 2 hours, These drugs achieve higher concentrations in the skin than first-generation antihistamines, and a single dose can suppress the wheal-and-flare reaction from 1 to 24 hours. Regular use prolongs this effect; for example, 6 days of daily cetirizine use results in 7 days of wheal-and-flare suppression.[11-15]

The second-generation antihistamines—loratadine, acrivastine, mizolastine, ebastine, and oxatomide—are metabolized in the liver via the hepatic enzyme CYP 3A4. Cetirizine, fexofenadine, levocabastine, desloratadine, and levocetirizine undergo minimal hepatic metabolism, which reduces the likelihood of interactions with other drugs. In general, most of these antihistamines are excreted in the urine and thus dosages need to be adjusted for patients with renal insufficiency.[1,4]

In healthy adults, cetirizine and levocetirizine reach peak concentrations approximately 1 hour after administration, with elimination half-lives of 6.5 to 10 hours. Fexofenadine generally reaches a peak concentration at 2 to 3 hours, with an elimination half-life of 14 hours.[5] While dosage adjustments are recommended for patients with decreased creatinine clearance, this is usually unnecessary for patients with hepatic disease because fexofenadine undergoes minimal hepatic metabolism.[1,4] Loratadine's half-life ranges on average from 8 to 24 hours, depending on hepatic function. Ebastine, which is metabolized to form its carboxylic acid metabolite, and carebastine, has a half-life of 15 hours.[1,4] In a single-dose study, normal subjects were treated with cetirizine (10 mg), fexofenadine (60 mg), or loratadine (10 mg) prior to repeated intradermal histamine injections over 24 hours. In the study, cetirizine proved to be more potent than fexofenadine, which was more effective than loratadine in suppressing these histamine reactions.[16] Similar studies also have demonstrated that levocetirizine (5 mg) and fexofenadine (180 mg) are more potent than desloratadine (5 mg) in suppressing histamine's effects in the skin.[17] Pharmacogenetics may also influence drug metabolism and clearance of antihistamines. In a series of pharmacokinetic studies, approximately 7% of all subjects and 20% of African Americans were slow metabolizers of desloratadine. Comparable differences may exist for other H_1 antihistamines.[4,18]

INDICATIONS

Table 189-2 outlines the indications for treatment with H_1 antihistamines.

H_1 antihistamines appear to be effective in treating up to 50% of patients with chronic idiopathic urticaria (CIU), angioedema, and dermatographism. They are not as effective in treating physical urticarias, hereditary and acquired angioedema, urticarial vasculitis, and pruritus unrelated to histamine. Comparative studies of different groups of first-generation H_1 antihistamines are few; however, in general, these agents appear to have equal efficacy in the treatment of CIU. If an agent from one class of H_1 antihistamines proves ineffective, then an agent from another antihistamine group should be considered.[4,19]

Studies comparing the efficacy of second-generation antihistamines, on the other hand, are numerous. Double-blind, placebo-controlled, or parallel studies, have demonstrated that low-sedating H_1 antihistamines (cetirizine, loratadine, fexofenadine, desloratadine, levocetirizine, acrivastine, mizolastine, azelastine, ebastine, and oxatomide) are superior to placebo in the treatment of urticaria and angioedema.[20-26] Trials comparing different second-generation antihistamines with one another have not shown any one agent to be consistently superior, although cetirizine and levocetirizine have fared best overall in comparative trials.[1,26-29]

Even though both first-generation and second-generation H_1 antihistamines are used to treat pruritus in patients with atopic dermatitis, their efficacy has not been proved by rigorous clinical trials. In the 18-month Early Treatment of the Atopic Child study, cetirizine afforded a steroid-sparing benefit to children with severe atopic dermatitis, but no consistent benefit was observed in children with moderate disease.[30,31] A meta-analysis of 16 studies conducted from 1966 through 1999 failed to demonstrate a major role for either first-generation or second-generation H_1 antihistamines in the treatment of atopic dermatitis.[31]

Mastocytosis represents an uncontrolled proliferation of tissue mast cells, and histamine is believed responsible for many of the symptoms associated with this disorder; H_1 antihistamines are commonly used to treat symptomatic mastocytosis patients.[32-34] In general, higher doses of H_1 antihistamines than normally employed for allergic disorders may be necessary for symptom control in mastocytosis patients. For example, fexofenadine 360 mg in the morning and cetirizine 40 mg at night may be necessary for some symptomatic mastocytosis patients.

DOSING REGIMENS

The H_1 antihistamines are considered first-line therapy in the treatment of CIU and physical urticarials, and may be useful in treating other conditions in which histamine-driven pruritus is a major feature. The lowest effective dosage is preferred to minimize dose-related side effects, such as sedation. Table 189-3 outlines the dosing regimens for H_1 antihistamines. After several days of therapy, the dosage may be increased if symptom control is inadequate. Occasionally, gradual escalation of dosing permits the development of tolerance to sedation, which allows higher dosages to be used to treat certain conditions, such as refractory CIU. Doses up to 4 times that normally recommended for second-generation H_1 antihistamines may be necessary in the treatment of some CIU patients.[19,35] In a retrospective study of 368 CIU patients treated with either first-generation or second-generation H_1 antihistamines, 276 (75%) increased their dose by 2 to 4 times the normal recommended dose. Half of these patients experienced a clinical benefit from the medication increase. Those patients treated with second-generation H_1 antihistamines also experienced less sedation and other side effects compared to patients treated with first-generation H_1 agents.[35]

Ingestion of the medication with food may alleviate the GI discomfort that sometimes can accompany antihistamine use. Patients, however, should be advised to avoid taking fexofenadine with antacids because this can interfere with drug absorption. Individuals with comorbid conditions, such as hepatic or renal disease, may require lower dosages as a result of impaired metabolism or excretion of these drugs. Certain special patient populations, including children,

TABLE 189-2
Indications for Treatment with H_1 Antihistamines

- Acute urticaria
- Chronic idiopathic urticarial
- Physical urticarias and dermatographism
- Pruritus associated with histamine release
- Symptoms of mastocytosis

TABLE 189-3
Dosing Regimens for H_1 Antihistamines[1,6,15,18,33,81]

DRUG	FORMULATION	DOSAGE	CONDITIONS REQUIRING DOSAGE ADJUSTMENT
First-generation H_1 Antihistamines			
Chlorpheniramine	2-, 4-, 8-, 12-mg tablet	Adult: 4 mg thrice daily, 4 times daily; 8-12 mg twice daily	Hepatic impairment
	2 mg/5 mL syrup	Age 6-11 years: 2 mg q4-6h	
Cyproheptadine	4-mg tablet	Adult: 4 mg thrice daily, 4 times daily	Hepatic impairment
	2 mg/5 mL syrup	Age 7-14 years: 4 mg twice daily, thrice daily	
Diphenhydramine	25-, 50-mg tablet	Adult: 25-50 mg q4-6h	Hepatic impairment
	12.5 mg/5 mL syrup	Age 6-12 years: 12.5-25 mg q4-6h	
	50 mg/15 mL syrup	Age <6 years: 6.25-12.5 mg q4-6h	
	6.25 mg/5 mL syrup		
	12.5 mg/5 mL syrup		
Hydroxyzine	10-, 25-, 50-, 100-mg tablet	Age ≥6 years: 25-50 mg q6-8h or at bedtime	Hepatic impairment
	10 mg/5 mL syrup	Age <6 years: 25-50 mg daily	
Tripelennamine	25-, 50-, 100-mg tablets	Adult: 25-50 mg q4-6h	Hepatic impairment
Second-generation H_1 Antihistamines			
Acrivastine[a]	8-mg tablet	Adult: 8 mg thrice daily	Renal impairment
Azelastine	2-mg tablet[b]	Adult: 2-4 mg twice daily	Renal and hepatic impairment
	0.1% nasal spray	Age 6-12 years: 1-2 mg twice daily	
		2 sprays/nostril twice daily	
Cetirizine	5-, 10-mg tablet	Age ≥6 years: 5-10 mg daily	Renal and hepatic impairment
	5 mg/mL syrup	Age 2-6 years: 5 mg daily	
		Age 6 months to 2 years: 2.5 mg daily	
Desloratadine	2.5-, 5-mg tablet	Age ≥12 years: 5 mg daily	Renal and hepatic impairment
	5 mg/mL syrup	Age 6-12 years: 2.5 mg daily	
		Age 1-6 years: 1.25 mg daily	
		Age 6-12 months: 1 mg daily	
Ebastine[b]	10-mg tablet	Age ≥6 years: 10-20 mg daily	Renal impairment
		Age 6-12 years: 5 mg daily	
		Age 2-5 years: 2.5 mg daily	
Fexofenadine	30-, 60-, 120-, 180-mg tablet	Age ≥12 years: 60 mg daily, twice daily; 120-180 mg daily	Renal impairment
		Age 6-12 years: 30 mg daily, twice daily	
Levocetirizine	5-mg tablet	Age ≥6 years: 5 mg daily	Renal and hepatic impairment
Loratadine	10-mg tablet	Age ≥6 years: 10 mg daily	Renal and hepatic impairment
	5 mg/mL suspension	Age 2-9 years: 5 mg daily	
Mizolastine[b]	10-mg tablet	Adult: 10 mg daily	Hepatic impairment

[a]Available in the United States only as a fixed-dose combination with pseudoephedrine hydrochloride, 120 mg.
[b]Not currently available in the United States.

the elderly, and pregnant or breastfeeding women, may also need antihistamine dosage adjustments (Table 189-4). Therapeutic end points are usually dictated by improvement in histamine-related signs and symptoms (eg, severity of pruritus; wheal number, size, and frequency). As for drug toxicity, no particular monitoring beyond the usual surveillance for adverse effects is required in most cases. Because of reports of hepatotoxicity, some sources recommend periodic liver transaminase evaluation when cyproheptadine is prescribed.[1,4,6]

RISKS AND PRECAUTIONS

Sedation is the most commonly reported problem, primarily with first-generation H_1 antihistamines

(Table 189-5).[1,4] The sedative effect is much more pronounced with first-generation H_1 antihistamines, especially in the ethanolamine and phenothiazine groups, and is less marked with the alkylamine group antihistamines. The use of first-generation H_1 antihistamines is associated with an increase in occupational injuries and automobile accidents.[36] Sedating H_1 antihistamines are sometimes used for their somnolent effects at night; however, these agents actually delay the onset of rapid eye movement sleep, leading to poor sleep quality and impaired memory, attention capabilities, and sensory-motor performance the following day.[37] Other CNS effects of sedating antihistamines include dizziness, tinnitus, disturbed coordination, inability to concentrate, blurred vision, and diplopia. Stimulatory CNS effects, which occur especially with the alkylamine group, include nervousness, irritability, insomnia, and tremor.[1,4] Most second-generation H_1 antihistamines, except for cetirizine and levocetirizine, are low sedating and thus better tolerated than first-generation agents.[37-41] Although far less soporific than its parent compound hydroxyzine, cetirizine causes sedation in approximately 10% to 15% of users, and appears to be dose dependent.[38,39] At doses of 10 mg and 20 mg, cetirizine occupies 12% and 25% of H_1 receptors in the human brain, respectively, as assessed by positron emission tomography scan.[40] Fexofenadine and loratadine/desloratadine, on the other hand, are least likely to enter the brain, and consequently have few if any CNS effects.[4,41]

Anticholinergic side effects are much more common with first-generation H_1 antihistamines as they have an affinity for cholinergic receptors.[4,42,43] These anticholinergic side effects include dry mucous membranes, urinary retention and hesitancy, postural hypotension, dizziness, erectile dysfunction, and constipation. These effects are often associated with the ethanolamine, phenothiazine, and piperazine groups. The anticholinergic effects of H_1 antihistamines preclude their use in patients with narrow-angle glaucoma and require close monitoring in patients with prostatic hypertrophy.[4,42] Most second-generation H_1 antihistamines are selective for H_1 receptors, and thus lack these anticholinergic side effects.[1,4,41]

GI complaints, including anorexia, nausea, vomiting, epigastric distress, diarrhea, and constipation, are uncommon side effects. The administration of these agents with food frequently reduces/eliminates these symptoms.[1,6]

Arrhythmias, particularly prolongation of the QT interval and torsades de pointes, are the most serious, but fortunately rare, cardiac side effects.[1,6] These dose-dependent effects are mediated through blockade of potassium channels unrelated to the H_1 histamine receptor. Transient hypotension may develop after intravenous therapy, especially if the drug is administered rapidly.[43] Two early second-generation H_1 antihistamines, terfenadine and astemizole, were removed from the world market because of risk of QT interval prolongation and torsades de pointes. Other second-generation agents have an approximately 1000-fold lower affinity for cardiac ion channels than terfenadine and astemizole. Evidence for ventricular arrhythmias have been extensively investigated and found to be absent in the newer second-generation H_1 antihistamines currently available in the United States.[4,5,42]

The occurrence of cutaneous reactions after the administration of oral H_1 antihistamines is extremely uncommon. Reported reactions include eczematous dermatitis, allergic contact dermatitis, urticaria, petechiae, fixed drug eruptions, and photosensitivity. Some of these reactions may be secondary to excipients in the drug.[44]

DRUG INTERACTIONS

The H_1 antihistamines may interact with other drugs metabolized by the hepatic CYP system, such as imidazole antifungals, cimetidine, and macrolide antibiotics.[4,6] The first-generation H_1 antihistamines—diphenhydramine, chlorpheniramine, clemastine, promethazine, hydroxyzine, and tripelennamine—inhibit the hepatic enzyme CYP 2D6 in vitro.[45,46] In vivo, diphenhydramine has been noted to increase levels of other drugs metabolized by the CYP 2D6

TABLE 189-4
Factors for Risk-to-Benefit Assessment of First-generation H_1 Antihistamine Therapy

- Risks
  - History of cardiac arrhythmias, particularly ventricular arrhythmias
  - First trimester of pregnancy
  - Prostatic hypertrophy
- Contraindications
  - Narrow-angle glaucoma
  - Concomitant use of monoamine oxidase inhibitors

TABLE 189-5
Adverse Effects of H_1 Antihistamines

- Sedation[a]
- Other CNS disturbances[a]
  - Dizziness
  - Tinnitus
  - Blurred vision
  - Irritability or nervousness
  - Insomnia
  - Tremor
- GI complaints (rare)[a]
  - Nausea and vomiting
  - Diarrhea or constipation
  - Anorexia
- Anticholinergic effects[a]
  - Dry mucous membranes
  - Urinary retention
  - Postural hypotension
- Cardiac arrhythmias (particularly prolongation of the QT interval, ventricular arrhythmias, torsades de pointes) (rare)[a]
- Hypersensitivity reactions (rare)

[a]More common in first-generation H_1 antihistamines.

system, including metoprolol and venlafaxine. First-generation H_1 antihistamines are contraindicated for patients receiving monoamine oxidase inhibitors as these medications may interfere with the metabolism of monoamine oxidase inhibitors.[6,46,47]

Central depressive effects may be accentuated when sedating H_1 antihistamines are combined with alcohol or other CNS depressants such as benzodiazepines. These interactions are generally not observed with second-generation H_1 antihistamines. In rare circumstances, antihistamines of the phenothiazine group may block and reverse the vasopressor effect of epinephrine. If individuals receiving a phenothiazine require a vasopressor agent, norepinephrine or phenylephrine should be used.[1,6,42]

SPECIAL PATIENT POPULATIONS

CHILDREN

Many of the sedating and low-sedating H_1 antihistamines can be safely used in children with appropriate dosing. Children may be more susceptible to certain side effects, such as excitation and insomnia, especially with first-generation H_1 antihistamines. Acute poisoning may develop with first-generation agents, but this is rare. Hallucinations, ataxia, incoordination, athetosis, and convulsions are the major features. The second-generation H_1 antihistamines cetirizine, levocetirizine, and loratadine have been extensively studied in children from 6 to 36 months of age with long-term safety profiles equal to placebo.[4,48,49]

ELDERLY

Caution should be used when treating elderly patients who may have renal insufficiency, cardiac disease, chronic hepatic disease, and/or CNS or balance comorbidities with first-generation H_1 antihistamines. Older individuals may be more susceptible to anticholinergic effects, particularly urinary retention and hesitancy, constipation, and postural hypotension.[4,6,42]

PREGNANT WOMEN

There are limited guidelines for the use of H_1 antihistamines in pregnant women. Most H_1 antihistamines are classified as U.S. Food and Drug Administration (FDA) pregnancy category B or category C. Based on earlier reports linking H_1 antihistamines to fetal malformations, particularly cleft palate defects, these agents have been customarily avoided in the first trimester of pregnancy. However, newer studies, including a metaanalysis of 200,000 first-trimester exposures to first-generation antihistamines, did not demonstrate an increased risk of congenital malformations.[50] In a prospective trial, astemizole administered to pregnant women was not associated with intrauterine growth retardation or perinatal complications, and the rate of congenital abnormalities was identical to the control group and general population.[51-53]

BREASTFEEDING WOMEN

No formal studies have been performed on the safety of H_1 antihistamines during breastfeeding. Theoretically, these drugs may diminish milk supply via anticholinergic effects. Clemastine, diphenhydramine, promethazine, triprolidine, cetirizine, loratadine, fexofenadine, desloratadine, and levocetirizine are all known to be excreted in breastmilk; however, their effects on the nursing infants has not been studied. When antihistamine therapy is necessary for the nursing mother, second-generation agents, which have fewer side effects and toxicities, are preferred.[4,6,52]

H_2 ANTIHISTAMINES

MECHANISM OF ACTION

H_2 antihistamines also are inverse agonists and include cimetidine, ranitidine, famotidine, and nizatidine. These agents bind to H_2 receptors located throughout the body, including epithelial cells, endothelial cells, and chondrocytes, as well as lymphocytes, neutrophils, eosinophils, monocytes, mast cells and dermal dendritic cells. In addition to their association with gastric acid secretion, H_2 receptors, and thus H_2 antihistamines, appear to play some role in antigen presentation, cellular recruitment, cutaneous vascular permeability, and local release of inflammatory mediators.[54] These complex immune events, however, remain poorly defined.

PHARMACOKINETICS

H_2 antihistamines are rapidly absorbed from the GI tract with peak levels occurring between 1 and 2 hours after administration. They are eliminated primarily unchanged through renal excretion with only 10% to 35% undergoing hepatic metabolism. The half-life of cimetidine in plasma is 2 hours, and approximately 70% is excreted unchanged in the urine.[54,55] The plasma half-life of ranitidine is 2 to 3 hours in healthy adults, and longer in elderly individuals and those with liver or kidney disease.[55,56] Famotidine has a plasma half-life of 3 to 8 hours, but may exceed 20 hours in patients with renal failure.[57] Nizatidine has a plasma half-life of 1 to 2 hours, and its duration of action is up to 10 hours.[51] The oral bioavailability of nizatidine is not affected by food and this antihistamine is primarily eliminated by the kidneys within 16 hours. In general, H_2 antihistamines have limited penetration of the blood–brain barrier.[55-58]

INDICATIONS IN DERMATOLOGY

There are few data from controlled studies supporting the use of H_2 antihistamines to treat dermatologic conditions (Table 189-6). Several studies demonstrate that H_2 antihistamines have a limited role in blocking histamine-induced wheal-and-flare reactions in the skin. Compared to H_1 antihistamines alone, the addition of an H_2 antihistamine further reduces this reaction by only 5% to 15%.[59] Most often, H_2 antihistamines are used in combination with H_1 agents in refractory cases of CIU and angioedema. In a double-blind crossover study, greater reductions in pruritus and wheal number, size, and severity were observed when cimetidine was combined with hydroxyzine versus hydroxyzine alone.[59] Similar observations have been made for when cimetidine was combined with chlorpheniramine.[60] Combination H_1 and H_2 antihistamine therapy also may be helpful in reducing GI symptoms associated with mastocytosis.[34] High doses of cimetidine also have been reported successful in the treatment of verruca vulgaris in some individuals.[61]

INITIATION OF THERAPY

For treatment of dermatologic conditions, H_2 antihistamines are generally used following an unsuccessful trial of H_1 antihistamines alone. In most cases, treatment with H_2 antihistamines may be initiated without any particular laboratory screening. The inhibition of the hepatic CYP system and the potential for drug interactions is usually the greatest concern, and patients' medication lists should be reviewed carefully before initiating therapy. Ranitidine is less inhibitory of the CYP system than cimetidine and may be the preferred H_2 antihistamine in situations in which drug interactions are a particular concern.[56] Also, patients with decreased creatinine clearance may require dosage adjustments.[62] In patients taking the cardiac drug dofetilide, cimetidine is contraindicated because of the risk of prolongation of the QT interval and life-threatening cardiac arrhythmias.[63] Therapeutic end points for H_2 antihistamines are determined by improvements in histamine-related signs and symptoms (eg, pruritus; flushing, wheal size/frequency/intensity). Table 189-7 lists the dosing regimens for H_2 antihistamines.

TABLE 189-6
Dermatologic Indications for Treatment with H_2 Antihistamines

- Acute allergic reactions
- Chronic urticaria (as a second-line agent)
- Systemic symptoms associated with mastocytosis (especially GI related)

RISKS AND PRECAUTIONS

In general, H_2 antihistamines are safe and rarely cause significant side effects. However, in patients with hepatic or renal disease, there is a greater risk for adverse effects. H_2 antihistamines may have CNS effects, including confusion, headache, and dizziness (Table 189-8). These effects seem to be partly dose-related. Other, less-common side effects include drowsiness, malaise, muscular pain, diarrhea, and constipation. There are rare reports of granulocytopenia.[56-58] For patients with a history of thrombocytopenia, a complete blood count may be warranted once H_2 antihistamine therapy is initiated, because thrombocytopenia has been reported as an idiosyncratic effect in a few individuals.[64] By their suppression of gastric acid secretion, H_2 antihistamines

TABLE 189-7
Dosing Regimens for H_2 Antihistamines[46,47,50,82]

DRUG	FORMULATION	DOSAGE	CONDITIONS REQUIRING DOSAGE ADJUSTMENT
Cimetidine	100-, 200-, 300-, 400-, 800-mg tablet	Adult: 400-800 mg twice daily	Renal or hepatic impairment
	300 mg/5 mL syrup		
	200 mg/20 mL syrup		
Ranitidine	75-, 150-, 300-mg tablet	Adult: 75-150 mg twice daily	Renal impairment
	15 mg/5 mL syrup	Pediatric: 5-10 mg/kg/day divided in 2 doses	
	150-mg granules		
Famotidine	10-, 20-, 40-mg tablet	Adult: 20-40 mg twice daily	Renal impairment
	40 mg/5 mL syrup	Age 1-16 years: 1 mg/kg/day	
		Divided in 2 doses, up to 40 mg twice daily	
Nizatidine	150-, 300-mg capsule	Age ≥12 years: 150 mg daily, twice daily	Renal impairment
	15 mg/5 mL syrup		

TABLE 189-8
Adverse Effects of H₂ Antihistamines

- CNS disturbances
  - Confusion
  - Dizziness
  - Drowsiness
  - Headache
- GI effects
  - Abdominal pain
  - Diarrhea or constipation
  - Increased transaminases and hepatitis (rare)
  - Nausea or vomiting
- Gynecomastia
- Hematologic (rare)
  - Anemia
  - Thrombocytopenia
- Hypersensitivity to H₂ (uncommon)
- Drug interactions
- Cardiac effects (with concomitant administration of dofetilide; dofetilide use is therefore a contraindication)

may facilitate oral infections and increase the risk of pneumonia in immunocompromised individuals.[65] As a class, these drugs may mask symptoms of gastric carcinoma. Also, cimetidine and ranitidine inhibit alcohol dehydrogenase activity, which can lead to increased blood alcohol levels.[56]

Uncommon side effects of cimetidine include gynecomastia with or without elevated prolactin levels in men; galactorrhea with elevated prolactin levels in women; and loss of libido, impotence, and reduction of sperm counts in young men.[56] Modest elevations in serum creatinine levels and hepatic transaminase levels have been reported and are reversible after the drug is withdrawn.[56,66] Rare dermatologic adverse effects, including alopecia and urticarial vasculitis, also have been reported.[66-68]

Ranitidine does not bind to androgen receptors and unlike cimetidine, does not enhance cell-mediated immune responses.[56] Ranitidine may affect the cardiovascular system by altering parasympathetic and sympathetic control functions. This altered cardiac sympathovagal balance may lead to a susceptibility to arrhythmias, particularly bradyarrhythmias, after intravenous infusion.[68]

Famotidine and nizatidine are associated with few side effects. They cause less inhibition of the CYP system, and therefore have fewer reported drug interactions.[57,58]

DRUG INTERACTIONS

Through inhibition of the CYP system, cimetidine increases the serum levels of numerous drugs, including some commonly prescribed medications.[68,69] Cimetidine increases levels of warfarin potentially leading to an increased risk of bleeding. This agent also interacts with cardiac drugs, including β blockers, calcium channel blockers, amiodarone, and antiarrhythmic agents. As already mentioned, cimetidine use is contraindicated in patients taking dofetilide. Both cimetidine and ranitidine also can reduce the urinary excretion of procainamide and quinidine. Other common drugs with which cimetidine interacts are phenytoin, benzodiazepines, metformin, sulfonylureas, and selective serotonin reuptake inhibitors.[56,68,69]

Although ranitidine interacts with other medications less frequently than cimetidine, significant interactions with fentanyl, metoprolol, midazolam, nifedipine, theophylline, and warfarin have been observed. Ranitidine may decrease the absorption of diazepam and reduce its plasma concentration by 25%.[56]

SPECIAL PATIENT POPULATIONS

CHILDREN

Of the H₂ antihistamines, ranitidine and famotidine have pharmacokinetics that have been relatively well studied in children, and these drugs have acceptable safety profiles with appropriate dosing. Cimetidine and nizatidine are not recommended for children for uses other than reducing gastric acidity. One adverse effect unique to children is an uncommon but drug class–wide risk of necrotizing enterocolitis in neonates.[70]

ELDERLY

Older patients may require a reduction in dosage to accommodate decreased renal function, as well as careful review of medication lists. Elderly patients also appear more susceptible to H₂ antihistamine–induced CNS disturbances, such as confusion and dizziness.[56-58]

PREGNANT WOMEN

The H₂ antihistamines are classified as FDA pregnancy category B drugs. Cimetidine, ranitidine, famotidine, and nizatidine are all excreted in breastmilk; however, the potential effects on the nursing infant have not been studied.[56-58]

OTHER THERAPEUTIC AGENTS WITH ANTIHISTAMINIC ACTIVITY

TRICYCLIC ANTIDEPRESSANTS

Tricyclic antidepressants bind to both H₁ and H₂ receptors. The tricyclic antidepressant most commonly used in dermatology is doxepin, which is 800 times more potent than diphenhydramine.[71] Oral doxepin has been used successfully in the treatment of refractory CIU, physical urticarials, and pruritus associated with systemic conditions.[72,73] In a double-blind, crossover study, doxepin proved more efficacious than diphenhydramine in the treatment of CIU.[72] Topical doxepin cream has proven effective for the treatment of pruritus in patients with atopic dermatitis and lichen simplex chronicus.[73]

Sedation is the most common adverse effect with both oral and topical doxepin, although some patients may develop tolerance with regular use.[72-74] Oral doxepin has been classified by the FDA as a pregnancy category C drug; topical doxepin is classified as a pregnancy category B drug.[74] Use of both oral and topical forms is contraindicated during breastfeeding. The safety and efficacy of doxepin therapy in children younger than age 12 years has not been established. This drug also should be used with caution in elderly patients, who may be more susceptible to its anticholinergic effects, including urinary retention and blurred vision. Doxepin should not be used concurrently with monoamine oxidase inhibitors, and all patients with underlying depression should be closely monitored for signs of suicidal ideation when initiating therapy. Doxepin also can cause a sudden increase in intraocular pressure and should not be used in patients with glaucoma.[71-74] Although doxepin has the potential to alter myocardial function, several studies have shown this medication to be safe in depressed patients with and without underlying heart disease.[75]

KETOTIFEN

Ketotifen, a benzocycloheptathiophene derivative, is an H_1 antihistamine with additional mast cell– and basophil-stabilizing properties.[3,76,77] Ketotifen has been used successfully in the treatment of CIU, physical urticaria, and symptoms associated with mastocytosis.[76-79] In a double-blind trial in CIU patients, ketotifen alleviated pruritus more effectively than clemastine or placebo.[79] Studies comparing ketotifen with low-sedating H_1 antihistamines have not been performed. Sedation and atropine-like side effects have been reported with this medication.[80] There are no studies evaluating the safety of ketotifen in pregnant or breastfeeding women. Ketotifen is available in the United States only as an ophthalmic solution.[80]

REFERENCES

1. Simons FE. Advances in H_1-antihistamines. *N Engl J Med*. 2004;351:2203-2217.
2. Parsons ME, Ganellin R. Histamine and its receptors. *Br J Pharmacol*. 2006;147:S127-S135.
3. Leurs R, Church MK, Taglialatela M. H_1 antihistamines: inverse agonism, anti-inflammatory actions and cardiac effects. *Clin Exp Allergy*. 2002;32:489.
4. Simons EF, Simons KJ. Histamine and H_1 antihistamines: celebrating a century of progress. *Clin Rev Allergy Immunol*. 2011;128:1139-1150.
5. Simons EF, Simons KJ. H_1 antihistamines. Current status and future directions. *World Allergy Organ J*. 2008;1:145-155.
6. Passalacqua G, Canonica GW. Structure and classification of H_1-antihistamines and overview of their activities. In: Simons FER. *Histamine and H_1-Antihistamines in Allergic Disease*, 2nd ed. New York, NY: Marcel Dekker; 2002:65.
7. Jinquan T, Reimert CM, Deleuran B, et al. Cetirizine inhibits the in vitro and ex vivo chemotactic response of T lymphocytes and monocytes. *J Allergy Clin Immunol*. 1995;95(5, pt 1):979-086.
8. Marone G, Granata F, Spadaro G, et al. Antiinflammatory effects of oxatomide. *J Investig Allergol Clin Immunol*. 1999;9(4):207-214.
9. el-Shazly AE, Masuyama K, Samejima Y, et al. Inhibition of human eosinophil chemotaxis in vitro by the antiallergic agent emedastine difumarate. *Immunopharmacol Immunotoxicol*. 1996;18(4):587-595.
10. Agrawal DK, et al. Desloratadine attenuation of eosinophil chemotaxis, adhesion, and superoxide generation. *Allergy*. 2000;55(suppl 63):276.
11. Jansen B, Graselli U, Dallinger S, et al. Pharmacokinetics and pharmacodynamics of the novel H_1-receptor antagonist emedastine in healthy volunteers. *Eur J Clin Pharmacol*. 2000;55(11-12):837-841.
12. Deschamps C, Dubruc C, Mentre F, et al. Pharmacokinetic and pharmacodynamic modeling of mizolastine in healthy volunteers with an indirect response model. *Clin Pharmacol Ther*. 2000;68(6):647-657.
13. Grant JA, Riethuisen JM, Moulaert B, et al. A double-blind, randomized, single-dose, crossover comparison of levocetirizine with ebastine, fexofenadine, loratadine, mizolastine, and placebo: suppression of histamine-induced wheal-and-flare response during 24 hours in healthy male subjects. *Ann Allergy Asthma Immunol*. 2002;88(2):190-197.
14. Devalia JL, De Vos C, Hanotte F, et al. A randomized, double-blind, crossover comparison among cetirizine, levocetirizine, and ucb 28557 on histamine-induced cutaneous responses in healthy adult volunteers. *Allergy*. 2001;56(1):50-57.
15. Cetirizine. In: DRUGDEX System. Greenwood Village, CO: Thomson Micromedex [updated periodically].
16. Grant JA, Danielson L, Rihoux JP, et al. A double-blind, single-dose, crossover comparison of cetirizine, ebastine, epinastine, fexofenadine, terfenadine and loratadine versus placebo: suppression of histamine-induced wheal and flare response during 24 hours in healthy male subjects. *Allergy*. 1999;54:700-707.
17. Meltzer EO, Gillman SA. Efficacy of fexofenadine versus desloratadine in suppressing histamine-induced wheal and flare. *Allergy Asthma Proc*. 2007;28:67-73.
18. Geha RS, Meltzer EO. Desloratadine: a new, nonsedating, oral antihistamine. *J Allergy Clin Immunol*. 2001;107:751.
19. Morgan M, Khan DA. Therapeutic alternatives for chronic urticaria: an evidence-based review, part 1. *Ann Allergy Asthma Immunol*. 2008;100:403-412.
20. Breneman D, Bronsky EA, Bruce S, et al. Cetirizine and astemizole therapy for chronic idiopathic urticaria: A double-blind, placebo-controlled comparative trial. *J Am Acad Dermatol*. 1995;33(2, pt 1):192-198.
21. Ring J, Hein R, Gauger A, et al. Once-daily desloratadine improves the signs and symptoms of chronic idiopathic urticaria: a randomized, double-blind, placebo-controlled study. *Int J Dermatol*. 2001;40(1):72-76.
22. Leynadier F, Duarte-Risselin C, Murrieta M. Comparative therapeutic effect and safety of mizolastine and loratadine in chronic idiopathic urticaria: URTILOR

22. study group. *Eur J Dermatol.* 2000;10:205.
23. Lorette G, Giannetti A, Pereira RS, et al. One-year treatment of chronic urticaria with mizolastine: Efficacy and safety. URTOL study group. *J Eur Acad Dermatol Venereol.* 2000;14(2):83-90.
24. Camarasa JM, Aliaga A, Fernández-Vozmediano JM, et al. Azelastine tablets in the treatment of chronic idiopathic urticaria. Phase III, randomised, double-blind, placebo and active controlled multicentric clinical trial. *Skin Pharmacol Appl Skin Physiol.* 2001;14(2):77-86.
25. LaRosa M, Leonardi S, Marchese G, et al. Double-blind multicenter study on the efficacy and tolerability of cetirizine compared to oxatomide in chronic idiopathic urticaria in preschool children. *Ann Allergy Asthma Immunol.* 2001;87(1):48-53.
26. Breneman DL. Cetirizine versus hydroxyzine and placebo in chronic idiopathic urticaria. *Ann Pharmacother.* 1996;30:1075.
27. Potter PC, Kapp A, Maurer M, et al. Comparison of the efficacy of levocetirizine 5 mg and desloratadine 5 mg in chronic idiopathic urticaria patients. *Allergy.* 2009;64(4):596-604.
28. Handa S, Dogra S, Kumar B. Comparative efficacy of cetirizine and fexofenadine in the treatment of chronic idiopathic urticaria. *J Dermatolog Treat.* 2004;15(1):55-57.
29. Garg G, Thami GP. Comparative efficacy of cetirizine and levocetirizine in chronic idiopathic urticaria. *J Dermatolog Treat.* 2007;18:23.
30. Diepgen TL; Early Treatment of the Atopic Child Study Group. Long-term treatment with cetirizine of infants with atopic dermatitis: a multi-country, double-blind, randomized, placebo-controlled trial (the ETAC trial) over 18 months. *Pediatr Allergy Immunol.* 2002;13(4):278-286.
31. Klein PA, Clark RA. An evidence-based review of the efficacy of antihistamines in relieving pruritus in atopic dermatitis. *Arch Dermatol.* 1999;135(12):1522-1555.
32. Tefferi A, Pardanani A. Clinical, genetic, and therapeutic insights into systemic mast cell disease. *Curr Opin Hematol.* 2004;11:58.
33. Frieri M, Alling DW, Metcalfe DD. Comparison of the therapeutic efficacy of cromolyn sodium with that of combined chlorpheniramine and cimetidine in systemic mastocytosis. Results of a double-blind clinical trial. *Am J Med.* 1985;78:9.
34. Friedman BS, Santiago ML, Berkebile C, et al. Comparison of azelastine and chlorpheniramine in the treatment of mastocytosis. *J Allergy Clin Immunol.* 1993;92(4):520-526.
35. Weller K, Ziege C, Staubach P, et al. H_1 antihistamine up dosing in chronic spontaneous urticaria: patients' perspective of effectiveness and side effects—a retrospective study. *PLoS One.* 2011;6(9):e23931.
36. Casale TB, Blaiss MS, Gelfand E, et al. First do no harm: managing antihistamine impairment in patients with allergic rhinitis. *J Allergy Clin Immunol.* 2003;111(5):S835-S842.
37. Kay GG, Berman B, Mockoviak SH, et al. Initial and steady-state effects of diphenhydramine and loratadine ion sedation, cognition, mood and psychomotor performance. *Arch Intern Med.* 1997;157:2350-2356.
38. Aaronson DW. Evaluation of cetirizine in patients with allergic rhinitis and perennial asthma. *Ann Allergy Asthma Immunol.* 1996;76:440.
39. Mansmann HC Jr, Altman RA, Berman BA, et al. Efficacy and safety of cetirizine therapy in perennial allergic rhinitis. *Ann Allergy.* 1992;68(4):348-353.
40. Tashiro M, Kato M, Miyake M, et al. Dose dependency of brain histamine H_1 receptor occupancy following oral administration of cetirizine hydrochloride measured using PET with [11C]doxepin. *Hum Psychopharmacol.* 2009;24:540-548.
41. Horak F, Stübner UP. Comparative tolerability of second generation antihistamines. *Drug Saf.* 1999;20:385.
42. Church DS, Church MK. Pharmacology of antihistamines. *World Allergy Organ J.* 2011;4:S22-S27.
43. Lauria JI, Markello R, King BD. Circulatory and respiratory effects of hydroxyzine in volunteers and geriatric patients. *Anesth Analg.* 1968;47:378.
44. Sharkouri AA, Bahan SL. Hypersensitivity to antihistamines. *Allergy Asthma Proc.* 2013;34:488-496.
45. Mann RD, Pearce GL, Dunn N, et al. Sedation with "non-sedating" antihistamines: four prescription-event monitoring studies in general practice. *BMJ.* 2000;320(7243):1184-1186.
46. Hamelin BA, Bouayad A, Drolet B, et al. In vitro characterization of cytochrome P450 2D6 inhibition by classic histamine H_1 receptor antagonists. *Drug Metab Dispos.* 1998;26(6):536-539.
47. Hamelin BA, Bouayad A, Méthot J, et al. Significant interaction between the nonprescription antihistamine diphenhydramine and the CYP2D6 substrate metoprolol in healthy men with the high or low CYP2D6 activity. *Clin Pharmacol Ther.* 2000;67(5):466-477.
48. Simons FE; Early Prevention of Asthma in Atopic Children (EPAAC) Study Group. Safety of levocetirizine treatment in young atopic children; an 18-month study. *Pediatr Allergy Immunol.* 2007;18:535-542.
49. Church MK, Maurer M, Simons FE, et al. Risk of first generation H_1 antihistamines: a GA(2)LEN position paper. *Allergy.* 2010;65(4):459-466.
50. Gilbert C, Mazzotta P, Loebstein R, et al. Fetal safety of drugs used in the treatment of allergic rhinitis: a critical review. *Drug Saf.* 2005;28(8):707-719.
51. Seto A, Einarson T, Koren G. Pregnancy outcome following first trimester exposure to antihistamines: meta-analysis. *Am J Perinatol.* 1997;14:119.
52. Pastuszak A, Schick B, D'Alimonte D, et al. The safety of astemizole in pregnancy. *J Allergy Clin Immunol.* 1996;98(4):748-750.
53. Gilboa SM, Alles EC, Rai RP, et al. Antihistamines and birth defects; a systemic review of the literature. *Expert Opin Drug Saf.* 2014;13:1667-1698.
54. Panula P, Chazot PL, Cowart M, et al. International union of basic and clinical pharmacology. XCVVIII. Histamine receptors. *Pharmacol Rev.* 2015;67:601-655.
55. Simons FE, Sussman GL, Simons KJ. Effect of the H_2-antagonist cimetidine on the pharmacokinetics and pharmacodynamics of the H_1-antagonists hydroxyzine and cetirizine in patients with chronic urticaria. *J Allergy Clin Immunol.* 1995;95:685.
56. Cimetidine, Ranitidine. In: DRUGDEX System. Greenwood Village, CO: Thomson Micromedex [updated periodically].
57. Famotidine. In: DRUGDEX System. Greenwood Village, CO: Thomson Micromedex [updated periodically].
58. Nizatidine. In: DRUGDEX System. Greenwood Village, CO: Thomson Micromedex [updated periodically].
59. Thomas RH, Browne PD, Kirby JD. The influence of

59. ranitidine, alone and in combination with clemastine, on histamine-mediated cutaneous weal and flare reactions in human skin. *Br J Clin Pharmacol.* 1985;20:377-382.
60. Bleehen SS, Thomas SE, Greaves MW, et al. Cimetidine and chlorpheniramine in the treatment of chronic idiopathic urticaria: a multi-centre randomized double-blind study. *Br J Dermatol.* 1987;117(1):81-88.
61. Leman JA, Benton EC. Verrucas. Guidelines for management. *Am J Clin Dermatol.* 2000;1:143.
62. Drayer DE, Romankiewicz J, Lorenzo B, et al. Age and renal clearance of cimetidine. *Clin Pharmacol Ther.* 1982;31(1):45-50.
63. Yamreudeewong W. Potentially significant drug interactions of class III antiarrhythmic drugs. *Drug Saf.* 2003;26:421.
64. Gafter U, Zevin D, Komlos L, et al. Thrombocytopenia associated with hypersensitivity to ranitidine: possible cross-reactivity with cimetidine. *Am J Gastroenterol.* 1989;84(5):560-562.
65. Laheij RJ, Sturkenboom MC, Hassing RJ, et al. Risk of community-acquired pneumonia and use of gastric acid-suppressive drugs. *JAMA.* 2004;292(16):1955-1960.
66. Tullio CJ, Roberts MA. Cimetidine-induced alopecia. *Clin Pharm.* 1985;4:145.
67. Nault MA, Milne B, Parlow JL. Effects of the selective H_1 and H_2 histamine receptor antagonists loratadine and ranitidine on autonomic control of the heart. *Anesthesiology.* 2002;96:336.
68. Penston J, Wormsley KG. Adverse reactions and interactions with H_2 receptor antagonists. *Med Toxicol.* 1986;3:192-216.
69. Jensen RT, Collen MJ, Pandol SJ, et al. Cimetidine-induced impotence and breast changes in patients with gastric hypersecretory states. *N Engl J Med.* 1983;308(15):883-887.
70. Guillet R, Stoll BJ, Cotten CM, et al. Association of H_2-blocker therapy and higher incidence of necrotizing enterocolitis in very low birth weight infants. *Pediatrics.* 2006;117(2):e137-e142.
71. Richelson E. Tricyclic antidepressants and histamine H_1 receptors. *Mayo Clin Proc.* 1979;54:669-674.
72. Greene SL, Reed CE, Schroeter AL. Double-blind crossover study comparing doxepin with diphenhydramine for the treatment of chronic urticaria. *J Am Acad Dermatol.* 1985;12:669.
73. Drake LA, Fallon JD, Sober A. Relief of pruritus in patients with atopic dermatitis after treatment with topical doxepin cream. The Doxepin Study Group. *J Am Acad Dermatol.* 1994;31:613.
74. Doxepin. In: DRUGDEX System. Greenwood Village, CO: Thomson Micromedex [updated periodically].
75. Veith RC, Raskind MA, Caldwell JH, et al. Cardiovascular effects of tricyclic antidepressants in depressed patients with chronic heart disease. *N Engl J Med.* 1982;306:954-59.
76. Egan C, Rallis TM. Treatment of chronic urticaria with ketotifen. *Arch Dermatol.* 1997;133:147.
77. Phanuphak P. Double-blind, placebo-controlled study of ketotifen in chronic urticaria. *Immunol Allerg Pract.* 1987;9:138.
78. Mansfield LE, Taistra P, Santamauro J, et al. Inhibition of dermographia, histamine, and dextromethorphan skin tests by ketotifen. A possible effect on cutaneous vascular response to mediators. *Ann Allergy.* 1989;63(3):201-206.
79. Kamide R, Niimura M, Ueda H, et al. Clinical evaluation of ketotifen for chronic urticaria: Multicenter double-blind comparative study with clemastine. *Ann Allergy.* 1989;62(4):322-325.
80. Ketotifen. In: DRUGDEX System. Greenwood Village, CO: Thomson Micromedex [updated periodically].
81. Simons FE, Simons KJ. Clinical pharmacology of H_1-antihistamines. In: Simons FE, ed. *Histamine and H_1-Antihistamines in Allergic Disease.* 2nd ed. New York, NY: Marcel Dekker; 2002:141.
82. Lessard E, Yessine MA, Hamelin BA, et al. Diphenhydramine alters the disposition of venlafaxine through inhibition of CYP2D6 activity in humans. *J Clin Psychopharmacol.* 2001;21(2):175-184.

Chapter 190 :: Cytotoxic and Antimetabolic Agents :: Jeremy S. Honaker & Neil J. Korman

第一百九十章
细胞毒性和抗代谢药

中文导读

细胞毒性和抗代谢药物用于治疗严重或难治性皮肤病，因这些药物的毒性显著，必须与它们的治疗优势相平衡。在治疗皮肤病时，这些药物大多以较低的免疫调节剂量而不是较高的细胞毒性剂量使用，通过抑制细胞生长发育来调节炎症细胞和其他细胞的行为，特定的细胞毒性药物可能在细胞周期的不同阶段有效。皮肤科常用的细胞毒性药物分为抗代谢药和烷基化剂。抗代谢药模仿自然分子，在DNA合成（S相）时最活跃。烷基化剂通过与DNA的物理化学相互作用发挥作用，通常与细胞周期无关。本章将该类药物分为3组：抗增殖、细胞毒性和免疫抑制/抗感染，分别介绍了其相关内容。

首先介绍了抗增殖的细胞毒性和抗代谢药物，重点介绍了甲氨蝶呤和羟基脲的作用机制、药代动力学、给药方案、启动治疗、监护疗法、风险及防范措施、不良反应及药物相互作用等。

接下来介绍了免疫抑制剂/抗感染药，重点介绍了硫唑嘌呤、硫鸟嘌呤的霉酚酸和霉酚酸酯的作用机制、药代动力学、给药方案、启动治疗、监护疗法、风险及防范措施、不良反应及药物相互作用，同时简单提及了霉酚酸和霉酚酸酯、环孢霉素、他克莫司和沙利度胺的作用机制和临床应用。

最后介绍了细胞毒性药物，主要介绍了环磷酰胺、氯霉素、氯霉素、蒽环类药物的作用机制、药代动力学、给药方案、启动治疗、监护疗法、风险及防范措施、不良反应及药物相互作用。

〔粟 娟〕

AT-A-GLANCE

- Cytotoxic and antimetabolic agents are used in dermatology to treat serious, life-threatening, and recalcitrant disease.
- Methotrexate and azathioprine are commonly used in dermatology whereas thioguanine, hydroxyurea, cyclophosphamide, chlorambucil, and liposomal doxorubicin are occasionally used.
- Methotrexate is U.S. Food and Drug Administration (FDA) approved for treatment of psoriasis and advanced mycosis fungoides, whereas cyclophosphamide is FDA approved for advanced mycosis fungoides only, and liposomal doxorubicin is approved for AIDS-related Kaposi sarcoma; other uses of the agent in this chapter occur on an "off-label" basis.
- Cytotoxic and antimetabolic agents act through inhibition and/or interruption of the cell cycle.
- Side effects and complications with these potentially dangerous medications are numerous, and close clinical followup and laboratory evaluation is necessary.
- Cytotoxic agents used in dermatology, as well as those initiated for other purposes, may yield distinctive cutaneous eruptions and cutaneous sequelae.

Cytotoxic and antimetabolic agents may be used to treat severe or refractory skin disease. The toxicities of such agents are significant and must be balanced against their therapeutic advantages. In treating skin disease, most of these agents are utilized at the lower immunomodulatory doses rather than at the higher cytotoxic doses.

Cytotoxic and antimetabolic drugs modulate the behavior of inflammatory and other cells through inhibition of cell growth and development. The cell cycle represents a conceptual schema for the sequence of growth experienced by essentially all cells (Chap. 5). Specific cytotoxic drugs may be effective at different stages of the cell cycle.

The cytotoxic drugs commonly used in dermatology fall into 2 classes: (1) antimetabolites and (2) alkylating agents. Antimetabolites mimic natural molecules and are most active while DNA is being synthesized (S phase). Alkylating agents exert effect through physicochemical interactions with DNA, such as alkylation, crosslinking, and carbamylation. The effects of alkylating agents are generally independent of the cell cycle.

The immunosuppressive properties of cytotoxic agents (see also Chap. 192) provide benefit in immunologically mediated disease, yet these agents may predispose to infection as well. Potentially lethal infections may arise quickly in an immunosuppressed patient. Those placed on cytotoxic agents should be queried at each visit for symptoms of infection, such as fever, chills, sweating, shortness of breath, cough, headache, dysuria, and arthritis. Prompt reporting of symptoms should be encouraged.

We have organized these medications into 3 groups, Antiproliferative, Cytotoxic, and Immunosuppressive/antiinflammatory.

ANTIPROLIFERATIVE AGENTS

METHOTREXATE

Methotrexate (MTX) is one of the most frequently employed antimetabolic agents in dermatology. An impressive record of safety with MTX has accumulated, though patient selection and monitoring is crucial for its safe use.

Discovered in 1948, MTX was initially used as a chemotherapeutic agent to treat hematologic malignancies. In dermatology, low doses of MTX are given for the treatment of nonneoplastic diseases including psoriasis, psoriatic arthritis, and dermatomyositis. It also has been used for the treatment of a wide variety of cutaneous disease (Table 190-1), including sarcoidosis, lymphomatoid papulosis, and pyoderma gangrenosum, among others.

In the treatment of psoriasis and psoriatic arthritis, MTX is considered the "gold standard" for the treatment of severe psoriasis and psoriatic arthritis. Based on a meta-analysis of several studies of psoriasis patients treated with MTX, approximately 45% of patients reach a 75% improvement in their Psoriasis Area and Severity Index (PASI) score.[1] Furthermore, the combination of MTX with biologics in the

---

TABLE 190-1

Uses for Methotrexate in Dermatology

- U.S. Food and Drug Administration–approved indications
  - Severe psoriasis (± psoriatic arthritis)
  - Mycosis fungoides
- "Off-label" uses
  - Dermatomyositis
  - Cutaneous lupus erythematosus
  - Scleroderma
  - Pemphigus vulgaris
  - Bullous pemphigoid
  - Mucous membrane pemphigoid
  - Cutaneous polyarteritis nodosa
  - Behçet disease
  - Pyoderma gangrenosum
  - CD30+ lymphoproliferative disease lymphomatoid papulosis; anaplastic large cell lymphoma
  - Pityriasis lichenoides et varioliformis acuta
  - Pityriasis rubra pilaris
  - Sarcoidosis
  - Alopecia areata
  - Atopic dermatitis
  - Lichen planus

treatment of psoriasis has improved efficacy compared to either drug alone.[2]

MECHANISM OF ACTION

MTX is a synthetic analog of folate that competitively and irreversibly inhibits dihydrofolate reductase, thereby inhibiting folic acid metabolism and acting as an immunosuppressant/antiinflammatory medication (Fig. 190-1). MTX also partially inhibits thymidylate synthetase. Inhibition of these enzymes reduces availability of purine nucleotides and thymidylate, required for RNA and DNA synthesis. Of note, it was recently discovered that MTX also can inhibit DNA methylation via decreasing cellular levels of S-adenyl methionine.[3]

All folate antagonists (eg, trimethoprim-sulfamethoxazole) share the same basic properties as MTX and concomitant use may potentiate the toxicity of MTX (see section "Drug Interactions").

PHARMACOKINETICS

Oral MTX is absorbed rapidly through the GI tract. In children, absorption is decreased by concurrent ingestion of food and milk, but this has not been observed in adults. In adults, the mean bioavailability is 67% of the administered dose. Peak plasma levels occur 1 to 3 hours after administration and remain greater than 0.1 μM, the level at which inhibition of protein synthesis ends, for about 6 hours. The half-life of the drug is 4 to 5 hours. For doses higher than 20 mg/wk, GI absorption is more erratic, and subcutaneous (SC) dosing is recommended.[4] A head-to-head, randomized, crossover study of oral versus SC MTX in 47 patients with rheumatoid arthritis revealed that SC administration had a 14% to 40% higher bioavailability than oral MTX, with a linear dose-proportional increase up to 25 mg/wk.[5] Therefore, patients treated with MTX may have improved efficacy with SC MTX, in comparison to oral MTX, due to improved bioavailability.

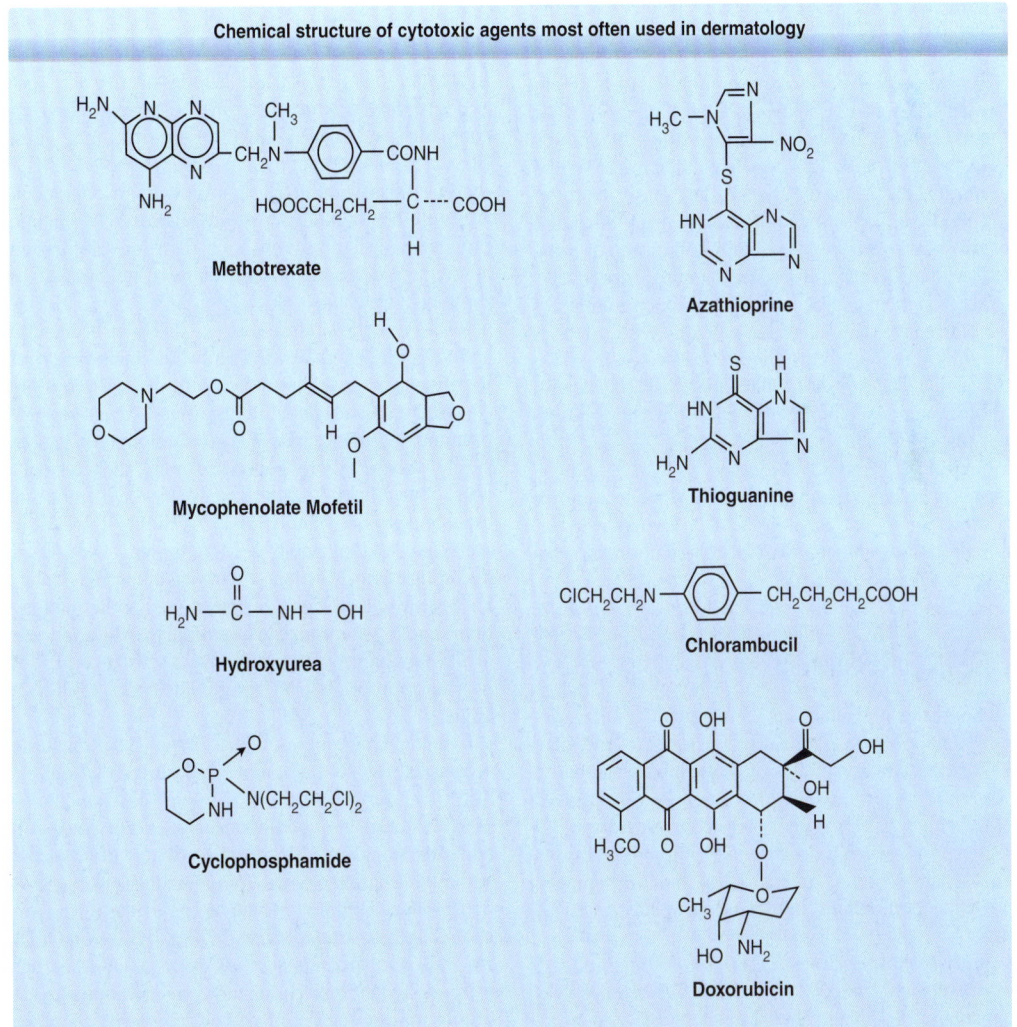

Figure 190-1 Chemical structure of cytotoxic agents most often used in dermatology.

Methotrexate is eliminated chiefly by the kidneys, with 60% to 95% excreted unchanged. Decreases in glomerular filtration or tubular secretion may lead to MTX toxicity. Approximately 50% of MTX within the blood is protein bound. Weak organic acids, such as aspirin or many other nonsteroidal antiinflammatory agents, may displace MTX, altering blood levels and renal excretion (see section "Drug Interactions").

INDICATIONS

Methotrexate may be used for several diseases in dermatology (Table 190-1), but its chief indication is for treatment of severe psoriasis and psoriatic arthritis. The effects of MTX in psoriasis were first recognized in the late 1950s and 1960s,[6] and in 1972, MTX was approved by the U.S. Food and Drug Administration (FDA) for psoriasis at the same time the initial psoriasis guidelines were published. The listed indication was for the treatment of severe, recalcitrant, disabling psoriasis.[7] By the later 1980s, more than one-half of dermatologists reported using MTX to treat severe psoriasis.[8] MTX has been used to treat all of the psoriasis subtypes, including plaque, guttate, pustular, and erythrodermic forms of the disease.

The impact of an increasing number of systemic treatments for psoriasis (the "biologics"; Chap. 193) on the use of MTX has not been fully studied, although MTX is significantly less expensive than the biologics, even after including the costs of laboratory monitoring and liver biopsies.[9] Unfortunately many insurance companies require an inadequate response to or intolerance to MTX as a prerequisite to biologic approval.

Many patients with lymphomatoid papulosis are treated with MTX.[10] Fewer patients with mycosis fungoides/Sezary syndrome are treated with MTX, but higher doses of MTX have been associated with improvements in all primary CD30+ lymphoproliferative disorders.[11]

Topical MTX is available; its successful use has been reported in stage IA or IB mycosis fungoides and in lymphomatoid papulosis (1% MTX compounded in a hydrophilic gel containing laurocapram to enhance percutaneous absorption).[12]

DOSING REGIMEN

Methotrexate is available in 2.5-mg tablets. Subcutaneous solution (25 mg/mL) is less expensive, and may have better efficacy and less adverse effects compared with the oral form. Although a single weekly dose of MTX is the typical regimen used, some prefer the older regimen of a weekly dose divided into 3 equal parts and separated by 12 hours. These dosing regimens are equally efficacious, but split dosing may lessen GI upset.

Typical oncologic doses of MTX (100-250 mg/m^2/wk) are cytotoxic; however, lower doses (7.5-25.0 mg/wk) are immunomodulatory. In dermatology, MTX doses are typically less than 30 mg/wk; most psoriasis patients are controlled and tolerate 15 mg/wk. For CTCL, MTX is usually administered at a dose of 10 to 25 mg per week, although higher doses have been used.[11] Lymphomatoid papulosis is sensitive to MTX and may respond well to weekly doses as low as 5 mg.[10] Higher doses (60-240 mg^2/m^2 IV) of MTX, given with folinic acid (leucovorin) to minimize damage to normal tissues, have been used to treat advanced mycosis fungoides.[11]

Despite its longstanding use in CTCL patients, relatively few clinical studies of MTX have been published. The response of patients with mycosis fungoides to low-dose MTX (defined commonly as <100 mg/wk but often limited to <30 mg/wk) ranges from "definite improvement" in 9 of 16 patients to an overall response in 17 of 29 patients with erythrodermic MF and 20 of 60 with plaque MF (median dose of 25 mg/wk).[13]

Cumulative dose should be tracked and recorded, as this may impact monitoring (particularly liver function) with continued use (see section "Monitoring Therapy").

INITIATING THERAPY

Evaluation before MTX use includes a careful history and physical examination, and assessment of concomitant conditions or medications that may limit MTX use. Exclusion of patients inappropriate for MTX therapy is an important first step in management. Absolute contraindications to the use of MTX include pregnancy, lactation, and bone marrow suppression as evidenced by significant anemia, leukopenia, or thrombocytopenia.

Relative contraindications to MTX use include abnormalities in renal or liver function (including viral hepatitis), cirrhosis, excessive alcohol consumption, concomitant use of hepatotoxic drugs, active infection, immunosuppression, recent vaccination with a live vaccine, obesity (body mass index >30), diabetes mellitus, poor reliability, and an active desire to conceive (men and women) (Table 190-2).[7] Although the elderly are often less amenable to MTX therapy because of declining renal function, elderly patients may tolerate MTX at lower doses, and titration of the medication should be approached cautiously. Although use of MTX is typically avoided in the setting of HIV, it may be appropriate in select circumstances; caution is advised.[14]

Baseline laboratory studies (Table 190-3) include a complete blood cell count with differential (CBC/diff), liver function testing, serologic assessment for hepatitis B and C antibodies, renal function assessment, and pregnancy and HIV screening (where indicated).[14] Although a baseline screen for tuberculosis using purified protein derivative (PPD) or one of the interferon gamma release assays (such as QuantiFERON GOLD) is not expressly mandated, the Centers of Disease Control and Prevention recommends consideration of such testing for any patient placed on long-term immunosuppressive medication.[15]

TABLE 190-2
Risks and Precautions With Methotrexate Use

- Absolute contraindications
  - Pregnancy (category X)
  - Lactation
  - Significant anemia, leukopenia, or thrombocytopenia
- Relative contraindications
  - Renal dysfunction (dose may be reduced)
  - Hematologic disease (dose may be reduced)
  - Hepatic disease or hepatic dysfunction
  - Unreliable patient
  - Excessive alcohol consumption
  - Diabetes mellitus and/or obesity
  - Active infection and/or potential reactivation of infection (tuberculosis)
  - HIV infection
  - Man or woman contemplating impending conception
- Common adverse effects
  - GI distress (minimized with folate supplementation)
  - Myelosuppression (acute)
  - Toxic hepatitis
  - Liver fibrosis/cirrhosis (chronic)

Initiation of MTX therapy in a psoriasis patient typically involves use of a single 2.5- to 5-mg test dose, which is particularly important in patients with declining renal function or other risk factors for hematologic toxicity.[16] Repeat laboratory studies, a skin examination, and a review of systems are conducted 1 week later. Performance of repeat laboratory studies sooner than 5 to 6 days after dosing yields only expected elevated liver transaminases and may confound interpretation.

If the test dose is tolerated and laboratory studies are unremarkable, weekly therapy may commence using a typical starting dose of 5 to 15 mg/wk, depending on the severity of disease, overall health, and ideal body weight of the patient. The dose may be increased by 2.5 to 5.0 mg every 4 to 8 weeks until adequate control is achieved or toxicity ensues up to a dose of 25 mg per week as a maximum (management of toxicity discussed below).[7] When improvement has stabilized, the dose may be tapered in 2.5-mg decrements to a point at which disease activity is stable. For those patients in whom the plan is to treat with long-term MTX, the goal is to allow for mild- or low-grade psoriasis to minimize the cumulative dose. It is important to discuss this expectation with the patient. Concomitant topical therapy may also lower the MTX dose needed for satisfactory control.

If a patient does not demonstrate satisfactory improvement on a dose of 20 to 25 mg/wk, consideration of alternative agents is indicated. Some patients with refractory disease may respond better to SC MTX. In psoriasis, MTX can be combined with ultraviolet B (UVB) phototherapy, or biologics to enhance efficacy.[7]

MONITORING THERAPY

It can take 4 to 8 weeks to see a response to changes in MTX dosage.[7] Ongoing laboratory evaluation during MTX therapy (Table 190-3) should include a CBC with differential and liver function tests weekly for 2 to 4 weeks for the first few months, then every 1 to 3 months.[7] It is recommended to repeat testing with any decreased oral intake, dose escalation or intercurrent illness. Liver function testing should not be performed earlier than 5 days after dosing to avoid confounded results. Renal function tests should be performed every 1 to 2 months,[7] or with any suspicion of altered renal function.

For patients without risk factors for liver injury (Table 190-2), current recommendations suggest consideration of liver biopsy after 3.5 to 4 g total cumulative dosage. However, for patients with risk factors for MTX-induced liver injury, a delayed baseline liver biopsy should be considered (after 2-6 months of use, when it is apparent the medication is efficacious, well tolerated, and likely to be continued), and again at a cumulative dose of 1.0 to 1.5 g.

The gold standard for assessing MTX-induced liver fibrosis is percutaneous needle biopsy. The procedure is not without risk; minor bleeding occurs in 1 in 1000 patients, and the risk of death is estimated at 1 in 10,000.[17] Liver specimens are assessed for lobular architecture, inflammation and fibrosis, and fat infiltration and graded using a scale of I to IV (Table 190-4). Patients with grades I and II histology may continue MTX, those with grade IIIA histology may continue with a repeat liver biopsy in 6 months, and those with grades IIIB and IV histology (moderate to severe fibrosis or cirrhosis) should discontinue MTX.[7]

Noninvasive serum biomarkers, including procollagen (PIIINP) and FibroTest/FibroSURE, and ultrasound diagnostics have been used to evaluate liver fibrosis as an alternative to liver biopsy. Measurement of the amino terminal peptide of procollagen III (PIIINP) is popular in some European countries, but the test is not approved in the United States.[7] Serum

TABLE 190-3
Laboratory Monitoring for Methotrexate[a]

CBC, platelets	7-14 d after drug initiation, then every 2-4 wk for the first few months, then every 1-3 mo, depending on leukocyte count and patient stability
Renal function studies	Serum BUN and Cr levels at 1- to 2-mo intervals: GFR for patients at risk for decreased renal function
Liver chemistries: AST, ALT alkaline phosphatase, serum albumin	Every 4-8 wk (more frequent liver chemistry monitoring in lieu of an initial liver biopsy for patients with hepatic risk factors)
Pregnancy test	Women of childbearing potential

[a]More frequent monitoring may be required under certain circumstances such as dosage changes or if there are concomitant medications.
Adapted from Kalb RE, Strober B, Weinstein G, et al. Methotrexate and psoriasis: 2009 National Psoriasis Foundation Consensus Conference. J Am Acad Dermatol. 2009;60(5):824-837.

TABLE 190-4
Guidelines for MTX Therapy Based on Roenigk Scale for Histopathologic Evaluation for Liver Biopsy Findings

Roenigk Scale for Histopathologic Evaluation of liver biopsy findings	Guidelines for MTX therapy
Grade 1: Normal; fatty infiltration, mild; nuclear variability, mild; portal inflammation, mild	Continue MTX
Grade 2: Fatty infiltration, moderate to severe; nuclear variability, moderate to severe; portal tract expansion, portal tract inflammation and necrosis, moderate to severe	Continue MTX
Grade IIIA: Fibrosis, mild (portal fibrosis here denotes formation of fibrotic septa extending into the lobules; slight enlargement of portal tracts without disruption of limiting plates or septum formation does not classify the biopsy as grade III)	Continue MTX Repeat biopsy after approximately 6 mo of MTX therapy Consider alternate prescription
Grade IIIB: Fibrosis, moderate to severe	Stop MTX. Exceptional circumstances may require continued MTX with thorough followup liver biopsies.
Grade IV: Cirrhosis (regenerating nodules as well as bridging of portal tracts must be demonstrated)	Stop MTX. Exceptional circumstances, however, may require continued MTX therapy with thorough followup liver biopsies

Adapted from Kalb RE, Strober B, Weinstein G, Lebwohl M. Methotrexate and psoriasis: 2009 National Psoriasis Foundation Consensus Conference. *J Am Acad Dermatol.* 2009;60(5):824-837, with permission. Copyright © American Academy of Dermatology.

assay of the PIIINP may suggest fibrosis; however, specificity is limited. PIIINP is a marker of fibrogenesis, and it may be elevated in any organ system PIIINP as it is a marker of fibrogenesis.[18-21] It is unreliable in patients with psoriatic arthritis. The FibroTest, also known as FibroSURE in the United States, uses a patented validated artificial intelligence algorithm of indirect serum markers for fibrosis that is corrected for age and sex. The 5 serum markers used in the FibroSURE test are γ-glutamyltranspeptidase, total bilirubin, haptoglobin, apolipoprotein A-I, and $α_2$-macroglobulin. The composite FibroSURE score ranges from 0-1 with higher scores associated with higher levels of liver fibrosis.[22] A systemic review of studies evaluating the use of FibroTest in hepatitis C–related fibrosis revealed a specificity and sensitivity of 90% and 47%, respectively.[23]

In addition to serum markers, ultrasonography of the liver has been used to monitor hepatotoxicity without any helpful results.[24,25] However, transient elastography (TE), which is measured by using pulse-echo ultrasonography of the liver, is capable of one-dimensional evaluation of liver fibrosis by measuring the propagation and velocity of the wave in the liver. A meta-analysis of 9 TE studies for the detection of liver fibrosis in hepatitis C patients identified a sensitivity of 87% and specificity of 91%.[26] Although a few small studies comparing TE to liver biopsy have been conducted in psoriasis patients treated with MTX,[22,27,28] the consensus finding is that TE, when used in conjunction with other biomarkers (FibroSURE, PIIINP), may be helpful in monitoring for liver toxicity, and therefore reduce unnecessary liver biopsies. However, at present, percutaneous liver biopsy remains the gold standard for evaluation when MTX-induced liver disease is suspected.[29,30]

RISKS AND PRECAUTIONS

Absolute and relative contraindications and common adverse effects of MTX are summarized in Table 190-2.

COMPLICATIONS

Adverse reactions to MTX can range from the trivial to life threatening.[1]

Hematologic Effects: The most important acute adverse effect of MTX is myelosuppression. Neutropenia with life-threatening bone marrow toxicity can occur. Leukocyte and platelet counts are decreased maximally approximately 7 to 10 days after treatment. Risk factors for bone marrow toxicity include advanced age, poor renal function, hypoalbuminemia, lack of folate supplementation, and concurrent administration of conflicting medications (see section "Drug Interactions"). Blood counts should be monitored after changes in therapy, especially in patients with impaired renal function (eg, the elderly). Trimethoprim-sulfamethoxazole and other folate antagonists should be avoided entirely as they compete with MTX for renal tubular secretion and when coadministered with MTX are commonly associated with severe toxicity.

GI Effects: Nausea and vomiting with oral administration is common (10%-30% of all patients) and dose-related. Such effects may be seen with parenteral dosing as well. Symptoms may even occur before dosing or 24 to 36 hours afterward, suggesting a psychosomatic or anticipatory basis in select cases. Supplementation with folate (1-5 mg/d) reduces GI symptoms without compromising efficacy.[31-34] A study on folate supplementation (5 mg daily) suggested a slight decrease in MTX efficacy,[35] but others questioned the methodology,[16] and most authorities continue to advocate strongly for supplementation.[7]

Hepatic Effects: MTX is hepatotoxic, and induction of liver fibrosis is a major concern with long-term MTX use. The drug should be avoided in patients with liver disease and active alcoholics. Some elevation in liver transaminases is expected with use; these occur near the time of drug administration. Therefore, monitoring labs should be performed at least 5 to 6 days after the last dose. These elevations are not strictly predictive of those predisposed to fibrosis. Dose reduction is indicated if transaminases exceed 2- to 3-fold normal values and discontinuance is indicated if transaminases exceed 5-fold normal values when measured at least 5 to 6 days after the last dose. It is recommended to withhold MTX for 1 to 2 weeks and then repeating liver function tests before reintroducing the drug. Indications for liver biopsy are described before ("Monitoring therapy").

Mucosal and Cutaneous Effects: Oral ulcerations or stomatitis may occur with MTX use. Skin ulceration, particularly of the lower legs, may herald bone marrow suppression. In patients treated with MTX for psoriasis, rapid ulceration of psoriatic plaques may also suggest toxicity.[36] Laboratory studies and dose reduction or complete discontinuance is indicated when mucocutaneous ulcerations or skin ulcerations develop, respectively. Methotrexate may also engender a cutaneous "recall reaction" in areas of prior irradiation or recent sunburn.[25] In patients with coexistent renal failure, MTX excretion is reduced and can lead to prolonged blood and skin levels of MTX. Mild alopecia may uncommonly occur with MTX use. "Methotrexate-induced rheumatoid papular eruption" occurs in patients with rheumatoid arthritis and presents with erythematous indurated papules usually on the proximal extremities that develop shortly after MTX administration and resolve upon MTX discontinuation.[37] Other cutaneous manifestations include acral erythema, epidermal necrosis, and vasculitis.

Carcinogenicity: It is not clear that MTX increases the risk for malignancy or lymphoproliferative disease. One study showed that MTX was associated with a small increased risk of nonmelanoma skin cancers in rheumatoid arthritis and psoriatic arthritis patients.[38] Another study of patients taking MTX for rheumatoid arthritis demonstrated a 50% increased risk of malignancy relative to the general population, with a 3-fold increased risk in melanoma, a 5-fold increased risk in non-Hodgkin lymphoma, and a nearly 3-fold increase in lung cancer.[39] Conversely, another study revealed a slight increase in lymphoma among psoriatic patients, but use of MTX was not discriminatory.[40] A systematic review of 88 studies revealed there was insufficient evidence to fully evaluate the risk of lymphoma and malignancies, but there was no strong evidence of increased risk identified.[41] Furthermore, a nested case control of 5,757 rheumatoid arthritis patients treated with MTX found that high disease activity, but not MTX dose, was a risk factor for lymphoproliferative disorders.[42]

Mutagenicity and Teratogenicity: MTX is a category X agent during pregnancy and administration is absolutely contraindicated (Table 190-2). Reliable contraception is requisite while taking MTX.[7] Pregnancies that occur after the discontinuation of MTX appear unaffected, but it is generally advocated that men wait 3 months after discontinuance before attempting conception and women wait 1 complete menstrual cycle.[7]

Pulmonary Effects: Acute pneumonitis and pulmonary fibrosis have been reported with MTX use in psoriasis, although such reactions are more common in rheumatoid arthritis patients.[43] Pulmonary toxicity likely represents an idiosyncratic reaction. MTX-induced lung injury can be sudden and severe with a 17% mortality rate.[44] However, the process is usually subacute and presents as a new onset of cough and shortness of breath. A meta-analysis demonstrated that MTX was not associated with an increased risk of adverse respiratory events, respiratory infections, or noninfectious respiratory events in those with psoriasis, psoriatic arthritis, and inflammatory bowel disease.[45] The strongest predictors of lung injury are older age, diabetes, rheumatoid pleuropulmonary involvement, hypoalbuminemia, and previous use of disease-modifying antirheumatic drugs (DMARDs). A chest radiograph should be performed in those with symptoms of pneumonitis. Discontinuance is recommended if examination findings are concerning. Pulmonary function testing is not helpful in screening for the detection or prevention of pulmonary toxicity.[46]

Opportunistic Infections: Opportunistic infections (eg, *Pneumocystis* pneumonia, cryptococcosis, and histoplasmosis) have been reported in otherwise healthy individuals receiving low-dose MTX.[47-51] However, affected patients were often being concurrently treated with other immunosuppressive medications as well, with prednisone being the most common agent.

Anaphylaxis: Systemic anaphylaxis with low-dose MTX has been reported.[52] Many patients with anaphylaxis had received MTX before, at comparable doses, without untoward effects.

Folate and Folinic Acid Supplementation: Daily supplementation with 1 to 5 mg of folate has reduced adverse effects and toxicities without compromising the efficacy of MTX.[28,31] Nausea, vomiting, diarrhea, alopecia, stomatitis and oral ulceration, elevated transaminases, and mild myelosuppression may be prevented. Folic acid supplementation ranges from 1 to 5 mg daily or skipped on the day MTX is taken.[53] Elevated homocysteine levels—common with MTX use and an independent risk factor for coronary artery disease—are decreased with folate supplementation.[54] Pneumonitis and moderate to severe myelosuppression are not mitigated by folate supplementation.

Folinic acid (leucovorin) also may be used if folic acid does not sufficiently control MTX toxicities. Folinic acid should be given at least 24 hours after the dose of weekly MTX, because unlike folate, it competes with MTX for cellular uptake. Folinic acid is prescribed as 5 mg by mouth every 12 hours for 3 doses.[55]

One theoretical risk that may occur with folate supplementation is the potential masking of vitamin B_{12} deficiency (macrocytosis). Progressively increasing mean corpuscular volume is common in patients on MTX and signals the onset of macrocytic anemia.

Overdose: MTX overdose should be treated promptly (within 24-36 hours after overdose) with folinic acid (leucovorin). Folinic acid is metabolized in vivo to tetrahydrofolate in the absence of dihydrofolate reductase, providing an alternative supply of

DNA and RNA precursors.

Folinic acid should be given early, preferably within the first 24 to 36 hours after overdose. Folinic acid itself has very little toxicity. An oral dose of 10 mg/m², or 15 to 25 mg every 6 hours for 6 to 10 doses should be given on first suspicion of MTX overdose without delay for a serum assay.[7] If serum assay is available, oral or parenteral doses may be continued every 6 hours until the serum concentration of MTX falls to less than 10^{-8} M.

Drug Interactions: Although any drug that may enhance MTX toxicity should be avoided during therapy, there are several near-absolute contraindications (Table 190-5), including aspirin, many nonsteroidal antiinflammatory agents, probenecid, and trimethoprim-sulfamethoxazole.[56] Conversely, many cyclooxygenase-2 selective inhibitors, such as celecoxib, do not impact the pharmacokinetics of MTX.[7] Patients with psoriatic arthritis can be safely treated with ketoprofen, flurbiprofen, and piroxicam. In addition, patients receiving warfarin should have plasma prothrombin times monitored.

HYDROXYUREA

Hydroxyurea is an antiproliferative medication. Hydroxyurea was first synthesized in 1869 and has been used to treat hematologic malignancies, sickle cell anemia, and psoriasis among others.

MECHANISM OF ACTION

Hydroxyurea impairs DNA synthesis through inhibition of ribonucleotide diphosphate reductase, an enzyme that reduces nucleotides to deoxynucleotides. This inhibition limits the supply of DNA bases available for synthesis; strand breakage and cell death result. Hydroxyurea also prevents cells from repairing damage from UV or ionizing radiation, acting as a radiosensitizer. Finally, hydroxyurea yields hypomethylation of genes, altering expression,[57] and this may contribute to normalization of psoriatic skin through improved keratinocyte differentiation. Hydroxyurea is most active in cells with a high proliferative index. It is preferentially concentrated within leukocytes.

PHARMACOKINETICS

Hydroxyurea is a small molecule that is well absorbed after oral administration. Serum levels peak within 2 hours of dosing. Hydroxyurea has a rapid onset of action, with tissue effects noted within 5 hours. The metabolism of hydroxyurea is incompletely understood, but at least 80% is excreted by the kidney. With 24 hours of dosing, negligible amounts of hydroxyurea remain in the body.

INDICATIONS

In dermatology, hydroxyurea has been used chiefly for the treatment of psoriasis (Table 190-6) but also has been used as an adjuvant treatment in metastatic melanoma and in the treatment of erythromelalgia. Although there are no randomized clinical trials on hydroxyurea's use in psoriasis, studies suggest it has a beneficial effect. Efficacy has been demonstrated in plaque, pustular, and erythrodermic forms.

In 2 large series of 60 and 85 patients treated with hydroxyurea for severe psoriasis, 50% to 60% achieved a response.[58] One study compared use of MTX (15-20 mg/wk) and lower dose hydroxyurea (3-4.5 g/wk) and found a 77% reduction versus a 49% reduction in the PASI score, respectively.[59] In another nonrandomized study of 31 patients with recalcitrant psoriasis, 75% of patients treated with 1 to 1.5 g/d of hydroxyurea showed at least a 35% reduction in PASI score and 55% had a more than 70% reduction in PASI.[60] When hydroxyurea is effective, a response generally occurs within 2 to 3 weeks, with maximal improvement at 6 to 8 weeks. Because hydroxyurea has relatively little hepatotoxicity, it may be a viable alternative for those with liver disease, which precludes use of MTX.

TABLE 190-5
Drug Interactions of Methotrexate

- Aspirins[a]
- Nonsteroidal antiinflammatory agents[a]
- Probenecid[a]
- Trimethoprim-sulfamethoxazole
- Sulfonamides
- Penicillins
- Minocycline
- Ciprofloxacin
- Thiazide diuretics
- Furosemide
- Phenytoin
- Sulfonylureas
- Barbiturates
- Phenytoin
- Dipyridamole
- Ethanol
- Trimethoprim-sulfamethoxazole[a]

[a]Near absolute contraindications.

TABLE 190-6
Uses for Hydroxyurea in Dermatology

- U.S. Food and Drug Administration–approved indications
  - Squamous cell carcinoma of the head and neck (rare use)
  - Metastatic melanoma and GI melanoma (rare use)
- "Off-label" uses
  - Severe psoriasis (often an option for those with liver disease that limits other options)
  - Pyoderma gangrenosum
  - Sweet syndrome
  - Cryoglobulinemia
  - Scleromyxedema
  - Hypereosinophilic syndrome update

DOSING REGIMEN

Hydroxyurea is available as 200-, 400-, and 500-mg tablets. Typical doses range from 1 to 2 g daily, usually as a divided dose. Doses above 2 g daily are unlikely to yield additional benefit and are increasingly toxic.[61] Hydroxyurea is usually well tolerated, but if dyspepsia occurs, it may be taken with food, milk, or antacids. There is limited data on the use of hydroxyurea in the pediatric population.

INITIATING THERAPY

Patients placed on hydroxyurea should have a complete history and physical examination. Exclusion of patients with severe comorbidities or active infections is indicated. All women of childbearing age should receive a pregnancy test. Baseline laboratory evaluation should include a CBC with differential, a serum chemistry evaluation, and urinalysis. Older patients and those with renal impairment are more susceptible to toxicity with hydroxyurea and should receive starting doses of only 500 mg/d.

MONITORING THERAPY

It is recommended that CBC with differential should be repeated weekly during the first month of therapy until stable, then monthly; this may be increased to biweekly, and, later, to monthly if results remain stable. Liver function studies and serum chemistry should be monitored monthly until stable, then every 3 to 6 months. Close surveillance for nonmelanoma skin cancer at followup visits is indicated. Discontinuance of hydroxyurea is indicated if a satisfactory response is not achieved with 8 weeks of therapy. Safety guidelines used during hydroxyurea therapy are summarized in Table 190-7.

RISKS AND PRECAUTIONS

Absolute and relative contraindications and common adverse effects of hydroxyurea are summarized in Table 190-8.

COMPLICATIONS

Approximately 18% of patients discontinued hydroxyurea because of side effects whereas 57% of patients experienced no side effects.[62] All patients on hydroxyurea develop megaloblastosis. Between 10% and 35% of patients given hydroxyurea develop anemia, whereas approximately 7% develop leukopenia, and 2% to 3% develop thrombocytopenia. Hydroxyurea should be discontinued if the hemoglobin declines by more than 3 g or the WBC declines to <4000 to 4500 cells/mm, or the platelet count declines to <100,000.[6] The most common adverse effect with hydroxyurea is myelosuppression. Myelosuppression due to hydroxyurea usually resolves rapidly on discontinuation.

TABLE 190-7
Safety Monitoring for Hydroxyurea Use

- Initial evaluation
  1. Careful history and physical examination
  2. Identification of proper patient characteristics and risk factors
- Survey for interacting medications (cytarabine)
- Baseline laboratory tests:
  1. CBC with differential/platelets
  2. Basic serum chemistry profile
  3. Urinalysis
  4. Renal function testing (creatinine/blood urea nitrogen)
- Ongoing laboratory monitoring
  1. CBC with differential/platelets
     Perform weekly initially, then
     a. transition to biweekly or monthly after 1 mo,
     b. perform testing with any dose escalation, and
     c. decrease/discontinue if hemoglobin decreases by 3 g/dL, white blood cell count <4000/mm^3, or platelets <100,000/mm^3
  2. Serum chemistry
     Perform monthly initially, then
     a. transition to every 3-6 mo if stable,
     b. perm testing with any dose escalation, and
     c. physical exam (focus on SCCs in particular)

CBC, complete blood cell count.

Transient, reversible hepatitis occurs occasionally and is associated with an acute "flulike" syndrome. Sporadic elevations of blood urea nitrogen (BUN) and serum creatinine have been reported, but frank renal failure is rare.

Cutaneous side effects include diffuse reversible hyperpigmentation including the buccal mucosa and tongue) and ulcers over pressure points, often on the malleolus or tibial crest and on the back. Nail changes consist of longitudinal transverse or diffuse melanonychia, lunular pigmentation. The drug is also associated with hydroxyurea-associated vascular occlusion in patients with myeloproliferative disease. Other side effects include dermatomyositis-like eruptions.[63,64] lichenoid drug eruptions, ulcerations of the lower leg, alopecia, cutaneous vasculitis, photosensitivity, and radiation recall. In patients treated with hydroxyurea for myeloproliferative disorders, nonmelanoma skin cancer has

TABLE 190-8
Risks and Precautions With Hydroxyurea Use

- Absolute contraindications
  1. Hypersensitivity to hydroxyurea
- Relative contraindications
  1. Pregnancy/lactation (category D)
  2. History of hepatovenular occlusive disease
  3. Chronic anemia
  4. Renal disease
- Common adverse effects
  1. Myelosuppression (most common side effect)
  2. Dermatomyositis-like eruption
  3. Renal toxicity (elevated creatinine/blood urea nitrogen, hematuria, proteinuria)
  4. Increased risk of secondary hematologic malignancies when used for polycythemia vera

been reported as an association.[65,66] Patients on hydroxyurea with atrophie-blanch-like lesions may need a trial off the drug, because hydroxyurea can mimic this syndrome through unknown mechanisms. Hydroxyurea may cause serpentine supravenous hyperpigmentation.

Other reported side effects of hydroxyurea include lupus erythematosus, mild GI distress (anorexia, nausea, vomiting, diarrhea, and constipation), and secondary malignancies when used in patients with primary hematologic disorders, such as polycythemia vera. Elevations in transaminases have been observed. A rare but important adverse effect of hydroxyurea is fever with a flulike illness. Hydroxyurea is a category D agent during pregnancy, and its use should be avoided. Males should use adequate contraception.

Drug Interactions: Hydroxyurea appears to have few significant drug interactions, with the exception of coadministration with other myelosuppressive agents and cytarabine. Use of such agents with hydroxyurea may lead to additive bone marrow toxicity.

IMMUNOSUPPRESSIVE/ ANTIINFLAMMATORY AGENTS

AZATHIOPRINE

Azathioprine is a synthetic analog of natural purine bases used in RNA and DNA synthesis (Fig. 190-1). Although many thiopurine derivatives exist, azathioprine is the agent most often used in dermatology.

MECHANISM OF ACTION

Azathioprine is a prodrug that is metabolized to 6-mercaptopurine (6-MP) and acts as an immunosuppressant/antiinflammatory. It was first synthesized in the 1950s and has better availability when given by mouth than 6-MP. 6-MP is further anabolized via hypoxanthine-guanine phosphoribosyl transferase (HGPRT), ultimately to a purine analog, 6-thioguanine (6-TG), which inhibits RNA and DNA synthesis and repair, yielding immunosuppression. HGPRT activation is critical. Interestingly, however, patients with Lesch-Nyhan syndrome (HGPRT deficiency) experience no immunosuppression or untoward effects while taking azathioprine.[67]

PHARMACOKINETICS

Azathioprine and its metabolite, 6-MP, are equally potent when administered parenterally, but azathioprine has improved bioavailability, with 88% of the oral dose being absorbed through the GI tract. After absorption, azathioprine is converted to 6-MP, mostly within erythrocytes. The fate of 6-MP is determined by one of 3 competing metabolic pathways: (1) it may be anabolized to an ultimate active form (6-TG) via HGPRT, (2) it may be catabolized to an inactive form via xanthine oxidase (XO), or (3) it may be catabolized to an inactive form by thiopurine methyltransferase (TPMT).[68]

Elucidation of the TPMT-dependent catabolic pathway has revolutionized the clinical use of azathioprine. In humans, expression of TPMT is variable as a result of genetic polymorphisms. Patients may be categorized into 3 subgroups: (1) a large majority possesses high levels of TPMT expression (~90%), (2) intermediate expression is found in ~10%, and (3) less than 1% demonstrate very low TPMT activity (about 1 in 300 persons).[69] Commercial assays for TPMT activity allow for graduated azathioprine dosing, with improved efficacy and a lesser incidence of unforeseen side effects (see section "Dosing Regimen").[70,71]

XO is another enzyme involved in the catabolism of 6-MP. Allopurinol, used in the treatment of gout, is a potent inhibitor of XO; toxicity may result in those taking both medications.[72] Unlike TPMT, there is very little genetic variation in XO expression, and it is unnecessary to assess innate XO expression before azathioprine dosing. A careful medication history, however, is critical (see section "Drug Interactions").

INDICATIONS

Azathioprine is licensed for 3 major indications: pemphigus vulgaris, systemic lupus erythematosus, and dermatomyositis. It is used for many other dermatologic conditions "off-label" (Table 190-9).[73] A randomized clinical trial in adjuvant immunosuppressants in the treatment of pemphigus vulgaris, azathioprine was the most efficacious of the immunosuppressive medications.[74] Of the 4 medications (mycophenolate mofetil, azathioprine, cyclophosphamide, prednisolone), azathioprine remains a common regimen among practicing dermatologists.[75] Another study found no difference between mycophenolate mofetil (MMF)

TABLE 190-9

Uses for Azathioprine in Dermatology

- U.S. Food and Drug Administration–approved indications
    - Dermatomyositis
    - Pemphigus vulgaris
    - Systemic lupus erythematosus
- "Off-label" uses
    - Scleroderma
    - Atopic dermatitis
    - Psoriasis
    - Bullous pemphigoid
- Mucous membrane pemphigoid
    - Pityriasis rubra pilaris
    - Wegener granulomatosis
    - Cutaneous vasculitis
    - Relapsing polychondritis
    - Behçet disease
    - Sarcoidosis
    - Lichen planus
    - Polymorphous light eruption

and azathioprine efficacy in the treatment of bullous pemphigoid, yet MMF had a lower liver toxicity profile.[76] In addition to bullous pemphigoid, azathioprine has been shown to be effective in treating moderate-to-severe, refractory atopic dermatitis.[77,78]

DOSING REGIMEN

Azathioprine is supplied as 50-mg tablets and also as an injectable solution for subcutaneous delivery. It is strongly recommended that dosing be based on the patient's TPMT expression (Table 190-10).[70,79] Acute severe neutropenia is the most feared complication and may occur in 86% of patients receiving a standard dosing of azathioprine in patients with 2 TPMT variant alleles.[80] Patients with one variant allele also may be at risk for greater toxicity, but this is controversial.[80] Dosing azathioprine should be approached with caution because of the potential for great toxicity in the following conditions: older adults, impaired renal or hepatic function, and concomitant treatment with allopurinol.[80]

Insufficient data exists to recommend an optimal dose, duration of therapy, or to predict the relapse rate upon discontinuation in the pediatric population. Doses up to 3 mg/kg/d have been used. TPMT levels should be repeated in cases of nonresponse or change in response. For pediatric patients with atopic dermatitis, safe and successful treatment has been described with a recommended starting dose of 2.0 to 2.5 mg/kg (1.0-1.5 mg/kg when TPMT levels are reduced).[81,82]

INITIATING THERAPY

Azathioprine can be initiated as monotherapy; however, concomitant bridge therapy with prednisone is often used in steroid-responsive bullous disorders.[80] Azathioprine should not be used in patients with severe comorbidities, active infections, or the possibility of reactivation of an infection (tuberculosis).

Baseline laboratory tests include a CBC with differential, renal and liver function testing, and an erythrocyte TPMT activity assay. Mycobacterial infections have occurred in patients taking azathioprine. Tuberculin skin testing or QuantiFERON gold should be considered in high-risk populations prior to initiating therapy.

MONITORING THERAPY

During therapy, a CBC with differential should be obtained biweekly for the first 2 months, monthly for the next 2 months, and every 2 months thereafter; liver function testing should occur every month for 3 months and then bimonthly thereafter, unless abnormalities are noted.[83] Laboratory monitoring may not need to be this frequent. Additional laboratory evaluation to rule out hepatitis B and C, HIV, and tuberculosis is also recommended.

Additional laboratory testing is necessary with dosage increases or if an initial TPMT level cannot be determined. Biannual physical examinations should pay particular attention to evidence of possible lymphoreticular disease and skin cancer, particularly squamous cell carcinoma (SCC). Safety guidelines used during azathioprine therapy are summarized in Table 190-11.

RISK FACTORS AND PRECAUTIONS

Absolute and relative contraindications and common adverse effects of azathioprine are summarized in Table 190-12.

TABLE 190-10
Dosing of Azathioprine Based on Thiopurine Methyltransferase (TPMT) Enzyme Assay

TPMT ERYTHROCYTE ASSAY	DOSING RANGE
>19.0 U (high expression)	2.0-3.0 mg/kg
13.7-19.0 U (intermediate expression)	1.0-1.5 mg/kg
5.0-13.7 U (low expression)	Could consider 0.5 mg/kg or select alternative medication
<5.0 U (very low expression)	Do not use

TABLE 190-11
Safety Monitoring for Azathioprine Use

- Initial evaluation
- Careful history and physical examination
- Identification of proper patient characteristics and risk factors
- Survey for interacting medications (allopurinol, aminosalicylates)
- Baseline laboratories:
  - Thiopurine methyltransferase erythrocyte assay
  - CBC with differential
  - Basic serum chemistry profile
  - Liver function tests
  - Urinalysis
  - Pregnancy testing for women of child-bearing age
  - Tuberculin testing (if indicated)
  - Consider TPMT genotype assay if borderline intermediate/high expression by erythrocyte measurement
- Ongoing laboratory monitoring
  - CBC with differential
  - Biweekly for 2 mo, monthly for 2 mo, then bimonthly thereafter
- Liver function testing
  - Monthly for 3 mo, then bimonthly monthly thereafter
- Consider erythrocyte 6-TG level, repeat TPMT (to check for induction)
- Followup clinical evaluation
  - Biannual complete physical examinations
  - Particular attention to possible lymphoreticular disease (adenopathy)
  - Careful survey for nonmelanoma skin cancer (squamous cell carcinoma)

CBC, complete blood cell count.

TABLE 190-12
Risks and Precautions With Azathioprine Use

- Absolute contraindications
  - Hypersensitivity to azathioprine
  - Active or ongoing infection
- Relative contraindications
  - Pregnancy/lactation (category D, but myelosuppression of fetus/infant common—avoid)
  - Allopurinol use (dose must be reduced by 75%)
  - Prior lymphoproliferative disease or prior use of alkylating agents
- Common adverse effects
  - GI distress (minimized by administration with food)
  - Myelosuppression
  - Possible increased risk of lymphoproliferative disease or skin cancer
  - Possible opportunistic infections

COMPLICATIONS

With careful monitoring, azathioprine is generally safe. Adverse effects tend to occur in those patients with lower TPMT activity levels, higher doses of azathioprine, or concomitant use of allopurinol. Specifically, overall adverse reactions and bone marrow toxicity have been found to be associated with TMPT polymorphisms, but hepatotoxicity has not.[84]

Hematologic Effects: Myelosuppression is a major side effect of azathioprine use. Higher rates of myelosuppression have been seen in patients without *TMPT* variations; therefore, pretreatment TPMT measurement should not be a substitute for regular hematologic surveillance during azathioprine treatment. In a large prospective study, the probability of myelotoxicity in the normal TPMT activity group was 3.5% compared with 14.3% in the intermediate TPMT activity group (95% CI 1.37-14.99, OR 4.5).[85] Generalized depression of all blood cell lines is most common,[86] but depression of any single lineage may be observed. Thrombocytopenia is a common initial presentation of bone marrow toxicity. Bone marrow suppression tends to occur at higher doses,[87] and in those with lower TPMT expression. Discontinuance usually results in complete marrow recovery.

Infections: Most patients treated with azathioprine also receive large doses of glucocorticoids. Therefore, it is often difficult to quantify the independent role of azathioprine in any predisposition toward infection. Herpes virus infections, human papilloma infection among others, have been reported in patients taking azathioprine.[87] However, there is not a general increased incidence of infection in cohorts of inflammatory bowel disease or atopic dermatitis patients.[88] Nevertheless, proper screening and selection of patients is warranted because of potential risk.

GI Effects: GI side effects are the most common side effects leading to drug discontinuation and are dose dependent.[89] Patients receiving high doses of azathioprine may experience nausea, vomiting, and diarrhea. Such symptoms are not usually treatment limiting and may be reduced by gradual dose escalation over weeks, administration with food, splitting the daily dose, or concomitant dosing with antiemetics. Pancreatitis is a separate established adverse effect, is rare, and is limited to patients with Crohn disease.[80]

Hepatic Effects: Mild imbalances in liver transaminases, bilirubin, and alkaline phosphatase are not uncommon, may be transient, and are typically without serious clinical implications. Toxic hepatitis (drug-induced hepatotoxicity, nodular regenerative hyperplasia) has developed in approximately 1% of patients treated with azathioprine for rheumatoid arthritis, and it is usually reversible.[90] Other adverse effects include hepatic veno-occlusive disease and associated pancreatitis. Discontinuation is warranted with evidence of liver toxicity.

Anaphylaxis: Azathioprine-induced shock and hypersensitivity reactions have been reported in patients with cutaneous disease. In most cases, hypotensive collapse occurred within hours of the initial dose. Several cases of drug fever also have been reported with azathioprine (Chap. 45).

Carcinogenesis: Azathioprine has been associated with increased risk for skin cancer and lymphoma. The increased number and aggressive behavior of SCCs may occur because of increased absorption of UVA radiation by 6-TG. As a result of increased UVA radiation absorption, increased reactive oxygen species develop and result in mutagenic DNA damage that is conducive for skin cancer development.[91-93] One small case series confirmed a reduced minimal erythema dose to UVA irradiation with coadministration of azathioprine.[91] Azathioprine increases the risk of squamous cell carcinoma by 56% (95% CI 1.11-2.18, OR 1.56),[94] and is associated with >12 months of use in patients with inflammatory bowel disease (95% CI 3.1-6.0, OR 4.3).[95] As UVA radiation is an important carcinogenic hazard for patients taking azathioprine, efforts (sun avoidance, broad spectrum sunscreen) to mitigate UVA exposure are paramount. Furthermore, for organ transplant patients, skin cancer screening at baseline and every 6 months, is advised. For patients who are developing multiple SCC, switching from azathioprine to medications with lower photocarcinogenesis potential (such as mycophenolate mofetil or sirolimus) may be considered.[80]

An increased risk of lymphoproliferative disease occurs in renal transplant recipients, rheumatoid arthritis patients, and inflammatory bowel disease patients treated with chronic azathioprine.[96-98] In one study, the relative risk was increased 10- to 13-fold, or 1 lymphoma per 1000 patient-years of azathioprine treatment. Dermatologic doses of azathioprine are often lower and the duration of treatment shorter than those used in other conditions, suggesting that the risk of lymphoma is probably lower in those treated for cutaneous disease. However, a meta-analysis of patients treated with azathioprine for inflammatory bowel disease who developed lymphoma included those on "low-dose" regimens.[98] In light of this information, it seems prudent to inform patients that the exact magnitude of any increased risk for lymphoma with "low-dose" azathioprine is not known.

Mutagenicity and Teratogenicity: Azathioprine is a category D agent during pregnancy. The prodrug and the active metabolites readily cross the placenta. The rate of congenital malformation is low (4.3%), but myelosuppression and immunosuppression are significant occurrences in neonates and breastfed infants. Fertility of men or women appears unaffected by azathioprine.[99]

Drug Interactions: A major drug interaction occurs between azathioprine and allopurinol. When allopurinol must be used concurrently with azathioprine, the azathioprine dose should be decreased by 75%. The aminosalicylates may inhibit TPMT activity, and it is prudent to minimize or avoid such medications in patients using azathioprine.

THIOGUANINE

Thioguanine (Fig. 190-1) is a less used member of the thiopurine family of drugs. It is the natural metabolite of AZA and appears to be more effective than its parent compound. It has a metabolism and mechanism of action similar to that of azathioprine.

MECHANISM OF ACTION

Thioguanine is a prodrug and member of the thiopurine family; its metabolism and mechanism of action is via inhibition of purine synthesis. Thioguanine produces nucleotide analogs that ultimately yield cytotoxic activity via incorporation into cellular DNA. Apoptosis is induced preferentially against activated T lymphocytes.[100]

PHARMACOKINETICS

Thioguanine is given orally, but it has incomplete and unpredictable absorption with variations of 10-fold seen in plasma concentrations. Peak plasma concentrations occur 2 to 4 hours after ingestion.[101]

INDICATIONS

In dermatology, thioguanine has been used chiefly for the treatment of psoriasis, particularly in those with recalcitrant disease or with contraindications to other systemic therapies (Table 190-13). A small retrospective study of patients with recalcitrant psoriasis, demonstrated that 14 of 18 patients experienced significant improvement with thioguanine, including patients with psoriatic arthritis, palmoplantar disease, or scalp involvement.[102] Two additional open-label studies on the drug used in psoriasis showed response rates of 78% and 49%, respectively,[103,104] In a longer-term study, 58% of 76 patients with psoriasis were effectively maintained at 24 months, and the drug was safely used up to 145 months. Thioguanine has been used effectively, although infrequently, to treat lupus and atopic dermatitis. There is limited data available regarding the use of thioguanine in the pediatric population.

TABLE 190-13

Uses for Thioguanine in Dermatology

- U.S. Food and Drug Administration–approved indications
  - None
- "Off-label" uses
  - Severe psoriasis
  - Severe cutaneous lupus erythematosus
  - Severe atopic dermatitis

DOSING REGIMEN

Thioguanine is supplied as 40-mg tablets. Guidelines suggest beginning with a dose of 80 mg twice weekly with possible advancement by 20 mg every 2 to 4 weeks, to a maximum dose of 160 mg 3 times weekly.[83]

Similar to azathioprine, use of commercial assays for TPMT activity improves thioguanine dosing. The latest review of thioguanine use in severe psoriasis recommends an assessment of TPMT levels before treatment so as to guide the selection of an adequate starting dose.[102]

Pulse dosing, either twice or 3 times per week (120 mg twice per week up to 160 mg 3 times per week), may confer a reduced risk of bone marrow toxicity, as compared to daily dosing.[83]

INITIATING THERAPY

Patients with severe comorbidities, particularly hematologic disturbances, active infection, or who are pregnant or wish to become pregnant should be excluded, and males must also use adequate contraception. Recommended baseline laboratory studies include a CBC with differential, liver function studies, and a TPMT activity assay.

MONITORING THERAPY

Repeat blood counts and liver function tests should be followed weekly at first, transitioning to biweekly as the dose stabilizes, then monthly for 3 months, and quarterly thereafter and always with dose escalation (Table 190-14).

RISKS AND PRECAUTIONS

Absolute and relative contraindications and common adverse effects of thioguanine are summarized in Table 190-15.

TABLE 190-14
Safety Monitoring for Thioguanine Use

- Initial evaluation
  - Careful history and physical examination
  - Identification of proper patient characteristics and risk factors
  - Survey for interacting medications (aminosalicylates)
- Baseline laboratories:
  - Thiopurine methyltransferase erythrocyte assay
  - CBC with differential/platelets
  - Liver function tests
  - Renal function testing (creatinine/blood urea nitrogen)
- Ongoing laboratory monitoring
- CBC with differential/platelets and liver function tests
  - Perform weekly initially, then
    - Transition to biweekly as the dose stabilizes, then
    - Monthly for 3 mo and quarterly thereafter
  - Perform laboratory testing with any dose escalation

CBC, complete blood cell count.

COMPLICATIONS

Common adverse effects of thioguanine include myelosuppression and GI disturbances. In the largest series of patients using thioguanine for psoriasis, 49% experienced myelosuppression, yet only 20% required complete discontinuance.[104] In one series, thrombocytopenia was the earliest indicator of myelosuppression.[102] Pulsed dosing of thioguanine has been associated with a lower rate of myelosuppression, but TPMT testing was not performed in this study.[105]

GI disturbances include nausea, excessive flatulence, taste changes, esophageal reflux, and diarrhea, symptoms that are often tolerated without discontinuance. In a single study, elevated liver transaminases occurred in 25% of patients, but many had been taking MTX prior to the study.[104] Generally, thioguanine is not considered particularly hepatotoxic; liver biopsy is not indicated during treatment. Rare cases of toxic hepatic veno-occlusive disease have occurred in patients using thioguanine for psoriasis.[106] Low-dose thioguanine use in pregnant women has been reported with inflammatory bowel disease; however, use during pregnancy is generally avoided.[107]

TABLE 190-15
Risks and Precautions With Thioguanine Use

- Absolute contraindications
  - Hypersensitivity to thioguanine
- Relative contraindications
  - Pregnancy/lactation (category D)
  - History of hepatovenular occlusive disease
  - Hematologic disorders
- Common adverse effects
  - Myelosuppression (most common side effect)
  - GI distress (often tolerated)
  - Toxic hepatitis (less common than with other cytotoxic agents)

Drug Interactions: Thioguanine metabolism is not dependent on XO; it may be administered concurrently with allopurinol without dose reduction. Aminosalicylates may inhibit TPMT activity, and it is prudent to minimize or avoid such medications in patients taking thioguanine.

MYCOPHENOLIC ACID AND MYCOPHENOLATE MOFETIL

Mycophenolic acid (MPA) (Fig. 190-1) is a lipid-soluble, weak organic acid with antifungal, antibacterial, antiviral, and immunosuppressive properties. MPA was first used as an oral agent for moderate-to-severe psoriasis in the 1970s, but use was discontinued because of intolerability. Mycophenolate mofetil (MMF) represents a derivative of MPA, with greater bioavailability, improved tolerance, and enhanced immunosuppression. Properties and use of this agent are discussed in detail in Chap. 192.

CYCLOSPORINE

Cyclosporine is a neutral cyclic peptide that suppresses T lymphocyte function via inhibition of intracellular calcineurin, resulting in decreased IL-2 and interferon γ production. As a result of decreased IL-2 and interferon γ production, there is decreased activation and proliferation of helper and cytotoxic lymphocytes. Cyclosporine was discovered while searching for new antifungal agents and it was later found to have potent immunosuppressive effects. Although cyclosporine is not routinely used by most US dermatologists, it is approved for the treatment of psoriasis and also has been used to treat many other inflammatory dermatoses. Properties and use of this agent are discussed in detail in Chap. 192.[108,109]

TACROLIMUS

Tacrolimus is a macrolide that inhibits calcineurin by binding to the FK506 binding protein. As a result of binding the FK506 binding protein, gene encoding via calcineurin is inhibited leading to decreased IL-2 and interferon γ production.[110] This leads to decreased proliferation and activation of T lymphocytes. Tacrolimus is available in topical and oral formulations. Although oral tacrolimus is commonly used in the prevention of organ transplant rejection, topical tacrolimus is indicated for the treatment of atopic dermatitis and also has been used to treat many other inflammatory dermatoses. Properties and use of this agent is discussed in detail in Chap. 192.[110]

THALIDOMIDE

Thalidomide is a nonpolar glutamic acid derivative with hypnosedative, immunomodulatory, and neural/vascular tissue effects. Initially removed from the market because of severe teratogenic effects (phocomelia) in 1961, thalidomide was later found to be effective in treating erythema nodosum leprosum.[111] The FDA approval of thalidomide for erythema nodosum leprosum resulted in the opportunity for off-label use treating dermatoses including AIDS-related Kaposi sarcoma, pyoderma gangrenosum, bullous pemphigoid, prurigo nodularis, uremic pruritus, and Jessner lymphocytic infiltrate of the skin among others. The mechanism of action of thalidomide is not well understood. Properties and use of this agent is discussed in detail in Chap. 195.[111]

CYTOTOXIC AGENTS

CYCLOPHOSPHAMIDE

Cyclophosphamide (Fig. 190-1) was originally derived from nitrogen mustard in 1958, then combined with phosphoric acid in an effort to make an inert drug capable of entering and releasing active nitrogen mustard within target cells.[77] Cyclophosphamide is an alkylating agent and acts primarily by crosslinking DNA. In oncology, cyclophosphamide is used as an antineoplastic agent. In dermatology, it is used as an immunosuppressive and steroid-sparing agent, particularly for autoimmune blistering disorders and systemic vasculitis.

MECHANISM OF ACTION

Cyclophosphamide is a classic cell cycle–nonspecific drug; its cytotoxic effect is independent of the proliferative index. Active metabolites of cyclophosphamide form covalent bonds with the nucleophilic centers of DNA. This alkylation leads to DNA crosslinking, abnormal base-pair formation, imidazole ring cleavage with depurination, and chain scission. Ultimately, these mutations lead to cell death and possibly mutagenesis and carcinogenesis. Cyclophosphamide has a greater effect on B lymphocytes than T lymphocytes and a greater effect on suppressor T cells than helper T cells.[112] Resistance to cyclophosphamide may occur as a result of decreased cellular penetration, increased competition from other nucleophilic substances, improved DNA repair, or increased drug metabolism.

PHARMACOKINETICS

Oral cyclophosphamide has a bioavailability of 74%. Peak plasma levels are achieved within 1 hour of administration. The half-life of the drug is between 2 and 10 hours. Cyclophosphamide is initially inactive, but undergoes hepatic metabolism via the cytochrome P_{450} (CYP) system into the active metabolite nitrogen mustard, which can then be converted into the other active metabolite phosphoramide mustard.[93] It is first converted to 4-hydroxycyclophosphamide, an active molecule that exists in equilibrium with aldophosphamide. Aldophosphamide may be cleaved to phosphoramide mustard, another active metabolite, and acrolein, an inactive metabolite. Aldehyde dehydrogenase may also convert aldophosphamide into a second inactive metabolite, carboxyphosphamide. The kidneys excrete just 10% to 20% of the drug unchanged but excrete 50% of the active metabolites.

INDICATIONS

In dermatology, cyclophosphamide is used as a steroid-sparing agent in only the most serious diseases. In particular, patients with pemphigus vulgaris may be treated with cyclophosphamide in combination with steroids, and evidence supports its steroid-sparing benefits.[113] Cyclophosphamide also has been used for the treatment of mucous membrane pemphigoid and has been inconsistently reported as beneficial in Stevens–Johnson syndrome and toxic epidermal necrolysis.[114,115]

Other diseases that may respond to cyclophosphamide include pyoderma gangrenosum, necrobiotic xanthogranuloma, cutaneous amyloidosis, lichen myxedematosus, giant cell reticulohistiocytoma, primary cutaneous diffuse large B-cell lymphoma, and mycosis fungoides. However, with the availability of safer immunosuppressive agents, cyclophosphamide is not an agent that is routinely used for the enormous majority of cutaneous inflammatory diseases.

DOSING REGIMEN

Cyclophosphamide is available as 25- and 50-mg tablets and also in an injectable form. Oral doses are typically 1 to 3 mg/kg/d either divided or as a single morning dose. Intravenous pulse dosing of 0.5 to 1.0 g/m² monthly provides an alternative therapeutic approach that has been associated with fewer side effects than daily oral dosing. Vigorous hydration, beginning 24 hours before and continuing throughout therapy, is recommended to minimize bladder toxicity. Although pulse dosing may be efficacious in achieving disease control in pemphigus vulgaris, bullous pemphigoid, systemic sclerosis, and ANCA positive vasculitis, patients may have a slightly increased risk of disease relapse in comparison to oral cyclophosphamide following completion of therapy.[116]

INITIATING THERAPY

Patients being considered for cyclophosphamide therapy should have a thorough history and physical examination. Cyclophosphamide is contraindicated in patients with a history of transitional cell carcinoma of the bladder.[117] Patients with a history of a lymphoproliferative disorder must be treated with extreme caution. Use in pregnant or lactating patients is contraindicated. Baseline laboratory evaluations should include a CBC with differential, serum chemistry profile, liver function testing, and urinalysis. Initiation of cyclophosphamide therapy is contraindicated if the total white blood cell count is less than 5000/mm^3 or if the absolute neutrophil is less than 1000/mm^3.[116]

MONITORING THERAPY

Blood counts and urinalysis with microscopic examination to look for red blood cells in the urine should be repeated weekly initially but may be reduced to biweekly or monthly over the first few months as long as the results remain in the normal range. Liver function testing should be performed monthly, but over time if the results remain in the normal range liver function testing may be reduced to every 2 to 3 months. Urine cytology is indicated when the cumulative dose exceeds 50 g and every 6 months thereafter, or on any occasion of hemorrhagic cystitis. Some authorities recommend a chest radiograph every 6 months. Followup physical examination should pay particular attention for any evidence of lymphoproliferative disease (lymphadenopathy). Patients taking cyclophosphamide should have all age-appropriate cancer screening, including stool guaiac examination and Papanicolaou smears for women. Safety guidelines used during cyclophosphamide therapy are summarized in Table 190-16.[116]

TABLE 190-17
Risks and Precautions With Cyclophosphamide Use

- Absolute contraindications
  - Hypersensitivity to cyclophosphamide (can cross-react with chlorambucil)
- Relative contraindications
  - Pregnancy/lactation (category D; fetal loss common)
  - History of transitional cell carcinoma of the bladder
  - Depressed bone marrow function
  - Impaired hepatic or renal function
- Common adverse effects
  - GI distress (minimized with antiemetic medications)
  - Myelosuppression (often dose limiting)
  - Hemorrhagic cystitis due to elimination of toxic metabolites (minimized with mesna)
  - Carcinogenicity (transitional cell carcinoma of bladder, lymphoproliferative disease)
  - Reproductive consequences (amenorrhea, azoospermia, gonadal failure)

RISKS AND PRECAUTIONS

Absolute and relative contraindications and common adverse effects of cyclophosphamide are summarized in Table 190-17.

COMPLICATIONS

Because of its activity independent of the cell cycle, the toxic effects of cyclophosphamide are significant and numerous.

GI Effects: Nausea and vomiting are the most common GI side effects associated with cyclophosphamide use. Coadministration of ondansetron and dexamethasone reduces these side effects. The addition of aprepitant to this combination therapy may provide even greater antiemetic action.[118]

Hematologic Effects: Hematologic disturbances are frequent with cyclophosphamide, especially leukopenia and thrombocytopenia. A nadir in blood counts occurs 8 to 12 days after initiation of therapy. Myelosuppression is not requisite to immunosuppression, but it often represents a dose-limiting side effect.

Genitourinary Effects: Bladder toxicity is a well-recognized consequence of cyclophosphamide use. Patients should be counseled to ensure vigorous hydration throughout the day and to empty their bladder before bed and cyclophosphamide should be given in the early morning to allow for vigorous hydration throughout the day.[116] Hemorrhagic cystitis can occur in up to 40% of patients treated with oral cyclophosphamide.[119] This cystitis occurs during therapy and is believed to be caused by the metabolite, acrolein. A scavenging agent, mesna (sodium 2-mercaptoethane sulfonate), binds acrolein in the bladder and may be used to reduce the incidence of cystitis. Mesna is used primarily with high-dose

TABLE 190-16
Safety Monitoring for Cyclophosphamide Use

- Initial evaluation
  - Careful history and physical examination
  - Identification of proper patient characteristics and risk factors
  - Survey for interacting medications (allopurinol, cimetidine)
- Baseline laboratories:
  - CBC with differential
  - Basic serum chemistry profile
  - Urinalysis with microscopic exam for red blood cells in the urine
  - Renal function testing (creatinine/blood urea nitrogen)
- Ongoing laboratory monitoring
- CBC with differential and urinalysis with microscopic exam for red blood cells
  - Perform weekly initially, then
  - Transition to biweekly or monthly after 2-3 mo
  - Perform testing with any dose escalation
  - Decrease/discontinue if white blood cell count <4000/mm^3, or platelets <100,000/mm^3
  - Discontinue and refer to urologist if red blood cells appear in urine
- Basic serum chemistry and liver function tests
  - Perform monthly initially, then
  - Transition to every 2-3 mo if stable
- Urine cytology testing
  - Perform when cumulative dose >50 g or if patient has hemorrhagic cystitis

CBC, complete blood cell count.

intravenous cyclophosphamide regimens, but it also may be used in low-dose oral cyclophosphamide therapy.[120] Mesna may be administered orally or intravenously. In the rheumatologic literature, a cumulative dose of >36 g, concomitant hemorrhagic cystitis during treatment and untreated bladder toxicity are thought to be responsible for the markedly increased risk of transitional cell carcinoma of the bladder (8- to 10-fold increased risk) among those taking chronic oral cyclophosphamide. Bladder cancer may arise years after cyclophosphamide therapy, and ongoing monitoring of the lower urinary tract (by urinalysis and cystoscopy when necessary) should be considered.[116]

Infectious Disease: Because of the potent immunosuppressant effects of cyclophosphamide, patients may be at an increased risk of developing opportunistic infections, including *Pneumocystis jirovecii* (formerly *Pneumocystis carinii*) pneumonia, especially when patients are treated with additional immunosuppressive medications (eg, systemic corticosteroids). Prophylaxis should be considered based on a cumulative dose of cyclophosphamide (>7.5 g) and concomitant therapy with other immunosuppressive medications. Prophylactic treatment options to prevent *P. jirovecii* include trimethoprim-sulfamethoxazole, aerosolized pentamidine, oral dapsone, or oral atovaquone).[116]

Carcinogenicity: Treatment with cyclophosphamide has been associated with an increased risk of various solid organ tumors, non-Hodgkin lymphoma, leukemia, transitional cell carcinoma of the bladder, and squamous cell carcinoma. Most of these associations are derived from organ transplant and oncology patients who have been exposed to chronic use or higher doses of cyclophosphamide, and who often are on other concurrent immunosuppressive agents. There is also a slight increased risk of non-Hodgkin lymphoma in patients with rheumatologic disorders who are treated with cyclophosphamide.[121,122] Because cyclophosphamide dosing tends to be of shorter duration and of lower dose for patients who are receiving the drug for dermatologic disorders than for patients with organ transplants, cancer, or rheumatologic disorders, it seems reasonable to conclude that the risk of cancer is likely lower in dermatology patients than in patients who receive cyclophosphamide for other indications.

Cutaneous Effects: Anagen effluvium can occur in up to 30% of those treated with cyclophosphamide.[123] This alopecia typically resolves after therapy is completed. Diffuse brown hyperpigmentation of the skin and mucosa, as well as transverse, longitudinal, or diffuse melanonychia, may occur. Cutaneous hyperpigmentation usually resolves within 6 to 12 months after therapy is discontinued. Toxic acral erythema of chemotherapy has been described, as well as radiation recall.[124] Similar to other chemotherapeutic agents that are secreted in the eccrine glands, cyclophosphamide may induce neutrophilic eccrine hidradenitis.[125] Urticaria, dermatomyositis, cutaneous vasculitis, and induction of Stevens–Johnson syndrome may occur.[88]

Mutagenicity and Teratogenicity: Cyclophosphamide is a category D agent during pregnancy. Therefore, adequate contraception is necessary while on cyclophosphamide. Four pregnant women exposed to cyclophosphamide during treatment for systemic lupus resulted in pregnancy loss in all cases.[126] Azoospermia and amenorrhea may also occur with cyclophosphamide use. Amenorrhea may occur in up to 60% of women treated with cyclophosphamide, with up to 80% of those experiencing premature ovarian failure.[127] Age and cumulative dose are most determinative of the risk of gonadal failure. In men, testosterone administration may lessen the risk of gonadal failure, whereas in women, leuprolide acetate may provide a similar partial protection.[128,129] These observations make it clear that cyclophosphamide should not be a first-line therapy for men or women who wish to conceive after treatment.

Cardiac/Pulmonary Toxicity: Cardiac and pulmonary are rare complications that typically only occur when cyclophosphamide is used in high doses for chemotherapy.[116]

Drug Interactions: Because the microsomal enzyme system responsible for activation of cyclophosphamide is involved in the metabolism of many other drugs, the potential for multiple drug interactions exists. Allopurinol, cimetidine, and chloramphenicol all increase cyclophosphamide toxicity. The effects of succinylcholine are potentiated by cyclophosphamide. Digoxin absorption is diminished with coadministration of oral cyclophosphamide.

CHLORAMBUCIL

Chlorambucil is another alkylating agent derived from nitrogen mustard. In comparison to cyclophosphamide, chlorambucil is used infrequently in dermatology.

MECHANISM OF ACTION

Like cyclophosphamide, chlorambucil exerts its effects independent of the cell cycle through crosslinking of DNA.

PHARMACOKINETICS

Chlorambucil is well absorbed, with 87% bioavailability after oral administration. The drug is 99% protein bound in plasma. It has a plasma half-life of approximately 1.5 hours. Less than 1% of the drug is excreted by the kidney. Although the drug is extensively metabolized by the liver, it does not require hepatic activation. In comparison to cyclophosphamide, chlorambucil has a slower onset of effect.

INDICATIONS

Isolated reports detail use of chlorambucil as a steroid-sparing agent in pemphigus vulgaris, bullous

TABLE 190-18
Uses for Chlorambucil in Dermatology

- U.S. Food and Drug Administration–approved indications
  - None
- "Off-label" uses
  - Granulomatosis with polyangiitis (Wegener)
  - Lymphomatoid granulomatosis
  - Dermatomyositis
  - Scleroderma
  - Relapsing polychondritis
  - Severe cutaneous lupus erythematosus
  - Pemphigus vulgaris
  - Bullous pemphigoid
  - Epidermolysis bullosa acquisita
  - Pyoderma gangrenosum
  - Langerhans cell histiocytosis
  - Necrobiotic xanthogranuloma with paraproteinemia
  - Sarcoidosis
  - Severe disseminated granuloma annulare

TABLE 190-19
Safety Monitoring for Chlorambucil Use

- Initial evaluation
  - Careful history and physical examination
  - Identification of proper patient characteristics and risk factors
  - Survey for interacting medications (vaccinations, other immunosuppressives)
- Baseline laboratories:
  - CBC with differential
  - Serum chemistry profile
  - Urinalysis
  - Renal function testing (creatinine/blood urea nitrogen)
- Ongoing laboratory monitoring
  - Complete blood count with differential and urinalysis
  - Perform weekly initially, then
    - Transition to biweekly or monthly after 2-3 mo
    - Repeat with any dose escalation
    - Decrease or discontinue dosing if white blood cell count <4000/mm^3, or platelets <100,000/mm^3
- Basic serum chemistry and liver function tests
  - Perform monthly initially, then
    - Transition to every 3-6 mo if stable

pemphigoid, primary cutaneous B-cell lymphoma, aggressive pyoderma gangrenosum, and Behçet disease (Table 190-18). Chlorambucil use also has been described in erythrodermic cutaneous T-cell lymphoma and necrobiotic xanthogranuloma.[130,131] Complicating management decisions, the U.S. FDA–approved package insert states that chlorambucil should not be used for nonmalignant diseases.

DOSING REGIMEN

Chlorambucil is supplied as 2-mg tablets. The recommended dosage is 0.05 to 0.2 mg/kg/d. Doses for cutaneous disease should remain toward the lower end of this range.

INITIATING THERAPY

Patients being considered for chlorambucil therapy should have a thorough history and physical examination. When considering chlorambucil use, patients with a history of a lymphoproliferative disorder must be approached with extreme caution. Use in pregnant or lactating patients is contraindicated. Baseline laboratory evaluations should include a CBC with differential, serum chemistry profile, liver function testing, and urinalysis.

MONITORING THERAPY

Blood counts should be repeated weekly initially but may be reduced to biweekly or monthly over time in patients whose blood counts remain stable. Liver function testing and urinalysis should continue monthly but may be reduced to every 3 months if stable. Some authorities recommend a chest radiograph every 6 months. followup physical examination should pay particular attention to any evidence of lymphoproliferative disease (lymphadenopathy). Patients taking chlorambucil should have all age-appropriate cancer screening, including stool guaiac examinations and Papanicolaou smears for women. Safety guidelines during chlorambucil therapy are summarized in Table 190-19.

RISKS AND PRECAUTIONS

Absolute and relative contraindications and common adverse effects of chlorambucil are summarized in Table 190-20.

COMPLICATIONS

Common side effects of chlorambucil include nausea and vomiting, azoospermia, amenorrhea, pulmonary fibrosis, seizures, anemia, thrombocytopenia, neutropenia, pancytopenia, and hepatotoxicity. Chlorambucil

TABLE 190-20
Risks and Precautions With Chlorambucil Use

- Absolute contraindications
  - Hypersensitivity to chlorambucil (can cross-react with cyclophosphamide)
- Relative contraindications
  - Pregnancy/lactation (category D)
  - Active infection (dependent on severity)
  - Impaired hepatic function
  - Childhood (possible increased risk of seizures)
- Common adverse effects
  - Myelosuppression (often dose-limiting)
  - GI distress (minimized with antiemetic medications)
  - Carcinogenicity (lymphoproliferative disease, squamous cell carcinoma)
  - Reproductive consequences (amenorrhea, azoospermia)

increases the risk of lymphoproliferative disorders and squamous cell carcinoma of the skin among organ transplant recipients. Other cutaneous side effects include alopecia, a morbilliform rash, urticaria, and mucosal ulcerations. Chlorambucil is pregnancy category D.

Drug Interactions: Through strong immunosuppression, chlorambucil may decrease the efficacy of viral vaccinations. Concomitant use of additional immunosuppressive drugs may potentiate any risk of infection or carcinogenesis.

ANTHRACYCLINES

Anthracyclines are antibiotic molecules that possess potent antineoplastic properties.

These agents act specifically during the S phase of cell division. Pegylated liposomal doxorubicin (PLD) (Fig. 190-1) is an anthracycline that is sometimes used in the treatment of Kaposi sarcoma.[132,133]

MECHANISM OF ACTION

Anthracyclines, such as doxorubicin, are intercalated within DNA and RNA. Through template disorder and steric obstruction, this incorporation leads to defective synthesis. Cell death typically results, but mutagenesis and carcinogenesis may also occur.

PHARMACOKINETICS

PLD has pharmacokinetic properties similar to standard doxorubicin; however, the liposomal formulation results in improved tolerance. Encapsulating liposomes have a diameter of approximately 100 nm and are designed to prevent phagocytosis of the agent by the reticuloendothelial system. The result is a plasma half-life of more than 55 hours and improved tumor penetrance.

INDICATIONS

PLD is approved by the U.S. FDA for the treatment of AIDS-related Kaposi sarcoma. PLD also has been used to treat cutaneous T-cell lymphoma mycosis fungoides and Sezary syndrome types.

DOSING REGIMEN

PLD is administered at a dose of 20 to 30 mg/m^2 infused intravenously over 30 to 60 minutes once every 2 to 3 weeks.

INITIATING THERAPY

A thorough history and physical examination is required before initiation of therapy with PLD. Prior use of anthracyclines is an indication for caution, as additive cardiotoxicity may occur. Physical evidence of existing cardiac failure should be sought. Baseline laboratory studies should include a complete blood count with differential, a CD4 count, an HIV viral load assay, and liver function studies, including a total bilirubin.

MONITORING THERAPY

Before each dose of PLD, all patients should have a repeat blood count, CD4 count, and liver function tests with total bilirubin. Specific tests for cardiotoxicity, such as a multiple-gated acquisition scan, are indicated for cumulative doses greater than 450 mg/m^2 or if signs or symptoms of congestive heart failure develop.

RISKS AND PRECAUTIONS

Absolute and relative contraindications and common adverse effects of doxorubicin are summarized in Table 190-21.

COMPLICATIONS

Myelosuppression is the most common side effect of PLD. A nadir in blood counts is expected during the second week of therapy. Neutropenia should be treated with granulocyte-macrophage colony-stimulating factor or granulocyte colony-stimulating factor. The HIV viral load does not change substantially during treatment, but CD4 counts may be lowered slightly. Abrupt or precipitous decreases in a CD4 count may require treatment discontinuation.

Although it is known that PLD has myocardial toxicity, it seems to have less cardiotoxicity with non-liposomal forms of doxorubicin. Although testing for congestive heart failure with cumulative doses in excess of 450 mg/m^2 is suggested, multiple studies show no adverse cardiac impact with cumulative doses of up to 1040 mg/m^2. Hepatotoxicity may occur with PLD, and this may be additive to any such toxicity caused by antiretroviral medications. Nausea and vomiting with dosing is also common. Doxorubicin is pregnancy category D. It is embryotoxic and an abortifacient and should be avoided in women who are pregnant or who are planning to conceive during treatment.

TABLE 190-21
Risks and Precautions With Doxorubicin Use

- Absolute contraindications
  - Hypersensitivity to anthracyclines
- Relative contraindications
  - Pregnancy/lactation (category D)
- Common adverse effects
  - Myelosuppression
  - GI distress
  - Toxic hepatitis
  - Hyperpigmentation of the skin and nails

A small percentage of patients may experience an initial infusion reaction, which typically resolves and does not occur with later dosing. Other effects include hyperpigmentation of the skin and nails, alopecia, acral erythema and dysesthesias, urticaria, radiation recall reactions, or a pustular psoriasiform drug eruption.

Drug Interactions: Although no drug interaction studies have been conducted with PLD, it is reasonable to conclude it may interact with drugs known to interact with conventional doxorubicin, which includes digoxin, cyclosporine, calcium channel blockers, and ciprofloxacin.

Despite continued introduction of highly targeted immunomodulating drugs ("biologics"; (Chap. 194), cytotoxic agents remain as important medications in the therapeutic arsenal of dermatologists. Table 190-22 summarizes the major indications, principal mechanism of action, and common toxicities of these agents.

MUCOCUTANEOUS REACTIONS TO CYTOTOXIC AGENTS

Specific cytotoxic agents may be used by dermatologists for the treatment of severe and recalcitrant dermatologic disease, but typically only certain agents are employed, and dosages are typically less than those used for other indications. Mucocutaneous reactions to these medications initiated by other providers are commonly seen in patients during consultation. A morphologic approach to those reactions is useful. To this end, subcategories of mucocutaneous reactions to various cytotoxic agents are examined, paying particular attention to those that may provoke characteristic mucocutaneous reactions.

HAIR FOLLICLE COMPLICATIONS

Alopecia: One of the most widely recognized cutaneous effects of cytotoxic agents is alopecia. Cytotoxic agent–induced alopecia is a form of anagen effluvium caused by interruption of the rapidly dividing cells of the hair matrix. The particular agent, dose, schedule, and route of administration impact the degree of hair loss, yet at equivalent dosages, intravenous administration is generally more deleterious than oral administration. Numerous cytotoxic agents produce alopecia, but doxorubicin, cyclophosphamide, and vincristine are most often implicated (Table 190-23).[134,135]

Cytotoxic agent–induced alopecia usually begins 2 to 4 weeks after therapy and may progress for several months. Up to 85% to 90% of the hair may be lost; the remaining fraction spared is that normally in telogen. Loss of hair on the scalp and eyebrows is most noticeable, but eyelashes and body hair may be shed as well (Fig. 190-2). The alopecia typically resolves with cessation of treatment, although regrowth may occur with a different color, quality, or texture. Permanent alopecia has occurred most often with high-dose busulfan.[136]

TABLE 190-22
Summary of Cytotoxic Agents Commonly Used in Dermatology

DRUG	COMMON INDICATIONS	MECHANISM OF ACTION	TYPICAL DOSE	KEY SIDE EFFECTS
Methotrexate	Psoriasis Connective tissue disease	Inhibition of dihydrofolate reductase	7.5-25	Myelosuppression Toxic hepatitis Liver fibrosis/cirrhosis
Azathioprine	Bullous disorders Connective tissue disease	Forms purine analogs that interrupt DNA/RNA synthesis	0.5-3.0 mg/kg/d (dependent on innate TPMT expression)	Myelosuppression GI distress Increased risk of malignancy
Thioguanine	Psoriasis	Forms purine analogs that interrupt DNA/RNA synthesis	80-120 mg/d or 120-160 mg 3×/wk (dependent on innate TPMT expression)	Myelosuppression
Hydroxyurea	Psoriasis	Inhibition of ribonucleotide diphosphate reductase	1-2 g/d	Myelosuppression Dermatomyositis-like reaction
Cyclophosphamide	Vasculitis Connective tissue disease Advanced cutaneous T-cell lymphoma	Metabolites undergo physiochemical reactions with DNA (alkylation)	1-3 mg/kg/d or 0.5-1.0 g/monthly	GI distress Myelosuppression Hemorrhagic cystitis Bladder carcinogenesis
Chlorambucil	Vasculitis Connective tissue disease	Physiochemical reactions with DNA (alkylation)	0.05-0.2 mg/kg/d	GI distress Myelosuppression Increased risk of malignancy
Doxorubicin (liposomal)	AIDS-related Kaposi sarcoma	Intercalation into DNA with termination of synthesis	20-30 mg/m² every 2-3 wk	GI distress Toxic hepatitis Possible cardiotoxicity Infusion site reactions

TPMT, thiopurine methyltransferase.

TABLE 190-23
Cytotoxic Agents Associated With Alopecia

- Bleomycin
- Busulfan (significant risk of permanent loss)
- Cytarabine
- Dacarbazine
- Daunorubicin
- Docetaxel
- **Doxorubicin**
- Etoposide
- Fluorouracil
- **Hydroxyurea**
- **Methotrexate**
- Nitrogen mustard derivatives (**cyclophosphamide, chlorambucil**)
- Nitrosoureas
- Paclitaxel
- Procarbazine
- Thiotepa
- Vinca alkaloids

Agents in bold represent medications more often used by dermatologists in treating patients with skin disease.

TABLE 190-24
Cytotoxic Agents Associated With Nail Plate Malformations (Dystrophy)

- Bleomycin
- **Cyclophosphamide**
- Daunorubicin
- Docetaxel
- **Doxorubicin**
- Fluorouracil
- **Hydroxyurea**
- Mitoxantrone

Scalp cooling has been used with limited success to minimize hair loss, likely by reducing biochemical activity, but it may create a haven for malignant cells and it therefore remains a controversial intervention, particularly for hematologic malignancies.[134,137] Topical minoxidil shortened the duration of alopecia in breast cancer patients receiving adjuvant chemotherapy and in patients with gynecologic malignancies who received cyclophosphamide, doxorubicin, or cis-platinum, but it did not induce significant regrowth in patients with permanent alopecia due to busulfan or cyclophosphamide.[134,138]

Acneiform Eruption: Classic cytotoxin-induced folliculitis begins as erythematous macules, followed in days by the appearance of papules, and then pustules. Lesions predominate on the face and upper trunk. The eruption typically resolves over 2 weeks, but comedones may persist, or postinflammatory hyperpigmentation may result. Simple acne vulgaris also may be aggravated by androgens used in conjunction with chemotherapeutic agents in some multidrug regimens. Folliculitis is most often associated with actinomycin D and less often with MTX or cisplatin.[139]

NAIL COMPLICATIONS

Malformed Nail Plates (Dystrophy): Nail changes may sometimes occur in patients treated with cytotoxic agents (Table 190-24). Mild nail reactions produce Beau lines, for example, typically seen following trauma. Severe reactions may produce onycholysis or onychomadesis (Fig. 190-3). The great toenail is most

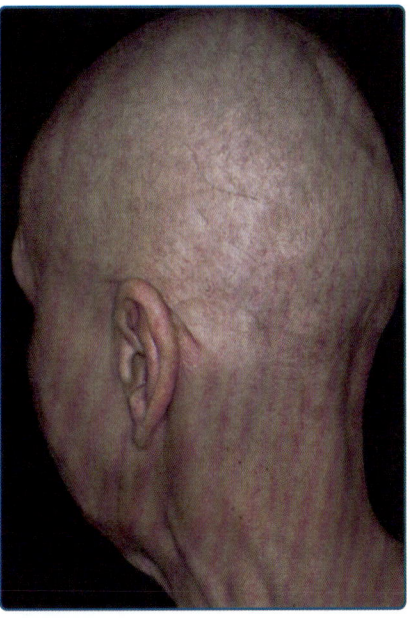

Figure 190-2 Alopecia after the administration of combined chemotherapy with cyclophosphamide, doxorubicin, and vincristine.

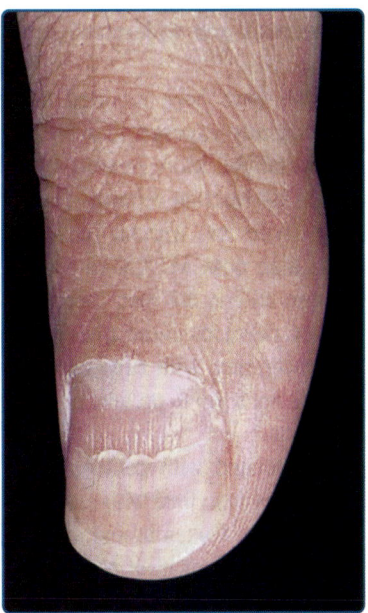

Figure 190-3 Presence of proximal indented Beau line and distal band of leukonychia due to cyclophosphamide 3 months after bone marrow transplantation.

often affected.[104] Less common nail problems caused by cytotoxic drugs include nail bed pain, thickening or thinning of the nail plate, and splinter hemorrhage or subungual hemorrhage. Anthracyclines (doxorubicin) and taxanes (paclitaxel, docetaxel) most often yield onychodystrophy, with paclitaxel and docetaxel producing nail changes in up to 30% to 40% of those treated.[135,140]

Nail Pigmentation: Treatment with cytotoxic agents may lead to leukonychia or hyperpigmentation of the nail plate. Leukonychia is characterized by a white discoloration in the nail; although the mechanism is unknown, it is presumed to be cytotoxic in nature. Mees lines is a type of patterned leukonychia that was described in 1919 as transverse white lines after arsenic exposure.[141] Cytotoxic agents that most often lead to leukonychia include doxorubicin, vincristine, cyclophosphamide, MTX, and 5-fluorouracil.[142]

Nail hyperpigmentation usually develops weeks or months after chemotherapy. Hyperpigmentation of the nail may be oriented longitudinally, horizontally, diffusely, or in a perilunar fashion.[143] Various mechanisms have been proposed, including genetic predisposition, toxic effect on the nail matrix, photosensitization, or focal stimulation of melanocytes. Blacks are more often affected, presumably due to increased numbers of melanocytes within the nail matrix.[144] Cyclophosphamide, doxorubicin, hydroxyurea, and bleomycin are most often implicated in nail hyperpigmentation.[145] Typically, leukonychia or nail hyperpigmentation due to cytotoxic agents resolves with cessation of therapy.

ECCRINE GLAND COMPLICATIONS

Neutrophilic Eccrine Hidradenitis: Neutrophilic eccrine hidradenitis (NEH) consists of tender, erythematous macules, papules, and plaques on the trunk, neck, and extremities that develop after exposure to cytotoxic agents (Fig. 190-4).[146,147] Lesions resolve spontaneously over a period of days. Histologic changes include a characteristically perieccrine

TABLE 190-25
Cytotoxic Agents Associated With Adnexal Toxicity

NEUTROPHILIC ECCRINE HIDRADENITIS	ECCRINE SYRINGOSQUAMOUS METAPLASIA
Bleomycin	Bleomycin
Chlorambucil	Cytarabine (common)
Cytarabine (common)	Daunorubicin
Daunorubicin	**Doxorubicin**
Doxorubicin (common)	Mitoxantrone
Mitoxantrone	Suramin
Vincristine	

Agents in bold represent medications more often used by dermatologists in treating patients with skin disease.

neutrophilic infiltrate. Apocrine gland involvement also has been identified.[148] Concentration of the cytotoxic agent within sweat is the likely mechanism of injury. NEH is most often associated with cytarabine, but other agents have been implicated (Table 190-25). A similar condition unassociated with cytotoxic agents is recognized, suggesting the lesions represent a final common pathway of adnexal injury. In a single case report, prophylactic dosing of dapsone prevented NEH in a patient who had had multiple prior eruptions due to lomustine, an alkylating agent.[149]

Syringosquamous Metaplasia: Chemotherapy-induced syringosquamous metaplasia (CISM) is closely related to NEH. Like neutrophilic hidradenitis, direct cytotoxic injury of sweat ducts is implicated. Clinically, CISM presents as erythematous papular eruptions, similar to miliaria, which erupt 2 to 39 days after administration of the cytotoxic agent.[150,151] The papules resolve approximately 4 weeks after discontinuance. Histologic examination demonstrates prominent squamous metaplasia of the upper sweat duct, with necrotic ductal epithelial cells; inflammation is minimal. On occasion, CISM may even mimic SCC.[152] Cytarabine has been most often associated with CISM.

CHEMOTHERAPY-INDUCED EPIDERMAL COMPLICATIONS

Acral Erythema: Multiple cytotoxic agents may yield a distinct cutaneous reaction known as toxic *acral erythema*. The reaction usually develops 4 to 23 days after initiation of chemotherapy as painful, sharply demarcated erythema of the palmoplantar surfaces, with associated edema (Fig. 190-5).[153] In severe cases, large bullae may extend over the dorsum of the hands and feet.[154] Pain may limit ambulation or use of the hands. Therapy is limited mostly to analgesics and emollients, although pyridoxine supplementation may improve dysesthesias. The reaction is self-limited and resolves over 2 to 4 weeks. Recurrence with subsequent exposure is highly variable. Although the etiology of acral erythema is unknown, the elevated levels

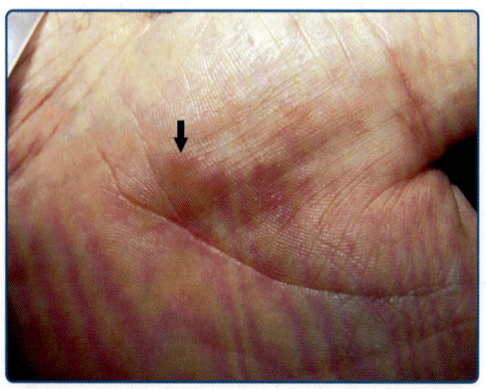

Figure 190-4 Neutrophilic eccrine hidradenitis (*arrow*). (From the Archives of Fitzsimmons Army Medical Center.)

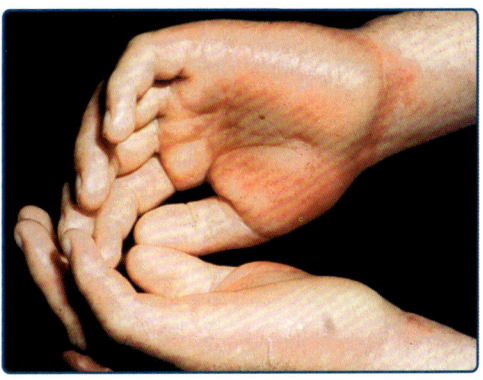

Figure 190-5 Cytarabine-induced painful acral erythema with edema.

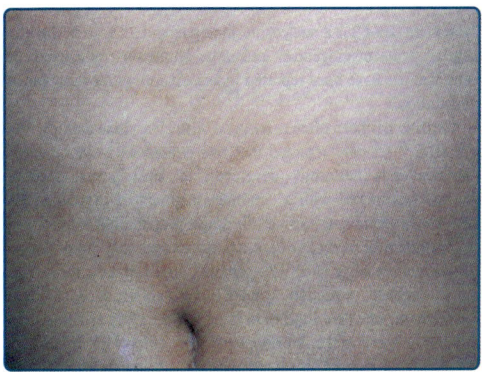

Figure 190-6 Flagellate hyperpigmentation occurs 2 weeks after administration of bleomycin.

of cytotoxic agents within eccrine glands of acral skin has been proposed to play a role. In support of such a theory, coexistent syringosquamous metaplasia has been demonstrated.[155,156] Acral erythema is most common with cytarabine, doxorubicin, fluorouracil, and MTX (Table 190-26). Long-term hydroxyurea therapy may produce a unique form of acral erythema that is linear and resembles dermatomyositis, without any corresponding muscle findings (drug-induced pseudo-dermatomyositis); rarely, the face may be involved.[63,157]

Inflammation of Actinic Keratoses:
A number of different cytotoxic agents and chemotherapeutic protocols yield inflammation of actinic keratoses. Systemic fluorouracil is the most common cause of inflamed actinic keratoses, and this should come as no surprise to dermatologists.[158] The reaction usually develops within 1 week of initiating chemotherapy. The actinic keratoses may resolve or remain after completion of the therapy. A similar reaction within seborrheic keratoses has been reported to occur with cytarabine and may mimic the sign of Leser-Trélat or herpes zoster.[159,160]

Cutaneous Hyperpigmentation:
Bleomycin may produce a unique form of flagellate (linear) hyperpigmentation of the skin in those exposed; typically after cumulative doses of 90 to 285 mg.[157,161] Lesions begin as linear, erythematous, pruritic lesions that are slowly replaced by hyperpigmentation and are present hours to weeks after dosing (Fig. 190-6). The eruption usually resolves without treatment over weeks to months. The pathogenesis of bleomycin-induced flagellate hyperpigmentation is unknown.

Bleomycin may also produce patchy pigmentation in areas of pressure, within the palmar creases, or within striae distensae. Other unique forms of cutaneous hyperpigmentation are recognized, such as the serpentine supravenous hyperpigmentation that may accompany fluorouracil infusions[162] or the polycyclic bands of pigmentation on the scalp occurring with daunorubicin.[144]

Many antineoplastic drugs may lead to other forms of hyperpigmentation, including patchy, acral, photoaccentuated, polycyclic, occlusion-accentuated, pressure-accentuated (Fig. 190-7), or generalized patterns (Table 190-27).[139] Although the cause of cutaneous hyperpigmentation is unknown, postulated mechanisms include a toxic effect on melanocytes, increased drug deposition due to increased blood flow,

TABLE 190-26
Cytotoxic Agents Associated With Acral Erythema

- Bleomycin
- **Cyclophosphamide**
- Cytarabine
- Daunorubicin
- Docetaxel
- **Doxorubicin**
- Etoposide
- Fluorouracil
- **Hydroxyurea** (dermatomyositis-like eruption possible)
- Lomustine
- Mercaptopurine
- **Methotrexate**
- Paclitaxel
- Suramin
- Vinblastine

Agents in bold represent medications more often used by dermatologists in treating patients with skin disease.

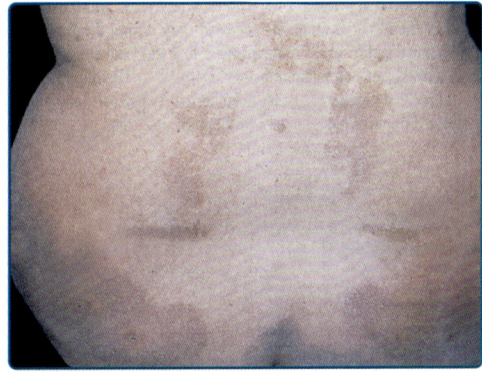

Figure 190-7 Hyperpigmentation at sites of occlusion during administration of thiotepa.

TABLE 190-27
Cytotoxic Agents Associated With Skin Hyperpigmentation

DRUG	PATTERN OF PIGMENTATION
Bleomycin	Flagellate
Busulphan	Dusky, may appear similar to Addison disease
Cisplatin	Pressure-induced
Cyclophosphamide	May be localized to palms, soles, or nails
Dactinomycin	Diffuse
Daunorubicin	Sun-exposed areas
Doxorubicin	Diffuse, particularly nails
Etoposide	Occluded areas
Fluorouracil	Sun-exposed areas, areas of prior irradiation, nails
Hydroxyurea	Diffuse, particularly nails
Ifosfamide	Hands, feet, and occluded areas
Methotrexate	Sun-exposed areas, hair may develop "flag sign"
Nitrosoureas	Occluded areas
Paclitaxel	Localized
Plicamycin	Localized
Procarbazine	Diffuse
Tamoxifen	Hair pigmentation
Thiotepa	Occluded areas
Vinca alkaloids	Localized

Agents in bold represent medications more often managed by dermatologists in treating patients with skin disease.

TABLE 190-28
Cytotoxic Agents With Radiation Reactions

- Photosensitivity
  - Dacarbazine
  - Fluorouracil
  - **Hydroxyurea**
  - **Methotrexate**
  - Mitomycin
  - **Thioguanine**
  - Vinblastine
- Radiation enhancement
  - Bleomycin
  - Cisplatin
  - Dactinomycin
  - **Doxorubicin**
  - Fluorouracil
  - **Hydroxyurea**
  - **Methotrexate**
- Radiation recall reaction
  - Bleomycin
  - Cytarabine (common)
  - Dactinomycin
  - **Doxorubicin**
  - Etoposide 1
  - Fluorouracil
  - **Hydroxyurea**
  - Lomustine
  - **Methotrexate**
  - Melphalan
  - Mitomycin
  - Paclitaxel
- Sunburn recall reaction
  - **Methotrexate**
  - Suramin

Agents in bold represent medications more often used by dermatologists in treating patients with skin disease.

local toxicity due to concentration in sweat, associated endocrinologic abnormalities, and drug-induced depletion of tyrosinase inhibitors.[143]

Photosensitivity: Most chemotherapy-induced photosensitivity is phototoxic rather than photoallergic in nature (Table 190-28; see also Chap. 97). Phototoxic reactions begin rapidly after administration and often mimic sunburns, with burning, erythema, and even vesicles or bullae. Photoallergic reactions typically present as an eczematous process whereas photoallergic processes are dependent on sensitization and may be delayed weeks or months after an initial exposure.

Radiation Recall Reaction: Recall reactions consist of erythema confined to an area of prior radiation exposure or sunburn. Severe cases may develop vesiculation (Fig. 190-8). Radiation recall may occur years after irradiation, and the pathogenesis is unknown. It has been postulated that radiation-damaged keratinocytes are further damaged by the administration of the cytotoxic agent (Table 190-28).[163] Methotrexate often engenders a unique recall reaction to sunburn when dosed 1 to 3 days after exposure.[164] Folinic acid supplementation (leucovorin rescue) does not prevent UV sunburn recall reactions due to MTX.

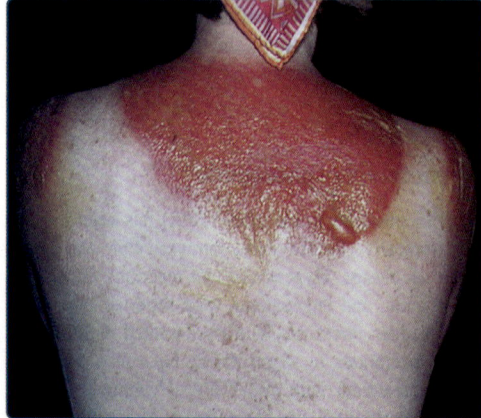

Figure 190-8 Reactivation of solar erythema 2 days after high-dose methotrexate administration to a young woman with choriocarcinoma. (From Bronner AK, Hood AF. Cutaneous complications of chemotherapeutic agents. J Am Acad Dermatol 1983;9:645, with permission.)

Radiation Enhancement Reactions: Radiation enhancement is a synergistic reaction between an antineoplastic agent and irradiation. This radiosensitization is often desired in antineoplastic treatment, but it may lead to adverse effects on the skin. The result may be radiation dermatitis that presents initially as pain and erythema followed by desquamation and hyperpigmentation. Although a number of chemotherapeutic agents may produce this reaction, doxorubicin and dactinomycin are most often implicated (Table 190-28).[139]

CHEMOTHERAPY-INDUCED DERMAL COMPLICATIONS

Local Injury: Extravasation of chemotherapeutic agents may occur in up to 6% of adults treated with infusions and is likely an even more common occurrence among pediatric patients.[143,165] As expected, the degree of injury is related to the drug used, the rate of delivery, the concentration of the agent, and the amount extravasated.

Agents with minimal toxicity on extravasation may produce only a chemical cellulitis or phlebitis and are classified as irritants. Chemical cellulitis manifests as erythema, induration, and pain at the injection site. Sometimes it may follow the course of a vein. It is often of short duration and resolves without treatment. Chemotherapy-induced phlebitis manifests as linear cords, often with accompanying discomfort.

Vesicants are agents, which on extravasation yield direct-tissue necrosis. Chemotherapy-induced tissue necrosis can be a devastating complication. Extravasation should always be treated by immediate discontinuance of the infusion and the application of either hot or cold packs. Cold packs are used for all chemotherapeutic agents except vinca alkaloids to localize the drug and promote degradation. Vinca alkaloids are treated with hot packs because application of cold promotes tissue necrosis.[166] Doxorubicin is perhaps the most dangerous of all vesicants, and extravasation of this agent may yield ulcers that progress for months that may even erode into tendon or bone (Fig. 190-9). Severe ulcerations caused by extravasation of doxorubicin may require wide excision and skin grafting.

Other treatments advocated for specific situations include (1) topical dimethyl sulfoxide (DMSO); (2) local injection of hyaluronidase; or (3) potent topical, intralesional, or oral steroids. DMSO is a topical solvent that has free radical scavenging and antioxidant properties; it may hasten removal of extravasated drugs. Topical DMSO may have benefit in anthracycline-induced skin ulceration.[167,168] Hyaluronidase degrades hyaluronic acid, breaking down subcutaneous tissue, and promoting drug diffusion through the interstitial space. It appears effective in vinca alkaloid, epipodophyllotoxin, and paclitaxel extravasations, but should not be used in anthracycline extravasation.[169,170] Hyaluronidase is contraindicated in sites involved with malignancy or superinfection. Finally, histologic examination of extravasation injuries has demonstrated surprisingly few inflammatory cells in areas of tissue damage, perhaps explaining why corticosteroids are, in general, of little value in management.[167,170]

Sclerotic Dermal Reactions: Bleomycin and docetaxel produce sclerotic tissue reactions that may be localized, regional, or diffuse in extent.[171,172] Localized tissue reactions may mimic morphea or systemic sclerosis. Melphalan may produce a unique form of reticulate scleroderma after limb perfusion. The mechanism of tissue sclerosis is unknown. Biopsies of cytotoxic agent–induced dermal sclerosis may be indistinguishable from morphea or systemic sclerosis. In some cases, the sclerosis resolved after withdrawal of the offending agent.

Raynaud Phenomenon: Secondary Raynaud phenomenon, with or without digital ulceration, is most often associated with bleomycin, vincristine, cisplatin, or cisplatin with gemcitabine.[173-175] This reaction may occur with systemic chemotherapy or after intralesional injection to treat verruca vulgaris. The mechanism of development is unknown, but bleomycin is known to be toxic to endothelial cells. In one study of 90 patients receiving bleomycin for testicular cancer, 37% developed Raynaud phenomenon, with 7% having transient disease.[173] Risk factors for the development of Raynaud phenomenon include combination therapy with vinblastine or high cumulative doses of bleomycin.

CHEMOTHERAPY-INDUCED MUCOSAL COMPLICATIONS

Oral complications may occur in up to 40% of those receiving chemotherapy. Because of a high inherent proliferative index, the mucosa is susceptible to the effects of multiple cytotoxic agents. Young patients and those with preexisting oral disease appear even more susceptible.[143]

Mucositis/Stomatitis: A wide range of cytotoxic agents may induce stomatitis (Table 190-29). Patients with cytotoxic agent–induced stomatitis usually

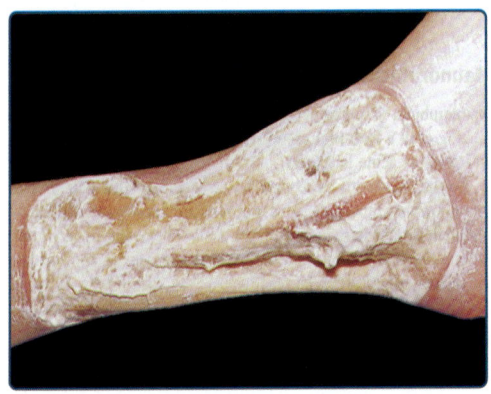

Figure 190-9 Severe tissue necrosis after extravasation of doxorubicin.

TABLE 190-29
Cytotoxic Agents Associated With Mucositis

- Bleomycin
- **Cyclophosphamide**
- Cytarabine
- Dactinomycin
- Daunorubicin
- Docetaxel
- **Doxorubicin**
- Fluorouracil
- **Hydroxyurea**
- Mercaptopurine
- **Methotrexate**
- Mitomycin
- Nitrosoureas
- Paclitaxel
- Plicamycin
- Procarbazine
- Vinblastine

Agents in bold represent medications more often used by dermatologists in treating patients with skin disease.

experience burning and mucosal erythema days after administration. Painful erosions and ulcerations often follow (Fig. 190-10). The mouth is most often affected, especially the buccal mucosa and tongue, but any mucosal surface may be involved. Mucositis may be complicated by secondary bacterial or fungal infection. Meticulous, but not overly aggressive, hygiene may reduce the incidence of secondary infection, and antibiotics and antifungal agents are often used. A meta-analysis of treatments for cytotoxic agent–induced mucositis suggested that simple modalities, such as ice chips, had equivalent benefit as more aggressive interventions.[176,177] Oral hemorrhage may be secondary to chemotherapy-induced thrombocytopenia, and a careful clinical examination is always required.

Mucosal Hyperpigmentation: Many cytotoxic agents induce mucosal hyperpigmentation. Mucosal hyperpigmentation may manifest as various patterns, including linear, patchy, and macular forms. Some agents tend to affect certain anatomic areas such as the gingival margin (cyclophosphamide) or tongue (fluorouracil). The mechanism of mucosal hyperpigmentation is not well understood. Typically, cytotoxic agent–induced hyperpigmentation resolves slowly over weeks to months after discontinuance. One notable exception is mucosal hyperpigmentation caused by cyclophosphamide, which may be permanent. Cyclophosphamide may also produce a permanent pigmented band on the teeth.

ACKNOWLEDGMENTS

We would like to thank Drs Aieska De Souza, Megan M. Moore, and Bruce E. Strober, the authors of the previous version of this chapter. Many of the display items have been reused from the previous version.

REFERENCES

1. West J, Ogston S, Foerster J. Safety and efficacy of methotrexate in psoriasis: a meta-analysis of published trials. *PLoS One.* 2016;11(5):e0153740.
2. Armstrong AW, Bagel J, Van Voorhees AS, et al. Combining biologic therapies with other systemic treatments in psoriasis: evidence-based, best-practice recommendations from the Medical Board of the National Psoriasis Foundation. *JAMA Dermatol.* 2015; 151(4):432-438.
3. Cronstein BN. The mechanism of action of methotrexate. *Rheum Dis Clin North Am.* 1997;23(4):739-755.
4. Said S, Jeffes EW, Weinstein GD. Methotrexate. *Clin Dermatol.* 1997;15(5):781-797.
5. Schiff MH, Jaffe JS, Freundlich B. Head-to-head, randomised, crossover study of oral versus subcutaneous methotrexate in patients with rheumatoid arthritis: drug-exposure limitations of oral methotrexate at doses ≥15 mg may be overcome with subcutaneous administration. *Ann Rheum Dis.* 2014;73(8):1549-1551.
6. Rees RB, Bennett JH. Methotrexate vs. aminopterin for psoriasis. *Arch Dermatol.* 1961;83:970-972.
7. Kalb RE, Strober B, Weinstein G, et al. Methotrexate and psoriasis: 2009 National Psoriasis Foundation Consensus Conference. *J Am Acad Dermatol.* 2009; 60(5):824-837.
8. Peckham PE, Weinstein GD, McCullough JL. The treatment of severe psoriasis. A national survey. *Arch Dermatol.* 1987;123(10):1303-1307.
9. Beyer V, Wolverton SE. Recent trends in systemic psoriasis treatment costs. *Arch Dermatol.* 2010; 146(1):46-54.
10. Newland KM, McCormack CJ, Twigger R, et al. The efficacy of methotrexate for lymphomatoid papulosis. *J Am Acad Dermatol.* 2015;72(6):1088-1090.
11. Wood GS, Wu J. Methotrexate and Pralatrexate. *Dermatol Clin.* 2015;33(4):747-755.
12. Demierre M-F, Vachon L, Ho V, et al. Phase 1/2 pilot study of methotrexate-laurocapram topical gel for the treatment of patients with early-stage mycosis fungoides. *Arch Dermatol.* 2003;139(5):624-628.
13. Zackheim HS, Kashani-Sabet M, McMillan A. Low-dose methotrexate to treat mycosis fungoides:

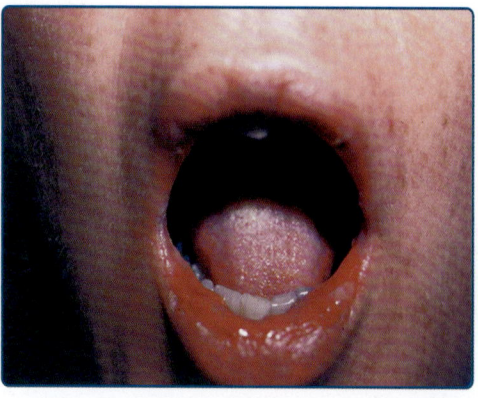

Figure 190-10 Stomatitis induced by combined chemotherapy with cytarabine, doxorubicin, and methotrexate. (Used with permission from Allan C. Harrington, MD.)

a retrospective study in 69 patients. *J Am Acad Dermatol*. 2003;49(5):873-878.
14. Menon K, Van Voorhees AS, Bebo BF, et al. Psoriasis in patients with HIV infection: from the medical board of the National Psoriasis Foundation. *J Am Acad Dermatol*. 2010;62(2):291-299.
15. Targeted Tuberculin Testing and Treatment of Latent Tuberculosis Infection ATS/CDC Statement Committee on Latent Tuberculosis Infection Membership List. https://www.cdc.gov/mmwr/preview/mmwrhtml/rr4906a1.htm.
16. Gutierrez-Ureña S, Molina JF, García CO, et al. Pancytopenia secondary to methotrexate therapy in rheumatoid arthritis. *Arthritis Rheum*. 1996;39(2):272-276.
17. Tugwell P, Bennett K, Bell M, et al. Methotrexate in rheumatoid arthritis. Feedback on American College of Physicians guidelines. *Ann Intern Med*. 1989;110(8):581-583.
18. Zachariae H, Aslam HM, Bjerring P, et al. Serum aminoterminal propeptide of type III procollagen in psoriasis and psoriatic arthritis: relation to liver fibrosis and arthritis. *J Am Acad Dermatol*. 1991;25(1, pt 1):50-53.
19. Nagy Z, Czirják L. Increased levels of amino terminal propeptide of type III procollagen are an unfavourable predictor of survival in systemic sclerosis. *Clin Exp Rheumatol*. 2005;23(2):165-172.
20. Teppo A-M, Törnroth T, Honkanen E, et al. Urinary amino-terminal propeptide of type III procollagen (PIIINP) as a marker of interstitial fibrosis in renal transplant recipients. *Transplantation*. 2003;75(12):2113-2119.
21. dos Santos Moreira C, Serejo F, Alcântara P, et al. Procollagen type III amino terminal peptide and myocardial fibrosis: a study in hypertensive patients with and without left ventricular hypertrophy. *Rev Port Cardiol*. 2015;34(5):309-314.
22. Lynch M, Higgins E, McCormick PA, et al. The use of transient elastography and FibroTest for monitoring hepatotoxicity in patients receiving methotrexate for psoriasis. *JAMA Dermatol*. 2014;150(8):856-862.
23. Shaheen AAM, Wan AF, Myers RP. FibroTest and FibroScan for the prediction of hepatitis C-related fibrosis: a systematic review of diagnostic test accuracy. *Am J Gastroenterol*. 2007;102(11):2589-2600.
24. Coulson IH, Mckenzie J, Neild VS, et al. A comparison of liver ultrasound with liver biopsy histology in psoriatics receiving long-term methotrexate therapy. *Br J Dermatol*. 1987;116(4):491-495.
25. Miller JA, Dodd H, Rustin MH, et al. Ultrasound as a screening procedure for methotrexate-induced hepatic damage in severe psoriasis. *Br J Dermatol*. 1985;113(6):699-705.
26. Talwalkar JA, Kurtz DM, Schoenleber SJ, et al. Ultrasound-based transient elastography for the detection of hepatic fibrosis: systematic review and meta-analysis. *Clin Gastroenterol Hepatol*. 2007;5(10):1214-1220.
27. Berends MA, Snoek J, de Jong EM, et al. Biochemical and biophysical assessment of MTX-induced liver fibrosis in psoriasis patients: FibroTest predicts the presence and Fibroscan predicts the absence of significant liver fibrosis. *Liver Int*. 2007;27(5):639-645.
28. Bray AP, Barnova I, Przemioslo R, et al. Liver fibrosis screening for patients with psoriasis taking methotrexate: a cross-sectional study comparing transient elastography and liver biopsy. *Br J Dermatol*. 2012;166(5):1125-1127.
29. Zachariae H. Liver biopsies and methotrexate: a time for reconsideration? *J Am Acad Dermatol*. 2000;42(3):531-534.
30. Osuga T, Ikura Y, Kadota C, et al. Significance of liver biopsy for the evaluation of methotrexate-induced liver damage in patients with rheumatoid arthritis. *Int J Clin Exp Pathol*. 2015;8(2):1961-1966.
31. Endresen GK, Husby G. Folate supplementation during methotrexate treatment of patients with rheumatoid arthritis. An update and proposals for guidelines. *Scand J Rheumatol*. 2001;30(3):129-134.
32. Ortiz Z, Shea B, Suarez-Almazor ME, et al. The efficacy of folic acid and folinic acid in reducing methotrexate gastrointestinal toxicity in rheumatoid arthritis. A metaanalysis of randomized controlled trials. *J Rheumatol*. 1998;25(1):36-43.
33. Duhra P. Treatment of gastrointestinal symptoms associated with methotrexate therapy for psoriasis. *J Am Acad Dermatol*. 1993;28(3):466-469.
34. Morgan S l, Alarcón GS, Krumdieck CL. Folic acid supplementation during methotrexate therapy: it makes sense. *J Rheumatol*. 1993;20(6):929-930.
35. Salim A, Tan E, Ilchyshyn A, et al. Folic acid supplementation during treatment of psoriasis with methotrexate: a randomized, double-blind, placebo-controlled trial. *Br J Dermatol*. 2006;154(6):1169-1174.
36. Pearce HP, Wilson BB. Erosion of psoriatic plaques: an early sign of methotrexate toxicity. *J Am Acad Dermatol*. 1996;35(5)(pt 2):835-838.
37. Goerttler E, Kutzner H, Peter HH, et al. Methotrexate-induced papular eruption in patients with rheumatic diseases: a distinctive adverse cutaneous reaction produced by methotrexate in patients with collagen vascular diseases. *J Am Acad Dermatol*. 1999;40(5, pt 1):702-707.
38. Scott FI, Mamtani R, Brensinger CM, et al. Risk of nonmelanoma skin cancer associated with the use of immunosuppressant and biologic agents in patients with a history of autoimmune disease and nonmelanoma skin cancer. *JAMA Dermatol*. 2016;152(2):164-172.
39. Buchbinder R, Barber M, Heuzenroeder L, et al. Incidence of melanoma and other malignancies among rheumatoid arthritis patients treated with methotrexate. *Arthritis Rheum*. 2008;59(6):794-799.
40. Gelfand JM, Berlin J, Van Voorhees A, et al. Lymphoma rates are low but increased in patients with psoriasis: results from a population-based cohort study in the United Kingdom. *Arch Dermatol*. 2003;139(11):1425-1429.
41. Salliot C, van der Heijde D. Long-term safety of methotrexate monotherapy in patients with rheumatoid arthritis: a systematic literature research. *Ann Rheum Dis*. 2009;68(7):1100-1104.
42. Shimizu Y, Nakajima A, Inoue E, et al. Characteristics and risk factors of lymphoproliferative disorders among patients with rheumatoid arthritis concurrently treated with methotrexate: a nested case-control study of the IORRA cohort. *Clin Rheumatol*. 2017;36(6):1237-1245.
43. McKenna KE, Burrows D. Pulmonary toxicity in a patient with psoriasis receiving methotrexate therapy. *Clin Exp Dermatol*. 2000;25(1):24-27.
44. Kremer JM, Alarcón GS, Weinblatt ME, et al. Clinical, laboratory, radiographic, and histopathologic features of methotrexate-associated lung injury in patients with rheumatoid arthritis: a multicenter

study with literature review. *Arthritis Rheum.* 1997;40(10):1829-1837.
45. Conway R, Low C, Coughlan RJ, et al. Risk of liver injury among methotrexate users: a meta-analysis of randomised controlled trials. *Semin Arthritis Rheum.* 2015;45(2):156-162.
46. Cottin V, Tébib J, Massonnet B, et al. Pulmonary function in patients receiving long-term low-dose methotrexate. *Chest.* 1996;109(4):933-938.
47. Basile A, Simzar S, Bentow J, et al. Disseminated *Strongyloides stercoralis*: hyperinfection during medical immunosuppression. *J Am Acad Dermatol.* 2010;63(5):896-902.
48. Kaneko Y, Suwa A, Ikeda Y, et al. *Pneumocystis jiroveci* pneumonia associated with low-dose methotrexate treatment for rheumatoid arthritis: report of two cases and review of the literature. *Mod Rheumatol.* 2006;16(1):36-38.
49. Duncan KO, Imaeda S, Milstone LM. *Pneumocystis carinii* pneumonia complicating methotrexate treatment of pityriasis rubra pilaris. *J Am Acad Dermatol.* 1998;39(2, pt 1):276-278.
50. Witty LA, Steiner F, Curfman M, et al. Disseminated histoplasmosis in patients receiving low-dose methotrexate therapy for psoriasis. *Arch Dermatol.* 1992;128(1):91-93.
51. Altz-Smith M, Kendall LG, Stamm AM. Cryptococcosis associated with low-dose methotrexate for arthritis. *Am J Med.* 1987;83(1):179-181.
52. Alkins SA, Byrd JC, Morgan SK, et al. Anaphylactoid reactions to methotrexate. *Cancer.* 1996;77(10):2123-2126.
53. Menting SP, Dekker PM, Limpens J, et al. Methotrexate dosing regimen for plaque-type psoriasis: a systematic review of the use of test-dose, start-dose, dosing scheme, dose adjustments, maximum dose and folic acid supplementation. *Acta Derm Venereol.* 2016;96(1):23-28.
54. van Ede AE, Laan RF, Blom HJ, et al. Homocysteine and folate status in methotrexate-treated patients with rheumatoid arthritis. *Rheumatology (Oxford).* 2002;41(6):658-665.
55. Strober BE, Menon K. Folate supplementation during methotrexate therapy for patients with psoriasis. *J Am Acad Dermatol.* 2005;53(4):652-659.
56. Thomas DR, Dover JS, Camp RD. Pancytopenia induced by the interaction between methotrexate and trimethoprim-sulfamethoxazole. *J Am Acad Dermatol.* 1987;17(6):1055-1056.
57. Nyce J, Liu L, Jones PA. Variable effects of DNA-synthesis inhibitors upon DNA methylation in mammalian cells. *Nucleic Acids Res.* 1986;14(10):4353-4367.
58. Moschella SL, Greenwald MA. Psoriasis with hydroxyurea. An 18-month study of 60 patients. *Arch Dermatol.* 1973;107(3):363-368.
59. Ranjan N, Sharma NL, Shanker V, et al. Methotrexate versus hydroxycarbamide (hydroxyurea) as a weekly dose to treat moderate-to-severe chronic plaque psoriasis: a comparative study. *J Dermatol Treat.* 2007;18(5):295-300.
60. Kumar B, Saraswat A, Kaur I. Rediscovering hydroxyurea: its role in recalcitrant psoriasis. *Int J Dermatol.* 2001;40(8):530-534.
61. Smith CH. Use of hydroxyurea in psoriasis. *Clin Exp Dermatol.* 1999;24(1):2-6.
62. Layton AM, Sheehan-Dare RA, Goodfield MJ, et al. Hydroxyurea in the management of therapy resistant psoriasis. *Br J Dermatol.* 1989;121(5):647-653.
63. Elliott R, Davies M, Harmse D. Dermatomyositis-like eruption with long-term hydroxyurea. *J Dermatol Treat.* 2006;17(1):59-60.
64. Dacey MJ, Callen JP. Hydroxyurea-induced dermatomyositis-like eruption. *J Am Acad Dermatol.* 2003;48(3):439-441.
65. Pata O, Tok CE, Yazici G, et al. Polycythemia vera and pregnancy: a case report with the use of hydroxyurea in the first trimester. *Am J Perinatol.* 2004;21(3):135-137.
66. Callot-Mellot C, Bodemer C, Chosidow O, et al. Cutaneous carcinoma during long-term hydroxyurea therapy: a report of 5 cases. *Arch Dermatol.* 1996;132(11):1395-1397.
67. Chan GL, Canafax DM, Johnson CA. The therapeutic use of azathioprine in renal transplantation. *Pharmacotherapy.* 1987;7(5):165-177.
68. Lennard L. The clinical pharmacology of 6-mercaptopurine. *Eur J Clin Pharmacol.* 1992;43(4):329-339.
69. Weinshilboum RM, Sladek SL. Mercaptopurine pharmacogenetics: monogenic inheritance of erythrocyte thiopurine methyltransferase activity. *Am J Hum Genet.* 1980;32(5):651-662.
70. Jackson AP, Hall AG, McLelland J. Thiopurine methyltransferase levels should be measured before commencing patients on azathioprine. *Br J Dermatol.* 1997;136(1):133-134.
71. Snow JL, Gibson LE. A pharmacogenetic basis for the safe and effective use of azathioprine and other thiopurine drugs in dermatologic patients. *J Am Acad Dermatol.* 1995;32(1):114-116.
72. Kennedy DT, Hayney MS, Lake KD. Azathioprine and allopurinol: the price of an avoidable drug interaction. *Ann Pharmacother.* 1996;30(9):951-954.
73. Schram ME, Borgonjen RJ, Bik CMJM, et al. Off-label use of azathioprine in dermatology: a systematic review. *Arch Dermatol.* 2011;147(4):474-488.
74. Chams-Davatchi C, Esmaili N, Daneshpazhooh M, et al. Randomized controlled open-label trial of four treatment regimens for pemphigus vulgaris. *J Am Acad Dermatol.* 2007;57(4):622-628.
75. Bystryn JC, Steinman NM. The adjuvant therapy of pemphigus. An update. *Arch Dermatol.* 1996;132(2):203-212.
76. Beissert S, Werfel T, Frieling U, et al. A comparison of oral methylprednisolone plus azathioprine or mycophenolate mofetil for the treatment of bullous pemphigoid. *Arch Dermatol.* 2007;143(12):1536-1542.
77. Berth-Jones J, Takwale A, Tan E, et al. Azathioprine in severe adult atopic dermatitis: a double-blind, placebo-controlled, crossover trial. *Br J Dermatol.* 2002;147(2):324-330.
78. Meggitt SJ, Gray JC, Reynolds NJ. Azathioprine dosed by thiopurine methyltransferase activity for moderate-to-severe atopic eczema: a double-blind, randomised controlled trial. *Lancet.* 2006;367(9513):839-846.
79. Relling MV, Gardner EE, Sandborn WJ, et al. Clinical pharmacogenetics implementation consortium guidelines for thiopurine methyltransferase genotype and thiopurine dosing: 2013 update. *Clin Pharmacol Ther.* 2013;93(4):324-325.
80. Meggitt SJ, Anstey AV, Mohd Mustapa MF, et al. British Association of Dermatologists' guidelines for the safe and effective prescribing of azathioprine 2011. *Br J Dermatol.* 2011;165(4):711-734.
81. Fuggle NR, Bragoli W, Mahto A, et al. The adverse effect profile of oral azathioprine in pediatric atopic

dermatitis, and recommendations for monitoring. *J Am Acad Dermatol.* 2015;72(1):108-114.
82. Sidbury R, Davis DM, Cohen DE, et al. Guidelines of care for the management of atopic dermatitis: section 3. Management and treatment with phototherapy and systemic agents. *J Am Acad Dermatol.* 2014;71(2):327-349.
83. Menter A, Korman NJ, Elmets CA, et al. Guidelines of care for the management of psoriasis and psoriatic arthritis: section 4. Guidelines of care for the management and treatment of psoriasis with traditional systemic agents. *J Am Acad Dermatol.* 2009;61(3):451-485.
84. Liu Y-P, Xu H-Q, Li M, et al. Association between thiopurine S-methyltransferase polymorphisms and azathioprine-induced adverse drug reactions in patients with autoimmune diseases: a meta-analysis. *PLoS One.* 2015;10(12):e0144234.
85. el-Azhary RA, Farmer SA, Drage LA, et al. Thioguanine nucleotides and thiopurine methyltransferase in immunobullous diseases: optimal levels as adjunctive tools for azathioprine monitoring. *Arch Dermatol.* 2009;145(6):644-652.
86. Bacon BR, Treuhaft WH, Goodman AM. Azathioprine-induced pancytopenia. Occurrence in two patients with connective-tissue diseases. *Arch Intern Med.* 1981;141(2):223-226.
87. Younger IR, Harris DW, Colver GB. Azathioprine in dermatology. *J Am Acad Dermatol.* 1991;25(2, pt 1):281-286.
88. Lawson DH, Lovatt GE, Gurton CS, et al. Adverse effects of azathioprine. *Adverse Drug React Acute Poisoning Rev.* 1984;3(3):161-171.
89. Pasadhika S, Kempen JH, Newcomb CW, et al. Azathioprine for ocular inflammatory diseases. *Am J Ophthalmol.* 2009;148(4):500-509.e2.
90. Whisnant JK, Pelkey J. Rheumatoid arthritis: treatment with azathioprine (Imuran(R)). Clinical side-effects and laboratory abnormalities. *Ann Rheum Dis.* 1982;41(suppl 1):44-47.
91. Perrett CM, Walker SL, O'Donovan P, et al. Azathioprine treatment photosensitizes human skin to ultraviolet A radiation. *Br J Dermatol.* 2008;159(1):198-204.
92. Brem R, Li F, Karran P. Reactive oxygen species generated by thiopurine/UVA cause irreparable transcription-blocking DNA lesions. *Nucleic Acids Res.* 2009;37(6):1951-1961.
93. O'Donovan P, Perrett CM, Zhang X, et al. Azathioprine and UVA light generate mutagenic oxidative DNA damage. *Science.* 2005;309(5742):1871-1874.
94. Jiyad Z, Olsen CM, Burke MT, et al. Azathioprine and risk of skin cancer in organ transplant recipients: systematic review and meta-analysis. *Am J Transplant.* 2016;16(12):3490-3503.
95. Long MD, Herfarth HH, Pipkin CA, et al. Increased risk for non-melanoma skin cancer in patients with inflammatory bowel disease. *Clin Gastroenterol Hepatol.* 2010;8(3):268-274.
96. Wilkinson AH, Smith JL, Hunsicker LG, et al. Increased frequency of posttransplant lymphomas in patients treated with cyclosporine, azathioprine, and prednisone. *Transplantation.* 1989;47(2):293-296.
97. Silman AJ, Petrie J, Hazleman B, et al. Lymphoproliferative cancer and other malignancy in patients with rheumatoid arthritis treated with azathioprine: a 20 year follow up study. *Ann Rheum Dis.* 1988;47(12):988-992.
98. Kandiel A, Fraser AG, Korelitz BI, et al. Increased risk of lymphoma among inflammatory bowel disease patients treated with azathioprine and 6-mercaptopurine. *Gut.* 2005;54(8):1121-1125.
99. Roubenoff R, Hoyt J, Petri M, et al. Effects of antiinflammatory and immunosuppressive drugs on pregnancy and fertility. *Semin Arthritis Rheum.* 1988;18(2):88-110.
100. Murphy FP, Coven TR, Burack LH, et al. Clinical clearing of psoriasis by 6-thioguanine correlates with cutaneous T-cell depletion via apoptosis: evidence for selective effects on activated T lymphocytes. *Arch Dermatol.* 1999;135(12):1495-1502.
101. LePage GA, Whitecar JP. Pharmacology of 6-thioguanine in man. *Cancer Res.* 1971;31(11):1627-1631.
102. Mason C, Krueger GG. Thioguanine for refractory psoriasis: a 4-year experience. *J Am Acad Dermatol.* 2001;44(1):67-72.
103. Zackheim HS, Maibach HI. Treatment of psoriasis with 6-thioguanine. *Australas J Dermatol.* 1988;29(3):163-167.
104. Zackheim HS, Glogau RG, Fisher DA, et al. 6-Thioguanine treatment of psoriasis: experience in 81 patients. *J Am Acad Dermatol.* 1994;30(3):452-458.
105. Silvis NG, Levine N. Pulse dosing of thioguanine in recalcitrant psoriasis. *Arch Dermatol.* 1999;135(4):433-437.
106. Romagosa R, Kerdel F, Shah N. Treatment of psoriasis with 6-thioguanine and hepatic venoocclusive disease. *J Am Acad Dermatol.* 2002;47(6):970-972; author reply 972.
107. de Boer NKH, Van Elburg RM, Wilhelm AJ, et al. 6-Thioguanine for Crohn's disease during pregnancy: thiopurine metabolite measurements in both mother and child. *Scand J Gastroenterol.* 2005;40(11):1374-1377.
108. Amor KT, Ryan C, Menter A. The use of cyclosporine in dermatology: part I. *J Am Acad Dermatol.* 2010;63(6):925-946; quiz 947-948.
109. Ryan C, Amor KT, Menter A. The use of cyclosporine in dermatology: part II. *J Am Acad Dermatol.* 2010;63(6):949-972; quiz 973-974.
110. Nghiem P, Pearson G, Langley RG. Tacrolimus and pimecrolimus: from clever prokaryotes to inhibiting calcineurin and treating atopic dermatitis. *J Am Acad Dermatol.* 2002;46(2):228-241.
111. Tseng S, Pak G, Washenik K, et al. Rediscovering thalidomide: a review of its mechanism of action, side effects, and potential uses. *J Am Acad Dermatol.* 1996;35(6):969-979.
112. Rapini RP. Cytotoxic drugs in the treatment of skin disease. *Int J Dermatol.* 1991;30(5):313-322.
113. Martin LK, Werth V, Villanueva E, et al. Interventions for pemphigus vulgaris and pemphigus foliaceus. *Cochrane Database Syst Rev.* 2009;(1):CD006263.
114. Sacher C, Hunzelmann N. Cicatricial pemphigoid (mucous membrane pemphigoid): current and emerging therapeutic approaches. *Am J Clin Dermatol.* 2005;6(2):93-103.
115. Trautmann A, Klein CE, Kämpgen E, et al. Severe bullous drug reactions treated successfully with cyclophosphamide. *Br J Dermatol.* 1998;139(6):1127-1128.
116. Kim J, Chan JJ. Cyclophosphamide in dermatology. *Australas J Dermatol.* 2017;58(1):5-17.
117. Volkmer BG, Seidl-Schlick EM, Bach D, et al. Cyclophosphamide is contraindicated in patients with a history of transitional cell carcinoma. *Clin Rheumatol.* 2005;24(4):319-323.
118. Herrstedt J, Muss HB, Warr DG, et al. Efficacy and tolerability of aprepitant for the prevention of

chemotherapy-induced nausea and emesis over multiple cycles of moderately emetogenic chemotherapy. *Cancer.* 2005;104(7):1548-1555.
119. Foad BS, Hess EV. Urinary bladder complications with cyclophosphamide therapy. *Arch Intern Med.* 1976;136(5):616-619.
120. Martin-Suarez I, D'Cruz D, Mansoor M, et al. Immunosuppressive treatment in severe connective tissue diseases: effects of low dose intravenous cyclophosphamide. *Ann Rheum Dis.* 1997;56(8):481-487.
121. Baltus JA, Boersma JW, Hartman AP, et al. The occurrence of malignancies in patients with rheumatoid arthritis treated with cyclophosphamide: a controlled retrospective follow-up. *Ann Rheum Dis.* 1983;42(4):368-373.
122. Baker GL, Kahl LE, Zee BC, et al. Malignancy following treatment of rheumatoid arthritis with cyclophosphamide. Long-term case-control follow-up study. *Am J Med.* 1987;83(1):1-9.
123. DeSpain JD. Dermatologic toxicity of chemotherapy. *Semin Oncol.* 1992;19(5):501-507.
124. Borroni G, Vassallo C, Brazzelli V, et al. Radiation recall dermatitis, panniculitis, and myositis following cyclophosphamide therapy: histopathologic findings of a patient affected by multiple myeloma. *Am J Dermatopathol.* 2004;26(3):213-216.
125. Wenzel FG, Horn TD. Nonneoplastic disorders of the eccrine glands. *J Am Acad Dermatol.* 1998;38(1):1-17; quiz 18-20.
126. Clowse MEB, Magder L, Petri M. Cyclophosphamide for lupus during pregnancy. *Lupus.* 2005;14(8):593-597.
127. Wetzels JFM. Cyclophosphamide-induced gonadal toxicity: a treatment dilemma in patients with lupus nephritis? *Neth J Med.* 2004;62(10):347-352.
128. Masala A, Faedda R, Alagna S, et al. Use of testosterone to prevent cyclophosphamide-induced azoospermia. *Ann Intern Med.* 1997;126(4):292-295.
129. Somers EC, Marder W, Christman GM, et al. Use of a gonadotropin-releasing hormone analog for protection against premature ovarian failure during cyclophosphamide therapy in women with severe lupus. *Arthritis Rheum.* 2005;52(9):2761-2767.
130. Coors EA, von den Driesch P. Treatment of erythrodermic cutaneous T-cell lymphoma with intermittent chlorambucil and fluocortolone therapy. *Br J Dermatol.* 2000;143(1):127-131.
131. Torabian SZ, Fazel N, Knuttle R. Necrobiotic xanthogranuloma treated with chlorambucil. *Dermatol Online J.* 2006;12(5):11.
132. Hengge UR, Esser S, Rudel HP, et al. Long-term chemotherapy of HIV-associated Kaposi's sarcoma with liposomal doxorubicin. *Eur J Cancer.* 2001;37(7):878-883.
133. Di Lorenzo G, Kreuter A, Di Trolio R, et al. Activity and safety of pegylated liposomal doxorubicin as first-line therapy in the treatment of non-visceral classic Kaposi's sarcoma: a multicenter study. *J Invest Dermatol.* 2008;128(6):1578-1580.
134. Trüeb RM. Chemotherapy-induced alopecia. *Semin Cutan Med Surg.* 2009;28(1):11-14.
135. Hussain S, Anderson DN, Salvatti ME, et al. Onycholysis as a complication of systemic chemotherapy: report of five cases associated with prolonged weekly paclitaxel therapy and review of the literature. *Cancer.* 2000;88(10):2367-2371.
136. Tosti A, Piraccini BM, Vincenzi C, et al. Permanent alopecia after busulfan chemotherapy. *Br J Dermatol.* 2005;152(5):1056-1058.
137. Grevelman EG, Breed WP. Prevention of chemotherapy-induced hair loss by scalp cooling. *Ann Oncol.* 2005;16(3):352-358.
138. Duvic M, Lemak NA, Valero V, et al. A randomized trial of minoxidil in chemotherapy-induced alopecia. *J Am Acad Dermatol.* 1996;35(1):74-78.
139. Koppel RA, Boh EE. Cutaneous reactions to chemotherapeutic agents. *Am J Med Sci.* 2001;321(5):327-335.
140. Nicolopoulos J, Howard A. Docetaxel-induced nail dystrophy. *Australas J Dermatol.* 2002;43(4):293-296.
141. Rümke CL. An observation in Broek in Waterland in 1919 [in Dutch]. *Ned Tijdschr Geneeskd.* 1985;129(51):2469-2471.
142. Benatti C, Gnocchi M, Travaglino E, et al. Chemotherapy-induced leukonychia. *Haematologica.* 2004;89(7):EIM16.
143. Susser WS, Whitaker-Worth DL, Grant-Kels JM. Mucocutaneous reactions to chemotherapy. *J Am Acad Dermatol.* 1999;40(3):367-398; quiz 399-400.
144. Anderson LL, Thomas DE, Berger TG, et al. Cutaneous pigmentation after daunorubicin chemotherapy. *J Am Acad Dermatol.* 1992;26(2, pt 1):255-256.
145. Dave S, Thappa DM. Peculiar pattern of nail pigmentation following cyclophosphamide therapy. *Dermatol Online J.* 2003;9(3):14.
146. Flynn TC, Harrist TJ, Murphy GF, et al. Neutrophilic eccrine hidradenitis: a distinctive rash associated with cytarabine therapy and acute leukemia. *J Am Acad Dermatol.* 1984;11(4, pt 1):584-590.
147. Thorisdottir K, Tomecki KJ, Bergfeld WF, et al. Neutrophilic eccrine hidradenitis. *J Am Acad Dermatol.* 1993;28(5, pt 1):775-777.
148. Brehler R, Reimann S, Bonsmann G, et al. Neutrophilic hidradenitis induced by chemotherapy involves eccrine and apocrine glands. *Am J Dermatopathol.* 1997;19(1):73-78.
149. Shear NH, Knowles SR, Shapiro L, et al. Dapsone in prevention of recurrent neutrophilic eccrine hidradenitis. *J Am Acad Dermatol.* 1996;35(5, pt 2):819-822.
150. Bhawan J, Malhotra R. Syringosquamous metaplasia. A distinctive eruption in patients receiving chemotherapy. *Am J Dermatopathol.* 1990;12(1):1-6.
151. Valks R, Fraga J, Porras-Luque J, et al. Chemotherapy-induced eccrine squamous syringometaplasia. A distinctive eruption in patients receiving hematopoietic progenitor cells. *Arch Dermatol.* 1997;133(7):873-878.
152. El Darouti MA, Marzouk SA, El Hadidi HA, et al. Eccrine syringosquamous metaplasia. *Int J Dermatol.* 2001;40(12):777-781.
153. Burgdorf WH, Gilmore WA, Ganick RG. Peculiar acral erythema secondary to high-dose chemotherapy for acute myelogenous leukemia. *Ann Intern Med.* 1982;97(1):61-62.
154. Werchniak AE, Chaffee S, Dinulos JGH. Methotrexate-induced bullous acral erythema in a child. *J Am Acad Dermatol.* 2005;52(5)(suppl 1):S93-S95.
155. Rongioletti F, Ballestrero A, Bogliolo F, et al. Necrotizing eccrine squamous syringometaplasia presenting as acral erythema. *J Cutan Pathol.* 1991;18(6):453-456.
156. Tsuboi H, Yonemoto K, Katsuoka K. A case of bleomycin-induced acral erythema (AE) with eccrine squamous syringometaplasia (ESS) and summary of reports of AE with ESS in the literature. *J Dermatol.* 2005;32(11):921-925.
157. Guillet G, Guillet MH, de Meaux H, et al. Cutaneous pigmented stripes and bleomycin treatment. *Arch Dermatol.* 1986;122(4):381-382.

158. Omura EF, Torre D. Inflammation of actinic keratoses due to systemic fluorouracil therapy. *JAMA*. 1969;208(1):150-151.
159. Patton T, Zirwas M, Nieland-Fisher N, et al. Inflammation of seborrheic keratoses caused by cytarabine: a pseudo sign of Leser-Trelat. *J Drugs Dermatol*. 2004;3(5):565-566.
160. Williams JV, Helm KF, Long D. Chemotherapy-induced inflammation in seborrheic keratoses mimicking disseminated herpes zoster. *J Am Acad Dermatol*. 1999;40(4):643-644.
161. Kumar R, Pai V. Bleomycin induced flagellate pigmentation. *Indian Pediatr*. 2006;43(1):74-75.
162. Jain V, Bhandary S, Prasad GN, et al. Serpentine supravenous streaks induced by 5-fluorouracil. *J Am Acad Dermatol*. 2005;53(3):529-530.
163. Yeo W, Johnson PJ. Radiation-recall skin disorders associated with the use of antineoplastic drugs. Pathogenesis, prevalence, and management. *Am J Clin Dermatol*. 2000;1(2):113-116.
164. Westwick TJ, Sherertz EF, McCarley D, et al. Delayed reactivation of sunburn by methotrexate: sparing of chronically sun-exposed skin. *Cutis*. 1987;39(1):49-51.
165. Ener RA, Meglathery SB, Styler M. Extravasation of systemic hemato-oncological therapies. *Ann Oncol*. 2004;15(6):858-862.
166. Dorr RT, Alberts DS. Vinca alkaloid skin toxicity: antidote and drug disposition studies in the mouse. *J Natl Cancer Inst*. 1985;74(1):113-120.
167. Dorr RT. Antidotes to vesicant chemotherapy extravasations. *Blood Rev*. 1990;4(1):41-60.
168. Svingen BA, Powis G, Appel PL, et al. Protection against adriamycin-induced skin necrosis in the rat by dimethyl sulfoxide and alpha-tocopherol. *Cancer Res*. 1981;41(9, pt 1):3395-3399.
169. Laurie SW, Wilson KL, Kernahan DA, et al. Intravenous extravasation injuries: the effectiveness of hyaluronidase in their treatment. *Ann Plast Surg*. 1984;13(3):191-194.
170. Bertelli G. Prevention and management of extravasation of cytotoxic drugs. *Drug Saf*. 1995;12(4):245-255.
171. Cohen IS, Mosher MB, O'Keefe EJ, et al. Cutaneous toxicity of bleomycin therapy. *Arch Dermatol*. 1973;107(4):553-555.
172. Hassett G, Harnett P, Manolios N. Scleroderma in association with the use of docetaxel (Taxotere) for breast cancer. *Clin Exp Rheumatol*. 2001;19(2):197-200.
173. Berger CC, Bokemeyer C, Schneider M, et al. Secondary Raynaud's phenomenon and other late vascular complications following chemotherapy for testicular cancer. *Eur J Cancer*. 1995;31A(13-14):2229-2238.
174. Gottschling S, Meyer S, Reinhard H, et al. First report of a vincristine dose-related Raynaud's phenomenon in an adolescent with malignant brain tumor. *J Pediatr Hematol Oncol*. 2004;26(11):768-769.
175. Vanhooteghem O, Richert B, de la Brassinne M. Raynaud phenomenon after treatment of verruca vulgaris of the sole with intralesional injection of bleomycin. *Pediatr Dermatol*. 2001;18(3):249-251.
176. Worthington HV, Clarkson JE, Bryan G, et al. Interventions for preventing oral mucositis for patients with cancer receiving treatment. *Cochrane Database Syst Rev*. 2011;(4):CD000978.
177. Riley P, Glenny A-M, Worthington HV, et al. Interventions for preventing oral mucositis in patients with cancer receiving treatment: oral cryotherapy. *Cochrane Database Syst Rev*. 2015;(12):CD011552.

Chapter 191 :: Antiviral Drugs
:: Zeena Y. Nawas, Quynh-Giao Nguyen, Khaled S. Sanber, & Stephen K. Tyring

第一百九十一章

抗病毒药

中文导读

艾滋病毒（HIV）的流行加快了新型抗病毒药物的研发步伐，目前在病毒性疾病的分子生物学和发病机制的认识方面取得了可喜的进展。本章重点介绍了皮肤科医生常用的抗病毒药物，以及那些引起皮肤副作用的药物。按抗病毒药物的适应证分为5个部分，首先介绍了治疗疱疹病毒感染的药物，包括阿昔洛韦、伐昔洛韦、泛昔洛韦、喷昔洛韦、三氟尿苷，接下来介绍了治疗巨细胞病毒感染的药物，包括更昔洛韦/缬更昔洛韦、磷甲酸钠、西多福韦，随后特别介绍了治疗艾滋病毒感染的药物和目前治疗丙型肝炎和乙型肝炎的试验药物，主要介绍了这些药物的作用机制、药代动力学、给药方案、启动治疗、监护疗法、风险及防范措施、不良反应及药物相互作用等。本章还简单提及了其他病毒感染的治疗药物。

〔粟 娟〕

AT-A-GLANCE

- Antivirals are approved for treatment of a variety of viral infections.
- Antiviral resistance is a growing concern, especially in the treatment of HIV infection.
- Antivirals work in a number of different ways, and their spectra of activity can be very specific (amantadine) or quite broad (ribavirin).
- The use of prodrugs of acyclovir and ganciclovir has greatly increased the oral bioavailability of these agents, which allows outpatient treatment of many herpesvirus infections.

The pace of development of new antiviral drugs has been accelerated by the HIV (HIV) epidemic. Progress in our understanding of the molecular biology and pathogenesis of viral diseases has been remarkable. This chapter focuses on the antiviral drugs most likely to be used by dermatologists, as well as those that cause cutaneous side effects. The age of effective antiviral therapy is here, and they are used throughout all disciplines of medicine. We need to be prepared to evaluate patients on a wide variety of antiviral drugs, especially those currently used to treat HIV.

DRUGS FOR THE TREATMENT OF HERPESVIRUS INFECTIONS

See Chaps. 164 and 165.

ACYCLOVIR

MECHANISM OF ACTION

See Fig. 191-1. Acyclovir, 9-[(2-hydroxyethoxy)methyl] guanine, was the first orally available drug to be widely used for the treatment of herpes simplex virus (HSV) and varicella-zoster virus (VZV) infections. The triphosphate form of the drug is the active form, which has a potent inhibitory effect on herpesvirus-induced DNA polymerases but relatively little effect on host cell DNA polymerase. As such, it has a tremendous margin of safety when used to treat herpetic infections. Acyclovir triphosphate causes premature termination of the nascent viral DNA chain. HSV- and VZV-induced thymidine kinases result in efficient phosphorylation of acyclovir to acyclovir monophosphate, the first step in drug metabolism. This step is not accomplished efficiently by normal cellular kinases, resulting in greater concentrations of active drug in infected cells.

PHARMACOKINETICS

Although acyclovir is available in oral, IV, and topical formulations, the oral bioavailability is only in the range of 15% to 30%, with the topical even less. Excretion is almost entirely renal, with approximately 62% of the drug remaining unmetabolized. Because of its reliance on renal excretion, the dose

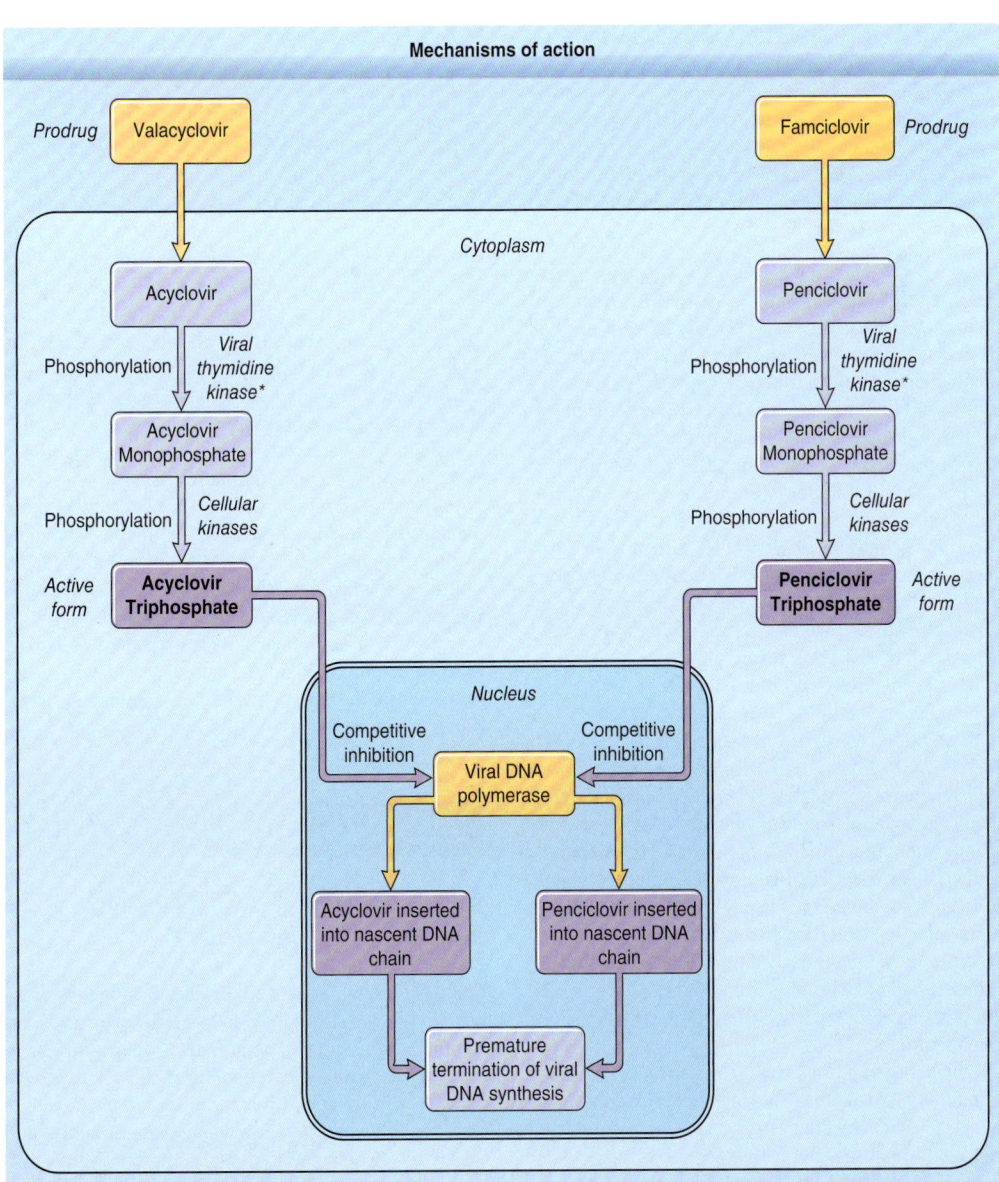

Figure 191-1. Mechanisms of action.

must be reduced for patients with a creatinine clearance of less than 50 mL/min. Acyclovir is water-soluble and distributes widely throughout the body, including into the contents of vesicles, cerebrospinal fluid (1:2 ratio from serum concentration), and vaginal secretions. Its half-life is 4 hours in neonates, 2 to 3 hours in children 1 to 12 years old, 2 to 3.5 hours in adults, and approximately 5 hours in hemodialysis patients.

INDICATIONS

- Symptomatic primary or recurrent HSV1/2 infections
- Chronic suppression of HSV1/2 infections
- HSV encephalitis
- Primary VZV infection, including HIV associated acute retinal necrosis
- Herpes zoster (shingles)
- Prevention of perinatal and treatment of neonatal HSV infection
- HSV gingivostomatitis and orolabial cold sores (off-label)
- Prevention of HSV, CMV, or VZV reactivation in hematopoietic stem cell transplant and HIV patients (off-label)
- New onset Bell palsy (off-label)

Acyclovir is indicated for a variety of infections, including that of primary HSV1/2 as well as VZV. In general, treatments for herpes viral infections are most effective when initiated as early as possible, within 24 hours for varicella and 72 hours for herpes zoster onset. A buccal tablet formulation of acyclovir was approved by the FDA in 2013 for treatment of recurrent herpes labialis in immunocompetent adults. Acyclovir given in late pregnancy to women with recurrent genital herpes has been shown to decrease the frequency of genital lesions, though there is some evidence that suggests standard oral dosing of acyclovir results in insufficient levels to prevent viral shedding on delivery.[1] As a result, acyclovir treatment is still recommended to neonates of mothers with recent genital HSV infection.

In addition, acyclovir has been shown to select for HIV-1 V85I reverse transcriptase variant in vitro,[2] which suggests a possible role in reducing HIV viral load. However, it was shown that acyclovir did not significantly prevent transmission of HIV despite a reduction of 0.25log(10) copies per milliliter in HIV RNA in those treated for genital HSV.[3] In fact, herpes virus infections in HIV patients is not yet well understood, and the only indicated treatment for HSV that is independent of HIV status is that of HSV encephalitis. All other indications, while useful on many occasions, remain off-label.

Despite its high efficacy, resistance to acyclovir remains an issue with herpes infections. Data from corneal HSV-1 isolates suggests that infections commonly represent mixtures of acyclovir-sensitive and resistant viruses with different *thymidine kinase* gene sequences. The acyclovir-resistant HSV-1 can establish latency and reactivate intermittently to cause acyclovir-refractory disease.[4]

DOSING REGIMENS

Treatment regimens with acyclovir vary depending on the indication and route of administration. An IV dose of 5 mg per kg every 8 hours or oral dose of 400 mg 3 times daily is generally recommended and more successful for patient compliance than 200 mg 5 times daily.[5] Chronic suppression requires an oral dose of 400 mg 3 times daily for up to 12 months (Table 191-1A).[6] The dose should be adjusted for patients with a creatinine clearance level of less than 50 mL/min, but drug level assays are not routinely performed. Data for pediatric dosing for <12 years of age is limited but available, particularly recommended for HSV-related neonatal and encephalitis infections (Table 191-1B).[7]

SIDE EFFECTS AND PRECAUTIONS

Acyclovir is generally very well tolerated with uncommon reactions such as renal impairment (5% incidence). The major risk for impairment is renal tubular crystallization with rapid IV administration, though interstitial nephritis also has been reported. CNS toxicity is uncommon, but may manifest as lethargy, tremors, or seizures. Patients with these side effects commonly have underlying diseases involving the CNS. Thrombophlebitis is a known complication of infusion, and appears to be related to the high pH of the reconstituted solution (pH 11).

It should be warned that acyclovir crosses the human placenta and is excreted in breastmilk. However, it has been determined safe for use (pregnancy category B; see Table 191-2) and recommended for herpes treatment during pregnancy. The drug is also safe for administration during active breast-feeding, so long as the nursing mother does not have active lesions near or on the breast.[8] It has been shown to increase the risk of toxicity of foscarnet, mycophenolate, tenofovir, and zidovudine and decrease the therapeutic effects of talimogene laherparepvec, varicella vaccine, and zoster vaccine.

VALACYCLOVIR

MECHANISM OF ACTION AND PHARMACOKINETICS

See Fig. 191-1. Valacyclovir, the L-valine ester of acyclovir, was developed to provide increased oral bioavailability of the active drug acyclovir.[9] Valacyclovir is readily absorbed from the GI tract and almost entirely converted to acyclovir by intestinal and hepatic esterases. The mechanism of action and spectrum of activity of valacyclovir are identical to those of acyclovir, though improved from its predecessor. Valacyclovir has an oral bioavailability of

TABLE 191-1A
Commonly Used Dosing Regimens for Acyclovir—Adults and Adolescents ≥12 Years

CONDITION	DOSAGE	ROUTE	DURATION
Primary HSV infection, immunocompetent host	5 mg/kg every 8 h	IV	5-7 d
	or		
	400 mg 3×/d	Oral	7-10 d
Recurrent genital HSV infection, immunocompetent host	400 mg 3×/d	Oral	5 d
	or		
	800 mg 3×/d	Oral	2 d[a]
Recurrent oral labial HSV infection, immunocompetent host	400 mg 5×/d	Oral	5 d
	or		
	5% cream 6×/d	Topical	7 d
Mucocutaneous HSV infection, immunocompromised host[6]	5 mg/kg every 8 h	IV	7 d
	or		
	400 mg 5×/d	Oral	14-21 d
Perinatal HSV infection	10-20 mg/kg every 8 h	IV	10-21 d
Chronic suppression of HSV infection	400 mg 2×/d	Oral	<12 mo
	or		
	800 mg every day		
HSV encephalitis	10 mg/kg every 8 h	IV	14-21 d
Varicella: adolescent >40 kg/adult	800 mg 4×/d	Oral	5 d
Varicella: pneumonia or third-trimester pregnancy	800 mg 5×/d	Oral	5 d
	or		
	10 mg/kg every 8 h	IV	5 d
Herpes zoster: normal host or not severe disease in immunocompromised host	800 mg 5×/d	Oral	7-10 d
Herpes zoster: severe disease or immunocompromised host	10-12 mg/kg every 8 h	IV	7-14 d

55%. Following a 1-g oral dose of valacyclovir, peak plasma concentrations of acyclovir in the range of 5.7 μg/mL are achieved in 1.75 hours, and area-under-the-curve (AUC) concentrations are similar to those achieved with 5 mg/kg of acyclovir given IV. Its half-life ranges from 1.3 to 2.5 hours in children to approximately 30 minutes in adults. Excretion is primarily renal, with 89% metabolized to acyclovir. Like

TABLE 191-1B
Commonly Used Dosing Regimens for Acyclovir—Pediatrics <12 Years

CONDITION	DOSAGE	ROUTE	DURATION
Primary HSV infection, immunocompetent host	40-80 mg/kg divided into 3-4 doses	Oral	5-10 d
Recurrent genital HSV infection, immunocompetent host[7]	20-25 mg/kg 2×/d	Oral	—
Primary HSV, immunocompromised host	20 mg/kg 3×/d	Oral	5-10 d
	or		
	5-10 mg/kg every 8 h	IV	
Mucocutaneous HSV infection, immunocompromised host[6]	5 mg/kg every 8 h	IV	7 d
	or		
	400 mg 5×/d	Oral	14-21 d
Neonatal HSV infection	20 mg/kg every 8 h	IV	14-21 d
Chronic suppression of HSV infection	20 mg/kg 2×/d	Oral	5-14 d
HSV encephalitis	10-15 mg/kg every 8 h	IV	14-21 d
Varicella: >1 y old and <41 kg	20 mg/kg 4×/d	Oral	5 d
Herpes zoster:	10 mg/kg every 8 h	Oral	7-10 d
<1 y old	or		
≥1 y old	500 mg every 8 h		

HSV, herpes simplex virus.

TABLE 191-2
Pregnancy Categories of Systemic Antiviral Agents

AGENT	PREGNANCY CATEGORY
Acyclovir	B
Valacyclovir	B
Famciclovir	B
Ganciclovir and valganciclovir	C
Foscarnet	C
Cidofovir	C

acyclovir, the dose must be adjusted for those with underlying renal impairment.

INDICATIONS

- Initial and recurrent HSV genital infections
- Suppression and reduction of transmission of genital HSV infections
- Herpes zoster (shingles)
- Herpes labialis (cold sores)
- Varicella (chickenpox)

Valacyclovir therapy should be initiated at the earliest symptom of an HSV or VZV infection, within 72 hours of first diagnosis or 24 hours of onset of recurrent episode. It is preferred by patients due to its oral efficacy, compared to acyclovir, and ease of use in the outpatient setting. Treatment with valacyclovir has been suggested to decrease the frequency of clinical outbreaks as well as the incidence of viral shedding. Early studies showed a 30% reduction in viral shedding from valacyclovir-treated genital herpes compared to placebo-treated ($P <.001$).[10,11] Recent data showed even more promising results, where valacyclovir given 1 g daily resulted in a 78% reduction in viral shedding compared to placebo, and 79% of subjects had no clinical recurrences while receiving valacyclovir compared with 52% of subjects receiving placebo ($P <.01$).[12] Though less commonly, the drug has further been used to suppress recurrence of ocular herpes disease.[13]

In the setting of oral herpes simplex, valacyclovir has been used alone or combined with oral corticosteroids. In one study, there were more aborted lesions in the valacyclovir-clobetasol arm than in the placebo group (50% vs 15.8%, $P = .04$),[14] but further study is needed to assess the independent contribution of the corticosteroid.

Valacyclovir demonstrates in vitro activity against Epstein-Barr virus (EBV). It is being studied in the settings of infectious mononucleosis, hepatitis, encephalopathy, and posttransplant lymphoproliferative disease. Unfortunately, in a recent trial, valacyclovir treatment was not effective in decreasing peripheral blood EBV viral loads in pediatric liver transplantation patients.[15] In healthy volunteers, long-term administration of valacyclovir effectively reduces the number of EBV-infected B cells, although it does not reduce the number of EBV DNA copies per B cell.[16]

DOSING REGIMENS

Standard doses for adults with herpetic infections range from 0.5 to 1 g 2 to 3 times daily, as listed in Table 191-3.[17] The drug also has been evaluated in children with malignancy.[18] In this setting, valacyclovir (15 mg/kg) was well tolerated and demonstrated excellent bioavailability.[19] Those less than 3 months of age demonstrate decreased clearance of the drug. Among children 3 months through 11 years of age, a 20-mg/kg dose of an extemporaneously compounded valacyclovir oral suspension produced favorable acyclovir blood levels and was well tolerated. The authors noted that among children 2 through 5 years of age, a dose increase from 20 to 25 mg/kg resulted in near doubling of the peak concentration [C(max)] and the area under the curve (AUC).[20]

SIDE EFFECTS AND PRECAUTIONS

Most adverse effects are similar to those with acyclovir, including a potential for acute renal failure as well as CNS effects of agitation, hallucinations, seizures, and encephalopathy.[21] Additionally, the drug has been reported to produce both immediate hypersensitivity and a symmetrical drug-related intertriginous and flexural exanthem.[22,23] Severe effects of thrombotic thrombocytopenic purpura/hemolytic uremic syndrome (TTP/HUS) have been reported in patients with AIDS as well as in transplant recipients receiving dosages of 8 g/d. TTP/HUS has not been reported in patients in

TABLE 191-3
Dosing Regimens for Valacyclovir

CONDITION	DOSAGE	ROUTE	DURATION
Primary HSV infection, immunocompetent host	1000 mg 2x/d	Oral	10 d
Recurrent genital HSV infection, immunocompetent host	500 mg 2x/d	Oral	3 d
Recurrent oral labial HSV infection, immunocompetent host	2000 mg 2x/d	Oral	1 d
Oral labial HSV infection, immunocompromised host	500 mg 2x/d	Oral	5-10 d
Chronic suppression of HSV infection	1000 mg every day	Oral	Undefined/indefinite
Varicella: adolescent/adult	1000 mg 3x/d	Oral	5 d
Herpes zoster: normal host or not severe disease in immunocompromised host	1000 mg 3x/d	Oral	7 d

HSV, herpes simplex virus.

patients taking conventional dosages (up to 3 g/d) of valacyclovir. It is labeled as pregnancy category B risk.

Valacyclovir has been shown to precipitate in renal tubules and should be used with caution in those with renal impairment. Its most severe effects have been observed in elderly and immunocompromised patients, for which it is recommended to give the lowest dose possible. Given its metabolism to acyclovir, which can be detected in breastmilk, breast-feeding mothers should be aware that their nursing infants may receive small, though clinically insignificant, amounts of acyclovir. Common drug interactions include increased toxicity risk of foscarnet, mycophenolate, tenofovir, zidovudine, and decreased therapeutic effects of talimogene laherparepvec, varicella vaccine, and zoster vaccine.

FAMCICLOVIR AND PENCICLOVIR

MECHANISM OF ACTION

See Fig. 191-1. Famciclovir, [9-(4-hydroxy-3-hydroxymethylbut-1-yl)guanine], is biotransformed to the active compound penciclovir, [9-(4-hydroxy-3-hydroxy-3-hydroxymethylbut-1-yl)guanine], which is phosphorylated to penciclovir triphosphate to eventually inhibit HSV-2 polymerase. The initial phosphorylation of penciclovir to penciclovir monophosphate is efficiently carried out by HSV- or VZV-induced thymidine kinases with subsequent phosphorylation to diphosphate and triphosphate forms occurring via cellular kinases. The mechanism by which penciclovir triphosphate competitively inhibits viral DNA polymerases is similar to that of acyclovir, though more DNA chain extension may occur with penciclovir because of its hydroxyl group on the acyclic side chain.

PHARMACOKINETICS

Famciclovir is marketed as an oral formulation, which is converted to penciclovir by deacetylation and oxidation in the liver and intestine. The bioavailability of oral famciclovir is 77%, with a peak plasma concentration of 3.3 µg/mL reached 1 hour after oral administration of 500 mg of famciclovir. The plasma half-life of the converted penciclovir is 2 to 4 hours, with 60% to 70% of the drug excreted in urine unchanged. As with acyclovir, the dose of penciclovir should be reduced in patients with advanced renal dysfunction. Compared with the intracellular half-life of acyclovir triphosphate, that of penciclovir triphosphate is markedly prolonged in both HSV-infected cells (10 to 20 hours) and VZV-infected cells (7 hours), allowing the drug to be administered 2 to 3 times daily. Penciclovir is available as a 1% ointment for the treatment of recurrent oral HSV. At least in some vehicles, topical penetration of penciclovir is superior to that of acyclovir.[24] Microemulsion and nanoparticle formulations investigations concluded that these could be a promising vehicle for topical delivery of penciclovir.[25-27]

INDICATIONS

- Initial and recurrent HSV genital infections
- Suppression of frequently recurring genital HSV infections
- Initial and recurrent HSV labialis (cold sores) infections
- Herpes zoster (shingles)
- Varicella infection (chickenpox) in HIV patients (off-label)

As with acyclovir and valacyclovir, famciclovir and penciclovir should be initiated as soon as possible after diagnosis, ideally within 72 hours of rash onset. Famciclovir also has been shown to be an effective, well-tolerated option for the suppression of genital herpes among individuals with multiple recurrences.[28] Famciclovir is also equivalent to acyclovir for treatment of ophthalmic zoster.[29]

DOSING REGIMENS

Famciclovir is available as an oral agent and penciclovir as a topical cream. Standard adult doses are given in Table 191-4.[30] Pediatric doses are generally of increased treatment duration though with similar amount per dose, for example, 500 mg twice daily. In one study

TABLE 191-4
Dosing Regimens for Famciclovir and Penciclovir

CONDITION	DOSAGE	ROUTE	DURATION
Primary HSV infection, immunocompetent host	250 mg 3×/d	Oral	7-10 d
Recurrent genital HSV infection, immunocompetent host	125 mg 2×/d or 1000 mg 2×/d	Oral Oral	5 d 1 d
Recurrent oral labial HSV infection, immunocompetent host	1500 mg every day or 1% penciclovir cream every 2 h	Oral Topical	1 d 5 d or until lesions healed
Oral labial HSV infection, immunocompromised host	500 mg 2×/d	Oral	7 d
Chronic suppression of HSV infection	250 mg 2×/d	Oral	Up to 1 y
Varicella: adolescent/adult	500 mg 3×/d	Oral	5-7 d
Herpes zoster: normal host or not severe disease in immunocompromised host	500 mg 3×/d	Oral	7 d

HSV, herpes simplex virus.

of recurrent genital HSV, a 2-day course of 500 mg initially, then 250 mg twice daily, was noninferior to the standard 5-day course of 125 mg twice daily.[31] In another study, single-day famciclovir (1000 mg administered twice daily) was similar in efficacy to 3-day valacyclovir (500 mg administered twice daily) for the treatment of recurrent genital herpes.[32] Single-day treatment is associated with high patient satisfaction.[33] Some data suggest that suppressive treatment may be superior to episodic treatment.[34] Studies in children are ongoing, and currently the drug is used less commonly in this population.[35,36] Although famciclovir has shown efficacy in general populations, one study of patient-initiated episodic treatment of recurrent genital herpes in immunocompetent black patients showed efficacy similar to that of placebo.[37]

SIDE EFFECTS AND PRECAUTIONS

Like acyclovir and valacyclovir, famciclovir is generally well tolerated.[38] The dose should be reduced for patients with a creatinine clearance less than 60 mL/min. The drug has been used safely along with hydration in patients with prior renal toxicity related to acyclovir.[39] Leukocytoclastic vasculitis has been reported with the drug.[40] Common side effects include:

- headache,
- nausea,
- diarrhea, and
- dizziness.

Serious toxicity is uncommon and the drug is labeled a pregnancy risk factor B. Famciclovir has been shown to diminish the therapeutic effect of talimogene laherparepvec, varicella virus vaccine, and zoster vaccine.

TRIFLURIDINE

MECHANISM OF ACTION AND PHARMACOKINETICS

Trifluridine, 5-trifluoromethyl-2′-deoxyuridine, is a pyrimidine nucleoside analog. Trifluridine monophosphate acts as an irreversible competitive inhibitor of thymidylate synthetase, and trifluridine triphosphate inhibits HSV DNA polymerase. Trifluridine triphosphate also inhibits cellular DNA polymerases, although it does so to a lesser extent than viral DNA polymerases. Because of its mechanism, it is considered a potent drug with expected response to treatment within 2 to 7 days. Because of systemic toxicity, trifluridine is approved only for topical application in the form of a 1% ophthalmic aqueous solution. The elimination half-life for the ophthalmic solution is 12 minutes.

INDICATIONS

- Primary and recurrent HSV keratoconjunctivitis, keratitis
- Acyclovir-resistant mucocutaneous HSV infections in patients with AIDS (off-label)

Trifluridine is indicated for the treatment of primary keratoconjunctivitis and recurrent epithelial keratitis caused by HSV types 1 and 2. It also has been suggested to benefit acyclovir-resistant HSV infections in AIDS patients. The drug offers a unique and effective delivery route that has similar efficacy to others of its class. A meta-analysis data from 99 randomized trials of 5363 total participants showed no significant difference between topical trifluridine, vidarabine, acyclovir, or ganciclovir in treatment of dendritic epithelial keratitis within 1 week of therapy.[41] A 2010 systematic review of 106 trials found that use of any of 4 topical antiviral agents (trifluridine, acyclovir ganciclovir, or brivudine) were equally effective and resulted in healing of 90% of the eyes within 2 weeks.[42] However, other authors have suggested that although the drug is effective, it may result in delays in reepithelialization of corneal ulcers.[43] As a result, there may be additional benefit from topical interferon in those treated with this agent.[44]

DOSING REGIMENS

Standard dosing regimens consist of 1 drop of 1% solution every 2 hours until reepithelialization of ulcer occurs, followed by 1 drop every 4 hours for another 7 days. Regimens are provided in Table 191-5. It is recommended to consider another form of therapy if no clinical improvement is seen at 7 to 14 days.

TABLE 191-5
Dosing Regimens for Trifluridine

CONDITION	DOSAGE	ROUTE	DURATION
HSV keratoconjunctivitis/ keratitis	Induction: 1 drop every 2 h (maximum, 9 drops/24 h) Maintenance: 1 drop every 4 h (maximum, 6 drops/24 h)	Topical	Maximum, 21 d
Acyclovir-resistant HSV infection in AIDS	1 drop every 8 h	Topical	10-14 d or until lesions resolve

HSV, herpes simplex virus.

SIDE EFFECTS AND PRECAUTIONS

Adverse reactions to trifluridine are generally minor, mainly manifesting as transient local burning or stinging (5%), palpebral edema (3%), epithelial and punctate keratopathy, and stromal edema. It is considered a pregnancy category C risk with systemic application, but the amount available systemically following topical application of the ophthalmic drops has been considered negligible.

DRUGS FOR THE TREATMENT OF CYTOMEGALOVIRUS INFECTIONS

GANCICLOVIR AND VALGANCICLOVIR

MECHANISM OF ACTION AND PHARMACOKINETICS

Ganciclovir, 9-(1,3-dihydroxy-2-propoxymethyl)guanine, is phosphorylated by viral kinases to a substrate that competitively inhibits the binding of deoxyguanosine triphosphate to DNA polymerase, thereby inhibiting viral DNA synthesis. It is effective in treating cytomegalovirus infections intravenously, though oral bioavailability is only 5%. Valganciclovir, L-valine 2-[(2-amino-1,6-dehydro-6-*oxo*-9*H*-purin-9-yl)methoxy]-3-hydroxypropyl ester, is the L-valyl ester of ganciclovir that is more bioavailable. After oral administration, valganciclovir is converted to ganciclovir by intestinal and hepatic esterases with an oral availability of approximately 60% that is increased by 30% when administered with a high-fat meal. After a 900-mg dose of valganciclovir, the maximum plasma concentration of ganciclovir is 5.61 µg/mL, and the plasma concentration–time curve is similar to that achieved with ganciclovir given intravenously at a dose of 5 mg/kg. The elimination half-life is approximately 4 hours, though delayed in those with renal impairment.

INDICATIONS

- CMV retinitis in immunocompromised patients
- Suppression and prevention of CMV disease in transplant recipients
- CMV esophagitis, colitis, or neurologic disease in HIV patients (off-label)

Intravenous ganciclovir and oral valganciclovir are both approved for use in the treatment of cytomegalovirus in immunocompromised patients as well as in prevention of CMV disease in transplant patients.[45-47]

DOSING REGIMENS

Standard dosing regimens include 5 mg/kg/dose of ganciclovir every 12 hours for induction followed by every 24 hours for maintenance therapy. The equivalent dosing of valganciclovir is 900 mg twice daily induction followed by once-daily maintenance. Dosing summary is provided in Table 191-6. Pediatric dosing regimens also have been published and are similar to adult dosing.[48]

SIDE EFFECTS AND PRECAUTIONS

Potential side effects include a variety of GI (ie, diarrhea, nausea, and loss of appetite) as well as hematologic side effects (ie, anemia, thrombocytopenia, neutropenia, bone marrow aplasia, and aplastic anemia). Acute renal failure may occur, for which doses should be immediately adjusted to half the regular dose. Nonspecific adverse reactions include headache, dizziness, confusion, nervousness, vivid dreams, tremor, weakness, peripheral edema, and pain at the injection site.

Known drug interactions include potentiation of imipenem, mycophenolate, probenecid, reverse transcriptase inhibitors, and tenofovir. It is labeled as pregnancy category C and recommended to use contraception during and 30 to 90 days post treatment. Breast-feeding is not recommended, since it is not known if ganciclovir or valganciclovir are excreted into breastmilk.

FOSCARNET

MECHANISM OF ACTION

Foscarnet, trisodium phosphonoformate, is a pyrophosphate-containing antiviral drug that noncompetitively inhibits viral DNA polymerases at the pyrophosphate binding site. In contrast to the nucleoside analogs, foscarnet does not require phosphorylation and is therefore active against many strains of virus that are resistant to acyclovir, famciclovir, or

TABLE 191-6
Dosing Regimens for Ganciclovir/Valganciclovir

CONDITION	DOSAGE	ROUTE	DURATION
CMV retinitis	Induction:		
	900 mg 2×/d	Oral	21 d
	5 mg/kg every 12 h	IV	14-21 d
	Maintenance:		
	900 mg every day	Oral	Until CD4 count >100 after 6 mo of HAART
	5 mg/kg every day	IV	

CMV, cytomegalovirus; HAART, highly active antiretroviral therapy.

ganciclovir as a result of absent or reduced kinase activity.[49-51] Salvage therapy with foscarnet plus a thymidine analog has been shown to be effective in patients with advanced-stage HIV disease and viruses harboring multiple drug-resistance mutations including thymidine-associated mutations.[52] Unfortunately, resistance to combined ganciclovir and foscarnet therapy has been reported in the setting of dual-strain cytomegalovirus coinfection.[53] Valproic acid has been reported to impair the antiviral activity of ganciclovir, cidofovir, and foscarnet.[54]

PHARMACOKINETICS

Foscarnet is available as an IV preparation that has poor solubility and must be administered by an infusion pump in a dilute solution over 1 to 2 hours. The drug has a half-life of 3 to 4 hours initially with a terminal component of 88 hours or longer, for which up to 20% of the cumulative dose may be deposited in bone. Twenty-eight percent of the dose is excreted unaltered by the kidney.

INDICATIONS

- CMV retinitis
- Acyclovir-resistant HSV infections
- CMV esophagitis or colitis (off-label)
- Ganciclovir-resistant CMV infections (off-label)

DOSING REGIMENS

Standard dosing schedules consist of induction therapy of 40 to 90 mg/kg/dose every 8 to 12 hours followed by maintenance therapy of 90 to 120 mg/kg/d. Specific regimens are provided in Table 191-7. The dose must be adjusted accordingly in patients with renal dysfunction.

SIDE EFFECTS AND PRECAUTIONS

Renal toxicity (30%) is the major risk with foscarnet, for which close monitoring of renal function is required. Impairment of renal function typically occurs during the second week of induction therapy and is reversible within 1 week following dose adjustment or discontinuation of therapy. Saline hydration before administration and slow infusion of the drug may reduce nephrotoxicity risk. In addition, the drug has been associated with electrolyte and metabolic abnormalities including hypocalcemia, hyper/hypophosphatemia, hypomagnesaemia, and hypokalemia, described with up to 48% incidence. Other common adverse reactions include nausea/vomiting with diarrhea (<47%), anemia (33%), granulocytopenia (17%), fever (65%), and headache (26%).

Careful monitoring for renal impairment and seizures is recommended because of foscarnet's effects on renal function and electrolytes, respectively. Because of its sodium content, foscarnet use is cautioned in patients with underlying heart failure. It has been determined as pregnancy category C risk, for which ultrasonographic monitoring of amniotic fluid volumes is recommended after 20 weeks to detect oligohydramnios. It not known whether foscarnet is excreted in breastmilk. Known drug interactions include potentiation of adverse side effects of acyclovir/valacyclovir, aminoglycosides, amphotericin B, cyclosporine, QTc-prolonging agents, methotrexate, and tacrolimus. Conversely, loop diuretics and pentamidine have been shown to enhance the toxic effect of foscarnet.

CIDOFOVIR

MECHANISM OF ACTION AND PHARMACOKINETICS

Cidofovir, (S)-1-[3-hydroxy-2(phosphonylmethoxy)-propyl]cytosine, is a phosphonate nucleotide analog.[55] Unlike other nucleoside analogs, it does not require initial phosphorylation by virus-induced kinases and can be converted by host cell enzymes to cidofovir diphosphate, a competitive inhibitor of viral DNA polymerases. Cidofovir is officially approved for IV administration, though a topical formulation can be compounded for off-label usage. It has a volume of distribution of 0.31 L per kg with low CSF penetration; therefore, an IV dose of 5 mg/kg results in a peak plasma concentration of 11.5 µg/mL. Plasma half-life is approximately 2.6 hours with markedly longer intracellular half-life of 24 to 87 hours. Excretion is mainly renal, which can be facilitated by the addition of concomitant probenecid.

INDICATIONS AND CONTRAINDICATIONS

- CMV retinitis
- Acyclovir-resistant HSV infections (off-label)

TABLE 191-7
Dosing Regimens for Foscarnet

CONDITION	DOSAGE	ROUTE	DURATION
CMV retinitis	Induction: 90 mg/kg every 12 h	IV	14-21 d
	Maintenance: 90 mg/kg every 24 h	IV	Until CD4 count >100 on 6 mo of HAART
Acyclovir-resistant HSV infection	40 mg/kg every 8 h or	IV	14-21 d
	60 mg/kg every 12 h		2-3 wk or until clinical resolution
CMV esophagitis/colitis	90 mg/kg every 12 h	IV	21-42 d or until clinical resolution

CMV, cytomegalovirus; HAART, highly active antiretroviral therapy; HSV, herpes simplex virus.

Cidofovir is approved for IV treatment of CMV retinitis particularly in those with AIDS, though it has been shown in multiple incidences to be effective in acyclovir-resistant HSV infections,[5,56] both via IV and topical routes, as well as in topical treatments for human papillomavirus infections, Kaposi sarcoma, and molluscum contagiosum.[57-65] Given its significant renal metabolism, cidofovir is contraindicated in those with preexisting renal impairment, as evidenced by serum creatinine >1.5 or >2+ proteinuria.

DOSING REGIMENS

For adults, cidofovir may be given at an induction dose of 5 mg/kg once weekly for the first 2 weeks, followed by a 5-mg/kg dose once every 2 weeks (Table 191-8). Data regarding the use in pediatric patients are accumulating.[66]

SIDE EFFECTS AND PRECAUTIONS

Common adverse effects consist of renal impairment (59% incidence), which consists of:

- renal tubular damage,
- dose-dependent proximal tubular injury (Fanconi-like),
- proteinuria, and
- elevated serum creatinine levels.

Other common effects include nausea (48%), alopecia (16%), rash, fever, myalgias, asthenia, headache, abdominal pain, diarrhea, nausea, dyspepsia, flatulence, increased creatinine, pancreatitis, and hypophosphatemia. The incidence of nephrotoxicity can be reduced by vigorous hydration before and after infusion, in addition to coadministration of probenecid. In addition to close monitoring of renal function, the drug should not be used concurrently with tenofovir disoproxil fumarate (TDF) because of a risk of increased tenofovir levels and toxicity. The following rare but possible effects can occur: squamous cell carcinoma associated with intralesional injection of cidofovir to treat human papillomavirus (HPV)–related recurrent respiratory papillomatosis,[67-69] and herpes simplex stomatitis associated with prophylactic cidofovir therapy.[70]

TABLE 191-8
Dosing Regimens for Cidofovir

CONDITION	DOSAGE	ROUTE	DURATION
CMV retinitis	Induction: 5 mg/kg every week	IV	2 wk
	Maintenance: 5 mg/kg every 2 wk	IV	Until CD4 count >00 after 6 mo on HAART

CMV, cytomegalovirus; HAART, highly active antiretroviral therapy.
Note: Cidofovir IV administration must be accompanied by prehydration and probenecid.

Cidofovir has been labeled pregnancy category C, suggesting possible teratogenic risk. It is thus recommended that women of childbearing potential use effective contraception during and for 1 month following treatment and that men use barrier contraception during and for 3 months following treatment. The indications for treating CMV retinitis during pregnancy are the same as in nonpregnant HIV-infected women; however, therapy with cidofovir should be avoided during the first trimester when possible. It is not known whether cidofovir is excreted in breastmilk, but generally breast-feeding on cidofovir is not recommended because of the potential for serious adverse reactions in the nursing infant.

OTHER INFECTIONS

MECHANISM OF ACTION

Interferons are cytokines derived from a variety of cells that interact through high-affinity cell surface receptors. They have broad antiviral and immunomodulating effects that include induction of gene transcription, inhibition of cellular growth, interference with oncogene expression, alteration of cell surface antigen expression, increased phagocytic activity of macrophages, and cytotoxicity of lymphocytes.

PHARMACOKINETICS

Interferon is commonly given subcutaneously, but also may be administered intravenously, intralesionally, or intramuscularly. It has a plasma half-life of 2 to 3 hours after IV administration, and 4 to 6 hours after subcutaneous or intramuscular administration. A prolonged half-life can be obtained with pegylated interferon.

INDICATIONS

Interferon therapy has been approved for a variety of viral infections (IFN-alpha), for multiple sclerosis (IFN-beta), for chronic granulomatous disease (IFN-gamma), as well as for a number of neoplastic diseases (IFN-alpha), including melanoma. It also has been useful as off-label therapies for chronic myelogenous leukemia, cutaneous T-cell lymphoma, Behçet disease, desmoid tumor, multiple myeloma, neuroendocrine tumors, renal cell carcinoma, and West Nile virus. In the setting of viral infections, interferon-α has been studied most extensively and includes alphacon-1, alpha-2a/b, and alpha-n3.

VIRAL DISEASES TREATED WITH INTERFERON

- Condylomata acuminata (intralesional)
- Chronic hepatitis C infection +/− in combination with ribavirin (IM, subcutaneous [SC])

- Chronic hepatitis B infection (IM, SC)
- AIDS-related Kaposi sarcoma (IM, SC)

DOSING REGIMENS

Common dosing regimens are provided in Table 191-9. Pediatric dosing is adjusted by one-third to one-half of adult dosing with recommendation to consider acetaminophen premedication prior to interferon administration to reduce the incidence of some adverse reactions.

SIDE EFFECTS AND PRECAUTIONS

Side effects with interferon are common and often result in discontinuation of the drug. In a majority of patients, flulike symptoms of fever, chills, tachycardia, malaise, myalgia, and headache may occur within 1 to 2 hours of administration. The most common cutaneous side effects include injection site reactions, alopecia, psoriasis, fixed drug eruptions, eczematous drug reactions, sarcoidosis,[71] lupus, pigmentary changes, and lichenoid eruptions.[72,73] Other adverse effects include bone marrow suppression as well as GI- and hepatotoxicity for which blood counts and metabolic panels should be monitored. Interferon-α has further been shown to cause or aggravate neuropsychiatric events for which patients should be monitored for depression psychosis, cognitive changes, and suicidal and homicidal ideation. Interferon-α should not be used to treat hepatitis B–related cirrhosis or decompensated liver disease because hepatitis flares could lead to further decompensation.

Precaution should be taken in prescribing interferon to patients with underlying eye, autoimmune, cardiovascular, ischemic, infectious, or lung disease. Alone, interferon is labeled as pregnancy risk factor C. Combination therapy of interferon-α with ribavirin is associated with birth defects (category X) and is contraindicated in pregnant women as well as males of pregnant partners. Interferon may enhance the activity of aldesleukin, clozapine, deferiprone, dypnone, methadone, ribavirin, theophylline, tizanidine, zidovudine, and telbivudine.

DRUGS FOR THE TREATMENT OF HIV INFECTION

Drug treatment of HIV infection requires specialized training and experience. The US Department of Health and Human Services (HHS) and the World Health Organization (WHO) publish guidelines for the treatment of HIV. Both sets of guidelines are updated regularly as evidence from ongoing clinical trials emerges and therefore should be consulted routinely. The DHHS guidelines are available at http://aidsinfo.nih.gov/guidelines, and the WHO guidelines are available at http://www.who.int/hiv/pub/guidelines.

INTRODUCTION

HIV infection is treated with antiretroviral therapy (ART) which involves the use of multidrug regimens to reduce HIV-associated morbidity, prolong the duration and quality of survival, and prevent HIV transmission.

As of June 2016, there are more than 25 available antiretroviral (ARV) drugs in 6 major classes (Table 191-10). Multiple comparative clinical trials have shown that combination therapy involving multiple drugs from different classes is most effective. However, eradication of HIV infection cannot be achieved with available ARV regimens, primarily because the pool of latently infected CD4 T cells is established during the earliest stages of acute HIV infection and persists with a long half-life.[74]

ARV drugs work by blocking the virus at various points in its 7-stage life cycle. The stages of the HIV life cycle and the classes of ARV drugs that block them are as follows[74,75]:

TABLE 191-9
Dosing Regimens for the Interferons

CONDITION	DOSAGE	ROUTE	DURATION
Kaposi sarcoma	IFNα-2b 30 million units 3×/wk	IM, Subcutaneous	Dependent on response
Condyloma acuminata	IFNα-2b 1 million units 3×/wk or	Intralesional	3 wk
	IFNα-n3 250k units 2×/wk		Up to 8 wk
Chronic hepatitis C (with ribavirin)	PEG-IFNα-2a 180 μg once a week or PEG-IFNα-2b 1.5 μg/kg once a week or	Subcutaneous	Dependent on response and genotype
	IFN-alfacon-1 15 μg/d or		Up to 48 wk
	IFNα-2b 3 million units 3×/wk	IM, Subcutaneous	18-24 mo
Chronic hepatitis B	PEG-IFNα-2a 180 μg once a week or	Subcutaneous	48 wk
	IFNα-2b 10 million units 3×/wk	IM, Subcutaneous	16 wk

IFN, interferon; PEG-IFN, peginterferon.

TABLE 191-10
Available Antiretroviral Therapy and Their Abbreviations

Entry Inhibitor
  Maraviroc (MVC)

Fusion Inhibitor
  Enfuvirtide (T-20)

Nucleoside and Nucleotide Reverse Transcriptase Inhibitors (NRTIs)
  Abacavir (ABC)
  Didanosine (ddI)
  Emtricitabine (FTC)
  Lamivudine (3TC)
  Stavudine (d4T)
  Tenofovir disoproxil fumarate (TDF)
  Zidovudine (ZDV, AZT)

Nonnucleoside Reverse Transcriptase Inhibitors (NNRTIs)
  Delavirdine (DLV)
  Efavirenz (EFV)
  Etravirine (ETR)
  Nevirapine (NVP)
  Rilpivirine (RPV)

Integrase Strand Transfer Inhibitors (INSTIs)
  Dolutegravir (DTG)
  Elvitegravir (EVG)
  Raltegravir (RAL)

Protease Inhibitors (PIs)
  Atazanavir (ATV)
  Atazanavir/ritonavir (ATV/r)
  Atazanavir/cobicistat (ATV/c)
  Darunavir (DRV)
  Darunavir/cobicistat (DRV/c)
  Fosamprenavir (FPV)
  Indinavir (IDV)
  Lopinavir/ritonavir (LPV/r)
  Nelfinavir (NFV)
  Saquinavir (SQV)
  Tipranavir (TPV)

Pharmacokinetic Enhancers/Boosters
  Ritonavir (RTV)
  Cobicistat (COBI)

1. Binding (also called Attachment): The viral envelope glycoprotein binds to the host receptors (CD4) and coreceptors (CC-chemokine receptor 5 (CCR5) or CXC-chemokine receptor 4 (CXCR4)). Entry inhibitors target this stage. The only FDA-approved drug that targets this stage is a CCR5 inhibitor.
2. Fusion: The HIV envelope and the host cell membrane fuse enabling the entry of the viral capsid in the host cell. Fusion inhibitors target this stage.
3. Reverse Transcription: The viral reverse transcriptase converts its genetic material (HIV RNA) into HIV double-stranded DNA. Nucleoside/nucleotide analog reverse transcriptase inhibitors (NRTIs) and nonnucleoside reverse transcriptase inhibitors (NNRTIs) target this stage.
4. Integration: The viral integrase integrates the viral DNA into the host DNA. Integrase strand transfer inhibitors (INSTIs) target this stage.
5. Replication: HIV protein chains and RNA are produced using the host cell machinery.
6. Assembly: The newly replicated proteins and RNA move to the surface of the host cell and assembly into immature virions.
7. Budding and Maturity: The newly formed virion buds out of the host cell and releases protease that breaks up the viral protein chains, ultimately resulting in mature virions. Protease inhibitors (PIs) target this stage, which results in inhibition of reverse transcription and possibly other downstream stages in the life cycle, including integration.

In addition, 2 drugs are pharmacokinetic (PK) enhancers/boosters used solely to improve the pharmacokinetic profiles of some ARV. These are listed in Table 191-10.[74]

ART was shown to reduce HIV-related morbidity and mortality, and reduce perinatal and behavior-associated transmission of HIV. HIV suppression with ART may also decrease inflammation and immune activation thought to contribute to higher rates of cardiovascular and other end-organ damage reported in HIV-infected cohorts. Maximal and durable suppression of plasma viremia delays or prevents the selection of drug-resistance mutations, preserves CD4 T-cell numbers, and confers substantial clinical benefits, all of which are important treatment goals.[74]

THERAPY INITIATION RECOMMENDATIONS

Antiretroviral therapy (ART) is recommended for all HIV-infected individuals to reduce the risk of disease progression, regardless of CD4 count, age group or pregnancy/lactation. Both the HHS and WHO expanded the recommendation of ART to *all* HIV-infected individuals in 2015. In January 2016, based on new findings, the HHS gave the highest strength and evidence rating for this recommendation.[74,76,77]

For most patients, ART is initiated soon after the initial diagnosis. However, several conditions increase the urgency for therapy, these include pregnancy, presence of HIV-related complications, opportunistic infections, chronic hepatitis B and C infection, acute symptomatic HIV infection, and CD4 ≤200 cells/μL, rapidly declining CD4 counts, and higher viral loads (eg, >100,000 copies/mL).[74]

THERAPY REGIMEN RECOMMENDATIONS

The initial ART regimen for a treatment-naive patient generally consists of 2 NRTIs, combined with an INSTI, an NNRTI, or a pharmacologically boosted PI. This strategy has resulted in decreased HIV RNA and increase in CD4 T lymphocyte (CD4) cell in most patients. However, on the basis of individual patient characteristics and needs, an alternative regimen

TABLE 191-11
Preferred and Alternative First-Line ART Regimens

POPULATION	PREFERRED FIRST-LINE REGIMEN	ALTERNATIVE FIRST-LINE REGIMENS
Adults	TDF + 3TC (or FTC) + EFV	AZT + 3TC + EFV (or NVP)
		TDF + 3TC (or FTC) + DTG
		TDF + 3TC (or FTC) + EFV
		TDF + 3TC (or FTC) + NVP
Pregnant/breastfeeding women	TDF + 3TC (or FTC) + EFV	AZT + 3TC + EFV (or NVP)
		TDF + 3TC (or FTC) + NVP
Adolescents	TDF + 3TC (or FTC) + EFV	AZT + 3TC + EFV (or NVP)
		TDF (or ABC) + 3TC (or FTC) + DTG
		TDF (or ABC) + 3TC (or FTC) + EFV
		TDF (or ABC) + 3TC (or FTC) + NVP
Children 3 y to less than 10 y	ABC + 3TC + EFV	ABC + 3TC + NVP
		AZT + 3TC + EFV (or NVP)
		TDF + 3TC (or FTC) + EFV (or NVP)
Children less than 3 y	ABC (or AZT) + 3TC + LPV/r	ABC (or AZT) + 3TC + NVP

Note: For expansions of the abbreviations used, please refer to Table 191-10.

may in some instances be the optimal regimen.[74,76] Table 191-11 shows the recommended and alternative first-line regimens based on the latest WHO guidelines.

Given the large number of excellent options for initial therapy, selection of a regimen for a particular patient should be guided by factors such as viral load, CD4 count, virologic efficacy, side-effect profile, toxicity, pill burden, dosing frequency, previous exposure to drugs, drug–drug interaction potential, resistance testing results, comorbid conditions, and cost. When initiating a combination ART, all drugs should be started simultaneously rather than sequentially.[74]

When initial suppression is not achieved or is lost, rapidly changing to a new regimen with at least 2 active drugs is required. Thus, when prescribing a first-line regimen, second- and third-line strategies should be formulated, keeping in mind the high-level cross-resistance seen among the same class of drugs. Indiscriminate use of the drugs will lead to minimal options for the future. The increasing number of drugs and drug classes makes viral suppression below detection limits an appropriate goal in all patients.[74]

Viral load reduction to below limits of assay detection in an ART-naive patient usually occurs within the first 12 to 24 weeks of therapy.[74]

PREVENTION

PREEXPOSURE PROPHYLAXIS (PrEP)

Oral PrEP of HIV is the use of ARV drugs by HIV-negative people before potential exposure to prevent infection.[78] The WHO recommends oral PrEP containing TDF for all populations with substantial risk of HIV infection (defined by an incidence of HIV infection in the absence of PrEP greater than 3%). For such populations, oral PrEP should be offered as an additional prevention choice as part of combination of prevention approaches, including regular HIV testing and counseling, provision of condoms, screening and treatment for sexually transmitted infections, and adherence counseling.[74,78] Furthermore, HIV testing is required before PrEP is offered and regularly while PrEP is taken. Renal function testing using serum creatinine testing is preferred before starting PrEP and quarterly during PrEP use for the first 12 months then annually thereafter. These populations may include people engaging in high-risk sexual behaviors, people who inject drugs, people in prisons and closed settings, and sex workers.[78,79] Table 191-12 shows the WHO's recommend regimen for PrEP.

TABLE 191-12
WHO Guidelines for Use of ARV Drugs for HIV Prevention

PROPHYLAXIS TYPE	POPULATION	REGIMEN			
Preexposure prophylaxis (PrEP)	All populations at substantial risk	TDF (alone or in combination with FTC)			
		Recommended 2-Drug Regimen	Alternative 2-Drug Regimen	Preferred Additional 3rd Drug	Preferred Additional 3rd Drug Alternative
Postexposure prophylaxis (PEP)	Adults and adolescents	TDF + 3TC (or FTC)	N/A	LPV/r or ATV/r	RAL, DRV/r or EFV
	Children	ZDV + 3TC	ABC + 3TC	LPV/r	Age-appropriate selection from ATV/r, RAL, DRV, EFV, and NVP
			TDF + 3TC (or FTC)		

Note: For expansions of the abbreviations used, please refer to Table 191-10.

POSTEXPOSURE PROPHYLAXIS (PEP)

PEP of HIV is the use of ARV drugs by HIV-negative people after exposure to a known or suspected (high-risk) source of HIV infection. PEP should be prescribed following occupational exposure to HIV by health workers and following non-occupational exposures, including unprotected sexual exposure, injecting drug use and exposure following sexual assault. The WHO recommends at least a 2-drug PEP regimen, but prefers 3 drugs. A full 28-day prescription of antiretrovirals should be provided for HIV PEP following initial risk assessment, and enhanced adherence counseling is suggested for all individuals initiating HIV PEP. Data from animal studies suggest that the efficacy of PEP in preventing transmission is time dependent, and every effort should be made to provide PEP as soon as possible following exposure.[79] Table 191-13 shows the WHO's recommended regimens for PEP.

ADVERSE EFFECTS

Adverse effects have been reported with the use of all antiretroviral (ARV) drugs and are among the most common reasons cited for switching or discontinuing therapy and for medication nonadherence. Fortunately, newer ARV regimens are less toxic than regimens used in the past. Generally less than 10% of antiretroviral therapy (ART)-naive patients enrolled in randomized trials have treatment-limiting adverse events.[74]

Several factors may predispose individuals to adverse effects of ARV medications, these include[74]

- concomitant use of medications with overlapping and additive toxicities,
- comorbid conditions that increase the risk of or exacerbate adverse effects,
- drug–drug interactions that may lead to an increase in drug toxicities, and
- genetic factors that predispose patients to abacavir (ABC) hypersensitivity reaction.

In general, the overall benefits of ART outweigh its risks and that some non–AIDS-related conditions (eg, anemia, cardiovascular disease, renal impairment) may be more likely in the absence of ART.[74]

DRUG INTERACTIONS

Pharmacokinetic (PK) drug–drug interactions between antiretroviral (ARV) drugs and concomitant medications are common, and may lead to increased or decreased drug exposure. In some instances, changes in drug exposure may increase toxicities or affect therapeutic responses. When prescribing or switching one or more drugs in an ARV regimen, clinicians must consider the potential for drug–drug interactions—both those that affect ARVs and those that ARVs affect on other drugs a patient is taking. The magnitude and significance of interactions are difficult to predict when several drugs with competing metabolic pathways are prescribed concomitantly. When prescribing interacting drugs is necessary, clinicians should be vigilant in monitoring for therapeutic efficacy and/or concentration-related toxicities.[74]

The following gives an overview of the pharmacology, mechanism of action, and side effects, particularly mucocutaneous adverse effects, of each class of drugs.

ENTRY INHIBITOR

The only FDA-approved fusion inhibitor is maraviroc.

PHARMACOLOGY AND MECHANISM OF ACTION

Maraviroc selectively binds to the human chemokine receptor CCR5 present on the cell membrane, preventing the interaction of HIV-1 gp120 and CCR5 necessary for CCR5-tropic HIV-1 to enter cells. Maraviroc is a substrate of CYP3A and P-glycoprotein (P-gp) and its pharmacokinetics are likely to be modulated by inhibitors and inducers of these enzymes/transporters.

TABLE 191-13
WHO Guidelines for Postexposure Prophylaxis

POPULATION	RECOMMENDED 2-DRUG REGIMEN	ALTERNATIVE 2-DRUG REGIMEN	PREFERRED ADDITIONAL THIRD DRUG	PREFERRED ADDITIONAL THIRD DRUG ALTERNATIVE
Adults and adolescents	TDF + 3TC (or FTC)	N/A	LPV/r or ATV/r	RAL, DRV/r, or EFV
Children	ZDV + 3TC	ABC + 3TC TDF + 3TC (or FTC)	LPV/r	Age-appropriate selection from ATV/r, RAL, DRV, EFV, and NVP

Note: For expansions of the abbreviations used, please refer to Table 191-10.

SIDE EFFECTS AND PRECAUTIONS

Mucocutaneous Side Effects: Severe and potentially life-threatening skin and hypersensitivity reactions have been reported in patients taking maraviroc. This includes cases of Stevens–Johnson syndrome, hypersensitivity reaction, and toxic epidermal necrolysis.

Other Side Effects:

- Abdominal pain
- Cough
- Dizziness
- Musculoskeletal symptoms
- Pyrexia
- Upper respiratory tract infections
- Hepatotoxicity, which may be preceded by severe rash or other signs of systemic allergic reactions
- Orthostatic hypotension, especially in patients with severe renal insufficiency

FUSION INHIBITOR

The only FDA-approved fusion inhibitor is enfuvirtide.

PHARMACOLOGY AND MECHANISM OF ACTION

Enfuvirtide is a synthetic peptide that mimics a portion of glycoprotein 41 (gp41), HR1, an HIV envelope glycoprotein required for fusion of the viral envelope with the host cell membrane.[80] The drug blocks the formation of a 6-helix bundle structure that is critical for the fusion process.

Enfuvirtide is administered via subcutaneous injection. Pharmacokinetics are linear up to a dose of 180 mg. Enfuvirtide does not influence concentrations of drugs metabolized by CYP 3A4, CYP 2D6, or N-acetyltransferase, and has only minimal effects on those metabolized by CYP 1A2, CYP 2E1, or CYP 2C19.

SIDE EFFECTS AND PRECAUTIONS

Mucocutaneous Side Effects:

- Local injection site reactions
- Induration
- Erythema
- Nodules
- Cysts

Other Side Effects:

- GI upset
- Increased risk of bacterial pneumonias

Injection site reactions occur in nearly all patients. Patients should be alert for signs or symptoms of pneumonia.

NUCLEOSIDE AND NUCLEOTIDE REVERSE TRANSCRIPTASE INHIBITORS (NRTIs)

FDA-approved NRTIs are abacavir, didanosine, emtricitabine, lamivudine, stavudine, tenofovir disoproxil fumarate, and zidovudine.

PHARMACOLOGY AND MECHANISM OF ACTION

NRTIs compete with the naturally occurring deoxynucleoside substrates for binding to reverse transcriptase (RT). After diffusing into the cytoplasm, they are phosphorylated by intracellular kinases to their active triphosphate forms. The triphosphate form is incorporated into DNA, resulting in chain termination. This group of agents demonstrates activity against HIV-1 and HIV-2, as well as other retroviruses.

NRTIs are well absorbed from the GI tract, although there are differences in bioavailability when they are administered with and without food as well as differences in both serum and intracellular half-lives. The volume of distribution, metabolism, and excretion also vary considerably among the different agents.

SIDE EFFECTS AND PRECAUTIONS

Mucocutaneous Side Effects: Serious and sometimes fatal hypersensitivity reactions can occur with abacavir. Patients who carry the HLA-B*5701 allele are at a higher risk of experiencing a hypersensitivity reaction to abacavir.

Fat redistribution has been seen in some patients taking emtricitabine. These changes may include an increased amount of fat in the upper back and neck ("buffalo hump"), breast, and around the trunk. Loss of fat from the legs, arms, and face may also happen. Hyperpigmentation primarily of palms and/or soles, but also possibly the tongue, arms, lip, and nails, also have been seen with this medication. Rash is common and includes hypersensitivity reaction, maculopapular rash, pustular rash, and vesiculobullous rash.

Rash, pruritus, xerostomia, alopecia, lipodystrophy, Stevens–Johnson syndrome, and vasculitis can occur with didanosine.

Alopecia, rash, pruritus, and fat redistribution can be seen with lamivudine.

Fat redistribution can be seen with stavudine.

Rash, including macular, papular, pustular, vesiculobullous, or urticarial, as well as pruritus and diaphoresis, can be seen with tenofovir.

Lipodystrophy, skin/nail pigmentation changes (blue), Stevens–Johnson syndrome, toxic epidermal necrolysis, urticarial, and morbilliform eruption can be seen with zidovudine.

Other Side Effects: The hallmark toxicity of the NRTI class is mitochondrial toxicity, which may manifest as hepatic steatosis, peripheral neuropathy, pancreatitis, dyslipidemia, fat maldistribution, and lipoatrophy. All NRTIs have "black box" warnings in their product labeling regarding the possibility of lactic acidosis syndrome, which is potentially fatal.

Common side effects of zidovudine include bone marrow suppression and GI intolerance. Stavudine is associated with lipoatrophy and lactic acidosis. Didanosine can cause pancreatitis and peripheral neuropathy, whereas abacavir is associated with life-threatening hypersensitivity reactions. Tenofovir is associated with headache and nausea. It can elevate didanosine levels and lower those of atazanavir. Lamivudine is generally well tolerated but may produce neutropenia. Onset of bullous pemphigoid has been reported with the combination of lamivudine + didanosine + nelfinavir.[81]

NONNUCLEOSIDE REVERSE TRANSCRIPTASE INHIBITORS (NNRTIs)

FDA-approved NNRTIs are delavirdine, efavirenz, etravirine, nevirapine, and rilpivirine.

PHARMACOLOGY AND MECHANISM OF ACTION

Drugs in this class are structurally different from the NRTIs. The NNRTIs bind near the catalytic site of reverse transcriptase and alter the enzymes' ability to change conformation. This increased enzyme rigidity prevents its normal polymerization function and therefore the replication rate of the virus reduces.

Nevirapine has greater than 90% bioavailability and a plasma half-life of 24 hours. It is metabolized in the liver and induces its own metabolic pathway. As the metabolism of the drug increases, the dose is increased from once a day during the first 2 weeks to twice per day thereafter. Delavirdine has a bioavailability of 85%. It requires an acidic environment for absorption and should not be given with antacids, H_2 blockers, or proton pump inhibitors. Its plasma half-life is 6 hours, and it is metabolized in the liver.

The absorption of efavirenz is increased by food. However, it is generally administered on an empty stomach to minimize side effects. The half-life of efavirenz is 40+ hours, and it is metabolized in the liver.[82]

SIDE EFFECTS AND PRECAUTIONS

Mucocutaneous Side Effects: Nevirapine is associated with rash in about 20% of patients and may cause Stevens–Johnson syndrome.[83,84] Among HIV-infected patients with CD4 counts <250 cells/μL, higher baseline counts are associated with a higher incidence of rash, requiring discontinuation of the drug.[85] The rash appears to be related to the quinone methide formed in the skin by sulfation of the 12-OH metabolite followed by loss of the sulfate.[86] Mucosal side effects include whitish plaques, burning, taste disturbance, and xerostomia.[87] Treatment with nevirapine should be initiated slowly to minimize the incidence of cutaneous reactions. If the rash is extensive, or if mucous membranes are involved, the drug should be discontinued. Nevirapine is generally not recommended for women with CD4+ T-cell counts higher than 250 cells/mm³ or for men with CD4+ T-cell counts above 400/mm³ because of an increased risk of hepatitis in these patients.

Etravirine is associated with a self-limiting rash in 19% of patients.[88] Delavirdine is also commonly associated with drug rash.

Other Side Effects:

- Hepatitis
- CNS abnormalities
- Efavirenz is teratogenic

INTEGRASE STRAND TRANSFER INHIBITORS (INSTIs)

FDA-approved INSTIs are dolutegravir, elvitegravir, and raltegravir.

PHARMACOLOGY AND MECHANISM OF ACTION

INSTIs inhibit HIV integrase and thus prevent the integration of HIV-1 DNA into host genomic DNA, blocking the formation of the HIV-1 provirus and propagation of the viral infection.

SIDE EFFECTS AND PRECAUTIONS

Mucocutaneous Side Effects: Severe, potentially life-threatening and fatal skin reactions have been reported with the use of raltegravir. This includes cases of Stevens–Johnson syndrome, hypersensitivity reaction, and toxic epidermal necrolysis.

Hypersensitivity reactions characterized by rash, constitutional findings, and sometimes organ dysfunction, including liver injury, have been reported with the use of dolutegravir.

Other Side Effects: The most common adverse reactions include insomnia, headache, dizziness, nausea, diarrhea, and fatigue.

PROTEASE INHIBITORS (PIs)

FDA-approved protease inhibitors are atazanavir, atazanavir-cobicistat, darunavir, darunavir-cobicistat, fosamprenavir, indinavir, lopinavir/ritonavir boosting, nelfinavir, ritonavir (used as a pharmacokinetic boosting agent), saquinavir, and tipranavir.

PHARMACOLOGY AND MECHANISM OF ACTION

Protease inhibitors target an enzyme responsible for the proteolytic cleavage of viral polypeptide precursors. They demonstrate activity against HIV-1 and HIV-2 and may be active against other viruses as well.

Oral bioavailability and first-pass hepatic metabolism vary among the protease inhibitors and formulations have been altered to provide greater absorption. Saquinavir and lopinavir have poor oral availability and are administered in combination with low-dose ritonavir to improve drug levels. Ritonavir has good oral bioavailability, but side effects limit the dose in most patients. It is often used at low doses to boost blood levels of other protease inhibitors.

All protease inhibitors are metabolized via the hepatic cytochrome P_{450} (CYP) system. This makes them prone to interactions with drugs that induce, inhibit, or are themselves metabolized by CYP enzymes. Ritonavir is used primarily for its CYP effect to inhibit the metabolism of other agents and thus raise their blood levels.

SIDE EFFECTS AND PRECAUTIONS

Mucocutaneous Side Effects: The most common side effect of the protease inhibitors to present to dermatologists is lipodystrophy.[89,90] The lipodystrophy may relate to inhibition of ZMPSTE24, an enzyme that removes the farnesylated tail of prelamin A. Buildup of this protein appears to be related to acquired lipodystrophy, possibly through an interaction with a transcription factor called sterol regulatory element–binding protein 1.[91] Fat distribution may improve with L-acetylcarnitine therapy, and fillers have been employed to reduce the social stigma associated with therapy.[92]

Other mucocutaneous side effects:

- Morbilliform rash, generalized erythema, SJS
- Striae
- Paronychia, ingrown toenails
- Pruritus, xerosis
- Desquamative cheilitis
- Icterus (especially with atazanavir as it is associated with unconjugated hyperbilirubinemia)

Other Adverse Effects:

- GI upset
- Nausea
- Vomiting
- Diarrhea
- Hepatitis
- Occasional hepatic failure
- Dyslipidemias (except atazanavir)
- Alteration in glucose metabolism
- Significant drug–drug interactions

INVESTIGATIONAL DRUGS

The guidelines are continuously being adjusted and improved based on the latest available research. The currently available drugs are safer, simpler to use, and more potent than previous drugs. These improvements are expected to continue given the current crop of investigational drugs. Table 191-14 summarizes the current investigational drugs.

DRUGS FOR THE TREATMENT OF HEPATITIS C

Hepatitis C virus (HCV) infection is a major global health problem with 130 to 150 million people estimated to be chronically infected individuals worldwide.[93] Up to 85% of patients with acute HCV infection are unable to clear the infection, and become chronically infected if left untreated. For these patients, the risk of progression to liver cirrhosis is estimated to be 15% to 30% within 20 years. These patients are at higher risk of subsequently developing hepatocellular carcinoma.[94]

HCV belongs to the Flaviviridae family. It is an enveloped, positive-sense RNA virus.[95] The lack of a proofreading mechanism during the replication of the HCV RNA genome leads to significant variation. Thus, HCV has been divided into 7 genotypes with distinct geographic distribution. Genotype 1 is the most common genotype worldwide and in the United States. Genotypes 1, 2, 4, and 5 are endemic in Africa, whereas genotypes 3 and 6 are mostly found in Asia. Genotype 7 was only recently identified and is thought to have originated in Africa.[96]

Knowledge of the HCV life cycle paved the way for the development of direct-acting antivirals (DAAs)

TABLE 191-14
Investigational Drugs

DRUG CLASS	DRUG NAME	MECHANISM OF ACTION
Entry inhibitor	AMD-070	Selective, reversible, small molecule CXCR4 chemokine coreceptor antagonist
	Cenicriviroc	Small-molecule CCR5 coreceptor antagonist
	Fostemsavir	Binds to the viral envelope gp120 and interfering with virus attachment to the host CD4 receptor
	INCB-9471	Small-molecule CCR5 coreceptor antagonist
	Ibalizumab	Humanized monoclonal antibody that binds to extracellular domain 2 of the CD4 receptor and causes conformational changes
	Monomeric DAPTA	Selective CCR5 coreceptor antagonist
	PRO-140	Humanized IgG4 monoclonal antibody (mAb) that binds to hydrophilic extracellular domains on CCR5
	Vicriviroc	Reversible, small-molecule CCR5 coreceptor antagonist
Nucleoside reverse transcriptase inhibitors (NRTIs)	Amdoxovir	Inhibits the activity of HIV-1 reverse transcriptase
	Apricitabine	
	Censavudine	
	Elvucitabine	
	PSI-5004	
	Tenofovir Alafenamide	A prodrug of the nucleotide analog tenofovir
Nonnucleoside reverse transcriptase inhibitor (NNRTI)	Doravirine	Noncompetitive inhibitors of HIV-1 reverse transcriptase
Integrase strand transfer inhibitors (INSTI)	Cabotegravir	Prevents viral DNA integration into the host genome
Protease Inhibitor (PI)	TMC-310v911	PIs bind the HIV-1 protease enzyme to inhibit cleavage of viral Gag and Gag-Pol polyproteins, thereby preventing the formation of mature, infectious virus particles.[5-7] TMC-310911 is characterized as having a broader in vitro resistance profile than that of currently approved PIs, including darunavir.
Maturation Inhibitor	BMS-955176	Binds to HIV-1 Gag, inhibiting the final protease-mediated cleavage event
Gene Therapy Product	SB-728-T	May provide HIV-infected individuals with a reproducible pool of CD4 T cells permanently resistant to HIV entry, potentially improving immune restoration and leading to functional control of HIV
Histone deacetylase inhibitors	Valproic Acid	HDAC inhibitors reactivate latent HIV within resting CD4 T cells. When latent HIV is reactivated, it is once again able to produce new virus and replicate. It is hoped that after latent HIV is reactivated, the CD4 T cells in which the virus was hiding are more likely to die off on their own or be recognized and killed by the body's immune system.[8,9] In addition, any new virus that is produced during reactivation can then be prevented from infecting other cells with the use of ongoing ART.[8,9] Recent research has shown that additional therapies, together with HDAC inhibitors, may be needed to fully eliminate latent HIV from the body.
	Vorinostat	
Immune modulator	Tucaresol	Enhances costimulatory signaling to CD4-positive T cells
Microbicides	Astodrimer	Blocks HIV attachment to and entry into host CD4 cells
	Dapivirine	Developed as a preexposure prophylaxis. Topical microbicide that inhibit the infection process at the vaginal or rectal mucosa and directly interfere with the HIV replication cycle
	Tenofovir	

that have revolutionized the treatment of HCV infection. Briefly, the HCV life cycle consists of the following steps[97]:

1. Attachment: This involves the binding of HCV particles onto hepatocytes and is mediated by multiple cellular factors and components of the enveloped virions.
2. Cell entry: Clathrin-mediated endocytosis allows the HCV particles to enter early endosomes.
3. Fusion: pH-dependent membrane fusion is induced by the acidic environment in early endosomes. This releases the HCV genome into the cytosol.
4. Translation and Replication: The viral genome in the cytosol becomes available for translation by cellular ribosomes into a single polyprotein that is subsequently cleaved by cellular and viral proteases (NS2, NS3/4A) into the 10 mature viral proteins including structural proteins (core, E1, E2, p7) and nonstructural proteins (NS2, NS3, NS4A, NS4B, NS5A, and NS5B). The replication complex is subsequently assembled at the cellular ER membrane in association with the viral genomic RNA and nonstructural viral proteins (a process thought to be coordinated by NS4B and NS5A). Viral RNA replication is thought to occur at these complexes where NS5B (the viral RNA–dependent RNA polymerase) uses the viral genomic RNA as a template to synthesize a negative-sense intermediate strand. The negative sense intermediate strand is then used as a template to synthesize

nascent genomic RNA strands that can be translated into viral proteins, used as templates for further RNA replication, or assembled in virions.
5. Assembly: This step is not fully understood but is thought to be dependent on cellular lipid metabolism as well as viral proteins.
6. Release: HCV virions are released as lipoviral particles with associated apoE and/or apoB, which are essential for viral infectivity.

DAAs target specific viral proteins with the aim of interrupting critical stages of the HCV life cycle. Approved DAAs as of this writing can be classified based on their mechanism of action as follows:

1. Protease (NS3/4A) inhibitors: boceprevir (discontinued), telaprevir (discontinued), paritaprevir, simeprevir, elbasvir, grazoprevir
2. NS5A inhibitors: daclatasvir, ledipasvir, ombitasvir
3. Polymerase (NS5B) inhibitor, nucleot(s)ide analog: sofosbuvir
4. Polymerase (NS5B) inhibitor, nonnucleoside analog: dasabuvir

The goal of HCV is sustained virologic response (SVR), which is defined as undetectable HCV RNA levels at a specified end point after completion of therapy. This end point has historically been set at 24 weeks from completion of therapy, but SVR at 12 weeks post-treatment has been shown to correlate closely to that at 24 weeks.[98] Thus, SVR at 12 weeks has been adopted as the primary efficacy endpoint in more recent clinical trials and clinical practice.[99]

The exact treatment chosen depends several factors that can affect responses, which include genotype, coinfection with HIV-1, comorbidities, cirrhosis, and prior treatment. This is an area of active research and as new results from clinical trials become available, guidelines outlining the preferred regimens for different patient populations are being updated.[93,100] The following website is a useful resource: http://www.hepatitisc.uw.edu/page/treatment/drugs.

PEG-IFNα AND RIBAVIRIN COMBINATION THERAPY

HCV virus is able to suppress the innate and adaptive immune and proinflammatory responses of the host by various mechanisms. Exogenous PEG-IFNα is used in an attempt to counteract that suppression. Ribavirin has an unclear mechanism of action against HCV, but there is evidence to suggest that it may have an immunomodulatory effect that mediates increased sensitivity to PEG-IFNα.[101]

PEG-IFNα is administered subcutaneously and is associated with localized injection site reactions in the majority of treated patients. These include erythema, tenderness, pruritus, and rashes at the site of injection.[102] The latter most commonly present as pruritic, erythematous patches or plaques with ill-defined borders. These reactions usually resolve spontaneously without treatment. Less commonly (<4%), cutaneous necrosis can occur at the injection site, which can be managed with local wound care and usually resolve in 1 to 2 months. Alternative injection sites can be used for future doses. Other miscellaneous localized skin reactions have been reported, including blistering reactions, granulomatous and suppurative dermatitis, lupus-like reactions, embolia cutis medicamentosa, and localized alopecia.[103]

Generalized dermatologic adverse events also have been associated with the use of PEG-IFNα, and the addition of ribavirin further increases their incidence. These adverse events can affect compliance and may lead to premature discontinuation of antiviral therapy. The most commonly encountered generalized dermatologic adverse events seen with the combination of PEG-IFNα and ribavirin include alopecia (28% to 36%) and skin rash (21%).[104] The skin rash most commonly seen with PEG-IFNα and ribavirin combination therapy has been characterized as eczematous dermatitis (erythematous papules and microvesicles often with excoriation) that is predominantly located over friction sites on the extremities and trunk. It can be associated with generalized pruritus and xerosis. Symptomatic patients can be treated with topical steroids and emollients without discontinuation of antiviral treatment. Steroids can be tapered off once the rash resolves. Systemic anti-histamines and hydroxyzine also can be used for pruritus.[102,103]

Other forms of dermatitis also have been reported including nummular dermatitis and Meyerson phenomenon, an eczematous eruption centered around preexisting melanocytic nevi. Fixed drug eruptions and lichenoid eruptions (most commonly lichen planus) also have been described in association with PEG-IFNα and ribavirin therapy in HCV-infected patients.

PEG-IFNα and ribavirin also have been associated with the exacerbation or unmasking of various autoimmune disorders, many of which have skin manifestations that are important to recognize. These disorders include psoriasis, alopecia aerata, vitiligo, sarcoidosis, systemic lupus erythematosus, systemic sclerosis, polyarteritis nodosa. Some of these conditions were successfully treated with systemic corticosteroids but they often necessitate the discontinuation of antiviral therapy. Topical options for the treatment of psoriasis include steroids, calcipotriol, and PUVA.[103]

Other side effects of PEG-IFNα include flulike symptoms, fatigue, bone marrow suppression/cytopenias, and mood disturbances. Interferon is contraindicated for patients with liver failure and should be used with caution in patients with compensated cirrhosis. Other contraindications for PEG-IFNα include cytopenias, severe cardiac disease, uncontrolled seizures, uncontrolled psychiatric disease, and pregnancy.

Ribavirin also has "black box" warnings for hemolytic anemia and teratogenicity. The former can be severe and most often occurs within 1 to 2 weeks after starting therapy. Therefore, hemoglobin/hematocrit level should be checked at baseline and then 2 and 4 weeks after starting therapy. Given its teratogenicity, ribavirin is contraindicated in pregnancy and in male partners of pregnant women. Pregnancy should also be avoided (by using 2 forms of contraception) during therapy with ribavirin and for at least 6 months after completion of therapy (WHO).

FIRST-GENERATION DAAs

The first-generation protease inhibitors include boceprevir and telaprevir. They were initially used for the treatment of genotype 1 in combination with PEG-IFNα and ribavirin, since they were associated with higher SVR rates. However, compared to PEG-IFNα plus ribavirin alone, these agents were more expensive and were associated with a higher incidence of clinically significant adverse events leading to poor adherence and higher rates of premature discontinuation of therapy. This can subsequently lead to higher rates of resistance and treatment failure.[99] Therefore, these regimens are no longer recommended by the most recent guidelines as they have been replaced by safer and more efficacious second-generation DAAs.[100]

The most notable adverse events with boceprevir were anemia, neutropenia, and dysgeusia. However, the latter was not a common cause of discontinuation of therapy. When compared to PEG-IFNα and ribavirin alone, the use of boceprevir was not associated with a significantly increased incidence of serious skin rash.

On the other hand, the most notable adverse events associated with telaprevir were rash, pruritus, anorectal discomfort, diarrhea, and anemia. Around 6% to 7% of patients receiving telaprevir discontinued therapy due to skin rash. The rash can occur at any time during treatment with telaprevir, but 50% of the cases occurred within the first 4 weeks of initiation of therapy. Around 90% were classified as Grade 1 or 2 and did not progress. The rash most commonly associated with telaprevir was described as eczematous dermatitis that usually resolved with the discontinuation of therapy. However, telaprevir has been associated with more serious dermatologic adverse reactions, including drug rash with eosinophilia and systemic symptoms (DRESS) and Stevens–Johnson syndrome (SJS).

Therefore, patients receiving telaprevir should be instructed to report any skin or mucosal lesions, and any patient with such lesions should be questioned about systemic symptoms. In patients with systemic symptoms or involvement of mucous membranes or a significant portion of body surface area then discontinuation of therapy should be considered. Although the efficacy has not been fully established, mild to moderate rash can be managed with topical steroids and/or oral antihistamines. Systemic corticosteroids should be avoided.[105,106]

SECOND-GENERATION DAAs

Different combinations of the second-generation DAAs have been approved for HCV treatment.[93] There is a trend toward using interferon-free and, whenever possible, ribavirin-free regimens for the shortest effective treatment duration. Indicated and preferred treatment regimens are being actively updated as results of recent and ongoing trials get reported (useful resource: http://www.hepatitisc.uw.edu/page/treatment/drugs). This section attempts to provide an account of the dermatologic adverse events (exclusive of infectious complications like cellulitis) as well as the most common adverse events reported in recent clinical trials using FDA-approved DAA-based regimens without ribavirin when used over a duration of 12 weeks. It should be noted that the dermatologic side effects previously associated with ribavirin (including rash and pruritus) had higher incidence in patients who received DAA-based regimens that included ribavirin (mostly for treatment-experienced patients with cirrhosis).

- Simeprevir (Olysio): It is only indicated in combination with sofosbuvir or PEG-IFNα plus ribavirin. The most common adverse events associated with simeprevir were rash, photosensitivity, pruritis, nausea, and transient hyperbilirubinemia. However, the rates of discontinuation of therapy were comparable to those with PEG-IFNα plus ribavirin alone. The skin rash can develop at any time during treatment but most commonly begins within 4 weeks from the initiation of therapy. A photosensitivity reaction with skin rash can also occur and patients should be instructed to minimize exposure to sunlight.[107,108]
- Sofosbuvir (Sovaldi): When used in combination with PEG-IFNα plus ribavirin, the most common adverse events include fatigue, nausea, anemia, and neutropenia. There was no significant increase in rate of discontinuation of therapy when compared with PEG-IFNα plus ribavirin alone. When used in combination with ribavirin alone, the most common adverse effects reported were fatigue, headache, nausea and pruritis. However, the rate of discontinuation of this regimen was relatively low (≤1%).[107]
- Ledipasvir and sofosbuvir (Harvoni): The most common adverse events were fatigue, headache, nausea, and diarrhea. In the ION-1 Study, up to 7% of patients had rash.[109] Mild rash and pruritus were reported in 1% to 2% of patients in the ION-2 and 3 studies.[110,111] However, none of the dermatologic adverse events required discontinuation of treatment. No rash was reported in ION-4 study wherein Harvoni was used to treat patients with HCV/HIV-1 coinfection.[112]
- Daclatasvir (Daklinza) and sofosbuvir: The most common adverse events were fatigue, headache, nausea, and diarrhea. This combination can also cause bradycardia in patients taking amiodarone (especially if they also take a beta-blocker). Rash was reported in 2% and pruritis in 5% of patients in the 12-week treatment groups.[113]
- Elbasvir and grazoprevir: The most common adverse observed in patients were fatigue, headache, and nausea. Skin rash (that did not require

discontinuation of therapy) was reported in 2 of 33 patients (6%) in the group receiving elbasvir and grazoprevir without ribavirin.[114,115]
- Ombitasvir-paritaprevir-ritonavir and dasabuvir (Viekira Pak): The most common adverse events were fatigue and nausea. Pruritus was reported in 5% to 6% of patients, and skin rash was reported in up to 4% to 5% of patients. The latter did not warrant discontinuation of therapy in any of the treated patients.[116,117]
- Sofosbuvir and velpatasvir (Epclusa): The most common adverse effects were headache, fatigue, and nausea. Pruritus was reported in 3% to 4% of patients. However, there were no reports of serious skin rash after 12 weeks of treatment with sofosbuvir and velpatasvir in the clinical trials that have been published as of this writing.[118,119]

DRUGS FOR THE TREATMENT OF HEPATITIS B

Hepatitis B virus (HBV) infection is most commonly treated with a nucleoside/tide reverse transcriptase inhibitor (NRTI). Generally, these agents are mostly given orally once daily, with dose adjustment for patients with impaired renal function (creatinine clearance <50 mL/min). NRTIs act by inhibiting the polymerase activity of HBV. However, their low-level activity against the human mitochondrial DNA polymerase gamma and can lead to mitochondrial toxicity, for which a "Black Box" warning is included in the product labeling of all NRTIs. This may be manifested as myopathy, peripheral neuropathy, hepatic steatosis, pancreatitis, dyslipidemia, lipoatrophy, and lactic acidosis.[120]

Currently, the preferred agents for HBV treatment are either entecavir or tenofovir based on a favorable side effect profile and lower rates of resistance. The other NRTIs approved for treatment of HBV include lamivudine, adefovir, and telbivudine. Tenofovir and adefovir have been associated with nephrotoxicity and Fanconi syndrome as well as rashes with variable morphology (including maculopapular, urticarial, vesiculobullous, pustular, and lichenoid rashes). Telbivudine has been reported to cause myopathy and peripheral neuropathy. Pancreatitis has been reported with lamivudine. Entecavir is generally well tolerated.[121,122]

PEG-IFNα-2a also can be used in patients without cirrhosis who are HBeAg positive with good efficacy (27% rate of seroconversion at 1 year) but poor tolerability due to side effects as discussed previously. Of note, PEG-IFNα-2a is contraindicated in patients with decompensated cirrhosis, cytopenias, severe cardiac disease, uncontrolled seizures, and uncontrolled psychiatric disease. It should be used with caution in patients with compensated cirrhosis.

For persons with HDV coinfection, the only effective treatment is PEG-IFNα. For persons with HIV coinfection, treatment of HBV and HIV need to be coordinated to utilize drugs active against both viruses (tenofovir, entecavir, lamivudine, and telbivudine).[121]

Indications for initiation of treatment include the following:

1. ALF or decompensated cirrhosis (NRTIs only)
2. The presence of significant liver injury or fibrosis, as reflected by elevated ALT levels or biopsy-proven inflammation and/or fibrosis plus active HBV viremia (HBV DNA >2000 IU/mL if HBeAg negative, or >20,000 IU/mL if HBeAg positive).
3. Immunosuppressive therapy.

For patients treated with PEG-IFNα, the recommended duration of treatment is 48 weeks. For patients treated with NRTIs, the exact duration of therapy varies and depends on multiple factors including HBeAg status, duration of HBV DNA suppression, and presence of cirrhosis/decompensation (AASLD Guidelines for Treatment of Chronic Hepatitis B). If seroconversion of HBeAg or hepatitis B surface antigen (HBsAg) is observed, then treatment can be discontinued. However, the latter is only rarely observed.[121,123]

DRUGS TO TREAT OTHER VIRAL INFECTIONS

Neuraminidase inhibitors can be used to treat patients presenting with severe influenza infection or those at high risk for severe infection or complications (such as pregnant women and elderly patients). Neuraminidase inhibitors include oseltamivir, zanamivir, and peramivir. Oseltamivir and peramivir have been associated with serious skin adverse events, including cases of Stevens–Johnson syndrome and erythema multiforme. Other skin side effects have been reported with peramivir including urticaria and maculopapular rash.

Ribavirin is used to treat respiratory syncytial virus infection. The dermatologic side effects were discussed in the HCV section.

ACKNOWLEDGMENTS

The authors thank Drs Hay, Reichman, and Elston for their work on this chapter in previous editions. The authors also thank M. Liu for her contribution to this chapter.

REFERENCES

1. Leung DT, Henning PA, Wagner EC, et al. Inadequacy of plasma acyclovir levels at delivery in patients with genital herpes receiving oral acyclovir suppressive therapy in late pregnancy. *J Obstet Gynaecol Can.* 2009;31(12):1137-1143.
2. Vanpouille C, Lisco A, Margolis L. Acyclovir: a new use for an old drug. *Curr Opin Infect Dis.* 2009;22(6):583-587.
3. Celum C, Wald A, Lingappa JR, et al. Acyclovir and transmission of HIV-1 from persons infected with HIV-1 and HSV-2. *N Engl J Med.* 2010;362(5):427-439.
4. Duan R, de Vries RD, van Dun JM, et al. Acyclovir sus-

ceptibility and genetic characteristics of sequential herpes simplex virus type 1 corneal isolates from patients with recurrent herpetic keratitis. *J Infect Dis.* 2009;200(9):1402-1414.
5. Workowski KA, Bolan GA; Centers for Disease Control and Prevention (CDC). Sexually transmitted diseases treatment guidelines, 2015. *MMWR Recomm Rep.* 2015;64(RR-03):1-137.
6. Leflore S, Anderson PL, Fletcher CV. A risk-benefit evaluation of acyclovir for the treatment and prophylaxis of herpes simplex virus infections. *Drug Saf.* 2000: 23(2):131-142.
7. Bradley JS, Nelson JD, Kimberlin DK, et al, eds. *Nelson's Pocket Book of Pediatric Antimicrobial Therapy*. 18th ed. Philadelphia, PA: Lippincott Williams & Wilkins; 2011.
8. Gartner LM, Morton J, Lawrence RA, et al. Breastfeeding and the use of human milk. *Pediatrics.* 2005; 115(2):496-506.
9. Yadav M, Upadhyay V, Singhal P, et al. Stability evaluation and sensitive determination of antiviral drug, valacyclovir and its metabolite acyclovir in human plasma by a rapid liquid chromatography-tandem mass spectrometry method. *J Chromatogr B Analyt Technol Biomed Life Sci.* 2009;877(8-9):680-688.
10. Corey L, Wald A, Patel R, et al. Once-daily valacyclovir to reduce the risk of transmission of genital herpes. *N Engl J Med.* 2004;350(1):11-20.
11. Sperling RS, Fife KH, Warren TJ, et al. The effect of daily valacyclovir suppression on herpes simplex virus type 2 viral shedding in HSV-2 seropositive subjects without a history of genital herpes. *Sex Transm Dis.* 2008;35(3):286-290.
12. Martens MG, Fife KH, Leone PA, et al. Once daily valacyclovir for reducing viral shedding in subjects newly diagnosed with genital herpes. *Infect Dis Obstet Gynecol.* 2009;2009:105376.
13. Miserocchi E, Modorati G, Galli L, et al. Efficacy of valacyclovir vs acyclovir for the prevention of recurrent herpes simplex virus eye disease: a pilot study. *Am J Ophthalmol.* 2007;144(4):547-551.
14. Hull C, McKeough M, Sebastian K, et al. Valacyclovir and topical clobetasol gel for the episodic treatment of herpes labialis: a patient-initiated, double-blind, placebo-controlled pilot trial. *J Eur Acad Dermatol Venereol.* 2009;23(3):263-267.
15. Ozçay F, Arslan H, Bilezikçi B, et al. The role of valacyclovir on Epstein-Barr virus viral loads in pediatric liver transplant patients. *Transplant Proc.* 2009;41(7): 2878-2880.
16. Hoshino Y, Katano H, Zou P, et al. Long-term administration of valacyclovir reduces the number of Epstein-Barr virus (EBV)-infected B cells but not the number of EBV DNA copies per B cell in healthy volunteers. *J Virol.* 2009;83(22):11857-11861.
17. Aoki FY. Contemporary antiviral drug regimens for the prevention and treatment of orolabial and anogenital herpes simplex virus infection in the normal host: four approved indications and 13 off-label uses. *Can J Infect Dis.* 2003;14(1):17-27.
18. Zeng L, Nath CE, Blair EY, et al. Population pharmacokinetics of acyclovir in children and young people with malignancy after administration of intravenous acyclovir or oral valacyclovir. *Antimicrob Agents Chemother.* 2009;53(7):2918-2927.
19. Bomgaars L, Thompson P, Berg S, et al. Valacyclovir and acyclovir pharmacokinetics in immunocompromised children. *Pediatr Blood Cancer.* 2008;51(4):504-508.
20. Kimberlin DW. Pharmacokinetics and safety of extemporaneously compounded valacyclovir oral suspension in pediatric patients from 1 month through 11 years of age. *Clin Infect Dis.* 2010;50(2):221-228.
21. Asahi T, Tsutsui M, Wakasugi M, et al. Valacyclovir neurotoxicity: clinical experience and review of the literature. *Eur J Neurol.* 2009;16(4):457-460.
22. Daito J, Hanada K, Katoh N, et al. Symmetrical drug-related intertriginous and flexural exanthema caused by valacyclovir. *Dermatology.* 2009;218(1):60-62.
23. Ebo DG, Bridts CH, De Clerck LS, et al. Immediate allergy from valacyclovir. *Allergy.* 2008;63(7): 941-942.
24. Hasler-Nguyen N, Shelton D, Ponard G, et al. Evaluation of the in vitro skin permeation of antiviral drugs from penciclovir 1% cream and acyclovir 5% cream used to treat herpes simplex virus infection. *BMC Dermatol.* 2009;9:3.
25. Zhu W, Guo C, Yu A, et al. Microemulsion-based hydrogel formulation of penciclovir for topical delivery. *Int J Pharm.* 2009;378(1-2):152-158.
26. Lv Q, Yu A, Xi Y, et al. Development and evaluation of penciclovir-loaded solid lipid nanoparticles for topical delivery. *Int J Pharm.* 2009;372(1-2):191-198.
27. Zhu W, Yu A, Wang W, et al. Formulation design of microemulsion for dermal delivery of penciclovir. *Int J Pharm.* 2008;360(1-2):184-90.
28. Tyring SK, Diaz-Mitoma F, Shafran SD, et al. Oral famciclovir for the suppression of recurrent genital herpes: the combined data from two randomized controlled trials. *J Cutan Med Surg.* 2003;7(6):449-454.
29. Tyring S, Berger T, Yen-Moore A, et al. Single-day therapy for recurrent genital herpes. *Am J Clin Dermatol.* 2006;7(4):209-211.
30. Harpaz R, Ortega-Sanchez IR, Seward JF; Advisory Committee on Immunization Practices (ACIP) Centers for Disease Control and Prevention (CDC). Prevention of herpes zoster: recommendations of the Advisory Committee on Immunization Practices (ACIP). *MMWR Recomm Rep.* 2008;57(RR-5):1-30.
31. Bodsworth N, Bloch M, McNulty A, et al; Australo-Canadian FaST Famciclovir Short-Course Herpes Therapy Study Group. 2-day versus 5-day famciclovir as treatment of recurrences of genital herpes: Results of the FaST study. *Sex Health.* 2008;5(3):219-225.
32. Abudalu M, Tyring S, Koltun W, et al. Single-day, patient-initiated famciclovir therapy versus 3-day valacyclovir regimen for recurrent genital herpes: a randomized, double-blind, comparative trial. *Clin Infect Dis.* 2008;47(5):651-658.
33. Aoki FY. The continuing evolution of antiviral therapy for recurrent genital herpes: 1-day patient-initiated treatment with famciclovir. *Herpes.* 2007;14(3):62-65.
34. Bartlett BL, Tyring SK, Fife K, et al. Famciclovir treatment options for patients with frequent outbreaks of recurrent genital herpes: The RELIEF trial. *J Clin Virol.* 2008;43(2):190-195.
35. Ogungbenro K, Matthews I, Looby M, et al. Population pharmacokinetics and optimal design of paediatric studies for famciclovir. *Br J Clin Pharmacol.* 2009;68(4):546-560.
36. Sáez-Llorens X, Yogev R, Arguedas A, et al. Pharmacokinetics and safety of famciclovir in children with herpes simplex or varicella-zoster virus infection. *Antimicrob Agents Chemother.* 2009;53(5): 1912-1920.
37. Leone P, Abudalu M, Mitha E, et al. One-day famciclovir vs. placebo in patient-initiated episodic treatment

of recurrent genital herpes in immunocompetent Black patients. *Curr Med Res Opin.* 2010;26(3):653-661.
38. Tyring S, Richwald G, Hamed K. Single-day therapy: an expert opinion on a recent development for the episodic treatment of recurrent genital herpes. *Arch Gynecol Obstet.* 2007;275(1):1-3.
39. Htwe TH, Bergman S, Koirala J. Famciclovir substitution for patients with acyclovir-associated renal toxicity. *J Infect.* 2008;57(3):266-268.
40. Te CC, Le V, Allee M. Famciclovir-induced leukocytoclastic vasculitis. *Ann Pharmacother.* 2008;42(9):1323-1326.
41. Wilhelmus KR. Therapeutic interventions for herpes simplex virus epithelial keratitis. *Cochrane Database Syst Rev.* 2008;(1):CD002898.
42. Wilhelmus KR. Antiviral treatment and other therapeutic interventions for herpes simplex virus epithelial keratitis. *Cochrane Database Syst Rev.* 2010;(12):CD002898.
43. Kaufman HE, Varnell ED, Gebhardt BM, et al. Efficacy of a helicase-primase inhibitor in animal models of ocular herpes simplex virus type 1 infection. *J Ocul Pharmacol Ther.* 2008;24(1):34-42.
44. Guess S, Stone DU, Chodosh J. Evidence-based treatment of herpes simplex virus keratitis: a systematic review. *Ocul Surf.* 2007;5(3):240-250.
45. Perrottet N, Manuel O, Lamoth F, et al. Variable viral clearance despite adequate ganciclovir plasma levels during valganciclovir treatment for cytomegalovirus disease in D+/R- transplant recipients. *BMC Infect Dis.* 2010;10(1):2.
46. Perrottet N, Decosterd LA, Meylan P, et al. Valganciclovir in adult solid organ transplant recipients: pharmacokinetic and pharmacodynamic characteristics and clinical interpretation of plasma concentration measurements. *Clin Pharmacokinet.* 2009;48(6):399-418.
47. Simon P, Sasse M, Laudi S, et al. Two strategies for prevention of cytomegalovirus infections after liver transplantation. *World J Gastroenterol.* 2016;22(12):3412-3417.
48. Marshall BC, Koch WC. Antivirals for cytomegalovirus infection in neonates and infants: focus on pharmacokinetics, formulations, dosing, and adverse events. *Paediatr Drugs.* 2009;11(5):309-321.
49. Duan R, de Vries RD, Osterhaus AD, et al. Acyclovir-resistant corneal HSV-1 isolates from patients with herpetic keratitis. *J Infect Dis.* 2008;198(5):659-663.
50. Hatchette T, Tipples GA, Peters G, et al. Foscarnet salvage therapy for acyclovir-resistant varicella zoster: report of a novel thymidine kinase mutation and review of the literature. *Pediatr Infect Dis.* 2008;27(1):75-77.
51. Wang H, Zhu L, Xue M, et al. Low-dose foscarnet preemptive therapy for cytomegalovirus viremia after haploidentical bone marrow transplantation. *Biol Blood Marrow Transplant.* 2009;15(4):519-520.
52. Charpentier C, Laureillard D, Sodqi M, et al. Foscarnet salvage therapy efficacy is associated with the presence of thymidine-associated mutations (TAMs) in HIV-infected patients. *J Clin Virol.* 2008;43(2):212-215.
53. Rodriguez J, Casper K, Smallwood G, et al. Resistance to combined ganciclovir and foscarnet therapy in a liver transplant recipient with possible dual-strain cytomegalovirus coinfection. *Liver Transpl.* 2007;13(10):1396-1400.
54. Michaelis M, Ha TA, Doerr HW, et al. Valproic acid interferes with antiviral treatment in human cytomegalovirus-infected endothelial cells. *Cardiovasc Res.* 2008;77(3):544-550.

55. De Clercq E. Emerging antiviral drugs. *Expert Opin Emerg Drugs.* 2008;13(3):393-416.
56. Andrei G, Fiten P, Goubau P, et al. Dual infection with polyomavirus BK and acyclovir-resistant herpes simplex virus successfully treated with cidofovir in a bone marrow transplant recipient. *Transpl Infect Dis.* 2007;9(2):126-131.
57. Jesus DM, Costa LT, Gonçalves DL, et al. Cidofovir inhibits genome encapsidation and affects morphogenesis during the replication of vaccinia virus. *J Virol.* 2009;83(22):11477-11490.
58. Sonvico F, Colombo G, Gallina L, et al. Therapeutic paint of cidofovir/sucralfate gel combination topically administered by spraying for treatment of orf virus infections. *AAPS J.* 2009;11(2):242-249.
59. Van Pachterbeke C, Bucella D, Rozenberg S, et al. Topical treatment of CIN 2+ by cidofovir: results of a phase II, double-blind, prospective, placebo-controlled study. *Gynecol Oncol.* 2009;115(1):69-74.
60. Coremans G, Snoeck R. Cidofovir: clinical experience and future perspectives on an acyclic nucleoside phosphonate analog of cytosine in the treatment of refractory and premalignant HPV-associated anal lesions. *Expert Opin Pharmacother.* 2009;10(8):1343-1352.
61. Calista D. Topical 1% cidofovir for the treatment of vulvar intraepidermal neoplasia (VIN1) developed on lichen sclerosus. *Int J Dermatol.* 2009;48(5):535-536.
62. Amine A, Rivera S, Opolon P, et al. Novel anti-metastatic action of cidofovir mediated by inhibition of E6/E7, CXCR4 and Rho/ROCK signaling in HPV tumor cells. *PLoS One.* 2009;4(3):e5018.
63. Field S, Irvine AD, Kirby B. The treatment of viral warts with topical cidofovir 1%: our experience of seven paediatric patients. *Br J Dermatol.* 2009;160(1):223-224.
64. De Socio GV, Simonetti S, Rosignoli D, et al. Topical cidofovir for severe warts in a patient affected by AIDS and Hodgkin's lymphoma. *Int J STD AIDS.* 2008;19(10):715-716.
65. Cusack C, Fitzgerald D, Clayton TM, et al. Successful treatment of florid cutaneous warts with intravenous cidofovir in an 11-year-old girl. *Pediatr Dermatol.* 2008;25(3):387-389.
66. Bhadri VA, Lee-Horn L, Shaw PJ. Safety and tolerability of cidofovir in high-risk pediatric patients. *Transpl Infect Dis.* 2009;11(4):373-379.
67. Tchernev G. Sexually transmitted papillomavirus infections: epidemiology pathogenesis, clinic, morphology, important differential diagnostic aspects, current diagnostic and treatment options. *An Bras Dermatol.* 2009;84(4):377-389.
68. Lott DG, Krakovitz PR. Squamous cell carcinoma associated with intralesional injection of cidofovir for recurrent respiratory papillomatosis. *Laryngoscope.* 2009;119(3):567-570.
69. Donne AJ, Hampson L, He XT, et al. Potential risk factors associated with the use of cidofovir to treat benign human papillomavirus-related disease. *Antivir Ther.* 2009;14(7):939-952.
70. Dvorak CC, Cowan MJ, Horn B, et al. Development of herpes simplex virus stomatitis during receipt of cidofovir therapy. *Clin Infect Dis.* 2009;49(8):e92-e95.
71. Shuja F, Kavoussi SC, Mir MR, et al. Interferon induced sarcoidosis with cutaneous involvement along lines of venous drainage in a former intravenous drug user. *Dermatol Online J.* 2009;15(12):4.

72. Mistry N, Shapero J, Crawford RI. A review of adverse cutaneous drug reactions resulting from the use of interferon and ribavirin. *Can J Gastroenterol.* 2009;23(10):677-683.
73. Sato M, Sueki H, Iijima M. Repeated episodes of fixed eruption 3 months after discontinuing pegylated interferon-alpha-2b plus ribavirin combination therapy in a patient with chronic hepatitis C virus infection. *Clin Exp Dermatol.* 2009;34(8):e814-e817.
74. Panel on Antiretroviral Guidelines for Adults and Adolescents. Guidelines for the use of antiretroviral agents in HIV-1-infected adults and adolescents. https://aidsinfo.nih.gov/contentfiles/lvguidelines/adultandadolescentgl.pdf. Accessed June 21, 2016.
75. Laskey SB, Siliciano RF. A mechanistic theory to explain the efficacy of antiretroviral therapy. *Nat Rev Micro.* 2014;12(11):772-780.
76. WHO. *Policy Brief: Consolidated Guidelines on the Use of Antiretroviral Drugs for Treating and Preventing HIV Infection: What's New.* Geneva, Switzerland: WHO; 2015. http://www.who.int/hiv/pub/arv/policy-brief-arv-2015/en/.
77. Panel on Antiretroviral Therapy and Medical Management of HIV-Infected Children. Guidelines for the use of antiretroviral agents in pediatric HIV infection. https://aidsinfo.nih.gov/contentfiles/lvguidelines/pediatricguidelines.pdf. Accessed January 14, 2016.
78. WHO. *Guideline on When to Start Antiretroviral Therapy and on Pre-exposure Prophylaxis for HIV.* Geneva, Switzerland: WHO; 2015. http://www.who.int/hiv/pub/guidelines/earlyrelease-arv/en/.
79. United States Public Health Service, Centers for Disease Control and Prevention (US), National Center for HIV/AIDS, Viral Hepatitis, STD, and TB Prevention (US), et al. Preexposure prophylaxis for the prevention of HIV infection—2014: a clinical practice guideline. http://stacks.cdc.gov/view/cdc/23109.
80. WHO. *News and Events Topics Publications Data and Statistics About US Guidelines on Post-exposure Prophylaxis for HIV and the Use of Co-trimoxazole Prophylaxis for HIV-Related Infections among Adults, Adolescents and Children.* Geneva, Switzerland: WHO; 2014. http://www.who.int/hiv/pub/guidelines/arv2013/arvs2013upplement_dec2014/en/.
81. Atzori L, Pinna AL, Pilloni L, et al. Bullous skin eruption in an HIV patient during antiretroviral drugs therapy. *Dermatol Ther.* 2008;21(suppl 2):S30-S34.
82. Maggiolo F. Efavirenz: a decade of clinical experience in the treatment of HIV. *J Antimicrob Chemother.* 2009;64(5):910-928.
83. Vemula S, Kerr S, Pancharoen C, et al. Incidence and risk factors for non-nucleoside reverse transcriptase inhibitors (NNRTI)-related rash in Thai children with HIV infection. *J Med Assoc Thai.* 2007;90(11):2437-2441.
84. Hall DB, Macgregor TR. Case-control exploration of relationships between early rash or liver toxicity and plasma concentrations of nevirapine and primary metabolites. *HIV Clin Trials.* 2007;8(6):391-399.
85. Manosuthi W, Sungkanuparph S, Tansuphaswadikul S, et al. Incidence and risk factors of nevirapine-associated skin rashes among HIV-infected patients with CD4 cell counts <250 cells/microL. *Int J STD AIDS.* 2007;18(11):782-786.
86. Chen J, Mannargudi BM, Xu L, et al. Demonstration of the metabolic pathway responsible for nevirapine-induced skin rash. *Chem Res Toxicol.* 2008;21(9):1862-1870.
87. Moura MD, Senna MI, Madureira DF, et al. Oral adverse effects due to the use of Nevirapine. *J Contemp Dent Pract.* 2008;9(1):84-90.
88. Fulco PP, McNicholl IR. Etravirine and rilpivirine: nonnucleoside reverse transcriptase inhibitors with activity against human immunodeficiency virus type 1 strains resistant to previous nonnucleoside agents. *Pharmacotherapy.* 2009;29(3):281-294.
89. Mercier S, Gueye NF, Cournil A, et al. Lipodystrophy and metabolic disorders in HIV-1-infected adults on 4- to 9-year antiretroviral therapy in Senegal: a case-control study. *J Acquir Immune Defic Syndr.* 2009;51(2):224-230.
90. Sarni RO, Souza FI, Battistini TR, et al. Lipodystrophy in children and adolescents with acquired immunodeficiency syndrome and its relationship with the antiretroviral therapy employed [in Portuguese]. *J Pediatr (Rio J).* 2009;85(4):329-334.
91. Goulbourne CN, Vaux DJ. HIV protease inhibitors inhibit FACE1/ZMPSTE24: A mechanism for acquired lipodystrophy in patients on highly active antiretroviral therapy? *Biochem Soc Trans.* 2010;38(pt 1):292-296.
92. Benedini S, Perseghin G, Terruzzi I, et al. Effect of L-acetylcarnitine on body composition in HIV-related lipodystrophy. *Horm Metab Res.* 2009;41(11):840-845.
93. World Health Organization. *Guidelines for the Screening Care and Treatment of Persons with Chronic Hepatitis C Infection: Updated Version.* Geneva: World Health Organization; 2016.
94. Webster DP, Klenerman P, Dusheiko GM. Hepatitis C. *Lancet.* 2015;385(9973):1124-1135.
95. Simmonds P. Reconstructing the origins of human hepatitis viruses. *Philos Trans R Soc Lond B Biol Sci.* 2001;356(1411):1013-1026.
96. Smith DB, Bukh J, Kuiken C, et al. Expanded classification of hepatitis C virus into 7 genotypes and 67 subtypes: updated criteria and genotype assignment web resource. *Hepatology.* 2014;59(1):318-327.
97. Kim CW, Chang KM. Hepatitis C virus: virology and life cycle. *Clin Mol Hepatol.* 2013;19(1):17-25.
98. Yoshida EM, Sulkowski MS, Gane EJ, et al. Concordance of sustained virological response 4, 12, and 24 weeks post-treatment with sofosbuvir-containing regimens for hepatitis C virus. *Hepatology.* 2015;61(1):41-45.
99. FakhriRavari A, Malakouti M, Brady R. Interferon-free treatments for chronic hepatitis C genotype 1 infection. *J Clin Transl Hepatol.* 2016;4(2):97-112.
100. AASLD/IDSA HCV Guidance Panel. Hepatitis C guidance: AASLD-IDSA recommendations for testing, managing, and treating adults infected with hepatitis C virus. *Hepatology.* 2015;62(3):932-954.
101. Chung RT, Gale M Jr, Polyak SJ, et al. Mechanisms of action of interferon and ribavirin in chronic hepatitis C: summary of a workshop. *Hepatology.* 2008;47(1):306-320.
102. Negro F. Adverse effects of drugs in the treatment of viral hepatitis. *Best Pract Res Clin Gastroenterol.* 2010;24(2):183-192.
103. Mistry N, Shapero J, Crawford RI. A review of adverse cutaneous drug reactions resulting from the use of interferon and ribavirin. *Can J Gastroenterol.* 2009;23(10):677-683.
104. Fried MW. Side effects of therapy of hepatitis C and their management. *Hepatology.* 2002;365(suppl 1):S237-S244.
105. Cacoub P, Bourlière M, Lübbe J, et al. Dermatological side effects of hepatitis C and its treatment: patient

management in the era of direct-acting antivirals. *J Hepatol.* 2012;56(2):455-463.
106. Jacobson IM, Pawlotsky JM, Afdhal NH, et al. A practical guide for the use of boceprevir and telaprevir for the treatment of hepatitis C. *J Viral Hepat.* 2012;19(suppl 2):1-26.
107. Kohli A, Shaffer A, Sherman A, et al. Treatment of hepatitis C: a systematic review. *JAMA.* 2014;312(6):631-640.
108. Manns MP, Fried MW, Zeuzem S, et al. Simeprevir with peginterferon/ribavirin for treatment of chronic hepatitis C virus genotype 1 infection: pooled safety analysis from Phase IIb and III studies. *J Viral Hepat.* 2015;22(4):366-375.
109. Afdhal N, Zeuzem S, Kwo P, et al. Ledipasvir and sofosbuvir for untreated HCV genotype 1 infection. *N Engl J Med.* 2014;370(20):1889-1898.
110. Afdhal N, Reddy KR, Nelson DR, et al. Ledipasvir and sofosbuvir for previously treated HCV genotype 1 infection. *N Engl J Med.* 2014;370(16):1483-1493.
111. Kowdley KV, Gordon SC, Reddy KR, et al. Ledipasvir and sofosbuvir for 8 or 12 weeks for chronic HCV without cirrhosis. *N Engl J Med.* 2014;370(20):1879-1888.
112. Naggie S, Cooper C, Saag M, et al. Ledipasvir and sofosbuvir for HCV in Patients Coinfected with HIV-1. *N Engl J Med.* 2015;373(8):705-713.
113. Sulkowski MS, Gardiner DF, Rodriguez-Torres M, et al. Daclatasvir plus sofosbuvir for previously treated or untreated chronic HCV infection. *N Engl J Med.* 2014;370(3):211-221.
114. Lawitz E, Gane E, Pearlman B, et al. Efficacy and safety of 12 weeks versus 18 weeks of treatment with grazoprevir (MK-5172) and elbasvir (MK-8742) with or without ribavirin for hepatitis C virus genotype 1 infection in previously untreated patients with cirrhosis and patients with previous null response with or without cirrhosis (C-WORTHY): a randomised, open-label phase 2 trial. *Lancet.* 2015;385(9973):1075-1086.
115. Sulkowski M, Hezode C, Gerstoft J, et al. Efficacy and safety of 8 weeks versus 12 weeks of treatment with grazoprevir (MK-5172) and elbasvir (MK-8742) with or without ribavirin in patients with hepatitis C virus genotype 1 mono-infection and HIV/hepatitis C virus co-infection (C-WORTHY): a randomised, open-label phase 2 trial. *Lancet.* 2015;385(9973):1087-1097.
116. Andreone P, Colombo MG, Enejosa JV, et al. ABT-450, ritonavir, ombitasvir, and dasabuvir achieves 97% and 100% sustained virologic response with or without ribavirin in treatment-experienced patients with HCV genotype 1b infection. *Gastroenterology.* 2014;147(2):359-365.e1.
117. Ferenci P, Bernstein D, Lalezari J, et al. ABT-450/r-ombitasvir and dasabuvir with or without ribavirin for HCV. *N Engl J Med.* 2014;370(21):1983-1992.
118. Feld JJ, Jacobson IM, Hézode C, et al. Sofosbuvir and velpatasvir for HCV Genotype 1, 2, 4, 5, and 6 Infection. *N Engl J Med.* 2015;373(27):2599-2607.
119. Foster GR, Afdhal N, Roberts SK, et al. Sofosbuvir and Velpatasvir for HCV Genotype 2 and 3 Infection. *N Engl J Med.* 2015;373(27):2608-2617.
120. Fontana RJ. Side effects of long-term oral antiviral therapy for hepatitis B. *Hepatology.* 2009;49(5 suppl):S185-S195.
121. Terrault NA, Bzowej NH, Chang KM, et al; American Association for the Study of Liver Diseases. AASLD guidelines for treatment of chronic hepatitis B. *Hepatology.* 2016;63(1):261-283.
122. Borras-Blasco J, Navarro-Ruiz A, Borras C, et al. Adverse cutaneous reactions associated with the newest antiretroviral drugs in patients with human immunodeficiency virus infection. *J Antimicrob Chemother.* 2008;62(5):879-888.
123. Trepo C, Chan HL, Lok A. Hepatitis B virus infection. *Lancet.* 2014;384(9959):2053-2063.

Chapter 192 :: Immunosuppressive and Immunomodulatory Drugs
:: Drew Kurtzman, Ruth Ann Vleugels, & Jeffrey Callen

第一百九十二章

免疫抑制药和免疫调节药

中文导读

目前在抗炎治疗领域取得的关键进展是早期或同时采用免疫抑制或免疫调节药,成功地减少了系统性皮质类固醇的使用。

本章首先在前言中介绍了免疫抑制药和免疫调节药的特点与区别。免疫抑制药的特点是治疗指数较低(治疗和毒性范围之间的窗口较窄)和个体内及个体间的药代动力学变化显著。免疫调节药具有更广泛的治疗指数,更大的安全边际,更可预测的药代动力学特性,以及更少的个体间差异。并提到了免疫治疗的首要目标是安全性和有效性。接下来重点介绍了关键的药理学特性以及皮肤病学中使用的一些主要免疫抑制药和免疫调节药,包括霉酚酸酯、钙调神经磷酸酶抑制药(环孢素、他克莫司和吡美莫司)和雷帕霉素抑制药依维莫司的作用机制、药代动力学、给药方案、不良反应等。而其他免疫抑制药和细胞毒性剂已经在第一百九十章进行了讨论。

〔粟 娟〕

AT-A-GLANCE

- Immunosuppressants and immunomodulators represent an indispensable group of antiinflammatory medications that are capable of treating a wide array of inflammatory skin conditions.
- The immunosuppressive and immunomodulatory drugs covered in this chapter include mycophenolate mofetil, the calcineurin inhibitors (cyclosporine, tacrolimus, and pimecrolimus), and the mammalian target of rapamycin (mTOR) inhibitor everolimus.
- The primary goal of therapy with immunosuppressants and immunomodulators is to effectively treat an inflammatory condition while maintaining patient safety.
- By working in an additive or synergistic fashion, combination regimens have the potential for greater efficacy and may allow for decreased doses of individual drugs, which may enhance overall safety and reduce medication-related side effects.
- A comprehensive understanding of the pathophysiology of the disease being treated as well as the pharmacokinetic and pharmacodynamic properties of each immunosuppressant and immunomodulator is fundamental to favorable patient outcomes.

INTRODUCTION

There has been significant progress in the field of anti-inflammatory therapy. A critical advance has been the successful effort to reduce the use of systemic corticosteroids by the early or concomitant introduction of immunosuppressive or immunomodulatory therapy (or both). Before a detailed discussion of these agents is provided, an important distinction between immunosuppressants and immunomodulators must be made. Immunosuppressants are characterized by a low therapeutic index (narrow window between the therapeutic and toxic range) and significant intra- and interindividual pharmacokinetic variability. These shortcomings are circumvented by precise drug dosing (based on ideal or lean body weight) as well as by screening for end-organ toxicity and, in some cases, close monitoring of plasma drug levels (parent or metabolite peak and trough levels). Immunomodulators, by contrast, have a wider therapeutic index, a greater safety margin, more predictable pharmacokinetic properties, and less interindividual variability. In addition, although immunosuppressants appear to globally impair the host immune response typically in a dose-dependent fashion, immunomodulators may act more selectively by targeting only specific portions of the immune system and therefore pose a lower risk of complications related to immune dysfunction. Whether immunosuppressants or immunomodulators are selected, the primary goals of immunotherapy are safety and efficacy. These goals are best accomplished by using the lowest effective drug doses to achieve disease remission and, in certain scenarios, by using combination therapy (Fig. 192-1).[1,2] Among dermatologists, immunosuppressants and immunomodulators are frequently used as corticosteroid-sparing agents.[3] This chapter reviews the key pharmacologic properties and prescribing principles of some of the major immunosuppressants and immunomodulators used in dermatology, including mycophenolate mofetil (MMF), the calcineurin inhibitors (CNIs; cyclosporine, tacrolimus, and pimecrolimus), and the mammalian target of rapamycin (mTOR) inhibitor everolimus. Other immunosuppressants, antimetabolites, and cytotoxic agents are discussed in Chap. 190.

MYCOPHENOLATE MOFETIL

MMF is an ethyl ester of its active metabolite, mycophenolic acid (MPA), a biological product of several *Penicillium* species. Because of its enhanced bioavailability, MMF is the more widely available drug formulation.

PHARMACOLOGY AND MECHANISM OF ACTION

MECHANISM OF ACTION

MPA reversibly inhibits the type II isoform of inosine monophosphate dehydrogenase, which is a key enzyme in the de novo purine synthesis pathway. As a result, the proliferation of both T and B lymphocytes is selectively reduced because of their impaired ability to use the hypoxanthine-guanine phosphoribosyl transferase–dependent purine salvage pathway. Decreased delayed hypersensitivity reactions and immunoglobulin levels have been observed in individuals treated with MMF, which is attributable to its effect on T and B lymphocytes, respectively.

ABSORPTION, DISTRIBUTION, METABOLISM, AND EXCRETION

MMF is rapidly absorbed after oral administration and is presystemically hydrolyzed to form MPA, the active metabolite. At clinically relevant concentrations, 97% of MPA is bound to plasma albumin. MPA is metabolized by hepatic glucuronyl transferases to form the inactive glucuronide of MPA (MPAG), which is almost exclusively excreted by the kidneys. In the setting of renal failure, increased serum levels of MPAG displace MPA from albumin binding sites and lead to elevated free concentrations of MPA, which can result in supratherapeutic drug concentrations. Secondary peaks of serum MPA levels are seen 6 to 12 hours after ingestion, suggesting that enterohepatic circulation contributes to steady-state serum MPA concentrations. As with other immunosuppressive agents, doses of MMF up to 20% higher may be required in children because of increased hepatic metabolism. An enteric-coated oral formulation of mycophenolate (MP-EC) is available and exhibits fewer gastrointestinal (GI) side effects than MMF. This formulation is as effective as MMF at the following conversion rate: 250 mg of MMF is equivalent to 180 mg of MP-EC, and 500 mg of MMF is equivalent to 360 mg of MP-EC.

A modified, median-effect formula

$$CI = \frac{A \text{ combined with } B}{A} + \frac{B \text{ combined with } A}{B}$$

CI: index inhibition (eg, immunglobulins, disease activity)

CI: = 1 additive
    < 1 synergistic
    > 1 antagonistic

Figure 192-1 A modified, median-effect formula is widely used in organ transplantation, which helps in finding the therapeutic windows of immunosuppressive drugs as well as the synergistic, additive, or antagonistic effect of a postulated drug combination. CI, combination index. (Data from Chou TC, Talalay P. Quantitative analysis of dose-effect relationships: the combined effects of multiple drugs or enzyme inhibitors. *Adv Enzyme Regul.* 1984;22:274.)

INDICATIONS AND CONTRAINDICATIONS

INDICATIONS

There are currently no licensed indications for MMF in dermatology. However, MMF is frequently used to treat immunobullous disorders (especially pemphigus), connective tissue diseases (including cutaneous lupus erythematosus, dermatomyositis, and systemic sclerosis), papulosquamous disorders (including lichen planus, lichen planopilaris, and psoriasis), pyoderma gangrenosum, cutaneous vasculitis, sarcoidosis, and chronic atopic dermatitis, among other conditions.[3-5] Despite the wide spectrum of inflammatory disorders effectively treated with MMF, high-quality studies supporting its use for these conditions are limited. MMF may be combined with other immunosuppressants and immunomodulators, but an increased risk of infection, malignancy, and other serious adverse effects may discourage this practice. Combination regimens, however, may allow for dose reduction of individual drugs and may decrease the incidence of dose-dependent adverse side effects.

CONTRAINDICATIONS

Absolute contraindications to using MMF include known hypersensitivity and pregnancy. Relative contraindications include severe renal dysfunction and deficiency of the hypoxanthine-guanine phosphoribosyl transferase enzyme (see Other Considerations).

DOSING REGIMEN

Depending on the condition being treated, dosing of MMF varies (Table 192-1). Most patients with skin disease respond to 1 to 1.5 g given twice daily. In pediatric patients, the recommended starting dose of MMF is 600 mg/m^2. Children with a body surface area of 1.5 m^2 or greater should receive adult-equivalent doses or more, particularly if augmented hepatic metabolism is a concern.

MMF is frequently and safely co-prescribed with corticosteroids and can be continued while corticosteroid therapy is tapered or withdrawn. Depending on the condition being treated, MMF may display a steroid-sparing effect. The full therapeutic benefit of MMF is seen after 3 months of use, and judging its success should be reserved until after adequate time on medication has been allotted.

THERAPEUTIC MONITORING

No guidelines for preventing or screening for MMF toxicity exist. At the outset of therapy, blood counts and serum chemistries, including liver and kidney function testing, should be obtained on a regular basis. When patients are receiving stable doses and have no signs of toxicity, the frequency of monitoring can be extended to 3-month intervals.

Measuring serum MPA concentrations to achieve a target trough level has been advocated for in the transplantation literature because this practice appears to improve allograft survival in transplant recipients receiving MMF therapy.[6,7] Small prospective studies have shown similar benefit of monitoring serum MPA levels for systemic lupus erythematosus and certain systemic vasculitides.[8,9] A major hindrance to routinely measuring serum MPA levels is the time-sensitive nature of the assay—trough levels need to be taken 12 hours after the last dose, which is not always feasible for patients, and drug kinetics are highly influenced by enterohepatic recirculation, which may vary by individual and is affected by certain medications. The utility of monitoring serum MPA levels has not been established for any dermatologic condition and is therefore not presently recommended.

SIDE EFFECTS AND PRECAUTIONS

Dose-dependent GI side effects, occasionally with intractable diarrhea, are common, but in the vast majority of cases, these symptoms diminish with continuation of therapy. Further dividing the total daily dose (eg, three or four times a day) and taking the medication with food may improve tolerability. If such measures fail, switching to MP-EC is recommended. An increased risk of herpes zoster virus reactivation is seen during treatment with MMF, particularly among older adult patients.

SERIOUS ADVERSE EFFECTS (TABLE 192-2)

Significant cytopenias rarely complicate treatment with MMF but are more common when maximum dose therapy is used in conjunction with other immunosuppressants. An increased incidence of lymphoma and skin cancer has been reported in MMF users and appears to be related to the intensity and duration of immunosuppression. In children using MMF, lymphoproliferative disorders have also occurred. The risk of serious infection is increased during treatment with MMF, and some infections (eg, JC virus–associated

TABLE 192-1
Mycophenolate Mofetil Dosing Regimen[a]

	DAILY ORAL DOSE (mg/kg)
Cytotoxic T cell–mediated diseases	25–35
Antibody-mediated diseases	35–55

[a]180 mg of enteric-coated mycophenolate sodium is the equivalent of 250 mg of mycophenolate mofetil; 360 mg of enteric-coated mycophenolate sodium is the equivalent of 500 mg of mycophenolate mofetil.

TABLE 192-2
Serious Adverse Effects of Mycophenolate Mofetil
Embryotoxicity
Lymphoma and other malignancies
Serious and opportunistic infections, including progressive multifocal leukoencephalopathy
Severe cytopenias, including neutropenia and pure red cell aplasia
Skin cancer

progressive multifocal leukoencephalopathy [PML]) may have fatal outcomes.

DRUG INTERACTIONS

Simultaneous administration of MMF with antacids, cholestyramine, and proton pump inhibitors (PPIs) decreases its absorption. Whereas cholestyramine disrupts enterohepatic circulation, PPIs impair absorption by increasing gastric pH. Spacing the administration of PPIs by a period of 2 hours before or after MMF may circumvent this interaction. Cyclosporine also interferes with the enterohepatic circulation of MPA, and coadministration of the two agents may result in decreased serum concentrations of MPA, although the clinical significance of this specific interaction has not been shown to be meaningful.[10] There is no increase in nephrotoxicity, hepatotoxicity, hypertension, or neurotoxicity when MMF is combined with cyclosporine and corticosteroids. Despite an unknown influence on the ovulation-suppressing actions of certain oral contraceptives, MMF has been shown to decrease mean plasma concentrations of levonorgestrel and ethinylestradiol. For this reason, reliable forms of contraception are recommended in women of childbearing potential who use MMF (see Other Considerations).

OTHER CONSIDERATIONS

Because MMF decreases host immunity, age-appropriate vaccinations are recommended before starting and during therapy, but live attenuated vaccines should be avoided after treatment has been initiated. Individuals with preexisting renal disease might require lower doses of MMF as a result of impaired drug excretion, and more frequent toxicity monitoring may be necessary in these instances. Judicious use of MMF is warranted in the setting of hepatic insufficiency, although even in cases of advanced liver disease (eg, alcoholic cirrhosis), conversion to active MPA and enterohepatic recirculation appear unaffected. MMF is a Pregnancy Category D medication because it has been shown to increase the risk of first trimester pregnancy loss and cause congenital malformations. Therefore, women of reproductive potential using MMF require contraception, and because of an unknown effect on the efficacy of oral contraceptive pills, if a hormone-based contraceptive is selected, concurrent use of a barrier contraceptive is recommended.[10] Active contraception should continue for 6 to 8 weeks after discontinuation of MMF. Because MMF inhibits the de novo synthesis of purines, deficiency of hypoxanthine-guanine phosphoribosyl transferase (eg, Lesch-Nyhan syndrome) is a relative contraindication to its use.

CALCINEURIN INHIBITORS

The CNIs are a versatile class of immunomodulators that were originally discovered as microorganism fermentation products. The CNIs selectively suppress T-cell responses and have synergistic therapeutic effects when they are combined with most other immunosuppressive drugs.[1,2] Despite established efficacy for a number of inflammatory conditions, the use of cyclosporine and other systemic CNIs to treat skin disease has declined with the advent of biologic agents that exert more targeted effects.

CYCLOSPORINE

Cyclosporine is a lipophilic cyclic polypeptide metabolite produced by the fungal species *Beauveria nivea*.

PHARMACOLOGY AND MECHANISM OF ACTION (FIG. 192-2)

Mechanism of Action: Cyclosporine, also known as cyclosporine A (CsA), and other CNIs inhibit T-cell activation by several mechanisms. Of these, disruption of T-cell receptor signaling is the best understood mechanism and is thought to be the most important in terms of antiinflammatory activity.[11] Cyclosporine binds the intracytoplasmic, high-affinity immunophilin receptor cyclophilin and forms a drug–receptor complex that binds to calcineurin, a serine/threonine protease composed of two subunits, CnA and CnB. CnA constitutes the catalytic unit possessing binding sites for CnB and calmodulin (Fig. 192-2). Cyclophilin activity strongly correlates with increased interleukin (IL)-2 production via activation of the CD3 domain of the T-cell receptor. Cyclophilin is also involved in the induction of apoptosis and degranulation of cytotoxic T-lymphocytes. Experimental data has shown that the CsA–cyclophilin complex inhibits the nuclear translocation of the nuclear factor of activated T cells (NFAT) molecule by blocking its dephosphorylation. This is thought to be a key step by which CsA and other CNIs uncouple T-cell receptor activation from IL-2 and other inflammatory cytokine transcription.

In summary, CsA inhibits T-cell activation mediated by antigens by blocking the downstream signaling cascade of the T-cell receptor, but it does not inhibit the early phases of T-lymphocyte signal transduction. The immunosuppressive effects of CsA and the CNIs are intricate and subject to constant discoveries. A simplified explanation of the mechanism of action of these drugs is illustrated in Fig. 192-2.

Absorption, Distribution, Metabolism, and Excretion: After oral administration, absorption of CsA follows a predictable trajectory but is heavily influenced by the formulation chosen as well as patient-specific characteristics. Peak plasma drug concentrations occur 1 to 4 hours after administration, but co-ingestion with food can delay or even reduce total drug absorption. After entry into the circulation, CsA distributes into a variety of tissues and displays a large volume of distribution (13 L/kg). Notably, unlike most other medications, CsA binds to cellular elements of whole blood, including lymphocytes, granulocytes, and erythrocytes, and only a fraction remains bound to plasma lipoproteins. If monitoring drug levels, whole blood levels are preferred to plasma measurements because of the drug's accumulation in erythrocytes and leukocytes.[12] Cyclosporine is metabolized into more than 30 partially active byproducts primarily by the hepatic cytochrome P450 3A4 enzyme (CYP3A4).[13,14] Medications that compete for binding to CYP3A4 will increase CsA levels, and drugs that induce P450 will accelerate its metabolism and decrease blood levels (see Drug Interactions and Table 192-3). In addition, certain foods rich in bioflavonoids, such as grapefruit, appear to increase CsA bioavailability through an interaction with hepatic and enteric cytochromes. The elimination half-life of CsA is 6 to 12 hours in the absence of severe hepatic disease, and biliary excretion accounts for more than 90% of its elimination. Renal failure does not substantially alter CsA clearance.

A microemulsion formulation of CsA (Neoral, Novartis) is available and has greater bioavailability than the standard formulation.[12] Because the two preparations are not bioequivalent, lower doses of microemulsion CsA appear to have comparable efficacy to standard doses of the nonemulsified formulation. An intravenous preparation of CsA is also available. Topical CsA solution has limited utility for treating inflammatory skin conditions, owing to its poor penetration across cornified epithelia, but recently, a liposomal gel of CsA was developed and has shown efficacy for treating plaque psoriasis.[15] Further studies are needed to determine whether CsA gel is useful for other inflammatory skin conditions.

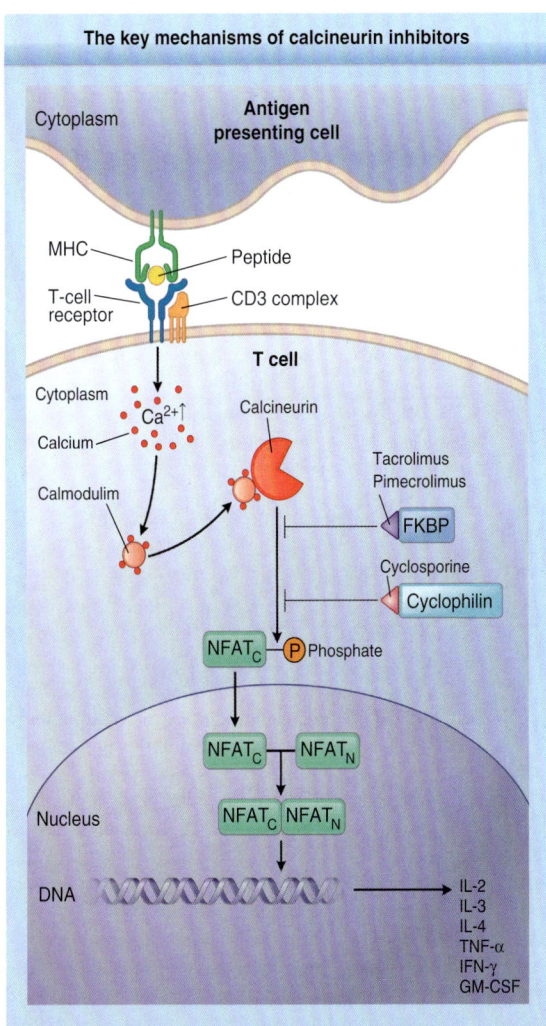

Figure 192-2 The key mechanisms by which calcineurin inhibitors disrupt T-cell activation triggered by the presentation of antigen via the T-cell receptor (TCR). The first step in antigen presentation involves the presentation of a peptide that is bound within the peptide-binding groove of the major histocompatibility complex (MHC) class II molecule. This complex is then presented to the TCR. This causes transmembrane signaling that increases intracellular calcium concentrations. The liberated calcium, bound to calmodulin, interacts with calcineurin, a calcium-dependent serine/threonine phosphatase that dephosphorylates nuclear factor of activated T cells (shown here as NFATc), and this causes NFAT to translocate to the nucleus. There it binds to other nuclear components of NFAT (shown here as NFATn). This complex regulates the transcription of many cytokine genes, shown in the diagram. Cyclosporine, tacrolimus, and pimecrolimus diffuse freely into the cytoplasm of T cells and bind with their respective immunophilins (eg, cyclosporine with cyclophilin, and tacrolimus/pimecrolimus with FK506 binding protein [FKBP-506] or macrophilin 506). This drug–immunophilin complex binds to calcineurin and blocks its ability to dephosphorylate NFAT, preventing translocation into the nucleus and blocking the production of cytokines, chemokines, and growth factors (eg, interleukin [IL]-2, IL-3, IL-4, tumor necrosis factor-α [TNF-α], interferon-γ [IFN-γ], granulocyte macrophage colony-stimulating factor [GM-CSF]) that would normally be induced after T-cell activation via the TCR. APC, antigen-presenting cell. (Figure modified from Nghiem P, Pearson G, Langley RG. Tacrolimus and pimecrolimus: from clever prokaryotes to inhibiting calcineurin and treating atopic dermatitis. *J Am Dermatol*. 2002;46:228-241.)

INDICATIONS AND CONTRAINDICATIONS

Indications: Cyclosporine is approved for treating moderate to severe plaque psoriasis. The dosage for optimal disease control is 4 to 5 mg/kg/day. The use of CsA in combination with methotrexate appears beneficial, but combination with biologics (eg, tumor necrosis factor-α [TNF-α] inhibitors and IL-12/23 and IL-17 blockers) has not been adequately studied and should be avoided, apart from short periods of overlap when de-escalation followed by discontinuation of CsA is planned. Although approved for psoriasis, use of CsA has decreased owing to the availability of more targeted agents as well as the predictable toxicity associated with long-term administration.

Although CsA is only licensed for psoriasis, it appears efficacious for treating a variety of dermatologic conditions, including pyoderma gangrenosum, pemphigus and its variants, palmoplantar pustulosis, lichen planus, atopic dermatitis, Behçet disease, alopecia areata, and epidermolysis bullosa acquisita, among others.[16-18] Despite historically mixed outcomes, more recent data supports that CsA may improve mortality in patients with Stevens-Johnson syndrome and toxic epidermal necrolysis.[19]

Contraindications: Contraindications to using CsA include known hypersensitivity, severe renal dysfunction, uncontrolled hypertension, and malignancy. Patients with psoriasis who are receiving CsA should not undergo phototherapy because of an increased risk of cutaneous malignancy.

DOSING REGIMEN (TABLE 192-4)

The recommended starting dosage of CsA is 2.5 mg/kg/day, which can be increased by 0.5 to 1.0 mg/kg/day at 2-week intervals until the desired outcome is achieved. If rapid disease control is needed, initiation of CsA at 4 to 5 mg/kg/day is acceptable because most patients with dermatologic conditions respond to doses within this range. Dosages greater than 5 mg/kg/day are not advisable other than for very short periods of time. Dose reductions are permissible at any time, although judicious decreases are recommended to prevent a disease flare. Intravenous CsA can be infused slowly over a period of 2 to 6 hours at about one third of the usual oral dose, or about 2 mg/kg/day. Because nephrotoxicity complicates long-term use, courses of CsA should typically not exceed 6 to 12 months.

Therapeutic Monitoring: Before initiating CsA, baseline laboratory studies should be obtained, including blood counts; comprehensive serum chemistries, including tests for renal function and electrolytes (including magnesium); uric acid; lipids; and urinalysis. These studies should be repeated every 2 weeks at the outset of therapy, and if stable, the assessment intervals can be extended at the discretion of the prescriber. During CsA therapy, if serum creatinine increases 25% above the pretreatment level on two consecutive occasions, the CsA dose should be reduced, and if it remains persistently elevated despite dose modification, CsA should be discontinued (Fig. 192-3). Blood pressure measurements should also be performed before and regularly during treatment with CsA because elevations in blood pressure may be the first sign of nephrotoxicity.

Although targeting a specific trough level is useful for preventing organ rejection in transplant recipients, this practice has not been shown to be beneficial in individuals with psoriasis or other inflammatory skin conditions who receive CsA and is therefore not recommended. In patients who are not responsive to CsA or drug compliance is in question, checking a trough level may be warranted because it can distinguish

TABLE 192-3
Drugs that Interact with Cyclosporine[a]

DRUG CLASS	SPECIFIC DRUGS
Drugs That May Increase the Risk of Nephrotoxicity	
Antibiotics	Ciprofloxacin, gentamycin, tobramycin, vancomycin, trimethoprim with sulfamethoxazole
Antimetabolites	Melphalan
Antifungals	Amphotericin B, ketoconazole
Antiinflammatory drugs	Colchicine, diclofenac, naproxen, sulindac
Gastrointestinal agents	Cimetidine, ranitidine
Immunosuppressives	Tacrolimus
Other drugs	Fibrates, methotrexate
Drugs That Increase Cyclosporine Concentrations	
Calcium channel blockers	Diltiazem, nicardipine, verapamil
Antibiotics	Azithromycin, clarithromycin, erythromycin, quinupristin–dalfopristin
Antifungals	Fluconazole, itraconazole, ketoconazole, voriconazole
Antivirals	Boceprevir, indinavir, nelfinavir, ritonavir, telaprevir, saquinavir
Glucocorticoids	Methylprednisolone
Other drugs and supplements	Allopurinol, amiodarone, bromocriptine, colchicine, danazol, grapefruit juice, imatinib, metoclopramide, oral contraceptives
Drugs That Decrease Cyclosporine Concentrations	
Antibiotics	Nafcillin, rifampin
Anticonvulsants	Carbamazepine, oxcarbazepine, phenobarbital, phenytoin
Other drugs and supplements	Bosentan, octreotide, orlistat, sulfinpyrazone, St. John's wort, terbinafine, ticlopidine

[a]Neoral (cyclosporine) prescribing information. [Medication prescribing guide]. 2015; https://www.pharma.us.novartis.com/sites/www.pharma.us.novartis.com/files/neoral.pdf.

TABLE 192-4
Calcineurin Inhibitor Dosing Regimen

DRUG	ADULT DOSAGE	PEDIATRIC DOSAGE[a]
Cyclosporine—oral	2.5–5.0 mg/kg/day	5–7 mg/kg/day
Cyclosporine—intravenous	2–3 mg/kg/day	3–5 mg/kg/day
Tacrolimus—oral	150–200 µg/kg/day	200–300 µg/kg/day
Tacrolimus—intravenous	25–50 µg/kg/day	50–100 µg/kg/day
Tacrolimus—topical	2×/day	2×/day[b]
Pimecrolimus—topical	2×/day	2×/day

[a]Initiating therapy at adult-equivalent doses may be the most prudent approach with dose escalation as tolerated or to effect.
[b]Only the 0.03% ointment is approved for children.

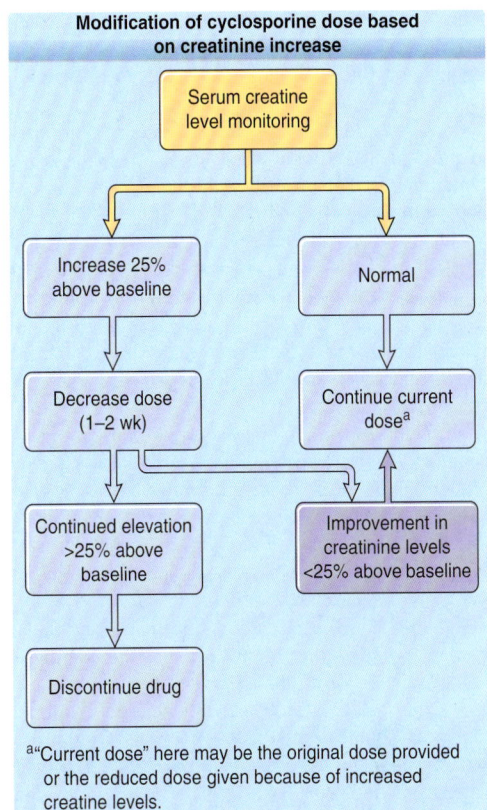

Figure 192-3 Modification of cyclosporine dose based on creatinine increase.

between primary noncompliance and lack of efficacy. The two most common commercially available assays—high-performance liquid chromatography (HPLC) and radioimmunoassay—are performed on EDTA (ethylenediaminetetraacetic acid)-containing whole blood.

SIDE EFFECTS AND PRECAUTIONS

Nausea, vomiting, anorexia, and diarrhea are common side effects of CsA. These symptoms tend to subside with ongoing use, although dose reduction may be necessary. Headache is another common side effect of CsA, especially in patients with a history of migraine. Cyclosporine-induced seizures are uncommon but are associated with hypomagnesemia and the concomitant use of systemic corticosteroids. For this reason, serum magnesium levels should be monitored closely during treatment, and caution should be exercised in individuals receiving CsA and corticosteroids. Lethargy, confusion, tremors, and paresthesias are uncommon side effects of CsA.[20]

Overall, one in four patients taking CsA develops clinical or laboratory evidence of altered renal function. Two types of CsA-induced nephrotoxicity are seen. The first type typically begins within 2 to 3 weeks after drug initiation, and it is associated with high CsA blood levels. A decrease in glomerular filtration rate is seen, along with hypertension and tubular dysfunction. Upon dose reduction or discontinuation, there is complete reversal of this type of nephrotoxicity. The second type of CsA-associated nephrotoxicity is likely a result of cumulative, subclinical chronic renal toxicity. This type tends to occur with long-term therapy (>6 months) and is typically irreversible. Notably, it may occur in the absence of any detectable elevation of creatinine or blood pressure. When individuals experience this form of chronic nephrotoxicity, kidney biopsies characteristically show interstitial fibrosis, tubular atrophy, and vasculopathy. The pathogenesis underlying both types of CsA-mediated nephrotoxicity is poorly understood, but several mediators, including endothelin-1, angiotensin II, osteopontin, and transforming growth factor-β, have been implicated. Calcium channel blockers; angiotensin-converting enzyme inhibitors; angiotensin receptor blockers; and newer drugs, including endothelin A receptor blockers (eg, bosentan) and renin inhibitors (eg, aliskiren), appear to be beneficial for attenuating CsA-induced hypertension and nephrotoxicity.[20] Because of the risk of nephrotoxicity, diuretics and other nephrotoxic drugs should be used cautiously in individuals treated with CsA (see Table 192-3). Importantly, in patients undergoing long-term CsA therapy, serum creatinine and its clearance may not be reliable indicators of altered renal function, and more sensitive tests (eg, renal biopsy) may be needed to detect deleterious changes.

There is evidence of impaired fibrinolysis and endothelial damage and proliferation after CsA use. Hypercoagulability seems to contribute to the progression of atherosclerosis and glomerular damage in CsA-treated patients. In addition to renal artery vasoconstriction, CsA may cause peripheral vasoconstriction and precipitate attacks of Raynaud phenomenon.

Hypercholesterolemia, elevation of low-density lipoproteins, and hypertriglyceridemia may be seen during treatment with CsA. Electrolyte perturbations, most commonly hypomagnesemia and hyperkalemia (less so, hypokalemia), occur in up to 15% of CsA users. Close electrolyte monitoring is needed, particularly if medications that alter potassium balance (eg, triamterene and spironolactone) are co-prescribed. Hyperuricemia can also be seen during CsA therapy, and CsA should therefore be administered cautiously in individuals with a known history of gout. Hyperuricemia may also be an early indicator of CsA-induced nephrotoxicity.

Osteoporosis can complicate CsA treatment and appears to result from its action on osteoblasts and osteoclasts and from its ability to alter lymphocyte-derived cytokines. Myopathy has been reported in transplant recipients receiving high doses of CsA; therefore, caution should be exercised with the concomitant use of statins.

Mucocutaneous side effects from CsA therapy are common. Hypertrichosis occurs in virtually all patients on long-term CsA. It is not limited to androgen-dependent, hair-bearing areas and shows no tendency for spontaneous remission. Gingival hypertrophy is reported in up to 70% of CsA users. It is more common in children; in individuals with poor oral hygiene; and with the concomitant use of calcium channel blockers, particularly nifedipine. Improvement of this complication can be seen with the administration of oral metronidazole or azithromycin. An acneiform eruption, indistinguishable from that seen in steroid-induced acne, is frequently reported with CsA use. Disseminated comedonal or cystic acneiform eruptions can also occur. Keratosis pilaris, sebaceous hyperplasia, warts, and epidermal inclusion cysts occur in up to one third of CsA-treated patients. Eruptive nevi may also develop during CsA use.[21]

Serious Adverse Effects (Table 192-5):
Significant cytopenias rarely occur during treatment with CsA. An uncommon but serious adverse complication is the development of thrombotic microangiopathy–hemolytic uremic syndrome, the risk of which is greatest in allogeneic bone marrow transplant patients receiving CsA for acute graft-versus-host disease (GVHD).[22] Hepatotoxicity with a risk of liver failure is rare but appears to be more common in patients with significant comorbidities and in those concurrently taking hepatotoxic medications.

As in other patients receiving immunosuppressants, individuals treated with CsA have a higher risk of malignancy, particularly lymphoma and skin cancers. Cyclosporine-treated transplant recipients have a relative risk of all skin cancers of 6.8 compared with 2.2 to 5.5 in those receiving other immunosuppressants, such as azathioprine. Cyclosporine-treated dermatologic patients also have an elevated risk of skin cancer, including squamous cell carcinoma, basal cell carcinoma, human papilloma virus–associated anogenital carcinoma, and Kaposi sarcoma. Approximately 25% of nonvisceral Kaposi sarcomas that develop in the setting of CsA use can be expected to undergo complete or partial remission following cessation or reduction of CsA. Epstein-Barr virus–associated post-transplant lymphoproliferative disorder (PTLD) is exceedingly rare among individuals receiving CsA for inflammatory skin conditions. PTLD frequently fails to respond to chemotherapy, but it may regress after reduction or cessation of immunosuppression. The incidence of lymphoma in CsA-treated dermatologic patients appears to be less than 0.2%, and lymphomas developing in CsA-treated patients appear to have a better prognosis despite having a shorter latency period. Other neoplasms, such as melanoma, have also been reported in patients on CsA, although their true incidence is unknown.

Patients receiving CsA are at risk for serious and opportunistic infections, which can have fatal outcomes. JC virus-associated PML and polyoma virus–associated nephropathy have been reported in renal, hepatic, and cardiac transplant recipients receiving CsA.

Neurotoxicity, including serious complications such as cortical blindness and hemiplegia, has been reported in association with CsA use. The posterior reversible encephalopathy syndrome (PRES), which is characterized by impaired consciousness, visual changes, movement disorders, and psychiatric disturbance, has been described in postmarketing reports. Hypomagnesemia and the concomitant use of high-dose systemic corticosteroids appear to be associated with these serious neurotoxic sequelae.

Drug Interactions:
A variety of drugs interact with CsA and either increase or decrease its therapeutic effect by inhibiting or accelerating CYP3A4-mediated metabolism, respectively. Table 192-3 provides a detailed list of drugs that interact with CsA.

Other Considerations:
During treatment with CsA, vaccination may be less effective, and live attenuated vaccines should be avoided. Children and adults have similar bioavailability of oral CsA, but children usually exhibit a higher degree of renal clearance and have shorter blood level half-lives. Children may therefore require higher doses of CsA or more frequent administration to achieve comparable serum drug concentrations and beneficial therapeutic outcomes. Cyclosporine is a Pregnancy Category C medication, so it should only be used when the potential benefits outweigh the risks.[12] It does not appear to be mutagenic or teratogenic, although there is a higher than expected incidence of preterm birth, fetal growth retardation, abortions, preeclampsia, and hypertension in mothers taking CsA during pregnancy. There are no

TABLE 192-5
Serious Adverse Effects of Cyclosporine
Fulminant hepatotoxicity
Hyperkalemia
Lymphoma and other malignancies, including skin cancer
Nephrotoxicity
Neurotoxicity
Serious and opportunistic infections, including polyoma virus infection (eg, progressive multifocal leukoencephalopathy)
Thrombotic microangiopathy/hemolytic uremic syndrome

reports of neonatal complications in children born to fathers taking CsA. Adequate contraceptive measures are recommended in women of childbearing potential. Cyclosporine is excreted in breast milk and should be avoided in nursing mothers.

TACROLIMUS

Tacrolimus, a CNI formerly known as FK506, is a macrolide immunosuppressant that was first isolated from *Streptomyces tsukubaensis*.

PHARMACOLOGY AND MECHANISM OF ACTION

Mechanism of Action (see Fig. 192-2): The postulated mechanism of action of tacrolimus is similar to that of CsA. Instead of binding to cyclophilin, however, tacrolimus binds to FK506 binding protein (FKBP), but the downstream effect is similar—inhibition of the calcium-dependent phosphatase, calcineurin, which disrupts nuclear translocation of NFAT and uncouples T-cell receptor activation from inflammatory cytokine transcription (eg, IL-2, IL-3, IL-4, IL-12, and TNF-α).[11]

Absorption, Distribution, Metabolism, and Excretion: Tacrolimus can be administered orally, topically, and intravenously. The pharmacokinetics of systemic tacrolimus are understood as a two-compartment model with a rapid initial drop in plasma concentrations after entry into the circulation followed by a long elimination half-life of 12 to 21 hours when equilibrium is achieved. Tacrolimus is primarily metabolized by the hepatic cytochrome P450 system (CYP3A4), and less than 1% of the drug is excreted unchanged in the urine. Tacrolimus has not demonstrated superiority to CsA for the prophylaxis of organ rejection or for treating inflammatory conditions, but it appears to have better bioavailability, higher potency, and a lower molecular weight, the latter of which confers enhanced skin penetration. These pharmacologic properties provided the rationale for experiments that demonstrated attenuation of contact hypersensitivity after topical application of tacrolimus and subsequent development of tacrolimus ointment for atopic dermatitis.[23,24]

Pharmacokinetic studies of topical tacrolimus have shown low percutaneous absorption in individuals with atopic dermatitis. Although the initial systemic absorption may be as high as 10% to 20%, blood levels become undetectable by 1 week as healing and reestablishment of the skin barrier occurs. In clinical trials, detection of blood levels of tacrolimus greater than 2 ng/mL were exceedingly rare, in contrast with trough levels of 5 to 15 ng/mL in transplant patients receiving oral tacrolimus.[25] The notable exception is when topical tacrolimus is used in patients with Netherton syndrome, in whom blood levels within or above the established therapeutic trough range for oral tacrolimus in organ transplant recipients may be observed, owing to poor barrier function inherent to this syndrome.[26]

INDICATIONS AND CONTRAINDICATIONS

Topical Indications: Tacrolimus ointment (Protopic, Astellas), available in 0.03% and 0.1%, is approved by the U.S. Food and Drug Administration (FDA) for use in adults with moderate to severe atopic dermatitis. In children aged 2 to 15 years with moderate to severe atopic dermatitis, only the 0.03% ointment is approved.

Off-label use of tacrolimus ointment has been employed for a number of other inflammatory skin conditions, including seborrheic dermatitis, cutaneous lupus erythematosus, pyoderma gangrenosum, and vitiligo, among others.

Oral and Intravenous Indications: There are no labeled indications for the use of systemic tacrolimus for any dermatologic condition. It is currently approved only for the prophylaxis of organ rejection in renal, hepatic, and cardiac transplant recipients. Its mechanism of action suggests that any patient who is responsive to CsA will also respond to tacrolimus. Beneficial outcomes using tacrolimus have been reported for psoriasis, pyoderma gangrenosum, lupus erythematosus, GVHD, and atopic dermatitis, among others.

Contraindications: Tacrolimus is contraindicated in individuals with known hypersensitivity, and the intravenous formulation should be avoided in those with allergy to hydrogenated castor oil because it represents the main excipient. Other contraindications to systemic tacrolimus are similar to CsA and include active infection, malignancy, and severe hepatic or renal dysfunction. Topical tacrolimus is contraindicated in patients with Netherton syndrome.

DOSING REGIMEN (SEE TABLE 192-4)

The recommended doses of topical and systemic tacrolimus are outlined in Table 192-4. The use of topical tacrolimus deserves special mention. Currently, there is an FDA-issued boxed warning for topical tacrolimus that outlines a lack of long-term safety data and that new malignancies (eg, skin cancer and lymphoma) have been reported in individuals treated with topical tacrolimus. In light of this warning, initiation of tacrolimus and other topical CNIs should begin by addressing parental and patient concerns. These agents should be considered second-line treatments and are typically indicated when standard therapy, including emollients and topical corticosteroids, have failed or resulted in deleterious side effects. Topical CNIs should be applied sparingly to affected areas of skin twice daily using the smallest effective amount. Therapy should be discontinued where signs of prior skin inflammation have subsided. Adjunctive measures, such as emollients, should be continued. When the skin barrier is restored and inflammation is quiescent, two or three weekly applications to sites of prior involvement appear to decrease the requirement for topical steroid use.[27] Importantly, the application of tacrolimus ointment should be restricted to small areas of inflamed skin because large application quantities have been associated with increased percutaneous absorption and a higher risk of systemic side effects.[28] Application under occlusion should be avoided, except for short periods when rapid disease control is desired.

Therapeutic Monitoring: Monitoring for adverse effects and end-organ toxicity with an approach similar to that used for CsA (eg, blood counts, hepatic and renal function tests, electrolytes [including magnesium], uric acid levels, and lipid panels) is strongly recommended for individuals receiving systemic tacrolimus. In renal, hepatic, and cardiac transplant recipients, measuring trough levels to a target plasma concentration between 5 and 15 ng/mL is recommended to prevent organ rejection during treatment with oral tacrolimus. This practice has not been established for any dermatologic condition.

During treatment with topical tacrolimus, patients should be evaluated for signs of cutaneous infection with particular vigilance for eczema herpeticum, the risk of which is increased among atopic patients treated with topical tacrolimus. Any evidence of lymphadenopathy should be documented and closely followed. Skin examinations for cutaneous malignancy should also be conducted at regular intervals, although a causal link between topical tacrolimus use and skin cancer development has not been established. No routine serologic monitoring is necessary. If there is clinical evidence of systemic absorption, serum levels of tacrolimus, as assessed by enzyme-linked immunosorbent assay or HPLC on whole blood, should be obtained.

SIDE EFFECTS AND PRECAUTIONS

The side effects of tacrolimus are similar to those of CsA (see earlier discussion). Neurotoxicity and glucose intolerance are somewhat higher than with CsA, however, so close monitoring of magnesium and glucose levels is strongly recommended. Nephrotoxicity, as with CsA, is a predictable side effect, particularly when high doses or prolonged courses are used. Acute nephrotoxicity appears to be the result of afferent renal arteriole vasoconstriction and is characterized by elevated serum creatinine, hyperkalemia, or a decrease in urine output and is typically reversible.[29] Chronic nephrotoxicity from tacrolimus, which is a result of long-term use, is progressive and irreversible. Caution should be exercised when administering other nephrotoxic agents with tacrolimus. Mucocutaneous side effects appear to be less frequent with tacrolimus than CsA.

Users of topical tacrolimus may experience application site stinging and burning, which is typically more pronounced in excoriated skin. Efforts to limit exposure to denuded areas by pretreating with a topical steroid may ameliorate this side effect and improve adherence to therapy. Pretreatment with oral aspirin before application of tacrolimus has also been shown to reduce symptoms of skin irritation.[30] Refrigeration before application may also mitigate these side effects. Topical tacrolimus has been associated with exacerbations of rosacea, including the granulomatous subtype, and it should therefore be used cautiously in individuals with this condition.[31] Tacrolimus ointment should be avoided on premalignant skin lesions, on infected skin, and in those receiving phototherapy, owing to a theoretically increased susceptibility to skin cancer.

SERIOUS ADVERSE EFFECTS (REFER TO TABLE 192-4)

Similar to CsA, the use of systemic tacrolimus has been associated with lymphoma and other malignancies; serious infections, including those secondary to opportunistic organisms (eg, polyoma virus); irreversible nephrotoxicity; severe neurotoxicity; and pure red cell aplasia as well as other clinically significant cytopenias. Notably, tacrolimus may have a reduced risk for predisposition to skin cancer compared with CsA because in vitro studies have shown that CsA facilitates malignant keratinocyte survival, an attribute that tacrolimus has failed to demonstrate.[32] Tacrolimus may prolong the QT interval and result in torsades de pointes and should therefore be avoided in patients with long QT syndrome. GI perforation has been reported as a rare complication of tacrolimus use.

Drug Interactions: Hepatic cytochrome CYP3A4 enzymes metabolize tacrolimus, and therefore medications or other substances that inhibit or induce these enzymes may increase or decrease whole blood concentrations of tacrolimus, respectively. The relevant food and drug interactions are similar to those for CsA (see Table 192-3) and include grapefruit juice, certain antivirals (eg, protease inhibitors), azole antifungals, calcium channel blockers, select antibiotics, anticonvulsants, and St. John's wort. Understanding these interactions is critical to avoid supratherapeutic or subtherapeutic blood concentrations of tacrolimus. Tacrolimus should not be combined with CsA because their mechanisms of action and toxicity profiles overlap. Unlike CsA, tacrolimus does not interfere with enterohepatic circulation, so lower doses of MMF should be used when the two medications are co-prescribed.

Other Considerations: Individuals with impaired hepatic function should receive a reduced dose of systemic tacrolimus, concordant with the degree of liver dysfunction. Closer monitoring of tacrolimus trough levels may be warranted in such scenarios. Because tacrolimus is minimally metabolized and excreted by the kidneys, dose adjustments are typically not necessary in individuals with preexisting renal disease, but increased surveillance for tacrolimus-induced nephrotoxicity is recommended. Tacrolimus is a Pregnancy Category C medication, and its use in pregnant women should be restricted to scenarios in which known or perceived benefit outweighs its risk. Similar to CsA, tacrolimus is excreted in breast milk, so caution is advised in nursing mothers. Live attenuated vaccines should be avoided during treatment with systemic tacrolimus.

PIMECROLIMUS

Pimecrolimus is a topical, synthetic CNI modified from the macrolide immunosuppressant, ascomycin. Pimecrolimus is formulated exclusively in a cream vehicle (Elidel, Valeant).

PHARMACOLOGY AND MECHANISM OF ACTION

After topical application, pimecrolimus remains largely confined to the skin and has poor percutaneous absorption. In the rare event that clinically significant systemic absorption occurs, as with other CNIs, pimecrolimus is metabolized and excreted primarily by the liver.

Mechanism of Action: Pimecrolimus acts similarly to the other CNIs and functions by inhibiting calcineurin, uncoupling T-cell receptor activation from inflammatory cytokine production (see Fig. 192-2 and Mechanism of Action for CsA and tacrolimus for more detail). The clinical efficacy of pimecrolimus is slightly lower than that of topical tacrolimus as a result of decreased binding avidity to FKBP.[33]

INDICATIONS AND CONTRAINDICATIONS

Indications: Pimecrolimus 1% cream is indicated as a second-line treatment for mild to moderate atopic dermatitis in individuals aged 2 years and older.

Contraindications: Pimecrolimus is contraindicated in patients with a known hypersensitivity. As with topical tacrolimus, pimecrolimus is also contraindicated in patients with Netherton syndrome.

DOSING REGIMEN (SEE TABLE 192-4)

Pimecrolimus should be applied to affected areas of skin twice daily, using the smallest effective amount, and it should be discontinued after cutaneous inflammation has subsided. Emollients should be continued even after cessation of pimecrolimus. Continuous long-term use of pimecrolimus is not recommended. Selecting pimecrolimus over topical tacrolimus is often a matter of prescriber and patient preference because pimecrolimus and tacrolimus are formulated in different vehicles, which may influence compliance. Furthermore, because of its occlusive vehicle, topical tacrolimus appears to have greater potency than pimecrolimus, which may also influence which drug is preferred.

SIDE EFFECTS AND PRECAUTIONS

In general, pimecrolimus is very well tolerated. Intense burning and itching may occur at application sites, particularly in areas of eroded or excoriated skin. If these symptoms develop, they tend to subside with continued use and may also be ameliorated with refrigeration before use. Acneiform eruptions may develop in areas of application. Uncommonly, cutaneous infections complicate its use, and a slightly increased risk of eczema herpeticum has been observed in atopic patients treated with topical pimecrolimus compared with the baseline incidence typically seen in atopic patients. Pimecrolimus should not be applied to premalignant or malignant skin lesions, in areas of active infection, or to skin exposed to phototherapy. Rarely, flulike symptoms and headache may develop and may be a result of systemic absorption.[23] If percutaneous absorption does occur, pimecrolimus appears to have little systemic immunosuppressive effects, and therefore a wider margin of safety compared with other CNIs.

Serious Adverse Effects (Table 192-6): Similar to topical tacrolimus, the labeling of pimecrolimus contains an FDA-issued boxed warning regarding rare reports of malignancy developing during use. Treatment with topical pimecrolimus, therefore, should be limited to short treatment periods with the least amount of drug used to attain a clinical response. A recent case-control study evaluated the association between topical immunomodulator therapy and lymphoma in a

TABLE 192-6
Serious Adverse Effects of Tacrolimus and Pimecrolimus

FORMULATION	SPECIFIC SIDE EFFECTS
Tacrolimus	
Systemic	Hyperkalemia
	Lymphoma and other malignancies
	Nephrotoxicity
	Neurotoxicity
	QT prolongation
	Serious and opportunistic infections
	Severe cytopenias, including pure red cell aplasia
Topical	Theoretical risk of lymphoma and skin malignancy[a]
Pimecrolimus	
	Theoretical risk of lymphoma and skin malignancy[a]

[a]Long-term safety data have not been established, although there are studies that refute this theoretical risk (see text for full details).

cohort of patients with atopic dermatitis and found no increased risk with the use of topical CNIs.[34]

Drug Interactions: Because percutaneous absorption is limited, there are no substantial drug interactions with topical pimecrolimus.

Other Considerations: There are insufficient studies reporting pregnancy outcomes in women using topical pimecrolimus, but as with other medications, use during pregnancy should be approached circumspectly and, if used, the potential benefit should outweigh any perceived risk.

mTOR INHIBITORS

EVEROLIMUS

Everolimus belongs to a class of medications that inhibit mTOR, a key serine-threonine kinase in the PI3K/AKT pathway that governs cellular metabolism, differentiation, and proliferation. Rapamycin (sirolimus) was the first mTOR inhibitor discovered and was first isolated from *Streptomyces hygroscopicus*. Everolimus and temsirolimus are synthetic rapamycin analogues with greater bioavailability.

PHARMACOLOGY AND MECHANISM OF ACTION

Mechanism of Action (Fig. 192-4): Everolimus and other mTOR inhibitors bind to the intracellular protein FKBP-12 (macrophilin-12) to form an aggregate with mTOR complex 1 (mTORC1) that disrupts mTOR kinase activity. In mammalian cells, mTOR inhibitors abrogate the activity of S6 ribosomal protein kinase (S6K) and eukaryotic initiation factor 4E-binding protein (4E-BP1), which are downstream effectors of mTOR involved in protein synthesis.[35] In T lymphocytes, mTOR inhibitors also block cell cycle progression from G1 to S phase and therefore exhibit potent immunosuppressive effects.[36]

Absorption, Distribution, Metabolism, and Excretion: After oral administration, peak serum everolimus concentrations occur within 1 to 2 hours. Consumption with high fat meals appears to reduce total drug absorption.[35] Approximately 75% of everolimus is protein bound within the circulation, and the majority of drug metabolism occurs in the liver because it is a substrate for the hepatic cytochrome CYP3A4 enzyme. Importantly, everolimus is also a competitive inhibitor of CYP3A4 and may increase the concentration of medications that are also metabolized by this enzyme (see Drug Interactions). After conversion into inactive moieties, excretion occurs primarily in the feces, with only 5% of drug excreted unchanged in the urine.

INDICATIONS AND CONTRAINDICATIONS

Indications: There are no labeled dermatologic indications for everolimus. Everolimus is currently indicated to treat hormone receptor–positive breast cancer; neuroendocrine tumors of pancreatic, GI, or lung origin; advanced renal cell carcinoma; and angiomyolipoma and subependymal giant cell astrocytoma that develop in individuals with tuberous sclerosis complex (TSC). Off-label use of everolimus has shown efficacy for treating psoriasis, atopic dermatitis, Kaposi sarcoma, chronic GVHD, and morphea.[37-42] Topical everolimus has also been used to treat facial angiofibromas in individuals with TSC.[43] This beneficial outcome is not surprising, given that constitutive mTOR signaling represents the key pathogenic perturbation underlying TSC. Of note, compared with CNIs, especially CsA, when used as allograft-preserving immunosuppressants, mTOR inhibitors, including

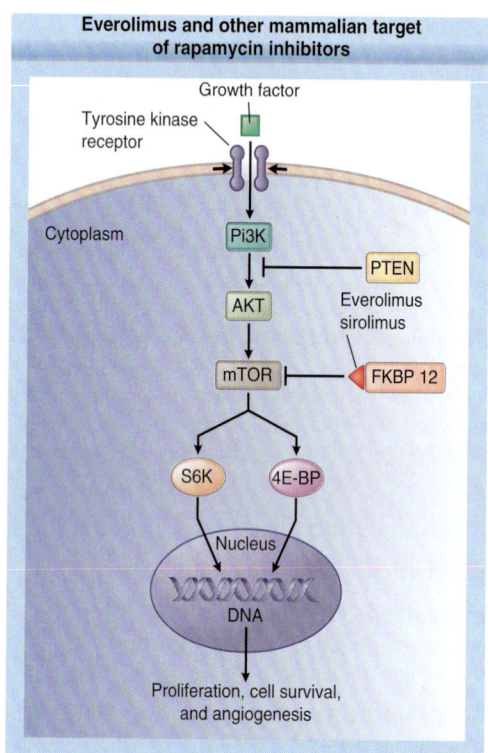

Figure 192-4 Everolimus and other mammalian target of rapamycin (mTOR) inhibitors (eg, sirolimus) bind to FK binding protein (FKBP)-12, forming a complex that inhibits mTOR kinase activity. The downstream effect is reduced activity of S6 ribosomal protein kinase (S6K) and eukaryotic initiation factor 4E–binding protein (4E-BP), which results in decreased cellular proliferation, survival, and angiogenesis. In T cells, mTOR inhibitors also block cell cycle progression from G1 to S phase. AKT, serine/threonine kinase; Pi3K, phosphatidylinositol-3-kinase; PTEN, phosphate and tensin homolog. (Adapted by permission from Springer Nature: Atkins MB, Yasothan U, Kirkpatrick P. Everolimus. *Nat Rev Drug Discov*. 2009;8:535-536. Copyright © 2009.)

everolimus, appear to reduce the long-term risk of cutaneous malignancy in transplant recipients.[44,45]

Contraindications: Everolimus is contraindicated in individuals with known hypersensitivity to the active ingredient or any of its excipients.

DOSING REGIMEN

No established dosing regimen for treating dermatologic conditions exists, although everolimus dosages between 0.5 and 1.5 mg twice daily have been reportedly successful for controlling certain inflammatory and neoplastic skin diseases.

Therapeutic Monitoring: Routine laboratory testing, including blood counts, serum chemistries, assessment of hepatic and renal function, and lipid quantification, is recommended during treatment with everolimus.

Titrating drug doses to achieve a trough concentration between 5 and 15 ng/mL is recommended for individuals receiving everolimus for certain malignancies,[35] but this practice has not been established for any dermatologic condition.

SIDE EFFECTS AND PRECAUTIONS

Mucocutaneous side effects are common during everolimus treatment and tend to occur within the first month of initiating therapy. Common reactions include aphthous stomatitis, acneiform and morbilliform eruptions, folliculitis, and pruritus; less common reactions include erythroderma, onychodystrophy, cutaneous small vessel vasculitis, and symmetrical drug-related intertriginous and flexural exanthema (SDRIFE).[46,47] Other side effects from everolimus are diarrhea, fatigue, headache, peripheral edema, and impaired wound healing. Treatment-induced diabetes mellitus is an uncommon but important potential side effect of everolimus.

mTOR inhibitors should be used cautiously when co-prescribed with MMF or CNIs. Cytopenias, hypercholesterolemia, electrolyte disturbances, elevation of liver enzymes, and thrombotic microangiopathy–hemolytic uremic syndrome are observed more frequently when these drugs are coadministered.

Serious Adverse Effects (Table 192-7): Noninfectious pneumonitis is a potentially serious side effect seen during treatment with everolimus. Nonspecific signs and symptoms such as cough, dyspnea, and hypoxia should raise suspicion for the possibility of this complication, and treatment should be discontinued if radiologic imaging is confirmatory. Corticosteroid therapy may be required if symptoms are severe. Everolimus has been associated with serious, potentially fatal infections, including opportunistic infections. In addition, severe renal and hepatic dysfunction may complicate everolimus therapy. Of note, malignancy is a much less common adverse effect seen during everolimus therapy, likely related to the antiproliferative and antineoplastic properties of mTOR inhibitors. Capillary leak syndrome has been observed during oral sirolimus treatment for psoriasis, but this complication has never been reported for everolimus.[48]

Drug Interactions: Everolimus is both a substrate for and a competitive inhibitor of CYP3A4. Therefore, plasma concentrations of everolimus and drugs metabolized by this enzyme may be affected by concurrent use and should be cautiously co-prescribed. Whereas medications that inhibit CYP3A4 activity (eg, ketoconazole, erythromycin, verapamil) increase plasma concentrations of everolimus, CYP3A4 inducers (eg, rifampin, St. John's wort) reduce concentrations.[35]

Other Considerations: Renal impairment does not influence the metabolism or excretion of everolimus, and therefore no dosage adjustment is necessary for individuals with renal dysfunction. Liver dysfunction, however, appears to increase drug levels, and reduced doses of everolimus are warranted in such scenarios, commensurate with the degree of hepatic impairment. Based on preclinical and small clinical studies, everolimus appears to cause fetal harm and is therefore categorized as a Pregnancy Category D medication. It should not be used during pregnancy, but its use may be justified in very limited clinical settings when known benefit outweighs the risk. Although it is unknown whether everolimus passes into breast milk, lactating women should avoid nursing while using everolimus. Everolimus may acutely impair both male and female fertility, although its long-term effect on fertility has not been established.[35]

TABLE 192-7
Serious Adverse Effects of Everolimus

Embryotoxicity
Hepatotoxicity
Nephrotoxicity
Noninfectious pneumonitis
Serious and opportunistic infections

REFERENCES

1. Madan V, Griffiths CE. Systemic ciclosporin and tacrolimus in dermatology. *Dermatol Ther*. 2007;20(4): 239-250.
2. Kahan BD, Kramer WG. Median effect analysis of efficacy versus adverse effects of immunosuppressants. *Clin Pharmacol Ther*. 2001;70(1):74-81.
3. Kalajian AH, Van Meter Jr, Callen JP. Sarcoidal anemia and leukopenia treated with methotrexate and mycophenolate mofetil. *Arch Dermatol*. 2009;145(8):905-909.
4. Edge JC, Outland JD, Dempsey JR, et al. Mycophenolate mofetil as an effective corticosteroid-sparing therapy for recalcitrant dermatomyositis. *Arch Dermatol*. 2006;142(1):65-69.

5. Eaton PA, Callen JP. Mycophenolate mofetil as therapy for pyoderma gangrenosum. *Arch Dermatol*. 2009;145(7):781-785.
6. Figurski MJ, Pawinski T, Goldberg LR, et al. Pharmacokinetic monitoring of mycophenolic acid in heart transplant patients: correlation the side-effects and rejections with pharmacokinetic parameters. *Ann Transplant*. 2012;17(1):68-78.
7. Le Meur Y, Buchler M, Thierry A, et al. Individualized mycophenolate mofetil dosing based on drug exposure significantly improves patient outcomes after renal transplantation. *Am J Transplant*. 2007;7(11):2496-2503.
8. Djabarouti S, Breilh D, Duffau P, et al. Steady-state mycophenolate mofetil pharmacokinetic parameters enable prediction of systemic lupus erythematosus clinical flares: an observational cohort study. *Arthritis Res Ther*. 2010;12(6):R217.
9. Djabarouti S, Lazaro E, Breilh D, et al. Lower 12-hour trough concentrations of mycophenolic acid in patients with active systemic vasculitides taking mycophenolate mofetil. *J Rheumatol*. 2012;39(11):2222-2223.
10. CellCept (mycophenolate mofetil) prescribing information. [Medication prescribing guide]. 2015; https://http://www.gene.com/download/pdf/cellcept_prescribing.pdf.
11. Nghiem P, Pearson G, Langley RG. Tacrolimus and pimecrolimus: from clever prokaryotes to inhibiting calcineurin and treating atopic dermatitis. *J Am Acad Dermatol*. 2002;46(2):228-241.
12. Neoral (cyclosporine) prescribing information. [Medication prescribing guide]. 2015; https://http://www.pharma.us.novartis.com/sites/www.pharma.us.novartis.com/files/neoral.pdf.
13. Kovarik JM, Mueller EA, Richard F, et al. Evidence for earlier stabilization of cyclosporine pharmacokinetics in de novo renal transplant patients receiving a microemulsion formulation. *Transplantation*. 1996;62(6):759-763.
14. Lee CS KJ. Cyclosporine. In: Wolverton S, ed. *Comprehensive Dermatologic Drug Therapy*. 2nd ed. Philadelphia: Elsevier; 2007:219-237.
15. Kumar R, Dogra S, Amarji B, et al. Efficacy of novel topical liposomal formulation of cyclosporine in mild to moderate stable plaque psoriasis: a randomized clinical trial. *JAMA Dermatol*. 2016;152(7):807-815.
16. Matis WL, Ellis CN, Griffiths CE, et al. Treatment of pyoderma gangrenosum with cyclosporine. *Arch Dermatol*. 1992;128(8):1060-1064.
17. Mendes D, Correia M, Barbedo M, et al. Behcet's disease—a contemporary review. *J Autoimmun*. 2009;32(3-4):178-188.
18. Lebwohl M, Ellis C, Gottlieb A, et al. Cyclosporine consensus conference: with emphasis on the treatment of psoriasis. *J Am Acad Dermatol*. 1998;39(3):464-475.
19. Lee HY, Fook-Chong S, Koh HY, et al. Cyclosporine treatment for Stevens-Johnson syndrome/toxic epidermal necrolysis: retrospective analysis of a cohort treated in a specialized referral center. *J Am Acad Dermatol*. 2017;76(1):106-113.
20. Dubertret L. Retinoids, methotrexate and cyclosporine. *Curr Probl Dermatol*. 2009;38:79-94.
21. Lopez V, Molina I, Martin JM, et al. Eruptive nevi in a patient receiving cyclosporine A for psoriasis treatment. *Arch Dermatol*. 2010;146(7):802-804.
22. Woo M, Przepiorka D, Ippoliti C, et al. Toxicities of tacrolimus and cyclosporin A after allogeneic blood stem cell transplantation. *Bone Marrow Transplant*. 1997;20(12):1095-1098.
23. Hanifin JM, Paller AS, Eichenfield L, et al. Efficacy and safety of tacrolimus ointment treatment for up to 4 years in patients with atopic dermatitis. *J Am Acad Dermatol*. 2005;53(2 suppl 2):S186-S194.
24. Saripalli YV, Gadzia JE, Belsito DV. Tacrolimus ointment 0.1% in the treatment of nickel-induced allergic contact dermatitis. *J Am Acad Dermatol*. 2003;49(3):477-482.
25. Pascual JC, Fleisher AB. Tacrolimus ointment (Protopic) for atopic dermatitis. *Skin Therapy Lett*. 2004;9(9):1-5.
26. Allen A, Siegfried E, Silverman R, et al. Significant absorption of topical tacrolimus in 3 patients with Netherton syndrome. *Arch Dermatol*. 2001;137(6):747-750.
27. Breneman D, Fleischer AB Jr, Abramovits W, et al. Intermittent therapy for flare prevention and long-term disease control in stabilized atopic dermatitis: a randomized comparison of 3-times-weekly applications of tacrolimus ointment versus vehicle. *J Am Acad Dermatol*. 2008;58(6):990-999.
28. Teshima D, Ikesue H, Itoh Y, et al. Increased topical tacrolimus absorption in generalized leukemic erythroderma. *Ann Pharmacother*. 2003;37(10):1444-1447.
29. PROGRAF (tacrolimus) prescribing information. Medication prescribing guide. 2015; https://www.astellas.us/docs/prograf.pdf.
30. Mandelin J, Remitz A, Reitamo S. Effect of oral acetylsalicylic acid on burning caused by tacrolimus ointment in patients with atopic dermatitis. *Arch Dermatol*. 2010;146(10):1178-1180.
31. Hu L, Alexander C, Velez NF, et al. Severe tacrolimus-induced granulomatous rosacea recalcitrant to oral tetracyclines. *J Drugs Dermatol*. 2015;14(6):628-630.
32. Norman KG, Canter JA, Shi M, et al. Cyclosporine A suppresses keratinocyte cell death through MPTP inhibition in a model for skin cancer in organ transplant recipients. *Mitochondrion*. 2010;10(2):94-101.
33. Paller AS, Lebwohl M, Fleischer AB Jr, et al. Tacrolimus ointment is more effective than pimecrolimus cream with a similar safety profile in the treatment of atopic dermatitis: results from 3 randomized, comparative studies. *J Am Acad Dermatol*. 2005;52(5):810-822.
34. Arellano FM, Wentworth CE, Arana A, et al. Risk of lymphoma following exposure to calcineurin inhibitors and topical steroids in patients with atopic dermatitis. *J Invest Dermatol*. 2007;127(4):808-816.
35. AFINITOR (everolimus) prescribing information. Medication prescribing guide. 2016; https://http://www.pharma.us.novartis.com/sites/www.pharma.us.novartis.com/files/afinitor.pdf.
36. Magnuson B, Ekim B, Fingar DC. Regulation and function of ribosomal protein S6 kinase (S6K) within mTOR signalling networks. *Biochem J*. 2012;441(1):1-21.
37. Frigerio E, Colombo MD, Franchi C, et al. Severe psoriasis treated with a new macrolide: everolimus. *Br J Dermatol*. 2007;156(2):372-374.
38. Van Velsen SG, Haeck IM, Bruijnzeel-Koomen CA. Severe atopic dermatitis treated with everolimus. *J Dermatolog Treat*. 2009;20(6):365-367.
39. Wei KC, Lai PC. Combination of everolimus and tacrolimus: a potentially effective regimen for recalcitrant psoriasis. *Dermatol Ther*. 2015;28(1):25-27.
40. Mourah S, Porcher R, Battistella M, et al. Paradoxical simultaneous regression and progression of lesions in a phase II study of everolimus in classic Kaposi sarcoma. *Br J Dermatol*. 2015;173(5):1284-1287.

41. Jedlickova Z, Burlakova I, Bug G, et al. Therapy of sclerodermatous chronic graft-versus-host disease with mammalian target of rapamycin inhibitors. *Biol Blood Marrow Transplant*. 2011;17(5):657-663.
42. Frumholtz L, Roux J, Bagot M, et al. Treatment of generalized deep morphea with everolimus. *JAMA Dermatol*. 2016;152(10):1170-1172.
43. Dill PE, De Bernardis G, Weber P, et al. Topical everolimus for facial angiofibromas in the tuberous sclerosis complex. A first case report. *Pediatr Neurol*. 2014;51(1):109-113.
44. Feldmeyer L, Hofbauer GF, Boni T, et al. Mammalian target of rapamycin (mTOR) inhibitors slow skin carcinogenesis, but impair wound healing. *Br J Dermatol*. 2012;166(2):422-424.
45. Holdaas H, De Simone P, Zuckermann A. Everolimus and malignancy after solid organ transplantation: a clinical update. *J Transplant*. 2016;2016:4369574.
46. Campistol JM, de Fijter JW, Flechner SM, et al. mTOR inhibitor-associated dermatologic and mucosal problems. *Clin Transplant*. 2010;24(2):149-156.
47. Kurtzman DJ, Oulton J, Erickson C, et al. Everolimus-Induced Symmetrical Drug-Related Intertriginous and Flexural Exanthema (SDRIFE). *Dermatitis*. 2016; 27(2):76-77.
48. Kaplan MJ, Ellis CN, Bata-Csorgo Z, et al. Systemic toxicity following administration of sirolimus (formerly rapamycin) for psoriasis: association of capillary leak syndrome with apoptosis of lesional lymphocytes. *Arch Dermatol*. 1999;135(5):553-557.

Chapter 193 :: Immunobiologics: Targeted Therapy Against Cytokines, Cytokine Receptors, and Growth Factors in Dermatology

:: Andrew Johnston, Yoshikazu Takada, & Sam T. Hwang

第一百九十三章
免疫生物制剂：皮肤病学中针对细胞因子、细胞因子受体和生长因子的靶向治疗

中文导读

免疫生物制剂是指通过与特定生物靶点相互作用诱导或改变免疫反应的活生物体产生的抗体和蛋白质，包括重组细胞因子、生长因子、基于抗体的试剂和融合蛋白。已知许多细胞因子在最常见的皮肤病中起关键作用，截至本文撰写之时，已经或即将批准10多种免疫生物制剂，主要是人源化单克隆抗体。

本章分别介绍了白介素1（IL-1）、白介素18、白介素33、白介素36、Th17轴细胞因子（IL-17、IL-22、IL-12，IL-23）、肿瘤坏死生长因子α和生长因子在生物或免疫过程中的基本作用，然后介绍了目前针对各靶点的生物制剂，同时也介绍了各种重组细胞因子和生长因子、其他免疫生物制剂，并且指出了生物制剂特有的副作用，靶向免疫系统可能会增加感染和患恶性肿瘤的风险。

〔栗 娟〕

AT-A-GLANCE

- Immunobiologics are drugs defined as antibodies and proteins engineered from living organisms that induce or alter immune responses by interacting with specific biologic targets.
- Those used to treat cutaneous disease and cancer include recombinant cytokines and growth factors, monoclonal antibodies, and fusion proteins.
- Targeting the immune system with biologics may result in an increased risk of infections and malignancies.

Immunobiologics are compounds synthesized in living organisms that exhibit immune modulatory properties for therapeutic purposes. They consist of recombinant cytokines, growth factors, antibody-based agents, and fusion proteins. Many cytokines are known to play critical roles in the most common of dermatologic conditions, including psoriasis and atopic dermatitis, and, as of this writing, more than 10 immunobiologic agents, mostly humanized monoclonal antibodies, have been approved or will soon be approved for these conditions since the last version of this chapter. Herein, we briefly discuss cytokines as it is difficult to discuss immunobiologics that target specific cytokines without understanding the fundamental role of the cytokine in biologic or immunologic processes. Besides tumor necrosis factor (TNF)-α, interleukin (IL)-4, and IL-1, some of the first cytokines to be recognized as central to immunopathogenesis of common skin diseases, cytokines such as IL-18, IL-22, and IL-23, are now seen to play critical roles in Still disease (IL-18), epidermal psoriatic hyperproliferation (IL-22), and T-helper cell type 17 (Th17) maintenance (IL-23). We emphasize the newer cytokines and treatments that are in development and refer to excellent reviews to highlight the clinical usefulness of older agents. Lastly, we point out some of the unique side effects that are sometimes observed with the new biologic agents as these (often rare) side effects take time to recognize and to characterize in the literature. When possible, we depict the cellular events that mediate cutaneous inflammation and identify the molecular interactions affected by specific immunobiologic agents in relevant figures.

INTERLEUKIN 1

IL-1 was the first cytokine to be detected in skin[1] and is now regarded as the prototypical member of a family of 11 structurally related cytokines (Fig. 193-1). IL-1 is a fundamental cytokine for directing epidermal responses to injury and infection. Although pro-IL-1α is active as a cell membrane–associated cytokine, under conditions of cell stress, cytoplasmic pro-IL-1α also can be rapidly processed and secreted.[2,3] In contrast, pro-IL-1β is inactive and always requires the action of a protease for activity. A diverse array of stimuli, including cell stress, infection, and local danger signals, trigger the assembly of macromolecular inflammasome complexes that activate caspase-1, which then cleaves pro-IL-1β to its active form.[4] Once activated, both IL-1α and IL-1β can bind IL-1 receptor 1 (R1) on the surface on target cells, driving signal transduction (Fig. 193-2). A decoy receptor, IL-1R2, that has a shorter cytoplasmic tail devoid of signaling domains and unable to initiate signal transduction, can be expressed on the cell surface. IL-1 signaling is also controlled by the expression of the IL-1 receptor antagonist (IL-1Ra), which limits IL-1 receptor activation by competitive inhibition (Fig. 193-2). Once secreted, IL-1α and IL-1β have similar functions, acting on keratinocytes, fibroblasts, vascular endothelium, and lymphocytes. IL-1 has rapid and profound effects on keratinocytes, inducing a range of gene transcripts involved in inflammatory and antimicrobial responses. IL-1 also appears to be a key cytokine in the development of Th17 T-cell responses.[5]

A critical step in the activation of IL-1β is the assembly of inflammasome complexes, which are a combination of a molecular sensor (eg, MEFV [pyrin], NLRP1, NLRP3 [cryopyrin], NLRP12, and AIM2), combined with an adaptor molecule (apoptosis-associated speck-like protein containing a CARD [ASC]), and an effector molecule (caspase-1). These complexes transduce the detection of a variety of cellular danger signals into IL-1 cytokine activity. A number of sterile autoinflammatory conditions are associated with mutations in genes encoding inflammasome components.[6] In particular, the cryopyrin-associated periodic syndromes,

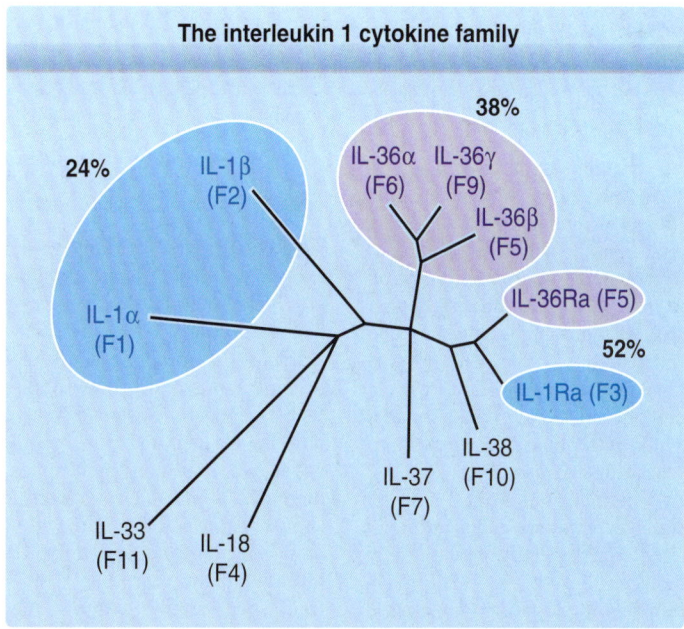

Figure 193-1 The interleukin (IL)-1 family consists of 11 cytokine ligands. A high degree of homology is shared between IL-1α/β, IL-36α/β/γ, and their respective receptor antagonists.

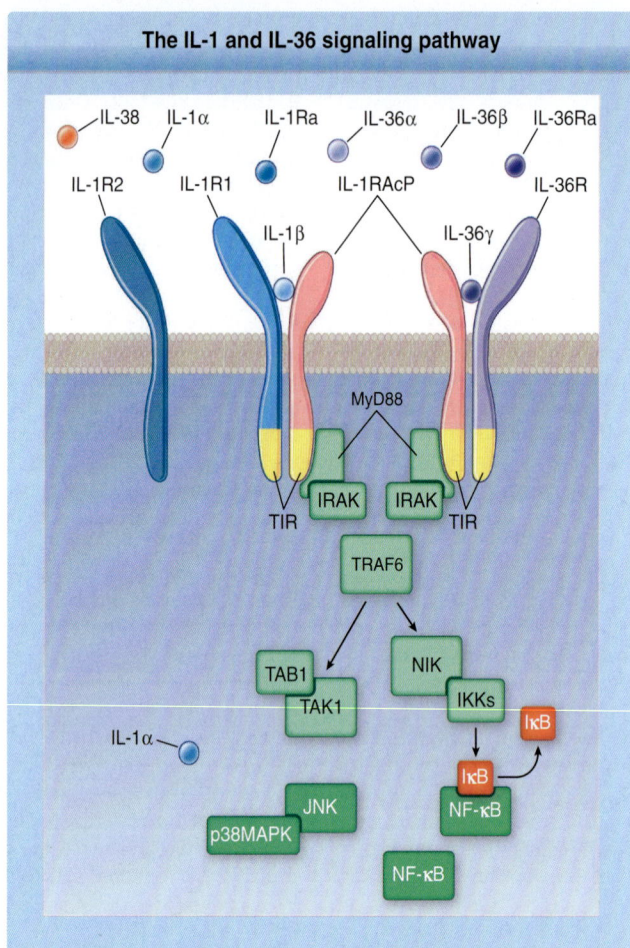

Figure 193-2 The interleukin (IL)-1 and IL-36 signaling pathways. IκB, inhibitor of nuclear factor κB; IKK, inhibitor of nuclear factor κB kinase; IRAK, interleukin-1 receptor-associated kinase; JNK, c-Jun N-terminal kinase; MyD88, myeloid differentiation 88; NF-κB, nuclear factor κB; NIK, nuclear factor κB–inducing kinase; TIR, Toll interleukin-1 receptor; TRAF, tumor necrosis factor receptor-associated factor.

a collection of diseases including familial cold autoinflammatory syndrome, Muckle-Wells syndrome, and neonatal-onset multisystem inflammatory disorder (also known as chronic infantile neurologic cutaneous and articular syndrome) are associated with gain-of-function mutations in *NLRP3*, encoding cryopyrin, leading to increased inflammasome activation and IL-1β processing and activity.[7,8] Pyrin (*MEFV*) mutations are the cause of familial Mediterranean fever[9] and the recently described disease, pyrin-associated autoinflammation with neutrophilic dermatosis.[10]

Another condition arising because of elevated IL-1 activity is caused by a deficiency of the IL-1 receptor antagonist, an autosomal recessive, genetic, autoinflammatory syndrome resulting from mutations in *IL1RN*.[11] The mutations result in an abnormal protein that is not secreted, exposing the cells to unopposed IL-1 activity. This results in pustular rash, joint swelling, oral mucosal lesions, multifocal osteomyelitis, and periostitis.[11]

ANAKINRA

Anakinra was the first biologic developed to specifically target IL-1. It is a recombinant, nonglycosylated version of IL-1Ra that competitively inhibits both IL-1α and IL-1β activity at the IL-1 receptor. Anakinra has proved useful in treating a number of joint, bone, and muscle diseases.[12] Several case reports and clinical trials have demonstrated the efficacy of anakinra for treating the cryopyrin-associated periodic syndromes and deficiency of the IL-1 receptor antagonist.[11] Anakinra has a short half-life of 4 to 6 hours and therefore requires daily subcutaneous injections. IL-1β is elevated in hidradenitis suppurativa,[13] and encouraging data from small studies support the use of anakinra for hidradenitis suppurativa.[14,15] Several reports describe the use of anakinra to treat pustular psoriasis where anakinra appears to induce a rapid normalization of systemic inflammatory symptoms followed by improvement of the pustular skin eruption. However, the response in the skin tends to be incomplete with erythema and hyperkeratosis remaining in some cases.[16-18] Clinical trials to assess the efficacy of anakinra for pustular skin diseases are ongoing (NCT01794117).

RILONACEPT

Rilonacept is a dimeric fusion protein consisting of the IL-1-binding domains of the extracellular portions of human IL-1R1 and IL-1RAcP fused to the Fc portion of human immunoglobulin (Ig) G_1. Thus rilonacept functions as a soluble IL-1 decoy receptor binding IL-1α and IL-1β. Rilonacept is indicated for the treatment of cryopyrin-associated periodic syndromes, including familial cold autoinflammatory syndrome and Muckle-Wells syndrome.[19,20]

CANAKINUMAB

Canakinumab is a fully human monoclonal IgG$_1$ antibody that neutralizes IL-1β. Canakinumab is U.S. Food and Drug Administration (FDA) approved for use in cryopyrin-associated periodic syndromes[20] and recently approved for tumor necrosis factor receptor–associated periodic syndrome, hyperimmunoglobulin D syndrome/mevalonate kinase deficiency, and familial Mediterranean fever. Canakinumab has a been used in cases of pustular psoriasis[21]; however, the relevance of using IL-1 antagonism to tackle a disease that may be primarily driven by deviations in IL-36 signaling, particularly when *IL36RN* mutations are present, has been questioned.[22]

INTERLEUKIN-18

IL-18 is an IL-1 family member and like IL-1β, IL-18 always requires posttranslational cleavage of the pro protein for activity either by caspase-1,[23] mast cell chymase,[24] or granzyme B.[25] IL-18 is broadly expressed by epithelia, blood mononuclear cells, and keratinocytes.[26] IL-18 acts via its dimeric receptor, IL18Rα-IL18Rβ, to induce p38 mitogen-activated protein kinase and AP-1 signaling, but unlike IL-1, no nuclear factor κB (NF-κB) activation.[27] IL-18 activity is mainly regulated by the expression of soluble IL-18 binding protein (IL-18BP). IL-18 is best understood for its ability, in combination with IL-12, for the induction of Th1 T-cell responses.[28] However, since pro-IL-18 is also activated by inflammasomes, a contributing role for IL-18 in the cryopyrin-associated periodic syndromes has been suggested.[29] Increased IL-18 expression is seen in acute atopic dermatitis and psoriasis,[30] and heightened responses of keratinocytes to IL-18 have been observed in cutaneous lupus erythematosus lesions, thus roles for IL-18 in chronic or autoimmune inflammatory skin conditions have been proposed.[31] Elevated levels of free IL-18 (not bound to neutralizing IL-18BP) have been detected in the serum of patients with adult-onset Still disease,[32] thus following Phase II trials, tadekinig alfa, a recombinant human IL-18BP, was granted orphan drug and breakthrough therapy status by the FDA in 2017 for adult-onset Still disease.

INTERLEUKIN-33

IL-33 is an IL-1 family cytokine broadly expressed by endothelia and epithelia, but typically absent from leukocytes. IL-33 signals through a complex containing the receptor ST2 (IL-33R) coupled with IL-1RAcP,[33] and like IL-1, IL-33 signaling activates NF-κB, as well as c-Jun N-terminal kinase and p38 mitogen-activated protein kinase.[28] IL-33 activity is controlled by a soluble alternatively spliced form of ST2 forming a decoy receptor[34] and also a single immunoglobulin IL-1-related receptor, an IL-1 family receptor that interacts with ST2 on the cell surface to reduce responses to IL-33.[35] Unlike IL-1β and IL-18, IL-33 is not a substrate for caspase-1 activation; rather, IL-33 is inactivated by the apoptosis-associated caspases 3 and 8, as a means of reducing cell death-related inflammation.[36] Likely as a consequence of its ability to promote Th2 responses, disruptions in IL-33 or soluble ST2 expression have been linked with allergic inflammation,[37] but there are no ongoing clinical trials assessing the use of IL-33 or ST2.

INTERLEUKIN-36

The cytokines IL-36α, IL-36β, and IL-36γ are a trio of homologous proinflammatory cytokines, and due to their sequence similarities to IL-1α and IL-1β, are members of the IL-1 superfamily (see Fig. 193-1). The 3 IL-36 cytokines are expressed primarily by epithelial tissues, including skin, with IL-36α and IL-36β expression detectable only in inflamed skin, whereas IL-36γ expression is present in normal skin and strongly upregulated in inflammatory skin conditions, including psoriasis,[38-40] hidradenitis suppurativa,[41] and pustular disease.[42] All 3 IL-36 isoforms are highly inducible by proinflammatory stimuli such as IL-1, TNF, and IL-17A,[39] and work synergistically with these cytokines.[43] The IL-36 cytokines are overexpressed in both chronic plaque and pustular psoriasis skin lesions[38,39,42,44] where they drive keratinocyte inflammatory responses,[39] synergize with other proinflammatory cytokines,[43] and promote activation of dendritic cells,[45,46] macrophages and Langerhans cells.[47] Like IL-1β and IL-18, the IL-36 cytokines require posttranslational N-terminal peptide cleavage for full activity,[48] with recent data indicating the activity of the neutrophil proteases elastase and cathepsin G,[42,49] as well as keratinocyte-derived cathepsin S,[50] may be critical for IL-36 activation. Once activated, IL-36 has powerful effects on epithelial cell gene expression, with the induction of a range of chemokine and proinflammatory cytokines by keratinocytes, and as such may help drive the vicious inflammatory cycle seen in a number of skin diseases. IL-36 cytokines signal via the IL-36R coupled to the IL-1RAcP (see Fig. 193-2), which appear to be widely expressed in tissues, including lung epithelium, dendritic cells, keratinocytes, fibroblasts, and some endothelia.

Analogous to IL-1β, IL-36 activity is limited by the presence of the IL-36 receptor antagonist (IL-36RA) encoded by *IL36RN*. Missense mutations in *IL36RN* are associated with a number of inflammatory skin diseases,[51] including the severe episodic skin disease generalized pustular psoriasis (GPP),[52,53] impetigo herpetiformis,[54] and acute generalized exanthematous pustulosis.[55,56] Mutations in *IL36RN* account for between 46% and 82% of cases of GPP without concomitant plaque psoriasis.[57] The disease-associated missense mutations in *IL36RN* affect the structure and function of IL-36RA, leading to unchecked activity at the IL-36 receptor. In skin, this results in keratinocyte IL-1β, IL-6, IL-8, and chemokine production, promoting neutrophil infiltration.[52,53] The identification of a role for the IL-36 cytokines in inflammatory skin diseases has prompted interest in targeting this pathway therapeutically and clinical trials of IL-36 receptor antagonists may be on the horizon in the near future.[58]

IL-37 and IL-38 data are scarce but these cytokines appear to be antiinflammatory in nature,[59,60] although their receptors, disease associations, and mechanisms of action have yet to be defined.

CYTOKINES OF THE TH17 AXIS (IL-17A, IL-22, AND IL-23)

INTERLEUKIN-17

The homodimeric cytokine IL-17A is the best-studied of the 6-member IL-17 cytokine family (IL-17A through IL-17F, and reviewed by Monin and Gaffen[61]) and is the signature cytokine of Th17 cells, a T-cell phenotype recognized both for being essential for immune defense at epithelial barriers and implicated in a number of inflammatory immune diseases,[62] including psoriasis,[63] rheumatic diseases,[64] and systemic lupus erythematosus.[65] IL-17A has wide-ranging proinflammatory effects and it induces the secretion of cytokines such as IL-6, IL-8, CCL20, and granulocyte-macrophage colony-stimulating factor by keratinocytes and fibroblasts, resulting in recruitment of T cells, macrophages, and neutrophils to the skin. Furthermore, IL-17A synergizes with other proinflammatory cytokines such as interferon (IFN)-γ,[5,66] TNF-α,[67-69] and IL-36,[43] among others. There are multiple cellular sources of IL-17A in the skin. Immunohistochemistry demonstrates that the major portion of staining for IL-17A in lesional psoriasis skin is associated with mast cells and neutrophils,[70] CD4+ and CD8+ T cells,[71] mucosal-associated invariant T cells[72] and Type 3 innate lymphoid cells.[73] Around 50% of epidermal T cells are capable of secreting IL-17A.[5] IL-17A signals via ubiquitously expressed IL-17RA–IL-17RC receptor complexes transducing signals via ACT1/ tumor necrosis factor receptor-associated factor-6 and activate multiple pathways including NF-κB, extracellular signal-regulated kinase, p38, and c-Jun N-terminal kinase.[61] Mutations in a number of components of this pathway are associated with chronic mucocutaneous candidiasis[74] and variants in several genes involved in IL-17A responses are associated with increased genetic risk for psoriasis[75,76] revealing critical roles for IL-17A in psoriasis.

SECUKINUMAB

Secukinumab is a fully human anti–IL-17A IgG$_1$κ monoclonal antibody that, following demonstration of efficacy in 2 Phase III trials[77] became the first anti–IL-17A biologic FDA approved for plaque psoriasis.[78] The proportion of patients attaining a 75% reduction in their disease from baseline (ie, PASI75 [Psoriasis Area and Severity Index 75] response) at week 12 of treatment was greater than 80% (ERASURE [Efficacy of Response and Safety of Two Fixed Secukinumab Regimens in Psoriasis] study NCT01365455) and greater than 70% (FIXTURE [Full Year Investigative Examination of Secukinumab vs Etanercept Using Two Dosing Regimens to Determine Efficacy in Psoriasis] study NCT01358578) showing better efficacy than etanercept (44% of etanercept recipients achieved a PASI75 response) or placebo (<5%).[77] Secukinumab also rapidly improves both systemic and skin symptoms in GPP patients.[79-81] A recent study of secukinumab for moderate to severe palmoplantar pustulosis demonstrated a 50% improvement in disease severity and significant improvements in quality-of-life scores.[81] Secukinumab is also undergoing, as of this writing, clinical trials for hidradenitis suppurativa (NCT03099980), psoriatic arthritis (NCT02854163, NCT02745080, NCT01989468), and allergic contact dermatitis (NCT02778711).

IXEKIZUMAB

Ixekizumab is a humanized IgG$_4$ monoclonal antibody that neutralizes IL-17A. Data from 3 Phase III clinical trials (UNCOVER-1, UNCOVER-2, and UNCOVER-3) indicate that ixekizumab 80 mg every 2 or 4 weeks, is effective for plaque psoriasis with more than 80% of patients achieving PASI75 at 12 weeks.[82,83] These Phase III trials also indicated that ixekizumab was superior to the anti-TNF agent etanercept for plaque psoriasis[84] and had beneficial effects on scalp involvement,[85] nail involvement,[86] and itch.[87] A recent small trial also suggested that ixekizumab may be useful for treating erythrodermic psoriasis and GPP.[88] Clinical trials are ongoing for psoriatic arthritis (NCT01695239, NCT03151551, NCT02349295, NCT02584855), rheumatoid arthritis (NCT00966875), and bullous pemphigoid (NCT03099538).

BRODALUMAB

Brodalumab, is a human anti–IL-17RA monoclonal antibody targeting the IL-17 receptor A chain. Brodalumab was recently FDA approved for moderate-to-severe plaque psoriasis in adult patients who are candidates for systemic therapy or phototherapy and have failed to respond or have lost response to other systemic therapies. Three Phase III studies have been conducted and generated some very promising results for plaque psoriasis (AMAGINE-1, AMAGINE-2 and AMAGINE-3).[89,90] At week 12, 60% (brodalumab 140 mg) and 83% (brodalumab 210 mg) versus 3% (placebo) patients achieved a PASI75 (AMAGINE-1[89]). In the second 2 trials, at week 12, the PASI75 response rates were 86% (210 mg) and 67% (140 mg) versus 8% (placebo) (AMAGINE-2) and 85% (210 mg) and 69% (140 mg) versus 6% (placebo) (AMAGINE-3).[90] Moreover, brodalumab 210 mg every 2 weeks was shown to be superior to ustekinumab and placebo in treating plaque psoriasis.[90] In a smaller study, brodalumab was also shown to induce clinical improvement in 11 (92%) of 12 GPP patients.[91] There are also ongoing clinical trials examining the efficacy of brodalumab for psoriatic arthritis (NCT02029495, NCT02024646).

INTERLEUKIN-22

IL-22 is a member of the IL-10 family of cytokines (along with IL-19, IL-20, IL-24, and IL-26), members of which are related by their sequence and structural similarities as well as their shared receptor usage. Each IL-10 family cytokine uses a heterodimeric receptor with IL-22 using the ubiquitously expressed IL-10R2 in conjunction with IL-22R1, a receptor with a highly specific tissue expression pattern, being expressed only by the skin, lung, and gut epithelia, and liver and pancreas cells, but not lymphocytes.[92] IL-22 production has been detected from Th1 and Th17 T-cells, as well as Tc22 (IL-22+ CD8+) T cells, Th22 cells that produce IL-22 in the absence of IFN-γ, IL-4, or IL-17.[93] In addition, several phenotypes of innate immune cells have been reported to produce IL-22, including natural killer (NK) cells, γδ T cells, lymphoid tissue inducer cells, and Type 3 innate lymphoid cells. As such, Th17, Th22, Tc22 T cells, Type 3 innate lymphoid cells, and NK cells (reviewed in Sabat et al[92]) have all been reported to be increased in number in psoriasis plaques. IL-22 has profound effects on epidermal keratinocytes, driving hyperplasia, keratinocyte migration, and disruption of epidermal differentiation.[94] IL-22, along with the other IL-20 subfamily members is abundantly overexpressed in lesional psoriasis epidermis, as well as in the blood of psoriasis patients,[95] and is restored back to normal levels during effective treatments.[96] Consequently, IL-22 has long been suspected of playing a crucial role in the development of psoriasis skin lesions. The effects of IL-22 on skin are further heightened by powerful synergies with IL-17 and TNF, promoting IL-22 as an attractive cytokine target for inflammatory skin diseases. A number of targeted IL-22/IL-22R therapeutics have been investigated for psoriasis and atopic dermatitis, but as of this writing there are no agents approved nor in ongoing trials.

INTERLEUKIN-12

IL-12 is a heterodimeric cytokine composed of IL-12p35 and IL-12p40 subunits. IL-12 is a major inducer of IFN-γ-producing (Th1) T cells (Fig. 193-3), activates NK and CD8+ T cells, and has the ability to induce skin-homing characteristics (cutaneous lymphocyte-associated antigen expression) on memory T cells.[97] Activated antigen-presenting cells are the chief source of IL-12 and skin macrophages are the main source of IL-12 in psoriasis,[98] but the functional role of IL-12 in psoriasis is uncertain in light of the dominance of the Th17 pathway in this disease. IL-12 uses the dimeric receptor IL-12Rβ1–IL-12Rβ 2, signaling via Jak2/Tyk2 promoting the formation of STAT4 homodimers. IL-12 expression is increased in psoriasis lesions[98] and chronic, but not acute, atopic dermatitis skin.[99] Several genetic polymorphisms conferring risk or protection for psoriasis have been identified near the *IL12B* gene,[100-102] which may enhance Th1 T-cell responses in psoriasis.[103]

USTEKINUMAB

Ustekinumab is an IgG$_1$κ human monoclonal antibody directed at IL-12p40 (the shared subunit of IL-12 and IL-23) that is FDA approved for use in psoriasis, psoriatic arthritis, and Crohn disease. Phase III clinical trial data for plaque psoriasis highlighted the efficacy of ustekinumab with more than 66% of patients using ustekinumab 45 mg and more than 75% of patients using ustekinumab 90 mg attaining a PASI75 by week 12.[104,105] Although ustekinumab is effective, subsequent research identified IL-23, rather than IL-12, as the more important driver of psoriasis pathogenesis, leading to a focus on specifically blocking the IL-23/IL-17 inflammatory axis, detailed below (see "Interleukin-23"). A number of case reports and a small uncontrolled study show the potential of ustekinumab for treating hidradenitis suppurativa[106] although TNF antagonists have shown greater efficacy.[107] The efficacy of ustekinumab in severe atopic dermatitis was suggested from multiple case reports, however data from recent randomized controlled trials do not support this use.[108-110]

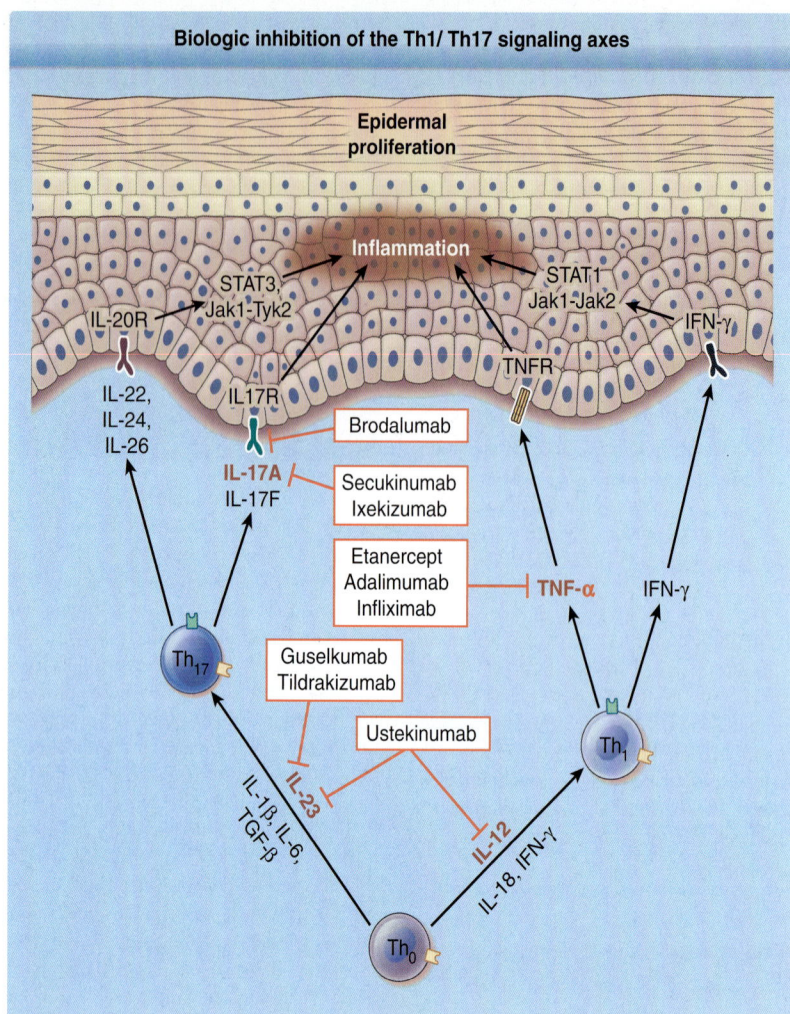

Figure 193-3 Biologic inhibition of the IL-23/IL-17 (Th1/Th17) signaling axes. IFN, interferon; IL, interleukin; STAT, signal transducer and activator of transcription; TGF, transforming growth factor; Th, T-helper; TNFR, tumor necrosis factor receptor.

INTERLEUKIN-23

IL-23 is a heterodimeric cytokine composed of 1 IL-23p19 and 1 IL-12p40 subunit; the IL-12p40 subunit is also used by IL-12 (IL-12p40 + IL-12p35). IL-23 is expressed by dendritic cells[111] and epidermal keratinocytes.[112] IL-23 binds the dimeric receptor IL-23R–IL-12Rβ1 (shared with IL-12) on the cell surface and signals via Jak2/Tyk2, and signal transducer and activator of transcription (STAT) 3/STAT4 heterodimers.[113] The importance of IL-23 in immune-mediated inflammatory skin diseases stems from its key functions as a master regulator of Th17 T-cell responses.[114,115] This role is highlighted by several disease-associated polymorphisms in *IL23R* encoding one of the IL-23 receptor subunits in Crohn disease, psoriasis, and psoriatic arthritis.[100-102,116] Targeting IL-23 is attractive as it is deemed upstream of the Th17 cells implicated in multiple inflammatory diseases (see Fig. 193-3). A number of biologics designed to inhibit IL-23 are, as of this writing, showing promise in the clinic. Approaches targeting the IL-23 receptor itself are also in development.[117,118] The first biologic used to target IL-23 was the anti–IL-12p40 biologic ustekinumab (see "Ustekinumab"), which has been used with success for treating psoriasis.[104,105]

GUSELKUMAB

Specific targeting the IL-23p19 subunit with guselkumab, a fully human IgG₁λ antibody, is showing clinical promise. Guselkumab (see Fig. 193-3) was FDA approved in 2017 for the treatment of moderate to severe plaque psoriasis after the completion of 2 Phase III clinical trials.[119,120] Both clinical trials used guselkumab 100 mg, at weeks 0 and 4 and then every 8 weeks, and found this was superior to placebo at week 16 as more than 70% of patients reached a 90% improvement in their disease (PASI90). Guselkumab was also found to be superior to the anti-TNF agent adalimumab with respect to PASI90 measurements at weeks 16 (73.3% vs 49.7%), week 24 (80.2% vs 53.0%), and week 48 (76.3% vs 47.9%).[120] Guselkumab is, as of this writing, also in Phase III trials for palmoplantar pustulosis (NCT02641730), GPP, and erythrodermic psoriasis (NCT02343744), and Phase IIa trials for psoriatic arthritis (NCT02319759), although results of a Phase II study on rheumatoid arthritis treated with guselkumab were negative.[121]

TILDRAKIZUMAB

Tildrakizumab is a humanized monoclonal $IgG_1\kappa$ antibody targeting IL-23p19 (see Fig. 193-3). Results from multicenter Phase III trials (reSURFACE 1 and reSURFACE 2) for moderate-to-severe chronic plaque psoriasis showed tildrakizumab (100 and 200 mg) effective with more than 60% of patients achieving a PASI75 compared with placebo (6%) and the anti-TNF agent etanercept (48%).[122]

RISANKIZUMAB

Risankizumab is a fully human IgG1 monoclonal antibody against IL-23p19. Results from a Phase II trial (NCT02054481) with moderate-to-severe chronic plaque psoriasis are promising, with 77% of risankizumab-treated patients (pooled 90-mg and 180-mg treated groups) attaining a PASI90 at week 12, compared with 40% of patients at PASI90 with ustekinumab (45 or 90 mg).[123] In addition, a Phase III trial examining risankizumab for GPP or erythrodermic psoriasis is, as of this writing, ongoing in Japan (NCT03022045).

TUMOR NECROSIS FACTOR-α

TNF-α is a homotrimeric cytokine expressed by a wide array of cell types, including most phenotypes of activated T cells, neutrophils, mast cells, NK cells, antigen-presenting cells, adipocytes, fibroblasts, and keratinocytes.[124] TNF triggers its effects by binding to its p55 and p75 receptors expressed primarily on the surface of keratinocytes, neutrophils, endothelial cells, and fibroblasts. TNF has strong synergistic interactions with other proinflammatory cytokines such as IL-17A.[67] TNF is regarded as a central cytokine in the development of several autoimmune diseases, including psoriatic arthritis, rheumatoid arthritis, and inflammatory bowel disease. TNF-α is a significant participant in skin inflammation, involved in the recruitment of immune cells to the cutaneous microenvironment,[125,126] inhibiting keratinocyte apoptosis, and promoting keratinocyte proliferation in psoriasis.[124,127] Following the successful targeting TNF-α in arthritis,[128] this approach was taken in psoriasis where treatments targeting TNF-α (such as etanercept, adalimumab, and infliximab) were shown to be effective. Although all 3 drugs inhibit TNF-α, they are structurally different and have unique pharmacodynamic and pharmacokinetic profiles. Furthermore, not all psoriasis patients show a significant response to the anti-TNF biologics,[129] suggesting that there may be differences in inflammatory signaling in skin lesions possibly as a consequence of heterogeneity in genetic background.[130] Some loss of efficacy of the anti-TNF biologics has been reported over time,[131] even with fully humanized antibodies, suggesting the production of antiidiotype antibodies.[132,133] Other TNF inhibitors, without dermatologic indications, also have been approved by the FDA, including golimumab (for the treatment of rheumatoid arthritis, psoriatic arthritis, and ankylosing spondylitis) and certolizumab pegol (for the treatment of Crohn disease and rheumatoid arthritis).

ETANERCEPT

Etanercept is a fusion protein consisting of the Fc region of IgG_1 fused to the soluble TNF receptor 2 (p75 TNFR) extracellular domain. Etanercept is FDA approved for rheumatoid arthritis, polyarticular juvenile idiopathic arthritis, psoriatic arthritis, ankylosing spondylitis, and plaque psoriasis. Psoriasis dosing is 50 mg twice weekly for 3 months, followed by 50 mg once weekly.

ADALIMUMAB

Adalimumab is a recombinant humanized monoclonal antibody engineered with a human variable domain (compared with infliximab's mouse variable domain [see "Infliximab" below]). Adalimumab is FDA approved for plaque psoriasis, Crohn disease, ulcerative colitis, and uveitis. For psoriasis, the initial dose is 80 mg, followed by 40 mg every 2 weeks starting 1 week after the initial dose. There is mounting evidence of the efficacy of adalimumab for hidradenitis suppurativa,[134] and the drug is now FDA approved for this indication.

INFLIXIMAB

Infliximab is a chimeric monoclonal antibody containing a mouse variable domain. Infliximab is FDA approved for plaque psoriasis, psoriatic arthritis, Crohn disease, ulcerative colitis, ankylosing spondylitis, and rheumatoid arthritis. Psoriasis dosing is 5 mg/kg given as an IV infusion, followed by additional doses at 2 and 6 weeks after the first infusion, then every 8 weeks thereafter. Of the 3 TNF biologics in use for plaque psoriasis, infliximab has most commonly been used for pustular forms of psoriasis[135,136] and as such has become one of the recommended treatment options for severe acute GPP despite the lack of adequate clinical trials.[137] Infliximab has been reported to have a rapid effect, with systemic inflammation and skin pustules starting to recede in as little as 2 days from the first infusion. The risk of development of antidrug antibodies is higher with infliximab than with other anti-TNF agents because of the presence of the mouse variable domain.

PARADOXICAL PSORIASIS

Although TNF antagonists are effective for the treatment of various rheumatic and nonrheumatic diseases, including psoriasis, there are many case reports describing several paradoxical cutaneous adverse effects during their use. New-onset or exacerbation of cutaneous psoriasis, a lupus-like syndrome,[138] cutaneous vasculitis, and sarcoidosis have been described,[139] with increased IFN-α production[140] and disruption in the cytokine balance in the skin implicated in its pathogenesis.[141]

INFECTIONS

TNF inhibitors are associated with serious infections, including pneumonia, sepsis, tuberculosis, histoplasmosis, coccidioidomycosis, and other invasive fungal infections. Labeling also indicates that for patients who have resided in regions where histoplasmosis and coccidioidomycosis are endemic, the risks and benefits of TNF inhibitor therapy should be carefully considered. A metaanalysis of rheumatoid arthritis patients treated with infliximab or adalimumab in randomized controlled trials suggested that use of these agents result in 1 excess serious infection for every 59 patients treated for a period of 3 to 12 months.[142] Use of etanercept with anakinra is associated with an increased risk of serious infections; consequently, it is recommended that anakinra not be used concurrently with any TNF inhibitor. One prospective study reported an increased incidence of herpes zoster among rheumatoid arthritis patients treated with anti-TNF monoclonal antibodies (adalimumab, infliximab) compared to conventional disease-modifying antirheumatic drugs.[143] A metaanalysis addressing the risk of serious infections (infection requiring antibiotic treatment and/or hospitalization) among rheumatoid arthritis patients treated with adalimumab and infliximab reported a significantly increased risk for such infections compared to placebo.[142] Another metaanalysis addressing the risk of serious infections among rheumatoid arthritis patients treated with adalimumab, etanercept, or infliximab, with and without adjustment for exposure, reported no increased risk of serious infection at manufacturer-recommended doses; however, there was a twofold increased risk of serious infection among patients treated with higher doses (2 to 3 times the recommended dose).[144]

MALIGNANCY

A metaanalysis of data from 9 randomized controlled trials of 3493 rheumatoid arthritis patients treated with adalimumab or infliximab demonstrated an increased risk of solid-organ malignancies.[142] This increased risk proved to be dose dependent. Nonmelanoma skin cancers accounted for the majority of reported malignancies followed by lymphoma in this study. Infliximab was associated with aggressive hepatosplenic T-cell lymphomas in postmarketing surveillance of patients with Crohn disease treated with concomitant azathioprine or 6-mercaptopurine. Additionally, aggressive cutaneous T-cell lymphomas have been reported in patients receiving TNF inhibitors.[145] A metaanalysis of data from 18 randomized control trials, involving 8808 rheumatoid arthritis patients, reported no increased risk for lymphoma, nonmelanoma skin cancer, and melanoma among patients treated with adalimumab, etanercept, and infliximab.[144] The largest observational study as of this writing suggests a slightly higher risk of lymphoma associated with adalimumab and infliximab compared to etanercept.[146] It remains unclear whether the excess risk of lymphoma reported in observational studies is a result of the TNF inhibitor or the severity of the underlying disease (eg, rheumatoid arthritis), which itself may portend a greater risk of lymphoma. Psoriasis patients may also have an increased risk of lymphoma, independent of biologic therapy, making additional studies necessary to determine if long-term exposure to biologics impacts lymphoma risk in psoriasis patients.[147]

RECOMBINANT CYTOKINES AND GROWTH FACTORS

Cytokines, including the interleukins, are low-molecular-weight polypeptides that exhibit paracrine and/or autocrine activity in the mediation of immune responses. They may act as growth factors by inducing the proliferation of specific immune cell populations. A particular cytokine may also influence the production of other cytokines and the behavior of cellular populations that express its receptor. Since the molecular cloning of the first cytokines in the early 1980's, recombinant cytokines have proven to be invaluable for the treatment of conditions in which immunologic aberrations exist or among which some clinical benefit might be derived from augmentation or suppression of the host immune response.

RECOMBINANT INTERLEUKINS AND INTERFERONS

INTERLEUKIN-2

IL-2 is a Th1 cytokine with antitumor activity produced by CD4+ lymphocytes in response to activation by antigen-presenting cells.[148] IL-2 promotes the proliferation and maintenance of helper T-cell populations, but is also key to the proliferation and activation of regulatory T cells. In addition, it enhances both NK cell cytotoxicity and lymphokine-activated cell activity.[149] In the dermatologic setting, recombinant human IL-2 has been used for the treatment of melanoma. Although described as the first true immunotherapy,[148] its use as a single agent has been largely supplanted by checkpoint inhibitors such as anti-CTLA4 and anti-PD1/PD-L1, as well as by drugs such as vemurafenib (which is FDA-approved for melanoma) and dabrafenib, which target small molecules. IL-2 may have a role in stimulating autoreactive antitumor T cells in vitro to proliferate prior to reintroducing these cells back into patients, after which IL-2 is administered to maintain proliferation of the adoptively transferred antitumor T cells in vivo.

Several studies, particularly those that combine IL-2 with adoptive cell transfer, have reported durable clinical responses among melanoma patients, and it has FDA approval for the treatment of patients with metastatic disease.[150]

At high doses, serious adverse effects associated with infused IL-2 include fever, chills, hypotension, thrombocytopenia, vascular leak syndrome, pulmonary edema, cardiac arrhythmias, renal compromise, and exfoliative erythroderma.[151,152]

INTERFERONS

Interferons are small proteins produced by many cells in response to viral and other injury. Key components of the innate immune response, they have cytostatic and immunoregulatory properties in addition to interfering with viral replication. Three major types of IFN—α, β, and γ—are commercially approved by the FDA for treatment of a number of indications, primarily in the treatment of cancers and lymphomas. IFN-α and IFN-β bind the same receptor and are termed Type I IFN, whereas IFN-γ binds to a different receptor and is classified as a Type II IFN.[153]

IFN-α and IFN-β, Type I interferons, are produced by a variety of leukocytes as well plasmacytoid dendritic cells. Imiquimod, a potent Toll-like receptor 7 agonist that is used for the treatment of viral warts and skin cancer, stimulates the production of IFN-α by plasmacytoid dendritic cells in the skin. IFN-α is useful in the treatment of hepatitis C but has good activity in the treatment of cutaneous T-cell lymphomas (CTCLs), including mycosis fungoides and Sézary syndrome.[153] Until 2009 both recombinant IFN-α2a (Roferon) and IFN-α2b (Intron-A) were available in the United States, but as of this writing only the Intron-A is available in the United States. Similar in structure, they have similar biologic properties. Pegylated, longer-lasting formations (once a week) of IFN-α are also available.[154]

The interferons help to reverse some of the immune dysfunction that are found in CTCL, which have been reported to be increased Th2 cytokine activity (increased IL-4 and IL-13) and function (increased eosinophilia) that is triggered by the malignant, pathogenic CD4+ helper T cells. The interferons stimulate a Th1-mediated immune environment by activation of CD8+ T cells and shifting the Th2 environment toward a Th1 environment that has increased levels of IFN-γ and IL-12. IL-5, a potent stimulator of eosinophil proliferation, levels decrease in the blood of patients who are treated with Type I interferons.[155] Indeed type I interferons have been recognized as key cytokines that portend effective antitumor responses.

There has been abundant experience using interferons in CTCL.[153] Recombinant IFN is generally administered via subcutaneous or IM injection from 1 to 3 times a week at doses ranging from 1 to 3 million units. It appears to be particularly effective in Sézary syndrome where it can be highly effective in reducing pruritus, and clinical responses up to 75% have been observed in CTCL patients at various stages of disease. Combining IFN with other agents, such as bexarotene and psoralen and ultraviolet A therapy, may increase the overall efficacy of the Type I interferons. Side effects, particularly at the high dosing ranges, are common and include "flu-like" symptoms (arthralgia and myalgia), which can be managed by acetaminophen, and fatigue. Other common side effects include weight loss, sexual dysfunction, and depression. Laboratory monitoring, particularly at the initiation of therapy and with increased dosing, that includes hepatic function tests (aspartate aminotransferase/alanine aminotransferase) and complete blood cell count is commonly performed in light of abnormalities that include leukopenia. Care should be exercised in using interferons in patients with preexisting autoimmune disease because these agents may worsen or precipitate a number of autoimmune events, including thyroid disease and connective tissue disorders. IFN-α has been reported to worsen CD8+ CTCL, an uncommon variant of CTCL, perhaps because of its ability to enhance Th1 immunity.

IFN-α has also had wide application as adjuvant therapy for high-risk melanoma in which patients may not have detectable systemic disease, but have known high-risk biomarkers such as tumor depth and regional lymph node metastases. Despite initial enthusiasm for the use of this agent, large clinical trials have not conclusively demonstrated a clinical benefit for IFN and its use in the adjuvant setting is decreasing.[156] Besides CTCL and melanoma, the ability of the Type I interferons to stimulate antiviral and antitumor immunity have resulted in a large number of non–FDA-approved uses, including viral warts, Behçet disease, Kaposi sarcoma, and nonmelanoma skin cancer.[157]

The use of IFN-γ for CTCL and other dermatologic conditions has been reported but not at the level of the Type I interferons. Approved by the FDA for chronic granulomatous disease and osteoporosis, IFN-γ1b (Actimmune) is the only form available. Mechanistically, IFN-γ is a hallmark Th1 cytokine and potently stimulates Th1 immunity against cancer cells and virally infected cells. It can enhance the ability of macrophages and dendritic cells to produce costimulatory molecules and present viral and other antigens on their cell surface. In the context of CTCL, it tips the balance of the immune environment toward a Th1 environment and possibly enhances adaptive immune responses against CTCL cells.

IFN-γ1b is administered similarly to IFN-α1a and IFN-α1b, via subcutaneous injection. Dosing is based on body surface area, and this agent is usually given 1 to 3 times a week. A limited number of studies involving small numbers of patients between 1990 and 2013 (delivered IV)[158] suggest that high-dose IFN-γ1b can have objective responses in 30% to 66% of patients, depending on the stage of the patient. In general, early-stage (IA to IIA) patients had an impressive partial response rate of approximately 90% in the 2013 study.[158] In general, the adverse effects of IFN-γ1b are similar to those of recombinant Type I interferons, although it may have less of a tendency to impair the mood or cognitive faculties of older patients.[159]

GROWTH FACTORS

THE EPIDERMAL GROWTH FACTOR RECEPTOR FAMILY

The epidermal growth factor receptor (EGFR; ErbB1; HER1 in humans), a member of the ErbB family of receptors, is a transmembrane protein that is a receptor for members of the epidermal growth factor (EGF) family of extracellular protein ligands.[160] Mutations affecting EGFR expression or activity can result in cancer.[161]

EGFR ligands are initially synthesized as membrane-bound precursors consisting of an EGF motif flanked by an N-terminal extension and a C-terminal membrane-anchoring region. The EGF-like domain, characterized by a consensus sequence composed of 6 conserved cysteines forming 3 intramolecular disulfide bonds, can be cleaved (shed) to release the mature, circulating form. Seven EGFR ligands (amphiregulin, betacellulin, heparin-binding EGF-like growth factor, transforming growth factor [TGF]-α, epiregulin, epigen, and EGF) bind to EGFR.

Ligand binding to EGFR induces the formation of receptor homodimers (EGFR/EGFR) and heterodimers with other ErbB family members (EGFR/ErbB2, EGFR/ErbB3, and EGFR/ErbB4), and the activation of the intrinsic kinase domain, resulting in phosphorylation of specific tyrosine residues within the cytoplasmic tail. Phosphorylated tyrosine residues act as binding sites for a variety of intracellular signal inducers, and stimulate multiple pathways of signal transduction including the Ras/Raf/mitogen activated protein/extracellular signal-related kinase kinase (MEK)/extracellular signal-regulated kinase, the phospholipase Cγ/protein kinase C, the phosphoinositide-3 kinase (PI3K)/AKT, STAT, and NF-κB cascades (Fig. 193-4).[162] Thus, the EGF receptor/ligand system comprises expression of EGFR-ligand precursors, their processing by metalloproteases, ligand binding to EGFR, and subsequent activation of EGFR signaling.

RELEVANCE OF EPIDERMAL GROWTH FACTOR RECEPTOR SIGNALING TO HUMAN SKIN HOMEOSTASIS AND DISEASES

EGFR signaling is essential for epidermal and hair follicle homeostasis, and dysregulation of the EGFR/ligand system and aberrant activation of EGFR signaling is involved in nonmelanoma skin cancer and chronic inflammatory disorders, such as psoriasis, atopic dermatitis, and allergic contact dermatitis.[163-165] Excessive activation of EGFR signaling by overexpression of, or mutations in, EGFR is also found in various types of human tumors, making EGFR a target for cancer therapy (see Fig. 193-4). Although humanized neutralizing antibodies and synthetic small compounds against EGFR are in clinical use today, these drugs are known to cause a variety of skin toxicities, including acneiform skin rash, skin dryness (xerosis), itching (pruritus), paronychia, nail changes, hair abnormalities, mucositis, and increased growth of the eyelashes (trichomegaly) or facial hair.[166] These side effects derive from the impairment of the multiple EGFR-dependent homeostatic functions of the skin. EGFR signaling is involved in reepithelialization of epidermal wound healing[163] and proliferation of keratinocyte stem cells in vivo.[167]

Reduced expression of EGFR or its ligand TGF-α results in impaired epidermal and hair follicle differentiation, delayed hair development, and multiple hair shaft abnormalities.[165] Reduced expression of TGF-α leads to impaired wound healing, wavy hair, curly whiskers, defective outer root sheath (ORS), altered hair follicle structure, and impaired early wound epithelialization.[165] Although mutations that lead to EGFR overexpression (known as upregulation) or overactivity are associated with many cancers, including squamous cell carcinoma of the lung (80% of cases) and anal cancers,[168] aberrant EGFR signaling is implicated in psoriasis, eczema, and atherosclerosis.[169]

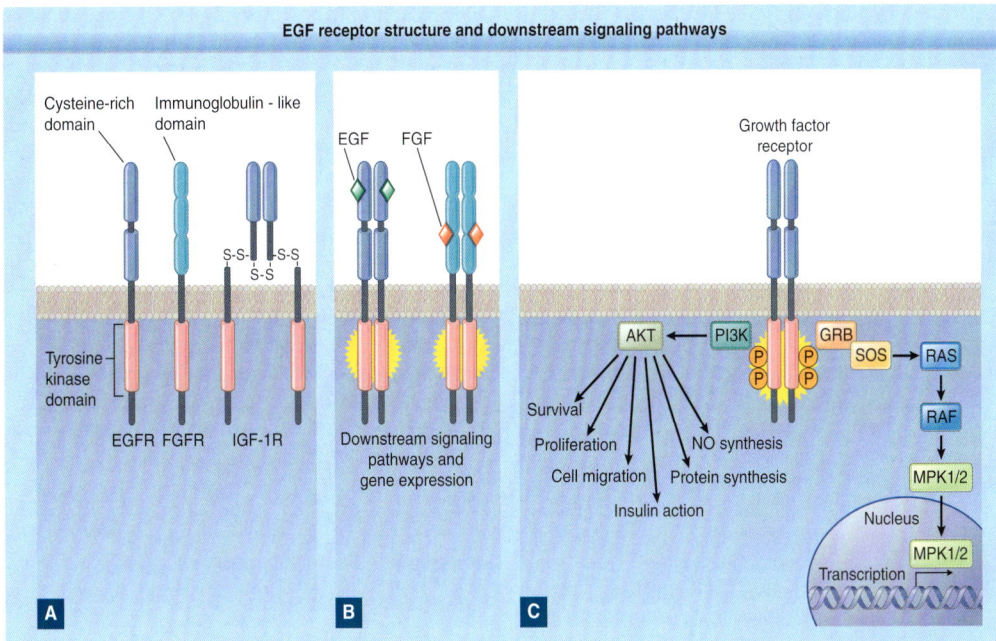

Figure 193-4 Growth factor receptor tyrosine kinases and signaling cascades. **A** and **B,** Epidermal growth factor receptor (EGFR) and fibroblast growth factor receptor (FGFR) are monomeric and upon binding to growth factors they dimerize and the kinase domains phosphorylate to each other (transphosphorylation). Insulin-like growth factor (IGF)-1R and insulin receptor are ααββ tetrameric and it has not been fully established how growth factor binding to the ectodomain induces kinase activation. **C,** Ligand binding to receptor tyrosine kinases (RTK), including EGFR and FGFR, induces kinase activation and subsequently induces signaling pathways inside the cells through signaling cascades (eg, PI3K/AKT and MAPK pathways), leading to cell proliferation, survival, transcription and many other biologic processes. GRB, growth factor receptor bound protein; PI3K, phosphoinositide 3 kinase; MAPK, mitogen-activated protein kinase; NO, nitrous oxide; SOS, son of sevenless.

CLINICAL USE OF EPIDERMAL GROWTH FACTOR LIGANDS AND ANTAGONISTS

Recombinant human EGF (Heberprot-P) is used to treat diabetic foot ulcers, with preliminary data showing improved wound healing.[170] It can be given by injection into the wound site,[171] or may be used topically.

The ErbB receptors are aberrantly activated in a wide range of human tumors, and as such they are excellent candidates for selective anticancer therapies. Several antibodies directed against the extracellular domain of ErbBs and tyrosine kinase inhibitors that target the kinase domain are in clinical use or at advanced developmental stages. The treatment of tumor cells with these agents affects many of the intracellular pathways that are essential for cancer development and progression. In preclinical models, treatment of tumor cells with ErbB-targeted tyrosine kinase inhibitors and antibodies rapidly downregulates PI3K/AKT, mitogen-activated protein kinase, Src, and STAT signaling, and blocks the proliferation of tumor cell lines and xenografts in nude mice.[172]

Cetuximab and panitumumab are examples of monoclonal antibody inhibitors. Other monoclonals in clinical development are zalutumumab, nimotuzumab, and matuzumab. The monoclonal antibodies block the extracellular ligand-binding domain. With the binding site blocked, signal molecules can no longer attach there and activate the tyrosine kinase.

Another method is using small molecules to inhibit the EGFR tyrosine kinase, which is on the cytoplasmic side of the receptor. Without kinase activity, EGFR is unable to activate itself, which is a prerequisite for binding of downstream adaptor proteins. Ostensibly by halting the signaling cascade in cells that rely on this pathway for growth, tumor proliferation and migration is diminished. Gefitinib, erlotinib, brigatinib, and lapatinib (mixed EGFR and ErbB2 inhibitor) are examples of small-molecule kinase inhibitors. Many patients, however, develop resistance via mutations in the *EGFR* gene.

The most common adverse effect of EGFR inhibitors, found in more than 90% of patients, is a papulopustular rash that spreads across the face and torso. The rash's presence is correlated with the drug's antitumor effect.[173] In 10% to 15% of patients the effects can be serious and require treatment.

FIBROBLAST GROWTH FACTORS

Fibroblast growth factors (FGFs) are a family of growth factors with members involved in angiogenesis, wound healing, embryonic development, and various endocrine-signaling pathways. The FGFs are heparin-binding proteins and interactions with cell-surface-associated heparan sulfate proteoglycans are essential for FGF signal transduction. FGFs are key players in developmental processes that include mesoderm induction, anteroposterior patterning, limb development, neural induction, and neural development, and in mature tissues/systems, angiogenesis, keratinocyte organization, and wound healing processes.

The mammalian FGF receptor family has 4 members: FGFR1, FGFR2, FGFR3, and FGFR4. The FGFRs consist of 3 extracellular immunoglobulin-type domains (D1 to D3), a single-span transmembrane domain, and an intracellular tyrosine kinase domain. FGFs interact with the D2 and D3 domains, with the D3 interactions primarily responsible for ligand-binding specificity.[174,175] Alternate messenger RNA splicing gives rise to "b" and "c" variants of FGFRs 1, 2, and 3. Through this mechanism 7 different signaling FGFR subtypes can be expressed at the cell surface. Each FGFR binds to a specific subset of the FGFs. Similarly, most FGFs can bind to several different FGFR subtypes. FGF1 is sometimes referred to as the "universal ligand" as it activates all 7 different FGFRs. In contrast, FGF7 (keratinocyte growth factor) binds only to FGFR2b (keratinocyte growth factor receptor), and FGF5 binds to FGFR1. The signaling complex at the cell surface is believed to be a ternary complex formed between 2 identical FGF ligands, 2 identical FGFR subunits, and either 1 or 2 heparan sulfate chains.

FGF1 through FGF10 (called *paracrine FGF*) all bind FGFRs. FGF1 is also known as acidic, and FGF2 is also known as *basic fibroblast growth factor*. FGF1 and FGF2 promote endothelial cell proliferation and the physical organization of endothelial cells into tube-like structures. They thus promote angiogenesis, the growth of new blood vessels from the preexisting vasculature. FGF1 and FGF2 are more potent angiogenic factors than vascular endothelial growth factor or platelet-derived growth factor. FGF1 has been shown in clinical experimental studies to induce angiogenesis in the heart. Exogenous FGF2 stimulates migration and proliferation of endothelial cells in vivo, has antiapoptotic activity, and encourages mitogenesis of smooth muscle cells and fibroblasts, which induces the development of large collateral vessels with adventitia. Gene therapy using FGF1 in nonviral expression vector has been studied in diabetic limb ischemia patients in clinical trials.[176]

As well as stimulating blood vessel growth, FGFs are important players in wound healing. FGF1 and FGF2 stimulate angiogenesis and the proliferation of fibroblasts that give rise to granulation tissue, which fills up a wound space/cavity early in the wound-healing process. FGF7 (keratinocyte growth factor) and FGF10 (keratinocyte growth factor-2) stimulate the repair of injured skin and mucosal tissues by stimulating the proliferation, migration, and differentiation of epithelial cells, and they have direct chemotactic effects on tissue remodeling. Dysregulation of the FGF signaling system underlies a range of diseases, where inhibitors of FGF signaling have shown clinical efficacy. Some FGF ligands (particularly FGF2) enhance tissue repair (eg, skin burns and ulcers) in a range of clinical settings.[177]

FGF4 plays a particularly unique role in the hair cycle. This gene was initially identified as an oncogene, which confers transforming potential when transfected into mammalian cells. Targeted disruption of the homolog of this gene in mouse resulted in the phenotype of abnormally long hair, which suggested a function as an inhibitor of hair elongation. The disruption of FGF5 expression in mammals increases the length of the anagen (growth) phase of the hair cycle, resulting in a phenotype of extremely long hair in many species, including humans. Blocking FGF5 in the human scalp (by applying herbal extract that blocked FGF5) extends the hair cycle, resulting in less hair fallout and increased hair length.[178]

INSULIN-LIKE GROWTH FACTOR/INSULIN

The insulin-like growth factor (IGF)/insulin family consists of insulin, IGF-1, and IGF-2. IGF-1 is specific to IGFR Type I (IGF-1R); insulin is specific to insulin receptor (IR); and IGF-2 bind to IGF-1R; and IR. Insulin is composed of B-chain and A-chain, which are disulfide-linked. IGF-1 and IGF-2 have B-chain, A-chain, and C-chain, which connects B-chains and A-chains. B-chains and A-chains are involved in receptor binding. Insulin is synthesized as a single chain with the C-peptide (B-C-A) (proinsulin). The C-peptide is cleaved upon maturation. Insulin is released when any of several stimuli are detected. These stimuli include ingested protein and glucose in the blood produced from digested food.

IGF-1 is produced primarily by the liver as an endocrine hormone, as well as in target tissues in a paracrine/autocrine fashion. Production is stimulated by growth hormone. IGF-1 is always bound to 1 of 6 binding proteins (IGF-BP). IGF-BP3, the most abundant protein, accounts for 80% of all IGF binding. IGF-1 binds to IGF-BP3 in a 1:1 molar ratio.

IGF-2 is imprinted, with expression resulting favorably from the paternally inherited allele. The major role of IGF-2 is as a growth-promoting hormone during fetal development. IGF-2 exerts its effects by binding to the IGF-1 receptor and to the short isoform of the IR (IR-A).

Insulin is produced by the beta cells of the pancreatic islet. It regulates the metabolism of carbohydrates, fats and protein by promoting the absorption of, especially, glucose from the blood into fat, liver, and skeletal muscle cells.

IR, under normal insulin stimulation, activates 2 major intracellular signaling cascades. The PI3K/AKT pathway has a predominant metabolic effect and is activated by the IR phosphorylation of IR substrate 1/2. The Ras/Raf/MEK/extracellular signal-regulated kinase pathway has predominant mitogenic effects and is activated by the IR phosphorylation of Shc. When the metabolic signaling pathway is partially impaired (insulin resistance), a compensatory increase of insulin occurs to maintain the metabolic homeostasis. Under this condition, the mitogenic pathway, which is not affected by specific impairment, is over stimulated.

Diabetes mellitus is one of the most common and best-known metabolic disorders affecting the wound healing process. Hyperglycemia reduces collagen deposits and delays wound remodeling. Wounds of diabetic patients respond poorly to conventional treatment. This delay in wound healing has been associated with increased morbidity and mortality rates in this patient population. The use of local injection of long-acting insulin-zinc suspension accelerates wound healing without any major side effects. Intralesional insulin administration restores collagen synthesis and formation of granulation tissue to normal values when administered during the early stages of the healing process.[179]

OTHER IMMUNOBIOLOGIC AGENTS

ALEFACEPT

Alefacept is a bioengineered protein consisting of the human IgG$_1$ antibody Fc region fused to the first extracellular domain of human lymphocyte function-associated antigen-3 (CD58). Lymphocyte function-associated antigen-3 is a member of the immunoglobulin superfamily and is expressed on the surface of antigen presenting cells. It normally binds to CD2, which is preferentially expressed on the surface of effector/memory T cells, an interaction that plays an important role in the activation of T cells in response to antigen. Although alefacept was the first biologic agent FDA-approved for the treatment of psoriasis in 2003, monoclonal antibodies that target TNF-α or components of the IL-17 signaling pathway (see section "Cytokines of the Th17 axis (IL-17A, IL-22, and IL-23)" above) have better efficacy (50% to 90% PASI75 vs. 21% PASI75 for alefacept) and thus dominate the therapeutic agents that are used for psoriasis.

DENILEUKIN DIFTITOX

Denileukin diftitox (DAB389–IL-2) is a ligand-toxin fusion protein consisting of a fragment of diphtheria toxin fused to IL-2. DAB389–IL-2 is believed to associate with malignant cells expressing the high-affinity IL-2 receptor. Upon binding to the receptor, it is internalized within endosomes, where its adenosine diphosphate–ribosyltransferase region is cleaved and translocated into the cytoplasm. In the cytoplasm, it interrupts protein synthesis, eventually leading to apoptosis of the affected cell.

CD25 is the α chain of the IL-2 receptor, which, when bound to the β and common γ chain, forms the high-affinity IL-2 receptor. CD25 serves both as a marker of activated T cells, as well as for regulatory CD4+ T cells that express the transcription factor, FoxP3 (ie, CD4+CD25+FoxP3+ T-regs). Naturally occurring T-regs exhibit immunosuppressive properties and have been shown to play an important role in the induction of immune tolerance. Thus, elimination of T-reg cells may increase antitumor immunity, similar to the concept employed by checkpoint inhibitors such as anti–PD-1. Because of its ability to deplete CD25+ T cells, DAB389–IL-2 may contribute to antitumor immunity by eliminating T-reg cells in addition to malignant cells that express the CD25 component of the IL-2 receptor.

While clinical data do not indicate that DAB389-IL-2 is helpful in the treatment of metastatic melanoma, use of this agent resulted in a 10% complete response rate in heavily pretreated CTCL patients. Patient numbers, however, were small, but the relatively long mean duration of response (9 months) in complete responders suggests that this agent may be useful in some patients with CTCL.[180] These data led to the approval by the FDA for DAB389–IL-2 in patients with detectable CD25 expression. Isolated reports have also suggested that this agent may be useful in some patients with psoriasis although it is not approved for this indication.

DAB389–IL-2 is administered IV over at least 15 minutes. Doses at 9 μg/kg/day and 18 μg/kg/day have been used for the treatment of CTCL. Infusion reactions represent the most common adverse effect associated with DAB389–IL-2 treatment, but reversible transaminitis and vascular leak syndrome and morbilliform skin rash also represent known adverse effects.

MOGAMULIZUMAB (ANTI-CCR4)

Chemokines are small (approximately 10 kDa) chemoattractant cytokines that are released by keratinocytes, endothelial cells, leukocytes, dendritic cells, and many other cell types. As their name implies, the binding of a chemokine (3 principal structural classes with approximately 50 known chemokines) to its appropriate cell surface receptor (approximately 20 known receptors) triggers a G-protein–coupled signaling pathway that affects cellular migration as well as multiple other complex intracellular signals via PI3K and AKT.

CCR4 is a chemokine receptor (binds to CCL22 and CCL17) that is highly expressed by skin-homing T cells (Th2 > Th1 cells) at the cell surface.[181] CCR4+ skin-homing T cells are abundant in many inflammatory skin conditions, including CTCLs such as mycosis fungoides and Sézary syndrome. With that in mind, mogamulizumab is a humanized, defucosylated monoclonal antibody that binds to CCR4 and induces antibody-dependent cellular cytotoxicity of the target cell. In the case of CTCL, that target cell is frequently a clonal CCR4+, CD4+ T-cell population with Th2 characteristics.

In Japan, mogamulizumab is already approved for the treatment of adult T-cell leukemia/lymphoma. A Phase I/II clinical trial of IV administered agent in previous treated mycosis fungoides and Sézary syndrome patients revealed an overall 37% response rate with better response rates among the Sézary syndrome patients.[182] Treatment side effects consisted of nausea (31%) and other nonspecific events that were mostly grade 1 or grade 2 in severity, suggesting that this agent has a good safety profile. Interestingly, several patients on this agent have exhibited a morbilliform skin eruption. This may be related to the high expression of CCR4 on regulatory skin T cells. Depletion of this population of cells may increase the possibility of inflammatory, and potentially antitumor, skin responses that are suppressed by skin T-regs, adding another mechanism of action for its therapeutic benefit in CTCL.[183]

RITUXIMAB

Rituximab is a humanized chimeric monoclonal antibody against CD20, a cell surface protein expressed by mature and pre-B cells. It induces the depletion of B cells in vivo. CD20 expression is lost during the differentiation of B cells to plasma cells. Aside from playing a crucial role in antibody production, B cells may also serve as antigen-presenting cells and provide costimulatory signals, which promote CD4+ T-cell expansion and effector cell function.[184]

Rituximab is FDA approved for the treatment of patients with moderate-to-severe rheumatoid arthritis and for the treatment of relapsed or chemorefractory (low-grade or follicular) CD20+ non-Hodgkin B-cell lymphomas, and transiently reduces the population of CD20+ cells in the circulation.[185] This effect is achieved by its ability to enhance antibody and complement-mediated cytotoxicity, and promote the apoptosis of malignant CD20+ cells.[186] Aside from its role in the treatment of lymphoma and rheumatoid arthritis, rituximab is increasingly used off-label for the management of other autoimmune diseases. More specifically, reports have suggested its efficacy for the treatment of paraneoplastic and refractory pemphigus, autoimmune hemolytic anemia, granulomatosis with polyangiitis (Wegener) hypocomplementemic urticarial vasculitis, systemic lupus erythematosus, cutaneous B-cell lymphoma, chronic graft-versus-host disease, and epidermolysis bullosa acquisita.

Caution, however, should be taken before initiating therapy with rituximab for off-label use. Two cases of progressive multifocal leukoencephalopathy were reported to the FDA in 2006 involving patients who received rituximab for the treatment of systemic lupus erythematosus.[85] Recent reports have also noted marked progression of Kaposi sarcoma among patients treated for autoimmune hemolytic anemia and Castleman disease.[187,188]

In a case series of patients receiving rituximab for autoimmune bullous disorders (pemphigus vulgaris, bullous pemphigoid, and mucous membrane pemphigus), severe adverse reactions were noted in 3 (43%) of 7 patients.[189] These reactions, which consisted of serious infections, enteropathy, and pulmonary embolism, were thought to be associated with concurrent high-dose adjuvant immunosuppression and underlying malignancy among the affected individuals. In a study involving 11 patients with refractory pemphigus vulgaris treated with rituximab and IV immunoglobulin, no infections or other clinically significant adverse effects were noted.[190] Additionally, no severe adverse effects were reported in case series and open-label studies among patients treated with intralesional and/or IV rituximab for cutaneous B-cell lymphoma and dermatomyositis.[191] A study addressing the safety of rituximab for the treatment of diffuse cutaneous systemic sclerosis (among 15 patients) reported mild infusion reactions (affecting 7 [46%] patients), urinary tract infection and a dental abscess affecting a single patient, and 1 case of prostate cancer at 6-month followup.[192]

INDICATIONS

Rituximab is FDA approved for the treatment of CD20+ non-Hodgkin B-cell lymphomas and moderate-to-severe rheumatoid arthritis.

INITIATING THERAPY AND MONITORING

No specific dosing regimen has been established for the off-label use of this medicine in the dermatologic setting. Rituximab is usually administered at a standard dose of 375 mg/m² body surface area at weekly intervals. Premedication with acetaminophen and antihistamines should be considered to decrease the risk for infusion reactions. Monitoring of blood cell counts and serum antibody levels may be pursued every 2 to 3 months while on therapy. A rapid depletion of CD20+ B cells occurs after treatment and may last from 2 to 6 months before recovery. Live vaccines should not be administered to patients prior to and during therapy.

Rituximab is a pregnancy category C medication with unknown safety during lactation.

RISKS, PRECAUTIONS, AND COMPLICATIONS

Reported adverse effects associated with rituximab therapy include fatal infusion reactions, vasculitis, hepatitis B reactivation, tumor lysis syndrome, renal toxicity, severe mucocutaneous reactions, cardiac arrhythmias/angina and bowel obstruction/perforation. Cases of progressive multifocal leukoencephalopathy have been reported among patients with lymphoid malignancies and systemic lupus erythematosus treated with rituximab.[92]

Besides efficacy in pemphigus vulgaris[190] and foliaceus,[193] rituximab is reported to be beneficial in immune thrombocytopenia[194] and antineutrophilic cytoplasmic antibody–associated vasculitis, a historically difficult-to-control disease with potentially very significant skin ulceration.[195] Regarding antineutrophilic cytoplasmic antibody–associated vasculitis, a 2014 study compared the efficacy of azathioprine with rituximab to maintain patients in remission following treatment with cyclophosphamide and glucocorticoids. Importantly, only 5% of the patients in the rituximab group (vs 29% of patients in the azathioprine group) relapsed during the followup period, suggesting that anti-CD20 therapy is more effective in keeping patients in remission. Side effects were similar in both arms.[195]

Other anti-CD20 therapies also in development as of this writing include ocrelizumab, ofatumumab, and obinutuzumab, with obinutuzumab having glycosylation properties that increase antibody-dependent cellular cytotoxicity.[196]

DUPILUMAB

While treatment of psoriasis with biologic agents has made great strides with the development of agents such as etanercept, adalimumab, and infliximab, the use of biologics to treat eczematous and atopic disorders has lagged far behind. This has changed with the development of dupilumab, a humanized monoclonal antibody that targets the IL-4Rα subunit that is shared between the IL-4 and the IL-13 receptors (Fig. 193-5). Because this target is critical for both IL-4 and IL-13 signaling, dupilumab is expected to block the binding and signaling of both these classic Th2 cytokines. Even though the efficacy of dupilumab suggests that IL-4 and IL-13 have critical roles in asthma and atopic disease, IL-4 itself may be a counterregulatory cytokine in other diseases, such as psoriasis, as local injection of IL-4 in human psoriatic plaques results in reduction of skin inflammation by silencing IL-23 in antigen-presenting cells.[197]

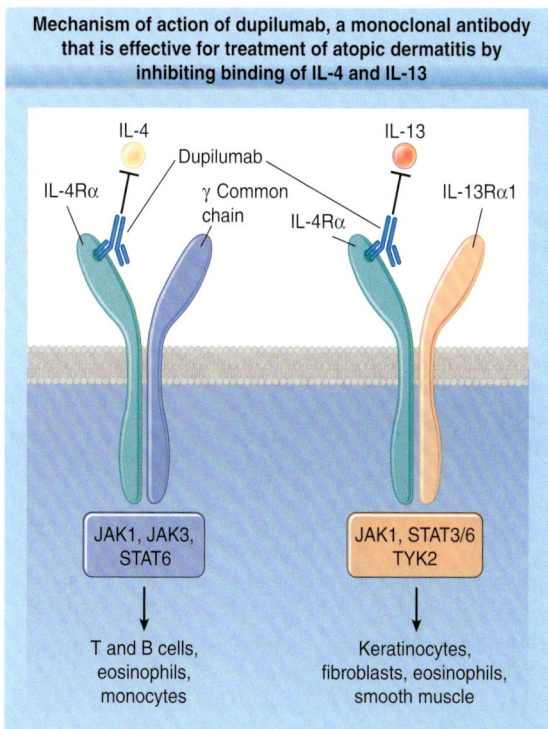

Figure 193-5 Dupilumab blocks a cell member receptor subunit that is essential for signaling via interleukin (IL)-4 as well as IL-13. The IL-4 and IL-13 receptors are 2 subunit receptors that share the common IL-4Rα subunit, which is the target for dupilumab. Downstream signaling through Janus kinase (JAK) and signal transducer and activator of transcription (STAT) proteins are attenuated in the presence of dupilumab. Note that the IL-4 and IL-13 receptors are distributed among different cell types that are likely to play roles in both skin and airway allergic inflammation and asthma. TYK, tyrosine kinase.

Dupilumab was initially approved for asthma, but in early 2017 the FDA approved it as the first biologic agent for the treatment of moderate-to-severe atopic dermatitis that is not adequately controlled by topical treatments. Although structural integrity via a defect in the keratinocyte protein, filaggrin, clearly does play a role in a sizeable proportion of patients with atopic dermatitis, a shift in the immune environment toward a Th2-skewed milieu has been observed in acute atopic dermatitis, although a Th1 alteration in chronic atopic dermatitis also has been reported.

Traditional treatments for atopic dermatitis include ultraviolet-B light, topical steroids, cyclosporine, and calcineurin inhibitors. In patients with severe disease, none of these agents can uniformly achieve desirable results. The largest clinical trial as of this writing enrolled 380 patients with at least moderate disease, assigning them to either dupilumab at one of several dosing schemes or placebo. Patients receiving the highest doses (300 mg) either once a week or every 2 weeks achieved a reduction in a standardized atopic dermatitis EASI score of at least 68% versus only 17% for patients on placebo. Interestingly, itching, a primary component of atopic dermatitis symptoms, was reduced very quickly in many patients on active drug and the greatest improvement in symptoms was seen in just 4 weeks of treatment. In terms of safety, patients in the dupilumab group had the same frequency of adverse events. Importantly the number of infectious adverse events, except for an increase in herpes virus infection in the dupilumab group, was similar and low in both groups. The safety profile of this agent thus is at least as good as, if not better than, systemic agents such as cyclosporine.

BRENTUXIMAB VEDOTIN

CD30 is a cell-surface activation marker that is frequently expressed by malignant B cells in Hodgkin disease as well as in T-cell neoplasms such as most anaplastic large-cell lymphoma (systemic as well as

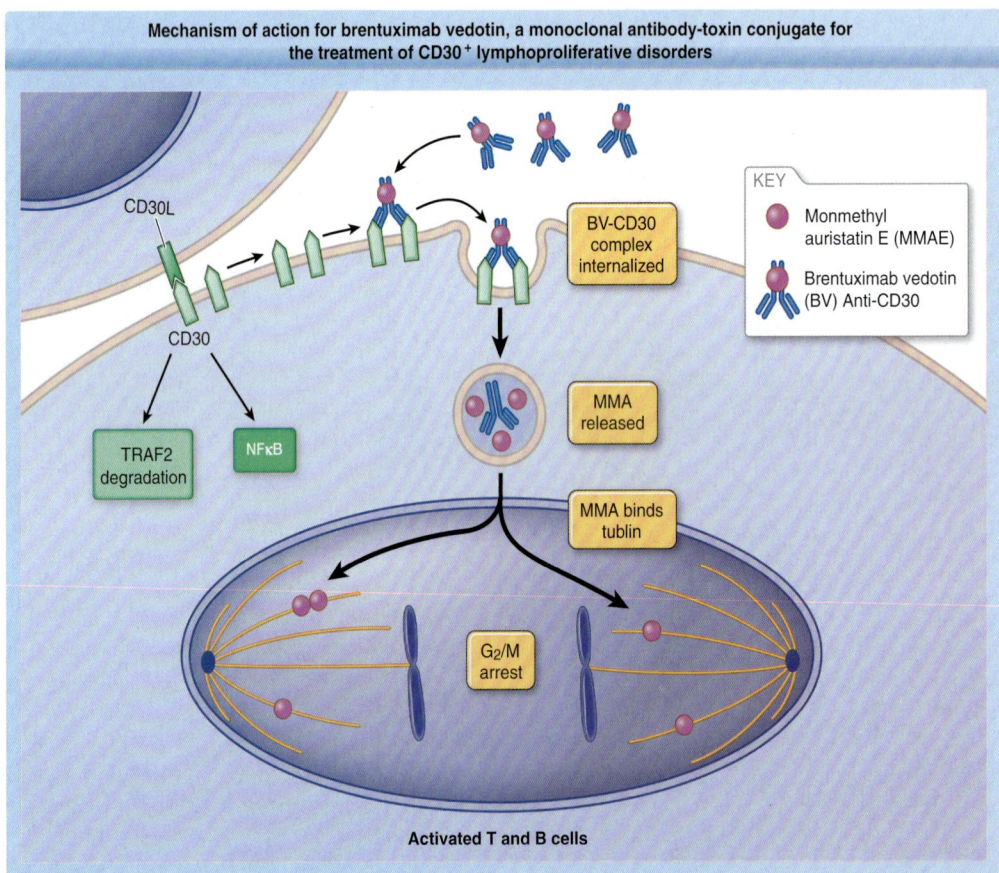

Figure 193-6 CD30 as a biologic target in cutaneous T-cell lymphoma (CTCL). Activated T and B cells express CD30. Brentuximab vedotin (BV) is conjugated to a potent microtubule disruptor, monomethyl auristatin E (MMAE). Following binding of BV to CD30, it is internalized, and eventually MMAE is released from CD30 in lysosomes. MMAE then binds tublin and causes G_2/M arrest and cell death. CD30L, CD30 ligand; NFκB, nuclear factor κB; TRAF, tumor necrosis factor receptor-associated factor.

primary skin-localized), a minority of mycosis fungoides neoplasms and indolent cutaneous lymphoid proliferation such as lymphomatoid papulosis. The CD30 engagement to its ligand, CD30L, is thought to normally lead to cellular inactivation via NF-κB pathways and tumor necrosis factor receptor-associated factor-2 degradation, perhaps explaining why lymphomatoid papulosis has a waxing-and-waning characteristic. It has been proposed that CD30, however, does not function in this manner in anaplastic large-cell lymphoma, but instead causes further cell activation and proliferation.[198]

Brentuximab vedotin is a novel biologic agent in which a monoclonal antibody to CD30 is conjugated to monomethyl auristatin E, a potent disruptor of cell microtubules (Fig. 193-6).[199] Binding of this agent to the cell surface results in internalization and eventual release of the toxin intracellular, resulting in cell division arrest and cell death.[199] Brentuximab vedotin was found to be very effective in CD30+ Hodgkin disease, and it was also very effective in a small number of CD30+ anaplastic large-cell lymphoma patients.[200] Based on that positive result, it was tested in a large clinical trial of mycosis fungoides and anaplastic large-cell lymphoma patients who compared it to a physician's choice of either bexarotene or methotrexate.[201] Interestingly, there was very little correlation with CD30 expression levels (ie, some patients had only 10% detectable CD30+ cells) and efficacy, suggesting that specific depletion of other CD30+ cells (possibly a CD30+ regulatory T cell[202]) besides the tumor cells may contribute to this agent's mechanism of action.[201] Treatment with 1.8 mg/kg once every 3 weeks with brentuximab vedotin yielded impressive results, with almost 5 times as many patients who were assessed with an objective global response lasting at least 4 months compared to the other arm of standard agents. Even though 1 on-study death was attributed to this agent in the brentuximab group (none in the other group), serious grade 3 to grade 4 adverse events were fewer in the brentuximab group, and overall side effects were similar. Peripheral neuropathy, an adverse event related to the monomethyl auristatin, was frequently observed, but reversible, in most of the patients who developed it.[201] Given the poor response of patients with advanced CTCL to many chemotherapies and biologic agents, the remarkable and somewhat durable response that was observed with brentuximab vedotin make it a promising agent for patients who have failed other therapies.

TOCILIZUMAB

IL-6 is a pleiotropic, 21 kDa (in humans), single-chain, nonglycosylated protein cytokine with diverse functions in inflammation, neurologic function, and endocrine activity.[203] Depending on the cell type and the timing of exposure to IL-6, it can act as both a proinflammatory and an antiinflammatory cytokine.

It is produced by T cells and macrophages (often in response to pathogen-associated molecular patterns) following infection, injury, and burns and helps to mobilize neutrophils from the bone marrow. Its functions in skin are many but help shape the inflammatory response to viral, parasitic, and particularly bacterial infections. For example, it has been reported that individuals who develop autoantibodies to IL-6 have repeated episodes of staphylococcal cellulitis and skin abscesses.[204]

The IL-6 receptor is comprised of a specific 80-kDa chain known as IL-6R that is required to bind IL-6 and a widely expressed universal signaling subunit known as gp130, or CD130, that is organized as a dimeric structure. Neutrophils also express the IL-6 receptor, which when engaged, stimulates production of key Th17 cytokines such as IL-17 and IL-23.

Tocilizumab, a humanized monoclonal antibody, targeted at IL-6R, has shown efficacy in rheumatoid arthritis, juvenile arthritis, and other conditions. IL-6 is undoubtedly involved in our cutaneous response to pathogens as well as in a number of inflammatory skin disease including lupus, and its pleotropic contributions to skin inflammation are complex, which can be illustrated from human psoriasis and murine models.[205] IL-6 and STAT3 polymorphisms have been found that link predisposition with the development of psoriasis as well as predict response to TNF antagonists.[205] Clinically, IL-6 serum levels correlate with skin disease activity in psoriasis,[206] and IL-6 knockout mice have reduced dermal inflammation and epidermal hyperplasia in response to IL-23.[207] IL-6 is a downstream cytokine produced by a number of cells, particularly keratinocytes, in the skin in response to Th17 cytokines such as IL-1, IL-17, and IL-36, as well as TNF-α. Together with IL-17, IL-6 likely contributes to neutrophil recruitment in psoriasis vulgaris, as well as in pustular psoriasis. Despite the evidence, however, that IL-6 is easily detectable in skin and blood of psoriasis patients, clinical trials with tocilizumab have not shown sufficient efficacy to warrant treatment of patients with psoriasis vulgaris, although it has been reported that a limited number of patients with the pustular psoriasis variant have responded to this agent.[208]

SUMMARY

Table 193-1 summarizes the immunobiologic agents discussed above.

ACKNOWLEDGMENTS

The authors wish to thank and acknowledge Drs. Stephen K. Richardson and Dr. Joel M. Gelfand for their excellent chapter on immunobiologics, cytokines, and growth factors in dermatology in the 8th edition of this text, which helped to shape this chapter for the 9th edition.

TABLE 193-1
A Summary of Immunobiologic Agents

DRUG	PROTEIN STRUCTURE	INDICATIONS	MECHANISM OF ACTION	DOSE[a]	COMMON SIDE EFFECTS & SPECIAL CONSIDERATIONS
Interleukin-1 Inhibitors					
Anakinra	Recombinant, nonglycosylated IL-1RA	- CAPS[b] - DIRA - Pustular psoriasis[c] - Hidradenitis suppurativa	Competitive inhibition of IL-1α and IL-1β activity at IL-1 receptor level	Off-label use	- Injection-site reaction - Upper respiratory tract infection - Headache - Diarrhea - Flu-like symptoms - Abdominal pain[1]
Rilonacept	Dimeric fusion protein	- CAPS - FCAS - MWS	Soluble IL-1 decoy receptor binding IL-1α and IL-1	Off label use	- Injection site reactions - Upper respiratory tract infections[2]
Canakinumab	Human monoclonal IgG$_1$ antibody	- CAPS - FCAS - MWS[3] - TRAPS - HIDS - MKD - FMF - Pustular psoriasis	Neutralizes IL-1β	Off-label use	- Nasopharyngitis - Diarrhea - Influenza - Headache - Nausea[3]
Interleukin-17					
Secukinumab	Human anti–IL-17A IgG$_1$κ monoclonal antibody	- Plaque psoriasis - Psoriatic arthritis - Ankylosing spondylitis[4] - Generalized pustular psoriasis - palmoplantar pustulosis	Anti–IL-17A IgG$_1$κ	Plaque Psoriasis: 300 mg SQ weekly for 4 weeks and then every 4 weeks thereafter[4]	- Increased risk for serious infections, tuberculosis - Inflammatory bowel disease - Nasopharyngitis - Diarrhea - Upper respiratory tract infection[4]
Ixekizumab	Humanized IgG$_4$ monoclonal antibody	- Plaque psoriasis - Erythrodermic psoriasis - Generalized pustular psoriasis	Neutralizes IL-17A	Plaque Psoriasis: two 80-mg (total dose: 160 mg) SQ injections every 2 to 4 weeks, then 80 mg every 4 weeks[5]	- Increased risk for serious infections, tuberculosis - Inflammatory bowel disease - Injection-site reactions - Nausea - Upper respiratory tract infection[5]
Brodalumab	Human anti–IL-17RA monoclonal antibody	- Moderate to severe plaque psoriasis	Targets IL-17 receptor A chain	Plaque psoriasis: 210 mg SQ at weeks 0, 1, and 2, followed by 210 mg every 2 weeks[6]	- Suicidal ideation - Increased risk for serious infections, tuberculosis - Crohn disease - Arthralgia - Headache - Injection-site reactions - Neutropenia[6]
Interleukin-12					
Ustekinumab	IgG$_1$κ human monoclonal antibody	- Psoriasis - Psoriatic arthritis - Crohn disease	Targets IL-12p40 subunit	Plaque psoriasis: 45 to 90 mg SQ and 4 weeks later, followed by 45 mg administered SQ every 12 weeks[7]	- Increased risk for serious infections, tuberculosis - Malignancies - Hypersensitivity reactions - Reversible posterior leukoencephalopathy syndrome[7]

(Continued)

TABLE 193-1
A Summary of Immunobiologic Agents (Continued)

DRUG	PROTEIN STRUCTURE	INDICATIONS	MECHANISM OF ACTION	DOSE[a]	COMMON SIDE EFFECTS & SPECIAL CONSIDERATIONS
Interleukin-23					
Guselkumab	Human IgG$_1$λ antibody	• Moderate to severe plaque psoriasis	Targets IL-23p19 subunit	Psoriasis: 100 mg SQ at weeks 0 and 4, then every 8 weeks	• Increased risk for infection, tuberculosis • Upper respiratory tract infections • Headache • Injection-site reactions[B]
Tildrakizumab	Humanized monoclonal IgG$_1$λ antibody	• *Moderate to severe chronic plaque psoriasis*	Targets IL-23p19 subunit	Psoriasis: 100 mg at weeks 0 and 4 and then every 12 weeks thereafter	
Risankizumab	Fully human IgG$_1$ monoclonal antibody	• *Moderate to severe plaque psoriasis* • *Generalized pustular psoriasis* • *Erythrodermic psoriasis*	Targets IL-23p19 subunit	Psoriasis: 90 and 180 mg[d]	
Tumor Necrosis Factor-α					
Etanercept	Fusion protein (Fc region of IgG$_1$ fused to soluble TNF receptor 2)	• Rheumatoid arthritis • Polyarticular juvenile idiopathic arthritis • Psoriatic arthritis • Ankylosing spondylitis • Plaque psoriasis	Binds to TNF-α and inhibits activity	Psoriasis: 50 mg twice weekly × 3 months, followed by 50 mg once weekly	• New-onset/exacerbation of cutaneous psoriasis • Lupus-like syndrome • Cutaneous vasculitis • Sarcoidosis • Infections (pneumonia, sepsis, tuberculosis, histoplasmosis, coccidioidomycosis, invasive fungal infection) • Solid-organ malignancies (dose-dependent risk)
Adalimumab	Recombinant humanized monoclonal antibody with a human variable domain	• Plaque psoriasis • Crohn disease • Ulcerative colitis • Uveitis • Hidradenitis suppurativa	Binds to TNF-α and inhibits activity	Psoriasis: 80 mg initial dose, then 40 mg every 2 weeks starting 1 week after initial dose	
Infliximab	Chimeric monoclonal antibody containing a mouse variable domain	• Plaque psoriasis • Psoriatic arthritis • Crohn disease • Ulcerative colitis • Ankylosing spondylitis • Rheumatoid arthritis • *Generalized pustular psoriasis*	Binds to TNF-α and inhibits activity	Psoriasis: 5 mg/kg IV, followed by additional doses at 2 and 6 weeks after the first infusion, then every 8 weeks thereafter	
Recombinant Interleukins and Interferons					
IL-2	Recombinant interleukin	• Metastatic melanoma	Antitumor activity; promotes proliferation and maintenance of helper and regulatory T cells; enhances NK cell cytotoxicity	Metastatic melanoma: 600,000 IU/kg every 8 hours for not more than 14 doses; course repeated after 9 days rest, for a maximum of 28 doses per course[g]	• Fever, chills, hypotension • Thrombocytopenia, vascular leak syndrome • Pulmonary edema • Cardiac arrhythmias • Renal compromise • Exfoliative erythroderma

(Continued)

TABLE 193-1
A Summary of Immunobiologic Agents (Continued)

DRUG	PROTEIN STRUCTURE	INDICATIONS	MECHANISM OF ACTION	DOSE[a]	COMMON SIDE EFFECTS & SPECIAL CONSIDERATIONS
- IFN-α - IFN-α2a - IFN-α2b - Pegylated IFN-α	Recombinant interferon	- Hepatitis C - CTCL: Mycosis fungoides; Sézary syndrome - Viral warts - Behçet disease - Kaposi sarcoma - Nonmelanoma skin cancer	Stimulate Th1-mediated immune environment, activate CD8+ T cells and shift the Th2 environment toward a Th1 environment	CTCL: 1 to 3 million units SQ or IM 1 to 3 times/week	- Flu-like symptoms (arthralgia, myalgia) - Fatigue - Weight loss - Sexual dysfunction - Depression - Leukopenia - Worsening of preexisting autoimmune disease (thyroid, connective tissue disorders)
- IFN-γ - IFN-γ1b	Recombinant interferon	- Chronic granulomatous disease[10] - CTCL	Stimulates Th1 immunity against cancer cells and virally infected cells	Off-label use	- Exacerbation of preexisting cardiac conditions - Bone marrow toxicity - Hepatic toxicity - Renal toxicity - Flu-like symptoms[10]
Epidermal Growth Factor Ligands and Antagonists					
Cetuximab	Monoclonal antibody inhibitors	- Head and neck cancers - Colorectal cancers[11] - Tumors (especially nonmelanoma skin cancers)	Blocks the extracellular ligand-binding domain and inhibits activation of tyrosine kinase; blocks tumor growth and proliferation via these pathways	Off-label use	- Acneiform papulopustular rash (facial, trunk) - Xerosis - Pruritus - Paronychia - Nail changes - Hair abnormalities - Mucositis - Trichomegaly (eyelashes) - Facial hair
Panitumumab	Monoclonal antibody inhibitors	- Metastatic colorectal carcinoma[12]	Blocks the extracellular ligand-binding domain and inhibits activation of tyrosine kinase	Off-label use	
Other Agents					
Alefacept	Human IgG₁ antibody Fc region fused to LFA-3, CD58	- Psoriasis	Disrupts activation of effector/memory T cells	Psoriasis: 15 mg once weekly as IM injection for 12 weeks[13]	- Lymphopenia - Increased risk of serious infections - Pharyngitis[13]
Denileukin Diftitox	Ligand toxin fusion protein	- CTCL with CD25 expression - Metastatic melanoma	Associates with malignant cells expressing IL-2	CTCL: 9 to 18 μg/kg/day IV over 15 minutes	- Infusion reactions - Reversible transaminitis - Vascular leak syndrome - Morbilliform skin rash
Mogamulizumab (anti-CCR4)	Humanized, defucosylated monoclonal antibody	- CTCL - Adult T-cell leukemia/lymphoma	Binds to CCR4, induced antibody-dependent cellular cytotoxicity of the target cell		- Nausea - Morbilliform skin eruption
Rituximab	Humanized chimeric monoclonal antibody against CD20	- Moderate to severe rheumatoid arthritis - CD20+ non-Hodgkin B-cell lymphomas - Paraneoplastic and refractory pemphigus - Autoimmune hemolytic anemia - Granulomatosis	Induces depletion of B cells in vivo	Off-label use	- Infusion reactions - Vasculitis - Hepatitis B reactivation - Tumor lysis syndrome - Renal toxicity

(Continued)

TABLE 193-1
A Summary of Immunobiologic Agents (Continued)

DRUG	PROTEIN STRUCTURE	INDICATIONS	MECHANISM OF ACTION	DOSE[a]	COMMON SIDE EFFECTS & SPECIAL CONSIDERATIONS
		▪ Wegener polyangiitis ▪ Hypocomplementemic urticarial vasculitis ▪ Systemic lupus erythematosus ▪ Cutaneous B-cell lymphoma ▪ Chronic GVHD ▪ EBA			▪ Severe mucocutaneous reactions ▪ Cardiac arrhythmias/angina ▪ Bowel obstruction/perforation ▪ PML
Dupilumab	Humanized monoclonal antibody	▪ Moderate to severe atopic dermatitis ▪ Asthma	Targets IL-4Rα subunit	Moderate to severe atopic dermatitis: 300 mg once a week or every 2 weeks	▪ Increased risk for herpes virus infection
Brentuximab vedotin	Monoclonal antibody to CD30 conjugated to monomethyl auristatin E	▪ CD30+ Hodgkin disease ▪ Mycosis fungoides ▪ Anaplastic large-cell lymphoma	Binding to cell surface results in internalization and eventual release of the toxin intracellularly, leading to cell division arrest and cell death	Mycosis fungoides: 1.8 mg/kg once every 3 weeks	▪ Peripheral neuropathy (reversible) ▪ Neutropenia ▪ Infusion reactions ▪ PML[14]
Tocilizumab	Humanized monoclonal antibody	▪ Rheumatoid arthritis ▪ Juvenile arthritis ▪ *Pustular psoriasis*	IL-6 receptor binding with effects on cutaneous inflammation	*Off-label use*	▪ Increased risk for serious infections ▪ Increased liver function enzymes ▪ Nasopharyngitis ▪ Hypertension[15]

[a]Recommended doses are based on U.S. Food and Drug Administration (FDA)-approved indications.
[b]Underlining indicates FDA approved.
[c]Italicizing indicates small trials and/or case reports.
[d]Final FDA-approved dosing interval not yet available.

[1]https://www.accessdata.fda.gov/drugsatfda_docs/label/2016/103950s5175lbl.pdf
[2]https://www.accessdata.fda.gov/drugsatfda_docs/label/2008/125249lbl.pdf
[3]https://www.accessdata.fda.gov/drugsatfda_docs/label/2012/125319s047lbl.pdf
[4]https://www.accessdata.fda.gov/drugsatfda_docs/label/2016/125504s001s002lbl.pdf
[5]https://www.accessdata.fda.gov/drugsatfda_docs/label/2016/125521s000lbl.pdf
[6]https://www.accessdata.fda.gov/drugsatfda_docs/label/2017/761032lbl.pdf
[7]https://www.accessdata.fda.gov/drugsatfda_docs/label/2016/761044lbl.pdf
[8]https://www.accessdata.fda.gov/drugsatfda_docs/label/2017/761061s000lbl.pdf
[9]https://www.accessdata.fda.gov/drugsatfda_docs/label/2012/103293s5130lbl.pdf
[10]https://www.accessdata.fda.gov/drugsatfda_docs/label/2015/103836s5182lbl.pdf
[11]https://www.accessdata.fda.gov/drugsatfda_docs/label/2012/125084s0228lbl.pdf
[12]https://www.accessdata.fda.gov/drugsatfda_docs/label/2009/125147s080lbl.pdf
[13]https://www.accessdata.fda.gov/drugsatfda_docs/label/2012/125036s0144lbl.pdf
[14]https://www.accessdata.fda.gov/drugsatfda_docs/label/2011/125388s000,125399s000lbl.pdf
[15]https://www.accessdata.fda.gov/drugsatfda_docs/label/2013/125276s092lbl.pdf

CAPS, cryopyrin-associated periodic syndromes; CTCL, cutaneous T-cell lymphoma; DIRA, deficiency of interleukin-1-receptor antagonist; EBA, epidermolysis bullosa acquisita; FCAS, familial cold autoinflammatory syndrome; FMF, familial Mediterranean fever; GVHD, graft-versus-host-disease; HIDS, hyperimmunoglobulin D syndrome; IFN, interferon; Ig, immunoglobulin; IL, interleukin; IM, intramuscular; LFA, leukocyte function–associated antigen; MKD, mevalonate kinase deficiency; MWS, Muckle-Wells syndrome; NK, natural killer; PML, progressive multifocal leukoencephalopathy; SQ, subcutaneous; TNF, tumor necrosis factor; TRAPS, tumor necrosis factor receptor-associated periodic syndrome.

REFERENCES

1. Luger TA, Stadler BM, Luger BM, et al. Murine epidermal cell-derived thymocyte-activating factor resembles murine interleukin 1. *J Immunol*. 1982;128(5):2147-2152.
2. Kondo S, Sauder DN, Kono T, et al. Differential modulation of interleukin-1 alpha (IL-1 alpha) and interleukin-1 beta (IL-1 beta) in human epidermal keratinocytes by UVB. *Exp Dermatol*. 1994;3(1):29-39.
3. Afonina IS, Tynan GA, Logue SE, et al. Granzyme B-dependent proteolysis acts as a switch to enhance the proinflammatory activity of IL-1α. *Mol Cell*. 2011;44(2):265-278.
4. Franchi L, Eigenbrod T, Muñoz-Planillo R, et al. The inflammasome: a caspase-1-activation platform that regulates immune responses and disease pathogenesis. *Nat Immunol*. 2009;10(3):241-247.
5. Kryczek I, Bruce AT, Gudjonsson JE, et al. Induction of IL-17+ T cell trafficking and development by IFN-gamma: mechanism and pathological relevance in psoriasis. *J Immunol*. 2008;181(7):4733-4741.
6. Broderick L, De Nardo D, Franklin BS, et al. The inflammasomes and autoinflammatory syndromes. *Annu Rev Pathol*. 2015;10:395-424.
7. Aksentijevich I, Nowak M, Mallah M, et al. De novo CIAS1 mutations, cytokine activation, and evidence for genetic heterogeneity in patients with neonatal-onset multisystem inflammatory disease (NOMID): a new member of the expanding family of pyrin-associated autoinflammatory diseases. *Arthritis Rheum*. 2002;46(12):3340-3348.
8. Hoffman HM, Mueller JL, Broide DH, et al. Mutation of a new gene encoding a putative pyrin-like protein causes familial cold autoinflammatory syndrome and Muckle-Wells syndrome. *Nat Genet*. 2001;29(3):301-305.
9. Ancient missense mutations in a new member of the RoRet gene family are likely to cause familial Mediterranean fever. The International FMF Consortium. *Cell*. 1997;90(4):797-807.
10. Masters SL, Lagou V, Jéru I, et al. Familial autoinflammation with neutrophilic dermatosis reveals a regulatory mechanism of pyrin activation. *Sci Transl Med*. 2016;8(332):332ra45.
11. Aksentijevich I, Masters SL, Ferguson PJ, et al. An autoinflammatory disease with deficiency of the interleukin-1-receptor antagonist. *N Engl J Med*. 2009;360(23):2426-2437.
12. Dinarello CA, van der Meer JW. Treating inflammation by blocking interleukin-1 in humans. *Semin Immunol*. 2013;25(6):469-484.
13. van der Zee HH, de Ruiter L, van den Broecke DG, et al. Elevated levels of tumour necrosis factor (TNF)-α, interleukin (IL)-1β and IL-10 in hidradenitis suppurativa skin: a rationale for targeting TNF-α and IL-1β. *Br J Dermatol*. 2011;164(6):1292-1298.
14. Leslie KS, Tripathi SV, Nguyen TV, et al. An open-label study of anakinra for the treatment of moderate to severe hidradenitis suppurativa. *J Am Acad Dermatol*. 2014;70(2):243-251.
15. Zarchi K, Dufour DN, Jemec GB. Successful treatment of severe hidradenitis suppurativa with anakinra. *JAMA Dermatol*. 2013;149(10):1192-1194.
16. Rossi-Semerano L, Piram M, Chiaverini C, et al. First clinical description of an infant with interleukin-36-receptor antagonist deficiency successfully treated with anakinra. *Pediatrics*. 2013;132(4):e1043-e1047.
17. Huffmeier U, Wätzold M, Mohr J, et al. Successful therapy with anakinra in a patient with generalized pustular psoriasis carrying IL36RN mutations. *Br J Dermatol*. 2014;170(1):202-204.
18. Viguier M, Guigue P, Pagès C, et al. Successful treatment of generalized pustular psoriasis with the interleukin-1-receptor antagonist anakinra: lack of correlation with IL1RN mutations. *Ann Intern Med*. 2010;153(1):66-67.
19. McDermott MF. Rilonacept in the treatment of chronic inflammatory disorders. *Drugs Today (Barc)*. 2009;45(6):423-430.
20. Kone-Paut I, Galeotti C. Current treatment recommendations and considerations for cryopyrin-associated periodic syndrome. *Expert Rev Clin Immunol*. 2015;11(10):1083-1092.
21. Skendros P, Papagoras C, Lefaki I, et al. Successful response in a case of severe pustular psoriasis after interleukin-1β inhibition. *Br J Dermatol*. 2017;176(1):212-215.
22. Tauber M, Viguier M, Le Gall C, et al. Is it relevant to use an interleukin-1-inhibiting strategy for the treatment of patients with deficiency of interleukin-36 receptor antagonist? *Br J Dermatol*. 2014;170(5):1198-1199.
23. Dinarello CA, Novick D, Kim S, et al. Interleukin-18 and IL-18 binding protein. *Front Immunol*. 2013;4:289.
24. Omoto Y, Tokime K, Yamanaka K, et al. Human mast cell chymase cleaves pro-IL-18 and generates a novel and biologically active IL-18 fragment. *J Immunol*. 2006;177(12):8315-8319.
25. Omoto Y, Yamanaka K, Tokime K, et al. Granzyme B is a novel interleukin-18 converting enzyme. *J Dermatol Sci*. 2010;59(2):129-135.
26. Naik SM, Cannon G, Burbach GJ, et al. Human keratinocytes constitutively express interleukin-18 and secrete biologically active interleukin-18 after treatment with pro-inflammatory mediators and dinitrochlorobenzene. *J Invest Dermatol*. 1999;113(5):766-772.
27. Lee JK, Kim SH, Lewis EC, et al. Differences in signaling pathways by IL-1beta and IL-18. *Proc Natl Acad Sci U S A*. 2004;101(23):8815-8820.
28. Smith DE. The biological paths of IL-1 family members IL-18 and IL-33. *J Leukoc Biol*. 2011;89(3):383-392.
29. Brydges SD, Broderick L, McGeough MD, et al. Divergence of IL-1, IL-18, and cell death in NLRP3 inflammasomopathies. *J Clin Invest*. 2013;123(11):4695-4705.
30. Ohta Y, Hamada Y, Katsuoka K. Expression of IL-18 in psoriasis. *Arch Dermatol Res*. 2001;293(7):334-342.
31. Wittmann M, Macdonald A, Renne J. IL-18 and skin inflammation. *Autoimmun Rev*. 2009;9(1):45-48.
32. Girard C, Rech J, Brown M, et al. Elevated serum levels of free interleukin-18 in adult-onset Still's disease. *Rheumatology (Oxford)*. 2016;55(12):2237-2247.
33. Schmitz J, Owyang A, Oldham E, et al. IL-33, an interleukin-1-like cytokine that signals via the IL-1 receptor-related protein ST2 and induces T helper type 2-associated cytokines. *Immunity*. 2005;23(5):479-490.
34. Hayakawa H, Hayakawa M, Kume A, et al. Soluble ST2 blocks interleukin-33 signaling in allergic airway inflammation. *J Biol Chem*. 2007;282(36):26369-26380.

35. Bulek K, Swaidani S, Qin J, et al. The essential role of single Ig IL-1 receptor-related molecule/Toll IL-1R8 in regulation of Th2 immune response. *J Immunol.* 2009;182(5):2601-2609.
36. Luthi AU, Cullen SP, McNeela EA, et al. Suppression of interleukin-33 bioactivity through proteolysis by apoptotic caspases. *Immunity.* 2009;31(1):84-98.
37. Smith DE. IL-33: a tissue derived cytokine pathway involved in allergic inflammation and asthma. *Clin Exp Allergy.* 2010;40(2):200-208.
38. Debets R, Timans JC, Homey B, et al. Two novel IL-1 family members, IL-1 delta and IL-1 epsilon, function as an antagonist and agonist of NF-kappa B activation through the orphan IL-1 receptor-related protein 2. *J Immunol.* 2001;167(3):1440-1446.
39. Johnston A, Xing X, Guzman AM, et al. IL-1F5, -F6, -F8, and -F9: a novel IL-1 family signaling system that is active in psoriasis and promotes keratinocyte antimicrobial peptide expression. *J Immunol.* 2011;186(4):2613-2622.
40. D'Erme AM, Wilsmann-Theis D, Wagenpfeil J, et al. IL-36γ (IL-1F9) is a biomarker for psoriasis skin lesions. *J Invest Dermatol.* 2015;135(4):1025-1032.
41. Thomi R, Kakeda M, Yawalkar N, et al. Increased expression of the interleukin-36 cytokines in lesions of hidradenitis suppurativa. *J Eur Acad Dermatol Venereol.* 2017;31(12):2091-2096.
42. Johnston A, Xing X, Wolterink L, et al. IL-1 and IL-36 are dominant cytokines in generalized pustular psoriasis. *J Allergy Clin Immunol.* 2017;140(1):109-120.
43. Carrier Y, Ma HL, Ramon HE, et al. Inter-regulation of Th17 cytokines and the IL-36 cytokines in vitro and in vivo: implications in psoriasis pathogenesis. *J Invest Dermatol.* 2011;131(12):2428-2437.
44. Blumberg H, Dinh H, Trueblood ES, et al. Opposing activities of two novel members of the IL-1 ligand family regulate skin inflammation. *J Exp Med.* 2007;204(11):2603-2614.
45. Foster AM, Baliwag J, Chen CS, et al. IL-36 promotes myeloid cell infiltration, activation, and inflammatory activity in skin. *J Immunol.* 2014;192(12):6053-6061.
46. Mutamba S, Allison A, Mahida Y, et al. Expression of IL-1Rrp2 by human myelomonocytic cells is unique to DCs and facilitates DC maturation by IL-1F8 and IL-1F9. *Eur J Immunol.* 2012;42(3):607-617.
47. Dietrich D, Martin P, Flacher V, et al. Interleukin-36 potently stimulates human M2 macrophages, Langerhans cells and keratinocytes to produce proinflammatory cytokines. *Cytokine.* 2016;84:88-98.
48. Towne JE, Renshaw BR, Douangpanya J, et al. Interleukin-36 (IL-36) ligands require processing for full agonist (IL-36α, IL-36β and IL-36γ) or antagonist (IL-36Ra) activity. *J Biol Chem.* 2011;286(49):42594-42602.
49. Henry CM, Sullivan GP, Clancy DM, et al. Neutrophil-derived proteases escalate inflammation through activation of IL-36 family cytokines. *Cell Rep.* 2016;14(4):708-722.
50. Ainscough JS, Macleod T, McGonagle D, et al. Cathepsin S is the major activator of the psoriasis-associated proinflammatory cytokine IL-36γ. *Proc Natl Acad Sci U S A.* 2017;114(13):E2748-E2757.
51. Setta-Kaffetzi N, Navarini AA, Patel VM, et al. Rare pathogenic variants in IL36RN underlie a spectrum of psoriasis-associated pustular phenotypes. *J Invest Dermatol.* 2013;133(5):1366-1369.
52. Marrakchi S, Guigue P, Renshaw BR, et al. Interleukin-36-receptor antagonist deficiency and generalized pustular psoriasis. *N Engl J Med.* 2011;365(7):620-628.
53. Onoufriadis A, Simpson MA, Pink AE, et al. Mutations in IL36RN/IL1F5 are associated with the severe episodic inflammatory skin disease known as generalized pustular psoriasis. *Am J Hum Genet.* 2011;89(3):432-437.
54. Sugiura K, Oiso N, Iinuma S, et al. IL36RN mutations underlie impetigo herpetiformis. *J Invest Dermatol.* 2014;134(9):2472-2474.
55. Navarini AA, Valeyrie-Allanore L, Setta-Kaffetzi N, et al. Rare variations in IL36RN in severe adverse drug reactions manifesting as acute generalized exanthematous pustulosis. *J Invest Dermatol.* 2013;133(7):1904-1907.
56. Nakai N, Sugiura K, Akiyama M, et al. Acute generalized exanthematous pustulosis caused by dihydrocodeine phosphate in a patient with psoriasis vulgaris and a heterozygous IL36RN mutation. *JAMA Dermatol.* 2015;151(3):311-315.
57. Capon F. IL36RN mutations in generalized pustular psoriasis: just the tip of the iceberg? *J Invest Dermatol.* 2013;133(11):2503-2504.
58. Ganesan R, Raymond EL, Mennerich D, et al. Generation and functional characterization of anti-human and anti-mouse IL-36R antagonist monoclonal antibodies. *MAbs.* 2017;9(7):1143-1154.
59. Dinarello CA, Nold-Petry C, Nold M, et al. Suppression of innate inflammation and immunity by interleukin-37. *Eur J Immunol.* 2016;46(5):1067-1081.
60. van de Veerdonk FL, Stoeckman AK, Wu G, et al. IL-38 binds to the IL-36 receptor and has biological effects on immune cells similar to IL-36 receptor antagonist. *Proc Natl Acad Sci U S A.* 2012;109(8):3001-3005.
61. Monin L, Gaffen SL. Interleukin 17 family cytokines: signaling mechanisms, biological activities, and therapeutic implications. *Cold Spring Harb Perspect Biol.* 2018;10(4).
62. Beringer A, Noack M, Miossec P. IL-17 in chronic inflammation: from discovery to targeting. *Trends Mol Med.* 2016;22(3):230-241.
63. Lowes MA, Suarez-Farinas M, Krueger JG. Immunology of psoriasis. *Annu Rev Immunol.* 2014;32:227-255.
64. Lubberts E. The IL-23-IL-17 axis in inflammatory arthritis. *Nat Rev Rheumatol.* 2015;11(7):415-429.
65. Li D, Guo B, Wu H, et al. Interleukin-17 in systemic lupus erythematosus: a comprehensive review. *Autoimmunity.* 2015;48(6):353-361.
66. Teunissen MB, Koomen CW, de Waal Malefyt R, et al. Interleukin-17 and interferon-gamma synergize in the enhancement of proinflammatory cytokine production by human keratinocytes. *J Invest Dermatol.* 1998;111(4):645-649.
67. Chiricozzi A, Guttman-Yassky E, Suárez-Fariñas M, et al. Integrative responses to IL-17 and TNF-α in human keratinocytes account for key inflammatory pathogenic circuits in psoriasis. *J Invest Dermatol.* 2011;131(3):677-687.
68. Wang CQF, Akalu YT, Suarez-Farinas M, et al. IL-17 and TNF synergistically modulate cytokine expression while suppressing melanogenesis: potential relevance to psoriasis. *J Invest Dermatol.* 2013;133(12):2741-2752.
69. Johnston A, Guzman AM, Swindell WR, et al. Early tissue responses in psoriasis to the antitumour necrosis factor-α biologic etanercept suggest reduced interleukin-17 receptor expression and signalling. *Br J Dermatol.* 2014;171(1):97-107.

70. Lin AM, Rubin CJ, Khandpur R, et al. Mast cells and neutrophils release IL-17 through extracellular trap formation in psoriasis. *J Immunol*. 2011;187(1):490-500.
71. Res PC, Piskin G, de Boer OJ, et al. Overrepresentation of IL-17A and IL-22 producing CD8 T cells in lesional skin suggests their involvement in the pathogenesis of psoriasis. *PLoS One*. 2010;5(11):e14108.
72. Teunissen MBM, Yeremenko NG, Baeten DLP, et al. The IL-17A-producing CD8+ T-cell population in psoriatic lesional skin comprises mucosa-associated invariant T cells and conventional T cells. *J Invest Dermatol*. 2014;134(12):2898-2907.
73. Villanova F, Flutter B, Tosi I, et al. Characterization of innate lymphoid cells in human skin and blood demonstrates increase of NKp44+ ILC3 in psoriasis. *J Invest Dermatol*. 2014;134(4):984-991.
74. Okada S, Puel A, Casanova JL, et al. Chronic mucocutaneous candidiasis disease associated with inborn errors of IL-17 immunity. *Clin Transl Immunology*. 2016;5(12):e114.
75. Elder JT, Bruce AT, Gudjonsson JE, et al. Molecular dissection of psoriasis: integrating genetics and biology. *J Invest Dermatol*. 2010;130(5):1213-1226.
76. Das S, Stuart PE, Ding J, et al. Fine mapping of eight psoriasis susceptibility loci. *Eur J Hum Genet*. 2015;23(6):844-853.
77. Langley RG, Elewski BE, Lebwohl M, et al. Secukinumab in plaque psoriasis—results of two phase 3 trials. *N Engl J Med*. 2014;371(4):326-338.
78. Armstrong AW, Papp K, Kircik L. Secukinumab: review of clinical evidence from the pivotal studies ERASURE, FIXTURE, and CLEAR. *J Clin Aesthet Dermatol*. 2016;9(6)(suppl 1):S7-S12.
79. Bohner A, Roenneberg S, Eyerich K, et al. Acute generalized pustular psoriasis treated with the IL-17A antibody secukinumab. *JAMA Dermatol*. 2016;152(4):482-484.
80. Imafuku S, Honma M, Okubo Y, et al. Efficacy and safety of secukinumab in patients with generalized pustular psoriasis: a 52-week analysis from phase III open-label multicenter Japanese study. *J Dermatol*. 2016;43(9):1011-1017.
81. Gottlieb A, Sullivan J, van Doorn M, et al. Secukinumab shows significant efficacy in palmoplantar psoriasis: results from GESTURE, a randomized controlled trial. *J Am Acad Dermatol*. 2017;76(1):70-80.
82. Gordon KB, Blauvelt A, Papp KA, et al. Phase 3 trials of ixekizumab in moderate-to-severe plaque psoriasis. *N Engl J Med*. 2016;375(4):345-356.
83. Farahnik B, Beroukhim K, Zhu TH, et al. Ixekizumab for the treatment of psoriasis: a review of phase III trials. *Dermatol Ther (Heidelb)*. 2016;6(1):25-37.
84. Griffiths CE, Reich K, Lebwohl M, et al. Comparison of ixekizumab with etanercept or placebo in moderate-to-severe psoriasis (UNCOVER-2 and UNCOVER-3): results from two phase 3 randomised trials. *Lancet*. 2015;386(9993):541-551.
85. Reich K, Leonardi C, Lebwohl M, et al. Sustained response with ixekizumab treatment of moderate-to-severe psoriasis with scalp involvement: results from three phase 3 trials (UNCOVER-1, UNCOVER-2, UNCOVER-3). *J Dermatolog Treat*. 2017;28(4):282-287.
86. van de Kerkhof P, Guenther L, Gottlieb AB, et al. Ixekizumab treatment improves fingernail psoriasis in patients with moderate-to-severe psoriasis: results from the randomized, controlled and open-label phases of UNCOVER-3. *J Eur Acad Dermatol Venereol*. 2017;31(3):477-482.
87. Kimball AB, Luger T, Gottlieb A, et al. Impact of ixekizumab on psoriasis itch severity and other psoriasis symptoms: results from 3 phase III psoriasis clinical trials. *J Am Acad Dermatol*. 2016;75(6):1156-1161.
88. Saeki H, Nakagawa H, Ishii T, et al. Efficacy and safety of open-label ixekizumab treatment in Japanese patients with moderate-to-severe plaque psoriasis, erythrodermic psoriasis and generalized pustular psoriasis. *J Eur Acad Dermatol Venereol*. 2015;29(6):1148-1155.
89. Papp KA, Reich K, Paul C, et al. A prospective phase III, randomized, double-blind, placebo-controlled study of brodalumab in patients with moderate-to-severe plaque psoriasis. *Br J Dermatol*. 2016;175(2):273-286.
90. Lebwohl M, Strober B, Menter A, et al. Phase 3 studies comparing brodalumab with ustekinumab in psoriasis. *N Engl J Med*. 2015;373(14):1318-1328.
91. Yamasaki K, Nakagawa H, Kubo Y, et al. Efficacy and safety of brodalumab in patients with generalized pustular psoriasis and psoriatic erythroderma: results from a 52-week, open-label study. *Br J Dermatol*. 2017;176(3):741-751.
92. Sabat R, Ouyang W, Wolk K. Therapeutic opportunities of the IL-22–IL-22R1 system. *Nat Rev Drug Discov*. 2014;13(1):21-38.
93. Duhen T, Geiger R, Jarrossay D, et al. Production of interleukin 22 but not interleukin 17 by a subset of human skin-homing memory T cells. *Nat Immunol*. 2009;10(8):857-863.
94. Boniface K, Bernard FX, Garcia M, et al. IL-22 inhibits epidermal differentiation and induces proinflammatory gene expression and migration of human keratinocytes. *J Immunol*. 2005;174(6):3695-3702.
95. Boniface K, Guignouard E, Pedretti N, et al. A role for T cell-derived interleukin 22 in psoriatic skin inflammation. *Clin Exp Immunol*. 2007;150(3):407-415.
96. Wolk K, Sabat R. Interleukin-22: a novel T- and NK-cell derived cytokine that regulates the biology of tissue cells. *Cytokine Growth Factor Rev*. 2006;17(5):367-380.
97. Sigmundsdóttir H, Johnston A, Gudjónsson JE, et al. Differential effects of interleukin 12 and interleukin 10 on superantigen-induced expression of cutaneous lymphocyte-associated antigen (CLA) and alphaEbeta7 integrin (CD103) by CD8+ T cells. *Clin Immunol*. 2004;111(1):119-125.
98. Yawalkar N, Karlen S, Hunger R, et al. Expression of interleukin-12 is increased in psoriatic skin. *J Invest Dermatol*. 1998;111(6):1053-1057.
99. Hamid Q, Naseer T, Minshall EM, et al. In vivo expression of IL-12 and IL-13 in atopic dermatitis. *J Allergy Clin Immunol*. 1996;98(1):225-231.
100. Capon F, Di Meglio P, Szaub J, et al. Sequence variants in the genes for the interleukin-23 receptor (IL23R) and its ligand (IL12B) confer protection against psoriasis. *Hum Genet*. 2007;122(2):201-206.
101. Cargill M, Schrodi SJ, Chang M, et al. A large-scale genetic association study confirms IL12B and leads to the identification of IL23R as psoriasis-risk genes. *Am J Hum Genet*. 2007;80(2):273-290.
102. Nair RP, Ruether A, Stuart PE, et al. Polymorphisms of the IL12B and IL23R genes are associated with psoriasis. *J Invest Dermatol*. 2008;128(7):1653-1661.
103. Johnston A, Xing X, Swindell WR, et al. Susceptibility-associated genetic variation at IL12B enhances

Th1 polarization in psoriasis. *Hum Mol Genet.* 2013;22(9):1807-1815.
104. Papp KA, Langley RG, Lebwohl M, et al. Efficacy and safety of ustekinumab, a human interleukin-12/23 monoclonal antibody, in patients with psoriasis:52-week results from a randomised, double-blind, placebo-controlled trial (PHOENIX 2). *Lancet.* 2008;371(9625):1675-1684.
105. Leonardi CL, Kimball AB, Papp KA, et al. Efficacy and safety of ustekinumab, a human interleukin-12/23 monoclonal antibody, in patients with psoriasis:76-week results from a randomised, double-blind, placebo-controlled trial (PHOENIX 1). *Lancet.* 2008;371(9625):1665-1674.
106. Blok JL, Li K, Brodmerkel C, et al. Ustekinumab in hidradenitis suppurativa: clinical results and a search for potential biomarkers in serum. *Br J Dermatol.* 2016;174(4):839-846.
107. Eisen DB. Ustekinumab, another biologic with potential to help patients with hidradenitis suppurativa? *Br J Dermatol.* 2016;174(4):718-719.
108. Weiss D, Schaschinger M, Ristl R, et al. Ustekinumab treatment in severe atopic dermatitis: down-regulation of T-helper 2/22 expression. *J Am Acad Dermatol.* 2017;76(1):91-97; e3.
109. Khattri S, Brunner PM, Garcet S, et al. Efficacy and safety of ustekinumab treatment in adults with moderate-to-severe atopic dermatitis. *Exp Dermatol.* 2017;26(1):28-35.
110. Saeki H, Kabashima K, Tokura Y, et al. Efficacy and safety of ustekinumab in Japanese patients with severe atopic dermatitis: a randomized, double-blind, placebo-controlled, phase II study. *Br J Dermatol.* 2017;177(2):419-427.
111. Hoebeeck J, van der Luijt R, Poppe B, et al. Rapid detection of VHL exon deletions using real-time quantitative PCR. *Lab Invest.* 2005;85(1):24-33.
112. Piskin G, Sylva-Steenland RM, Bos JD, et al. In vitro and in situ expression of IL-23 by keratinocytes in healthy skin and psoriasis lesions: enhanced expression in psoriatic skin. *J Immunol.* 2006;176(3):1908-1915.
113. Robinson RT. IL12Rbeta1: the cytokine receptor that we used to know. *Cytokine.* 2015;71(2):348-359.
114. Di Meglio P, Nestle FO. The role of IL-23 in the immunopathogenesis of psoriasis. *F1000 Biol Rep.* 2010;2.
115. Langrish CL, McKenzie BS, Wilson NJ, et al. IL-12 and IL-23: master regulators of innate and adaptive immunity. *Immunol Rev.* 2004;202:96-105.
116. Nair RP, Duffin KC, Helms C, et al. Genome-wide scan reveals association of psoriasis with IL-23 and NF-kappaB pathways. *Nat Genet.* 2009;41(2):199-204.
117. Desmet J, Verstraete K, Bloch Y, et al. Structural basis of IL-23 antagonism by an Alphabody protein scaffold. *Nat Commun.* 2014;5:5237.
118. Quiniou C, Domínguez-Punaro M, Cloutier F, et al. Specific targeting of the IL-23 receptor, using a novel small peptide noncompetitive antagonist, decreases the inflammatory response. *Am J Physiol Regul Integr Comp Physiol.* 2014;307(10):R1216-R1230.
119. Reich K, Armstrong AW, Foley P, et al. Efficacy and safety of guselkumab, an anti-interleukin-23 monoclonal antibody, compared with adalimumab for the treatment of patients with moderate to severe psoriasis with randomized withdrawal and retreatment: results from the phase III, double-blind, placebo- and active comparator-controlled VOYAGE 2 trial. *J Am Acad Dermatol.* 2017;76(3):418-431.
120. Blauvelt A, Papp KA, Griffiths CE, et al. Efficacy and safety of guselkumab, an anti-interleukin-23 monoclonal antibody, compared with adalimumab for the continuous treatment of patients with moderate to severe psoriasis: results from the phase III, double-blinded, placebo- and active comparator-controlled VOYAGE 1 trial. *J Am Acad Dermatol.* 2017;76(3):405-417.
121. Smolen JS, Agarwal SK, Ilivanova E, et al. A randomised phase II study evaluating the efficacy and safety of subcutaneously administered ustekinumab and guselkumab in patients with active rheumatoid arthritis despite treatment with methotrexate. *Ann Rheum Dis.* 2017;76(5):831-839.
122. Reich K, Papp KA, Blauvelt A, et al. Tildrakizumab versus placebo or etanercept for chronic plaque psoriasis (reSURFACE 1 and reSURFACE 2): results from two randomised controlled, phase 3 trials. *Lancet.* 2017;390(10091):276-288.
123. Papp KA, Blauvelt A, Bukhalo M, et al. Risankizumab versus ustekinumab for moderate-to-severe plaque psoriasis. *N Engl J Med.* 2017;376(16):1551-1560.
124. LaDuca JR, Gaspari AA. Targeting tumor necrosis factor alpha. New drugs used to modulate inflammatory diseases. *Dermatol Clin.* 2001;19(4):617-635.
125. Indhumathi S, Rajappa M, Chandrashekar L, et al. Pharmacogenetic markers to predict the clinical response to methotrexate in south Indian Tamil patients with psoriasis. *Eur J Clin Pharmacol.* 2017;73(8):965-971.
126. Gottlieb AB, Masud S, Ramamurthi R, et al. Pharmacodynamic and pharmacokinetic response to anti-tumor necrosis factor-alpha monoclonal antibody (infliximab) treatment of moderate to severe psoriasis vulgaris. *J Am Acad Dermatol.* 2003;48(1):68-75.
127. Hancock GE, Kaplan G, Cohn ZA. Keratinocyte growth regulation by the products of immune cells. *J Exp Med.* 1988;168(4):1395-1402.
128. Keffer J, Probert L, Cazlaris H, et al. Transgenic mice expressing human tumour necrosis factor: a predictive genetic model of arthritis. *EMBO J.* 1991;10(13):4025-4031.
129. Papp KA, Poulin Y, Bissonnette R, et al. Assessment of the long-term safety and effectiveness of etanercept for the treatment of psoriasis in an adult population. *J Am Acad Dermatol.* 2012;66(2): e33-e45.
130. Tsoi LC, Spain SL, Knight J, et al. Identification of 15 new psoriasis susceptibility loci highlights the role of innate immunity. *Nat Genet.* 2012;44(12):1341-1348.
131. Gniadecki R, Bang B, Bryld LE, et al. Comparison of long-term drug survival and safety of biologic agents in patients with psoriasis vulgaris. *Br J Dermatol.* 2015;172(1):244-252.
132. Carrascosa JM, van Doorn MB, Lahfa M, et al. Clinical relevance of immunogenicity of biologics in psoriasis: implications for treatment strategies. *J Eur Acad Dermatol Venereol.* 2014;28(11):1424-1430.
133. van Schouwenburg PA, van de Stadt LA, de Jong RN, et al. Adalimumab elicits a restricted anti-idiotypic antibody response in autoimmune patients resulting in functional neutralisation. *Ann Rheum Dis.* 2013;72(1):104-109.
134. Ingram JR. Interventions for hidradenitis suppurativa: updated summary of an original Cochrane review. *JAMA Dermatol.* 2017;153(5):458-459.
135. Elewski BE. Infliximab for the treatment of severe pustular psoriasis. *J Am Acad Dermatol.* 2002;47(5):796-797.

136. Newland MR, Weinstein A, Kerdel F. Rapid response to infliximab in severe pustular psoriasis, von Zumbusch type. *Int J Dermatol.* 2002;41(7):449-452.
137. Robinson A, Van Voorhees AS, Hsu S, et al. Treatment of pustular psoriasis: from the Medical Board of the National Psoriasis Foundation. *J Am Acad Dermatol.* 2012;67(2):279-288.
138. Williams VL, Cohen PR. TNF alpha antagonist-induced lupus-like syndrome: report and review of the literature with implications for treatment with alternative TNF alpha antagonists. *Int J Dermatol.* 2011;50(5):619-625.
139. Viguier M, Richette P, Bachelez H, et al. Paradoxical adverse effects of anti-TNF-alpha treatment: onset or exacerbation of cutaneous disorders. *Expert Rev Clin Immunol.* 2009;5(4):421-431.
140. Collamer AN, Battafarano DF. Psoriatic skin lesions induced by tumor necrosis factor antagonist therapy: clinical features and possible immunopathogenesis. *Semin Arthritis Rheum.* 2010;40(3):233-240.
141. Swindell WR, Xing X, Stuart PE, et al. Heterogeneity of inflammatory and cytokine networks in chronic plaque psoriasis. *PLoS One.* 2012;7(3):e34594.
142. Bongartz T, Sutton AJ, Sweeting MJ, et al. Anti-TNF antibody therapy in rheumatoid arthritis and the risk of serious infections and malignancies: systematic review and meta-analysis of rare harmful effects in randomized controlled trials. *JAMA.* 2006;295(19):2275-2285.
143. Strangfeld A, Listing J, Herzer P, et al. Risk of herpes zoster in patients with rheumatoid arthritis treated with anti-TNF-alpha agents. *JAMA.* 2009;301(7):737-744.
144. Leombruno JP, Einarson TR, Keystone EC. The safety of anti-tumour necrosis factor treatments in rheumatoid arthritis: meta and exposure-adjusted pooled analyses of serious adverse events. *Ann Rheum Dis.* 2009;68(7):1136-1145.
145. Adams AE, Zwicker J, Curiel C, et al. Aggressive cutaneous T-cell lymphomas after TNFalpha blockade. *J Am Acad Dermatol.* 2004;51(4):660-662.
146. Mariette X, Tubach F, Bagheri H, et al. Lymphoma in patients treated with anti-TNF: results of the 3-year prospective French RATIO registry. *Ann Rheum Dis.* 2010;69(2):400-408.
147. Gelfand JM, Shin DB, Neimann AL, et al. The risk of lymphoma in patients with psoriasis. *J Invest Dermatol.* 2006;126(10):2194-2201.
148. Rosenberg SA. IL-2: the first effective immunotherapy for human cancer. *J Immunol.* 2014;192(12):5451-5458.
149. Asadullah K, Sterry W, Trefzer U. Cytokine therapy in dermatology. *Exp Dermatol.* 2002;11(2):97-106.
150. Goff SL, Dudley ME, Citrin DE, et al. Randomized, prospective evaluation comparing intensity of lymphodepletion before adoptive transfer of tumor-infiltrating lymphocytes for patients with metastatic melanoma. *J Clin Oncol.* 2016;34(20):2389-2397.
151. Rook AH, Kuzel TM, Olsen EA. Cytokine therapy of cutaneous T-cell lymphoma: interferons, interleukin-12, and interleukin-2. *Hematol Oncol Clin North Am.* 2003;17(6):1435-1448, ix.
152. Holman DM, Kalaaji AN. Cytokines in dermatology. *J Drugs Dermatol.* 2006;5(6):520-524.
153. Spaccarelli N, Rook AH. The use of interferons in the treatment of cutaneous T-cell lymphoma. *Dermatol Clin.* 2015;33(4):731-745.
154. Schiller M, Tsianakas A, Sterry W, et al. Dose-escalation study evaluating pegylated interferon alpha-2a in patients with cutaneous T-cell lymphoma. *J Eur Acad Dermatol Venereol.* 2017;31(11):1841-1847.
155. Suchin KR, Cassin M, Gottleib SL, et al. Increased interleukin 5 production in eosinophilic Sezary syndrome: regulation by interferon alfa and interleukin 12. *J Am Acad Dermatol.* 2001;44(1):28-32.
156. Sabel MS, Sondak VK. Pros and cons of adjuvant interferon in the treatment of melanoma. *Oncologist.* 2003;8(5):451-458.
157. Stadler R. Interferons in dermatology. Present-day standard. *Dermatol Clin.* 1998;16(2):377-398.
158. Sugaya M, Tokura Y, Hamada T, et al. Phase II study of i.v. interferon-gamma in Japanese patients with mycosis fungoides. *J Dermatol.* 2014;41(1):50-56.
159. Olsen EA, Rook AH, Zic J, et al. Sezary syndrome: immunopathogenesis, literature review of therapeutic options, and recommendations for therapy by the United States Cutaneous Lymphoma Consortium (USCLC). *J Am Acad Dermatol.* 2011;64(2):352-404.
160. Herbst RS. Review of epidermal growth factor receptor biology. *Int J Radiat Oncol Biol Phys.* 2004;59(2)(suppl):21-26.
161. Zhang H, Berezov A, Wang Q, et al. ErbB receptors: from oncogenes to targeted cancer therapies. *J Clin Invest.* 2007;117(8):2051-2058.
162. Bublil EM, Yarden Y. The EGF receptor family: spearheading a merger of signaling and therapeutics. *Curr Opin Cell Biol.* 2007;19(2):124-134.
163. Pastore S, Mascia F, Mariani V, et al. The epidermal growth factor receptor system in skin repair and inflammation. *J Invest Dermatol.* 2008;128(6):1365-1374.
164. Sibilia M, Kroismayr R, Lichtenberger BM, et al. The epidermal growth factor receptor: from development to tumorigenesis. *Differentiation.* 2007;75(9):770-787.
165. Schneider MR, Werner S, Paus R, et al. Beyond wavy hairs: the epidermal growth factor receptor and its ligands in skin biology and pathology. *Am J Pathol.* 2008;173(1):14-24.
166. Lacouture ME. Mechanisms of cutaneous toxicities to EGFR inhibitors. *Nat Rev Cancer.* 2006;6(10):803-812.
167. Nanba D, Toki F, Barrandon Y, et al. Recent advances in the epidermal growth factor receptor/ligand system biology on skin homeostasis and keratinocyte stem cell regulation. *J Dermatol Sci.* 2013;72(2):81-86.
168. Walker F, Abramowitz L, Benabderrahmane D, et al. Growth factor receptor expression in anal squamous lesions: modifications associated with oncogenic human papillomavirus and human immunodeficiency virus. *Hum Pathol.* 2009;40(11):1517-1527.
169. Jost M, Kari C, Rodeck U. The EGF receptor—an essential regulator of multiple epidermal functions. *Eur J Dermatol.* 2000;10(7):505-510.
170. Yang S, Geng Z, Ma K, et al. Efficacy of topical recombinant human epidermal growth factor for treatment of diabetic foot ulcer: a systematic review and meta-analysis. *Int J Low Extrem Wounds.* 2016;15(2):120-125.
171. Berlanga J, Fernández JI, López E, et al. Heberprot-P: a novel product for treating advanced diabetic foot ulcer. *MEDICC Rev.* 2013;15(1):11-15.
172. Hynes NE, Lane HA. ERBB receptors and cancer: the complexity of targeted inhibitors. *Nat Rev Cancer.* 2005;5(5):341-354.
173. Liu HB, Wu Y, Lv TF, et al. Skin rash could predict the response to EGFR tyrosine kinase inhibitor and the prognosis for patients with non-small cell lung

174. Ornitz DM, Xu J, Colvin JS, et al. Receptor specificity of the fibroblast growth factor family. *J Biol Chem.* 1996;271(25):15292-15297.
175. Zhang X, Ibrahimi OA, Olsen SK, et al. Receptor specificity of the fibroblast growth factor family. The complete mammalian FGF family. *J Biol Chem.* 2006;281(23):15694-15700.
176. Belch J, Hiatt WR, Baumgartner I, et al. Effect of fibroblast growth factor NV1FGF on amputation and death: a randomised placebo-controlled trial of gene therapy in critical limb ischaemia. *Lancet.* 2011;377(9781):1929-1937.
177. Nunes QM, Li Y, Sun C, et al. Fibroblast growth factors as tissue repair and regeneration therapeutics. *PeerJ.* 2016;4:e1535.
178. Maeda T, Yamamoto T, Isikawa Y. Sanguisorba officinalis root extract has FGF-5 inhibitory activity and reduces hair loss by causing prolongation of the anagen period. *Nishi Nihon Hifuka.* 2007;69(1):81-86.
179. Martínez-Jiménez MA, Aguilar-García J, Valdés-Rodríguez R, et al. Local use of insulin in wounds of diabetic patients: higher temperature, fibrosis, and angiogenesis. *Plast Reconstr Surg.* 2013;132(6):e1015-e1019.
180. Olsen E, Duvic M, Frankel A, et al. Pivotal phase III trial of two dose levels of denileukin diftitox for the treatment of cutaneous T-cell lymphoma. *J Clin Oncol.* 2001;19(2):376-388.
181. Gehad A, Al-Banna NA, Vaci M, et al. Differing requirements for CCR4, E-selectin, and α4β1 for the migration of memory CD4 and activated T cells to dermal inflammation. *J Immunol.* 2012;189(1):337-346.
182. Duvic M, Pinter-Brown LC, Foss FM, et al. Phase 1/2 study of mogamulizumab, a defucosylated anti-CCR4 antibody, in previously treated patients with cutaneous T-cell lymphoma. *Blood.* 2015;125(12):1883-1889.
183. Ni X, Langridge T, Duvic M. Depletion of regulatory T cells by targeting CC chemokine receptor type 4 with mogamulizumab. *Oncoimmunology.* 2015;4(7):e1011524.
184. Dorner T, Burmester GR. The role of B cells in rheumatoid arthritis: mechanisms and therapeutic targets. *Curr Opin Rheumatol.* 2003;15(3):246-252.
185. Edwards JC, Cambridge G. Sustained improvement in rheumatoid arthritis following a protocol designed to deplete B lymphocytes. *Rheumatology (Oxford).* 2001;40(2):205-211.
186. Cerny T, Borisch B, Introna M, et al. Mechanism of action of rituximab. *Anticancer Drugs.* 2002;13(suppl 2):S3-S10.
187. Marcelin AG, Aaron L, Mateus C, et al. Rituximab therapy for HIV-associated Castleman disease. *Blood.* 2003;102(8):2786-2788.
188. Clifford KS, Demierre MF. Progression of classic Kaposi's sarcoma with rituximab. *J Am Acad Dermatol.* 2005;53(1):155-157.
189. Schmidt E, Seitz CS, Benoit S, et al. Rituximab in autoimmune bullous diseases: mixed responses and adverse effects. *Br J Dermatol.* 2007;156(2):352-356.
190. Ahmed AR, Spigelman Z, Cavacini LA, et al. Treatment of pemphigus vulgaris with rituximab and intravenous immune globulin. *N Engl J Med.* 2006;355(17):1772-1779.
191. Kerl K, Prins C, Saurat JH, et al. Intralesional and intravenous treatment of cutaneous B-cell lymphomas with the monoclonal anti-CD20 antibody rituximab: report and follow-up of eight cases. *Br J Dermatol.* 2006;155(6):1197-1200.
192. Lafyatis R, Kissin E, York M, et al. B cell depletion with rituximab in patients with diffuse cutaneous systemic sclerosis. *Arthritis Rheum.* 2009;60(2):578-583.
193. Loh TY, Paravar T. Rituximab in the management of juvenile pemphigus foliaceus. *Dermatol Online J.* 2017;23(6).
194. Salama A. Emerging drugs for immune thrombocytopenia (ITP). *Expert Opin Emerg Drugs.* 2017;22(1):27-38.
195. Guillevin L, Pagnoux C, Karras A, et al. Rituximab versus azathioprine for maintenance in ANCA-associated vasculitis. *N Engl J Med.* 2014;371(19):1771-1780.
196. Maverakis E, Kim K, Shimoda M, et al. Glycans in the immune system and The Altered Glycan Theory of Autoimmunity: a critical review. *J Autoimmun.* 2015;57:1-13.
197. Guenova E, Skabytska Y, Hoetzenecker W, et al. IL-4 abrogates T(H)17 cell-mediated inflammation by selective silencing of IL-23 in antigen-presenting cells. *Proc Natl Acad Sci U S A.* 2015;112(7):2163-2168.
198. El-Mallawany NK, Frazer JK, Van Vlierberghe P, et al. Pediatric T- and NK-cell lymphomas: new biologic insights and treatment strategies. *Blood Cancer J.* 2012;2(4):e65.
199. Berger GK, McBride A, Lawson S, et al. Brentuximab vedotin for treatment of non-Hodgkin lymphomas: a systematic review. *Crit Rev Oncol Hematol.* 2017;109:42-50.
200. Younes A, Bartlett NL, Leonard JP, et al. Brentuximab vedotin (SGN-35) for relapsed CD30-positive lymphomas. *N Engl J Med.* 2010;363(19):1812-1821.
201. Prince HM, Kim YH, Horwitz SM, et al. Brentuximab vedotin or physician's choice in CD30-positive cutaneous T-cell lymphoma (ALCANZA): an international, open-label, randomised, phase 3, multicentre trial. *Lancet.* 2017;390(10094):555-566.
202. de Kleer I, Vercoulen Y, Klein M, et al. CD30 discriminates heat shock protein 60-induced FOXP3+ CD4+ T cells with a regulatory phenotype. *J Immunol.* 2010;185(4):2071-2079.
203. Hunter CA, Jones SA. IL-6 as a keystone cytokine in health and disease. *Nat Immunol.* 2015;16(5):448-457.
204. Puel A, Picard C, Lorrot M, et al. Recurrent staphylococcal cellulitis and subcutaneous abscesses in a child with autoantibodies against IL-6. *J Immunol.* 2008;180(1):647-654.
205. Saggini A, Chimenti S, Chiricozzi A. IL-6 as a druggable target in psoriasis: focus on pustular variants. *J Immunol Res.* 2014;2014:964069.
206. Neuner P, Urbanski A, Trautinger F, et al. Increased IL-6 production by monocytes and keratinocytes in patients with psoriasis. *J Invest Dermatol.* 1991;97(1):27-33.
207. Lindroos J, Svensson L, Norsgaard H, et al. IL-23-mediated epidermal hyperplasia is dependent on IL-6. *J Invest Dermatol.* 2011;131(5):1110-1118.
208. Younis S, Rimar D, Slobodin G, et al. Tumor necrosis factor-associated palmoplantar pustular psoriasis treated with interleukin 6 blocker. *J Rheumatol.* 2012;39(10):2055-2056.

Chapter 194 :: Molecular Targeted Therapies
:: David Michael Miller, Bobby Y. Reddy, & Hensin Tsao

第一百九十四章
分子靶向治疗

中文导读

2000年以来，随着分子遗传学、细胞生物学和药理学的进展，人类疾病的治疗策略发生了巨大的变化，针对特定分子靶点相互作用的治疗学得以发展。本章重点介绍了有皮肤科适应证的分子靶向治疗的适应证、禁忌证和注意事项，其中包括了酪氨酸激酶的BCR-ABL、c-KIT、PDGFR；表皮生长因子受体抑制药；SMO抑制药；组蛋白脱乙酰基酶抑制药；MAP激酶途径抑制药的靶向治疗。最后简单介绍了AKT和ERK抑制药是黑色素瘤未来的治疗方向。

〔粟 娟〕

The treatment strategy for human disease has evolved dramatically since 2000 as a result of advances in molecular genetics, cell biology, and pharmacology. Increased understanding of molecular pathophysiology has allowed for the development of therapeutics that interact with specific molecular targets associated with disease. Agents that are the product of rational drug design, in which compounds are deliberately designed to interact with a biologic target, are often referred to as "targeted therapy" and form one of the cornerstones of "precision medicine." The potential of targeted therapy is perhaps best exemplified with oncologic disease, but the promise of rational drug design is beginning to be seen across all fields of medicine.

Discussing all targeted therapies in medicine is beyond the scope of this chapter. Consequently, we focus on those molecular targeted therapies that have the most overlap with dermatology in either their indication or the adverse effects caused by their use (Table 194-1). Thus we review targeted therapies designed to interact with the tyrosine kinases BCR-ABL, c-KIT, PDGFR and EGFR; smoothened; histone deacetylases; and proteins of the MAP kinase pathway. We finish with a section on the future directions in melanoma targeting AKT and ERK proteins.

Of note, marketing indications, contra-indications and warnings are dynamic and constantly evolving. Thus, those covered in this chapter are current as of the writing. Please refer to the FDA product label for the most up-to-date information.

KIT, BCR-ABL, AND PDGFR INHIBITORS

AT-A-GLANCE

- The small-molecule tyrosine kinase inhibitors imatinib, nilotinib, dasatinib, bosutinib, and ponatinib are indicated for Philadelphia chromosome–positive leukemia.
- Imatinib also has indications for dermatofibrosarcoma protuberans, a soft-tissue sarcoma, driven in part by alterations in platelet-derived growth factor receptor signaling.
- Cutaneous adverse effects of these multityrosine kinase inhibitors include edema, morbilliform eruptions, bullous eruptions, dyspigmentation, keratosis-pilaris–like eruptions and neutrophilic dermatoses.

TABLE 194-1
Molecular Target Therapies

GENERIC NAME	BRAND NAME	MOLECULAR TARGET	INDICATION
Imatinib	Gleevec	BCR-ABL, c-KIT, PDGFR	Ph+-CML, GIST, ASM, DFSP, Ph+-ALL, HES/CEL
Nilotinib	Tasigna	BCR-ABL, c-KIT, PDGFR	Ph+-CML
Dasatinib	Sprycel	BCR-ABL, c-KIT, PDGFR	Ph+-CML, Ph+-ALL
Bosutinib	Bosulif	BCR-ABL	Ph+-CML
Ponatinib	Iclusig	BCR-ABL, c-KIT, PDGFR	Ph+-CML, Ph+-ALL
Cetuximab	Erbitux	EGFR	CRC, SCCHN
Panitumumab	Vectibix	EGFR	CRC
Gefitinib	Iressa	EGFR	NSCLC
Erlotinib	Tarceva	EGFR	EGFR-mutated NSCLC, Pancreatic Cancer
Afatinib	Gilotrif	EGFR	EGFR-mutated NSCLC
Osimertinib	Tagrisso	EGFR	EGFR-mutated (T790M) NSCLC
Vismodegib	Erivedge	SMO	BCC
Sonidegib	Odomzo	SMO	BCC
Vorinostat	Zolinza	HDACs	CTCL
Romidepsin	Istodax	HDACs	CTCL, PTCL
Belinostat	Beleodaq	HDACs	PTCL
Panobinostat	Farydak	HDACs	Multiple Myeloma
Vemurafenib	Zelboraf	BRAF^{V600E}	Melanoma
Dabrafenib	Tafinlar	BRAF^{V600E}	Melanoma
Trametinib	Mekinist	MEK	Melanoma
Cobimetinib	Cotellic	MEK	Melanoma

ASM, aggressive systemic mastocytosis; BCC, basal cell carcinoma; CEL, chronic eosinophilic leukemia; CRC, colorectal cancer; CTCL, cutaneous T-cell lymphoma; DFSP, dermatofibrosarcoma protuberans; EGFR, epidermal growth factor receptor; GIST, GI stromal tumor; HDAC, histone deacetylases; HES, hypereosinophilic syndrome; NSCLC, non-small cell lung cancer; PDGFR, platelet-derived growth factor receptor; Ph+-ALL, Philadelphia chromosome-positive acute lymphoblastic leukemia; Ph+-CML, Philadelphia chromosome-positive chronic myeloid leukemia; PTCL, peripheral T-cell lymphoma; SCCHN, squamous cell carcinoma, head and neck; SMO, smoothened.

BACKGROUND

Tyrosine kinases are key components of numerous cellular pathways involved in cell growth, proliferation, migration, angiogenesis, differentiation, and survival. Drug development focusing on tyrosine kinases began after the initial discovery in 1980 that the oncogene associated with Abelson murine leukemia virus, ABL1, was a tyrosine kinase.[1] This finding led to the understanding that a fusion protein, which resulted from a translocation of the *Abl1* gene on chromosome 9 to a part of the breakpoint cluster region (*BCR*) gene on chromosome 22, was the driving event in the majority of chronic myeloid leukemias (CMLs).[2] The protein product of this fusion oncogene, known as the Philadelphia chromosome, was one of the first targets for rational drug design. Cells that express the Philadelphia chromosome are transformed as a result of constitutive activation of the BCR-ABL kinase, which mediates oncogenesis through a variety of transduction pathways including the mitogen-activated protein kinase (MAPK), Janus kinase (JAK)/signal transducer and activator of transcription (STAT), and phosphatidylinositol-4,5-bisphosphate 3-kinase (PI3K) (Fig. 194-1).

One of the earliest proof of principles of "targeted therapy" came via the demonstration that a small molecular inhibitor of the BCR-ABL fusion oncoprotein—imatinib mesylate—inhibited the growth of BCR-ABL–expressing cells[3] and exhibited substantial clinical activity in patients with Philadelphia chromosome–expressing CML and acute lymphoblastic leukemia.[4,5] These data revolutionized the approach to cancer therapy and shifted the drug development paradigm toward identifying disease-causing targets. In dermatofibrosarcoma protuberans, a fusion between the collagen gene (COL1A1) and the platelet-derived growth factor (PDGFR) β-chain gene produces a constitutively active mitogen driven by paracrine and autocrine ligands.[6] Imatinib inhibits the tyrosine kinase associated with PDGFRβ and its use in patients with dermatofibrosarcoma protuberans yields a clinical benefit.[7]

Despite the breakthrough impact that imatinib has had on the field of oncology in general and in several malignancies in particular, nearly one-third of patients with CML require other therapies. Most commonly the reason for alternate treatment is the development of resistance mutations in BCR-ABL1 that affect

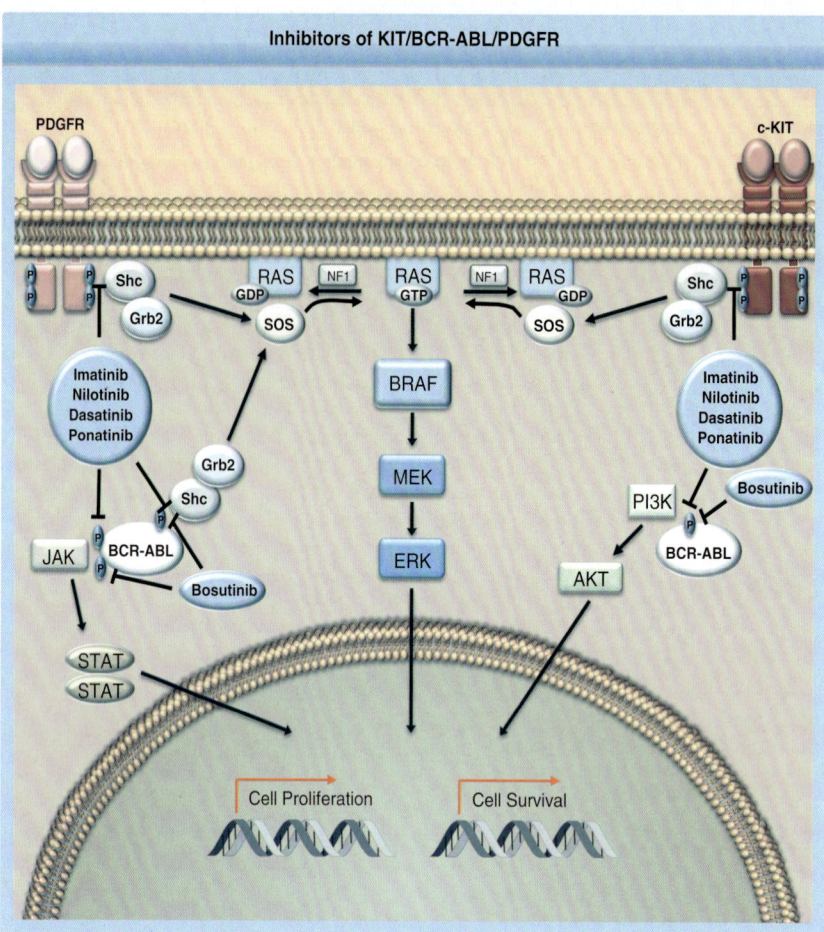

Figure 194-1 Inhibitors of KIT/BCR-ABL/PDGFR. Imatinib, nilotinib, dasatinib, and ponatinib are multi–tyrosine kinase inhibitors that modulate autophosphorylation of tyrosine residues associated with BCR-ABL (breakpoint cluster region–Abelson murine leukemia virus), c-KIT, and PDGFR (platelet-derived growth factor receptor). c-KIT and PDGFR are receptor tyrosine kinases and BCR-ABL is a nonreceptor tyrosine kinase. Bosutinib is an inhibitor of BCR-ABL, but not of c-KIT or PDGFR. The signal transduction pathways downstream of these tyrosine kinases, such as MAPK (mitogen-activated protein kinase) cascade, Janus kinase (JAK)/signal transducer and activator of transcription (STAT), and phosphatidylinositol-4,5-bisphosphate 3-kinase (PI3K) regulate the expression of genes involved in cell growth, proliferation, and cell survival.

the ability of imatinib to interact with the adenosine triphosphate (ATP)-binding pocket. Consequently, second-generation and third-generation tyrosine kinase inhibitors (TKIs) have been developed with enhanced affinity for BCR-ABL. These TKIs include nilotinib, dasatinib, bosutinib, and ponatinib.

amino]-phenyl]benzamide methanesulfonate, has the molecular formula $C_{29}H_{31}N_7O \cdot CH_4SO_3$ and a molecular weight of 589.7 daltons. Figure 194-2 shows its structure.

Metabolism: Imatinib is predominantly metabolized by cytochrome P450 (CYP) 3A4 and the main active metabolite is a N-demethylated piperazine

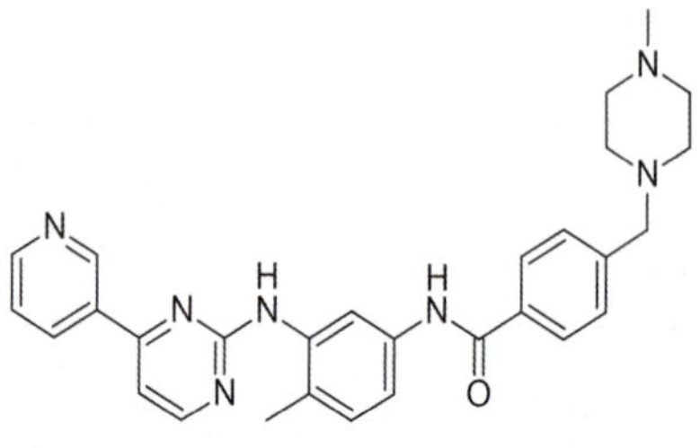

IMATINIB MESYLATE (GLEEVEC)

PHARMACOLOGY AND MECHANISM OF ACTION

Structure: Imatinib, 4-[(4-methyl-1-piperazinyl)methyl]-N-[4-methyl-3-[[4-(3-pyridinyl)-2-pyrimidinyl]

Figure 194-2 Structure of Imatinib.

derivative. The drug and its metabolites are primarily excreted in the feces. The elimination half-life is approximately 18 hours for the unchanged form and 40 hours for the N-desmethyl derivative.[8]

Absorption and Distribution: Imatinib is absorbed orally with bioavailability of 98%. The compound has high levels of binding to circulating plasma proteins, mainly albumin and α_1-acid glycoprotein.

Mechanism of Action: Imatinib mesylate is a small-molecule TKI with activity against BCR-ABL, c-KIT, and PDGFR (see Fig. 194-1). Imatinib binds near the ATP-binding site of the inactive, unphosphorylated confirmation of these kinases, inhibiting the enzyme activity of the protein. In cells with constitutively active BCR-ABL, imatinib induces apoptosis and inhibits proliferation. Imatinib also downregulates cell proliferation triggered by aberrant c-KIT and platelet-derived growth factor (PDGF) signaling.

TABLE 194-2
Dosing for Imatinib

DISEASE	DOSE
Chronic myeloid leukemia, chronic phase	400 mg daily
Chronic myeloid leukemia, accelerated phase or blast crisis	600 mg daily
GI stromal tumors	400 mg daily
Dermatofibrosarcoma protuberans	400 mg twice daily
Aggressive systemic mastocytosis	400 mg daily
Myelodysplastic/myeloproliferative diseases	400 mg daily
Relapsed/refractory Philadelphia chromosome–positive acute lymphocytic leukemia	600 mg daily
Hypereosinophilic syndrome/chronic eosinophilic leukemia	400 mg daily
Melanoma[a]	400 mg twice daily

[a]Use of imatinib for melanoma is not FDA approved; off-label dosing based on NCT00470470.[11]

INDICATIONS AND CONTRAINDICATIONS

Imatinib mesylate was initially approved in 2001 for use in CML. In 2002, the label was updated to include advanced or metastatic GI stromal tumors. In 2006, the U.S. Food and Drug Administration (FDA) further expanded the approval to include dermatofibrosarcoma protuberans, aggressive systemic mastocytosis, myelodysplastic/myeloproliferative diseases with PDGFR gene rearrangements, relapsed/refractory Philadelphia chromosome–positive acute lymphocytic leukemia, and hypereosinophilic syndrome/chronic eosinophilic leukemia with FIP1L1-PDGFR fusion kinase rearrangements.

Off-label uses of imatinib have been reported for melanomas harboring KIT alterations, which occur at a higher frequency in melanomas arising from mucosal, acral and chronically sun-damaged skin. Data from several newer trials suggest a modest clinical benefit as a single agent in c-KIT–mutated melanoma and newer National Comprehensive Cancer Network (NCCN) guidelines include imatinib as a treatment option for metastatic melanoma.[9-11] Clinical activity of imatinib is also being investigated for desmoid tumors and for advanced or metastatic chordomas expressing PDGFRβ and/or PDGFβ.

There are no contraindications on the manufacturer's label.

DOSING REGIMEN

Table 194-2 outlines the dosing regimens for imatinib.

Dosing adjustments for hepatic and renal impairment are recommended. For patients with mild renal impairment (creatinine clearance [CrCl] = 40 to 59 mL/min), doses of greater than 600 mg are not recommended. A 50% reduction in the starting dose is recommended for patients with moderate renal impairment (CrCl = 20 to 39 mL/min), with subsequent dose increases given as tolerated to a maximum recommended dose of 400 mg. Use imatinib with caution in patients with several renal impairment (CrCl <20 mL/min); no specific recommendations have been defined. Dose reductions of 25% are recommended for patients with severe hepatic impairment (total bilirubin >3 times to 10 times the upper limits of normal [ULN]).

SIDE EFFECTS AND PRECAUTIONS

Adverse Effects: The most common adverse effects include edema, nausea, vomiting, muscle cramps, myalgias, diarrhea, bone pain, fatigue, and abdominal pain. Less common but serious adverse effects include severe fluid retention (eg, pericardial effusion, pulmonary edema, pleural effusions, and ascites), hematologic toxicity (eg, anemia, neutropenia, and thrombocytopenia), congestive heart failure, liver failure, and hemorrhage.

A wide variety of cutaneous side effects have been reported in patients taking imatinib, including periorbital edema, dyspigmentation, morbilliform eruption, pityriasis rosea-like eruption, acute generalized exanthematous pustulosis, exacerbation of psoriasis, drug rash with eosinophilia and systemic symptoms, pseudoporphyria, mycosis fungoides–like eruption, acute neutrophilic dermatosis, erythroderma, Stevens-Johnson syndrome, perforating folliculitis, and urticaria.[12]

Women of reproductive age should be counseled that imatinib is a pregnancy category D drug as it was teratogenic when tested in rodents and there have been postmarket reports of congenital anomalies from pregnant women on imatinib. Thus, patients should be advised to use highly effective contraception and avoid pregnancy while taking imatinib.

Nursing mothers should be counseled that imatinib and its metabolites have been detected in human breastmilk and nursing infants could receive up to 10%

of the maternal dose. Given the risk to infants, breast-feeding is not recommended while taking imatinib.

Drug Interactions: Because of its metabolism by CYP3A4, drug concentrations of imatinib are affected by agents that inhibit or induce CYP3A4. Furthermore, studies demonstrate that imatinib is a moderate inhibitor of CYP3A4 and weakly inhibits CYP2D6; therefore, caution should be used when prescribing imatinib with CYP3A4 and CYP2D6 substrates with a narrow therapeutic window.

Please see the Gleevec package insert for full drug–drug interactions and adverse effects.[8]

NILOTINIB (TASIGNA)

PHARMACOLOGY AND MECHANISM OF ACTION

Structure: Nilotinib, 4-methyl-*N*-[3-(4-methyl-1H-imidazol-1-yl)-5-(trifluoromethyl)phenyl]-3-[[4-(3-pyridinyl)-2-pyrimidinyl]amino]-benzamide, monohydrochloride, monohydrate, has the molecular formula $C_{28}H_{22}F_3N_7O \cdot HCl \cdot H_2O$ and molecular weight of 584 daltons. Figure 194-3 shows the structure of nilotinib.

Metabolism: Nilotinib is metabolized by CYP3A4 and metabolism is predominantly by oxidation and hydroxylation. The vast majority of the dose (93%) is eliminated in the feces. The elimination half-life is estimated at 17 hours.[13]

Absorption and Distribution: Nilotinib is absorbed orally and absorption is increased when given 30 minutes after a meal. Of the circulating compound, 98% is bound to serum protein.

Mechanism of Action: Similar to its forerunner imatinib, nilotinib is a multityrosine kinase inhibitor. The compound binds and stabilizes the inactive conformation of the kinase domain of its target proteins (BCR-ABL, KIT, PDGFR, discoidin domain receptor). It was rationally designed based on the structure of its predecessor to overcome resistance in CML to imatinib. Rational designs of the compound yield a significantly higher affinity and inhibitor activity of nilotinib against BCR-ABL compared with imatinib, while maintaining its activity against PDGFR and KIT.

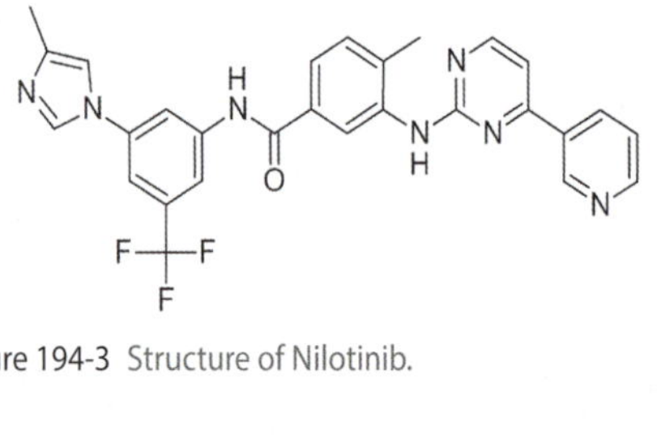

Figure 194-3 Structure of Nilotinib.

INDICATIONS AND CONTRAINDICATIONS

Nilotinib is indicated for adult patients with either newly diagnosed Philadelphia chromosome–positive (Ph⁺) CML in chronic phase or accelerated-phase CML that is resistant or intolerant to prior treatment with imatinib. Nilotinib does not have any current FDA-approved indications for dermatologic disease.

However, the results with imatinib in c-KIT–mutated melanoma have provided the rationale for early phase trials exploring the usefulness of nilotinib in these subsets. Similar to imatinib, the results have been modest. In one trial, 7 (16.7%) of 42 patients with metastatic KIT-altered melanoma achieved a response with single-agent nilotinib.[14] In a second trial of patients with advanced melanoma harboring KIT mutations or amplifications who had received prior KIT inhibitor therapy, 4 (21%) of 19 patients experienced a response.[15]

Nilotinib is contraindicated for use in patients with long QT syndrome, hypokalemia, or hypomagnesemia.

DOSING REGIMEN

The recommended dose for newly diagnosed Ph⁺ chronic-phase CML is 300 mg by mouth twice daily; for resistant or intolerant Ph⁺ chronic-phase CML and accelerated-phase CML, 400 mg by mouth twice daily is recommended.

Nilotinib should not be taken with food. It is recommended to avoid food for at least 2 hours before and 1 hour after the dose is taken. Foods that inhibit CYP3A4 should be avoided.

Dose adjustments are recommended for a variety of indications, including impaired hepatic function, QT interval, and hematologic toxicity. See the Tasigna product label for full dose adjustment recommendations.

SIDE EFFECTS AND PRECAUTIONS

Adverse Effects: The most common adverse effects include cutaneous toxicities (see below), thrombocytopenia, neutropenia, anemia, constipation, nausea, vomiting, hyperbilirubinemia, fatigue, elevated lipase, and elevated transaminases.

Serious adverse effects include a boxed warning for QT prolongation and sudden death. Thus, nilotinib is not recommended for use in patients with hypokalemia, hypomagnesemia, or long QT syndrome. Medications known to prolong the QT interval or that strongly inhibit CYP3A4 should also be avoided. Potassium, calcium, magnesium, phosphate, or sodium electrolyte abnormalities should be corrected prior to initiation and should be periodically monitored during therapy.

In the initial trial of nilotinib in CML, cutaneous toxicities were the most common adverse effects noted and included rash (specific morphologies not described), pruritus, dry skin, and alopecia. Postmarket reports have included a case of bullous Sweet syndrome.[12]

Nilotinib is a pregnancy category D drug, based on its mechanism of action and data in animal studies that the compound may cause fetal harm. Women with reproductive potential should be advised to use highly effective contraception during therapy. Findings in animal studies demonstrate that nilotinib may be unsafe during nursing. It is recommended to consider alternatives to breastfeeding or to weigh the risks against the benefits of use during nursing.

Drug Interactions: As nilotinib is a substrate of CYP3A4, inhibitors and inducers of CYP3A4 may affect serum concentrations. Nilotinib is an inhibitor of CYP3A4, CYP2C8, CYP2C9, and CYP2D6, and may also induce CYP2B6, CYP2C8, and CYP2C9. Thus, coadministration of nilotinib with substrates of these enzymes may affect the serum concentrations.

See the Tasigna product label for full drug–drug interactions and adverse effects.[13]

DASATINIB (SPRYCEL)

PHARMACOLOGY AND MECHANISM OF ACTION

Structure: Dasatinib, N-(2-chloro-6-methylphenyl)-2-[[6-[4-(2-hydroxyethyl)-1-piperazinyl]-2-methyl-4-pyrimidinyl]amino]-5-thiazolecarboxamide, monohydrate, has the molecular formula $C_{22}H_{26}ClN_7O_2S \cdot H_2O$, which corresponds to a formula weight of 506.02 daltons for the monohydrate form and 488.01 daltons for the anhydrous free base.[16] Figure 194-4 shows the structure of dasatinib.

Metabolism: Dasatinib is predominantly metabolized by CYP3A4. Dasatinib metabolites are also produced by uridine diphosphate-glucuronosyltransferase (UGT) and flavin-containing monooxygenase 3 (FMO-3) enzymes. The estimated elimination half-life is 3 to 5 hours. Dasatinib is primarily excreted through the feces.

Absorption and Distribution: Following oral administration, peak plasma concentrations are reached between 30 minutes and 6 hours. The apparent volume of distribution is 2505 L.

Mechanism of Action: Dasatinib is a small molecule kinase inhibitor. It inhibits numerous kinases, including BCR-ABL, c-KIT, PDGFRβ, SRC family (SRC, LCK, YES, FYN), and EPHA2. In preclinical in vitro studies, dasatinib inhibited the growth of BCR-ABL overexpressing CML and acute lymphoblastic leukemia (ALL) cell lines.[16] In these assays, dasatinib was effective in cell lines that possess BCR-ABL kinase mutations that conferred resistance to imatinib.

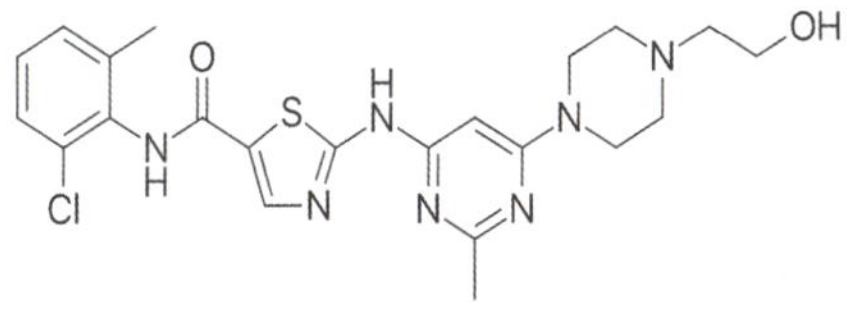

INDICATIONS AND CONTRAINDICATIONS

Dasatinib has FDA approval for adults with (a) newly diagnosed Ph+ chronic-phase CML, (b) chronic, accelerated, or myeloid or lymphoid blast-phase Ph+-CML with intolerance or resistance to previous therapy including imatinib, and (c) adults with Ph+-ALL with intolerance or resistance to previous therapy.

In melanoma, early-phase investigations with dasatinib have shown only a modest clinical benefit when used a monotherapy[17] or in combination with systemic chemotherapy.[18]

There are no contraindications listed on the manufacturer's label.

DOSING REGIMEN

The recommended oral dose is 100 mg daily for chronic-phase CML and 140 mg once daily for accelerated-phase CML, myeloid or lymphoid blast-phase CML, or Ph+-ALL.

Please see the manufacturer's label for dose modification for neutropenia, thrombocytopenia, and concomitant use of CYP3A4 modifiers. Studies were not performed in patients with impaired renal function, thus there are no specific dose modifications for patients with renal impairment.

SIDE EFFECTS AND PRECAUTIONS

Adverse Effects: For newly diagnosed chronic-phase CML, the most common adverse effects are myelosuppression, diarrhea, and fluid retention. Patients who have previously progressed, or were intolerant to prior imatinib therapy, commonly experience myelosuppression, fluid retention, diarrhea, headache, fatigue, dyspnea, nausea, hemorrhage, musculoskeletal pain, and skin toxicity.

Cutaneous adverse effects include neutrophilic dermatosis,[19] keratosis pilaris–like lesions and pustules, white keratotic papules, and milia.[20]

Drug Interactions: Caution is advised when dasatinib is used concomitantly with strong CYP3A4 inducers (including, but not limited to phenytoin, rifampin, phenobarbital, carbamazepine, dexamethasone, rifabutin) and strong CYP3A4 inhibitors (ketoconazole, voriconazole, itraconazole, atazanavir, nelfinavir, indinavir, ritonavir, saquinavir, nefazodone, telithromycin, and clarithromycin). It is recommended to avoid St. John's wort and grapefruit juice while taking dasatinib.

It is recommended to advise women of reproductive potential to avoid pregnancy during treatment with dasatinib and for at least 30 days following the final dose. Breastfeeding is not recommended while taking dasatinib and for at least 2 weeks after the final dose.

Figure 194-4 Structure of Dasatinib.

Use with caution in patients with hepatic impairment. See the Sprycel package insert for full drug–drug interactions and adverse effects.[16]

BOSUTINIB (BOSULIF)

PHARMACOLOGY AND MECHANISM OF ACTION

Structure: Bosutinib, 3-Quinolinecarbonitrile, 4-[(2,4-dichloro-5-methoxyphenyl)amino]-6-methoxy-7-[3-(4-methyl-1-piperazinyl) propoxy]-, hydrate (1:1), has the chemical formula $C_{26}H_{29}Cl_2N_5O_3 \cdot H_2O$ (monohydrate); its molecular weight is 548.46 (monohydrate), equivalent to 530.46 (anhydrous).[21] Figure 194-5 shows the structure of bosutinib.

Metabolism: Bosutinib is predominantly metabolized by CYP3A4 and primarily excreted through the feces.

Absorption and Distribution: Oral bioavailability is 34% when taken with food and following oral administration; peak plasma concentrations are reached between 4 and 6 hours. The apparent volume of distribution is 6080 L ± 1230 L.

Mechanism of Action: Bosutinib is a small-molecular-weight kinase inhibitor. It inhibits numerous kinases, including BCR-ABL and the SRC family kinases SRC, LCK, and FYN. In preclinical in vitro studies, bosutinib inhibited the growth of 16 of 18 BCR-ABL overexpressing murine myeloid cell lines that were resistant to imatinib. Bosutinib did not inhibit the mutant cell lines that expressed the T315I and V299L resistance mutations.[21]

INDICATIONS AND CONTRAINDICATIONS

Bosutinib has FDA approval for adults with chronic-phase, accelerated-phase, or blast-phase Ph+-CML with intolerance or resistance to previous therapy. Bosutinib does not have any current FDA-approved indications for dermatologic disease.

Bosutinib is contraindicated in patients with a known hypersensitivity to the drug.

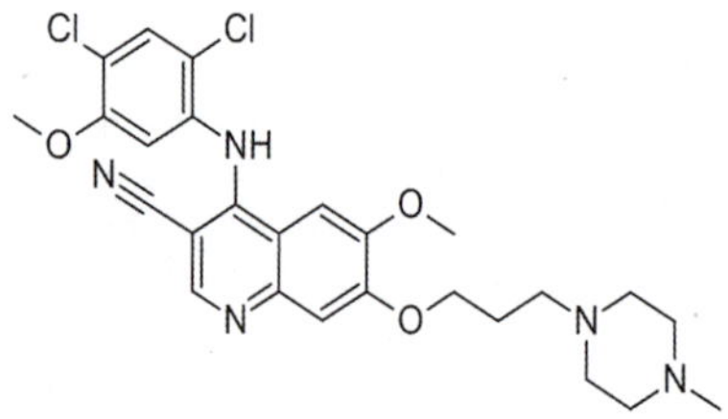

Figure 194-5 Structure of Bosutinib.

DOSING REGIMEN

The recommended oral dose is 500 mg once daily with food.

See the manufacturer's label for dose modifications for neutropenia, thrombocytopenia, renal impairment, hepatic impairment, and concomitant use of CYP3A4 modifiers.

SIDE EFFECTS AND PRECAUTIONS

Adverse Effects: The most common adverse effects are diarrhea, nausea, thrombocytopenia, vomiting, abdominal pain, rash (not otherwise specified), anemia, pyrexia, and fatigue.

Bosutinib is a pregnancy category D drug, and it is recommended to advise women of reproductive potential to avoid pregnancy during treatment. As to breastfeeding, bosutinib may be excreted in human milk and thus the risk of harm to a nursing infant must be weighed with the importance of the drug to the mother.

Drug Interactions: Caution is advised when bosutinib is used concomitantly with strong CYP3A4 inducers (including, but not limited to, phenytoin, rifampin, phenobarbital, carbamazepine, dexamethasone, rifabutin) and strong CYP3A4 inhibitors (ketoconazole, voriconazole, itraconazole, atazanavir, nelfinavir, indinavir, ritonavir, saquinavir, nefazodone, telithromycin, and clarithromycin). It is recommended to avoid St. John's wort and grapefruit juice while taking bosutinib. Proton pump inhibitors can reduce exposure to bosutinib and should be avoided if possible. Consider H_2 blockers or short-acting antacids.

See the Bosulif package insert for full drug–drug interactions and adverse effects.[21]

PONATINIB (ICLUSIG)

PHARMACOLOGY AND MECHANISM OF ACTION

Structure: Ponatinib, 3-(imidazo[1,2-b]pyridazin-3-ylethynyl)-4-methyl-N-{4-[(4-methylpiperazin-1-yl)methyl]-3-(trifluoromethyl)phenyl}benzamide hydrochloride, has the chemical formula $C_{29}H_{28}ClF_3N_6O$, which corresponds to a molecular weight of 569.02 daltons.[22] Figure 194-6 shows the structure of ponatinib.

Metabolism: Ponatinib is metabolized by CYP3A4, and to a lesser degree by CYP2C8, CYP2D6, and CYP3A5. It is also metabolized by amidases and/or esterases. Ponatinib is primarily excreted through the feces.

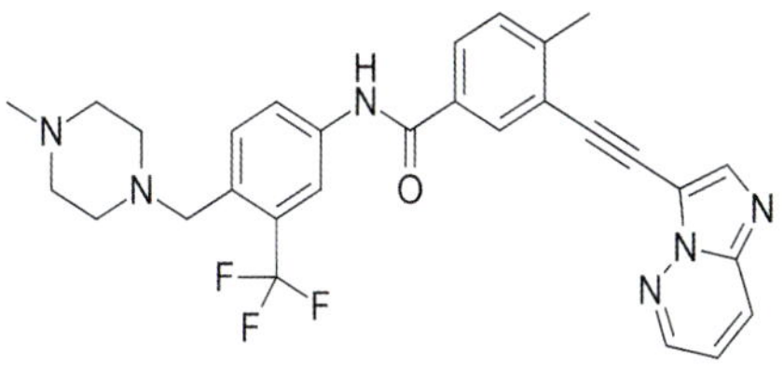

Figure 194-6 Structure of Ponatinib.

Absorption and Distribution: Following oral administration, peak plasma concentrations are reached within 6 hours. The apparent volume of distribution is 1223 L.

Mechanism of Action: Ponatinib is a small-molecular-weight kinase inhibitor. It inhibits a variety of kinases, including BCR-ABL, VEGFR (vascular endothelial growth factor receptor), PDGFR, FGFR (fibroblast growth factor receptor), EPH (ephrin), KIT, RET, TIE2 (TEK receptor tyrosine kinase), FLT3 (fms-related tyrosine kinase 3), and the SRC family kinases. Ponatinib also inhibits the T315I mutation that confers resistance to imatinib.

INDICATIONS AND CONTRAINDICATIONS

Ponatinib has FDA approval for adults with T315I-mutant-positive chronic-phase, accelerated-phase, or blast-phase CML or T315I-mutant-positive Ph+-ALL. It is also approved for adults with chronic-phase, accelerated-phase, or blast-phase CML or Ph+-ALL in which no other TKI treatment is indicated. Ponatinib does not have any current FDA-approved indications for dermatologic disease.

There are no contraindications listed on the manufacturer's label.

DOSING REGIMEN

The recommended oral dose is 45 mg once daily taken with or without food.

Please see the manufacturer's label for dose modification for neutropenia, thrombocytopenia, renal impairment, hepatic impairment, and concomitant use of CYP modifiers.

SIDE EFFECTS AND PRECAUTIONS

Adverse Effects: The most common nonhematologic adverse effects include hypertension, rash (not otherwise specified), fatigue, xerosis, headache, abdominal pain, constipation, nausea, arthralgia, and pyrexia. Hematologic toxicities include myelosuppression including leukopenia, neutropenia and thrombocytopenia, anemia, and lymphopenia.

Ponatinib has a boxed warning for vascular occlusion, including arterial and venous thrombosis, which occurred in at least 27% of patients, heart failure and hepatotoxicity.

Ponatinib is a pregnancy category D drug and it is recommended to advise women of reproductive potential to avoid pregnancy during treatment. With considerations to breastfeeding, it is unknown if ponatinib is excreted in human milk and thus the risk of harm to a nursing infant must be weighed with the importance of the drug to the mother.

Drug Interactions: Caution is advised when ponatinib is used concomitantly with strong CYP3A inducers and inhibitors.

See the Iclusig package insert for full drug–drug interactions and adverse effects.[22]

EPIDERMAL GROWTH FACTOR RECEPTOR INHIBITORS

AT-A-GLANCE

- The epidermal growth factor receptor (EGFR) is found on the cell surface of a variety of epithelial cells and is dysregulated in numerous malignancies.
- Monoclonal antibodies that block epidermal growth factor binding to EGFR and small-molecular-weight inhibitors of the EGFR intracellular tyrosine kinase have been approved as therapy for several types of cancer.
- Although there are no FDA-approved dermatologic indications at the time of publication of this book, clinical investigations in cutaneous oncology are ongoing.
- EGFR inhibitors commonly have skin toxicities that include papulopustular eruptions, pruritus, xeroderma, and paronychia.

BACKGROUND

Drug development focused on the EGFR (also known as ErbB1 or HER1) showcases the potential of targeted therapy, rational drug design and personalized medicine. Although agents that inhibit EGFR signaling do not currently have any FDA-approved dermatologic indications, investigations into their use in cutaneous malignancy are ongoing. In addition these agents, which include cetuximab, panitumumab, gefitinib, erlotinib, afatinib, and osimertinib have significant cutaneous adverse effects and thus knowledge of their indication, mechanism of action, and associated toxicities is relevant to all dermatologists.

EGFR is a member of the ErbB family of tyrosine kinase receptors, which also includes ErbB2 (HER2/neu), ErbB3 (HER3), and ErbB4 (HER4). These cell-surface proteins possess an extracellular ligand-binding domain, a transmembrane domain and an intracellular tyrosine kinase domain (Fig. 194-7). EGFR, which is found on a variety of cell types, including keratinocytes and cells of various solid tumors, is activated following binding of epidermal growth factor (EGF) and other growth factors. Ligand binding to the extracellular domain of EGFR results in dimerization in which the receptor either binds with another EGFR protein or heterodimerizes with an additional monomer of the ErbB family. Dimerization triggers the intracellular tyrosine kinase to autophosphorylate several tyrosine residues. Subsequent recognition of the phosphorylated tyrosine residues on the C-terminal domain of the receptor by various adaptor proteins initiates downstream signal transduction signaling. EGFR activation can trigger networks involved in tumor growth and proliferation, inhibition of apoptosis and metastases such as the MAPK, STAT, PI3K, and phospholipase pathways.

Dysregulation of EGFR signaling is common in several epithelial cancers and can occur through multiple mechanisms including gene amplification and activating mutations. In 2004, the discovery of in-frame activating deletions in exon 19 and the L858R substitution in exon 21 of EGFR profoundly changed the therapeutic landscape in non–small-cell lung cancer (NSCLC) and provided an additional early rationale for precision medicine in oncology.[23,24]

Two distinct mechanisms have been developed to interrupt EGFR signaling as a therapeutic strategy in

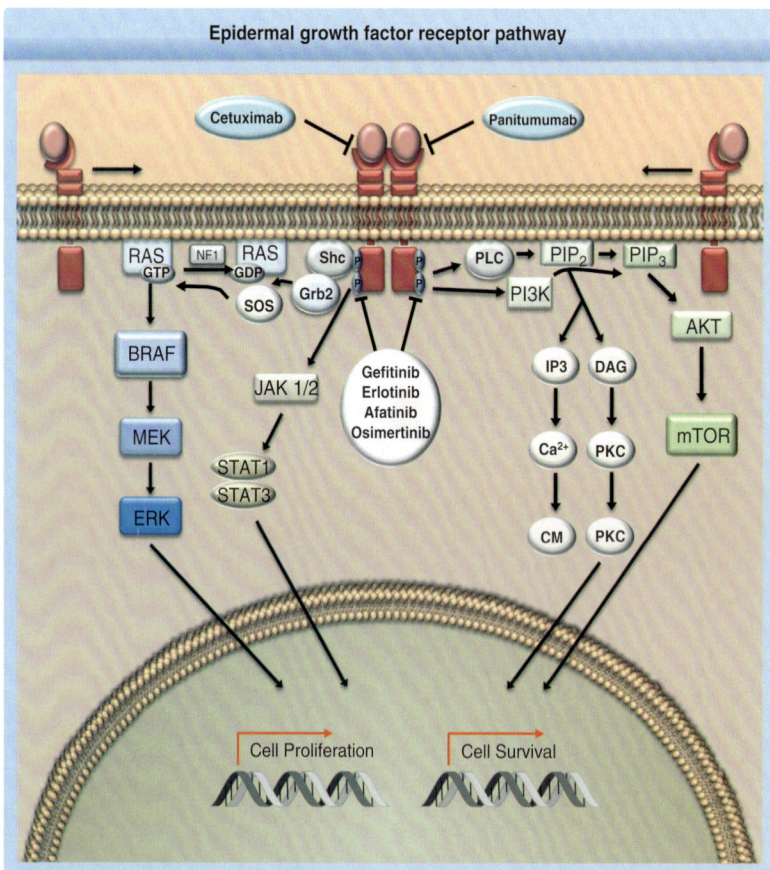

Figure 194-7 Epidermal growth factor receptor (EGFR) pathway. The human epidermal growth receptor is a cell-surface protein comprised of an extracellular ligand-binding domain, a transmembrane domain, and an intracellular tyrosine kinase domain. Binding of the epidermal growth factor and other ligands to the extracellular domain results in dimerization in which the receptor either binds with another EGFR protein (seen above) or heterodimerizes with an additional monomer of the ErbB family. Dimerization triggers the intracellular tyrosine kinase to autophosphorylate several tyrosine residues. Subsequent recognition of the phosphorylated tyrosine residues on the C-terminal domain of the receptor by various adaptor proteins initiates downstream signal transduction signaling. EGFR activation can trigger networks involved in cell proliferation, cell survival and metastases such as the mitogen-activated protein kinase (MAPK), Janus kinase(JAK)/signal transducer and activator of transcription (STAT), phosphatidylinositol-4,5-bisphosphate 3-kinase (PI3K), and phospholipase C (PLC) pathways.

cancer: (a) targeting of the extracellular ligand binding domain via monoclonal antibodies and (b) inhibition of intracellular tyrosine kinase via small molecules.

The monoclonal antibodies cetuximab and panitumumab have demonstrated efficacy in several carcinomas. Cetuximab holds approval for colorectal and head and neck cancer and panitumumab is indicated in combination with systemic chemotherapy for colorectal cancer.

During the 1990s a concerted effort began to develop small-molecular-weight compounds that inhibit various tyrosine kinases. The first-generation TKIs against EGFR, gefitinib and erlotinib, were designed as competitive inhibitors of ATP binding to the intracellular kinase domain. Despite promising preclinical data, early clinical studies in lung cancer with gefitinib were discouraging as ISEL (Iressa Survival Evaluation in Lung Cancer), a large trial of unselected, heavily pretreated patients, did not show an overall survival benefit in patients with NSCLC.[25] Interestingly, subgroup analysis revealed that never-smokers and Asian patients achieved better overall survival with gefitinib. Translational studies subsequently demonstrated the importance of the exon 19 and exon 21 EGFR mutations as predictive biomarkers. These somatic mutations, which encode the tyrosine kinase domain of EGFR (encoded by exons 18 to 24), occur at higher frequency in adenocarcinomas, nonsmokers, and Asians. These alterations reduce the affinity of the tyrosine kinase to ATP and thus confer enhanced sensitivity to EGFR TKIs. Followup studies in NSCLC with gefitinib and erlotinib incorporating EGFR-mutation biomarkers have demonstrated superior clinical benefit in patients with exon 19 and exon 21 alterations.[26,27] As a result, erlotinib and the second-generation TKI afatinib are indicated only for NSCLC patients with tumors that possess exon 19 or exon 21 alterations.

Despite initial response to monotherapy EGFR TKI, resistance emerges for the majority of patients within the first 1 to 2 years following initiation of treatment. Secondary mutations in the tyrosine kinase domain of EGFR are associated with the development of resistance to reversible TKIs in the majority of patients. The most clinically relevant secondary mutation, the T790M of exon 20, has been detected in nearly 60% of patients who have become resistant while taking gefitinib or erlotinib.[28] The T790M mutation replaces threonine with a larger methionine residue, simultaneously enhancing the affinity of the EGFR kinase for ATP and sterically impeding drug binding.[29] Showcasing the success of rational drug development, osimertinib, a small molecule inhibitor with activity against EGFR possessing T790M, was shown to be highly active in lung cancer patients with the T790M resistance mutation.[30] This sequence of developmental successes, beginning with the identification a disease-causing protein, demonstrating the clinical efficacy with disruption of that target, followed by second-generation and third-generation modifications of therapies to overcome mechanisms of resistance, exemplifies the goal of targeted therapy.

CETUXIMAB (ERBITUX)

PHARMACOLOGY AND MECHANISM OF ACTION

Structure: Cetuximab is a recombinant, human/mouse chimeric monoclonal antibody. It is a composite of the Fv region of a murine anti-EGFR antibody with a human immunoglobulin G_1 heavy-chain and kappa light-chain constant regions.[31] It has an approximate molecular weight of 152,000 daltons.

Metabolism: The estimated elimination half-life of cetuximab is approximately 112 hours. Clearance of cetuximab appears to be similar to pathways of metabolism for other biologics, including internalization of the ligand-receptor complex with subsequent removal from the circulation.[32]

Absorption and Distribution: Cetuximab is administered intravenously and exhibits nonlinear pharmacokinetics. The volume of distribution appeared to be independent of dose and approximated 2 to 3 L/m^2. Cetuximab reaches steady-state plasma concentrations by the third weekly infusion.

Mechanism of Action: Cetuximab is a monoclonal antibody with affinity for the extracellular ligand-binding portion of EGFR. Cetuximab acts as a competitive inhibitor for EGF and other ligands on normal epithelium as well as tumor cells. Preclinical studies have demonstrated that cetuximab binding to EGFR precludes receptor-associated kinase activation and downregulates signal transduction pathways associated with cell growth, proliferation, angiogenesis, and metastases.[31]

INDICATIONS AND CONTRAINDICATIONS

Cetuximab is FDA approved for use in colorectal and head and neck cancer. Initial approval in 2004 was granted for use in metastatic colorectal cancer (mCRC) in combination with irinotecan in patients who are refractory to irinotecan-based therapy. On March 1, 2006, the FDA expanded approval for use in combination with radiotherapy for patients with local or regionally advanced squamous cell carcinoma of the head and neck (SCCHN) or as monotherapy for patients with recurrent or metastatic SCCHN whose tumors were refractory to platinum-based chemotherapy. In 2011, cetuximab was approved for patients with recurrent locoregional or metastatic SCCHN in combination with platinum-based therapy plus 5-fluorouracil. On July 6, 2012, the FDA granted approval to cetuximab for first-line therapy in combination with FOLFIRI (irinotecan, 5-fluorouracil, and leucovorin) in patients with wildtype K-ras mCRC that expresses EGFR. Erbitux is not indicated for use in patients with RAS-mutated colorectal cancer.

Cetuximab has been investigated for use in cutaneous squamous cell carcinoma (cSCC), although the totality of the efficacy data to date are limited. A Phase II, uncontrolled trial of 36 chemotherapy-naïve patients with unresectable or metastatic cSCC who were treated with an initial dose of 400 mg/m² body surface area of cetuximab, followed by weekly doses of 250 mg/m² for at least 6 weeks, was published in 2011.[33] This small study reported a complete response in 2 (6%), a partial response in 8 (22%), and stable disease in 15 (42%) of the 36 patients at 6 weeks. Nevertheless, responses were limited in duration, with the median duration of response for the responders of 5 months. Additional prospective studies with larger number of patients are needed to better assess the efficacy of cetuximab in cSCC.

There are no contraindications on the manufacturer's label.

DOSING REGIMEN

Cetuximab is given as an IV infusion. The initial dose is 400 mg/m² infused over 120 minutes, followed by weekly infusions at 250 mg/m². See the manufacturer's label for premedication recommendations and additional dose and infusion rate modifications.

SIDE EFFECTS AND PRECAUTIONS

Adverse Effects: The most common adverse reactions are cutaneous toxicity, headache, diarrhea, and infection. Cetuximab carries a boxed warning for serious, potentially fatal, infusion reactions that occurred in approximately 3% of patients and for cardiopulmonary arrest and/or sudden death. Close monitoring of serum electrolytes during and after infusion is strongly recommended. Other serious adverse effects include interstitial lung disease and hypomagnesemia.

Similar to other agents that disrupt EGFR signaling, skin toxicities are common with cetuximab and include a papulopustular eruption, xerosis, pruritus, mucositis, alopecia, trichomegaly, paronychia, and onycholysis.[34] The development of an acne-like eruption occurs typically within 1 to 2 weeks of initiation of cetuximab therapy and also is associated with improved clinical outcomes.[35]

Cetuximab is a pregnancy category C drug, and should be used during pregnancy only if the potential harms to the fetus are outweighed by the potential benefit to the mother. Immunoglobulin G antibodies, such as cetuximab, are secreted in human milk; consequently, breastfeeding should be avoided during and at least up to 60 days after treatment, if possible, to prevent potential adverse reactions to nursing infants.

Drug Interactions: No drug interactions are listed on the manufacturer's label.

PANITUMUMAB (VECTIBIX)

PHARMACOLOGY AND MECHANISM OF ACTION

Structure: Panitumumab is a recombinant, human immunoglobulin G_2 kappa monoclonal antibody with a molecular weight of 147,000 daltons.[36] It is engineered in Chinese hamster ovary cells.

Metabolism: The mean estimated elimination half-life is 7.5 days.

Absorption and Distribution: Administration of the recommended dose will result in reaching steady-state concentrations by the third infusion.

Mechanism of Action: Panitumumab is a monoclonal antibody with affinity for the extracellular ligand-binding portion of EGFR. Panitumumab, like cetuximab, functions as a competitive inhibitor for EGF and other ligands on both normal epithelium and tumor cells. Preclinical studies have demonstrated that binding to EGFR by panitumumab decreases receptor-associated kinase activation, resulting in downregulated signal transduction pathways that are associated with cell growth, proliferation, angiogenesis, and metastases.

INDICATIONS AND CONTRAINDICATIONS

Panitumumab is indicated for the treatment of mCRC that is wildtype for KRAS as determined by an FDA-approved test. It has FDA approval as first-line therapy in combination with FOLFOX and as monotherapy following progression after treatment with a regimen incorporating fluoropyrimidine, oxaliplatin, and irinotecan. Panitumumab is not approved for use in mCRC patients who possess a KRAS mutation or for whom the mutation status of KRAS is unknown.

Panitumumab is currently in development for head and neck cancer.

Use of panitumumab has been reported in locally advanced cSCC with promising results. The successful use of panitumumab in an elderly patient who had an anaphylactic reaction to cetuximab[37] and in a small Phase II trial of 16 patients who produced a best overall response rate by RECIST criteria of 31% have been reported.[38] Although promising, pivotal Phase III trials are needed to confirm these early investigational results.

There are no contraindications on the manufacturer's label.

DOSING REGIMEN

Panitumumab is administered as an IV infusion and the recommended dose is 6 mg/kg every 14 days.

There are no specific dosing adjustments for renal or hepatic impairment.

SIDE EFFECTS AND PRECAUTIONS

Adverse Effects: The most common adverse effects are skin toxicity, fatigue, nausea, and diarrhea. Serious adverse effects include electrolyte disturbance, infusion reactions, pulmonary fibrosis/interstitial lung disease, and keratitis. Panitumumab carries a box warning for dermatologic toxicity. Skin adverse events were common in the registration trial, with 90% of patients experiencing toxicity of any grade, while 15% suffered from severe skin toxicity. The cutaneous manifestations include, but are not limited to, papulopustular eruptions, exfoliation, pruritus, erythema, photosensitivity, xeroderma, and paronychia. Fatal bullous disease and life-threatening necrotizing fasciitis, abscesses and sepsis have been observed in patients on panitumumab.[36]

Panitumumab is a pregnancy category C drug. No studies have been performed in pregnant women, although Cynomolgus monkeys treated with 1.25 to 5 times the recommended human dose did demonstrate evidence of embryo lethality and abortions. Consequently, extreme caution is recommended with administration during pregnancy and the risks to the fetus must be weighed against the potential benefit to the mother.

It is recommended that breastfeeding by avoided during treatment of at least 2 months following completion of treatment.

Drug Interactions: No specific drug interactions are listed on the manufacturer's label.

GEFITINIB (IRESSA)

PHARMACOLOGY AND MECHANISM OF ACTION

Structure: Gefitinib, 4-quinazolinamine N-(3-chloro-4-uorophenyl)-7-methoxy-6-[3-(4-morpholinyl) propoxy], has the molecular formula $C_{22}H_{24}ClFN_4O_3$ and a molecular mass of 446.9 daltons.[39] Figure 194-8 shows the structure of gefitinib.

Metabolism: Gefitinib is metabolized predominantly by CYP3A4 and to a lesser degree by CYP2D6. The estimated elimination half-life is 48 hours after intravenous administration.

Absorption and Distribution: The oral bioavailability of gefitinib is approximately 60% and peak plasma levels are reached 3 to 7 hours after dosing.

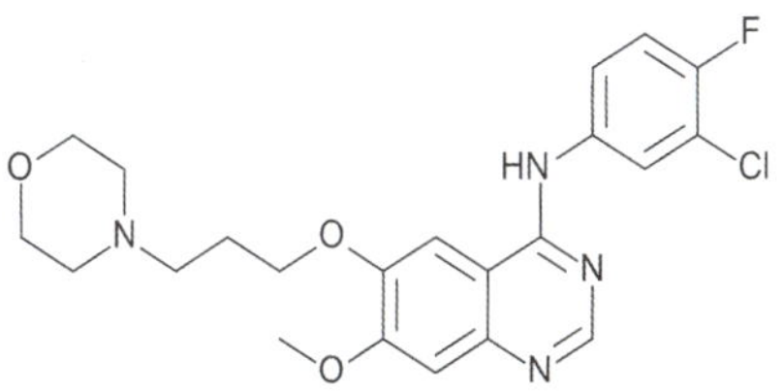

Figure 194-8 Structure of gefitinib.

Food does not significantly affect absorption. The volume of distribution is 1400 L.

Mechanism of Action: Gefitinib is a small-molecule TKI. It reversibly binds and inhibits the kinase domain of EGFR. Gefitinib has a higher affinity for EGFR harboring exon 19 deletions or the exon 21 point mutation L858R, as compared with the wild-type EGFR protein.

INDICATIONS AND CONTRAINDICATIONS

Gefitinib has limited indication in the United States to patients with NSCLC who are currently receiving and benefitting from gefitinib or have previously benefited from therapy with gefitinib. Gefitinib was initially granted accelerated approval by the FDA in May 2003 for patients with NSCLC tumors that were refractory to a platinum-based regimen and docetaxel. However, after 2 studies demonstrated a lack of efficacy, the FDA changed the label in 2005, withdrawing approval for new patients. Subsequent studies have demonstrated clinical effectiveness of gefitinib in patients with tumors harboring EGFR mutations and the drug is indicated for use in advanced NSCLC in Europe. Gefitinib does not have any current FDA-approved indications for dermatologic disease.

There are no contraindications on the manufacturer's label.

DOSING REGIMEN

Recommended dosing is 250 mg once daily by mouth, with or without food.

SIDE EFFECTS AND PRECAUTIONS

Adverse Effects: Skin toxicities and diarrhea are the most common adverse effects. Cutaneous toxicities are common and share the characteristics of other agents targeting EGFR. A papulopustular eruption, xeroderma, and pruritus are all common. The papulopustular eruption typically develops 1 to 2 weeks following treatment initiation and has been associated with improved overall survival.[40] Other adverse cutaneous manifestations include photosensitivity, mucositis as well as nail and hair changes. Nail effects include onycholysis, paronychia, and pyogenic granulomalike lesions of the nailfold. Hair changes include alopecia, trichomegaly and hirsutism.[12]

Based on preclinical animal studies, gefitinib may produce fetal harm when administered to pregnant women. Thus, it is recommended to strongly advise avoidance of gefitinib during pregnancy. Gefitinib has been detected in rat milk and thus lactating women should be made aware of the potential harm to infants during nursing.

Drug Interactions: Caution is advised when gefitinib is administered concomitantly with inhibitors and inducers of CYP3A4. It is also recommended to avoid compounds that can affect gastric pH such as proton pump inhibitors. Close monitoring of the prothrombin time and/or international normalized ratio when used with warfarin is warranted.

See the Iressa package insert for full drug–drug interactions and adverse effects.[39]

ERLOTINIB HYDROCHLORIDE (TARCEVA)

PHARMACOLOGY AND MECHANISM OF ACTION

Structure: Erlotinib, N-(3-ethynylphenyl)-6,7-bis(2-methoxyethoxy)-4-quinazolinamine, has the molecular formula $C_{22}H_{23}N_3O_4 \cdot HCl$ and a molecular weight of 429.90 daltons.[41] Figure 194-9 shows the structure of erlotinib.

Metabolism: Erlotinib is predominantly metabolized by CYP3A4 and to a lesser degree by CYP1A2 and CYP1A1. The elimination half-life is estimated to be 36.2 hours. Time to steady-state in the plasma is 7 to 8 days.

Absorption and Distribution: Peak plasma levels are reached after 4 hours of an oral dose. Oral absorption is 60%, which is increased to approximately 100% if administered with food. The volume of distribution is 232 L.

Mechanism of Action: Erlotinib is a reversible small-molecule inhibitor of EGFR. It competes with the binding of ATP to the intracellular domain of EGFR, thus preventing autophosphorylation of the tyrosine residues and precluding downstream signal transduction. Erlotinib exhibits preferential binding to EGFR proteins that possess the exon 19 deletion or exon 21 (L858R) mutations as compared to the wildtype EGFR protein.

INDICATIONS AND CONTRAINDICATIONS

Erlotinib has FDA approval for use in NSCLC and pancreatic carcinoma. In NSCLC its approval extends to first-line, maintenance, or second-line or greater therapy after progression following at least 1 regimen of chemotherapy in patients with metastatic tumors that possess either exon 19 deletions or exon 21 (L858R) substitution mutations in EGFR, as detected by an FDA-approved test.

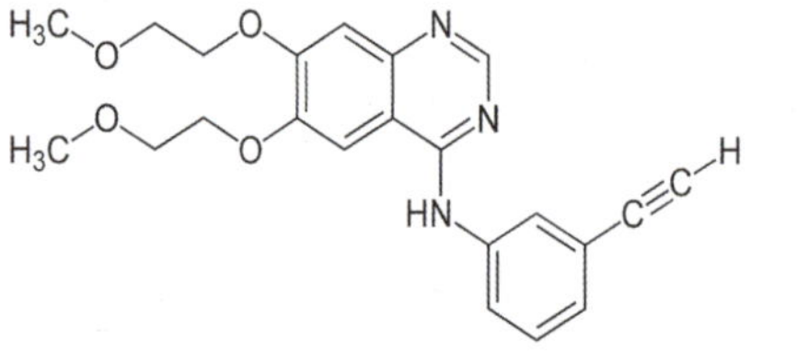

Erlotinib is also indicated for patients with locally advanced, unresectable or metastatic pancreatic carcinoma as frontline therapy in combination with gemcitabine.

Erlotinib is being investigated in combination with radiotherapy and other systemic agents in cSCC. In melanoma, a Phase II trial of erlotinib and bevacizumab for patients with metastatic disease demonstrated disappointing results, with a progression-free survival (PFS) of only 2 months.[42]

There are no contraindications listed on manufacturer's label.

DOSING REGIMEN

For NSCLC, the recommended dose of erlotinib is 150 mg by mouth administered once daily until disease progression or unacceptable toxicity. The dose for pancreatic cancer is 100 mg once daily, in combination with gemcitabine, until disease progression or unacceptable toxicity. It is recommended that erlotinib be taken on an empty stomach.

No dose adjustments are provided in the manufacturer's labeling during initial treatment in patients with renal impairment. Monitoring of renal function is recommended while taking erlotinib and the drug should be stopped in patients developing renal impairment until toxicity has resolved.

Specific dosing for hepatic impairment has not been defined. See the manufacturer's label for adjustments in patients with baseline liver abnormalities.

SIDE EFFECTS AND PRECAUTIONS

Adverse Effects: The most common adverse effects include cutaneous toxicity, diarrhea, fatigue, anorexia, dyspnea, cough, nausea, and vomiting. Serious drug toxicities include interstitial lung disease, which occurs in 1.1% of patients who are taking erlotinib, hepatotoxicity, GI perforations, myocardial ischemia/infarction, microangiopathic hemolytic anemia, cerebrovascular accident, corneal perforations/ulcerations, and persistent severe keratitis.

Skin toxicities are very common and occur to some degree in most patients receiving erlotinib. The most common include the development of a papulopustular eruption, xeroderma, and pruritus. The papulopustular eruption often develops 1 to 2 weeks following treatment initiation and has been associated with improved overall survival.[40] Other adverse cutaneous manifestations include bullous eruptions, photosensitivity, and mucositis, as well as nail and hair changes. Nail effects include onycholysis, paronychia, and pyogenic granuloma-like lesions of the nailfold. Hair changes include alopecia, trichomegaly, and hirsutism.[12]

Erlotinib can cause fetal harm and women of reproductive potential should be advised to use highly effective contraception. In regards to breastfeeding,

Figure 194-9 Structure of erlotinib.

it is not known if erlotinib is found in breastmilk, but based on the potential for serious harm, it is recommended that the risks and benefits of taking Tarceva be weighed carefully.

Drug Interactions: Caution should be advised when erlotinib is administered with inhibitors or inducers of CYP3A4 and CYP1A2 as they can affect the plasma concentrations. Cigarette smoking can accelerate clearance of erlotinib, potentially decreasing its antitumor effects. Caution is also advised with concomitant use of compounds such as proton pump inhibitors, H_2-receptor antagonists, and antacids, which increase gastric pH and can decrease erlotinib plasma concentrations.

See the Tarceva package insert for full drug–drug interactions and adverse effects.

AFATINIB DIMALEATE (GILOTRIF)

PHARMACOLOGY AND MECHANISM OF ACTION

Structure: Afatinib dimaleate, 2-butenamide, N-[4-[(3-chloro-4-fluorophenyl)amino]-7-[[(3S)-tetrahydro-3-furanyl]oxy]-6-quinazolinyl]-4-(dimethylamino)-,(2E)-,(2Z)2-butenedioate (1:2), has the molecular formula $C_{32}H_{33}ClFN_5O_{11}$ and a molecular weight of 718.1 daltons.[43] Figure 194-10 shows the structure of afatinib.

Metabolism: Enzymatic metabolism of afatinib is minimal and the compound is principally excreted in the feces following covalent adducts to circulating proteins. The elimination half-life is estimated to be 37 hours. Time to steady-state in the plasma is approximately 8 days.

Absorption and Distribution: Peak plasma levels are reached 2 to 5 hours after an oral dose. Oral absorption is approximately 92%, and a high-fat meal decreased maximal plasma concentrations by 50%.

Mechanism of Action: Afatinib is a second-generation small-molecule kinase inhibitor with activity against all 4 ErbB family members. Unlike the first-generation EGFR TKIs gefitinib and erlotinib, which reversibly inhibit EGFR, afatinib covalently binds the kinase domain of the receptor. Consequently, afatinib irreversibly inhibits autophosphorylation of associated tyrosine residues, resulting in downregulation of cell growth and survival signal transduction pathways.

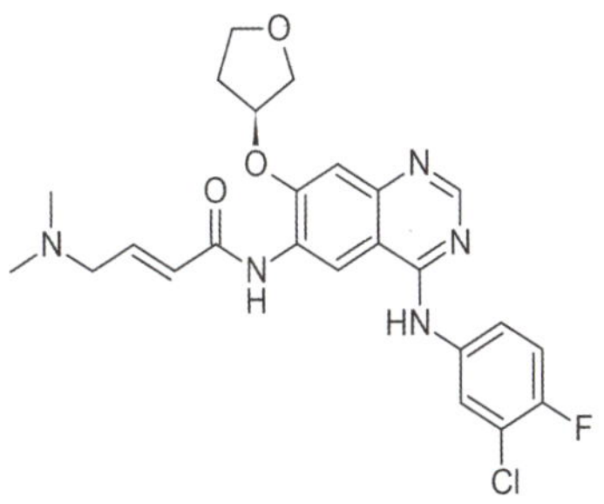

INDICATIONS AND CONTRAINDICATIONS

Afatinib has FDA approval for use as a first-line agent in metastatic NSCLC that possesses either exon 19 deletions or exon 21 (L858R) substitution mutations in EGFR, as detected by an FDA-approved test. Afatinib does not have any current FDA-approved indications for dermatologic disease.

There are no contraindications listed on manufacturer's label.

DOSING REGIMEN

The recommended dose for afatinib is 40 mg by mouth administered once daily until disease progression or unacceptable toxicity. It is recommended that afatinib be taken at least 1 hour before or 2 hours after a meal.

For patients with renal impairment (estimated glomerular filtration rate: 15 to 29 mL/min), a reduction to 30 mg by mouth daily is recommended. Afatinib has not been studied in patients with glomerular filtration rates of <15 mL/min; consequently, no specific dose adjustments are recommended.

Afatinib has not been studied in patients with severe (Child-Pugh grade C) hepatic impairment. For patients with mild-to-moderate hepatic impairment, no specific dose modifications are given.

SIDE EFFECTS AND PRECAUTIONS

Adverse Effects: The most common adverse effects of afatinib include diarrhea, cutaneous toxicity, anorexia, nausea, and vomiting. Serious drug toxicities include interstitial lung disease, which occurs in 1.6% of patients who are taking afatinib, hepatotoxicity, keratitis, and embryofetal toxicity.[43]

Skin toxicities are common and include the development of a papulopustular eruption, xeroderma, pruritus, stomatitis, and nail changes. Correlative studies suggest that the development of the papulopustular eruption might be predictive of tumor response, similar to that seen in other EGFR inhibitors.[44] When compared to gefitinib and erlotinib, afatinib has been shown to induce paronychia at a higher frequency and with accelerated onset.[45] Although the mechanism for this difference has not been elucidated, the fact that afatinib is an irreversible inhibitor while both gefitinib and erlotinib are both reversible inhibitors, has been cited as a possible explanation.[45] There is a report of afatinib-associated Stevens-Johnson syndrome.[46]

Figure 194-10 Structure of afatinib.

Other cutaneous effects include hypertrichosis of the eyelashes and eyebrows.[47]

Afatinib can cause fetal harm and women of reproductive potential should be recommended to use highly effective contraception during treatment and for at least 2 weeks after the last dose. In regards to breastfeeding, it is not known if afatinib is found in human breastmilk, but based on the potential for serious harm, it is recommended that breastfeeding be avoided in women taking Gilotrif and for 2 weeks following the final dose.

Drug Interactions: Caution is advised when afatinib is used with agents that modify P-glycoprotein. Coadministration of inhibitors of P-glycoprotein—including, but not limited to, ketoconazole, itraconazole, ritonavir, cyclosporine, tacrolimus, erythromycin, verapamil, quinidine, nelfinavir, saquinavir, and amiodarone—can increase afatinib concentrations. Conversely, afatinib exposure can be decreased when coadministered with inducers of P-glycoprotein, such as phenytoin, rifampicin, phenobarbital, carbamazepine, and St. John's wort.[43]

See the Gilotrif package insert for full drug–drug interactions and adverse effects.

OSIMERTINIB (TAGRISSO)

PHARMACOLOGY AND MECHANISM OF ACTION

Structure: Osimertinib (AZD9291), N-(2-{2-dimethylaminoethyl-methylamino}-4-methoxy-5-{[4-(1-methylindol-3-yl)pyrimidin-2-yl]amino}phenyl) prop-2-enamide mesylate salt, has the molecular formula $C_{28}H_{33}N_7O_2 \cdot CH_4O_3S$, and the molecular weight of 596 daltons.[48] Figure 194-11 shows the structure of osimertinib.

Metabolism: Osimertinib is metabolized primarily by oxidation via CYP3A and dealkylation. It is excreted primarily in the feces and the estimated elimination half-life is 48 hours.

Absorption and Distribution: Following administration, the median time to maximum concentration is 6 hours, with a range of 3 to 24 hours. The mean volume of distribution at steady-state is 986 L.

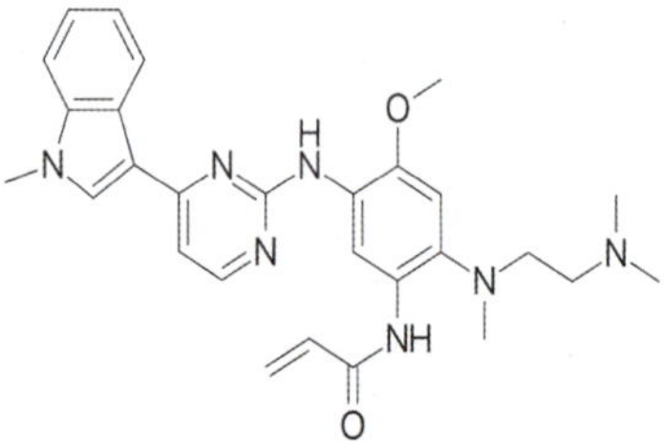

Mechanism of Action: Osimertinib is a small-molecule kinase inhibitor of the EGFR. It binds irreversibly to certain mutant forms of EGFR, such as T790M, L858R, and exon 19 deletion, and with a higher affinity as compared with the wildtype EGFR protein. In vitro, osimertinib has been shown to inhibit ACK1, BLK, and HER2, HER3, and HER4, the other 3 ERbB members.

INDICATIONS AND CONTRAINDICATIONS

Osimertinib received accelerated approval in November 2015 for patients with metastatic NSCLC that possess a T790M mutation in EGFR and have progressed on prior EGFR TKI therapy. Approval was based on data from the 2 AURA Phase II studies (AURA extension and AURA2). These were multicentered single-arm trials of 411 patients with T790M-mutant EGFR NSCLC who had progressed on prior EGFR TKI therapy and in aggregate osimertinib-treated patients had a 59% overall objective response rate.[30] Osimertinib does not have any current FDA-approved indications for dermatologic disease. In 2018, the FDA granted an approval for first-line treatment in patients with metastatic NSCLC with exon 19 deletions or exon 21 L858R mutations.

There are no contraindications on the manufacturer's label.

DOSING REGIMEN

The recommended dosing in patients with a confirmed T790M EGFR mutation is 80 mg once daily by mouth, with or without food.

SIDE EFFECTS AND PRECAUTIONS

Adverse Effects: Similar to other EGFR kinase inhibitors, osimertinib commonly causes diarrhea, rash, xerosis, nail changes, nausea, and anorexia. Serious toxicities include interstitial lung disease/pneumonitis, QTc interval prolongation, cardiomyopathy, and embryofetal toxicity.

Based on the mechanism of action and animal studies, osimertinib can cause harm to a developing fetus when administered to a pregnant woman. It is recommended to advise females of reproductive age to use effective contraception during treatment and for 6 weeks after the final dose of osimertinib. Additionally, it is recommended to advise males to use highly effective contraception for 4 months after the final dose if they are sexually active with females of reproductive potential.

Breastfeeding while taking osimertinib and for the 2 weeks following the final dose is not recommended.

Drug Interactions: Caution is advised when osimertinib is administered concomitantly with strong inducers of CYP3A (eg, phenytoin, rifampin, carbamazepine, St. John's wort). Coadministering osimertinib with rosuvastatin (a breast cancer resistance protein [BRCP] substrate) increased plasma concentrations

Figure 194-11 Structure of osimertinib.

of rosuvastatin, whereas coadministration with simvastatin (a CYP3A4 substrate) had no clinically significant effect on simvastatin concentrations. Thus, close monitoring for adverse effects is recommended when osimertinib is used with BRCP substrates (eg, rosuvastatin, sulfasalazine, topotecan).

See the Tagrisso package insert for full drug–drug interactions and adverse effects.

SMOOTHENED INHIBITORS

AT-A-GLANCE

- The hedgehog pathway is disrupted in the vast majority of basal cell carcinomas.
- Loss of the tumor-suppressor PTCH1 or activating mutations in smoothened leads to unregulated cell growth and oncogenesis.
- The small molecules vismodegib and sonidegib are inhibitors of smoothened and are approved for the treatment of unresectable and advanced basal cell carcinoma.
- Vismodegib and sonidegib carry boxed warnings for embryofetal toxicity.

BACKGROUND

The hedgehog (HH) pathway, a cascade vital for embryonic development, is now known to be critical in the molecular pathogenesis of basal cell carcinoma (BCC). In the 1990s, mutations in the tumor-suppressor patched 1 (*PTCH1*) gene were found in both BCCs arising in basal cell nevus syndrome[49] and in sporadic cases.[50] Loss of *PTCH1*, an inhibitor of the downstream protein smoothened (SMO), results in constitutive upregulation of HH signaling and overexpression of genes responsible for cell survival, growth, proliferation, vascularization and healing (Fig. 194-12). Nearly all sporadic BCCs have a disease-promoting mutation in HH signaling, with approximately 90% possessing a loss of at least 1 allele PTCH1 and 10% having activating mutations in SMO.[51] Molecularly targeted therapy for BCC emerged in 2012 with the first-in-class SMO inhibitor vismodegib (Erivedge). In 2015, the second-in-class inhibitor sonidegib (Odomzo) was approved.

VISMODEGIB (ERIVEDGE)

PHARMACOLOGY AND MECHANISM OF ACTION

Structure: Vismodegib, 2-Chloro-*N*-[4-chloro-3-(2-pyridinyl)phenyl]-4-(methylsulfonyl)benzamide, has the molecular formula $C_{19}H_{14}Cl_2N_2O_3S$ and molecular weight of 421.3 g/mol.[52] Figure 194-13 shows the structure of vismodegib.

Metabolism: Vismodegib is metabolized via oxidation and glucuronidation primarily by CYP2C9 and CYP3A4/5, although it is excreted predominantly in its unchanged form.[52] The estimated half-life is 12 days following a single dose and 4 days with continuous daily dosing.

Absorption and Distribution: Vismodegib is absorbed orally and has a bioavailability of 31.8%. The volume of distribution is 16.4 L to 26.6 L. Vismodegib binds to serum albumin and α_1-acid glycoprotein.

Mechanism of Action: Vismodegib is a first-in-class small-molecule inhibitor of the 7-pass transmembrane protein SMO, a key member of the HH signal-transduction pathway. Inhibition of SMO precludes activation and translocation of the transcription factor GLI (glioma-associated oncogene homolog), thereby decreasing the induction of genes involved with cell proliferation and survival.

INDICATIONS AND CONTRAINDICATIONS

Vismodegib was approved by the FDA on January 30, 2012, for treatment of adult patients with metastatic or unresectable BCC. Approval stemmed from data from the ERIVANCE BCC trial, a multicenter, Phase II, single-arm, two-cohort, open-label II trial of 104 patients with locally advanced (n = 63) or metastatic BCC (n = 33).[53] Vismodegib taken orally produced objective responses in 10 (30.3%) patients with metastatic BCC and 27 (42.8%) patients with locally advanced BCC. Median duration of response was 7.6 months.

There are no contraindications on the manufacturer's label.

DOSING REGIMEN

Recommended dosing for vismodegib is 150 mg daily by mouth for metastatic and locally advanced BCC. It is usually continued until disease progression or the development of unacceptable adverse effects. The safety and effectiveness of vismodegib has not been established in patients with hepatic or renal impairment.

SIDE EFFECTS AND PRECAUTIONS

Adverse Effects: Treatment-emergent adverse effects are commonly experienced with vismodegib. In the STEVIE (Safety Events in Vismodegib) study, a multicenter, open-label trial of 499 patients with metastatic BCC or locally advanced BCC, 491 patients had at least 1 adverse effect.[54] Common adverse effects include muscle spasms, dysgeusia, asthenia, decrease in weight, fatigue, nausea, decrease in appetite, and diarrhea. Cutaneous adverse effects are common. Alopecia occurs in the majority of patients (58% to 63%).[55] Keratoacanthomas and well-differentiated

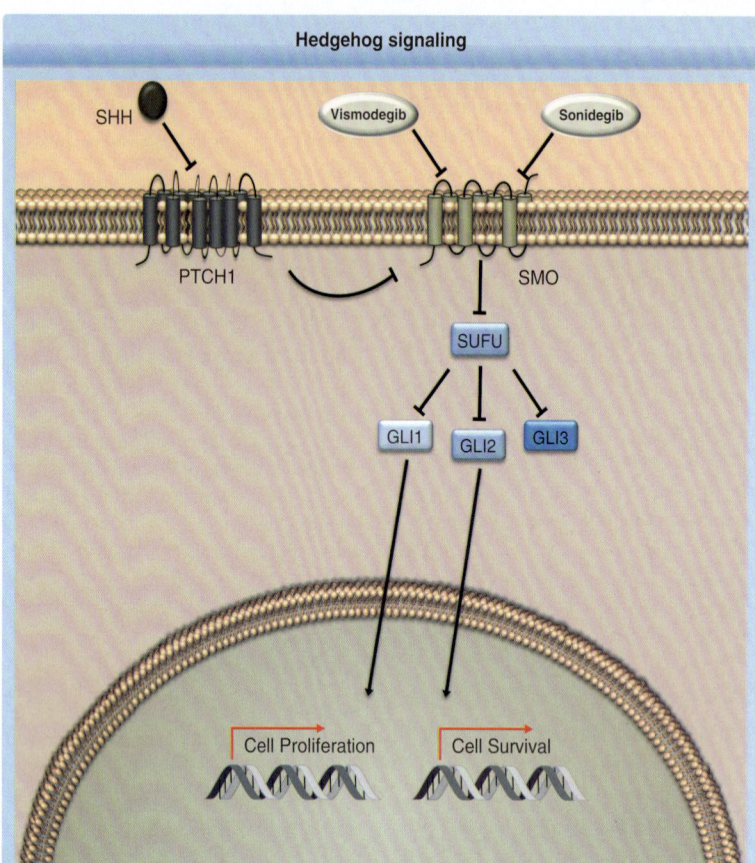

Figure 194-12 Hedgehog signaling. Hedgehog (HH) signaling is initiated by binding of 1 of 3 extracellular HH ligands, sonic hedgehog (SHH), Indian hedgehog (IHH) and desert hedgehog (DHH). These ligands bind to 12-pass transmembrane protein receptors Patched 1 (PTCH1) and Patched 2 (PTCH2). When unbound, Patched receptors interact and inhibit the 7-pass transmembrane transduction protein Smoothened (SMO). Following ligand binding to Patched, the inhibition of SMO is relieved and transduction through a series of interacting proteins, including suppressor of fused (SUFU), results in translocation of the glioma-associated oncogene homolog (GLI) transcription factors: GLI1, GLI2, and GLI3. GLI1 functions exclusively as an activator of transcription, while the actions of GLI2 and GLI3 are dependent on the signaling context. In the absence of HH ligands, GLI3 functions as the primary repressor of the transduction cascade. Following nuclear translocation, GLI transcription factors modulate the expression on numerous cell programs including those involved in cell growth, proliferation, epithelial–mesenchymal transition, angiogenesis, inhibition of apoptosis, and stem cell maintenance. The small molecules vismodegib and sonidegib bind to SMO and impair signaling through the HH pathway.

squamous cell carcinomas occurring during treatment also have been described.[55] Roughly one-third of patients in STEVIE discontinued treatment because of unacceptable toxicity. Grade 5 adverse effects have been reported in patients using vismodegib, although according to the trial investigators, those events were thought to be unrelated to vismodegib.[53,54] Premature fusion of the epiphyses has been reported in pediatric patients exposed to Erivedge, and in some cases, the fusion progressed after discontinuation of the drug.[52]

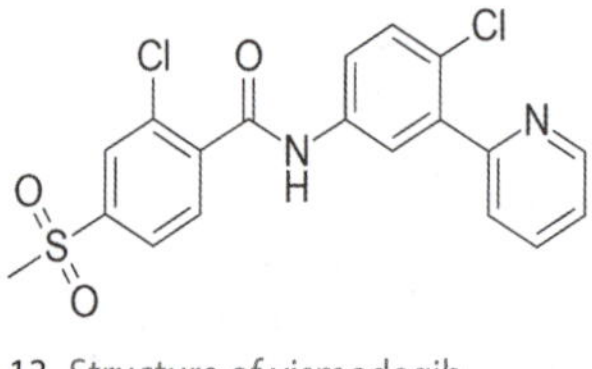

Animal reproductive studies demonstrated that vismodegib is teratogenic, embryotoxic, and fetotoxic. In rats, doses approximately 0.2 times the area under the curve of the recommended dose in humans resulted in malformation, retardations, or variations in skeletal and visceral structures. As a result, the Erivedge product label contains a boxed warning of embryofetal toxicity. Women should be screened for pregnancy 7 days prior to starting and it is recommended that females avoid pregnancy during treatment and for up to 24 months after the last dose. It is recommended that male patients use condoms with spermicide during treatment and for 3 months after discontinuation. Women should be counseled not to breastfeed during treatment and for 24 months after the last dose.

Figure 194-13 Structure of vismodegib.

Patients are advised not to donate blood products during treatment and for 24 months after completing treatment.

Drug Interactions: There is little definitive evidence at this time of drug interactions with vismodegib. Data indicates that vismodegib is a substrate of the P-glycoprotein efflux transporter; consequently, coadministration with inhibitors of P-glycoprotein, such as macrolide antibiotics, may increase drug levels and systemic toxicity. Medications that affect gastric pH may reduce the drug's bioavailability, but there are no formal studies evaluating the effect of pH-altering drugs on vismodegib.

See the Erivedge package insert for full drug–drug interactions and adverse effects.[52]

SONIDEGIB (ODOMZO)

PHARMACOLOGY AND MECHANISM OF ACTION

Structure: Sonidegib, N-[6-(cis-2,6-dimethylmorpholin-4-yl)pyridine-3-yl]-2-methyl-4'-(trifluoromethoxy)[1,1'-biphenyl]-3-carboxamide diphosphate, has the molecular formula $C_{26}H_{26}F_3N_3O_2 \cdot 2H_3PO_4$ and molecular weight of 681.49 daltons. Figure 194-14 shows the structure of sonidegib.

Metabolism: Sonidegib is metabolized by CYP3A, and the compound and its metabolites are primarily excreted via the enterohepatic circulation. The elimination half-life is approximately 28 days and 70% of the absorbed dose is eliminated in the feces and 30% is excreted in the urine.[56]

Absorption and Distribution: When given orally, less than 10% of the dose is absorbed. Consumption of a high-fat meal results in an increased systemic exposure of the drug. Steady-state volume of distribution is 9166 L with the compound exhibiting high binding to plasma proteins.

Mechanism of Action: Sonidegib, like vismodegib, is a small-molecule inhibitor of the 7-pass, transmembrane protein SMO. Consequently, exposure to the compound is thought to attenuate the expression of HH signaling genes involved with cell proliferation and survival.

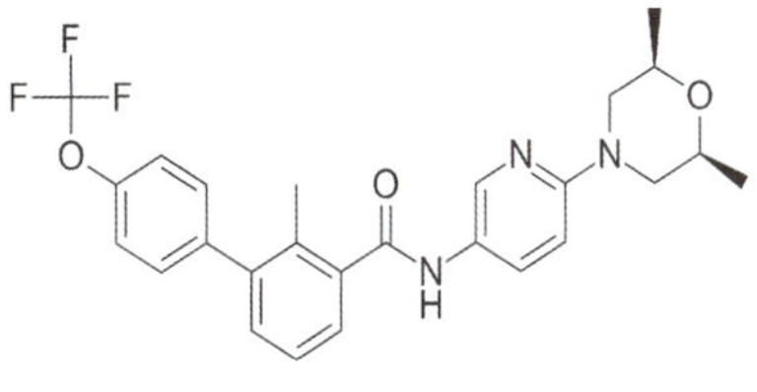

Figure 194-14 Structure of sonidegib.

INDICATIONS AND CONTRAINDICATIONS

Sonidegib was approved by the FDA on July 24, 2015, for treatment of adults patients with locally advanced BCC that recurs following surgical excision or radiotherapy, and for those patients who are not candidates for surgery or radiotherapy. The approval was based on data from the BOLT (Basal Cell Carcinoma Outcomes With LDE225 Treatment) trial, an international multicenter, randomized, 2-arm, noncomparative trial of 230 patients.[57] Daily administration of 200 mg of sonidegib produced objective responses in 43% of patients, and 800 mg daily achieved objective responses of 38%.

The drug has no contraindications on the product label.

DOSING REGIMEN

Recommending dosing is 200 mg by mouth daily, taken at least 1 hour prior to or 2 hours after a meal, until disease progression or unacceptable adverse effects.

Prior to starting treatment, it is recommended to obtain verification of the pregnancy status of women with reproductive potential, and serum creatinine kinase and kidney function tests for all patients.

There are no recommended dose adjustments for patients with mild-to-moderate renal impairment (CrCl 30 to 59 mL/min) or for patients with mild hepatic impairment. Data is lacking in patients with more significant liver impairment.

SIDE EFFECTS AND PRECAUTIONS

Adverse Effects: The most common adverse events include muscle spasms, alopecia, dysgeusia, nausea, elevated creatinine kinase, fatigue, weight loss, anorexia, myalgia, headache, and pruritus. Adverse effects limit the duration of treatment in roughly one-third of patients. One case of rhabdomyolysis was reported by the study investigators, although upon independent review, the case was deemed not to be consistent with rhabdomyolysis. Nevertheless, baseline creatinine kinase levels are suggested and dose interruptions are recommended for the first occurrence of serum creatinine kinase elevation between 2.5 and 10 times the ULN.

Although there are no data from pregnant women, animal toxicity studies demonstrated that sonidegib, like vismodegib, is teratogenic, embryotoxic, and fetotoxic. As a result, there is a boxed warning on the Odomzo package label for embryofetal toxicity. Consequently, women with childbearing potential should be warned of the potential embryofetal death and severe birth defects and should be advised to avoid pregnancy during treatment and for at least 20 months after the last dose. Although the concentration of sonidegib in semen has not been evaluated, it is recommended that male patients use condoms with spermicide during treatment and for at least 8 months after discontinuation. There is inadequate literature to assess the safety of sonidegib in regards to lactation; consequently, it is recommended that women avoid breastfeeding during treatment with sonidegib for at least 20 months after the last dose. There are no data regarding the effects of sonidegib on human reproduction; however, the compound did decrease fertility in female rodents at doses 1 to 2 times the recommended human dose.

Patients are advised not to donate blood products during treatment and for 20 months after completing treatment.

Drug Interactions: Given that sonidegib is metabolized by CYP3A, inhibitors and inducers of CYP3A can affect drug concentrations and such agents should be used with caution. Preclinical studies suggest that sonidegib inhibits CYP2B6 and CYP2C9 and thus can affect drug levels of those substrates.

See the Odomzo package insert for full drug–drug interactions and adverse effects.[56]

HISTONE DEACETYLASE INHIBITORS

AT-A-GLANCE

- Histone modification is a key epigenetic phenomena that regulates gene expression.
- Abnormalities in the acetylation of histone proteins is a common occurrence in several malignancies.
- Regulation of histone acetylation is controlled by histone acetyltransferases and histone deacetylases (HDACs).
- Inhibitors of HDACs have demonstrated efficacy as cancer therapy and their administration is thought to induce differentiation, cell-cycle arrest and apoptosis through restoration of normal acetylation of histone and nonhistone proteins.
- Of the 4 HDAC inhibitors currently approved, 2—vorinostat and romidepsin—have FDA approval for the treatment of cutaneous T-cell lymphoma.

BACKGROUND

Dysregulated gene expression is a hallmark of oncogenesis. Aberrant expression of genes can result from mutations of the DNA nucleotide sequence or via epigenetic modulations, such as chromatin modification. DNA and histone complexes form the basic structural unit of chromatin, the nucleosome. The conformational structure of nucleosomes and chromatin is regulated, in part, by acetylation of histone proteins. In its condensed form, negatively charged DNA is wrapped tightly around positively charged histone proteins, limiting the ability of transcription factors to access DNA promoter regions. The acetylation of lysine residues in the tails of histones by histone acetyltransferases neutralizes the positive charge on histones (Fig. 194-15). This results in a more relaxed structure for chromatin and permits greater access to gene promoters by transcription factors, facilitating gene expression. In contrast, the activity of histone deacetylases (HDACs) promotes an underacetylated state, contributing to transcriptional silencing by impairing nucleosome accessibility. The fine balance between acetylation and deacetylation is disrupted in several human diseases. In cancer cells, histone deacetylation is associated with the downregulation of proapoptotic genes as well as of genes critical for differentiation.[58] In addition to chromatin modulation, histone acetyltransferases and HDACs have been shown to be involved in the regulation of nonhistone proteins involved in oncogenesis, such as p53, nuclear factor κB, E2F, and hypoxia-inducible factor 1α.[58,59] Consequently, inhibitors of HDACs have been developed for therapeutic use and have shown promise in several malignancies, including cutaneous T-cell lymphoma. Although the exact therapeutic mechanism is unknown, drugs that inhibit HDACs are thought to induce differentiation, cell-cycle arrest and apoptosis through restoration of normal acetylation.[58] The FDA has approved 4 HDAC inhibitors for cancer therapy: vorinostat, romidepsin, belinostat, and panobinostat. Vorinostat and romidepsin have approval for use in cutaneous T-cell lymphoma, while romidepsin and belinostat are indicated to treat peripheral T-cell lymphoma. Panobinostat is approved for use in multiple myeloma.

VORINOSTAT (ZOLINZA)

PHARMACOLOGY AND MECHANISM OF ACTION

Structure: Vorinostat, suberanilohydroxamic acid or N-hydroxy-N'-phenyloctanediamide, is a hydroxamic acid derivative with the empirical formula $C_{14}H_{20}N_2O_3$ and molecular weight of 264.32 daltons. Figure 194-16 shows the structure of vorinostat.

Metabolism: Glucuronidation and hydrolysis are the major metabolic pathways of vorinostat. There is negligible biotransformation by CYP. The mean terminal half-life is approximately 2 hours.

Absorption and Distribution: When taken orally with a high-fat meal, the median time to maximum concentration is 4 hours. Steady-state concentrations after multiple doses in the fed-state are achieved in 4 hours (range: 0.5 to 14 hours).

Mechanism of Action: Vorinostat is an inhibitor of the several HDACs including HDAC1, HDAC2, HDAC3, and HDAC6. In vitro, vorinostat results in the accumulation of acetylated histones, and in some transformed cells, induces apoptosis and/or arrest of the cell cycle.[60]

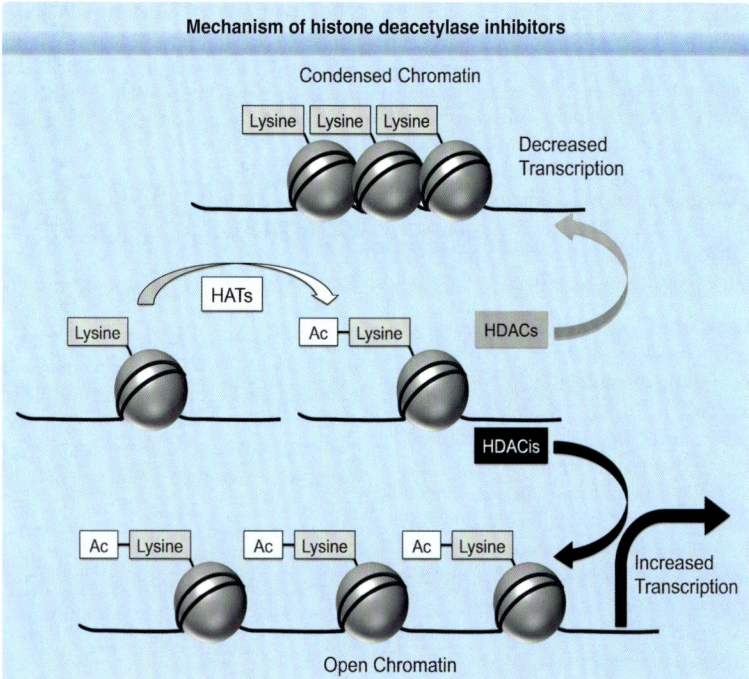

Figure 194-15 Mechanism of histone deacetylase inhibitors. In its condensed form, negatively charged DNA (*black lines*) is wrapped tightly around positively charged histone proteins (*gray spheres*), limiting the ability of transcription factors to access DNA promoter regions. Histone acetyltransferases (HATs) neutralize the positive charge on histones by the addition of acetyl groups to the lysine residues in the tails of histones. Acetylation of these residues results in a more relaxed structure for chromatin and permits greater access to gene promoters by transcription factors, facilitating gene expression. In contrast, the activity of histone deacetylases (HDACs) promotes an underacetylated state, contributing to transcriptional silencing by impairing nucleosome accessibility (*upper panel*). Agents that inhibit HDACs (HDACis) are thought to restore normal acetylation, resulting in increased transcription of genes that regulate differentiation, cell-cycle arrest, and apoptosis (*bottom panel*).

INDICATIONS AND CONTRAINDICATIONS

Vorinostat was approved in 2006 for treatment of cutaneous T-cell lymphoma in patients with persistent, recurrent, or progressive disease on or following 2 systemic therapies. Approval was based on 2 Phase II trials that demonstrated overall objective response rates ranging from 24% to 30% in heavily pretreated patients.[61,62] Improvement in baseline pruritus was also noted in 32% to 45% of patients.[61,62] Although vorinostat demonstrates efficacy in patients with refractory disease, it is typically regarded as beyond second-line therapy.

There are no specific contraindications on the drug label.

DOSING REGIMEN

The recommended dose of vorinostat is 400 mg by mouth once daily with food.

Vorinostat has not been adequately studied in patients with renal impairment. Although renal excretion does not play a role in the elimination of vorinostat, caution is advised in patients with preexisting renal impairment.

Compared to patients with normal renal function, patients with mild (bilirubin >1 to 1.5 times ULN or aspartate aminotransferase > ULN but bilirubin ≤ ULN) and moderate (bilirubin 1.5 to ≤3 times ULN) hepatic impairment has mean area-under-the-curve levels that were increased by 50%. Therefore, it is recommended to reduce the dose in patients with mild-to-moderate hepatic impairment, although no specific recommendations are made on the package label because of insufficient data.

SIDE EFFECTS AND PRECAUTIONS

Adverse Effects: The most common adverse reactions (incidence ≥20%) are fatigue, diarrhea, nausea, dysgeusia, thrombocytopenia, anorexia, and weight loss. Alopecia was observed in 18.6% of patients in the clinical trials leading to the drug's approval.[60] The most common serious adverse reactions in the clinical

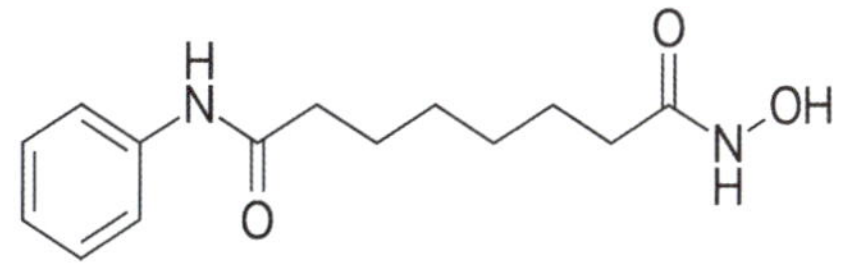

Figure 194-16 Structure of vorinostat.

trials that led to approval were pulmonary embolism, squamous cell carcinoma, and anemia.

Vorinostat is a pregnancy category D medication. Although there are no adequate studies in pregnant women, preclinical animal studies demonstrated that vorinostat may cause fetal harm. Thus, it is recommended to advise avoidance of vorinostat during pregnancy. The safety of vorinostat during breastfeeding is unknown. However, because it is possibly unsafe for use, lactating women should be made aware of the potential harm to infants during nursing.

Drug Interactions: GI bleeding and severe thrombocytopenia have been observed when vorinostat is used concurrently with other HDAC inhibitors such as valproic acid.

Prolongation of prothrombin time and international normalized ratio were observed when vorinostat was coadministered with coumarin-derivative anticoagulants. Close monitoring of prothrombin time and international normalized ratio is recommended with concurrently administered vorinostat and coumarin derivatives such as warfarin.

See the Zolinza package insert for full drug–drug interactions and adverse effects.[60]

ROMIDEPSIN (ISTODAX)

PHARMACOLOGY AND MECHANISM OF ACTION

Structure: Romidepsin, (1S,4S,7Z,10S,16E,21R)-7-ethylidene-4,21-bis(1-methylethyl)-2-oxa-12,13-dithia-5,8,20,23-tetraazabicyclo[8.7.6]tricos-16-ene-3,6,9,19,22-pentone, has the empirical formula $C_{24}H_{36}N_4O_6S_2$ and a molecular weight of 540.71 daltons.[63] Figure 194-17 shows the structure of romidepsin.

Metabolism: Romidepsin is principally metabolized by CYP3A4 with partial contribution by CYP3A5, CYP2B6, CYP2C19, and CYP1A1. The elimination half-life is approximately 3 hours.

Absorption and Distribution: When given intravenously in concentrations ranging from 1 to 24 mg/m^2 romidepsin exhibits linear pharmacokinetics. The drug is a substrate for the P-glycoprotein ABCB1 efflux transporter.

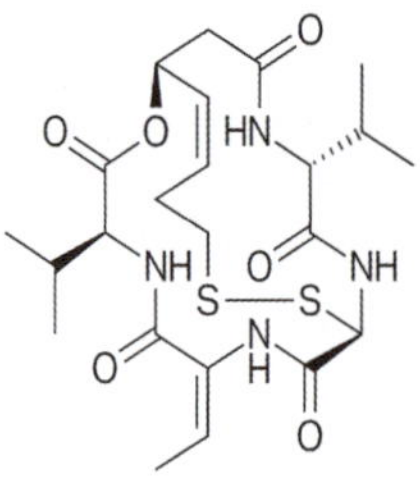

Figure 194-17 Structure of romidepsin.

Mechanism of Action: Romidepsin acts as a HDAC inhibitor. In preclinical studies, romidepsin was shown to induce cell-cycle arrest and apoptosis in some cancer cell lines.[63] The full mechanism of action, however, has not been fully elucidated.

INDICATIONS AND CONTRAINDICATIONS

Romidepsin was approved by the FDA in 2009 for treatment of cutaneous T-cell lymphoma in patients who have received at least 1 previous systemic therapy. Approval was based on 2 Phase II clinical trials. Clinical benefit was noted across all stages of disease, with overall response rates of 34%, including 38% in patients with advanced disease (Stage IIB or greater). Complete responses were noted in 5.6% to 7% of patients.[64,65]

In 2011, the FDA expanded approval for treatment of peripheral T-cell lymphoma in patients who have received at least 1 prior therapy.

There are no specific contraindications on the drug label.

DOSING REGIMEN

Romidepsin is administered as an IV infusion. The recommended dose is 14 mg/m^2 given over 4 hours on days 1, 8, and 15 of a 28-day cycle. Cycles are repeated for as long as the patient tolerates the treatment and continues to demonstrate a clinical benefit.

Although there have been no dedicated hepatic or renal impairment studies with romidepsin, caution is advised in patients with moderate-to-severe hepatic impairment and endstage renal impairment.

SIDE EFFECTS AND PRECAUTIONS

Adverse Effects: The most common adverse effects are nausea, asthenia/fatigue, thrombocytopenia, vomiting, diarrhea, diarrhea, pyrexia, constipation, neutropenia, and electrocardiogram T-wave changes. The most common serious adverse effect observed in trials leading to romidepsin's approval was infection. Additional serious adverse effects that occurred in at least 2% of patients included pyrexia, vomiting, cellulitis, deep vein thrombosis, febrile neutropenia, abdominal pain, chest pain, pulmonary embolism, dyspnea, and dehydration. One case of grade IV "dermatitis medicamentosa" and a single case of oral candidiasis were noted in the pivotal Phase II trial.[65] Several treatment-emergent changes in the morphology of electrocardiograms were observed in the clinical studies. Thus, the package label recommends considering cardiovascular monitoring in patients with congenital long QT syndrome, patients taking QT-prolonging medications, and in patients with a history of significant cardiovascular disease.

Based on the mechanism of action and preclinical animal studies, romidepsin may produce fetal harm when administered to pregnant women. Thus, it is recommended to advise avoidance of romidepsin during pregnancy. Romidepsin is possibly unsafe for use during breastfeeding, and lactating women should be made aware of the potential harm to infants during nursing.

Drug Interactions: Concomitant use of strong CYP3A4 inducers such as rifampin is not recommended. Close monitoring of toxicities is recommended when coadministering strong CYP3A4 inhibitors and warfarin and coumarin derivatives.

See the Istodax package insert for full drug–drug interactions and adverse effects.[63]

BELINOSTAT (BELEODAQ)

PHARMACOLOGY AND MECHANISM OF ACTION

Structure: Belinostat, (2E)-N-hydroxy-3-[3-(phenylsulfamoyl)phenyl]prop-2-enamide, has the molecular formula $C_{15}H_{14}N_2O_4S$ and the molecular weight is 318.35 g/mol.[66] Figure 194-18 shows the structure of belinostat.

Metabolism: Belinostat is primarily metabolized by UGT1A1, but also undergoes hepatic metabolism by CYP3A4, CYP2A6, and CYP2C9. The elimination half-life is 1.1 hours.

Absorption and Distribution: After intravenous injection, the mean volume of distribution of belinostat approaches total body water.

Mechanism of Action: Belinostat inhibits the activity of HDACs. In preclinical studies, belinostat was shown to induce cell-cycle arrest and apoptosis in some cancer cells. Compared to normal cells, belinostat demonstrates preferential cytotoxicity to transformed cells.[66]

INDICATIONS AND CONTRAINDICATIONS

Beleodaq was granted FDA approval in 2014 for treatment of relapsed or refractory peripheral T-cell lymphoma. Approval was based on a pivotal Phase II trial of 120 patients with relapsed or refractory disease. Overall response rates were 25.8%, including a complete response in 13 patients (10.8%).[67]

There are no specific contraindications on the drug label.

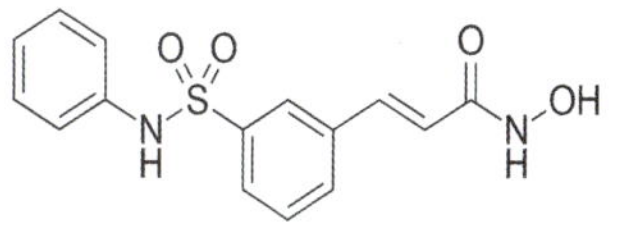

DOSING REGIMEN

The recommended dosing and schedule of Beleodaq is 1000 mg/m² administered IV on days 1 to 5 of a 21-day cycle.

Patients with moderate-to-severe hepatic impairment were not included in the pivotal clinical trials; as a result, there is insufficient data to recommend a dose of Beleodaq in patients with hepatic impairment.

The exposure to Beleodaq was not altered in patients with a CrCl of greater than 39 mL/min. There is insufficient data to recommend a dose of Beleodaq in patients with a CrCl of less than 39 mL/min.

SIDE EFFECTS AND PRECAUTIONS

Adverse Effects: The most common adverse effects of belinostat are nausea, fatigue, pyrexia, anemia, vomiting, constipation, diarrhea, dyspnea, rash, and peripheral edema. The most common serious adverse effects include pneumonia, pyrexia, infection, anemia, increased creatinine, thrombocytopenia, and multiorgan failure.

Belinostat is a pregnancy category D medication. It may cause embryofetal lethality as it targets actively dividing cells and is genotoxic.[66] Thus, it is recommended to advise avoidance of belinostat during pregnancy. The safety of belinostat during breastfeeding is unknown. However, because it is possibly unsafe for use, nursing women should be made aware of the potential harm to infants during breastfeeding.

Drug Interactions: It is recommended to avoid concomitant use of belinostat with strong UGT1A1 inhibitors.

See the Beleodaq package insert for full drug–drug interactions and adverse effects.[66]

PANOBINOSTAT (FARYDAK)

PHARMACOLOGY AND MECHANISM OF ACTION

Structure: Panobinostat, (2E)-N-hydroxy-3-[4-[[[2-(2-methyl-1H-indol-3-yl)ethyl]amino]methyl]phenyl]-2-propenamide, has the molecular formula $C_{21}H_{23}N_3O_2 \cdot C_3H_6O_3$ and molecular weight of 439.51 daltons (as a lactate), which is equivalent to 349.43 of free base.[68] Figure 194-19 shows the structure of panobinostat.

Figure 194-18 Structure of belinostat.

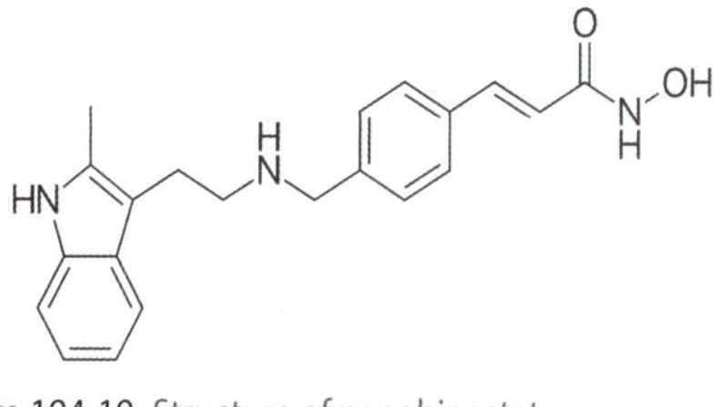

Figure 194-19 Structure of panobinostat.

Metabolism: Panobinostat is metabolized via oxidation, reduction, hydrolysis, and glucuronidation. Approximately 40% of the compound is metabolized by CYP3A. Minor contributions come via CYP2D6 and CYP2C19. Glucuronidation occurs via UGT1A1, UGT1A3, UGT1A7, UGT1A8, UGT1A9, and UGT2B4. The elimination half-life is approximately 37 hours.

Absorption and Distribution: The oral bioavailability of panobinostat is approximately 21% and peak plasma concentrations are achieved within 2 hours of oral administration. In vitro, panobinostat is approximately 90% bound to plasma proteins.

Mechanism of Action: Panobinostat is an HDAC inhibitor. In vitro, panobinostat was shown to induce cell-cycle arrest and apoptosis in some transformed cells. Panobinostat demonstrates preferential cytotoxicity to transformed cells compared to normal cells.

INDICATIONS AND CONTRAINDICATIONS

Farydak was approved by the FDA in 2015 for use in combination with bortezomib and dexamethasone as treatment of multiple myeloma in patients who have received at least 2 prior regimens. Panobinostat does not have any current FDA-approved indications for dermatologic disease, although there is an ongoing Phase Ib/II trial exploring the treatment of resistant metastatic melanoma with panobinostat and the epigenetic modifier decitabine along with temozolomide (NCT00925132).

There are no specific contraindications on the drug label.

DOSING REGIMEN

The recommended dose of panobinostat is 20 mg, taken by mouth once every other day for 3 doses per week (on days 1, 3, 5, 8, 10, 12) of weeks 1 and 2 of each 21-day cycle for 8 cycles.

It is recommended to reduce the starting dose of panobinostat to 15 mg for patients with mild hepatic impairment and to 10 mg in patients with moderate hepatic impairment. Use in patients with severe hepatic impairment is not recommended.

The exposure to Farydak was not altered in patients with mild or severe renal impairment. It was not studied in patients with end stage renal disease or those on dialysis.

Dose and/or schedule modifications of Farydak may be required based on toxicity. See the Farydak package insert for the appropriate dose reduction.

SIDE EFFECTS AND PRECAUTIONS

Adverse Effects: The most common adverse effects (incidence of at least 20%) in clinical studies are diarrhea, fatigue, nausea, peripheral edema, anorexia, pyrexia, and vomiting. The most common hematologic adverse effects (≥60% incidence) include thrombocytopenia, lymphopenia, leukopenia, neutropenia, and anemia. Electrolyte abnormalities, such as hypophosphatemia, hypokalemia, and hyponatremia, occur in 40% or more of patients. Farydak possesses a boxed warning for severe diarrhea and severe and fatal cardiac ischemic events, severe arrhythmias, and electrocardiogram changes. Severe diarrhea occurred in 25% of patients receiving Farydak. Fatal and serious cases of GI and pulmonary hemorrhage have been reported.

Farydak may cause fetal harm if administered during pregnancy. In preclinical studies, panobinostat was teratogenic in rabbits and rats. Patients should be advised to avoid getting pregnant while taking Farydak. It is also recommended that women use highly effective contraception for at least 1 month after the last dose of Farydak. Men should be advised to use condoms while on treatment and for 3 months after the last dose of Farydak. The safety of panobinostat during breastfeeding is unknown. However, because it is possibly unsafe for use, nursing women should be made aware of the potential harm to infants during breastfeeding.

Drug Interactions: It is recommended to avoid concomitant use of Farydak with strong inducers of CYP3A4, CYP2D6 substrates, and antiarrhythmic/QT-prolonging drugs. The dose of Farydak should be reduced with concomitant use of strong inhibitors of CYP3A4.

See the Farydak package insert for full drug–drug interactions and adverse effects.[68]

MITOGEN-ACTIVATED PROTEIN KINASE INHIBITORS

AT-A-GLANCE

- Between 75% and 85% of melanomas harbor oncogenic mutations in the mitogen-activated protein kinase (MAPK) pathway, including BRAF (v-raf murine sarcoma viral oncogene homolog B), RAS, and neurofibromin 1 (NF1).
- Activating mutations in BRAF, such as V600E and V600K, can trigger unregulated cell growth and promote melanocyte transformation.
- Vemurafenib and dabrafenib are inhibitors of certain mutated forms of BRAF, including V600E and V600K.
- Trametinib and cobimetinib are inhibitors of mitogen-activated extracellular signal-regulated kinase (MEK).

- Combination BRAF and MEK inhibition can lead to clinical benefit, including improved overall survival, in patients with unresectable or metastatic melanoma in patients harboring BRAF V600E or V600K mutations.

BACKGROUND

Melanomagenesis results from the dysregulation of a number of cellular circuits including the PI3K pathway, telomerase promoter, the retinoblastoma pathway, and the MAPK pathway. Targeted therapy in melanoma became a possibility following the 2002 discovery that activating mutations of the protooncogene v-raf murine sarcoma viral oncogene homolog B (BRAF) drive nearly half of melanomas.[69] BRAF, a serine-threonine kinase in the MAPK pathway, is normally activated by RAS, resulting in signal transduction via the phosphorylation of mitogen-activated extracellular signal-regulated kinase (MEK) (Fig. 194-20). Mutations in BRAF—usually V600E, but occasionally V600K and other substitutions—result in constitutive activation of the kinase domain, leading to RAS-independence and hyperactivation of downstream mediators such as MEK and extracellular signal-regulated kinase (ERK). Aberrant activation of the MAPK pathway can lead to cell-cycle dysregulation, resistance to apoptosis, immune evasion, and increased invasion and metastases. The discovery that gain-of-function alterations in BRAF were a key determinant in melanomagenesis drove the development of therapeutic strategies to intervene at multiple nodes in the MAPK pathway.

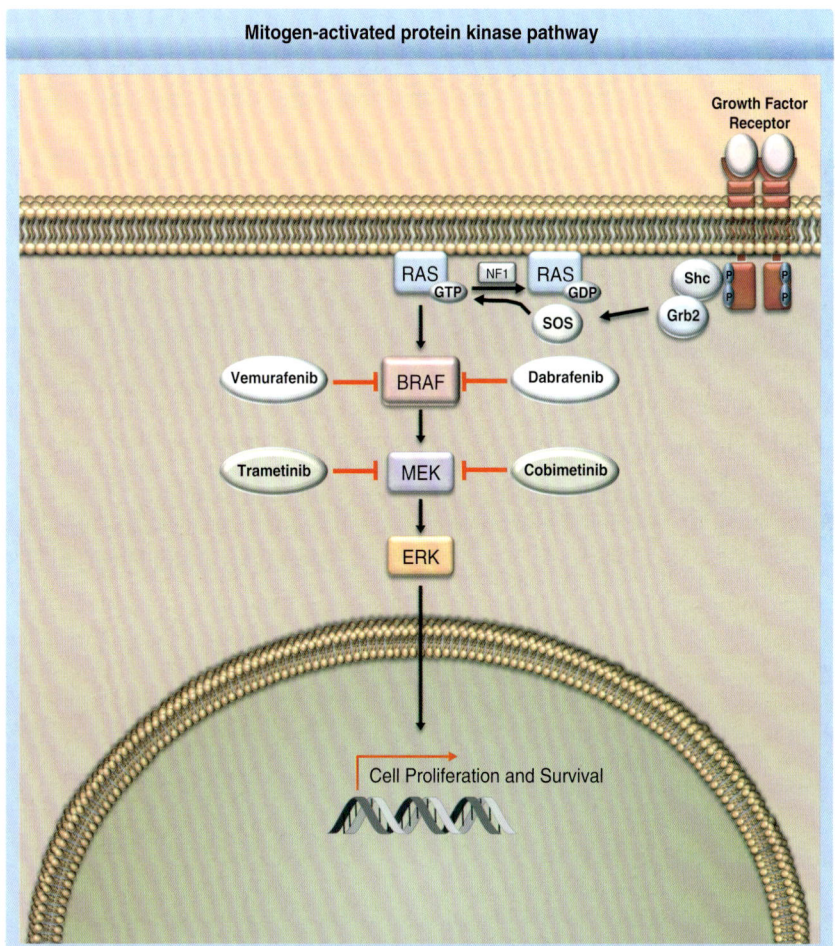

Figure 194-20 Mitogen-activated protein kinase (MAPK) pathway. Activation of receptor tyrosine kinases, such as c-KIT initiates signaling through the MAPK pathway. The action of guanine nucleotide exchange factors (GEFs), such as son of sevenless (SOS), accelerates the exchange of guanosine diphosphate (GDP) for guanosine triphosphate (GTP) by RAS. Activated RAS triggers the MAPK cascade, which includes BRAF, MEK, and ERK, leading to cell proliferation and survival. The activity of RAS is attenuated by guanosine triphosphatase–activating proteins such as neurofibromin 1 (NF1). The small molecules vemurafenib and dabrafenib inhibit the activity of BRAF, whereas trametinib and cobimetinib inhibit MEK.

Precision medicine in melanoma became a possibility with the demonstration that the small-molecule inhibitors of mutant BRAF, vemurafenib and dabrafenib, could prolong disease-free and overall survival when used as monotherapy.[70-72] In addition, inhibition of MEK with trametinib monotherapy improves PFS in patients with BRAF-mutant melanoma.[73] Although initially promising, it became evident that the acquisition of resistance to single-agent therapy precludes durable responses in advanced disease. Building off of preclinical data that showed dual-targeting of BRAF and MEK cooperate to reduce MAPK output, clinical trials have subsequently validated the safety and superior efficacy of combined BRAF/MEK inhibition in BRAF-mutant melanoma.[74-77] Indeed, many of the dermatologic toxicities seen with single-agent BRAF inhibition, such as cSCC and keratoacanthomas, are attenuated with dual BRAF inhibition/MEK inhibition. However, despite reducing many of the adverse effects and delaying the emergence of therapeutic resistance, combined BRAF inhibition/MEK inhibition does not entirely circumvent mechanisms of resistance and the vast majority of patients progress on treatment. In addition, 20% to 25% of patients have mutations in MAPK signaling proteins that are not currently druggable, such as RAS and neurofibromin 1. Consequently, additional targets and approaches are being explored such as AKT and ERK, as well as immune checkpoint blockade.

VEMURAFENIB (ZELBORAF)

PHARMACOLOGY AND MECHANISM OF ACTION

Structure: Vemurafenib, propane-1-sulfonic acid {3-[5-(4-chlorophenyl)-1H-pyrrolo[2,3-b]pyridine-3-carbonyl]-2,4-difluoro-phenyl}-amide, has the molecular formula $C_{23}H_{18}ClF_2N_3O_3S$ and molecular weight of 489.92 daltons. Figure 194-21 shows the structure of vemurafenib.

Metabolism: In vitro studies demonstrate that vemurafenib is a substrate of CYP3A4. Following oral administration, 94% of the dose of vemurafenib was recovered in the feces, while approximately 1% was found in the urine. The median elimination half-life is 57 hours.[78]

Absorption and Distribution: The bioavailability of vemurafenib has not been determined; however, following multiple doses, the median time to maximum plasma concentration was approximately 3 hours. In the clinical trials leading to its approval, Zelboraf was taken without regard to food.

Mechanism of Action: Vemurafenib is a small-molecular-weight inhibitor of certain mutated forms of the serine-threonine kinase BRAF, including V600E. In addition, vemurafenib inhibits wildtype BRAF, CRAF, ARAF, SRMS, ACK1, MAP4K5, and FGR. In cells with V600E-mutated BRAF, vemurafenib has antitumor effects.

INDICATIONS AND CONTRAINDICATIONS

The FDA approved Zelboraf in 2011 for use as monotherapy in the treatment of unresectable or metastatic melanoma with the $BRAF^{V600E}$ mutation, as detected by an FDA-approved test. Approval was based on 2 trials that demonstrated improved response rates and survival rates as compared to dacarbazine.[70,71] The median PFS was 5.3 months and 1.6 months, and the objective response rates were 48% and 5% in the vemurafenib-treated and dacarbazine-treated groups, respectively.[71] The median overall survival in patients treated with vemurafenib was 15.9 months in the single-arm Phase II trial.[70]

When used in combination with the MEK inhibitor cobimetinib (Cotellic), vemurafenib demonstrated improved efficacy, achieving an overall response rate of 68% and a PFS of 9.9 months.[77]

Zelboraf is also indicated to treat patients with Erdheim-Chester disease harboring V600 mutations. There are no contraindications listed on the drug label.

DOSING REGIMEN

The recommended dose of vemurafenib is 960 mg, taken by mouth with or without a meal, twice daily administered approximately 12 hours apart.

No formal studies have been conducted to evaluate the effects of renal or hepatic impairment on the pharmacokinetics of Zelboraf. No dose adjustments are recommended for patients with mild and moderate renal or hepatic impairment. Caution is advised for severe renal or hepatic impairment.

SIDE EFFECTS AND PRECAUTIONS

Adverse Effects: The most common noncutaneous adverse effects of Zelboraf include arthralgia, fatigue, and nausea. Zelboraf is associated with a variety of skin toxicities, including rash, alopecia, photosensitivity, pruritus, and new primary malignancies. Skin eruptions occurred in up to 68% of the patients taking vemurafenib.[70,71,79] The rashes have been described as folliculocentric, toxic erythema–like,

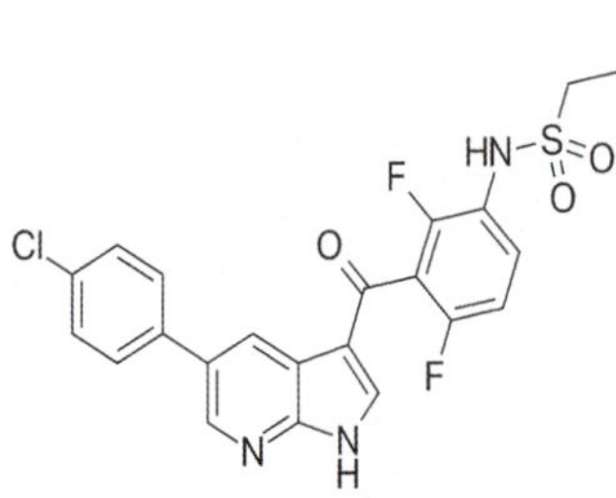

Figure 194-21 Structure of vemurafenib.

or exaggerated keratosis pilaris–like.[80] The toxic erythema–like rash has been described as having a morphology similar to a classic maculopapular drug hypersensitivity rash with histopathologic features suggestive of an exanthematous drug eruption.[80] Squamous proliferations ranging from benign papillomas and verrucous keratoses to keratoacanthomas and squamous cell carcinomas are commonly seen in patients taking single-agent vemurafenib. Papillomas were reported in 29% of patients and cSCCs and keratoacanthomas were described in 26% of patients in the Phase II trial.[70] In a newer prospective study of the cutaneous adverse effects of vemurafenib, verrucous papillomas occurred in 79% of patients, with nearly half of the patients developing between 4 and 20 efflorescent and verruciform lesions.[81] A hand–foot skin reaction characterized by hyperkeratotic plaques located on pressure points of the sole was observed in 60% of patients.[81] Additional skin toxicities that have been described with monotherapy include hair growth modification, hyperkeratotic follicular rash, xerosis, cystic lesions, facial erythema, cheilitis, nipple hyperkeratosis, Stevens-Johnson syndrome, toxic epidermal necrolysis, drug rash with eosinophilia and systemic symptoms syndrome, nevi efflorescence, and radiodermatitis.[81] Several of the cutaneous adverse effects appear to be dependent on MEK output via paradoxical activation of MAPK signaling, as concomitant use of the MEK inhibitor cobimetinib was associated with lower rates of keratoacanthomas, cSCCs, and alopecia.[77]

Additional adverse effects of Zelboraf include hepatoxicity, QT prolongation, uveitis, photophobia, and renal injury, including interstitial nephritis and acute tubular necrosis.

Based on its mechanism of action, Zelboraf may cause fetal harm and women should be made aware of the potential risk to a fetus. It is recommended that women of reproductive age be advised to use highly effective contraception during treatment and for 2 weeks after the final dose of Zelboraf. Although there is no information available regarding the presence of vemurafenib in human milk, the potential for harm to nursing infants exists; therefore, women should be advised to avoid breastfeeding during treatment and for at least 2 weeks following the last dose of Zelboraf.

Drug Interactions: It is recommended to avoid concomitant use of strong CYP3A4 inhibitors or inducers and CYP1A2 substrates with a narrow therapeutic window.

See the Zelboraf package insert for full drug–drug interactions and adverse effects.[78]

DABRAFENIB (TAFINLAR)

PHARMACOLOGY AND MECHANISM OF ACTION

Structure: Dabrafenib mesylate, N-{3-[5-(2-amino-4-pyrimidinyl)-2-(1,1-dimethylethyl)-1,3-thiazol-4-yl]-2-fluorophenyl}-2,6-difluorobenzene sulfonamide, methanesulfonate salt, has the molecular formula $C_{23}H_{20}F_3N_5O_2S_2 \cdot CH_4O_3S$ and a molecular weight of 615.68 daltons.[82] Figure 194-22 shows the structure of dabrafenib mesylate.

Metabolism: Dabrafenib is primarily metabolized by CYP2C8 and CYP3A4. Excretion through the feces is the main route of elimination (71%) of dabrafenib, while urinary excretion accounts for 23% of its elimination. After oral administration, the half-life of dabrafenib is 8 hours.

Absorption and Distribution: Dabrafenib exhibits 95% bioavailability and peak plasma concentrations are reached in 2 hours after oral administration; 99.7% of dabrafenib is bound to plasma proteins and its volume of distribution is 70.3 L.

Mechanism of Action: Dabrafenib is a small-molecular-weight inhibitor of certain mutated forms of the BRAF, including V600E, V600K, and V600D. It is a reversible ATP-competitive inhibitor, with a concentration required for 50% inhibition that is 5 times lower for $BRAF^{V600E}$ than for wildtype BRAF.[72] In addition, dabrafenib inhibits wildtype BRAF, CRAF, SIK1, NEK11, and LIMK1. In melanoma cells with V600-mutated BRAF, dabrafenib inhibits cell growth.

INDICATIONS AND CONTRAINDICATIONS

Tafinlar was given FDA approval in 2013 for treatment of unresectable or metastatic melanoma with BRAF V600E mutation, as detected by an FDA-approved test. Approval was based on data from a multicenter, open-label, randomized trial of 250 patients that demonstrated improved PFS as compared to dacarbazine (5.1 months vs. 2.7 months).[72] Tafinlar was also given accelerated approval in 2014 and full approval in 2015 for use in combination with the MEK inhibitor trametinib (Mekinist) in unresectable or metastatic BRAF V600E or V600K mutated melanoma. Approval was given after the combination demonstrated objective response rates of 64% to 76% and PFS of 9.3 to 11.4 months.[74-76] Long-term followup of patients from that cohort demonstrated on overall survival of 25 months and a 3-year overall survival of 38%.[83]

Tafinlar is also indicated in combination with Mekinist as: 1) adjuvant treatment for patients with V600 mutant melanoma involving lymph nodes following complete resection; 2) treatment for metastatic V600

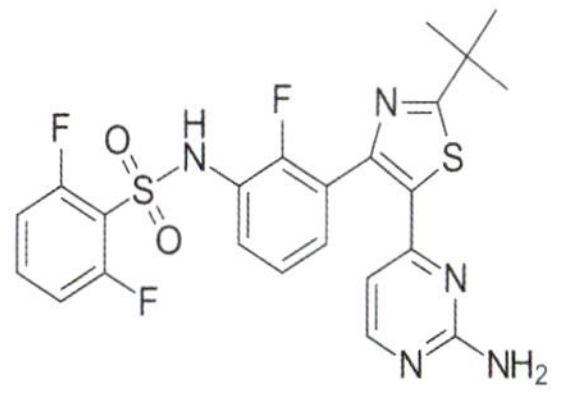

Figure 194-22 Structure of dabrafenib.

mutant NSCLC; and 3) metastatic or locally advanced V600 mutant anaplastic thyroid cancer with no satisfactory locoregional treatment options. There are no specific contraindications on the drug label.

DOSING REGIMEN

The recommend dose of Tafinlar is 150 mg taken by mouth twice daily at least 1 hour before or at least 2 hours after a meal. An FDA-approved test must be performed that confirms either the presence of a BRAF V600E mutation prior to monotherapy with Tafinlar, or the presence of a BRAF V600E or V600K mutation prior to combined therapy with trametinib.

No formal studies have been conducted to evaluate the effects of renal or hepatic impairment on the pharmacokinetics of Tafinlar. No specific dose adjustments are recommended for patients with mild hepatic or mild or moderate renal impairment. An appropriate dose has not been determined for moderate to severe hepatic or severe renal impairment.

Dose modifications of Tafinlar may be required based on toxicity. See the Tafinlar product label for the appropriate dose reduction.

SIDE EFFECTS AND PRECAUTIONS

Adverse Effects: The most common noncutaneous adverse effects include headache, pyrexia, and arthralgia. Cutaneous toxicities are similar to those seen with vemurafenib and include verruciform keratotic squamoproliferative lesions, papillomas, alopecia, rash, Grover disease, plantar hyperkeratosis, cSCC, keratoacanthoma, increased incidence of melanoma, seborrheic dermatitis–like eruption and palmar-plantar erythrodysesthesia syndrome.[82,84] New primary malignancies, cutaneous and noncutaneous, have been reported during treatment with Tafinlar. Additional toxicities include hemorrhage, cardiomyopathy, uveitis (including iritis and iridocyclitis), hyperglycemia, and hemolytic anemia in patients with glucose-6-phosphate dehydrogenase deficiency.

Based on data from animal studies and its mechanism of action, Tafinlar may cause fetal harm and women should be made aware of the potential risk to a fetus. It is recommended that women of reproductive age be advised to use highly effective contraception during treatment and for 2 weeks after the final dose of Tafinlar. Although there is no information available regarding the presence of dabrafenib in human milk, there is a potential for serious adverse reactions to nursing infants; consequently, women should be advised to avoid breastfeeding during treatment and for at least 2 weeks following the last dose of Tafinlar.

Drug Interactions: It is recommended to avoid concurrent use of strong inhibitors or inducers of CYP3A4 or CYP2C8. Coadministration of compounds that are sensitive substrates of CYP3A4, CYP2B6, CYP2C8, CYP2C9, or CYP2C19 may result in decreased efficacy of these agents.

See the Tafinlar package insert for full drug–drug interactions and adverse effects.[82]

TRAMETINIB (MEKINIST)

PHARMACOLOGY AND MECHANISM OF ACTION

Structure: Trametinib dimethyl sulfoxide, or acetamide, N-[3-[3-cyclopropyl-5-[(2-fluoro-4-iodophenyl)amino]-3,4,6,7-tetrahydro-6,8-dimethyl-2,4,7-trioxopyrido[4,3-d]pyrimidin-1(2H)-yl]phenyl]-, compound with 1,1′-sulfinylbis[methane] (1:1), has the molecular formula $C_{26}H_{23}FIN_5O_4 \bullet C_2H_6OS$ and molecular mass of 693.53 daltons. Figure 194-23 shows the structure of trametinib dimethyl sulfoxide.

Metabolism: Trametinib is primarily metabolized by non–CYP-mediated deacetylation alone or in combination with monooxygenation or glucuronidation biotransformation pathways. The estimated elimination half-life is 3.9 to 4.8 hours. Greater than 80% is excreted through the feces, while less than 20% is eliminated through the urine.

Absorption and Distribution: Trametinib is 72% bioavailable and the volume of distribution is 214 L.

Mechanism of Action: Trametinib is a reversible, small-molecule inhibitor of activation and kinase activity of MEK1 and MEK2.[85] Trametinib inhibits the in vitro and in vivo cell growth of BRAF V600 mutation-positive melanoma.

INDICATIONS AND CONTRAINDICATIONS

Mekinist is indicated for use as a single agent or in combination with dabrafenib for the treatment of unresectable or metastatic BRAF V600E–mutated or BRAF V600K–mutated melanoma, as determined by an FDA-approved test. Approval as monotherapy was given in 2013 based on the Phase III METRIC (MEK Versus Dacarbazine [DTIC] or Paclitaxel [Taxol] in Metastatic Melanoma) study which demonstrated improved PFS in patients receiving trametinib 2 mg once daily (4.8 months) as compared to those receiving either dacarbazine or paclitaxel (1.5 months).[73]

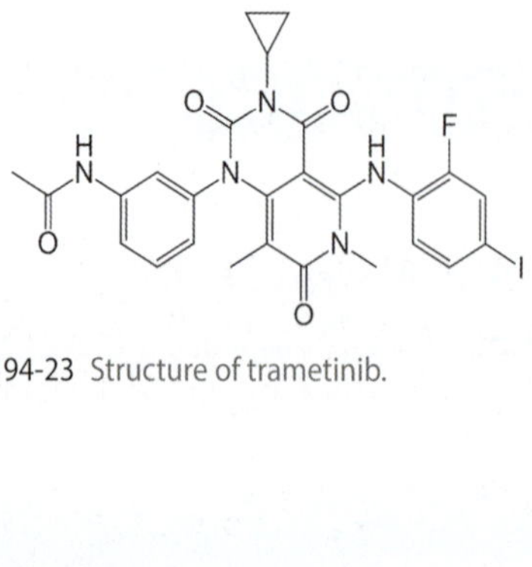

Figure 194-23 Structure of trametinib.

As stated above, Mekinist is synergistic when used in combination with Tafinlar resulting in superior objective response rates (64% to 76%) and PFS (9.3 to 11.4 months) compared to monotherapy.[74-76]

Mekinist is also indicated in combination with Tafinlar as: 1) adjuvant treatment for patients with V600 mutant melanoma involving lymph nodes following complete resection;2) treatment for metastatic V600 mutant NSCLC; and 3) metastatic or locally advanced V600 mutant anaplastic thyroid cancer with no satisfactory locoregional treatment options.

There are no specific contraindications on the product label.

DOSING REGIMEN

The recommend dose of trametinib is 2 mg taken by mouth once daily at least 1 hour before or at least 2 hours after a meal.

No dedicated studies have been conducted to evaluate the effects of renal or hepatic impairment on the pharmacokinetics of Mekinist. No specific dose adjustments are recommended for patients with mild hepatic or mild or moderate renal impairment. An appropriate dose of Mekinist has not been determined for moderate to severe hepatic or severe renal impairment.

Dose modifications of Mekinist may be required based on toxicity. See the Mekinist package insert for the appropriate dose reduction.

SIDE EFFECTS AND PRECAUTIONS

Adverse Effects: The most common adverse effects include rash, diarrhea, and lymphedema. When used in combination with Tafinlar, the most common toxicities include pyrexia, nausea, rash, diarrhea, vomiting, chills, hypertension, and peripheral edema. The most common cutaneous toxicity is a papulopustular eruption similar to those seen with inhibitors of EGFR, occurring in 40% to 93% of patients.[86] Other skin changes include pruritus, xerosis, alopecia, paronychia, and eruptions described as maculopapular and urticarial-to-targetoid with central duskiness.[86] Other adverse effects include venous thromboembolism, cardiomyopathy, retinal vein occlusion, retinal pigment epithelial detachment, interstitial lung disease, and hyperglycemia.

Based on data from animal studies and its mechanism of action, Mekinist may cause fetal harm and women should be made aware of the potential risk to a fetus. It is recommended that women of reproductive age be advised to use highly effective contraception during treatment and for 4 months after the final dose of Mekinist. Increased follicular cysts and decreased corpora lutea were observed in animal studies; thus, women should be advised that Mekinist may impair fertility. Although there is no information available regarding the presence of trametinib in human milk, there is a potential for serious adverse reactions to nursing infants; consequently, women should be advised to avoid breastfeeding during treatment and for at least 4 months following the last dose of Mekinist.

Drug Interactions: Trametinib is not a substrate of CYP enzymes and at the clinically relevant systemic concentration of 0.04 µM, it is not an inhibitor of CYP1A2, CYP2A6, CYP2B6, CYP2C9, CYP2C19, CYP2D6, or CYP3A4.

See the Mekinist package insert for full drug–drug interactions and adverse effects.[82]

COBIMETINIB (COTELLIC)

PHARMACOLOGY AND MECHANISM OF ACTION

Structure: Cobimetinib fumarate, (S)-[3,4-difluoro-2-(2-fluoro-4-iodophenylamino)phenyl] [3-hydroxy-3-(piperidin-2-yl)azetidin-1-yl]methanone hemifumarate, has the molecular formula $C_{46}H_{46}F_{6}I_{2}N_{6}O_{8}$ and molecular mass of 1178.71 daltons. Figure 194-24 shows the structure of cobimetinib fumarate.

Metabolism: Cobimetinib is primary metabolized by oxidization via CYP3A and glucuronidation by way of UGT2B7. The elimination half-life following oral administration is 44 hours. Excretion is primarily via the fecal route (76%).

Absorption and Distribution: The bioavailability of cobimetinib is 46% and its volume of distribution is 806 L.

Mechanism of Action: Cobimetinib fumarate is a reversible inhibitor of MEK1 and MEK2. The compound inhibits BRAF V600E–mutant murine cells transplanted into mice.[87]

INDICATIONS AND CONTRAINDICATIONS

Cotellic is indicated for the treatment of unresectable or metastatic BRAF V600E–mutant or BRAF V600K–mutant melanoma, in combination with vemurafenib. Approval was based on results from the coBRIM (Cobimetinib Combined with Vemurafenib in Advanced BRAF V600–mutant Melanoma) trial which showed that the combination of vemurafenib and cobimetinib produced improved PFS and

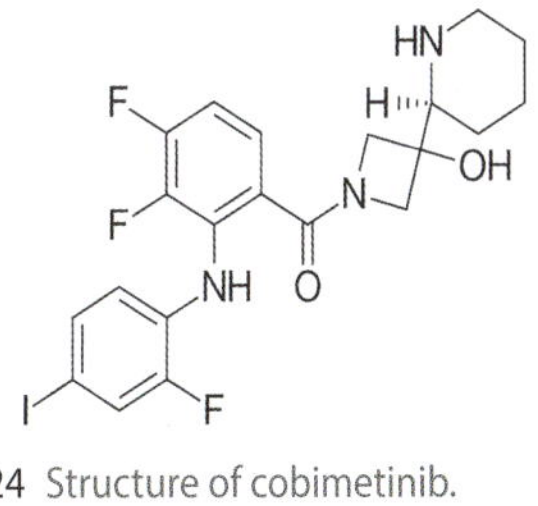

Figure 194-24 Structure of cobimetinib.

response rates compared to single-agent vemurafenib in patients with previously untreated, unresectable or metastatic BRAF V600 mutation-positive melanoma (PFS: 9.9 months vs. 6.2 months; objective response rate 68% vs. 45%).[77]

There are no specific contraindications on the product label.

DOSING REGIMEN

The recommended dose of Cotellic is 60 mg by mouth once daily, with or without food, for the first 21 days of a 28-day cycle.

No dedicated studies have been conducted to evaluate the effects of renal or hepatic impairment on the pharmacokinetics of Cotellic. No specific dose adjustments are recommended for patients with mild hepatic or mild or moderate renal impairment. An appropriate dose of Cotellic has not been determined for moderate to severe hepatic or severe renal impairment.

Dose modifications of Cotellic may be required based on toxicity. See the Cotellic package insert for the appropriate dose reduction.[87]

SIDE EFFECTS AND PRECAUTIONS

Adverse Effects: The most common adverse reactions for Cotellic are diarrhea, photosensitivity reaction, nausea, pyrexia, and vomiting. The most common grade 4 event (4%) was elevated creatinine kinase, a known class effect of MEK blockade.[77] Other serious laboratory abnormalities include increased γ-glutamyl transferase, hypophosphatemia, increased alanine aminotransferase and aspartate aminotransferase, lymphopenia, increased alkaline phosphatase, and hyponatremia. Although squamoproliferative events are seen with combination therapy, cSCC and keratoacanthomas appear to be less common with the dual therapy cobimetinib and vemurafenib compared with single-agent vemurafenib.[77] A grade 3 to grade 4 rash was seen in 16% of patients receiving dual therapy compared with 17% receiving single agent vemurafenib. Other noncutaneous adverse effects include cardiomyopathy, hemorrhage, noncutaneous malignancies, retinopathy, and rhabdomyolysis.

Based on data from animal studies and its mechanism of action, Cotellic may cause fetal harm and women should be made aware of the potential risk to a fetus. It is recommended that women of reproductive age be advised to use highly effective contraception during treatment and for 2 weeks following the final dose of Cotellic. Patients should be advised that Cotellic may impair fertility in both females and males. Although there is no information available regarding the presence of cobimetinib in human milk, there is a potential for serious adverse reactions to nursing infants; therefore, women should be advised to avoid breastfeeding during treatment and for at least 2 weeks following the last dose of Cotellic.

Drug Interactions: Moderate or strong inhibitor or inducers of CYP3A should be avoided when taking Cotellic.

See the Cotellic package insert for full drug–drug interactions and adverse effects.

FUTURE DIRECTIONS IN MELANOMA: AKT AND ERK INHIBITION

AKT INHIBITORS

PI3K–AKT–mTOR (mammalian target of rapamycin) signaling is an important oncogenic pathway in melanoma development and progression. The hyperactivation of this pathway is associated with activation of receptor tyrosine kinases, somatic mutations in key signaling genes such as *PIK3CA*, or inactivation of the tumor-suppressor gene *PTEN*.[88] Preclinical studies with AKT inhibitors have demonstrated the usefulness of AKT inhibitors in melanoma treatment. Conjunctival melanoma is a rare, but deadly, variant of melanoma with limited effective treatment options. Preclinical in vitro studies demonstrate that the AKT inhibitor, MK2206, suppresses growth in conjunctival melanoma cell lines, and furthermore, a synergistic effect was observed when combined with the MEK inhibitor MEK162.[89] These preliminary findings have supported the rationale for a recently initiated Phase II clinical trial studying the efficacy of the MEK inhibitor trametinib, with or without the AKT inhibitor GSK2141795, for treatment of patients with stage IV uveal melanoma (NCT01979523). Also, in a Phase I trial investigating the oral AKT inhibitor MK2206 combined with chemotherapy for solid tumors, 2 patients with stage IV *BRAF WT* melanoma tolerated and experienced disease-free progression with MK2206 combined with carboplatin and paclitaxel.[90]

More recently, another Phase I study revealed that the AKT inhibitor ipatasertib (GDC-0068) is capable of safe and robust targeting of AKT in patients with solid tumors.[91] These preliminary studies are paving the way for larger randomized, controlled clinical trials, which may result in the addition of AKT inhibitors to the armamentarium of therapeutics for advanced melanoma.

EXTRACELLULAR SIGNAL-REGULATED KINASE INHIBITORS

The MAPK (RAS-RAF-MEK-ERK) pathway is hyperactivated in more than 90% of melanomas.[92] RAF and MEK inhibitors were the first clinically available therapeutics aimed at targeting the MAPK pathway for advanced melanoma patients. However, acquired resistance to BRAF and MEK inhibitors proves to be a major limitation to sustainable outcomes.[93] One well-characterized mechanism of resistance is the reactivation of the downstream MAPK pathway target ERK; hence, investigators are focusing on the development of ERK inhibitors.[93] Preclinical studies show that ERK inhibition is more effective, compared to MEK inhibition, in suppressing MAPK activity and tumor growth in multiple BRAF inhibitor–resistant melanoma cell lines.[94] Also, in vitro data demonstrates that MEK inhibitor–resistant melanoma cell lines are sensitive to ERK inhibition, and that combined treatment with MEK and ERK inhibitors is synergistic and overcomes acquired resistance to MEK inhibition.[95] Although the preclinical data is promising, ERK inhibitors are capable of targeting a wide range of kinases, hence a potential narrow therapeutic index is a major concern. Currently, there are Phase I clinical trials underway exploring safety and tolerability of the ERK inhibitors, BVD-523 and LTT462, in patients with advanced solid malignancies (NCT01781429, NCT02711345).

REFERENCES

1. Goff SP, Gilboa E, Witte ON, et al. Structure of the Abelson murine leukemia virus genome and the homologous cellular gene: studies with cloned viral DNA. *Cell.* 1980;22(3):777-785.
2. Ben-Neriah Y, Daley GQ, Mes-Masson AM, et al. The chronic myelogenous leukemia-specific P210 protein is the product of the bcr/abl hybrid gene. *Science.* 1986;233(4760):212-214.
3. Druker BJ, Tamura S, Buchdunger E, et al. Effects of a selective inhibitor of the Abl tyrosine kinase on the growth of Bcr-Abl positive cells. *Nat Med.* 1996;2(5):561-566.
4. Druker BJ, Sawyers CL, Kantarjian H, et al. Activity of a specific inhibitor of the BCR-ABL tyrosine kinase in the blast crisis of chronic myeloid leukemia and acute lymphoblastic leukemia with the Philadelphia chromosome. *N Engl J Med.* 2001;344(14):1038-1042.
5. Druker BJ, Talpaz M, Resta DJ, et al. Efficacy and safety of a specific inhibitor of the BCR-ABL tyrosine kinase in chronic myeloid leukemia. *N Engl J Med.* 2001;344(14):1031-1037.
6. Simon MP, Pedeutour F, Sirvent N, et al. Deregulation of the platelet-derived growth factor B-chain gene via fusion with collagen gene COL1A1 in dermatofibrosarcoma protuberans and giant-cell fibroblastoma. *Nat Genet.* 1997;15(1):95-98.
7. McArthur GA, Demetri GD, van Oosterom A, et al. Molecular and clinical analysis of locally advanced dermatofibrosarcoma protuberans treated with imatinib: Imatinib Target Exploration Consortium Study B2225. *J Clin Oncol.* 2005;23(4):866-873.
8. *Gleevec (imatinib)* [package insert]. Stein, Switzerland: Novartis; 2016.
9. Guo J, Si L, Kong Y, et al. Phase II, open-label, single-arm trial of imatinib mesylate in patients with metastatic melanoma harboring c-Kit mutation or amplification. *J Clin Oncol.* 2011;29(21):2904-2909.
10. Hodi FS, Corless CL, Giobbie-Hurder A, et al. Imatinib for melanomas harboring mutationally activated or amplified KIT arising on mucosal, acral, and chronically sun-damaged skin. *J Clin Oncol.* 2013;31(26):3182-3190.
11. Carvajal RD, Antonescu CR, Wolchok JD, et al. KIT as a therapeutic target in metastatic melanoma. *JAMA.* 2011;305(22):2327-2334.
12. Macdonald JB, Macdonald B, Golitz LE, et al. Cutaneous adverse effects of targeted therapies: part I: inhibitors of the cellular membrane. *J Am Acad Dermatol.* 2015;72(2):203-218; quiz 219-220.
13. *Tasigna (nilotinib)* [package insert]. Stein, Switzerland: Novartis; 2010.
14. Lee SJ, Kim TM, Kim YJ, et al. Phase II trial of nilotinib in patients with metastatic malignant melanoma harboring KIT gene aberration: a multicenter trial of Korean Cancer Study Group (UN10-06). *Oncologist.* 2015;20(11):1312-1319.
15. Carvajal RD, Lawrence DP, Weber JS, et al. Phase II study of nilotinib in melanoma harboring KIT alterations following progression to prior KIT inhibition. *Clin Cancer Res.* 2015;21(10):2289-2296.
16. *Sprycel (dasatinib)* [package insert]. Princeton, NJ: Bristol-Myers Squibb Company; 2016.
17. Kluger HM, Dudek AZ, McCann C, et al. A phase 2 trial of dasatinib in advanced melanoma. *Cancer.* 2011;117(10):2202-2208.
18. Algazi AP, Weber JS, Andrews SC, et al. Phase I clinical trial of the Src inhibitor dasatinib with dacarbazine in metastatic melanoma. *Br J Cancer.* 2012;106(1):85-91.
19. Ainechi S, Carlson JA. Neutrophilic dermatosis limited to lipo-lymphedematous skin in a morbidly obese woman on dasatinib therapy. *Am J Dermatopathol.* 2016;38(2):e22-e26.
20. Drucker AM, Wu S, Busam KJ, et al. Rash with the multitargeted kinase inhibitors nilotinib and dasatinib: metaanalysis and clinical characterization. *Eur J Haematol.* 2013;90(2):142-150.
21. *Bosulif (bosutinib)* [package insert]. New York, NY: Pfizer Inc; 2016.
22. *Iclusig (ponatinib)* [package insert]. Cambridge, MA: Ariad Pharmaceuticals, Inc; 2016.
23. Paez JG, Janne PA, Lee JC, et al. EGFR mutations in lung cancer: correlation with clinical response to gefitinib therapy. *Science.* 2004;304(5676):1497-1500.
24. Lynch TJ, Bell DW, Sordella R, et al. Activating mutations in the epidermal growth factor receptor underlying responsiveness of non-small-cell lung cancer to gefitinib. *N Engl J Med.* 2004;350(21):2129-2139.
25. Thatcher N, Chang A, Parikh P, et al. Gefitinib plus best supportive care in previously treated patients with refractory advanced non-small-cell lung cancer: results from a randomised, placebo-controlled, multicentre study (Iressa Survival Evaluation in Lung Cancer). *Lancet.* 2005;366(9496):1527-1537.
26. Fukuoka M, Wu YL, Thongprasert S, et al. Biomarker analyses and final overall survival results from a phase III, randomized, open-label, first-line study of gefitinib versus carboplatin/paclitaxel in clinically selected patients with advanced non-small-cell lung cancer in Asia (IPASS). *J Clin Oncol.* 2011;29(21):2866-2874.
27. Rosell R, Carcereny E, Gervais R, et al. Erlotinib versus standard chemotherapy as first-line treatment for European patients with advanced EGFR mutation-positive non-small-cell lung cancer (EURTAC):

28. Yu HA, Arcila ME, Rekhtman N, et al. Analysis of tumor specimens at the time of acquired resistance to EGFR-TKI therapy in 155 patients with EGFR-mutant lung cancers. *Clin Cancer Res.* 2013;19(8):2240-2247.
29. Carrera S, Buque A, Azkona E, et al. Epidermal growth factor receptor tyrosine-kinase inhibitor treatment resistance in non-small cell lung cancer: biological basis and therapeutic strategies. *Clin Transl Oncol.* 2014;16(4):339-350.
30. Janne PA, Yang JC, Kim DW, et al. AZD9291 in EGFR inhibitor-resistant non-small-cell lung cancer. *N Engl J Med.* 2015;372(18):1689-1699.
31. *Erbitux (cetuximab)* [package insert]. Branchburg, NJ: ImClone LLC; 2012.
32. Tan AR, Moore DF, Hidalgo M, et al. Pharmacokinetics of cetuximab after administration of escalating single dosing and weekly fixed dosing in patients with solid tumors. *Clin Cancer Res.* 2006;12(21):6517-6522.
33. Maubec E, Petrow P, Scheer-Senyarich I, et al. Phase II study of cetuximab as first-line single-drug therapy in patients with unresectable squamous cell carcinoma of the skin. *J Clin Oncol.* 2011;29(25):3419-3426.
34. Garden BC, Wu S, Lacouture ME. The risk of nail changes with epidermal growth factor receptor inhibitors: a systematic review of the literature and metaanalysis. *J Am Acad Dermatol.* 2012;67(3):400-408.
35. Perez-Soler R, Saltz L. Cutaneous adverse effects with HER1/EGFR-targeted agents: is there a silver lining? *J Clin Oncol.* 2005;23(22):5235-5246.
36. *Vectibix (panitumumab)* [package insert]. Thousand Oaks, CA: Amgen Inc; 2015.
37. Marti A, Fauconneau A, Ouhabrache N, et al. Complete remission of squamous cell carcinoma after treatment with panitumumab in a patient with cetuximab-induced anaphylaxis. *JAMA Dermatol.* 2016;152(3):343-345.
38. Foote MC, McGrath M, Guminski A, et al. Phase II study of single-agent panitumumab in patients with incurable cutaneous squamous cell carcinoma. *Ann Oncol.* 2014;25(10):2047-2052.
39. *Iressa (gefitinib)* [package insert]. Wilmington, DE: AstraZeneca Pharmaceuticals LP; 2015.
40. Wacker B, Nagrani T, Weinberg J, et al. Correlation between development of rash and efficacy in patients treated with the epidermal growth factor receptor tyrosine kinase inhibitor erlotinib in two large phase III studies. *Clin Cancer Res.* 2007;13(13):3913-3921.
41. *Tarceva (erlotinib)* [package insert]. Northbrook, IL: OSI Pharmaceuticals, LLC; 2016.
42. Mudigonda TV, Wyman K, Spigel DR, et al. A phase II trial of erlotinib and bevacizumab for patients with metastatic melanoma. *Pigment Cell Melanoma Res.* 2016;29(1):101-103.
43. *Gilotrif (afatinib dimaleate)* [package insert]. Ridgefield, CT: Boehringer Ingelheim International GmbH; 2016.
44. Kudo K, Hotta K, Bessho A, et al. Development of a skin rash within the first week and the therapeutic effect in afatinib monotherapy for EGFR-mutant non-small cell lung cancer (NSCLC): Okayama Lung Cancer Study Group experience. *Cancer Chemother Pharmacol.* 2016;77(5):1005-1009.
45. Chen KL, Lin CC, Cho YT, et al. Comparison of skin toxic effects associated with gefitinib, erlotinib, or afatinib treatment for non-small cell lung cancer. *JAMA Dermatol.* 2016;152(3):340-342.
46. Doesch J, Debus D, Meyer C, et al. Afatinib-associated Stevens-Johnson syndrome in an EGFR-mutated lung cancer patient. *Lung Cancer.* 2016;95:35-38.
47. Miguel-Gomez L, Vano-Galvan S, Garrido-Lopez P, et al. Afatinib-induced hypertrichosis of the eyelashes and eyebrows. *Indian J Dermatol Venereol Leprol.* 2016;82(2):192-193.
48. *Tagrisso (osimertinib mesylate)* [package insert]. Wilmington, DE: AstraZeneca Pharmaceuticals LP; 2016.
49. Johnson RL, Rothman AL, Xie J, et al. Human homolog of patched, a candidate gene for the basal cell nevus syndrome. *Science.* 1996;272(5268):1668-1671.
50. Gailani MR, Stahle-Backdahl M, Leffell DJ, et al. The role of the human homologue of *Drosophila* patched in sporadic basal cell carcinomas. *Nat Genet.* 1996;14(1):78-81.
51. Epstein EH. Basal cell carcinomas: attack of the hedgehog. *Nat Rev Cancer.* 2008;8(10):743-754.
52. *Erivedge (vismodegib)* [package insert]. South San Francisco, CA: Genetech; 2016.
53. Sekulic A, Migden MR, Oro AE, et al. Efficacy and safety of vismodegib in advanced basal-cell carcinoma. *N Engl J Med.* 2012;366(23):2171-2179.
54. Basset-Seguin N, Hauschild A, Grob JJ, et al. Vismodegib in patients with advanced basal cell carcinoma (STEVIE): a preplanned interim analysis of an international, open-label trial. *Lancet Oncol.* 2015;16(6):729-736.
55. Macdonald JB, Macdonald B, Golitz LE, et al. Cutaneous adverse effects of targeted therapies: part II: inhibitors of intracellular molecular signaling pathways. *J Am Acad Dermatol.* 2015;72(2):221-236; quiz 237-228.
56. *Odomzo (sonidegib)* [package insert]. East Hanover, NJ: Novartis; 2016.
57. Migden MR, Guminski A, Gutzmer R, et al. Treatment with two different doses of sonidegib in patients with locally advanced or metastatic basal cell carcinoma (BOLT): a multicentre, randomised, double-blind phase 2 trial. *Lancet Oncol.* 2015;16(6):716-728.
58. Minucci S, Pelicci PG. Histone deacetylase inhibitors and the promise of epigenetic (and more) treatments for cancer. *Nat Rev Cancer.* 2006;6(1):38-51.
59. Lane AA, Chabner BA. Histone deacetylase inhibitors in cancer therapy. *J Clin Oncol.* 2009;27(32):5459-5468.
60. *Zolinza (vorinostat)* [package insert]. Whitehouse Station, NJ: Merck & Co., Inc; 2015.
61. Duvic M, Talpur R, Ni X, et al. Phase 2 trial of oral vorinostat (suberoylanilide hydroxamic acid, SAHA) for refractory cutaneous T-cell lymphoma (CTCL). *Blood.* 2007;109(1):31-39.
62. Olsen EA, Kim YH, Kuzel TM, et al. Phase IIb multicenter trial of vorinostat in patients with persistent, progressive, or treatment refractory cutaneous T-cell lymphoma. *J Clin Oncol.* 2007;25(21):3109-3115.
63. *Istodax (romidepsin)* [package insert]. Summit, NJ: Celgene Corporation; 2016.
64. Piekarz RL, Frye R, Turner M, et al. Phase II multiinstitutional trial of the histone deacetylase inhibitor romidepsin as monotherapy for patients with cutaneous T-cell lymphoma. *J Clin Oncol.* 2009;27(32):5410-5417.
65. Whittaker SJ, Demierre MF, Kim EJ, et al. Final results from a multicenter, international, pivotal study of romidepsin in refractory cutaneous T-cell lymphoma. *J Clin Oncol.* 2010;28(29):4485-4491.

66. *Beleodaq (belinostat)* [package insert]. Irvine, CA: Spectrum Pharmaceuticals; 2014.
67. O'Connor OA, Horwitz S, Masszi T, et al. Belinostat in patients with relapsed or refractory peripheral T-cell lymphoma: results of the pivotal phase II BELIEF (CLN-19) study. *J Clin Oncol*. 2015;33(23):2492-2499.
68. *Farydak (panobinostat)* [package insert]. East Hanover, NJ: Novartis Pharmaceuticals Corporation; 2015.
69. Davies H, Bignell GR, Cox C, et al. Mutations of the BRAF gene in human cancer. *Nature*. 2002;417(6892):949-954.
70. Sosman JA, Kim KB, Schuchter L, et al. Survival in BRAF V600-mutant advanced melanoma treated with vemurafenib. *N Engl J Med*. 2012;366(8):707-714.
71. Chapman PB, Hauschild A, Robert C, et al. Improved survival with vemurafenib in melanoma with BRAF V600E mutation. *N Engl J Med*. 2011;364(26):2507-2516.
72. Hauschild A, Grob JJ, Demidov LV, et al. Dabrafenib in BRAF-mutated metastatic melanoma: a multicentre, open-label, phase 3 randomised controlled trial. *Lancet*. 2012;380(9839):358-365.
73. Flaherty KT, Robert C, Hersey P, et al. Improved survival with MEK inhibition in BRAF-mutated melanoma. *N Engl J Med*. 2012;367(2):107-114.
74. Robert C, Karaszewska B, Schachter J, et al. Improved overall survival in melanoma with combined dabrafenib and trametinib. *N Engl J Med*. 2015;372(1):30-39.
75. Flaherty KT, Infante JR, Daud A, et al. Combined BRAF and MEK inhibition in melanoma with BRAF V600 mutations. *N Engl J Med*. 2012;367(18):1694-1703.
76. Long GV, Stroyakovskiy D, Gogas H, et al. Combined BRAF and MEK inhibition versus BRAF inhibition alone in melanoma. *N Engl J Med*. 2014;371(20):1877-1888.
77. Larkin J, Ascierto PA, Dreno B, et al. Combined vemurafenib and cobimetinib in BRAF-mutated melanoma. *N Engl J Med*. 2014;371(20):1867-1876.
78. *Zelboraf (vemurafenib)* [package insert]. South San Francisco, CA: Genentech; 2016.
79. Flaherty KT, Puzanov I, Kim KB, et al. Inhibition of mutated, activated BRAF in metastatic melanoma. *N Engl J Med*. 2010;363(9):809-819.
80. Sinha R, Edmonds K, Newton-Bishop JA, et al. Cutaneous adverse events associated with vemurafenib in patients with metastatic melanoma: practical advice on diagnosis, prevention and management of the main treatment-related skin toxicities. *Br J Dermatol*. 2012;167(5):987-994.
81. Boussemart L, Routier E, Mateus C, et al. Prospective study of cutaneous side-effects associated with the BRAF inhibitor vemurafenib: a study of 42 patients. *Ann Oncol*. 2013;24(6):1691-1697.
82. *Tafinlar (dabrafenib)* [package insert]. East Hanover, NJ: Novartis Pharmaceuticals Corporation; 2016.
83. Long GV, Weber JS, Infante JR, et al. Overall survival and durable responses in patients with BRAF V600-mutant metastatic melanoma receiving dabrafenib combined with trametinib. *J Clin Oncol*. 2016;34(8):871-878.
84. Anforth RM, Blumetti TC, Kefford RF, et al. Cutaneous manifestations of dabrafenib (GSK2118436): a selective inhibitor of mutant BRAF in patients with metastatic melanoma. *Br J Dermatol*. 2012;167(5):1153-1160.
85. *Mekinist (trametinib)* [package insert]. East Hanover, NJ: Novartis Pharmaceuticals Corporation; 2015.
86. Patel U, Cornelius L, Anadkat MJ. MEK inhibitor-induced dusky erythema: characteristic drug hypersensitivity manifestation in 3 patients. *JAMA Dermatol*. 2015;151(1):78-81.
87. *Cotellic (cobimetinib)* [package insert]. South San Francisco, CA: Genentech; 2015.
88. Jokinen E, Koivunen JP. MEK and PI3K inhibition in solid tumors: rationale and evidence to date. *Ther Adv Med Oncol*. 2015;7(3):170-180.
89. Cao J, Heijkants RC, Jochemsen AG, et al. Targeting of the MAPK and AKT pathways in conjunctival melanoma shows potential synergy. *Oncotarget*. 2016.
90. Molife LR, Yan L, Vitfell-Rasmussen J, et al. Phase 1 trial of the oral AKT inhibitor MK-2206 plus carboplatin/paclitaxel, docetaxel, or erlotinib in patients with advanced solid tumors. *J Hematol Oncol*. 2014;7:1.
91. Saura C, Roda D, Rosello S, et al. A first-in-human phase I study of the ATP-competitive Akt inhibitor ipatasertib (GDC-0068) demonstrates robust and safe targeting of Akt in patients with solid tumors. *Cancer Discov*. 2017;7(1):102-113.
92. Wellbrock C, Arozarena I. The complexity of the ERK/MAP-kinase pathway and the treatment of melanoma skin cancer. *Front Cell Dev Biol*. 2016;4:33.
93. Welsh SJ, Rizos H, Scolyer RA, et al. Resistance to combination BRAF and MEK inhibition in metastatic melanoma: where to next? *Eur J Cancer*. 2016;62:76-85.
94. Carlino MS, Todd JR, Gowrishankar K, et al. Differential activity of MEK and ERK inhibitors in BRAF inhibitor resistant melanoma. *Mol Oncol*. 2014;8(3):544-554.
95. Hatzivassiliou G, Liu B, O'Brien C, et al. ERK inhibition overcomes acquired resistance to MEK inhibitors. *Mol Cancer Ther*. 2012;11(5):1143-1154.

Chapter 195 :: Antiangiogenic Agents
:: Adilson da Costa, Michael Y. Bonner, & Jack L. Arbiser

第一百九十五章

抗血管生成抑制药

中文导读

本章首先介绍了抗血管生成的作用在临床中被认识，是源于1971年Judah Folkman发表的一篇具有里程碑意义的论文，他假设所有肿瘤的生长都依赖于血管生成，因此血管生成抑制药可用于治疗癌症。随后证明抗血管生成抑制药不仅在肿瘤治疗中，而且在其他各种疾病治疗中都有好的前景。本章中介绍了多种抗血管生成抑制药，包括贝卡普勒明、贝伐单抗、硼替佐米、西妥昔单抗、糖皮质激素、厄洛替尼、依维莫司、咪喹莫特、干扰素α-2B、帕尼曲单抗、培加他尼、普萘洛尔、雷尼珠单抗、西罗莫司、苏尼替尼、替西罗莫司、沙利度胺、曲妥珠单抗等，并介绍了这些药物的机制、适应证、初始治疗、风险、预防措施及并发症等。

〔粟 娟〕

AT-A-GLANCE

- "Direct" antiangiogenic agents act directly on untransformed endothelial cells to prevent proliferation, migration, and survival.
- "Indirect" antiangiogenic agents inhibit tumor-produced oncogene proteins that promote a proangiogenic state.
- Antiangiogenic agents are a promising class of drugs because they are effective against slow-growing tumors.

In 1971, Judah Folkman published a landmark paper hypothesizing that all tumor growth is dependent on angiogenesis and that inhibitors of angiogenesis could be used to treat cancers.[1] The ensuing years have proven him correct and have seen the development of new agents that, either alone or in adjunct, have shown promise not only in oncology but in a variety of dermatologic conditions as well.[2]

Antiangiogenic drugs can be classified as either "direct" or "indirect;" the direct act directly on untransformed endothelial cells to prevent proliferation, migration, or survival, a process that normally occurs upon stimulation by proangiogenic molecules; the indirect act indirectly by inhibition of tumor-produced oncogenic protein products that promote proangiogenic states. Angiogenesis inhibitors as a drug class provide a unique approach to cancer treatment because they are also effective against slow-growing tumors, whereas traditional therapies, such as chemotherapy and radiation, work best on rapidly-dividing cells. In the future, the switch to an angiogenic phenotype may be able to be blocked in clinically undetectable cancers, thereby preventing disease progression using therapies directed, in part, by angiogenesis biomarkers.[3,4] Although application of these agents center so far on oncologic and ophthalmologic diseases, promising and new dermatologic indications are sure to come.[2]

Figure 195-1 better illustrates the mechanisms of action of some of the drugs described in this chapter, helping to elucidate how they work as antiangiogenic agents.

BECAPLERMIN (REGRANEX)

With the rise in incidence of diabetes and the increasingly aging population, chronic wounds have become increasingly prevalent. Treatment of these wounds is particularly challenging because normal wound-healing processes have been disrupted.[2]

MECHANISM OF ACTION

Becaplermin (recombinant human platelet-derived growth factor BB) is the first FDA-approved angiogenesis-stimulating therapy. Endogenous platelet-derived growth factor (PDGF) is chemotactic for several cell types necessary for wound healing, and is also a mitogen for fibroblasts, the source for extracellular matrix components like glycosaminoglycans and fibronectin. Thus, PDGF is an important factor in the formation of granulation tissue.[5]

INDICATIONS

Becaplermin gel is currently indicated for the treatment of lower extremity, diabetic, neuropathic ulcers which must be adequately vascularized and reach to at least the level of subcutaneous tissue.[5-7] Off-label uses include the application of becaplermin to ulcerated hemangiomata, surgical wounds, grafts, pyoderma gangrenosum, calciphylaxis, ulcerated necrobiosis lipoidica, and flaps.[8-11] However, cost-effectiveness of this form of therapy in the treatment of diabetic foot ulcers is also outlined.[12]

CONTRAINDICATIONS

Becaplermin gel is contraindicated in patients with known cancer within the treatment area or a history of hypersensitivity.[2] Efficacy has not been established

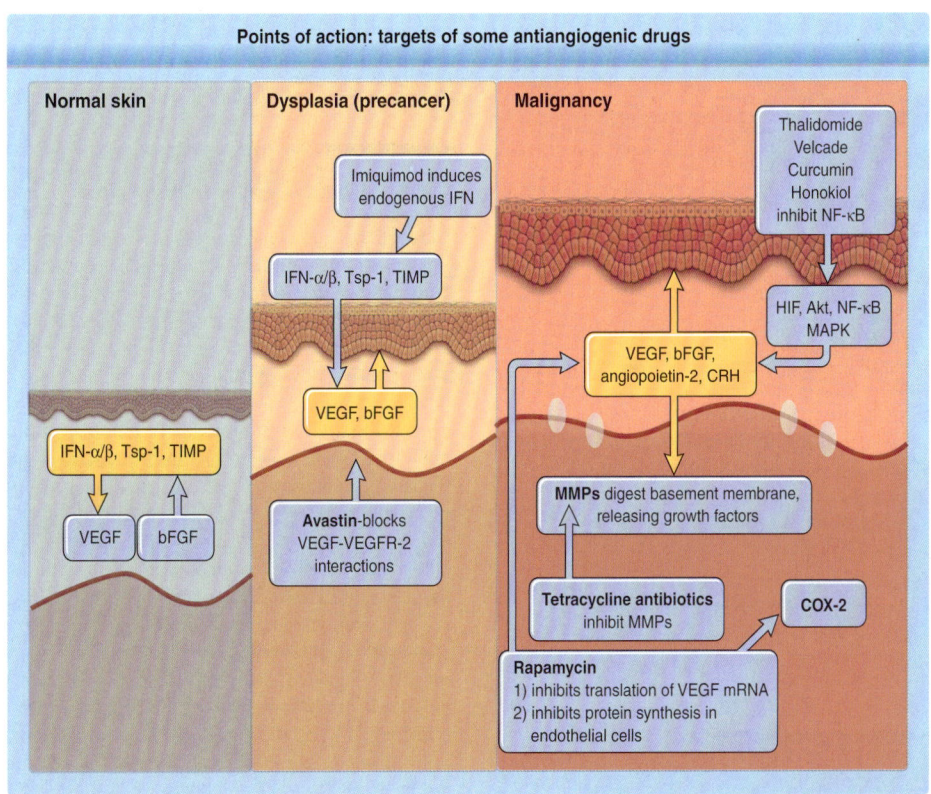

Figure 195-1 Points of action of some of the antiangiogenic drugs. Schematic depiction of the key points of action of some of the antiangiogenic drugs discussed in this chapter in normal skin, precancerous lesions, and malignancy. bFGF, basic fibroblast growth factor; COX-2, cyclooxygenase 2; CRH, corticotropin-releasing hormone; HIF, histoplasma inhibitory factor; IFN, interferon; MAPK, mitogen-activated protein kinase; MMP, matrix metalloproteinase; mRNA, messenger RNA; NF-κB, nuclear factor κB; TIMP, tissue inhibitor of metalloproteinases; Tsp-1, thrombospondin 1; VEGF, vascular endothelial growth factor; VEGFR-2, vascular endothelial growth factor receptor 2.

for pressure and venous stasis ulcers. Efficacy has also not been evaluated for diabetic neuropathic ulcers that do not extend through the dermis into subcutaneous tissue or for ischemic diabetic ulcers.[5]

DOSING REGIMEN

Becaplermin gel should be applied topically once daily with dose depending on the size of the lesion; generally, every square inch of ulcer requires two-thirds inch of gel from a 15-g tube or one-and-one-third inches of gel from a 2-g tube. After application, the area should be covered with a saline-moistened dressing, then left in place for approximately 12 hours. The dose should be recalculated every 1 to 2 weeks to ensure accurate dosing as the wound changes size. Becaplermin gel should be used in conjunction with standard proper ulcer care.[5]

MONITORING THERAPY

If there is less than a 30% decrease in size after 10 weeks or if the wound has not completely healed after 20 weeks of treatment, the treatment plan should be reevaluated.[5]

RISKS AND PRECAUTIONS[5,13,14]

- Because becaplermin gel is nonsterile, it should not be applied to wounds closed by primary intention.
- An increased rate of mortality because of malignancy has been observed in patients treated with 3 or more tubes of becaplermin gel. Consequently, caution should be used in patients with a known history of malignancy. However, a newer cohort study has shown that such malignancy association is not yet completely established.
- *Pregnancy category:* C.
- The safety and efficacy of becaplermin have not been evaluated in children younger than 16 years of age.

COMPLICATIONS (SOME EXAMPLES)[5]

- Rash
- Hypersensitivity reaction (most often to the paraben or m-cresol components)
- Ulcer-related complications (incidence was similar in becaplermin vs placebo groups)

BEVACIZUMAB (AVASTIN)

MECHANISM OF ACTION

Bevacizumab is a recombinant, humanized immunoglobulin G_1 monoclonal antibody against vascular endothelial growth factor (VEGF). VEGF is a growth factor that promotes angiogenesis by supporting endothelial cell replication and survival as well as vascular permeability. This potent proangiogenic molecule is upregulated in a majority of human tumors and serves to alter tumor vasculature.[2]

Binding of bevacizumab to VEGF is direct and specific. The antibody also competitively binds VEGF receptor 1 (VEGFR-1) and VEGFR-2, preventing VEGF from binding to its receptors and initiating the signaling cascade. It also reduces and normalizes tumor vascularity.[15] In addition, changes in interleukin (IL)-8 or soluble VEGFR-2 levels at second cycle appear predictive for response.[16] Specifically talking about metastatic colorectal cancer, a recent report suggests that NOTCH1 hyperexpression is a detrimental prognostic factor in patients treated with chemotherapy plus bevacizumab.[17]

INDICATIONS

In February 2004, bevacizumab became the first antiangiogenesis drug approved by the U.S. Food and Drug Administration (FDA) for first-line treatment of metastatic colorectal carcinoma when given in combination with intravenous 5-fluorouracil–based chemotherapy. Bevacizumab also has indications for non–small-cell lung cancer, cervical cancer (including metastatic), glioblastoma, ovarian (epithelial), fallopian tube, primary peritoneal cancer (platinum-resistant/sensitive recurrent), metastatic renal cell carcinoma, head and neck squamous cell carcinoma, gastric cancer, and renal carcinoma.[18-25] Bevacizumab, in combination either with other antiangiogenic agents or with chemotherapy, even if isolated, is currently being investigated in metastatic melanoma, hemangioendothelioma, angiosarcoma, metastatic colorectal cancer, age-related macular degeneration, retinoblastoma, corneal neovascularization, and ovary tumor.[17,18,26-32] Other than a history of hypersensitivity, no known contraindications to bevacizumab therapy exist.[18] Bevacizumab-induced inhibition of angiogenesis promotes a more homogeneous intratumoral distribution of paclitaxel, improving the antitumor response.[33] In general, bevacizumab prolongs progression-free survival and overall survival, and increases the 1-year survival rate in cancer patients as compared with control therapy.[34]

COMPLICATIONS (SOME EXAMPLES)[18,35,36]

- GI perforation with associated intraabdominal abscess or fistula formation.
- Wound dehiscence (incisions should be healed completely before treatment initiation; drug should be held for at least 28 days prior to elective surgery).
- Serious hemorrhagic events including hemoptysis, GI bleeding, CNS hemorrhaging, epistaxis, vaginal bleeding, and pulmonary hemorrhage. Use in patients with active hemorrhaging or recent history of hemoptysis is not advised.
- Arterial thromboembolic events, including cerebral infarction, transient ischemic attacks, myocardial infarction, and angina.
- Reversible posterior leukoencephalopathy syndrome, a neurologic disorder characterized by headache, seizure, lethargy, confusion, blindness, and other visual or neurologic disturbances, that is diagnosed and confirmed by MRI.
- Hypertension (monitoring every 2 to 3 weeks during course of treatment is advised).
- Proteinuria.
- Infusion reactions.

BORTEZOMIB (VELCADE)

MECHANISM OF ACTION

Bortezomib is the first proteasome inhibitor to gain FDA approval. This novel class of drugs acts by impairing the ability of the proteasome to degrade a variety of ubiquitinated proteins. Proteasome inhibitors may promote a proapoptotic state by preventing the degradation of tumor-suppressor proteins, such as p53 and inhibitors of nuclear factor κB (NF-κB). NF-κB upregulates the transcription of genes involved in neoplastic progression including VEGF.[37] Bortezomib also acts directly to inhibit chemotaxis, capillary formation, and transcription of VEGF, IL-6, insulin-like growth factor-1, ang-1, and ang-2.[38,39] Because it has been shown to correlate with NF-κB activity, chemoresistance might also be lessened in the presence of bortezomib. Moreover, bortezomib inhibits the angiogenesis mediated by mesenchymal stem cells.[40]

INDICATIONS

Bortezomib is currently indicated for the treatment of recurrent or refractory multiple myeloma and mantle cell lymphoma.[38] Investigational applications include cutaneous T-cell lymphoma, squamous cell carcinoma, and metastatic melanoma.[41] It has been reported that the combination of bortezomib, melphalan, dexamethasone, and intermittent thalidomide is an effective regimen for relapsed/refractory myeloma and is associated with improvement of abnormal bone metabolism and angiogenesis.[42] Good results can be obtained when bortezomib is combined with bevacizumab to treat temozolomide-resistant malignant gliomas.[43]

CONTRAINDICATIONS[39]

- Hypersensitivity to bortezomib, boron, or mannitol.

COMPLICATIONS (SOME EXAMPLES)[39]

- Hypotension
- Peripheral neuropathy
- Acute respiratory distress syndrome
- Blood dyscrasias (neutropenia, thrombocytopenia)
- Fatigue, malaise, and weakness
- Cytochrome P450 (CYP) 3A4 drug metabolism interactions
- Skin rash

CETUXIMAB (ERBITUX)

MECHANISM OF ACTIONS

Cetuximab is a chimeric, human–murine monoclonal antibody against the epithelial growth factor receptor (EGFR), and, as such, competitively inhibits the binding of epithelial growth factor (EGF), transforming growth factor, and other associated ligands. Downstream signaling blockade results in myriad antitumor properties, including decreased proliferation, cellular motility, and invasive potential via downregulation of signaling molecules such as basic fibroblast growth factor (bFGF, a product of keratinocytes) and IL-8.[44,45] Angiogenesis is also inhibited through decreased EGFR-mediated VEGF expression. When combined with irinotecan, cetuximab has synergistic antiangiogenesis and anti-invasion activities mediated by downregulation of phosphatidylinositol-3-kinase (PI3K)/Akt and mitogen-activated protein kinase/extracellular signal-regulated kinase (ERK) pathways[46]; such combination seems to induce a sudden, long-lasting reduction in VEGF-circulating levels, as well as an increase in interferon (IFN)-γ.[44] In addition, cetuximab may inhibit tumor growth and angiogenesis induced by ionizing radiation.[47]

INDICATIONS

Cetuximab is currently indicated for the treatment of metastatic colorectal carcinoma and squamous cell carcinoma of the head and neck, either alone or in combination with radiation or chemotherapy.[48] Additionally, its use in squamous cell carcinoma of the skin is currently under investigation. Given the demonstrated role of EGFR in melanoma, cetuximab may also play an eventual role in melanoma treatment. Be aware, however, that EGFR inhibitors are contraindicated in organ transplantation, as they can stimulate immunity. The subconjunctival use of cetuximab and bevacizumab to inhibit corneal angiogenesis has been reported in the literature.[29]

COMPLICATIONS (SOME EXAMPLES)[48]

- Serious infusion reactions
- Acneiform neutrophilic folliculitis—appearance correlates with clinical response
- Pruritus
- Electrolyte disturbances
- Abdominal pain and upset
- Infections associated with neutropenia

CORTICOSTEROIDS

The role of corticosteroids in angiogenesis is a bit of a mixed picture, with neutral, antiangiogenic, and proangiogenic effects having been observed in various cases. In the setting of uveal melanoma, El Filali and colleagues demonstrated no significant differences in levels of VEGF, PDGF, or thrombospondin 1 (TSP-1) in in vitro models treated with triamcinolone acetate.[49] In vivo and in vitro models of prostate cancer have shown potentiation of antiangiogenesis by docetaxel when concurrently exposed to dexamethasone as measured by levels of VEGF, IL-8, and chemokine ligand-1.[50] Contrastingly, sequential delivery of dexamethasone followed by VEGF showed an increase in vascularity in a biosensor-model implant into murine subcutaneous fat.[51] Whatever the ultimate mechanism and role, the clinical usefulness of steroids as antiinflammatory and antiangiogenic agents is readily apparent.

ERLOTINIB (TARCEVA)

MECHANISM OF ACTION

Erlotinib is a small-molecule phosphorylation inhibitor that specifically inhibits the EGFR tyrosine kinase. Acting intracellularly, erlotinib downregulates the expression of VEGF via the PI3K/Akt signaling pathway.[2] When combined with cisplatin, erlotinib inhibits growth and angiogenesis through c-MYC and hypoxia inducible factor (HIF)-1α in EGFR-mutated lung cancer.[52]

INDICATIONS

Erlotinib is currently indicated for the treatment of non–small-cell lung cancer and pancreatic cancer.[53] There is an ongoing clinical trial investigating using the combination of erlotinib and bevacizumab in stage 4 melanoma. Other than a history of hypersensitivity, there are no known contraindications.[2] Preliminary clinical trials have shown that association of erlotinib with pazopanib, an oral angiogenesis inhibitor, can work perfectly together to obtain better results against angiogenesis.[54]

COMPLICATIONS (SOME EXAMPLES)[53]

- Acneiform rash
- GI upset
- CYP450, CYP1A2, and CYP3A4 drug metabolism interactions

EVEROLIMUS (AFINITOR)

MECHANISM OF ACTION

Everolimus is another mammalian target of rapamycin (mTOR) inhibitor classified as semisynthetic because it is derived from sirolimus; it has a shorter half life than sirolimus, but better oral bioavailability and less frequent toxic side effects.[55] This agent also complexes with FK-binding protein 2 to inhibit mTOR, suppress HIF-1α, and block VEGF-mediated vascular endothelial cell stimulation, bFGF-induced angiogenesis, and T-cell activation and proliferation.[56,57] Nevertheless, a few years ago, everolimus was linked with lymphangiogenesis, after causing hyperexpression of prospero homeobox protein 1, podoplanin, VEGFR-C, and VEGFR-3 in chick chorioallantoic membranes treated with it.[58]

INDICATIONS

Everolimus is indicated for the treatment of advanced renal cell carcinoma after failure of sunitinib or sorafenib, and as an agent in drug-eluting stents.[59] Everolimus is approved for astrocytoma and breast, neuroendocrine, renal angiomyolipoma with tuberous sclerosis complex, and renal cancers.[58,59] Some other commercial brands are also approved for liver and renal transplantation.[59] Dermatologic, off-label applications are limited to a case report of its use in psoriasis.[60] Recently, it was shown that immune modulatory oligonucleotide, a toll-like receptor 9 agonist, cooperates with everolimus in renal cell carcinoma by interfering with tumor growth and angiogenesis.[61]

COMPLICATIONS (SOME EXAMPLES)[59]

- Noninfectious pneumonitis
- Susceptibility to infections
- Oral ulceration and mucositis
- Blood dyscrasias
- Musculoskeletal pain
- CYP3A4 drug metabolism interactions

IMIQUIMOD (ALDARA)

MECHANISM OF ACTION

Imiquimod (imidazoquinoline) is both the first immune response modifier and the first topical antiangiogenic agent for dermatologic use. Imiquimod acts by inducing the activation of toll-like receptor 7 in immune cells. Toll-like receptor 7 activation enhances the innate immune response by increasing endogenous IFN and interleukin production, including IFN-α, IFN-β, IFN-γ, IL-10, IL-12, and IL-18; these cytokines also function as endogenous angiogenesis inhibitors.[62,63] The upregulation of these cytokines, as well as of other endogenous angiogenesis inhibitors, such as IFN-inducible protein 10, tissue inhibitor of metalloproteinases, and TSP-1, is the basis for imiquimod's antiangiogenic activity.[64] Additionally, imiquimod also downregulates proangiogenic factors such as bFGF and matrix metalloproteinase 9. In vivo, imiquimod has been shown to inhibit angiogenesis in human bowenoid papulosis, hemangioendothelioma, cutaneous melanoma, and murine lung sarcoma cells.[64-66] A topical combination therapy of imiquimod and gentian violet for cutaneous melanoma metastases has been reported[67]; recently, we have observed that such combination can be helpful for plantar warts as well (unpublished data).

INDICATIONS

Imiquimod is currently approved for the treatment of clinically typical, nonhyperkeratotic, nonhypertrophic actinic keratosis on the face or scalp, and biopsy-confirmed, primary, superficial basal cell carcinoma located on the trunk, neck, or extremities (maximum tumor diameter of 2 cm) in immunocompetent adults. It is also approved for the treatment of external genital and perianal condyloma acuminata.[68] Several studies have shown efficacy in squamous cell carcinoma, lentigo maligna, hemangiomas, Kaposi sarcoma, pyogenic granuloma, discoid lupus erythematosus, and port-wine stain in combination with pulsed-dye laser.[69-74] Other than a history of hypersensitivity, there are no known contraindications.[2]

PHARMACOKINETICS

Imiquimod is only minimally absorbed transdermally, with less than 0.9% of the topical dose being excreted in the urine or feces.[68]

DOSING REGIMEN[68]

- *Actinic keratosis:* Patients are to apply the cream 2 times per week to the face or scalp but not both concurrently, preferably before sleeping hours. The area should be washed with a mild soap and water and allowed to dry before application. After approximately 8 hours following application, the area should again be washed with mild soap and water to remove the agent. Treatment should continue for a full 16 weeks, and should not be extended because of missed doses or skip periods.
- *Superficial basal cell carcinoma:* Following biopsy confirmation, patients are to apply the cream 5 times per week to the affected area plus 1 cm around the lesion, preferably before sleeping hours. The area should be washed with a mild soap and water and allowed to dry before application. After approximately 8 hours following application, the area should again be washed with mild soap and water to remove the agent.
- *External genital and perianal condyloma acuminate:* Patients are to apply the cream 3 times per week to the affected area, preferably before sleeping hours. The area should be washed with a mild soap and water and allowed to dry before application. After approximately 6 to 10 hours following application, the area should again be washed with mild soap and water to remove the agent. Treatment should continue until the lesion(s) completely resolve or until a maximum course of 16 weeks.

RISKS AND PRECAUTIONS[68]

- *Immunosuppression:* The safety and efficacy of imiquimod has not been established in immunosuppressed patients.
- *Photosensitivity:* Patients should be instructed to avoid or minimize exposure to sunlight or sunlamps during the treatment course.

- *Pregnancy class:* C.
- *Pediatrics:* The safety and efficacy of imiquimod has not been established in the treatment of external genital and perianal condyloma acuminate in children younger than 12 years of age, or in the treatment of actinic keratosis or superficial basal cell carcinoma in children younger than 18 years of age.

COMPLICATIONS (SOME EXAMPLES)[68]

- *Local skin toxicities:* Frequency of local skin toxicities include: erythema (97%), flaking/scaling/dryness (93%), scabbing crusting (79%), induration (78%), edema (71%), erosion/ulceration (54%), vesicles (29%), and weeping or exudates (22%). Patients should be instructed to contact their health care provider if they experience any sign or symptom in the treatment area that restricts or prohibits daily activity or makes continued application of the cream difficult; a rest period of a few days may be necessary. Additionally, to reduce the likelihood of an adverse reaction, the agent should not be applied under occlusion other than porous gauze or cotton underwear. Health care providers should evaluate for possible bacterial superinfection when assessing reactions to imiquimod.
- *Decreased wound healing:* Recent wounds should be allowed to heal completely prior to initiating treatment.
- GI upset.
- Upper respiratory tract infection, coughing, sinusitis.
- Musculoskeletal pain.
- Headache.

INTERFERON-α2b (INTRON A)

IFN-α made history in 1988 as the first antiangiogenic therapy used in humans for the successful treatment of pulmonary hemangiomatosis in a pediatric patient. IFN-α2b is a synthetic cytokine made from the bacterium *Escherichia coli* transformed with recombinant DNA and has similar actions to its natural endogenous counterpart, IFN-α, a type I IFN produced endogenously by the immune system.[2]

MECHANISM OF ACTION

The IFNs act through the Janus kinase–signal transducers and activators of transcription (JAK-STAT) pathway. IFN-α, which is both a direct-on-endothelial-cells agent, including impairment of their proliferation and migration[75] as a result of delayed progression from the S-phase to the G_2-phase of the cell cycle and resulting in the inhibition of Cdc2 kinase activity,[76] and an indirect-on-endothelial-cells antiangiogenic agent, was first observed to impair capillary endothelial cell migration. Its properties as an indirect antiangiogenic agent include the ability to decrease tumor cell production of bFGF, which may explain its success in treating hemangiomata.[4] Further actions, such as downregulation of IL-8 and VEGF gene expression,[75] work together to interfere with both blood vessels and tumor cell proliferation, leading to regression of tumors without necrosis.[75] IFN-α has well-known antiviral activity and antitumor activity, which may be mediated in part by upregulating major histocompatibility complex Class I antigen expression, activating natural killer cells, controlling progression through cell-cycle checkpoints, and activating apoptosis.[2] In vitro assays also demonstrate ability for IFN-α to inhibit osteoclast differentiation and renal cell carcinoma-induced angiogenesis by reducing calcium-phosphate resorption activity and expression of proteoclastic transcription factor c-Fos; by inhibiting bone endothelial cell proliferation and the expression of FGF-2; and by inhibiting secretion of FGF-2.[77]

INDICATIONS

INF-α2b is currently indicated for the treatment of chronic hepatitis B (which may be chemopreventive against hepatocellular carcinoma), chronic hepatitis C, AIDS-associated Kaposi sarcoma, and condylomata acuminata. It is also indicated in malignant melanoma (adjuvant to surgical therapy in patients who are at high-risk of systemic recurrence; must be administered within 56 days postoperatively), hairy cell leukemia, and follicular lymphoma.[78] Off-label uses in dermatology include cutaneous T-cell lymphoma (mycosis fungoides) and basal and squamous cell skin cancers. It also has been used in the treatment of infantile hemangiomas along with corticosteroids or in the event of corticosteroid resistance; however, given rising concerns over the risk of spastic diplegia (especially in children younger than 1 year of age), its usefulness in this setting has been somewhat tempered.[79] Early reports had shown that combination therapy of IFN-α and 5-fluorouracil inhibits tumor angiogenesis in human hepatocellular carcinoma cells by regulating VEGF and angiopoietins.[76]

CONTRAINDICATIONS[78]

- Hypersensitivity to IFN-α or any drug components
- Combination IFN-α and ribavirin therapy in pregnancy or in males whose female partners are pregnant
- Autoimmune hepatitis

- Personal history of a hemoglobinopathy (eg, sickle cell disease, thalassemia major)
- Renal insufficiency (creatinine clearance <50 mL/min)

PHARMACOKINETICS

IFN-α2b comes as a powder that, upon reconstitution, should be used immediately but may be stored up to 24 hours at 2°C to 8°C (36°F to 46°F). It can be given by subcutaneous, IM, IV, or intralesional routes. Its half-life is 3 to 12 hours when given subcutaneously or IM and 30 minutes when given IV. The drug is likely metabolized by the kidneys. Polyethylene glycol IFN-α2b has a 10-fold increase in half life, decreased toxicity, and increased compliance.[78,80] Table 195-1 outlines dosing regimens.

COMPLICATIONS (SOME EXAMPLES)[78,79]

- Flu-like symptoms (headache, fatigue, fever, chills, tachycardia, myalgia, and anorexia)
- Depression (new-onset depression or worsening of preexisting depression; patients should be monitored during therapy for severe depression, and therapy should be discontinued if necessary)
- Sarcoidosis (observed in combination IFN-α-ribavirin therapy)
- Spastic diplegia (a form of cerebral palsy that is a neuromuscular condition characterized by hypertonia and spasticity in the muscles of the lower extremities; Little disease)

INITIATING THERAPY

Hemoglobin, complete blood cell count with differential, electrolytes, liver function tests, thyroid-stimulating hormone, chest radiography, and eye examination should be obtained before initiation of and during therapy on a routine basis. Patients with prior cardiac disease or advanced cancer require a baseline electrocardiogram and routine reevaluation thereafter. Therapy should not be initiated in patients with a history of depression or severe psychiatric disorder because of the risk of worsening psychiatric symptoms and suicide. Patients with thyroid disorders that cannot be corrected with medication should not be treated. The development of spastic diplegia in patients with hemangiomas who are taking IFN seems to correlate with age and severe hypothyroidism (caused by the presence of ectopic thyroxine–degrading enzymes produced by the hemangiomas). Thus, thyroid monitoring is mandatory in all patients with large hemangiomas.[78,79]

MONITORING THERAPY

Treatment should be discontinued if the absolute neutrophil count reaches less than 0.5×10^9/L or the platelet count reaches less than 25×10^9/L. Other symptoms warranting discontinuation include new-onset or worsening eye symptoms, the development of thyroid dysfunction not correctable by medication, and the development of severe depression or other psychiatric disorder during therapy.[78]

RISKS AND PRECAUTIONS[78]

- *Pregnancy category:* C.
- *Pediatrics:* The safety and efficacy in children have not established for any indications other than chronic hepatitides B and C.

PANITUMUMAB (VECTIBIX)

MECHANISM OF ACTION

Panitumumab is an entirely human monoclonal antibody directed against EGFR. Like cetuximab, it blocks ligand interactions associated with the EGFR (EGF, transforming growth factor) and downstream signaling molecules like VEGF, bFGF, and IL-8; however, because panitumumab is not chimeric, the hypoth-

TABLE 195-1
Interferon-α2b Dosing[78,81]

DISEASE	DOSE
Malignant melanoma high-dose regimen	Induction: 20 million IU/m² IV infusion over 20 minutes, 5 consecutive days/week for 4 weeks
	Maintenance: 10 million IU/m² subcutaneously 3 times/week for 48 weeks
Malignant melanoma adjuvant low-dose regimen (in clinical trials)	Maintenance: 3 million IU/m² subcutaneously 3 times/week for 1 year
AIDS-related Kaposi sarcoma	30 million IU/m² subcutaneously or IM 3 times/week until disease progression or maximal response has been achieved after 16 weeks
Condylomata acuminata	1 million IU per lesion (maximum of 5 lesions per course) 3 times/week on alternate days for 3 weeks; may administer additional courses at 12- to 16-week intervals
Hemangiomas	3 million U/m²/day for at least 6 months

esized benefit is better overall efficacy and immunologic tolerance.[82]

INDICATIONS

Panitumumab is currently indicated for progressing, metastatic colorectal carcinoma in combination with or as a single agent following chemotherapy.[83] No known dermatologic uses or investigations into potential uses exist at this time, but, given its similarity to cetuximab, possible investigations into panitumumab's usefulness in cutaneous squamous cell carcinoma and melanoma are warranted. Other than a history of hypersensitivity, there are no known contraindications.[2]

COMPLICATIONS (SOME EXAMPLES)[83]

- Severe dermatologic toxicities (acneiform dermatitis, pruritus, erythema, rash, skin exfoliation, paronychia, dry skin, skin fissures)
- Photosensitivity
- Pulmonary fibrosis
- Electrolyte disturbances
- Infusion reactions

PEGAPTANIB (MACUGEN)

MECHANISM OF ACTION

Pegaptanib is a short peptide strand, or aptamer, directed against a specific isomer of secreted VEGF, namely, VEGF165, which is thought to play a particular role in endothelial cell proliferation.[84]

INDICATIONS

Like ranibizumab, pegaptanib is currently indicated for the treatment of neovascular, or wet, age-related macular degeneration[85-87]; however, no known dermatologic uses or investigations into potential uses exist at this time.[2] New reports have presented benefits in other oculovasculopathies, for instance, ischemic diabetic macular edema,[88,89] choroidal neovascularization,[90] retinal ischemic diseases,[91] and myopic choroidal neovascularization.[92]

CONTRAINDICATIONS[85]

- Ocular or periocular infection

COMPLICATIONS (SOME EXAMPLES)[85]

- Endophthalmitis, retinal detachment, and traumatic cataract formation associated with intravitreal administration
- Hypertension
- Dizziness, headache, and vertigo

PROPRANOLOL (HEMANGEOL)

MECHANISM OF ACTION

The effectiveness of propranolol in the treatment of hemangioma was discovered by chance in 2008[93] and is considered relatively safe for this usage.[94] Given to infants who are at least 5-weeks old, propranolol, a beta-blocker, can be used in the treatment of infantile hemangioma (Fig. 195-2).[95,96] Propranolol is not only successfully used for cutaneous hemangioma, but also for liver infantile hemangioma;[97] some incomplete responses have been described, such as in focal subglottic hemangioma.[98] In general, beta-blockers, whether systemic or topical, have better long-term results when compared to corticosteroids,[99-101] but when beta-blockers and corticosteroids are used together, there is a faster positive outcome.[102]

Propranolol works in the treatment of hemangioma, by blocking both β_1- and β_2-adrenergic receptors in hemangioma endothelial cells; it also reduces levels without transactivating VEGF-2 signaling, and without promoting G_0/G_1-phase cell-cycle arrest—indeed, G_0/G_1-phase cell-cycle arrest has been associated with decreased cyclin D_1, CDK-4, CDK-6, phospho-Rb expression, and with cessation of cell proliferation.[35] Moreover, propranolol reduces the expression of HIF-1α in a dose-dependent and a time-dependent manner, mainly by acting on β_2-adrenergic receptors, in addition to blocking both STAT-3 and proapoptotic Bcl-2 pathways.[103] In fact, newer studies point to better results when propranolol is prescribed to infants older than 6 months of age; propranolol also reduces plasma VEGF levels in a posttreatment long-term manner.[104]

INDICATIONS[95]

- Tremors
- Angina
- Hypertension
- Heart rhythm disorders
- Treatment and prevention of myocardial infarction
- Reduction of the severity and frequency of migraine
- Infantile hemangioma

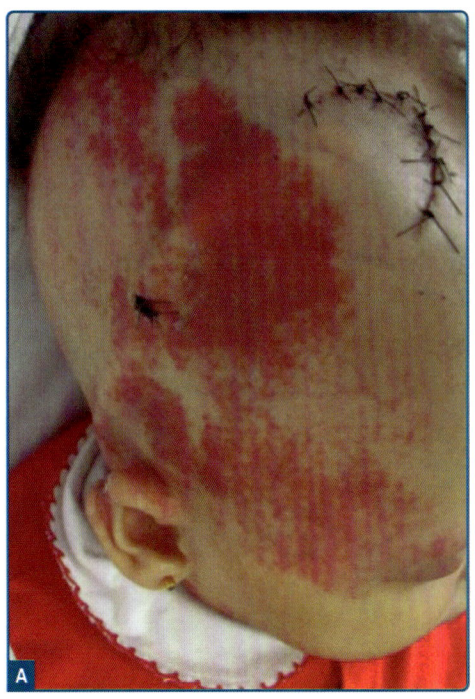 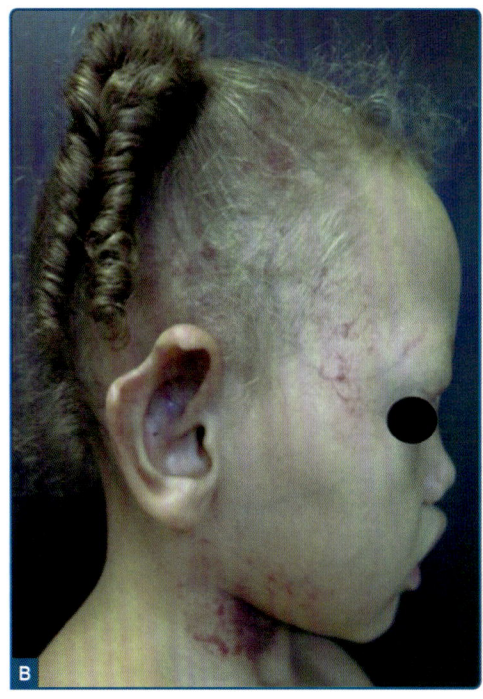

Figure 195-2 Posterior fossa brain malformations, hemangiomas of the face, arterial anomalies, cardiac anomalies, and eye abnormalities (PHACE) syndrome patient whose cranial hemangioma was treated with systemic propranolol. **A,** Patient before treatment, at age 45 days; (**B**) same patient at age 5 years. (Images used with permission from Dr. Caroline Romanelli Tiburcio Alves Zelenika, Pontifical Catholic University of Campinas, Campinas/SP, Brazil.)

CONTRAINDICATIONS[95]

- Muscle disorder
- Bronchitis, emphysema, or other breathing disorders
- Low blood glucose or diabetes
- Slow heartbeats, low blood pressure
- Congestive heart failure
- Depression
- Liver or kidney disease
- Thyroid disorder
- Pheochromocytoma
- Problems with circulation (eg, Raynaud syndrome)

DOSING REGIMEN

Chapter 118 provides dosing regimen information for propranolol.

COMPLICATIONS (SOME EXAMPLES)[95]

- Nausea, vomiting, diarrhea, constipation, or stomach cramps
- Decreased sex drive, impotence, or difficulty having an orgasm
- Sleep problems (insomnia)
- Tired feeling
- Hypoglycemia
- Asthma attack

RANIBIZUMAB (LUCENTIS)

MECHANISM OF ACTION

Ranibizumab is an antibody fragment related to bevacizumab that similarly competitively binds VEGF and inhibits its interactions with VEGFR-1 and VEGFR-2; it acts to block endothelial proliferation and survival. Smaller in size than bevacizumab (a full-length antibody), ranibizumab is thought to have better tissue absorption and fewer inflammatory reactions.[105]

INDICATIONS

Ranibizumab is currently indicated for the treatment of patients with neovascular, or wet, age-related macular degeneration, as well as diabetic retinopathy, macular edema, and choroidal neovascularization secondary to pathologic myopia;[28,106-108] clinical trials looking into its use in combination with pulsed-dye laser in cutaneous neurofibroma and port-wine stain are ongoing.[2]

CONTRAINDICATIONS[106]

- Ocular or periocular infection
- Hypersensitivity

COMPLICATIONS (SOME EXAMPLES)[106]

- Endophthalmitis and retinal detachment associated with intravitreal administration
- Increase in intraocular pressures
- Arterial thromboembolic events

SIROLIMUS (RAPAMUNE)

MECHANISM OF ACTION

Isolated from the bacterium *Streptomyces hygroscopicus*, sirolimus is a macrocyclic lactone antibiotic with immunosuppressant, antifungal, and antineoplastic properties. After forming a complex with FK-binding protein-12, sirolimus acts by inhibiting the interaction of the mTOR with its substrates; mTOR is a serine–threonine protein kinase activated by several growth factors whose downstream targets affect cell-cycle control and angiogenesis in normal and neoplastic cells.[109] Sirolimus decreases levels of hypoxia HIF-1α and significantly inhibits VEGF-mediated vascular endothelial cell stimulation, bFGF-induced angiogenesis, and T-cell activation and proliferation.[110] By suppressing mTOR complex 2, sirolimus also inhibits Akt activation.[111] Of the drugs used in the solid-organ transplantation setting, including cyclosporine and tacrolimus, rapamycin has the greatest antiangiogenic activity. To that effect, it may be useful for the prevention of squamous cell carcinoma and lymphoma in the immunosuppressed transplantation population.[2]

INDICATIONS

Rapamycin is currently approved for prophylaxis against renal transplant rejection as well as lymphangioleiomyomatosis.[112] Off-label uses in dermatology include the treatment of psoriasis, Kaposi sarcoma, tuberous sclerosis, and angiofibromatosis.[113-117] There are also case reports of its efficacy in nephrogenic systemic fibrosis, scleroderma, and dermatomyositis.[118-120] Ongoing clinical trials are looking into the usefulness of sirolimus in the prevention of nonmelanoma skin cancer in patients following kidney transplantation, that of topical sirolimus in basal cell nevus syndrome (Gorlin-Goltz syndrome), and in combination with pulsed-dye laser in port-wine stain. Other than a history of hypersensitivity to it or other rapamycin derivatives, there are no known contraindications.[2] A new generation of sirolimus-based compounds, phosphorus-containing sirolimus (FIM-A), inhibit the angiogenesis and proliferation of osteosarcomas, as they arrest cells in the G_1-phase of the cell cycle, accompanied by reduction of VEGF and HIF-1α; as well as they also inhibit mTORC1 signaling as demonstrated by decreased phosphorylation of p70S6K1 and 4E-BP1.[121]

COMPLICATIONS (SOME EXAMPLES)[112,122]

- *Systemic toxicities:* Complications that may occur include headache, thrombocytopenia, arthralgia, interstitial pneumonitis, and hypercholesterolemia.
- *Cutaneous toxicities:* Cutaneous side effects of therapy include angioedema, leukocytoclastic vasculitis, xerosis, and aphthous ulceration, which all resolve with discontinuation of therapy.
- Increased susceptibility to infections and malignancies.

SORAFENIB (NEXAVAR)

MECHANISM OF ACTION

Sorafenib is a small-molecule, phosphorylation inhibitor of several tyrosine kinase receptors, including PDGF-β, VEGFR-1, VEGFR-2, VEGFR-3, and RAF kinase,[123,124] thereby contributing to RAF/MEK/ERK pathway blockage.[125,126] Like sunitinib, sorafenib inhibition of multiple points of downstream signaling by tyrosine kinase receptors results in tumor growth inhibition and regression.[2] Furthermore, it has been reported, in preclinical models, that sorafenib blocks tumor growth, angiogenesis, and metastatic potential of osteosarcoma through a mechanism potentially involving the inhibition of the ERK1/ERK2, MCL-1, and ezrin pathways.[127]

INDICATIONS

Sorafenib is currently indicated for the treatment of advanced renal cell carcinoma, unresectable hepatocellular carcinoma, and differentiated thyroid cancer.[128] Ongoing clinical trials are looking into the use of sorafenib in the treatment of metastatic melanoma, both alone and in combination with chemotherapy (carboplatin and paclitaxel). Other than a history of hypersensitivity, there are no known contraindications.[128]

It has been observed in patients who use sorafenib for cancer treatment that progression-free survival was significantly shorter in patients with high levels of Ang-2, granulocyte colony-stimulating factor, hematopoietic growth factor, and leptin.[129] Interestingly, expression levels of many angiogenesis-related genes in the cutaneous metastasis of sarcomatoid-changed and rhabdoid features of an advanced renal cell carcinoma were relatively higher than those of the primary sorafenib-resistant tumor.[130]

A plethora of different sorafenib derivatives with good clinical and in vitro profiles have been presented in recent years. DCT015, a new sorafenib derivate, inhibits tumor growth and angiogenesis in gastric cancer models by inhibiting proliferation, inducing the morphologic changes of apoptosis, increasing the apoptosis percentage, as well as increasing the sub-G_1 population in gastric cancer cells, once it inhibits both MEK/ERK and PI3K/Akt signaling pathways, VEGF-induced migration, and tube formation in human umbilical vein endothelial cells. In addition, DCT015 downregulates VEGF-induced VEGFR-2 phosphorylation with the decreased phosphorylation of the downstream key protein.[131] Such suppression of VEGFR-2/EGFR–mediated angiogenesis can be also observed with NSK-01105, another novel sorafenib derivative, in human prostate tumor growth.[132] Another sorafenib derivative, SL1122-37, has greater effects than sorafenib on human hepatocellular carcinoma growth and prevention of angiogenesis.[133]

COMPLICATIONS (SOME EXAMPLES)[128]

- Dermatologic toxicities (rash, hand–foot syndrome, alopecia, pruritus)
- Multiple blood dyscrasias
- Hypertension, cardiac ischemia
- GI upset, perforation
- CYP2B6, CYP2C8, and CYP3A4 drug metabolism interactions
- Nephrotic syndrome[134]

SUNITINIB (SUTENT)

MECHANISM OF ACTION

Sunitinib is a small-molecule, phosphorylation inhibitor of several tyrosine kinase receptors, including PDGF-α, PDGF-β, VEGFR-1, VEGFR-2, and VEGFR-3; tumor growth inhibition and tumor regression result due to a variety of downstream mechanisms.[55,135,136]

INDICATIONS

Sunitinib is currently indicated for the treatment of GI stromal tumors, advanced renal cell carcinoma, and pancreatic neuroendocrine tumors.[137] Indeed, patients with AA/AC alleles of the VEGFR-1 single-nucleotide polymorphism rs9582036 as well as expression of phosphorylated VEGFR-2 in tumor stroma may carry a good prognosis for sunitinib-treated metastatic renal cell carcinoma.[138,139] Clinical trials are ongoing as to the efficacy of sunitinib in metastatic melanoma, but case reports exist of sunitinib efficacy in treating metastatic melanomas, as well as in treating skin ulcers associated with angioosteohypertrophy syndrome (or Klippel-Trénaunay syndrome, hemangiectatic hypertrophy).[140] Other than a history of hypersensitivity, there are no known contraindications.[2]

COMPLICATIONS (SOME EXAMPLES)[137,141]

- Dermatologic toxicities (rash, skin discoloration, hand–foot syndrome, alopecia)
- Hypertension
- Adrenal insufficiency
- CYP3A4 drug metabolism interactions (monitor with concurrent use of CYP3A4 inducers and/or inhibitors)

TEMSIROLIMUS (TORISEL)

MECHANISM OF ACTION

Like sirolimus, temsirolimus is an mTOR inhibitor that downregulates production of HIF-1α and blocks VEGF-mediated vascular endothelial cell stimulation, bFGF-induced angiogenesis, and T-cell activation and proliferation. The increased water solubility of temsirolimus allows for both oral and IV administration.[55]

INDICATIONS

Temsirolimus is currently indicated for the treatment of advanced renal cell carcinoma[142] and is being evaluating in clinical trials for the treatment of metastatic melanoma in combination with either sorafenib or bevacizumab.[2] Preliminary data show that metformin, another mTOR inhibitor, might enhance temsirolimus activity.[136] Preclinical studies show that good synergistic effect can be obtained by combining temsirolimus and cetuximab in head and neck squamous cell carcinoma,[143] in which baseline detection of caspase-3 activity may be useful for early identification of therapy success.[144] Promising results may also be obtained when temsirolimus is combined with bevacizumab and cetuximab for solid tumor treatment.[145] Other than a history of hypersensitivity to it or other rapamycin derivatives, there are no known contraindications.[2]

COMPLICATIONS (SOME EXAMPLES)[142]

- Rash
- Mucositis, GI upset, and bowel perforation
- Metabolic derangements (hyperglycemia, hyperlipidemia)
- Interstitial lung disease
- Renal toxicity
- CYP3A4 drug metabolism interactions
- Diarrhea and stomatitis[146]
- Fatigue[147]

THALIDOMIDE (THALOMID)

Thalidomide was first released in Europe and several other regions in the late 1950s and quickly became a popular sedative used for the treatment of nausea in pregnancy. It was not approved in the United States at that time because of its questionable safety in pregnancy and emerging evidence of peripheral neuropathy as a side effect; the drug was, however, approved for use in clinical trials in the United States and was given to more than a thousand physicians in the United States for this purpose before its eventual banning. It was soon discovered that thalidomide caused severe embryopathy, resulting in phocomelia, amelia, or other severe birth defects when taken during pregnancy. The tragic experience with thalidomide prompted dramatic changes in drug regulation and approval.[2] Recently, it was shown in zebrafish and chickens that thalidomide teratogenicity occurs due to thalidomide binding to the *cereblon (CRBN)* gene, which inhibits ubiquitin ligase activity.[148]

In 1965, Sheskin prescribed thalidomide for psychosis in one of his patients and accidentally discovered that thalidomide effectively treated her erythema nodosum leprosum. The FDA approved thalidomide in 1998 for the treatment of erythema nodosum leprosum and currently classifies it as an orphan drug.[2]

As interest in thalidomide's ability to treat a wide variety of refractory diseases grows, a promising class of drugs named IMiDs (thalidomide and its derivatives lenalidomide and pomalidomide) or immunomodulatory thalidomide analogs, are under development and investigation. One member of this new class of drugs, lenalidomide (CC-5013, Revlimid), has been approved for the treatment of multiple myeloma, myelodysplastic syndromes, and chronic lymphocytic leukemia. However, Phase III clinical studies of lenalidomide for the treatment of metastatic melanoma did not show a significant effect.[149]

MECHANISM OF ACTION

Thalidomide exhibits a wide range of effects in vitro and in vivo. Its mechanisms of action are still unclear, but, exhibiting antineoplastic, immunomodulatory, and antiangiogenic properties, thalidomide downregulates the expression of VEGF, bFGF, and possibly tumor necrosis factor-α, IFN-α insulin-like growth factor-1, NF-κB, IL-6, IL-12, IL-8, and matrix metalloproteinase-2.[150-152] Recently, it was described that Slit2/Robo1 endothelial signaling plays a role in angiogenesis, which can be blocked by thalidomide, once it blocks the PI3K/Akt pathway.[153] Thalidomide's antiangiogenic properties may be the basis for its antineoplastic activity, but its myriad other effects likely account for its teratogenicity.[154] Apart from its hypnosedative properties, thalidomide's eventual effects on the immune system result in a reduction in the helper T-cell–to–suppressor T-cell ratio, and a decrease in leukocyte chemotaxis and in monocyte phagocytosis.[155] Additionally, human keratinocytes demonstrate increased migration and proliferation when exposed to thalidomide.[156]

INDICATIONS

Thalidomide is currently approved and considered first-line therapy for the acute treatment of the cutaneous manifestations of moderate to severe erythema nodosum leprosum as well as maintenance therapy for prevention and suppression of the cutaneous manifestations of erythema nodosum leprosum recurrence. In combination with dexamethasone, thalidomide is also approved for the treatment of newly-diagnosed multiple myeloma.[157] Off-label uses include Kaposi sarcoma, hemangioendotheliomas, severe aphthous stomatitis (especially in patients with AIDS), psoriasis, and a variety of other dermatologic conditions.[151]

CONTRAINDICATIONS[157]

- *Pregnancy class:* X
- Hypersensitivity to the drug or its components

PHARMACOKINETICS

Thalidomide has low water solubility and slow absorption from the GI tract, reaching peak plasma levels 0.5 to 4 hours after administration; it is only available in an oral form. A delay in absorption of up to 2 hours may occur if given in conjunction with foods high in fat.[157]

Thalidomide's half-life is approximately 5 to 7 hours, with renal clearance estimated to be 1.15 mL/min. Thalidomide's main route of elimination remains unknown, but it undergoes nonenzymatic hydrolysis in the serum to a variety of metabolites. Because hepatic metabolism appears to play an insignificant role, thalidomide is unlikely to affect levels of CYP-metabolized drugs such as oral contraceptives. Acetylcholine, prostaglandins, histamine, and serotonin are antagonized by thalidomide in vitro; alcohol, barbiturates, chlorpromazine, and reserpine have enhanced hypnosedative activity in the presence of thalidomide.[157]

DOSING REGIMEN

Because thalidomide may induce drowsiness, guidelines for dosing include initiation at 100 to 300 mg/day with a full glass of water at bedtime or at least 1 hour after the evening meal. Therapy should be continued until improvement is noted, at which point the physician can begin tapering the dose by 50 mg every 2 to 4 weeks. In the case of maintenance therapy, an attempt at tapering should occur every 3 to 6 months (Table 195-2).[157]

TABLE 195-2
Thalidomide Dosing for Selected Dermatologic Diseases[157,159]

DISEASE	DOSE
Erythema nodosum leprosum	Initial dose: 100-300 mg/day, preferably 1 hour after the evening meal with a full glass of water Maintenance dose: 50-100 mg/day Tapering recommendations: 50-mg decrements every 2-4 weeks once symptoms subside (usually after 2 weeks); in patients requiring prolonged treatment, attempt tapering schedule every 3-6 months
Severe cutaneous erythema nodosum leprosum reaction	Initial dose: 400 mg/day
Chronic graft-versus-host disease	Initial dose: 100 mg 4 times daily Maintenance dose: 200 to 400 mg 4 times daily Pediatric dose: 3-9.5 mg/kg twice daily to 4 times daily
Cutaneous lupus erythematosus	Initial dose: 400 mg/day Maintenance dose: 25-50 mg/day
Recurrent aphthous stomatitis	100 mg/day
Behçet syndrome	Initial dose: 400 mg/day Maintenance dose: 200 mg/day

INITIATING THERAPY

Thalidomide therapy should be reserved for patients with debilitating, serious diseases that have proven refractory to other therapies. The manufacturer of thalidomide has developed a restricted distribution program called System for Thalidomide Education and Prescribing Safety (S.T.E.P.S.), which requires both prescribers and dispensing pharmacists to be registered. It is mandatory for patients to be informed about the program, adhere to its requirements, and demonstrate in writing an understanding of these warnings. Female patients of childbearing potential (defined by the program as sexually mature women who have not undergone a hysterectomy or who have not been postmenopausal for at least 24 consecutive months) must have a negative pregnancy test (with a β-human chorionic gonadotropin sensitivity of at least 50 mU/mL) within 24 hours of treatment initiation. Patients must use reliable contraception (2 effective methods unless using the abstinence method) for a period of at least 1 month before initiating therapy and must continue this practice during and for 1 month after therapy is completed. Male patients are required to use latex condoms, including those patients who have had a vasectomy.[157]

MONITORING THERAPY

S.T.E.P.S. requires patient monitoring during therapy. Strict guidelines for pregnancy testing are outlined for males and females of childbearing potential to prevent possible fetal damage. If, during the course of therapy, a patient becomes pregnant, the drug should be stopped immediately and the exposure reported to the FDA and the manufacturer (Celgene; Summit, New Jersey, USA). Patients should then see an obstetrician/gynecologist with experience in reproductive toxicity.[157]

RISKS AND PRECAUTIONS[157]

- Hypersensitivity
- Bradycardia
- Stevens-Johnson syndrome and toxic epidermal necrolysis
- Seizures
- *Pregnancy category:* X

COMPLICATIONS (SOME EXAMPLES)

- *Teratogenicity:* Thalidomide's embryopathy is well documented. Thalidomide is pregnancy category

X, and patients selected for therapy must follow strict contraceptive measures as directed by the program. Thalidomide-induced defects in limb formation may be a consequence of bFGF inhibition, as bFGF induces embryologic limb formation.[158]
- *Peripheral neuropathy:* Thalidomide is neurotoxic and may result in a sensory, symmetrical distal polyneuropathy, which may later evolve to include motor symptoms as well. Neurotoxicity can be permanent. Incidence of peripheral neuropathy in patients receiving thalidomide ranges from 0.5% to 25%. Patients with preexisting peripheral neuropathy should not begin treatment. Baseline nerve conduction studies should be obtained before treatment initiation along with monthly monitoring during the first 3 months decreasing to 6-month intervals thereafter during treatment. A 40% decrease in nerve conduction necessitates treatment discontinuation.[157]
- *Neutropenia:* Because of the risk of neutropenia, baseline measurements should be obtained (including a white blood cell count with differential) and monitored regularly during the treatment course. Treatment should not be initiated in patients with an absolute neutrophil count of less than 750/mm.[157]
- *Other side effects:* Other side effects include drowsiness, orthostatic hypotension, rash, fever, and increases in HIV viral loads.[157,159]

TRASTUZUMAB (HERCEPTIN)

MECHANISM OF ACTION

Trastuzumab is a human, monoclonal antibody directed against the human estrogen receptor 2 (HER-2). Blockade of HER-2 results in downregulation of angiopoeitin-1, plasminogen-activator inhibitor-1, VEGF, and transforming growth factor-α but upregulation of TSP-1, an inhibitor of angiogenesis.[160]

INDICATIONS

Trastuzumab is currently indicated for the treatment of HER-2 overexpression, lymph node–positive breast cancer, or breast cancer that is node-negative and is estrogen receptor/progesterone receptor–negative or has 1 high-risk feature,[2] sometimes associated with another chemotherapy, such as paclitaxel, doxorubicin, cyclophosphamide, or docetaxel, as well as for treatment of metastatic gastric or gastroesophageal junction adenocarcinoma (in combination with cisplatin and either capecitabine or 5-fluorouracil).[161]

No known dermatologic uses or investigations into potential uses exist at this time. Other than a history of hypersensitivity, there are no known contraindications.[2]

COMPLICATIONS (SOME EXAMPLES)[161]

- Cardiomyopathy (requires a baseline measurement of left ventricular ejection fraction and monitoring every 3 months during treatment)
- Pulmonary toxicities (interstitial pneumonitis, acute respiratory distress syndrome)
- Worsening of chemotherapy-induced neutropenia
- Infusion reactions

Table 195-3 summarizes the most important aspects of some experimental drugs that are still in experimental use and that may be helpful as antiangiogenic agents in the future.

TABLE 195-3
Antiangiogenic Properties of Selected Experimental Drugs

DRUG	ANTIANGIOGENIC EFFECTS
ABT-510	Synthetic TSP-1 analog; inhibits actions of VEGF-A, VEGF-C, and bFGF[162-166]
Calcium dobesilate	Binds and antagonizes bFGF[167,168]
Curcumin (diferuloylmethane)	Decreases proangiogenic factors, decreases endothelial cell proliferation, decreases neovascularization[169-173]
Fulvene-5	Fulvene-5 inhibits Nox4 and NADP-oxidase, as well as downregulates expression of ANG-2[174]
Gentian violet	Triphenylmethane dye; downregulates expression of ANG-2[175]
Honokiol	Inhibits VEGFR-2 autophosphorylation, blocks activation of Rac (necessary for endothelial cell migration and proliferation) in response to vascular endothelial growth factor, interferes with the expression of Bcl-2, caspase-3, and TNF-α[176-178]
Interleukin-12	Decreases bFGF-mediated angiogenesis, stimulates natural killer cells to exhibit cytotoxicity against endothelial cells, acts through interferon-γ to induce interferon-inducible protein 10, an antiangiogenic chemokine, and downregulates matrix metalloproteinase synthesis[179]

ANG, angiopoietin; bFGF, basic fibroblast growth factor; NADP, nicotinamide adenine dinucleotide phosphate; TNF, tumor necrosis factor; TSP, thrombospondin; VEGFR, vascular endothelial growth factor receptor.

ACKNOWLEDGMENTS

We thank Ricard L. Berrios, MD, and Jonathan Hofmekler, BSc, who contributed to the equivalent chapter in the 7th edition.

REFERENCES

1. Folkman J. Tumor angiogenesis: therapeutic implications. *N Engl J Med*. 1971;285(21):1182-1186.
2. Berrios RL, Bonner MY, Hofmekler J, et al. Antiangiogenic agents. In: Goldsmith LA, Katz SI, Gilchrest BA, et al. *Fitzpatrick's Dermatology in General Medicine*. 7th ed. New York, NY: McGraw-Hill; 2008:2827-2833.
3. Folkman J. Angiogenesis. *Annu Rev Med*. 2006;57:1-18.
4. Kerbel R, Folkman J. Clinical translation of angiogenesis inhibitors. *Nat Rev Cancer*. 2002;2(10):727-739.
5. Drugs.com. Becaplermin. http://www.drugs.com/ppa/becaplermin.html. Accessed March 2016.
6. Goldman R. Growth factors and chronic wound healing: past, present, and future. *Adv Skin Wound Care*. 2004;17(1):24-35.
7. Gilligan AM, Waycaster CR, Motley TA. Cost-effectiveness of becaplermin gel on wound healing of diabetic foot ulcers. *Wound Repair Regen*. 2015;23(3):353-360.
8. Cohen MA, Eaglstein WH. Recombinant human platelet-derived growth factor gel speeds healing of acute full-thickness punch biopsy wounds. *J Am Acad Dermatol*. 2001;45(6):857-862.
9. Metz BJ, Rubenstein MC, Levy ML, et al. Response of ulcerated perineal hemangiomas of infancy to becaplermin gel, a recombinant human platelet-derived growth factor. *Arch Dermatol*. 2004;140(7):867-870.
10. Twu O, Mednik S, Scumpia P, et al. Use of becaplermin for nondiabetic ulcers: pyoderma gangrenosum and calciphylaxis. *Dermatol Ther*. 2016;29(2):104-108.
11. Tauveron V, Rosen A, Khashoggi M, et al. Long-term successful healing of ulcerated necrobiosis lipoidica after topical therapy with becaplermin. *Clin Exp Dermatol*. 2013;38(7):745-747.
12. Fang RC, Galiano RD. A review of becaplermin gel in the treatment of diabetic neuropathic foot ulcers. *Biologics*. 2008;2(1):1-12.
13. Ziyadeh N, Fife D, Walker AM, et al. A matched cohort study of the risk of cancer in users of becaplermin. *Adv Skin Wound Care*. 2011;24(1):31-39.
14. Papanas N, Maltezos E. Benefit-risk assessment of becaplermin in the treatment of diabetic foot ulcers. *Drug Saf*. 2010;33(6):455-461.
15. Jain RK, Duda DG, Clark JW, et al. Lessons from phase III clinical trials on anti-VEGF therapy for cancer. *Nat Clin Pract Oncol*. 2006;3(1):24-40.
16. Lam SW, Nota NM, Jager A, et al. Angiogenesis- and hypoxia-associated proteins as early indicators of the outcome in patients with metastatic breast cancer given first-line bevacizumab-based therapy. *Clin Cancer Res*. 2016;22(7):1611-1620.
17. Paiva TF Jr, de Jesus VH, Marques RA, et al. Angiogenesis-related protein expression in bevacizumab-treated metastatic colorectal cancer: NOTCH1 detrimental to overall survival. *BMC Cancer*. 2015;15:643.
18. Drugs.com. Bevacizumab. http://www.drugs.com/ppa/bevacizumab.html. Accessed March 2016.
19. Tredan O, Lacroix-Triki M, Guiu S, et al. Angiogenesis and tumor microenvironment: bevacizumab in the breast cancer model. *Target Oncol*. 2015;10(2):189-198.
20. Rinne ML, Lee EQ, Nayak L, et al. Update on bevacizumab and other angiogenesis inhibitors for brain cancer. *Expert Opin Emerg Drugs*. 2013;18(2):137-153.
21. Veytsman I, Aragon-Ching JB, Swain SM. Bevacizumab and angiogenesis inhibitors in the treatment of CNS metastases: the road less travelled. *Curr Mol Pharmacol*. 2013 [Epub ahead of print].
22. Yamatodani T, Holmqvist B, Kjellen E, et al. Using intravital microscopy to observe bevacizumab-mediated anti-angiogenesis in human head and neck squamous cell carcinoma xenografts. *Acta Otolaryngol*. 2012;132(12):1324-1333.
23. Seystahl K, Weller M. Is there a world beyond bevacizumab in targeting angiogenesis in glioblastoma? *Expert Opin Investig Drugs*. 2012;21(5):605-617.
24. Deguchi T, Shikano T, Kasuya H, et al. Combination of the tumor angiogenesis inhibitor bevacizumab and intratumoral oncolytic herpes virus injections as a treatment strategy for human gastric cancers. *Hepatogastroenterology*. 2012;59(118):1844-1850.
25. Gerger A, El-Khoueiry A, Zhang W, et al. Pharmacogenetic angiogenesis profiling for first-line Bevacizumab plus oxaliplatin-based chemotherapy in patients with metastatic colorectal cancer. *Clin Cancer Res*. 2011;17(17):5783-5792.
26. Hu CC, Chaw JR, Chen CF, et al. Controlled release bevacizumab in thermoresponsive hydrogel found to inhibit angiogenesis. *Biomed Mater Eng*. 2014;24(6):1941-1950.
27. Kuo CN, Chen CY, Chen SN, et al. Inhibition of corneal neovascularization with the combination of bevacizumab and plasmid pigment epithelium-derived factor-synthetic amphiphile INTeraction-18 (p-PEDF-SAINT-18) vector in a rat corneal experimental angiogenesis model. *Int J Mol Sci*. 2013;14(4):8291-8305.
28. Dursun A, Arici MK, Dursun F, et al. Comparison of the effects of bevacizumab and ranibizumab injection on corneal angiogenesis in an alkali burn induced model. *Int J Ophthalmol*. 2012;5(4):448-451.
29. Tunik S, Nergiz Y, Keklikci U, et al. The subconjunctival use of cetuximab and bevacizumab in inhibition of corneal angiogenesis. *Graefes Arch Clin Exp Ophthalmol*. 2012;250(8):1161-1167.
30. Del Vecchio M, Mortarini R, Canova S, et al. Bevacizumab plus fotemustine as first-line treatment in metastatic melanoma patients: clinical activity and modulation of angiogenesis and lymphangiogenesis factors. *Clin Cancer Res*. 2010;16(23):5862-5872.
31. Lee SY, Kim DK, Cho JH, et al. Inhibitory effect of bevacizumab on the angiogenesis and growth of retinoblastoma. *Arch Ophthalmol*. 2008;126(7):953-958.
32. Tao X, Sood AK, Deavers MT, et al. Anti-angiogenesis therapy with bevacizumab for patients with ovarian granulosa cell tumors. *Gynecol Oncol*. 2009;114(3):431-436.
33. Cesca M, Morosi L, Berndt A, et al. Bevacizumab-induced inhibition of angiogenesis promotes a more homogeneous intratumoral distribution of paclitaxel, improving the antitumor response. *Mol Cancer Ther*. 2016;15(1):125-135.
34. Su Y, Yang WB, Li S, et al. Effect of angiogenesis inhibitor bevacizumab on survival in patients with cancer: a meta-analysis of the published literature. *PLoS One*. 2012;7(4):e35629.
35. Chen XL, Lei YH, Liu CF, et al. Angiogenesis inhibitor bevacizumab increases the risk of ischemic heart

36. Ranpura V, Hapani S, Chuang J, et al. Risk of cardiac ischemia and arterial thromboembolic events with the angiogenesis inhibitor bevacizumab in cancer patients: a meta-analysis of randomized controlled trials. *Acta Oncol.* 2010;49(3):287-297.
37. Ludwig H, Khayat D, Giaccone G, et al. Proteasome inhibition and its clinical prospects in the treatment of hematologic and solid malignancies. *Cancer.* 2005;104(9):1794-1807.
38. Roccaro AM, Hideshima T, Raje N, et al. Bortezomib mediates antiangiogenesis in multiple myeloma via direct and indirect effects on endothelial cells. *Cancer Res.* 2006;66(1):184-191.
39. Drugs.com. Bortezomib. http://www.drugs.com/ppa/bortezomib.html. Accessed March 2016.
40. Wang X, Zhang Z, Yao C. Bortezomib inhibits the angiogenesis mediated by mesenchymal stem cells. *Cancer Invest.* 2012;30(9):657-662.
41. Zinzani PL, Musuraca G, Tani M, et al. Phase II trial of proteasome inhibitor bortezomib in patients with relapsed or refractory cutaneous T-cell lymphoma. *J Clin Oncol.* 2007;25(27):4293-4297.
42. Terpos E, Kastritis E, Roussou M, et al. The combination of bortezomib, melphalan, dexamethasone and intermittent thalidomide is an effective regimen for relapsed/refractory myeloma and is associated with improvement of abnormal bone metabolism and angiogenesis. *Leukemia.* 2008;22(12):2247-2256.
43. Bota DA, Alexandru D, Keir ST, et al. Proteasome inhibition with bortezomib induces cell death in GBM stem-like cells and temozolomide-resistant glioma cell lines, but stimulates GBM stem-like cells' VEGF production and angiogenesis. *J Neurosurg.* 2013;119(6):1415-1423.
44. Vincenzi B, Santini D, Russo A, et al. Angiogenesis modifications related with cetuximab plus irinotecan as anticancer treatment in advanced colorectal cancer patients. *Ann Oncol.* 2006;17(5):835-841.
45. Perrotte P, Matsumoto T, Inoue K, et al. Anti-epidermal growth factor receptor antibody C225 inhibits angiogenesis in human transitional cell carcinoma growing orthotopically in nude mice. *Clin Cancer Res.* 1999;5(2):257-265.
46. Pham MH, Delestre L, Dewitte A, et al. Synergistic effect of SN-38 in combination with cetuximab on angiogenesis and cancer cell invasion. *Anticancer Res.* 2015;35(11):5983-5991.
47. Pueyo G, Mesia R, Figueras A, et al. Cetuximab may inhibit tumor growth and angiogenesis induced by ionizing radiation: a preclinical rationale for maintenance treatment after radiotherapy. *Oncologist.* 2010;15(9):976-986.
48. Drugs.com. Cetuximab. http://www.drugs.com/ppa/cetuximab.html. Accessed March 2016.
49. El Filali M, Homminga I, Maat W, et al. Triamcinolone acetonide and anecortave acetate do not stimulate uveal melanoma cell growth. *Mol Vis.* 2008;14:1752-1759.
50. Wilson C, Scullin P, Worthington J, et al. Dexamethasone potentiates the antiangiogenic activity of docetaxel in castration-resistant prostate cancer. *Br J Cancer.* 2008;99(12):2054-2064.
51. Sung J, Barone PW, Kong H, et al. Sequential delivery of dexamethasone and VEGF to control local tissue response for carbon nanotube fluorescence based micro-capillary implantable sensors. *Biomaterials.* 2009;30(4):622-631.
52. Lee JG, Wu R. Erlotinib-cisplatin combination inhibits growth and angiogenesis through c-MYC and HIF-1alpha in EGFR-mutated lung cancer in vitro and in vivo. *Neoplasia.* 2015;17(2):190-200.
53. Drugs.com. Erlotinib. http://www.drugs.com/ppa/erlotinib.html. Accessed March 2016.
54. Dy GK, Infante JR, Eckhardt SG, et al. Phase Ib trial of the oral angiogenesis inhibitor pazopanib administered concurrently with erlotinib. *Invest New Drugs.* 2013;31(4):891-899.
55. Nguyen A, Hoang V, Laquer V, et al. Angiogenesis in cutaneous disease: part I. *J Am Acad Dermatol.* 2009;61(6):921-942; quiz 943-944.
56. Bianco R, Garofalo S, Rosa R, et al. Inhibition of mTOR pathway by everolimus cooperates with EGFR inhibitors in human tumours sensitive and resistant to anti-EGFR drugs. *Br J Cancer.* 2008;98(5):923-930.
57. Cejka D, Preusser M, Woehrer A, et al. Everolimus (RAD001) and anti-angiogenic cyclophosphamide show long-term control of gastric cancer growth in vivo. *Cancer Biol Ther.* 2008;7(9):1377-1385.
58. Ceausu RA, Cimpean AM, Dimova I, et al. Everolimus dual effects of an area vasculosa angiogenesis and lymphangiogenesis. *In Vivo.* 2013;27(1):61-66.
59. Drugs.com. Everolimus. http://www.drugs.com/ppa/everolimus.html. Accessed March 2016.
60. Frigerio E, Colombo MD, Franchi C, et al. Severe psoriasis treated with a new macrolide: everolimus. *Br J Dermatol.* 2007;156(2):372-374.
61. Damiano V, Rosa R, Formisano L, et al. Toll-like receptor 9 agonist IMO cooperates with everolimus in renal cell carcinoma by interfering with tumour growth and angiogenesis. *Br J Cancer.* 2013;108(8):1616-1623.
62. Testerman TL, Gerster JF, Imbertson LM, et al. Cytokine induction by the immunomodulators imiquimod and S-27609. *J Leukoc Biol.* 1995;58(3):365-372.
63. Majewski S, Marczak M, Mlynarczyk B, et al. Imiquimod is a strong inhibitor of tumor cell-induced angiogenesis. *Int J Dermatol.* 2005;44(1):14-19.
64. Hesling C, D'Incan M, Mansard S, et al. In vivo and in situ modulation of the expression of genes involved in metastasis and angiogenesis in a patient treated with topical imiquimod for melanoma skin metastases. *Br J Dermatol.* 2004;150(4):761-767.
65. Miller RL, Gerster JF, Owens ML, et al. Imiquimod applied topically: a novel immune response modifier and new class of drug. *Int J Immunopharmacol.* 1999;21(1):1-14.
66. Suzuki H, Wang B, Shivji GM, et al. Imiquimod, a topical immune response modifier, induces migration of Langerhans cells. *J Invest Dermatol.* 2000;114(1):135-141.
67. Arbiser JL, Bips M, Seidler A, et al. Combination therapy of imiquimod and gentian violet for cutaneous melanoma metastases. *J Am Acad Dermatol.* 2012;67(2):e81-e83.
68. Drugs.com. Imiquimod cream (Aldara). http://www.drugs.com/pro/imiquimod.html. Accessed March 2016.
69. Ezzell TI, Fromowitz JS, Ramos-Caro FA. Recurrent pyogenic granuloma treated with topical imiquimod. *J Am Acad Dermatol.* 2006;54(5)(suppl):S244-S245.
70. Li VW, Li WW, Talcott KE, et al. Imiquimod as an antiangiogenic agent. *J Drugs Dermatol.* 2005;4(6):708-717.
71. Sidbury R, Neuschler N, Neuschler E, et al. Topically applied imiquimod inhibits vascular tumor growth in vivo. *J Invest Dermatol.* 2003;121(5):1205-1209.
72. Gul U, Gonul M, Cakmak SK, et al. A case of generalized discoid lupus erythematosus: success-

72. ful treatment with imiquimod cream 5%. *Adv Ther.* 2006;23(5):787-792.
73. Chang CJ, Hsiao YC, Mihm MC Jr, et al. Pilot study examining the combined use of pulsed dye laser and topical Imiquimod versus laser alone for treatment of port wine stain birthmarks. *Lasers Surg Med.* 2008;40(9):605-610.
74. Tremaine AM, Ortiz A, Armstrong J, et al. Combined therapy for enhanced microvascular destruction in port wine stains: pulsed dye laser photothermolysis and imiquimod. *Lasers Surg Med.* 2009:22-23.
75. Indraccolo S. Interferon-alpha as angiogenesis inhibitor: learning from tumor models. *Autoimmunity.* 2010;43(3):244-247.
76. Rosewicz S, Detjen K, Scholz A, et al. Interferon-alpha: regulatory effects on cell cycle and angiogenesis. *Neuroendocrinology.* 2004;80(suppl 1):85-93.
77. Avnet S, Cenni E, Perut F, et al. Interferon-alpha inhibits in vitro osteoclast differentiation and renal cell carcinoma-induced angiogenesis. *Int J Oncol.* 2007;30(2):469-476.
78. Drugs.com. Interferon alfa-2b. http://www.drugs.com/ppa/interferon-alfa-2b.html. Accessed March 2016.
79. Michaud AP, Bauman NM, Burke DK, et al. Spastic diplegia and other motor disturbances in infants receiving interferon-alpha. *Laryngoscope.* 2004;114(7):1231-1236.
80. Tagliaferri P, Caraglia M, Budillon A, et al. New pharmacokinetic and pharmacodynamic tools for interferon-alpha (IFN-alpha) treatment of human cancer. *Cancer Immunol Immunother.* 2005;54(1):1-10.
81. Arbiser JL. Antiangiogenic therapy and dermatology: a review. *Drugs Today (Barc).* 1997;33(10):687-696.
82. Cohenuram M, Saif MW. Panitumumab the first fully human monoclonal antibody: from the bench to the clinic. *Anticancer Drugs.* 2007;18(1):7-15.
83. Drugs.com. Panitumumab. http://www.drugs.com/ppa/panitumumab.html. Accessed March 2016.
84. Ferrara N, Houck KA, Jakeman LB, et al. The vascular endothelial growth factor family of polypeptides. *J Cell Biochem.* 1991;47(3):211-218.
85. Drugs.com. Pegaptanib sodium. http://www.drugs.com/ppa/pegaptanib-sodium.html. Accessed March 2016.
86. Manresa N, Mulero J, Losada M, et al. Effect of pegaptanib and ranibizumab on plasma and vitreous homocysteine in patients with exudative age-related macular degeneration. *Retina.* 2015;35(9):1765-1771.
87. Inoue M, Kadonosono K, Arakawa A, et al. Long-term outcome of intravitreal pegaptanib sodium as maintenance therapy in Japanese patients with neovascular age-related macular degeneration. *Jpn J Ophthalmol.* 2015;59(3):173-178.
88. Kiire CA, Morjaria R, Rudenko A, et al. Intravitreal pegaptanib for the treatment of ischemic diabetic macular edema. *Clin Ophthalmol.* 2015;9:2305-2311.
89. Basile AS, Hutmacher MM, Kowalski KG, et al. Population pharmacokinetics of pegaptanib sodium (Macugen(®)) in patients with diabetic macular edema. *Clin Ophthalmol.* 2015;9:323-335.
90. Lytvynchuk L, Sergienko A, Lavrenchuk G, et al. Antiproliferative, apoptotic, and autophagic activity of ranibizumab, bevacizumab, pegaptanib, and aflibercept on fibroblasts: implication for choroidal neovascularization. *J Ophthalmol.* 2015;2015:934963.
91. Hussain RM, Harris A, Siesky B, et al. The effect of pegaptanib (Macugen(®)) injection on retinal and retrobulbar blood flow in retinal ischaemic diseases. *Acta Ophthalmol.* 2015;93(5):e399-e400.
92. Rinaldi M, Chiosi F, Dell'Omo R, et al. Intravitreal pegaptanib sodium (Macugen) for treatment of myopic choroidal neovascularization: a morphologic and functional study. *Retina.* 2013;33(2):397-402.
93. Delmotte N, Curti C, Montana M, et al. News on infantile hemangioma therapy by beta-blocker [in French]. *Therapie.* 2012;67(3):257-265.
94. Chang L, Ye X, Qiu Y, et al. Is propranolol safe and effective for outpatient use for infantile hemangioma? A prospective study of 679 cases from one center in China. *Ann Plast Surg.* 2016;76(5):559-563.
95. Drugs.com. Propranolol. http://www.drugs.com/propranolol.html. Accessed March 2016.
96. Phillips CB, Pacha O, Biliciler-Denkta G, et al. A review of beta antagonist treatment for infantile hemangioma. *J Drugs Dermatol.* 2012;11(7):826-829.
97. Marsciani A, Pericoli R, Alaggio R, et al. Massive response of severe infantile hepatic hemangioma to propranolol. *Pediatr Blood Cancer.* 2010;54(1):176.
98. Canadas KT, Baum ED, Lee S, et al. Case report: treatment failure using propranolol for treatment of focal subglottic hemangioma. *Int J Pediatr Otorhinolaryngol.* 2010;74(8):956-958.
99. Xu SQ, Jia RB, Zhang W, et al. Beta-blockers versus corticosteroids in the treatment of infantile hemangioma: an evidence-based systematic review. *World J Pediatr.* 2013;9(3):221-229.
100. Chinnadurai S, Fonnesbeck C, Snyder KM, et al. Pharmacologic interventions for infantile hemangioma: a meta-analysis. *Pediatrics.* 2016;137(2):1-10.
101. Sawa K, Yazdani A, Rieder MJ, et al. Propranolol therapy for infantile hemangioma is less toxic but longer in duration than corticosteroid therapy. *Plast Surg (Oakv).* 2014;22(4):233-236.
102. Aly MM, Hamza AF, Abdel Kader HM, et al. Therapeutic superiority of combined propranolol with short steroids course over propranolol monotherapy in infantile hemangioma. *Eur J Pediatr.* 2015;174(11):1503-1509.
103. Li P, Guo Z, Gao Y, et al. Propranolol represses infantile hemangioma cell growth through the beta2-adrenergic receptor in a HIF-1alpha-dependent manner. *Oncol Rep.* 2015;33(6):3099-3107.
104. Ozeki M, Nozawa A, Hori T, et al. Propranolol for infantile hemangioma: effect on plasma vascular endothelial growth factor. *Pediatr Int.* 2016;58(11):1130-1135.
105. Million RP. Therapeutic area crossroads: anti-angiogenesis. *Nat Rev Drug Discov.* 2008;7(2):115-116.
106. Drugs.com. Ranibizumab. http://www.drugs.com/ppa/ranibizumab.html. Accessed March 2016.
107. Figurska M, Robaszkiewicz J, Wierzbowska J. Safety of ranibizumab therapy in wet AMD and the role of vascular endothelial growth factors in physiological angiogenesis. *Klin Oczna.* 2010;112(4-6):147-150.
108. Barzelay A, Lowenstein A, George J, et al. Influence of non-toxic doses of bevacizumab and ranibizumab on endothelial functions and inhibition of angiogenesis. *Curr Eye Res.* 2010;35(9):835-841.
109. Rao RD, Buckner JC, Sarkaria JN. Mammalian target of rapamycin (mTOR) inhibitors as anti-cancer agents. *Curr Cancer Drug Targets.* 2004;4(8):621-635.
110. Kwon YS, Kim JC. Inhibition of corneal neovascularization by rapamycin. *Exp Mol Med.* 2006;38(2):173-179.
111. Sarbassov DD, Ali SM, Sengupta S, et al. Prolonged rapamycin treatment inhibits mTORC2 assembly and Akt/PKB. *Mol Cell.* 2006;22(2):159-168.
112. Drugs.com. Sirolimus. http://www.drugs.com/ppa/sirolimus.html. Accessed March 2016.
113. Chumsri S, Zhao M, Garofalo M, et al. Inhibition of the

114. mammalian target of rapamycin (mTOR) in a case of refractory primary cutaneous anaplastic large cell lymphoma. *Leuk Lymphoma*. 2008;49(2):359-361.
115. Zhang Q, Nowak I, Vonderheid EC, et al. Activation of Jak/STAT proteins involved in signal transduction pathway mediated by receptor for interleukin 2 in malignant T lymphocytes derived from cutaneous anaplastic large T-cell lymphoma and Sezary syndrome. *Proc Natl Acad Sci U S A*. 1996;93(17):9148-9153.
116. Saggar S, Zeichner JA, Brown TT, et al. Kaposi's sarcoma resolves after sirolimus therapy in a patient with pemphigus vulgaris. *Arch Dermatol*. 2008;144(5):654-657.
117. Hofbauer GF, Marcollo-Pini A, Corsenca A, et al. The mTOR inhibitor rapamycin significantly improves facial angiofibroma lesions in a patient with tuberous sclerosis. *Br J Dermatol*. 2008;159(2):473-475.
118. Reitamo S, Spuls P, Sassolas B, et al. Efficacy of sirolimus (rapamycin) administered concomitantly with a subtherapeutic dose of cyclosporin in the treatment of severe psoriasis: a randomized controlled trial. *Br J Dermatol*. 2001;145(3):438-445.
119. Swaminathan S, Arbiser JL, Hiatt KM, et al. Rapid improvement of nephrogenic systemic fibrosis with rapamycin therapy: possible role of phospho-70-ribosomal-S6 kinase. *J Am Acad Dermatol*. 2010;62(2):343-345.
120. Lapidoth M, Ben-Amitai D, Bhandarkar S, et al. Efficacy of topical application of eosin for ulcerated hemangiomas. *J Am Acad Dermatol*. 2009;60(2):350-351.
121. Nadiminti U, Arbiser JL. Rapamycin (sirolimus) as a steroid-sparing agent in dermatomyositis. *J Am Acad Dermatol*. 2005;52(2)(suppl 1):17-19.
122. Liu WN, Lin JH, Cheng YR, et al. FIM-A, a phosphorus-containing sirolimus, inhibits the angiogenesis and proliferation of osteosarcomas. *Oncol Res*. 2013;20(7):319-326.
123. Warino L, Libecco J. Cutaneous effects of sirolimus in renal transplant recipients. *J Drugs Dermatol*. 2006;5(3):273-274.
124. Ng R, Chen EX. Sorafenib (BAY 43-9006): review of clinical development. *Curr Clin Pharmacol*. 2006;1(3):223-228.
125. Plaza-Menacho I, Mologni L, Sala E, et al. Sorafenib functions to potently suppress RET tyrosine kinase activity by direct enzymatic inhibition and promoting RET lysosomal degradation independent of proteasomal targeting. *J Biol Chem*. 2007;282(40):29230-29240.
126. Liu L, Cao Y, Chen C, et al. Sorafenib blocks the RAF/MEK/ERK pathway, inhibits tumor angiogenesis, and induces tumor cell apoptosis in hepatocellular carcinoma model PLC/PRF/5. *Cancer Res*. 2006;66(24):11851-11858.
127. Murphy DA, Makonnen S, Lassoued W, et al. Inhibition of tumor endothelial ERK activation, angiogenesis, and tumor growth by sorafenib (BAY43-9006). *Am J Pathol*. 2006;169(5):1875-1885.
128. Pignochino Y, Grignani G, Cavalloni G, et al. Sorafenib blocks tumour growth, angiogenesis and metastatic potential in preclinical models of osteosarcoma through a mechanism potentially involving the inhibition of ERK1/2, MCL-1 and ezrin pathways. *Mol Cancer*. 2009;8:118.
129. Drugs.com. SORAfenib. http://www.drugs.com/ppa/sorafenib.html. Accessed March 2016.
130. Miyahara K, Nouso K, Tomoda T, et al. Predicting the treatment effect of sorafenib using serum angiogenesis markers in patients with hepatocellular carcinoma. *J Gastroenterol Hepatol*. 2011;26(11):1604-1611.
131. Karashima T, Fukuhara H, Tamura K, et al. Expression of angiogenesis-related gene profiles and development of resistance to tyrosine-kinase inhibitor in advanced renal cell carcinoma: characterization of sorafenib-resistant cells derived from a cutaneous metastasis. *Int J Urol*. 2013;20(9):923-930.
132. Wang W, Wang H, Ni Y, et al. DCT015, a new sorafenib derivate, inhibits tumor growth and angiogenesis in gastric cancer models. *Tumour Biol*. 2016;37(7):9221-9232.
133. Yu P, Ye L, Wang H, et al. NSK-01105, a novel sorafenib derivative, inhibits human prostate tumor growth via suppression of VEGFR2/EGFR-mediated angiogenesis. *PLoS One*. 2014;9(12):e115041.
134. Qin Y, Lu Y, Wang R, et al. SL1122-37, a novel derivative of sorafenib, has greater effects than sorafenib on the inhibition of human hepatocellular carcinoma (HCC) growth and prevention of angiogenesis. *Biosci Trends*. 2013;7(5):237-244.
135. Overkleeft EN, Goldschmeding R, van Reekum F, et al. Nephrotic syndrome caused by the angiogenesis inhibitor sorafenib. *Ann Oncol*. 2010;21(1):184-185.
136. Roskoski R Jr. Sunitinib: a VEGF and PDGF receptor protein kinase and angiogenesis inhibitor. *Biochem Biophys Res Commun*. 2007;356(2):323-328.
137. Cabebe E, Wakelee H. Sunitinib: a newly approved small-molecule inhibitor of angiogenesis. *Drugs Today (Barc)*. 2006;42(6):387-398.
138. Drugs.com. Sunitinib malate. http://www.drugs.com/ppa/sunitinib-malate.html. Accessed March 2016.
139. Dornbusch J, Walter M, Gottschalk A, et al. Evaluation of polymorphisms in angiogenesis-related genes as predictive and prognostic markers for sunitinib-treated metastatic renal cell carcinoma patients. *J Cancer Res Clin Oncol*. 2016;142(6):1171-1182.
140. del Puerto-Nevado L, Rojo F, Zazo S, et al. Active angiogenesis in metastatic renal cell carcinoma predicts clinical benefit to sunitinib-based therapy. *Br J Cancer*. 2014;110(11):2700-2707.
141. Nguyen S, Franklin M, Dudek AZ. Skin ulcers in Klippel-Trenaunay syndrome respond to sunitinib. *Transl Res*. 2008;151(4):194-196.
142. Zhu X, Stergiopoulos K, Wu S. Risk of hypertension and renal dysfunction with an angiogenesis inhibitor sunitinib: systematic review and meta-analysis. *Acta Oncol*. 2009;48(1):9-17.
143. Drugs.com. Temsirolimus. http://www.drugs.com/ppa/temsirolimus.html. Accessed March 2016.
144. Lattanzio L, Milano G, Monteverde M, et al. Schedule-dependent interaction between temsirolimus and cetuximab in head and neck cancer: a preclinical study. *Anticancer Drugs*. 2016;27(6):533-539.
145. John K, Rosner I, Keilholz U, et al. Baseline caspase activity predicts progression free survival of temsirolimus-treated head neck cancer patients. *Eur J Cancer*. 2015;51(12):1596-1602.
146. Liu X, Kambrick S, Fu S, et al. Advanced malignancies treated with a combination of the VEGF inhibitor bevacizumab, anti-EGFR antibody cetuximab, and the mTOR inhibitor temsirolimus. *Oncotarget*. 2016;7(17):23227-23238.
147. Abdel-Rahman O, Fouad M. Risk of oral and gastrointestinal mucosal injury in patients with solid tumors treated with everolimus, temsirolimus or ridaforolimus: a comparative systematic review

and meta-analysis. *Expert Rev Anticancer Ther.* 2015;15(7):847-858.
147. Abdel-Rahman O, Fouad M. Risk of fatigue in patients with solid tumors treated with everolimus, temsirolimus or ridaforolimus: a comparative meta-analysis. *Expert Rev Anticancer Ther.* 2015;15(4):477-486.
148. Ito T, Ando H, Suzuki T, et al. Identification of a primary target of thalidomide teratogenicity. *Science.* 2010;327(5971):1345-1350.
149. Bartlett JB, Tozer A, Stirling D, et al. Recent clinical studies of the immunomodulatory drug (IMiD) lenalidomide. *Br J Cancer.* 2005;93(6):613-619.
150. Li X, Liu X, Wang J, et al. Thalidomide down-regulates the expression of VEGF and bFGF in cisplatin-resistant human lung carcinoma cells. *Anticancer Res.* 2003;23(3B):2481-2487.
151. Rosenbach M, Werth VP. Dermatologic therapeutics: thalidomide. A practical guide. *Dermatol Ther.* 2007;20(4):175-186.
152. Gelati M, Corsini E, Frigerio S, et al. Effects of thalidomide on parameters involved in angiogenesis: an in vitro study. *J Neurooncol.* 2003;64(3):193-201.
153. Li Y, Fu S, Chen H, et al. Inhibition of endothelial Slit2/Robo1 signaling by thalidomide restrains angiogenesis by blocking the PI3K/Akt pathway. *Dig Dis Sci.* 2014;59(12):2958-2966.
154. D'Amato RJ, Loughnan MS, Flynn E, et al. Thalidomide is an inhibitor of angiogenesis. *Proc Natl Acad Sci U S A.* 1994 26;91(9):4082-4085.
155. Fuchida SI, Shimazaki C, Hirai H, et al. The effects of thalidomide on chemotactic migration of multiple myeloma cell lines. *Int J Lab Hematol.* 2008;30(3):220-229.
156. Nasca MR, O'Toole EA, Palicharla P, et al. Thalidomide increases human keratinocyte migration and proliferation. *J Invest Dermatol.* 1999;113(5):720-724.
157. Drugs.com. Thalidomide. http://www.drugs.com/ppa/thalidomide.html. Accessed March 2016.
158. Stephens TD, Bunde CJ, Fillmore BJ. Mechanism of action in thalidomide teratogenesis. *Biochem Pharmacol.* 2000;59(12):1489-1499.
159. Faver IR, Guerra SG, Su WP, et al. Thalidomide for dermatology: a review of clinical uses and adverse effects. *Int J Dermatol.* 2005;44(1):61-67.
160. Izumi Y, Xu L, di Tomaso E, et al. Tumour biology: Herceptin acts as an anti-angiogenic cocktail. *Nature.* 2002;416(6878):279-280.
161. Drugs.com. Trastuzumab. http://www.drugs.com/ppa/trastuzumab.html. Accessed March 2016.
162. Hoekstra R, de Vos FY, Eskens FA, et al. Phase I safety, pharmacokinetic, and pharmacodynamic study of the thrombospondin-1-mimetic angiogenesis inhibitor ABT-510 in patients with advanced cancer. *J Clin Oncol.* 2005;23(22):5188-5197.
163. Markovic SN, Suman VJ, Rao RA, et al. A phase II study of ABT-510 (thrombospondin-1 analog) for the treatment of metastatic melanoma. *Am J Clin Oncol.* 2007;30(3):303-309.
164. Baker LH, Rowinsky EK, Mendelson D, et al. Randomized, phase II study of the thrombospondin-1-mimetic angiogenesis inhibitor ABT-510 in patients with advanced soft tissue sarcoma. *J Clin Oncol.* 2008;26(34):5583-5588.
165. Punekar S, Zak S, Kalter VG, et al. Thrombospondin 1 and its mimetic peptide ABT-510 decrease angiogenesis and inflammation in a murine model of inflammatory bowel disease. *Pathobiology.* 2008;75(1):9-21.
166. Anderson JC, Grammer JR, Wang W, et al. ABT-510, a modified type 1 repeat peptide of thrombospondin, inhibits malignant glioma growth in vivo by inhibiting angiogenesis. *Cancer Biol Ther.* 2007;6(3):454-462.
167. Arbiser JL, Byers HR, Cohen C, et al. Altered basic fibroblast growth factor expression in common epidermal neoplasms: examination with in situ hybridization and immunohistochemistry. *J Am Acad Dermatol.* 2000;42(6):973-977.
168. Lameynardie S, Chiavaroli C, Travo P, et al. Inhibition of choroidal angiogenesis by calcium dobesilate in normal Wistar and diabetic GK rats. *Eur J Pharmacol.* 2005 7;510(1-2):149-156.
169. Arbiser JL, Klauber N, Rohan R, et al. Curcumin is an in vivo inhibitor of angiogenesis. *Mol Med.* 1998;4(6):376-383.
170. Sharma RA, Gescher AJ, Steward WP. Curcumin: the story so far. *Eur J Cancer.* 2005;41(13):1955-1968.
171. Wang F, He Z, Dai W, et al. The role of the vascular endothelial growth factor/vascular endothelial growth factor receptors axis mediated angiogenesis in curcumin-loaded nanostructured lipid carriers induced human HepG2 cells apoptosis. *J Cancer Res Ther.* 2015;11(3):597-605.
172. Zhang JR, Lu F, Lu T, et al. Inactivation of FoxM1 transcription factor contributes to curcumin-induced inhibition of survival, angiogenesis, and chemosensitivity in acute myeloid leukemia cells. *J Mol Med (Berl).* 2014;92(12):1319-1330.
173. Das L, Vinayak M. Long term effect of curcumin in regulation of glycolytic pathway and angiogenesis via modulation of stress activated genes in prevention of cancer. *PLoS One.* 2014;9(6):e99583.
174. Bhandarkar SS, Jaconi M, Fried LE, et al. Fulvene-5 potently inhibits NADPH oxidase 4 and blocks the growth of endothelial tumors in mice. *J Clin Invest.* 2009;119(8):2359-2365.
175. Perry BN, Govindarajan B, Bhandarkar SS, et al. Pharmacologic blockade of angiopoietin-2 is efficacious against model hemangiomas in mice. *J Invest Dermatol.* 2006;126(10):2316-2322.
176. Bai X, Cerimele F, Ushio-Fukai M, et al. Honokiol, a small molecular weight natural product, inhibits angiogenesis in vitro and tumor growth in vivo. *J Biol Chem.* 2003;278(37):35501-35507.
177. Ma L, Chen J, Wang X, et al. Structural modification of honokiol, a biphenyl occurring in *Magnolia officinalis*: the evaluation of honokiol analogues as inhibitors of angiogenesis and for their cytotoxicity and structure-activity relationship. *J Med Chem.* 2011;54(19):6469-6481.
178. Li Z, Liu Y, Zhao X, et al. Honokiol, a natural therapeutic candidate, induces apoptosis and inhibits angiogenesis of ovarian tumor cells. *Eur J Obstet Gynecol Reprod Biol.* 2008;140(1):95-102.
179. Yao L, Sgadari C, Furuke K, et al. Contribution of natural killer cells to inhibition of angiogenesis by interleukin-12. *Blood.* 1999;93(5):1612-1621.

Chapter 196 :: Other Topical Medications
:: Shawn G. Kwatra & Manisha Loss

第一百九十六章

其他外用药

中文导读

本章介绍了用于治疗皮肤病的外用药物，包括止痛药、抗感染药、抗菌药、抗寄生虫药、止汗剂、止痒剂和收敛剂、漂白剂和角膜溶解剂、病毒疣外用药物、复合制剂等，并介绍了它们的作用机制、适应证及注意事项等。

〔粟　娟〕

AT-A-GLANCE

Topical medications discussed in this chapter include:
- Analgesics
- Antiinflammatory agents
- Antimicrobial and antiparasitic agents
- Antiperspirants, antipruritics, and astringents
- Bleaching and keratolytic agents
- Topical psoriasis and wart therapies
- Compounding medications

This chapter reviews topical therapies that are used to treat dermatologic diseases but that are not discussed elsewhere in the text. When applied to large areas of skin, particularly in the presence of skin disease, or to infants and children, all topical medications have the potential to cause systemic side effects.

ANALGESICS

CAPSAICIN

Capsaicin is the active ingredient responsible for the "hotness" in chili peppers. Initial topical application results in itching, pricking, and burning as a result of activation of the transient receptor potential vanilloid-1.[1] Repeated application depletes substance P from cutaneous nerve endings and leads to desensitization of epidermal nerve fibers, thereby producing hypoalgesia.

Topical capsaicin has been used to treat postherpetic neuralgia, diabetic neuropathy, reflex sympathetic dystrophy, Raynaud phenomenon, osteoarthritis, plantar warts, and diabetic neuralgia.[2] A recent metaanalysis of 6 randomized controlled trials found high efficacy of topical capsaicin in the treatment of postherpetic neuralgia.[3] In addition, capsaicin is also an effective antipruritic agent for localized areas of pruritus of neuropathic origin, such as in brachioradial pruritus and notalgia paresthetica.[4]

The chief side effect of capsaicin is irritation and an intense burning sensation. Thus, capsaicin should not be applied to a large area of the body and may not be tolerated by children.

TOPICAL ANESTHETICS

Numerous topical anesthetic formulations are available. Eutectic mixture of local anesthetics (EMLA) cream and topical lidocaine are two of the most frequently employed topical anesthetics and are discussed in further detail below.

EUTECTIC MIXTURE OF LOCAL ANESTHETICS CREAM

EMLA cream contains the sodium channel-blocking amide anesthetics lidocaine 2.5% and prilocaine 2.5%.

Application under occlusion to intact skin or genital mucous membranes for at least 1 hour before performance of a painful procedure, including debridement of venous leg ulcers,[5] can provide local anesthesia that may persist for up to 2 hours. In addition, EMLA is effective in cases of postburn pruritus[6] and notalgia paresthetica.

The cream may cause transient local blanching followed by transient local erythema. Like all products containing lidocaine, it should not be used in patients with hypersensitivity to amide anesthetics. Side effects to EMLA are usually limited to mild skin reactions. Rare severe complications include CNS toxicity, cardiotoxicity, and methemoglobinemia.[7] The prilocaine component of EMLA has been linked to cases of methemoglobinemia in patients for whom applications exceeded the recommended dose, application area, or application time.[8] Those particularly susceptible to methemoglobinemia include patients who are very young, those with glucose-6-phosphate dehydrogenase deficiency, and those taking oxidizing drugs such as sulfonamides and antimalarials.

Caution regarding dosing should also be used in patients susceptible to systemic effects of lidocaine or prilocaine, including acutely ill, debilitated, and elderly patients. In addition, factors that increase risk of systemic toxicity include application of excessive amounts of EMLA, longer application time, and application to inflamed skin.[7] Finally, as EMLA is ototoxic, it should not be used if there is a concern that it could penetrate or migrate beyond the tympanic membrane to the middle ear. EMLA is a pregnancy category B drug.

LIDOCAINE

Various topical anesthetic products contain only lidocaine, typically at concentrations of 4% or 5%, which may be applied with or without occlusion. Lidocaine 5% medicated plaster is commonly used to treat localized neuropathic pain, in particular postherpetic neuralgia and diabetic polyneuropathy.[9]

Lidocaine can result in local skin irritation, such as erythema, edema, or bruising. Systemic toxicity from topical lidocaine prepared in a 30% concentration has been reported. Systemic effects may include CNS and cardiac effects, including seizure, coma, arrhythmia, apnea, and death. Lidocaine is a pregnancy category B drug.

ANTIINFLAMMATORY AGENTS

COAL TAR

Coal tar has been used in the treatment of inflammatory dermatoses, including psoriasis and atopic dermatitis. In 1925, Goeckerman pioneered the concomitant use of coal tar and ultraviolet B therapy for psoriasis. Coal tar inhibits DNA synthesis and mitosis in epidermal cells, an effect potentiated by ultraviolet A exposure.[10]

Coal tar also has antiinfective, antipruritic, photosensitizing, and vasoconstrictive effects. Coal tar works by activating the aryl hydrocarbon receptor, which results in induction of epidermal differentiation. Coal tar also counteracts T-helper type-2 cytokine-mediated downregulation of skin barrier proteins.[11]

Coal tar has historically been messy to use, has an unpleasant odor, and can stain clothing, making its use challenging for some. Newer formulations may be better tolerated. Systemic adverse effects are uncommon, whereas local adverse effects can include tar folliculitis, acneiform eruptions, irritant dermatitis, burning, stinging, allergic contact dermatitis, atrophy, telangiectases, pigmentation, exfoliative dermatitis, and keratoacanthomas.[12] Although animal experiments have shown coal tar to induce skin cancers, a large cohort study among patients with psoriasis and eczema revealed that coal tar is not associated with an increased risk of skin cancer.[13]

WOOD TAR

Wood tar (or pine tar) is produced by distillation of wood and roots of pine under controlled conditions, and can be added to arachis oil (peanut oil) or other bases. Wood tar is thought to work through reducing DNA synthesis and mitotic activity and has been found to have antibacterial, antiinflammatory, antifungal, and antipruritic activity. Wood tar can be used for atopic dermatitis, psoriasis (especially of the scalp), and seborrheic dermatitis, among other inflammatory skin conditions. Although most commonly derived from juniper (oil of cade), wood tar also may be derived from beech, birch, and pine. Wood tar may result in contact sensitivity.

SHALE OIL

Shale oil (also referred to as *ammonium bituminosulfonate*, *ichthyol*, *ichthammol*, or *black salve*) is derived from oil shale, a sulfur-rich sedimentary rock. Further processing of extracted shale oil yields light-colored and dark-colored components. Shale oil decreases inflammation by inhibiting leukotriene B_4 lipoxygenase.[14,15] A randomized, controlled trial showed that pale sulfonated shale oil cream 4% is more effective than placebo in the treatment of mild to moderate atopic dermatitis.[16] Pale sulfonated shale oil also has been used to treat venous leg ulcers, acne, psoriasis, seborrhea, eczema, rosacea, and pruritus.[17] Shale oil is generally well tolerated and the most common side effect is skin irritation.

CRISABOROLE

Crisaborole is a boron-containing, novel, small molecule that reduces skin inflammation by inhibiting phosphodiesterase 4. Two double-blind, randomized, controlled trials found crisaborole to be more effective than vehicle in reducing disease severity and improving pruritus in patients with mild to moderate atopic dermatitis.[18] Crisaborole is generally well tolerated and no severe adverse effects have been reported as of this writing.

ANTIMICROBIAL AGENTS

Table 196-1 outlines the topical antimicrobials and astringents discussed in this section of the chapter.

CHLORHEXIDINE

Chlorhexidine gluconate is a bisbiguanide with rapid onset that binds to the stratum corneum. Chlorhexidine provides sustained fungicidal and broad-spectrum bactericidal activity (Gram-negative and Gram-positive organisms). Although it does not kill bacterial spores or mycobacteria, it does inhibit their growth. Chlorhexidine has residual activity for longer than 6 hours, even when wiped from the field. A metaanalysis found chlorhexidine had reduced bacterial colonization and surgical site infections as compared to povidone iodine.[19] Because chlorhexidine does not lose its effectiveness in the presence of organic material, such as whole blood, it is an important antiseptic, disinfectant, antibacterial dental rinse, and preservative. Because of ototoxicity and the risk of conjunctivitis and corneal ulceration, chlorhexidine is not recommended for preoperative preparation of the face or head.

DYES

Dyes are useful topical treatments because they are inexpensive and chemically and physically stable. The topical antiseptic dyes used in dermatology—gentian violet (methylrosaniline chloride), brilliant green, malachite green, and fuchsine—are all derivatives or metabolites. The dyes are effective against *Candida* species and several aerobic Gram-positive bacteria, including methicillin-resistant *Staphylococcus aureus*. Gentian violet is a known contact sensitizer and may cause skin necrosis in concentrations greater than 2% aqueous solution or when used undiluted in skin folds.[20]

HYDROGEN PEROXIDE

Hydrogen peroxide has been used for a number of years as a cleansing agent and for the removal of debris. It has antibacterial properties against both Gram-positive and Gram-negative bacteria, and its effervescent quality helps debride wounds.

IODINATED COMPOUNDS

Iodine solution is bactericidal, sporicidal, and viricidal. Iodophors are complexes of iodine with a carrier that slowly liberates inorganic iodine on contact with reducing substances. This preserves the antimicrobial activities of iodine while minimizing the irritant effects of the free tincture. Iodophors must be applied to dry skin as they are inactivated by contact with blood and sputum.

POVIDONE-IODINE

Povidone iodine has a wide spectrum of in vitro activity against Gram-negative and Gram-positive bacteria, fungi, and viruses. Systemic absorption can occur with resultant renal and thyroid dysfunction if large or prolonged quantities are used.

CLIOQUINOL

Clioquinol, 5-chloro-8-hydroxy-7-iodoquinoline, is weakly antifungal and antibacterial. It is effective alone or combined with a topical steroid to treat inflammatory dermatoses, especially in intertriginous areas. Adverse reactions include a yellowish discoloration on clothing or skin, delayed contact hypersensitivity, and contact dermatitis. In the early 1970s, it was linked to subacute myelooptic neuropathy in Japan,[21] and was banned in many countries, including the United States. This link was questioned by subsequent epidemiologic studies,[22] but product labeling still warns of possible irreversible optic atrophy and peripheral neuromuscular disease.

METRONIDAZOLE

Metronidazole is an imidazole with activity against anaerobic bacteria and protozoa that is most often used in dermatology for rosacea. In addition to its antibiotic properties, its mode of action in rosacea may involve the impedance of leukocyte chemotaxis and selective suppression of cellular immunity.

MUPIROCIN

Mupirocin was initially isolated by *Pseudomonas fluorescens* and is bactericidal at the concentration achieved with topical application to the skin and mucous membranes. As mupirocin has a unique mechanism of action, in which it prevents the incorporation of isoleucine into proteins by inhibiting bacterial isoleucyl-tRNA synthetase, there is no cross-resistance with other antimicrobials. It has activity against staphylococci, streptococci, and certain Gram-negative bacteria, but is not effective against *Pseudomonas* and is inactive against much of the normal skin flora. It is the

TABLE 196-1
Topical Antimicrobials and Astringents

DRUG	GROUP	ANTIBACTERIAL MECHANISM	ANTIMICROBIAL SPECTRUM	MAJOR SIDE EFFECTS OR CONTRAINDICATIONS	USE (SELECTED)	U.S. FOOD AND DRUG ADMINISTRATION PREGNANCY CATEGORY
Chlorhexidine	Bisbiguanide	(1) Binds to negatively charged bacterial cell wall and cytoplasmic components leading to altered osmotic equilibrium (2) Precipitation of cytoplasmic components	Gram-positive, Gram-negative bacteria, enveloped viruses, and fungi	Keratitis, ototoxicity	Antiseptic surgical hand scrub and surgical site preparation	B
Gentian violet	Dye	Unknown	Some vegetative Gram-positive bacteria (eg, *Staphylococcus* sp.) and yeast	Potential skin necrosis at high concentrations or when occluded; stains skin and clothing; tattooing when applied over granulation tissue; mutagenic	Impetiginized eczema; mycotic skin infections; oral candidiasis; superficial skin infections	C
Brilliant green	Dye	Unknown	Similar to gentian violet	Potential skin necrosis; stains skin and clothing	Similar to gentian violet	Not used in Western medicine
Hydrogen peroxide	Peroxide	Oxidizes microbial molecules	Broad-spectrum antimicrobial	Avoid in abscesses; bleaches hair	Cleansing of wounds, suppurating ulcers, and local infections	—
Povidone-iodine	Iodophor	Oxidation and release of free iodine	Gram-positive, Gram-negative, enveloped viruses, fungi, sporicidal, *Mycobacterium tuberculosis*	Caution in patients with thyroid disorders; potential systemic toxicity in neonates or when applied to large body surface area; neutralized by blood, serum proteins, and sputum	Antiseptic surgical hand scrub, prevention or treatment of topical site infection associated with surgery, burns, minor cuts/scrapes	C
Clioquinol	Iodophor	Oxidation and release of free iodine; chelates bacterial surface and trace metals needed for bacterial growth	Gram-positive, Gram-negative, enveloped viruses, fungi, sporicidal, *M. tuberculosis*	Possible irreversible optic atrophy and peripheral neuropathy (oral); contraindicated in children <2 years of age; contraindicated for diaper rash; stains skin yellow; neutralized by blood, serum proteins, and sputum	Approved for fungal infections; also used for pyoderma, folliculitis, and impetigo	—
Metronidazole	Imidazole	Creation of reduced intermediate compounds and free radicals	Anaerobes, protozoa, and microaerophilic bacteria	Contraindicated during first trimester of pregnancy	Rosacea	B

(Continued)

TABLE 196-1
Topical Antimicrobials and Astringents (Continued)

DRUG	GROUP	ANTIBACTERIAL MECHANISM	ANTIMICROBIAL SPECTRUM	MAJOR SIDE EFFECTS OR CONTRAINDICATIONS	USE (SELECTED)	U.S. FOOD AND DRUG ADMINISTRATION PREGNANCY CATEGORY
Mupirocin	Fermentation product of *Pseudomonas fluorescens*	Inhibits bacterial isoleucyl-tRNA synthetase	Gram-positive, some Gram-negative, spares normal flora	Potentially toxic amounts of polyethylene glycol contained in vehicle may be absorbed in patients with extensive burns or open wounds	Nonbullous impetigo, eradication of nasal carriage of *Staphylococcus aureus*	B
Retapamulin	Pleuromutilin	Inhibits 50S subunit of prokaryotic ribosome	Gram-positive	Allergic contact dermatitis	Nonbullous impetigo	B
Azelaic acid	Dicarboxylic acid	Possibly through inhibition of microbial respiratory chain	*Propionibacterium acnes* and *Staphylococcus epidermidis*	Hypopigmentation	Acne	B
Benzoyl peroxide	Peroxide	Oxidizes microbial molecules	Broad-spectrum antimicrobial	Bleaches dark clothing	Acne	C
Aluminum salts	Astringent	Coagulation of proteins	Broad-spectrum antimicrobial	Do not use under impervious material to prevent evaporation	Weeping, impetiginized skin disorders	—
Potassium permanganate	Astringent	Oxidizes microbial molecules	Broad-spectrum antimicrobial	Skin discoloration; caustic at high concentrations or with contact of undissolved crystals	Weeping, impetiginized skin disorders	—
Silver nitrate	Astringent	Precipitation of bacterial proteins by free silver ions	Gram-positive and Gram-negative bacteria	Black skin discoloration, caustic at high concentrations; potential methemoglobinemia	Weeping, impetiginized skin disorders, cauterization of wounds, removal of granulation tissue, aseptic prophylaxis of burns	C

treatment of choice for nonbullous impetigo, and is effective in the elimination of *S. aureus* nasal colonization. Mupirocin is a pregnancy category B drug.

RETAPAMULIN

Retapamulin is a member of the pleuromutilin class of antibiotics and is derived from *Clitopilus scyphoides*. It is bacteriostatic and inhibits the elongation phase of protein synthesis through selective binding to the 50S subunit of prokaryotic ribosomes. It is effective against certain Gram-positive bacteria and is approved by the U.S. Food and Drug Administration (FDA) for the treatment of methicillin-sensitive *S. aureus* and *Streptococcus pyogenes*. It is prescribed as a 1% topical ointment. Side effects can include irritant and contact dermatitis. Retapamulin is a pregnancy category B drug.

AZELAIC ACID

Azelaic acid is a naturally occurring aliphatic dicarboxylic acid that is a competitive inhibitor of tyrosinase. Azelaic acid is a reversible inhibitor of cytochrome P450 reductase and 5α-reductase in microsomes as well as a reversible inhibitor of some enzymes in the respiratory chain. In vitro azelaic acid has antimicrobial effects against *Propionibacterium acnes* and *Staphylococcus epidermidis*. Its efficacy against acne and rosacea is attributed to activity against *P. acnes*, normalization of keratinization, and a direct antiinflammatory effect. Azelaic acid is a pregnancy category B drug and is often a preferred treatment of acne or rosacea in pregnant patients.

BENZOYL PEROXIDE

Benzoyl peroxide is an organic compound that is commonly used in the treatment of acne vulgaris. Benzoyl peroxide functions by reducing and decreasing the size of comedones, increasing the sebum excretion rate, and through its bactericidal effects. Benzoyl peroxide is directly toxic to *P. acnes* and effective against resistant strains of *P. acnes*. To limit antibiotic resistance, it is suggested that topical benzoyl peroxide be added when a long-term oral antibiotic is used.[23] In addition, benzoyl peroxide is frequently combined with topical antibiotics, as combination therapy may reduce the development of antibiotic resistance by *P. acnes*. Benzoyl peroxide is a pregnancy category C drug.

ANTIPARASITIC AGENTS

Table 196-2 outlines the topical antiparasitic agents discussed in this section. Chapter 178 provides detailed discussions of scabies, other mites, and pediculosis.

CROTAMITON

Crotamiton (crotonyl-*N*-ethyl-*o*-toluidine) is a colorless or pale yellow oil used in the treatment of scabies, pediculosis capitis, and, occasionally, pruritus. Its mode of action is unknown. Other antiparasitic formulations, such as topical permethrin and ivermectin cream, have been found in head-to-head controlled trials to be superior to crotamiton in the treatment of scabies.[24,25] It is approved for use in infants and children, but is a pregnancy category C drug.

LINDANE (γ-BENZENE HEXACHLORIDE)

Lindane, also known as *γ-benzene hexachloride* or *hexachlorocyclohexane*, is a chlorinated hydrocarbon pesticide that is effective against lice, scabies, and fleas as a 1% lotion or shampoo. There are multiple side effects of topical lindane application, including CNS toxicity, seizures, and aplastic anemia. The use of lindane is limited given this potential for lindane toxicity, in addition to the fact that safer and more effective alternative agents

TABLE 196-2
Topical Antiparasitic Agents

TREATMENT	GROUP OR COMPOSITION	MECHANISM	MAJOR SIDE EFFECTS OR CONTRAINDICATIONS	USE	U.S. FOOD AND DRUG ADMINISTRATION PREGNANCY CATEGORY
Permethrin (1% or 5%)	Synthetic pyrethroid	Inhibits nerve cell sodium ion influx	Itching and stinging on application; contraindicated for infants <2 months of age	Lice and scabies; used on clothing as an insect repellant	B
Ivermectin	Avermectin	Binding to glutamate- and γ-aminobutyric acid–gated chloride ion channels	Skin irritation upon application	Scabies, head lice, rosacea	C
Synergized pyrethrins	Natural botanical	Pyrethrins inhibit nerve cell sodium ion influx; piperonyl butoxide inhibits cytochrome P450	Itching and stinging on application; ragweed or chrysanthemum allergy	Lice	C
Malathion (0.5%)	Organophosphate	Cholinesterase inhibitor	Flammable; not approved for children <6 years of age	Lice	B
Crotamiton (10%)	Crotonyl-*N*-ethyl-*o*-toluidine	Unknown	Poor efficacy	Scabies	C
Lindane (1%)	Organochlorine	Cholinesterase inhibitor	May cause seizures, muscle spasms, aplastic anemia; not for use in children <3 years of age, pregnant or breast-feeding women, patients with underlying neurologic disorders, or over broken skin	Lice and scabies	C
Spinosad (0.9%)	Fermentation product	Generalized CNS excitation leading to paralysis	No major side effects in preclinical trials	Lice	Not rated

are available.[26] Patients with seizure disorders, children who weigh less than 50 kg, and patients with acutely inflamed or raw skin should avoid using lindane.

IVERMECTIN

Ivermectin is a derivative of the avermectin family of macrocyclic lactone parasiticides. It is a broad-spectrum anti parasitic agent and also displays antiinflammatory properties. Ivermectin's antiparasitic mechanism of action is through binding to glutamate-gated and γ-aminobutyric acid–gated chloride ion channels of parasite nerve and muscles cells, leading to increased permeability of chloride ions and later paralysis and death. Topical ivermectin can be used to treat scabies, head lice, as well as rosacea. Topical 1% ivermectin was found to be as effective as 2.5% permethrin cream in scabies patients when applied with 2 applications and a 1-week interval between applications.[27] Two multi-site, randomized, double-blinded studies showed that a single, 10-minute, at-home application of topical 0.5% ivermectin is effective in eliminating head-louse infestations.[28] For the treatment of rosacea, in an investigator-blinded, randomized trial, once-daily ivermectin 1% cream displayed superior efficacy to twice-daily metronidazole 0.75% cream in the treatment of inflammatory lesions in patients with moderate to severe papulopustular rosacea.[29]

MALATHION

Malathion is an organophosphate insecticide that acts by irreversibly binding to acetylcholinesterase. It is approved in the United States as a 0.5% lotion for the treatment of head and body lice and is an alternative agent for the treatment of scabies. The lotion, containing 78% isopropyl alcohol, is flammable. Safety for children younger than 6 years of age has not been established, and it is a pregnancy category B drug.

PERMETHRIN

Permethrin is a synthetic pyrethroid modeled after the natural insecticide found in the pyrethrum flower, *Chrysanthemum cinerariifolium*. It acts by disabling sodium transport channels on parasitic nerve cell membranes, causing paralysis and death. It is available as a nonprescription 1% cream rinse, which is left on dry hair for 10 minutes. There is a lack of safety data for its use in children younger than 2 months of age, and in pregnant and breastfeeding women. Prescription-strength permethrin 5% cream is also effective against pediculosis capitis resistant to the 1% cream, pediculosis pubis, and scabies. The 5% cream is applied to dry skin from the neck down with a repeat application 1 week later. Application of 5% permethrin cream twice (1 week apart) was found to be superior to a single dose of oral ivermectin in scabies patients. In addition, permethrin-treated patients recovered earlier.[30] Permethrin is a pregnancy category B drug.

PYRETHRINS

Pyrethrins are the naturally occurring esters of chrysanthemumic acid. In combination with piperonyl butoxide, it is available as a liquid, gel, oil, aerosol spray, foam, and shampoo, and is used in the treatment of lice. Pyrethrins are neurotoxins, and piperonyl butoxide inhibits pyrethrin metabolism, potentiating the effects of pyrethrins. It is also effective against fleas, mosquitoes, and houseflies. As it is derived from the extract of chrysanthemums, individuals who are sensitive to chrysanthemum or ragweed should avoid this medication. The aerosol spray should never be prescribed to patients with a history of asthma.

SPINOSAD

Spinosad is a fermentation product of the soil bacterium *Saccharopolyspora spinosa* that causes widespread excitation of the insect CNS and leads to paralysis. In particular, spinosad disrupts acetylcholine transmission and acts as a γ-aminobutyric acid agonist. Spinosad 0.9% cream was found to be superior to 1% permethrin cream in the treatment of head lice and is both pediculicidal and ovicidal with a 10-minute application.[31]

ANTIPERSPIRANTS

ALUMINUM COMPOUNDS

Aluminum chloride solutions are typically used as a first-line therapy for hyperhidrosis in 15% to 20% solutions in the axilla and up to 30% on the palms and soles. Aluminum chloride is thought to work though obstructing the distal portion of eccrine sweat gland ducts. The solution is applied topically for 1 week at night, when eccrine glands are less active, and if tolerated up to twice daily. After control is achieved, it can be applied every 1 to 3 weeks as maintenance therapy. Skin irritation is a common adverse effect with aluminum chloride that may limit its use. Application to dry skin may reduce local irritation from aluminum chloride.

GLYCOPYRROLATE

Glycopyrrolate is an anticholinergic agent that blocks muscarinic receptors and inhibits cholinergic transmission. It is often used as a systemic therapy for hyperhidrosis. Topical glycopyrrolate is increasingly being used as a therapy, particularly for facial and axillary hyperhidrosis. A 2% glycopyrrolate spray applied twice daily to the axillae was found to have similar efficacy as a single session of botulinum toxin type-A injection when the two treatments were evaluated at 6 weeks.[32] In addition, 2% topical glycopyrrolate impregnated in cotton pads significantly reduced sweat production on the forehead as compared to placebo in a split-face, randomized, double-blinded study.[33]

IONTOPHORESIS

Iontophoresis is a procedure in which electric current is used to transport ions through the skin. The mechanism by which iontophoresis acts to decrease sweating is not fully understood, although there are several hypotheses. The hypotheses include a disruption of ion channels resulting in obstruction of the sweat gland, inhibition of sympathetic nerve transmission, and local alterations in pH that affect the sweat gland.[34] In an iontophoretic treatment, a hyperhidrotic area of skin to be treated is covered with lukewarm tap water. Electrodes are then inserted into the water and a direct current delivered, usually at 8 to 20 amperes. The amperage is increased until a tingling sensation is experienced and then applied for 10 to 20 minutes 3 to 4 times weekly. The effect of iontophoresis can be enhanced with the addition of glycopyrrolate to the trays before initiation of iontophoresis. Iontophoresis works best on palmar and plantar surfaces. Adverse effects may include irritation, hyperesthesia, and blisters.

ANTIPRURITIC AGENTS

Table 196-3 outlines the topical antipruritics discussed in this section.

DOXEPIN

Doxepin is a tricyclic antidepressant that is a potent antagonist of histamine H_1 and histamine H_2 receptors. Doxepin's antipruritic effects also may be secondary to modulation of adrenergic, muscarinic, and serotonergic receptors. In its topical form, 5% doxepin cream may be effective in treating neuropathic itch, lichen simplex chronicus, and nummular eczema. Exposure to topical doxepin cream has been reported to result in systemic contact dermatitis upon exposure to oral doxepin.[35]

MENTHOL

Menthol is a highly lipid-soluble cyclic terpene alcohol that is often used with camphor. It is derived from

TABLE 196-3
Topical Antipruritics

DRUG	GROUP	MECHANISM	PRECAUTIONS	U.S. FOOD AND DRUG ADMINISTRATION PREGNANCY CATEGORY
Diphenhydramine	Antihistamine	Local anesthesia; histamine antagonism	Significant percutaneous absorption; potential sensitization with cross-sensitization to oral diphenhydramine and related compounds	B
Doxepin	Tricyclic antidepressant	Histamine antagonism, interference with neuronal synaptic communication; decreased awareness through production of drowsiness	Potential contact sensitization; significant systemic absorption resulting in drowsiness and drug interactions; contraindicated in patients taking monoamine oxidase inhibitors	B
Menthol	Cyclic terpene alcohol	Counter irritant. Cooling sensation in the skin via transient receptor potential melastatin 8 (TRPM8) receptors in the skin	—	C when combined with camphor (ie, Sarna)
Phenol	—	Local anesthesia	Avoid in pregnant women and infants; irritant in diaper area and skin folds	Should be avoided
Pramoxine hydrochloride	Surface anesthetic	Local anesthesia	—	C

naturally occurring plant oils or prepared synthetically. Menthol is a counterirritant that, by induction of a cool sensation via transient receptor potential melastatin 8 (TRPM8) receptors in the skin, overwhelms the sensation of itch.

PHENOL

Phenol in low concentrations (0.5% to 2%) acts as an antipruritic agent through its anesthetic effect. It is percutaneously absorbed and should be avoided in pregnant women and infants. In higher concentrations, it is caustic and is used for deep chemical peels.

PRAMOXINE HYDROCHLORIDE

Pramoxine hydrochloride is effective in cases of mild to moderate pruritus. As with other local anesthetics, it inhibits conduction of nerve impulses by altering the cell membrane permeability to ions. The onset of action of pramoxine products is 2 to 5 minutes. A double-bind, randomized-controlled trial showed that pramoxine 1% lotion significantly decreased itch as compared to a control lotion in patients with uremic pruritus and hemodialysis-dependent end-stage renal disease.[36]

ASTRINGENTS

In medical practice, astringents are agents that cause contraction or shrinking of the tissues, arrest of secretion, or control of bleeding.

ALUMINUM SALTS

Aluminum acetate tablets diluted 1:10 to 1:40 (Burow solution) are an effective astringent and germicidal agent. Nonprescription aluminum sulfate and calcium acetate (Domeboro) are available and, when dissolved in water, a chemical reaction occurs forming aluminum acetate and a precipitate of calcium sulfate (modified Burow solution). These solutions may be used as wet dressings, compresses, or soaks, and can be used in a variety of skin conditions, such as insect bites and poison ivy, oak, sumac, and allergic contact dermatitis.

POTASSIUM PERMANGANATE

Potassium permanganate is an oxidizing agent, astringent, antiseptic, and antifungal that may be used to clean or deodorize wounds. Solutions of 1:4000 to 1:16,000 may be used as wet compresses to reduce weeping, or at 1:25,000 as a medicated bath. This agent may cause permanent staining of clothing and ceramics and temporary brown or bright purple staining of the skin, which may be removed with a weak solution of oxalic acid or sodium thiosulfate.

SILVER NITRATE

Silver nitrate in 0.5% aqueous solution is an astringent and antimicrobial that is applied as a wet dressing in the treatment of infected eczema, gravitational ulcers, and other weeping and/or infected skin lesions caused by Gram-positive or Gram-negative bacteria. It is also available in a solid form that may be used as a hemostat. At low concentration (0.5% formulation, used clinically), it is bacteriostatic, while bactericidal at higher concentrations (10%). As methemoglobinemia has been noted secondary to topical treatment, methemoglobin levels should be followed with prolonged use.[37]

BLEACHING AGENTS

HYDROQUINONE

Usually used in concentrations of 2% to 5%, hydroquinone decreases pigmentation by inhibiting tyrosinase, thereby blocking the conversion of dopa to melanin. It may also act by inhibiting DNA and RNA synthesis, degrading melanosomes, and destroying melanocytes.[38] Combination therapy consisting of hydroquinone, a retinoid, and a topical steroid has shown efficacy in the treatment of melasma. In particular, once-daily application of hydroquinone 4% in combination with tretinoin 0.05% and fluocinolone acetonide 0.01% showed superior efficacy as compared to twice-daily application of hydroquinone 4% cream in the treatment of moderate to severe facial melasma.[39] Side effects include irritant dermatitis, contact dermatitis, postinflammatory pigmentation, and cutaneous ochronosis.

TRETINOIN (RETINOIC ACID)

Tretinoin's mechanism of action involves inhibition of transcription of tyrosinase, stimulation of keratinocyte turnover, and decreased melanosome transfer,[38] leading to decreased pigmentation.[40] It is typically used in concentrations of 0.05% to 0.1% to treat melasma. Local adverse effects include erythema and desquamation; postinflammatory hyperpigmentation has been reported. Adapalene may be used as an alternative, milder retinoid for patients who do not tolerate tretinoin.[38]

AZELAIC ACID

Azelaic acid is a dicarboxylic acid derived from *Pityrosporum ovale*. It is a weak, competitive, reversible inhibitor of tyrosinase.[41] Treatment of melasma is typically with concentrations of 15% to 20%. Side effects include burning, itching, and erythema.

MONOBENZYL ETHER OF HYDROQUINONE

Occasionally used to depigment skin in individuals with widespread vitiligo, monobenzyl ether of hydroquinone typically causes irreversible depigmentation by causing melanocyte necrosis.[42]

KERATOLYTIC AGENTS

Table 196-4 outlines the topical keratolytic agents discussed in this section.

Keratolytics are agents that cause keratolysis, or peeling, of the epidermis. At low concentrations, most keratolytics act as humectants, or moisturizing agents, and can be used to soften keratin.

α-HYDROXY ACIDS

Chapter 213 discusses chemical peels and dermabrasion in greater detail.

α-Hydroxy acids (lactic acid, glycolic acid, citric acid, glucuronic acid, and pyruvic acid) reduce the thickness of the hyperkeratotic stratum corneum by an incompletely understood mechanism wherein the acids may directly solubilize the protein components of desmosomes or activate endogenous hydrolytic enzymes by changing the pH of the stratum corneum, resulting in keratolysis. Also, by diffusing into the stratum corneum and binding water, the acids act as humectants increasing the water content of the stratum corneum. This decreases the formation of dry scales on the skin surface and allows gentle rubbing of the skin during bathing to mechanically remove cornified tissue. The concentration of α-hydroxy acid, pH of the preparation, and composition of the base in which it is compounded are important in determining their efficacy. In general, more anhydrous preparations are less irritating, allowing higher concentrations of acid to be tolerated.

PROPYLENE GLYCOL

Propylene glycol is a humectant, occlusive, and keratolytic agent. It is often combined with other medications to enhance their penetration. A combination of 20% propylene glycol with 5% lactic acid in a semiocclusive cream base is used as a highly effective and

TABLE 196-4
Topical Keratolytic Agents

AGENT	DOSAGE	INDICATIONS (SELECTED)	SIDE EFFECTS/ COMMENTS	U.S. FOOD AND DRUG ADMINISTRATION PREGNANCY CATEGORY
α-Hydroxy acids	2% to 20% as nonpeeling agent, >20% as peeling agent	Photoaging, scaling, hyperkeratosis, acne, hyperpigmentation	Increased photosensitivity	Not contraindicated in pregnancy
Propylene glycol	40% to 60% under occlusion at bedtime; may be combined with salicylic acid (Keralyt gel) or lactic acid (Epilyt); 2% vehicle in many preparations	Ichthyosis, hyperkeratosis, psoriasis	Enhances absorption of other topical agents; possible CNS effects	—
Salicylic acid	Scaly dermatoses: FDA-approved twice daily to 4 times daily at 1.8% to 3%; calluses, corns, and warts: FDA-approved at 12% to 40% for plaster vehicles, 12% to 17.6% in collodion-like vehicles	Hyperkeratosis, scaling	Salicylism (headache, drowsiness, and tinnitus); maximum topical dose of 2 g/24 hours in adults	C
Urea	Twice daily to 4 times daily in 10% to 40% creams and lotions	Xerosis, pruritus, hyperkeratosis, eczema, ichthyosis, psoriasis, nail avulsion	Some patients experience burning; enhances absorption of other topical agents	C
Lactic acid (an α-hydroxy acid)	Twice daily to 4 times daily in 5% to 12% preparations	Ichthyosis, xerosis, eczema, photoaging	Hypothetical risk of metabolic acidosis	Not contraindicated in pregnancy

well-tolerated keratolytic in patients with lamellar ichthyosis and may be used in various other hyperkeratotic diseases.[43]

SALICYLIC ACID

Salicylic acid has been used in concentrations ranging from 0.5% to 60% in almost any base. In concentrations of 3% to 6%, it causes shedding of scales by softening the stratum corneum, dissolving the intracellular matrix, and loosening connections between corneocytes. In concentrations higher than 6%, salicylic acid is destructive to tissue. Salicylism has been reported with widespread and prolonged use, especially in children, who should apply no more than 2 g (33 mL of a 6% solution) to their skin in a 24-hour period. Sensitization is rare, and irritation can be minimized if introduced at lower concentrations. Salicylic acid is often used to treat warts, psoriasis, and acne.

UREA

Urea is a humectant that is proteolytic at high concentrations. Urea has been added to some topical glucocorticoid preparations to possibly increase their penetration. Urea preparations have been used to treat psoriasis, dry skin, onychomycosis, and eczema.

LACTIC ACID

Lactic acid is a humectant and keratolytic that is available at concentrations up to 12%. In addition to being a keratolytic, lactic acid increases ceramide production by keratinocytes, improving water barrier function.[44]

CALCIPOTRIENE

Calcipotriol is a vitamin D analog that inhibits epidermal proliferation, induces epidermal differentiation, and exerts antiinflammatory effects. Hypercalcemia may occur if more than 100 g is used per week. It is applied initially twice daily, and maximal improvement can be expected within 6 to 8 weeks. Cutaneous irritation may occur in up to 20% of patients, particularly when used on the face or in intertriginous areas. Of note, calcipotriene and betamethasone dipropionate are more effective when combined together than either is individually when treating scalp and body psoriasis.[40]

Please see Chap. 28 for additional information on calcipotriene.

WART THERAPIES

CANTHARIDIN

Cantharidin is a naturally occurring terpenoid that is secreted by blister beetles. Cantharidin application causes acantholysis and blistering of the skin. Cantharidin solutions are used to treat warts and molluscum contagiosum. Cantharidin is a pregnancy category C drug.

DIPHENYLCYCLOPROPENONE

Diphenylcyclopropenone (DPCP), also known as *diphencyprone*, is a potent contact allergen used in the treatment of viral warts and alopecia areata. Theories for its mechanism of action include alterations in cytokine levels, nonspecific inflammation causing wart regression, and binding of DPCP to wart protein inducing a specific immune response.[45] Many clinics recommend avoiding DPCP in children younger than 12 years of age, although children with alopecia areata who are younger than 12 years of age have been successfully treated with DPCP.[45]

SQUARIC ACID DIBUTYL ESTER

Squaric acid dibutyl ester is a potent topical sensitizer with a similar mechanism of action and use as DPCP. It has been used in the treatment of warts and alopecia areata and involves the production of an allergic dermatitis. As squaric acid functions through eliciting an inflammatory response, the most common side effects include eczematous reactions, blistering, and swelling of regional lymph nodes.[46]

DINITROCHLOROBENZENE

Dinitrochlorobenzene is a potent sensitizer with a similar mechanism of action and use as DPCP and squaric acid. Of note, dinitrochlorobenzene is not commonly used given the agent was found to be mutagenic by the Ames test and genotoxic through the exchange of sister chromatids in human fibroblasts.[47]

FORMALDEHYDE

Formaldehyde is a powerful disinfectant that causes anhidrosis, desiccation, and, sometimes, hypersensitivity when applied to skin. It can cause hardening and fissuring of the skin, so normal surrounding skin should be protected from it by petrolatum, zinc paste, or meticulous application. Individuals with eczema or allergies should avoid formaldehyde as sensitization is problematic given that it is a ubiquitous component of many personal products.

GLUTARALDEHYDE

Glutaraldehyde is viricidal. It also combines chemically with keratin-producing polymers that harden the wart surface thereby facilitating paring.

IMIQUIMOD

Imiquimod is a topically applied medication that stimulates the innate immune system through toll-like receptor 7. Imiquimod is used to treat genital warts, actinic keratoses, and superficial basal cell carcinoma. Side effects commonly include local skin irritation and systemic reactions are uncommon but can include symptoms such as fever and fatigue. Imiquimod is a pregnancy category C drug.

MONOCHLOROACETIC, DICHLOROACETIC, AND TRICHLOROACETIC ACIDS

Monochloroacetic acid, dichloroacetic acid, and trichloroacetic acid in concentrations of 50% to 90% are all effective in the management of warts. Trichloroacetic acid is also commonly used at lower concentrations (10% to 35%) for facial peels. Anal and vaginal lesions are occasionally treated with trichloroacetic acid, whereas monochloroacetic acid is most commonly used on plantar warts under salicylic acid plaster occlusion. The application needs to be repeated at 1- to 2-week intervals until complete resolution.

PODOFILOX

Podofilox is podophyllotoxin, the active ingredient of podophyllin, and is used to treat warts and molluscum contagiosum. It should not be used during pregnancy unless the potential benefit justifies the potential risk to the fetus.

SALICYLIC ACID

The effectiveness of salicylic acid in treating warts is thought to be related to keratolysis and local irritation of the skin in which the virus is present. Salicylic acid is the most established agent in terms of consistency of data regarding efficacy as well as safety in the treatment of viral warts.[48]

SINECATECHINS

Sinecatechins originate from green tea leaves of *Camellia sinensis*. A 15% sinecatechins ointment is available for the treatment of external genital warts and is applied 3 times daily until all warts are cleared, for up to a maximum of 16 weeks.[49] The mechanism of clearance may be related to the immunostimulatory, antiproliferative, antiangiogenic, and antitumor properties of catechins within the sinecatechins ointment. It appears to have a clinical efficacy comparable to other currently available topical therapies for external genital warts.[50]

COMPOUNDING MEDICATIONS

Compounding medications allows physicians to tailor a specific mixture of an active drug or drugs to an appropriate vehicle. While pharmaceutical companies decide how to compound standardized topical agents, there are instances where it may be appropriate to compound different formulations based on individual patient needs or if there is treatment failure to respond to commercially available products.

ACKNOWLEDGMENTS

The authors would like to acknowledge Drs. Craig Burkhart and Kenneth Katz for their contributions to a previous version of this chapter.

REFERENCES

1. Caterina MJ, Schumacher MA, Tominaga M, et al. The capsaicin receptor: a heat-activated ion channel in the pain pathway. *Nature.* 1997;389(6653):816-824.
2. Bode AM, Dong Z. The two faces of capsaicin. *Cancer Res.* 2011;71(8):2809-2814.
3. Yong YL, Tan LT, Ming LC, et al. The effectiveness and safety of topical capsaicin in postherpetic neuralgia: a systematic review and meta-analysis. *Front Pharmacol.* 2016;7:538.
4. Steinke S, Gutknecht M, Zeidler C, et al. Cost-effectiveness of an 8% capsaicin patch in the treatment of brachioradial pruritus and notalgia paraesthetica, two forms of neuropathic pruritus. *Acta Derm Venereol.* 2017;97(1):71-76.

5. Briggs M, Nelson EA, Martyn-St James M. Topical agents or dressings for pain in venous leg ulcers. *Cochrane Database Syst Rev.* 2012;11:Cd001177.
6. Kopecky EA, Jacobson S, Bch MB, et al. Safety and pharmacokinetics of EMLA in the treatment of postburn pruritus in pediatric patients: a pilot study. *J Burn Care Rehabil.* 2001;22(3):235-242.
7. Tran AN, Koo JY. Risk of systemic toxicity with topical lidocaine/prilocaine: a review. *J Drugs Dermatol.* 2014;13(9):1118-1122.
8. Guay J. Methemoglobinemia related to local anesthetics: a summary of 242 episodes. *Anesth Analg.* 2009;108(3):837-845.
9. de Leon-Casasola OA, Mayoral V. The topical 5% lidocaine medicated plaster in localized neuropathic pain: a reappraisal of the clinical evidence. *J Pain Res.* 2016;9:67-79.
10. Stoughton RB, DeQuoy P, Walter JF. Crude coal tar plus near ultraviolet light suppresses DNA synthesis in epidermis. *Arch Dermatol.* 1978;114(1):43-45.
11. van den Bogaard EH, Bergboer JG, Vonk-Bergers M, et al. Coal tar induces AHR-dependent skin barrier repair in atopic dermatitis. *J Clin Invest.* 2013;123(2):917-927.
12. Paghdal KV, Schwartz RA. Topical tar: back to the future. *J Am Acad Dermatol.* 2009;61(2):294-302.
13. Roelofzen JH, Aben KK, Oldenhof UT, et al. No increased risk of cancer after coal tar treatment in patients with psoriasis or eczema. *J Invest Dermatol.* 2010;130(4):953-961.
14. Rabe KF, Perkins RS, Dent G, et al. Inhibitory effects of sulfonated shale oil fractions on the oxidative burst and Ca++ mobilization in stimulated macrophages. *Arzneimittelforschung.* 1994;44(2):166-170.
15. Diezel W, Schewe T, Rohde E, et al. Ammonium bituminosulfonate (Ichthyol). Anti-inflammatory effect and inhibition of the 5-lipoxygenase enzyme [in German]. *Hautarzt.* 1992;43(12):772-774.
16. Korting HC, Schollmann C, Cholcha W, et al. Efficacy and tolerability of pale sulfonated shale oil cream 4% in the treatment of mild to moderate atopic eczema in children: a multicentre, randomized vehicle-controlled trial. *J Eur Acad Dermatol Venereol.* 2010;24(10):1176-1182.
17. Boyd AS. Ichthammol revisited. *Int J Dermatol.* 2010;49(7):757-760.
18. Paller AS, Tom WL, Lebwohl MG, et al. Efficacy and safety of crisaborole ointment, a novel, nonsteroidal phosphodiesterase 4 (PDE4) inhibitor for the topical treatment of atopic dermatitis (AD) in children and adults. *J Am Acad Dermatol.* 2016;75(3):494-503.e494.
19. Privitera GP, Costa AL, Brusaferro S, et al. Skin antisepsis with chlorhexidine versus iodine for the prevention of surgical site infection: a systematic review and meta-analysis. *Am J Infect Control.* 2017;45(2):180-189.
20. Balabanova M, Popova L, Tchipeva R. Dyes in dermatology. *Clin Dermatol.* 2003;21(1):2-6.
21. Tsubaki T, Honma Y, Hoshi M. Neurological syndrome associated with clioquinol. *Lancet.* 1971;1(7701):696-697.
22. Meade TW. Subacute myelo-optic neuropathy and clioquinol. An epidemiological case-history for diagnosis. *Br J Prev Soc Med.* 1975;29(3):157-169.
23. Walsh TR, Efthimiou J, Dreno B. Systematic review of antibiotic resistance in acne: an increasing topical and oral threat. *Lancet Infect Dis.* 2016;16(3):e23-e33.
24. Pourhasan A, Goldust M, Rezaee E. Treatment of scabies, permethrin 5% cream vs. crotamiton 10% cream. *Ann Parasitol.* 2013;59(3):143-147.
25. Goldust M, Rezaee E, Raghifar R. Topical ivermectin versus crotamiton cream 10% for the treatment of scabies. *Int J Dermatol.* 2014;53(7):904-908.
26. Koch E, Clark JM, Cohen B, et al. Management of head louse infestations in the United States—a literature review. *Pediatr Dermatol.* 2016;33(5):466-472.
27. Goldust M, Rezaee E, Raghifar R, et al. Treatment of scabies: the topical ivermectin vs. permethrin 2.5% cream. *Ann Parasitol.* 2013;59(2):79-84.
28. Pariser DM, Meinking TL, Bell M, et al. Topical 0.5% ivermectin lotion for treatment of head lice. *N Engl J Med.* 2012;367(18):1687-1693.
29. Taieb A, Ortonne JP, Ruzicka T, et al. Superiority of ivermectin 1% cream over metronidazole 0.75% cream in treating inflammatory lesions of rosacea: a randomized, investigator-blinded trial. *Br J Dermatol.* 2015;172(4):1103-1110.
30. Goldust M, Rezaee E, Hemayat S. Treatment of scabies: comparison of permethrin 5% versus ivermectin. *J Dermatol.* 2012;39(6):545-547.
31. Stough D, Shellabarger S, Quiring J, et al. Efficacy and safety of spinosad and permethrin creme rinses for pediculosis capitis (head lice). *Pediatrics.* 2009;124(3):e389-e395.
32. Baker DM. Topical glycopyrrolate reduces axillary hyperhidrosis. *J Eur Acad Dermatol Venereol.* 2016;30(12):2131-2136.
33. Hyun MY, Son IP, Lee Y, et al. Efficacy and safety of topical glycopyrrolate in patients with facial hyperhidrosis: a randomized, multicentre, double-blinded, placebo-controlled, split-face study. *J Eur Acad Dermatol Venereol.* 2015;29(2):278-282.
34. Grabell DA, Hebert AA. Current and emerging medical therapies for primary hyperhidrosis. *Dermatol Ther (Heidelb).* 2017;7(1):25-36.
35. Brancaccio RR, Weinstein S. Systemic contact dermatitis to doxepin. *J Drugs Dermatol.* 2003;2(4):409-410.
36. Young TA, Patel TS, Camacho F, et al. A pramoxine-based anti-itch lotion is more effective than a control lotion for the treatment of uremic pruritus in adult hemodialysis patients. *J Dermatolog Treat.* 2009;20(2):76-81.
37. Chou TD, Gibran NS, Urdahl K, et al. Methemoglobinemia secondary to topical silver nitrate therapy—a case report. *Burns.* 1999;25(6):549-552.
38. Sheth VM, Pandya AG. Melasma: a comprehensive update: part II. *J Am Acad Dermatol.* 2011;65(4):699-714; quiz 715.
39. Ferreira Cestari T, Hassun K, Sittart A, et al. A comparison of triple combination cream and hydroquinone 4% cream for the treatment of moderate to severe facial melasma. *J Cosmet Dermatol.* 2007;6(1):36-39.
40. Kin KC, Hill D, Feldman SR. Calcipotriene and betamethasone dipropionate for the topical treatment of plaque psoriasis. *Expert Rev Clin Pharmacol.* 2016;9(6):789-797.
41. Kim YJ, Uyama H. Tyrosinase inhibitors from natural and synthetic sources: structure, inhibition mechanism and perspective for the future. *Cell Mol Life Sci.* 2005;62(15):1707-1723.
42. Hariharan V, Klarquist J, Reust MJ, et al. Monobenzyl ether of hydroquinone and 4-tertiary butyl phenol activate markedly different physiological responses in melanocytes: relevance to skin depigmentation. *J Invest Dermatol.* 2010;130(1):211-220.
43. Ganemo A, Virtanen M, Vahlquist A. Improved topical treatment of lamellar ichthyosis: a double-blind study of four different cream formulations. *Br J Dermatol.* 1999;141(6):1027-1032.
44. Rawlings AV, Davies A, Carlomusto M, et al. Effect of

lactic acid isomers on keratinocyte ceramide synthesis, stratum corneum lipid levels and stratum corneum barrier function. *Arch Dermatol Res.* 1996;288(7):383-390.
45. Buckley DA, Du Vivier AW. The therapeutic use of topical contact sensitizers in benign dermatoses. *Br J Dermatol.* 2001;145(3):385-405.
46. Micali G, Cicero RL, Nasca MR, et al. Treatment of alopecia areata with squaric acid dibutylester. *Int J Dermatol.* 1996;35(1):52-56.
47. DeLeve LD. Dinitrochlorobenzene is genotoxic by sister chromatid exchange in human skin fibroblasts. *Mutat Res.* 1996;371(1-2):105-108.
48. Kwok CS, Gibbs S, Bennett C, et al. Topical treatments for cutaneous warts. *Cochrane Database Syst Rev.* 2012(9):Cd001781.
49. Tatti S, Swinehart JM, Thielert C, et al. Sinecatechins, a defined green tea extract, in the treatment of external anogenital warts: a randomized controlled trial. *Obstet Gynecol.* 2008;111(6):1371-1379.
50. De Clercq E, Li G. Approved antiviral drugs over the past 50 years. *Clin Microbiol Rev.* 2016;29(3):695-747.

Chapter 197 :: Photoprotection
Jin Ho Chung

第一百九十七章

光保护剂

中文导读

太阳辐射包括紫外线（UV）、可见光和红外线。UVB占到达地球表面的紫外线的5%~10%，能量很高，可引起红斑。UVA1是低能量的，在到达地球表面的紫外线中占95%，一般不引起红斑，但容易引起色素沉着，参与皮肤光老化。红外线也会通过升高皮肤温度来影响皮肤并引发皮肤老化。本章介绍了目前可用的常用的光防护措施以及越来越受到关注的口腔光防护措施、光敏性皮肤病的光防护护理。

〔粟　娟〕

AT-A-GLANCE

- Photoprotection measures include seeking shade during the peak ultraviolet (UV) B hours of 10:00 AM to 2:00 PM and the use of high sun protection factor (SPF) broad spectrum sunscreen, clothing, wide-brimmed hat, and sunglasses.
- UV induces skin aging and skin cancer, but using sunscreen may slow down skin aging and reduce the risk of developing skin cancer.
- Photoprotection in children is essential and its importance should be taught from childhood.
- Although oral photoprotection cannot substitute for topical sunscreen, it may serve as a secondary measure to prevent skin damage from solar radiation.
- UV protection factor is a UV protection rating for fabrics. Several chemical treatments can increase a fabric's natural UV protection factor.
- Many types of glass have very good UVA2 and UVA1 protection (up to 380 nm).
- Sunglass standards, mandatory in Australia and voluntary in the United States, specify a maximum percentage of light allowed to be transmitted and a minimum vertical dimension of sunglasses.

The earth is constantly exposed to radiation from the sun, which is indispensable for life. Radiation includes ultraviolet, visible, and infrared rays. Ultraviolet (UV) light B, which accounts for 5% to approximately 10% of the UV light that reaches the surface of the earth, is high in energy and induces erythema. UVA is composed of UVA2 (320 nm to approximately 340 nm) and UVA1 (340 nm to approximately 400 nm). UVA1 is low energy and accounts for 95% of the UV that reaches the surface of the earth because it can penetrate through clouds and glass windows, and is not obstructed by the ozone layer For this reason, UVA1 is present all the time, regardless of cloud cover or other obstruction. Although UVA1 may not cause erythema, it is more likely to cause pigmentation than any other wavelength. In addition, it induces reactive oxygen species (ROS), which cause damage to blood vessels, collagen fibers, and elastic fibers located deep under the skin, and are involved in skin aging. Infrared rays also affect skin and trigger skin aging by increasing skin temperature.[1]

With increased attention to physical fitness and outdoor recreational activities, daily exposure to sunlight is common. In addition, longer life expectancy has increased the amount of lifetime exposure to sunlight. Although sun exposure may have beneficial effects, such as mood elevation and vitamin D_3 photosynthesis, unwanted effects are well known. Acute effects of sun exposure include sunburn and delayed tanning. Acute responses to sunlight result from the direct influence on biologic chromophores like DNA. These responses release proinflammatory cytokines, enzymes, and immunosuppressive factors. These effects are mediated by ROS, which are generated by UVB, UVA and visible light as well as and infrared rays. Chronic responses to sunlight are a result of accumulation of damage and decreased ability to repair. Chronic sun exposure is strongly associated with photoaging, actinic keratoses, and skin cancers. Complete avoidance of sun exposure is neither necessary, practical, nor would it be generally acceptable to the general public. As such, behavioral modifications such as seeking shade during peak UVB hours of 10:00 AM and 2:00 PM, the use of photoprotective measures, such as sunscreen, clothing, wide-brimmed hat, and sunglasses, and, when appropriate, intake of vitamin D supplements, have become the public health message to deliver. This chapter discusses the currently available (as of this writing), commonly used photoprotective measures, as well as oral photoprotection, which is gaining increasing attention.

AVOIDANCE OF SUN EXPOSURE

An ideal photoprotection method is to avoid sunlight. Therefore, it is recommended to stay indoors when the UV rays are strong. The amount of UV that reaches human skin is influenced by the changes in environment. Sunlight is absorbed when entering the atmosphere. The ozone (O_3) layer, the stratosphere layer at 10 to 50 km above the surface of the earth, absorbs all of the UVC, most of the UVB and barely any UVA. When the sun is at its highest above the horizon, the distance UV penetrates the atmosphere is relatively shorter, and thus less is absorbed in the atmosphere and more reaches the surface of the earth. Therefore, between 10:00 AM and 2:00 PM, when UV is strongest, the sun is best avoided. Also, UV decreases by 3% as the latitude increases by 1°. Because atmosphere becomes thinner as altitude increases, UV increases by 4% every 300 meters from the horizon. Snow, sand, and metal can reflect up to 90% of UV. UV is reduced by 50% to approximately 95% under the shade; hence, one should stay in the shade if possible.

SUNSCREEN

Sunscreen is used to prevent the detrimental effects of UV, and should not be used to prevent sunburn simply to stay longer outside under the sun. People generally apply sunscreen less than the recommended amount, and do not reapply it every 2 hours. Furthermore, the amount of UV required for DNA damage is far less than the amount of UV needed to induce erythema. Therefore, application of sunscreen does not preclude sun damage, and one should continuously take all measures to prevent UV irradiation.

HISTORY

The first UVB filter, PABA (*para*-aminobenzoic acid), was patented in 1943, and the first UVA filter, a benzophenone, was introduced in 1962. In 1972, the U.S. Food and Drug Administration (FDA) reclassified sunscreens from cosmetics to nonprescription drugs, resulting in more stringent regulation. In 1979, long UVA filters, dibenzoylmethane derivatives, became available. In the 1990s, the need for protection against UVA, as well as against UVB, was recognized, which led to further development of UVA filters. In 2001, the FDA defined 16 active sunscreen ingredients with maximum concentrations, and in 2011, established labeling and effectiveness testing for broad-spectrum protection and water resistance.[2]

SUN PROTECTION FACTOR

The sun protection factor (SPF) was first developed by an Austrian, Franz Greiter, in 1962, and was adopted by the FDA in 1978.[3] Current FDA guidelines specifically require that products be tested using a solar simulator with emission spectrum covering the wavelength range of 290 nm to 400 nm, and that the sunscreen product be applied at a concentration of 2 mg/cm^2.

By definition, SPF is the ratio of the minimal erythema dose (MED) of a subject's sunscreen-protected skin over the MED of the unprotected skin:

$$SPF = \frac{\text{MED of sunscreen-protected skin}}{\text{MED of unprotected skin}}$$

Because the end point is erythema, SPF is a reflection of sun protection against the biologic effect of UVB (290 nm to 320 nm), and, to a lesser extent, UVA2 (320 nm to 340 nm). In other words, SPF15 does not mean that the exposure time to solar radiation is extended by 15 times, but that the amount of radiation required to cause erythema is increased by 15 times after the use of sunscreen. Figure 197-1 shows the effect of sunscreens with different SPFs on the transmission of erythemogenic rays.[4] If an individual develops slight erythema after 10 minutes of sun exposure, 30 minutes of unprotected sun exposure will result in a 3 MED sunburn. In contrast, when wearing an SPF15 or SPF30 sunscreen, the same 30-minute exposure would result in only 20% or 10%, respectively, of an MED. With chronic exposure, the added protection from an SPF30 sunscreen halves the cumulative UV damage compared to the SPF15 sunscreen, even though both products prevent sunburn.

The concentration of sunscreen specified for SPF testing (2 mg/cm^2) is the equivalent of 1 oz (30 mL) of sunscreen to cover the entire body surface. Studies of the actual sunscreen usage by individuals have consistently demonstrated that the amount of sunscreen applied is closer to 0.5 to 0.8 mg/cm^2, so that the actual

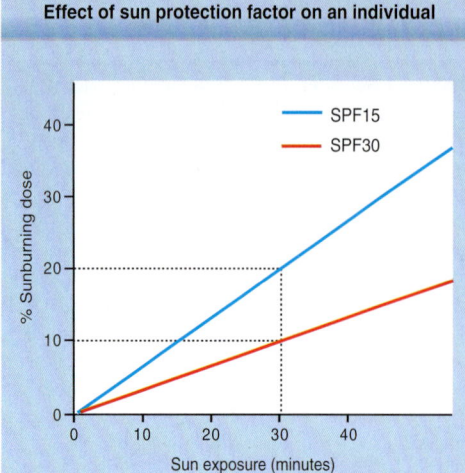
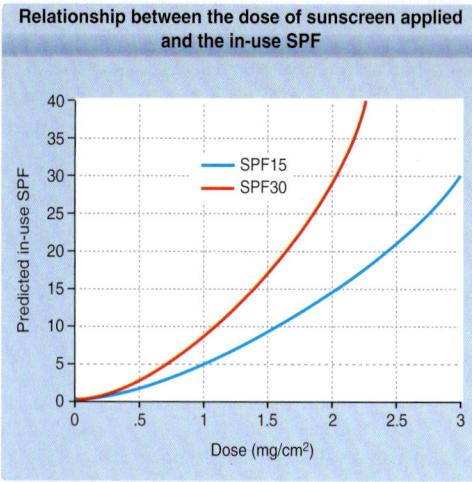

Figure 197-1 Effect of sun protection factor (SPF) 15 and SPF-30 sunscreens on an individual who would develop minimal erythema after 10 minutes of unprotected sun exposure. After a 30-minute sun exposure, 20% of a sunburning dose is achieved after the application of SPF15 sunscreen; after the application of SPF30 sunscreen, only 10% of a sunburning dose reaches the skin.

Figure 197-2 Relationship between the dose of sunscreen applied and the in-use sun protection factor (SPF). (Used with permission from JF Nash, Procter & Gamble, Cincinnati, OH.)

in-use SPF is significantly lower than the label SPF.[5] The relationship is not linear, and an SPF30 product (at 2 mg/cm^2) has an SPF of only 3 if applied at 0.5 mg/cm^2 (Fig. 197-2).[6]

SPF2 products absorb 50% of the UVB when applied at 2 mg/cm^2 and the other 50% is absorbed into skin. SPF15 blocks 93.3% of UVB and 6.7% is absorbed into skin. SPF30 blocks 96.7% of UVB and 3.3% is absorbed into skin. It may appear that this difference is not significant as SPF15 blocks 93.3% and SPF30 blocks 96.7% of UVB; however, this is not true. In fact, the important factor in photoprotection is not how much is blocked by sunscreen, but how much is prevented from being absorbed into skin. For SPF15, 6.7% is absorbed into skin, whereas for SPF30, 3.3% is absorbed, which is only half the amount. Also, the amount of UVB needed to cause DNA damage that results in skin cancer is less than the amount needed to cause erythema. Moreover, the amount of sunscreen people use is always less than 2 mg/cm^2. Therefore, it is more helpful to choose sunscreen with the highest SPF available.

ASSESSMENT OF ULTRAVIOLET A PROTECTION

SPF is accepted as the worldwide standard for the assessment of protection against the erythemogenic effects of UVB and UVA2. Among the several methods to evaluate protection against UVA, the persistent pigment darkening (PPD) method has become the most widely used in the past years.[6,7] In the PPD method, the dose of UVA required to induce PPD observed 2 to 24 hours after exposure of sunscreen-protected skin is compared to that of sunscreen-unprotected skin; the ratio is then expressed as the UVA protection factor. In many countries, including Japan and Korea, the UVA protection of sunscreen products is then classified as PA+, PA++, or PA+++ (where PA indicates protection for UVA). The European Union requires UVA protection factor to be at least one-third of the labeled SPF, with the PPD method as the assessment of the UVA protection. For example, a SPF30 sunscreen must have a UVA protection factor of at least 10.[8]

In June 2011, the FDA decided to use an in vitro critical wavelength test (broad-spectrum test) to assess UVA protection of sunscreens sold in the United States.[9] The broad-spectrum test measures a sunscreen product's absorbance of UV radiation across both the UVA and UVB regions of the spectrum. To label a sunscreen product as "broad spectrum," it should have a critical wavelength of at least 370 nm. The critical wavelength is the wavelength at which the area-under-the-absorbance-curve represents 90% of the total area-under-the-curve in the UV region. For SPF15 or higher sunscreen products that are broad spectrum, use of the following statement is optional: "if used as directed with other sun protection measures, decreases the risk of skin cancer and early skin aging caused by the sun." In addition, in vivo PPD testing is no longer required in the United States according to this rule.

IMMUNE PROTECTION FACTOR

SPF for a sunscreen product correlates poorly with its ability to protect against immunosuppression. This has resulted in the development of the concept of immune protection factor to quantify the ability of sunscreen products to prevent immunosuppression.[10] Several different methods have been used, including contact sensitization and intradermal injection, all of which are quite laborious and time consuming to perform. Until a simple and reliable method that can be easily performed in a large number of test persons is developed, it is unlikely that immune protection factor will be used to rate commercial products.

ULTRAVIOLET FILTERS

There are 3 different nomenclatures used by the sunscreen industry and regulatory agencies around the world: (a) International Nomenclature of Cosmetic Ingredients (INCI), (b) United States Adopted Name (USAN), and (c) trade name. USAN is the nomenclature used in the FDA Sunscreen Monograph. For example, for a widely used UVA1 filter, the INCI name is butyl methoxydibenzoylmethane, the USAN is avobenzone, and a trade name is Parsol 1789. In this chapter, when available, the USAN nomenclature is used.

The term *sunblock* is commonly used to refer to sunscreens and their active ingredients, but it is a misnomer, and the FDA Sunscreen Monograph does not sanction the term. All sunscreen active ingredients are filters that absorb part of the incident UV radiation, but a portion of the radiation is always transmitted. Microfine inorganic filters additionally reflect and scatter UV radiation.

In the United States, all active sunscreen ingredients are regulated by the FDA as nonprescription drugs.[9] Only UV filters listed in the Sunscreen Monograph issued by the FDA may be marketed in the United States (16 active ingredients; Table 197-1). In addition, filters approved by the FDA as active ingredients of final products through the New Drug Application (NDA) process also can be marketed in the United States, as was done for the latest UVA filter available in the U.S. market, ecamsule (Mexoryl SX). In 2002, the FDA instituted the Time and Extend Application process as an alternate to filing the NDA.[11] With the Time and Extend Application process, data generated outside the United States can, for the first time, be used for the application, provided that the sunscreen product has been marketed for nonprescription purchase for a minimum of 5 years in the country where testing was performed. In the European Union, South America, many Asian countries, and Africa, sunscreens are regulated as cosmetics, resulting in a simpler and more expeditious approval process compared to the United States, usually resulting in approval within 1 to 2 years of filing. Currently, there are at least 34 approved active ingredients in Australia and 26 in the European Union.

UV filters can be divided into 2 categories: *organic* and *inorganic*. These terms are recommended by the FDA to replace the terms *chemical* and *physical* filters, respectively. Organic filters can be subdivided further into UVB filters and UVA filters. The most widely used UVB filter worldwide is octinoxate (ethylhexyl methoxycinnamate), whereas the most widely used UVA filter is oxybenzone (benzophenone-3).

Titanium dioxide (TiO_2) and zinc oxide (ZnO) are inorganic filters that are snowy white in color and insoluble in water. They are photostable and do not react with organic filters. When their size is larger than 200 nm, inorganic filters can protect skin from all the wavelengths of UV. Also, visible rays and infrared rays may be reflected and scattered. Depending on the size, the properties of reflection or absorption change. Inorganic filters are not allergenic and do not react with skin, and are thus recommended for children and adults with allergies. However, inorganic filters are not preferred and are restricted in use because they leave a white coating behind. If applied too often, they may be comedogenic. On the other hand, micronized titanium dioxide is 10 nm to 100 nm in size. Because titanium dioxide scatters less visible light, it does not leave a white coating behind. However, its ability to block UV radiation decreases, leading to declined effect of photoprotection. Also, titanium dioxide may have negative effects on health if absorbed into skin. Therefore, more studies are required to elucidate whether inorganic filters actually penetrate into the skin, especially if they are used on inflamed skin or infants.

Sunscreen products combine ingredients in a variety of combinations to produce a product that confers stability and optimal UV protection. Currently, unless products are approved as new drugs through the NDA process, the FDA guidelines do not allow avobenzone to be combined with PABA, padimate O, or inorganic filters (titanium dioxide, zinc oxide).

ULTRAVIOLET FILTERS AND PHOTOSTABILITY

Avobenzone (butyl methoxydibenzoylmethane; Parsol 1789) is an excellent UVA1 filter but is photounstable and degrades during UV exposure. There are several other UV filters with this characteristic, including UVB filters padimate O (ethylhexyl dimethyl PABA) and octinoxate (ethylhexyl methoxycinnamate).[12] It is possible to incorporate other agents to increase the photostability of the final product (Fig. 197-3). Most of these agents are photostable UV filters (eg, octocrylene, salicylates, oxybenzone) that absorb photons to minimize the effect on the photounstable UV filter; they also serve as receptor molecules for energy transfer from excited state photounstable filter, hence minimizing the photodegradation of the latter (Fig. 197-3).[5,13]

In vitro, sunscreens containing photostabilized avobenzone have been shown to retain up to 90% of the active filter following 25 MED (50 J/cm^2) of solar-simulated radiation, the equivalent of approximately 5 hours of sun exposure.[13] Under ideal circumstance this would allow the user to apply sunscreen only once daily. However, it should be noted that sunscreens do

TABLE 197-1
Ultraviolet (UV) Filters Listed in the U.S. Food and Drug Administration Sunscreen Monograph

U.S. ADOPTED NAME[a]	INTERNATIONAL NOMENCLATURE OF COSMETIC INGREDIENTS	λ_{max} (nm); OR ABSORPTION RANGE	COMMENT
Organic Filters: UVB			
▪ PABA derivatives			
▪ PABA	PABA	283	Stains clothing; not widely used
▪ Padimate O	Ethylhexyl dimethyl PABA	311	Most commonly used PABA derivative; photounstable
▪ Cinnamates			
▪ Octinoxate	Ethylhexyl methoxycinnamate	311	Most widely used UVB filter; photounstable
▪ Cinoxate	Cinoxate	289	—
▪ Salicylates			
▪ Octisalate	Ethylhexyl salicylate	307	Weak UVB absorbers; improves photostability of other filters
▪ Homosalate	Homosalate	306	
▪ Trolamine salicylate	Triethanolamine salicylate	260 to 355	Weak UVB absorbers; good substantivity—used in water-resistant sunscreens and hair-care products
▪ Others			
▪ Octocrylene	Octocrylene	303	Photostable; improves photostability of photolabile filters
▪ Ensulizole	Phenylbenzimidazole sulfonic acid	310	Water soluble; enhances sun protection factor of the final product
Organic Filters: UVA			
▪ Benzophenones			
▪ Oxybenzone	Benzophenone-3	288, 325	Most commonly used UVA filter; most common cause of photoallergic contact dermatitis to UV filters
▪ Sulisobenzone	Benzophenone-4	366	—
▪ Dioxybenzone	Benzophenone-8	352	—
▪ Others			
▪ Avobenzone	Butyl methoxydibenzoylmethane	360	Photounstable; enhances the photodegradation of octinoxate
▪ Meradimate	Menthyl anthranilate	340	A weak UVA filter; no sensitization reaction reported
Inorganic Filters			
▪ Titanium dioxide	Titanium dioxide	See below[b]	No report of sensitization reaction; photostable; used to enhance photostability of the final product; micronized zinc oxide has better UVA1 protection compared to microfine titanium dioxide; micronized zinc oxide has lower refractive index compared to microfine titanium dioxide and thus appears less white; commonly coated with dimethicone or silica to maintain effectiveness as sunscreen
▪ Zinc oxide	Zinc oxide	See below[b]	

[a]This is the name used by the U.S. Food and Drug Administration in the listing.
[b]λ_{max} ranges from visible to UVA to UVB range, depending on the particle size. As titanium dioxide is micronized (10 nm to 50 nm in diameter), λ_{max} shifts toward UVB; microfine zinc oxide maintains a flat absorption profile spanning from UVB to UVA.
PABA, *para*-aminobenzoic acid.
Data from Kullavanijaya P, Lim HW. Photoprotection. *J Am Acad Dermatol.* 2005;52:937; and Department of Health and Human Services, Food and Drug Administration. Sunscreen drug products for nonprescription human use; final monograph. *Fed Regist.* 1999;64:27666.

migrate on the skin surface toward follicular orifices, resulting in an uneven distribution of UV filters; furthermore, sunscreens do get removed by rubbing and from water or sweat exposure. This is the reason that the FDA, in the final rule, advises that sunscreen should be reapplied every 2 hours.[9]

ULTRAVIOLET FILTERS AND PHOTOALLERGY

Octocrylene, oxybenzone (benzophenonone-3), and avobenzone (butyl methoxydibenzoylmethane) are the most common causes of UV filter photoallergy.[14] It

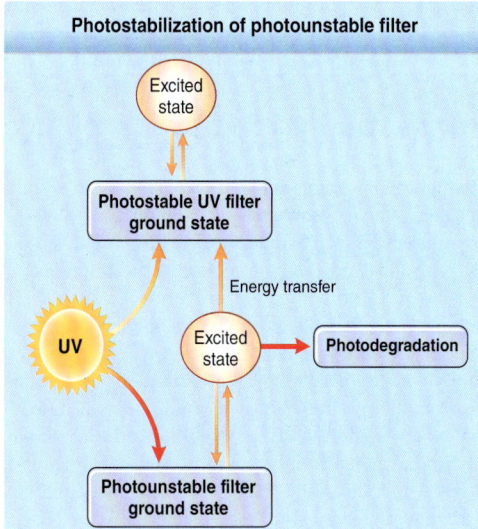

Figure 197-3 Photostabilization of photounstable filter. Photostable ultraviolet (UV) filter absorbs a portion of incident photons, hence decreasing the number of photons absorbed by the photounstable filter. Photostable UV filter also serves as a receptor for energy transfer from the excited-state photounstable filter, minimizing the photodegradation of the latter.

should be noted that although UV filters are the most common cause of photoallergy in many studies in the United States and the United Kingdom, considering the number of individuals using sunscreens, the prevalence of photoallergy to UV filters is very low (much less than 1%). No photoallergy has been reported with inorganic UV filters (titanium dioxide and zinc oxide).

SUNSCREEN USE IN CHILDREN

Because of the concern about percutaneous absorption of sunscreens, the 1999 FDA Sunscreen Monograph recommends that the physician should be consulted on the use of sunscreens in children younger than age 6 months.[9] For this group of patients, it is prudent to use other means of photoprotection, such as clothing.[15] Children younger than 2 years old should use inorganic sunscreen rather than organic sunscreen.

SUNSCREEN USE IN PREGNANCY

During pregnancy, sunscreen is also recommended to prevent skin damage from UV radiation, such as pigmentary disorders, especially melasma. Sunscreen has been proven safe by toxicology tests, including teratogenic tests; however, studies regarding safety of nanoparticulate inorganic ingredients during pregnancy are not available.[16]

CONTROVERSIES

POTENTIAL SYSTEMIC ABSORPTION

Organic Ultraviolet Filters: Systemic absorption of some organic UV filters following topical application to the skin has been reported.[17] In humans, up to 2% of an applied dose of benzophenone-3 and its metabolites were excreted in the urine following topical application of a commercially available product. The chemical characteristics of organic UV filters, such as molecular weight and solubility in fluids, as well as vehicle and viscosity of the sunscreen products, influence skin penetration.

Inorganic Nanoparticles: Metal oxide inorganic UV filters (titanium dioxide and zinc oxide) have been widely used in the form of nanoparticles. This is to minimize the reflection of visible light, thereby enhancing the aesthetic appearance of the final product. Nanoparticles are defined as particles less than 100 nm. In vitro, these particles can induce free radical formation in the presence of UV radiation, resulting in cell damage. Multiple studies have shown that neither nanostructured titanium dioxide nor zinc oxide penetrates beyond the stratum corneum of skin.[18] The risk for humans from using sunscreens that contain nanostructured titanium dioxide or zinc oxide is considered negligible.

NONMELANOMA SKIN CANCER AND MELANOMA

Although there have been questions in the past, the protective role of sunscreens in the prevention of skin cancer development has now been established. In a 4.5-year study with an 8-year followup of more than 1600 individuals in Australia, it was shown that the group that was assigned to use SPF16 broad-spectrum sunscreen had a decreased incidence of squamous cell carcinoma and basal cell carcinoma by 38% and 25%, respectively.[19] In a 10-year followup, 11 melanomas developed in the sunscreen group, compared to 22 in the control group.[20]

VITAMIN D

Another area of controversy is the concern that photoprotection may compromise health by decreasing a person's serum vitamin D level, specifically the level of the highly variable "storage form" (25-OH-vitamin D) that is the precursor to the tightly regulated active form [1,25-$(OH)_2$-vitamin D]. There are only 3 sources of vitamin D. Exposure to the UVB spectrum of sunlight converts 7-dehydrocholesterol in the skin to previtamin D by photoisomerization. Also, previtamin D converts to vitamin D by heat isomerization. Subsequently, vitamin D is hydroxylated in the liver and kidneys to its active form. The peak action spectrum for previtamin D synthesis is 300 ± 5 nm. However, previtamin D_3 and vitamin D_3 are sensitive to UV radiation. If they are constantly exposed to sunlight in the skin, they will be photodegraded and become inactive. Therefore, continuous exposure to sunlight does not produce vitamin D proportionally. It is the reason why vitamin D intoxication does not occur with excessive sun exposure. The amount of UVB required to produce daily needed vitamin D in humans is not so much; exposure of 0.33 or 0.5 MED 2 or 3 times a week to arms, hands, and face is sufficient. In other words, a person with skin type II who lives in Boston needs only 5 minutes at noon in July.[21] According to another study, arms and legs can create 3000 IU by being exposed to 0.5 MED of UVB. Therefore, light-skinned people can produce sufficient vitamin D by staying under midday sunlight for 5 to approximately 30 minutes, twice a week.[22]

Another source is dietary intake, although only a few naturally-occurring foods contain a significant amount of vitamin D (eg, oily salt water fish [herring, salmon, and sardines], cod liver oil, and egg yolk). In the United States, milk, orange juice, margarine, butter, cereals, and chocolate mixes are fortified with vitamin D. Lastly, vitamin D supplements are readily available as vitamin D_3 (cholecalciferol, the form produced in skin) or vitamin D_2 (ergocalciferol); as of this writing, vitamin D_3 is more commonly used than vitamin D_2 because vitamin D_3 is considered to be more stable.[22]

The effect of application of sunscreens on vitamin D levels has been evaluated. A relatively recent review of all the published evidence concluded that normal usage of sunscreens does not generally result in vitamin D insufficiency.[23] This is primarily a result of the inadequate application of sunscreens—applying an insufficient amount of sunscreen or not reapplying sunscreen every 2 hours—and sunscreen users may expose themselves to more sun than nonusers. Hence, in these cases, even when sunscreen is applied, daily required UVB for vitamin D production is achieved. However, among patients who practiced diligent photoprotection (eg, those with lupus erythematosus or erythropoietic protoporphyria), a large percentage were found to have inadequate serum vitamin D levels.[24,25] A comprehensive review by the U.S. Institute of Medicine, released in November 2010, concluded that the strongest evidence for the beneficial effect of vitamin D on health is for bone health; in contrast, for extraskeletal outcomes, the Institute of Medicine review indicated that the current evidence is inconsistent and inconclusive and as such is insufficient to make public health recommendation.[26] Because the action spectrum for cutaneous vitamin D synthesis (ie, UVB) is the same as for DNA damage and photocarcinogenesis, it is not advisable to use sun exposure as a means of obtaining vitamin D. For those individuals who are concerned or are at risk for vitamin D insufficiency, a balanced diet and a daily 600 IU vitamin D_3 supplement, along with 1 g of calcium, is recommended.[26] This recommendation applies especially to elderly individuals who are homebound dark-skinned individuals with modest sun exposure, and those who practice rigorous photoprotection.

ORAL PHOTOPROTECTION

Oral photoprotection refers to consumption of one or more active ingredients to minimize skin damage caused by solar radiation. However, by definition an oral substance cannot replace topical sunscreen, because consumption of the substance is incapable of physically blocking UVR penetration into skin. Instead, it can be used as a complement to prevent or reduce skin damage caused by solar radiation absorption. Oral photoprotection is convenient and useful, assuming that it is effective. It is not influenced by external environments, such as swimming and sweating, and it is not affected by the need to penetrate through the horny layer of skin. However, systemic adverse effects may be present. The action mechanisms by which active ingredients for oral photoprotection prevent skin damage from UV radiation are diverse. The substances react with various targets in UV-induced signaling pathways, exerting antioxidant, antiinflammatory, and immunomodulating actions. The most common substance used for oral photoprotection is an antioxidant, which should be stable and highly capable of eliminating ROS. Its end products after reaction as an antioxidant should not be converted into free radicals.

Oral photoprotection alone, without topical sunscreen, is insufficient to adequately protect skin from solar radiation. Nevertheless, its effectiveness is evident. Vitamins, such as vitamin C and vitamin E, as well as extracts or purified substances from certain plants (phytochemicals) can prevent skin damage from solar radiation. Hence, they may be used topically or as oral supplements to maintain healthy skin. Such active phytochemicals include polyphenols, which are either flavonoids or nonflavonoids, and nonpolyphenols, such as carotenoids and caffeine (Table 197-2).

VITAMINS

L-ASCORBIC ACID (VITAMIN C)

Because of its water soluble properties L-ascorbic acid is the most important antioxidant in the hydrophilic phase. As it is not naturally synthesized in humans, daily intake is best be achieved through food. Studies have not yet proven that oral supplementation of vitamin C alone can protect human skin from sunlight exposure. However, some studies have demonstrated that combined use of vitamin C and vitamin E has positive effects.[27]

TOCOPHEROL (VITAMIN E)

Along with vitamin C, tocopherol is a natural antioxidant, but is lipid soluble. Having affinity mainly with cell membrane lipids and intercellular cement lipids,

TABLE 197-2
Active Ingredients for Oral Photoprotection

Vitamins
- L-Ascorbic acid (vitamin C)
- Tocopherol (vitamin E)
- Nicotinamide

Polyphenol
- Flavonoids
  - Catechins
  - Isoflavones (genistein, silymarin)
  - Proanthocyanidins
- Nonflavonoids
  - Phenolic acid (benzoic, gallic, and cinnamic [caffeic, ferulic, and p-coumaric] acids)
  - Resveratrol

Nonpolyphenols
- Carotenoids
  - Beta-carotene
  - Lycopene
  - Astaxanthin
- Caffeine

tocopherol plays an important role in protection from oxidative damage by eliminating ROS. α-Tocopherol is oxidized to tocoferoxyl radical by ROS and, in turn, regenerated by vitamin C. Along with vitamin C, glutathione and coenzyme Q10 can recycle tocopherol. Although controversial, high dose oral vitamin E appears effective at reducing UVB-induced damage in human skin.[28]

NICOTINAMIDE

Nicotinamide (or niacinamide) is an amide form of vitamin B_3, which is an essential water-soluble vitamin. Oral nicotinamide is photoprotective. Nicotinamide prevents adenosine triphosphate depletion induced by UV radiation, thereby boosting cellular energy and enhancing DNA repair. Oral nicotinamide is safe and effective in reducing the rates of new nonmelanoma skin cancers and actinic keratoses in high-risk patients.[29]

POLYPHENOL

Polyphenols are mainly found in fruits, vegetables, coffee, tea, red wine, nuts, cereal, and chocolate. Polyphenols are chemicals that have more than one phenolic ring per molecule. A phenolic ring has a hydroxyl group bound to an aromatic ring. The intrinsic antioxidant activity of polyphenols resides in this hydroxyl (–OH) group that acts as a hydrogen or electron donor to a free radical or other reactive species. The typical classification of these molecules depends on the number and type of phenolic rings, which determine their biologic properties. Polyphenols are classified as flavonoids or nonflavonoids and are being proven effective for cutaneous inflammation, oxidative stress, UV-induced DNA damage, and carcinogenesis in vivo.[30]

FLAVONOIDS

The flavonoids include catechins, isoflavones, and proanthocyanidins.

Catechins: The catechins are mainly present in tea leaves and are made up of catechin, epicatechin, galactocatechin, epicatechingallate, and epigallocatechin-3-gallate. A double-blind, placebo-controlled study revealed that consuming green tea polyphenols decreased UV-induced erythema in women.[31]

Isoflavones: The most well-known isoflavones are genistein, derived from soybean, and silymarin, derived from the milk thistle (*Silybum marianum*). Genistein exerts a photoprotective effect in animal models.[32] The major active component of silymarin is silibinin, which has been shown to protect against photocarcinogenesis in animals.[33]

Proanthocyanidins: The proanthocyanidins are also known as condensed tannins; this is a group of substances widely present in grape seeds. Oral administration of an extract of grape seeds is effective in preventing the UV-induced pigmentation of guinea pig skin[34] and inhibiting tumor induction in response to UV radiation in mice.[35]

NONFLAVONOIDS

The nonflavonoids include the phenolic acids and resveratrol.

Phenoic Acid: The phenolic acids include benzoic, gallic, and cinnamic (caffeic, ferulic, and p-coumaric) acids. They appear mostly in red wine and tea. They exhibit antioxidant properties. Caffeic acid has been shown to protect against UVA-induced photodamage by ROS in mice.[36]

Resveratrol: Resveratrol, a stilbene found in grapes, red wine, and nuts, is also a potential polyphenolic antioxidant. Resveratrol suppresses UV-induced malignant tumor progression in mice.[37]

NONPOLYPHENOLS

The nonpolyphenolic phytochemicals include carotenoids and caffeine.

CAROTENOIDS

Carotenoids, which are vitamin A derivatives, include beta-carotene, lycopene, and astaxanthin. They are effective antioxidants for photoprotection. Lycopene and beta-carotene are relatively abundant in the human skin.[38]

Beta-Carotene: Fruits and vegetables (eg. carrot, pumpkin, sweet potato, mango) are rich in beta-carotene. As an endogenous photoprotector, it prevents erythema formation resulting from UV radiation.[39] The effect of photoprotection is dependent on treatment dosages and duration.

Lycopene: Lycopene, a bright red carotenoid pigment, exists in tomatoes and red vegetables or fruits, such as red carrots, watermelons, and papayas, and is a very efficient singlet oxygen quencher. Research has proven its effectiveness in reduction of erythema resulting from UV radiation.[40]

Astaxanthin: Microalgae, salmon, trout, shrimp, and crayfish contain astaxanthin. Astaxanthin has proven photoprotective activity against UVA.[41]

GARMENTS

CLOTHING AS A PHOTOPROTECTIVE MEASURE

Clothing, including hats, is an integral part of photoprotection. Compared to sunscreens, clothing is easy to put on, durable, and a social necessity. However, in most cultures, there are body sites that are infrequently covered by clothing, such as the face, the V area of the neck, and the dorsal hands. During hot (and sunny) weather, garments tend to cover even less skin.

When performing outdoor activities, it is crucial that one wear clothing that provides protection against the sun, especially children. Parents should educate their children about proper clothing before going outdoors. A wide-brimmed hat is highly recommended as it can protect wider areas, including the forehead, eyes, and nose.

ULTRAVIOLET PROTECTION FACTOR

UV protection factor (UPF) is the in-vitro measurement used in many countries, including the United States, Australia, and the European Union, to quantify the ability of fabrics to protect against UV. The amount to which 290 to 400-nm wavelengths penetrate through clothing is measured by spectrophotometric technique. The higher UPF, the less UV penetrates through fabrics. Because erythema is the factor considered, similar to the SPF, UPF is a better reflection of UVB than UVA protection.[42] In the United States, garments are classified as having good protection (UPF15 to UPF24), very good protection (UPF25 to UPF39), or excellent protection (UPF40 to UPF50+).

Several factors affect the UV protectiveness of garments.[5,42] Polyester fibers are the best UV absorber, whereas cotton and rayon are the poorest. Laundering garments made from cotton or rayon increases the UPF because of shrinkage, causing a decrease in the porosity of the fabrics. Wetness decreases the UV protection of a light-colored (especially white) garment. This is because the protective effect of white cotton fabric is mainly from light-scattering at the fiber–air interface: when wet, the fabric no longer scatters light and the garment becomes more transparent to both UV and visible light. In contrast, dark-colored garments absorb light and thus do not become see-through or provide less UV protection when wet. Chemical treatments include the incorporation of UV absorbers in fabrics during the manufacturing (mill finishing) process; the addition of UV absorber as laundry additives, and the addition of optical whitening agents, which are widely incorporated in many laundry detergents in the United States and Europe. These optical whitening agents absorb UV radiation at 360 nm and convert it to a visible light wavelength of 430 nm, thereby decreasing UV transmission through the fabric. The emission of visible light from the fabric makes the fabric look "brighter."

It is a common misperception that color of the fabric linearly correlates with the UPF. In experiments with cotton fabric with a UPF of 4.1, red fabric with the same dye concentration had UPF of 41, 31, and 20, depending on the type of red dye used. A yellow fabric had UPF of 25, whereas a violet one had UPF of 24.[42] This is because color is a reflection of the *visible light* that the eye would see and the brain would perceive; it does not necessarily correlate with the transmission of UV rays through the fabric.

GLASS

GLASS USED IN BUILDINGS AND CARS

Transmission of UV radiation through windows depends on glass type, thickness, and color. It is well known that UVB is effectively filtered by glass. Many types of glass now also have very good UVA2 and UVA1 protection (up to 380 nm). It should be noted that car windshields are made of laminated glass, which allows less than 1% of UV (300 nm to 380 nm) to pass through, whereas side and rear windows are usually made from nonlaminated glass that allows a higher level of UVA transmission. This explains why common sites of involvement for patients with a photodermatosis are the side of the face and forearm closest to the side window of the car.[43]

SUNGLASSES

Sunglasses protect eyes and skin near eyes from the sunlight, as UV radiation damages cornea, conjunctiva, lens, and retina. Acute UV damage includes photokeratitis, mainly caused by UVB, and solar retinitis, caused by visible light. Chronic damage include cataract, pterygium, and macular degeneration. Mainly UVB is absorbed by the cornea to damage it; in addition, UVA, the longer UV wavelengths, damages the lens and further provokes cataracts. Visible and infrared rays impair the retina. Consequently to protect the retina, yellow-colored or red-colored sunglasses, which can block blue or purple light, are preferred.[44] Sunglasses are especially important for children because their clear ocular lenses transmit more visible light when compared to adult lenses.[45] Lenses with darker colors may induce greater exposure to UV as a consequence of pupil dilation, unless the lenses offer good UV protection. Also, the shape of the lenses should such that they block light entering from the side. Sunglasses are also recommended during morning and afternoon hours when sunlight is parallel with eye levels. The time of maximum UV exposure to the eye is not from 10:00 AM to 2:00 PM as in the case of the skin, but is between 8:00 and 10:00 AM and 2:00 and 4:00 PM, when solar radiation is parallel to the eye.[46]

Australia has led the world in sunglass standards, developing the world's first national mandatory standard for sunglasses for general use in 1971; it was last revised in 2003 (AS/NZ 1067:2003). The amount of visible light transmitted through the lens is called *luminous transmittance*; a lens with 20% luminous transmittance would allow 20% of the visible light to pass through. Lenses are grouped into 5 categories (0 to 4), ranging from fashion sunglasses (lens category 0) to special-purpose sunglasses for very high sun-glare reduction (lens category 4); category 4 lenses are not to be worn during driving. Category 0 lenses are allowed to have luminous transmission of 80% to 100%, whereas category 4 transmission is limited to 3% to 8%. The standard requires that the UVB transmittance be 5% of the luminous transmittance. Specifically, if the luminous transmittance is 20%, then the allowed UVB transmittance is 5% of 20%, which is 1%. The UVA transmittance for lens categories 0 to 2 must be no more than the luminous transmittance, while for lens categories 3 and 4, it must be no more than 50% of the luminous transmittance. The standard also mandates that the minimum vertical diameter for adult sunglasses is 28 mm, and for children, 24 mm. The 2003 Australian Standard is similar to the European Standard EN 1836:2005. The 2 standards differ in the maximum amount of UVB transmission allowed and the definition of UVA.[47]

The U.S. sunglass standard was first published in 1972 by the American National Standards Institute (ANSI) and last revised in 2010 (ANSI Z80.3). However, unlike the Australian standard, compliance with the U.S. standard is voluntary and is not followed by all manufacturers. The U.S. standard classified sunglasses as *Normal Use* (eg, from home to the car to the office) or *High* or *Prolonged Exposure* (eg, at the beach, fishing, skiing). Lenses are classified by intended function as cosmetic purpose, general purpose, special purpose very dark, and special purpose strongly colored.[47] For example, for general purpose sunglasses, ANSI Z80.3 requires less than 1% of the wavelengths below 310 nm to be transmitted. No minimum vertical dimension of the sunglasses is stated in the U.S. standard.

PHOTOPROTECTIVE CARE FOR PHOTOSENSITIVE SKIN DISEASES

Photosensitivity is generally defined as an abnormal reaction of the skin to sunlight and other sources of UV light. In patients with photosensitive skin diseases, it is important to provide them with specific instructions and guidelines regarding how to incorporate photoprotection in daily life (Table 197-3). Individuals with limited sun exposure because of rigorous practice of photoprotection and patients with photosensitive skin diseases are known to be at risk for vitamin D insufficiency. In a newer study with cutaneous lupus erythematosus patients, 25-hydroxyvitamin D levels were found to be significantly lower among sun avoiders and daily sunscreen users than among individuals who did not avoid the sun.[24] Dietary supplementation with at least 400 IU/day of vitamin D_3 (cholecalciferol) is thus recommended for all patients with photosensitive disorders who avoid sun and use sunscreens. Vitamin D_3 (cholecalciferol, the natural form produced endogenously) is superior to vitamin D_2 (ergocalciferol).

LUPUS ERYTHEMATOSUS

As UV-induced skin lesions in patients with cutaneous lupus erythematosus could develop up to several weeks after UV exposure, a relationship between sun exposure and exacerbation of cutaneous lupus erythematosus does not seem obvious to the patient. Consequently, patients must be informed about the relationship of UV exposure to their disease. The use of a broad-spectrum sunscreen with high UVB and UVA protection factors prevents skin lesions in all patients with photosensitive cutaneous lupus erythematosus.[48]

TABLE 197-3
Ultraviolet Protection in Patients with Photosensitive Diseases

- Strict avoidance of sunlight exposure and other sources of ultraviolet
- Physical protection including clothing, hat, umbrella, and sunglasses
- Broad-spectrum sunscreens (sun protection factor ≥50)
- Oral antioxidants
- Removal of photosensitizing drugs
- Vitamin D supplementation

XERODERMA PIGMENTOSUM

Xeroderma pigmentosum is a rare autosomal recessive disease of DNA repair, characterized by severe UV sensitivity with greatly increased risk for skin cancer. The goal of UV protection is to significantly lessen the amount of UV radiation reaching the skin and eyes of xeroderma pigmentosum patients. Special UV-blocking clothing treated with UV absorbers and blockers is recommended. Xeroderma pigmentosum patients should wear large-brimmed sun hats (made with UV blocking material), and may use a UV-blocking plastic shield attached to the hat that covers the whole face. Xeroderma pigmentosum patients should wear UVA-blocking and UVB-blocking sunglasses that provide full eye coverage, as well as a highly effective sunscreen on a daily basis. During the day, sunscreen should be reapplied every 2 to 3 hours.

ERYTHROPOIETIC PROTOPORPHYRIA

Erythropoietic protoporphyria is a rare, autosomal recessive inborn error of metabolism that is associated with severe painful photosensitivity. When the skin is exposed to sunlight, the accumulated phototoxic protoporphyrin is activated by blue light, resulting in singlet oxygen free radical reactions that lead to severe neuropathic pain, often followed by swelling and redness. Although several treatments (including beta-carotene, N-acetyl-L-cysteine, and vitamin C) have been described in the literature, a systematic review of more than 20 studies showed little to no benefit.[49] Afamelanotide (analog of human α-melanocyte–stimulating hormone) provided safe and effective photoprotection through eumelanin synthesis in patients with erythropoietic protoporphyria.[50]

ACKNOWLEDGMENTS

This chapter has been revised from its previous version written by Dr. Henry W. Lim.

REFERENCES

1. Krutmann J, Morita A, Chung JH. Sun exposure: what molecular photodermatology tells us about its good and bad sides. *J Invest Dermatol*. 2012;132(3, pt 2):976-984.
2. Department of Health and Human Services, Food and Drug Administration. Labeling and effectiveness testing; sunscreen drug products for over-the-counter human use. Final rule. *Fed Regist*. 2011;76(117):35620-35665.
3. Department of Health, Education and Welfare, Food and Drug Administration. Sunscreen drug products for over-the-counter human use. *Fed Regist*. 1978;43:38206-38269.
4. Australian/New Zealand Standard. Sunscreen products—evaluation and classification. AS/NZS 2604; 1998.https://www.scribd.com/document/102213663/As-NZS-2604-1998-Sunscreen-Products-Evaluation-and-Classification.
5. Kullavanijaya P, Lim HW. Photoprotection. *J Am Acad Dermatol*. 2005;52(6):937-958.
6. Diffey BL, Ferguson J. Assessment of photoprotective properties of sunscreens. In: Lim HW, Draelos ZD, eds. *Clinical Guide to Sunscreens and Photoprotection*. New York, NY: Informa Healthcare; 2009:53-63.
7. Lim HW, Naylor M, Honigsmann H, et al. American Academy of Dermatology Consensus Conference on UVA protection of sunscreens: summary and recommendations. *J Am Acad Dermatol*. 2001;44(3):505-508.
8. Jansen R, Osterwalder U, Wang SQ, et al. Photoprotection: part II. Sunscreen: development, efficacy, and controversies. *J Am Acad Dermatol*. 2013;69(6):867.e1-e14; quiz 881-882.
9. Wang SQ, Lim HW. Current status of the sunscreen regulation in the United States: 2011 Food and Drug Administration's final rule on labeling and effectiveness testing. *J Am Acad Dermatol*. 2011;65(4):863-869.
10. Fourtanier A, Moyal D, Maccario J, et al. Measurement of sunscreen immune protection factors in humans: a consensus paper. *J Invest Dermatol*. 2005;125(3):403-409.
11. Department of Health and Human Services, Food and Drug Administration. Additional criteria and procedures for classifying over-the-counter drugs as generally recognized as safe and effective and not misbranded. *Fed Regist*. 2002;67(15):3060-3076.
12. Maier H, Schauberger G, Brunnhofer K, et al. Change of ultraviolet absorbance of sunscreens by exposure to solar-simulated radiation. *J Invest Dermatol*. 2001;117(2):256-262.
13. Cole CA, Vollhardt J, Mendrok C. Formulation and stability of sunscreen products. In: Lim HW, Draelos ZD, eds. *Clinical Guide to Sunscreens and Photoprotection*. New York, NY: Informa Healthcare; 2009:39-51.
14. European Multicentre Photopatch Test Study (EMCPPTS) Taskforce. A European multicentre photopatch test study. *Br J Dermatol*. 2012;166(5):1002-1009.
15. Quatrano NA, Dinulos JG. Current principles of sunscreen use in children. *Curr Opin Pediatr*. 2013;25(1):122-129.
16. Schalka S, Steiner D, Ravelli FN, et al. Brazilian consensus on photoprotection. *An Bras Dermatol*. 2014;89(6)(suppl 1):1-74.
17. Gonzalez H. Percutaneous absorption with emphasis on sunscreens. *Photochem Photobiol Sci*. 2010;9(4):482-488.
18. Burnett ME, Wang SQ. Current sunscreen controversies: a critical review. *Photodermatol Photoimmunol Photomed*. 2011;27(2):58-67.
19. van der Pols JC, Williams GM, Pandeya N, et al. Prolonged prevention of squamous cell carcinoma of the skin by regular sunscreen use. *Cancer Epidemiol Biomarkers Prev*. 2006;15(12):2546-2548.
20. Green AC, Williams GM, Logan V, et al. Reduced melanoma after regular sunscreen use: randomized trial follow-up. *J Clin Oncol*. 2011;29(3):257-263.

21. Holick MF. Sunlight "D"ilemma: risk of skin cancer or bone disease and muscle weakness. *Lancet*. 2001;357(9249):4-6.
22. Holick MF. Vitamin D deficiency. *N Engl J Med*. 2007;357(3):266-281.
23. Norval M, Wulf HC. Does chronic sunscreen use reduce vitamin D production to insufficient levels? *Br J Dermatol*. 2009;161(4):732-736.
24. Cusack C, Danby C, Fallon JC, et al. Photoprotective behaviour and sunscreen use: impact on vitamin D levels in cutaneous lupus erythematosus. *Photodermatol Photoimmunol Photomed*. 2008;24(5):260-267.
25. Holme SA, Anstey AV, Badminton MN, et al. Serum 25-hydroxyvitamin D in erythropoietic protoporphyria. *Br J Dermatol*. 2008;159(1):211-213.
26. Ross AC, Manson JE, Abrams SA, et al. The 2011 report on dietary reference intakes for calcium and vitamin D from the Institute of Medicine: what clinicians need to know. *J Clin Endocrinol Metab*. 2011;96(1):53-58.
27. Placzek M, Gaube S, Kerkmann U, et al. Ultraviolet B-induced DNA damage in human epidermis is modified by the antioxidants ascorbic acid and D-alpha-tocopherol. *J Invest Dermatol*. 2005;124(2):304-307.
28. Eberlein-Konig B, Ring J. Relevance of vitamins C and E in cutaneous photoprotection. *J Cosmet Dermatol*. 2005;4(1):4-9.
29. Chen AC, Martin AJ, Choy B, et al. A phase 3 randomized trial of nicotinamide for skin-cancer chemoprevention. *N Engl J Med*. 2015;373(17):1618-1626.
30. Nichols JA, Katiyar SK. Skin photoprotection by natural polyphenols: anti-inflammatory, antioxidant and DNA repair mechanisms. *Arch Dermatol Res*. 2010;302(2):71-83.
31. Heinrich U, Moore CE, De Spirt S, et al. Green tea polyphenols provide photoprotection, increase microcirculation, and modulate skin properties of women. *J Nutr*. 2011;141(6):1202-1208.
32. Terra VA, Souza-Neto FP, Frade MA, et al. Genistein prevents ultraviolet B radiation-induced nitrosative skin injury and promotes cell proliferation. *J Photochem Photobiol B*. 2015;144:20-27.
33. Mallikarjuna G, Dhanalakshmi S, Singh RP, et al. Silibinin protects against photocarcinogenesis via modulation of cell cycle regulators, mitogen-activated protein kinases, and Akt signaling. *Cancer Res*. 2004;64(17):6349-6356.
34. Yamakoshi J, Otsuka F, Sano A, et al. Lightening effect on ultraviolet-induced pigmentation of guinea pig skin by oral administration of a proanthocyanidin-rich extract from grape seeds. *Pigment Cell Res*. 2003;16(5):629-638.
35. Mittal A, Elmets CA, Katiyar SK. Dietary feeding of proanthocyanidins from grape seeds prevents photocarcinogenesis in SKH-1 hairless mice: relationship to decreased fat and lipid peroxidation. *Carcinogenesis*. 2003;24(8):1379-1388.
36. Yamada Y, Yasui H, Sakurai H. Suppressive effect of caffeic acid and its derivatives on the generation of UVA-induced reactive oxygen species in the skin of hairless mice and pharmacokinetic analysis on organ distribution of caffeic acid in ddY mice. *Photochem Photobiol*. 2006;82(6):1668-1676.
37. Kim KH, Back JH, Zhu Y, et al. Resveratrol targets transforming growth factor-beta2 signaling to block UV-induced tumor progression. *J Invest Dermatol*. 2011;131(1):195-202.
38. Scarmo S, Cartmel B, Lin H, et al. Significant correlations of dermal total carotenoids and dermal lycopene with their respective plasma levels in healthy adults. *Arch Biochem Biophys*. 2010;504(1):34-39.
39. Kopcke W, Krutmann J. Protection from sunburn with beta-carotene—a meta-analysis. *Photochem Photobiol*. 2008;84(2):284-288.
40. Stahl W, Heinrich U, Aust O, et al. Lycopene-rich products and dietary photoprotection. *Photochem Photobiol Sci*. 2006;5(2):238-242.
41. Yoshihisa Y, Rehman MU, Shimizu T. Astaxanthin, a xanthophyll carotenoid, inhibits ultraviolet-induced apoptosis in keratinocytes. *Exp Dermatol*. 2014;23(3):178-183.
42. Hatch KL, Block L, Gies P. Photoprotection by fabric. In: Lim HW, Draelos ZD, eds. *Clinical Guide to Sunscreens and Photoprotection*. New York NY: Informa Healthcare; 2009:223-241.
43. Hampton PJ, Farr PM, Diffey BL, et al. Implication for photosensitive patients of ultraviolet A exposure in vehicles. *Br J Dermatol*. 2004;151(4):873-876.
44. Wu J, Seregard S, Algvere PV. Photochemical damage of the retina. *Surv Ophthalmol*. 2006;51(5):461-481.
45. Roberts JE. Ultraviolet radiation as a risk factor for cataract and macular degeneration. *Eye Contact Lens*. 2011;37(4):246-249.
46. Sasaki H, Sakamoto Y, Schnider C, et al. UV-B exposure to the eye depending on solar altitude. *Eye Contact Lens*. 2011;37(4):191-195.
47. Almutawa F, Vandal R, Wang SQ, et al. Current status of photoprotection by window glass, automobile glass, window films, and sunglasses. *Photodermatol Photoimmunol Photomed*. 2013;29(2):65-72.
48. Kuhn A, Gensch K, Haust M, et al. Photoprotective effects of a broad-spectrum sunscreen in ultraviolet-induced cutaneous lupus erythematosus: a randomized, vehicle-controlled, double-blind study. *J Am Acad Dermatol*. 2011;64(1):37-48.
49. Minder EI, Schneider-Yin X, Steurer J, et al. A systematic review of treatment options for dermal photosensitivity in erythropoietic protoporphyria. *Cell Mol Biol (Noisy-le-grand)*. 2009;55(1):84-97.
50. Langendonk JG, Balwani M, Anderson KE, et al. Afamelanotide for erythropoietic protoporphyria. *N Engl J Med*. 2015;373(1):48-59.

# Physical Treatments PART 29

第二十九篇 物理治疗

Chapter 198 :: Phototherapy
:: Tarannum Jaleel, Brian P. Pollack, & Craig A. Elmets

第一百九十八章
光疗

中文导读

光疗是应用可见光或不可见光防治疾病的方法，是皮肤科常用的一种治疗方式，应用广泛。本章共分为4节：①光疗机制；②光疗设备；③光疗的安全性；④光疗的临床应用。全面介绍了光疗在皮肤科的应用以及治疗机制。

第一节介绍了光疗的治疗机制。用于光疗的不同波长的紫外线辐射具有不同的穿透深度，并可与特定范围的分子相互作用。故每种形式的光疗在功效、副作用和有效的疾病方面都具有独特的光化学和光生物学特性。该节分别介绍了光疗对免疫系统、肥大细胞、胶原蛋白、角质细胞以及黑素细胞的作用。

第二节介绍了光疗设备和光疗的具体治疗流程。光疗设备可通过将电能转换为电磁能来产生光，而不同波长和光剂量的光疗，作用机制和临床应用场景也不同。本节主要介绍了宽带紫外线B和窄带紫外线B、补骨脂素和紫外线A、靶向光疗等几种光疗方法。本节还讨论了规避和管理光毒性反应。

第三节介绍了光疗的安全性相关内容。光疗通常是比较安全可靠的，但仍存在一定的治疗风险。本节分别阐述了紫外线B、补骨脂素和紫外线A、紫外线的相关风险，并提出了针对艾滋病患者、儿童、孕妇、老年人的注意事项。

第四节介绍了光疗的临床应用。涉及的疾病包括银屑病、特应性皮炎、T淋巴细胞瘤、白癜风、硬化性皮肤病、瘙痒、慢性荨麻疹等，讨论了通过光疗治疗上述疾病的光源选择、具体治疗方案、联合用药、临床疗效等内容。

〔赵 爽〕

AT-A-GLANCE

The main wavelengths used for phototherapy include broadband ultraviolet B (BB-UVB), narrowband UVB (NB-UVB), ultraviolet A (UVA) 1, and UVA for psoralen photochemotherapy (PUVA); these have different depths of penetration and interact with a specific range of molecules rendering unique photobiologic properties with respect to potency, side effects, and diseases in which they are effective.

Targeted therapy devices can deliver distinct wavelengths of ultraviolet radiation to only lesional skin. Such devices that can deliver wavelengths of UVR at or close to those that are most effective at clearing localized atopic dermatitis, psoriasis, vitiligo, and cutaneous T-cell lymphoma have been evaluated, and are being used clinically.

Sunburn-like reactions are the most common short term adverse effect of phototherapy. UVB phototoxicity usually peaks at 12 to 24 hours and PUVA reaction manifests at 24 to 48 or even 72 hours. Importantly, except for PUVA therapy for which formal long term follow up studies established an increased risk of lentigines, squamous cell carcinoma, and possibly melanoma, other forms of phototherapy appear to be remarkably safe.

MECHANISMS OF PHOTOTHERAPY

Phototherapy is the use of ultraviolet radiation or visible light for therapeutic purposes. Its beneficial effects in vitiligo were first recognized thousands of years ago in India and Egypt and its activity is now well-established for a variety of other dermatologic conditions. The enduring appeal of phototherapy is based on its relative safety coupled with an ongoing interest in its molecular and biologic effects. The expanded use of phototherapy for dermatologic and nondermatologic conditions can be attributed to the following factors: identification of photosensitizers with unique photochemical properties; development of novel methods for the delivery of light to cutaneous and noncutaneous surfaces; and manufacture of light sources that emit selective wavelengths of radiant energy. The main phototherapeutic devices that are in use today (aside from lasers, high-output incoherent light sources, and visible light sources employed for photodynamic therapy) include broadband ultraviolet B (BB-UVB), narrowband UVB (NB-UVB), ultraviolet A (UVA) 1, and UVA for psoralen photochemotherapy (PUVA). Ideally, these devices used for therapeutic ultraviolet radiation (UVR) should be safe, efficient, and cost-effective. Therefore, understanding the basic principles of these devices is important for dermatologists and other providers using phototherapy for the management of dermatologic diseases.[1,2]

The distinct wavelengths of UVR used for phototherapy have different depths of penetration and interact with a specific range of molecules. As a consequence, each form of phototherapy has unique photochemical and photobiologic properties with respect to potency, side effects, and diseases in which they are effective (Fig. 198-1).

Most UVB radiation (290 to 320 nm) is absorbed superficially by the epidermis and superficial dermis (Fig. 198-2). In white skin, less than 10% of UVB radiation is transmitted beyond 14 microns.[3] This particular wavelength of radiant energy produces many different types of DNA damage, including pyrimidine dimers and 6,4-pyrimidine-pyrimidone photoproducts. These by-products are thought to be particularly important for both UVB's efficacy and toxicity.[4] UVB also causes photochemical changes in *trans*-urocanic acid, converting it into the *cis* form of the molecule. Urocanic acid is a breakdown product of histidine and is present in large amounts in the stratum corneum. Originally considered to be a natural photoprotectant, there is now substantial evidence that *cis*-urocanic acid is a mediator of UVB-induced immunosuppression.[5] In addition, urocanic acid levels can also affect vitamin D production. Specifically, upon NB-UVB exposure, there is an accompanied increase in hydroxyvitamin D synthesis that inversely correlates with the baseline levels of *trans*-urocanic acid.[6] A third direct target of UVB radiation is the amino acid tryptophan. UVB converts tryptophan into 6-formylindololo[3,2-b]carbazole, which binds to the intracellular aryl hydrocarbon hydroxylase receptor, initiating a series of events that culminates in activation of signal transduction pathways. One such pathway results in expression of cyclooxygenase-2, an enzyme required for synthesis of prostaglandin E_2.[7] Finally, there is evidence that UVB exposure leads to the generation of reactive oxygen intermediates, which has downstream effects such as DNA damage in the form of 8-oxo-deoxyguanosine, lipid peroxidation, activation of signal transduction pathways, and stimulation of cytokine production.[8]

In contrast to UVB radiation which has a relatively superficial depth of penetration, UVA radiation (320 to 400 nm) can reach the mid- or lower dermis to a depth of 140 microns (see Fig. 198-2).[3] It is therefore more effective than UVB for skin diseases in which the cutaneous pathology lies deeper than the superficial dermis. Like UVB, UVA radiation can produce pyrimidine dimers in DNA, but, on a per-photon basis, it is much less effective at doing so.[9] In most situations, the major biologic effects of UVA radiation are from the generation of reactive oxygen intermediates.[10] Following UVA exposure, reactive oxygen intermediates are formed in mitochondrial enzyme complexes during oxidative phosphorylation. Although the skin contains antioxidants, reactive oxygen intermediates formed during phototherapy exceed the amount that can be neutralized by endogenous photoprotective activities. UVA-induced oxidants are capable of harming DNA, lipids, structural and nonstructural proteins, and organelles such as mitochondria. The generation of oxidants following UV exposure also has been implicated in photoaging of the skin and skin cancer. Interestingly, animal studies show that exposure to UVA's longer

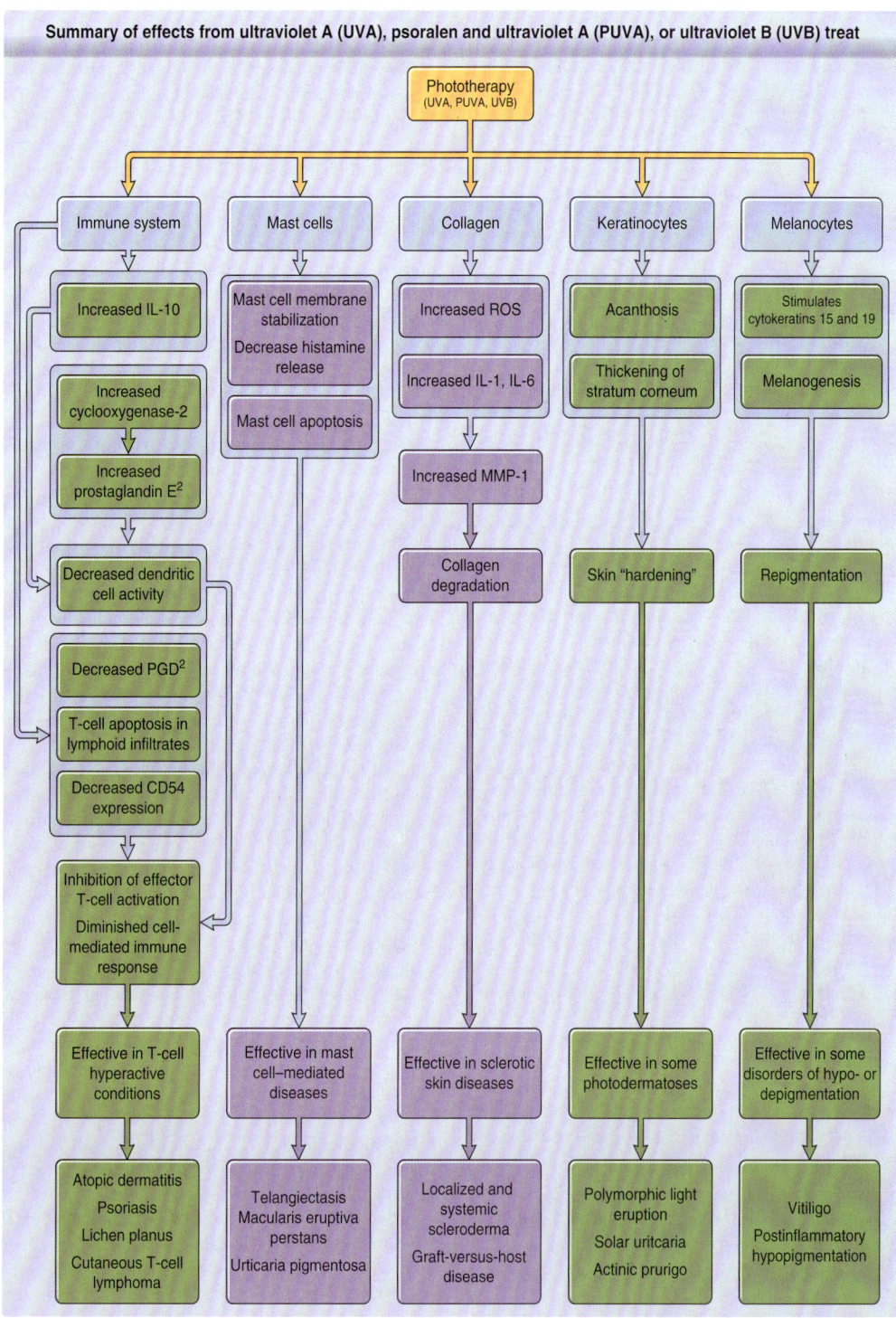

Figure 198-1 Summary of effects from ultraviolet A (UVA), psoralen and ultraviolet A (PUVA), or ultraviolet B (UVB) treatment. Detailed discussion in text. Boxes in *purple* indicate effects of either UVA and/or PUVA only, boxes in *green* indicate effects of both UVB and UVA and/or PUVA. The bottom two rows of boxes indicate clinical relevance of and application of skin changes induced by phototherapy. IL, interleukin; MMP, matrix metalloproteinase; PGD_2, prostaglandin D_2; ROS, reactive oxygen species.

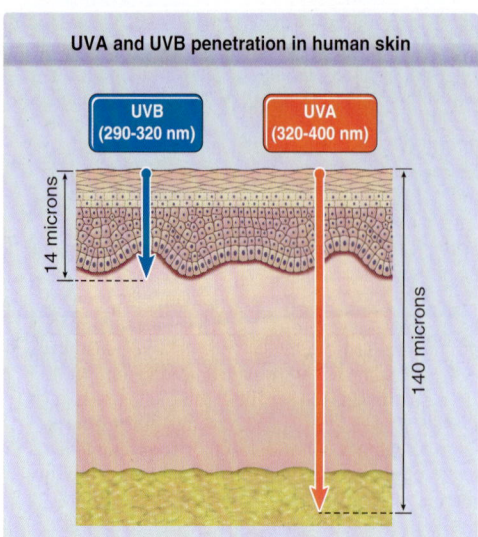

Figure 198-2 Depth of penetration in human skin for ultraviolet B (UVB) and ultraviolet A (UVA).

wavelength (UVA1, 340-400 nm) has immunoprotective properties via the generation of heme oxygenase-1, which exerts antioxidant and antiinflammatory effects while also decreasing UVB-induced damage.[11]

In psoralen photochemotherapy, psoralen photosensitizers are activated by UVA radiation, and the depth of penetration of PUVA is the mid-dermis. The major photochemical effect of psoralen photochemotherapy is damage to DNA. Psoralen photochemotherapy–induced changes in DNA differ from those of UVB and UVA without psoralens.[12] Psoralens used for photochemotherapy have 2 double bonds that can absorb UVA radiation. When administered to an individual, these compounds intercalate with DNA. Following UVA exposure, they form a single adduct with DNA and then become a bifunctional adduct, crosslinking the DNA strands in the double helix, when a second photon is absorbed. There is also some evidence that photochemotherapy augments the production of reactive oxygen intermediates such as singlet oxygen. This effect has been implicated in induction of the cyclooxygenase enzyme and activation of arachidonic acid pathways.[13]

EFFECTS ON THE IMMUNE SYSTEM

The photoimmunologic effects of phototherapy are thought to provide an explanation, at least in part, for phototherapy's efficacy in cutaneous diseases in which T-cell hyperactivity predominates (eg, psoriasis, atopic dermatitis, lichen planus). Under normal circumstances, both effector and regulatory T cells are generated, with the overall intensity of the immune response dependent on the relative proportion of effector and regulatory T-cell populations that are present. UVB exposure inhibits activation of effector T cells, whereas it leaves the development of regulatory T cells unaltered.[14] Consequently, the equilibrium of effector and regulatory T cells is biased toward a diminished cell-mediated immune response. This perturbation in the balance of effector and regulatory T cells reflects disruption of the activities of dendritic cells within the skin, the major function of which is to present antigen to T-lymphocytes. This is a result of the direct effects of UVB on dendritic cells and indirectly through the production of interleukin (IL)-10 and prostaglandin E_2, both of which diminish the capacity of dendritic cells to present antigen to effector T cells leading to suppressed T-cell responses.[15] Increased levels of IL-10 have been found after UVB, UVA1, and PUVA exposure. Prostaglandin E_2 production occurs through UVB effects on keratinocytes[16-18]; UVB is an inductive stimulus for cyclooxygenase-2, which is important for prostaglandin E_2 production. UV exposure also significantly lowers levels of immunomodulatory factors such as prostaglandin D_2, possibly reflecting a loss of Langerhans cells from the epidermis upon UV exposure.[19]

Other immunosuppressive soluble mediators that are reported to be increased following UVB exposure include agonists of the platelet activating factor receptor,[20] melanocyte-stimulating hormone, and calcitonin gene–related peptide.[21] In addition, in the setting of inflammation, FoxP3-positive regulatory T cells can convert into IL-17–producing cells and lose FoxP3. UVB radiation, however, increases FoxP3 expression by binding the transcription factor, p53, and stabilizing the FoxP3-positive regulatory T-cell population.[22,23] The epidermal growth factor–like growth factor amphiregulin influences the activity of regulatory T cells and basophil-derived amphiregulin is implicated in mediating UVB-induced immune suppression in murine models, which supports the notion that growth factors have immunomodulatory properties relevant to skin biology and disease.[24,25]

PUVA has effects that are similar to UVB with respect to antigen-presenting cells within the skin, the balance between effector and regulatory T cells, and the production of soluble immunosuppressive mediators.[14] However, there is limited information on the effect of UVA1 on antigen-presenting cells and on effector and regulatory T cells. In acute skin lesions of atopic dermatitis, UVA1 appears to increase IL-4 and thymus-regulated and activation-regulated chemokine messenger RNA expression, but has little effect on expression of human beta defensin-1, thymic stromal lymphopoietin, IL-5, IL-10, IL-13, or IL-31.[26,27]

In addition to its actions on cutaneous antigen-presenting cells, phototherapy causes cell death by apoptosis of T cells in cutaneous lymphoid infiltrates. This has been demonstrated for UVA1 phototherapy in the lymphocytic infiltrate in atopic dermatitis,[28] and for NB-UVB in psoriasis.[29] Another immunologic effect of phototherapy is on expression of CD54 (intercellular adhesion molecule-1) and other adhesion molecules. Intercellular adhesion molecule-1 is not normally present on epidermal keratinocytes, but can be induced in a variety of inflammatory skin conditions. It facilitates

T-cell binding to keratinocytes, through its interaction with lymphocyte function–associated antigen-1 that is present on T cells. Because UVB, UVA1, and PUVA all interfere with keratinocyte expression of CD54, this effect of phototherapy may contribute to phototherapy's efficacy in diseases that have increased keratinocyte CD54 expression.[14]

EFFECTS ON MAST CELLS

Both UVA1 and PUVA have deleterious effects on mast cells, although the mechanisms of action differ.[30,31] PUVA is not cytotoxic for mast cells, and because of this, there is little reduction in mast cell concentrations in the dermis. However, PUVA does stabilize mast cell membranes and, as a result, limits the release of histamine and other mediators when these cells are stimulated to degranulate.[31] In contrast, chronic therapy with UVA1 results in apoptosis of mast cells with a marked reduction in their concentrations that can last for several months.[30] Both PUVA and UVA1 have been employed to treat selective mast cell–mediated diseases.

EFFECTS ON COLLAGEN

One of the downstream effects of UVA-induced generation of reactive oxygen intermediates is activation of matrix metalloproteinase (MMP)-1,[32,33] the major biologic activity of which is degradation of collagen. UVA radiation increases the production of IL-1 and IL-6, which are stimuli for MMPs.[34] PUVA also increases MMPs.[35] These effects of UVA1 and PUVA on MMP-1 and collagen degradation provide the rationale for its use in sclerotic skin diseases.

EFFECTS ON KERATINOCYTES

UVB, PUVA, and UVA all cause acanthosis of the epidermis and thickening of the stratum corneum.[36] This effect accentuates light scattering and increases its absorption by the upper levels of the epidermis. Therefore, phototherapy treatment doses must be progressively increased so that an equivalent number of photons can reach the lower levels of the epidermis and dermis where therapeutic targets lie. Alternatively, this attribute of phototherapy has been exploited for the management of chronic photosensitivity disorders because this "hardens" the skin, permitting individuals afflicted with these disorders to tolerate greater amounts of sun exposure.

EFFECTS ON MELANOCYTES

Exposure to UVR is also known to stimulate melanogenesis,[37] which is, at least in part, a consequence of DNA damage and/or its repair.[38-41] Experimental studies have shown that treatment of melanocytes with DNA repair enzymes increases the melanin content of melanocytes,[42] and application of small fragments of thymidine dinucleotides to guinea pig skin produces a tanning response.[39-41] The stimulatory effects on melanogenesis decrease the efficacy of phototherapy unless the doses of UVR are gradually increased, but in patients with some photosensitivity disorders, this biologic effect can be exploited therapeutically, allowing them to tolerate greater amounts of ambient sun exposure.

Narrowband UVB and PUVA are also employed to repopulate vitiliginous skin with melanocytes. The mechanism by which phototherapy stimulates repigmentation of vitiliginous skin is incompletely understood, but may involve stimulation of hair follicle melanocyte proliferation and migration.[43] Cytokines and other inflammatory mediators released from other cells, such as keratinocytes, are thought to stimulate inactive melanocytes in the outer root sheath of hair follicles to proliferate, mature, and migrate to repopulate the interfollicular epidermis.[44] Increased expression of cytokeratins 15 and 19, markers for stem cell activation in the follicular and interfollicular epithelium, is also seen in response to phototherapy.[45]

PHOTOTHERAPY DEVICES

In an ideal situation, the wavelengths that are most effective for the treatment (ie, the action spectrum) for every dermatologic condition would be known and there would be a device capable of delivering those wavelengths specifically to lesional skin. For some skin diseases, such as psoriasis, great strides have been made toward this ideal; targeted therapy using devices that can deliver wavelengths of UVR at or close to those that are most effective at clearing psoriatic plaques have been evaluated and are being used clinically. Unfortunately, for most dermatologic conditions this information is still unknown. However, the increased availability of improved phototherapy devices and novel treatment approaches is providing new options for patients and clinicians. In addition, as studies are conducted that use phototherapy, there is a better understanding of how best to use these technologies. Many different types of phototherapy devices exist and more are currently under development. Phototherapy devices are varied and can be booth-like devices that patients enter to receive their treatment, smaller stationary devices that can deliver UVR to a specific anatomic region (such as the hands and/or feet) while sparing uninvolved areas, or handheld devices that can be maneuvered to deliver UVR to lesional skin. The type of device used needs to be individually tailored to a given patient. Some patients may have trouble standing for the required amount of time needed for therapy, whereas others may have difficulty maneuvering themselves. It is important to note that phototherapy can be delivered in the setting of a dermatology practice or in the home. Numerous changes are being made to phototherapy devices to make them safer and more convenient. For example, a "digital phototherapy device" has been developed that integrates a camera, computer hardware and software, a digital mirror device, and other components that only delivers UVR specifically to diseased skin while sparing surrounding normal skin.[46,47]

BASIC PRINCIPLES OF PHOTOTHERAPY DEVICES AND TYPES OF LAMPS

Phototherapy devices generate light by the conversion of electrical energy into electromagnetic energy. Filters and fluorophores are used to modify the output such that the desired wavelengths are emitted. There are several types of lamps (or bulbs) used to generate therapeutic UVR. These include incandescent lamps, arc lamps, and fluorescent lamps.

Incandescent lamps generate UVR by passing an electric current through a thin tungsten filament, which, in turn, generates heat and light. Because much of the electrical energy is converted to heat, these lamps are relatively inefficient light sources and have relatively short life spans. By sealing the tungsten filament in a quartz envelope that contains a halogen (bromine or iodine), the filament can be made to emit more energetic photons without reducing the longevity of the bulb. These lamps are called quartz halogen lamps and can emit wavelengths within the UV, visible, and infrared ranges. In clinical dermatology, these lamps are employed primarily in situations that require visible light such as phototesting and photodynamic therapy.

Arc or gas discharge lamps were the first effective artificial UVR sources used for phototherapy. Arc lamps take advantage of the fact that when a high voltage is passed across 2 electrodes in the presence of a gas, the electrons of the gas atoms become excited. The "arc" of an arc lamp refers to the electric arc generated when the gas is ionized (ionized gas is also known as plasma) by a high electric current. When the gas electrons return to their ground state, light is emitted. The type of gas incorporated into the lamp determines the wavelengths that are emitted (ie, spectral output). The output of arc lamps can be modulated by altering the gas pressure within the bulb such that at high pressures, the peak wavelength output broadens. High-pressure arc lamps typically contain mercury or xenon gas, whereas low-pressure arc lamps use fluorescent material. In addition to altering the gas pressure to modify the spectral output of arc discharge lamps,

the addition of metal halides broadens the output spectrum such that it becomes nearly continuous across the UV spectrum. For example, when mercury arc lamps are operated at high pressures, they have output emission peaks (so-called mercury lines) seen at 297, 302, 313, 334, and 365 nm. In contrast, if a metal halide is added to the mercury, the output between these peaks is increased and is thus more continuous. The use of optical filters can then further refine the output of these lamps such that only the desired wavelengths are emitted. The advantage of metal halide lamps is the high output that allows for shorter treatment times. However, they are costlier and more difficult to operate than fluorescent lamps. One example of a metal halide lamp currently in clinical use is the UVA1 light source.

Fluorescent lamps are the most commonly used sources of therapeutic UVR. These lamps take advantage of the fact that chemicals called phosphors (a specific type of chromophore also called a fluorophore) absorb and then reemit light. The light that is reemitted is of lower energy (and thus longer wavelength) than the inciting light. Using this principle, the ultraviolet C irradiation (which peaks at 254 nm) generated from a low-pressure mercury lamp can be converted to the longer UVB and UVA wavelengths of light that are desirable for phototherapy. The final output of a fluorescent lamp is dictated by the specific phosphor of the bulb. An important advance in photodermatology came with the development of a modified fluorescent lamp that emits largely at 311 nm.[48] Broadband UVB and UVA light sources used for PUVA are other examples of fluorescent lamps.

Because different forms of phototherapy are used to treat different diseases, it is important and practical to divide devices based upon wavelength. Devices that deliver BB-UVB, 311-nm NB-UVB, UVA (for use in psoralen photochemotherapy), and UVA1 (340 to 400 nm) are available in the United States and in most other countries. In addition to differing by spectral output, phototherapy devices range in the surface area that they are designed to treat (whole body, localized regions, or only lesional skin). Devices used for large body surface areas resemble booths, which patients enter for each treatment. These devices come in a variety of styles, from round cylinders to folding units that can be unfolded for treatments and then collapsed while not in use. Devices have been developed to treat more limited areas (such as the palms and soles) and are substantially smaller in size. Finally, targeted therapy uses devices that can deliver therapeutic UVR only to lesional skin range in size from small handheld units to larger devices with a handheld wand attached.

BROADBAND AND NARROWBAND ULTRAVIOLET B

Originally used for psoriasis therapy, artificial sources of BB-UVB have been used therapeutically since the early 20th century. In particular, UVB combined with the topical application of coal tar (as developed initially by William Goeckerman) had been a mainstay of psoriasis treatment for many decades.[49] With the development and availability of NB-UVB, some dermatologists have concluded that BB-UVB is obsolete.[50] However, BB-UVB is still widely used in the United States for a variety of conditions.

The most commonly employed devices that deliver BB-UVB use fluorescent lamps. These devices emit UVR over a broad spectral range. Approximately two-thirds of the output is in the UVB range and the rest is primarily in the UVA. Because wavelengths within the UVB spectrum have higher energy than those within the UVA, the UVA component generally contributes little to the therapeutic efficacy, assuming the patient is not taking a photosensitizing medication. BB-UVB and NB-UVB devices are specifically designed to limit output below 290 nm (ie, in the ultraviolet C range).

The wavelengths that most efficiently clear psoriasis are approximately around 313 nm.[51] In contrast, wavelengths less than 300 nm are the most efficient at causing erythema and nonmelanoma skin cancer. Based on this knowledge, light sources, termed NB-UVB, have been produced.[48] These light sources emit only wavelengths between 308 and 313 nm, and have largely supplanted BB-UVB UV radiation sources for phototherapy. Although originally employed to treat psoriasis, they are now used to treat several other inflammatory skin diseases as well.

The initial starting dose of both BB-UVB and NB-UVB is determined in one of two ways (Tables 198-1 and 198-2). In the first, the minimal erythema dose (MED) is determined by exposing six 1-cm^2 areas of skin on the inner aspect of the forearm or lower back to gradually increasing amounts of UV radiation from the same device that will be used for phototherapy. Twenty-four hours later, the UV-exposed areas of skin are examined and phototherapy is initiated at 50% to 70% of the smallest UV dose that results in uniform erythema over the entire area (ie, the MED). A semi-automated handheld device to determine MED has shown high correlation with the conventional method with low interobserver variability. This may be a faster, more reproducible alternative to conventional MED testing.[52] Alternatively, the initial dose of phototherapy is established empirically based on Fitzpatrick skin phototype (Tables 198-1 and 198-2). Subsequent exposures are given 2 to 5 times per week and the dose is increased at each treatment, assuming the patient has not developed an erythema response. If an erythema response has occurred, then, depending on its severity, the dose is either reduced or the treatment is delayed (Tables 198-1 and 198-2). Interestingly, NB-UVB is considerably less photoadaptive in comparison to BB-UVB, demonstrating the importance of wavelength on epidermal thickening and need for higher subsequent MEDs when treated with BB-UVB in comparison to NB-UVB.[53] The maximum NB-UVB dose that should be administered is 2000 to 5000 mJ/cm^2, depending on the photoreactive skin type. If patients miss treatments, dosage modifications should be made to avoid a phototoxic response (see Table 198-5).

PSORALEN AND ULTRAVIOLET A

PUVA photochemotherapy combines the oral ingestion or topical application of psoralens with exposure to UVR in the UVA range. Although psoralens and sunlight had been employed for thousands of years for the treatment of vitiligo, it was not until 1947 that PUVA in its modern form was described, initially for the treatment of vitiligo, and subsequently for the treatment of psoriasis.[54]

Three forms of psoralen are used in photochemotherapy regimens: 8-methoxypsoralen (8-MOP), 5-methoxypsoralen (5-MOP), and 4,5',8-trimethylpsoralen. In the United States, only 8-MOP is available. There are 2 oral formulations of 8-MOP, a micronized form that is typically given at a dose of 0.6 mg/kg 120 minutes prior to UVA exposure or a dissolved form that is given at a dose of 0.4 to 0.6 mg/kg 90 minutes before UVA exposure. Because the dissolved preparation is absorbed faster and yields higher and more reproducible serum levels, it is more commonly employed in PUVA phototherapy regimens.

The most common sources of radiation for PUVA therapy are UVA fluorescent lamps, which have a maximum emission at 352 nm, near the absorption maximum for psoralens. For oral PUVA therapy, UVA radiation is usually initiated at a dose that corresponds

TABLE 198-1
Narrowband Ultraviolet B Phototherapy

I. MED based
   A. MED determination
      Expose 1-cm^2 areas on the lower back or inner aspect of the forearm to 200, 400, 600, 800, 1000, 1200 mJ/cm^2; read at 24 hours
   B. Initial exposure: 50% to 70% of MED
   C. Subsequent exposures: 2 to 5 times per week
      Increase UV dose by 10% to 20% with each treatment

II. Skin phototype based
   Initial exposure based on Fitzpatrick skin phototype; subsequent exposures as above

SKIN PHOTOTYPE	INITIAL NB-UVB DOSE (MJ/CM^2)	MAXIMUM DOSE (MJ/CM^2)
I	130	2000
II	220	2000
III	260	3000
IV	330	3000
V	350	5000
VI	400	5000

MED, minimal erythema dose; NB-UVB, narrowband ultraviolet B.
Modified from Menter et al[1] and Krutmann et al.[374]

TABLE 198-2
Broadband Ultraviolet B Phototherapy

I. MED based
   A. MED determination
      Expose 1-cm² areas on the lower back or inner aspect of the forearm to 20, 40, 60, 80, 100, 120 mJ/cm²; read at 24 hours
   B. Initial exposure: 50% to 70% of MED
   C. Subsequent exposures: 2 to 5 times per week
      Increase UV dose by 25% with each treatment for the first 10 treatments; 10% per treatment thereafter

II. Skin phototype based
   Initial exposure based on Fitzpatrick skin phototype; subsequent exposures as above

SKIN PHOTOTYPE	INITIAL BB-UVB DOSE (MJ/CM²)
I	20
II	25
III	30
IV	40
V	50
VI	60

MED, minimal erythema dose; BB-UVB, broadband ultraviolet B.
Modified from Menter et al[1] and Krutmann et al.[374]

immersion, and other topical PUVA forms have been published by the British Photodermatology Group.[55] A cost-effectiveness analysis of data collected across 4 centers in Scotland revealed that courses of both bath PUVA and other topical PUVA treatments were consistently more expensive than oral PUVA.[55] This is related predominantly to the increased nursing time required.

More recently, cream PUVA has been developed which can be used to treat local and more widespread disease.[55A] Thirty minutes following the application of a psoralen-containing cream, patients are exposed to UVA irradiation.

AVOIDANCE AND MANAGEMENT OF PHOTOTOXIC REACTIONS

Sunburn-like reactions are the most common short-term adverse effect of phototherapy. UVB phototoxicity usually peaks at 12 to 24 hours and PUVA reaction manifests at 24 to 48 or even 72 hours. Severe burns over a large portion of the skin surface produce systemic toxicity with fever and malaise in addition to pain. Severe PUVA burns, which extend well into the dermis, can lead to epidermal sloughing and are an indication for admission to a burn care hospital facility.

to either the skin phototype or to 50% to 70% of the minimum phototoxic dose (Table 198-3). The minimum phototoxic dose is determined by having the patient take the dose of the oral psoralen to be used for the photochemotherapy treatment and exposing six 1-cm² areas of skin to the gradually increasing doses of UVA. The minimum phototoxic dose is evaluated 72 hours after UVA exposure and is the lowest amount of UVA that produces a uniform erythema over the entire area. In the United States, it is more common to initiate therapy based on the skin phototype (Table 198-3). Treatments are usually given 2 to 4 times per week, avoiding consecutive days. The amount of UVA that is to be given is increased with each treatment. UVA dose modifications are made if an erythema response develops or if treatments are missed (Table 198-3).

Delivery of psoralens in bathwater is popular in some areas of the world because it provides a uniform drug distribution over the skin surface, is associated with very low psoralen plasma levels, and results in a rapid elimination of free psoralens from the skin. This form of psoralen delivery circumvents GI side effects and possible phototoxic hazards to the eyes that are associated with the oral form. Skin psoralen levels are highly reproducible, and photosensitivity lasts for no more than 2 hours. Bath PUVA consists of 15 to 20 minutes of whole-body immersion in solutions of 1 mg 8-MOP per liter of body temperature bathwater (Table 198-4). 5-MOP and trimethylpsoralen are also employed for bath PUVA. Irradiation is performed immediately after bathing, as photosensitivity decreases rapidly. Bath PUVA is started at 30% of the minimum phototoxic dose. Treatments are typically given twice weekly. Guidelines for bath, local

TABLE 198-3
Oral Psoralen and Ultraviolet A Photochemotherapy

I. Psoralen dose
   8-MOP micronized   0.6 mg/kg; 120 minutes before UVA
   8-MOP dissolved   0.4-0.6 mg/kg; 90 minutes before UVA
   MPD based
   A. MPD determination
      Expose 1 cm² areas on the lower back or inner aspect of the forearm to 0.5, 1, 2, 3, 4, 5 J/cm² UVA; read 72 hours after UVA exposure
   B. Initial exposure: 50% to 70% of MPD
   C. Subsequent exposures: 2 to 4 times per week
      Increase UVA dose per table entries each week (not each exposure)

II. Skin phototype based
   A. Initial exposure based on Fitzpatrick skin phototype; subsequent exposures as above

SKIN PHOTOTYPE	INITIAL PUVA DOSE (J/CM²)	DOSE INCREASES (PER WEEK AFTER THE FIRST WEEK)
I	0.5	0.5
II	1.0	0.5
III	1.5	1.0
IV	2.0	1.0
V	2.5	1.5
VI	3.0	1.5

8-MOP, 8-methoxypsoralen; MPD, minimum phototoxic dose; PUVA, psoralen and ultraviolet A; UVA, ultraviolet A.
Modified from Menter et al[1] and Krutmann et al.[374]

TABLE 198-4
Bath Psoralen and Ultraviolet A Photochemotherapy

I. Psoralen dose
   8-MOP dissolved in bath water for a final concentration of 1 mg/L
   Bath water is at body temperature (37°C [98.6°F])
   Duration of bath is 15 to 20 minutes
II. UVA Exposure
   A. MPD Determination
      Expose 1-cm² areas on the lower back or inner aspect of the forearm; read 72 hours after UVA exposure
      Skin phototype I or II: 0.5, 1, 2, 3, 4, and 5 J/cm² UVA
      Skin phototype III or IV: 1, 2, 4, 6, 8, or 10 J/cm² UVA
   B. UVA exposure immediately after bathing
   C. Initial exposure: 30% of MPD
   D. Subsequent exposures: 2 times per week
                               Increase UVA dose by 20% each week

8-MOP, 8-methoxypsoralen; MPD, minimum phototoxic dose; PUVA, psoralen and ultraviolet A; UVA, ultraviolet A.
Modified from Menter et al[1] and Krutmann et al.[374]

TABLE 198-5
Modification of Phototherapy Dose for Erythema or Missed Sessions

REASON FOR MODIFICATION	MODIFICATION OF DOSE
No erythema	Increase by 25%
Erythema with no pain	No increase
Erythema with pain	Hold treatment until symptoms subside
Erythema with pain and blistering	Hold treatment until symptoms subside and then reduce dose by 50% from last dose
Modification of Phototherapy Dose for Missed Treatments	
<1 week	No increase in dose
1 to 2 weeks	Decrease dose by 50% (BB-UVB) or 25% (NB-UVB or PUVA)
2 to 3 weeks	Decrease dose by 75% (BB-UVB) or 50% (NB-UVB or PUVA)
>3 weeks	Restart at initial exposure dose

BB-UVB, broadband ultraviolet B; NB-UVB, narrowband ultraviolet B; PUVA, psoralen and ultraviolet A.
Modified from Menter et al[1] and Krutmann et al.[374]

To avoid exacerbating a still-developing PUVA burn it is recommended that PUVA treatments not be given on consecutive days. Table 198-5 specifies the UVB or UVA dose adjustments in the event of a burn reaction during phototherapy. A burn reported by the patient at the next visit, even if no longer visible, should be managed in the same manner as a still-visible reaction. Burns over limited body areas, such as just the face or breasts, can be managed by local application of an appropriate sunscreen before or part way through subsequent treatments, especially if the area is not affected by the disease being treated. However, care must be taken to consistently protect the same area(s) to avoid a sudden full treatment to previously shielded skin.

Repeated UV-irradiated skin develops tolerance to subsequent exposures, allowing and, indeed, mandating progressively larger doses for optimal therapeutic effect. However, this tolerance is rapidly lost when exposures cease, requiring downward adjustments of dose after as little as 1 week (see Table 198-5) to avoid burns.

ULTRAVIOLET A1

Because of its longer wavelength, UVA1 phototherapy (340 to 400 nm) can penetrate deeper into the skin than UVB or shorter-range UVA called UVA2 (ie, 320 to 340 nm). The first report describing a device capable of emitting UVA1 occurred in 1981.[56] It was not until 1992 when the therapeutic benefit of UVA1 was demonstrated for atopic dermatitis that greater interest in its therapeutic properties occurred.[57,58] Initially, one obstacle to the widespread use of first-generation UVA1 devices was the intense heat that they produced. Although not widely available in the United States, these light sources are useful for the management of a variety of dermatologic conditions for which other forms of phototherapy are not helpful.[59,60]

UVA1 is administered 3 to 5 times per week. Three dosing regimens have been used: low dose (10 to 30 J/cm²), medium dose (40 to 70 J/cm²), and high dose (130 J/cm²). In general, patients are started at 20 to 30 J/cm² and increased to the full dose within 3 to 5 treatments. The risk of burns is far less than with UVB or PUVA therapy.

TARGETED PHOTOTHERAPY

Targeted phototherapy is also called focused phototherapy, concentrated phototherapy, and microphototherapy. Unlike the previously described phototherapy devices that expose both lesional and uninvolved skin to UVR, targeted phototherapy delivers therapeutic doses of UVR only to lesional skin. Several devices are available to deliver targeted phototherapy, including both monochromatic (1 wavelength) and polychromatic systems. As of this writing, there is also a new therapeutic device in development that provides digital UV phototherapy that can be used to institute either targeted UVA or UVB therapy.[47] There are several advantages to targeted phototherapy. These devices spare normal skin, thereby allowing higher fluences to be delivered to diseased skin while decreasing the risk of acute and chronic side effects to normal skin. Targeted therapy can be used on treatment-resistant lesions and in difficult anatomic locations (such as the scalp, chin, and nails). The handheld nature of a targeted phototherapy device may have increased feasibility for young children compared to receiving treatments in a phototherapy booth that can be large and intimidating. The limitations of targeted phototherapy are device expense and that it may not be practical to treat for patients with greater than 10% to 20% body surface area involvement.

Targeted phototherapy devices have been used to administer targeted therapy to patients with psoriasis, vitiligo, and cutaneous T-cell lymphoma.[61,62] Monochromatic light sources, which include excimer lasers, monochromatic UVA1 lasers,[63] and nonlaser devices known as monochromatic excimer light devices, have been developed for this purpose. They differ in several respects. Lasers typically treat smaller areas, but can emit higher amounts of radiation over a shorter period. In contrast, monochromatic excimer light devices deliver monochromatic irradiation to a larger area but with a lower power density. There are also several devices that emit polychromatic UVA or UVB (BB-UVB or NB-UVB) to targeted areas. These devices typically use fiberoptic systems coupled with UVB-generating sources. They have spot sizes from 1 to 3 cm. In addition, these devices have multiple delivery programs and automatic calibration which makes treatment with predetermined dosages possible. These devices are smaller, less expensive, and have fewer maintenance problems than lasers.[64,65] Treatment protocols with targeted phototherapy vary depending on the type of device that is employed. A novel cream that selectively filters solar UVB may be a cheaper and more convenient alternative to traditional phototherapy in certain cases. This cream has been shown to improve symptoms of chronic pruritus after 3 months of treatment (3 sessions per week).[66]

SAFETY OF PHOTOTHERAPY

Safety principles are common to most phototherapy devices. Equipment should be checked on a regular basis by the clinical staff or the manufacturer's engineer, since bulb output may change over time and internal dosimetry components may fail. While phototherapy is usually delivered without incident, the risk of overtreatment is real, although the exact incidence of adverse events attributable to phototherapy is unknown and varies depending on the device. Importantly, except for PUVA therapy for which formal long-term followup studies established an increased risk of lentigines, squamous cell carcinoma, and possibly melanoma, other forms of phototherapy appear to be remarkably safe.[62,67] Newer therapies, such as NB-UVB and UVA1 appear to be relatively safe especially compared to nonphototherapeutic options for the same diseases.

ULTRAVIOLET B

Repeated exposure of the skin to UV irradiation does result in cumulative actinic damage regardless of the source. With respect to nonmelanoma skin cancer, most studies show that there is little risk beyond that associated with habitual sun exposure with either BB-UVB or NB-UVB phototherapy.[68,69] More than 300 BB-UVB treatments is associated with a modest, but significant, increase in squamous cell carcinoma (SCC) and basal cell carcinoma.[70] However, the carcinogenic risk of a single PUVA treatment is approximately 7 times greater than a single UVB treatment.[71] As a result of its safety profile and efficacy, NB-UVB has emerged as a leading therapy for a number of skin diseases. Several studies also show that long-term exposure to BB-UVB combined with topical tar preparations is not associated with an increased risk of SCC.[72]

PSORALEN AND ULTRAVIOLET A

ACUTE SIDE EFFECTS

Potential side effects of PUVA include drug intolerance in addition to the adverse reactions resulting from the combined action of psoralens plus UVA radiation. Oral 8-MOP may cause nausea (10% of patients) and vomiting, which occasionally necessitates discontinuation of treatment. These side effects are more common with liquid preparations than with crystalline preparations, probably because of higher psoralen serum levels. The nausea may be minimized or avoided by instructing the patient to take 8-MOP with milk, food, or ginger, or to divide the dose into 2 portions, taken approximately 30 minutes apart. Other reported effects include nervousness, insomnia, and depression. With 5-MOP, nausea is rare, even with doses up to 1.8 mg/kg/body weight.

Following exposure to UVA, approximately 10% of patients undergoing PUVA therapy will experience pruritus. In most cases, this can be alleviated by bland emollients. Some patients with severe pruritus require systemic treatment. A stinging pain may rarely occur; the mechanism for this is unknown. These symptoms are usually unresponsive to antihistamines, and, in most instances, subside when the treatment is discontinued.

Mild and often transient focal erythema after PUVA therapy occurs frequently. Any area showing erythema with tenderness or blistering should be shielded during subsequent UVA exposures until the erythema has resolved. As noted above, erythema appearing within 24 hours may signal a potentially severe phototoxic reaction, and may worsen progressively over the next 24 hours, as peak erythema with PUVA characteristically occurs at least 48 hours after the treatment. In that situation, patients should be protected from further UVA exposures and sunlight, and should be monitored closely until the erythema has resolved.

Very rare side effects of PUVA include polymorphous light eruption-like rashes, acneiform eruptions, subungual hemorrhages caused by phototoxic reactions of the nail beds, onycholysis, and occasionally hypertrichosis of the face. These disappear when treatment is discontinued. Analysis of laboratory data in several large studies revealed no significant abnormal findings in patients receiving PUVA over prolonged periods of time.[73-75]

CHRONIC ACTINIC DAMAGE

Chronic exposure to PUVA may result in skin changes that resemble photoaging, which is aggravated by chronic natural sun exposure. PUVA lentigines are small brown macules with irregular borders and uneven pigmentation[76] and are histologically characterized by proliferation of large melanocytes.[77] In contrast to solar lentigines, melanocytes in PUVA lentigines often display an increased size of melanosomes, clustering and binucleation with nuclear hyperchromatism, and cellular pleomorphism. BRAF (v-raf murine sarcoma viral oncogene homolog B) mutations have been found to be present in PUVA lentigines,[78] but the full significance of this is not yet understood, as both cutaneous malignant melanoma and benign melanocytic nevi often have BRAF mutations.[79-82] The presence of these lesions is directly related to the number of PUVA treatments and total UVA dose that has been administered. The absence of PUVA lentigines serves as a useful indicator of a lower risk of PUVA malignancy.[83]

CARCINOGENESIS

Cutaneous malignancies are the major concern of long-term and repeated PUVA treatments. The risk of nonmelanoma skin cancer and possibly malignant melanoma increases in a dose-dependent manner. In laboratory animals, 8-MOP and 5-MOP have unequivocally induced skin cancer at levels of drug and UVA irradiation comparable to those used in PUVA therapy.[84] Cancer development is thought to stem from both DNA damage and downregulation of the immune system. The PUVA Follow-up Study, which evaluated 1380 patients who began PUVA treatment for psoriasis in 1975 and 1976 has documented major health events in these individuals in a prospective manner. Overall, patients who were treated with at least 337 PUVA treatments exhibited a 100-fold increased risk of SCC compared to that expected from population incidence rates.[85] Moreover, almost 4% of patients with SCC developed metastases, most commonly originating in the genital area. There is uncertainty about PUVA being the sole factor as many of the patients in the long-term followup studies also had significant exposure to sunlight and to treatments with carcinogenic potential, including arsenic, UVB, and methotrexate. The risk of developing SCC with PUVA may be further potentiated by the use of cyclosporine and for this reason cyclosporine is contraindicated in individuals who have been treated with PUVA.[86] Oral retinoids used concurrently with PUVA, on the other hand, reduce the risk of SCC.[87]

Individuals treated with PUVA are at increased risk of cutaneous malignancies of the genitalia, and this has led to standard protection of the genitalia during phototherapy.[88] The risk is dose-dependent, with a 90-fold increased risk of genital tumors among patients exposed to high doses of PUVA compared with that expected in the general population. Men treated with high-dose exposures to both PUVA and topical tar/UVB have the greatest risk of genital tumors.[88,89] There is currently no standardized regimen for genital shielding. Commonly used protective agents include commercially available pouches for genital shielding, surgical masks, paper towels, blue surgical towels, and underwear. The efficacy of these materials has been studied, and surgical masks were found to provide insufficient protection against UV irradiation, most likely because of increased porosity (looser weave) and decreased mass.[90]

The relationship between PUVA and melanoma also has been examined in detail. The PUVA Follow-Up Study has provided evidence that individuals with at least 250 treatments and at least 15 years from the first PUVA treatment were at increased risk of developing melanoma.[91] Patients who developed a phototoxic reaction more easily were at higher risk for melanoma than those with darker skin.[92] As a result of those studies, a personal or family history of melanoma or a history of more than 200 PUVA treatments is considered to be a relative contraindication to further PUVA therapy.[92]

In patients employing PUVA therapy in combination with methotrexate for at least 36 months, the incidence of lymphoma was more than 7 times higher than that of cohort members earlier in the study who had not taken methotrexate.[93]

OPHTHALMOLOGIC EFFECTS

UVA is absorbed in the lens and in the presence of UVA, psoralens can bind protein, DNA, and RNA. Because the lens never sheds its cells, protein-bound 8-MOP accumulates in the lens, increasing the risk of irreversible opacification.[94] There have been reports of various ocular problems in patients on PUVA including cataracts,[95,96] conjunctival hyperemia,[97] and decreased lacrimation.[97]

A 25-year prospective study[98] sought to evaluate the effect of PUVA on the eyes. Participants were instructed to use UVA-blocking eyewear when outside or looking outside through window glass during daylight for a minimum of 12 hours, although current labeling calls for 24 hours of eye protection. This study found no relationship between increasing numbers of PUVA sessions and visual impairment or cataracts, and demonstrates that increasing exposure to PUVA does not increase cataract risk among middle-aged and older persons using eye protection as practiced by this cohort.[98] Other smaller studies also have found no increase in cataract formation or visual impairment.[99-102]

ULTRAVIOLET A1

UVA1 phototherapy is generally well tolerated.[103,104] Reported side effects include intense tanning, erythema, pruritus, urticaria, tenderness, a burning sensation, polymorphous light eruption, eczema herpeticum, and bacterial superinfection.[59,60,105] However, because UVA1 phototherapy has only been available since the 1990s', the long-term effects are still under investigation.

SPECIAL CONSIDERATIONS

HIV

The safety of phototherapy and photochemotherapy in HIV-positive patients has been debated. UVR may activate HIV by the induction of nuclear factor κB,[106-108] and UVB therapy increases HIV-1 gene expression in the skin.[109-111] However, BB-UVB phototherapy does not appear to affect plasma HIV levels nor does it have an effect on CD4 counts.[110,112,113] In general, phototherapy is thought to be safe for HIV patients.[114] A consensus statement published by the American Academy of Dermatology in 2010 concluded that for moderate to severe psoriasis in HIV-positive patients, phototherapy and antiretrovirals are the recommended first-line therapeutic agents.[115]

CHILDREN

NB-UVB is now preferred to PUVA in children for most skin conditions, because of concern about PUVA side effects, including phototoxicity, carcinogenicity, photoaging, and the potential development of cataracts.

PREGNANCY

NB-UVB in a high mean cumulative dose (>118.16 J/cm^2 in 36 treatments) and BB-UVB (110 to 220 mJ/cm^2 in 7 to 22 treatments) can cause a proportionate decrease in serum folic acid levels. Although there are no specific guidelines, dermatologists should consider measuring folic acid levels intermittently, especially during the first trimester.[116-118]

ELDERLY

Phototherapy should be considered in patients older than 65 years of age if there are no physical and cognitive disabilities impairing use of phototherapy. However, it is important to be aware that UVB-induced erythema lasts longer and peaks later in the elderly.[119] Also, photoadaptation may be decreased in the elderly secondary to decreased epidermal turnover, melanocyte number, and tanning response. Hence, it is important to consider initiating phototherapy at a lower dose and increasing dose levels more slowly to limit the number of phototoxic events.[120]

MISCELLANEOUS

Patients who have had arsenic exposure are at increased risk for cutaneous malignancies and should avoid phototherapy. Transplantation patients have a much higher risk of skin cancer compared to the general population because of the medications they are taking to prevent rejection of their transplanted organ. Consequently, there is a relative contraindication to phototherapy in transplantation patients. Photosensitizing medications should theoretically be avoided during phototherapy treatment, although in practice many patients receive phototherapy while taking tetracycline, hydrochlorothiazide, or other photosensitizing drugs without adverse consequences. There are reports of an association between chronic use of voriconazole and the development of aggressive cutaneous malignancies, including melanoma.[121-123]

DISEASES AMENABLE TO PHOTOTHERAPY

Table 198-6 summarizes the diseases amenable to phototherapy.

TABLE 198-6
Diseases Amenable to Phototherapy

	NB-UVB/BB-UVB	PUVA	UVA1
Aquagenic pruritus	−	+	−
Atopic dermatitis	+	+	+ (acute flares)
Cholestatic pruritus	+	−	−
Chronic graft-versus-host disease	+	+	+
Chronic hand eczema	+	+	+
Chronic urticaria	+	+/−	+/−
Cutaneous T-cell lymphoma	+	+	+
Granuloma annulare	−	+	+
Indolent systemic mastocytosis	+	+	+
Lichen planus	+	+	+
Localized and systemic scleroderma	−	+	+
Lymphomatoid papulosis	−	+	+
Perforating disorders	+	+	−
Photodermatoses	+	+	+
Pityriasis lichenoides	+	+	+
Pruritus of chronic renal failure	+	−	−
Pruritus of polycythemia vera	+	+	−
Psoriasis	+	+	−
Telangiectasis macularis eruptiva perstans	−	+	+
Urticaria pigmentosa	−	+/−	+
Vitiligo	NB-UVB	+	−

BB-UVB, broadband ultraviolet B; NB-UVB, narrowband ultraviolet B; PUVA, psoralen and ultraviolet A; UVA, ultraviolet A.

PHOTOTHERAPY OF PSORIASIS

BROADBAND AND NARROWBAND ULTRAVIOLET B

Both BB-UVB and NB-UVB have been employed to treat psoriasis. Their presumptive mechanisms of action in this disease include its effects on DNA, antimicrobial actions that may alter the microbial flora of the skin,[124] induction of anti-inflammatory and immunosuppressive cytokines,[125-127] augmentation of vitamin D levels,[128,129] alterations in antimicrobial peptides,[129] modulation of vascular endothelial growth factor expression,[130] restoration of Th17/Treg imbalance as well as function,[131] suppression of Type I interferon signaling,[132] a reduction in C-reactive protein,[133] and decrease in serum plasmin.[134]

Clinical trials[48] supporting the research findings[51] that wavelengths in the range of 313 nm are most effective at clearing psoriasis have led to broad use of NB-UVB for psoriasis (Fig. 198-3). NB-UVB has thus become first-line therapy for chronic plaque psoriasis, and is considered to be superior to conventional BB-UVB with respect to both clearing and remission times.[48,135] The difference in efficacy may be related to more efficient clearing of T cells by NB-UVB from the epidermis and dermis of psoriatic plaques compared with conventional BB-UVB.[29] The end point of phototherapy is complete clearance of all psoriatic skin lesions. Psoriasis, however, is a chronic disease and the remission induced by UVB phototherapy is often short-lived. In a randomized, prospective, multicentered trial, investigators found that continuing UVB phototherapy, after initial clearing, contributes to control of the disease and is justified for many patients.[136] The frequency of UVB treatments is reduced while maintaining the last dose given at the time of clearing. NB-UVB can be used safely in pregnancy and in children.

Other agents (topical and oral) combined with UVB phototherapy may clear psoriatic skin lesions in a shorter period of time. Combined therapies may thus allow for fewer treatments and potentially less photoaging and fewer other risks. Often combination regimens are administered when phototherapy alone is no longer effective. Oral retinoids, such as acitretin,[137] increase efficacy, particularly in patients with chronic plaque-type psoriasis.[138-140] Addition of oral acitretin to either NB-UVB or the Goeckerman regimen (see next paragraph) reduces the total number of treatments necessary.[141] Although fewer sessions may be required with combination therapy, the rate of relapse may be slightly higher. Methotrexate (15 mg/week) administered 3 weeks before starting NB-UVB can also enable quicker results in fewer phototherapy sessions.[142] Biologic therapies are being evaluated in conjunction with phototherapy. Treatment with NB-UVB significantly accelerated the clearance of psoriatic lesions in patients responding slowly to etanercept.[143]

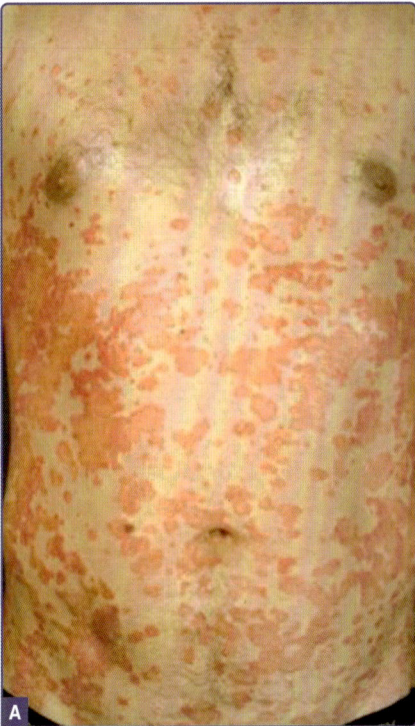 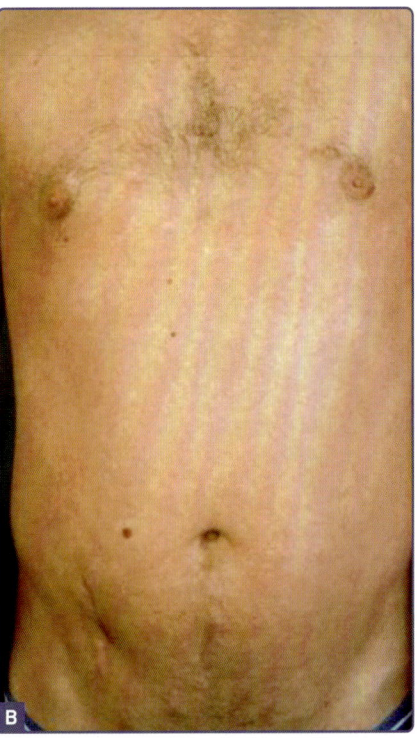

Figure 198-3 **A,** Psoriasis prior to narrowband ultraviolet B (NB-UVB) phototherapy. **B,** At the completion of NB-UVB therapy. (Photos used with permission from Herbert Hönigsmann, MD.)

BB-UVB and NB-UVB phototherapy can be combined with topical agents to achieve higher clearance rates, longer disease-free intervals, and a lower risk of side effects. The Goeckerman regimen consists of the application of tar-containing topical agents with subsequent UV irradiation. The use of liquid carbonis detergens with NB-UVB is one example of a modified form of this regimen. The regimen is safe, convenient, effective, and leads to a more rapid improvement of psoriasis than light therapy alone.[144] The antipsoriatic vitamin D analogs calcipotriol and calcitriol, used in conjunction with NB-UVB, provide additional benefit compared to either the drugs or the phototherapy alone.[145-150] Application of calcipotriol prior to phototherapy leads to unwanted degradation of vitamin D_3, and calcipotriene increases the MED in patients, suggesting that it has a photoprotective effect.[151] For these reasons, when used in combination with phototherapy, vitamin D analogs must be applied after the light treatment. Tazarotene 0.1% gel has an additive or synergistic effect when combined with NB-UVB.[152] Because retinoids can cause photosensitivity, it is common practice to initiate phototherapy at 50% to 75% of the usual starting dose when tazarotene is used with UVB.[153] Topical bexarotene gel 1% also has been combined with NB-UVB for the treatment of psoriasis and has greater efficacy than either alone.[154] By decreasing scatter from scales in the stratum corneum, lubricants improve transmission of UVB, and a combination of topical lubricants with UVB therapy increases efficacy.[155-157] The use of topical salicylic acid with UVB has not been found to increase the efficacy of UVB phototherapy because it blocks UVB penetration.[157A]

TARGETED PHOTOTHERAPY

Targeted phototherapy using a monochromatic 308-nm excimer laser or monochromatic excimer light is effective and safe for psoriasis. A large, multicenter study found that fewer patient visits were required with targeted phototherapy compared to conventional phototherapy.[158] The use of monochromatic excimer compared to cream PUVA has been found to have equivalent efficacy for palmoplantar psoriasis.[159] Calculating the dose that induces blistering on a psoriatic plaque and treating the plaques at just below that dose can lead to clearance in significantly fewer sessions.[160]

PSORALEN AND ULTRAVIOLET A PHOTOCHEMOTHERAPY

Oral PUVA has consistently induced remission of psoriasis in clinical studies.[73,161,162] At least a 75% improvement in the Psoriasis Area and Severity Index score can be expected after 12 weeks of PUVA treatments in 60% of patients.[161] In some studies, oral PUVA has been observed to be more efficacious in clearing plaque psoriasis than NB-UVB, and the duration of remission is more prolonged,[162] whereas other studies have found the 2 treatments to be comparable, particularly when NB-UVB is administered 3 times per week.[163-166] It must be noted here that unlike drug administration, the success of PUVA and phototherapy generally depends in large part on physician-determined patient-specific subtle modifications of the regimen, such as dose increments between treatments, that optimize therapeutic response while avoiding burns or other adverse effects. Hence, the response to phototherapy may vary greatly among studies and among practitioners. Additionally, polymorphisms in genes encoding glutathione S-transferases are associated with PUVA sensitivity and these may have implications for treatment response.[167]

Repeated exposures are required to clear PUVA-responsive diseases, with gradual increments in dose as pigmentation and epidermal thickness increase. Upon clearing, patients are often transitioned to maintenance therapy, during which the frequency of treatments is gradually reduced. There are various maintenance algorithms. One regimen consists of 1 month of twice-weekly treatments, at the last UVA dose used for clearing, followed by another month of once-weekly exposures.

A combination of PUVA and methotrexate can reduce the duration of treatment, number of exposures, and total UVA dose required for clearing. It is also effective in clearing patients unresponsive to PUVA alone.[168] This combination appears to be safe if used during the clearing phase. However, long-term methotrexate, defined as 36 or more months of use, in combination with PUVA may increase the risk of lymphoma.[93]

The combination of cyclosporine with PUVA is not recommended because of the greatly increased risk of squamous cell carincoma.[86] There are no published clinical trials combining PUVA with biologic agents.

PUVA therapy is more efficacious when combined with a daily oral retinoid (etretinate, acitretin, isotretinoin; 1 mg/kg), a treatment regimen that has been referred to as RePUVA. The addition of an oral retinoid can bring patients into remission, even if they have not responded to PUVA alone.[169] The oral retinoid is typically administered 5 to 10 days before initiating PUVA, and is continued throughout the clearing phase. RePUVA can often reduce the number of PUVA exposures by one-third and the total cumulative UVA dose by more than one-half. Oral retinoids when combined with PUVA have been shown to reduce the risk of SCC by 30%, although it does not alter the incidence of basal cell carcinoma.[87] The mechanism of the synergistic action of retinoids and PUVA is unknown, but has been postulated to result in part from accelerated desquamation that optimizes the optical properties of the skin.

Topical tazarotene gel 0.1% combined with oral PUVA accelerates the response to treatment.[170] This may decrease exposure to UVA and thus the long-term hazards associated with PUVA therapy. Because of the photosensitizing effect to tazarotene, it is recommended that PUVA therapy be initiated at slightly lower doses than usual.[153] Topical tazarotene plus PUVA bath therapy is also clinically and statistically superior to vehicle plus PUVA bath therapy.[171]

The application of salicylic acid in petrolatum just before PUVA therapy is not recommended as it may hinder the penetration of UVA.[172] When calcipotriol is used with PUVA, it should not be applied within 2 hours of phototherapy.

TOPICAL AND BATH PSORALEN AND ULTRAVIOLET A FOR PSORIASIS

Application of 8-MOP in creams, ointments. or lotions followed by UVA irradiation is effective in clearing psoriasis, but may result in nonuniform distribution on the skin surface. This may induce unpredictable phototoxic erythema reactions and irregular patches of cosmetically unacceptable hyperpigmentation. Furthermore, the application of the medication is potentially labor intensive. For these reasons, topical psoralens are used most commonly in psoriasis for limited plaque psoriasis and palmoplantar disease.

PHOTOSENSITIVE PSORIASIS

Interestingly, UVA and UVB are both capable of triggering or aggravating psoriatic plaques in predisposed patients. This phenomenon appears to be linked to certain genetic traits, female gender and susceptibility to photosensitive disorders such as polymorphous light eruption. In predisposed individuals, there is a tendency toward creating a microenvironment that is inflammatory rather than immunosuppressive upon exposure to UVR, resulting in worsening of psoriatic disease.[173] However, even though there are anecdotal reports of developing polymorphous light eruption secondary to NB-UVB treatment for psoriasis, NB-UVB can still be a viable treatment option in these patients. The strategy is to temporarily discontinue phototherapy until the lesions resolve and to restart at a much lower NB-UVB dose. NB-UVB should be increased slowly, which allows for treatment of psoriatic plaques with simultaneous photohardening that leads to resolution of polymorphous light eruption.[174]

PHOTOTHERAPY OF ATOPIC DERMATITIS

NARROWBAND ULTRAVIOLET B

Studies evaluating NB-UVB as a treatment for severe atopic dermatitis have shown that it improves severity scores, reduces potent topical steroid use, and provides a long-term benefit for most patients.[175-178] Compared with bath PUVA, using half-body UVB versus UVA comparisons, NB-UVB and bath PUVA are both highly effective. Most patients, however, prefer NB-UVB. Relief of pruritus usually occurs in the first 2 weeks, prior to visible resolution of the cutaneous lesions.[179] Additionally, improvements can be maintained months after phototherapy is stopped. NB-UVB can also be used sequentially following cyclosporine, to avoid relapse of disease.[180]

There is little information regarding the use of NB-UVB in children, and long-term data on the safety of this therapy are still needed. However, those studies that have examined NB-UVB for atopic dermatitis and other skin diseases in children have found that it is well-tolerated and produces excellent responses with no serious side effects.[181-185] When side effects are mentioned, erythema is the most common[182]; other adverse reactions, such as herpes simplex reactivation, are rarely reported.[183] In some cases, UVA combined with NB-UVB appears to provide added benefit.[186]

Long-term studies in animal models evaluating the carcinogenic potential of tacrolimus (0.03% and 0.1%) and pimecrolimus 1% did not find an increase in the incidence of UV-induced skin tumor growth.[187] There are no studies evaluating the safety or efficacy of combined phototherapy with topical calcineurin inhibitors for atopic dermatitis in humans.

EXCIMER LASER AND ATOPIC DERMATITIS

The 308-nm xenon-chloride monochromatic excimer light has been evaluated in localized atopic dermatitis and has been shown to be efficacious in reducing its severity, and in diminishing its pruritus with lasting results.[70,188-190] In extensive atopic dermatitis, this treatment is impractical, but it is particularly useful for atopic dermatitis involving the hands,[70] and in situations in which there is an interest in limiting the use of topical steroids.

PSORALEN AND ULTRAVIOLET A

Oral PUVA is highly effective for the treatment of atopic dermatitis.[191-194] In contrast to psoriasis, the number of treatments required for clearance of atopic dermatitis may be relatively high. Additionally, a rebound effect may occur in a high percentage of patients if the phototherapy is not combined with other therapies or if maintenance therapy is not instituted.[191] Bath PUVA is also used for atopic dermatitis, primarily in Europe, and is a very effective treatment.[195-197]

ULTRAVIOLET A1

UVA1 phototherapy is a highly effective, nonsteroidal, therapeutic alternative for treatment of acute exacerbations of atopic dermatitis and is almost devoid of uncomfortable side effects.[57,103,105,198] Doses of UVA1 (60 to 130 J/cm² per day) over a 3-week period reduce the clinical severity of atopic dermatitis. However, effectiveness is short term and is followed by recurrence of symptoms in a majority of patients.[104,199] In one study, NB-UVB provided a greater therapeutic effect than UVA1 for chronic atopic dermatitis.[200]

PHOTOTHERAPY OF CUTANEOUS T-CELL LYMPHOMA

PSORALEN AND ULTRAVIOLET A

PUVA photochemotherapy has been a successful therapeutic option for cutaneous T-cell lymphoma (CTCL) since the 1970s'.[201,202] Complete clearing may be induced when malignant cells are confined to the epidermis and the superficial dermis, within the depth of UVA penetration. For the clearing phase, treatment schedules and dosimetry are essentially the same as for psoriasis. The treatment consists of 3 phases: a clearing phase, a maintenance phase, and monitoring off therapy. Maintenance therapy is not standardized; patients benefit most from individualized schedules.[203] Therapy is discontinued after a variable period of time and patients are monitored. Relapses tend to respond as well as initially when PUVA is resumed. Patients with tumor-stage CTCL (IIB or greater) exhibit a high rate of early recurrences, which require permanent maintenance treatment. In these cases, PUVA typically is combined with other modalities to produce complete responses. Prolonged remissions have been observed with combinations of PUVA and interferon-α2a[204] or low-dose interferon-α2b.[205] In later stages of CTCL, PUVA has been employed as a palliative treatment, reducing the tumor-cell burden and acting synergistically with other treatments.[202] For example, there has been success combining PUVA and oral bexarotene for the treatment of advanced CTCL (Sézary syndrome).[206]

Bathwater PUVA therapy with 8-MOP is a valuable phototherapeutic alternative, which can be considered for patients in whom systemic psoralen cannot be used. Excellent responses have been reported in patients with early stage mycosis fungoides[207] and in children.[208] There is also evidence of efficacy in patients with superficial folliculotropic mycosis fungoides.[209] Cream PUVA with 8-MOP as a form of targeted UV therapy can be considered in patients with high risk of skin cancer.[46]

NARROWBAND ULTRAVIOLET B

NB-UVB may be as effective as PUVA for early stage CTCL.[210-218] Some authors advocate starting with NB-UVB because of its more favorable safety and side-effect profile.[211] Clinical remissions are reported to last for 3[216] to 24.5[211] months; maintenance therapy tends to prolong remission.[217] NB-UVB also has been used successfully in conjunction with oral bexarotene.[219]

PHOTOTHERAPY OF VITILIGO

PUVA and NB-UVB are two of the leading treatments for vitiligo. NB-UVB decreases IL-17 and IL-22 levels that are usually elevated in vitiligo and also increases FoxP3-expressing cells, restoring the balance between Th17 and regulatory T cells.[220] It also appears to restore the balance of oxidant and antioxidants relieving oxidative stress that is considered to play a role in the pathogenesis of vitiligo.[221] When employed for vitiligo, NB-UVB is typically administered 3 times per week.[222] The earliest sign of response to therapy is perifollicular repigmentation. Cosmetically acceptable treatment success, defined as greater than or equal to 75% repigmentation, has been achieved in 12.5%[223] to more than 75%[224,225] of patients. Factors that predict how a patient will respond to NB-UVB include ethnic background, skin phototype, the areas treated,[224-230] and the type of vitiligo.[228] There does not appear to be an association between response to treatment and patients' sex, age, family history of vitiligo, or the extent of body surface involvement.[229-231] Patients who show early initial repigmentation are more likely to have a higher percentage of final repigmentation.[223,229] In individuals with Fitzpatrick skin types IV and V, vitiliginous areas have been noted to repigment slightly darker than the surrounding skin. This resolves after a few months, resulting in a cosmetically acceptable outcome.[222,229] Although data is somewhat limited, relapse rates may be anywhere from 25% to 84% after 1 year.[229,232,233] Those who relapse tend to respond to another course of phototherapy.

When NB-UVB is used in combination with topical tacrolimus 0.3% ointment, the therapeutic efficacy is higher than with NB-UVB alone.[234] This synergistic effect is mediated through upregulation of MMP-2 and MMP-9 resulting in enhanced melanocyte migration.[235] However, combination therapy is not effective in typical UV therapy–resistant sites such as the hands and feet.[236] Pseudocatalase cream has been used in conjunction with NB-UVB. Whether pseudocatalase increases the efficacy of NB-UVB is controversial.[237-239] In difficult-to-treat areas, laser dermabrasion in combination with topical steroids and NB-UVB twice weekly has been significantly more effective than just topical steroids and NB-UVB. Despite significant improvement in repigmentation rates, the procedure is poorly tolerated because of pain and there are risks of delayed wound healing and hypertrophic scarring.[240] A novel approach using afamelanotide, an analog of melanocyte-stimulating hormone, combined with NB-UVB has shown significant improvement compared to NB-UVB monotherapy especially in patients with Fitzpatrick skin types IV through VI.[236]

Targeted phototherapy with a 308-nm excimer laser also is reported to be effective in vitiligo and should be considered first-line therapy in localized vitiligo.[241-245] Sessions are performed 2 to 3 times weekly, with the ultimate rate of repigmentation dependent on the total number of sessions rather than the frequency.[246,247] The treatments are well-tolerated and side effects are minimal. Excimer laser achieved the same grade of repigmentation as NB-UVB, but at a lower total cumulative dose.[248] Because the laser is monochromatic, it can deliver higher energy exclusively to the affected areas while minimizing side effects. Similar to standard NB-UVB therapy, lesions on the face, neck, and trunk respond better than those on the extremities. The hands and feet have the least-favorable outcome.[241,244,249-252] Combining a topical antioxidant gel with the excimer laser appears to have higher efficacy in terms of repigmentation than excimer laser alone.[253] Monochromatic excimer light also is effective in patients with vitiligo, even if they have not previously responded to NB-UVB.[61]

Although PUVA was first used for vitiligo, it is used less often for that indication since the introduction of NB-UVB. Responses have been achieved in up to 70% of patients.[254] Combination therapy of PUVA and a medium-potency topical corticosteroid is 3 times more effective than either treatment alone.[255] In contrast to NB-UVB and PUVA, UVA1 does not cause repigmentation and only accentuates the difference in color between normal and vitiliginous areas by tanning the normal skin.

SCLEROTIC SKIN DISEASES

LOCALIZED AND SYSTEMIC SCLERODERMA

UVA1 has been reported to decrease lesional skin thickness, improve skin elasticity, reduce sclerotic plaques, and increase passive range of motion in localized scleroderma.[256-258] There have been varying opinions as to the best dose and treatment regimen.[259-261] In most studies, UVA1 has been administered at a dose of 60 to 130 J/cm² 5 times per week, although lower doses (20 J/cm²) also have been reported to be effective. When doses of 20 J/cm² and 70 J/cm² were compared, the higher dose caused greater improvement.[259] However, when 130 J/cm² was administered 3 times per week, the tanning response produced by the UVA1 treatment interfered with its ability to soften the sclerodermatous patches, implying that medium dose and less-frequent treatments would be more effective.[261] The recurrence after successful UVA1 treatment was dependent on the duration of morphea prior to treatment rather than morphea subtypes, Fitzpatrick skin type, or medium-to-high-dose regimens implying that a medium-high dose of UVA1 is adequate in terms of prevention of recurrence.[262]

The mechanism of action is at least partly through induction of MMP-1,[263] and downregulation transforming growth factor-β through the SMAD (Sma- and Mad-related protein) signaling pathway.[264-266] UVA1 downregulates human beta-defensin, IL-6, and IL-8, which correlates with clinical improvement.[267]

UVA1 also has been used to treat acrosclerosis in patients with systemic scleroderma.[268] Marked improvement was noted with softening of affected skin and increased finger movement. It also improved microstomia.[269] Oral and topical PUVA also have been used for this disease, with improvement in range of motion and contractures.[270] Oral PUVA has been used to treat disabling, extensive morphea in children.[271-274]

GRAFT-VERSUS-HOST DISEASE

In chronic graft-versus-host disease, NB-UVB has been employed as a second-line treatment in children[275] and adults[276] who are resistant to or have relapsed on standard immunosuppressive regimens. Oral PUVA,[277-281] topical PUVA,[282,283] and UVA1[284-286] also have been employed. Bath PUVA in combination with isotretinoin is another option for sclerodermoid graft-versus-host disease.[287] If phototherapy is to be employed for these patients, it is important to examine the patients regularly, as they already have an increased risk of skin cancer from their immunosuppressive therapies. There are anecdotal reports of successful treatment of sclerotic graft-versus-host disease with NB-UVB treatment.[288]

OTHER SCLEROTIC SKIN DISEASES

UVA1 has led to modest improvement in the degree of induration, and, at times, in mobility of the hands and legs in nephrogenic systemic fibrosis.[121,289] Total treatments have ranged from 22 treatments (with a cumulative dose of 1855 J/cm²) to 50 treatments (3850 J/cm²). There are also anecdotal reports of its use in scleredema, vulvar lichen sclerosis and stiff skin syndrome, as well as radiation-induced morphea.[60]

PRURITUS

UVB phototherapy is an option for the pruritus associated with chronic renal failure. Approximately 80% to 90% of patients improve within 2 to 5 weeks.[290-292] If symptoms recur, they commonly respond to retreatment with UVB. For this disorder, phototherapy works on a systemic level rather than locally, because BB-UVB exposure to one-half of the body improves pruritus in both the exposed and unexposed sites.[291] Some patients respond well to BB-UVB, but are less responsive to NB-UVB.[293]

Phototherapy is considered by some to be the most effective treatment for cholestatic pruritus.[294-296] UVB phototherapy also has been combined with cholestyramine.[297]

PUVA has resulted in improvement in aquagenic pruritus in several patients, but maintenance treatments may be required.[298-300]

Treatment with NB-UVB 3 times a week,[301] UVA in combination with UVB,[302] and PUVA[303-305] have been reported to improve the pruritus associated with polycythemia vera.

NB-UVB, BB-UVB, and PUVA have been used safely and effectively to treat eosinophilic folliculitis in HIV-positive patients.[306-310]

CHRONIC URTICARIA

NB-UVB should be considered in patients who have failed first-line antihistamine regimens. It appears to be effective and well-tolerated. BB-UVB has a higher relapse rate. The observed efficacy of NB-UVB may be partly from the greater penetration into the dermis and relatively larger systemic immunosuppressive effects of NB-UVB in comparison to BB-UVB. PUVA or UVA therapy shows some efficacy but results are inconsistent.[311]

PHOTODERMATOSES

NB-UVB[312-314] and oral PUVA[315,316] are useful methods for preventing outbreaks of moderate to severe polymorphous light eruption. "Hardening" is obtained by exposing the individual to low levels of phototherapy while, at the same time, placing them prophylactically on oral corticosteroids to prevent the rash. Proposed mechanisms by which phototherapy induces tolerance to sunlight include thickening of the stratum corneum, hyperpigmentation, and cutaneous immune modulation by normalizing UV-induced inflammatory cytokines such as IL-1β,[317] restoring impaired neutrophil chemotaxis,[318] increasing regulatory T cells,[319] and transiently decreasing Langerhans cells in the epidermis while increasing the mast cell recruitment into the papillary dermis.[320] Although NB-UVB is currently used more commonly than PUVA, PUVA has the advantage of a rapid and intense pigment induction at relatively low UVA doses that usually remain well below the threshold for eliciting an outbreak. Approximately 10% of patients will develop typical polymorphous light eruption lesions during the initial phase of PUVA, but these usually disappear with continued treatment. Phototherapy is typically initiated 1 month before the first anticipated intense sun exposure, such as a sunny midwinter vacation. Once "hardening" has been induced, it must be maintained by frequent exposure to ambient sunlight. Novel home UVB low-intensity phototherapy devices that can be used each day for 6 minutes have shown better acceptance by patients while providing the same efficacy as a BB-UVB hospital treatment.[321]

Lesions of solar urticaria also can be prevented with phototherapy. The regimen involves induction of tolerance by repeatedly exposing the patient to graded doses of the causative wavelengths.[322-324] Successful treatment has been achieved with repeated exposures to NB-UVB,[325] UVA, or PUVA.[322,324-327] PUVA may result in a response of greater duration. A condensed type of phototherapy called "rush hardening" also has been used.[328] In rush hardening patients are exposed to quarter- or half-body UVA irradiation at 50% of the determined minimal urticarial dose with hourly increases in body surface area irradiation and dose.[328] "Hardening" or "desensitization" has been reported to occur in as few as 3 days. The most important parameter in rush hardening is to determine the minimal urticarial dose and action spectra immediately before starting therapy and initiating the treatment at a dose lower than the minimal urticarial dose to minimize exacerbations.[329] The disadvantage of this modality is that tolerance is lost quickly if the treatments are not continued every few days. For unexplained reasons, UVA1, which has effects on mast cells, is not particularly effective in preventing solar or other forms of urticaria.

Chronic actinic dermatitis and actinic prurigo are other photosensitive disorders that are reported to benefit from controlled, low doses of UV irradiation.[190,330,331] In contrast to polymorphous light eruption, an extended duration of treatment is often required for chronic actinic dermatitis.

OTHER DISEASES

LICHEN PLANUS

NB-UVB therapy has been used for recalcitrant lichen planus and is typically administered 3 times per week on nonconsecutive days. A complete response in 70% of patients has been reported after an average time of 10 weeks.[332-334] Improvement in pruritus can be expected before disappearance of skin lesions. Oral and topical PUVA[335] are other alternatives. In general, lichen planus tends to be more resistant to PUVA than psoriasis when treated with a similar schedule. A regimen of RePUVA may accelerate clearing, but has been reported to cause transient hyperpigmentation.[336] NB-UVB produces similar outcomes, but some have reported a better initial clinical response with PUVA.[337] Followup of patients who have cleared on PUVA shows that the disease reoccured at a higher frequency compared to non-PUVA group, raising the possibility that the treatment may prolong the disease.[335] Although exceedingly rare, PUVA has been reported to induce lichen planus[338] and lichen planus pemphigoides[339] in patients undergoing the therapy for other skin diseases. In a small series, the excimer laser has successfully treated erosive oral lichen planus.[340] However, the long-term effects of this form of radiant energy on the oral mucosa, which may also have been exposed to tobacco products, are unknown. Consequently, phototherapy for oral lichen planus should not be a first-line therapy for this form of the disease.

CHRONIC HAND ECZEMA

NB-UVB and local bath PUVA have been successful treatments for dyshidrotic eczema and chronic palmoplantar eczema.[341-343] Bath PUVA may be less effective in smokers with dyshidrotic eczema.[344] Oral PUVA is preferable for patients with hyperkeratotic eczema and bath PUVA is more beneficial for dyshidrotic eczema,[345] although oral PUVA also is effective for dyshidrotic eczema.[346]

Localized UVA1 has been used for dyshidrosis[347,348] and has the same efficacy when compared to cream PUVA for chronic vesicular dyshidrotic eczema.[347] Because the long-term effects of UVA1 are unknown, it has been recommended that courses of localized UVA1 phototherapy be performed no more than twice annually.

PITYRIASIS LICHENOIDES

NB-UVB and BB-UVB are safe and effective for both pityriasis lichenoides chronica[349,350] and pityriasis lichenoides et varioliformis acuta.[351] A complete response has been reported to occur with NB-UVB in 65% of pityriasis lichenoides et varioliformis acuta patients and a partial response in the rest.[351] NB-UVB also led to a complete response in more than 85% of pityriasis lichenoides chronica patients.

LYMPHOMATOID PAPULOSIS

Oral PUVA has been used for patients with lymphomatoid papulosis,[352,353] but relapse may occur upon cessation of therapy.[353] Bath PUVA is effective in lymphomatoid papulosis in children.[354,355] Some patients have also responded to targeted phototherapy with the 308-nm excimer laser.[356] UVA1 (60 J/cm²) also has been employed,[357] but relapses are common.

TELANGIECTASIA MACULARIS ERUPTIVE PERSTANS

Oral PUVA is reserved for telangiectasia macularis eruptiva perstans patients with severe disease, because other therapies, such as laser treatment, may be safer long-term, and because the response is often temporary.[358-360]

URTICARIA PIGMENTOSA

UVA1 phototherapy ameliorates both the objective and subjective symptoms of urticaria pigmentosa in adult patients, and long-term remission can be achieved in many cases.[30,361,362] Although lesions may not respond completely with UVA1 therapy, the symptoms of pruritus are often relieved. Urinary histamine levels also decrease in response to UVA1. In some patients, systemic manifestations, such as diarrhea and migraine headaches, also have been reported to improve. In 1 patient with bone marrow infiltration, mast cell numbers decreased continuously after high-dose UVA1, which may have resulted from modulation of soluble cytokine production by UVA1-treated skin.[30] PUVA does not decrease mast cell numbers, which may explain its limited benefit in many patients.[363]

INDOLENT SYSTEMIC MASTOCYTOSIS

In a small case series, NB-UVB phototherapy resulted in complete and long-term remission of cutaneous lesions and pruritus after approximately 40 total treatments and a total median cumulative dose of 51.4 J/cm².[364] Even though the number of treatments needed to achieve improvement in symptoms was lower with PUVA therapy, the average total exposure was higher with PUVA. In the case series, serum tryptase levels trended downward in patients receiving phototherapy and potentially may be used as a surrogate marker for response in some patients.[365]

GRANULOMA ANNULARE

Patients with widespread granuloma annulare treated with PUVA have had complete clearance of their disease.[366] Maintenance therapy may result in prolonged disease-free intervals. Bath and cream PUVA also is reported to be useful for granuloma annulare.[367-369] Although the mechanism of action of PUVA in granuloma annulare is unclear, selective elimination of pathogenic cells may be one explanation. UVA1 phototherapy provides good or excellent results in the majority of patients, but discontinuation of treatment is followed by early reoccurrence of disease.[370] There are anecdotal reports of NB-UVB successfully treating disseminated granuloma annulare.[371]

PERFORATING DISORDERS

There has been some success in treating perforating disorders with NB-UVB phototherapy.[372] There are anecdotal reports that PUVA also is effective.[373] Patients are treated 2 to 3 times weekly, with lesions and symptoms clearing after 10 to 15 treatments. The mechanism by which improvement occurs is unknown.

REFERENCES

1. Menter A, Korman NJ, Elmets CA, et al. Guidelines of care for the management of psoriasis and psoriatic arthritis: section 5. Guidelines of care for the treatment of psoriasis with phototherapy and photochemotherapy. *J Am Acad Dermatol.* 2010;62:114-135.
2. Taylor DK, Anstey AV, Coleman AJ, et al. Guidelines for dosimetry and calibration in ultraviolet radiation therapy: a report of a British Photodermatology Group workshop. *Br J Dermatol.* 2002;146:755-763.
3. Kochevar IE. Photobiology. Basic science. *Dermatol Clin.* 1986;4:171-179.

4. Yoon JH, Lee CS, O'Connor TR, et al. The DNA damage spectrum produced by simulated sunlight. *J Mol Biol*. 2000;299:681-693.
5. Gibbs NK, Tye J, Norval M. Recent advances in urocanic acid photochemistry, photobiology and photoimmunology. *Photochem Photobiol Sci*. 2008;7:655-667.
6. Landeck L, Jakasa I, Dapic I, et al. The effect of epidermal levels of urocanic acid on 25-hydroxyvitamin D synthesis and inflammatory mediators upon narrowband UVB irradiation. *Photodermatol Photoimmunol Photomed*. 2016;32:214-223.
7. Fritsche E, Schäfer C, Calles C, et al. Lightening up the UV response by identification of the arylhydrocarbon receptor as a cytoplasmatic target for ultraviolet B radiation. *Proc Natl Acad Sci U S A*. 2007;104:8851-8856.
8. Heck DE, Vetrano AM, Mariano TM, et al. UVB light stimulates production of reactive oxygen species: unexpected role for catalase. *J Biol Chem*. 2003;278:22432-22436.
9. Freeman SE, Hacham H, Gange RW, et al. Wavelength dependence of pyrimidine dimer formation in DNA of human skin irradiated in situ with ultraviolet light. *Proc Natl Acad Sci U S A*. 1989;86:5605-5609.
10. Grether-Beck S, Felsner I, Brenden H, et al. Mitochondrial cytochrome c release mediates ceramide-induced activator protein 2 activation and gene expression in keratinocytes. *J Biol Chem*. 2003;278:47498-47507.
11. Xiang Y, Liu G, Yang L, et al. UVA-induced protection of skin through the induction of heme oxygenase-1. *Biosci Trends*. 2011;5:239-244.
12. Diffey BL, Kochevar IE. Basic principles of photobiology. In: Lim HW, Hönigsmann H, Hawk JLM, eds. *Photodermatology*. New York, NY: Informa Healthcare; 2007:15-27.
13. Averbeck D. Recent advances in psoralen phototoxicity mechanism. *Photochem Photobiol*. 1989;50:859-882.
14. Krutmann J, Morita A, Elmets CA. Mechanisms of photo(chemo)therapy. In: Krutmann J, Hönigsmann H, Elmets CA, eds. *Dermatological Phototherapy and Photodiagnostic Methods*. 2nd ed. Berlin, Germany: Springer-Verlag; 2009:63-77.
15. Shreedhar V, Giese T, Sung VW, et al. A cytokine cascade including prostaglandin E2, IL-4, and IL-10 is responsible for UV-induced systemic immune suppression. *J Immunol*. 1998;160:3783-3789.
16. Pentland A, Needleman P. Modulation of keratinocyte proliferation in vitro by endogenous prostaglandin synthesis. *J Clin Invest*. 1986;77:246-261.
17. Pentland AP, Mahoney M, Jacobs SC, et al. Enhanced prostaglandin synthesis after ultraviolet injury is mediated by endogenous histamine stimulation. *J Clin Invest*. 1990;86:566-574.
18. Rodriguez-Burford C, Tu JH, Mercurio M, et al. Selective cyclooxygenase-2 inhibition produces heterogeneous erythema response to ultraviolet irradiation. *J Invest Dermatol*. 2005;125:1317.
19. Pilkington SM, Gibbs NK, Costello P, et al. Effect of oral eicosapentaenoic acid on epidermal Langerhans cell numbers and PGD2 production in UVR-exposed human skin: a randomised controlled study. *Exp Dermatol*. 2016;25(12):962-968.
20. Zhang Q, Yao Y, Konger RL, et al. UVB radiation-mediated inhibition of contact hypersensitivity reactions is dependent on the platelet-activating factor system. *J Invest Dermatol*. 2008;128:1780-1787.
21. Seiffert K, Granstein RD. Neuropeptides and neuroendocrine hormones in ultraviolet radiation-induced immunosuppression. *Methods*. 2002;28:97-103.
22. Zhang D, Chen Y, Chen L, et al. Ultraviolet irradiation promotes FOXP3 transcription via p53 in psoriasis. *Exp Dermatol*. 2016;25:513-518.
23. Buhl T, Schon MP. Peeking into immunoregulatory effects of phototherapy. *Exp Dermatol*. 2016;25:511-512.
24. Meulenbroeks C, van Weelden H, Schwartz C, et al. Basophil-derived amphiregulin is essential for UVB irradiation-induced immune suppression. *J Invest Dermatol*. 2015;135:222-228.
25. Zaiss DM, van Loosdregt J, Gorlani A, et al. Amphiregulin enhances regulatory T cell-suppressive function via the epidermal growth factor receptor. *Immunity*. 2013;38:275-284.
26. Bogaczewicz J, Malinowska K, Sysa-Jedrzejowska A, et al. Medium-dose ultraviolet A1 phototherapy and mRNA expression of TSLP, TARC, IL-5, and IL-13 in acute skin lesions in atopic dermatitis. *Int J Dermatol*. 2016;55:856-863.
27. Bogaczewicz J, Malinowska K, Sysa-Jedrzejowska A, et al. Medium-dose ultraviolet A1 phototherapy improves SCORAD index and increases mRNA expression of interleukin-4 without direct effect on human beta defensin-1, interleukin-10, and interleukin-31. *Int J Dermatol*. 2016;55:e380-e385.
28. Morita A, Werfel T, Stege H, et al. Evidence that singlet oxygen-induced human T helper cell apoptosis is the basic mechanism of ultraviolet-A radiation phototherapy. *J Exp Med*. 1997;186:1763-1768.
29. Ozawa M, Ferenczi K, Kikuchi T, et al. 312-nanometer ultraviolet B light (narrow-band UVB) induces apoptosis of T cells within psoriatic lesions. *J Exp Med*. 1999;189:711-718.
30. Stege H, Schopf E, Ruzicka T, et al. High-dose UVA1 for urticaria pigmentosa. *Lancet*. 1996;347:64.
31. Vella Briffa D, Eady R, James M, et al. Photochemotherapy (PUVA) in the treatment of urticaria pigmentosa. *Br J Dermatol*. 1983;109:67-75.
32. Scharffetter K, Wlaschek M, Hogg A, et al. UVA irradiation induces collagenase in human dermal fibroblasts in vitro and in vivo. *Arch Dermatol Res*. 1991;283:506-511.
33. Petersen MJ, Hansen C, Craig S. Ultraviolet A irradiation stimulates collagenase production in cultured human fibroblasts. *J Invest Dermatol*. 1992;99:440-444.
34. Wlaschek M, Heinen G, Poswig A, et al. UVA-induced autocrine stimulation of fibroblast-derived collagenase/MMP-1 by interrelated loops of interleukin-1 and interleukin-6. *Photochem Photobiol*. 1994;59:550-556.
35. Brenner M, Herzinger T, Berking C, et al. Phototherapy and photochemotherapy of sclerosing skin diseases. *Photodermatol Photoimmunol Photomed*. 2005;21:157-165.
36. Young AR. Damage from acute vs. chronic solar exposure. In: Giacomoni PU, ed. *Biophysical and Physiological Effects of Solar Radiation on Human Skin*. London, UK: RSC Publishing; 2007:3-23.
37. Brenner M, Hearing VJ. The protective role of melanin against UV damage in human skin. *Photochem Photobiol*. 2008;84:539-549.
38. Parrish JA, Jaenicke KF, Anderson RR. Erythema and

38. melanogenesis action spectra of normal human skin. *Photochem Photobiol.* 1982;36:187-191.
39. Eller MS, Gilchrest BA. Tanning as part of the eukaryotic SOS response. *Pigment Cell Res.* 2000;13(suppl 8):94-97.
40. Gilchrest BA, Eller MS. DNA photodamage stimulates melanogenesis and other photoprotective responses. *J Investig Dermatol Symp Proc.* 1999;4:35-40.
41. Eller MS, Ostrom K, Gilchrest BA. DNA damage enhances melanogenesis. *Proc Natl Acad Sci U S A.* 1996;93:1087-1092.
42. Gilchrest BA, Zhai S, Eller MS, et al. Treatment of human melanocytes and S91 melanoma cells with the DNA repair enzyme T4 endonuclease V enhances melanogenesis after ultraviolet irradiation. *J Invest Dermatol.* 1993;101:666-672.
43. Passeron T, Ostovari N, Zakaria W, et al. Topical tacrolimus and the 308-nm excimer laser: a synergistic combination for the treatment of vitiligo. *Arch Dermatol.* 2004;140:1065-1069.
44. Abdel-Naser MB, Hann SK, Bystryn JC. Oral psoralen with UV-A therapy releases circulating growth factor(s) that stimulates cell proliferation. *Arch Dermatol.* 1997;133:1530-1533.
45. Saleh FY, Awad SS, Nasif GA, et al. Epithelial expression of cytokeratins 15 and 19 in vitiligo. *J Cosmet Dermatol.* 2016;15(4):312-317.
46. Reidel U, Bechstein S, Lange-Asschenfeldt B, et al. Treatment of localized mycosis fungoides with digital UV photochemotherapy. *Photodermatol Photoimmunol Photomed.* 2015;31:333-340.
47. Werfel T, Holiangu F, Niemann KH, et al. Digital ultraviolet therapy: a novel therapeutic approach for the targeted treatment of psoriasis vulgaris. *Br J Dermatol.* 2015;172:746-753.
48. van Weelden H, De La Faille HB, Young E, et al. A new development in UVB phototherapy of psoriasis. *Br J Dermatol.* 1988;119:11-19.
49. Perry HO, Soderstrom CW, Schulze RW. The Goeckerman treatment of psoriasis. *Arch Dermatol.* 1968;98:178-182.
50. Schneider LA, Hinrichs R, Scharffetter-Kochanek K. Phototherapy and photochemotherapy. *Clin Dermatol.* 2008;26:464-476.
51. Parrish JA, Jaenicke KF. Action spectrum for phototherapy of psoriasis. *J Invest Dermatol.* 1981;76:359-362.
52. Lynch M, Carroll F, Kavanagh A, et al. Comparison of a semiautomated hand-held device to test minimal erythema dose before narrowband ultraviolet B phototherapy with the conventional method using matched doses. *J Eur Acad Dermatol Venereol.* 2014;28:1696-1700.
53. Darne S, Stewart LC, Farr PM, et al. Investigation of cutaneous photoadaptation to narrowband ultraviolet B. *Br J Dermatol.* 2014;170:392-397.
54. Parrish JA, Fitzpatrick TB, Tanenbaum L, et al. Photochemotherapy of psoriasis with oral methoxsalen and longwave ultraviolet light. *N Engl J Med.* 1974;291:1207-1211.
55. Halpern SM, Anstey AV, Dawe RS, et al. Guidelines for topical PUVA: a report of a workshop of the British Photodermatology Group. *Br J Dermatol.* 2000;142:22-31.
55A. Pozo-Román T, González-López A, Velasco-Vaquero ME, et al. Psoralen cream plus ultraviolet A photochemotherapy (PUVA cream): our experience. *J Eur Acad Dermatol Venereol.* 2006 Feb;20(2):136-142. Available at https://www.ncbi.nlm.nih.gov/pubmed/16441619.
56. Mutzhas MF, Holzle E, Hofmann C, et al. A new apparatus with high radiation energy between 320-460 nm: physical description and dermatological applications. *J Invest Dermatol.* 1981;76:42-47.
57. Krutmann J, Czech W, Diepgen T, et al. High-dose UVA1 therapy in the treatment of patients with atopic dermatitis. *J Am Acad Dermatol.* 1992;26(2, pt 1):225-230.
58. Krutmann J, Morita A. Mechanisms of ultraviolet (UV) B and UVA phototherapy. *J Investig Dermatol Symp Proc.* 1999;4:70-72.
59. Dawe RS. Ultraviolet A1 phototherapy. *Br J Dermatol.* 2003;148:626-637.
60. Tuchinda C, Kerr HA, Taylor CR, et al. UVA1 phototherapy for cutaneous diseases: an experience of 92 cases in the United States. *Photodermatol Photoimmunol Photomed.* 2006;22:247-253.
61. Leone G, Iacovelli P, Paro Vidolin A, et al. Monochromatic excimer light 308 nm in the treatment of vitiligo: a pilot study. *J Eur Acad Dermatol Venereol.* 2003;17:531-537.
62. Nguyen T, Gattu S, Pugashetti R, et al. Practice of phototherapy in the treatment of moderate-to-severe psoriasis. *Curr Probl Dermatol.* 2009;38:59-78.
63. Babino G, Giunta A, Esposito M, et al. UVA1 Laser in the treatment of vitiligo. *Photomed Laser Surg.* 2016;34:200-204.
64. Toll A, Velez-Gonzalez M, Gallardo F, et al. Treatment of localized persistent plaque psoriasis with incoherent narrowband ultraviolet B phototherapy. *J Dermatolog Treat.* 2005;16:165-168.
65. Lotti TM, Menchini G, Andreassi L. UV-B radiation microphototherapy. An elective treatment for segmental vitiligo. *J Eur Acad Dermatol Venereol.* 1999;13:102-108.
66. Zanardelli M, Kovacevic M, McCoy J, et al. Management of chronic pruritus with a UV filtering topical cream. *Dermatol Ther.* 2016;29:101-103.
67. Lee E, Koo J, Berger T. UVB phototherapy and skin cancer risk: a review of the literature. *Int J Dermatol.* 2005;44:355-360.
68. Weischer M, Blum A, Eberhard F, et al. No evidence for increased skin cancer risk in psoriasis patients treated with broadband or narrowband UVB phototherapy: a first retrospective study. *Acta Derm Venereol.* 2004;84:370-374.
69. Hearn RM, Kerr AC, Rahim KF, et al. Incidence of skin cancers in 3867 patients treated with narrowband ultraviolet B phototherapy. *Br J Dermatol.* 2008;159:931-935.
70. Aubin F, Vigan M, Puzenat E, et al. Evaluation of a novel 308-nm monochromatic excimer light delivery system in dermatology: a pilot study in different chronic localized dermatoses. *Br J Dermatol.* 2005;152:99-103.
71. Lim JL, Stern RS. High levels of ultraviolet B exposure increase the risk of non-melanoma skin cancer in psoralen and ultraviolet A-treated patients. *J Invest Dermatol.* 2005;124:505-513.
72. Stern RS, Laird N. The carcinogenic risk of treatments for severe psoriasis. *Cancer.* 1994;73:2759-2764.
73. Melski JW, Tanenbaum L, Parrish JA, et al. Oral methoxsalen photochemotherapy for the treatment of psoriasis: a cooperative clinical trial. 1977. *J Invest Dermatol.* 1989;92:153S; discussion 154S-156S.

74. Henseler T, Wolff K, Honigsmann H, et al. Oral 8-methoxypsoralen photochemotherapy of psoriasis. The European PUVA study: a cooperative study among 18 European centres. *Lancet.* 1981;1:853-857.
75. Honigsmann H. Psoralen photochemotherapy—mechanisms, drugs, toxicity. *Curr Probl Dermatol.* 1986:15:52-66.
76. Basarab T, Millard TP, McGregor JM, et al. Atypical pigmented lesions following extensive PUVA therapy. *Clin Exp Dermatol.* 2000;25:135-137.
77. Rhodes AR, Harrist TJ, Momtaz TK. The PUVA-induced pigmented macule: a lentiginous proliferation of large, sometimes cytologically atypical, melanocytes. *J Am Acad Dermatol.* 1983;9:47-58.
78. Lassacher A, Worda M, Kaddu S, et al. T1799A BRAF mutation is common in PUVA lentigines. *J Invest Dermatol.* 2006;126:1915-1917.
79. Brose MS, Volpe P, Feldman M, et al. BRAF and RAS mutations in human lung cancer and melanoma. *Cancer Res.* 2002;62:6997-7000.
80. Gorden A, Osman I, Gai W, et al. Analysis of BRAF and N-RAS mutations in metastatic melanoma tissues. *Cancer Res.* 2003;63:3955-3957.
81. Pollock PM, Harper UL, Hansen KS, et al. High frequency of BRAF mutations in nevi. *Nat Genet.* 2003;33:19-20.
82. Poynter JN, Elder JT, Fullen DR, et al. BRAF and NRAS mutations in melanoma and melanocytic nevi. *Melanoma Res.* 2006;16:267-273.
83. Lever LR, Farr PM. Skin cancers or premalignant lesions occur in half of high-dose PUVA patients. *Br J Dermatol.* 1994;131:215-219.
84. Dunnick JK, Forbes PD, Eustis SL, et al. Tumors of the skin in the HRA/Skh mouse after treatment with 8-methoxypsoralen and UVA radiation. *Fundam Appl Toxicol.* 1991;16:92-102.
85. Stern RS, Liebman EJ, Vakeva L. Oral psoralen and ultraviolet-A light (PUVA) treatment of psoriasis and persistent risk of nonmelanoma skin cancer. PUVA Follow-up Study. *J Natl Cancer Inst.* 1998;90:1278-1284.
86. Marcil I, Stern RS. Squamous-cell cancer of the skin in patients given PUVA and ciclosporin: nested cohort crossover study. *Lancet.* 2001;358:1042-1045.
87. Nijsten TE, Stern RS. Oral retinoid use reduces cutaneous squamous cell carcinoma risk in patients with psoriasis treated with psoralen-UVA: a nested cohort study. *J Am Acad Dermatol.* 2003;49:644-650.
88. Stern RS. Genital tumors among men with psoriasis exposed to psoralens and ultraviolet A radiation (PUVA) and ultraviolet B radiation. The Photochemotherapy Follow-up Study. *N Engl J Med.* 1990;322:1093-1097.
89. Stern RS, Bagheri S, Nichols K. The persistent risk of genital tumors among men treated with psoralen plus ultraviolet A (PUVA) for psoriasis. *J Am Acad Dermatol.* 2002;47:33-39.
90. Abdulla FR, Breneman C, Adams B, et al. Standards for genital protection in phototherapy units. *J Am Acad Dermatol.* 2010;62:223-226.
91. Stern RS, Nichols KT, Vakeva LH. Malignant melanoma in patients treated for psoriasis with methoxsalen (psoralen) and ultraviolet A radiation (PUVA). The PUVA Follow-Up Study. *N Engl J Med.* 1997;336:1041-1045.
92. Lindelof B. Risk of melanoma with psoralen/ultraviolet A therapy for psoriasis. Do the known risks now outweigh the benefits? *Drug Saf.* 1999;20:289-297.
93. Stern RS. Lymphoma risk in psoriasis: results of the PUVA Follow-Up Study. *Arch Dermatol.* 2006;142:1132-1135.
94. Andley UP, Chylack LT Jr. Recent studies on photodamage to the eye with special reference to clinical phototherapeutic procedures. *Photodermatol Photoimmunol Photomed.* 1990;7:98-105.
95. Woo TY, Wong RC, Wong JM, et al. Lenticular psoralen photoproducts and cataracts of a PUVA-treated psoriatic patient. *Arch Dermatol.* 1985;121:1307-1308.
96. Boukes RJ, van Balen AT, Bruynzeel DP. A retrospective study of ocular findings in patients treated with PUVA. *Doc Ophthalmol.* 1985;59:11-19.
97. Calzavara-Pinton PG, Carlino A, Manfredi E, et al. Ocular side effects of PUVA-treated patients refusing eye sun protection. *Acta Derm Venereol Suppl (Stockh).* 1994;186:164-165.
98. Malanos D, Stern RS. Psoralen plus ultraviolet A does not increase the risk of cataracts: a 25-year prospective study. *J Am Acad Dermatol.* 2007;57:231-237.
99. Abdullah AN, Keczkes K. Cutaneous and ocular side-effects of PUVA photochemotherapy—a 10-year follow-up study. *Clin Exp Dermatol.* 1989;14:421-424.
100. Stern RS, Parrish JA, Fitzpatrick TB. Ocular findings in patients treated with PUVA. *J Invest Dermatol.* 1985;85:269-273.
101. Ronnerfalt L, Lydahl E, Wennersten G, et al. Ophthalmological study of patients undergoing long-term PUVA therapy. *Acta Derm Venereol.* 1982;62:501-505.
102. Glew WB, Nigra TP. Psoralens and ocular effects in humans. *Natl Cancer Inst Monogr.* 1984;66:235-239.
103. Krutmann J, Diepgen TL, Luger TA, et al. High-dose UVA1 therapy for atopic dermatitis: results of a multicenter trial. *J Am Acad Dermatol.* 1998;38:589-593.
104. Tzaneva S, Seeber A, Schwaiger M, et al. High-dose versus medium-dose UVA1 phototherapy for patients with severe generalized atopic dermatitis. *J Am Acad Dermatol.* 2001;45:503-507.
105. von Kobyletzki G, Pieck C, Hoffmann K, et al. Medium-dose UVA1 cold-light phototherapy in the treatment of severe atopic dermatitis. *J Am Acad Dermatol.* 1999;41:931-937.
106. Cavard C, Zider A, Vernet M, et al. In vivo activation by ultraviolet rays of the human immunodeficiency virus type 1 long terminal repeat. *J Clin Invest.* 1990;86:1369-1374.
107. Stein B, Kramer M, Rahmsdorf HJ, et al. UV-induced transcription from the human immunodeficiency virus type 1 (HIV-1) long terminal repeat and UV-induced secretion of an extracellular factor that induces HIV-1 transcription in nonirradiated cells. *J Virol.* 1989;63:4540-4544.
108. Yamagoe S, Kohda T, Oishi M. Poly(ADP-ribose) polymerase inhibitors suppress UV-induced human immunodeficiency virus type 1 gene expression at the posttranscriptional level. *Mol Cell Biol.* 1991;11:3522-3527.
109. Vogel J, Cepeda M, Tschachler E, et al. UV activation of human immunodeficiency virus gene expression in transgenic mice. *J Virol.* 1992;66:1-5.
110. Zmudzka BZ, Miller SA, Jacobs ME, et al. Medical UV exposures and HIV activation. *Photochem Photobiol.* 1996;64:246-253.
111. Breuer-McHam J, Simpson E, Dougherty I, et al. Activation of HIV in human skin by ultraviolet B radiation and its inhibition by NFkappaB blocking agents. *Photochem Photobiol.* 2001;74:805-810.
112. Breuer-McHam J, Marshall G, Adu-Oppong A, et al. Alterations in HIV expression in AIDS patients with psoriasis or pruritus treated with phototherapy. *J*

113. Gelfand JM, Rudikoff D, Lebwohl M, et al. Effect of UV-B phototherapy on plasma HIV type 1 RNA viral level: a self-controlled prospective study. *Arch Dermatol.* 1998;134:940-945.
114. Akaraphanth R, Lim HW. HIV, UV and immunosuppression. *Photodermatol Photoimmunol Photomed.* 1999;15:28-31.
115. Menon K, Van Voorhees AS, Bebo BF Jr, et al. Psoriasis in patients with HIV infection: from the medical board of the National Psoriasis Foundation. *J Am Acad Dermatol.* 2010;62:291-299.
116. Juzeniene A, Stokke KT, Thune P, et al. Pilot study of folate status in healthy volunteers and in patients with psoriasis before and after UV exposure. *J Photochem Photobiol B.* 2010;101:111-116.
117. El-Saie LT, Rabie AR, Kamel MI, et al. Effect of narrowband ultraviolet B phototherapy on serum folic acid levels in patients with psoriasis. *Lasers Med Sci.* 2011;26:481-485.
118. Park KK, Murase JE. Narrowband UV-B phototherapy during pregnancy and folic acid depletion. *Arch Dermatol.* 2012;148:132-133.
119. Gloor M, Scherotzke A. Age dependence of ultraviolet light-induced erythema following narrow-band UVB exposure. *Photodermatol Photoimmunol Photomed.* 2002;18:121-126.
120. Powell JB, Gach JE. Phototherapy in the elderly. *Clin Exp Dermatol.* 2015;40:605-610.
121. Cowen EW, Nguyen JC, Miller DD, et al. Chronic phototoxicity and aggressive squamous cell carcinoma of the skin in children and adults during treatment with voriconazole. *J Am Acad Dermatol.* 2010;62: 31-37.
122. Vanacker A, Fabre G, Van Dorpe J, et al. Aggressive cutaneous squamous cell carcinoma associated with prolonged voriconazole therapy in a renal transplant patient. *Am J Transplant.* 2008;8:877-880.
123. McCarthy KL, Playford EG, Looke DF, et al. Severe photosensitivity causing multifocal squamous cell carcinomas secondary to prolonged voriconazole therapy. *Clin Infect Dis.* 2007;44:e55-e56.
124. Fluhr JW, Gloor M. The antimicrobial effect of narrow-band UVB (313 nm) and UVA1 (345-440 nm) radiation in vitro. *Photodermatol Photoimmunol Photomed.* 1997;13:197-201.
125. Hruza L, Pentland A. Mechanisms of UV-induced inflammation. *J Invest Dermatol.* 1993;100:S35-S41.
126. Beissert S, Schwarz T. Role of immunomodulation in diseases responsive to phototherapy. *Methods.* 2002;28:138-144.
127. Walters IB, Ozawa M, Cardinale I, et al. Narrowband (312-nm) UV-B suppresses interferon gamma and interleukin (IL) 12 and increases IL-4 transcripts: differential regulation of cytokines at the single-cell level. *Arch Dermatol.* 2003;139:155-161.
128. Vahavihu K, Ala-Houhala M, Peric M, et al. Narrowband UVB treatment improves vitamin D balance and alters antimicrobial peptide expression in skin lesions of psoriasis and atopic dermatitis. *Br J Dermatol.* 2010;163(2):321-328.
129. Vahavihu K, Ylianttila L, Kautiainen H, et al. Narrowband ultraviolet B course improves vitamin D balance in women in winter. *Br J Dermatol.* 2010;162: 848-853.
130. Zhu JW, Wu XJ, Lu ZF, et al. Role of VEGF receptors in normal and psoriatic human keratinocytes: evidence from irradiation with different UV sources. *PLoS One.* 2013;8:e55463.
131. Furuhashi T, Saito C, Torii K, et al. Photo(chemo)therapy reduces circulating Th17 cells and restores circulating regulatory T cells in psoriasis. *PLoS One.* 2013;8:e54895.
132. Gui J, Gober M, Yang X, et al. Therapeutic elimination of the type 1 interferon receptor for treating psoriatic skin inflammation. *J Invest Dermatol.* 2016;136:1990-2002.
133. Coimbra S, Oliveira H, Reis F, et al. C-reactive protein and leucocyte activation in psoriasis vulgaris according to severity and therapy. *J Eur Acad Dermatol Venereol.* 2010;24(7):789-796.
134. Metwally D, Sayed K, Abdel Hay R, et al. Reduction in tissue plasmin: a new mechanism of action of narrowband ultraviolet B in psoriasis. *Clin Exp Dermatol.* 2015;40:416-420.
135. Green C, Ferguson J, Lakshmipathi T, et al. 311 nm UVB phototherapy—an effective treatment for psoriasis. *Br J Dermatol.* 1988;119:691-696.
136. Stern RS, Armstrong RB, Anderson TF, et al. Effect of continued ultraviolet B phototherapy on the duration of remission of psoriasis: a randomized study. *J Am Acad Dermatol.* 1986;15:546-552.
137. Lebwohl M, Drake L, Menter A, et al. Consensus conference: acitretin in combination with UVB or PUVA in the treatment of psoriasis. *J Am Acad Dermatol.* 2001;45:544-553.
138. Iest J, Boer J. Combined treatment of psoriasis with acitretin and UVB phototherapy compared with acitretin alone and UVB alone. *Br J Dermatol.* 1989;120:665-670.
139. Green C, Lakshmipathi T, Johnson BE, et al. A comparison of the efficacy and relapse rates of narrowband UVB (TL-01) monotherapy vs. etretinate (re-TL-01) vs. etretinate-PUVA (re-PUVA) in the treatment of psoriasis patients. *Br J Dermatol.* 1992;127:5-9.
140. Lebwohl M. Acitretin in combination with UVB or PUVA. *J Am Acad Dermatol.* 1999;41: S22-S24.
141. Caliskan E, Tunca M, Açıkgöz G, et al. Narrow band ultraviolet-B versus Goeckerman therapy for psoriasis with and without acitretin: a retrospective study. *Indian J Dermatol Venereol Leprol.* 2015;81:584-587.
142. Asawanonda P, Nateetongrungsak Y. Methotrexate plus narrowband UVB phototherapy versus narrowband UVB phototherapy alone in the treatment of plaque-type psoriasis: a randomized, placebo-controlled study. *J Am Acad Dermatol.* 2006;54:1013-1018.
143. Kircik L, Bagel J, Korman N, et al. Utilization of narrow-band ultraviolet light B therapy and etanercept for the treatment of psoriasis (UNITE): efficacy, safety, and patient-reported outcomes. *J Drugs Dermatol.* 2008;7:245-253.
144. Bagel J. LCD plus NB-UVB reduces time to improvement of psoriasis vs. NB-UVB alone. *J Drugs Dermatol.* 2009;8:351-357.
145. Ashcroft DM, Li Wan Po A, Williams HC, et al. Combination regimens of topical calcipotriene in chronic plaque psoriasis: systematic review of efficacy and tolerability. *Arch Dermatol.* 2000;136:1536-1543.
146. Koo J. Calcipotriol/calcipotriene (Dovonex/Daivonex) in combination with phototherapy: a review. *J Am Acad Dermatol.* 1997;37(3, pt 2):S59-S61.
147. Kragballe K. Combination of topical calcipotriol (MC 903) and UVB radiation for psoriasis vulgaris. *Dermatologica.* 1990;181:211-214.
148. Bourke JF, Iqbal SJ, Hutchinson PE. The effects of

148. UVB plus calcipotriol on systemic calcium homeostasis in patients with chronic plaque psoriasis. *Clin Exp Dermatol.* 1997;22:259-261.
149. Hecker D, Lebwohl M. Topical calcipotriene in combination with UVB phototherapy for psoriasis. *Int J Dermatol.* 1997;36:302-303.
150. Woo WK, McKenna KE. Combination TL01 ultraviolet B phototherapy and topical calcipotriol for psoriasis: a prospective randomized placebo-controlled clinical trial. *Br J Dermatol.* 2003;149, 146-150.
151. Youn JI, Park BS, Chung JH, et al. Photoprotective effect of calcipotriol upon skin photoreaction to UVA and UVB. *Photodermatol Photoimmunol Photomed.* 1997;13:109-114.
152. Koo JY, Lowe NJ, Lew-Kaya DA, et al. Tazarotene plus UVB phototherapy in the treatment of psoriasis. *J Am Acad Dermatol.* 2000;43(5, pt 1):821-828.
153. Hecker D, Worsley J, Yueh G, et al. Interactions between tazarotene and ultraviolet light. *J Am Acad Dermatol.* 1999;41:927-930.
154. Magliocco MA, Pandya K, Dombrovskiy V, et al. A randomized, double-blind, vehicle-controlled, bilateral comparison trial of bexarotene gel 1% versus vehicle gel in combination with narrowband UVB phototherapy for moderate to severe psoriasis vulgaris. *J Am Acad Dermatol.* 2006;54:115-118.
155. Lebwohl M, Martinez J, Weber P, et al. Effects of topical preparations on the erythemogenicity of UVB: implications for psoriasis phototherapy. *J Am Acad Dermatol.* 1995;32:469-471.
156. Hoffmann K, Kaspar K, Gambichler T, et al. Change in ultraviolet (UV) transmission following the application of Vaseline to non-irradiated and UVB-exposed split skin. *Br J Dermatol.* 2000;143:532-538.
157. Berne B, Blom I, Spangberg S. Enhanced response of psoriasis to UVB therapy after pretreatment with a lubricating base. A single-blind controlled study. *Acta Derm Venereol.* 1990;70:474-477.
157A. Kristensen B, Kristensen O. *Acta Derm Venereol.* 1991;71(1):37-40. Topical salicylic acid interferes with UVB therapy for psoriasis. Available at https://www.ncbi.nlm.nih.gov/pubmed/1676212.
158. Feldman SR, Mellen BG, Housman TS, et al. Efficacy of the 308-nm excimer laser for treatment of psoriasis: results of a multicenter study. *J Am Acad Dermatol.* 2002;46:900-906.
159. Vongthongsri R, Konschitzky R, Seeber A, et al. Randomized, double-blind comparison of 1 mg/L versus 5 mg/L methoxsalen bath-PUVA therapy for chronic plaque-type psoriasis. *J Am Acad Dermatol.* 2006;55:627-631.
160. Debbaneh MG, Levin E, Sanchez Rodriguez R, et al. Plaque-based sub-blistering dosimetry: reaching PASI-75 after two treatments with 308-nm excimer laser in a generalized psoriasis patient. *J Dermatolog Treat.* 2015;26:45-48.
161. Sivanesan SP, Gattu S, Hong J, et al. Randomized, double-blind, placebo-controlled evaluation of the efficacy of oral psoralen plus ultraviolet A for the treatment of plaque-type psoriasis using the Psoriasis Area Severity Index score (improvement of 75% or greater) at 12 weeks. *J Am Acad Dermatol.* 2009;61:793-798.
162. Yones SS, Palmer RA, Garibaldinos TT, et al. Randomized double-blind trial of the treatment of chronic plaque psoriasis: efficacy of psoralen-UV-A therapy vs narrowband UV-B therapy. *Arch Dermatol.* 2006;142:836-842.
163. Markham T, Rogers S, Collins P. Narrowband UV-B (TL-01) phototherapy vs oral 8-methoxypsoralen psoralen-UV-A for the treatment of chronic plaque psoriasis. *Arch Dermatol.* 2003;139:325-328.
164. Tanew A, Radakovic-Fijan S, Schemper M, et al. Narrowband UV-B phototherapy vs photochemotherapy in the treatment of chronic plaque-type psoriasis: a paired comparison study. *Arch Dermatol.* 1999;135:519-524.
165. Van Weelden H, Baart de la Faille H, Young E, van der Leun JC. Comparison of narrow-band UV-B phototherapy and PUVA photochemotherapy in the treatment of psoriasis. *Acta Derm Venereol.* 1990;70:212-215.
166. Gordon PM, Diffey BL, Matthews JN, et al. A randomized comparison of narrow-band TL-01 phototherapy and PUVA photochemotherapy for psoriasis. *J Am Acad Dermatol.* 1999;41:728-732.
167. Ibbotson SH, Dawe RS, Dinkova-Kostova AT, et al. Glutathione S-transferase genotype is associated with sensitivity to psoralen-ultraviolet A photochemotherapy. *Br J Dermatol.* 2012;166:380-388.
168. Morison WL. Phototherapy and photochemotherapy. *Adv Dermatol.* 1992;7:255-270; discussion 271.
169. Honigsmann H, Wolff K. Results of therapy for psoriasis using retinoid and photochemotherapy (RePUVA). *Pharmacol Ther.* 1989;40:67-73.
170. Tzaneva S, Honigsmann H, Tanew A, et al. A comparison of psoralen plus ultraviolet A (PUVA) monotherapy, tacalcitol plus PUVA and tazarotene plus PUVA in patients with chronic plaque-type psoriasis. *Br J Dermatol.* 2002;147:748-753.
171. Behrens S, von Kobyletzki G, Gruss C, et al. PUVA-bath photochemotherapy (PUVA-soak therapy) of recalcitrant dermatoses of the palms and soles. *Photodermatol Photoimmunol Photomed.* 1999;15:47-51.
172. Birgin B, Fetil E, Ilknur T, et al. Effects of topical petrolatum and salicylic acid upon skin photoreaction to UVA. *Eur J Dermatol.* 2005;15:156-158.
173. Wolf P, Weger W, Patra V, et al. Desired response to phototherapy versus photo-aggravation in psoriasis: what makes the difference? *Exp Dermatol.* 2016;25(12):937-944.
174. Nakamura M, Bhutani T, Koo JY. Narrowband UVB-induced iatrogenic polymorphous light eruption: a case and suggestions to overcome this rare complication. *Dermatol Online J.* 2016;22(6).
175. George SA, Bilsland DJ, Johnson BE, et al. Narrow-band (TL-01) UVB air-conditioned phototherapy for chronic severe adult atopic dermatitis. *Br J Dermatol.* 1993;128:49-56.
176. Grundmann-Kollmann M, Behrens S, Podda M, et al. Phototherapy for atopic eczema with narrow-band UVB. *J Am Acad Dermatol.* 1999;40:995-997.
177. Hudson-Peacock MJ, Diffey BL, Farr PM. Narrow-band UVB phototherapy for severe atopic dermatitis. *Br J Dermatol.* 1996;135:332.
178. Reynolds NJ, Franklin V, Gray JC, et al. Narrow-band ultraviolet B and broad-band ultraviolet A phototherapy in adult atopic eczema: a randomised controlled trial. *Lancet.* 2001;357:2012-2016.
179. Der-Petrossian M, Seeber A, Honigsmann H, et al. Half-side comparison study on the efficacy of 8-methoxypsoralen bath-PUVA versus narrow-band ultraviolet B phototherapy in patients with severe chronic atopic dermatitis. *Br J Dermatol.* 2000;142:39-43.
180. Brazzelli V, Prestinari F, Chiesa MG, et al. Sequential

treatment of severe atopic dermatitis with cyclosporin A and low-dose narrow-band UVB phototherapy. *Dermatology*. 2002;204:252-254.
181. Clayton TH, Clark SM, Turner D, et al. The treatment of severe atopic dermatitis in childhood with narrowband ultraviolet B phototherapy. *Clin Exp Dermatol*. 2007;32:28-33.
182. Ersoy-Evans S, Altaykan A, Sahin S, et al. Phototherapy in childhood. *Pediatr Dermatol*. 2008;25:599-605.
183. Jury CS, McHenry P, Burden AD, et al. Narrowband ultraviolet B (UVB) phototherapy in children. *Clin Exp Dermatol*. 2006;31:196-199.
184. Tay YK, Morelli JG, Weston WL. Experience with UVB phototherapy in children. *Pediatr Dermatol*. 1996;13:406-409.
185. Sidbury R, Davis DM, Cohen DE, et al. Guidelines of care for the management of atopic dermatitis: section 3. Management and treatment with phototherapy and systemic agents. *J Am Acad Dermatol*. 2014;71:327-349.
186. Pasic A, Ceović R, Lipozencić J, et al. Phototherapy in pediatric patients. *Pediatr Dermatol*. 2003;20: 71-77.
187. Lerche CM, Philipsen PA, Poulsen T, et al. Topical pimecrolimus and tacrolimus do not accelerate photocarcinogenesis in hairless mice after UVA or simulated solar radiation. *Exp Dermatol*. 2009;18:246-251.
188. Nistico SP, Saraceno R, Capriotti E, et al. Efficacy of monochromatic excimer light (308 nm) in the treatment of atopic dermatitis in adults and children. *Photomed Laser Surg*. 2008;26:14-18.
189. Baltás E, Csoma Z, Bodai L, et al. Treatment of atopic dermatitis with the xenon chloride excimer laser. *J Eur Acad Dermatol Venereol*. 2006;20:657-660.
190. Mavilia L, Mori M, Rossi R, et al. 308 nm monochromatic excimer light in dermatology: personal experience and review of the literature. *G Ital Dermatol Venereol*. 2008;143:329-337.
191. Atherton DJ, Carabott F, Glover MT, et al. The role of psoralen photochemotherapy (PUVA) in the treatment of severe atopic eczema in adolescents. *Br J Dermatol*. 1988;118:791-795.
192. Morison WL, Parrish J, Fitzpatrick TB. Oral psoralen photochemotherapy of atopic eczema. *Br J Dermatol*. 1978;98:25-30.
193. Uetsu N, Horio T. Treatment of persistent severe atopic dermatitis in 113 Japanese patients with oral psoralen photo-chemotherapy. *J Dermatol*. 2003;30:450-457.
194. Sheehan MP, Atherton DJ, Norris P, et al. Oral psoralen photochemotherapy in severe childhood atopic eczema: an update. *Br J Dermatol*. 1993;129:431-436.
195. de Kort WJ, van Weelden H. Bath psoralen-ultraviolet A therapy in atopic eczema. *J Eur Acad Dermatol Venereol*. 2000;14:172-174.
196. Ogawa H, Yoshiike T. Atopic dermatitis: studies of skin permeability and effectiveness of topical PUVA treatment. *Pediatr Dermatol*. 1992;9:383-385.
197. Yoshiike T, Sindhvananda J, Aikawa Y, et al. Topical psoralen photochemotherapy for atopic dermatitis: evaluation of two therapeutic regimens for inpatients and outpatients. *J Dermatol*. 1991;18: 201-205.
198. Kowalzick L, Kleinheinz A, Weichenthal M, et al. Low dose versus medium dose UV-A1 treatment in severe atopic eczema. *Acta Derm Venereol*. 1995;75: 43-45.
199. Abeck D, Schmidt T, Fesq H, et al. Long-term efficacy of medium-dose UVA1 phototherapy in atopic dermatitis. *J Am Acad Dermatol*. 2000;42:254-257.
200. Legat FJ, Hofer A, Brabek E, et al. Narrowband UV-B vs medium-dose UV-A1 phototherapy in chronic atopic dermatitis. *Arch Dermatol*. 2003;139:223-224.
201. Gilchrest BA, Parrish JA, Tanenbaum L, et al. Oral methoxsalen photochemotherapy of mycosis fungoides. *Cancer*. 1976;38:683-689.
202. Herrmann JJ, Roenigk HH Jr, Honigsmann H. Ultraviolet radiation for treatment of cutaneous T-cell lymphoma. *Hematol Oncol Clin North Am*. 1995;9:1077-1088.
203. Honigsmann H. Phototherapy for psoriasis. *Clin Exp Dermatol*. 2001;26:343-350.
204. Stadler R, Otte HG, Luger T, et al. Prospective randomized multicenter clinical trial on the use of interferon-2a plus acitretin versus interferon-2a plus PUVA in patients with cutaneous T-cell lymphoma stages I and II. *Blood*. 1998;92:3578-3581.
205. Rupoli S, Goteri G, Pulini S, et al. Long-term experience with low-dose interferon-alpha and PUVA in the management of early mycosis fungoides. *Eur J Haematol*. 2005;75:136-145.
206. McGinnis KS, Shapiro M, Vittorio CC, et al. Psoralen plus long-wave UV-A (PUVA) and bexarotene therapy: An effective and synergistic combined adjunct to therapy for patients with advanced cutaneous T-cell lymphoma. *Arch Dermatol*. 2003;139:771-775.
207. Weber F, Schmuth M, Sepp N, et al. Bath-water PUVA therapy with 8-methoxypsoralen in mycosis fungoides. *Acta Derm Venereol*. 2005;85:329-332.
208. Pabsch H, Rütten A, Von Stemm A, et al. Treatment of childhood mycosis fungoides with topical PUVA. *J Am Acad Dermatol*. 2002;47:557-561.
209. Pavlotsky F, Hodak E, Ben Amitay D, et al. Role of bath psoralen plus ultraviolet A in early-stage mycosis fungoides. *J Am Acad Dermatol*. 2014;71:536-541.
210. Ponte P, Serrao V, Apetato M. Efficacy of narrowband UVB vs. PUVA in patients with early-stage mycosis fungoides. *J Eur Acad Dermatol Venereol*. 2010;24(6):716-721.
211. Diederen PV, van Weelden H, Sanders CJ, et al. Narrowband UVB and psoralen-UVA in the treatment of early-stage mycosis fungoides: a retrospective study. *J Am Acad Dermatol*. 2003;48:215-219.
212. Gokdemir G, Barutcuoglu B, Sakiz D, et al. Narrowband UVB phototherapy for early-stage mycosis fungoides: evaluation of clinical and histopathological changes. *J Eur Acad Dermatol Venereol*. 2006;20:804-809.
213. Ahmad K, Rogers S, McNicholas PD, et al. Narrowband UVB and PUVA in the treatment of mycosis fungoides: a retrospective study. *Acta Derm Venereol*. 2007;87:413-417.
214. Ghodsi SZ, Hallaji Z, Balighi K, et al. Narrow-band UVB in the treatment of early stage mycosis fungoides: report of 16 patients. *Clin Exp Dermatol*. 2005;30:376-378.
215. Xiao T, Xia LX, Yang ZH, et al. Narrow-band ultraviolet B phototherapy for early stage mycosis fungoides. *Eur J Dermatol*. 2008;18:660-662.
216. Gathers RC, Scherschun L, Malick F, et al. Narrowband UVB phototherapy for early-stage mycosis fungoides. *J Am Acad Dermatol*. 2002;47:191-197.
217. Boztepe G, Sahin S, Ayhan M, et al. Narrowband

ultraviolet B phototherapy to clear and maintain clearance in patients with mycosis fungoides. *J Am Acad Dermatol.* 2005;53:242-246.
218. Brazzelli V, Antoninetti M, Palazzini S, et al. Narrowband ultraviolet therapy in early-stage mycosis fungoides: study on 20 patients. *Photodermatol Photoimmunol Photomed.* 2007;23:229-233.
219. D'Acunto C, Gurioli C, Neri I. Plaque stage mycosis fungoides treated with bexarotene at low dosage and UVB-NB. *J Dermatolog Treat.* 2010;21(1):45-48.
220. Hegazy RA, Fawzy MM, Gawdat HI, et al. T helper 17 and Tregs: a novel proposed mechanism for NB-UVB in vitiligo. *Exp Dermatol.* 2014;23:283-286.
221. Karsli N, Akcali C, Ozgoztasi O, et al. Role of oxidative stress in the pathogenesis of vitiligo with special emphasis on the antioxidant action of narrowband ultraviolet B phototherapy. *J Int Med Res.* 2014;42:799-805.
222. Scherschun L, Kim JJ, Lim HW. Narrow-band ultraviolet B is a useful and well-tolerated treatment for vitiligo. *J Am Acad Dermatol.* 2001;44:999-1003.
223. Chen GY, Hsu MM, Tai HK, et al. Narrow-band UVB treatment of vitiligo in Chinese. *J Dermatol.* 2005;32:793-800.
224. Kanwar AJ, Dogra S, Parsad D, et al. Narrow-band UVB for the treatment of vitiligo: an emerging effective and well-tolerated therapy. *Int J Dermatol.* 2005;44:57-60.
225. Kanwar AJ, Dogra S. Narrow-band UVB for the treatment of generalized vitiligo in children. *Clin Exp Dermatol.* 2005;30:332-336.
226. Brazzelli V, Antoninetti M, Palazzini S, et al. Critical evaluation of the variants influencing the clinical response of vitiligo: study of 60 cases treated with ultraviolet B narrow-band phototherapy. *J Eur Acad Dermatol Venereol.* 2007;21:1369-1374.
227. Westerhof W, Nieuweboer-Krobotova L. Treatment of vitiligo with UV-B radiation vs topical psoralen plus UV-A. *Arch Dermatol.* 1997;133:1525-1528.
228. Anbar TS, Westerhof W, Abdel-Rahman AT, et al. Evaluation of the effects of NB-UVB in both segmental and non-segmental vitiligo affecting different body sites. *Photodermatol Photoimmunol Photomed.* 2006;22:157-163.
229. Nicolaidou E, Antoniou C, Stratigos AJ, et al. Efficacy, predictors of response, and long-term follow-up in patients with vitiligo treated with narrowband UVB phototherapy. *J Am Acad Dermatol.* 2007;56:274-278.
230. Hamzavi I, Jain H, McLean D, et al. Parametric modeling of narrowband UV-B phototherapy for vitiligo using a novel quantitative tool: the Vitiligo Area Scoring Index. *Arch Dermatol.* 2004;140:677-683.
231. Njoo MD, Bos JD, Westerhof W. Treatment of generalized vitiligo in children with narrow-band (TL-01) UVB radiation therapy. *J Am Acad Dermatol.* 2000;42:245-253.
232. Natta R, Somsak T, Wisuttida T, et al. Narrowband ultraviolet B radiation therapy for recalcitrant vitiligo in Asians. *J Am Acad Dermatol.* 2003;49:473-476.
233. Sitek JC, Loeb M, Ronnevig JR. Narrowband UVB therapy for vitiligo: does the repigmentation last? *J Eur Acad Dermatol Venereol.* 2007;21:891-896.
234. Nordal EJ, Guleng GE, Ronnevig JR. Treatment of vitiligo with narrowband-UVB (TL01) combined with tacrolimus ointment (0.1%) vs. placebo ointment, a randomized right/left double-blind comparative study. *J Eur Acad Dermatol Venereol.* 2011;25:1440-1443.
235. Lee KY, Jeon SY, Hong JW, et al. Endothelin-1 enhances the proliferation of normal human melanocytes in a paradoxical manner from the TNF-α-inhibited condition, but tacrolimus promotes exclusively the cellular migration without proliferation: a proposed action mechanism for combination therapy of phototherapy and topical tacrolimus in vitiligo treatment. *J Eur Acad Dermatol Venereol.* 2013;27:609-616.
236. Dang YP, Li Q, Shi F, et al. Effect of topical calcineurin inhibitors as monotherapy or combined with phototherapy for vitiligo treatment: a meta-analysis. *Dermatol Ther.* 2016;29:126-133.
237. Schallreuter KU, Wood JM, Lemke KR, et al. Treatment of vitiligo with a topical application of pseudocatalase and calcium in combination with short-term UVB exposure: a case study on 33 patients. *Dermatology.* 1995;190:223-229.
238. Bakis-Petsoglou S, Le Guay JL, Wittal R. A randomized, double-blinded, placebo-controlled trial of pseudocatalase cream and narrowband ultraviolet B in the treatment of vitiligo. *Br J Dermatol.* 2009;161:910-917.
239. Schallreuter KU, Salem MA, Holtz S, et al. Basic evidence for epidermal H2O2/ONOO(-)-mediated oxidation/nitration in segmental vitiligo is supported by repigmentation of skin and eyelashes after reduction of epidermal H2O2 with topical NB-UVB-activated pseudocatalase PC-KUS. *FASEB J.* 2013;27:3113-3122.
240. Bayoumi W, Fontas E, Sillard L, et al. Effect of a preceding laser dermabrasion on the outcome of combined therapy with narrowband ultraviolet B and potent topical steroids for treating nonsegmental vitiligo in resistant localizations. *Br J Dermatol.* 2012;166:208-211.
241. Choi KH, Park JH, Ro YS. Treatment of Vitiligo with 308-nm xenon-chloride excimer laser: therapeutic efficacy of different initial doses according to treatment areas. *J Dermatol.* 2004;31:284-292.
242. Baltás E, Nagy P, Bónis B, et al. Repigmentation of localized vitiligo with the xenon chloride laser. *Br J Dermatol.* 2001;144:1266-1267.
243. Spencer JM, Nossa R, Ajmeri J. Treatment of vitiligo with the 308-nm excimer laser: a pilot study. *J Am Acad Dermatol.* 2002;46:727-731.
244. Taneja A, Trehan M, Taylor CR. 308-nm excimer laser for the treatment of localized vitiligo. *Int J Dermatol.* 2003;42:658-662.
245. Alhowaish AK, Dietrich N, Onder M, et al. Effectiveness of a 308-nm excimer laser in treatment of vitiligo: a review. *Lasers Med Sci.* 2013;28:1035-1041.
246. Passeron T, Ortonne JP. Use of the 308-nm excimer laser for psoriasis and vitiligo. *Clin Dermatol.* 2006;24:33-42.
247. Hofer A, Hassan AS, Legat FJ, et al. Optimal weekly frequency of 308-nm excimer laser treatment in vitiligo patients. *Br J Dermatol.* 2005;152:981-985.
248. Linthorst Homan MW, Spuls PI, Nieuweboer-Krobotova L, et al. A randomized comparison of excimer laser versus narrow-band ultraviolet B phototherapy after punch grafting in stable vitiligo patients. *J Eur Acad Dermatol Venereol.* 2012;26:690-695.
249. Ostovari N, Passeron T, Zakaria W, et al. Treatment of vitiligo by 308-nm excimer laser: an evaluation of variables affecting treatment response. *Lasers Surg Med.* 2004;35:152-156.

250. Esposito M, Soda R, Costanzo A, et al. Treatment of vitiligo with the 308 nm excimer laser. *Clin Exp Dermatol.* 2004;29:133-137.
251. Hofer A, Hassan AS, Legat FJ, et al. The efficacy of excimer laser (308 nm) for vitiligo at different body sites. *J Eur Acad Dermatol Venereol.* 2006;20: 558-564.
252. Hadi S, Tinio P, Al-Ghaithi K, et al. Treatment of vitiligo using the 308-nm excimer laser. *Photomed Laser Surg.* 2006;24:354-357.
253. Soliman M, Samy NA, Abo Eittah M, et al. Comparative study between excimer light and topical antioxidant versus excimer light alone for treatment of vitiligo. *J Cosmet Laser Ther.* 2016;18:7-11.
254. Grimes PE, Minus HR, Chakrabarti SG, et al. Determination of optimal topical photochemotherapy for vitiligo. *J Am Acad Dermatol.* 1982;7:771-778.
255. Westerhof W, Nieuweboer-Krobotova L, Mulder PG, et al. Left-right comparison study of the combination of fluticasone propionate and UV-A vs. either fluticasone propionate or UV-A alone for the long-term treatment of vitiligo. *Arch Dermatol.* 1999;135: 1061-1066.
256. Andres C, Kollmar A, Mempel M, et al. Successful ultraviolet A1 phototherapy in the treatment of localized scleroderma: a retrospective and prospective study. *Br J Dermatol.* 2010;162:445-447.
257. Kreuter A, Hyun J, Stücker M, et al. A randomized controlled study of low-dose UVA1, medium-dose UVA1, and narrowband UVB phototherapy in the treatment of localized scleroderma. *J Am Acad Dermatol.* 2006;54:440-447.
258. Kerscher M, Volkenandt M, Gruss C, et al. Low-dose UVA phototherapy for treatment of localized scleroderma. *J Am Acad Dermatol.* 1998;38:21-26.
259. Sator PG, Radakovic S, Schulmeister K, et al. Medium-dose is more effective than low-dose ultraviolet A1 phototherapy for localized scleroderma as shown by 20-MHz ultrasound assessment. *J Am Acad Dermatol.* 2009;60:786-791.
260. Morita A, Kobayashi K, Isomura I, et al. Ultraviolet A1 (340-400 nm) phototherapy for scleroderma in systemic sclerosis. *J Am Acad Dermatol.* 2000;43:670-674.
261. Wang F, Garza LA, Cho S, et al. Effect of increased pigmentation on the antifibrotic response of human skin to UV-A1 phototherapy. *Arch Dermatol.* 2008;144:851-858.
262. Vasquez R, Jabbar A, Khan F, et al. Recurrence of morphea after successful ultraviolet A1 phototherapy: a cohort study. *J Am Acad Dermatol.* 2014;70: 481-488.
263. Gruss C, Reed JA, Altmeyer P, et al. Induction of interstitial collagenase (MMP-1) by UVA-1 phototherapy in morphea fibroblasts. *Lancet.* 1997;350: 1295-1296.
264. Kreuter A, Hyun J, Skrygan M, et al. Ultraviolet A1 phototherapy decreases inhibitory SMAD7 gene expression in localized scleroderma. *Arch Dermatol Res.* 2006;298:265-272.
265. Gambichler T, Skrygan M, Tomi NS, et al. Significant downregulation of transforming growth factor-beta signal transducers in human skin following ultraviolet-A1 irradiation. *Br J Dermatol.* 2007;156:951-956.
266. Quan T, He T, Kang S, et al. Ultraviolet irradiation alters transforming growth factor beta/smad pathway in human skin in vivo. *J Invest Dermatol.* 2002;119:499-506.
267. Kreuter A, Hyun J, Skrygan M, et al. Ultraviolet A1-induced downregulation of human beta-defensins and interleukin-6 and interleukin-8 correlates with clinical improvement in localized scleroderma. *Br J Dermatol.* 2006;155:600-607.
268. von Kobyletzki G, Uhle A, Pieck C, et al. Acrosclerosis in patients with systemic sclerosis responds to low-dose UV-A1 phototherapy. *Arch Dermatol.* 2000;136: 275-276.
269. Tewari A, Garibaldinos T, Lai-Cheong J, et al. Successful treatment of microstomia with UVA1 phototherapy in systemic sclerosis. *Photodermatol Photoimmunol Photomed.* 2011;27:113-114.
270. Kanekura T, Fukumaru S, Matsushita S, et al. Successful treatment of scleroderma with PUVA therapy. *J Dermatol.* 1996;23:455-459.
271. Scharffetter-Kochanek K, Goldermann R, Lehmann P, et al. PUVA therapy in disabling pansclerotic morphoea of children. *Br J Dermatol.* 1995;132:830-831.
272. Todd DJ, Askari A, Ektaish E. PUVA therapy for disabling pansclerotic morphoea of children. *Br J Dermatol.* 1998;138:201-202.
273. Morita A, Sakakibara S, Sakakibara N, et al. Successful treatment of systemic sclerosis with topical PUVA. *J Rheumatol.* 1995;22:2361-2365.
274. Grundmann-Kollmann M, Ochsendorf F, Zollner TM, et al. PUVA-cream photochemotherapy for the treatment of localized scleroderma. *J Am Acad Dermatol.* 2000;43:675-678.
275. Brazzelli V, Grasso V, Muzio F, et al. Narrowband ultraviolet B phototherapy in the treatment of cutaneous graft-versus-host disease in oncohaematological paediatric patients. *Br J Dermatol.* 2010; 162:404-409.
276. Grundmann-Kollmann M, Martin H, Ludwig R, et al. Narrowband UV-B phototherapy in the treatment of cutaneous graft versus host disease. *Transplantation.* 2002;74:1631-1634.
277. Vogelsang GB, Wolff D, Altomonte V, et al. Treatment of chronic graft-versus-host disease with ultraviolet irradiation and psoralen (PUVA). *Bone Marrow Transplant.* 1996;17:1061-1067.
278. Jampel RM, Farmer ER, Vogelsang GB, et al. PUVA therapy for chronic cutaneous graft-vs-host disease. *Arch Dermatol.* 1991;127:1673-1678.
279. Wiesmann A, Weller A, Lischka G, et al. Treatment of acute graft-versus-host disease with PUVA (psoralen and ultraviolet irradiation): results of a pilot study. *Bone Marrow Transplant.* 1999;23:151-155.
280. Eppinger T, Ehninger G, Steinert M, et al. 8-Methoxy-psoralen and ultraviolet A therapy for cutaneous manifestations of graft-versus-host disease. *Transplantation.* 1990;50:807-811.
281. Atkinson K, Weller P, Ryman W, et al. PUVA therapy for drug-resistant graft-versus-host disease. *Bone Marrow Transplant.* 1986;1:227-236.
282. Hoffner MV, Carrizosa Esquivel A, Pulpillo Ruiz A, et al. Two cases of cutaneous chronic graft versus host disease in treatment with psoralen plus ultraviolet-A-bath photochemotherapy. *J Drugs Dermatol.* 2009; 8:1027-1029.
283. Leiter U, Kaskel P, Krähn G, et al. Psoralen plus ultraviolet-A-bath photochemotherapy as an adjunct treatment modality in cutaneous chronic graft versus host disease. *Photodermatol Photoimmunol Photomed.* 2002;18:183-190.
284. Calzavara Pinton P, Porta F, Izzi T, et al. Prospects for ultraviolet A1 phototherapy as a treatment for

285. Wetzig T, Sticherling M, Simon JC, et al. Medium dose long-wavelength ultraviolet A (UVA1) phototherapy for the treatment of acute and chronic graft-versus-host disease of the skin. *Bone Marrow Transplant.* 2005;35:515-519.
286. Ziemer M, Thiele JJ, Gruhn B, et al. Chronic cutaneous graft-versus-host disease in two children responds to UVA1 therapy: improvement of skin lesions, joint mobility, and quality of life. *J Am Acad Dermatol.* 2004;51:318-319.
287. Ghoreschi K, Thomas P, Penovici M, et al. PUVA-bath photochemotherapy and isotretinoin in sclerodermatous graft-versus-host disease. *Eur J Dermatol.* 2008;18:667-670.
288. Sorenson E, McAndrew R, Patel V, et al. Narrowband UV-B phototherapy for steroid-refractory sclerotic chronic cutaneous graft-vs-host disease. *JAMA Dermatol.* 2015;151:635-637.
289. Kreuter A, Gambichler T, Weiner SM, et al. Limited effects of UV-A1 phototherapy in 3 patients with nephrogenic systemic fibrosis. *Arch Dermatol.* 2008;144:1527-1529.
290. Gilchrest BA, Rowe JW, Brown RS, et al. Relief of uremic pruritus with ultraviolet phototherapy. *N Engl J Med.* 1977;297:136-138.
291. Gilchrest BA. Ultraviolet phototherapy of uremic pruritus. *Int J Dermatol.* 1979;18:741-748.
292. Simpson NB, Davison AM. Ultraviolet phototherapy for uraemic pruritus. *Lancet.* 1981;1:781.
293. Hsu MM, Yang CC. Uraemic pruritus responsive to broadband ultraviolet (UV) B therapy does not readily respond to narrowband UVB therapy. *Br J Dermatol.* 2003;149:888-889.
294. Hanid MA, Levi AJ. Phototherapy for pruritus in primary biliary cirrhosis. *Lancet.* 1980;2:530.
295. Perlstein SM. Phototherapy for primary biliary cirrhosis. *Arch Dermatol.* 1981;117:608.
296. Person JR. Ultraviolet A (UV-A) and cholestatic pruritus. *Arch Dermatol.* 1981;117:684.
297. Cerio R, Murphy GM, Sladen GE, et al. A combination of phototherapy and cholestyramine for the relief of pruritus in primary biliary cirrhosis. *Br J Dermatol.* 1987;116:265-267.
298. Holme SA, Anstey AV. Aquagenic pruritus responding to intermittent photochemotherapy. *Clin Exp Dermatol.* 2001;26:40-41.
299. Menage HD, Norris PG, Hawk JL, et al. The efficacy of psoralen photochemotherapy in the treatment of aquagenic pruritus. *Br J Dermatol.* 1993;129:163-165.
300. Goodkin R, Bernhard JD. Repeated PUVA treatment of aquagenic pruritus. *Clin Exp Dermatol.* 2002;27:164-165.
301. Baldo A, Sammarco E, Plaitano R, et al. Narrowband (TL-01) ultraviolet B phototherapy for pruritus in polycythaemia vera. *Br J Dermatol.* 2002;147:979-981.
302. Hernandez-Nunez A, Dauden E, Cordoba S, et al. Water-induced pruritus in haematologically controlled polycythaemia vera: response to phototherapy. *J Dermatolog Treat.* 2001;12:107-109.
303. Jeanmougin M, Rain JD, Najean Y. Efficacy of photochemotherapy on severe pruritus in polycythemia vera. *Ann Hematol.* 1996;73:91-93.
304. Swerlick RA. Photochemotherapy treatment of pruritus associated with polycythemia vera. *J Am Acad Dermatol.* 1985;13:675-677.
305. Morison WL, Nesbitt JA 3rd. Oral psoralen photochemotherapy (PUVA) for pruritus associated with polycythemia vera and myelofibrosis. *Am J Hematol.* 1993;42:409-410.
306. Kuwano Y, Watanabe R, Fujimoto M, et al. Treatment of HIV-associated eosinophilic pustular folliculitis with narrow-band UVB. *Int J Dermatol.* 2006;45:1265-1267.
307. Misago N, Narisawa Y, Matsubara S, et al. HIV-associated eosinophilic pustular folliculitis: successful treatment of a Japanese patient with UVB phototherapy. *J Dermatol.* 1998;25:178-184.
308. Ho MH, Chong LY, Ho TT. HIV-associated eosinophilic folliculitis in a Chinese woman: a case report and a survey in Hong Kong. *Int J STD AIDS.* 1998;9:489-493.
309. Parker SR, Parker DC, McCall CO. Eosinophilic folliculitis in HIV-infected women: case series and review. *Am J Clin Dermatol.* 2006;7:193-200.
310. Ellis E, Scheinfeld N. Eosinophilic pustular folliculitis: a comprehensive review of treatment options. *Am J Clin Dermatol.* 2004;5:189-197.
311. Aydogan K, Karadogan SK, Tunali S, et al. Narrowband ultraviolet B (311 nm, TL01) phototherapy in chronic ordinary urticaria. *Int J Dermatol.* 2012;51:98-103.
312. Dummer R, Ivanova K, Scheidegger EP, et al. Clinical and therapeutic aspects of polymorphous light eruption. *Dermatology.* 2003;207:93-95.
313. Boonstra HE, van Weelden H, Toonstra J, et al. Polymorphous light eruption: a clinical, photobiologic, and follow-up study of 110 patients. *J Am Acad Dermatol.* 2000;42:199-207.
314. Bilsland D, George SA, Gibbs NK, et al. A comparison of narrow band phototherapy (TL-01) and photochemotherapy (PUVA) in the management of polymorphic light eruption. *Br J Dermatol.* 1993;129:708-712.
315. Murphy GM, Logan RA, Lovell CR, et al. Prophylactic PUVA and UVB therapy in polymorphic light eruption—a controlled trial. *Br J Dermatol.* 1987;116:531-538.
316. Gschnait F, Honigsmann H, Brenner W, et al. Induction of UV light tolerance by PUVA in patients with polymorphous light eruption. *Br J Dermatol.* 1978;99:293-295.
317. Wolf P, Gruber-Wackernagel A, Rinner B, et al. Phototherapeutic hardening modulates systemic cytokine levels in patients with polymorphic light eruption. *Photochem Photobiol Sci.* 2013;12:166-173.
318. Gruber-Wackernagel A, Heinemann A, Konya V, et al. Photohardening restores the impaired neutrophil responsiveness to chemoattractants leukotriene B4 and formyl-methionyl-leucyl-phenylalanin in patients with polymorphic light eruption. *Exp Dermatol.* 2011;20:473-476.
319. Schweintzger N, Gruber-Wackernagel A, Reginato E, et al. Levels and function of regulatory T cells in patients with polymorphic light eruption: relation to photohardening. *Br J Dermatol.* 2015;173:519-526.
320. Wolf P, Gruber-Wackernagel A, Bambach I, et al. Photohardening of polymorphic light eruption patients decreases baseline epidermal Langerhans cell density while increasing mast cell numbers in the papillary dermis. *Exp Dermatol.* 2014;23:428-430.
321. Franken SM, Genders RE, de Gruijl FR, et al. Skin hardening effect in patients with polymorphic light

eruption: comparison of UVB hardening in hospital with a novel home UV-hardening device. *J Eur Acad Dermatol Venereol*. 2013;27:67-72.
322. Dawe RS, Ferguson J. Prolonged benefit following ultraviolet A phototherapy for solar urticaria. *Br J Dermatol*. 1997;137:144-148.
323. Ryckaert S, Roelandts R. Solar urticaria. A report of 25 cases and difficulties in phototesting. *Arch Dermatol*. 1998;134:71-74.
324. Ramsay CA. Solar urticaria treatment by inducing tolerance to artificial radiation and natural light. *Arch Dermatol*. 1977;113:1222-1225.
325. Calzavara-Pinton P, Zane C, Rossi M, et al. Narrowband ultraviolet B phototherapy is a suitable treatment option for solar urticaria. *J Am Acad Dermatol*. 2012;67:e5-e9.
326. Bernhard JD, Jaenicke K, Momtaz TK, et al. Ultraviolet A phototherapy in the prophylaxis of solar urticaria. *J Am Acad Dermatol*. 1984;10:29-33.
327. Parrish JA, Jaenicke KF, Morison WL, et al. Solar urticaria: treatment with PUVA and mediator inhibitors. *Br J Dermatol*. 1982;106:575-580.
328. Beissert S, Stander H, Schwarz T. UVA rush hardening for the treatment of solar urticaria. *J Am Acad Dermatol*. 2000;42:1030-1032.
329. Roelandts R. Diagnosis and treatment of solar urticaria. *Dermatol Ther*. 2003;16:52-56.
330. Crouch R, Foley P, Baker C. Actinic prurigo: a retrospective analysis of 21 cases referred to an Australian photobiology clinic. *Australas J Dermatol*. 2002;43:128-132.
331. Honigsmann H. Mechanisms of phototherapy and photochemotherapy for photodermatoses. *Dermatol Ther*. 2003;16:23-27.
332. Pavlotsky F, Nathansohn N, Kriger G, et al. Ultraviolet-B treatment for cutaneous lichen planus: our experience with 50 patients. *Photodermatol Photoimmunol Photomed*. 2008;24:83-86.
333. Taneja A, Taylor CR. Narrow-band UVB for lichen planus treatment. *Int J Dermatol*. 2002;41:282-283.
334. Saricaoglu H, Karadogan SK, Baskan EB, et al. Narrowband UVB therapy in the treatment of lichen planus. *Photodermatol Photoimmunol Photomed*. 2003;19:265-267.
335. Helander I, Jansen CT, Meurman L. Long-term efficacy of PUVA treatment in lichen planus: comparison of oral and external methoxsalen regimens. *Photodermatol*. 1987;4:265-268.
336. Carlin CS, Florell SR, Krueger GG. Induction of dramatic hyperpigmentation in a patient with generalized lichen planus treated with re-PUVA. *J Cutan Med Surg*. 2002;6:125-127.
337. Wackernagel A, Legat FJ, Hofer A, et al. Psoralen plus UVA vs. UVB-311 nm for the treatment of lichen planus. *Photodermatol Photoimmunol Photomed*. 2007;23:15-19.
338. Nanda S, Grover C, Reddy BS. PUVA-induced lichen planus. *J Dermatol*. 2003;30:151-153.
339. Kuramoto N, Kishimoto S, Shibagaki R, et al. PUVA-induced lichen planus pemphigoides. *Br J Dermatol*. 2000;142:509-512.
340. Kassem R, Yarom N, Scope A, et al. Treatment of erosive oral lichen planus with local ultraviolet B phototherapy. *J Am Acad Dermatol*. 2012;66:761-766.
341. Sezer E, Etikan I. Local narrowband UVB phototherapy vs. local PUVA in the treatment of chronic hand eczema. *Photodermatol Photoimmunol Photomed*. 2007;23:10-14.

342. Schempp CM, Muller H, Czech W, et al. Treatment of chronic palmoplantar eczema with local bath-PUVA therapy. *J Am Acad Dermatol*. 1997;36:733-737.
343. Behrens S, Grundmann-Kollmann M, Peter RU, et al. Combination treatment of psoriasis with photochemotherapy and tazarotene gel, a receptor-selective topical retinoid. *Br J Dermatol*. 1999;141:177.
344. Douwes KE, Karrer S, Abels C, et al. Does smoking influence the efficacy of bath-PUVA therapy in chronic palmoplantar eczema? *Photodermatol Photoimmunol Photomed*. 2000;16:25-29.
345. Tzaneva S, Kittler H, Holzer G, et al. 5-Methoxypsoralen plus ultraviolet (UV) A is superior to medium-dose UVA1 in the treatment of severe atopic dermatitis: a randomized crossover trial. *Br J Dermatol*. 2010;162(3):655-660.
346. LeVine MJ, Parrish JA, Fitzpatrick TB. Oral methoxsalen photochemotherapy (PUVA) of dyshidrotic eczema. *Acta Derm Venereol*. 1981;61:570-571.
347. Petering H, Breuer C, Herbst R, et al. Comparison of localized high-dose UVA1 irradiation versus topical cream psoralen-UVA for treatment of chronic vesicular dyshidrotic eczema. *J Am Acad Dermatol*. 2004;50:68-72.
348. Schmidt T, Abeck D, Boeck K, et al. UVA1 irradiation is effective in treatment of chronic vesicular dyshidrotic hand eczema. *Acta Derm Venereol*. 1998;78:318-319.
349. Ersoy-Evans S, Hapa AA, Boztepe G, et al. Narrowband ultraviolet-B phototherapy in pityriasis lichenoides chronica. *J Dermatolog Treat*. 2009;20:109-113.
350. Pavlotsky F, Baum S, Barzilai A, et al. UVB therapy of pityriasis lichenoides—our experience with 29 patients. *J Eur Acad Dermatol Venereol*. 2006;20:542-547.
351. Aydogan K, Saricaoglu H, Turan H. Narrowband UVB (311 nm, TL01) phototherapy for pityriasis lichenoides. *Photodermatol Photoimmunol Photomed*. 2008;24:128-133.
352. Lange-Wantzin G, Thomsen K, Hou-Jensen K. Lymphomatoid papulosis: a follow-up study. *Acta Derm Venereol*. 1984;64:46-51.
353. Thomsen K, Wantzin GL. Lymphomatoid papulosis. A follow-up study of 30 patients. *J Am Acad Dermatol*. 1987;17:632-636.
354. Hoetzenecker W, Guenova E, Hoetzenecker K, et al. Successful treatment of recalcitrant lymphomatoid papulosis in a child with PUVA-bath photochemotherapy. *Eur J Dermatol*. 2009;19:646-647.
355. Volkenandt M, Kerscher M, Sander C, et al. PUVA-bath photochemotherapy resulting in rapid clearance of lymphomatoid papulosis in a child. *Arch Dermatol*. 1995;131:1094.
356. Kontos AP, Kerr HA, Malick F, et al. 308-nm excimer laser for the treatment of lymphomatoid papulosis and stage IA mycosis fungoides. *Photodermatol Photoimmunol Photomed*. 2006;22:168-171.
357. Calzavara-Pinton P, Venturini M, Sala R. Medium-dose UVA1 therapy of lymphomatoid papulosis. *J Am Acad Dermatol*. 2005;52:530-532.
358. Sotiriou E, Apalla Z, Ioannides D. Telangiectasia macularis eruptive perstans successfully treated with PUVA therapy. *Photodermatol Photoimmunol Photomed*. 2010;26:46-47.
359. Martin LK, Romanelli P, Ahn YS, et al. Telangiectasia macularis eruptiva perstans with an associated myeloproliferative disorder. *Int J Dermatol*.

2004;43:922-924.
360. Metcalfe DD. The treatment of mastocytosis: an overview. *J Invest Dermatol.* 1991;96:S55-S56; discussion S56-S59, S60-S65.
361. Gobello T, Mazzanti C, Sordi D, et al. Medium- versus high-dose ultraviolet A1 therapy for urticaria pigmentosa: a pilot study. *J Am Acad Dermatol.* 2003;49:679-684.
362. Rombold S, Lobisch K, Katzer K, et al. Efficacy of UVA1 phototherapy in 230 patients with various skin diseases. *Photodermatol Photoimmunol Photomed.* 2008;24:19-23.
363. Kolde G, Frosch PJ, Czarnetzki BM. Response of cutaneous mast cells to PUVA in patients with urticaria pigmentosa: histomorphometric, ultrastructural, and biochemical investigations. *J Invest Dermatol.* 1984;83:175-178.
364. Brazzelli V, Grasso V, Manna G, et al. Indolent systemic mastocytosis treated with narrow-band UVB phototherapy: study of five cases. *J Eur Acad Dermatol Venereol.* 2012;26:465-469.
365. Brazzelli V, Grassi S, Merante S, et al. Narrow-band UVB phototherapy and psoralen-ultraviolet A photochemotherapy in the treatment of cutaneous mastocytosis: a study in 20 patients. *Photodermatol Photoimmunol Photomed.* 2016;32(5-6):238-246.
366. Kerker BJ, Huang CP, Morison WL. Photochemotherapy of generalized granuloma annulare. *Arch Dermatol.* 1990;126:359-361.
367. Szegedi A, Begany A, Hunyadi J. Successful treatment of generalized granuloma annulare with polyethylene sheet bath PUVA. *Acta Derm Venereol.* 1999;79:84-85.
368. Batchelor R, Clark S. Clearance of generalized papular umbilicated granuloma annulare in a child with bath PUVA therapy. *Pediatr Dermatol.* 2006;23:72-74.
369. Grundmann-Kollmann M, Ochsendorf FR, Zollner TM, et al. Cream psoralen plus ultraviolet A therapy for granuloma annulare. *Br J Dermatol.* 2001;144:996-999.
370. Schnopp C, Tzaneva S, Mempel M, et al. UVA1 phototherapy for disseminated granuloma annulare. *Photodermatol Photoimmunol Photomed.* 2005;21:68-71.
371. Solano-Lopez G, Concha-Garzon MJ, de Argila D, et al. Successful treatment of disseminated granuloma annulare with narrowband UV-B phototherapy. *Actas Dermosifiliogr.* 2015;106:240-241.
372. Ohe S, Danno K, Sasaki H, et al. Treatment of acquired perforating dermatosis with narrowband ultraviolet B. *J Am Acad Dermatol.* 2004;50:892-894.
373. Serrano G, Aliaga A, Lorente M. Reactive perforating collagenosis responsive to PUVA. *Int J Dermatol.* 1988;27:118-119.
374. Krutmann J, Hönigsmann H, Elmets C, eds. *Dermatological Phototherapy and Photodiagnostic Methods.* 2nd ed. Berlin, Germany: Springer-Verlag; 2009.

Chapter 199 :: Photochemotherapy and Photodynamic Therapy
:: Herbert Hönigsmann, Rolf-Markus Szeimies, & Robert Knobler

第一百九十九章
光化学疗法和光动力疗法

中文导读

光化学疗法和光动力疗法作为一种美观和疗效兼具的物理治疗方法，已经被广泛应用于各种皮肤疾病治疗。本章共分为8节：①光化学疗法的背景；②光化学疗法的作用机制；③光化学疗法的治疗方案；④光化学疗法的适应证；⑤光化学疗法的副作用；⑥光化学疗法的禁忌证；⑦光动力疗法；⑧总结与展望。详细介绍了光化学疗法，并对光动力疗法进行了简单介绍。

第一节主要介绍了光化学疗法的背景，光化学疗法主要指口服或局部使用补骨脂素（一种光敏化合物，psoralens，缩写为P）与紫外线A辐射（UVA）联用的治疗方法，称为PUVA。PUVA主要通过补骨脂素进入细胞后吸收光子以产生光化学反应，从而改变细胞的结构和功能等，达到治疗疾病的目的。该光化学治疗已成功应用了40多年，疗效显著且副反应相对可控，是治疗银屑病和白癜风的常规治疗，而且目前也广泛应用于治疗其他多种疾病。

第二节介绍了PUVA治疗银屑病的作用机制，可能是补骨脂素等光敏化合物在光照射下发生光化学反应，抑制了表皮细胞的有丝分裂、DNA合成和细胞增殖。同时，PUVA可以影响免疫效应细胞功能，例如淋巴细胞、角质形成细胞或多核巨细胞等，从而起到治疗作用。另外，PUVA能使黑色素细胞增加酪氨酸酶活力，促进黑色素生成，从而治疗白癜风。

第三节罗列了3种常见光化学疗法的治疗方案，分别是局部外用、光化学浴和口服疗法。局部外用补骨脂素乳膏、药膏或洗剂，因为其治疗范围的局限性和相对高的光毒性反应，目前仅用于局限性的斑块状银屑病和掌跖疾病。光化学浴和口服疗法的治疗效果更为显著，应用更为广泛。PUVA浴需要全身浸泡15到20分钟，毒副反应相当低。口服疗法则需要在光照前1~3小时口服8-MOP。由于存在光毒性等副作用，表199-2提出了PUVA沐浴疗法和口服疗法在剂量上的建议，对不同方案的光化学疗法提供指导。

第四节介绍了光化学疗法的适应证。光化学疗法适用于银屑病、特异性皮炎、皮肤T细胞淋巴瘤、扁平苔藓、慢性移植物抗宿主病、白癜风、HIV感染和其他光线诱导的皮肤病等。一般而言，所有类型的银屑病对PUVA都有效，而对于红皮病型银屑病和继发性脓疱型银屑病的疗效相对差一点。根据目前临床试验发现，PUVA口服疗法或联合疗法对银屑病治疗更有意义，其中联合疗法主要包括联合外用糖皮质激素、蒽醌和焦油制剂等。

第五节指出PUVA光化学疗法的常见急性副作用包括药物不耐受反应、严重的延迟性红斑反应和瘙痒等。药物不耐受反应包括了恶心、呕吐等，是PUVA常见的不良反应。当大面积皮肤受到影响时，可能会出现全身光毒性症状，如发烧和全身不适。非甾体抗炎药物和局部或全身糖皮质类固醇药物可以减轻症状，必须尽早给予。

第六节介绍了光化学疗法的禁忌证，并对此进行分情况讨论：鉴于PUVA潜在的短期和长期危害，患者治疗方案的选择，应该基于对风险和患者受益的综合考虑。同时有指南指出，建议女性在使用PUVA时采取避孕措施，因为PUVA具有致畸的风险。严重的肝肾功能损害通常被认为是PUVA的禁忌证，对于红斑狼疮、卟啉症和色素性干皮病等也禁用。

第七节对光动力疗法进行了简介，光动力疗法（Photodynamic therapy，PDT）是指在氧气存在的条件下，光敏剂（通常为卟啉类）在肿瘤等组织特异性高表达，被可见光激发，从而产生活性氧，对靶细胞产生直接或间接细胞毒性作用。目前PDT已有效地用于癌前和皮肤恶性肿瘤，以及尖锐湿疣等。

第八节对光化学疗法进行了总结与展望。PUVA是治疗银屑病等多种皮肤病的有效疗法；同时，PDT作为一种新的无创治疗，目前已经在治疗尖锐湿疣等病毒性疾病、光化性角化病、Bowen病和浅表BCC中有明确的疗效。期待未来随着科技的进步，更多更安全有效的光敏剂和设备将被研发，应用于临床，造福患者。

〔赵　爽〕

AT-A-GLANCE

- Photochemotherapy (psoralen and ultraviolet A light [PUVA]) has been successfully used for more than 40 years. Its effectiveness has profoundly influenced dermatologic therapy in general, providing treatment for many diverse disorders besides psoriasis and vitiligo.
- PUVA can be combined with topical treatments and with some systemic agents (retinoids, methotrexate, and, perhaps, biologics) to enhance efficacy and to reduce the number of exposures.
- The most important adverse effects of oral PUVA consist of an increased risk of squamous cell carcinoma and a possible risk of melanoma. No such increased risk was found so far with bath-PUVA.
- Extracorporeal photochemotherapy (ECP) was introduced in the 1980s for the palliative treatment of erythrodermic cutaneous T-cell lymphoma.
- ECP appears to have a major impact in the treatment of graft-versus-host disease after allogeneic bone marrow transplantation where it allows progressive reduction or even discontinuation of the concomitant immunosuppressive therapy without an increase in graft-versus-host disease activity. Several other indications are under investigation.
- No serious side effects have been reported with ECP.
- Photodynamic therapy (PDT) for skin tumors started with the introduction of topical photosensitization by a porphyrin precursor (5-aminolevulinic acid or its methyl ester) that would avoid generalized light sensitivity over many weeks.
- Current experience with PDT of epithelial cancers and precancerous conditions suggests that actinic keratoses, Bowen disease, superficial and nodular basal cell carcinomas, and early squamous cell carcinomas can be treated curatively.
- Cosmetic outcomes following PDT are excellent; therefore, it is also used for rejuvenation purposes, frequently in combination with laser treatment.
- The only significant side effect of topical PDT is a stinging pain during and shortly after irradiation. With daylight-mediated PDT, pain is no longer an issue. PDT has neither mutagenic nor carcinogenic potential.

PHOTOCHEMOTHERAPY

Photochemotherapy with psoralens combines the use of oral or topical psoralens (P) and ultraviolet A radiation (UVA), termed *PUVA*. Psoralens are phototoxic compounds that enter cells and then absorb photons to produce photochemical reactions that alter the function of cellular constituents.[1] This interaction results in a beneficial therapeutic effect after repeated controlled phototoxic reactions. Psoralens can be administered orally or applied topically to the skin in the form of solutions, creams, or baths. This therapy is currently used in the treatment of several common and uncommon skin diseases.

HISTORICAL BACKGROUND

In the 1970s, it was shown that orally administered 8-methoxypsoralen (8-MOP) and subsequent irradiation with artificial UVA was a highly effective treatment for psoriasis.[2,3] Psoralen baths (soaking in a dilute psoralen solution) and subsequent UVA exposure (bath-PUVA), which originated in Scandinavia,[4] is also being used in many European institutions. The effectiveness of all variants of PUVA has been widely confirmed and has profoundly influenced dermatologic therapy, in general, providing treatment for numerous disorders in addition to psoriasis (Table 199-1). A major advance in phototherapy was the development of fluorescent bulbs that emitted narrowband UVB radiation at 311 to 313 nm in the mid-1980s. This narrow spectrum is slightly inferior in clearing psoriasis or mycosis fungoides. However, because it is easier to perform and possibly safer than PUVA, it is now more frequently used in many phototherapy centers. Narrowband UVB phototherapy is also beneficial for a variety of other dermatoses that were previously treated with PUVA. Nevertheless, PUVA has remained the mainstay for recalcitrant diseases.

PRINCIPLES OF PHOTOCHEMOTHERAPY

The rationale for PUVA therapy is to induce remissions of skin diseases by repeated, controlled phototoxic reactions. These reactions occur only when psoralens are photoactivated by UVA. Because of the penetration characteristics of UVA, absorption of photons is confined to the skin. However, there is also some evidence that PUVA may exert systemic effects through circulating lymphocytes affected while transiting through the skin. Clinically, PUVA-induced phototoxic reactions are characterized by a delayed sunburn-like erythema and inflammation.

PSORALENS

Three psoralens are used in PUVA therapy. Methoxsalen or 8-methoxysporalen (8-MOP), obtained from the seeds of a plant called *Ammi majus*, is most widely used and the only psoralen available in the United States. Bergapten or 5-methoxypsoralen (5-MOP) and trioxsalen or 4,5′,8-trimethylpsoralen (TMP) are available in Europe and elsewhere.

TABLE 199-1
Phototherapy-Responsive Diseases

THERAPY OF DISEASE	PREVENTION OF DISEASE SYMPTOMS
- Psoriasis	- Polymorphous light eruption
- Palmoplantar pustulosis	- Hydroa vacciniforme[a]
- Mycosis fungoides (stages IA, IB)	- Solar urticaria
- Vitiligo	- Erythropoietic protoporphyria[a]
- Atopic dermatitis	- Chronic actinic dermatitis[a]
- Generalized lichen planus	- Polymorphous light eruption
- Urticaria pigmentosa	- Hydroa vacciniforme[a]
- Cutaneous graft-versus-host disease	- Solar urticaria
- Generalized granuloma annulare	- Erythropoietic protoporphyria[a]
- Pityriasis lichenoides*	- Chronic actinic dermatitis[a]
- Lymphomatoid papulosis[a]	
- Pityriasis rubra pilaris[a]	
- Localized scleroderma[a]	
- Psoriasis	
- Palmoplantar pustulosis	
- Mycosis fungoides (stages IA, IB)	
- Vitiligo	
- Atopic dermatitis	

[a]Experience limited to small number of patients.

PSORALEN PHOTOCHEMISTRY[5-7]

Psoralens intercalate between apposing DNA base pairs in the double helix in the absence of UV radiation. Absorption of photons in the UVA range results in the formation of a 3,4- or 4,5-cyclobutane addition product (adduct) with pyrimidine bases of native DNA. In the first step of this photochemical reaction, a monofunctional adduct with thymine or cytosine is formed. Some psoralens, including 8-MOP, TMP, and 5-MOP, can absorb a second photon, and this reaction leads to the formation of a bifunctional adduct with a 5,6-double bond of the pyrimidine base of the opposite strand, thus producing an interstrand crosslink of the double helix (Fig. 199-1). This intercalation of psoralens with epidermal DNA suppresses both DNA synthesis and cell division, and it was originally assumed that this was the therapeutic mechanism in psoriasis. However, crosslinking does not appear to be a prerequisite for the therapeutic effect,[7] and successful PUVA treatment of other skin diseases is unlikely to be directly caused by this molecular reaction; psoralens also react with RNA, proteins, and other cellular components, and indirectly modify proteins and lipids via singlet oxygen-mediated reactions or by generating free radicals.[7] Perhaps these mechanisms contribute to

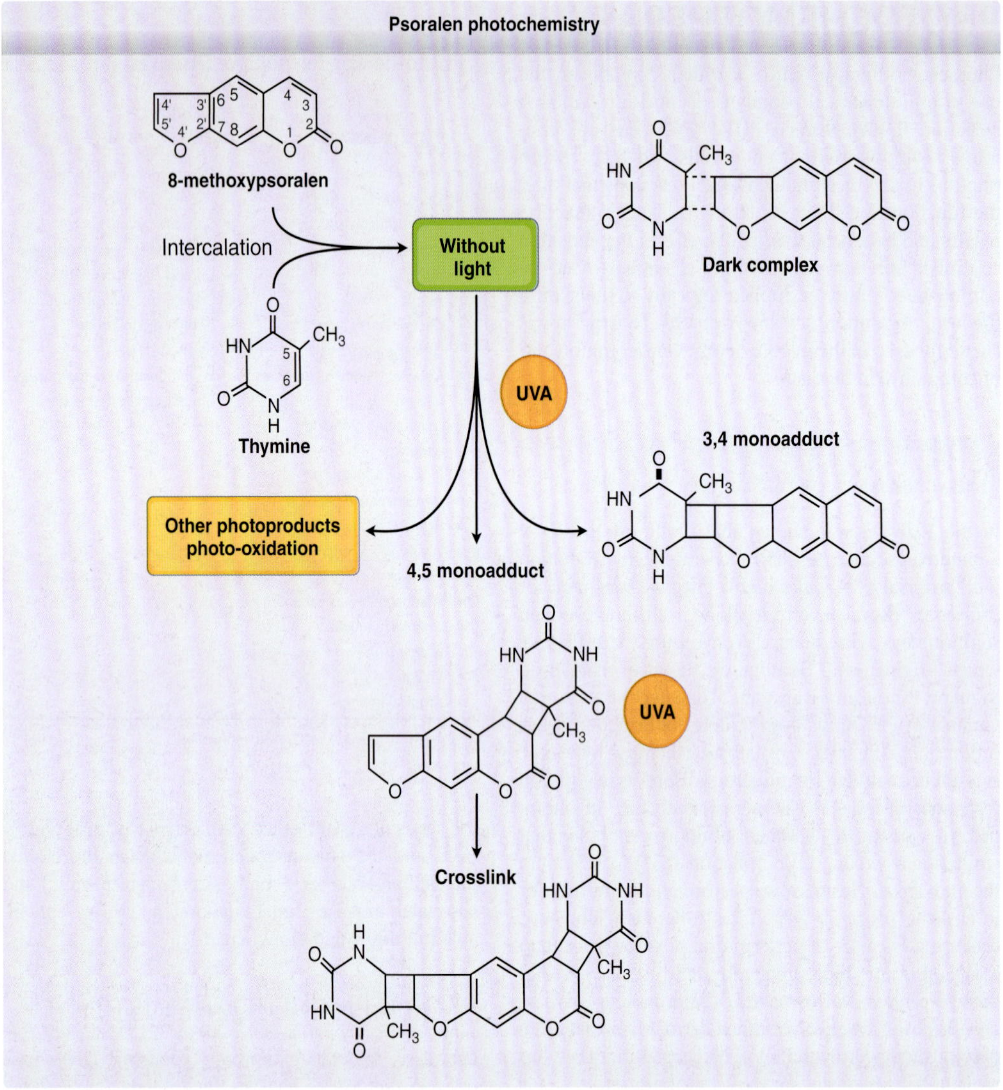

Figure 199-1 Psoralen photochemistry. Psoralens intercalate between apposing DNA base pairs forming a "dark complex." Absorption of ultraviolet A (UVA) photons leads to a 3,4- or 4,5-cyclobutane monoadduct with pyrimidine bases of native DNA. The absorption of a second photon results in a bifunctional adduct, producing an interstrand crosslink of the double helix.

the effects of PUVA in diseases that are not hyperproliferative in nature.

The formation of mono- and bifunctional photoadducts in DNA results in the immediate inhibition of DNA synthesis. The interstrand crosslinks are believed to be largely responsible for eliciting skin photosensitization reactions of linear psoralens such as 8-MOP. Excessive production of these cyclobutane adducts causes cell death. Mutation and skin carcinogenesis also result from photoconjugation of psoralens to DNA because the cells surviving this DNA damage tend to repair it through an error-prone repair process.[7]

In Type II reactions (Chap. 17), reactive oxygen species ($^1O_2$, O_2, or OH) induce the oxidation of cellular lipoprotein membrane lipids and destruction of membrane-bound cytochrome P450. The membrane-damaging events activate the arachidonic acid metabolism pathway, which results in an increase of secondary oxidation products that contribute to the increased synthesis of eicosanoids. Furthermore, the reactive oxygen species can directly damage DNA by generating DNA strand breaks.[7]

MECHANISMS OF PHOTOCHEMOTHERAPY

Hypotheses about the mechanism of action in psoriasis are based on the known photoconjugation of psoralens to DNA with subsequent suppression of mitosis, DNA synthesis, and cell proliferation, expected to revert increased cell proliferation rates in psoriasis to normal.

However, PUVA also alters the expression of cytokines and cytokine receptors, downregulates certain lymphocyte and antigen-presenting cell functions, influences adhesion molecule expression, and diminishes Langerhans cell numbers within the epidermis. In addition, PUVA affects immune effector cells such as lymphocytes or polymorphonuclear leukocytes. Because there is evidence that psoriasis is caused primarily by the action of blood-derived immunocytes, it is reasonable to speculate that PUVA therapy may act by affecting immune function through a direct phototoxic effect on lymphocytes in skin infiltrates. This is consistent with the observation that several other disorders that are not hyperproliferative in nature but immunomediated also respond well to PUVA. PUVA can revert pathologically altered patterns of keratinocyte differentiation and reduce the number of proliferating epidermal cells. Infiltrating lymphocytes are strongly suppressed by PUVA, with variable effects on different T-cell subsets. Lymphocytes are far more likely to undergo apoptosis than keratinocytes[8] in response to PUVA, which may explain the high efficacy in cutaneous T-cell lymphoma (CTCL), as well as in inflammatory skin diseases including psoriasis that is now recognized to be in part T-cell mediated as well as hyperproliferative. Although much is known about pathways and mechanisms of psoralen photosensitization, the interactions and relative contributions to the clearing of a specific disease are not well understood.

Psoralens also stimulate melanogenesis. This involves the photoconjugation of psoralens to DNA in melanocytes, mitosis, and subsequent proliferation of melanocytes, an increased formation and melanization of melanosomes, an increased transfer of melanosomes to keratinocytes, and activation and increased synthesis of tyrosine mediated in part by stimulation of cAMP activity.

PHARMACOKINETICS

The important steps between the ingestion of a psoralen and its arrival at the site of action include absorption, first-pass effect, blood transportation, and tissue distribution. The absorption rate of a psoralen from the gut depends mainly on the physical characteristics of the preparation and the fat content of the concomitant food intake. Liquid preparations of 8-MOP and 5-MOP give higher and earlier peak serum levels than do crystalline formulations. In addition, peak serum levels are achieved by liquid preparations after a relatively reproducible time interval in all subjects, whereas wide time variability occurs with crystalline formulations. Before reaching the skin via the circulation, psoralens are metabolized during passage through the liver. Plasma levels of 8-MOP administered orally at different doses show a strong nonlinearity, indicating a saturable first-pass effect. The unpredictable pharmacokinetic behavior is probably due to inter- and intraindividual variations of intestinal absorption, first-pass effect, blood distribution in the body, metabolism, and elimination of the drug.

Within the same individual, serum levels of 8-MOP correspond fairly well with skin reactivity, the peak of skin phototoxicity coinciding with peak serum levels. However, phototoxic responses to PUVA show large interindividual variations. Hence, measurement of serum psoralens is a research tool and not used to monitor clinical therapy.

The pharmacokinetics of 8-MOP after topical treatment depend on the method of application. 8-MOP topically applied as a 0.15% emulsion or solution leads to plasma levels comparable to those found with oral treatment if large areas of the body are treated. In contrast, plasma levels after bath-PUVA treatment of almost the total body surface are very low. Bathwater-delivered psoralens are readily absorbed in the skin but are promptly eliminated without cutaneous accumulation.[8]

ULTRAVIOLET A RADIATION

UVA sources commonly used for PUVA therapy are fluorescent lamps or high-pressure metal halide lamps. The typical fluorescent PUVA lamp has an emission peak at 352 nm and emits approximately 0.5% in the UVB range. UVA doses are given in Joules per centimeter-squared, usually measured with a photometer with a maximum sensitivity at 350 to 360 nm. Although the action spectrum of antipsoriatic activity and phototoxic erythema peaks at 335 nm, longer wavelengths have proved equally effective for clearing psoriasis if delivered in an adequate dose to obtain an equal erythemogenic response.[9]

PHOTOSENSITIVITY EFFECTS OF PHOTOCHEMOTHERAPY

PUVA treatment produces an inflammatory response that manifests as delayed phototoxic erythema, proportional to the dose of both drug and UVA and to the individual's sensitivity to phototoxic reactions. 8-MOP dose changes within individuals, over a narrow but clinically relevant range, appears to significantly alter the threshold for PUVA erythema, but not the rate of increase in erythema intensity with increasing UVA dose.[10] Importantly, the time course of PUVA erythema differs from sunburn or UVB erythema that appears after 4 to 6 hours and peaks 12 to 24 hours after exposure. PUVA erythema does not appear before 24 to 36 hours and peaks at 72 to 96 hours, or even later. Hence, daily PUVA treatments can result in unexpected severe delayed cumulative phototoxicity. PUVA erythema has a shallower dose-response curve than UVB erythema (by a factor of approximately 2), and this difference is maintained even at the point of maximum erythema.[11] Severe PUVA reactions may lead to blistering and to superficial skin necrosis. Overdoses of UVA are frequently followed by swelling, intense pruritus, and, sometimes, by a stinging sensation in the affected skin area, possibly as a consequence of damage of superficial nerve endings. Erythema is at present the only available parameter that allows an assessment of the magnitude of the PUVA reaction; thus, it represents an important criterion for dose adjustments.[9]

Pigmentation is the second important effect of PUVA. It may develop without clinically evident erythema, especially when oral 5-MOP or TMP is used; this is particularly important in the treatment of vitiligo and for the preventive therapy of certain photodermatoses. In unaffected skin, PUVA pigmentation is maximal approximately 7 days after a PUVA exposure and may last from several weeks to months. As with sun-induced pigmentation, the individual's ability to tan is genetically determined, but the dose-response curve is much steeper. A few PUVA exposures result in a much deeper tan than that produced by multiple exposures to solar radiation.

TREATMENT PROTOCOLS

TOPICAL TREATMENT

Application of 8-MOP in creams, ointments, or lotions followed by UVA irradiation is effective in clearing psoriasis but has several disadvantages. The nonuniform distribution on the skin surface induces unpredictable phototoxic erythema reactions and irregular patches of cosmetically unacceptable hyperpigmentation. Furthermore, if numerous lesions are present, the application is laborious and time consuming, and the treatment does not prevent the development of new active lesions in previously unaffected, untreated areas. Therefore, topical PUVA with psoralen creams, ointments, or lotions is now used only for limited plaque psoriasis and for palmoplantar disease.

BATH PHOTOCHEMOTHERAPY

The use of bathwater delivery of psoralens provides for a uniform drug distribution over the skin surface, very low psoralen plasma levels, and rapid elimination of free psoralens from the skin. Bathwater delivery of 8-MOP circumvents GI side effects and possible phototoxic hazards to the eyes because there is no systemic photosensitization. Skin psoralen levels are highly reproducible, and photosensitivity lasts no more than 2 hours. The higher incidence of unwanted burn reactions can be prevented by a lower starting dose (50% of the minimal phototoxic dose [MPD]) and a more cautious dosimetry in the initial treatment phase. A major drawback in many treatment facilities is the requirement for a bathtub. Originally, bath-PUVA was performed with TMP, but 8-MOP and 5-MOP are now being used as well. Bath-PUVA consists of 15 to 20 minutes of whole-body immersion in solutions of 0.5- to 5.0-mg 8-MOP per liter of bathwater. Irradiation needs to be performed immediately, as photosensitivity decreases rather rapidly. TMP is more phototoxic after topical application and is used at lower concentrations than 8-MOP. Minimal phototoxicity dose (MPD) determination for bath-PUVA must consider that the phototoxic threshold declines during the early treatment phase,[8] in contrast to oral PUVA. Guidelines for bath, local immersion, and other topical PUVA forms have been published by the British Photodermatology Group and are based, where possible, on the results of controlled studies, or otherwise on consensus.[12]

ORAL TREATMENT

In oral PUVA, 8-MOP is administered orally (0.6-0.8 mg/kg body weight) 1 to 3 hours before exposure, depending on the absorption characteristics of the particular drug brand. Liquid drug preparations are absorbed faster and yield higher and more reproducible serum levels than microcrystalline forms. For 5-MOP, the usual dosage is 1.2- to 1.8-mg/kg body weight.

The initial UVA doses are determined by either the patient's skin type[13-15] or by MPD testing.[9] The MPD is defined as the minimal dose of UVA that produces a barely perceptible, but well-defined, erythema when template areas of the skin are exposed to increasing doses of UVA. Erythema readings are performed 72 hours after testing, at which time the psoralen phototoxicity reaction usually reaches its peak. The MPD test should be performed on previously nonexposed skin (eg, buttocks). Although the MPD test is more time-consuming than phototyping, it allows for more accurate and higher UVA doses during initial treatment. Table 199-2 shows recommendations for dosimetry in bath and oral PUVA.

Repeated exposures are required to clear PUVA-responsive diseases, with gradual dose increments as pigmentation develops. Lower doses quite frequently result in failure of treatment except in those diseases in which induction of pigmentation is the desired

TABLE 199-2

Recommended Treatment Schedule for Photochemotherapy[a]

DETERMINATION OF MPD	READING	AFTER 96-120 H (BATH-PUVA) AFTER 72-96 H (ORAL PUVA)
Start of treatment	First therapeutic dose	30% of MPD (bath-PUVA) 50%-70% of MPD (oral PUVA)
Treatments 2 to 4 times weekly	No erythema, good response	Increase once weekly by 30%
	No erythema, no response	Increase by 30% per session
	Minimal erythema	No increase
	Persistent asymptomatic erythema	No increase
	Painful erythema (with or without blistering)	No treatment until symptoms subside
Resumption of treatment after missed sessions	After resolution of symptoms	Reduction of last dose by 50%; next increase by 10%

[a]Exact practices vary between the United States and Europe and among practitioners in specific locales, based on historical teaching and individual experiences.

MPD, minimal phototoxic dose; PUVA, psoralen and ultraviolet A light.

objective. In most dermatoses amenable to PUVA, the frequency of treatments is reduced after satisfactory clearing of disease, and the last UVA dose is used as a maintenance dose, if maintenance treatment is planned. The duration of this maintenance phase and the frequency of treatments depend on the particular disease being treated and its propensity to relapse.

INDICATIONS FOR PHOTOCHEMOTHERAPY

PHOTOCHEMOTHERAPY FOR PSORIASIS

Basically, all types of psoriasis respond to PUVA (Figs. 199-2 and 199-3), although the management of erythrodermic or generalized pustular psoriasis is more difficult.[8] The effectiveness of oral PUVA in inducing and maintaining remission of psoriasis has been widely documented and confirmed by large-scale clinical trials (Figs. 199-2 and 199-3).

Administration: Three studies have compared bathwater delivery of 8-MOP with oral administration.[8] In 2 reports, initial doses were determined by skin typing, and treatments were given 2 to 3 times weekly. Dose increments were instituted with every treatment in one study, whereas smaller increments were given every third treatment in the other. In the third report, patients were treated according to the standard European regimen for oral PUVA, which is still in use (treatments 4 times weekly with an intermission on Wednesdays until clearing). This showed the lowest incidence of treatment failures and overdose phenomena, despite the potential burn risk of back-to-back PUVA treatments. Compared with oral 8-MOP, bath-PUVA showed equal clearing rates with fewer exposures.[8] The greater therapeutic efficacy could be because of a higher penetration of psoralens through the abnormal stratum corneum overlying psoriatic plaques, as compared with healthy perilesional skin where phototoxicity is monitored during the therapy. The incidences of erythema and pruritus were similar or lower compared with oral therapy. Systemic intolerance, such as nausea and vomiting, were not observed.

Oral 5-MOP–PUVA represents an alternative to oral 8-MOP–PUVA. Psoriatic lesions are cleared with a comparable number of treatments, but at the expense of significantly higher cumulative UVA doses. This difference may be due to the lower phototoxicity potential of 5-MOP and of its higher tanning activity. However, 5-MOP–PUVA therapy is not associated with nausea and vomiting and has a lower incidence of pruritus and severe phototoxic erythema.[8]

On complete clearing, patients are often assigned to maintenance therapy, during which the frequency of treatments is gradually reduced. The purpose of maintenance therapy is to achieve longer remission. Maintenance therapy in the original European regimen consisted of 1 month of twice-weekly treatments, with the last UVA dose used for clearing, followed by another month of once-weekly exposures. According to other recommendations,[16] maintenance treatment should be considered only on rapid relapses, because patients with a stable remission may be overtreated, and long-term risks of PUVA are related to the total cumulative phototoxic doses. In one recent left–right comparison study with psoriatics, PUVA maintenance treatment over 2 months did not increase the length

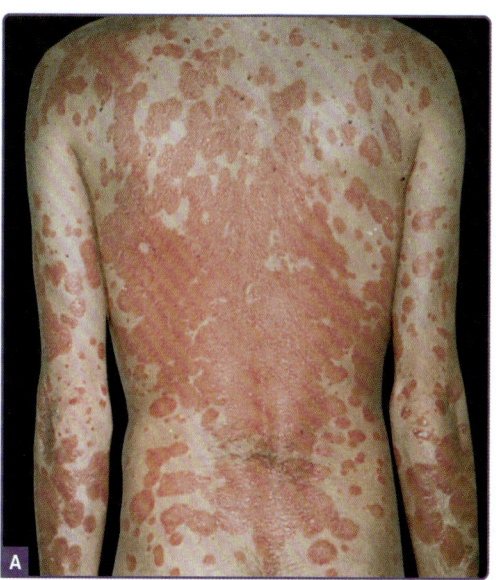
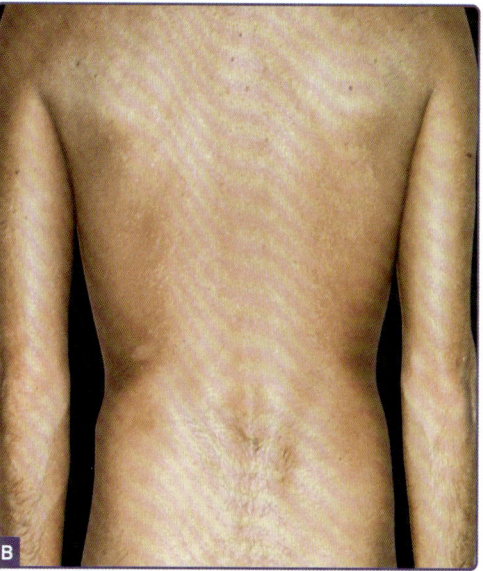

Figure 199-2 Twenty-three-year-old patient with generalized psoriasis (seborrheic type). **A,** Before photochemotherapy treatment. **B,** After treatment. (From Wolff K, et al. Photochemotherapie bei Psoriasis. Klinische Erfahrungen bei 152 Patienten. *Dtsch Med Wochenschr.* 1975;100:2471, with permission.)

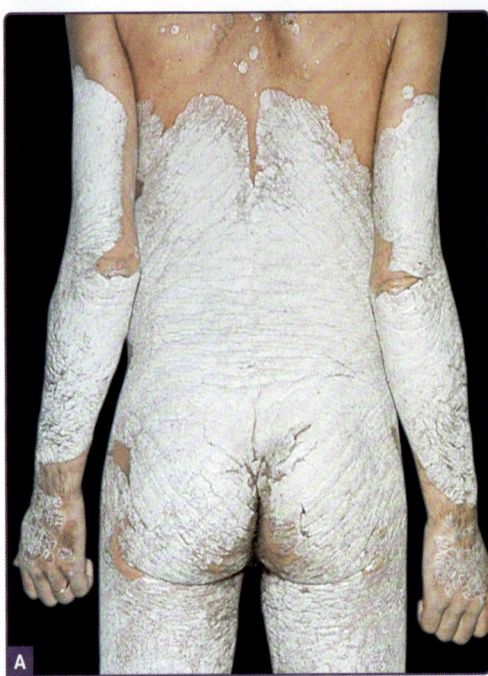 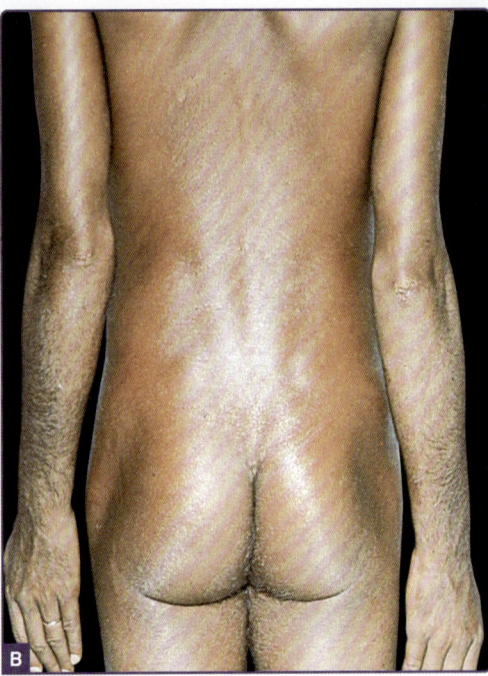

Figure 199-3 Twenty-three-year-old patient with generalized psoriasis (plaque-type). **A,** Before photochemotherapy treatment. **B,** After treatment. (From Wolff K, Hönigsmann H. Clinical aspects of photochemotherapy. *Pharmacol Ther.* 1981;12:381, with permission.)

of remission.[17] Thus, maintenance treatment should be given only in selected cases.

Erythrodermic and generalized pustular psoriasis (von Zumbusch type) respond to PUVA (Fig. 199-4), but the time required to induce remission is considerably longer, more treatments are needed, and higher failure rates are reported, compared with plaque or guttate varieties. Pustular eruptions of palms and soles are quite recalcitrant to treatment, regardless of whether they are true localized pustular psoriasis, nonpsoriatic palmoplantar pustulosis or pustular psoriasis, or pustular eczema. Oral PUVA alone can produce a slow but definite remission in many cases, but a considerable number of patients require adjunctive therapy for clearing. As mentioned above, the combination with topically applied 8-MOP can be beneficial, but bath-PUVA appears to be also quite effective in such cases.

PUVA alone can produce definite remissions in many patients with psoriasis, but a considerable number require additional therapies for clearing. Such combination therapy improves efficacy and may reduce side effects.

Combination Treatments: *Topical combinations:* Topical adjuvant therapies with glucocorticoids, anthralin, and tar preparations, and, more recently, with calcipotriol and tazarotene, have yielded good results. However, adjunctive topical therapy is unacceptable to some patients.

Methotrexate: A combination of PUVA and methotrexate can reduce the duration of treatment, number of exposures, and total UVA dose and is also effective in clearing patients unresponsive to PUVA or UVB alone.[18] This combination appears to be safe if used during the clearing phase only. However, if used for long-term treatment, PUVA and methotrexate may act synergistically in the development of skin cancers.[19]

Cyclosporine: Cyclosporine plus PUVA dramatically enhances skin carcinogenesis. This is in keeping with the observation of a greatly increased risk of cutaneous squamous cell carcinomas in patients with solid organ transplants maintained on this immunosuppressant. Thus, this combination should be definitely discouraged.[8,20-22]

Retinoids: The therapeutic efficacy of PUVA therapy is dramatically increased by daily oral retinoid (etretinate, acitretin, isotretinoin; 1 mg/kg) administration beginning 5 to 10 days before the initiation of PUVA, and continued throughout the clearing phase. This so-called *RePUVA* characteristically reduces the number of exposures by one-third and the total cumulative UVA dose by more than one-half. RePUVA also often clears "poor responders" who are not brought into complete remission by PUVA alone.[23]

The mechanism of the synergistic action of retinoids and PUVA is unknown, but may be a result of the accelerated desquamation that optimizes the optical properties of the skin and reduction of the inflammatory infiltrate. As an additional theoretic benefit, etretinate and other retinoids may protect against long-term carcinogenic effects of PUVA. In one study, patients with psoriasis treated with PUVA in combination with systemic retinoids showed a reduced risk of squamous cell carcinoma but not a significantly altered incidence of

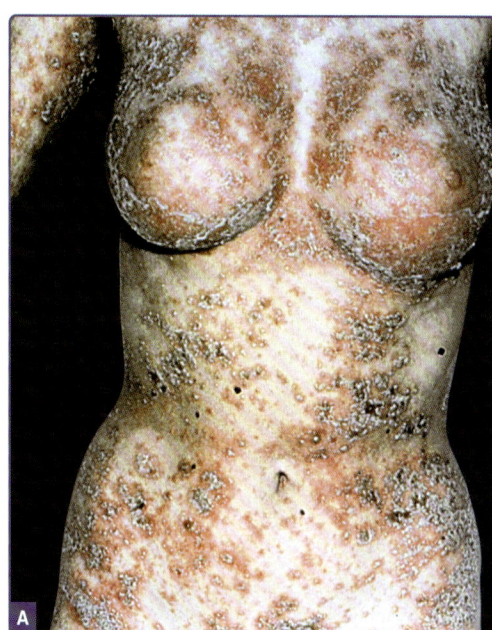 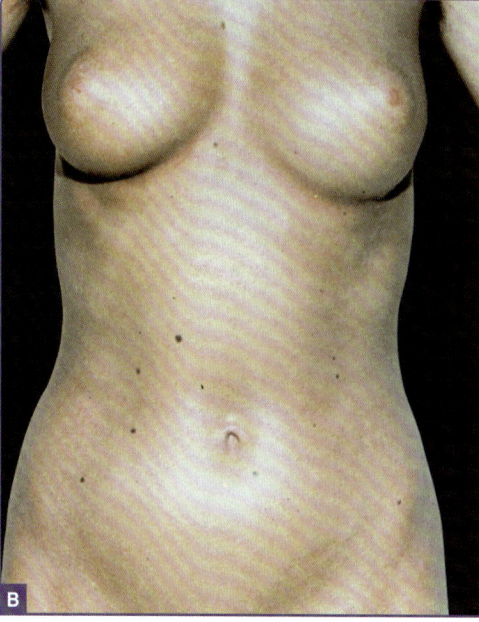

Figure 199-4 Eighteen-year-old patient with pustular psoriasis (von Zumbusch type). **A,** Before photochemotherapy treatment. **B,** After treatment. (From Hönigsmann H et al. Photochemotherapy for pustular psoriasis (von Zumbusch). *Br J Dermatol.* 1977;97:119, with permission. Copyright © 1977 John Wiley & Sons.)

basal cell carcinoma (BCC).[24] Although retinoid toxicity is generally not a concern because the administration is limited to the clearing phase, the potential teratogenicity of retinoids represents a serious concern for women of childbearing age. In these patients, the use of isotretinoin is advisable because contraception is necessary for only 1 month after discontinuation of therapy, in contrast to etretinate and acitretin, which require 2 years of contraception because of their slower elimination.[8]

Biologics: The mechanism of action of biologic agents suggests that there may be additive effects in treating psoriasis with PUVA, but this remains to be further defined in clinical trials.[25,26] Presently, there are no long-term studies evaluating the safety and efficacy of the combination of any biologics with PUVA.

PUVA FOR CUTANEOUS T-CELL LYMPHOMA (CTCL, MYCOSIS FUNGOIDES)

Since the first promising results with PUVA in CTCL in 1976,[27] numerous investigators from the United States and Europe have confirmed the efficacy of PUVA for CTCL.[28] Treatment schedules and dosimetry are essentially the same as for psoriasis. The treatment consists of a clearing phase (Fig. 199-5), a maintenance phase consisting of 2 exposures per week for 1 month and 1 exposure per week for another month, and a followup phase without therapy. Remission should be confirmed by histologic examination of previously involved skin sites. After therapy is discontinued, the patient is monitored monthly and later bimonthly. If a relapse occurs, the patient is again subjected to a full PUVA course. Some investigators advocate permanent maintenance treatment consisting of treatments once monthly or every other month. However, the course of CTCL varies considerably from patient to patient, and clinical experience suggests that patients benefit most from individualized treatment schedules.[8]

Relapses often respond as well as the initial lesions when PUVA is resumed. Clinical remissions appear to be directly related to phototoxic destruction of the malignant lymphocytes that infiltrate the skin. Thus, complete clearing may be induced when the cells are confined to the epidermis and superficial dermis, the depth of effective UVA penetration into the skin.

Present knowledge indicates that PUVA is an excellent treatment option that may induce long-lasting disease-free intervals in CTCL if used in the early stages of the disease.[28] In later stages, PUVA may reduce the tumor cell burden and thus may act synergistically with other treatment. It improves the quality of life and may prolong survival when used in combination with more aggressive treatment modalities. Prolonged remissions were observed with combinations of PUVA with retinoids, bexarotene,[29,30] or interferon-α 2a.[31-33]

Patients with tumor-stage CTCL exhibit a high rate of early recurrences and, therefore, require indefinite maintenance treatment. PUVA causes complete tumor resolution only when used in combination with local x-ray treatment and/or systemic chemotherapy. Most followup studies have demonstrated that the great majority of patients with early disease can be kept in remission with or without maintenance therapy for several years, but tumor-stage patients (IIB) usually experience multiple recurrences despite aggressive combination therapies and eventually die within a few

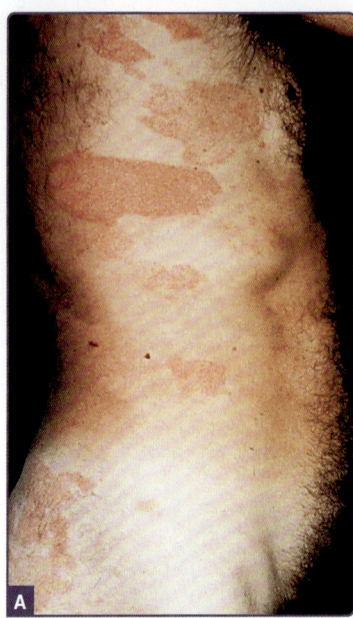 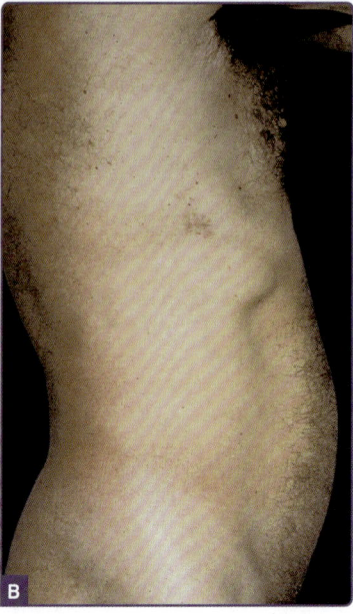

Figure 199-5 Forty-six-year-old patient with cutaneous T-cell lymphoma (mycosis fungoides) stage IB. **A,** Before photochemotherapy treatment. **B,** After treatment (clearing phase).

years.[28] Currently, no therapeutic regimen is known to alter the disease course of CTCL. Psoralen UV-A is an effective treatment for MF, inducing long-term remissions and perhaps in some cases disease "cure." Thirty percent to 50% of patients remain disease free for 10 years, but late relapses occur.[34]

Successful treatment of erythrodermic CTCL (Sézary syndrome) has been reported with extracorporeal PUVA (photopheresis) (see section "Extracorporeal Photochemotherapy [Photopheresis]"). Possible long-term hazards related to frequent PUVA treatments are better justified for patients with CTCL, compared with patients with benign conditions.

PHOTOTHERAPY FOR ATOPIC DERMATITIS

Many patients with atopic eczema can benefit from PUVA therapy.[35] The treatment guidelines are the same as for psoriasis. However, the condition is more difficult to treat, and quite often a higher number of treatments are required to clear the eczema. There is a high and early recurrence rate, requiring frequent maintenance exposures. However, in a recent study, PUVA provided a better short- and long-term response than medium-dose UVA1 in patients with severe atopic eczema.[36] A combination of PUVA with topical glucocorticoids appears to be superior to PUVA alone in maintaining remissions. Because the average patient is young, long-term maintenance therapy is problematic; and combination of PUVA with topical immune modulators (tacrolimus, pimecrolimus), although effective, cannot be recommended until more data are available. The mechanism of action of PUVA in atopic eczema is unclear; current concepts support an alteration of lymphocytes in the dermal infiltrate.

PHOTOTHERAPY FOR LICHEN PLANUS

In generalized lichen planus, PUVA can provide an effective alternative to systemic glucocorticoid treatment, although it appears to be more resistant to PUVA than psoriasis when treated according to a similar schedule. More exposures and higher cumulative UVA doses are required for clearing, and not all patients respond satisfactorily. An exacerbation during PUVA treatment has been reported in a few patients. In patients who clear, relapses respond equally well when PUVA is resumed. Bath-PUVA can also clear lichen planus, and combined PUVA-etretinate regimen may be considered.[37]

PHOTOCHEMOTHERAPY FOR CUTANEOUS MASTOCYTOSIS

In cutaneous mastocytosis (urticaria pigmentosa), PUVA leads to a temporary involution of skin lesions[38] probably because of chronic degranulation of the mast cells. The treatment results in loss of Darier sign, relief of itching, and flattening and even complete disappearance of cutaneous papules and macules. Surprisingly, even systemic symptoms such as histamine-induced migraine and flushing improve gradually as treatment is continued.[38] In most patients, the manifestations of the disease recur several months after discontinuation of PUVA, but the recurrences respond as well as the original lesions.

Because treatment of cutaneous mastocytosis has been unrewarding with other modalities, the use of PUVA, although not curative, seems to be warranted in patients when the disease is causing severe distress.

PHOTOTHERAPY FOR MISCELLANEOUS DERMATOSES

Both acute and chronic pityriasis lichenoides[37] respond to PUVA, and favorable results have been reported for lymphomatoid papulosis.[39] However, the experience with these conditions is limited to a few anecdotal cases. In pityriasis rubra pilaris, the results are quite inconsistent. Some cases seem to respond well, others may flare, and some require combination treatment with retinoid or methotrexate therapy. Generalized granuloma annulare has been reported to clear completely, but long-term maintenance treatment was required to maintain remissions.[40] Regrowth of hair was noted in alopecia areata with either topical or systemic PUVA exposures localized to the alopecia areas. Followup studies of larger patient groups concluded that PUVA is generally not an effective treatment for alopecia areata.[41] The experience of the present authors has also not been encouraging. Localized scleroderma and pansclerotic morphea have been successfully treated with bath-PUVA and oral PUVA.[42,43]

PHOTOCHEMOTHERAPY FOR CHRONIC GRAFT-VERSUS-HOST DISEASE

Acute and chronic cutaneous graft-versus-host disease (GVHD) have become indications of increasing importance. Because of the clinical and histologic similarities of idiopathic lichen planus and lichenoid GVHD, PUVA treatment was evaluated for the latter.[44] PUVA cleared or improved this lichen planus–like eruption in patients who had not responded to conventional immunosuppressive therapy alone. PUVA can also improve acute GVHD,[45] although results of PUVA treatment for scleroderma-like variants of cutaneous GVHD are controversial. According to our own experience, the more circumscribed, localized forms appear to respond to PUVA with softening of the fibrotic, sclerotic connective tissue, but more widespread, disseminated lesions hardly respond.

Improvement of mucosal erosions followed by healing, observed during treatment of chronic lichenoid GVHD with PUVA, suggests that PUVA may exert both local and systemic effects, but this is not proven. There is no improvement of GVHD of other organs, such as the liver. The therapeutic regimen used for the treatment of chronic GVHD is basically the same as for psoriasis. UVA doses should not be increased too aggressively, to avoid erythema and possible (re)activation of GVHD. In general, increase of the UVA dosage by 0.5 J/cm^2 at maximum after every second to fourth exposure is recommended. Patients are exposed to UVA radiation 3 to 4 times weekly. After clearing of skin lesions, the frequency of exposures is reduced.

Because there appears to be an overall increased risk of secondary malignancies for all bone marrow/peripheral stem cell recipients, patients should be examined on a regular basis for the development of cutaneous malignancies, independent of whether they have been treated with PUVA.

PHOTOCHEMOTHERAPY FOR VITILIGO

Vitiligo was the first disease treated with an ancient form of psoralen PUVA in India and Egypt. PUVA in its modern form stimulates melanogenesis, melanocyte proliferation, and migration, and *can* reconstitute the normal skin color in *many* vitiligo patients, *although the actual response rate has still not been defined*. However, it is less used now since narrowband UVB phototherapy has been shown to be an effective and possibly safer alternative for repigmentation of this condition.

To induce maximal repigmentation, patients need long-term therapy with 100 to 200 exposures given twice or thrice weekly. Approximately 70% of patients respond after 12 to 24 months (Fig. 199-6), defined as the development of perifollicular macules of repigmentation. If there is no response after 6 months or approximately 50 treatments (as defined as perifollicular macules of repigmentation), PUVA should be terminated. If treatment is discontinued, this newly acquired repigmentation may be lost. The permanency of PUVA-induced repigmentation in vitiligo is poorly documented. Some investigators have reported continuing pigment loss following PUVA, while others have reported the repigmentation to be long lasting.[46]

Patient selection appears to be particularly important in vitiligo treatment. Lips, distal dorsal hands, tips of fingers and toes, areas of bony prominences, palms, soles, and nipples are very refractory to treatment, and patients with involvement limited to these areas should be excluded. Segmental vitiligo tends to show a variable response. Because of the different response in different body areas, total repigmentation is only rarely achieved, and some 30% of patients do not respond at all despite many months of therapy. Duration of the disease before PUVA therapy does not affect response rate.[46] It should be mentioned here that in a recent trial of nonsegmental vitiligo, narrowband-UVB therapy resulted in a better color match than oral PUVA.[47]

The mechanisms by which PUVA induces repigmentation in vitiligo skin are speculative. However, PUVA's known effect on a number of immunologic reactions suggests a suppression of the autoimmune stimulus for melanocyte destruction.

PHOTOCHEMOTHERAPY AS PREVENTION FOR PHOTODERMATOSES

Tolerance to sunlight can be induced in several photodermatoses by PUVA therapy.[48] In polymorphous light eruption, the most common photodermatosis,

PUVA is the most effective preventive treatment.[49] In approximately 70% of patients with this condition, a 3- to 4-week PUVA course of 2 to 3 treatments per week suffices to suppress the disease on subsequent exposure to sunlight such as a holiday trip or the arrival of summer. The initial exposure and dose increments during therapy should be performed according to the guidelines outlined for psoriasis. PUVA has the advantage of a rapid and intense pigment induction at relatively low UVA doses that usually remain well below the threshold doses for eliciting the rash. Approximately 10% of patients develop typical lesions during the initial phase of PUVA, but these usually disappear when treatment is continued. The authors' treatment schedule consists of 3 to 4 treatments per week for 3 to 4 weeks in early spring. PUVA protects only temporarily, but subsequent sun exposures usually maintain protection and many patients remain protected for 2 to 3 months even after their pigmentation has faded.

The mechanism by which phototherapy induces tolerance to sunlight is not clear. Hyperpigmentation and thickening of the stratum corneum may be important factors, but other mechanisms, such as modulations of cutaneous immune function, also may be involved.[49]

There is also some experience with PUVA prophylaxis of other photodermatoses. In solar urticaria, PUVA therapy appears to be the most effective preventive treatment available and is certainly better than antihistamines. Tolerance to sunlight can be increased 10-fold or more after a single treatment course.[50] The suppressive effect may last throughout the summer if the patients have regular sunlight exposures, which seems to be necessary to maintain tolerance. Problems may arise during the first PUVA exposures, because, in some patients, the urticaria threshold dose is very low. In these cases, careful conditioning by stepwise UVA irradiation of single quadrants of the body surface a few hours before each PUVA treatment has proved use-

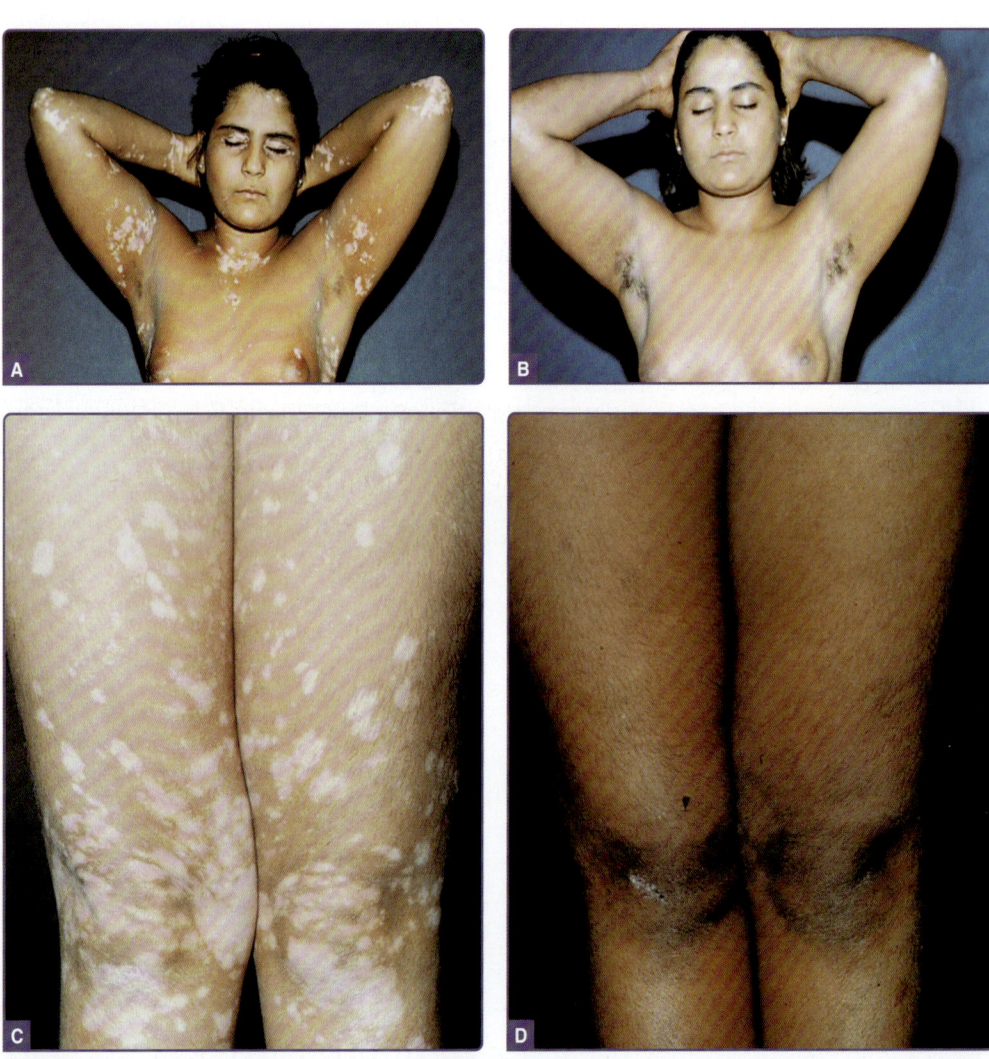

Figure 199-6 Twelve-year-old patient with generalized vitiligo of 4 years' duration. **A** and **C,** During the initial phases of photochemotherapy treatment. **B** and **D,** One month after treatment (8-methoxypsoralen + artificial ultraviolet A) with thrice-weekly exposures for 10 months.

ful. Treatments with PUVA are then given during the refractory period of presumed mast cell degranulation.

Successful PUVA therapy also has been reported in occasional cases of chronic actinic dermatitis and hydroa vacciniforme. Limited experience in patients with erythropoietic protoporphyria indicates that with a very cautious approach and in combination with beta-carotene, PUVA may increase light tolerance considerably.[51,52]

Extended treatment is usually not required in polymorphous light eruption but may be necessary in solar urticaria and chronic actinic dermatitis. There exist no ready-to-use schedules for these latter conditions, and PUVA is usually just one part of the management.[51]

PHOTOCHEMOTHERAPY IN HIV-INFECTED PATIENTS

The use of phototherapy and PUVA in HIV-infected patients with skin diseases is controversial. Both therapies can induce systemic immune suppression and may modify the immune status of the patient in a way that would worsen HIV disease.[53] Both UV radiation and psoralen photosensitization activate the HIV promoter, which could boost viral gene transcription and, eventually, virus production,[54] although available data and theoretic considerations indicate that UVB is more likely to be a hazard than PUVA in an HIV-infected population.[55,56] Nevertheless, oral PUVA treatment of psoriasis does not detectably accelerate progression of HIV disease or increase PUVA side effects, and hence PUVA is not considered contraindicated for HIV-positive patients with responsive skin diseases.[57]

SIDE EFFECTS AND TOXICITY OF PHOTOCHEMOTHERAPY

ACUTE SIDE EFFECTS

The side effects of PUVA include drug intolerance reactions as well as side effects of the combined action of psoralens plus UVA radiation (Table 199-3). Oral 8-MOP (0.6-0.8 mg/kg) has a high incidence of nausea (30% of patients) and vomiting (10% of patients), and this may occasionally require discontinuation of the treatment. The mechanism of this adverse effect is unknown. These side effects are more common with liquid preparations than with crystalline preparations, probably because of higher psoralen serum levels. With 5-MOP, nausea occurs rarely, even with doses of up to 1.8 mg/kg body weight.

Undesired acute effects of the combined action of psoralens and UVA include unexpectedly severe delayed erythema reactions. Severe burns with blistering can occur and may rarely require hospitalization. When large areas of skin are affected, systemic

TABLE 199-3
Side Effects and Toxicity of Photochemotherapy

Acute Side Effects	
Drug intolerance	Nausea, vomiting with oral MOP, but not with 5-MOP.
UVA overdosage	Can range from an increased delayed erythema reaction to severe burns with blistering. When large areas of skin are affected, systemic symptoms of excess phototoxicity, such as fever and general malaise, can occur.
Pruritus	Some patients experience persistent pruritus during photochemotherapy (PUVA) treatment, particularly after slight UVA overdosage.
Laboratory data	No significant abnormal findings in patients receiving PUVA over prolonged periods of time.
Potential Long-term Risks	
Chronic actinic damage	Chronic exposure to PUVA may produce changes in the skin that resemble photoaging. PUVA lentigines and generalized PUVA lentiginosis result from repeated and prolonged treatment and are commonly associated with high cumulative doses of UVA and a large number of treatments. So far, no increased risk of cutaneous melanoma associated with these lentigines has been recorded.
Carcinogenesis	The risk of squamous cell carcinoma, but not of basal cell carcinoma, is significantly increased in comparison with matched controls, and the magnitude of the increase appears to be dose-dependent. There is still uncertainty about PUVA being the sole factor—many of the affected patients had previous exposure to excessive sunlight and to treatments with carcinogenic potential, including arsenic, UVB, cyclosporine, and antimetabolite therapy. No increased risk was found so far with bath-PUVA.
Melanoma	Stern et al. reported from patients enrolled in the PUVA Follow-up Study (16-Center Study[69]) that, beginning 15 years after first exposure to PUVA, an increased risk of melanoma was observed. This risk was greater in patients exposed to high doses of PUVA and appeared to be increasing with the passage of time. The conclusions of this study have been questioned, and the authors now agree that the observed risk of melanoma does not represent an absolute contraindication to PUVA or that PUVA therapy should be abandoned. Rather, the risks of both melanoma and squamous cell carcinoma in PUVA should be weighed against the substantial efficacy of PUVA and the risks of other therapies.
Ophthalmologic effects	Several studies have shown no indication that psoralen-induced cataracts occur in patients undergoing long-term photochemotherapy, even in patients who neglected eye protection.

MOP, 8-methoxypsoralen; PUVA, psoralen and ultraviolet A light.

symptoms of excess phototoxicity, such as fever and general malaise, may occur. Nonsteroidal anti-inflammatory drugs and topical and systemic corticosteroids may be required to alleviate the symptoms but must be given early. Some patients experience persistent pruritus during PUVA treatment, particularly after slight UVA overdosage, and, in rare cases, a stinging pain may develop in circumscribed areas. The mechanism is unknown although a phototoxicity reaction affecting cutaneous nerves is postulated, and the symptoms are unresponsive to antihistamines. These complaints usually subside on continuation of treatment. Overdosage phenomena occur mostly in body areas not usually exposed to natural sunlight. Cautious dosimetry can minimize these side effects. The danger of overdosage is much less with 5-MOP than with 8-MOP.

Very rare side effects of PUVA include polymorphous light eruption-like rashes, acnelike eruptions, subungual hemorrhages caused by phototoxic reactions in the nail beds, and occasional hypertrichosis of the face. These disappear when treatment is discontinued. Single case reports note exacerbation of systemic lupus erythematosus and bullous pemphigoid during PUVA.

LABORATORY DATA

Analysis of laboratory data in several large-scale studies showed no significant abnormal findings in patients receiving PUVA over prolonged periods of time.[13,14,58] Serial laboratory examinations performed over a period of several years have not revealed any substantial evidence for impairment of hepatic function. Liver biopsies after 1 year of therapy did not reveal hepatotoxicity.[59] No evidence exists suggesting impairment of renal function.[13] Several large-scale studies have negated a suggested relation between PUVA therapy and the occurrence of antinuclear antibodies.[60]

POTENTIAL LONG-TERM RISKS OF PHOTOCHEMOTHERAPY

CHRONIC ACTINIC DAMAGE

Repeated photodamage to the skin can be expected to result in cumulative injury regardless of whether it is induced by sunlight, artificial UV radiation, or PUVA. Chronic exposure to PUVA may produce changes that resemble photoaging and that may compound the injury induced by sunlight.

PUVA lentigines and generalized PUVA lentiginosis result from repeated and prolonged treatment and are commonly associated with high cumulative doses of UVA and a large number of treatments.[14] The lentigines exhibit irregular borders and uneven pigmentation. No increased risk of cutaneous melanoma has been associated with these lentigines, but the cosmetic effect may be quite disturbing.

CARCINOGENESIS

Cutaneous carcinogenicity is the major concern for long-term PUVA treatment associated with high cumulative UVA doses. PUVA is a photocarcinogen (Chap. 19). In laboratory animals, 8-MOP and 5-MOP have been unequivocally shown to induce skin cancer at levels of drug and UVA irradiation comparable to those used in PUVA therapy.[61,62] This risk is related to DNA damage, but PUVA-induced downregulation of immune responses may play an additional role. This risk must be assessed against the potential therapeutic benefit.

Long-term followup PUVA studies are confounded by the fact that patients, particularly those with severe psoriasis, are likely to have been exposed previously to other carcinogenic treatments, such as ionizing radiation, UVB therapy, methotrexate, tar, or arsenic, and accurate exposure data are often lacking.

In PUVA patients, the risk of squamous cell carcinoma, but not of BCC, is significantly increased in comparison with matched controls and the magnitude of the increase appears to be dose dependent.[19,62] However, there is uncertainty about PUVA being the sole factor—many of the affected patients had previous exposure to excessive sunlight and to treatments with carcinogenic potential, including arsenic, UVB, and antimetabolite therapy.[63] Particularly, high levels of UVB exposure appear to increase the risk of nonmelanoma skin cancer in PUVA-treated patients.[64] An increased risk of any skin cancer with oral PUVA has not been shown in the nonwhite population.[65] According to one study, the genitalia in men previously treated with tar and UVB appeared to be particularly susceptible to PUVA carcinogenesis,[66] but in a separate population the risk seemed not to be increased if only PUVA was used.[67] In a retrospective study from France comprising 5400 patients treated with PUVA between 1978 and 1998, no case of genital skin cancer was found, despite the fact that the genital area had not been protected.[68] This makes it unlikely that genital shielding is absolutely necessary.

Carcinogenicity of 5-MOP–UVA therapy in PUVA-treated patients is not documented, but 5-MOP has shown mutagenicity like 8-MOP in model systems.

Stern et al reported that of the cohort of 1380 patients enrolled in the 16-Center PUVA Follow-up Study, 23 patients have developed 26 invasive or in situ cutaneous melanomas over a period of roughly 25 years. Beginning 15 years after first exposure to PUVA, this constituted an increased risk of melanoma.[69,70] This risk was greater in patients exposed to high doses of PUVA and appeared to increase with the passage of time. Still, the authors conclude that the observed risk of melanoma does not represent an absolute contraindication to PUVA. Rather, the risks of both melanoma and squamous cell carcinoma in PUVA should be weighed against the substantial efficacy of PUVA and the risks of other therapies.[70,71] As well, no increased risk of melanoma has been observed so far in any large-scale study from Europe; and several other US studies did not show an increased risk of melanoma in patients treated with PUVA.[72,73] Of note, PUVA's long-term risks have been subject to much greater scrutiny than the risks of other therapies advocated for severe psoriasis, such as methotrexate and, particularly, immunosuppressive therapies such as cyclosporine. These latter therapies greatly increase cancer risk in populations less likely to have substantial exposures to other known cutaneous carcinogens such as UVB than are patients with severe psoriasis. Early detection through careful, long-term followup and education of PUVA patients may reduce the long-term morbidity and mortality associated with this therapy, as can low cumulative dosage regimens.[74]

Studies of 944 Swedish and Finnish patients[75] and 158 Finnish patients[76] with psoriasis showing no association between cutaneous cancer and TMP or 8-MOP bath-PUVA, respectively, are also reassuring. Mathematic model studies indicate that the observed risk of squamous cell carcinoma is much higher with PUVA than with UVB,[77] but the carcinogenic risk of narrow-band UVB in comparison with PUVA is unknown, and it will be crucial to monitor its long-term effects in psoriatics.

OPHTHALMOLOGIC EFFECTS

Data from animal studies indicate a risk of premature cataract formation due to PUVA, but clinical evaluation suggests no increase in lens opacities, even in patients who neglect careful eye protection during long-term PUVA.[78,79]

PATIENT SELECTION AND CONTRAINDICATIONS

In view of the potential short-term and long-term hazards of PUVA, the assignment of patients should be based on consideration of the risks and the benefit for the individual patient. If only a short-term course of therapy is planned, as, for example, in prevention of photodermatoses, the benefit very probably outweighs the risk. In the treatment of a malignant condition such as CTCL, long-term risks may be discounted because other treatment options bear even greater long-term risks. The major concerns relate to long-term treatment of psoriasis, by far the most common indication for PUVA. Careful patient selection is mandatory, bearing in mind that long-term risks of alternative therapies may simply be less well documented rather than less. Guidelines have been published.[15]

PUVA is not recommended during pregnancy, and women should be advised to use contraceptive measures while on PUVA. This precaution is only for reasons of absolute safety as there is no evidence that 8-MOP alone is teratogenic, and UVA does not penetrate through the abdominal and uterine walls. Further, a retrospective study in 256 deliveries among the cohort of the 16-Center PUVA Follow-up Study revealed no birth defects.[80] However, it should be emphasized that RePUVA bears the risk of retinoid teratogenicity.

Severe impairment of hepatic and renal functions is usually considered a contraindication to PUVA because metabolism and excretion of psoralens may be inadequate. PUVA is also contraindicated in patients with known light-aggravated or light-induced diseases such as lupus erythematosus, porphyria (but, as mentioned earlier, light tolerance can be induced by PUVA in erythropoietic protoporphyria), and xeroderma pigmentosum. Pemphigus vulgaris and bullous pemphigoid may be exacerbated by PUVA. Patients with chronic actinic damage and a history of skin cancers may be at higher risk for the development of new cancers. Previous arsenic intake and previous treatment with ionizing radiation also seem to increase the risk of nonmelanoma skin cancers. Immunosuppressed patients should probably not receive PUVA, although this is not yet clearly defined. As outlined earlier, PUVA can be used in HIV-positive patients. Cataracts and aphakia are not contraindications if adequate eye protection is employed.

CONCLUSIONS AND PERSPECTIVES

PUVA is a highly effective treatment for several dermatologic diseases. Although there exists comprehensive clinical experience documenting PUVA's short-term safety when used according to standardized methods, potential long-term sequelae are still being studied. Thus, treatment decisions should take into account whether other equally effective forms of therapy that carry a lower risk are available. Risk-versus-benefit varies with the disease being treated.

Severe widespread psoriasis is a devastating disease that may impair professional, social, and private life. After more than 3 decades of experience with PUVA for the treatment of psoriasis, it is evident that this therapy offers innumerable patients the chance to resume a normal life. For disabling psoriasis, the choice of therapies lies not between risk and safety but among modalities (methotrexate, cyclosporine, UVB, and biologics), none of which is absolutely safe.[71]

EXTRACORPOREAL PHOTOCHEMOTHERAPY (PHOTOPHERESIS)

Extracorporeal PUVA (ECP) was introduced in the 1980s for the palliative treatment of erythrodermic CTCL,[81] a disorder characterized by circulating malignant lymphocytes. Its efficacy was subsequently confirmed by several clinical trials and approved in 1988 by the U.S. Food and Drug Administration for this indication. At the International Consensus Conference on Staging and Treatment Recommendations for CTCL in 1994[82] and at the European Organization for Research and Treatment of Cancer Consensus Recommendations in 2006,[83] ECP was recommended as the first line of treatment for patients with erythrodermic CTCL.

Attempts to better characterize those CTCL patients likely to respond to ECP revealed a significant association between response and CD4:CD8 ratio. Patients with a ratio less than 10 are more likely to respond than patients with a ratio greater than 10. There is also a marginally significant association between response and lactic acid dehydrogenase (LDH) level, with patients whose LDH is not elevated at the start of treatment responding better than patients with an elevated LDH.[84]

Besides CTCL, ECP also plays an important role in the treatment of chronic GVHD after allogeneic bone marrow transplantation with excellent response rates. ECP also has been used in uncontrolled studies in several other autoimmune diseases including systemic sclerosis, acute allograft rejection among cardiac, lung, and renal transplant recipients[85-87] and Crohn disease, with some success.

TREATMENT METHOD

ECP originally involved the oral administration of 8-MOP followed by phlebotomy at the time of peak photosensitization passage of blood fractions from one arm vein through a photopheresis machine and back. A discontinuous flow cell separator harvests peripheral blood mononuclear cells (PBMCs) in a buffy coat collection and returns the red cell fraction to the patient without further treatment. The collection of PBMC is then exposed to 2.0 J/cm^2 of UVA using a photopheresis device that ensures exposure of individual PBMC in a thin film to the light source and then reinfused into the patient. More recently, 8-MOP is administered directly to the heparinized plasma and buffy coat fraction as it flows through a UVA exposure system, thereby avoiding 8-MOP-induced nausea and unintended phototoxicity with subsequent incidental sun exposure.[88] This treatment is customarily repeated on 2 successive days at 2- to 4-week intervals.

MECHANISM OF ACTION

The mode of action of ECP remains unknown. The PUVA exposures likely induce apoptosis of circulating malignant lymphocytes. However, it also has been shown that infusion of autologous haptenated cells in which apoptosis had been initiated by 8-MOP/UVA induces immunologic tolerance. This tolerance is likely due primarily to regulatory T cells because transfer can be achieved in an animal model. Induction of regulatory T cells could also explain why ECP exerts a beneficial effect in a wide variety of immune-mediated diseases and why generalized immunosuppression does not occur with ECP.[89,90]

SIDE EFFECTS

No serious side effects have been reported with ECP. With oral ingestion of 8-MOP, transient nausea is not uncommon (as in oral PUVA therapy) and, rarely, episodes of hypotension and vasovagal reflex due to volume shifts during treatments have been noted. However, these events usually do not interfere with the treatment.

TREATMENT RESULTS

CUTANEOUS T-CELL LYMPHOMA

Erythrodermic CTCL (Sézary syndrome) was the first disease for which ECP was evaluated. A response occurs in up to 75% of the patients, with complete remissions in up to 25%. In Sézary syndrome patients who do not sufficiently respond to ECP alone, ongoing studies are evaluating possible synergistic effects with other treatments such as interferon-α, methotrexate, bexarotene, and total-skin electron-beam therapy.[91-94]

GRAFT-VERSUS-HOST DISEASE AND ALLOGRAFT REJECTION

ECP appears to have a major impact in the treatment of GVHD after allogeneic bone marrow transplantation.[95,96] In patients with either acute or chronic GVHD, ECP allows reduction or even discontinuation of immunosuppressive therapy without an increase in GVHD activity. More than 450 patients with chronic (even steroid-refractory cases), GVHD treated with ECP have been reported, with mean response rates of 63% (range 29%-100%). Responses were highest for those patients with cutaneous or mucous membrane involvement. Positive results also have been published for acute GVHD.[87,97] ECP is especially useful for patients affected by GVHD resistant to conventional treatment.

As mentioned above, ECP is effective in the treatment of acute allograft rejection among lung, cardiac, and renal transplant recipients. ECP is effective for patients resistant to conventional treatments, particularly if started early. Benefit is obtained without the complications typically encountered with immunosuppressive regimens used to control organ rejection.[98,99] Table 199-4 shows indications for photopheresis as currently approved by regulatory agencies.

TABLE 199-4
Indications for Photopheresis (as Seen by Regulatory Agencies in 2017)

Sufficient Evidence Available

Erythrodermic cutaneous T-cell lymphoma	Chronic graft-versus-host disease
Acute graft-versus-host disease	Organ transplant rejection

Experimental and Investigational

Scleroderma	Nephrogenic fibrosing dermopathy
Bullous dermatoses	Lichen planus
Crohn disease	Multiple sclerosis

PHOTODYNAMIC THERAPY

Photodynamic therapy (PDT) aims to destroy the desired target selectively, thereby minimizing damage to normal tissue. The photodynamic reaction consists of the excitation of photosensitizers (usually porphyrins) by visible light in the presence of oxygen, resulting in the generation of reactive oxygen species, particularly singlet oxygen. These reactive oxygen species mediate cellular and vascular effects, depending on the tissue localization of the photosensitizer, and results in a direct or indirect cytotoxic effect on the target cells.[100] In dermatology, PDT has been used effectively for precancerous and malignant conditions such as actinic keratosis, BCC, Bowen disease, and superficial squamous cell carcinoma, as well as for inflammatory and infectious dermatoses such as localized scleroderma, acne vulgaris, and leishmaniasis. A relatively new approach is the treatment of ageing skin with PDT (photochemorejuvenation).

PRINCIPLES OF PHOTODYNAMIC THERAPY

PHOTOSENSITIZERS

The ideal photosensitizer for PDT in dermatology should meet the following criteria: (1) chemical purity, (2) high singlet-oxygen quantum yield, (3) significant light absorption at wavelengths that penetrate the skin sufficiently deeply, (4) high tissue selectivity, and (5) efficacy after topical application.

Porfimer sodium (Photofrin), a systemically administered mixture of several hematoporphyrin derivative (HpD) ethers and esters, has a low selectivity for skin tumors, and leads to long-lasting photosensitivity; consequently, it is far from ideal for dermatologic use. In contrast, 5-aminolevulinic acid (ALA), an intermediate in heme biosynthesis or its methyl ester (MAL) leads to synthesis of photosensitizing protoporphyrin IX in the target tissue.[101] In this case, the concentration of the photosensitizer depends on the metabolic status of the diseased tissue with photosensitization greatest in precancerous or malignant tissue. ALA in combination with blue light, ALA in combination with red light, and MAL in combination with red light are approved by the US Food and Drug Administration for the treatment of actinic keratoses. In Europe, New Zealand, Australia, and South America, ALA and MAL also have been registered for superficial and nodular BCCs, and MAL also for Bowen disease.

Most photosensitizers generate singlet oxygen with a quantum yield between 5% and 20%. A high quantum yield means that less sensitizer is required in the target tissue to induce sufficient PDT effects. The light absorption maxima of the current sensitizers are in the visible range (400-700 nm). In this range, light penetration in tissue is only up to 3 mm, limiting PDT to superficial tumors unless interstitial light propagation is used. A high selectivity for sensitizer accumulation in target tissue is necessary to avoid damage to surrounding normal tissue, and this is particularly important when larger areas are treated (eg, actinic keratoses). ALA and MAL show reasonably high selectivity after topical application, with the ratio of porphyrin induction in skin tumors to the surrounding tissue higher than 10:1,[102] likely due to a combination of enhanced ALA-MAL penetration through an abnormal stratum corneum and altered metabolism and accumulation within the premalignant or malignant cells.

LIGHT SOURCES AND DOSIMETRY

Light penetration into skin increases with longer wavelengths up to 1100 nm. Although porphyrins absorb maximally in the Soret band (400-410 nm, blue light), there are minor absorption peaks at longer visible light wavelengths. To increase depth of penetration while matching the absorption maxima of porphyrin photosensitizers, wavelengths around 630 nm are often used. Lasers are effective but they are quite expensive, require regular maintenance, and have a small treatment aperture. Hence, simpler incoherent light sources represent a valuable alternative. Fluorescent lamps or light-emitting diodes (LEDs) with appropriate red or blue light emission are commercially available and designed for treatment of large surface areas. Also, intense pulsed-light sources are used for dermatologic PDT. Dosimetry depends on the photosensitizer and light source used, as well as on the condition to be treated. For PDT of epithelial cancer, photosensitization must be sufficient to induce necrosis or apoptosis. With current incoherent light sources (lamps, LED), the treatment duration, apart from of ALA-MAL incubation time, is approximately 10 to 15 minutes. For treating inflammatory dermatoses, significantly lower doses suffice because the goal appears not to be cell death but rather sublethal damage or modulation of cellular functions.

A relatively new approach that is already registered in Europe, South America, Canada, and Australia is the combination of MAL application to AK lesions on the skin (face, scalp), followed by subsequent exposure to daylight for 120 min. This procedure is called daylight-mediated photodynamic therapy (DL-PDT).[103]

MECHANISM OF ACTION

PDT-induced effects are mediated by photo-oxidative reactions. During irradiation, the photosensitizer absorbs light (energy) and is converted to an excited (triplet) state. The energy can then be transferred to molecular oxygen (Type II photo-oxidative reaction), resulting in the generation of reactive oxygen species, mainly singlet oxygen. The biologic effects can be divided into primary cellular and secondary vascular damage. With HpD, early visible damage consists of cell membrane defects as a consequence of lipid peroxidation with consequent cell lysis. Depending on the intracellular localization of the photosensitizers, damage to subcellular structures, such as mitochondria, lysosomes, or endoplasmic reticulum, also occurs, whereas DNA is not a primary target. These direct effects probably play a key role in topical PDT, whereas vascular effects after systemic administration of photosensitizers appear to be the decisive event. These effects consist of vasoconstriction, blood stasis, and thrombosis of tumor vessels leading to tumor ischemia and subsequent necrosis.[104]

TABLE 199-5
Current Indications for Photodynamic Therapy

ONCOLOGIC	NONONCOLOGIC (ALL OFF-LABEL USES)
- Actinic keratosis[a#]	- Localized scleroderma
- Bowen disease[b]	- Human papillomavirus–associated dermatoses
- Actinic cheilitis[b]	• Epidermodysplasia verruciformis
- Superficial BCC[b]	• Verrucae vulgaris
- Nevoid BCC syndrome (off-label use)	• Condylomata acuminata
- Keratoacanthoma (off-label use)	- Leishmaniasis
- Superficial SCC (off-label use)	- Acne vulgaris
- Kaposi sarcoma (off-label use)	- Rosacea
- Cutaneous metastases (off-label use)	- Photochemorejuvenation of sun-damaged skin
- Cutaneous T-cell lymphoma (off-label use)	

[a]Approved in the Americas, European Union, Australia–New Zealand.
[b]Approved in the European Union, Australia–New Zealand, and Brazil.
[#]Approval for classical PDT with blue or red light (ALA, MAL) and daylight-mediated PDT (MAL).
BCC, basal cell carcinoma; SCC, squamous cell carcinoma.

PHOTODYNAMIC THERAPY IN DERMATOLOGY

Table 199-5 lists current applications for PDT described in the literature. In contrast to other organs, the skin can be sensitized by either intravenous, topical, or intralesional routes of administration of the photosensitizer.

SYSTEMIC PHOTODYNAMIC THERAPY

PDT after systemic administration of HpD and porfimer sodium has been used for both skin cancers and inflammatory dermatoses. Standard therapeutic procedures do not yet exist.

Systemic Photodynamic Therapy for Oncologic Indications: Systemic PDT with porfimer sodium for Bowen disease is very effective,[105] but invasive squamous cell carcinomas respond less well, with recurrence rates of up to 50% within 6 months. Systemic PDT for BCCs, first used in 1981,[106] has been reported by Oseroff and coworkers[107] to give initial complete responses in 92.2% of 77 patients with sporadic BCC or nevoid BCC syndrome.[107] In these patients, the 5-year recurrence rate was 15%.

Benzoporphyrin-derivative monoacid ring A (verteporfin), registered for the ophthalmologic indication of age-related macular degeneration, is also under investigation for PDT of BCC and offers a duration of cutaneous photosensitization of less than 72 hours, significantly shorter than that of porfimer sodium.[108]

Systemic Photodynamic Therapy for Nononcologic Indications: The use of PDT with HpD was reported for the treatment of psoriasis as early as 1937; better results were reported using red light instead of UVA,[109] and systemic PDT with verteporfin was also investigated in a Phase I study of 15 patients in whom clinical severity scores for psoriatic plaques improved after 5 weekly treatments.[110]

TOPICAL PHOTODYNAMIC THERAPY

Small hydrophilic molecules like ALA or MAL penetrate well into the skin, particularly if the stratum corneum is abnormal, as is the case in some epidermal tumors.[101] In addition, epidermal cells and the pilosebaceous unit synthesize porphyrins to a much greater extent than fibroblasts, myocytes, or endothelial cells[102]; epithelial tumors generally synthesize much higher amounts of protoporphyrin IX than the surrounding tissue and can therefore be destroyed without equivalent damage to healthy skin (Fig. 199-7).[101,111] Topical ALA-MAL-induced photosensitivity thus preferentially affects the target area. Systemic porphyrin induction is not observed after topical application.[112] The only significant side effect of topical ALA-MAL PDT is a stinging pain during and shortly after irradiation, proportional to the intensity of the phototoxicity reaction. In contrast to classical ALA/MAL PDT with red light, DL-PDT is not painful,[103] because of its different mode of action. With conventional PDT, PPIX formation is continuously induced during the incubation period (between 3 and 18 hours); PPIX

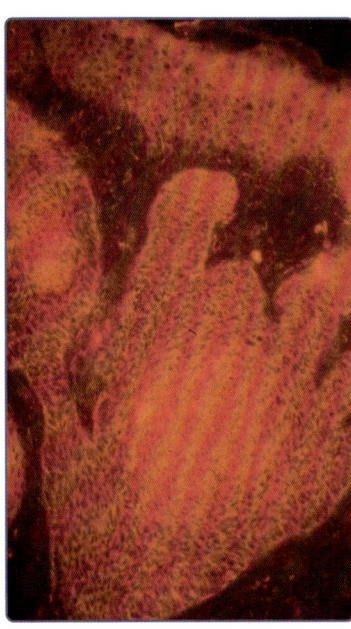

Figure 199-7 Endogenous porphyrin fluorescence after topical application of 20% aminolevulinic acid formulation to a solid basal cell carcinoma. Twelve hours after aminolevulinic acid application, there was strong fluorescence of the tumor-bearing areas, and weak to no fluorescence of the surrounding dermis. Also visible is fluorescence in the overlying epidermis. (From Szeimies RM, Sassy T, Landthaler M. Penetration potency of topical applied & alpha-aminolevulinic acid for photodynamic therapy of basal cell carcinoma. *Photochem Photobiol.* 1994;59:73. Copyright © 1977 John Wiley & Sons.)

therefore leaves the subcellular compartments of the cell and is excreted extracellularly to sustain cellular homeostasis. The consequence is photosensitization of free nerve endings in the epidermis. Upon illumination within the PDT procedure, direct ROS formation within and near those nerve fibers is responsible for the pain perception.[113,114] With DL-PDT, continuous illumination for 2 hours starts within 30 minutes following photosensitizer application. Newly formed PPIX then is still within the intracellular mitochondria of diseased keratinocytes (in the case of AK treatment) so that no PPIX or ROS reaches nerve fibers.[114]

Topical Photodynamic Therapy for Oncologic Indications[115-124]: The experience with treatment of epithelial cancers and precancerous conditions with PDT as of this writing suggests that actinic keratoses,[103,115,116] Bowen disease (Fig. 199-8),[117] superficial and nodular BCCs,[118-120] (tumor thickness less than 2 mm) are suitable for topical ALA/MAL-PDT. For this purpose, both photosensitizers are applied topically for variable incubation periods, with or without occlusion, followed by visible light exposure.

Actinic keratoses have been studied most extensively and respond to PDT as readily as to local cryotherapy or to broad-area 5-fluorouracil (Chap. 190) or imiquimod therapy (Chap. 192) administered over weeks to months. Topical application of a 20% ALA solution for 14 to 18 hours followed by irradiation with blue light (417 nm) for 1000 seconds (10 J/cm^2) clears more than 80% of actinic keratoses after 1 to 6 months,[116] and 90% complete clearance at 1 and 5 months was observed after one full face treatment using a 1- to 3-hour incubation period.[116] DL-PDT with MAL for mild to mod-

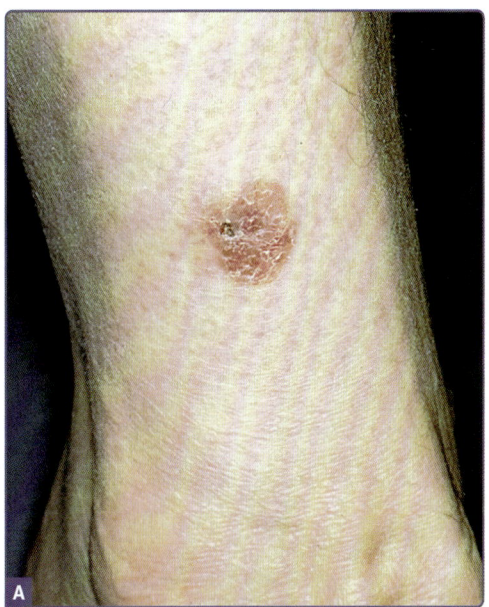
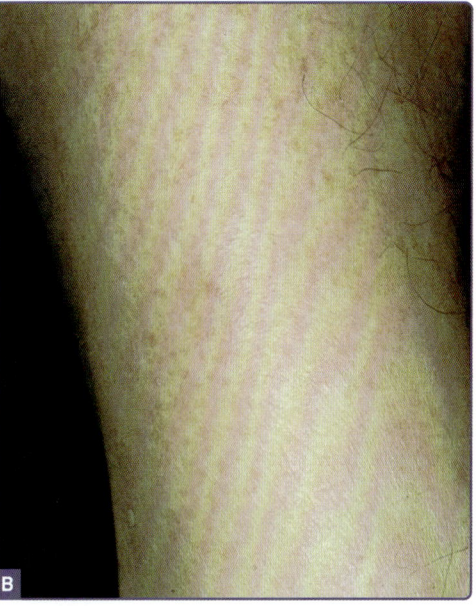

Figure 199-8 Bowen disease. **A,** Lesion located on the right lower leg. **B,** Twelve months after topical aminolevulinic acid–photodynamic therapy (10% aminolevulinic acid ointment, application for 4 hours, irradiation with argon-pumped dye laser [175 mW/cm^2; 180 J/cm^2]), clinically and histologically, there were no signs of tumor residue.

erate AK is equally efficacious to conventional PDT with red LED light.[103,121] However, cutaneous metastases of malignant melanoma, pigmented BCC, and sclerodermiform variants of BCC respond poorly to ALA-PDT, probably because of insufficient porphyrin synthesis and/or penetration of light within the lesions.[111] Treatment efficacy is enhanced by repeated treatment sessions[121] or by lesion pretreatment with either fractionated ablative laser devices[122] (Er:YAG, CO_2) (Chap. 209) or microneedling.[122,123]

In superficial and nodular BCCs, 2 randomized phase-III studies have been reported so far comparing MAL-PDT with either surgery or cryotherapy. After an observation period of 60 months, MAL-PDT for superficial BCC showed a similar recurrence rate as cryotherapy (22% vs 20%). In nodular BCC, MAL-PDT was compared with simple excision; recurrence rates after 60 months were 14% and 4%, respectively. In both studies, the cosmetic outcome was considered superior for the PDT-treated groups.[118,119] Indeed, these and other reports[120,121] suggest that a major theoretical benefit of ALA/MAL-PDT is elimination of skin cancers without scarring, as well as prevention of such lesions in high-risk patients treated periodically with broad-area PDT.

CTCL (mycosis fungoides) also responded in 8 single case reports to ALA-MAL PDT after several treatment sessions. Controlled investigations are currently not available, and, as with PUVA treatment of single lesions, this treatment would not be expected to prevent the appearance of new lesions in other areas.[124]

Topical Photodynamic Therapy for Non-oncologic Indications[125-141]: Few data are available regarding the treatment of inflammatory and proliferative skin conditions. These include psoriasis, localized scleroderma, human papilloma virus (HPV)–associated conditions, leishmaniasis, acne, and rosacea.

ALA/MAL-PDT is also effective for acne and rosacea, although optimal protocols have not been developed. In 2 separate studies,[134,135] 22 patients with mild to moderate acne on the back received 20% ALA cream under occlusion for 3 hours. The areas were then exposed to broadband (550-700 nm) or laser light (635 nm) using various protocols. The authors observed a significant reduction in inflammatory acne lesion counts compared with baseline that persisted at least 20 weeks in some patients.[134] One study found a reduction in sebaceous gland size and sebum secretion, as well as reduced fluorescence attributable to *Propionibacterium acnes*,[134] although the other did not.[135]

PDT with ALA or MAL also has been demonstrated to enhance the treatment of photodamaged skin with a variety of lasers and light sources (also Chaps. 209 and 210). Improvement of global appearance, fine lines, tactile skin roughness, mottled hyperpigmentation, and telangiectasias has been described.[138-145] Mode of action is based on the degradation of altered collagen and elastotic material and the formation of newly synthesized collagen directly underneath the epidermis.[142-144] The combination with daylight exposure also seems possible.[146]

PERSPECTIVES

The efficacy of PDT in the treatment of superficial neoplastic skin lesion, particularly actinic keratoses, Bowen disease, and superficial BCCs, has been sufficiently documented. PDT may also find a place in the treatment of selected patients with inflammatory dermatoses. Nonetheless, the limitations of both systemic and topical PDT have to be kept in mind. Crucial issues are the depth of the penetration of light, as well as of the sensitizer, into the skin, and inability to ensure complete eradication of malignancy by histologic criteria.

REFERENCES

1. Pathak MA, Fitzpatrick TB. The evolution of photochemotherapy with psoralens and UVA (PUVA): 2000 BC to 1992 AD. *J Photochem Photobiol B Biol*. 1992; 14(1-2):3-22.
2. Parrish JA, Fitzpatrick TB, Tanenbaum L, et al. Photochemotherapy of psoriasis with oral methoxsalen and long wave ultraviolet light. *N Engl J Med*. 1974; 291(23):1207-1211.
3. Wolff K, Fitzpatrick TB, Parrish JA, et al. Photochemotherapy for psoriasis with orally administered methoxsalen. *Arch Dermatol*. 1976;112(7):943-950.
4. Fischer T, Alsins J. Treatment of psoriasis with trioxsalen baths and dysprosium lamps. *Acta Derm Venereol*. 1976;56(5):383-390.
5. Dall'Acqua F. Principles of psoralen photosensitization. In: Hönigsmann H, Jori G, Young AR, eds. *The Fundamental Bases of Phototherapy*. Milano: OEMF; 1996:1-16.
6. Schmitt IM, et al. Photobiology of psoralens. In: Hönigsmann H, Jori G, Young AR, eds. *The Fundamental Bases of Phototherapy*. Milan: OEMF; 1996:17.
7. Averbeck D. Recent advances in psoralen phototoxicity mechanism. *Photochem Photobiol*. 1989;50(6):859-882.
8. Hönigsmann H. Phototherapy for psoriasis. *Clin Exp Dermatol*. 2001;26(4):343-350.
9. Wolff K, Gschnait F, Hönigsmann H, et al. Phototesting and dosimetry for photochemotherapy. *Br J Dermatol*. 1977;96(1):1.
10. Ibbotson SH, Dawe RS, Farr PM. The effect of methoxsalen dose on ultraviolet-A-induced erythema. *J Invest Dermatol*. 2001;116(5):813-815.
11. Ibbotson SH, Farr PM. The time-course of psoralen ultraviolet A (PUVA) erythema. *J Invest Dermatol*. 1999;113(3):346-350.
12. Halpern SM, Anstey AV, Dawe RS, et al. Guidelines for topical PUVA: a report of a workshop of the British photodermatology group. *Br J Dermatol*. 2000; 142(1):22-31.
13. Melski JW, Tanenbaum L, Parrish JA, et al. Oral methoxsalen photochemotherapy for the treatment of psoriasis: a cooperative clinical trial. *J Invest Dermatol*. 1977;68(6):328-335.
14. Henseler T, Wolff K, Hönigsmann H, et al. Oral 8-methoxypsoralen photochemotherapy of pso-

riasis. The European PUVA study: a cooperative study among 18 European centres. *Lancet.* 1981; 1(8225):853-857.
15. Menter A, Korman NJ, Elmets CA, et al. Guidelines of care for the management of psoriasis and psoriatic arthritis Section 5. Guidelines of care for the treatment of psoriasis with phototherapy and photochemotherapy. *J Am Acad Dermatol.* 2010;62(1): 114-135.
16. Anonymous. British Photodermatology Group guidelines for PUVA. *Br J Dermatol.* 1994;130(2):246-255.
17. Radakovic S, Seeber A, Hönigsmann H, et al. Failure of short-term psoralen and ultraviolet A light maintenance treatment to prevent early relapse in patients with chronic recurring plaque-type psoriasis. *Photodermatol Photoimmunol Photomed.* 2009;25(2):90-93.
18. Morison WL. Phototherapy and photochemotherapy. *Adv Dermatol.* 1992;7:255-270; discussion 271.
19. Stern RS, Laird N. Photochemotherapy follow-up study: the carcinogenic risks of treatments for severe psoriasis. *Cancer.* 1994;73(11):2759-2764.
20. Marcil I, Stern RS. Squamous-cell cancer of the skin in patients given PUVA and ciclosporin: nested cohort crossover study. *Lancet.* 2001;358(9287):1042.
21. Molin L, Larkö O. Cancer induction by immunosuppression in psoriasis after heavy PUVA treatment [letter]. *Acta Derm Venereol.* 1997;77(5):402.
22. van de Kerkhof PC, De Rooij MJ. Multiple squamous cell carcinomas in a psoriatic patient following high-dose photochemotherapy and cyclosporin treatment: response to long-term acitretin maintenance. *Br J Dermatol.* 1997;136(2):275-278.
23. Hönigsmann H, Wolff K. Results of therapy for psoriasis using retinoid and photochemotherapy (RePUVA). *Pharmacol Ther.* 1989;40:67.
24. Nijsten TEC, Stern RS. Oral retinoid use reduces cutaneous squamous cell carcinoma risk in patients with psoriasis treated with psoralen-UVA: a nested cohort study. *J Am Acad Dermatol.* 2003;49:644.
25. Ortonne JP, Khemis A, Koo JY, et al. An open-label study of alefacept plus ultraviolet B light as combination therapy for chronic plaque psoriasis. *J Eur Acad Dermatol Venereol.* 2005;19(5):556-563.
26. Lebwohl M. Combining the new biologic agents with our current psoriasis armamentarium. *J Am Acad Dermatol.* 2003;49(suppl 2):S118-S124.
27. Gilchrest BA, Parrish JA, Tanenbaum L, et al. Oral methoxsalen photochemotherapy of mycosis fungoides. *Cancer.* 1976;38(2):683-689.
28. Baron ED, Stevens SR. Phototherapy for cutaneous T-cell lymphoma. *Dermatol Ther.* 2003;16(4):303-310.
29. Zhang C, Duvic M. Retinoids: therapeutic applications and mechanisms of action in cutaneous T-cell lymphoma. *Dermatol Ther.* 2003;16(4):322-330.
30. Singh F, Lebwohl MG. Cutaneous T-cell lymphoma treatment using bexarotene and PUVA: a case series. *J Am Acad Dermatol.* 2004;51(4):570-573.
31. Tanew A, Hönigsmann H. Ultraviolet B and psoralen plus UVA phototherapy for cutaneous T-cell lymphoma. *Dermatol Ther.* 1997;4:38.
32. Stadler R, Otte HG, Luger T, et al. Prospective randomized multicenter clinical trial on the use of interferon-2a plus acitretin versus interferon-2a plus PUVA in patients with cutaneous T-cell lymphoma stages I and II. *Blood.* 1998;92(10):3578-3581.
33. Stadler R. Optimal combination with PUVA: rationale and clinical trial update. *Oncology (Williston Park).* 2007;2(suppl 1):29-32.
34. Querfeld C, Rosen ST, Kuzel TM. Long-term followup of patients with early-stage cutaneous T-cell lymphoma who achieved complete remission with psoralen plus UV-A monotherapy. *Arch Dermatol.* 2005;141(3):305-311.
35. Morison WL. *Phototherapy and Photochemotherapy of Skin Disease.* 2nd ed. New York, NY: Raven; 1991:148.
36. Tzaneva S, Kittler H, Holzer G, et al. 5-Methoxypsoralen plus ultraviolet (UV) A is superior to medium-dose UVA1 in the treatment of severe atopic dermatitis: a randomized crossover trial. *Br J Dermatol.* 2010; 162(3):655-660.
37. Honig B, Morison WL, Karp D. Photochemotherapy beyond psoriasis. *J Am Acad Dermatol.* 1994;31(5, pt 1): 775-790.
38. Christophers E, Hönigsmann H, Wolff K, et al. PUVA-treatment of urticaria pigmentosa. *Br J Dermatol.* 1978; 98(6):701-702.
39. Lange-Wantzin G, Thomsen K. PUVA-treatment in lymphomatoid papulosis. *Br J Dermatol.* 1982; 107(6):687-690.
40. Kerker BJ, Huang CP, Morison WL. Photochemotherapy of generalized granuloma annulare. *Arch Dermatol.* 1990;126(3):359-361.
41. Taylor CR, Hawk JLM. PUVA treatment of alopecia areata partialis, totalis and universalis: audit of 10 years' experience at St. John's Institute of Dermatology. *Br J Dermatol.* 1995;133(6):914-918.
42. Kerscher M, Volkenandt M, Meurer M, et al. Treatment of localised scleroderma with PUVA bath photochemotherapy. *Lancet.* 1994;343(8907):1233.
43. Scharffetter-Kochanek K, Goldermann R, Lehmann P, et al. PUVA therapy in disabling pansclerotic morphoea of children. *Br J Dermatol.* 1995;132(5):830-831.
44. Volc-Platzer B, Hönigsmann H, Hinterberger W, et al. Photochemotherapy improves chronic cutaneous graft-versus-host disease. *J Am Acad Dermatol.* 1990; 23(2, pt 1):220-228.
45. Kunz M, Wilhelm S, Freund M, et al. Treatment of severe erythrodermic acute graft-versus-host disease with photochemotherapy. *Br J Dermatol.* 2001; 144(4):901-902.
46. Kwok YK, Anstey AV, Hawk JL. Psoralen photochemotherapy (PUVA) is only moderately effective in widespread vitiligo: a 10-year retrospective study. *Clin Exp Dermatol.* 2002;27(2):104-110.
47. Yones SS, Palmer RA, Garibaldinos TM, et al. Randomized double blind trial of treatment of vitiligo. *Arch Dermatol.* 2007;143(5):578-584.
48. Hönigsmann H. Mechanisms of phototherapy and photochemotherapy for photodermatoses. *Dermatol Ther.* 2003;16(1):23-27.
49. Hönigsmann H. Polymorphous light eruption. *Photodermatol Photoimmunol Photomed.* 2008;24(3):155.
50. Roelandts R. Diagnosis and treatment of solar urticaria. *Dermatol Ther.* 2003;16(1):52-56.
51. Tanew A, Ferguson J. Phototherapy and photochemotherapy of the idiopathic photodermatoses. In: Krutmann J, Hönigsmann H, Elmets C, eds. *Dermatological Phototherapy and Photodiagnostic Methods.* 2nd ed. Berlin: Springer; 2009:119.
52. Roelandts R. Photo(chemo)therapy and general management of erythropoietic protoporphyria. *Dermatology.* 1995;190(4):330-331.
53. Ullrich SE. Does exposure to UV radiation induce a shift to a Th-2-like immune reaction? *Photochem Photobiol.* 1996;64(2):254-258.

54. Morrey JD, Bourn SM, Bunch TD, et al. In vivo activation of human immunodeficiency virus type 1 long terminal repeat by UV type A (UV-A) light plus psoralen and UV-B light in the skin of transgenic mice. *J Virol*. 1991;65(9):5045-5051.
55. Zmudzka BZ, Miller SA, Jacobs ME, et al. Medical UV exposures and HIV activation. *Photochem Photobiol*. 1996;64(2):246-253.
56. Morison WL. PUVA therapy is preferable to UVB phototherapy in the management of HIV-associated dermatoses. *Photochem Photobiol*. 1996;64(2):267-268.
57. Menon K, Van Voorhees AS, Bebo BF Jr, et al; for the National Psoriasis Foundation. Psoriasis in patients with HIV infection: from the medical board of the National Psoriasis Foundation. *J Am Acad Dermatol*. 2010;62(2):291-299.
58. Hönigsmann H. Psoralen photochemotherapy—mechanisms, drugs, toxicity. *Curr Probl Dermatol*. 1986;15:52-66.
59. Nyfors A, Dahl-Nyfors B, Hopwood D. Liver biopsies from patients with psoriasis related to photochemotherapy (PUVA): findings before and after 1 year of therapy in twelve patients. A blind study and review of literature on hepatotoxicity of PUVA. *J Am Acad Dermatol*. 1986;14(1):43-48.
60. Calzavara-Pinton PG, Franceschini F, Rastrelli M, et al. Antinuclear antibodies are not induced by PUVA treatment with uncomplicated psoriasis. *J Am Acad Dermatol*. 1994;30(6):955-958.
61. Dunnick JK, Forbes PD, Eustis SL, et al. Tumors of the skin in the HRA/Skh mouse after treatment with 8-methoxypsoralen and UVA radiation. *Fundam Appl Toxicol*. 1991;16(1):92-102.
62. Stern RS, Liebman EJ, Vakeva L. Oral psoralen and ultraviolet-A light (PUVA) treatment of psoriasis and persistent risk of nonmelanoma skin cancer. PUVA Follow-up Study. *J Natl Cancer Inst*. 1998;90(17):1278.
63. Henseler T, Christophers E, Hönigsmann H, et al. Skin tumors in the European PUVA study. Eight year follow-up of 1643 patients treated with PUVA for psoriasis. *J Am Acad Dermatol*. 1987;16(1, pt 1):108-116.
64. Lim JL, Stern RS. High levels of ultraviolet B exposure increase the risk of nonmelanoma skin cancer in psoralen and ultraviolet A-treated patients. *J Invest Dermatol*. 2005;124(3):505-513.
65. Murase JE, Lee EE, Koo J. Effect of ethnicity on the risk of developing nonmelanoma skin cancer following long-term PUVA therapy. *Int J Dermatol*. 2005;44(12):1016-1021.
66. Stern RS; Members of the Photochemotherapy Follow-up Study. Genital tumors among men with psoriasis exposed to psoralens and ultraviolet A (PUVA) radiation and ultraviolet B radiation. *N Engl Med J*. 1990;322(16):1093-1097.
67. Wolff K, Hönigsmann H. Genital carcinomas in psoriasis patients treated with photochemotherapy. *Lancet*. 1991;337(8738):439.
68. Aubin F, Puzenat E, Arveux P, et al. Genital squamous cell carcinoma in men treated by photochemotherapy. A cancer registry-based study from 1978 to 1998. *Br J Dermatol*. 2001;144(6):1204-1206.
69. Stern RS; The PUVA follow-up study. The risk of melanoma in association with long-term exposure to PUVA. *J Am Acad Dermatol*. 2001;44(5):755-761.
70. Stern RS, Nichols KT, Vakeva LH. Malignant melanoma in patients treated for psoriasis with methoxsalen (psoralen) and ultraviolet A radiation (PUVA). The PUVA follow-up study. *N Engl J Med*. 1997;336(15):1041-1045.
71. Wolff K. Should PUVA be abandoned? [editorial]. *N Engl J Med*. 1997;336(15):1090-1091.
72. Forman AB, Roenigk HH Jr, Caro WA, et al. Long-term follow-up of skin cancer in the PUVA-48 cooperative study. *Arch Dermatol*. 1989;125(4):515-519.
73. Chuang TY, Heinrich LA, Schultz MD, et al. PUVA and skin cancer: a historical cohort study on 492 patients. *J Am Acad Dermatol*. 1992;26(2, pt 1):173-177.
74. Young AR. Photochemotherapy and skin carcinogenesis: a critical review. In: Hönigsmann H, Jori G, Young AR, eds. *The Fundamental Bases of Phototherapy*. Milan: OEMF; 1996:77.
75. Hannuksela-Svahn A, Sigurgeirsson B, Pukkala E, et al. Trioxsalen bath PUVA did not increase the risk of squamous cell skin carcinoma and cutaneous malignant melanoma in a joint analysis of 944 Swedish and Finnish patients with psoriasis. *Br J Dermatol*. 1999;141(3):497-501.
76. Hannuksela-Svahn A, Pukkala E, Koulu L, et al. Cancer incidence among Finnish psoriasis patients treated with 8-methoxypsoralen bath PUVA. *J Am Acad Dermatol*. 1999;40(5, pt 1):694-696.
77. Young AR. Carcinogenicity of UVB phototherapy assessed. *Lancet*. 1995;345(8962):1431-1432.
78. Stern RS. Ocular lens findings in patients treated with PUVA. Photochemotherapy follow-up study. *J Invest Dermatol*. 1994;103(4):534-538.
79. Malanos D, Stern RS. Psoralen plus ultraviolet A does not increase the risk of cataracts: a 25-year prospective study. *J Am Acad Dermatol*. 2007;57(2):231-237.
80. Stern RS, Lange R. Outcomes of pregnancies among women and partners of men with a history of exposure to methoxsalen photochemotherapy (PUVA) for the treatment of psoriasis. *Arch Dermatol*. 1991;127(3):347-350.
81. Edelson R, Berger C, Gasparro F, et al. Treatment of cutaneous T-cell lymphoma. *N Engl J Med*. 1987;316(6):297-303.
82. Demierre MF, Foss F, Koh H. Proceedings of the International Consensus Conference on cutaneous T-cell lymphoma (CTCL): treatment recommendations. *J Am Acad Dermatol*. 1997;36(3, pt 1):460-466.
83. Trautinger F, Eder J, Assaf C, et al. European Organisation for Research and Treatment of Cancer consensus recommendations for the treatment of mycosis fungoides/Sézary syndrome—update 2017. *Eur J Cancer*. 2017;77:57-74.
84. Knobler E, Warmuth I, Cocco C, et al. Extracorporeal photochemotherapy—the Columbia Presbyterian experience. *Photodermatol Photoimmunol Photomed*. 2002;18(5):232-237.
85. Scarisbrick J. Extracorporeal photopheresis: what is it and when should it be used? *Clin Exp Dermatol*. 2009;34(7):757-760.
86. Knobler R, Barr ML, Couriel DR, et al. Extracorporeal photopheresis: past, present, and future. *J Am Acad Dermatol*. 2009;61(4):652-665.
87. McKenna KE, Whittaker S, Rhodes LE, et al. Evidence-based practice of photopheresis 1987-2001: a report of a workshop of the British Photodermatology Group and the U.K. Skin Lymphoma Group. *Br J Dermatol*. 2006;154(1):7-20.
88. Knobler RM, Trautinger F, Graninger W, et al. Parenteral administration of 8-methoxypsoralen in photopheresis. *J Am Acad Dermatol*. 1993;28(4):

89. Maeda A, Schwarz A, Kernebeck K, et al. Intravenous infusion of syngeneic apoptotic cells by photopheresis induces antigen-specific regulatory T-cells. *J Immunol.* 2005;174(10):5968-5976.
90. Maeda A, Schwarz A, Bullinger A, et al. Experimental extracorporeal photopheresis inhibits the sensitization and effector phases of contact hypersensitivity via two mechanisms: generation of IL-10 and induction of regulatory T cells. *J Immunol.* 2008;181(9):5956-5962.
91. Knobler R, Girardi M. Extracorporeal photochemoimmunotherapy in cutaneous T-cell lymphomas. *Ann N Y Acad Sci.* 2001;941:123-138.
92. Zic JA, Stricklin GP, Greer JP, et al. Long-term follow-up of patients with cutaneous T-cell lymphoma treated with extracorporeal photochemotherapy. *J Am Acad Dermatol.* 1996;35:935-945.
93. Gottlieb SL, Wolfe JT, Fox FE, et al. Treatment of cutaneous T-cell lymphoma with extracorporeal photopheresis monotherapy and in combination with recombinant interferon alfa: a 10-year experience at a single institution. *J Am Acad Dermatol.* 1996;35(6):946-957.
94. Shapiro M, Rook AH, Lehrer MS, et al. Novel multimodality biologic response modifier therapy, including bexarotene and long-wave ultraviolet A for a patient with refractory stage IVa cutaneous T-cell lymphoma. *J Am Acad Dermatol.* 2002;47(6):956-961.
95. Greinix HT, Volc-Platzer B, Rabitsch W, et al. Successful use of extracorporeal photochemotherapy in the treatment of severe acute and chronic graft-versus-host disease. *Blood.* 1998;92(9):3098-3104.
96. Foss FM, DiVenuti GM, Chin K, et al. Prospective study of extracorporeal photopheresis in steroid-refractory or steroid-resistant extensive chronic graft-versus-host disease: analysis of response and survival incorporating prognostic factors. *Bone Marrow Transplant.* 2005;35(12):1187-1193.
97. Greinix HT, Knobler RM, Worel N, et al. The effect of intensified extracorporeal photochemotherapy on long-term survival in patients with severe acute graft-versus-host disease. *Haematologica.* 2006;91(3):405-408.
98. Dall'Amico R, Murer L. Extracorporeal photochemotherapy: a new therapeutic approach for allograft rejection. *Transfus Apher Sci.* 2002;26(3):197-204.
99. Kumlien G, Genberg H, Shanwell A, et al. Photopheresis for the treatment of refractory renal graft rejection. *Transplantation.* 2005;79(1):123-125.
100. Pass HI. Photodynamic therapy in oncology: mechanisms and clinical use. *J Natl Cancer Inst.* 1993;85(6):443-456.
101. Kennedy JC, Pottier RH. Endogenous protoporphyrin IX, a clinically useful photosensitizer for photodynamic therapy. *J Photochem Photobiol B Biol.* 1992;14(4):275-292.
102. Fritsch C, Batz J, Bolsen K, et al. Ex vivo application of α-aminolevulinic acid induces high and specific porphyrin levels in human skin tumors: possible basis for selective photodynamic therapy. *Photochem Photobiol.* 1997;66(1):114-118.
103. Fitzmaurice S, Eisen DB. Daylight photodynamic therapy: what is known and what is yet to be determined. *Dermatol Surg.* 2016;42(3):286-295.
104. Penning LC, Dubbelman TM. Fundamentals of photodynamic therapy: cellular and biochemical aspects. *Anticancer Drugs.* 1994;5(2):139-146.
105. Jones CM, Mang T, Cooper M, et al. Photodynamic therapy in the treatment of Bowen's disease. *J Am Acad Dermatol.* 1992;27(6, pt 1):979-982.
106. Dougherty TJ. Photoradiation therapy for cutaneous and subcutaneous malignancies. *J Invest Dermatol.* 1981;77(1):122-124.
107. Oseroff AR, Blumenson LR, Wilson BD, et al. A dose ranging study, of photodynamic therapy with porfimer sodium (Photofrin®) for treatment of basal cell carcinoma. *Lasers Surg Med.* 2006;38(5):417-426.
108. Lui H, Anderson RR. Photodynamic therapy in dermatology. *Arch Dermatol.* 1992;128(12):1631-1636.
109. Weinstein GD, McCullough JL, Nelson JS, et al. Low-dose photofrin II photodynamic therapy of psoriasis. *Clin Res.* 1991;39:509A.
110. Boehncke WH, Elshorst-Schmidt T, Kaufmann R. Systemic photodynamic therapy is a safe and effective treatment for psoriasis. *Arch Dermatol.* 2000;136(2):271-272.
111. Szeimies RM, Sassy T, Landthaler M. Penetration potency of topical applied α-aminolevulinic acid for photodynamic therapy of basal cell carcinoma. *Photochem Photobiol.* 1994;59(1):73-76.
112. Fritsch C, Verwohlt B, Bolsen K, et al. Influence of topical photodynamic therapy with 5-aminolevulinic acid on porphyrin metabolism. *Arch Dermatol Res.* 1996;288(9):517-521.
113. Warren CB, Karai LJ, Vidimos A, et al. Pain associated with aminolevulinic acid-photodynamic therapy of skin disease. *J Am Acad Dermatol.* 2009;61(6):1033-1043.
114. Wang B, Shi L, Zhang YF, et al. Gain with no pain? Pain management in dermatological photodynamic therapy. *Br J Dermatol.* 2017;177(3):656-665.
115. Szeimies RM, Karrer S, Sauerwald A, et al. Topical photodynamic therapy with 5-aminolevulinic acid in the treatment of actinic keratoses: a first clinical study. *Dermatology.* 1996;192:246-251.
116. Jeffes EW, McCullough JL, Weinstein GD, et al. Photodynamic therapy of actinic keratosis with topical 5-aminolevulinic acid. *Arch Dermatol.* 1997;133(6):727-732.
117. Morton CA, Whitehurst C, Moseley H, et al. Comparison of photodynamic therapy with cryotherapy in the treatment of Bowen's disease. *Br J Dermatol.* 1996;135(5):766-771.
118. Basset-Seguin N, Ibbotson SH, Emtestam L, et al. Topical methyl aminolaevulinate photodynamic therapy versus cryotherapy for superficial basal cell carcinoma: a 5 year randomized trial. *Eur J Dermatol.* 2008;18(5):547-553.
119. Rhodes LE, de Rie M, Enström Y, et al. Photodynamic therapy using topical methyl aminolevulinate vs. surgery for nodular basal cell carcinoma: results of a multicenter randomized prospective trial. *Arch Dermatol.* 2004;140(1):17-23.
120. Szeimies RM, Ibbotson S, Murrell DF, et al. A clinical study comparing methyl aminolevulinate photodynamic therapy and surgery in small superficial basal cell carcinoma (8-20 mm), with a 12-month follow-up. *J Eur Acad Dermatol Venereol.* 2008;22(11):1302-1311.
121. Morton C, Szeimies RM, Sidoroff A, et al. European Dermatology Forum Guidelines on topical photodynamic therapy. *Eur J Dermatol.* 2015;25(4):296-311.
122. Bay C, Lerche CM, Ferrick B, et al. Comparison of physical pretreatment regimens to enhance protoporphyrin IX uptake in photodynamic therapy: a randomized clinical trial. *JAMA Dermatol.* 2017;153(4):270-278.

123. Torezan L, Chaves Y, Niwa A, et al. A pilot split-face study comparing conventional methyl aminolevulinate-photodynamic therapy (PDT) with microneedling-assisted PDT on actinically damaged skin. *Dermatol Surg.* 2013;39(8):1197-1201.
124. Zane C, Venturini M, Sala R, et al. Photodynamic therapy with methylaminolevulinate as a valuable treatment option for unilesional cutaneous T-cell lymphoma. *Photodermatol Photoimmunol Photomed.* 2006;22(5):254-258.
125. Weinstein GD, McCullough JL, Jeffes EW. Photodynamic therapy (PDT) of psoriasis with topical delta aminolevulinic acid (ALA): a pilot dose ranging study. *Photodermatol Photoimmunol Photomed.* 1994;10:92.
126. Radakovic-Fijan S, Blecha-Thalhammer U, Schleyer V, et al. Topical aminolaevulinic acid based photodynamic therapy as a treatment option for psoriasis? Results of a randomized, observer-blinded study. *Br J Dermatol.* 2005;152(2):279-283.
127. Schleyer V, Radakovic-Fijan S, Karrer S, et al. Disappointing results and low tolerability of photodynamic therapy with topical 5-aminolevulinic acid in psoriasis. A randomized, double-blind phase I/II study. *J Eur Acad Dermatol Venereol.* 2006;20(7):823-828.
128. Karrer S, Abels C, Landthaler M, et al. Topical photodynamic therapy for localized scleroderma. *Acta Dermatol Venereol.* 2000;80(1):26-27.
129. Karrer S, Bosserhoff AK, Weiderer P, et al. Keratinocyte-derived cytokines after photodynamic therapy and their paracrine induction of matrix metalloproteinases in fibroblasts. *Br J Dermatol.* 2004;151(4):776-783.
130. Frank RG, Bos JD. Photodynamic therapy for condylomata acuminata with local application of 5-aminolevulinic acid. *Genitourin Med.* 1996;72(1):70-71.
131. Karrer S, Szeimies RM, Abels C, et al. Epidermodysplasia verruciformis treated using topical 5-aminolevulinic acid photodynamic therapy. *Br J Dermatol.* 1999;140(5):935-938.
132. Stender IM, Na R, Fogh H, et al. Photodynamic therapy with 5-aminolaevulinic acid or placebo for recalcitrant foot and hand warts: randomized double-blind trial. *Lancet.* 2000;355(9208):963-966.
133. Asilian A, Davami M. Comparison between the efficacy of photodynamic therapy and topical paromomycin in the treatment of Old World cutaneous leishmaniasis: a placebo-controlled, randomized clinical trial. *Clin Exp Dermatol.* 2006;31(5):634-637.
134. Hongcharu W, Taylor CR, Chang Y, et al. Topical ALA-photodynamic therapy for the treatment of acne vulgaris. *J Invest Dermatol.* 2000;115(2):183-192.
135. Pollock B, Turner D, Stringer MR, et al. Topical aminolaevulinic acid-photodynamic therapy for the treatment of acne vulgaris: a study of clinical efficacy and mechanism of action. *Br J Dermatol.* 2004;151(3):616-622.
136. Bhardwaj SS, Rohrer TE, Arndt K. Lasers and light therapy for acne vulgaris. *Semin Cutan Med Surg.* 2005;24(2):107-112.
137. Nybaek H, Jemec GBE. Photodynamic therapy in the treatment of rosacea. *Dermatology.* 2005;211(2):135-138.
138. Dover JS, Bhatia AC, Stewart B, et al. Topical 5-aminolevulinic acid combined with intense pulsed light in the treatment of photoaging. *Arch Dermatol.* 2005;141(10):1247-1252.
139. Gold MH, Bradshaw VL, Boring MM, et al. Split-face comparison of photodynamic therapy with 5-aminolevulinic acid and intense pulsed light versus intense pulsed light alone for photodamage. *Dermatol Surg.* 2006;32(6):795-801.
140. Ruiz-Rodriguez R, Sanz-Sanchez T, Cordoba S. Photodynamic photorejuvenation. *Dermatol Surg.* 2002;28(8):742-744; discussion 744.
141. Touma DJ, Gilchrest BA. Topical photodynamic therapy: a new tool in cosmetic dermatology. *Semin Cutan Med Surg.* 2003;22(2):124-130.
142. Orringer JS, Hammerberg C, Hamilton T, et al. Molecular effects of photodynamic therapy for photoaging. *Arch Dermatol.* 2008;144(10):1296-1302.
143. Szeimies RM, Torezan L, Niwa A, et al. Clinical, histopathological and immunohistochemical assessment of human skin field cancerization before and after photodynamic therapy. *Br J Dermatol.* 2012;167(1):150-159.
144. Kohl E, Torezan LA, Landthaler M, et al. Aesthetic effects of topical photodynamic therapy. *J Eur Acad Dermatol.* 2010;24(11):1261-1269.
145. Szeimies RM, Lischner S, Philipp-Dormston W, et al. Photodynamic therapy for skin rejuvenation: treatment options—results of a consensus conference of an expert group for aesthetic photodynamic therapy. *J Dtsch Dermatol Ges.* 2013;11(7):632-636.
146. Philipp-Dormston WG, Sanclemente G, Torezan L, et al. Daylight photodynamic therapy with MAL cream for large-scale photodamaged skin based on the concept of "actinic field damage": recommendations of an international expert group. *J Eur Acad Dermatol Venereol.* 2016;30(1):8-15.

Chapter 200 :: Radiotherapy
:: Roy H. Decker & Lynn D. Wilson

第二百章

放疗

中文导读

放疗是利用放射线治疗病变的一种局部治疗方法，目前普遍用于癌前病变和恶性病变。本章共分为7节：①辐射方法；②放疗方案的制定；③作用机制；④剂量与分割；⑤放射性皮炎；⑥回忆反应；⑦临床应用。全面介绍了放疗的流程、在皮肤科的运用以及治疗机制。

第一节介绍了放疗中的多种辐射方式，以及如何选择具体的辐射方式。利用射线的放疗主要包括基于γ射线和X射线的放疗，而基于带电粒子的放疗则主要使用到电子和质子。选择具体的辐射方式需要根据病灶的解剖位置和大小、肿瘤生物学特性、周围组织的结构性质等。

第二节介绍了制定放疗方案所涉及的一系列内容：放射能量、辐射方向、患者位置以及治疗设备的选择等。放疗设备的正确选择有利于增加对目标结构的辐射剂量，并避免或减少正常组织的辐射暴露。除此之外，本节着重介绍了等效组织填充物在放疗中的应用。

第三节介绍了放疗的机制。以临床中最常使用的基于X射线和γ射线的放疗为例，电离辐射通过发射出外轨电子，将能量传递给目标组织，在目标组织的细胞内形成自由基，损伤DNA从而达到杀死目标部位细胞的作用。

第四节介绍了确定放疗剂量和分割方案的原则以及常见皮肤疾病的放疗剂量和分割方案。

第五节介绍了放疗后皮肤的变化，具体的病理改变与放疗剂量、时间相关，同时也存在个体差异。在这一部分详细介绍了放射性皮炎相关的临床和分子学内容。

第六节介绍了放疗的回忆反应，即应用某些药物后发生于既往接受放射治疗部位的炎性反应，皮肤是发生放疗回忆反应最常见的部位。

第七节从良性皮肤疾病和恶性皮肤疾病两个方面介绍了放疗的临床应用。随着替代疗法的改进以及人们对放射疗法副作用认识的深化，放疗在良性疾病中的使用已大大减少，且必须遵守一些原则。对于放疗在恶性疾病中的应用，主要涉及了以下几种疾病：基底细胞癌与鳞状细胞癌、黑色素瘤和皮肤淋巴瘤，并阐述了运用放射疗法治疗上述三种恶性疾病的机制、具体方案和治疗效果。

〔赵　爽〕

AT-A-GLANCE

- Radiotherapy is a collection of versatile treatment modalities that includes brachytherapy and external-beam radiation.
- The clinical effects of radiotherapy include acute and late skin changes:
  - Acute effects include an inflammatory reaction and desquamation.
  - Late effects include fibrotic changes and atrophy of skin adnexa.
  - Radiation-induced malignancy is a rare but serious side effect, which presents at a median of 10 years after treatment.
- Radiotherapy is indicated for selected benign, proliferative diseases after more conservative measures have failed.
- Radiotherapy is a valuable option for primary or adjuvant therapy for malignant skin disease.

The first documented use of radiation as a therapeutic treatment was for a cutaneous malignancy, in a patient with squamous cell cancer of the nose, in 1900. Over the next century, radiotherapy was widely used in the treatment of both malignant and benign disorders of the skin, in both adults and children. As the long-term consequences of radiotherapy became evident, particularly the risk of radiation-induced malignancy, its use in the treatment of benign diseases declined, particularly in children. Radiotherapy continues to have a small but important role in the management of benign proliferative diseases of the skin, but is more commonly used as a valuable adjunct or alternative to surgery for both premalignant and malignant lesions.

RADIATION MODALITIES

There are several choices for radiation modalities, some commonly available and others only in specialized centers. The selection is made on the basis of the anatomic location and size of the target, tumor biology, the nature of critical surrounding structures, and availability. In particular, with respect to the cutaneous targets, the depth of the lesion plays a large role in determining the optimal therapy.

High-energy photons, in the form of γ- or X-rays, are most commonly produced by a linear accelerator (LINAC) and are available in a spectrum of energies. Incident radiation deposits its energy as it passes through matter, becoming attenuated as a function of depth and the density of the tissue. Higher energy beams deliver increased doses at depth in tissue, and proportionally less at the surface (often referred to as "skin sparing"). Lower energy radiation deposits the dose primarily at the target surface, sparing deeper tissue. The most commonly available treatment energies in general oncology practice are in the megavoltage range (6 to 18 megavolts),[1] depositing their dose at a range practical for the treatment of internal targets in human tissue. Such beams were designed to relatively spare surface structures such as skin in the interest of delivering a higher dose to deeper target structures and sparing the skin from toxicity. This is in contrast to lower radiation energy beams in the kilovoltage range (commonly referred to as "superficial radiation therapy"), which are often more appropriate for cutaneous targets. Figure 200-1A shows the depth dose curves demonstrating the absorption of X-rays as a function of their energy.

Orthovoltage X-rays refer to lower-energy photons with maximum energy in the range of 125 to 400 kilovolts, often used in dermatologic applications because the dose at the skin surface is maximized. The dose is then rapidly attenuated as the beam penetrates deeper into soft tissue. Half of the incident energy is absorbed within the first few centimeters, and full dose is only delivered to a depth of a few millimeters. Consequently, the most appropriate use is for very superficial tumors. Importantly, lower doses continue to penetrate fairly deeply, so critical structures can still be exposed to a significant exit dose. Orthovoltage X-rays are produced by specialized treatment units that are far smaller than higher-energy machines. Because of their small size and the lower shielding requirements, they are much easier to install in medical offices or even in portable applications.

Grenz rays are even lower-energy X-rays in the range of 5 to 15 kilovolts, and therefore deposit their dose at shallower depths than orthovoltage. Historically, Grenz rays were used to treat superficial, benign skin disease. In these cases, the majority of the target processes occur within 1 mm of the skin surface. Grenz rays are no longer recommended as first-line therapy for routine treatment of benign cutaneous disease.

Charged particle therapy is also commonly used in cancer treatment, and includes both electrons, which are commonly available, and protons, which are available at select regional centers. Electrons are the product of the same linear accelerators used to produce megavoltage energy photons. Electron beams are commonly used in dermatologic applications because they deliver a high skin-surface dose and, unlike photons, the deposited dose rapidly falls to negligible values at depth in tissue. Different electron energies can be used to deliver therapeutic doses from 1 to 5 cm deep in tissue, and deeper tissues can be completely spared. Figure 200-1B describes the depth dose characteristics of electrons.

Protons are charged particles that are the product of large and expensive cyclotrons or synchrotrons, and are available at a small number of specialized centers. Proton therapy is generally several times more expensive than photon or electron therapy, because of the very high capital outlay required to establish a center, although this cost is falling with the development of smaller treatment units. One consequence of a proton's relatively large mass is little side scatter during penetration of a proton beam. The dose is largely delivered within a few millimeters of the end of the particle range (the *Bragg peak*), rather than at shallower

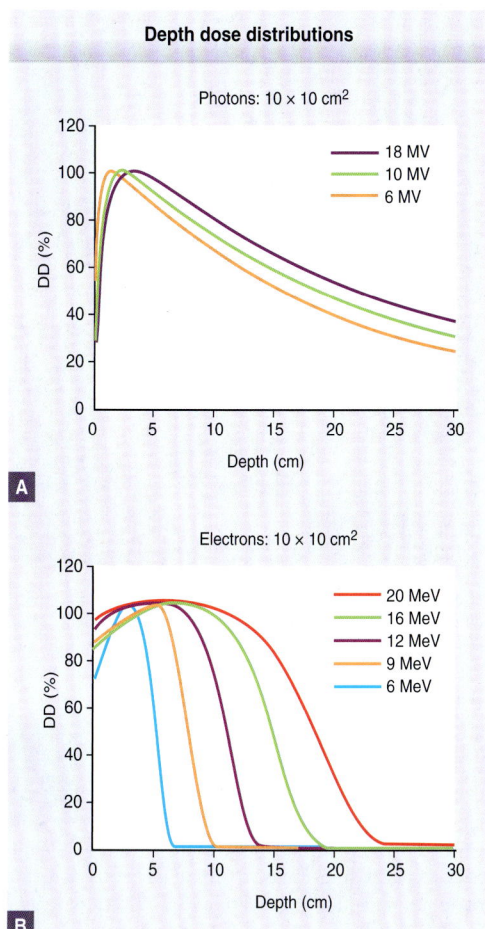

Figure 200-1 Depth dose distributions. **A,** The percent of the maximum radiation dose (DD) deposited at depth in tissue (in cm), as a function of the photon (X-ray) energy. As photon energy increases, the percent dose at superficial depth decreases, and the percent dose in deeper tissue increases. MV, megavolt. **B,** A similar relationship for electron therapy. In contrast to photons, the percent dose deposited at both superficial and deep tissue increases with electron energy. Note the difference in scale; electron energy is almost completely absorbed at shallower depths, compared to photons. MeV, million electron volts.

modality, radiation energy, beam orientation, patient positioning, and the choice of treatment devices. The choice of device can help increase the radiation dose to targeted structures and block or reduce radiation exposure of normal tissue. "Bolus" is tissue-density material commonly used in radiation treatment of superficial skin malignancies. It can be custom designed in varying thicknesses and applied to the patient's skin during daily treatment. It serves several potential purposes: for higher-energy X-rays (eg, megavolt energy), or low-energy electrons, the surface dose is low compared to that in deeper tissue. By using the appropriate thickness of bolus, the skin dose can be raised to therapeutic levels (Fig. 200-2). Another function of bolus is to attenuate the incident beam to lower the dose that reaches deeper structures; for example, during treatment of a skin cancer on the temple, the dose that reaches the underlying brain is decreased. Bolus material also can be used to compensate for complex topography and to smooth the dose distribution for treatment of the skin around the nose and ears (Fig. 200-3).

Beams can be shaped by a variety of devices depending on their energy. Megavoltage treatment beams may be shaped by custom-designed, 7-cm thick, lead alloy blocks to conform to the desired shape; most modern linear accelerators have a multileaf collimator (MLC), which contains sliding leaves of tungsten that conform to the desired treatment aperture. Electron-beam radiation is normally blocked with custom-made lead or lead alloy blocks. Orthovoltage radiation is blocked or deeper depths. By modulating the energy of the proton beam, radiation absorption can be more precisely delivered to deep tumor targets, with less incidental radiation of surrounding normal tissue. Like electrons, protons have a negligible exit dose, but unlike electrons, protons can be delivered to deep targets while sparing the overlying skin.

MODULATION OF EXTERNAL-BEAM RADIATION

Radiation treatment planning involves a complex set of decisions regarding the appropriate radiation

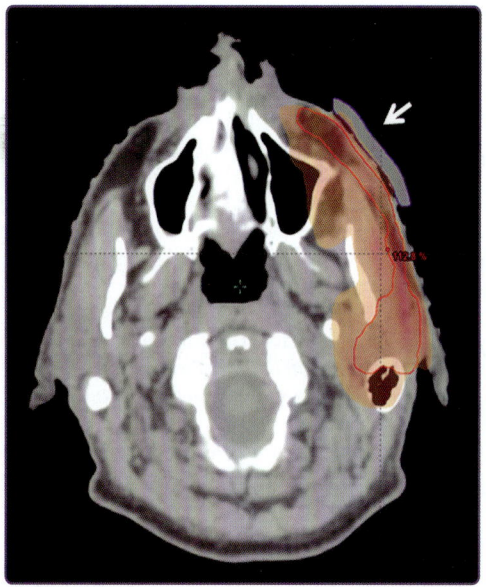

Figure 200-2 Bolus to increase the skin dose. A 61-year-old male underwent resection of a deeply invasive squamous cell carcinoma overlying the zygoma with involvement of parotid lymph nodes and facial nerve. The tumor bed was treated, along with the remaining parotid gland and course of the facial nerve, using megavoltage photons. A tissue-density bolus (*white arrow*) was placed over the tumor bed to increase the skin dose to 100% in that area.

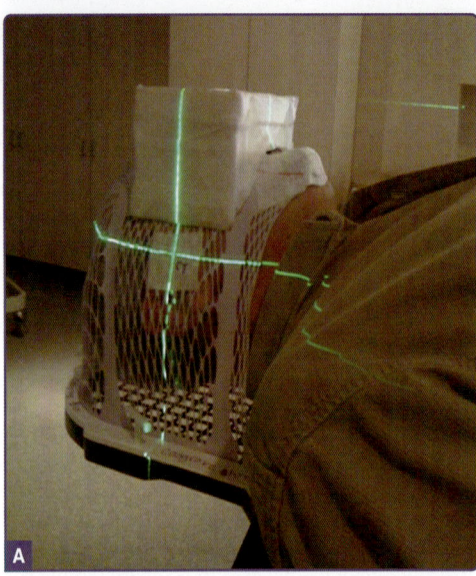 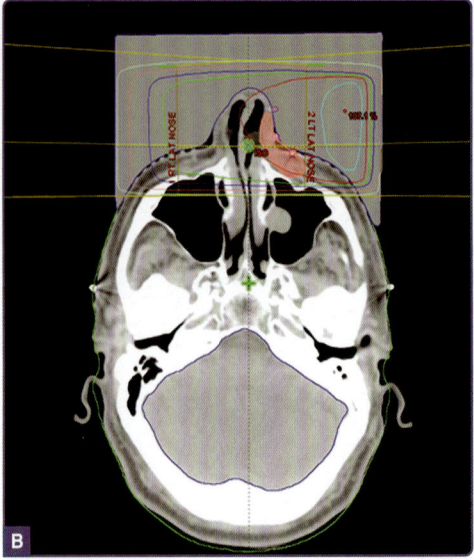

Figure 200-3 Bolus as a tissue compensator. A deeply invasive basal cell carcinoma was excised from the left nasal ala. **A,** The patient was immobilized for treatment in a thermoplastic mask. A rectangular, tissue-density box was constructed to overlay the nose and compensate for the irregular tissue contours in this area. **B,** The patient was treated with right and left lateral megavoltage photon beams, weighted left greater than right. The 100% isodose line (*red line*) covers the tumor bed (*red-shaded area*) with full dose at the skin surface and good dose homogeneity.

using much thinner custom lead shielding, typically placed on the patient's skin. Figure 200-4 shows an example of a custom blocking device for superficial radiation.

Traditionally, external-beam radiation beams are designed using blocks or static MLCs to conform to a target that is delineated clinically or using CT or other imaging. Multiple beams, beam angles, and energies are chosen to avoid specific normal structures, and the dose is calculated with iterative changes until an acceptable plan was generated. An "inverse planned" method is now increasingly used when the tumor target lies in proximity to a dose-limiting structure. Intensity-modulated radiation therapy incorporates individual radiation beams that are not static; the aperture changes during the treatment to finely adjust beam fluence. This requires a dynamic MLC, in which the leaves slide during beam-on time. During the pretreatment planning phase, the treating physician contours the target volume and those of the normal tissue organs at risk. Dose constraints for each contoured structure are chosen, and the physician, physicist, and dosimetry staff use dedicated treatment planning software algorithms to optimize the treatment plan. This is a time-intensive, expensive technique that can generate plans to treat complex-shaped tumor targets and spare adjacent, critical, normal tissue structures.

MECHANISM OF ACTION

The most common forms of radiotherapy used in clinical practice are X-rays and γ-rays. Both represent photon particles or electromagnetic waves that differ only in the method of their generation: γ-rays are emitted by nuclear reactions, whereas X-rays are emitted by energy transitions in orbital electrons. Ionizing radiation includes that part of the electromagnetic spectrum of sufficient energy to impart energy to target tissue by the ejection of orbital electrons. This is the primary means of energy absorption in human tissue

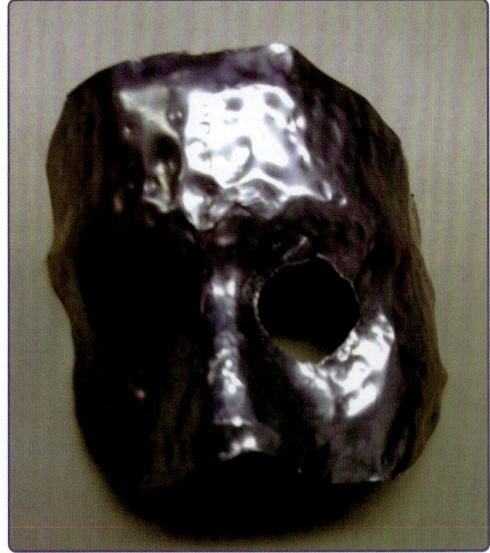

Figure 200-4 A custom lead shield that would be placed on the patient's face, with a cutout to allow orthovoltage treatment of a cutaneous malignancy of the left lower eyelid.

following exposure to therapeutic radiation. As cells are largely composed of water, it is in water molecules that the majority of the ionization occurs, which results in the generation of short-lived free radicals such as hydroxyl radicals. Consequently, the effectiveness of radiation in tissue is dependent upon the availability of oxygen. This is clinically manifest in the reduced radiation response in hypoxic tissue, and is the reason that higher radiation doses are used in the postoperative setting when there is diminished microcirculation.

The primary mediator of cell death in response to ionizing radiation, in both tumor and normal tissue, is damage to DNA by indirect ionization by radiation-induced free radicals.[2] Indirect DNA damage is characteristic of sparsely ionizing radiation, including not only X-rays, but also commonly used charged particles such as electron and proton therapy. In contrast, densely-ionizing radiation (eg, neutrons, α particles) with a higher linear energy transfer deposit their energy densely along their incident tracks, and more commonly induce double-strand DNA breaks directly, without the intermediate ionization of cellular water.

The initial deposition of radiation energy in tissue and the resulting DNA damage occur within thousandths of a second of exposure. The biologic response to DNA damage includes modulation of cell death, differentiation, survival pathways, and activation of DNA repair. These biologic processes occur orders of magnitude more slowly than the initial DNA damage. The ultimate cellular response to radiation can be repair, senescence, differentiation, or cell death. Cell death may occur via apoptosis, a relatively rapid process, but more commonly occurs as mitotic cell death. Misrepair of double-strand DNA breaks generates chromosomal abnormalities, and cells die during failed mitosis, often several generations later.

DOSE AND FRACTIONATION SCHEDULE

The Systéme International d'Unites (SI) unit of radiation dose is the *gray* (Gy), which is defined as 1 joule (J) of energy absorbed per kilogram of tissue. An alternate unit of absorbed dose, largely replaced by the gray, is the rad (an acronym for *radiation absorbed dose*); 1 Gy is equal to 100 rads. Dose is specified to the target volume as defined by the treating radiation oncologist. Most epithelial malignancies are treated to a total dose in the range of 50 to 80 Gy; lymphoid malignancies typically respond to doses of 15 to 40 Gy. Select benign conditions can be treated with lower doses; hypertrophic scars and keloids are commonly prescribed doses in the range of 4 to 20 Gy.

Fractionation refers to the delivery of specified radiation dose in temporally separate treatments, and is recommended to both increase the efficacy of effects on target tissue and to allow normal irradiated tissue to repair radiation damage. Thus, the schedule of radiation fractionation can be used to both increase efficacy of the dose to the target and minimize radiation damage to normal tissue. Common fractionation schemes using conventional radiotherapy deliver treatments at intervals ranging from twice daily to once per week.

The effectiveness of radiation treatment is highly dependent upon the treatment schedule; both the total number of days over which the treatment is spread and the fraction size. The common daily fraction size is 1.8 to 2 Gy per day, given 5 days per week. Different fractionation schedules can be compared using a mathematical conversion to a biologically effective dose (BED), using a formula that accounts for the number of fractions, fraction size, and the DNA-repair characteristics of the target tissue. Commonly used dose-fractionation schedules for cutaneous malignancies include 60 Gy in 30 fractions, and 48 Gy in 12 fractions. The BED to the tumor is similar, but the dose of 48 Gy in 12 fractions would be expected to have more-severe acute and late side effects.

CLINICAL AND MOLECULAR ASPECTS OF RADIATION DERMATITIS

Skin changes after radiation exposure follow a predictable course dictated by radiation dose, timing, and the biology of the human inflammatory reaction.[3] The earliest reaction is erythema that may occur and resolve within hours, and is normally only evident after relatively high-dose exposure. The threshold dose is 2 Gy or greater skin dose, and is not normally noted after daily fractionated treatment of visceral organs with skin-sparing megavoltage radiation. This effect is noted in therapeutic courses aimed at cutaneous targets, where the skin receives full dose, or during treatment regimens that use large fraction sizes. Microscopically, there is a vasodilation and a transiently increased capillary permeability that results in mild erythema and edema at 2 to 24 hours following exposure. Prior to the adoption of SI units of radiation dose, skin erythema dose (SED) was used as a crude clinical measure of patient radiation exposure. This transient acute reaction is no longer commonly noted because of the increased use of high-energy, relatively skin-sparing radiation energies, and the increased use of lower fraction sizes. Acute, transient skin erythema is still reported following interventional diagnostic and therapeutic procedures with prolonged fluoroscopy times.

The more sustained, common, and relevant reactions take place over a matter of weeks during and even shortly after fractionated radiation therapy. Acute radiation dermatitis progresses through characteristic stages of severity based on the accumulation of radiation-induced changes to dermal vasculature, appendageal structures, epidermal stem cells, and the activation of inflammatory pathways. Radiation dermatitis is a distinct adverse event graded by the

National Cancer Institute's *Common Terminology Criteria for Adverse Events* (CTCAE). This scale is graded on severity, and primarily describes the acute reaction of skin exposed to therapeutic radiation. Chronic skin changes may occur months to years after exposure, and include a spectrum of changes characterized by fibrosis and atrophy. Table 200-1 summarizes the common acute and late adverse events attributable to radiation.

Grade 1 dermatitis first manifests as faint skin erythema within the treatment area. Erythema is seen in two contexts: first, there may be a transient vasodilation in the hours after a single fraction skin exposure of 2 Gy or higher. More commonly, erythema or hyperpigmentation develops over the first 2 to 3 weeks of fractionated radiation with accumulated exposure. Vasodilation and increasing vascular permeability occur early, and the resulting perivascular inflammation results in clinically characteristic erythema and edema. Moderate-to-brisk erythema is grade 2.

With continuing or higher-dose radiation exposure, damage to the basal cells in the epidermis may progress until this stem cell population is lost in localized areas, which results in dry desquamation (CTCAE grade 1). Further damage to the basal layer leads to more widespread desquamation, and the production of a fibrinous exudate resulting from increased arteriole permeability, loss of basement membrane integrity, and edema in the underlying dermis. This is characteristic of moist desquamation. The CTCAE differentiates moist desquamation based on whether it is patchy and localized to areas subject to trauma such as skin folds (grade 2), or confluent and present in a more widespread area (grade 3). Radiation damage to the underlying dermis may lead to ulceration, bleeding, and/or necrosis (grade 4). Skin adnexal cells are relatively radiosensitive and may not regenerate following exposure.

The process of epilation begins within days of radiation exposure. Sebaceous glands have similar sensitivity, and eccrine sweat glands become dysfunctional shortly afterward in a fractionated radiation treatment course. Histologically, these glandular structures demonstrate apoptosis, necrosis, and loss of normal mitotic activity. Chronically, there can be fibrotic replacement and loss of the supporting microvasculature. This leads to both acute and chronic hypohidrosis or anhidrosis.

Regeneration of areas of desquamation occurs through replacement of epidermal basal cells, either from islands of intact cells within the epidermis or by the migration of such cells from adjacent, uninvolved areas. Normal healing of the radiation wound becomes clinically evident approximately 2 weeks after exposure, consistent with the basal cell turnover time. Widespread confluent moist desquamation (grade 3), or more severe toxicity, such as necrosis of the epidermis or underlying dermis, may not undergo complete regeneration of the structural and adnexal elements. Instead, there can be prolonged inflammation, fibroblast activation, and collagen deposition. This fibrosis is often termed a consequential late effect, because it is a consequence of the severity of the acute reaction. It is in contrast to the more common late fibrosis, which arises following the regeneration of relatively normal-appearing skin and can occur years after treatment.

Late radiation toxicity occurs months to years following exposure, following a period during which the skin may not exhibit significant abnormalities. The risk and severity of true late skin changes are a function of the irradiation dose and volume. A landmark study of normal tissue radiation tolerance determined that the risk of grade 4 or greater toxicity (ie, ulceration or necrosis) was 5% when 10 cm^2 of skin was treated to 70 Gy, or when 30 cm^2 was treated to 60 Gy.[4] Comorbid medical disease may exacerbate this risk; clinical risk

TABLE 200-1
Commonly-Observed Adverse Events Attributable to Radiation

ADVERSE EVENT	GRADE 1	GRADE 2	GRADE 3	GRADE 4	GRADE 5
Radiation dermatitis	Faint erythema	Moderate-to-brisk erythema	Moist desquamation (other than skin folds and creases)	Skin necrosis	Death
	Dry desquamation	Patchy moist desquamation (mostly confined to skin folds and creases)	Bleeding induced by minor trauma or abrasion	Ulceration of full thickness of dermis	
		Moderate edema		Spontaneous bleeding	
Alopecia	Visible on close inspection	Hair loss ≥50% of normal	—	—	—
Atrophy	Associated with telangiectasia or pigmentation changes	Striae or adnexal structure loss	Ulceration	—	—
Induration or fibrosis	Mild, able to pinch skin	Moderate, able to slide skin but unable to pinch	Severe, unable to slide or pinch, limiting self-care	Generalized, impaired breathing or feeding	Death

factors associated with increased symptom severity include advanced patient age, diabetes, peripheral vascular disease, and tobacco use.[5] The concurrent administration of radiosensitizing drugs significantly increases the severity of acute radiation dermatitis and prolongs healing of the radiation wound. Collagen vascular diseases with a fibrotic cutaneous component (eg, scleroderma and systemic lupus erythematosus) are associated with a pronounced and often debilitating late subcutaneous fibrosis following radiation treatment.[6,7] Certain genetic syndromes, particularly inherited defects in DNA damage repair (eg, ataxia-telangiectasia), predispose to a severe, acute, and late radiation response in exposed normal tissue.

The late skin toxicity with the most functional consequence is subcutaneous fibrosis. Replacement of the subcutaneous adipose tissue with fibrous tissue leads to loss of normal range of motion, contraction, pain, and poor cosmesis. Even in cases where dermal and subcutaneous fibrosis is not clinically evident, there may be atrophy of skin adnexa. Hair follicles as well as sebaceous and sweat glands may be absent in previously-irradiated skin, because these are not regenerated during normal radiation wound repair. Loss of glandular elements leads to anhidrosis when extensive skin areas are irradiated, such as in total-skin electron therapy. The microvasculature of the dermis and subcutis may exhibit abnormal myointimal proliferation, leading to hypoperfusion. Tortuosity within small vessels and microthrombi result in visible telangiectasia. Irregular regeneration of the basal layer of the epidermis may be evident as dyspigmentation. Paradoxically, there may be a decrease in the population of resident skin fibroblasts in atrophic skin, resulting in loss of the normal collagen structure leading to impaired tissue remodeling, increased skin fragility, and poor wound healing.

The pathophysiologic mechanism of late changes, particularly fibrosis, in response to radiation is incompletely understood.[8,9] Transforming growth factor-beta (TGF-β) is a secreted protein that serves a complex regulatory role in normal tissue inflammation and remodeling by controlling proliferation, differentiation, and secretory function. TGF-β levels are increased within hours of radiation exposure, and this elevation has been correlated with late fibrotic changes. Abrogation of downstream mediator SMAD3 (Sma- and Mad-related protein 3), a proinflammatory signaling molecule induced in response to TGF-β, appears to protect tissue from late fibrotic changes after radiation exposure in laboratory models. TGF-β is a complex regulator of inflammation that increases fibroblast proliferation, differentiation, and activation, thereby increasing secretion of extracellular matrix components. TGF-β promotes its own secretion by fibroblasts in a self-amplifying cascade and decreases the production of matrix proteinases. Epithelial cell proliferation is diminished, and there is chemotaxis of mast cells and macrophages. The result is increasing production, processing, and deposition of collagen (fibrosis) and loss of epithelial reconstitution of normal tissue structure.

The initiating event in TGF-β activation in response to radiation is poorly understood. Latent TGF-β in the extracellular matrix may be activated by proteolytic enzymes that act in the presence of radiation-induced reactive oxygen species. Other potential sources of TGF-β include endothelial cells, fibroblasts, epithelial cells, and tissue macrophages, which may release TGF-β in direct response to radiation or as a generalized response to tissue damage.

RADIATION RECALL REACTIONS

Radiation recall is a phenomenon that was first described several decades ago. Radiation recall is a cutaneous reaction, in response to specific systemic agents, in the area of previous radiation exposure. The most commonly cited chemotherapeutic agents are anthracyclines, taxanes, and gemcitabine. Other systemic agents implicated in radiation recall reactions include standard chemotherapeutic agents, newer targeted therapeutics, and hormonal agents as well as nononcologic medications; Table 200-2 lists these agents based on case reports.

The clinical manifestations of radiation recall occur with the initial administration of the systemic agent—within minutes to days with IV drug, or days to weeks with oral medication. The timing of presentation may be related to the drug dose, and both the severity and timing of the reaction may be related to the prior radiation dose. The duration of the response may range from weeks to months. Interestingly, readministration of the same systemic agent does not consistently lead to recurrence of the phenomenon.[10]

Although a recall reaction can occur in any organ, skin is the most common site. It occurs in a well-demarcated area defined by the borders of the previous treatment field and can occur despite the lack of any clinically significant skin reaction during the previous radiation treatment. The clinical signs and symptoms mimic an acute radiation dermatitis, ranging from erythema to desquamation and necrosis. A localized maculopapular rash, characteristic of a hypersensitivity reaction, also has been described.

The pathogenesis of radiation recall is not well understood. An early hypothesis was that tissue stem cells remained depleted long after radiation, making the tissue more sensitive to cytotoxics. This does not explain, however, radiation recall reactions elicited by noncytotoxics or, in some cases, the lack of a reaction to subsequent drug exposure. The clinicopathologic manifestations are best explained by a localized, acquired hypersensitivity reaction. Prior radiation therapy may alter the normal dermal immunologic response by changing basal and stimulated cytokine production. This is consistent with histologic findings of acute inflammation (eg, vasodilation, infiltration of inflammatory cell mediators) in affected tissue. Radiation recall dermatitis responds to treatment with topical or oral corticosteroids.

TABLE 200-2
Radiation Recall Reactions

Agents implicated in inducing a radiation recall reaction include chemotherapy drugs, targeted and hormonal agents, and nononcologic medications.

- Chemotherapy
  - Arsenic trioxide
  - Bleomycin
  - Capecitabine
  - Cyclophosphamide
  - Cytarabine
  - Dacarbazine
  - Dactinomycin
  - Daunorubicin
  - Docetaxel
  - Doxorubicin
  - Epirubicin
  - Etoposide
  - Fluorouracil
  - Gemcitabine
  - Hydroxyurea
  - Idarubicin
  - Lomustine
  - Melphalan
  - Methotrexate
  - Paclitaxel
  - Vinblastine
- Targeted anticancer drugs
  - Bevacizumab
  - Pemetrexed
- Hormonal agents
  - Tamoxifen
- Nononcologic drugs
  - Gatifloxacin
  - Isoniazid
  - Levofloxacin
  - Simvastatin

CLINICAL APPLICATIONS OF RADIATION

BENIGN DISEASE

The use of ionizing radiation for benign disease has decreased considerably, because of improvements in alternative therapy and an increasing awareness of the rare, but serious, side effects of radiotherapy.[11] Rare but serious side effects include fibrotic changes in the affected skin and, more significantly, a risk of secondary malignancy. It is estimated that the relative risk of malignancy following radiation treatment increases by 10% to 50%; the absolute risk, however, remains very low. These malignancies occur at a median of 10 years following treatment. The risk appears to be greater in younger patients, and in those patients whose treatment was targeted to anatomic areas at highest risk for malignancy (eg, breast or thyroid tissue). For this reason, radiotherapy should be (a) considered in benign disease only after other therapeutic options have been exhausted; (b) avoided when possible in children and young adults; and (c) delivered with attention to sparing radiation exposure to sensitive normal tissue.

Radiotherapy is effective for symptomatic treatment of several inflammatory dermatoses, including eczema, psoriasis, and lichen planus, at relatively low-dose exposures (ie, less than 10 Gy of fractionated treatment). Inflammatory dermatoses are rarely treated with radiation, given the number of other antiinflammatory options. Benign lymphoproliferative disorders are sensitive in a similar fashion, and disorders such as lymphomatoid papulosis, lymphoid hyperplasia, and lymphocytoma cutis have an excellent response to radiotherapy. These may be treated with radiation after other options have been exhausted, and are approached using lymphoma regimens. Other benign proliferative processes that can be treated with radiotherapy include keratoacanthomas and hemangiomas. Table 200-3 lists the diagnoses for which radiotherapy may be indicated.

A number of large series and one randomized trial have examined the efficacy of localized, low-dose irradiation for the prevention of recurrence of hypertrophic scars or keloids following excision.[12-14] This should be undertaken after failure of more conservative therapies. The most common treatment regimen is to use kilovoltage X-rays or electrons to a total dose of 10 to 20 Gy delivered over several days. The treatment is usually initiated within 24 to 48 hours of excision. The recurrence risk after surgery and radiation is approximately 20% or less. The use of radiation without excision on existing keloids is not as effective.

TABLE 200-3
Cutaneous Indications for Primary or Adjuvant Radiotherapy[a]

Benign	Malignant
Eczema	Squamous carcinoma
Psoriasis	Basal cell carcinoma
Lichen planus	Melanoma
Benign lymphoid hyperplasia	Merkel cell carcinoma
Keratoacanthoma	Eccrine and apocrine carcinoma
Keloids/hypertrophic scars	Cutaneous T-cell and B-cell lymphomas
	Kaposi sarcoma
	Angiosarcoma
Premalignant	
Actinic keratoses	
Lentigo melanoma	
Bowen disease	
Erythroplasia of Queyrat	
Lymphocytoma cutis	

[a]Radiotherapy is not recommended as first-line therapy for all the listed indications, particularly the benign disorders.

MALIGNANT DISEASE

BASAL CELL CARCINOMA AND SQUAMOUS CELL CARCINOMA

Radiation has been used as primary treatment for basal and squamous cell carcinoma, as an alternative to excision, with local control rates of 90% or greater for small lesions.[15] There is concern for progressive late skin atrophy and necrosis decades after radiation, and for this reason surgical excision is usually thought to be a better option in younger patients (ie, those younger than age 55 years). The control rate for primary treatment is a function of tumor size and T stage. For small lesions, radiation is thought to offer local control that approximates the control seen with excision.

Radiation is also an effective adjuvant treatment, following excision or Mohs micrographic surgery. The clearest indication for adjuvant treatment is a positive surgical margin; other considerations include tumor depth greater than 4 mm in the case of squamous cell cancer or tumor size greater than 2 cm. Involvement of cartilage or bone is a strong predictor of local recurrence and consensus guidelines recommend adjuvant treatment. Perineural invasion correlates with both local and nodal recurrence following excision and is a relative indication for treatment.[16,17] Involvement of large, named nerves should prompt consideration of extension of the clinical target volume to include the proximal nerve tract. Other relative indications for treatment include poorly-differentiated tumors, adenosquamous subtype, and limitations imposed on excision by anatomic location. Patient factors include the presence of neurologic symptoms, implying underlying nerve involvement, and immunosuppressed host status. For squamous cell carcinoma, locally-advanced lesions may have a significant risk of nodal metastasis. In patients being treated adjuvantly or definitively for locally-advanced primaries with risk factors, draining lymphatics should be electively included.

Dose fractionation schemes represent a balance between patient convenience and the relative risk of poor cosmesis. A total of 60 to 66 Gy in 2-Gy fractions is appropriate for gross disease, with higher doses indicated for lesions larger than 2 to 4 cm. Published experience with relatively hypofractionated treatment has shown equivalent locoregional control after 45 to 50 Gy in 2.5-Gy fractions, or radiobiologically equivalent doses in fraction sizes of 3 or 4 Gy.

Tumors or postoperative areas that are at superficial depth may be treated with orthovoltage radiation to spare the deeper normal tissue. An alternative is electron therapy with the appropriate bolus to maximize the surface dose. When the target volume is deeper, then megavoltage X-rays, with appropriate bolus, may be required. Target structures such as lymph node basins or nerve tracts, in close proximity to critical normal structures, may require intensity-modulated radiation therapy.

MELANOMA

The role of radiotherapy in the management of localized melanoma has not been conclusively established. Radiotherapy is frequently used for palliation of unresectable lesions, and there is evidence that selected patients at increased risk of local or regional failure may reduce that risk with adjuvant radiation.[18] Risk factors predictive of local relapse after wide excision include tumor thickness greater than 4 mm, ulceration, satellitosis, positive surgical margins, mucosal origin, perineural invasion, and desmoplastic histology. Patients with positive lymph nodes at high risk of recurrence after node dissection may benefit from postoperative radiation directed at the nodal basin.[19,20]

Melanomas are frequently treated with hypofractionated radiation, with fraction sizes of 4 to 6 Gy (ie, 30 Gy in 5 fractions) using megavoltage X-rays. The recurrence risk for melanoma after radiation is significantly higher than that for squamous or basal cell carcinoma.

CUTANEOUS LYMPHOMAS

Cutaneous T-cell lymphomas include numerous subtypes, the most common of which are mycosis fungoides (MF) and anaplastic large-cell lymphoma. MF is exquisitely sensitive to radiotherapy and patients may present with localized or disseminated skin disease. Anaplastic large-cell lymphoma (CD30-positive) is also a common cutaneous T-cell lymphoma, but has a lower incidence than MF. The clinical presentation is also somewhat different, and these cells generally demonstrate a CD4-positive phenotype (which can be seen in MF), and also express cutaneous lymphocyte antigen. As opposed to MF, these cells are typically not epidermotropic and do stain positive for CD30. Lymphomatoid papulosis is also CD30 positive and may be associated with anaplastic large-cell lymphoma. Anaplastic lymphoma kinase is usually not overexpressed in patients suffering specifically from cutaneous lymphoma of the CD30-positive variety, though it may be expressed in patients with noncutaneous anaplastic large-cell lymphoma.

There are also a variety of subtypes of cutaneous B-cell lymphoma, but the most commonly encountered are diffuse large B-cell, marginal zone, and follicular center cell. Diffuse large B-cell lymphoma may express CD20 and CD79, and lesions involving the lower extremities may express BCL-2, BCL-6, and MUM-1. Marginal zone lymphoma can be identified via expression of CD20 and CD79 and often BCL-2, but typically BCL-6 is not noted as a marker in this case. The follicular center cell variant may express CD20 and CD79, but expression of BCL-2 and MUM-1 is unusual.

Localized radiotherapy fields may be incorporated into the management of patients with limited disease, but in some cases, patients have extensive areas of skin which are involved and a total skin electron beam therapy (TSEBT) technique may be incorporated for adequate disease control.

Localized radiotherapy is typically provided using an electron technique and bolus material is applied to the skin in an effort to maintain an appropriate deposition of dose at the skin surface. Typically the 90% isodose curve is used to provide homogeneous coverage of the skin area in question and margins of 2 to 3 cm radially are incorporated into the treatment plan. Doses of 20 to 30 Gy in 2-Gy fractions are used. With this type of regimen for most cutaneous B-cell lymphomas, the complete response (CR) rate is greater than 95% with 5-year local control of approximately 75%.[21,22] Some patients may not be able to logistically receive daily therapy over several weeks, but are in need of palliation of lesions that are bleeding, uncomfortable, unsightly, or impairing function. Such patients may be candidates for an abbreviated regimen of 2 Gy × 2 for a total of 4 Gy, which has been found to provide excellent response rates with reasonable durability in selected patients with low-grade cutaneous B-cell lymphoma.[23]

TSEBT is significantly more complicated to provide and is typically used in patients suffering from extensive MF. TSEBT provides excellent response rates for patients with various levels of disease and also has been successful in patients with tumors of the skin, assuming that a supplemental boost is provided to the region involved by tumor. MF patches and plaques have an excellent response rate of 100% to TSEBT. The CR rate is variable and decreases with the degree of thickness associated with cutaneous lesions. Historically, the course of therapy is provided over approximately 8 to 10 weeks and, based on a Stanford technique, involves 36 fractions to the total skin using 6 fields with blocking of the eyes, hands, fingernails, and feet based on dosimetric parameters resulting from the individualized treatment program.[24] Newer data demonstrating excellent results with only 12 Gy have been published.[25] An advantage is that the course is much shorter and toxicities decreased compared with the 36-Gy regimen. The patient is treated in a variety of standing positions. Given its degree of complexity, TSEBT is best performed in centers that have a significant amount of experience with the technique. An important feature to be considered following response to TSEBT is a maintenance program, and such maintenance can be provided in a variety of forms. For MF patients with T1-level and T2-level disease, effective regimens, which have been documented in the literature, include the use of psoralen and ultraviolet A and mechlorethamine.

Both cutaneous T-cell and B-cell lymphomas are very sensitive to radiotherapy, and it is generally accepted that all lesions will respond and that localized cutaneous B-cell lymphoma lesions have a CR rate approaching 100%. Cutaneous T-cell lymphoma lesions have CR rates that are also excellent but are more dependent on extent of disease.

REFERENCES

1. Khan FM. *The Physics of Radiation Therapy*. 4th ed. Philadelphia, PA: Lippincott Williams & Wilkins; 2010.
2. Hall EJ, Giaccia AJ. *Radiobiology for the Radiologist*. 6th ed. Philadelphia, PA: Lippincott Williams & Wilkins; 2006:ix, 546.
3. Hymes SR, Strom EA, Fife C. Radiation dermatitis: clinical presentation, pathophysiology, and treatment 2006. *J Am Acad Dermatol*. 2006;54(1):28-46.
4. British Thoracic Society; Society of Cardiothoracic Surgeons of Great Britain and Ireland Working Party. BTS guidelines: guidelines on the selection of patients with lung cancer for surgery. *Thorax*. 2001;56(2):89-108.
5. Chon BH, Loeffler JS. The effect of nonmalignant systemic disease on tolerance to radiation therapy. *Oncologist*. 2002;7(2):136-143.
6. Holscher T, Bentzen SM, Baumann M. Influence of connective tissue diseases on the expression of radiation side effects: a systematic review. *Radiother Oncol*. 2006;78(2):123-130.
7. Lin A, Abu-Isa E, Griffith KA, et al. Toxicity of radiotherapy in patients with collagen vascular disease. *Cancer*. 2008;113(3):648-653.
8. Rodemann HP, Blaese MA. Responses of normal cells to ionizing radiation. *Semin Radiat Oncol*. 2007;17(2):81-88.
9. Lehnert S. *Biomolecular Action of Ionizing Radiation (Series in Medical Physics and Biomedical Engineering)*. New York, NY: Taylor & Francis; 2008.
10. Azria D, Magné N, Zouhair A, et al. Radiation recall: a well recognized but neglected phenomenon. *Cancer Treat Rev*. 2005;31(7):555-570.
11. Lahaniatis JE, Farzin F, Brady LW, et al. Radiation treatment for benign disease. A survey of current treatment programs. *Front Radiat Ther Oncol*. 2001;35:1-17.
12. Kovalic JJ, Perez CA. Radiation therapy following keloidectomy: a 20-year experience. *Int J Radiat Oncol Biol Phys*. 1989;17(1):77-80.
13. Lo TC, Seckel BR, Salzman FA, et al. Single-dose electron beam irradiation in treatment and prevention of keloids and hypertrophic scars. *Radiother Oncol*. 1990;19(3):267-272.
14. Sclafani AP, Gordon L, Chadha M, et al. Prevention of earlobe keloid recurrence with postoperative corticosteroid injections versus radiation therapy: a randomized, prospective study and review of the literature. *Dermatol Surg*. 1996;22(6):569-574.
15. Locke J, Karimpour S, Young G, et al. Radiotherapy for epithelial skin cancer. *Int J Radiat Oncol Biol Phys*. 2001;51(3):748-755.
16. McCord MW, Mendenhall WM, Parsons JT, et al. Skin cancer of the head and neck with clinical perineural invasion. *Int J Radiat Oncol Biol Phys*. 2000;47(1):89-93.
17. McCord MW, Mendenhall WM, Parsons JT, et al. Skin cancer of the head and neck with incidental microscopic perineural invasion. *Int J Radiat Oncol Biol Phys*. 1999;43(3):591-595.
18. Ballo MT, Ang KK. Radiotherapy for cutaneous malignant melanoma: rationale and indications. *Oncology (Williston Park)*. 2004;18(1):99-107.
19. Ballo MT, Ross MI, Cormier JN, et al. Combined-modality therapy for patients with regional nodal metastases from melanoma. *Int J Radiat Oncol Biol Phys*. 2006;64(1):106-113.
20. Gyorki DE, Ainslie J, Joon ML, et al. Concurrent adjuvant radiotherapy and interferon-alpha2b for resected high risk stage III melanoma—a retrospective single centre study. *Melanoma Res*. 2004;14(3):223-230.
21. Cotter GW, Baglan RJ, Wasserman TH, et al. Palliative radiation treatment of cutaneous mycosis fungoides—a dose response. *Int J Radiat Oncol Biol Phys*. 1983;9(10):1477-1480.

22. Wilson LD, Kacinski BM, Jones GW. Local superficial radiotherapy in the management of minimal stage IA cutaneous T-cell lymphoma (mycosis fungoides). *Int J Radiat Oncol Biol Phys*. 1998;40(1):109-115.
23. Neelis KJ, Schimmel EC, Vermeer MH, et al. Low-dose palliative radiotherapy for cutaneous B- and T-cell lymphomas. *Int J Radiat Oncol Biol Phys*. 2009;74(1):154-158.
24. Chen Z, Agostinelli AG, Wilson LD, et al. Matching the dosimetry characteristics of a dual-field Stanford technique to a customized single-field Stanford technique for total skin electron therapy. *Int J Radiat Oncol Biol Phys*. 2004;59(3):872-885.
25. Harrison C, Young J, Navi D, et al. Revisiting low-dose total skin electron beam therapy in mycosis fungoides. *Int J Radiat Oncol Biol Phys*. 2011;81:e651-e657.

Dermatologic Surgery PART 30

第三十篇 皮肤外科

Chapter 201 :: Cutaneous Surgical Anatomy
:: Arif Aslam & Sumaira Z. Aasi

第二百零一章
皮肤外科解剖学

中文导读

皮肤外科学是指采用有创手段进行诊治的皮肤病学分支学科，它又是一门交叉学科，融合了皮肤病学理论和许多外科、成形美容技术。皮肤外科的技术范畴有广义和狭义两种。从广义上讲它涵盖了手术、激光、物理治疗（冷冻、电解等）、毛发移植、吸脂与脂肪移植、肉毒杆菌毒素注射、填充注射等多种治疗手段和技术。因此了解并掌握解剖学，是皮肤外科的基础。本章共分为7节：①解剖知识介绍；②介绍浅表肌腱膜系统；③介绍局部解剖学和美容单位；④介绍游离缘；⑤介绍手术中的危险区域；⑥介绍手术中易受损伤的面部运动神经；⑦介绍头颈部肌肉、血管、淋巴等概念，全面介绍了与皮肤外科密切相关的头颈部解剖知识。

第一节简单介绍了解剖学知识。

第二节解释了浅表肌腱膜系统（SMAS）这一重要概念，它是连接面部肌肉的胸肌层，是一层浅筋膜，将面部表情肌肉相互包裹并与上面的皮肤联系起来。

第三节介绍了面部的局部解剖学和美容单位，美容单位是具有相同皮肤特征的组织区域，如颜色、质地、毛皮脂质、毛孔大小和光化暴露程度。

第四节引入游离缘（Free Margin）的概念，它是任何当施加张力时容易扭曲的解剖结构。眼睑边缘、鼻翼、唇红部位和耳廓都是游离缘。当这些区域受到张力时，由此产生的不对称可能会引起美容不对称和功能畸形等。

第五节强调在头颈部进行手术时，有三个主要的危险区域是至关重要的。这些区域中的每一个都涉及运动神经及其支配的肌肉，这些是面神经的颞支和下颌缘支（颅神经Ⅶ）和脊神经副神经（颅神经Ⅺ）（表201-1）。在这些区域进行手术之前，需要确认这些神经和肌肉的解剖，同时尽可能保护面神经的分支不受损。而值得注意的是，在老年患者的某些部位，如太阳穴和其他部位，脂肪层的厚度可能是最小的，需要提高警惕，注意保护。

第六节详细地描述了这些面神经在面部的位置和损伤会导致的后果。面神经的颞支（或额支）支配额肌、眼轮匝肌上纤维、上睑皱肌、耳前肌和耳上肌。面神经颞支的损伤会导致容貌和功能的丧失、额头变平、皱纹和皮肤紧张线的可见性减弱。随着时间的推移，随着失神经肌肉的萎缩，患者会出现眉毛和眼睑下垂，这可能会导致视野障碍，可能需要做眉毛提升和眼睑成形术来纠正这个问题。下颌缘神经：面神经下颌缘支在颌角处出腮腺，在这个位置可能很薄，特别是在老年人面部，手术时需要注意。脊髓副神经：颈部的后三角由胸锁乳突肌的后缘、斜方肌的前缘和锁骨界定。提出通过画一条连接下颌角和乳突的线，可以推测出脊髓副神经的位置。脊髓副神经损伤会导致斜方肌瘫痪、肩胛骨抽动、肩膀下垂、无法耸肩、手臂外展困难，以及慢性肩痛。感觉神经：三叉神经（颅神经V）提供面部的大部分感觉神经（图201-5和201-6以及表201-2）。

第七节最后详细地讲述了面部表情肌肉、血管解剖学、淋巴管引流等概念；面部表情肌肉各司其职控制面部运动（图201-7）。面部的血液供应几乎全部来自颈外动脉的分支（图201-8）。面部淋巴管一般由浅向深、内侧向外侧和尾侧引流。虽然这里描述了一般的引流模式，但可能会发生变化。后头部和颈部的淋巴结最终汇入一系列末端结节（颈深淋巴结），最后汇入外侧颈内静脉链。

〔赵　爽〕

AT-A-GLANCE

- The superficial musculoaponeurotic system (SMAS) is a fibromuscular layer connecting the facial muscles. Incisions and undermining within the subcutaneous fat above SMAS will not result in damage to motor nerves.
- When planning reconstruction, the surgeon should consider cosmetic units, junctional lines, and resting skin tension lines to optimize the final aesthetic result.
- The three branches of the trigeminal nerve (cranial nerve V) provide sensory innervation to the face.
- The three main danger zones are areas where the temporal and marginal mandibular branches of the facial nerve and spinal accessory nerve lie superficial and can be easily injured. Damage to the temporal branch of the facial nerve may result in an ipsilateral eyebrow ptosis and obscuring of the superolateral visual field. The marginal mandibular branch of the facial nerve is vulnerable to damage along the inferior edge of the body of the mandible. Damage to the marginal mandibular branch of the facial nerve results in an asymmetrical smile. The spinal accessory nerve lies in the posterior triangle of the neck and may be identified by Erb's point.
- The rich vascular supply to the face from both the external and internal carotid ensures the reliable healing potential and viability of flaps and grafts in head and neck surgery.

INTRODUCTION TO CUTANEOUS SURGICAL ANATOMY

Factors such as the increasing incidence of skin cancer, the desire to maintain a youthful appearance in an aging population that is living longer, and the financial pressure to perform procedures in less invasive and more cost-effective ways have made surgery a cornerstone of the practice of dermatology. Knowledge of anatomy is critical for a number of reasons, including communicating precisely with colleagues, performing safe and efficient procedures, achieving aesthetic and functional reconstruction, understanding the lymphatic drainage, and anticipating metastatic spread of cutaneous malignancies. Because the vast majority of these procedures are performed on the head and neck, this chapter focuses on the anatomy of this critical region.

This chapter focuses on five important concepts in head and neck anatomy, which are

- The superficial musculoaponeurotic system (SMAS)
- Topography and cosmetic units
- Free margins
- Relaxed skin tension lines (RSTL)
- Facial motor nerves susceptible to damage during dermatologic surgery

THE SUPERFICIAL MUSCULOAPONEUROTIC SYSTEM

An important concept in understanding head and neck anatomy is the SMAS, a layer of superficial fascia that envelopes and links the facial expression muscles with each other and with the overlying skin.

It stretches over the cheeks between the temporalis and frontalis muscles above and the platysma muscle below. The SMAS also attaches to the orbicularis oculi muscles anteriorly and the trapezius muscle posteriorly and includes the fascia of the forehead and galea of the scalp.

Most of the superficial muscles of the scalp and face insert into the skin either directly through fibrous bands running in the subcutaneous tissue or indirectly by attachment to the SMAS, which in turn is attached to the skin. In the lateral areas of the face, the SMAS is organized and more visible but becomes less discrete medially. Because of its attachment to the skin superficially and muscles deep, the SMAS coordinates a wide range of facial expressions. In addition, the SMAS is an important landmark because most major arteries and nerves run within or deep to it. Dissection above the SMAS allows the dermatologic surgeon to safely avoid neurovascular structures.

TOPOGRAPHIC ANATOMY AND COSMETIC UNITS

Cosmetic units are zones of tissue that share cutaneous features such as color, texture, pilosebaceous quality, pore size, and degree of actinic exposure. These cosmetic units are demarcated by junction lines that can be discrete (eyebrows) or subtle (nasofacial sulcus). The forehead, temples, eyelids, nose, cheeks, upper and lower lips, chin, and ears represent the major cosmetic units of the face. Cosmetic units can also be further divided into subunits. Because of the tissue similarity, it is often best to reconstruct a surgical defect within a cosmetic unit or subunit or borrow tissue from nearby units. In addition, scar lines can be hidden easily in junction lines between the cosmetic units. Scars that cross cosmetic units are more noticeable and cosmetically less pleasing.

The more complex regions of the face that have multiple subunits include the nose, ears, and lips (Figs. 201-1 and 201-2).

Topographic anatomy and cosmetic units help localize areas of the face accurately for purposes of communication with colleagues and to perform the surgery itself. For instance, it is more helpful to describe a lesion on the face if it is said to be located on the "left nasal sidewall" versus left nose or "right triangular fossa" versus right ear. The subunits of the nose include the glabella (the area between the eyebrows), the root (the deep sulcus below the glabella and uppermost portion of the nose), the dorsum or bridge (the area overlying

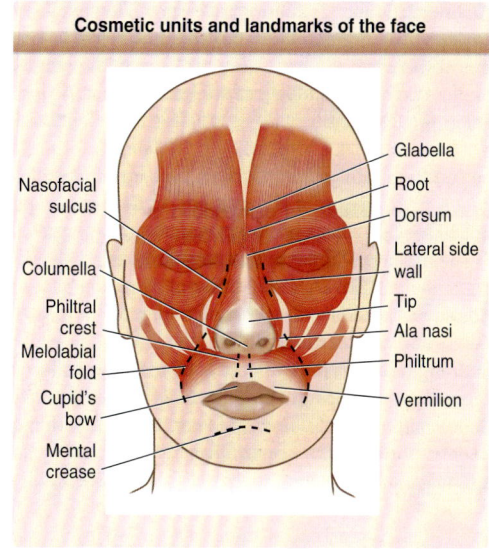

Figure 201-1 Cosmetic units and landmarks of the face.

the nasal bone), lateral sidewalls (the sides of the nose), the nasal tip, the nasal ala (the nostril), the alar groove and nasolabial crease (the grooves that demarcate the alae superiorly from the lateral nasal sidewall and alae inferiorly from the lip, respectively), and the columella (the mobile linear structure separating the alae inferiorly) (see Fig. 201-1).

The lateral surface of the ear is rimmed by the helix, a curved cartilaginous structure that begins at the crus just above the external auditory canal and continues around the ear to end at the fleshy lobule. The central concavity within which the external auditory meatus lies is the concha. The concha is divided by the crus of the helix into a superior portion; the cymba; and an inferior portion, the cavum. The posterior border of the concha is formed by another cartilaginous structure called the *antihelix*. Superiorly, the antihelix originates from two legs (*crus* is Latin for *leg*): (1) the

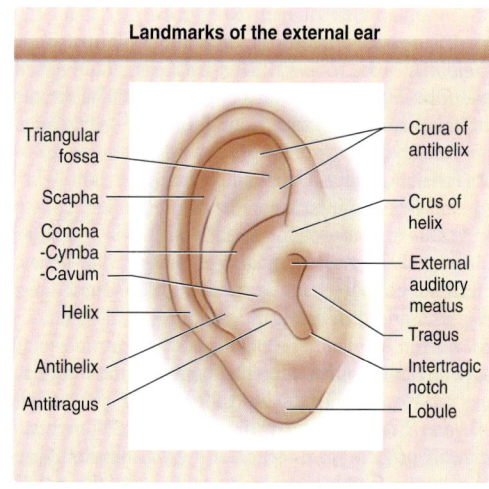

Figure 201-2 Landmarks of the external ear.

superior crus and (2) inferior crus. The region between the crura is referred to as the triangular fossa. The groove between the helix and antihelix is the scaphoid fossa. The triangulated cartilaginous structure just anterior to the auditory canal is called the *tragus*, and just posterior to this is the triangulated end of the antihelix, referred to as the *antitragus*. The inferior region between the tragus and antitragus is the intertragic notch (see Fig. 201-2).

The cutaneous upper lip has a concave depression in the center, called the *philtrum*, which is bounded by two ridges, the philtral crests. There is a prominent crease, the mental crease, which divides the cutaneous lower lip from the chin. The boundary between the red mucosal surface of the lips and the cutaneous surface is called the vermillion border. The raised contoured area of the inferior portion of the philtrum is a critical aesthetic landmark known as the *Cupid's bow* (see Fig. 201-1).

FREE MARGINS

A free margin is any anatomical structure that can be easily distorted when tension is placed on it. The eyelid margin, alar rim, lip vermillion, and helical rim are free margins. When these regions become distorted, the resulting asymmetry can cause cosmetic and functional concerns. An ectropion can result in epiphora, as well as conjunctival and corneal exposure leading to corneal scarring. An eclabium may result in altered speech, an asymmetrical smile, or drooling. The nasal ala does not have cartilage and is composed of fibrofatty tissue, thus making it quite vulnerable to distortion when tension is placed on it.

It is important for dermatologic surgeons to appreciate the tension vectors during wound closure to avoid free margin distortion.

RELAXED SKIN TENSION LINES

RSTLs are another characteristic of the face that help guide surgical reconstruction and allow the structural camouflage of scar lines. RSTLs are creases on the face that form over time because of factors such as loss of elastic tissue tone, lengthening of the collagenous fibrous septae that connect the dermis to the underlying facial muscles, development of excessive skin, gravity, and ultraviolet radiation exposure (see Fig. 201-3). RSTLs are most obvious on the face because unlike other muscles in the body that connect tendons and bones, facial muscles attach to the overlying skin. These lines can be induced by facial muscle movement in young people but inevitably become more pronounced with age. RSTLs usually run perpendicular to the underlying muscles. In most situations, the long axis of the excision should be placed parallel to the RSTL because they are often in the direction of the least tension for a scar. It is preferable to design flaps such that the majority of the scar lines fall within the RSTL.

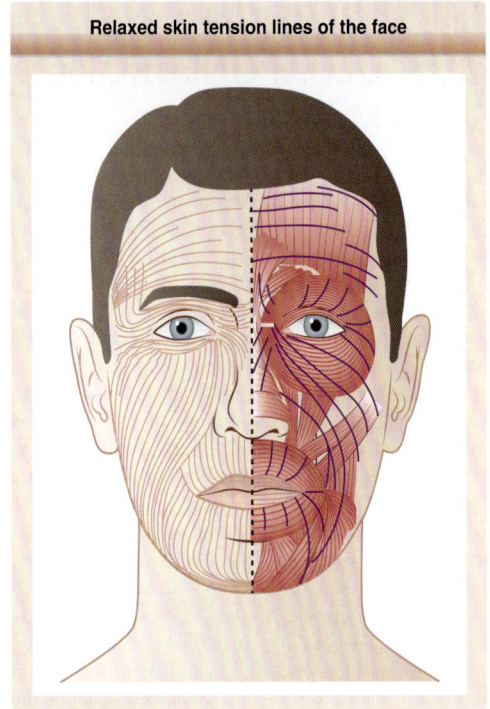

Figure 201-3 Relaxed skin tension lines of the face.

FACIAL MOTOR NERVES SUSCEPTIBLE TO DAMAGE DURING DERMATOLOGIC SURGERY

There are three main danger zones that are critical to understand while performing surgical procedures on the head and neck. Each of these zones involves a motor nerve and the muscles it innervates. These are the *temporal* and *marginal* mandibular branches of the facial nerve (cranial nerve VII) and the *spinal accessory nerve* (cranial nerve XI) (Table 201-1). These will be discussed in more detail below. It is important to confirm the baseline function of these nerves and muscles before performing a procedure in these areas so that it can be readily determined whether an injury occurred during surgery.

The facial nerve exits the skull through the stylomastoid foramen near the earlobe and immediately gives off the posterior auricular branch, which provides motor innervation to the occipital and posterior auricular muscles. It then enters the parotid gland at the midpoint of a line connecting the tragus with the angle of the mandible. Within the parotid gland, the facial nerve divides into the temporofacial and cervicofacial rami from which five branches arise. The well-known mnemonic "to Zanzibar by motor car" can be used to remember the five main branches: (1) temporal, (2) zygomatic, (3) buccal, (4) mandibular, and (5) cervical.

After leaving the parotid gland, the branches of the facial nerve lie deep to the SMAS and enter the

TABLE 201-1
Danger Zones of the Face

NERVE AT RISK	MUSCLE AFFECTED	LOCATION	DAMAGE
Temporal branch of the facial nerve	Frontalis, upper fibers of the orbicularis oculi, corrugator supercilii, anterior and superior auricular muscles	Facial nerve as it crosses the middle third of the zygomatic arch	Flattening of forehead, diminished wrinkles, skin tension lines, eyebrow and eyelid ptosis, visual field disturbance
Marginal mandibular branch of the facial nerve	Depressor anguli oris, depressor labii inferioris, mentalis, part of orbicularis oris	Inferior border of the mandible, as the nerve crosses the angle of the mandible at the inferoanterior border of the masseter	Contralateral and upward pull on the mouth; ipsilateral side presents with lip droop
Spinal accessory nerve	Trapezius	Posterior triangle of the neck, from the midpoint of the posterior border of the sternocleidomastoid	Paralysis of trapezius, winging of the scapula, shoulder drop, inability to shrug the shoulder, difficulty with arm abduction, chronic shoulder pain

Figures from Robinson JK, Hanke CW, Siegel DM, et al, eds. *Surgery of the Skin*, 3rd ed. St. Louis: Elsevier Saunders; 2015; with permission. Copyright © Elsevier.

muscles of facial expression from their deep surface. The branches of the facial nerve are therefore well protected during surgical procedures that are no deeper than fat. However, it is important to note that there can be minimal thickness of the fat layer at certain sites such as the temple and at other sites in older adult patients.

The two branches of the facial nerve most susceptible to injury during dermatologic surgery are the temporal branch as it crosses the zygomatic arch and the marginal mandibular branch along the inferior border of the mandible. The buccal and zygomatic branches form an interconnecting network across the midface, and although damage to these nerves may occur during surgical procedures, any injury is less debilitating than an injury to the temporal nerve because of the multiple rami in the buccal and zygomatic branches. Damage to the cervical branch is of minimal clinical importance because it innervates the platysma muscle, which also receives nerve fibers from the marginal mandibular nerve.

TEMPORAL BRANCH OF THE FACIAL NERVE

The temporal (or frontal) branch of the facial nerve innervates the frontalis, the upper fibers of the orbicularis oculi, the corrugator supercilii, and the anterior and superior auricular muscles. After emerging from the parotid gland, the nerve travels diagonally across the temple, where it lies between the superficial temporal fascia (a component of SMAS) and the deep temporal fascia. The temporal branch of the facial nerve divides into three to five rami as it crosses the middle third of the zygomatic arch. At this point, the nerve is most superficial and susceptible to damage and it is critical in this area to undermine just beneath the dermis in the superficial fat above the fascia. The approximate course of the temporal branch of the facial nerve can be projected on the skin by a line drawn from the earlobe to the lateral edge of the eyebrow and another line from the tragus to just above the and behind the highest forehead crease (Fig. 201-4).

Damage to the temporal branch of the facial nerve results in cosmetic and functional loss. Flattening of the forehead with diminished visibility of wrinkles and skin tension lines becomes easily noted. Over time, as the denervated muscle atrophies, patients develop eyebrow and eyelid ptosis, which may lead to visual field disturbance. A brow lift and blepharoplasty may be required to correct this problem.

MARGINAL MANDIBULAR NERVE

The marginal mandibular branch of the facial nerve exits the parotid gland at the angle of the jaw. It divides into two or more rami and travels anteriorly along the

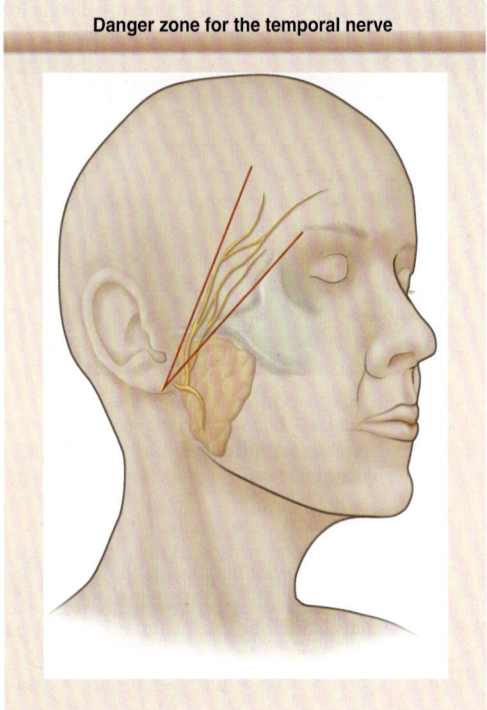

Figure 201-4 Danger zone for the temporal nerve.

ramus of the mandible to supply the depressor anguli oris, the depressor labii inferioris, the mentalis, and part of the orbicularis oris. As it crosses the angle of the mandible at the inferoanterior border of the masseter, the marginal mandibular nerve is covered only by skin, subcutaneous fat, and fascia, which may be thin in this location, particularly in older adults. Damage to the marginal mandibular nerve results in contralateral and upward pull on the mouth while the affected ipsilateral side of the mouth is fixed in a grimace with a lip droop.

SPINAL ACCESSORY NERVE

The posterior triangle of the neck is defined by the posterior border of the sternocleidomastoid, the anterior border of the trapezius, and the clavicle. The spinal accessory nerve enters the posterior triangle of the neck from under the posterior border of the sternocleidomastoid, roughly at its midpoint. It then crosses the floor of the posterior triangle, before leaving the posterior triangle under the trapezius. In the posterior triangle of the neck, the spinal accessory nerve occupies a relatively superficial location between the superficial and prevertebral layers of the deep cervical fascia.

One can anticipate the location of the spinal accessory nerve by drawing a line connecting the angle of the mandible with the mastoid process. A vertical line is then drawn from the midpoint of this line 6 cm inferiorly. The point at which this line intersects the posterior border of the sternocleidomastoid muscle is Erb's point. This landmark indicates the location of several important sensory nerves, including the transverse cervical, lesser occipital, and great auricular nerves, but most important, the point at which the spinal accessory nerve emerges from behind the sternocleidomastoid.

Injury to the spinal accessory nerve leads to the paralysis of the trapezius with winging of the scapula, shoulder drop, inability to shrug the shoulder, difficulty with abducting the arm, and chronic shoulder pain.

SENSORY NERVES

The trigeminal nerve (cranial nerve V) provides the majority of the sensory innervation of the face (Figs. 201-5 and 201-6 and Table 201-2). It exits the skull via three foramina located bilaterally in the midpupillary line, the supraorbital, infraorbital, and mental foramina. The first branch, the ophthalmic nerve (V_1), has several branches that supply the innervation to the superior portion of the face: the supraorbital, supratrochlear, infratrochlear, external nasal, and lacrimal nerves. The supraorbital (lateral) and supratrochlear (medial) nerves supply the forehead and anterior scalp and are branches of the frontal nerve (the largest branch of the ophthalmic nerve). They exit from two

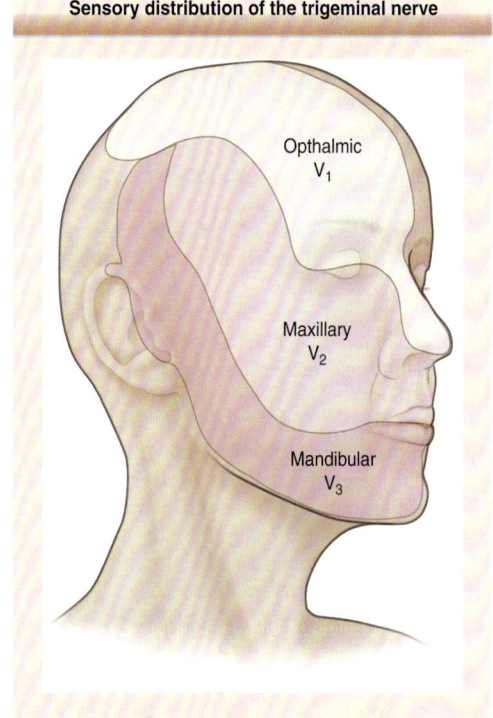

Figure 201-5 Sensory distribution of the trigeminal nerve.

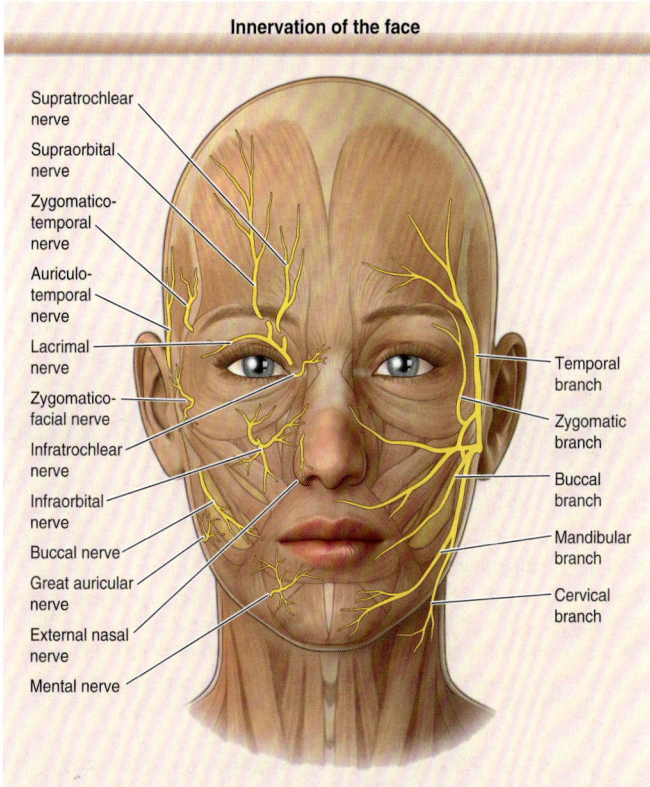

Figure 201-6 Nerves in the face. **A,** Sensory nerve supply to the skin of the face. **B,** Branches of the seventh cranial nerve to muscles of facial expression.

TABLE 201-2
Branches of the Trigeminal Nerve

BRANCH		AREA INNERVATED
V1 (Ophthalmic Nerve)		
Supraorbital (lateral) nerve		Forehead, anterior scalp
Supratrochlear (medial) nerve		Forehead, anterior scalp
Infratrochlear nerve (nasociliary)		Glabella, nasal root, nose bridge
External nasal nerve (dorsal nasal)		Anterior ethmoidal nerve, dorsal nose
Lacrimal nerve		Upper eyelid
V2 (Maxillary Nerve)		
Zygomatic nerve	Zygomaticofacial	Lateral canthus
	Zygomaticotemporal	Anterior temporal region
Infraorbital nerve		Eyelid, superior cheek
V3 (Mandibular Nerve)		
Auriculotemporal		Most of the temple, temporoparietal scalp, anterior ears, external ear canal, tympanic membrane
Buccal		Buccinators, buccal mucosa, gingiva
Mental		Lower lip, chin

notches along the orbital rim: (1) the supraorbital foramen or notch laterally and (2) the supratrochlear notch medially. The infratrochlear branch (of the nasociliary nerve) supplies the glabella, nasal root, and bridge. The external nasal branch (or the dorsal nasal nerve) is a branch of the anterior ethmoidal nerve of the nasociliary branch of V_1. The external nasal branch supplies the dorsal nose and provides the anatomical explanation of Hutchinson sign that can occur in some cases of herpes zoster of the ophthalmic nerve. Vesicles on the nasal tip indicate that the eye may be involved because the nasociliary branch of V_1 sends branches both to the nasal tip and the cornea. The lacrimal branch supplies sensation to the upper eyelid.

The second branch of the trigeminal nerve is the maxillary nerve (V_2). The maxillary nerve supplies sensation to the lateral nose, lower eyelid, superior cheek, and anterior temple. The maxillary nerve gives off two main branches that supply the skin of the face. The zygomatic branch of the maxillary nerve gives rise to the zygomaticofacial nerve, which exits the skull through the lateral zygomatic bone and supplies a small area of the lateral canthus. In addition, the zygomatic branch also gives rise to the zygomaticotemporal nerve, which exits the skull through the anterior temporal fossa and supplies skin of the anterior temporal region. The largest branch of the maxillary nerve is the infraorbital nerve that exits the skull through the infraorbital foramen of the maxilla. This supplies sensation to the eyelid and superior cheek.

The third branch of the trigeminal nerve is the mandibular nerve (V_3). Its branches provide sensory innervation to the lower lip, chin, mandibular and preauricular cheek, anterior ear, and central temporal scalp. The mandibular nerve gives off three major cutaneous branches: the (1) auriculotemporal, (2) buccal, and (3) mental nerves. The auriculotemporal nerve innervates most of the temple, the temporoparietal scalp, the anterior ears, parts of the external ear canal, and the tympanic membrane. The buccal nerve lies deep to the parotid gland and supplies the skin over the buccinators, the buccal mucosa, and the gingiva. The mental nerve exits through the mental foramen and is a continuation of the inferior alveolar nerve. The mental nerve supplies sensation to the lower lip and chin.

MUSCLES OF FACIAL EXPRESSION

The scalp has two muscles overlying it, the frontalis anteriorly and the occipitalis posteriorly. These muscles are joined by a thick fascia centrally over the scalp, the galea aponeurotica. The frontalis muscle also covers the forehead and elevates the eyebrows. The eyebrows move medially and downward with contraction of the corrugator supercilii muscles. The procerus lies between the supercilii muscles and draws the skin of the forehead inferiorly to create the horizontal creases at the root of the nose. The orbicularis oculi muscle surrounds the eye and consists of an orbital and palpebral portion. The orbicularis oculi muscle serves to close the eyes with the palpebral part with both reflexive and voluntary control and the orbital part with voluntary control. The central sphincter-like muscle around the mouth is the orbicularis oris. This muscle helps purse the lips to form certain sounds and whistle. The lip depressors are depressor anguli oris, depressor labii inferioris, and the mentalis. The lip elevators are the zygomaticus major, zygomatic minor, levator anguli oris, levator labii superioris, and levator superioris alaeque nasi. The risorius helps retract the corner of the mouth. The buccinators and masseter muscles help with mastication (Fig. 201-7).

VASCULAR ANATOMY

The blood supply of the face is almost entirely derived from branches of the external carotid artery (Fig. 201-8). Just posterior and medial to the angle of the mandible, the facial artery branches off the external carotid artery. The facial artery continues anteriorly and superiorly toward the angle of the mouth, giving off the inferior labial artery and superior labial arteries that supply the lips. The continuation of the facial artery in the nasofacial sulcus is called the *angular artery*. The angular artery continues superiorly to enter the orbit immediately over the medial canthal tendon, where it anastomoses with the ophthalmic artery, a branch of the internal carotid artery. After giving off the facial artery, the external carotid artery then passes deep to

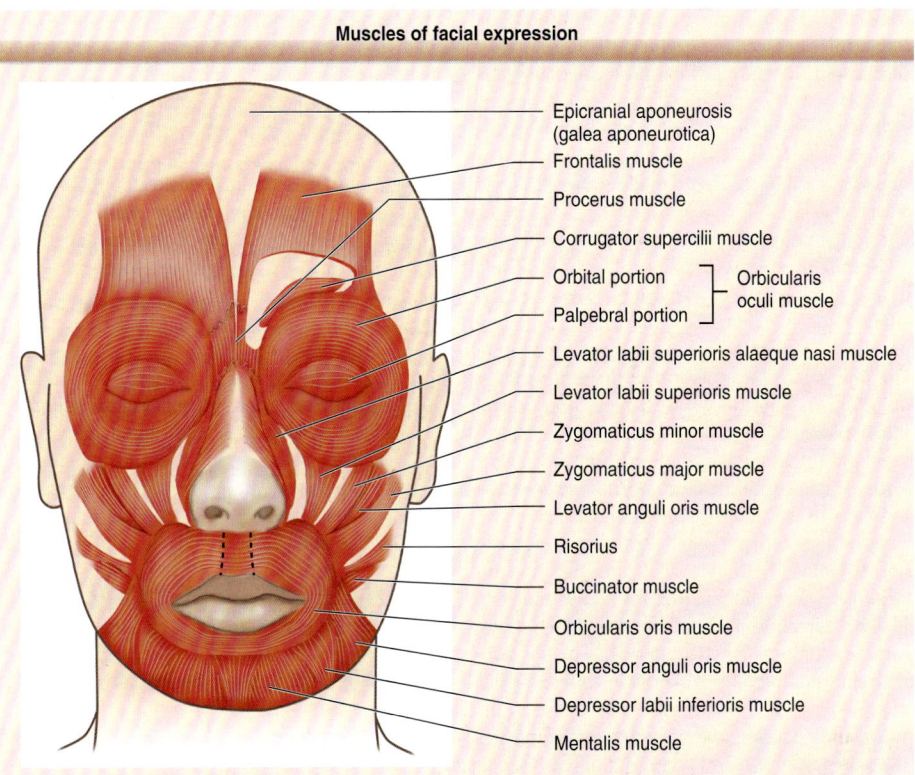

Figure 201-7 Muscles of facial expression.

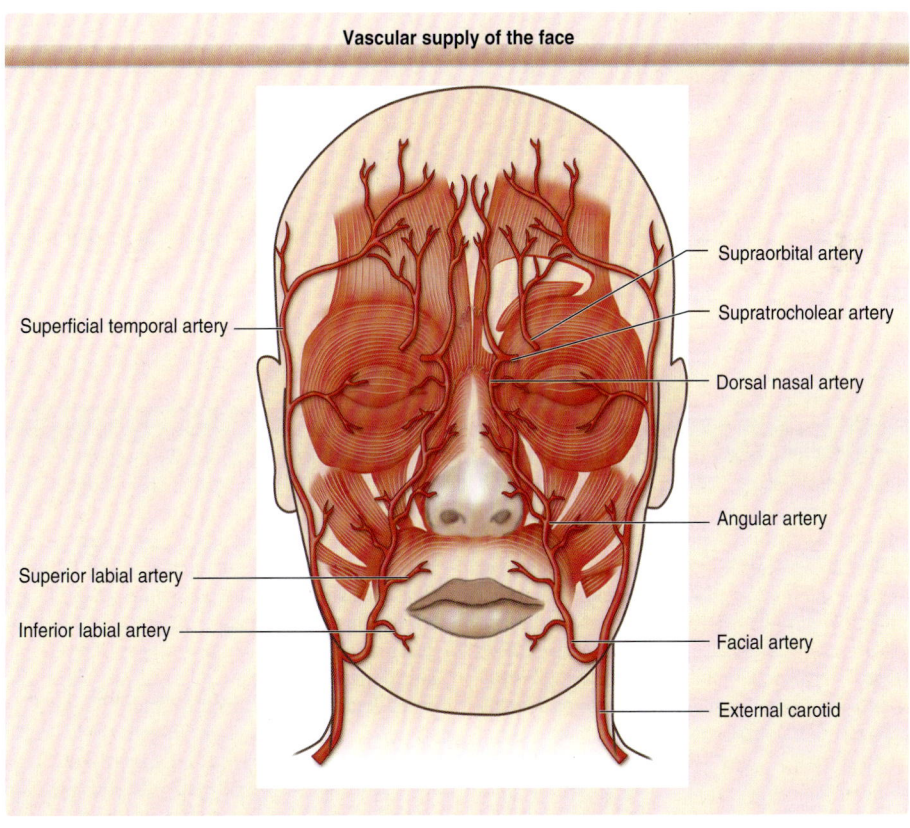

Figure 201-8 Vascular supply of the face.

the sternocleidomastoid muscle and enters the body of the parotid gland, where it gives off the posterior auricular artery that supplies the postauricular scalp, the maxillary artery, and the superficial temporal artery. The terminal branch of the maxillary artery exits the infraorbital foramen with the infraorbital nerve as the infraorbital artery to supply the lower eyelids and infraorbital cheek.

The terminal branches of the internal carotid artery are the ophthalmic artery branches, the supraorbital artery, and the supratrochlear artery. The supraorbital artery emerges from the supraorbital foramen, whereas the supratrochlear artery emerges more medially. The internal and external carotid systems join in two places: (1) where the supratrochlear branch and the dorsal nasal artery anastomose with the angular artery and (2) where the forehead branches of the supraorbital and supratrochlear arteries anastomose with branches of the superficial temporal artery.

The veins of the face are parallel and lie posterior to the arteries. Unlike the veins of the trunk and extremities, facial veins have no valves. This allows blood to flow in either direction. Thus, in the central face where there are anastomoses between branches of the ophthalmic vein and of the angular vein, infection has easy access to travel along the ophthalmic vein to the cavernous sinus. The angular vein also communicates with the deep facial vein and pterygoid plexus.

LYMPHATICS

The lymphatic vessels of the face generally drain from superficial to deep and medial to lateral and caudad. Although the general drainage patterns are described here, variations can occur. The posterior scalp drains to the postauricular and occipital nodes. The lateral and superior face, the forehead, and the lateral eyelids drain to the parotid nodes. The medial and inferior face, including the medial eyelids and lateral lips, drain to the submandibular nodes. The middle two-thirds of the lower lip and the chin drain to the submental nodes. These nodes can be optimally palpated by performing a bimanual examination with a gloved hand feeling through the floor of the mouth.

The lymph nodes of the head and neck eventually drain into a terminal series of nodes (deep cervical nodes) and finally into the lateral internal jugular chain.

ACKNOWLEDGMENTS

We acknowledge and are grateful to Brent Pennington, MD, coauthor of the previous edition of this chapter.

Chapter 202 :: Perioperative Considerations in Dermatologic Surgery
Noah Smith, Kelly B. Cha, & Christopher Bichakjian

第二百零二章
皮肤科手术的围手术期注意事项

中文导读

　　皮肤外科手术的量比其他科手术更多，因此在日常皮外手术中，除了需要精通外科手术技术，医生还必须考虑各种围手术期的注意事项，以最大程度地提高治疗效果并最大程度地减少并发症。本章共分为3节：①术前评估；②手术注意事项和流程；③术后注意事项。全面地讨论了皮肤科手术的围手术期注意事项。

　　第一节介绍了术前评估是确保安全、成功的手术过程的关键组成部分。还介绍了抗生素在皮肤科手术中应用的重要性；如果患者有可植入电子设备，需要改变术中止血方法；在计划进行外科手术时，必须重视对抗凝、抗血栓治疗以及糖皮质激素治疗的重要性；以及妊娠患者的药物使用注意事项。

　　第二节介绍了手术注意事项和流程，包括术前的知情同意书、生命体征的观察、局部麻醉、备皮、患者体位、设备、手术和缝合等各个阶段的注意事项，并详细介绍了局部麻醉的优点、作用机制及局麻药的使用注意事项、副作用。还介绍了根据手术过程、解剖位置和患者伤口的情况选择缝合材料和技术。

　　第三节介绍了术后注意事项，适当的围手术期护理对于降低并发症的风险至关重要，手术后应对伤口进行加压包扎以及在合适的时间拆除缝合。最后对术后并发症进行了介绍。

〔赵　爽〕

AT-A-GLANCE

- Preoperative assessment includes a thorough medical and social history, and physical examination.
- The choice and route of anesthesia are determined by the nature and duration of the procedure, and by patient-dependent factors.
- Suture material and technique are selected based on the surgical procedure, anatomical location, and patient-related qualities of the wound.
- Proper perioperative care is essential to decrease risk of complications.

Dermatologists likely perform more cutaneous surgical procedures than any other medical or surgical specialty.[1] In addition to mastery of the technical aspects of a surgical procedure, the provider must also navigate a variety of perioperative considerations to maximize treatment efficacy and minimize complications. This chapter outlines the preoperative, operative, and postoperative considerations in dermatologic surgery.

PREOPERATIVE ASSESSMENT

Preoperative assessment is a critical component of ensuring a safe and successful surgical procedure. A detailed review of a patient's history, including past medical and surgical history, medications, allergies, and social history, should be conducted. This serves to identify and enable appropriate planning around factors that may contribute to increased potential for intraoperative and postoperative complications.

HISTORY AND PHYSICAL EXAMINATION

PAST MEDICAL AND SURGICAL HISTORY

Common conditions such as hypertension and diabetes may impact surgical outcome. Hypertension may increase the risk of bleeding both during and after surgery, while uncontrolled diabetes may result in delayed wound healing and increased risk of infection. Patients with inherited bleeding disorders may require administration of clotting factors.

Cardiac history, including valve replacement and history of joint replacement, may impact the decision to prescribe prophylactic antibiotics. The presence and proximity of implantable electronic devices, such as a pacemaker or defibrillator, may require a modification of the intraoperative approach to hemostasis to reduce risk of adversely affecting the function of such a device.

Antibiotic Prophylaxis: Antibiotics have an important role in the setting of dermatologic surgery. A wound infection following surgery may increase symptoms including pain, and can result in complications, including poor wound healing. The presence of skin microflora at baseline results in some level of bacterial contamination of a surgical wound following compromise of the epidermal barrier during surgery. Therefore, careful attention to maintaining as close to a sterile procedural field as possible during surgery is imperative to minimize the risk of postsurgical wound infection. Additional factors that may increase risk of infection include microbial pathogenicity, length of surgery, the presence of foreign material including suture or dead space, poor suturing or reconstructive technique, poor vascular supply, and host immunity.

As routine use of antibiotics may promote antibiotic resistance, the judicious use of antibiotics surrounding surgery is essential. Table 202-1 provides examples of clinical scenarios in which prophylactic antibiotics should be considered to prevent surgical site infection. The most common organism resulting in infection following cutaneous surgery is *Staphylococcus aureus*, and initiation of a first-generation cephalosporin (or clindamycin, if patient is penicillin or cephalosporin allergic) should be considered when indicated. Initiation of an antibiotic preoperatively or within 2 to 3 hours postoperatively is important in modifying infection risk as maximal protection against infection occurs when antibiotics are given prior to bacterial colonization of the wound.

A distinct indication for the use of prophylactic antibiotics in dermatologic surgery is the prevention of infection at a distant site as a result of an infected surgical wound or surgically-induced bacteremia. The 2 major concerns are infective endocarditis and prosthetic joint infection. According to the revised *Guidelines* of the American Heart Association, antimicrobial prophylaxis for the prevention of bacterial endocarditis is only indicated for patients with cardiac conditions that confer the highest risk of adverse outcome from infective endocarditis.[2] Table 202-2 lists the high-risk cardiac conditions for which antibiotic prophylaxis is suggested. However, there is no convincing evidence that antimicrobial prophylaxis provides significant benefit

TABLE 202-1
Risk Factors for Surgical Site Infection

- Inflamed or infected skin close to surgical site
- Flap reconstruction on the nose
- Wedge excision of the lip or ear
- Skin graft repair
- Mucosal, anogenital, or lower leg procedure site
- High-tension closure
- Multiple simultaneous procedures or prolonged procedure time
- Immunocompromised status

Adapted from Wright TI, Baddour LM, Berbari EF, et al. Antibiotic prophylaxis in dermatologic surgery: advisory statement 2008. *J Am Acad Dermatol.* 2008;59(3):464-73.

TABLE 202-2
Cardiac Conditions Associated with the Highest Risk of Adverse Outcome from Endocarditis

- History of infective endocarditis
- Prosthetic heart valve or prosthetic material used for cardiac valve repair
- Congenital heart disease (CHD)
- Unrepaired cyanotic CHD, including palliative shunts and conduits
- Completely repaired congenital heart defect with prosthetic material or device, whether placed by surgery or by catheter intervention, during the first 6 months after the procedure
- Repaired CHD with residual defects at the site or adjacent to the site of a prosthetic patch or prosthetic device (which inhibit endothelialization)
- Cardiac transplantation recipients who develop cardiac valvulopathy

Adapted from Wilson W, Taubert KA, Gewitz M, et al. Prevention of infective endocarditis: guidelines from the American Heart Association: a guideline from the American Heart Association Rheumatic Fever, Endocarditis and Kawasaki Disease Committee, Council on Cardiovascular Disease in the Young, and the Council on Clinical Cardiology, Council on Cardiovascular Surgery and Anesthesia, and the Quality of Care and Outcomes Research Interdisciplinary Working Group. J Am Dent Assoc. 2007;138(6):739-45, 747-60.

in terms of prevention of infective endocarditis, which is much more likely to result from random bacteremia associated with daily activities such as tooth brushing. Moreover, the risk of antibiotic-associated side effects may exceed the benefit, if any, from prophylactic therapy. The risk of infective endocarditis is generally considered to be the highest for dental procedures and is extrapolated to patients undergoing a surgical procedure of infected skin or skin structure.

In 2013, the American Dental Association (ADA) and American Academy of Orthopaedic Surgeons (AAOS) published a joint guideline on the prevention of orthopedic implant infections in patients undergoing dental procedures. The guideline states that there is no convincing evidence to support routine use of prophylactic antibiotics in patients with prosthetic joints who undergo dental procedures.[3] The conclusion is based on the observation that there is no convincing clinical or experimental evidence to suggest a link between bacteremia induced by a dental procedure and prosthetic joint infections. While the ADA/AAOS guideline also states that prophylactic antibiotics are not generally recommended for patients with prosthetic joints who are undergoing cystoscopy or GI endoscopies, no specific recommendations are made with regard to dermatologic procedures. However, given the low risk of bacteremia as a result of clean dermatologic procedures, it is reasonable to extrapolate from the ADA/AAOS guideline that the routine use of prophylactic antibiotics to prevent prosthetic joint infections is not recommended. However, this should be considered a general recommendation for healthy, immunocompetent patients, and the decision to prescribe prophylactic antibiotics must be made on an individual basis. Preoperative prophylactic antibiotics may be appropriate in select patients, including, but not limited to, patients with a history of previous prosthetic joint infection or individuals with high-risk comorbidities including immunosuppression.

For those patients who meet the criteria for endocarditis or prosthetic joint infection prophylaxis, administration of cephalexin (2 g by mouth for nonoral sites) or amoxicillin (2 g by mouth for oral sites) 1 hour prior to a cutaneous surgical procedure is considered adequate. Alternative regimens for individuals with a penicillin allergy include clindamycin 600 mg by mouth or azithromycin 500 mg by mouth, 1 hour prior to surgery.[2]

Known nasal carriers of methicillin-resistant *S. aureus* (MRSA) also can be considered for preoperative antibiotic therapy. MRSA has been observed in an increasing number of wounds, and a 4-fold increased risk of MRSA wound infection has been reported following a surgical procedure in nasal carriers of MRSA.[4] Treatment of the nasal vestibule with mupirocin 2% ointment prior to surgery may decrease risk of MRSA wound infection, although MRSA resistance to mupirocin ointment has been reported in up to 12% of individuals.[5,6]

Implantable Electronic Devices: The use of implantable electronic devices (IEDs) to manage various cardiac and neurologic disorders continues to expand. IEDs that may be encountered include cardiac and gastric pacemakers, implantable cardioverter defibrillators (ICDs), cochlear implants, and stimulators, including deep brain, vagal nerve, phrenic nerve, spinal cord, and bone. Electromagnetic interference (EMI) with the use of electrocautery during surgical procedures has been reported to result in malfunctioning of IEDs. The majority of outpatient cutaneous surgical procedures use an external, electrically powered energy source for hemostasis, whether in the form of electrocautery or electrosurgery. To select the appropriate method of hemostasis that minimizes EMI and maximizes patient safety, IED history must be elicited prior to the procedure.

Heat electrocautery functions by converting electrical energy into thermal energy at a metal tip, which produces hemostasis when directly contacting tissue. Even though it is less effective than electrosurgery in hemostatic capability, electrocautery is the safest method of hemostasis in patients with IEDs with high risk of EMI as no electric current is passed to the patient. Additionally, an advantage of electrocautery is its ability to function in a wet environment.

Electrosurgery consists of a high-frequency alternating current through an unheated electrode. Current can be delivered either monopolarly, in which current is delivered to the surgical site through 1 electrode, or bipolarly, in which current is delivered to tissue between 2 adjacent electrodes. The use of monopolar electrosurgery without a grounding pad is a common method of obtaining hemostasis during office-based dermatologic procedures, as it is useful for both coagulation and dissection. Although generally safe, ungrounded, monopolar electrosurgery has the potential to cause EMI in a patient with an IED, as electrical current flows beyond the surgical site and disperses through the body. In contrast to monopolar electrosurgery, bipolar electrosurgery is useful only for coagulation and not dissection.

As electrical current passes only across the tips of the bipolar instrument, there is minimal risk of EMI with bipolar electrocautery in a patient with an IED.

For patients with a pacemaker or ICD, heat electrocautery or bipolar electrosurgery are considered optimal methods of hemostasis given their minimal risk for EMI. Should a dermatologist proceed with ungrounded monopolar electrosurgery in a patient with an IED, the use of minimum power settings and short, intermittent, irregular bursts of less than 1 second are highly encouraged. An in vitro study conducted on pacemakers and ICDs with a hyfrecator used at settings typical of in-office dermatologic surgical procedures suggested that a hyfrecator can safely be used for dermatologic procedures outside a 5-cm device perimeter without causing EMI.[7] For a patient with a pacemaker or ICD on the left upper chest, the three-dimensional 5-cm perimeter would include the left upper back, left shoulder, and left aspect of the neck. Device interrogation should be performed after the procedure if any change of device function or settings is suspected.

For patients with a cochlear implant or a stimulator such as a deep brain, vagal nerve, phrenic nerve, spinal cord, or bone, referring to specific manufacturer recommendations regarding electrosurgery precautions is recommended when available. Electrosurgical instruments are capable of producing voltages that can result both in direct damage to a cochlear implant and in necrosis of vital cells of the basilar membrane of the cochlea, potentially rendering reimplantation ineffective. Generally, thermal electrocautery is preferred for cochlear implant or stimulator devices as it has the lowest associated risk of EMI if used at sufficient distance from the device.[8] For additional information on electrosurgery, see Chap. 206 ("Cryosurgery and Electrosurgery").

MEDICATIONS

A review of current prescription and nonprescription medications is important to identify medications that may contribute to intraoperative or postoperative complications as well as potential interactions if prescribing perioperative medications.

Anticoagulants: Anticoagulants are medications commonly prescribed to prevent thrombotic events in patients with atrial fibrillation, a history of stroke, or other predisposing conditions. When planning any type of surgical procedure, it is important to elicit the use of anticoagulant therapy, including warfarin, clopidogrel, aspirin, dipyridamole, and the novel oral anticoagulants such as dabigatran, rivaroxaban, and apixaban. Historically, anticoagulants were routinely discontinued prior to surgical procedures. However, recent studies focused on dermatologic surgery suggest that continuation of such medications, including novel oral anticoagulants, rarely results in significant adverse outcomes.[9] Most importantly, while bleeding complications are inconvenient and should be minimized, they do not outweigh the morbidity and mortality associated with thrombotic or embolic events, such as stroke or pulmonary embolism, which may result from discontinuation of anticoagulant therapy.[10] It has become standard practice to continue medically-indicated anticoagulants throughout the perioperative period, unless discontinuation is considered necessary because of a procedure-specific risk and directly cleared with the prescribing health care provider.

Elective nonprescription medications or supplements with antithrombotic properties for general or preventive health maintenance without the direct recommendation of a physician must also be considered in the perioperative setting. Examples include aspirin, nonsteroidal antiinflammatory drugs, and dietary or herbal supplements with antithrombotic properties, such as fish oil, garlic, ginger, *Ginkgo biloba*, ginseng, and vitamin E.[11] Alcohol also prolongs coagulation. Discontinuation of these substances 7 to 14 days prior to cutaneous surgery may be considered to decrease the risk of hemorrhagic complications. Table 202-3 lists several medications and supplements that inhibit platelet function.

Systemic Corticosteroids: Medical immunosuppression with systemic corticosteroids, particularly when used chronically in solid-organ transplant recipients or in patients with autoimmune disease, may result in delayed or poor surgical wound healing.[12]

ALLERGIES

Prior knowledge of a history of allergies to local anesthetics, including associated preservatives; other procedure-related allergens, such as topical antiseptics; and topical or oral antibiotics is important when selecting perioperative medications and surgical supplies. An allergy to latex mandates latex-free gloves and procedural products. Intolerance to adhesive tapes and bandages can be ameliorated by bandages with paper tape or by elastic compression dressings.

TABLE 202-3
Medications That Inhibit Platelet Function

- Persantine
- Trental
- Sulfinpyrazone
- Clofibrate
- Salicylates
- Aspirin
- Sulfasalazine
- Vitamin E
- Plavix
- Herbs
    - *Ginkgo biloba*
    - Garlic
    - Feverfew
    - Ginger
    - Ginseng
    - Turmeric
- Nonsteroidal antiinflammatory drugs

SOCIAL HISTORY

Alcohol: Chronic excessive alcohol consumption may result in increased bleeding risk through platelet dysfunction and reduced platelet count, in addition to coagulation abnormalities that can manifest in the setting of liver disease. The consumption of alcohol should preferably be limited for 7 to 14 days preoperatively and postoperatively.

Smoking and Nicotine: Smoking tobacco is associated with reduced tissue oxygenation and a prolonged effect on inflammatory and reparative cellular functions, resulting in impaired wound healing.[13] Smoking history is particularly relevant when considering a complex surgical reconstruction as smoking may increase the likelihood of flap or graft failure. Smoking cessation should be encouraged with all patients, for a minimum of 1 week preoperatively and postoperatively. Nicotine alone also is associated with impaired wound healing secondary to vasoconstriction.[14] This is important to note, as the use of electronic nicotine devices, or e-cigarettes, as an alternative to traditional cigarette smoking, is increasingly common. Discontinuation of e-cigarette use may be considered perioperatively.

Functional Status and Support System: A patient's mental status, mobility, ability to conduct activities of daily living, availability of transportation, and support system have critical practical implications related to a surgical procedure. Examples range from a patient's ability to reach a procedure site for routine cleaning and dressing changes to transportation for postoperative followup. Coordination of appropriate assistance may be warranted for debilitated patients who lack necessary resources in the postoperative period.

PREGNANCY

Special considerations are indicated when planning a surgical procedure in a pregnant patient. If a perioperative antibiotic is indicated, use pregnancy category B medications, which include β-lactam antibiotics (cephalosporins and penicillins) and azithromycin. Mupirocin ointment is also pregnancy category B. Notably, tetracyclines and sulfamethoxazole-trimethoprim are pregnancy category D and should be avoided. With regard to topical antiseptics, chlorhexidine is pregnancy category B. Hexachlorophene, a possible teratogen, and povidone-iodine, which carries a theoretical risk of impairing thyroid function if used extensively and long-term or as part of a procedure involving a low-birthweight neonate, are both pregnancy category C.[15] Isopropyl alcohol and ethyl alcohol have not been classified by the U.S. Food and Drug Administration, but are considered low risk as typically used during a routine dermatologic procedure. The majority of local anesthetics are pregnancy category C, with the exception of lidocaine, prilocaine, and etidocaine, which are pregnancy category B. The addition of epinephrine (pregnancy category C) to a local anesthetic has historically been avoided in pregnancy over concern for theoretical decreased uterine blood flow. While the effect on placental perfusion at the concentrations used in local anesthesia is unclear, epinephrine is generally considered safe when used judiciously and in relatively low volume.[16,17]

PHYSICAL EXAMINATION

Assessment of existing scars, including those from previous surgical procedures or at a body site similar to the planned procedure, is helpful in assessing a patient's propensity for scarring, particularly hypertrophic scarring and keloid formation. In such situations, it is reasonable to preoperatively discuss the concept of scar revision, including intralesional triamcinolone acetonide injection or ablative laser therapy, should a symptomatic or cosmetically-undesirable scar develop. The risk of hypertrophic scarring should specifically be discussed when performing surgery on anatomic sites with higher levels of tension and a predilection for hypertrophic scars, such as the upper trunk, shoulders, and upper arms. Identification of these features in existing scars can serve to educate a patient on expectations of future scarring in a personalized manner.

OPERATIVE CONSIDERATIONS AND PROCEDURE

INFORMED CONSENT

After a preoperative assessment has been completed and prior to performing a surgical procedure, a comprehensive informed consent that confirms the patient's identity, diagnosis, surgical site, planned procedure, and possible associated risks should be reviewed with and signed by the patient. Specifically, 2 recognized patient identifiers, such as full legal name and birthdate, should be reviewed with the patient as a safeguard against performing the procedure on the wrong patient. Additionally, the surgical site should be outlined with a skin marker and agreed upon with the patient, with the assistance of one or two mirrors for visualization as needed, to minimize likelihood of wrong-site surgery. General surgical risks should be discussed, including pain and discomfort, bleeding, bruising, hematoma formation, wound infection, nerve damage, recurrence of the lesion, and the expectation of a scar.

VITAL SIGNS

Vital signs, specifically heart rate and blood pressure, should be measured prior to initiating and upon completion of a dermatologic procedure. Although hypertension may be observed secondary to anxiety surrounding a procedure, it is important to identify as uncontrolled hypertension may increase bleeding risk, both intraoperatively and postoperatively. Additionally, use of epinephrine may require further consideration in a patient with arrhythmia. For patients with severe hypertension or in whom untreated or unknown arrhythmia is identified, deferment of surgery until the condition can be evaluated and managed by an appropriate health care provider may be indicated.

LOCAL ANESTHESIA

Compared with general anesthesia, local anesthesia is effective, fast acting, low cost, and relatively simple to employ. The selection of the appropriate method and agent is based upon such factors as desired route of administration, rapidity of onset, and anticipated procedure length (Table 202-4). For dermatologic procedures, tissue infiltration is the most common route of administration of local anesthetic, and lidocaine, with its rapid onset of action and duration of 1 to 2 hours, is the most commonly used local anesthetic agent.

Local anesthetics function by impairing neuronal transmission of sensory input, including pain and heat. Specifically, the chemical structure of the anesthesia serves to block neuronal sodium channels, thereby inhibiting depolarization and impairing formation of an action potential across the nerve axon, resulting in an inability for signal to be relayed to the CNS. Smaller, unmyelinated C-type nerve fibers, which transmit heat and pain sensation, are blocked by local anesthetics more rapidly and effectively than larger, myelinated, Aδ-type nerve fibers, which transmit pressure sensation and innervate skeletal muscle fibers. Smaller volumes of local anesthetics therefore tend to block transmission of pain and heat stimuli, while preserving sensation of pressure and motor function. At higher volumes or with increased tissue infiltration, pressure sensation and motor function also may be impaired.

The function of a local anesthetic is determined by its chemical structure. All local anesthetics are composed of three subunits: a lipophilic aromatic ring, a terminal amine group, and an intermediate linking chain that connects the hydrophobic and hydrophilic groups. Local anesthetics are characterized by the structure of this intermediate linking chain, which is either an amide or ester group.

Onset of action is related to the ionization constant (pK_a) of the anesthetic. The terminal amine group may exist in an uncharged, lipid soluble form or in a cationic, hydrophilic form. While the amine group is in the cationic, hydrophilic form to maintain its solubility in solution, the anesthetic penetrates the neuron when the amine group is in its uncharged, lipid soluble form. When the environmental pH is less than the pK_a, an increasing proportion of the amine group is in the

TABLE 202-4
Local Anesthetics

GENERIC NAME	PRIMARY USE	RELATIVE POTENCY	ONSET	DURATION[a] PLAIN	MAXIMUM[b] DOSE PLAIN (mg)	MAXIMUM[b] DOSE WITH EPINEPHRINE (mg)
Amides						
Bupivacaine	Infiltration	8	2 to 10 minutes	3 to 10 hours	175	250
Dibucaine	Topical	—	Rapid	Short	—	—
Etidocaine	Infiltration	6	3 to 5 minutes	3 to 10 hours	300	400
Lidocaine	Infiltration/topical	2	Rapid	1 to 2 hours	300	500 (3,850 dilute[c])
Mepivacaine	Infiltration	2	3 to 20 minutes	2 to 3 hours	300	400
Prilocaine	Infiltration	2	Rapid	2 to 4 hours	400	600
Prilocaine/lidocaine	Topical	—	30 to 120 minutes	Short	—	—
Esters						
Benzocaine	Topical	—	Rapid	Short	—	—
Chloroprocaine	Infiltration	1	Rapid	0.5 to 2 hours	600	—
Cocaine	Topical	—	2 to 10 minutes	1 to 3 hours	200	—
Procaine	Infiltration	1	Slow	1 to 1.5 hours	500	600
Proparacaine	Topical	—	Rapid	Short	—	—
Tetracaine	Infiltration	8	Slow	2 to 3 hours	20	—
Tetracaine	Topical	—	Rapid	Short	—	—

[a]In clinical practice, the duration of anesthesia appears to be less than stated above, especially for head and neck areas, and addition of epinephrine prolongs anesthesia by a factor of 2.

[b]Maximum doses are for a 70-kg person.

[c]Maximum safe dosage of tumescent lidocaine for 70-kg individual at 55 mg/kg.

cationic, hydrophilic form; when the environmental pH is greater than the pK_a, an increasing proportion of the amine group is in the uncharged, lipid soluble form. The pK_a of all local anesthetics is greater than the physiologic pH of 7.4, meaning that less than half of the amine groups in the anesthetic are in the lipid-soluble form, capable of penetrating the neuron when injected into tissue with a normal physiologic pH of 7.4. When injected into the acidic environment associated with inflamed tissues, even fewer of the amine groups are in the lipid soluble form, potentially explaining in part why inflamed or infected tissues are more difficult to anesthetize than normal-appearing skin. Buffering of an epinephrine-containing anesthetic solution, from the acidic pH at which it is often prepared to a pH closer to physiologic pH and the pKa of the anesthetic, may result in more rapid onset of action upon injection.

The lipid solubility of the lipophilic aromatic ring determines the potency of an anesthetic through its ability to diffuse through nerve sheaths and neural membranes of individual axons. The duration of action is proportional to the plasma protein binding properties of the anesthetic, as this correlates with affinity for binding within sodium channels, which corresponds to time of neural blockade.[18]

Amide anesthetics include lidocaine, prilocaine, bupivacaine, mepivacaine, and etidocaine. Amide anesthetics are metabolized by hepatic microsomal cytochrome P450 enzymes. Following dealkylation and hydrolysis in the liver, metabolites are ultimately excreted renally. An alternative to an amide anesthetic may be considered in patients with liver failure or in those taking medications such as propranolol, which may prolong the half-life of the anesthetic by inhibiting the activity of cytochrome P450 enzymes.

Ester anesthetics include procaine, benzocaine, tetracaine, and cocaine. Ester anesthetics are metabolized through hydrolysis by plasma pseudocholinesterases with subsequent renal excretion.

EPINEPHRINE

All local anesthetics are vasodilators, with the exception of cocaine, which is a vasoconstrictor. Even though local anesthetics afford the necessary blockade of pain sensation to allow for surgical procedures to be conducted, this vasodilatory effect results in increased intraoperative bleeding. By adding epinephrine to local anesthetics, typically at a concentration ranging between 1:100,000 and 1:500,000, the vasoconstrictive property of epinephrine is used to counteract the vasodilatory properties of local anesthetics and reduce intraoperative bleeding. The local vasoconstriction caused by epinephrine also serves to concentrate the anesthesia at the site of injection, resulting in increased duration and efficacy of anesthesia by up to 150% while reducing the potential for systemic absorption and toxicity.

As a potent α-adrenergic and β-adrenergic receptor agonist, the use of epinephrine as a component of local anesthetics has several contraindications. Its use is absolutely contraindicated in patients with pheochromocytoma or hyperthyroidism as it may result in hypertensive crisis. Relative contraindications include severe coronary artery disease, peripheral vascular disease, uncontrolled hypertension, acute angle glaucoma, and pregnancy, given the concern for decreased uterine blood flow. Epinephrine may also potentiate the effects of medications such as monoamine oxidase inhibitors, phenothiazines, and tricyclic antidepressants. Importantly, the use of epinephrine in patients taking medications of the β-adrenergic blocking (β-blocker) class may result in unopposed stimulation of α-adrenergic receptors, putting patients at risk of severe hypertension. Epinephrine should be used judiciously in patients taking such medications.

The use of epinephrine on distal anatomic regions with less-robust collateral circulation, such as the digits, nasal tip, and penis, has historically been cautioned against over concern that the vasoconstrictive properties of epinephrine could result in ischemia and tissue necrosis. More recently, ischemia and necrosis at distal anatomic sites have been attributed to use of excessive volume, resulting in a physical tamponade effect on the local vasculature. When used judiciously, a small volume of local anesthetic containing epinephrine can typically be used to safely anesthetize distal anatomic sites such as the digits, nasal tip, and penis. For patients with severe peripheral vascular disease, the use of an anesthetic without epinephrine or a lower concentration of epinephrine (1:500,000) may be warranted.

Systemic side effects associated with epinephrine are self limited and include feelings of anxiety and fear, tremor, heart palpitations, tachycardia, and hypertension. While exceedingly rare when used as part of conventional cutaneous surgery in an appropriate patient population, severe systemic side effects of excessive epinephrine dosing may include heart arrhythmias, cardiac arrest, and cerebrovascular hemorrhage.

TOPICAL ANESTHETICS

Topical administration of local anesthetic provides an alternative route to infiltration of tissue by injection. This may provide a suitable level of anesthesia for minor dermatologic procedures, such as shave biopsy, or when a significant skin surface area requires anesthesia, such as prior to laser therapy. Topical anesthetics also may be considered when performing a procedure on an anxious patient, such as a child or patient with fear of needles. Sufficient penetration of the stratum corneum by the topical anesthetic, often requiring prolonged application time in combination with occlusion, is required for maximum efficacy.

Commonly used topical anesthetics include L-M-X (lidocaine hydrochloride) and EMLA (eutectic mixture of local anesthetics) creams. L-M-X cream consists of lidocaine delivered in a liposomal vehicle and is available in 4% (L-M-X4) or 5% (L-M-X5) concentrations. It is most effective when applied 30 minutes prior to a procedure; it may be occluded at the discretion of the provider and as tolerated by the patient. EMLA cream consists of a mixture of the amide anesthetics lidocaine and prilocaine, each at 2.5% concentration. EMLA is most effective when applied under occlusion 1 hour prior to a procedure with data suggesting equal efficacy to L-M-X cream applied 30 minutes prior to a procedure without occlusion. Both L-M-X and EMLA creams have been shown to be more effective than tetracaine 4% topical gel and a mixture of prilocaine and lidocaine in a liquid paraffin ointment vehicle. Importantly, prilocaine-containing topical preparations, including EMLA cream, have the potential to induce methemoglobinemia in infants and when applied to an impaired skin barrier, and should therefore be used with caution in such clinical scenarios. Allergic contact dermatitis to topical ester anesthetics such as benzocaine and tetracaine may occur.

Topical anesthetics are effective in providing anesthesia to mucosal membrane surfaces as they are readily absorbed in the absence of a stratum corneum. Tetracaine or proparacaine preparations may be used on the ocular surface prior to insertion of eye shields. Topical benzocaine and lidocaine are effective in anesthetizing oral mucosal surfaces prior to surgical procedures or to increase patient comfort while performing intraoral nerve blocks.

Cold may be used to offer transient anesthesia to diminish pain sensation as needed. A cryogen, such as ethyl chloride, may be delivered in a topical spray to a concentrated area of the skin prior to injection or nerve block. An ice cube or ice pack also may be held temporarily on a procedure site prior to needle insertion.

PERIPHERAL NERVE BLOCKAGE

When a cutaneous procedure involves a significant surface area of the skin, multiple injections to achieve a satisfactory level of anesthesia may be undesirable and lead to significant patient discomfort. Infiltration of a large volume of anesthetic at the procedure site may also distort anatomic structures while increasing the risk of anesthetic toxicity. In such a scenario, appropriate execution of a regional peripheral nerve block, based on comprehensive knowledge of regional anatomy, may be a useful tool when the anatomic region lies within a particular sensory nerve distribution. By injecting a small volume of anesthesia at the proximal aspect of a sensory nerve root, sensory anesthesia of the region supplied by that nerve can be effectively achieved. Caution is warranted as direct trauma to a nerve during blockage may result in neurapraxia, which may last 6 weeks or longer.

Nerve blockade is usually performed with a standard anesthetic such as lidocaine (1%) with epinephrine (1:100,000), using a 1-inch, small-diameter (30-gauge) needle. If extended effect is desired based upon the anticipated length of the procedure, a longer-acting anesthetic such as bupivacaine also may be used.

Nerve blockage in dermatologic surgery is particularly useful when performing procedures on the face or digits. Sensory input from the face is transmitted primarily via the trigeminal nerve (cranial nerve V), the branches of which are readily accessible for peripheral nerve blockage. Nerve blockade of the digits prior to digital or nail surgery allows for effective anesthesia with minimal volume, which is particularly important as injection of more than 1 mL around a digit may increase the risk for digital vascular tamponade with subsequent ischemia and necrosis.

Branches of the ophthalmic division (cranial nerve V1) of the trigeminal nerve include the supraorbital, supratrochlear, and infratrochlear nerves. The supraorbital nerve exits the skull via the supraorbital foramen, a bony prominence that is palpable at the orbital rim, just medial to the midpupillary line. The supratrochlear branch exits the skull approximately 1.5 cm medial to the supraorbital notch along the orbital rim. The infratrochlear nerve exits the skull just superior to the medial canthus. Nerve blockade of these 3 branches can be accomplished with a single injection and provides anesthesia to the ipsilateral forehead, frontal scalp, upper eyelid, medial canthus, and superior nasal sidewall and root. Blockade of these nerves is performed by inserting the needle 2 to 3 mm lateral to the supraorbital notch and advancing medially through the subcutaneous tissue to the medial canthus, followed by slow withdrawal of the needle while simultaneously injecting the medication along the path that the needle travels.

The maxillary division (cranial nerve V2) of the trigeminal nerve gives rise to several branches including the infraorbital nerve, which provides sensation to the ipsilateral lower eyelid, medial cheek, nasal ala, upper lip, and upper teeth. Nerve blockade of the infraorbital nerve with resulting anesthesia of these structures can be achieved using either a percutaneous or an intraoral approach. The infraorbital nerve exits the skull through the infraorbital foramen, which is located approximately 1 cm below the infraorbital rim along the midpupillary line. Percutaneous blockade of the infraorbital nerve is performed by inserting the needle perpendicularly into the skin at the infraorbital foramen and advancing the needle directly down to the maxillary bone, where the anesthetic is injected. The intraoral approach to infraorbital nerve blockade consists of palpating the sulcus just superior and lateral to the canine tooth, and inserting the needle at the superior portion of this sulcus. The needle should be advanced superiorly approximately 1 cm in the midpupillary line, where the anesthetic should be slowly injected. The intraoral approach is typically less painful than the percutaneous one, and may be even better tolerated if a topical anesthetic such as lidocaine or benzocaine is applied to the oral mucosa prior to injection.

Branches of the mandibular division (cranial nerve V3) of the trigeminal nerve include the mental nerve, which supplies sensation to the ipsilateral lower lip and chin. The mental nerve exits the skull through the mental foramen, which is located along the mandible, just medial to the midpupillary line. The mental nerve is located opposite of the first bicuspid on the buccal mucosa of the lower lip, and can sometimes be visualized as a thin, white, glistening strand. Blockade of this nerve may be performed using an intraoral approach, with insertion of the needle at the inferior portion of the nerve along the buccal mucosa of the lower lip, just opposite the first bicuspid.

In addition to the above branches, there are other branches of the trigeminal nerve that are amenable to regional nerve blocks. These include the buccal, auriculotemporal, anterior ethmoidal (external nasal branches), and zygomaticotemporal nerves. A block of the greater auricular nerve off the cervical plexus provides anesthesia to the posterior auricle and angle of the mandible.

When performing digital or nail procedures, digital nerve blockade is readily possible based upon the longitudinal orientation of the digital sensory nerve along either lateral surface of the digit. A needle is inserted at the proximal aspect of the digit perpendicular to the lateral surface and advanced to the lateral aspect of the underlying digital bone. Injection of a small volume of anesthetic at this site can accomplish satisfactory anesthesia of the digit with minimal risk of tamponade effect.

SIDE EFFECTS

The most common side effect of local anesthetics is pain during administration, which is the result of acidity of the anesthetic preparation and injection technique. Epinephrine is more stable at an acidic pH, and premixed epinephrine-containing local anesthetics are typically prepared at an acidic pH between 3 and 5. The difference between the acidity of the solution and physiologic pH of 7.4 results in significant discomfort upon injection. Adjustment to a more basic pH closer to physiologic pH can be accomplished by addition of sodium bicarbonate to the solution, for example, 1 part 8.4% sodium bicarbonate mixed with 10 parts lidocaine. While this buffered solution causes less pain with injection, it should be noted that it increases the rate at which epinephrine degrades to approximately 25% per week. An alternative approach to preparing a more neutral solution is mixing epinephrine with the anesthetic at the time of the procedure.

Injection components including needle and syringe size, needle orientation to the skin, rate of tissue infiltration, and anatomic placement of anesthesia significantly impact the degree of discomfort experienced by the patient. Use of a small-diameter needle, such as 27-gauge or 30-gauge, is better tolerated with less pain during injection. Rapid injection of a large volume of anesthetic into tissue is also painful. Slow injection with a low-volume syringe, between 1 and 3 mL, allows for optimal control of the rate of tissue infiltration and minimization of pressure at the injection site. Insertion of the needle through a pore or at an orientation perpendicular to the skin may be better tolerated.[19] Injection of anesthesia at the subcutaneous layer is less painful than intradermal injection; however, intradermal injection results in more rapid onset and longer duration of action as compared to injection into the subcutaneous tissue. When anesthetizing a larger area, initiate anesthesia at the proximal aspect of the nerve distribution and insert subsequent needles within the anesthetized periphery to decrease overall pain. A nerve block could also be considered to provide regional anesthesia with fewer injections and lower volume of anesthesia. Additional techniques for lessening discomfort and anxiety of injection include cold or vibration at or near the site of needle insertion and distraction techniques ranging from social conversation to handheld devices with applications interesting to the patient.

Vasovagal reaction may occur during any portion of a dermatologic procedure. To decrease risk of vasovagal reaction, pain and anxiety should be minimized. The patient should be placed in a recumbent or Trendelenburg position prior to injection for local anesthesia and throughout the procedure. Signs and symptoms that herald vasovagal reaction include pallor, weakness, bradycardia, hypotension, nausea, and diaphoresis. Diaphoresis also may be observed in the settings of hypoglycemia or angina. Seizure can (rarely) occur in the context of a vasovagal reaction and is typically short lived. Should a vasovagal reaction occur, the patient should be placed in Trendelenburg position, which usually leads to resolution within minutes; standard surgical positioning in recumbent or Trendelenburg position facilitates this and mitigates the risk of adverse events such as falls. Cool compresses also can be soothing.

Allergic reactions to local anesthetics can occur. These are typically Type I, immunoglobulin E–mediated reactions that may manifest as angioedema, urticaria, bronchospasm, tachycardia, hypotension, and even cardiovascular collapse. Less commonly, Type IV, delayed hypersensitivity reactions presenting as allergic dermatitis may be observed. Allergy to ester anesthetics is far more common than to amide anesthetics, and typically occurs secondary to para-aminobenzoic acid (PABA), which is an intermediate metabolite of ester anesthetics. Importantly, cross-reactions to both injected and topical ester anesthetics can occur in individuals with allergies to para-phenylenediamine, sulfonamides, para-aminosalicylic acid, azo dyes, and PABA sunscreens.[20] Amide local anesthetics are not metabolized to a PABA derivate, and allergy to amide anesthetics is far less common. However, it is important to note that methylparaben, a preservative used in amide anesthetics, is structurally similar to PABA, and cross-reactivity to the aforementioned allergens may occur. Additionally, metabisulfite, an antioxidant that is often added to epinephrine-containing local anesthetics as a stabilizer of epinephrine, may result in allergy and cross-react in individuals allergic to sulfites and bisulfites. Referral for allergy testing prior to surgery should be considered in patients who report a history or suspicion of allergy to local anesthetic or an associated preservative. In patients with documented or observed allergy to local anesthetics, alternative methods of local anesthesia for a simple dermatologic procedure include intradermal injection of diphenhydramine hydrochloride solution or bacteriostatic (0.9%) normal saline, although the efficacy of these methods is limited. Intradermal injection of diphenhydramine solution may result in classic antihistamine side effects, including significant drowsiness. The anesthetic effect of normal saline is likely related to a combination of tamponade effect on local nerves and a mild anesthetic effect of the preservative benzoyl alcohol.

Risk of anesthetic toxicity should be considered when performing large dermatologic procedures requiring significant volume of local anesthesia. Maximum dosage should be kept under 4.5 mg/kg of plain lidocaine without epinephrine, 7 mg/kg of lidocaine with 1:100,000 epinephrine, and for tumescent anesthesia, 55 mg/kg of 0.05% to 0.1% lidocaine with 1:1,000,000 epinephrine. Initial symptoms of anesthetic toxicity include circumoral and distal extremity numbness and tingling, tinnitus, lightheadedness, and nausea. More-severe manifestations of anesthetic toxicity that occur with increasing dose include CNS depression accompanied by hallucinations, seizures, and respiratory depression, followed by cardiovascular toxicity, including hypotension, arrhythmias, and cardiac arrest. Intraarterial and intravenous injection of local anesthetic results in increased serum levels of anesthetic and, therefore, increased risk of anesthesia toxicity. Drawing back on the syringe plunger after needle insertion and prior to infiltration of the anesthetic will reveal a flash of blood if the needle is within the lumen of a vessel, which warrants repositioning the needle. Of note, patients with liver disease are at increased risk of amide anesthetic toxicity secondary to reduced metabolism of amide anesthetic. Therefore, dose reduction of an amide local anesthetic or use of an ester anesthetic is recommended for a patient with liver disease undergoing an extensive dermatologic procedure requiring a significant volume of local anesthetic.

SKIN PREPARATION

Normal skin flora primarily consists of aerobic cocci, including *Streptococcus* and *Staphylococcus* (*aureus* and *epidermidis*), with *S. aureus* serving as the most common pathogen in cutaneous infection following dermatologic surgery. Other bacteria, including *Pseudomonas, Propionibacterium*, and micrococci, are commonly identified on the skin. *Pseudomonas* is a common pathogen related to infections of surgical sites involving cartilage, such as on the ear. An aseptic approach to cutaneous surgery involves preparation of the skin with an antiseptic solution to minimize the bacterial flora at the surgical site, followed by diligent surgical technique with a goal of minimizing microbial contamination of the surgical site during the procedure. However, as some bacteria reside in the pilosebaceous unit, complete sterilization of the skin with a topical antiseptic solution is not possible.

The area that is prepared with topical antiseptic should include the planned incision site with a wide margin of normal skin to provide an adequate surgical field for visualization, tissue handling, and path for suture material. Sterile towels or drapes should be placed at the edge of the prepared surgical field, and can be fixed in place with towel clamps, as needed. Every effort should be made to maintain patient positioning and orientation of the surgical field once the procedure is initiated to minimize the possibility of contamination of the surgical site. For nonglabrous surgical sites that require hair removal to optimally conduct a procedure, clipping hairs or using depilatory agents is favored over shaving. The use of a razor for hair removal prior to surgery may be associated with increased risk of surgical site infection, likely by causing microabrasions that serve as reservoirs for bacteria and promote infection.[21]

TOPICAL ANTISEPTICS

Characteristics that are considered when selecting an antiseptic include breadth of microbicidal or microbiostatic activity, rapidity of onset, duration of effect, potential for irritation, allergic sensitization, and toxicity including teratogenicity. Antiseptics commonly utilized in invasive skin procedures include iodophors, chlorhexidine, and isopropyl alcohol.

The most commonly used iodophor in cutaneous surgery is povidone-iodine. The mechanism of action through which iodophors act as antiseptics is through oxidation of microbial cell membranes by free iodine. Iodophors display broad antimicrobial activity against both Gram-positive and Gram-negative bacteria, fungi, mycobacteria, and viruses. The onset of action of povidone-iodine is usually within 1 to 3 minutes. The needle should be advanced superiorly approximately 1 cm in the midpupillary line, once the antiseptic has dried. The duration of microbicidal activity following application is on the order of hours, although contact with blood or serum results in attenuation and loss of microbicidal activity. Side effects include allergic contact dermatitis, irritant contact dermatitis, and risk of tissue necrosis in wounds with prolonged exposure to significant volume of iodophors.

Chlorhexidine, another commonly used topical antiseptic in cutaneous surgery, also disrupts cell membranes. It has broad antimicrobial activity including Gram-positive and Gram-negative coverage, with some antiviral coverage. It does not display suitable antimicrobial effect against fungi or mycobacteria. Advantages of chlorhexidine over povidone-iodine include an almost instant onset of action, sustained activity for many hours after application, additive effect with repeated applications, and superior decontamination of the skin with lower rates of postoperative infection.[22] Potential side effects of chlorhexidine include keratitis or corneal ulceration, if direct contact with the cornea occurs, and cochlear and vestibular toxicity, if a perforation in the tympanic membrane allows chlorhexidine to reach the inner ear. These site-specific side effects limit the use of chlorhexidine on surgical sites near the ears and eyes. Additionally, tissue toxicity may occur as a side effect of prolonged exposure to chlorhexidine.

Isopropyl alcohol and ethyl alcohol are commonly used antiseptic agents for cutaneous procedures as they display broad antimicrobial activity against Gram-positive and Gram-negative bacteria, mycobacteria, viruses, and fungi, although to a lesser extent than iodophors or chlorhexidine. The mechanism of action is denaturation of microbial proteins. An advantage of isopropyl or ethyl alcohol is rapid onset of activity; however, this antimicrobial activity is not persistent. Additionally, as alcohols are highly flammable, they should be used with caution during procedures requiring electrosurgery.

Hexachlorophene is an antiseptic solution with excellent antimicrobial activity against Gram-positive bacteria; however, it possesses limited activity against Gram-negative bacteria and fungi. Additionally, hexachlorophene has neurotoxic properties and is readily absorbed through the skin, resulting in side effects in health care providers who frequently handle the medication and in infant patients. Importantly, hexachlorophene also may be teratogenic in individuals who frequently handle the antiseptic.

PATIENT POSITIONING

When positioning a patient for surgery, 4 aspects should be considered: (a) patient comfort; (b) accessibility and exposure of the surgical site; (c) tissue toxicity to surrounding tissue from the topical antiseptic; and (d) surgeon posture and comfort.

A position should be established that allows access and exposure of the intended surgical site and is comfortable for the patient to maintain throughout the duration of the procedure. This may be accomplished by a combination of table positioning and the use of arm rests and pillows of various shapes and sizes.

While cleansing with antiseptic, it is critically important to position the patient such that the risk of contact with vulnerable sites is minimized. If chlorhexidine is used on the head and neck region, contact with the eyes or external ear canal should be avoided.

Finally, the patient should ideally be positioned to optimize an ergonomic approach from the standpoint of the surgeon. Specifically, the table should be elevated to an appropriate height and the patient positioned such that the angles of back flexion and cervical neck flexion of the surgeon are both less than 15 degrees. Operating with a back flexion angle or cervical neck flexion angle greater than 15 degrees significantly increases long-term risk of disability associated with back and neck injury.

EQUIPMENT

Procedure room equipment typically consists of a mechanically-adjustable patient table, overhead adjustable procedure lights, hyfrecator, vital signs monitor, Mayo stand, waste receptacle for contaminated material, and suction device, as indicated.

Surgical tray setup, in terms of instruments and layout, may vary based upon factors including planned procedure and surgeon preference. However, it is important to maintain a consistent layout with regards to placement of surgical sharps in an attempt to minimize inadvertent injury and exposure to contaminated materials by the primary surgeon or other members of the surgical team.

Instruments that are commonly included as part of a basic excisional surgery tray are a curette; No. 3 or No. 7 scalpel handle with a blade; small forceps (eg, Bishop-Harmon) and/or smooth-toothed Adson forceps; delicate standard skin hook or double-prong skin hook; curved iris scissors; blunt-tipped undermining scissors; a hemostat; towel clamps; a needle holder; and suture scissors. Common blades are No. 15 and No. 10, with the No. 10 often used for large excisions on anatomic sites with a thicker dermis such as the back. Special procedures will require additional instruments, such as additional hemostats or skin hooks for larger procedures such as skin flaps, or a dermatome when a split-thickness skin graft is used during repair. Disposable material often included on a surgical tray includes suture, marking pen, gauze sponges, cotton tip applicator sticks, scratch pad for electrocautery tip, electrocautery hand piece and tip, surgical drapes, and foam or magnetic pad for discarded sharps, including blades and needles.

SURGICAL PROCEDURE

After the patient has provided informed consent for the procedure, the patient is properly positioned, and the surgery site is appropriately anesthetized and prepared, a final verification "time out" should be completed immediately prior to the skin incision. A "time out" consists of verbal confirmation of the correct patient, surgical procedure, surgical site, and when applicable, implanted devices. For additional information on surgical procedures, see Chap. 203, "Excisional Surgery and Repair, Flaps, and Grafts."

SUTURING

Repair of a surgical defect should maximize cosmetic and functional outcomes. For sutured repairs, the choice of appropriate suture material and the use of meticulous suturing technique are critical.

SUTURE MATERIALS

Selection of the proper suture material matches sutures with appropriate intrinsic characteristics to the anatomic location and anticipated tension of the planned repair. Table 202-5 summarizes the characteristics of suture material commonly used in dermatologic surgery.

Sutures are categorized most generally as absorbable and nonabsorbable, with an absorbable suture defined as losing half of its tensile strength within 2 months of placement. Absorbable sutures are typically used for approximation of the dermal and subcutaneous layers of the skin. They provide the key function of wound stabilization during the earliest period of scar formation, as a scar has only 5% to 10% of the original strength of the skin at 2 weeks postprocedure. Thus, the absorbable suture gradually loses its tensile strength as the scar gains intrinsic strength. Nonabsorbable sutures are most commonly used for external epidermal approximation, rather than significant structural support. They are typically removed within 1 to 2 weeks of the procedure.

Suture structure may be either monofilament or multifilament. Monofilament sutures are composed of a single, homogeneous strand, whereas multifilament sutures are composed of multiple identical strands that are arranged in a braided or twisted configuration. Monofilament sutures possess a low coefficient of friction, meaning that they pull through tissue with relative ease, and have low capillarity, resulting in both low tissue reactivity and low risk of infection. Monofilaments tend to have high memory, which describes the tendency of a suture to revert back to its original shape despite handling. As a result, a monofilament suture has lower knot security because of its tendency to unravel, and requires that additional knots be tied to minimize risk of wound dehiscence. Multifilament sutures tend to have low memory, resulting in increased knot security and requiring fewer ties. Multifilament sutures are structurally porous as a result of their braided or twisted configuration. This increased capillarity is associated with trapping of fluid and bacteria, thus increasing tissue reactivity and risk of infection.

Categorization of suture diameter is based upon the USP (United States Pharmacopeia) scale. For dermatologic surgery, suture size is typically between 3-0 and 6-0 (Table 202-6), with suture diameter being inversely related to the first digit of the USP designation. As tensile strength is directly related to the diameter of a suture, a USP 3-0 suture possesses a larger diameter and greater tensile strength than a 4-0 suture, and a 6-0 suture possesses a smaller diameter and lesser tensile strength than a 5-0 suture. The smallest suture diameter that provides adequate tensile strength for a repair should be selected. Typically, 5-0 sutures are used on anatomic sites of relatively low tension such as the face and ears; 6-0 suture may be used on or near sites of even less tension, such as the eyelid. Anatomic sites of higher tension, such as the trunk and scalp, typically require 4-0, and sometimes 3-0, suture. Depending on the dermal thickness and degree of photodamage of an individual's neck, 4-0 or 5-0 sutures are typically

TABLE 202-5
Suture Materials

	TYPE	MEMORY	TISSUE REACTIVITY	KNOT STRENGTH	TENSILE STRENGTH HALF-LIFE
Nonabsorbable					
Cotton	Twisted	Low	Very high	—	—
Nylon	Monofilament	High	Low	Poor	—
Nylon	Braided	Low	Low	Fair	—
Polybutester	Monofilament	High	Low	Good	—
Polyester, uncoated	Braided	Low	Low	Very good	—
Polyester, coated	Braided	Low	Low	Good	—
Polypropylene	Monofilament	Very high	Very low	Poor	—
Silk	Braided/twisted	Very low	High	Excellent	—
Stainless steel	Monofilament/braided/twisted	Very high	Very low	—	—
Absorbable					
Catgut, fast absorbing/mild chromic	Twisted	Very high	High	Poor	2 days
Catgut	Twisted	Very high	High	Poor	4 days
Catgut, chromic	Twisted	Very high	High	Fair	1 wk
Polyglactin 910	Braided	Very low	Low	Good	2 wks
Polyglycolic acid	Braided	Very low	Low	Good	2 wks
Poliglecaprone 25	Monofilament	Low	Very low	Very good	1 wk
Polyglyconate	Monofilament	Low	Very low	Very good[a]	1 mo
Polydioxanone	Monofilament	High	Very low	Poor	1 mo

[a]For further reading on polyglyconate suture, see Fong ED, Bartlett AS, Malak S, Anderson IA. Tensile strength of surgical knots in abdominal wound closure. ANZ J Surg. 2008 Mar;78(3):164-6. doi: 10.1111/j.1445-2197.2007.04394.x.

Data from Melton JL, Hanke WC. Wound closure materials. In: Lask GP, Moy RI, eds. *Principles and Techniques of Cutaneous Surgery*. New York, NY: McGraw-Hill; 1996:77; Garrett AB. Wound closure materials. In: Wheel RG, ed. *Cutaneous Surgery*. Philadelphia, PA: WB Saunders; 1994:199; and Srivastava D, Taylor RS. Suturing technique and other closure materials. In: Robinson JK, Hanke CW, Siegel DM, et al, eds. *Surgery of the Skin*. 3rd ed. Philadelphia, PA: WB Saunders; 2015:193-213.

TABLE 202-6
Recommended Diameter and Time to Removal of Absorbable Suture According to Anatomical Site

ANATOMICAL SITE	RECOMMENDED SUTURE DIAMETER	LENGTH OF TIME PRIOR TO SUTURE REMOVAL
Eyelids	6-0	5 to 7 days
Face and ears	5-0	5 to 7 days
Neck	4-0, 5-0	7 days
Scalp	3-0, 4-0	7 to 14 days
Trunk and extremities	3-0, 4-0	10 to 14 days[a]

[a]High-tension sites or sites with poor wound healing may require sutures to remain in place longer.

suitable. Dermatologic surgical procedures are generally best performed with needles intended for plastic or cosmetic surgery.

SUTURING TECHNIQUE

Appropriate suturing technique and careful suture placement are critical for maximizing cosmesis while minimizing complications. An ideal wound closure consists of meticulous wound edge approximation and eversion. As wound contraction normally occurs during healing, wound edge eversion at the time of closure promotes the development of a flat, smooth, cosmetically-appropriate scar. If the wound edge is not sufficiently everted during wound closure, wound contraction may increase the risk of a depressed or spread scar. An ideal wound closure also minimizes tension and dead space; maintains or restores anatomic contours with respect to cosmetic subunits; and avoids permanent suture track marks adjacent to the suture line, particularly in cosmetically sensitive areas.

Interrupted Sutures: Variants of interrupted sutures utilized in dermatologic surgery include the simple interrupted suture, the horizontal mattress suture, the half-buried horizontal mattress suture, and the vertical mattress suture.

Simple interrupted sutures are commonly used in dermatologic surgery as both buried and epidermal sutures. Properly placed, absorbable, buried, interrupted sutures are critical to a successful, layered wound closure. They reduce tension along the wound edges while providing necessary tensile support during the early stages of wound healing, minimizing risk of wound dehiscence. Eversion of the wound edges is best achieved by placing sutures in the deep dermis and subcutis in a heart-shaped configuration (Fig. 202-1), where the initial entry point of the needle on one side and the final exit point of the suture on the contralateral side are deepest relative to the skin surface. Placement of more superficial dermal sutures may be used as part of the layered wound closure of deeper wound defects to reduce dead space and further facilitate wound eversion.

Epidermal, nonabsorbable, simple interrupted sutures may be placed to precisely align the wound edges following cutaneous surgery. Although more time-consuming to place than a continuous, running suture, they may be considered in areas of high wound

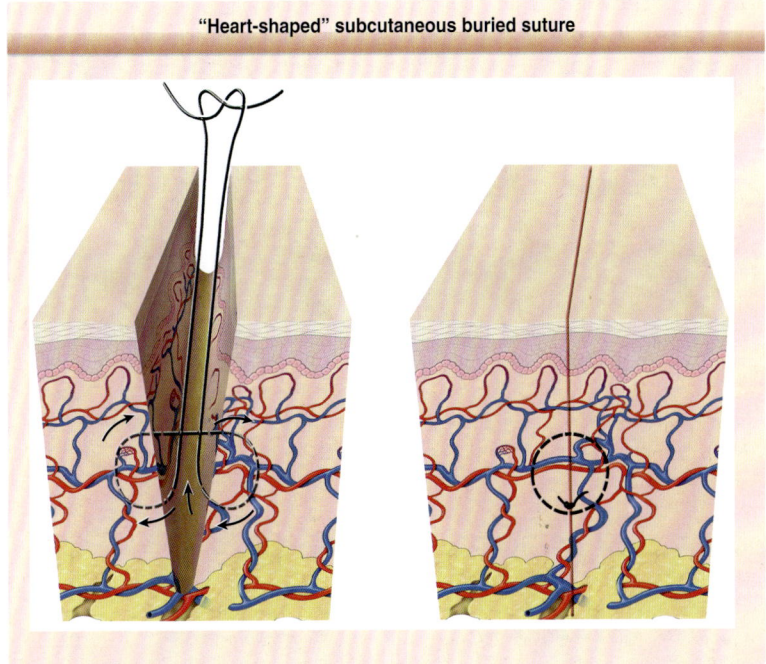

Figure 202-1 "Heart-shaped" subcutaneous buried suture.

tension where wound dehiscence is a concern. Simple interrupted sutures allow for alternating sutures to be removed in stages over time, providing additional tensile support as needed to minimize risk of wound dehiscence. Interrupted sutures may also cause less edema and impaired microcirculation than a running suture, and may be considered when there is a concern for impaired wound healing. In the event that the placement of buried, dermal sutures results in uneven approximation of the epidermal edge with a "stepped" appearance, simple interrupted epidermal sutures can be used to evenly approximate the epidermal edge by placing the suture more superficially at the elevated epidermal edge and more deeply at the depressed epidermal edge.

The horizontal mattress suture (Fig. 202-2) may be used to reduce persistent tension along wound edges following placement of buried sutures. This technique also provides the added benefits of hemostasis and wound edge eversion, and may be utilized in cosmetically-sensitive areas. Horizontal mattress sutures also may be used as temporary bridging sutures as part of high-tension closures to offset tension and temporarily approximate wound edges, facilitating the ease with which subcutaneous or dermal sutures may be placed, after which time the bridging sutures may be removed. Alternatively, the bridging sutures may be left in place for several days to permit wound edge healing under reduced tension. The risk of wound-edge necrosis can be minimized by placing the suture at least a few millimeters from the wound edge. Affixing bolsters on either side of the wound edge can also reduce the risk of tissue necrosis.

The half-buried horizontal mattress suture, also referred to as a Gillies corner stitch or 3-point corner stitch, may be used in a variety of local flap closures, such as M-plasty, V-Y plasty, or rotation flaps, to approximate the flap tips to recipient wound corners. It may decrease flap tip necrosis by minimizing interference with the dermal vascular plexus of the flap tip.[23]

The vertical mattress suture (Fig. 202-3) can provide wound edge eversion, minimize dead space, and minimize tension. It acts as a combination of a buried dermal and interrupted epidermal suture. The initial entry and exit points of the suture are farther from the wound edge, followed by reentry and final exit points closer to the wound edge. The risk of tissue necrosis increases when the suture is placed under excessive tension. Care should be taken to remove the suture as soon as reasonable, as paired suture track mark scars may develop as this high-tension suture becomes embedded in the skin.

Running Sutures: Variants of a running suture include the simple running suture, the running locking suture, and the running subcuticular suture.

The simple, continuous running suture can be used to efficiently approximate wound edges of equal thickness under minimal tension. It is most useful when buried sutures were used to close the wound and eliminate dead space and tension. It allows for only 2 knots to be tied, thereby limiting the amount of suture material that rests against the skin and potentially minimizing the development of suture track mark scars. It is also useful in areas of thin skin, such as the eyelids, ears, neck, and scrotum, and to attach full-thickness or split-thickness skin grafts to the recipient wound edges. Fine adjustments along the suture line are more difficult to make with the simple running suture. When used on lax or thin skin, such as eyelid skin, the simple running suture may be more likely to pucker and cut into tissue. Avoidance of unnecessary tension when approximating wound edges and tying the end knots over small bolsters can reduce this risk.

The running locking suture may be useful when approximating wound edges of equal thickness under moderate tension and to aid in hemostasis of well-vascularized wounds such as on the scalp. It is a variant of the simple, continuous running suture in which the needle is passed through the previous loop prior to

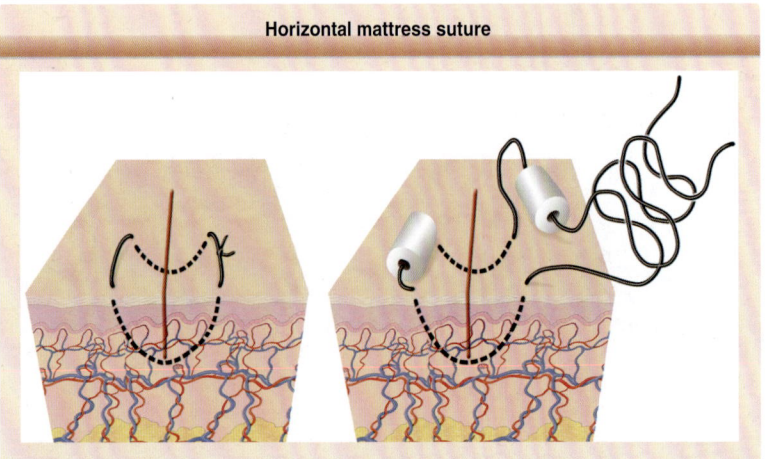

Figure 202-2 Horizontal mattress suture.

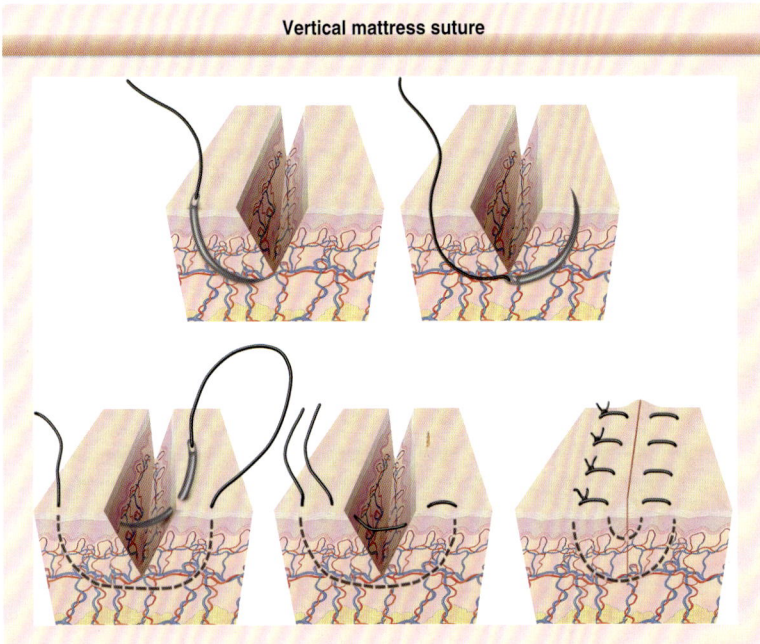

Figure 202-3 Vertical mattress suture.

placing the next loop. It is best used at anatomic sites without a tendency for inversion. While the running locking suture is stronger than the simple running suture, there is an increased risk of wound-edge necrosis if the suture is placed too tightly or if significant postoperative wound swelling develops.

The running subcuticular suture is a buried running suture placed at the level of the superficial dermis that allows for wound edge approximation and decreases risk of suture track scarring in situations in which the suture will be left in place longer than typically recommended. It does not provide significant approximation of the wound edge, and is therefore best reserved for wound edges of relatively equal thickness that have already been closely approximated with deep, buried sutures. Either absorbable or nonabsorbable suture material may be used. Absorbable suture material, which should be monofilament and nonreactive, may be left in place until it is absorbed. Nonabsorbable suture, such as polypropylene, also may be used to minimize tissue reactivity and suture breakage within the wound. Nonabsorbable sutures will require removal at a future date; if left in place indefinitely to reduce scar stretching, a clear suture is best selected (Table 202-6).

STAPLE CLOSURE

Closure of a wound with staples rather than sutures can sometimes be considered, particularly for a long wound or a wound under very high tension. Advantages of staple closure include quick placement, high tensile strength of wound closure, easy removal with a surgical staple remover, minimal tissue reactivity, and potentially lower risk of infection of contaminated wounds compared to closure with sutures. A disadvantage is less precise wound edge approximation. A common site for staple closure of a surgical defect is on the scalp, where suturing may be technically more challenging if minimal hair removal around the surgical site is desired, and the suture line and potential track marks are hidden by the hair on the scalp. When more precise wound edge approximation is desired, closure should be performed with sutures.

HEALING BY SECOND INTENTION

Healing by second intention may be a reasonable, or even preferable, consideration for select surgical defects, based on the size, depth, and location of the defect as well as an individual patient's preferences, comorbidities, and postoperative activities. It is important to counsel the patient regarding the expected duration of the healing process and appearance of a granulating wound during that time. Wounds for which healing by second intention may be considered include relatively small and superficial defects on concave surfaces of the face including the nasal root, the temple, the preauricular region, the fossae and conchal bowl of the ear, the posterior helix, and the postauricular sulcus. It is important to consider the site of a defect and nearby free margins, such as the eyelid, nasal ala, or lip, which may be adversely affected by wound contraction that occurs during healing by second intention. This allows for anticipation and avoidance of potential functional impairment such as ectropion or eclabium. Defects on the scalp and superficial wounds on the trunk and extremities also may be suitable for healing by second intention.

POSTOPERATIVE CONSIDERATIONS

IMMEDIATE POSTOPERATIVE CARE

Upon completion of a surgical procedure, a pressure bandage should be applied to the surgical site and left intact for 24 to 48 hours. An effective pressure dressing minimizes risk of postoperative bleeding and typically consists of petrolatum jelly applied directly to the wound, a nonadherent dressing, and a layer of cotton, all held under tension by surgical tape. Verbal and written instructions regarding home wound care, appropriate activity restrictions, and signs and symptoms of hemorrhage and wound infection should be reviewed with and provided to the patient prior to discharge, along with physician contact information should any questions or concerns arise. Patients treated for cutaneous malignancy should be counseled regarding recommended time frame for followup and skin surveillance.

After removal of the pressure dressing, the wound should be gently cleansed with mild soap and water once to twice daily, followed by reapplication of petrolatum jelly and a nonadherent dressing. An occluded wound reepithelializes and heals more rapidly than a dry wound, and petrolatum serves as an inert, nontoxic, nonirritating, and nonsensitizing occlusive wound dressing.[24] Petrolatum is generally preferred to topical antibiotic ointments, which are associated with a significant risk of allergic contact dermatitis. It has been demonstrated that topical antibiotics are not superior to petrolatum in preventing wound infection. The nonadherent dressing serves to immobilize the wound and reduce the chance of wound dehiscence. Cleansing with a dilute acetic acid (vinegar) solution can be considered for wounds at sites prone to *Pseudomonas* infection, such as the ear. Hydrogen peroxide can be used to debride significantly crusted wounds; however, prolonged use of hydrogen peroxide can result in tissue toxicity and impair wound healing. Alternative wound dressings such as gauze, films, hydrocolloids, hydrogels, and alginates may be considered for wounds with higher than typical levels of drainage.

FOLLOWUP

Recommended timing of nonabsorbable suture removal is based upon anatomic site and relative tension across a surgical defect. Leaving sutures in place for a longer period of time allows for increased wound healing, including reepithelialization, and lowers the risk of wound dehiscence. However, reepithelialization occurring around an epidermal suture may result in the development of permanent suture track marks adjacent to the suture line. Therefore, a balance must be struck between function and cosmesis. Sutures are removed more quickly from wounds in anatomic areas with abundant circulation and minimal tension, such as on the head and neck. Sutures on the face and ears should typically be removed in 5 to 7 days, on the eyelids in 5 to 7 days, on the neck in 7 days, and on the scalp in 7 to 14 days. On anatomic sites such as the trunk and extremities where tension is higher, increasing risk of dehiscence, sutures are typically left in place for 10 to 14 days. For particularly high-tension closures, such as on the lower legs, sutures may be left in place for up to 21 days after the procedure.

COMPLICATIONS

COMPLICATIONS IN THE IMMEDIATE POSTOPERATIVE PERIOD

Infection: Despite meticulous aseptic preparation and procedural technique, wound infection may occasionally occur. The most common culprits in cutaneous surgery include *Streptococcus pyogenes* and *S. aureus*. *Streptococcus* infection typically occurs within 24 to 48 hours of surgery, and presents clinically as tender, expanding erythema around the surgery site. *Staphylococcus* infection often appears as erythema and purulent drainage at 2 to 5 days following surgery. Treatment of wound infection with cephalexin 500 mg by mouth 3 to 4 times daily is often a first-line approach. Doxycycline 100 mg by mouth twice daily may be considered in the setting of penicillin allergy or MRSA infection. Wound culture should be considered for speciation and antibiotic sensitivity studies should a wound infection not respond to typical first-line antibiotic agents.[25]

Less commonly, wound infection by *Mycobacterium* species, including *Mycobacterium fortuitum* and *Mycobacterium chelonae*, may occur following cutaneous surgery. It typically presents weeks after the time of surgery as pyogenic abscess formation with local erythema, induration, and sinus formation. These infections may also display sporotrichoid spread suggestive of local lymphatic dissemination.

Contact Dermatitis: Wound dressing with an ointment such as petrolatum jelly is typically recommended following cutaneous surgery. Alternatively, antibiotic ointments such as neomycin or bacitracin are sometimes used; however, allergic contact dermatitis to the antibiotic component of these ointments is not uncommon (Fig. 202-4).[26] Physical examination will reveal bright-red erythema, edema, or vesiculation in the general distribution of application. Pruritus is

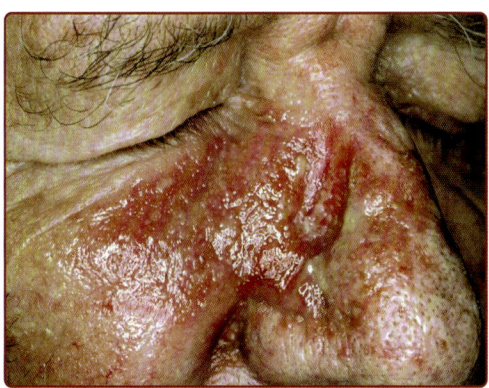

Figure 202-4 Contact dermatitis to antibiotic ointment near skin flap.

more common than pain. Contact dermatitis also may be observed secondary to topical antiseptics, such as iodinates and chlorhexidine, or adhesives in bandage materials, which may be allergic or irritant in etiology.

Pain: Postoperative pain following cutaneous surgery is typically minimal and well-controlled with measures to reduce swelling, such as minimizing physical activity and icing the wound, and acetaminophen as an analgesic. Rarely, more significant pain may be experienced when surgery involves larger areas or a complex repair. In such instances, a short course of analgesics may be considered. Acetaminophen alternating with ibuprofen has shown similar efficacy to acetaminophen with codeine for postoperative pain relief after dermatologic surgical procedures.[27]

Bleeding and Hematoma Formation:

Bleeding in the postoperative period may occur despite best efforts to obtain meticulous hemostasis. Epinephrine used as a component of local anesthesia acts as a vasoconstrictor and provides temporary hemostatic effect during and immediately following the procedure. However, increased bleeding may occur after epinephrine is metabolized. When postoperative bleeding occurs, the patient should be instructed to apply firm, continuous pressure at the site of bleeding in an attempt to obtain hemostasis. For a wound healing by second intention, isolation and hyfrecation of the focus of bleeding may be all that is necessary to obtain hemostasis.

Ongoing bleeding beneath a sutured wound may result in formation of a hematoma (Fig. 202-5A). Management of a hematoma depends on the time of detection. When identified within 24 hours of surgery, management typically consists of removal of the sutures necessary to expose the source of bleeding (Fig. 202-5B), followed by efforts to obtain hemostasis, whether by hyfrecation or ligation of an identifiable vessel, and finally by resuturing of the wound (Fig. 202-5C). Final cosmesis is typically unaltered (Fig. 202-5D). If a patient presents with a hematoma more than 24 hours following surgery, aspiration of the hematoma using a large-bore needle may be attempted to reduce swelling and facilitate wound healing. If the hematoma recurs, suture removal may be required to obtain hemostasis. Narrow excision of the wound edges followed by resuturing will improve outcome.

Necrosis: Tissue necrosis may occur following a dermatologic procedure if there is inadequate blood supply at the procedure site. This most commonly occurs in the setting of a skin graft or flap repair (Fig. 202-6); it is less often observed in the setting of a primary closure, unless extremely tight epidermal approximating sutures are placed.

Intrinsic factors associated with the procedure itself that may impact wound healing and increase the risk of tissue necrosis include excessive wound tension, hematoma formation, and infection. Skin graft necrosis and failure may occur in the setting of excessive skin graft thickness, which may result in inadequate nutrient supply to the tissue, or inadvertent shearing forces or trauma to the graft. Partial or complete flap necrosis may occur due to incorrect flap design resulting in a pedicle of insufficient size to provide the required vascular supply, a flap that is too thin, excessive kinking of a flap, or excessive tension at the flap's leading edge, which may compromise its vascular supply.

Extrinsic factors that may contribute to the development of tissue necrosis in the postoperative period include impaired vascular or cardiac function, history of radiation to the involved skin, poorly-controlled diabetes, and smoking. As previously discussed, smoking tobacco and nicotine use may impair wound healing by causing vasoconstriction and decreasing vascular supply to the wound.

Dehiscence: Wound dehiscence may occur in the setting of primary wound closure under high tension, or if wound healing is complicated by infection or tissue necrosis. If dehiscence occurs within 24 hours of suture placement, resuturing of the wound may be performed without modification of the wound edge. However, if wound dehiscence occurs greater than 48 hours after initial wound closure, excision of approximately 1 mm of normal skin at the wound edge should be performed prior to resuturing the wound. If wound dehiscence occurs in the setting of infection or tissue necrosis, healing by second intention rather than resuturing the wound may be preferable. Leaving epidermal sutures in place for 2 to 3 weeks prior to suture removal may minimize the risk of wound dehiscence at anatomic sites of high wound tension, such as the back, and sites with relatively slow wound healing, such as the lower leg.

COMPLICATIONS IN THE DISTANT POSTOPERATIVE PERIOD

Milia or Keratinous Cysts: Milia cysts sometimes develop within or adjacent to a suture line following cutaneous surgery. They can be removed with needle incision and a comedone extractor. If a cystic lesion is not easily removed or recurs, biopsy should be considered to rule out skin cancer recurrence.

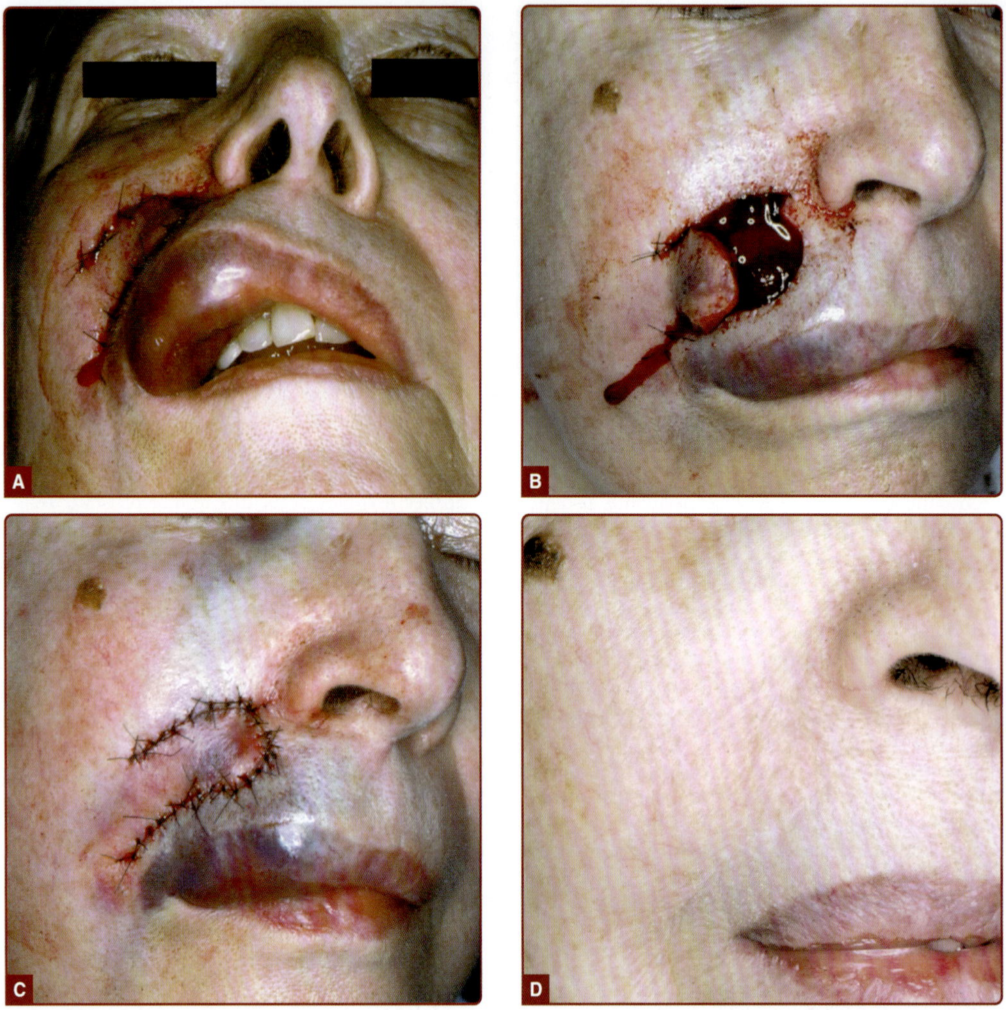

Figure 202-5 **A,** Swelling of right upper lip 2 hours after a skin flap procedure. **B,** Flap unsutured, exposing blood coagulated below. Arteriole bleeder found and tied off. **C,** Flap immediately resutured. **D,** Healed flap 3 months later.

Suture Track Marks: Suture track marks can occur when suture material cuts into tissue because of tension or remains in place long enough to allow reepithelialization (Fig. 202-7A). Wound edge approximation with polypropylene, which possesses plasticity after being stretched and reduces the risk of suture cutting into swollen tissue. The risk of track mark formation can be reduced by using an alternative

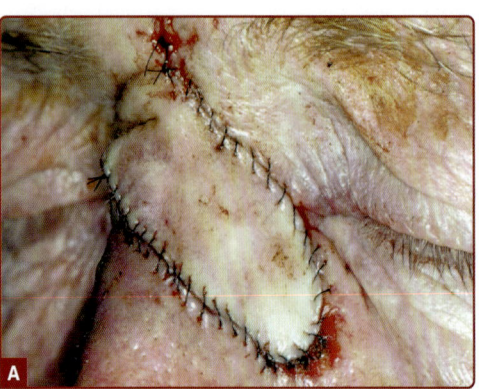
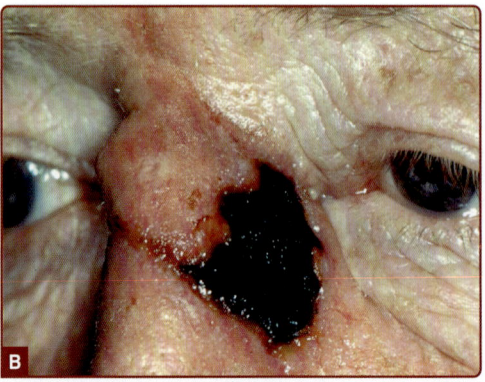

Figure 202-6 **A,** Flap from glabella to left dorsal nose. **B,** Necrosis in flap 1 week postoperatively.

suturing method such as a running suture, which evenly distributes tension along the wound length, or a running intradermal subcuticular suture. Dermabrasion can be used within 1 to 2 months of suture track formation to ameliorate the appearance (Fig. 202-7B and C).

Scar Formation: Scarring is an expected outcome that should be discussed with patients prior to any surgical procedure. Some scars require intervention to improve the cosmetic and functional outcome. These may include hypertrophic and keloid scars, depressed or furrow-like scars, and spread scars.

Hypertrophic scars are characterized by an elevated or thickened scar that is confined within the boundaries of the original defect (Fig. 202-8A). Anatomic sites with higher levels of tension, such as the upper trunk, shoulders, and upper arms, are more likely to develop hypertrophic scars. Keloid scars differ from hypertrophic scars in that they consist of expansile scar development with finger-like projections beyond the original wound boundaries (Fig. 202-9). Keloid scar formation is more common among patients with Fitzpatrick skin phototypes III to VI. Table 202-7 outlines key differences between hypertrophic and keloid scars. Hypertrophic and keloid scars may improve with intralesional triamcinolone acetonide injection, typically at a starting concentration of 10 mg/mL with dose increases up to 40 mg/mL as needed (Fig. 202-8B). Application of silicone gel or gel sheeting may result in reduced scar thickness and improvement in scar erythema; however, the available evidence is limited.[28] Additional treatment modalities with variable efficacy include surgical excision, intralesional 5-flourouracil or interferon-α, cryosurgery, radiotherapy, and laser therapy.[29,30]

Anatomic sites with an abundance of sebaceous glands, such as the nasal tip, are at increased risk of tissue tearing and separation at the wound edge, resulting in the development of a depressed or furrow-like scar. A depressed scar may be excised with undermining of the fresh wound edges and resutured with

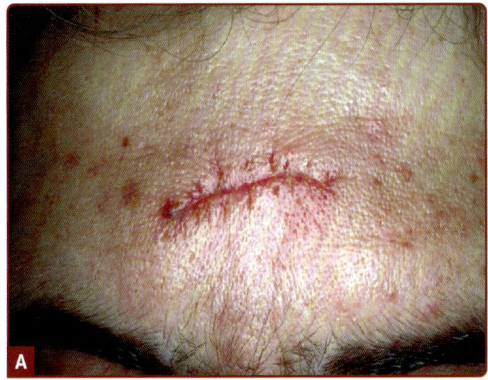
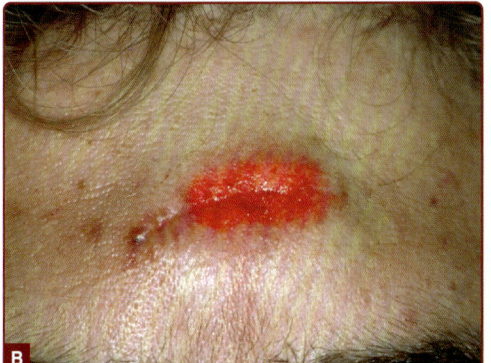
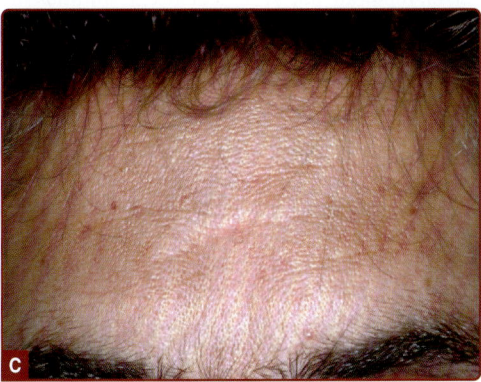

Figure 202-7 **A,** Suture track marks around forehead scar. **B,** Dermabrasion of scar at 5 weeks after being sutured. **C,** Healed scar 2 months later. Suture track marks have disappeared.

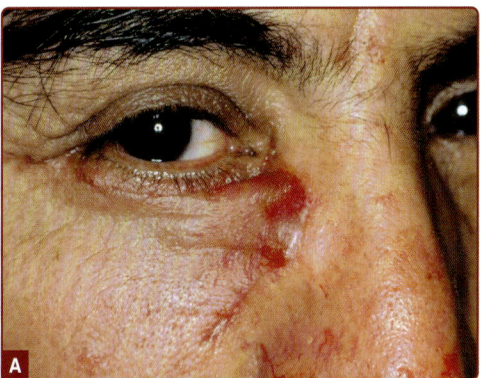
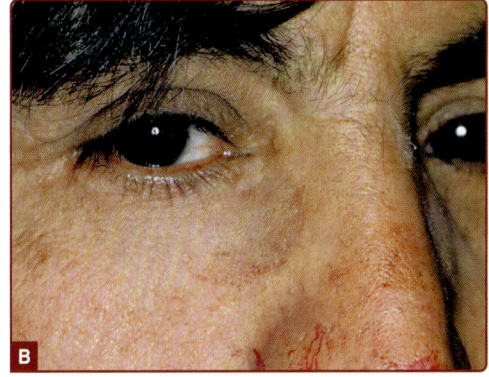

Figure 202-8 **A,** Hypertrophic flap on right nose and cheek. Treated with intralesional triamcinolone acetonide, 10 mg/mL. **B,** Flap 2 months later.

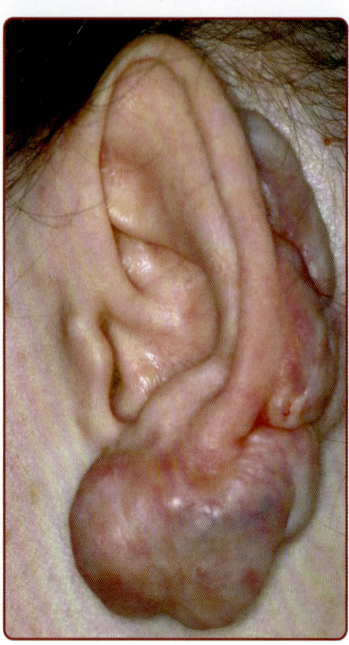

Figure 202-9 Keloid of earlobe and posterior auricular sulcus. Patient underwent an ear pinning procedure.

scalp, upper trunk, shoulders, and upper arms, may predispose to spread scars.

Buried Suture Extrusion ("Spitting Suture"):
Buried, dissolvable sutures are not uncommonly observed to extrude through the sutured wound edge around 3 to 4 weeks following surgery, resulting in localized erythema, swelling, and sometimes sterile pustule formation. The partially-extruded suture material can be clipped at the wound edge, followed by gentle drainage of purulent material that may be present.

Erythema and Telangiectasia:
Wound erythema is expected and generally improves within 3 to 12 months with appropriate photoprotection with broad-spectrum sunscreen or photoprotective barrier. Sun exposure may result in prolonged wound erythema or hyperpigmentation of a scar, particularly in individuals with darker skin types.

Telangiectasia formation adjacent to a sutured wound or associated with a flap or graft commonly occurs, perhaps more so in women secondary to estrogenic effects, and typically improves over time. If erythema or telangiectasia are cosmetically bothersome to the patient, a vascular laser, such as a 585-nm to 595-nm pulsed-dye laser or 532-nm potassium-titanyl-phosphate (KTP) laser, may be used to expedite the resolution of the erythema.

Hypopigmentation:
Hypopigmentation of scars may occur as initial erythema gradually resolves. Hypopigmentation of skin grafts also may be observed. Scar hypopigmentation may be particularly noticeable if contrasted against a background of erythema in the setting of rosacea. If desired, laser treatment of erythema can soften the contrast and improve cosmesis.

Sensory Anesthesia:
Sensory anesthesia at the site of cutaneous surgery is common, particularly following a flap or graft repair. It is typically self limited, often with complete resolution within 3 to 18 months, depending on the size and location of surgery. Notably, if one transects the supraorbital nerve while operating on the forehead, diminished or absent sensation to the central upper eyelid, ipsilateral forehead, and scalp may result. Additionally, if the greater auricular nerve is severed while operating at the Erb point on the lateral neck, potentially permanent anesthesia of the inferior aspect of the ipsilateral ear may result.

Motor Function Loss:
Brief motor loss of facial muscles resulting from temporary anesthesia effects on superficial motor nerves, such as the temporal or marginal mandibular branches of the facial nerve, may be observed at the time of surgery, and should be discussed with the patient prior to performing a surgical procedure in these regions. Permanent motor loss may occur when nerve branches are transected during surgery. Diligent and careful surgical technique should be employed when operating in the region of the temporal or marginal mandibular branches of the facial nerve, as well as the spinal accessory nerve, to avoid this undesirable complication.

buried sutures and placement of vertical or horizontal mattress sutures. Sutures with a 5-0 USP designation or larger diameter should be used to appropriately evert the wound edges and minimize the risk of developing another depressed scar.

Spread, or widened, scars may occur when there is significant tension along a wound edge. Closure of wounds on anatomic sites of high tension, such as the

TABLE 202-7
Comparison of Hypertrophic Scar and Keloid

	HYPERTROPHIC SCAR	KELOID
Incidence	Common	Uncommon
Race	All	Usually Fitzpatrick skin phototypes III to VI
Preceding injury	Yes	Sometimes
Location	Anywhere, especially perpendicular to maximal skin tension lines on the upper trunk, shoulders, and upper arms	Common at earlobes and trunk; rare on the central face
Growth	Within initial wound boundaries	Beyond initial wound boundaries
Improves with time	Typically	Typically not
Recurs with excision	Typically not	Typically

REFERENCES

1. Roenigk RK. Dermatologists perform more skin surgery than any other specialist: implications for health care policy, graduate and continuing medical education. *Dermatol Surg*. 2008;34(3):293-300.
2. Wilson W, Taubert KA, Gewitz M, et al. Prevention of infective endocarditis: guidelines from the American Heart Association: a guideline from the American Heart Association Rheumatic Fever, Endocarditis and Kawasaki Disease Committee, Council on Cardiovascular Disease in the Young, and the Council on Clinical Cardiology, Council on Cardiovascular Surgery and Anesthesia, and the Quality of Care and Outcomes Research Interdisciplinary Working Group. *J Am Dent Assoc*. 2007;138(6):739-745, 747-760.
3. Watters W 3rd, Rethman MP, Hanson NB, et al. Prevention of orthopaedic implant infection in patients undergoing dental procedures. *J Am Acad Orthop Surg*. 2013;21(3):180-189.
4. Safdar N, Bradley EA. The risk of infection after nasal colonization with *Staphylococcus aureus*. *Am J Med*. 2008; 121(4):310-315.
5. Jones JC, Rogers TJ, Brookmeyer P, et al. Mupirocin resistance in patients colonized with methicillin-resistant Staphylococcus aureus in a surgical intensive care unit. *Clin Infect Dis*. 2007;45(5):541-547.
6. Zoumalan RA, Rosenberg DB. Methicillin-resistant *Staphylococcus aureus*–positive surgical site infections in face-lift surgery. *Arch Facial Plast Surg*. 2008; 10(2):116-123.
7. Weyer C, Siegle RJ, Eng GG. Investigation of hyfrecators and their in vitro interference with implantable cardiac devices. *Dermatol Surg*. 2012;38(11):1843-1848.
8. Voutsalath MA, Bichakjian CK, Pelosi F, et al. Electrosurgery and implantable electronic devices: review and implications for office-based procedures. *Dermatol Surg*. 2011;37(7):889-899.
9. Chang TW, Arpey CJ, Baum CL, et al. Complications with new oral anticoagulants dabigatran and rivaroxaban in cutaneous surgery. *Dermatol Surg*. 2015;41(7):784-793.
10. Alam M, Goldberg LH. Serious adverse vascular events associated with perioperative interruption of antiplatelet and anticoagulant therapy. *Dermatol Surg*. 2002;28(11):992-998; discussion 998.
11. Chang LK, Whitaker DC. The impact of herbal medicines on dermatologic surgery. *Dermatol Surg*. 2001; 27(8):759-763.
12. Sbitany H, Xu X, Hansen SL, et al. The effects of immunosuppressive medications on outcomes in microvascular free tissue transfer. *Plast Reconstr Surg*. 2014;133(4):552e-558e.
13. Sorensen LT. Wound healing and infection in surgery: the pathophysiological impact of smoking, smoking cessation, and nicotine replacement therapy: a systematic review. *Ann Surg*. 2012;255(6):1069-1079.
14. Davies CS, Ismail A. Nicotine has deleterious effects on wound healing through increased vasoconstriction. *BMJ*. 2016;353:i2709.
15. Aitken J, Williams FL. A systematic review of thyroid dysfunction in preterm neonates exposed to topical iodine. *Arch Dis Child Fetal Neonatal Ed*. 2014; 99(1):F21-F28.
16. Richards KA, Stasko T. Dermatologic surgery and the pregnant patient. *Dermatol Surg*. 2002;28(3):248-256.
17. Sweeney SM, Maloney ME. Pregnancy and dermatologic surgery. *Dermatol Clin*. 2006;24(2):205-214, vi.
18. Becker DE, Reed KL. Essentials of local anesthetic pharmacology. *Anesth Prog*. 2006;53(3):98-108; quiz 109-110.
19. Martires KJ, Malbasa CL, Bordeaux JS. A randomized controlled crossover trial: lidocaine injected at a 90-degree angle causes less pain than lidocaine injected at a 45-degree angle. *J Am Acad Dermatol*. 2011;65(6):1231-1233.
20. LaBerge L, Pratt M, Fong B, et al. A 10-year review of *p*-phenylenediamine allergy and related para-amino compounds at the Ottawa Patch Test Clinic. *Dermatitis*. 2011;22(6):332-334.
21. Tanner J, Norrie P, Melen K. Preoperative hair removal to reduce surgical site infection. *Cochrane Database Syst Rev*. 2011(11):CD004122.
22. Darouiche RO, Wall MJ Jr, Itani KM, et al. Chlorhexidine-alcohol versus povidone-iodine for surgical-site antisepsis. *N Engl J Med*. 2010;362(1):18-26.
23. Kandel EF, Bennett RG. The effect of stitch type on flap tip blood flow. *J Am Acad Dermatol*. 2001;44(2):265-272.
24. Winter GD, Scales JT. Effect of air drying and dressings on the surface of a wound. *Nature*. 1963;197:91-92.
25. Hutcheson AC, Lang PG. Atypical mycobacterial infections following cutaneous surgery. *Dermatol Surg*. 2007;33(1):109-113.
26. Alavi A, Sibbald RG, Ladizinski B, et al. Wound-related allergic/irritant contact dermatitis. *Adv Skin Wound Care*. 2016;29(6):278-286.
27. Sniezek PJ, Brodland DG, Zitelli JA. A randomized controlled trial comparing acetaminophen, acetaminophen and ibuprofen, and acetaminophen and codeine for postoperative pain relief after Mohs surgery and cutaneous reconstruction. *Dermatol Surg*. 2011;37(7): 1007-1013.
28. O'Brien L, Jones DJ. Silicone gel sheeting for preventing and treating hypertrophic and keloid scars. *Cochrane Database Syst Rev*. 2013(9):CD003826.
29. Gold MH, Berman B, Clementoni MT, et al. Updated international clinical recommendations on scar management: part 1—evaluating the evidence. *Dermatol Surg*. 2014;40(8):817-824.
30. Gold MH, McGuire M, Mustoe TA, et al. Updated international clinical recommendations on scar management: part 2—algorithms for scar prevention and treatment. *Dermatol Surg*. 2014;40(8):825-831.

Chapter 203 :: Excisional Surgery and Repair, Flaps, and Grafts
:: Adele Haimovic, Jessica M. Sheehan, & Thomas E. Rohrer

第二百零三章
肿物切除术和修复、皮瓣和皮片移植

中文导读

任何皮肤外科手术的目的都是以适当的切除病灶，并尽可能少留下明显的疤痕为目的，皮瓣和皮片的应用正是根据这一需求，可以改善大型创口的愈合后美观度。本章共分为8节：①背景；②设备；③切除手术；④皮瓣；⑤皮片；⑥术后护理；⑦并发症；⑧监测与随访。全面讨论了切除手术与修复、皮瓣和皮片移植在皮肤科的应用场景、流程及注意事项。

第一节介绍了手术切除和闭合手术切口时的一些原则。应在最小张力下闭合手术切口，应使得手术疤痕沿着美容单元连接处或皮肤张力线，且不会变形关键的解剖结构和标志。

第二节介绍了获取皮瓣和皮片时需要的设备。基本设备包括仪器机械台、强大的头顶操作灯、电灼、生命体征监护仪、用于处理受污染废物和尖锐仪器的容器等，尤其需要谨慎选择缝合线，这对于伤口愈合和美观效果至关重要。

第三节介绍了三种切除方法的适用范围、具体操作步骤和缝合的注意事项。三种切除手术方法包括：适用于切除小至中等大小的良性或恶性肿瘤，以及活检和疤痕修复术的椭圆形切除法；无法确定松弛的皮肤张力线和最小张力的精确方向的情况下使用的圆锥形切除法；椭圆切口的变式切除法，包括菱形/切线-圆形切除、曲椭圆切口、S成形术、M成形术、部分闭合、连续切除等。

第四节介绍了皮瓣的概念、类型以及皮瓣修复皮肤缺损的具体操作。皮瓣是从供区获取的转移到手术缺损中的全层皮肤和皮下组织，其通过保留与供皮部相连的血管蒂保持血液供应。可根据其血液供应和具体操作对皮瓣进行分类。皮瓣修复缺损涉及的两个操作是：将皮瓣放入缺损处（主要）和对供区的修复（次要）。

第五节介绍了皮片的概念、应用和主要分类。皮片通常用于去除皮肤恶性肿瘤后的皮肤重建，其完全从供区脱离，并从受区的伤口床上吸收营养。皮片的3种基本类型是全厚皮片（FTSG）、中厚皮片（STSG）和复合皮片，也按其供体来源分为自体皮片、同种异体皮片和异种皮片。本节详细介绍了3种基本类型皮片的应用和切取方法。

第六节介绍了皮瓣或皮片移植的术后护理。皮瓣和皮片的术后出血可能会危害组织的存活并增加感染的风险，应当注意保持伤口清洁，定期更换敷料以提高皮片或皮瓣的存活率。

第七节介绍了各种形式的皮肤手术和闭合术的并发症，以及相应的处理方案。早期并发症是出血、疼痛和感染。感染的迹象通常会在手术后的第一周内出现，包括疼痛加剧、红斑和伤口周围发热、化脓和时有引流恶臭以及发烧。疤痕的形成也是在手术预期结果内的，应提前向患者说明。其他并发症有移植失败、皮瓣坏死等。

第八节介绍了术后监测和随访的流程。应在术后3～4个月内对患者进行随访，再次评估手术部位，以确保伤口正常愈合。

〔赵　爽〕

AT-A-GLANCE

- Excisional surgery is one of the most common surgical procedures in dermatology.
- The goal of excisional surgery is to remove the lesion with appropriate margins and obtain the best cosmetic result.
- The planning and execution of dermatologic surgery procedures must balance risk and benefit and consider all options to achieve an optimal outcome. Wounds should be closed under minimal tension, with scars placed along cosmetic unit junctions or skin tension lines, contained within as few single cosmetic units as possible, without distorting critical anatomic structures and landmarks.
- The closure must preserve sensory and motor nerve function.
- An elliptical or fusiform excision is the fundamental procedure in dermatologic surgery and typically allows for a linear, side-to-side closure.
- Flap or graft repair may be considered when linear closure is not feasible.
- Flaps are commonly classified according to their primary movement as advancement, rotation, transposition, or interpolation.
- The 3 basic types of skin grafts are full-thickness, split-thickness, and composite.

BACKGROUND

The goal of any excisional surgery is to remove the lesion with appropriate margins and leave the least noticeable scar possible. To consistently attain aesthetically pleasing results, time must be taken long before the first incision to appropriately plan the procedure. Although excisional surgery is as much an art form as it is a science, there are many principles to keep in mind when planning the surgical excision and closure. Wounds should be closed under minimal tension, with scars placed along cosmetic unit junctions or skin tension lines, without distorting critical anatomic structures and landmarks (eyelid, eyebrow, nose, lip, hairline, etc). Biologically, the closure must be such that the mobilized skin and associated adnexal structures are viable, and there is maximal preservation of sensory and motor nerve function.

Knowledge of underlying anatomy is critical in both the design and execution of the excision (Chap. 201).

The planning and execution of dermatologic surgery procedures varies from case to case. A skilled surgeon evaluates the risks and benefits of various options in each patient and anticipates potential complications. The main risks of excisional surgery include pain and discomfort, bleeding, bruising, hematoma formation, nerve damage, wound infection, wound dehiscence, and undesirable scar or contracture. Key elements of dermatologic surgery procedures include proper patient selection and preparation; comprehension of risks and necessary precautions; obtaining effective local anesthesia; use of sterile or clean technique; informed procedure design and meticulous technique in performing the incision and repair; diligent postoperative wound care and patient education (Chap. 202).

EQUIPMENT

Prior to surgery, it is essential to have all the necessary instruments and equipment available and set up in an organized, accessible, and safe manner.

PROCEDURE ROOM

- Basic: mechanical table, powerful overhead procedure lights, electrocautery, vital signs monitor, Mayo stand (1 or 2), receptacle for contaminated waste, and a sharps container.
- Optional: depending on the location and scope of the procedure, suction may be needed.

SURGICAL TRAY

The specific instruments selected depend on the scope of the procedure and personal preference of the surgeon. It is helpful to set up the basic elements on the tray in the same layout each time. Consistency in place-

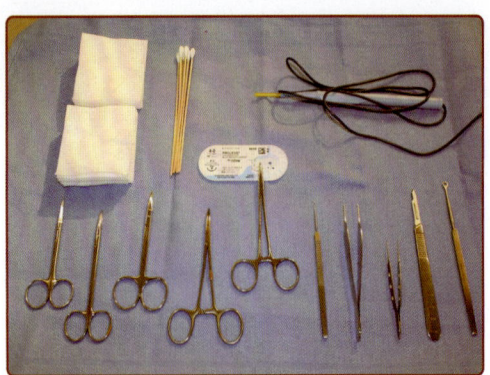

Figure 203-1 Surgical tray: a surgical tray should be equipped with high-quality delicate instruments. This tray has a scalpel, small skin hook, Bishop Harmon forceps, larger Adson forceps, 5-mm curette, curved iris scissors, blunt curved Metzenbaum scissors, delicate needle holder, suture scissors, gauze, and cotton-tipped applicators.

ment of sharps prevents inadvertent injury with contaminated instruments to the surgeon or the assistant.

A basic excisional surgery tray (Fig. 203-1) contains:

- Instruments: curette, No. 3 or No. 7 Bard-Parker scalpel handle with a No. 15 or No. 10 blade or Beaver blade, small forceps (eg, Bishop-Harmon) and/or smooth-toothed Adson forceps, delicate standard skin hook or double-prong skin hook, curved iris scissors, blunt-tipped undermining scissors, hemostat, towel clamps, needle holder, suture scissors. For larger procedures, such as flaps, additional hemostats or hooks may be needed. Special procedures will need other instruments added to this tray (eg, split-thickness skin grafts require a dermatome).
- Disposable material: marking pen, gauze sponges, cotton tip applicator sticks, scratch pad for electrocautery tip, electrocautery hand piece and tip, surgical drapes, foam or magnetic pad for discarded needles
- Suture: Proper suture selection is critical for optimal wound healing and aesthetic result (Chap. 202).

EXCISIONAL SURGERY

ELLIPTICAL EXCISION

Excisional surgery is one of the most frequently performed dermatologic surgery procedures. The elliptical or fusiform excision allows for a linear, side-to-side closure. The commonly referred to elliptical excision is actually fusiform in shape as the edges are pointed and not rounded as in a true ellipse.[1] Mastery of elliptical excision and closure is fundamental to more advanced procedures, including variations on the ellipse itself and planning and executing more complex flaps. An elliptical excision is indicated for the removal of small- to moderate-sized benign or malignant neoplasms as well as for excisional biopsy and scar revision.

PLANNING THE ELLIPSE

In planning the excision, the lesion to be excised must first be identified and confirmed by the patient. Using an appropriate marker, a circle is drawn around the lesion with the appropriate margins. The size of the surgical margin is dependent on the nature of the lesion.[2]

Once the margins of the lesion have been marked, the ellipse is planned. When planning a fusiform excision with linear closure, one must consider several factors, including the impact of the procedure on form and function. In addition to ensuring that an adequate reservoir of surrounding tissue or skin laxity is present, the surgeon must take great care to preserve free margins, minimize tension, and maintain skin contour.[3]

FREE MARGINS

Free margins, such as the eyelid margin, alar rim, and lip vermillion are of primary concern as they provide minimal to no opposition to the tension created from nearby tissue movement. Any distortion of a free margin will be aesthetically unacceptable and may even impact function. To prevent distortion, closures should be planned such that tension vectors are perpendicular to free margins.

RELAXED SKIN TENSION LINES

For optimal cosmetic results and maximum scar strength, the long axis of the fusiform excision should be oriented along relaxed skin tension lines.[4] Relaxed skin tension lines are generally perpendicular to the direction of the pull of the underlying muscle (Fig. 203-2). These lines should be identified while the patient is sitting upright, and may be highlighted by asking the patient to make certain facial expressions. If the relaxed skin tension lines are not obvious, the direction of laxity may be identified by manipulating tissue manually. Relaxed skin tension lines rarely follow published diagrams, and closures should mimic the subtle arcs in the facial lines of expression.

COSMETIC UNITS

When possible, excisions should be restricted to one of the major cosmetic units. Within each cosmetic unit the skin shares a common color, thickness, texture, sebaceous quality and hair density. The major cosmetic units of the face include the forehead, periorbital area, nose, lips and perioral area, chin, and cheeks and can be further divided into smaller subunits (Fig. 203-3). Placing the incision line at the junction of the cosmetic units, or contour lines, also minimizes the appearance of the resultant scar as it will be hidden in a natural transition zone where the eye expects to see a change.[5]

When the elliptical excision and closure cannot include these conditions consideration must be given to other forms of repair such as flaps, grafts, partial purse sting closures, or healing by second intention.

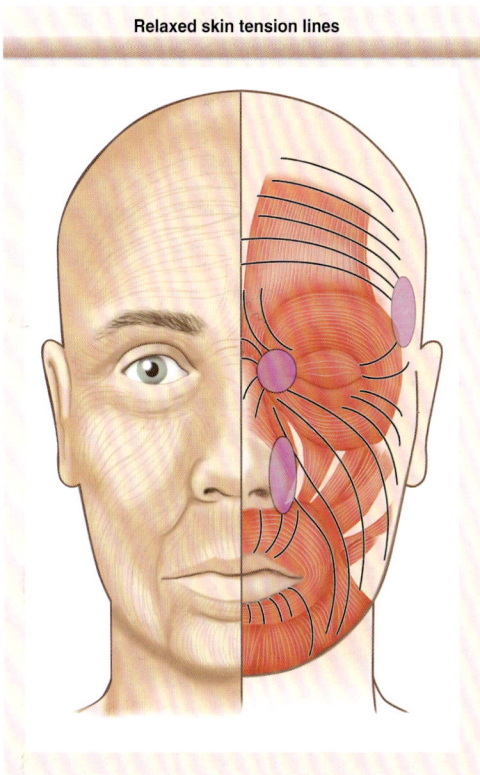

Figure 203-2 Relaxed skin tension lines. Relaxed skin tension lines generally form perpendicular to underlying muscles of facial expression. Closure lines heal better and with a thinner, less noticeable scar when placed in relaxed skin tension lines.

The simple ellipse is based on an optimal length-to-width ratio of 3.5:1 to minimize the formation of redundant tissue at the apices, otherwise known as "dog-ears" or "standing tri-cones." The ratio may be increased to 4:1 or greater in locations with less tissue distensibility and in convex surfaces. Likewise, it may be decreased to 3:1 or less in concave surfaces or in areas where the tissue is more lax and a lower tendency to produce cones.[3] The apical angle between the 2 arciform incisions ranges from 37° to 74°, depending on the length-to-width ratio.[6] As the ratio becomes larger, the apical angle decreases; thus, for a ratio of 5:1, which may be needed for scalp surgery, the apical angle approaches 30° (Fig. 203-4). Standing cones will form if the sides of the closure are of unequal length, with redundant tissue developing on the longer side.

It is important to note that as a wound is closed in a linear fashion, the length of the resultant scar will be longer than the distance between the 2 distal points drawn out in the preoperative design of the ellipse. The arc of the 2 sides of the closure that are brought together is necessarily longer than a straight line drawn between the distal points of the ellipse. Mathematically, with the angles used in excisional surgery, the arcs are roughly 20% longer than the straight line drawn down the middle of the ellipse. In most cases this becomes irrelevant as there is contraction along the long axis of a scar and the tissue around the closure distends and absorbs this small difference without any noticeable distortion. In areas such as the upper lip, however, this small difference may be enough to distort the lip margin inferiorly and be disfiguring. Lengthening the elliptical closure to bring it around the lip past the wet mucosal margin will often help hide this potential distortion.

TECHNIQUE

After the ellipse is planned and drawn, the field is anesthetized, prepped, draped, and the first incision is made using a scalpel (Fig. 203-5). In most instances, a No. 15 blade is used to score the epidermis or to cut

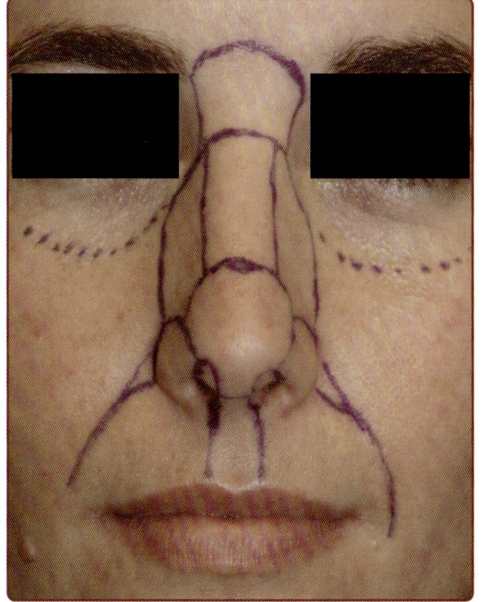

Figure 203-3 Cosmetic units. The face can be divided into many cosmetic units. The cosmetic units are differentiated from each other by alterations in skin texture, color, or contour. Incisions hide very well when placed in cosmetic unit junctions.

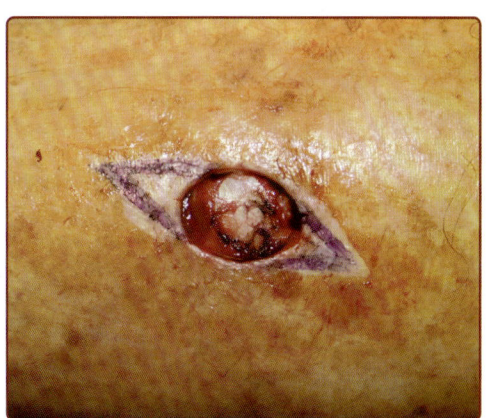

Figure 203-4 Acute apical angle. Certain areas such as the convex surface of an extremity or the nasal dorsum require a length-to-width ratio greater than 3:1.

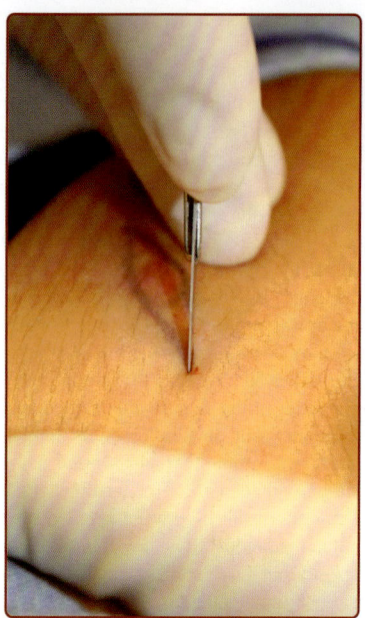

Figure 203-5 Incision. Incisions should be made 90° (perpendicular) to the skin surface and continued down through the dermis into the subcutaneous tissue.

through to the fat on the first pass; however, thick back skin may require the use of a No. 10 blade. The surgery begins with the point of the blade at the apex distal from the surgeon's position. As the incision progresses toward the arc of the ellipse, the belly of the blade is held perpendicular to the skin surface, preventing a beveled incision. As the opposite apex of the incision is approached, the blade rocks back up onto its tip, which allows the surgeon to clearly see the apex of the incision under the advancing hand. This prevents extending the incision beyond the planned apex. To prevent bunching of the tissue ahead of the pressure exerted by the blade, traction on the surrounding skin is held with the nondominant hand; in addition, an assistant may aid with traction. The depth of the excision is, again, dependent on the nature of the neoplasm being excised. When a side-to-side closure is planned, the depth of the incision must be full thickness into the superficial subcutaneous fat. The proximal apex of the ellipse is grasped gently with a toothed forceps or skin hooks to elevate the tissue. The base of the specimen is dissected in an even plane with a scalpel or scissors. The depth at the apices should be the same as the depth at the center; there is a tendency to remove the specimen with the depth at the apices more superficially. When the depth of the excision is not uniform, a more noticeable standing cone of tissue may surround the tips as the wound is closed.

CLOSURE

Undermining is performed to increase mobility of the surrounding tissue, aid in wound eversion, decrease tension on the wound edges, and diffuse scar contraction.[7] The subcutaneous tissue is undermined at the same level around all edges of the wound, including the apices, utilizing iris or blunt-tipped scissors. The tissue may be snipped or bluntly dissected by inserting the tip of the scissors and spreading. Electrosurgery is a common undermining technique performed in other surgical subspecialties. The plane of undermining will vary depending on body site but should be uniform in depth at all edges (Chap. 201). Knowledge of anatomy is extremely important and careful attention must be given to surrounding vital structures.

Although undermining is critical for dermatologic surgery, there are risks associated with extensive undermining. Such risks include but are not limited to inadvertent damage to structures such as nerves and vessels, vascular compromise for flaps, and the creation of large dead spaces with an increased chance for hematoma or seroma development.[8] Patients receiving anticoagulants or with reduced platelet number or function may benefit by limiting the extent of undermining as the risk of bleeding and hematoma formation is decreased.

Electrocoagulation or electrocautery is employed to attain meticulous hemostasis of the bed of the wound. A skin hook is used to gently elevate the wound edges to expose vessels injured during the excision or undermining. Blood that accumulates in the wound must be cleared with gauze or cotton swabs to allow for visualization of pinpoint bleeding and to allow for a relatively dry field. The cautery tip may be applied directly to the vessel until bleeding ceases. Alternatively, indirect coagulation is achieved using small forceps to grasp the vessel and applying the cautery tip to the forceps. Indirect cautery limits the residual thermal damage surrounding the cauterization and may speed wound healing and reduce the risk of infection. No matter which method is used, care should be taken to stop all significant bleeding while minimizing cautery char. Larger, more high-pressured arteries can require ligation with absorbable suture.

Suturing technique (Chap. 202) reduces and redistributes wound tension, everts the skin edge, eliminates dead space, and maintains or restores natural anatomic contours, while minimizing the formation of permanent suture marks on the skin surface. Most wounds are closed in 2 layers: (1) absorbable deep sutures and (2) nonabsorbable superficial sutures. Deeper wounds or those with significant dead space may benefit from a third, deep layer in the subcutaneous fat or fascia.

Ideally, the wound is closed by first placing the deep sutures using the rule of halves to minimize the formation of dog-ears (Fig. 203-6). The first suture is placed in the center of the wound. Each half of the remaining defect is closed in a similar manner, which is repeated until a suitable numbers of sutures have been placed. A wound gains only 7% of its final strength after 2 weeks.[9] As most skin sutures are removed within 1 to 2 weeks of placement, absorbable buried sutures are an important part of a layered wound closure.[10] Buried sutures typically dissolve over the course of months and provide support for the wound until

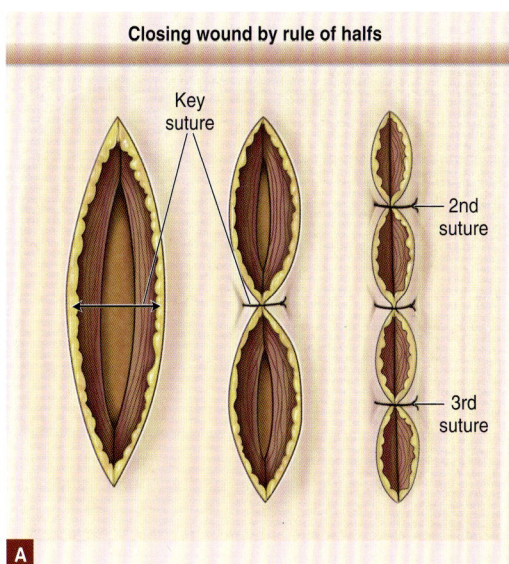
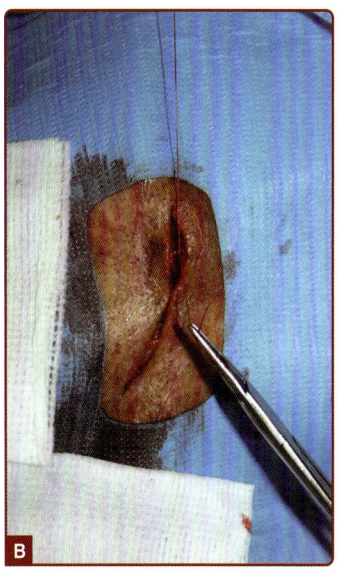

Figure 203-6 **A** and **B**, Closing wound by rule of halves. Sutures are placed at the midpoint of any open area of the defect.

epidermal tensile strength has increased sufficiently to prevent wound dehiscence.

Buried vertical-mattress sutures mechanically aid significantly in wound eversion and in doing so reduce or eliminate tension on the wound edge and produce thinner less noticeable scars (Fig. 203-7). This type of buried suture should be used in nearly all closures.

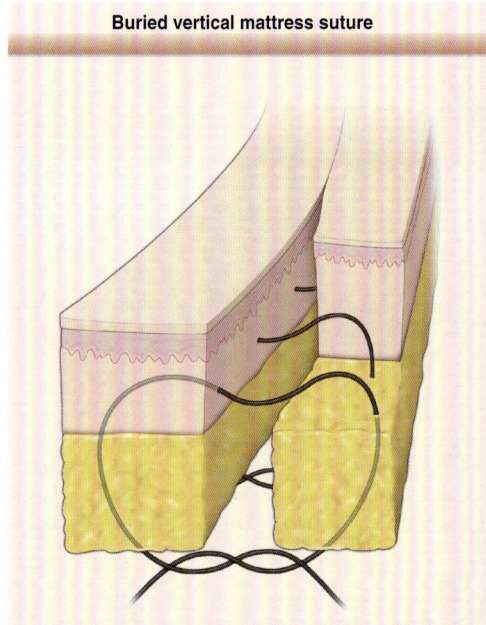

Figure 203-7 Buried vertical mattress suture. The buried vertical mattress suture gives excellent eversion to the wound edge and should be used for most if not all subcutaneous sutures.

Subcutaneous sutures help minimize or eliminate dead space and align deep structures such as skeletal muscle or fascia. They also can be used to anchor overlying tissue to underlying fixed structures, such as periosteum, to prevent distortion of free margins or maintain proper facial contour and function. This is exemplified by anchoring a melolabial flap to the maxillary periosteum. When tying a buried suture, it is important not only to keep both free ends of the suture on the same side of the loop created, but also to tie the suture in such a manner that draws the knot down on the same side so it will tuck up under the loop and not get hung up on it (Fig. 203-8). Buried sutures should align the wound edges such that they are perfectly approximated with good wound eversion before the placement of epidermal sutures.

Epidermal sutures are placed to approximate the margins of the skin edge. They should be evenly spaced and placed at roughly the same distance from the wound edge as the combined dermal–epidermal depth. Therefore, sutures placed on the eyelid will be much closer together than those placed on the thick skin of the back. Most practitioners use a running nonabsorbable minimally reactive monofilament suture, such as polypropylene or nylon, that requires subsequent removal.[11] Alternatives include running absorbable fast-acting gut,[12] absorbable or nonabsorbable running subcuticular sutures,[13] simple interrupted nonabsorbable sutures, and polymethylmethacrylate tissue glue. Simple interrupted sutures are more time-consuming to place and remove than a running suture. In settings where wound healing may be impaired due to the patient's advanced age or underlying disease, interrupted sutures may be preferred, as interrupted sutures may have, with all other factors being equal, greater tensile strength and less potential to pull through thin skin or impair microcirculation.[14]

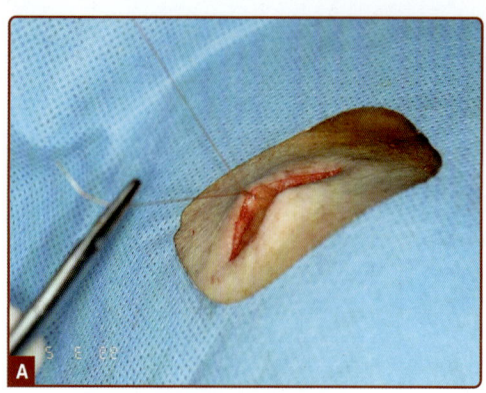 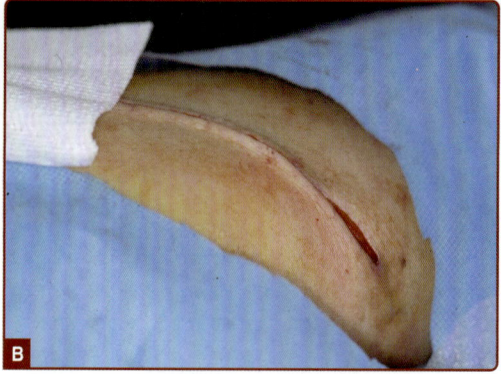

Figure 203-8 **A** and **B,** Tying deep sutures. When tying the knot, it is important to keep the 2 free ends on the same side of loop. The needle driver should be placed between the 2 free ends in the center of the wound. The loose end with the needle is then wrapped around the head of the needle driver and a knot is formed. Keeping the free ends on the same side of the loop will allow the knot to slip under the loop and draw the wound edges together. The wound should be together with skin edges nicely opposed and everted.

SUTURE REMOVAL

The risk of crosshatch marks across the suture line can be minimized by removing the sutures within a week of placement, before the formation of epithelial suture tracks. On the face and ears, most skin sutures are removed within 5 to 7 days. Neck sutures should be removed in 7 days and scalp sutures in 7 to 10 days. On the trunk and extremities, risk of wound dehiscence mandates that epidermal sutures may be left in place longer, typically 10 to 14 days, to provide additional support. In repairs under high tension or when dehiscence is likely, sutures may be left in place for 3 to 4 additional days. However, if sufficient buried sutures have been placed and the wound is well approximated at 7 to 10 days, epidermal sutures may be removed. The use of a running subcuticular suture for well-approximated wounds will prevent the formation of suture tracks and should be used in most cases that require sutures be left in for more than 7 days.

REVISION OF STANDING CONES OF TISSUE

Under certain circumstances, a circular excision may be performed when the orientation of the ellipse is difficult to anticipate. This may occur when the precise direction of relaxed skin tension lines and least tension is difficult to determine, when the length of the ellipse for an optimal outcome is unclear, or when alternative repairs may be considered, such as a local flap. Nonelliptical defects require revision of the cones or dog-ears. First, the wound is closed with a few centrally placed sutures; bilateral standing cones of excess tissue form on either side of the central closure. In addition, tissue redundancies may persist at one or both ends of a planned fusiform excision if the apical angle is too wide, if the sides are of unequal lengths, or on convex surfaces and the techniques for addressing these redundancies are similar under both clinical circumstances. Skillful repair of the redundant standing cones extend the incision line by removing an additional triangle of tissue at the tip (Fig. 203-9). The apex of the standing cone is lifted with forceps or a skin hook and manipulated to determine where to place the incision that releases the redundant tissue. The incision is made with a scalpel and the dog-ear is undermined. The free end of the cone is pulled over the incision and the remaining incision is made such that the resultant wound edges lie flat. The freed cone is termed a *Burow's triangle*. This technique results in a linear extension of the scar. Variations on the revision of tissue cones include a curved extension, an angled extension, and an M-plasty.

VARIATIONS OF THE ELLIPSE

RHOMBIC/TANGENT-TO-CIRCLE EXCISION

In a traditional fusiform excision, the lines connecting the 2 ends are curved. However, in a rhombic or tangent-to-circle excision, straight lines radiating in opposite directions connect the tips. This leads to the formation of 2 triangles that enclose the defect and form a rhombic shape. The advantages are simpler design, easier excision for the surgeon, and removal of less healthy tissue. The main disadvantage is notching or a gap can develop in the center of the defect where the 2 triangles peak.[1]

CURVED ELLIPSE

The classic fusiform excision creates a linear scar. At times, it is aesthetically preferable to create a curvilinear scar. The curvilinear repair is useful on the cheek and around the chin. The curved ellipse is created by

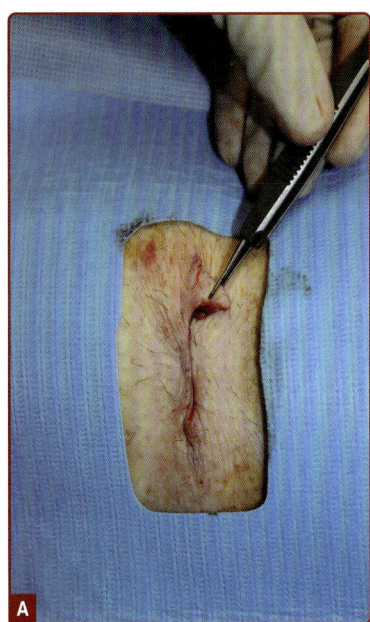 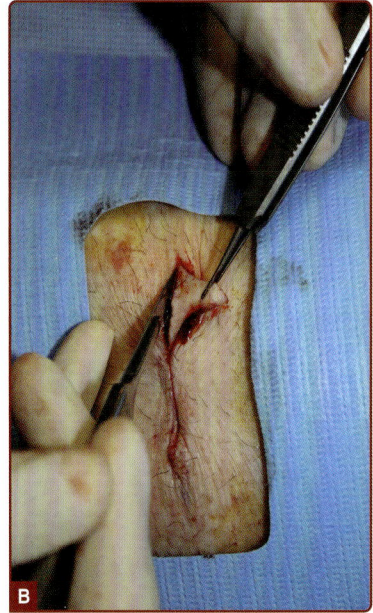

Figure 203-9 **A** and **B**, Standing cones. Redundant tissue may be removed by incising one side, draping the excess skin over the wound, and excising the resultant triangle.

intentionally designing it with one side longer than the other. The wound is closed by the rule of halves.

S-PLASTY

An S-shaped repair is useful on convex surfaces such as the extremities where a linear repair may result in persistent standing cones or indentations. The tension vectors of a standard elliptical incision are perpendicular to the long axis of the ellipse. Because wounds contract along their long axis, designing the closure with an S-plasty displaces the tension over a greater length and a variety of angles (Fig. 203-10) and does not create a contracting in one direction with resulting indentation over a convex surface such as an extremity.

M-PLASTY

An M-plasty allows the length of a scar to be shortened. Rather than extending the end of an ellipse or removing a Burow's triangle, the redundant tissue may be excised inward, forming a M-shaped scar. The long axis of the incision is reduced by the length equivalent to the inverted triangle that makes the center of the M. This technique is useful for confining a scar to a single cosmetic unit or when an incision approaches a free margin. The scar may be camouflaged in locations where rhytides bifurcate, such as the crow's feet in the periorbital area or around the lips. It is important to advance the inverted triangle up into the rest of the ellipse to take full advantage of the scar-shortening effect. A half-buried horizontal mattress suture, also known as a tip stitch, may help prevent necrosis of the central tip.

PARTIAL CLOSURE

Partial closure is used when more extensive repairs are limited by lack of local tissue reservoirs or the patient's health or coagulation status. The wound is closed from the ends toward the center. When wound tension prevents further closure, the area remains open to heal by second intention. The final scar is usually linear and may resemble a spread scar in the middle. Alternatively, a purse-sting suture is placed around the wound and the tissue is drawn together circumferentially. The purse-string suture is closed just to the point of minimal tissue buckling. Additional guiding sutures may then be placed across the partially closed wound to attain better alignment and even further closure.

SERIAL EXCISION

In some cases, the length of an ellipse required to excise a lesion with a 3 or 4:1 ratio is too long for an acceptable cosmetic or functional outcome. In such instances, the lesion may be removed with a series of staged excisions. A partial excision is performed, ideally an ellipse that accommodates the full length of the lesion, with primary linear closure. During the following months, the surrounding tissue stretches and the tension in the area decreases. Additional excisions are performed in a similar manner, removing the remaining lesion as well as the scar or scars created from the first steps of the procedure. This is typically used to minimize the length of the final scar in large circumference neoplasms that are benign or low risk.

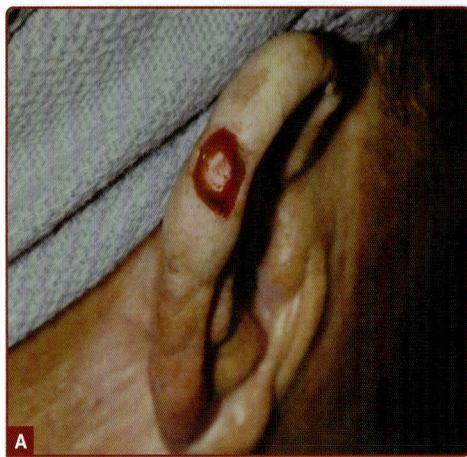
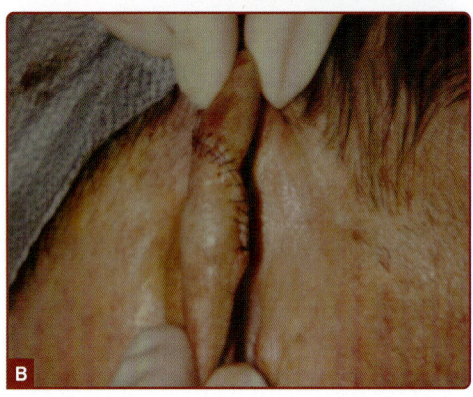
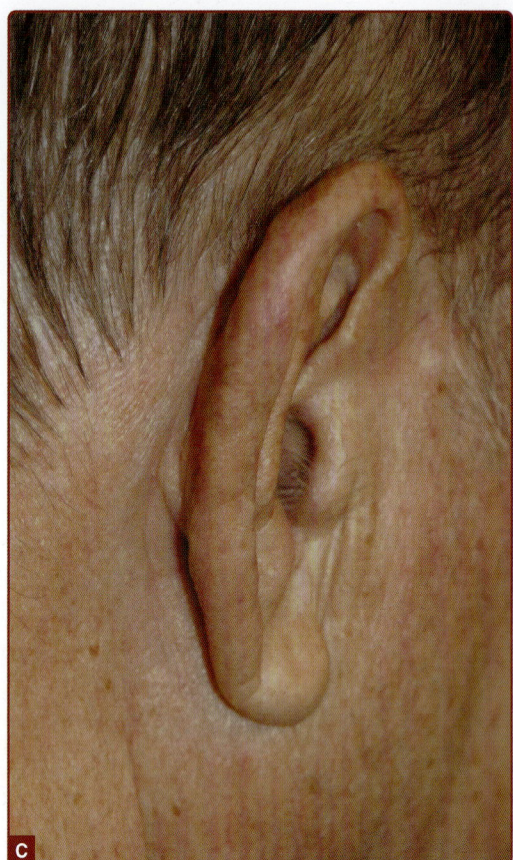

Figure 203-10 A-C, S-plasty closures are often used to give a wound a curvilinear line and to alter the tension vectors so they do not all pull along the long axis of the wound and cause noticeable contraction. The S-plasty is especially useful on convex surfaces where wound contraction may cause the scar to sink down and appear depressed.

EXCISION WITHOUT CLOSURE

There are certain locations and situations where allowing a wound to heal by secondary intention is the preferred method of closure. Wounds in patients who are poor surgical risks for reconstructive surgery, where there is relatively minimal tissue mobility (scalp, distal lower extremities), where there is a high risk of infection, or when the patient requests minimal down-time healing by secondary intention may be indicated.

Wounds located in concave areas such as the medial canthus, ear concha, alar crease (if small), temple region, and postauricular sulcus lend themselves well to healing by secondary intention.[15] Second intention wounds heal by both contraction and reepithelialization. First, a wound contracts to its maximum capacity, and then the remainder of the wound is filled in with scar tissue.[16] Contraction contributes to approximately 50% to 70% of the final wound closure and scar tissue fills out the remaining wound.[16] In general, increased wound contraction and decreased scar tissue will have a better cosmetic outcome; however, scar location, specifically contour of the lesion location, is the most important factor for cosmetic result.[15,16] Superficial wounds heal very well. Therefore, a very superficial wound, even on a convex surface such as the forehead or the nose, can potentially heal well. Because all wounds contract to some degree, it is important that there be no free margin along one side of the wound that can be elevated during wound contracture and cause distortion at the site. This may be encountered along the eyelid margins, ear margins, eyebrow, nasal ala, and lip vermillion border. These areas are almost always better managed with appropriate reconstructive surgery.

When a lesion is excised with the intention of allowing the wound to heal by secondary intention, appropriate margins should be included and the resulting defect will typically be circular in nature. The incision through the skin is beveled inward to provide exposure of the base of the wound. The depth need not reach the subcutaneous fat if the lesion can be removed satisfactorily by transecting the dermis.

Wounds that are allowed to granulate are more resistant to infection and do not form hematomas. In addition, the size of the final scar is kept to a minimum by negating the need to remove standing cones. These wounds, however, require more time to heal than those that are closed primarily and exhibit increased contracture. In some cases, there is an unpredictable cosmetic result. Employing a purse-string suture, a running suture that is placed circumferentially around a wound and then pulled taut, can significantly decrease the circumference of a wound and abbreviate the healing time considerably.[17]

FLAPS

When simple primary closure cannot be done because a wound is too large, there is excessive tension, or an unacceptable functional or cosmetic result would ensue from a linear scar, a tissue-movement procedure, such as a flap or a graft, should be considered. A local skin flap is a portion of full-thickness skin and subcutaneous tissue transferred from an adjacent donor site into the surgical defect. The flap maintains its blood supply via a vascular pedicle that remains connected to the donor site.

Flaps may be categorized based on their blood supply. Axial pattern flaps depend on a named artery for their blood supply. In contrast, random pattern flaps, the most widely used in dermatologic surgery, are supported by the small arterioles and capillaries of the subdermal vascular plexus found in the mid-to-superficial fat. Therefore, undermining and flap mobilization must be done at or below this level to ensure adequate blood supply. If undermining occurs too superficially, the intradermal vasculature alone will often not be able to support a flap. In certain areas other than the face, the perfusion pressure of even the subdermal vascular plexus is often not sufficient to support a random pattern flap. Fortunately, the blood supply of the face is rich, estimated to be 10 times greater than necessary to support the skin's basic metabolic needs so it can support a wide variety of random pattern flaps.

The vascular perfusion pressure, that is, the force of blood flow through a vessel, is greatest at the proximal end of a vessel and decreases steadily as it travels more distal into the flap. To ensure flap survival, the perfusion pressure must be great enough to keep the distal capillaries of the flap open. If the pressure falls below a critical level, the capillaries close and insufficient blood is supplied to the distal end of the flap.

For years, it was believed that the viable length of a flap was directly proportional to the width of the pedicle. In 1970, Milton discovered that axial flaps in a pig model under the same conditions of blood supply survive only to a finite length regardless of width.[18] Daniel and Williams, as well as Stell, confirmed Milton's findings and concluded that there was an upper limit of flap length that cannot be increased by increasing the pedicle width.[19,20] The maximal flap length is determined by vascular supply, not simply pedicle width. The greater the perfusion pressure in the flap pedicle, the longer the flap can be without undergoing necrosis. In addition, the greater the perfusion pressure in the pedicle, the narrower the pedicle may be. Axial pattern flaps have the highest perfusion pressure at the base and therefore can support very narrow long flaps (generally greater than a 4:1 length-to-width ratio). Musculocutaneous flaps have the next greatest vascular perfusion pressure, followed by fasciocutaneous flaps, and finally random pattern flaps. Stell discovered that the greatest length of a viable axial flap was 60% greater than that of a random pattern flap. In general, random pattern flaps on the face should have a maximal length-to-width ratio of 3:1.[21] This is however only a rough guideline, and individual patient characteristics such as tobacco use, sebaceous nature of skin, prior radiation or surgical procedures, and precise location all affect vascular perfusion. To help ensure flap survival, the pedicle length-to-width ratios should not exceed 2:1 on the trunk and extremities.

The 2 movements involved in repairing a defect with a flap are the primary movement, which is the action of placing the flap into the defect and the secondary movement of tissue in the donor area, which closes the secondary defect and facilitates primary flap movement. Both movements are important in terms of distributing tension in the proper direction and over a larger area so as to minimize tension on the flap itself, which might compromise its survival.[22] Flaps are commonly classified according to their primary movement—advancement flaps, rotation flaps, transposition flaps, and interpolation flaps. This classification underplays the reality that many flaps have more than one primary movement, eg, a rotation flap usually has a component of advancement to fill the distal portion of a wound. Therefore, another way to classify flaps is by whether the primary movement is sliding, which displaces tissue redundancy at a site distant from the defect (advancement and rotation) or lifting, where a flap is moved over intact skin, reorienting wound tension (transposition and interpolation).

Flaps should only be placed over defects that are neoplasm free as it is difficult to detect tumor growth under a healthy flap and the neoplasm can continue to grow for an extended period of time before detection.

As with elliptical excisions, the flap should be planned paying attention to the concepts discussed above, such as free margins, skin laxity, relaxed skin tension lines, cosmetic units, and attention to function. The flap and possible resultant Burow's triangles should be drawn out with a marking pen while the patient is in an upright position. It is advisable to plan the flap prior to administering anesthesia, as the injected volume may distort the tissue and alter its movement.

Flap incisions should be made perpendicular to the skin, and the recipient wound edges should similarly be squared off. The thickness of the flap should be uniform and should approximate the thickness of the wound edge. The area around the flap should be widely undermined.

ADVANCEMENT FLAPS

The primary movement of an advancement flap is the one-dimensional sliding of tissue directly into a defect. In essence, incisions are made tangentially to the defect to free up neighboring tissue. With the wound edge acting as the free margin of the flap, the tissue is advanced into place, the key suture is placed at the advancing edge, and the tissue cones become apparent. Although some adjacent tissue laxity may be tapped into with an advancement flap, the tension vectors of the closure remain the same and therefore the primary advantage of an advancement flap is the displacement of closure lines into more cosmetically acceptable locations. All advancement flaps are random-pattern flaps; they do not rely on a specific named vessel, but rather adequate tissue laxity, for survival.[23]

SINGLE ADVANCEMENT

The simplest example of a pure advancement flap is the *U-plasty*, whereby double, parallel incisions are made tangential to what is most often a round defect. The flap is undermined, advanced into the defect, and secured with sutures, creating a U-shaped scar (Fig 203-11). Redundant tissue cones may be sewn out using the rule of halves or removed as Burow's triangles at the base of the flap. Although the U-plasty is occasionally used to make the majority of lines in the repair of a forehead defect run in the horizontal direction with the natural skin tension lines, the fact that it does not alter tension vectors and does not significantly free tissue up limits its usefulness.

An *L-plasty* or A-to-L or O-to-L advancement is a single tangent flap where an incision is made at one end of a defect extending outward for some length, and the tissue mobilized is then advanced into the defect (Fig. 203-12). Tissue redundancy is created on the side

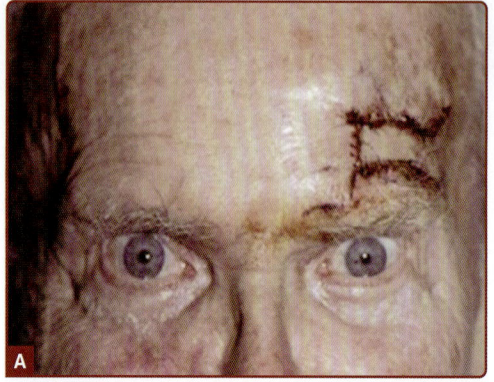
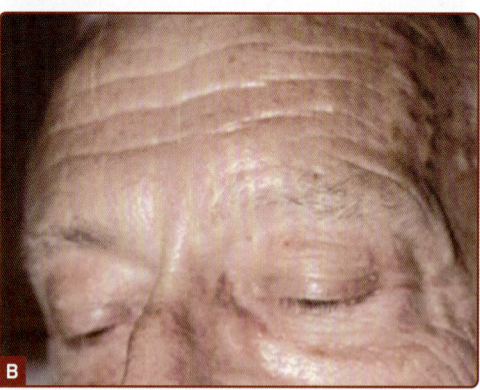

Figure 203-11 A and **B,** U-shaped advancement flap. Although advancement flaps do not necessarily change the vectors of tension of a closure, they do change the direction of the incisions and resultant scar line.

of the defect opposite the flap incision and must be removed. Although this type of advancement flap may tap into some distant laxity, it is generally minimal. Advancement flaps also do not change the tension vectors of the closure. Advancement flaps spread the

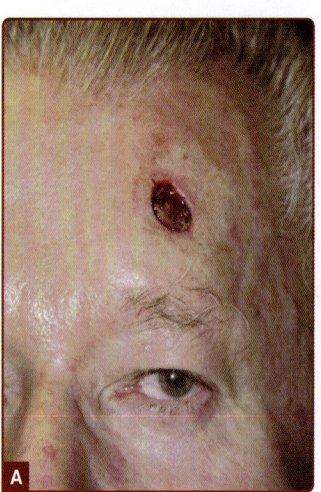
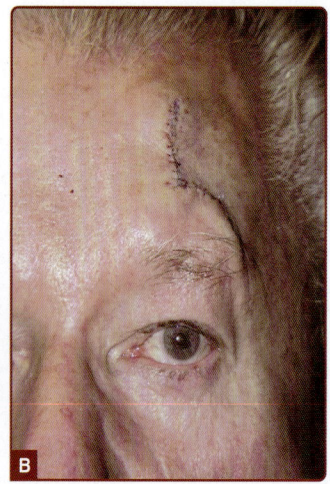
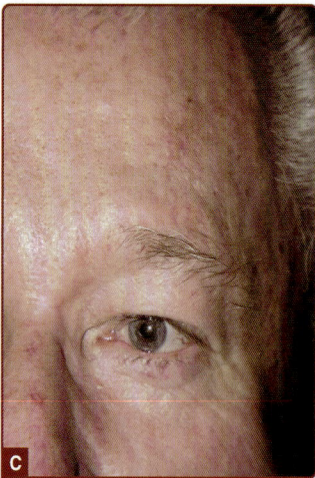

Figure 203-12 A-C, A to L advancement flap. Here, one line of the closure is drawn and incised perpendicular to the closure.

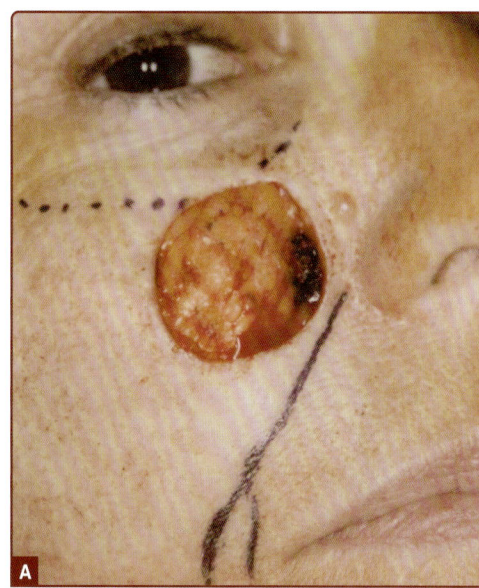

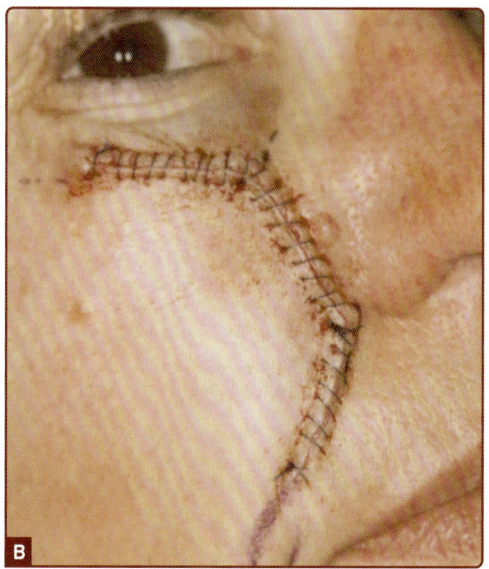

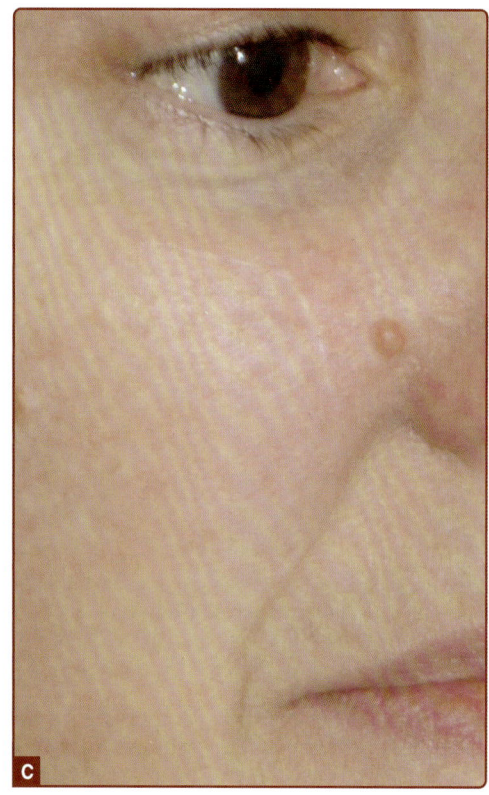

Figure 203-13 **A-C,** Cheek advancement flap. Tissue laxity of the cheek is advanced medially into the defect.

tension out over a longer distance and offer some of the closure line to be perpendicular to the vector of tension. O-to-L advancement flaps are particularly useful with defects where the limb of the flap may be incorporated into RSTLs or cosmetic unit junctions or where a linear closure may otherwise cross a free margin or cosmetic unit junction, as may be the case on the eyebrow, nose, or upper lip.

A larger single advancement flap is the *cheek advancement flap*, used to repair medium-to-large defects of the medial cheek and/or lateral nose (Fig. 203-13). The incision may be placed in the alar crease or nasolabial fold by removing tissue above and below the defect to allow the cheek to advance into the nasofacial sulcus. It is usually advantageous to tack the leading edge of a cheek advancement flap into periosteum at the nasal sidewall cheek junction, even if the defect is on the nasal sidewall. Tacking the flap to periosteum at the nasal sidewall cheek junction will take pressure off the leading edge and re-create the natural concave surface of the area and prevent unnatural webbing. When a defect involves both the cheek and the ala, a cheek advancement flap may be used to cover the defect on the cheek and a full-thickness skin graft may be used to repair the alar part of the defect (Fig. 203-14). This will keep the cosmetic units separate and place the scar lines along the cosmetic unit junctions.

Helical rim advancement flaps may be used to repair defects of the helix, utilizing the tissue laxity of the lobule. Traditionally, this flap was created with a through-and-through incision inferior to the defect along the scaphoid fossa, terminating in the lobule, and creating

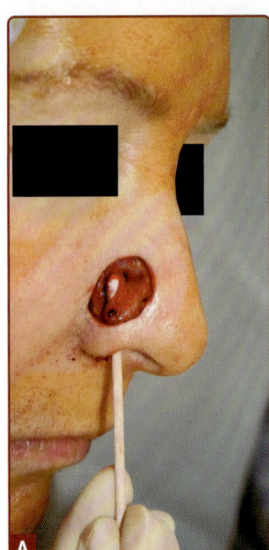 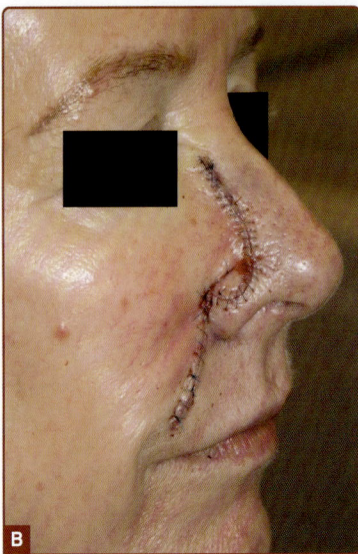 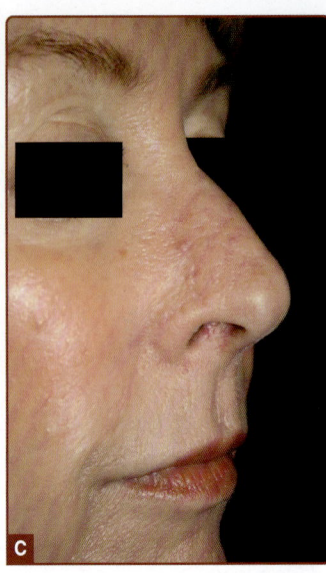

Figure 203-14 **A-C**, Cheek advancement flap with full-thickness skin graft. When the defect involves both the cheek and the ala, it is often best to utilize separate closures for each of the cosmetic units. Here a cheek advancement flap was used to close the part of the defect on the cheek, and a conchal bowl full-thickness skin graft was used to close the alar aspect of the defect.

a narrow pedicle to be advanced (conceptually similar to the U-plasty). The survivability of this flap is proportional to the length-to-width ratio and could only be performed on inferior helical defects where this ratio will not exceed 3 to 4:1. A more popular modification of this flap is to use a single tangent incision along the scaphoid fossa, leaving the posterior auricular skin intact[24] (conceptually analogous to the L-plasty) (Fig. 203-15). This allows for the maintenance of a more reliable blood supply via the tissue inferiorly and posteriorly and permits the repair of defects more distant from the lobule.

It is important to have good eversion when closing this flap at the helical rim as forces of contraction during healing will tend to invert the wound edge and create an aesthetically unpleasant notch.

BILATERAL ADVANCEMENT

If 2 sets of parallel incisions are made symmetrically on both edges of the defect, a bilateral advancement flap, termed an *H-plasty*, has been created. This flap is essentially a bilateral U-plasty and is occasionally used

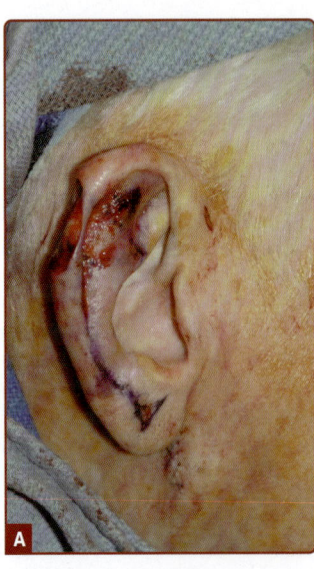 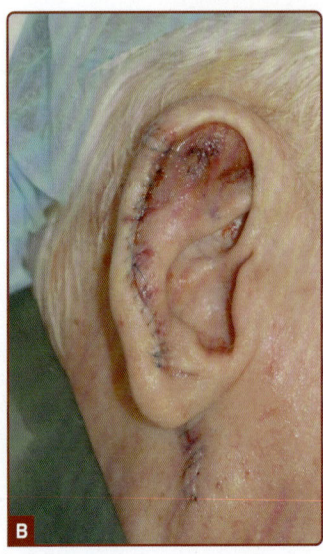 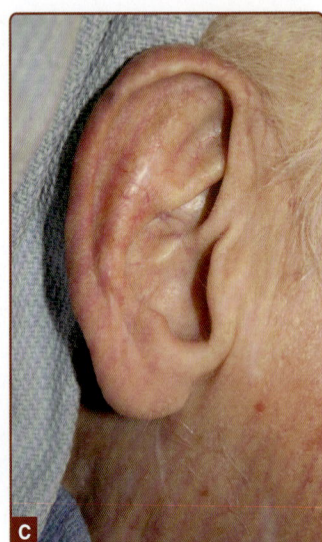

Figure 203-15 **A-C**, Helical rim advancement flap. An incision is made along the anterior helical rim down to the ear lobule. A "dog ear" is taken out on the posterior aspect of the ear. The helix is advanced superiorly to close the defect with everting sutures. This allows for consistent reconstruction of the helical rim.

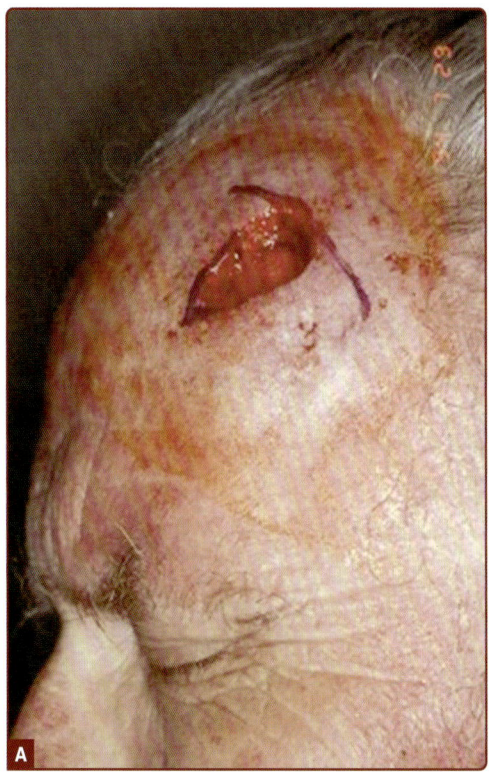 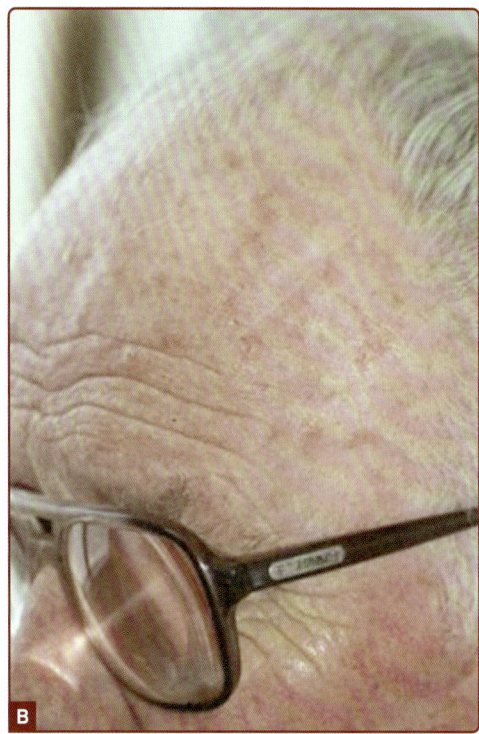

Figure 203-16 **A** and **B,** This flap can be considered a bilateral O to L advancement flap.

on the forehead, eyebrow, glabella, and upper lip to hide incision lines along relaxed skin tension lines and cosmetic unit junctions.

Another commonly employed bilateral advancement flap is an O-to-T flap, also termed an A-to-T or a *T-plasty* (Fig. 203-16), analogous to a bilateral L-plasty. This flap is essentially a bilateral O to L flap. The standing cone is removed from one end of the defect, creating a triangle, or transforming an "O" into an "A." Single incisions extend from the base of this triangular defect, and the 2 sides of the triangle slide together along this baseline. This flap allows for redistribution of tension to 2 advancing edges. The T-plasty is best performed with the broad base along a free margin or cosmetic unit junction (eg, lip, eyebrow).

CRESCENTIC ADVANCEMENT FLAP

The crescentic advancement flap utilizes the removal of a small crescent of tissue along an advancement flap to either better hide the scar line or increase the length of the line to prevent distortion. This flap is particularly useful for the repair of upper lip and perialar defects. The superior standing cone is removed in a crescentic shape around the ala such that the superior scar line is placed in the perinasal sulcus (Fig. 203-17).[25] For defects on the upper cutaneous lip, the inferior cone is removed along relaxed skin tension lines and extended through the vermilion border and around to the wet mucosa to prevent a downward distortion of the vermilion. A modification of the crescentic advancement includes the repair of a small, perialar defect of the medial cheek where both cones are removed around the ala, and the entire scar line is placed in the nasal sulcus, similar to the cheek advancement. Another modification includes incorporating a crescent along the vermilion border to an advancement flap closing a defect just superior to the vermilion border. Removing a crescent here increases the length of flap and helps minimize the differences in length between the flap and the total length of the closure (flap + defect). This will take some of the horizontal tension off the flap and minimize distortion of the lip and modiolus (Fig. 203-18).

V-TO-Y FLAP (FORMERLY REFERRED TO AS AN ISLAND PEDICLE FLAP)

A subcutaneous V-to-Y advancement flap may be considered as a variation of an advancement flap that has had all of its connections to the epidermis and dermis severed, maintaining its blood supply through a subcutaneous tissue pedicle (Fig. 203-19).[26] The flap is designed within cosmetic units when possible and, as with all repairs, it is optimal for the incision lines to run along cosmetic junctions. The V-to-Y flap is frequently used on nasal and perioral closures where free margins are at risk for distortion. The tension vectors of an island pedicle flap are primarily in the same direction as that of a primary closure; however, they

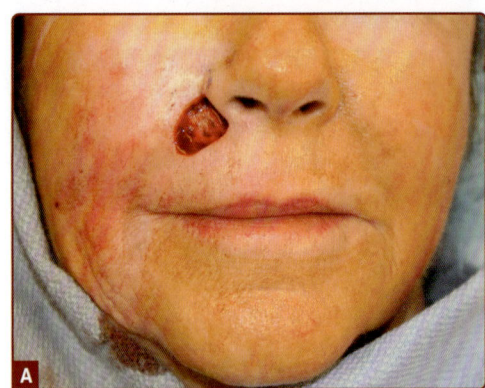

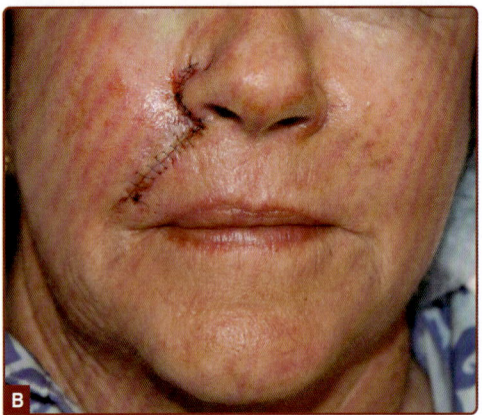

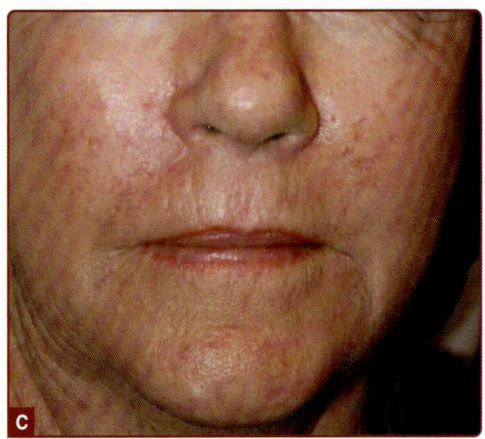

Figure 203-17 **A-C,** Crescentic advancement flap. A crescent of tissue is removed around the lateral aspect of the ala and the cheek is advanced medially.

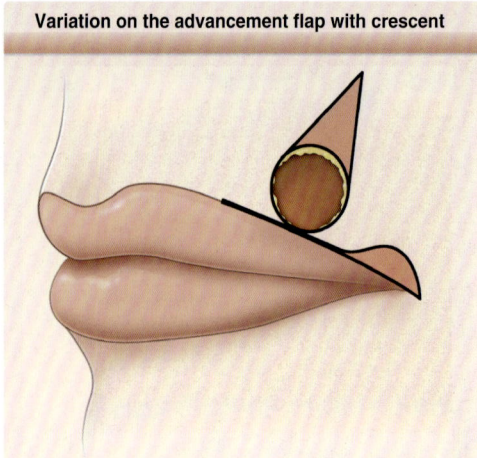

Figure 203-18 Variation on the advancement flap with crescent. Removing the crescent of tissue elongates the incision and compensates for the length mismatch of the incision versus the incision + defect.

are displaced distal to the wound (ie, superior to the nasal tip, superior or lateral to the vermilion border) and help avoid distortion of the area around the defect.

The V-to-Y flap is created by extending 2 nonparallel tangential incisions to meet at an approximate 30° angle, similar to when planning a Burow's triangle. The difference is that the incision lines stay parallel for a short distance before converging, creating a slightly larger triangle than would be created with a Burow's triangle. This extra length gives tissue that closely approximates the size of the defect and minimizes local distortion. The triangle may be designed larger or smaller depending on how much tension sharing is desired. The incisions are made just to the superficial subcutaneous tissue. The tip and sides of the flap are undermined widely extending outward from the flap in the subcutaneous plane. The triangular flap is also undermined slightly to help mobilize it. The flap is then advanced into the defect and sutured into place. For the flap to fit properly into a circular defect, either the corners of the flap must be trimmed or the defect squared off. The flap must be undermined with attention both to the mobility of the tissue and to the maintenance of a subcutaneous vascular pedicle. Although the initial design should have a broad pedicle, if mobility is limited the pedicle may be progressively diminished (particularly at the trailing tip of the flap).

When closing defects on the nasal dorsum and tip, a muscular flap is often created laterally on one or both sides. For this musculocutaneous island pedicle flap, undermining is performed both above and below the nasalis muscle. If there is not enough laxity to close the defect without upward tension on the nasal tip, the muscular flap is released horizontally at the superior and inferior edge to create a muscular sling that advances with the flap into place. The muscular attachment gives a robust blood supply to the flap and helps ensure its survival.

EAST–WEST FLAP

The east–west flap is an advancement flap used for small to medium-sized defects (up to 1.5 cm) of the lateral nasal supratip.[27] Two triangles are removed in the vertical axis. The superior one is adjacent to the defect and parallel to the long axis of the nose. The inferior triangle is midline, toward the columella. Removal of

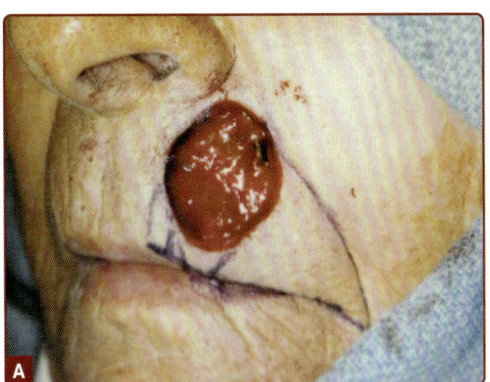
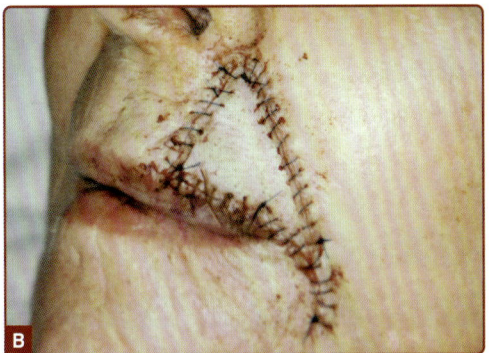
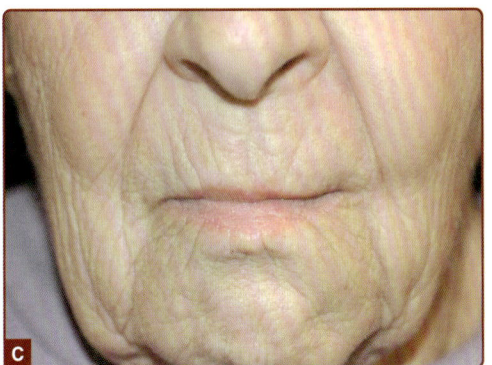

Figure 203-19 **A-C,** V to Y flap-A triangular shaped flap is incised through the dermis and advanced into the defect while a pedicle of tissue is left intact deep to the flap, which supplies a rich vascular network and aids in survival.

both triangles allows for an easy lateral sliding movement and closure (Fig. 203-20). This flap permits reconstruction without significant nasal distortion or excess tension,[27] and allows for excellent tissue match.

RINTALA FLAP

The Rintala flap is a superior based advancement flap for large defects on the nasal dorsum.[28] A rectangular flap from the nasal dorsum and glabella is elevated in the supraperiosteal plane and advanced downward to cover the defect. Burrows triangles are created proximal to the alar groove or on the forehead. Thorough undermining must be performed to avoid nasal tip elevation.[28]

ROTATION FLAPS

In a rotation flap, skin moves into the defect by rotating around a pivot point (Fig. 203-21). This is classically used to close relatively large defects on the cheek, temple, or scalp. The design of the traditional rotation flap uses a curvilinear incision along an arc adjacent to the primary defect. Adjacent lax tissue is recruited while the closure tension is redirected in multiple directions away from the primary defect. The flap is designed with attention to its length and curvature.[29] Rotation flaps often require long incision lines, as a larger arc of the rotation vector allows closure with minimal tension on the flap's tip while simultaneously decreasing the width of the secondary defect. The ideal arc of a rotation flap extends up to 5 times the width of the defect and makes up approximately one-quarter of the circumference of a circle.

As the flap is raised and undermined, the adjacent tissue laxity allows the flap to rotate into the primary defect. The key stitch closes the primary defect and a burrows triangle usually forms at the base. The rotation flap has a large vascular pedicle and therefore has a lower risk of tissue necrosis. The stiffness about the pivot point may hinder the flap's movement,[29] and undermining the area of pivotal restraint improves flap mobility. If restraint of motion keeps the tip from moving into the distal defect, a back cut can increase tissue movement in areas of limited tissue laxity, such as the nose. However, caution must be taken as the back-cut may decrease the pedicle width, interfering with blood flow into the flap.

DORSAL NASAL ROTATION FLAP

Also known as the *Rieger flap*, this flap is employed to repair nasal defects involving the distal dorsum or tip.[30] The tissue reservoir of the nasal root and glabella allows for the movement of the dorsal nasal skin superior to the defect. A long, sweeping arc is created that extends into the nasofacial sulcus and terminates in the glabella. A back cut in the glabella improves the rotational mobility of this flap and is termed a *hatchet flap* (Fig. 203-22). If the arc of this flap is not long enough or there is too much tension on the leading edge of the flap, elevation of the nasal tip will result. Wide undermining at the level of the perichondrium is required.

BILATERAL ROTATION FLAP

At times, the size of the defect or the tension on the flap mandates a bilateral rotation flap, in which tissue is rotated into a defect from 2 opposite sides. The vectors

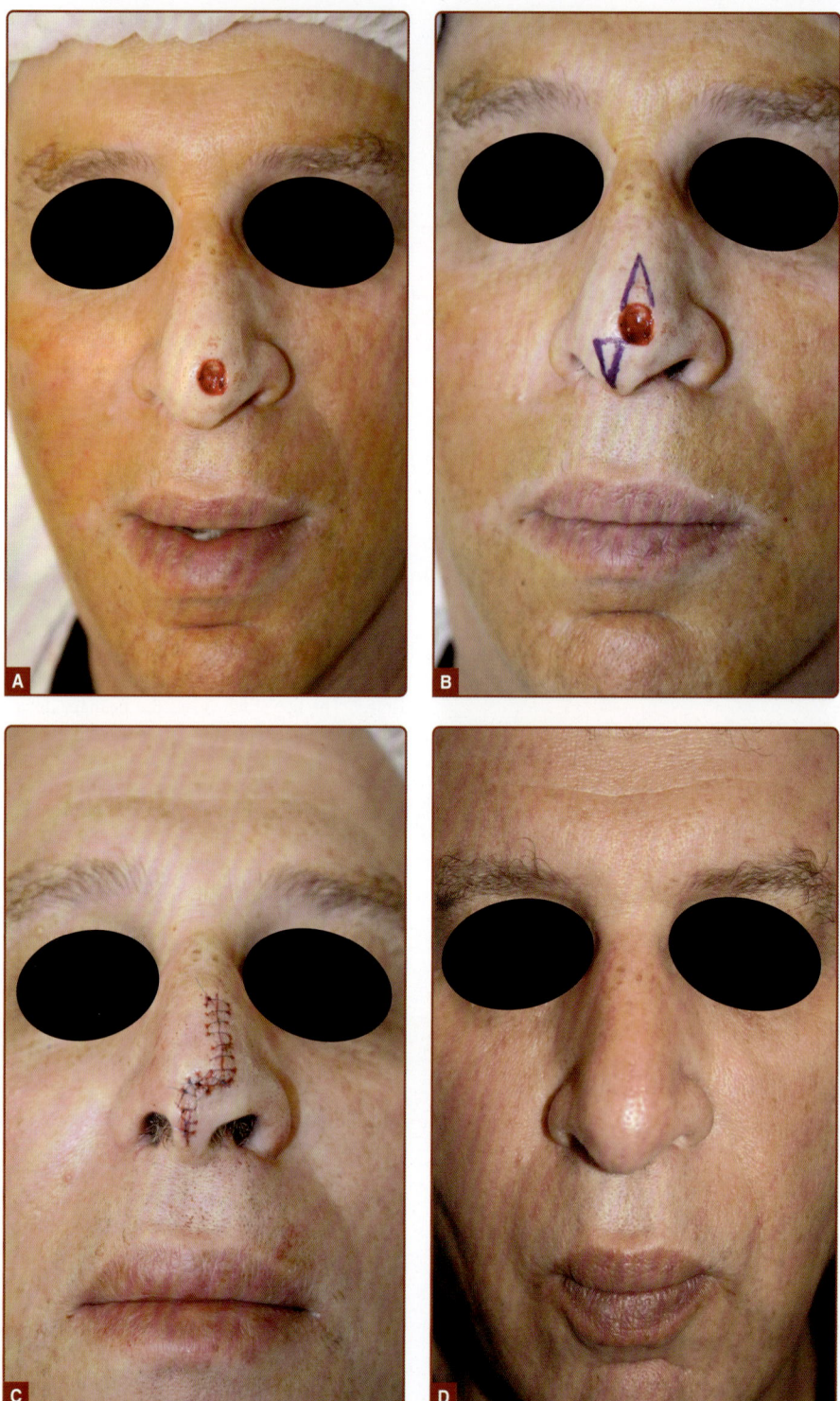

Figure 203-20 **A-D,** East–west flap. The east–west advancement flap is used for small to medium-sized defects on the nasal tip. It allows for excellent tissue match and minimal nasal distortion.

of rotation may be mirror images of each other, recapitulating the premise of the A–T advancement flap. This may be utilized for large defects on the scalp and larger defects on the lower lip (Fig. 203-23). The vectors of movement also may be in opposition, creating an O-to-Z flap.

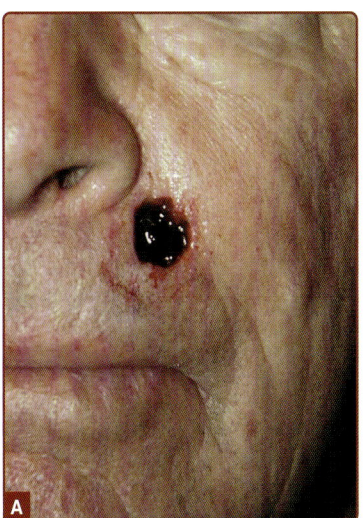
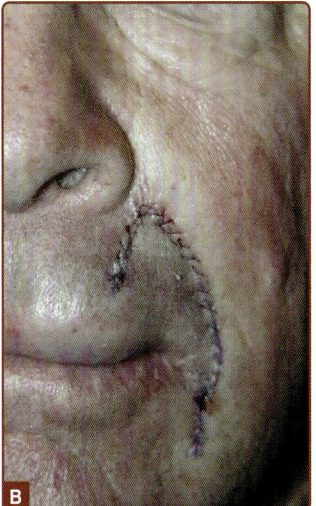
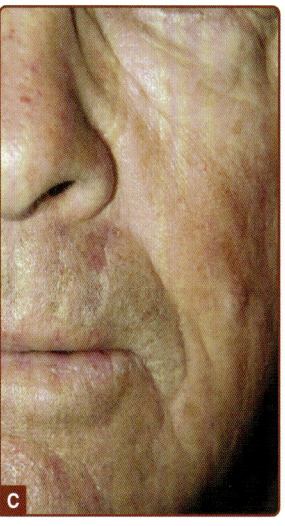

Figure 203-21 **A-C,** Rotation flap. An arcuate incision is made from one end of the defect and the flap is rotated into the defect. Rotation flaps help spread tension vectors out in multiple directions radiating from the arc.

PERIOCULAR ROTATION FLAPS

Defects of the lower eyelid and infraorbital cheek are at high risk for ectropion. To prevent this complication, the tension must be parallel to the lid margin. Both the *Mustarde flap* and the modified *Tenzel flap* are rotation flaps that can help prevent ectropion. A Mustarde flap is useful for larger defects on the lower lid/periorbital cheek. The flap extends laterally from the defect, arches superiorly to the lateral canthus and temple and ends in the preauricular area. The flap is undermined extensively and transposed over the defect. The Tenzel flap is a semicircular flap for a lower lid defect that rotates the skin and orbicularis muscle from the lateral canthal area. Additionally, the lateral canthal tendon is cut for increased tissue mobility. Both of these flaps must be anchored to the periosteum at the lateral orbital rim to help minimize downward tension on the eyelid and risk of ectropion.[31,32]

SPIRAL FLAP

The Spiral flap has been shown to be effective for the reconstruction of small to medium-sized partial-thickness defects of the nasal ala and inferior nasal sidewall. It is a modified rotation flap with a 180° arc. The tip is advanced and rotated into the wound and sutured into the proximal aspect of the wound, the body of the flap follows creating a spiral (Fig. 203-24). With this flap, the cosmetic unit is preserved, there is no shortening of the nasal ala, and a standing cone does not form, therefore decreasing the risk of alar distortion.[33]

TRANSPOSITION FLAPS

A transposition flap is a random pattern flap, which borrows skin laxity from an adjacent area to fill a

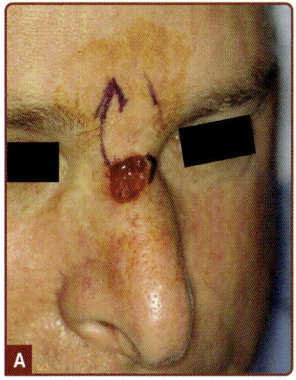
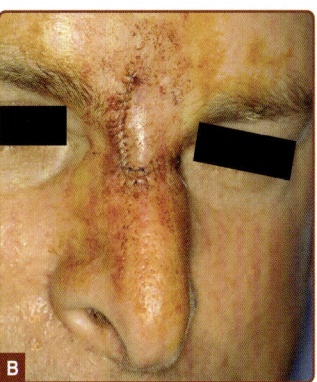
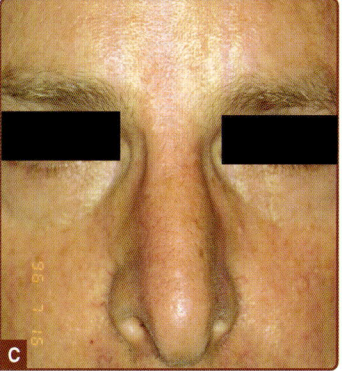

Figure 203-22 **A-C,** Hatchet flap. The hatchet flap is a rotation flap with a cutback. The cutback gives the flap extra length and aids in its movement.

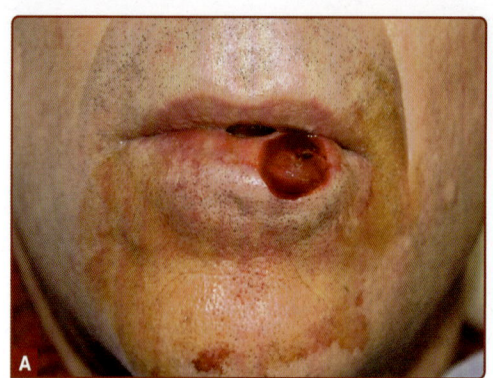
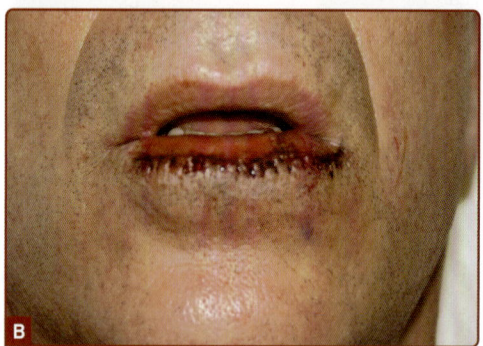
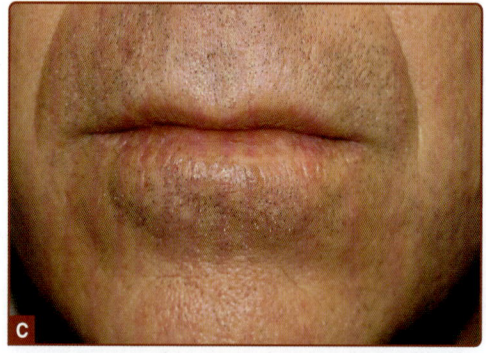

Figure 203-23 A-C, Bilateral rotation flap of the lip. Incisions are made bilaterally along the vermillion border and a redundant tricone of tissue is removed posteriorly into the wet mucosal lip. Both wings of the flap are rotated together and sutured with braided suture.

defect in an area with little or no skin laxity. In its travel from the donor site to the recipient site, the flap is lifted or "transposed" over a segment of intervening tissue. When the secondary defect is closed, the transposition flap pushes tissue into a defect rather than pulling it, as with the advancement and rotation flaps. While moving to the recipient site, the flap actually follows a rotational path and must be designed so it does not rotate too far and pull too tightly on its pedicle.

Transposition flaps have several advantages over other closures. Their primary function is to redistribute and redirect tension. This is useful in the closure of defects which would otherwise close under high tension or distort a nearby anatomical structure leading to functional or aesthetic impairment. Transposition flaps are usually smaller in overall size than advancement and rotation flaps. The resulting scars are geometric broken lines that may be less noticeable than longer linear closures in certain areas. This geometric broken line scar, however, may be thought of as a disadvantage as they are difficult to completely place along a relaxed skin tension line or cosmetic unit junction. One of the major advantages of transposition flaps is that they utilize adjacent skin and provide an excellent color and textural match.

The most common transposition flaps in cutaneous surgery include rhombic flaps (and their variations), bilobed flaps, and banner flaps such as the nasolabial flap. Knowledge of the tissue dynamics used in these 3 basic transposition flaps can be carried over to the planning and execution of the numerous variations of these flaps.

RHOMBIC FLAP

First described by Lindberg in 1963 is a single-lobed transposition flap. The classic rhombic flap was designed to create a secondary defect perpendicular to the primary defect.[34] When closed, it would not only provide tissue to the primary defect, but also redirect the tension vector by 90°. This allowed the primary defect to be closed under almost no wound edge tension. Subsequent modifications by DuFourmentel and Webster provide more tension sharing between the primary and secondary defects. These modifications are useful in situations where some laxity around the primary defect is available.[35]

The classic Lindberg rhombic flap is designed by conversion of the primary defect into a 4-sided parallelogram with each side of equal length and tip angles of 60° and 120°.[34] This rhombus forms the recipient site for the flap as well as the template on which to plan the flap incisions. In its classic configuration (Fig. 203-25), the incisions are designed by extending a line (line a–b) outward from one of the obtuse tips for a length equal to that of one side of the rhombus. From the free end of the extended line (point b), a second line (line b–c) is drawn. The tip angle in this configuration is 60°. The flap is lifted and transposed into place. The tension vector is redirected from that of closing the primary defect, to that of closing the new secondary defect created in the design of the flap. This allows the tension vector to be shifted and redirected by 90°.

There are 4 possible flap designs off of the short axis of any rhomboid defect (Fig. 203-26). Which of these 4 flap configurations is selected depends on several factors that affect the final outcome. These factors include adjacent anatomic structures, adjacent skin type, and where the scar line will be best hidden. Though the classic rhombic transposition flap can be designed and executed off of the long axis of the rhombus, there are 2 advantages to designing it off of the short axis of the defect. First, it keeps the flap as small as possible while filling the defect completely. Second, it minimizes the

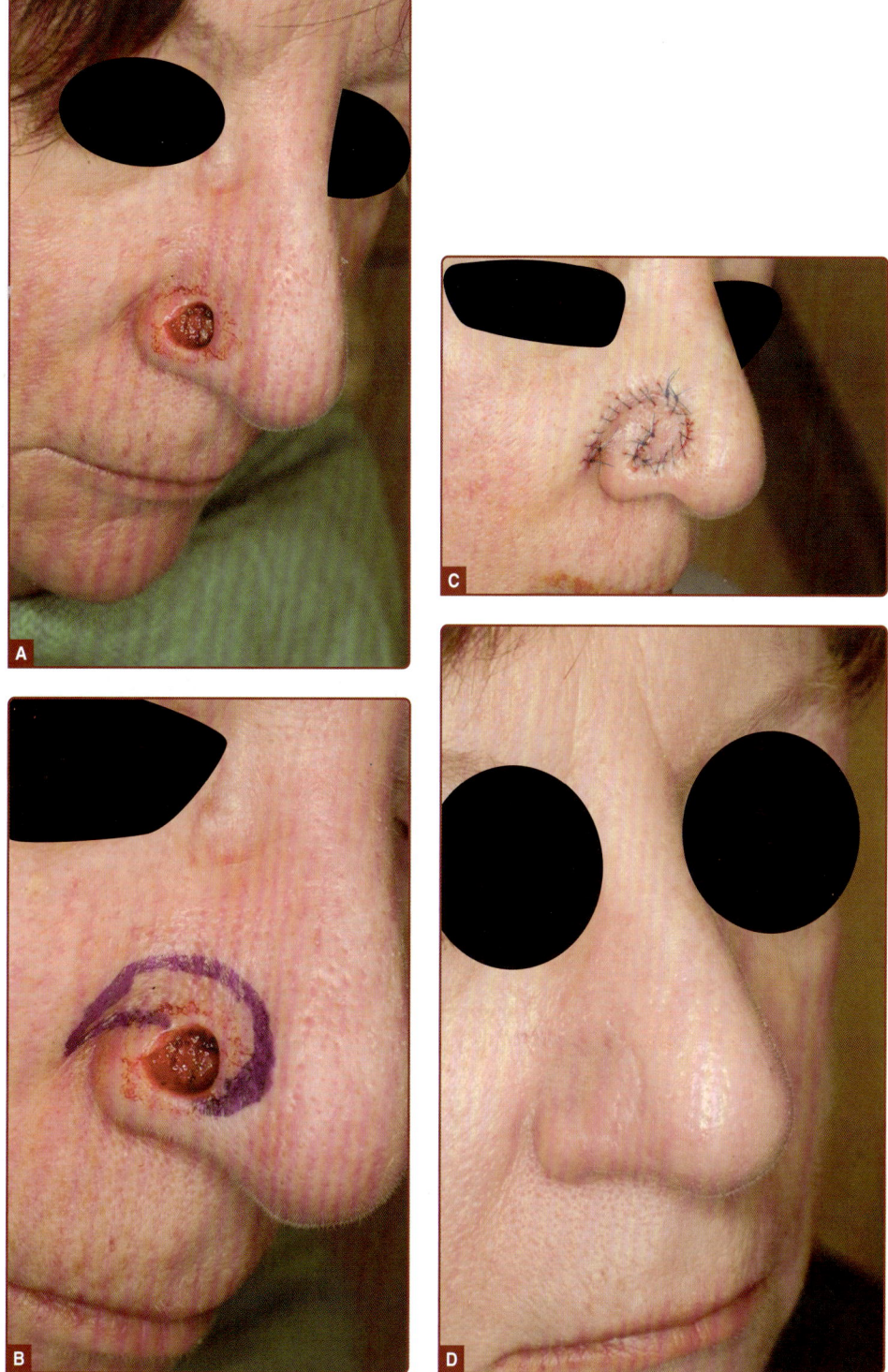

Figure 203-24 A-D, Spiral flap. The spiral flap is a modified rotation flap that can be used to repair defects of the nasal ala and alar groove. The flap is incised, undermined, and rotated into the wound with no alar distortion.

arc through which the flap must rotate to fit into the defect.

In designing the flap from the circular defect, the length of the line extended out from the defect should be drawn longer than the diameter of the circular defect. This will account for the fact that the diameter of the circular defect is shorter than the short axis of a rhombus drawn around the defect. A second line

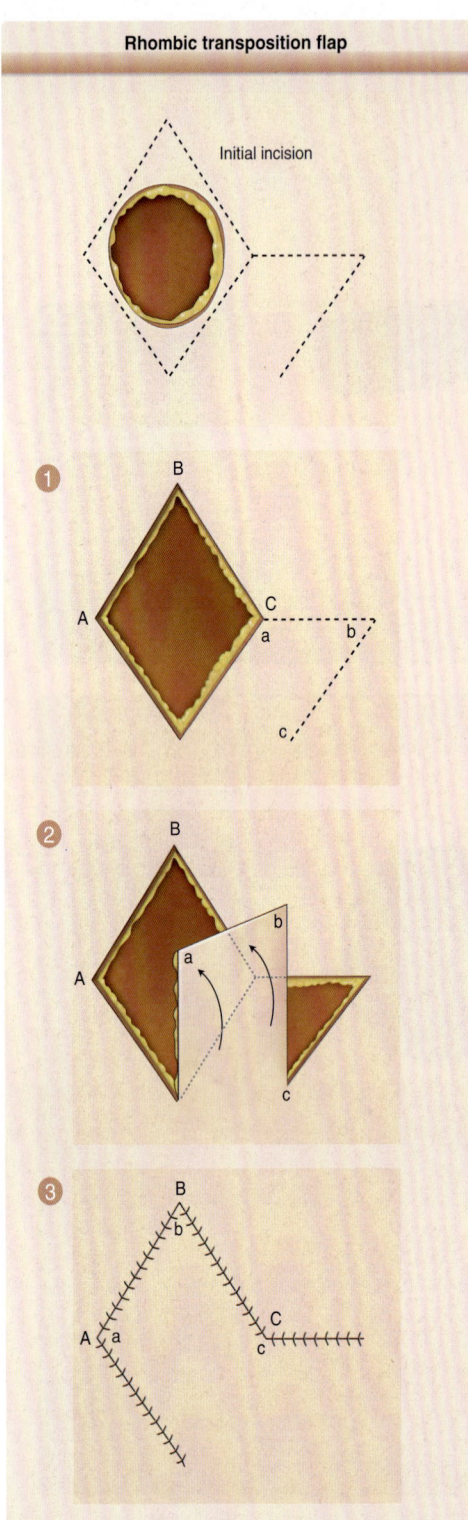

Figure 203-25 Rhombic transposition flap. Classic rhombic flaps alter the vectors of tension in a closure by 90° and leave a broken geometric scar shape. The tension is taken completely by the closure of the secondary defect as the flap is pushed into the primary defect.

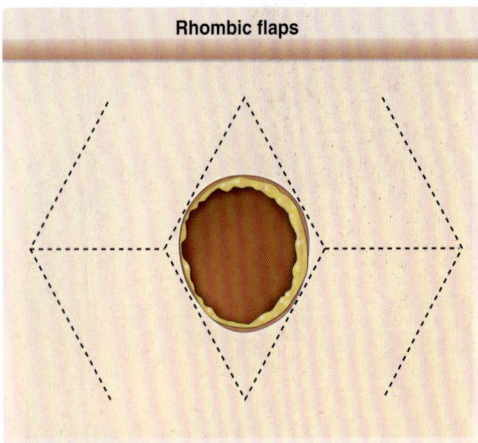

Figure 203-26 Rhombic flaps may be drawn in any of 4 directions off of the short axis of any rhomboid-shaped defect.

of the same length is drawn, keeping the tip angle at 60° to complete the flap. The triangle of tissue redundancy created by the rotation of the transposition flap is removed by trimming a Burow's triangle at the pivot point. The transposed tissue may be rounded to fit the circular defect, or the defect may be squared off to accommodate the angular flap. This choice can be made based on which option yields the best aesthetic result (Fig. 203-27).

As with any closure, understanding the tension forces is essential to the planning, execution, and outcome of the repair. There are 2 main tension forces associated with the classic rhombic flap. The first set of tension forces are realized during the approximation and closure of the secondary defect. The second set of tension forces are generated at the tip of the flap when moving it into the primary defect. These forces are due to the resistance to rotation at the flap's pedicle as well as shortening of the length of the flap during rotation into the recipient site. Dzubow describes these forces as pivotal restraint.[29] Securing the flap into the recipient site under high tension is not advised because it may lead to tip ischemia and necrosis. Two modifications in design can be utilized to assist in minimizing the shortening of the flap and subsequent tension at the flap tip.

- By lengthening both the leading edge and the secondary limb of the flap, the flap can be enlarged and lengthened. This lengthening can compensate for the shortening resulting from pivoting at the base, thus reducing tension at the tip when secured in the recipient defect.
- An alternate method to lengthen the flap is by designing the flap with a slightly more obtuse (greater than 120°) flap angle. Widely undermining around the flap also assists in the redistribution of tension vectors as well as redistribution of contractile forces during the healing phase.

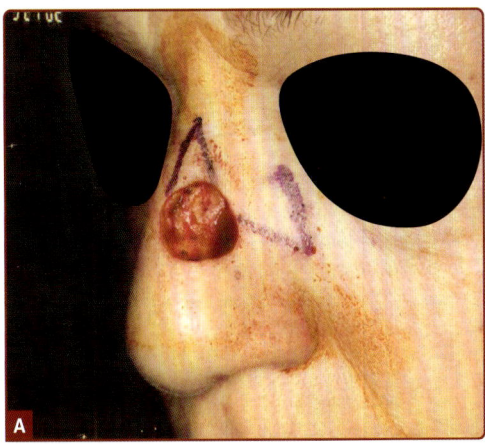
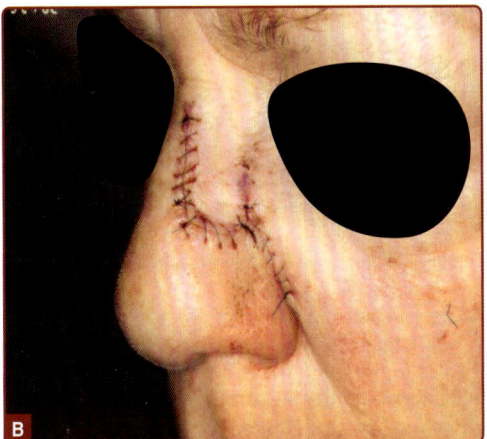
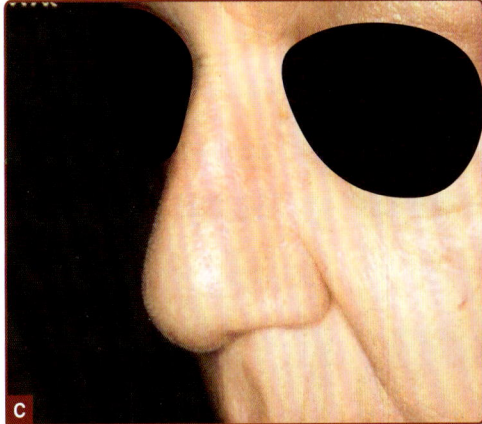

Figure 203-27 **A-C,** A modified rhombic flap allows for closure of circular defects. A standing cone is excised at the pivot point. The tissue is then transposed into the defect and the wound closure tension is redirected.

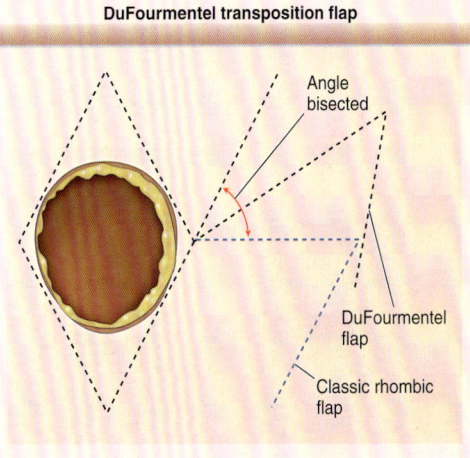

Figure 203-28 DuFourmentel transposition flap. The flap is designed with a narrower tip angle and a shorter arc of rotation. This allows easier closure of the secondary defect and allows some sharing of tension between the primary and secondary defects. The vectors of tension are altered by 45° not the full 90° seen in a classic rhombic flap.

The DuFourmentel Flap: The DuFourmentel flap modification differs from the classic rhombic transposition flap (Fig. 203-28) in that it utilizes a narrower flap tip angle and a shorter arc of rotation, allowing easier closure of the secondary defect, and some sharing of the tension between the primary and secondary defects. Given that there is generally some tissue laxity at the site of the surgical defect, the DuFourmentel modification is utilized by this author more than the classic rhombic flap.

As with the classic rhombic flap, it is designed by extending the first line from the short axis of the rhomboid defect. However, the angle at which the first line is extended differs from the classic rhombic flap in that it bisects the angle formed by the first line of the classic rhombic flap (which extends straight out from the short axis of the rhombic defect) and the line formed by extending one of the sides of the rhombus from the same corner of the rhombus. The length of the first line is equal to that of a side length of the rhombus. The second line originates from the free end of the first line, and is drawn parallel to the long axis of the rhombus. This second line's orientation results in a slightly widened pedicle, a decrease in the tip volume, and a decrease in the degree of rotation necessary to execute the flap. The tissue redundancy at the base of the leading edge of the flap can be removed by taking a slightly larger Burrow's triangle.

The 30ç-Angle Webster Flap: The 30°-angle Webster modification of the classic rhombic flap utilizes a more acute angle than other rhombic transposition flaps, allowing for even greater tension sharing between the primary and secondary defects. A Webster 30°-angle flap is planned similarly to the DuFourmentel flap; however, its distal tip angle is designed to be 30° (Fig. 203-29). This gives the flap a slimmer design and narrower pedicle. The flap area is only 50% of the area of the primary defect; therefore, it only relieves half of the tension from the primary defect. This modification is used in situations where a fair amount of laxity exists in the horizontal axis of the rhombic shaped defect. Because this design places more tension on the

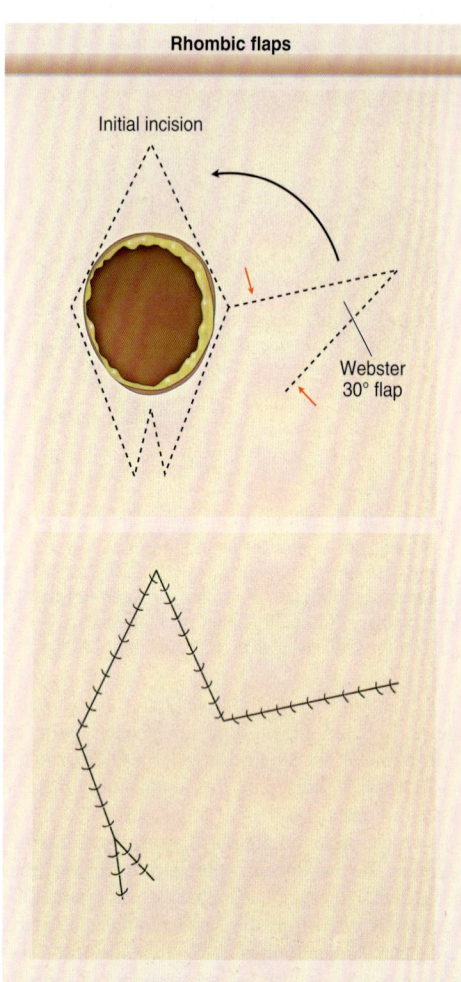

Figure 203-29 30° Webster flap. The angle of the rhombic flap is made even more acute, and more of the closure tension is shared with the primary defect.

primary defect, care must be taken not to close with too much lateral tension or distort adjacent anatomic structures.

Rhombic transposition flaps are very versatile and may be used to reconstruct a variety of defects. Transposition flaps are generally used when there is insufficient laxity in the immediate surrounding area of closure and/or the tension vectors need to be redirected. This is particularly important when repairing defects near free margins such as the eyelids and the nose. The most common areas they are employed include the nasal dorsum, nasal sidewall, medial and lateral canthus, lateral forehead, temple, cheek, perioral region, inferior chin, and the dorsal hand.

THE BANNER FLAP

Banner-type flaps are random-pattern finger-shaped cutaneous flaps that, like other transposition flaps, tap into adjacent skin to borrow laxity and fill a defect.[36] This flap is most commonly planned as a melolabial transposition to repair defects of the nasal ala or from the pre- or postauricular area to close defects on the ear. For an optimal cosmetic result, the scar is generally placed at the junction of 2 cosmetic units, providing excellent camouflage (in the nasolabial fold or preauricular sulcus) (Fig. 203-30).

The fundamental design of the banner flaps consists of a finger-shaped flap drawn with a width that is equal to the width of the defect and a length equal to the distance from the pivot point to the far edge of the defect. The flap is transposed and rotated in an arc around the pivot point to fill the defect. Because this is a long random-pattern flap with a narrow pedicle, the risk of vascular compromise may be high if the entire length of the flap is used and its pedicle originates from an area of minimal vascularity. To minimize risk of vascular compromise, the flap is typically designed

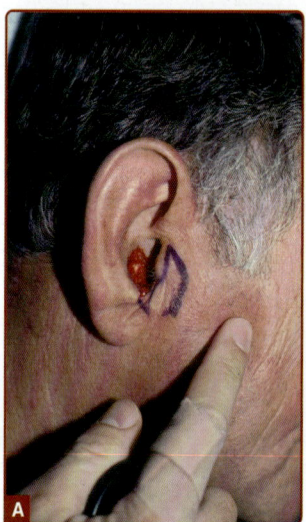 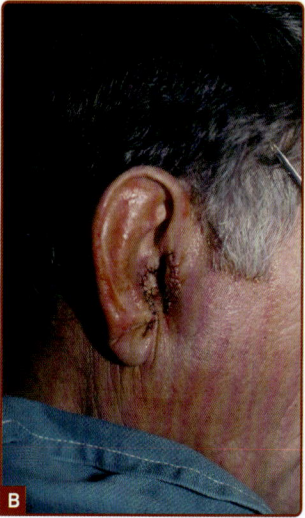 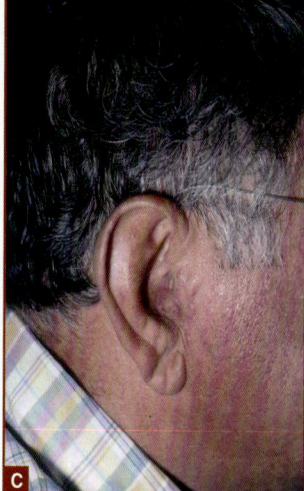

Figure 203-30 A-C, Banner transposition flap. A finger-shaped flap is incised and draped into the primary defect. These closure lines are generally placed along cosmetic unit junctions such as the preauricular sulcus.

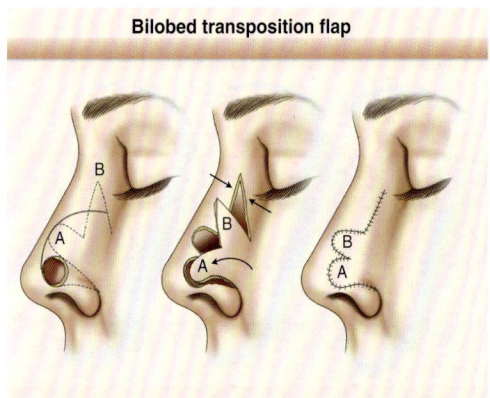

Figure 203-31 Bilobed transposition flap. The bilobed flap is designed with 2 adjacent transposition flaps elevated and rotated into position. The Zitelli modification (shown here) is designed placing the lobes over a 90° arc.

to rotate through an angle of 60° to 120° instead of the originally described 180°. Additionally, when designing the backcut and removing the redundancy at the base of the flap, it should be designed in a direction away from the pedicle of the flap to avoid further narrowing of the pedicle, thereby maximizing flap viability. Typical locations for use of Banner-type flaps include the nasal ala, the superior helix of the ear, and the medial anterior ear.

BILOBED FLAP

The bilobed flap used today is a highly evolved transposition flap. The bilobed flap was first described by Esser in 1918. It became a workhorse flap only after the modifications described by Zitelli were published in 1989 (Fig. 203-31).[37] The design of the bilobed flap actually consists of 2 transposition flaps executed in succession, which follow the same direction of rotation over intervening tissues. The basic premise of this flap is to fill the defect with the primary lobe, while filling the secondary defect with the secondary lobe, leaving a triangle-shaped tertiary defect to be closed primarily. The key suture closes the tertiary defect. This series of transposition flaps allows the surgeon to further the reach of the flap, and borrow laxity from donor sites at a greater distance from the defect while decreasing the arc of rotation of the pedicle.

The Zitelli modification of the bilobed flap is designed by placing the lobes over a 90° arc from the center of the defect, with the primary lobe rotating from a pivot point that is created by removing a Burow's triangle at one pole of the defect.[37] The width of the primary lobe should be equal to the width of the defect and should be long enough to just extend past the edge of the defect. The secondary lobe must be trimmed to match the secondary defect left by the transposition of the primary lobe.

As with the rhombic flap, the bilobed flap redirects the principal tension vector and takes advantage of tissue laxity of the donor site. This flap is predominantly used for small to medium-sized defects of the lower nose as the tension is redirected to a near vertical vector, preventing distortion of the alar rim (Fig. 203-32).

TRILOBE FLAP

This flap is very similar to the bilobed flap; however, it is able to use tissue that is further from the primary defect. The key suture closes the quaternary defect. In general, the primary lobe should be equal to the defect diameter, the secondary lobe should be 85% to 90% of the defect size, and the tertiary lobe should be 75% to 80% of the defect size. The trilobed flap is useful for defects on the distal tip of the nose and nasal ala.

Z-PLASTY

The Z-plasty is a transposition flap that improves the functional and cosmetic appearance of a scar by realigning a scar, camouflaging a scar, or most commonly increasing the scar length after contraction. The classic Z-plasty has 60° angles and will lengthen the scar by 75%. However, there are multiple variations based off of the classic Z-plasty. In a traditional Z-plasty there are 2 incisions of equal lengths, referred to as limbs, and 1 central incision. The limbs form 60° angles with the central incision. This leads to the formation of 2 triangular flaps that are transposed to redirect the tension vector and lengthen the central limb direction. This results in a new central incision that is perpendicular to the original central incision and ideally within relaxed skin tension lines.[38]

INTERPOLATION FLAPS

Interpolation flaps are more complex repairs that import pedicle-based tissue from a site distant to the defect. They are typically used on defects that are either too wide or too deep to reconstruct with local flaps or grafts. Many interpolation flaps may be classified as axial flaps if their vascular pedicle is based on a large, named artery. They are also commonly referred to as staged flaps as more than one stage is required to complete the repair. Interpolation flaps require careful planning, substantial time in executing, and significant, albeit temporary, disfigurement of the patient.

The first stage of an interpolation flap involves the design and creation of the flap, including repair of the secondary defect. The flap is designed around a substantial artery and therefore is able to support a larger mass of tissue than random flaps. Because the flap is used to repair defects distant from the donor site, the vascular pedicle must temporarily be left in place to ensure adequate blood supply. The distal end of the flap is thinned to match the depth of the defect and sutured in place. The area is bandaged

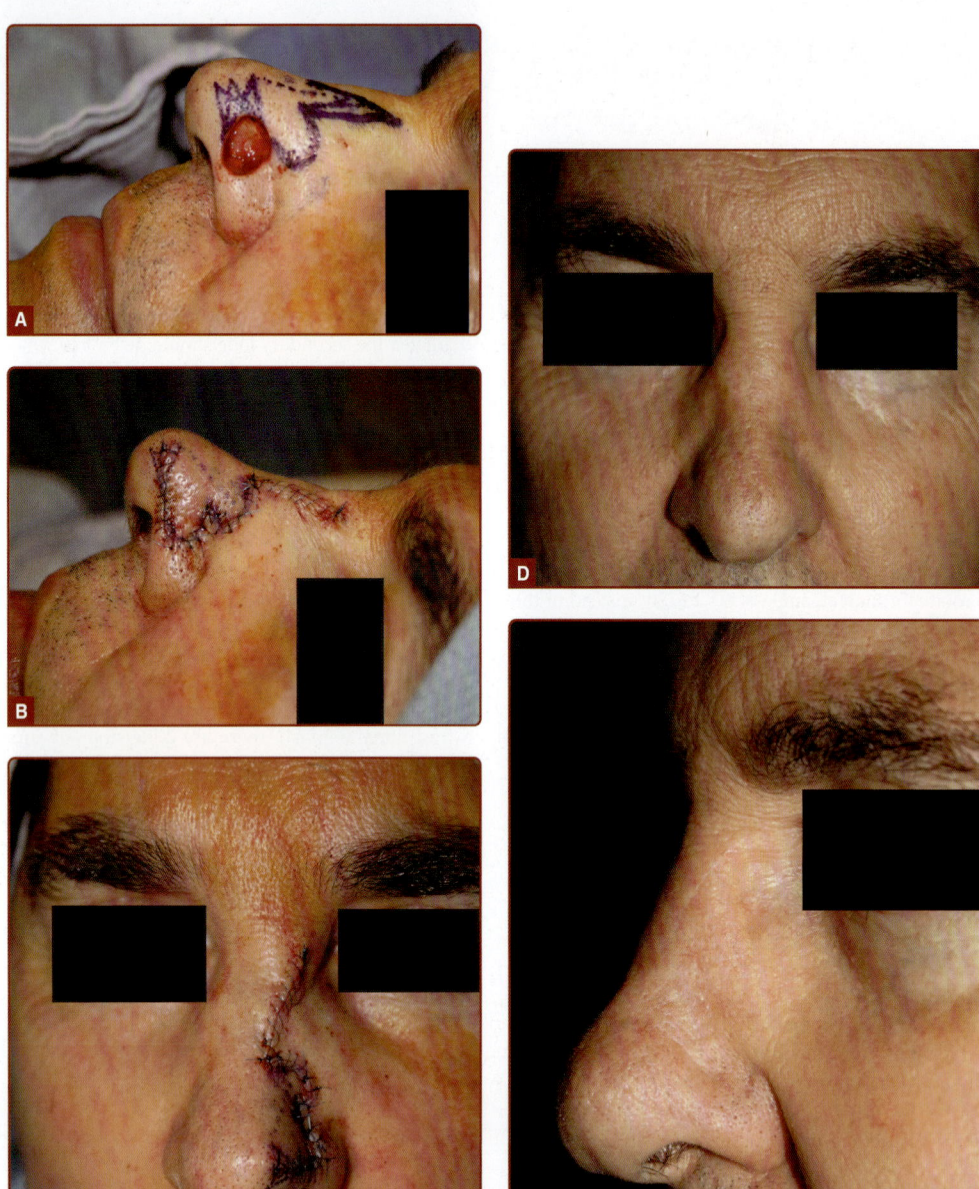

Figure 203-32 A-E, Execution of a medially based bilobed transposition flap. The tertiary defect is closed side to side, the secondary defect is filled with the second lobe of the flap, and the primary defect is filled with the first lobe of the flap. When used in this location, mobility and flap survival are improved when the flap is undermined below the nasalis muscle.

and kept moist. The second stage generally takes place 2- to 3-weeks later, by which time the flap has established a local blood supply from the donor site. The pedicle is then divided from the donor site and the proximal portion of the flap is secured into the original defect. Because of granulation tissue formation, this portion of the flap may need to be thinned out subcutaneously to approximate the depth of the defect. The pedicle is also separated from the donor site, which will then require further steps for complete repair.

PARAMEDIAN FOREHEAD FLAP

The paramedian forehead flap is useful to repair large, deep nasal defects that may or may not require cartilage grafts. Tissue is mobilized from the forehead, based on one of the supratrochlear arteries, and transposed to repair large distal nasal defects with the pedicle remaining attached in the glabellar region (Fig. 203-33). The supratrochlear artery is located at the medial border of the eyebrow, approximately 1.5 to 2 cm from the midline.

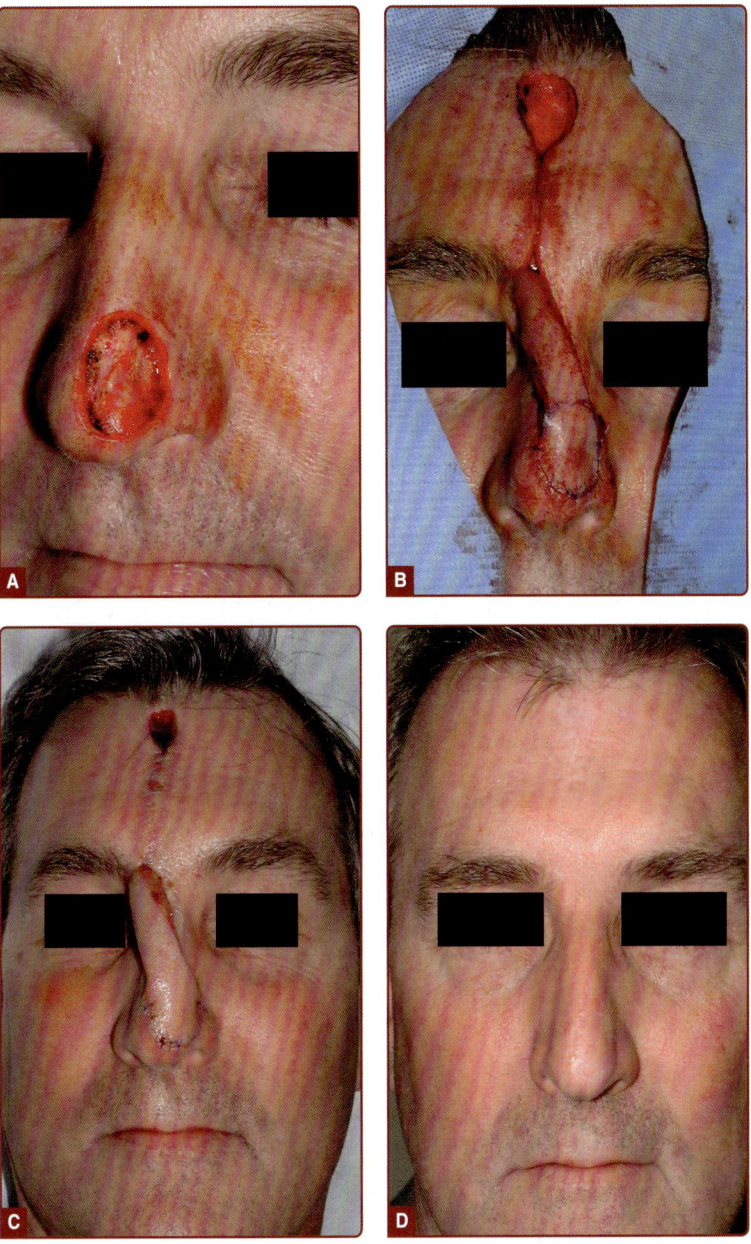

Figure 203-33 **A-D,** Paramedian forehead flap. For deep defects on the nose, a pedicled flap is created on the forehead based on the hearty vasculature of the supratrochlear arterial system and rotated down into place. The pedicle is divided and removed approximately 3 weeks after the inset of the flap (**C**).

The aesthetics of the repair are often improved when the defect is enlarged to include the total cosmetic subunit. The portion of the flap that will fill the defect is the superior portion closest to the hairline; the width here should be equal to the widest portion of the defect, although the pedicle itself need be no wider than 1 to 1.5 cm. Its height must be equal to the distance from the base of the flap to the distal edge of the defect. In designing the flap, it is important that the vertical height of the forehead is able to accommodate the necessary length of the flap. The tissue is rotated approximately 180° around its pedicle and should be rotated medially as to minimize obscuration of the medial visual field of the ipsilateral eye; therefore, the flap will require less rotation if it is harvested from the forehead supplied by the supratrochlear artery contralateral to the defect.

The donor site is undermined and closed primarily as far superiorly as it will close. The distal aspect of the flap is debulked to the depth of the defect and secured at the distal margin with sutures. The proximal margin, by design, cannot be secured until the pedicle is

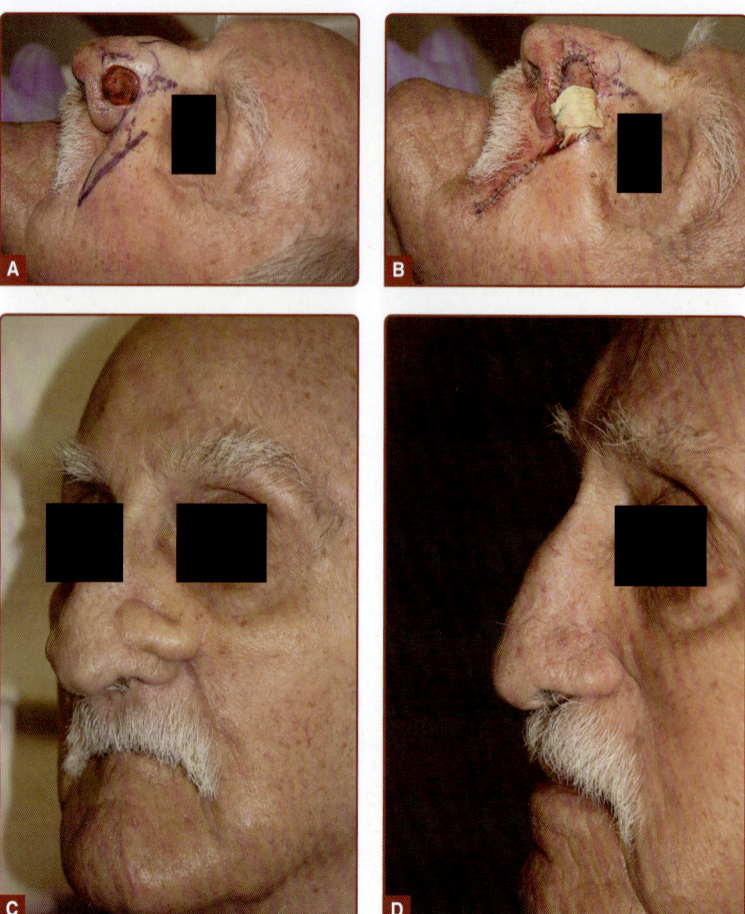

Figure 203-34 **A-D,** Nasolabial interpolation flap. The pedicle is created from excess skin lateral to the nasolabial fold and rotated into the defect. The pedicle is divided and removed approximately 3 weeks after the inset of the flap (c).

divided. The donor site is repaired with a side-to-side closure, resulting in a long linear scar. The superior portion of the defect will be the widest, as it is here that the width of the defect must be accommodated, and thus, generally this portion of the wound is too tight to be closed and is left to heal by secondary intention. The pedicle should be circumferentially wrapped with Vaseline or Xeroform gauze or Surgicel to prevent desiccation.

The second stage takes place 3 weeks subsequently. The pedicle is separated from the brow, the wound edges are freshened, and the donor defect is closed. After the pedicle is separated from the defect, the tissue is further debulked and trimmed, and the remaining edge is secured.

NASOLABIAL INTERPOLATION FLAP

This flap is used to repair complex defects of the ala, particularly in instances when cartilage grafting is also required to restore the structural integrity of the alar rim. The flap is harvested from the medial cheek and nasolabial fold and is based on branches of the angular artery (Fig. 203-34).

The aesthetics of the repair is often improved when the defect is enlarged to include the entire alar lobule. The flap is designed around a pedicle that will be placed at the alar groove, extending as an ellipse that will be easily closed in the nasolabial fold. Through-and-through nasal defects will require the repair of the mucosa, and thus, the width of the flap must take this into account. This myocutaneous flap is dissected from the donor site, rotated downwardly, debulked and trimmed, and secured to the widely undermined defect.

As with the paramedian forehead flap, the pedicle may be wrapped with Vaseline or Xeroform gauze or Surgicel. Three weeks later, the pedicle is separated, the wound edges are freshened, and the donor defect is closed. After the pedicle is separated from the defect, the tissue is further debulked and trimmed, and the remaining edge is secured.

The reverse nasolabial flap, also known as a *Spear's flap*, is employed when the defect involves the entire ala. The motion of this flap is an upward rotation, opposite of the traditional nasolabial interpolation flap.

ABBÉ FLAP

The Abbé flap is also known as the *lip-switch flap* and is reserved for repair of large, deep defects, typically of the upper lip. It is particularly useful for defects that involve up to half of the lip without crossing the midline and those that penetrate into the muscularis. The Abbé flap is harvested from the ipsilateral lower lip and is based on the inferior labial artery. This artery is located deep to or within the orbicularis oris muscle and runs along the mucosal aspect of the vermillion border.[39]

The vermillion border and flap design must be properly marked out. The defect should be full thickness (including muscularis and oral mucosa) and may be enlarged to encompass the total cosmetic unit, which includes the ipsilateral upper cutaneous lip. The flap, also designed to be full-thickness to fill the enlarged defect, is rotated upon a vascular pedicle that makes up the lateral aspect of the flap. The inferior labial artery will be visualized as it is transected at the mobilized (medial) edge of the flap. The pedicle itself should be about 1 cm thick, containing the robust blood supply.

The donor site is undermined and closed first to facilitate the movement of the flap. It should be closed in layers as in the repair of a lip wedge resection: mucosa, muscularis, subcutaneous, then cutaneous. The flap is rotated superiorly and also inset with a layered closure. Careful attention should be given to aligning the vermillion borders at the donor site and defect.

The pedicle of the Abbé flap should not be circumferentially wrapped, but kept moist with occlusive ointment. As with other interpolation flaps, the pedicle will remain in place for at least 3 weeks. During this time, the oral aperture will be significantly distorted, and the patient must be counseled. The pedicle is divided and the final repair takes place, again with careful attention to the placement of the vermillion borders.

RETROAURICULAR FLAP

The retroauricular flap is a 2-staged interpolation flap useful for large defects of the helix. Defects in this location typically involve the perichondrium and are not suitable for grafts. This flap is considered a random flap as it is not based on a large named artery. It is harvested from the richly vascularized skin of the postauricular scalp and is advanced over intervening intact skin to fill the helical defect; the pedicle remains attached to the posterior scalp (Fig. 203-35). The flap should be thinned to match the depth of the defect and carefully sewn into place. The pedicle is circumferentially dressed, and the patient is warned of likely postoperative bleeding and discomfort. The donor site is not repaired until pedicle take-down and often, because of its inconspicuous location, is allowed to heal secondarily.

GRAFTS

Skin grafts are transplanted skin from a donor to recipient site with the goal of closing a surgical defect or wound. They are typically used in reconstruction after removal of a cutaneous malignancy; however, they are also used in the treatment of chronic skin ulcerations, full-thickness burns, epidermolysis bullosa, and vitiligo. Grafts are completely detached from the donor site and receive all nutrients from the wound bed of the recipient site. The 3 basic types of skin grafts are full-thickness skin grafts (FTSG), split-thickness skin grafts (STSG), and composite grafts. FTSGs consist of epidermis with full-thickness dermis and preserved adnexa. STSGs consist of epidermis with partial-thickness dermis with loss of adnexa. Composite grafts are full-thickness skin grafts with cartilage attached to the graft.

Skin grafts are also categorized by their donor origin. These include autografts (donor = recipient), allografts (human to human), and xenografts (animal to human). Autografts are most commonly used in dermatology. Allografts and xenografts serve to protect and debride the wound and stimulate healing. They are commonly used for burn and chronic wounds.

Because the graft is completely separated from its blood source, it is essential for the transferred tissue to develop a new vascular supply from the recipient wound bed.

STAGES OF WOUND HEALING IN GRAFTS

- *Plasma Imbibition:* First 24 hours—plasmatic imbibition or ischemia: the graft affixes to the recipient bed via fibrinous material
- *Inosculation:* 48 to 72 hours—anastomosis and proliferation of preexisting vessels of the graft and recipient wound base
- *Revascularization:* 4 to 7 days—growth and proliferation of vessels from the base. Blood and lymphatic flow begin, leading to the reestablishment of full circulation.
- *Reinnervation:* 2 weeks to 1 year—sensory reinnervation occurs from the periphery to the center of the graft, and may never be fully restored.

Stress on the wound should be avoided to provide the best results. Overstimulation of the patient may lead to increased blood flow to graft site leading to fluid overload and disruption of vascularity. The patient should be advised not to undergo strenuous activity for at least 1 to 2 weeks. Mechanical shear

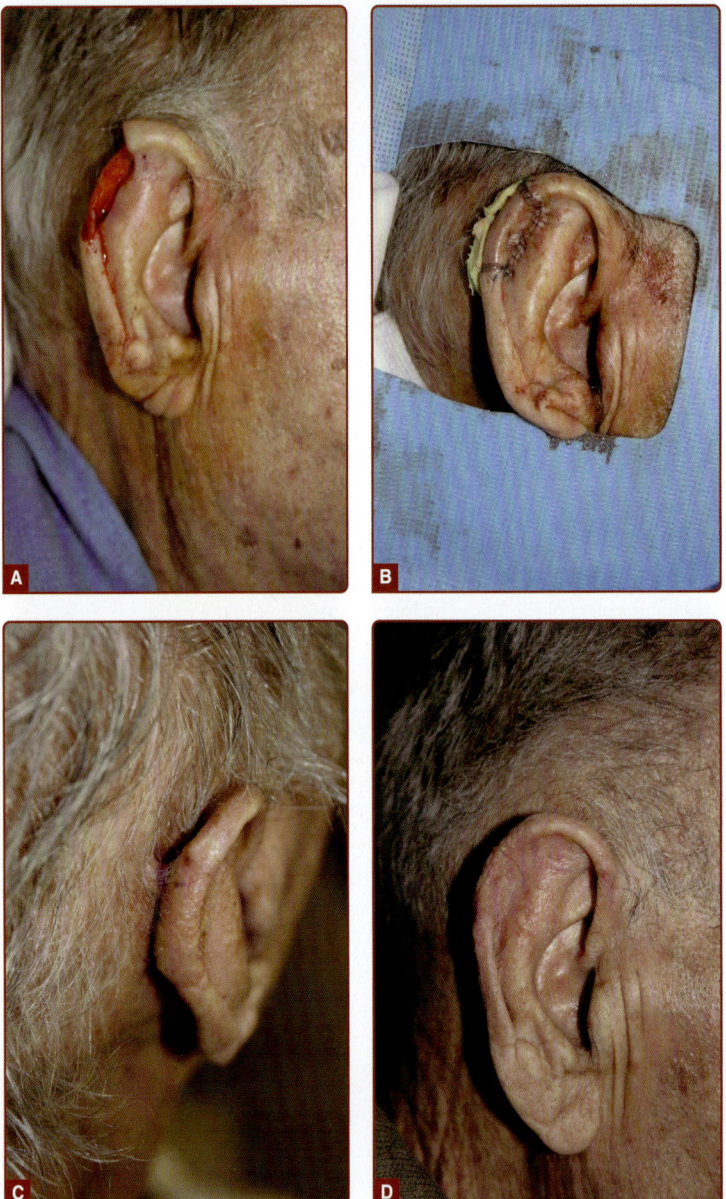

Figure 203-35 **A-D,** Retroauricular pedicle flap. A pedicled flap is developed posterior to the ear in a shape similar to the U-shaped advancement flap. The flap is advanced over the postauricular sulcus and over the auricular cartilage of the helix and sutured into place. The pedicle is divided and set back into place 3 weeks after the inset of the flap (**C**). The area surrounding the postauricular sulcus is allowed to heal in by second intention.

forces, hematoma, seroma, or infection may prevent essential vascular growth and increase the rate of graft failure.

FULL-THICKNESS SKIN GRAFTS

FTSGs are useful for defects in which complex linear closures or a flap would not be suitable, where close monitoring of the site is advisable, and in certain areas where they provide optimal aesthetic reconstruction. When possible, FTSGs are chosen over STSGs because of their similarity in thickness and texture to surrounding skin and their relative lack of significant wound contraction. Because STSGs generally result in a depressed, hypopigmented, scar without normal epidermal texture, they are reserved for larger wounds that cannot be covered with FTSGs. When wounds are too deep for even an FTSG to cover without creating a depression (when the depth of the wound exceeds the thickness of a graft),

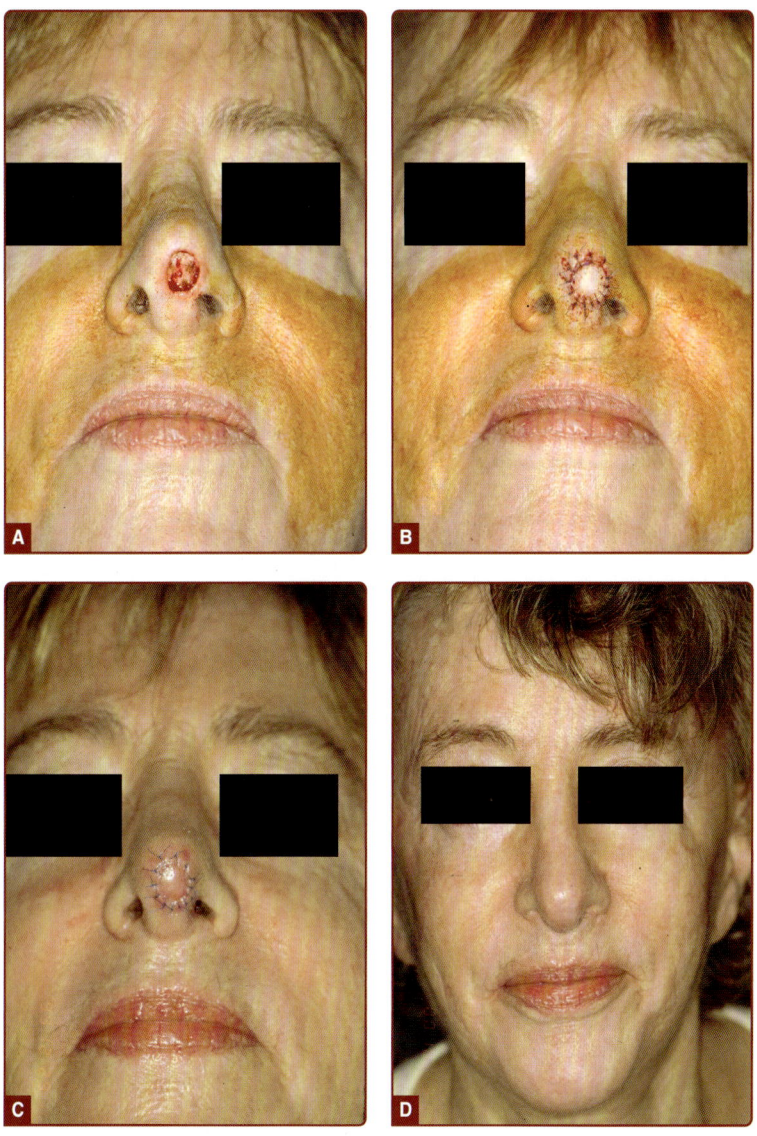

Figure 203-36 **A-D,** Conchal bowl full-thickness skin graft. The graft is harvested from the conchal bowl because, like the skin of the nasal tip and ala, the sebaceous density in the conchal bowl is high. The defect in the conchal bowl is allowed to heal by second intention.

secondary intention healing may be employed for a period of time to build the base of the wound up to the point where an FTSG would completely fill the defect.

FTSGs have essential nutrient requirements and, therefore, should not be placed at a site where the vascular supply is poor. FTSGs will not survive if transplanted directly over bone, cartilage, or tendon.

DETERMINING DONOR SITE

When planning your graft, there are many factors to be taken into consideration. The donor site should be well matched to the skin surrounding the defect in terms of thickness, texture, sun exposure, and adnexal structures.[40] Donor sites can be differentiated by thickness, for example, thin (eyelids, postauricular sulcus), medium thickness (preauricular, conchal, cervical), and thick (supraclavicular, clavicular, nasolabial fold, forehead). However, examining for tissue similarity, such as adnexal structures and sun exposure, is also pertinent.

Common sites for FTSGs for nasal defects include preauricular, postauricular, nasolabial fold, forehead, and conchal bowl skin. Preauricular skin can be used to repair most nasal defects, has similar sun exposure and skin quality, and heals with minimal scar visibility.[41,42] Conchal bowl grafts are particularly well matched for nasal tip and alar defects because of the similarity in texture and concentration of sebaceous glands (Fig. 203-36) as well as the ability to allow the donor site to heal by secondary intention.[43] Nasolabial fold and forehead skin offer excellent matches but leave secondary scars in more visible areas. Common donor sites for larger defects on the scalp and forehead include the supraclavicular region, lateral neck, or inner arm.

HARVESTING

Once the donor site has been established, the graft is harvested. To ascertain the size and shape of the graft needed to fill a given defect, many surgeons will create a template using a nonstick dressing, pressing it against defect. The template is cut out and then traced with a marking pen onto the donor skin. Although some authors have recommended grafts be designed 10% to 20% larger than the defect to accommodate contraction of the graft skin once it is removed,[44] oversizing grafts can lead to unsightly pincushioning. For this reason, the authors size their grafts at or just under the size of the defect. If the donor site is to be closed primarily, an ellipse is planned around the designed graft (see section "Excisional Surgery").

Defatting the graft before securing it to the recipient bed is critical. The subcutaneous tissue is poorly vascularized and, therefore, hinders graft survival. Defatting can be performed with an iris scissors by trimming away the yellow fat to expose the shiny white dermis. If the area being repaired is uneven, thin areas of fat may be left on the graft to more closely approximate the natural contours. Alternatively, at times, it may be necessary to thin the dermis slightly to ensure similar thickness between graft and donor tissue. If this is the case, minimal thinning is recommended to avoid structural damage of adnexae. Once the graft has been prepared, it should be placed in the recipient bed as soon as possible. The recipient bed should have good hemostasis without devitalizing the tissue with overuse of cautery.

Grafts generally need to be trimmed at the edges to ensure a perfect match to the donor site. Survival of the graft is also dependent on the surgical technique during placement. The graft must be manipulated and grasped gently.

Small-caliber nonabsorbable or fast-absorbing cat gut sutures are commonly used for FTSGs on the face. Insertion of sutures should be from graft to recipient tissue to minimize graft movement and best approximate wound edges. It is helpful to place the initial 4 sutures at intervals of approximately 90° from each other to ensure proper placement and to secure the graft. These are followed by interrupted sutures or, at times, running sutures to complete closure. When grafts are large or placed over concave areas, basting sutures help keep good graft to bed contact. This will stabilize the graft and minimize shearing forces. Several authors recommend the use of bolster dressings. Although bolster dressings may assist in prevention of hematomas and seromas, they also compromise vascularity and can increase the risk of necrosis.

For larger defects or those with exposed bone or cartilage at the periphery, a purse-string approach may be introduced. A purse-string suture is placed subdermally along the defect edges, then tightened to advance edges into the defect circumferentially. This technique helps protect exposed tissue as well as reduce the defect size, thereby allowing the surgeon to use a smaller graft.

Sutures should be removed in 1 week for grafts on the face. Healthy grafts are pink in color. Although a purple color indicates relative hypoxia, most grafts with this color will survive. A white color on the surface of a graft generally represents maceration and may do fine when no longer occluded. If the white color is full thickness, it may represent necrosis. Black grafts are necrotic. Gentle wound care without debridement is the best treatment for graft necrosis. The necrotic graft will act as a biologic wound dressing, promote dermal healing, and generally avoid contraction. Antibiotics should also be started to minimize the risk of infection.

BUROW'S/REGIONAL GRAFT

Burow's or regional grafts essentially use the Burow's triangle or dog-ear, often from a partial linear closure, to act as an FTSG (Fig. 203-37). This utilizes removed skin that might otherwise have been thrown away and eliminates the need for removing tissue from a separate donor site. Because these are often local grafts, the tissue match is generally excellent. Since a circular defect has a much larger surface area than a standard triangle taken in an elliptical closure, the triangle must be designed more like that of a V-to-Y advancement flap (island pedicle flap) with a wider and longer body.

SPLIT-THICKNESS SKIN GRAFTS

STSGs are composed of epidermis and partial dermis. Because these grafts are much thinner than FTSGs, they have a less rigorous demand for vascular support and have an increased survivability profile. Unfortunately, because they lack the full thickness of dermis and dermal appendageal structures, STSGs appear more like scar tissue than skin; they are depressed, hypopigmented, and have a shiny texture. They are used to cover large defects unable to be closed by other methods, to allow better wound bed surveillance, to line tubed pedicle flaps, or to resurface mucosa. STSGs are often harvested from the upper inner arm, thigh, or buttock. If small, STSGs may be harvested with a blade by hand. When they are larger, STSGs are harvested with a dermatome, which provides a more precise width and depth. Once the graft is obtained, it is placed in sterile saline on the meshing plate.

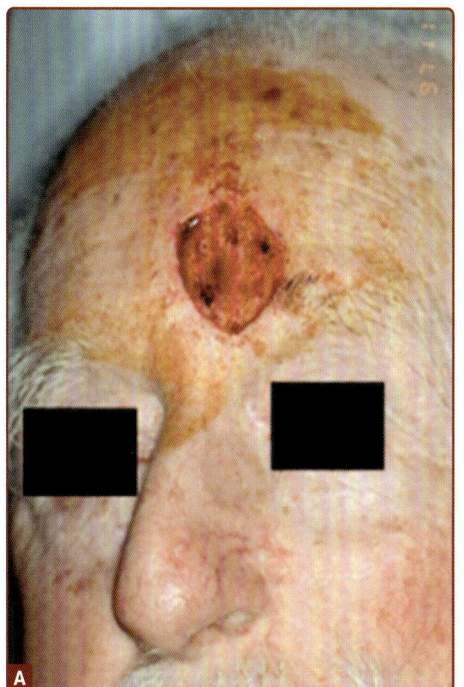
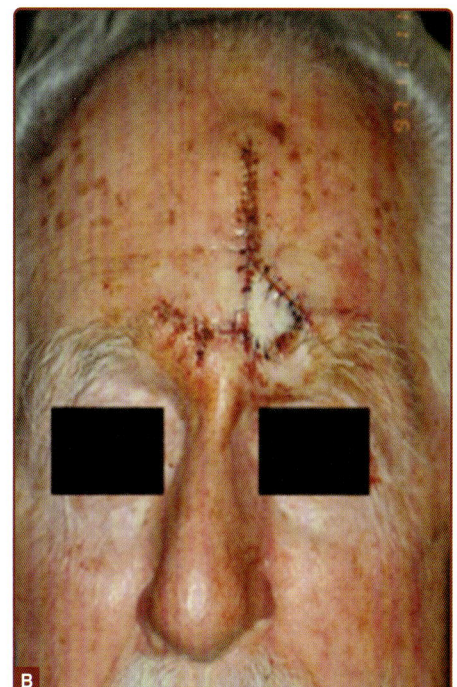
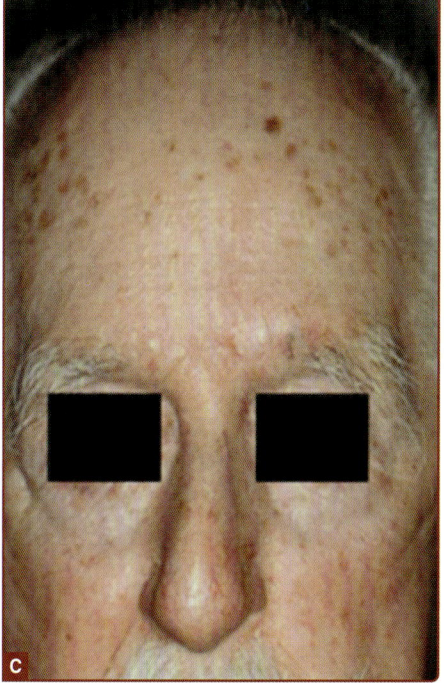

Figure 203-37 **A-C,** Regional full-thickness skin graft. A triangular shape of tissue is removed from adjacent skin and placed in the defect. The graft donor site is closed primarily. The concept is very similar to an island pedicle flap without a vascular pedicle. Another triangular area was also removed from the right glabella of this patient.

Meshing is beneficial because it expands the donor tissue, allows wound exudate to drain preventing seroma and hematoma formation, and has been found to increase graft survival. Increased wound contraction and decreased cosmesis, however, are associated with meshing. After harvesting is complete, STSGs are placed over the defect and secured similarly to FTSG. For larger defects, surgical staples are often used to secure the graft.

STSG size can vary. They are categorized as thin

(0.013-0.033 cm), medium (0.033-0.046 cm), or thick (0.046-0.076 cm). The amount of dermis present determines the chance of survival of the graft on a poor vascular bed. Generally, the thinner the graft, the higher the "take rate" but the poorer cosmesis. The donor site reepithelializes rapidly and relatively painlessly with the use of bio-occlusive dressings.

The main advantage of an STSG is that it survives even in locations with poor vascularization, such as over bone or cartilage. It also allows for early detection of tumor recurrence. Cosmetically, the final outcome of this graft is suboptimal with absent appendages, poor color match, and frequent wound contracture under the graft. For this reason, secondary intention healing and skin substitutes are often employed for defects once covered with STSGs. These methods avoid the wound care and generally unsightly appearance of the STSG harvest site.

PUNCH AND PINCH GRAFTS

A subset of STSGs includes punch and pinch grafts. These are useful for accelerating the healing phase of a chronic ulcer. Several grafts are harvested from a donor site and placed in the wound bed. Instruments used are a 4-mm punch for punch grafts or a scalpel (Weck knife) for pinch grafts. The rate of survival of these grafts is good if the site has meticulous postoperative care; however, the cosmetic outcome is suboptimal because of the variable thickness throughout the wound.

COMPOSITE GRAFTS

Composite grafts consist of 1 or more adjacent tissues, often involving a typical FTSG with underlying cartilage. Small full-thickness defects of the nasal ala and helical rim most commonly require such a graft. Donor sites for composite grafts frequently include the helix and conchal bowl. It is desirable to harvest the graft in a manner that allows the underlying cartilage to extend beyond overlying tissue. This extension allows for the cartilage to insert under the surrounding defect margins. Two small pockets are generally made across from each other at a level below the dermis in the recipient site to accommodate the cartilaginous wings on the composite graft. The cartilage may or may not be sutured, and the remaining FTSG is sutured and secured as described earlier in this section. After being sutured into place, a composite graft with cartilage at its base receives its blood supply from its lateral margins only. Therefore, composite grafts should remain less than 2 cm^2, as a larger graft will not receive sufficient nutrients to allow its central portion to survive.[45] These grafts have the highest metabolic demand and therefore the highest rate of failure. Oral antibiotics against streptococcus and staphylococcus are recommended due to the high bacterial load of the nares.

Pseudomonal coverage is often recommended for grafts performed on the ear.

FREE CARTILAGE GRAFTS

Free cartilage grafts consist of cartilage and perichondrium. They are commonly used to reconstruct defects on free margins such as the nasal tip, nasal ala, ear, and eyelid.[46] This type of graft assists in structural support (eg, prevent nasal valving) and retention of natural facial contours (eg, ala and helical rim). Elastic cartilage from the ear, versus hyaline cartilage from the nose, is the best for recontouring. A strip or disc of cartilage is usually harvested through an incision in the postauricular sulcus or conchal bowl. As is done with a composite graft, the strip of cartilage harvested is slightly longer than the size of the defect and the edges are inserted into pockets made under the dermis. The cartilage is sutured lightly into place with absorbable sutures. The site is then typically closed with a flap. Full-thickness skin grafts may be placed over very thin cartilage struts but as the size of the cartilage increases, the vascular supply to the graft becomes increasingly compromised and decreases graft survival. The addition of cartilage helps with structural support such as preventing collapse of the nasal valves, which results in disruption of air flow. It also helps retain the patient's original facial contours and prevents concavity and/or contraction of the repair.

SKIN SUBSTITUTES

Tissue that has been cultured or processed prior to grafting is known as a *skin substitute*. In addition to postsurgical wounds, they are being used for the treatment of burns and chronic ulcers to augment wound healing. There are 3 main types of skin substitutes: epidermal, dermal, and composite (combination of epidermal and dermal). They can be further categorized as autologous, allogenic, or xenogenic. Cost and shelf-life should be considered when using a skin substitute.[47]

Dermal xenografts, most commonly porcine xenografts, are frequently used in the dermatologic surgery. They are helpful for the repair of large defects, may decrease postoperative pain, and have a long shelf-life.[47] The dressings promote granulation and need minimum post-operative care, therefore are often helpful in elderly or debilitated patients. Dermal allogenic skin substitutes are developed from cadaver skin or neonatal foreskin-harvested allogenic fibroblasts. These are helpful in replacing the dermis in a defect, minimize wound contraction, and can be covered by an STSG. They can be helpful for the treatment of full thickness non-healing ulcers, fasciotomy wounds and other chronic wounds.

Autologous epidermal skin substitutes are derived by culturing the patient's own keratinocytes. These dressings are good for covering a wound and stimulating the healing process. Allogenic epidermal skin substitutes are keratinocytes from human foreskin or cadavers, they provide superficial and temporary coverage.

Composite skin substitutes, are bilayered, containing both epidermis and dermis and are made from allogenic neonatal foreskin-derived fibroblasts and keratinocytes and bovine collagen. They are useful for protection of large wounds where donor tissue is insufficient to cover.

POSTOPERATIVE CARE

Meticulous postoperative wound care is necessary to ensure an optimal outcome. Attention must be made to limit postoperative bleeding of all surgical wounds, particularly flaps and grafts, as hemorrhage or hematoma formation may jeopardize tissue survival and increase the risk of infection. Meticulous intraoperative hemostasis and good postoperative compression dressings are very important in minimizing postoperative bleeding. A pressure dressing should be applied and left intact for 24 to 48 hours. This dressing includes a layer of ointment applied directly to the wound, a nonstick bandage such as Telfa, gauze for pressure, and surgical tape. Finally, elastic dressing materials, such as Flexinet or Coban, may be helpful for wounds on the scalp or extremities.

For the aforementioned procedures, it is important that the wound be kept clean, moist, and covered until suture removal. This will eliminate desiccation and promote reepithelialization, reduce bacterial contamination, and aid in hemostasis. Verbal and written instructions regarding home wound care should be reviewed and then provided in writing to the patient. After removal of the pressure dressing, the wound should be cleaned once or twice daily with attention to gently removing any crust and debris that may form. This is followed by a layer of ointment. A bland, nonmedicated ointment such as petrolatum or aquaphor is preferred over topical antibiotic products such as neomycin. The use of these topical antibiotics following cutaneous surgery increases the risk of contact dermatitis[48] without imparting a significant reduction in infection rates.[49] The patient should be advised to limit activity for 1 to 2 weeks after surgery, particularly, movement that stretches or adds tension to the wound area and may result in wound dehiscence or a widened scar.

The signs and symptoms of hemorrhage and wound infection should be reviewed as early intervention can reduce serious complications. To better prepare patients, it is helpful to educate him or her about what to expect during normal wound healing. The patient should be provided with the physician's contact information and should be encouraged to call with any questions or concerns.

COMPLICATIONS OF DERMATOLOGIC SURGERY

Early complications of all forms of cutaneous surgery and closure are bleeding, pain, and infection. Bleeding typically occurs in the first 24 hours after surgery and must be addressed promptly. Low-flow ooze may be treated by compression. Patients should be instructed to apply direct pressure for at least 20 minutes without peeking to see if it is working. Frank arterial hemorrhage or large hematoma formation will require partial or complete suture removal, evacuation of clot, and exploration of the wound to allow visualization and closure of the bleeding vessel. Patients should be instructed to call if they see an enlarging mass below or around the wound.

Pain is usually manageable with nonnarcotic pain relievers such as acetaminophen. Acetaminophen may be administered at the time of surgery and continued for 24 hours to reduce the risk of postoperative discomfort. It is generally easier to get ahead of pain than it is to catch up to it. Patients should be instructed to avoid nonprescribed nonsteroidal anti-inflammatory medication for up to 48 hours postoperatively to reduce bruising and bleeding from platelet dysfunction. Although more severe pain may require the administration of prescription pain medication, it should be investigated to be sure more significant issues such as infection or hematoma are not occurring.

Signs of infection usually will occur within the first week after surgery and include increased pain, erythema, and heat around the wound, purulent and sometimes foul-smelling drainage, and fever. When wound infection is suspected, a culture must be obtained for pathogen identification and antibiotic susceptibility, and treatment with a broad-spectrum antibiotic should be initiated. Common pathogens on skin and mucosal surfaces are gram-positive cocci, notably staphylococci or, less commonly, streptococci. However, gram-negative aerobes and anaerobic bacteria contaminate skin in the groin/perineal areas. Gram-negative bacilli also may be cultured from ear and lower leg wounds, particularly in diabetic patients. Methicillin-resistant *Staphylococcus aureus* (MRSA) infections are increasing dramatically in frequency and should be vigilantly watched for.[50]

An expected consequence of surgery is the formation of a scar. Although the goal of reconstructive surgery is to minimize the appearance of the resultant scar, at times they may widen, or even become hypertrophic. With time, hypertrophic scars tend to flatten and soften. Their course may be hastened with the administration of intralesional steroids or 5-fluorouracil and a variety of fractional and vascular laser devices. In areas under tension and/or motion, such as the upper back and arms over the deltoids, scars may spread or become atrophic. Although scar spread may become less noticeable with time as the initial dark pink color fades, the width generally does not change significantly. Erythema and telangiectasia often form around scars during the healing phase and may persist for extended periods of time. Highly vascular areas (rosacea) and those under high tension are more likely to develop persistent erythema and telangiectasia. This can be effectively treated with lasers, such as the pulsed dye laser, KTP, or intense pulsed light.

Spitting sutures or suture granulomas from buried sutures may occur. Placing the buried dermal sutures in the appropriate plane will help minimize the occurrence. If the spitting suture becomes visible it may be trimmed out, but it is unadvisable to aggressively go after these as a scar may result.

In the case of a flap repair, additional complications may be encountered. In the early postoperative period, partial or complete flap necrosis may occur. This may be due to inadequate blood supply from the wound bed, which is more commonly encountered in smokers, or when an underlying hematoma is present. Flap design may also lead to vascular compromise and flap necrosis, as when the pedicle is too narrow to support the mass of the flap, when there is too much torque, or when there is too much tension at the flap's leading edge. Areas of partial necrosis will heal secondarily and may lead to a less appealing scar, which can be revised after wound healing is complete. Later in the postoperative period, a trapdoor deformity may occur in which the center of the flap becomes elevated and the suture line becomes depressed. It may resolve spontaneously over a period of 6–12 months. However, if the trapdoor effect or pin-cushioning persists, it may respond to intralesional steroids, 5-fluorouracil, flap elevation with flap thinning, and/or fractional ablative lasers or dermabrasion. The risk of forming a trapdoor may be minimized with wide undermining around the primary defect, proper thinning and sizing of the flap, and the use of a sharp geometric shape for the flap (not rounded edges).

Complications of grafting include graft failure in the early postoperative period and results from inadequate nutrient supply to the tissue. This is often due to poor vascular health of the wound bed as encountered in smokers or diabetics, inadvertent shearing forces or trauma to the graft, hematoma or seroma formation, or infection. Later complications typically are attributed to the cosmetic appearance of the graft, usually related to mismatch of thickness, color, or texture. If the cosmetic result is unsatisfactory, fractional ablative or nonablative treatment or dermabrasion may be considered 6 to 12 weeks after graft placement. Contraction may be considerable, particularly with thinner grafts, which may result in the distortion of free margins.

MONITORING AND FOLLOWUP

If nonabsorbable epidermal sutures are placed, the patient should return for suture removal at the appointed time. If the defect has been left to heal secondarily, the wound should be checked in approximately 4 weeks. The surgical site should then again be evaluated 3 to 4 months postoperatively to ensure wound healing is progressing as expected. Patients who have been treated for malignancy should be counseled regarding proper followup for full skin examination to monitor for new or recurrent skin cancers.

ACKNOWLEDGMENTS

We would like to thank Melanie Kingsley, MD, for her help and contributions with earlier versions of this chapter.

REFERENCES

1. Goldberg LH, Alam M. Elliptical excisions: variations and the eccentric parallelogram. *Arch Dermatol*. 2004; 140:176-180.
2. Brodland DG, Zitelli JA. Surgical margins for excision of primary cutaneous squamous cell carcinoma. *J Am Acad Dermatol*. 1992;27:241-248.
3. Sobanko JF. Optimizing design and execution of linear reconstructions on the face. *Dermatol Surg*. 2015; 41(suppl 10):S216-S228.
4. Borgstrom S, Sandblom P. Suture technic and wound healing; an investigation based on animal experiments. *Ann Surg*. 1956;144:982-990.
5. Chow S, Bennett RG. Superficial head and neck anatomy for dermatologic surgery: critical concepts. *Dermatol Surg*. 2015;41(suppl 10):S169-S177.
6. Moody BR, McCarthy JE, Sengelmann RD. The apical angle: a mathematical analysis of the ellipse. *Dermatol Surg*. 2001;27:61-63.
7. Boyer JD, Zitelli JA, Brodland DG. Undermining in cutaneous surgery. *Dermatol Surg*. 2001;27:75-78.
8. Chen DL, Carlson EO, Fathi R, et al. Undermining and hemostasis. *Dermatol Surg*. 2015;41(suppl 10): S201-S215.
9. Harris DR. Healing of the surgical wound. I. Basic considerations. *J Am Acad Dermatol*. 1979;1:197-207.
10. Zitelli JA, Moy RL. Buried vertical mattress suture. *J Dermatol Surg Oncol*. 1989;15:17-19.
11. Wong NL. Review of continuous sutures in dermatologic surgery. *J Dermatol Surg Oncol*. 1993;19:923-931.
12. Guyuron B, Vaughan C. A comparison of absorbable and nonabsorbable suture materials for skin repair. *Plast Reconstr Surg*. 1992;89:234-236.
13. Alam M, Posten W, Martini MC, et al. Aesthetic and functional efficacy of subcuticular running epidermal closures of the trunk and extremity: a rater-blinded randomized control trial. *Arch Dermatol*. 2006; 142:1272-1278.
14. Speer DP. The influence of suture technique on early wound healing. *J Surg Res*. 1979;27:385-391.
15. Zitelli JA. Wound healing by secondary intention. A cosmetic appraisal. *J Am Acad Dermatol*. 1983;9: 407-415.
16. Mott KJ, Clark DP, Stelljes LS. Regional variation in wound contraction of Mohs surgery defects allowed to heal by second intention. *Dermatol Surg*. 2003; 29:712-722.

17. Lam TK, Lowe C, Johnson R, et al. Secondary intention healing and purse-string closures. *Dermatol Surg*. 2015; 41(suppl 10):S178-S186.
18. Milton SH. Pedicled skin-flaps: the fallacy of the length: width ratio. *Br J Surg*. 1970;57:502-508.
19. Daniel RK, Williams HB. The free transfer of skin flaps by microvascular anastomoses. An experimental study and a reappraisal. *Plast Reconstr Surg*. 1973;52: 16-31.
20. Stell PM. The pig as an experimental model for skin flap behaviour: a reappraisal of previous studies. *Br J Plast Surg*. 1977;30:1-8.
21. Heniford BW, Bailin PL, Marsico RE. Field guide to local flaps. *Dermatol Clin*. 1998;16:65-74.
22. Dzubow LM. Flap dynamics. *J Dermatol Surg Oncol*. 1991;17:116-130.
23. Kruter L, Rohrer T. Advancement flaps. *Dermatol Surg*. 2015;41(suppl 10):S239-S246.
24. Antia NH, Buch VI. Chondrocutaneous advancement flap for the marginal defect of the ear. *Plast Reconstr Surg*. 1967;39:472-477.
25. Mellette JR, Harrington AC. Applications of the crescentic advancement flap. *J Dermatol Surg Oncol*. 1991; 17:447-454.
26. Tomich JM, Wentzell JM, Grande DJ. Subcutaneous island pedicle flaps. *Arch Dermatol*. 1987;123: 514-518.
27. Goldberg LH, Alam M. Horizontal advancement flap for symmetric reconstruction of small to medium-sized cutaneous defects of the lateral nasal supratip. *J Am Acad Dermatol*. 2003;49:685-689.
28. Onishi K, Okada E, Hirata A. The Rintala flap: a versatile procedure for nasal reconstruction. *Am J Otolaryngol*. 2014;35:577-581.
29. Dzubow LM. The dynamics of flap movement: effect of pivotal restraint on flap rotation and transposition. *J Dermatol Surg Oncol*. 1987;13:1348-1353.
30. Rieger RA. A local flap for repair of the nasal tip. *Plast Reconstr Surg*. 1967;40:147-149.
31. Subramanian N. Reconstructions of eyelid defects. *Indian J Plast Surg*. 2011;44:5-13.
32. LoPiccolo MC. Rotation flaps—principles and locations. *Dermatol Surg*. 2015;41(suppl 10):S247-S254.
33. Humphreys TR. Use of the "spiral" flap for closure of small defects of the nasal ala. *Dermatol Surg*. 2001; 27:409-410.
34. Limberg AA. Design of local flaps. *Mod Trends Plast Surg*. 1966;2:38-61.
35. Bray DA. Clinical applications of the rhomboid flap. *Arch Otolaryngol*. 1983;109:37-42.
36. Masson JK, Mendelson BC. The banner flap. *Am J Surg*. 1977;134:419-423.
37. Zitelli JA. The bilobed flap for nasal reconstruction. *Arch Dermatol*. 1989;125:957-959.
38. Hove CR, Williams EF, Rodgers BJ. Z-plasty: a concise review. *Facial Plast Surg*. 2001;17:289-294.
39. Schulte DL, Sherris DA, Kasperbauer JL. The anatomical basis of the Abbé flap. *Laryngoscope*. 2001; 111:382-386.
40. Ratner D. Skin grafting. *Semin Cutan Med Surg*. 2003; 22:295-305.
41. Breach NM. Pre-auricular full-thickness skin grafts. *Br J Plast Surg*. 1978;31:124-126.
42. Corwin TR, Klein AW, Habal MB. The aesthetics of the preauricular graft in facial reconstruction. *Ann Plast Surg*. 1982;9:312-315.
43. Rohrer TE, Dzubow LM. Conchal bowl skin grafting in nasal tip reconstruction: clinical and histologic evaluation. *J Am Acad Dermatol*. 1995;33:476-481.
44. Hill TG. Contouring of donor skin in full-thickness skin grafting. *J Dermatol Surg Oncol*. 1987;13:883-888.
45. Konior RJ. Free composite grafts. *Otolaryngol Clin North Am*. 1994;27:81-90.
46. Adams C, Ratner D. Composite and free cartilage grafting. *Dermatol Clin*. 2005;23:129-140, vii.
47. Cronin H, Goldstein G. Biologic skin substitutes and their applications in dermatology. *Dermatol Surg*. 2013; 39:30-34.
48. Gette MT, Marks JG, Maloney ME. Frequency of postoperative allergic contact dermatitis to topical antibiotics. *Arch Dermatol*. 1992;128:365-367.
49. Smack DP, Harrington AC, Dunn C, et al. Infection and allergy incidence in ambulatory surgery patients using white petrolatum vs bacitracin ointment. A randomized controlled trial. *JAMA*. 1996;276:972-977.
50. Cruse PJ, Foord R. The epidemiology of wound infection. A 10-year prospective study of 62,939 wounds. *Surg Clin North Am*. 1980;60:27-40.

Chapter 204 :: Mohs Micrographic Surgery
:: Sean R. Christensen & David J. Leffell

第二百零四章

莫氏显微外科

中文导读

莫氏显微外科手术（Mohs），是皮肤外科常用术种之一，具有治愈率高，能最大程度地保留正常组织的优势，已成为治疗高危非黑素瘤性皮肤癌的标准治疗，目前在黑素瘤中的应用也不断增加。本章共分为7节：①手术介绍；②手术流程；③手术适应证；④手术后皮肤重建；⑤术后不良反应；⑥非黑色素瘤皮肤癌的手术治疗；⑦总结。全面介绍了莫氏显微外科手术在皮肤科的应用以及治疗机制。

第一节介绍了莫氏手术的限制因素、历史和手术当前在美国的使用率及适应证，并提及在今天，被称为莫氏显微外科的技术被用于治疗美国大约五分之一的皮肤癌。

第二节详细介绍了莫氏手术的整个手术流程，将莫氏手术和常规切除手术进行对比，并强调手术医师和病理医师联手合作的重要性。作者首先将莫氏手术和常规切除手术进行对比，并强调莫氏手术的基本优势是对整个手术切缘进行显微分析，这是标准的切除和病理处理无法完成的。

第三节提出了莫氏手术的适应证，包括基底细胞癌、鳞状细胞癌、黑素瘤、其他皮肤细胞癌（隆突性纤维肉瘤、大汗腺和外分泌癌、平滑肌肉瘤、默克尔细胞癌、黏液癌和其他罕见的皮肤恶性肿瘤）。

第四节提出莫氏手术造成的缺损可能特别适合在不重建的情况下愈合，因为该手术通常会产生浅深度的伤口，这可能有助于二次愈合。强调莫氏手术最大限度地保存正常的非癌组织有助于肿瘤切除后创面的愈合。在适当选择的患者中，二次修复莫氏手术缺损可使患者满意，相当于一次手术修复。然后作者提及术后重建的重要性，随着冷冻切片取代原位化学固定和莫氏手术成为鼻子、嘴唇和眼睑等解剖敏感部位的标准护理，使用整形和美容外科技术进行重建已成为该技术不可或缺的一部分。

第五节用数据证实Mohs手术是一种非常安全的手术，并发症发生率很低。最常见的不良事件是感染、伤口愈合不良（包括裂开和坏死）以及术后出血或血肿。老年患者、心脏疾病患者、接受抗凝治疗患者并不是莫氏手术禁忌证的对象。

第六节介绍了莫氏手术被广泛应用于非黑色素瘤皮肤癌的治疗，已被证明是最有效的皮肤癌根治方法。

第七节总结了莫氏手术是皮肤癌切除的一种特殊形式，它依赖于分期切除，并立即对整个深部和外围手术边缘进行组织病理学检查。最常用于治疗基底细胞癌和鳞状细胞癌患者，并已被证明优于其他形式的癌症治疗。

〔赵 爽〕

AT-A-GLANCE

- Mohs micrographic surgery is a specialized form of skin cancer excision in which one physician functions as surgeon and pathologist, verifying surgical margins intraoperatively in successive stages.
- Mohs surgery achieves the highest cure rate and is the treatment of choice for basal cell and squamous cell carcinoma with high risk of recurrence or progression and for tumors in anatomic areas where tissue sparing is critical.
- Mohs surgery may also be used for treatment of melanoma in situ and other skin cancers in which pathologic margins can be verified on frozen sections.
- Mohs surgery optimizes functional and cosmetic outcomes after skin cancer removal, has a low rate of postoperative complications, and is highly cost-effective for appropriately selected tumors.

INTRODUCTION AND BACKGROUND

Complete surgical removal is the cornerstone of therapy for solid tumors. This is particularly true for nonmelanoma skin cancers, which have a low risk of metastasis. Complete surgical removal may be difficult to achieve, however, for skin cancers with extensive subclinical spread and for lesions adjacent to vital structures such as the eye. Staged excision or intraoperative pathologic examination of margin status have been used to help ensure adequate surgical margins, but these techniques are limited by logistical hurdles in coordination and communication between the surgeon and pathologist, the inability to precisely map areas of positive margins in three dimensional space, and the inherent limitation of standard pathologic specimen processing, which only examines a small, noncontiguous fraction of the surgical margin. In the 1930s and 1940s, Dr. Frederic Mohs developed a novel method of skin cancer excision using zinc chloride paste to chemically fix the tissue in situ on the patient followed by staged excision with rapid pathologic examination of the surgical margins by the operating physician.[1] The procedure was originally named *chemosurgery* because of the use of a chemical fixative (chemotherapy was not used). In his seminal report, Dr. Mohs reported an overall cure rate of 93% in 425 cases of nonmelanoma skin cancer, many of which were advanced lesions not amenable to standard surgical excision.

In the 1970s and 1980s, the use of chemical fixative was gradually replaced with frozen section analysis of unfixed (fresh) tissue, which allowed the procedure to be completed in hours rather than days. Application of the technique grew rapidly in subsequent years, as the superiority of the procedure over other forms of treatment was established in the peer-reviewed medical literature. Today, the technique known as Mohs micrographic surgery (MMS) is used for treatment of approximately one in five skin cancers in the United States.[2] It is the standard of care for basal cell carcinoma (BCC) and squamous cell carcinoma (SCC) with a high risk of recurrence or in sensitive anatomic locations or where clinical margins are difficult to ascertain. It is routinely indicated for treatment of other cutaneous malignancy as well. The inherent advantages of complete microscopic surgical margin analysis and precise tumor mapping allow for the highest possible cure rate while maximizing tissue preservation and optimizing cosmetic and functional outcomes. Additionally, because MMS is an office-based procedure, the high cost of hospital-based or ambulatory surgery center treatment is avoided, and patient satisfaction is enhanced.

OPERATIVE TECHNIQUE

The fundamental advantage of MMS is the microscopic analysis of the complete surgical margin, which cannot be accomplished with standard excision and pathologic processing. The thoroughness of the Mohs method is facilitated by the use of tangential, or beveled, excision. With standard excision, the skin is incised with the scalpel blade held perpendicular to the skin, creating a right angle between the peripheral and deep margin (Fig. 204-1A). Although this facilitates optimal wound closure, it prevents histopathologic analysis of the deep and peripheral margins in the same plane. In contrast, with the Mohs technique, incision of the skin is made at a 45-degree angle, creating a beveled, or sloping, surface to the excised specimen (Fig. 204-1B). After tissue is excised with a beveled edge, it is processed for histopathologic analysis with en face sections that are cut parallel to the surgical margin. This is another critical difference from standard excision, in which the excised specimen is most often sectioned perpendicular to the surgical margins in a "bread-loaf" fashion. Perpendicular sections allow for histopathologic examination of the central bulk of the tumor but cannot practically examine the entire surgical margin because each section only visualizes a few micrometers of margin length. Thousands of sections would be required to examine a few centimeters of surgical margin in its entirety, and thus representative sections are often examined at intervals of 1 to 2 mm. This results in examination of less than 1% to 3% of the length of the surgical margin. For many skin cancers with irregular subclinical extension, areas of malignancy may be missed on representative sections, resulting in false-negative margins and potential tumor recurrence (Fig. 204-2A). Beveled excision coupled with en face sections in Mohs surgery examines the entire deep and peripheral surgical margin in a single plane, permitting detection of focal areas of tumor extension as small as a few malignant cells (Fig. 204-2B). This difference is clinically relevant because perpendicular

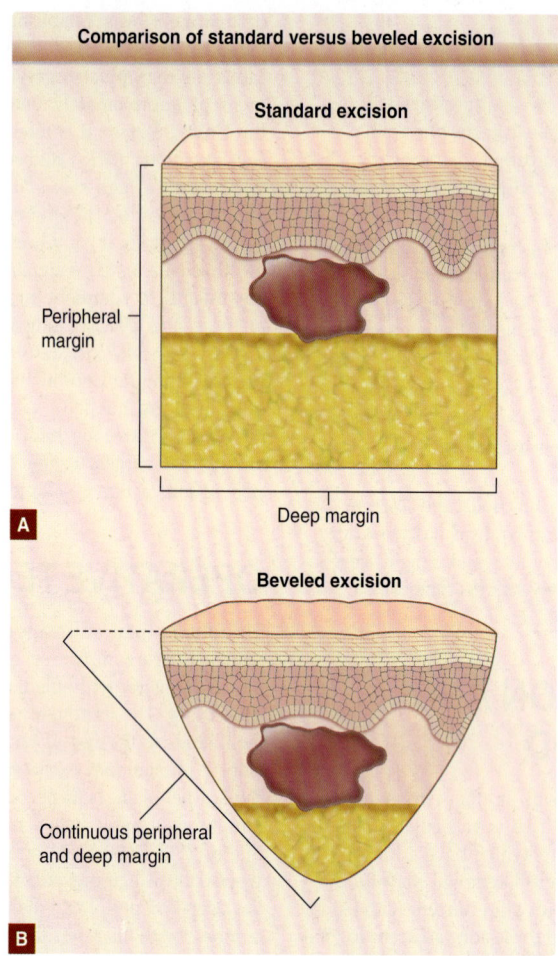

Figure 204-1 Comparison of standard versus beveled excision. **A,** With standard surgical excision, the incision is made perpendicular to the skin surface with a 90-degree angle between the peripheral and the deep margin. **B,** With beveled excision, the incision is made at a 45-degree angle with the skin surface, creating a continuous peripheral and deep margin on the same plane.

sections at intervals of 1 mm may miss up to 42% of irregular tumor extensions.³

MMS, like every surgical procedure, begins with a consultation between the surgeon and the patient. This allows the surgeon to confirm the pathologic diagnosis of skin cancer before surgery, examine the patient to evaluate tumor location and size, and assess for signs or symptoms of extensive subclinical extension such as paresthesia or motor nerve dysfunction. If there is uncertainty about the pathologic diagnosis (eg, from an inconclusive biopsy) or if malignant invasion of critical deep structures is suspected, further evaluation may be warranted before surgery. The patient must also be informed of the likely extent of the cancer, the implications for function and cosmesis, expectations for wound healing, and other associated risks and benefits of the procedure. After informed consent has been documented, the procedure can be scheduled or initiated.

Mohs surgery is almost universally performed as an office-based procedure under local anesthesia. Facility requirements include treatment rooms equipped to ensure patient comfort, optimal tissue excision, hemostasis, and reconstruction. The on-site histology laboratory for processing, sectioning, and staining the surgical specimens is a fundamental requirement of the Mohs technique. In addition to the surgeon, who also functions as the pathologist in reading intraoperative histopathology specimens, the procedure requires trained nursing staff and a histotechnician experienced in processing frozen sections. Because the procedure relies on accurate interpretation of histopathologic margin status, optimal histologic processing with robust quality control is essential.

The Mohs procedure commences with accurate identification of the lesion to be treated (Fig. 204-3A) and confirmation of the site by the patient using a mirror. Photographic records from the time of the diagnostic biopsy may be extremely helpful in cases of patient uncertainty or when wound healing and the passage of time have obscured the precise location of

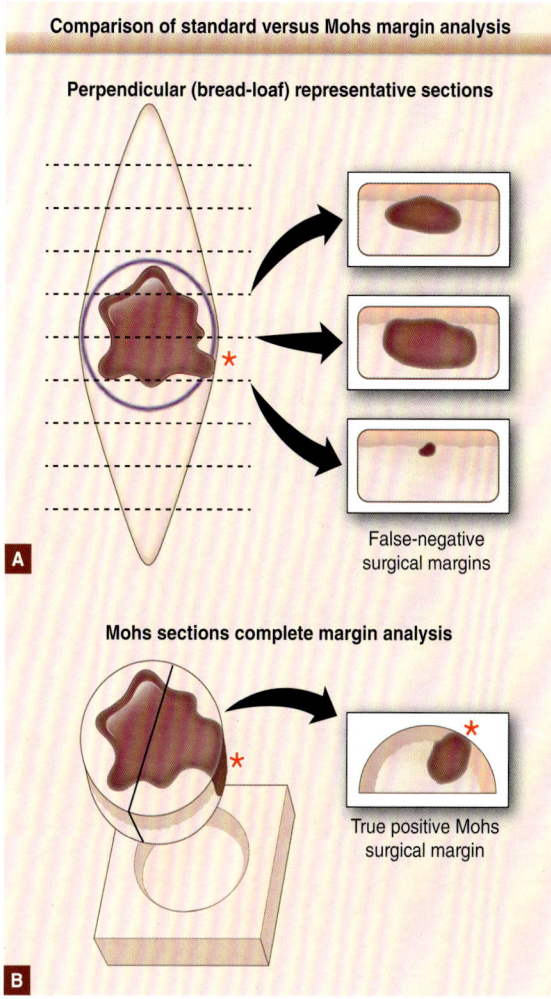

Figure 204-2 Complete margin analysis with Mohs surgical technique. **A,** With typical perpendicular or "bread-loaf" sections, representative cross sections, indicated by dashed lines, are examined at regular intervals along the excised tissue. Arrows indicate histopathologic visualization of tumor (red) with apparently clear margins in these sections. An irregular projection of tumor (*red asterisk*) at the margin is not detected in between these sections. **B,** In Mohs surgery, beveled excision specimens are examined with en face sections, permitting visualization of the entire deep and peripheral margin and identification of any tumor projections at the surgical margin (*red asterisk*). By definition, any tumor visible with en face sections is present at the surgical margin.

the lesion. The patient is then positioned on the surgical table and the site is infiltrated with local anesthetic. The grossly visible tumor is debulked by curettage or blade if appropriate. The tendency of the semi-sharp curette to dislodge friable tumor aggregates while sparing normal skin helps to define the deep and lateral extent of the tumor. The skin lesion is then excised with a 1- to 2-mm margin around the curettage area, taking care to excise the tissue with a beveled edge at a level deep enough to ensure an adequate margin below the initial curettage (Fig. 204-3B). This may be at the intradermal, subcutaneous, muscular, or fascial layer, depending on the nature of the cancer and the anatomic site. Before removing the lesion, one or more score marks may be placed across the specimen and onto the surrounding skin to serve as anatomic markers for subsequent stages. Hemostasis is then obtained, a temporary bandage is placed over the wound, and the ambulatory patient waits in a comfortable waiting room while the specimens are processed for histopathologic examination.

The excised tissue from the first stage is transported by hand to the adjacent histology laboratory. The tissue is divided into appropriately sized specimens using the score marks made at the time of excision. The anatomic orientation relative to surrounding landmarks on the patient is preserved, each piece is marked with at least two colors of indelible ink (to designate laterality or sidedness), and a "map" is drawn to represent the specimen and precisely locate any areas of positive margins (Fig. 204-3C). The tissue is frozen, mounted, and sectioned by the technician with en face sections such

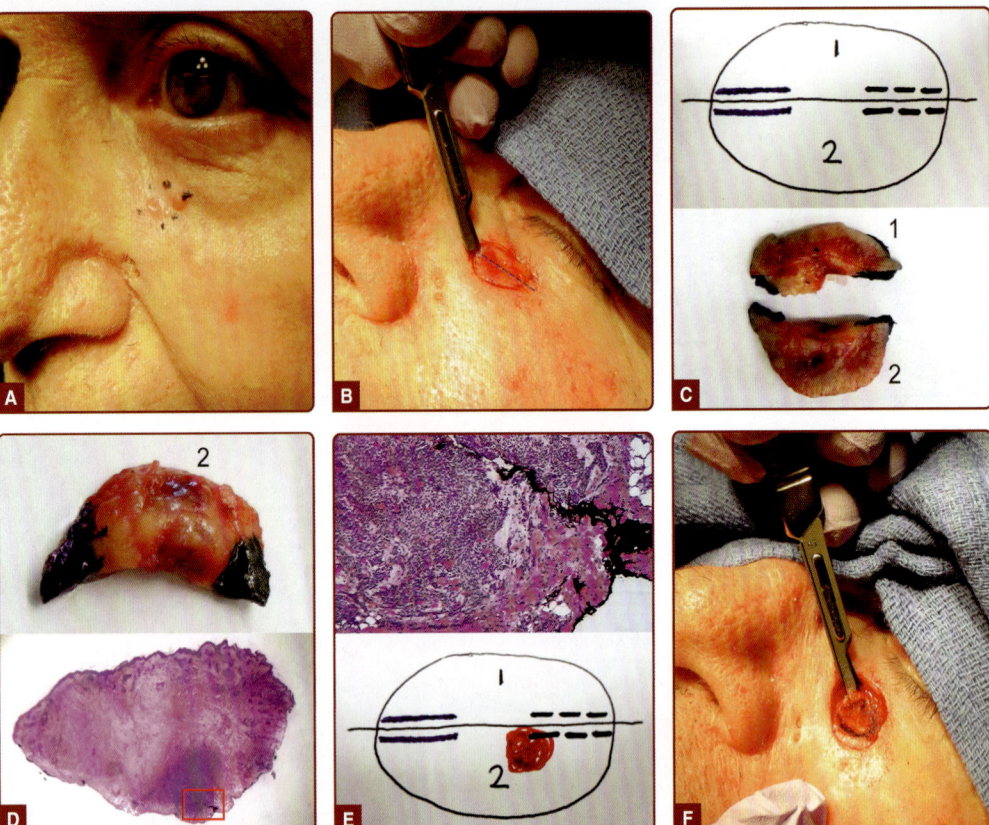

Figure 204-3 Mohs surgery procedure. **A,** A biopsy-confirmed basal cell carcinoma (BCC) is identified and marked on the left cheek overlying the inferior orbital rim. **B,** After curettage to remove gross carcinoma and define the clinical margins, the lesion is excised in the first stage with a narrow margin and a beveled edge, holding the scalpel at a 45-degree angle to the skin surface. A score mark (blue dashed line) is made on the excised specimen and extended onto the surrounding skin to preserve anatomic orientation. **C,** A map is drawn of the excised tissue (upper panel) and the specimen, shown with the epidermal surface facing up, is bisected along the score mark (lower panel). Indelible ink is used to mark the marginal surface blue on the left and black on the right. **D,** Piece 2 is shown flipped over with the deep marginal surface facing up, revealing the blue and black indelible ink (upper panel). Histopathologic sections are cut from the marginal surface and stained with hematoxylin and eosin (lower panel), revealing the epidermal peripheral margin and the subcutaneous deep margin in a single plane. The red box at the deep margin is shown at higher magnification in panel E. **E,** Higher magnification reveals persistent BCC at the deep margin near the black ink (upper panel). The area of carcinoma at the margins is marked on the map in red (lower panel). **F,** The area of residual carcinoma is excised in a second stage, again with a beveled edge to allow complete margin examination. This process is repeated until clear margins are obtained.

that the peripheral and deep margin are visualized on the histopathologic slides (Fig. 204-3D). The slides are then stained, often with standard hematoxylin and eosin stains. Inspection of the slides prepared in this fashion reveals the true surgical margin, and any areas of carcinoma that are noted represent tumor extension to the margin. If present, these areas of persistent malignancy in stage 1 are marked in their precise location on the map in relation to the inked edges (Fig. 204-3E).

If carcinoma is detected at the microscopically examined surgical margins, the patient is returned to the procedure room for ongoing staged excision. The fact that the Mohs surgeon functions as the pathologist in detecting and mapping any areas of positive surgical margins ensures the most focused and precise reexcision when subsequent stages are necessary. These subsequent stages are generally incised with a beveled edge to facilitate complete margin examination and may involve excision of epidermis and dermis from the peripheral margin; subcutis, muscle, fascia, or cartilage from the deep margin; or a combination of these depending on the location and extent of residual tumor (Fig. 204-3F). Subsequent stages are inked, mapped, processed, sectioned, and stained as described earlier, and the surgical margin is again examined microscopically by the surgeon. This iterative process continues until the surgical margins are free of carcinoma and a tumor-free plane has been achieved. When all surgical margins are clear, the patient is evaluated for consideration of immediate surgical repair or healing of the defect by second intent.

The staged nature of Mohs surgery allows optimal flexibility in surgical treatment. Because no a priori assumptions are made about required surgical margins, small lesions can be treated with a minimal surgical defect, and highly invasive lesions, even if not grossly evident, can be completely excised over multiple stages. In general, each stage takes 20 to 45 minutes to process in our laboratory; about half of patients achieve clear margins after a single stage, and approximately 90% are clear after two stages.[4] Skin cancers requiring four to six stages are uncommon. It is important to note that the Mohs technique does not examine the central portion of an excised tumor. In selected cases when additional information about histopathologic risk factors such as perineural invasion or poor differentiation is required, the frozen tissue can be thawed and submitted for standard perpendicular section processing through the bulk of the tumor. For the majority of BCCs and SCCs treated with Mohs surgery, this additional pathologic examination is not necessary.

INDICATIONS FOR MOHS SURGERY

BASAL CELL CARCINOMA

BCC is the most common human malignancy, with more than 2 million cases per year in the United States.[5] Although BCC rarely leads to metastasis or death, it can be highly destructive and result in significant morbidity and functional impairment. Given the disproportionate incidence of BCC on anatomically sensitive sites such as the nose, ears, and periocular skin, Mohs surgery has been performed for BCC more than any other skin cancer. Mohs surgery is particularly beneficial for facial BCC because of the tendency of this malignancy to exhibit subclinical extension (Fig. 204-4). Several risk factors have been identified to predict microscopic tumor extension beyond the grossly visible margin of the tumor, including poorly defined clinical margins; diameter greater than 2 cm; and location on the high-risk, or "H" zone of the face, encompassing the nose, eyelids, eyebrows, temples, lips, ear, and periauricular skin.[6-8] Histologic subtype of BCC is also a critical determinant of subclinical extension. Although most nodular BCC are completely excised with surgical margins of 4 mm, infiltrative and micronodular subtypes, when excised with the Mohs technique, were found to require surgical margins of 5 to 10 mm for complete clearance and were more likely to require excision of underlying muscle, cartilage, and periosteum.[9,10]

As it became clear that Mohs surgery could offer superior treatment outcomes for high-risk BCC, systematic studies of the procedure focused on this subgroup of tumors. Dr. Mohs himself published the largest series of cases of BCC of the eyelids: among 1124 primary BCC and 290 recurrent BCC with 5-year follow-up, the cure rates after Mohs surgery were an exceptional 99.4% and 92.4%, respectively.[11]

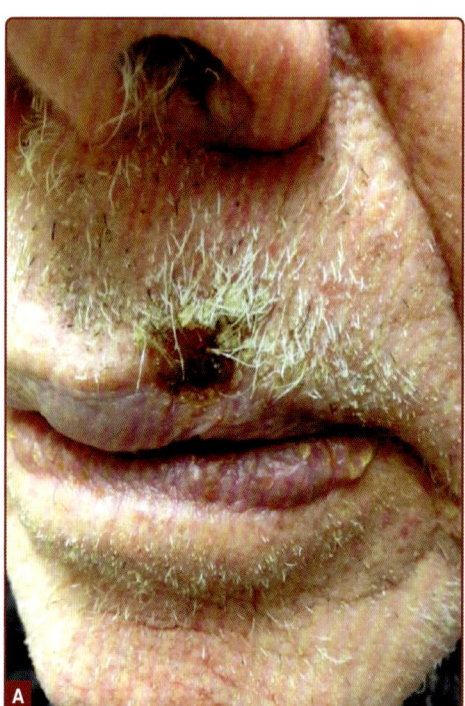 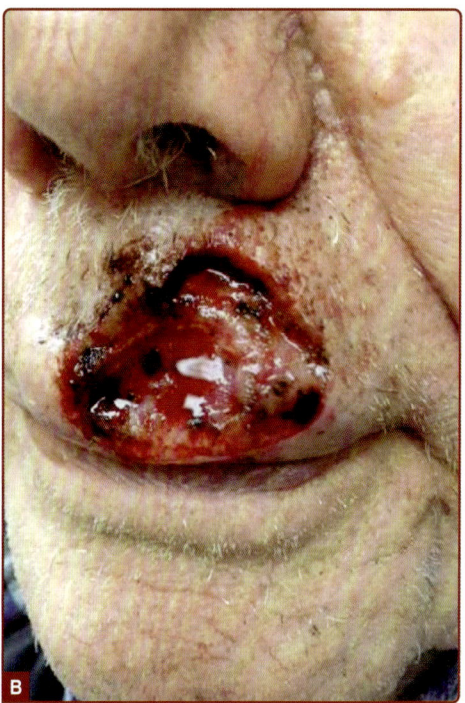

Figure 204-4 Basal cell carcinoma (BCC) subclinical extension. An apparently small BCC of the upper lip (**A**) was found to extend broadly over the cutaneous and mucosal lip and invade into the orbicularis oris muscle (**B**). Clear margins were obtained after three stages of Mohs surgery and the defect was repaired with a local skin flap.

Subsequent studies in thousands of patients have confirmed a long-term recurrence rate of 1% to 4% after Mohs surgery for primary BCC with high-risk features and a higher recurrence rate of 4% to 8% for recurrent BCC, which are likely to have greater subclinical invasion that could be masked by scarring from prior treatment.[12,13]

The durable cure rates obtained with Mohs surgery are superior to those obtained with standard excision as documented in several retrospective studies and one randomized clinical trial (Table 204-1). A pair of meta-analyses of published data on over ten thousand patients reported that Mohs surgery results in a recurrence rate that is three- to fourfold lower than standard excision,[14,15] and a more recent observational study confirmed that although standard excision provides a high rate of cure for cancers on low-risk anatomic locations, Mohs surgery affords at least as high of a cure rate when selectively used on tumors with high-risk features.[16] Yet interpretation of these studies is hampered by their retrospective nature and lack of appropriate controls. More recently, 10-year follow up data from a prospective, randomized trial has now provided high-level evidence that Mohs surgery is superior to standard excision for BCC at high risk of recurrence.[17] Both primary and recurrent BCC with high-risk features (>1-cm diameter and location on the H zone or with an infiltrative or micronodular histologic pattern) were found to have a more than twofold reduction in recurrence rate after Mohs surgery, although statistical significance was only reached for recurrent BCC. In contrast, small, primary BCC without aggressive histologic features on low-risk anatomic locations such as the trunk are unlikely to have significant benefit from the Mohs technique compared with other forms of surgical treatment.

SQUAMOUS CELL CARCINOMA

SCC is the second most common human malignancy, although recent evidence suggests that SCC incidence is increasing and may be approaching that of BCC.[5] Like BCC, SCC is effectively treated with Mohs surgery, facilitating identification and complete excision of irregular branches of subclinical tumor extension. Also like BCC, the differential efficacy of Mohs surgery over standard excision is most pronounced for tumors in the H zone of the face, and for tumors greater than 2 cm in diameter or with aggressive histologic features.[18] These tumors, as well as those recurring after previous treatment, exhibit an increased propensity for subclinical extension and an increased risk of incomplete excision in the absence of the complete margin assessment of Mohs surgery.[19] Particularly on the chronically sun-exposed scalp, SCC may exhibit an infiltrative histology with broad involvement of the fascia and periosteum that is not evident on examination of the skin surface (Fig. 204-5). Overall, the reported rates of recurrence of primary cutaneous SCC are up to 8.1% after standard excision and 3.1% after Mohs surgery.[20] The risk of recurrence for previously treated SCC is increased to 23.3% after standard excision and 10.0% after Mohs surgery.

Unlike BCC, SCC has a significant risk of regional and distant metastasis, particularly for certain subsets of SCC. Treatment is therefore focused not only on preventing local recurrence but on complete tumor extirpation to prevent metastasis. Four factors that appear most strongly associated with adverse outcomes in SCC are diameter greater than 2 cm, depth of invasion below the subcutaneous adipose, perineural invasion, and

TABLE 204-1
Recurrence of Basal Cell Carcinoma

REFERENCE	TYPE OF STUDY	BCC (n)	FOLLOW-UP PERIOD (yr)	LOCATION	RECURRENCE AFTER STANDARD EXCISION (%)	RECURRENCE AFTER MOHS SURGERY (%)	P VALUE
Primary Basal Cell Carcinoma							
van Loo et al[17] (2014)	Prospective randomized trial	397	10	Facial, high risk	12.2	4.4	0.1
Chren et al[16] (2013)	Retrospective observational	1127	5	Any[a]	3.5	2.1	> 0.1
Rowe et al[14] (1989a)	Meta-analysis	10,276	5	Any[b]	10.1	1.0	Not reported
Recurrent Basal Cell Carcinoma							
van Loo et al[17] (2014)	Prospective randomized trial	202	10	Facial, high risk	13.5	3.9	0.023
Rowe et al[15] (1989b)	Meta-analysis	3531	5	Any[c]	17.4	5.6	NR

[a]A total of 26% of excisions and 65% of Mohs were in high-risk anatomic sites (nose, eyelids, eyebrows, lips, temple, and ears and periauricular skin); 27% of all lesions were squamous cell carcinoma (SCC), not basal cell carcinoma (BCC).
[b]Data were derived from 12 separate reports; location was not reported (NR).
[c]Data were derived from 9 separate reports; location was not reported.

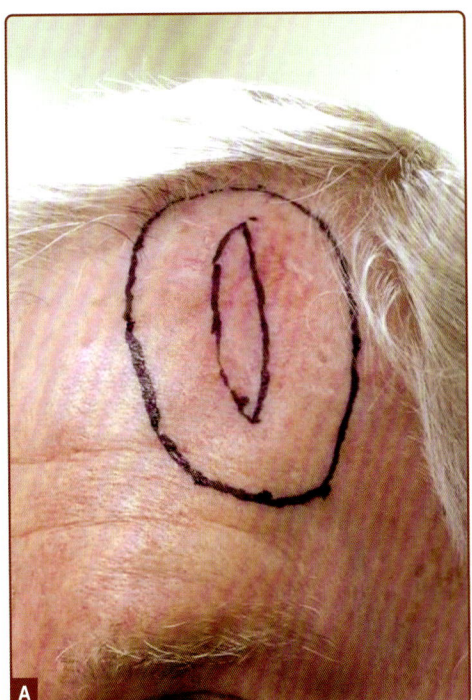 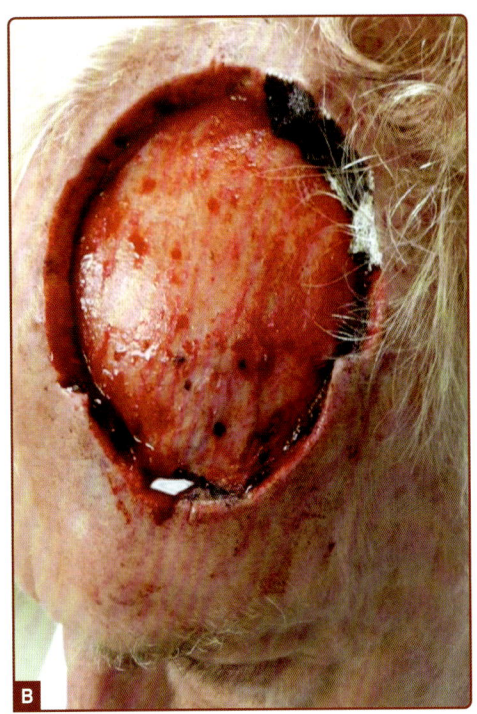

Figure 204-5 Squamous cell carcinoma (SCC) subclinical extension. SCC of the forehead and scalp with infiltrative histology and positive deep and lateral margins after initial excision and linear repair (**A**). A broad, 2-cm margin was excised as the initial stage of Mohs surgery (outer black line), but carcinoma was found infiltrating the fascia and periosteum at the surgical margins. Clear margins were obtained after the second stage of Mohs surgery. The defect measured 8.4 cm and extended to the exposed frontal bone (**B**); it was repaired with a delayed full-thickness skin graft.

poor histologic differentiation. In a large retrospective review, the presence of one of these factors increased local recurrence from 0.6% (no risk factors) to 5% (one risk factor) and 21% (two or three risk factors), and increased nodal metastasis from 0.1% (no risk factors) to 3% (one risk factor) and 21% (two or three risk factors).[21] Importantly, effective local control with Mohs surgery may decrease the risk of subsequent metastasis because SCC with perineural invasion was found to metastasize in 47% of cases after standard excision compared with 8.3% of cases after Mohs surgery.[20] Even with complete verification of the histopathologic margin status, however, SCC with perineural invasion or poor differentiation still presents a significant risk of local or regional recurrence. Adjuvant therapy such as radiation may be considered after Mohs surgery to decrease this risk, although high-quality evidence to support the benefit of this approach is lacking. Other risk factors for adverse outcomes of SCC that may benefit from Mohs surgery include host immunosuppression and location on the lip, ear, and temple. SCC arising on penile skin has also been reported to have a high rate of local and regional recurrence, and Mohs surgery is an effective treatment for penile SCC as well.[22]

SCC in situ can also be effectively treated with Mohs surgery. The reported cure rate for SCC in situ after Mohs surgery is 93.7%, which compares favorably with standard excision.[23] Although SCC in situ has been reported to progress to invasive SCC, the risk of progression in appropriately treated lesions appears to be very low. Moreover, a histopathologic study of depth of invasion of SCC in situ found that in 54 tumors, the maximum depth of invasion was only 0.82 mm.[24] Thus, with the exception of high risk lesions such as those within the H zone of the face or lesions with the clinical suggestion of invasive disease, other forms of treatment besides Mohs surgery should be considered for SCC in situ.

MELANOMA

Dr. Mohs first reported the use of margin-controlled excision for invasive melanoma in 1950 using the *chemosurgery* approach of in situ tissue fixation with zinc chloride, although this was not widely adopted.[25] The transition from in situ fixed tissue to fresh frozen tissue processing for Mohs surgery brought new controversy to the field because it was noted that artifacts introduced on frozen sections complicated the detection of intraepidermal melanocytes and decreased the sensitivity of melanoma detection.[26] The more recent development of immunohistochemical stains on frozen sections has brought the potential for more sensitive melanocyte detection and melanoma diagnosis at the microscopic margins but has not resolved the controversy.

Currently, Mohs surgery using immunohistochemical stains for melanoma antigen recognized by T cells

(MART-1) on rapidly processed frozen sections is the most common technique, although it is only used by a minority of Mohs surgeons, and its use is limited to melanoma in situ and superficially invasive melanoma (Breslow depth <1 mm) with a minimal risk of metastasis. The largest study to date on clinical outcomes with this technique reported a remarkably low 5-year local recurrence rate of less than 1% in more than 2000 melanomas; half of these cases were on the head and neck, 60% were in situ melanoma, and 30% were invasive with a Breslow depth of less than 1 mm.[27] Because of concerns about the accuracy of en face frozen sections for melanoma diagnosis and the potential for undetected invasive disease in unexamined tissue from the center of the tumor, other investigators have proposed staged excision with formalin-fixed sections or a combination of perpendicular (bread-loaf) and en face frozen sections during Mohs surgery, both of which can achieve high cure rates of greater than 95%.[28,29] Importantly, there has not yet been a direct comparison of Mohs surgery with standard wide excision for superficial melanoma in an appropriately matched cohort of patients, and additional study is required to determine the relative efficacy of these treatments. It is likely that some form of staged excision will provide significant benefit for patients with superficial melanoma on chronically sun-exposed skin because nearly 20% of these tumors will have subclinical extension beyond the recommended 5-mm margin of grossly uninvolved skin.[27] Ongoing investigation of the adaptation of the Mohs technique for melanoma treatment illustrates how technologic innovations in tissue processing and staining can be incorporated into surgical treatment, but how these innovations could improve outcomes remains to be determined.

OTHER SKIN CANCERS

Dermatofibrosarcoma protuberans (DFSP) is a rare cutaneous malignancy for which Mohs surgery may be particularly effective. DFSP is a slowly progressive tumor that rarely metastasizes but frequently has broad subclinical extension and a historically high recurrence rate after conventional excision. DFSP originates within the dermis or dermal–subcutaneous junction and frequently invades muscle or fascia, requiring accurate assessment of both peripheral and deep surgical margins (Fig. 204-6). The characteristic spindled cells of DFSP can be readily identified on frozen sections, and complete margin assessment with Mohs surgery facilitates identification of the irregular projections of the tumor that may be missed with standard perpendicular section processing. A meta-analysis of published studies on DFSP, none of which were randomized trials, found that whereas local recurrence after conventional excision was approximately 6%, this rate decreased to 1% after Mohs surgery.[30] For cases in which Mohs surgery is not practical, staged excision

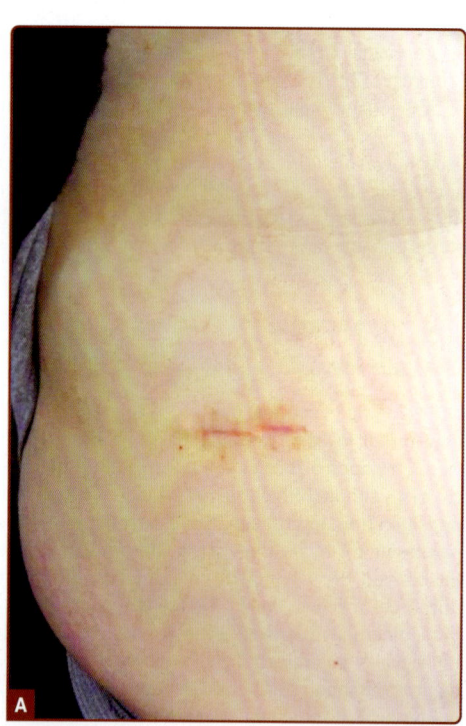
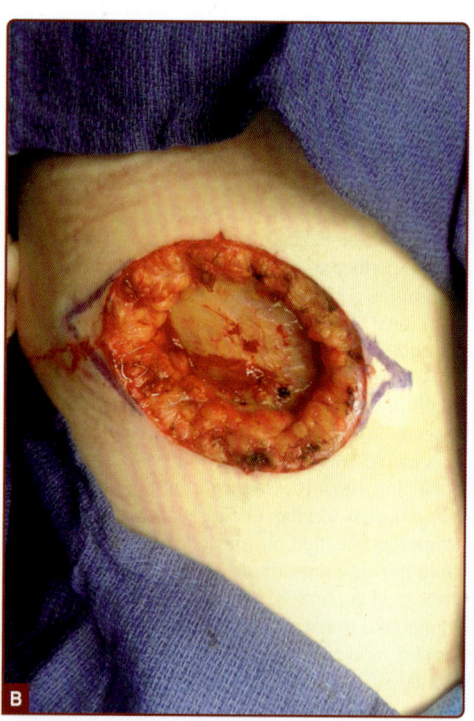

Figure 204-6 Dermatofibrosarcoma protuberans (DFSP). A subtle clinical lesion on the abdomen at the site of a biopsied DFSP (**A**) was found to extend over a broad area with penetration to the deep subcutis overlying the fascia of the abdominal wall musculature (**B**). Clear margins were obtained after three stages of Mohs surgery, and the defect was repaired with a linear closure.

with appropriate pathologic verification of clear margins can also be an effective treatment for DFSP.[31]

In principle, any solid cancer with contiguous growth (as opposed to discontiguous spread or satellite lesions) that can be identified on frozen histopathologic sections and is accessible from the external surface of the body can be treated with Mohs surgery. Mohs surgery is likely to provide the most therapeutic benefit for tumors with broad and unpredictable subclinical extension, such as microcystic adnexal carcinoma,[32] or tumors arising in anatomic locations for which tissue sparing is critical, such as sebaceous carcinoma of the eyelid or extramammary Paget disease (EMPD) of the genitalia. Although EMPD may be multifocal in some cases, a review of published observational studies found that Mohs surgery may result in a lower recurrence rate than standard excision.[33] Atypical fibroxanthoma is an uncommon spindle cell cancer of chronically sun-exposed skin with a behavior similar to high-risk cutaneous SCC that is effectively treated with Mohs surgery. The technique has also been used for treatment of adnexal carcinoma, apocrine and eccrine carcinoma, leiomyosarcoma, Merkel cell carcinoma, mucinous carcinoma, and other rare cutaneous malignancies.[34]

HEALING AND RECONSTRUCTION

Maximal conservation of normal, noncancerous tissue with Mohs surgery facilitates wound healing after tumor extirpation. With the use of in situ chemical fixation originally described by Dr. Mohs, immediate primary surgical repair was often not feasible because of the residual effects of the chemical fixative. Thus, nearly all of the 440 cases originally described by Dr. Mohs were allowed to heal by second intent, or granulation without surgical repair.[1] The continued use of second intent healing for defects after Mohs surgery, even after the transition to non–chemically fixed tissue, was a significant contribution to the surgical literature and established second intent healing as a viable option for selected wounds. Defects resulting from Mohs surgery may be particularly suited to healing without reconstruction because the procedure often creates wounds of shallow depth that may be conducive to second intent healing. This is in contrast to traditional surgical excision, which is routinely performed to the depth of the subcutaneous adipose or connective tissue. Other wounds with reliable functional and cosmetic results after second intent healing include wounds on thin skin such as the eyelid or ear and wounds on concave surfaces such as the medial canthus, anterior surface of the ear, and the temple (Fig. 204-7). Although Mohs surgical defects on convex surfaces such as the nasal tip, malar cheek, and central forehead can also heal with acceptable functional results, the resulting scars in these areas are more likely to be depressed and cosmetically conspicuous. In appropriately selected patients, healing of Mohs surgical defects by second intent results in patient satisfaction that is equivalent to primary surgical repair.[35]

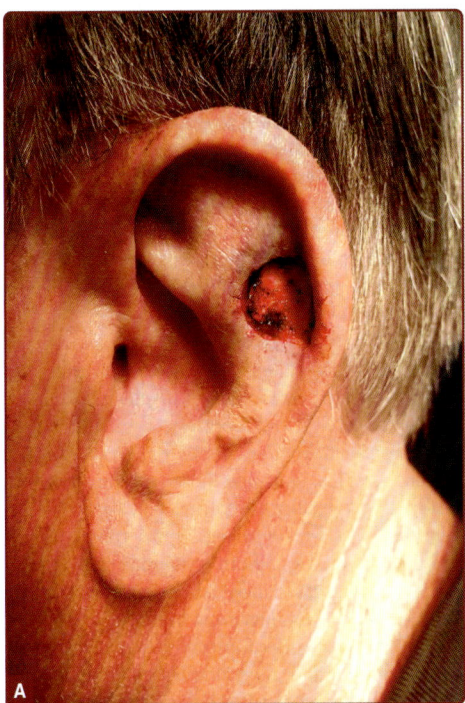 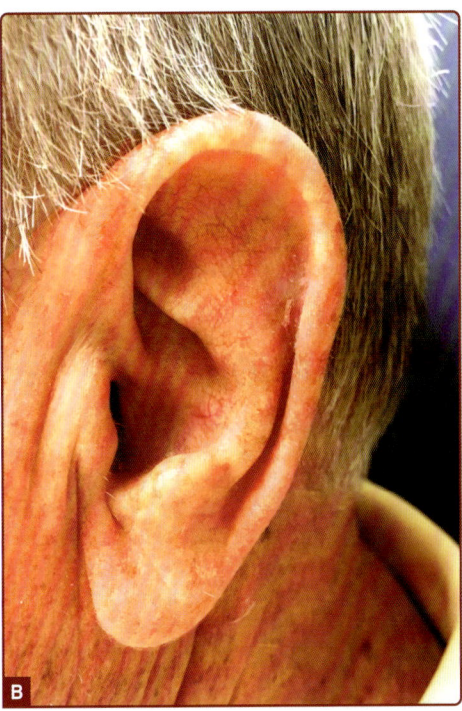

Figure 204-7 Healing by second intent. A 1.6-cm defect of the left scapha and antihelix after Mohs surgical extirpation of a basal cell carcinoma of the ear was allowed to heal by second intent (**A**). After 6 weeks, the wound is fully healed with an excellent cosmetic and functional result (**B**).

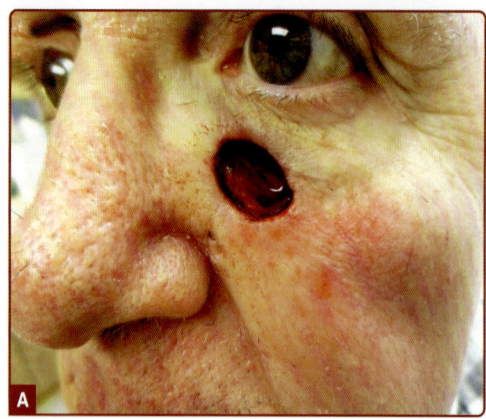 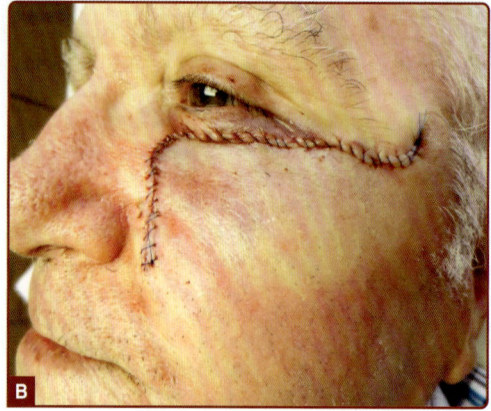

Figure 204-8 Local skin flap reconstruction. After two stages of Mohs surgery, the basal cell carcinoma shown in Fig. 204-3 was completely excised, leaving a 1.6-cm defect of the left cheek and lower eyelid (**A**). The defect was repaired with an advancement flap from the lateral lower eyelid and temple to avoid distortion of the free margin of the lower eyelid (**B**).

Pathologic verification of complete tumor extirpation after Mohs surgery also facilitates immediate surgical reconstruction because the Mohs technique provides the lowest possible risk of residual or recurrent cancer. As the use of frozen sections replaced in situ chemical fixation and Mohs surgery became the standard of care for anatomically sensitive areas such as the nose, lips, and eyelids, reconstruction with plastic and aesthetic surgical techniques has become an integral part of the technique. In fact, several advances in cutaneous reconstruction were described and popularized by Mohs surgeons, including the use of the buried vertical mattress suture, the modern bilobe transposition skin flap on the nose, and the use of cartilage grafts and multistaged interpolation flaps as office based-procedures under local anesthesia.[36-39] Immediate surgical repair with linear closure, skin grafts, or skin flaps from adjacent or interpolated tissue reservoirs is now used more often than second intent healing for Mohs surgical defects and permits optimal restoration of function and cosmesis in critical areas such as the eyelid and nose (Fig. 204-8).

RISKS AND COMPLICATIONS

Although no surgical procedure is without risk, Mohs surgery is a remarkably safe procedure with low complication rates. A multicenter prospective study of adverse events in 20,821 Mohs surgical procedures identified an overall adverse event rate of 0.72% and a serious adverse event rate of 0.02% (4 cases of 20,821).[40] The most common adverse events were infections (0.40% event rate), impaired wound healing including dehiscence and necrosis (0.14% event rate), and postoperative bleeding or hematoma (0.11% event rate). The four serious adverse events in this study were all infections requiring hospitalization, and no deaths or life-threatening cardiovascular complications were reported. Smaller studies have confirmed similarly low rates of complications (minor bleeding in 1.2% and infection in 0.9%) and reported mild postoperative pain scores (mean of 1.99 on a 0–10 scale of pain).[41] The use of local anesthetic rather than general anesthesia or conscious sedation, as well as the lack of significant volume shift or cardiovascular stress after cutaneous surgery likely contribute to the safety of the Mohs procedure.

The documented safety of office-based Mohs surgery allows the procedure to be performed with minimal risk on a wide range of patients, including octa- and nonagenarians and patients with comorbid conditions including stable cardiac disease. Nevertheless, preoperative evaluation to determine the relative risks and benefits of the procedure and to identify modifiable risk factors is critical. Patients with relatively indolent skin cancers who have limited life expectancy because of another terminal condition may not sufficiently benefit from the procedure to justify even small risks of complications. Patients on anticoagulant therapy such as aspirin, warfarin, or direct factor Xa inhibitors such as rivaroxaban or apixaban have a modestly increased risk of minor bleeding complications (1.7% vs 0.7% in one study[41]), but this is not a contraindication to Mohs surgery, and patients are generally advised to continue their prescribed anticoagulation therapy during and after surgery.

Antibiotic prophylaxis is generally not required before Mohs surgery, with a few notable exceptions. The American Heart Association and American College of Cardiology recommend prophylactic antibiotic therapy only for patients at highest risk of complications of infective endocarditis, including those with prosthetic heart valves, a prior history of infective endocarditis, cardiac transplant recipients with significant valvular disease, and patients with significant cyanotic congenital heart disease. Even in these high-risk patients, antibiotic prophylaxis is only recommended in cases with breach of the oral mucosa; surgical procedures on intact skin or gastrointestinal and genitourinary procedures are not clear indications for antibiotic prophylaxis.[42] Patients with total knee or hip replacements may be at increased risk of hematogenous total joint infection after Mohs surgery, and prophylaxis may be considered for these patients as well. However, there is no evidence to support the use of antibiotic prophylaxis with routine surgical or dental procedures in these patients, and recent guidelines from the American Academy of Orthopedic Surgeons and the American Dental Association do not provide specific recommendations for prophylaxis after prosthetic joint replacement.[43] In general, Mohs surgeons use antibiotic prophylaxis sparingly and only in patients at highest risk for hematogenous or surgical site infections.

COST AND APPROPRIATE USE

Mohs surgery is widely used for treatment of non-melanoma skin cancers and has been shown to be the most effective method of skin cancer eradication. The increasing use of Mohs surgery, however, has prompted concerns about the cost of this procedure relative to other surgical treatments. Cost analysis based on procedure codes and typical reimbursements indicates that the immediate cost of skin cancer treatment, including tumor removal, pathologic examination, and repair of the surgical defect, is approximately 25% greater for Mohs surgery than for standard surgical excision with permanent pathologic section analysis in the outpatient setting.[44] This cost differential is reversed, however, when immediate frozen section margin analysis is performed with non-Mohs surgical excision, raising the cost to nearly double that of Mohs surgery. Moreover, when Mohs surgery is limited to high-risk skin cancers or critical anatomic locations such as the H zone of the face, when the use of second intent healing instead of surgical repair is considered with selected Mohs surgery cases, and when the increased rate of recurrence is accounted for with standard surgical excision, the overall costs of Mohs surgery may be 20% to 30% less than standard excision.[45]

To ensure that Mohs surgery is reserved for clinical scenarios in which the procedure will be most cost-efficient and provide the greatest benefit over other forms of treatment, the American Academy of Dermatology, the American College of Mohs Surgery, the American Society for Dermatologic Surgery, and the American Society for Mohs Surgery jointly published appropriate use criteria (AUC) in 2012.[34] The appropriate use criteria define tumor-specific and patient-specific factors for which Mohs surgery is deemed to be either appropriate, uncertain, or inappropriate in most situations (Table 204-2). A central factor in the AUC is anatomic location, owing to the critical need for tissue sparing with Mohs surgery in certain locations as well as the increased risk of subclinical extension and recurrence of skin cancers in these areas. High-risk areas include the H zone of the face (eyelids, eyebrows, nose, lips, chin, ears and periauricular skin, and temples; Fig. 204-9), genitalia, hands, feet, ankles, and nipple and areola region. Medium-risk areas are the remainder of the face (cheeks, forehead, and jawline), scalp, neck, and pretibial surfaces. The trunk and the remainder of the extremities are considered low-risk areas. The AUC primarily focuses on specific clinical scenarios for BCC and SCC but also notes that Mohs surgery can be appropriate for melanoma in situ and other, more rare tumors. It is important to note that the AUC does not encompass all clinical scenarios nor does it imply that Mohs surgery is required for all tumors deemed appropriate. Individual clinical judgment must always be used to ensure optimal management of cutaneous malignancy, and the AUC are likely to be modified as further research and clinical experience can refine the recommendations.

TABLE 204-2
Mohs Surgery Appropriate Use Criteria[a]

DIAGNOSIS	RISK AREA[b]	CLINICAL DIAMETER (cm)			
		<0.5	0.6–1	1.1–2	>2
Primary nodular BCC	High	A	A	A	A
	Medium	A	A	A	A
	Low	I	I	U	A
Primary aggressive BCC[c]	High	A	A	A	A
	Medium	A	A	A	A
	Low	U	A	A	A
Primary superficial BCC	High	A	A	A	A
	Medium	U	A	A	A
	Low	I	I	I	I
Recurrent BCC (not superficial)	Any	A	A	A	A
Recurrent superficial BCC	High	A	A	A	A
	Medium	A	A	A	A
	Low	I	I	I	I
Primary SCC without high-risk features[d]	High	A	A	A	A
	Medium	A	A	A	A
	Low	I	I	U	A
Primary SCC with high-risk features[d]	Any	A	A	A	A
Primary SCC in immunocompromised patient	High	A	A	A	A
	Medium	A	A	A	A
	Low	U	U	A	A
Recurrent SCC (invasive)	Any	A	A	A	A
Primary SCC in situ	High	A	A	A	A
	Medium	A	A	A	A
	Low	I	I	U	A

[a]The most common clinical scenarios are presented. Each scenario is scored as appropriate (A) or inappropriate (I) for Mohs surgery or uncertain (U).
[b]High-risk area: central face, eyelids, eyebrows, nose, lips, chin, ears and periauricular skin, temples, genitalia, hands, feet, ankles, and nipple and areola. Medium-risk area: cheeks, forehead, scalp, neck, jawline, and pretibial surface. Low-risk area: trunk and remainder of extremities.
[c]Aggressive basal cell carcinoma (BCC) includes pathologic subtypes of infiltrative, morpheaform or sclerosing, micronodular, and metatypical or keratotic or with perineural invasion.
[d]High risk features for squamous cell carcinoma (SCC) include poor differentiation, perineural or intravascular invasion, spindle cell or infiltrative features, Breslow depth >2 mm, and Clark level IV or greater.

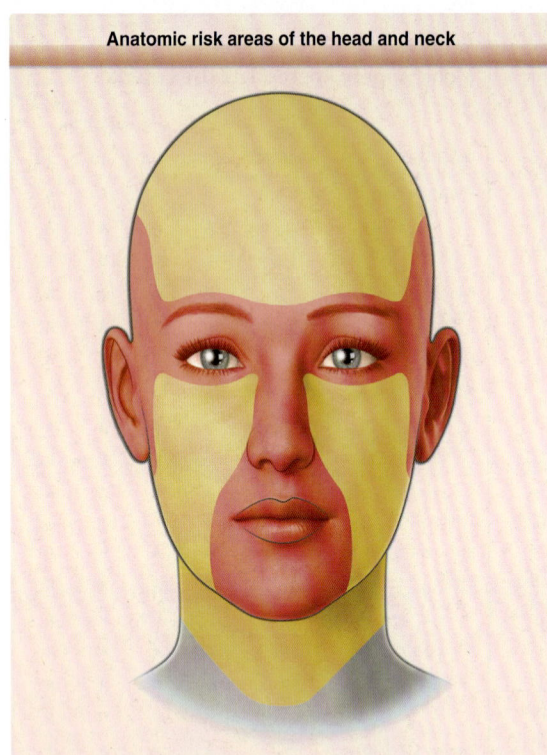

Figure 204-9 Mohs surgery appropriate use criteria anatomic risk areas of the head and neck. High-risk areas on the central face, eyelids, eyebrows, nose, lips, chin, ears, periauricular skin, and temples are shown in red. Medium-risk areas on the cheeks, forehead, scalp, neck and jawline are shown in yellow. Not shown are high-risk areas on the hands, feet, ankles, genitalia, and nipple and areola, as well as medium-risk areas on the pretibial surface.

CONCLUSIONS

Mohs surgery is a specialized form of skin cancer extirpation that relies on staged excision with immediate histopathologic examination of the entire deep and peripheral surgical margin. Mohs surgery is most often used to treat patients with BCCs and SCCs and has been shown to be superior to other forms of treatment for cancers at increased risk of recurrence. The versatility of the Mohs procedure allows for maximal tissue conservation while ensuring complete tumor removal and facilitates optimal wound healing, whether by immediate surgical reconstruction or by second intent. The procedure is the accepted standard of care for appropriately selected cancers as defined by the AUC. Ongoing investigation and technological advances will continue to refine the indications for Mohs surgery, which may include expanded use for superficial melanoma or other less common tumors.

REFERENCES

1. Mohs FE. Chemosurgery: a microscopically controlled method of cancer excision. *Arch Surg.* 1941;42(2):279-295.
2. Reeder VJ, Gustafson CJ, Mireku K, et al. Trends in Mohs surgery from 1995 to 2010: an analysis of nationally representative data. *Dermatol Surg.* 2015;41(3):397-403.
3. Kimyai-Asadi A, Katz T, Goldberg LH, et al. Margin involvement after the excision of melanoma in situ: the need for complete en face examination of the surgical margins. *Dermatol Surg.* 2007;33(12):1434-1439; discussion 1439-1441.
4. Donaldson MR, Coldiron BM. Mohs micrographic surgery utilization in the Medicare population, 2009. *Dermatol Surg.* 2012;38(9):1427-1434.
5. Rogers HW, Weinstock MA, Feldman SR, et al. Incidence estimate of nonmelanoma skin cancer (keratinocyte carcinomas) in the U.S. population, 2012. *JAMA Dermatol.* 2015;151(10):1081-1086.
6. Wolf DJ, Zitelli JA. Surgical margins for basal cell carcinoma. *Arch Dermatol.* 1987;123(3):340-344.
7. Batra RS, Kelley LC. Predictors of extensive subclinical spread in nonmelanoma skin cancer treated with Mohs micrographic surgery. *Arch Dermatol.* 2002;138(8):1043-1051.
8. Song SS, Goldenberg A, Ortiz A, et al. Nonmelanoma skin cancer with aggressive subclinical extension in immunosuppressed patients. *JAMA Dermatol.* 2016;152(6):683-690.
9. Hendrix JD Jr, Parlette HL. Duplicitous growth of infiltrative basal cell carcinoma: analysis of clinically undetected tumor extent in a paired case-control study. *Dermatol Surg.* 1996;22(6):535-539.
10. Hendrix JD Jr, Parlette HL. Micronodular basal cell carcinoma. A deceptive histologic subtype with frequent clinically undetected tumor extension. *Arch Dermatol.* 1996;132(3):295-298.
11. Mohs FE. Micrographic surgery for the microscopically controlled excision of eyelid cancers. *Arch Ophthalmol.* 1986;104(6):901-909.
12. Smeets NW, Kuijpers DI, Nelemans P, et al. Mohs' micrographic surgery for treatment of basal cell carcinoma of the face—results of a retrospective study and review of the literature. *Br J Dermatol.* 2004;151(1):141-147.

13. Leibovitch I, Huilgol SC, Selva D, et al. Basal cell carcinoma treated with Mohs surgery in Australia II. Outcome at 5-year follow-up. *J Am Acad Dermatol.* 2005;53(3):452-457.
14. Rowe DE, Carroll RJ, Day CL Jr. Long-term recurrence rates in previously untreated (primary) basal cell carcinoma: implications for patient follow-up. *J Dermatol Surg Oncol.* 1989;15(3):315-328.
15. Rowe DE, Carroll RJ, Day CL Jr. Mohs surgery is the treatment of choice for recurrent (previously treated) basal cell carcinoma. *J Dermatol Surg Oncol.* 1989;15(4):424-431.
16. Chren MM, Linos E, Torres JS, et al. Tumor recurrence 5 years after treatment of cutaneous basal cell carcinoma and squamous cell carcinoma. *J Invest Dermatol.* 2013;133(5):1188-1196.
17. van Loo E, Mosterd K, Krekels GA, et al. Surgical excision versus Mohs' micrographic surgery for basal cell carcinoma of the face: a randomised clinical trial with 10 year follow-up. *Eur J Cancer.* 2014;50(17):3011-3020.
18. Brodland DG, Zitelli JA. Surgical margins for excision of primary cutaneous squamous cell carcinoma. *J Am Acad Dermatol.* 1992;27(2 Pt 1):241-248.
19. Schell AE, Russell MA, Park SS. Suggested excisional margins for cutaneous malignant lesions based on Mohs micrographic surgery. *JAMA Facial Plast Surg.* 2013;15(5):337-343.
20. Rowe DE, Carroll RJ, Day CL Jr. Prognostic factors for local recurrence, metastasis, and survival rates in squamous cell carcinoma of the skin, ear, and lip. Implications for treatment modality selection. *J Am Acad Dermatol.* 1992;26(6):976-990.
21. Karia PS, Jambusaria-Pahlajani A, Harrington DP, et al. Evaluation of American Joint Committee on Cancer, International Union Against Cancer, and Brigham and Women's Hospital tumor staging for cutaneous squamous cell carcinoma. *J Clin Oncol.* 2014;32(4):327-334.
22. Machan M, Brodland D, Zitelli J. Penile squamous cell carcinoma: penis-preserving treatment with Mohs micrographic surgery. *Dermatol Surg.* 2016;42(8):936-944.
23. Hansen JP, Drake AL, Walling HW. Bowen's disease: a four-year retrospective review of epidemiology and treatment at a university center. *Dermatol Surg.* 2008;34(7):878-883.
24. Christensen SR, McNiff JM, Cool AJ, et al. Histopathologic assessment of depth of follicular invasion of squamous cell carcinoma (SCC) in situ (SCCis): Implications for treatment approach. *J Am Acad Dermatol.* 2016;74(2):356-362.
25. Mohs FE. Chemosurgical treatment of melanoma; a microscopically controlled method of excision. *Arch Derm Syphilol.* 1950;62(2):269-279.
26. Barlow RJ, White CR, Swanson NA. Mohs' micrographic surgery using frozen sections alone may be unsuitable for detecting single atypical melanocytes at the margins of melanoma in situ. *Br J Dermatol.* 2002;146(2):290-294.
27. Valentin-Nogueras SM, Brodland DG, Zitelli JA, et al. mohs micrographic surgery using MART-1 immunostain in the treatment of invasive melanoma and melanoma in situ. *Dermatol Surg.* 2016;42(6):733-744.
28. de Vries K, Greveling K, Prens LM, et al. Recurrence rate of lentigo maligna after micrographically controlled staged surgical excision. *Br J Dermatol.* 2016;174(3):588-593.
29. Etzkorn JR, Sobanko JF, Elenitsas R, et al. Low recurrence rates for in situ and invasive melanomas using Mohs micrographic surgery with melanoma antigen recognized by T cells 1 (MART-1) immunostaining: tissue processing methodology to optimize pathologic staging and margin assessment. *J Am Acad Dermatol.* 2015;72(5):840-850.
30. Foroozan M, Sei JF, Amini M, et al. Efficacy of Mohs micrographic surgery for the treatment of dermatofibrosarcoma protuberans: systematic review. *Arch Dermatol.* 2012;148(9):1055-1063.
31. Goldberg C, Hoang D, McRae M, et al. A strategy for the successful management of dermatofibrosarcoma protuberans. *Ann Plast Surg.* 2015;74(1):80-84.
32. Leibovitch I, Huilgol SC, Selva D, et al. Microcystic adnexal carcinoma: treatment with Mohs micrographic surgery. *J Am Acad Dermatol.* 2005;52(2):295-300.
33. Bae JM, Choi YY, Kim H, et al. Mohs micrographic surgery for extramammary Paget disease: a pooled analysis of individual patient data. *J Am Acad Dermatol.* 2013;68(4):632-637.
34. Ad Hoc Task F, Connolly SM, Baker DR, et al. AAD/ACMS/ASDSA/ASMS 2012 appropriate use criteria for Mohs micrographic surgery: a report of the American Academy of Dermatology, American College of Mohs Surgery, American Society for Dermatologic Surgery Association, and the American Society for Mohs Surgery. *J Am Acad Dermatol.* 2012;67(4):531-550.
35. Stebbins WG, Gusev J, Higgins HW 2nd, et al. Evaluation of patient satisfaction with second intention healing versus primary surgical closure. *J Am Acad Dermatol.* 2015;73(5):865-867;e861.
36. Zitelli JA, Moy RL. Buried vertical mattress suture. *J Dermatol Surg Oncol.* 1989;15(1):17-19.
37. Zitelli JA. The bilobed flap for nasal reconstruction. *Arch Dermatol.* 1989;125(7):957-959.
38. Sage RJ, Leach BC, Cook J. Antihelical cartilage grafts for reconstruction of mohs micrographic surgery defects. *Dermatol Surg.* 2012;38(12):1930-1937.
39. Jellinek NJ, Nguyen TH, Albertini JG. Paramedian forehead flap: advances, procedural nuances, and variations in technique. *Dermatol Surg.* 2014;40(Suppl 9):S30-S42.
40. Alam M, Ibrahim O, Nodzenski M, et al. Adverse events associated with mohs micrographic surgery: multicenter prospective cohort study of 20,821 cases at 23 centers. *JAMA Dermatol.* 2013;149(12):1378-1385.
41. Merritt BG, Lee NY, Brodland DG, et al. The safety of Mohs surgery: a prospective multicenter cohort study. *J Am Acad Dermatol.* 2012;67(6):1302-1309.
42. Nishimura RA, Otto CM, Bonow RO, et al. 2014 AHA/ACC guideline for the management of patients with valvular heart disease: a report of the American College of Cardiology/American Heart Association Task Force on Practice Guidelines. *J Am Coll Cardiol.* 2014;63(22):e57-e185.
43. Watters W 3rd, Rethman MP, Hanson NB, et al. Prevention of orthopaedic implant infection in patients undergoing dental procedures. *J Am Acad Orthop Surg.* 2013;21(3):180-189.
44. Rogers HW, Coldiron BM. A relative value unit-based cost comparison of treatment modalities for nonmelanoma skin cancer: effect of the loss of the Mohs multiple surgery reduction exemption. *J Am Acad Dermatol.* 2009;61(1):96-103.
45. Ravitskiy L, Brodland DG, Zitelli JA. Cost analysis: Mohs micrographic surgery. *Dermatol Surg.* 2012;38(4):585-594.

Chapter 205 :: Nail Surgery
:: Robert Baran & Olivier Cogrel

第二百零五章
甲部手术

中文导读

甲部手术的主要目的是甲组织活检诊断、治疗感染、减轻疼痛、去除局部肿瘤并确保获得性和先天性异常的最佳美容效果。由于指板坚硬且甲部结构复杂，需要具体细致的指南作为指导。本章共分为5节：①围手术期注意事项；②指甲撕脱术；③指甲活检；④甲部不同组织的手术方法；⑤嵌甲。详细介绍了甲部手术的相关事项。

第一节从术前、术中、术后三个阶段介绍了围手术期注意事项。术前需要为患者进行手术说明、术后发病率等常规准备事项。术前及术中采集患处照片并仔细记录病史，尤其注意患者使用药物史。紧接着作者详细介绍了甲部的解剖学、手术器材。其中着重讲解了术前麻醉，多采用1%或2%的利多卡因。大多数甲外科手术均在严格的外科手术缺血下进行，以避免出血影响手术视野，接着介绍了止血带的应用方法（图205-6）。术后需要进行细致的敷料选择和护理，使用敷料时必须考虑到渗漏、疼痛和敏感性，为防止感染应每隔一天或每天更换敷料。

第二节介绍了指甲撕脱术。指甲撕脱是将甲板与其下面的附属器分开，此方法协助探查并治疗甲下病变或切除病理性甲板。介绍了四种入路的具体操作方法，分别为远端入路、近端入路、指甲局部撕脱、撕裂活动甲板。

第三节介绍了三种甲部活检方法。由于甲部的特殊性，进行活检可以确定病变组织的病理学特征或阐明不确定的临床诊断。一般采用侧面纵切活检或梭形切除，图205-10至图205-12展示了远端甲母质活检方法，图205-14对应甲床组织活检，图205-15对应近端甲襞活检。

第四节以甲部不同组织作为分类标准，详细介绍了甲部不同组织的手术方法。对于甲母质手术来说，主要包括3种方式：①减小其宽度或长度；②使用外科手术来清除肿瘤；③2～3毫米的打孔活检。另外，完全的基质切除术——即消融指甲形成组织，会永久性地失去指甲，因此很少进行（图205-16、图205-18）。最后根据甲母质肿瘤的不同位置，提供了不同的治疗方案。

第五节专门介绍了嵌甲这种常见的甲相关疾病。嵌甲是一种甲板向远处的真皮组织或外侧的甲槽内嵌而产生的疾病，主要包括远端趾甲嵌入、逆生甲、幼年（皮下）嵌甲、钳状甲、侧面甲皱肥大、先天性大脚趾甲等。远端趾甲嵌入可以通过在远端指骨周围进行梭形切除处理（图205-24）；逆生甲可以撕开指甲，使其角质层重叠（图205-25）。在最后，介绍了两种无创嵌甲治疗方法——锚带、丙烯酸固定钩形甲。这两种方法已在治疗嵌甲方面取得了良好的效果，尤其是在儿童中。

〔赵　爽〕

AT-A-GLANCE

- Nail surgery requires careful patient selection to prevent unnecessary complications.
- The technique used for anesthesia depends on the type of surgery. Distal digital block with ropivacaine 2 mg/mL is usually the best option.
- Partial nail avulsion allows the exploration and/or the treatment of a subungual lesion or the removal of a pathologic nail plate. Total nail plate avulsion should be discouraged to prevent nail bed shrinking and distal embedding.
- Nail biopsies are performed to determine the histopathologic features of a lesion or to clarify an uncertain clinical diagnosis.
- Lateral longitudinal biopsy is the best technique for inflammatory disorders or lateral longitudinal melanonychia.
- Punch biopsy less than 3 mm in the distal matrix does not produce serious dystrophy.
- Tangential shave excision is the best option for superficial matrix tumors such as wide longitudinal melanonychia or superficial epithelial benign tumors.

BACKGROUND

The main objectives of nail surgery are to aid diagnosis by biopsy, to treat infection, to alleviate pain, to remove local tumors, and to ensure the best cosmetic results in acquired and congenital abnormalities.

PERIOPERATIVE CONSIDERATIONS

PATIENT SELECTION

Providing the patient with an exact illustration of the operation is helpful to give the patient insight into the procedure and its expected outcome. A thorough discussion regarding postoperative morbidity is essential.

RISKS AND PRECAUTIONS

Preoperative photographs as well as any taken during surgery may be useful medicolegally. Careful history taking may reveal systemic disease such as diabetes mellitus, blood dyscrasia, vascular disease, vascular collagen disease (scleroderma), allergy, chronic pulmonary disease, or immune impairment. Any of these may at times be relative contraindications to surgery, may be associated with severe complications (infection, necrosis), or may call for alteration of the technique to be used. Surgery of the nail is not recommended in patients with high-risk conditions. A history of concurrent use of drugs may be relevant, because these drugs may affect anesthesia (eg, monoamine oxidase inhibitors or phenothiazines), prolong bleeding (eg, aspirin and anticoagulants), delay healing (eg, glucocorticoids), or have toxic effects on the nail apparatus (eg, retinoids). There may be a history of allergy to lidocaine or mepivacaine or to parabens contained in both as a preservative. A magnifying lens and dermoscopy are useful to observe the color, surface, and structure of the periungual tissue and to compare the unaffected contralateral digit. It may be necessary to probe to localize pain, to obtain a radiograph to rule out underlying bone involvement, or to ask for ultrasonography and MRI when a tumor is suspected. The basic requirements for nail surgery include a detailed knowledge of the anatomy and physiology of the nail apparatus on the part of the surgeon. Full aseptic conditions, regional block anesthesia, and local hemostasis are indispensable.

ANATOMY[1] (CHAP. 8)

The nail plate is the permanent product of the nail matrix. Its normal appearance and growth depend on the integrity of the perionychium and the bony phalanx (Fig. 205-1). The nail is a semihard horny plate covering the dorsal aspect of the tip of the digit. The nail is inserted proximally in an invagination that is practically parallel to the upper surface of the skin and laterally in the lateral nail grooves. This pocket-like invagination has a roof, the proximal nail fold, and a floor, the matrix from which the nail is derived. The matrix extends approximately 6 mm under the proximal nail fold, and its distal portion is only visible as the white semicircular lunula. The general shape of the matrix is a crescent, concave in its posteroinferior portion. The lateral horns of this crescent are more developed in the great toe and are located at the coronal plane of the bone. The ventral aspect of the proximal nail fold encompasses both a lower portion, which continues the matrix, and an upper portion (roughly three-quarters of its length), called the *eponychium* (Fig. 205-2). The germinal matrix forms the bulk of the nail plate. The proximal element forms the superficial third of the nail plate, whereas the distal element provides its inferior two-thirds. The ventral surface of the proximal nail fold adheres closely to the nail for a short distance and forms a gradually desquamating tissue, the cuticle, made of the stratum corneum of both the dorsal and the ventral sides of the proximal nail fold. The cuticle seals and protects the nail cul-de-sac. The nail plate is bordered by the proximal nail fold, which is continuous with the similarly structured lateral nail fold on each side. The nail bed extends from the lunula to the hyponychium. It has parallel, longitudinal rete

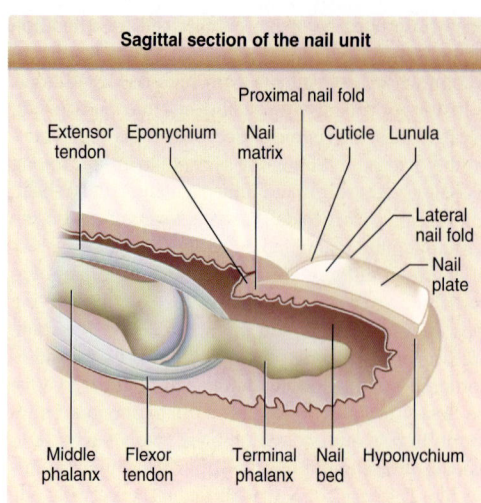

Figure 205-1 Sagittal section of the nail unit.

ridges. In contrast to the matrix, the nail bed has a firm attachment to the nail plate. Colorless but translucent, this highly vascular connective tissue, containing glomus organs, transmits a pink color through the nail. Avulsion of the overlying nail plate denudes the nail bed. Distally, adjacent to the nail bed, lies the hyponychium, an extension of the volar epidermis under the nail plate, which marks the point at which the nail separates from the underlying tissue. The distal nail groove, which is convex anteriorly, separates the hyponychium from the fingertip. The circulation of the nail apparatus is supplied by 2 digital arteries that course along the digits and give off branches to the distal and proximal arches. The sensory nerves to the distal phalanx of the 3 middle fingers are derived from fine, oblique, dorsal branches of the volar collateral nerves. Longitudinal branches of the dorsal collateral nerves supply the terminal phalanx of the fifth digit

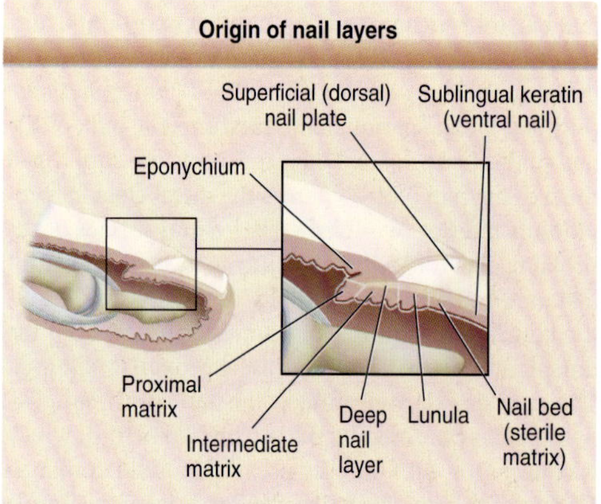

and also the thumb. Among its multiple functions, the nail provides counterpressure to the pulp that is essential to the tactile sensation involving the fingers and to the prevention of hypertrophy of the nail bed.

INSTRUMENTS AND DRAPING

The instruments used in nail surgery are, in general, the same as those used in cutaneous surgery with the addition of the instruments listed in Table 205-1.

Draping is accomplished by means of a sterile surgical drape or a sterile glove on the involved hand. The tip of the glove is cut off on the finger that is to undergo surgery. The remaining open finger of the glove is then rolled back down the digit. This exsanguinates the digit and provides a tourniquet when it reaches the proximal part of the finger. Disinfection is extremely important to avoid contamination of the wound with consecutive infection. Isopropyl alcohol scrub and chlorhexidine have proven to be superior to povidone iodine washing.

ANESTHESIA

Local anesthesia should be administered while the patient is reclining or in a supine position. Lidocaine 1% or 2% is widely used because the incidence of allergy to this agent is very low as well as for its low cost. Buffered 2% lidocaine and ropivacaine are characterized by quick absorption and near instantaneous anesthesia. Applying Emla or LMD under occlusion 2 hours prior to the injection may lessen the pain especially in children. For anxious patients, administering a fast-acting benzodiazepine orally (midazolam, alprazolam or diazepam) 2 hours before anesthesia can considerably reduce the fear of the injection.[2] Ropivacaine 2 mg/mL is another agent that can be used and offers the advantage of a rapid onset and a long duration, usually between

Figure 205-2 Origin of the nail layers. (Used with permission from P. Kechijian, MD.)

TABLE 205-1
Instruments Required for Nail Surgery

- Nail elevators
- Single- or double-pronged skin hooks
- Double-action nail splitter (bone rongeur)
- Clippers, splitting scissors, English nail splitter
- Pointed scissors (Gradle scissors), curved iris scissors
- Small-nosed hemostats
- Disposable biopsy punches
- Penrose drains
- Luer-Lok syringe, 30-gauge needles

8 and 12 hours. The use of local anesthesia in conjunction with epinephrine for surgery on digits is no longer contraindicated and offers the advantage of vasoconstriction and thus a less bloody surgical field. However, caution is warranted for patients with risk factors predisposing for local circulatory insufficiency. Buffering and warming the local anesthetic coupled with a slow rate of injection and small needle size, all drastically reduce the pain of injection. Buffering is accomplished with the use of 1 part 7.5% bicarbonate with 9 parts. Anesthetics are administered via a 30-gauge needle for fingernails or a 27-gauge needle for toenails on a Luer-Lock syringe using either a proximal digital block or, better, a distal digital block (wing block) procedure. Other techniques, such as median distal anesthesia or transthecal block, have not replaced the classic routes of anesthesia. Although emergencies related to minor surgery occur rarely, the ready availability of resuscitative equipment and expertise is essential.

PROXIMAL DIGITAL BLOCK

This is the more traditionally used block. Although less painful than the distal block procedure, the anesthesia takes 5 to 10 minutes to become established. The hand is laid down flat, with the fingers spread, so that 1 to 2 mL of anesthetic can be administered by a dorsal injection, with a thin needle inserted and directed tangentially to the sides of the bony phalanx at the base of the involved finger and as far as the lateral side of the flexor tendon (Fig. 205-3). A tourniquet effect may inadvertently be produced by injecting more than 5 mL of anesthetic and should be avoided. The absence of blood reflux in the syringe should be verified before injection if a nondental syringe is used. When the operation is strictly localized to a lateral region, a block limited to the nerves ipsilateral to the lesion suffices, as in the case of a partial distolateral nail avulsion.

DISTAL DIGITAL BLOCK

The distal digital block procedure is more painful than the proximal block procedure, but anesthesia occurs immediately. As such, it is our preferred method of anesthesia in the absence of a digital bacterial infection. For a distal digital block, the needle is inserted just behind the junction of the proximal nail fold and a lateral nail fold and a few 10ths of a milliliter of anesthetic is injected, which whitens the region. The injection is continued by aiming the needle toward the pad. One then returns to the initial area to inject the proximal fold transversely. Finally, at the junction of the proximal fold with the lateral fold on the opposite side, one proceeds as described earlier (Fig. 205-4). The anesthesia is almost immediate, and when the procedure is done correctly, injections rarely have to be extended to the distal area of the finger. Median distal administration is relatively simple and quick (Fig. 205-5). The needle is introduced at a 30° angle into the middle of the proximal nail fold and advanced distally into the underlying matrix. Anesthetic is injected slowly as the needle pierces first the nail plate, then the matrix, and finally the adjacent nail bed. The nail plate is soft and offers little resistance. Blanching confirms the delivery of anesthetic to the nail matrix and bed. Pain is brief and anesthesia nearly instantaneous. This method is suitable for most procedures performed on the proximal half of the nail unit. It is not suitable for matricectomy or complete nail avulsion.

TRANSTHECAL BLOCK

The flexor tendon sheath may be used as an avenue for introducing anesthetic to the core of the digit. Through centrifugal anesthetic diffusion all 4 digital nerves are anesthetized rapidly. This technique involves palmar percutaneous injection of 2 mL of lidocaine or ropivicaine into the potential space of the flexor tendon sheath at the level of the palmar flexion crease using a 3-mL syringe and a 25-gauge hypodermic needle.

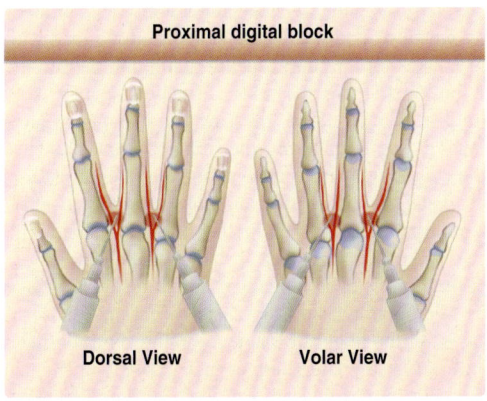

Figure 205-3 Proximal digital block.

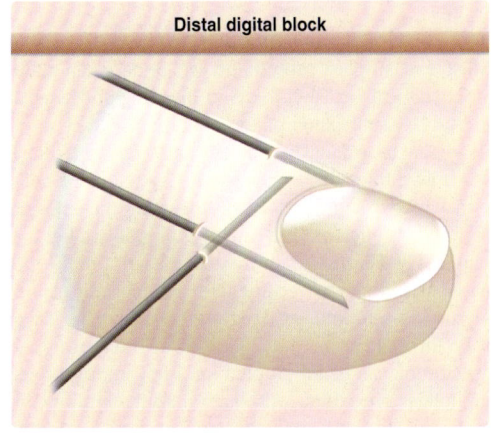

Figure 205-4 Distal digital block.

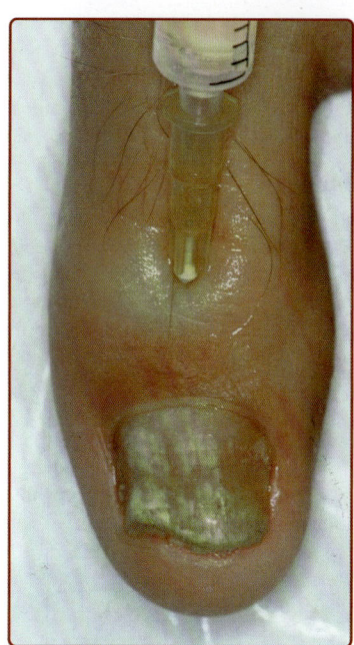

Figure 205-5 Median distal block.

Postoperative pain may be more severe than with other techniques.

REGIONAL BLOCKS AND GENERAL ANESTHESIA

These are used mainly in more extensive and painful surgeries or in circumstances under which it is useful to have anesthesia of more than 1 digit at the same time. For instance, it may be appropriate in the surgical treatment of numerous warts and in the infiltration of more than 1 finger with triamcinolone in the treatment of nail unit psoriasis. General anesthesia is also indicated for nail rotation of congenital malalignment of the big toe nail in children.

TOURNIQUETS

Most nail surgery procedures are undertaken with strict surgical ischemia to avoid bleeding and enable a correct visualization of the operative field. Use of the digital tourniquet is relatively safe and efficacious. For brief intraoperative hemostasis (eg, nail avulsion, punch biopsy of the nail bed), squeezing the sides of the digits is effective. If a prolonged bloodless field is required, a Penrose drain may be placed around the base of the digit and secured with a hemostatic clamp for use as a tourniquet. It is preferable not to leave it on for more than 15 to 20 minutes. The tourniquet application can be interrupted for a few minutes during longer procedures. Although it seems intuitive, it is essential to never forget the tourniquet on, as several cases of digital necrosis following forgotten tourniquet

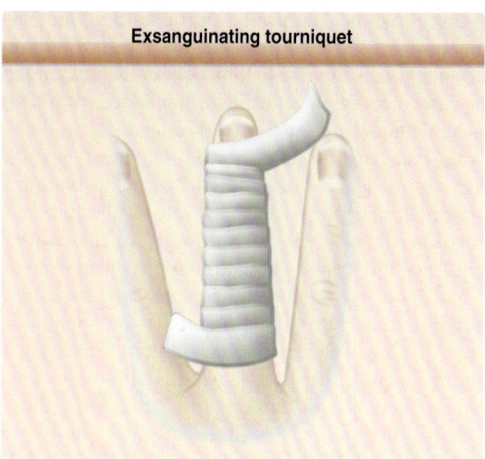

Figure 205-6 Exsanguinating tourniquet.

have been reported.[3]

To facilitate establishment of a bloodless field, the use of an exsanguinating tourniquet is recommended[1] before anesthesia. A wide Penrose drain is wound tightly in loops that overlap in a distal to proximal fashion, with an exposed loose end left distally (Fig. 205-6). This "milks" the blood from the digit. The loose end is then grasped and the drain unwound, again from distal to proximal, until the nail unit is exposed with the final proximal loop. In the absence of contraindication, the addition of epinephrine to lidocaine, for example, may reduce the need for a tourniquet and produce better and longer pain control perioperatively.

DRESSING AND POSTOPERATIVE CARE

DRESSING

At the end of the operation, either the digit is cleansed with sterile 10% hydrogen peroxide solution and sprayed with a colorless disinfectant or an antiseptic with hemolytic action is applied. The nail area is then covered with an antiseptic or antibiotic ointment on gauze or pads. Dressing must be done in a way that takes into account oozing, pain, and sensitivity. A bulky dressing provides a cushion against local trauma. Compressive dressing is mandatory and must not be removed in the first 48 hours following the procedure. The compression must be applied to the distal part of the digit and not proximally to avoid a tourniquet effect. Then, the dressings should be changed every other day or daily if there is infection. Several layers of sterile gauze should be kept in place by Micropore (2.5-cm) tape placed first on the dorsal aspect of the finger or toe, then on the ventral aspect, and last on the lateral edges in a U shape (a circular dressing should never be applied in the first week). Finally, use of an X-span tube dressing or Surgitube will give the patient more freedom to use the hand, but care must be taken that dressings do not constrict blood flow. During the first 48 hours, the arm must be kept in a sling. Stitches are removed after 7 to 12 days. When the feet are treated, daily chlorhexidine baths precede the care just described. For all operations involving the toes, the patient should wear an appropriate shoe or sandal after the dressing has been applied. The patient should be recumbent for 24 to 48 hours, with the foot elevated to 30°.

POSTOPERATIVE COMPLICATIONS

BLEEDING

Bleeding seen after the tourniquet is removed is not worrisome as the compressive dressing will stop it. In case of persistent bleeding, 35% aluminium chloride solution or an oxidized cellulose application (Gelfoam) should be applied. Alternatively, an extra injection of lidocaine + epinephrine bilaterally will stop the bleeding through compression of the vessels.

PAIN

Pain threshold varies based on the procedure and from patient to patient. CO_2 laser vaporization of warts and chemical matricectomy are the least painful procedures whereas larger excisions require the use of more potent postoperative painkillers. While the dressing is being put in place, the patient must be told what precautions to take. Providing a supply of moderately potent oral analgesics will help the patient feel in control of any pain. Elevating the extremity during the first 48 hours is advised to prevent swelling and decreases the experienced postoperative pain. Weak opioids can be prescribed in the presence of moderately perceived pain as well as nonsteroidal antiinflammatory drugs while strong opioids are restricted to intense pain. Pulsating pain beginning after 36 to 48 hours may indicate an infection, which should be treated according to the results of bacterial culture of the organism. Any bulky dressing that is blood stained after 24 hours should be changed.

DYSESTHESIA

Occurrence of postoperative long-term dysesthesia after nail surgery is well known. Complete or partial resolution may be noted after 6 to 12 months.

INFECTION

Prophylactic antibiotic treatment is mandatory for patients with prosthetic valve and in prevention of joint prosthesis infection. Peripheral vascular disease and young age (in childhood, the nail matrix is extremely fragile and behavior is less sanitary) are further indications. Tetanus toxoid for lesions of the toes should be discussed and advised especially in farmers, for example. If there are ragged surfaces to the nail, which makes thorough preoperative cleaning difficult, antibiotics may prevent wound infection. Postoperative infection may be caused by preoperative colonization or infection. Culture of preoperative swab specimens will indicate the best choice of drug after initial coverage with a broad-spectrum antibiotic. Attention to detail is important. Carelessness may result in serious infectious complications in the soft tissue and occasionally in bone. Routine or preoperative nail cleansing softens the nail plate and keeps contamination to a minimum. In the event of an infection, broad-spectrum antibiotics should be initiated.

ACQUIRED NAIL MALALIGNMENT[4]

Development of malalignment of the nail plate may result from lateral longitudinal biopsy in excess of the routine 3 mm.

RELAPSE

Relapse will depend on the nature of the lesion treated. Warts, ingrown nails, and myxoid cysts can be difficult to eradicate.

RESIDUAL DYSTROPHY

Residual dystrophies are not unusual when surgery involves the proximal area of the matrix. Nail spicules can be observed after lateral longitudinal excision, lateral matricectomies, or total removal of the nail apparatus.

UNPREDICTABLE COMPLICATIONS

- Necrosis can result from too tight stiches.
- Hypertrophic scars and keloids are rare.
- Implantation epidermoid cysts may occur in operation scars.
- Reflex sympathetic dystrophy now known as "Complex regional pain syndrome" Type I is rare. It presents with pain sensitive and motor disturbances along with autonomic and even soft tissue trophic changes.

NAIL AVULSION

A nail avulsion consists of separating the nail plate from its underlying attachments. It allows the exploration and/or the treatment of a subungual lesion or the removal of a pathologic nail plate. The nail is strongly adherent to its underlying bed and less adherent at the level of the distal matrix and the lateral nail folds. An avulsion is therefore easier to perform either a proximal or lateral approach. The removal of the nail plate can be carried out using distal or proximal approaches. In both techniques, inserting the blunt instrument back and forth between the horny layer of the proximal nail fold and the nail plate loosens the proximal nail fold adherence. Anesthesia is mandatory except in case of preexisting onycholysis.

DISTAL APPROACH

In the more commonly used distal approach, a Freer septum elevator or a dental spatula is inserted between the nail plate and nail bed (Fig. 205-7A). The nail is separated from its nail-bed attachment using proximal force applied in anterior–posterior movements so as not to injure the longitudinal ridges of the nail bed. The detachment is completed by firmly pushing the instrument into the posterolateral corners of the nail plate. Then, one of the lateral edges is grasped with a sturdy hemostat, and extracted with an upward and circular movement to accomplish the removal of the nail plate.

PROXIMAL APPROACH

The advantage of a proximal approach for nail avulsion is to prevent an injury to the distal nail bed and hyponychium through the insertion of the Freer septum. The

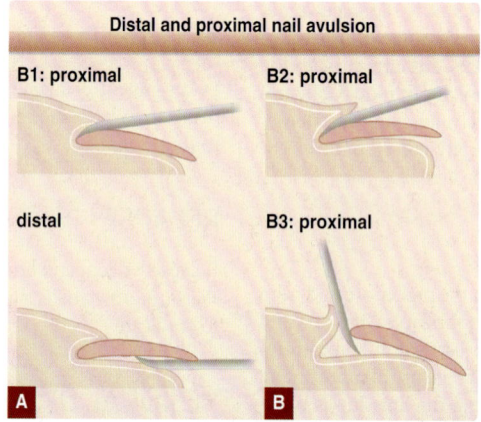

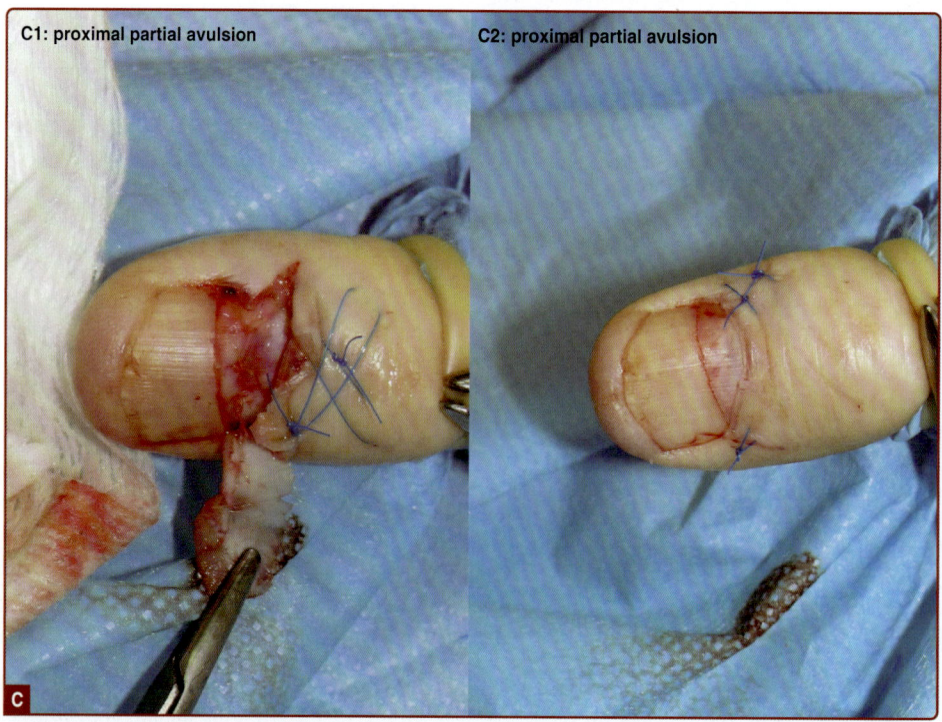

Figure 205-7 **A,** Distal nail avulsion. **B,** Proximal nail avulsion. **C,** Partial avulsions.

spatula is then used to reflect the proximal nail fold, and is delicately inserted under the base of the nail plate where adherence is normally weak (Fig. 205-7B). The instrument is advanced distally following the natural cleavage plane, and this operation is repeated on the entire width of the subungual region. After the last attachments are freed, the nail plate is easily pulled out.

Total surgical removal should be discouraged, however, because the distal nail bed may shrink and become dislocated dorsally. In addition, the loss of counterpressure produced by the removal of the nail plate allows expansion of the distal soft tissue, and the distal edge of the regrowing nail then embeds itself. In patients at high risk, nonsurgical removal of the nail plate should be considered when necessary. This can be accomplished by applying 40% urea paste directly to the nail after protecting the surrounding skin. Urea acts on the bond between nail keratin and diseased nail plate, sparing only the normal nail tissue.

PARTIAL NAIL AVULSION

The problems that can arise after total nail avulsion may be overcome by partially avulsing the nail. Partial distal avulsion requires only separation of the nail from the distal nail bed. This procedure can be performed under local anesthesia in selected patients, when, for instance, a fungal infection is of limited extent. An affected portion of the nail plate may be removed in one session, even when the disease has reached the deeper regions of the subungual tissue beneath the proximal nail fold. Commonly, an English anvil nail splitter or a double-action bone rongeur is used for this procedure. Partial surgical section of the lateral and/or medial segment of the nail plate may be sufficient for the treatment of distal lateral subungual onychomycosis (Fig. 205-7C). In the toe, this procedure leaves enough normal nail to counteract the upward forces exerted on the distal soft tissue when walking, and this will prevent the appearance of a distal nail wall. In proximal subungual onychomycosis, removal of the nonadjacent base of the nail plate, cut transversely, leaves the distal portion of the nail in place (Fig. 205-8), which decreases discomfort. Similarly, an acute paronychia that does not respond to appropriate antibiotics within 48 hours should be treated surgically by removing the base of the nail plate. Moreover, in cases of nail matrix procedures, a partial proximal avulsion prevents damaging the distal nail while allowing for an excellent visualization of the matrix and the cul-de-sac. The proximal nail plate is usually cut at its proximal third, lifted up, and always pulled back into its initial position at the end of the procedure.

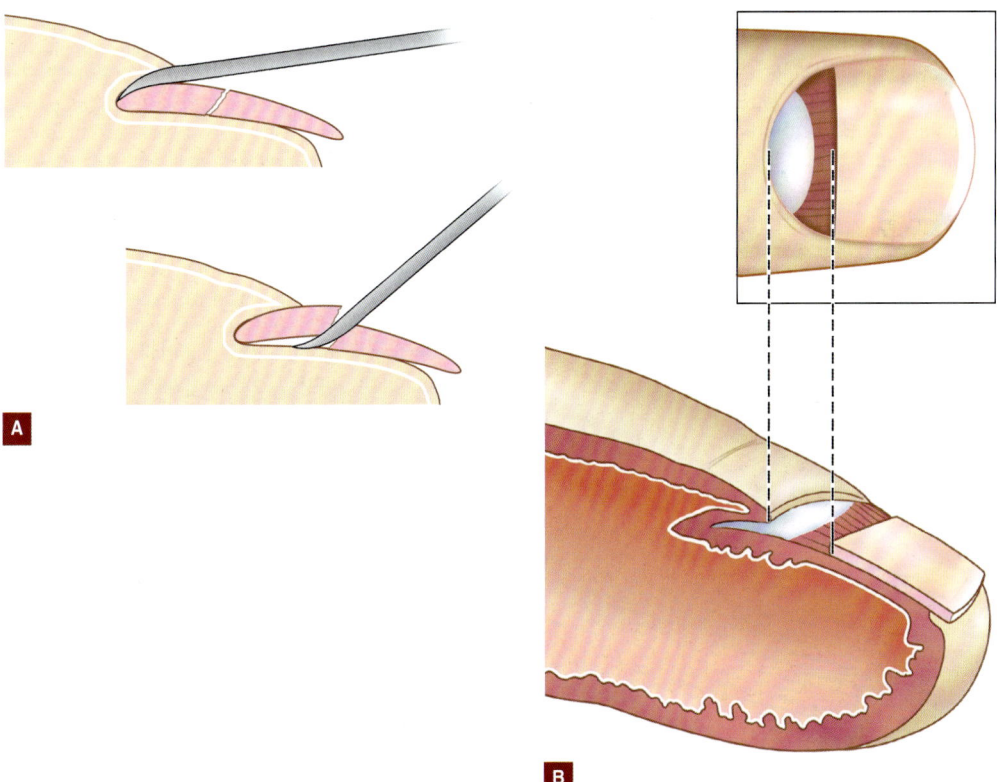

Figure 205-8 **A** and **B,** Technique of removal of the base of the nail plate.

TRAP DOOR NAIL AVULSION

This technique minimizes trauma in nail surgery when accessing the nail bed and matrix. Trap door nail plate avulsion entails separation of all periungual attachments except for that between the dorsum of the nail and the ventral aspect of the proximal nail fold. Both are then reflected en bloc in the manner of a trap door, utilizing the same oblique incisions normally made for reflection of the PNF alone. A partial medial trap door nail avulsion is also recommended for medial longitudinal excision.

NAIL BIOPSIES

Biopsies are performed to determine the histopathologic features of a lesion or to clarify an uncertain clinical diagnosis. Techniques depend on the location of the lesion.

LATERAL LONGITUDINAL BIOPSY OR LATERAL FUSIFORM EXCISION

It gives information of the entire nail organ and therefore represents the best technique for the diagnosis of inflammatory disorders as lichen planus or psoriasis when all the subunits of the nail apparatus are involved. Lateral longitudinal biopsy is also advised when longitudinal melanonychia[3] is located in the lateral part of the nail plate (Fig. 205-9). An elliptical incision may be made on either side of the nail plate and proximal nail fold. For the most part, the incisions parallel the lateral edge of the nail plate. Beginning in the lateral nail groove, the incisions should include a 3- to 4-mm nail segment reaching to the bone. (See Video 205-1 at mhprofessional.com/fitzderm9evideos) This ensures that a full-thickness fragment of the matrix with its lateral horn is obtained. Slightly curved iris scissors are useful for separating the tissue from the bone. Starting at the tip of the digit, one proceeds proximally while maintaining contact with the bony phalanx. Backstitches for the lateral nail folds avoid their flattening. It is helpful, especially for thick toenails, to soften the nail before the procedure by soaking it in warm water for 5 minutes.

BIOPSY OF THE DISTAL NAIL MATRIX [5-7]

A 3-mm punch biopsy may be performed through the nail plate into the distal matrix. Three millimeters is the maximum size that does not produce serious dystrophy, although even biopsies of this size can cause such effects if carried out in the most proximal portion of the nail matrix. When a punch biopsy is used to sample longitudinal melanonychia of less than 3 mm in width, the circumferential incision is made around the origin of the band, through the nail plate (Fig. 205-10A). This area may be distal enough to be reached by pushing back the cuticle (Fig. 205-10B), but if it is more proximal, the proximal nail fold may have to be reflected using a posterolateral incision. The next step is to remove the proximal third of the nail plate (Figs. 205-10B and C), while leaving the cylinder of tissue containing the origin of the longitudinal melanonychia still in place. This technique allows the surgeon to inspect the surrounding nail matrix and bed with a magnifying lens to determine whether the pigment extends around the punch incision (Figs. 205-10C and D) and facilitates the removal of the cylinder of biopsy tissue with a Gradle scissors. (See Video 205-2 at mhprofessional.com/fitzderm9evideos.)

For transverse biopsy (Fig. 205-11), 2 small oblique incisions are made on each side of the proximal nail fold. The fold is then reflected to expose the matrix area. The proximal third of the nail plate is avulsed. Then, the lesion is removed by excising an elliptical or crescent-shaped wedge of tissue with the convex portion of the crescent paralleling the anterior border of the lunula. When longitudinal melanonychia lies within the midportion of the nail plate, the potential for postoperative dystrophy is great, and selection of the optimal biopsy method is difficult (Fig. 205-12) (Haneke's releasing flap technique derived from Schernberg's releasing flat method). It is important to establish the matrix origin (proximal or distal) of longitudinal melanonychia preoperatively, because the more proximal the origin, the greater the risk of nail dystrophy.[5] The origin of pigmentation may be determined by dermoscopy of the free edge of the nail.[8]

Tangential matrix biopsy (Fig. 205-13) for wide longitudinal melanonychia is a good option. Cutting, then reclining the proximal portion of the nail plate (1), after reflecting the proximal nail fold (2), the pigmented lesion is exposed. An incision is made around

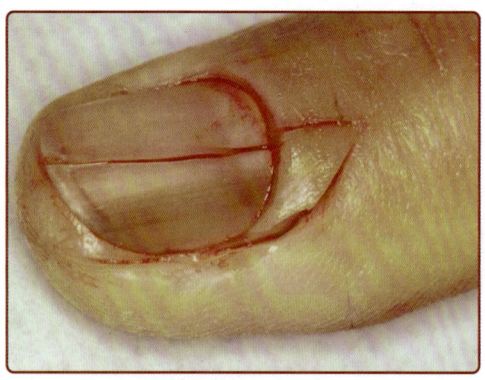

Figure 205-9 Lateral longitudinal biopsy of longitudinal melanonychia located within the lateral third of the nail plate.

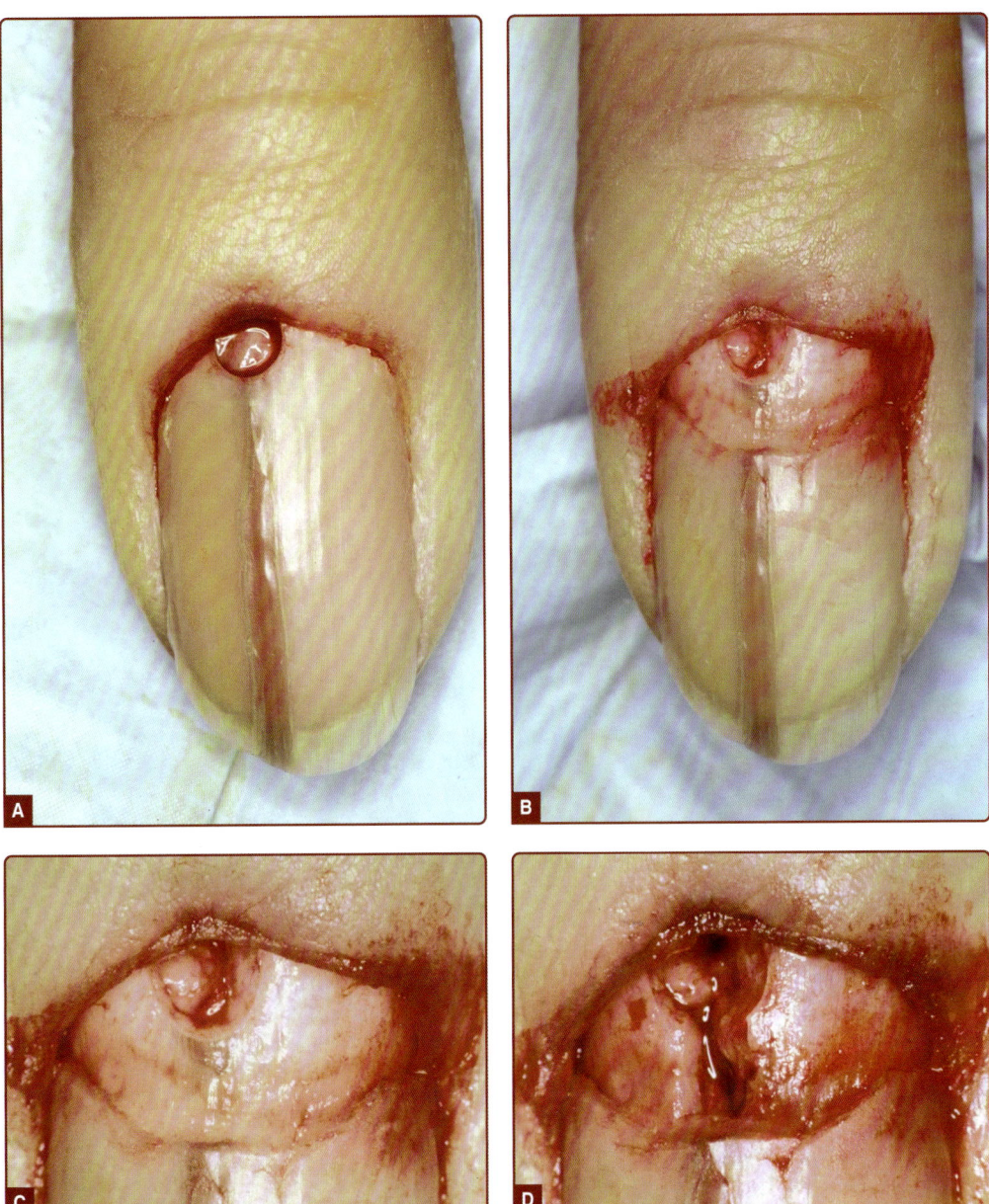

Figure 205-10 A, Punch biopsy of longitudinal melanonychia of width less than 3 mm. **B–D,** Removal of the base of the nail plate (**B**) to allow easy removal of the biopsied cylinder of matrix tissue (**C**), and pigment left distally (**D**).

the lesion, followed by its tangential removal. Finally, the proximal nail plate is replaced and the oblique incisions of the proximal nail fold are maintained by micropore. This technique is claimed to give the best cosmetic results.

NAIL BED BIOPSY

Biopsy (Fig. 205-14) may be useful in any pathologic condition involving the nail bed. Punch biopsy is done with a 3- or 4-mm-diameter punch, which is driven perpendicularly into the nail plate in a circular motion down to the bone. However, it is not always easy to extract the cylinder cut with an area this small. One useful technique is to perforate the nail plate with a 6-mm punch without injuring the underlying tissue (Fig. 205-14A). The covering nail is then detached by using the tip of the scalpel to remove the disk of nail, and the biopsy is performed easily by using the 4-mm punch to the bone. The tissue can then be released from its tether with fine scissors. It is advisable to replace the 6-mm disk of nail keratin, after cleaning with 10% hydrogen peroxide, to cover the hole. If the nail plate is thick, rotating grinders can

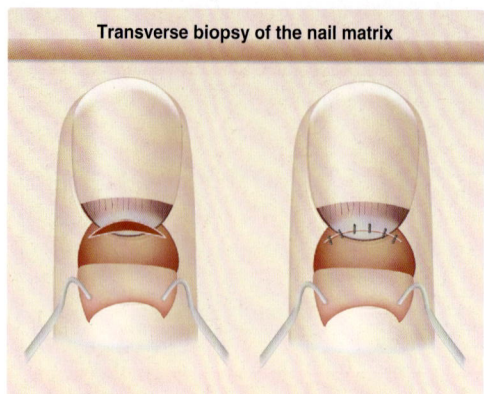

Figure 205-11 Transverse biopsy of the nail matrix.

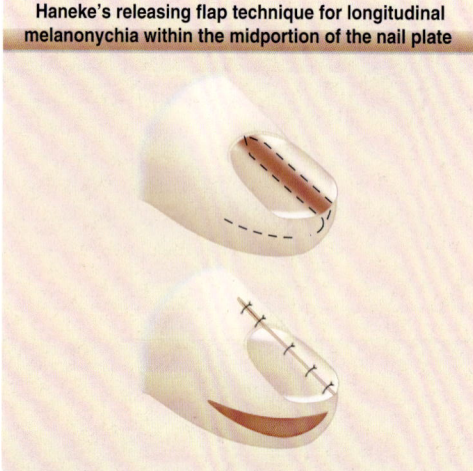

Figure 205-12 Haneke's releasing flap technique for longitudinal melanonychia within the midportion of the nail plate.

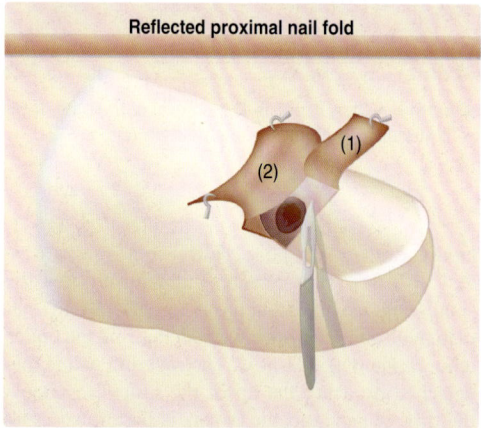

Figure 205-13 Reflected proximal nail fold and removal of the proximal portion of the nail plate exposing the pigmented lesion. Around the latter is made an incision followed by its tangential removal Haneke's matrix tangential biopsy technique.

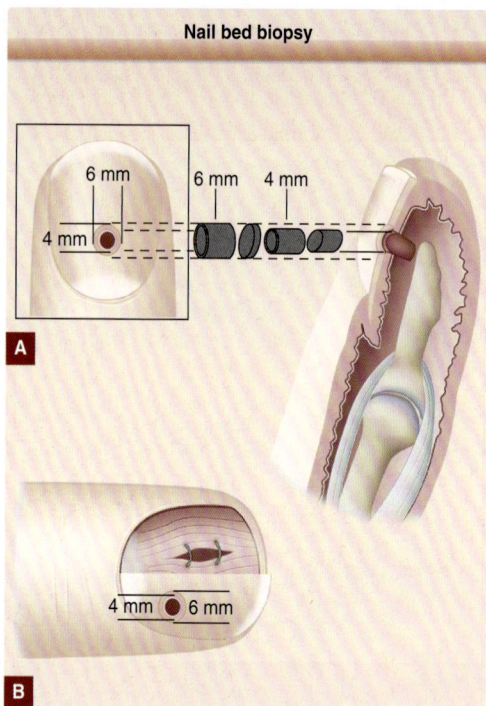

Figure 205-14 Nail bed biopsy. **A,** Punch biopsy. **B,** Fusiform biopsy.

be used to thin it down and facilitate the transungual biopsy.

PROXIMAL NAIL FOLD BIOPSY

A 2- to 3-mm punch may be used for biopsy of a tumor. A blister may be completely removed by shave biopsy using half a razor blade (Fig. 205-15). Excision of a 3-mm crescent-shaped tissue segment in the proximal region of the lateral nail folds may be helpful in the evaluation of collagen disease.

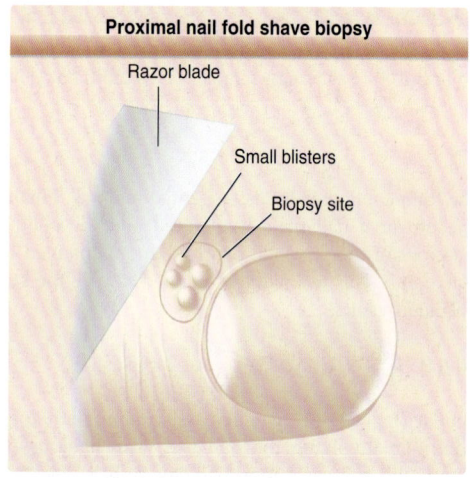

Figure 205-15 Proximal nail-fold shave biopsy.

APPLICATION TO THE DIFFERENT TISSUES OF THE NAIL APPARATUS

NAIL MATRIX PROCEDURES

When surgery involves the nail matrix, there are 3 primary approaches, including (1) a reduction in its width or (2) its length for removal of tumors, for instance, by using a cold steel procedure or (3) a 2- to 3-mm punch biopsy. In contrast to these 3 procedures, complete matricectomy, that is, ablation of the nail-forming tissue, is rarely performed because the nail is permanently lost (Fig. 205-16).

After reduction of the nail matrix width, one is left with a narrower nail and after reduction of the length, with a diminution in the thickness of the nail. Reduction of the matrix width is a useful and/or necessary procedure in the following major circumstances: need for lateral-longitudinal biopsy, lateral nail splitting, benign or malignant tumor in the lateral third of the nail apparatus, longitudinal melanonychia in a lateral location, ingrown nail, racquet nail. Destruction of lateral horn of the matrix can be performed surgically for lateral tumors or chemically with a solution of 88% phenol, 80% trichloroacetic acid, or 10% sodium hydroxide for nail splitting, ingrowing nail, or racquet nail (cf infra).

Reduction of the matrix length is necessary only in limited cases: to obtain a transverse elliptical biopsy specimen, to treat tumors that are 3 mm wide or larger, and to thin thick nails in patients with dystrophic congenital and/or hereditary disorders.

NAIL MATRIX TUMORS

If the tumor is located within the lateral third of either portion of the nail, especially when it is close to the lateral margin, the best method is the technique recommended for lateral longitudinal nail biopsy, that is, the removal of the lateral portion of the nail with the defect. If the tumor is located in the middle region, the proximal nail fold is carefully freed from the underlying nail plate, obliquely incised at both sides, and reflected to expose the whole matrix area. For distal matrix tumors, excision is performed as a transverse biopsy except for very superficial epithelial tumors or wide longitudinal melanonychia that can be removed by tangential shave excision. (See Video 205-3 at mhprofessional.com/fitzderm9evideos.) For tumors located underneath the matrix, incision should be done parallel to the anterior border of the lunula.

If the tumor is located to the proximal nail matrix and too deep to allow a tangential excision, an alternative approach is the formation of a Schernberg nail bed–matrix flap with an L-shaped incision of the lateral aspect of the finger (Fig. 205-17). A technique slightly modified by E. Haneke.

NAIL ABLATION AND ISOLATED MATRICECTOMY

Nail ablation (Fig. 205-16A) is the definitive removal of the entire nail organ and matricectomy (Fig. 205-16B), the complete extirpation of the nail matrix, which results in permanent nail loss. The principle of nail ablation is the complete removal of the nail unit

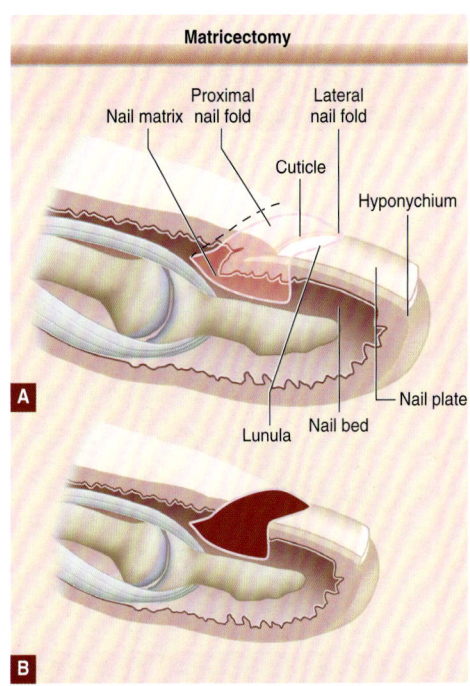

Figure 205-16 Matricectomy. **A,** Area of excision. **B,** Remaining defect.

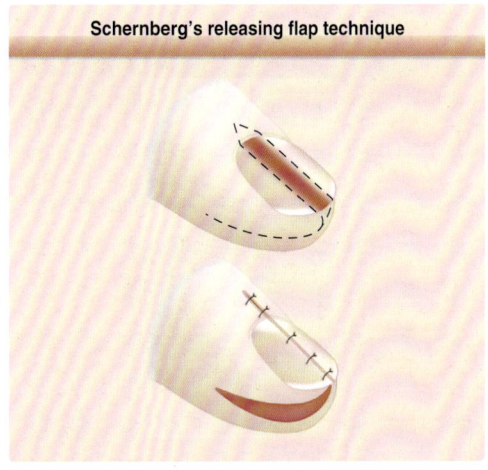

Figure 205-17 Schernberg's releasing flap method.

with hyponychium, nail bed, matrix, and lateral and proximal nail folds. Except for treatment of malignant tumors of the nail apparatus, nail ablation is rarely indicated. It may be necessary in the case of an excessively painful nail treated several times without success, but this should be an exception. Scalpel excision is strongly advocated whenever the surgical specimen needs histopathologic examination. If periungual pigmentation is associated with longitudinal melanonychia or if the latter is wider than 6 mm or the full thickness of the nail is pigmented, a large portion of the matrix would necessarily be involved. Under these circumstances, the underlying disease process is unlikely to be benign. The entire portion of the involved nail apparatus has to be excised en bloc.

The defect from nail ablation (Fig. 205-18B) may be covered with a free graft (split-thickness, full-thickness, reversed dermal graft), which usually takes on the bone in this particular location. A cross-finger flap is an alternative to a free graft. The use of the skin from the intermediate phalanx of a neighboring finger is more convenient for the patient than skin from the thenar area of the palm.

If only permanent nail matrix removal is necessary, the procedure is less extensive.

In cases in which pathologic examination of the removed tissue is unnecessary, phenol cautery, rather than scalpel excision, is the preferred technique for matricectomy. Most patients return to normal ambulation and activity as early as 1 day after the operation.

NAIL-BED PROCEDURES

Nail-bed surgery is performed for biopsy, removal of tumors, and treatment of subungual hematoma or nail dystrophies such as onychogryphosis. If a larger nail bed fragment is needed, fusiform biopsy with a major longitudinal axis can be performed after partial avulsion of the lateral half of the nail (Fig. 205-14B; see Video 205-4 at mhprofessional.com/fitzderm9evideos) or after total avulsion if the fragment is central. After excision, the nail bed is undermined to facilitate reapproximation of both sides. The suture needle is used generously on these fragile subungual tissues. The wound is stitched with 6-0 resorbable thread. It is sometimes useful to make relaxing incisions at the most lateral margins of the nail bed.

SUBUNGUAL HEMATOMA

In cases of subungual hematoma, acute trauma with severe pain is always remembered by the patient. Depending on the site and intensity of the injury, the hematoma may be visible almost immediately or it may grow out from under the proximal nail fold within a few weeks.

When the hematoma is partial (less than 25% of the visible portion of the nail), it should be drained with a pointed scalpel or by hot paperclip cautery over the center of the dark spot (Fig. 205-19). This will produce relief from pain. Sometimes the nail sloughs as the new nail regenerates beneath the old one. Small hematomas may be included in the nail, but they cannot be degraded to hemosiderin, and results of the Prussian blue test will be negative. Therefore, to demonstrate the nature of the blackish pigment, scrapings are boiled in a small test tube with Hemostix, which gives a positive benzidine result. A hematoma involving more than 25% of the visible portion of the nail is a sign of significant nail bed injury. A radiograph is mandatory, because the phalanx may be fractured. The nail plate

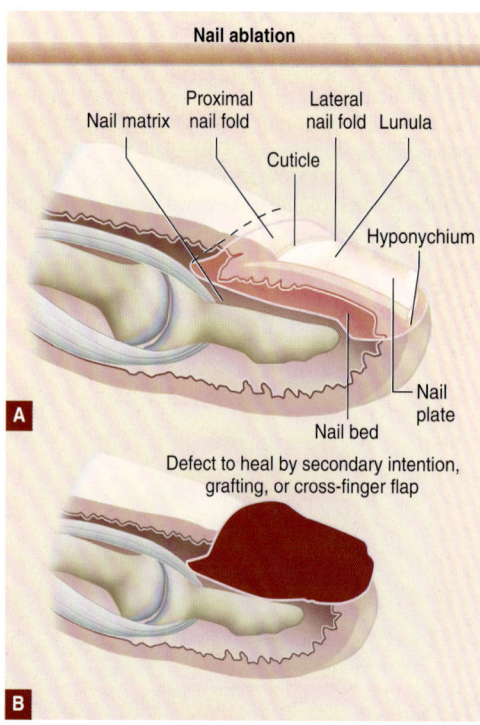

Figure 205-18 Nail ablation. **A,** Area of excision. **B,** Remaining defect.

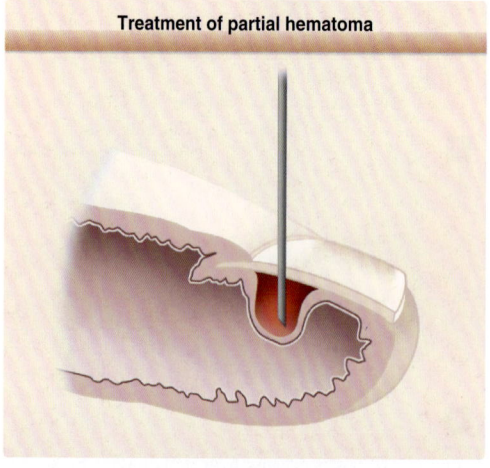

Figure 205-19 Treatment of partial hematoma.

is carefully removed and the hematoma evacuated. Traumatic nail bed laceration or wounds need a surgical approach to avoid delayed complications. Nail bed lacerations can be sutured after thorough cleaning with antiseptics, using 6-0 resorbable monofilament material. The avulsed nail plate should be put back to cover the wound and then kept in place by suturing to the lateral nail folds or the fingertip. Nail bed defects larger than 4 mm can be repaired using a split-thickness graft taken either from the nail bed of the same digit or from the nail bed of a great toe. The torn nail bed should be sutured with 6-0 resorbable thread, and large bites of tissue should be taken so that the suture material does not pull through when it is tied. The nail plate is cleaned, shortened, and slightly narrowed, and then replaced with sutures into the lateral nail folds. The stitches are left in for 2 weeks. Chronic hematomas are usually painless and are caused mainly by repeated microtrauma from either ill-fitting footwear or sporting activities. A notch is made with a scalpel blade at the distal and proximal border of the pigmented spot. Observation over a 3-week period will demonstrate whether the nail grows independently of the pigmentation or with it. However, chronic hematoma may resemble subungual melanoma and pose a distressing problem, and nonmigrating hematoma should be ruled out.

PROXIMAL NAIL FOLD PROCEDURES

RECALCITRANT CHRONIC PARONYCHIA

Presence of a foreign body (eg, hair) under the proximal nail fold is the main cause of recalcitrant chronic paronychia. The disorder manifests as a red swelling that is painless except when pressed, with secondary retraction of the paronychial tissue whose cuticle has disappeared and with recurrent episodes of acute paronychial inflammation.

For crescentic excision, a Freer septum elevator is inserted under the proximal nail fold to protect the matrix and extensor tendon. A No. 15 Bard-Parker blade is used to excise, en bloc, a crescent-shaped full-thickness skin segment, 4 mm at its greatest width that extends from one lateral nail fold to the other. Use of a beveled incision prevents accidental damage to the proximal nail matrix and the most proximal portion of the proximal nail fold, which is responsible for the normal shine of the nail plate (Fig. 205-20). In patients who experience repeated acute flares associated with chronic paronychia, additional removal of the base of the nail is useful.

The drawback of this technique is that the PNF is usually slightly retracted giving rise to a longer nail. This can be avoided by reclining the PNF in order to remove the fibrous under surface and suture it back to its original position.[9]

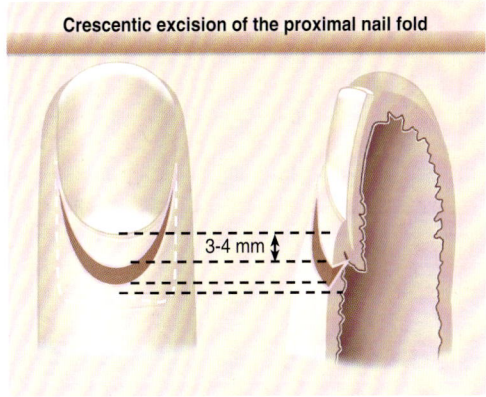

Figure 205-20 Crescentic excision of the proximal nail fold.

TUMORS OF THE PROXIMAL NAIL FOLD

Different techniques can be used to treat tumors of the proximal nail fold, depending on the nature of the tumor, its location, and the length of its long axis.

Crescentic excision is useful for small distal tumors. The crescent should not exceed 4 mm at its greatest width.

Tumors of the proximal nail fold that are situated in a median position and have a longitudinal axis longer than 4 to 5 mm can be excised with a wedge of proximal nail fold whose base is located at the free margin and whose apex points proximally (Fig. 205-21A). Two relaxing lateral incisions are then made in the proximal nail fold to allow suturing of the wedge-shaped defect after the undersurface of the proximal nail fold has been released from the nail plate (Fig. 205-21B).

The resulting symmetric narrow defects on both sides heal rapidly by secondary intention.

A small tumor on the lateral part of the proximal nail fold may be treated using a wedge-shaped excision

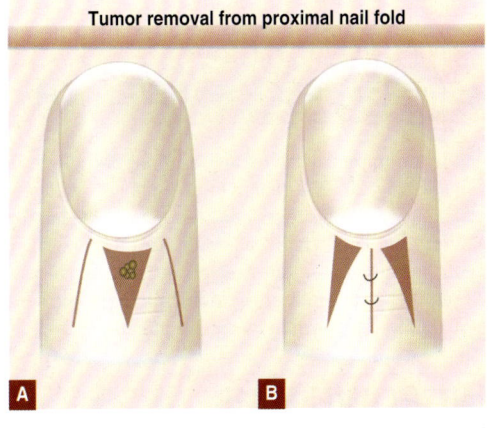

Figure 205-21 **A,** Tumor of the proximal nail fold situated in a median position. **B,** Suturing of the defect after relaxing lateral incisions are made and the proximal nail fold has been released from the nail plate.

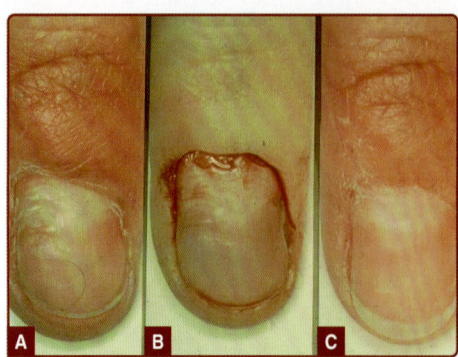

Figure 205-22 **A,** Irregular shape of the distal border of the proximal nail fold. **B,** Crescenting wedge-shaped excision of the proximal nailfold. **C,** Two months after healing.

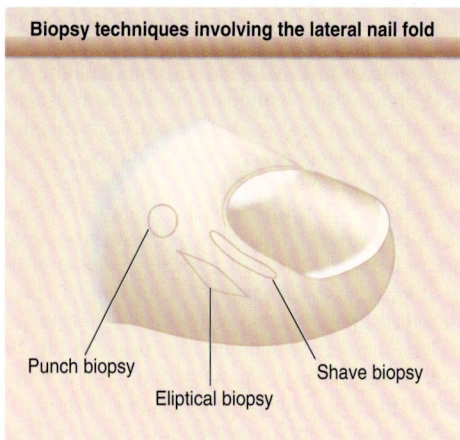

Figure 205-23 Biopsy techniques involving the lateral nail fold.

(Fig. 205-22). Only one lateral relaxing incision is made at the opposite region of the proximal nail fold. To obtain better healing of the secondary defect, which is wider than in the procedure using 2 relaxing incisions, the surgery may be supplemented by making a relaxing crescent-shaped incision in the proximal nail fold.

A dorsal flap can be raised from the proximal nail fold by using 2 dorsolateral incisions and a horizontal one proximal to the cuticle. This gives complete exposure of subcutaneous tumors.

RECONSTRUCTION OF THE PROXIMAL NAIL FOLD

Reconstruction of the proximal nail fold may be necessary after any injury (accident, burn, avulsion caused by rapidly rotating belts and sanders, etc.). If the irregular tissue is excised, it is sometimes possible to recreate the distal curve of the proximal nail fold, which may produce a nearly perfect restoration. The proximal nail fold also may be restored by using 2 long, narrow, V-shaped transposition flaps from the lateral aspects of the terminal phalanx.

LATERAL NAIL FOLD PROCEDURES

A 2- to 4-mm punch can remove a tumor of the lateral nail fold (Fig. 205-23). Benign tumors may be removed by taking an elliptical wedge of tissue from the lateral nail fold and lateral nail wall. Malignant tumors, such as in Bowen disease, are treated by excision of the whole lateral nail fold or by Mohs micrographic surgery followed by healing by second intention.

INGROWN NAIL

Ingrown nail is a condition that occurs mainly in the great toe. It is created by impingement of the nail plate into the dermal tissue distally or into the distolateral nail groove. Irrespective of the initial cause, the condition finally presents with a nail bed that is too narrow for its nail plate. Logical treatment is therefore aimed at correcting this disparity.

DISTAL TOENAIL EMBEDDING

Surgical avulsion or the loss of the toenail from trauma, such as tennis toe, may initiate the pathology. The distal subungual tissues released from the physiologic counterpressure of the nail plate become hypertrophic, and the newly formed nail plate abuts this distal wall. To treat the condition, a crescentic wedge-shaped excision is made around the distal phalanx (Fig. 205-24). The wedge should be 4 mm at its greatest width and must be dissected from the bone. The defect is closed with 5-0 monofilament sutures, which should be removed after 12 to 14 days.

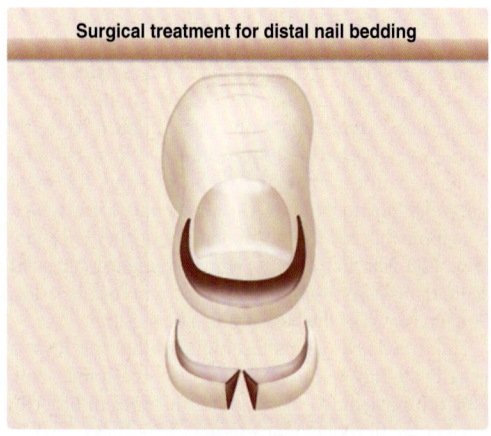

Figure 205-24 Surgical treatment for distal nail embedding.

RETRONYCHIA

Retronychia represents proximal regrowth of the nail that occurs when the nail embeds backwards into the proximal nail fold. This condition involves usually big toenails but also, rarely, fingernails. There is a thickening of the proximal portion of the yellowish nail plate as well as a painful paronychia. There is an embedding of the nail into the proximal nail groove following an acute insulte of fingers or toes. There is a characteristic triade: disruption of the linear nail growth, subacute paronychia, with lifting at the rear of the nail due a double or triple-layered proximal nail plate associated with frequent xanthonychia. A longitudinal overcurvature may be seen. Proximal granulation tissue, inflammatory subungual exsudate and onycholysis are often observed.

Ultrasound shows the pathognomonic sign: the shortening of the distance between the proximal edge of the nail and the distal interphalangial joint. Surgical treatment consists of avulsing the nail showing superimposed layers of keratin (Fig. 205-25).[10,11]

JUVENILE (SUBCUTANEOUS) INGROWN NAILS

Juvenile or subcutaneous embedded nail is the most common type of ingrown nail. The nail is usually embedded medially, but both sides are often affected. In an effort to relieve the pain, the patient often tries to cut off the offending corner under the inflamed and swollen soft tissue. The remaining portion gives rise to a nail spicule piercing the epithelium of the lateral nail groove, which produces secondary infection and excessive granulation tissue.

Treatment at the early stage must be conservative but demands a high degree of patient compliance. The foot is soaked in warm water with povidone-iodine soap; then, under local anesthesia, the nail spicule is removed and a wisp of cotton wool is placed between the nail and the lateral nail groove. It should be moistened repeatedly with a disinfectant.

For definitive cure, surgical excision or, better, chemical suppression of the lateral horn of the nail matrix permanently narrows the nail. The lateral fifth of the nail plate is freed with a nail elevator from the proximal nail fold and the subungual tissues. It is then cut longitudinally with an English nail splitter or nail-splitting scissors and extracted using a sturdy hemostat. The lateral matrix horn is cauterized with a freshly made solution of liquefied phenol (88% solution) (Fig. 205-26). Above all, a bloodless field is needed, because blood inactivates phenol. Hemostasis is therefore accomplished with a tourniquet, and the blood is carefully cleaned from the space under the proximal nail fold using sterile gauze. The surrounding skin is protected with petroleum jelly. The phenol is rubbed onto the matrix epithelium for 30 seconds, 3 times with a cotton-tipped swab that is changed each time. Postoperative pain

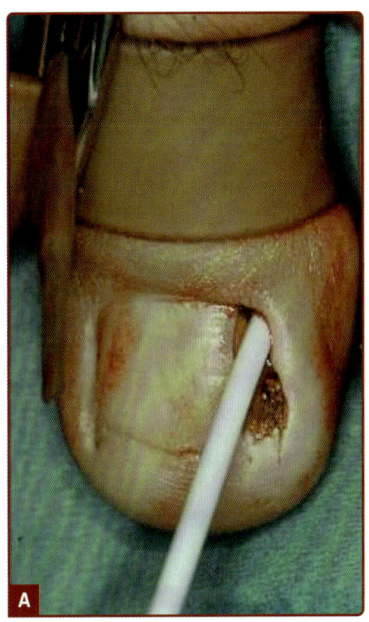

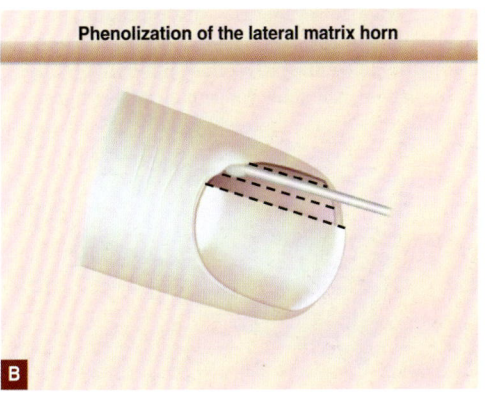

Figure 205-26 **A,** Juvenile ingrown nail with excessive granulation tissue. **B,** Phenolization of the lateral matrix horn.

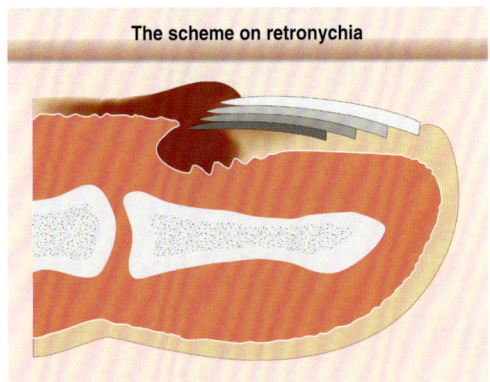

Figure 205-25 The scheme on retronychia.

is minimal because phenol has a local anesthetic action and is antiseptic. The matrix epithelium is sloughed off, and oozing is usual for 2 to 6 weeks. Daily warm foot baths with povidone-iodine soap accelerate healing.

Besides phenol and 10% sodium hydroxide, 80% trichloracetic acid also has been performed for partial matricectomy. The wound almost always heals within 2 weeks without prolonged exudative discharge. Pain is mild but transient.

PINCER NAIL[12]

Overcurvature of the nails may affect the great toe alone or all the digits. This condition may be so painful that even contact with a bedsheet becomes unbearable.

When the condition is mild, the nail brace technique aims at correcting the inward distortion of the nail by maintaining continuous tension on the nail plate. A stainless steel wire brace is fitted to the nail plate. A series of adjustments adapted to the gradual decrease of curvature is made over a period of 6 months and results in a painless correction of the pincer nail. Because the underlying bone pathology remains untreated, however, relapse is usual. Therefore, the definitive cure—the use of phenol cautery on the lateral matrix horns—is undoubtedly the simplest effective treatment modality.

HYPERTROPHY OF THE LATERAL NAIL FOLD

Hypertrophic lateral nail folds are usually the result of long-standing ingrown nails. Inflammation may range from the subclinical to the severe. For treatment, approximately one-fifth of the nail digging into the lateral nail fold is removed. Then an elliptical wedge of tissue is taken from the lateral nail wall of the toe, down to the bone (Fig. 205-27). Suturing of the defect pulls the lateral nail fold away from the offending lateral nail edge. In severe cases, this procedure may be combined with phenol cautery of the lateral horn of the matrix. In contrast to adult-acquired hypertrophy of the lateral nail fold, congenital lateral hypertrophic lips disappear progressively and spontaneously within 12 months.

CONGENITAL MALALIGNMENT OF THE GREAT TOENAIL[13]

In congenital malalignment of the nail of the great toe, typically the nail is malaligned laterally, with transverse furrows on a thick brownish or greenish nail.

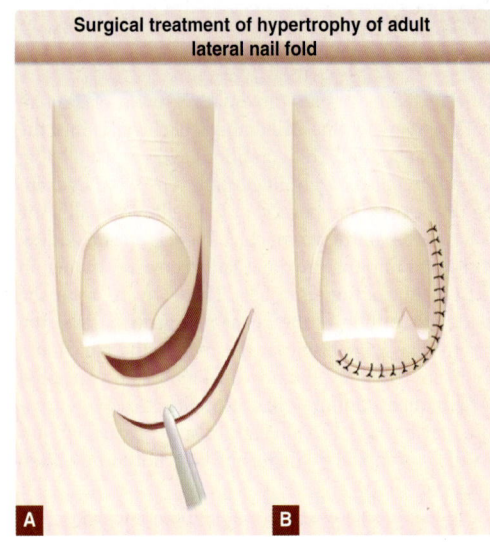

Figure 205-27 Surgical treatment of hypertrophy of adult lateral nail fold.

In 50% of cases, this condition corrects itself without therapy before the age of 10. If the appearance is extreme, surgery diminishes the risk of permanent dystrophy.

Treatment requires rotation of a bulky nail unit flap, including the entire nail, nail bed, and matrix (Fig. 205-28). This demands creation of an external Burow's triangle. An eccentric crescent-shaped excision is made to undermine the nail unit, with the maximum width located on the internal side of the foot, corresponding to the side to which the nail needs to be redirected. This crescent ends on each side 3 to 4 mm behind the most proximal part of the proximal nail fold. The nail bed and the matrix are then undermined and lifted until the fibers of the extensor tendon are visible on its bony insertion, and the dorsal expansion of the lateral ligament of the distal interphalangeal joint is cut.

Suturing the edges of the excised triangle together reduces the loss of cutaneous substance. The nail unit

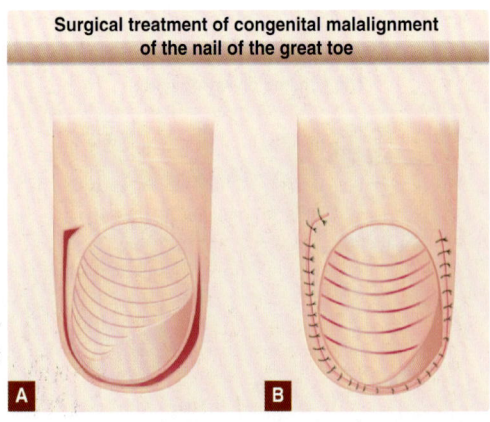

Figure 205-28 Surgical treatment of congenital malalignment of the nail of the great toe.

is rotated inwardly, because the maximum cutaneous resection is mostly distal and medial.

NONINVASIVE TREATMENT FOR INGROWN NAILS

Anchor taping, acrylic affixed gutter splint sculptered nail and others have obtained good results for treating ingrown nails, especially in children. Most ingrown nail cases are noninvasively cured by the combination of anchor-taping and acrylic affix gutter splint methods and do not require invasive surgery.[14]

REFERENCES

1. Fleckman P. Surgical anatomy of the nail unit. *Dermatol Surg*. 2001;27:257-260.
2. Jellinek N, Velez NF. Nail surgery: best way to obtain effective anesthesia. *Dermatol Clin*. 2015;33:265-271.
3. Durrant C, Townley WA, Ramkumar S, et al. Forgotten digital tourniquet: salvage of an ischaemic finger by application of medicinal leeches. *Ann R Coll Surg Engl*. 2006;88:462-464.
4. De Berker D, Baran R. Acquired malalignment: a complication of lateral longitudinal biopsy. *Acta Derm Venereol*. 1993;78:468-470.
5. Rich P. Nail biopsy: indications and methods. *Dermatol Surg*. 2001;27:229.
6. Baran R, Perrin C, Thomas L, et al. The melanocyte system of the nail and its disorders. In: Nordlung JJ, Boissy RE, Hearing VJ, et al., eds. *The Pigmentary System*. 2nd ed. Oxford: Blackwell; 2006:1057-1068.
7. Haneke E, Baran R. Longitudinal mélanonychie. *Dermatol Surg*. 2001;27:580.
8. Braun, Baran R, Saurat JH, et al. Surgical pearl: dermoscopy of the free edge of the nail determine the level of nail plate pigmentation and the location of its probable origin in the proximal or distal nail matrix. *J Am Acad Dermatol*. 2006;55:512-513.
9. Ferreira Vieira d'Almeida L, Papaiordanou F, Araujo Machado E, et al. Chronic paronychia treatment: Square flap technique. *JAAD*. 2016;75:398-403.
10. De Berker DAR, Richert B, Duhard E, et al. Retronychia: proximal ingrowing of the nail plate. *JAAD*. 2018;58:978-983.
11. Wortman X, Calderon P, Baran R. Finger retronychias detected early by 3D ultrasound examination. *JEADV*. 2012;2:254-256.
12. Baran R, Haneke E. Pincer nails. Definition and surgical treatment. *Dermatol Surg*. 2001;27:261-266.
13. Baran R, Haneke E. Etiology and treatment of nail malalignment. *Dermatol Surg*. 1998;24:719-721.
14. Arai H, Haneke E. Noninvasive treatment of ingrowing nails. In Baran R, Hadj-Rabia S, Silverman R. Pediatric nails disorders. *CRC Press*. 2017;263-274.

Chapter 206 :: Cryosurgery and Electrosurgery
:: Justin J. Vujevich & Leonard H. Goldberg

第二百零六章

冷冻疗法和电疗法

中文导读

本章中主要涉及了两种外科常用的治疗方法——冷冻疗法与电疗法，并从背景、技术、围手术期注意事项和临床应用等方面具体介绍了这两种治疗方法的相关内容。本章共分为12节：①冷冻疗法概述；②冷冻剂；③冷冻疗法围手术期注意事项；④冷冻疗法风险与并发症；⑤冷冻治疗的技术；⑥冷冻疗法在良性皮肤疾病中的应用；⑦冷冻疗法在恶性皮肤疾病中的应用；⑧电疗法的概述及分类；⑨电疗法的围手术期注意事项；⑩电疗法的风险及并发症；⑪电疗法的具体操作技术；⑫电疗法的临床应用。前7节介绍了冷冻疗法的相关内容，后5节则针对与多种电疗法有关的内容展开讨论。

第一节介绍了冷冻疗法的发展历史与治疗机制。冷冻疗法是一种使用极低温度来破坏异常或患病组织细胞的治疗方法，其造成组织破坏是通过直接细胞损伤、血管内血流淤滞和局部炎症反应来实现的。冷冻的过程主要是血流淤滞，组织缺血缺氧造成损伤；而解冻的过程则是短暂的充血导致水肿和炎症反应。

第二节介绍了冷冻疗法中的冷冻剂。液氮是皮肤科最常用的冷冻剂，其具有方便贮存、易于使用、环保、不易燃、价格低廉等优势。

第三节介绍了冷冻疗法的围手术期注意事项，包括患者选择、解剖位置注意事项、治疗禁忌证、风险及潜在的并发症、麻醉和护理这六个方面，其中着重介绍的内容是风险与并发症。

第四节介绍了冷冻疗法的风险和并发症，主要包括疼痛、出血、色素沉着、神经损伤、瘢痕形成和脱发等，同时阐述了各并发症常发生的情况和相关的处理措施。

第五节介绍了几种冷冻疗法的技术，其中最常用的方法是喷雾法，该方法使用到的设备是带有指尖扳机的手持式冷冻外科设备。冷冻的时间和手术部位范围需要根据具体的病变情况来选择。而封闭式接触治疗使用的设备是铜制低温探针，适用于治疗细小、界限分明的病变或在狭窄部位的病变。棉签法则是没有冷冻喷雾设备时的一种替代方法，用蘸取了少量液氮的棉签紧压病灶来进行冷冻。

第六节介绍了冷冻疗法在脂溢性角化病、疣、日光性黑子、瘢痕疙瘩和肥大性瘢痕、皮肤纤维瘤和皮脂腺增生这六类良性疾病中的应用。

第七节介绍了冷冻疗法在恶性皮肤疾病中的应用，列举了6种疾病，分别是光化性角化病、鲍温病、基底细胞癌、鳞状细胞癌、恶性雀斑样痣和Kaposi肉瘤。

第八节介绍了电疗法的基本内容和分类。电疗法是一种利用电力来切除组织、破坏组织和烧灼血管的技术。对于皮肤手术，电疗法可根据电力产生原理的不同细分为6种不同的治疗方式：电灼、电击、电凝、电切和电解。

第九节介绍了电疗法围手术期的注意事项，包括电疗法患者的选择、并发症、麻醉和护理相关的内容，重点阐述了电疗法可能带来的不良反应和并发症。

第十节介绍了电疗法常见的风险和并发症，包括对起搏器/植入式心脏除颤器的干扰、烧伤、手术室着火、电击伤、感染和致突变性。其中，作者详细介绍了电疗法对起搏器/植入式心脏除颤器的干扰，并给出了对植入式心脏除颤器患者的建议。

第十一节介绍了电疗法的具体操作技术。电疗法可以使用直流电也可以使用交流电，电疗法治疗设备可以是单极或双极的，单双极指的是设备电极末端（含组织尖端）的数量。患者应仰卧或俯卧在手术台上。

第十二节介绍了电疗法在止血、良性皮肤疾病和恶性肿瘤治疗中的应用。其中止血是电疗法在手术中最常见的应用，介绍了用于止血的几种不同的电疗法技术。根据不同的皮肤疾病，可以选择不同的电疗法。

〔赵　爽〕

AT-A-GLANCE

- With a boiling point of −195.8 Celsius, liquid nitrogen is the cryogen of choice for treating benign and malignant neoplasms.
- Melanocytes and fibroblasts are the cells that are most and least sensitive to the destructive effects of cryosurgery.
- Tumors that require histopathology for diagnosis and recurrent nonmelanoma skin cancers are contraindications for treatment with cryosurgery.
- Several cryosurgery techniques exist to treat benign and malignant neoplasms.
- Electrosurgery can be categorized into electrofulguration, electrodessication, electrocoagulation, electrosection, electrocautery, and electrolysis (Table 206-4).
- Electrosurgical devices have a low risk of interfering with cardiac and non cardiac implanted electronic devices (IEDs).
- Perioperative and intraoperative safety considerations should be made when performing electrosurgery on patients with IEDs.
- Curettage and electrodessication is an acceptable definitive treatment for malignant tumors.

CRYOSURGERY

BACKGROUND

Cryosurgery refers to the use of extreme cold to destroy cells of abnormal or diseased tissue. The earliest use of a cold refrigerant in medicine is attributed to White, a New York dermatologist, in 1899.[1,2] Using a cotton-tipped applicator dipped into liquefied air, he successfully treated warts, nevi, and precancerous and cancerous lesions. In 1907, Whitehouse, another New York dermatologist, reported the use of the spray method in the cryosurgical treatment of skin cancers.[3]

Cryobiology refers to the study of the effects of subzero temperature on living systems. Tissue destruction from cryotherapy results from direct cell injury, vascular stasis, and the local inflammatory response.

Freezing cells convert water to ice (crystallization). Rapid freezing causes intracellular ice crystal formation with the disruption of electrolytes and pH changes, whereas slow freezing causes extracellular ice formation and less cell damage. Therefore, tissue effects and cell death are most readily achieved when tissue is frozen rapidly.[4]

During thawing, recrystallization occurs when ice crystals fuse to form large crystals that disrupt cell membranes. As the ice melts further, the extracellular environment becomes hypotonic, causing water to infuse into cells and cause cell lysis.[5] The longer the thawing time, the greater the damage to cells because of increased solute effect and greater recrystallization.

After freezing, stasis within the vasculature occurs. This loss of circulation and resultant anoxia is a major mechanism of injury from cryosurgery. As the tissue thaws at temperatures higher than 0°C (32°F), a brief hyperemic response ensues with resultant edema and inflammation.[5]

TARGETS OF CRYOSURGERY

Table 206-1 lists targets of cryosurgery with associated cell death temperatures. Melanocytes are the

TABLE 206-1
Tissue Target Cell Death Temperatures

CELL	TEMPERATURE (°C/°F)
Melanocytes	−4 to −7 (24.8 to 19.4)
Keratinocytes	−20 to −30 (−4 to −22)
Fibroblasts	−30 to −35 (−22 to −31)

TABLE 206-2
Cryogens Used in Cryosurgery

AGENT	BOILING POINT (°C/°F)
Freon	−40.8/−41.4
Solid CO_2	−79.0/−110.2
Nitrous oxide	−89.5/−129.1
Liquid nitrogen	−195.8/−320.4

most sensitive to cryosurgery, with cell destruction at temperatures of −4°C to −7°C (24.8°F to 19.4°F).[6] As a result, depigmentation may occur, especially in darkly pigmented individuals. Keratinocytes require longer freezing to temperatures of −20°C to −30°C (−4°F to −22°F) until cell death and are more resistant to cooling effects. Fibroblasts are the most resistant to freezing and do not undergo cell death until −30°C to −35°C (−22°F to −31°F). A temperature of −50°C to −60°C (−58°F to −76°F) is needed for destruction of malignant lesions, whereas lesser degrees of freezing are needed for benign lesions.

CRYOGENS

Liquid nitrogen is the cryogen of choice in dermatology. It is easy to store in an insulated unit, easy to use, environmentally friendly, nonflammable, inexpensive, and, at −195.8°C (−320.4°F), has the lowest temperature of all the common cryogens, causing rapid freeze of treated tissue.

Other available cryogens include fluorinated hydrocarbons, solid carbon dioxide, and nitrous oxide (Table 206-2). Fluorinated hydrocarbons are used as topical sprays to provide temporary anesthesia before the removal of skin lesions and the administration of vaccinations. Cryogen spray cooling is also used to reduce the pain of laser surgery and eliminate overheating of the epidermis.[7]

PERIOPERATIVE CONSIDERATIONS

PATIENT SELECTION

Cryosurgery is one of several destruction modalities used for benign and malignant skin neoplasms. Several factors, including lesion type, size, depth, border, location, and patient skin type, should be considered when cryosurgery is a treatment choice.

ANATOMICAL SITE PRECAUTIONS

The cryosurgeon should be aware of certain anatomical locations where cryosurgery may lead to complications. Caution should be undertaken when treating lesions overlying nerves, such as the postauricular nerve on the neck or digital nerves on medial and lateral fingers and toes. Damage may result in regional paresthesia or motor dysfunction. In addition, cryosurgery at anatomical sites such as the eyelids, mucosa, nasal ala, and auditory canal, may result in scarring with retraction after treatment. As skin melanocytes are easily prone to destruction by freezing, the cryosurgeon should treat darkly-pigmented skin with caution as cryosurgery may result in hypopigmentation at treated sites.

TREATMENT CONTRAINDICATIONS

Absolute contraindications to cryosurgery include lesions that require histopathology for diagnosis and recurrent nonmelanoma skin cancers. Relative contraindications to cryosurgery include patients with cold urticaria, abnormal cold intolerance, cryoglobulinemia, or cryofibrinogenemia, or tumors with indistinct borders or darkly pigmented features (Table 206-3).

RISKS AND POTENTIAL COMPLICATIONS

Pain: In addition to pain during freezing, patients will experience some discomfort several hours post-treatment. Typically, pain is controlled with acetaminophen. Lesions such as periungual warts, digital lesions, or mucous membrane lesions may require stronger analgesics because of intense swelling and throbbing.

Bleeding: Patients on anticoagulant therapy should be warned of bruising resulting from tissue necrosis. If painful hemorrhagic bullae form, they may

TABLE 206-3
Contraindications to Cryosurgery

- Lesions that require histopathology for diagnosis[a]
- Recurrent nonmelanoma skin cancers[a]
- Cold urticaria
- Abnormal cold tolerance
- Cryoglobulinemia
- Cryofibrinogenemia
- Tumors with indistinct borders or darkly pigmented features

[a]Absolute contraindication.

be drained with an 18-gauge needle inserted into the lateral blister skin. Care should be undertaken not to remove the surface of the bullae, as this tissue acts as a natural wound dressing.

Pigmentation Changes: Hypopigmentation or hyperpigmentation is the most disconcerting complication following cryosurgery. As shown in Table 206-1, pigmented cells are highly susceptible to freezing at temperatures of −4°C to −7°C (24.8°F to 19.4°F). Although pigmentation changes are usually transient, prolonged freezing for longer than 30 seconds may result in permanent pigment loss. Topical steroids, glycolic acids, retinoids, and hydroquinone may aid in reducing the incidence of hypopigmentation.

Nerve Damage: Treatment of lesions overlying nerves, such as the postauricular nerve on the neck or digital nerves on medial and lateral fingers and toes, may result in regional paresthesia or motor dysfunction. Digital neuropathy occurring after cryosurgery of digital warts has been reported.[8]

Scarring: Fibroblasts are the most resistant to freezing and do not undergo cell death until −30°C to −35°C (−22°F to −31°F). Therefore, most benign and premalignant lesions treated with cryotherapy heal with little scarring. Soft, contracted linear scars resulting from second intention may occur in malignancies treated with cryosurgery.

Alopecia: Freeze times longer than 20 seconds may result in alopecia. This is especially true when treating malignant lesions.

Insufflation of Soft Tissue: During freezing nitrogen gas may escape into perilesional skin, producing crepitus. Pressure on the crepitated area will expel the gas. The use of a cone surrounding the biopsy site prevents crepitus from occurring.

ANESTHESIA

For the majority of patients, anesthesia is not necessary prior to a cryosurgical procedure. However, cryosurgery is painful, especially in children. For short cryosurgery treatment times, 1% lidocaine with 1:100,000 epinephrine may be locally injected prior to treatment. For longer cryosurgery treatment times, such as treatment of skin neoplasms (up to 30 seconds), local anesthesia is mandatory. Topical anesthesia can be applied approximately 1 hour prior to the procedure to minimize pain. A single-center, double-blinded, randomized, placebo-controlled, parallel-group trial comparing a cream containing 5% lidocaine and 5% prilocaine applied 1 hour prior to cryosurgery for warts, however, did not demonstrate a statistically significant difference in pain during the procedure.[9] For longer cryosurgery treatment times, such as treatment of skin neoplasms (up to 30 seconds), 1% lidocaine with 1:100,000 epinephrine can be locally injected prior to treatment.

PERIOPERATIVE CARE

Patients should be given simple verbal and written wound care instructions posttreatment. Edema, vesicles, bullae, and weeping should be expected from treated areas within 24 hours posttreatment. Treated sites may be rinsed with soap and water and patted dry with a towel daily. If actively weeping, the wound site may be bandaged.

Benign and premalignant lesion-treated sites heal typically in 1 to 2 weeks, with malignant lesion-treated sites requiring 3 to 4 weeks of healing. Clinically-suspicious actinic keratoses not responsive to cryosurgery should be biopsied to rule out invasive skin cancer.

CRYOSURGERY TECHNIQUES

There are several cryosurgical techniques that can be used in treating skin lesions. The open spray method is most frequently used. This method uses a handheld cryosurgical unit with fingertip trigger (Fig. 206-1). Patients may be seated or lying on an examination table at an angle. The canister should be held upright when treating the patient as tilting the canister sideways will result in the sudden release of a vapor from the canister. Spray tips with varying-sized apertures are attached to the unit, emitting a stream of liquid nitrogen toward the lesion from a distance of 1 to 2 cm.

Although freeze times vary for lesion types, an intermittent spray in a solid, circular, or paintbrush pattern is normally used. Longer spray times are required for thicker, keratotic lesions or malignant lesions; shorter times are required for thinner, atrophic, or benign lesions. The intermittent spray helps to localize

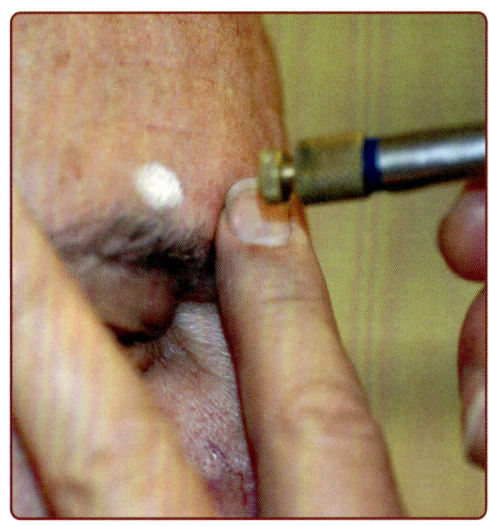

Figure 206-1 Actinic keratosis on forehead treated with liquid nitrogen.

treatment to the lesion with a small freeze halo, thus minimizing collateral normal tissue damage. This is particularly important when treating lesions around the orbital, nasal, auricular, genital, or periungual regions.

As the lesion is treated, a lateral freeze spreads beyond the margins of the lesion. The measurement of the surface radius of the freeze is equal to the central depth of the freeze into the skin.[5] Temperature gradients exist within the freeze, with colder temperatures in the middle and warmer temperatures toward the periphery. In general, superficial lesions should have a clinical freeze margin of 2 to 3 mm, and malignant or deeper lesions should have a clinical freeze margin of 5 mm to ensure successful treatment.

The closed technique uses a copper cryoprobe that is attached to the cryosurgical unit. Once the metal probe is pressed against a lesion on the skin, the trigger of the unit is squeezed, and liquid nitrogen leaves the unit through a conduit line that maintains it in a closed system. This technique is useful for treating small, well-circumscribed lesions or lesions found in confined locations.

Similarly, a metal, cone-sized chamber can be attached to the cryosurgical unit and held in contact with the lesion. This allows liquid nitrogen spray to enter the cone and rapidly freeze the lesion. Another cone apparatus option includes holding an otoscope cover tip against the lesion with one hand while freezing with the cryosurgical unit held in the other hand. Treatment times using the cone method should be decreased because the final temperature at the orifice of the cone is obtained faster, when compared with an open spray.

If a cryospray unit is not available, the dipstick technique can be used. First, a small amount of liquid nitrogen is poured into a polystyrene cup or other insulated container. Cotton-tipped swabs are placed tip-down in the container and cooled. Using firm pressure, the cotton tips are placed against the lesion until a 2-mm to 3-mm halo forms around the treated lesion. This method treats lesions on the body where surrounding tissue must be spared, such as periorbital, mucosal, nail, and genital regions.

Alternatively, tissue forceps can be placed in the container and allowed to cool. This method is useful for treating filiform lesions such as verrucae and skin tags. The metal forceps cool rapidly, so insulated gloves should be worn while holding the forceps to prevent freeze injury to the practitioner's fingers.

APPLICATIONS FOR COMMON BENIGN LESIONS

SEBORRHEIC KERATOSIS

The spray technique is an effective modality for treating this common lesion. Although longer freeze times of 10 to 15 seconds with a 1-mm to 2-mm halo are required for these raised growths, too aggressive freezing may result in scarring or hyperpigmentation. For cosmetic purposes and to prevent pigmentation changes, a lighter freeze followed by curettage may be preferential. Forewarn patients that a second treatment may be required, especially for thicker seborrheic keratoses.

VERRUCAE

Warts are a common problem, with a high prevalence in the population.[10] Although cryosurgery for warts has sustained a common practice in dermatology, varying techniques have been offered with regard to freezing method, number of freeze–thaw cycles, and frequency of treatment sessions. Cryosurgery using the spray technique is probably the most common method because of its quick, convenient use and ease of obtaining a freeze halo around the lesion (Fig. 206-2). The cotton-tip applicator technique is cheaper and may be less frightening to the patient, particularly if the patient is a child. Care must be undertaken not to cross-contaminate by reintroducing the cotton-tip applicator into a common flask.

Combination therapy with cryosurgery also has been advocated to treat verrucae. Berth-Jones and Huchinson[11] demonstrated a 52% cure rate at 3 months with the combination of cryotherapy, keratolytic wart paint, and paring. The authors also noted that paring the wart before cryotherapy improved the cure rates for plantar warts, but not hand warts.

SOLAR LENTIGO

As described in Table 206-1, pigmented cells are highly susceptible to freezing. Therefore, these lesions require a shorter freeze time of 3 to 5 seconds with minimal halo. For darker-skinned individuals, care must be taken not to induce hypopigmentation at treatment sites. Consequently, a test site in a cosmetically less noticeable region may be performed first before treating multiple lesions on sun-exposed areas. In addition, sunscreen with ultraviolet A and ultraviolet B protection should be advocated pretreatment and posttreatment.

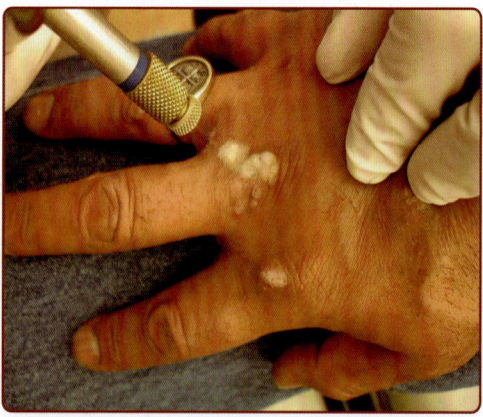

Figure 206-2 Warts on hand treated with liquid nitrogen.

KELOIDS AND HYPERTROPHIC SCARS

Treatment of keloids and hypertrophic scars is frequently unsatisfactory. Cryosurgery is a less common but effective means of treating these recalcitrant lesions. Freeze times of 30 seconds are required monthly until flattening is achieved. Zouboulis and colleagues reported a prospective study of 93 keloids and hypertrophic scars treated with 30-second freeze times over 1 to 3 sessions.[12] Improved responses were seen in patients treated with 3 or more sessions (79%), compared with subjects treated once or twice (33%).

DERMATOFIBROMA

Dermatofibroma treatment times may require cryosurgery up to 60 seconds because of the fibrotic nature of the lesion and the need to treat cells located in the deep dermis. Torre reported a series of 79 dermatofibromas treated with cryosurgery. Out of the 79 that were followed, 61 were no longer palpable post treatment.[13]

SEBACEOUS HYPERPLASIA

These benign lesions can be a cosmetic concern for patients. Freeze times of 5 to 10 seconds are required, using the cryoprobe technique with the probe applied directly into the central punctum of the lesion. Patients must be advised that retreatment is frequently necessary.

APPLICATIONS FOR PREMALIGNANT AND MALIGNANT LESIONS

Cryosurgery appears useful in well-defined lesions for situations where surgery is less favorable, either for technical or cosmetic reasons, or when the patient prefers this treatment option. The goal of cryosurgery is to cure the patient by destroying the lesion in a single treatment.

ACTINIC KERATOSIS

Cryosurgery is an effective modality for the treatment of actinic keratoses (AKs). The open spray technique, using a single freeze–thaw cycle of 8 to 10 seconds, is the treatment of choice. Hypertrophic AKs require longer freeze times, whereas atrophic AKs and AKs on thin-skinned regions require shorter freeze times. A 1-mm to 2-mm freeze margin around the lesion is adequate. For thicker lesions, pretreatment of emollients or curetting may shorten freezing times.

Although cryosurgery is widely used in dermatology for treatment of AKs, there are few well-designed studies assessing cure rates. Lubritz and Smolewski[14] treated 1018 AKs on 70 patients with cryosurgery with 20- to 45-second thaw times. At 1-year posttreatment, they reported a cure rate of 99%. Another prospective, multicenter study of 421 AKs larger than 5 mm in diameter on the face and scalp demonstrated a complete response of 39% with a 5-second freeze, 69% for a 5- to 20-second freeze, and 83% for a 20-second freeze.[15]

In patients with diffuse actinic damage, extensive cryosurgery, or cryopeeling, may be useful. Chiarello[16] reported cryopeeling was twice as effective as 5-fluorouracil in the reduction of actinic keratoses and the formation of squamous cell carcinomas at 1 and 3 years post-cryopeeling.

BOWEN DISEASE

Ahmed and colleagues[17] treated 26 Bowen disease patients using 3-mm clinical margins and spray technique with two 5- to 10-second freeze–thaw cycles. Two years after treatment, 50% of the treated lesions were still present at the same site. The average healing time was 46 days, with lesions on the lower leg taking longer to heal (90 days). Although the cure rate using cryosurgery for Bowen disease was low in this study, the authors did use a lower freeze time to minimize side effects postprocedure.

BASAL CELL CARCINOMA

Several studies have reported treating basal cell carcinomas (BCCs) with cryosurgery with cure rates ranging between 95% and 99%.[18-20] Although excellent cure rates have been claimed, few studies have demonstrated histologically that the BCC is no longer present posttreatment. Furthermore, there are no good studies comparing cryosurgery with other known treatment modalities, such as Mohs surgery, excision with clinical margins, and electrodesiccation and curettage.

Postsurgical cosmetic appearance is a concern to patients. Kokoszka and Scheinfeld[21] reported good cosmetic results in their review of the literature. Thissen and colleagues,[22] however, compared the cosmetic results of surgical excision compared with cryosurgery for BCCs of the head and neck and concluded that cosmetic results after excision are better than after cryosurgery.

SQUAMOUS CELL CARCINOMA

Similar cure rates to BCCs are evident when treating squamous cell carcinomas (SCCs) with cryosurgery. In a study of 563 primary SCCs, of which most were between 0.5 and 1.2 cm in diameter, Graham and Clark[23] reported a cure rate of 97.3%. Treatment technique with cryosurgery for SCCs is the same as for BCCs.

LENTIGO MALIGNA

With proper patient selection, cryosurgery can be an effective treatment option for lentigo maligna because of the sensitivity of melanocytes to cold. With the aid of a Wood lamp, a clinical margin of 5 mm is drawn around the visible borders of the lesion. The lesion is subsequently treated with a double freeze–thaw cycle of 30 to 60 seconds each cycle. Because atypical melanocytes may extend along the length of the hair follicles, treatment must freeze the tissue to this depth.

Stevenson and Ahmed[24] reviewed cure rates from more than 200 lentigo maligna patients treated with cryotherapy, with an overall recurrence rate of less than 9%. However, the recurrence rates in these studies ranged from 0% to 50%.

Advantages of cryotherapy for lentigo maligna include its efficiency and avoidance of large surgical scars. One major disadvantage of cryosurgery is the inability to assess whether the lesion has been completely destroyed. In addition, because no tissue is obtained for definitive confirmation of cancer removal, the chance exists that recurrent melanoma may develop and that it may be invasive. Overlying scars may conceal the cancer.

KAPOSI SARCOMA

Although not commonly used, Tappero and colleagues reported the treatment of Kaposi sarcoma using a double freeze–thaw cycle every 3 weeks.[25] An average of 3 treatments were required.

ELECTROSURGERY

Electrosurgery is a technique that uses the transmission of electricity to cut tissue, destroy tissue, and cauterize vessels. Variations in current wavelength result in different biologic effects on tissue. For cutaneous procedures, electrosurgery can be categorized into 6 different treatment modalities: electrofulguration, electrodessication, electrocoagulation, electrosection, electrocautery, and electrolysis (Table 206-4).

MODALITIES OF ELECTROSURGERY

ELECTROFULGURATION

Electrofulguration uses a damped sine wave, high-voltage, low-amperage alternating current to generate a spark from a monoterminal electrode to the tissue via the air. There is no contact between the electrode and the tissue. This modality is the least tissue damaging of all of the high-frequency electrosurgery techniques, and results in rapid tissue healing. Most of the tissue damage is superficial, primarily involving the epidermis.

TABLE 206-4
Modalities of Electrosurgery

	DAMPING	VOLTAGE & AMPERAGE	CURRENT	NUMBER OF TERMINALS	DESCRIPTION	CIRCUIT LOOP INVOLVES PATIENT
Electrofulguration	Damped sine wave	High-voltage, low-amperage	AC	Spark from monoterminal electrode to tissue through air; no direct contact	Least damaging modality; epidermis primarily affected	Yes
Electrodessication	Damped sine wave	High-voltage, low-amperage	AC	Direct contact from monoterminal electrode to tissue	Greater than electrofulguration, but damage is superficial	Yes
Electrocoagulation	Moderately damped sine wave	Low-voltage, high-amperage	AC	Direct contact from a biterminal node to tissue	Deeper tissue damage than electrofulguration and electrodessication; provides tissue coagulation	Yes
Electrosection	Undamped or slightly damped sine wave	Low-voltage, high-amperage	AC	Direct contact	Cuts tissue with minimal peripheral heat damage	Yes
Electrocautery		Low-voltage, high-amperage	DC	Heat is transferred from filament to tissue	Protein denaturation and coagulation	No[a]
Electrolysis		Low-voltage, low-amperage	DC	Negative electrode is applied to target tissue; acids are produced at the positive electrode	Tissue liquefaction (negative electrode); tissue coagulation (positive electrode)	Yes

[a]Therefore, this technique is useful for patients with pacemakers or in nonconductive tissues of the body.
AC, alternating current; DC, direct current.

ELECTRODESSICATION

Electrodessication uses a damped sine wave, high-voltage, low-amperage alternating current to generate a current from direct contact of a monoterminal electrode to the tissue. Superficial tissue damage occurs as heat is transferred to tissue, causing cell death. The extent of tissue damage is directly related to electrode contact time with the skin. Although skin injury is greater with electrodessication compared to electrofulguration, most of the tissue damage remains superficial.

ELECTROCOAGULATION

Electrocoagulation uses a moderately damped sine wave, low-voltage, high-amperage alternating current to generate a current from direct contact of a biterminal electrode to the tissue. Tissue damage is deeper than with electrofulguration and electrodessication, providing tissue coagulation through the generation of heat in the tissue.

Another distinguishing feature of electrocoagulation is the involvement of the patient within the circuit. This allows the use of a lower voltage and higher amperage to generate more coagulation.

ELECTROSECTION

Electrosection uses an undamped or slightly damped sine wave, low-voltage, high-amperage alternating current to cut tissue with minimal peripheral heat damage. The "Bovie" knife incorporates a blended undamped and damped sine wave that provides both cutting and coagulation at the same time.

ELECTROCAUTERY

Electrocautery uses a heating filament tip connected to a low-voltage, high-amperage direct current, usually a battery. Heat is transferred from the filament to the target tissue, causing protein denaturation and tissue coagulation. There is no electric current transfer to the target tissue, and the patient is not part of the circuit loop.

Electrocautery is most used for patients with pacemakers or implantable cardiac defibrillators (ICDs) who are high-risk candidates for receiving electrosurgery. In addition, because patients are not part of the circuit loop, electrocautery is useful for nonconductive tissue areas of the body, such as the cartilage, bone, and nails.

ELECTROLYSIS

Electrolysis uses low-voltage, low-amperage direct current from a negative electrode to the positive electrode. The negative electrode is applied to the target tissue where electrons are released. The electrons interact with the tissue to produce sodium hydroxide and hydrogen gas resulting in tissue liquefaction. Acids are produced at the positive electrode resulting in tissue coagulation. The main use of electrolysis is for hair removal.

PERIOPERATIVE CONSIDERATIONS

PATIENT SELECTION

Patients commonly present for cutaneous surgery with either a cardiac pacemaker or an ICD. When taking preoperative history for surgery, patients should be asked if they have a device. Although technologic advances, such as titanium shielding, have provided safeguards against electromagnetic interference, electrosurgical devices may cause these cardiac devices to malfunction.

RISKS AND POTENTIAL COMPLICATIONS

Interference with Pacemakers/Implantable Cardiac Defibrillators: ICDs deliver an electrical response to an abnormal ventricular rhythm. Some ICDs have a combination of a pacemaker and defibrillator to respond to both bradycardia and tachycardia. Electromagnetic interferences from electrosurgical devices may mimic a cardiac arrhythmia and cause the unit to discharge. Alternatively, the ICD may also respond by inhibiting cardioversion or pacing.

Complications resulting from using electrosurgery for cutaneous surgery in patients with pacemakers or ICDs are uncommon. Matzke and colleagues published a 3-year retrospective review of 173 patients with pacemakers and 13 patients with ICDs who underwent dermatologic surgery and reported no documented complications from electrosurgery.[26] El-Gamal and colleagues reported a rate of 0.8 cases per 100 years of surgical practice from 166 completed surveys from members of the American College of Mohs Surgery and Cutaneous Oncology.[27] In this study, the types of interferences reported were skipped beats, reprogramming of a pacemaker, firing of an ICD, asystole, bradycardia, and depletion of pacemaker battery life. Weyer and colleagues[28] developed an ex vivo simulation device for assessing disruption of an implanted cardiac device. When electrosurgery was performed using normal (10W) and maximum (30W) power settings, the simulated devices only demonstrated interference at a distance of 1 cm with normal power settings and 3 cm at maximum power settings.

Safety and Recommendations for Patients with Implantable Cardiac Defibrillators: Recommendations have been published for the preoperative and intraoperative management of patients with pacemakers and ICDs during dermatologic surgery.[29-33] Patients should be asked when scheduling surgery if they have one of these devices. If present, a preoperative evaluation by the patient's cardiologist should be arranged before the surgical procedure. For management of patients with pacemakers or ICDs undergoing surgical procedures, consider the following recommendations.

- Obtain cardiology consultation to determine if any perioperative actions need to be planned.
- Provide continuous electrocardiography monitoring throughout the procedure.
- Have advanced cardiac life support staff and crash-cart equipment available.
- Consider the use of alternative means of hemostasis such as patient-applied manual pressure[34] or electrocautery.
- Place the dispersing electrode in a location that directs the current pathway away from the cardiac device.
- Use a bipolar forceps device to maintain the electrical circuit between the forceps tips.
- Use minimal power and short electrosurgical bursts of 5 seconds or less.
- Do not discharge the electrosurgical electrode on the skin directly over the pacemaker power source.

Patients may also present with noncardiac implanted electronic devices (IEDs) such as deep brain stimulators and cochlear implants. Noncardiac IEDs have a battery-powered pulse generator with electrodes that end in the targeted tissue. Risks and recommendations for noncardiac IEDs are similar to cardiac IEDs.[35] In some cases, the devices may be turned off, however, the clinical effects on the patient after turning off the device must be taken into consideration.

Burns: There are several situations in which burns may occur with electrosurgery. Thermal injury can occur if there is inadequate contact between the patient and the dispersing electrode plate, when there is inadvertent contact between the dispersing electrode and the patient or surgeon, and if the patient or surgeon may "ground" himself or herself by touching a metal component of the table. Metal jewelry near the electrosurgical site should also be removed.

Fire: Electrosurgical current will ignite flammable substances like alcohol. When prepping the patient before electrosurgery, nonflammable disinfectants such as iodine or chlorhexidine should be used. If an alcohol-based disinfectant is used, the surgical area must be allowed to dry for at least 90 seconds prior to electrosurgery. In addition, electrosurgery should not be used near the presence of nasal cannulas, masks, or endotracheal anesthesia administering oxygen. Finally, care should be taken not to ignite paper surgical drapes in the surgical field.

Channeling: High-frequency electrosurgical current can be conducted along neurovascular bundles, causing pain and tissue damage distant to the local electrosurgical site. Using low-current settings or bipolar forceps may minimize this.

Infection and Mutagenicity: A plume of smoke is generated during electrosurgery. This traveling plume has been shown to contain carbonized tissue and blood, airborne particles, and various chemicals and gases. A review of the literature by Lewin and colleagues[36] reported that electrocautery produces a plume of smoke composed of at least 38 chemical contents, including hydrocarbons, phenols, nitriles, fatty acids, carbon monoxide, acrylonitrile, and hydrogen cyanide. In addition, smoke created from treating lesions such as warts may contain bacteria and viruses, such as human papillomavirus, which may transmit infection.[37]

No known long-term risk for neoplasia or infection is known. The Occupational Safety and Health Administration recommends that surgical smoke be removed and properly filtered by a smoke evacuation system as close to the surgical site as possible.[38] Furthermore, protective equipment, such as face shields and respiratory masks, should be worn during electrosurgery.

ANESTHESIA

During electrosurgery, local anesthesia such as lidocaine with epinephrine is required for patient's comfort.

PERIOPERATIVE CARE

For all treatment groups, wound areas should be covered with a pressure bandage consisting of a topical petroleum product directly on the wound, an overlying nonstick bandage, and firmly applied gauze with adhesive tape.

The pressure bandage is removed 24 to 48 hours posttreatment, and the wound site is cleaned with tap water or saline, gently rinsing over the wound. Petroleum jelly and bandage are changed daily after rinsing, for 3 to 4 weeks or until healed.

ELECTROSURGERY TECHNIQUES

EQUIPMENT

Electrosurgical equipment uses either direct or alternating current. In direct current, electrons flow in one direction, whereas in alternating current, electron flow reverses direction. With the exception of electrocautery or electrolysis, electrosurgical units used in dermatologic procedures have high-frequency alternating current.

Electrosurgical units can be *monopolar* or *bipolar*, referring to the number of tissue-containing tips at the end of a surgical electrode. Monopolar denotes 1 tip, and bipolar denotes 2 tips.

Monoterminal refers to the use of a treatment electrode without an indifferent or dispersing electrode. *Biterminal* refers to the use of both treatment and indifferent electrodes.

POSITIONING

Patients should be supine or prone on the examination table. The dispersing electrode (grounding pad) should be placed in a location that directs the current pathway away from the cardiac device (usually the right lower leg). If a pedal is used, it should be placed near the surgeon's feet.

ELECTROSURGERY APPLICATIONS

HEMOSTASIS

The most common application of electrosurgery is its use in maintaining hemostasis in the operative field. Different techniques of electrosurgery can be used based on the type of electrosurgical unit used during surgical procedures. Coagulation can be achieved using electrofulguration, electrodessication, or electrocoagulation by direct application of the electrode to the bleeding vessel. This provides conduction of heat to the vessel, resulting in tissue coagulation (Fig. 206-3).

Alternatively, vessels can be grasped by a forceps or hemostat, followed by application of the active electrode. When electrical current is placed against the metal instrument, heat is transferred from the electrode through the metal tip to the vessel. This technique is best used when the surgical field cannot be visualized because of bleeding (Fig. 206-4).

ELECTROSURGERY OF BENIGN TUMORS

Electrodessication is an effective treatment modality for papular or plaque-like tumors of the epidermis, such as seborrheic keratoses, verrucae, dermatosis papulosis nigra, molluscum, or flat warts. First, the area around the lesion is anesthetized with lidocaine containing epinephrine. Then, the lesion is touched with the low-power electrode until a gray, superficial, charred layer involves the entire lesion. The charred tissue is removed from the treated lesion by wiping with a sterile gauze or curetting. The process is repeated until the lesion is removed at the level of the surrounding skin. This method results in minimal bleeding and scarring because just the epidermal components are removed.

CURETTAGE AND ELECTRODESSICATION OF MALIGNANT TUMORS

Curettage and electrodessication (C+D) is a commonly used treatment option for BCCs and SCCs. Certain tumor characteristics, however, should be present to ensure high cure rates and acceptable cosmetic outcome. Tumors should be primary; have distinct clinical borders; be located on sites of low recurrence, such as the trunk, extremities, or non-"H"-zone regions of the face; have a superficial or nodular histologic subtype; and have a diameter of less than 1 cm on the face and less than 2 cm on the trunk and extremities. In addition, C+D is a viable treatment option for patients with high morbidity cofactors that make surgical excision too risky, and for patients who cannot make regular followup visits.

Tumors not acceptable for C+D include those with indistinct borders, tumors on the "H"-zone of the face, tumors with an aggressive histologic pattern, tumors with high metastatic potential, and tumors that require histologic diagnosis. For patients with cardiac pacemakers or ICDs, electrocautery may be substituted for electrodessication.

The tumor outline should be marked, and lidocaine with epinephrine should be injected to provide

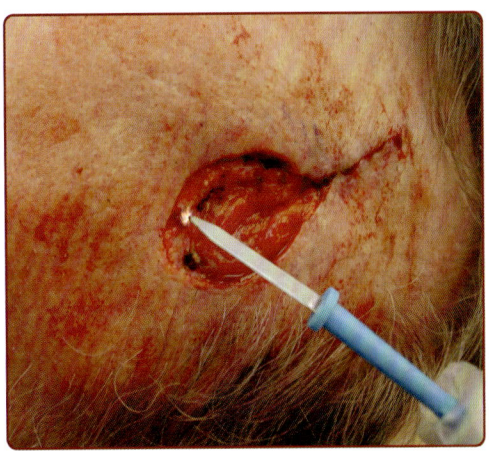

Figure 206-3 Electrodessication of bleeding vessel during Mohs surgery.

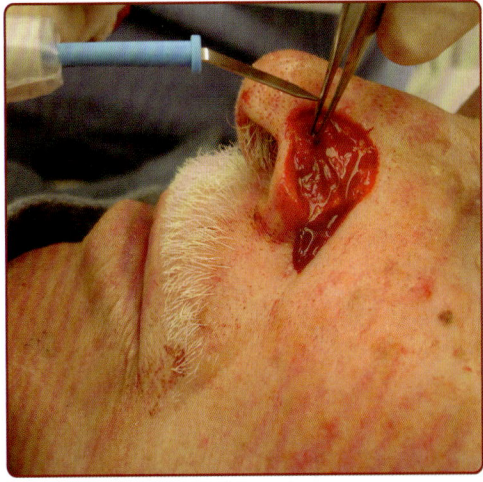

Figure 206-4 Electrocurrent applied to forceps to cauterize bleeding vessel during Mohs surgery.

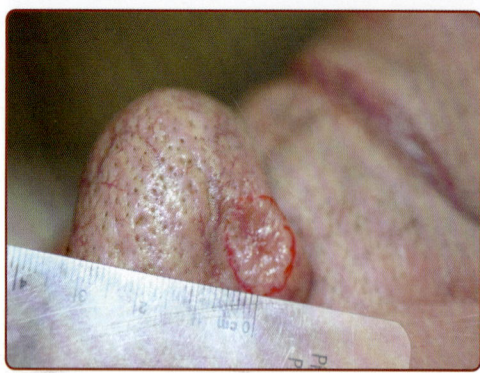

Figure 206-5 Clinical outline of skin tumor before curettage and electrodessication.

adequate local anesthesia (Fig. 206-5). With firm counterpressure, the lesion is then curetted in a checkerboard pattern until the clinical appearance of the lesion is removed (Fig. 206-6). This is followed by electrodessication on high power of the base and periphery of the lesion (Fig. 206-7). This C+D procedure is repeated up to 2 more times until a resultant atrophic defect without clinical evidence of residual tumor is achieved. Some advocate the inclusion of a 2-mm to 4-mm rim of clinically normal skin during the C+D procedure, and individual variations of the protocol are established. If curettage of the BCC extends into subcutis, then an extensive invasion of a BCC has occurred, and excision should be performed.

The advantages of treatment with C+D include time efficiency, ease of surgical technique, and minimal posttreatment morbidity. Disadvantages of treating with C+D include nonconfirmation of histologic tumor clearance, practitioner-dependent efficacy, and potentially long (3- to 4-week) healing times via second intention healing. Furthermore, the cosmetic result may show hypopigmentation, atrophy, persistent erythema, and hypertrophic scarring.

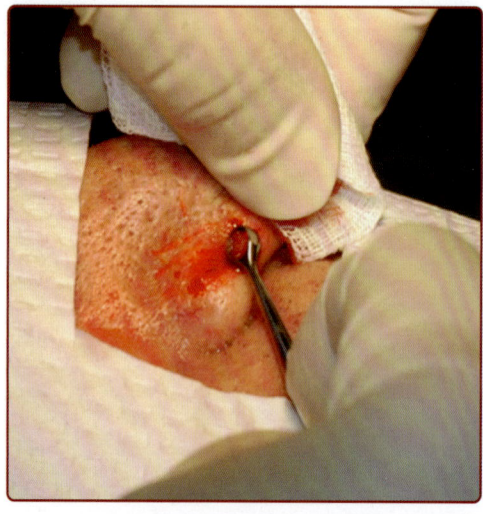

Figure 206-6 Curettage of skin tumor during curettage and electrodessication procedure.

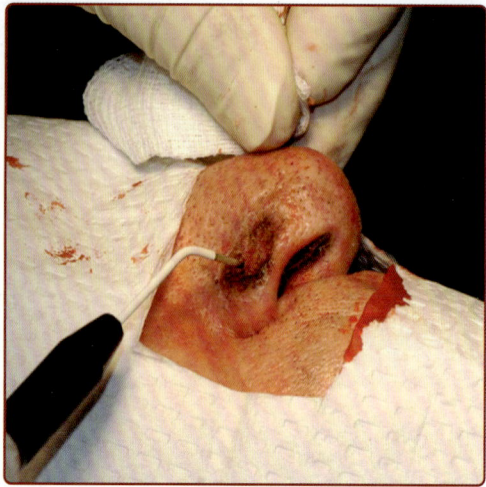

Figure 206-7 Electrodessication of skin tumor during curettage and electrodessication procedure.

OUTCOME ASSESSMENTS OF CURETTAGE AND ELECTRODESSICATION

The 5-year cure rates for C+D have been reported to be 74% to 100% for BCCs[39-49] and 96% to 100% for SCCs.[39] Although some authors have reported that 20% to 40% of tumors remain immediately following C+D, the 5-year cure rates demonstrate an additional factor may be contributing to the destruction of the treated malignancy. Some authors have speculated that the inflammatory response or a specific antitumor humoral response following electrosurgery may be responsible for the low recurrence rate.[50,51]

C+D in combination with other topical treatments may have a synergistic effect in tumor clearance. In a double-blinded, placebo-controlled pilot study by Spencer,[52] 10 BCCs were treated with C+D and 10 patients were treated with C+D followed by 1 month of daily, topically-applied imiquimod cream. The author reported a substantially reduced frequency of residual BCC and improved cosmetic appearance in the C+D-imiquimod group compared with the C+D-alone group. Another study by Wu and colleagues[53] reported excellent efficacy and cosmetic results for nodular BCCs of the trunk and limbs treated with curettage (no electrodessication) followed by daily topical application of imiquimod cream for 6 to 10 weeks. In that study, 32 (94%) of 34 lesions demonstrated no residual histologic evidence of tumor.

REFERENCES

1. Mikhail GR. The application of chemosurgery in cancer. *Henry Ford Hosp Med J.* 1969;17:217-224.
2. White AC. Liquid air in medicine and surgery. *Med Rec.* 1899;56:109.

3. Whitehouse HH. Liquid air in dermatology: its indications and limitations. *JAMA*. 1907;49:371.
4. Mazur P. Freezing of living cells: mechanisms and implications. *Am J Physiol*. 1984;247:125-142.
5. Gage AA, Baust J. Mechanisms of tissue injury in cryosurgery. *Cryobiology*. 1998;37:171-186.
6. Gage AA, Meenaghan M. Sensitivity of pigmented mucosa and pigmented cells in skin due to freezing injury. *Cryobiology*. 1979;16:348-361.
7. Waldorf HA, Alster TS, McMillan K, et al. Effect of dynamic cooling on 585-nm pulse dye laser treatment of port-wine stain birthmarks. *Dermatol Surg*. 1997;24:657-662.
8. Nix TW Jr. Liquid nitrogen neuropathy. *Arch Dermatol*. 1965;92:185.
9. Gupta AK, Koren G, Shear NH. A double-blind, randomized, placebo-controlled trial of eutectic lidocaine/prilocaine cream 5% (EMLA) for analgesia prior to cryotherapy of warts in children and adults. *Pediatr Dermatol*. 1998;15:129-133.
10. Kilkenny M, Merlin K, Young R, et al. The prevalence of common skin conditions in Australian school students. *Br J Dermatol*. 1998;138(5):840-845.
11. Berth-Jones J, Hutchinson PE. Modern treatment of warts: cure rates at 3 and 6 months. *Br J Dermatol*. 1992;127:262-265.
12. Zouboulis CC, Blume U, Buttner P, et al. Outcomes of cryosurgery in keloids and hypertrophic scars. A prospective consecutive trial of case series. *Arch Dermatol*. 1993;129:1146-1151.
13. Torre D. Dermatological cryosurgery: a progress report. *Cutis* 1973;11:782.
14. Lubritz RR, Smolewski SA. Cryosurgery cure rate of actinic keratosis. *J Am Acad Dermatol*. 1982;7:631-632.
15. Thai KE, Fergin P, Freeman M, et al. A prospective study of the use of cryosurgery for the treatment of actinic keratoses. *Int J Dermatol*. 2004;43:687-692.
16. Chiarello SE. Cryopeeling (extensive cryosurgery) for treatment of actinic keratoses: an update and comparison. *Dermatol Surg*. 2000;26:728-732.
17. Ahmed I, Berth-Jones J, Charles-Holmes S, et al. Comparison of cryotherapy with curettage in the treatment of Bowen's disease: a prospective study. *Br J Dermatol*. 2000;143:759-766.
18. Kuflik EG, Gage AA. The five-year cure rate achieved by cryosurgery for skin cancer. *J Am Acad Dermatol*. 1991;24:1002-1004.
19. Torre D. Cryosurgery of basal cell carcinoma. *J Am Acad Dermatol*. 1986;15:917-929.
20. Kurlick EG. Cryosurgery for skin cancer: 30-year experience and cure rates. *Dermatol Surg*. 2004;30:297-300.
21. Kokoszka A, Scheinfeld N. Evidence-based review of the use of cryosurgery in treatment of basal cell carcinoma. *Dermatol Surg*. 2004;29:566-571.
22. Thissen MR, Nieman FH, Ideler AH, et al. Cosmetic results of cryosurgery versus surgical excision for primary uncomplicated basal cell carcinomas of the head and neck. *Dermatol Surg*. 2000;26:759-764.
23. Graham G, Clark L. Statistical analysis in cryosurgery of skin cancer. *Clin Dermatol*. 1990;8:101-107.
24. Stevenson O, Ahmed I. Lentigo maligna: prognosis and treatment options. *Am J Clin Dermatol*. 2005;6:151-164.
25. Tappero JW, Berger TG, Kaplan LD, et al. Cryotherapy for cutaneous Kaposi's sarcoma associated with acquired immune deficiency syndrome: a phase II trial. *J Acquir Immune Defic Syndr*. 1991;4:839.
26. Matzke TJ, Christenson LJ, Christenson SD, et al. Pacemakers and implantable cardiac defibrillators in dermatologic surgery. *Dermatol Surg*. 2006;32:1155-1162.
27. El-Gamal HM, Dufresne RG Jr, Saddler K. Electrosurgery, pacemakers and ICDs: a survey of precautions and complications experienced by cutaneous surgeons. *Dermatol Surg*. 2001;27:385-390.
28. Weyer C, Siegle RJ, Eng GG. Investigation of hyfrecators and their in vitro interference with implantable cardiac devices. *Dermatol Surg*. 2012;38:1843-1848.
29. Krull KA, Pickard SD, Hall JC. Effects of electrosurgery on cardiac pacemakers. *J Dermatol Surg*. 1975;1:43-45.
30. Riordan AT, Gamache C, Fosko SW. Electrosurgery and cardiac devices. *J Am Acad Dermatol*. 1997;37:250-255.
31. Burke MC, Knight BP. Management of implantable pacemakers and defibrillators at the time of noncardiac surgery. *ACC Curr J Rev*. 2005;14:52-55.
32. LeVasseur JG, Kennard CD, Finley EM, et al. Dermatologic electrosurgery in patients with implantable cardioverter-defibrillators and pacemakers. *Dermatol Surg*. 1998;24:233-240.
33. Fader DJ, Johnson TM. Medical issues and emergencies in the dermatology office. *J Am Acad Dermatol*. 1997;36:1-16.
34. Behroozen DS, Petersen R, Goldberg LH. Surgical pearl: patient applied manual pressure for hemostasis. *J Am Acad Dermatol*. 2005;53:871-872.
35. Howe N, Cherpelis B. Obtaining rapid and effective hemostasis. Part II. Electrosurgery in patients with implantable cardiac devices. *J Am Acad Dermatol*. 2013;69:677-685.
36. Lewin JM, Brauer JA, Ostad A. Surgical smoke and the dermatologist. *J Am Acad Dermatol*. 2011;65:636-641.
37. Sawchuk WS, Weber PJ, Lowry DR, et al. Infectious papillomavirus in the vapor of warts treated with carbon dioxide laser or electrocoagulation: detection and protection. *J Am Acad Dermatol*. 1989;21:41-49.
38. Centers for Disease Control and Prevention (CDC). *Control of Smoke from Laser/Electric Surgical Procedures*. US Department of Health and Human Services (DHHS), National Institute for Occupational Safety and Health (NIOSH) Publication No. 96-128 (Hazard Controls 11). 1996. https://www.cdc.gov/niosh/docs/hazardcontrol/hc11.html.
39. Knox JM, Lyles TW, Shapiro EM, et al. Curettage and electrodessication in the treatment of skin cancer. *Arch Dermatol*. 1960;82:197-204.
40. Silverman MK, Kopf AW, Grin CM, et al. Recurrence rates of treated basal cell carcinomas. Part 2: curettage-electrodessication. *J Dermatol Surg Oncol*. 1991;17:720-726.
41. Freeman RG, Knox JM, Heaton CL. The treatment of skin cancer. *Cancer*. 1964;17:535.
42. Tromovitch TA. Skin cancer: treatment by curettage and desiccation. *Calif Med*. 1965;103:107.
43. McCallum DI, Kinmont PC. Basal cell carcinoma: an analysis of cases seen at a combined clinic. *Br J Dermatol*. 1966;78:141.
44. Simpson JR. The treatment of rodent ulcers by curettage and cauterization. *Br J Dermatol*. 1966;78:147.
45. Knox JM, Freeman RG, Duncan WC, et al. Treatment of skin cancer. *South Med J*. 1967;60(3):241-246.
46. Shanoff LB, Spira M, Hardy SB. Basal cell carcinoma: a statistical approach to rational management. *Plast Reconstr Surg*. 1967;39:619.
47. Dubin N, Kopf AW. Multivariate risk score for recurrence of cutaneous basal cell carcinomas. *Arch Dermatol*. 1983;119:373.
48. Spiller WF, Spiller RF. Treatment of basal-cell carcino-

mas by a combination of curettage and cryosurgery. *J Dermatol Surg Oncol*. 1984;11:808.
49. Sweet RD. The treatment of basal cell carcinoma by curettage. *Br J Dermatol*. 1963;75:137.
50. Spencer JM, Tannenbaum A, Sloan L, et al. Does inflammation contribute to the eradication of basal cell carcinoma following curettage and electrodessication? *Dermatol Surg*. 1997;23:625-631.
51. Nouri K, Spencer JM, Taylor JR, et al. Does wound healing contribute to the eradication of basal cell carcinoma following curettage and electrodessication? *Dermatol Surg*. 1999;25:183-188.
52. Spencer JM. Pilot study of imiquimod 5% cream as adjunctive therapy to curettage and electrodessication for nodular basal cell carcinoma. *Dermatol Surg*. 2006;32:63-69.
53. Wu J, Oh C, Strutton G, et al. An open-label, pilot study examining the efficacy of curettage followed by imiquimod 5% cream for the treatment of primary nodular basal cell carcinoma. *Aust J Dermatol*. 2006;47:46-48.

Cosmetic Dermatology PART 31

第三十一篇 美容皮肤学

Chapter 207 :: Cosmeceuticals and Skin Care in Dermatology
:: Leslie Baumann

第二百零七章
化妆品和皮肤护理

中文导读

本章共分为10节：①皮肤科医生应提供护肤建议；②正确识别皮肤问题；③油性或干性皮肤；④敏感性皮肤；⑤皮肤色素沉着；⑥皮肤老化；⑦最理想的皮肤类型；⑧皮肤表型诊断；⑨选择最有效的产品；⑩结论。

第一、第二节介绍了皮肤科医生应提供护肤建议且正确识别皮肤问题。

第三节介绍了油性或干性皮肤保湿问题，并从双层脂膜皮肤屏障、皮脂的生成、天然保湿因子、糖胺聚糖、水通道蛋白-3（AQP3）5个方面介绍皮肤屏障。接下来作者阐述了油性或干性皮肤的7种护理方法：①清洁剂；②去角质剂；③保湿霜；④润肤剂；⑤遮盖剂；⑥保湿剂；⑦药物治疗。最后总结以上情况，指出基本护肤是洁面剂和保湿剂的选择，并指明油性或干性皮肤需使用的护肤产品。

第四节介绍了敏感性皮肤，并把敏感性皮肤分为四个亚型：痤疮型、玫瑰痤疮型、刺痛型、过敏型。作者再从清洁剂和保湿剂两方面讲述了敏感性皮肤的护理：清洁剂中提出需要注意的事项及各型对应的清洁剂，同样对于保湿剂成分的选择也提出了一些建议，包括一些舒缓的抗炎成分、血管收缩成分，并配合一些处方药使用。最后提出敏感性皮肤的护理治疗是取决于其亚型的，而在治疗多种亚型的敏感皮肤时，应首先去除过敏原，然后添加抗炎成分，最后进行痤疮药物治疗。

第五节介绍了皮肤色素沉着，并从6个方面陈述减少皮肤色素沉着的方法：①防晒霜；②酪氨酸酶抑制药；③PAR-2阻断药；④去角质；⑤木质素过氧化物酶；⑥抗氧化剂。

最后总结皮肤色素沉着的护理治疗。以黄褐斑作为例子，分为治疗方案和维持治疗方案。作者讲述了治疗方案和维持治疗方案所包括的内容、时间，以及两者来回循环的治疗周期。

第六节介绍了皮肤老化问题，首先从防晒霜、清洁剂、保湿剂及其他方面简述了抗衰老技术以及可能的作用机制。最后总结抗衰老的重要方法，即每天使用防晒霜、维甲酸和抗氧化剂，结合健康的生活习惯，尽量减少糖基化、紫外线暴露和自由基的产生。

第七节介绍了皮肤表型诊断，即将皮肤分为4个不同的情况来评估：干（D）或油性（O）；敏感（S）或抗性（R）；色素（P）或非色素（N）；易皱（W）或紧（T）。这4个皮肤情况可以结合起来形成16种不同的皮肤表型，也称为鲍曼皮肤类型（图207-4），从而让皮肤科医生更好地提出护肤方案。

第八节介绍了最理想的皮肤类型，并提出最理想的皮肤表型是鲍曼皮肤类型中的ORNT或油性、具有抵抗能力、无皮肤色素沉着且紧实的皮肤。

第九节介绍了如何选择最有效的产品，主要介绍了成分的选择、产品的选择、应用各产品的顺序问题（分为早和晚两种情况，并列于表207-7）、对于患者的教育、长期随访。

第十节介绍了本章的大致内容，强调皮肤科医生对于皮肤护理的重要作用。

〔简　丹〕

AT-A-GLANCE

- Dermatologists have the most training and scientific knowledge to understand cosmeceuticals and skin care products.
- Using a diagnostic skin typing system helps identify underlying skin issues and facilitates product matching and patient education.
- Cosmeceuticals and skin care products can be a source of a range of adverse reactions, including irritation and allergy; therefore, proper selection and patient compliance is critical for improved outcomes.

DERMATOLOGISTS ROUTINELY PROVIDE SKIN-CARE ADVICE

According to recent data, sales in the United States of skin-care cosmeceuticals approach $6.5 billion annually and international sales surpass $10 billion, with forecasts of steady continued growth.[1-3] A plethora of skin-care products are currently available to account for this substantial business volume. The vast variety of products, and the often exaggerated associated claims, is so complex that physicians and consumers are often confused about their indications and effectiveness. Dermatologists are uniquely positioned to decipher the product claims and supportive data (or lack thereof) and can guide their patients. They are trained in acne, rosacea, eczema, and many other skin concerns and therefore understand the underlying science of skin care, even if they choose not to sell skin-care products in their offices. Most dermatologists are too busy to spend time discussing skin care with patients. Using a diagnostic methodology to streamline the skin-care prescribing process and educate staff and patients is one approach. The methodology should include routine skin-care advice for facial skin as well as specific instructions for the treatment and healthy maintenance of body skin. Educating the patient on the proper use of sunscreen and medications, such as those for psoriasis, eczema, fungal infections, and wound healing, and how to use those medications in combination with cleansers and moisturizers improves patient compliance and outcomes. This chapter will focus on the issues that should be considered when developing a methodology to prescribe skin-care regimens to treat facial skin issues, but the concept can be easily extended to body skin.

IDENTIFYING FACIAL SKIN ISSUES

The process of properly diagnosing a patient's skin issues can be cumbersome and time consuming. One method is by assigning the skin a diagnosis such as acne, rosacea, melasma, contact/irritant dermatitis, eczema, psoriasis, or actinic keratosis and treating it accordingly. However, in many cases, the patient has more than one issue occurring concurrently. For example, many acne patients develop irritant dermatitis from acne medications. The focus here is caring for the skin from a phenotypic approach, which is a simplified way to discuss the various issues that need to be considered when prescribing the proper skin-care regimen. The phenotypic approach focuses on 4 main facial skin issues: skin hydration, inflammation, pigmentation, and skin aging risk factors.

SKIN HYDRATION

OILY VERSUS DRY

Xerosis, or "dry skin," is characterized by dull color (usually gray white), rough texture, and an elevated number of ridges, and may be associated with a sensation of tightness or itching.[4] Patients complain that their "skin is no longer radiant" because its rough surface is a poor reflector of light. Although the etiology of dry skin is multifactorial, the most significant factor in the development of xerosis is the role of the *stratum corneum (SC)* skin barrier and its capacity to retain water.

BILAYER LIPID MEMBRANE SKIN BARRIER

Rawlings et al. showed that patients with dry skin have a perturbation in the lipid bilayer of the SC.[5] The SC skin barrier is composed of a bilayer lipid membrane formed from 3 primary groups of compounds: (1) ceramides, (2) fatty acids, and (3) cholesterol. When present in the proper amount and ratio (1:1:1), these components help to protect the skin and keep it watertight (Figs. 207-1 and 207-2).[6] When the barrier is impaired, the skin develops an inability to retain water, which leads to dehydration if interventions to retard water evaporation are not implemented. Defects or deficiencies in this barrier layer of the skin cause a spike in water evaporation, known as transepidermal water loss (TEWL). TEWL leads to decreased water content in the SC and abnormal desquamation of corneocytes. Desmosomes remain intact at higher levels of the SC,[7] and desmoglein I levels remain elevated in the superficial SC of individuals with dry skin as compared to controls. This occurs because the enzymes necessary for desmosome digestion are impaired when the water level is insufficient, which spurs abnormal desquamation resulting in visible "clumps" of keratinocytes that leave the skin appearing rough and dry.[8] Recent studies suggest that both the initial cohesion and the ultimate desquamation of corneocytes from the SC surface may be orchestrated by localized changes in pH, which selectively activate different classes of extracellular proteases in a pH-dependent fashion.[9] For this reason, the pH of skin-care products should be taken into account when designing a skin-care regimen for a patient with dry skin. Impairment of the lipid bilayer of the SC can be engendered by various exogenous factors such as ultraviolet (UV) radiation, detergents, acetone, chlorine, and prolonged water immersion. Skin barrier impairment is often caused by an incorrect choice of skin cleansers and moisturizers or overzealous use of exfoliating methods. Although skin barrier function is the most important issue to consider when approaching dehydrated skin, there are other factors to take into account that affect the perception of skin hydration.

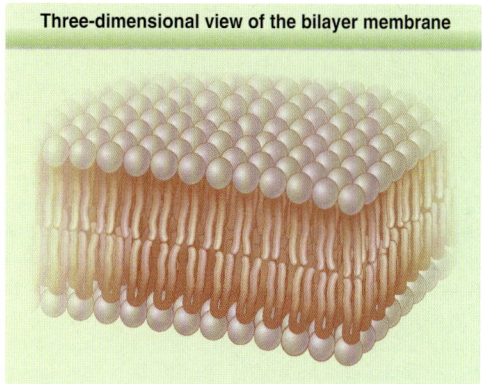

Figure 207-2 Three-dimensional view of the bilayer membrane.

SEBUM PRODUCTION

Sebum production plays a role in dry skin because it provides an occlusive layer on the surface of the skin that retards TEWL. When assessing the face for the presence of sebum, it is important to wait 20 minutes after the patient washes because that is how long it takes the sebaceous glands to generate enough sebum to be visualized and accurately measured on the skin's surface. The oily secretion of the sebaceous glands contains wax esters, sterol esters, cholesterol, di- and triglycerides, squalene,[10] and the antioxidant vitamin E and is thought to confer protection to the

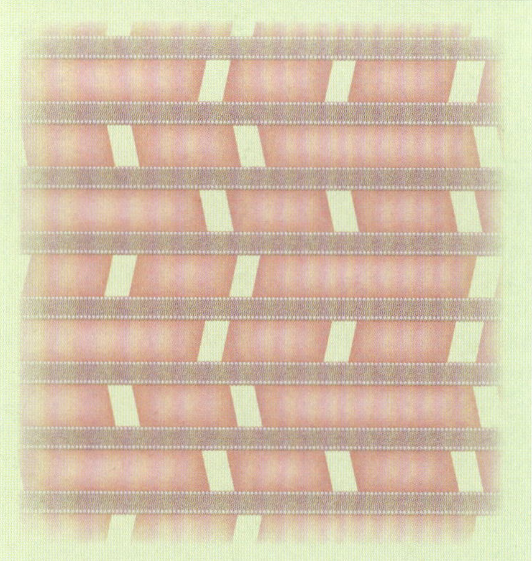

Figure 207-1 Brick-and-mortar structure of the epidermis. The pink bricks represent the keratinocytes and the blue represents the bilayer membrane layer.

skin from environmental insults such as free radicals.[11] Lipids from modified sebaceous glands in the eye, called meibomian glands, help prevent dry eyes by hindering tear evaporation.[12,13] It is important to note that sebaceous gland–impoverished skin, such as the lips and the skin in prepubertal children, may be at a higher risk for free radical and other environmental damage. Sebum production changes at different stages of life. It is well understood that an age-related change is seen in sebaceous gland activity, with levels typically low during childhood, rising in the mid- to late teens, and generally remaining stable for decades until trailing off in the seventh and eighth decades as endogenous androgen production declines.[14] Children between 2 and 9 years of age commonly display eczematous patches (pityriasis alba) on the face and trunk that disappear with the onset of sebaceous gland activation. The level of sebum production is influenced by diet, stress, hormone production, exercise, and genetics. In a study of 20 pairs each of identical and nonidentical like-sex twins, the identical twins exhibited essentially the same sebum excretion rates, with significantly divergent acne severity, whereas the nonidentical twins differed significantly according to both parameters, implying both the genetic influence of sebum and the mediation of exogenous factors in lesion development.[15]

The presence of sebum on the face does not exclude a skin barrier defect but often compensates for it. In fact, an adequate or increased amount of sebum production can mask a deficient skin barrier. This is the reason that some patients state that they have combination skin that is oily in the t-zone and dry along the sides of the face. In the case of this t-zone type of combination skin, the patient should be treated as an oily facial skin type because the barrier repair moisturizers will feel too heavy and cosmetically displeasing to them. However, they need to be treated with a barrier repair moisturizer in areas with few sebaceous glands such as the arms and legs.

NATURAL MOISTURIZING FACTOR

Natural moisturizing factor (NMF) provides intracellular hydration. It is derived from the breakdown of the protein filaggrin, which provides structural support and strength in the lower layers of the SC. It is broken down in the higher levels (stratum compactum) of the SC into free amino acids, including histidine, glutamine (glutamic acid), and arginine.[16] These osmotically active amino acids remain inside the keratinocyte and avidly bind to water. The pace at which filaggrin is broken down into NMF is thought to be regulated by aspartate protease (cathepsin), which initiates this cascade and determines the amount of NMF that is present.[17] Interestingly, this putative aspartate protease (cathepsin) is regulated by changes in external humidity. In other words, in low-humidity environments, the pace of NMF production increases. This acclimation process typically occurs over the course of several days,[18] and cannot yet be regulated artificially via products or procedures.

GLYCOSAMINOGLYCANS

Glycosaminoglycans (GAGs), such as heparan sulfate and hyaluronic acid, bind and hold water, providing skin hydration and structural integrity.[19] Although their role in skin hydration and aging is poorly understood, much research is ongoing to look at effects of aging on the characteristics of these and other important GAGs.[20] These GAGs are found in skin-care products that target dry and aged skin.

Hyaluronic Acid (HA): HA, which can bind 1000 times its weight in water, is a glycosaminoglycan found in the extracellular matrix and thought to give the skin its volume and plumpness. HA is produced mainly by fibroblasts and keratinocytes in the skin, and has an estimated turnover rate of 2 to 4.5 days in mammals.[21] HA is localized not only in the dermis but also in the epidermal intercellular spaces, especially the middle spinous layer, but not in the SC or stratum granulosum.[22] Aged skin, which is less plump than youthful skin, is characterized by decreased levels of HA. The exact contribution of HA in skin hydration is not clear. Studies have been conflicting about the penetration of HA into the skin on topical application,[23] but the size of the molecule plays an important role.[24] HA has been added to various drug formulations to increase drug delivery because it seems to play a role in enhancing penetration of other ingredients through a poorly understood mechanism.[25] Oral glucosamine supplements have been shown to increase production of HA in the skin and joints.[26,27]

Heparan Sulfate (HS): HS and heparan sulfate proteoglycans (HSPGs), such as syndecan, glypican, and perlecan, are the most common constituents of the cell surface and extracellular matrix, including the basement membrane. These glycans bind ligands at the cell surface and modulate key processes in the skin such as cell proliferation, migration, communication, and activation because of their capacity to bind, store, present, degrade, and amplify key secreted signaling molecules such as growth factors and cytokines. A decreased detection of endogenous HS and HSPGs in the skin has been linked to aging, resulting in deterioration of the mechanical properties of the dermis.[28] Increasing the amount of HS in the skin may provide an important target for skin rejuvenation by not only increasing the skin's ability to hold onto water but also restoring skin homeostasis. Endogenous HS is too large and highly polar to penetrate into skin when applied topically because it is rapidly degraded on the skin surface. Therefore, it serves primarily as a humectant, which brings water onto the surface of the skin. Studies are being conducted with an HS analog that has been shown to penetrate into skin to improve hydration and lower TEWL as well as improve wrinkles and even skin tone.[29]

AQUAPORIN-3

Aquaporin-3 (AQP3) is a member of a family of homologous aquaporin water channels that facilitate fluid transport. AQP3 is a member of a subclass of aquaporins called aquaglyceroporins, which transport not only water but also glycerol and possibly other small solutes. Researchers have found that AQP3 is expressed at the plasma membrane of epidermal keratinocytes in human skin.[30] There is evidence for a high concentration of solutes (Na^+, K^+ and Cl^-) and a low concentration of water (13%-35%)[31] in the superficial SC, producing in the steady-state gradients of both solutes and water from the skin surface to the viable epidermal keratinocytes.[32,33] It has been proposed that AQP3 might facilitate transepidermal water permeability to protect the SC against desiccation by evaporative water loss from the skin surface and/or to dissipate water gradients in the epidermal keratinocyte cell layer.[30] A study looking at skin phenotype in transgenic mice lacking AQP3 showed significantly reduced water and glycerol permeability in AQP3 null mice proving that AQP3 is functional as a plasma membrane water/glycerol transporter in the epidermis.[34] Conductance measurements showed remarkably reduced SC water content in AQP3 null mice in most areas of the skin. However, epidermal cell water permeability is probably not a major determinant of SC hydration because water movement across AQP3 is markedly slow compared with other tissues.[35] Pharmacologic manipulation of AQP3 may be used in the future to treat skin disorders of excess and decreased hydration. At this time, the only cosmeceutical ingredients that have demonstrated a role in regulating AQP3 are Ajuga turkestanica[36] and glycerin.[37]

SKIN CARE FOR THE OILY–DRY PARAMETER

In the context of the oily–dry parameter, ideal skin is typically characterized by balanced sebum secretion, an intact SC with an unbroken barrier, sufficient levels of NMF and GAGs, and normal expression of AQP3. Skin-care products should be chosen with ingredients to meet these goals (Table 207-1).

Cleansers: The choice of cleanser is crucial because cleansers have a significant effect on the lipid contents of the skin, which affects skin barrier function. In the case of oily skin (excess sebum), a foaming cleanser that contains surfactants to remove the excess lipid is preferable. Oily skin types prefer the clean feeling that these give to the skin. For dry skin types, a nonfoaming cleanser such as an oil, cream, or milk cleanser is preferable. Choose nonfoaming cleansers that deposit fatty acids on the skin, thereby repairing the skin barrier. Good choices include stearic acid (a component of shea butter), which has straight nonpolar hydrophobic tails that stack closely together in the cell membrane giving optimal barrier repair. Linoleic acid, found in safflower oil, argan oil, and others, is also a good choice because of its antiinflammatory capabilities; however, its barrier repair properties are not as strong as those of stearic acid. Avoid oleic acid, found in olive oil, which can cause membrane disruption because its fatty acid hydrophobic tails project at an angle that disrupts the bilayer membrane's natural structure (Fig 207-3).[38] The pH of the cleanser also plays a role in skin barrier function. Soap cleansers

TABLE 207-1

Types of Ingredients in Moisturizers for Topical Skin Care

Barrier Repair
- Ceramides
- Cholesterol
- Fatty acids
- MLE technology

Occlusives
- Oils
  - Argan
  - Safflower
  - Grape seed
  - Mineral
  - Jojoba
  - Flax seed
  - Lanolin
- Silicones
- Petrolatum
- Squalene
- Soybean oil
- Propylene glycol
- Wax
- Plastic wrap
- Fabrics or patches

Humectants
- α-Hydroxy acids
- Glycerin
- Heparan sulfate
- Hyaluronic acid
- Propylene glycol
- Sugars
- Urea

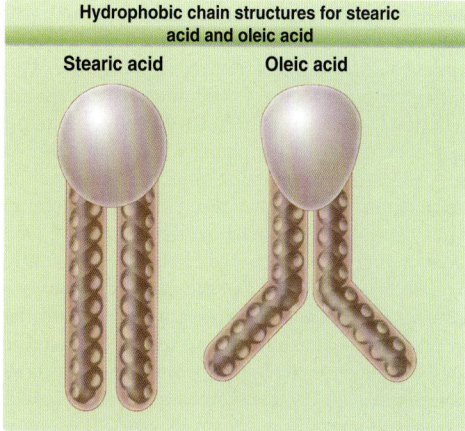

Figure 207-3 Stearic acid has straight hydrophobic "legs," whereas the hydrophobic chains of oleic acid stick out at an angle that precludes close packing of the membrane lipids.

that exhibit a high pH have been consistently shown to perturb the skin barrier. Dry skin types need a neutral or acidic cleanser while oily types that do not exhibit a propensity for inflammation can tolerate a higher-pH soap-type cleanser. Cleansers are the most commonly used skin-care product, so their impact on oily and dry skin cannot be overemphasized.

Exfoliants: Exfoliants, which are often found in exfoliating cleansers, aid in desquamation of the superficial layer of the SC, leading to a smoother surface and greater light-reflecting abilities. Exfoliants can be mechanical as in the case of crushed shells, sugar or rice grains, aluminum particles, rotating brushes, or rough fabrics. These promote an immediate visual improvement of the skin but overuse can lead to barrier impairment. Hydroxy acids represent the family of chemical exfoliants.[39] α-Hydroxy acids such as lactic and glycolic acids have humectant properties, whereas β-hydroxy acids such as salicylic acid extract lipids from the skin and have drying properties. Exfoliants are often used by skin-care companies to show the immediate benefit of their product on the skin, but these benefits are short-lived and deceiving if the exfoliant products are not combined with barrier repair moisturizers.

Moisturizers: Moisturizers play an import role in treating dry and oily skin. Oily skin types make their own moisturizer because, by definition, they produce an adequate or excess amount of sebum to provide surface occlusion to help retard TEWL. The oily sensation that sebum causes on the skin may make people with oily skin types less likely to use sun protection because many sunscreen products are made with silicones and oil-soluble ingredients that render an oily feel. For this reason, very oily skin types should use a sunscreen in lieu of a moisturizer and slightly oily types should use a lighter lotion or serum-type moisturizer. The choice of cleanser will influence the need for a moisturizer. Oily types should avoid oils and heavy cream moisturizers and will likely prefer humectant-containing moisturizers such as those with hyaluronic acid and heparan sulfate analog. Dry skin types should all use a barrier repair moisturizer containing the proper ratio of ceramides, fatty acids, and cholesterol, which is 1:1:1.[40] Historically, ceramides have been derived from animals, but new technologies using a pseudoceramide formulated in a multilamellar emulsion (MLE) have been shown to mimic the skin's natural 3-dimensional barrier structure.[41] Only barrier repair moisturizers will help correct underlying defects in the skin so that skin health can improve; however, there are other classes of ingredients that are included in moisturizers as a temporary solution. These ingredients are popular because their effects are more rapidly observable than barrier repair ingredients, which may take 4 or more days to yield noticeable results.[42]

Emollients: Emollients are substances added to immediately soften and smooth the skin. They function by filling the spaces between desquamating corneocytes to create a smooth surface, which makes the skin reflect light better and impart immediate visible improvement.[43] Emollients provide increased cohesion that causes a flattening of the curled edges of the individual corneocytes.[4] This leads to a smoother surface with less friction and greater light refraction. Many emollients have barrier repair, humectant, and occlusive properties as well as smoothing emollient properties.

Occlusives: Occlusives, such as naturally occurring sebum and exogenously applied ingredients, often contain lipids and coat the surface of the skin. Plastic wrap, patches, and masks are examples of occlusion technologies used in skin-care regimens. The occlusive coating provides an emollient effect, helps increase penetration of previously applied ingredients, and decreases TEWL. Ingredients with the highest occlusive properties are petrolatum and oils. Petrolatum, for example, has a water vapor loss resistance 170 times that of olive oil.[44] However, petrolatum has a greasy feeling that may make agents containing it cosmetically unacceptable to many patients. Other commonly used occlusive ingredients include paraffin, squalene, dimethicone, soybean oil, grapeseed oil, propylene glycol, lanolin, and beeswax.[45] These agents are only effective while present on the skin; once removed, the TEWL returns to the previous level. Decreasing TEWL by more than 40% can lead to maceration and increased levels of bacteria; therefore, there is a limit to the amount of occlusive ingredients that can be used.[46]

Humectants: Humectants are ingredients with high water absorption capabilities that are able to attract water from the atmosphere. They are most effective when the atmospheric humidity is greater than 80%. Although humectants may draw water from the environment to help hydrate the skin, in low-humidity conditions they may absorb water from the deeper epidermis and dermis, leading to increased skin dryness.[47] For this reason, they are more effective when combined with occlusives. Humectants rapidly draw water into the skin, causing a slight swelling of the SC that gives the perception of smoother skin with fewer wrinkles. Examples of commonly used humectants include glycerin, sorbitol, sodium hyaluronate, urea, propylene glycol, α-hydroxy acids, and sugars. The effects of humectants are temporary, usually lasting less than 24 hours. However, the barrier repair properties of glycerin (also known as glycerol and glycerine) and its ability to traverse AQP3 channels give it longer-lasting effects than other humectants.[48]

Medications: Medications can affect skin type by changing sebum production rates or by perturbation of the skin barrier by disrupting lipid production. Oral ketoconazole,[49] oral spironolactone,[50] oral contraceptives, oral retinoids,[51] and injected botulinum toxin type A[52] have been shown to decrease sebum secretion. Statins and other cholesterol-lowering medications may increase the risk of dry skin but studies are conflicting.

SUMMARY OF SKIN CARE FOR DRY AND OILY SKIN TYPES

The basic care of dry and oily skin types begins with the choice of a cleanser and a moisturizer. At this time there are no skin-care ingredients known to increase NMF production and there are minimal data on ingredients that affect AQP3 function. Topical products have not been reliably shown to decrease sebum production. Humectants, occlusives, and exfoliants only offer temporary improvement. For this reason, oily skin types should be treated with a foaming cleanser and either a light moisturizer or no moisturizer at all. Dry skin types should be treated with lipid-sparing cleansers such as nonfoaming cleansers and barrier repair moisturizers. Humectant-, occlusive-, and exfoliant-containing cleansers and moisturizers can be added to the basic skin-care regimen to treat other issues such as pigmentation and wrinkles and to increase compliance by demonstrating a more rapid visible result on the skin.

SKIN SENSITIVITY

SENSITIVE VERSUS RESISTANT

Resistant skin is defined as skin that rarely exhibits signs of sensitivity, which include acne lesions, redness, itching, flushing, stinging, and urticaria. Sensitive skin, on the other hand, is characterized by frequent incidence of these characteristics of inflammation. There are 4 distinct variations of sensitive skin that should be considered independently when customizing a skin-care regimen. The 4 types of sensitive skin are (1) acne type (prone to developing acne lesions such as papules, pustules, comedones, and cysts); (2) rosacea type (featuring a tendency toward recurrent flushing, facial redness, and experiencing hot sensations); (3) stinging type (predilection to stinging or burning sensations); and (4) allergic type (more likely to exhibit erythema, pruritus, and skin flaking on contact with allergens and irritants). A review of 27,485 patient results from the Baumann Skin Type Indicator (BSTI) Questionnaire[53] taken by patients in 30+ different dermatology offices showed that 73% of patients who presented to these offices reported having sensitive skin (unpublished data). See Table 207-2 for the breakdown of sensitive subtypes in these patients. Each of these subtypes of sensitive skin can occur alone or in combination with other types of sensitive skin. Although all 4 types benefit from the addition of antiinflammatory ingredients,[54] each subtype has unique skin-care needs.

TABLE 207-2
The Subtype Breakdown of 27,485 Patients Seen by Dermatologists in 32 Practices in the USA (20,019 Patients Reported Sensitive Skin)[a]

	# PATIENTS	% PATIENTS
Acne	11,563	58%
Rosacea	9779	49%
Stinging	2970	15%
Allergic	10,990	55%
Acne and rosacea	4909	25%
Acne and stinging	1678	8%
Acne and allergic	5284	26%
Rosacea and stinging	1931	10%
Rosacea and allergic	4991	25%
Stinging and allergic	2135	11%

[a]Many patients exhibited more than 1 type of sensitive skin concurrently.

ACNE TYPE

Sensitive skin acne subtypes are characterized by recurring papules, pustules, comedones, and cysts and exhibit an increased amount of fluorescence from the porphyrins produced by *Propionibacterium acnes* bacteria when seen under various types of light. There are 3 primary factors in the pathogenesis of acne: (1) inflammation, (2) disordered keratinization, and (3) the presence of the bacteria *P. acnes*. In many acne cases, elevated sebum production is seen but this is not a requirement to develop acne. In fact, patients with dry skin and acne are more difficult to treat than those with oily skin and acne because many of the medications used to treat acne lead to dryness of the skin. Although acne has various causal pathways and contributing factors, the essential pathognomonic feature is abnormal keratinization of the SC with adherence of desquamated skin cells in the hair follicles. These skin cells combine with sebum and clog the follicle, creating a comedone. The bacteria *P. acnes* migrates into the hair follicle, causing a cascade of events including activation of Toll-like receptor 2. This stimulates the release of cytokines and other inflammatory factors that trigger the inflammatory response. Goals of treatment include lowering *P. acnes* levels, blocking inflammatory pathways, and normalizing keratinization. Skin-care regimens for acne take about 8 to 12 weeks to yield results, so patients should be educated about the delay to improve compliance. Camera imaging such as the Canfield Visa CA can be used to visualize the amount of *P. acnes* on the skin. This helps determine the amount of bacteria at baseline, tracks improvement, and encourages the patient to return for followup visits to check progress. Decreased bacterial counts are often seen in the camera before the acne lesions clear, showing the patient that progress is occurring. Regimens should be divided into treatment and maintenance programs. The treatment regimen should be implemented for the first 12 weeks, which is geared to speed healing of active

> **TABLE 207-3**
> **Nonprescription Acne Treatments**
>
> Normalize keratinization-
>   Hydroxy acids
>   Retinol
> Decrease *P. acnes*
>   Benzoyl peroxide
>   Silver
>   Blue light (415 nm)
>   Antimicrobials
> Antiinflammatories (see Table 207-4)

lesions in addition to preventing new lesions. Use acne medications such as benzoyl peroxide, clindamycin, salicylic acid, and retinoids but they should be combined with nonfoaming cleansers and noncomedogenic barrier repair ingredients in dry types. Acne treatment visits should be scheduled at weeks 4, 8, and 12 to improve compliance. Studies have shown that compliance improves around the time of the patient visit[55]; therefore, monthly visits are suggested until the acne medications are being tolerated and acne has significantly improved. After the acne has cleared, switch the patient to a retinoid-containing maintenance regimen geared to prevent recurrence (Table 207-3).

ROSACEA TYPE

Rosacea is characterized by facial redness and flushing that may include inflammatory papules and telangiectasias. Topical skin care for rosacea is primarily geared toward vasoconstrictive, antimicrobial, and antiinflammatory ingredients to decrease redness and prevent progression. Many types of antiinflammatory ingredients are found in skin-care products (Table 207-4). These should be combined with prescription medications and vascular laser (595 nm) treatments for maximal results. However, special thought needs to be given to what these types of patients should *not* use.

> **TABLE 207-4**
> **Antiinflammatory Ingredients**
>
> - Aloe vera
> - Argan oil
> - Arnica
> - Bisabolol
> - Caffeine
> - Chamomile
> - Colloidal oatmeal
> - Cucumber
> - Feverfew
> - Green tea
> - Hamamelis (witch hazel)
> - Licorice extract
>
> Niacinamide (also known as nicotinamide)
> - Oxymethazoline
> - Salicylic acid
> - Zinc

Vigorous exfoliation should be avoided. Triggers such as cold and heat could contribute to this pathology if the patient uses extreme temperatures of water or has frequent facials that often include facial steaming. The choice of cleansers, moisturizers, and sunscreens should include some form of antiinflammatory ingredient. If retinoids are to be used, they should be started slowly to avoid exacerbation of rosacea. Decreasing the dose and frequency by applying a low-strength retinoid on top of an antiinflammatory moisturizer every third night is often tolerated by rosacea patients. The dose and frequency can be increased as they adjust.

STINGING TYPE

Burning, stinging, or itching caused by application of a cosmetic or topical medicament without detectable visible or microscopic change is termed *sensory irritation*. The afferent limb of this reaction is carried by C nerve fibers that are present throughout the dermis and viable epidermis. The stinging occurs on the face within an hour of application in susceptible individuals. Patients with this subtype of sensitive skin do not have a higher incidence of atopy or dry skin, but do report frequent adverse reactions to cosmetics. Several tests such as the lactic acid stinging test have been devised to identify patients with the stinging propensity; however, there is no universally accepted test because different ingredients sting different people. Patients with rosacea and patients experiencing retinoid dermatitis often report stinging even with contact to only water. The stinging sensation is not necessarily associated with erythema as many patients feel stinging without experiencing redness or irritation.[56] Most often patients with the stinging subtype of sensitive skin feel stinging upon application of the following ingredients: α-hydroxy acids (particularly glycolic acid), benzoic acid, bronopol, cinnamic acid compounds, Dowicel 200, formaldehyde, lactic acid, propylene glycol, quaternary ammonium compounds, sodium lauryl sulfate, sorbic acid, urea, ascorbic acid, and witch hazel. Use of antiinflammatory ingredients may help lessen stinging but the best therapy is avoidance of products with stinging ingredients.

ALLERGIC/IRRITANT TYPE

The allergic/irritant subtype is more likely to develop a dermatitis upon exposure to various allergens and irritants. This subtype also has been called "status cosmeticus" by Fisher,[57] contact urticaria when a wheal and flare response occurs,[58] "cosmetic intolerance syndrome" when it occurs with cosmetics, and more commonly contact or irritant dermatitis. This subtype can be due to an increased immune response in the case of contact dermatitis or an impaired skin barrier that allows allergens and irritants to more easily enter the skin.[59] Various studies reveal that approximately 10% of patch-tested dermatologic patients are allergic to at least one ingredient common in cosmetic products.[60] Fragrances and preservatives are the most

TABLE 207-5
Frequently Identified Cosmetic Ingredients Causing Allergic Contact Dermatitis

- Benzyl alcohol
- Bisabolol
- Calendula (marigold)
- Cetyl alcohol
- Cinnamon
- Essential oils
- Fragrances
- Glyceryl thioglycolate
- Lanolin
- Niacinamide
- Paraphenylenediamine (PPD)
- Peppermint
- Preservatives
- Propylene glycol
- Sorbitan
- Sunscreens
- Toluene sulfonamide/formaldehyde resin
- Triclosan
- Vitamin E

common allergens (Table 207-5). New emerging allergens include sorbitan, the preservatives methylisothiazolinone and sodium dehydroacetate, cetyl alcohol, bisabolol, peppermint, and the red pigment carmine. The first step in treating these patients is to try and identify the allergen by patch testing or a detailed history. In some cases, a patient diary will reveal the culprit. The popularity of organic and natural ingredients has resulted in an increase in exposure to plant-derived allergens. Skin care should aim for avoidance of the allergen and fortification of the skin barrier with barrier repair ingredients. There are also cosmeceutical products that coat the skin to protect against nickel and other allergen contact.

CLEANSERS

Sensitive skin types are more prone to inflammation, so they should avoid extremes of temperature. Washing with tepid water is prudent. Avoiding exfoliants is particularly important including scrubs, facial cloths, and rotating brushes, which all can cause dermatographism, flushing, and other forms of inflammation in these susceptible types. In fact, friction has been associated with an increase in acne breakouts. Soothing cleansers that contain antiinflammatory ingredients are preferred. Hydroxy acid cleansers may irritate stinging and rosacea types but will help decrease *P. acnes* counts by lowering the pH and preventing and treating comedones in acne types. Salicylic acid is a good choice of hydroxy acids for acne skin types because it is lipophilic, able to enter the pilar unit, and exhibits the antiinflammatory properties of salicylates. Patients with the allergic/irritant subtype should avoid foaming cleansers that can disturb the skin barrier, facilitating entry of foreign substances into the skin.

MOISTURIZERS

Patients with acne are often hesitant about moisturizer use but at least one study has demonstrated improvement of acne with moisturizer use alone.[61] Moisturizers that do not contain comedogenic ingredients such as isopropyl myristate, isopropyl palmitate, and coconut oil (although not all forms of coconut extract are acnegenic) should be chosen. Patients with the rosacea type of sensitive skin do well with soothing antiinflammatory ingredients such as argan oil, chamomile, niacinamide, colloidal oatmeal, feverfew, licorice extract, green tea, and chamomile. These should be combined in the regimen with prescription rosacea medications such as azelaic acid, metronidazole, brimonidine, ivermectin, and oxymetazoline. Oxymetazoline and brimonidine have α-adrenoreceptor agonist activity that results in vasoconstriction, causing a rapid improvement in facial redness. Brimonidine has selective α_2 activity,[62] whereas oxymetazoline has effects on both α_1 and α_2 adrenergic receptors. Using these vasoconstrictive prescription products may improve compliance by showing rapid and noticeable results. Brimonidine has been associated with rebound redness, and therefore should be combined with other antiinflammatory ingredients. Oxymetazoline seems to confer some antiinflammatory benefits in addition to the vasoconstrictive effects.[63] If retinoids are used in rosacea-prone skin, they should be introduced slowly and in conjunction with antiinflammatory ingredients. Patients with stinging-type skin should avoid retinoids and ingredients with a low pH such as acids whereas patients with allergic- and irritant-prone skin should avoid known allergens and any harsh ingredients.

SUMMARY OF SKIN CARE FOR SENSITIVE SKIN TYPES

Treatment of sensitive skin depends upon the subtype. Many people have more than one type of sensitive skin. In that case, it is important to know which subtype is predominant. The allergic/irritant subtype is the most important because the treatment includes avoiding inciting factors. Use of a hypoallergenic skin-care line is preferred in the case of this type of skin. Products should be added one at a time with a week in between each addition so that if the patient has a reaction, it is easier to identify the culprit. The second form of sensitive skin that trumps acne and stinging skin types is the rosacea type of skin. Patients who have inflammation and redness from rosacea need to have antiinflammatory ingredients added to their regimen and should be given about 4 weeks for the inflammation to calm down before adding any acne treatment ingredients. If the patient has concurrent stinging with the redness, in many cases the stinging will clear with the same antiinflammatory ingredients used for the rosacea regimens. Once the redness and stinging have improved and allergens have been identified, then the patient can be placed on an acne regimen with less risk of side effects. In summary, when treating sensitive skin with multiple subtypes, remove the allergens first, then add antiinflammatory ingredients, and finally proceed with acne medications. The more subtypes of sensitive skin the patient has, the more closely they should be monitored. Acne patients may feel frustrated by the delay in resolution so it is important to explain the process to them. Addition of oral medications or blue light can hasten the process of acne treatment without compromising this stepwise routine. As with other skin issues, once the skin type has reverted to a resistant type, the patient can be placed on a maintenance regimen to keep the symptoms of the sensitive subtypes at bay.

TABLE 207-6
Cosmeceuticals to Reduce Skin Pigmentation

- Arbutin
- Hydroquinone
- Hydroxy acids
- Kojic acid
- Licorice extract
- Mulberry extract
- Niacinamide
- Pycnogenol
- Resorcinol
- Retinol
- Soy (with estrogenic components removed)
- Topical steroids
- Vitamin C (ascorbic acid)

SKIN PIGMENTATION

PIGMENTED VERSUS NONPIGMENTED

The third primary skin characterization parameter is based on the presence or absence of uneven skin tone caused by hyperpigmentation or dyschromia on the face. The dyschromia may be in the form of melasma, solar lentigines, or postinflammatory hyperpigmentation.

Skin pigment (melanin) is produced by melanocytes, which transfer the pigment via melanosomes to keratinocytes. Melanin is derived from the enzymatic breakdown of tyrosine by tyrosinase into 3,4-dihydroxyphenylalanine, which yields 2 forms of melanin (eumelanin and pheomelanin).[64] Four primary mechanisms can be employed to impede the development of skin pigmentation: sunscreen use and sun avoidance, inhibiting the tyrosinase enzyme, preventing melanosome transfer into keratinocytes by blocking the PAR-2 receptor, and increasing desquamation of the SC. Treatments work best if all of these 4 strategies are employed. Patient education is crucial because patient habits can greatly contribute to dyspigmentation, especially melasma. For example, stress, estrogen use, heat exposure, melatonin supplements, over exfoliation leading to skin inflammation, and lack of SPF use in cars and indoors can all contribute to melanocyte activation.

SUNSCREEN

Sunscreen should be a routine part of the skin regimen every morning even if the patient stays indoors. There are many new SPF formulations that block infrared and other forms of light that can worsen melasma. If the patient has oily skin, then the SPF can be used in lieu of a moisturizer. Acne-prone patients should be treated with a noncomedogenic sunscreen. Oral sun-protective supplements such as polypodium leukotomes and pycnogenols offer extra protection but should not be used as a replacement for sunscreen.

TYROSINASE INHIBITORS

Tyrosinase inhibitors block the production of melanin and include vitamin C, hydroquinone, kojic acid, arbutin, mulberry extract, and licorice extract (Table 207-6). Many authors recommend a "holiday" from tyrosinase inhibitors every 3 to 6 months to prevent tachyphylaxis although the need for this is anecdotal.[65,66] Ascorbic acid is a tyrosinase inhibitor that has a different structure than the others so it can be used during the holiday period. Hydroquinone is the most effective tyrosinase inhibitor but unfounded public concerns about hydroquinone safety[67] have popularized the use of similar derivatives such as kojic acid and arbutin. Hydroquinone has been found to be efficacious in combination with a retinoid and a steroid in the "Kligman formula" because retinoids and steroids such as fluocinolone inhibit tyrosinase. This triple combination agent combines hydroquinone with retinoids, which prevent the skin-thinning effects of steroids, and steroids that mitigate the inflammation from retinoids and hydroquinone.

PAR-2 BLOCKERS

Small proteins present in soy, such as soybean trypsin inhibitor and Bowman-Birk inhibitor, exhibit depigmenting activity and prevent UV-induced pigmentation both in vitro and in vivo.[68] These soy proteins inhibit the cleavage of the 7 transmembrane G-protein coupled receptor known as protease-activated receptor 2 (PAR-2). It is expressed in keratinocytes at intersection points with melanocytes and functions like a key opening a lock allowing the melanosomes to transfer from the melanocyte into the keratinocyte. Both soy and niacinamide, a derivative of vitamin B_3, have been shown to inhibit melanosome movement from melanocytes to keratinocytes.[69]

EXFOLIANTS

Removing the top layer of the SC induces the cell cycle to speed up, which hastens desquamation of melanosome-laden keratinocytes. The melanocytes cannot make the pigment fast enough to keep the keratinocytes full of melanosomes, so less pigmentation is seen at the cell surface. Exfoliants work much better when combined with tyrosinase inhibitors and PAR-2 blocking agents in addition to sunscreen. Exfoliants can be mechanical such as microdermabrasion, scrubs, rotating brushes, or rough fabrics, or chemical such as hydroxy acids. Retinoids also serve the purpose of accelerating desquamation. These ingredients can be added into the skin-care regimen or applied as an in-office procedure to treat dyschromia. However, overuse or misuse can result in inflammation, which would stimulate the melanocytes to make more melanin and worsen the problem. For this reason, exfoliants should be used with extreme caution and patients should be educated about the harms of overexfoliating. Using exfoliating cleansers such as hydroxy acid cleansers is a low-risk way to add exfoliants into the skin-care regimen. In-office peels can be used but with caution and only by experienced users because peels can easily exacerbate melasma.

LIGNIN PEROXIDASE

Lignin peroxidase is an enzyme synthesized by the white-rot tree fungus *Phanerochaete chrysosporium* that breaks down lignin in decaying trees.[70] It is used in the paper industry to whiten wood pulp and was found to break down eumelanin, which has a similar structure to lignin.[71] In topical preparations, lignin peroxidase has been found to be effective for the improvement of skin pigmentation due to an excess of eumelanin. Lignin peroxidase is commercially available as a glycoprotein known as ligninase (or Melanozyme), which functions best at a pH of 2 to 4.5. It has been found to be nonirritating and safe for use in all of the sensitive skin subtypes. It can be used during the holiday period when tyrosinase inhibitors are discontinued to help prevent rebound of melasma during the maintenance period.

ANTIOXIDANTS

Antioxidants play multiple roles in the treatment and prevention of dyschromia. Their actions may include one or more of the following: chelating copper, neutralizing free radicals, and decreasing inflammation. Tyrosinase requires copper to function, and many antioxidants such as flavonoids chelate copper. Free radicals can incite inflammatory pathways leading to increased melanocyte activity. Many antioxidant ingredients such as argan oil and green tea have antiinflammatory activities independent of their antioxidant capabilities. Some antioxidants prevent UV-induced pigmentation by affecting the p53 pigmentation pathway through the rate-limiting step of p53 phosphorylation at site 15.[72] This phosphorylation step is blocked by the plant-derived antioxidant phloretin.[73] Ascorbic acid (vitamin C) is a unique antioxidant in that it also has tyrosinase-inhibiting properties separate from its antioxidant properties. Antioxidants are formulated in serums, sunscreens, and moisturizers.

SUMMARY OF SKIN CARE FOR PIGMENTED AND NONPIGMENTED SKIN TYPES

Nonpigmented types should use a daily sunscreen to preserve even skin tone. Pigmented skin types should be prescribed and educated on 2 forms of skin-care regimens: the treatment regimen and the maintenance regimen. Melasma studies show a 1- to 2-grade improvement at 12 to 16 weeks in most cases. For this reason, the treatment regimen should last 3 to 4 months and the patient should be warned that it may take several treatment cycles depending on (1) severity of melasma, (2) compliance with regimen, (3) sun avoidance, and (4) presence of other factors such as stress and estrogen use. Compliance is a major factor in achieving success. Monthly visits with photography and mexameter or other objective measurements at each visit can improve compliance. Patients should be counseled that changes in these measurements and in photos are not usually seen until 12 weeks to prevent discouragement, which usually occurs at the week 8 visit. The treatment cycle should consist of (1) daily broad-spectrum SPF; (2) twice-daily tyrosinase inhibitor; (3) nightly retinoid; (4) a PAR-2 blocking agent in either a sunscreen, serum, or moisturizer; and (5) an exfoliating cleanser. To save regimen steps and improve efficacy, the evening product can be a triple combination of retinoid, tyrosinase inhibitor, and a steroid such as the "Kligman formula." After 4 months, or on clearance of the pigmentation disorder, the regimen should be changed to a maintenance regimen. The maintenance regimen should not have tyrosinase inhibitors (with the exception of ascorbic acid) but should include (1) daily broad-spectrum SPF; (2) an antioxidant such as ascorbic acid; (3) a PAR-2 blocking agent in either a sunscreen, serum, or moisturizer; (4) lignin peroxidase; and (5) an exfoliating cleanser. The maintenance regimen will be used for at least 1 month or until pigmentation begins to return, at which time the treatment regimen will be resumed for another 4 months. The back-and-forth cycle will continue until the dyspigmentation clears. This may take 1 to 6 treatment cycles but clearing will occur in almost all cases if the patient is compliant with the regimen and lifestyle advice.

SKIN AGING

WRINKLE-PRONE SKIN VERSUS NON–WRINKLE-PRONE SKIN ("TIGHT")

Aging of the skin is a complex chain of events reflecting natural intrinsic and extrinsic processes. Intrinsic aging is a function of individual heredity and results from the passage of time. This process is, of course, inevitable and beyond voluntary control. However, the largest percentage of skin aging is due to lifestyle factors such as sun exposure, tanning bed use, smoking, increased cortisol levels, increased blood sugar levels, lack of exercise, excessive use of drugs and alcohol, and poor diet. Use of daily sunscreen, retinoids, and other antiaging technologies can mitigate the risk of skin aging. Wrinkle-prone skin is found in patients over the age of 20 who do not use antiaging technologies to prevent wrinkles while also engaging in several deleterious lifestyle behaviors. There are many exaggerated claims about antiaging ingredient efficacy, but only a few have stood the test of scientific evaluation. Although many studies are ongoing, it is much too early for any technologies to manipulate gene expression and affect skin aging with one notable exception—retinoids. Retinoids, by definition, bind the retinoic acid receptor, which turns on and off various genes including the procollagen gene. The only antiaging technologies that have been proven in vivo to improve skin appearance with long-term use are daily sunscreen, hydroxy acids, ascorbic acid, and retinoids. Many other antiaging technologies are being studied that aim to improve the appearance of skin or slow aging by lengthening telomeres; neutralizing free radicals; affecting production of matrix metalloproteinases, growth factors, and cytokines; preventing glycation; increasing skin levels of hyaluronic acid, heparan sulfate, collagen, and elastin; preserving or improving mitochondrial or lysosome function; and upregulating sirtuin expression.[74] The focus here is on the technologies that have demonstrated efficacy and are more widely used by dermatologists and omits the overhyped and unproven technologies.

The dermatologic focus of antiaging skin care should be to prevent the formation of rhytides in the first place,[75] and to improve wrinkles and a thinning dermis once this occurs. Prevention of aging is difficult to prove but the goal is to halt the degradation of the main structural components of the skin—collagen, elastin, heparan sulfate, and HA—all of which are known to be diminished in aged skin. The treatment of aging skin, usually judged by visual analysis of wrinkles, is much easier to prove but harder to achieve without using deceptive measures such as photography and use of humectants that immediately plump the skin. For this reason, placebo-controlled trials are vital to substantiate wrinkle improvement claims. Ingredients that have data to substantiate claims of wrinkle *prevention* include sunscreens and retinoids. Ingredients that have plausible claims that they prevent skin aging include ascorbic acid, through its collagen-stimulating and antioxidant properties, and green tea because of its antioxidant and antiinflammatory properties. The only ingredients that have convincing peer-reviewed data about their *ability to improve wrinkles* are hydroxy acids, ascorbic acid, and retinoids. Ingredients that have qualities that suggest they improve skin aging but need more proof include growth factors such as transforming growth factor-β, epidermal-derived growth factor, hyaluronic acid, and heparan sulfate. Ingredients that have minimal to no published peer-reviewed scientific data on photoaging include stem cells, collagen, products to prevent or reverse glycation, and ingredients that claim to upregulate sirtuin or lengthen telomeres. It is important to note that an antiaging claim can be made on any product that contains sunscreen.

SUNSCREENS

UV exposure results in skin damage through several mechanisms including sunburn cell formation, creation of thymine dimers, collagenase production, and provoking an inflammatory response. Signaling through p53 following telomere disruption is also a common feature observed in aging as well as photodamage.[76] Although much remains to be learned about the mechanisms through which UV irradiation unleashes a chain of cascading health effects, photoaging, photocarcinogenesis, and photo-immunosuppression are well-known results of UV exposure.[77] Every antiaging regimen should consist of a daily SPF. The most important factor to consider when choosing a sunscreen is patient compliance. Oily types will not wear a heavy oil-based product, whereas acne-prone types often suspect their SPF as the cause of breakouts. Chemical sunscreen agents often precipitate allergic dermatitis in susceptible sensitive skin subtypes. Patients should be educated on the major points of sunscreen use because many do not use enough SPF and do not reapply it.

CLEANSERS

Cleansers prepare the skin by removing sweat, dirt, and debris that can decrease the penetration of skin-care ingredients. Penetration of ingredients in their active form is a major issue for most antiaging products because the skin barrier prevents penetration of large and/or charged molecules. This barrier to penetration affects the efficacy of peptides, hyaluronic acid, growth factors, antioxidants, and many other ingredients. Cleansers can change the pH and other factors on the skin's surface that affect both penetration and the chemical structure and efficacy of the compounds that are placed on the skin after cleansing. For example, a low-pH cleanser such as a hydroxy acid will lower the skin's surface pH, increasing penetration of ascorbic acid, which penetrates more readily at a pH of 2 to 2.5.[78] A low pH would also improve the efficacy of lignin peroxide preparations and render the skin less hospitable for acne bacteria. Soap, on the other hand, increases the skin's pH.[79] The choice of an antiaging cleanser depends directly on skin hydration, presence of a sensitive subtype, and choice of therapeutic products to be used on the skin after cleansing.

MOISTURIZERS AND SERUMS

The main goal of antiaging skin care is to preserve and increase dermal levels of collagen, heparan sulfate, hyaluronic acid, and elastin. Of these, elastin is the most elusive as no ingredients have been able to increase levels of mature functional elastin. To protect and/or encourage production of these components, antiaging serums and moisturizers should contain a retinoid at a minimum. Collagen synthesis has been shown to be increased through the use of retinoids.[80] Retinoids also have been demonstrated in animal models to increase production of HA[81] and have been shown in multiple studies to improve photoaged skin.[82-84] Not all patients, especially dry skin types and sensitive skin types with the rosacea subtype, can tolerate a retinoid. Retinoids penetrate easily into the skin and can incite a reaction known as retinoid dermatitis. Starting the patient accordingly on a regimen directed to barrier repair and/or decreasing inflammation for 4 weeks may increase patient tolerance of retinoids and prevent retinoid dermatitis. Retinoids should be started with a low dose and used sparingly. One suggested regimen is a pea-size amount of product applied over moisturizer every third night. The amount and frequency can be adjusted as the patient's dryness and inflammation improve. Oily and resistant skin types usually have no trouble tolerating retinoids.

Antioxidants are commonly used in antiaging regimens to neutralize free radicals that damage DNA and cell membranes leading to increased aging, and induce glycation that causes damage to collagen strands.[85] Free radicals can act directly on growth factor and cytokine receptors in keratinocytes and dermal cells, leading to skin inflammation. The direct effects of free radicals on the aging process are beginning to be understood. In 1998, investigators demonstrated that free radical activation of the mitogen-activated protein kinase pathways resulted in production of collagenase, which led to degradation of collagen.[86] Another study by Kang and colleagues on human skin supported this concept. They showed that when human skin was pretreated with the antioxidants genistein and N-acetyl cysteine, the UV induction of the cJun-driven enzyme collagenase was blocked.[87] Antioxidants may block the process of glycation, but more data are needed before this hypothesis is proven. Many antioxidants are available in skin-care products, including argan oil, vitamins C and E, ferulic acid, coenzyme Q_{10}, green tea, phloretin, pycnogenol, resveratrol, silymarin, and idebenone. Vitamin C is a particularly interesting antioxidant because it has the added ability to induce fibroblasts to produce collagen.[88]

Hydroxy acids have been shown in multiple studies to improve fine lines and skin texture.[89] Present in cleansers, moisturizers, masks, in-office peels, and several other modalities, they function by increasing desquamation of the SC cells, which stimulates the stem cells in the skin to begin to produce various important cell components including collagen and hyaluronic acid. Hydroxy acids must be formulated at the proper pH to be effective, with the most acidic versions causing the most exfoliation but with increased side effects. Hydroxy acids can affect the efficacy of other ingredients applied at the same time, so their order in the regimen should be carefully considered.

SUMMARY OF SKIN CARE FOR WRINKLE-PRONE SKIN TYPES

The goal of antiaging skin care is daily use of sunscreen, retinoids, and antioxidants combined with healthy lifestyle habits to minimize glycation, UV light exposure, and free radical production. Antioxidants should be obtained by a myriad of sources, including food, beverages, supplements, and topical products. There is no one best antioxidant, and studies support the fact that they work better in combination than alone.[90]

COMBINING THE 4 SKIN PARAMETERS TO ASSIGN A PHENOTYPE DIAGNOSIS

The 4 skin parameters can be combined to form 16 distinct skin phenotypes also known as Baumann Skin Types (Fig 207-4).[91-93] Diagnosing the skin type allows the dermatologist to more easily prescribe a skin-care regimen taking into account the issues discussed in this chapter. It is more efficient to use a methodology to preset customized skin-care regimens based on a skin type diagnosis than to develop a de novo skin-care regimen for each patient. In addition, this allows the physician to more easily track results and efficacy.

All facial skin, regardless of age or gender, can be assessed by evaluating the skin and assigning it to 4 different parameters by choosing one of the following: dry (D) or oily (O); sensitive (S) or resistant (R); pigmented (P) or nonpigmented (N); and wrinkle prone (W) or tight (T) [or non–wrinkle prone]. One of each of the 2 options is chosen, so for example, the facial skin would be considered dry (D) or oily (O).

Once the skin has been assigned one of each of the 4 parameters, these 4 parameters are combined and the skin is diagnosed as one of 16 distinct skin phenotypes. For example, an individual may exhibit dry, sensitive, pigmented, wrinkle-prone skin and be referred to as a DSPW skin type. This person would require significantly different skin-care products compared to someone with oily, sensitive, pigmented, and wrinkled skin (OSPW). In many cases, historical data are necessary to properly identify the skin phenotype. The Baumann Skin Type Indicator questionnaire was developed to speed the skin phenotype diagnostic process. It aids physicians in identifying a patient's skin type, factoring in sebum secretion, skin hydration, propensity for inflammation—such as acne and contact dermatitis—as well as uneven skin pigmentation on the face and habits that increase the risk for cutaneous aging and skin cancer.[53,94] The Baumann Skin Type Indicator is a 3- to 5-minute questionnaire that is administered in the waiting room prior to the patient consultation. It has been tested in all ethnicities and genders and in ages 14 and older to diagnose skin phenotype. Its use

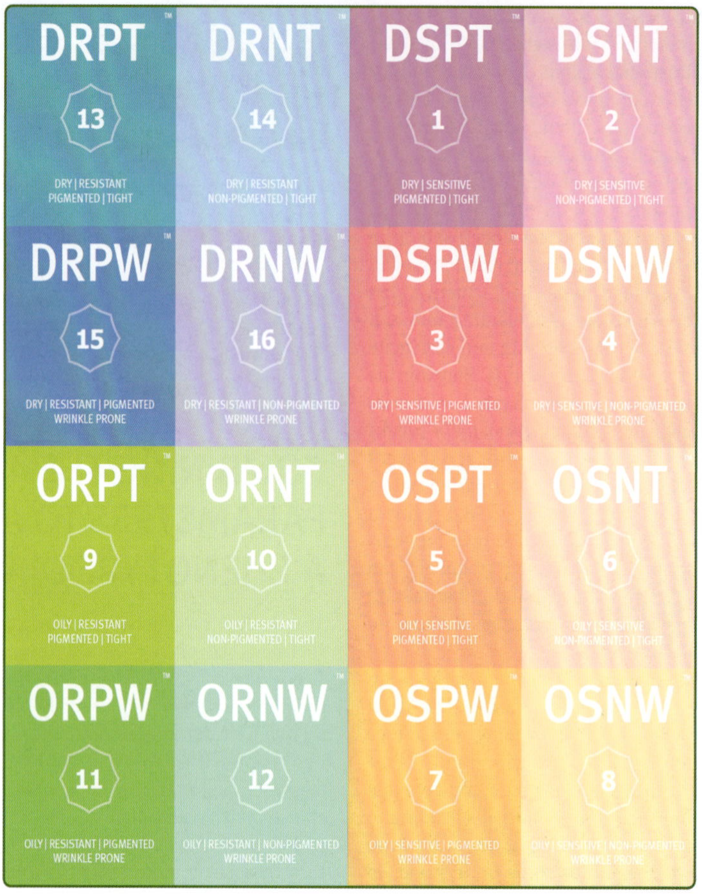

Figure 207-4 Sixteen distinct Baumann skin types based on the designations Oily vs Dry; Sensitive vs Resistant; Pigmented vs Nonpigmented; and Wrinkled vs Tight. (The image herein is © Copyright 2016 MetaBeauty Inc. and is used with permission.)

has been validated in studies in white, Chinese, and Korean populations.[95]

Once the skin phenotype has been determined, certain extrinsic or intrinsic factors, such as a move to a different climate, a change in stress levels, pregnancy, menopause, aging, disease, and other stressors, can result in a skin type change. The Baumann Skin Type Indicator, a questionnaire developed to determine skin type, is helpful in assessing skin type initially and again after major life events.[96]

THE HEALTHIEST SKIN TYPE

The goal of a prescribed skin-care regimen is to improve the skin's appearance and health through proper lifestyle choices and daily use of topical and oral cosmeceuticals and medications. The healthiest skin type would manifest an adequate amount of sebum production to protect the skin from TEWL, free radicals, and allergens and irritants. This idealized healthy skin type would have a robust skin barrier, inflammatory pathways that are only activated when provoked, normalized melanocytic function to provide even skin tone, strong defenses against aging, and good lifestyle choices. This skin phenotype is ORNT or oily, resistant, nonpigmented, and tight. Although the baseline genetic Baumann Skin Type may exhibit various characteristics, consistent use of a proper regimen and therapeutic treatments can change the skin to the desirable characteristics of ORNT skin.

IDENTIFYING THE MOST EFFICACIOUS PRODUCTS

There is no one ingredient or product that is ideal for all skin types. Each skin type has individual needs that should be taken into account when choosing products and which ones to combine to maximize efficacy. There are other variables to consider when selecting a skin-care product for patients including the quality and choice of ingredients, product formulation, manufacturing, packaging, storage, and shipping. Counterfeit products have become a huge problem in the online retail world, so patients need guidance about what brands to use and where to purchase them. When treatment regimens consisting of cosmeceuticals and/or medications do not work, patients will have poor outcomes, resulting in diminished trust that mars the physician–patient relationship.

CHOOSING INGREDIENTS

It is important to understand the characteristics of various ingredients and match formulations to a patient's skin type. Take into account which prescription medications will be combined in the regimen and how they will be affected by the cosmeceuticals. For example, hyaluronic acid–containing preparations may accelerate penetration of medications,[25] and the pro-oxidant activity of benzoyl peroxide can lessen the efficacy of other ingredients. The order of application and the combination of ingredients affects stability, efficacy, safety, and the chemical structure of the formulation, and there is really no such thing as an inactive ingredient (or excipient). Ingredients can modulate penetration, enhance the activity of other ingredients, or inactivate them depending on the order in which ingredients are used on the skin. For example, olive oil increases penetration of other ingredients because it has a high content of oleic acid, whereas safflower oil can reduce penetration by strengthening the skin barrier. It is imperative to know which ingredients work well together and which do not. The order in which ingredients are placed on the skin is also significant, because products can inactivate each other and affect absorption.

CHOOSING PRODUCTS

A brand-agnostic approach is recommended, choosing the best products from each brand and combining and testing them on various skin types to see which products and what combinations of products work best. The formulation recipe and the entire spectrum of production can affect efficacy. The "formulation recipe" refers to the order in which ingredients are added in the formulation process, the pH, the amount of each ingredient, the temperature at which the ingredient is added, and many other important factors that determine the final chemistry. Ingredients like vitamin C, green tea, and retinol are more expensive when formulated properly. Many "copycat" brands use the same ingredients, but they cannot use the patented recipe; therefore, the end product is qualitatively different.

How a product is made and packaged is pivotal. For example, retinol decomposes when exposed to light and air. If it is stirred in an open vat it loses its efficacy and therefore must be formulated in a closed system. The process of packaging the completed product is also important. The formulation can be exposed to air and light when the bottles, pumps, or jars are filled. A product may be formulated in one place and shipped to another location for final packaging—and many ingredients can lose their potency during transit. Once the product is filled and packaged, how it is stored and how long it is stored can also affect efficacy. Many sunscreens, antioxidants, and retinoids will lose efficacy when stored in high heat. This concern extends to how the products are stored in the warehouse, how they are shipped through the mail, how they are stored in the retail space, and where the patient stores the product once it is purchased. The container itself is also a significant consideration as air and light can enter tubes, affecting the efficacy of the formulation. Air and heat are the primary culprits for unstable ingredients such as retinoids and ascorbic acid; therefore, these should be packaged in amber bottles or airless pumps to minimize light and air exposure.

DESIGNING THE REGIMEN AND ORDER OF APPLICATION OF PRODUCTS

Once a doctor has identified a patient's skin type and properly matched products to her or his skin type, it is necessary to decide the order of the products. Table 207-7 gives an example of a basic structure of a skin-care regimen. The cleanser is the obvious first step in the morning and evening regimen to clear the skin of dirt and debris. The eye product is applied next to protect the thin skin from the third regimen step, which is the medication or treatment product. Examples include rosacea, acne, melasma, or seborrheic dermatitis medications. The fourth step is a moisturizer. In the morning, the fifth step is a sunscreen whereas in the evening the fifth step is a retinoid. The retinoid is applied last to limit penetration.

PATIENT EDUCATION

It is crucial to instruct the patient exactly *how* to apply the products. The order in which products are applied makes a difference. Ingredient interactions, ingredient

TABLE 207-7
A Typical Structure for a Skincare Regimen That Suits the Majority of Skin Types

MORNING	EVENING
Step 1: Cleanser	Step 1: Cleanser
Step 2: Eye product	Step 2: Eye product
Step 3: Treatment product or medication	Step 3: Treatment product or medication
Step 4: Moisturizer	Step 4: Moisturizer
Step 5: Sunscreen	Step 5: Retinoid

penetration times and cross reactions, and skin type factors such as the condition of the skin barrier, sebum production, thickness of the stratum corneum, and sun exposure and bathing habits should be considered. Providing a printed regimen with step-by-step instructions for morning and night can be beneficial to patients.

If possible, explain to patients the basis for each product selection because this can greatly enhance patient compliance and, thus, outcomes. Training your staff to facilitate this is a key component in patient education. Preprinted, web-based, or automatically emailed educational newsletters or fact sheets can be utilized, particularly in a busy practice. This information helps keep patients engaged and educates them about new technologies and products that are appropriate for their skin type.

ENCOURAGE COMPLIANCE

A followup visit after 1 month is recommended to check on patient progress. Studies have shown that routine followup improves compliance. In addition, any side effects can be mitigated. For example, a prescribed retinoid may have induced irritation, prompting the patient to stop using it. An imaging system in the office also can be useful as baseline, and followup photos help illustrate progress and encourage vigilance and compliance. The importance of a followup visit should be emphasized at the initial appointment. Ideally, visits should be every month until the skin condition has improved or the ideal ORNT skin type has been achieved.

CONCLUSION

Dermatologists have the scientific background and knowledge of skin pathology to develop and prescribe efficacious skin-care regimens. However, the many product choices and time pressure in the dermatology clinic make this process difficult. When patients choose the wrong skin-care products, they may experience less efficacy with prescription medications, so there is value in dermatologists taking the time to review every product that the patient places on their skin. Keeping the staff up-to-date on the latest technologies and implementing these in a busy medical practice is challenging. A standardized and scientific methodology using a diagnostic system to classify skin types can be used to facilitate the patient skin-care regimen prescribing process. This methodology should be easy to implement and speed patient consult times rather than slow them. Taking time to train the staff and providing educational handouts for patients can streamline the process and make it more effective, resulting in improved patient outcomes. Incorporating staff training and patient education is mandatory to improve patient compliance. Using monthly followup appointments and analyses such as photography and instrumentation to show progress to patients keeps them interested and motivated to improve the health of their skin.

REFERENCES

1. http://www.ibisworld.com/industry/cosmeceutical-skincare-production.html. Accessed August 6, 2016.
2. http://www.freedoniagroup.com/Cosmeceuticals.html. Accessed August 6, 2016.
3. http://www.wdrb.com/story/32522329/surge-in-sales-of-physician-dispensed-cosmeceuticals-expected-as-demand-for-skincare-products-among-aged-people-rises-reports-tmr. Accessed August 6, 2016.
4. Chernosky ME. Clinical aspects of dry skin. *J Soc Cosmet Chem*. 1976;27:365-376.
5. Rawlings AV, Hope J, Rogers J, et al. Skin dryness—what is it? *J Invest Dermatol*. 1993;100:510.
6. Bouwstra JA, Dubbelaar FE, Gooris GS, et al. The lipid organization in the skin barrier. *Acta Derm Venereol Suppl (Stockh)*. 2000;208:23-30.
7. Wildnauer RH, Bothwell JW, Douglass AB. Stratum corneum biomechanical properties. I. Influence of relative humidity on normal and extracted human stratum corneum. *J Invest Dermatol*. 1971;56(1):72-78.
8. Orth D, Appa Y. Glycerine: a natural ingredient for moisturizing skin. In: Loden M, Maibach H, eds. *Dry Skin and Moisturizers*. Boca Raton, FL: CRC Press; 2000:214.
9. Ekholm IE, Brattsand M, Egelrud T. Stratum corneum tryptic enzyme in normal epidermis: a missing link in the desquamation process? *J Invest Dermatol*. 2000;114(1):56-63.
10. Thiboutot D. Regulation of human sebaceous glands. *J Invest Dermatol*. 2004;123(1):1-12.
11. Clarys P, Barel A. Quantitative evaluation of skin surface lipids. *Clin Dermatol*. 1995;13(4):307-321.
12. Mathers WD, Lane JA. Meibomian gland lipids, evaporation, and tear film stability. *Adv Exp Med Biol*. 1998;438:349-360.
13. Tiffany JM. The role of meibomian secretion in the tears. *Trans Ophthalmol Soc UK*. 1985;104(pt 4):396-401.
14. Pochi PE, Strauss JS, Downing DT. Age-related changes in sebaceous gland activity. *J Invest Dermatol*. 1979;73(1):108-111.
15. Walton S, Wyatt EH, Cunliffe WJ. Genetic control of sebum excretion and acne—a twin study. *Br J Dermatol*. 1988;118(3):393-396.
16. Elias PM. The epidermal permeability barrier: from the early days at Harvard to emerging concepts. *J Invest Dermatol*. 2004;122(2):xxxvi-xxxix.
17. Scott IR, Harding CR. Filaggrin breakdown to water binding compounds during development of the rat stratum corneum is controlled by the water activity of the environment. *Dev Biol (Basel)*. 1986;115(1):84-92.
18. Sato J, Denda M, Chang S, et al. Abrupt decreases in environmental humidity induce abnormalities in permeability barrier homeostasis. *J Invest Dermatol*. 2002;119(4):900-904.
19. Gallo RL, Trowbridge J. Proteoglycans and glycosaminoglycans of skin. In: Freedberg IM, Eisen AZ, Wolff K, et al, eds. *Fitzpatrick's Dermatology in General Medicine*. 6th ed. New York, NY: McGraw-Hill; 2003:210-216.
20. Lee DH, Oh JH, Chung JH. Glycosaminoglycan and proteoglycan in skin aging. *J Dermatol Sci*. 2016;83(3):174-181.

21. Tammi R, Säämänen AM, Maibach HI, et al. Degradation of newly synthesized high molecular mass hyaluronan in the epidermal and dermal compartments of human skin in organ culture. *J Invest Dermatol*. 1991;97(1):126-130.
22. Sakai S, Yasuda R, Sayo T, et al. Hyaluronan exists in the normal stratum corneum. *J Invest Dermatol*. 2000;114(6):1184-1187.
23. Brown TJ, Alcorn D, Fraser JR. Absorption of hyaluronan applied to the surface of intact skin. *J Invest Dermatol*. 1999;113(5):740-746.
24. Rieger M. Hyaluronic acid in cosmetics. *Cosm Toil*. 1998;113(3):35-42.
25. Brown MB, Jones SA. Hyaluronic acid: a unique topical vehicle for the localized delivery of drugs to the skin. *J Eur Acad Dermatol Venereol*. 2005;19(3):308-318.
26. Baumann L. Skin ageing and its treatment. *J Pathol*. 2007;211(2):241-251.
27. Murad H, Tabibian MP. The effect of an oral supplement containing glucosamine, amino acids, minerals, and antioxidants on cutaneous aging: a preliminary study. *J Dermatolog Treat*. 2001;12(1):47-51.
28. Maquart F-X, Brézillon S, Wegrowski Y. Proteoglycans in skin aging. In: Farage MA, Miller KW, Maibach HI, eds. *Textbook of Aging Skin*. Berlin: Springer-Verlag; 2010:109.
29. Gallo RL, Bucay VW, Shamban AT, et al. The potential role of topically applied heparin sulfate in the treatment of photodamage. *J Drugs Dermatol*. 2015;14(7):669-674.
30. Sougrat R, Morand M, Gondran C, et al. Functional expression of AQP3 in human skin epidermis and reconstructed epidermis. *J Invest Dermatol*. 2002;118(4):678-685.
31. Takenouchi M, Suzuki H, Tagami H. Hydration characteristics of pathologic stratum corneum—evaluation of bound water. *J Invest Dermatol*. 1986;87(5):574-576.
32. Warner RR, Bush RD, Ruebusch NA. Corneocytes undergo systematic changes in element concentrations across the human inner stratum corneum. *J Invest Dermatol*. 1995;104(4):530-536.
33. Warner RR, Myers MC, Taylor DA. Electron probe analysis of human skin: element concentration profiles. *J Invest Dermatol*. 1988;90(1):78-85.
34. Ma T, Hara M, Sougrat R, et al. Impaired stratum corneum hydration in mice lacking epidermal water channel aquaporin-3. *J Biol Chem*. 2002;277(19):17147-17153.
35. Yang B, Verkman AS. Water and glycerol permeabilities of aquaporins 1-5 and MIP determined quantitatively by expression of epitope-tagged constructs in Xenopus oocytes. *J Biol Chem*. 1997;272(26):16140-16146.
36. Dumas M, Gondran C, Barre P, et al. Effect of an *Ajuga turkestanica* extract on aquaporin 3 expression, water flux, differentiation and barrier parameters of the human epidermis. *Eur J Dermatol*. 2002;12(6):XXV-XXVI.
37. Hara M, Verkman AS. Glycerol replacement corrects defective skin hydration, elasticity, and barrier function in aquaporin-3-deficient mice. *Proc Natl Acad Sci U S A*. 2003;100(12):7360-7365.
38. Naik A, Pechtold LARM, Potts RO, et al. Mechanism of oleic acid-induced skin penetration enhancement in vivo in humans. *J Control Release*. 1995;37(3):299-306.
39. Kim TH, Choi EH, Kang YC, et al. The effects of topical alpha-hydroxyacids on the normal skin barrier of hairless mice. *Br J Dermatol*. 2001;144(2):267-273.
40. Zettersten EM, Ghadially R, Feingold KR, et al. Optimal ratios of topical stratum corneum lipids improve barrier recovery in chronologically aged skin. *J Am Acad Dermatol*. 1997;37(3, pt 1):403-408.
41. Park BD, Youm JK, Jeong SK, et al. The characterization of molecular organization of multilamellar emulsions containing pseudoceramide and type III synthetic ceramide. *J Invest Dermatol*. 2003;121(4):794-801.
42. Lodén M, Bárány E. Skin-identical lipids versus petrolatum in the treatment of tape-stripped and detergent-perturbed human skin. *Acta Derm Venereol* 2000;80(6):412-415.
43. Draelos Z. Moisturizers. *Atlas of Cosmetic Dermatology*. New York, NY: Churchill Livingstone; 2000:85.
44. Spruit D. The interference of some substances with the water vapour loss of human skin. *Dermatologica*. 1971;142(2):89-92.
45. Draelos Z. Moisturizers. *Atlas of Cosmetic Dermatology*. New York, NY: Churchill Livingstone; 2000:83.
46. Wehr RF, Krochmal L. Considerations in selecting a moisturizer. *Cutis*. 1987;39(6):512-515.
47. Idson B. Dry skin: moisturizing and emolliency. *Cosmet Toiletr*. 1992;107:69.
48. Fluhr JW, Gloor M, Lehmann L, et al. Glycerol accelerates recovery of barrier function in vivo. *Acta Derm Venereol*. 1999;79(6):418-421.
49. De Pedrini P, Rapisarda R, Spano G. The effect of ketoconazole on sebum secretion in patients suffering from acne and seborrhoea. *Int J Tissue React*. 1988; 10(2):111-113.
50. Goodfellow A, Alaghband-Zadeh J, Carter G, et al. Oral spironolactone improves acne vulgaris and reduces sebum excretion. *Br J Dermatol*. 1984;111(2): 209-214.
51. Goldstein JA, Socha-Szott A, Thomsen RJ, et al. Comparative effect of isotretinoin and etretinate on acne and sebaceous gland secretion. *J Am Acad Dermatol*. 1982;6(4, pt 2, suppl):760-765.
52. Rose AE, Goldberg DJ. Safety and efficacy of intradermal injection of botulinum toxin for the treatment of oily skin. *Dermatol Surg*. 2013;39(3, pt 1):443-448.
53. Baumann L. Understanding and treating various skin types: the Baumann Skin Type Indicator. *Dermatol Clin*. 2008:26(3):359-373.
54. Baumann L. Anti-inflammatory agents. In: Baumann L, ed. *Cosmeceuticals and Cosmetic Ingredients*. New York, NY: McGraw-Hill; 2015:227-228.
55. Feldman SR, Camacho FT, Krejci-Manwaring J, et al. Adherence to topical therapy increases around the time of office visits. *J Am Acad Dermatol*. 2007;57(1): 81-83.
56. Basketter DA, Griffiths HA. A study of the relationship between susceptibility to skin stinging and skin irritation. *Contact Dermatitis*. 1993;29(4):185-188.
57. Fisher AA. "Status cosmeticus": a cosmetic intolerance syndrome. *Cutis*. 1990;46(2):109-110.
58. Amin S, Maibach HI. Immunologic contact urticaria definition. In: Amin S, Lahti A, Maibach HI, eds. *Contact Urticaria Syndrome*. Boca Raton, FL: CRC Press; 1997:11.
59. Jovanovic M, Poljacki M, Duran V, et al. Contact allergy to Compositae plants in patients with atopic dermatitis. *Med Pregl*. 2004;57(5-6):209-218.
60. Orton DI, Wilkinson JD. Cosmetic allergy: incidence, diagnosis, and management. *Am J Clin Dermatol*. 2004;5(5):327-337.
61. Chularojanamontri L, Tuchinda P, Kulthanan K, et al. Moisturizers for acne: what are their constituents? *J Clin Aesthet Dermatol*. 2014;7(5):36-44.
62. Piwnica D, Rosignoli C, de Ménonville ST, et al. Vasoconstriction and anti-inflammatory properties of the selective α-adrenergic receptor agonist brimonidine. *J Dermatol Sci*. 2014;75(1):49-54.

63. Tuettenberg A, Koelsch S, Knop J, et al. Oxymetazoline modulates proinflammatory cytokines and the T-cell stimulatory capacity of dendritic cells. *Exp Dermatol* 2007;16(3):171-178.
64. Freedberg IM, Eisen AZ, Wolff K, et al, eds. *Fitzpatrick's Dermatology in General Medicine*. 5th ed. New York, NY: McGraw-Hill; 1999:996.
65. Woolery-Lloyd H, Kammer JN. Treatment of hyperpigmentation. *Semin Cutan Med Surg*. 2011;30(3):171-175.
66. Sofen B, Prado G, Emer J. Melasma and post inflammatory hyperpigmentation: management update and expert opinion. *Skin Ther Lett*. 2016;21(1):1-7.
67. Levitt J. The safety of hydroquinone: a dermatologist's response to the 2006 Federal Register. *J Am Acad Dermatol*. 2007;57(5):854-872.
68. Paine C, Sharlow E, Liebel F, et al. An alternative approach to depigmentation by soybean extracts via inhibition of the PAR-2 pathway. *J Invest Dermatol*. 2001;116(4):587-595.
69. Hakozaki T, Minwalla L, Zhuang J, et al. The effect of niacinamide on reducing cutaneous pigmentation and suppression of melanosome transfer. *Br J Dermatol*. 2002;147(1):20-31.
70. Baumann L. Lignin peroxidase. In: Baumann L, ed. *Cosmeceuticals and Cosmetic Ingredients*. New York, NY: McGraw-Hill; 2015:123-124.
71. Woo S, Cho J, Lee B, et al. Decolorization of melanin by lignin peroxidase from *Phanerochaete chrysosporium*. *Biotechnol Bioprocess Eng*. 2004;9:256-260.
72. Cui R, Widlund HR, Feige E, et al. Central role of p53 in the suntan response and pathologic hyperpigmentation. *Cell*. 2007;128(5):853-864.
73. Oresajo C, Stephens T, Hino PD, et al. Protective effects of a topical antioxidant mixture containing vitamin C, ferulic acid, and phloretin against ultraviolet-induced photodamage in human skin. *J Cosmet Dermatol*. 2008;7(4):290-297.
74. Baumann L. Overview of aging. In: Baumann L, ed. *Cosmeceuticals and Cosmetic Ingredients*. New York, NY: McGraw-Hill; 2015:317-321.
75. Baumann L. How to prevent photoaging? *J Invest Dermatol*. 2005;125(4):xii-xiii.
76. Kosmadaki MG, Gilchrest BA. The role of telomeres in skin aging/photoaging. *Micron*. 2004;35(3):155-159.
77. Marrot L, Belaïdi JP, Meunier JR. Importance of UVA photoprotection as shown by genotoxic related endpoints: DNA damage and p53 status. *Mutat Res*. 2005;571(1-2):175-184.
78. Pinnell SR, Yang H, Omar M, et al. Topical L-ascorbic acid: percutaneous absorption studies. *Dermatol Surg*. 2001;27(2):137-142.
79. Ananthapadmanabhan KP, Moore DJ, Subramanyan K, et al. Cleansing without compromise: the impact of cleansers on the skin barrier and the technology of mild cleansing. *Dermatol Ther (Heidelb)*. 2004;17(suppl 1):16-25.
80. Varani J, Warner RL, Gharaee-Kermani M, et al. Vitamin A antagonizes decreased cell growth and elevated collagen-degrading matrix metalloproteinases and stimulates collagen accumulation in naturally aged human skin. *J Invest Dermatol*. 2000;114(3):480-486.
81. Margelin D, Medaisko C, Lombard D, et al. Hyaluronic acid and dermatan sulfate are selectively stimulated by retinoic acid in irradiated and nonirradiated hairless mouse skin. *J Invest Dermatol*. 1996;106(3):505-509.
82. Weiss JS, Ellis CN, Headington JT, et al. Topical tretinoin improves photoaged skin. A double-blind vehicle-controlled study. *JAMA*. 1988;259(4):527-532.
83. Kafi R, Kwak HS, Schumacher WE, et al. Improvement of naturally aged skin with vitamin A (retinol). *Arch Dermatol*. 2007;143(5):606-612.
84. Cho S, Lowe L, Hamilton TA, et al. Long-term treatment of photoaged human skin with topical retinoic acid improves epidermal cell atypia and thickens the collagen band in papillary dermis. *J Am Acad Dermatol*. 2005;53(5):769-774.
85. Baumann L. Antioxidants. In: Baumann L, ed. *Cosmeceuticals and Cosmetic Ingredients*. New York, NY: McGraw-Hill; 2015:135-136.
86. Fisher GJ, Talwar TS, Lin JY, et al. Retinoic acid inhibits induction of c-Jun protein by ultraviolet irradiation that occurs subsequent to activation of mitogen-activated protein kinase pathways in human skin in vivo. *J Clin Invest*. 1998;101(6):1432-1440.
87. Kang S, Chung JH, Lee JH, et al. Topical *N*-acetyl cysteine and genistein prevent ultraviolet-light-induced signaling that leads to photoaging in human skin in vivo. *J Invest Dermatol*. 2003;120(5):835-841.
88. Nusgens BV, Humbert P, Rougier A, et al. Topically applied vitamin C enhances the mRNA level of collagens I and III, their processing enzymes and tissue inhibitor of matrix metalloproteinase 1 in the human dermis. *J Invest Dermatol*. 2001;116(6):853-859.
89. Ditre CM, Griffin TD, Murphy GF, et al. Effects of alpha-hydroxy acids on photoaged skin: a pilot clinical, histologic, and ultrastructural study. *J Am Acad Dermatol*. 1996;34(2, pt 1):187-195.
90. Lin JY, Selim MA, Shea CR, et al. UV photoprotection by combination topical antioxidants vitamin C and vitamin E. *J Am Acad Dermatol*. 2003;48(6):866-874.
91. Baumann L. Cosmetics and skin care in dermatology. In: Wolff K, ed. *Fitzpatrick's Dermatology in General Medicine*. 7th ed. New York, NY: McGraw-Hill; 2008: 2357-2364.
92. Baumann L. The Baumann skin typing system. In: Farage MA, Miller KW, Maibach HI, eds. *Textbook of Aging Skin*. Berlin, Germany: Springer-Verlag; 2010: 929-944.
93. Baumann L. The importance of skin type: the Baumann skin type system. In: Baumann L, ed. *Cosmeceuticals and Cosmetic Ingredients*. New York, NY: McGraw-Hill; 2015:1-4.
94. Baumann L, Penfield R, Clarke J, et al. A validated questionnaire for quantifying skin oiliness. *J Cosmet Dermatol Sci Appl*. 2014;4(2):78-84.
95. Baumann L. Validation of a questionnaire to diagnose the Baumann skin type in all ethnicities and in various geographic locations. *J Cosmet Dermatol Sci Appl*. 2016;6(1):34-40.
96. Baumann L. *The Skin Type Solution*. New York, NY: Bantam Dell; 2006.

Chapter 208 :: Fundamentals of Laser and Light-Based Treatments
:: Omer Ibrahim & Jeffrey S. Dover

第二百零八章
激光原理和光学治疗

中文导读

激光（Laser）是受激释放并放大的光。本章共分为9节：①激光原理；②强脉冲光原理；③光辐射基本参数；④激光能量传输；⑤激光-组织相互作用；⑥选择性光热作用；⑦局灶性光热作用；⑧皮肤冷却；⑨激光安全。

第一节介绍了光的一般特征及激光的单色性、相干性、平行性、高能量性的物理特性，再列出皮肤科常使用的可见光范围至近红外光谱范围内的激光及其靶标、效果、脉冲时间、临床应用（表208-1）。接下来介绍了激光器械的构成，再通过图208-1、2、3详细讲述了光子在激光器械里发生的受激释放过程。

第二节介绍了强脉冲光原理，作者指出强脉冲光（IPL）不是激光，产生的是420 nm~1200 nm的非相干光，它是多色的、宽带的、发散的。并提出滤光片在IPL中的应用。

第三节介绍了光辐射基本参数：波长（nm）、功率（w）、辐射度（w/cm²）、照射时间（s）和能量密度或剂量（J/cm²），并提出影响以上参数的因素。

第四节介绍了关节臂、光纤、微型操作器、光纤激光技术四种激光的传输技术。

第五节介绍了激光与组织间可能经历反射、透射、吸收和散射（图208-6），其中吸收作用是比较重要的，并通过吸收系数来判断组织吸收光子的能力，作者总结了不同波长的激光对应皮肤中不同色基（氧合血红蛋白、黑色素、水）的吸收系数（图208-7），及IPL在不同滤光片下色基的吸收情况（图208-8）。接下来作者提出，色基吸收后产生几种相互作用，包括光化学反应、机械作用、光热作用，之后变为激活态，最后产生生物学效应，其中光热作用是大多数激光的作用机制，并举出了具体激光的例子。紧接着，就光热效应可能产生的周围组织热损伤展开讨论，并提出不同温度下组织的发生发展变化（图208-9）。最后，通过能量=功率×脉冲持续时间的公式，提出激光促使目标组织气化和周围组织凝固性坏死之间的矛盾（图208-10）。

第六节介绍了选择性光热作用，即选择一个波长的激光，被特定的色基吸收后，当脉冲持续时间或照射时间短于热弛豫时间时，此时周围组织的损伤将被最小化。其中热弛豫时间是指靶标冷却到其被加热温度一半时所需要的时间，并通过公式提出热弛豫时间的决定因素。选择性光热作用需要注意的两个方面，包括选择激光波长、选择正确的脉冲持续时间。

第七节介绍了点阵激光的局灶性光热作用治疗原理，即产生显微治疗区（MTZ），产生柱状损伤，从而减少愈合时间并将不良影响降到最低的优点。并把点阵激光分为气化型和非气化型。

第八节介绍了皮肤冷却可以减少激光对

于表皮不必要的伤害，同时向下输送足够的能量。提出了两种冷却方法：接触冷却（整体冷却）和非接触冷却，并总结于表208-3。

第九节介绍了关于激光的潜在危险，及安全措施的实施是至关重要的，包括皮肤安全、眼部安全及维持激光的安全使用三个方面。

〔简　丹〕

AT-A-GLANCE

- Lasers and flashlamps harness the power of light to precisely treat a myriad of cutaneous disorders and conditions.
- Laser light is monochromatic, coherent, and collimated; whereas, intense pulsed light (IPL) is polychromatic, broadband, and divergent.
- Upon light's impact with skin, several tissue interactions occur including reflection, transmission, scattering, and absorption.
- Laser parameters such as fluence, pulse duration, wavelength, and spot size can be adjusted to safely deliver energy to the skin to achieve desired therapeutic effects.
- In general, within the visible spectrum longer-wavelength light penetrates more deeply.
- Laser and light delivered though a larger spot size penetrates more deeply into tissue and is scattered less than with smaller spot sizes.
- Selective photothermolysis allows lasers and light sources to target specific chromophores in the skin to achieve certain effects while minimizing injury to surrounding structures.
- Fractional photothermolysis creates evenly distributed zones of microthermal injury in skin to produce columns of injury in the epidermis and dermis, leaving intervening columns of unaltered skin, thereby decreasing healing time and minimizing adverse effects.
- Knowledge of the potentially hazardous effects of lasers and flashlamps, and implementation of safety measures, are essential to maintain a safe environment for the practitioner, staff, and patient.

INTRODUCTION

Light is a fundamental form of energy that is harnessed in the form of lasers and pulsed light sources that has countless applications in modern medicine. In 1900, Max Planck described that light is released, transferred, and absorbed in specific amounts of energy called quanta.[1] In 1917, Einstein published "The Quantum Theory of Radiation" in which he suggested that most atoms exist in a ground-energy state, and upon absorbing energy are converted to higher energy levels. When these excited atoms return to their ground state, they release energy as photons or electromagnetic waves. Einstein also discovered that when a photon of a specific wavelength collides with an excited atom, 2 photons are released concurrently with equal frequencies, a phenomenon otherwise known as "stimulated emission."[2,3]

Laser is an acronym for *light amplification by the stimulated emission of radiation*. Theodore Maiman created the first laser in 1960 by using an energy source to energize solid ruby crystals.[4] Since this seminal discovery, the variety and applications of lasers in medicine has expanded dramatically over the ensuing decades. Because of its accessibility, the skin was the object of many of the early experiments that sought to harness this powerful modality, and as a result over the years lasers have revolutionized the treatment of numerous cutaneous disorders.

LASER PRINCIPLES

In its simplest form, a laser device creates energy in the form of a beam of light that interacts with its target tissue. Light and other forms of electromagnetic radiation are composed of photons that travel at a constant velocity, or speed of light ($c = 2.998 \times 10^8$ m/s) in a vacuum.[5] The major properties of radiation are wavelength λ and frequency ν, which are correlated: $c = \lambda \cdot \nu$. The energy of a photon is proportional to its frequency, such that the energy of radiation increases with increasing frequency (and decreasing wavelength). Visible light represents a relatively small portion of the electromagnetic spectrum, ranging from 390 nm (violet) to 700 nm (red), and can be seen by the human eye.[5] Most lasers used in dermatology fall within the visible-light range and the near infrared spectrum (Table 208-1).

Natural light and spontaneously emitted light such as that from a light bulb are created as a result of excited atoms that emit photons at different times, in any direction and usually with different wavelengths. This electromagnetic radiation is incoherent, divergent and spectrally broadband. In contrast, lasers are fundamentally different. All laser devices are composed of an energy source and an optical resonator. The energy source is what is used to bring atoms and electrons to an excited energy state, and can take the form of an electrical current, flashlamp, or even another laser.[6] The resonator is composed of a medium enclosed

TABLE 208-1
Commonly Used Dermatologic Lasers

LASER	WAVELENGTH	TARGET	EFFECT IN TARGET	MODE (PULSE DURATION)	APPLICATIONS
Excimer	308 nm	DNA, proteins	Photochemical reactions	Pulsed (µs)	Comparable to narrow-band UVB[311]
Argon	488/514 nm	Vascular lesions	Semiselective coagulation	Pulsed (ms)	Telangiectases, spider nevi, venous lakes
		Tissue	Coagulation		Syringoma, xanthelasma, epidermal nevi
Frequency-doubled Nd:YAG (KTP)	532 nm	Vascular lesions	Selective coagulation	Pulsed (ms)	Telangiectases, spider nevi, venous lakes
Frequency doubled Nd:YAG	532 nm	Pigmented lesions and tattoos	Selective and fast heating (explosion)	Pulsed (ns, ps)	Ephelides, lentigines, tattoos (red)
Flashlamp pumped pulsed dye	585-600 nm	Vascular lesions	Selective coagulation	Pulsed (ms)	Port-wine stains, telangiectases, rosacea, spider nevi
		Tissue			Scars, keloids, warts, photoaging
Ruby	694 nm	Pigmented lesions and tattoos	Selective and fast heating (explosion)	Pulsed (ns, ps)	Benign melanin-containing lesions, tattoos (black, blue, green), dermal melanocytoses
Alexandrite	755 nm	Vascular lesions	Selective coagulation	Pulsed (ms)	Large vessels (leg veins, hypertrophic port-wine stains)
		Tissue			Hair removal
		Pigmented lesions and tattoos	Selective and fast heating (explosion)	Pulsed (ns, ps)	Benign melanin-containing lesions, tattoos (black, blue, green) Dermal melanocytoses
Diode	810 nm	Vascular lesions	Selective coagulation	Pulsed (ms)	Large vessels (leg veins, hypertrophic port-wine stains)
		Tissue			Hair removal
Nd:YAG	1064 nm	Vascular lesions	Unspecific coagulation	Continuous wave (cw)	Vascular malformations, tumors
		Vascular lesions	Selective coagulation	Pulsed (ms)	Large vessels (leg veins, hypertrophic port-wine stains)
		Tissue			Hair removal
		Pigmented lesions	Selective and fast heating (explosion)	Pulsed (ns, ps)	Benign melanin-containing lesions, tattoos (black, blue, green), dermal melanocytoses
Erbium glass	1540 nm	Tissue	Selective coagulation (nonablative)	Pulsed (ms)	Skin remodeling, photoaging
Diode	1450-1550 nm	Tissue	Selective coagulation	Pulsed (ms)	Skin remodeling, photoaging
Thulium	1927 nm	Tissue	Selective coagulation (nonablative)	Pulsed (ms)	Skin remodeling, photoaging
Er:YAG	2940 nm	Tissue	Selective and fast heating (ablation)	Pulsed (ms)	Skin resurfacing, epidermal ablation
CO_2	10,600 nm	Tissue	Nonspecific coagulation (vaporization)	Continuous wave (cw)	Vaporization of tissue
			Selective and fast heating ablation	Pulsed (ms)	Skin resurfacing, epidermal ablation

CO_2, carbon dioxide; Er:YAG, erbium-doped yttrium aluminum garnet; KTP, potassium titanyl phosphate; Nd:YAG, neodymium-doped yttrium aluminum garnet; UVB, ultraviolet B.

within a tube that contains 2 parallel mirrors, one of which is completely opaque and the other is partially transmissible. The medium can be a solid, liquid, liquid crystal, or gas. The medium determines the resultant wavelength and properties of the laser. The energy source drives the electrons in the medium to an excited state. After excitation, or "pumping," the atoms or molecules return from the excited to the ground state and thereby emit photons with a specific wavelength λ_L that is determined by the energy difference ΔE of the excited and the ground state with

$$\Delta E = hc/\lambda_L$$

The combination of such identical transitions and photons with the same wavelength λ_L in a confined volume (laser medium) allows another process to occur: the stimulated emission of photons, as described by Albert Einstein[2] (Fig. 208-1). If an electron in an excited state encounters another photon of the same energy, it releases another photon of the same wavelength (Fig. 208-2). Therefore, one photon stimulates the next atom or molecule to emit a photon. The resulting 2 photons stimulate the next 2 atoms or molecules, and that results in 4 photons and so on. The photons move back and forth between the parallel mirrors, colliding with and exciting other atoms in the process. This chain reaction does not change the energy of photons but increases their number exponentially. Once the number of excited atoms outweighs the number of atoms in the ground state, this is referred to as inversion. Ultimately, the photons that are traveling in a perfectly parallel direction exit the resonator through the partially transmissible mirror at the distal end of the resonator as a laser beam (Fig. 208-3).

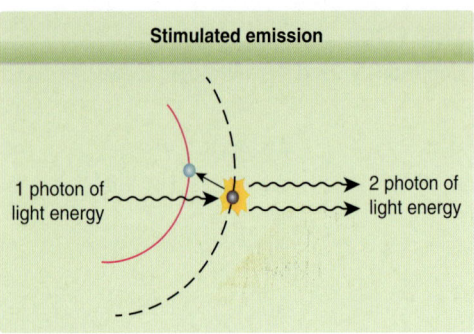

Figure 208-2 When an excited atom collides with a photon of light of the same wavelength that it has previously absorbed, it returns to its resting state and emits 2 photons of light energy of the same wavelength traveling coherently and in parallel direction. This is referred to as stimulated emission. (Used with permission from Dover JS, Arndt KA. *Illustrated Cutaneous Laser Surgery: A Practitioner's Guide*. Norwalk, CT: Appleton & Lange; 1990. Copyright © McGraw-Hill Education.)

The resulting beam possesses a number of unique traits that distinguishes it from natural or incandescent light; lasers emit light that is monochromatic, coherent, and collimated (Fig. 208-4).[5] The monochromatic nature of laser describes its temporal coherence: laser light is composed of a single wavelength, as opposed to natural

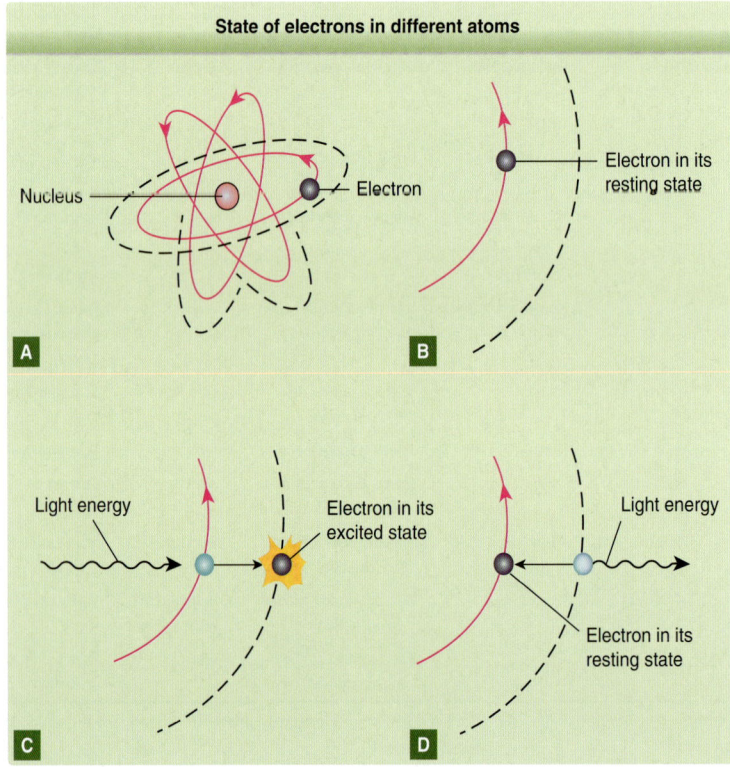

Figure 208-1 A, B, A diagram of an atom with its electron in its resting state. **C,** Upon absorption of light energy, the atom's electron transitions from its resting state to its excited state. **D,** When the electron returns to its resting state, energy is released as electromagnetic radiation (light), a process otherwise referred to as spontaneous emission. (Used with permission from Dover JS, Arndt KA. *Illustrated Cutaneous Laser Surgery: A Practitioner's Guide*. Norwalk, CT: Appleton & Lange; 1990. Copyright © McGraw-Hill Education.)

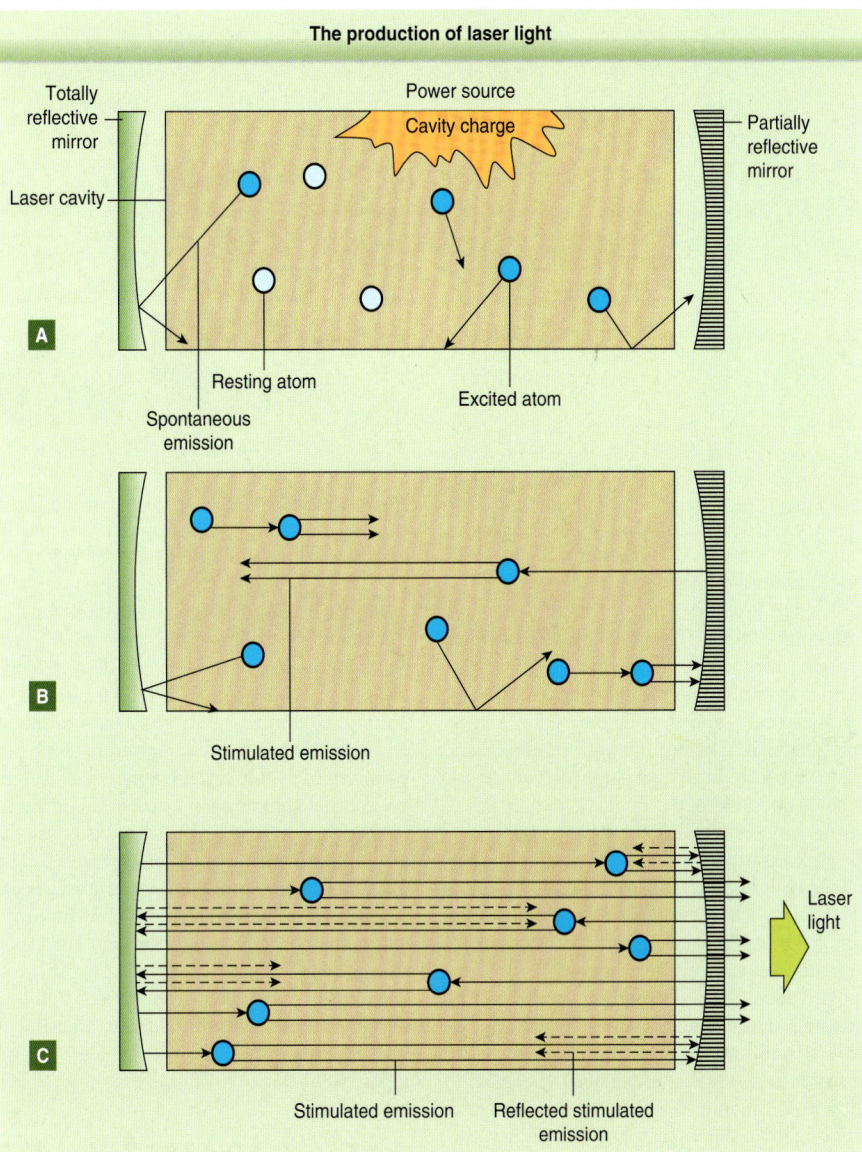

Figure 208-3 The production of laser light: **A,** The charge in the cavity pumps the electrons to an excited state. **B,** Emitted photons of light energy collide with excited atoms and produce stimulated emission. **C,** The light reflects back and forth within the cavity, promoting further stimulated emission and amplifying the process. Finally, a small portion of the laser light passes through the partially transmissible mirror as a laser beam. (Used with permission from Dover JS, Arndt KA. *Illustrated Cutaneous Laser Surgery: A Practitioner's Guide*. Norwalk, CT: Appleton & Lange; 1990. Copyright © McGraw-Hill Education.)

or incandescent light that emits light across the entire visible spectrum. This property of laser light is important therapeutically as it allows for the selective absorption of the laser by specific chromophores (light-absorbing compounds). Laser light is also coherent, in that the waves are in phase in space and time. The crests and troughs of the light wave are synchronous and therefore the laser beam exhibits minimal divergence, allowing the beam to travel larger distances without substantial loss of intensity. Finally, laser light is collimated, in that all the photons are parallel to each other. Collimation not only allows the light to travel long distances with minimal distortion and dispersion, but also allows the dense packing of energy into a relatively small volume of light.

The temporal behavior of the laser emission depends on the temporal behavior of the excitation of the atoms or molecules. That is, when the energy supply to the laser medium is continuous, the emission of the laser is considered continuous-wave emission. Continuous-wave lasers produce a continuous beam of laser light with little or no variation in power output over time. Shutters may be opened or closed to either permit or obstruct the laser beam from exiting the device. Shutters can be set to open for a few milliseconds to several seconds, depending on the treatment goal.

When the energy supply of the laser is limited to a certain time interval by gas discharge or flashlamp, this is referred to as pulsed excitation, and the laser

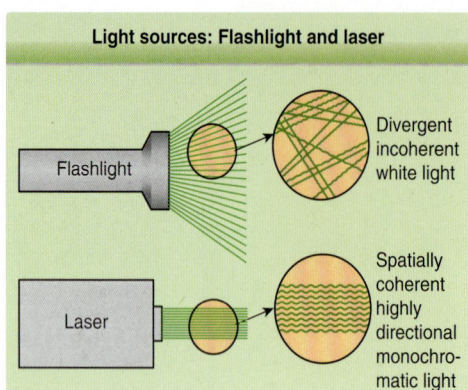

Figure 208-4 An ordinary light source such as a flashlight produces light that is divergent, coherent, and polychromatic (above), whereas a laser emits light that is spatially collimated, coherent, and monochromatic. (Used with permission from Dover JS, Arndt KA. *Illustrated Cutaneous Laser Surgery: A Practitioner's Guide*. Norwalk, CT: Appleton & Lange; 1990. Copyright © McGraw-Hill Education.)

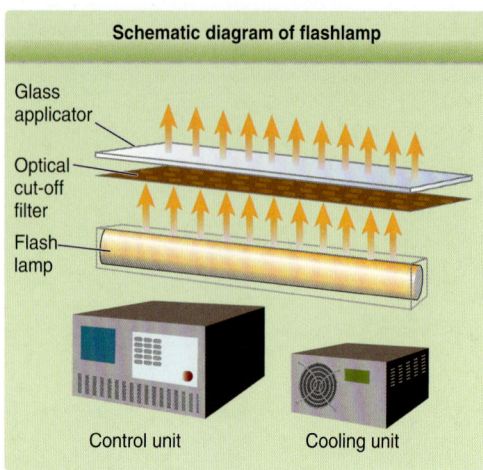

Figure 208-5 The flashlamp of intense pulsed light (IPL) emits radiation that is filtered by a cut-off filter. The control unit operates radiant exposure and pulse duration.

emits pulses accordingly. These laser pulse durations can vary from microseconds to milliseconds, and the energy within the pulse of a pulsed beam is not constant; it builds, peaks, and then tapers within a very short time. The peak power outputs of pulsed lasers are often greater than the maximum output of continuous-wave lasers by up to 100-fold.

To achieve very short pulse durations in the nanosecond or picosecond range, the resonator is additionally equipped with an optical polarizer and a nonlinear crystal. The polarizer sets the linear polarization of the laser beam that passes through the crystal. However, if an appropriate electrical voltage is applied to the crystal, the polarization of the photons is changed inside the crystal and subsequently blocked by the optical polarizer. This prevents photons from running back and forth inside the resonator (oscillation), which hampers light amplification and which is equivalent to a low circuit quality of the resonator. In such a case, the stimulated emission is minimized and the pumping of the laser medium produces a maximum number of excited atoms or molecules in the laser medium. When this maximum number is achieved, the electrical voltage of the crystal is switched off within nanoseconds and the photons can easily pass the crystal, which is equivalent to a high circuit quality of the resonator. Now, the laser oscillation immediately starts and the light amplification yields a very high number of photons per time unit because of the high number of excited atoms or molecules in the laser medium. The outcome of this circuit quality switch (Q-switch) is a very intense laser pulse with pulse durations in the range of nanoseconds to picoseconds.

INTENSE PULSED LIGHT PRINCIPLES

Intense pulsed light (IPL) devices are not lasers, but rather contain a flashlamp that produces noncoherent light of a broad spectrum of wavelengths that can be tuned and set to different wavelengths, fluences, and pulse durations.[7] IPL technology delivers noncoherent light from about 420 nm to the far-infrared spectrum around 1200 nm (Fig. 208-5). Different cutoff filters and separate handpieces are used to "tune" the broad spectrum of light to certain desired wavelengths to target specific chromophores and to tailor the treatment to specific skin types. The filter cuts off emitted light, allowing only wavelengths longer than a certain threshold value to pass through. For example, a 560-nm filter is used to treat vascular lesions, allowing wavelengths longer than 560 nm to pass through, corresponding to the vascular absorption peak of 585 to 595 nm.[7] Longer-wavelength cutoff filters may be used to treat pigment in darker individuals. In addition, adjustments of the fluence, pulse duration, and cooling system can be made on the device to optimize treatment.

BASIC PARAMETERS OF OPTICAL RADIATION

The main parameters of optical radiation are wavelength, optical power, intensity, the exposure time and radiant exposure or fluence. The unit for energy is Joule (J); optical power Watt (W); intensity (W/cm^2); radiant exposure (J/cm^2); the exposure time second (s); and the area of irradiation on the skin surface (cm^2). After being transported through a glass fiber or articulated arm, laser radiation is usually applied as a circular spot to the skin surface by means of a lens in a holder. The spot size and the energy of the laser beam determine the radiant exposure (J/cm^2). The IPL applicator directly contacts the skin through an ultrasonic gel. Thus, the radiant exposure of IPL emission is determined by the size of the applicator and the energy of radiation (J/cm^2).

To achieve various therapeutic objectives, exposure times ranging from picoseconds to seconds are employed. Continuous wave lasers use exposure times in the range of fractions of a second to seconds, correlating to the length of time the switch is activated. In most medical treatments, individual laser or light pulses are used. The exposure time is predefined by the pulse duration of a single laser or IPL pulse. In the case of pulsed radiation, the exposure time is equivalent either to a single pulse or to a train of single pulses. The broad range of pulse durations implies a broad range of intensities and applications.

The most frequently modified parameter in laser treatments is the radiant exposure or fluence. It is the product of light intensity and exposure time. When taking the total range of medical treatments into account, the radiant exposure varies from about 1 to 400 J/cm^2 for pulsed radiation. This range can be exceeded for continuous-wave applications.

LASER ENERGY DELIVERY

ARTICULATED ARMS

The delivery of laser energy from the optical resonator to the tissue is accomplished through several methods. First, the incorporation of articulated arms into laser systems have facilitated the delivery of energy from the laser cavity to the desired location. Energy is transferred through a series of hollow, interconnected tubes with reflecting mirrors at each connection.[8] Each mirror reflects the desired wavelength of laser such that collimation and coherence are preserved. The energy beam is then focused through a lens in the attached handpiece. Although more recently designed lasers have articulated arms that are less bulky and rigid, the arms can still be cumbersome and difficult to navigate through extremely flexible and spatially constrained situations. Despite their inherent rigidity, articulated arms remain the mainstay in CO_2 lasers, as CO_2 cannot be transmitted through fiber optics.[8]

FIBER OPTICS

Fiber optics are fine flexible fibers most commonly composed of quartz that also have revolutionized the transmission of laser energy to tissue. Most visible and some invisible continuous-wave laser light can be transmitted through fiber optics. Unlike articulated arms, fiber optics fibers are flexible, but also associated with some loss of energy and coherence, thereby limiting the ability to focus the beam.[8] In addition, fiber optic extensions require extra care and precaution as overstretching the handpiece away from the laser console may result in fiber breakage and further loss of energy and coherence.

MICROMANIPULATORS

Micromanipulators can be used to couple articulated arms and fiber optics through a microscope, allowing precise movement of the laser across tissue. This technology is mainly used by gynecologists to treat cervical lesions and by otolaryngologists for laryngeal and inner ear surgery.

FIBER LASERS

Fiber laser technology is the latest advent in laser engineering that has paved the way for more precise, highly reliable, and highly flexible lasing capabilities.[9-12] As discussed, in the traditional design of a laser, stimulated emission and laser beam generation occur within the resonator, and the articulated arm or fiber optic tube transmits the beam to the handpiece. Depending on the system, the beam may undergo loss of energy and coherence. In contrast, fiber lasers have harnessed the ability to generate a highly efficient and highly precise laser beam within the transmitting fiber tube itself. Fiber lasers are composed of glass tubes doped with rare-earth elements such as erbium (1550 nm) or thulium (1927 nm). A power source, most commonly a diode, provides the initial pumping of atoms within the cavity. The photons then travel through the metal-doped tube eventually coalescing into a monochromatic, coherent, and collimated beam of energy once they reach the distal handpiece.[9-12] Fiber lasers can be relatively compact and adaptable as a result of the bendability and flexibility of their fibers, and they can provide highly reliable, highly precise, efficient outputs of energy.

LASER–TISSUE INTERACTIONS

When laser light reaches tissue a number of different responses may occur. The light beam may undergo reflection, transmission, absorption, and scatter (Fig. 208-6).[8] The fundamental effect of the laser light depends on the absorption of the light beam. Absorption is described as the conversion of laser energy to heat when its photons strike the target chromophore. Reflection occurs when the laser beam strikes the surface at an oblique angle and a portion of the beam bounces off the surface in a different direction. Because of the inherent reflective property of the stratum corneum, even laser beams perfectly perpendicular to the skin undergo about 5% reflectance.[5] Reflection of the beam, even with perfect operator technique, necessitates the use of safety goggles. Scattering of laser occurs when the light passes through the stratum corneum, but deviates once in the tissue due to contact with small molecules in the skin. This process is more likely to occur with shorter wavelengths. The size of the scattering objects ranges from a few nanometers (small cell organelles, cell membranes) to a few microns (large cell organelles, cells, collagen fibers) to hundreds of microns (hair follicle, sweat glands). Scattering of the beam changes the focus of the laser and increases the spatial distribution of the light within tissue, thereby increasing the effective irradiated area.

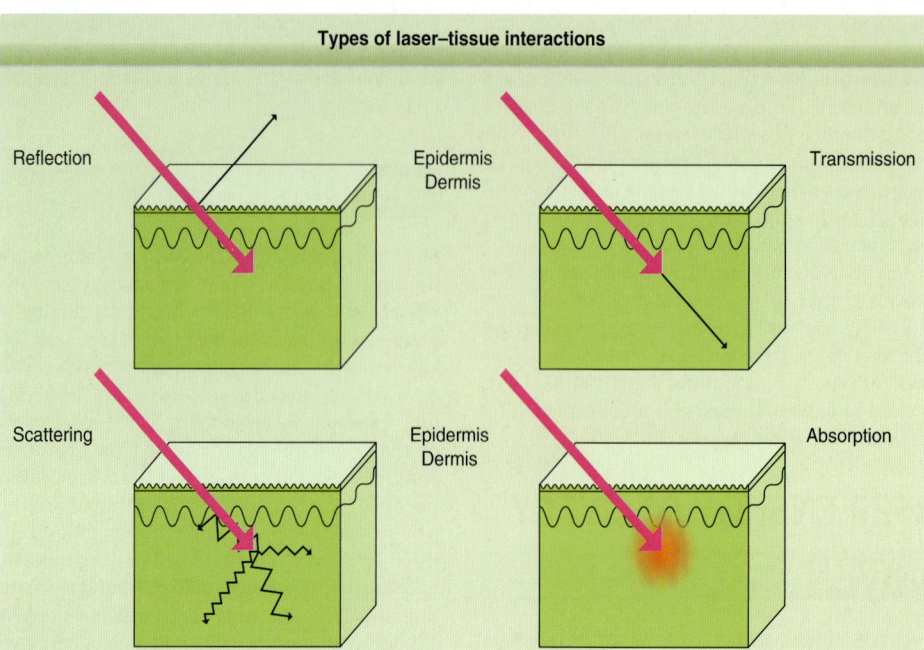

Figure 208-6 Types of laser–tissue interactions: Reflection, transmission, scattering, and absorption. (Used with permission from Franck P, Henderson PW, Rothaus KO. Basics of Lasers: History, Physics, and Clinical Applications. *Clin Plast Surg.* 2016;43[3]:505-513. Copyright © Elsevier.)

Finally, transmission of the laser occurs when the beam is not absorbed by the target chromophore and is conducted to deeper structures. This is more likely to occur with longer wavelengths and larger spot sizes.[5] For example, ultraviolet B radiation (around 300 nm) penetrates skin up to only a few tenths of a millimeter, whereas infrared radiation achieves a penetration depth of up to a few millimeters. However, the increase in penetration depth with increasing wavelength reverses for wavelengths longer than about 1100 nm because radiation is increasingly absorbed by water in skin.

For monochromatic lasers, photons of a single wavelength are absorbed according to the absorption coefficient of the respective chromophores (absorbing targets in the skin) at this wavelength (Fig. 208-7). The absorption of broadband radiation of IPL is more complex given the polychromatic nature of the light. Photons of different wavelengths are absorbed by different chromophores, thereby necessitating the use of cut-off filters when specific effects or actions are required of the IPL system (Fig. 208-8).

When laser or IPL light is absorbed by a chromophore, several types of interactions ensue: chemical (photochemical), mechanical (photoacoustic or photodisruptive), or thermal.[5] An example of a photochemical effect is the use of low-level laser therapy in the treatment of hair loss, in which photons are presumed to be absorbed by mitochondria and activate the cellular respiratory chain to induce hair growth.[13] Photoacoustic effects can be exemplified by the use of nanosecond or picosecond lasers in the treatment of pigmented lesions and tattoos: high-energy photons absorbed by pigment generate acoustic waves within the particles leading to their break up.[14]

Photothermal effects, the mechanism on which most lasers rely, describe the transformation of light energy into heat when absorbed by a chromophore, causing direct damage to adjacent cells, tissues, and structures. The neodymium-doped yttrium aluminum garnet (Nd:YAG) laser (1064 nm frequency doubled to 532 nm) and pulsed dye lasers (585–600 nm) preferentially interact with oxyhemoglobin. Radiation of ruby lasers (694 nm), alexandrite lasers (755 nm), and diode lasers (around 810 nm) are less well absorbed by oxyhemoglobin and more suitable for pigmented chromophores in benign pigmented lesions and for hair removal. Radiation of the Nd:YAG laser (1064 nm) is minimally absorbed by all skin chromophores. Nevertheless, at high radiant exposures, this laser can be used for nonspecific coagulation of tissue as a continuous wave, or for pigmented or vascular lesions as a short or long pulse. Infrared lasers such as the erbium-doped yttrium aluminum garnet (Er:YAG) and carbon dioxide (CO_2) lasers interact solely with water heating up tissue for vaporization or ablation. These ablative lasers induce thermal damage to the epidermis and dermis to stimulate neocollagenesis, tissue rejuvenation, and skin tightening. In contrast, nonablative lasers (1440, 1540, 1550, 1565, and 1927 nm) target dermal tissue to induce bulk heating of dermal collagen and avoid damage to the epidermis. Ablative and nonablative laser principles are discussed in further detail later.

Unlike photochemical effects such as low-level laser therapy, which occurs at very low energy levels, photothermal reactions necessitate relatively high energy

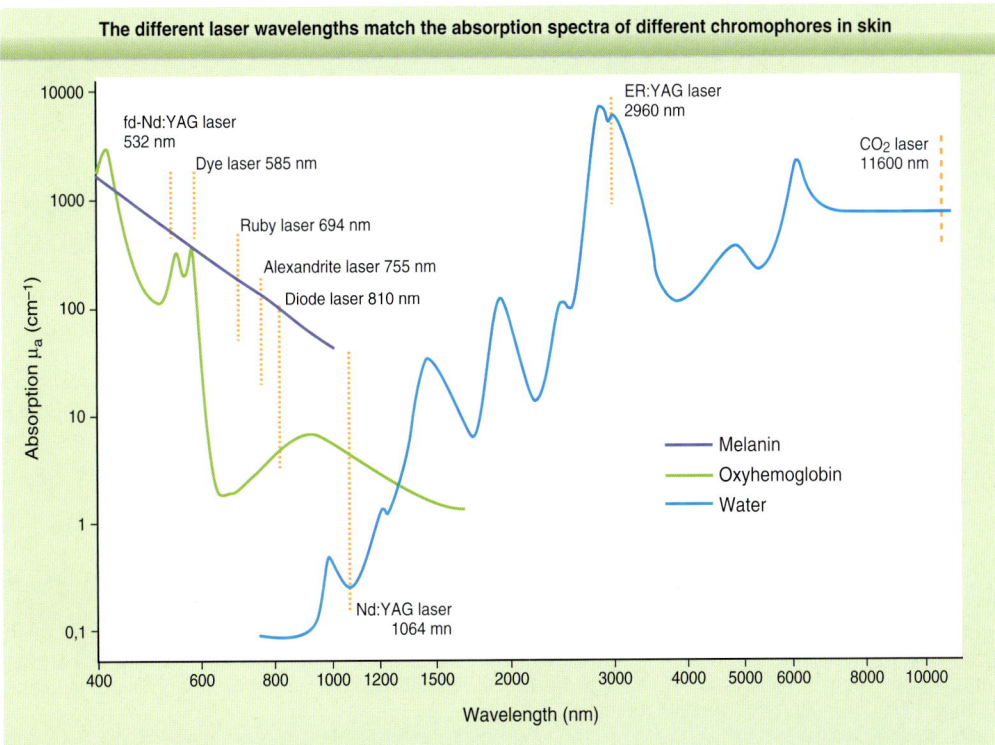

Figure 208-7 The different laser wavelengths match the absorption spectra of different chromophores in skin.

levels. After being absorbed by the target chromophore (eg, oxyhemoglobin in a blood vessel), the energy of the photons causes an increase in temperature inside the target. Concurrently, some heat flows to the tissue adjacent to the target, thereby limiting the temperature increase to a maximum value.[15]

At low intensities and long exposure times (pulse duration), laser or IPL radiation causes moderate temperature increases. At temperatures below 50°C, reversible thermal damage, local vasodilation, and inflammatory cascade activation are produced.[16] At temperatures between 50°C and 100°C, tissue and its proteins undergo irreversible coagulation or denaturation (Fig. 208-9). Reaching temperatures in this range even for as short as 1 millisecond results in coagulative necrosis of tissue. The extent of thermal damage depends on wavelength, intensity, and duration of exposure.[15]

At temperatures greater than 100°C, tissue vaporization occurs, generating plume containing water vapor and tissue components (Fig. 208-9).[16] The use of short CO_2 laser pulses heats up tissue very quickly, leading to rapid vaporization. This effect causes precise small holes with minimal thermal damage of the adjacent tissue. With sufficiently high energy levels at temperatures greater than 100°C, steam can be formed deep within tissue cavities. This can lead to explosion and mechanical damage to tissue. The Nd:YAG laser penetrates deeply into tissue and can generate these deep-seated steam cavities, leading to tissue explosion and eventual ulceration. Because the total energy of the laser pulse is limited, ablation and explosion can be restricted to a very small volume. Such high intensities at short pulse durations are accomplished only with lasers and not with IPL.

As a general rule, the higher the intensity (W/cm²) and the shorter the pulse duration, the higher the maximum temperature inside the targeted volume. By changing the intensity and pulse duration parameters, the temperature can be modulated to achieve coagulation,

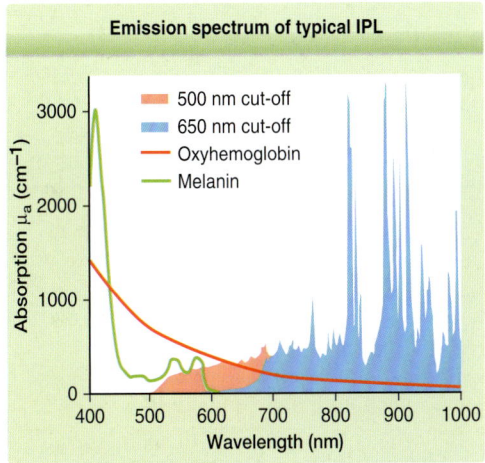

Figure 208-8 The emission spectrum of a typical intense pulsed light (IPL) is broad. Filters with a 500-nm cut-off provide an overlap with the absorption of oxyhemoglobin; filters with a 650-nm cut-off provide an overlap with the absorption of melanin.

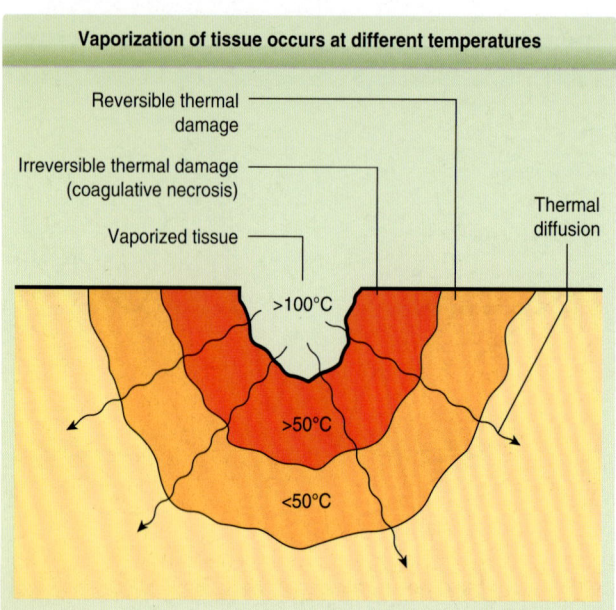

Figure 208-9 At temperatures greater than 100°C, vaporization of tissue occurs. At temperatures between 50°C and 100°C, irreversible thermal coagulation occurs. At temperatures below 50°C, tissue undergoes reversible thermal damage. (Used with permission from Dover JS, Arndt KA. *Illustrated Cutaneous Laser Surgery: A Practitioner's Guide*. Norwalk, CT: Appleton & Lange; 1990. Copyright © McGraw-Hill Education.)

vaporization, or explosion of a specific target in skin. The total amount of energy is proportional to both the power and the pulse duration, where E (Joules) = P (watts) × t (seconds).[8] Therefore, to maintain a constant energy output, a decrease in power requires an increase in pulse duration. However, the tissue effects can be vastly different. For example, using higher power and shorter pulse duration results in more tissue vaporization and less surrounding coagulative necrosis, while lower power and longer pulse widths results in less vaporization and more coagulative necrosis at the edge of the vaporized tissue (Fig. 208-10).

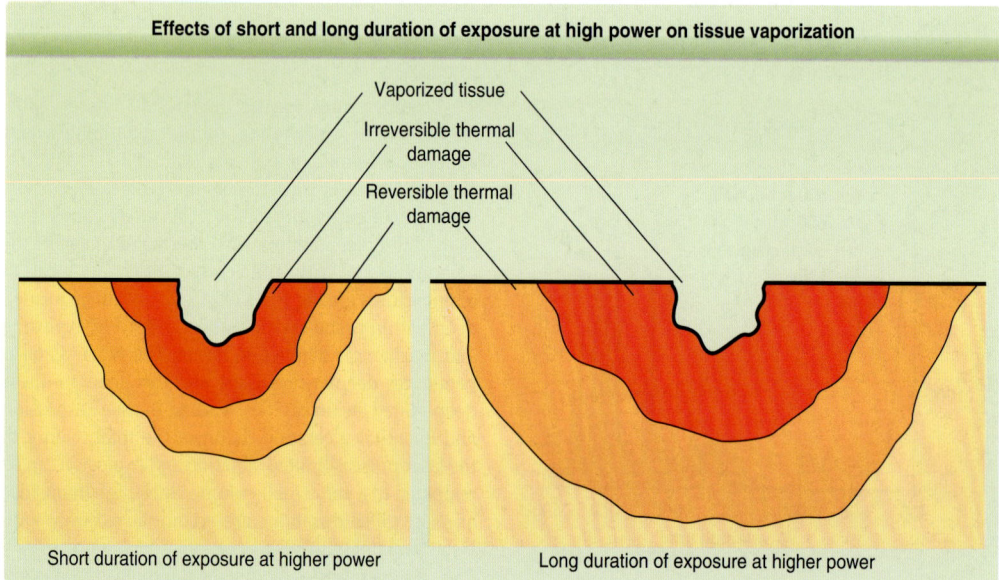

Figure 208-10 A high power with shorter pulse duration results in more tissue vaporization and less surrounding coagulative necrosis, while a high or a relatively lower power and longer pulse width results in less vaporization and more coagulative necrosis at the edge of the vaporized tissue. (Used with permission from Dover JS, Arndt KA. *Illustrated Cutaneous Laser Surgery: A Practitioner's Guide*. Norwalk, CT: Appleton & Lange; 1990. Copyright © McGraw-Hill Education.)

SELECTIVE PHOTOTHERMOLYSIS

In the 1980s, Anderson and Parrish described the model of selective photothermolysis that revolutionized how lasers can be used to safely treat specific ailments of the skin.[17] Using a 577-nm wavelength for vessels and 351-nm wavelength for pigment, they demonstrated that by selecting a wavelength that can be delivered to a specific chromophore with a pulse duration or exposure time shorter than the thermal relaxation time, the damage to the peripheral tissue would be minimized. The thermal relaxation time is defined as the time needed for the irradiated tissue to cool down to half of its heated temperature.[18] The keys to this theory are twofold: laser light must be absorbed by the target by selecting a wavelength absorbed by the chromophore in the target, and the correct pulse duration is essential for spatial confinement of heat in the target.

The pulse duration should be comparable to the thermal relaxation time (t_R), which mainly depends on the diameter of the target (D)

$$t_R = \rho c/(16k) \times D^2$$

where ρ, c, k are thermal parameters of the target. The thermal relaxation time is roughly proportional to the square of the mean diameter of the target. Therefore, the larger the chromophore, the longer the required pulse duration, and the greater the overall heating.

WAVELENGTH

The major chromophores in skin in order of depth of location are water, melanin, and hemoglobin. The CO_2 laser (10,600-nm) is absorbed by tissue water, limiting penetration into skin to less than 0.1 mm.[19] The beam can be delivered with a large spot size and low power density or focused with great power density. The CO_2 laser can be used to vaporize and cut tissue while coagulating blood vessels. The Er:YAG laser (2940 nm) is also preferentially absorbed by water. Argon-ion lasers (488 and 514 nm), KTP lasers (532nm), and pulsed dye lasers (585-595 nm) may be absorbed by both hemoglobin and melanin. Ruby lasers (694 nm) are absorbed mainly by melanin pigment although a small amount of hemoglobin absorption also occurs. Alexandrite lasers (755 nm) are preferentially absorbed by melanin, and therefore useful for pigmented lesions and hair. As mentioned earlier, although there is no specific chromophore for the Nd:YAG laser (1064 nm), this wavelength is absorbed, albeit less than with other visible wavelengths, by hemoglobin and melanin and at higher fluences it can be used to treat pigmented or vascular lesions.

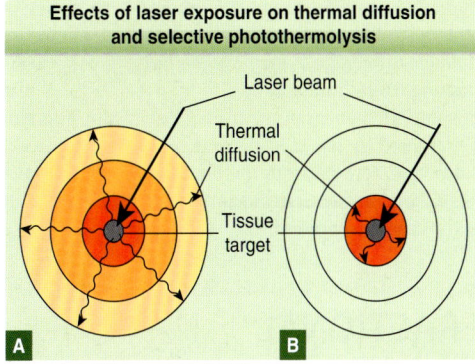

Figure 208-11 A, Longer laser exposure time results in increased thermal diffusion out of the target and damage to adjacent structures. **B,** Collateral thermal injury can be reduced by choosing a wavelength that is specifically absorbed by the target chromophore and by maintaining a pulse duration that is shorter than the thermal relaxation (cooling) time of the target. This is referred to as selective photothermolysis. (Used with permission from Dover JS, Arndt KA. *Illustrated Cutaneous Laser Surgery: A Practitioner's Guide*. Norwalk, CT: Appleton & Lange; 1990. Copyright © McGraw-Hill Education.)

PULSE DURATION

The pulse duration determines the size of target that will be selectively damaged. Coagulation of small blood vessels with diameters of 50–150 μm require pulse durations in the millisecond range.[20-22] Initially, only the temperature in the vessel increases, coagulating the vessel. Because of the temperature increase, however, heat begins to diffuse to the adjacent dermis. At this point, the radiation pulse should be terminated to achieve selective vessel destruction. Pulse durations longer than the thermal relaxation time result in excessive heat flow to the dermis, which may cause unnecessary adverse reactions (Fig. 208-11). The same range of pulse durations is applied for the treatment of large vessels such as leg veins.[23]

The pulse duration necessary to effectively treat pigment in hair, epidermal and dermal melanocytic lesions, and tattoos depends on the size (and therefore the thermal relaxation time) of the target chromophore (Table 208-2). Hair follicles are 0.02 to 0.2 millimeters

TABLE 208-2
Target Chromophores, Size, and Pulse Duration

TARGET	APPROXIMATE SIZE OF TARGET	PULSE DURATION
blood vessels	50-150 μm	ms
Hair follicles	0.02-0.2 μm	10-50 ms
Melanocytes	7 μm	ms to ns
Melanosomes	1.5 μm	ns to ps
Tattoo pigment particles	100 nm (0.1 μm)	ns to ps

in diameter and are targeted by pulses in the range of 10 to 50 milliseconds.[24] Melanocytes are a few μm in diameter (average 7 μm) and require pulse widths ranging from milliseconds to nanoseconds. Melanosome diameter ranges from 1 to 1.5 μm and can be targeted by nanosecond and picosecond pulses.[25] Tattoo pigment particles are on average 100 nanometers (0.1 μm) in diameter and are targeted by nanosecond and picosecond pulses.[26]

FRACTIONAL PHOTOTHERMOLYSIS: ABLATIVE VS NONABLATIVE FRACTIONATION

In the late 1980s and 1990s, ablative lasers (CO_2 and erbium) gained rapid popularity for the treatment of facial photodamage and skin laxity. Although the results were dramatic, so were the potential side effects. Prolonged recovery times and the potential for serious adverse effects were its ultimate downfall, and the nonablative lasers of the time fell short of the dramatic results that ablative ones offered. In response to these dilemmas, the concept of fractional photothermolysis emerged.[27] Fractional photothermolysis creates spatially distributed columns of microthermal injury within the treatment area, called microscopic treatment zones (MTZs). These are generated in the skin by focused laser irradiation. There is enough energy in each column of MTZ to induce thermal heating or ablation without spread to adjacent tissue. Fractional irradiation allows relatively deeper penetration of the laser beam into the dermis, causing controlled denaturation, transepidermal elimination of the coagulated debris, and reactive collagen remodeling, while maintaining the integrity of the epidermis, shortening healing times, and decreasing side effects.[19]

Fractional photothermolysis can be performed in either ablative (CO_2 and erbium) or nonablative (1440, 1540, 1550, 1565, and 1927 nm) mode. In ablative fractionation, there is controlled vaporization of thin columns of both epidermis and dermis alike. In nonablative fractionation, the heating is concentrated within the dermis, leaving the epidermis relatively or absolutely spared.[27,28] The theory is that intense heating of columns within the dermis with intervening normal skin can induce enough protein denaturation and collagen remodeling and synthesis. Overall, nonablative fractional lasers allow for higher levels of intense heat within the dermis, and therefore better results, in comparison to the older nonfractionated, nonablative lasers that merely created a homogenous layer of dermal heat.[27] As expected, nonablative fractional photothermolysis is much better tolerated, with fewer side effects and shorter healing time. However, results may not be as impressive as ablative fractional resurfacing. Fractional photothermolysis can be used to treat a myriad of dermatologic conditions including photoaging, acne scarring, traumatic scarring, skin laxity, and dyschromias.[28] Fractionation has also helped pave the way for laser-assisted topical drug delivery.[29-32]

SKIN COOLING

Laser and light therapy requires the delivery of high radiant exposure to targets within the dermis or the dermal–epidermal junction, while minimizing injury to the epidermis. To reach these targets, photons must traverse the epidermis, which can itself absorb radiation. In addition, the buildup of heat within the dermis can diffuse to epidermal structures causing unintended damage. To circumvent unwanted injury, skin cooling systems have been developed to protect the epidermis while delivering sufficient heat to the dermis.[33]

Cooling can be achieved before, during, or after treatment, referred to as precooling, parallel cooling, and postcooling.[33] There are 2 types of cooling methods: contact cooling, sometimes known as bulk cooling, and noncontact cooling (Table 208-3). Contact cooling can be active or passive. Active contact cooling employs copper or sapphire tips integrated into the laser handpiece, and passive contact cooling involves the use of ice or cold aqueous gels. In contact cooling, heat is transferred from the warm skin to the cooling agent. In passive cooling, heat is transferred through diffusion from the cutaneous surface to the ice or gel. In active cooling, the tip actively removes heat by thermoelectric elements or flowing liquid cooling agents.[33] Noncontact cooling can be achieved with cryogen spray or forced cold air. The first device used for spray cooling was liquid nitrogen spray held at a certain distance from skin during laser treatment. This technique was operator-dependent, imprecise, and came with risks of cryonecrosis. The development of the dynamic cooling device (DCD) integrated within the laser system has revolutionized epidermal cooling.[34-36] The inbuilt software allows the user to set specific DCD spray and delay settings. The device sprays the cryogen, usually the nontoxic 1,1,1,2-tetrafluoroethane, at −15°C immediately before the application of the laser. The DCD allows for uniform, precise, and reproducible cooling with every laser pulse.[33] Forced cold air (Zimmer Cryo; Zimmer Medizin Systems, Irvine, CA) can deliver cooling before, during, and after laser application without interfering with the laser beam.

TABLE 208-3
Cooling Methods in Cutaneous Laser Surgery

CONTACT COOLING	NONCONTACT COOLING
Active (copper, sapphire tips)	Cryogen spray (liquid nitrogen)
Passive (ice)	Pulsed cryogen spray (dynamic cooling device)
Passive (aqueous gels)	Forced refrigerated air (Zimmer Cryo, Zimmer Medizin Systems, Irvine, CA)

The device minimizes pain and unwanted thermal injury during laser and light treatment.

LASER SAFETY

The use of lasers and intense pulsed light sources requires knowledge and application of many safety measures to reduce the risk of temporary or permanent tissue damage (Table 208-4). The organizations that regulate laser operations are the International Electrotechnical Commission (IEC), the American National Standards Institute (ANSI), the Center for Devices and Radiological Health (CDRH) of the US FDA, the Department of Labor's Occupational Safety and Health Administration (OSHA), and the Council of Radiation Control Program Directors (CRCPD).[37] The ANSI Z136.3 is a regulatory document that provides guidance for the safe use of lasers in medicine. These regulations are implied, and compliance is mandated by the individual institution or organization.[38] Prior to any laser or light-based procedure, possible side effects should be discussed with the patient in detail, to protect the patient and provider alike.

SKIN SAFETY

Radiation of any wavelength can pose a risk to any human tissue, and in particular the eyes and skin.[39,40] Cutaneous injuries are the most common complications of dermatologic laser surgery and the most common cause of laser-related litigation.[41] In one study, laser hair removal was the most frequently implicated procedure in lawsuits, likely as a result of the high number of procedures done per year. The second most commonly litigated procedure was rejuvenation, including fully ablative carbon dioxide resurfacing, ablative and nonablative fractional resurfacing, and intense pulsed light treatments.[41] Reported cutaneous injuries included burns, scars, and pigmentary changes.

TABLE 208-4
Principles of Laser Safety

- Set patient realistic expectations
- Discuss, in-detail, the procedure and possible side effects
- Select correct device for target chromophore and patient skin type
- Lower fluences, longer pulse durations, longer wavelengths, higher cutoff filters decrease risk in darker skin types
- Precooling, cooling during procedure, postprocedural cooling
- When using radiofrequency energy, avoid patients with implantable devices or pacemakers
- Lowest risk lasers are vascular, pigment-specific, and nonablative types
- Ablative lasers are higher risk, with greater chances of infection and scarring
- Appropriate eye protection is essential; eye protection is device-specific
- When used for tissue vaporization, plumes must be evacuated to avoid infectious material

Avoidance of cutaneous injuries requires appropriate laser selection and realistic expectations. Selecting the correct laser/light device demands careful consideration of the target chromophore as well as the patient's natural skin color, while keeping in mind that more aggressive treatment to achieve results may increase the risk of pigmentary alteration, burns, and scars. Lower fluences, longer pulse durations, and longer wavelengths or higher cutoff filters decrease the risk of injury to darker skin types. Appropriate pre-cooling, cooling during the procedure, and post-procedural cooling all provide additional epidermal protection.[38] When using devices that employ radiofrequency energy and may have less deleterious effects on the epidermis, patients with implantable devices or pacemakers should be avoided and caution should be taken in areas with tattoos or overlying metal implants, hardware, and braces.[42]

Overall, the risk of cutaneous injuries is lower with pigment-specific, vascular, and nonablative lasers. Ablative lasers lead to epidermal and dermal destruction, albeit controlled, that increases the risk of infection and scarring.[38] Fractionally ablative lasers have minimized this risk significantly.

EYE SAFETY

Ocular injuries arise from direct or indirect (reflected) laser light, and 70% of ocular injuries result from inappropriate or lack of use of eye protection. Types of ocular injuries are wavelength-specific, and severity is dependent on energy level, beam size, and exposure time.[38] Radiation between 380 and 1400 nm is transmitted by the eye and absorbed by the retina.[43] The refractive media of the eye gathers and focuses this spectrum onto the retina and increases the irradiance by a factor of more than 10,000 above the irradiance at the cornea.[43] Thus, even a small amount of energy from low-power lasers can still inflict significant damage on the retina. Photons of wavelengths shorter than 380 nm are absorbed by organic molecules in the cornea, thereby causing injury or cataract formation. Light of wavelengths longer than 1000 to 1400 nm is readily absorbed by water, does not penetrate deeply, and therefore may cause corneal injury, even ablation or vaporization, by a thermal process.[43]

The pulse duration and energy level determine the type of ocular injury: thermal, mechanical, or photochemical. Thermal damage occurs when energy is absorbed by the chromophore, such as melanin in the retina, at a pulse ranging from microseconds to seconds. Heat is generated faster than it can be dissipated, thereby denaturing proteins resulting in cell death and tissue necrosis. Mechanical injury is caused when energy is rapidly absorbed at pulse durations ranging from picoseconds to nanoseconds. A rapid absorption of energy and therefore rapid increase in temperature strips electrons from atoms, disintegrating tissue to a pool of ions and electrons, or plasma. Concomitant vaporization of water results in a compressive pressure pulse, or explosion, that disrupts surrounding tissue. Photochemical damage results from energy at relatively lower levels and longer pulse durations, more than a few seconds. The slow delivery of energy does not deliver enough heat to induce thermal damage. However, single photons can break molecular bonds in nucleic acids and proteins. Retinal cells can recover from this type of damage over a period of weeks, but over a certain threshold damage can be irreversible.[43]

In response to visible light, the macula activates the blink reflex within 150 to 250 milliseconds. Additionally, the "aversion response," or turning away of the head from the light source, is another natural defense mechanism against harmful visible radiation. However, these reflexes are not rapid enough to protect from most laser systems, which possess pulse durations shorter than 250 milliseconds. Also, the aversion response to radiation at the retinal periphery can lead to an instinctive turning of the head towards the light source and result in further damage.[44] Furthermore, injuries from lasers of invisible, longer wavelength radiation such as the Nd:YAG and carbon dioxide lasers can occur entirely unnoticed.

Complete protection from laser injury requires adequate knowledge of the properties and mode of employment of the instrument in use. The universal safety precaution in place to prevent eye injuries is the use of proper eyewear. Safety goggles are composed of filters that either reflect or absorb specific wavelengths of light, while allowing sufficient light of other wavelengths to be transmitted. Laser goggles are rated by optical density (OD) at various wavelengths, and an OD of at least 4 is considered safe. The important parameters of the radiation sources are wavelength, pulse duration, intensity, and radiant exposure. These parameters of a laser or IPL system determine the characteristics of the safety goggles. Each laser or IPL requires special safety goggles that are labeled for their use, including wavelength range of protection, laser mode, and scale number of protection. The manufacturer of lasers or IPL must provide sufficient information about the appropriate safety goggles, which can be found in the handbook of each laser or IPL device. The main limitation of these devices is the reluctance of personnel to wear them. It is also important to pair the correct eyewear with the correct corresponding laser device, and in the age of multiwavelength lasers, the laser operator must remember to switch goggles if need be when switching from wavelength to wavelength.

MAINTAINING LASER SAFETY

When employing a medical laser, it is mandatory to appoint a laser safety officer (LSO). This person possesses the authority to draft, maintain, and enforce the laser safety guidelines and controls to ensure the proper employment of lasers in the medical setting. The LSO administers the overall laser safety program where the duties include items such as confirming the classification of lasers and ensuring that the proper control measures are in place, approving substitute controls and conducting medical surveillance. The LSO should receive detailed training, including laser fundamentals, laser bioeffects, exposure limits, classifications, control measures (including area controls, eye wear, barriers, etc), and medical surveillance requirements.

To maintain the safety of all persons in the vicinity of a laser or light device, safety checklists can be used. In a controlled environment such as a dermatology clinic, updated checklists and compliant personnel can significantly reduce adverse events and morbidity by ensuring adherence to crucial checkpoints such as confirming eyewear placement and proper setup of the laser.[45] Checklists can be of 2 forms, depending on the complexity of the task. READ-DO checklists demand that users perform each step as they check them off. DO-CONFIRM checklists require that users perform the tasks from memory but then pause to make sure all facets of the checklist were met prior to treatment. Safety checklists are able to make potentially risky procedures safer and less error prone.

ACKNOWLEDGMENTS

We extend our sincerest gratitude to Michael Landthaler, Wolfgang Bäumler, and Ulrich Hohenleutner for their indispensable work "Lasers and Flashlamps in Dermatology" in *Fitzpatrick's Dermatology*, 8th edition.

REFERENCES

1. Dicke RH. Coherence in spontaneous radiation processes. *Phys Rev*. 1954;93:99-110.
2. Einstein A. Zur Quantentheorie der Strahlung. *Phys Zeitschrift*. 1917;18:121-128.
3. Azadgoli B, Baker RY. Laser applications in surgery. *Ann Transl Med*. 2016;4(23):452.
4. Maiman TH. Stimulated optical radiation in ruby. *Nature*. 1960;187:493-494.
5. Franck P, Henderson PW, Rothaus KO. Basics of lasers: history, physics, and clinical applications. *Clin Plast Surg*. 2016;43(3):505-513.
6. De Felice E. Shedding light: laser physics and mechanism of action. *Phlebology*. 2010;25(1):11-28.
7. Raulin C, Greve B, Grema H. IPL technology: a review. *Lasers Surg Med*. 2003;32(2):78-87.
8. Dover JS, Arndt KA. *Illustrated Cutaneous Laser Surgery: A Practitioner's Guide*. Norwalk, CT: Appleton & Lange; 1990.
9. Rahman Z, Alam M, Dover JS. Fractional Laser treatment for pigmentation and texture improvement. *Skin Therapy Lett*. 2006;11(9):7-11.
10. Wanner M, Tanzi EL, Alster TS. Fractional photothermolysis: treatment of facial and nonfacial cutaneous photodamage with a 1,550-nm erbium-doped fiber laser. *Dermatol Surg*. 2007;33(1):23-28.
11. Chiu RJ, Kridel RW. Fractionated photothermolysis: the Fraxel 1550-nm glass fiber laser treatment. *Facial Plast Surg Clin North Am*. 2007;15(2):229-237, vii.

12. Thongsima S, Zurakowski D, Manstein D. Histological comparison of two different fractional photothermolysis devices operating at 1,550 nm. *Lasers Surg Med*. 2010;42(1):32-37.
13. Gupta AK, Foley KA. A critical assessment of the evidence for low-level laser therapy in the treatment of hair loss. *Dermatol Surg*. 2017;43(2):188-197.
14. Ho DD, London R, Zimmerman GB, et al. Laser-tattoo removal—a study of the mechanism and the optimal treatment strategy via computer simulations. *Lasers Surg Med*. 2002;30(5):389-397.
15. Bogdan Allemann I, Kaufman J. Laser principles. *Curr Probl Dermatol*. 2011;42:7-23.
16. Herd RM. Basic laser principles. *Dermatol Clin*. 1997;15:355-372.
17. Anderson RR, Parish JA. Selective photothermolysis: precise microsurgery by selective absorption of pulsed radiation. *Science*. 1983;220:524-527.
18. Goldman L, Wilson RG, Hornby P, et al. Radiation from Q-switched ruby laser: effect of repeated impacts of power output of 10 megawatts on a tattoo of man. *J Invest Dermatol*. 1964;44:69-71.
19. Borges J, Manela-Azulay M, Cuzzi T. Photoaging and the clinical utility of fractional laser. *Clin Cosmet Investig Dermatol*. 2016;9:107-114.
20. Brightman LA, Geronemus RG, Reddy KK. Laser treatment of port-wine stains. *Clin Cosmet Investig Dermatol*. 2015;8:27-33.
21. Morton LM, Smith KC, Dover JS, et al. Treatment of purpura with lasers and light sources. *J Drugs Dermatol*. 2013;12(11):1219-1222.
22. Franca K, Chacon A, Ledon J, et al. Lasers for cutaneous congenital vascular lesions: a comprehensive overview and update. *Lasers Med Sci*. 2013;28(4):1197-1204.
23. Meesters AA, Pitassi LH, Campos V, et al. Transcutaneous laser treatment of leg veins. *Lasers Med Sci*. 2014;29(2):481-492.
24. Zandi S, Lui H. Long-term removal of unwanted hair using light. *Dermatol Clin*. 2013;31(1):179-191.
25. Thong HY, Jee SH, Sun CC, et al. The patterns of melanosome distribution in keratinocytes of human skin as one determining factor of skin colour. *Br J Dermatol*. 2003;149(3):498-505.
26. Hogsberg T, Loeschner K, Lof D, et al. Tattoo inks in general usage contain nanoparticles. *Br J Dermatol*. 2011;165(6):1210-1218.
27. Manstein D, Herron GS, Sink RK, et al. Fractional photothermolysis: a new concept for cutaneous remodeling using microscopic patterns of thermal injury. *Lasers Surg Med*. 2004;34(5):426-438.
28. Saedi N, Jalian HR, Petelin A, et al. Fractionation: past, present, future. *Semin Cutan Med Surg*. 2012;31(2):105-109.
29. Waibel JS, Wulkan AJ, Shumaker PR. Treatment of hypertrophic scars using laser and laser assisted corticosteroid delivery. *Lasers Surg Med*. 2013;45(3):135-140.
30. Rkein A, Ozog D, Waibel JS. Treatment of atrophic scars with fractionated CO_2 laser facilitating delivery of topically applied poly-L-lactic acid. *Dermatol Surg*. 2014;40(6):624-631.
31. Waibel JS, Mi QS, Ozog D, et al. Laser-assisted delivery of vitamin C, vitamin E, and ferulic acid formula serum decreases fractional laser postoperative recovery by increased beta fibroblast growth factor expression. *Lasers Surg Med*. 2016;48(3):238-244.
32. Haak CS, Hannibal J, Paasch U, et al. Laser-induced thermal coagulation enhances skin uptake of topically applied compounds. *Lasers Surg Med*. 2017;49(6):582-591.
33. Das A, Sarda A, De A. Cooling devices in laser therapy. *J Cutan Aesthet Surg*. 2016;9(4):215-219.
34. Waldorf HA, Alster TS, McMillan K, et al. Effect of dynamic cooling on 585-nm pulsed dye laser treatment of port-wine stain birthmarks. *Dermatol Surg*. 1997;23:657-662.
35. Anvari B, Milner TE, Tanenbaum BS, et al. A comparative study of human skin thermal response to sapphire contact and cryogen spray cooling. *IEEE Trans Biomed Eng*. 1998;45:934-941.
36. Nahm WK, Tsoukas MM, Falanga V, et al. Preliminary study of fine changes in the duration of dynamic cooling during 755-nm laser hair removal on pain and epidermal damage in patients with skin types III-V. *Lasers Surg Med*. 2002;31:247-251.
37. US Department of Labor, Occupational Safety and Health Administration website. OSHA Technical Manual, Section III, Chapter 6. https://www.osha.gov/dts/osta/otm/otm_iii/otm_iii_6.html. Accessed February 9, 2017.
38. Lolis M, Dunbar SW, Goldberg DJ, et al. Patient safety in procedural dermatology: part II. Safety related to cosmetic procedures. *J Am Acad Dermatol*. 2015;73(1):15-24; quiz 25-26.
39. Goldman L. Progress in laser safety in biomedical installations. *Arch Environ Health*. 1970;20(2):193-196.
40. Powell CH, Goldman L. Recommendations of the Laser Safety Conference. *Arch Environ Health*. 1969;18(3):448-452.
41. Jalian HR, Jalian CA, Avram MM. Common causes of injury and legal action in laser surgery. *JAMA Dermatol*. 2013;149(2):188-193.
42. Rongsaard N, Rummaneethorn P. Comparison of a fractional bipolar radiofrequency device and a fractional erbium-doped glass 1,550-nm device for the treatment of atrophic acne scars: a randomized split-face clinical study. *Dermatol Surg*. 2014;40(1):14-21.
43. Barkana Y, Belkin M. Laser eye injuries. *Surv Ophthalmol*. 2000;44(6):459-478.
44. Boldrey EE, Little HL, Flocks M, et al. Retinal injury due to industrial laser burns. *Ophthalmology*. 1981;88(2):101-107.
45. Hamilton HK, Dover JS. Using checklists to minimize complications from laser/light procedures. *Dermatol Surg*. 2014;40(11):1173-1174.

Chapter 209 :: Laser Skin Resurfacing: Cosmetic and Medical Applications
:: Bridget E. McIlwee & Tina S. Alster

第二百零九章
激光皮肤表皮重建：美容和医疗应用

中文导读

激光表皮重建（LSR）越来越受到人们的关注。本章共分为7节：①概述三种表皮重建技术；②治疗设备；③适应证、禁忌证及病人的选择；④治疗流程和技术；⑤疗效的评估；⑥副作用及并发症；⑦对激光表皮重建激光治疗的未来展望。

第一节介绍了剥脱型、非剥脱型、局灶性表皮重建。剥脱型表皮重建中CO_2或Er:YAG激光是代表，其治疗原理是引起物理愈合反应，最终导致伤口重塑和表皮修复。非剥脱型表皮重建术后预后良好，副作用少，但需多次治疗。局灶性光热作用和局灶性表皮重建产生的热损伤局限于显微治疗区（MTZ），其治疗区域较小，可快速修复。

第二节介绍了治疗设备，表209-1总结了可用于表皮重建的光治疗设备，并分为三类：剥脱型激光、非剥脱型激光、点阵激光设备。剥脱型激光包括CO_2、Er:YAG及两者组合的激光设备。非剥脱型激光包括强脉冲光、Nd:YAG（1064和1320 nm）、二极管（980和1450 nm）及铒-玻璃激光（1540 nm）。点阵激光是治疗区域限于柱状显微治疗区（MTZ）的激光技术。

第三节介绍了激光表皮重建可用于治疗光损伤皮肤、萎缩疤痕和各种表皮和真皮病变，并总结于表209-2。接着就CO_2、Er:YAG及点阵激光分别进行适应证的讲述。其充分的术前患者评估和教育对于优化临床治疗效果至关重要，其中表209-3列出医生治疗前需考虑的9个问题，主要包括病人的选择、风险和预防措施。作者还强调Fitzpatrick皮肤分型I或II型的患者是理想的治疗对象，之后指出最重要的是要和患者充分沟通后才能进行治疗。关于激光表皮重建的禁忌证，包括皮肤感染的活跃期（绝对禁忌证）、皮肤附件异常、使用异维A酸和系统用维甲酸、有瘢痕疙瘩史、Fitzpatrick皮肤分型属于III至VI的患者。

第四节介绍了术前护理、麻醉、流程、术后护理及建议四个方面。作者推荐所有表皮重建的患者术前采用抗病毒治疗。之后提到了局部使用利多卡因乳膏或其他麻醉制剂、局部神经阻滞和静脉镇静药物。流程中最重要的是需注意仪器使用安全。术后即刻正确的伤口护理对激光皮肤修复的成功至关重要。由于皮肤伤口在潮湿的环境中可以更有效地愈合，所以作者提出了医学敷料的重要性。除伤口护理以外，还有抗炎、止痛药物等治疗也很重要。

第五节介绍了疗效的评估方法并以CO_2激光表皮重建为例，从临床和组织学两方面进行阐述。最后通过引用实验研究对比CO_2激光和Er:YAG激光的差异，突出不同激光治疗后有不同的生理组织紧缩机制。

第六节介绍了副作用及并发症，并把副作用及并发症分为四类：可预期的、轻度的、中度及重度的，并按此顺序分开讲述。红斑和水肿是最为常见的并发症。轻度：包括粟丘疹的形成、痤疮的恶化、接触性皮炎、色素沉着或色素减退都有可能产生。中度：最常见的是单纯疱疹病毒感染，尤其在唇部。所以术前口服抗病毒药物如阿昔洛韦、泛昔洛韦和伐昔洛韦十分必要。表皮重建术后最严重的并发症是增生性瘢痕形成和睑外翻。

第七节介绍了对激光表皮重建激光治疗的未来展望。

〔简　丹〕

AT-A-GLANCE

- Several ablative and nonablative laser technologies are available for the treatment of cosmetic concerns including photodamage, rhytides, and scarring.
- Fractional laser technology has increased clinical applications and reduced postoperative recovery and side-effect profiles of laser skin resurfacing.
- Individual patient characteristics and expectations, as well as the risks and benefits inherent to each treatment modality, should be considered prior to laser selection.

AN OVERVIEW

Years of damaging ultraviolet light exposure manifests clinically with skin dyspigmentation, roughened surface texture, and variable degrees of wrinkling and laxity. Other imperfections, such as scars from trauma, past surgical procedures, or acne, also affect the appearance of the skin. Histologically, the effects of aging and trauma are usually limited to the epidermis and upper papillary dermis, levels that are easily targeted by a variety of ablative and nonablative lasers.

The selection of lasers available to treat cutaneous photodamage, textural irregularities, and cosmetic imperfections continues to grow. Progress over the past few decades has led to a great increase in the number of laser skin resurfacing procedures with options that cater to a diverse patient population. The spectrum ranges from fully ablative resurfacing with pulsed and scanned carbon dioxide (CO_2) and erbium:yttrium aluminum garnet (Er:YAG) lasers, to newer nonablative and fractional laser devices.[1-3] Determining the most appropriate laser system requires consideration of the severity of the photodamage, scarring, or other imperfection to be treated, the expertise of the dermatologic surgeon, and the expectations and lifestyle of the individual patient. Thorough preoperative patient evaluation and preparation, intraoperative technical expertise, and close postoperative care and followup are all essential to optimizing clinical outcomes while preventing and minimizing the risk of complications.

ABLATIVE LASER RESURFACING

The mechanism of action of either the CO_2 or Er:YAG system for laser skin resurfacing (LSR) involves the absorption of infrared wavelengths by water-containing tissue. Treatment with these laser systems causes tissue vaporization and dermal collagen denaturation, which results in tissue contraction and subsequent stimulation of neocollagenesis.[4,5] Ablative LSR treatment thus causes removal of the entirety of the epidermis and a portion of the dermis.[6]

Ablative laser wounds induce a cascade of physiologic healing responses, ultimately leading to cutaneous remodeling and the desirable aesthetic results of laser resurfacing. After ablative LSR, it is thought that progenitor cells dwelling within the pilosebaceous units play a key role in repopulating the epidermis as well as recruiting other cells to the area to aid in various wound-healing processes. For this reason, the use of ablative LSR is not advocated on nonfacial skin as the relative paucity of pilosebaceous units in such areas hampers postoperative healing and may lead to increased risk of adverse events.[7]

Tissue ablation results in significant postoperative recovery for patients with serosanguinous discharge and crusting during the 7- to 10-day reepithelialization process. The risk of complications is highest during the reepithelialization stage when infection, erythema, and swelling can lead to permanent skin dyspigmentation and scarring if left unattended.[8]

For many years, the pulsed ablative CO_2 laser was considered the gold standard in skin resurfacing. Developed in the mid-1990s, a variety of pulsed and scanned CO_2 laser systems were used for LSR that demonstrated excellent efficacy for the treatment of rhytides, photodamage, and scars.[1-3] The subsequent development of pulsed and scanned Er:YAG lasers, as well as combination CO_2 and Er:YAG laser systems, were also highly effective for skin resurfacing and resulted in reduced damage to normal tissue surrounding treatment areas.[1-3,9,10]

NONABLATIVE LASER RESURFACING

Despite the clinical advantages of advanced ablative lasers, the prolonged postoperative recovery and potential complications associated with their use eventually led to a decrease in their popularity.[8,11,12] Nonablative laser devices were subsequently introduced with the goal of stimulating dermal neocollagenesis without inducing epidermal injury or requiring significant postoperative recovery. Although demonstrable changes in dermal collagen could be achieved with nonablative laser skin treatment and the postoperative management was favorable with few side effects, clinical improvement was modest and multiple treatments were necessary to obtain satisfactory results.[13]

A continued desire for superior clinical results while maintaining a manageable recovery and side-effect profile gave rise to a number of ablative laser devices that adhere to the concept of fractional photothermolysis.

FRACTIONAL PHOTOTHERMOLYSIS AND FRACTIONAL RESURFACING

A novel concept in skin treatment, termed *fractional photothermolysis*, was described and developed by Manstein and colleagues in 2004.[14] Fractional photothermolysis involves the creation of laser-induced small thermal injuries or microscopic treatment zones (MTZs) in water-containing skin with sparing of normal healing skin around each MTZ. The intact, nontreated skin forms bridges between the MTZs, thereby leading to more rapid healing.

The process of cutaneous healing after fractional photothermolysis differs in several ways from the healing required after fully ablative laser techniques. First, histologic evaluation of skin immediately after fractional laser irradiation reveals thermal injury sharply confined to the MTZ, which extends from the epidermis to the mid-dermis. Because the undamaged, intact epidermal tissue between MTZs contains viable transient amplifying cells capable of rapid reepithelialization, healing after fractional laser ablation progresses quite rapidly. The degenerated, necrotic dermal and epidermal debris from the MTZ is incorporated into columns and then eliminated transepidermally. This production of microscopic epidermal necrotic debris appears to be unique to the process of fractional photothermolysis.[14] Microscopic epidermal necrotic debris are naturally exfoliated within days of treatment.

Ablative lasers that adhere to the concept of fractional photothermolysis for ablative fractional resurfacing (AFR) include CO_2, Er:YAG, and erbium:yttrium scandium gallium garnet (Er:YSGG) lasers. The pedicles of thermally induced coagulation produced by these systems extend to far greater dermal depths than those delivered by nonablative devices. AFR thereby induces greater tissue contraction and neocollagenesis than nonablative lasers while leading to rapid reepithelialization and a more favorable side-effect profile than fully ablative lasers.[3,15,16] Because of the less-invasive nature of AFR, nonfacial areas, such as the neck, chest, and dorsal hands, can be more safely treated.[17,18] The technical characteristics of AFR reduce recovery time, postoperative discomfort, and complications associated with traditional multipass ablative LSR.[15]

EQUIPMENT

Table 209-1 identifies the available skin resurfacing lasers and light-based devices.

ABLATIVE LASERS

CARBON DIOXIDE

The first system developed for ablative cutaneous laser resurfacing was the CO_2 laser, which was approved by the U.S. Food and Drug Administration in 1996. The 10,600-nm wavelength emitted by CO_2 lasers is absorbed by water-containing tissue. Because of their efficacy in ameliorating severe photodamage, rhytides, and laxity, CO_2 lasers remain the gold standard in ablative LSR.[13] The earliest systems were continuous-wave CO_2 lasers, which were highly effective for gross lesional destruction; however, these systems could not reliably ablate fine layers of tissue because of their prolonged tissue-dwell times and unacceptably high rates of scarring and dyspigmentation.[19] With the subsequent development of high-energy pulsed CO_2 lasers, higher energy densities could be applied with exposure times shorter than the thermal relaxation time of water-containing tissue, thereby lowering the risk of injury to surrounding, nontargeted tissue.[4,5]

TABLE 209-1
Skin Resurfacing Lasers and Light-Based Devices

LASER TYPE	MEDIUM	WAVELENGTH
Ablative pulsed/scanned	CO_2	10,600 nm
	Er:YAG	2940 nm
	CO_2/Er:YAG	10,600/2940 nm
Nonablative	IPL	500-1200 nm
	Nd:YAG	1064 nm, 1320 nm
	Diode	980 nm, 1450 nm
	Er:Glass	1540 nm
Fractionated (ablative)	CO_2	10,600 nm
	Er:YAG	2940 nm
	Er:YSGG	2790 nm
Fractionated (nonablative)	Erbium fiber	1550 nm
	Thulium	1927 nm

CO_2, carbon dioxide; Er:YAG, erbium:yttrium aluminum garnet; Er:YSGG, erbium:yttrium scandium gallium garnet; IPL, intense pulsed light; Nd:YAG, neodymium:yttrium aluminum garnet.

The initial laser systems (Ultrapulse, SilkTouch) emitted either individual pulses (ranging from 600 microseconds to 1 millisecond [msec]) or microprocessor-directed scans that limited tissue dwell-time to less than 1 msec. The peak fluences (4 to 5 J/cm^2) delivered per pulse or scan vaporized water-containing tissue to a depth of 20 to 60 μm with a zone of thermal damage ranging from 20 to 150 μm, depending on the number of laser passes delivered.[4-6,20,21]

ERBIUM:YTTRIUM ALUMINUM GARNET

Er:YAG lasers emit 2940 nm light with a much higher water absorption coefficient (12,800 cm^{-1}) than CO_2 lasers (800 cm^{-1}), thereby rendering Er:YAG laser energy 12 to 18 times more efficiently absorbed by water-containing tissue than is CO_2 laser energy.[22,23] At typical treatment parameters, the Er:YAG laser ablates 2 to 4 μm of tissue per J/cm^2 and produces narrow zones of thermal necrosis (20 to 50 μm).[22-24] Its short pulse duration (mean: 250 microseconds) decreases thermal diffusion (with less-effective hemostasis and increased intraoperative bleeding), and along with its shallow dermal penetration, often hampers deeper dermal treatment and significant collagen contraction.[10] The major disadvantage of short-pulsed Er:YAG laser treatment (reduced thermal tissue effect) leads to a significant advantage: a shorter postoperative recovery.[25] Technologic advancements led to the subsequent development of modulated Er:YAG lasers systems that emit a combination of short and long coagulative pulses to achieve deeper tissue ablation depths and coagulative zones of thermal injury (comparable to CO_2) to improve hemostasis and increase collagen remodeling.[26-29]

HYBRIDS

More recently, Er:YAG-CO_2 hybrid laser systems have been devised to simultaneously deliver both ablative Er:YAG and coagulative CO_2 laser pulses. The Er:YAG component of these hybrid lasers generates fluences as high as 28 J/cm^2 with a 350-microsecond pulse duration; hemostasis is concomitantly provided by the CO_2 component (programmed to deliver 1-msec to 100-msec pulses at 1 to 10 W of power). Depending on the treatment parameters used, these hybrid systems produce significant zones of thermal necrosis (50 μm) with measurable increases in posttreatment collagen thickness.[1]

NONABLATIVE LASERS

Most of the nonablative systems emit light in the infrared portion of the electromagnetic spectrum, including the intense pulsed light (500 to 1200 nm), neodymium:yttrium aluminum garnet (Nd:YAG) (1064 and 1320 nm), diode (980 and 1450 nm), and Er:Glass (1540 nm) lasers. These nonablative laser systems target dermal water, which leads to collagen heating and subsequent dermal remodeling, but without production of an external wound because of concomitant application of epidermal cooling that prevents tissue vaporization.

Because nonablative lasers have limited thermal tissue effect, treatments are commonly delivered in a series of 3 or more monthly sessions to produce mild clinical results.

FRACTIONAL LASERS

Since the introduction, in 2004, of the first fractional laser using the concept of fractional photothermolysis, a wide range of fractional ablative and nonablative lasers has become available. The mid-infrared wavelengths of these fractional systems target water-containing tissue to produce skin photocoagulation at depths of 200 to 500 μm with spacing between each microthermal zone of 200 to 300 μm.[30] Compared to fully ablative LSR, only 15% to 25% of treated skin is ablated during a typical fractional photothermolysis treatment. Differences in depth of ablation and coagulation, variation in available spot size and shape, application of energy (stamped vs rolling), and ergonomics of the laser handpiece distinguish one fractional device from another, but few differences in overall clinical improvement have been demonstrated.[2,3]

INDICATIONS AND CONTRAINDICATIONS FOR LASER SKIN RESURFACING

INDICATIONS

Pulsed, scanned, and fractional lasers have been used to successfully treat photodamaged skin, atrophic scars, and a variety of epidermal and dermal lesions (Figs. 209-1 to 209-3; Table 209-2).[1-3,9,16,31] Pulsed and scanned CO_2 lasers typically demonstrate 50% to 80% improvement of facial rhytides and acne scars after 1 skin resurfacing treatment.[9,21] The clinical results are longstanding and have been shown to improve for 18 months after treatment.[32] Although Er:YAG LSR also leads to substantive (>50%) improvement of photodamaged skin and scars, the modulated (variable pulsed Er:YAG) and hybrid (Er:YAG-CO_2) systems more closely mirror the clinical results obtained with CO_2 laser.[13,29] Similar clinical results can be obtained with the ablative fractionated lasers, but often more than one laser treatment is necessary.[2,3] Moderate to severe acne scarring in patients with a wide range of skin phototypes (I to V) shows significant (50% to 75%) clinical improvement in scar depth after 2 or 3 fractional CO_2 laser treatments.[33] Quantitative image analysis of nonacne atrophic traumatic or surgical

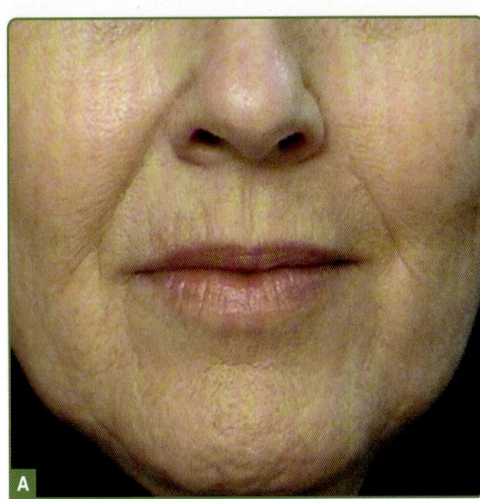
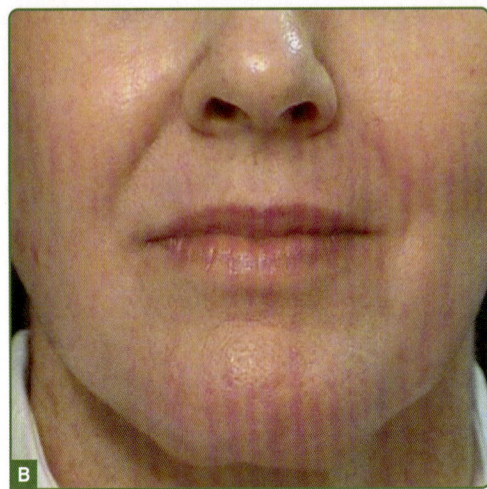

Figure 209-1 Facial photodamage and rhytides before (**A**) and several months after (**B**) ablative CO_2 laser skin resurfacing.

scars 6 months after fractional CO_2 laser treatments demonstrated clinical and volumetric improvement with mean reduction of scar volume and depth by 38% (traumatic scars) and 36% (surgical scars).[34]

One of the biggest advantages of fractional laser treatment is its ability to be safely and effectively applied to nonfacial as well as physiologically impaired skin with fewer pilosebaceous glands (eg, burn scars). As such, fractionated lasers can be used for a much wider range of skin conditions, including extensive body scars and photodamaged skin on the arms and legs.[3] In addition, fractionated lasers have shown usefulness

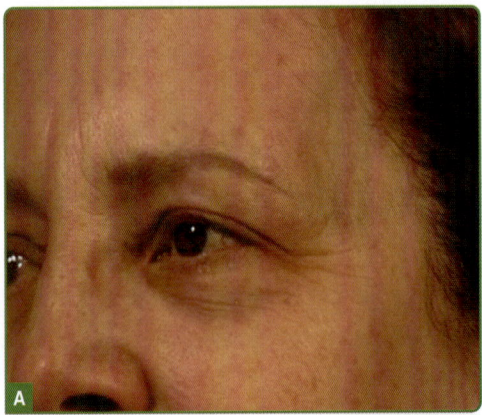
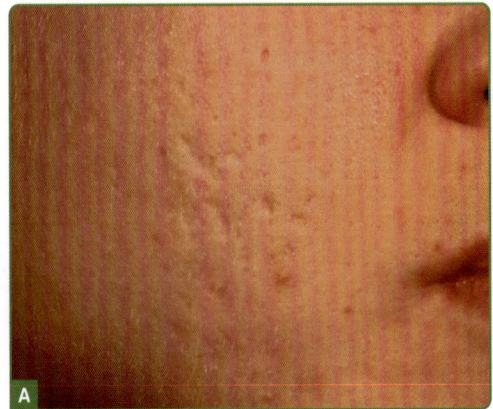
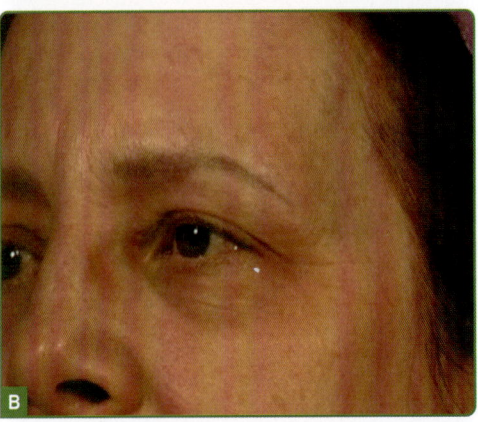
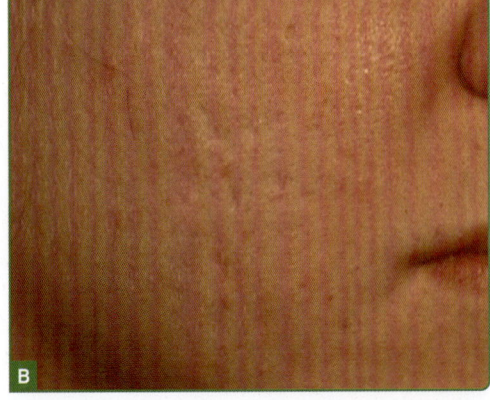

Figure 209-2 Facial photodamage and rhytides before (**A**) and 6 months after (**B**) fractional ablative CO_2 laser skin resurfacing.

Figure 209-3 Atrophic scars before (**A**) and 6 months after (**B**) fractional ablative CO_2 laser skin resurfacing.

TABLE 209-2
Lesions and Conditions Amenable to Laser Skin Resurfacing

- Actinic damage
  - Actinic cheilitis
  - Actinic keratoses
  - Facial rhytides (superficial and deep)
  - Superficial dyschromia (lentigines, melasma)
  - Superficial nonmelanoma skin cancer (squamous or basal cell carcinomas)
- Atrophic scars (acne, surgical, traumatic)
- Epidermal lesions
  - Seborrheic keratosis
  - Epidermal nevi
  - Verrucae
- Benign hyperplasias/neoplasms
  - Adnexal tumors (syringomas, angiofibromas)
  - Lymphangioma
  - rhinophyma
  - Sebaceous hyperplasia
  - Xanthomas, xanthelasma
- Miscellaneous dermatologic conditions
  - Balanitis xerotica obliterans
  - Chondrodermatitis nodularis helicis
  - Colloid milia
  - Eruptive hair cysts
  - Hailey-Hailey disease
  - Keratoderma
  - Lichen sclerosus
  - Onychodystrophy
  - Porokeratosis

TABLE 209-3
Laser Skin Resurfacing: Patient Selection, Risks, and Precautions

- Are the lesions amenable to laser skin resurfacing?
  - All suspicious (malignant) lesions require biopsy before treatment.
- Has the patient *ever* had the areas treated before?
  - Laser skin resurfacing can unmask hypopigmentation or fibrosis produced by prior dermabrasion, cryosurgery, or phenol peels.
  - Patients with prior lower blepharoplasties using an external approach are at greater risk of ectropion formation after infraorbital ablative skin resurfacing.
- What is the patient's skin phototype?
  - After laser skin resurfacing, patients with lighter skin tones (skin phototype I or II) have a lower incidence of postoperative hyperpigmentation than patients with darker skin tones.
- Does the patient have a history of herpes labialis?
  - Prophylactic antiviral medication for patients undergoing perioral laser skin resurfacing is advised because reactivation and/or dissemination of prior herpes simplex virus infection can occur.
  - Laser-deepithelialized skin is particularly susceptible to primary inoculation by herpes simplex virus.
- Does the patient have evidence of inflammation (acne, psoriasis, eczema) or infection?
  - Avoidance of treatment in patients with active skin inflammation will reduce the risk of prolonged postoperative healing and disseminated infection.
- Does the patient have an immunologic deficiency or autoimmune disease?
  - Intact immunologic function and collagen repair mechanisms are necessary to optimize the tissue healing response during the recovery period.
- Is the patient taking any medications that are contraindicated?
  - Oral retinoids (eg, isotretinoin) have been shown to have a detrimental effect on wound healing and collagenesis leading many practitioners to delay treatment for 6 months after retinoid discontinuation; however, recent research has revealed no greater risk of postoperative hypertrophic scar formation with concomitant ingestion of oral retinoids and laser skin resurfacing.
- Does the patient have a tendency to form hypertrophic scars or keloids?
  - Patients with a propensity to scar abnormally will be at greater risk of scar formation after laser skin resurfacing, independent of laser selectivity and operator expertise.
- Does the patient have realistic expectations of the procedure and will the patient adhere to postoperative instructions?
  - Those who cannot physically or emotionally tolerate the postoperative recovery period should be dissuaded from pursuing ablative laser skin resurfacing procedures.

in improving CO_2 laser–induced hypopigmentation, residua from infantile hemangioma, and topical drug delivery.[2,18]

PATIENT SELECTION

The ideal patient for cutaneous laser resurfacing has a fair complexion (Fitzpatrick skin phototype I or II) with photodamaged or scarred facial skin. Patients with darker skin tones (phototypes III to VI) are best treated with fractionated systems because of their lower postoperative dyspigmentation profile.[15] Importantly, the patient should have realistic expectations of the treatment process and the anticipated clinical results. Adequate preoperative patient evaluation and education are essential to optimize the clinical outcomes (Table 209-3). Because ablative LSR can be complicated by a prolonged postoperative recovery, pigmentary alteration, or an unexpected side effect, proper patient selection is paramount. The patient's emotional ability to tolerate an extended convalescence is an important factor in determining the most appropriate choice of laser for treatment.

Although CO_2 or modulated Er:YAG ablative LSR produces the most dramatic clinical results, some patients may be unable to tolerate the intensive recovery periods required. Ablative LSR postoperative recovery involves 7 to 10 days of intense wound healing during the reepithelialization process, followed by intense erythema for several additional weeks. For patients who are unable to commit to an extended recovery process, nonablative or fractional LSR may be a more appropriate choice. After AFR, intense erythema and serosanguinous drainage are evident for 2 to 3 days, followed by complete reepithelialization and diminution of erythema by day 6 or 7. Nonablative lasers typically produce mild erythema and edema, which spontaneously resolve within 24 hours. In contrast to ablative systems, nonablative and fractionated lasers can be safely applied to nonfacial areas because there is no epidermal disruption and, thus, areas with a relative paucity of pilosebaceous glands necessary for reepithelialization (such as the neck and anterior chest) can be safely treated.

CONTRAINDICATIONS

When considering a patient for LSR, there are several contraindications of which the physician must be cognizant. First and foremost, patients must be counseled adequately such that their expectations are in line with the clinical results that can be reasonably expected from the LSR procedure.

Active skin infections—whether bacterial, viral, or fungal—are absolute contraindications to laser resurfacing procedures. Furthermore, as ablated skin heals from progenitor cells contained within the pilosebaceous units, patients with adnexal abnormalities may have significant issues with postoperative wound healing, and should not undergo ablative LSR. This subset of patients includes those who have previously undergone therapeutic skin irradiation which often compromises local adnexa.

As isotretinoin and other systemic retinoids affect the function of sebaceous units, the issue of pursuing ablative LSR in patients who have received isotretinoin therapy remains controversial. Although many experts in the field of laser surgery advocate a washout period of at least 6 months,[8,11-13] newer published research demonstrates normal reepithelialization and lack of scar formation in patients undergoing ablative LSR while on concomitant isotretinoin therapy.[35]

Patients who have a history of keloid or hypertrophic scar formation should be carefully counseled and considered, as these types of scars can potentially result from LSR. Patients with a history of extensive electrolysis or aggressive chemical peels and/or dermabrasion may have cutaneous adnexal structures that are damaged or absent, leading to impaired postoperative healing and unfavorable results. Patients with a history of skin grafts and previous ablative laser resurfacing procedures also fall into this category. Certainly, patients who have had prior treatments can undergo LSR, but laser parameters might need adjustments based on the observed intraoperative laser-tissue interaction.

Darker-skinned patients (skin phototypes III to VI) should be informed regarding the risk of hypopigmentation or hyperpigmentation after ablative LSR that may be permanent in some cases. In these patients, it may be prudent to perform a spot test on an inconspicuous area (eg, an area of the face normally obscured by the patient's hair). If no dyspigmentation is observed in the area several weeks to months after application, full-face treatment may be more comfortably pursued.

If a patient has a history of herpes labialis [herpes simplex virus (HSV)], the prophylactic antiviral regimen may be modified with earlier initiation of treatment and/or extension of the typical 7-day post-treatment course.[36]

PROCEDURE AND TECHNIQUE

PREOPERATIVE CARE

Currently, no consensus has been reached regarding the most appropriate preoperative medical regimen for LSR patients. The use of topical retinoic acid compounds, hydroquinone bleaching agents, or α-hydroxy acids for several weeks before cutaneous resurfacing has been touted by some as a means of speeding recovery and decreasing the incidence of postinflammatory hyperpigmentation; others, however, have reported that these regimens do little to affect, in particular, postoperative pigmentation.[37] Although topical tretinoin accelerates postoperative reepithelialization after dermabrasion and deep chemical peels, laser-induced wounds are intrinsically different from those created by other destructive methods, and, thus, laser skin penetration and postoperative healing are not typically affected by topical tretinoin application.[36]

Because of the moist, deepithelialized state of ablative laser-resurfaced skin and the potential for bacterial contamination and overgrowth, many laser surgeons advocate oral antibiotic prophylaxis. This practice remains controversial, particularly as a controlled study demonstrated no significant change in post-LSR infection rates with prophylactic antibiotic use.[38]

In contrast, given the susceptibility of LSR-treated skin to viral infection, antiviral prophylaxis is recommended for all ablative LSR patients regardless of prior HSV history. Oral prophylaxis is often started on the day of, or prior to, treatment and continues until reepithelialization is complete (7 to 10 days).[36]

ANESTHESIA

Most LSR procedures are delivered in outpatient office settings or ambulatory surgery facilities. Topical lidocaine cream or other anesthetic preparations are often applied for an hour prior to treatment in order enhance tissue hydration and anesthetic penetration prior to laser irradiation.[39] Regional nerve blockade and IV sedation may be used to provide more complete anxiolysis, amnesia, and sedation during ablative LSR procedures.[40]

PROCEDURE

SAFETY PRECAUTIONS

Standard protective health equipment and precautions should be observed. All patients, physicians, and staff in the room during LSR must wear appropriate protective eyewear throughout the entirety of the procedure. Furthermore, a smoke evacuator should be used to protect patient and staff from inhalation of the ablative laser plume as it may contain both carcinogens and infectious particles. If the patient has been anesthetized with IV sedation and oxygen is in use, additional precautions must be taken to prevent combustion of the oxygen or other flammable substances by high-powered laser energy.

TECHNIQUE

After appropriate informed consent is obtained, eye protection is in place, and anesthesia or sedation is employed, laser treatment can begin. Ablative LSR is typically advised for the entire face to avoid postoperative discrepancy between treated and untreated skin in adjacent cosmetic units. Conversely, nonablative and fractional laser treatment can be performed on separate facial and nonfacial cosmetic units without fear of prolonged healing and mismatched skin. Regardless of laser system used, meticulous laser technique with nonoverlapping scans will minimize excessive thermal damage to skin during treatment. Additional laser passes are delivered perpendicular to previous passes until the desired clinical effect has been achieved. Optimal laser settings vary depending upon the laser system employed and the severity of the condition being treated.

Carbon Dioxide Ablative Laser Skin Resurfacing: The objective of ablative LSR is to vaporize unwanted skin lesions as deep as the papillary dermis. Limiting the depth of penetration decreases the risk of scarring and permanent pigmentary alteration. When choosing treatment parameters, several factors should be considered, including site to be resurfaced, the skin phototype of the patient, and previous skin treatments administered.[7,36] Anatomic location can guide selection of treatment parameters; for example, thinner skin (eg, periorbital) requires fewer laser passes than thicker facial skin, and laser resurfacing of nonfacial skin (eg, neck, chest) should be avoided because of the relative paucity of pilosebaceous units in these areas.[7,36]

The depth of ablation (usually restricted to the epidermis and upper papillary dermis) correlates directly with the number of passes performed.[41] "Stacking" laser pulses by treating an area with multiple passes in rapid succession or by using a high-overlap setting on a scanning device leads to excessive thermal injury with increased risk of scarring and should, thus, be avoided.[8,42] After several overlapped laser passes, an ablative plateau is reached, tissue ablation becomes less effective, and tissue heating (eg, thermal damage) is greatly increased.[42] To reduce the risk of excessive thermal injury during multipass LSR procedures, partially desiccated tissue should be removed manually with wet gauze after each pass to expose the underlying dermis to subsequent laser passes.[42]

In an attempt to address many of the difficulties associated with multipass CO_2 LSR, refinements in surgical technique have been developed. A minimally-traumatic single-pass CO_2 LSR procedure has been described that results in faster postoperative reepithelialization and an improved side-effect profile as compared to the multipass technique.[43] During this single-pass protocol, partially desiccated tissue is not removed (as is standard during multipass procedures); rather, the lased skin is left intact to serve as a biologic wound dressing. Additional laser passes can then be applied focally to areas of more extensive photodamage in order to limit unnecessary thermal and mechanical trauma to less-involved skin. Numerous reports have substantiated the improved side-effect profile of this less-aggressive protocol.[44-46]

Er:YAG Ablative Laser Skin Resurfacing: The short-pulsed Er:YAG laser fluences used most often range from 5 to 15 J/cm^2 depending on the degree of photodamage and anatomic location. Because of an improved absorption coefficient—10 times greater than CO_2 lasers—thermal energy conveyed during Er:YAG procedures is confined to the targeted tissue with minimal collateral thermal damage. Very little thermal tissue necrosis is produced with each pass of the short-pulsed Er:YAG laser, making manual removal of desiccated tissue between passes often unnecessary; however, it takes 3 to 4 times as many Er:YAG passes to achieve similar depths of penetration as the CO_2 laser at typical treatment parameters.[7] Treatment of deep dermal lesions or areas of the face with extensive photodamage may require up to 9 or 10 passes of the short-pulsed Er:YAG laser, whereas the CO_2 laser would affect similar levels of tissue ablation in only 2 or 3 passes.[7,10] Modified Er:YAG laser systems provide improved hemostasis and visualization of the treatment area, as well as enhanced collagen contraction because of the added thermal effects on the tissue.[13] As such, modified and hybrid systems are generally delivered as single treatments with clinical outcomes similar to pulsed or scanned CO_2 lasers.

Ablative Fractional Skin Resurfacing: Fractional CO_2 laser systems typically involve delivery of 70 to 100 mJ energies with 20% to 30% coverage to achieve depths of penetration of 200 to 1600 μm. Treatment of periocular skin (thinner) and neck skin (fewer pilosebaceous units) require a decrease in both energy and coverage density. Although clinical results and, thus, patient satisfaction may improve with the use of higher fluences, higher treatment energies increase the risk of adverse events such as pain, erythema, and postoperative dyspigmentation.[47] Ablative fractional lasers generally require only 1 treatment to achieve patient satisfaction. However, reappraisal of photodamage, rhytides, or scarring can be performed 6 to 12 months postoperatively to assess if additional treatments are clinically warranted.

Nonablative Laser Skin Resurfacing: Significant improvement of facial and nonfacial rhytides, scars, and dyspigmentation has been demonstrated using a wide range of different nonablative laser systems. Treatments are typically delivered in a series of 3 or more monthly sessions with clinical improvement averaging 30% to 50%. By increasing the energy delivered, greater depth of dermal penetration (and tissue effect) is achieved. Similarly, increasing the density (or area of coverage) also serves to increase clinical effect without significantly altering postoperative recovery. In general, nonablative laser skin treatment of facial skin has shown superior results to nonfacial (eg, neck, chest, dorsal hand) skin; however, good clinical outcomes have been achieved in a variety of conditions and treatment areas (including traumatic scars and abdominal striae). Clinical assessment scores corresponding to 50% to 75% improvement or more are typically reported after a series of 3 or more treatments on facial rhytides.[48] Similarly, atrophic acne scars have shown remarkable improvement (50% and higher) after a treatment series using either a 1550-nm erbium-doped fiber laser or a number of other fractionated diode and Nd:YAG lasers (1410 nm to 1540 nm).[49-51] Additionally, nonablative fractionated lasers have been used with success to improve the appearance of large pores and hypertrophic scars from a variety of causes.[52-54]

POSTOPERATIVE CARE AND PATIENT INSTRUCTIONS

Proper wound care during the immediate postoperative period is vital to the successful recovery of laser-resurfaced skin. Partial-thickness cutaneous wounds heal more efficiently and with a reduced risk of scarring when maintained in a moist environment. The presence of a dry crust or scab impedes keratinocyte migration. Although there is consensus among laser surgeons on this principle, disagreement exists regarding the optimal dressing for the laser-ablated wound. Either an open or a closed wound dressing may be prescribed. The "open" dressing technique involves frequent application of thick healing ointment to the deepithelialized skin surface, whereas the "closed" technique calls for the placement of occlusive or semiocclusive dressings directly on the lased skin. Although the open technique facilitates wound visualization, the closed technique requires less patient involvement and may also decrease postoperative pain. Increased patient comfort, decreased erythema and edema, increased rate of reepithelialization, and decreased requirement for patient effort in wound care are among other advantages of closed wound dressings, but their use involves additional expense and a higher infection risk.[55]

In addition to wound care, postoperative ice pack application and the administration of antiinflammatory medications should be prescribed. Pain medication during the first few postoperative days is particularly important for patients undergoing fully ablative LSR. Comparatively, although pinpoint bleeding, serosanguinous drainage, and edema can be significant during the first 24 to 36 hours after AFR, minimal (if any) discomfort is present.

OUTCOMES ASSESSMENT

There are many clinical and histologic benefits of cutaneous laser resurfacing. The greatest advantages associated with CO_2 LSR are excellent tissue contraction, hemostasis, prolonged neocollagenesis, and collagen remodeling. Histologic examination of CO_2 laser-treated skin demonstrates replacement of epidermal cellular atypia and dysplasia with normal, healthy epidermal cells from adjacent follicular adnexal structures.[20] The most profound effects occur in the papillary dermis, where coagulation of disorganized masses of actinically-induced elastotic material are replaced with normal compact collagen bundles arranged in parallel to the skin's surface.[56] Immediately after CO_2 laser treatment, a normal inflammatory response is initiated with granulation tissue formation, neovascularization, and increased recruitment of macrophages and fibroblasts.[56]

After ablative CO_2 LSR, most studies have shown at least a 50% improvement over baseline skin tone and wrinkle severity.[3,6,7] Persistent collagen shrinkage and dermal remodeling are responsible for much of the continued clinical benefits observed after treatment and are influenced by several factors.[28,57] Thermal effects of laser skin irradiation result in collagen fiber contraction through disruption of interpeptide bonds at temperatures ranging from 55°C to 62°C (131°F to 143.6°F). This results in a conformational change of collagen's basic triple-helical structure, thereby shortening the molecule to approximately one-third of its normal length.[58] These laser-remodeled collagen fibers may act as the contracted scaffold for neocollagenesis. Fibroblasts that migrate into laser wounds after resurfacing may upregulate the expression of immune-modulating factors that serve to further enhance collagen shrinkage and ongoing neocollagenesis.[59]

Investigators have compared collagen tightening induced by the CO_2 laser to that induced by the CO_2–Er:YAG hybrid laser system.[60] Intraoperative contraction of approximately 43% was produced after three passes of the CO_2 laser, compared to 12% contraction after Er:YAG irradiation. At 4 weeks, however, the CO_2 laser-treated and Er:YAG laser-treated sites were contracted to the same degree. This highlights the different mechanisms of physiologic tissue tightening observed after various laser treatments. Immediate thermal-induced collagen tightening is the predominant response seen after CO_2 irradiation, whereas modulated Er:YAG laser resurfacing induces slow and progressive rather than immediate collagen tightening.[60-62]

Significant clinical improvement of rhytides and atrophic scars following fractional ablative LSR has been demonstrated in several published studies.[18,33,34,59] Moderate to marked (50% to 75%) improvement is typical, with better results obtained when higher energies and density coverage are implemented. Not surprisingly, the use of more-aggressive laser parameters tends to yield better clinical outcomes, but also longer postoperative recovery.[18]

SIDE EFFECTS AND COMPLICATIONS

Side effects associated with LSR vary and are related to the expertise of the operator, the anatomic location treated, the skin phototype of the patient, underlying skin conditions, the aggressiveness of the laser procedure, postoperative wound care, and several other variables (Table 209-4).

When most ablative LSR techniques are compared (single-pass CO_2 vs multipass, long-pulsed Er:YAG), postoperative healing times and complication profiles are comparable, even in patients with darker skin phototypes.[45] In a retrospective review and analysis of 100 consecutively-treated patients, investigators found that average time to reepithelialization was 5.5 days with single-pass CO_2 and 5.1 days with long-pulsed Er:YAG laser resurfacing.[46]

COMMON POSTOPERATIVE REACTIONS

Erythema and edema are expected in the immediate postoperative period and are not considered adverse events. The duration, incidence, and severity of erythema can vary between and among different CO_2 and Er:YAG systems.[11,12] The degree of erythema correlates directly with the depth of ablation and the number of laser passes performed.[7] In an extended evaluation of 50 patients, postoperative erythema averaged 4.5 weeks in duration after single-pass CO_2 laser treatment and 3.6 weeks after long-pulsed Er:YAG laser treatment.[46] A split-face comparison of pulsed CO_2 and variable-pulsed Er:YAG LSR revealed decreased erythema and edema with faster healing on the Er:YAG laser-treated facial half as compared to CO_2.[46]

TABLE 209-4
Side Effects and Complications of Ablative and Nonablative Laser Skin Resurfacing

Expected
- Erythema
- Edema
- Pruritus

Mild
- Prolonged erythema
- Milia
- Acne
- Allergic or irritant contact dermatitis

Moderate
- Infection (bacterial. viral, fungal)
- Transient hyperpigmentation

Severe
- Permanent hypopigmentation
- Hypertrophic scarring
- Ectropion

While postoperative erythema also may be aggravated by underlying rosacea or dermatitis, most erythema will resolve spontaneously. Application of topical ascorbic acid after reepithelialization may serve to decrease the degree of cutaneous inflammation.[62] Light-emitting diode photomodulation also has been shown to improve postlaser erythema and to help patients recover more quickly post-LSR.[63] Potentially irritating topicals, such as retinoic acid derivatives, glycolic acid, fragrance-containing or chemical-containing cosmetics, and chemical sunscreens should be strictly avoided in the early postoperative period until substantial reepithelialization has occurred.

MINOR SIDE EFFECTS

Mild side effects of ablative LSR include milia formation and worsening of acne which may be exacerbated by the postoperative use of occlusive dressings and ointments. Milia and acne usually resolve spontaneously as healing progresses and the application of thick emollient creams and occlusive dressings ceases. For acne flares that do not respond to topical preparations, oral antibiotics may be prescribed.

Contact dermatitis, either irritant or allergic, can develop in response to various topical medications, soaps, and moisturizers used postoperatively. Most of these reactions are irritant in nature, due in part to the decreased barrier function of newly resurfaced skin.[64]

Hyperpigmentation is one of the more common side effects of ablative LSR and occurs to some degree in all treated patients with darker skin tones.[7,11,15,65] The hyperpigmentation is generally transient, but resolution can be hastened by the postoperative use of a variety of topical agents, including hydroquinone as well as retinoic, azelaic, kojic, and glycolic acids. Daily sunscreen use is also important to prevent further skin darkening during the healing process.

Hypopigmentation is often not observed for several months postoperatively. Estimates vary, but postoperative hypopigmentation may occur in upwards of 10% to 20% of patients after ablative LSR.[66] Its incidence is markedly reduced with use of fractionated lasers. Hypopigmentation is of particular concern because it is often refractory to treatment and may be permanent. The use of an excimer laser or topical photochemotherapy to stimulate repigmentation has proven successful in some patients.[66,67] Others report improvement of hypopigmentation after the use of a non-AFR laser.[68]

MODERATE SIDE EFFECTS

The most common infection following ablative laser resurfacing is reactivation of labial HSV infection, most likely encouraged by thermal tissue injury and epidermal disruption.[11,15] After CO_2 LSR, approximately 7% of all patients develop a localized or disseminated form of HSV infection.[11,15,65] Evidence of HSV infection typically presents within the first postoperative week and, because of the denuded condition of newly lased skin, can present as erosions without intact vesicles. Even with appropriate antiviral prophylaxis, it is possible for a herpetic outbreak to occur. To prevent dissemination or scarring, HSV infection should be treated aggressively.[7] Oral antiviral agents such as acyclovir, famciclovir, and valacyclovir are effective against HSV infection, although IV therapy may be required in severe (disseminated) cases. Because many patients may be unaware of their HSV status and because laser-ablated skin is susceptible to inadvertent exposure to HSV, most practitioners advocate the use of oral prophylaxis during the postoperative period until reepithelialization is complete (7 to 10 days).[8]

Other postoperative wound infections associated with ablative LSR include *Staphylococcus* and *Pseudomonas* infections as well as cutaneous candidiasis. All postoperative infections should be treated aggressively with the appropriate systemic antibiotic or antifungal agent.[55]

There have been rare reports of koebnerization of lesions (psoriasis, keratoacanthomas) after ablative LSR.[69] It is, thus, imperative to perform a full skin examination and obtain a complete medical and family history to determine whether a predilection for this undesirable side effect is present.

SEVERE COMPLICATIONS

The most severe complications associated with ablative cutaneous laser resurfacing are hypertrophic scarring and the formation of ectropion.[11,12] While the risk of scarring is low, inadvertent pulse stacking or scan overlapping and incomplete removal of desiccated tissue between laser passes can cause excessive thermal injury leading to fibrosis. Ablative laser resurfacing of skin with absent, poorly functioning, or decreased pilosebaceous units (eyelids, neck, chest) can also increase the likelihood of hypertrophic scar formation.

Postoperatively, focal areas of bright erythema with associated pruritus, particularly along the mandible, may signal impending scar formation.[15] Potent topical corticosteroid preparations should be applied to these areas to decrease the inflammatory response. Pulsed-dye laser treatment can be used to improve the appearance and symptoms of such scars.[70]

Ectropion of the lower eyelid is rarely seen after periorbital LSR; however, if encountered, it often requires surgical correction. Ectropion is more likely to occur in patients who have had previous lower blepharoplasty or other surgical manipulation of the periorbital region. Preoperative examination is essential to determine eyelid laxity and skin elasticity. If the infraorbital skin does not return briskly to its normal resting position after a manual downward pull ("snap test"), then ablative laser resurfacing near the lower eyelid margin should be avoided. In general, lower fluences and fewer laser passes should be used in the periorbital area to decrease the risk of fibrosis and lid eversion.

SIDE EFFECTS OF ABLATIVE FRACTIONAL LASER SKIN RESURFACING

The main advantages of ablative fractional lasers—as compared to fully ablative LSR techniques—are their excellent side-effect profiles and low incidence of complications.[15] Postoperative recovery is quicker and more predictable after AFR treatment, with pinpoint bleeding and serosanguinous discharge resolving within 24 to 48 hours. Intense erythema and crusting are typically seen for 3 to 6 days postoperatively. Moderate erythema lasts days to weeks, standing in sharp contrast to the months of erythema often experienced after traditional ablative LSR. Post-AFR erythema may be slower to resolve in patients with skin phototype I or II and in those who received more-aggressive treatments. Even with fractional resurfacing, particular care must be taken when treating anatomic sites with a relative paucity of pilosebaceous units such as the eyelids, neck, and chest. Excessive thermal injury in these areas can result in subsequent hypertrophic scarring. With proper technique, however, excellent clinical results can be achieved, accompanied by a quicker convalescence as compared to traditional ablative LSR and a much lower risk of scarring and dyspigmentation.

NEW AND FUTURE DEVELOPMENTS USING ABLATIVE LASERS

Ablative fractional lasers create microscopic vertical holes through the epidermis. In addition to stimulating the physiologic effects responsible for antiaging results, these microscopic holes can serve as channels through which topically applied drugs can gain access to the dermis.[71] Initial histologic studies have shown that the microthermal zones created by ablative fractional lasers penetrate to depths of at least 300 μm and diameters of 100 μm. The ability of a variety of different drugs, including topical methyl 5-aminolevulic acid, 5-aminolevulinic acid, lidocaine, platelet-rich plasma, autologous cells, corticosteroids, and ascorbic acid, to penetrate skin using laser-assisted delivery systems has been studied.[72] Dermal penetration of each of these drugs has uniformly been increased when applied to ablative fractional laser–treated skin. Because physicochemical properties of a particular drug greatly influence its ability to permeate tissues (even after stratum corneum penetration), the number, size, and depth of laser-induced channels affect drug delivery. AFR-assisted drug delivery promises to be an important dermatologic therapy in the future and numerous investigations are being conducted to evaluate appropriate drug-specific channel density and depth parameters for a wide variety of topical medications. In addition, fractional ablative lasers combined with other laser technology have been shown to amplify clinical results and shorten recovery times in the treatment of pigmented lesions and tattoos.[73] Clinical trials are underway to elucidate the safety and effectiveness of these and other combination treatments using ablative and fractional laser technology.

REFERENCES

1. Alexiades-Armenakas M, Dover JS, Arndt KA. The spectrum of laser skin resurfacing: nonablative, fractional, and ablative laser resurfacing. *J Am Acad Dermatol*. 2008;58:719-737.
2. Brightman LA, Brauer JA, Anolik R, et al. Ablative and fractional ablative lasers. *Dermatol Clin*. 2009;27:479-489.
3. Aslam A, Alster TS. Evolution of laser skin resurfacing: from scanning to fractional technology. *Dermatol Surg*. 2014;40:1163-1172.
4. Walsh JT, Flotte TJ, Anderson RR, et al. Pulsed CO_2 laser tissue ablation: effect of tissue type and pulse duration on thermal damage. *Lasers Surg Med*. 1988;8:108-118.
5. Walsh JT, Deutsch TF. Pulsed CO_2 laser tissue ablation: measurement of the ablation rate. *Lasers Surg Med*. 1988;8:264-275.
6. Ross EV, McKinlay JR, Anderson RR. Why does carbon dioxide resurfacing work? *Arch Dermatol*. 1999;135:444-454.
7. Alster TS. Cutaneous resurfacing with CO_2 and erbium:YAG lasers: preoperative, intraoperative, and postoperative considerations. *Plast Reconstr Surg*, 1999;103:619-632.
8. Treatment of complications of laser skin resurfacing. *Arch Facial Plast Surg*. 2000 Oct-Dec;2(4):279-84.
9. Alster TS, Lupton JR. An overview of cutaneous laser resurfacing. *Clin Plast Surg*. 2001;28:37-52.
10. Alster TS, Lupton JR. Erbium:YAG cutaneous laser resurfacing. *Dermatol Clin*. 2001;19:453-466.
11. Nanni CA, Alster TS. Complications of carbon dioxide laser resurfacing: an evaluation of 500 patients. *Dermatol Surg*. 1998;24:315-320.
12. Alster TS, Doshi S. Ablative and non-ablative laser skin resurfacing. In Burgess C (ed). *Cosmetic Dermatology*. Heidelberg: Springer-Verlag, 2005: 111-126.
13. Alster TS, Tanzi EL. Laser skin resurfacing: ablative and nonablative. In: Robinson J, Sengelman R, Siegel DM, et al, eds. *Surgery of the Skin*. Philadelphia, PA: Elsevier; 2005:611-624.
14. Manstein D, Herron GS, Sink RK, et al. Fractional photothermolysis: a new concept for cutaneous remodeling using microscopic patterns of thermal injury. *Lasers Surg Med*. 2004;34:426-438.
15. Metelitsa AI, Alster TS. Fractionated laser skin resurfacing treatment complications: a review. *Dermatol Surg*. 2010;36:299-306.
16. MacGregor JL, Alster TS. Fractional resurfacing lasers: ablative and non-ablative. In: Nouri K, ed. *Dermatologic Surgery: Step by Step*. Oxford, England UK: Blackwell; 2013: 349-358.
17. Tierney EP, Kouba DJ, Hanke CW. Review of fractional photothermolysis: treatment indications and efficacy. *Dermatol Surg*. 2009;5:1445-1461.
18. Hunzeker CM, Weiss ET, Geronemus RG. Fractionated CO_2 laser resurfacing: our experience with more than 2000 treatments. *Aesthet Surg J*. 2009;29:317-322.
19. Lanzafame RJ, Naim JO, Rogers DW, et al. Comparisons of continuous-wave, chop wave, and superpulsed laser wounds. *Lasers Surg Med*. 1988;8:119-124.
20. Alster TS, Kauvar ANB, Geronemus RG. Histology of high-energy pulsed CO_2 laser resurfacing. *Semin Cutan Med Surg*. 1996;15:189-193.
21. Alster TS, Nanni CA, Williams CM. Comparison of four carbon dioxide resurfacing lasers: a clinical and histopathologic evaluation. *Dermatol Surg*. 1999;25:153-159.
22. Hibst R, Kaufmann R. Effects of laser parameters on pulsed ErYAG laser ablation. *Lasers Med Sci*. 1991;6:391-397.
23. Hohenleutner U, Hohenleutner S, Baumler W, et al. Fast and effective skin ablation with an Er:YAG laser: determination of ablation rates and thermal damage zones. *Lasers Surg Med*. 1997;20:242-247.
24. Alster TS. Clinical and histologic evaluation of six erbium:YAG lasers for cutaneous resurfacing. *Lasers Surg Med*. 1999;24:87-92.
25. Tanzi EL, Alster TS. Side effects and complications of variable-pulsed erbium:yttrium-aluminum-garnet laser skin resurfacing: extended experience with 50 patients. *Plast Reconstr Surg*. 2003;111:1524-1529.
26. Pozner JM, Goldberg DJ. Histologic effect of a variable pulsed Er:YAG laser. *Dermatol Surg*. 2000;26:733-736.
27. Ross EV, McKinlay JR, Sajben FP, et al. Use of a novel erbium laser in a Yucatan minipig: a study of residual thermal damage (RTD), ablation, and wound healing as a function of pulse duration. *Lasers Surg Med*. 1999;26:15-17.
28. Fitzpatrick RE, Rostan EF, Marchell N. Collagen tightening induced by carbon dioxide laser versus erbium:YAG laser. *Lasers Surg Med*. 2000;27:395-403.
29. Rostan EF, Fitzpatrick RE, Goldman MP. Laser resurfacing with a long pulse erbium:YAG laser compared to the 950 ms pulsed CO_2 laser. *Lasers Surg Med*. 2001;29:136-141.
30. Waibel J, Beer K, Narurkar V, et al. Preliminary observations on fractional ablative resurfacing devices: clinical impressions. *J Drugs Dermatol*. 2009;8:481-485.
31. Hruza GJ. Laser treatment of epidermal and dermal lesions. *Dermatol Clin*. 2002;20:147-164.
32. Walia S, Alster TS. Prolonged clinical and histologic effects from CO_2 laser resurfacing of atrophic acne scars. *Dermatol Surg*. 1999;25:926-930.
33. Walgrave SE, Ortiz AE, MacFalls HT, et al. Evaluation of a novel fractional resurfacing device for treatment of acne scarring. *Lasers Surg Med*. 2009;41:122-127.
34. Weiss ET, Chapas A, Brightman L, et al. Successful treatment of atrophic postoperative and traumatic scarring with carbon dioxide ablative fractional resurfacing: quantitative volumetric scar improvement. *Arch Dermatol*. 2010;146:133-140.
35. Alster TS, Khoury R. Treatment of laser complications. *Facial Plast Surg*. 2009;25:316-323.
36. Alster TS. Preoperative preparation for CO_2 laser resurfacing. In: Coleman WP, Lawrence N, eds. *Skin Resurfacing*. Baltimore, MD: Williams & Wilkins; 1998:171-179.
37. Alster TS, Tanzi EL. Complications in laser and light surgery. In: Goldberg DB, ed. *Laser Skin Surgery*. Vol. 2. Philadelphia, PA: Elsevier;2005:103-118.
38. Walia S, Alster TS. Cutaneous CO_2 laser resurfacing infection rate with and without prophylactic antibiotics. *Dermatol Surg*. 1999;25:857-861.
39. Kilmer SL, Chotzen V, Zelickson BD, et al. Full-face laser resurfacing using a supplemented topical anesthesia protocol. *Arch Dermatol*. 2003;139:1279-1283.

40. Bing J, McAuliffe MS, Lupton JR. Regional anesthesia with monitored anesthesia care for dermatologic laser surgery. *Dermatol Clin.* 2002;20:123-134.
41. Ruback BW, Schroenrock LD. Histological and clinical evaluation of facial resurfacing using a carbon dioxide laser with the computer pattern generator. *Arch Otolaryngol Head Neck Surg.* 1997;123:929-934.
42. Fitzpatrick RE, Smith SR, Sriprachya-anunt S. Depth of vaporization and the effect of pulse stacking with a high-energy, pulsed carbon dioxide laser. *J Am Acad Dermatol.* 1999;40:615-622.
43. David L, Ruiz-Esparza J. Fast healing after laser skin resurfacing: the minimal mechanical trauma technique. *Dermatol Surg.* 1997;23:359-361.
44. Ruiz-Esparza J, Barba Gomez JM. Long-term effects of one general pass laser resurfacing: a look at dermal tightening and skin quality. *Dermatol Surg.* 1999;25:169-174.
45. Alster TS, Hirsch RJ. Single-pass CO_2 laser skin resurfacing of light and dark skin: extended experience with 52 patients. *J Cosmet Laser Ther.* 2003;5:39-42.
46. Tanzi EL, Alster TS. Single-pass carbon dioxide versus multiple-pass Er:YAG laser skin resurfacing: a comparison of postoperative wound healing and side-effect rates. *Dermatol Surg.* 2003;29:80-84.
47. Kono T, Chan HH, Groff WF, et al. Prospective direct comparison study of fractional resurfacing using different fluences and densities for skin rejuvenation in Asians. *Lasers Surg Med.* 2007;39:311-314.
48. Wanner M, Tanzi EL, Alster TS. Fractional photothermolysis: treatment of facial and non-facial cutaneous photodamage with a 1,550 nm erbium-doped fiber laser. *Dermatol Surg.* 2007;33:23-28.
49. Alster TS, Tanzi EL, Lazarus M. The use of fractional laser photothermolysis for the treatment of atrophic scars. *Dermatol Surg.* 2007;33:295-299.
50. Hu S, Chen MC, Lee MC, et al. Fractional resurfacing for the treatment of atrophic facial acne scars in Asian skin. *Dermatol Surg.* 2009;35:826-832.
51. Chan NP, Ho SG, Yeung CK, et al. The use of non-ablative fractional resurfacing in Asian acne scar patients. *Lasers Surg Med.* 2010;42:710-715.
52. Kunishige JH, Katz TM, Goldberg LH, et al. Fractional photothermolysis for treatment of surgical scars. *Dermatol Surg.* 2010;36:538-541.
53. Waibel J, Wulkan AJ, Lupo M, et al. Treatment of burn scars with the 1,550 nm nonablative fractional erbium laser. *Lasers Surg Med.* 2012;44:441-446.
54. Saedi N, Petrell K, Arndt K, et al. Evaluating facial pores and skin texture after low-energy nonablative fractional 1440-nm laser treatments. *J Am Acad Dermatol.* 2013;68:113-118.
55. Sriprachya-anunt S, Fitzpatrick RE, Goldman MP, et al. Infections complicating pulsed carbon dioxide laser resurfacing for photo-aged facial skin. *Dermatol Surg.* 1997;23:527-536.
56. Ratner D, Viron A, Puvion-Dutilleul F, et al. Pilot ultrastructural evaluation of human preauricular skin before and after high-energy pulsed carbon dioxide laser treatment. *Arch Dermatol.* 1998;134:582-587.
57. Ross E, Naseef G, Skrobal M, et al. In vivo dermal collagen shrinkage and remodeling following CO_2 laser resurfacing. *Lasers Surg Med.* 1996;18:38-43.
58. Flor PJ, Spurr OK. Melting equilibrium for collagen fibers under stress: elasticity in the amorphous state. *J Am Chem Soc.* 1960;83:1308.
59. Alster TS. On: increased smooth muscle actin, factor XIIIa, and vimentin-positive cells in the papillary dermis of carbon dioxide laser-debrided porcine skin. *Dermatol Surg.* 1998;24:155.
60. Ross VE, Miller C, Meehan K, et al. One-pass CO_2 versus multiple-pass Er:YAG laser resurfacing in the treatment of rhytides: a comparison side-by-side study of pulsed CO_2 and Er:YAG lasers. *Dermatol Surg.* 2001;27:709-715.
61. Zachary CB. Modulating the Er:YAG laser. *Lasers Surg Med.* 2002;26:223-226.
62. Alster TS, West TB. Effect of topical vitamin C on postoperative carbon dioxide resurfacing erythema. *Dermatol Surg.* 1998;24:331-334.
63. Alster TS, Wanitphakdeedecha R. Improvement of post-fractional laser erythema with light-emitting diode photomodulation. *Dermatol Surg.* 2009;35:813-815.
64. Fisher AA. Lasers and allergic contact dermatitis to topical antibiotics, with particular reference to bacitracin. *Cutis.* 1996;58:252-254.
65. Manuskiatti W, Fitzpatrick RE, Goldman MP. Long-term effectiveness and side effects of carbon dioxide laser resurfacing for photoaged facial skin. *J Am Acad Dermatol.* 1999;40:401-411.
66. Friedman PM, Geronemus RG. Use of the 308-nm excimer laser for postresurfacing leukoderma. *Arch Dermatol.* 2001;137:824-825.
67. Grimes PE, Bhawan J, Kim J, et al. Laser resurfacing-induced hypopigmentation: histologic alteration and repigmentation with topical photochemotherapy. *Dermatol Surg.* 2001;27:515-520.
68. Glaich AS, Rahman Z, Goldberg LH, et al. Fractional resurfacing for the treatment of hypopigmented scars: a pilot study. *Dermatol Surg.* 2007;33:289-294.
69. Mamelak AJ, Goldberg LH, Marquez D, et al. Eruptive keratoacanthomas on the legs after fractional photothermolysis: report of two cases. *Dermatol Surg.* 2009;35:513-518.
70. Alster TS, Nanni CA. Pulsed-dye laser treatment of hypertrophic burn scars. *Plast Reconstr Surg,* 1998;102:2190-2195.
71. Haedersdal M, Erlendsson AM, Paasch U, et al. Translational medicine in the field of ablative fractional laser (AFXL)-assisted drug delivery: a critical review from basics to current clinical status. *J Am Acad Dermatol.* 2016;74:981-1004.
72. Bloom BS, Brauer JA, Geronemus RG. Ablative fractional resurfacing in topical drug delivery: an update and outlook. *Dermatol Surg.* 2013;39:839-848.
73. Weiss ET, Geronemus RG. Combining fractional resurfacing and Q-switched ruby laser for tattoo removal. *Dermatol Surg.* 2011;37:97-99.

Chapter 210 :: Nonablative Laser and Light-Based Therapy: Cosmetic and Medical Indications
:: Jeffrey S. Orringer

第二百一十章
非剥脱激光和以光为基础的治疗：美容和医学适应证

中文导读

本章共分为5节：①背景；②围手术期注意事项；③设备类型；④应用；⑤结论。

第一节介绍了非剥脱激光的历史背景。提出非剥脱激光和以光为基础的治疗在产生开放创口，且术后恢复快，并发症少。

第二节介绍了围手术期注意事项，从病人的选择、风险和潜在的并发症、安全措施、麻醉、围手术期的护理五个方面进行阐述。

第三节介绍了非剥脱激光设备的类型，分为可见光、红外线、强脉冲光、射频和超声进行阐述。

第四节介绍了此激光的应用。分为5个方面：①血管性疾病；②色素性疾病；③脱毛；④纹身；⑤皮肤质地。其中闪光灯脉冲染料激光器（PDL）是鲜红斑痣治疗金标准，血管瘤常用PDL治疗，而毛细血管扩张、血管瘤、静脉湖治疗手段较多，如KTP、Nd:YAG激光脉冲染料激光、IPL等。良性色素性病变的治疗通常使用各种波长的Q开关（QS）激光，但也提到了IPL的治疗。脱毛治疗激光，包括长脉冲紫翠宝石（755 nm）、半导体（810 nm）、Nd:YAG（1064 nm）激光及IPL等。作者还指出各种波长的Q开关激光被用来选择性地作用于不同颜色的纹身颗粒，强调了含有二氧化钛（通常为白色或粉红色色块）的纹身颗粒在激光治疗后纹身变黑和人体对纹身颗粒的过敏反应。

第五节总结了以上5个方面其各自对应非剥脱激光的选择、治疗后的副作用及特殊的处理，列于表210-1中。

〔简　丹〕

> **AT-A-GLANCE**
>
> - Nonablative treatments produce no clinical wounds.
> - Nonablative procedures are associated with minimal social downtime and a low risk of complications.
> - Several visible light and infrared wavelengths may be used for nonablative applications.
> - Nonablative devices may be used for a variety of conditions including benign pigmented lesions, vascular lesions, hair removal, tattoo removal, scarring, and wrinkles.

BACKGROUND

Much of modern laser therapy is based on the principle of selective photothermolysis, first detailed by Anderson and Parrish in 1983.[1] In short, this principle states that with the use of a wavelength of light that is preferentially absorbed by a cutaneous target applied over an appropriate pulse duration, a skin structure may be selectively destroyed if adequate energy is delivered. This principle opened the door to a revolution in laser and light-based therapy for a wide variety of both medical and cosmetic applications.

Laser and light-based therapy may be categorized as nonablative when a biologic change is produced without the creation of a clinically relevant wound. Thus, as opposed to ablative laser techniques, nonablative treatments tend to necessitate minimal postprocedure wound care and are associated with a highly favorable risk profile. Although nonablative devices in general may produce results that are sometimes less dramatic than ablative techniques for some indications, they are the clear treatment of choice for a number of aesthetic and medical conditions. For some indications, serial nonablative procedures may produce results that approach or even surpass those that may be obtained from more invasive procedures.

Nonablative lasers may be further categorized as those utilizing visible light or infrared light. In addition, light-based devices that involve a broad band of wavelengths are often referred to as intense pulsed light (IPL) systems. Other energy-based devices that are used in a nonablative fashion such as radiofrequency devices and focused ultrasound systems may also have a variety of aesthetically oriented applications, and these will be reviewed in greater detail elsewhere in the text (Chap. 211). Another increasingly critical subcategory of energy-based systems is that of fractionated or fractional devices. Based on the principle of fractional photothermolysis first reported by Manstein and colleagues in 2004, a fractionated application of laser energy involves numerous microscopically small laser beams applied to the skin with sparing of a percentage of intervening skin surface area.[2] The resulting columns of thermally altered tissue are called microscopic treatment zones (MTZs).[3] These MTZs form the basis of clinical changes while the intervening untreated skin facilitates relatively rapid healing. In this way, patient safety is enhanced while social downtime is minimized.

PERIOPERATIVE CONSIDERATIONS

PATIENT SELECTION

There has been a significant trend in aesthetic medicine toward treatments that produce clear results but minimize interruptions in patients' lives. Nonablative laser therapy is generally associated with the need for rather brief social downtime, but patients must be counseled about the expected healing process. With nonablative treatments for many conditions such as certain vascular lesions and benign pigmented lesions, results are often dramatic and fairly rapid in onset. Alternatively, achieving optimal outcomes for some other indications such as acne scarring and rhytides may require serial procedures and results may be more subtle and develop very gradually. Thus, ideal patients for nonablative laser therapy are those who are willing and able to handle the resulting brief social downtime and who are willing to accept potentially more subtle results for some conditions. Potential candidates for nonablative treatments are generally attracted to the very favorable risk profile of many such procedures.

Patients of any age are reasonable candidates for some forms of nonablative laser therapy, while in other cases, elderly patients or those with severe photodamage may not be ideal patients. For example, nonablative laser resurfacing may produce results that are too subtle for a patient with deep rhytides and profound skin laxity to appreciate a meaningful clinical difference. Patients of either gender are likely to respond to nonablative treatments, and men are now increasingly among those seeking noninvasive laser therapy and other aesthetic procedures.[4]

Particular care must be taken when performing some forms of nonablative laser and light-based procedures on patients with darker skin tones due to an increased risk of postinflammatory dyspigmentation. Although many infrared lasers are essentially "color blind" and may be safely used for patients of any Fitzpatrick skin type, the use of some shorter-wavelength visible-light devices must be undertaken only with great care in patients with more pigmented skin using lower fluences and often with the use of perioperative topical therapies such as hydroquinone. In such cases, initial treatment of small test areas is recommended.

RISKS AND POTENTIAL COMPLICATIONS

Nonablative therapies have become extremely popular in part because of the very low risk of complications associated with the proper use of these devices.[5] However, it is vital to recall that these procedures may, in fact, produce significant complications and a detailed and thorough knowledge of skin optics and cutaneous physiology is necessary to mitigate against these risks.[6-8] Patients must be counseled that infection, scarring, and temporary or even permanent skin discoloration may result from these procedures. In fact, a survey from the American Society for Dermatologic Surgery notes that some nonablative procedures such as laser hair removal result in significant numbers of complications annually—particularly when performed by nonphysicians.[9]

Although many nonablative procedures may create no apparent surface changes in the skin, others may produce some degree of crusting requiring topical therapy such as emollients. Other potential complications include ocular injuries which may be prevented with the use of wavelength-appropriate eyewear and patient safety goggles or corneal shields. Localized tissue reactions such as edema and erythema are associated with many nonablative treatments.

SAFETY

A detailed knowledge of laser safety regulations and procedures is required to optimize the safety of not only patients but also clinical personnel. Basic safety precautions demand the use of wavelength-specific eye protection and the posting of device-specific warning signs on the treatment room door. All windows must be appropriately covered and smoke evacuators used when there are concerns about the formation of a laser plume. Reflective surfaces adjacent to the treatment site should be covered and care must be taken to avoid circumstances that increase the risk of an electrical fire. Many institutions have specific laser privileging processes and policies regarding the potential delegation of any laser treatment. Device-specific in-service training of laser support personnel is required. All safety measures taken should ideally be in accordance with the American National Standards Institute (ANSI) guidelines that describe best practice laser safety methods in health care facilities.

ANESTHESIA

Although media descriptions of various nonablative procedures may suggest that such treatments are virtually painless, pain of variable intensity is often associated with nonablative therapy.[10] Many nonablative procedures may be tolerated without the use of anesthetic techniques whereas others may require a variety of interventions such as the use of topical anesthetic creams, ice applications, forced chilled air, local anesthesia, oral or injectable analgesics, and/or regional nerve blocks. There is great variability in patient tolerance for these treatments, and it is critical to work with each patient to understand his or her needs and expectations to optimize patient comfort. The latter is a critical part of patient satisfaction.

PERIOPERATIVE CARE

Most nonablative laser procedures do not require a specific perioperative topical regimen, but patients with darker Fitzpatrick skin types may be treated with hydroquinone or other agents intended to minimize the risk of postinflammatory dyspigmentation. Commonly, patients are asked to apply petrolatum to treated skin to facilitate healing after laser therapy, particularly when surface changes such as crusting occur. Although the use of antibacterial antibiotics is usually not required, patients with a strong history of herpes simplex may benefit from prophylactic perioperative antiviral medications in some cases. Because many nonablative laser procedures generate significant erythema and edema, topical application of ice and elevation of treated body sites are often advised.

TYPES OF DEVICES

VISIBLE AND INFRARED LASERS AND INTENSE PULSED LIGHT

There is a wide variety of laser systems available for dermatologic uses. Although many lasers, such as the argon, copper vapor, and krypton lasers, are of primarily historical significance in dermatology, others are widely used for a number of applications. The flashlamp-pumped pulsed dye laser, now most commonly used at a wavelength of 595 nm, remains the gold standard device for several applications including the treatment of port-wine stains and a variety of benign vascular conditions that are of significant cosmetic concern to patients. The 532-nm-wavelength potassium titanyl phosphate (KTP) laser is commonly used to treat vascular conditions such as discrete telangiectases and facial hypervascularity. The long-pulsed 1064-nm-wavelength neodymium yttrium-aluminum-garnet (Nd:YAG) laser is commonly used for facial vessels, "spider veins" of the legs, and hair removal, whereas diode lasers (810 nm) are one of the more commonly used systems for hair removal. Another commonly used wavelength, 755 nm, is used by a variety of long-pulsed alexandrite laser systems, with common applications including the treatment of vascular lesions and hair removal. The ruby (694-nm) laser was the first laser used for dermatologic applications, and this wavelength is still employed by some systems in the treatment of both pigment-related and vascular conditions. Carbon dioxide (10,600 nm) and erbium:YAG (2940 nm) lasers are most frequently used for resurfacing applications, but these are considered ablative devices for most applications. However, several other infrared laser systems have been used for nonablative dermal remodeling including both fractionated and nonfractionated systems. Examples of nonfractionated devices include the 1320-nm-wavelength novel Nd:YAG laser, the 1450-nm-wavelength diode laser, and the 1540-nm-wavelength erbium-doped phosphate glass laser. Fractionated nonablative devices include the 1550-nm-wavelength erbium-doped fiber laser as well as a variety of other systems using several other wavelengths (1440, 1540, and 1927 nm, for example). The excimer laser (308-nm) is an ultraviolet light source sometimes used to treat conditions such as psoriasis and vitiligo. Some of the laser wavelengths noted above may be used in Q-switched mode with brief nanosecond-range pulse durations (and more recently with even shorter picosecond pulse durations) to treat pigmented lesions such as lentigines and tattoos. Finally, there are multiple systems available that produce a broad band of visible and infrared light. Although these devices are not truly lasers, such IPL systems have overlapping applications in the treatment of such conditions as vascular lesions, pigmentation, and unwanted hair. These IPL systems usually generate a band of light with wavelengths ranging from about 500 to 1200 nm. Filters are used with these systems to narrow the spectrum of light applied to the skin and to, thereby, more specifically target certain skin chromophores.

The advent of various cooling techniques that are intended to protect the epidermis has, in some cases, allowed for the safe and effective use of higher fluences.[11-13] The most common cooling techniques involve a dynamic cryogen spray, direct contact cooling such as with the use of a chilled sapphire tip, or bulk cooling with the use of a forced cold air chiller unit. By chilling the surface of the skin, the epidermis is cooled even as dermal structures are targeted and complications such as blistering and crusting are often avoided.

RADIOFREQUENCY AND ULTRASOUND SYSTEMS

Several commercially available devices use radiofrequency energy and focused ultrasound waves to create cutaneous changes. In most cases, these systems are used to heat the dermis and and/or subcutaneous structures in a nonablative fashion. Applications include skin tightening, decreasing adipose tissue, and skin rejuvenation via dermal remodeling. These devices and procedures will be reviewed in greater detail in Chap. 211, "Noninvasive Body Contouring."

APPLICATIONS

TREATMENT OF VASCULAR LESIONS

Numerous cosmetic and medical vascular conditions are responsive to nonablative laser therapy. Efficacious devices use wavelengths near peaks in the absorption spectrum for oxygenated hemoglobin. Selective targeting of hemoglobin results in thermal damage to blood vessels within the treated lesions, including coagulation of vessel walls.

PORT-WINE STAINS

Port-wine stains (PWSs) or capillary vascular malformations are relatively common, generally congenital lesions that usually present as pink or red patches at birth (Fig. 210-1). Over a period of years, PWSs grow in proportion to the patient and, because of progressive ectasia of the vessels, may gradually darken such that many are dark red or purple in color by adulthood. Many such lesions also become hypertrophic and may develop discrete vascular papules within them that are a potential source of bleeding.[14] In rare cases, PWSs may be acquired during adolescence or adulthood and their development may be related to trauma to the affected skin.[15,16] In other instances, PWSs may be associated with multisystem conditions such as Sturge-Weber syndrome or Klippel-Trenaunay syndrome (Chap. 147). PWSs may be functionally, psychosocially, and aesthetically impactful, and laser therapy is the treatment of choice for the vast majority of capillary vascular malformations.

A number of continuous-wave lasers such as the argon laser were initially applied to the treatment of PWSs, but complications such as scarring and dyspigmentation due to bulk heating limited their use.[17] With the introduction of pulsed laser systems in the 1980s, the flashlamp-pumped pulsed dye laser (PDL) emerged as the gold standard treatment for PWSs. PDL systems involve a high-power flashlamp whose energy excites organic rhodamine dye. This leads to the production of yellow light of a specific wavelength. Earlier systems used 585-nm-wavelength laser light, whereas more recent PDLs have used a wavelength of 595 nm, thought to be preferable in the treatment of PWSs because of the comparatively increased tissue penetration of the longer wavelength. Relatively short pulse durations (0.45-1.5 msec) are generally used in the treatment of PWSs.[18] This leads to purpura that lasts for approximately 1 to 2 weeks posttreatment. The advent of dynamic cryogen spray cooling to protect the epidermis has allowed for the use of higher fluences, potentially leading to more pronounced results and a decreased risk of complications. A series of treatments, sometimes with progressively higher fluences, is generally required for optimal results. Although only a small minority of have been employed in the treatment of PWSs with varying results. The long-pulsed alexandrite (755-nm) laser and the long-pulsed Nd:YAG (1064-nm) laser have proven useful in treating the exophytic papules that may develop within PWSs. The latter tend to produce less purpura than do PDL systems, but the use of the Nd:YAG laser in the treatment of PWSs has been associated with a relatively increased risk of scarring as compared to the PDL.[20]

The anatomic location of the PWS and its size may impact final clinical results with laser therapy.[21] In general, facial lesions clear more easily at the lateral aspects of the face whereas central facial PWSs of the cheeks and upper lip tend to be more resistant. Larger lesions of the extremities, and in particular of the legs, may be less treatment responsive than those of the trunk or head and neck.[21,22] In addition, smaller lesions tend to clear with laser therapy more completely than do larger PWSs. Some advocate early treatment starting before one year of age, although positive results may be achieved at any age.[22-25]

HEMANGIOMAS

Infantile hemangiomas (IHs) are common benign vascular tumors that generally appear in the first month of life and tend to initially present as a circumscribed erythematous telangiectatic plaque (Chap. 118).[26] These benign proliferations of endothelial tissue undergo a period of growth lasting several months before stabilizing in appearance and then eventually gradually involuting over a period of years.[27] Although many IHs do not require active intervention, others are associated with complications such as bleeding, ulceration, infection, and impingement on vital structures. Such lesions may be treated with a variety of topical or systemic medications and/or laser therapy. The ability of transcutaneous lasers to improve deeper hemangiomas is limited, but PDL treatments do speed re-epithelialization of ulcerated IHs and may halt the growth of some superficial lesions.[26,28] Because of the potential for side effects from the laser therapy itself, treatment should be considered carefully given the natural history of IHs and the expectation of spontaneous involution over time.

Following maximal involution of IHs, about 50% of patients have no trace of the lesion remaining whereas many others are left with residual fibrofatty tissue and telangiectases.[29] PDL treatments (or those using other vascular devices such as IPL or the KTP laser) are quite effective at improving the residual superficial hypervascularity. Fibrofatty tissue has traditionally been treated with surgical excision, but fractionated laser resurfacing has more recently been used to address this issue with promising results.[30]

TELANGIECTASES, ANGIOMAS, VENOUS LAKES

Particularly among patients with lighter skin tones, prominent facial telangiectases are a very common

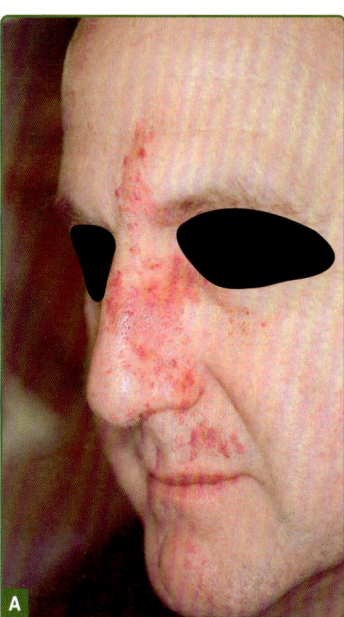

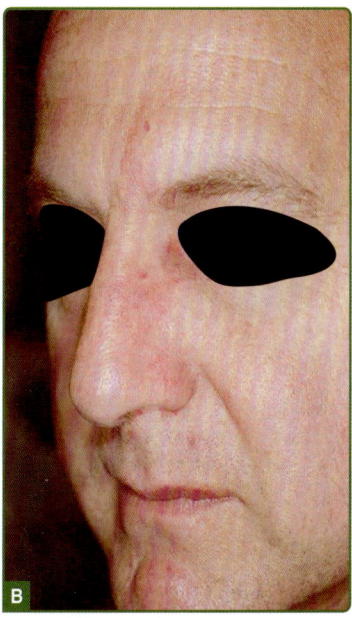

Figure 210-1 Capillary vascular malformation (port-wine stain) of the central face, before (**A**) and after (**B**) serial pulsed dye laser therapy.

PWSs respond completely to laser therapy, the vast majority (more than 85% of patients) demonstrate significant improvement with lightening of at least 50% or better.[18] Some degree of clinical recurrence is fairly common as residual vessels undergo gradual dilation in accordance with the natural history of these lesions.[19] Periodic laser therapy may thus be required to maintain improvements achieved with the initial treatment series.

Other devices including KTP lasers, Nd:YAG lasers, combined PDL/Nd:YAG lasers, and IPL systems also reason for which patients seek cosmetic intervention (Fig. 210-2). Whether based on photodamage, rosacea, autoimmune disorders, or other causes, telangiectasia may be aesthetically problematic. Individual vessels are efficiently treated with KTP and Nd:YAG lasers, usually without resulting purpura. For broad areas of hypervascularity in the setting of photodamage or rosacea, the pulsed dye laser is often highly effective. Newer systems with programmable extended pulse durations (≥6 msec) generally allow for purpura-free treatments. Multiple passes and/or pulse stacking techniques may sometimes be used to enhance efficacy.[31,32] Hypervascular poikiloderma of Civatte may similarly respond well to PDL treatments. IPL treatments are a commonly used and effective alternative for the treatment of facial redness.

A variety of other common benign vascular lesions may be effectively addressed with nonablative laser therapy. Angiomas and venous lakes in particular are common aesthetic issues that are handled nicely with pulsed dye, KTP, or Nd:YAG laser treatments. Typically, only 1 or 2 treatment sessions result in the complete resolution of these lesions. Although surgery or endovenous techniques are generally required for true varicose veins of the legs, smaller prominent vessels may be effectively treated transcutaneously with a variety of systems including the Nd:YAG, alexandrite, diode (940-nm), and pulsed dye lasers. See Chap. 212 for more information on the treatment of leg veins.

TREATMENT OF PIGMENTED LESIONS

Treatment of benign pigmented lesions is frequently performed with Q-switched (QS) lasers of a variety of wavelengths.[33] Care must be taken to appropriately diagnose pigmented lesions to avoid the inadvertent treatment of premalignant or malignant lesions. Laser therapy may lighten the color of such lesions and thereby potentially impede the diagnosis of a pigmented malignancy. Only lesions felt to have no increased risk of malignant degeneration should be treated with laser therapy.[34,35]

LENTIGINES AND SEBORRHEIC KERATOSES

Lentigines are among the most common reasons for patients to seek a cosmetic dermatology consultation. These lesions may be effectively treated with QS-alexandrite, QS-ruby, and frequency doubled (532-nm) QS-Nd:YAG lasers. The latter may more frequently cause some purpura in association with the treatment, but all of these devices are quite effective. Immediately following QS laser treatment, a white frosting of the epidermis transiently appears at the treatment sites. This represents intraepidermal water vapor and the

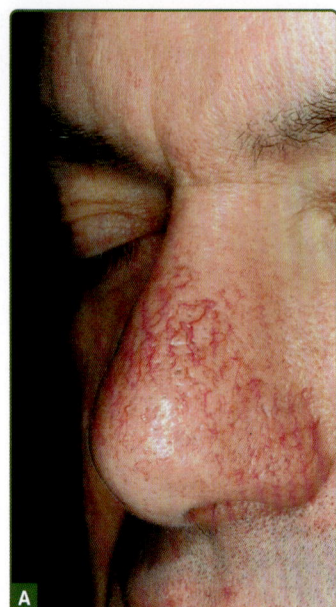
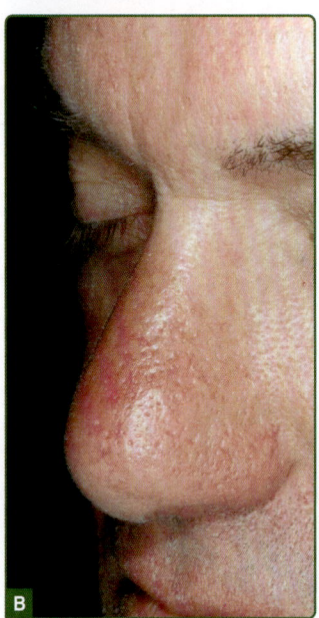

Figure 210-2 Telangiectatic vessels of the nose, before (**A**) and after (**B**) potassium titanyl phosphate (KTP) laser therapy.

whitening effect fades within several minutes. Facial lesions ultimately typically become a bit darker and scaly or develop superficial crusting for approximately 5 days postprocedure, whereas those located on the trunk or extremities may require longer periods (often 1-2 weeks) for healing. IPL is another potentially efficacious treatment for lentigines, although results with this modality are sometimes more gradual and require multiple treatments. Thin seborrheic keratoses also respond nicely to QS laser therapy, with the advantage over cryotherapy of a significantly decreased risk of hypopigmentation and a more predictably favorable outcome.

CAFÉ-AU-LAIT MACULES AND BECKER NEVI

QS lasers using various wavelengths (532, 694, 755, and 1064 nm) are potentially effective for café-au-lait macules and for Becker nevi (Fig. 210-3). The latter respond less consistently. Both types of lesions should initially be treated with test spots of various wavelength lasers to determine which, if any, is most likely to provide a positive outcome. Recurrence of these lesions is possible even after apparent clinical resolution. Even if the pigment within a Becker nevus is only partially responsive to QS laser therapy, the density of hair often seen within these lesions may be reduced with laser hair removal. Hair reduction may provide a significant cosmetic benefit when hypertrichosis is a striking feature.[36]

NEVUS OF OTA AND NEVUS OF ITO

Nevi of Ota and Ito are more commonly seen among Asian patients, with the former located on the face and the latter seen on the neck. These melanocytic lesions are benign but may be aesthetically disfiguring. Given the depth of pigmentation in nevi of Ota and Ito, relatively deeper-penetrating laser wavelengths are generally used. The QS ruby, alexandrite, and Nd:YAG lasers all may be effective for these lesions.[37] Multiple treatments are usually required for maximal correction.

MELASMA

This common but poorly understood condition is often resistant to QS laser and IPL treatments. More recently, nonablative fractionated laser therapy used with conservative energy levels has been performed for this condition with somewhat more encouraging yet variable results.[38,39] New protocols using low-fluence QS 1064-nm-wavelength Nd:YAG lasers are being developed and studied for the treatment of melasma.[40,41] Mainstays of treatment continue to include topical therapies and avoidance of factors including ultraviolet light that tend to exacerbate melasma.

HAIR REMOVAL

Laser hair removal has become among the most commonly performed cosmetic procedures. Lasers or light-based devices work to remove hair by injuring the follicular unit following absorption of energy by its melanin-containing structures. Thermal damage to the follicle ensues, thus preventing new hair growth. There is some controversy as to the exact mechanism(s) of action of laser hair removal in that various authors have proposed the need to destroy cells of the hair bulge and/or the hair bulb to achieve long-term hair removal.[42,43]

Although most patients seek photoepilation for cosmetic reasons, others undergo laser hair removal for medical reasons such as pseudofolliculitis barbae. Patients with excessive hair growth, in particular those with signs of an endocrinopathy, should be evaluated by an endocrinologist. Regardless of the etiology or patient motivation for hair removal, treatment is not effective for white or blond hair because the lack of eumelanin content in such hair does not facilitate adequate absorption of laser energy. Similarly, thick or coarse hair is generally easier to remove than fine hair because there is simply less target chromophore in the more wispy hair seen among some patients. The use of longer-wavelength devices such as the 1064-nm Nd:YAG laser has allowed patients with darker skin tones to be candidates for safe and effective laser hair removal.[44,45] The relatively less pronounced absorption of longer wavelengths by epidermal melanin content decreases the chances of complications such as dyspigmentation, yet the energy is still absorbed well enough by deeper pigment-containing structures in the hair follicle to allow for adequate efficacy.[46] In addition, the use of longer pulse durations in laser hair removal for patients with darker skin tends to heat skin structures more slowly and thus further decreases the risks of hypopigmentation and/or hyperpigmentation. For all patients undergoing laser hair removal, strict

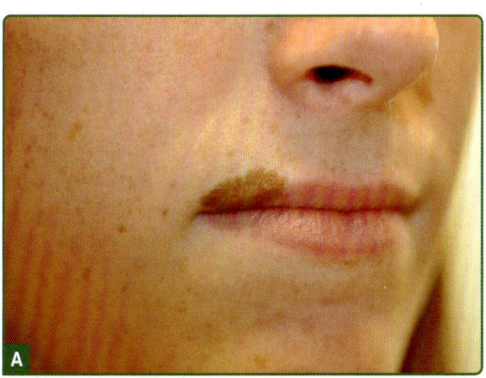

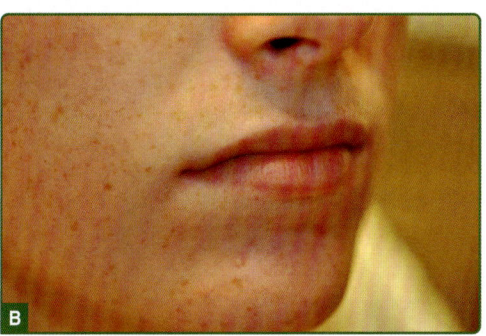

Figure 210-3 Café-au-lait macule of the right upper lip, before (**A**) and after (**B**) Q-switched alexandrite laser therapy.

perioperative sun precautions are necessary to avoid dyspigmentation. Patients must also be instructed to avoid alternative hair removal treatments such as waxing, threading, and plucking that actually remove the target chromophore and render photoepilation ineffective. Shaving unwanted hair is acceptable and, in fact, is routinely performed prior to treatment to allow maximal penetration of laser energy without significant absorption at the surface of the skin. This may help avoid burns due to singeing of surface hair.

Laser or IPL-based hair removal is generally performed as a series of treatments and there is often the need for some degree of maintenance therapy even when long-term hair reduction is achieved. Direct comparative studies seem to indicate that the long-pulsed alexandrite (755-nm) and diode (810-nm) lasers are among the most effective devices for this indication.[46] However, excellent results also have been demonstrated for both the Nd:YAG (1064-nm) laser and several IPL systems. Most devices used for photoepilation include a cooling system to minimize epidermal damage and decrease the potential for complications. Patients can usually expect erythema and perifollicular edema following each treatment, but the need for significant social downtime is uncommon with this procedure. One complication of photoepilation that may be unique to laser hair removal is paradoxical new hair growth in the area surrounding the treatment site.[47] This is more commonly seen in patients of Fitzpatrick types III or IV skin, with new hair formation tending to occur at the margins of treated skin—especially on the face or neck.

TATTOO REMOVAL

The incidence of tattoo acquisition is on the rise and with this trend there is also a growing demand for tattoo removal. In addition to decorative tattoos, other types of tattoos such as embedded graphite pencil material, old radiation markers, gunpowder from explosives, and other material such as gravel from biking or motor vehicle accidents may sometimes be effectively removed with laser therapy. Traditional methods of tattoo removal such as excision and dermabrasion are fraught with the potential for significant scarring. However, in more recent years, QS lasers of various wavelengths have been used to selectively target specific ink colors and thereby lighten or remove tattoos (Fig. 210-4).[48,49] Working via photoacoustic and photomechanical effects, QS devices force exogenous tattoo material within lysosomes to be expelled into the extracellular space. Altered ink particles are then taken up by the lymphatic system. With respect to the principle of selective photothermolysis (Chap. 208), the nanosecond-range pulse durations of QS lasers match nicely with the tiny subcellular ink particles that comprise most tattoos, making for efficient clearance of the ink. More recently, promising results also have been demonstrated with the treatment of tattoos using lasers with pulse widths in the picosecond range.[50,51]

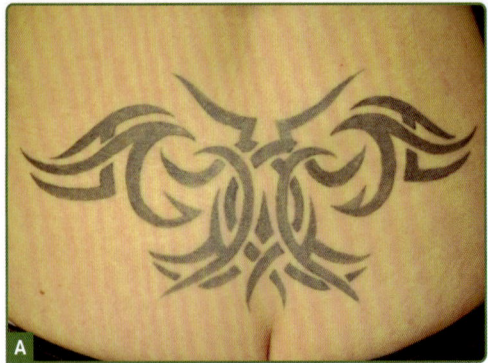
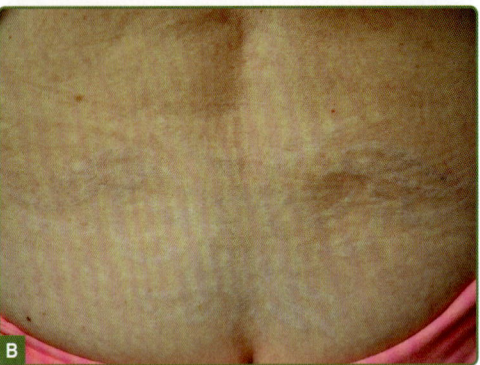

Figure 210-4 Decorative tattoo, before (**A**) and after (**B**) serial Q-switched Nd:YAG laser therapy.

Although there is some variability based on the specific mixture of inks in a given tattoo, in general, black and dark blue ink is addressed well with the QS Nd:YAG (1064-nm) laser, the QS alexandrite (755-nm) laser, or the QS ruby (694-nm) laser. Blue and green inks may be challenging to remove in some cases, but excellent results have been reported with the use of the QS alexandrite and QS ruby lasers as well as the newer picosecond-based devices. Red ink may respond well to the frequency-doubled QS Nd:YAG (532 nm) laser while purple and orange colors are often successfully treated with either the 532-nm- or the 755-nm-wavelength devices. Yellow ink may be difficult to eliminate, but it may respond the QS 532-nm laser.

Treatments may be painful and often require topical or local anesthetics, although some patients tolerate treatments without anesthesia. Edema, blistering, crusting, and pinpoint bleeding are all rather common after laser-mediated tattoo removal, requiring topical applications of petrolatum to speed healing. In many cases, numerous treatment sessions may be necessary to maximally lighten a tattoo, and some colors (yellow, light green, etc) may be particularly resistant. Recently, the so-called R20 treatment method has been proposed. This involves multiple treatment passes performed on the same day but separated by several minutes.[52] Preliminary results imply the potential to decrease the time to tattoo clearance by minimizing the required number of treatment sessions, although practical matters of clinic flow may limit the use of this method in

TABLE 210-1
Nonablative Laser Treatment for Common Dermatologic Indications

	PREFERRED LASERS	POSTTREATMENT EFFECTS AND SPECIAL CONSIDERATIONS
Vascular Lesions		
Port-wine stains	PDL (595 nm) KTP (532 nm) Alexandrite[a] (755 nm) Nd:YAG[a] (1064 nm)	PDL: purpura 1-2 wk posttreatment Nd:YAG: less purpura; slightly increased risk of scarring
Infantile hemangiomas[b]	PDL (595 nm) IPL KTP (532 nm)	PDL can speed re-epithelialization of ulcerated IH
Telangiectases, angiomas, venous lakes	KTP (532 nm) Nd:YAG (1064 nm) PDL (595 nm)	Purpura may occur Multiple passes and/or pulse stacking with the PDL or KTP laser may enhance efficacy
Pigmented Lesions		
Lentigines and seborrheic keratoses	QS alexandrite (755 nm) QS ruby (694 nm) QS frequency-doubled Nd:YAG (532 nm) IPL	Transient white frosting of the epidermis Lesions may darken with superficial crusting ~5 days postprocedure (facial lesions) or 1-2 wk (truncal lesions). Frequency-doubled Nd:YAG: purpura may occur IPL: more gradual improvement with more treatments required
Café-au-lait macules, Becker nevi	QS frequency-doubled Nd:YAG (532 nm) QS ruby (694 nm) QS alexandrite (755 nm) QS Nd:YAG (1064 nm)	Lesions may recur Becker nevi: laser hair removal also may be considered
Nevus of Ota, Nevus of Ito	QS ruby (694 nm) QS alexandrite (755 nm) QS Nd:YAG (1064 nm)	Multiple treatments needed
Melasma	QS Nd:YAG (1064 nm)	Use at low fluences only for melasma Topical therapies are still the mainstay of treatment
Hair Removal		
	Nd:YAG laser (1064 nm) IPL Alexandrite (755 nm) Diode (800-810 nm)	Erythema and perifollicular edema following each treatment Multiple sessions needed Nd:YAG: Safer and effective for darker skin types IPL: Gradual hair reduction but maintenance therapy needed
Tattoo Removal		
Black/dark blue	QS Nd:YAG (1064 nm) QS alexandrite (755 nm) QS ruby (694 nm)	Edema Blistering Crusting Pinpoint bleeding Multiple sessions needed
Blue and green	QS alexandrite (755 nm) QS ruby (694 nm)	
Red ink	QS frequency-doubled Nd:YAG (532 nm)	
Purple and orange	QS frequency-doubled Nd:YAG (532 nm) Alexandrite (755 nm)	
Yellow	QS frequency-doubled Nd:YAG (532 nm)	
Treatment of Textural Changes[c]		
Striae rubra; hypervascular scars	PDL	

[a]Effective for exophytic lesions in port-wine stains.
[b]Laser treatment options covered more extensively in Chap. 118.
[c]Textural changes are further addressed in Chap. 209.
IPL, intense pulsed light; KTP, potassium titanyl phosphate; Nd:YAG, neodymium-doped yttrium aluminum garnet; PDL, pulsed dye laser; QS, Q-switched.

some practices. Initial reports of the use of picosecond lasers to treat tattoos also suggest that clearance may be achieved in fewer treatments for some ink colors.[50] In predicting the outcome of laser treatment of a tattoo, patients may be counseled that large, newer, multicolored professionally placed tattoos are the most difficult to adequately eliminate. Alternatively, small, older, amateur tattoos of a single color tend to respond best.

In addition to standard concerns about complications such as hypopigmentation or scarring, laser treatment of tattoos may also result in a few potential side effects that are unique to this procedure. Some inks may undergo an oxidization reaction when laser energy is applied, resulting in an immediate darkening effect that may or may not respond to additional treatments with alternative devices and wavelengths.[53] Inks containing titanium dioxide (often white or pink colors) are particularly susceptible to this phenomenon. When treating colors of tattoo ink that are known to be at a higher risk for this problem, small test areas should initially be treated and assessed. Some patients may develop an allergic response to the ink within their own tattoo. When this occurs, QS laser treatment of the tattoo is generally to be avoided to mitigate against the possibility of creating a wider spread localized or even systemic allergic reaction.[54] When signs of an allergic response (pruritus, induration, erythema) within a tattoo are noted, patients are often counseled to have the offending ink excised or otherwise treated. Finally, patients who have received systemic gold therapy are at risk for developing localized chrysiasis when treated with a QS laser. A blue-gray discoloration of the skin develops at the sites of laser therapy due to structural alterations in dermal gold deposits.[55]

TREATMENT OF TEXTURE (RHYTIDES, STRIAE, AND SCARS)

Laser treatment of textural changes in the skin is primarily accomplished with the use of ablative or nonablative resurfacing devices, often applied in a fractional manner.[56] This issue is extensively addressed in Chap. 209, "Laser Resurfacing: Cosmetic and Medical Applications." Briefly, by targeting water as the chromophore, both ablative and nonablative systems have been shown to induce dermal remodeling and neocollagenesis that lead to improvements in the quality and texture of skin.[57-59] In addition to devices that are designed to specifically produce alterations in the dermal matrix and collagen, some vascular-specific lasers may also play a role in the treatment of erythematous striae (striae rubra) and hypervascular scars. Pulsed dye lasers are frequently used to target the telangiectatic vessels within scar tissue and stretch marks.[60] Serial treatment is often required for optimal results and, in the case of hypertrophic scars, laser therapy may be combined with intralesional injections of corticosteroids or 5-fluorouracil.

CONCLUSIONS

Nonablative laser therapy provides physicians with an array of tools to treat myriad conditions that are of medical and aesthetic concern to patients (Table 210-1). Advancements in laser design and therapeutic strategies are making laser therapy increasingly effective and safe, but optimal use of these devices requires extensive training and experience. Although highly effective for many indications, even nonablative laser procedures may produce significant complications whose occurrence may be mitigated against by the use of meticulous technique and an extensive knowledge of laser–tissue interactions. The evolution of laser therapy promises to facilitate the treatment of an ever-increasing number of cutaneous problems.

REFERENCES

1. Anderson RR, Parrish JA. Selective photothermolysis: precise microsurgery by selective absorption of pulsed radiation. *Science*. 1983;220(4596):524-527.
2. Manstein D, Herron GS, Sink RK, et al. Fractional photothermolysis: a new concept for cutaneous remodeling using microscopic patterns of thermal injury. *Lasers Surg Med*. 2004;34(5):426-438.
3. Laubach HJ, Tannous Z, Anderson RR, et al. Skin responses to fractional photothermolysis. *Lasers Surg Med*. 2006;38(2):142-149.
4. Rossi AM. Men's aesthetic dermatology. *Semin Cutan Med Surg*. 2014;33(4):188-197.
5. Alam M, Kakar R, Nodzenski M, et al. Multicenter prospective cohort study of the incidence of adverse events associated with cosmetic dermatologic procedures: lasers, energy devices, and injectable neurotoxins and fillers. *JAMA Dermatol*. 2015;151(3):271-277.
6. Graber EM, Tanzi EL, Alster TS. Side effects and complications of fractional laser photothermolysis: experience with 961 treatments. *Dermatol Surg*. 2008;34(3):301-305; discussion 305-307.
7. Hirsch R. Iatrogenic laser complications. *Clin Dermatol*. 2011;29(6):691-695.
8. Setyadi HG, Jacobs AA, Markus RF. Infectious complications after nonablative fractional resurfacing treatment. *Dermatol Surg*. 2008;34(11):1595-1598.
9. Brody HJ, Geronemus RG, Farris PK. Beauty versus medicine: the nonphysician practice of dermatologic surgery. *Dermatol Surg*. 2003;29(4):319-324.
10. Orringer JS, Kovarik HY, Chubb H, et al. A gender-based comparison of pain tolerance during pulsed dye laser therapy. *J Cosmet Laser Ther*. 2014;16(5):253-257.
11. Kao B, Kelly KM, Aguilar G, et al. Evaluation of cryogen spray cooling exposure on in vitro model human skin. *Lasers Surg Med*. 2004;34(2):146-154.
12. Klavuhn KG, Green D. Importance of cutaneous cooling during photothermal epilation: theoretical and practical considerations. *Lasers Surg Med*. 2002;31(2):97-105.

13. Svaasand LO, Randeberg LL, Aguilar G, et al. Cooling efficiency of cryogen spray during laser therapy of skin. *Lasers Surg Med*. 2003;32(2):137-142.
14. Cantatore JL, Kriegel DA. Laser surgery: an approach to the pediatric patient. *J Am Acad Dermatol*. 2004;50(2):165-184; quiz 185-188.
15. Adams BB, Lucky AW. Acquired port-wine stains and antecedent trauma: case report and review of the literature. *Arch Dermatol*. 2000;136(7):897-899.
16. Smoller BR, Rosen S. Port-wine stains. A disease of altered neural modulation of blood vessels? *Arch Dermatol*. 1986;122(2):177-179.
17. Stratigos AJ, Dover JS. Overview of lasers and their properties. *Dermatol Ther*. 2000;13:2-16.
18. Reyes BA, Geronemus R. Treatment of port-wine stains during childhood with the flashlamp-pumped pulsed dye laser. *J Am Acad Dermatol*. 1990;23(6, pt 1):1142-1148.
19. Nelson JS, Geronemus RG. Redarkening of port-wine stains 10 years after laser treatment. *N Engl J Med*. 2007;356(26):2745-2746; author reply 2746.
20. Willey A, Anderson RR, Azpiazu JL, et al. Complications of laser dermatologic surgery. *Lasers Surg Med*. 2006;38(1):1-15.
21. Renfro L, Geronemus RG. Anatomical differences of port-wine stains in response to treatment with the pulsed dye laser. *Arch Dermatol*. 1993;129(2):182-188.
22. Morelli JG, Weston WL, Huff JC, et al. Initial lesion size as a predictive factor in determining the response of port-wine stains in children treated with the pulsed dye laser. *Arch Pediatr Adolesc Med*. 1995;149(10):1142-1144.
23. Ashinoff R, Geronemus RG. Flashlamp-pumped pulsed dye laser for port-wine stains in infancy: earlier versus later treatment. *J Am Acad Dermatol*. 1991;24(3):467-472.
24. Mariwalla K, Dover JS. The use of lasers in the pediatric population. *Skin Ther Lett*. 2005;10(8):7-9.
25. van der Horst CM, Koster PH, de Borgie CA, et al. Effect of the timing of treatment of port-wine stains with the flash-lamp-pumped pulsed-dye laser. *N Engl J Med*. 1998;338(15):1028-1033.
26. Ashinoff R, Geronemus RG. Failure of the flashlamp-pumped pulsed dye laser to prevent progression to deep hemangioma. *Pediatr Dermatol*. 1993;10(1):77-80.
27. Drolet BA, Esterly NB, Frieden IJ. Hemangiomas in children. *N Engl J Med*. 1999;341(3):173-181.
28. David LR, Malek MM, Argenta LC. Efficacy of pulse dye laser therapy for the treatment of ulcerated haemangiomas: a review of 78 patients. *Br J Plast Surg*. 2003;56(4):317-327.
29. Bruckner AL, Frieden IJ. Hemangiomas of infancy. *J Am Acad Dermatol*. 2003;48(4):477-493; quiz 494-496.
30. Laubach HJ, Anderson RR, Luger T, et al. Fractional photothermolysis for involuted infantile hemangioma. *Arch Dermatol*. 2009;145(7):748-750.
31. Rohrer TE, Chatrath V, Iyengar V. Does pulse stacking improve the results of treatment with variable-pulse pulsed-dye lasers? *Dermatol Surg*. 2004;30(2, pt 1):163-167; discussion 167.
32. Tanghetti EA, Sherr EA, Alvarado SL. Multipass treatment of photodamage using the pulse dye laser. *Dermatol Surg*. 2003;29(7):686-690; discussion 690-691.
33. Saedi N, Green JB, Dover JS, et al. The evolution of quality-switched lasers. *J Drugs Dermatol*. 2012;11(11):1296-1299.
34. Jones CE, Nouri K. Laser treatment for pigmented lesions: a review. *J Cosmet Dermatol*. 2006;5(1):9-13.
35. Polder KD, Landau JM, Vergilis-Kalner IJ, et al. Laser eradication of pigmented lesions: a review. *Dermatol Surg*. 2011;37(5):572-595.
36. Lapidoth M, Adatto M, Cohen S, et al. Hypertrichosis in Becker's nevus: effective low-fluence laser hair removal. *Lasers Med Sci*. 2014;29(1):191-193.
37. Chan HH, Kono T. Nevus of Ota: clinical aspects and management. *Skinmed*. 2003;2(2):89-96; quiz 87-88.
38. Halachmi S, Haedersdal M, Lapidoth M. Melasma and laser treatment: an evidenced-based analysis. *Lasers Med Sci*. 2014;29(2):589-598.
39. Rivas S, Pandya AG. Treatment of melasma with topical agents, peels and lasers: an evidence-based review. *Am J Clin Dermatol*. 2013;14(5):359-376.
40. Alsaad SM, Ross EV, Mishra V, et al. A split face study to document the safety and efficacy of clearance of melasma with a 5 ns q switched Nd YAG laser versus a 50 ns q switched Nd YAG laser. *Lasers Surg Med*. 2014;46(10):736-740.
41. Kauvar AN. Successful treatment of melasma using a combination of microdermabrasion and Q-switched Nd:YAG lasers. *Lasers Surg Med*. 2012;44(2):117-124.
42. Grossman MC, Dierickx C, Farinelli W, et al. Damage to hair follicles by normal-mode ruby laser pulses. *J Am Acad Dermatol*. 1996;35(6):889-894.
43. Orringer JS, Hammerberg C, Lowe L, et al. The effects of laser-mediated hair removal on immunohistochemical staining properties of hair follicles. *J Am Acad Dermatol*. 2006;55(3):402-407.
44. Ismail SA. Long-pulsed Nd:YAG laser vs. intense pulsed light for hair removal in dark skin: a randomized controlled trial. *Br J Dermatol*. 2012;166(2):317-321.
45. Rao K, Sankar TK. Long-pulsed Nd:YAG laser-assisted hair removal in Fitzpatrick skin types IV-VI. *Lasers Med Sci*. 2011;26(5):623-626.
46. Bouzari N, Tabatabai H, Abbasi Z, et al. Laser hair removal: comparison of long-pulsed Nd:YAG, long-pulsed alexandrite, and long-pulsed diode lasers. *Dermatol Surg*. 2004;30(4, pt 1):498-502.
47. Alajlan A, Shapiro J, Rivers JK, et al. Paradoxical hypertrichosis after laser epilation. *J Am Acad Dermatol*. 2005;53(1):85-88.
48. Choudhary S, Elsaie ML, Leiva A, et al. Lasers for tattoo removal: a review. *Lasers Med Sci*. 2010;25(5):619-627.
49. Kilmer SL, Anderson RR. Clinical use of the Q-switched ruby and the Q-switched Nd:YAG (1064 nm and 532 nm) lasers for treatment of tattoos. *J Dermatol Surg Oncol*. 1993;19(4):330-338.
50. Brauer JA, Reddy KK, Anolik R, et al. Successful and rapid treatment of blue and green tattoo pigment with a novel picosecond laser. *Arch Dermatol*. 2012;148(7):820-823.
51. Saedi N, Metelitsa A, Petrell K, et al. Treatment of tattoos with a picosecond alexandrite laser: a prospective trial. *Arch Dermatol*. 2012;148(12):1360-1363.
52. Kossida T, Rigopoulos D, Katsambas A, et al. Optimal tattoo removal in a single laser session based on the method of repeated exposures. *J Am Acad Dermatol*. 2012;66(2):271-277.
53. Anderson RR, Geronemus R, Kilmer SL, et al. Cosmetic tattoo ink darkening. A complication of Q-switched and pulsed-laser treatment. *Arch Dermatol*. 1993;129(8):1010-1014.
54. Bernstein EF. A widespread allergic reaction to black tattoo ink caused by laser treatment. *Lasers Surg Med*. 2015;47(2):180-182.
55. Trotter MJ, Tron VA, Hollingdale J, et al. Localized

chrysiasis induced by laser therapy. *Arch Dermatol.* 1995;131(12):1411-1414.
56. Alexiades-Armenakas MR, Dover JS, Arndt KA. The spectrum of laser skin resurfacing: nonablative, fractional, and ablative laser resurfacing. *J Am Acad Dermatol.* 2008;58(5):719-737; quiz 738-740.
57. Orringer JS, Kang S, Johnson TM, et al. Connective tissue remodeling induced by carbon dioxide laser resurfacing of photodamaged human skin. *Arch Dermatol.* 2004;140(11):1326-1332.
58. Orringer JS, Rittie L, Baker D, et al. Molecular mechanisms of nonablative fractionated laser resurfacing. *Br J Dermatol.* 2010;163(4):757-768.
59. Orringer JS, Voorhees JJ, Hamilton T, et al. Dermal matrix remodeling after nonablative laser therapy. *J Am Acad Dermatol.* 2005;53(5):775-782.
60. Alster TS. Improvement of erythematous and hypertrophic scars by the 585-nm flashlamp-pumped pulsed dye laser. *Ann Plast Surg.* 1994;32(2):186-190.

Chapter 211 :: Noninvasive Body Contouring :: Murad Alam

第二百一十一章
无创塑形

中文导读

本章先对无创塑形概念进行讲述，再指出本章主要讲述的三种无创式塑形手段：①皮肤紧致；②减脂；③脂肪团治疗（CELLULITE REMOVAL）。

第一节介绍皮肤紧致，首先告知什么样的皮肤情况和人群适合皮肤紧致，如轻度至中度皮肤松弛而无严重下垂的患者（25～55岁）及对皮肤紧致术反应灵敏的皮肤区域，也讲述了不适用此治疗的皮肤情况。接下来介绍常用皮肤紧致的设备，包括红外激光、射频、高频超声。紧接着是对以上三种治疗的皮肤收缩机制及治疗方式进行简单介绍，其中射频治疗的方式是需多次的低能量治疗，且需紧密排列真皮热损伤区域，插入式射频则需要将一排细小的微针插入皮肤，还简述了二氧化碳（10,600纳米）激光和Nd:YAG（钕:钇铝石榴石）激光紧致皮肤的机制及治疗方法。而对于并发症的治疗管理，作者提出其并发症大部分很轻微，一般是红斑水肿，而射频针可能会留下点状痕迹，二氧化碳激光的副作用则相对较多。根据解剖部位、皮肤类型和反应程度调整治疗方法也是很重要的，治疗躯干和四肢比治疗头颈部时需要更大的能量和更深的穿透深度，但却很少根据皮肤类型改变治疗方案（而二氧化碳激光则需调整）。关于病人对治疗的反映情况，作者根据疼痛感、第一次治疗后的疗效来调整治疗及间歇时间。最后讲述的是预期疗效，通过图211-3展示了在额头和上脸皮肤紧致后眉毛的抬高，再提到了不同身体部位紧致后的皮肤表现。

第二节介绍无创式和微创式减脂，类似上述讲述顺序，作者也是首先告知无创式和微创式减脂的适应证及人群，它最适合饮食及运动后还不能减去的那些多余脂肪，但它无法去除多余的皮肤，即皮肤褶皱。接下来介绍常用减脂技术，无创式包括射频、超声和低温脂解，微创减脂包括化学脂肪溶解、激光脂肪溶解和肿胀法吸脂术。紧接着是对以上减脂技术作用机制的讲述，其中射频和热型超声加热脂肪细胞，机械超声通过传播声波冲击波将脂肪细胞分开，冷冻会破坏脂肪，化学脂肪细胞溶解技术中的化学试剂可乳化脂肪细胞。且并发症较为少见，但也会有术中疼痛感，术后身体外型不对称，低温脂解治疗后可出现局部感觉异常和麻木，化学注射脂肪细胞溶解术会导致治疗后水肿、暂时性下颌边缘神经功能障碍和麻痹，激光脂解可导致皮肤烧灼和血清肿。接着，作者讲述无创式和微创式减脂可广泛应用于身体的各个部位，且适用于所有Fitzpatrick皮肤类型。最后，作者陈述可能达到的预期疗效，局部脂肪减少甚至去除，但不排除将来体重增加和脂肪堆积的情况，并且指出减脂不会收紧皮肤或去除色素。

第三节介绍脂肪团的治疗，先通过图

211-7解释脂肪团是臀部和大腿上部的皮肤凹陷，陈述脂肪团在女性中更常见的原因（图211-8）及脂肪团治疗的预期，并指出理想的病人是20～50岁体重正常且在臀部有局部脂肪团的女性。接下来介绍常用脂肪团治疗技术，包括皮下注射、激光和机械设备、光照和按摩设备。再分别介绍了皮下注射、带有热尖端的侵入式激光设备、非侵入式激光设备、减肥、体育锻炼对脂肪团的作用。脂肪团治疗后最常见的并发症是瘀伤，其对应的处理作者也有描述。最后，作者指出治疗后可能的效果：臀部和大腿皮肤凹陷的改善，但不排除将来会产生脂肪团的可能。

最后指出无创塑形总体疗效可能不如有创的手术治疗，所以无创塑形技术的反复治疗及多种无创塑形技术联合治疗可以最大程度地改善治疗效果。

〔简　丹〕

AT-A-GLANCE

- Noninvasive body contouring includes skin tightening, fat reduction, and cellulite treatment.
- Noninvasive body-contouring treatments are associated with minimal intraoperative risk, postoperative discomfort, and recovery time, but overall effectiveness may be less than for more invasive procedures.
- Improvement in body contouring may be maximized when noninvasive modalities are repeated or used in combination.

BACKGROUND

WHAT IS NONINVASIVE BODY CONTOURING?

In dermatology, body contouring is defined in contradistinction to more superficial skin remodeling. Change in the fine skin texture is thus not considered amenable to treatment by body-contouring methods. On the other hand, body contouring can correct change in skin elevation, shape, and drape associated with full-thickness dermal aging or injury, as well as such change secondary to alteration in the morphology or size of the subcutaneous layer.

Whether a method of body contouring is classified as noninvasive or invasive is predicated on the degree of manual or device-based macroscopic injury to the skin that use of this method entails. This can be a subtle determination. Noninvasive body contouring may be defined by exclusion as typically not requiring scalpel incision or excision, manual dissection of the skin tissue planes, or insertion of devices (eg, suction cannulas, drains, sutures) that are of sufficient size and bore to elicit scarring upon healing. In general, noninvasive procedures are associated with less postoperative discomfort and briefer recovery, requiring minimal time away from work and social activities.

MAJOR TYPES OF NONINVASIVE BODY CONTOURING

Noninvasive body contouring is a rapidly evolving field. As such, the nosology of clinical conditions requiring body contouring remains fluid and subject to change. Currently, the 3 widely recognized therapeutic subtypes of noninvasive body contouring are skin tightening, fat reduction, and cellulite treatment. As is obvious, these treatments are designed to address excess or sagging skin (skin tightening), pockets of unwanted fat (fat reduction), and dimpling of the thighs and buttocks (cellulite treatment). There may be overlap. That is, noninvasive body-contouring modalities used to target a particular condition may favorably impact other skin contour problems at the same anatomic site, albeit to a lesser extent.

PHYSICIAN AND PATIENT PREFERENCE FOR NONINVASIVE BODY CONTOURING

Physicians and patients both have reasons for preferring noninvasive body contouring to invasive contouring procedures. Patients may perceive noninvasive interventions as less "frightening," or safer, and also less drastic or vain than surgery. Those who wish to avoid even the smallest visible scars, or to minimize postoperative downtime, also may be attracted to noninvasive options.

From a physician's standpoint, noninvasive body contouring offers the promise of fewer complications to manage. It is also less time intensive from a provider standpoint, as in some cases much of the work is accomplished by devices that are positioned or injected over the treatment area rather than by direct physician manipulation. Finally, more patients are good candidates for noninvasive body-contouring approaches, which are routinely used to correct minor conditions for which an invasive procedure may be excessive or not indicated.

TYPES OF BODY CONTOURING

SKIN TIGHTENING[1-14]

INDICATIONS AND PATIENT SELECTION

Noninvasive skin tightening is most appropriate for patients with mild to moderate skin laxity without severe sagging. In patients with Fitzpatrick skin types I to III, this usually correlates to ages in the 25 to 55 years range. Focal facial anatomic areas that are responsive to noninvasive tightening include the forehead and brows, the midface, and the neck and jowls. Off the head and neck, skin can be tightened on the upper arms, décolletage area, abdomen, knees, and other areas. Patients appropriate for this procedure expect the possibility of modest improvement, but clearly understand that complete resolution, a so-called home-run, is unlikely except in selected cases of mild skin laxity.

Some types of cosmetic complaints will not resolve with skin tightening. Crepe-like skin with fine superficial textural change will generally not respond. Pigmentary abnormalities must be addressed by vascular or pigment devices, not skin-tightening devices. Extremely saggy skin, with underlying loss of substructure and fat-pad integrity, will not return to its youthful contour after noninvasive tightening. Patients with severe photodamage or severe sagging who would like the gold standard treatment are typically dissuaded from receiving skin tightening. For such concerns, nonablative or ablative resurfacing procedures with or without excisional lifting approaches, such as rhytidectomy, brow lift, or blepharoplasty, may be more successful.

TYPES OF DEVICES AND TECHNOLOGIES

Several distinct technologies have been adapted for skin tightening. These include light-based devices, notably infrared lasers and light sources. Additionally, radiofrequency devices, including monopolar and bipolar devices, as well as more exotic configurations, are in widespread use. Recently, there has been a proliferation of insertional needle and injectable radiofrequency skin tightening devices that skirt the boundary between noninvasive and minimally invasive. High-frequency ultrasound is also commonly used for skin tightening. Devices that have other primary indications, but secondarily induce skin tightening, include ablative resurfacing devices, particularly carbon dioxide laser, as well as insertional infrared laser-tipped devices used in laser lipolysis.

MODES OF ACTION

Fully noninvasive skin tightening spares the epidermis and superficial dermis, and directs energy into the deep dermis and subcutis. This energy, which can be infrared light, radiofrequency, or ultrasound, heats the skin. Precisely directed heat injury results in numerous small volumetric zones of thermal necrosis. The immediate mechanisms of shrinkage include collagen contraction resulting from collagen denaturation, and shrinkage of the fibrous septae of the fat lobules, which compresses the subcutis (Fig. 211-1). It has been suggested that heat-induced shrinkage may also effect superficial muscular aponeurotic system shrinkage, in a manner akin to surgical plication in a facelift, but this is highly speculative and unproven. Longer-term, over a period of 30 to 90 days, neocollagenesis may result in additional skin tightening.

Based on experience with the index device for noninvasive skin tightening, a monopolar radiofrequency[1,2,9-12] device introduced in 2002, several treatment paradigms have been adopted across devices. First, to avoid the risk of skin burns or localized fat atrophy manifesting as configurated skin depressions, several to many lower-energy passes rather than 1 to 2 high-energy passes are typically performed. Second, to maximize effectiveness, zones of thermal necrosis are placed close together, very densely. As many focal necrosis zones as feasible are created in each plane of the dermis, with 2 to 3 such planes not being uncommon. The objective is to maximize the cumulative volumetric injury because this is believed to coincide with the degree of tissue tightening. Of course, some skin must be spared between zones of thermal injury so as to allow prompt, reliable, and scarless wound healing.

Ultrasound[3,4,6,14] is useful for skin tightening because it is a form of energy that can be configured to penetrate arbitrarily deeply into the skin without causing injury to overlying structures. As such, ultrasound for skin tightening can be readily configured to create zones of thermal necrosis at several different levels in the dermis (Fig. 211-2).

Insertional radiofrequency needles[5] penetrate into the skin, with an array of fine microneedles delivering heat to an adjustable depth of less than 1 mm to several millimeters. In this manner, insertional hot needles can achieve many of the same benefits of microfocused ultrasound. Insulated needles may be used to propagate heat just from the needle tips; noninsulated

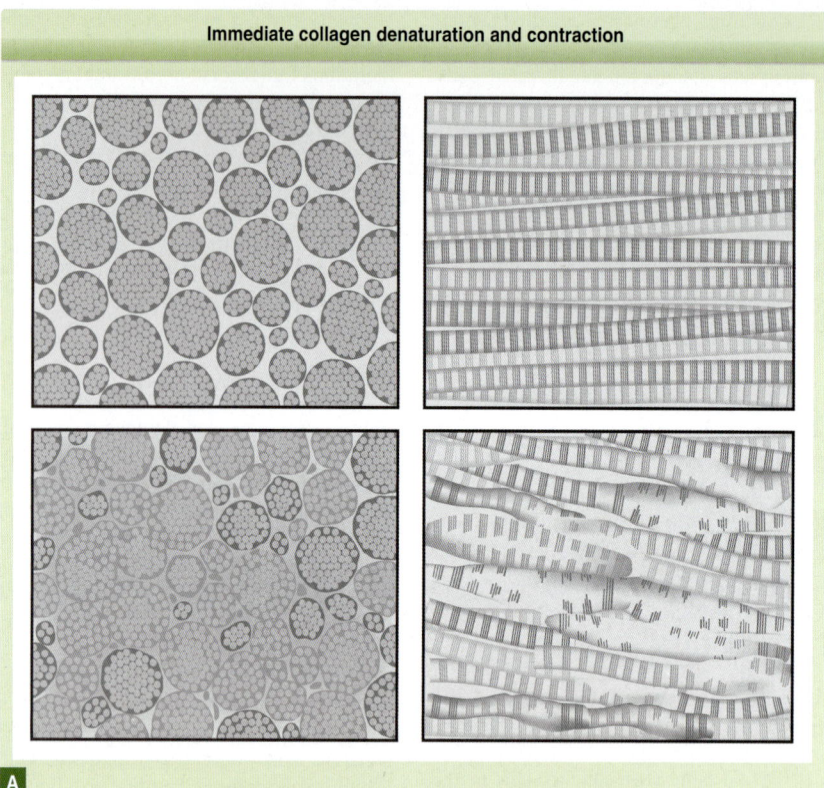

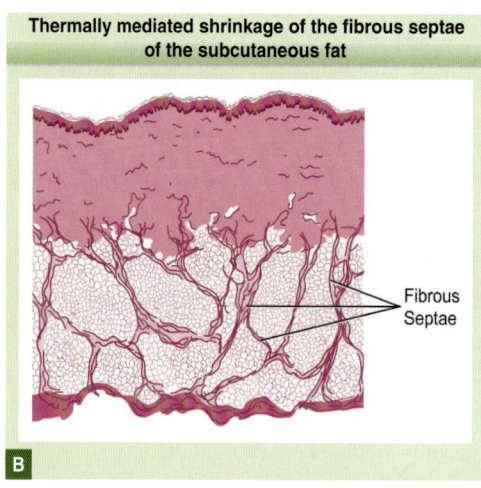

Figure 211-1 Immediate collagen denaturation and contraction (**A**), as well as thermally-mediated shrinkage of the fibrous septae of the subcutaneous fat (**B**), are among the mechanisms of noninvasive skin tightening.

needles leak heat along their whole length, thus potentially causing more tightening at the cost of more of a visible epidermal and superficial dermal injury.

Carbon dioxide (10,600 nm) laser[7,13] ablates the epidermis and partial thickness dermis. Immediate tissue tightening is seen as a result of collagen denaturation. Laser lipolysis operates under the skin surface, as a fine laser fiber encased in a protective metal sleeve is introduced via a skin puncture into the subcutis. The hot laser tip, traditionally an Nd:YAG (neodymium:yttrium aluminum garnet) laser, protrudes from the sheath and is moved back and forth under the dermis to induce heat-related contraction. A handheld temperature gun can be held over the skin by an assistant to ensure that the peak temperature adjacent to the laser tip does not exceed the 40°C to 42°C (100°F to 107.6°F) at which full-thickness injury or burn can occur. In this manner, laser lipolysis can

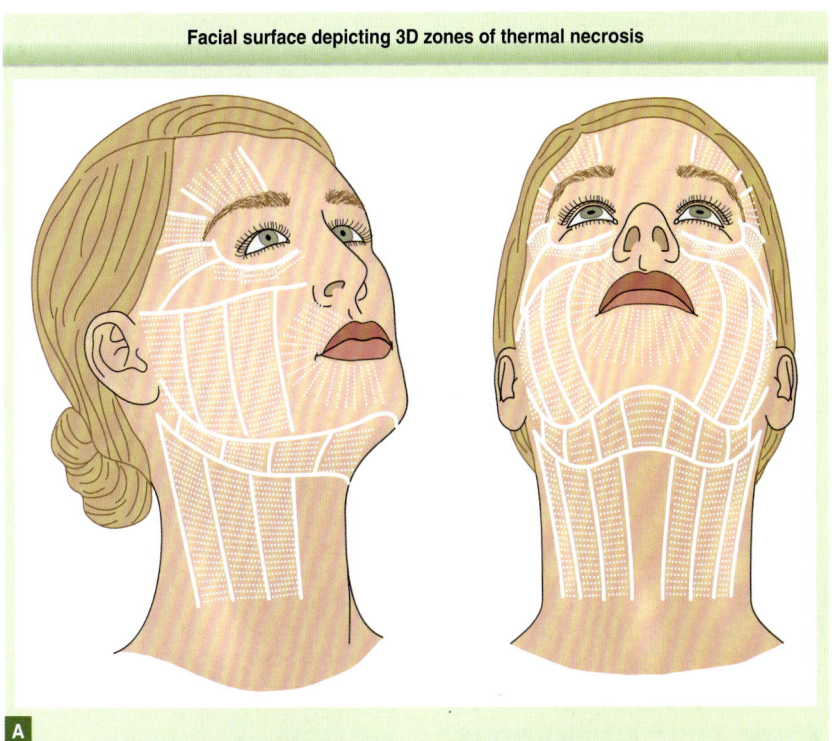

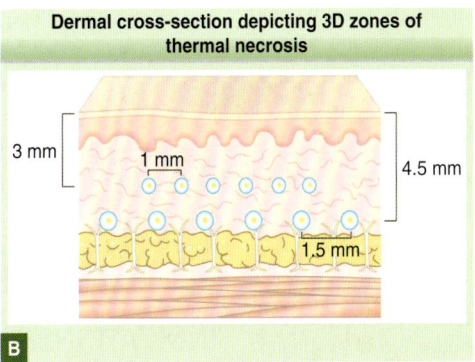

Figure 211-2 Noninvasive skin tightening proceeds by creating minute 3-dimensional zones of thermal necrosis in the dermis, with skin tightening the sum of immediate contraction and collagen remodeling over the ensuing months. Over time, these zones of thermal necrosis are placed ever more densely across the face (**A**) and in multiple planes in the skin (**B**), as demonstrated in these schematics of the facial surface and dermal cross section, respectively.

augment liposuction, which reduces fat but does not tighten skin. Similar radiofrequency wands can be used for skin tightening at multiple sites on the body.

AVOIDING AND MANAGING COMPLICATIONS

Noninvasive skin tightening is generally very safe, with anticipated mild sequelae. Expected posttreatment tissue effects are erythema and edema, lasting from several hours to 1 to 2 days. Intraoperative discomfort can be managed with topical anesthesia or, in some cases, with oral benzodiazepines and analgesics. Because treatment paradigms have moved away from very-high-energy passes, burns and fat atrophy have become rare. Repeated treatment of the same size can very rarely result in heat stacking culminating in white, wheal-like skin plaques, which resolve with time and topical steroids. Scars and pigmentary change are exceedingly rare.

Radiofrequency needling may result in punctate marks on the skin, which resolve over 1 to 2 days. Pinpoint bleeding may also occur with some devices. Rare indented scarring has been reported.

Carbon dioxide laser is routinely associated with more protracted downtime: 1 week for fractional resurfacing and 2 to 3 weeks for traditional full-face resurfacing. Persistent erythema, edema, crust, and serous drainage is common, particularly after full-face resurfacing. Overtreatment and heat stacking with carbon dioxide laser can result in significant adverse events, notably hypopigmentation that does not resolve and scarring.

Laser lipolysis is usually uncomplicated, requiring only healing of the entry sites, which may also have been used for liposuction. Burns, including those associated with full-thickness tears in the skin, can occur if the laser tip is held subdermally at one anatomic location for too long. Overtreatment can also result in seromas, which must be drained promptly. Radiofrequency wands comparable in effect to lipolysis lasers have been optimized for skin tightening, with built-in temperature monitoring that can help prevent burns.

ADAPTING TREATMENTS FOR ANATOMIC AREAS, SKIN TYPES, AND DEGREE OF RESPONSE[15]

A certain minimum density of zones of thermal necrosis is required to elicit the best result. As such, patients with larger faces or bodies may require more total treatment spots or lines. Pain response is subjective and also varies across individuals. Even though noninvasive skin-tightening procedures are always performed with the patient awake, some patients may require anxiolytics or analgesics. There is a very low treatment-associated risk of pigmentary abnormality in patients with darker-pigmented skin; consequently, treatment regimens are not usually adjusted for skin type. Greater care is taken when treating off the head and neck. On truncal and extremity sites, posttreatment healing is slower, and handpieces are adapted to be larger and to deliver energy deeper, as the dermis is thicker.

Depending on treatment response, repeat treatments may be indicated. If a patient is among the minority who experience no or very minimal response, additional treatments may be deferred as they may be similarly futile. Should the patient be willing to try again and incur further costs, then despite the heightened risk of failure, it is reasonable to proceed. More commonly, an observable benefit is obtained after the first treatment. In this case, a patient may receive additional treatments to improve upon this outcome. The average number of treatments per course varies by device and technology, from as few as 1 or 2, to as many as 4 to 6 or more. In some cases, it may be prudent to wait for 2 or 3 months before retreating to allow new collagen to form, as these newly laid-down fibers may be relatively more amenable to subsequent energy-mediated contraction.

Carbon dioxide laser, laser lipolysis, and radiofrequency wand tightening are often single procedures, as their longer-associated postoperative downtime is counterbalanced by greater effectiveness. Carbon dioxide procedures, and to a lesser extent insertional radiofrequency needles, should be used with some caution in patients with darker-pigmented skin so as to minimize the risk of hyperpigmentation. Indeed, the risk of such pigmentation in darker skin types is almost 100% with carbon dioxide laser. Laser lipolysis and subdermal radiofrequency wand tightening are less concerning in darker skin types because they deliver energy under the skin and do not directly injure the epidermis and papillary dermis.

EXPECTED OUTCOMES

After treatment of the forehead and upper face, 1 to 2 mm of brow elevation is commonly seen at 60 to 90 days (Fig. 211-3). Treatments on the lower face may result in modestly more defined jawline or neck contour with slightly reduced skin excess. Midface treatments may result in more subtle skin tightening.

Off the face, outcomes are even more variable. Successful skin tightening on the abdomen, upper and lower knees, décolletage area, and upper arms has been reported. Treatment parameters are modified for these indications.

The degree of tightening or wrinkle reduction is generally modest. Patients with significant skin excess may be better served by a surgical tightening or skin-reduction procedure, or by a minimally-invasive form of skin tightening like carbon dioxide laser, laser lipolysis, or subdermal wand radiofrequency. Alternatively, such patients should be prepared to undergo numerically more treatments of energy-based noninvasive skin tightening for an incrementally greater degree of improvement.

NONINVASIVE AND MINIMALLY INVASIVE FAT REDUCTION[16-31]

INDICATIONS AND PATIENT SELECTION

Noninvasive fat reduction is most appropriate for treatment of small pockets of excess fat resistant to diet and exercise. Treatments with energy-based modalities may result in permanent reduction of such pockets. Early data with cryolipolysis showed that so-called love handles, or protrusions of abdominal fat on either side of the flanks, were particularly responsive to treatment (Fig. 211-4). More recent experience has confirmed that even large subcutaneous collections of abdominal and truncal fat will remit with noninvasive fat reduction, although many serial treatments may be needed.

Noninvasive fat reduction does not reduce excess skin, and may worsen the appearance of skin folds if a substantial quantity of fat is removed because normal skin elasticity is insufficient to retract the skin adequately. For example, after fat-reduction treatment, patients seeking correction of sagging upper arms may observe even more hanging skin. When faced with the

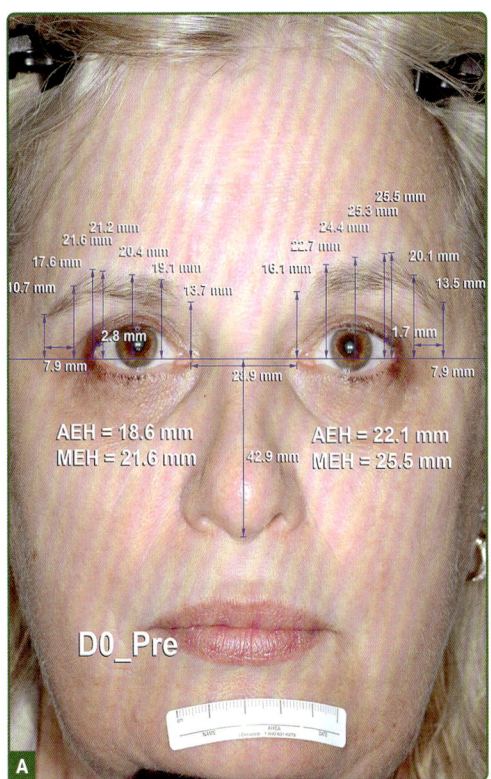
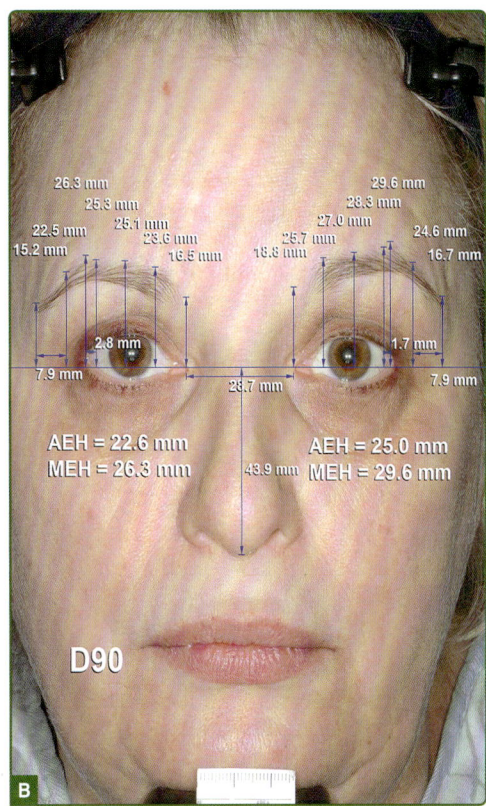

Figure 211-3 Noninvasive skin tightening was first quantitatively demonstrated for brow elevation, which is relatively easier to measure given the availability of anatomic landmarks. More recently, skin tightening has been used on the lower face, neck, and other parts of the body. (From Alam M, White LE, Martin N, et al. Ultrasound tightening of facial and neck skin: a rater-blinded prospective cohort study. *J Am Acad Dermatol*. 2010;62(2):262-69, Fig. 5, with permission.)

risk of exacerbating excess skin, physicians consulting with patients requesting fat reduction should explain the risks. Ideally, susceptible patients should be prepared to undergo, if necessary, a subsequent skin-reduction procedure, such as an elliptical excision to resect upper arm skin. Thermal fat-reduction methods may be slightly more effective in shrinking skin, but the aforementioned constraints still apply.

Fat-reduction treatments do not smooth the appearance of cellulite. Cellulite, or dimpling of the thighs and buttocks, is discussed further in the next section.

TYPES OF DEVICES AND TECHNOLOGIES

Fat reduction can be accomplished with physical modalities, including radiofrequency energy, therapeutic ultrasound, and cryolipolysis. In the United States, cryolipolysis was the first widely used noninvasive treatment for fat, and is the most used and best described approach for this indication. Minimally-invasive approaches include injection chemical adipocytolysis and laser lipolysis. Tumescent liposuction, which accesses fat through tiny apertures that reepithelialize without sutures into barely visible punctate scars also may be considered a form of minimally-invasive fat reduction, but it is incorrectly often considered more invasive than it is. Liposuction is discussed in depth elsewhere in this text.

MODES OF ACTION

The different technologies for noninvasive and minimally-invasive fat reduction span a range of modes of action. As a group, the energy-based modalities[16-21] are more similar than different. Radiofrequency and ultrasound energy targeting fat are configured to direct energy deeper and more diffusely than necessary for tightening skin. Ultrasound fat reduction devices can be further subdivided into thermal and mechanical types. Thermal ultrasound heats adipocytes, as does radiofrequency used for fat destruction, and mechanical ultrasound breaks fat cells apart by propagating an acoustic shock wave.

Cryolipolysis[22-25] is predicated on the mechanism of popsicle panniculitis (Fig. 211-5). Fat is destroyed by freezing while the overlying dermis and epidermis are spared (Fig. 211-6B).

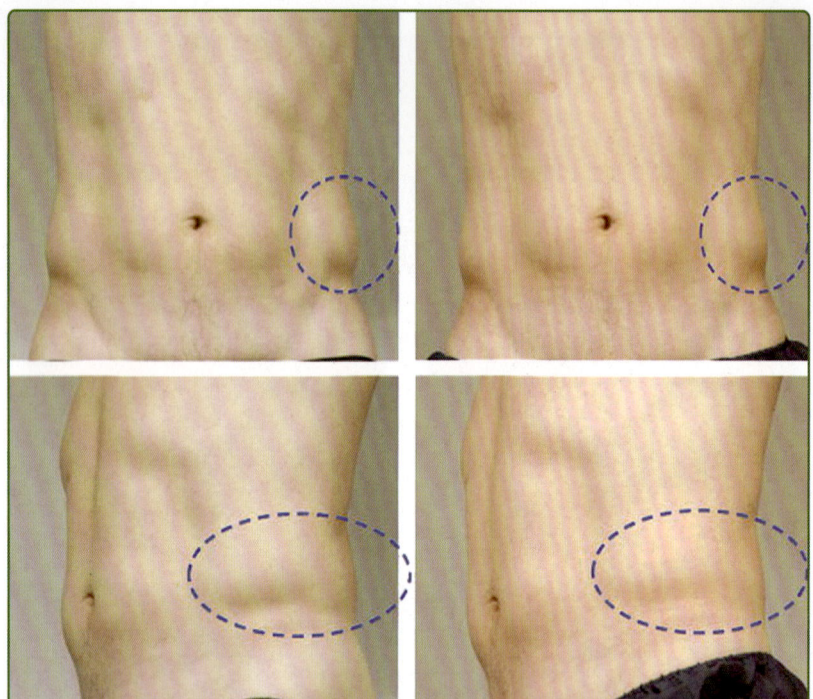

Figure 211-4 Fat reduction by cryolipolysis was first demonstrated to reduce the small fat pockets in the "love handles," as shown in this figure. Noninvasive fat-reduction methods have since been also used to treat larger areas of subcutaneous fat and fat accumulations in the submental area on the neck, using modified handpieces and repeated treatments. (Reprinted by permission from Springer: Coleman SR, Sachdeva K, Egbert BM, et al. Clinical efficacy of noninvasive cryolipolysis and its effects on peripheral nerves. *Aesth Plast Surg.* 2009;33(4):482-488, Fig. 1. Copyright © 2009.)

Chemical adipocytolysis[26-29] employs deoxycholate, a detergent, to emulsify fat cells. It is currently only U.S. Food and Drug Administration (FDA) approved for submental fat reduction (Fig. 211-6A). Laser lipolysis,[30,31] discussed in depth in the previous section on skin tightening, can also melt fat by direct heat injury.

In all cases of noninvasive and minimally invasive fat reduction, fat cells are lysed, with the constituent fatty acids then resorbed into the systemic circulation. For modalities that have proceeded through the FDA premarket approval process, the FDA has requested data regarding blood lipid levels following treatments. Such analyses have shown the absence of a cotemporaneous sharp elevation in lipid levels. This may be attributable to the small quantity of fat cells lysed per treatment, the high intrinsic biologic clearance capacity for fatty acids, or the slow rate at which the products of adipocytolysis are mobilized over many hours to days.

AVOIDING AND MANAGING COMPLICATIONS

Like nonsurgical skin tightening, noninvasive and minimally-invasive fat reduction are safe procedures. Intraoperative tenderness can be managed with oral anxiolytics and analgesics. Tenderness requiring medication is less common with cryolipolysis, as the associated cold sensation inherent to the procedure results in intraoperative pain relief after a few minutes. With heat and shockwave–based modalities, treatment over bony prominences, surgical scars, or hernias is avoided to prevent injury to these structures.

After each treatment of cryolipolysis, local paresthesia and numbness are expected to persist for several weeks before gradually resolving completely. There are extremely rare reports of cryolipolysis actually stimulating fat growth, which then can be corrected by liposuction; these episodes are idiosyncratic and cannot be planned for, predicted, or actively circumvented.

Fat-reduction treatments can result in asymmetry. Similarly, they can result in too much fat being removed, which can lead to a skeletonized, unattractive appearance. The risk of both these outcomes is minimized by carefully mapping the distribution of pretreatment fat. Pinching the fat to be treated can provide the operator with information regarding the quantity and relative distribution of fat. Treatment intensity, duration, and frequency can then be adjusted to meet specific patient needs, and to correct preexisting asymmetries.

It is preferred that patients be at or above their normal weight before a fat reduction treatment regimen. If they diet to a level below their baseline weight prior to treatment, they will likely eventually regain weight after treatment. This new gain may manifest in unexpected areas, as treated pockets of fat will be depleted of

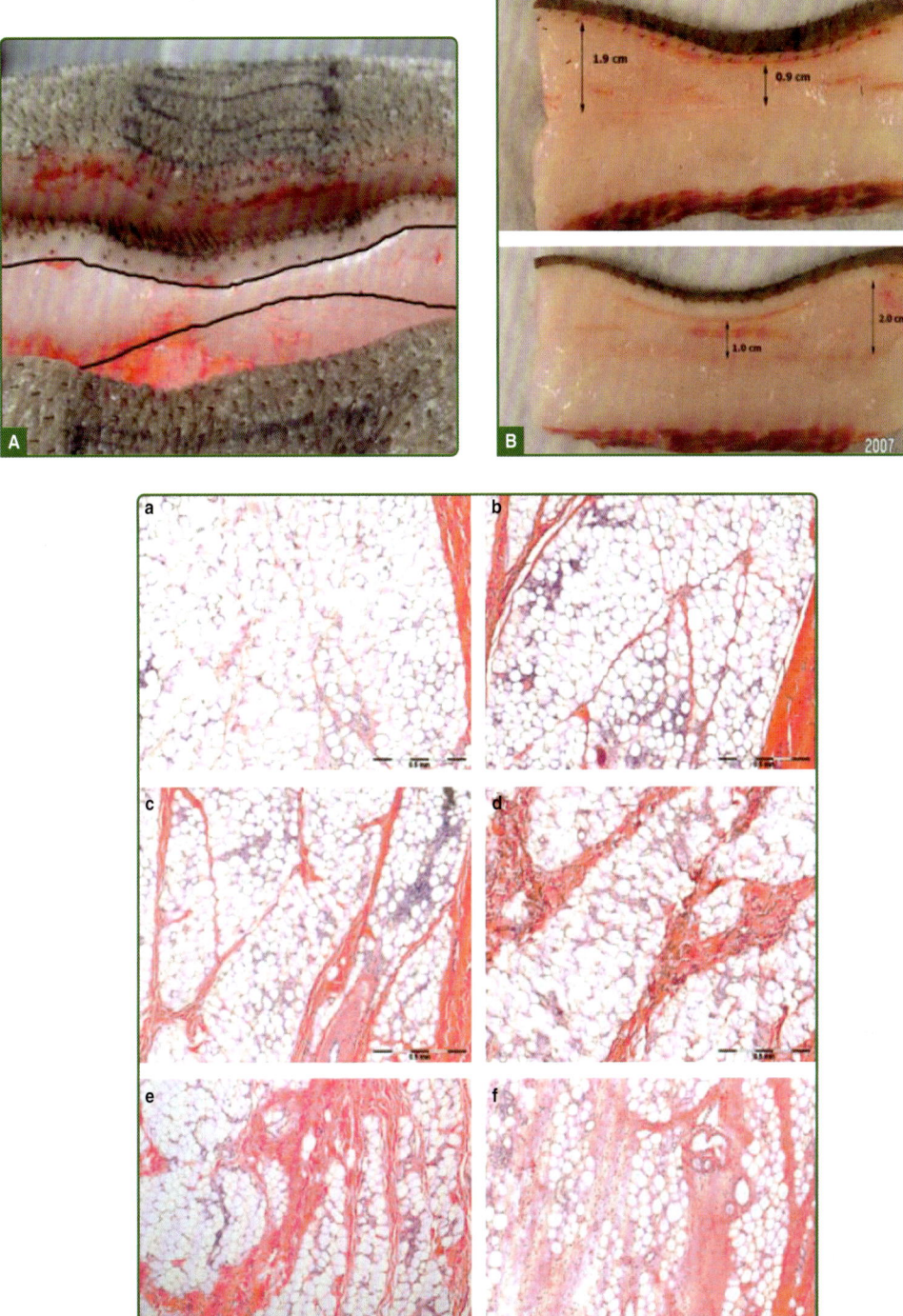

Figure 211-5 Fat shrinkage secondary to cryolipolysis creates a band of cold-mediated injury in the deep subcutis, with this causing shrinkage of the fat layer, in vivo (**A**) and ex vivo (**B**), as shown in this porcine model. Concurrently, there is an inflammatory reaction (**C**) that is easily seen from day 3 (*top left*) to day 90 (*bottom right*). (From Zelickson B, Egbert BM, Preciado J, et al. Cryolipolysis for noninvasive fat cell destruction: initial results from a pig model. *Dermatol Surg*. 2009;35(10):1462-70, Figs. 4, 6, and 8, with permission. © 2009 by the American Society for Dermatologic Surgery, Inc. Published by Wiley Periodicals, Inc.)

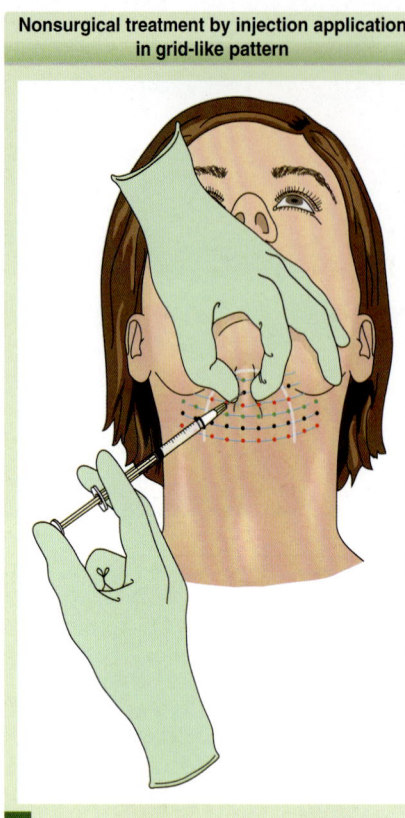 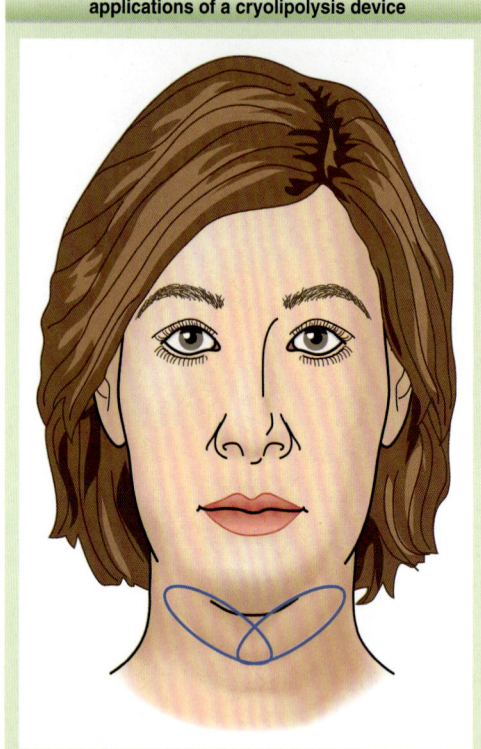

Figure 211-6 Nonsurgical treatment of submental fat can be accomplished by injection of deoxycholate in a grid-like pattern (**A**), or by 2 overlapping applications of a cryolipolysis device (**B**). The marginal mandibular nerve is avoided in both cases.

adipocytes and less able to accommodate future weight gain.

Chemical injection adipocytolysis routinely results in extreme posttreatment edema. Patients receiving such treatment to the submental area may have a "bull frog"–like double-chin and underneck swelling for several days. This can be tender and warm. Injections are best avoided over the course of the marginal mandibular nerve. In a small proportion of cases, chemical injection adipocytolysis results in temporary marginal mandibular nerve dysfunction and palsy, but this resolves completely over several weeks.

Laser lipolysis can result in burns and seromas. These are discussed further in the section on skin tightening.

ADAPTING TREATMENTS FOR ANATOMIC AREAS AND SKIN TYPES

Noninvasive and minimally invasive fat reduction modalities can be safely and effectively applied at a wide range of anatomic sites. Common treatment areas include the neck and submental area, upper arms, upper and lower abdomen, flanks and love handles, thighs, and knees. The feasibility of treatments at a particular site can be limited by the size and shape of available handpieces. For instance, in recent years, specialized cryolipolysis handpieces have been developed to conform to the submental area, thighs, and other areas.

One to several noninvasive or minimally-invasive fat reduction treatments may be needed to reach the desired outcome. Multiple treatments are the norm.

Fat reduction without surgery is appropriate for patients of all Fitzpatrick skin types. Pigmentary abnormality typically does not occur at a higher rate in darker-skinned patients.

EXPECTED OUTCOMES

Fat-reduction treatments can result in partial or complete permanent resolution of small pockets of excess subcutaneous fat that is diet and exercise resistant. Visceral fat, which can be associated with health risks, is not reduced. Patients should be aware that fat-reduction treatments will not tighten skin or erase cellulite, and may even worsen loose skin in older patients.

Repeated treatments with noninvasive modalities can eliminate larger reservoirs of fat for patients willing to tolerate many consecutive treatments as well as the attendant financial cost. Given the intervals between treatments, treatments of large accumulations of fat

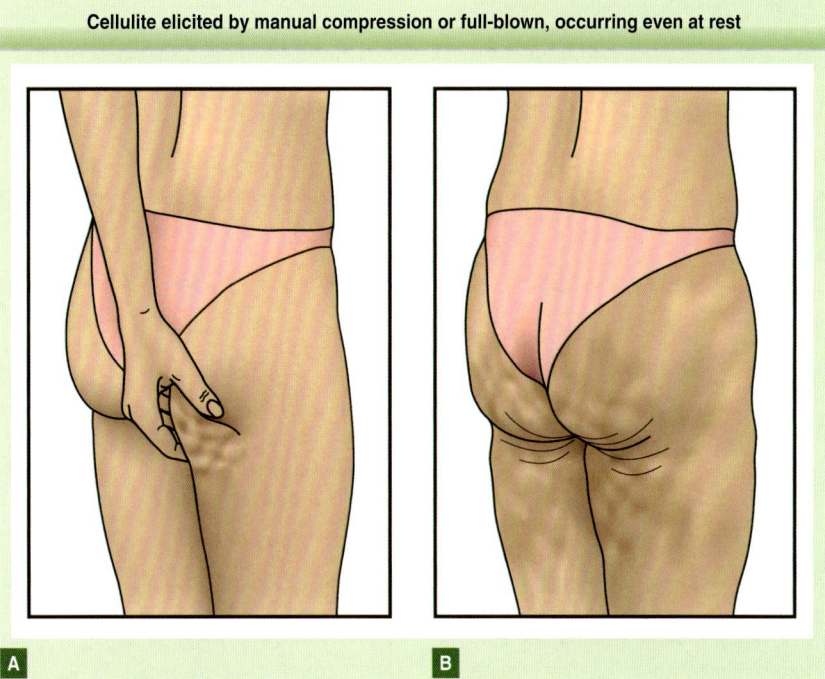

Figure 211-7 Cellulite is the dimpling of the skin on the thighs and buttocks, and can be incipient, elicited by manual compression (**A**) or full-blown, occurring even at rest (**B**).

may require many months or even years to complete. A more efficient one-time procedure like liposuction may be a reasonable alternative. Needless to say, and as discussed before, regardless of the modality used, successful fat removal does not preclude future weight gain, including fat accumulation at untreated anatomic sites.

CELLULITE REMOVAL[32-40]

INDICATIONS AND PATIENT SELECTION

Cellulite was historically a popular rather than a technical term, but is now also in common usage in clinical and research medicine, and serves both functions. Simply, cellulite is skin dimpling of the buttocks and upper thighs (Fig. 211-7). It is more common in women, and may worsen with aging. There is no strong association between overall body weight and cellulite, which is seen frequently in non-overweight individuals.

Cellulite removal technologies are best suited for patients with localized dimpling of the affected areas. Widespread skin rippling, deep creases, and severe excess fat of the upper thighs and buttocks are not corrected with current therapies for cellulite. Younger people tend to respond better, as they often do not suffer from the concurrent issues of skin excess and skin sagging.

It is unclear why cellulite is more common in women than in men (Fig. 211-8). One hypothesis, borne of anatomic studies, is that men have fascial bands in the affected area comprised of crisscrossed rather than parallel fibers. Presumably, these bands are more impermeable to fat herniation, and hence dimpling, than the parallel bands in most women. Whatever the cause, cellulite is markedly more common in women, who also tend to be more bothered by it, and more likely to seek treatment.

Patients seeking cellulite treatment should understand that this will not prevent the formation of new cellulite dimples in the future. Some dimples may not respond at all, and cellulite treatment will not result in fat reduction or a buttock or thigh lift. Multiple treatments may be necessary. A physical exercise regimen also may be recommended as adjunctive therapy. The ideal patient is a 20- to 50-year-old woman of normal weight with a few localized areas of cellulite, mostly on the buttock.

TYPES OF DEVICES AND TECHNOLOGIES

There are several specific therapies for cellulite. Many of these are predicated on the concept of subcision, pioneered for treatment of acne scars by the late Norman Orentreich, a pioneering New York dermatologist who also discovered the scientific basis for hair transplantation. Hypodermic needles, lasers, and mechanical

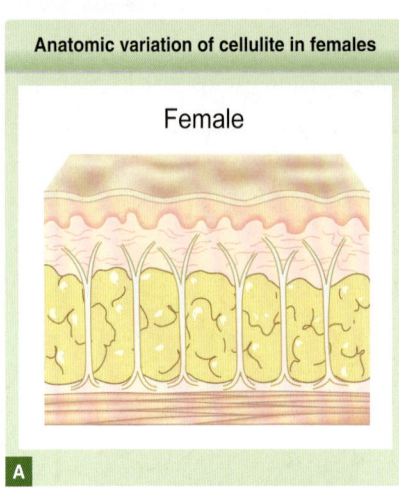
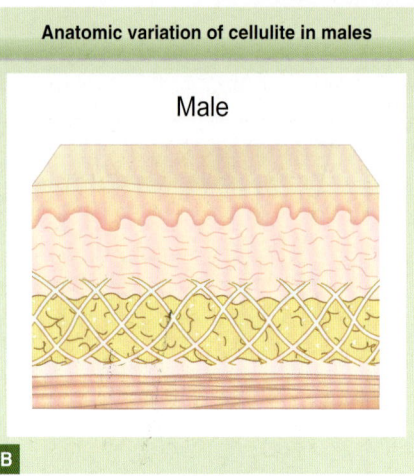

Figure 211-8 Cellulite is believed to be potentiated by anatomic variation, particularly by the parallel fascial bands more characteristic in women (**A**). The fascial bands more typical in men, which are believed to be a more crisscross pattern (**B**), may be more resistant to subcutaneous fat herniation.

devices have been used to correct cellulite. Temporary improvement in the appearance of cellulite can be obtained by noninvasive light and massage devices. Nondevice interventions include physical exercise, but weight loss is less helpful.

MODES OF ACTION

Subcision entails inserting a metal implement with a sharp end through the skin, and then moving it back and forth subdermally in a fanning motion to sever fascial bands and release fibrous attachments around pockets of subcutaneous fat depression or herniation (Fig. 211-9A). This results in elevation of the depressed area by mechanical release. Trauma associated with the procedure can secondarily induce collagen remodeling as well as capillary leaks that culminate in fibrotic plugs that further elevate the depressed area.

Subcision with a hypodermic needle similar to that used for acne scar subcision was shown to be effective for cellulite by Doris Hexsel, a Brazilian dermatologist. Limiting factors were routine bleeding and bruising, and risk of hematoma.

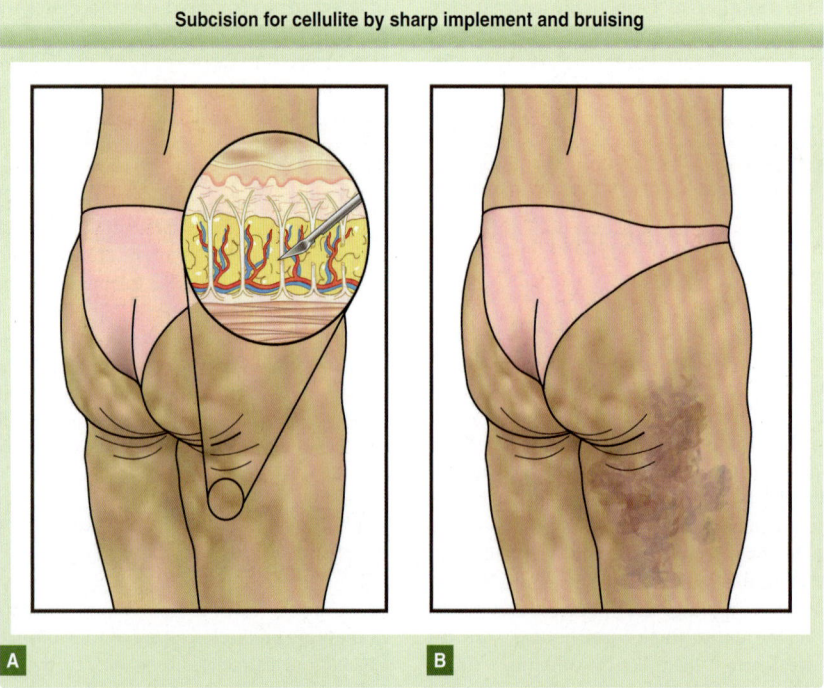

Figure 211-9 Subcision for cellulite entails release of skin dimpling by using a sharp implement in a rasping, fanning motion under the dermis to sever restrictive subcutaneous fibrous septae and fascial bands (**A**). Preoperative infiltration of tumescent anesthesia can mitigate bruising (**B**). More modern device-based variants of this technique are less operator-dependent and less likely to cause pain or bruising.

To make subcision[32-36] for cellulite better tolerated, specific devices have been developed. These aim to minimize disfiguring bleeding and bruising, and to reduce the sensitivity of the procedure to minor differences in operator technique. An insertional Nd:YAG laser device with a hot tip has been used to separate fascial bands and melt fat, while cauterizing small vessels to reduce bleeding. More recently, a device has been developed to mechanically elevate and hold the dermal–subcutaneous junction in place, after which standardized cold needles separate the fascia using a fanning motion. Remaining in the same plane mitigates the risk of injuring peripheral vessels. Device-based subcision for cellulite uses injection of dilute local anesthesia, so-called tumescent anesthesia, to protect skin structures by inflating the skin layers and inducing preoperative vasoconstriction.

Noninvasive laser and light devices, often with multiple heads, have been used to treat cellulite. The FDA guidance for these devices notes that they[37-40] may temporarily improve the appearance of cellulite. The primary mode of action appears to be the induction of edema, which camouflages cellulite dimples. There also may be some degree of mechanical disruption of the cellulite, but this is speculative and has not been definitely shown.

Weight loss does not improve cellulite, which is a condition of the superficial subcutis and not of the deeper fat. Liposuction, by reducing superficial fat, can exacerbate cellulite, although in most cases liposuction is performed to avoid superficial suctioning and therefore has no net effect on cellulite. Physical exercise can improve cellulite by increasing muscle mass. Muscle growth increases the size of the compartment under the fat, pressing the fascia against the subcutis and dermis, and thus flattening cellulite.

AVOIDING AND MANAGING COMPLICATIONS

Bruising is the common, annoying but not serious complication of subcision-based techniques for cellulite reduction. Apart from being tender and impeding social activities in which the affected skin is exposed, bruising can be troublesome, if it resolves with persistent hyperpigmentation. This is more common in patients with darker-pigmented skin, who also may be left with dark marks caused at the point of needle or device insertions.

Bruising in cellulite treatment can be minimized. Sharp injury to small vessels that results in bleeding and bruising can be reduced by employing devices that either cauterize or stabilize the skin tissue during the procedure (Fig. 211-9B). Allowing tumescent anesthesia to set for approximately 30 minutes or longer before the procedure ensures adequate vasoconstriction.

Hematomas and seromas have been reported infrequently and appear to be relatively more likely after application of hot-tipped laser treatments that may induce copious focal trauma. If such fluid accumulation occurs, it needs to be decompressed by syringe extraction or surgical drainage. A preventive strategy is limiting the number of dimples treated at one time in a given contiguous anatomic area.

Like bleeding and bruising, discomfort during the procedure can be managed by application of tumescent anesthesia. Such anesthesia also inflates the skin mechanically, reducing the risk of inadvertent injury to deeper structures and vessels.

ADAPTING TREATMENTS FOR ANATOMIC AREAS AND SKIN TYPES

In general, subcision-based treatments for cellulite are safe for all skin types. Patients with Fitzpatrick skin Type IV and higher may develop hyperpigmentation at the site of ecchymoses or entry sites. Buttock dimpling appears more amenable to treatment than cellulite of the thighs.

EXPECTED OUTCOMES

Treatment of cellulite can result in improvement of small skin dimples of the buttocks and thighs. Several treatments are typically required, and not all dimples will resolve. Better demarcated round dimples will improve more than larger, irregular ones, and buttock dimples may respond better than thigh dimples.

Postoperative bruising and pinpricks at the site of insertion sites may be visible and tender for several days to 2 weeks. Hyperpigmentation in localized patches is possible, but uncommon, and is a greater risk in darker-skinned patients.

Current treatments do not reduce the future risk of developing more cellulite. Physical exercise and stable, normal weight levels may improve cellulite, or at least slow its exacerbation.

MEANS OF OPTIMIZATION

REPEAT THERAPIES

Treatments for skin tightening, fat reduction, and cellulite removal are often performed repeatedly for best effect. The likely number of treatments is dependent on the degree of the problem to be corrected, a discussion with the patient regarding their preference, and practical constraints, like the time required, patient tolerance of discomfort,[41] and aggregate cost. There is increasing evidence that performing many treatments for skin tightening or fat reduction can result in marked and continuous improvement. Treatments are frequently spaced 1 to 3 months apart to allow for wound healing and collagen remodeling prior to retreatment.

COMBINATION THERAPIES

In some cases, improvement may be maximized by using different modalities in combination for the same indication. For instance, several different technologies may be used for fat reduction for optimal effect. Different molecular mechanisms associated with these treatments may augment the cumulative improvement. Again, this requires planning, discussion with the patient, and communication of reasonable expectations.

SUMMARY

Noninvasive body-contouring methods, including skin tightening, fat reduction, and cellulite removal, are emerging technologies. Adverse events are minimal and posttreatment recovery time is brief. Younger to middle-aged adult patients with limited overall skin laxity and sagging are the best candidates. Effectiveness continues to improve and is further enhanced by repeat and combination treatments. Even though some single-intervention invasive surgical procedures for similar indications may be as, or even more, effective, patients are increasingly averse to the risk, scarring, and sense of invasiveness associated with these.

REFERENCES

1. Beasley KL, Weiss RA. Radiofrequency in cosmetic dermatology. *Dermatol Clin*. 2014;32(1):79-90.
2. Weiss RA. Noninvasive radio frequency for skin tightening and body contouring. *Semin Cutan Med Surg*. 2013;32(1):9-17.
3. MacGregor JL, Tanzi EL. Microfocused ultrasound for skin tightening. *Semin Cutan Med Surg*. 2013;32(1):18-25.
4. Minkis K, Alam M. Ultrasound skin tightening. *Dermatol Clin*. 2014;32(1):71-77.
5. Tanaka Y. Long-term three-dimensional volumetric assessment of skin tightening using a sharply tapered non-insulated microneedle radiofrequency applicator with novel fractionated pulse mode in Asians. *Lasers Surg Med*. 2015;47(8):626-633.
6. Gold MH, Sensing W, Biron J. Use of microfocused ultrasound with visualization to lift and tighten lax knee skin (1.). *J Cosmet Laser Ther*. 2014;16(5):225-229.
7. Dainichi T, Kawaguchi A, Ueda S, et al. Skin tightening effect using fractional laser treatment: I. A randomized half-side pilot study on faces of patients with acne. *Dermatol Surg*. 2010;36(1):66-70.
8. Goldberg DJ, Hussain M, Fazeli A, et al. Treatment of skin laxity of the lower face and neck in older individuals with a broad-spectrum infrared light device. *J Cosmet Laser Ther*. 2007;9(1):35-40.
9. Alam M, Levy R, Pajvani U, et al. Safety of radiofrequency treatment over human skin previously injected with medium-term injectable soft-tissue augmentation materials: a controlled pilot trial. *Lasers Surg Med*. 2006;38(3):205-210.
10. Nahm WK, Su TT, Rotunda AM, et al. Objective changes in brow position, superior palpebral crease, peak angle of the eyebrow, and jowl surface area after volumetric radiofrequency treatments to half of the face. *Dermatol Surg*. 2004;30(6):922-928; discussion 928.
11. Vega JM, Bucay VW, Mayoral FA. Prospective, multicenter study to determine the safety and efficacy of a unique radiofrequency device for moderate to severe hand wrinkles. *J Drugs Dermatol*. 2013;12(1):24-26.
12. Carruthers J, Fabi S, Weiss R. Monopolar radiofrequency for skin tightening: our experience and a review of the literature. *Dermatol Surg*. 2014;40(suppl 12):S168-S173.
13. Ortiz AE, Goldman MP, Fitzpatrick RE. Ablative CO_2 lasers for skin tightening: traditional versus fractional. *Dermatol Surg*. 2014;40(suppl 12):S147-S151.
14. Alam M, White LE, Martin N, et al. Ultrasound tightening of facial and neck skin: a rater-blinded prospective cohort study. *J Am Acad Dermatol*. 2010;62(2):262-269.
15. Alam M. What devices to use or not use in skin of color. *Semin Cutan Med Surg*. 2016;35(4):218-222.
16. Robinson DM, Kaminer MS, Baumann L, et al. High-intensity focused ultrasound for the reduction of subcutaneous adipose tissue using multiple treatment techniques. *Dermatol Surg*. 2014;40(6):641-651.
17. Adatto MA, Adatto-Neilson RM, Morren G. Reduction in adipose tissue volume using a new high-power radiofrequency technology combined with infrared light and mechanical manipulation for body contouring. *Lasers Med Sci*. 2014;29(5):1627-1631.
18. Adatto MA, Adatto-Neilson R, Novak P, et al. Body shaping with acoustic wave therapy AWT(®)/EPAT(®): randomized, controlled study on 14 subjects. *J Cosmet Laser Ther*. 2011;13(6):291-296.
19. Jewell ML, Baxter RA, Cox SE, et al. Randomized sham-controlled trial to evaluate the safety and effectiveness of a high-intensity focused ultrasound device for noninvasive body sculpting. *Plast Reconstr Surg*. 2011;128(1):253-262.
20. Nassar AH, Dorizas AS, Shafai A, et al. A randomized, controlled clinical study to investigate the safety and efficacy of acoustic wave therapy in body contouring. *Dermatol Surg*. 2015;41(3):366-370.
21. Saedi N, Kaminer M. New waves for fat reduction: high-intensity focused ultrasound. *Semin Cutan Med Surg*. 2013;32(1):26-30.
22. Zelickson BD, Burns AJ, Kilmer SL. Cryolipolysis for safe and effective inner thigh fat reduction. *Lasers Surg Med*. 2015;47(2):120-127.
23. Munavalli GS, Panchaprateep R. Cryolipolysis for targeted fat reduction and improved appearance of the enlarged male breast. *Dermatol Surg*. 2015;41(9):1043-1051.
24. Garibyan L, Cornelissen L, Sipprell W, et al. Transient alterations of cutaneous sensory nerve function by noninvasive cryolipolysis. *J Invest Dermatol*. 2015;135(11):2623-2631.
25. Wanitphakdeedecha R, Sathaworawong A, Manuskiatti W. The efficacy of cryolipolysis treatment on arms and inner thighs. *Lasers Med Sci*. 2015;30(8):2165-2169.
26. Jones DH, Carruthers J, Joseph JH, et al. REFINE-1, a multicenter, randomized, double-blind, placebo-controlled, phase 3 trial with ATX-101, an injectable drug for submental fat reduction. *Dermatol Surg*. 2016;42(1):38-49.
27. Ascher B, Hoffmann K, Walker P, et al. Efficacy, patient-reported outcomes and safety profile of ATX-101 (deoxycholic acid), an injectable drug for the reduction of unwanted submental fat: results from a phase

III, randomized, placebo-controlled study. *J Eur Acad Dermatol Venereol*. 2014;28(12):1707-1715.
28. Salti G, Ghersetich I, Tantussi F, et al. Phosphatidylcholine and sodium deoxycholate in the treatment of localized fat: a double-blind, randomized study. *Dermatol Surg*. 2008;34(1):60-66; discussion 66.
29. Rotunda AM, Weiss SR, Rivkin LS. Randomized double-blind clinical trial of subcutaneously injected deoxycholate versus a phosphatidylcholine-deoxycholate combination for the reduction of submental fat. *Dermatol Surg*. 2009;35(5):792-803.
30. Leclère FM, Moreno-Moraga J, Mordon S, et al. Laser-assisted lipolysis for cankle remodelling: a prospective study in 30 patients. *Lasers Med Sci*. 2014;29(1):131-136.
31. Alexiades-Armenakas M. Combination laser-assisted liposuction and minimally invasive skin tightening with temperature feedback for treatment of the submentum and neck. *Dermatol Surg*. 2012;38(6):871-881.
32. Green JB, Cohen JL, Kaufman J, et al. Therapeutic approaches to cellulite. *Semin Cutan Med Surg*. 2015;34(3):140-143.
33. Zerini I, Sisti A, Cuomo R, et al. Cellulite treatment: a comprehensive literature review. *J Cosmet Dermatol*. 2015;14(3):224-240.
34. Luebberding S, Krueger N, Sadick NS. Cellulite: an evidence-based review. *Am J Clin Dermatol*. 2015;16(4):243-256.
35. Hexsel DM, Mazzuco R. Subcision: a treatment for cellulite. *Int J Dermatol*. 2000;39(7):539-544.
36. Kaminer MS, Coleman WP 3rd, Weiss RA, et al. Multicenter pivotal study of vacuum-assisted precise tissue release for the treatment of cellulite. *Dermatol Surg*. 2015;41(3):336-347.
37. Russe-Wilflingseder K, Russe E, Vester JC, et al. Placebo controlled, prospectively randomized, double-blinded study for the investigation of the effectiveness and safety of the acoustic wave therapy (AWT(®)) for cellulite treatment. *J Cosmet Laser Ther*. 2013;15(3):155-162.
38. Hexsel D, Siega C, Schilling-Souza J, et al. Noninvasive treatment of cellulite utilizing an expedited treatment protocol with a dual wavelength laser-suction and massage device. *J Cosmet Laser Ther*. 2013;15(2):65-69.
39. Truitt A, Elkeeb L, Ortiz A, et al. Evaluation of a long pulsed 1064-nm Nd:YAG laser for improvement in appearance of cellulite. *J Cosmet Laser Ther*. 2012;14(3):139-144.
40. Mlosek RK, Woźniak W, Malinowska S, et al. The effectiveness of anticellulite treatment using tripolar radiofrequency monitored by classic and high-frequency ultrasound. *J Eur Acad Dermatol Venereol*. 2012;26(6):696-703.
41. Kakar R, Ibrahim O, Disphanurat W, et al. Pain in naïve and non-naïve subjects undergoing nonablative skin tightening dermatologic procedures: a nested randomized control trial. *Dermatol Surg*. 2014;40(4):398-404.

Chapter 212 :: Treatment of Varicose Veins and Telangiectatic Lower-Extremity Vessels
:: Daniel P. Friedmann, Vineet Mishra, & Jeffrey T. S. Hsu

第二百一十二章
下肢静脉曲张和毛细血管扩张的治疗

中文导读

本章介绍了静脉解剖和生理学、流行病学和诱发因素、静脉病理生理学、病史与体格检查、硬化治疗、微创手术治疗静脉曲张。

第一节介绍了深静脉系统、浅表静脉系统，及两者的交通支，并通过图212-1直观展示出来。90%的静脉血从腿部的深静脉系统回流，并重点介绍了浅静脉系统中大隐静脉（GSV）及小隐静脉（SSV）的解剖结构，其中大隐静脉的主要属支见表212-1，而交通支的作用是连接深浅静脉，下肢主要交通支见表212-2。

第二节提出疾病的危险因素，如年龄、性别、妊娠史、家族史、日常行为习惯等与慢性静脉功能不全患病率的关系。提示有妊娠史的中老年女性是易感因素，静脉疾病家族史阳性的患病率更高，并强调疾病严重程度与GSV有关，与SSV无关。

第三节提到静脉病理生理学，分为三个方面讲述，包括静脉瓣膜功能不全、静脉血管壁改变、血流动力学的变化，最终导致静脉高压。

第四节指出病史和体格检查对于了解特定患者的静脉功能不全的性质至关重要，首先是病史的采集，如静脉曲张家族史、妇科疾病，并把静脉曲张治疗的绝对和相对禁忌总结于表212-3。然后，强调体格检查应360度旋转式检查整个患侧下肢，并通过临床-病因-解剖-病理生理学（CEAP）分类工具进行疾病诊断和严重程度的评估（表212-4）。作者提到了诊断此病的金标准——双重超声检查（DUS），它用于定位病变的皮下网状静脉、了解潜在交通支的回流情况、静脉手术之前、诊断性评估及相关鉴别诊断时。

第五节分别介绍三种硬化剂：①洗涤硬化剂；②高渗硬化剂；③化学硬化剂。洗涤硬化剂主要介绍了POL、STS、月桂酸钠及乙醇胺油酸酯，高渗硬化剂介绍高渗盐水、葡萄溶液及甘油，化学硬化剂包括聚碘化碘、乙醇、铬化甘油。并把常用硬化剂的并发症（注射疼痛、色素沉着、坏死、过敏反应）发生情况进行对比，列于表212-5。

还强调治疗最好按顺序进行，最大、最高压的回流源（如隐静脉）应首先处理，最小、最低压的血管（如网状静脉和毛细血管扩张）应最后处理（图212-6），还应注意病人治疗时的体位、注射器的大小，及医生在注射时应该注意的事项。并根据静脉内径

来决定最适合治疗的硬化剂类别和浓度（表212-6）

紧接着，提出了内径大于1mm静脉的标准治疗方法：泡沫硬化疗法联合洗涤剂硬化剂。并指出硬化治疗术后使用腿部弹力袜的重要性，及可能的术后并发症，包括物理性荨麻疹、血凝块的形成、色素沉着及促发因素（表212-7）、毛细血管扩张（Telangiectatic Matting）、皮肤坏死/溃疡、浅静脉血栓性静脉炎、深静脉血栓形成（DVT）、注射剂进入动脉、神经症状，并分别陈述其处理方法。

第六节介绍微创手术治疗静脉曲张，从静脉内消融术/闭塞术、非固定静脉切除术、激光及光治疗三个方面介绍。首先讲述静脉内消融术/闭塞术相对于手术治疗的优点，及作用机制，并提出消融或导致血管闭塞的两种治疗：射频和激光治疗，接着介绍非固定静脉切除术，最后通过血管内血红蛋白对光的吸收峰及选择性光热作用引出激光、IPL等光相关治疗方法。

〔简　丹〕

AT-A-GLANCE

- Reverse venous flow (reflux) is exceedingly common in the general population.
- Age, pregnancy, body mass, and a family history of varicose leg veins all increase the incidence of venous reflux in patients.
- Duplex ultrasound examination can rapidly, effectively, and reproducibly map the superficial venous pathways of the lower extremities and identify sources of reflux in a noninvasive fashion.
- Sclerotherapy is the gold standard treatment for spider veins, although lasers may play an important adjuvant or alternative role.
- Varicose veins are often treated with a combination of endovenous ablation and sclerotherapy or phlebectomy, depending on their underlying cause.

Abnormal lower-extremity veins, from unsightly telangiectasias ("spider veins") to symptomatic varicose veins, affect millions of people worldwide. Although telangiectasias and reticular veins are often considered solely a cosmetic nuisance, they are, like varicose veins, an early manifestation of chronic venous disease (CVD) and may foreshadow the development of advanced CVD, termed chronic venous insufficiency (CVI). Signs and symptoms of CVI have high socioeconomic costs, including reduced quality of life and millions of work days lost per year, in the United States and Western Europe.[1,2]

While telangiectasias and reticular veins may be treated with sclerotherapy or long-pulsed vascular lasers, varicose veins require sclerotherapy (typically with the aid of duplex ultrasound guidance), ambulatory phlebectomy, or endovenous thermal ablation. Successful treatment of lower-extremity venous disease is predicated on the fundamental understanding of venous anatomy, physiology, and patterns of insufficiency; methods of diagnosing venous disease; uses and actions of sclerosing solutions; and the proper use of posttreatment compression.

VENOUS ANATOMY AND PHYSIOLOGY

The venous system of the lower extremities is an intricate, variable network of vessels divided into 3 compartments (superficial, deep, and perforating) that allow for outflow of blood back to the heart and local tissue drainage and thermoregulation (Fig. 212-1). One-way valves are present in veins of all 3 systems, ensuring unidirectional blood flow against gravity, toward the heart.

DEEP VENOUS SYSTEM

The veins of the deep venous compartment lie beneath muscular (aka deep aponeurotic) fascia and act as a conduit for approximately 90% of venous return from the leg. Deep venous blood flow is regulated by the physiologic alternate contraction–relaxation of the calf flexor–extensor skeletal muscles that act as a peristaltic pump. During calf muscle contraction, rising pressure in the deep compartment (up to 250 mm Hg) propels blood through the deep system in a proximal direction with an ejection fraction of 65%.[3] This and the fact that these high pressures close valves of deep and perforating veins prevent retrograde blood flow.

The deep vein system begins in the foot, where the digital and metatarsal veins drain into the deep plantar venous arch or pedal vein, which, in turn, drain into the posterior and anterior tibial veins at the ankle. The tibial veins and peroneal vein actually contribute little

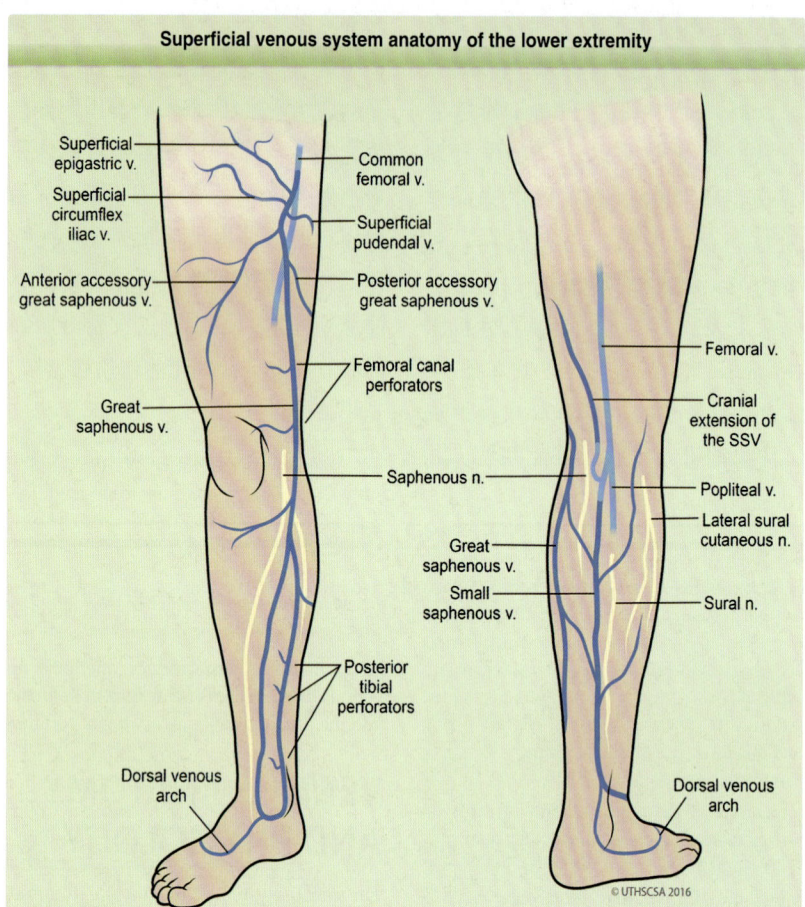

Figure 212-1 Superficial and (pertinent) deep venous system anatomy of the lower extremity. n, Nerve; SSV, small saphenous vein; v, vein. (Reproduced with permission from UT Health Science Center at San Antonio. © UTHSCSA.)

to the calf muscle pump. Instead, it is the large, spiral-shaped gastrocnemius and sural veins that are critical members of the calf muscle pump, directly emptying venous sinuses within the belly of calf muscles. The confluence of these multiple calf veins forms the popliteal vein at or immediately below the knee. The small saphenous vein (SSV) may drain into the popliteal vein at this point, forming the saphenopopliteal junction. The deep femoral regularly communicates with the popliteal vein as well, either directly (38% of cases) or via a tributary (48% of cases).[3]

The popliteal vein becomes the femoral vein at the upper margin of the popliteal fossa and courses through the adductor canal in the middle third of anteromedial thigh.[4] Approximately 9 cm distal to the inguinal ligament, the femoral vein joins the deep femoral vein, creating the common femoral vein.[5] The common femoral vein has multiple veins that drain into it immediately below the inguinal ligament; the most important of these is the great saphenous vein (GSV), forming the saphenofemoral junction (SFJ). The common femoral vein ultimately becomes the external iliac vein at the level of the inguinal ligament.

SUPERFICIAL VENOUS SYSTEM

The cutaneous microcirculation and subcutaneous saphenous truncal veins (and associated veins) comprise the superficial venous network. A network of subdermal reticular veins runs parallel to the skin surface, helping to drain dermal and subcutaneous tissue.

The GSV and SSV are circumscribed by a thin saphenous sheath, which merges with muscular fascia to form the saphenous compartment (Fig. 212-2).[4] Accessory veins are saphenous-like and ascend parallel with saphenous veins, while tributary veins are tortuous and varicose in nature; do not course with saphenous veins; and are a conduit between the saphenous system and reticular vein network. Unlike the GSV and SSV, which are found entirely within the saphenous compartment, accessory and tributary veins lie outside of (ie, superficial to) the saphenous compartment within subcutaneous tissue. The primary exception to this rule is the anterior accessory of the GSV,

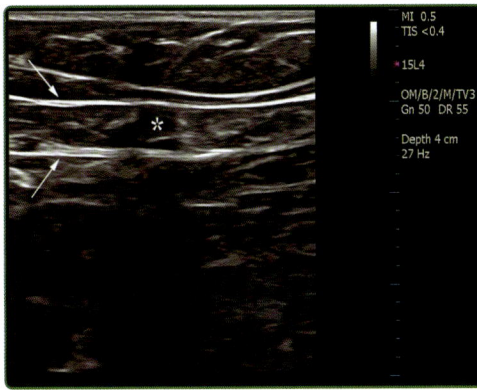

Figure 212-2 Thigh segment of the great saphenous vein (*asterisk*) within the saphenous compartment (*arrows*).

TABLE 212-1
Major Great Saphenous Vein Tributary Veins

LOCATION	NAME	COURSE/FUNCTION
Saphenofemoral junction	Superficial circumflex iliac vein	Drains blood from the groin
	Superficial epigastric vein	Drains blood from abdominal wall
	Superficial/external pudendal vein	Drains blood from the pelvis
	AAGSV	Courses anterolateral to the GSV, aligned over the femoral artery/vein in the proximal thigh
	PAGSV	Courses posterior to the GSV; rarer than the AAGSV
Proximal thigh	Anterior thigh circumflex vein	Ascends obliquely in the anterior thigh, draining into GSV or AAGSV
	Posterior thigh circumflex vein	Ascends obliquely in the posterior thigh, draining into GSV or PAGSV. May originate in SSV or its thigh extension
Leg	Posterior arch vein	Below the knee segment of the PAGSV

AAGSV, anterior accessory of the great saphenous vein; GSV, great saphenous vein; PAGSV, posterior accessory of the great saphenous vein.

which can course anterior to the GSV within its own layer of hyperechoic fascia in the proximal thigh.[5] Nevertheless, the GSV may penetrate the saphenous fascia at the level of the mid or distal thigh, becoming more superficial. True duplication of the GSV is present in the thigh in 8% of cases, and in the calf in 25% of cases, with both vessels lying within the saphenous sheath; unlike the GSV, the SSV is rarely duplicated.[3,6]

The GSV originates in the dorsal foot from the dorsal venous arch and internal marginal vein. It courses anterior to the medial malleolus, ascends the medial calf within the triangle formed by the tibia and medial gastrocnemius, and continues in the anteromedial thigh. Anatomical variations of the GSV and its tributary and accessory veins in the knee and thigh are common.[7,8] The GSV terminates at the SFJ approximately 3 cm inferior to the inguinal ligament (and 3 to 4 cm inferior and lateral to the pubic tubercle), at the level of the groin skin crease (Fig. 212-3).[9,10] The SFJ extends from the termination of the GSV to its preterminal valve and is bound proximally by the suprasaphenic and distally by the infrasaphenic valves of the common femoral vein.[5] Multiple tributaries (Table 212-1) drain into the GSV at the SFJ, with the majority of these doing so within the SFJ between the terminal valve (1 to 2 mm from GSV termination) and preterminal valve (2 to 5 cm distal to the terminal valve) (Fig. 212-4).[11] The preterminal valve ensures that reflux into these tributaries does not occur when the terminal valve is closed.[5]

The saphenous nerve lies anteriorly to the GSV within the saphenous compartment from the medial foot to 2 to 3 cm distal and medial to the tibial tuberosity, supplying cutaneous sensation to the medial aspects of the leg, ankle, and foot. It can run intimately with the vein more than 80% of the time in the distal

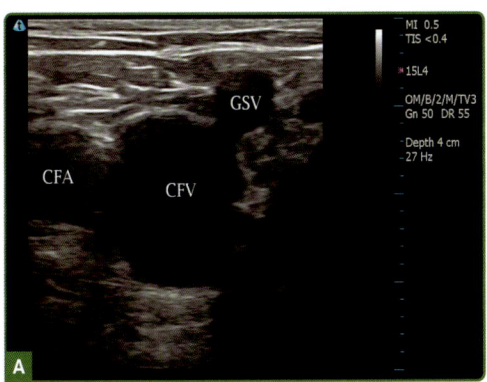
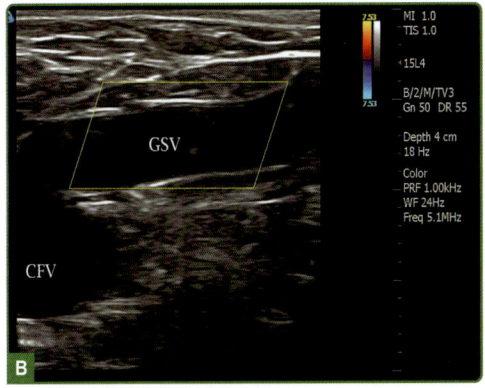

Figure 212-3 The saphenofemoral junction in transverse (**A**) and longitudinal (**B**) views. Note the "Mickey Mouse sign" produced by the relationship of the 3 vessels in transverse view (**A**). CFA, common femoral artery; CFV, common femoral vein; GSV, great saphenous vein.

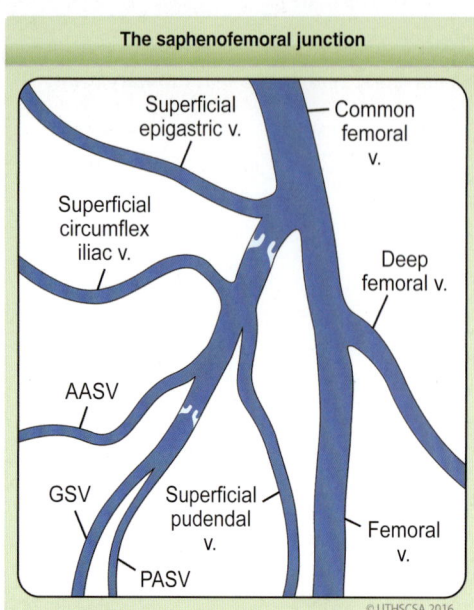

Figure 212-4 The saphenofemoral junction (SFJ). The great saphenous vein (GSV) drains into the common femoral vein at the SFJ, immediately below the inguinal ligament. Numerous tributaries drain into the GSV, primarily between the terminal valve and preterminal valve. AAGSV, anterior accessory of the great saphenous vein; PAGSV, posterior accessory of the great saphenous vein; v, vein. (Reproduced with permission from UT Health Science Center at San Antonio. © UTHSCSA.)

third of the leg (often with the nerve perineum histologically attached to the vein adventitia) and nearly 60% of the time in the middle third of the leg.[12]

The SSV originates in the lateral foot from the dorsal venous arch, coursing posterior to the lateral malleolus and between gastrocnemius muscles in the posterior calf. SSV termination, however, is variable. Sixty percent of the time it drains into the popliteal vein at the saphenopopliteal junction within 5 cm of the popliteal skin crease, with junctional anatomy analogous to that of the SFJ.[10] One-third of the time it drains into the popliteal vein above the knee joint, and below the knee joint in the remaining 5% to 10%.[6] Yet, it may also terminate above the popliteal fossa in another deep vein or thigh GSV, communicate with the popliteal vein but terminate in the thigh GSV, or terminate below the popliteal fossa in another deep vein or leg GSV. When it terminates at the saphenopopliteal junction, the proximal segment of the SSV may actually pierce and lie deep to the deep fascia in order to reach the popliteal fossa, the only significant exception among vessels of the superficial venous system. A proximal SSV segment deep to the deep fascia cannot become grossly incompetent.

A cranial extension of the SSV may continue into the thigh. If it communicates with the GSV in the medial thigh via the posterior thigh circumflex vein, it is often referred to as the *Giacomini vein*. This intersaphenous communicating vein may be significantly more common in patients with combined GSV and SSV incompetence. The sural nerve lies just lateral to the SSV within the saphenous compartment primarily in the distal third of the leg (but may do so as far up as the apex of the calf), after which it travels below the muscular fascia.[3,13] The SSV may also travel in close proximity to the tibial nerve in the popliteal fossa before its termination in the popliteal vein.[14] The tibial nerve provides motor to medial and lateral plantar muscles, while the sural nerve provides cutaneous sensation to the posterolateral leg and lateral foot.

The subdermic lateral venous system of the lateral thigh is often considered the third primary territory of the superficial venous system. It represents the remnant of the embryonic vena marginalis lateralis and is a high-risk area for vein development. A popliteal fossa vein (aka posterior fossa vein) also may be found ascending the upper calf and posterior knee in up to 3% of patients, piercing the deep fascia and emptying into the popliteal vein at a separate junction.[11] Its presence may correlate with a higher propensity for incompetence of the GSV, its tributaries, and adjacent perforating veins.[15]

PERFORATING VENOUS SYSTEM

Perforating veins course through the deep fascia to connect the superficial and deep systems.[16] Perforating veins of the ankle, leg, knee, and thigh direct flow in a *superficial to deep* direction. During calf muscle pump contraction, perforator valves close, preventing flow into the superficial system; when calf muscle relaxation occurs, deep venous pressure is reduced and perforator valves open, resuming flow into the deep system.[3,17] Valvular insufficiency in these veins can thereby lead to outward flow (or sometimes bidirectional flow) into lower pressure saphenous or reticular veins and is frequently associated with reflux in the superficial system.[3,18] Perforating veins of the foot are the exception, normally directing flow toward superficial veins.

Although perforating veins are highly variable in arrangement, connection, size, and distribution, they are best grouped on the basis of their topography.[4] The 4 clinically important locations for perforators are the thigh, knee fold, and upper medial and lower medial leg.[17] Table 212-2 lists these and other perforators. The number and size of competent and the number of incompetent perforating veins correlate directly with the severity of CVD.[18]

EPIDEMIOLOGY AND PREDISPOSING FACTORS

A number of epidemiologic studies provide information regarding telangiectatic and varicose lower-extremity veins and predisposing factors associated with their development. The Edinburgh Vein Study found that in

TABLE 212-2
Major Perforating Veins of the Lower Extremity

LOCATION	SUBLOCATION	NAME	CONNECTION/ROLE
Thigh	Medial thigh	Perforators of the femoral canal (formerly known as the Dodd or Hunterian perforators)	GSV to the proximal popliteal vein in the distal thigh or the femoral vein in the mid thigh
		Inguinal perforators	GSV to the femoral vein in the proximal thigh
	Posterior thigh	Posteromedial and posterolateral thigh, sciatic, and pudendal perforators	
	Other areas	Anterior and lateral thigh perforators	
Knee	Popliteal fossa	Popliteal fossa perforator	SSV to the popliteal vein
	Other areas	Medial knee, lateral knee, suprapatellar, and infrapatellar perforators	
Leg	Medial leg	Paratibial perforators (formerly known as the Boyd perforator)	GSV to the posterior tibial veins in the upper third of the medial leg
		Posterior tibial perforators (formerly known as Cockett perforators)	Posterior accessory GSV of the leg (*posterior arch vein*) to the posterior tibial veins in the mid-to-distal third of the medial leg
	Posterior leg	Medial and lateral gastrocnemius perforators	SSV to the gastrocnemius vein
		Intergemellar perforators	SSV to the soleal vein
		Para-Achillean perforators	SSV to fibular veins
	Other areas	Anterior leg perforators	GSV to anterior tibial vein
		Lateral leg perforators	

GSV, great saphenous vein; SSV, small saphenous vein.

a random sample of 1566 people 16 to 64 years of age, 1316 people (84%) had telangiectasias (88% of women and 79% of men).[19] Of these, 92% of the telangiectasias were graded as mild in severity and were primarily located in the posteromedial aspects of the thigh, popliteal fossa, and proximal calf. Subjects with telangiectasias were significantly more likely to be female (89.7%), more advanced in age (mean: 56.6 vs 34.4 years; $p < 0.001$), and have had a history of pregnancy. Advancing grade of telangiectasia was significantly associated with the presence and severity of varicose veins and increasing incompetence in proximal and distal GSV segments ($p < 0.001$), but not the SSV.[20]

The prevalence of superficial and deep venous reflux increases with age.[21] While segmental venous reflux may be found in superficial and deep veins in subjects without varicosities, the presence of superficial and combined superficial and deep reflux correlate with varicose vein severity.[22] A study of GSV reflux in women with varicose veins also demonstrated progression from segmental to multisegmental reflux over time.[23]

The Edinburgh Vein Study reported rates of GSV incompetence above and below the knee of 2.9% and 7.2% in patients without evidence of CVD, 28.0% and 35.8% in those with varicosities but no signs of CVI, and 51.7% to 55.6% and 44.4% to 68.9% in those with CVI. SSV incompetence prevalence rates in those same categories were 1.7%, 10.8%, and 10.3% to 11.1%, respectively.[24] SSV prevalence rates approaching 30% (alone or in combination with other areas of reflux) have been reported and are likely subject to referral bias.[25,26] The presence of SSV reflux also has been positively correlated with an increased incidence of concurrent deep (popliteal greater than femoral) venous reflux.[6,25]

Long-term followup (mean: 13.4 years) showed disease progression in 193 (57.8%) of 334 patients with varicose veins or CVI at baseline.[27] Risk factors for progression included having both varicose veins and CVI at baseline (63.6% vs 40% with only varicose veins; $p = 0.002$); history of deep vein thrombosis (DVT; 4 times as likely); and family history of varicose veins (nearly twice as likely). In patients with only varicose veins at baseline, disease progression increased with age ($p = 0.04$), with patients older than age 55 years being almost 4 times as likely as those 18 to 34 years old. Family history of varicose veins and overweight/obesity also significantly increased the risk of CVI development twofold. Although men were more likely to have saphenous varicose veins at baseline (39.7% vs 32.2%), the incidence of varicose veins and CVI was not significantly different between genders, increasing proportionately with age.[28,29] Garcia-Gimeno and colleagues,[30] however, found that female gender also increased the frequency (by 1.3 times) of more-severe CVI. Although prolonged standing, dietary intake, and smoking have been postulated to be risk factors for developing varicose veins, evidence is lacking.[31]

Subjects with baseline superficial venous reflux were at twofold risk of ipsilateral clinical progression, with the rate of progression increasing by 1.7 times per refluxing venous segment, 2.6 times with combined superficial and deep reflux, and nearly 5 times with the presence of SSV reflux.[27] Of 306 patients free from reflux at baseline, the incidence of developing reflux over this same followup time was 12.7% (annual incidence of 0.9%). Reflux developed most commonly in the GSV, particularly the lower third of the thigh (8.1% incidence).[32]

A study of 5187 Italian patients demonstrated a

77.3% prevalence of CVD.[33] Men had significantly higher rates of saphenous varicose veins than women (27.4% vs 19.5%; $p < 0.0001$). The rate of saphenous vein incompetence increased rapidly with advancing age, with venous reflux found in 53% of patients older than age 50 years and saphenous varicose veins being 5.9 times more likely than in younger subjects. The prevalence of lower-extremity veins and venous incompetence were significantly higher in subjects with a positive family history of venous disease.

Like in the Edinburgh Vein Study, men demonstrated lower rates of telangiectasias than women (33.4% vs 69.9%), with women being 4 times more likely than men to develop telangiectasia if nulliparous and 5.5 times more likely after having 1 or more children.[34] Women with more than 3 children demonstrated a greater prevalence than nulliparous females with regard to telangiectasias (75.7% vs 63.4%; $p < 0.0001$), saphenous varicose veins (35.5% vs 12.0%; $p < 0.0001$), and non-saphenous varicose veins (50.5% vs 19.6%; $p < 0.0001$).

A history of hormone replacement therapy was significantly more likely in patients with telangiectasias than with no lower-extremity veins in the Edinburgh Vein Study. Interestingly, women without clinically evident leg veins were more likely to have used oral contraceptives than those with telangiectasias (84.4% vs 44.0%; $p < 0.001$). A study of 3590 women by Jukkola and colleagues[35] confirmed that advanced age and higher parity are associated with varicose veins, but found that hormone replacement therapy or oral contraceptive use does not increase their risk.

The most frequent presenting symptom of CVD in the Italian vein study was tired, heavy legs.[33] Tingling, heat sensation, pain, and swelling were also common. Apart from tingling, all were more common in women compared to men but not necessarily age related. Multiparity significantly increased the prevalence and onset of these subjective symptoms in female subjects.

VENOUS PATHOPHYSIOLOGY

Dysfunction of either the superficial, deep, or perforating venous system can create widespread venous hypertension, leading to the abnormal dilation, tortuosity, and dysfunction of superficial veins. Increased deep venous pressure can also result from arteriovenous malformations, pelvic masses, obesity, or sources of intraabdominal pressure.[36] Other potential contributing factors for venous hypertension include combined venous outflow obstruction (DVT or thrombophlebitis) and reflux, calf muscle pump failure, or congenital absence of valves.[37]

The venous system of the lower extremity relies on the interdependent functionality of valves, vein walls, and flow hemodynamics. Disruption of one of these components interferes with the integrity of the others, creating a positive feedback loop that eventuates in pathologic retrograde flow (referred to as reflux), prolonged venous hypertension, and varicose vein formation. Although primary valvular incompetence (disruption or loss) was once thought to be the inciting event for this disease process, recent evidence demonstrates that vein wall alterations precede valvular damage and insufficiency and are thus the primary event.[38] Recent studies suggest that given the frequent occurrence of normal saphenous veins in patients with varicose veins, varicose disease may progressively extend in an antegrade fashion, with a centripetal progression from saphenous tributaries associated with varicose veins toward saphenous veins.[39]

Varicose veins demonstrate significant structural and biochemical defects in cellular and extracellular connective tissue matrix components of all layers of the vein wall, altering venous tone and weakening its structure.[37,38] These include increased collagen, decreased elastin, increased tissue inhibitor of metalloproteinases activity, increased or decreased matrix metalloproteinase activity, and elevated transforming growth factor-β1 and fibroblast growth factor-β, promoting a state of extracellular connective tissue matrix accumulation.[40] These abnormalities are thought to be a product of hemodynamic stresses (eg, hypoxia, mechanical stretch, and low shear stress) and subsequent inflammatory cascades brought on by prolonged venous hypertension and stasis.[41,42]

Valvular incompetence is often multicentric, developing simultaneously in discontinuous venous segments. The hormone-induced and volume-induced venous distensibility and elevated deep venous pressures generated by pregnancy can produce valvular incompetence. Vein diameter and valve closure time of the common femoral vein, femoral vein, popliteal vein, GSV, and SSV significantly increase from the second to the end of the third trimester of pregnancy in primigravid women ($p = 0.001$), reverting to baseline in most cases within 3 months of delivery.[43] Primary valvular insufficiency resulting from degenerative disease with age or thrombophlebitis associated with DVT can affect any venous system.

HISTORY AND EXAMINATION

A thorough history and physical examination is essential to understand the nature of venous insufficiency in a given patient. Past or present signs and symptoms of CVD should be noted, ranging from subjective and nonspecific (eg, discomfort, aching, cramps, fatigue, and heaviness) to objective (eg, edema, dermatitis, pigmentation, and ulceration). A family history of large varicose veins denotes a greater likelihood of truncal varicosities, even when presenting with telangiectasias alone.[44] Symptoms of pelvic congestion syndrome (pelvic pain, aching or heaviness, and dyspareunia) should be ruled out in premenopausal women with varicose veins. Exacerbation of signs and symptoms with menstrual periods should also be documented.

Table 212-3 lists the relative and absolute contraindications to treatment of the superficial venous system.

TABLE 212-3
Contraindications to Treatment of Lower Extremity Veins

RELATIVE CONTRAINDICATIONS[a]	ABSOLUTE CONTRAINDICATIONS
History of SVT, DVT or hypercoagulability	Acute SVT, DVT, or hypercoagulability
Mild PAD	Advanced PAD
Breastfeeding	Pregnancy (1st and 2nd trimester)
Diabetes	Concurrent general anesthesia
Obesity	Immobilized state
Inability to tolerate compression	Prior anaphylaxis to a proposed sclerosing agent
History of lower-extremity trauma	Infection localized to the treatment area or severe generalized infection

[a]Relative contraindications may require evaluation with duplex ultrasound or therapeutic control prior to treatment.
DVT, deep venous thrombosis; PAD, peripheral artery disease; SVT, superficial venous thrombosis.

TABLE 212-4
Clinical-Etiologic-Anatomic-Pathophysiologic (CEAP) Classification Tool

Clinical class	C0	No signs of venous disease
	C1	Telangiectasias or reticular veins
	C2	Varicose veins
	C3	Edema of venous origin
	C4a	Hemosiderin pigmentation or eczematous changes
	C4b	Lipodermatosclerosis or atrophie blanche
	C5	Healed venous ulcer
	C6	Active venous ulcer
Etiology	Ec	Congenital
	Ep	Primary
	Es	Secondary
	En	No venous cause identified
Anatomic Distribution	As	Superficial veins
	Ap	Perforating veins
	Ad	Deep veins
	An	No venous location identified
Pathophysiology	Pr	Reflux
	Po	Obstruction
	Pr,o	Reflux and obstruction
	Pn	No venous pathophysiology identifiable

Although treatment of varicose veins is contraindicated during the first and second trimesters of pregnancy, extremely painful or bleeding varicose veins may be safely treated in the third trimester by endovenous ablation. Treatment is typically postponed, however, as varicosities and telangiectasias may resolve spontaneously within 1 to 6 months postpartum. A history of migraines or a known congenital heart defect should be noted and included in informed consent for sclerotherapy.

Physical examination involves inspection of the entire affected lower extremity in a 360-degree rotation. Telangiectasias ("spider veins") are red to dark blue vessels measuring 1 mm or less in diameter, while reticular veins are deeper, larger (1 to 3 mm), and exhibit a blue or greenish hue. Varicose veins measure 4 mm or larger and are bulging, dilated, and tortuous in nature.[36] Although varicose veins and other cutaneous signs of venous insufficiency are best evaluated with the patient in a standing position; reticular veins are most easily visible when lying prone or supine. The use of transillumination is also helpful in detailing the relationship and extent of reticular veins to telangiectasias. Palpation along saphenous vein distributions helps rule out early varicose veins that are not yet visible. Cutaneous hallmarks of CVD typically appear on the lower leg and medial malleolus and include edema, stasis dermatitis, hemosiderin pigmentation, lipodermatosclerosis, and cutaneous ulceration.[40] The clinical-etiologic-anatomic-pathophysiologic (CEAP) classification system is a descriptive tool that may aid in diagnosis and severity assessment (Table 212-4).[45]

Patients with superficial venous disease limited to scattered telangiectasias and reticular veins without evidence of CVI or associated varicose veins on visual examination do not require further workup. Preoperative duplex ultrasonography (DUS) is not typically required for these aesthetic concerns. However, DUS may still have value in localizing reflux in incompetent subcutaneous reticular veins or underlying perforating veins associated with extensive, treatment-resistant thigh telangiectasias.[46-48] Previous venous surgery also warrants DUS before performing additional treatment.

Asymptomatic or symptomatic varicose veins in a saphenous system distribution, such as the mid or distal thigh, anteromedial calf, extending distally from the popliteal fossa, or extending into the groin require diagnostic evaluation with DUS to evaluate for primary sources of retrograde flow.[10,49] It also may be useful in patients without visible varicosities who have signs and symptoms of venous hypertension suggestive of saphenous vein incompetence, as well as for identifying nonsaphenous sources of reflux caused by incompetent perforators.[50]

DUS remains the gold standard diagnostic study because of its noninvasive, reliable, and cost-effective venous imaging, providing far greater diagnostic accuracy than continuous-wave Doppler ultrasound.[49] Progressive improvements in the ease-of-use and portability of DUS devices have allowed them to largely supersede the use of more invasive, limited, and outdated diagnostic options, such as venography and plethysmography. Current DUS devices can superimpose Doppler information on areas of blood flow within a grayscale B-mode (time-delay) image as a graduated color scale (red and blue) based on

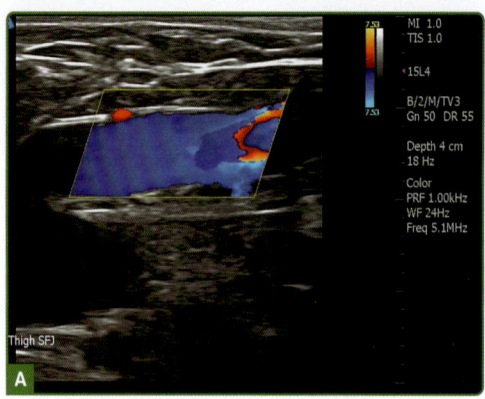 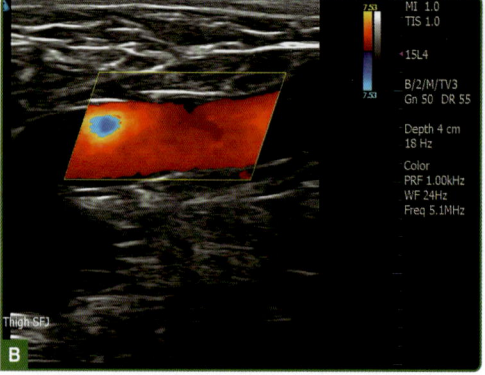

Figure 212-5 Duplex ultrasound examination of the saphenofemoral junction. **A,** Manual compression at the apex of the calf increases antegrade blood flow in the saphenofemoral junction. Blood flow should cease almost immediately upon release. **B,** Retrograde blood flow (reflux) time greater than 500 msec is abnormal. Blue and red colors represent bidirectional flow relative to a stationary duplex ultrasound transducer.

direction and speed. Detection of physiologic reflux is best evaluated with the patient standing upright or in 45-degree reverse Trendelenburg position (tilted-table technique). The deep vein system is first evaluated to rule out obstruction. Failure to fully compress a vein with downward pressure along with the presence of intraluminal echogenicity is highly suspicious for thrombus. The superficial venous system is then evaluated for obstruction and reflux. Manual compression at the apex of the calf increases antegrade blood flow that should cease almost immediately upon release. Valsalva maneuver may additionally be used to elicit reflux at the SFJ. Reflux times greater than 500 msec are considered to be abnormal (Fig. 212-5). Mean and maximal vein diameter should also be documented.[51]

SCLEROTHERAPY

Derived from the Greek word for *hard*, the term *sclerotherapy* describes the introduction of a foreign substance into the lumen of a vessel, causing endothelial damage (endosclerosis) and transient vasospasm with subsequent fibrotic occlusion and eventual obliteration.[52] The fitting term *endovascular chemoablation* also has been proposed. Sclerotherapy remains an excellent primary treatment option for cutaneous veins of all sizes and adjuvant therapy to endovenous procedures for saphenous veins and ambulatory phlebectomy for saphenous tributaries and varicose veins.[53]

HISTORICAL ASPECTS

Although sclerotherapy was first attempted in 1682, when Zollikofer of St. Gallen, Switzerland, injected an acid intravenously to produce a thrombus, the foundations of modern sclerotherapy began in the early 20th century. Scharff (1910) first reported venous thrombosis and sclerosis from the use of mercuric chloride for the intravenous treatment of syphilis.[54] Linser confirmed these findings and began using 20% hypertonic saline (HS) in 1921. Biegeleisen reported the first treatment of telangiectasias in the 1930s using sodium morrhuate. Although McAusland first popularized sclerotherapy in the United States in 1939, it was not until a safe synthetic sclerosing agent, sodium tetradecyl sulfate (STS), was developed in 1946 that sclerotherapy began to be seriously studied in the country. Renewed interest in sclerotherapy developed in the 1970s, with Duffy promoting the use of polidocanol (POL) and HS as safe and effective sclerosing solutions among dermatologists in the 1980s. The double-syringe technique developed by Tessari in 2000 increased the popularity of foam sclerotherapy worldwide.[55]

Another key to the success and acceptance of sclerotherapy was the addition of elastic compression, whose ease of use and popularity were facilitated by the discovery of a vulcanization process for increasing the elasticity and durability of rubber followed by the creation of synthetic, latex-free elastomers in the mid-19th century.[56]

SCLEROSING AGENTS

The ideal sclerosing agent would be selective against damaged endothelium (ie, abnormal blood vessels) with minimal to no reversible damage to surrounding tissue, be painless to inject, and have no adverse events.[57] Unfortunately, an ideal sclerosing agent does not yet exist. Currently available sclerosing agents are classified into 3 groups based on chemical structure and mechanism of action: detergent, hyperosmotic (hypertonic), and chemical (irritant).[58] A 2011 Cochrane review demonstrated that the available evidence does not suggest superior efficacy or subject satisfaction for any one sclerosing agent class for the treatment of lower extremity telangiectasias.[59] Table 212-5 describes the relative complications for each sclerosing agent.

TABLE 212-5
Complications by Sclerosing Agent

SCLEROSING AGENT	PAIN WITH INJECTION	PIGMENTATION	NECROSIS	ALLERGIC REACTIONS
Polidocanol	0	+/++	+	+
Sodium tetradecyl sulfate	+	++	+	+
Glycerin	+	0	0	0
Chromated glycerin	++	0	0	+
Hypertonic saline	+++	+	+++	0
Hypertonic saline/dextrose	++	+	+	0

0, none; +, minimal; ++, moderate; +++, significant/severe.

DETERGENT SCLEROSING AGENTS

Detergent sclerosing agents are long-chain fatty acids that aggregate into micelles, interfering with endothelial cell surface lipids and proteins.[60] By decreasing endothelial cell surface tension, they cause plaques of endothelial desquamation within seconds of injection. The ability to be foamed gives detergent solutions a noted advantage over the other sclerosant groups. Foaming increases the potency of detergents twofold to fourfold by mechanically displacing blood and maximizing endothelial contact.[57]

POL (Asclera, Merz North America, Inc., Raleigh, NC; Aethoxysklerol, Chemische Fabrik Kreussler & Co., Wiesbaden, Germany) is composed of hydroxy-polyethoxydodecane dissolved in distilled water with a 5% ethanol stabilizer that was originally developed as an anesthetic, but was subsequently found to sclerose small-diameter vessels after intradermal injection.[57] POL gained popularity worldwide for treating smaller-diameter dermal vessels because of its painless intravascular injection and extremely low incidence of cutaneous necrosis with extravasation. The U.S. Food and Drug Administration (FDA) has approved POL for sclerosis of uncomplicated veins whose diameter is less than 1 mm (0.5% solution) and for those whose diameter is from 1 to 3 mm (1% solution). Decades of combined experience with POL inside and outside the United States has confirmed its safety and efficacy as a sclerosing agent.[61,62]

STS (Sotradecol, Mylan Institutional LLC, Canonsburg, PA; Fibrovein, STD Pharmaceuticals, Hereford, United Kingdom) is an anionic surfactant that is FDA approved for uncomplicated varicose veins of the lower extremities in 1% and 3% concentrations. In repeated studies, both POL and STS have been found to be largely equivalent in terms of efficacy.[63] Like with POL, the risk of postsclerotherapy hyperpigmentation (PSH) with STS is directly proportional to concentration injected, and a relatively high incidence of PSH has been reported at inappropriately high doses (1% STS).[64] However, a study by Goldman and colleagues showed that STS and POL injected at equivalent concentrations had no significant difference in PSH.[63,65] Cutaneous necrosis risk with STS is low with concentrations less than 1%, but increases significantly at higher concentrations.

Sodium morrhuate is a 5% solution of the salts of saturated and unsaturated fatty acids in cod liver oil, although approximately 10% of its fatty acid composition is unknown. Sodium morrhuate should not be used for cutaneous sclerotherapy given the significant potential for cutaneous necrosis and the highest risk of anaphylaxis among sclerosing agents.

Ethanolamine oleate is a synthetic sclerosing agent for varicose veins that, like sodium morrhuate, should not be used for cutaneous sclerotherapy. Also like sodium morrhuate, ethanolamine oleate was exempted from FDA approval because of its common use prior to FDA safety requirements. Ethanolamine oleate is associated with anaphylaxis, cutaneous necrosis, pulmonary toxicity, and nonspecific red blood cell (RBC) hemolysis.[58]

HYPEROSMOTIC SCLEROSING AGENTS

This class of off-label sclerosing agents produces endothelial cell surface protein denaturation by means of concentration-dependent osmotic dehydration leading to fibrin deposition and thrombus formation. Although hyperosmotic sclerosing agents have been used off label for telangiectasias, they have numerous disadvantages, including rapid dilution in blood, transient pain and muscle cramping from extravascular diffusion or extravasation, and nonspecific collateral damage of RBCs and perivascular tissue. Appropriately so, their usage has steadily declined with the growing worldwide popularity of synthetic detergents with far superior side-effect profiles.[66]

Hypertonic saline, wrought with shortcomings and FDA approved only as an abortifacient, is still commonly used in the United States in concentrations from 10% to 30% to treat telangiectasias (most often 23.4% or diluted to 11.7% for smaller telangiectasias). The only advantages of HS are its low cost and lack of allergenicity when unadulterated. Given the significant pain associated with the intravascular injection of HS, lidocaine is often added to the solution, potentially increasing the risk of allergic reaction. HS 23.4% carries the highest risk of cutaneous necrosis from injection-site extravasation, particularly when injecting very close to the skin surface. Injection of hyaluronidase into sites of extravasation may significantly reduce the incidence of cutaneous necrosis with HS.[67]

HS and dextrose (Sclerodex, Omega Laboratories Ltd, Montreal, Canada) is a viscous mixture of 10% HS and 25% dextrose in propylene glycol and phenethyl alcohol. The decreased osmolarity of HS in HS and dextrose produces less pain and muscle cramping, and an ulceration risk less than that of 23.4% HS. Allergic reactions have been reported, potentially because of the phenethyl alcohol component of the solution. Given its relatively weak sclerosant properties, it is best reserved for the treatment of small telangiectasias.

Glycerin (50% to 100%, but most often 72%) is a weak hyperosmotic sclerosing agent that is an excellent treatment option for telangiectasias given its exceedingly rare risks of PSH, telangiectatic matting, and cutaneous necrosis.[68] Its high viscosity and transient pain with injection are both reduced with the addition of lidocaine.[69] Although no allergic reactions have been reported with glycerin, the addition of lidocaine may theoretically increase this risk. Epinephrine is often added to glycerin as well, increasing vasospasm and potentially enhancing efficacy. Glycerin is used off label in the United States, but is FDA approved for relief of intracranial pressure resulting from acute glaucoma or cerebral edema. The volume injected per session should not exceed 10 mL, as larger amounts may induce transient hematuria from ureteral colic or hemoglobinuria from RBC hemolysis. Glycerin is best avoided in diabetic patients because of the risk of iatrogenic secondary hyperglycemia.

CHEMICAL SCLEROSING AGENTS

Chemical irritant sclerosing agents lead to dissolution of intimal intracellular bonds and subsequent endothelial dysfunction and death.[57] The resulting exposed subendothelial connective tissue and elastic lamina also triggers thrombus formation. Like hyperosmotic sclerosing agents, their off-label therapeutic effects are limited by rapid dilution in blood and inactivation by blood proteins. Polyiodinated iodine is a strong chemical sclerosant that is rarely used because of a high risk of cutaneous necrosis with perivascular injection. Ethanol is also rarely used for dermatologic indications, being reserved for arteriovenous malformations and other high-flow vascular abnormalities.

Chromated glycerin (72% solution) possesses combined osmotic and chemical mechanisms of action. The addition of a chromium alum to glycerin increases its sclerosing power, which may impart a greater risk of PSH; it prevents hematuria and ureteral colic. Unfortunately, chromated glycerin has no FDA label and therefore has poor availability in the United States.

SCLEROTHERAPY TECHNIQUE

Despite 150 years of sclerotherapy, there is still no absolute, irrefutable technique to achieve flawless results. No quote is more fitting than that of Henry Faxon, an assistant in surgery at Harvard Medical School in 1933, who, upon thorough review of cases performed at the peripheral circulatory clinic of the Massachusetts General Hospital, stated:

> "We feel from our three and one-half years' experience that the surgeon who believes that there is nothing more required than a syringe, some solution, and a patient to effect permanent obliteration of varicose veins, still has much to learn."[70]

Nevertheless, there are basic principles and guidelines that experienced practitioners should follow to optimize efficacy and mitigate adverse events. First, treatment should proceed from points of highest to lowest pressure reflux, progressing from the largest varicosities to telangiectasias in stepwise fashion. Patients with saphenous vein reflux must have their saphenous disease addressed prior to sclerotherapy for saphenous tributaries and varicose veins. Likewise, sclerotherapy for reticular veins and telangiectasias should proceed only after varicose veins and larger sources of reflux have been addressed (Fig. 212-6).

Injection of telangiectasias is simultaneously performed with injection of reticular veins, with the goal of maximizing treatment efficacy and reducing the number of treatments necessary for complete clearance.[71] Weiss and Weiss[46] showed an association between telangiectasias and the presence of reflux in adjacent reticular veins on the lateral thighs. When no clear feeder vessel is visualized, transillumination with a light-emitting diode (Veinlite, Translite LLC, Sugar Land, TX) or fiber optic device (Sam's Light, Wagner Medical, Middlebourne, WV) may help identify a "feeding" reticular vein. When no associated reticular vein is present, then the point at which the telangiectasias begin to branch out or arborize is the ideal site at which to begin injecting. The use of a magnified cross-polarized light device (Syris Scientific, LLC, Grey, ME) can dramatically improve visualization of fine telangiectasias.

The patient should be positioned lying flat, either supine or prone, depending on the area of the lower extremities being treated. The goal of treatment is to inject intravascularly with minimal pressure, so as to minimize extravasation and prevent vessel rupture.[72] As injection pressure is inversely proportional to the square of the syringe piston radius, the smaller the vein, the larger the syringe that should be used. Therefore, although a 3-mL syringe can be used for reticular veins, telangiectasias are best treated with a 5- to 6-mL syringe.[71] Both types of veins should be treated with a 30-gauge half-inch needle. Given that telangiectasias are extremely superficial (subepidermal), bending the

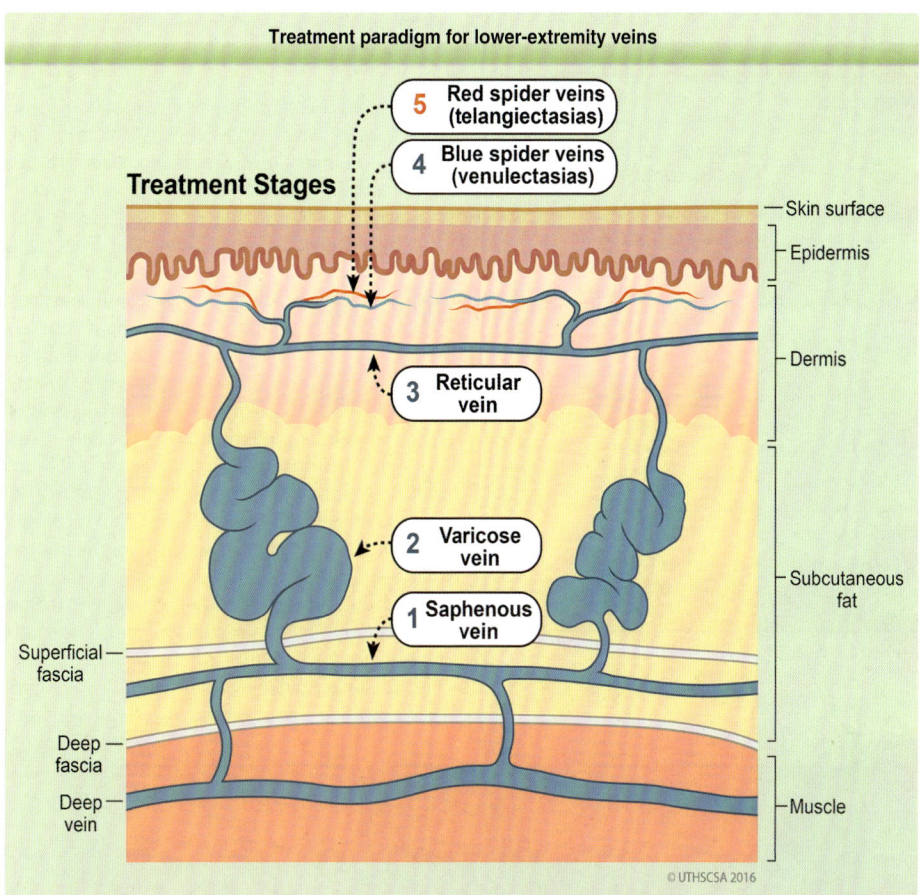

Figure 212-6 Treatment paradigm for lower extremity veins. Treatment is best approached sequentially. The largest, highest-pressure sources of reflux (eg, saphenous veins) should be treated first, with the smallest, lowest-pressure vessels (eg, venulectasias and telangiectasias) treated last. (Reproduced with permission from UT Health Science Center at San Antonio. © UTHSCSA.)

needle to an angle of 10 to 30 degrees with the bevel up, placed on the skin so that the needle is parallel to the skin surface, facilitates treatment. The syringe should be held between the index and middle fingers, with the thumb on the plunger, while the fourth and fifth fingers support the practitioner's hand against the patient's lower extremity in a fixed position to stabilize the hand. The practitioner's nondominant hand or the hands of an assistant can simultaneously be used to stretch the skin in the treatment area (Fig. 212-7).

Venous diameter is the critical factor for determining which sclerosing agent class and concentration is most appropriate for treatment (Table 212-6). The lowest sufficient concentration should always be used.[73] Vessel diameter also predicts treatment success. Vessels with a diameter of 0.3 mm or less are likely to require multiple treatments, while those with a diameter of 0.5 mm or more may require only a single treatment. The volume of sclerosing agent injected per site should be limited to 1 mL and is typically 0.5 mL or less. Although a conservative limit for total liquid sclerosant volume is approximately 10 mL, significantly larger volumes can be used safely over large areas as long as the volume per injection remains small. Treatment intervals vary, but allowing 3 months for maximal clearance following a sclerotherapy session, helps minimize the number of retreatments (Figs. 212-8 and 212-9). When ineffective sclerosis is evident at followup, the concentration of sclerosing agent, *not* the volume per site, ought to be increased.

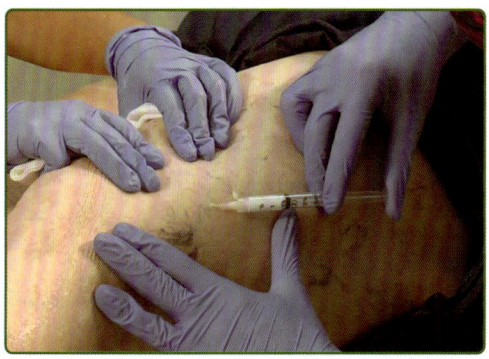

Figure 212-7 Proper sclerotherapy injection technique.

TABLE 212-6
Sclerosing Agent Class and Concentration by Vessel Size

VESSEL SIZE	APPROPRIATE SCLEROSING AGENT CONCENTRATION
<1 mm (spider veins)	• 0.1% to 0.25% STS liquid • 0.25% to 0.5% POL liquid • 72% Glycerin mixed 2:1 with 1% lidocaine ± epinephrine

1 to 3 mm (reticular veins)	• Small (1 to 2 mm)
	  ■ 0.25% STS foam or 0.5% STS liquid
	  ■ 0.5% POL foam or 1% POL liquid
	• Large (3 mm)
	  ■ 0.5% STS foam
	  ■ 1% POL foam

>3 mm (varicose veins, incompetent saphenous tributary veins)	• 1% POL foam • 0.5% to 1% STS foam
>5 mm (incompetent saphenous veins or their tributaries)	• 3% POL foam • 1% to 3% STS foam

POL, polidocanol; STS, sodium tetradecyl sulfate.

FOAM SCLEROTHERAPY

Foam sclerotherapy with detergent sclerosing agents has become a standard treatment of veins larger than 1 mm.[74] Foam microbubbles mechanically displace blood within targeted veins, maximizing endothelial contact time, decreasing sclerosing agent dilution, and increasing detergent potency at least twofold.[75] Foam sclerotherapy can thereby enhance treatment efficacy and reduce the overall number of sessions for complete clearance.[76] This method also enables the use of lower sclerosing agent concentrations and volumes, decreasing potential adverse events and risks of systemic toxicity. An additional advantage of foam is its echogenicity, making it easily visualized on duplex ultrasound. Use of foam sclerotherapy, however, should be approached cautiously in vessels smaller than 1 mm because of an increased risk of vessel rupture and associated pigmentation and matting.[77]

Agitating a detergent sclerosing agent with a gas, most commonly air, produces a foam. The most commonly used techniques for foam sclerotherapy are the Tessari (double-syringe with 3-way stopcock) and modified Tessari (double-syringe with Luer-to-

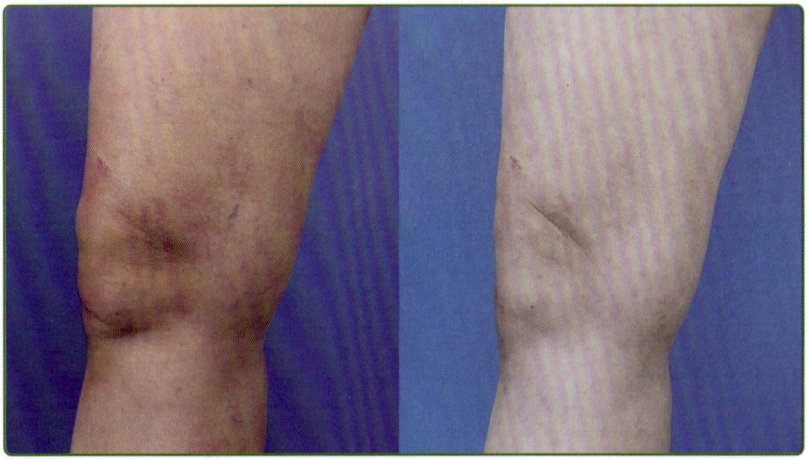

Figure 212-8 Before (*left*) and 3 months after (*right*) 2 sessions of sclerotherapy performed 3 months apart. Sodium tetradecyl sulfate foam 0.25% and glycerin 72% were used for reticular veins and telangiectasias, respectively.

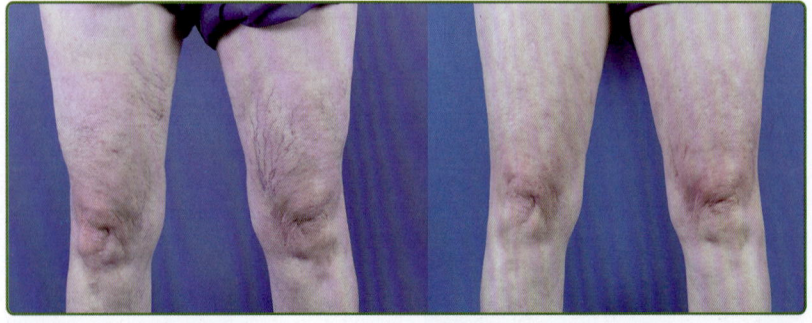

Figure 212-9 Before (*left*) and 3 months after (*right*) 2 sessions of sclerotherapy performed 3 months apart. Sodium tetradecyl sulfate 0.25% foam and glycerin 72% were used for reticular veins and telangiectasias, respectively.

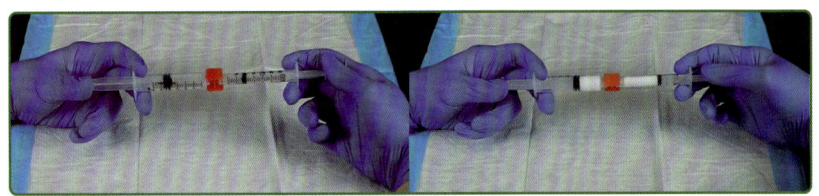

Figure 212-10 Double-syringe system with Luer-to-Luer connector for foaming a detergent sclerosing agent with room air (1:4 liquid-to-gas ratio).

Luer connector) methods.[78] In either method, 1 sterile syringe is filled with room air, while the other is filled with a detergent sclerosing agent, with an optimal liquid-to-gas dilution ratio of 1:4. The contents of the syringes are quickly shifted back and forth approximately 10 to 20 times; the turbulent flow generates homogeneous foam (Fig. 212-10). The foamed solution should be used immediately (injected via the 3-mL syringe) because it degrades within 60 to 90 seconds. Commercially prepared POL microfoam has a smaller, narrower bubble size distribution and slower degradation rate, which may enhance results, compared to physician-compounded POL foam.[79]

POSTSCLEROTHERAPY COMPRESSION

There are multiple reasons why compression following sclerotherapy enhances results and mitigates adverse events. First and foremost, compression promotes sclerophlebitis and eliminates thrombophlebitis (Fig. 212-11).[80] Decreasing the extent of thrombus formation in treated veins may significantly decrease the risk of recanalization, PSH, and even telangiectatic matting. Compression also can augment the direct

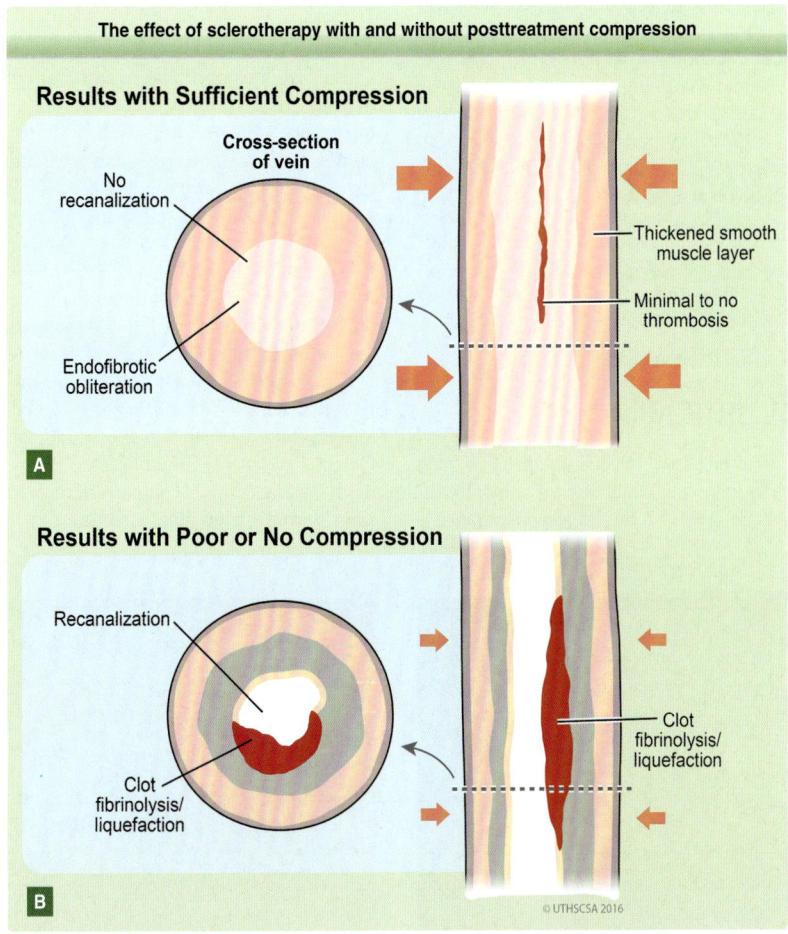

Figure 212-11 The effect of sclerotherapy with and without posttreatment compression. **A,** Proper compression promotes endofibrosis, leading to complete venous occlusion. **B,** Poor to no compression enables thrombosis, which impedes endofibrosis and results in recanalization. (Reproduced with permission from UT Health Science Center at San Antonio. © UTHSCSA.)

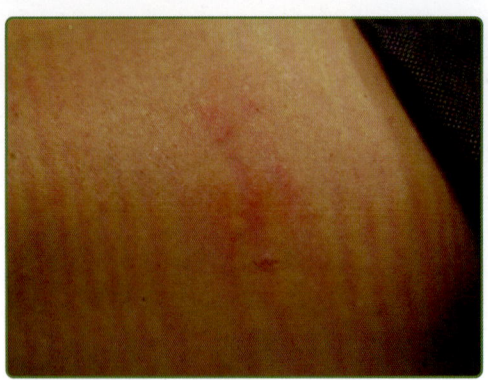

Figure 212-12 Physical urticaria within minutes of injecting 0.25% sodium tetradecyl sulfate for reticular veins.

apposition of treated vein walls, leading to more effective intraluminal fibrosis. It also likely serves a role in enhancing the function of the calf muscle pump and decreasing the extent and duration of bruising and edema posttreatment.[81]

As graduated elastic compression stockings should cover the entire treated area, thigh-high stockings are most commonly prescribed postsclerotherapy.[82] The class and duration of compression following sclerotherapy remains a point of contention between practitioners.[58] Although 7 days is superior to 3 days of compression, compression for 3 days leads to significantly greater improvement and fewer adverse events than no compression at all.

SIDE EFFECTS AND COMPLICATIONS

PHYSICAL URTICARIA

Physical urticaria localized to sites of injection may occur transiently following treatment with any sclerosing agent, even HS (Fig. 212-12).[83] Their appearance is likely a consequence of endothelial irritation and histamine release from perivascular mast cells. The intensity of urticaria may increase with greater sclerosing agent concentrations or repeat treatment sessions.

COAGULUM

Coagulum formation is not uncommon following sclerotherapy and represents focal thrombus formation resulting from incomplete occlusion of the vascular lumen during treatment. These thrombi incite a subacute perivenulitis with RBC extravasation. Coagula present clinically as mildly tender indurated dermal or subcutaneous nodules (depending on what type of vein was treated) that may persist for months. It is best to evacuate coagula at approximately 2 weeks postsclerotherapy using a 21- to 25-gauge needle and bimanual expression (Fig. 212-13).[84]

POSTSCLEROTHERAPY HYPERPIGMENTATION

PSH is defined as the temporary appearance of linear pigmentation along the course of a treated vein of any size (Fig. 212-14). It is initially related to perivascular hemosiderin deposition from the superficial dermal extravasation of RBCs secondary to dilation or rupture of treated vessels; however, over time, the hemosiderin may be replaced by melanin.[85] The incidence of pigmentation is directly related to the type and concentration of sclerosing agent, as well as to the diameter of treated vessel.[86] Table 212-7 lists the factors that increase the risk of PSH.[87,88] Weak sclerosing agents, such as glycerin and chromated glycerin, have the lowest risk of PSH. Vessels with diameters smaller than 1 mm also rarely (if ever) develop PSH.[86]

Pigmentation clears spontaneously in 70% of patients within 6 months but rarely persists for longer than a year.[86] Nanosecond or picosecond Q-switched lasers (694-nm ruby, 755-nm alexandrite, or 1064-nm Nd:YAG [neodymium:yttrium aluminum garnet]) are often effective for clearing PSH,

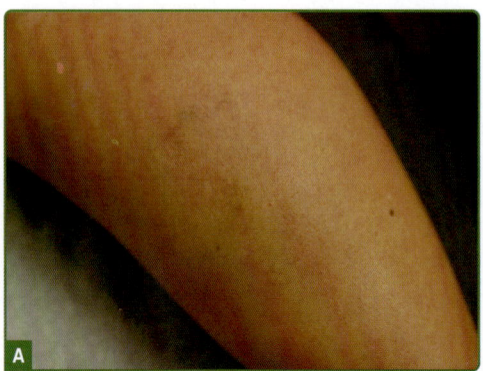
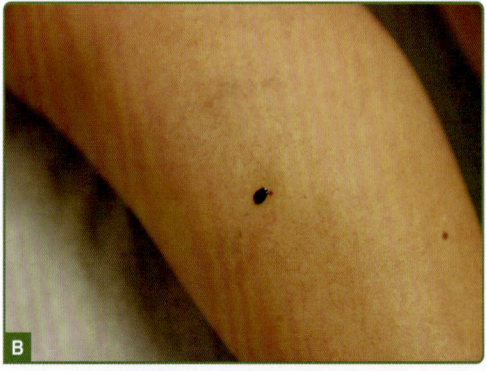

Figure 212-13 **A,** Postsclerotherapy coagulum 2 weeks after sclerotherapy. **B,** Evacuation of coagulum (thrombectomy) following puncture with a 25-gauge needle and bimanual compression.

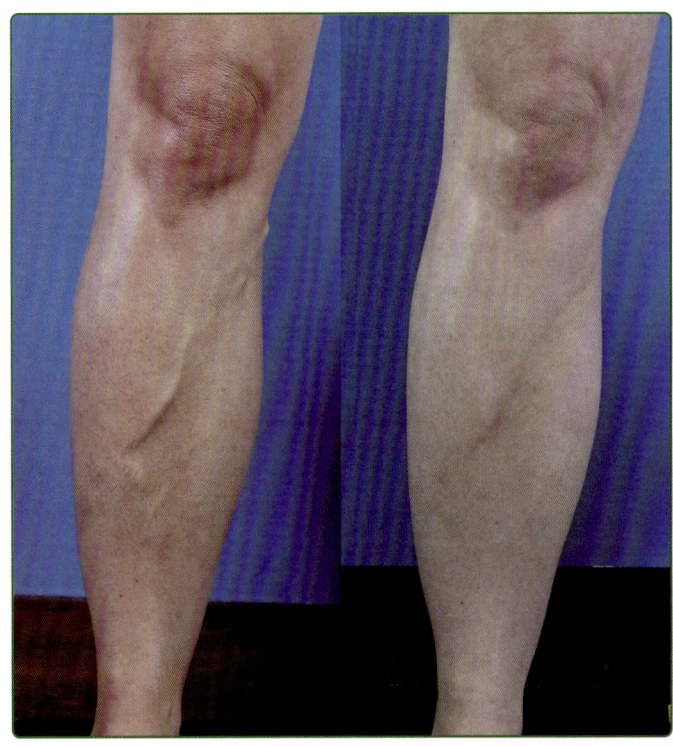

Figure 212-14 Before (*left*) and 6 months after (*right*) 1320-nm endovenous laser ablation of the thigh segment of the great saphenous vein with sclerotherapy for the associated medial knee and anteromedial leg varicose veins using 0.5% sodium tetradecyl sulfate foam. Note the mild residual postsclerotherapy hyperpigmentation at followup.

although low fluences should be used in darker-skinned patients to avoid causing hypopigmentation or worsening hyperpigmentation.[89,90] Picosecond 532-nm frequency-doubled Nd:YAG laser treatment may be useful for PSH, but only in very light-skinned patients.

TABLE 212-7 Risk Factors for Postsclerotherapy Hyperpigmentation	
Patient-related	Skin Type V or VI (hemosiderin and inflammatory cascade may stimulate cutaneous melanocytes)
	Periprocedural minocycline use (perivascular deposition of iron complexes or hemosiderin and minocycline moieties)
	Increased vessel fragility (decreased capillary strength) 2 days after ovulation and 3 to 5 days before menstruation
Procedure-related	Excessive sclerosing agent concentrations (lead to excessive inflammation) and injection pressures (cause vessel rupture and extravasation)
	Lack of graduated compression
	Excessive ecchymosis
	Untreated coagulum

TELANGIECTATIC MATTING

Telangiectatic matting is the blush-like, grouped appearance of fine (<0.2 mm) red telangiectasias replacing or adjacent to an area of prior sclerotherapy or surgical vein ligation. Angiogenic and inflammatory pathophysiologic mechanisms have been implicated.[88] Inflammatory-mediated endothelial injury from sclerosing agents can lead to the release of mast cell heparin, whose affinity for endothelial growth factors can trigger microvascular proliferation via capillary endothelial cell proliferation and angiogenesis. Excess inflammation and thrombus formation with sclerotherapy may create a hypermetabolic state that incites reactive blood vessel growth. Angiogenesis also may be a direct response to targeted vessel closure produced by sclerotherapy. Dilation of existing subclinical blood vessels is thought to play a combinatory or alternative role.[88]

Although the most common area for telangiectatic matting is the medial thigh, it may also appear in the medial ankle and medial or lateral calf.[88] Predisposing factors include obesity, a family history of leg veins, a prolonged history of telangiectasias, hyperestrogenic states, such as pregnancy, and use of oral contraceptives or hormonal therapy.[91] As the incidence of telangiectatic matting may be proportional to the degree of inflammation and thrombus formation, weak sclerosing agents are thought unlikely to cause telangiectatic matting.

A retrospective study of more than 2100 patients reported a telangiectatic matting incidence of 16% in patients treated with HS and POL.[91] Spontaneous resolution usually occurs within 3 to 12 months of onset, with 70% to 80% of cases resolving within the first 6 months.[86,88] Telangiectatic matting can be treated with a weak hypertonic sclerosing agent or 585-nm to 595-nm pulsed-dye laser.[92] The treatment of any residual feeding reticular veins may also quicken its resolution.

CUTANEOUS NECROSIS/ULCERATION

Cutaneous ulceration may occur with any sclerosing agent. However, the risk from perivenous dermal extravasation of detergent (POL, STS) or weak hypertonic (glycerin, chromated glycerin) sclerosing agents is very unlikely with typical product concentrations and small injection volumes. If extravasation occurs, one should stop injecting and massage the dermal bleb to minimize prolonged blanching of the area.

Cutaneous necrosis may also occur by a number of other mechanisms.[93] Rapid or large-volume injection into a telangiectasia associated with an arteriole by means of an arteriovenous anastomosis can produce localized ulceration.[94] Reactive arterial vasospasm can occur from puncture of a nearby artery without injection of sclerosing agent, leading to a porcelain-white injection site that progresses to hemorrhagic bulla formation. Prolonged nongraduated compression greater than 30 to 40 mm Hg can also induce tissue anoxia.

SUPERFICIAL VENOUS THROMBOPHLEBITIS

In contrast, to a coagulum, which is a focal and mildly tender lesion resulting from proper sclerotherapy, superficial venous thrombophlebitis (SVT) presents clinically as a markedly tender, indurated, linear erythematous cord (Fig. 212-15). Signs of symptoms

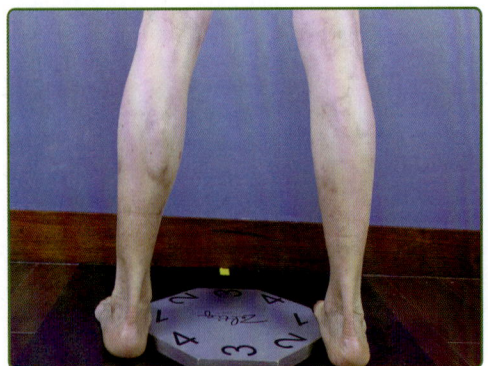

Figure 212-15 Superficial venous thrombophlebitis 2 weeks postsclerotherapy. Signs and symptoms resolved with graduated compression and nonsteroidal antiinflammatory medications.

of SVT may develop even weeks posttreatment. The incidence of SVT postsclerotherapy is variable and was recently found to be 4.7% in a large-scale review of foam sclerotherapy for varicose veins.[95] However, a subsequent survey of 1605 French patients only found 2 occurrences of SVT that were caused by foam POL or STS.[62] Treatment consists of leg elevation, compression, and nonsteroidal antiinflammatory drugs. Extension of superficial thrombophlebitis into the deep venous system is extremely rare.

DEEP VENOUS THROMBOSIS (DVT)

DVT following sclerotherapy is relatively rare (incidence < 1%) and may be a result of sclerosing agent migration into the deep venous system resulting from excessive injection volumes (>1 mL) at a single site and from the use of foam sclerotherapy.[58,62] Patients with preexisting hypercoagulable states, difficulty mobilizing, or undergoing a concomitant surgical procedure are likely to be at higher risk. Pulmonary emboli, however, are extremely rare. Suspicion for DVT or pulmonary emboli should prompt duplex ultrasound imaging and referral for possible anticoagulation.[58] Transient, self-limited chest tightness, shortness of breath, or coughing may occur in a minority of patients immediately following treatment with foam sclerotherapy and should not be confused with pulmonary emboli.

INTRAARTERIAL INJECTION

This dreaded medical emergency is, fortunately, extremely rare. Intraarterial injection of a sclerosing agent produces a sludge embolus from denatured endothelial cells and blood that obstructs microcirculation, leading to secondary thrombosis and necrosis.[96] Consequently, the extent of cutaneous necrosis is related to the amount of sclerosing agent injected. Highest-risk areas for intraarterial injection are the popliteal fossa, dorsal foot, and medial malleolus.

Warning signs immediately following injection usually include a continuous intense burning pain (far beyond normal) and bone-white cutaneous blanching in an arterial pattern. Progression to a sharply-demarcated area of cyanosis within minutes is typical. This may eventuate in wide areas of skin necrosis and damage to underlying subcutaneous tissue and muscle. Rarely, cutaneous signs and symptoms following arterial injection may not be seen for up to 24 hours; these cases may be from leakage of sclerosant into the arterial circulation via an arteriovenous anastomosis.[93]

Treatment involves the immediate initiation of a vasodilatory protocol (massage, aspirin, warm compresses, and oxygen); flushing the inadvertently injected artery with normal saline or heparin; and vascular surgery consultation for intravenous anticoagulation with heparin. Infiltration with 1% to 3% procaine is recommended to inactivate STS, if used.

NEUROLOGIC SYMPTOMS

Rare reports of headaches and visual disturbances, and exceedingly rare accounts of transient ischemic attack and stroke, have been described postsclerotherapy and are associated with the presence of a patent foramen ovale or a history of migraine with aura.[97] Although they may more commonly occur with injection of foam, they also have been reported with liquid sclerotherapy and in patients without patent foramen ovale.[98] Given the latter and the fact that asymptomatic patients can demonstrate cerebrovascular microemboli, other factors, including endothelin release from damaged endothelial cells and genetic susceptibility, may play a role.[99]

MINIMALLY-INVASIVE SURGICAL APPROACHES FOR VARICOSE VEINS

The Swiss surgeon Rima was the first to recognize the critical role of saphenofemoral reflux in the pathogenesis of varicose veins in the late 18th century. Although he performed the first high ligation of the GSV, Trendelenburg advanced the procedure in 1890.[100,101] Saphenous stripping was developed by Mayo in 1904 and advanced during the early 20th century.

However, the postoperative morbidity, potential for scarring, and need for general or epidural anesthesia associated with traditional surgical management established the need for minimally-invasive methods of treating saphenous reflux. In March 1999, the first endovenous radiofrequency ablation (RFA) device was cleared by the FDA.[102] Endovenous laser ablation (EVLA) followed soon thereafter.[103] Dermatologic surgeons were instrumental in developing these endovenous techniques.

ENDOVENOUS ABLATION/OCCLUSION TECHNIQUES

Endovenous ablation has largely replaced traditional surgical management in industrialized countries such as the United States and England, given the decreased morbidity, more rapid recovery, and improved cosmetic outcomes with RFA and EVLA compared to surgical methods.[104,105] Postoperative pain, wound infection, and hematoma formation are also particularly far less common.[106] Endovenous techniques have likewise been found to improve patient quality of life, while significantly decreasing patient and societal costs of managing venous disease relative to surgery.[107] Large-scale reviews have found no significant long-term differences in primary failure, recurrence, or neovascularization rates between RFA, EVLA, and surgical intervention.[106,108,109]

Endovenous therapy is typically performed *prior* to addressing superficial varicosities, reticular veins, or telangiectasias, as part of a proximal to distal (highest to lowest pressure) treatment approach. The radiofrequency catheter or laser fiber are introduced into the target vein under duplex ultrasound guidance and then advanced to 2 to 3 cm from the SFJ or saphenopopliteal junction termination (Fig. 212-16A). Dilute lidocaine is infiltrated into the perivenous saphenous compartment immediately prior to treatment, which acts as a heat sink, physically distances the vein from surrounding tissue, and induces circumferential apposition of the vein wall onto the catheter or

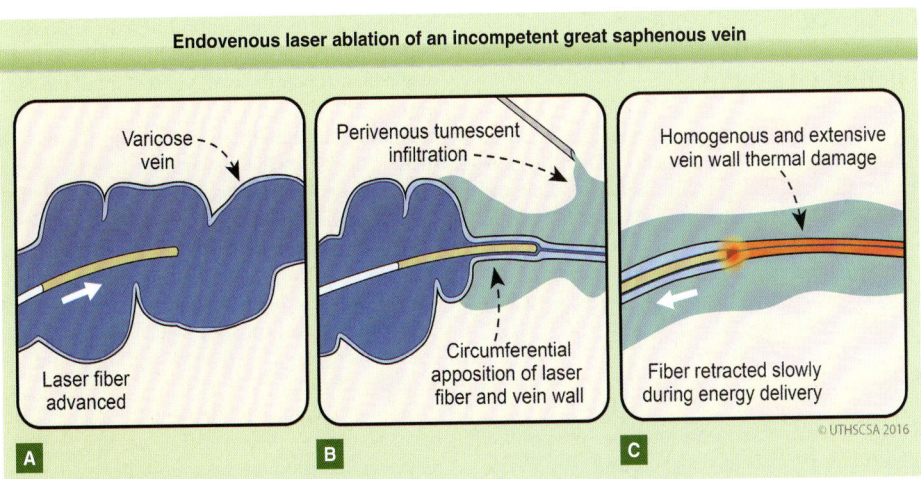

Figure 212-16 Endovenous laser ablation of an incompetent great saphenous vein (GSV). **A,** The GSV is accessed under duplex ultrasound and a laser fiber is advanced to 2 to 3 cm from the saphenofemoral junction. **B,** Dilute lidocaine solution is infiltrated into the perivenous space (ie, the saphenous compartment) under ultrasound guidance. **C,** Transmural thermal damage is produced as the fiber is retracted at a fixed pull-back speed. (Reproduced with permission from UT Health Science Center at San Antonio. © UTHSCSA.)

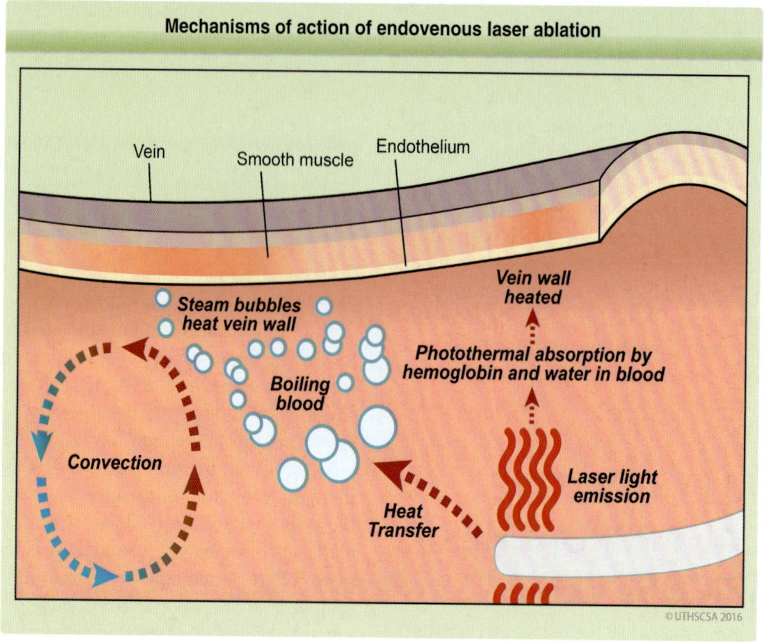

Figure 212-17 Mechanisms of action of endovenous laser ablation. Vessel injury is produced from the heating of residual blood immediately surrounding the laser fiber, leading to secondary damage of the vessel wall. Residual blood heating occurs as a result of (a) heat transfer from a hot fiber tip and (b) photothermal absorption of hemoglobin and water. Both may lead to steam bubble formation. (Reproduced with permission from UT Health Science Center at San Antonio. © UTHSCSA.)

fiber (Fig. 212-16B). Tumescent anesthesia with this procedure reduces postoperative pain and allows for immediate ambulation postprocedure, mitigating the risk for DVT.[110]

Energy is delivered to the target saphenous vessel as the catheter or fiber is slowly withdrawn from the patient (see Fig. 212-16C). Thermal damage causes destruction of the intima and collagen denaturation of the media within the vein wall, leading to fibrotic vascular occlusion.[111,112]

RADIOFREQUENCY

The efficacy for radiofrequency elimination of reflux is 90% at 2 years and 80% at 5 years.[108] The RFA catheter comes in direct contact with the vessel wall and produces resistive heating (impedance) by means of a high-frequency, electrode-mediated alternating current. As impedance decreases with increasing tissue coagulation, the amount of heat that can be generated is inherently limited.

LASER

Irreversible thermal damage of the inner vein wall, a requirement for permanent vessel occlusion by EVLA, can be achieved by a number of devices and wavelengths. It was originally assumed that intravascular coagulation occurs by selective photothermolysis of either hemoglobin in RBCs of intraluminal blood using shorter wavelengths (810, 940, 980, and 1064 nm) or water in the vein wall using longer wavelengths (1320, 1470, 1500 nm, and higher).[113,114] However, recent mathematical models show that irreversible thermal damage of the inner vein wall is *not* dependent on competitive direct photothermal absorption by hemoglobin or water.[115,116] Instead, thermal damage is primarily achieved by the combined effects of heat transfer through a small residual layer of intraluminal blood from an extremely hot layer coating the fiber tip and photothermal absorption by both chromophores within that blood layer (Fig. 212-17).[115] Both mechanisms may act on the wall via steam bubble diffusion as well.[116,117]

Limiting the amount of residual intraluminal blood thereby decreases the distance for heat transfer to the vein wall and enhances efficacy. This is achieved by reducing vein diameter during treatment with Trendelenburg positioning and perivenous tumescent fluid infiltration.[118] The extent of thermal injury to the vessel wall is also strongly dependent on the amount and duration of heat exposure, which is a factor of both laser power (energy delivered over time) and the rate of fiber pullback.

Despite having a fundamentally identical mechanism of action, newer EVLA devices with longer wavelengths produce less postoperative pain and potentially have greater efficacy than their older counterparts with shorter wavelengths. However, this may simply be a factor of the pulsed-wave energy delivery, decreased power,[119,120] faster pullback velocity,[121] and protected fiber tip design[122] that are now the stan-

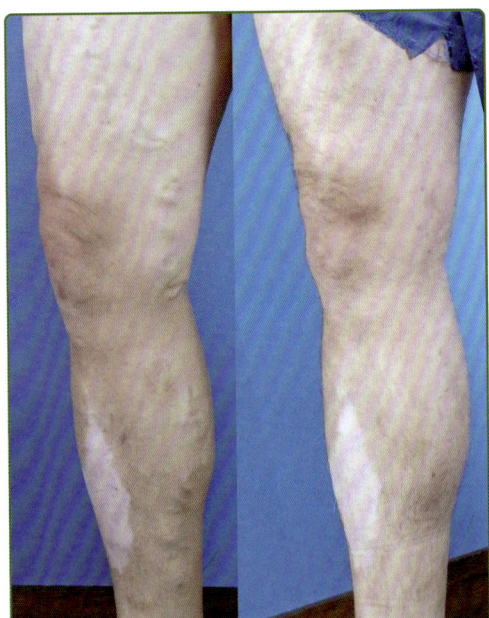

Figure 212-18 Before (*left*) and 1 year after (*right*) 1320-nm endovenous laser ablation of the thigh segment of the great saphenous vein (GSV), combined with ultrasound-guided foam sclerotherapy for the below-the-knee segment of the GSV and anterior accessory GSV (1% sodium tetradecyl sulfate) and ambulatory phlebectomy of associated anteromedial thigh and medial leg varicose veins.

dard with longer wavelength device treatments.[113,123] Regardless of the device, long-term closure rates with EVLA match, if not exceed, those of RFA. Typical results of EVLA combined with foam sclerotherapy or ambulatory phlebectomy are shown in Figs. 212-14 and 212-18, respectively. Both subjects were treated with a 1320-nm device using 12 W, 50 Hz, and a 2 mm/sec pull-back speed.

AMBULATORY PHLEBECTOMY

The first documented case of surgical removal of varicose veins, described by Plutarch, was performed on the Roman Consul Gaius Marius (157-186 BC) without anesthesia. The field advanced slowly in Ancient Rome and Greece, with Celsus (25 BC-30 AD) detailing primitive stripping and cauterization, contemporaries Antyllus and Galen (second century AD) describing ligation and vein removal with hooks, and Paulus of Aegina (660 AD) performing ligation and stripping.[100] Modern-day ambulatory phlebectomy originated with Swiss dermatologist Robert Muller in the late 1960s and was refined and popularized worldwide by Ramelet, Ricci, Georgiev, and Goldman.[101]

Ambulatory phlebectomy is an outpatient procedure to remove varicose veins through tiny incisions and small hooks using only local anesthesia (Fig. 212-19).[124,125] Ambulatory phlebectomy is often combined with endovenous ablation techniques for treatment of the SFJ or saphenopopliteal junction and sclerotherapy for treatment of associated reticular networks and telangiectasias. Varicose veins or saphenous tributaries that are resistant to foam sclerotherapy are also particularly suitable for ambulatory phlebectomy.

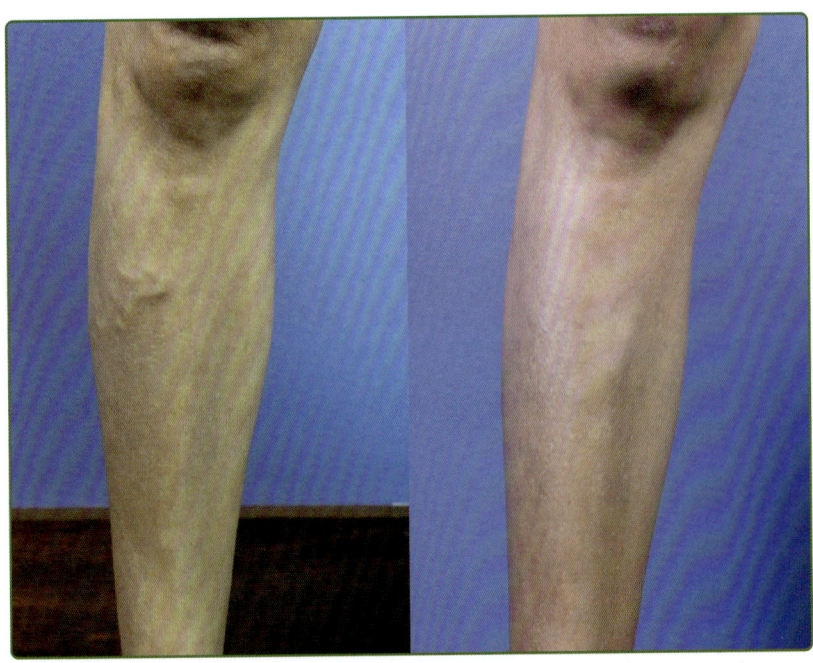

Figure 212-19 Before (*left*) and 1 year following (*right*) a single session of ambulatory phlebectomy.

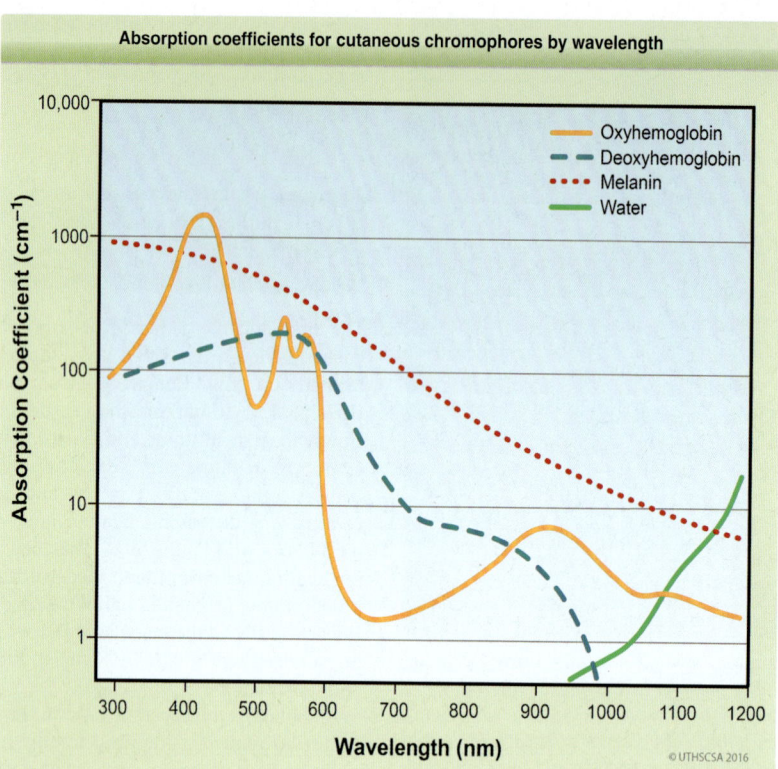

Figure 212-20 Absorption coefficients for cutaneous chromophores by wavelength. (Reproduced with permission from UT Health Science Center at San Antonio. © UTHSCSA.)

Compared to sclerotherapy for varicose veins, ambulatory phlebectomy may have a lower risk of SVT, DVT, PSH, and cutaneous necrosis.[126]

LASER AND LIGHT SOURCES

Although sclerotherapy remains the gold standard for superficial, small-caliber vessels of the lower extremities, laser devices may be a valuable alternative or adjunct treatment option. Patients with vessels with diameters too small to cannulate with a 30-gauge needle, a history of needle phobia, or an unwillingness to wear graduated compression stockings may all benefit from laser therapy.[127]

Selective thermal damage of a pigmented cutaneous chromophore can be achieved by delivering a wavelength within its absorption spectrum at an appropriate fluence and pulse duration.[128] The primary chromophore of cutaneous blood vessels is intravascular oxyhemoglobin, with some influence from deoxyhemoglobin as well. Oxyhemoglobin has 3 absorption peaks at 418, 540, and 575 to 580 nm, while deoxyhemoglobin peaks at 550 to 560 nm (Fig. 212-20). Current pulsed-dye laser (585 to 595 nm) and frequency-doubled Nd:YAG (532 nm) devices match these absorption peaks and can effectively target telangiectasias (Fig. 212-21).[129] Intense pulsed light devices (515 to 1200

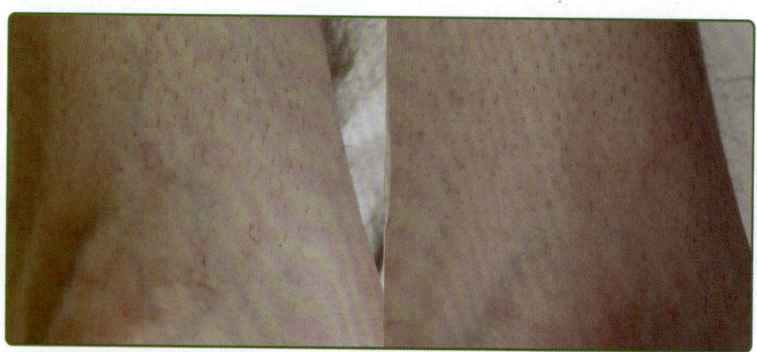

Figure 212-21 Before (*left*) and 1 month following (*right*) a single treatment of 585- to 595-nm pulsed-dye laser for isolated telangiectasias of the medial malleolus.

nm) also can be used for photothermal sclerosis of telangiectasias.[130,131]

Near-infrared wavelengths at 800 to 1100 nm match a small, yet broad peak for oxyhemoglobin.[132] Devices emitting 810 and 940 nm have been shown to improve lower-extremity veins.[133,134] Long-pulsed Nd:YAG devices (1064 nm) allow for thermocoagulation of larger, deeply situated vessels (eg, reticular veins) up to 3.7 mm in depth.[135] The minimal melanin absorption of 1064 nm energy makes this wavelength ideal for darker or suntanned skin types. However, laser therapy for reticular veins must be performed with care because of the treatment-related pain, high rates of recurrence with incomplete treatment, and the risk of blistering or ulceration from improper technique.

REFERENCES

1. Rabe E, Pannier F. Societal costs of chronic venous disease in CEAP C4, C5, C6 disease. *Phlebology.* 2010;25(suppl 1):64-67.
2. Onida S, Davies AH. Predicted burden of venous disease. *Phlebology.* 2016;31(1)(suppl):74-79.
3. Meissner MH. Lower extremity venous anatomy. *Semin Intervent Radiol.* 2005;22(3):147-156.
4. Caggiati A, Bergan JJ, Gloviczki P, et al. Nomenclature of the veins of the lower limbs: an international interdisciplinary consensus statement. *J Vasc Surg.* 2002;36(2):416-422.
5. Caggiati A, Bergan JJ, Gloviczki P, et al. Nomenclature of the veins of the lower limb: extensions, refinements, and clinical application. *J Vasc Surg.* 2005;41(4):719-724.
6. O'Donnell TF, Iafrati MD. The small saphenous vein and other "neglected" veins of the popliteal fossa: a review. *Phlebology.* 2007;22(4):148-155.
7. Ricci S, Cavezzi A. Echo-anatomy of long saphenous vein in the knee region: proposal for a classification in five anatomical patterns. *Phlebology.* 2002;16(3):111-116.
8. Ricci S, Caggiati A. Echoanatomical patterns of the long saphenous vein in patients with primary varices and in healthy subjects. *Phlebology.* 1999;14(2):54-58.
9. Gillespie D, Glass C. Importance of ultrasound evaluation in the diagnosis of venous insufficiency: guidelines and techniques. *Semin Vasc Surg.* 2010;23(2):85-89.
10. Oguzkurt L. Ultrasonographic anatomy of the lower extremity superficial veins. *Diagn Interv Radiol.* 2012;18(4):423-430.
11. Cavezzi A, Labropoulos N, Partsch H, et al. Duplex ultrasound investigation of the veins in chronic venous disease of the lower limbs—UIP consensus document. Part II. Anatomy. *Eur J Vasc Endovasc Surg.* 2006;31(3):288-299.
12. Murakami G, Negishi N, Tanaka K, et al. Anatomical relationship between saphenous vein and cutaneous nerves. *Okajimas Folia Anat Jpn.* 1994;71(1):21-33.
13. Ricci S, Moro L, Antonelli Incalzi R. Ultrasound imaging of the sural nerve: ultrasound anatomy and rationale for investigation. *Eur J Vasc Endovasc Surg.* 2010;39(5):636-641.
14. Tuveri M, Borsezio V, Argiolas R, et al. Ultrasonographic venous anatomy at the popliteal fossa in relation to tibial nerve course in normal and varicose limbs. *Chir Ital.* 2009;61(2):171-177.
15. Delis KT, Knaggs AL, Hobbs JT, et al. The nonsaphenous vein of the popliteal fossa: prevalence, patterns of reflux, hemodynamic quantification, and clinical significance. *J Vasc Surg Venous Lymphat Disord.* 2006;44(3):611-619.
16. Mozes G, Gloviczki P. New discoveries in anatomy and new terminology of leg veins: clinical implications. *Vasc Endovascular Surg.* 2004;38(4):367-374.
17. van Neer PA, Veraart JC, Neumann HA. Venae perforantes: a clinical review. *Dermatol Surg.* 2003;29(9):931-942.
18. Labropoulos N, Mansour MA, Kang SS, et al. New insights into perforator vein incompetence. *Eur J Vasc Endovasc Surg.* 1999;18(3):228-234.
19. Ruckley CV, Evans CJ, Allan PL, et al. Telangiectasia in the Edinburgh Vein Study: epidemiology and association with trunk varices and symptoms. *Eur J Vasc Endovasc Surg.* 2008;36(6):719-724.
20. Ruckley CV, Allan PL, Evans CJ, et al. Telangiectasia and venous reflux in the Edinburgh Vein Study. *Phlebology.* 2012;27(6):297-302.
21. Evans CJ, Allan PL, Lee AJ, et al. Prevalence of venous reflux in the general population on duplex scanning: the Edinburgh vein study. *J Vasc Surg.* 1998;28(5):767-776.
22. Allan PL, Bradbury AW, Evans CJ, et al. Patterns of reflux and severity of varicose veins in the general population—Edinburgh Vein Study. *Eur J Vasc Endovasc Surg.* 2000;20(5):470-477.
23. Engelhorn CA, Manetti R, Baviera MM, et al. Progression of reflux patterns in saphenous veins of women with chronic venous valvular insufficiency. *Phlebology.* 2012;27(1):25-32.
24. Ruckley CV, Evans CJ, Allan PL, et al. Chronic venous insufficiency: clinical and duplex correlations. The Edinburgh Vein Study of venous disorders in the general population. *J Vasc Surg.* 2002;36(3):520-525.
25. Lin JC, Iafrati MD, O'Donnell TF, et al. Correlation of duplex ultrasound scanning-derived valve closure time and clinical classification in patients with small saphenous vein reflux: Is lesser saphenous vein truly lesser? *J Vasc Surg.* 2004;39(5):1053-1058.
26. Myers KA, Ziegenbein RW, Zeng GH, et al. Duplex ultrasonography scanning for chronic venous disease: patterns of venous reflux. *J Vasc Surg.* 1995;21(4):605-612.
27. Lee AJ, Robertson LA, Boghossian SM, et al. Progression of varicose veins and chronic venous insufficiency in the general population in the Edinburgh Vein Study. *J Vasc Surg Venous Lymphat Disord.* 2015;3(1):18-26.
28. Evans CJ, Fowkes FG, Ruckley CV, et al. Prevalence of varicose veins and chronic venous insufficiency in men and women in the general population: Edinburgh Vein Study. *J Epidemiol Community Health.* 1999;53(3):149-153.
29. Robertson L, Lee AJ, Evans CJ, et al. Incidence of chronic venous disease in the Edinburgh Vein Study. *J Vasc Surg Venous Lymphat Disord.* 2013;1(1):59-67.
30. García-Gimeno M, Rodríguez-Camarero S, Tagarro-Villalba S, et al. Reflux patterns and risk factors of primary varicose veins' clinical severity. *Phlebology.* 2013;28(3):153-161.
31. Robertson L, Evans C, Fowkes FG. Epidemiology of chronic venous disease. *Phlebology.* 2008;23(3):103-111.

32. Robertson LA, Evans CJ, Lee AJ, et al. Incidence and risk factors for venous reflux in the general population: Edinburgh Vein Study. *Eur J Vasc Endovasc Surg.* 2014;48(2):208-214.
33. Chiesa R, Marone EM, Limoni C, et al. Chronic venous insufficiency in Italy: the 24-cities cohort study. *Eur J Vasc Endovasc Surg.* 2005;30(4):422-429.
34. Chiesa R, Marone EM, Limoni C, et al. Demographic factors and their relationship with the presence of CVI signs in Italy: the 24-cities cohort study. *Eur J Vasc Endovasc Surg.* 2005;30(6):674-680.
35. Jukkola TM, Mäkivaara LA, Luukkaala T, et al. The effects of parity, oral contraceptive use and hormone replacement therapy on the incidence of varicose veins. *J Obstet Gynaecol.* 2006;26(5):448-451.
36. Goldman MP, Weiss RA, Bergan JJ. Diagnosis and treatment of varicose veins: a review. *J Am Acad Dermatol.* 1994;31(3):393-413.
37. Naoum JJ, Hunter GC. Pathogenesis of varicose veins and implications for clinical management. *Vascular.* 2007;15(5):242-249.
38. Lim CS, Davies AH. Pathogenesis of primary varicose veins. *Br J Surg.* 2009;96(11):1231-1242.
39. Pittaluga P, Chastanet S. Saphenous vein preservation: is the new gold standard? In: Becquemin JP, Alimi YS, eds. *Updates and Controversies in Vascular Surgery.* Turin, Italy: Minerva Medica; 2007:392-399.
40. Bergan JJ, Schmid-Schönbein GW, Smith PD, et al. Chronic venous disease. *N Engl J Med.* 2006;355(5):488-498.
41. Naoum JJ, Hunter GC, Woodside KJ, et al. Current advances in the pathogenesis of varicose veins. *J Surg Res.* 2007;141(2):311-316.
42. Bergan JJ, Pascarella L, Schmid-Schönbein GW. Pathogenesis of primary chronic venous disease: insights from animal models of venous hypertension. *J Vasc Surg Venous Lymphat Disord.* 2008;47(1):183-192.
43. Asbeutah AM, Al-Azemi M, Al-Sarhan S, et al. Changes in the diameter and valve closure time of leg veins in primigravida women during pregnancy. *J Vasc Surg Venous Lymphat Disord.* 2015;3(2):147-153.
44. Sadick NS. Predisposing factors of varicose and telangiectatic leg veins. *J Dermatol Surg Oncol.* 1992;18(10):883-886.
45. Rabe E, Pannier F. Clinical, aetiological, anatomical and pathological classification (CEAP): gold standard and limits. *Phlebology.* 2012;27(suppl 1):114-118.
46. Weiss RA, Weiss MA. Doppler ultrasound findings in reticular veins of the thigh subdermic lateral venous system and implications for sclerotherapy. *J Dermatol Surg Oncol.* 1993;19(10):947-951.
47. Weiss RA, Weiss MA. Continuous wave venous Doppler examination for pretreatment diagnosis of varicose and telangiectatic veins. *Dermatol Surg.* 1995;21(1):58-62.
48. Schuller-Petrović S, Pavlović MD, Schuller S, et al. Telangiectasias resistant to sclerotherapy are commonly connected to a perforating vessel. *Phlebology.* 2013;28(6):320-323.
49. Khilnani NM, Min RJ. Duplex ultrasound for superficial venous insufficiency. *Tech Vasc Interv Radiol.* 2003;6(3):111-115.
50. Malgor RD, Labropoulos N. Diagnosis and follow-up of varicose veins with duplex ultrasound: how and why? *Phlebology.* 2012;27(suppl 1):10-15.
51. Coleridge-Smith P, Labropoulos N, Partsch H, et al. Duplex ultrasound investigation of the veins in chronic venous disease of the lower limbs—UIP consensus document. Part I. Basic principles. *Eur J Vasc Endovasc Surg.* 2006;31(1):83-92.
52. Duffy DM. Cosmetic applications of sclerotherapy. *G Ital Dermatol Venereol.* 2012;147(1):45-63.
53. Friedmann DP, Liolios AM, Goldman MP. An update on the treatment of lower extremity veins. *Curr Dermatol Rep.* 2014;3(2):113-121.
54. Hach W. How sublimate of mercury for syphilis led to sclerotherapy for varicose veins. *Phlebologie.* 2013;42(4):213-218.
55. Wollmann J. The history of sclerosing foams. *Dermatol Surg.* 2004;30(5):694-703.
56. Partsch H. Use of compression therapy. In: Goldman MP, Guex JJ, Weiss RA, eds. *Sclerotherapy: Treatment of Varicose and Telangiectatic Leg Veins.* 5th ed. Philadelphia, PA: Saunders Elsevier; 2011:123-155.
57. Duffy DM. Sclerosants: a comparative review. *Dermatol Surg.* 2010;36(suppl 2):1010-1025.
58. Weiss MA, Hsu JT, Neuhaus I, et al. Consensus for sclerotherapy. *Dermatol Surg.* 2014;40(12):1309-1318.
59. Schwartz L, Maxwell H. Sclerotherapy for lower limb telangiectasias. *Cochrane Database Syst Rev.* 2011;12:CD008826.
60. Parsi K. Interaction of detergent sclerosants with cell membranes. *Phlebology.* 2015;30(5):306-315.
61. Rabe E, Pannier F. Sclerotherapy of varicose veins with polidocanol based on the guidelines of the German Society of Phlebology. *Dermatol Surg.* 2010;36(suppl 2): 968-975.
62. Guex J, Schliephake DE, Otto J, et al. The French polidocanol study on long-term side effects: a survey covering 3,357 patient years. *Dermatol Surg.* 2010;36(suppl 2):993-1003.
63. Goldman MP. Treatment of varicose and telangiectatic leg veins: double-blind prospective comparative trial between aethoxyskerol and sotradecol. *Dermatol Surg.* 2002;28(1):52-55.
64. Rabe E, Schliephake D, Otto J, et al. Sclerotherapy of telangiectases and reticular veins: a double-blind, randomized, comparative clinical trial of polidocanol, sodium tetradecyl sulphate and isotonic saline (EASI study). *Phlebology.* 2010;25(3):124-131.
65. Rao J, Wildemore JK, Goldman MP. Double-blind prospective comparative trial between foamed and liquid polidocanol and sodium tetradecyl sulfate in the treatment of varicose and telangiectatic leg veins. *Dermatol Surg.* 2005;31(6):631-635.
66. Dietzek CL. Sclerotherapy: introduction to solutions and techniques. *Perspect Vasc Surg Endovasc Ther.* 2007;19(3):317-324.
67. Zimmet SE. The prevention of cutaneous necrosis following extravasation of hypertonic saline and sodium tetradecyl sulfate. *J Dermatol Surg Oncol.* 1993;19(7):641-646.
68. Ghaznavi AM, Nakamura M, Tepper D. An analysis of 72% chromated glycerin used for sclerotherapy: sterility, potency, and cost after extended shelf life. *Dermatol Surg.* 2015;41(1):121-125.
69. Friedmann DP. Commentary on an analysis of 72% chromated glycerin used for sclerotherapy. *Dermatol Surg.* 2015;41(2):277-278.
70. Clinical methods for sclerotherapy of varicose veins. In: Goldman MP, Guex JJ, Weiss RA, eds. *Sclerotherapy: Treatment of Varicose and Telangiectatic Leg Veins.* 5th ed. Philadelphia, PA: Saunders Elsevier; 2011:238-281.
71. Goldman MP. My sclerotherapy technique for tel-

71. angiectasia and reticular veins. *Dermatol Surg.* 2010;36(suppl 2):1040-1045.
72. Mann MW. Sclerotherapy: it is back and better. *Clin Plast Surg.* 2011;38(3):475-487, vii.
73. Sadick NS. Choosing the appropriate sclerosing concentration for vessel diameter. *Dermatol Surg.* 2010;36(suppl 2):976-981.
74. Alder G, Lees T. Foam sclerotherapy. *Phlebology.* 2015;30(2)(suppl):18-23.
75. Bergan J. Sclerotherapy: a truly minimally invasive technique. *Perspect Vasc Surg Endovasc Ther.* 2008;20(1):70-72.
76. Uncu H. Sclerotherapy: a study comparing polidocanol in foam and liquid form. *Phlebology.* 2010;25(1):44-49.
77. Stücker M, Kobus S, Altmeyer P, et al. Review of published information on foam sclerotherapy. *Dermatol Surg.* 2010;36(suppl 2):983-992.
78. Cavezzi A, Tessari L. Foam sclerotherapy techniques: different gases and methods of preparation, catheter versus direct injection. *Phlebology.* 2009;24(6):247-251.
79. Carugo D, Ankrett DN, Zhao X, et al. Benefits of polidocanol endovenous microfoam (Varithena®) compared with physician-compounded foams. *Phlebology.* 2016;31(4):283-295.
80. Goldman MP. Compression in the treatment of leg telangiectasia: theoretical considerations. *J Dermatol Surg Oncol.* 1989;15(2):184-188.
81. Weiss RA, Sadick NS, Goldman MP, et al. Postsclerotherapy compression: controlled comparative study of duration of compression and its effects on clinical outcome. *Dermatol Surg.* 1999;25(2):105-108.
82. Goldman MP. How to utilize compression after sclerotherapy. *Dermatol Surg.* 2002;28(9):860-862.
83. Guex JJ. Complications and side-effects of foam sclerotherapy. *Phlebology.* 2009;24(6):270-274.
84. Scultetus AH, Villavicencio JL, Kao T, et al. Microthrombectomy reduces postsclerotherapy pigmentation: multicenter randomized trial. *J Vasc Surg.* 2003;38(5):896-903.
85. Goldman MP, Kaplan RP, Duffy DM. Postsclerotherapy hyperpigmentation: a histologic evaluation. *J Dermatol Surg Oncol.* 1987;13(5):547-550.
86. Weiss RA, Weiss MA. Incidence of side effects in the treatment of telangiectasias by compression sclerotherapy: hypertonic saline vs. polidocanol. *J Dermatol Surg Oncol.* 1990;16(9):800-804.
87. Clemetson CA, Blair L, Brown AB. Capillary strength and the menstrual cycle. *Ann N Y Acad Sci.* 1962;93:279-299.
88. Goldman MP, Sadick NS, Weiss RA. Cutaneous necrosis, telangiectatic matting, and hyperpigmentation following sclerotherapy. Etiology, prevention, and treatment. *Dermatol Surg.* 1995;21(1):19-29.
89. Tafazzoli A, Rostan EF, Goldman MP. Q-switched ruby laser treatment for postsclerotherapy hyperpigmentation. *Dermatol Surg.* 2000;26(7):653-656.
90. Moore M, Mishra V, Friedmann DP, et al. Minocycline-induced postsclerotherapy pigmentation successfully treated with a picosecond alexandrite laser. *Dermatol Surg.* 2016;42(1):133-134.
91. Davis LT, Duffy DM. Determination of incidence and risk factors for postsclerotherapy telangiectatic matting of the lower extremity: a retrospective analysis. *J Dermatol Surg Oncol.* 1990;16(4):327-330.
92. Cavezzi A, Parsi K. Complications of foam sclerotherapy. *Phlebology.* 2012;27(suppl 1):46-51.
93. Bergan JJ, Weiss RA, Goldman MP. Extensive tissue necrosis following high-concentration sclerotherapy for varicose veins. *Dermatol Surg.* 2000;26(6):535-541.
94. Bihari I, Magyar E. Reasons for ulceration after injection treatment of telangiectasia. *Dermatol Surg.* 2001;27(2):133-136.
95. Jia X, Mowatt G, Burr JM, et al. Systematic review of foam sclerotherapy for varicose veins. *Br J Surg.* 2007;94(8):925-936.
96. Parsi K, Hannaford P. Intra-arterial injection of sclerosants: report of three cases treated with systemic steroids. *Phlebology.* 2016;31(4):241-250.
97. Rush JE, Wright DD. More on microembolism and foam sclerotherapy. *N Engl J Med.* 2008;359(6):656-657.
98. Gillet JL. Neurological complications of foam sclerotherapy: fears and reality. *Phlebology.* 2011;26(7):277-279.
99. Duffy DM. Prevention of excessive endothelin-1 release in sclerotherapy: in vitro and in vivo studies. *Dermatol Surg.* 2014;40(12):1306-1308.
100. Introduction. In: Goldman MP, Guex JJ, Weiss RA, eds. *Sclerotherapy: Treatment of Varicose and Telangiectatic Leg Veins.* 5th ed. Philadelphia, PA: Saunders Elsevier; 2011:ix-xiv.
101. Caggiati A, Allegra C. Historical introduction. In: Bergan JJ, Bunke-Paquette N, eds. *The Vein Book.* 2nd ed. Oxford, UK: Oxford University Press; 2014:1-14.
102. Goldman MP. Closure of the greater saphenous vein with endoluminal radiofrequency thermal heating of the vein wall in combination with ambulatory phlebectomy: preliminary 6-month follow-up. *Dermatol Surg.* 2000;26(5):452-456.
103. Weiss RA. Comparison of endovenous radiofrequency versus 810 nm diode laser occlusion of large veins in an animal model. *Dermatol Surg.* 2002;28(1):56-61.
104. Brown K, Moore CJ. Update on the treatment of saphenous reflux: laser, RFA or foam? *Perspect Vasc Surg Endovasc Ther.* 2010;21(4):226-231.
105. Nesbitt C, Eifell RK, Coyne P, et al. Endovenous ablation (radiofrequency and laser) and foam sclerotherapy versus conventional surgery for great saphenous vein varices. *Cochrane Database Syst Rev.* 2011;10:CD005624.
106. Siribumrungwong B, Noorit P, Wilasrusmee C, et al. A systematic review and meta-analysis of randomised controlled trials comparing endovenous ablation and surgical intervention in patients with varicose vein. *Eur J Vasc Endovasc Surg.* 2012;44(2):214-223.
107. Kelleher D, Lane TR, Franklin IJ, et al. Socio-economic impact of endovenous thermal ablation techniques. *Lasers Med Sci.* 2014;29(2):493-499.
108. Merchant RF, Pichot O. Long-term outcomes of endovenous radiofrequency obliteration of saphenous reflux as a treatment for superficial venous insufficiency. *J Vasc Surg.* 2005;42(3):502-509.
109. Miyazaki K, Nishibe T, Sata F, et al. Long-term results of treatments for varicose veins due to greater saphenous vein insufficiency. *Int Angiol.* 2005;24(3):282-286.
110. Memetoğlu ME, Kurtcan S, Kalkan A, et al. Combination technique of tumescent anesthesia during endovenous laser therapy of saphenous vein insufficiency. *Interact Cardiovasc Thorac Surg.* 2010;11(6):774-777.
111. Navarro L, Min RJ, Boné C. Endovenous laser: a new minimally invasive method of treatment for varicose veins—preliminary observations using an 810 nm diode laser. *Dermatol Surg.* 2001;27(2):117-122.
112. Manfrini S, Gasbarro V, Danielsson G, et al. Endove-

nous management of saphenous vein reflux. Endovenous Reflux Management Study Group. *J Vasc Surg*. 2000;32(2):330-342.
113. Weiss RA, Weiss MA, Eimpunth S, et al. Comparative outcomes of different endovenous thermal ablation systems on great and small saphenous vein insufficiency: long-term results. *Lasers Surg Med*. 2015;47(2):156-160.
114. Lee JM, Jung IM, Chung JK. Clinical and duplex-sonographic outcomes of 1,320-nm endovenous laser treatment for saphenous vein incompetence. *Dermatol Surg*. 2012;38(10):1704-1709.
115. Poluektova AA, Malskat WS, van Gemert MJ, et al. Some controversies in endovenous laser ablation of varicose veins addressed by optical-thermal mathematical modeling. *Lasers Med Sci*. 2014;29(2):441-452.
116. van Ruijven PW, Poluektova AA, van Gemert MJ, et al. Optical-thermal mathematical model for endovenous laser ablation of varicose veins. *Lasers Med Sci*. 2014;29(2):431-439.
117. Proebstle TM, Sandhofer M, Kargl A, et al. Thermal damage of the inner vein wall during endovenous laser treatment: key role of energy absorption by intravascular blood. *Dermatol Surg*. 2002;28(7):596-600.
118. Vuylsteke ME, Martinelli T, Van Dorpe J, et al. Endovenous laser ablation: the role of intraluminal blood. *Eur J Vasc Endovasc Surg*. 2011;42(1):120-126.
119. Proebstle TM, Moehler T, Gül D, et al. Endovenous treatment of the great saphenous vein using a 1,320 nm Nd:YAG laser causes fewer side effects than using a 940 nm diode laser. *Dermatol Surg*. 2005;31(12):1678-1683.
120. Vuylsteke M, De Bo T, Dompe G, et al. Endovenous laser treatment: is there a clinical difference between using a 1500 nm and a 980 nm diode laser? A multicenter randomised clinical trial. *Int Angiol*. 2011;30(4):327-334.
121. Kabnick LS. Outcome of different endovenous laser wavelengths for great saphenous vein ablation. *J Vasc Surg*. 2006;43(1):88.e1-88.e7.
122. Doganci S, Demirkilic U. Comparison of 980 nm laser and bare-tip fibre with 1470 nm laser and radial fibre in the treatment of great saphenous vein varicosities: a prospective randomised clinical trial. *Eur J Vasc Endovasc Surg*. 2010;40(2):254-259.
123. Malskat WS, Poluektova AA, van der Geld CW, et al. Endovenous laser ablation (EVLA): a review of mechanisms, modeling outcomes, and issues for debate. *Lasers Med Sci*. 2014;29(2):393-403.
124. Ramelet AA. Müller phlebectomy. A new phlebectomy hook. *J Dermatol Surg Oncol*. 1991;17(10):814-816.
125. Smith SR, Goldman MP. Tumescent anesthesia in ambulatory phlebectomy. *Dermatol Surg*. 1998;24(4):453-456.
126. Ramelet AA. Complications of ambulatory phlebectomy. *Dermatol Surg*. 1997;23(10):947-954.
127. Meesters AA, Pitassi LH, Campos V, et al. Transcutaneous laser treatment of leg veins. *Lasers Med Sci*. 2014;29(2):481-492.
128. Anderson RR, Parrish JA. Selective photothermolysis: precise microsurgery by selective absorption of pulsed radiation. *Science*. 1983;220(4596):524-527.
129. McCoppin HH, Hovenic WW, Wheeland RG. Laser treatment of superficial leg veins: a review. *Dermatol Surg*. 2011;37(6):729-741.
130. Goldman MP, Eckhouse S. Photothermal sclerosis of leg veins. ESC Medical Systems, LTD Photoderm VL Cooperative Study Group. *Dermatol Surg*. 1996;22(4):323-330.
131. Fodor L, Ramon Y, Fodor A, et al. A side-by-side prospective study of intense pulsed light and Nd:YAG laser treatment for vascular lesions. *Ann Plast Surg*. 2006;56(2):164-170.
132. Ross EV, Domankevitz Y. Laser treatment of leg veins: physical mechanisms and theoretical considerations. *Lasers Surg Med*. 2005;36(2):105-116.
133. Klein A, Bäumler W, Koller M, et al. Indocyanine green-augmented diode laser therapy of telangiectatic leg veins: a randomized controlled proof-of-concept trial. *Lasers Surg Med*. 2012;44(5):369-376.
134. Kaudewitz P, Klövekorn W, Rother W. Treatment of leg vein telangiectases: 1-year results with a new 940 nm diode laser. *Dermatol Surg*. 2002;28(11):1031-1034.
135. Kunishige JH, Goldberg LH, Friedman PM. Laser therapy for leg veins. *Clin Dermatol*. 2007;25(5):454-461.

Chapter 213 :: Chemical Peels and Dermabrasion
:: Gary Monheit & Bailey Tayebi

第二百一十三章
化学剥脱术和磨削术

中文导读

本章分别介绍了化学剥脱和物理磨削术，并按照作用深度由浅至深列出常见皮肤重建术的治疗手段于表213-1。

第一节介绍了化学剥脱术围手术期注意事项。首先提到化学剥脱术的适应证可包括色素性、光照性和结构异常，病人选择方面尤其需要注意根据Fitzpatrick皮肤光照类型进行化学剥脱的治疗，因为深色皮肤类型治疗后色素改变的风险增加，所以不同Fitzpatrick皮肤类型对应不同深度的化学剥脱治疗（表213-2），还需询问病人的皮肤疾病并对应表213-3判断病人是否具有剥脱术的禁忌证，尤其是中、深程度的化学剥脱。紧接着介绍围手术期的护理，包括术前和术后的药物治疗及注意事项（表213-4）。

第二节介绍了化学剥脱术的技术流程，从术前患者清洁卸妆面部、治疗体位、术中麻醉剂、清洁剂、吸收剂、剥脱剂、术后的冷却、生理盐水的使用、防晒和润肤都有讲述，并且强调各流程中的注意事项，如眼部的保护。作者还强调角质层凝固，表现为皮肤表面一层白色霜样物质，通常被认为是理想的临床治疗终点。

第三节介绍化学剥脱术。作者先总结：浅表剥脱去除角质层并损伤表皮，中等深度的剥脱达到真皮网状层上部，深层剥脱会损伤真皮网状层的大部分，从而产生新的胶原蛋白和基质，并通过图213-3表示。接下来作者逐一介绍以上三种深度的化学剥脱治疗。

浅表化学剥脱适用于痤疮，尤其是粉刺性痤疮、毛孔扩大、炎症后色素沉着、黄褐斑、轻度皮肤损伤和细微的皮肤质地改变，并举例常见的试剂，如10%～20%三氯醋酸（TCA）、Jessner溶液、间苯二酚、14%水杨酸和α-羟基酸等，并突出水杨酸亲脂、抗炎及对色素治疗的特性，并用图213-6展示了不同化学剥脱剂的抗炎效果。中等深度的化学剥脱用于治疗轻度至中度光老化、色素紊乱、雀斑样痣（lentigines）、表皮过度生长、皱纹和光化性角化病，包括45%～60%的TCA、70%乙醇酸等，并介绍使用TCA治疗的情况及术后注意事项。最后是深层化学剥脱，它适用于深层皱纹、严重光老化，而萎缩性疤痕需使用70%到100%的TCA进行治疗。

第四节介绍了化学剥脱术的术后护理——使用0.25%的醋酸每日清洁皮肤四次并日常润肤。

第五节介绍化学剥脱术的并发症，其分为术中和术后两种情况，术中并发症可有：不正确的剥脱浓度、使用过期的产品、溶液错放以及未能正确中和剥脱试剂，而术后并发症包括感染、红斑、瘙痒、色素改变、接触性皮炎、粟丘疹/痤疮、潜在皮肤疾病恶化、瘢痕、炎症后色沉，并提到相对应的预防及治疗措施。

第六节介绍了三种物理磨削术：微晶磨削术、手动磨削术和电动剥脱术。此三种剥脱术是治疗瘢痕的有效方法。

〔简　丹〕

AT-A-GLANCE

- Chemexfoliation agents are broadly classified into superficial, medium, and deep peeling agents according to their depth of penetration and histologic injury.
- Preoperative evaluation of skin type, degree of photoaging, and underlying skin disorders is critical in safeguarding against potential complications.
- Appropriate patient selection and choice of procedure are critical to success.
- Keratocoagulation, evidenced by a white frosting of the skin, is generally regarded as the desired clinical end point of chemical peeling with trichloroacetic acid.
- Mechanical resurfacing, which includes microdermabrasion, manual dermasanding, and motorized dermabrasion, is an effective method for treatment of scars.
- Infection, prolonged erythema, pigmentary alterations, and scarring are potential complications of resurfacing procedures.

BACKGROUND

Resurfacing procedures, including chemical, mechanical, and laser resurfacing, wound the skin in a controlled and predictable manner so as to promote the growth of new skin with improved texture and quality. The art of chemical peeling dates back to ancient Egyptian times when the use of animal oils, salt, and lactic acid in sour milk were used to cosmetically enhance the appearance of skin. Mechanical exfoliation was first described in Greek and Roman literature using compounds containing mustard, sulfur, and limestone. In the mid-1800s, Viennese dermatologist Ferdinand Hebra used various peeling agents to treat pigmentary abnormalities. These early exfoliative agents included tinctures of iodine and lead, croton oil, cantharides, and various acids, including sulfuric, acetic, hydrochloric, and nitric acids. Tilbury Fox first introduced phenol to the topical dermatology arena in 1871. A decade later, P. G. Unna reported on the use of salicylic acid, resorcinol, phenol, and trichloroacetic acid (TCA) as peeling agents. Over the next century, several physicians worked to modify peeling agent formulations, combinations, and procedures. In the 1980s, Samuel Stegman identified the depth of injury associated with various peeling agents, which enabled later categorization into superficial, medium, and deep chemical peels. Today, chemexfoliation, or chemical peeling, involves the application of a chemical exfoliant aimed to wound and subsequently regenerate the epidermis and/or dermis to remove superficial skin lesions, improve pigmentary abnormalities and photodamage, and address textural concerns (Table 213-1).[1]

PERIOPERATIVE CONSIDERATIONS

The perioperative evaluation is a critical component of every chemical resurfacing procedure. The physician should seek a thorough understanding of patient treatment goals, expectations, and allotted down time prior to initiation of the procedure. The physician should also assess the patient's level of compliance and need for preprocedural and/or postprocedural adjuvant treatments.[2] Patients should be instructed to avoid depilatory procedures, such as waxing and shaving, prior to the procedure, as well as ultraviolet light exposure before and after the date of the chemical peel. Lastly, preoperative photographs should be taken to serve as a benchmark with which to grade clinical results.

INDICATIONS

Chemexfoliation indications can be classified into pigmentary (eg, postinflammatory hyperpigmentation, melasma), photoinduced (eg, actinic keratoses), and textural abnormalities (eg, epidermal growths, rhytides, scarring, acne vulgaris).[2]

PATIENT SELECTION

The perioperative evaluation should assess the patient's skin type, degree of photoaging, and whether or not the patient has underlying skin disorders. When evaluating skin type, it is useful to classify patients according to their Fitzpatrick skin phototype (SPT). In general, darker skin types (SPT IV to SPT VI) have an increased risk of pigmentary alterations following chemical peels. While superficial peels tend to be well tolerated by all skin types, deep peels are commonly avoided in patients with SPT IV to SPT VI skin because of the higher risks of postprocedural pigmentary change and scarring (Table 213-2).[2-4]

TABLE 213-1
Resurfacing Procedures

	PEELING	DERMABRASION	LASER
Superficial	Glycolic Jessner solution Salicylic acid	Microdermabrasion	–
Medium depth	Jessner solution + 35% trichloroacetic acid	Manual dermasanding	Erbium laser
Deep	Baker phenol peel	Mechanical dermabrasion	CO_2 laser

The patient's degree of photodamage assists the physician in electing the appropriate rejuvenation procedure necessary to achieve clinically significant results. The Glogau system, which classifies patients into categories I through IV based on whether the patient has mild, moderate, advanced, or severe photodamage, is a useful categorization tool for this purpose. In general, both category I and category II photodamage will improve with more superficial peeling agents (Fig. 213-1). Category III will respond to medium-depth peels, while category IV will require deep peeling agents possibly in combination with mechanical and/or laser resurfacing procedures[3] (Fig. 213-2).

Lastly, inquiring about a patient's underlying skin disorders allows the physician to safeguard against potentially-devastating complications such as infection and scarring. The physician should inquire about a history of atopy, rosacea, isotretinoin therapy, poor wound healing, connective tissue disease, and hypertrophic or keloid scar formation as chemical resurfacing may be contraindicated in these patients.[4] Additionally, a history of recurrent infections, including bacterial, fungal, and viral, should be elicited in the preoperative consultation. A patient with recurrent herpes simplex virus should be prophylactically treated with an antiviral agent prior to the procedure. Common pretreatment regimens include acyclovir 400 mg thrice daily and valacyclovir 500 mg twice daily starting on the day of the peel and continued until reepithelialization has occurred (Table 213-3).[3,5]

SIDE EFFECTS

The perioperative consultation is also an appropriate time to review the risks and benefits of chemical peeling. Expected intraoperative side effects include stinging, burning, and/or itching. In the immediate postoperative period, erythema, edema, and desquamation may be experienced.[2]

PERIOPERATIVE PREPARATIONS

Chemical peeling agents can penetrate to predictable histologic depths; however, the physician can augment this depth with the use of certain preoperative preparations.[6-8] Topical pretreatment with retinoic, glycolic, or lactic acid alone, or in combination, will increase the absorption of the wounding agent and promote a more even penetration of the peel. Pretreatment should begin 2 to 4 weeks before the procedure and be discontinued approximately 2 to 3 days prior to the peel date.[2,6] Pretreatment with a topical retinoid may also speed the healing process (Table 213-4).[4]

Topical medications such as 2% to 5% hydroquinone may be applied to the skin preoperatively and postoperatively to minimize the risk of postinflammatory hyperpigmentation. Pretreatment should be considered in patients with SPT III to SPT VI, and in those treated for problems of hyperpigmentation.[6] Application of hydroquinone, in addition to a ultraviolet A/ultraviolet B protective sunscreen (sun protection factor 30 or higher), should be initiated 2 to 4 weeks prior to the date of the peel and resumed once reepithelialization has occurred postoperatively. As a rule, patients prone to dyschromias should adhere to a policy of strict sun avoidance in the perioperative period.

TABLE 213-2
Fitzpatrick Skin Phototypes and Peel Indications

SKIN PHOTOTYPE	SKIN REACTION	PEEL SUPERFICIAL	PEEL MEDIUM	PEEL DEEP
I	Always burn, never tan	+	+	–
II	Always burn, sometimes tan	+	+	–
III	Sometimes burn, always tan	+	+	–
IV	Never burn, always tan	+	+	±
V	Moderate pigmented skin	+	±	–
VI	Darkly pigmented skin	+	±	–

–, no; +, yes; ±, either.

PROCEDURAL TECHNIQUE

Following informed consent, instruct the patient to remove any makeup with a gentle facial cleanser. The patient is then placed in the supine position on the operating table with the head elevated to a 30-degree angle.[9] This position minimizes the risk of solution inadvertently dripping toward the eyes and allows the physician to visualize the complete treatment area.

In general, more superficial chemical peels do not require sedation or other forms of anesthesia. Medium

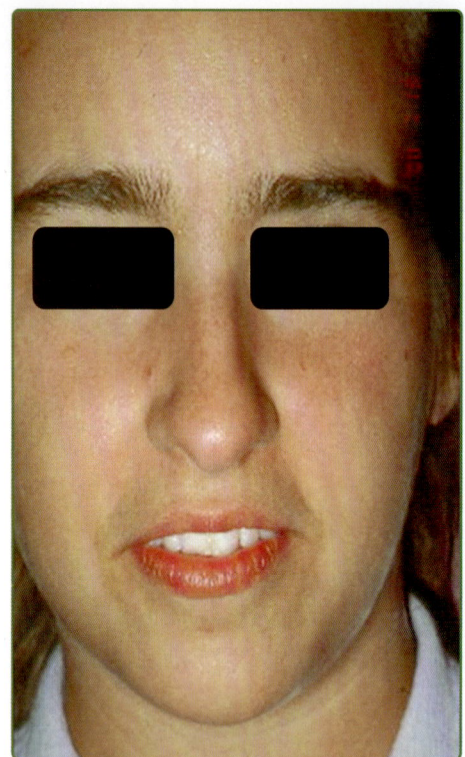
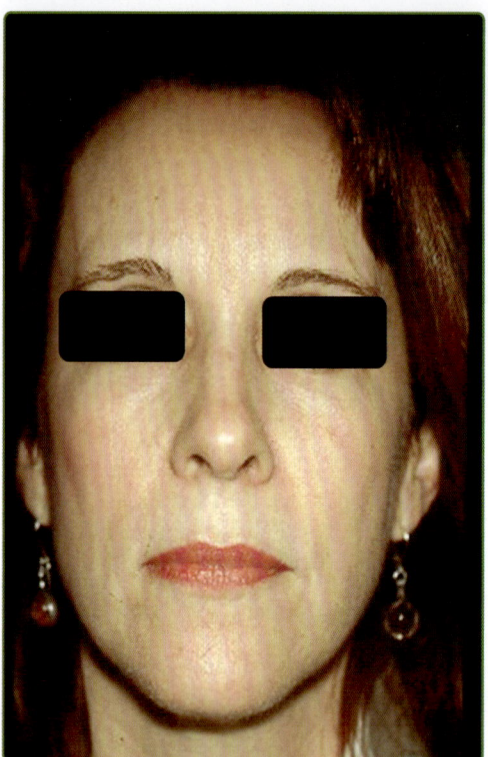

Figure 213-1 Glogau photoaging types I and II. Indications for superficial peeling.

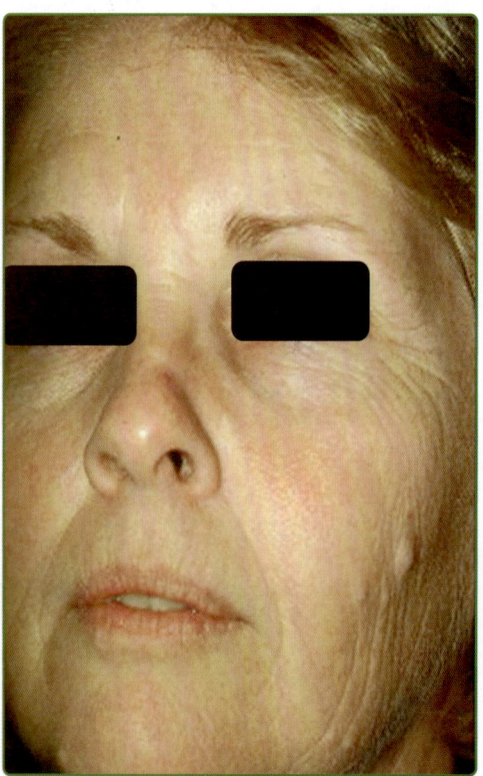
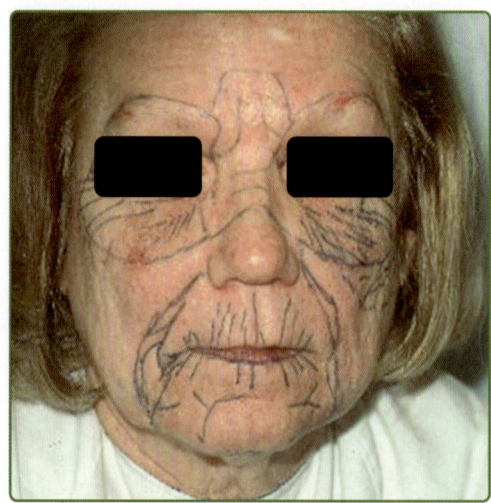

Figure 213-2 Glogau photoaging types III and IV. Indications for medium and deep chemical peeling.

TABLE 213-3
Contraindications to Medium and Deep Peels

RELATIVE CONTRAINDICATIONS	ABSOLUTE CONTRAINDICATIONS
Active skin disease	Open wounds, excoriations
Recent facial surgery	Isotretinoin within last 6 months
History of facial keloids	Pregnancy
History of postinflammatory hyperpigmentation	Unrealistic expectations
Radiation to head and neck	Poor patient–physician relationship
Active skin infection • Bacterial • Viral	

and deep peeling agents, however, are associated with significantly more operative discomfort and may require sedative and pain medications and/or local nerve blocks. Such blocks commonly include anesthetizing the supraorbital, infraorbital, temporal, and mental nerves.[9]

Once the patient has been positioned and the appropriate level of anesthesia has been undertaken, the skin is vigorously cleansed and degreased. A variety of cleansing agents may be used for this purpose including hexachlorophene, acetone, rubbing alcohol, chlorhexidine, or some combination of these agents.[3,6,7,9] An even application can be achieved with a 4-inch × 4-inch gauze. The skin should then be rinsed and dried prior to application of the chemexfoliant.

TABLE 213-4
Preoperative and Postoperative Care for Chemical Peels

Preparation (Weeks to Days Before Peel)
- Topical pretreatment with a retinoid, glycolic or lactic acid solution (begin 2 to 4 weeks prior, discontinue 2 to 3 days before peel date)
- Consider topical 2% to 5% hydroquinone preoperatively and postoperatively, if postinflammatory hyperpigmentation is a concern (2 to 4 weeks prior)
- Sun avoidance, especially in individuals at risk for dyschromias
- Consider pretreatment with acyclovir 400 mg thrice daily or valacyclovir 500 mg twice daily on the day of peel and until reepithelization

Preprocedural Care (Immediately Prior to Peel)
- Cleanse skin with gentle facial cleanser
- Position patient with head up at a 30-degree angle
- Consider sedative/pain medications or local nerve blocks for medium to deep peels
- Degrease skin with acetone, hexachlorophene, rubbing alcohol, or chlorhexidine
- Rinse and dry skin prior to application of chemexfoliant

Postprocedural Care
- Cleanse skin up to 4 times/day
- Dilute 0.25% acetic acid (1 tbsp vinegar in 1 pint water) as cleansing agent
- Pat dry, apply bland emollient
- Daily sunscreen use
- Avoidance of excessive sun exposure

This cleansing regimen will remove all oil and debris and promote even penetration of the wounding agent while minimizing the risk of a spotty or ineffective peel.

For medium-depth peeling, an absorbing agent may be applied to the skin to increase the effectiveness or penetration depth of the peeling agent. In 1986, Brody and Hailey applied solid carbon dioxide (CO_2) in combination with acetone prior to application of 35% TCA to disrupt the epidermal barrier and achieve a more even peel at a greater histologic depth.[3] Later, in 1989, Monheit described a similar technique using Jessner solution prior to application of 35% TCA. Acting as an absorbing agent, Jessner solution removes the stratum corneum allowing for deeper penetration of TCA. Coleman similarly demonstrated greater wounding depths with use of 70% glycolic acid prior to application of 35% TCA.[3,9] Use of absorbing agents such as these offers improved safety, minimizes the risk of pigmentary alterations and scarring, and creates clinical results comparable to a deep 50% TCA peel.

The peeling agent is then applied. This is commonly done with cotton-tipped applicators or 4-inch × 4-inch/2-inch × 2-inch gauze. The face is peeled sequentially by anatomic location starting on the forehead, followed by the temples, cheeks, and finally the lips and eyelids.[3] Feathering of the solution into the hairline, brows, and jawline helps to conceal lines of demarcation between peeled and nonpeeled areas.[9] Alternatively, a superficial peeling agent may be applied to such areas as neck and décolleté to assist in blending treated and untreated cosmetic units. Special care is taken to protect the eyes during a chemical peel. A semidry applicator should be used to carry the solution within 2 to 3 mm of the lid margin. Furthermore, tears are wicked away with a dry cotton-tipped applicator to prevent peel solution from traveling to the puncta and eye via capillary action.[9] Should peel solution inadvertently enter the eye, initiate aggressive irrigation with normal saline flushes immediately.

During the procedure, the physician is able to ensure even application of the peeling agent by the demonstration of even frosting. Frosting is representative of underlying keratocoagulation, or denaturation of epidermal keratin proteins.[9] Although true frosting does not occur with each and every peeling agent, frosting is generally regarded as the desired end point. Level I frosting is defined as erythema with blotchy or spotty frosting. This is often seen with light chemical peels. Level II frosting is commonly seen in medium-depth chemical peels and is achieved when a white coating is evident with a slight erythematous background showing through. Level III frosting is attained when a solid white enamel-like frosting is demonstrated on the skin. This is seen in deeper chemical peels and is indicative of peel penetration into the papillary dermis.[3]

Immediately following the procedure, cool saline compresses are applied for 5 to 10 minutes. This is for comfort as the reaction is complete after frosting. Only glycolic acid peels require neutralization. A bland emollient as well as a broad-spectrum sunscreen are then gently massaged into the skin.

CHEMICAL RESURFACING PROCEDURES

Chemical peeling involves the application of a chemical agent that wounds the epidermis and/or dermis and stimulates collagen remodeling and new epidermal growth, thus achieving a cosmetic benefit. The degree of penetration, destruction, and inflammation determines the level of peeling.[3] Superficial peeling agents remove the stratum corneum and wound the epidermis.[8,9] Destruction of the entire epidermis defines a full superficial peel. Medium-depth peels penetrate through the papillary dermis to the upper reticular dermis.[3,8] Deep peeling agents wound a greater portion of the reticular dermis resulting in production of new collagen and ground substances (Fig. 213-3).[3,8,9]

SUPERFICIAL CHEMICAL PEELING

Superficial chemical peels are indicated for acne, particularly comedonal acne, enlarged pores, postinflammatory hyperpigmentation, melasma, mild photodamage, and fine textural concerns.[2,4,10] Superficial exfoliants include 10% to 20% TCA (20% to 35% TCA achieves a complete epidermal peel), Jessner solution (14% salicylic acid, 14% lactic acid, and 14% resorcinol in ethanol), resorcinol, salicylic acid, and α-hydroxy acids such as glycolic acid.[2,6] Superficial peeling agents disrupt corneocyte adhesion and lead to regeneration of a thickened epidermis, normalization of the basal cell layer, and dispersal of melanin. Superficial agents may also enact dermal change including increased dermal collagen and improved quality of elastic fibers.[11,12] Complete recovery is expected in 2 to 4 days (Fig. 213-4).[4,6]

Salicylic acid is a naturally occurring β-hydroxy acid derived from the bark of the willow tree. It is regarded as a safe peel in all skin types for the treatment of acne, melasma, and postinflammatory hyperpigmentation. As described by Grimes, salicylic acid exhibits a lipophilic nature that allows for effective dissolution of the stratum corneum as well as comedolysis.[13] Therefore,

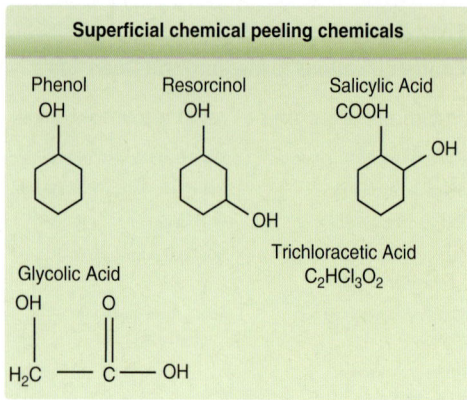

Figure 213-4 Superficial chemical peeling chemicals.

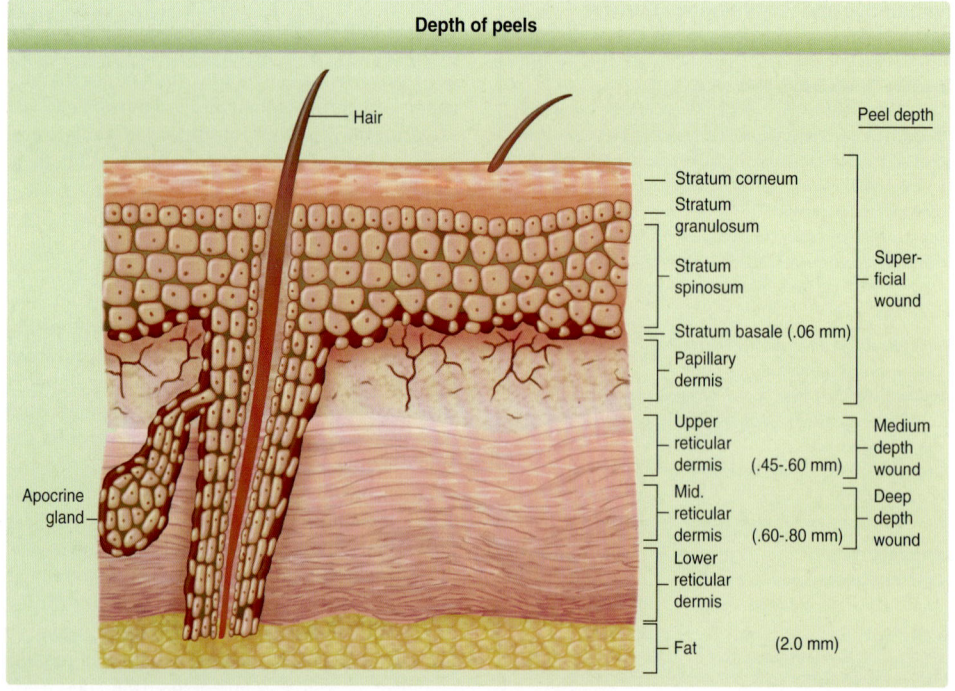

Figure 213-3 Depth of peels.

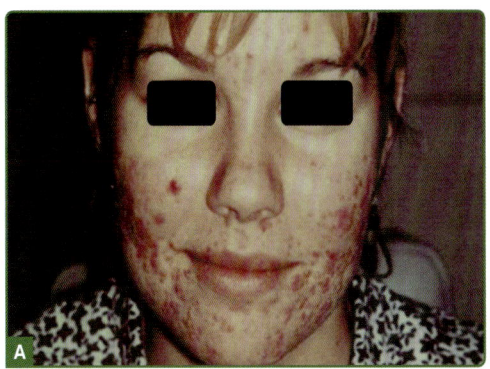

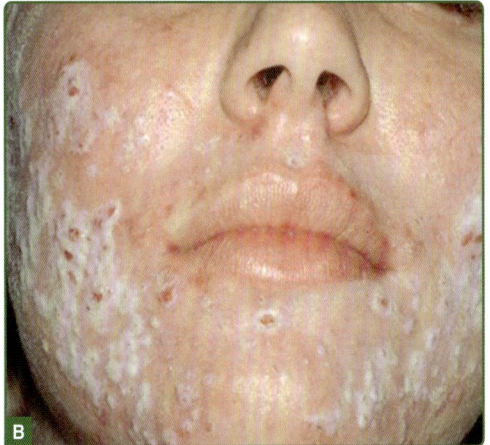

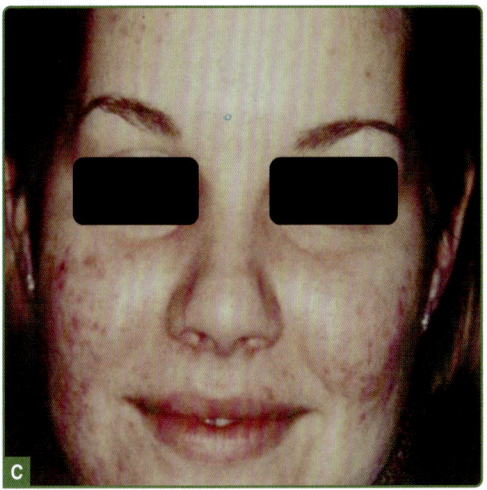

Figure 213-5 Salicylic acid peel for acne. **A,** Pretreatment. **B,** Perifollicular frosting. **C,** After 3 treatments.

treatment of dyschromias. In a pilot study by Grimes, 88% of patients with SPT V and SPT VI demonstrated improvement in dyschromias, with 4% hydroquinone pretreatment followed by a graduated series of 20% and 30% salicylic acid peels.[10] Salicylic acid is a preferential peeling agent for dyschromia as it is the least inflammatory of peeling agents. It has the least risk of producing postinflammatory hyperpigmentation (Fig. 213-6).

α-Hydroxy acids include glycolic acid along with several other naturally, occurring, nontoxic agents such as lactic, citric, malic, and tartaric acid.[2,6] Glycolic acid concentrations of 10% to 70% are frequently used in the treatment of acne, dyschromias, and mild signs of photoaging, and are safe in most skin types. Unlike other superficial peeling agents, the action of glycolic acid is time dependent and must be neutralized with normal saline, water, or sodium bicarbonate. α-Hydroxy acids wound the skin via loss of keratinocyte cohesion within the epidermis. Peels using 70% glycolic acid can also result in increased fibroblast proliferation, collagen and elastic fiber formation, and melanin dispersion.[2,15]

MEDIUM-DEPTH CHEMICAL PEELING

Medium-depth chemical peels are indicated for the treatment of mild to moderate photoaging, pigmentary disorders, lentigines, epidermal growths, rhytides, and actinic keratoses.[9] Peeling agents include 45% to 60% TCA as well as combination peels such as Jessner solution with 35% TCA (Monheit peel), 70% glycolic acid with 35% TCA (Coleman peel), and solid CO_2 with 35% TCA (Brody peel).[3,6,9] Fifty percent TCA is not used any longer because of the risk of scar from deeper penetration of the agent in the dermis. Combination peels are the preferred medium-depth peels because of their lower risk of postprocedural dyschromias and scarring.[3,9] Histologically, medium-depth chemical peels are associated with diminished solar elastosis, fibroblast proliferation, increased collagen formation, and reorganization of elastic fibers (see Fig. 213-3; Table 213-5).[8,12]

TCA is a crystalline inorganic compound that results in keratocoagulation, or protein denaturation, and resultant cell death, as indicated by a white frosting on the skin. Effects of this self-neutralizing peeling agent are cumulative with each application penetrating deeper than the last. TCA may be relatively quantitated with utilization of 1 to 4 cotton-tipped applicators. Loose or wrinkled skin should be stretched to achieve an even application of the solution and prevent pooling of the solution in folds. A level II to level III frosting is generally complete within 30 seconds to 2 minutes of TCA application; however, thicker epidermal growths may require additional applications.[2,9] Moreover, areas of poor frosting may require careful reapplication of the peeling agent.[3] At the completion of the peel, cool

salicylic acid proves beneficial in the treatment of comedonal and papular/pustular acne.[2,4,13,14] A split-face study by Meguid and colleagues reported that treatment of inflammatory acne lesions with the use of 30% salicylic acid was superior to treatment using 25% TCA, although an improvement in total lesions, including both comedonal and inflammatory, occurred in 95% of patients on the salicylic acid–treated side (Fig. 213-5).[14] Salicylic acid peels are also effective in the

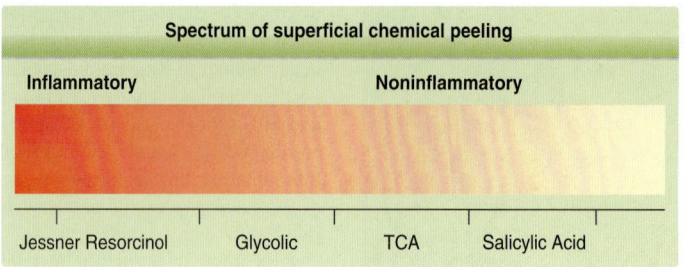

Figure 213-6 Spectrum of superficial chemical peeling. TCA, trichloroacetic acid.

saline compresses are placed on the skin. A bland emollient and sunscreen are then applied. Expected side effects include erythema, edema, and desquamation. Edema of the eyelids may be severe enough that it closes the lids. As the skin heals, erythema intensifies as desquamation comes to an end within 3 to 4 days. New skin is evident within 6 to 7 days, and healing is complete within 7 to 10 days. At this point, the erythema is reminiscent of a sunburn and is expected to resolve within 3 to 4 weeks.[9] TCA should be used cautiously in SPT IV to SPT VI. One should never "overcoat" TCA once the frosting is complete as accumulated TCA will produce a deeper peel (Fig. 213-7).

DEEP CHEMICAL PEELING

Deep chemical peels are indicated for deep rhytides and severe photoaging (Glogau categories III and IV) and include peeling agents such as Baker phenol.[9] The phenol is diluted to a concentration of 45% to 55% with croton oil, hexachlorophene, and water, and is referred to as the Baker-Gordon phenol peel. Two variations, an occluded and unoccluded, exist in clinical practice. In the occluded phenol peel, zinc oxide tape is placed over the skin after the peeling solution has been applied so as to increase absorption. The unoccluded method, described by McCollough, requires application of higher volumes of peeling solution; however, depth of penetration is diminished as compared to the occluded technique. Both variations of the Baker-Gordon phenol peel possess inherent risks and require monitoring and IV fluid administration because of potential cardiac, renal, and hepatic toxicities.[3,16,17] Baker-Gordon deep chemical peeling is a more aggressive procedure with inherent risks, but is the most permanent skin rejuvenation of all resurfacing procedures.

High concentrations of TCA are used in the treatment of atrophic scars in a procedure known as TCA chemical reconstruction of skin scars (TCA CROSS). In this procedure, first described by Lee and colleagues, TCA is applied with a sharp-tipped wooden applicator pressed firmly against the base of the scar until a white frost is apparent. Because high concentrations (70% to 100%) of TCA penetrate to the deep dermis, histologic remodeling also occurs at this level. Such remodeling consists of dermal expansion with increased collagen proliferation that results in elevation of depressed, atrophic scars.[18,19] Agarwal and colleagues reported successful use of 70% TCA applied with standard TCA CROSS technique in the treatment of boxcar, rolling, and ice pick scars in SPT IV and SPT V. In this study, postinflammatory hyperpigmentation was reported but improved with time and use of "depigmenting" creams; formation of keloids, persistent erythema, and reactivation of herpes simplex virus were not seen.[19]

Medium-depth and deep peeling agents result in significant inflammation and wounding within the deep reticular dermis and heal with 4 characteristic stages, including inflammation, coagulation, reepithelialization, and fibroplasia. Inflammation and coagulation occur within hours of application of the peeling agent. Reepithelialization then begins on day 3 and continues through days 10 to 14. Fibroplasia is the last stage of the healing process and persists for 3 to 4 months. This stage includes neoangiogenesis and collagen proliferation.[3] In a histologic and biochemical analysis by Butler and colleagues, reorganization of dermal collagen and elastic fiber networks was prominently seen following 50% TCA and phenol peels.[12] These dermal changes allow for the improvement in rhytides and other signs of photoaging seen clinically following deep chemical peels.

POSTOPERATIVE CARE

Following a chemical peel, patients are instructed to cleanse the skin up to 4 times daily to prevent infection and debride the necrotic exfoliation. Dilute 0.25% acetic acid (1 tablespoon vinegar in 1 pint water) is a commonly recommended cleansing agent because of its antibacterial action against *Pseudomonas* and other Gram-negative bacterial organisms.[3,5,9] After cleansing, the skin is patted dry and a bland emollient is applied.

TABLE 213-5
Medium-Depth Wounding

- Trichloroacetic acid (TCA) 50%
- Liquified phenol USP (U.S. Pharmacopoeia) 88%
- Solid carbon dioxide + TCA 35% to 50%
- Jessner solution + TCA

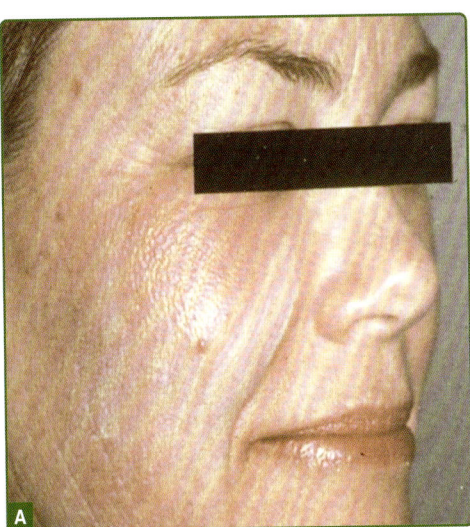

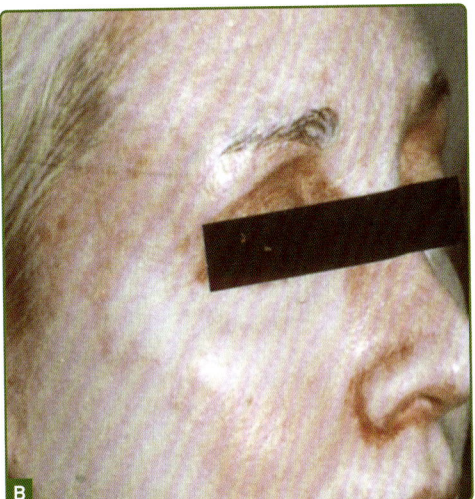

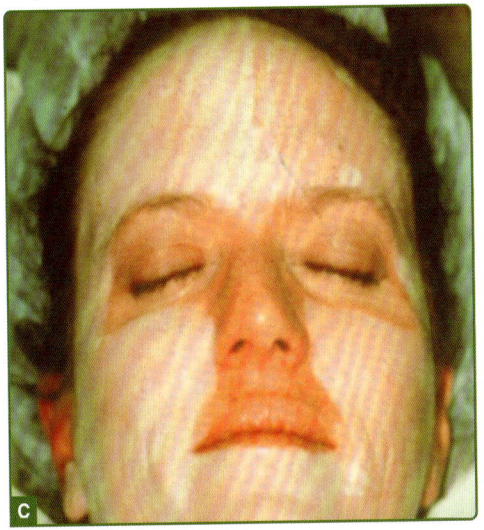

Figure 213-7 Levels of frosting. **A,** Level I: erythema with streaky frosting—superficial epidermal. **B,** Level II: white frosting with visible erythema—full-thickness epidermal. **C,** Level III: white enamel frosting—epidermal or dermal.

COMPLICATIONS

Complications can occur either intraoperatively or postoperatively.[3] Intraoperative complications include, but are not limited to, incorrect peel concentrations, use of expired products, accidental solution misplacement, and failure to properly neutralize the peel solution. Such errors may be prevented with care taken to check concentrations and dates of expiration. As removal of intact peeling agent crystals from the storage bottle may lead to higher concentrations placed on the skin, the physician should pour the peeling solution into a secondary container prior to initiation of the procedure. Furthermore, solution should never be passed over the face or allowed to actively drip onto the skin. Neutralizing solutions should be identified properly (eg, sodium bicarbonate for glycolic acid peels) and kept at the patient's bedside for quick placement following completion of the peel.

Postoperative complications include infection (bacterial, viral, fungal), prolonged erythema, pruritus, pigmentary alterations, contact dermatitis, milia/acne, exacerbation of an underlying skin disease, and scarring.[3,9] Frequent postoperative visits and early recognition of complications are critical, especially for medium and deep chemical peels in which risks of scarring are inherently higher. Delayed wound healing and persistent erythema are signs that skin is not healing normally and are indicative of scarring potential. Delayed healing is evident with the appearance of friable, stellate erosions on the skin at the time reepithelialization is expected. As erosions may be indicative of infectious etiologies, all such wounds should be cultured. Erosions should be treated with artificial wound dressings and topical or systemic corticosteroids.[5] Persistent erythema is defined as erythema lasting longer than 3 to 5 days for a superficial peel, 15 to 30 days for a medium-depth peel, and 60 to 90 days for a deep chemical peel.[3] Etiologies include underlying skin disorders such as rosacea and atopy, contact dermatitis or sensitivity to the peeling agent, and aggressive peeling techniques.[20] Persistent erythema should be treated promptly with topical and/or systemic corticosteroids (Fig. 213-8).[3,5,20]

Postinflammatory hyperpigmentation and other pigmentary dyschromias are more common in SPT IV to SPT VI with medium and deep chemical peels presenting a greater risk than superficial peels. Hyperpigmentation is also more common

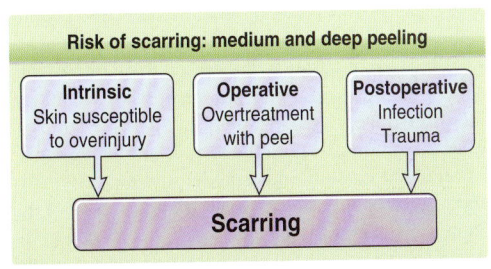

Figure 213-8 Risk of scarring: medium and deep peeling.

in individuals on hormonal therapies including oral contraceptive pills and photosensitizing medications.[5] In general, superficial peels should be elected in individuals with darker skin types. The physician may recommend treatment with hydroquinone, with or without a retinoid, in the perioperative period to minimize risks of hyperpigmentation.[2,4,5] Hypopigmentation, on the other hand, can be a complication associated with phenol peels. The resulting coloration of the skin is comparable to the natural appearance of sun-protected sites, such as the axillae and postauricular skin, and is directly proportional to the amount of phenol applied.[5] Deeper penetration can efface the papillary dermis creating a much lighter appearance with an "alabaster" texture.

MECHANICAL RESURFACING PROCEDURES

MICRODERMABRASION

Developed by Marini and Lo Brutto in 1985, microdermabrasion is a closed-system mechanical resurfacing procedure using abrasive aluminum oxide crystals to ablate the superficial epidermis.[21-23] The machine operates by discharging crystals onto the skin from a compression source. Crystals wound the superficial epidermis, removing keratinocytes and sebum, and are then returned to a waste container via vacuum suction. The ablative strength of the procedure is dependent on the strength of the vacuum and contact time with the skin. Depth of injury and clinical results are generally comparable to that of superficial chemical peels. Histologic investigation by Freedman and colleagues demonstrated return of a "basket-weave" stratum corneum, thickening of the epidermis and dermis, and increased collagen and elastic fibers following a series of microdermabrasion treatments.[24]

Microdermabrasion is regarded as a safe procedure in most skin types. The procedure is well tolerated and does not require anesthesia. Indications include enlarged pores, fine rhytides, mild photodamage, and acne scarring. Multiple treatments are usually necessary to achieve appreciable clinical results. Side effects are minimal and short-lived including erythema, petechiae/purpura, and tenderness. Complications such as persistent erythema, telangiectases, and postinflammatory hyperpigmentation are uncommon; however, microdermabrasion is best avoided in patients with underlying rosacea, and aggressive technique should be discouraged in patients with SPT V and SPT VI. Rare complications to the technician involve inhalation of the crystals and include pulmonary fibrosis and foreign-body granuloma, which are a result of the aluminum oxide crystals used in the procedure. To minimize such risks, eye protection and masks should be worn by the operators.[23,25]

TABLE 213-6
Manual vs Motorized Dermabrasion

MANUAL DERMABRASION	MOTORIZED DERMABRASION
• Minimal cost of equipment, no maintenance, disposable	• High cost of machine; gas sterilization of burrs and fraises required; face shields, draping required
• No aerosolization of blood and infectious particles	
• Difficult to perform in concavities (alar groove, nasolabial fold)	• Aerosolization of blood and infectious particles
• Longer procedure time	• Specialized burr shapes provide ease of use in smaller units or concavities
• Depending on material used, risk for granuloma formation if inadequate postprocedural cleaning	• Shorter procedure time
	• No risk for granuloma formation

Data from Gillard M, Wang T, Boyd C. Conventional diamond fraise vs manual spot dermabrasion with drywall sanding screen for scars from skin cancer surgery. *JAMA Dermatol.* 2002;138(8):1035-39.

MANUAL DERMASANDING

Manual dermabrasion (Table 213-6), or dermasanding, uses sterile sandpaper of varying grades to ablate the epidermis and portions of the dermis. Two hundred or 400 grit-grade sandpaper wrapped around gauze or a cotton-tipped applicator is used to abrade the skin until punctate bleeding is evident. This cost- and time-effective procedure is frequently elected for the treatment of surgical scars. A split-scar study by Poulos and colleagues reported improvement in the appearance of surgical scars, particularly that of scar color and elevation, following manual dermabrasion performed 6 to 8 weeks postoperatively.[26] It is important to rinse the abraded skin thoroughly to remove the silica-carbide crystals as they can become imbedded in the skin and create granulomas or tattoos (Fig. 213-9).

MOTORIZED DERMABRASION

Motorized dermabrasion (see Table 213-6) is a mechanical resurfacing technique in which handheld devices using burrs of varying degrees of coarseness are used to remove layers of the epidermis and/or dermis.[25] Biopsies of dermabraded skin demonstrate normalization of the rete ridge pattern, increased type I collagen, and increased elastic fibers.[27,28]

Motorized dermabrasion is indicated for moderate to severe photodamage, including textural changes, rhinophyma, and scar revision. Patients with SPT IV to SPT VI should be treated cautiously because of the potential for postprocedural pigmentary alterations. To minimize such risks, pretreatment and posttreatment with a topical retinoid or hydroquinone may be elected.

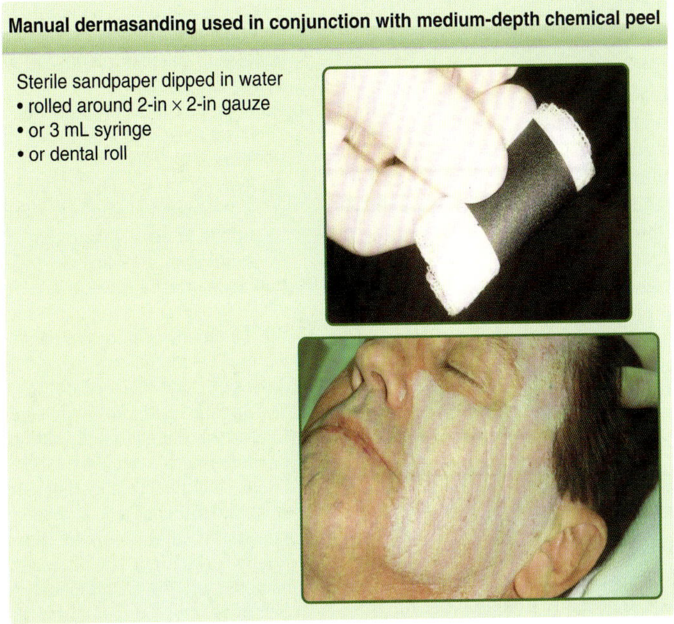

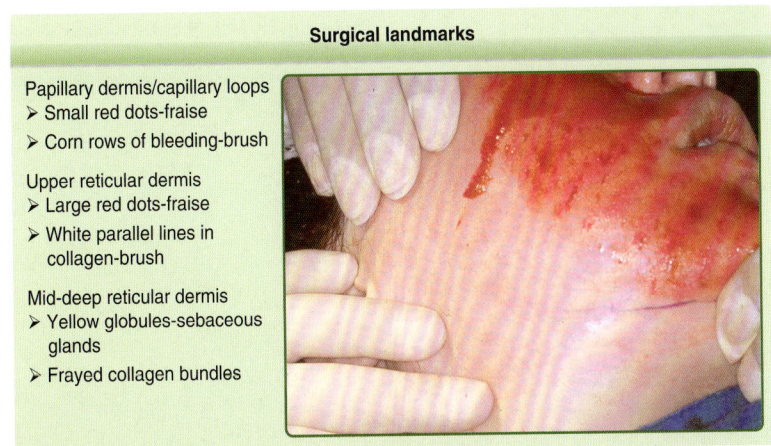

Figure 213-9 Manual dermasanding can be used in conjunction with medium-depth chemical peel to provide selective deeper resurfacing.

Prior to the procedure, the treatment area is injected with local anesthesia. Regional nerve blocks also may be done to improve patient comfort. For larger treatment areas, sedative medications and/or general anesthesia may be required. The physician and assistants should wear gowns and eye protection because of aerosolization of skin particles and blood during the procedure.

The proper burr should then be selected for the treatment area and desired clinical result. Commonly-used burrs include diamond fraises and wire brushes. The physician is able to control the depth of destruction by means of the amount of pressure applied and the selected speed of the dermabrader. Punctate bleeding is indicative of wounding to the level of the papillary dermis while more confluent bleeding is seen with wounding to the level of the reticular dermis. To minimize the risk of adverse events including scarring, treatment should never extend below the mid-reticular dermis (Fig. 213-10).

At the conclusion of the procedure, cool saline-soaked gauze is applied to the skin followed by application of a bland emollient. The patient is instructed to cleanse the treated skin with 0.25% acetic acid daily and keep the affected skin moist with a bland emollient until reepithelialization has occurred at approximately 7 to 10 days. Ultraviolet radiation should be strictly avoided and broad-spectrum sunscreens should be applied daily. Healing generally occurs in 2 to 4 weeks and postprocedural erythema is expected to resolve in 1 to 2 months.[25]

Figure 213-10 Surgical landmarks.

CONCLUSIONS

Chemical and mechanical resurfacing procedures serve as effective treatments for a multitude of pigmentary, textural, and photodamage-related concerns. A vast variety of procedures exist, each targeting a specific depth of wounding and repair and each with its own inherent risks and benefits. It is prudent for the physician to have a broad knowledge base regarding these procedures so as to ensure treatment success and safeguard against untoward complications. Likewise, the proper selection of patients and choice of procedure are critical. With appropriate usage, resurfacing procedures can be a gratifying part of dermatologic practice.

REFERENCES

1. Brody HJ, Monheit GD, Resnik SS, et al. A history of chemical peeling. *Dermatol Surg*. 2000;26:405-409.
2. Salam A, Dadzie OE, Galadari H. Chemical peeling in ethnic skin: an update. *Br J Dermatol*. 2013;169:82-90.
3. Monheit GD. Chemical peels. *Skin Therapy Lett*. 2004;9(2):6-11.
4. Berson DS, Cohen JL, Rendon MI, et al. Clinical role and application of superficial chemical peels in today's practice. *J Drugs Dermatol*. 2009;8(9):803-811.
5. Brody HJ. Complications of chemical resurfacing. *Dermatol Clin*. 2001;19(3):427-438.
6. Coleman WP III, Brody HJ. Advances in chemical peeling. *Dermatol Clin*. 1997;15(1):19-26.
7. Brody HJ. Trichloroacetic acid application in chemical peeling. *Oper Tech Plast Reconstr Surg*. 1995;2(2):127-128. https://www.sciencedirect.com/science/article/pii/S1071094905800071
8. Nelson BR, Fader DJ, Gillard M, et al. Pilot histologic and ultrastructural study of the effects of medium-depth chemical facial peels on dermal collagen in patients with actinically damaged skin. *J Am Acad Dermatol*. 1995;32(3):472-478.
9. Monheit GD. The Jessner's + TCA peel: a medium-depth chemical peel. *J Dermatol Surg Oncol*. 1989;15(9):945-950.
10. Grimes PE. The safety and efficacy of salicylic acid peels in darker racial-ethnic groups. *Dermatol Surg*. 1999;25(1):18-22.
11. Ditre CM, Griffin TD, Murphy GF, et al. Effects of α-hydroxy acids on photoaged skin: a pilot clinical, histological, and ultrastructural study. *J Am Acad Dermatol*. 1996;34:187-195.
12. Butler PE, Gonzalez S, Randolph MA, et al. Quantitative and qualitative effects of chemical peeling on photoaged skin: an experimental study. *Plast Reconstr Surg*. 2001;107:222-228.
13. Grimes PE. The safety and efficacy of salicylic acid chemical peels in darker racial-ethnic groups. *Dermatol Surg*. 1999;25:18.
14. Abdel Meguid AM, Elaziz Ahmed Attallah DA, Omar H. Trichloroacetic acid versus salicylic acid in the treatment of acne vulgaris in dark-skinned patients. *Dermatol Surg*. 2015;41:1398-1404.
15. Kubiak M, Mucha P, Debowska R, et al. Evaluation of 70% glycolic peels versus 15% trichloroacetic peels for the treatment of photodamaged facial skin in aging women. *Dermatol Surg*. 2014;40:883-891.
16. Alt TH. Occluded Baker-Gordon chemical peel: review and update. *J Dermatol Surg Oncol*. 1989;15(9):980-993.
17. Landau M. Cardiac complications in deep chemical peels. *Dermatol Surg*. 2007;33:190-193.
18. Lee JB, Chung WG, Kwahck H, et al. Focal treatment of acne scars with trichloroacetic acid: chemical reconstruction of skin scars method. *Dermatol Surg*. 2002;28:1017-1021.
19. Agarwal N, Gupta LK, Khare AK, et al. Therapeutic response of 70% trichloroacetic acid CROSS in atrophic acne scars. *Dermatol Surg*. 2015;41:597-604.
20. Maloney BP, Millman B, Monheit G, et al. The etiology of prolonged erythema after chemical peel. *Dermatol Surg*. 1998;24:337-341.
21. Tsai R, Wang C, Chan H. Aluminum oxide crystal microdermabrasion: a new technique for treating facial scarring. *Dermatol Surg*. 1995;21:539-542.
22. Bhalla M, Thami GP. Microdermabrasion: reappraisal and brief review of literature. *Dermatol Surg*. 2006;32:809-814.
23. Shim EK, Barnette D, Hughes K, et al. Microdermabrasion: a clinical and histopathologic study. *Dermatol Surg*. 2001;27:524-530.
24. Freedman BM, Rueda-Pedraza E, Waddell SP. The epidermal and dermal changes associated with microdermabrasion. *Dermatol Surg*. 2001;27:1031-1034.
25. Kim EK, Hovsepian RV, Mathew P, et al. Dermabrasion. *Clin Plast Surg*. 2011;38:391-395.
26. Poulos E, Taylor C, Solish N. Effectiveness of dermasanding (manual dermabrasion) on the appearance of surgical scars: a prospective, randomized, blinded study. *J Am Acad Dermatol*. 2003;48:897-900.
27. Benedetto AV, Griffin TD, Benedetto EA, et al. Dermabrasion: therapy and prophylaxis of the photoaged face. *J Am Acad Dermatol*. 1992;27(3):439-447.
28. Nelson BR, Metz RD, Majmudar G, et al. A comparison of wire brush and diamond fraise superficial dermabrasion for photoaged skin. *J Am Acad Dermatol*. 1996;34(2):235-243.

Chapter 214 :: Liposuction Using Tumescent Local Anesthesia
:: C. William Hanke, Cheryl J. Gustafson, William G. Stebbins, & Aimee L. Leonard

第二百一十四章
局部麻醉下的肿胀吸脂术

中文导读

肿胀技术是用大量的特殊配方液体注射至皮下脂肪组织，注射过的部位被麻醉，同时使脂肪组织扩大，便于精细吸脂的技术。本章主要介绍了：病人的选择、术前评估、风险防范及措施、病人体位、治疗设备、麻醉、技术流程、结果评估、并发症、患者教育及术后长期随访跟踪调查，最后简单介绍了其在其他方面的应用。

理想的候选者是接近个人理想体重的健康人，并有不相称的局部脂肪沉积，且此脂肪对饮食和运动减脂无明显反应。术前评估需考虑治疗部位、周围重要解剖结构及插管深度。作者提出吸脂术具有安全性高、病人恢复快、满意度高、术后发病率低的特点。其术后并发症包括常见外科手术并发症（如血肿、感染）和人体美学上的并发症（如皮肤表面不规则等）。

〔简 丹〕

AT-A-GLANCE

- Liposuction is one of the most commonly performed cosmetic procedures practiced by dermatologic surgeons.
- The tumescent technique of local anesthesia is one of the most important innovations in liposuction surgery.[1]
- Liposuction performed with tumescent local anesthesia allows for the removal of large volumes of fat safely and effectively.
- Liposuction is characterized by unparalleled safety, rapid patient recovery, and low postoperative morbidity.
- Importantly, liposuction is very safe to perform in the office setting, the preferred venue for the procedure when carried out by dermatologic surgeons.

PATIENT SELECTION

Liposuction should be regarded not as a method of weight reduction or an alternative to diet and exercise, but as a body-contouring procedure. The ideal candidate is a healthy patient near his or her ideal body weight who has disproportionate, localized adipose deposits resistant to diet and exercise. Liposuction should be avoided in patients with unrealistic treatment goals and those with emotional or psychological instability (ie, presence of an eating disorder or body dysmorphic disorder). A comprehensive preoperative consultation that includes a screening questionnaire is used to identify patients who are appropriate candidates. During the consultation, the risks, goals, anticipated results, and expected postoperative course are discussed.

TABLE 214-1
Preoperative Preparation

- Drug intake review:
  - Discontinue all anticoagulant medications and nonprescription supplements that may augment bleeding (at least 2 weeks prior to procedure)
  - Discontinue all medications that may interfere with lidocaine metabolism (drugs metabolized through cytochrome P450 3A4) at least 2 weeks prior to procedure
- Preoperative laboratory testing:
  - Complete blood count with differential and platelet count
  - Prothrombin time
  - Partial thromboplastin time
  - Chemistry panel with liver function tests
  - Serologic testing for HIV, hepatitides B and C
  - Serum pregnancy test for females
  - Electrocardiogram if >60 years of age, or otherwise indicated

PREOPERATIVE EVALUATION

Table 214-1 outlines preoperative preparation. Taking a thorough medical history will screen for patients who may be poor surgical candidates for liposuction (see the section "Risks and Precautions"). Patients at risk for complications should receive medical clearance before surgery.[2,3] A careful review of all medications is essential. All anticoagulant medications, including vitamins and herbal supplements, should be discontinued 2 weeks before surgery. Use of medically-necessary anticoagulant therapy is a contraindication for tumescent liposuction. Medications that are metabolized by the hepatic cytochrome P450 3A4 enzyme system should be identified. These medications may interfere with the hepatic metabolism of lidocaine, which leads to the potential for toxicity. They should be discontinued or tapered off 2 weeks before surgery if permitted by the prescribing physician. For patients who are unable to interrupt therapy, a lower maximum dose of lidocaine may be used (ie, less than 35 mg/kg).

Preoperative laboratory testing includes complete blood count with differential and platelet count, prothrombin time, partial thromboplastin time, and chemistry panel (including liver function tests); serologic testing for HIV and hepatitides B and C viruses; and, for females, a serum pregnancy test.[2] An electrocardiogram may be considered when the patient is older than the age of 60 years or when indicated based on the patient's history or a review of systems.

RISKS AND PRECAUTIONS

Table 214-2 identifies the risks of liposuction and the precautions that should be taken.

PATIENT POSITIONING

Proper patient positioning is essential for safe and effective removal of adipose tissue. Specific positioning maneuvers differ by anatomic target site and are used to avoid important anatomic structures and optimize cannula access to fatty deposits.

EQUIPMENT

Liposuction requires the following equipment (Figs. 214-1 and 214-2):

- Tumescent local anesthetic solution
- Infiltration needles and/or cannulas
- Intravenous or peristaltic pump tubing
- Infiltration pump
- Liposuction cannulas (manual and/or powered)
- Aspiration tubing
- Aspiration pump with aspirate receptacles
- Monitoring device and emergency equipment

TABLE 214-2
Risks and Precautions for Liposuction

- Contraindications to liposuction
  - Severe cardiovascular disease
  - Severe coagulation disorders, including hemophilia
  - Pregnancy
- Conditions that put patients at risk for complications
  - History of bleeding diathesis, thrombophlebitis, or emboli (fat or thrombotic)
  - History of infectious disease (including hepatitis and HIV infection)
  - Poor wound healing
  - Diabetes mellitus
  - Immunosuppression
  - Prior extensive abdominal surgery
  - Hepatic disease
  - Renal disease
  - Morbid obesity
  - Underlying systemic disease with functional limitations
  - Use of anticoagulant medications, vitamins, or herbal supplements
  - Use of medications metabolized by cytochrome P450 3A4 enzyme system

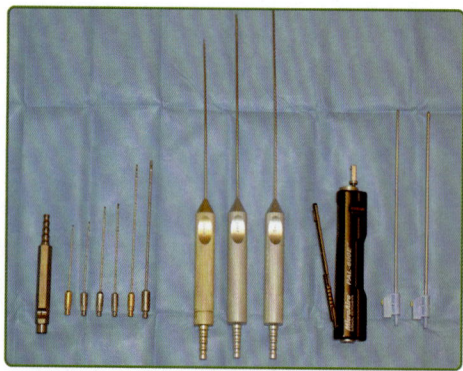

Figure 214-1 A selection of liposuction cannulas, including hand cannulas (*left*) and powered cannulas (*right*). (Used with permission from C. William Hanke, MD.)

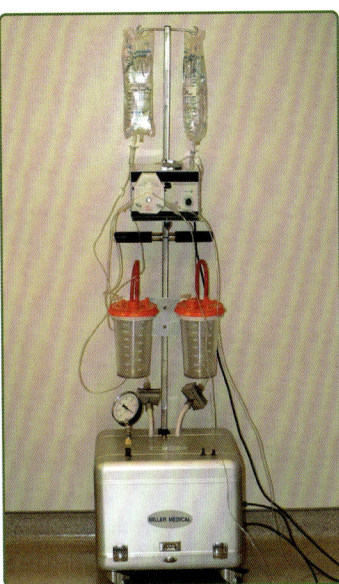

Figure 214-2 Liposuction equipment including (*from top to bottom*) tumescent anesthetic solution, infiltration pump and tubing, aspirate receptacles, and aspiration pump. (Used with permission from C. William Hanke, MD.)

ANESTHESIA

Lidocaine is the preferred anesthetic for tumescent liposuction.[2] The maximum dose reported to be safe is 55 mg/kg.[4] Normal saline (0.9% sodium chloride) is typically used as a vehicle. Sodium bicarbonate is used to buffer the solution, and epinephrine is added to augment hemostasis and slow the absorption of lidocaine. Table 214-3 outlines the compositions of tumescent lidocaine solutions of 0.05%, 0.075%, and 0.1%. Using the highest concentration liposuction solution (0.1% lidocaine) provides better analgesia and is useful in treating small or sensitive areas. In comparison, the lower concentrations (0.075% and 0.05% lidocaine) provide adequate anesthesia and are used when treating large or multiple areas. Accurate recordkeeping of tumescent anesthetic solution preparation and administration is critical to avoid lidocaine toxicity.

TECHNIQUE

With the patient standing, the target areas for treatment as well as entry sites for cannula insertion are outlined with a permanent marker. The patient is brought to the procedure table and undergoes sterile preparation. Entry sites are anesthetized locally using 1% lidocaine with 1:100,000 epinephrine. These sites are then incised with a No. 11 blade. A blunt-tipped infiltration cannula or 21-gauge needle is inserted, and tumescent anesthesia fluid is delivered to the subcutaneous space. Rates of infiltration and amounts of fluid delivered vary depending on target area and patient tolerance.

Liposuction aspiration cannulas vary in diameter, tip style, and tip configuration. One innovation is powered liposuction using a motorized cannula. In general, larger cannulas with tapered tips and multiple distal apertures allow easier fat removal but also increase tissue injury. The choice of cannula depends on anatomic site as well as surgeon preference and experience. The cannula is inserted into entry sites with the tip apertures facing downward, away from the dermis. Tunneling with the cannula is performed in linear, even strokes with the surgeon's dominant hand; the nondominant hand, or "smart hand," controls the cannula tip position at all times. The majority of suctioning should be aimed parallel to the axis of lymphatic drainage to minimize tissue trauma. Uneven or overly aggressive suctioning can lead to contour irregularities and should be avoided. End points can be measured as the time spent in a given area, the amount of fat suctioned, patient discomfort, and assessment of the target area by palpation. The transition from yellow adipocyte-rich aspirate into fat-sparse serosanguineous tumescent fluid is an additional end point. Comparative suctioned aspirate volumes and vital signs are also recorded throughout the procedure.

OUTCOMES ASSESSMENT

Several studies support the excellent safety profile and high rates of patient satisfaction observed with tumescent liposuction. A 1995 survey of dermatologic surgeons who performed tumescent liposuction on 15,336 patients found no fatalities or serious complications. There were no adverse events that necessitated hospitalization.[5] In 2002, Housman and colleagues reported a serious adverse event rate of 0.68 per 1000 cases in a survey of 267 dermatologic surgeons who performed 66,570 liposuction procedures; no deaths were reported.[6] In a prospective study involving 688 liposuction patients, Hanke and colleagues found a major complication rate of only 0.14% and a minor complication rate of 0.57%. Eighty-four percent of patients reported high levels of satisfaction with the procedure (Figs. 214-3 and 214-4).[7]

COMPLICATIONS

The majority of medical and surgical complications from tumescent liposuction, such as bleeding, hematoma, infection, and lidocaine toxicity, can be avoided by comprehensive perioperative patient evaluation and adherence to published guidelines of care. Aesthetic complications, such as surface irregularities, persistent edema, and suboptimal target area fat

TABLE 214-3 Tumescent Liposuction Solutions			
	0.1%	0.075%	0.05%
Sodium chloride 0.9%	1000 mL	1000 mL	1000 mL
Lidocaine 1%	100 mL	75 mL	50 mL
Epinephrine 1:1000	1 mL	1 mL	1 mL
Sodium bicarbonate 8.4%	10 mL	10 mL	10 mL

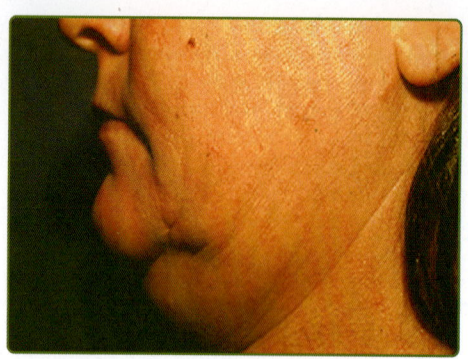

Figure 214-3 Liposuction of the neck, preoperative. (Used with permission from C. William Hanke, MD.)

reduction, can be minimized by proper patient selection, patient education, and good technique. Dermatologic surgeons performing liposuction should be knowledgeable about the prevention and management of all potential intraoperative and postoperative complications.

PATIENT INSTRUCTIONS

Anticipated sequelae of tumescent liposuction include copious drainage from cannula entry sites, ecchymoses, edema, soreness, postural dizziness, and temporary dysesthesia. Proper education and instructions regarding diet, activity, and use of compression garments prepare the patient for the postoperative period. The patient must be discharged to the care of a family member or friend. The patient is encouraged to ambulate and avoid immobilization. Heavy exercise and hot baths and showers should be avoided.

MONITORING AND FOLLOWUP

A series of followup visits is scheduled to assist the patient through the immediate postoperative period and to assess the long-term surgical outcome. Postoperative healing from liposuction is characterized by a protracted period of edema resolution followed by subsequent skin contracture, which leads to a delayed final treatment result. Taking preoperative and postoperative photographs and weight measurements is essential to address patient concerns and assess treatment response. Patients are encouraged to wait at least 6 months before judging the final cosmetic result. The performance of touchup procedures in a treated area should be deferred for at least 1 year.

OTHER USES

In addition to being an aesthetic procedure, tumescent local anesthesia is being used for symptomatic breast reduction and lipedema.

Excess, heavy breast tissue can have a significant impact on various aspects of one's quality of life. From a physical perspective, women with heavy, large breasts often experience chronic neck, back, and/or shoulder pain, as well as discomfort from bra straps. Also, the bulky breast tissue can impair one's physical mobility. For instance, many women with bulky breasts report difficulty exercising because of the weight and volume of their breast tissue. Additionally, the enlarged breast size can make it challenging to find appropriate-fitting athletic gear. As a result, their desire and ability to exercise regularly are often reduced, which not only impacts their physical well-being, but also their emotional and psychological well-being.

Likewise, women with large breasts often have difficulty finding clothing that properly fits as their chest circumference may be out of proportion to other body measurements. As a result, these women often wear larger clothing sizes to compensate for the enlarged breast tissue. Hence, these patients may report self-consciousness, embarrassment, and/or depressive symptoms related to their heavy, enlarged breast tissue. Therefore, it is important for health care providers to be aware of the impact that enlarged, heavy breasts can have on the patient's quality of life, including physical, emotional, and psychological.

Excision is one of the most common methods of breast reduction. Usually this procedure is done under general anesthesia. Common complications from excision include postoperative pain, scarring, necrosis of the nipple–areolar complex, and prolonged healing. Habbema and colleagues evaluated the use of liposuction with tumescent local anesthesia for breast reduction in 151 women. The average volume reduction was 415 mL per breast (41% of the preoperative volume). In addition to reducing breast volume, tumescent liposuction significantly reduced breast ptosis. Prior to liposuction, the average preoperative value of breast sagging was 6.5 cm. At 6 weeks postliposuction, the average value for ptosis was 3.6 cm.[8]

Of the 151 patients, all but 1 (0.7%) were mostly (21.8%) or very (77.5%) satisfied with the results of tumescent liposuction. None of the patients requested or required a secondary "touchup" procedure. Breast reduction had a significant impact on patients' quality of life, as many experienced improvement or com-

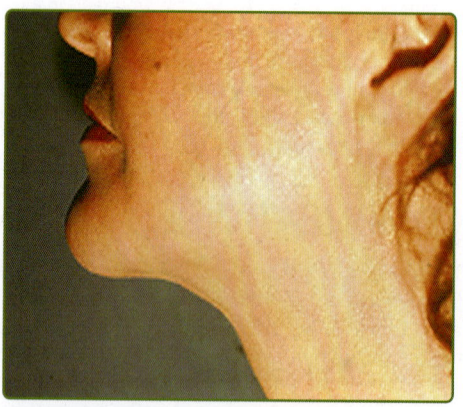

Figure 214-4 Liposuction of the neck, postoperative. (Used with permission from C. William Hanke, MD.)

plete resolution of chronic shoulder, neck, or back pain. Additionally, patients reported fewer physical restrictions when exercising. Many of the women also reported the ability to wear more attractive, well-fitting clothing. Overall, most patients experienced improvement in their self-confidence following the procedure. In conclusion, Habbema and colleagues found tumescent liposuction to be an effective, safe, and minimally invasive procedure for breast reduction in women.

Men with enlarged breasts from excess fat (pseudogynecomastia) and/or hypertrophic ductal and stromal tissue (gynecomastia) are good candidates for tumescent liposuction. In a published study, 38 male patients (ages 23 to 64 years) with enlarged breast tissue underwent liposuction using tumescent local anesthesia.[9] A single entry site was made in each axillary fossa to allow insertion of the microcannula. In addition to removing undesired excess adipose tissue, excess ductal and stromal tissue were effectively removed using this minimally-invasive procedure. There were no early postoperative complications, such as infection, hematoma, or seroma. From an aesthetic perspective, there were no treatment-induced asymmetries or contour deformities. Additionally, patients were very satisfied with the final outcome as none required open excision or skin-reduction procedures. Overall, tumescent liposuction was found to be a safe and effective procedure for gynecomastia.

Lipedema is a chronic, painful disorder of subcutaneous adipose tissue and lymphatics. It clinically manifests as symmetrical fatty swelling of the bilateral waist, hips, and legs (Fig. 214-5). Unlike the "normal" fatty tissue of obesity, the adipose tissue in lipedema cannot be reduced with diet and exercise; consequently, liposuction using tumescent local anesthesia is being used in the management of lipedema. In a German study by Rapprich and colleagues, 25 lipedema patients underwent tumescent liposuction of the lower extremities. The average reduction in leg volume was 6.9%. Leg pain was significantly reduced from an average score of 7.2 preprocedure to 2.1 postprocedure. Patients also reported a significant improvement in quality of life (8.7 to 3.6).[10]

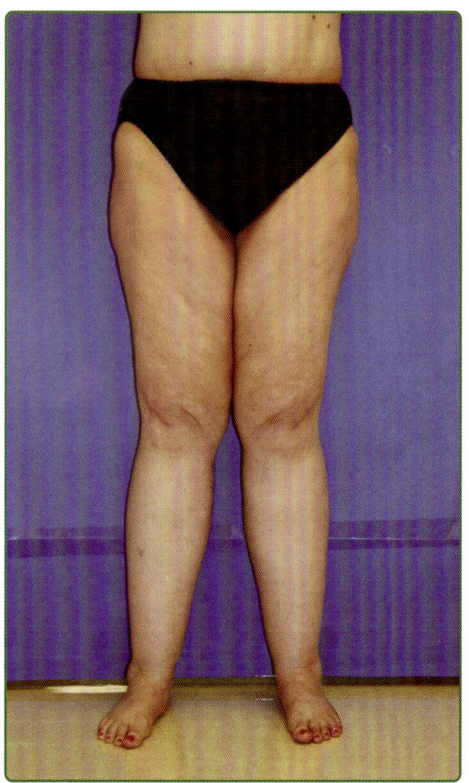

Figure 214-5 Female patient with significant lipedema. Note the significant bilateral fatty swelling of the lower extremities that ends at the level of the ankles. (Used with permission from C. William Hanke, MD.)

REFERENCES

1. Klein JA. The tumescent technique for liposuction surgery. *Am J Cosmet Surg*. 1987;4:263. Available at http://journals.sagepub.com/doi/10.1177/074880688700400403.
2. Hanke CW, Sattler G. *Liposuction*. Philadelphia, PA: Elsevier; 2005.
3. Svedman KJ, Coldiron B, Coleman WP 3rd, et al. ASDS guidelines of care for tumescent liposuction. *Dermatol Surg*. 2006;32(5):709-716.
4. Ostad A, Kageyama N, Moy RL. Tumescent anesthesia with a lidocaine dose of 55 mg/kg is safe for liposuction. *Dermatol Surg*. 1996;22(11):921-927.
5. Hanke CW, Bernstein G, Bullock S. Safety of tumescent liposuction in 15,336 patients. National survey results. *Dermatol Surg*. 1995;21(5):459-462.
6. Housman TS, Lawrence N, Mellen BG, et al. The safety of liposuction: results of a national survey. *Dermatol Surg*. 2002;28(11):971-978.
7. Hanke CW, Cox SE, Kuznets N, et al. Tumescent liposuction report performance measurement initiative: national survey results. *Dermatol Surg*. 2004;30(7):967-977.
8. Habbema L. Breast reduction using liposuction with tumescent local anesthesia and powered cannulas. *Dermatol Surg*. 2009;35(1):41-50; discussion 50-52.
9. Boni R. Tumescent power liposuction in the treatment of the enlarged male breast. *Dermatology*. 2006;213(2):140-143.
10. Rapprich S, Dingler A, Podda M. Liposuction is an effective treatment for lipedema—results of a study with 25 patients. *J Dtsch Dematol Ges*. 2011;9(1):33-40.

Chapter 215 :: Soft-Tissue Augmentation
:: Lisa M. Donofrio & Dana L. Ellis

第二百一十五章
软组织填充术

中文导读

软组织填充术主要用于治疗皮肤皱纹、凹陷、折痕等年轻化治疗。作者首先大致讲述注射的方法，并总结不同填充剂于表215-1、表215-2，再按照适应人群、剂型或配方、麻醉、方法技术、术后处理及并发症、填充剂使用寿命来介绍填充剂。

第一节介绍软组织填充术的方法与技术，包括线状沉积式Threading、停顿式Depot、扇形式Fanning、交叉式Crosshatching、推进式Push-ahead五种不同的注射方式，并展示于图215-1。

第二节介绍了胶原蛋白，重点介绍了一种不可吸收（永久）的填充材料——聚甲基丙烯酸甲酯。

第三节介绍了透明质酸是位于细胞外的一种多糖。用于注射的透明质酸根据来源分为动物源性和非动物源性，并常用于鼻唇沟、面颊中部、唇部、唇颏部、眶周区域的填充。注射时一般需用利多卡因进行局部麻醉。接下来作者讲述了不同注射部位常使用的注射技术及注意事项。注射治疗完成后应立即冰敷，并密切注意病人情况。术后并发症除了常见的出血或瘀伤，还可出现透明质酸注射部位过浅导致皮肤蓝色变（Tyndall效应）、产生过敏反应形成肉芽肿等特有并发症。作者最后指出交联性更强的透明质酸在皮肤内的"寿命"相对更长。

第四节介绍了可生理降解的填充剂：多聚-L-乳酸（PLLA）和羟磷灰石钙（CaHA）。多聚-L-乳酸（PLLA）不是一种直接的填充剂，而是一种生物刺激剂，在数月的治疗过程中会通过启动异物组织反应（免疫反应）引起组织增厚，所以服用免疫抑制剂或抗炎药的患者是不适用的。作者还提到了PLLA的储存及配置，尤其在注射时对于上、下面部的注射有提到相应的注意事项。注射后，必须立即对治疗部位进行按摩，使注射液均匀地分布在组织中。作者还提到了多聚-L-乳酸（PLLA）注射术后特殊的并发症是丘疹的形成。而PLLA在皮肤内的"寿命"一般为2年甚至更长。羟磷灰石钙（CaHA）类似PLLA，也是一种生物刺激剂，当注射到真皮深处后会刺激胶原的生长，一般用于鼻唇沟、唇颏皱褶、面颊、手背萎缩、萎缩性痤疮疤痕、鼻缺损、乳头重建等。在注射时为减小不适感，多使用利多卡因局部麻醉，并根据注射部位选择不同的注射方法。CaHA治疗后也会出现常见的肿胀、瘀斑和结节，当CaHA注射部位过浅，可导致CaHA可视。最后，作者提出CaHA临床寿命为6～18个月。

第五节介绍了自体脂肪填充（AFT），它是从人体自身某些部位吸取多余的皮下脂肪，然后经过处理，再移植到自身需要进行脂肪填充的部位，所以那些自身脂肪含量低的人群不适用。此技术流程包括术前准备、麻醉、脂肪获取及脂肪的转移，脂肪获取部位要尽可能不影响美观。术后常见肿胀和瘀斑。最后，作者提出AFT成功后，可以是永久性的。

第六节介绍了硅胶注射，可用于艾滋病毒相关的脂肪萎缩、瘢痕及其他凹陷萎缩，微量注射液态硅树脂，一般不需要麻醉，术后也几乎没有不适，且注射后产生的填充效果几乎是永久性的。

第七节总结以上所有填充剂可能出现的并发症。常见的并发症包括淤血、水肿、填充物的挤压或漂移、异物反应、色素改变、注射部位瘢痕、填充过度、填充不足、错误填充和感染。作者强调血管阻塞是最具破坏性的并发症，还可因为血管阻塞导致失明和大脑中动脉梗塞。

〔简 丹〕

AT-A-GLANCE

- Soft-tissue fillers are used for multiple cosmetic and therapeutic indications.
- A wide variety of injectable soft-tissue fillers are available for clinical use, including biodegradable products such as hyaluronic acid, collagen, calcium hydroxylapatite, and poly-L-lactic acid; products that remain indefinitely in tissue, such as polymethylmethacrylate microspheres, hydrogel polymers, and silicone; and viable autologous fat.
- Adequate clinician training in the use of these agents is essential for the prevention of adverse events.

As we age, lines, grooves, and creases become more apparent. Superficial rhytides are largely caused by solar damage, characterized by the loss of collagen at the epidermal–dermal junction and an increased elastosis in the reticular dermis. Repetitive facial movement over the years produces pronounced rhytides in the most active areas of the face, such as the forehead, glabella, periorbital and perioral areas, and nasolabial folds. Rhytides tend to appear deeper in the nasolabial and melolabial creases with the compounding feature of soft-tissue atrophy.[1]

Facial rejuvenation comes in many forms; its primary stake being replacement of soft-tissue volume by an assortment of augmentation techniques. Two major categories are subcutaneous volumizers and dermal fillers. Although subcutaneous volumizers tend to provide more long-lasting results, with improvements in dermal fillers over the past several years, these products have become increasingly popular and are now widely used. When deciding which technique(s) to use in the correction of facial soft-tissue atrophy, an accurate diagnosis of the level(s) of volume loss must be made. In younger patients, dermal fillers may be adequate for treatment, while in a more advanced aging face, a combination of the two above categories may be necessary to obtain optimal results.[1]

METHOD AND TECHNIQUE

Dermal filler use began in the mid 1980s and has since become the cornerstone of facial filling in the office setting.[1] There are several dermal fillers approved for use in the United States (Table 215-1). Soft-tissue fillers (Table 215-2) are either injected through a sharp needle or blunt cannula. The level of injection into the skin and the length of the needle chosen depend on the type of filler injected, the properties of the filler, the area injected, and the desired result. Threading is a technique in which the needle is inserted into the skin and the filler is deposited in a linear fashion along the track of the needle as it is being withdrawn. Fanning is a type of threading in which, instead of inserting the needle into a new area each time, the needle is just withdrawn so that a new track can be made radially adjacent to the last. In the "push-ahead" technique, an injection is made in an anterograde direction, so that the injectable material flows from the tip of the needle and hydrodissects the tissues as it flows. This technique is often used in areas where bruising is more likely to occur along the needle track, such as the upper lid and brow. In the depot method of injection, small "pearls" of material are deposited serially, usually along a fold or deep by bone. Crosshatching is an approach used to diffusely cover an area with the injected material. In this method, linear threads are lined up in succession and a second series of rows is then layered at right angles to the first. Some of the more viscous fillers on the U.S. market are injected in a deep subcutaneous bolus through a blunt cannula or large-bore needle. Figure 215-1 illustrates the different injection techniques. Whichever technique is chosen, care should be taken in highly vascular areas to avoid intravascular injection of filling material. With each injection, the plunger of the syringe should be drawn back to check for blood flow, and if it is found, the needle should be withdrawn and repositioned.

TABLE 215-1
U.S. Food and Drug Administration–Approved and Available Dermal Fillers

TRADE NAME	MATERIAL
Restylane Silk	Hyaluronic acid with lidocaine
ArteFill (no longer available)	Polymethylmethacrylate beads, collagen, lidocaine
Bellafill	Polymethylmethacrylate beads, collagen, lidocaine
Fibrel (no longer available)	Collagen
Sculptra	Poly-L-lactic acid
Sculptra Aesthetic	Poly-L-lactic acid
Restylane Injectable Gel	Hyaluronic acid
Restylane-L Injectable Gel	Hyaluronic acid with lidocaine
Restylane Lyft with Lidocaine	Hyaluronic acid with lidocaine
CosmoDerm 1 Human-Based Collagen (no longer available)	Collagen
Captique Injectable Gel	Hyaluronic acid
Prevelle Silk	Hyaluronic acid with lidocaine
Hylaform	Modified hyaluronic acid (avian source)
Belotero Balance	Hyaluronic acid
Zyplast (no longer available)	Collagen
Evolence Collagen Filler (no longer available)	Collagen
Radiesse	Hydroxylapatite
Elevess	Hyaluronic acid with lidocaine
Juvederm	Hyaluronic acid
Juvederm Voluma XC	Hyaluronic acid with lidocaine
Zyderm Collagen Implant (no longer available)	Collagen
Revanesse Versa	Hyaluronic acid
Juvederm Vollure XC	Hyaluronic acid
Juverderm Volbella XC	Hyaluronic acid with lidocaine
Restylane Refyne	Sodium hyluronate
Restylane Defyne	Sodium hyluronate

COLLAGENS

Once considered the "gold standard" of dermal fillers, collagens (bovine, human, and porcine) are no longer available on the U.S. market.

NONABSORBABLE (PERMANENT) MATERIALS

One collagen-containing product worth mentioning is polymethylmethacrylate (PMMA) microspheres. PMMA is a nonbiodegradable, biocompatible, synthetic polymer that is often used in other medical devices, such as bone cement and intraocular lenses.[1] PMMA beads are minuscule, round, smooth particles that are not absorbed by the body. When used as a soft-tissue filler, these beads are suspended in a gel-like solution that contains cow (bovine) collagen and are injected into the face. A few months after it is injected, the collagen gel breaks down and natural collagen fills out the residual space. This dermal filler is considered semipermanent, and is most often used to treat medium-to-deep rhytides and folds, particularly the nasolabial creases. It is also used by some to fill pitted scars and to augment the lips.

HYALURONIC ACIDS

PATIENT SELECTION

Hyaluronic acid–derived fillers are a good choice for patients who desire a long period of correction or more volume enhancement. They are currently approved for augmentation of the nasolabial folds, mid cheeks, and lips, but other common areas of treatment include the labiomental crease and periorbital areas. Patients often feel that the hyaluronic acid fillers are softer and more natural in appearance than the collagens were, but they need to be warned about the risk of increased erythema, edema, and bruising associated with these products.

FORMULATIONS

Hyaluronic acid is a polysaccharide and a normal extracellular component of most mammalian tissues including the dermis. Hyaluronic acid polymers offer superb biocompatibility and provide the same structural and mechanical properties of normal subcutaneous tissue. Injectable U.S. Food and Drug Administration (FDA)-approved forms include non–animal-derived stabilized hyaluronic acid products made through a bacterial fermentation process and an avian-derived version isolated from cocks' combs. Brands of injectable hyaluronic acids differ not only in their derivation but also in their concentration of hyaluronic acid per milliliter of product, type of crosslinking or stabilizing agents, viscosity, and particle size. In its native form, hyaluronic acid has a short life span. However, crosslinking increases its longevity. As the proportion and degree of crosslinking increases, the gel becomes more and more like a solid, is more resistant to degradation by enzymes and free radicals, and as such, tends to persist longer in tissue. Injection of crosslinked hyaluronic acid into the deep dermis also has been shown to increase de novo collagen synthesis by fibroblast stretching, resulting in even longer-lasting correction.[1] Some hyaluronic acid products exist as biphasic gels containing both crosslinked and uncrosslinked particles, and some as monophasic

TABLE 215-2
Clinical Features of Soft-Tissue Fillers

FILLER	USES	TYPE	PLACEMENT	COMPLICATIONS	LONGEVITY
Hyaluronic acid	Treatment of medium-to-deep folds, lips, acne scars, periorbital hollows, facial contouring	Non–animal-derived stabilized hyaluronic acid	Mid-to-deep dermis or superficial subcutis	Allergic reaction or inflammation, blue discoloration, misplacement, lumps	6 to 12 months
Calcium hydroxylapatite	Treatment of deep folds, nipple reconstruction, nasal reconstruction, jawline, malar augmentation	Calcium hydroxylapatite	Deep dermis to superficial subcutis	Nodules (especially in lips and periorbitally), misplacement with demarcation of product	6 to 18 months
Poly-L-lactic acid	Treatment of HIV lipoatrophy, nasolabial fold, cheek, and temple hollows	Poly-L-lactic acid	Superficial subcutis	Visible and palpable papules	2 years or longer
Autologous fat	Pan-facial filling, especially periorbital area	Autologous fat	Subcutaneous tissue	Bumps, vascular occlusive events with injudicious placement	5 years or longer
Silicone	Treatment of scars, HIV lipoatrophy, lips, deep folds	Silicone oil	Deep dermis	Delayed granuloma formation, migration	—

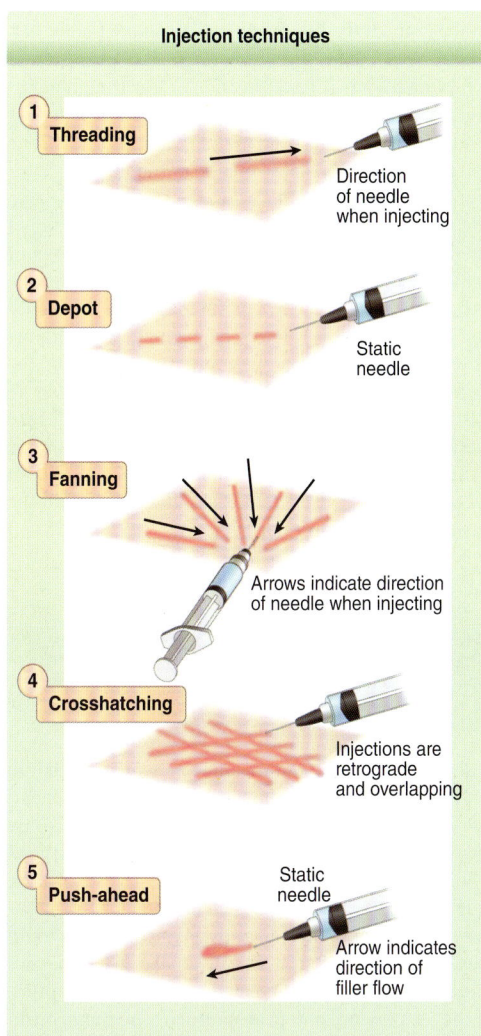

Figure 215-1 Injection techniques.

gels containing only crosslinked particles. The biphasic non–animal-derived stabilized hyaluronic acid products are made en bloc initially and then passed through a sieve to create particles ranging in size from 10,000 per mL to 100,000 per mL with a hyaluronic acid concentration of 20 mg/mL. The smaller particle size permits injection through smaller-gauge needles into finer wrinkles and the larger particle size is best for volumetric filling. The small amount of non-crosslinked hyaluronic acid allows for smooth flow with low injection pressures. Monophasic hyaluronic acid gels are produced by varying the amount of high- and low-molecular weight hyaluronic acid, producing a hydrogenous gel. The monophasic product is available in 2 formulations, one containing 24 mg/mL of hyaluronic acid and one containing 30 mg/mL of hyaluronic acid. The crosslinking agent used in both the monophasic and biphasic products is BDDE (1,4-butanediol diglycidyl ether). The avian-derived hyaluronic acid, contains 6 mg/mL of hyaluronic acid highly crosslinked with divinyl sulfide. The hydrophilic nature of hyaluronic acid allows it to create larger volumes relative to its mass. This property makes hyaluronic acid fillers especially useful for soft-tissue augmentation. The hyaluronic acid fillers have an excellent tolerability profile and can be used without the need for skin testing.[1]

ANESTHESIA

As a consequence of their high viscosity, hyaluronic acid products can cause significant discomfort on injection so most hyaluronic acids on the market are combined with lidocaine. As such, it is often beneficial

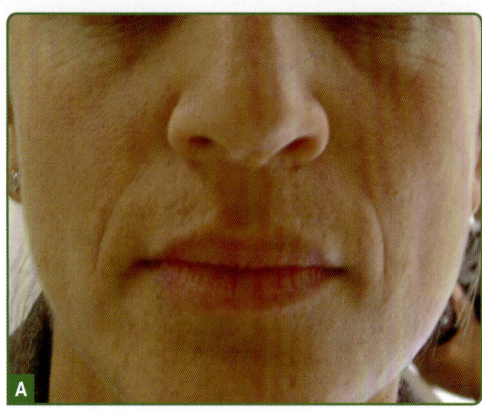 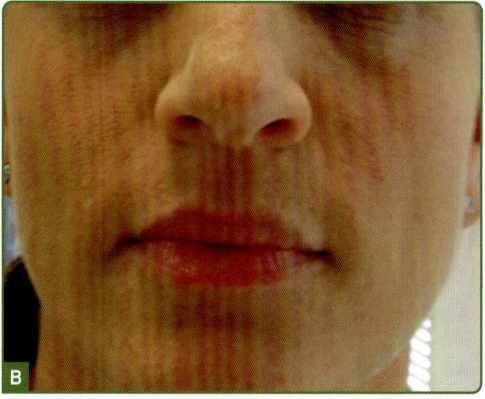

Figure 215-2 Thirty-five-year-old woman before (**A**) and after (**B**) infiltration of Restylane into the nasolabial folds.

to inject antegrade (in addition to retrograde), as placement of the lidocaine-containing product ahead of the needle tip, can help decrease the associated pain. Topical anesthetic also can be applied before injection. This usually results in adequate anesthesia for periorbital, nasolabial fold, and labiomental crease injections; however, if lips or perioral rhytides are being treated, an ancillary local infiltration of 1% lidocaine or segmental nerve block may be indicated.

TECHNIQUE

Hyaluronic acids should be injected with the patient in a position that elicits the defect or creases to be treated and offers ease of injection to the operator. This is best accomplished by reclining the patient to a 45-degree angle. All the hyaluronic acid products come with a needle in the gauge of choice for ease of injection and preservation of the physical properties of the gel. However, because of their viscoelastic properties, the hyaluronic acids can often be injected through needles tailored to the area or level of injection. For instance, a 32-gauge needle allows for more precise injection of vertical lip rhytides and a 1.5-inch needle may facilitate injection into distal sites. Hyaluronic acids are injected in most areas via threading, depot, or fanning. They are particularly amenable to crosshatching in areas where a greater density of augmentation is desired. In particular, when hyaluronic acid is injected into the nasolabial fold it is important to span the width of the fold with a serial threading technique and then crosshatch at right angles. This gives structural integrity to the fold and prevents the undesirable result of merely moving the fold medially (Fig. 215-2). In addition, it is often necessary to "suspend" the fold by augmenting the cheek. This is usually done with a deep bolus injection of a high density hyaluronic acid. The labiomental crease can be injected similarly to the nasolabial fold, again blending the product so as not to move the fold medially. Lip injections are made using a depot or threading technique, either along the vermilion border, in the body of the lip, or in a combination of both. Perhaps one of the most exciting off-label applications of hyaluronic acids is the correction of tear trough deformity or suborbital hollows. Injections are made either under the orbicularis oculi muscle near the orbital bone or subdermally above the muscle. Intramuscular injections are to be avoided as the movement in this area increases the risk of lumping of the product. A depot method of injection in which very small amounts of hyaluronic acid are deposited on each pass is preferred, but threading also can be helpful to ensure even blending into neighboring areas. The push-ahead technique is preferred for the sub-brow area. After injection, the periorbital area should be vigorously massaged to disperse the product and minimize aggregation of gel particles. Although periorbital injection of hyaluronic acid results in high levels of patient satisfaction, it is an advanced injection method best left to those with the greatest injecting experience.

POSTPROCEDURE INSTRUCTIONS

The application of ice immediately after the procedure and periodically throughout the day is recommended after the injection of hyaluronic acid. Patients are instructed to avoid manipulation of the treated area and extremes of temperature for the first 48 hours after injection. If the lips were treated in a patient with a history of cold sores, then an antiviral medication should be administered prophylactically on the day of the procedure. Patients are instructed to return to the office if they experience any problem such as redness, purulence, or nodule formation.

UNIQUE COMPLICATIONS

Common side effects of dermal fillers include bleeding or bruising during and following the procedure. Patients should expect some degree of pain during injections. As recommended above, the application of ice to the injection sites can decrease these symptoms. Most additional complications result from improper application of the product. Placement of this clear gel too superficially results in a blue discoloration, known as the Tyndall effect. This occurs as superficial injection allows for more water binding in the dermis, which selectively reflects the blue wavelength of light, making it appear darker than the surrounding skin. Placement of too large an aliquot can result in a noninflammatory bump. Most ill-placed hyaluronic acid can be removed by incising with a 20-gauge needle and expressing the material. An important characteristic of the hyaluronic acid products is their ability to break down with the use of an enzyme known as hyaluronidase. This enzyme breaks the crosslinks by hydrolysis of the glucosamine and glucuronic acid moiety. A few hyaluronidase products are commercially available in the United States in 200 units/mL and 150 units/mL vials. Approximately 15 to 20 units of hyaluronidase can be injected directly into a pea-sized volume of hyaluronic acid, leading to its degradation within minutes to hours.

Hyaluronic acid products also contain small amounts of impurities that can cause hypersensitivity reactions; true allergic reactions, however, are exceedingly rare. Patients can react to sterile bacterial proteins or avian proteins by forming sterile abscesses or granulomatous inflammatory nodules. It has been shown that these nodules, which appear clinically to be granulomas, may in fact be small foci of infection. Treatment with an antistaphylococcal antibiotic is the initial treatment of choice. If no resolution occurs, dilute intralesional corticosteroids can be administered, or hyaluronidase can be injected to cause rapid dissolution of the product.[2] It is also important to be aware that excess water absorption by many of the hyaluronic acid fillers can cause immediate swelling that will often decrease over days.

LONGEVITY

In general, the longevity of augmentation is greater for the more highly crosslinked or stabilized forms and is also directly proportional to filler viscosity and particle size. Naturally occurring hyaluronic acid is metabolized by lymphatic clearance and is eventually degraded in the liver to carbon dioxide and water. Hyaluronic acid–based products are broken down via isovolemic degradation; they maintain a constant volume throughout their degradation because of their ability to bind water. This property makes possible a very long-lasting product.

BIODEGRADABLE MICROPARTICLE INJECTABLE IMPLANTS

POLY-L-LACTIC ACID

PATIENT SELECTION

Poly-L-lactic acid (PLLA) was approved by the FDA in 2004 for correction of HIV-related facial atrophy and is also approved for the cosmetic correction of shallow-to-deep contour deficiencies. Currently in the United States, PLLA is well known as a no-downtime, long-lasting filler with a wide range of applications. PLLA's uniqueness lies in the fact that it is not a direct filling agent but rather a biostimulatory agent, eliciting tissue thickening over the course of many months and many treatment sessions. It is, therefore, the ideal filler for someone desiring a gradual, subtle change. Because PLLA works by initiating a foreign-body tissue response, it is not suited for patients taking immunosuppressive or antiinflammatory drugs, and it appears to work most efficiently in younger patients with robust immune responses. PLLA can be used for volume enhancement in the nasolabial fold, labiomental crease, chin, jawline, buccal hollows, and temples. Some practitioners have found it efficacious for filling for the dorsum of aging hands, however there is a moderate risk of nodule formation in this area. It is not recommended for use in the lips and should be used with care in the periorbital area.

FORMULATION

PLLA is supplied as a vial (367.5 mg) of freeze-dried powder of synthetic L-polymer of polylactic acid (from the α-hydroxy acid family), sodium carboxymethylcellulose, and mannitol. Injection of PLLA on repeated occasions presumably initiates an immune response that eventually leads to fibroblast activation and collagen deposition. High-level ultrasonographic images taken before and after a series of treatments in study patients confirms the presence of a zone of dermal thickening, but the exact mechanism is unknown.

ANESTHESIA

PLLA must be reconstituted at least 2 hours in advance of use; however, current standard of care is reconstitution at least 8 hours before treatment to fully suspend and hydrate the microparticles of PLLA. The package insert recommends reconstitution with 3 to 5 mL of sterile water, but the consensus of physicians currently using the product is to reconstitute with a minimum of 5 mL of diluent. It is possible to reconstitute the product in advance with 4 mL or more of sterile water and immediately before injection to add 1 mL of 1% lidocaine to the bottle. This tempers the pain

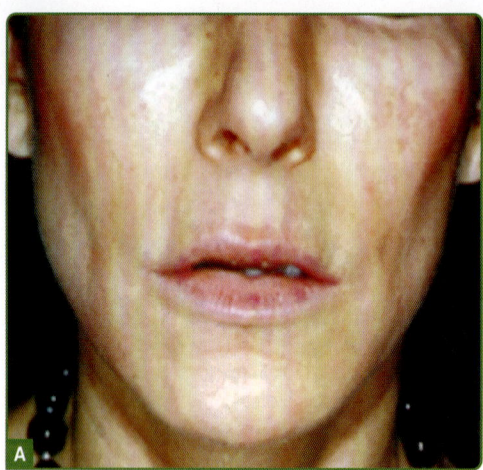 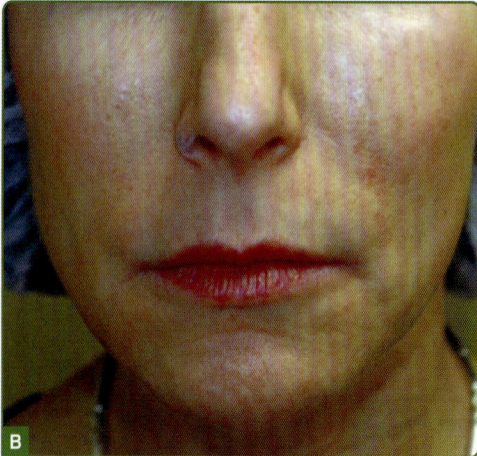

Figure 215-3 Thirty-nine-year-old woman before (**A**) and 4 months after (**B**) the last of 2 Sculptra treatments to the lower face.

on injection. In addition, patients may want to apply a topical anesthetic containing either 4% lidocaine or 20% tetracaine in advance of treatment.

TECHNIQUE

Because of the diffuse panfacial nature of PLLA injections, it is helpful to inject the patient in a supine position. PLLA is injected through a 25- to 26-gauge needle. Because of the risk of particle clumping, the bottle must be agitated frequently throughout the course of treatment. The operator must maintain maximum control over injection amounts, so drawing the material up into 1-mL syringes is highly recommended. The injection technique used when infiltrating PLLA is diffuse cross-hatching and threading. Depot deposition of product is not recommended. The principle is to inject PLLA into areas that will eventually display a direct impact from local volume change or affect neighboring areas by filling and suspending tissues upstream. Lower-face injections are performed diffusely over a wide surface area and involve the placement of 0.1-mL linear threads of solution 2 mm apart. The recommended technique is to inject across folds to distend them, rather than filling them directly. No attempt at volumetric correction is made during treatment; rather, the intent is to place the PLLA solution diffusely. The level of injection in the lower face (cheek, nasolabial fold, jawline, labiomental crease, chin) is subdermal (Fig. 215-3). In the upper face (temples and periorbital area) treatment is via diffuse threading of 0.05 mL of PLLA solution under or close to periosteum. No more than 0.5 mL total should be distributed in this fashion. If clogging of the needle occurs, it should be withdrawn and either changed or cleared before proceeding. Many practitioners have found that the use of long needles (1.5 inches) better facilitates even dispersion of the product.

POSTPROCEDURE INSTRUCTIONS

Immediately after injection, treated areas must be vigorously massaged to distribute the suspension evenly into the tissues. No blebs of material should be palpable. When the practitioner is satisfied that this is the case, the massage may then be continued in a gentler manner by an assistant for the next 5 minutes. Ice is then applied to the face for 20 minutes. The patient may then apply makeup and resume normal activities. The patient should massage the areas of injection for 5 minutes, 5 times a day for 5 days. Because minimal augmentation is achieved in each session, patients are instructed to return at 6-week intervals for additional treatments. The motto "treat, wait, assess" is an important one to follow when using PLLA. Resultant augmentation can take 4 months or longer to occur, so patience is necessary to avoid overcorrection. For the average patient with cosmetic concerns, between 3 and 6 treatments will be required for ample augmentation to occur. For patients with severe lipoatrophy, a minimum of 6 sessions will be required, often with injection of 2 vials per session.

UNIQUE COMPLICATIONS

Superficial injection of PLLA most often results in visible papule formation.

Reconstitution with inadequate amounts of fluid may also increase this risk. Delayed formation of subcutaneous papules has been reported in the literature. These papules although palpable are most often nonvisible, asymptomatic, and noninflammatory, and require no treatment. If they are of concern to the patient, an attempt can be made to break apart the papules by injecting sterile water into them or by teasing them apart with a 27-gauge needle. Results of an 8-year injectable filler safety study found evidence to support a decreased risk of nodules with increasing dilutions.[3] Rarely, large visible nodules can be seen as a late-onset side effect. Intralesional cortisone may be of help since they are often inflammatory or granulomatous in nature. Surgical removal is also an option for large unresponsive or deforming nodules.

LONGEVITY

The results from PLLA infiltration are thought to last 2 years or longer, with gradual resorption and breakdown of the product to lactic acid over the course of 2 to 3 years.

CALCIUM HYDROXYLAPATITE

PATIENT SELECTION

Patients requiring augmentation of the nasolabial folds, labiomental crease, mandibular ramus, cheeks, or prejowl sulcus, or those with age-related atrophy of the dorsal hands are candidates for treatment with calcium hydroxylapatite (CaHA). CaHA also has been used with success in the correction of atrophic acne scars, in the recontouring of nasal defects, and in nipple reconstruction after failed nipple areolar reconstruction. Because of the risk of nodule formation, CaHA is not recommended for lip augmentation and should be used judiciously in the periorbital area.

FORMULATION

Originally approved for use by the FDA as a radiographic marker and for the correction of oral and maxillofacial defects and the treatment of vocal cord insufficiency, CaHA has since gained approval for treatment of the nasolabial folds and dorsal hands. All other areas mentioned above are common off-label uses. The microspheres of CaHA, once injected into the deep dermis, form a scaffold to support the growth of autologous collagen so there is overlap with this product as not only a temporary filler, but also as a biostimulatory agent. CaHA contains smooth spheres of 30% CaHA between 25 and 45 microns and 70% carboxymethylcellulose gel suspension, which serves to hold the microspheres in place until it is resorbed and neocollagenesis takes place.[1] CaHA contains no animal or human tissues, so allergy testing is not indicated. This filler is unique in that the standard syringe volume is 1.5 mL of material, making it the largest packaged syringe by volume.[1]

ANESTHESIA AND TECHNIQUE

Injection of CaHA is quite uncomfortable, so it is almost always necessary to anesthetize the area first with 1% lidocaine. For facial injections, a current popular practice is to mix 0.2 mL of 1% lidocaine with the CaHA via a female–female adapter. This not only provides adequate anesthesia, but also thins the product to allow for smoother injection. Because of its viscosity, CaHA must be injected through a 27- to 28-gauge needle. Placing the patient supine or at 45 degrees, a threading technique is used, with infiltration staying at the dermal–subcutaneous junction in the area of the nasolabial fold and at the deep fat or supraperiosteal region in the areas of the cheek and mandible. CaHA appears to work best if patients undergo retreatment or touchup at 3 months. For injections to the dorsal hands, the patient should be placed in a comfortable position with the hands faced prone on a flat surface. The FDA approved method of injecting CaHA in the hands, involves using 1.3 mL of the CaHA-injectable implant mixed with 0.2 mL of 2% lidocaine HCl. Using a 27-gauge needle, several 0.2- to 0.5-mL aliquots are injected subdermally in the space bound laterally between the first and fifth metacarpals, proximally by the dorsal wrist crease, and distally by the metacarpophalangeal joints. This is followed by gentle massaging of the injected areas to blend the product evenly across the dorsal hand. The number of injection points is left to the discretion of the treating physician, based on the amount of correction needed. No more than 3 mL of the CaHA implant is to be injected per hand. Some clinicians prefer to use cannulas for CaHA injection in the dorsal hands using either a bolus or threading technique.

POSTPROCEDURE INSTRUCTIONS

There can be marked swelling and bruising after the injection of CaHA, so posttreatment icing is recommended. Many physicians advocate immediate postinjection massage but others believe that continued massage is unwarranted.

UNIQUE COMPLICATIONS

CaHA is not a mucopolysaccharide and therefore does not rely on water binding for its persisting clinical effect and it does not carry the risk of producing the Tyndall effect in the skin. However, if CaHA is injected too superficially or at appropriate levels in thin skin, its opacity can be seen. Because it contains microspheres of CaHA and collagen forms around these particles, these physical properties can lead to more palpability in the soft subcutaneous tissues. The majority of complications with CaHA (nodules) are seen in the lips, but it is possible for nodules lasting 1 to 2 years to occur anywhere the substance is injected. These nodules are supposedly noninflammatory, and often the material can be extruded from a puncture incision. Persistent nodules may have to be surgically removed. Demarcation of product is especially evident in the periorbital area, as is prolonged erythema.

LONGEVITY

In a 12-month, multicenter prospective randomized split face trial comparing CaHA to non–animal-derived stabilized hyaluronic acid in the nasolabial folds, CaHA was found to provide significantly greater correction at all time points. In practice, though, longevity appears variable, with effects lasting anywhere between 6 and 18 months.[4]

AUTOLOGOUS FAT TRANSFER

PATIENT SELECTION

Autologous fat transfer (AFT) is a practical option for patients who desire a more dramatic global change in facial appearance. Recent anatomic research suggests that facial fat is delineated in discreet fat compartments that change morphologically over time.[5] Therefore, using fat as a filler is done with the intent of restoring the youthful architecture to these fat compartments. This provides broader rejuvenation to the aging face affected by volume loss. Fat is a versatile filler, effective in the periorbital area as well as the lips. Because it is autologous, it is the filler of choice for patients with collagen vascular disease or proven allergic reactions to collagens or hyaluronic acids. AFT is a more involved surgical procedure than the injection of the other fillers previously discussed. There are a subset of patients in whom AFT is not indicated. These patients include those with very low body fat, such as long distance runners, the elderly, and those with HIV-associated lipodystrophy, patients on concomitant anticoagulant treatment, and those who are of poor health.

TECHNIQUE

PREPARATION AND ANESTHESIA

For 2 weeks before the initial AFT procedure, the patient must stop taking all nonsteroidal antiinflammatory drugs, vitamin E, ω-3 fatty acid supplements, and ginkgo, ginger, or ginseng supplements. The patient is instructed to begin therapy with an appropriate antistaphylococcal antibiotic starting the day before the procedure. On the day of the procedure, the donor fat site and the face are both washed with an antibacterial soap. The physician then delineates the area to be suctioned with a marking pen. Every attempt should be made to choose a donor site that benefits a patient aesthetically. The outer thighs and hips in women and the flanks in men are usually good sites for fat harvesting.

In preparation for fat transfer, a pattern is drawn on the face delineating the areas in which fat is to be placed and highlighting any scars or baseline asymmetry. The patient is then placed on a sterile, draped operating table and the areas requiring fat suctioning are infiltrated with dilute local anesthesia until turgid (tumescent technique; Table 215-3; see Chap. 214).

It takes at least 20 minutes for the epinephrine in the tumescent fluid to achieve hemostasis. The face is then anesthetized diffusely with dilute 0.5% lidocaine with epinephrine 1:200,000, and segmental nerve blocks are established where appropriate. For safety, the total lidocaine dose in the tumescent fluid should not exceed 35 mg/kg of body weight.

FAT HARVESTING

Suctioning of the fat used for transplantation should be done by hand with an open-tipped harvesting cannula attached to a 10-mL syringe. After a hole is made with a 1.5-mm punch or No. 11 blade, the cannula is inserted into the deep fat and moved back and forth while the plunger on the syringe is retracted. Fat collection usually occurs quite rapidly and, due to the vasoconstrictive properties of the tumescent fluid, is nearly bloodless. After fat extraction, the syringes may be placed into a centrifuge and spun at 3400 revolutions per minute for 20 seconds or left to stand for 20 minutes to allow separation of the hydrophilic tumescent fluid from the lipophilic fat. The infranate of tumescent fluid should then be decanted before the fatty layer is transferred to 1-mL syringes in preparation for injection into the face. Any supranate of ruptured fat cells (triglycerides and free fatty acids) should be discarded.

FAT TRANSFER

All AFT to the face is performed with the patient fully supine using an 18-gauge or smaller blunt cannula for infiltration. Incision sites can be made with an 18-gauge needle, a NoKor needle (Becton, Dickinson and Co., USA), or the tip of a No. 11 blade scalpel. Fat is infiltrated in a retrograde manner; that is, fat is injected only as the cannula is withdrawn. Injection is in small aliquots of 0.1 mL or less using a threading or depot method. Placement of fat always starts closest to bone when possible and then proceeds up through muscle and into subcutaneous fat. Fat is deposited in a crosshatched three-dimensional lattice and thus imparts structure as well as augmentation to the tissues. All areas of the face should be addressed to achieve filling both laterally and anteriorly. The goal

TABLE 215-3
Tumescent Anesthesia Solution

- 1 L Normal saline
- 50 mg Lidocaine
- 0.5 to 1 mg Epinephrine
- 12.5 mEq Sodium bicarbonate

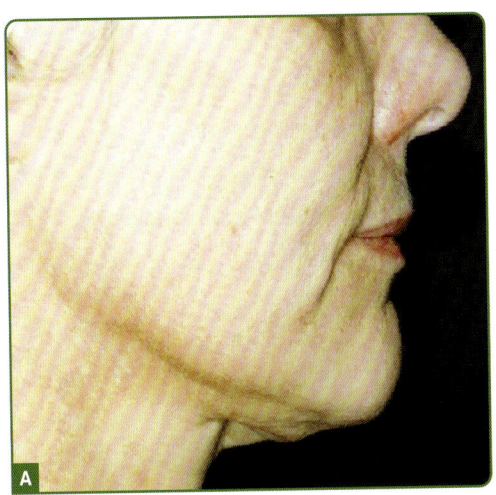 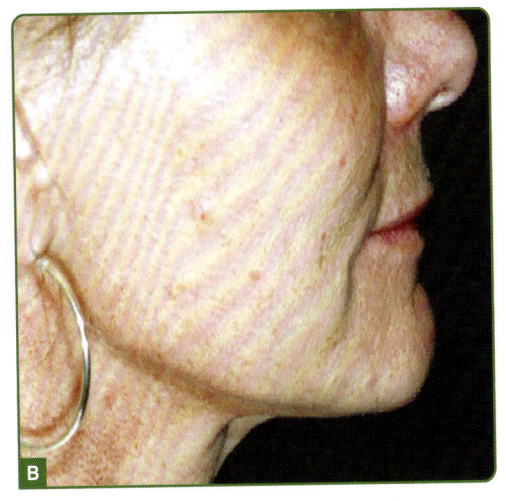

Figure 215-4 Fifty-five-year-old woman before (**A**) and 20 months after (**B**) full-face fat transfer treatment series.

is to advance tissues forward and elevate them away from the bone, fill in areas of shadow, and restore youthful contours.

POSTPROCEDURE INSTRUCTIONS

Immediately after the procedure and on-and-off for the next 2 days, ice should be applied to the face. The area suctioned is dressed with absorbent pads, and a snug garment is applied. Incision sites on the body and face are left unsutured. The patient is instructed not to submerge the body in water until all incisions are healed (approximately 1 week). Antibiotics must be continued for 6 days after the initial procedure. Intramuscular triamcinolone may be given to reduce postoperative edema.

UNIQUE COMPLICATIONS

Postoperative edema and ecchymoses are common and last for approximately 2 weeks. Undercorrection with a gradual decrease in augmentation is common and usually represents a decline in edema rather than absorption of the fat. For this reason, fat transfer should never be recommended as a one-time procedure, but rather as a series of treatments with cumulative augmentation and long-term results. Small, persistent lumps can occur that represent either fat cysts or accumulation of fat. They can be treated, usually to resolution, with intralesional injection of triamcinolone (2 to 4 mg/mL). If a larger fat lump is present, the best option is to feather it into the surrounding tissues with an infiltration cannula. Irregularities can also occur at the harvest site, but operator experience and judicious removal of fat makes this a highly unlikely event. Rarely, infections, such as atypical mycobacteria, can be seen and should be in the differential diagnosis for any nodules occurring up to 1 year following AFT.

LONGEVITY

Many authors using a standardized, multilevel microinjection technique have published photodocumentation of long-term followup demonstrating persistence of autologous fat (Fig. 215-4).[6] When AFT is done with proper technique, the results are permanent. Successful grafting really depends on the precise performance of four important aspects: collecting, processing, injecting and protecting.

INJECTABLE SILICONE

PATIENT SELECTION

Injectable silicone is categorically a permanent filler with a wide range of applications. It appears to provide permanent, cosmetically superior augmentation for treatment of HIV lipoatrophy, plantar defects, and scars. Historically, silicone injection has been associated with disfiguring tissue distortions and migration of product. These side effects can almost always be traced to the use of large-volume injections or non–medical-grade silicone. Because of the controversial nature of silicone augmentation, patient selection for cosmetic indications is complex, and use of the procedure should be reserved for those physicians who have extensive experience in the injection of silicone as a filler and who understand the concepts outlined in the "Technique" section.

Patients with a known history of autoimmune disease, and those with chronic or active infections should be excluded from treatment.

FORMULATION

Injectable silicone has both inspired a loyal following and provoked vehement opposition. There is no approved silicone for soft-tissue skin augmentation. However, off-label uses of ophthalmologic preparations of silicone have been adapted for use, especially in the treatment of HIV-associated lipoatrophy and other clinical conditions of facial volume loss. One formulation, PMS-350, has European approval for treatment of glabellar lines, nasolabial folds, perioral lines, lip augmentation, and scarring disorders. Silicone oil varies in chemical structure, physical properties, purity, sterility, and biocompatibility. Medical-grade silicone oil contains long polymers of dimethylsiloxanes.[7] It is noncarcinogenic and does not appear to be associated with arthritic disease in mice. Viscosity of silicone oil is measured in centistokes (cs), which is a unit of kinematic viscosity. After injection, silicone is encapsulated in collagenous fibrous tissue, so that final augmentation is a result of both volume of injected silicone and host tissue response.

ANESTHESIA

Currently available forms of silicone do not contain an anesthetic solution, because such small volumes are injected on each visit an ancillary anesthesia is not often required. If desired, a topical anesthetic agent containing 4% lidocaine or 20% tetracaine may be applied before the procedure.

TECHNIQUE

Improper technique in the injection of silicone oil will almost always guarantee permanent adverse sequelae. Consequently, it is absolutely necessary that a physician considering its use apprentice with an experienced practitioner. Silicone (1000 cs) is highly viscous and must be injected through either a 26-gauge needle on a 1-mL syringe or a 30-gauge needle on a 0.3-mL syringe. Use of a microinjection technique is paramount to success with silicone, so large-bore needles are never to be used. The microdroplet injection technique involves injecting 0.01 mL of silicone oil, with the needle bevel down, into the deep dermis in a depot fashion at 1- to 3-mm intervals. Note that 100 droplets are therefore required to empty a 1-mL syringe. Except in the treatment of HIV cheek atrophy, it is rare to use more than 0.3 mL total per injection session. Treated areas are always undercorrected, and patients are instructed to return for multiple injection sessions at monthly intervals until full augmentation occurs.

POSTPROCEDURE INSTRUCTIONS

There is very little postoperative discomfort, edema, or ecchymosis after microinjection with liquid silicone. Ice may be applied if needed to lessen the risk of postinjection ecchymosis. Patients may apply makeup and pursue their daily activities as usual after injection.

UNIQUE COMPLICATIONS

Most authorities on silicone use agree that the incidence of serious complications after the proper use of medical-grade silicone is very low. In an FDA-authorized study involving 1400 patients over a 20-year period, 2 patients experienced serious side effects: one case involved migration of silicone after treatment with large volumes, and the second involved inflammation and necrosis in a patient with concomitant Weber-Christian disease and rheumatoid arthritis. Local granulomatous nodularities can occur many years after the cessation of treatment and are usually preceded by a systemic infection. Treatment regimens for granulomas include intralesional or systemic steroids, minocycline, topical imiquimod and, if necessary, surgical excision.[8]

LONGEVITY

The augmentation derived from liquid silicone injection is permanent. Many authors have published reports of long-term studies, some with 30-year followup, showing persistence of improvement. Patients receiving liquid silicone injections will continue to age, and, for this reason, additional augmentation may be required should neighboring areas of age-related atrophy develop.

COMPLICATIONS ASSOCIATED WITH THE USE OF ALL FILLERS

Vascular occlusion is perhaps the most devastating complication associated with the use of all fillers. This can manifest as local necrosis, CNS infarction, or blindness. Blindness and middle cerebral artery infarction have been described most often after fat transfer, but vascular occlusion with ensuing sequelae has occurred after the use of collagen and hyaluronic acid fillers as well. In theory, the central occlusive events have occurred from high-pressure injections with retrograde flow into arterioles that connect with the internal carotid system. It is, therefore, of utmost importance to keep the needle or cannula moving during withdrawal while depositing filler and to exert as little pressure as possible on the syringe. For similar reasons, when fat transfer is performed, only blunt cannulas should be used for infiltration.

Other complications common to the use of all fillers include ecchymosis, edema, extrusion or drifting of the filling substance, foreign-body reactions, pigmentary alteration, injection site scarring, overcorrection, undercorrection, misplacement, and infection.

REFERENCES

1. Newman J. Review of soft tissue augmentation in the face. *Clin Cosmet Investing Dermatol.* 2009;2:141-150.
2. Lowe NJ, Maxwell CA, Patnaik R. Adverse reactions to dermal fillers: review. *Dermatol Surg.* 2005;31:1616.
3. Rossner F, Rossner M, Hartmann V, et al. Decrease of reported adverse events to injectable polylactic acid after recommending an increased dilution: 8-year results from the injectable filler safety study. *J Cosmet Dermatol.* 2009;8:14-18.
4. Moers-Carpi MM, Tefet JO. Calcium hydroxylapatite versus nonanimal stabilized hyaluronic acid for the correction of the nasolabial folds: a 12 month, multicenter, prospective, randomized, controlled, split-face trial. *Dermatol Surg.* 2009;34:210-221.
5. Rohrich RJ, Pessa JE. The fat compartments of the face: anatomy and clinical implications for cosmetic surgery. *Plast Reconstr Surg.* 2007;119:2219-2227.
6. Donofrio LM. Panfacial volume restoration with fat. *Dermatol Surg.* 2005;31:1496.
7. Narins RS, Beer K. Liquid injectable silicone: a review of its history, immunology, technical considerations, complications and potential. *Plast Reconstr Surg.* 2006;118:77-84.
8. Duffy DM. Liquid silicone for soft tissue augmentation. *Dermatol Surg.* 2005;31:1530.

Chapter 216 :: Botulinum Toxin
:: Richard G. Glogau

第二百一十六章
肉毒杆菌毒素

中文导读

肉毒杆菌毒素是神经毒素的一种，能使肌肉麻痹、腺体分泌能力下降，现已广泛应用于皮肤美容科。本章从6个方面介绍：①商业市场及近期发展；②药理学；③适应证；⑤副作用和并发症；⑥肉毒杆菌毒素的其他应用。

第一节简单介绍了肉毒杆菌毒素应用历史，目前可观的产品销售额及市场规模，FDA相继批准的几种肉毒杆菌毒素，并指出"肉毒杆菌"这一术语正走向大众。举例近期肉毒素研究有A型毒素—daxibotulinumtoxinA、NDS™、ANT-1207、AI-09等。

第二节从毒素的结构、发挥生物作用的机制及机体对其免疫的情况进行介绍。肉毒杆菌神经毒素目前分为7种不同的血清型。目前市场上可获得的血清型有A型和B型。毒素通过与表面蛋白受体结合进入神经，并通过内吞作用进入内在化的囊泡。轻链被释放到神经细胞质中，SNARE（可溶性n-乙基马来酰亚胺敏感因子附着蛋白受体）蛋白复合物被裂解以抑制神经递质如乙酰胆碱的分泌（图216-2），最终导致局部骨骼肌活动丧失或靶器官（如汗腺）的自主控制能力下降。随着时间的推移，原神经突触周围长出新的侧突触并建立新的联系，此时肌肉活动、腺体分泌逐渐恢复，当原先被阻断的突触恢复后，侧突触又逐渐消失，最终原先被阻断的突触重新连接并发挥作用。

第三节介绍适应证：常用于面部上三分之一的动态皱纹及腋下多汗症，较少用于下面部及四肢。

第四节介绍肉毒杆菌毒素治疗，包括眉间纹、水平前额纹、外眦纹（鱼尾纹）、多汗症及联合治疗。在面部治疗前需熟悉面部肌肉解剖位置（图216-4），并介绍了治疗不同部位时需注意的事项，如对皱纹的正确识别、进针位点、治疗后处理和治疗间隔时间等，防止产生眉毛下垂、眉弓丧失、眼睑松弛、颧肌麻痹、嘴角下垂等情况的发生。

而联合治疗主要指软组织填充面中下部，联合神经毒素治疗面上三分之一。肉毒杆菌毒素对于多汗症的治疗包括局灶性腋下多汗症、手掌多汗症，其中局灶性腋下多汗症的治疗相对成功，而手掌多汗症的治疗由于毒素难以扩散、疼痛及治疗后手部无力限制了它的应用。

第五节提到了副作用和并发症，主要关注眉间注射后眼睑下垂、过度治疗额肌引起的眉毛下垂、眼周注射引起的短暂性眼睑浮肿、注射面部上三分之一后出现的头痛、多汗症注射后手掌无力及其相对应的解决办法。

第六节提到肉毒杆菌毒素的其他应用（FDA未批准），临床医生发现肉毒杆菌毒素除应用于眉间纹和鱼尾纹外，还可以用于其他部位，如额肌、口轮匝肌、鼻翼肌肉、下颌部位甚至颈部肌肉。

〔简　丹〕

COMMERCIAL MARKET

When Drs. Jean and Alastair Carruthers made the critical leap from ophthalmologist Dr. Alan Scott's seminal use of botulinum as an alternative to strabismus surgery to the cosmetic use of the toxin to treat the glabellar frown lines, no one could have predicted the explosive growth of this agent in the commercial market.[1] On April 15, 2002, the US Food and Drug Administration (FDA) approved Allergan, Inc.'s Botox Cosmetic* (botulinum toxin type A) for "temporary improvement in the appearance of moderate-to-severe glabellar lines in adult men and women 65 or younger." This was the first elective cosmetic indication for which any commercially available botulinum toxin in the US market had been approved.

The toxin had previously been approved and was marketed as Botox® for the treatment of strabismus, blepharospasm, and cervical dystonia but existing off-label cosmetic use of the toxin had already propelled annual sales to $250 million per year by 2002. With FDA recognition of the cosmetic indication, sales of both Botox® and Botox Cosmetic® surpassed $1 billion per year by the end of 2009. The last half of 2015 and first half of 2016 produced $2.6 billion in sales. Analysts anticipate a $3 billion annual market for Botox® and Botox Cosmetic® in 2017-2018.

Allergan's product in the US market has equaled the brand name equity of Pfizer's product Viagra® (sildenafil citrate). "Botox" is now part of the daily vernacular, used to refer to a class of biologic neurotoxins in much the same way as the well-known trademarks Coke® and Kleenex® are used to refer to carbonated beverages and facial tissue. The clinical utility of the neurotoxin is so widely known today that the word *Botox* has become a generic term in the public mind for all agents used in cosmetic neurotoxin therapy, although the term is properly reserved for Allergan's trademarked commercial version of the type A neurotoxin complex.

In April 2009, the FDA approved a third commercial neurotoxin, a serotype A product, Dysport® (Ipsen [UK]/Medicis [US]) to join Allergan's Botox®/Botox Cosmetic® and a previously approved serotype B product, Myobloc® (Solstice Neurosciences [US]). In July 2011, the FDA approved a fourth commercial neurotoxin for the US market, a serotype A product, Xeomin® (Merz Pharma GmbH [Germany]). To emphasize the noninterchangeability of these biologic toxins, the FDA in August 2009 required the manufacturers to adopt new drug names: onabotulinumtoxinA (Botox®/Botox Cosmetic®), abobotulinumtoxin A (Dysport®), rimabotulinum toxin B (Myobloc®), and incobotulinum toxin A (Xeomin®).

Another serotype A toxin in development in 2011, at the time the last edition was written, was called PurTox® (Mentor [US]). This toxin is purportedly a "naked" toxin, that is, without complexing proteins, and probably with a molecular weight similar to that of Xeomin®. Johnson & Johnson acquired Mentor in 2009 and decided in 2014 to walk away from the neurotoxin portion of their investment represented by PurTox®. The development of this toxin is apparently at an end, all production having ceased, and with some of the intellectual property reportedly having been sold off. The $16-million manufacturing facility that Mentor had built in Madison, Wisconsin, was deemed redundant by Johnson & Johnson and was donated to a private–public research foundation based at University of Wisconsin.

In 2014, Allergan spent $65 million (with potential milestone bonuses of another $180 million) to acquire worldwide licensing rights (exclusive of Korea) for the neurotoxin products produced by Medy-Tox [Korea], which are marketed outside the United States under the names Meditoxin® or Neuronox®. The Medy-Tox product is produced in liquid form. Some clinicians have suggested that the liquid formulation may provide a stable, prefilled syringe as a convenience for those practitioners who would like to avoid the required dilution of the lyophilized forms of botulinum toxin such as Botox Cosmetic® and Dysport®. Others speculate that Allergan simply made this licensure agreement to stave future competition for Botox® in the US commercial space.

Korea has been the center of another commercial botulinum toxin product, Botulax®, which was released in Korea and Japan in 2010. It has been used for blepharospasm and glabellar lines. It is an A-type toxin that has a molecular weight of about 900 kDa, similar to Allergan's product, with the accessory complexing protein structure wrapped around the central 150-kDa core toxin like Botox®. Botulax® is made by Hugel Pharma and is made from the Clostridium strain CBFC26.

The American company ALPHAEON (Irvine, CA) acquired Evolus, Inc (Santa Barbara, CA) in 2013 and, as a result of that acquisition, entered into licensure agreement with Daewoong Pharmaceutical (Seoul, Korea) to develop a 900-kDa A toxin for the US and other international markets. This toxin is named Evosyal® and has been known as either DWP-450 or Nabota® in the Korean markets. Evosyal® has completed Phase II and III trials in the US and is awaiting FDA approval.

---

*It is the editors' policy not to use trade names in this book. However, in certain instances, the editors had to depart from this policy to avoid confusion.

Another serotype of A toxin in use outside of the United States (Asia, South America) is Hengli®/Prosigne® (Lanzhou [China]). The hurdles to entry into the US market, particularly given the FDA's rigorous manufacturing standards, may ultimately forestall entry of the Chinese product into the US market. At the time of this writing, there are no particular plans reportedly afoot to bring Hengli® into the US market.

RECENT DEVELOPMENTS

An A-type toxin manufactured by Revance Therapeutics (Newark, CA), daxibotulinumtoxinA, was initially formulated as a topical gel (RT001™) and then as formula for injection (RT002™). Although early Phase II trials showed promise for the topical formulation in the treatment of hyperhidrosis and crow's feet, in June 2016, the company announced that the RT001 phase 3 trial for crow's feet had failed to meet its primary endpoints and that future efforts would center on the phase 3 trials of the injectable RT002 for glabellar lines and Phase II trials for cervical dystonia. Earlier, Phase II trials of the RT002 injectable suggested a statistically significant increase in duration of action that would merit confirmation studies in phase 3.

In January 2016, Allergan announced the purchase of Anterios, Inc, a biopharmaceutical firm that purported to have a proprietary technology that permits delivery of neurotoxins through the skin. The transport system, called NDS™, was apparently developed with intellectual property from the University of Massachusetts, and involves surrounding the target molecule with nano-particles that permit movement of the molecule across the skin barriers. The topical A-type toxin, ANT-1207, has completed Phase II clinical trials in lateral canthal lines, acne, and hyperhidrosis in March 2016, but results were unpublished at the time of this writing. An additional formulation of A-type toxin in liquid form, AI-09, is in preclinical development as an injectable form of the A toxin.

PHARMACOLOGY

TOXIN STRUCTURE

Botulinum neurotoxins are currently categorized into 7 distinct serotypes: A, B, C1, D, E, F, and G.[2] The molecules vary in their biosynthesis, size, cellular sites of action, binding kinetics, duration of effect, and stability. The serotypes currently commercially available, serotypes A and B, are derived from different strains of *Clostridium botulinum*. They both have 150-kDa dichain polypeptides with a heavy chain and light chain linked by disulfide bonds. During biosynthesis, the molecules of A and B can be surrounded by proteins to form a neurotoxin complex, ranging from 500 to 900 kDa (Fig. 216-1). Xeomin® (incobotulinumtoxin A) consists of the 150-kDa dichain without accessory proteins.

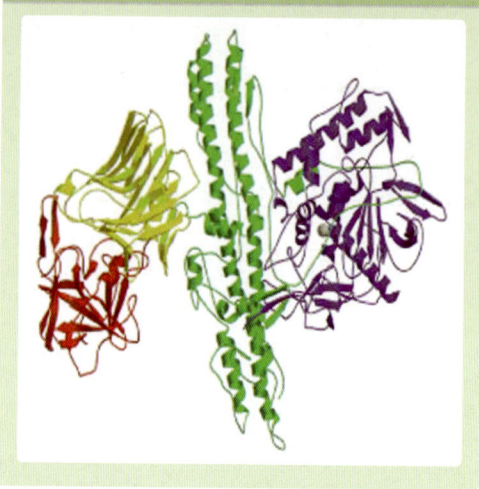

Figure 216-1 Schematic of the botulinum complex showing the binding domain with the N-terminus (*yellow*) and the C-terminus (*red*), together with the translocation domain (*green*) and the light chain (*blue*). (Used with permission from Turton K, Chaddock JA, Acharya KR. Botulinum and tetanus neurotoxins: structure, function and therapeutic utility. *Trends Biochem Sci*. 2002;27:554. Copyright © Elsevier.)

MECHANISM OF ACTION

The toxin enters the nerves by binding to surface protein receptors and undergoing endocytosis into internalized vesicles. The light chain is released into the nerve cytosol, and the SNARE (soluble *N*-ethylmaleimide-sensitive factor attachment protein receptor) protein complex is cleaved to inhibit exocytosis of the neurotransmitters such as acetylcholine (Fig. 216-2). Type A toxin cleaves SNAP-25 (synaptosome-associated protein of 25 kDa), whereas type B cleaves VAMP (vesicle-associated membrane protein), also called *synaptobrevin* (Fig. 216-3). These proteins are necessary for the release of acetylcholine from vesicles within the cytoplasm of the motor nerve endings. The binding characteristics of each serotype dictate the locus of action on the intracellular SNARE protein complex (Table 216-1).

The end result is a chemodenervation of the cholinergic neurons, either motor nerves or autonomic nerves, leading to localized absence of skeletal muscle activity or autonomic control of target organs such as the eccrine sweat glands. The way in which the nerves escape the effect of the neurotoxin is partially understood.[3] The chemodenervated nerve endings develop collateral sprouting near the primary terminus of the nerve. These sprouts eventually make proximate contact with the targets, either muscle or gland, and begin to overcome the loss of neurotransmitter at the end organ synaptic junctions.

Once these sprouts have reestablished chemical contact with their targets, muscles resume activity and glands begin to secrete. Simultaneously, the original

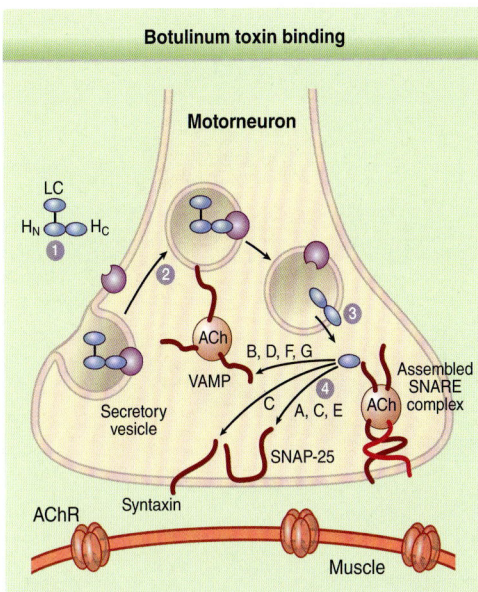

Figure 216-2 The heavy-chain domain of the botulinum neurotoxin complex binds to the plasma membrane receptor (1), and the complex is internalized (2). The light-chain fragment is then released into the cytoplasm (3), where it cleaves the SNARE (soluble *N*-ethylmaleimide-sensitive factor attachment protein receptor) protein complex at a site determined by the neurotoxin serotype (4). This disruption of the SNARE complex prevents exocytosis of acetylcholine (ACh) into the synaptic space of the neuromuscular junction n. A through G, neurotoxin serotypes; AChR, acetylcholine receptor; LC, light chain; H_C, heavy chain C-terminus; H_N, heavy chain N-terminus; SNAP-25, synaptosome-associated protein of 25 kDa; VAMP, vesicle-associated membrane protein. (Used with permission from Turton K, Chaddock JA, Acharya KR. Botulinum and tetanus neurotoxins: Structure, function and therapeutic utility. *Trends Biochem Sci*. 2002;27:555. Copyright © Elsevier.)

chemodenervated terminal nerve ending begins to degrade the blocked SNARE proteins and develop new proteins to resume the chemical exocytosis of acetylcholine. While these repairs are under way, and while the original terminal nerve ending reacquires communication with the target organ, the collateral sprouts begin to slowly resorb until anatomically nothing is left but the original terminal ending with restored junctional activity.

Four commercially available preparations of botulinum neurotoxin were on the market in the United States and Europe in late 2016, and one was pending approval (Table 216-2). All but one are serotype botulinum toxin A, and one is a serotype botulinum toxin B. The products differ in their methods of manufacture, commercial form, and biologic profiles. Various other toxins are available outside of the US or are in current development. These are summarized, compared, and contrasted in Table 216-3.

The units by which these products are described are not interchangeable because of the nature of the assays used to determine their potency. The mouse assays used differ in the diluents used and are not comparable. There is no such thing as a standard neurotoxin unit; hence, there is no "International Unit" for neurotoxin. Thus, there is no way of standardizing neurotoxin units to compare serotype A products to each other, let alone to other serotype B products.

Although the molecule complexes are unique, similar uses are based on clinical observations. For example, in the glabellar frown line pivotal trials, 20 units of Botox® or Xeomin® and 50 units of Dysport® were used.[4] Botox® is generally diluted with either 1.0, 2.0, or 2.5 mL of saline per 100 units, producing concentrations of either 10 units per 0.1 mL, 5 units per 0.1 mL, or 4 units per 0.1 mL, respectively. Xeomin® is diluted with 2.5 mL per 100-unit vial. Allergan's pivotal trial used the 4 unit per 0.1 mL dilution.

Dysport® is usually diluted with 1.5 mL of saline per 300-unit vial producing a concentration of 10 units in 0.05 mL as used in the pivotal trial. Notice that the Dysport® pivotal trial used injection volumes that were half those used in the Allergan trial: 0.05 mL (10 U) per injection point (Dysport®) versus 0.1 mL (4 U) per injection site (Botox®). It is unclear whether such differences in volume may contribute to behavioral differences between the 2 products in terms of diffusion and persistence. At some point, a larger volume might increase diffusion but probably decrease persistence since less drug would saturate the receptors in a given area.

The use of sterile saline with preservative (benzyl alcohol) as a diluent appears to lessen the sting of injection with Botox® and Dysport®. Myobloc®, the B serotype, causes more discomfort on injection because of its low pH, but it is stable in liquid form at room temperature for many months.

In addition to the drug name changes, which the FDA required of the manufacturers in 2009, the agency instituted a Risk Evaluation and Mitigation Strategy (REMS), and a boxed warning for these products that warned of the possibility of spread distant from the injection site with potentially life-threatening consequences. Emphasizing the noninterchangeability of these commercial products, the FDA wished to minimize the possibility of medication errors as well as draw attention to the need for tailoring specific doses of each toxin product to specific situations.

IMMUNOLOGY

The possibility of antibody-mediated resistance appears to be largely theoretical. Original Botox® batch No. 79-11, widely used in ophthalmology and neurology for years, produced rare cases of nonresponse in the treatment of torticollis and blepharospasm. Newer batches introduced in 1997, No. 91223US and No. BCB2024, have significantly less protein load. Although cases of primary nonresponse may be rarely encountered, immunologic resistance to Botox® and Botox Cosmetic® does not appear to be clinically relevant in dermatology, even at the dosages used to treat

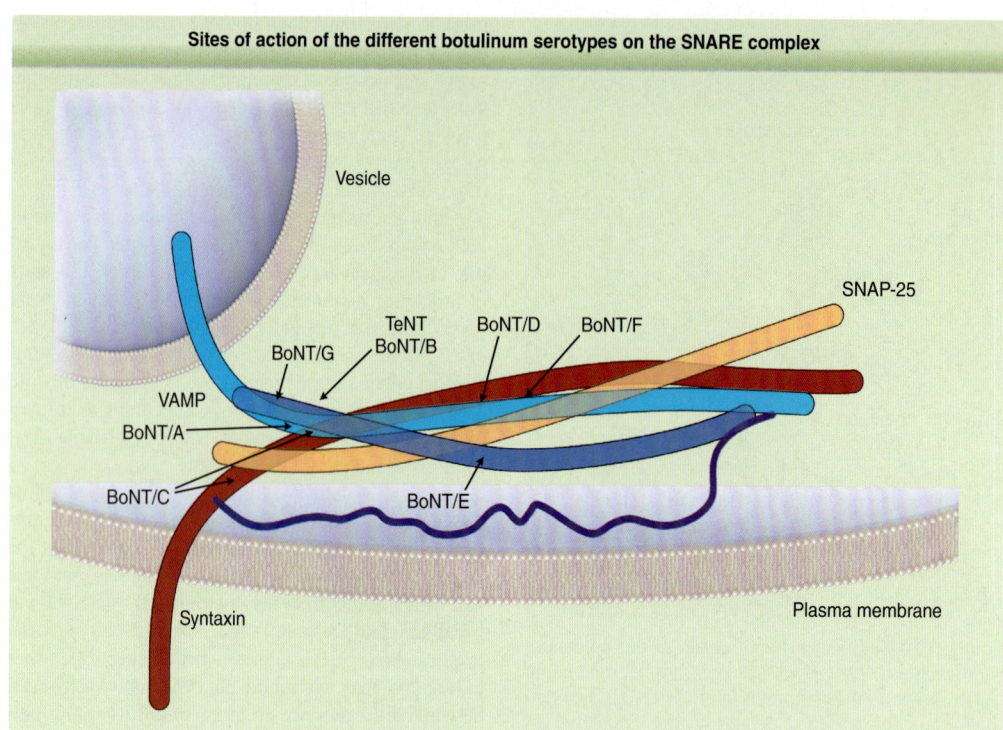

Figure 216-3 Schematic representation showing the sites of action of the different botulinum serotypes on the intracellular protein complex known as the SNARE (soluble *N*-ethylmaleimide-sensitive factor attachment protein receptor) proteins responsible for exocytosis of acetylcholine from the nerve. Botulinum A serotype cleaves SNAP-25 (synaptosome-associated protein of 25 kDa). Other serotypes impact VAMP (vesicle-associated membrane protein), synaptobrevin, or syntaxin. BoNT/A through BoNT/G, botulinum neurotoxin serotypes A through G; TeNT, tetanus neurotoxin.

hyperhidrosis, which can average 400 units per treatment session. In addition, the treatment interval does not appear to be a significant factor in clinical resistance for the newer batches and at the smaller dosages used in cosmetic facial treatment, although exposure to the toxin at increasingly shorter intervals may theoretically be associated with development of neutralizing antibodies. In clinical practice, the reality of induced resistance on the basis of development of neutralizing antibodies is extremely rare, a fact bolstered by the difficulty in trying to purposefully induce resistance to the toxin through repeated vaccination.

INDICATIONS

Botulinum toxin is used in cosmetic dermatology primarily for the treatment of dynamic expression lines in the upper third of the face (the glabellar brow furrow, horizontal frontalis forehead lines, periocular rhytides aka crow's feet) and for the treatment of axillary hyperhidrosis. Less common and therapeutically more challenging indications are platysmal banding in the neck, perioral rhytides, marionette lines at the corners of the mouth from the action of the depressor anguli oris, shaping the lower face with masseter volume reduction, postsurgical synkinesis in the lower face, and palmar/plantar and forehead/scalp hyperhidrosis.

TREATMENT

GLABELLAR LINES (BROW FURROWS)

A firm understanding of the underlying facial anatomy is the sine qua non of successful aesthetic therapy with botulinum toxin. Depending on the muscle

TABLE 216-1
Binding Sites in the Snare Protein Complex of the 7 Known Botulinum Toxin Serotypes

SEROTYPE	INTRACELLULAR PROTEIN
A	SNAP-25
B	VAMP/synaptobrevin
C1	SNAP-25 and syntaxin
D	VAMP/synaptobrevin
E	SNAP-25
F	VAMP/synaptobrevin
G	VAMP/synaptobrevin

SNAP-25, synaptosome-associated protein of 25 kDa; SNARE, soluble *N*-ethylmaleimide-sensitive factor attachment protein receptor; VAMP, vesicle-associated membrane protein.

TABLE 216-2
Comparison of the Properties of the Commercially Available Forms of Botulinum Toxin in Current Medical Use in the United States (4) and Pending (1)

PROPRIETARY NAME	BOTOX® BOTOX® COSMETIC	DYSPORT®	XEOMIN®	MYOBLOC®	RT001 TOPICAL RT002 INJECTABLE
Non-proprietary Name (FDA)	Onabotulinum-toxin A	Abobotulinumtoxin A	Incobotulinumtoxin A	Rimabotulinumtoxin B	Daxibotulinumtoxin A
First approval	1989 (US) 2002 (US)	1991 (UK)	2010 (US)	2000 (US)	Pending
Manufacturer	Allergan (US)	Ipsen (UK)	Merz (Germany)	Solstice Neurosciences (US)	Revance Therapeutics (US)
Commercial US	Yes	Yes	Pending US	Yes	Pending US
Serotype	A	A	A	B	A
Strain	Hall (Allergan)	Hall	Hall	Bean	Hall
Process	Crystallization	Chromatography	Chromatography	Chromatography	Chromatography
Excipients	HSA (500 µg) Sodium chloride	HSA (125 µg) Lactose	HSA (1 mg/vial) Sucrose (5 mg/vial)	HSA (500 µg/mL) Sodium succinate Sodium chloride	HSA
Receptor/Target	SV2/SNAP-25	SV2/SNAP-25	SV2/SNAP-25	Syt II/VAMP	SV2/SNAP-25
Complex molecular weight uniformity	~900 kDa homogeneous	~500 kDa heterogeneous	~150 kDa	~700 kDa homogeneous	~150 kDa
Stabilization Solubilization pH	Vacuum dried Normal saline ~7	Lyophilization Normal saline ~7	Vacuum dried Normal saline ~7.4	Solution N/A 5.6	Lyophilization Normal saline ~7
Package (units per vial)	100, 200	300, 500	100	2500/5000/10,000	50
Neurotoxin protein per vial (ng/vial)	~5 (100-U vial)	4.35 (500-U vial)	0.6 (100-U vial)	25/50/100	1 (100-U vial)

mass present and the degree of atrophy from prior treatment, 20 to 35 units of Botox® or Xeomin® or 50 to 75 units of Dysport® may be placed in 5 separate injection points to treat the corrugators and procerus muscle in the average brow (Fig. 216-4). A 30-gauge, 31-gauge, or even 32-gauge needle and a tuberculin or diabetic syringe are used to minimize the trauma of the intramuscular injections. The corrugator injections are placed (1) just at or above the medial brow and (2) in or just medial to the midpupillary line, at least 1 cm above the bony orbital rim (see Fig. 216-4). The fifth injection is placed in the procerus at the midline at a point just above the horizontal creases created in the glabella at the bridge of the nose. Figure 216-5 shows the results of the procedure.

Based on earlier experience with ophthalmologic periocular injections for treatment of muscle spasms, patients have been instructed to remain upright for 2 to 3 hours to limit the incidence of eyelid ptosis, which occurs with diffusion of the toxin down into the levator muscles of the lid (Fig. 216-6). With operator experience, the incidence of ptosis after injection of the brow should be less than 2%.

Temporary stimulation of Müller muscle in the lid can be achieved with 0.5% apraclonidine or 2.5% phenylephrine eyedrops or even naphazoline hydrochloride 0.025%/pheniramine maleate 0.3% eyedrops (Naphcon A® available over the counter) (see Fig. 216-6). These will produce 2 to 3 mm of elevation of the lash margin, and administration may be repeated at intervals of 4 to 6 hours as needed until the distant diffusion effect of the botulinum toxin on the levator muscle disappears, usually in 2 to 3 weeks.

HORIZONTAL FOREHEAD LINES

The frontalis is treated at the horizontal equator of the forehead or above to avoid inactivation of the lower third of the frontalis muscle, which is responsible for suspension and movement of the eyebrows (see Figs. 216-4 and 216-7). Twelve to 20 units of Botox® or 20 to 50 units of Dysport® are placed in 4 or 5 divided doses equidistantly along the forehead equator. If too large a dose is applied or injection sites are placed too low, brow ptosis and loss of brow arch are produced, which leads to an unpleasant, heavy sensation in the brow as well as an aesthetically unattractive appearance in females.

Unlike in the treatment of eyelid ptosis, there is no comparable adrenergic agent available to reverse brow ptosis induced by botulinum, and the patient

TABLE 216-3

Comparison of the Properties of Some Commercial Forms of Botulinum Toxin in Use Outside the United States or Pending US Approval

PROPRIETARY NAME	PURTOX®	MEDITOXIN® NEURONOX®	DWP-450, EVOSYAL®, NABOTA®	BOTULAX®	HENGLI®/ PROSIGNE®	ANT-1207 TOPICAL AI-09 INJECTABLE
Non-proprietary Name (FDA)	Not named	Licensed to Allergan Outside Korea	Outside US only	Outside US only	Outside US only	In trials US
First approval	No approval	2006 (Korea)	2013 (Korea)	2010 (Korea, Japan)	1993 (China)	Pending US
Manufacturer	Mentor (J&J) (US)	Medy-Tox (Korea)	Daewoong Pharma (Korea), Alphaeon (US), Evolus, Inc. (US)	Hugel Pharma (Korea)	Lanzhou (China)	Anterios (US) Acquired by Allergan 2016
Commercial US	No approval	No	Pending	No	No	Pending
Serotype	A	A	A	A	A	A
Strain	Hall	Hall	Hall	Clostridium CBFC26	Hall	Hall
Process	Chromatography	Chromatography	Chromatography	Chromatography	Crystallization	Chromatography
Excipients	HSA Trehalose	HSA (500 µg) Sodium chloride	HSA (500 µg) Sodium chloride	HSA (500 µg) Sodium chloride	Porcine gelatin 5 mg Dextran 25 mg Sucrose 25 mg	Unpublished; Proprietary NDS technology
Receptor/target	SV2/SNAP-25	SV2/SNAP-25	SV2/SNAP-25	SV2/SNAP-25	SV2/SNAP-25	SV2/SNAP-25
Complex molecular weight uniformity	~150 kDa	~150 kDa	? ~150 kDa	900 kDa	~500 kDa heterogeneous	? 150 kDa
Stabilization Solubilization pH	Lyophilization Normal saline ~7	Lyophilization	Lyophilization	Freeze Dried 6.5 ± 0.5	Lyophilization	Liquid
Package (units per vial)	100	50/100	100	50/100/200	100	Unpublished
Neurotoxin protein per vial (ng/vial)	1 (100-U vial)	?	?	<2.5 / <5.0 / <10	?	Unpublished

must wait several weeks for the effect to wear off. In a patient who has never received botulinum toxin before, it is wise to separate the glabellar area from the forehead area and to wait a couple of weeks between treating the two to avoid the possibility of overtreatment and brow ptosis. Many patients find even the smallest drop in brow position very bothersome, and great care should be taken to avoid this complication of aesthetic treatment.

LATERAL CANTHAL LINES (CROW'S FEET)

The rhytides at the corners of the eye respond favorably to injections of toxin; however, patients frequently confuse true crow's feet rhytides with the dynamic expression lines that appear across the malar eminence laterally in conjunction with smiling and contraction of the zygomaticus muscles. Toxin may successfully ameliorate true crow's feet, which radiate directly from the lateral canthus and are associated with contraction of the orbicularis oculi muscles by themselves. But the "smile lines" that appear over the malar eminence often lie in wait for the unwary injector. Placing toxin at or below the malar eminence in an attempt to weaken these lines may lead to paralysis of the zygomaticus muscles and a drooping corner of the mouth that cannot spontaneously be raised, so that the patient may acquire a poststroke appearance.

To safely approach crow's feet, the toxin is usually placed at 1 to 3 injection points approximately 1 cm lateral to the lateral canthus. Some practitioners place all of the drug at one point, and others distribute the dose evenly among 3 points. Typical doses range from 10 to 18 units of Botox® or 25 to 30 units of Dysport® depending on the estimate of muscle mass and activity.

Great care must be taken to make the injections into the skin only, raising wheals or blebs that can be gently massaged down. Intramuscular injection in this area will reliably produce unwanted bruising because of the rich venous plexus underlying the skin in this region. The toxin will readily diffuse from the blebs into the underlying orbicularis muscle, relaxing

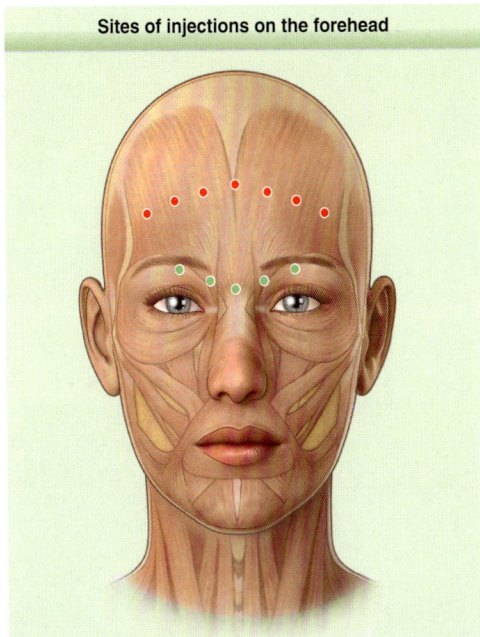

Figure 216-4 Sites of injections on the forehead. The corrugator and procerus muscles are weakened by carefully positioning 5 injections of botulinum toxin of 5 units each (Botox®) (*green circles*). If Dysport® is used, 10 units would be placed in the 3 central injection points but the lateral corrugator injection points (represented by the red circles) are a little medial and slightly higher than the lateral injection points used for Botox,® in most cases, according to Ascher.[15] Forceful knitting of the brow is prevented. To weaken the frontalis muscle, injections are placed in 5 or more divided doses along the forehead equator (*red circles*).

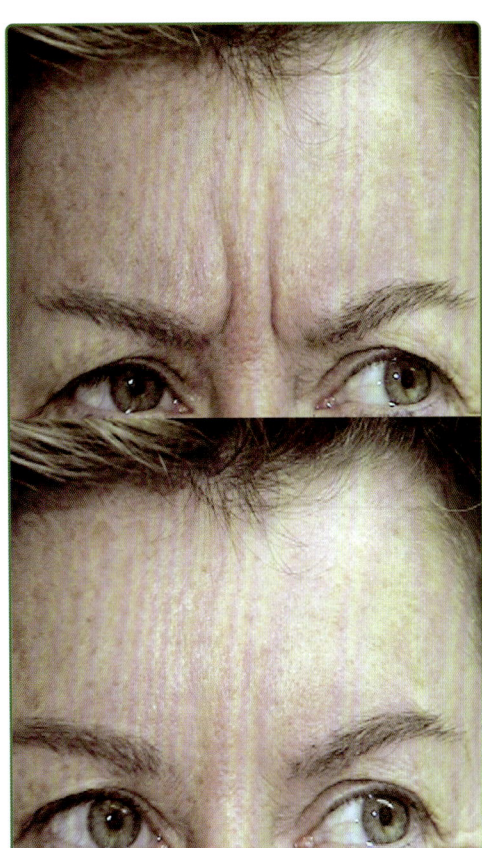

Figure 216-5 Before botulinum toxin treatment of the corrugator and procerus muscles (*upper panel*) and 1 week after treatment (*lower panel*).

the grip on the overlying skin and smoothing out the wrinkles. As previously mentioned, care must be taken to avoid injecting too low down onto the malar eminence, where diffusion may affect the zygomaticus major muscle and disrupt the symmetrical movement of the corner of the mouth in smiling.

The patient being treated for crow's feet should have good lower eyelid tarsal tone to avoid the appearance of senile ectropion from too much laxity of the lower eyelid. Pretreatment of the crow's feet area is very useful as an adjunctive technique before laser resurfacing. It prevents the problem of rhytides being readily re-formed by repeated squinting during the postoperative healing period, in which case the resurfacing may give rise to more noticeable lines than existed before the resurfacing.

COMBINATION THERAPY

As clinical experience accumulated with these commercial botulinum toxin products, experts in soft-tissue augmentation soon recognized that a synergy exists between soft-tissue fillers and neurotoxins.[5] Concomitant with the rise in the use of botulinum neurotoxin for cosmetic applications, the marketplace for soft-tissue augmentation expanded with the introduction of injectable hyaluronic acid gels (Chap. 215). These agents provided the first new directions in cosmetic therapy since the introduction of solubilized bovine collagen in the mid-1970s. The ability to control both muscles of expression and their secondary lines and folds, and to repair age-related volume changes in subcutaneous tissue has revolutionized minimally invasive cosmetic techniques.

Many patients have eagerly embraced simultaneous treatment with both fillers and botulinum toxin to achieve a natural look and forego more traditional incisional surgery.[6] As an example, patients frequently combine treatment of the upper third of the face (glabellar frown lines, horizontal forehead lines, and crow's feet) with volume restoration of the lower and middle face (lip enhancement, filling of nasolabial fold and marionette lines, chin and cheek augmentation) (Chap. 215).

HYPERHIDROSIS

Focal axillary hyperhidrosis is successfully treated with botulinum toxin by using Minor starch-iodine test to map out the extent of surface area in the axillary vault

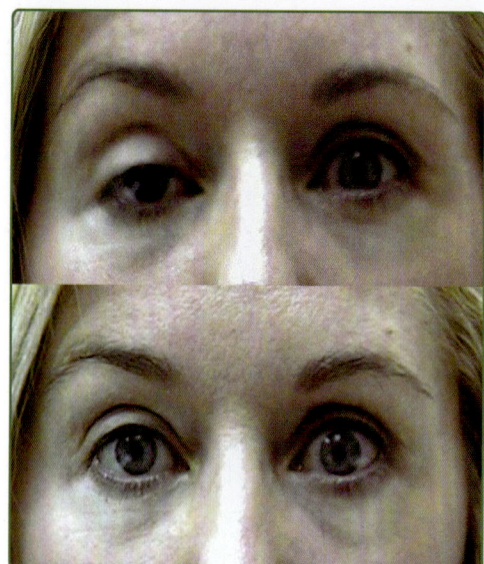

Figure 216-6 Patient who developed ptosis of the right upper eyelid due to diffusion of the botulinum toxin from the area above the midbrow down into the levator muscle of the upper eyelid. The lower photograph shows the patient approximately 1 minute after instillation of 2 drops of apraclonidine 0.5% ophthalmic solution into the right eye. Direct adrenergic stimulation of Müller muscle occurs, which lifts the lid temporarily. The drops may be administered every 4 hours as needed. The botulinum-induced ptosis resolves spontaneously, usually in 3 weeks or less.

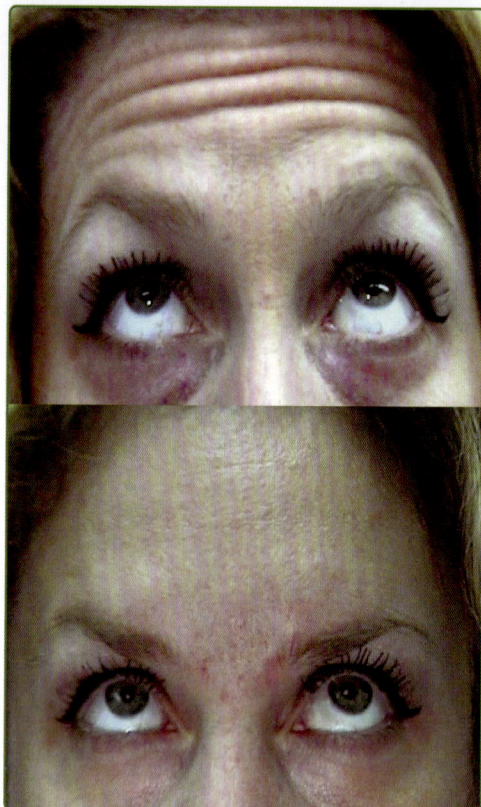

Figure 216-7 The upper half of the frontalis muscle is weakened by injecting 4 or 5 sites equidistantly along the equator of the forehead with a total of 16 to 20 units of Botox® or 30 to 50 units of Dysport®. Patient is shown before treatment (*upper panel*) and 1 week after treatment (*lower panel*).

that is affected. Anesthesia may be achieved with a eutectic mixture of local anesthetics but is usually not needed because of the relative insensitivity of the axillary skin. Doses of 2.5 to 4.0 units of Botox® are placed every 1 to 2 cm as intradermal injections in axillary skin. Reliable anhidrosis is produced within 72 hours and will last for 8 to 12 months with doses of 50 to 100 units of Botox® per axilla (Fig. 216-8). The duration of effect appears to be dose related, and doses of up to 200 units (Dysport®) per axilla have been reported to produce dryness for up to 29 months.[7] Aside from insignificant bruising from the needle trauma, there are no apparent side effects. Compensatory hyperhidrosis is not a clinically significant side effect, probably because of the relatively small surface area of the axillary vaults in contrast to the much larger surface areas affected by the surgical interruption of the nerves that occurs with endoscopic cervical sympathectomy, where compensatory hyperhidrosis is a real concern in up to a third of patients treated.

Palmar hyperhidrosis (Fig. 216-9) is more challenging to treat because of (1) the more limited diffusion of the toxin in palmar skin, (2) the pain on injection, and (3) the generally predictable incidence of temporary weakness in the hand. Anesthesia is achieved with regional wrist blocks of the median, ulnar, and radial nerves using lidocaine 1% to 2% without epinephrine. Approximately, 100 to 150 units of Botox® are needed to treat a single palm, divided into 50 to 60 intradermal injections of 2 to 3 units each. Onset of anhidrosis peaks in 5 to 7 days and is accompanied by minor weakness of the intrinsic muscles of the hand, which makes tasks requiring strength and stability (eg, pushing a button through a buttonhole) difficult to perform. The weakness usually subsides within 3 weeks, whereas the anhidrosis persists for several months. There is wider variation in response to palmar treatment than to axillary treatment, with anhidrosis lasting from 4 to 12 months, which probably reflects the technical difficulties in achieving even dispersion of the toxin through the palmar skin.

SIDE EFFECTS AND COMPLICATIONS

Minor needle trauma and bruising on injection with a 30-gauge needle are insignificant short-term complications of botulinum toxin injection, and use of a smaller-gauge needle (31 gauge or 32 gauge) will minimize needle trauma. Minor discomfort can be made more tolerable in some patients by pretreating the injection site areas with topical anesthetic and using sterile saline with preservative as a diluent, which greatly reduces the sensation of injection.

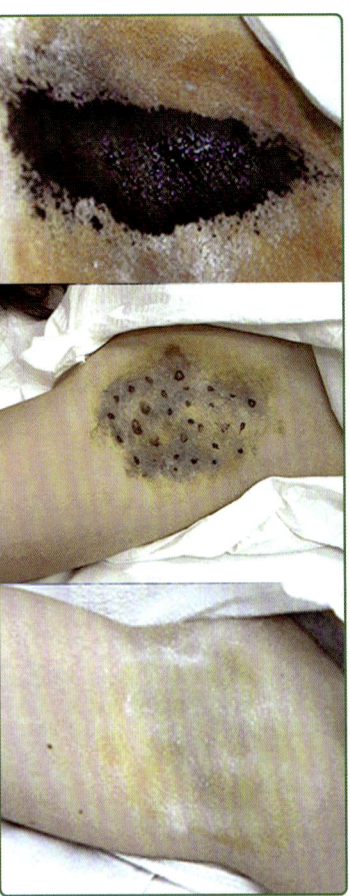

Figure 216-8 Minor starch-iodine test is used to demonstrate the area of axillary sweating (*top panel*). The pattern of intradermal botulinum toxin injections is shown with the starch-iodine material in place to highlight the injection points (*middle panel*). One week later, the treated axilla shows a negative result on the starch-iodine test (*bottom panel*).

The more problematic complications to consider are eyelid ptosis, which can occur after injections in the glabellar brow (see Fig. 216-6); brow ptosis from overzealous treatment of the frontalis muscle; transient lid edema from periocular injections; headaches after injections anywhere in the upper third of the face; and palmar weakness after injections for hyperhidrosis.

Antibody-mediated resistance appears to be an exceedingly rare event and of little clinical consequence in cosmetic dermatologic uses of botulinum toxin. Although millions of doses have been given as of this writing, there is no well-documented evidence of the development of immunologic resistance in patients treated with cosmetic doses. Resistance continues to be observed in patients treated for cervical dystonia, albeit at much lower rates than in the early years, probably because of the lower protein content of current formulations.

Eyelid ptosis is thought to be best avoided by carefully placing the midbrow injections at a minimal distance of 1 cm from the superior orbital rim, keeping the injection rate slow and gentle, and having the patient avoid prone positions and sleeping for 2 hours after injection.

Restricting injections to the upper two-thirds of the frontalis and reducing doses to the minimum necessary to produce the desired clinical effect may minimize brow ptosis. Unopposed muscle groups may trigger headaches as a rebound phenomenon after facial injections of botulinum toxin, but their etiology is unclear. Usually nonsteroidal anti-inflammatory agents are sufficient to treat them, unless the patient experiences migraines, in which case the patient's usual migraine medication will be required.

In hyperhidrosis, palmar weakness is a predictable consequence of injecting the palms. It is transient and dealt with by clear preinjection counseling. There is no similar effect of any clinical significance in either the axillae or the feet.

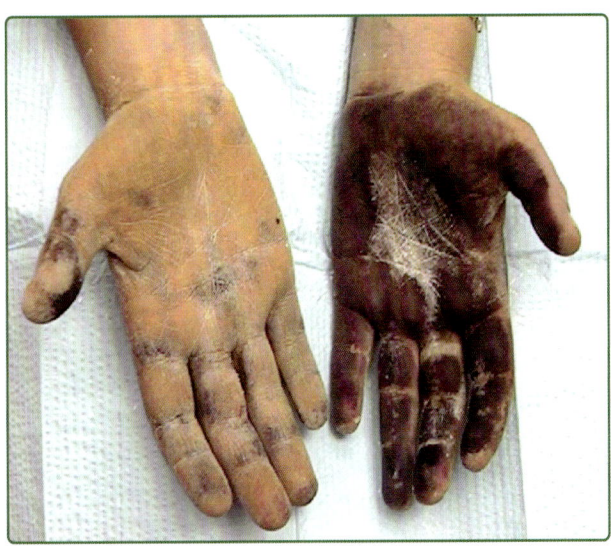

Figure 216-9 Hands showing response to Minor starch-iodine test. The left hand was not treated. The right hand received 100 units of intradermal Botox® 1 week before the photograph was taken.

COSMETIC USES "OFF-LABEL"

At the present time, the only FDA-approved indications for cosmetic botulinum toxin are the glabellar frown lines and the lateral canthal lines or crow's feet. But clinicians have described a variety of different anatomic locations that can benefit from carefully dosed botulinum toxin. These include the horizontal lines on the forehead (frontalis muscle),[8,9] the vertical rhytides of the upper lip (orbicularis),[10,11] the rhytides from nasalis muscles ("bunny lines"),[12] the melomental folds at the corners of the mouth (depressor anguli oris),[13,14] the deep mental crease on the chin and pebbly or peau d'orange chin (mentalis),[15] hypertrophy of the masseters (squared lower face),[16,17] and horizontal neck lines and bow-string bands of the neck (platysma).[18,19] The techniques and doses for these indications have been widely discussed, but few have been systematically studied.

SUMMARY

The development of botulinum toxin treatment has brought great creativity and capability to cosmetic dermatologic therapy. Further evolution will occur as new serotypes come to market and greater therapeutic synergies evolve as developers of soft-tissue augmentation systems strive to achieve similar effect and elegance. The high degree of efficacy and safety in the use of botulinum toxins in cosmetic dermatology has produced a great level of satisfaction in patients and physicians alike.

REFERENCES

1. Carruthers JD, Carruthers, JA. The evolution of botulinum neurotoxin type A for cosmetic applications. *J Cosmet Laser Ther*. 2007;9:186.
2. Aoki KR. Pharmacology and immunology of botulinum toxin serotypes. *J Neurol*. 2001;248(suppl 1):3-10.
3. Meunier FA, Lisk G, Sesardic D, et al. Dynamics of motor nerve terminal remodeling unveiled using SNARE-cleaving botulinum toxins: the extent and duration are dictated by the sites of SNAP-25 truncation. *Mol Cell Neurosci*. 2003;22(4):454-466.
4. Carruthers A, Carruthers J, Coleman WP 3rd, et al. Multicenter, randomized, phase III study of a single dose of incobotulinumtoxinA, free from complexing proteins, in the treatment of glabellar frown lines. *Dermatol Surg*. 2013;39(4):551-558.
5. Carruthers JD, Glogau RG, Blitzer A; Facial Aesthetics Consensus Group F. Advances in facial rejuvenation: botulinum toxin type a, hyaluronic acid dermal fillers, and combination therapies—Consensus recommendations. *Plast Reconstr Surg*. 2008;121(5)(suppl): 5S-30S; quiz 31S-36S.
6. Molina B, David M, Jain R, et al. Patient satisfaction and efficacy of full-facial rejuvenation using a combination of botulinum toxin type A and hyaluronic acid filler. *Dermatol Surg*. 2015;41(suppl 1):S325-S332.
7. Glogau RG. Hyperhidrosis and botulinum toxin A: patient selection and techniques. *Clin Dermatol*. 2004; 22(1):45-52.
8. Carruthers A, Carruthers J. Botulinum treatment of forehead wrinkles. *Plast Reconstr Surg*. 2006;117(4):1354; author reply 1355.
9. Steinsapir KD, Rootman D, Wulc A, et al. Cosmetic microdroplet botulinum toxin A forehead lift: a new treatment paradigm. *Ophthal Plast Reconstr Surg*. 2015; 31(4):263-268.
10. Barton FE Jr, Carruthers J, Coleman S, et al. The role of toxins and fillers in perioral rejuvenation. *Aesthet Surg J*. 2007;27(6):632-640.
11. Semchyshyn N, Sengelmann RD. Botulinum toxin A treatment of perioral rhytides. *Dermatol Surg*. 2003; 29(5):490-495; discussion 495.
12. Tamura BM, Odo MY, Chang B, et al. Treatment of nasal wrinkles with botulinum toxin. *Dermatol Surg*. 2005; 31(3):271-275.
13. Braz AV, Louvain D, Mukamal LV. Combined treatment with botulinum toxin and hyaluronic acid to correct unsightly lateral-chin depression. *An Bras Dermatol*. 2013;88(1):138-140.
14. Choi YJ, Kim JS, Gil YC, et al. Anatomical considerations regarding the location and boundary of the depressor anguli oris muscle with reference to botulinum toxin injection. *Plast Reconstr Surg*. 2014;134(5):917-921.
15. Papel ID, Capone RB. Botulinum toxin A for mentalis muscle dysfunction. *Arch Facial Plast Surg*. 2001; 3(4):268-269.
16. Ahn J, Horn C, Blitzer A. Botulinum toxin for masseter reduction in Asian patients. *Arch Facial Plast Surg*. 2004; 6(3):188-191.
17. Chang CS, Kang GC. Achieving ideal lower face aesthetic contours: combination of tridimensional fat grafting to the chin with masseter botulinum toxin injection. *Aesthet Surg J*. 2016;36(10):1093-1100.
18. Brandt FS, Boker A. Botulinum toxin for the treatment of neck lines and neck bands. *Dermatol Clin*. 2004; 22(2):159-166.
19. Kane MA. Nonsurgical treatment of platysma bands with injection of botulinum toxin a revisited. *Plast Reconstr Surg*. 2003;112(5)(suppl):125S-126S.

Chapter 217 :: Hair Transplantation
:: Robin H. Unger & Walter P. Unger

第二百一十七章

毛发移植

中文导读

　　本章分为13节：①背景；②选择适合毛发移植的病人；③风险和预防措施；④病人体位；⑤设计毛发受体区；⑥决定毛发供体区；⑦切除毛发供体区；⑧移植物的处理；⑨受体区准备；⑩移植物植入；⑪修复手术；⑫毛发移植手术副作用和并发症；⑬脱发区切除术。

　　第一节提到大多数接受毛发移植的患者多是雄激素性脱发病人，包括男性型脱发（MPB）和女性型脱发（FPHL）。男性脱发的汉密尔顿-诺伍德分型（HAMILTON-NORWOOD型）见图217-1、图217-2，女性脱发的路德维希型（LUDWIG型）见图217-3。并列出各年龄和65岁以上MPB汉密尔顿-诺伍德各型发病率，分别见表217-1和表217-2，指出男性中老年发病率较高。接着作者提出MPB毛发移植应由四个区域组成：前额区域、头皮中部区域、顶点区域及邻近上述三个主要区域的脱发区。通常，每次移植治疗三个主要区域中的一个，加上相邻的脱发区。

　　第二节中提到病人选择。首先要排除暂时脱发或药物引起脱发的患者，接下来评估毛发受体和供体部位的情况，然后是对毛发特征进行评估（表217-3列出了理想毛发移植的情况），关于性别、年龄及脱发阶段，作者认为没有严格的限制。

　　第三节风险和预防措施：不仅需要完备的仪器（表217-4），还需要排除病人其他疾病，尤其是病人的凝血功能，这些都与治疗风险相关。

　　第四节提到病人体位：一般为仰卧位。

　　第五节提到设计毛发受体区，应在术前勾勒出目标移植区，并对MPB毛发移植的前额区域、头皮中部区域、顶点区域的要点分别进行讲述。

　　第六节提到决定毛发供体区。这是非常关键的一步，作者提出对于第一次手术，通常选择边缘发质最稠密区域的中部作为供体区域，男性供体区域为颞区，而女性供体区域为耳后，可通过湿润头发和头发密度器进行头发密度判断，并提到减少供体区手术瘢痕的方法。

　　第七节提到切除毛发供体区。作者指出带状切除和以毛囊为单位进行切除（FUE）是目前主要使用的两种方法，并分别讲述了这两种方法。

　　带状切除可以一次采集大量毛发，仍然是最常用的毛发移植方法。此治疗一般需镇静剂及局部麻醉，接下来是收集供体区毛发，一般根据头皮松弛度来确定合适的宽度，通常宽度是8~15 mm，作者还讲述了手术刀的切除方向、角度、终止切割的部位及供体区缝合的技术，并且指出不同次数的手术中，其切割深度是不同的，一般后一次手术切割更深，还提到了如何减少瘢痕形成的方法。

　　以毛囊为单位进行切除（FUE）的优点是产生的瘢痕为点状，比带状切除的线状瘢痕更小更窄，但FUE也有不足之处：当脱发较为严重时，毛发供体区可能超出"安全供体区（SDA）"。因此可能导致移植后的毛发不是永久性的，且从SDA以外获取毛发可能导致此处出现虫蚀样外观。接着作者还提到FUE过程中毛囊单位（FU）可能出现的横断现象。于是作者提出了带状切除和以毛囊为单位进行切除（FUE）的联合治疗方法来进一步减少不良反应增加疗效。最后，作者认为从头皮以外的部位，如胡须、胸部进行FUE也是值得考虑的。

第八节提到移植物的处理，带状切除后的移植物条带需切割细分为单个FU，或几个FU组成的"FU家族"，并让离体移植物保持低温，而供体组织需始终保持湿润。而FUE得到的即为单个FU，此时涉及受损FU的去除。最后作者指出必须确保移植物保持湿润和冷却，以保持其生存能力。

第九节指出受体区准备。需用皮下针头或小刀片切割受体区，用以匹配移植物的大小，以及术中需要的麻醉、止血药物、手术刀的切割方向和角度都是重要因素。随后，作者强调受体区处于合适的压力是较为合适的，当密度过高外观不自然甚至此处毛发存活率会出现下降，切口、压力太大毛发存活率也会下降。

第十节指出移植物获取后需要医生判断不同FU应该放置的位置，植入的方向和角度，植入前、植入时需要使用的药物及植入成功与否的判断。作者还提出了一种可以减少毛发创伤的植发器，未来有很大的应用前景。

第十一节提出修复手术。如果毛囊太粗太多或不恰当的植入，则需要修复手术治疗，如用切除较大FU、瘢痕切除术等进行改善。

第十二节介绍毛发移植手术的副作用和并发症。作者先把潜在副作用和并发症列于表217-8，再详细阐述了水肿、感染、出血、供体区瘢痕、植入后植入物密度低、术后恶臭等各自产生的原因及处理方法。

第十三节提到脱发区切除术是较少使用的治疗手段。目前，该技术被用于修复效果欠佳的毛发移植术，切除瘢痕性脱发区域或发际线。

〔简　丹〕

AT-A-GLANCE

- Most patients undergoing surgical procedures for hair loss have either male pattern baldness (MPB) or female pattern hair loss (FPHL).
- Surgical techniques used to treat hair loss include hair transplantation, alopecia reduction, and transposition flaps. The latter 2 techniques are rarely used currently.
- Follicular units (FUs) are the building blocks of modern hair transplantation (follicular unit transplanting [FUT]).
- The 2 main methods of donor harvest are strip harvesting and follicular unit excision (FUE). The latter may be achieved using a variety of techniques and devices.
- Minoxidil or finasteride may arrest or partially reverse MPB and FPHL, so a trial of treatment is often appropriate prior to surgery, or concurrent with surgery.
- Additional innovations of potential benefit include bio-enhanced storage solutions and platelet-rich plasma (PRP)

BACKGROUND

Hamilton and Norwood described the degrees of severity of male pattern baldness (MPB) from a mild Type I to a severe Type VII[1-3] (Fig. 217-1). Fortunately, a large majority of male patients do not progress past Types VI: Norwood found that at age 79 only 11% of men have Type VII MPB (Table 217-1), and Unger found that among 328 men older than 65 only 13.7% have Type VII MPB[4] (Table 217-2). Thus, if one treats all or most patients as if they will develop Type VI MPB, one is being reasonably cautious. Exceptions are individuals with earlier than usual onset of significant degrees of MPB or Diffuse Unpatterned Alopecia especially if there is a family history of Type VII MPB, in which case it is wiser to plan on an evolution to Type VII MPB.

Ludwig described 3 degrees of female pattern hair loss (FPHL),[5] whereas Olsen developed a distinct classification system based on her observation of a "Christmas-tree" pattern of hair loss[6] (Fig. 217-3). According to Hamilton's study, 79% of postpubertal females develop at least a mild Hamilton/Norwood pattern of hair loss.[2] Most female patients do not have a sufficiently large and/or high-density donor area to surgically treat all of the eventually affected alopecic

The Hamilton-Norwood classification of MPB

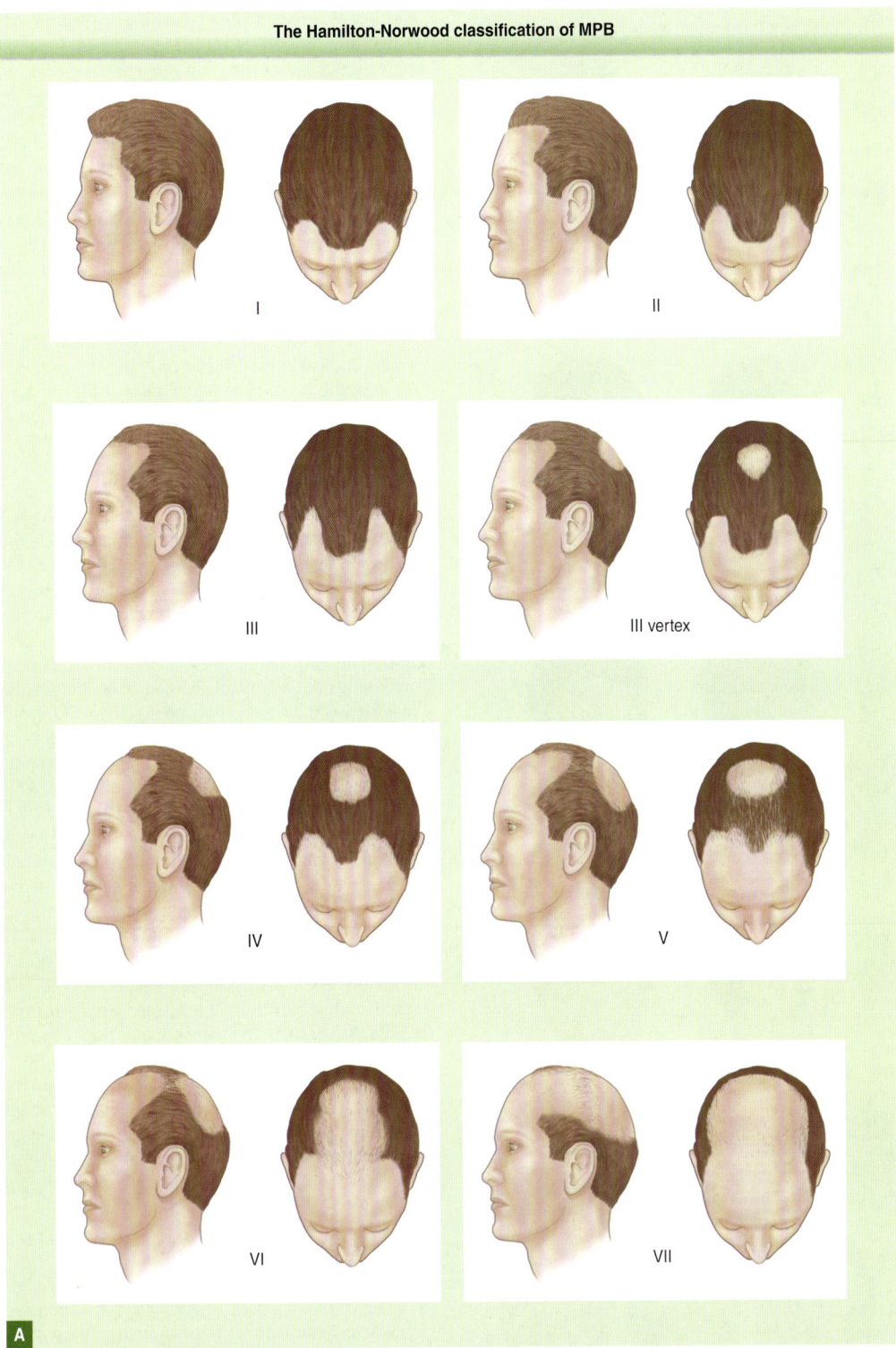

Figure 217-1 A, The Hamilton-Norwood classification of MPB. **B,** The Norwood classification for Type A variant MPB. **C,** Ludwig pattern of hair loss in females.

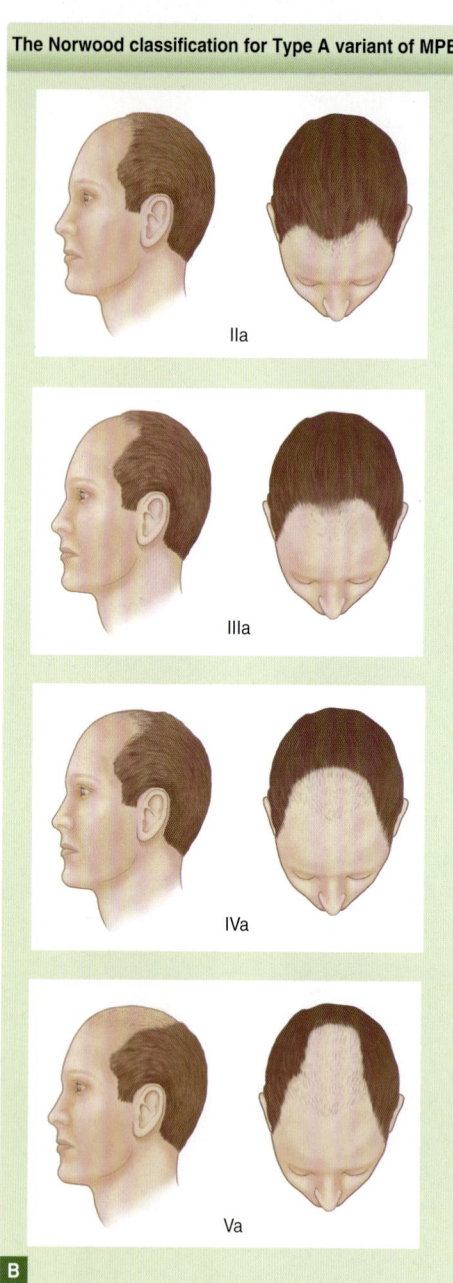
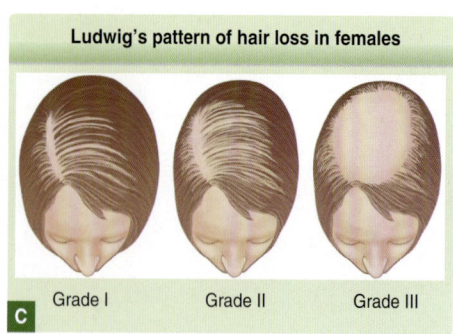

Figure 217-1 (continued)

areas. For this reason, some practitioners believe that women are "rarely" candidates for hair restoration surgery (HRS)—a view promulgated by the media and therefore shared by the general public! However, in the authors' experience, and in a survey of experts, the opposite appears to be the case.[7] A less than optimal donor/recipient ratio does not preclude surgery but does require a treatment plan that focuses on cosmetically strategic areas. In women, this most often corresponds to the frontal area and the part-line, which is usually a 5-mm-wide anteroposterior corridor (Fig. 217-2). The thickened hair in these areas can then be styled in a way that camouflages untreated areas. When this is done, the cosmetic improvement is significant, and patient satisfaction is high.[8]

In men, the transplantation of areas of MPB should be conceptualized as consisting of 4 areas: (1) a frontal area extending from the proposed hairline to a coronal line drawn perpendicularly between the tragus of each ear; (2) a midscalp area extending from the posterior border of the frontal area to a point where the caudal scalp changes its orientation from parallel to the ground to more or less vertical; (3) a vertex area that consists of the remainder of the alopecic regions; and finally (4) evolving areas of alopecia adjacent to the aforementioned 3 major areas, which on close inspection contain hair that appears likely to be temporary. Commonly, each transplant session treats one of the 3 major areas, plus adjacent evolving areas. Occasionally, the treatment of evolving areas of hair loss is deferred to a later session to transplant a larger proportion of already existing more obvious areas of hair loss. In such cases, sufficient numbers of grafts must be left in reserve to permit the future treatment of these areas, unless an "isolated frontal forelock" is the ultimate goal.

In Unger's study of 328 males older than 65 years, he delineated an area within the zone of rim hair that contained 8 or more hairs per 4-mm circle.[4] He referred to this as the "safe" donor area; later to the "safest" donor area (SDA). For most patients, the equivalent of 3 to 5 strips, each of which is 10 mm, can be excised from the SDA during their lifetime. Each of those strips produces 1500 to 2750 follicular units (FUs) (Fig. 217-3), depending on the density of the donor hair. Current methods of follicular unit excision (FUE) allow slight expansion upon Unger SDA, although *not* as extensively as some practitioners are claiming.

PATIENT SELECTION

During the initial consultation, surgeons must clarify whether the hair loss is temporary or responsive to medical treatment. Dermoscopy may be a very useful method to evaluate the underlying etiology of hair loss.[9] A comprehensive discussion of this subject is available elsewhere in this textbook. Provided this is not the case, the first step in the surgical evaluation of a patient is to assess the current and anticipated future size of the donor and recipient areas. An accurate assessment of the donor/recipient ratio depends

TABLE 217-1
Hamilton Study of Incidence of MPB (Norwood-Hamilton Scale) by Age

	AGE (y)						
	18–29	30–39	40–49	50–59	60–69	70–79	≥80
Type I	110 (60%)	60 (36%)	55 (33%)	45 (28%)	29 (19%)	18 (17%)	12 (16%)
Type II	52 (28%)	43 (26%)	38 (22%)	32 (20%)	24 (16%)	20 (19%)	11 (14%)
Type III	14 (6%)	30 (18%) (3V)[a]	37 (20%) (15V)[a]	34 (23%) (15V)[a]	22 (15%) (10V)[a]	16 (16%) (7V)[a]	12 (16%) (8V)[a]
Type IV	4 (3%)	16 (10%)	15 (10%)	21 (9%)	17 (12%)	13 (13%)	9 (12%)
Type V	3 (2%)	10 (6%)	13 (8%)	15 (10%)	22 (15%)	13 (13%)	9 (12%)
Type VI	2 (1%)	4 (3%)	7 (4%)	10 (7%)	19 (13%)	11 (11%)	10 (13%)
Type VII	0	2 (1%)	5 (3%)	4 (3%)	16 (10%)	11 (11%)	14 (17%)
Total	185 (100%)	165 (100%)	165 (100%)	156 (100%)	149 (100%)	102 (100%)	77 (100%)

[a]Numbers in parentheses under Type III represent Type III Vertex individuals.

on professional experience, the family history of patterned hair loss, and most importantly the patient's age. The second step is to evaluate hair characteristics. Table 217-3 lists the hair characteristics of the best hair transplant candidates. Not all of these characteristics are necessary for a satisfactory result, but each one improves the final cosmetic appearance.

The authors do not follow any strict rules on patient selection with respect to the stage of hair loss, age, or gender. For example, in regard to the stage of hair loss, it is important to note that the recipient area does not need to be completely alopecic to successfully operate. In fact, there are important advantages to transplanting at an earlier stage of MPB, although treating such areas demands a high degree of skill. Many surgeons have resorted to shaving the recipient areas for ease of surgery; the authors do not find this necessary and it certainly helps patients to seamlessly resume regular life shortly after surgery. Similarly, there are no definite age requirements, although younger patients, especially those under the age of 25, should have more conservative treatment plans. As part of this planning, such patients are encouraged to use medical treatment to delay or partially reverse the progression of MPB. In addition, surgeons should leave enough hair in the SDA to permit at least 1 future surgery in the event of unexpected areas of hair loss.

With respect to gender, it is worth mentioning again that women are more often than generally thought acceptable candidates for hair restoration surgery, despite the strong disagreement of a few surgeons. In an effort to discern the consensus opinion, the authors informally polled a group of leading experts in the field. From among this group, a majority (13 of 22) felt that more than 50% of women had enough donor hair to permit *at least* 1 transplant. In the authors' opinion, the percentage is even higher provided that the patient's expectations are commensurate with what is

TABLE 217-2
Unger Study of Incidence of MPB (Norwood-Hamilton Scale) in Men Older Than 65

	AGE (years)			
TYPE	65–69	70–74	75–79	80+
I	2 (3.6%)	5 (6.2%)	4 (5.5%)	2 (1.7%)
II	9 (16.4%)	7 (8.6%)	7 (9.6%)	12 (10.1%)
III	4 (7.3%)	15 (18.5%)	18 (24.7%)	11 (9.2%)
IV	10 (18.2%)	16 (19.8%)	8 (11.0%)	10 (8.4%)
V	6 (10.9%)	7 (8.6%)	10 (13.7%)	16 (13.4%)
VI	13 (23.6%)	19 (23.5%)	16 (21.9%)	37 (31.1%)
VII	11 (20.0%)	12 (14.8%)	10 (13.7%)	31 (26.1%)
Total	55 (100%)	81 (100%)	73 (100%)	119 (100%)

Note:
- In age group 65–69, if one excludes Type I and II, 33 of the remaining 44 (75%) have Types III–VI (83.3% Norwood);
- In age group 70–74, if one excludes Type I and II, 57 of the remaining 69 (82.6%) have Types III–VI (82.8% Norwood);
- In age group 75–79, if one excludes Type I and II, 52 of the remaining 62 (83.9%) have Types III–VI;
- In age group 80+, if one excludes Type I and II, 74 of the remaining 105 (70.5%) have Types III–VI (74.0% Norwood).

TABLE 217-3
Ideal Hair Characteristics

- High-density hair in the safe donor area
- A mixture of fine and coarse hair
- Minimal contrast between the skin and the hair color
- Wave or curl

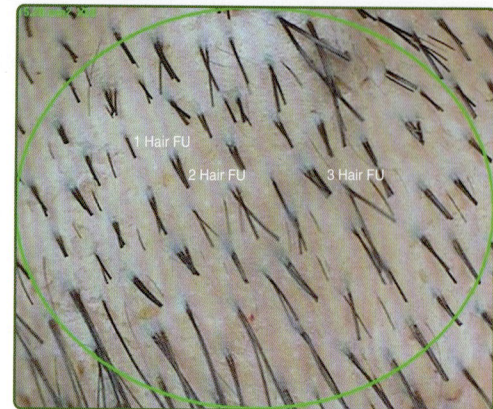

Figure 217-3 A relatively small number of single hairs emerge from the scalp. Most often, hairs grow in small groupings of 2 to 5, as shown in the above photo. These groupings are referred to as *follicular units*.

realistically possible given their anticipated eventual donor/recipient ratio and hair characteristics. A strategically planned surgery, with a focus on transplanting the frontal zone and part-line, usually produces a cosmetically significant improvement, and typically leaves female patients very satisfied.[10]

Although hair transplantation surgery is predominantly used to treat patients with MPB or FPHL, it also can be used to correct surgical scars, (Fig. 217-4), treat congenital areas of hair loss such as temporal triangular alopecia, and change hairlines. With appropriate care, it has also successfully improved areas of cicatricial alopecia such as end-stage central centrifugal cicatricial alopecia or areas of alopecia resultant from radiation therapy. Although predominantly used for the scalp, hair transplantation also can be performed on other sites such as the eyebrows and beard area in select cases.

RISKS AND PRECAUTIONS

Before proceeding with surgery, the patient's physician is contacted to discuss any areas of major medical concern. Basic instruments and supplies needed for surgery are listed in Table 217-4. For safety, the operating room should be equipped with the medications and equipment needed for basic monitoring and advanced life support. Although rarely necessary, the authors prefer operating with an anesthetist or anesthesiologist when patients have significant underlying health risks, including serious cardiovascular conditions, certain respiratory problems, and seizure disorders. Table 217-5 presents a list of significant (but rare) potential intraoperative complications.

Whenever possible, the patient should also be free of all medications that may negatively influence bleeding or healing properties. This includes blood thinners such as acetyl salicylic acid, nonsteroidal anti-inflammatory medications, and natural supplements that may create bleeding problems such as garlic, and Ginkgo biloba. Patients are also encouraged to stop alcohol consumption 10 days before surgery as this may prolong bleeding time.

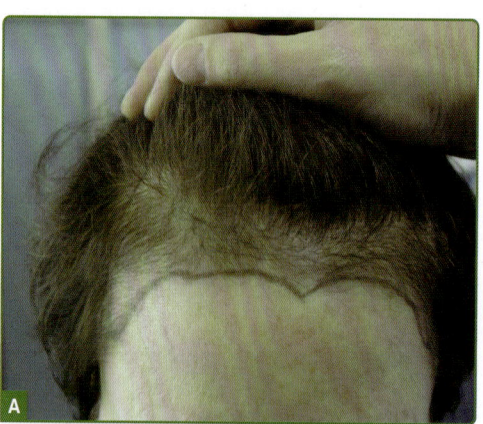

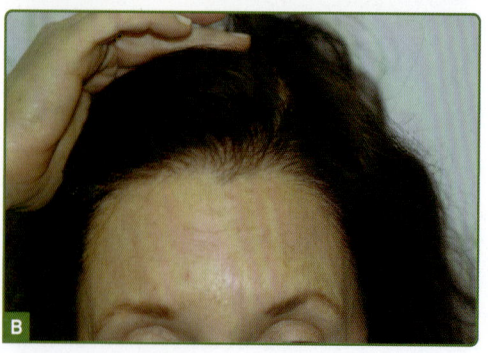

Figure 217-2 A, A 54-year-old female patient with significant hair loss in the hairline and temple regions. **B,** The same patient 2½ years after a session of 1248 FUs and 264 DFUs. The frontal view shows the effect that can be achieved for the overall appearance.

PATIENT POSITIONING

When removing the donor strip, the authors' patients are placed in a prone position, with their head in a "doughnut" ("prone") pillow that allows them to breathe comfortably. During the creation of the recipient sites and the insertion of the grafts, patients remain in a semisupine position except when working on the inferior portion of the vertex, in which case a prone position facilitates the work of both the surgeon and technicians.

RECIPIENT AREA DESIGN[11]

On the morning of the surgery, a grease pencil is used to outline the treatment area. The frontal recipi-

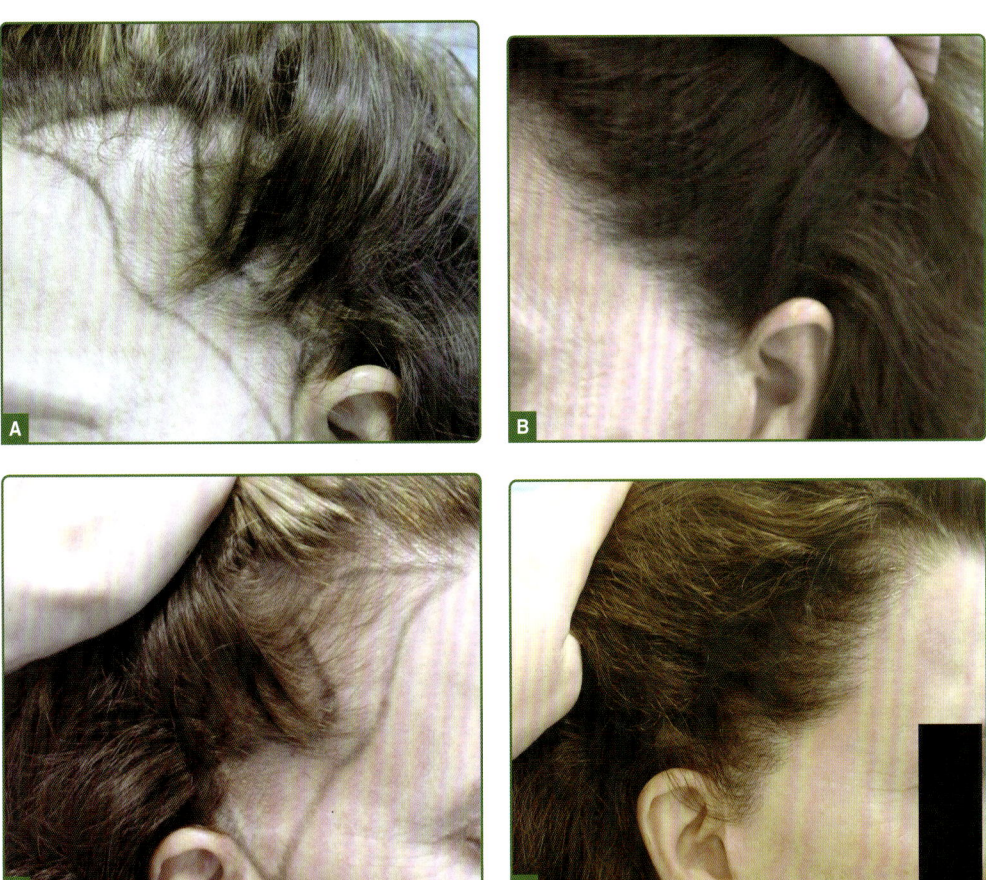

Figure 217-4 Transplanting hair to alopecic areas after a facelift procedure showing before (**A** and **C**) and after (**B** and **D**) photos.

ent area is designed by drawing the proposed hairline. The midline, anteriormost point of the hairline should be as superior as acceptable to the patient, but nearly always lies within the area in which the vertical forehead changes into the essentially horizontal caudal scalp.

The lateral borders are determined by outlining the supratemporal "humps"—semihemispheric areas containing only temporary hair and that are in the superior temporal areas (with the exception of those with existing Type VII MPB). Some of this area may or may not have initially persisting original hair but, regardless, should sooner (or later) usually be transplanted. The lateral ends of the proposed hairline are then joined to the supratemporal humps with a slight flare, to produce a rounded corner that creates a natural shape, but that usually leaves patients with a mature-looking hairline that includes frontotemporal recessions. In some patients, the anterior border of temporal hair is significantly receded, and it may need to be re-created at the same time as the anterior supratemporal humps are being transplanted. The posterior border of the frontal area is completed with an arc that helps create a natural pattern of hair loss in the event that the patient decides not to transplant any further posteriorly, or does not have sufficient donor hair to do so. When transplanting the midscalp, the posterior aspects of the supratemporal humps are included, and the posterior border of the transplant is similarly finished in an arc. For the vertex area, either the entire region or its anticipated eventual periphery can be transplanted, depending on the available donor supply and patient goals.

For less experienced surgeons, it may be useful to consider using a premade grid template with 1-cm^2 boxes to estimate the surface area of the target treatment area and use this to determine the number of grafts necessary to cover the proposed treatment area. This will also help the surgeon determine the ideal, achievable graft density.

DONOR AREA DETERMINATION

Choosing the optimal location and width of the donor strip is one of the most important decisions

TABLE 217-4
Instruments and Supplies Needed in Hair Transplantation

INSTRUMENTS AND SUPPLIES	STRIP HARVESTING	FUE
Preoperative Surgical Planning and Setup		
▪ Aluminum rat tail comb	✓	✓
▪ Curved Metzenbaum scissors	✓	✓
▪ China marker grease pencil	✓	✓
▪ Prone pillow	✓	✓
Anaesthesia		
▪ Syringes (various sizes)	✓	✓
▪ Short-acting local anaesthesia (eg, lidocaine)	✓	✓
▪ Long-acting local anaesthesia (eg, bupivacaine)	✓	✓
▪ Epinephrine (1 in 100,000 dilution)	✓	✓
Harvesting Follicular Units		
▪ Double-bladed cutting knife handle	✓	
▪ No. 10 scalpel blade	✓	
▪ No. 15 scalpel blade	✓	
▪ Small curved surgical scissors	✓	
▪ Small straight Iris scissors	✓	
▪ Hyfrecator	✓	
▪ Smoke evacuation system	✓	
▪ Needle driver	✓	
▪ Suture material	✓	
▪ Toothed curved forceps	✓	
▪ Straight Adson forceps	✓	
▪ Stainless steel bowls	✓	✓
▪ FUE extraction devices (eg, manual punch, motorized device, robotic system)		✓
▪ Aid to Extraction instrument for FUE		✓
Processing and Storage of Follicular Units		
▪ Stereoscopic microscope with under-lighting	✓	✓
▪ Clear plastic cutting boards	✓	✓
▪ Double-sided razor blades	✓	✓
▪ Razor blade holder	✓	✓
▪ Divided Petri dishes	✓	✓
▪ Holding solution (eg, hypothermasol)	✓	✓
▪ Electric chilling device or ice packs	✓	✓
Recipient Site Creation		
▪ Hypodermic needles (18G, 19G, and 20G)	✓	✓
▪ Cut to size blades	✓	✓
Graft Insertion		
▪ No. 5 planting jeweler's forceps	✓	✓
▪ No. 2 jeweler's forceps	✓	✓
▪ Ring graft storage	✓	✓
▪ Implanters (used either as sharp implanter or for loading into premade sites)	✓	✓
▪ Magnifying loupes	✓	✓
Other Consumables		
▪ Gauze	✓	✓
▪ Telfa pads	✓	✓
▪ Kerlix dressing	✓	✓
▪ Povidone-iodine solution	✓	✓
▪ Hydrogen peroxide solution	✓	✓

TABLE 217-5
Major Intraoperative Risks

- Lidocaine toxicity
- Respiratory depression secondary to sedatives or narcotics
- Excessive intraoperative bleeding

made during hair transplanting. For the first surgery, the authors typically choose a donor area that lies in the middle of the densest zone of the fringe hair, and extends into the temporal region in males, but ends posterior to the ears in females. This location is the most logical, because hair is progressively lost from the superior and inferior borders of the fringe hair in MPB, and hence this position provides the greatest degree of likelihood that transplanted hair is permanent. Each subsequent harvest includes any scar from prior session(s), as well as donor hair immediately superior and inferior to it. This results in the presence of only 1 scar, regardless of the number of sessions carried out (Fig. 217-5). To determine the location of the densest zone, it is sometimes helpful to wet the hair to determine the superior and inferior margins of current areas that are already thinning somewhat. Another useful adjunct that can be employed is a hand-held densitometer. This allows the practitioner to more objectively quantify the patient's donor density and estimate the total number of grafts that can be safely obtained from the donor area and help in the surgical planning. Once the donor area is identified, hair in a 10- to 18-mm-wide zone is clipped to approximately 2-mm length and cleansed with alcohol- and typically an iodine-based antiseptic. FUE harvest may be taken from a slightly expanded SDA, but the surgeon still needs to be wary of going too far outside of it. Subsequent harvests will result in the small punctuate scars becoming more numerous and closer together; thus, the surgeon needs to be particularly careful with choosing extraction sites location and density during the first and any subsequent harvesting in the same areas. To limit this problem, some FUE surgeons recommend "splitting individual multi-hair FU in vivo" with the punch being utilized; this technique has not yet been shown to produce good hair survival in both the recipient and donor areas.

DONOR SITE EXCISION[12]

Strip harvesting and follicular unit excision are currently the 2 main methods being used by hair restoration surgeons for the purpose of donor harvest (Fig. 217-6). In recent years, there has been a rising tide of hair restoration surgeons who are promoting the "superiority" and benefits of FUE. FUE in our opinion, however, remains optimally indicated in only a select group of patients, whereas strip harvesting remains a method that still has significant and more long-term proven benefits. In particular, the frequent promotion of FUE as "minimal incision surgery" is completely unwarranted (Table 217-6). Notwithstanding the preceding, it is the authors' opinion that all good hair restoration practices should include surgeons skilled in both techniques, and be able to offer both option to patients, after taking into account patient long-term donor/recipient area ratios, hair characteristics, and lifestyle.

STRIP HARVESTING

Strip harvesting (also called the unified tissue harvest technique) is the most commonly employed method by the majority of hair restoration surgeons for donor harvest. This has been the mainstay for donor harvesting following the old punch graft harvesting methods, and has allowed large numbers of grafts to be taken from the densest region of the "safest donor area" while retaining a single linear scar that is typically unnoticeable when carried out by good hair restoration surgeons.

ANESTHESIA

Oral sedatives (eg, diazepam and lorazepam) are given to the patient approximately half an hour prior to commencing the surgery. In some patients who may have additional anxiety and have difficulty tolerating a prolonged procedure, an anesthetist or anesthesiologist can be employed to facilitate surgery with conscious sedation.

Once the donor area is identified and clipped, the surgeon proceeds with administering local anesthesia, usually 1% or 2% lidocaine with 1 in 100,000 epinephrine along the inferior and lateral edges of the clipped donor area. Subsequently, longer-acting anesthesia such as bupivacaine is administered before the initial lidocaine becomes ineffective.

STRIP REMOVAL

Effectiveness of the anesthetic block is verified directly prior to strip harvesting. Scalp laxity is clinically assessed to determine the appropriate width of the donor strip, which in the authors' practice is typically 8 to 15 mm wide and is usually wider in the middle section and narrower toward the temporal regions. A prudent decision is to take a *slightly* narrower strip than the examination suggests is possible, thus permitting a margin of error that will minimize the possibility of a high-tension donor closure, and hence production of a wider than optimal scar.

Immediately prior to donor tissue excision, the donor area is tumesced with 10 to 40 mL of normal saline. This increases tissue turgor, thereby minimizing bleeding, but also limiting distortion of the follicle that might otherwise result in FU transection. The authors typically use a single-blade scalpel to cut donor tissue parallel to the exit angle of the hair. Occasionally, if the follicles are particularly long, the superficial epidermis is scored and blunt dissection may be used to increase the depth of incision. The incision begins and ends approximately 2 cm lateral to the ends of the clipped donor area. To reduce the likelihood of "dog ears" forming, the 2 ends are tapered to a 30° angle using a No. 15 scalpel. The depth of the incision can vary significantly. In the first surgery, the blades are placed in high subcutaneous fat, to minimize underlying neurovascular damage. In subsequent surgeries, where fibrous scar tissue has formed deep to the original donor site, the depth of

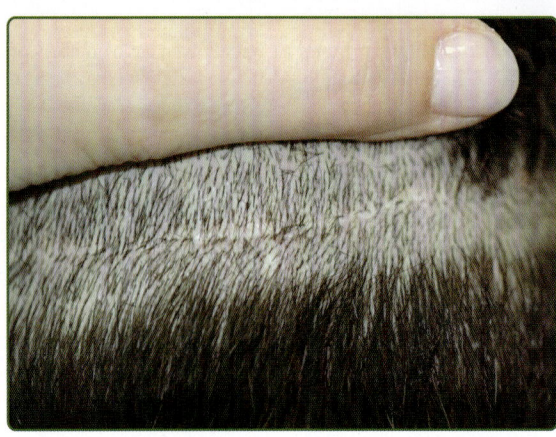

Figure 217-5 The hair was clipped short in the donor area before the surgery. The narrow scar that can be seen in this photo is the only scar he is going to have as we typically excise any scar from a prior surgery as part of the subsequent donor strips. Scars are usually 0.2 to 1.5 mm wide regardless of the number of strips that have been excised. We believe that this is mainly because we nearly always try to choose strip widths that create wounds that that will close with what we call "minus 1" (-1) to minus 2 (-2) tension, that is, we believe we could have taken a strip that was 1.0 to 2.0 mm wider than what was actually excised.

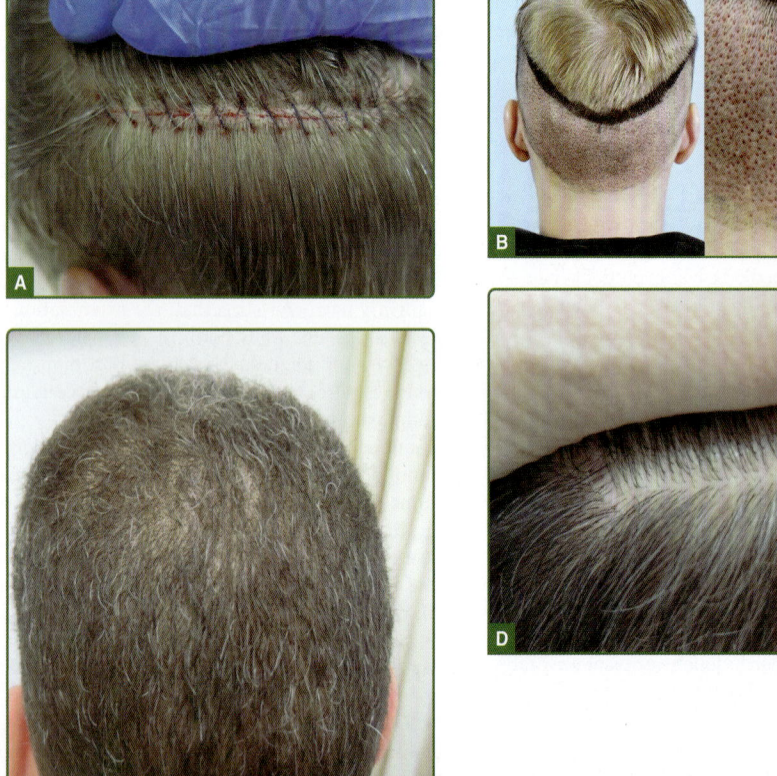

Figure 217-6 FUE. **A,** The donor area is shown after suturing. **B,** The donor area shows the sites of extraction during FUE. **C,** At 6 months after surgery, the scars are not visible and the overall appearance of the donor is not different from before the FUE. **D,** Fully healed donor strip.

TABLE 217-6
FUE "Minimal Incision Surgery"?

	DONOR AREA	
	FUE punch (2000 0.9 mm diameter)	STRIP (24-cm strip length)
Total incision length	2πr × 2000 sites 2000 (0.9 mm) diameter (2 × 3.14 × 0.45) × 2000 = 565.2 cm	24 cm × 2 (sides) = 48 cm
Area of scar	πr² × 2000 (3.14) (0.45²) × 2000 = 12.72 cm²	24 cm × 0.1 cm (at most) = 2.4 cm²

Typical strip harvesting produces a far smaller total incision length and total area of scar than does typical FUE when a 1 mm diameter punch is used for the latter. (If a 0.9-mm punch or 0.8-mm punch was used, the total incision lengths and area of scars would be, respectively, 565.2 cm and 12.71 cm² for the 0.9-mm punch and 502.4 cm and 10.048 cm² for the 0.8-mm punch). Yet FUE is often promoted as "minimal incision surgery"?!!

the incision may be increased to permit its removal. This is important because scar tissue is avascular, space occupying, and tethers the edges of the wound, thereby increasing donor closing tension and interfering with wound healing. At the same time, care is observed to prevent the creation of a depression in the tissue.

Importantly, the entire strip is removed in 3 sections, each sutured before reassessing scalp laxity in the remaining unharvested section(s). This provides greater control of bleeding and a more accurate guide to the optimal width of the next section of the strip to be excised. Vessels with exuberant bleeding are cauterized using a unipolar hyfrecator. The wound sections are closed either with a single-layer running suture or with a bi-layered closure. The bi-layered closure is typically employed if the authors feel that there is greater than optimal closing tension or if there is hyperlaxity in the scalp. In practice, the authors use an absorbable No. 3.0 PDS II suture for their subcutaneous interrupted sutures, and a No. 2.0 to 4.0 Prolene or Supramid for the superficial closing suture. Other surgeons sometimes close the donor site with staples, but at this point, the authors prefer sutures for greater precision in wound edge approximation, and a more comfortable postoperative patient experience.

Occasionally, the authors will employ a "trichophytic closure" to minimize scar visibility in individuals who have previously (and rarely) healed with a wider than usual scar or in patients who wear their hair very short and who have a strong contrast in the color of their skin and hair. In such instances, a very thin slice of the epidermis (<1 mm from the edge) on the inferior wound edge is removed prior to donor closure, using either curved scissors or a bent razor blade. This creates a purposeful controlled transection of the upper portion of hair follicles, and when the 2 edges of the wound are apposed, most of these transected follicles will lie under the line of closure. If properly done, these hairs then grow *through* the middle of the donor scar, thus reducing the noticeability of scar tissue. The potential disadvantages of a trichophytic closure include temporary folliculitis, an alteration in the direction of hair growing through the scar, and a change in the density of hair follicles within the scar that could be more visible than a thin scar in patients who wear very short hair. It should also be avoided in patients with tighter than average scalps as it results in a minimal increase in wound tension (if the same width strip is taken).

FOLLICULAR UNIT EXCISION

FUE is an alternative method of donor harvesting and as mentioned earlier is widely gaining popularity among hair restoration surgeons and patients for a variety of reasons; in fact, many young surgeons use only this method of harvesting. Using this technique, each individual FU is harvested directly from the scalp, rather than from a strip of donor tissue.[13,14] FUs are excised using a small, sharp cylindrical punch (generally 0.8-1.2 mm in diameter), which superficially incises the skin around each FU. The FU can then be carefully removed with forceps and gentle traction. The donor wounds are left to heal by secondary intention over the course of 7 to 10 days, finally leaving multiple small white scars over the harvested area.

On the one hand, this technique offers distinct advantages. Most importantly, it does not leave a linear scar. The resultant punctate scars are minimally noticeable, even with the hair closely cropped (Fig. 217-7). Thus, this is a useful procedure for individuals who want to wear exceptionally short hairstyles, those who have a tendency to heal with wider scars, and patients with a strong dislike or fear of linear scars. It is also an excellent technique to provide additional grafts after strip harvest surgery is for variable reasons no longer a good option. On the other hand, FUE is associated with important disadvantages. Chief among them, if a patient is destined to develop greater than Type V MPB, and therefore will need more than 6000 transplanted FUs; many of these grafts would need to be harvested from areas outside the boundaries of the SDA (Fig. 217-7). This is because in most patients FUE involves the extraction of every third or fourth FU (depending on patient ages, donor hair density, caliber, color contrast with the skin, etc.), and therefore the donor area would have to be 3 to 4 times as large as the donor area required for strip harvesting and would necessitate extension beyond the SDA. The hair within many of these FUs is therefore less likely to be permanent and may ultimately disappear in the future. Also, as the fringe hair beyond the SDA is progressively lost and/or miniaturized, the small hypopigmented scars from the FUE harvest may become exposed. In a worse-case scenario, overharvesting could result in a moth-eaten appearance that is difficult to rectify.

Equally important to consider are the transection rates during graft harvesting. Most hair restoration surgeons who practice both strip harvesting and FUE still find that transection rates are higher for FUE than for strip excision. Although improvement in FUE instrumentation has led to a significant decrease in FUE transection rates compared to its early days, there is still skepticism regarding equivalent transection rates in FUE reported by some practitioners. In FUE, each FU is at risk of transection when it is extracted blindly from the scalp. In contrast, in strip harvesting, only grafts at the edges of the strip are vulnerable, because other FUs are prepared with magnified, direct visualization (see below). Also, the FU grafts obtained through FUE tend to be more skeletonized with less surrounding supportive tissue. Contrast this with the grafts that are created from strip harvesting, which tend to have more protective tissue surrounding each follicle (Fig. 217-8). This is believed to lend greater protection to the FU and is likely to contribute to higher survival rates and hence better growth from strip harvest surgeries. The use of implanters, which minimize handling of grafts, may help minimize the trauma associated with implanting FUE grafts and improve their survival. As of this writing, there are very few survival studies to assess the growth of FUE grafts, and the few that have been completed indicate lower survival.[15]

FUE also may be suggested on occasion as a first surgery in the occasional young patient who wants to preserve the option of stopping hair transplants and switching to a short "buzzed look." The authors most often recommend FUE be used to complement strip harvesting, not to replace it, except in select patients for whom the benefits outweigh the drawbacks. In particular, FUE may be helpful in thinning the bushy temple regions in some patients and it can be utilized to obtain FU for placement into linear scars produced by strip harvesting. This is desirable when the scar is wider than average or when no further strip harvesting is planned. Such an approach combines the main advantage of strip harvesting—the maximization of the number of permanent hairs that can be harvested via the strip method—with the main advantage of FUE, the lack of a linear scar. For this purpose, we recommend that patients with a poorer prognosis (ie, MPB Type VI or VII) start with sessions using strip harvesting followed by FUE. This will maximize the number of available permanent hairs for harvesting over the patient's lifetime. In some situations, a combination approach with both a strip harvest and FUE also can be carried out on the same day in select patients. This approach is employed when the patient has had previous surgeries that have resulted in a tight, limited donor area due to underlying scarring, as performing FUE around the strip harvest scar can theoretically help in increasing the laxity of the scalp. Additional points of comparison between FUE and strip harvesting are outlined in Table 217-7.

ANESTHESIA

Just like in strip harvesting, oral sedation is given on the morning of the surgery and local anesthesia is employed by way of a ring block around the determined harvest area once this area is shaved and cleansed with usually povidone iodine.

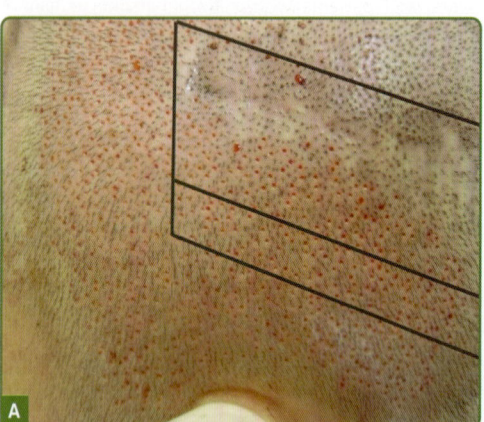 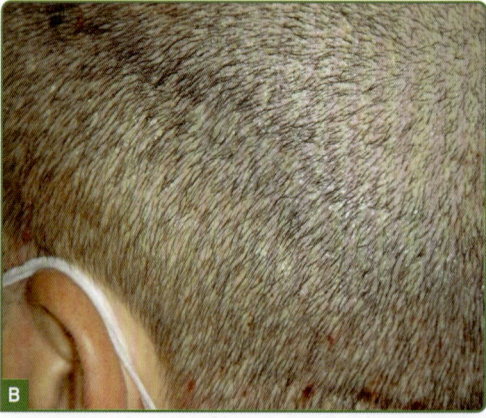

Figure 217-7 **A,** This is an intraoperative photo of a patient who had a linear scar from prior conventional strip harvesting, and who was undergoing FUE with the intention of placing grafts within the linear scar, and in areas of alopecia. The FUE was carried out by another surgeon. The round holes are the sites of FU extraction. The superimposed rectangle outlines the safe donor area (SDA). Many of the FUE sites were outside of the SDA, and the hair in these harvested grafts will likely be lost with time as MPB progresses. **B,** A photo taken 9 months postoperatively demonstrates the most important, immediately recognizable advantage of FUE, namely, the ability for the patient to cut the donor area to any length without visible scarring. The previous linear scar has been effectively concealed with grafting.

INSTRUMENTATION AND ROBOTICS

FUE is a surgeon (and his or her surgical team) AND instrument dependent procedure and there are an increasing number of devices that are being developed to increase both efficiency as well as accuracy of the method. A range of instruments have been developed and marketed, from simple manual FUE punches to motorized FUE devices (with a variety of distinguishing features ranging from whether a sharp or dull tip is employed, to whether the device uses a rotatory head or an oscillatory head) and entire robotic systems.[16] The most important properties of the instrument chosen include the amount of surrounding tissue left intact around the grafts, the rate of transection, the size of the resultant punctuate scars, and flexibility in tissue characteristics. It is difficult to find a good objective overview of the benefits and drawbacks of each instrument but, fortunately, as with all innovations, the field continues to evolve.[17]

BODY FUE

Body to scalp FUE can be used if the patient has insufficient donor hair in the scalp. The highest growth rates have been observed in hairs harvested from the beard and chest areas. However, the hair in these areas

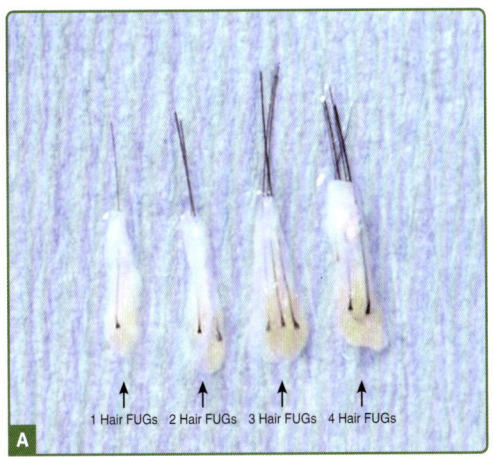
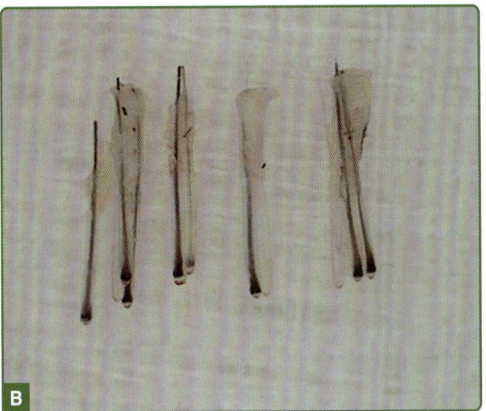
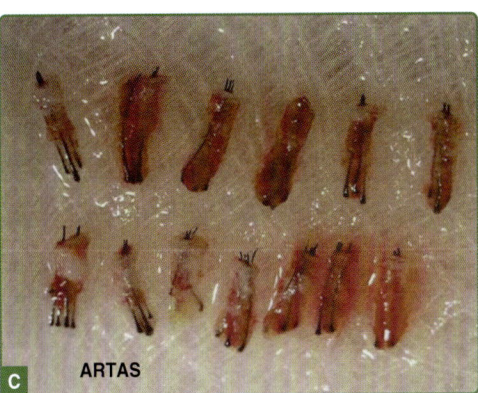

Figure 217-8 Comparison of grafts obtained through 3 different techniques. **A,** Grafts are harvested using the strip method. The grafts are trimmed into a "tear drop" shape preserving the appendages and leaving enough fat tissue to protect the follicle. **B,** Grafts are harvested by FUE using a motorized punch. Grafts are skeletonized and "naked," losing their accompanying appendages and devoid of fat tissue for added protection. Note also that there is a more than desired amount of epidermis that needs to be trimmed, which makes the grafts more skeletonized. **C,** Grafts harvested by FUE using the ARTAS robot.

TABLE 217-7
Advantages And Disadvantages Of Follicular Unit Extraction

Advantages
- Reduced postoperative pain
- Fairly rapid donor healing
- Fewer limits on postoperative activity, which is beneficial for patients who need a quick return to activity
- No suturing required
- Absence of linear scar
- Ideal for patients who prefer to wear their hair short (<2 mm)
- Ability to selectively choose FUs according to desired size or texture
- Ability to utilize body hair in patients with insufficient scalp donor hair
- Ideal for donor scar repair
- Requires a smaller team of technicians

Disadvantages
- Difficult to obtain large numbers of grafts without exceeding the limits of the safe donor area
- Higher follicular transection rates
- Skeletonized grafts with potentially lower survival rates due to increased vulnerability and trauma during placing
- More difficult postoperative camouflage because hair needs to be shaved short for harvesting of significant number of grafts
- Longer operative times
- Scarring of donor area makes subsequent FUE sessions more challenging and limited

have different growth rates than from scalp and also has a different curl and caliber/coarseness. Hence, it is not recommended for transplantation into the hairline area, which is more visible and should be created using fine scalp hair. However, the body hair can be mixed posterior to transplanted scalp hair to lend increased density, or to camouflage scars.

GRAFT PREPARATION

STRIP HARVESTING

The preparation of grafts from a strip harvest is accomplished using either stereoscopic microscopes or magnifying loupes or glasses. After removal of a donor strip, the first step is "slivering" the donor strip, in which slices, one FU wide, are carefully produced from the strip, much like cutting a loaf of bread into individual slices. These "slivers," composed of 4 to 10 FUs, are then further divided into individual FUs. FUs naturally occur in clusters of 1 to 4 hairs, with the average white FU containing an average of 2.3 hairs (other races usually have lower hair density, and hairs/FUs as well as different hair characteristics described elsewhere in this chapter). Occasionally, 2 very closely spaced FUs are combined into an individual "follicular family" (FF) small enough to fit into a typical FU recipient site. Compared with larger multi-FU grafts, FUs and FFs are far more susceptible to injury during graft preparation, storage, and insertion.[18] Therefore, technicians must have thorough and prolonged training, excellent manual dexterity, and ongoing supervision.

The ideal FU has most of its epidermis removed and is tear shaped, with the tapered end near the epidermis and the bulkier end in the subcutaneous tissue (Fig. 217-8A). This results in an FU wherein the dermal and subcutaneous tissue remains surrounding the follicle isthmus, hair bulge, and dermal papilla. The donor tissue is kept moist at all times, and prepared FUs are stored in a sectioned Petri dish filled with a storage solution.[19] It is important to ensure that the grafts remain cool throughout the procedure; hence the Petri dish constantly rests on icepacks or an electric chilling device. Within the sectioned dish, FUs are distributed into labeled compartments depending on the number and caliber of hairs. In this way, the individuals planting grafts can immediately find the type of graft that they need for a particular recipient site. Hairs that are partially transected are not discarded, provided that the distal two-thirds or proximal half is intact. They are, however, placed in less cosmetically important regions, because hair growth from these grafts is unpredictable.

FOLLICULAR UNIT EXCISION

As individual units are harvested directly from the donor area, processing of the grafts typically involves primarily removing damaged follicles from partially transected FUs, as well as segregating the FU according to number of hair follicles.

GRAFT STORAGE

Today, hair transplantation surgery is largely a full-day procedure as larger sessions involving thousands of small grafts have replaced the smaller older sessions involving far fewer and larger grafts. As such, it is important to ensure graft viability by storing them in the best possible way once they are out of the body. The technical team must ensure that the grafts remain moist and chilled from the point of harvesting to the point of graft insertion. Survival of transplanted grafts has been found to decrease over the length of time that they are out of the body, with negative factors being ischemia-induced hypoxemia, adenosine triphosphate (ATP) depletion, and ischemia-reperfusion injury. There are various types of storage media being developed, and practitioners are increasingly using hypothermic tissue–holding solutions (eg, Hypo-Thermosol) to replace intravenous fluids (eg, lactated Ringer). Some practitioners also add liposomal ATP to the holding solution as ATP depletion has been found to negatively influence graft survivability.[20]

RECIPIENT SITE CREATION[22]

Recipient sites are created using hypodermic needles or small blades cut to match the size of grafts. Prior to the creation of recipient sites, local anesthesia typically using 1% lidocaine with 1 in 100,000 epinephrine, is administered as a ring block surrounding the area to be treated. As necessary subsequently, a 1 in 50,000 epinephrine solution or normal saline is injected intermittently and superficially into the recipient area to provide better hemostasis. Such infiltration offers the additional advantage of spreading any existing recipient area hairs farther apart, thus minimizing the risk of injury when making incisions. Furthermore, as the solutions dissipate, the recipient sites move closer together, which ultimately produces higher hair density.

The authors stress that all incisions should be made at the same angle and direction as any persisting terminal or vellus hairs (Fig. 217-9). Much of the art of hair transplanting resides in the ability of the surgeon to do this, as both angle and direction vary considerably from patient to patient, and between different areas of the scalp. If one fails to do this, the resultant appearance will be unnatural and preexisting hair in the recipient area can be lethally damaged. Therefore, recipient site creation should be done slowly and carefully to ensure accurate angling and direction (Fig. 217-10). Typically, it will take between 1½ and 2½ hours to make 2000 to 2500 sites, depending on the density of preexisting hair in the recipient area and the amount of bleeding.

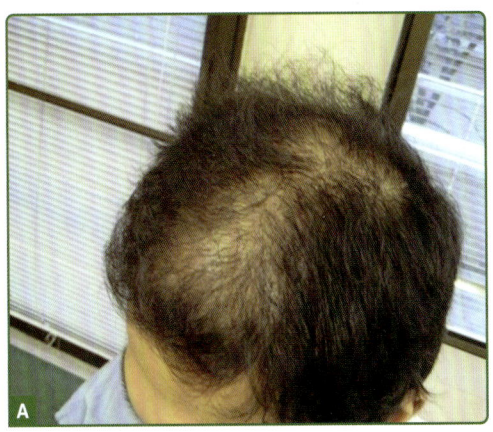
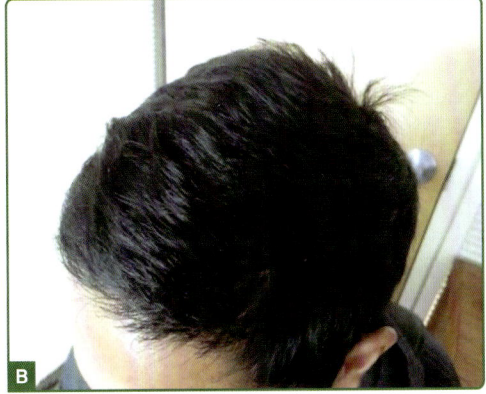
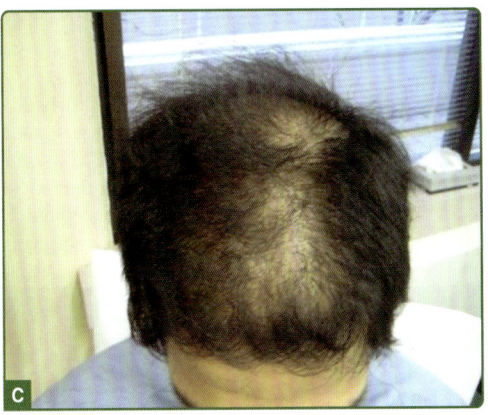
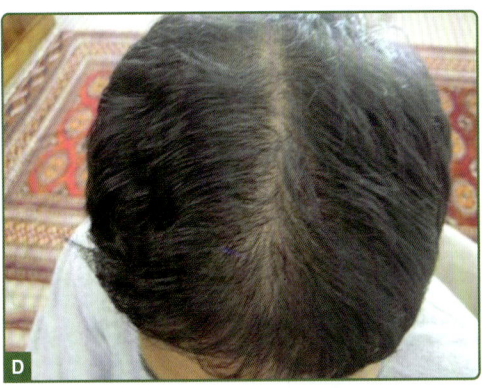

Figure 217-9 Transplanting hair to areas with preexisting hair. **A** and **C** show the areas with preexisting hair before the surgery and the result after transplanting as shown in **B** and **D**.

Recipient sites also can be created in either a perpendicular (coronal) or parallel (sagittal) fashion, relative to the hair direction and angle. The authors typically make most sites in a sagittal fashion and create coronal sites in temporal areas and in eyebrows, where it is ideal and natural to have the transplanted hairs lie flat.

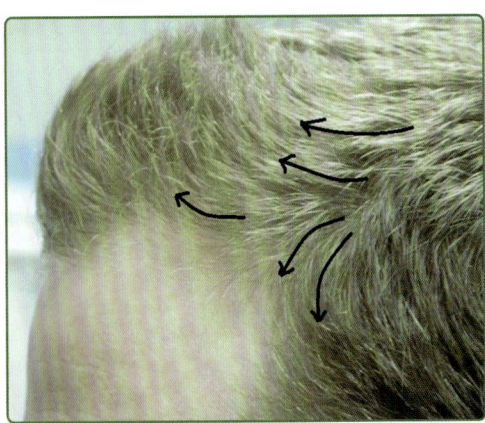

Figure 217-10 Although various directions and angles of hairs in different areas have been described, none of these generalities apply to all patients. Hair directions and angles can change dramatically in relatively small areas. The surgeon should follow what he or she observes rather than any general rule concerning hair angle and direction.

GRAFT DENSITY

If hair survival is high, a density of 20 to 30 FUs/cm^2 produces very good cosmetic results while preserving donor hair for future areas; consequently, this is the density that the authors prefer (Fig. 217-11). Higher-density grafting is limited to small cosmetically strategic areas of the recipient area, including an oval area in the anterior midline of the frontal area. Greater density in this particular area gives an impression of higher density across the entire frontal area. The authors believe that it is a significant mistake to create an overly dense hairline, which is not natural, and that better results can be achieved by creating a higher-density area behind the anterior hairline. The hairline should also be created with macro- and micro-irregularities to create a natural appearance and not a too straight and dense line that does not occur in nature.

A second reason for grafting at 20 to 30 FUs/cm^2 is that most studies on hair survival have demonstrated a

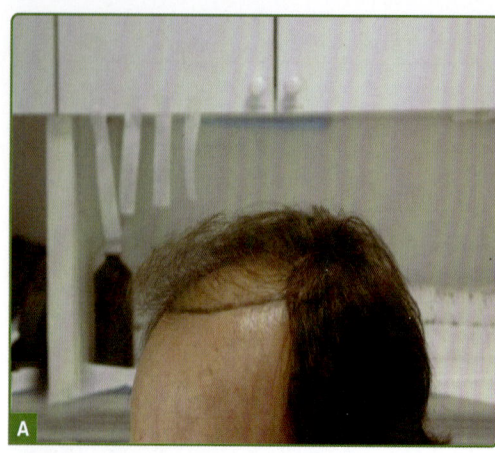
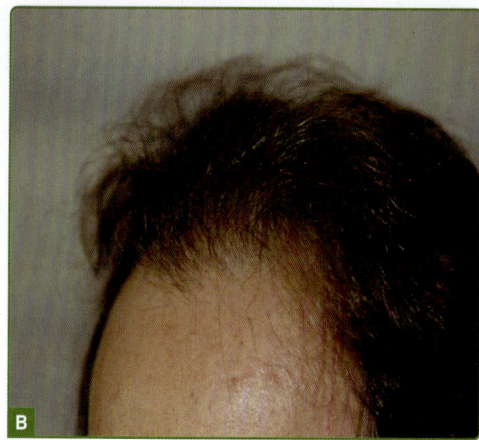

Figure 217-11 **A,** Before. Objective was more hair but subtle enough to increase likelihood of not being noticed by others. **B,** 12 months after 1 session at 15 to 20 cm².

tendency for unacceptable decreases in hair survival at higher FU densities, especially when the total incision length exceeds 3.0 cm/cm².[21-23] In part, this is because of increased competition for a limited blood supply and also may be because higher densities require smaller recipient sites and, therefore, more graft handling. Although hair survival at high FU densities has improved substantially in the last few years, good cosmetic results can be achieved with 20 to 30 FUs/cm² (Fig. 217-12), and thus higher densities are reserved for individuals with small areas of alopecia and publicly visible professions. For other individuals, especially

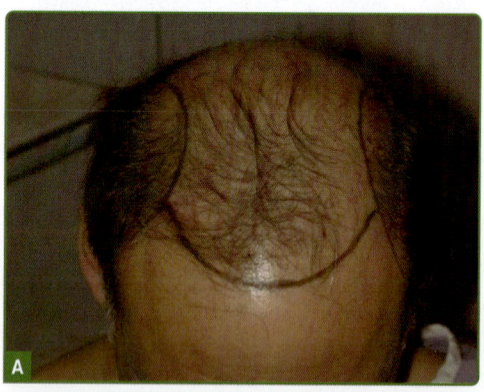
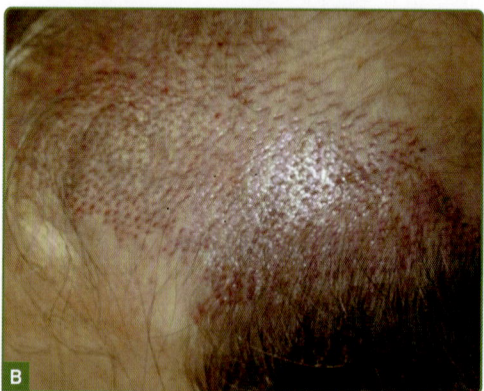
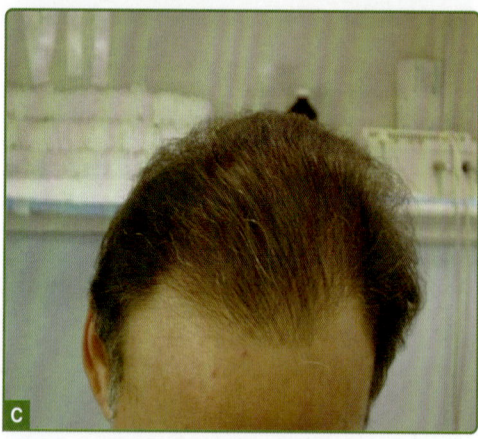
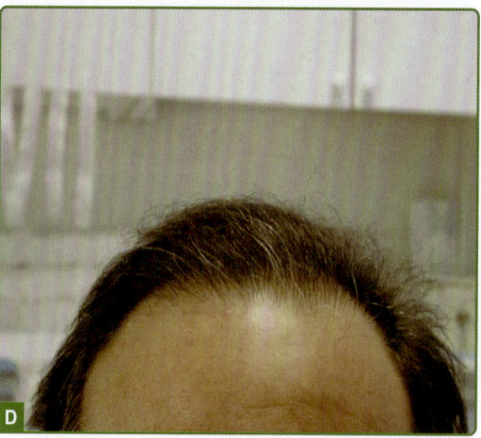

Figure 217-12 **A, B,** and **C,** A patient before treatment (**A** and **B**) and 9 months after the second of 2 transplants (**C**)—the first to the frontal area and the second to the midscalp area with a total of 3864 FUs and a relatively low density of approximately 20 to 30 FUs/cm². **D,** A frontal view of the same patient taken at the same time as **C**. Note that the hair appears thicker in this view than in **C**.

younger patients with uncertain long-term donor/recipient ratios, it is often an inappropriate use of a limited resource. The authors believe that it is important to create a natural appearance with maximal cosmetic improvement using the minimum number of hairs to meet the patient's density objectives (Fig. 217-13). This approach will allow the hair restoration surgeon to treat more of the alopecic areas that will develop over the patient's lifetime, rather than depleting the patient's finite number of donor grafts by overcommitting to a higher density than is required.

With regard to "mega-sessions" of 3000 to 5000 FUs, it should be pointed out that the average recipient site is 1 mm long, and while 1 mm seems quite small, the *total* length of a 3000-, 4000-, or 5000-graft session is respectively 9.99, 13.33, and 16.67 ft. Obviously, the larger the area treated, the more worrisome any given number of incisions and the resulting vascular damage. It seems reasonable to be cautious about creating 10 to 16 ft of incisions on the scalp until high hair survival rates in such sessions have been confirmed.

To determine the optimal size of the recipient site, several grafts containing varying numbers of hairs are tested in different sized incisions. The needle or blade size is adjusted accordingly. In general, the hair restoration surgeon should try to create the smallest recipient sites into which the grafts can be easily placed as this minimizes vascular disruption. Typically, 1-hair FU and fine 2-hair FU fit into sites made with 20-G needles, higher caliber 2-hair FUs fit into 19G sites, and 3- and 4-hair FUs fit into sites made with 18-G needles. On the other hand, the ideal graft fit is one that is "snug," and not made too small and tight to require significant handling during insertion. Though a mixture of 1, 2, and 3 or more hairs is used in all areas, in general, sites for 1 or 2 fine-haired FUs are created in the hairline zone, and sites for 2 or 3 coarse-haired FUs are created in areas that need greater hair density.

GRAFT INSERTION

After the recipient sites have been created, the surgeon reviews with their assistants the locations where the various sized FUs should be placed. Usually, 2 or 3 technicians work on a single patient simultaneously. Prior to graft insertion, platelet-rich plasma (PRP) and ACell is injected into the recipient sites and a small amount of the mixture is reserved for bathing grafts in

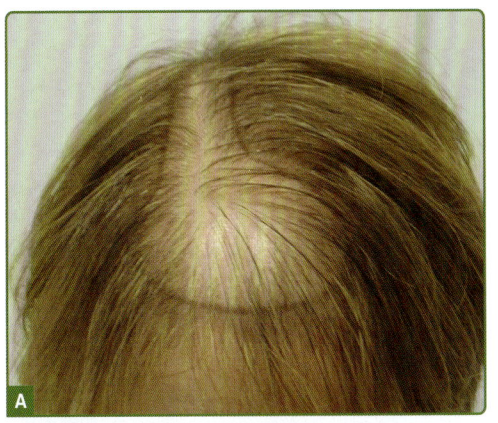
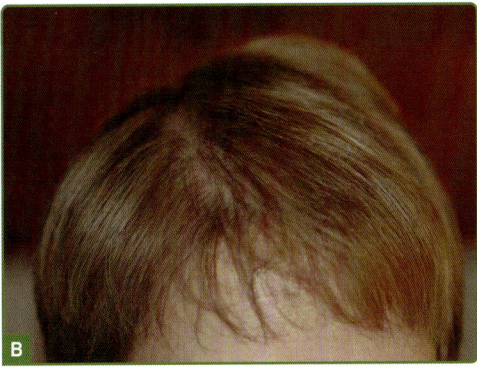
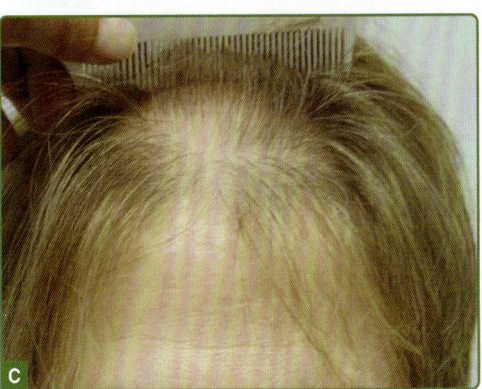
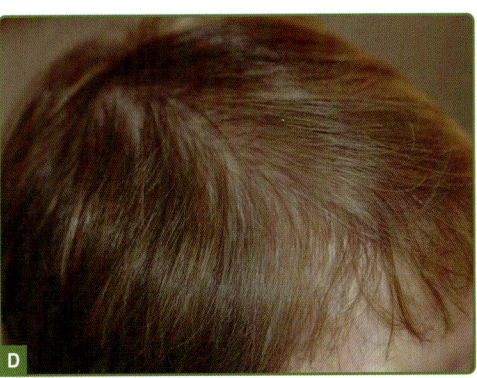

Figure 217-13 The "Christmas tree" pattern of hair loss as described by Olsen. Before surgery and after 1 surgery in a patient with a limited donor density. Concentrating grafts along the part-line and frontal block created an excellent cosmetic improvement.

before their placement. A group of grafts is removed from the fluid-filled wells of the Petri dish, placed in a "ring" filled with PRP and ACell on the finger, and from there placed in its recipient site. In this way, grafts are kept constantly moist. The skilled technician minimizes trauma to the follicles by handling only the subcutaneous tissue along the base of the graft rather than the grafts themselves. The long axis of each incision tells the technician the direction in which the graft should be inserted, and the graft typically slides in easily at the angle with which the site was made with 1 or 2 swift movements. The recipient area is kept clean by regularly spraying a mixture of saline (90%) and peroxide (10%), and the grafts are left slightly elevated to help in identifying sites that have not yet been filled. At the end of the procedure, grafts are repositioned to the level of the epidermis, or left slightly elevated, but never below the skin surface as this can cause pitting, or depressions, in the perifollicular skin.

HAIR IMPLANTERS

In some countries, for example Korea, the use of hair implanters has largely replaced the forceps technique of placing grafts. When used properly, hair implanters enhance graft viability by minimizing mechanical trauma to the follicle because the graft is pulled into the device by grasping its hair(s) and the crucial hair bulge and dermal papilla are not touched while loading the implanters as well as during implantation. Furthermore, some implantation devices enable the surgeon to simultaneously place the grafts into the sites as they are being made by the implanter, thus reducing the overall time for the procedure.

Because FUE grafts are both more skeletonized and vulnerable to trauma, some practitioners believe that using hair implanters in FUE cases has a significant advantage since the implanters not only fit more easily into the hollow needle of the implanter than into the skin, but their use also concurrently minimizes graft trauma during handling. Some physicians also find greater success rates when using implanters in Asian patients than in patients of other races. This could be because, as noted earlier, the Asian hair shaft diameter is generally greater than in whites and straighter, making it easier to properly load into the implanter. Implanters will likely develop further and become more important for all types of hair in the near future.

REPAIR SURGERY

The appearance of the recipient area of patients who have easily visible, unnatural grafting from prior surgeries, in particular from multi–follicular unit (MFU) grafting, can be greatly improved with modern hair transplanting techniques, primarily by placing FUs anterior and peripheral to these larger grafts.[24] If FUs with too many hairs or too coarse hairs have been inappropriately placed in the hairline zone, these can be dealt with similarly, by surrounding them with properly selected FUs. For larger grafts, the excision of all or a portion of any larger grafts also may be useful in minimizing "plugginess," while providing additional hair that can be transplanted elsewhere in the recipient area (Figs. 217-14 and 217-15). For patients in whom poor planning resulted in the unnatural placement of grafts, for example, a hairline that is too far anteriorly, the grafts can be excised either individually or by employing an "en bloc" excision.

In the donor area, multiple rows of scarring can often be reduced by excising a strip of tissue that contains 2 rows of scar tissue and an intervening zone of hair-bearing skin. This converts 2 scars into a single scar, while providing additional hair for use in the recipient area. It is important, however, that the removed strip is not so wide as to prevent a tension free closure. Alternatively,

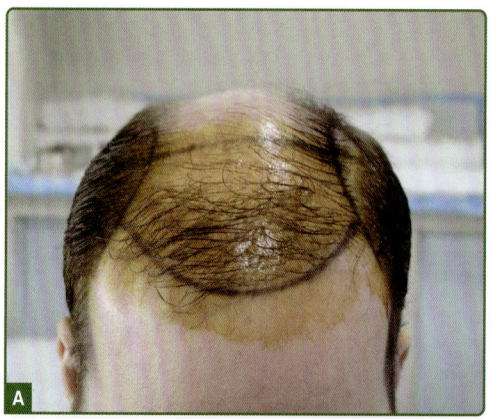

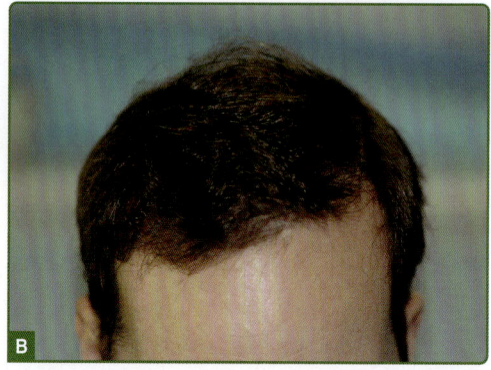

Figure 217-14 **A,** This 39-year-old patient had an "FUT" procedure carried out by another physician 3 years before this photograph was taken. A number of errors have been made. These included a failure to transplant into evolving areas of hair loss, and the placement of grafts that contained too many hairs, or too coarse a texture, in the hairline zone. The black crayon outlines the area that we proposed to treat. **B,** The patient returned 9 months after his first repair consisting of 1973 FUs. A new hairline had been created using finely textured 1- and 2-haired grafts. The rest of the frontal area was repaired by surrounding prior grafts with FUs, and by extending the transplant into adjacent areas of evolving hair loss. A third session, this time to the midscalp, was carried out 2 months after this photo was taken.

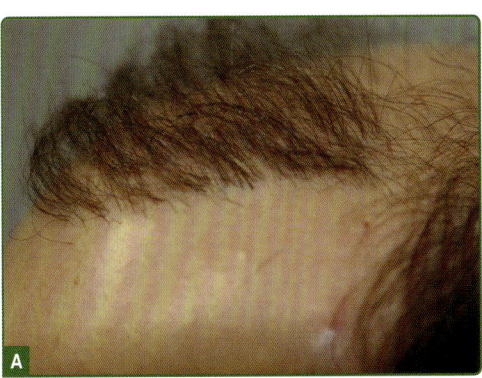

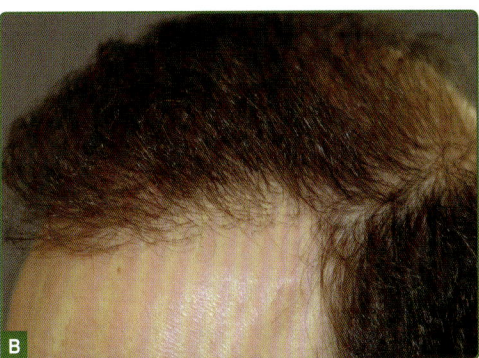

Figure 217-15 A, This patient had a procedure done by another surgeon using round grafts. The grafts contained too many hairs, and too many coarse hairs are seen especially in the hair line zone. Another hair transplant procedure was done using the strip method to correct the hairline and add density to the scalp extending the treatment to areas of possible future loss. **B,** The patient is seen after 1 year showing refined hairline and increased density of hair and coverage of the scalp.

TABLE 217-8
Side Effects and Complications

Side Effects
- Minor bleeding
- Scalp hypoesthesia
- Edema
- Crusting
- Pruritus
- Postoperative telogen effluvium

Medical Complications
- Wound Infection
- Wound dehiscence
- Neuralgia and neuromas
- Arteriovenous fistulas
- Central recipient area necrosis
- Folliculitis

Aesthetic Complications
- Visible scarring
- Hypertrophic and keloid scarring
- Unnatural appearance
- Poor density

donor scarring can be improved by transplanting FUs, often obtained via FUE, into abnormally wide scars.

SIDE EFFECTS AND COMPLICATIONS

The potential side effects and complications of hair restoration surgery are listed in Table 217-8.[25] Below we elaborate on a few of them:

1. Edema: Severe postoperative edema is unusual, but can be unsightly if it occurs in the frontal region, or interfere with healing if it occurs in the donor area. The risk is minimized by prescribing perioperative corticosteroids, by proper postoperative patient positioning, and by using ice compresses adjacent to but not on the actual operative sites.
2. Infection: Although rare, infection can present as early folliculitis in the recipient area, or more seriously wound dehiscence in the donor area. A number of measures such as prophylactic perioperative antibiotics reduce the risk of superficial surgical site infection.
3. Bleeding: Minor donor area bleeding can occur in the first few days postoperatively. Usually this resolves with firmly applied pressure, but rarely extra suturing is required.
4. Donor area scarring: In the authors' office, significant attention is given to measures that minimize the likelihood of wide donor scarring: the wound is closed with the absolute minimum of tension; postoperative edema is minimized through the aforementioned measures; and postoperative care is meticulous. Although this prevents wide scars in most patients, intrinsic poor wound-healing characteristics and severe scarring from old surgeries can result in wider than average scars. In such situations, grafts harvested from FUE can be transplanted into the scar, or alternatively trichophytic closures or double-layer suturing can be carried out during subsequent strip excisions.
5. Poor density: This may reflect poor hair survival, suboptimal graft distribution, or poor postoperative care. This problem is probably entirely avoidable.
6. Postoperative effluvium: This problem may occur in hair-bearing areas in the recipient or donor areas. It is presumably due to the interruption of blood supply and is always temporary. Approximately 10% to 20% of male patients and 50% of females experience some degree of postoperative effluvium.

PATIENT FOLLOWUP

In the authors' practice, all patients are seen the day after surgery for bandage removal. The hair and scalp are thoroughly washed and the occasional dislodged graft can be adjusted. Postoperative instructions are also reviewed at this point and a clean cap is used to cover the surgical area before sending the patient home. Unless contraindicated, the patients in our practice are also given a tapering course of oral corticosteroids to minimize postoperative swelling.

All patients are seen 8 to 12 days postoperatively to check the surgical area and remove sutures. A followup appointment is also generally booked for 4 to 6 weeks postoperatively to check that healing is progressing along the normal course and again at 9 to 12 months to assess the surgical results and determine any need for further treatment.

ALOPECIA REDUCTION

Alopecia reduction, or scalp reduction, is defined as the excision of an area of alopecia or future alopecia.[26] In the past, the technique was used in conjunction with hair transplantation as a means of reducing the size of the prospective recipient area, and thus conserving grafts for cosmetically vital areas of the scalp. Unfortunately, the technique is technically demanding, and the high frequency of medical and aesthetic complications, in inexperienced hands, led to the procedure falling out of favor. Currently, the technique is used to repair aesthetically unsatisfactory hair transplanting, to excise areas of cicatricial alopecia, or for hairline advancement.

Despite the cosmetic improvement offered by the procedure, alopecia reduction is rarely used and it does come with its own set of complications. These include postoperative bleeding, infection, nerve damage, persistent hair thinning or loss in the fringe areas, disorientation of hair direction, stretch back, and poor scars which can all be minimized if the procedure is done properly.

CONCLUSION

The evolution of hair transplanting, over the last 10 to 15 years, has resulted in a remarkable increase in the number of patients who are candidates for the procedure and an even more impressive improvement in the naturalness of the results. Unfortunately, these new techniques also require far more skill and patience from not only the surgeon but also their surgical team. Additionally, hair restoration surgeons are not miracle workers, and individuals must be educated as to what they can realistically expect from hair transplanting. When this is done, the reward is nearly always a satisfied and grateful patient.

ACKNOWLEDGMENTS

We would like to acknowledge Dr Mark A. Unger, who contributed to the version of this chapter that was included in the previous edition.

REFERENCES

1. Unger W, Shapiro R. Commentary on Russell Knudsen's effect of medical therapy on surgical planning. In: Unger WP, Shapiro R, eds. *Hair Transplantation*. 4th ed. New York, NY: Marcel Dekker; 2004:148-151.
2. Hamilton JB. Patterned loss of hair in men: types and incidence. *Ann N Y Acad Sci*. 1951;53(3):708-728.
3. Norwood OT. Classification and incidence of male pattern baldness. In: Norwood OT, Sheill R, eds. *Hair Transplant Surgery*. 2nd ed. Springfield, IL: Charles C. Thomas; 1984:3-14.
4. Unger WP, Cole J. Donor harvesting. In: Unger WP, Shapiro R, eds. *Hair Transplantation*. 4th ed. New York, NY: Marcel Dekker; 2004:301-334.
5. Ludwig E. Classification of the types of androgenetic alopecia (common baldness) occurring in the female sex. *Br J Dermatol*. 1977;97(3):247-254.
6. Olsen EA. Female pattern hair loss: clinical features and potential hormonal factors. *J Am Acad Dermatol*. 2001;4(3)(suppl 1):S70-S80.
7. Unger WP, Unger RH. Hair transplanting: an important but often forgotten treatment for female pattern hair loss. *J Am Acad Dermatol*. 2003;49(5):853-860.
8. Unger RH. Female Hair Restoration. *Facial Plast Surg Clin North Am*. 2013;21(3):407-441.
9. Tosti A. *Dermoscopy of the Hair and Scalp Disorders With Clinical and Pathological Correlations*. London: Informa Healthcare; 2007.
10. Unger WP. Unger's technique for anesthesia. In: Unger WP, Shapiro R, eds. *Hair Transplantation*. 4th ed. New York, NY: Marcel Dekker; 2004:250-254.
11. Unger WP. Planning and organizing the recipient area. In: Unger WP, Shapiro R, Unger RH, et al, eds. *Hair Transplantation*. 5th ed. New York, NY: Informa USA; 2011:106-152.
12. Devroye JM. An overview of the donor area. In: Unger WP, Shapiro R, Unger RH, et al, eds. *Hair Transplantation*. 5th ed. New York, NY: Informa USA; 2011:247-261.
13. Rassman WR, Bernstein R, McLellan R, et al. Follicular unit extraction: minimally invasive surgery for hair transplantation. *Dermatol Surg*. 2002;28(8):720-728.
14. Harris J. Conventional FUE. In: Unger WP, Shapiro R, Unger RH, et al, eds. *Hair Transplantation*. 5th ed. New York, NY: Informa USA; 2011:291-295.
15. Beehner ML. FUE vs FUT-MD: Study of 1,780 follicles in four patients. *Hair Transplant Forum Intl*. 2016; 26(4):160-161.
16. Rose PT, Nusbaum B. Robotic hair restoration. *Dermatol Clin*. 2014;32(1):97-107.
17. Devroye J. Powered FU. Extraction with the Short-Arc-Oscillation Flat Punch FUE System (SFFS). *Hair Transplant Forum Intl*. 2016;26(4):129, 134-136.
18. Beehner M. Comparison of survival of FU grafts trimmed chubby, medium, and skeletonized. *Hair Transplant Forum Intl*. 2010;20(1):6.
19. Cooley J. Ischemia reperfusion injury and graft storage solutions. *Hair Transplant Forum Intl*. 2009;13(4):121.
20. Cooley J. Bio-enhanced hair restoration. *Hair Transplant Forum Intl*. 2014;24(4).
21. Unger WP, Shapiro R. The hairline. In: Unger WP, Shapiro R, Unger RH, et al, eds. *Hair Transplantation*. 5th ed. New York, NY: Informa USA; 2011:372-372.

22. Mayer M, Keene S, Perez-Meza D. Follicular unit density and hair yield. Paper presented at: Annual Meeting of the International Society of Hair Restoration Surgery, Sydney, Australia; October 2005.
23. Beehner M. Studying the effect of FU planting density on hair survival. *Hair Transplant Forum Intl*. 2006; 16(1):247-248.
24. Vogel JE. Correction of cosmetic problems secondary to hair transplanting. In: Unger WP, Shapiro R, Unger RH, et al, eds. *Hair Transplantation*. 5th ed. New York, NY: Informa USA; 2011:473-478.
25. Cooley J. Complications of hair transplantation. In: Unger WP, Shapiro R, eds. *Hair Transplantation*. 4th ed. New York, NY: Marcel Dekker; 2004:568-573.
26. Marzola M. Alopecia reductions. In: Unger WP, Shapiro R, Unger RH, et al, eds. *Hair Transplantation*. 5th ed. New York, NY: Informa USA; 2011:483-489.

图书在版编目（CIP）数据

菲兹帕里克皮肤病学：第9版：双语版：汉、英文. 下册 /[美] 康斯文（Sewon Kang）等主编；陈翔，粟娟等编译.—长沙：湖南科学技术出版社，2020.10
（西医经典名著集成）
ISBN 978-7-5710-0760-7

Ⅰ.①菲… Ⅱ.①康… ②陈… ③粟…Ⅲ.①皮肤病学－汉、英文 Ⅳ.①R751

中国版本图书馆 CIP 数据核字(2020)第 189071 号

Sewon Kang, Masayuki Amagai, Anna L. Brucker, Alexander H. Enk, David J. Margolis, Amy J. McMichael, Jeffrey S. Orringer
Fitzpatrick's Dermatology, Ninth Edition, 2-Volume Set
ISBN9780071837795
Copyright ©2019 by McGraw-Hill Education.

All Rights reserved. No part of this publication may be reproduced or transmitted in any form or by any means, electronic or mechanical, including without limitation photocopying, recording, taping, or any database, information or retrieval system, without the prior written permission of the publisher.

This authorized Bilingual edition is jointly published by McGraw-Hill Education and Hunan Science & Technology Press. This edition is authorized for sale in the People's Republic of China only, excluding Hong Kong, Macao SAR and Taiwan.

Translation Copyright © 2020 by McGraw-Hill Education and Hunan Science & Technology Press.

版权所有。未经出版人事先书面许可，对本出版物的任何部分不得以任何方式或途径复制或传播，包括但不限于复印、录制、录音，或通过任何数据库、信息或可检索的系统。

本授权双语版由麦格劳-希尔教育出版公司和湖南科学技术出版社合作出版。此版本经授权仅限在中华人民共和国境内（不包括香港特别行政区、澳门特别行政区和台湾省）销售。

翻译版权©2020 由麦格劳-希尔教育出版公司与湖南科学技术出版社所有。

本书封面贴有 McGraw-Hill Education 公司防伪标签，无标签者不得销售。
著作权合同登记号 18-2020-188

西医经典名著集成
FEIZIPALIKE PIFUBINGXUE
菲兹帕里克皮肤病学　第9版（双语版）下册

主　　编：	[美]康斯文（Sewon Kang），[日]天谷正之（Masayuki Amagai），[美]安娜 L.布鲁克纳（Anna L. Brucker），[德]亚历山大 H.恩（Alexander H. Enk），[美]大卫 J.马戈利斯（David J. Margolis），[美]艾美 J.麦克迈克尔（Amy J. McMichael），[美]杰弗里 S.奥林格（Jeffrey S. Orringer）
编译者：	陈翔，粟娟等
责任编辑：	李　忠　杨　颖
出版发行：	湖南科学技术出版社
社　　址：	长沙市湘雅路 276 号
	http://www.hnstp.com
印　　刷：	湖南凌宇纸品有限公司
厂　　址：	长沙市长沙县黄花镇黄花工业园
邮　　编：	410137
版　　次：	2020 年 10 月第 1 版
印　　次：	2020 年 10 月第 1 次印刷
开　　本：	787mm×1092mm　1/16
印　　张：	96
字　　数：	4990 千字
书　　号：	ISBN 978-7-5710-0760-7
定　　价：	1050.00 元（上、中、下册）

（版权所有 • 翻印必究）